NURSE ANESTHESIA

FOURTH EDITION

John J. Nagelhout, PhD, CRNA, FAAN
Director, School of Anesthesia
Kaiser Permanente/California State University, Fullerton
Southern California Permanente Medical Group
Pasadena, California

Karen L. Plaus, PhD, CRNA, FAAN
Executive Director
National Board on Certification and Recertification of Nurse Anesthetists
Park Ridge, Illinois

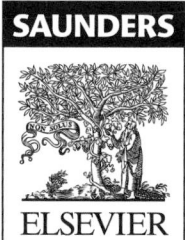

SAUNDERS

ELSEVIER

BP45

SAUNDERS
ELSEVIER

11830 Westline Industrial Drive
St. Louis, Missouri 63146

NURSE ANESTHESIA   ISBN: 978-1-4160-5025-4

Notice

Knowledge and best practice in this field are constantly changing. As new research and experience broaden our knowledge, changes in practice, treatment, and drug therapy may become necessary or appropriate. Readers are advised to check the most current information provided (i) on procedures featured or (ii) by the manufacturer of each product to be administered to verify the recommended dose or formula, the method and duration of administration, and contraindications. It is the responsibility of practitioners, relying on their own experience and knowledge of the patient, to make diagnoses, to determine dosages and the best treatment for each individual patient, and to take all appropriate safety precautions. To the fullest extent of the law, neither the Publisher nor the Authors assume any liability for any injury and/or damage to persons or property arising out of or related to any use of the material contained in this book.

The Publisher

Library of Congress Cataloging-in-Publication Data

Nurse anesthesia / [edited by] John J. Nagelhout, Karen L. Plaus. – 4th ed.
        p. ; cm.
    Includes bibliographical references and index.
    ISBN 978-1-4160-5025-4 (alk. paper)
  1. Anesthesia. 2. Operating room nursing. I. Nagelhout, John J. II. Plaus, Karen L.
    [DNLM: 1. Anesthesia–Nurses' Instruction. 2. Anesthetics–Nurses' Instruction. 3. Nurse Anesthetists. WO 200 N974 2010]
    RD82.N87 2010
    617.9'6–dc22   2008051376

Executive Publisher: Darlene Como
Editor: Tamara Myers
Associate Developmental Editor: Tina Kaemmerer
Publishing Services Manager: Anne Altepeter
Senior Project Manager: Cheryl A. Abbott
Designer: Paula Catalano

Printed in the United States of America

Last digit is the print number: 9   8   7   6   5   4   3   2   1

6/8/09

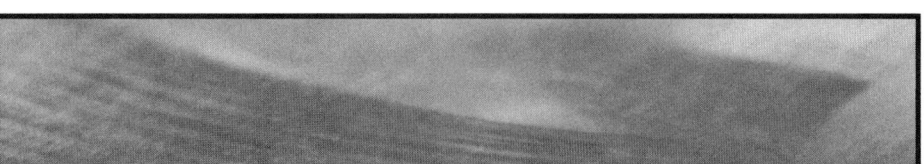

CONTRIBUTORS

John G. Aker, CRNA, MS
Staff Anesthetist
Department of Anesthesia
University of Iowa Hospitals and Clinics
Iowa City, Iowa

Charles R. Barton, CRNA, MSN, MEd
Director, Graduate Anesthesia Program
College of Nursing
The University of Akron
Akron, Ohio

Chuck Biddle, CRNA, PhD
Professor and Staff Anesthetist
Virginia Commonwealth University
Richmond, Virginia

Gregory Bozimowski, CRNA, MS
Assistant Professor
Graduate Program of Nurse Anesthesiology
University of Detroit Mercy
Detroit, Michigan

Charlene V. Brouillette, CRNA, MS, APRN
Kenner, Louisiana

Joseph F. Burkard, CRNA, DNSc
Associate Professor, USD DNP Program
Hahn School of Nursing
University of San Diego
San Diego, California

Anthony Chipas, CRNA, PhD
Division Director/Associate Professor
Medical University of South Carolina
Charleston, South Carolina

Gary D. Clark, CRNA, EdD
Associate Professor
Associate Director, Coordinator Special Projects
Nurse Anesthesia Program
Department of Biological Sciences
Webster University
St. Louis, Missouri

Theresa L. Culpepper, CRNA, PhD
Director, Clinical Anesthesia Services
Ida V. Moffett School of Nursing
Department of Nurse Anesthesia
Samford University
Birmingham, Alabama

Nicholas C. Curdt, CRNA, MS, BSN, RN
Northwest Anesthesia
St. Louis, Missouri

Michael P. Dosch, CRNA, MS
Associate Professor and Chair, Nurse Anesthesia
University of Detroit Mercy
Detroit, Michigan

Melydia J. Edge, CRNA, MSN
Clinical Associate Professor
Nurse Anesthesia Program
College of Nursing
East Carolina University
Greenville, North Carolina

Sass Elisha, CRNA, EdD
Assistant Director
Kaiser Permanente School of Anesthesia
Pasadena, California

Wayne E. Ellis, PhD, CRNA, ANP
Private Practice Anesthesia and Pain Management
Mountain State University
Beckley, West Virginia

Ladan Eshkevari, CRNA, MS, PhD(c)
Assistant Professor
Georgetown University
Washington, DC

Margaret Faut-Callahan, CRNA, PhD, FAAN
Dean and Professor
College of Nursing
Marquette University
Milwaukee, Wisconsin

Carmencita Ford-Fleifel, CRNA, MS
Staff Anesthetist and Clinical Instructor
St. John Macomb–Oakland Hospital
Macomb Center
Warren, Michigan

Judith A. Franco, MSN, ACNP, CRNA
Clinical Instructor of Anesthesiology
USC University Hospital
Los Angeles, California

Paul Gregg Gambrell, CRNA, MSN
Clinical Assistant Professor
College of Nursing
East Carolina University
Greenville, North Carolina

Francis Gerbasi, CRNA, PhD
Executive Director
Council on Accreditation of Nurse Anesthesia
  Educational Programs
American Association of Nurse Anesthetists
Park Ridge, Illinois

C. Wayne Hamm, CRNA, MSN, AP
Certified Registered Nurse Anesthetist
Medical Anesthesia Group
Memphis, Tennessee

Walter R. Hand, Jr., CRNA, PhD
Director of Corporate Education
Performance Anesthesia
Fort Bragg, North Carolina

Randolf R. Harvey, CRNA, BS
Chief of Anesthesia
Florida Eye Clinic/ASC
Altamonte Springs, Florida

Betty J. Horton, CRNA, PhD
Education Consultant
Tower Hill, Illinois

Donna M. Jasinski, CRNA, PhD
Georgetown University
Washington, DC

Joseph Anthony Joyce, CRNA, BS
Certified Registered Nurse Anesthetist
Moses Cone Health System
Wesley Long Community Hospital
Greensboro, North Carolina

Mary C. Karlet, CRNA, PhD
Samford University
Birmingham, Alabama

Bruce Evan Koch, CRNA, MSN
Adjunct Faculty
Kaiser Permanente School of Nurse Anesthesia
Pasadena, California

Mark A. Kossick, CRNA, DNSc, APN
Professor and Senior Fellow
School of Nursing
Union University
Jackson, Tennessee

Julie Ann Lowery, CRNA, MS, BSN
Certified Registered Nurse Anesthetist
University of North Carolina
Chapel Hill, North Carolina

Rex A. Marley, CRNA, MS, RRT
Chief Nurse Anesthetist
Northern Colorado Anesthesia Professional Consultants
Fort Collins, Colorado

John Maye, CRNA, PhD
Commander, United States Army
Uniformed Services University
Graduate School of Nursing
Nurse Anesthesia Program
Bethesda, Maryland

Maura S. McAuliffe, CRNA, PhD, FAAN
Professor and Director
Nurse Anesthesia Program
College of Nursing
East Carolina University
Greenville, North Carolina

Beth Ann Movinsky, CRNA, MS, MA
Clinical Coordinator
Navy Nurse Corps Anesthesia Program
San Diego, California

Anne Kiyomi Nishinaga, CRNA, MSN
Staff Nurse Anesthetist
Kaiser Permanente Medical Center
Panorama City, California

Jan Odom-Forren, MS, RN, CPAN, FAAN
Perianesthesia Consultant
Louisville, Kentucky

Michael P. O'Donnell, PhD
Didactic Director, Minneapolis School of Anesthesia
Professor, St. Mary's University of Minnesota
Minneapolis, Minnesota

R. Lee Olson, CRNA, MS
Director, Navy Nurse Corps Anesthesia Program
Bethesda, Maryland

Lisa A. Osborne, CRNA, PhD
Clinical Coordinator
Navy Nurse Corps Anesthesia Program
Naval School of Health Sciences
San Diego, California

Sandra Maree Ouellette, CRNA, MEd, FAAN
President, International Federation of Nurse Anesthetists
President, R&S Ouellette, Inc.
Winston-Salem, North Carolina

Timothy J. Palmer, CRNA, MS
Anesthesia Education Coordinator
Surgical Services Education
William Beaumont Hospital
Royal Oak, Michigan

Joseph E. Pellegrini, CRNA, PhD, DNP
Associate Professor and Assistant Director
Nurse Anesthesia Program
University of Maryland
Baltimore, Maryland

Brian P. Radesic, CRNA, MSN
Associate Director, Graduate Anesthesia Program
College of Nursing
The University of Akron
Akron, Ohio

Michael Rieker, CRNA, DNP
Director, Nurse Anesthesia Program
Wake Forest University Baptist Medical Center
Winston Salem, North Carolina

Bernadette T. Higgins Roche, CRNA, EdD
Administrative Director and Assistant Professor
NorthShore University HealthSystem
School of Nurse Anesthesia
De Paul University
Evanston, Illinois

Allan J. Schwartz, DDS, CRNA
Dentist-Certified Registered Nurse Anesthetist
Columbia, Missouri

Elizabeth Monti Seibert, CRNA, PhD
Associate Professor and Director of Doctoral Education
Department of Nurse Anesthesia
Virginia Commonwealth University
Richmond, Virginia

Julie A. Stone, CRNA, EdD
Northwest Anesthesia
St. Louis, Missouri

Henry C. Talley, V, CRNA, PhD
Program Director
College of Nursing
Michigan State University
East Lansing, Michigan

Lisa J. Thiemann, CRNA, MNA
Acting Senior Director, Professional Practice
American Association of Nurse Anesthetists
Park Ridge, Illinois

Charles A. Vacchiano, CRNA, PhD
Professor
Nurse Anesthesia Program
Duke University School of Nursing
Durham, North Carolina

Ronald L. Van Nest, CRNA, MA
Adjunct Assistant Professor
Van Nest and Associates, LLC
Davidsonville, Maryland

Edward Waters, CRNA, MN
Instructor
Kaiser Permanente School of Anesthesia
Pasadena, California

Mark D. Welliver, CRNA, DNPc
Assistant Professor
Nurse Anesthetist Program
School of Nursing
University of North Florida
Jacksonville, Florida

Wanda O. Wilson, CRNA, PhD
Associate Professor and Program Director
University of Cincinnati College of Nursing
Cincinnati, Ohio

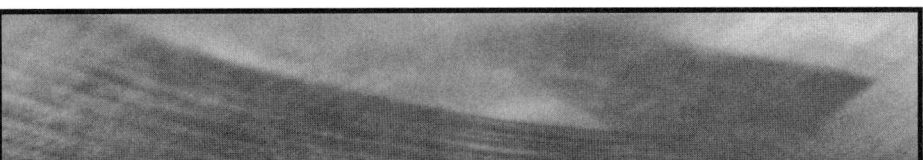

PREFACE

This textbook was conceived in the early 1990s to fill a need for a scientifically based, clinically oriented work on nurse anesthesia. At the time, we felt there was no single source that encompassed and outlined the tremendous contributions that nurse anesthetists make to improving patient care and advancing nursing research and education. With the advent of this fourth edition, we are tremendously gratified that this textbook has become the seminal work in our profession. Over the past decade, we have been included in the Library of Congress essential nursing textbooks, as well as receiving numerous other recognitions. The unique body of knowledge that nurse anesthetists bring to clinical practice now reaches an international audience.

Nurse anesthetists continue to lead clinical and academic nursing with their contributions to the advancement of safe, evidence-based patient care. Anesthesia practice continues to evolve, and the fourth edition reflects the newest information regarding a variety of practice areas. Each chapter has been extensively reviewed and revised to contain the most salient information available. This edition contains hundreds of new tables, figures, and boxes, which add to the written materials. Under Professional Issues, we have added a chapter on Nurse Anesthesia Education in the United States, as well as Legal Issues in Nurse Anesthesia pertinent to nurse anesthesia practice. We have been asked by many colleagues to expand the Chemistry and Physics of Anesthesia chapter to reflect the necessary material for a sound understanding of the chemical and physical principles underlying modern practice. This chapter has been totally redone to encompass the scientific knowledge necessary to ensure maximum performance in the highly technological modern operating suite. This chapter also provides the beginning anesthetist with the essential foundations of clinical anesthesia.

The section on Technology Related to Anesthesia Practice has been expanded to reflect the growing role of new monitoring modalities. We have divided Clinical Monitoring into three different chapters: Cardiovascular, Respiratory and Metabolic, and Neurologic systems. The essential chapters on Cardiovascular and Respiratory Anatomy, Physiology, Pathophysiology, and Anesthesia Management have been expanded to reflect the many advances in these two vital areas. An entirely new chapter on The Immune System and Anesthesia has been included to reflect the recent advances in this area. Clinical anesthesia continues to lead medicine and nursing in its safety profile. To further efforts in safety, we have included a new chapter on Anesthesia Complications as a way to reiterate the importance of continuous improvement efforts.

We are especially grateful to all of our returning and new authors, who bring a wealth of expertise and experience to their respective areas. The majority of clinical anesthesia continues to be provided by nurse anesthetists, and this textbook is a testament to the broad range of knowledge that we bring to the practice of anesthesia.

As we have with past editions, we have totally revised our companion handbook that accompanies this text. It provides essential information regarding pathophysiology, surgical procedures, and drugs that can be easily accessed in the clinical setting. Producing an educational resource of this size and complexity would not be possible without the tireless efforts of our authors and a broad array of experts. We would like to express our sincere gratitude to Retta Smith, who assisted in the production and editing of this textbook. Our medical illustrator, Steve Beebe, from Kaiser Permanente, has added dozens of new figures and illustrations that greatly clarify the information presented. A special thank you is sent to William Loechel, who illustrated the first edition of this textbook; many of those figures carry over to this edition. Special gratitude is expressed for the staff at Elsevier, including Tamara Myers, editor; Tina Kaemmerer, associate developmental editor; and Cheryl Abbott, senior project manager.

We are proud of the contributions that nurse anesthetists make to the practice of anesthesia and that we have been able, through this textbook, to be a part of the wonderful advancements that continue to be made in anesthesia practice and patient care.

John J. Nagelhout
Karen L. Plaus

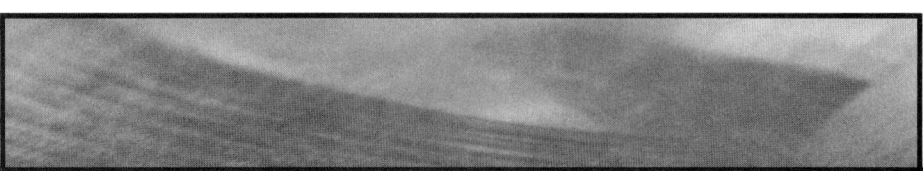

ACKNOWLEDGMENTS

We would like to thank the following authors for their contributions to the first, second, and third editions of this textbook.

Roy Alisoglu
Steve L. Alves
Anne E. Aprile
Victoria Base-Smith
Colleen M. Beauchamp
Donald Bell
Baher Boctor
Danny R. Bowman
Michael Boytim
Rick Brown
Joanne M. Cafarelli
Cynthia Cappello
Marge Chick
Angela Darsey
Diane Bleak Dayton
George G. DeVane
Lyle Dorman
Ronda L. Erway
Michael D. Fallacaro
Nadine A. Fallacaro
Michael A. Fiedler
Jan L. Frandsen
Donna J. Funke
Vance G. Gainer, Jr.
Silas N. Glisson
Ira P. Gunn
Richard E. Haas
Stanley M. Hall
Celestine Harrigan
Shelly Harthrong-Lethiot
Bernadette Henrichs
Don Hill
Frederick C. Hill, Jr.
Holly E. Holman
Maria Iacopelli

Jeanne M. Kachnij
Kenneth M. Kirsner
Jeffrey F. Kopecky
Michael J. Kremer
Gail LaPointe
Jeanne B. Learman
Kim Litwack
Janet Maroney
Denise Martin-Sheridan
John P. McDonough
Ann Misterovich
Michael P. Mitton
Diane Moniz
Ralph O. Morgan, Jr.
Julie A. Rigoni Neville
Howard J. Normile
Sherry Owens
DeAnna Powell
Richard S. Purdham
Janet Rojo
Linda Saber McIntosh
Susanna Sands
Elaine Sartain-Spivak
James Scarsella
Lisa A. Sebastian
Jeffrey P. Serwin
Barry Shaw
Jeffrey A. Sinkovich
Brent Sommer
Kathy Swender
Michael Troop
John Weisbrod
John R. Williams
Hilary V. Wong
E. Laura Wright

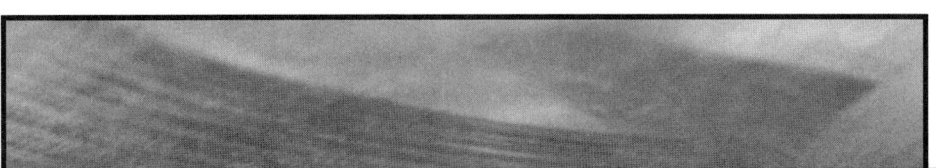

CONTENTS

CHAPTER

1

NURSE ANESTHESIA

A History of Challenge

Bruce Evan Koch

IT IS FITTING TO OPEN A TEXT ON NURSE ANESTHESIA WITH A HISTORY CHAPTER. NURSES HAVE
PROVIDED THE VAST MAJORITY OF ANESTHESIA IN THE UNITED STATES. NURSES HAVE CONTRIBUTED
GREATLY AND IN UNIQUE WAYS TO THE SAFETY, SCIENCE, EDUCATION, AND PUBLIC POLICY SUPPORT-
ING ANESTHESIA. ONCE WE LEARN WHAT EARLIER NURSE ANESTHETISTS ACCOMPLISHED, OFTENTIMES
AGAINST GREAT ODDS AND WITH FEW OR NONE OF THE RESOURCES AVAILABLE TO US TODAY, WE
GAIN A PROPER PERSPECTIVE AND RESPECT FOR THE PROFESSION AND OURSELVES.

IN PRIOR EDITIONS OF *NURSE ANESTHESIA*, IRA GUNN AUTHORED THIS CHAPTER. IRA IS OUR MOST
EMINENT HISTORIAN, AND I HAVE NOT ATTEMPTED TO ALTER MUCH OF HER WORK. INSTEAD, I HAVE
VALIDATED AND IN SOME AREAS EXPANDED IT WITH INFORMATION THAT HAS BECOME KNOWN SINCE
SHE LAST WROTE. I AM MOST GRATEFUL TO IRA FOR HER INSPIRATION AND MENTORING.

FOR THEIR ASSISTANCE AND SUPPORT, I WOULD ALSO LIKE TO THANK JEFF BEUTLER, KATHY KOCH,
AND LOREE E. PEERY.

The anesthetic properties of nitrous oxide and diethyl ether have
been known since the late 1700s. Priestley, Davy, and later
Faraday remarked on these properties and their possible use for
anesthesia during surgical operations. It was not until these two
drugs had become popular through their recreational use in
"laughing gas and ether frolics," however, that their application
as possible adjuncts to surgery was attempted. Before this time,
alcohol, ice, tourniquets, and even unconsciousness brought
about by blows to the head or strangulation were tried in the
effort to relieve the pain of surgical amputations and the drainage
of abscesses. For most lifesaving surgeries, however, strong men
were placed around patients to hold them down for the
surgeon.[1,2]

Crawford Long, a Georgia physician, first used diethyl ether
for the removal of a small cyst in 1842. Unfortunately he did
not report his findings. At least two other men, Massachusetts
physician Charles Jackson and Connecticut dentist Horace
Wells, experimented with ether or nitrous oxide. But it was
William T.G. Morton, a Boston-area dentist, who on October
16, 1846, conclusively demonstrated the use of ether for surgical
anesthesia in an operating room (now known as the "ether
dome") at Massachusetts General Hospital. After the procedure,
surgeon John Collins Warren reportedly exclaimed, "Gentlemen,
this is no humbug."[1] An observer who was an eminent surgeon
stated, "I have seen something today that will go around the
world."[1,3]

Over the grave of Dr. Morton, the citizens of Boston erected a
monument with the following inscription[1]:

Inventor and Revealer of Anaesthetic Inhalation
Before Whom, in All Time, Surgery was Agony
By Whom Pain in Surgery was Averted and Annulled
Since Whom Science Has Control of Pain

From the vantage point of the physician who wrote the
inscription, optimism seemed justified; however, another century
and a half would pass before the last line would be substantially
fulfilled. Long, Jackson, and Wells re-emerged to claim credit for
Morton's discovery. They battled for years and tainted what was
otherwise viewed as America's greatest contribution to health
care in the 19th century. For approximately the first 100 years
after Morton's demonstration, anesthesia was a mixed blessing in
other ways as well.

THE PERIOD OF THE FAILED PROMISE

In the early years, the discovery and application of anesthesia to
surgical procedures did not yield the promising results expected
for several reasons, principally the morbidity and mortality associated with both anesthesia and surgery. With surgery, the main
culprit was infection; with anesthesia, it was the unskilled work of
"occasional anesthetists."

The Problem of Infection

Justifying the greater use of surgery necessitated adequate
resolution of the problem of infection. Achievement of this
goal required Florence Nightingale (during the Crimean War,
1854-1856) and others to demonstrate that hospitals did
not have to be "pest houses." With cleanliness, good ventilation,
adequate nutrition, and care provided by a qualified staff,
patients could go into hospitals to get well rather than merely
to die. Oliver Wendell Holmes, a U.S. attorney who became a
physician, and Ignaz Philipp Semmelweis, a Viennese physician,
hypothesized that infection spread by the medical provider
was the major cause of the puerperal fever that resulted in
so many maternal deaths and that merely washing one's hands
between patients could reduce this morbidity and mortality.

Semmelweis developed his hypothesis while observing midwives, noting that their deliveries were associated with a lower incidence of infection and death than those assisted by medical students. The primary difference he observed was that the midwives washed their hands between patients; in contrast, the medical students often went from the autopsy rooms to the delivery wards without washing their hands or changing their clothes. Both Holmes and Semmelweis were severely criticized by their colleagues for their hypothesis.[1] At the time, the germ theory had been alluded to but had not been confirmed.

Before the medical establishment would accept the germ theory and the means of prevention of infection in the mid-1880s, Koch and Pasteur had to confirm the theory, and Lister and several German physicians had to advocate the concept of antisepsis through the use of germ-killing chemicals. Furthermore, it was up to Pasteur to introduce the heating of milk to eliminate the "germs" that it contained and, finally, to Koch and another German, von Bergmann, to demonstrate asepsis through physical and steam sterilization, respectively.[4,5] With the problem of infection greatly reduced (but not completely resolved), the problem of the occasional anesthetists became more apparent as a cause of surgical morbidity and mortality.

The Problem of the Occasional Anesthetists

Many have attributed the problem of the occasional anesthetists in part to the limited prestige and low pay they received for their work. For these reasons, physicians did not choose to specialize in anesthesia practice. Most physicians chose either medicine or surgery as their principal specialty, and if they did perform anesthesia, it was for the most part an effort to gain a front-row seat to surgery.[5] Often the patient was not afforded the continuous vigilance needed for balancing the two basic needs of every anesthetic procedure: patient safety and appropriate surgical conditions.

The 1890s were ushered in with scathing debates over the morbidity and mortality associated with anesthesia. Many surgeons and physicians began to understand the need for anesthesia providers who devoted their practice to the administration of anesthetics. These debates took place in Europe and the United States. In England, a physician model of anesthesia was chosen; in the United States, no particular model gained acceptance. However, history has shown that at the time of the debates, some surgeons took the problems associated with the "anesthetizer or narcotizer" to heart and were determined to develop an anesthesia specialty. Furthermore, they seemed to recognize the apparent need for anesthetists who, as Thatcher defined later, would "(1) be satisfied with the subordinate role that the work required, (2) make anesthesia their one absorbing interest, (3) not look on the situation of anesthetist as one that put them in a position to watch and learn from the surgeon's technic [sic], (4) accept the comparatively low pay, and (5) have the natural aptitude and intelligence to develop a high level of skill in providing the smooth anesthesia and relaxation that the surgeon demanded."[5]

As a result, as long ago as the mid-1870s, many surgeons began to encourage the Catholic Hospital Sisters and the new professional nurses who graduated from nursing schools patterned after the Nightingale plan to train as anesthetists.

HISTORICAL BEGINNINGS OF THE NURSE ANESTHETIST

In the United States, the first evidence of nurses administering anesthesia is found in accounts of the Civil War.

Catherine S. Lawrence, a native of Skaneateles, New York, wrote a 175-page autobiography in which she recorded practicing anesthesia as a Union Army nurse.[6,7] Lawrence wrote of her duties at a hospital outside Washington, D.C., during and after the Second Battle of Bull Run. She listed administering medications, resuscitating with restoratives like ginger, tying sutures around arteries, and administering chloroform. Lawrence wrote: "I rejoice that the time has arrived that our American nurses are being trained for positions so important. A skillful nurse is as important as a skillful physician." Elsewhere it was reported that a woman, Mrs. Harris, used chloroform and stimulants at the Battle of Gettysburg. It is not known whether Mrs. Harris was a nurse. In the military annals chronicling the war, one passage does connect a nurse with the use of chloroform. In a report of the care of a Private Budlinger of the 76th Ohio Unit, it was recorded that "after breathing it for a few minutes without any apparent effect, more chloroform was added and reapplied by a nurse in attendance."[8,9]

Thatcher[5] reported that both male and female nurses were taught to induce anesthesia and were used as anesthetists in the Franco-Prussian War (1870-1871). She also reported that during this period, patients were turned over to nurses who would drop more anesthetic agents onto patients' masks while anesthetizers went to start another anesthetic, a practice that was severely criticized in the 1890s. Therefore, the practice of using nurses for administering a part or all of an anesthetic was used on both sides of the Atlantic in the latter half of the 19th century, setting the stage for greater use of nurses for this purpose in times of peace and war. Health-care needs created by wars have often led to progress for medical therapeutics and health-care delivery modalities; this has been particularly true with regard to the historical confirmation of the use of nurses as anesthetists in the United States.

The First Nurse Anesthetists

Although early evidence of the use of nurses as anesthetists is somewhat fragmentary, reports of anesthesia provided by nurses became more and more frequent beginning in the 1880s. Sister Mary Bernard founded the Sisters of St. Joseph of Wichita, Kansas, and in 1877 entered St. Vincent's Hospital in Erie, Pennsylvania, to train as a nurse. A year later, she took over the anesthesia duties of the hospital.[5] Evidence abounds that this success was rapidly repeated in the Midwest. The Franciscan Sisters, who were active in the building and staffing of St. John's Hospital in Springfield, Illinois, were particularly successful in preparing Hospital Sisters as nurse anesthetists and sending them out to other midwestern hospitals for practice. Having been prepared by another community of the Sisters of St. Francis (Syracuse, New York), Sister Mary Erhard went to Hawaii in 1886, where she administered anesthesia and performed other nursing duties on the island of Maui for approximately 42 years.

The St. Mary's Experience

Another community of the Sisters of St. Francis in Rochester, Minnesota, contributed significantly to the rise of lay nurse anesthetists. The mother superior of this order went to Dr. William W. Mayo (who, along with his sons William and Charles, as well as other physicians, was destined to achieve international fame for his surgery after the advent of asepsis) and offered to build a hospital if Mayo would take charge of it. Mayo agreed, and St. Mary's Hospital was built and opened in 1889. It was planned that Edith and Dinah Graham, two hometown graduates of the School of Nursing at Women's Hospital in Chicago, would direct and supervise the new hospital's nursing service and administer anesthesia.[5]

Within a few weeks, the Catholic Sisters took on the nursing service positions and gave the jobs of anesthetist, office nurse, general bookkeeper, and secretary to the two trained nurses. Mayo, believing that there was no reason why intelligent nurses would not make good anesthetists, instructed both of these nurses in their anesthesia duties.[5] Dinah Graham administered anesthesia for only a short period of time, but Edith was active in its administration until she married Dr. Charles H. Mayo.[10] Her successor and friend Alice Magaw, a fellow graduate of the School of Nursing at Women's Hospital in Chicago, took over the anesthesia administration. The achievements of Alice Magaw (see box at top right), along with those of another nurse, Florence Henderson,[11] contributed significantly to the international fame enjoyed by the Mayos and St. Mary's Hospital for excellence in surgery and anesthesia. Principally, they were known for making anesthesia safer through vigilance. Henderson also contributed to the development of ether administration techniques and established assessment criteria for the anesthetized patient. It was Dr. Charles H. Mayo who gave Magaw the moniker "The Mother of Anesthesia."[5,12]

Having heard of the success of using nurses in anesthesia in Rochester or having observed it firsthand, many surgeons invited nurses to specialize in the field and become their anesthetists. In many places, the nurse anesthetist was employed by the hospital administrator and not placed under the authority of the nursing superintendent, so that the nurse's availability for providing anesthesia would be ensured. The pay of the nurse anesthetist often was equivalent to that of the nursing superintendent.

In the South, another practice pattern became prevalent: the nurse anesthetist was employed by the surgeon to serve as anesthetist and office nurse. This mode of practice was still in use in some parts of the United States in the early 1950s.

The Lakeside Experience

In 1900 Agatha Hodgins (see box at right), a Canadian nurse, went to Cleveland, Ohio, to work at Lakeside Hospital. Dr. George Crile chose her to become his anesthetist in 1908, and as such she became perhaps even more renowned than Alice Magaw. She is the founder of the American Association of Nurse Anesthetists (AANA). Like St. Mary's Hospital, Lakeside Hospital became an international showcase for its success in surgery and anesthesia and was the recipient of many requests for anesthetist training from both physicians and nurses. Its reputation grew from the work of the American Ambulance, a Lakeside Hospital surgical unit established in France before the United States' entry into World War I. This unit's staff included both Crile and Hodgins, who traveled to France in 1914 to conduct research. While in France, they took on the additional mission of training some English and French physicians and nurses in the art and science of anesthesia. It was after this experience that Crile, working with the General Medical Board of the Council for National Defense and the Red Cross to develop base hospitals for use in France during the war, ensured the placement of nurse anesthetists in these units, as well as their involvement (and that of some physicians) in the teaching and training of other physicians and nurses in the specialty.[5]

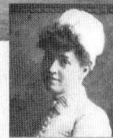

Alice Magaw

A scientist at heart, Alice Magaw saw the importance of observing, recording, analyzing, and publishing her findings concerning anesthesia practice at St. Mary's Hospital in Rochester, Minnesota. Her findings were published in various medical journals, including *Northwestern*, *The Lancet*, *St. Paul Medical Journal*, *Transactions of the Minnesota State Medical Association*, and *Surgery, Gynecology, and Obstetrics* in 1899, 1900, 1901, 1904, and 1906, respectively. In 1906 she reported the results of more than 14,000 anesthetic cases in which not a single death was attributed to anesthesia. In reporting her experiences and findings, Magaw advocated selected techniques and cited their advantages.[5]

Photo courtesy of the American Association of Nurse Anesthetists Archives.

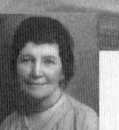

Agatha Hodgins

In addition to her practice, pedagogy, and organizational work, Agatha Hodgins was involved in the testing of some of the early anesthesia machines designed to administer a combination of nitrous oxide and oxygen. Working with surgeon George Crile, she pioneered the use of nitrous oxide–oxygen techniques for patients undergoing thyroid surgery for Graves disease.[5]

Photo courtesy of the American Association of Nurse Anesthetists Archives.

The Great War, a Small Battlefield

When America entered World War I, the Army Nurse Corps numbered 233 regular nurses; it would grow to 3524 nurses by 1918. Nurses were attached to the 50 base hospitals organized by the General Medical Board of the United States. The number of nurse anesthetists is unknown because at the time nurse anesthetists formed part of the general nursing staff.

Several outstanding World War I–era nurse anesthetists have been remembered because they wrote of their work. Nurse anesthetists spent countless hours etherizing wounded soldiers as they arrived in "ceaseless streams for days at a time after battles," wrote Mary J. Roche-Stevenson. "Work at a casualty clearing station came in great waves after major battles, with intervals between of very little to do. ... Barrages of gun fire would rock the sector for days, then convoys of wounded would begin to arrive by ambulance. Night and day this ceaseless stream kept coming on. ... The seriously wounded, especially the ones in severe shock, were taken to a special ward, given blood transfusions and other treatments in preparation for surgery later. From the receiving tent, the wounded were brought to the surgery, put on the operating tables stretcher and all given an anesthetic, operated upon, picked up on their stretcher, and loaded on hospital trains for evacuation to base hospitals."[13] Terri Harsch[14] described the works of Roche-Stevenson and others like Sophie Gran Winton; she reported that 272 nurses were killed during the war.

In a paper about Miss Nell Bryant, who was the sole nurse anesthetist for base hospital 26 from the Mayo Clinic,[15] we learn that chloroform and ether were in use, the physiology of shock was poorly understood, oxygen and nitrous oxide were given without controlled ventilation, and venipuncture involved a surgical cutdown.

Anne Penland was a nurse anesthetist with the Presbyterian Hospital of New York unit, Base Hospital Number 2. She had the honor of being the first U.S. nurse anesthetist to go officially to the British front, where she so won the confidence of British medical officers that the British decided to train their own nurses in anesthesia, ultimately relieving more than 100 physicians for medical and surgical work. Several hospitals were selected for this training of British nurses, including the American Base Hospital Number 2, with Penland as the instructor.[5]

One of the very poignant stories involving nurse anesthetists in World War I comes from Penland's diary. She was serving in a casualty clearing station, a small surgical unit usually made up of a surgeon, an anesthetist, an operating room nurse, and an orderly, situated close to the front in the Flanders section of Belgium. The casualties were heavy, and she was working the night shift and went on duty at 7 PM. Shortly after Penland arrived on duty, Lieutenant Osler, son of the distinguished professor of medicine Sir William Osler, was brought in with penetrating wounds of the chest, abdomen, and leg. Penland's surgeon, Major Darrasch, sent for Major Brewer, chief of surgery at Columbia College of Physicians and Surgeons; Major Crile from Lakeside Hospital in Cleveland; and Major Harvey Cushing, neurosurgeon from the Harvard Unit, all serving in casualty clearing stations within close proximity of one another. Penland writes the following:

All of them knew his father well. Major Crile brought his blood transfusion apparatus and Major Darrach operated, assisted by Major Brewer, Major Cushing kept his finger on the boy's pulse, and I gave a few drops of ether. It isn't often that in a small country-side, so many famous surgeons could be brought together in such a short span of time. The transfusion went beautifully, his pulse became perceptible, then gradually stronger, and his color became quite pink. The operation lasted thirty minutes; the abdomen was opened and found to have several perforations in the gut which were sutured. The chest and leg wounds were only dressed.

Thursday, August 20 [sic 30]. We were still operating at seven this morning when Major Darrach was sent for to see Lieut. Osler; his breathing had suddenly become embarrassed, and he died in a few minutes. It is a glorious thing to give one's life for one's country, but how unutterably sad; such numbers of lives being sacrificed in a strange land with no loved ones there. What grief and agony to those waiting at home!"[5]

Mary J. Roche-Stevenson, Nell Bryant, Ann Penland, Sophie Gran Jevne Winton, and many other nurse anesthetists like them demonstrated, without even intending to do so, that nurses could be exemplary anesthetists, even under the most dangerous and challenging circumstances. As a result, the world came to notice nurse anesthetists on a wider and larger scale.

The Proliferation of Nurse Anesthetists
Before World War I, surgeons and hospitals sought nurse anesthetists so enthusiastically that four formalized postgraduate programs were developed and implemented before the United States entered the war: at St. Vincent's Hospital in Portland, Oregon[16] (1909); at St. John's Hospital in Springfield, Illinois (1912); at New York Postgraduate Hospital in New York City (1912); and at Long Island College Hospital, Brooklyn, New York (1914).[5] Other nurse anesthesia programs were developed as a part of the undergraduate nursing curriculum as a specialty option. Isabel Adams Hampton Robb, a pioneer nursing leader and the first superintendent of the Johns Hopkins School of Nursing, which had opened in 1889, had in 1893 published a nursing textbook titled *Nursing: Its Principles and Practices for Hospital and Private Use*; this textbook included a chapter titled "The Administration of Anaesthetics."[5] By 1917, as a result of the "superior quality of anesthesia performed by nurse anesthetists," they were given the responsibility for surgical anesthesia at Johns Hopkins Hospital in Baltimore, where a training program was established under the direction of Ms. Olive Berger.[17]

The reputation gained by U.S. nurse anesthetists in World War I generated the climate for a great expansion of nurse anesthesia educational programs and an even greater demand for their graduates. But resistance to nurse anesthetists began to arise. A challenge to the program at Lakeside Hospital, however, brought this educational program to a halt until potential regulatory problems could be resolved.[5]

ANESTHESIA: MEDICINE, NURSING, DENTISTRY, OR WHAT?

Although few physicians chose to specialize in anesthesia before World War II, one such physician, Francis Hoeffer McMechan—a Cincinnati native—began a crusade to claim the field solely for physicians around 1911. Although McMechan had become disabled shortly after entering the field of medicine and was no longer able to practice, he and his wife undertook his mission through writing, publishing, and speaking on the issue. To what extent professional nurse anesthetists owe the Lakeside challenge in 1915 and the concomitant Kentucky challenge of nurse anesthetists to McMechan is unknown, but there can be little doubt that McMechan bore some responsibility for them.[5,18] These legal challenges were based on allegations that anesthesia was the practice of medicine and the administration of anesthesia by nurses was illegal because it constituted the practice of medicine. The two challenges, however, took separate forms.

The Lakeside challenge went to the Ohio Board of Medicine, which sent a letter to Crile in 1916. The board notified Crile of its position that no one other than a registered physician was permitted to administer anesthesia, and the state attorney general concurred with its position. Essentially, the board of medicine issued an order that Lakeside Hospital's School of Nursing was to cease its anesthesia program or lose its accreditation. Not wanting to be responsible for the loss of the school's accreditation, Crile obeyed the order, pending the outcome of a hearing conducted in 1917. At the hearing, Crile took the position that Lakeside Hospital was only following the lead of many of the major clinics in the country. Crile managed to persuade the board of medicine to lift its order, and he was able to reinstitute his nurse anesthesia educational program and his use of nurse anesthetists. Crile and supporting physicians took the additional step of petitioning the Ohio legislature to amend the state Medical Practice Act to ensure the legality of the nurse anesthetist's profession and activities by exception. The 1919 amendment essentially stated that nothing in the bill could be construed to prevent a registered nurse from administering anesthesia *under the supervision* and in the immediate presence of a physician, provided that such a nurse had taken a prescribed course in anesthesia at a hospital in good standing.[5] Physician supervision, first mentioned here, would recur many times over.

In the Kentucky challenge, the Louisville Society of Anesthetists passed a resolution proclaiming that only physicians should administer anesthesia, and it received a concurring opinion from the state attorney general in 1916. The Kentucky State Medical Association followed with a resolution stating that it was unethical for a physician to use a nonphysician anesthetist or to use a hospital that permitted nurses to administer anesthesia. This resolution led surgeon Louis Frank and his nurse anesthetist, Margaret Hatfield, to ask the state board of health to join them in a suit against the Kentucky State Medical Association.[5]

The attorney charged with representing the state board of health was the same attorney general who had issued the opinion in 1916 that prompted the medical association's actions. Frank and Hatfield lost at the lower court level but won on appeal.[5] In 1917 Judge Hurt of the Kentucky Court of Appeals, writing the opinion for the court, not only confirmed the right of nurses to administer anesthesia under the conditions that were in vogue at the time but also enunciated the following clear opinion with regard to the purpose and limits of state licensure of professionals:

[These] laws have not been enacted for the peculiar benefit of the members of such professions, further, than they are members of the general community, but they have been enacted for the benefit of the people.

While the practice of medicine is one of the most noble and learned professions, it is apparent that such a construction ought not to be given to the statute, which regulates the profession, that the effect of it would be to invade the province of the professions of pharmacy, dentistry or trained nursing, all of which are professions, which relate to the alleviation of the human family of sickness and bodily afflictions, and to make duties belonging to these professions, also "the practice of medicine" within the meaning of the statute.

Nor should such a construction be given to it as to deprive the people from all services, which could be rendered to them in sickness and affliction, except gratuitous services, or else by licensed physicians, unless the legislature intended that such should be the result of the enactment of the statute. We are of the opinion that, in the performance of the service by appellate Hatfield, in the way, and under the circumstances as agreed upon, as being the facts of this case, that she is not engaged in the practice of medicine within the meaning of the statute laws[5]

The results of these two challenges were not enough to deter the small group of physician anesthetists from other challenges. A California court case (1933 through 1936) in which Dagmar Nelson, a nurse anesthetist, was charged with the practice of medicine has been considered as the defining test case of whether nurse anesthetists are practicing medicine or nursing when they administer anesthesia. This case was decided in favor of Dagmar Nelson at each level of the California civil court system. The California Supreme Court ruled again that the functioning of the nurse anesthetist under the supervision and in the direct presence of the surgeon or the surgeon's assistants was the common practice in operating rooms; therefore the nurse anesthetist was not diagnosing and treating within the meaning of the medical practice act.[5,19]

ORGANIZATIONAL AND PROFESSIONAL SURVIVAL

Thatcher stated, "In times of prosperity, professional people give little thought to the principles of group survival and are satisfied with the most tenuous of bonds with their fellow workers. It is only when common problems become too big for individual solutions that the average professional person becomes conscious of the protection that can be found in organization."[5] Certainly, nurse anesthetists across the country were experiencing challenges. The hostility of physician anesthetists in California led to the development of a local organization of nurse anesthetists there in 1929. Other groups of nurse anesthetists often held meetings and in some instances met at the American Nurses Association (ANA) meetings. Some schools of anesthesia formed alumni associations, which served as the early model for nursing organizations.[5,20]

In 1926, Agatha Hodgins called together the Lakeside Hospital alumni group to form a national organization, with 133 names being submitted for membership; tentative bylaws were drawn up. Hodgins' concept of a national organization, however, did not take hold until 1931, after the Great Depression led physician anesthetists to exacerbate their challenges to nurse anesthetists in the interest of protecting their own incomes.[5] At approximately the same time, the ANA undertook an effort to consolidate the fields of office nursing and nurse anesthesia within the construct of organized nursing.

Hodgins maintained that nurse anesthetists were a highly specialized group of nurses. They were not exactly nurses, but they were not physicians either; rather, professionally they fell between the two. The concept of advanced practice nursing, although not by that title, was taking root in the forms of both the public health nurse and the nurse-midwife. Nurse-midwifery was emerging at the same time nurse anesthetists were seeking affiliation with the ANA.[21,22] Diers describes midwives (not nurse-midwives) as the "oldest of women healers, having been referred to in biblical times in the book of Genesis."[22] They were well established in Europe, and with the influx of immigrants into the United States and the urbanization of this country, midwives worked with public health nurses, caring for indigent populations that lived and worked in appalling conditions.[2]

The Sheppard-Towner Act of 1921 provided federal monies to public health nursing programs for the preparation and use of midwives. Midwives rapidly demonstrated their competence by lowering infant and maternal mortality rates and reducing the incidence of infant neonatal ophthalmia. As with the nurse anesthetists, physicians began to perceive midwives as threats to their livelihoods. They withdrew support for the Sheppard-Towner Act because public health nurses, along with midwives, were not under the direction of physicians. The legislation was permitted to lapse, and the funding was lost. Nurse-midwifery did not begin in the United States until 1925, when Mary Breckenridge, a British nurse and midwife, established the Frontier Nursing Service in Kentucky.[4,22]

The evolution of the nurse anesthesia profession and nurse-midwifery shared some common problems; as nursing specialties, both were somewhat ahead of their time and were not looked on with great favor by organized nursing as whole. To what extent they may have brought some of these intranursing problems on themselves will perhaps never be known. When organizing their specialty associations, neither group was able to work out agreeable conditions for merging with the ANA.[5,8]

As a result, the National Association of Nurse Anesthetists was established in 1931, and in 1933 the name was changed to the American Association of Nurse Anesthetists. The AANA developed a loose affiliation with the American Hospital Association, which furnished the AANA with its first office space. The AANA also held its national meetings in conjunction with the American Hospital Association. The AANA set as its first priority the establishment of standards for educating nurse anesthetists. It also filed its first amicus curiae brief in support of Dagmar Nelson of California. In establishing its educational standards, the AANA also recognized the need to certify nurse anesthetists on the basis of an examination after graduation from accredited educational programs. Unfortunately, World War II delayed these plans.[5]

WORLD WAR II AND NURSE ANESTHETISTS

Once again, nurse anesthetists distinguished themselves in time of war. According to Adriani,[23] when World War II broke out there were only seven anesthesiology residencies involving at least 1 year of training. Rosemary Stevens, a noted hospital historian, reports that in 1940 there were only 285 physicians in the full-time practice of anesthesiology, of whom only 30.2% were certified.[24] In another of her books, Stevens states that in 1942, nurse anesthetists outnumbered anesthesiologists by 17 to 1.[25] The military had to prepare both physicians and nurses in the specialty to meet its needs for anesthesia providers. By the end of World War II, the Army Nurse Corps had educated more than 2000 nurse anesthetists, using a 4- to 6-month curriculum patterned after that required by the AANA.[26] The shortage of nurse anesthetists could have been alleviated somewhat if U.S. law had not precluded male nurses from being commissioned and appointed in the Army and Navy Nurse Corps. A growing number of male nurses were specializing in anesthesia before World War II. They were also precluded from membership in the AANA at that time.[5]

Nurse anesthetists served at home and in all theaters of operation of World War II. They were serving in Hawaii when Pearl Harbor was attacked. Mildred Irene Clark, who was originally from North Carolina and later retired in Michigan, joined the U. S. Army in 1938. Under Army auspices, she became a student of and graduated from Hilda Salomon's nurse anesthesia educational program. Using her own military leave time, Clark went to the Mayo Clinic to observe and learn intravenous anesthesia techniques under Dr. John Lundy and Florence McQuillen, nurse anesthetist (Woodson MIC: personal oral communication, October 1994).

Clark was on assignment as a nurse anesthetist at the Schofield Barracks Hospital in Hawaii at the time of the attack on Pearl Harbor. Clark was among other nurse anesthetists on active duty who set up educational programs for preparing additional nurse anesthetists. Clark completed her illustrious career in 1967 as the Chief of the Army Nurse Corps, the first nurse anesthetist to hold this position.

Ann Mealor, another Army nurse anesthetist, was sent from Walter Reed Army Medical Center to the Philippines in 1941. She was assigned as chief nurse and chief nurse anesthetist of the hospital on Corregidor in September, just 3 months before the attack on Pearl Harbor. In addition to providing anesthesia services, she was responsible for a staff of 12 nurses.[5] Denny Williams, another Army nurse anesthetist, was assigned to the Philippines in 1936. She subsequently met and married a U.S.

engineer and terminated her Army career. (At that time and for some years to come, Army nurses could not be married and remain within the Army.) At the beginning of the war, Williams's husband was called up to join a U.S. Army battalion. Captain Maude Davidson, chief nurse of the Sternberg Army Hospital, Manila, requested that Williams be available for assisting the hospital in the provision of anesthesia services to the large number of casualties expected; Williams gladly agreed. When the Army nurses were ordered to Bataan and subsequently to Corregidor, Williams went with them. It was on Corregidor that Denny Williams, Ann Mealor, and two other Army nurse anesthetists, Doris Kehoe and Phyllis Arnold Iacobucci, were taken prisoner by the Japanese, along with some 62 other Army nurses. These nurses were interned at the Santo Tomas Internment Camp in Manila in May 1942. The prisoners of Santo Tomas were liberated by U.S. forces on February 3, 1945. All of the Army and Navy nurses who had been prisoners of war in the Philippines survived their ordeal despite starvation diets, deprivation, and tropical diseases. Throughout their imprisonment they provided nursing and anesthesia services for their fellow prisoners at the prison hospital, although access to drugs and equipment was severely limited. After Williams learned of her husband's death almost 3 years after his capture, she returned to the Army Nurse Corps and served on active duty as a nurse anesthetist until her retirement in the early 1960s.[27,28] Kehoe stayed in the Army, transferred later to the Air Force, and subsequently retired. Military nurse anesthetists served in U.S. hospitals wherever they went in support of U.S. troops, both on land and at sea on hospital ships. (The Air Force was established as a separate service of the military forces in 1949.)

Although male nurses were precluded from serving as nurses, they could and did serve in both enlisted and commissioned status, based on their educational qualifications. Some served as military medics and corpsmen. Ahead of many organizations, the AANA first accepted African American female nurse anesthetists as members in 1944, and male nurses in 1947. Hilda Salomon, the AANA's fourth president, had wanted to open up the membership to these groups during her presidency in the mid-1930s. However, at that time the recommendations were considered too radical.[5]

As World War II drew to a close, the AANA's plans for instituting a certification examination for membership were realized, and the first examination was given in June 1945. The examination was taken by 92 candidates. Provisions had been made for many nurse anesthetists to be grandmothered into the AANA on the basis of their education and experience before 1939. Of note, the title "Certified Registered Nurse Anesthetist" (CRNA) was not accepted for the identification of nurse anesthetist members of the AANA until 1957.[5]

A SHORT-LIVED PEACE FOR NURSE ANESTHETISTS AND THE NATION

Physicians and nurse anesthetists often worked in harmony to achieve their mission of providing high-quality anesthesia care to U.S. and Allied troops. World War II may be noted for alerting physicians to the potential of anesthesia as a specialty. The number of anesthesiology residencies greatly increased. The impact of World War II, as reported by Stevens,[24] resulted in an increase in the number of anesthesiologists from 285 full-time anesthesiologists in 1940, with 30.2% certified, to 1231 in 1949, with 38.3% certified. Beginning in early 1947, challenges once again faced nurse anesthetists.[5]

The American Society of Anesthesiologists (ASA) was founded in 1936* and declared its intention to make anesthesia an all-physician specialty. It changed the title "physician anesthetist" to "anesthesiologist" in an attempt to differentiate its members and eliminate the possibility of being confused by the public with "anesthetists." The ASA also promulgated member ethical guidelines that made working with and teaching nurse anesthetists unethical. Despite the ethical code of the ASA, many anesthesiologists, recognizing that the number of qualified anesthesia providers was insufficient to meet the nation's need, continued to participate in educating nurse anesthetists to work with them. John Adriani, chairman of the Anesthesiology Department at Charity Hospital in New Orleans, was among the more prominent of these.[5]

The historical problems between nurse anesthetists and physician anesthetists have been detailed in books by Thatcher[5] and Bankert[21] on the history of nurse anesthesia, as well as in Rosemary Stevens' history of hospitals and history of medical specialization.[24,25] Stevens[25] wrote the following:

> Since hospitals needed doctors in private practice to bring in hospital patients, the doctors had a strong power base of their own. Nevertheless, the traditional relationship between private practitioners and hospitals as the private doctor's workshop was difficult to justify and sustain by the late 1930s, for hospitals had obvious technologies of their own. Laboratories, x-ray, and anesthesia equipment could be operated by technicians and/or nurses, with or without the direct supervision of medical specialists.
>
> Anesthesia, often bitterly contested in a three-way tussle for control among surgeons, nurse anesthetists, and medical anesthesiologists, was the most dramatic case in point.... The employment of hospital based [medical] specialists became a major battleground for hospitals and doctors in the 1930s.... A leading anesthesiologist pressed for a propaganda campaign in the media in 1940 because he was tired, he said, of watching movies where dramatic operating scenes focused on the heroism and authority of the surgeon and represented anesthesiologists only in images of filling rubber bags and jiggling valves.

Even with the number of physician and nurse anesthetists prepared during World War II, particularly by the military, and the increasing number of anesthesiology residencies after the war, an acute and serious shortage of qualified anesthesia providers remained. Despite this shortage, some physician anesthetists, including some leaders among their specialty associations, set out to make anesthesia an all-physician specialty and initiated a public-relations campaign not directly aimed at surgeons, but rather aimed at destroying the confidence of the U.S. public in nurse anesthetists. This onslaught consisted of a series of articles, published principally in women's magazines, questioning the competence of nurse anesthetists and advocating the use of physician anesthetists. Surgeons and hospital administrators who had long experienced the achievements of nurse anesthetists came to the nurses' support. The American Medical Association, the American College of Surgeons, the Southern Surgical Association, and the American Hospital Association passed resolutions decrying the actions of these physicians and affirming their support of both physician and nurse anesthetists.[5]

The effort to make anesthesiology an all-physician specialty began before Beecher and Todd[29] completed and reported their findings in the first anesthesia outcome study in the United States. Beecher had been an anesthesiology consultant to the Army Surgeon General during World War II and had also worked previously with nurse anesthetists. After the war, Beecher and Todd performed a 5-year (1948 through 1952) prospective study of anesthesia outcomes in 10 university hospital settings. They reported the results in 1954. The results shocked and dismayed many anesthesiologists. After studying approximately 600,000 anesthetic procedures, they found that the mortality rates based on the providers were as follows: anesthesiologists, having done 62,200 cases, had a rate of 1:890; anesthesia residents, a category that included some medical and surgical residents on their anesthesia rotation, having done a total of 287,800 cases, had a rate of 1:1200; and nurse anesthetists, having done twice the number of cases as anesthesiologists, or 128,100 cases, had one half the mortality rate of anesthesiologists, or 1:1800. Furthermore, using a 7-point score for assessing patient physical status, Beecher and Todd found that there was no difference in this assessment across groups of providers. The findings were so surprising to physicians, they made assumptions that anesthesiologists were performing more complex surgical cases.[29] Perhaps this was true in some institutions, but the evidence in the literature demonstrates that in the time frame of this study, nurse anesthetists in university-type hospitals were pioneering anesthesia for specialty surgery. One such example was Olive Berger, Chief Nurse Anesthetist at Johns Hopkins Medical Center, who in 1948 reported on a series of 480 anesthetics administered to 475 patients who underwent surgery for cyanotic congenital heart disease, including procedures for tetralogy of Fallot. Of that series, physicians administered anesthesia in 41 cases, and in the remainder, anesthesia was administered by nurse anesthetists. Berger herself administered anesthesia in 289 of those cases. The patients ranged from 4 months to 45 years of age, with only 54 patients over age 20.[30] With regard to designing equipment and using cyclopropane for infants undergoing congenital heart repairs,[31] the pioneering work of Betty Lank, Chief Nurse Anesthetist at Boston's Children's Hospital, has been acknowledged by noted anesthesiologists Hamel and Lamont[32] and Smith.[33] Beecher and Todd's study had little or no effect on those anesthesiology leaders who were trying to claim the specialty solely for medicine. (Note that one must recognize the vast difference in the state of the art at the time of the study and that existing today to understand the magnitude and importance of these findings. Change in the health-care field as a result of advancing knowledge and technology, particularly in anesthesiology, has been logarithmic rather than linear.)

The national peace had been short lived when North Korea invaded South Korea in June 1950, and the United States committed its troops in support of South Korea. South Korea had been liberated from the Japanese after World War II, and the United States had troops there to help it rebuild. Again, nurse anesthetists lived up to their reputation as highly qualified and competent anesthesia professionals. The National Women's Press Club named the Army nurse as its Woman of the Year in 1953. An Army nurse anesthetist, Lieutenant Mildred Rush from Massachusetts, was designated to accept the award on behalf of all Army nurses.[5]

---

*The ASA has changed the date of its founding in recent years. Some small groups of physician anesthetists were formed earlier, as were some nurse anesthetist alumni associations. Earlier literature from the ASA, including its amicus curiae to the U.S. Supreme Court in the Hyde Case (October Term 1982), gives the 1936 date.

In 1951, U.S. Representative Frances Payne Bolton from Ohio introduced legislation to authorize the commissioning of male nurses as officers in the military nurse corps. It was not passed. However, in 1955, Public Law 294, also introduced by Representative Bolton, did pass, authorizing male nurses for reserve commissions. President Dwight D. Eisenhower signed it into law. Of note, the first male nurse commissioned in the Army Nurse Corps was a nurse anesthetist, Edward L.T. Lyon of New York. Representative Bolton attempted to correct the inequity of the 1955 law that restricted male nurses to reserve commissions by introducing legislation in 1961, 1963, and 1965. Representative Stratton of New York introduced a bill that was identical to Bolton's in 1965. The first and only male nurse draft in U.S. history was accomplished in April 1966; a bill authorizing male nurses for regular commissions in the Army, Navy, and Air Force was passed and signed into law in September 1966.[34] During the Korean War in 1952, the AANA began its accreditation program for nurse anesthetist education. (See Chapter 3.)

THE NEW AGE OF NURSE ANESTHESIA: THE 1960s

The decade of the 1960s was a transitional period in health care in general, as well as in anesthesiology. Passage of the Medicare and Medicaid legislation, with projections for a greater need for health services in the latter half of the decade, culminated in many meetings of various health-care professionals and specialists. The new legislation prompted the expansion of educational programs and the development of new programs for health professionals such as nurse practitioners and physician assistants, as well as the resurgence of nurse-midwifery. The increased federal funding for educating health professionals, for establishing additional academic health centers, and for research led to an escalation of new knowledge and new technology that pushed health-care delivery toward an ever-increasing degree of specialization.

Health care became even more hospital based and concentrated on acute care to the detriment of preventive and health-maintenance services. Public health services received less attention and, in many instances, fewer resources. The Medicaid program (designed to provide health-care services for the poor) was intended to supplant public health services, which had often been associated with indigent care. Unfortunately, the concomitant pursuit of new knowledge and new technology and the concentration on acute care were often funded at the expense of Medicaid and other public health programs. It was at this time that serious work in organ transplantation began; this work would lead to the development of artificial organs. As knowledge grew, so did specialization, with a spurt of subspecialization occurring in many medical fields. Subspecialization began to be seen in anesthesiology, which would peak in the 1980s and 1990s.

Anesthesiologists held meetings to define the future needs of anesthesiology. The meetings clearly delineated the philosophic differences among anesthesiologists concerning the ASA's goal to have an all-physician specialty and the practical reality that confronted many anesthesiologists in the 1960s, which made such a goal seem impossible. No consideration was given to calling a meeting with the AANA to jointly plan for the future.

Two schools of thought gained prominence in anesthesiology during the 1960s. Adherents of the first advocated rapprochement with nurse anesthesia and support of nurse anesthesia educational programs,[35] whereas adherents of the second supported the identification of another type of anesthesia

practitioner based on a physician assistant model and whom the anesthesiologist could control.[36,37] In 1962, Robert D. Dripps, a highly respected pioneer anesthesiologist from the University of Pennsylvania, wrote, "There are not now enough physician-specialists to administer all anesthetics in the country. It is unlikely that there ever will be. Who then will be available, how will they be trained, how *supervised and controlled?* The terms *nurse anesthetist* and *nurse technician* arouse strong emotional reaction in some quarters. Perhaps it is well to recognize this and to try to solve the problem of additional personnel in another way"[37] [emphasis added]. Dripps also suggested the preparation of persons in associate degree programs in community college settings.

At a 1967 meeting designed for debate of the manpower issue (after which a number of the papers were published in an issue of the quarterly *Clinical Anesthesia*), H.H. Bendixon, a renowned academician and research anesthesiologist, stated the following:

The total national anesthetic caseload cannot possibly at present or within the foreseeable future, be administered by trained physician anesthetists. We could not at present take the responsibility for the total anesthetic caseload, working with nurse anesthetists, because trained nurses are not available in sufficient numbers.... We need to increase the number of U.S. graduates in our residencies.... We should reduce sharply the recruitment of foreign physicians into technician service. This trend has been a mistake and a waste of valuable training.... I do not have the facilities or the time to predict our manpower needs for the next decade or two, but I offer the general observation that the shortage of nurses and technicians is far more serious than the physician shortage. We need to train more nurses and to assume responsibility for the work[35] [emphasis added].

In 1972, in his proposal to prepare anesthesiology assistants (a specialist type of physician assistant), John Steinhaus, chairman of the Department of Anesthesiology at Emory University, wrote the following:

There was general agreement at this conference [Crisis in Anesthesia Manpower 1965 Conference] that physician manpower should be increased and that programs in anesthesia research should be expanded. Although it was recognized that nurse anesthetists contribute a large portion of anesthesia service, there was no agreement as to the role this group should play in the future. The definition of the relationship between the physician and the nurse in general medicine has been difficult, [and] that between the anesthesiologists and the nurse anesthetist is even more so.[36]

This emphasis on "control," "supervision," and "assumption of responsibility for nurse anesthetist practice" was of no surprise to nurse anesthetists or to those who knew and understood the history of health care in the United States. Barbara Safreit, associate dean, Yale Law School, wrote the following in her 1992 monograph, *Health Care Dollars and Regulatory Sense: The Role of Advanced Practice Nursing:*

As Eliot Friedson has noted, in the mid-to-late 1800s, physicians rose from the ranks of previously undifferentiated occupations devoted to healing, and claimed preeminence through their highly organized effort to obtain the "exclusive right to practice." Having obtained that right, however, physicians also recognized their need for the services of other practitioners of healing, who were "useful to the physician and necessary to his practice, even if dangerous to his monopoly." Friedson concludes that, to solve this dilemma, physicians obtained from "the state control over those occupations' activities" so as to limit what they could do and to supervise or direct their activities.[38]

Having been the principal providers of anesthesia services since the late 1880s and often the anesthesia experts in operating rooms, nurse anesthetists had developed a strong sense of autonomy in their practice and were not inclined to give this up. Many had developed a conviction that was subsequently enunciated by the Ohio Supreme Court in a malpractice case. The court's legal opinion was that a physician's legal obligation to direct or supervise a nurse anesthetist's practice is not the same thing as control, and only when a physician actually exerts control over a nurse anesthetist's practice could he or she be held responsible for that practice.[39]

In fact, in the 1960s, nursing as a profession was coming of age. Nursing moved its education from hospital-based programs to institutions of higher education and was exerting efforts toward identification of its unique professional role. It also focused on determining its independent and collaborative roles with medicine and with other professionals. Some nurse educators perceived nursing as a dependent role, as did many physicians. Other nurses, particularly those moving into so-called "expanded" roles—like nurse anesthetists—asserted that they were engaged in collaborative practice with physicians and other health professionals. The women's movement attempted to remove restrictions of earnings, roles, and positions within the hierarchies of professions, industry, government, and universities. Although the number of men in nurse anesthesia was much greater than that in general nursing—probably because the former offered a higher degree of autonomy and greater remuneration—the same constraints that had been exerted on other traditionally "female" occupations and specialties continued to keep their numbers disproportionately small.

In 1964, the ASA and AANA established a liaison committee that met twice a year. C.R. Stephens, a noted anesthesiologist who had worked with nurse anesthetists for many years, wrote in a 1969 report to the ASA, "Progress has not been rapid, but the dialogue has enhanced understanding."[40]

The AANA and ASA developed and adopted a joint statement on anesthesia providers. It was published by both organizations in January 1972. This statement first recognized that both anesthesiologists and nurse anesthetists were needed in the field, and only those who were first prepared in total patient care should be prepared as anesthetists. It went on to recognize that "the ideal circumstances of qualified anesthesiologists and nurse anesthetists working together as an anesthesia care team may not be totally possible in the future."[41] By 1975, because of some substantive differences between the ASA and AANA, the ASA had withdrawn its support of the statement. Some within nurse anesthesia were happy to see its demise. The compromises made by both groups to achieve the statement had been too much for the purists and traditionalists of both professional groups. Among anesthesiologists were those of the traditional paradigm to which medicine was and is devoted. Nurse anesthetists were of two schools: the true traditionalists, who had worked exceedingly hard to overcome challenge after challenge, maintaining for the profession a relatively high degree of autonomy; and the newer nurse anesthetists, who had somewhat broader views regarding the happenings of the 1960s, saw the potential for change of the traditional health-care paradigm, and wanted to bring this change about sooner rather than later.

Some nurse anesthetists saw the need for nurse anesthesia to upgrade its educational programs and move into universities and colleges while retaining the hospital base for clinical education. The U.S. Army developed a graduate nurse anesthesia program in cooperation with the University of Hawaii School of Nursing in the fall of 1969. At about the same time, Kaiser Foundation Hospitals and the Southern California Permanente Medical Group launched a program in Los Angeles. John Garde, Ira Gunn, Joyce Kelly, and Sister Mary Arthur Schramm were the CRNAs who pioneered programs in the baccalaureate and then graduate frameworks in the early 1970s. From these beginnings, nurse anesthesia education has moved swiftly to include academically qualified faculty, a baccalaureate requirement for admission to accredited programs, and in 1988 a mandated requirement for all programs to offer a graduate degree.[42]

A little-known seed of the 1960s was the attempt by some state nurse anesthetist organizations to gain recognition by their states, either within the state nurse practice act or as a separate act. Codification in state practice acts was perceived not only as a matter of governmental recognition; more important, it provided a legal framework for public protection of patients who received nurse anesthesia services. Arizona was the first state to gain such inclusion in the nurse practice act in the mid-1960s. State codification has, in fact, become more of a necessity for advanced practice nurses (APNs) over the years. This has not been a problem for medicine because it claimed the whole of health care in its initial practice acts. Ever since, nurses and other health professionals have had to carve out their practices in state statutes to protect against charges of "practicing medicine" as the practice evolved. This expanded scope of practice, resulting from both evolutionary and revolutionary changes in health care and its delivery, made state codification of nurse anesthetists' roles even more important. California found codification necessary for its nurse anesthetists to reverse an attorney general's opinion that rendered it unlawful for nurses to provide regional anesthesia. The attorney general maintained that the California statute did not distinguish among types of nurses, and therefore opinions had to apply to all nurses.[43] To date, nurse anesthetists are addressed in one or more places within state statutes or regulations in all 50 states. Tobin[44] states, "Although it is clear that legitimacy of nurse anesthesia as a profession is widely accepted, the manner, type, and frequency of statutory and regulatory recognition of CRNA practice varies considerably." Historically and to the present day, state and federal regulations regarding nurse anesthetists and their practice have been battle sites where anesthesiologist–nurse anesthetist differences are publicly fought.

AMERICAN ASSOCIATION OF NURSE ANESTHETISTS' INCREASING FEDERAL INVOLVEMENT IN THE 1970s

The recognition of the AANA as the accreditor of nurse anesthesia programs by the U.S. Commissioner of Education in 1955 marked the AANA's first formalized relationship with federal agencies other than the military services and the Veterans Administration (VA). With the passage of federal Medicare and Medicaid legislation and subsequent legislation that provided for the funding of the education of additional health professionals, many nurse anesthetists saw the need for a federal presence for the AANA. In the late 1960s, a resolution was passed at an AANA business meeting that mandated the AANA to monitor federal legislation and to acquire a lobbyist. The signers of the resolution did not dream that the profession's governmental activities would grow sufficiently in the subsequent 20 years to require establishment of an AANA federal affairs office in Washington, D.C.

In 1970 the ASA procured a grant from the Bureau of Health Manpower of the U.S. Department of Health, Education, and Welfare (the forerunner of the current Department of Health and Human Services and the Department of Education) to perform a demographic study of anesthesia providers, both CRNAs and anesthesiologists. The Bureau of Health Manpower requested that the AANA furnish a listing of its membership with members' home or practice locations to use in the study. This was the extent to which the AANA was asked to participate in the study. When the study was completed and sent to the funding agency in 1972, it carried a notation that it had been conducted in cooperation with the AANA. As a result, governmental reviewers, in addressing its recommendations, did not think anything was amiss when one of the recommendations was for anesthesiologists to become more involved in the education and credentialing of nurse anesthetists.

This study was also made available by the ASA to the U.S. Office of Education's Department of Eligibility and Agency Evaluation, the group that reviewed accrediting agencies. John Profitt, director of this department, began communicating with the AANA on how this recommendation could best be implemented without knowing that the AANA had never been a party to the recommendation. This set the stage for a major confrontation between the ASA and AANA in the mid-1970s concerning which organization was going to control nurse anesthesia educational programs and credential their graduates. This very public challenge came at a time when major change was taking place in the criteria by which the Office of Education recognized accrediting agencies. These new criteria reflected many of the trends of the 1960s, including requirements defined in the civil rights legislation of that decade, such as public accountability, nondiscrimination, the involvement of the community of interests in decision making, students as the consumers of educational programs, requirements for due process, and grievance procedures to ensure fair and equitable treatment of students and faculty, as well as the typical educational standards concerning curriculum, instruction, and evaluation.

When these criteria were published in the *Federal Register* in August 1974, it became apparent that a great deal of change would have to be made in the AANA's educational standards, particularly as they related to the administration of accredited programs. It would also be necessary to change the organizational structure of the AANA to ensure that the accrediting groups' degree of autonomy would be maintained. It was decided that the body and mechanism for certification would be patterned after that planned for accreditation, in the belief that greater autonomy in private credentialing was the wave of the future. Ira Gunn spearheaded this process, together with Ruth P. Satterfield and Mary Cavagnaro (both AANA educational consultants) serving as principal advisors and assistants. Edward Kaleita was the newly appointed AANA educational director at that time.

After consultation with various educational and association leaders within the AANA, it became apparent that the time was right to implement new standards that incorporated not only the Office of Education's criteria but also those that set the stage for moving nurse anesthesia educational programs into university frameworks. Furthermore, with its accrediting mechanism under constant challenge by anesthesiologists, the AANA considered it necessary to demonstrate more definitive compliance with the Office of Education's criteria than did other accrediting agencies. These efforts resulted in the development of a credentialing council structure independent of the AANA.

Independent councils were first established as ad hoc structures in January 1975 because the AANA was one of the first accrediting agencies to be reviewed by the Office of Education under the new criteria in March 1975. The new organizational structure was confirmed with bylaw changes at the annual meeting in August 1975. Separate councils for accreditation (Council on Accreditation for Nurse Anesthesia Educational Programs and Schools) and certification (Council on Certification of Nurse Anesthetists) were established as multidisciplinary bodies composed of members of the communities of interest, including CRNAs, anesthesiologists, a hospital administrator, a student, and potential consumers of anesthesia services (i.e., the general public). These councils were given full autonomy in decision making concerning the credential that each council was authorized to confer. The Council on Practice was established to serve as an appeal body for the two councils, as well as to attend to matters that might be of public concern.

In 1979 the AANA membership established the Council on Recertification, which was responsible for the recertification program mandated in 1976 and implemented in 1978. Recertification has been and continues to be based primarily on continuing educational requirements and is required every 2 years. This program evolved from an AANA voluntary program implemented in 1968 for procuring certificates of excellence; the program was based on the acquisition of 100 contact hours of continuing education over a 5-year period. There is an evolving trend that could lead in the near future to a multifaceted approach for recertification, including the possibility of retesting.

The very public challenge leveled by the ASA against the AANA was answered, and recognition by the Office of Education was continued. It was this challenge that brought about the rapprochement between nurse anesthesia and the mainstream of nursing, a schism that had existed since the AANA's organization. Nursing believed that allowing physicians to take over the professional credentialing process of a long-standing nursing specialty could lead to other attempts by medicine to gain control over other nursing groups. Therefore, support for the AANA with regard to this challenge was forthcoming from the major players within the nursing community. The involvement of many CRNA practitioners, program directors, and students in acquiring letters of support for the AANA's credentialing mechanisms and their presence at Office of Education hearings also served as a training ground for subsequent lobbying of the federal government and of Congress. The Council on Accreditation has been recognized by the Council on Post-Secondary Accreditation (COPA), a private counterpart to governmental recognition since 1985. COPA has now evolved into the Council for Higher Education Accreditation.

The anesthesiologists' challenge of the AANA's credentialing prerogatives was a major one, disrupting many good relationships between individual CRNAs and anesthesiologists. This situation was further exacerbated by the AANA's first venture to seek legislation for direct reimbursement for CRNAs within the Medicare program in 1976. Medicine had long believed that physicians should be the only health-care professionals directly reimbursed for patient services and had been exceptionally active at the federal level in attempting to enforce this view in Medicare and Medicaid. The AANA was somewhat politically naive at this time, and the effort failed. However, the challenge before the Office of Education served to educate many CRNA leaders in the federal political and regulatory process, and these lessons were successfully drawn on when direct reimbursement was again on the AANA's legislative agenda in the 1980s.

Another change affecting nurse anesthetists and all professionals was the 1976 Supreme Court decision in the case of *Goldfarb v. Virginia State Bar*, 421 US 773 (1976), which ruled that members of learned professions were not exempt from federal antitrust laws. This decision was subsequently confirmed in the case of *National Society of Professional Engineers v. United States*, 435 US 679 (1978).

In both these cases, the U.S. Supreme Court indicated that in some circumstances, the attempts by professional groups to self-regulate the quality of their services or the ethics of their profession might be treated differently from other economic activities. However, the court in these and later decisions left little doubt that it would view these efforts with considerable suspicion and that exemption of the "learned professions," if extant at all, would be very narrowly defined.[45] Therefore, nurse anesthetists and other professionals are subject to antitrust laws. However, they also can use them when they are victims of a conspiracy to restrict their practices or another antitrust violation.

Although there have been many incidents in the education and practice of nurse anesthetists in which suspicion of antitrust violations has arisen, antitrust violations are often difficult to prove and are exceedingly lengthy and costly to pursue. The cases filed by two CRNAs, Tafford Oltz (*Oltz v. St. Peters Community Hospital*, 861 F2d 1440, 1450 [9th Cir 1988]) and Vinnie Bhan (*Bhan v. NME Hospitals, Inc.*, 84-2256, DC No. CV-S-83-295 LKK [October 2, 1985]), demonstrated these facts. Oltz had held clinical privileges and had worked as a private practitioner at St. Peters Community Hospital in Helena, Montana. His clinical privileges were terminated when the hospital gave an exclusive contract to a group of anesthesiologists. Oltz alleged, and the court agreed, that the hospital and the anesthesiologists had conspired to terminate his privileges so that the anesthesiologists would have access to his cases. Another factor involved in this case was that Oltz offered regional anesthesia as a part of his practice, and the anesthesiologists at St. Peters were not as interested in providing this type of anesthesia. Also, there were cost savings to the public when Oltz administered anesthesia, compared with when the anesthesiologists did. The court found that St. Peters Community Hospital had a significant enough market share within its service area, and by awarding the exclusive contract to the anesthesiologists and terminating Oltz's privileges, the hospital damaged competition. The verdict in favor of Oltz and the damages awarded were appealed by the hospital. (Oltz had previously settled with the anesthesiologists.) On appeal, the Ninth Circuit Court upheld the decision of the lower court with regard to the antitrust violation but remanded the case back to the lower court for retrial on the damages. Oltz again won in the retrial on damages, but the hospital once again appealed on a liability issue. Once again, Oltz won at the appellate court level, and the case was finally settled in August 1994, more than 12 years after it had been filed. Although nondisclosure was a condition of the final settlement of monetary damages in this case, the court awarded Oltz (the plaintiff) $1.6 million in attorney fees.[46]

The Bhan case was filed for similar reasons. However, the defendants challenged Bhan's standing—that is, his legal right to file an anticompetitive suit against NME, Inc. The anesthesiologists involved asserted that Bhan, who was licensed as a nurse and nurse anesthetist, could not legally compete with licensed physicians because of the differences in their legal scopes of practice. The defendant's argument prevailed at the lower court; however, the decision was reversed on appeal. The Circuit Court reasoned that "the issue is not whether the two groups perform identical services, but whether there is reasonable interchangeability of use or ... cross-elasticity of demand between the services provided by nurse anesthetists and by MD anesthesiologists."[46]

The Circuit Court concluded, *"No doubt the legal restrictions upon nurse anesthetists create a functional distinction between nurses and MD anesthesiologists. They do not, however, necessarily preclude the existence of a reasonable interchangeability of use or cross-elasticity of demand sufficient to constrain the market power of MD anesthesiologists and thereby to affect competition"* [emphasis added]. The court continued, stating that "as a matter of law, Bhan's allegations are sufficient to establish that he is a proper party to bring this antitrust action."[47]

Bhan lost his case because the hospital that terminated his privileges was ruled not to have sufficient market share in the community for the action to serve as a constraint on competition. The sine qua non of antitrust laws is the fact that they exist to protect competition, not competitors, and therefore the proof must be that competition within a defined economic market is adversely affected. However, the appellate court ruling that gave Bhan and CRNAs standing to sue anesthesiologists under antitrust laws sets a significant legal precedent for the profession.

FEDERAL LEGISLATIVE INITIATIVES IN THE 1980s

After the turbulent 1970s, it was hoped that a somewhat more peaceful environment would prevail in the 1980s. CRNAs were heavily recruited health-care professionals who practiced principally in three types of settings. The majority of civilian CRNAs worked as employees of hospitals or of anesthesiologists. In addition, a small but growing number of CRNAs were private practitioners. Their major problem at the time was an inability to gain direct reimbursement from many governmental programs, as well as from many private payers.

The private practitioners wanted the AANA to become more involved in assisting CRNAs to obtain direct reimbursement from both governmental and private payers for the anesthesia services CRNAs provided. Many of the contracts between CRNA private practitioners and hospitals for the provision of anesthesia services stipulated that the hospital serve as a billing service for them; this allowed the hospital to take a small percentage of the income generated from their services. These CRNAs believed that this arrangement was not to their advantage for a variety of reasons. First, some hospital administrators did not want the hospital to act as the billing agent and preferred the CRNA to be employed if they had to be the billing agent. Second, it was not always in the best interest of CRNAs for the hospital administrator to know the amount of income that the CRNAs were generating.

During 1980 and 1981, some AANA leaders were somewhat intimidated by the reaction of the anesthesiologists when the AANA first sought direct reimbursement for CRNAs. Therefore, direct reimbursement was not one of their priorities. Furthermore, the efforts and expenditures necessary to fight the challenges of the 1970s had depleted the AANA's treasury, and the leaders believed that the AANA needed time for retrenchment.

Every profession must attend to certain activities through its professional association; for CRNAs, these include monitoring and ensuring appropriate and timely standards of practice and education; establishing and enforcing ethical codes; issuing practice policies; ensuring the availability of malpractice insurance for its members; monitoring governmental regulations and those of private credentialing agencies, such as The Joint Commission; and intervening, whenever possible, in the interest of its members. Many of these areas also needed attention.

Although all professions have an inherent conflict of interest in terms of their obligations to the public versus those to their members, the implementation of the AANA's council structure freed the AANA to take a more vigorous stance with regard to protection of its members' interests. This was made possible by the AANA's provision of autonomy to the Councils on Accreditation, Certification, and Recertification and their appellate body, the Council on Public Interest, which eliminated the AANA's overt conflict of interest in credentialing for the public welfare while pursuing efforts aimed at members' benefit.

When the 1980s began, many CRNAs were tired of the challenges of the 1970s and wanted nothing better than a few peaceful years. Others recognized that many things were happening that would have direct impact on CRNAs and their practice and that the work ahead did not allow for rest. Among these issues were the federal and state governments' concerns regarding the cost of governmental health programs such as Medicare and Medicaid, the adequacy of the national health-care manpower mix, and the impact of the cost of health insurance on businesses and industry. Hospital costs had been singled out as a major problem, and studies were ongoing with regard to control of these costs. Because almost 50% of CRNAs were employed by hospitals at that time, anything aimed at controlling hospital costs could affect CRNAs. Many of the flaws in the system that related to cost escalation were based on incentives within health insurance or reimbursement mechanisms that actually promoted higher costs. Despite the AANA's many successes over the years, those AANA members who saw the increasing pressures building in society to address the emerging health-care problems believed that the AANA must change its operations to have a more proactive stance if CRNAs were to continue to meet future challenges successfully. In the election of AANA officers and board members in 1981 and 1982, CRNAs saw an opportunity to put into power a group of CRNAs willing and able to make every effort to move the AANA forward with regard to affairs of government, even if this action meant taking unpopular positions with physician colleagues.

Pat Fleming assumed the office of AANA president in August 1982. Although she had run for president in 1981 on the platform of "A Choice for Change," she did not realize the extent to which political events would influence her actions as president and set into motion a series of legislative initiatives that demanded the AANA's attention on a continuing basis throughout the subsequent years. The principal events during her presidency that necessitated priority action by the AANA were the Tax Equity and Fiscal Responsibility Act of 1982 (TEFRA), the decision to file an amicus curiae brief with the United States Supreme Court concerning the case of *Jefferson Parish Hospital District v. Hyde*, 104 SCt 1551 (1984), and the federal enactment into law of the Medicare Prospective Payment System (PPS) for Hospitals.

Tax Equity and Fiscal Responsibility Act of 1982

When the AANA first approached the Senate Finance Committee in 1976 and 1977 regarding direct reimbursement for CRNAs, the committee expressed concerns over the escalating Medicare costs for what formerly had been called *hospital-based services*, including anesthesiology, pathology, and radiology. At the time, the committee was exploring means for containing these costs. Despite the actions taken, by 1982 additional efforts were being made to constrain these costs. This effort took the form of the TEFRA legislation.

Before the passage of TEFRA in 1982, hospitals could bill Medicare under Part A for anesthesia services rendered by nurse anesthetists in hospitals and under Part B for anesthesia services rendered by nurse anesthetists in outpatient settings. The reimbursement was based on "a reasonable charge." The hospital also derived profits from the use of anesthesia drugs, supplies, and capital equipment.

Anesthesiologists could not bill for hospital-employed CRNAs' services, but they could bill for their own services in conjunction with medical direction of such CRNAs. This, however, was at a rate different from what they could bill for CRNAs they themselves employed. Although Medicare did not require anesthesiologists to actually be in the operating room with CRNAs to be reimbursed, its manual (4-76, 2050.2, Rev. 3-512, 2.21) did require that "the physician be close by and available to provide immediate and personal assistance and direction." The manual stated that availability by telephone would not constitute direct, personal, and continuous service.

However, in many instances during this period, anesthesiologists were billing for services when they were not present in the hospital or even in town. Some chose not to come out at night or on weekends to supervise care provided in emergencies, yet they billed as if they had been present. Anesthesiologist supervision or billing capability for concurrent cases was not limited to any specific fixed numbers, permitting abuse. During this time, some surgeons were openly critical of the number of fees being paid to anesthesiologists for concurrent services, particularly when the anesthesiologists were not available. A number of these surgeons and other providers complained to both private insurers and Medicare. As a result, some private payers began limiting reimbursement to not more than two concurrent procedures, and Medicare's Inspector General focused on anesthesia reimbursement in the search for potential fraud. Around this time, Richard Verville, the AANA's Washington counsel, stated that a source in the Inspector General's office of what was then the U.S. Department of Health, Education, and Welfare had told him that approximately 25% of Medicare fraud and abuse investigations concerned anesthesia services.

Among other things, TEFRA addressed anesthesia, radiology, and laboratory payments. The legislation indicated a need to ensure that anesthesiologists demonstrate that they provided certain services as a part of a given anesthetic procedure to qualify for payment. These services have been referred to as the *seven conditions for anesthesiologist payment when medically directing CRNAs*. They were initially those conditions specified by the ASA in its *Guidelines to the Ethical Practice of Anesthesiology* (adopted October 25, 1978, effective February 12, 1979) for anesthesiologists engaged in medically directing nonphysicians in an anesthesia care team (ACT) configuration. Therefore, the ASA has considered them standards of practice. Although changes have been made in the ASA's ethical guidelines, the last of which was in 2003, according to the online copy of the ethical code, these components of it have not been changed. (Available at http://www.asahq.org/publicationsAndServices/Standards/10.pdf.)

Subsequent to the enactment of the law, the Health Care Financing Administration (HCFA) proposed rules for implementation of TEFRA. The proposed rules separated reimbursement for anesthesiologists based on supervision or direction. Essentially the proposed rules called for anesthesiologist payments on the basis of direction to be limited to not more than two concurrent procedures administered by CRNAs. Such a payment took two forms, depending on the CRNA's employer. When the CRNAs were employed by the anesthesiologist, each service was billed as though the anesthesiologist had administered each case. When the CRNAs were hospital employees, the time units for the anesthesiologist were cut in half. When the anesthesiologist's service was supervision and not direction (i.e., supervising three or more CRNAs), the payment was to be made under Part A on the basis of reasonable charge. The hospital could still bill for the CRNA services of their own employees under Part A if the services were provided within the hospital and under Part B if the services were provided in a surgical center.

The AANA opposed the 2:1 ratio for the following reasons:
1. No research indicated differences in anesthesia outcomes based on fixed supervision or direction ratios in the provision of anesthesia services.
2. Because such ratios did not take into consideration the characteristics of the anesthesia workload or the population served within a given hospital, they were inappropriate for determining cost-effective personnel resources for a given facility.
3. Implementation of such ratios would significantly increase the cost of anesthesia services to individual Medicare beneficiaries and decrease the acceptance of Medicare assignment by anesthesiologists (which did not have a high assignment acceptance rate).
4. If the HCFA considered it necessary to differentiate between supervision and direction on the basis of an anesthesiologist's involvement, a 4:1 ratio would be more cost-effective in the long run, at least to beneficiaries, because anesthesiologists could derive greater income and would be more inclined to accept Medicare assignment. The AANA further stated that although the use of a ratio might be appropriate with regard to reimbursement, a ratio should never be used to imply a quality standard.

HCFA published final rules implementing TEFRA. HCFA chose the 4:1 ratio rather than the originally proposed 2:1 ratio. They also imposed the seven conditions an anesthesiologist must satisfy with regard to an anesthetic procedure if he or she is to obtain reimbursement for the medical direction of CRNAs[48]:
1. Perform a preanesthesia evaluation
2. Prescribe the anesthesia plan
3. Personally participate in induction and emergence and other demanding procedures in the plan
4. Monitor the course of anesthesia administration at frequent intervals
5. Remain physically available for the immediate diagnosis and treatment of emergencies
6. Provide needed postanesthesia care
7. Refrain from personally performing an anesthesia procedure when purporting to be engaged in medical direction

Over the years, various interpretations have somewhat loosened these conditions; for example, in an emergency, an anesthesiologist engaged in medically directing CRNAs may go to the obstetrics area and administer a regional anesthetic.

The HCFA also stated the following in the *Federal Register*: "*The distinction we are making is between physician services to providers and individuals, not between good and bad anesthesia services.... Therefore the criteria for 'medical direction' should not be interpreted as standards of practice or standards of quality, but rather as a description of those elements of common medical practice that are expected to be present when a physician has significant involvement with an individual patient*"[49] [emphasis added].

Nevertheless, what began as a means of controlling fraud and abuse within the complex payment mechanism for anesthesia services morphed into a standard of care.

Hyde v. Jefferson Parish Hospital District No. 2

The case of *Hyde v. Jefferson Parish Hospital District No. 2* centered on whether an exclusive contract by a group of anesthesiologists was per se a violation of the Sherman antitrust laws, because such a contract was the basis for denying Dr. Hyde clinical privileges in the East Jefferson Hospital, which was part of the larger Jefferson Parish Hospital District No. 2. At this hospital, a group of anesthesiologists who had an exclusive contract worked with hospital-employed CRNAs to cover anesthesia services. It was a fairly large hospital with a sizable workload. Dr. Hyde, who had clinical privileges at other hospitals in the area, decided he also wanted clinical privileges at East Jefferson Hospital. His request was denied solely on the basis of the exclusive contract. The legal question raised by the case was whether a patient who was admitted by his or her surgeon to East Jefferson Hospital for surgery in effect had any choice but to buy anesthesia from the hospital's exclusive group of anesthesiologists. It was alleged that this situation represented a tying arrangement, such as those previously found to be per se violations of the antitrust laws. (A tying arrangement would be similar to going to a store to buy bread but being unable to buy it by itself. Rather, one would be required to buy butter to get the bread, whether or not the purchaser used butter on bread.)

The Jefferson Parish Hospital District won the case at the lower court level. Dr. Hyde appealed to the U.S. Court of Appeals, which ruled in his favor. Jefferson Parish Hospital District then filed an appeal to the U.S. Supreme Court. This would ordinarily not be a case in which the AANA would consider filing an amicus curiae brief; however, in both the lower court and appellate court opinions, the judges cited some rather derogatory conclusions regarding nurse anesthetists that had been presented by anesthesiologists testifying for Dr. Hyde in an attempt to discredit the quality of anesthesia service provided by East Jefferson Parish Hospital. The AANA, in submitting its amicus curiae brief, chose not to take a position for or against exclusive contracts. It only wanted to "set the record straight" about the misrepresentation of nurse anesthetists and ensure that the Supreme Court in its decision did not perpetuate some of the myths cited by the other judges and was not swayed in its decision by such myths.

The AANA board of directors requested that the AANA legal counsel acquire permission to file such an amicus curiae brief and then to prepare it. Problems getting the AANA's legal counsel and law firm to follow the AANA's purpose for filing the amicus, identified only approximately 7 days before the due date of the brief, led President Fleming to turn the project over to Gene Blumenreich of the Fine and Ambrogne law firm in Boston. Blumenreich was legal counsel for the Massachusetts Association of Nurse Anesthetists at the time. Blumenreich was to be assisted by Richard Verville of Fine and Verville, the AANA's Washington, D.C., attorney, and by Susan Jenkins of Lyon and Kurz, also in the District of Columbia.

In the AANA amicus curiae brief, the Supreme Court was asked to decide the issue on very narrow grounds, ignoring the previous courts' opinions as they related to nurse anesthetists.

It stated that nurse anesthetists were not a party to the suit, had not had representation during any of the proceedings, and had certainly had no opportunity to counter erroneous testimony. The amicus masterfully corrected the record on nurse anesthetists.[49]

The ASA also filed an amicus curiae brief, but in support of Dr. Hyde. The ASA concluded their brief as follows:

ASA submits that this is hardly the case in which to reverse thirty-five years of consistent Supreme Court precedent applying the per se rule in tying cases. In the circumstances of this case, which involves the administration of lethal drugs to human beings under carefully controlled conditions, the elimination of competition through a classic tying arrangement is not simply a matter of dollars and cents. It can adversely affect the quality of medical care. ASA believes that in this setting it is particularly important that competition be allowed to reward superior performance and innovation, while exposing the indifference to quality that may too often be the hallmark of a monopoly.[50]

The Supreme Court, during its hearing on this case, gave evidence of noting the AANA's brief in its questioning of attorneys who argued the case. When the ruling came down, the Supreme Court had decided unanimously in favor of the hospital, not Dr. Hyde. The justices differed (five to four) as to why they decided in favor of the hospital. The majority opinion stated that the decision was based on the finding that "every refusal to sell two products separately cannot be said to restrain competition" and that no evidence had been presented to support the contention that the hospital had forced unwilling patients to buy this service. Because they found that this arrangement did not violate the per se rule, they applied the "rule of reason" and found no evidence of adverse effect on competition. East Jefferson Hospital did not have market power. The concurring opinion, written by Justice O'Connor and supported by three other justices, stated that it was time to abandon the per se rule and to focus on the adverse economic effects and the potential economic benefits of the exclusive contract. Finding no adverse competitive effects, and even citing a potential benefit from the exclusive contract in increasing a hospital's efficiency, these justices concurred that this exclusive contract was not a violation of the antitrust laws.[50]

The Hyde case is important not only for clarifying the law but also for its opportunity to correct the legal records concerning CRNAs. The Hyde case alerted the AANA to the need to revitalize its public relations program, continue its watch for attempts to discredit CRNAs or the profession, and take action either to correct or to prevent further damage.

Medicare Prospective Payment System for Hospital Services

In early 1983 the AANA was still dealing with TEFRA when, without much fanfare and with less media exposure than usually accompanies such legislation, the PPS legislation was passed in an effort to control the hospital costs of the Medicare program. Until that time, hospitals were allowed to submit their bills on a cost-plus basis to Medicare and therefore had no incentives for controlling their costs. The PPS was to be phased in over a 4-year period. Hospitals would be reimbursed for their services on the basis of prospective pricing for various diagnosis-related groups. Thus, if the hospital services did not cost as much as the hospital was paid, the hospital reaped a profit; if the services' actual costs were greater than the amount paid, the hospital had to absorb the loss.

The AANA developed an option paper that demonstrated the impact of the PPS legislation on nurse anesthetists, including its potential to result in higher costs for anesthesia services. AANA leaders believed that the only alternative for preventing the disincentives to using CRNA services found in the legislation was the acquisition of direct reimbursement rights for CRNAs under Medicare Part B or the placement of reimbursement for all anesthesia services (those provided by both anesthesiologists and CRNAs) under Medicare Part A. Based on its analysis and conclusions, the AANA's plans for resolving the problems the PPS had created for CRNAs also took into consideration the fact that making anesthesia a hospital-based service was not politically feasible at that time. The AANA proposed and eventually acquired the following provisions:

1. A temporary pass-through of hospitals' CRNA costs for a 3-year period, which would assure hospitals that they would not lose money on CRNA services for Medicare patients
2. A single exception to the unbundling provisions of the law for anesthesiologist-employed CRNAs, because it was questionable whether anesthesiologists could be reimbursed for CRNA services without such a provision
3. Direct reimbursement for all CRNAs under Medicare, because provisions 1 and 2 were temporary, and CRNAs needed a mechanism under Medicare that would pay for CRNA services

The AANA and CRNAs agreed to accept assignment as a condition for passage of the direct reimbursement legislation. In other words, CRNAs agreed they would not bill patients for that portion of services not paid by Medicare. As a part of the Omnibus Budget Reconciliation Act of 1986, direct reimbursement for CRNAs was enacted into law to become effective January 1, 1989, with the two temporary provisions being extended to the effective date of the legislation. The various practice configurations of CRNAs required the development of two payment schedules—one for CRNAs not medically directed by anesthesiologists and the other for CRNAs working under an anesthesiologist's direction. This latter payment schedule resulted in significantly higher Medicare prices for anesthesia services compared with prices for services provided either by anesthesiologists who administered their own anesthesia or by non–medically directed CRNAs. Furthermore, as a part of this legislation, Congress mandated a study of reimbursement mechanisms that would not serve as disincentives to the use of CRNAs.[51]

The success the AANA achieved with respect to Medicare during this period must be attributed to the commitment of the profession and its leaders to goals set during the Fleming administration. This required the commitment and concerted actions of the leaders of the succeeding AANA administrations—Patrick Downey, Barbara Adams, Richard Ouellette, Peggy McFadden, and Jan Mannino. Furthermore, AANA members owe much to Richard Verville, AANA's Washington attorney; Debbie Hardy, AANA lobbyist of Capitol Associates; and Jay Constantine, another lobbyist (who formerly had been the chief staff member of the Senate Finance Committee when the AANA first attempted to gain reimbursement), for expertise and untiring effort expended toward achieving these goals. Their commitment to this cause made them part of the AANA family, not merely retained experts.

Furthermore, these activities gave AANA members the opportunity to make certain their legislators knew who CRNAs were, how much they contributed to the provision and quality of anesthesia services in this country, and why such legislation was important to the nation, as well as to CRNAs—and they indeed met the challenge. Some of the legislators whom they were able to persuade to introduce and cosponsor AANA's direct reimbursement bills were Matsunaga (Democrat, Hawaii), Inouye (Democrat, Hawaii), Sasser (Democrat, Tennessee), Pell (Democrat, Rhode Island), Pressler (Republican, South Dakota), Humphrey (Republican, New Hampshire), Sarbanes (Democrat, Maryland), Melcher (Democrat, Montana), Burdick (Democrat, North Dakota), and Leahy (Democrat, Vermont) in the U.S. Senate and Barney Frank (Democrat, Massachusetts) and other cosponsors in the U.S. House of Representatives. Many of these legislators were fully aware that without nurse anesthetists, rural health care would have been nonexistent in many of their states. Nurse anesthetists, serving as the sole anesthesia providers in many of these areas, were also believed to be a key in retaining physicians in rural areas and in keeping hospitals in these areas open.

However, it is not enough to ensure that legislation is passed. Monitoring and intervention during the period of rule making must and did occur. Permanent rules were not in place until 1991.

The activism of the AANA at this time was thought to have been partially responsible for the ASA's issuance of practice policies that, if adhered to, would have restricted CRNA practice and severely limited obstetric patients' access to regional anesthesia. The ASA's policy that "only physicians should perform regional anesthesia" was the basis for the action of a Maine attorney general when anesthesiologists in Portland, Maine, revoked the right of CRNAs to perform regional blocks and to teach them to their students. The Maine attorney general obtained a consent decree from the anesthesiologists that reversed their decision regarding CRNAs' performance and teaching of regional blocks.

Quality-of-Care Studies

Despite the frequent challenges by the ASA, neither the AANA nor its members had given much time to considering the performance of quality-of-care studies relative to patient outcomes by CRNAs. There had been a constant market for nurse anesthesia services, and surgeons had provided them support and acclaim. There were no major indicators of any significant problems, although little question existed that studies demonstrating accountability in terms of patient outcomes were on the horizon. What was then called the *expanded role nurse* and now the *advanced practice nurse* essentially came on the health-care scene in the 1960s and 1970s. The nurse practitioner was the major new provider, along with the physician assistant, newly introduced by medicine. Certified nurse-midwives, who had existed in limited numbers before that time, began to expand their ranks and set up nurse-midwifery services. It was anticipated that these providers would offer many services previously restricted to physicians, and their practice and outcomes would be subjected to multiple studies. Because at that time nurse anesthetists quantitatively performed the greatest number of anesthetic procedures in the United States and few complaints were being heard, not much thought was given to studying their outcomes, except by a few physicians. Beecher and Todd's study, reported in 1954, had shown that nurse anesthetist mortality statistics were less than half those of anesthesiologists, even though the sample size for nurse anesthetists was twice that for anesthesiologists. Furthermore, the physical status of the patients in both groups was studied and found to be similar.[29]

A North Carolina retrospective study of anesthesia-related mortality during the period from 1969 to 1976 (performed by a committee from the North Carolina Society of Anesthesiologists) reported in 1981 that the findings based on providers (e.g., CRNAs working alone, anesthesiologists working alone, and CRNAs and anesthesiologists working together as a team) were similar. No test of significance was made in this study, because adequate data had not been collected to assess the likelihood that a variety of variables were factors in these cases.[51]

In the mid-1970s, amid major complaints about the VA health-care system, the U.S. House of Representatives mandated a study by the National Science Foundation regarding the care given to veterans. As a part of that study, physicians and surgeons reviewed a sample of VA medical facilities regarding the care being given. Most of the larger facilities were being used by medical schools both for medical student and graduate medical education. However, because of the shortfall of anesthesia residencies at that time, many nurse anesthetists were employed by the VA and worked in these facilities. The reviewers included surgery and anesthesia in their assessment and reported back to Congress in 1977 that there was no significant difference in the outcomes of anesthesia based on the provider of that care.[52]

In 1980 anesthesiologist W.H. Forrest reported and published a portion of an institutional differences study conducted by the Stanford Center for Health Care Research. In looking at hospitals and anesthesia outcomes, dividing the hospitals between those predominantly served by nurse anesthetists and those predominantly served by anesthesiologists, he also came to the conclusion—using conservative statistical methods—that there were no significant differences in anesthesia outcomes between the two hospital groups defined by their anesthesia provider.[53] (Ira Gunn spoke with Dr. Forrest regarding his study, and he mentioned that he had been castigated by his colleagues for reporting these results.)

It was apparent that physicians and anesthesiologists were conducting the studies and demonstrating that CRNAs were doing a commendable job. Furthermore, the fact that many anesthesiologists doubted studies performed by their own colleagues gave little reason to think these anesthesiologists would believe studies conducted by the AANA, whether the AANA chose to do them or paid to have someone else perform such studies.

Educational Funding for Nurse Anesthesia

In 1979 the AANA had been successful in acquiring passage of legislation that would have permitted funding for nurse anesthesia students. However, because the legislation was out of synchronization with the congressional appropriations cycle and because it ran up against some of the Reagan administration's policies, the funding was not available until 1983. By 1983, the AANA began to notice an increasing number of announcements concerning the closure of long-standing university-affiliated nurse anesthesia educational programs that had coexisted with anesthesiology residency programs. To be sure, the number of graduates of medical schools in the United States had more than doubled since the 1960s, and there was serious recruitment of graduates for anesthesiology residencies. The coming overall surplus of physicians, as identified by the Graduate Medical Education National Advisory Committee, along with its evidence that the field of anesthesiology demonstrated a shortage, added to the rapid influx of medical school graduates and physicians already certified in lower-paying specialty areas into anesthesiology residencies.[54]

The displeasure of many ASA leaders with the AANA's federal initiatives, along with concerns by some anesthesiologists that they were, in fact, participating in preparing their future competitors, led a sizable number of academic chairs to convert nurse anesthesia training slots into medical residency training spaces and close nurse anesthesia programs.[55,56] At this time, some anesthesiologist leaders expressed the belief that once again, the reality of an all-physician specialty might be possible. Strangely, the more anesthesiologists that were prepared, the more nurse anesthetists were being sought for employment by hospitals, surgical centers, and even anesthesiologists. It has been hypothesized that the decentralization of surgical facilities and the increasing specialization of health care, along with the aging of the population, are reflected in the increasing need for health professionals. Anesthesiology has been no exception.

The shortage of nurse anesthetists prompted salaries to rise to heights that our forebears never imagined. It also increased the workload of practically all CRNAs. The CRNA shortage prompted Congress to mandate a CRNA manpower study, which was reported in February 1990. It also prompted Richard Ouellette, a CRNA who was then serving a second term as association president, to appoint the National Commission on Nurse Anesthesia Education. Sandra Maree, a former AANA president and program director, was appointed to serve as its chairperson. The commission was multidisciplinary in nature, made up of leaders from nursing education, CRNA education, anesthesiology, hospital administration, managed care groups, health policy analysts, and health economists. Their charge was to study the problems concerning nurse anesthesia education and to advise and work with the association to increase its educational programs and the number of graduates from those programs. This study was reported in December 1990. The AANA implemented many of the commission's recommendations, with the consequence being a significant increase in the number of graduates from accredited programs.

Concomitant with the growing shortage of CRNAs were prevailing conditions favoring the possibility of some increases in federal funding for nurse anesthesia educational programs. These increases were tempered by the growing federal deficit, but funds were made available not only for student stipends but also for program development or for expansion and faculty development.

It was also in 1990 that the AANA's federal affairs department was moved to Washington, D.C., with the establishment of an AANA Washington office. A new team of lobbyists came on board to staff the Washington office.

THE CALL FOR HEALTH-CARE REFORM IN THE 1990s

Efforts Toward Cost Containment in Health Care

Health-care reform and cost containment in the delivery of care are important parts of nurse anesthesia history, because many issues involving nurse anesthetists have either evolved or been exacerbated as a result of this movement in which all health-care providers have a major interest. Understanding these issues within the context of nurse anesthesia history requires some explanation.

The escalating costs of health care precipitated by the passage and implementation of the Medicare and Medicaid programs; the increased federal and state support of health-care professional education in response to the anticipated increase in the number of patients seeking health care, particularly among the elderly and the poor; and the rapid advance of science and technology had led many national leaders to discuss the need for health-care reforms as early as 1972.[57] The 1992 election of Bill Clinton as president of the United States on a platform that promised health-care reform brought both hope and concern to the public and to health-care providers with regard to what actual reforms would be enacted as legislation and how those reforms would affect health professionals. More specifically to anesthesia providers, what would be the role of anesthesiologists and nurse anesthetists in such reform? The president's health-care reform package was aimed at universal coverage and reflected a major shift in health-care delivery toward managed care. A component of the legislation would have preempted state laws and thereby removed legal barriers to the practice of APNs, permitting them to more directly compete with their physician counterparts in efforts to reduce costs. This provision would also have provided the necessary legal authority for APNs to render services for which they were educationally qualified to all segments within the population without physician supervision (in some instances collaborating with or referring patients to physicians).

For a variety of reasons, Clinton's health-care plan was defeated, but in general it was believed to involve (1) too much change in too short a time, (2) too much governmental involvement and control and too many mandates, and (3) too high a cost, although spending caps were a part of its design. Large corporations, the health insurance industry, and in large measure, the American Medical Association (AMA) were able to influence enough legislators and the public via major television advertising to kill the plan. As soon as the plan was pronounced dead, the health insurance industry, in conjunction with the major businesses that provided health insurance to their employees, forced a "managed care" system on a large portion of the insured population. This managed care system did not have some of the patient or physician protections that were built into Clinton's proposed plan. However, because of the cost savings projected for a managed care system, the U.S. government offered Medicare beneficiaries certain incentives to move to managed care plans. Subsequently, some states begin to pattern their Medicaid programs after the managed care concept, permitting, in some instances, managed care groups to bid to cover Medicaid patients.

Managed care, in theory and in its pure form, was supposed to (1) move the health-care system from its acute-care orientation to a health-maintenance, disease-prevention system of care; (2) do away with some of the economic incentives found in the fee-for-service system—that is, the more services provided, the more money made—and thereby reduce unnecessary or minimally indicated health services (and concomitant procedures) that had been provided as a major component of the fee-for-service system that had been the major component of the health delivery system[58,59]; (3) promote a more ideal and less costly workforce mix, that is, more primary care providers and fewer specialists, fewer physicians and more nonphysician health professionals such as APNs; and (4) promote a shift from independent practice patterns to greater use of salaried personnel. In fact, in some of the incentives provided to physicians, particularly under capitation arrangements, it was also designed to encourage physicians to treat patients with less costly modalities, to reduce the number of screening and diagnostic tests performed, and to increasingly shorten the time patients spent in hospitals. Hospitals experimented with staffing patterns, in many instances reducing the number of nurses and employing more assistive personnel. Some anesthesiologist groups found their workload reduced by 40%.[60]

Health providers tried to find ways to cope with all the changes, and in some instances they were successful.

Managed care, as implemented, took many forms as physicians scrambled to protect their autonomy and their income, and patients sought to preserve some of their former health-care rights relative to the choice of provider. The traditional health maintenance organization (HMO) was considered a "one-stop shopping mall" for health-care needs. Kaiser Permanente's HMO was the classic example of a not-for-profit HMO model. It was designed principally to reduce costs by keeping people healthy or by picking up health problems early when they were less costly to correct.

The shift from the not-for-profit health-care organizations to for-profit organizations has also affected where health-care dollars are being spent. It has been reported that in for-profit managed care organizations, 30.9% of income on average is spent for administration, payment of merger debt, executive salaries, and stockholders' dividends. In Kaiser Permanente's not-for-profit HMO operation, administrative costs are reported to be approximately 3.5%, while excellent patient services and outcomes are maintained.[61] Data have consistently shown that the cost of health-care services has been higher in the for-profit sector. Data in 1999 showed that higher costs in for-profit facilities had persisted. Although managed care, overall, was thought to be responsible for slowing the escalating cost increases in the mid-1990s, it became obvious that in some organizations, much of that slowing was related to a reduction in services to patients, some of which were necessary and lifesaving; as a result, tragic stories hit the media. In some instances, costs were shifted to patients when they developed a need for emergency care and had to have health care away from their point of contact for health services. A cry went across the land for a patient's bill of rights, but partisan differences as to just what those rights should be has stalled development of a consensus and passage of such legislation.

Regardless of the method for delivering health care, the large amount of money involved has also attracted a large amount of fraud, not only associated with the Medicare and Medicaid programs but involving private payers as well. The fraud has taken a variety of forms, including setting up dummy health services providers and billing for services never rendered; up-coding patient diagnoses by hospitals to increase their reimbursement rate; double billing by physicians and hospitals; fraudulent billing practices by individual providers; and fraud on the part of Medicare intermediaries, which are Medicare-designated payers who are supposed to be watchdogs for fraud. When caught, some claim ignorance as the basis for what happened, although it is evident that most fraud has been purposeful and intentional. Even with the increasing surveillance for fraud and personnel devoted to its discovery, it is recognized that much has gone undetected. The result of such fraud can only be higher health-care premiums or a reduction in services provided to beneficiaries. In trying to come to grips with fraud, whistle-blower laws now permit private individuals or groups to pursue cases in court and receive a portion of the award should the case be won. Such was the case in one of two suits brought by the Minnesota Association of Nurse Anesthetists and a group of CRNAs against the Allina Health Systems and some anesthesiology groups after the transfer of hospital-employed CRNAs to anesthesiologist group employment, which resulted in some adverse effects for some of the CRNAs. After a 10-year-long fight over pretrial maneuvers, the CRNAs prevailed before going to trial.

For approximately 5 years, cost increases for health-care services slowed. However, in 1998 and 1999, health insurance premiums for managed care entities increased significantly, wiping out many of these cost savings. Furthermore, Medicare patients are being forced out of many managed care plans. Many managed care plans have gone bankrupt, and unrest within the health-care industry and among health professionals and consumers of health services is on the rise.

In summer 1999, two significant studies published in major journals indicated significant problems with the for-profit segment of the health-care industry, prompting some calls for another look at options for health-care reform. In one study, the quality of care in for-profit HMOs, as measured by 14 quality-of-care measures using the Health Plan Employer Data and Information Set (HEDIS) from the National Committee for Quality Assurance's Quality Compass, 1997, demonstrated that "investor-owned HMOs deliver lower quality of care than not-for-profit plans."[62] In the other study, the authors found that governmental spending "in for-profit areas was greater than in not-for-profit areas in each category of service examined . . . [but] the greatest increase in per capita spending between 1989 and 1995 [was] for hospital services . . . and home health care in areas where for-profit corporations dominated the scene."[62,63] Therefore, questions are beginning to be raised regarding efficacy of the current reforms wrought by the industrial giants and other health payers.[61-63]

Exacerbation of Tension and Conflict Between CRNAs and Anesthesiologists

The health-care reform environment has fostered insecurity among health providers and a realization that many advocate the greater use of lower-cost, highly qualified nonphysician health-care providers. This has led to exacerbation of tensions and open conflicts between groups of providers whose scopes of practice permit a significant degree of competition. State legislative agendas have been swamped by legislative proposals to either expand or restrict scopes of practices of various health providers, to gain direct reimbursement rights, to acquire nondiscriminatory language in the use or credentialing of health professionals based on one licensure, to codify the practice of groups, to gain prescriptive rights, and a multiplicity of other types of legislation affecting various players in health-care delivery, including the consumers of care.

These shifts in delivery and payment systems significantly affect CRNAs and anesthesiologists. Theoretically, they can have an even greater impact on anesthesiologists than on CRNAs, because the use of CRNAs has some definite cost advantages without compromise in the quality of care.[39,51-53,64,65] This impact is greatly affected by excess training of anesthesiologists since the early 1980s, when they began to convert the training slots of nurse anesthesia programs to medical residency training slots, causing many of the nurse anesthesia programs to close.[66-68] Although the AANA has worked to recoup the clinical training slots for CRNAs that had previously been lost, it has needed a dozen years to do so. In the meantime, the ratio of anesthesiologists to CRNAs, which in 1986 was 1:1.2,[64] was 1.2:1 in 1995.[69] In the mid-1990s, an excess of anesthesiologists resulted in the inability of a fair number of graduating residents to find positions. When publicized, this phenomenon elicited a response that included a significant drop in the number of graduates of U.S. medical schools who chose to enter the field of anesthesia and the transfer of some anesthesiology residents out of the specialty.

Many anesthesiology residencies cut some of their training spaces, but others resorted to accepting increasing numbers of international medical graduates. As a result, 55% of the current anesthesiology residents are international medical graduates, approaching the 58% that was the peak for such residencies in the early 1970s.[68]

It should be noted that nonphysician health providers capable of competing with physicians within the area of their overlapping scopes of practice require removal of at least two legal barriers to do so with relative ease: (1) they need a legal status with regard to autonomy that is sufficient to allow them to engage in such competition, and (2) they must have the capability to be reimbursed for their services. Efforts by these professionals to achieve these legal sanctions and others that facilitate their practice have presented significant threats to their physician counterparts. Such is the case between CRNAs and anesthesiologists.

Reimbursement Initiatives

Relationships between the AANA and the ASA have not improved significantly since the AANA sought direct reimbursement for CRNAs. Both organizations bear a responsibility to their individual memberships for their economic and professional welfare, and the welfare of CRNAs and that of anesthesiologists are not necessarily congruent. Therefore early in the 1990s, the two groups found themselves on opposing sides. When CRNAs won direct reimbursement rights in the mid-1980s, they had agreed to accept Medicare assignment, and the legislation called for a budget-neutral reimbursement methodology. Payment schedules were devised for anesthesiologists working alone, CRNAs working alone, and anesthesiologists medically directing CRNAs in the ACT practice setting. In the early 1990s, the "single-payment-for-anesthesia" issue arose as a result of a Government Accounting Office (GAO) study.[69] This study demonstrated that payments for anesthesia services under the medical direction model of delivery were 120% to 140% greater than those when CRNAs or anesthesiologists were administering their anesthetics alone. Although this greater cost to Medicare was not consistent with the legislative intent of Congress, it did serve as an economic incentive for anesthesiologists to employ or use more CRNAs. The GAO recommended that the payment model be changed and that only a single anesthesia fee, not more than what would be charged when an anesthesiologist performed the service alone, be reimbursed for each anesthetic procedure.[69] Furthermore, the payment for anesthetic procedures under the medical direction model was suggested to be reimbursed at 50% for the CRNA service and 50% for the anesthesiologist service, which significantly reduced both the anesthesiologist's and the CRNA's portion of the fee. (Payment for additional anesthesia providers would continue to be allowed if adequate justification based on patient-specific factors such as physical status and surgical complexity was submitted along with the bill.) The AANA chose to support the single-payment concept. Efforts to contain health-care costs were already being made by the federal government, and the AANA believed this change was consistent with the legislation it had initiated in gaining direct reimbursement for CRNAs. The ASA opposed it. The single-payment reimbursement plan was implemented, and tension between the two groups again was exacerbated.

ASA Anesthesia Care Team Statement

At the heart of many of the AANA-ASA differences has been the ASA's definition of the ACT concept, which has often reflected what appears to be a lingering desire to make anesthesia an all-physician specialty, albeit today with technical assistants. In the mid-1970s, the ASA appointed the Ad Hoc Anesthesia Care Team Committee, which fronted the effort by the ASA to take over the education and credentialing of CRNAs. In 1977 the ASA adopted a policy statement, *Suggestions to ASA Members for Delineation of Anesthesia Functions for Non-Physician Personnel*. This statement started with these words: "The provision of anesthesia by non-physician personnel should be under the direction of the physician responsible for the anesthesia."[70] It stated that the delineation of functions and local credentials should be based on the nonphysician's education, training, and experience. It ended as follows: "Qualified personnel under the direction of a physician should be competent to: (1) induce anesthesia; (2) maintain anesthesia at the required levels; (3) support life functions during the perioperative period; (4) recognize and take appropriate action for abnormal patient responses during anesthesia; and (5) provide professional observation and resuscitation until the patient has regained control of his vital functions."[70] (These guidelines were published before significant numbers of graduates of U.S. medical schools were choosing anesthesiology as their specialty.)

In 1982 the ASA unilaterally defined the ACT and announced its control by anesthesiologists. Although it did not call CRNAs technicians in its statement, it essentially assigned CRNAs a technician's role, and ASA leadership did not hesitate to verbally distinguish anesthesiologists and CRNAs by using the professional-technician categorization in public pronouncements. Furthermore, in the 1982 edition of the statement, such a team was to be in existence only until the ASA's goal of one-on-one anesthesia could be accomplished—that is, when enough anesthesiologists were available to personally provide each anesthesia service.[71]

In 1987 the ASA modified its ACT statement, removing the offensive paragraph cited previously.[72] In 1995 the ASA made another modification to its ACT statement, stating that "the Society believes that the involvement of an anesthesiologist in the care of every patient undergoing anesthesia is essential. This may be accomplished through personal provision of anesthesia care or by medical direction of the anesthesia care team." This was impractical, because in 1990 it had been estimated by the U.S. Office of Technology Assessment that approximately 25% of the U.S. population lived in rural areas. Further estimations indicated that up to 80% of the rural population received anesthesia services solely from CRNAs.[73] Furthermore, the majority of office anesthetic procedures in urban areas were also provided by CRNAs. Many health consumers needed CRNAs who were professionals, not merely technicians, and who were competent in a broad range of anesthesia and anesthesia-related modalities, including regional anesthesia techniques and resuscitation and stabilization. Their education prepared them as professionals, and their practice of anesthesia was the practice of professional nursing, not the practice of delegated medicine.

The AANA has recognized and continues to recognize the three basic practice patterns of CRNAs, including CRNAs working with anesthesiologists. Until the early 1980s, it was not unusual for CRNAs and anesthesiologists to work in the same institutions, yet not work together. CRNAs sometimes consulted these anesthesiologists or other medical specialists, but they did not work as a team in many settings. Furthermore, the AANA has always recognized that if CRNAs were required to work solely with or under the supervision or direction of anesthesiologists, millions of people would lose their access to anesthesia services. Rural America and in some instances other underserved populations have not drawn anesthesiologists to their location of health-care need, and for that matter many other medical specialists have not been drawn to those areas. CRNAs, working with primary care physicians and some surgeons, have been able to provide anesthesia for these populations because no state has required them to practice solely with anesthesiologists or under their supervision or direction.

Fruitful dialogue between the ASA and AANA has essentially been nonexistent since the mid-1980s because of stipulations placed on AANA-ASA dialogue by the ASA that the AANA must accept its ACT statement as a condition for such discussions. The AANA has not agreed with such stipulations for a variety of reasons, including the fact that it was never a party to the development of the statement. The ramifications, should the AANA adopt the ASA statement as a national position on anesthesia delivery, are unthinkable, primarily because this position would deny access to anesthesia services near the homes of some 20% to 25% of U.S. residents. Although the ASA and its leadership may sincerely believe in its position, it is also no less true that research data are inadequate to support such a position. Furthermore, the economic benefits derived by anesthesiologists if such a proposal were implemented present a serious conflict of interest that would be difficult for them to explain.

The AANA's position not to adopt the ASA's ACT statement has been long standing. According to AANA data, in 1998 approximately 37% of CRNAs were employed by anesthesiologists, and approximately the same percentage were employed by hospitals. Many hospital-employed CRNAs work with anesthesiologists who have privileges in those hospitals. The practice pattern of CRNAs working with anesthesiologists has long been one of those approved by the AANA. The question has never been whether the two groups of providers will work together in hospitals in which both groups practice, but rather how and under what conditions? Many CRNAs believe that the ASA's medical-direction model as defined demeans CRNAs, is restrictive of their practice, inhibits productivity of both providers, and is wasteful of anesthesia personnel. It is more costly than other models that recognize the full range of competencies of both providers and maximize these capabilities in practice, fostering a true collegial partnership.

In an article published November 8, 1999, the AMA News announced that the ASA's House of Delegates had approved an "educational affiliate membership" category for CRNAs and anesthesiologist associates. These providers would have to have their applications endorsed by two anesthesiologists, and "they would be required to sign on to the association's statements on ethics and the ACT, which advocates that anesthesiologists be in charge of the medical direction of all in providing anesthesia care."[74] To what extent anesthesiologist-employed CRNAs will be pressured or mandated by their employers to endorse these statements as a condition of employment will have to be evaluated with regard to potential for violation of antitrust or employment laws, both state and federal. The ACT statement has never been one on which the ASA has been willing to seek consensus, and this effort appears to attempt an end run around the AANA by declaring it a "nonissue." Such membership became available in 2001 and constitutes an issue to watch in the new millennium.[74]

State and Federal Regulations

Although the expanded-role movement for nurses got a major boost in the 1960s with the development of primary care nurse practitioners, it was not until the late 1980s that significant progress was made in removing some of the barriers to advanced nursing practice. States vary in their legal requirements concerning CRNA practice. If state laws or regulations mention any relationship with a physician, they specify it with phrases ranging from "under the supervision and/or direction of a physician" to "in collaboration with" or "with the consent of" a physician. Some 20 states now have no requirement for physician supervision of CRNAs in their medical practice acts, their nurse practice acts, or their hospital licensing regulations. Nine others have included a supervisory requirement only in their hospital licensing regulations. Some attorneys believe that regulating professionals through hospital licensing regulations may be unlawful if it conflicts with other legislation (e.g., giving authority to boards of nursing for regulating nurses and nursing practice).

In all states, it is a physician, usually the patient's attending physician or surgeon, who determines the patient's need for anesthesia or anesthesia-related services; therefore, anesthesiology has always been a referral service to anesthesiologists or CRNAs. It must be noted that the idiosyncratic language between doctors and nurses has reflected that referral over the years in the terminology of "ordering," for example, "an anesthetic." For the most part, such ordering has not been technique, drug, or device specific. It may have been as simple as posting a patient for anesthesia and surgery within the operating room. Historically, it has been accepted that each anesthesia provider knows what techniques, drugs, and devices are safest in his or her hands for a particular patient.

The changing regulatory scene regarding physician supervision and the continual complaints of CRNAs regarding the TEFRA regulations, which are believed by many CRNAs to adversely affect their ability to practice, came to a head in two additional initiatives pursued by the AANA in the 1990s. The HCFA requirement for physician supervision of CRNAs preempts state laws that permit them to practice without medical supervision. Furthermore, ASA leaders had started a campaign in the 1980s to convince surgeons who worked with CRNAs that the surgeons were legally liable for the CRNAs' practice. Many CRNAs thought this was an effort to discourage surgeons' use of CRNAs without anesthesiologist supervision. Physicians who employ CRNAs are legally liable for their employees under the master-servant legal doctrine, just as any other employer is liable for his or her employees. However, surgeons, who solely fulfill the legal requirement for supervision in states that require such supervision, are not automatically liable for the acts of CRNAs.[39] A surgeon may become liable under the following two conditions: (1) in cases in which the surgeon decides to control what the CRNA does, such as mandating a general anesthetic when the CRNA believes a regional anesthetic would be better; and (2) in instances in which hospital policies mandate a degree of supervision tantamount to control. (The early "captain of the ship" doctrine that made the surgeon responsible for everyone in the operating room has long since been nullified in the vast majority of states.) The inherent medical culture, including the emphasis that the ASA's leaders have placed on CRNA supervision, has led many anesthesiologists to believe that there are legal requirements for CRNAs to be supervised by a physician, even in states in which there are no such requirements. Many CRNAs believe anesthesiologists use this argument with hospital administrators and medical staff to create barriers for CRNAs who seek independent clinical privileges. Some CRNAs have expended tremendous time and effort to untangle the web the ASA and some of its members have been spinning. HCFA regulations that mandate physician supervision of CRNAs under Medicare policy are a barrier to practice, and many CRNAs believe the federal regulation needs changing. Therefore, the AANA began to work with the HCFA to propose elimination of the federal requirement for physician supervision and to defer to state laws, recognizing that even if the state permitted independent practice for CRNAs and other APNs, institutional credentialing policy could require physician supervision if the medical staff believed strongly that it was needed.

In December 1997 the HCFA published its proposal for major change in its *Hospital Conditions of Participation*, and it included the elimination of the supervisory requirement for CRNAs.[75,76] The immediate response by the ASA has led to a major political fight involving both organizations, the HCFA, and both houses of the U.S. Congress. As of the closing months of 1999, the matter had not been resolved, and the proposed HCFA rules were pending until 2001 when the issue was resolved. Again, the conflict is characterized by quality-of-care rhetoric on the part of the ASA and its leaders and charges of economic motivations on the part of the AANA and many of its members. Little question exists that the loss the ASA suffered to the AANA in the 1970s in its effort to take over CRNA education and credentialing fostered an intent not to lose again. Two unfortunate tactics on the part of the ASA and its leaders in this confrontation have been the attempt by ASA to frighten the elderly about the anesthesia care they would receive from unsupervised CRNAs and their use of research in inappropriate and misleading ways.

Of interest, within the medical literature in the 1990s, with the *British Medical Journal* and the American College of Physicians Journal Club taking the lead, serious questions have been raised regarding the quality and relevance of research being published, the peer review system, and the selection of articles for publication.[77] One report in 1993 concluded that 95% of the medical research being published in journals was either flawed or irrelevant.[78] This has been demonstrated in the misuse of research, not just within anesthesia over the CRNA supervision issue, but in the public media as well.[53,78-88]

In 1997 the AANA, ASA, and HCFA came to an agreement to revise the TEFRA rules and make them less onerous and less prone to fraud by anesthesiologists. Whether it was the change in ASA presidents or the hostilities over the supervision issue is unclear, but the ASA withdrew its support for the changes before the HCFA proposed and finalized them, negating the chance for change that both CRNAs and many anesthesiologists would have preferred.

In this age of cost containment in health-care services, the TEFRA rules preclude cost-effective use of both CRNAs and anesthesiologists without the anesthesiologists' risking a crossing of the line into fraudulent practice. Some anesthesia groups consisting of both types of providers have decided to eliminate TEFRA as a concern by billing for each provider's services as though the provider were practicing alone. This permits the group to configure its practice to be more productive while basing assignments on individual patient needs. These groups have, in effect, formed the collegial partnership arrangement that the AANA has fostered.

In all organizational and interprofessional affairs, it is easier for individual professionals to accommodate one another than it is for organizations to do the same when vital differences separate them. Such has been the case with nurse anesthetists and anesthesiologists throughout their history in the United States.

ENDING THE 20TH CENTURY

Nurse anesthetists were few in number but were making strong headway in this "new" nursing specialty as the 19th century closed and the 20th century began. They made great strides in that time, achieving what surgeons had requested of them back in the 19th century (i.e., making anesthesia safer for patients). In fact, although some physicians devoted their practice to anesthesia, it was not until after World War II that physicians in any significant numbers made it a full-time practice. The strides made in anesthesia practice at the end of the 20th century were attributable to all those who made it a life's work and contributed to its practice, research, and development. This includes CRNAs, surgeons, anesthesiologists, basic scientists, and engineers. As the 20th century closed, nurse anesthesia education had moved from hospital-based certificate programs (of which there were four before World War I) to graduate school programs in university settings offering master's or higher degrees to their graduates.

At the close of the millennium, the shifts in delivery and payment systems under managed care significantly affected both CRNAs and anesthesiologists. The use of CRNAs had some definite advantages with regard to cost, without a compromise in the quality of anesthesia care. Many teaching hospitals, whose anesthesia services were primarily provided by medical residents and the anesthesiologist teaching staff, were affected by the lingering decline in numbers of U.S. graduates who enter anesthesiology residencies, caused in part by some decline in graduate medical educational funding. Where the residencies were reduced in number, many such hospitals replaced residents with significant numbers of CRNAs. Some academic health centers that had had no CRNAs for 20 to 25 years began employing them. Although in the early 1990s there was some displacement of CRNAs in the workforce, by 2003 there was a shortage of CRNAs, and once again they were in high demand.

The efforts of proponents of managed care to reduce services that were not medically indicated did not reduce the need for anesthesia providers, as was expected. This resulted from the following:

1. The decentralization of services has invariably led to greater requirements for personnel resources. Anesthesia services are now required in hospitals, ambulatory surgi-centers, and physicians' offices (the fastest growing site for surgical procedures).
2. Subspecialization among anesthesiologists and even some CRNAs decreased the flexibility of these providers for use in a variety of settings, which also has resulted in the need for additional anesthesia providers.
3. In large hospitals there was a significant increase (22% to 66%) over the prior 15 years in the number of women seeking pain management during obstetric labor.[89] In larger hospitals this led to the staffing of obstetric services with anesthesia providers around the clock. Many CRNAs, 3% by one AANA estimate, devoted their practice to obstetric anesthesia, working with and without anesthesiologists. Furthermore, a significant proportion of a rural CRNA practice consists of obstetric anesthesia services.

4. The changing philosophy; advances in knowledge, methodologies, and technology; and greater recognition of the physical, emotional, social, economic, and personal benefits of pain management have led a large variety of professionals, including CRNAs and anesthesiologists, into acute and chronic pain management.

In addition, whereas the locum tenens business was seriously curtailed during the move into the managed care environment, such businesses boomed for both CRNAs and anesthesiologists. Some locum tenens CRNAs have been in the same facility for longer than a year and feel more secure being on contract than they would as employees.

Not all CRNAs benefited from these changes. Some have reported staying in their positions without wage increases for 4 to 6 years, after having their salaries and benefits reduced because of declining hospital revenues within their areas. Although some of these CRNAs could remedy their situation if they believed they were in a position to move, many have not done so. In addition, anesthesia was severely affected by the reduction of reimbursement rates for services by both governmental and private payers. CRNAs who were unaware of the income they generate for their employers feared loss of employment and therefore accepted lower pay. However, the variations in managed care penetration and other factors may also have played into the differences in CRNA income during the 1990s.

Many groups and individuals have advocated greater use of nurses, particularly APNs, as alternatives to physicians where their scopes of practice overlap and their practices have demonstrated quality.[38,90-92] It appears that organizational medicine may be fearing decline in its power, authority, and income with the many changes occurring in health-care delivery. Although it recognizes the value of APNs, the AMA is making efforts to increase the barriers to independent APN practice rather than removing them.[93-96] The AMA's passage of an ASA-submitted resolution declaring that anesthesiology is the practice of medicine and a public relations campaign and initiative to work with state medical boards to prevent any additional legislation and regulation that permits APNs and other nonphysician professionals more independence in practice are only the latest AMA efforts to avert increased competition.[94,96] They have moved back from a position they took in 1970—a position that has been confirmed by state courts and legislators—that recognizes functional or task overlaps in scopes of practice among health professionals; that is, when a task is performed by a physician, it is the practice of medicine, but when it is performed by another health professional, it is the practice of that professional (e.g., when performed by a nurse, it is nursing).[97] The Texas attorney general, in an opinion issued September 28, 1999, confirmed the concept of overlapping scopes of practice among health professionals and affirmed that state law does not require that CRNAs be supervised by physicians.[98,99]

A variety of reasons may explain why medicine is trying to reverse this well-accepted principle and fact. If what these professionals do is categorized as medicine, then the field of medicine can legally control them and their practice; and in an environment in which reimbursement for health professionals is declining, physicians can adjust payment to their employees for their own economic benefit. Much of the confusion over "delegation and ordering" stems from the late 19th century, when medicine claimed the whole of health care, necessitating other health professionals to legally carve their practices from

that claimed by medicine. However, it has become more recognized over time that although the purpose for which a profession is legally identified may be unique, state laws seldom give that profession a monopoly on practice modalities that are useful and included within the scope of practice of other professions.[99]

At the close of the previous century, several problems worked against resolution of the health-care-cost dilemma in the United States. Significant differences of opinion existed as to whether health care and its delivery could appropriately be subsumed under the market system of capitalism. With an excess of physician specialists, it became obvious that the laws of supply and demand had not worked to maintain health-care costs in an affordable range under the old fee-for-service delivery system. One of the major problems was that health-care needs of individuals and across populations are not as simple as those for food for sustenance or transportation for mobility. Another was that the greater the number of physicians, the greater the number of services provided, some of which may not be medically necessary.[57,59] Because health-care providers are legislatively regulated by the states and on occasion by the federal government, using funding and reimbursement as a basis, lower-cost providers were not allowed to compete significantly with physicians. The Pew Foundation's Health Professions Commission studied the health-care system and its delivery extensively during the 1990s. Some of the commission's findings and conclusions are detailed in its 1998 report *Strengthening Consumer Protection: Priorities for Health Care Workforce Regulation.*[92] These findings include the following vision as a basis for better serving of the public interest: (1) "a move from state standards to national standards"; (2) provision for "significant overlap of practice authority among the health professions"; (3) "new venues and participants for regulatory policy making" predicated on the concept that "legislatures may not be the best venue to decide technical professional matters as lobbying, campaign contributions and allegiance to constituents often distort rational policy development"; (4) "integration of regulatory systems that protect health care consumers"; and (5) "increased regulatory focus on quality of care and competence assurance."[91] The report also recommended that Congress establish "a national policy advisory body that will research, develop and publish national scopes of practice and continuing competency for state legislatures to implement."[92] The question remains as to whether there is sufficient legislative will to move beyond rhetoric, unrestrained campaign financing, and special interest influence to devise a health-care delivery system based on an appropriate, cost-effective health workforce mix that would have the potential to provide affordable health care to all.

THE NEW MILLENNIUM BEGINS

The old saying, "the more things change, the more they remain the same" is fully illustrated in the first few years of the new millennium. For instance, the use of U.S. military forces increased in the 1990s, including campaigns such as Desert Storm (to drive the Iraqis out of Kuwait) and smaller engagements in Somalia, Bosnia, and Kosovo (to stop internal ethnic and religious killings). Terrorists attacked the World Trade Center in New York in 1995. This was followed in 2001 by a major terrorist attack and the full destruction of the World Trade Center in New York and a section of the Pentagon in Washington, D.C. The result was a continuing war in Afghanistan, where many of these terrorists were trained. Additional terrorist bombings in Saudi Arabia and in the port waters of Yemen with U.S. losses eventually led to a preemptive repeat of the Iraq war of 1991 in 2003. The initiative was led by the United States and Great Britain and was based on stated concerns about nuclear, biologic, and chemical weapons and their potential to fall into the hands of terrorists. The United States did not have the degree of backing and support from the United Nations that it did in 1991 and therefore had to rely more on its own troops and support personnel. A sizable number of CRNAs have been called up, along with many reserve and national guard units, to supplement the active military force in caring for military and civilian casualties at home and abroad. The U.S. Army and Air Force use more CRNAs than anesthesiologists; these "call-ups," therefore, create additional CRNA shortages in many civilian and stateside military hospitals at a time when the surgical workload continues to escalate. To increase the total number of CRNAs available, many nurse anesthesia educational programs have increased the number of students they enroll, and a few new programs have been opened or are obtaining initial accreditation status, which allows them to accept students.

Further, the anesthesiologists' challenges to CRNAs and their professional association continued unabated. The HCFA passed new Medicare regulations that eliminated its requirement for physician supervision of nurse anesthetists on January 18, 2001 (66 FR No. 12. 4674-4686, 1/18/2001)[100] to take effect March 19, 2001. The unfortunate aspect of the issuance of these regulations was its occurrence late in President Clinton's terms of office, which allowed incoming president George W. Bush time to act on them before they went into effect. Bush did not single out the CRNA supervision regulation, but on the day he was sworn into office as President of the United States, he announced a 60-day moratorium on all regulations on which Clinton had signed off in his final days in office. The lobbying of the new President and his appointees began early and in earnest.

Bush's action was disappointing to CRNAs, although not surprising. Before taking further action on these regulations, Bush and Secretary Thompson of the U.S. Department of Health and Human Services changed the name of the HCFA to the Centers for Medicare and Medicaid Services (CMS). On July 5, 2001, Bush and the CMS proposed a new regulation that contained a provision allowing governors in those states in which no laws or regulations required physician supervision of CRNAs to opt out of the Medicare physician supervision requirement after discussions with the Boards of Medicine and Nursing. This moved the battle back to those states in which CRNAs had previously fought and won the supervision battle, requiring them to fight it again. Despite the ASA's fight to keep the original regulation that required physician supervision and the AANA's efforts to keep the Clinton regulation, the regulation proposed by Bush (66 FR 35395, 7/5/2001)[101] was adopted as the final regulation on November 13, 2001 (66 FR 56762, 11/13/2001). The public relations and lobbying battle had been fierce and financially costly to both organizations. In reality, neither side got all that it wanted. Michael Scott, ASA's director of Governmental and Legal Affairs, wrote the following: "What emerged from the Bush administration on the supervision issue was a compromise.... A more accurate characterization of what happened is that [the ASA's] ability to receive a fair hearing at [the Department of Health and Human Services] and the White House was enhanced by our relatively stronger support than AANA for [Republican] candidates in the 2000 and prior elections and by our early support in 2001 for the White House views

on patient protection liability issues. We also were measurably aided by urgings of key Senators and Representatives, on both sides of the aisle, who believed that a real anesthesia patient safety issue was at stake and were willing to stand up and be counted."[102] Scott's last sentence is of questionable accuracy, although the early part of his statement demonstrates that when dealing in governmental affairs, AANA members must know how and must be willing to be involved in and to pay the costs associated with public relations and lobbying.

It appeared to many that in the 20 states in which no legal provisions existed for physician supervision of CRNAs, the governors would be inclined to provide "opt-outs" in their states; however, this was not the case, for political reasons. To date, 14 state governors out of 20 have gone this route. These include Iowa, Nebraska, Idaho, Minnesota, New Hampshire, New Mexico, Kansas, North Dakota, Washington, Alaska, Wisconsin, South Dakota, Montana, and Oregon. Other state nurse anesthesia associations that have no state legal regulations requiring supervision of CRNA practice continue their efforts to get their governors to act on the "opt-out" provision.

Medicine developed its coalition to fight perceived incursions of its "turf" by nonphysician professionals in the late 1990s and has become better aligned to combat such initiatives at both the state and federal levels.[95] As a result, medicine has been more effective in blocking such initiatives,[103] which led nonphysician providers to strengthen their coalitions and get their own individual initiatives enacted into law.

During this period the ASA pursued other activities, perhaps in an attempt to intimidate CRNAs into discontinuing their efforts to eliminate physician supervision from their practice. The ASA revived a plan to open an affiliate membership category—the Educational Member—to CRNAs and anesthesiologist assistants (AAs) within its organization and also to support efforts to increase the number of AA programs. However, the ASA House of Delegates chose to open affiliate educational membership only to anesthesiologist assistants and anesthesiologist assistant students. The ASA has now opened educational membership status to AAs and CRNAs.[104]

After 30 years, in 2002 the ASA's Committee on the Anesthesia Care Team recommended to the ASA board of directors that the old statement on regional anesthesia be rescinded and a new one be adopted. The ASA's 1983 policy statement restricted the administration of regional anesthesia to anesthesiologists and other physicians. The ASA board of directors disapproved the recommendation pending action by the House of Delegates, which, after consideration, changed the statement to read that it was preferable for such techniques to be administered by anesthesiologists.[105] Despite the previous ASA regional anesthesia policy statement, many nurse anesthetists have been highly successful in incorporating regional techniques in their practice for years, dating back to World War II. Such techniques are preferable for some patients and some surgical procedures. Regional techniques are very frequently used for selected aspects of the management of pain, both acute and chronic. Experience with regional techniques also has become required in accredited nurse anesthesia educational programs.

The ASA has continued to claim that selected research shows that mortality is higher when CRNAs function without anesthesiologist supervision.[104] No such definitive research is available. A recently published study, performed by Pine, Holt, and Yu using Medicare data from over 400,000 patients from 22 states, found that patients were equally safe when undergoing anesthesia provided by CRNAs, anesthesiologists, or an ACT composed of a CRNA and an anesthesiologist.[106]

Despite the differences in supervision philosophy between CRNAs and anesthesiologists, these two groups of providers have functioned and continue to function collaboratively in many settings with a high degree of success; hospital administrators, surgeons, and patients who have access only to CRNAs are equally satisfied and have the same degree of anesthesia success as those who receive anesthesia service from other providers.

Two programs for training anesthesiologist assistants were established in 1974. One was developed as a master's program, primarily for premedical graduates who were not accepted into medical schools. This program has been in continuous existence. The other was developed as a baccalaureate program and closed after a few years. After its curriculum was revised into a graduate course of study, it was reactivated. CMS and state laws or regulations, where they exist, require that the graduates of these programs function under the supervision of anesthesiologists. They cannot practice where there are no anesthesiologists on duty in the operating room suite to supervise their practice. Thus anesthesiologist assistants have had little or no impact on the shortage of providers. There are only approximately 700 active practicing AAs. Although more have been graduated from these two schools in the past 30 years of their existence, approximately half of them have gone on to other pursuits, some to medical schools.

CRNA PRACTICE TODAY

Demographic information collected from CRNAs annually by AANA and confirmed by a study of CRNA supply and demand[107] indicates that in 2007 there were about 38,000 CRNAs in the United States. (Thirty-five thousand CRNAs, or 92%, belong to the AANA). The number of CRNAs grew 36% since 1997. The number of new graduates grew 56% in the same period, evidence of efforts to meet the growing demand for anesthesia nationwide. Because 40% of CRNAs have been practicing more than 20 years and will soon retire, it is predicted that demand for new CRNAs will continue to grow. In 2005, 20% of CRNAs worked in rural areas, 15% in hospitals performing fewer than 800 cases per year ("Critical Access Hospitals"). Ninety-seven percent of CRNAs reported they practice clinical anesthesia, whereas only 3% worked in management/administration and education. Most fulltime CRNAs (65%) administered 800 anesthetics in 2005, whereas 35% of CRNAs administered more than 1000 anesthetics in 2005. Median annual compensation for CRNAs, including salary and benefits, was $140,000. CRNAs worked in all states and in every clinical setting using every anesthetic modality (general, regional, sedation, pain management). The data point out that American CRNAs are very productive and make an enormous contribution to the care of patients under anesthesia.

The United States is currently a country at war, and so CRNA contributions to military anesthesia are particularly significant. Today the U.S. Army, Navy, and Air Force commission approximately 1100 CRNAs serving on active duty. Others work within the Department of Health and Human Services for the U.S. Public Health Service and Veterans Administration. Increased deployments of active duty CRNAs have disrupted the lives of many. A member of the AANA board of trustees, Lieutenant Colonel Brian Campbell, is one Army reservist who had to resign his position due to a prolonged deployment to Iraq.

CRNAs are proving to be very versatile, filling more than clinical duties in today's military. They are also leaders and in

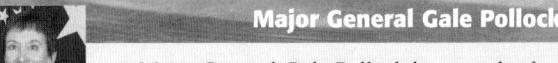
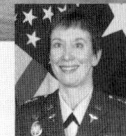

Major General Gale Pollock

Major General Gale Pollock became the first CRNA to serve as Interim Surgeon General of the United States in March 2007.

Photo courtesy of the U.S. Army.

some cases soldiers on the line. In 2003, Major General Gale Pollock, CRNA, (see box above) became the 22nd chief of the Army Nurse Corps and is today the acting Surgeon General of the Army. CRNAs Major Steve McColley and Captain Mitchell Bailey earned Bronze Star Medal nominations for acts of courage in Iraq. Major Jeffrey Roos, a CRNA stationed at Fort Benning, Georgia, earned a Bronze Star from the Army for his lifesaving efforts during Operation Anaconda, the first major U.S. offensive launched in Afghanistan after the September 11 attacks on the World Trade Center. A CRNA was in the news for extricating Private Jessica Lynch from a hospital in Iraq.

Deployments of CRNAs to Afghanistan and Iraq have reduced anesthesia staffs at stateside hospitals. No figures exist to describe the overall impact of the latest escalation on anesthesia services in stateside hospitals. However, the impact of deployments has been mitigated somewhat following a recent policy change in the Navy. Navy CRNAs are now considered "licensed independent practitioners" (LIPs), a term coined by The Joint Commission (TJC). According to Captain Annette Hasselbeck NC USN, LIP status has enabled the Navy's medical planners to use global sourcing of CRNAs. In other words, CRNAs are used interchangeably with anesthesiologists, based on skills, seniority, and availability. This had always been the practice pattern; but defining CRNAs as LIPs has kept practice in compliance with TJC policy. According to Captain Ron Van Nest NC USN (ret), the policy was changed in 2000 to reflect the facts that CRNAs very often deploy alone and capably make independent clinical decisions that affect anesthetic management. Recognizing CRNAs as LIPs has also kept morale high; all billets are filled and retention of Navy CRNAs is at 100%.

Wartime CRNA experiences are described in four new books.[108-111] The work of nurses, including CRNAs, throughout World War II is well documented by Evelyn Monahan and Rosemary Neidel-Greenlee in *And If I Perish: Frontline US Army Nurses in World War II*. CRNAs are present and accounted for in the North Africa and Italy campaigns, at the liberation of France, and the conquest of Germany. In her recently published memoir, *In Times of War: Memoirs of a World War II Nurse*, Isabelle Cook recounts her experiences in North Africa, Italy, and France. Nurse anesthetist CDR Cheryl L. Ruff has co-authored a riveting account of her experiences in Iraq titled: *Ruff's War: A Navy Nurse at the Frontline in Iraq*. Doris M. Sterner has also published *In and Out of Harm's Way: A History of the Navy Nurse Corps*.

A monument to military CRNAs, donated by AANA staff, was erected and dedicated at the Park Ridge AANA headquarters in November 2005. The monument is a "tranquil place of honor" consisting of a fountain, a plaque, and a flagpole. It is a small but significant reminder that America remains a nation at war.

Progress in Anesthesia

Progress in anesthesia has occurred in all areas of the discipline. "Discoveries of Distinction,"[112] a web page maintained by the AANA Foundation, lists and describes hundreds of recent and ongoing CRNA-led research projects. These projects range from basic and applied sciences to clinical anesthesia, education, and economics.

Particularly noteworthy strides have been made by CRNAs who have investigated the anesthesia workforce. In a number of studies, Fallacaro alone and together with others examined existing demographic databases to document and describe the inefficient urban/rural distribution of anesthesia providers. Not surprisingly, CRNAs were found to serve significantly more rural[113,114] and poor[115,116] communities. In 2001, Obst, Nauenberg, and Buck evaluated obstetric data in New York State and found an association between a woman's health insurance and her likelihood of receiving obstetric anesthesia.[117] Women without traditional insurance were less likely to receive an epidural for labor. Earlier studies by Fassett[118] and Stein[119] examined the costs and benefits of team-based anesthesia and questioned the value of the team approach to anesthesia care. Fagerlund[120] looked at the costs and benefits of CRNA education to students, academic institutions, hospitals, and taxpayers and found a strongly positive rate of return to all four groups. In other words, society as a whole benefits from CRNA education. At a time when the demand for anesthesia services is expanding and the pressure to reduce costs is so great, these studies may bring down barriers to CRNA practice. What is required is a societal commitment to provide access to cost-effective high quality anesthesia care regardless of the political fallout.

Anesthesia history has become a research interest among CRNAs. Other than historical research mentioned earlier in this chapter, recent examples include a book about strides in education, *A History of the Nurse Anesthesia Program Wake Forrest University-Baptist Medical Center*.[121]

Very importantly, CRNAs are advancing the field of clinician well-being. In October 2002, CRNAs were greatly dismayed when AANA past-president Jan Stewart died. Not long after her death, the Stewart family let it be known that her death had been caused by chemical dependency. The Stewarts urged the AANA to commemorate Jan by expanding the focus of its peer assistance activities in ways that would be constructive and would preserve Jan's faith in people moving forward together.

The AANA board responded favorably to the Stewarts' request. In 2003, it named a "blue ribbon" panel of experts to examine the problem of chemical dependency among anesthesia providers and to explore various options. The panel issued a lengthy report, which the AANA board accepted. At first a yearly lecture at the AANA Annual Meeting on a wellness-related topic was initiated in 2004. By the fall of 2005, a framework was established for building upon the already existing chemical dependency services of the AANA Peer Assistance program. Peer assistance efforts, which had consisted of a referral hotline, clearinghouse for information, and educational activities[122] grew to embrace more of the stress-related hazards of nurse anesthesia. These included compassion fatigue, burnout, sleep deprivation, and toxic work environments. The Wellness Program now resides within the Council for Public Interest in Anesthesia. Sandra Tunajek, CRNA, DNP was named executive secretary.[123] It offers access to an array of resources that foster and assist AANA members to seek an active, lifelong process of making choices that promote a healthier, more balanced, and fulfilling life.[124]

SUMMARY

Nurses were recruited into the field of anesthesia by surgeons in the latter half of the 19th century because inexpert clinical administration by physicians and others often resulted in morbidity and mortality. The Civil War was the earliest documented use of nurses as anesthetists, and it became a trend afterward. By the 1890s, nurse anesthesia was well established, having spread from midwestern Catholic hospitals to cities on both coasts. Before the turn of the 20th century, nurse anesthetists provided gratuitous training to others but recognized the need for formalized education in anesthesia. The first hospital-based anesthesia educational program opened in 1909. During World War I, nurse anesthetists were widely credited with significantly reducing combat-related surgical morbidity and mortality. By 1920, nurse anesthesia had become well established and well accepted.

Once nurses had established themselves in anesthesia practice, anti–nurse anesthetist activities began. First there were attempts to outlaw NAs based on the notion that anesthesia is the intellectual and financial property of medicine. These were followed by attempts to control anesthesia training and restrict scope of practice in numerous states. There have been continual attempts to frighten surgeons and the public against using nurse anesthetists. Anti–nurse anesthetist forces have also erected obstacles to educational resources, payment, insurance availability, and clinical privileges. Anti–nurse anesthetist activity has continued unabated and reached almost every level of government, business, education, and health-care institution. For a while it was the stated objective of the ASA to make anesthesia an all-physician specialty.

Against this backdrop, nurse anesthetists formed a national organization in 1931. Dedicating themselves to advancing anesthesia education and patient safety, nurse anesthetists implemented a number of firsts: annual meetings, a monthly bulletin, and a journal. In 1945 the first certification examination for graduates was implemented. As a result of service in the mid-century wars, nurse anesthetists earned officer's status, and men gained the right to join the military's nurse corps. When the military demanded that its nurse anesthetists pass the AANA certification examination, civilian hospitals soon followed suit. By the 1950s, nurse anesthetists worked with surgeons and engineers to pioneer anesthesia machinery, ventilators, and anesthesia for pediatric cardiovascular surgery. During this era, accreditation of anesthesia training programs was achieved.

The second half of the 20th century was marked by a closer involvement between the profession and government. As Medicare paid for a larger proportion of clinical anesthesia services, the government in turn exerted increasing control over how those services were rendered and at what cost to taxpayers. Because federal dollars also went for nursing education, government exerted a measure of control over accreditation. Independent councils on accreditation, certification, recertification, and public interest evolved from this.

In the 1960s and 1970s, state governments modernized nurse practice acts to account for new subspecialties in advanced practice nursing. CRNAs had to participate even though they had long predated other advanced practice nurses. The 1980s and 1990s brought on governmental efforts to "reform" health care by extending services and containing costs. Quality of care entered the debate, and CRNAs ultimately proved what had been shown 50 years earlier: anesthesia outcomes are no worse and perhaps better when a CRNA administers the anesthetic. For CRNAs, constant vigilance and a presence in federal and state government centers were essential because each of the aforementioned policy changes presented organized anesthesiologists with an opportunity to threaten nurse anesthesia.

As a result, state nurse anesthetist associations became stronger, and the AANA established an office in Washington, D.C.

Progress in nurse anesthesia has occurred over many decades and resulted in an extraordinary record of patient safety. Today all student nurse anesthetists are educated in a uniform curriculum with similar clinical exposures. All SRNA training programs are housed within universities and colleges, and all confer a master's degree. To be permitted to practice, all graduates must pass a national certifying exam, and in order to gain re-certification, all CRNAs must obtain continuing education biennially. There is a national learning center at AANA headquarters that sponsors continuing education programs for postgraduate CRNAs. CRNAs have undertaken hundreds of clinical, scientific, and policy research projects to further professional and public understanding of nurse anesthesia.

REFERENCES

1. Smith TC, Wollman H. History and principles of anesthesiology. In: Goodman LS et al, eds. *Goodman & Gilman's Pharmacological Basis of Therapeutics.* 7th ed. New York: Macmillan; 1985:260-275.
2. Fenster JM. *Ether Day: The Strange Tale of America's Greatest Medical Discovery and the Haunted Men Who Made It.* New York: Harper-Collins; 2001.
3. Nuland SB. *The Origins of Anesthesia.* Birmingham, AL: Classics of Medicine Library; 1983.
4. Donahue MP. *Nursing, the Finest Art: An Illustrated History.* St Louis: Mosby; 1985.
5. Thatcher V. *History of Anesthesia with Emphasis on the Nurse Specialist.* Philadelphia: Lippincott; 1953.
6. Lawrence CS. *Sketch of Life and Labors of Miss Catherine S. Lawrence.* Albany, NY: James B. Lyon, Printer; 1896.
7. Koch E. Catherine S. Lawrence: the world's first nurse anesthetist? part 2. *AANA NewsBull.* Nov-Dec 201. 2001;55:11, 14-15.
8. Otis GA, Huntington DL. *The Medical and Surgical History of the War of the Rebellion,* part III (vol II), "Surgical History." Washington, DC: US Government Printing Office; 1883:905.
9. Van Houten WC. Catherine S. Lawrence: civil war nurse. *Schoharie Cty Hist Rev.* Fall 1999:9.
10. Hartzell J. *Mrs. Charlie: The Other Mayo.* Gobles, MI: Arvi Books; 2000.
11. Harris N, Hunziker-Dean J. Florence Henderson, the art of open drop ether. *Nurs Hist Rev.* New York: Springer 2001;9:159-184.
12. Bennet LA, Jerabek BA. *Sophie Gran Jevne Winton: A Woman and Nurse Anesthetist Before Her Time, April 24, 1887—April 24, 1989* [thesis]. Rochester, MN: Mayo School of Health-Related Sciences; 1999.
13. Stevenson JMR. Front line anesthesia, *Bull AANA.* 1942;10:68-74.
14. Harsch TL. *Nurse Anesthetists in the United States Army Nurse Corps during World War II* [thesis]. Peoria, IL: Bradley University; 1993. [AANA Archives: WY 151 H25n].
15. Stoner D, Harris NA. *Miss Nell Bryant: World War I Nurse Anesthetist* (thesis). Rochester, MN: Mayo School of Health-Related Sciences; 1999. [AANA Archives: WZ 100 B915]; 1999.
16. Brown S. Nurse anesthesia in Oregon. In: Kendrick A, Klein R, eds. *The History of Anesthesia in Oregon.* Portland, OR: Oregon Trail. Publishing Col; 2004.
17. Harmel MH. Austin Lamont, MD (1905-1969). In: *Ralph Milton Waters MD: Mentor to a Profession.* Park Ridge, IL: Wood Library-Museum of Anesthesiology; 2004:107-111.
18. Sykes K. How Ralph Waters influenced the development of anaesthesia in the British Commonwealth and in Europe. In: *Ralph Milton Waters MD: Mentor to a Profession.* Park Ridge, IL: Wood Library-Museum of Anesthesiology; 2004:198.
19. Van Nest R. Imagining in time: the life and trial of Dagmar Nelson. *AANA J.* 2006;74(3):183-187;74(4):261-265.
20. Hanchett S. *Anesthesia Is Nursing: A Historic Review of the Chalmers-Francis v Nelson Case.* [thesis]. University of California, Los Angeles; 1995.
21. Bankert M. *Watchful Care: A History of America's Nurse Anesthetists.* New York: Continuum; 1989.
22. Diers D. Nurse-midwives and nurse anesthetists: the cutting edge in specialist practice, In: Aiken L, Fagin C, eds. *Charting Nursing's Future: Agenda for the 1990s.* Philadelphia: Lippincott; 1992:159.
23. Adriani J. Four decades of association with the pioneers of anesthesiology. *Anesth Analg.* 1972;51:665-667.
24. Stevens R. *American Medicine and the Public Interest.* Berkeley: Univ Calif Press; 1998.
25. Stevens R. *In Sickness and in Wealth: American Hospitals in the Twentieth Century.* New York: Basic Books; 1989.
26. Bellafaire J. *The Army Nurse Corps, a Commemoration of World War II Service* (CMH Publication No. 72-14). Washington, DC: US Army Center of Military History; 1991:6-7. Available at US Army Center of Military History Website. http://www2.army.mil/cmh/books/wwii/72-14/72-14.htm. Accessed April 7, 2008.
27. Williams D. *To the Angels.* San Francisco: Denson Press; 1985.
28. Norman E. *We Band of Angels: The Untold Story of American Nurses Trapped on Bataan by the Japanese.* New York: Random House; 1999.
29. Beecher HK, Todd DP. A study of deaths associated with anesthesia and surgery. *Ann Surg.* 1954;140:2-34.
30. Berger OL. Anesthesia for the surgical treatment of cyanotic congential heart disease. *Am J Assoc Nurse Anesth.* 1948;16:79-90.
31. Lank BE. Cyclopropane anesthesia in infant surgery. *J Am Assoc Nurse Anesth.* 1947;15:3-11.
32. Hamel MH, Lamont A. Anesthesia in the surgical treatment of congenital pulmonary stenosis. *Anesthesiology.* 1946;7:477-498.
33. Smith RM. Progress in paediatric anaesthesia in the United States. *Anesth Hist Assoc Newsl.* 1993;11:2.
34. Moore C, Feller C, eds. *Highlights in the History of the Army Nurse Corps* (CMH Publication No. 85-1). Washington, DC: US Army Center of Military History; 1995:27-28, 40.
35. Bendixon HH. Debate: Anesthesia manpower shortage—fact or fiction? *Fact Clin Anesth.* 1967;2:16-21.
36. Steinhaus JE et al. The physician assistant in anesthesiology. *Anesth Analg.* 1973;52:794-798.
37. Dripps RD. Decisions for the specialty. *Bull N Y Acad Med.* 1962;38:264-270.
38. Safreit BJ. Health care dollars and regulatory sense: the role of advanced practice nursing. *Yale J Regul.* 1992;9:417-487.
39. Blumenreich GA. The irrelevant issue of surgeon's liability. In: *AANA Journal Legal Briefs: 1984-86.* Park Ridge, IL: American Association of Nurse Anesthetists; 1987:16. (Reprinted from AANA J. 1985;53:5.)
40. Stephens CR. Nurses in anesthesia. In: *ASA Manpower Report.* Park Ridge, IL: American Society of Anesthesiologists; 1969.
41. American Society of Anesthesiologists, American Association of Nurse Anesthetists. Joint statement of the ASA and AANA concerning qualifications of individuals administering anesthetics. *AANA News Bull.* 1972;26:3.
42. Gunn IP. The history of nurse anesthesia education: highlights and influences. In: *Report of the National Commission on Nurse Anesthesia Education.* Park Ridge, IL: American Association of Nurse Anesthetists; 1990:33-41.
43. Wiseman E. Legislation: the California experience. *CRNA Forum.* 1986;2:3-10.
44. Tobin MH. Governmental regulation of nurse anesthesia practice. In: Foster SD, Jordan LM, eds: *Professional Aspects of Nurse Anesthesia Practice.* Philadelphia: FA Davis; 1994.
45. Wing KR. Government enforcement of competition: the antitrust laws. In: Wing KR, ed. *The Law and the Public's Health.* 2nd ed. Ann Arbor, MI: Health Administration Press; 1985.
46. Blumenreich GA, Markham JW Jr. *Bhan vs NME Hospital, Inc:* antitrust standing of CRNAs sustained. In: *AANA Journal Legal Briefs: 1984-86.* Park Ridge, IL: American Association of Nurse Anesthetists; 1987:14-15. (Reprinted from AANA J. 1985;53:6.)
47. US Department of Health and Human Services, Health Care Financing Administration. Final rules for the Tax Equity and Fiscal Responsibility Act, 1982. *Fed Regist.* 1983;48:8901-8951.
48. American Association of Nurse Anesthetists. Brief of Amicus Curiae No. 82-1031. *Jefferson Parish Hospital District No. 2 and East Jefferson Hospital Board, Petitioners v Edwin G. Hyde.* In the Supreme Court of the United States, October Term, 1982. Respondent, Counsel of Record: Phil David Fine.
49. American Society of Anesthesiologists. Brief of Amicus Curiae in Support of Respondent No. 82-1031. *Hyde v Jefferson Parish Hospital.* In the Supreme Court of the United States, October Term, 1982, 3. Respondent, Counsel of Record: John Lansdale Jr.
50. Garde JF. The case study involving the prospective payment system legislation, diagnostic related groups and CRNAs. *Nurs Clin North Am.* 1988;23:521-553.
51. Bechtold AA. Committee on anesthesia study of anesthesia-related deaths—1969-1976. *N C Med J.* 1981;42:253.

52. National Academy of Sciences, National Research Council. *Health Care for American Veterans (House Committee Print No. 36)*. Health Care for American Veterans;1977:156.
53. Forrest WH. Outcome—the effect of the provider, In: Wolman H, ed. *Health Care Delivery in Anesthesia*. Philadelphia: George F. Stickley; 1980.
54. Hardy-Havens D. Federal legislative and regulatory impact on funding of nurse anesthesia education. In: *Report of the National Commission on Nurse Anesthesia Education*. Park Ridge, IL: American Association of Nurse Anesthetists; 1990:123-129.
55. Zambricki C, Ouellette RG. On matters of concern about nurse anesthesia education. *AANA J*. 1987;55:499-505.
56. DePaolis-Lutzo MV. Factors influencing nurse anesthesia educational programs: 1982-1987. In: *Report of the National Commission on Nurse Anesthesia Education*. Park Ridge, IL: American Association of Nurse Anesthetists; 1990:46-51.
57. Ribicoff A, Danaceau P. *The American Medical Machine*. New York: Harper & Row; 1972.
58. Anders G. *Health Against Wealth: HMOs and the Breakdown of Medical Trust*. New York: Houghton Mifflin; 1996.
59. Blustein J, Marmor TR. Cutting waste by making rules: promises, pitfalls, and realistic prospects. In: Lee PR, Estes CL, eds. *The Nation's Health*. 4th ed. Boston: Jones & Bartlett; 1994:333.
60. American Society of Anesthesiologists. *Practice Management: Managed Care [videotape]*. Park Ridge, IL: American Society of Anesthesiologists; 1994.
61. Christensen KT. Ethically important distinctions among managed care organizations. *J Law Med Ethics*. 1995;23:223-229.
62. Himmelstein DU et al. Quality of care in investor-owned vs. not-for-profit HMOs. *JAMA*. 1999;282:159-163.
63. Silverman EM et al. The association between for-profit hospital ownership and increased Medicare spending. *N Engl J Med*. 1999;341:420-426.
64. Wiklund RA, Rosenbaum SH. Medical progress: anesthesiology (part 2). *N Engl J Med*. 1997;337(17):1215-1219.
65. American Association of Nurse Anesthetists Website. http://www.aana.com/resources.aspx?ucNavMenu_TSMenuTargetID=51&ucNavMenu_TSMenuTargetType=4&ucNavMenu_TSMenuID=6&id+666. Accessed April 7, 2008.
66. Himmelstein DU, Woolhandler S. When money is the mission—the high costs of investor-owned care [editorial]. *N Engl J Med*. 1999;341:444-446.
67. Reves JG. Anesthesiologist workforce projections. Paper presented at: American Association of Nurse Anesthetists' Assembly of States Meeting; November 11, 1995; St Louis.
68. Grogono AW. December 1998 update on residency composition 1960-1998. *ASA Newsl*. 1998. Available at: http://www.asahq.org/Newsletters/1998/12_98/Updater_1298.html. Accessed April 7, 2008.
69. US General Accounting Office, Human Resources Division, Report to Congressional Committees. *Medicare: Payments for Medically Directed Anesthesia Services Should Be Reduced (Publication RRD-92-25)*. Washington, DC: US General Accounting Office; 1992.
70. American Society of Anesthesiologists. *American Society of Anesthesiologists' Guidelines: Suggestions to ASA Members for Delineation of Anesthesia Functions for Non-physician Personnel*. Park Ridge, IL: American Society of Anesthesiologists; 1977.
71. American Society of Anesthesiologists. *American Society of Anesthesiologists' Guidelines: The Anesthesia Care Team*. Park Ridge, IL: American Society of Anesthesiologists; 1982.
72. American Society of Anesthesiologists. *American Society of Anesthesiologists' Guidelines: The Anesthesia Care Team*. 1987 rev ed. Park Ridge, IL: American Society of Anesthesiologists; 1987.
73. American Society of Anesthesiologists. *American Society of Anesthesiologists' Guidelines: The Anesthesia Care Team*. 1995 rev ed. Park Ridge, IL: American Society of Anesthesiologists; 1995.
74. Prager LO. Anesthesiologists decide to lay out the welcome mat. The American Society of Anesthesiologists proposed to create an educational arm for nurse anesthetists and others. But will the new affiliates attract any takers? *AMA News*. November 8, 1999. Available at: http://www.ama-assn.org/amednews/1999/pick_99/orga1108.htm.
75. Foster S. Comments of the American Association of Nurse Anesthetists on the proposed rule regarding the Medicare and Medicaid programs: hospital conditions of participation; provider and supplier approval [comments delivered to the U.S. Healthcare Financing Administration April 20, 1998], *AANA NewsBull* 1998;1).
76. Proposed rules, the Medicare and Medicaid programs: hospital conditions of participation. *Fed Regist*. 1997;62:66725-66763.
77. Godlee F. Getting evidence into practice [editorial], *BMJ*. 1998;317:6.
78. Haynes RB. Where's the meat in clinical journals? *ACP J Club*. 1993;119:A22-A23.
79. Abenstein JD, Warner MA. Anesthesia providers, patient outcomes, and costs. *Anesth Analg*. 1996;82:1273-1278.
80. Miller R. Perspective from the editor-in-chief: anesthesia providers, patient outcomes, and costs. *Anesth Analg*. 1996;82:1117-1278.
81. Zambricki CS. Anesthesia providers, patient outcomes, and costs. The AANA responds to the Abenstein and Warner article in the June 1996 *Anesthesia and Analgesia* [editorial]. *AANA J*. 1996;64:413-416.
82. Stoelting RK. Letters to the editor: anesthesia providers, patient outcomes and costs. *Anesth Analg*. 1996;83:1347.
83. Gaba DM. Anesthesia providers, patient outcomes and costs [letter]. *Anesth Analg*. 1996;83:1348.
84. Hanna K. Anesthesia providers, patient outcomes and costs [letter]. *Anesth Analg*. 1996;83:1348.
85. Kremer M. Anesthesia providers, patient outcomes and costs [letter]. *Anesth Analg*. 1996;83:1348-1349.
86. Abenstein JP, Warner MA. Anesthesia providers, patient outcomes and costs [letter]. *Anesth Analg*. 1996;83:1349-1350.
87. Martin-Sheridan D, Wing P. Anesthesia providers, patient outcomes, and costs: a critique. *AANA J*. 1996;64:528-534.
88. Boodman SG. Turf battle in the operating room. Does it matter who puts you to sleep—anesthesiologist or nurse anesthetists? *Washington Post*. May 5, 1998:Health 12-16.
89. Hawkins J. More women opt for pain relief during labor [press release]. Dallas: American Society of Anesthesiologists; October 12, 1999.
90. US Congress, Office of Technology Assessment. *Health Care in Rural America* (Publication OTA-H-434). Washington, DC: US Government Printing Office; 1990.
91. The Pew Foundation Health Professions Commission, Taskforce on Health Care Workforce Regulation. *Critical Challenges: Revitalizing the Health Professions for the 21st Century*. San Francisco: Pew Health Professions Commission; 1995.
92. Finnocchio LJ et al, Taskforce on Health Care Workforce Regulation. *Strengthening Consumer Protection: Priorities for Health Care Workforce Regulation*. San Francisco: Pew Health Professions Commission; 1998.
93. US Congress, Office of Technology Assessment. *Nurse Practitioners, Physician Assistants, and Certified Nurse Midwives: A Policy Analysis (Health Technology Case Study 37)* (Publication OTA-HCS-47). Washington, DC: US Government Printing Office; 1986.
94. American Medical Association House of Delegates. *Report 20 of the Board of Trustees: Supervision of Medical Care Delivered by Advanced Practice Nurses (Resolution 305, A-95)*. Adopted at the December 1995 meeting of the House of Delegates.
95. Greene J. The threat of the domino effect. The AMA plans to launch a Web-based advocacy campaign to help inform Federation members on efforts by nonphysician practitioners to expand scope of practice. *Am Med News*. June 21, 1999. Available at: http://www.ama-assn.org/amednews/1999/pick_99/prfa0621.htm. Accessed April 7, 2008.
96. AMA declares "Anesthesiology is the practice of medicine." *ASA Newsl*. February 1999. Available at: http://www.asahq-org/Newsletters/1999/02_99/AMA_0299.html. Accessed April 7, 2008.
97. AMA Committee on Nursing: Medicine and nursing in the 1970s: a position statement. *JAMA*. 1970;213:1882.
98. Texas Attorney General Opinion No. JC-0117, September 28, 1999. Available at: http://intranet1.oag.state.tx.us/opinions/jc/JC0117.pdf. Accessed September 29, 1999.
99. Blumenreich GA. The overlap between the practice of medicine and the practice of nursing. *AANA J*. 1998;66:11-15.
100. It's official! HCFA removes physician supervision requirement for nurse anesthetists [editorial]. *AANA Newsl*. January 2001. Available at: http://www.aana.com/members/newsbulletin/2001_01/cover.asp. Accessed April 7, 2008.
101. Administration puts politics before patients; implements cumbersome anesthesia care rule [editorial]. *AANA Capitol Corner*. November 13, 2001. Available at: http://www.aana.com/capcorner/finalrule_111301.asp. Accessed April 7, 2008.
102. Scott M. 2001: not shoes, nor ships, nor sealing wax. *ASA Newsl*. December 2001. Available at: http://www.asahq.org/Newsletters/2001/12_01/scott.htm. Accessed April 7, 2008.
103. American Society of Anesthesiologists. Board of Directors annual meeting summary, membership for anesthetists. *ASA Newsl*. October 1999. Available at: http://www.asahq.org/Newsletters/1999/10_99/board1099.html. Accessed April 7, 2008.
104. American Society of Anesthesiologists. Board of Directors annual meeting summary, educational affiliate membership. *ASA Newsl*. October 2001. Available at: http://www.asahq.org/Newsletters/2001/10_01/bodsumm.htm. Accessed April 7, 2008.

105. Silber JH et al. Anesthesiologist direction and patient outcomes. *Anesthesiology.* 2000;93:152-163.
106. American Society of Anesthesiologists. Board of Directors annual meeting summary, statement of regional anesthesia. *ASA Newsl.* October 2002. Available at: http://www.asahq.org/Newsletters/2002/10_02/article1.htm. Accessed April 7, 2008.
107. Merwin E et al. Supply, demand, and equilibrium in the market of CRNAs. *AANA J.* 2006;74:287-293.
108. Monohan EM, Neidel-Greenlee R. *And If I Perish: Frontline US Army Nurse in World War II.* New York: Knopf; 2003.
109. Cook I. *In Time of War: Memoirs of a World War II Nurse.* San Diego: Ivy; 1999.
110. Ruff CL, Roper KS. *Ruff's War: A Navy Nurse Anesthetist at the Frontline in Iraq.* Annapolis, MD: US Naval Institute; 2005.
111. Sterner DM. *In and Out of Harm's Way: A History of the Navy Nurse Corps.* Seattle, WA: Peanut Butter Publishing; 1997.
112. *Discoveries of Distinction,* American Association of Nurse Anesthetists Website. http://www.aana.com/ProfessionalDevelopment.aspx?ucNavMenu_TSMenuTargetID=137&ucNavMenu_TSMenuTargetType=4&ucNavMenu_TSMenuID=6&id=1315. Accessed April 7, 2008.
113. Fallacaro MD, Ruiz-Law R. Distribution of US anesthesia providers and services. *AANA J.* 2004;72(1):9-14.
114. Fallacaro MD. An inefficient mix: a comparative analysis of nurse and physician anesthesia providers across New York State. *J N Y State Nurses Assoc.* 1998;29(2):4-8.
115. Fallacaro MD. The practice and distribution of CRNAs in federally designated nurse shortage areas. *CRNA.* 1997;8(2):55-61.
116. Fallacaro MD et al. The national distribution of CRNAs across metropolitan and non-metropolitan settings. *AANA J.* 1996;64(3):237-242.
117. Obst TE et al. Maternal health insurance coverage as a determinant of obstetrical anesthesia care. *J Health Care Poor Underserved.* 2001;12(2):177-191.
118. Fassett S. *A Cost/Benefit Analysis of Medical Direction in a 2:1 Ratio* [thesis]. Los Angeles, CA: University of California; 1992.
119. Stein CS. *A Patient-Based Approach to Medical Direction within the Anesthesia Care Team* [thesis]. University of California, Los Angeles; 1994. [AANA Archives: WO 200 S30p]
120. Fagerlund K. An economic analysis of the investment in nurse anesthesia education. *AANA J.* 1998;66(2):153-160.
121. Quellette SM, Owens S. *A History of the Nurse Anesthesia Program.* Winston-Salem, NC: Wake Forest University-Baptist Medical Center; 2002.
122. Quinlan C. Peer Assistance: An Historical Perspective. *AANA NewsBull.* January 1996;15.
123. CPIA to set strategic framework for AANA Wellness Program. *AANA NewsBull.* 2005;59(9):7.
124. *AANA Wellness Program: Caring for Self and Others.* American Association of Nurse Anesthetists Website. http://www.aana.com/Resources.aspx?ucNavMenu_TSMenuTargetID=206&UCNavMenu_TSMenuTargetType=4&ucNavMenu_TSMenuID=6&id=6088. Accessed April 7, 2008.

CHAPTER 2

SPECIALTY PRACTICE OF NURSE ANESTHESIA

Betty J. Horton, Lisa J. Thiemann

In existence for more than 125 years, the specialty practice of nurse anesthesia has become one of the most challenging and rewarding areas of advanced nursing practice. Nurse anesthetists, together with their professional association, the American Association of Nurse Anesthetists (AANA), have been role models for members of other nursing groups and allied health organizations. The roles of the certified registered nurse anesthetist (CRNA) and the AANA are described in this chapter.

THE CERTIFIED REGISTERED NURSE ANESTHETIST

Definition

Founded in 1931, the AANA is a professional association that represents more than 36,000 CRNAs and students nationwide. More than 90% of CRNAs in the United States are members of the AANA.[1] CRNAs are anesthesia specialists who administer approximately 27 million anesthetics annually to patients in the United States. As an advanced practice nurse, a CRNA can serve in a variety of capacities in daily practice, such as clinician, educator, administrator, manager, and researcher. CRNAs administer anesthesia for all types of surgical and diagnostic cases, using all anesthetic techniques. They practice in every type of setting in which anesthesia is delivered, from university-based medical centers to freestanding surgical facilities located in private, public, and military facilities. CRNAs are the primary anesthesia providers in two thirds of hospitals in rural America.[2] In some states, they are the sole anesthesia providers in almost 100% of all rural hospitals, which enables these medical facilities to provide obstetric, surgical, diagnostic, and trauma stabilization services.[1]

Qualifications and Capabilities

The following are required for an individual to become a CRNA:
1. Current and unrestricted state licensure as a registered professional nurse
2. Graduation from a nurse anesthesia educational program accredited by the Council on Accreditation (COA) of Nurse Anesthesia Educational Programs or its predecessor
3. Successful completion of the certification examination administered by the Council on Certification of Nurse Anesthetists (CCNA) or its predecessor[2,3]

The Council on Recertification (COR) recertifies qualified CRNAs every 2 years. To become recertified, a CRNA must obtain a minimum of 40 hours of approved continuing education, document substantial anesthesia practice, maintain current state licensure, and certify that he or she has no conditions that could adversely affect the ability to practice anesthesia.[4]

Education

Nurse anesthesia educational programs range from 24 to 36 months of full-time study or the part-time equivalent.[5,6] All programs are required to award at least master's degrees to graduates who are entering nurse anesthesia practice. Those graduates, who already possess a master's degree prior to beginning their nurse anesthesia education training, may be awarded a post-master's certificate. Each accredited program provides an educationally sound curriculum that builds on prior nursing education and experience.

Courses of study leading to doctoral degrees also are available, and the number is projected to increase over the next 2 decades. The Council on Accreditation of Nurse Anesthesia Educational Programs reported in 2006 that 18 programs were planning to offer practice-oriented doctoral degrees. These programs would be in addition to four programs (two entry into practice and two post-master's) already accredited by COA to award either research- or practice-oriented doctoral degrees (Francis Gerbasi, CRNA, PhD, AANA director of Accreditation and Education, oral communication, August 7, 2007). This movement toward a higher-level degree was promoted by the AANA board of directors in a 2007 position statement in support of doctoral education for entry into nurse anesthesia practice by 2025.[7]

The master's level curriculum incorporates studies in the sciences, basic and advanced principles of anesthesia, research, and professional aspects of nurse anesthesia. Students acquire knowledge, skills, and competencies in patient safety, perianesthetic management, critical thinking, communication, and the professional role.[5] Students learn to integrate classroom content with direct application of state-of-the-art techniques in the provision of anesthesia care to all patient populations in all risk categories. Curricula for doctoral programs must meet additional accreditation requirements for both practice-oriented degrees and research-oriented degrees.

Clinical Curriculum Requirements. The clinical component of the nurse anesthesia curriculum focuses on preparing students for the full scope of current practice in a variety of work settings.[5] Each student must administer a minimum number of anesthetics involving a variety of procedures, techniques, and specialty cases. To meet this requirement, students provide anesthesia care under the supervision of qualified clinical instructors who are CRNAs or anesthesiologists. In most programs, the minimum requirements for clinical experience are far exceeded before graduation.[6]

Admission Prerequisites. Admission to nurse anesthesia educational programs is highly competitive. Applicants must meet specific admission criteria that include possession of a baccalaureate degree and current licensure as a registered nurse (RN) in the United States or its territories or protectorates. At least 1 year of experience as an RN in an acute care setting is also a prerequisite for admission.[5]

Most applicants have acquired extensive clinical experience in such settings as coronary, respiratory, postanesthesia, and surgical intensive care units and emergency departments or as members of a trauma or cardiac surgical team.[6] Such experiences attest to the high level of clinical skills possessed by licensed professional nurses who apply to nurse anesthesia programs.

Clinical Practice

Professional certification indicates that an individual has met predetermined criteria that measure the knowledge, skills, and abilities necessary for entry-level practice in a specialty area. Certification affords the public an awareness of the qualifications and capabilities of its health-care providers. The title *CRNA* signifies that the individual who holds it has fulfilled prescribed criteria and is qualified to provide, in a competent and compassionate manner, the services described within a CRNA's scope of practice. The standards for nurse anesthesia practice are listed in Box 2-1.

The AANA publishes a scope of practice for CRNAs[8] that includes but is not limited to the following tasks*:

1. Performing and documenting a preanesthetic assessment and evaluation of the patient, including requesting consultations and diagnostic studies; selecting, obtaining, ordering, and administering preanesthetic medications and fluids; and obtaining informed consent for anesthesia
2. Developing and implementing an anesthetic plan
3. Initiating the anesthetic technique, which may include general, regional, and local anesthesia and sedation
4. Selecting, applying, and inserting appropriate noninvasive and invasive monitoring modalities for continuous evaluation of the patient's physical status
5. Selecting, obtaining, and administering the anesthetics, adjuvant and accessory drugs, and fluids necessary to manage the anesthetic
6. Managing a patient's airway and pulmonary status using current practice modalities
7. Facilitating emergence and recovery from anesthesia by selecting, obtaining, ordering, and administering medications, fluids, and ventilatory support
8. Discharging the patient from a postanesthesia care area and providing postanesthesia follow-up evaluation and care
9. Implementing acute and chronic pain management modalities
10. Responding to emergency situations by providing airway management, administration of emergency fluids and drugs, and using basic or advanced cardiac life-support techniques

*Reprinted with permission from AANA August 29, 2007.

BOX **2-1**

Standards for Nurse Anesthesia Practice

I. Perform a thorough and complete preanesthesia assessment.

II. Obtain informed consent for the planned anesthetic intervention from the patient or legal guardian.

III. Formulate a patient-specific plan for anesthesia care.

IV. Implement and adjust the anesthesia care plan based on the patient's physiologic response.

V. Monitor the patient's physiologic condition as appropriate for the type of anesthesia and specific patient needs.
1. Monitor ventilation continuously.
2. Monitor oxygenation continuously by clinical observation, pulse oximetry, and if indicated, arterial blood gas analysis.
3. Monitor cardiovascular status continuously via electrocardiogram and heart sounds. Record blood pressure and heart rate at least every 5 minutes.
4. Monitor body temperature continuously on all pediatric patients receiving general anesthesia and when indicated, on all others.
5. Monitor neuromuscular function and status when neuromuscular blocking agents are administered.
6. Monitor and assess patient's positioning and protective measures, except for those aspects

that are performed exclusively by one or more other providers.

VI. There shall be complete, accurate, and timely documentation of pertinent information on the patient's medical record.

VII. Transfer the responsibility for care of the patient to other qualified providers in a manner that assures continuity of care and patient safety.

VIII. Adhere to appropriate safety precautions, as established within the institution, to minimize the risks of fire, explosion, electrical shock, and equipment malfunction. Document on the patient's medical record that the anesthesia machine and equipment were checked.

IX. Precautions shall be taken to minimize the risk of infection to the patient, the CRNA, and other health-care providers.

X. Anesthesia care shall be assessed to assure its quality and contribution to positive patient outcomes.

XI. The CRNA shall respect and maintain the basic rights of patients.

Adopted by the American Association of Nurse Anesthetists in 1974; revised in 1981, 1989, 1992, 1996, 2002, and 2005. Used with permission.

Other functions included in a CRNA's scope of practice are administrative and management-related activities, quality assessment, education, research, committee work, and interdepartmental liaison activities.[8]

Activities Outside the Operating Room

CRNAs are consulted on a 24-hour basis and are an integral part of the health-care team, lending their experience in airway management, respiratory care, management of fluid and electrolyte problems, pain management, resuscitative efforts, and other related clinical activities.[2] Many CRNAs are recognized by the American Heart Association as providers and instructors of advanced cardiac life support (ACLS), pediatric advanced life support (PALS), and neonatal advanced life support (NALS).

Nurse anesthesia education provides CRNAs with the theoretic and clinical foundation necessary for participating in pain management. Many CRNAs are involved in the administration of regional nerve blocks and assist physicians in the diagnosis of neurologic deficits or in the modification of pain. Pain management is an expanding area of nurse anesthesia practice and research. CRNAs serve on a variety of institutional committees and participate as instructors in staff development and continuing educational programs for both professional and nonprofessional staff members. Accreditation standards require that each nurse anesthesia program includes CRNAs with graduate degrees as program director and assistant director.[5] As teachers, CRNAs instruct student nurse anesthetists and mentor junior faculty members.

CRNAs hold and have held staff and committee appointments with state and federal governmental agencies such as state boards of nursing and the U.S. Food and Drug Administration. CRNAs also are actively involved in standard-setting organizations, including the American National Standards Institute, the National Fire Protection Association, the American Society of Testing and Materials International, and the Association of Professionals in Infection Control and Epidemiology.[2]

Administrative Role. Current data indicate that hundreds of CRNAs perform administrative functions for departments of anesthesia.[9] The services provided by these administrators are extremely important to the overall functioning of an anesthesia department and correlate directly with the efficiency and quality of service provided. These functions include department management, quality assurance, risk management, continuing education, and data and fiscal management.[8]

Research. Conducting and participating in departmental, hospital-wide, and university-sponsored research projects fall within the CRNA's scope of practice.[8] Historically, nurse anesthetists have been involved in research since the beginning of the 20th century. Early studies were generally descriptive in nature, whereas more recent investigations are scientifically designed quantitative and qualitative studies. Research findings have been published as theses and dissertations and in medical and nursing journals. CRNAs with doctoral degrees have qualified to be project directors or consultants for research projects, including those conducted in universities.[2]

Involvement in research activities is encouraged by the profession through the AANA Foundation and at AANA meetings. The Foundation sponsors a doctoral mentorship program as a support group for CRNAs involved in research. Educational sessions on scientific inquiry, poster presentations, and communication of research findings are frequently part of the agenda of AANA meetings.

Both CRNA and student researchers are eligible to apply for grants awarded by the Foundation. CRNAs have also competed successfully for private and governmental grants. Their research findings have been presented at national and international meetings sponsored by other nurses, physicians, physiologists, pharmacologists, and the government.[2]

Nurse Anesthesia Programs

In mid-2007, 106 nurse anesthesia programs were available in the United States, including two in Puerto Rico.[10] All of them offered master's degrees, and four offered optional doctoral degrees, reflecting a decision by the Council on Accreditation of Nurse Anesthesia Educational Programs to approve only graduate degree programs after January 1, 1998. In addition, all nurse anesthesia programs must meet specific accreditation standards, as outlined in the *Standards for Accreditation of Nurse Anesthesia Educational Programs*, to prepare students to take the national certification examination. On successful completion of the examination, the nurse anesthetist becomes a CRNA.

Practice Settings

The AANA has established professional standards of nurse anesthesia care, as well as guidelines for nurse anesthesia practice. These standards are published in the *AANA Professional Practice Manual for Certified Registered Nurse Anesthetists*, available from the AANA's national office. The standards and guidelines direct professional nurse anesthesia practice.[8]

CRNAs practice in urban hospitals, critical access designated hospitals, ambulatory surgical centers, and U.S. military, public health services, and Veterans Administration health-care facilities. CRNAs also practice in the offices of dentists, podiatrists, ophthalmologists, and plastic surgeons. CRNAs have a variety of employment possibilities available to them. The largest percentage of CRNAs are employed by hospital facilties; however, others are self-employed or employees of anesthesiologists, academic insitutions, military installations, or clinics. CRNAs provide anesthesia services in collaboration with other qualified practitioners, such as physicians (e.g., surgeons or anesthesiologists), dentists, or podiatrists.[8]

ROLE OF THE PROFESSIONAL ORGANIZATION

Historical Background

In 1926, at the first meeting of the Lakeside Hospital alumni group of nurse anesthetists, Agatha Hodgins announced her vision of a national association of nurse anesthetists. Although Hodgins maintained the philosophy that nurse anesthesia should not be considered a part of nursing service but rather a part of general hospital service, on several occasions she approached the American Nurses Association (ANA) to propose the recognition of nurse anesthetists within that group. However, the ANA did not approve the proposal and requested more study on the matter. Determined to form a group of nurse anesthetists, Hodgins called on CRNAs around the country to convene at Western Reserve University–Lakeside Hospital in Cleveland, Ohio, to try to organize their own group. In 1931, 53 CRNAs from 12 states agreed to form the National Association of Nurse Anesthetists (NANA) and to continue their efforts to affiliate with the ANA.[11]

In 1933 the American Hospital Association invited the NANA to present its first national meeting in conjunction with the older, more established organization. After this meeting, the NANA was confronted with one of the most important issues facing nurse anesthetists: education. NANA president Gertrude

Fife called for the creation of a committee to investigate all schools of nurse anesthesia with the objective of creating a list of accredited schools. In addition, she called for the establishment of a national board examination for nurse anesthetists. With this agenda set for NANA in 1933, the members continued to move forward. In 1939 the organization's name was changed to the American Association of Nurse Anesthetists.[11]

Organizational Structure and Function

The AANA (at that time, the NANA) was first incorporated in Ohio on March 12, 1932. It was reincorporated in the state of Illinois on October 17, 1939, and was designated as a tax-exempt organization in accordance with subsection 501(c) of the Internal Revenue Code. The AANA's Education and Research Foundation was incorporated on July 15, 1981, and was designated as a tax-exempt organization in accordance with the same subsection of the Internal Revenue Code. The name was changed to the AANA Foundation in 1994 (K. Koch, written communication, August 20, 2007).

The AANA's bylaws are essentially the AANA's working constitution, and they dictate how the association functions. The bylaws address areas such as the different classes of membership, decision-making procedures, the responsibilities of the AANA's elected officials, and the configuration of committees, as well as the functions of their members.[12] AANA bylaws also define the national organization's relationship with state nurse anesthesia associations.

National Headquarters

In 1937 the AANA executive office moved from Cleveland to Chicago.[11] After having been situated in downtown Chicago for more than 4 decades, in 1980 the AANA purchased and moved into its first building on Higgins Road in Park Ridge, Illinois, a northwestern suburb of Chicago. A satellite office for federal affairs was opened in Washington, D.C., in 1990; lobbyists there advocated for nurse anesthesia education and practice. By early 1990 the AANA had outgrown the executive office in Park Ridge because of an expanding staff and increase in services. A 43,000-square-foot building was purchased in 1992 on South Prospect Avenue in the downtown area of Park Ridge. This building nearly tripled the size of the AANA's national headquarters, allowing the housing of all member services and subsidiaries at one site. The site is also large enough to house a learning center, in which educational seminars are conducted for members on a variety of clinical and professional topics. By 2007, it was evident that continuing growth in membership—with a correlating increase in AANA staff and services—had resulted in the need to acquire more space (Jeffery Beutler, CRNA, MS, AANA executive director, oral communication, August 7, 2007).

Association Structure

The AANA employs approximately 110 professional and support staff between its Park Ridge and Washington, D.C., offices. The executive director is responsible for the administrative functions of the association and reports directly to the member-elected AANA board of directors. As outlined in AANA bylaws, the executive director is responsible for keeping minutes on file of all AANA board meetings, for attending meetings of the board of directors and the executive committee, and for participating in other activities designated by the president. The executive director has no voting privileges but provides advice and guidance on policy formulation to the AANA board of directors. Other duties are to maintain professional AANA staff, negotiate and renew necessary service contracts for the AANA, oversee all financial decisions for the national office with direction from the board, and provide leadership to educational, legal, and legislative entities of the AANA. The executive director also represents the AANA to external organizations.[12]

The daily activities of the association are managed by one or more of the current divisions (i.e., executive affairs, federal affairs, professional practice affairs, finance and administrative services, and communications). Each division is led by a senior director who reports directly to the executive director of the association. The executive affairs division handles issues related to governance and leadership, project management, and professional relations and provides state association management support. The federal affairs division focuses on issues relating to federal legislative and regulatory affairs, payment policy, and advocacy. The professional practice affairs division addresses issues having to do with clinical practice, state legislative and regulatory issues impacting the nurse anesthesia profession, and other nongovernmental regulatory areas. The finance and administrative services division handles issues concerning association finances, membership dues processing, and administrative and building services. The communications division encompasses the media and public relations areas, meetings and programs services, and various AANA publications. Staffing support for the AANA standing or ad hoc committees is also provided by the association.

Elected Leadership

The elected board of directors is responsible for managing the affairs of the AANA.[12] The board members include the president, the president-elect, the vice president, the treasurer, and seven regional directors. The officers are elected for 1-year terms and the regional directors for 2-year terms. Eligibility requirements for serving on the board include active involvement in state association activities, as well as proven leadership and interpersonal skills. A nominating committee oversees the recruitment and selection of individuals for the slate of candidates. All CRNAs are mailed a written ballot and are eligible to vote for candidates for all 11 positions.

The board of directors is the administrative authority for the AANA. It receives and considers the reports of the various committees and councils and makes recommendations as needed. Other responsibilities of the board include developing policy, overseeing the budget and related financial affairs, promulgating clinical standards and guidelines, participating in legislative activities, and serving as a liaison with external governmental and professional agencies.

In addition to maintaining the national office in Park Ridge, Illinois, and the federal affairs office in Washington, D.C., the AANA conducts business largely through meetings of its membership segments. These meetings include the Assembly of School Faculty, the Fall and Mid-Year Assemblies of States, and the Annual Meeting. All AANA members are invited to attend and fully participate in these activities.

Council Configurations and Relationships

Provisions within the AANA's bylaws have allowed the establishment of four separate autonomous councils that reside at the AANA's national office: the Council on Accreditation of Nurse Anesthesia Educational Programs (COA), the Council on

Certification of Nurse Anesthetists (CCNA), the Council on Recertification of Nurse Anesthetists (COR), and the Council for Public Interest in Anesthesia (CPIA). These councils are solely responsible for their own internal affairs, including the election of officers and the direction of financial activities. In accordance with the bylaws, membership on these councils includes CRNAs, students, physicians, hospital administrators, and members of the public.[12] CCNA and COR jointly incorporated in 2007 to form the National Board of Certification and Recertification of Nurse Anesthetists (NBCRNA).

The councils have been established with the intention of informing and assuring the public that accreditation, certification, recertification, and public interest activities are within the discipline of nurse anesthesia and are separate from and not unduly influenced by the national professional association. Communication between the AANA and the councils takes place through a formal liaison committee of council chairs and association officers that facilitates discussion of issues of mutual concern. A CRNA executive director serves each of the councils.

The COA consists of individuals who are involved in the accreditation process of educational programs and the promulgation of educational standards. The purpose of the council is to formulate and adopt standards, guidelines, procedures, and criteria for the accreditation of nurse anesthesia educational programs. This process is subject to review and comment from the AANA board of directors and from the larger community interested in nurse anesthesia.[12]

The CCNA consists of individuals who are involved in the process of certification of nurse anesthetists. The purpose of this council is to formulate and adopt the requirements, guidelines, and prerequisites for certification and eligibility for the certification examination.[12] The council is also responsible for administering the certification examination and for evaluating candidates' performance. The council grants initial certification to those candidates who successfully pass the examination and meet the other criteria for certification.

The COR consists of individuals who are involved in the evaluation and recertification of CRNAs.[4] Its purpose is to formulate, adopt, and continuously evaluate the eligibility criteria for recertification. CRNAs are recertified on the basis of their participation in approved continuing educational activities, documentation of practice, and registered nurse/advanced registered nurse practitioner (RN/ARNP) licensure. Certification is also required that no condition exists that might adversely affect the ability of a CRNA to administer anesthesia or provide safe care to patients.

The CPIA is a multidisciplinary body composed of anesthesia providers and representatives of the public concerned with issues that involve public safety in anesthesia care. It acts as an autonomous appellate body in the credentialing of nurse anesthetists and their educational programs. Its major activities are the monitoring of social and health care trends and issues from the viewpoint of the public; the provision of recommendations to the AANA board of directors, committees, and councils on matters pertaining to accreditation, certification, and recertification; and the application of a public perspective in the review of practice issues as requested by the AANA.[12] An additional responsibility was accepted by CPIA in 2005 for the AANA Wellness Program after it was launched in February 2004. The purpose of this program is to develop and implement strategies to promote healthy lifestyle choices pertaining to the physical, social, spiritual, emotional, occupational, and intellectual well-being of CRNAs and students.[13]

International Federation of Nurse Anesthetists

The International Federation of Nurse Anesthetists (IFNA) is a federation of national associations of nurse anesthetists. It is an affiliate member of the International Council of Nurses and a Nursing Partner of the World Health Organization. The IFNA represents more than 50,000 nurse anesthetists worldwide and is a growing organization with members in both developed and developing countries (S. Ouellette, written communication, August 10, 2007). The first organizational meeting was held in September 1988, and 11 countries were admitted as charter members in 1989. To date there are 34 member countries. The IFNA has developed international standards for education, standards of practice, standards for patient monitoring, and a code of ethics for nurse anesthetists.[14] A World Congress is held every 2 years and is hosted by a member country.

Subsidiary

The AANA owns one subsidiary, the AANA Association Management Services (AAMS), which provides non–dues-related sources of revenue, as well as services for the general membership. There are currently three divisions within the AAMS. These divisions provide services related to insurance, housing, and publishing to both internal and external clients (B. Yeo, CPA, BBA, AANA senior director, Finance and Administrative Services, oral communication, August 28, 2007).

SUMMARY

With the ongoing dedication of its members, volunteer leaders, and staff, the nurse anesthesia profession has been growing and evolving for well over a century. As they encounter the challenges resulting from health care growth and change, all CRNAs must take an active role in securing their future, because a profession is ultimately the sum of its members. As we look to the future, we can be guided by AANA's descriptions of its vision, mission, core values, and motto[15]:

Vision Statement: *Recognized leaders in anesthesia care.*
Mission Statement: *Advancing patient safety and excellence in anesthesia.*
Core Values: *Integrity, professionalism, advocacy, and quality.*
AANA Motto: *Supporting our members—protecting our patients.*

REFERENCES

1. American Association of Nurse Anesthetists. *Nurse Anesthetists at a Glance.* Park Ridge, IL: AANA; January 2007.
2. American Association of Nurse Anesthetists. *Qualifications and Capabilities of the Certified Registered Nurse Anesthetist.* Park Ridge, IL: AANA; 1999.
3. Council on Certification of Nurse Anesthetists. *Candidate Handbook.* Park Ridge, IL: the Council; 2007.
4. Council on Recertification of Nurse Anesthetists, *Criteria for Recertification of Certified Registered Nurse Anesthetists.* Park Ridge, IL: the Council; 2006.
5. Council on Accreditation of Nurse Anesthesia Educational Programs. *Standards for Accreditation of Nurse Anesthesia Educational Programs.* Park Ridge, IL: the Council; 2004.
6. American Association of Nurse Anesthetists. *Education of Nurse Anesthetists in the United States.* Park Ridge, IL: AANA; 2002.
7. American Association of Nurse Anesthetists: AANA adopts position on doctoral preparation of nurse anesthetists. *AANA NewsBull.* August 2007;61:16.
8. American Association of Nurse Anesthetists. *Scope and Standards for Nurse Anesthesia Practice.* Park Ridge, IL: AANA; 2005.

9. American Association of Nurse Anesthetists. *AANA 2005 Practice Profile Survey*. Park Ridge, IL: AANA; 2005.

10. American Association of Nurse Anesthetists. *AANA Annual Reports: Council on Accreditation of Nurse Anesthesia Educational Programs*. Park Ridge, IL: 2006-2007;12-13.

11. Garde JF. *The Nurse Anesthesia Profession: A Past*. Present, and Future Perspective. Park Ridge, IL: AANA; 1996.

12. American Association of Nurse Anesthetists. *Bylaws and Standing Rules of the American Association of Nurse Anesthetists*. Park Ridge, IL: AANA; 2006.

13. Tunajek, S. The wellness project is ahead of the curve. *AANA NewsBull*. December 2005;59:22-23.

14. International Federation of Nurse Anesthetists. *Educational Standards for Preparing Nurse Anesthetists* (rev June 23, 1999); *Standards of Practice* (rev May 18, 1996); *Code of Ethics* (adopted May 1992); *Monitoring Standards* (adopted June 1998), Villennes-sur-Seine, France: IFNA, 1999.

15. American Association of Nurse Anesthetists. *Strategic Plan Highlights*. Park Ridge, IL: AANA Board of Directors; 2004.

NURSE ANESTHESIA EDUCATION IN THE UNITED STATES

Francis Gerbasi, Betty J. Horton

The discovery of anesthesia to provide pain relief for surgery created a demand for nurses trained to be anesthetists. Early on-the-job training has evolved over time into a sophisticated educational process resulting in the award of graduate academic degrees to nurse anesthetists. Today the nurse anesthesia profession is known for its highly respected educational system and strong commitment to quality education. Many regulatory agencies view the nurse anesthesia accreditation and certification processes as the "gold standards."

As of January 1, 2008, 108 programs in the United States and its territories were affiliated with or operated by universities and offered a minimum of a master's degree upon completion. Approximately half of the programs are within schools of nursing, with the remainder housed within schools of health science and other appropriate graduate schools.[1] These nurse anesthesia graduate programs use more than 1600 clinical education sites. The programs range from 24 to 36 months in length, depending upon university requirements, and are at the master's degree level or higher. They provide more than 4000 enrolled students a graduate-level science foundation plus clinical anesthesia experience to prepare them to become competent nurse anesthesia providers.

HISTORY OF NURSE ANESTHESIA EDUCATION

The first nurse anesthetists were trained by surgeons to meet anesthesia manpower needs created by Morton's discovery of ether in 1846. Anesthesia provided surgeons with sufficient operating time on unconscious patients so that new surgical techniques could be developed. Lengthy periods of unconsciousness meant that someone needed to maintain the level of anesthesia and monitor the condition of the patient who could no longer maintain his own vital functions during surgery. It is reported that surgeons used the persons most conveniently available, whether they were medical students, nurses, physicians, or orderlies; however, a need was soon realized for a dedicated category of health-care worker to assume responsibility for the safety of anesthetized patients.[2] Because nurses were already experienced in providing care and protection to unconscious patients, anesthesia care soon became an added responsibility to the general duties of nurses in the United States.[3]

It was from the ranks of hospital-based nursing schools without academic degrees that the first nurse anesthetists were recruited by hospitals and surgeons. In fact, written reports provide some documentary evidence to support that nurse anesthetists preceded physician anesthetists in hospitals.[4] For example, Sister M. Bernard, the earliest known nurse anesthetist, practiced at St. Vincent's Hospital in Erie, Pennsylvania, in 1877. Alice Magaw, another nurse anesthetist, practiced at St. Mary's Hospital in Rochester, Minnesota, and was given the title "Mother of Anesthesia" by Dr. Mayo.[2]

Magaw could also have been titled "educator," as evidenced by the number of individuals who came to her from all over the world to learn anesthesia. According to Ira Gunn, CRNA, MN, some of her students were nurses from the U.S. Army who had been sent to Rochester to learn anesthesia before the United States entered World War I. Subsequently, U.S. nurse anesthetists taught French nurses and physicians how to administer anesthesia during this war, thereby freeing physicians for medical and surgical work (Ira Gunn, written communication, December 11, 1999).

Early Development of Formal Education for Nurse Anesthetists

The practice of training nurses to become anesthetists spread rapidly following the establishment of four schools in the early 20th century. Nurse anesthesia training was offered at St. Vincent's Hospital, Portland, Oregon, in 1909; St. John's Hospital in Springfield, Illinois, in 1912; the Post Graduate Hospital, New York City, in 1912; and the Long Island College Hospital, Brooklyn, New York, in 1914. Other nurse anesthesia schools quickly followed between 1915 and 1920 in Cleveland, Chicago, Milwaukee, Baltimore, Ann Arbor, St. Louis, and Minneapolis.[4]

THE PROFESSIONAL ORGANIZATION'S VISION FOR EDUCATION

Agatha Hodgins, an anesthetist and teacher, was the instructor for an early anesthesia school at Lakeside Hospital School of Anesthesia in Cleveland, Ohio, begun between 1912 and 1915. She was also the driving force in gaining national recognition for nurse anesthetists. In 1930, Hodgins presented her ideas regarding the essentials for a national organization of nurse anesthetists at the American Nurses Association's (ANA) meeting in Milwaukee, Wisconsin. Among her recommendations were the establishment of educational standards and improving the quality of work through study and research.[2] Her efforts to create a division for nurse anesthetists within the ANA were unsuccessful. She then turned her efforts to establishing the National Association of Nurse Anesthetists (NANA) as an independent association for which she served as the first president.

The foundation for the formal education of nurse anesthetists was embedded in the 1933 bylaws of the NANA (later renamed the American Association of Nurse Anesthetists [AANA]). The newly formed association was directed "to develop educational standards and technique[s] in the administration of anesthetic drugs," as specified in Article II, Objective 2.[5] This objective revealed the vision of early nurse anesthesia leaders for a formal educational process that has grown and matured throughout the 20th and early 21st centuries.

Policy decisions during the first 2 decades of the association's existence concerned developing the organizational structure, reviewing educational programs, writing a standard curriculum, and planning to credential nurse anesthetists by examination. Admission to membership in the association and admission to education programs was established during this time. Both required graduation from an accredited nursing school and state registration as a nurse.[4]

Setting Education Standards and Developing an Approval Process

By 1934 the NANA's Educational Committee had studied curricular outlines submitted to them by several schools of anesthesia as the basis for creating a standard curriculum that should be offered to all students. In addition to the detailed standard curricular outline, other guidelines for operating a school of anesthesia were developed, including the type of conducting institution, instructors, record keeping, and other activities.[6]

A recommendation was made to place a school of anesthesia within a hospital's department of anesthesia under the direction of the chief anesthetist. Further, it was recommended that the anesthesia department and its chief anesthetist should report directly to the chief surgeon or the medical director in hospitals if professional departments came under such direction.[6]

During the first decade of its existence, the Educational Committee worked on developing a list of schools of anesthesia and establishing an inspection process to evaluate whether the schools were offering the recommended standard curriculum. By 1939 a national survey of 106 hospitals and teaching institutions had been completed that identified 39 courses of instruction located in 18 states of the United States. There was also a plan to have a representative of the NANA visit all schools for the purpose of collecting information, coordinating training methods, and promoting quality education.

Helen Lamb's work on developing the initial method for approving schools led to a formal accreditation process.[6] Lamb, a former student of Hodgins, frequently addressed the value of a university education for nurse anesthetists. She was founder, then director of the Barnes School of Anesthesia in St. Louis, Missouri, from 1929 to 1951.[4] In 1980, the AANA established an annual award in Lamb's name to honor outstanding educators (Box 3-1).

With the advent of World War II, a shortage of anesthesia personnel became evident, and many hospitals began training anesthetists to meet their own needs. During this critical period, the professional organization encouraged the use of established schools of anesthesia that followed the association's standard curriculum to train anesthetists, rather than the development of new schools that might use substandard methods of training.[6]

The publication of the 1945 *Essentials of an Acceptable School of Anesthesiology for Graduate Registered Nurses* containing information on the proper training of nurses was partially in response to the establishment of new schools with questionable quality during the manpower shortage in World War II. A standard

---

BOX 3-1

Helen Lamb Outstanding Educator Award Recipients

1980—Joyce W. Kelly, CRNA, MA
1981—John F. Garde, CRNA, MS
1982—Virginia A. Gaffey, CRNA, BS
1983—Goldie D. Brangman, CRNA, MEd
1984—Leah Evans Katz, CRNA, EdD
1985—Celestine Harrigan, CRNA, PhD
1986—Hershel W. Bradshaw, CRNA, MEd (posthumously)
1987—Mary Alice Costello, CRNA
1988—Pauline C. Barbin, CRNA, MEd
1989—Betty L. Johnson, CRNA, MSN, USAF, NC
1990—Clarene A. Carmichael, CRNA, BS
1991—Sr. Mary Arthur Schramm, CRNA, PhD
1992—Michael J. Booth, CRNA, MA
1993—Betty J. Horton, CRNA, MSN, MA
1994—Shirley E. Bell, CRNA, MA
1995—Sr. M. Yvonne Jenn, CRNA, BS
1996—Helen P. Vos, CRNA, BSN
1997—Wynne R. Waugaman, CRNA, PhD
1998—Norman R. Wolford, CRNA, CNS, MA, MS, EdD
1999—Carmen E. Siejo, CRNA, BSN
2000—Agnes M. Hagan, CRNA, MS
2001—George P. Haag, CRNA, PhD
2002—Karen L. Zaglaniczny, CRNA, PhD, FAAN
2003—Denise Martin-Sheridan, CRNA, PhD
2004—Joseph Kanusky, CRNA, MS
2005—Sandra Kilde, CRNA, EdD
2006—Charles Reese, CRNA, PhD
2007—Cecil Drain, CRNA, PhD, FAAN
2008—Nancy Bruton-Maree, CRNA, MS

Reprinted from AANA Website with permission of C. Bettin 9-12-08.

---

curriculum was finally submitted to members of the board of trustees by the Educational Committee on July 11, 1945, for approval as part of the *Essentials*.[6]

The cost of inspection of schools was a concern for the new association, supported primarily by dues from a small membership; however, AANA expressed a desire to implement an approval program at whatever cost proved necessary. Initial approval of a school was to be based on a questionnaire, regarded as a temporary screening, to be followed later by an on-site inspection and final approval of the school by the AANA board of trustees. It was reported in 1949 that 14 curricula had been reviewed by the association's curriculum committee, with 7 of them meeting the requirements and 7 of them inadequate or deferred.[6]

The Formal Accreditation Process

The formal accreditation process for schools of nurse anesthesia was approved unanimously during the 17th Annual Meeting of the AANA in September 1950. Membership dues were also increased at that meeting to $20, with $5 of the assessment allocated for the accreditation program. The formal motion to approve the accreditation program included the rationale that the competency of past, present, and future graduate nurse anesthetists could be emphasized by having the schools of anesthesia inspected by qualified consultants, approved, and publicly endorsed. According to Helen Lamb, serving as chair of AANA's Advisory to the Approval Committee, "Such accreditation would vouch for the fact that graduate nurse anesthetists, who now occupy or who in the future enter our field from our standard courses of training, are irreproachably equipped, educationally and clinically, to meet the professional requirements and responsibilities that are inherent in the practice of our specialty."[6]

A workshop on accreditation was held prior to the 1951 AANA Annual Meeting in St. Louis, Missouri. This was one of four geographic regional conferences for directors of schools of anesthesia held in Chicago, New York, St. Louis, and Cleveland.[6] The following year, 1952, Mrs. Lucile Lovett was hired as AANA's first Educational Director. She was a graduate of the Postgraduate Hospital School of Anesthesia, Chicago, and of Millsaps College, Jackson, Mississippi.[6] Her employment at AANA provided the staff support necessary to implement a voluntary accreditation program through the Approval of Schools Committee. After the committee initiated the accreditation process in 1952, it gained federal recognition for the AANA in 1955 by getting it placed on the U.S. Office of Education's (later renamed the U.S. Department of Education) list of nationally recognized accrediting agencies.[6]

As part of the continued recognition process, the AANA submitted a routine petition in 1971 to the U.S. Department of Education. The response received was a request for AANA to explain why it should be retained as the accrediting agency for nurse anesthesia education programs because it had not satisfactorily demonstrated compliance with new federal regulations for accrediting agencies.[4] AANA engaged consultant Ira Gunn to draft any changes necessary to come into compliance with federal requirements so the association could remain recognized by the federal government. As a result, changes were made to the structure and functions within the association by creating the AANA's councils to avoid any potential conflicts of interest between an impartial process for the approval of schools and the interests of the profession. The accreditation process was also tightened to institute requirements such as programmatic self-studies.

The Council on Accreditation of Nurse Anesthesia Educational Programs (COA) is an outgrowth of the AANA's Approval of Schools Committee. Recognition was transferred from the AANA to the COA in 1975, following the delegation of specific responsibilities to AANA's councils. The formation of the original council structure with three separate councils for accreditation, certification, and practice was a major change in the operation of the professional organization.[4] From 1974 to 1977, COA instituted many new requirements for accredited programs to comply with significant changes in the U.S. Office of Education's (USOE) recognition criteria for accreditors.

Early Federal Funding for Education

Governmental awareness of an acute manpower shortage contributed to passage of the Bolton Act of 1943, one section of which offered financing of graduate nurses through established civilian schools of anesthesia.[4] Educational opportunities also became available for returning veterans when Public Law 293, commonly known as the GI Bill, was passed in 1946. Many anesthesia residencies for physicians were developed after World War II with this funding support.[7] The GI Bill was also important in supporting the education of military veterans as nurse anesthetists.

CHALLENGES FACING NURSE ANESTHESIA EDUCATION

Challenges from Anesthesiologists

With the growth in number of anesthesia residencies following World War II, the American Society of Anesthesiologists (ASA) board of directors disapproved the training of other than doctors of medicine in anesthesia during a meeting in June 1947. This ASA position challenged nurse anesthetists, who represented the majority of anesthesia providers in the United States at the time.[4]

Another historical event, the transfer of accrediting authority from AANA to the COA was also influenced by a challenge from anesthesiologists as to the appropriateness of the AANA controlling its own credentialing functions. The challenge included efforts to gain control of school accreditation from AANA. Letters of complaint were filed with the USOE in 1974 by anesthesiologists questioning AANA's capability to comply with new federal accreditation criteria. These ASA members alleged that nurse anesthesia educational programs lacked quality, and the entry requirements into programs were inadequate.[4]

Relinquishing control for accreditation decisions to other than a nurse anesthesia–controlled accrediting agency was strongly opposed by the AANA and COA, and the challenge was successfully resisted. The 1975 hearing before the USOE was attended by more than 100 nurse anesthetists, 15 anesthesiologists, and representatives of three major nursing organizations. Representatives from the ad hoc ASA Committee on the Anesthesia Care Team wanted equal representation with nurse anesthetists in accrediting activities, and a proposal for an alternative accreditation process by an anesthesiologists' sponsored group was introduced by E.S. Siker, a past president of the ASA; however, this proposal was not considered by USOE.[4]

The challenge from anesthesiologists to control accreditation provided advocates for university education an opportunity to initiate movement into academic centers. It also made nurse anesthetists highly aware of society's emerging value for academic degrees.[4] Control of education by universities moved control of many schools from anesthesiologist department chairmen to nurse anesthetists with academic credentials; however, the numbers of academically credentialed nurse anesthetists did not begin to increase until after revision of accreditation standards in 1980, when COA announced that an academic degree would be required for nurse anesthetist program directors in the near future.[6]

Another issue concerning anesthesiologists and nurse anesthesia education is depicted in a 1984 legal case in Portland, Maine. It was an antitrust case brought with reference to a nurse anesthesia educational program. Physicians had tried to keep the students from being prepared to administer all types of anesthesia techniques, thereby limiting their versatility in the market following graduation. The final court order prohibited the Portland anesthesiologist group from restricting the size of the nurse anesthesia class and limiting the students' clinical education.[4]

The issue of whether students should be required to learn the administration of regional anesthesia was opposed by many anesthesiologists, resulting in most schools not offering this experience. This situation was not corrected until 1993 when COA notified programs that all students must be taught the administration of regional anesthesia by 2000. Concern was expressed by some nurse anesthetist educators that such a requirement would limit the number of students that could be accepted into programs, because the administration of regional anesthesia was restricted to anesthesiologists in their clinical facilities. In spite of these concerns, the 2004 Standards for Accreditation of Nurse Anesthesia Educational Programs required that graduates of accredited programs must be prepared in the full scope of anesthesia practice, including the administration of regional anesthesia, insertion of catheters for various invasive monitors, and fiberoptic intubations.[6]

Program Closures

The number of nurse anesthesia graduates decreased significantly during the 1980s with the closure of 60 programs. A 1987 study by Mary DePaolis-Lutzo, CRNA, PhD, revealed reasons for the program closures as lack of support from hospital administration, lack of anesthesiologist support, reduced program funding, costs of program to the institution, and the belief that a future increased supply of anesthesiologists would decrease the need for nurse anesthetists. Another factor was a deteriorating political relationship between the AANA and ASA.[4]

In response to the program closures, the AANA board of directors appointed the National Commission on Nurse Anesthesia Education. The multidisciplinary commission was charged with studying the reasons for the closures and making recommendations to stop the trend. Another of its purposes was to make recommendations for increasing the number of CRNA faculty. The first commission report was published in December 1990 and its final report in 1994. Among its many accomplishments were the opening of several new programs and increased enrollments at many established programs.[8]

Following the commission's work, the trend in program closures continued during the 1990s but was counteracted by the opening of almost an equal number of new programs, many in colleges of nursing. This trend of program closures ended at the beginning of the 21st century to be replaced by a period of program growth.

UPGRADING NURSE ANESTHESIA EDUCATIONAL REQUIREMENTS

The upgrading of academic credentials for CRNA educators and their graduates has always been closely tied to the goals of the professional association to advance the art and science of anesthesia.[6] Nurse anesthesia leaders have been responsible for increasing requirements for curricular content, faculty qualifications, and academic credentials for graduates since early in the 20th century. Over time, schools of anesthesia have moved from apprenticeships at hospitals into degree-granting institutions fulfilling the vision of early anesthesia leaders for a university education for nurse anesthetists. This movement into academia required identifying the location of schools of anesthesia in the nation, determining the essential characteristics of better schools, agreeing on curricular requirements, inspecting schools, and developing a school approval process. A list of some critical events in nurse anesthesia education can be found in Box 3-2.

NURSE ANESTHESIA EDUCATION TODAY

Accredited nurse anesthesia programs are governed by the COA's *Standards for Accreditation of Nurse Anesthesia Educational Programs*.[9] The standards address governance, resources, program of study, program effectiveness, and accountability. All affected constituencies are invited to comment on any proposed standards prior to their adoption.

Nurse Anesthesia Program Requirements

Accredited programs are required to perform ongoing evaluation and assessment to determine their integrity and educational effectiveness. Each program continually monitors and evaluates its didactic and clinical curriculum, including curriculum content, admissions policies, faculty, and clinical sites used for

---

BOX 3-2

Critical Events in Nurse Anesthesia Education (1937-2007)

- Publication of the 1937 *Recommendations Regarding Schools of Anesthesia for Nurses* describing elements of education for curriculum, faculty, and students
- Publication of the 1945 *Essentials of an Acceptable School of Anesthesiology for Graduate Registered Nurses* containing information on the proper training for nurses stemming from the establishment of new schools with questionable quality during a World War II manpower shortage
- Establishment of a voluntary school approval process in 1949; accreditation process implemented in 1952 by the Approval of Schools Committee, with the AANA board of directors actually conferring the accreditation status
- AANA recognized in 1955 by the U.S. Commissioner of Education as the accrediting agency for nurse anesthesia education
- An official position statement adopted by the board of directors in 1982 declaring that education should be postbaccalaureate
- A mandate by COA in 1990 for a baccalaureate degree for entry into programs
- Notification from COA in 1990 that all programs had to offer graduate degrees (master's or higher) by 1998; all programs in the nation finally offered master's degrees on October 1, 1998
- Establishment of the National Commission on Nurse Anesthesia Education in 1989 to increase the number of anesthesia programs and nurse anesthetists in response to program closures and a severe drop in numbers of graduates
- Criteria published in the 2004 accreditation standards for optional doctoral programs
- Criteria published in the 2004 accreditation standards requiring that all students be prepared in the full scope of anesthesia practice, including the administration of regional anesthesia
- Official position statement adopted by the AANA board of directors in 2007 in support of practice doctorates for entry into practice by 2025

---

student educational experiences. These aspects of the program are evaluated periodically to determine their compliance with accreditation standards[9] and relevance to anesthesia practice. This process occurs through completion of a self-study and an on-site evaluation by anesthesia educators and practitioners at least every 10 years. Ongoing monitoring of an accredited program is accomplished through submission of annual reports and progress reports to COA for review. In addition, in 2002 the COA implemented the monitoring of programs' pass rates on the Council on Certification of Nurse Anesthetists' (CCNA) national certification examination (NCE). Programs must demonstrate that graduates take the NCE examination and pass it in accordance with the COA pass-rate requirement.[10] This stringent evaluation process helps to ensure the effectiveness of nurse anesthesia clinical and didactic education.

The administration of a nurse anesthesia program includes program management of faculty and students, fiscal program management, maintenance of COA accreditation and other higher-education accreditation requirements of the university, faculty continuing education, and program evaluation. The COA standards require that each nurse anesthesia program employ Certified Registered Nurse Anesthetists (CRNAs) with graduate degrees in the roles of program administrator and assistant program administrator. Each program must also be able to show organizationally that it provides an extensive, educationally sound curriculum combining both academic theory and clinical practice. Each program must devise policies and procedures using outcome criteria to promote student learning while enhancing the program's quality and integrity.

Admission to a nurse anesthesia program requires graduation from an accredited school of nursing, a baccalaureate degree, current licensure as a registered nurse, and at least 1 year of professional experience in an acute care setting. Most applicants have acquired extensive clinical experience in areas such as coronary, respiratory, postanesthesia, and surgical intensive care units.

Nurse Anesthesia Program Curriculum

The didactic curricula of nurse anesthesia programs are governed by COA standards and provide students the scientific, clinical, and professional foundation upon which to build sound and safe clinical practice. Most nurse anesthesia programs range from 60 to 75 graduate semester credits in courses pertinent to the practice of anesthesia.[1] The science curriculum of graduate nurse anesthesia programs includes courses in anatomy, physiology, pathophysiology, pharmacology, chemistry, biochemistry, physics, professional aspects, equipment, technology, pain management, research, and clinical conferences.[9] The accreditation standards identify the basic nurse anesthesia curriculum and prerequisite course requirements (Table 3-1). Courses in anesthesia practice provide content such as induction, maintenance, and emergence from anesthesia; airway management; anesthesia pharmacology; and anesthesia for special patient populations such as obstetrics, geriatrics, and pediatrics. Students are instructed in the use of anesthesia machines and other related biomedical monitoring equipment and are evaluated didactically using such traditional evaluation methods as examinations, presentations, and papers.

The methods used to provide education are changing as new technologies are being applied in higher education. Based on 2007 annual report data, more than 40% of nurse anesthesia programs use some form of distance education in providing didactic instruction.[1] The distance education offerings vary from several core nursing courses to programs in which the majority of the didactic curriculum is provided using distance education. In addition, the majority of nurse anesthesia programs incorporate some type of simulation (i.e., computer or full-body patient simulation).

The supervised clinical residency of nurse anesthesia education provides students the opportunity to incorporate didactic anesthesia education into the clinical setting. Nurse anesthetists are prepared to administer all types of anesthesia, including general, regional, selected local, and conscious sedation to patients of all ages for all types of surgeries. They are taught to use all currently available anesthesia drugs, manage fluid and blood replacement therapy, and interpret data from sophisticated monitoring devices. Other clinical responsibilities include the insertion of invasive catheters, the recognition and correction of complications that occur during the course of an anesthetic,

TABLE 3-1	Standards for Accreditation*
Minimum Curriculum Course Requirements	
Courses	**Minimum Contact Hours**
Pharmacology of anesthetic agents and adjuvant drugs, including concepts in chemistry and biochemistry	105
Anatomy, physiology, and pathophysiology	135
Professional aspects of nurse anesthesia practice	45
Basic and advanced principles of anesthesia practice, including physics, equipment, technology, and pain management	105
Research	30
Clinical Correlation Conferences	45

Note: 2004 Standards for Accreditation of Nurse Anesthesia Educational Programs.

the provision of airway and ventilatory support during resuscitation, and pain management. To meet COA standards and be eligible to take the NCE, a student must have performed a minimum of 550 anesthetics, which must include specialties such as pediatric, obstetric, cardiothoracic, and neurosurgical anesthesia.[9] This anesthesia experience includes the care of not only healthy but also critically ill patients of all ages for elective and emergency procedures. In most programs, this minimum is surpassed early in their clinical practicum, and the average number of anesthetics performed upon graduation is more than 800. Based on 2007 certification transcript data, nurse anesthesia programs provide an average of 1773 hours of hands-on clinical experience for each student.[11]

During their clinical anesthesia experience, students are supervised by CRNAs or anesthesiologists who provide instruction in the safe administration and monitoring of various techniques, including both general and regional anesthesia. The clinical faculty also evaluate the technical and critical thinking skills of students on a regular basis.

Doctoral Degrees

Beginning in the mid-1980s, the AANA and the COA have continually assessed the need for and feasibility of practice-oriented doctoral degrees for nurse anesthetists. In June 2005 the AANA board of directors convened an invitational summit meeting to discuss interests and concerns surrounding doctoral preparation for nurse anesthetists. Following the summit, the Task Force on Doctoral Preparation of Nurse Anesthetists (DTF) was formed and charged with developing options relative to doctoral preparation of nurse anesthetists that the AANA board could consider.[12] The DTF's final report and options were presented to the AANA board of directors in April 2007, and in June 2007 the board unanimously adopted the position of supporting doctoral education for entry into nurse anesthesia practice by the year 2025. This decision was based on more than 2 years of investigation to thoroughly explore the interests and concerns surrounding doctoral preparation of nurse anesthetists.

Numerous nursing schools are implementing doctorate nursing degree programs. As of September 1, 2008, several nurse anesthesia programs (i.e., Rush University College of Nursing Nurse Anesthesia Program, Virginia Commonwealth University Department of Anesthesia, University of Pittsburgh School of Nursing Nurse Anesthesia Program, and the Texas Wesleyan University Graduate Program of Nurse Anesthesia) offer post-master's doctorate degrees for nurse anesthetists. The first accredited program to replace its master's degree with an entry-level doctoral degree was the Charleston Area Medical Center School of Anesthesia in Charleston. West Virginia, under the leadership of Nancy Tierney, CRNA, MS. DMP, Program Director. The COA approved its doctor of management practice in nurse anesthesia (DMPNA) degree program in 2008. Continued growth in the number of programs offering post-master's and entry-level doctoral degrees is anticipated.

Scholarly Activities

With the evolution of nurse anesthesia educational programs into the graduate education framework, there has been an increase in program requirements for scientific inquiry, statistics, and faculty-guided student research. Professional advancement of numerous scholarly activities has been significantly supported by the AANA Foundation. Through the work of the foundation, clinical nurse anesthetists, faculty, and students have received support for 267 grants, 487 scholarships, and 86 fellowship program awards since 1982. Scholarly activities are presented annually at the national meeting in lectures and discussions, and to date, more than 850 posters have been presented.

Nurse anesthetist involvement in scholarly work includes a variety of research activities, such as quantitative research using descriptive and experimental design and qualitative research using valid research methods. Scholarly publications and scientific presentations have contributed to the overall foundations of nurse anesthesia practice. The move toward doctoral education for entry into practice will foster further involvement in scholarly activities.

SUMMARY

From the commencement of professional education in nursing, a minimum of 7 calendar years of education and training is involved in the preparation of a CRNA at the master's degree level. Graduates of accredited nurse anesthesia programs who pass the rigorous, psychometrically sound certification examination are qualified to practice as Certified Registered Nurse Anesthetists. Recertification, which includes a practice and continuing education requirements, must be met every 2 years. In the United States, nurse anesthesia education has flourished for more than a century by continuing to meet increasingly stringent educational standards. Today the profession and regulatory agencies set the standard of quality for nurse anesthesia education, which has maintained the long tradition of CRNAs delivering safe, high-quality anesthesia care to patients.

REFERENCES

1. Council on Accreditation of Nurse Anesthesia Educational Programs. *Annual Report Data.* Park Ridge, IL: COA; 2007.
2. Thatcher VS. *History of Anesthesia with Emphasis on the Nurse Specialist.* Philadelphia: Lippincott; 1953.
3. Robb I. *Nursing: Its Principles and Practices for Hospital and Private Use.* Toronto: Carveth & Co; 1893.
4. Stoll D. *The Emerging Role of the Nurse Anesthetist in Medical Practice* [dissertation]. Evanston, IL: Northwestern University; 1988.
5. The National Association of Nurse Anesthetists. *Constitution and By-laws.* Park Ridge, IL: AANA; 1933.
6. Horton BJ. Upgrading nurse anesthesia educational requirements (1933-2006)– part 1: setting standards. *AANA J,* 2007 Jun;75(3):167-70.
7. Starr P. *The Social Transformation of American Medicine.* New York: Harper Collins; 1982.
8. National Commission on Nurse Anesthesia Education. *Final Report of the Task Force.* Park Ridge, IL: AANA; 1994.
9. Council on Accreditation of Nurse Anesthesia Educational Programs. *Standards for Accreditation of Nurse Anesthesia Educational Programs.* Park Ridge, IL: COA; 2004.
10. Council on Accreditation of Nurse Anesthesia Educational Programs. *Accreditation Policies and Procedures.* Park Ridge, IL: COA; 2007.
11. Council on Certification of Nurse Anesthetists. *Report of the Assembly of School Faculty: Outcomes Related to Student/Graduate Performance on the Self-Evaluation Exam (SEE) and the National Certification Examination (NCE).* Park Ridge, IL: CCNA; 2008.
12. American Association of Nurse Anesthetists. *Report of the AANA Task Force on Doctoral Preparation of Nurse Anesthetists.* Park Ridge, IL: AANA; 2007.

CHAPTER 4

LEGAL ISSUES IN NURSE ANESTHESIA

Ronald L. Van Nest

THIS CHAPTER IS A BROAD OVERVIEW OF SOME CONCEPTS OF LAW THAT HAVE PERTINENCE TO
NURSE ANESTHESIA PRACTICE. IT IS NOT INTENDED TO GIVE LEGAL ADVICE. CRNAS SHOULD SEEK
LEGAL COUNSEL ON AN INDIVIDUAL BASIS.

SOURCES OF LAW

All of American law flows from the U.S. Constitution, which established (1) our government's structure and function, (2) the relationships of one branch of government with another, (3) the relationship of the states to the federal government, and (4) the relationship of the federal government with the governed.

Judicial Branch–Federal and State

Our judicial system, with its multiple tiers of courts, is probably the least understood branch of government. Our federal and state judicial system dates back to England before American independence. (Louisiana is an exception, basing much of its law on French Napoleonic concepts.) In some cases, our law dates back thousands of years.[1]

In pre-colonial times, most laws in England were made by judges. When a judge ruled on a case, the legal decision became law in that jurisdiction, and it had to be followed by all other judges in that jurisdiction who were inferior to it in the hierarchy of the court system. Those court rulings were passed on from judge to judge and became law by tradition, or **common law**.[1]

A court had authority to only overrule itself from a previous decision or overrule a decision of an inferior court in the same jurisdiction. Each case was looked upon as either unique or similar to a previously resolved court case. Either judges made rulings agreeing with prior law, accepting the precedent of the prior cases (a concept called **stare decisis**), or they created a new law. All such new laws were added to the body of the common law tradition.[2] The American colonists continued this concept in early America, but the state and federal legislatures were more active than their British counterparts, and most American laws had their birth in the legislatures; those laws are called **statutes**. Many laws that had their origins in common law have subsequently been codified by legislatures and are now statutes. In other cases, the legislatures disagreed with common law principles and modified them. A case involving that statute may later come before the state or federal court, and the court may affirm the statute in its ruling or overturn the statute and give the law a somewhat different interpretation. Court interpretations of the law have become vital to our society. The nature of the compromises and negotiations that take place in the various legislatures frequently results in laws that have been written to be intentionally vague. It is only when the law is challenged by two parties with opposing views in an open court that the court gives its judicial interpretation of how the law should be applied.

The concept of the court ruling on a statute did not occur in the United States until 1803 in the case of *Marbury v. Madison*.[3]

A court opinion affirming or overruling a law is only binding in the jurisdiction of that court. A state supreme court (called the court of appeals in some states) only affects the law in that state. If a case is heard in a Federal District court because of a violation of a federal law, and that court's ruling is appealed to a higher level in the federal judiciary, it may be heard in a U.S. Court of Appeals for that Federal Circuit. The court's ruling will be binding on the several states in that Federal Circuit, but only on those states. Rulings by one state's highest court or by a Federal Circuit Court of Appeals are frequently used to support an argument for a similar case in another jurisdiction. The final step in an appeal from any court is to the U.S. Supreme Court, whose decisions are binding on the entire country.[1]

In the early history of nurse anesthesia, few states had nurse practice acts, and those that did made no mention of the nurse's scope of practice. However, many states did have medical practice acts, and they were broadly written to give physicians vast power and authority, allowing them to level the charge of practicing medicine without a license against anyone who was not a licensed physician.[4]

In 1917, nurse anesthesia won its first court decision, establishing the legal right to practice. That case, *Frank v. South*[5] was in Kentucky. Margaret Hatfield was a licensed nurse in Louisville who had training in anesthesia and administered it exclusively for surgeon Louis Frank, a licensed physician. The suit was brought by John G. South, a member of the Kentucky Board of Health. The record is not clear as to what prompted this action. The lower court ruled against Frank and Hatfield, and they appealed to the Court of Appeals of Kentucky. In overturning the lower court decision, the court stated that to accept a broad definition of the practice of medicine would deprive all persons suffering an illness from the care of everyone but physicians. The court also noted that more than 100,000 anesthetics, invariably administered by trained nurses, had been administered at the Mayo Clinic in Rochester, Minnesota. In addition, the court stated that neither the state nursing board examination nor the medical board examination tested the knowledge and skills required of an anesthetist.[6]

In the 1930s, the practice rights of nurses to administer anesthesia was tested in California in the case of *Chalmers-Francis v. Nelson*.[7] In this case, physicians filed an injunction against nurse anesthetist Dagmar Nelson and her employing hospital, demanding she cease administering anesthesia, because by doing so she was practicing medicine without a license. Nelson won the case in the Los Angeles court. Chalmers-Francis appealed to the California Supreme Court, which affirmed the lower court: that Nelson, as a registered nurse, was not practicing medicine. Although Chalmers-Francis wanted to pursue the case further to the U.S. Supreme Court, he abandoned the effort because of insufficient financial backing.[8]

Legislative Branch Statutory Law

Health-care legislation is mainly an issue for the various states and not the federal government.[9]

Federal Legislation

Since Social Security of the 1930s and Medicare and Medicaid of the 1960s, the federal government has had an increasing role in health care, primarily as a very active third-party payer. Medicare policy is important to us because most commercial insurers and HMOs follow the Medicare model, and The Joint Commission inspects hospitals using Medicare requirements as its "go-by." When Medicare was created, it followed the Blue Cross–Blue Shield model: Medicare Part A—Blue Cross paying hospital bills; Medicare Part B—Blue Shield paying physician bills.

Medicare Part A. For hospitals to receive payment for their Medicare patients, they must comply with certain requirements, such as safety features, quantity, mix, and availability of certain services (e.g., pharmacy and nursing services). With regard to operating room services, Medicare Part A requires the **supervision** of CRNAs by a *physician*. Medicare does not define supervision; it permits the supervising physician to be the operating surgeon; it does not require the physician to have hospital "privileges" to supervise CRNAs; and it does not require CRNAs to be supervised by an anesthesiologist.[10]

Medicare permits physicians to bill Medicare for supervising CRNAs if the physicians have credentials in anesthesiology and are willing to certify that they have **medically directed** the anesthesia care.

The Tax Equity and Fiscal Responsibility Act (TEFRA) of 1982 requirements for medical direction describe what a physician must do to be paid by Medicare for medically directing a CRNA in the anesthesia care of a patient:

1. Perform a preanesthesia examination and evaluation
2. Prescribe the anesthesia plan
3. Personally participate in the most demanding aspects of the anesthesia plan, including, if applicable, induction and emergence
4. Ensure that any procedure in the anesthesia plan that he or she does not personally perform is performed by a qualified individual
5. Monitor the course of anesthesia administration at frequent intervals
6. Remain physically present and available for immediate diagnosis and treatment of emergencies
7. Provide indicated postanesthesia care

Since the implementation of this billing requirement, the American Society of Anesthesiologists (ASA) has made these requirements its "Standard of Care" in its "Anesthesia Care Team" model.

The Medicare supervision requirement has been altered, in that individual states are now given the opportunity to "opt out" of the supervision requirement.[11] As of April 2007, 14 states had taken that option.

The penalty for fraudulent billing of Medicare is enormous. Repayment must be made immediately, along with monetary penalties plus interest. Imprisonment is the penalty for particularly egregious offenses. Currently, many CRNAs sign over their billing rights to their hospital employers or anesthesia group employers. It is important that CRNAs have National Provider Identifier (NPI) numbers and that bills are submitted using the correct number. No cases should be billed by that number that were not personally performed by the owner of the number. For example, locum tenens CRNAs should use their own NPIs, not the NPIs of the CRNAs for whom they are covering.[12]

Medicare Part B. This pays physicians and some others, including CRNAs. There is no requirement in this section of the Medicare regulations for nurse anesthetists to be supervised or medically directed.

The Joint Commission. Although The Joint Commission, formerly the Joint Commission on the Accreditation of Healthcare Organizations (JCAHO), is neither a federal nor a state agency; it is mentioned here because it has achieved what is called **deemed status**. That is, it can serve as an inspector for compliance with Medicare regulations.

National Practitioner Data Bank. The Health Care Quality Improvement Act of 1986 created the National Practitioner Data Bank. It was originally designed to protect the public against poor-performing physicians who moved from state to state as a means of hiding a background of several malpractice actions. It has since been expanded to include other practitioners, including CRNAs.[13]

Insurance companies are required to report individuals to the National Practitioner Data Bank when any settlement of a malpractice claim is made. There is an $11,000 fine for not reporting. CRNAs in the Department of Defense can also be reported when the federal government makes a payment from a lawsuit.

A 2005 study noted that 5010 nurses have been reported to the National Practitioner Data Bank, of which 19.5% were nurse anesthetists.[14] The study made note of the fact that nurses have been entitled to due process by peer review groups, but there is no due process requirement for names being placed in the data bank. More than 70% of the reporting is done by malpractice insurance companies. This should be of concern in decisions CRNAs make when they decide to settle a lawsuit; the important matter of being subsequently listed in the data bank should be discussed with the insurance provider.

Individuals whose names are placed in the data bank may make an explanatory statement to be entered along with their name and record in the data bank. Individuals can view their own file, but only their own. Application can be made through the Internet site of the National Practitioner Data Bank.[13]

The data bank must be searched by employers and state nursing boards upon new license requests. It also reports new entries to each state's board of nursing. These boards may start an investigation of their own, leading to a "show cause" of why the CRNA should retain his/her *nursing license*. Thus an anesthesia bad outcome can have a significant affect on the future of a CRNA's practice. CRNAs may wish to consider using legal counsel who have experience in dealing with their state board of nursing.

State Legislation

States' legislatures have affected nurse anesthesia practice in many ways, including passage of legislation creating state boards of health, medical and nursing boards, and insurance commissions. State legislation is also responsible for "enabling laws," which give these boards authority to write regulations and enforce them.

The passage of nurse practice acts followed behind medical practice acts. The first medical practice act was written in Texas in 1873. Years later in West Virginia, a comparable act was challenged and upheld by that state's Supreme Court in *Dent v. W.V.* In the late 19th century, there were many traveling salespeople claiming to be physicians, who sold worthless products touted as cures for diseases. Medical and nursing practice acts were ostensibly written to protect an uneducated public from charlatans.

The first nursing "registry" act was passed in North Carolina in 1903. Like many nurse practice acts that followed, there was no mention of a scope of practice. The acts basically protected the title "Registered Nurse" and stated what was required to obtain the license.

Most states distinguish specialties within nursing, and some states require separate or additional licenses for CRNAs. Such nursing specialty licenses protect CRNAs from the charge of practicing medicine without a license.

All 50 states mention nurse anesthetists in at least one statute or regulation. Many states require a CRNA to remain "Certified" by active recertification through the Council on Re-Certification of Nurse Anesthetists. The Website of the American Association of Nurse Anesthetists (AANA) has more information on this subject.[15]

Executive Branch

The executive branch of a government is tasked with implementation and regulation of the law.

Federal

On the federal level, the executive branch influences nurse anesthetists through such departments and agencies as the Department of Health and Human Services, Department of Education, and Department of Justice.

The Department of Health and Human Services. This department oversees the Food and Drug Administration, which regulates anesthetic drug approval and labeling, and the National Institutes of Health, which has provided grants for anesthesia research and education. It also has under its charge the Centers for Medicare and Medicaid, which pays so much of the country's health care costs.[16]

The Department of Education. This department has ultimate approval of nurse anesthesia education program accreditation.[17]

The Department of Justice. This department houses the Drug Enforcement Agency, which monitors the flow of narcotics into the United States and has oversight of their handling and use.[18]

State

The state executive branch exerts its control of nurse anesthesia practice through the state board of health and its divisions of medical and nursing boards and hospital oversight panels. Each state board of medicine and state board of nursing is given authority by **enabling laws** that give the boards power to enforce laws and interpret and write rules and regulations regarding the practices of medicine and nursing, respectively.[19] These rules and regulations have the full impact of law.

Board of Nursing. The board of nursing, in addition to tracking CRNAs' licenses, controls CRNA practice through the nursing regulations of that state. As noted above, because the medical practice act gives vast authority to physicians, the nursing regulations are continually changing as new technology is introduced and nurses become more important in using that technology

for patient care. The scope of practice in nursing regulations has to be changed frequently to protect the nurse from the charge of practicing medicine without a license. In some states, advanced practice nurses such as nurse anesthetists have joint regulations, changes to which must be approved by both the medical and the nursing boards. CRNAs should be knowledgeable of the regulations that govern practice in their state. In many states, the members of the board of nursing are appointed by the governor.

LEGAL AREAS OF INTEREST TO THE NURSE ANESTHETIST

Because the law is complex, it has been categorized for easier study under headings such as Tort Law, Criminal Law, Contract Law, and Employment Law.

Tort Law

Tort law principles govern the rights of one person to seek compensation for an injury or harm caused by another person or entity. Over the many years of our country's history, some tort law has been codified in state and federal law by legislation. Much of tort law takes its origin from common law. Some laws have had their origin in tort but have been converted to crimes by legislative action.

In noncriminal cases, the party who alleges having been harmed is called the **plaintiff,** the accused is called the **defendant,** and the lawsuit is called an **action.** (In a criminal case, the state or federal government initiates the action because of a harm that was suffered by society for an alleged violation of the law. The person bringing this action is called the **prosecutor,** and the accused party is called the **defendant,** the same as in a tort action.)

Tort law has been created more by states than the federal government. Consequently, there may be as many as 50 different variations on the way tort law is enforced and interpreted.

Why Do We Have Tort Law?

Several reasons for the need for tort law have been proposed[20]:

1. To correct a wrong, whether committed by negligence or intention, the wrongdoer pays for the damage. It provides a legal way "to get even." It minimizes taking justice into one's own hands and settling matters by illegal methods. It may have given rise to calling one's attorney a "hired gun."

2. To deter certain activities from taking place or to deter certain products from being manufactured, such as mass production toxic gases and chemicals. Some products are worth the risk, however (e.g., steak knives and automobiles, which have a utility for society, but must be made and used safely).

3. To distribute loss. This is one of the principles of liability insurance: It is better to pay $100 on several occasions as a premium than one payment of many thousand: even though the probability of ever having to make that high payment is negligible.

4. To compensate the victim for loss or injury.

5. To address a social concern. Tort law provides a means for an average person to put a large, powerful organization on trial (e.g., asbestos lung injury, lead poisoning, pharmaceutical manufacturers, tobacco companies).

6. To punish and create an example. Punitive damages, sometimes called **exemplary damages,** are designed to punish the wrongdoer. They are usually very high monetary awards that draw notice and attention.

Goal of Tort Law

The goal of tort law is to restore the party who has suffered a damage to the condition that existed before the damage. The goal is not for the plaintiff to profit from the court action but to be made whole. (Note: A source of confusion when reading about court cases is the difference between *damage*, the harm the plaintiff suffered, and *damages*, the money the plaintiff is seeking for compensation for the harm.)

Categories of Torts

Tort law has three major subdivisions: **intentional torts,** which include such actions as assault, battery, and intentional infliction of emotional harm; **strict liability,** which includes product liability; and **negligence.** Some criminal offenses are also torts, so it is easy to get confused. The rules governing the evidence may be different, and the punishment certainly is different. Assault and battery, like many of the other intentional torts, are also criminal violations. A person who attacks another with a baseball bat may be charged in criminal court for battery and face a jail sentence.[21] That same person may be sued in civil court for the tort of battery, and the victim (plaintiff) may seek and receive a financial payment from the defendant for the harm and injury caused. A person may be acquitted in criminal court, yet an action can be brought by the victim under tort law. This is an example of courts being used to avoid vigilante justice or "taking the law into your own hands."

Negligence. The fundamental principle of negligence is that we all have a duty of reasonable care to one another; in other words, we have to act like a "reasonable person."[21] In the health-care professions and several other areas of society, we don't want to know how the "reasonable person" would have acted, because we don't want a reasonable *person* to administer our anesthetic, we want the reasonable *appropriately trained, licensed health-care professional* to administer our anesthetic. The courts, therefore, hold such professionals to a higher standard of care, and a violation of that standard of care is called **professional malpractice,** or simply **malpractice.**[22]

Anatomy of a Medical Negligence Action. In a negligence action, the plaintiff must prove to the court the following four elements. If *all* are not proved, the case should be dismissed.[21]

1. **Duty**—a patient/provider relationship exists, and reasonable care is expected. Reasonable care by a professional is defined by that profession's **Standard of Care.**
2. **Breach of duty**—failure to meet the Standard of Care. In court, an **expert witness** (one or more), usually of the same profession, defines that standard of care. The expert may provide evidence of the standard by presenting standards published by the professional organization (e.g., *The Professional Practice Manual* of the AANA),[23] hospital policy manuals, procedure manuals, nurse practice act standards, pertinent federal regulations, drug package inserts, and textbooks, among others. The opposing side may have expert witnesses who will give arguments that what has been presented does not violate the standard of care.
3. **Damage**—the plaintiff must have suffered some injury, physical or emotional.
4. **Cause**—the damage the plaintiff received was caused by actions of the defendant that deviated from the standard of care. There must be a direct or **actual cause** between the practitioner's actions and the damage the plaintiff suffered. The plaintiff must also prove **proximate cause,** which has been described as *foreseeable before the event took place.* In other words, it was foreseeable that if a certain action

would be taken, certain damage would occur. Some legal commentators describe proximate cause as *that which when viewed in retrospect is not thought of as extraordinary.*[22]

Professional Standards

The American Association of Nurse Anesthetists. Although the AANA does not write legally binding regulations, it is the only professional organization for nurse anesthetists in this country, and it writes and publishes standards and guidelines for the professional practice of CRNAs.[23] The Standards and Guidelines are helpful, influential, and suggestive, but not binding on state regulatory bodies and legislators. They are also presented in court as evidence to help establish the Standard of Care.

American Society of Anesthesiologists. The ASA's role for anesthesiologists is similar to the AANA's role for nurse anesthetists. Because of CRNAs' close working relationship with anesthesiologists, many of the ASA's standards and guidelines have influence on CRNAs' practice.

Concepts Used in Tort Law

Res Ipsa Loquitur. This Latin term refers to a presumption commonly used in negligence cases and especially in medical malpractice cases. It means "the thing speaks for itself" and dates to an 1863 incident in which a barrel rolled out of a warehouse and hit a pedestrian. The plaintiff asserted that it is not normal for barrels to roll out of a warehouse by themselves unless someone was negligent.

When the plaintiff asserts res ipsa loquitur, three elements must be proved:

1. The injury would not have occurred if someone were not negligent
2. The injury must be caused by something within the exclusive control of the defendant
3. The injury must not have been due to any voluntary action by the plaintiff[21]

Regarding the practice of anesthesia administration, res ipsa loquitur is particularly helpful to the plaintiff in complicated problems in which it is difficult to obtain all the facts, especially while the plaintiff was unconscious under general anesthesia. Although there are arguments to the contrary, this principle does somewhat reverse the concept of "innocent until proven guilty," because the defendant, at least to some extent, has to prove his or her innocence.

As an example of the importance the courts give to res ipsa loquitur, in the case of *Adams v. Family Planning Associates Medical Group, Inc., et al,* a patient suffered a cardiac arrest and died upon completion of an abortion. Despite expert testimony that the nurse anesthetist did not violate the Standard of Care, and despite the fact that the trial court ruled in favor of all defendants, the plaintiffs appealed on the grounds that the jury should have been instructed to consider res ipsa loquitur. An Illinois appellate court agreed, and a new trial was ordered.[24]

Informed Consent. Informed consent helps protect the health-care professional from charges of battery and negligent failure to warn. The important thing in the consent process is not the signature on the paper but the conversation and understanding that take place before signing. There are two different standards applied by the courts as to what to tell the patient. One is called the **professional standard,** in which the practitioner has to tell the patient what the reasonable practitioner would tell under the same or similar circumstances. The other standard is called the **material standard** or **patient standard,** in which the practitioner must tell all the material facts a reasonable patient, under the same or similar circumstances, would want to know.[25] The states are about evenly divided over which standard applies. Adding more confusion, some state supreme courts have also said the patient does not have to be told of something disastrous if its possibility is remote, whereas other courts have said the patient must be told if the matter is so material that if the patient had known it could occur, he or she would have had the choice of choosing not to have the procedure. In addition, some courts have also said that minor complications do not have to be discussed, even if the events are common.

Identifying who we are is also something to consider. A recent Ohio case that dealt with a ruptured esophagus (*Luettke v. St. Vincent Mercy Medical Center, et al.*) digressed slightly from the point of the lawsuit and made note of the manner of the identification of the student nurse anesthetist as a part of the informed consent.[26] The student had introduced herself by her first name and said she was a registered nurse in the anesthesia department, not that she was a nurse anesthesia *student*. She said that she was going to be helping a CRNA and an anesthesiologist with the anesthetic, when in fact she was going to be the one administering the anesthetic.

Assumption of the Risk. Some CRNAs have the mistaken belief that if the patient gives informed consent, it clears the CRNA of a later suit for negligence, because they warned the patient, and because the unfortunate event occurred as warned, the CRNA is excused of liability. This is a misunderstanding of the concept of assumption of risk. This theory of law is restricted to such foolhardy actions as "where one tries to beat a rapidly approaching train across the track, to engage in drag racing, or to walk upon a frozen pond where the ice is thin."[27] It has no application to consent for an anesthetic. The anesthesia consent provides a defense for the intentional tort of battery. By signing the consent, the patient gives permission to be touched.

Defenses. The best and easiest defense for negligence is to not have the problem at all: "First do no harm." But sometimes a CRNA can be pulled into a lawsuit because of the negligence of someone else, and the CRNA has to present evidence to the court to prove no causal relationship to the harm. This effort is normally started early in the multiple hearings that take place before the case goes to trial.

Another defense is to prove to the court that the CRNA did follow the standard of care, despite the poor outcome. Here the best evidence is a well-documented anesthesia record with a properly annotated preanesthesia evaluation. A good record provides the necessary material for a defense attorney and the expert witnesses. There are some who argue that it is better to say very little in the anesthesia record or patient chart. Plaintiff attorneys appreciate that behavior. They argue that what is not in the record was not done. In court it is difficult to convince a jury that one can remember what took place minute by minute during a case that took place 2 or more years ago. Therefore, make a complete record.

Some **jurisdictions** (geographic locations that are served by a particular court) allow a **contributory negligence** defense. Here the defendant presents evidence that the plaintiff contributed in some way to the bad outcome. Some considerations are, if appropriate, failure to comply with NPO guidelines; incomplete, intentional, or negligent failure to disclose significant information on preoperative questions and answers regarding previous medical

history; and noncompliance with drug dosing and scheduling preoperatively. In what are called "all-or-none" jurisdictions, the plaintiff will collect nothing in damages if anything is found to show that the plaintiff contributed to the problem. Such jurisdictions are in the minority. More commonly the jurisdiction will use some form of a **comparative negligence** theory, in which the damages awarded to the plaintiff will be reduced by a percentage of the role the plaintiff participated in his or her own problem.[21]

If the tort alleged is an intentional tort (like battery), the best defense is a properly executed informed consent.

The **statute of limitations** is another defense. All torts and most crimes have a time limit beyond which legal action may not be taken. The timer on the statute may begin from the time of the injury or the time of the discovery of the injury. Time periods vary among jurisdictions and by the offense. There are also different time periods when children are involved.

Spoliation of Evidence. Spoliation is the destruction, concealment or alteration of evidence. Sometimes the outcome of the surgical or obstetric case is so poor that a lawsuit seems inevitable. A common reaction is to review the anesthesia record and recognize some shortfalls in the documentation. This is NOT the time to delete, destroy, rewrite, or alter the record in any way. When medical records are subpoenaed and the anesthesia record is not included, the court gets suspicious that it has been intentionally withheld. Some records have appeared in court that are too good and too neat for the circumstances. In such cases, tampering with the record, which is now evidence, is looked at with a more critical eye; if alteration is discovered, the anesthesia record may discredit the entire defense. If the anesthesia record is not admitted into evidence, the CRNA has only memory to rely upon, and this will have little credibility with a jury. Some jurisdictions consider altering records as the **intentional tort** of **spoliation of evidence**.[28] Courts do not typically award punitive damages in negligence cases, recognizing that mistakes can happen. But when the offense is an intentional tort, in this case a "cover-up," punitive damages can be awarded.[21] Many liability insurance policies do not cover punitive damages. This is a serious issue that can cost millions of dollars. Spoliation of evidence is also a crime punishable by incarceration.

Liability Insurance. Liability insurance is designed to pay for the cost of the defense and the damages awarded by the court. During the 1980s, there was an explosion of malpractice claims the insurance industry could not afford to pay. All malpractice insurance at that time fell into the category of **Occurrence Policies,** which cover all acts that occur during the policy period, regardless of when the lawsuit is filed—even if the insured retired, moved, or chose to insure with another cheaper company. Back then, insurance companies were paying on claims against policy holders who were no longer paying premiums. Occurrence policies were soon replaced by **Claims Made** policies, limited to the period from the time the policy went into effect until the practitioner stopped making premium payments. (Thus practitioners would have to pay annually, even through retirement years, to avoid losing their life savings in a lawsuit.) Because this business practice was unpopular, insurers created an **Extended Reporting Period Endorsement,** commonly called **Tail coverage,** which will give the insured lifetime protection without making annual payments. Currently the cost of most tails approximates the cost of 200% of a year's premium.[29] (A mnemonic for remembering which policy is which is the abbreviation for October: OCT—Occurrence, Claims Made, Tail).

Criminal Law

Criminal law concerns itself with the duty a citizen owes to his government. The punishment for violation of criminal law is so severe (i.e., large fines or imprisonment), that the laws are precisely written, and the violation must be proved beyond a reasonable doubt. Nurse anesthetists do not normally get involved in this area of law in normal practice. However, areas outside of clinical practice may have a role here that can jeopardize the CRNA's nursing license.

Felony

A felony is a crime punishable by incarceration in a state prison for any period of time or in a local jail for 1 year or more. A felony conviction in many states is a basis for revocation of a nursing license. Therefore a nurse anesthetist who has a criminal entanglement could not only suffer the consequences of imprisonment but also a permanent loss of the right to practice anesthesia. This should be of particular concern during plea bargaining to avoid incarceration. A plea of nolo contendere to a felony is still considered a felony conviction.[30]

Gross Negligence

Negligence that has led to a death can trigger a criminal investigation. If the negligence is considered by the prosecutor to be gross negligence or a lawful act done without due caution or care, the prosecutor can pursue a conviction on the charge of **involuntary manslaughter,** the punishment for which includes imprisonment.[31]

Contract Law

Contract law is at the heart of our capitalist, business society. Contracts are promises people make to each other that the law will enforce. Contracts do not have to be in writing for the court to enforce them. Courts enforce contracts by (1) forcing a reluctant promisor to pay for damage incurred when a contractual promise is broken (**breach**), (2) forcing the party to do what was originally promised if it is still possible, or (3) requiring the party (by an **injunction**) to refrain from doing what he or she originally promised not to do. The compensatory damages the court awards in contract disputes can be much higher than is seen in tort cases. In contract disagreements, the court awards the **benefit of the bargain**—in other words, the lost profits resulting from the failure to perform on the contract.[32] CRNAs may meet contract law in employment and credentialing issues, but some attorneys also use contract law in malpractice situations as a means of pursuing a case beyond the shorter statute of limitations that usually apply to tort actions. They argue that CRNAs have an implied contract with their patients to provide safe anesthesia care.

Employment Contracts

There is more to employment contracts than salary and vacation time. An enjoyable workplace can become intolerable because a contract was created carelessly.

Know What You Sign. A basic principle of contract law holds that an adult who can read is bound by a contract that he or she signs, regardless of whether or not he or she has read it.[33] Remember, a pre-employment application form you sign may constitute a contract. You may be signing away your rights against your employer before you are even hired.

Parol Evidence Rule. A curiosity of contract law is the Parol Evidence Rule, which holds that promises not written into the contract but made orally before signing the contract are not admissible in court later.[34] Remember all the great promises made to you to entice you to work somewhere? If they are not written into the contract, you cannot enforce them later. If it is important enough for you to discuss with the prospective employer, it is important enough to insist that it be written into the contract. The best time to have a contract dispute is during its formation. If there cannot be a "meeting of the minds," either party is free to terminate negotiations. Once the contract is formed, disputes can become hostile and expensive to resolve.

Breach of Contract. Once a contract is signed, both parties are bound by its promises. Failure to comply with the contract terms is called a **breach of contract** and can result in a lawsuit to recover damages. Some CRNAs have signed contracts to work for a year or more and then have quit suddenly. This is a clear breach of contract, and the employer can sue for lost income that would have been derived by that CRNA's performance, the cost of advertising for a replacement, the cost of hiring a locum tenens replacement, and any other miscellaneous expenses.[35] Every contract should be fully understood before signing it.

Mitigation of Damage. When a person has suffered an injury, he or she has a duty to act to minimize the impact of that injury; this is called **mitigation**. For example, if someone negligently cuts you, you have a duty to clean the wound and take action to prevent an infection. You cannot take the situation as an opportunity to create a large lawsuit by allowing the wound to infect and cause a need for a later amputation. Likewise, if fired wrongfully from a job, the CRNA has a duty to seek other employment to mitigate the damage of the lost income and loss of clinical skills. The CRNA can still sue, and any damages awarded if the CRNA prevails will be offset by the supplementary wages received in the interim. If the CRNA made no effort to mitigate, the damages awarded may be offset by what the CRNA could have earned during the interim.

Interference with Contract. Interference with contract is an improper inducement of another to breach a contract. It is particularly egregious if coupled with threats, coercion, or even persuasion based on mutual interest.[21] This issue is discussed here under contracts, but it is actually a tort, for which damages may be sought, including punitive damages. In an atmosphere of intense competition for office practice sites, ambulatory surgery center contracts, and hospital group contracts, practitioners have to be careful that they do not overstep their offer to provide services when there is already an anesthesia practitioner in place.

Should You Have a Lawyer? When facing employment contracts, CRNAs may wish to have legal counsel. The employing hospital or employing physician group very likely has had legal counsel prepare the contract. In such a situation, it would be highly unlikely that the contract would have been worded with terms more favorable to the CRNA.

Employment Law
The Dead "Captain of the Ship" and "Borrowed Servants"

At the turn of the 20th century, most hospitals were either charity or government owned. They were underfunded and unable to protect themselves in liability action. Government hospitals were protected by government immunity, and legislatures protected the charity hospitals by granting them charitable immunity, leaving no one to pay for a malpractice action. At that time it was considered medically unethical for a physician to be an employee of anyone, and physician anesthetists refused to be employees of the hospital or the surgeons. Physicians were not employees of the hospital, but they had clinical privileges to admit patients and operate on them. By not being employees, they remained subject to liability action. During surgical procedures, charitable immunity did not transfer to the surgeon. All hospital employees working in the operating room, including employed CRNAs, became known as "borrowed servants," borrowed from the hospital to work for the surgeon during the procedure. The actions of the employees were under the control of the surgeon on a vicarious liability theory. It did not take too much imagination to see the surgeon in charge as liable and responsible for everything in the operating room and therefore looked upon as similar to the captain of a ship.[36]

Over time, hospitals have become big businesses. Thus most hospitals have lost their charitable immunity rights. Tort attorneys have nevertheless been reluctant to excuse the surgeon for any misadventure in the operating room, even if it was not caused by the surgeon. Under res ipsa loquitur, everyone in the operating room is named in a lawsuit. It is then up to each individual to clear himself or herself as not having caused the harm asserted. Because hospitals are insured, as are all professionals in the operating room, the "captain of the ship" now denies control of everyone else, and there is no need for borrowed servants.[37,38]

Respondeat Superior. By a legal principle called **vicarious liability,** one person may be liable for the actions of another based solely on the relationship between the two persons.[39,40] For example, a partner in a partnership can be liable for the actions of the other partner, parents can be held vicariously liable for the actions of their children, and employers can be liable for the actions of their employees.

For the employer to be held liable for the actions of an employee, the employee must be working within the course and scope of employment, whether or not the employer has the actual ability to control the employee's conduct. The courts historically interpret the scope of employment very broadly, allowing the injured plaintiff to seek compensation from the deep pockets of the employer rather than the shallow pockets of the employee. The opposite of an employee is an independent contractor. In determining which situation exists, the courts look at the right to control held by the employer.[41-45]

To escape liability, the employer will attempt to show that the employee was not working within the scope of employment. Employed CRNAs should be aware of what they are and are not permitted to do. There should be agreement among a CRNA's employment contracts, credentials, hospital policy manuals, department policy and procedure manuals, and any other local guidelines. Inconsistency between these and actual practice are difficult to justify in court.

To avoid having to pay costly health care benefits and disability insurance, among other things, employers may use independent contractors rather than employees.[46] Plaintiff attorneys are tenacious in finding employment relations when an independent contractor status was intended.[47]

Employees are not in the clear simply because their employer had to pay for their actionable activity. In addition to being fired, employees can be sued by an employer who had to make a payment on the liability of an employee under the principle of **indemnification**.[48] CRNAs who sign employment contracts should be watchful for indemnity clauses that are not easily understood.

AVOIDING A LAWSUIT

The adage "First, do no harm!" is never truer than in a malpractice action. Although a CRNA may be named in a malpractice action, the CRNA should not lose the suit if no harm or injury was caused, either directly or indirectly. Remember, one of the elements that must be proven by the plaintiff is that harm, injury, or damage was suffered. Practice safely, and do no harm.

Be Careful of Where You Work

Workplace safety is not typically a great concern for hospital-based CRNAs because of so many oversight regulations that must be followed, but ambulatory surgery centers and office practices can be a malpractice minefield. Many of these facilities are not accredited by any recognized agencies, and owners may cut corners on safety to reduce costs and increase profits. A fire in the building or even a cardiac arrest may not be related in any way to the anesthetic, but if the CRNA cannot get the anesthetized or sedated patient to safety or definitive care, the CRNA may be implicated. Consider egress of the anesthetized patient. Will the OR table roll? Will it or a stretcher fit on the elevator? Is there an elevator? How would fire and rescue personnel get your patient down stairs if that became essential? Is the building a modern facility, or is it a converted wood-frame apartment building? Does it have a sprinkler system? Is the building approved by the local fire department for the administration of general anesthesia? Is there central oxygen distribution? The first thing fire fighters want to do on arrival is turn off the central oxygen supply. Is there a ready source of portable oxygen tanks and ready tanks on the anesthesia machines?

Be Careful of the Employer

Some physicians operate in unaccredited and unlicensed facilities because they don't have a license themselves or can't get malpractice insurance because of a long history of bad outcomes and large payouts. Wherever CRNAs work, the employer will ask for credentials, proof of license, advanced cardiac life support (ACLS), and proof of liability insurance, among other things. CRNAs have the right to ask the same of surgeons. If there is a bad outcome, everyone will have to produce these for the court. *After* a lawsuit has been brought is not the time to find out that the surgeon has no insurance and lost his or her license to practice medicine 2 years ago. Some physicians balk at getting ACLS certified, but if the CRNA has a problem and needs to use ACLS protocols, the CRNA will need everyone around to be as proficient as possible to help, not the least of whom is the surgeon. In addition, the more surgeons know about the expectations and shortfalls of ACLS, the more discerning they may be in their selection of patients for this setting.

Evaluate the Nursing and Clinical Support Staff, Especially in the Office Setting

Many of these people have had no operating room experience at all and have no experience or understanding of what is required for the safety of an anesthetized patient. They may not have any formal or even informal education with regard to patient positioning, restraints, electrocautery, IV fluid handling, and sterile procedures. These people will be your extra pair of hands when you need them. Can they set up a second IV for you or give cricoid pressure?

Know the AANA Professional Standards and Guidelines

These will be the first things that a plaintiff's expert witness will present for evidence. This should not be the first time you have read them. Remember, there is no latitude with regard to standards of practice. You must follow them. Guidelines allow you to use a reasonable amount of discretion on a case-by-case basis.

Know Your State Nurse Practice Act

This is especially important if there are any provisions for CRNAs, particularly regarding scope of practice. If you are not practicing within your scope of practice you will be virtually defenseless.

Conduct a Proper Preanesthesia Evaluation

Production pressures and rapid turnover between cases are unfortunate facts of life. However, they are no excuse for an improperly conducted preanesthesia evaluation. While doing it, this is not only the time to establish rapport with the patient, it may be the only time to establish rapport with the patient's significant other. Before wheeling the patient into the operating room, the CRNA should be certain that both of them *know* that you genuinely care about your patient's safety and well-being during and after the anesthetic. If there is an unfortunate outcome, the CRNA may not see that significant other again until they meet in a courtroom. What was that person's last memory of you? Was it of someone who had to quickly fill out some paperwork, or was it of someone who genuinely cared?

Document, Document, Document

Some people actually believe that the anesthesia record should be intentionally brief and sketchy so as not to provide information that a plaintiff's attorney can use. The fact, however, is that the defense attorney and the CRNA's defense expert witnesses rely on what has been written. It is the plaintiff's attorney who relies on what is NOT there and attempts to prove to the jury that during those time gaps, nothing was being done to help the patient.

Time Medical Record Entries

Any time a documentation is made, either in a remarks section of the anesthesia record or in the progress notes, date and *time* the entry. Time can be critical, depending upon the event. A plaintiff's attorney can build an entire case on what took place during 2 minutes. Two years after the event, the CRNA may have to prove what took place at 0847 and not 0849.

Do Not Alter the Record

After the case is over, do not alter the anesthesia record. It is permissible to make notations in the progress notes that may add more narrative to what took place or rationale for your actions at a given moment, but date and time that entry. Do not remove the anesthesia record and rewrite it, no matter how sloppy and illegible it may be, not even if you record everything verbatim in the exact location on the new record. (See Spoliation of Evidence.)

IF YOU ARE SUED

Notify Your Insurance Company

If you have a bad outcome and think you may be sued, notify your insurance company immediately and take their advice. Don't be afraid you will lose your coverage because you report yourself. The more time your insurance company has to prepare your defense, the better for you *and* them, even if no lawsuit develops. If you had no suspicion of a suit and are served with a one by surprise, notify your insurance company immediately. Your insurance company will hire a defense attorney and pay the attorney fees.

Consider Hiring Your Own Attorney

If you are employed by a hospital or a large anesthesia group, the insurance company for them may decide to settle the case earlier than you wish or perhaps against your wish. You may want an attorney who will protect your interests only. It may be costly but worth it to you.

Board of Nursing Concerns

Whether you have successfully defended yourself or not, you may be investigated by the board of nursing. You may have to make a

statement and may have to testify to defend your right to retain your license. Boards of nursing are administrative agencies and work somewhat differently than courts. It may be wise to engage a lawyer who has experience in dealing with board of nursing issues to help you write answers to interrogatories and prepare your defense.

Consider Personal Counseling

An unfortunate outcome, especially one that also leads to a lawsuit, can cause self-doubt, heightened anxiety, isolation, anger, and fatigue and can lead to depression or Litigation Stress syndrome.[49] A personal counselor may help prevent these problems. If someone in your department has a bad outcome, moral support from a colleague can be very helpful. A summary of this section can be seen in Box 4-1.

BOX 4-1

Lawsuits

Avoiding a Lawsuit:
- First do no harm.
  - If the patient has suffered no harm or injury, there is no basis for a lawsuit.
- Be careful of *where* you work.
  - Particularly if in an office of small ambulatory surgery center.
  - Can patients be removed easily in the event of a fire or for transfer to a hospital?
  - Is the building itself a fire hazard?
  - Evaluate oxygen handling and storage.
  - Is there a sprinkler system?
  - Is the facility accredited by one of the national health-care accrediting agencies?
- Be careful of *who* you work for.
  - Are all of the surgeons board certified?
  - Do they all have liability insurance? And for how much?
  - Are the physicians ACLS certified?
- Be careful of who you work *with*.
  - What credentials do the nursing staff members have?
  - Remember that they will be your extra pair of hands in an emergency.
- Follow AANA Professional Standards and Guidelines, don't deviate.
- Take care of your patient; show genuine positive regard.
  - Give due regard to the patient's significant other as well.
- Document properly.
- Date and <u>time</u> all progress-note entries.
- Don't alter the record.

If You Are Sued:
- Contact your insurance company immediately in writing.
- Consider obtaining a personal attorney (especially if you are insured by the hospital or the anesthesia group and have not had your own liability policy).
- When the lawsuit is settled, good or bad, don't forget the board of nursing. It may conduct an investigation, and you may have to answer it as well. Consider an attorney experienced with board of nursing hearings.
- Consider personal counseling.

SUMMARY

Fortunately, anesthesia is safer than ever, and the number of lawsuits involving anesthesia care has decreased in the past several decades. Improvements in monitoring technology, drugs, and diagnostic tests and the greater knowledge and skill of anesthesia providers all play a role. When an untoward incident does happen, however, the consequences can be devastating for the patient, the family, and the provider. Patient safety should be a primary factor on a daily basis in every decision made and technique performed. Processes that incorporate safety into the workflow of the modern anesthesia department must be constantly reassessed and updated. This chapter has explained some of the current legal concepts underlying anesthesia practice.

It is important to remember that ignorance of the law is no excuse for improper practice judgments. Know the laws and regulations that govern your practice. Know and follow your professional standards and guidelines. Document accurately and in a timely manner.

Find a lawyer now that you can rely on; don't wait for a crisis to occur and not have time to conduct a thorough search. It is better to have an attorney and not need one than to *not* have an attorney and need one. Seek attorney advice before a problem arises.

REFERENCES

1. Mersky RM, Dunn DJ. *Fundamentals of Legal Research.* 2002 8th ed. New York: Foundation Press; 2002.
2. Holmes OW Jr. *The Common Law.* Available at: http://www.law.harvard.edu/library/collections/special/online-collections/common_law/Preface.php. Accessed April 6, 2007.
3. *Marbury v Madison,* 5 US (1 Cranch) 137 (1803).
4. See, e.g., The California Medical Act of 1876, Sect. 12 gave broad powers only to physicians to diagnosis and prescribe. Available at: http://history.library.ucsf.edu/imagelib/act1_pg2.gif. Accessed July 20, 2007.
5. *Frank v South,* 194 S.W. 375 (Ky 1917).
6. Frank, 194 S.W. at 377.
7. *Chalmers-Francis v Nelson,* 57 P2d 1312 (Cal 1936).
8. Van Nest RL. Imagining in time: the life and trial of Dagmar Nelson, part 2. *AANA J.* 2006;74(4):261-265.
9. U.S. Const. amend. X. "The powers not delegated to the United States by the Constitution, nor prohibited by it to the States, are reserved to the States respectively, or to the people."
10. 42 Code of Federal Regulations §482.52(a).
11. 42 Code of Federal Regulations §482.52(c).
12. CMS 1500 Form. Available at: http://www.cms.hhs.gov/CMSForms. Accessed July 21, 2007.
13. National Practitioner Data Bank regulations and background. Available at: http://www.npdb-hipdb.hrsa.gov. Accessed July 20, 2007.
14. Bolin JN. When nurses are reported to the national practitioner's, data bank. *J Nurs Law.* 2005;10:141-148.
15. American Association of Nurse Anesthetists. Available at: www.aana.com. Accessed July 20, 2007.
16. U.S. Department of Health and Human Services. Available at: http://www.hhs.gov. Accessed July 20, 2007.
17. American Association of Nurse Anesthetists. Available at: www.aana.com > credentialing > accreditation. Accessed July 20, 2007.
18. U.S. Department of Justice Drug Enforcement Agency. Available at: http://www.deadiversion.usdoj.gov/index.html. Accessed July 20, 2007.
19. *Dictionary of Legal Terms.* 3rd ed. Hauppauge, NY: Barrons; 1998.
20. Kenneth KS. *The Forms and Functions of Tort Law.* Westbury, NY: Foundation Press; 1997.
21. Keeton WP et al. *Prosser and Keeton on the Law of Torts.* 5th ed. St Paul, MN: West; 1971.
22. Finz S. *Torts* [audiotape]. Eagen, MN: West; 2000. Sum & Substance Audio Tape Series.
23. American Association of Nurse Anesthetists. *Professional Practice Manual for the Certified Registered Nurse Anesthetist.* Park Ridge, IL: AANA; 2007.
24. *Adams v Family Planning,* 844 N.E. 2d 35 (Ill 2005).
25. Richards RJ. How we got where we are: a look at informed consent in Colorado—past, present, and future. *North Ill Univ Law Rev.* 2005;26:69.
26. *Luettke v St. Vincent Mercy Medical Center,* 2006 Ohio 3872 (2006).
27. *Myers v Boleman,* 260 S.E.2d 359 at 363, (Ga1979).
28. Hoffman AC, Sanbar SS. Spoliation: record retention, destruction, and alteration. In: Sanbar SS, ed. *The Medical Malpractice Survival Handbook.* Philadelphia: Mosby; 2007.
29. American Association of Nurse Anesthetists Insurance Service. Available at: www.aana.com [follow link in member section]. Accessed April 19,2007.
30. Boyce RN et al. *Criminal Law and Procedure.* 9th ed. St Paul, MN: West; 2004.
31. LaFave WR. *Criminal Law.* 4th ed. St Paul, MN: West; 2003.
32. Rendleman D. *Cases and Material on Remedies.* 6th ed. St Paul, MN: West; 1999.
33. *Merit Music Service Inc v Sonneborn,* 245 Md 213, 225 A.2d 470 (1967).
34. Corbin AL. *Corbin on Contracts.* St Paul, MN: West; 1952.
35. Rendleman D. *Cases and Material on Remedies.* 6th ed. St Paul, MN: West; 1999.
36. *McConnell v Williams,* 65 A.2d 243 (Pa 1949).
37. *Tonsic v Wagner,* 329 A.2d 497 (Pa 1974).
38. *Baird v Sickler,* 433 N.E.2d 593 (Ohio 1982).
39. *Blacks Law Dictionary.* 6th ed. St Paul, MN: West; 1990.
40. *Tyler v Campbell,* 106 U.S. 322 (NY 1882).
41. Conviser RJ. *Agency, Partnership & Limited Liability Companies.* 5th ed. Chicago: Barbri Group; 2003.
42. Van Nest RL. Can a CRNA be medically directed and be an independent contractor for tax purposes at the same time? *AANA J.* 2006;74:89-92.
43. Blumenreich GA. CRNAs as independent contractors. *AANA J.* 2002;70:9-13.
44. Blumenreich GA. CRNA as employee. *AANA J.* 1994;62:102-105.
45. Internal Revenue Service. *IRS Publication No. 1779.* Available at: http://www.irs.gov/app/scripts/retriever.jsp. Accessed July 21, 2007.
46. Blumenreich GA. Another article on the surgeon's liability for anesthesia negligence. *AANA J.* 2007;75:89-93.
47. *Bird v United States,* 949 F.2d 1079 (Ok 1991).
48. Conard AF et al. *Agency, Associations, Employment and Partnerships.* 4th ed. Mineola, NY: Foundation Press; 1987.
49. Tunajek S. Dealing with litigation stress syndrome. *AANA NewsBull.* 2007;61(7):22-23.

CHAPTER

5

NURSE ANESTHESIA RESEARCH

Science of an Orderly, Purposeful, and Systematic Nature

Chuck Biddle

The certified registered nurse anesthetist (CRNA) brings a wealth of knowledge to the clinical arena. Although this knowledge comes from a variety of disciplines, including physiology, pharmacology, physics, nursing, medicine, and psychology, it should be appreciated that research and critical thinking first and foremost make this knowledge possible. Evidence-based practice greatly enhances credibility within the clinical setting.

Research represents a rational approach to the making of practice choices among initially plausible alternatives and provides direction and a means for validating these choices. Whether selecting one intravenous opioid over another or choosing one particular pediatric induction technique instead of another, CRNAs rely on research to provide a solid foundation for clinical decision making, thereby avoiding fads and inferior alternatives.

The impact of research on the day-to-day activities of the CRNA has become an especially relevant topic. Before the mid-1970s the vast majority of nurses functioned without much consideration of research or publication of their ideas. In the late 1970s, we experienced a period of punctuated evolution. Major driving forces behind this evolution included movement into a graduate educational framework, a more sophisticated appreciation of the scientific underpinnings of our specialty, recognition of the importance of evidence-based practice (EBP; see the discussion of this topic later in this chapter), national attention to issues of patient outcome and patient safety, and a growing self-awareness of nurse anesthetists not only as providers of excellent clinical care but also as active participants as scholars in the field.

Because CRNAs primarily function with a practice-oriented perspective, the recommendations of Brown and colleagues[1] seem especially relevant. These scholars suggested that four characteristics of research are essential for the development of a scientific knowledge base for a discipline such as nurse anesthesia. First, research should be actively conducted by the members of the discipline. Second, research should be focused on clinical problems encountered by members of the discipline. Third, the approach to these problems must be grounded in a conceptual framework—that is, it must be scientifically based, emphasizing selection, arrangement, and clarification of existing relationships. Finally, the methods used in studying the problems must be fundamentally sound.

WAYS OF KNOWING

The term *research* can be broadly defined as the application of a systematic approach to the study of a problem or question. However, we do not know all the things we claim to know on the basis of systematic inquiry. For example, tradition and custom are important sources of human knowledge. Those who live in the United States are raised in a democratic society and are taught that democracy is the best and most advanced form of government. This is a powerful and efficient route for communication of knowledge because it excuses individuals from initiating an independent effort to come to grips with the concept of democracy. In the absence of evaluation for validity, however, such a route may lead to blind acceptance.

Another source of our knowledge is authority. We know something to be true because an authoritative person such as a parent, educator, clergyman, physician, or teacher tells us it is true. Yet, despite the fact that authorities are fallible, the knowledge they pass on often remains unchallenged. Should we not ask the basis for what we are being told?

Personal experience (the trial-and-error method) represents a powerful source of knowledge. We make observations (e.g., that placing a hand on a hot stove causes a burn) and on their basis make predictions (e.g., that a stove may be hot) and future behavioral decisions (e.g., to avoid touching a stove). However, a risk remains: Not only are certain events perceived differently by different people, but one person's experience may be too narrow to serve as the basis for the development of a reasonable and unbiased understanding of a given phenomenon. Although this mechanism is a practical way of knowing, it is highly fallible and represents a coarse and inefficient way to gain knowledge.

Logical reasoning is yet another way of knowing. The reasoning method has two components: inductive reasoning and deductive reasoning. Inductive reasoning results in generalizations that are derived from specific observations. Consider the following line of reasoning using a character in many action and adventure movies, James Bond, for example. We observe that James Bond is mortal; we observe that a number of other people are mortal as well; on this basis, we conclude that all people are mortal. Deductive reasoning is the development of specific predictions from generalities. In this case, we see the following line of reasoning: we know that all men are mortal; we know that James Bond is a man; therefore we conclude that

James Bond is mortal. Both methods are useful, but the former offers no mechanism for evaluation or self-correction, and the latter is not in itself a source of new information.

Perhaps the most advanced way of knowing is reflected in the scientific method. Although it too is fallible, the scientific method is more reliable and valid than other methods. It provides for self-evaluation with a system of checks and balances that minimizes bias and faulty reasoning. In essence, it is a systematic approach to solving problems and enhancing our understanding of phenomena. It has, at its foundation, the gathering and interpretation of information without prejudice.

THE NATURE OF RESEARCH

Research is by definition a dynamic phenomenon. Whether it is directed purely at the acquisition of knowledge for knowledge's sake (basic research) or at the specific solution of problems (applied research), it is a process that can be conceptualized in terms of at least four characteristics.

First, research can assume many different forms. Second, research must be valid, both internally and externally (Box 5-1). Internal validity is necessary but not sufficient for ensuring external validity. Third, research must be reliable. *Reliability* refers to the extent to which data collection, analysis, and interpretation are consistent and to which the research can be replicated. Fourth, research must be systematic. The elements of a systematic approach include the identification of the problem or problems, the gathering and critical review of relevant information, the collection of data in a highly orchestrated manner, an analysis of the data appropriate to the problem or problems faced, and the development of conclusions within the study's framework.

Science is not a routine, cut-and-dried process. Rather, scientific knowledge emerges from an enterprise that is intensely human; as a consequence, it is subject to the full spectrum of human strengths and limitations. The scientific discovery and understanding that attend participation in research and its results can be professionally exhilarating and satisfying.

THE EIGHT CRITICAL STAGES IN THE RESEARCH PROCESS

Research accords several personal freedoms to those who engage in it: the freedom to pursue those opportunities in which one is interested, the freedom to exchange ideas with other interested colleagues, and the freedom to be a *deconstructionist*—that is, one who challenges existing knowledge. Yet, despite these freedoms, research must be logical, must progress in an orderly manner, and ultimately must be grounded within the framework of the scientific method. If research is a way of searching for truths, uncovering solutions to problems, and generating principles that result in theories, we must come to understand the process of research.

The research process can be described in many different ways. For purposes of simplicity, this process is defined as consisting of the following eight distinct stages:

1. Identification of the problem
2. Review of the relevant knowledge and literature
3. Formulation of the hypothesis or research question
4. Development of an approach for testing the hypothesis
5. Execution of the research plan
6. Analysis and interpretation of the data
7. Dissemination of the findings to interested colleagues
8. Evaluation of the research report

Stage 1: Identification of the Problem

The selection and formulation of the problem constitute an essential first step in the research process. The researcher decides the general subject of the investigation, guided principally by personal experience and by inductions and deductions based on existing sources of knowledge. The researcher makes the general subject manageable by narrowing of the focus of the problem.

BOX 5-1

Research Scenario: Internal versus External Validity

Internal Validity
The extent to which results can be accurately interpreted and the degree to which the independent variable (that which is manipulated) is responsible for a change in the dependent variable (that which is measured). For example, the patient's blood pressure is measured. A combination of propofol, midazolam, isoflurane, and a new muscle relaxant is used for induction of anesthesia. A postinduction blood pressure is recorded, and the researcher concludes that the new muscle relaxant lowers blood pressure.

Questions
Has the researcher isolated the effect of the muscle relaxant from those of the other agents?
Are there plausible or competing alternative explanations?

Analysis
Internal validity is low because the results cannot be interpreted with any degree of certainty.

External Validity
The extent to which the results can be generalized; this issue relates to the question "To whom can the results be applied?" For example, 35 obese men who are nonsurgical volunteers are anesthetized with a standard dose of a new induction drug. The clinical half-life of the drug is determined with plasma drug sampling and brain wave activity monitoring. The researcher concludes that future patients receiving the standard dose of the new drug will experience a clinical half-life of 11 minutes.

Questions
Is it reasonable to assume that obese patients might respond differently than their nonobese counterparts? Might women respond differently than men? Could surgical manipulation or other drug therapy have an impact on the pharmacokinetics of the new drug?

Analysis
External validity is low because the results cannot be generalized to any other individuals except those similar to the subjects in the study.

The following criteria must be met at this phase

x

The following criteria must be met at this phase of the research process:

1. The problem area should be of sufficient importance to merit study.
2. The problem must be one that is practical to investigate.
3. The researcher should be knowledgeable and experienced in the area from which the problem has emerged.
4. The researcher should be sincerely motivated and interested in studying the problem.

We constantly encounter problems and situations that can be studied. At clinical anesthesia conferences, one might hear remarks such as the following:

"It seems to me that a tiny dose of thiopental given just before propofol alleviates virtually any pain on injection."

"Do you think there is less nausea and vomiting in outpatients who are deliberately overhydrated?"

"I find that the use of the waveform generated by my pulse oximeter gives me valuable information about depth of anesthesia."

"I believe that the inspiratory pause mechanism on the Ohmeda 7810 ventilator significantly improves arterial oxygen tension in my patients with chronic obstructive pulmonary disease."

"I am convinced that sleepiness is a major cause of anesthesia accidents."

A study could emerge from each of these situations, built on ideas, hunches, or curiosity. A problem that lends itself to research often materializes from personal observations and in the sharing of ideas and experiences among those who are familiar with the phenomenon in question.

Once identified, the problem should be stated in terms that clarify the subject and restrict the scope of the study. Defining the terms involved in the problem statement also is critical, as demonstrated in Box 5-2.

The wording of the problem statement sets the stage for the type of study design used. Each step in the research process subsequently influences later steps, and this should be kept in mind at all times. A mistake made early inevitably creates difficulties at some later stage in the process. The novice researcher may be surprised to find that this first stage in the research process often consumes a large portion of the total time invested in the research effort. Yet the time is well spent, because research

should not commence until a problem has been identified and formulated in a thoughtful and useful manner.

Common Mistakes

At this stage of the process, pitfalls can include an overly ready acceptance of the first research idea that comes to mind and selection of a problem that is too broad or vague to allow effective study.

Stage 2: Review of the Relevant Knowledge and Literature

Once the problem has been identified, information is needed for putting the problem into proper context so that the research can proceed effectively. A well-conducted literature review provides the researcher with the following:

1. An understanding of what has already been accomplished in the area of interest
2. A theoretic framework within which the problem can be optimally stated, understood, and studied
3. An appreciation for gaps in current understanding of the phenomenon
4. Information for avoiding unanticipated difficulties
5. Examples of potentially useful or poorly constructed research designs and procedures
6. A background for interpreting the results of the proposed investigation

The knowledge that influences the problem originates from three general sources: personal files and experience, personal contacts with experts, and the library and Internet. Both manual indexes and computerized databases should provide the researcher with immediate and full access to the world's published literature. Additional literature searches may be required at different times throughout the research process.

Common Mistakes

At this stage in the research process, mistakes include hasty review of the literature, overly heavy reliance on secondary (book) rather than primary (journal) sources, lack of critical examination of the methods by which conclusions were reached, and incorrect copying of references so that they cannot be located again with ease.

Stage 3: Formulation of the Hypothesis or Research Question

In its most elemental form, a hypothesis is either a proposition of the solution to a problem or a stated relationship among variables. It establishes and defines the independent variable (the variable that is to be manipulated or is presumed to influence the outcome) and the dependent variable (the outcome that is dependent on the independent variable). The hypothesis is declarative in nature and assumes one of the following three forms:

1. A *directional hypothesis:* Patients premedicated with midazolam have less anxiety on arrival in the operating room than do those who were not premedicated.
2. A *nondirectional hypothesis:* Patients premedicated with midazolam experience a difference in anxiety on arrival in the operating room when compared with those who were not premedicated.
3. A *null hypothesis:* Patients premedicated with midazolam experience no difference in anxiety on arrival in the operating room compared with those who were not premedicated.

BOX 5-2

Research Scenario: Stating the Problem

Poor
I am unsure of the effectiveness of etomidate in patients.

Better
I am unsure at what dose etomidate induces unconsciousness in patients undergoing hysterectomy and what impact it has on heart rate, blood pressure, and vascular resistance.

Comments
- The problem should be focused.
- The terms should be clarified.
- The relationships should be understood.
- The problem should not be so narrow as to be trivial.

Research questions are generally reserved for investigations that are descriptive or exploratory in nature or for when the relationships among the variables are unclear. A research question might be more appropriate than a hypothesis in a study that proposes to determine the beliefs of anesthesia providers who interact with patients under specific circumstances. For example, consider the following research question: What are the attitudes of CRNAs in the northeastern United States who care for patients with acquired immunodeficiency syndrome (AIDS)?

Common Mistakes
At this point in the process, mistakes include use of a vague or unmanageable hypothesis and development of a research question that cannot be answered reasonably.

Stage 4: Development of an Approach for Testing the Hypothesis
After the research idea has taken shape in the form of a formal hypothesis or research question, a plan of attack is developed. The research proposal represents the stage at which the ideas of the project crystallize into a substantive form. The proposal includes the following:

1. A problem statement and clarification of the significance of the proposed study
2. The hypothesis or research question
3. A sufficient review of the literature for justification of the study
4. A description of the research design
5. A careful explanation of the sample to be studied
6. The type of statistical analysis to be applied

A research proposal is a useful and efficient way for the researcher to determine the completeness of the plan and is usually required if the researcher is to obtain departmental or institutional approval or is applying for financial support.

Research Methods
The research method is the way the truth of a phenomenon is coaxed from the world in which it resides and freed of the biases of the human condition. A variety of research methods are at our disposal, and researchers are not inflexibly wedded to any particular approach. Researchers do not follow a single scientific method but rather use a body of methods that are amenable to their fields of study.

Some of the methods available are highly recognizable, permanent components of the researcher's armamentarium, whereas others have evolved not only with respect to time, but also in response to the specific needs of a particular problem or discipline. The research method can be influenced by the way a researcher views a problem. For example, a researcher can test a hypothesis, search for a correlation, ask "why" or "how" questions, or probe a phenomenon on the basis of "what would happen if" suppositions.

The researcher can view the method on the basis of the fundamental task that it will accomplish. For example, two broad categories into which research efforts can be divided are basic research and applied research. Basic research adds to the existing body of knowledge and may not have immediate, practical use. Applied research is oriented toward solving an immediate, specific, and practical problem.

The research method can be characterized in terms of its temporal relationship to the problem. A retrospective study is the process of surveying the past; the thing in which we are interested has already occurred, and we are simply looking to see what did occur. In contrast, a prospective study looks forward to see what will happen in a given situation; here, the collection of data proceeds forward in time.

It is important to understand several terms fundamental to the research process. As mentioned previously, the dependent variable is the object of the study, or the variable that is being measured. The independent variable is the one that affects the dependent variable and is presumed to cause or influence it. Another way of looking at this relationship is that variables that are a consequence of or are dependent on antecedent variables are considered dependent variables.

Another set of variables consists of control variables, also known as *organismic*, *background*, or *attribute* variables. Control variables are not actively manipulated by the researcher, but because they might influence the relationships under study, they must be controlled, held constant, or randomized so that their effects are neutralized, canceled out, or at least considered by the researcher (Box 5-3).

The term *blinding* refers to the process of controlling for obvious and occult bias arising from subjects' or researchers' reactions to what is going on. In a single-blind design, the patients are unaware of which treatment or manipulation is actually being given to the subjects. In the double-blind design, neither the researcher nor the subject is aware of which treatment or manipulation the subject is receiving. Whereas randomization attempts to equalize the groups at the start of the study, blinding equalizes the groups by controlling for psychologic biases that might arise apart from any effect of the treatment. Many factors influence the decision to use a single-blind or a double-blind design. For example, in some situations, it may not be feasible to disguise a particular treatment or intervention.

Operationalization is the process of making the characteristics inherent in a given variable, condition, or process familiar or clear to others. If researchers do not operationalize the terms, phrases, and manipulations in the study, the net effect could be an ambiguous study. For example, in a study

---

BOX 5-3

Research Scenario: Understanding the Types of Variables

Study Group
A new intravenous drug that may be associated with fewer cardiovascular effects than thiopental during induction in pediatric patients is being studied. Fifty children ages 3 to 6 years undergoing intravenous inductions for hernia repair or eye muscle surgery are randomized to either the thiopental group or the new drug group. Blood pressure, heart rate, and rhythm are measured by a dedicated observer who is unaware of which drug the patients are receiving.

Analysis
The dependent variables are blood pressure, heart rate, and heart rhythm. The independent variable is the drug the child receives—either the thiopental or the new drug. A number of control variables are present, including sex, fluid status, time of day, underlying medical history, and concurrent drug therapy. With randomization, such control variables should be equated or neutralized for the two groups, but even randomization is not an absolute guarantee.

examining the effects of epidural anesthesia in critically ill patients, it would be essential to operationalize the terms *effects* and *critically ill patients*. Similarly, in a study comparing the quality of inhalation induction with isoflurane and sevoflurane in pediatric patients, it is essential that the researcher operationalize the terms *inhalation induction* and *quality*. Operationalization of terms clearly designates performable and observable acts or procedures in such a way that they can be replicated immutably.

Classifying Research on the Basis of Methodology

Although different authors use a variety of classification schemes, the following example provides a simple way for the researcher to select and classify a design. This scheme attends to the study's purpose and scope and to the nature of the problem at hand. Table 5-1 offers a simplified approach to classifying research design.

Quasi-experimental research differs from experimental research in that it is missing one or more of the key elements required for the experimental design. Either a control group or a randomization procedure may be absent from the design. For example, at an institution, outpatients may routinely receive ondansetron from a particular practitioner, whereas they routinely do not receive the drug from another practitioner. A prospective trial in which both practitioners use a standard anesthetic technique could be initiated. For example, isoflurane, an opioid, and cisatracurium could be administered; this would allow the two practitioners to use or not use ondansetron as they normally would. Outcome, measured in terms of the incidence of nausea and vomiting in the first 6 postoperative hours, is quantified, and the groups are compared. Although randomization is not achieved, a study that may not otherwise have been possible because of the inflexibility of the clinicians involved is successfully accomplished. Quasi-experiments, by yielding to one or more of the rigid criteria of the experimental design, offer an attractive alternative in certain circumstances.

Qualitative Research: An Alternative Paradigm

Up to this point, the traditional approach to a problem has been characterized by deductive reasoning, objectivity, manipulation, and control. An alternative approach involves a group of methods characterized by inductive reasoning, subjectivity, exploration, and process orientation. These methods fall under the rubric of qualitative research techniques.

Qualitative techniques include philosophic inquiry, histography, phenomenology, grounded theory, and ethnography. Generally speaking, *qualitative research* refers to systematic modes of inquiry directed principally at observing, describing, analyzing, interpreting, and understanding the patterns, themes, qualities, and meanings of specific contextual phenomena. Qualitative research seeks to gain insight by discovering the meanings associated with a given phenomenon and exploring the depth, richness, and complexity inherent in it.

For example, exploring how male and female CRNAs differ in the manner in which they deal with parental and child separation when a child is readied for induction of anesthesia might best be achieved through the use of a qualitative design. The actual experiences might be observed or videotaped. Those involved—anesthetists, parents, and children—might be interviewed immediately and at some time after the procedure. This study would be artificially constrained and disjointed if it were

TABLE **5-1**	Classifying Research by Method	
Type	**Qualities and Purpose**	**Example**
Experimental	At least one variable manipulated Random assignment to groups Dependent variable is measured Good for determining cause and effect Prospective in nature	Is there more or less pain on injection of one or the other drug? What did the manipulation do?
Ex post facto	Independent variable has already occurred Examines relationships by observing a consequence and looking back for associations Retrospective in nature (Latin for "from a thing done after")	Looking back over 5 years, did a relationship exist between the rate of myocardial infarction and the inhaled anesthetic that was administered?
Descriptive	Describes something as it occurred Incidence, relationships, and distributions are studied Deals more with "what-is?" than "why-is-it-so?" questions	What are the attitudes of CRNAs regarding the care of patients who have AIDS?
Historical	Describes "what was" rather than what effect variables had on others Events are described as accurately as possible through a process of critical inquiry	A test of the hypothesis is that Sister M. Bernard was the first nurse anesthetist

Qualitative
  Phenomenology
  Grounded theory
  Ethnography
	Experiences lived by people
	Perception is viewed as our access to that experience
	Discovers and conceptualizes the essence of complex processes
		What is the nature of the relationship of CRNAs and surgeons in private and in academic settings?

conducted in any setting other than the original one or if too many controls were brought to bear on the experiment.

The qualitative paradigm seems especially appropriate when the researcher does not want to artificially distance a study from its contextual richness or when there is not enough information available on a particular subject for the adequate development of sound and testable hypotheses. The treatise on qualitative approaches by Marshall and Rossman[2] is recommended to interested readers.

Sampling

Under most circumstances, studying everyone who might be affected by a particular study is impractical, if not impossible. For example, if we want to know how effective intravenous nitroglycerin is in minimizing the rise in blood pressure associated with laryngoscopy in hypertensive patients, we cannot realistically study all hypertensive patients who undergo laryngoscopy. Rather, we would hope to find a smaller group of subjects who are representative of the relevant population at large. By accessing certain information in the sample, we can credibly make inferences or generalizations regarding the population at large.

Similarly, if we want to know how often anesthesia machines in small community hospitals receive preventive maintenance, we cannot visit all the community hospitals in the nation. Instead, we might randomly select a number of hospitals in a number of different states, visit those locations, and inspect the maintenance records. By studying this representative sample, we can make some reasonable and safe generalizations regarding the phenomenon of preventive maintenance at large.

Consider the anecdote about the four blind people who encountered an elephant during one of their daily walks. Each person felt a different part of the elephant. When asked to describe what they had encountered, the first person replied, "a tree trunk" (the elephant's leg). The second reported feeling "a large snake" (the elephant's trunk). The third reported that it was "most definitely a wall" (the elephant's torso). The last person reported that it was "a large, frayed rope" (the elephant's tail). This analogy illustrates that a few discrete sampling points may not be adequate for describing a complex phenomenon. Not only is a random sample best, it also should be large enough and sample a sufficient number of points in the population that a truly representative perspective is gained.

Different sampling techniques can be used, depending on the research design used. In a true random sample (also known as *probability sampling*), all members of the population at large have a similar chance of being included in the study. This is rarely the case in clinical research, in which we are confined to dealing with those individuals who present themselves. In this situation, the sample is called a *convenience sample*. When a convenience sample is used in an experimental study, it is important to ensure that the subjects selected for the study are at least randomized when assigned to treatments or groups. In the ideal situation, the researcher aims for both random selection (from the population at large) and random assignment (to the different groups in the study).

For example, in a study designed to quantify the rate of arterial desaturation in pediatric patients who are transported to the postanesthesia care unit with and without supplemental oxygen, the researcher is limited to those patients who are undergoing surgery. It is difficult to obtain a sample from the pediatric population at large and subject them to anesthesia and surgery. Rather, a convenience sample of patients who are having an operation is used. However, the researcher should randomly assign the study participants to one of the two treatment groups—those who receive supplemental oxygen or those who do not receive supplemental oxygen.

Obtaining a random sample, especially in clinical research, is often a complicated process. Most important is the realization that the concept of randomness is essential to minimizing human biases associated with both selection and assignment.

Instrumentation and Measurement

Two important concepts essential to measurement are validity and reliability. Instrument validity is the degree to which an instrument, such as a blood pressure cuff or a personality inventory, measures what one believes it is measuring. *Instrument reliability* refers to the degree of consistency with which an instrument measures whatever it is measuring—that is, whether the same result is obtained on repeated trials.

Validity and reliability are often easily established for measures of certain physiologic phenomena but may be troublesome in behavioral or psychologic evaluations. Imagine trying to determine reliability and validity for a thermometer. Contrast this to trying to establish validity and reliability for a psychologic tool that professes to measure a CRNA's attitude toward euthanasia; obviously, the latter is a much more difficult undertaking. Although a measure must be reliable to be valid, it can be reliable without being valid. For example, a skin temperature probe might reliably (consistently) measure temperature even in a variety of extreme settings, although it would not be viewed as a valid indicator of core temperature. Both reliability and validity are discussed in degrees rather than in "all-or-nothing" terms.

Many published instruments have reliability and validity testing reported. When choosing an instrument for a study, it is critical to consider whether the instrument's reliability and validity have been established. For example, if an instrument measures evoked responses in the esophagus as an indicator of depth of anesthesia, it must be determined whether the reliability and validity of the instrument have been established under the conditions of the anesthetic protocol being used in the proposed study. Coefficients of reliability and validity are presented on a scale of 0 to 1, with 1 being perfect.

Occasionally the researcher may encounter no reasonable measures to use for a study. For example, instruments for measuring such phenomena as arterial oxygen tension, end-tidal anesthetic concentration, and opioid metabolic by-products are well established. A researcher may need to develop a totally new instrument (questionnaire) to determine perceptions regarding the propriety of a given manufacturer's high-pressure promotional campaigns for newly released pharmaceutical products. In developing such a tool, it is helpful to have an expert in the discipline look over the instrument and provide feedback to ensure that the instrument is appropriate.

Researchers have a variety of instruments for measuring phenomena. These include the following:
- Written tests
- Rating scales
- Questionnaires
- Chemical tests
- Physical tests
- Electrical tests
- Visual observation
- Auditory observation
- Psychologic inventories

TABLE 5-2	Characteristics of the Four Categories of Measurement	
Category	**Characteristics**	**Examples**
Nominal	Identifies	Male or female
		Diagnosis
Ordinal	Identifies	American Society of Anesthesiologists (ASA) class
	Orders	Order of race finish
Interval	Identifies	Intelligence
	Orders	Calendar years
	Equal intervals	Degrees Fahrenheit or Celsius
Ratio	Identifies	Blood pressure
	Orders	Reaction time
	Equal intervals	Weight
	Has a true zero	Distance
		Degrees Kelvin

Levels of Measurement. In designing a study, the researcher must decide how to measure a phenomenon such as anxiety level, blood pressure, attitude toward health care, or rate of complications. There are four levels or degrees of measurement: nominal, ordinal, interval, and ratio. The type of data measured determines the kind of statistical analysis that can be done. Table 5-2 characterizes the four levels of measurement.

Nominal level measurement allows categorization of data, but the only numeric data obtained are frequencies. For example, in a study assessing the educational level of CRNAs in the profession, only the frequency of each category (certificates, bachelor's degrees, master's degrees, doctorates) can be reported. No statement can be made concerning the amount of the characteristic.

Ordinal level measurement allows for data to be ordered or ranked. In a sense, numbers are used to indicate the magnitude of the observations. For instance, the American Society of Anesthesiologists' Physical Status system provides for a relative ranking system for patients on the basis of their pathophysiologic status.

Interval level measurement uses numeric data that are ordered and spaced equally, such as temperature on the Fahrenheit or centigrade scale, calendar years, or intelligence quotients derived from an intelligence performance test. Here, the distance between adjacent scores is highly meaningful.

Ratio level measurement uses numeric data that can be ordered and equally spaced. It is based on a scale with an absolute zero point, such as temperature on the Kelvin scale, reaction time, height, and blood pressure. Both interval and ratio level measures can be referred to as *continuous* in nature.

Measurement can also be defined in terms of four broad categories: cognitive, affective, psychomotor, and physiologic. Each can manifest as one of the levels noted earlier. *Cognitive measurement* addresses the test subjects' knowledge or achievement. For example, what actions should be taken in the face of unexplained bradycardia? *Affective measurements* determine interests, values, and attitudes, thereby providing behavioral insights. For example, how do CRNAs in different locations feel about anesthetizing patients with AIDS? *Psychomotor measurements* test the subjects' ability or

skill in performing specific tasks, such as evaluating performance with a new laryngoscopic design. *Physiologic measurements* look at the biologic functioning of the organism—for example, heart rate differences in men and women at basal conditions.

Although researchers sometimes develop unique instruments, which must be tested for reliability and validity, many published and acceptable instruments can be located in any number of sources.[3,4]

The Pilot Study
A pilot study is the implementation of a study on a small scale. It includes only a few subjects, who generally will not be included in the formal study. Its purpose is to troubleshoot the methodology for any anticipated design problems. The pilot study allows the researcher the opportunity to perform a dry run, ultimately facilitating the progression of the study.

Common Mistakes
At this point in the process, mistakes include failure to adequately operationalize definitions, failure to define the population or sample adequately, unrealistic expectations for subject recruitment and participation, underestimation of the difficulty of design execution, failure to establish instrument reliability and validity, and failure to appreciate the ethical dimensions of the investigation.

Stage 5: Execution of the Research Plan
Up to this point, the research process has involved the acquisition of knowledge regarding the subject, planning the project, and critical thinking about what is to occur. The next stage of the process involves actual data collection and the organization of the data into a format that allows data analysis.

The data collection must precisely follow the procedure the researcher specified previously. The real payoff in research comes with the drawing of useful and bona fide conclusions once the data have been collected and precisely analyzed within the framework of the research design. The goal of the previous step—namely, maximization of both internal and external validity—would not be achieved if the researcher were to deviate from the plan.

Maintaining careful records of what was done and what results were recorded is essential. The labeling and sorting of data into the respective categories or chronologies should be extremely precise. No data should be discarded until the researcher knows that they are absolutely unnecessary. Many researchers "stockpile" raw data and their notes, because additional uses for the information may not manifest for months or even years after the initial project's completion and publication.

Common Mistakes
The mistakes associated with this stage include drifting from the stated methodology for convenience or administrative purposes, placing excessive demands on subjects, allowing personal bias to creep into the research plan, using observers or research assistants who are improperly trained, failing to obtain a sufficient sample size, and improperly using measurement instruments.

Stage 6: Analysis and Interpretation of the Data
A few words on statistics are in order. Not only is proper analysis essential to the design, analysis, and interpretation of the investigation, it also is necessary for understanding and evaluating

TABLE 5-3	Frequency Distribution for Initial Systolic Blood Pressure
Interval (mm Hg)*	**Frequency†**
0-60	1
60-90	8
91-120	15
121-150	15
151-180	8
>180	3

*Interval equals the range or band into which a given measure is placed.
†Frequency equals the number of observations falling into that interval.

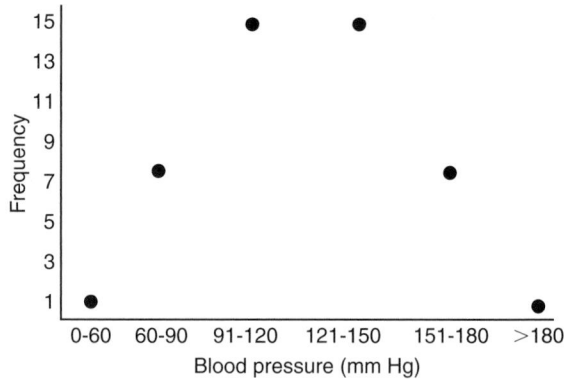

FIGURE **5-1** The frequency polygram. Note the bell-shaped configuration the plotted data have assumed; this typically is the "normal" distribution of biologic data (e.g., weight, heart rate, minimum alveolar concentration, intelligence).

research studies conducted by other investigators. Analysis has three general phases: the initial mechanical manipulation of the data, the analysis itself, and the thoughtful formulation of conclusions on the basis of the analysis.

For the purposes of this discussion, the following two questions are posed:

1. What is the rationale for the use of statistical analysis in research?
2. What are the more common statistical procedures used, and under what circumstances are they appropriate?

Descriptive Statistical Techniques

Once the data on the phenomenon under study have been collected, they often are categorized and described. For example, if the goal of a study is the determination of the incidence of headache and the change noted in blood pressure in 50 patients undergoing spinal anesthesia, the researcher would describe the demographics of the sample of patients in terms of sex, height, weight, or any other relevant variable.

The group or set of all the observations of the variable is called a *distribution*. The distribution yields information about the overall dispersion of the phenomenon within the sample, as well as the exact location of a given measure relative to the group as a whole. In the case of an interval- or ratio-level measurement, such as blood pressure, the distribution of values is probably Gaussian or bell shaped in nature (i.e., some pressures are low, most are intermediate, and some are high). By studying the distribution, the researcher can compare a particular measured value with all the values obtained for the phenomenon.

Alternatively, the researcher might use a technique that clusters data into rational blocks or intervals. For example, in the spinal anesthesia study, instead of listing all 50 initial blood pressures individually, the researcher could tabulate them according to frequency relative to a given interval. In this case, each measured blood pressure falls within a range, and the frequency of presentation in the sample is tabulated as shown in Table 5-3. Instead of using the tabular form, the researcher could arrange the same data in graphic form, indicating the frequency of the phenomenon on the vertical (y) axis and the blood pressure values on the horizontal (x) axis. In histograms and bar graphs, the width of each bar corresponds to the limits of the interval, and the height of the bar corresponds to the frequency or percent of the cases occurring in a specific interval. A frequency polygram also is a commonly used tool for displaying data. Points are plotted directly over the midpoint of each of the

intervals. The data given in Table 5-3 are presented in Figure 5-1 as a frequency polygram.

Other descriptive statistics include the *mean* (the arithmetic average of the sample); the *median* (the point below which one half of the measurements lie); and the *mode* (the value occurring most frequently). The range shows the dispersion data from the highest to the lowest value. *Variance* and *standard deviation* (SD) must be computed and are based on the concept of deviation (the difference between an observed score and the mean value in the distribution). Variance is the square of the sum of all of the deviations divided by the number of scores, and the SD is the positive square root of the variance. Because of variation, investigators describe the data not only in terms of the typical or average value but also the amount of variation that is present. With respect to quantitative data such as blood pressure, number of attempts at intubation, or amount of blood loss, this task is generally a matter of characterizing the distribution of the attribute in terms of its central tendency and dispersion. This is achieved by providing the mean and the SD. The SD is a tool for describing the variation of individual observations around the mean. *Standard error of the mean* (SEM) is linked to the SD by the following simple mathematical formula:

$$SEM = SD/n$$

where *n* is the number of observations in the sample.

The SEM describes the variation of the sample mean (that for the actual data collected) around the true, but unknown, population mean (that for all possible observations). The difficulty with using the SEM is that as the number of subjects or observations increases, the standard error of the mean decreases. In theoretic terms, as *n* approaches infinity, SEM approaches 0. Researchers are urged to consult with a biostatistician and to develop a rationale before deciding to use the SEM or SD.

In general, the higher the level of measurement used (i.e., ratio > interval > ordinal > nominal), the greater the flexibility in selecting a descriptive statistic. Using the data from the spinal anesthesia study noted earlier, it would be appropriate to compute the SD for initial systolic blood pressure (ratio-level data). However, such a computation would be meaningless for nominal-level information, such as whether subjects are male or female.

TABLE 5-4	Correlation Techniques Appropriate to Data Type	
Correlation	**Variable No. 1**	**Variable No. 2**
Product-moment	Interval or ratio	Interval or ratio
Spearman's rank	Ordinal	Ordinal
Point biserial	Nominal or ordinal	Interval or ratio
Phi	Dichotomy	Dichotomy
Contingency	Nominal	Nominal

Correlational Statistical Techniques

The correlation coefficient is generally used for describing the extent to which two variables are related to each other or for quantifying the degree of that relationship. For example, it would be useful if one were studying the extent to which the level of carbon monoxide in the blood is related to cigarette smoking. Calculated correlations vary from +1.0 (a perfect direct correlation) to −1.0 (a perfect inverse correlation). A correlation of 0 indicates no relationship. Researchers often display the correlations visually in the form of a scattergram, which shows the shape of a relationship between two variables. There are many types of correlational techniques (Table 5-4).

In the hypothetic study of carbon monoxide level and cigarette smoking, a researcher might decide to use the product-moment correlation technique. The numeric value for carbon monoxide in the blood has a true 0 (ratio-level data) and a numeric value (ratio-level data) for daily cigarette smoking. The correlation between these variables would probably be positive and very high (e.g., 0.8 or even higher), which suggests that heavy use of cigarettes is associated with a high carbon monoxide level in the blood.

Conversely, assume a study examines the relationship between gender (a nominal-level variable) and anesthetic minimum alveolar concentration (a ratio-level variable). In this example, the researcher using the point biserial correlation technique would expect to see a very low correlation, because gender has been found to not be associated in any meaningful way with anesthetic requirements.

Inferential Statistical Techniques

Inferential statistical procedures provide a set of techniques that allow the researcher to infer that the events observed in the sample will also occur in the larger unobserved population from which the sample was obtained. There are two basic reasons for using inferential techniques. First, they can assist the researcher who is testing a hypothesis and must decide whether to accept or reject it. For example, a researcher, having a particular value in mind, poses the question, "Is this value reasonable in light of the evidence from the sample?" Second, inferential techniques can be used for estimation. For example, a researcher may have no particular value in mind but wants to know what the population value is. The researcher draws a sample, studies it, and makes an inference about the population characteristic (Figure 5-2). These two classic situations as addressed by inferential techniques are as follows:

- *Testing a hypothesis* (Table 5-5). Is there a significant difference in the incidence of nausea between those patients given thiopental and those who receive propofol?

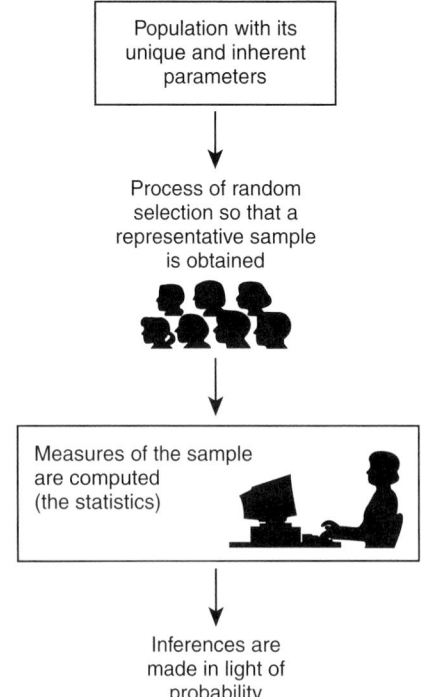

FIGURE **5-2** Conceptual model of inferential statistics.

- *Making an estimation.* What percentage of CRNAs perform a thorough machine check at the start of each day?

Researchers are seemingly preoccupied with the concept of significance. The level of significance (also designated as *alpha level* or P *value*) is a criterion used in making decisions regarding a hypothesis. For example, if P is less than 0.05, the probability that the difference observed between the samples was the result of chance alone is less than 5%. Accordingly, if P is less than 0.05, the probability that the difference between the samples was real (i.e., it resulted from the treatment) and not just the result of chance is greater than 95%. It is conventional to establish the alpha level before the data analysis is begun; however, there seems to be an increasing trend toward reporting calculated P values after hypotheses have been tested. Commonly used levels in research are P is less than 0.05 and P is less than 0.01; P is less than 0.10 is sometimes used in preliminary or descriptive studies. There is also a trend to simply report the calculated P value and leave the interpretations up to the reader.

In recent years, there has been growing resistance to exclusive use of the P value in interpreting research findings, despite the still widespread use of the P value in interpreting hypotheses. *Effect size* is a measure of the magnitude of the observed relationship(s) under consideration. The P value is a dimensionless value that is, in the best case, only an indicator of the direction of the effect and in no way speaks to the clinical meaningfulness of the relationship.

There are a number of standardized effect-size measures in use, and all have their unique place in the settings of reporting research findings. Although explanation and application illustrations are beyond the scope of this chapter, examples of these include but are not limited to Pearson's *r*, odds ratio, confidence intervals, and Cohen's *d*. The number needed to treat (NNT) is yet another example of a metric that provides clinically applicable "magnitude of effect" information. With these limitations involved, brief descriptions of some common statistical manipulations follow.

TABLE 5-5	Statistical Methods Used for Testing Hypotheses				
	Type of Experiment				
Scale of Measurement	**Two Treatment Groups Consisting of Different Individuals**	**Three or More Treatment Groups Consisting of Different Individuals**	**Before and After a Single Treatment in the Same Individual**	**Multiple Treatments in the Same Individual**	**Association Between Two Variables**
Interval (and drawn from normally distributed populations)*	Unpaired *t*-test	Analysis of variance	Paired *t*-test	Repeated-measures analysis of variance	Linear regression and Pearson product-moment correlation
Nominal	Chi-squared analysis of contingency table	Chi-squared analysis of contingency table	McNemar test	Cochrane Q	Contingency coefficient
Ordinal	Mann-Whitney rank sum test	Kruskal-Wallis statistic	Wilcoxon signed rank test	Friedman's statistic	Spearman rank correlation

Adapted with permission from Glantz SA. Primer of Biostatistics. 3rd ed. New York: McGraw-Hill; 1992.
If the assumption of normally distributed populations is not met, the observations should be ranked, and the methods for data measured on the ordinal scale should be used.

TABLE 5-6	Choice of Statistical Test Based on Assumptions	
	Parametric Procedures	**Nonparametric Procedures**
Nature of the assumptions	Data are interval or ratio level Each value is independent of the other values Value is normally distributed Groups have similar variance Usually work best with large population	Data are nominal or ordinal level Not necessarily distributed "normally" (i.e., data do not "fit" a bell-shaped curve)
Examples of tests	*t*-Test for independent groups* *t*-Test for dependent samples† Analysis of variance	Chi-squared test Mann-Whitney test Kruskal-Wallis test

For example, two totally unrelated groups are compared.
†*For example, a pretest and posttest comparison on one group of people.*

Selecting the Appropriate Statistical Procedure

There are two major categories of inferential procedures: parametric analyses and nonparametric analyses. The major factors that dictate which category should be selected involve the assumptions the investigator makes regarding the data. Tables 5-6 and 5-7 provide some guidelines for selecting a statistical procedure.

Power

The sensitivity of the planned experiment and analysis is known as its *power*. The concept of power is important to anyone planning a research project or evaluating a published paper. The estimate of an experiment's ability to accurately test the hypothesis under question should be computed before the research is begun. A researcher should ask the following two critical questions:

1. What is the chance I will incorrectly determine that my treatment had an effect when it really did not (type I error)?

2. What is the chance I will miss an effect that is actually present (type II error)?

Power estimates obtained during a study's design stage encourage investigators to thoughtfully enhance the study's sensitivity. Making such estimates forces the posing of questions regarding effect size (e.g., how potent is the effect of the independent variable on the dependent variable?) and sample size, both of which are essential in a study. Many adverse outcomes that occur as a result of anesthetic management are rare (e.g., death, postspinal hematoma, blindness, stroke), and studies proposing to measure such outcomes as a function of a particular interventional approach must be "powered" by a large sample size and other methodologic controls.

Established procedures and techniques can assist the researcher in determining what sample size must be used if a study is to have an acceptable chance of achieving its purpose (the testing of a given hypothesis). What is at stake is the issue of a trial's having sufficient rigor to detect whether a true difference between treatment groups exists. Other issues should be

TABLE 5-7	Choice of Statistical Test Based on Purpose
Test	**Goal**
t-Test, independent groups	To test the difference between the means of two independent groups
t-Test, dependent samples	To test for the difference between dependent, paired samples (e.g., pretreatment and posttreatment) outcome
Analysis of variance	To test the difference among the means of more than two independent groups or more than one independent variable
Chi-squared	To evaluate the difference between observed and expected frequencies
Correlation coefficient	To test whether a relationship exists between two variables (e.g., product-moment)
Simple linear regression	Used when one independent variable *(x)* is used to predict a dependent variable *(y)*
Multiple linear regression	To understand the effects of two or more independent variables on a dependent measure
Analysis of covariance	To test for differences between group means after adjustment of the scores on the dependent variable to eliminate the effects of the covariate
Factor analysis	To reduce a large set of variables into a smaller, more manageable set of measures
Canonical correlation	To analyze the relationship between two or more independent variables and two or more dependent variables
Discriminant analysis	To make predictions regarding membership in categories or groups, in contrast to using interval- or ratio-level measures

considered as well, and the reader is referred to the definitive text by Cohen[5] for further treatment of these issues. Careful attention to these issues may help prevent the commission of a type III error (conducting the wrong experiment). Most human subject committees and scientific journals require that study reports contain some discussion of power before they are seriously considered.

Data analysis allows the researcher to organize this information in a focused manner so the research question can be answered. Selecting the appropriate method of data analysis is essential to the proper execution of the research plan. Experienced and beginning researchers alike may need assistance when choosing an appropriate method for data analysis. Expert researchers, statisticians, and clinical nurse specialists may prove to be valuable resources for the beginning researcher.

Once the data collection and analysis have been completed, the researcher must interpret the results. These results are directly related to and should answer the research question or hypothesis. Researchers may find that the answers are different from those they were expecting. The answers, results, and outcomes should be interpreted and their implication for clinical practice described. The researcher also should discuss how the findings relate to other research studies and should present ideas for future practice.

Propensity Score

Mention should be made of an increasingly common analysis, the *propensity score*. This is particularly important in observational studies where bias may be a powerful confounder. Many factors influence the decision of how to treat a patient. In the randomized control trial, the bias inherent in assigning a particular patient to a particular treatment arm in the study is minimized by the study design itself. However, in an observational study, it is important to know the conditional probability of a particular subject receiving the intervention (treatment), given observed or measured covariates. The propensity score affords us the opportunity to do just that. If there is no hidden bias and treatment assignment is thus "random," the propensity score

should reveal that. There is some movement, using the propensity score, to elevate the "power" of observational studies to near that of the randomized trial. However, this is a somewhat contentious issue.

Common Mistakes

At this step in the research process, mistakes include selecting an inappropriate statistical procedure, using only one statistical procedure when several should be used, overstating the importance of small differences that are statistically significant but of little clinical importance, interpreting correlational research as evidence of cause-and-effect relationships, and overgeneralizing the findings of the investigation. Some common errors in statistical usage are noted in Box 5-4.

Stage 7: Dissemination of the Findings to Interested Colleagues

The research process is not complete until the results, conclusions, and implications have been adequately communicated to those likely to be interested in the study. Clearly, a study that has been completed but whose results have not been disseminated is of little value. Communication of the research findings can be done through a variety of routes, including publication in journals or newsletters, oral and poster presentations at formal symposia, or even discussion with others interested in the phenomenon.

Researchers fail to publish the results of their work for many reasons. These include such claims as "my findings were not significant," "my results were negative," and "the sample size was small." Negative or insignificant results can be as valuable as positive ones. For example, it has been found that in most circumstances, the by-product of atracurium breakdown, laudanosine, is unlikely to have significant clinical effects.[6] This is an important negative finding that has contributed substantively to clinical understanding.

Similarly, small sample sizes may provide an element of control over variables not present in larger studies or may indicate some preliminary direction as to how to approach a problem.

BOX **5-4**

Top 10 Common Errors in Statistical Usage

1. No justification for reporting statistical results
   - No control group (when one is possible)
   - Random sampling or random group assignment not performed (or reported)
   - Statistical test not specified
   - Obvious biases or threats to validity
   - No documentation of consent or institutional review board approval
2. Errors in use of the *t*-test
   - Multiple application without correction
   - Use of independent groups form for paired data and vice versa
   - Use for ordinal data
3. Negative conclusions when statistical test results are not significant
4. Use of a test for independent samples for paired data or repeated measures
5. Inappropriate or no follow-up to analysis of variance
6. Hypotheses generated by the data
7. Use of one-sided tests without justification (or disclosure)
8. Inadequate number for chi-squared analysis
9. Standard error of the mean used for specifying variability
10. Misinterpretation or misrepresentation of P value
    - Small P value called "highly significant"
    - No confidence intervals stated
    - Different interpretation of $P = 0.04$ and $P = 0.06$

An example is the finding that epidural anesthesia or analgesia in conjunction with light general anesthesia may be preferable to a purely general anesthesia technique and may be associated with lower mortality rates in critically ill patients.[7] Although the sample size in this particular investigation is relatively small, the overall design is acceptable and contributes to our understanding of the issue by stimulating other investigators to pursue answers to the questions raised.

Because the goal of nurse anesthesia research is the improvement of practice, the dissemination of research findings to clinicians is a major challenge faced by nurse anesthesia researchers. In a report directed at a highly research-oriented audience, the introduction is usually somewhat detailed, emphasizing the theoretic basis for the research. The introduction is followed by an extensive methodologic section that focuses on establishing the reliability and validity of the instruments used. The findings of the study are presented next, with emphasis on the statistical procedures employed. Finally, the conclusion focuses on the limitations and implications of the study's results.

Writing for a Clinically Oriented Audience

Generally, clinicians find research literature difficult to understand and its clinical application cumbersome. Both authors and journal editors can do much to make research more palatable to the clinical reader, thereby improving the chance that the research findings will be broadly disseminated and integrated into clinical situations. A recipe for successful clinical writing follows.

Clinical readers of research want to extract information applicable to clinical practice as quickly as possible. Therefore, the introduction of the research report should be brief, should establish the practical importance of the study, and should present a clear statement of the study's purpose. A deliberate effort should be made to connect the study with the realities of clinical practice.

With respect to the methods section, writing that "a quasi-experimental, Solomon three-group crossover design yielded data that were subjected to canonical and discriminant analysis" does little to satisfy the needs of the average clinical reader. Instead, stating how the subjects were obtained, what manipulations were made, how the measurements were taken, and how the statistical analysis was performed provides the reader with clear straightforward information, allowing him or her to put the study into a clinical context. The methods section should completely describe both the research design and the statistical procedures used, and it should indicate why this approach was selected.

The results of the study should focus on the relevant findings and describe them clearly and fully. Tables or figures, explicitly labeled and simple in design, should be used for representing the findings visually. Admittedly, the more complex the findings, the more difficult it is to avoid a statistical or technical focus.

In the discussion section, the implications of the investigation for theory and future research are somewhat less important to the clinical reader than are the implications for practice. For example, assume that a study demonstrates that the proposed intervention is not ready to be implemented in practice. In this situation, the discussion section should emphasize why this is so and what can be done about it. Encyclopedic comparisons of the results with those of other investigators at this point probably will not contribute materially to the report and may, paradoxically, deter the reader. Alternatively, if a researcher finds that a particular intervention, strategy, or assessment is ready to be introduced into clinical practice, the discussion section should emphasize how and for whom it should be used. It should include considerations such as efficiency and cost, as well as suggestions for clinical implementation.

This recipe for making research reports more palatable to primarily clinically oriented readers is not meant to diminish the importance of highly theoretic research-oriented writing. Many CRNAs continue to generate and publish valuable theoretic papers that contribute materially to a scientific basis for practice. Researchers and writers must keep the CRNA audience in mind as they develop and disseminate their findings.

All researchers must understand that the results of their studies, once published, become part of the general knowledge of the scientific community at large. However, the use of this knowledge requires acknowledgment of the original researchers; also, published results may be subject to copyright protection laws (i.e., their use may require permission from the publisher). It is not until the information becomes common knowledge that others may use it freely without acknowledgment.

Common Mistakes

At this stage of the research process, common mistakes include not keeping the study focused on the original problem, overwriting, generalizing the findings too broadly, and failing to address the clinical significance of the study.

Stage 8: Evaluation of the Research Report

Both clinicians (in their reading for application) and researchers (in their writing and analysis) are called on to evaluate research

Research Scenario: A Guide for Researchers* and Clinicians† in Evaluating Research for Completeness and Clinical Application

Problem
Is it lucid, researchable, justified, and practical?

Hypothesis
Is it clear, with the appropriate variables under consideration correctly identified?

Definitions
Are terms adequately defined and put into context?

Literature
Is it relevant, current, and organized?

Review
Is it logical, and does it justify the study?

Methods
Is the sample representative of the population being considered?
Is the sample large enough? If human subjects were used, was institutional approval granted? Is the instrumentation described and valid? Is the design compatible with the problem and the hypothesis or research question? Is there any evidence of drift from established procedure? Are the data-gathering procedures defined? Is there enough information for replication of the study, if desired? Are the statistical procedures described, and are they appropriate?

Results
Are results presented clearly, concisely, and without bias? Are they organized and displayed logically in tables or figures? Are they relevant to the problem or hypothesis?

Discussion
Is the discussion logically based on the results? Is it intimately grounded in the original problem or hypothesis? Is there overgeneralization of the findings? Is the writing impartial and scientific? How can this study be used in the practice setting? How similar is the study's environment to the real world? What are the risks associated with implementation of the recommendations?

*Researchers should benefit from this by critically asking themselves whether they have included answers to these questions in their report.
†Clinicians should benefit from this by judging the report on the basis of completeness and utility and by finding out whether it contains answers to these questions.

reports, despite the fact that many may not have received formal training in reading and interpreting professional literature. Evaluation is the process of appraising the quality of a phenomenon—in this case, the findings of research as they bear on the art and science of nurse anesthesia. Outside of the practice settings, humans evaluate hundreds of things every day: Are the apples on the grocery shelves to our liking? Does the description of the program in the television guide entice us to tune in? Is the weather too warm to wear a jacket? Have we cooked the eggs sufficiently? These seem trivial and informal compared with the

clinical evaluations the CRNA must perform daily: Is the patient's anesthesia too deep, too light, or about right? Should I administer more opioid? Is the patient dehydrated, or is the hematocrit level misleading me? Should I perform a rapid-sequence induction? What dose of which sleep agent do I use in this 80-year-old with a fractured hip? Both sets of questions, nonprofessional and professional, are highly evaluative and parallel the evaluative decision making that occurs when anesthesia research literature is read.

Systematic evaluation of the research, which influences the practice of nurse anesthesia, consists of a formal appraisal of the quality and value of the research. This essential step in the research process is multidimensional and can be approached in many ways. The approach outlined in the following subsections involves asking carefully orchestrated, critical questions. The answers to the suggested questions are not necessarily a dichotomous yes or no, but rather are qualitative in nature. An overview of this approach is detailed in Box 5-5.

Gaining Experience at Evaluation: the Journal Club
Most clinicians and researchers are familiar with the concept of the journal club, a common curricular component of many programs in the anesthesia community. A journal club offers a planned, periodic, and critical reading of anesthesia-oriented research and clinical articles pertaining directly to practice. Participants in a journal club are assigned to read selected articles; later, a discussion of the articles can proceed under the direction of an informed leader. Questions that should be asked during discussion and critique include the following:

1. What are the purposes and the research questions or hypotheses, and how does the related literature review bear on the purpose or problem?
2. What methods did the authors use to study or evaluate the problem?
3. How are the data presented, and in what manner are they analyzed?
4. What are the conclusions of the study, and what are the implications for practice?

Participation in a journal club can be a rewarding and intellectually stimulating activity that can be used for keeping one's knowledge of the field current and for gaining experience in evaluating the anesthesia-related literature.

Evaluating a Study: the Bottom Line
Ultimately, the nurse anesthetist evaluating a study is faced with the following three questions:

1. Do I disregard the study and its findings entirely, not applying them to either clinical practice or future analysis in any fashion?
2. Do I apply the study only in the sense of expanding my cognitive approach to anesthetic management? (In this scenario, although one may not materially or directly apply the study or its findings to practice, some intellectual growth or understanding is gained from the study, which subsequently is incorporated into one's repertoire.)
3. Do I make a direct application of the study to my practice?

Some questions to ask when one reads a study are listed in Box 5-6.

Common Mistakes
At this stage of the research process, mistakes include failing to adequately evaluate a study's methods and findings and in the

---

BOX 5-6

Questions to Ask in the Reading of a Study

Object or Hypothesis

What are the objectives of the study or the questions to be answered?

What is the population to which the investigators intend to refer their findings?

Design of the Investigation

Was the study an experiment, planned observations, or an analysis of records?

How was the sample selected? Do possible sources of selection exist that would make the sample atypical or nonrepresentative? If so, what provision was made for dealing with this bias?

What is the nature of the control group or standard of comparison?

Observations

Are there clear definitions of the terms used, including diagnostic criteria, measurements made, and criteria of outcome?

Was the method of classification or of measurement consistent for all the subjects and relevant to the objectives of the investigation? Do possible biases in measurement exist, and, if so, what provisions were made to deal with them?

Are the observations reliable and reproducible?

Presentation of Findings

Are the findings presented clearly, objectively, and in sufficient detail to enable the reader to judge them for herself or himself?

Are the findings internally consistent? That is, do the numbers add up properly, can different tables be reconciled, and so on?

Analysis

Are the data worthy of statistical analysis? If so, are the methods of statistical analysis appropriate to the source and nature of the data, and is the analysis correctly performed and interpreted?

Is analysis sufficient for determining whether "significant difference" may be the result of lack of comparability of the group in gender or age distribution, in clinical characteristics, or in other relevant variables?

Conclusions

Which conclusions are justified by the findings? Which are not?

Are the conclusions relevant to the questions posed by the investigators?

Constructive Suggestions

Assume you are planning an investigation to answer the questions put forth in this study. If they have not been clearly asked by the authors, frame them in an appropriate manner. Suggest a practical design, criteria for observations, and type of analysis that would provide reliable and valid information relevant to the questions under study.

Adapted from Colton T. Statistics in Medicine. Boston: Little, Brown; 1974. With permission from Little, Brown & Co, copyright 1974.

---

process, uncritically accepting into practice information that may be misleading or incorrect. Although articles in professional journals should undergo critical review by peers who can detect mistakes, omissions, and alternative explanations, the ultimate responsibility for evaluating a study and determining the pros and cons of the implementation of its recommendations rests with the clinical reader.

FRAUD, DECEIT, AND HUMAN ERROR IN SCIENTIFIC RESEARCH

Scientists are human and suffer from the inherent frailties of the human condition. Even the most scrupulous and compulsive scientist can make an honest mistake, and such mistakes are tolerated by the community at large. Errors are costly in a variety of ways. Not only might an error result in months or years of wasted effort if it is not identified and rectified, but it also can mislead others who attempt to use or build on the original, flawed work.

Unfortunately, not all errors are honest. Scientific and academic misconduct occurs in a variety of forms. Although the motives of the involved parties are not always identifiable, some researchers feel pressure to publish, whereas others simply are intent on gaining attention by compiling a long list of publications or presentations. The bottom line is that scientific misconduct ultimately erodes the foundation on which science is built and may result in the administration of inappropriate therapy to those in need of treatment. Common examples of scientific and academic misconduct include the following:

- Plagiarism
- Alteration of data so they conform to expectations
- Outright fabrication of data
- Intentional sloppiness in scientific work
- Selective publication of data with intent to support one's beliefs
- Coercing subordinates to acknowledge oneself unreasonably
- Unapproved use or misuse of human or animal subjects
- Not giving appropriate credit in collaborative research

Guidelines for Dealing with Errors or Suspected Misconduct

The nurse anesthetist who is personally involved with or suspects scientific or academic misconduct on the part of a colleague is morally and professionally compelled to take action as soon as possible. Box 5-7 lists guidelines to adhere to if such a situation occurs.

STUDIES INVOLVING HUMAN SUBJECTS

The process of making a research project a reality involves coordination between patients' needs and rights and the study's parameters and goals. This process is controlled in some respects by criteria set up by various governing agencies. The 1947 Nuremberg Code, the 1964 Helsinki Declaration, and the 1971 guidelines of the U.S. Department of Health, Education, and Welfare were drafted to reflect the concern for individuals participating in research. In 1979 the National Commission for the Protection of Human Subjects of Biomedical and Behavioral Research was established to continue work in this area. The culmination of that work, the Belmont report, defines the limits between research and practice and outlines the ethical guidelines to be considered for patient participation in research projects. According to the report, the difference between standard practice and research is defined in terms of design and outcomes. The phrase *medical practice* refers to diagnosis,

Dealing with Errors and Misconduct

If the Situation Has Resulted from Your Own Actions
Immediately acknowledge the error to your colleagues. If the error is in print, write to the journal editor or source in which the mistaken information was published.

If You Discover an Error in a Publication
Write a letter to the editor of the publication stating your case and supply any supportive materials you have.

If You Believe a Colleague Has Engaged in Misconduct
1. Discuss the situation with a trusted and experienced colleague, maintaining the anonymity of the accused. This will help you judge the motives of your own suspicions and establish the veracity of your charges.
2. Once the facts have been established, contact the colleague privately to determine whether the concern can be satisfactorily explained or rectified.
3. If resolution is not at hand, discuss the situation with the department director, chairperson, or dean, as indicated by the hierarchic administrative arrangement. Many institutions and universities have written procedures that carefully outline the process to be followed in such situations.
4. In situations in which resolution is still not achieved or if a definable administrative structure is not in place, consider contacting the National Academy of Sciences, Sigma Xi, the American Association for the Advancement of Science, the American Association of University Professors, or other scientific or professional organizations.

Adapted from Colton T. Statistics in Medicine. Boston: Little, Brown; 1974. With permission from Little, Brown & Co, copyright 1974.

treatment, and preventive health care whose purpose is the enhancement of the well-being of an individual. The term *research* refers to procedures whose purpose is the examination of a question or the testing of a hypothesis to expand the existing body of knowledge.

Institutional Review of Research That Involves Humans and Animals

All protocols involving the living must be submitted to a local institutional review board (IRB). The IRB is charged with the protection of each subject participating in the study. It is the responsibility of the IRB to ensure that informed consent is adequate, that no coercion is used in the recruitment of subjects, and that the risks to the subjects are minimal or no greater than necessary. To accomplish this, the IRB carefully reviews the study's protocol and consent forms, considering the study's design and patient selection.

A number of factors must be considered when a study calls for the involvement of human participants. The risk-benefit assessment compares the benefits of participating in a study with the potential risks generated by the study. Risks can involve the patient, the family, or the community. The risk-benefit balance should be justified by an analysis of information to be gained from the research, a description of the available treatment alternatives, and the measures to be taken to minimize risks and discomfort.

Vulnerable populations (e.g., children, pregnant women) require special considerations.

Providing a patient with the information necessary for making an informed decision about participation is fundamental. Informed consent should be easy to understand and include a description of the research and plan of treatment, the risks and benefits, the alternatives to participation in the study, confidentiality, costs, and compensation. Informed consent also must include an assertion of the voluntary nature of the study, a statement that the patient may withdraw at any time without penalty, and a commitment that during the course of the study, the discovery of any new findings that may affect the subject's participation will be disclosed. In most instances, a signed consent form from a participant is necessary; ultimately, however, the IRB decides whether such a form is necessary.

Virtually all institutions and funding agencies have model consent forms whose format researchers must follow when developing a study. Consent forms (written in lay terminology) should include a brief description of the study, a summary of the anticipated risks and benefits of participation in the study, a statement regarding the maintenance of the participant's confidentiality, a disclaimer obviating the host institution of financial responsibility for damages that might occur, and the names and telephone numbers of the researchers. Under most circumstances, the individual who has agreed to participate in the study signs the consent form in the presence of the researcher and a witness who cosigns the consent. A copy of the consent form is given to the participant for his or her records.

CONTROVERSIES IN ANIMAL RESEARCH

Biomedical institutions now operate under guidelines that mandate the humane treatment of animals used in research. The use of animals for research is a subject of controversy fueled by disagreements between people who are highly supportive of the use of animals and those who strongly oppose it, such as supporters of the People for the Ethical Treatment of Animals (PETA) and the Animal Liberation Front (ALF). Researchers contemplating the use of animals in their research should carefully consult with their local IRB for guidance in this area.

EVIDENCE-BASED PRACTICE: EMPOWERING DECISION MAKING THROUGH RESEARCH

Evidence-based practice is an approach to patient care founded on the belief that clinical decisions must be based on results obtained from rigorously controlled investigations. It cautions against using studies with low external validity (e.g., animal studies) or those based on uncontrolled observations (e.g., case reports, retrospective studies) in rendering decisions that influence or dictate patient care interventions.

Although many recipes for and approaches to EBP exist, the essential ingredients common to all include the following:
1. Defining the patient's problem
2. Proficiently searching the relevant literature
3. Critically appraising the discovered literature
4. Rationally applying the relevant literature in the context unique to the patient

At the core of EBP is the notion of critical thinking (appraisal) of the applicable literature. Here, intellectual rigor is balanced with clinical experience as the clinician determines whether the evidence is applicable to a particular patient's situation.

The dizzying array of studies in our field coupled with the complexities and vagaries of our patient population produce an informational tidal wave both frustrating and daunting to clinicians who endeavor to remain on the cutting edge with respect to patient care decisions. We all rely to one extent or another on reviews of primary research to assist us in coming to understand and apply clinical research findings. Whenever possible, we should endeavor to use systematic reviews. Systematic reviews are those that incorporate (1) a comprehensive study retrieval process that minimizes publication bias, (2) selection criteria that identify only relevant studies, (3) a critical appraisal of the emergent literature accomplished by knowledgeable and sophisticated clinicians and researchers, and (4) reproducible decisions regarding the relevance and methodologic rigor of the selected primary research.

Recently the metaanalysis has begun to appear in the anesthesia literature. A metaanalysis is a systematic review that includes a quantitative statistical analysis of the findings that have emerged from several (or many) discrete studies examining a similar phenomenon. Examples of anesthesia-based metaanalyses include those by Tramer, who examined ondansetron as an antiemetic; Ballantyne and colleagues, who studied pulmonary outcomes in patients who had epidural analgesia; Lee and colleagues, who looked at acupuncture and acupressure as alternative approaches in the management of postoperative emetic symptoms; and Biddle, who evaluated the use of nonsteroidal antiinflammatory drugs in the treatment of acute postoperative pain.[8-11]

When solid evidence evolves into sound clinical decision making, patients receive the best possible care; EBP helps us choose scientific evidence over confusing (or even unsound) opinion. In addition, EBP complements other foundational approaches to patient care and teaching. Some researchers argue that there is a crucial final step in the EBP model—namely, that clinicians self-evaluate their own EBP. In doing so, clinicians provide an ongoing process of evaluation and sensitivity testing for practice-based decisions.

Clinical research seeks to resolve, refine, and clarify the issues involved in the care and management of patients. Each day, we are faced with a host of common and uncommon patient scenarios that demand thoughtful, efficient decision making and resultant interventions. How we come to decide what course of action to take is in many cases as important as the action itself. Decisions involving the care of patients should be evidence based, a process of considerable complexity involving judging sources of information, evaluating the quality and relevance of information, recognizing the contextual elements that may alter the application of that information in a particular setting, and assessing its impact on the patient(s).

The Process of Evidence-Based Clinical Practice

What we do in a given circumstance is often more a matter of entrenched belief than a course of action firmly grounded in research. The published series *Clinical Evidence*, the international source of best available evidence related to common clinical interventions in various disease states, reveals that of 2500 treatments reviewed, 325 (13%) were rated "beneficial," 575 (23%) "likely to be beneficial," 200 (8%) as "a tradeoff between benefit and harm," 150 (6%) "unlikely to be beneficial," 100 (4%) "likely to be ineffective or harmful," and 1150 (46%) as having "unknown effectiveness." One might interpret this in many ways, but clearly it points to the theme that many treatment decisions are inadequately grounded in firm scientific rationale.[12]

The fundamentals of medicine and nursing have evolved from a time when the teaching and practice of authoritative figures (sages) were simply passed down and uncritically applied to patients. Advances came with clinical evolution, but primarily in the form of case reports, case series, editorials and other publications that were too often based on preconceived notions, and deliberate or unintentional bias. The advent of the randomized controlled clinical trial (RCT) some 6 decades ago set the stage for a new era in patient care. In the RCT, patients are randomized to treatment strategies, the effect of outside influences on outcome are considered, and there is methodologic precision, not only with regard to the interventions applied to patients but also to how outcomes are measured. Despite advances, practitioners, and nurses in particular, are often resistant about bringing research advances to the bedside.

Evidence-based practice (EBP) involves a series of consecutive, somewhat overlapping steps that follow.

Step 1: Asking a Question That Deserves an Answer

Should we anesthetize and perform elective surgery on a child who presents with an upper respiratory infection on the day of the scheduled procedure? What fluid and glucose management strategy should be used in the diabetic patient recovering from a major peripheral vascular procedure? Is it safe to use ketorolac in the fresh tonsillectomy patient? What can be done to minimize the risk of ventilator-acquired pneumonia in the postoperative patient receiving mechanical ventilation? Should all patients recovering from general anesthesia receive supplemental oxygen in the PACU? Should obstructive sleep apnea patients recovering from general anesthesia receive CPAP (continuous positive airway pressure) throughout their hospital stay if significant pulmonary hypertension is present? Such questions are common in practice and merit careful consideration in terms of intervention-related outcome, but relevant questions also apply to diagnosis, prognosis, and the potential for harm. It may seem like word play, but the answers to our questions are more likely to be important and valid if the questions posed are good. Questions should be focused to the extent that they are both applicable to the patients who are cared for and can be researched.

Steps 2 & 3: Searching for Relevant Evidence and Judging Its Worth

Once a question is at hand, the search for information begins, a process that can be both time consuming and challenging. Seeking evidence to address the question "What is the best antiemetic for the postoperative patient" is much different than asking "Is isopropyl alcohol inhalation more effective than ondansetron in managing post–general-anesthesia nausea in the postpartum tubal ligation patient?"

Although providers usually have an opinion about care-related questions, EBP demands that we critically evaluate researchable and meaningful information sources to best address a particular patient's care. *Index Medicus* and *MEDLINE* are familiar and excellent sources but are not applicable in all circumstances, especially if time is of the essence. A particularly valuable database specifically related to EBP is the Cochrane Collaboration, a collection of well-conducted clinical trials organized into specific topics. Established Websites, well-regarded (peer reviewed, authoritative) textbooks, or even colleagues with a more robust knowledge base than yours may suffice. But crucial to this is your level of confidence that your colleague, the database, or the book chapter is evidence based. The phrase "garbage in, garbage out" has particular application here.

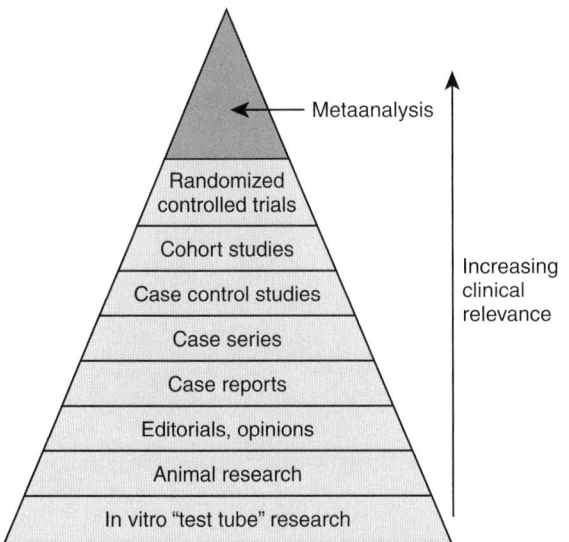

FIGURE **5-3**   The pyramid of evidence.

BOX **5-9**

Checklist for Evaluation of the Randomized Controlled Trial

- Is a clear objective for the study stated?
- Is the sample size adequate?
- Is the study population well described?
- Are the interventions clearly described?
- Are randomization and blinding procedures adequate?
- Are valid and reliable outcome measures used?
- Is attrition (dropouts) considered in the analysis?
- Are the statistical methods appropriate?
- Are both clinical and statistical significance reported?
- Are the results generalizable to clinical practice?

BOX **5-8**

Some Contextual Considerations in the Process of Evidence-Based Clinical Practice*

Considerations in Weighing the Application of a Therapy in a Particular Patient

- Age and gender
- Hydration status
- Smoking history
- Current drug therapy
- Duration of illness
- Severity of symptoms
- Cost of therapy
- Side effects
- Inpatient or outpatient
- Coexisting conditions
- Physician and staff familiarity and experience with intervention
- The degree of technical mastery necessary to perform the intervention
- Staff makeup (specialists, generalists)
- Type of hospital (community, medical center, urban, rural)
- Support personnel
- Is reasonable follow-up available to assess the intervention's outcome?

The list is partial and meant only to stimulate thinking regarding how factors may influence the application and outcome of a particular intervention.

Definitions of EBP abound; for its practicality and relevance, consider the following description: EBP is the conscientious and critical use of quality published evidence in making decisions related to the care of a particular patient, considering the caregiver's unique expertise and the setting in which the patient presents. It is important to recognize that not all evidence that is retrieved or brought to bear on a question has the same value.

Figure 5-3, the pyramid of evidence, demonstrates that the randomized, double-blind, controlled clinical trial has greater worth than the editorial or case report. This hierarchy of value is case and issue sensitive, because not all questions have relevant or applicable RCTs. On the other hand, when a number of RCTs are directed toward a similar issue, these can sometimes be combined, using rigorous methodology and a common set of statistical procedering, to produce a metaanalysis (or quantitative systematic review).

Step 4: Determining If the Evidence Applies to Your Particular Patient

Translating knowledge into practice is the next critical step. If you have determined the evidence is valid and important, you must now decide if you should apply it to the care of your patient. EBP then becomes an ongoing process of inquiry, asking "Why am I doing it this way?" and "Are there compelling reasons for me to do it differently to achieve a better outcome?" The factors influencing these decisions are complex. Ultimately the decision to implement an intervention is a blend of experience and science (evidence) as you carefully assess what value the evidence has in the context and setting of a particular patient. What is meant by *context*? Box 5-8 illustrates just a few of the contextual factors that we must consider in the process of EBP.

Step 5: Evaluating the Effect (Outcome) of the Evidence-Based Intervention

Absolutely vital to the process of EBP is evaluation. Here one determines if the evidence has altered the "usual" practice pattern. If so, has it been associated with improved efficiency and health outcome, and has it maintained the quality of care? Evaluation allows not only for deciding if the intervention "works" but also for determining if variations arise (e.g., dosing, timing, duration, complications, unexpected occurrences, etc.). In doing so, a kind of living, evolving document arises that can be used for purposes of assessing efficacy, quality assurance, and risk.

Conclusion

It is my belief that the questions we encounter may be compartmentalized into three fundamental areas: pain, critical care, and clinical anesthesia. EBP is a process that affords us the opportunity to explore, implement, and assess interventions that are applied to the patient. At the heart of EBP is the RCT. A brief overview/checklist is noted in Box 5-9 to help in judging the value of a particular RCT. In the culture of providing health care, EBP represents a shift away from basing decisions exclusively on opinion, past practice, and precedent, and toward making greater use of science, research, and evidence to guide clinical decision making. This is a train that has definitely left the station. All are invited to step aboard.

SUMMARY

Although CRNAs are only now becoming prepared to assume the role of primary researchers, all CRNAs are in a position to read about the latest advances in nurse anesthesia practice and incorporate validated interventions into their clinical practice. Nurse anesthesia research is grounded fundamentally in solving patient-care problems during the preoperative, intraoperative, and postoperative periods. Although much behavioral, educational, and product evaluation–oriented research has been conducted by nurse anesthesia researchers, all nurse anesthesia research is wedded inextricably to patient care. Research is essential to the professional evolution of nurse anesthesia as CRNAs become increasingly accountable for their own independent basis for practice.

A number of antiscience movements are operative in the world today. At the heart of all of these movements is the sophisticated use of the concept of proof by proclamation rather than proof by experimentation. As active consumers and producers of scientific knowledge, nurse anesthetists can do their part by resisting the integration of aberrant and ill-founded thinking into their discipline. This can be achieved if each CRNA understands the need to maintain a critical dialogue regarding what can be incorporated into nurse anesthesia practice.

All CRNAs are mandated to understand and use research in their practices. The American Nurses Association strongly urges even undergraduate nursing students to learn how to read, interpret, and evaluate published research for applicability to nursing practice. Although the evolution of nursing research—and that of nurse anesthesia research in particular—has lagged behind that of many other disciplines, tremendous strides are being made as greater numbers of nurse anesthetists are prepared at both the master's and doctoral levels. It is essential that nurse anesthetists recognize the need to promote nurse anesthesia as a science-based profession. There is no better way to achieve this end than to continue emphasizing the importance of the research process.

REFERENCES

1. Brown J et al. Nursing's search for scientific knowledge. *Nurs Res.* 1984; 33:26-32.
2. Marshall C, Rossman GB. *Designing Qualitative Research.* Newbury Park, CA: Sage; 1989.
3. Buros O: *Tests in Print.* Princeton, NJ: Gryphon Press; 1961.
4. Ward MJ, Lindeman C. *Instruments for Measuring Nursing Practice and Other Health Care Variables.* Denver: Western Interstate Commission for Higher Education; 1978.
5. Cohen J. *Statistical Power Analysis for the Behavioral Sciences.* 2nd ed. Hillsdale, NJ: Lawrence Erlbaum Associates; 1988.
6. Standaert FG. Magic bullets, science, and medicine. *Anesthesiology.* 1985;63: 577-578.
7. Yeager MP. Epidural anesthesia and analgesia in high-risk surgical patients. *Anesthesiology.* 1987;67:729-736.
8. Tramer MR. Does meta-analysis increase our knowledge in the management of postoperative nausea and vomiting? *Int Anesthesiol Clin.* 2003; 41(4):33-39.
9. Ballantyne JC et al. The comparative effects of postoperative analgesic therapies on pulmonary outcome: cumulative meta-analysis of randomized, controlled trials. *Anesth Analg.* 1998;86(3):1460.
10. Lee A, Done ML. The use of nonpharmacologic techniques to prevent postoperative nausea and vomiting: a meta-analysis. *Anesth Analg.* 1999; 88(6):1200-1202.
11. Biddle C. Meta-analysis of the effectiveness of nonsteroidal anti-inflammatory drugs in a standardized pain model. *AANA J.* 2002;70(2):111-114.
12. *BMJ Clinical Evidence:* Available at: http://www.clinicalevidence.bmj.com/ceweb/about/knowledge.jsp.

CHAPTER 6

GENERAL PRINCIPLES, PHARMACODYNAMICS, AND DRUG RECEPTOR CONCEPTS

John J. Nagelhout

The practice of anesthesia requires a full spectrum of drugs from which an anesthetic plan can be implemented to achieve the desired level of surgical anesthesia, analgesia, amnesia, and muscle relaxation. In addition to surgical anesthesia, pain medicine has evolved as a significant clinical practice component.[1-3] Now that the human genome has been mapped and the field of molecular and cellular proteomics is exploring new concepts, specific receptor-targeted drugs are envisioned as is a revolution in the way health care is delivered. Likewise, the methods used to provide anesthesia care will undergo a profound change based on this new knowledge. Already studies are challenging long-held concepts of pharmacodynamics and pharmacokinetics that guide the clinical use of anesthetic agents. Although the mechanism of action of the general anesthetics remains unknown, the primary site of anesthetic action is now considered to be membrane receptors and not the lipid bilayer surrounding the nerve cells.[4,5] Spinal cord receptors are being differentiated from receptors in the brain and targeted with specific drugs. A more in-depth knowledge of the concept of minimum alveolar concentration, which is used to define inhalation anesthetic dosing, is now coming to light.[6,7] Receptor superfamilies with definable amino acid subunits are the targets of new classes of anesthetic drugs such as α_2-agonists and analgesics.[8] The potentiation of the inhibitory γ-aminobutyric acid (GABA) receptors is considered a primary mechanism of action of inhalation and intravenous anesthetics.[9] The recovery from intravenous anesthesia is described in terms of context-sensitive half-time, which in addition to the usual concept of drug half-life takes into consideration the duration of anesthetic administration rather than just drug redistribution and elimination profiles.[10-12] The importance of the individual, with his or her unique genetic profile, is surfacing as a major determinant of anesthesia outcome.[13] The number of patients who now make up the portion of the population classified as elderly—those aged 60 to 90 years—is ever increasing. Clinical experience has shown that the response to anesthetic drugs in elderly patients differs from that in younger patients. Age-related change in drug pharmacokinetics (e.g., decreased total clearance) has been shown not to be responsible for the decrease in drug dose necessary to achieve anesthetic endpoints in elderly patients. Studies to date in elderly patients,

although limited, demonstrate an age-related decline in most receptor populations and an overall decrease in pharmacodynamic responses.[14-17] Preoperative assessment by the anesthetist may soon take on an entirely different meaning as patient information becomes more genetically oriented. The choice of anesthetic agents will be based on age-related receptor profiles and the patient's genetic ability to rapidly clear and recover from anesthetic drugs once their administration has been terminated.[18,19] Until that time, anesthetists will continue to administer anesthesia based on age-indexed population drug profiles adjusted for individual pathologies (i.e., general principles of pharmacology).

The current medical economic climate necessitates the optimum selection and use of anesthetic drugs based on their pharmacologic profiles. The term *pharmacology* refers to the processes by which a drug produces one or more measured physiologic responses. The concept of a drug-induced tissue response has changed little since Ehrlich first proposed it (circa 1905). What has changed, and continues to change, is our understanding of the processes involved in drug-receptor interactions.[20,21] Recent attention has focused on the biosphere, or the protein receptor site, as not only the locus of drug binding but also a primary regulator of the measured pharmacologic response. Secondary processes, including drug absorption, distribution, biotransformation, and excretion, also influence the pharmacologic response.[22]

RECEPTOR STRUCTURE

A *receptor* is a protein or other substance that binds to an endogenous chemical or a drug. This coupling causes a chain of events leading to an effect. Receptors have three common properties: sensitivity, selectivity, and specificity. These properties are characterized by the fact that a drug response occurs from a low concentration (sensitivity) produced by structurally similar chemicals (selectivity), and the response from a given set of receptors is always the same because the cells themselves determine the response (specificity). The bonds that form between drugs and receptors typically fall into these categories from weakest to strongest: van der Waals, hydrogen, ionic, and covalent.

Drug Receptors

The historic concept of a drug receptor complex considered the receptor to be a single protein to which the drug aligned and

The author would like to thank Dr. Silas Glisson for his contribution to this chapter in the previous editions.

attached itself. Four types of regulatory proteins are commonly drug receptors. These include (1) cell surface proteins, (2) enzymes, (3) carrier molecules (transporters), and (4) ion channels. Structural proteins may act as drug receptors, such as tubulin as the receptor for colchicine. Science once posited that the transduction of signal to tissue (the increased ion movement into or out of the cell or the activation of a coupled G protein) occurred at a site near the receptor. Current evidence identifies the receptor and transduction site as being the same.

Drug receptor proteins are located within the luminal membrane and at the surface of the ionic channel. A few are known to occupy intracellular sites. The drug lidocaine and other amide and ester local anesthetics act at intracellular receptor sites near the sodium channel. Studies of acetylcholine and its receptor at the neuromuscular junction indicate that less than 1% of the cell surface binds drug to receptor protein to achieve the tissue response.[13] Complete saturation of available receptors with drug molecules is not necessary for a desired tissue response to be elicited. With recent advances in molecular biology, many receptors have been extensively characterized, amino acid sequenced, and cloned. This is leading to new and better understanding of receptor pharmacology and new approaches to drug discovery.[23-25]

For intravenously administered drugs, sufficient drug for a maximal tissue response is delivered to the receptor site within the time required for a single complete circulation (approximately 1 minute), provided an adequate drug dose was administered initially. Current understanding of molecular pharmacology suggests that the delay recorded from initial drug administration to the onset of the tissue response reflects the time required for molecular orientation and attachment to the receptor—that is, the time course of the receptor protein conformational change and the tissue response time.[26] As long as both the drug and the receptor are hydrophobic, bonding occurs.[27] Intravenous anesthetics act by binding to membrane receptor channel proteins. The GABA$_A$ inhibitory receptor has been implicated and suggested as a primary site of intravenous anesthetic action, except in the case of ketamine.[28,29] Inhalation anesthetics have long been thought to produce their anesthetic action by dissolving in the lipid bilayer surrounding membrane ion channels and interfering with their ability to open and close. Recent electrophysiologic evidence, however, indicates that inhalation anesthetics, like intravenous anesthetics, bind to GABA$_A$ receptor proteins and cause inhibition of signal transduction by increasing the influx of chloride ions through membrane channels.[9,28,29]

Individual agonist drugs have at least three configuration points for attachment to their receptors. With more points of attachment, a more perfect drug-receptor fit occurs. Agonist drugs can induce receptor proteins to alter their topography to achieve a more exacting fit with the drug. The alignment of a drug with its receptor is aided by various bonding forces, of which van der Waals forces and ionic bonding are prominent. Volatile anesthetics (e.g., desflurane, sevoflurane, isoflurane, and nitrous oxide) bond to cell receptors by means of a nonspecific hydrophobic bonding mechanism.

Some endogenous proteins provide alternative drug-binding sites. These sites are more correctly termed *acceptors*; the acceptor reduces the amount of unbound drug available for receptor complexing. Albumin contains numerous acceptor sites and generally binds to acidic drugs. Alpha$_1$ acid glycoprotein and β-globulin favor basic drugs. Drug bound to these proteins are unavailable to interact with receptors, therefore reducing the available active drug concentration.

Types of Receptors

As noted earlier, a variety of receptor types have been isolated and investigated, including GABA, opioid, α$_2$, acetylcholine, benzodiazepine, histamine subtypes, and the pain-related capsaicin receptor, as well as numerous others.[30-35] The nicotinic and muscarinic cholinergic receptors that bind acetylcholine have been extensively studied.[36-38] The acetylcholine receptor protein is a pentamer of five peptide subunits conceptually forming a five-sided ring, with the central portion serving as the transduction ion channel. Only two of the five subunits are involved in acetylcholine binding. The remaining three peptide subunits participate in the signal transduction process that involves a protein conformational shift, allowing inward movement of sodium ions through the opened ion channel. It is interesting to note that the GABA$_A$ receptor also has been shown to be composed of five peptide subunits arranged to form a pentameric ring.[35,39-41]

Signal Transduction

In biology, *signal transduction* refers to processes by which a cell converts one kind of signal or stimulus into another. Most often, these involve ordered sequences or cascades of biochemical reactions inside the cell. They are commonly referred to as *second messenger pathways*. (Ligand drug binding to a receptor and subsequent signal transduction are shown in Figure 6-1).

Many of the actions of the common anesthetic drugs are transduced through cell-surface receptors that are linked to G protein-coupled receptors (GPCRs). Receptor signaling translated to changes to G proteins are then linked to a second messenger such as cyclic AMP or cyclic GMP. These second messengers regulate enzymes such as protein kinases and phosphatases, which drive their ultimate intracellular actions. Some examples of different types of receptors are given in Box 6-1.

Signal transduction for the GABA$_A$ receptor, for example, involves inward chloride ion movement through the opened central channel. The protein compositions of acetylcholine and GABA receptors are remarkably similar, despite their functional differences—specifically, acetylcholine and sodium ion transduce an excitatory signal, and GABA and chloride ion transduce an inhibitory signal.[42,43]

For many drugs, the composition of the receptor protein and the signal transduction process may be identical, even though the drug-induced tissue response is not. The primary difference among drug receptor proteins may be only the selective binding subunits and the ion species moving through the channel.[28,32,44-46] The specific peptide subunits are ultimately responsible for the pharmacologic properties of specificity, affinity, and potency.

Drug-Receptor Dynamics

The process by which the receptor protein undergoes a conformational shift to allow inward, and sometimes outward, ion movement is poorly understood. It may be more than mere chance that the pentameric ring structure of the receptor containing drug-specific peptide subunits is frequently met. Conceptually, when a drug binds to selective receptor peptide components, the outermost portion of the peptide ring may function as a backbone toward which the inner flexible surface is pulled.

By analogy, this "pulling" is similar to what occurs when a starfish opens its central mouth. The drug-induced conformational shift primarily involves a structural shortening of the protein filaments between the outer and inner surfaces. Such a process provides an open inner channel that allows the passage of ions through the receptor protein to achieve the intracellular response, thus initiating the dynamics of tissue response.

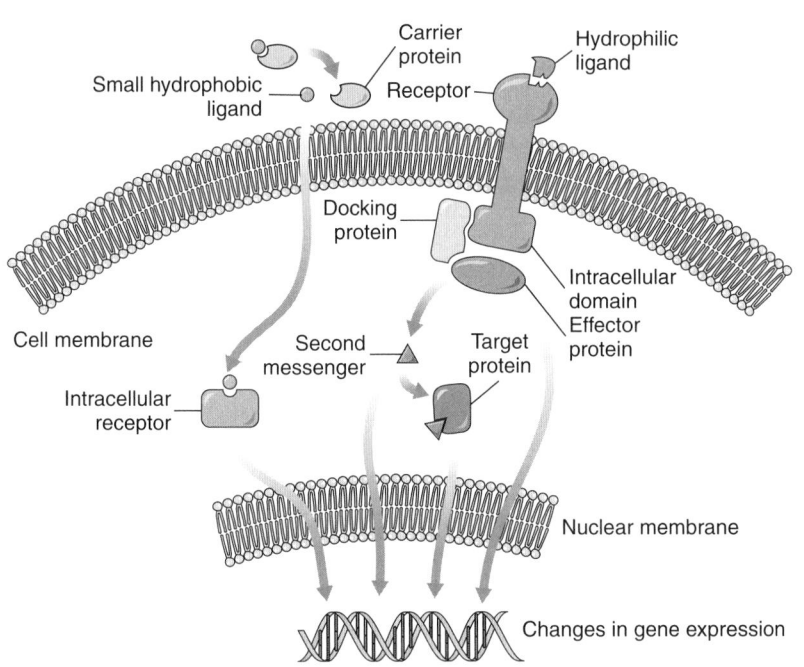

FIGURE **6-1**   Ligand-receptor interactions. (*Modified from Lodish H et al. Molecular Cell Biology. 3rd ed. New York: Freeman; 1995.*)

BOX 6-1

Receptor Classification

Cell Surface Receptors

G protein–coupled receptors (GPCRs)—receptors for hormones, neurotransmitters (biogenic amines, amino acids), and neuropeptides
Activate/inhibit adenylyl cyclase
Activate phospholipase C
Modulate ion channels
Ligand-gated ion channels—receptors for neurotransmitters (biogenic amines, amino acids, peptides)
Mediate fast synaptic transmission

Enzyme-Linked Cell Surface Receptors

Receptor guanylyl cyclases—receptors for atrial natriuretic peptide, *Escherichia coli* heat-stable enterotoxin
Receptor serine/threonine kinases—receptors for activin, inhibin, transforming growth factor (TGF)-β, müllerian inhibiting substance
Receptor tyrosine kinases—receptors for peptide growth factors
Tyrosine kinase-associated—receptors for cytokines, growth hormone, prolactin
Receptor tyrosine phosphates—ligands unknown in most cases

Intracellular Receptors

Steroid receptor superfamily—receptors for steroids, sterols, thyroxine (T_3), retinoic acid, and vitamin D

From Hemmings HC Jr, Hopkins PM. Foundations of Anesthesia: Basic Sciences for Clinical Practice. *2nd ed. Edinburgh: Mosby; 2006.*

Molecular pharmacology is rapidly identifying large numbers of specific cell binding sites involving etomidate, propofol, desflurane, and other anesthetics.[29,31] Drugs designed to bind only with selective sites to achieve a specific response are now available for clinical use (e.g., dexmedetomidine, S-ropivacaine, levobupivacaine, cisatracurium).[47,48]

DRUG RESPONSE EQUATION

The drug response equation is fundamental to pharmacologic principles.[26] It is derived from the law of mass action and is shown in the following equation, where drug (D) combines with receptor (R) to form a drug receptor complex (DRC) that elicits a tissue response (TR).

Equation 6-1

$$D + R \rightleftharpoons (DRC) \rightleftharpoons TR$$

What remains unique about this equation is that in most cases, the drug receptor complex represents a highly selective process. Yet the resultant tissue response tends to vary from individual to individual, reflecting each individual's receptor and genetic profile and physiologic state. The basic drug response relationship conceptually depends on a common pharmacologic theory of drug action. This is the *occupancy theory*. Simply stated, the magnitude of a drug's effect is proportional to the number of receptors occupied. Although it is understood that drug receptor interactions have more complexity than this theory accounts for, it serves as a useful background for many pharmacologic concepts.

POPULATION VARIABILITY

Because the objective of pharmacologic intervention is to achieve a desired therapeutic response, anesthetists recognize that a range of responses to a given drug and dosage is possible within a patient population. Therapeutic drug doses reflect average doses of a "normal" population of individuals. Specific therapeutic doses for population subsets (e.g., pediatric, neonatal, geriatric, patients with cardiac or other chronic diseases) are available, thereby narrowing the degree of response variability for a given drug and clinical population. The age, sex, body weight, body surface area, basal metabolic rate, pathologic state, and genetic profile of an individual directly influence the pharmacologic response.

Given the increasing median age of the population in the United States, studies of the influence of age on the responses to anesthetic drugs have increased. Steady-state plasma concentrations of hypnotic drugs such as midazolam and propofol and minimum alveolar concentrations (MAC) for inhaled anesthetics (e.g., desflurane, isoflurane, or sevoflurane) required to achieve desired anesthetic end-points decrease as age increases, independent of any age effect on drug pharmacokinetics.[14,17,49,50] In addition, the effective plasma concentration 50 (EC_{50}) needed to achieve sedation with midazolam infusion is reported to be decreased by 50% in elderly volunteers.[17] Unfortunately the specifics responsible for the observed age-related decrease in effective dose of anesthetic drugs is not presently known. Receptor changes associated with aging and kinetic differences in the elderly have been suggested as explanations for the response. Until a better understanding of the age-related changes exists, empirical dose reduction or the use of dosing algorithms for the elderly patient population is indicated.

Mean, Median, and Mode

A graphic description of the dose-response relationship is displayed in Figure 6-2. The theoretic normal distribution of quantal (desired) responses to increasing drug dose takes the shape of a Gaussian curve. Theoretically, the numbers of respondents on both sides of the mean (average dose) are equal, with the greatest percentage of individuals responding near the center of the curve. In a Gaussian distribution curve, the mean, median, and mode are equidistant from the two extremes.[51] Atypical responders fall at each end of the curve.

On the curve, the mean dose is the arithmetic average of the range of doses that produce a given response. The median dose is that dose on either side of which half of the responses occur. The mode dose is the dose representing the greatest percentage of responses. The mean, median, and mode doses are often close but are rarely the same in actual dose-response curves.

Standard Deviation

The terms *standard deviation* (SD) and *standard error of the mean* (SEM) describe population response variability.[52] The SD provides information regarding the actual responses measured and their difference from the calculated mean. In Figure 6-3, 1 SD makes up 68% of the responses (34% to the left and 34% to the

right of the mean value); 2 and 3 SDs constitute 95% and 99.7% of the responses, respectively. The greater the SD, the less the mean reflects the central tendency of responses.

Standard Error of the Mean

The SEM describes the variance of the mean. It is equivalent to the SD of the mean. By repeating the dose-response measurements on different, normally distributed populations, a slightly different mean dose value is obtained each time because the mean value is only an arithmetic average of the responses obtained. In Figure 6-4, 1 SEM represents the range within which the mean value would occur on repeat testing 68% of the time, and 2 and 3 SEMs (not shown) represent the range within which the mean value would occur 95% and 99.7% of the time, respectively. Both the SD and the SEM are important statistical descriptors of observed drug responses in patient care and in research and reflect pharmacologic principles of population variance.[52]

DRUG DOSE RESPONSE

The administration of drugs is largely determined by a mean therapeutic dose per kilogram of body weight or body surface area calculated from a previously determined average dose for

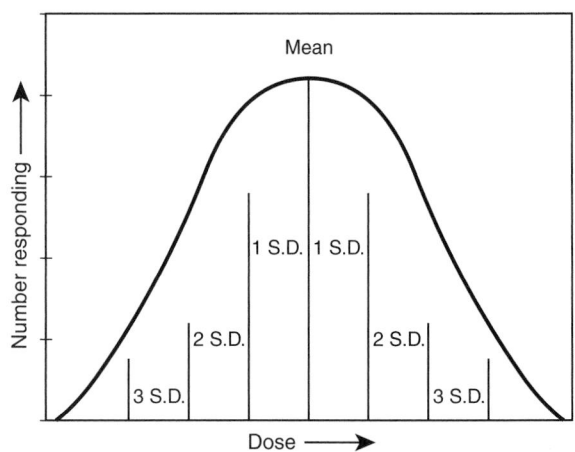

FIGURE **6-3**   A normal distribution curve showing the standard deviation (SD) in relation to the mean (average) dose value.

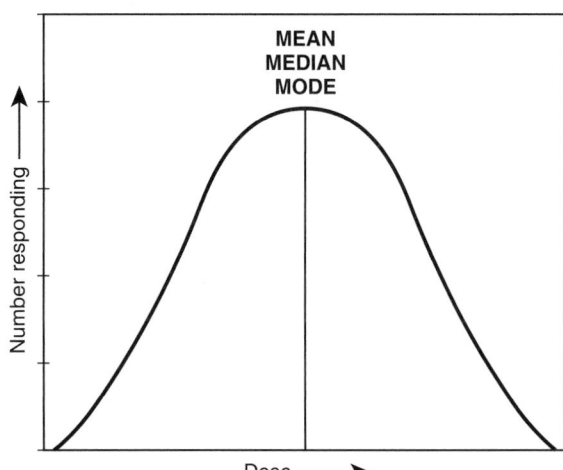

FIGURE **6-2**   The theoretic normal frequency distribution of a drug response in a normal population.

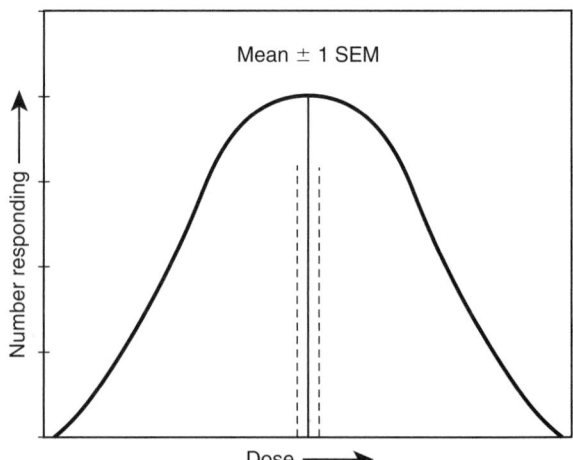

FIGURE **6-4**   A normal distribution curve showing the relationship of the standard error of the mean (SEM) to the mean (average) value.

the normal population. This approach may be responsible for underdosing and overdosing of patients, because population variability is not considered in the calculation. The individual therapeutic response to a fixed mean dose is frequently less than optimal.

Studies that used sensitive quantitative measurement techniques identified a response variability to given drug doses in the normal population that was far greater than previously demonstrated.[20] Clearly, the optimal dosing approach for patients when drugs are administered by the intravenous route is by titration until the desired therapeutic response is attained. This is particularly true in critical care and anesthesia patients, in whom drug onset and offset responses are relatively rapid.

Two types of dose-response curves—graded and quantal—describe average drug response and subject variability within a given population.

Graded Dose Response

The graded dose-response curve, which is plotted in linear fashion, characterizes the change in measured response as an administered dose is increased (Figure 6-5). The response curve has a hyperbolic shape, with the greatest change in response occurring to the left on a small portion of the x-axis. When plotted on a logarithmic scale, the graded dose-response curve takes an S shape; at the lowest dose, the measured response (e.g., vascular response to norepinephrine) is small or even nonexistent. At the highest doses, the response is maximal and approaches a plateau (Figure 6-6). Typically, at some point between 20% and 80% of the maximal response, the curve approaches a straight line because changes in dose and response reflect a proportional relationship.

Plotting on a semilogarithmic scale, with the dose in log units, provides a more detailed representation of the entire graded dose-response curve, especially at the two extremes.[20] From a semilogarithmic plot of graded dose responses, the potency of different agonist drugs with similar mechanisms of action (i.e., action through the same receptor) can be compared, or the ability of an antagonist drug to reduce the response to an agonist (e.g., in the alpha receptor blocker, phenoxybenzamine antagonism of norepinephrine-induced vasoconstriction) can be observed. It should be noted that "antagonist" drugs that do not bind to the agonist receptor are actually not antagonists. For example, neostigmine is not an antagonist of vecuronium, because it does not compete with vecuromium for the muscle

end-plate receptor site. Neostigmine inhibits acetylcholinesterase, which allows acetylcholine to compete effectively with vecuronium and other nondepolarizing muscle relaxants for the receptor, leading to a recovery of muscle tone. Therefore, its effect is at least a partial form of indirect antagonism. Sugammadex is the first and so far only drug in a new class of muscle relaxant reversal drugs. Known as a *selective relaxant binding agent* (SRBA), sugammadex offers a unique mechanism in that it encapsulates the muscle-relaxant molecule, rendering it inactive. The complex formed is eliminated. This is a form of chemical antagonism, because no direct receptor action is evident.[53]

Quantal Dose Response

Clinically, a quantal dose-response curve provides information on the frequency with which a given drug dose produces a desired therapeutic response in a patient population. The response is measured in an all-or-nothing fashion. The quantal response curve describes the variation in response to the threshold dose within a population of seemingly similar individuals (Figure 6-7). For example, with propofol induction of anesthesia, a small number of patients become unconscious after administration of

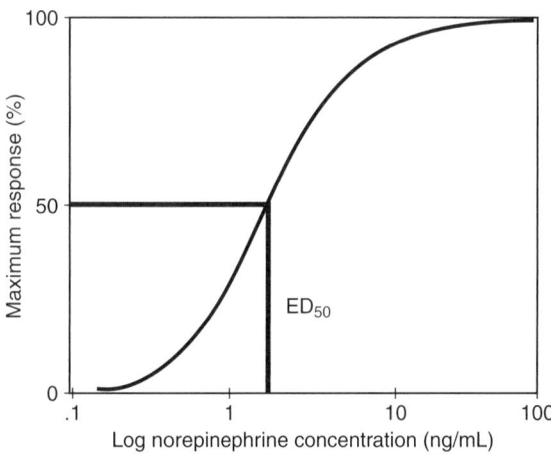

FIGURE **6-6** A logarithmic plot of the data from Figure 6-5 showing blood vessel constriction to increasing concentrations of norepinephrine. The median effective dose (ED$_{50}$) is identified.

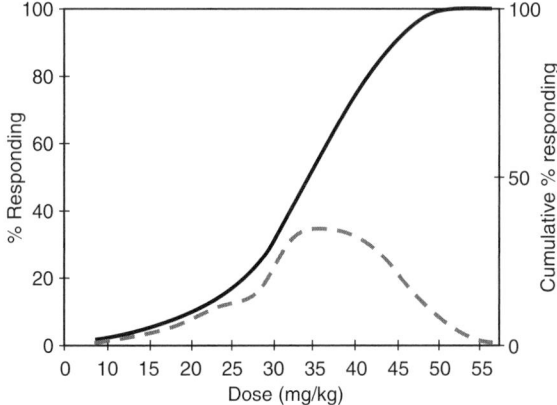

FIGURE **6-7** A quantal dose-response curve indicating the frequency of all-or-nothing dose responses. The *dashed line* represents a histogram of the number of responses measured at each dose. The *solid line* represents the cumulative response curve of the total number of responses up to and including each dose.

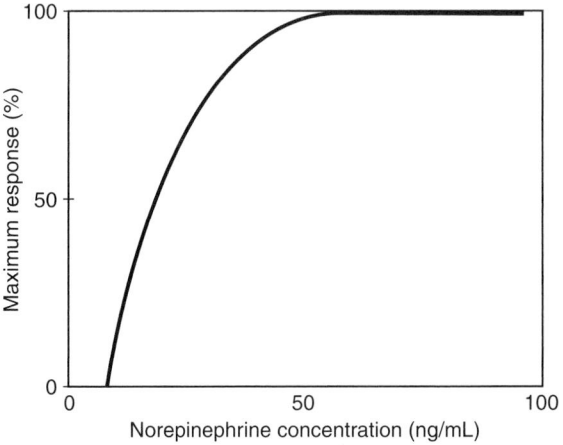

FIGURE **6-5** A linear arithmetic-graded response curve showing blood vessel constriction to increasing norepinephrine concentrations.

0.5 mg/kg, more after administration of 1 mg/kg, and virtually all after administration of 2 to 3 mg/kg. Plotting the cumulative number of patients with all-or-nothing responses over a range of doses produces an S-shaped response curve. However, the quantal dose S-shaped curve differs from the graded dose-response S-shaped curve because it reflects population variation for the threshold dose needed to produce a given all-or-nothing desired response.

Descriptive information about population dose-response characteristics can be obtained from quantal dose-response curves.[20] Descriptors such as effective dose, toxic dose, and lethal dose can be identified. The effective dose 99% (ED_{99}) and lethal dose 1% (LD_1) identify the therapeutic safety margin of a drug, as shown in the following equation.

Equation 6-2

$$Safety\ margin = LD_1 - ED_{99}/ED_{99} \times 100$$

When the therapeutic safety margin is great, the risk of drug-induced death is small, and the margin of therapeutic safety is wide. The opposite is true when the therapeutic safety margin is small.

The term *therapeutic index* (LD_{50}/ED_{50}) describes a drug's median therapeutic safety margin for a particular therapeutic effect.[20] For example, chemotherapeutic drugs have a very narrow margin of safety. Drugs that produce surgical depths of anesthesia, such as sevoflurane and other halogenated anesthetics, also have a relatively narrow margin of safety. Sevoflurane is administered clinically in an amount that is 1.3- to 1.4-fold the MAC, or the dose at which 50% of the patients do not move on surgical stimulation. The MAC can be lethal if the volume percentage delivered is increased to 1.7- to 2.0-fold and maintained for a prolonged period of time.

Another descriptor obtained from the quantal dose-response curve is the median effective dose (ED_{50})—the dose at which 50% of a population responds as desired. The ED_{50} is often used for comparing the potency of drugs within a class. Because the ED_{50} dose is derived from the linear portion of the quantal dose-response curve (20% to 80% of the responders), relatively accurate comparisons of drugs that cause similar responses can be made (see Figure 6-6). Important in each of these descriptions is the word *median*. Median ED_{50} dose values are derived average response doses from a population of patients.[20] Each individual within the population responds, more or less, to a median dose on the basis of his or her biologic variation or, specifically, genetic variations in drug-receptor protein. Confidence limits for a given median dose and its therapeutic response can be calculated. Typically, the proportion of subjects responding to an ED_{50} dose ranges from 45% to 55%. Derived median population dose values provide a point of reference for achieving an individual's optimum therapeutic dose.

For intravenously administered drugs used in anesthesia, the trend is toward drugs that have brief onset-offset times and can be administered by infusion, often with the use of a computer-controlled pump.[54,55] For example, the desired anesthetic response to propofol and remifentanil can be effectively titrated after an initial loading dose.

Future developments related to drugs will include the availability of indwelling drug-analyzing probes similar to the continuous mass spectrometers currently used for analysis of end-tidal anesthetic gas concentrations. Real-time analysis of drug concentration can incorporate feedback control to drug-infusion devices. These target-controlled infusions allow the dose to be set to patient response and automatically maintained with minimal

fluctuations in blood and effect site drug concentrations and the tissue response.[56,57] Currently, computer-controlled infusion pumps use programs based on pharmacokinetic modeling studies in an attempt to approximate the required effect site drug concentration to achieve and maintain a desired level of anesthesia in patients. The continuing development of ultrafast onset-offset anesthetic drugs such as remifentanil and propofol will simplify titration of the anesthetic end-point by the anesthetist and minimize undesired overdose effects.

DRUG RECEPTOR INTERACTIONS

Advances in molecular receptor pharmacology have provided a new understanding of patient drug responses.[21] The *drug receptor interaction* describes the formation of a single drug receptor complex, which leads to a fractional tissue response (FTR):

Equation 6-3

$$D + R \underset{k_2}{\overset{k_1}{\rightleftharpoons}} DR \overset{k_3}{\rightarrow} FT$$

The desired tissue response is observed when sufficient receptors have been occupied and activated by free drug. This process obeys the law of mass action: At steady state, equilibrium exists between bound and unbound drug receptors and the concentration of free unbound drug at the site. Specific characteristics of the drug and the receptor determine the association and dissociation of a drug with regard to its receptor and the kinetic, k, rates, which are constants.[14]

Drug Affinity and Efficacy

The terms *affinity* and *efficacy* (intrinsic activity) describe the degree of drug receptor interaction for a given drug and receptor protein population (e.g., $GABA_A$ and propofol). The observed tissue response reflects the quantity of drug receptor complexes intact at any given moment. Each drug receptor interaction elicits a quantum of excitation, and the summation of many individual quanta produces the tissue response.[52]

The time constant that describes the fractional tissue response after the drug receptor complex formation typically has been considered to be near zero or instantaneous. Until recently, the primary time constant thought to influence the onset of tissue response was the duration of the delay in the delivery of drug to the receptor sites. The phrase *pharmacokinetic analysis* of drug absorption and distribution describes onset time and magnitude of drug response. *Drug elimination kinetic analysis* describes the duration of the tissue response.

Drug-Receptor-Response Triad

Current understanding of receptor dynamics has added an additional and possibly the most descriptive component of the drug-receptor-response triad. When a drug combines with its receptor, a conformational change occurs in the receptor protein itself. No tissue response can occur without the structural shift. Evidence does suggest that events within the biosphere after drug association with the receptor are the principal regulatory variables of the response onset-offset time course.[52] An additional theory of drug action is referred to as the *two-state model*. In this model, the receptor is thought to exist in equilibrium between either an activated or inactivated state. Constitutively active receptors can exist and are shifted toward the activated state, even though no agonist or ligand is present. Receptors for benzodiazepines, cannabinoids, and serotonin are examples. Agonists shift the equilibrium toward activation. Antagonists

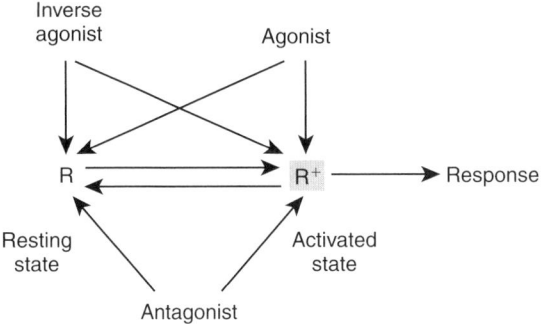

FIGURE **6-8** The two-state model. (*From Rang H et al: Rang and Dale's Pharmacology. 6th ed. Edinburgh: Churchill Livingstone; 2007.*)

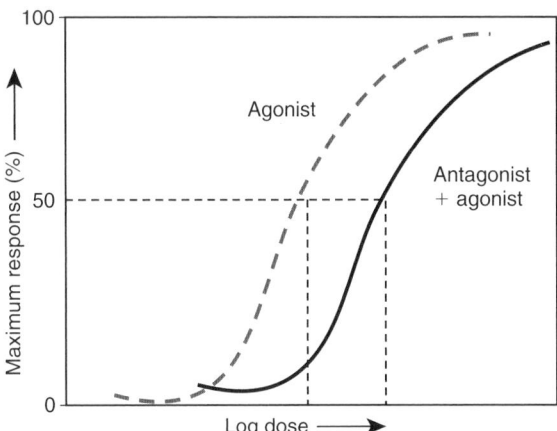

FIGURE **6-9** A logarithmic dose-response curve that shows an agonist drug response alone (*dashed line*) and in the presence of an antagonist drug (*solid line*).

freeze the equilibrium, and inverse agonists shift the equilibrium toward inactivation.[58,59] The two-state model is shown in Figure 6-8.

Until recently, the terms *drug absorption, distribution,* and *elimination* were used solely to describe the tissue-response time course.[60] However, the response may be more complex than was originally thought. It is now known that drug delivery sufficient to occupy 1% of the receptors is in many instances all that is required for a maximum tissue response to occur. Furthermore, the synthesis and destruction of receptor proteins occur at a much more rapid rate than was previously believed—within minutes rather than days. Receptor up-regulation and down-regulation can occur during drug infusion, with new receptor protein being synthesized in response to availability of free unbound drug.[20,21,61,62]

DRUG ANTAGONISM

Pure Antagonists

Pure pharmacologic antagonist drugs are similar in molecular structure to their corresponding agonist drugs. However, owing to the addition or subtraction of one or more chemical moieties, they are unable to initiate the receptor protein conformational shift necessary for eliciting a tissue response. Such antagonist drugs have receptor affinity but lack intrinsic activity or efficacy.

Antagonists that possess the property of weak affinity for the same receptor protein (e.g., atropine, esmolol) are competitive and may be displaced by an agonist. Noncompetitive antagonists, such as phenoxybenzamine and aspirin, have a strong affinity for the receptor protein, usually via covalent bonds, and cannot be displaced by the agonist.[63] New receptor protein must be synthesized if agonist receptor complexing is to occur.[62,63] As with agonist drugs, not all receptors are bound by antagonists. Antagonists cause a rightward shift in the drug dose-response curve. The extent of rightward shift reflects the number of available receptors occupied by the antagonist drug (Figure 6-9). Comparison of the ED_{50} doses in Figure 6-9 shows a reduced affinity of the agonist for its receptor when the antagonist is present.

Agonist-Antagonists

Agonist-antagonists are the second major type of antagonist drugs.[20] As the name implies, agonist-antagonist drugs have receptor protein affinity and intrinsic activity, but often only one tenth to one fiftieth the potency of the pure agonist. Narcotic antagonists often are of the nonpure, agonist-antagonist type, such as nalbuphine. The mechanism by which agonist-antagonist drugs elicit less of a tissue response is not fully understood. An incomplete receptor protein conformational shift has been suggested.

Physiologic Antagonism

Physiologic antagonism, another form of antagonism, involves two agonist drugs that bind to different receptors.[20] For competitive antagonism, the agonist and antagonist have affinity for the same receptor protein; in contrast, in physiologic antagonism, both drugs bind to specific unrelated receptor proteins, initiate a protein conformational shift, and elicit individual tissue responses. The responses, however, generate opposing forces such as are observed with isoproterenol-induced vasodilation and norepinephrine-induced vasoconstriction. The net effect on blood pressure is less than it would be if either drug were used by itself. The drug response that predominates depends on the intrinsic activity of each and on the extent of the tissue response that can be elicited.

Chemical Antagonism

Chemical antagonism occurs when a drug's action is blocked and no receptor activity is involved. For example, protamine is a positively charged protein that forms an ionic bond with heparin, thus rendering it inactive. Sugammadex, mentioned previously, is another example.

Receptor Regulation and Adaptation

Receptors not only initiate regulation of physiologic and biochemical functions but also are themselves subject to many regulatory and homeostatic controls. These controls include regulation of the synthesis and degradation of the receptor by multiple mechanisms, covalent modification, association with other regulatory proteins, and/or relocation within the cell. Modulating inputs may come from other receptors, directly or indirectly, and receptors are almost always subject to feedback regulation by their own signaling outputs.

Continued stimulation of cells with agonists generally results in a state of desensitization, also referred to as *refractoriness* or *down-regulation*, such that the effect that follows continued or subsequent exposure to the same concentration of drug is diminished. This phenomenon is very important in therapeutic situations; an example is attenuated response to the repeated use of β-adrenergic agonists as bronchodilators for the treatment of asthma. Clinically the patient experiences tolerance; increasing doses are required to achieve the same effect.

Chronic administration of an antagonist results in up-regulation as the number and sensitivity of the receptors increase

TABLE 6-1	Drug Interaction Terminology	
Drug Interaction	**Explanation**	**Viewed as an Equation**
Addition	The combined effect of two drugs acting via the same mechanism is equal to that expected by simple addition of their individual actions.	$1 + 1 = 2$
Synergism	The combined effect of two drugs is greater than the algebraic sum of their individual effects.	$1 + 1 = 3$
Potentiation	The enhancement of the action of one drug by a second drug that has no detectable action of its own.	$1 + 0 = 3$
Antagonism	The action of one drug opposes the action of another.	$1 + 1 = 0$

BOX 6-2

Pharmacodynamic Concepts

- **Agonist**. An agonist is a substance that binds to a specific receptor and triggers a response in the cell. It mimics the action of an endogenous ligand (such as hormone or neurotransmitter) that binds to the same receptor. In adequate concentrations, it can cause maximal activation of all receptors (a full agonist).
- **Antagonists**. An antagonist is a drug that has affinity for the receptor but no efficacy. It does not activate the receptor to produce a physiologic action. By occupying the receptor, it may block an endogenous chemical response, thereby producing a physiologic consequence. Antagonists commonly have a higher affinity for a given receptor than do agonists. Types of antagonism include pharmacologic, in which competitive is reversible and noncompetitive is irreversible, requiring syntheses of new receptors to reestablish homeostasis. Pharmacokinetic, chemical, and physiologic antagonism may also occur.
- **Affinity or potency**. When considering agonists, the term *potency* is used to differentiate between different agonists that activate the same receptor and can all produce the same maximal response (efficacy) but at differing concentrations. The most potent drug of a series requires the lowest dose.
- **Efficacy or intrinsic activity**. The efficacy of a drug is its ability to produce the desired response expected by stimulation of a given receptor population. It refers to the maximum possible effect that can be achieved with the drug. The term *intrinsic activity* is often used instead of efficacy, although this more accurately describes the relative maximum effect obtained when comparing compounds in a series.
- **Partial agonist**. A partial agonist activates a receptor but cannot produce a maximum response. It may also be able to partially block the effects of full agonists. It is postulated that partial agonists possess both agonist and antagonist properties, thus the term *agonist-antagonist* has been used. A partial agonist has a lower efficacy than a full agonist.
- **Inverse agonist**. A drug or endogenous chemical that binds to a receptor, resulting in the opposite action of an agonist. Using

the two-state model, they appear to bind preferentially to the inactivated receptor. They may have a theoretic advantage over antagonists in situations in which a disease state is partly due to an up-regulation* of receptor activity.
- **Spare receptor concept**. The relationship between the number of receptors stimulated and the response is usually nonlinear. A maximal or almost maximal response can often be produced by activation of only a fraction of the receptors present. A good example can be found in the neuromuscular junction. Occupation of more than 70% of the nicotinic cholinergic muscle receptors by an antagonist is necessary before there is a reduction in response, implying that a maximal response is obtained by activation of only 30% of the total number of receptors.
- **Tolerance**. Individual variation can result in a situation in which an increasing concentration of drug is required to produce a given response. This usually results from its chronic exposure to the agonist. Very rapid development of tolerance, frequently with acute drug administration, is referred to as *tachyphylaxis*. The underlying mechanism may not be clear. Common causes include up- or down-regulation, enzyme induction, depleted neurotransmitter, protein conformational changes, and changes in gene expression.
- **Ligand**. In biochemistry, a ligand is a molecule that is able to bind and form a complex with a receptor to produce a biologic response. Ligands are endogenous chemicals such as neurotransmitters and hormones that are exogenously administered drugs.
- **Quantal drug response**. Using dose response curves, the actions of drug can be quantified and expressed as the effective dose ED_{50}, toxic dose TD_{50} and lethal dose LD_{50}. The therapeutic index is the LD_{50}/ED_{50}.
- **Receptor adaptation or homeostasis**. The number and activity of a receptor population may increase or decrease in response to (usually) chronic drug administration.

*Up-regulation *is the process by which a cell increases the number of receptors to a given drug.* Down-regulation *is the process by which a cell decreases the number of receptors for a given drug in response to chronic stimulation. β-Adrenergic receptors, for example, up-regulate in the presence of antagonists and down-regulate in the presence of agonists.*

as a response to chronic blockade. Again the patient develops tolerance, requiring higher doses of the antagonist to counteract the increasing receptor number.

Drug Interaction Terminology

A drug interaction is an alteration in the therapeutic action of a drug by concurrent administration of other drugs or exogenous substances. The common classification is given in Table 6-1.

SUMMARY

The pharmacologic principles described in this chapter are essential to understanding drug responses in patients. The drug receptor subunit site now appears to be the primary regulator of onset-offset drug response. More and more evidence suggests that individual genetic variation in receptor proteins accounts for drug-response variation within seemingly normal populations. In clinical anesthesia, the range of patient responses to a given drug dose reflects this genetic variation. The trend toward dosing by titration with rapid onset and offset anesthetic drugs minimizes the response variability factor by optimizing the use of available receptor proteins. The age-related decline in anesthetic drug dose needed to achieve a desired anesthetic end-point is related to a change in both pharmacodynamics and pharmacokinetics.

The anesthetist uses pharmacologic intervention to elicit a desired patient response. The site of the intervention is the biosphere, or the protein drug receptor, which is the primary regulator of the therapeutic response. Observed variation in patient drug response reflects the functionality of the biosphere and genetics, as well as physiologic variability.

The mean, median, and mode typically describe the dose-response relationship of a "normally distributed" population. In anesthesia, the patient population is rarely "normal." The drug response of population subsets can be expected to vary around the mean dosage. The trend toward dose titration by infusion allows individualization of the desired drug response, with fewer resultant overresponses and underresponses. The SD, SEM, and median effective dose provide a description of a population's response to a drug. Such descriptors provide only an approximate dosage; the anesthetist must adjust this dosage for each patient to achieve the desired physiologic response. Viewed at the molecular level, the observed response to a drug represents countless individual drug responses at the biosphere. Each drug-receptor interaction at the protein receptor elicits a fractional tissue response, and the sum of the fractional responses provides the observed response. In accordance with the law of mass action, when free drug binds to a receptor, a conformational shift occurs in the receptor protein. This shift causes a central space or channel to open, allowing specific ions to enter or leave the cell or a G protein to be activated, resulting in a biochemical cascade yielding pharmacologic effects. The resultant tissue response continues until the drug dissociates from the receptor. Antagonist drugs also bind to the receptor but lack the ability to initiate the required protein conformational shift. The sum of fractional tissue responses elicited when an antagonist is present is inadequate for maintaining the desired tissue response. Some common pharmacodynamic concepts are given in Box 6-2.

Molecular pharmacology is identifying site-specific and age-related causes for the observed variation in patient drug response. Further investigation of the biosphere, genetics, and receptor protein subunits will provide a new understanding of pharmacodynamics for the anesthetist.

REFERENCES

1. Brown AK et al. Strategies for postoperative pain management. *Best Pract Res Clin Anaesthesiol.* 2004;18(4):703-717.
2. Viscusi ER. Emerging techniques in the management of acute pain: epidural analgesia. *Anesth Analg.* 2005;101(5 Suppl):S23-S29.
3. Block BM et al. Efficacy of postoperative epidural analgesia: a meta-analysis. *JAMA.* 2003;12:290(18):2455-2463.
4. Mashour GA et al. Mechanisms of general anesthesia: from molecules to mind. *Best Pract Res Clin Anaesthesiol.* 2005;19(3):349-364.
5. Eger EI, Sonner JM. Anaesthesia defined (gentlemen, this is not humbug). *Best Pract Res Clin Anaesthesiol.* 2006;20(1):23-29.
6. Sonner JM et al. Inhaled anesthetics and immobility: mechanisms, mysteries, and minimum alveolar anesthetic concentration. *Anesth Analg.* 2003;97:718-740.
7. Antognini JF, Carsten E. Measuring minimum alveolar concentration: more than meets the tail. *Anesthesiology.* 2005;103(4):679-680.
8. Fichna J et al. The endomorphin system and its evolving neurophysiological role. *Pharmacol Rev.* 2007;59:88-123.
9. Campana JA et al. Mechanisms of action of inhaled anesthesia. *N Engl J Med.* 2003;348:2110-2124.
10. Shafer SL, Varvel JR. Pharmacokinetics, pharmacodynamics, and rational opioid selection. *Anesthesiology.* 1991;74:53-63.
11. Hughes MA et al. Context-sensitive halftime in multicompartment pharmacokinetics models for intravenous anesthetic drugs. *Anesthesiology.* 1992;76:334-341.
12. Bailey JM. Technique for quantifying the duration of intravenous anesthetic effect. *Anesthesiology.* 1995;83:1095-1103.
13. Wakeling HG et al. Targeting effect compartment or central compartment concentration of propofol: what predicts loss of consciousness? *Anesthesiology.* 1999;90:92-97.
14. Jacob JR et al. Aging increases pharmacodynamic sensitivity to the hypnotic effects of midazolam. *Anesth Analg.* 1995;80:43-148.
15. Inoue M et al. Age-related reduction of extrastriatal dopamine D2 receptor measured by PET. *Life Sci.* 2001;69:1079-1084.
16. Kakiuchi T et al. Age-related changes in muscarinic cholinergic receptors in the living brain: a PET study using N- [11C] methyl-4-piperidyl benzilate combined with cerebral blood flow measurement in conscious monkeys. *Brain Res.* 2001;916:22-31.
17. Albrecht S et al. The effect of age on the pharmacokinetics and pharmacodynamics of midazolam. *Clin Pharmacol Ther.* 1999;65:630-639.
18. Allen PD. Anesthesia and the human genome project: the quest for accurate prediction of drug responses. *Anesthesiology.* 2005;102(3):494-495.
19. Palmer SN et al. Pharmacogenetics of anesthetic and analgesic agents. *Anesthesiology.* 2005;102(3):663-671.
20. Bourne HR, Von Zastrow M. Drug receptors and pharmacodynamics. In: Katzung BG, ed. *Basic and Clinical Pharmacology,* 10th ed. New York: McGraw-Hill; 2007:11-33.
21. Polllard BJ. Styles of drug action. In Hemming HC, Hopkins PM, eds. *Foundations of Anesthesia: Basic Sciences for Clinical Practice.* 2nd ed. Philadelphia: Mosby; 2006:91-100.
22. Rang HP et al. In: *Rang & Dale's Pharmacology.* 6th ed. Philadelphia: Churchhill Livingstone; 2007:8-23.
23. Zheng CJ et al. Trends in exploration of therapeutic targets. *Drug News Perspect.* 2005;18(2):109-127.
24. Sams-Dodd F. Drug discovery: selecting the optimal approach. *Drug Discov Today.* 2006;11(9-10):465-472.
25. Overington JP et al. How many drug targets are there? *Nat Rev Drug Discov.* 2006;5(12):993-996.
26. Bauer LA. Clinical pharmacokinetics & pharmacodynamics. In: Dipro JT et al, eds. *Pharmacology: A Pathophysiologic Approach.* 6th ed. New York: McGraw-Hill; 2005:51-74.
27. Calvey N, Williams N. Drug action. In: *Principles and Practice of Pharmacology for Anaesthetists.* 5th ed. Oxford: Blackwell; 2008:43-67.
28. Frank NP. Molecular targets underlying general anaesthesia. *Br J Pharmacol.* 2006;147(Suppl 1):S72-S81.
29. Bertaccini EJ et al. The common chemical motifs within anesthetic binding sites. *Anesth Analg.* 2007;104(2):318-324.
30. Waldhoer M et al. Opioid receptors. *Annu Rev Biochem.* 2004;73:953-990.

31. Thompson SA, Wafford K. Mechanism of action of general anaesthetics—new information from molecular pharmacology. *Curr Opin Pharmacol.* 2001;1(1):78-83.

32. Dilger JP. The effects of general anaesthetics on ligand-gated ion channels. *Br J Anaesth.* 2002;89(1):41-51.

33. Urban BW et al. Interactions of anesthetics with their targets: non-specific, specific or both? *Pharmacol Ther.* 2006;111(3):729-770.

34. Power BM et al. Pharmacokinetics of drugs used in critically ill adults. *Clin Pharmacokinet.* 1998;34:25-56.

35. Solt K, Forman SA. Correlating the clinical actions and molecular mechanisms of general anesthetics. *Curr Opin Anaesthesiol.* 2007;20(4):300-306.

36. Durieux ME. Muscarinic signaling in the central nervous system: recent developments and anesthetic implications. *Anesthesiology.* 1996;84:173-189.

37. Tassonyi E et al. The role of nicotinic acetylcholine receptors in the mechanisms of anesthesia. *Brain Res Bull.* 2002;57:133-150.

38. Hucho F et al. The emerging three-dimensional structure of a receptor: the nicotinic acetylcholine receptor. *Eur J Biochem.* 1996;239:539-557.

39. Drafts BC, Fisher JL. Identification of structures within GABA$_A$ receptor alpha subunits that regulate the agonist action of pentobarbital. *J Pharmacol Exp Ther.* 2006;318(3):1094-1101.

40. Bowery NG, Smart TG. GABA and glycine as neurotransmitters: a brief history. *BR J Pharmacol.* 2006;147(Suppl 1):S109-S119.

41. Michels G, Moss SJ. GABA$_A$ receptors: properties and trafficking. *Crit Rev Biochem Mol Biol.* 2007;42(1):3-14.

42. Tanelian DL et al. The role of the GABA$_A$ receptors/chloride channel complex in anesthesia. *Anesthesiology.* 1993;78:757-776.

43. Rabow LE et al. From ion currents to genomic analysis: recent advances in GABA$_A$ receptor research. *Synapse* 1998;21:189-274.

44. Plourde G. General anaesthetic action: ubiquity, complexity and relevance of neuroscience. *J Physiol.* 2007;580(Pt 1):5.

45. Alexander SP et al. Transmitter-gated channels. *Br J Pharmacol.* 2007;150(Suppl 1):S82-S95.

46. Pocock G, Richards CD. Excitatory and inhibitory synaptic mechanisms in anaesthesia. *Br J Anaesth.* 1993;71(1):134-147.

47. Nau C, Strichartz GR. Drug chirality in anesthesia. *Anesthesiology.* 2002;97(2):497-502.

48. Calvey TN. Isomerism and anaesthetic drugs. *Acta Anaesthesiol Scan Suppl.* 1995;106:83-90.

49. Schuttler J, Ihmsen HM. Population pharmacokinetics of propofol: a multicenter study. *Anesthesiology.* 2000;92:727-738.

50. Eger EI. Age, minimum alveolar anesthetic concentration, and minimum alveolar anesthetic concentration-awake. *Anesth Analg.* 2001;93:947-953.

51. Holfoard NGH. Pharmacokinetics and pharmacodynamics rational dosing and the time course of drug action. In: Katzung BG, ed. *Basic and Clinical Pharmacology.* 10th ed. New York: McGraw-Hill; 2007:24-49.

52. Lowe ES, Balis FM. Dose effect and concentration effect analysis. In: Atkinson AJ et al, eds. *Principles of Clinical Pharmacology.* 2nd ed. San Diego: Elsevier; 2007:289-301.

53. Bom A et al. Selective relaxant binding agents for reversal of neuromuscular blockade. *Curr Opin Pharmacol.* 2007;7(3):298-302.

54. Puri GD et al. Closed-loop anaesthesia delivery system (CLADS) using bispectral index: a performance assessment study. *Anaesth Intensive Care.* 2007;35(3):357-362.

55. Zaba Z et al. Spectral frequency index monitoring during propofol-remifentanil and propofol-alfentanil total intravenous anaesthesia. *CNS Drugs.* 2007;21(2):165-171.

56. Barakat AR et al. Effect site concentration during propofol TCI sedation: a comparison of sedation score with two pharmacokinetic models. *Anaesthesia.* 2007;62(7):661-666.

57. Wang LP et al. Low and moderate remifentanil infusion rates do not alter target-controlled infusion propofol concentrations necessary to maintain anesthesia as assessed by bispectral index monitoring. *Anesth Analg.* 2007;104(2):325-331.

58. Giraldo J et al. Assessing receptor affinity for inverse agonists: Schild and Cheng-Prusoff method revisited. *Curr Drug Targets.* 2007;8(1):197-202.

59. Kenakin T. Efficacy as a vector: the relative prevalence and paucity of inverse agonism. *Mol Pharmacol.* 2004;65(1):2-11.

60. Nierenberg DW, Melmon KL. Introduction to clinical pharmacology. In: Melmon KL, ed; *Clinical Pharmacology: Basic Principles in Therapeutics.* 4th ed. New York: McGraw-Hill; 2000;1-62.

61. von Zastrow M. Opioid receptor regulation. *Neuromolecular Med.* 2004;5(1):51-58.

62. Toews ML et al. Regulation of alpha-1B adrenergic receptor localization, trafficking, function, and stability. *Life Sci.* 2003;74(2-3):379-389.

63. Dogné JM et al. From the design to the clinical application of thromboxane modulators. *Curr Pharm Des.* 2006;12(8):903-923.

PHARMACOKINETICS

Ladan Eshkevari, Donna Jasinski

Pharmacokinetics is a term used to describe the study of the changes in the concentration of a drug during the processes of absorption, distribution, metabolism or biotransformation, and elimination from the body. Essentially, it is the study of what the body does to a drug once the agent has been introduced into the system. The knowledge of this discipline is important to the anesthetist because the pharmacokinetics of drugs are a major factor in their onset, time course, offset, and variability of responses from patient to patient, as well as in the determination of the amount of drug available to act at the effect site. Pharmacokinetic concepts also play a vital role in the delivery of serum concentrations that will result in desired effects without untoward side effects.

Regardless of the route of administration, the vascular system delivers the drug to various tissues. Therefore most kinetic concepts revolve around assessment of blood level over time, even if the correlation with the amount of drug at the effector site is poor. Once in the blood, the drug can either remain within the vascular system and body water, bound to proteins, or cross membranes to enter tissues. The unbound drug enters organs, muscles, fat, and, of greatest importance, the site of activity—the receptors. This transfer of drug to various sites depends on several intrinsic properties of the agent, such as molecular size, degree of ionization, lipid solubility, and protein binding. In addition to these drug properties, uptake also depends on the amount of blood flow to the tissue and the concentration gradient of the drug across membranes.

PROPERTIES THAT INFLUENCE PHARMACOKINETIC ACTIVITY

Molecular Size
The smaller the molecular size of an agent, the better it crosses the lipid barriers and membranes of tissues. When a drug is administered, it must be absorbed across biologic membranes that have very small openings or pores. Generally, molecules with molecular weights greater than 100 to 200 do not cross the cell membranes. Transport across the membranes can occur passively or actively. Passive transport does not require energy and involves transfer of a drug from an area of high concentration to an area of lower concentration. Active transport mechanisms are generally faster and require energy. This transport system uses carriers that form complexes with drug molecules on the membrane surface and can involve movement of the drug molecule against a concentration gradient from an area of low concentration to an area of high concentration.[1] Figure 7-1 depicts the movement of a drug across cell membranes.

Degree of Ionization and Lipid Solubility
Most drugs are salts of either weak acids or weak bases. When introduced into the body, they behave as a chemical in solution. As acids or bases they exist in solutions in both ionized and un-ionized forms. The charged (ionized) form is water soluble, and the uncharged (nonionized) form is lipophilic. Because the nonionized molecules are lipid soluble, they can diffuse across cell membranes such as the blood-brain, gastric, and placental barriers to reach the effect site. On the other hand, the ionized molecules are usually unable to penetrate lipid cell membranes easily because of their low lipid solubility. This results from the electric charges exerted by the ionized drug molecules. These charged drugs are repelled by those sections of the cell membranes with similar charges, preventing their diffusion across the membrane.[1] The higher the degree of ionization, the less access the drug has across tissues such as the gastrointestinal tract, the blood-brain and placental barriers, and liver hepatocytes. This is important in that ionized drugs are not absorbed well when taken orally and may not be metabolized by the liver to a significant extent. Instead, they commonly are excreted via the renal system.[2]

Whether acidic or basic, the degree of ionization of an agent at a particular site is determined by the dissociation constant (pK_a) of the agent and its pH gradient across the membrane. The pK_a is the negative log of the equilibrium constant for the dissociation of the acid or base. The relationship between the pK_a of the drug and the pH of the solution may be expressed by two equations. The first equation applies to drugs that are basic in nature:

Equation 7-1

$$pK_a = pH = \log\frac{(HA^+)}{(A^-)}$$

The second equation applies to acidic drugs:

Equation 7-2

$$pK_a = pH = \log\frac{(A^-)}{(HA^+)}$$

From these equations an estimate of the degree of drug absorption can be developed.[2,3] Acids are usually defined as proton donors, whereas bases are made up of molecules that can accept a proton. When the pH is equal to the pK_a, the two species exist in equal amounts; for example, because phenobarbital has a pK_a of 7.4 and blood has a pH of 7.4, in the bloodstream the drug is present in equal proportions of charged and uncharged forms.

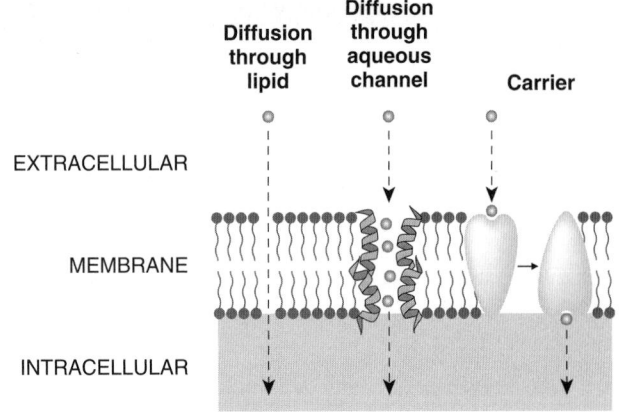

FIGURE **7-1** Routes by which solutes can traverse cell membranes. (*From Rang HP et al.* Pharmacology. *6th ed. Edinburgh: Churchill Livingstone; 2007.*)

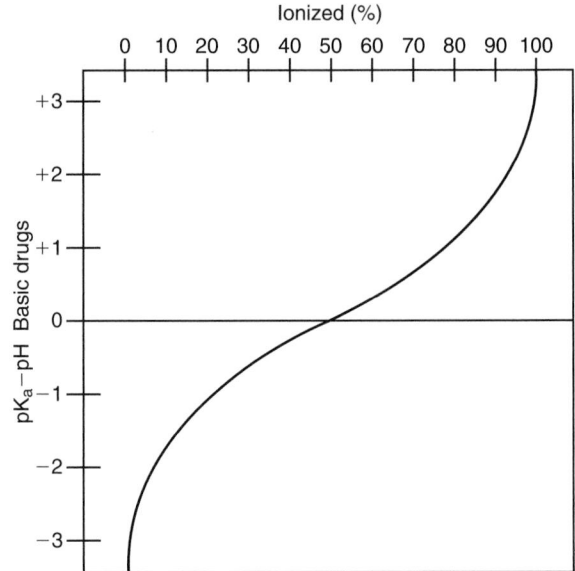

FIGURE **7-3** $pK_a - pH$ versus the percent ionized. The degree to which a basic drug remains in its nonionized state depends on the medium in which it is placed. pK_a is the dissociation constant (see text for further explanation).

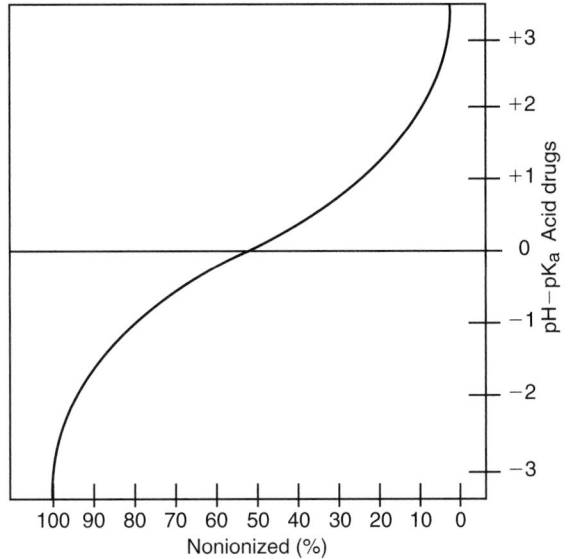

FIGURE **7-2** When acidic drugs are placed in physiologic solutions, the degree of nonionization is greater if the pH of the solution minus the pK_a of the drug ($pH - pK_a$) is less than zero. Conversely, when the $pH - pK_a$ is greater than zero, more of the drug exists in an ionized less absorbable form.

TABLE **7-1**	Relationship Between pH, pKa, and Ionization for Weak Acids and Weak Bases
Weak Base	
pH > pK_a	Un-ionized form predominates
pH = pK_a	Un-ionized equal to ionized
pH < pK_a	Ionized form predominates
Weak Acid	
pH > pK_a	Ionized form predominates
pH = pK_a	Un-ionized equal to ionized
pH < pK_a	Un-ionized form predominates

Modified with permission from Bovill JG, Howie MB. Clinical Pharmacology for Anaesthetists. *London: Saunders; 1999.*

It is of importance to note that relatively modest changes in the pH of the environment, when it is close to the pK, are more significant in changing the ratio of charged to uncharged forms than the same change in pH at some value far removed from the pK. For example, phenobarbital, with a pK of 7.4, is for the most part nondissociated and therefore is nonionized at a pH of 1.4. This results from the fact that the pH is well below the pK, and when phenobarbital is in a relatively strongly acidic environment with an abundance of protons, it does not give up its protons readily. If a drug is a weak acid and if the pH of the fluid environment is below the pK, most of the drug's protons are associated with the drug molecule, and the predominant species is uncharged and therefore lipid soluble (Figure 7-2). Conversely, if the pH is below the pK for a drug that is a weak base, an abundance of protons exists, and most of the drug tends to ionize as the proton is donated by the drug molecule, which results in a species that is highly charged and therefore lipid

insoluble[2] (Figure 7-3). The effects of pK_a and pH on ionization are summarized in Table 7-1.

Ion Trapping

Ion trapping has several anesthesia-related applications. Influences on oral absorption of drugs, maternal-fetal transfer, and central nervous system toxicity of local anesthetics are commonly cited. The degree of ionization for a specific agent can vary across a membrane that separates fluids with different pH values. For example, morphine sulfate, a base with a pK_a of 7.9 when present in the blood (pH 7.4), exists in appreciable amounts in both ionized and nonionized forms. The uncharged drug fraction moves freely across tissue membranes, and the charged fraction does not. As the drug enters the stomach, a very acidic environment with a pH of 1.9, morphine accepts protons and becomes ionized, and ion trapping occurs.[2] (Figure 7-4 illustrates this phenomenon using diazepam as an example.) The drug, however,

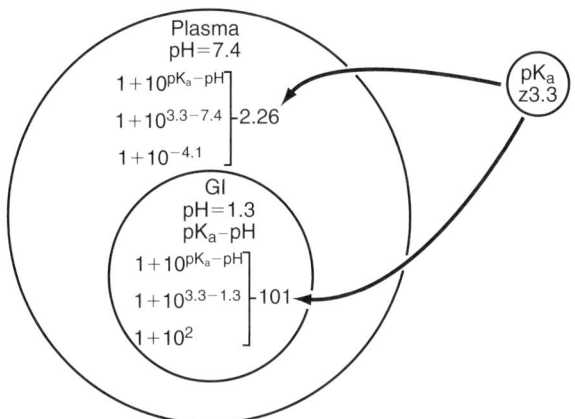

FIGURE **7-4** For both weak acids and weak bases, the total concentration of a drug is greater on the side of the membrane where it is more highly ionized. Diazepam, a basic drug with a pKa of 3.3, is more ionized at gastric pH than it is in plasma. Consequently it has a greater total concentration in the gastrointestinal compartment than it does in the plasma.

BOX **7-1**
Binding of Drugs to Plasma Proteins

- Plasma albumin is most important; β-globulin and α_1-acid glycoprotein also bind some drugs.
- Plasma albumin binds, for the most part, acidic drugs (approximately two molecules per albumin molecule). Basic drugs may be bound by β-globulin and α_1-acid glycoprotein.
- Saturable binding sometimes leads to a nonlinear relationship between dose and free (active) drug concentration.
- Extensive protein binding slows drug elimination (metabolism and excretion by glomerular filtration).
- Competition between drugs for protein binding rarely leads to clinically important drug interactions.

Modified with permission from Rang HP et al. Pharmacology. 6th ed. Edinburgh: Churchill Livingstone; 2007.

will be absorbed later, as stomach contents move farther down the gastrointestinal tract to the more basic and favorable environment of the small intestine.

A similar scenario occurs when agents are transferred between a mother and a fetus, where the placenta is the membrane separating fluids with varying pH values—that of the fetus is more acidic than that of the mother. Again, the lipid-soluble fraction of basic agents such as lidocaine (pK 7.9) crosses the placenta easily. However, once there, because of the lower pH of the fetus, the drug becomes more ionized and cannot easily cross the lipid bilayer of placenta, resulting in accumulation of drug in the fetus. Finally, ion trapping may occur in a local anesthetic overdose situation in which high concentrations of a basic local anesthetic agent have entered the central nervous system and caused toxicity. If the patient experiences respiratory arrest and hypoxia, the resulting acidosis may trap the drug in the brain, resulting in prolonged and possibly more intense toxicity. Ion trapping also plays a role in the use of bicarbonate solutions and carbonated local anesthetics. A discussion of the effects of ion trapping on local anesthetics can be found in Chapter 11, Box 11-2.

Protein Binding

Changes in protein binding have long been theorized to influence a drug's clinical effect. Two situations are commonly cited. The first involves a patient with a reduction in proteins, such as occurs with severe liver or kidney disease, with protein deficiencies caused by poor nutrition, and during the last trimester of pregnancy, when fluid shifts alter distribution volume. The second situation involves a drug interaction between two or more highly protein-bound drugs.

Potential clinical changes are conceptualized by the following phenomena. Some drugs are bound extensively to proteins in the plasma because of their innate affinity for the circulating and tissue proteins. The drug-protein molecule is too large to diffuse through blood vessel membranes and is therefore trapped within the circulatory system. Albumin is quantitatively the most abundant plasma protein, and although it is capable of binding basic, neutral, or acidic drugs, it favors acidic compounds. Two other proteins, α_1-acid glycoprotein (AAG) and β-globulin, favor binding to basic drugs.[4] Lipoproteins bind cyclosporine, and transcortin binds corticosteroids. Protein binding influences

how a drug is distributed, because protein-bound drug is not free to act on receptors. High protein binding prevents the drug from leaving the blood to enter into tissue, which results in high plasma concentrations. The degree of protein binding for a drug is proportional to its lipid solubility such that the more lipid soluble an agent, the more highly protein bound it tends to be.[5] See Box 7-1.

The number of potential binding sites on plasma proteins for drugs is finite; therefore the kinetics for binding behaves like any saturable process, in that protein binding can be overcome by adding more agent.[2] The bond between drug and protein is usually weak, and they can dissociate when the plasma concentration of the drug declines or a second drug that binds to the same protein is introduced. For example, when a drug has been in chronic use and is at steady state, an equilibrium will be reached between free and protein-bound drug. If a new drug with a high affinity for the same protein sites is introduced, the new drug competes with the chronic drug for binding sites. This leads to displacement of the first drug with an increase in free fraction of that agent. It is important to note that the displaced free drug does become available for biotransformation and elimination, so unless these clearance mechanisms are at capacity, a rise in free fraction will lead to a small change in free plasma concentrations.

Protein binding is expressed in terms of the percentage of total drug bound. Drugs with protein binding greater than 90%, such as warfarin, phenytoin, propranolol, propofol, fentanyl and its analogues, and diazepam, are conceptualized to have an unexpected intensification of their effect if they are displaced from plasma proteins.[6] Drugs that exhibit less than 90% binding have so little change in free active fractions that they are not a concern. The anticoagulant warfarin is commonly used as an example. Because warfarin is approximately 98% bound to plasma proteins, a reduction in bound fraction to 96% causes an increase in the free active fraction of the drug. Furthermore, when hypoalbuminemia exists, decreased albumin levels result in the availability of a greater amount of free drug. These theoretic concerns are rarely clinically relevant, as explained subsequently.

No clinically relevant examples of changes in drug disposition or effects can be clearly ascribed to changes in plasma protein binding. The idea that a drug displaced from plasma proteins increases the unbound drug concentration, increases the drug effect, and perhaps produces toxicity seems a simple and obvious mechanism. Unfortunately this simple theory, which is appropriate for a test tube, does not work in the body, which is an open system capable of eliminating unbound drug.

First, a seemingly dramatic change in the unbound fraction from 1% to 10% releases less than 5% of the total amount of drug in the body into the unbound pool because less than one third of the drug in the body is bound to plasma proteins, even in the most extreme cases (e.g., when warfarin is used). Drug displaced from plasma protein, of course, distributes throughout the volume of distribution, so a 5% increase in the amount of unbound drug in the body produces at most a 5% increase in pharmacologically active unbound drug at the site of action.

Second, when the amount of unbound drug in plasma increases, the rate of elimination increases (if unbound clearance is unchanged), and after four half-lives, the unbound concentration returns to its previous steady-state value. When drug interactions associated with protein binding displacement and clinically important effects have been studied, it has been found that the displacing drug is also an inhibitor of clearance, and it is the change in *clearance* of the *unbound* drug that is the relevant mechanism explaining the interaction.

The clinical application of plasma protein binding is only to help interpretation of measured drug concentrations. When plasma proteins are lower than normal, total drug concentrations are lowered, but unbound concentrations are not affected.[1]

Absorption

Routes of Drug Administration

An important variable in the bioavailability of drug at its effect site is the route by which the agent is administered. The route of administration determines how much of the drug is delivered to the systemic circulation. When the entire amount of drug given is delivered, the drug is said to have *100% bioavailability*. Many routes of drug administration are used; each has advantages and disadvantages (Table 7-2). The routes of drug administration are enteral (involves the gastrointestinal tract); parenteral (injected subcutaneously, intramuscularly, intravenously, intrathecally, or epidermally); pulmonary; and topical.[7] Absorption mechanisms of relevance to anesthesia are discussed in the following sections.

Enteral Administration. The oral route is the most common and convenient method for administration of drugs. It is relatively inexpensive, does not require sterile technique, and can be carried out with little skill. However, several disadvantages exist because many conditions—such as emotions, physical activity, and food intake—change the gastrointestinal environment. Therefore, orally administered drugs tend to have a lower bioavailability. The stomach has a large surface area, and the length of time a drug remains there is a significant factor in absorption. Because of the low pH in the stomach (1.5 to 2.5), drugs that are highly acidic, such as barbiturates, tend to remain nonionized and are highly absorbed. Basic drugs that remain intact in the stomach acids can pass through and are more readily absorbed in the intestine. The small intestine is highly vascular and has an alkaline environment (pH 7 to 8).[7]

The enteral route often results in failure of the drug to be absorbed into the systemic circulation. Alternatively, chemical alteration may occur before entry into the intestines. *Presystemic elimination* refers to the elimination of drug by the gastrointestinal system before the drug reaches the systemic circulation. This occurs by means of three mechanisms: the stomach acids hydrolyze the drug (e.g., penicillin); enzymes in the gastrointestinal wall deactivate the drug; or the liver biotransforms ingested drug before it reaches the effect site.[2] This liver activity is called *first-pass* hepatic effect. Drugs absorbed from the gastrointestinal tract after oral ingestion enter the portal venous blood and pass through the liver first, with subsequent delivery to the tissue receptors. In the liver they may undergo extensive hepatic extraction and metabolism before they have a chance to enter the systemic circulation (Box 7-2). Agents such as these exhibit large differences between oral and intravenous dosages. To have the desired effect, oral dosages must be exaggerated to

TABLE 7-2	Routes of Administration	
Route	**Bioavailability (%)**	**Comments**
Intravenous	100 (by definition)	Most rapid onset; allows for titration of doses; suitable for large volumes
Intramuscular	75 to 100	Moderate volumes feasible; may be painful
Subcutaneous	75 to 100	Smaller volumes than intramuscular; may be painful; suitable for implantation of pellets
Oral	5 to 100	Most convenient and economical; first-pass effect may be significant; requires patient cooperation
Rectal	30 to 100	Less first-pass effect than oral; useful in pediatric patients
Inhalation	5 to 100	Common anesthetic use for inhalation drugs, steroids, bronchodilators, and occasionally resuscitative drugs; very rapid onset (parallels intravenous administration)
Sublingual	60 to 100	Lack of first-pass effect; absorbed directly into systemic circulation
Intrathecal	Low (intentionally)	Specialized application, as with local anesthetics and analgesics, chemotherapy, and antibiotic administration; circumvents blood-brain barrier
Topical	80 to 100	Includes skin, cornea, buccal, vagina, and nasal mucosa; dermal application results in slow absorption; used for lack of first-pass effect; prolonged duration of action

compensate for the initial metabolism that occurs before the drug reaches the effect site.

The role transporters play in drug absorption and distribution should be further clarified. P-glycoprotein transporter is part of a larger family of efflux transporters found in the intestine, liver cells, renal proximal tubular cells, and capillary endothelial cells comprising the blood-brain barrier. Using ATP as an energy source, they transport substances against their concentration gradients. They appear to have developed as a mechanism to protect the body from harmful substances and can influence the ability of a drug to traverse barriers.

The sublingual and buccal routes of administration of drugs bypass the presystemic, portal system first-pass effect and are delivered rapidly to the superior vena cava for transport to the effect site.[1] Nitroglycerin is an example of a sublingual drug that is put under the tongue and absorbed by the rich blood supply there. If ingested, the drug would be hydrolyzed by the stomach; therefore sublingual administration is the ideal route for this agent. Protein hormones that would also be digested by the stomach are instead placed between the gum and cheek (buccal administration) and enter venous drainage without undergoing hepatic, presystemic elimination.[8,9]

Occasionally the rectal route of drug administration is the ideal route for prevention of emesis caused by irritation of the gastrointestinal mucosa by the drug. It is also a preferred method of drug delivery for patients in whom oral ingestion poses difficulty. For example, rectal acetaminophen is administered to infants and young children undergoing general anesthesia for postoperative pain control. Drugs placed in the proximal rectum are absorbed into the portal system via the superior hemorrhoidal vein. They will therefore undergo significant first-pass effect in the liver before entering the systemic circulation, leading to unpredictable responses.[1] Conversely, agents placed in the distal rectum do not undergo presystemic elimination and therefore have more predictable circulatory levels. The disadvantage historically associated with this route was the unpredictability of drug retention and absorption because of rectal contents. However, more recent studies have demonstrated that regardless of enema volume, agents are absorbed with consistent plasma concentrations within subjects.[10]

Parenteral Administration. *Parenteral administration* refers to administration by injection. The most rapid and predictable route to the systemic circulation is the parenteral route. With intramuscular injections, the drug is instilled deep into the muscle among the muscle fascicles.[2] Subcutaneous agents are placed under the skin. With both intramuscular and subcutaneous injections, the systemic absorption of the drug is dependent on the capillary blood flow to the area and the lipid solubility of the agent.[1] Conversely, intravenous injections allow for rapid and accurate delivery of drug into the systemic circulation. Parenteral administration is the route of choice for anesthetists, as it is an exact method of achieving the desired effect from agents delivered.

Pulmonary Administration. The lungs provide a large surface area for drugs administered by inhalation. Bronchodilators and antibiotics are administered via devices such as nebulizers, used to propel aerosols into the alveolar sacs.[10] Anesthetic gases are also effectively administered through the lungs, as described in detail in Chapter 8.

Transdermal (Topical) Administration. The transdermal route is usually chosen for administration of a sustained release agent, providing the patient with a steady therapeutic plasma concentration. Drugs that are administered via this route must possess several characteristics. They usually exist in a combined form—both water soluble and lipid soluble. The water solubility is necessary so the drug can penetrate the hair follicles and sweat ducts. Once in the system, the drug must be lipid soluble to traverse the skin and exert effect at the receptors. These agents must have a molecular weight of less than 1000, dose requirements less than 10 mg in a 24-hour period, and a pH of 5 to 9.[1] The area to which the drug is applied must have a relatively thin epidermis with a sufficient blood supply (Figure 7-5).

Bioavailability

Bioavailability is the extent to which a drug reaches its effect site after its introduction into the circulatory system. The rate at which systemic absorption occurs establishes a drug's duration of action and intensity. Many factors play a role in the bioavailability of agents, including lipid solubility, solubility in aqueous and organic solvents, molecular weight, pH, pK_a, and blood flow. For example, drugs given in aqueous solution are more rapidly absorbed than those given in oily solution or solid form because they mix more readily with the aqueous phase at the absorptive site.[11,12] A recent study demonstrated that propofol in the form of a water-soluble prodrug is metabolized to propofol with a longer half-life, increased volume of distribution, delayed onset, and greater potency.[13]

The environment into which the drug is introduced also has an impact on its bioavailability. The patient's age, sex, pathology, pH, blood flow, and temperature are all factors to consider. For example, pH plays a role when local anesthetic (a weak base) is injected into an infected wound (an acidic environment). In this instance, the local anesthetic is highly ionized (basic agent in acidic environment) and therefore cannot enter the lipid nerve membrane to reach the site of action. Some important concepts influencing absorption are listed in Box 7-3.

Distribution

Compartment Models. Compartment models depict the body as composed of distinct sections that represent theoretic spaces with calculated volumes and are used to describe the pharmacokinetics of agents. These models are useful for prediction of serum concentrations and changes in drug concentrations in other tissues. A single-compartment model represents the entire body, through which homogeneous distribution occurs (Figure 7-6A). Although a one-compartment model is sufficient to describe the

---

BOX **7-2**
Examples of Drugs That Undergo Substantial First-Pass Elimination
Aspirin Glyceryl trinitrate Isosorbide dinitrate Levodopa Lidocaine Metoprolol Morphine Propranolol Salbutamol Verapamil

Modified with permission from Rang HP et al. Pharmacology. 6th ed. Edinburgh: Churchill Livingstone; 2007.

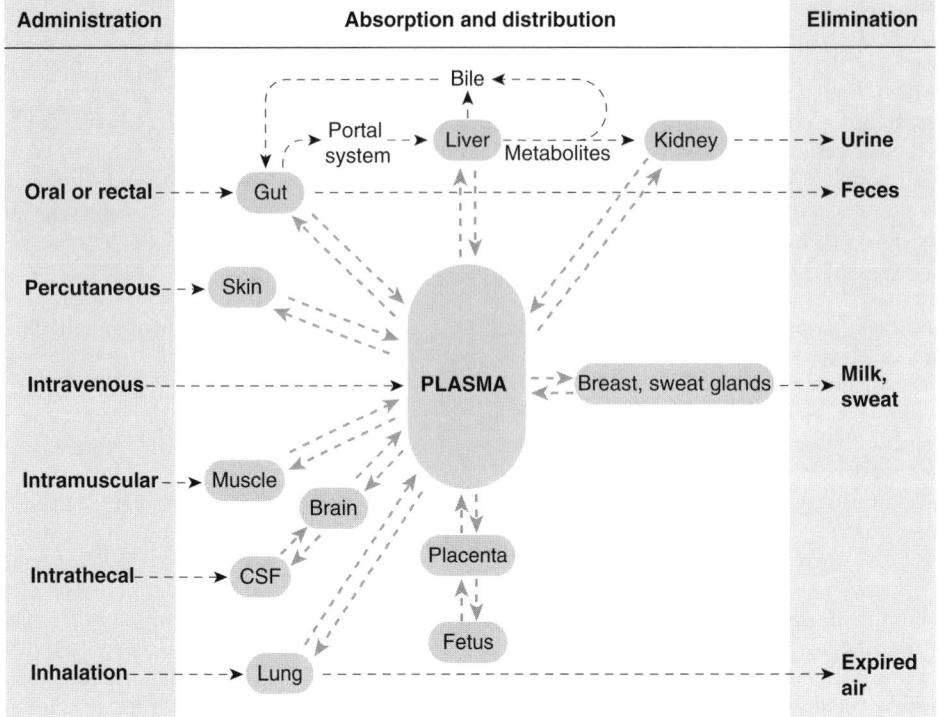

FIGURE **7-5** The main routes of drug administration and elimination. (*From Rang HP et al. Pharmacology. 6th ed. Edinburgh: Churchill Livingstone; 2007.*)

Movement of Drugs Across Cellular Barriers

- To traverse cellular barriers (e.g., gastrointestinal mucosa, renal tubule, blood-brain barrier, placenta), drugs must cross lipid membranes.
- Drugs cross lipid membranes mainly by passive diffusional transfer or by carrier-mediated transfer.
- The main factors that determine the rate of passive diffusional transfer across membranes are a drug's lipid solubility and the concentration gradient. Molecular weight is a less important factor.
- Drugs are weak acids or weak bases; their state of ionization varies with pH according to the Henderson-Hasselbalch equation.
- With weak acids or bases, only the uncharged species (the protonated form for a weak acid; the unprotonated form for a weak base) can diffuse across lipid membranes; this gives rise to pH partition or ion trapping.
- The term *pH partition* refers to the fact that weak acids tend to accumulate in compartments of relatively high pH, whereas weak bases tend to leave compartments of high pH.
- Carrier-mediated transport (e.g., in the renal tubule, blood-brain barrier, gastrointestinal epithelium) is important for some drugs that are chemically related to endogenous substances.
- Drugs of very low lipid solubility, including those that are strong acids or bases, are generally poorly absorbed from the gut.
- A few drugs (e.g., levodopa) are absorbed by carrier-mediated transfer.
- Absorption from the gut depends on many factors, including the following:
  - Gastrointestinal motility
  - Gastrointestinal pH
  - Particle size
  - Physicochemical interaction with gut contents (e.g., chemical interaction between calcium and tetracycline antibiotics)
- Bioavailability is the fraction of an ingested dose of a drug that gains access to the systemic circulation. It may be low because absorption is incomplete or because the drug is metabolized in the gut wall or liver before reaching the systemic circulation.
- Bioequivalence implies that if one formulation of a drug is substituted for another, no clinically untoward consequences will ensue.

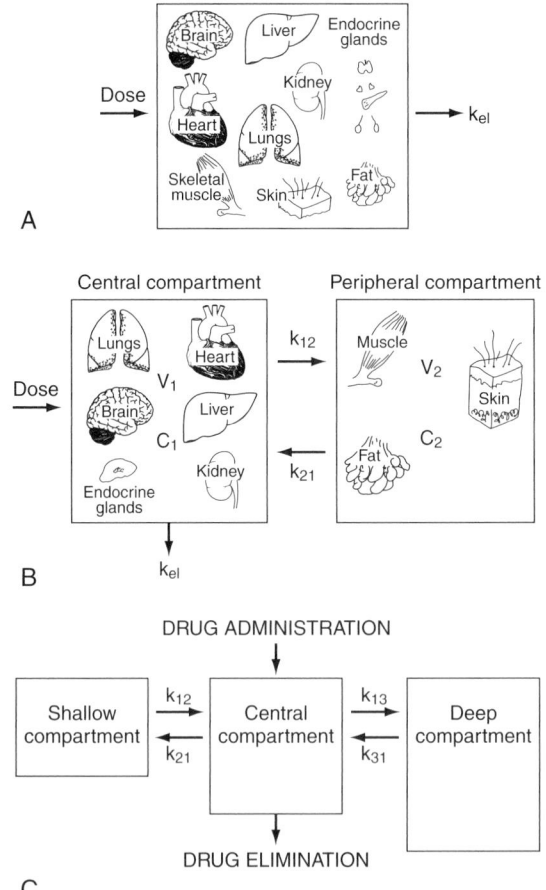

TABLE 7-3	Tissue Groups Based on Perfusion*			
Characteristic	**Vessel Rich**	**Muscle**	**Fat**	**Vessel Poor**
Percentage of body weight	10	50	20	20
Percentage of cardiac output	75	19	6	0
Perfusion (mL/min/100 g)	75	3	3	0

The vessel-rich group represents the central compartment, and the muscle, fat, and vessel-poor groups are peripheral compartments.

FIGURE 7-6 **A,** In the one-compartment model, a drug instantaneously and homogeneously is distributed throughout the fluids and tissues that constitute the compartment. When changes in drug concentration occur in any of these tissues, a corresponding quantitative change occurs in drug concentration in all the other tissues. **B,** In the two-compartment model, the body is assumed to be made up of two compartments: a central compartment (C_1) made up of a small apparent volume (V_1) and a peripheral compartment (C_2) made up of a larger apparent volume (V_2). **C,** The three-compartment model is depicted as having a central compartment into which the drug is administered and two peripheral compartments to which reversible drug distribution occurs. k_{12}, Rate of distribution of drugs to the peripheral compartment; k_{21}, rate of redistribution of drugs back to the central compartment; k_{el}, rate of drug removal or elimination from the body; k_{13}, rate of distribution of drugs from the central compartment to a shallow peripheral compartment; k_{31}, rate of distribution of drugs from the shallow peripheral compartment back to the central compartment (see text for further explanation).

action of many drugs, it is generally insufficient to explain the kinetics of lipid-soluble anesthetic drugs. A two-compartment model is typically used to simplify and explain pharmacokinetic concepts that can be extrapolated to more complex models.[14]

In the two-compartment model, the first compartment is termed the *central compartment* and is composed of intravascular fluid and the highly perfused tissues such as the heart, lungs, brain, liver, and kidneys (see Figure 7-6B). The central compartment represents only approximately 10% of body mass in an adult; however, it receives approximately 75% of the cardiac output and is also referred to as the *vessel-rich group*. The peripheral compartment (vessel-poor group) is composed of muscle, fat, and bone and represents 90% of body mass. This second compartment

receives approximately 25% of the cardiac output.[14] The terms *central* and *peripheral compartments* refer to differences in the size of the compartments and the rate at which a drug is distributed to them. In reality, the compartments are not true anatomic areas but conceptual representation of two separate volumes in which a quantitative change in drug concentration occurs.[15]

Drugs leave the central compartment in two phases. Drugs leave by distribution into the tissues or via metabolism and excretion. In the initial phase, after an intravenous bolus dose, those organs with the highest blood flow have the largest amount of drug delivered to them. These highly perfused tissues equilibrate with the initial high serum concentration and attain a high concentration of drug (Table 7-3). As blood flows through the less perfused organs, the drug begins to be deposited in those tissues as well.[11] However, the tissue levels rise more slowly and do not reach as high a concentration as in the vessel-rich group or central compartment, with extraction occurring to a lesser degree. As blood flows through the tissues, serum concentrations drop because of this distribution, and the fall in plasma concentration is described mathematically via the alpha half-life.[16] When the plasma concentration falls below the tissue concentration, the drug reemerges from the highly perfused tissue, enters the plasma serum, and is again redistributed. The drug enters the central compartment for clearance from the body. The degree to which drugs distribute and redistribute from the central compartment to the peripheral compartment, and the resultant concentration of the drug established before elimination occurs, allow for the calculation of the volume of distribution.

Volume of Distribution
The volume of distribution is a proportional expression that relates the amount of drug in the body to the serum concentration. It is the apparent volume in which the drug is distributed after it has been introduced into the system.[1] Essentially it is calculated by dividing the dose of the drug administered intravenously by the plasma concentration before elimination occurs. The volume of distribution is used to calculate the loading dose of a drug that will achieve a steady-state concentration.[14] In practice, a patient's volume of distribution is unknown, and an average volume of distribution is assumed and used to calculate a loading dose that will attain a therapeutic concentration rather than a steady-state concentration.

Equation 7-3

$$\text{Volume of distribution} = \frac{\text{Dose of drug}}{\text{Plasma concentration of drug}}$$

The volume of distribution is an independent variable and enables calculation of a loading dose if the desired plasma concentration is known. The volume of distribution is also of relevance in the drug's elimination from the body because drugs can be eliminated only by the body's organs of elimination, such as the kidneys and liver. Therefore a drug with a large volume of distribution has very low concentrations in the plasma, and very little drug would be available to the organs for elimination.[1]

The volume of distribution of a drug is affected by the physiochemical properties of that drug, such as lipid solubility, plasma protein binding, and molecular size.[2] Drugs that are free, unbound to plasma proteins, and lipid soluble easily cross membranes to tissues and therefore have large calculated volumes of distribution with low plasma concentrations. An example of a drug with a large volume of distribution is thiopental.[1] On injection of an induction dose, this highly lipid-soluble drug is distributed quickly to peripheral tissue, thereby ending its action much more rapidly than its elimination half-life would predict. The patient wakes up in just a few minutes because of redistribution from the brain (central compartment) to the peripheral compartment; however, the patient may feel sleepy for hours because of the long elimination half-life of the drug from the whole body (11.6 hours).[2]

The volume of distribution of a drug administered by bolus is also calculated by dividing the total dose administered by the area under the plasma concentration curve. The greater the area under the curve, the longer the drug acts and the drug intensity increases.[2] However, if the drug is infused or given in multiple doses and the amount given equals the amount eliminated, the central and peripheral compartments are in equilibrium. Therefore the volume of distribution at this steady state would differ if the agent were given as a bolus injection.[3]

Structure-Activity Relationship

The affinity of a drug for a specific macromolecular component of the cell and its intrinsic activity are intimately related to its chemical structure.[17] The relationship is frequently quite a rigid one, in that relatively minor modifications in the drug structure may result in major changes in pharmacologic properties. In fact, manipulation of structure-activity relationships often leads to the synthesis of therapeutic agents quite varied in their therapeutic effects, as well as their side effects. Changes in molecular configuration must occur in a manner that leads to alterations of all actions and effects of a drug equally. Therefore, it is sometimes possible to develop a congener with a more favorable ratio of therapeutic to toxic effects, enhanced selectivity among different cells or tissues, or more acceptable secondary characteristics than those of the parent drug.[17] Additionally, effective therapeutic agents have been developed by cultivating structurally related competitive antagonists of other drugs or of endogenous substances known to be important in biochemical or physiologic

function. Minor modifications of structure can also have profound effects on the pharmacokinetic properties of drugs. The structure of a drug can therefore occasionally supersede all of the above properties discussed and is of great importance in how a drug behaves in vivo. Important considerations in structure-activity relationships are enantiomerism and isomerism.

Stereochemistry

A carbon-containing compound usually exists as stereoisomers-molecules with the same chemical bonds but different configurations in their fixed spatial arrangements.[18] A specific configuration is achieved by either the presence of double bonds, where there is no freedom of rotation, or by chiral centers, around which varying groups are arranged in a specific sequence.[18] Chiral centers are therefore formed by a carbon atom with four different asymmetric substituents. A molecule with one chiral carbon can have two stereoisomers; however, as the number of carbons in a molecule increases, so does the number of its potential stereoisomers. Some stereoisomers are non-superimposable mirror images of each other called *enantiomers*. Free rotation about a chiral carbon is not possible, resulting in the existence of two stable forms of the molecule. These concepts become important in that interactions between biomolecules are stereospecific, and interface with biologic receptors can differ greatly between two enantiomers, even to the point of no binding. There are numerous examples among drug molecules in which only one isomer exhibits the desired pharmacology. Some isomers may even cause side effects or entirely different effects than their mirror image.[17] For instance, D(−) ephedrine, with a relative potency of 36, is used to a large extent as an antiasthmatic and, by an anesthesia professional, as a pressor amine to restore low blood pressure in the operating arena, whereas L(+) pseudoephedrine, with a relative potency of 7, is used primarily as a nasal decongestant (Figure 7-7). These drugs therefore have varying activities as well as potencies, rendering them ideal for varying situations. Cisatracurium, levobupivacaine, and ropivacaine are additional examples of select isomers with improved clinical properties.

Plasma Concentration Curve

A schematic depiction of the decline in plasma concentration of a drug with time after rapid intravenous injection into the central compartment is plotted on a logarithmic graph in Figure 7-8. The y-axis of the graph represents the plasma concentration, and the x-axis reflects the time after the dose is injected. The first phase of the curve is the α phase, or the distribution phase, which represents the initial dispersal of drug into the tissue compartments from the central compartment. This slope is usually steep with drugs that are highly lipid soluble, which demonstrates the ability of these agents to cross membrane

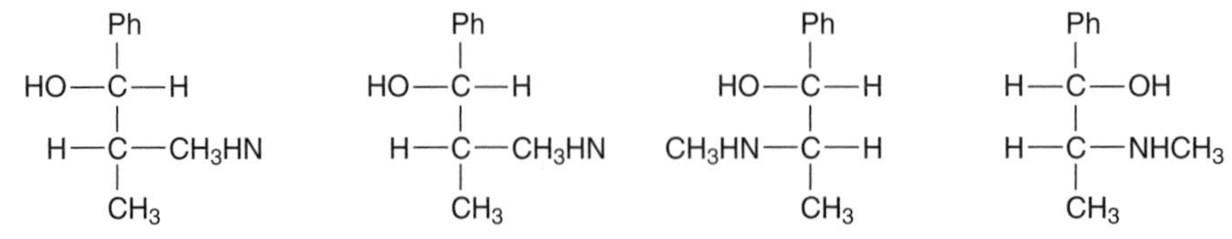

FIGURE **7-7**   Ephedrine has two chiral centers and four isomers with varying potencies.

lipid bilayers and be distributed to the peripheral compartment rapidly, leading to a rapid fall in plasma levels.[1]

The second phase of the curve is a logarithmic plot of the slower elimination, or β, phase of the plasma concentration curve. Once equilibrium has been reached, the concentration falls exponentially because of elimination. This portion of the graph is much less steep and has a plateau shape, illustrating the more gradual decline in the drug's plasma concentration. The slope is flatter because it reflects the elimination of the drug from the circulation by the hepatic, renal, and other systems, which is a more gradual process. The plasma concentration curve is an example of a biexponential decay curve, because

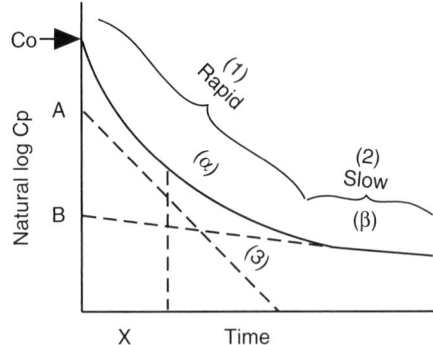

FIGURE **7-8**   The plot of the natural log of drug concentration. For drugs that conform to the two-compartment model, the plot of the natural log of the drug concentration is not linear along its entire length. Rather, it is curvilinear. The initial segment *(1)*, which represents the decline in drug concentration, is parabolic, then linear *(2)*. This decline in the drug concentration is also described as *biphasic*—a rapid phase, representing distribution (3), and a slow phase, representing elimination. The slope of the slow phase *(2)* is determined in a manner similar to that used for the elimination rate constant, k_{el}, in the one-compartment model.

two distinct components of decay exist—a steep slope that describes distribution and a second, less steep slope that depicts the elimination phase.[2]

The elimination phase of the plot is used to determine the elimination half-life of drugs, which becomes important with regard to dosing intervals.

Steady State

Theoretically, a steady state occurs when a stable plasma concentration of a drug is achieved. In this instance, all body compartments will have had ample opportunity to equilibrate with the circulating agent, and although tissue concentrations of the drug vary from organ to organ, they are not changing. At this point, drug elimination is equal to the rate at which the drug is made available, so the amount being eliminated in a given time equals the amount being added to the system at the same time.[19] This state is typically reached with chronic administration of a drug or by continuous intravenous administration. Some important distribution concepts are listed in Box 7-4.

Metabolism

Drug *metabolism* is synonymous with drug *biotransformation*. Metabolism is an enzyme-catalyzed change in the chemical structure of agents, and it usually involves more than one pathway. The main organ for drug metabolism is the liver, although metabolism can occur in the plasma, lungs, gastrointestinal tract, kidneys, heart, brain, and skin. The goal of metabolism is to change lipid-soluble agents into more water-soluble forms so the kidneys can then eliminate them from the body. Metabolism usually leads to transformation of active drugs into inactive metabolites; however, numerous consequences can occur. For example, a drug can be metabolized to an active drug with the same or new activity, or an agent can be converted from an inactive prodrug to its active form, as occurs with the metabolism of inactive enalapril to active enalaprilat. A new formulation of propofol, Aquavan, is

---

BOX **7-4**

Drug Distribution

The major compartments are as follows:
- Plasma (5% of body weight)
- Interstitial fluid (16%)
- Intracellular fluid (35%)
- Transcellular fluid (2%)
- Fat (20%)
- Volume of distribution (V_d) is defined as the volume of plasma that would contain the total body content of the drug at a concentration equal to that in the plasma.
- Water-soluble drugs are mainly confined to plasma and interstitial fluids; most do not enter the brain after acute dosing.
- Lipid-soluble drugs reach all compartments and may accumulate in fat.
- For drugs that accumulate outside the plasma compartment (e.g., in fat, or by being bound to tissues) V_d may exceed total body volume.
- For many drugs, disappearance from the plasma follows an exponential time course characterized by the plasma half-life.

- Plasma half-life, in the simple case, is directly proportional to the volume of distribution and inversely proportional to the overall rate of clearance.
- With repeated dosage or sustained delivery of a drug, the plasma concentration approaches a steady value within 4 or 5 plasma half-lives. Elimination of a drug also takes 4 or 5 half-lives.
- A two-compartment model is often needed. In this case the kinetics are biexponential. The two components roughly represent the processes of transfer between plasma and tissues or distribution (α phase) and elimination from the plasma (β phase).
- Some drugs show nonexponential "saturation" kinetics, with important clinical consequences, especially a disproportionate increase in steady-state plasma concentration when the dose is increased.

Modified with permission from Rang HP et al. Pharmacology. 6th ed. Edinburgh: Churchill Livingstone; 2007.

a prodrug that is converted by hydrolysis in the plasma by alkaline phosphatases to free propofol.[15]

For most drugs administered in therapeutic doses, metabolism occurs as a first-order process, in that the drug is cleared at a rate proportional to the amount of drug present in the plasma. Thus a constant fraction of total drug is metabolized in a set time period. The greatest amount of drug eliminated per unit time occurs when the concentration is highest.[20]

Drugs such as alcohol undergo zero-order kinetics at therapeutic doses. This means that even at therapeutic levels, they exceed the body's ability to excrete or metabolize them. In zero-order kinetics the available enzyme systems for elimination of drugs are saturated. For these agents a constant amount of drug is cleared regardless of the plasma concentration, as opposed to a constant percentage as occurs with first-order kinetics. The amount of agent cleared per unit time during zero-order kinetics is the same amount, independent of its plasma concentration.

Drug metabolism occurs in two phases. Phase I reactions are oxidation, reduction, and hydrolysis reactions and generally result in increased polarity of the molecule, transforming a lipid-soluble compound to a water-soluble one. Phase II reactions involve conjugation reactions, in which a drug or metabolite is conjugated with endogenous substrate such as glucuronic, sulfonic, or acetic acid.

Phase I Reactions

Oxidation reactions generally are reactions in which oxygen is introduced into the molecule or the oxidative state of a molecule is changed so that its relative oxygen content is increased. The molecule of oxygen is split; one atom oxidizes each molecule of drug, and the other is incorporated into a molecule of water. The loss of electrons results in oxidation. Oxidative metabolism reactions are catalyzed by the enzymes of the cytochrome P-450 system.[21] Reduction pathways of metabolism also use the cytochrome P-450 system. When insufficient amounts of oxygen are present to compete for electrons, these enzymes transfer electrons directly to a substrate rather than to oxygen. Reduction involves the gain of electrons.[22]

Hydrolysis is the addition of water to an ester or amide to break the bond and form two smaller molecules. Adding water to these compounds leads to an acid and alcohol, in the case of esters, and to an acid and an amine, in the case of amides. Amide drugs rarely undergo hydrolysis, even though they are formed by removing water. Steric hindrance limits the ability to add water to a drug (hydrolyze it) once the water has been removed. Examples of drugs that are hydrolyzed are listed in Box 7-5.

The end result of phase I reactions is typically a more polar compound that is easily excreted by the kidneys. It is also important to note that phase I reactions, by placing hydroxy or carboxy groups on drug molecules, enable phase II reactions to occur.[1]

Phase II Reactions

Phase II reactions are also referred to as *synthetic reactions* because the body actually synthesizes a new compound by donating a functional group usually derived from an endogenous acid. The new compound is the conjugate of the drug or the drug product of the phase I reaction with either glucuronic acid, sulfuric acid, glycine, acetic acid, or a methyl group.[19]

The products of phase II reactions almost always have little or no biologic activity. Conjugation always leads to a more polar compound that is more highly ionized at physiologic pH and therefore more easily extractable by the kidney via glomerular filtration. The conjugation proceeds by joining the body's donated group (during phase I reactions) with an OH, COOH,

---

BOX 7-5

Common Anesthesia-Related Drugs That Undergo Phase 1 Hydrolysis

Cholinesterase Catalyzed	Not Esterase Dependent
Succinylcholine	Remifentanil
Cocaine	Atracurium (partial pathway)
Procaine	Cisatracurium (partial pathway)
Chloroprocaine	Esmolol
Tetracaine	Aspirin
Neostigmine (partial pathway)	
Pyridostigmine (partial pathway)	
Edrophonium (partial pathway)	

---

or NH group to form an ester or amide bond. However, many drugs already possess an appropriate functional group for conjugation and therefore do not need to be modified by a prior phase I reaction in order to be conjugated.

Many intracellular sites exist for drug metabolizing enzymes, such as the endoplasmic reticulum, mitochondria, cytosol, lysosomes, and plasma membrane. Hepatic microsomal enzymes, responsible for biotransformation of numerous agents, reside mainly in the smooth hepatic endoplasmic reticulum. They are termed *microsomal enzymes* because microsomes are fragments of the endoplasmic reticulum that are obtained in vitro by physical disruption of the tissue and differential centrifugation. This microsomal fraction includes proteins called *cytochrome* (iron-containing hemoprotein) *P-450*, indicating its peak absorption at 450 nm, when it reacts with carbon monoxide. The cytochrome P-450 is also called the *mixed-function oxidase system* because it includes both oxidation and reduction steps and has low substrate specificity.[2] Some extrahepatic sites of the P-450 system exist, such as the kidneys, lungs, skin, and intestinal mucosa.

Six well-characterized forms, or isozymes, of the cytochrome P-450 system are involved in drug metabolism in humans: CYP1A2, CYP2D6, CYP2C19, CYP2E1, CYP2C9, and CYP3A.[23] The letters *CYP* stand for cytochrome P-450; the first number denotes genetic family, the next letter describes the genetic subfamily, and the second number stands for the specific gene or isozyme.

It is important to note some characteristics of these isozymes. It should be appreciated that small differences in amino acid sequences of the different isozymes lead to differences in drug metabolism and account for genetic variability among individuals' abilities to metabolize agents.[23] Therefore hepatic enzyme activity varies among individuals and is determined genetically. Genetic variability exists in the expression of CYP2C19, CYP2C9, and CYP2D6. It is possible to increase enzyme activity by stimulating the enzymes over a period of time. This is called *enzyme induction* and is usually produced by exposure to certain drug or chemical compounds. Alcohol is one such compound; when ingested chronically it induces enzymatic activity. The system can more quickly break down agents that use the same enzymatic system for biotransformation. Other drugs capable of enzyme induction include phenobarbital, phenytoin, rifampin, and carbamazepine. This increased capacity to clear drugs leads to reduction in half-lives of agents and is important with regard to dosing intervals.[24,25]

Microsomal enzymes also can be inhibited. This usually occurs through exposure to certain drugs and chemicals, leading to accumulation of the substrate agent, and can cause elevated plasma levels and potentially greater activity and toxicity. For example, erythromycin inhibits the metabolism of theophylline, and cimetidine inhibits metabolism of many drugs.[23] Box 7-6 contains a summary of important metabolic concepts. A list of cytochrome enzymes, metabolites, inducers, and inhibitors is given in Table 7-4.

Drug Elimination
Elimination Half-Life
The elimination half-life (t½) is the time necessary for the plasma content of a drug to drop to half of its prevailing concentration after a rapid bolus injection. It takes the same amount of time to reduce a drug's concentration from 100 to 50 mg/L as it does to decrease the concentration from 10 to 5 mg/L. The amount of drug remaining in the body is related to the number of elimination half-lives that have elapsed (Table 7-5). For practical purposes, a drug is regarded as being fully eliminated when approximately 95% has been eliminated from the body. This usually occurs when four or five half-lives have elapsed and is important with regard to dosing intervals because drug accumulation occurs if dosing intervals are shorter than this. The body has not been able to rid itself of the initial dose, and subsequent doses will lead to overdose and potential adverse effects. Instances can occur in which, although only 5% of the drug amount remains, it is still somewhat active; however, for the majority of agents, four half-lives is considered sufficient time for the drug's action to be terminated and the agent eliminated from the body. As noted earlier, most drugs leave the body at a constant rate or percentage over time. This is referred to as *first-order kinetics* or *dosage independence* and is the reason why half-life is constant. Other elimination rate kinetic models include zero-order (e.g., alcohol) elimination, in which a constant amount (not a percentage) is eliminated over time, and Michaelis-Menton models (e.g., phenytoin), which are dose dependent and follow zero order at high doses and first order once drug levels have fallen.[2]

BOX **7-6**

Drug Metabolism

- Phase I reactions involve oxidation, reduction, and hydrolysis—usually form more chemically reactive products; sometimes pharmacologically active, as with thiopental; toxic or carcinogenic
- Phase II reactions are conjugation (e.g., glucuronidation) of a reactive group (often inserted during phase I reaction) and usually form inactive and readily excretable products
- Some conjugated products are excreted via bile, are reactivated in the intestine, and then reabsorbed
- Induction of enzymes by other drugs and chemicals can greatly accelerate hepatic drug metabolism
- Some drugs show rapid "first-pass" hepatic metabolism and therefore poor oral bioavailability

Modified with permission from Rang HP et al. Pharmacology. *6th ed. Edinburgh: Churchill Livingstone; 2007.*

Context-Sensitive Half-Time
Deficiencies in the use of standard pharmacokinetic parameters such as half-life when describing anesthetic drug administration have led to a proposal for the introduction of a new model that accounts for continuous infusion or repeated dosing-induced changes in drug behavior.[26] Context-sensitive half-time was developed through use of computer simulations of typical anesthetic dosing practices to provide a more clinically relevant measure of drug concentrations, taking into consideration the method and duration of administration.[27] It is defined as the time to halving of the blood concentration after termination of drug administration by an infusion designed to maintain a constant concentration. It is believed that through incorporation of the effect compartment, the context-sensitive half-time of the pharmacodynamic effect can be modeled.[28] A flaw in the concept is that it describes only the time to a 50% decrease in central compartment concentration, which may not be the decrement in drug level required to achieve recovery.[29] Whether context-sensitive half-time is a useful secondary kinetic descriptor may await its more widespread application.

Clearance
The clearance of a drug is an independent value and is governed by the properties of the drug and the body's capacity to eliminate it. It is defined as the volume of plasma completely cleared of drug by metabolism and excretion per unit of time. Clearance is directly proportional to the dose and inversely related to the agent's half-life as well as its concentration in the central compartment. Clearance is a very important pharmacokinetic concept, because it influences the steady-state concentration for a given drug administered at repeated intervals or by infusion.

The two main organs for clearance are the liver and kidneys. The rate of clearance is determined by the blood flow to these organs, as well as by their ability to extract the drug from the bloodstream. Mathematically, clearance is equal to the product of the blood flow (Q) and extraction ratio (E):

Equation 7-4
$$\text{Clearance} = Q \times E$$

Total clearance is the sum of all organs' clearance values. The changes in clearance occur when blood flow to the liver or kidney is altered or when their extraction ratios are changed.

Hepatic Clearance. Drugs typically go through perfusion-dependent elimination or capacity-dependent elimination in the liver. Drugs that have a high extraction ratio of 0.7 or greater rely heavily on the perfusion of the liver to be cleared. These drugs are referred to as *high-clearance drugs*. Examples of high-clearance drugs are verapamil, morphine, and lidocaine. Hepatic blood flow for these agents far outweighs enzymatic activity in clearing them from the body, so a decrease in hepatic blood flow decreases the rate of clearance, and a high perfusion state leads to faster clearance. This is termed *perfusion-dependent* elimination.[1]

Capacity-dependent elimination occurs with agents that possess a low extraction ratio of 0.3 or lower. When a low extraction rate exists, only a small fraction of the agent is removed per unit time, and changes in hepatic perfusion do not have significant effect on hepatic clearance. Clearance of these drugs depends on hepatic enzymes and the degree of protein binding. Therefore alterations such as enzyme induction or suppression cause a change in the elimination of these drugs from the body. An increase in enzyme activity causes faster elimination from the body, and enzyme suppression has the opposite outcome. A decrease in protein binding (increase in availability of drug

TABLE 7-4	List of Cytochrome Enzymes, Metabolites, Inducers, and Inhibitors		
Isozyme	Metabolic Substrates	Inducers	Inhibitors
CYP1A2	Theophylline—has a narrow therapeutic range, so inhibition of its metabolism can lead to toxic levels Imipramine Propranolol Clozapine	Tobacco smoke—smokers may require higher doses of these drugs because their metabolism is increased	Ciprofloxacin Erythromycin
CYP2C19—absent in 20%-30% of Asians, who therefore need a reduced dose when these drugs are administered	Diazepam Phenytoin Omeprazole (proton pump inhibitor for ulcers)		Omeprazole Ketoconazole (antifungal agent) Isoniazid
CYP2C9—absent in approximately 1% of Caucasians	NSAIDs COX II inhibitors Warfarin Phenytoin		Fluconazole
CYP2D6—absent in approximately 7% of Caucasians; hyperactive in approximately 30% of East Africans (Ethiopians) because they have multiple copies of the gene	Codeine → morphine Some β-blockers Some tricyclic antidepressants		Fluoxetine Haloperidol Paroxetine Quinidine
CYP2E1	Acetaminophen Ethanol Some halogenated hydrocarbons such as halothane	Chronic ethanol Isoniazid	Disulfiram
CYP3A—present in GI tract and liver; responsible for a large amount of first-pass metabolism	Calcium channel blockers Most benzodiazepines HIV protease inhibitors HMG-CoA reductase inhibitors (lipid-lowering agents) Cyclosporine (immunosuppressant) Most nonsedating antihistamines Cisapride (gastric motility agent)	Carbamazepine Rifampin Rifabutin (to treat TB) Ritonavir (to treat HIV) St. John's wort (herbal product used for depression and menopause)	Azole antifungal agents such as itraconazole Ketoconazole Fluconazole Cimetidine (broad range P-450 inhibitor) Macrolide Antibiotics (but *not* azithromycin) Grapefruit juice

COX, *Cyclooxygenase*; GI, *gastrointestinal*; HIV, *human immunodeficiency virus*; HMG-CoA, *3-hydroxy-3-methylglutaryl coenzyme* A; NSAIDs, *nonsteroidal antiinflammatory drugs*; TB, *tuberculosis*.

TABLE 7-5	Relationship Between Half-Life and Drug Remaining in the Body	
Half-Life	Drug Eliminated (%)	Drug Remaining (%)
0	0	100
1	50	50
2	75	25
3	87.5	12.5
4	93.75	6.25
5	96.875	3.125

at hepatocytes) also leads to a greater rate of clearance. Examples of drugs with a low hepatic extraction ratio are thiopental, diazepam, and theophylline.[1]

Renal Clearance. The kidneys excrete water-soluble molecules with great ease. The excretion of drugs involves passive glomerular filtration, active tubular secretion, and some reabsorption. Selected substances that are actively secreted are noted in Box 7-7. The amount of drug made available to the renal tubule for elimination depends on the amount of free, unbound drug and the glomerular filtration rate. Water-soluble metabolites are filtered by the glomeruli and eliminated. The kidneys do not excrete lipid-soluble agents as efficiently as water-soluble compounds. For these agents, elimination depends on the liver for metabolism into water-soluble molecules. Indeed, increased water solubility reduces the volume of distribution of agents, leading to their excretion by the kidneys. Conversely, lipid-soluble

Important Drugs and Related Substances Actively Secreted into the Proximal Renal Tubule

Acids	Bases
ρ-Aminohippuric acid	Amiloride
Furosemide	Dopamine
Glucuronic acid	Histamine
conjugates	Mepacrine
Glycine conjugates	Morphine
Indomethacin	Meperidine
Methotrexate	Quaternary ammonium
Penicillin	compounds
Probenecid	Quinine
Sulphate	5-Hydroxytryptamine
conjugates	(serotonin)
Thiazide diuretics	Triamterene
Uric acid	

Modified with permission from Rang HP et al. Pharmacology. 6th ed. Edinburgh: Churchill Livingstone; 2007.

Elimination of Drugs by the Kidney

- Most drugs, unless highly bound to plasma protein, cross the glomerular filter freely.
- Many drugs, especially weak acids and weak bases, are actively secreted into the renal tubule and therefore are more rapidly excreted.
- Lipid-soluble drugs are passively reabsorbed by diffusion across the tubule and are not efficiently excreted in the urine.
- Because of pH partition, weak acids are more rapidly excreted in alkaline urine, and vice versa.
- Several important drugs are removed predominantly by renal excretion and are liable to cause toxicity in elderly persons and patients with renal disease.

Modified with permission from Rang HP et al. Pharmacology. 6th ed. Edinburgh: Churchill Livingstone; 2007.

molecules are reabsorbed from the renal tubules back into the systemic circulation. An example of a lipid-soluble drug that is almost completely reabsorbed (such that little or none of it is excreted unchanged) is thiopental.

The pH of the urine can also affect the elimination of drugs. Weak acids are better excreted in alkaline urine; conversely, weak bases are readily excreted in acid urine. The kidneys can use glomerular filtration for elimination of drugs that are highly polar (e.g., aminoglycoside antibiotics). Certain agents (e.g., penicillin) are eliminated via secretion. Some important clearance concepts are noted in Box 7-8.

OTHER FACTORS THAT INFLUENCE PHARMACOKINETICS

Age

Age plays an important role in the manner in which drug disposition occurs. Elderly patients have a decrease in renal function, resulting in impaired excretion of agents that are eliminated in the urine.[6] Creatinine clearance, as an indicator of renal function, parallels the kidneys' ability to excrete drugs and is a useful test in predicting renal pharmacokinetics in the elderly.[2] Liver blood flow decreases with age as well, decreasing the metabolism of agents with moderate to high extraction ratios. The elderly also have an increase in the fat compartment, leading to an increased volume of distribution, which can lead to accumulation of lipid-soluble agents.[9] Liver and renal function are also important in neonates. Elimination of drugs via the kidneys is altered in neonates because of poor renal function in the first year of life. Neonates and premature infants lack the ability to metabolize certain agents because of immature liver enzyme systems.[2] It is therefore important to consider extremes of age when administering any agent that may be highly lipid soluble with a high hepatic extraction ratio or that relies primarily on the kidneys for elimination.

Gender

Gender differences account for some variability in the pharmacokinetics of many agents. In a recent review of the literature, it was found that female patients had a 20% to 30% greater sensitivity to the muscle relaxant effects of vecuronium, pancuronium, and rocuronium.[13] It was also found that male patients were more sensitive to propofol than female patients and that it may be necessary to reduce propofol doses in male patients.[30] In 1999, Gan and co-workers studied emergence from general anesthesia with propofol, alfentanil, and nitrous oxide. Female patients emerged significantly more quickly than male patients. In fact, female patients were three times more likely than male patients to experience recall under general anesthesia.[31] Conversely, female patients were shown to be more sensitive to opioid receptor agonists, with their male counterparts requiring 30% to 40% more narcotics for management of pain.[30]

Temperature

Because temperature affects tissue metabolism and blood flow, it follows that the pharmacokinetics of agents are also affected by varying temperatures. In a 2002 study, Knibbe and colleagues examined the pharmacokinetics of long-term propofol sedation in critically ill patients. Temperature was a significant covariate for clearance of propofol. Warmer temperatures led to faster elimination of propofol, regardless of the concentration of the drug in solution.[32]

Disease States

Comorbidity accounts for some of the variability observed in drug pharmacokinetics. The pharmacokinetics of ropivacaine in patients with and without uremia after axillary brachial plexus block was examined. An enhanced absorption and larger total plasma concentrations of ropivacaine and its main metabolite were noted in the patients with uremia.[33] Conversely, Goyal and colleagues found a negative correlation of propofol dose with preoperative hemoglobin concentration in patients with renal failure. They concluded that the hyperdynamic state caused by anemia in these patients was responsible for their higher propofol dose requirement.[34]

Other disease states can cause variability, as illustrated by a recent study that found an increase in the volume distribution of ketamine disproportional to increases in clearance in spinal cord injury inpatients in the intensive care unit, leading to a longer than expected half-life for the drug, again placing the patients at

---

BOX 7-9

Summary of Pharmacokinetic Principles

- Clinical pharmacokinetics is the discipline that describes the absorption, distribution, metabolism, and elimination of drugs in patients who require drug therapy.
- Clearance is the most important pharmacokinetic parameter, because it determines the steady-state concentration for a given dosage rate. Physiologically, clearance is determined by blood flow to the organ that metabolizes or eliminates the drug and the efficiency of the organ in extracting the drug from the bloodstream.
- The dosage and clearance determine the steady-state concentration.
- The fraction of drug absorbed into the systemic circulation after extravascular administration is defined as its *bioavailability*.
- Pharmacokinetic models are useful for description of data sets, prediction of serum concentrations after several doses or different routes of administration, and calculation of pharmacokinetic constants such as clearance, volume of distribution, and half-life. The simplest case uses a single compartment to represent the entire body.
- The volume of distribution determines the loading dose.
- Half-life is the time required for serum concentration to decrease by one half after absorption and distribution are complete. Half-life is important because it determines the time required to reach steady state and the dosage interval. Half-life is a dependent kinetic variable because its value depends on the values of clearance and volume of distribution.

- The half-life determines the time to reach steady state and the time for "all" drug to be eliminated from the body.
- If a drug obeys first-order pharmacokinetics, a simple ratio of dosage to steady-state concentration can be used to estimate a new dosage, as long as the clearance has not changed.
- Phenytoin is an example of a drug that obeys Michaelis-Menton rather than first-order pharmacokinetics. In this case, as plasma concentration increases, the clearance decreases and the half-life becomes longer.
- *Cytochrome P-450* is a generic term for the group of enzymes responsible for most drug metabolism oxidation reactions. Several P-450 isozymes have been identified, including CYP1A2, CYP2C9, CYP2C19, CYP2D6, CYP2E1, and CYP3A4.
- Factors to be taken into consideration when deciding on the best drug dose for a patient include age, gender, weight, ethnic background, other concurrent disease states, and other drug therapy.
- The importance of transport proteins in drug bioavailability and elimination is now better understood. The principal transport protein involved in the movement of drugs across biologic membranes is P-glycoprotein. P-glycoprotein is present in many organs, including the gastrointestinal tract, liver, and kidney.

Modified from Dipiro JT et al, eds. Pharmacotherapy: A Pathophysiological Approach. *6th ed. New York: McGraw-Hill; 2005; and Helms RA et al, eds.* Textbook of Therapeutics: Drug and Disease Management. *8th ed. Philadelphia: Lippincott Williams & Wilkins; 2006.*

---

risk for overdose.[35] For a summary of some pharmacokinetic principles, see Box 7-9.

PHARMACOGENETICS AND PHARMACOGENOMICS

Definition

Pharmacogenetics is the study of variations in human genes that are responsible for different responses to drug therapy. These differences are identified in the pharmacodynamic and pharmacokinetic processes.[36] Pharmacogenomics is an evolution of pharmacogenetics research and involves the identification of drug response markers at the level of disease, drug metabolism, or drug target.[36]

Pharmacogenetics and pharmacogenomics take into account the genetic basis for the variability in an individual's drug response. Pharmacogenetics studies variations in genes suspected of affecting drug response, whereas pharmacogenomics encompasses the genome (all genes). The discipline of pharmacogenetics integrates biochemical and pharmacologic concepts and seeks to correlate phenotypic biomarkers such as toxicity with genetics via twin studies. Pharmacogenomics involves DNA sequencing and gene mapping to identify the genetic basis for variations in drug efficacy, metabolism, and transport.[37]

History

The history of pharmacogenetics goes back to the days of Pythagoras (510 BC) when he recognized only some people had fatal responses to ingestion of fava beans, but not all.[38]

Archibald Garrod's 1902 study of alcaptonuria in humans constituted the first genetic link to disease in humans. He later advanced the hypothesis that genetically determined differences in biochemical processes may be the reason for adverse drug reactions.[39]

Familial clustering of toxic drug responses led to suspicion of a biochemical genetic basis for the toxicities.[36,37] In a seminal article published in 1957, Motulsky outlined many genetic conditions associated with toxic reaction to a specific drug or chemical and proposed that inheritance of certain traits may explain individual variations in drug efficacy and toxic reactions.[40]

Early advances in the field of pharmacogenetics came from research into the biochemical and genetic basis for idiosyncratic drug responses. Several independent observations were made. For example, in the 1950s following reports of prolonged muscle relaxation following administration of succinylcholine during anesthesia, the variation in serum cholinesterase levels was found to be an inherited trait. Similarly, hemolytic anemia found in African-American male soldiers following administration of the antimalarial drug primaquine during World War II led to the discovery of a defect in the gene encoding glucose 6-phosphate dehydrogenase (G6PD).[37,41]

The term *pharmacogenetics* was coined by Vogel in 1959 and defined as "clinically important hereditary variation in response to drugs."[36] In 1962, Kalow wrote a text, *Pharmacogenetics: Heredity and the Response to Drugs.*[36,42]

In the 1960s, twin studies established the role of genetic factors in individual variations in rates of drug metabolism; however, they did not identify the specific genes involved. Gene identification emerged in the 1980s.[36] Currently, genomic techniques make it possible to identify associations between genetic markers and drug response within a population.[41]

Polymorphisms

Polymorphic genes relevant to pharmacokinetics (absorption, distribution, metabolism, and excretion) and pharmacodynamics (drug targets–receptors and enzymes) can have a significant impact on pharmacotherapy.[43] Pharmacotherapy may be affected by three types of genetic variation. These include variations in target proteins, enzyme metabolism, or idiosyncratic effects.[44]

Polymorphisms are defined as variations in the DNA sequences that occur in at least 1% of the population.[41] There are a number of different types of polymorphisms, but most attention has been focused on single nucleotide polymorphisms (SNPs—pronounced "snips") in which one nucleotide is exchanged for another in a given position.[38] Approximately 10 million SNPs exist, and they can occur anywhere on the genome, but only a fraction are likely to prove relevant to drug response.[41] To matter from a pharmacologic standpoint, the differences generally affect either the function or amount of target proteins involved in the biochemical pathways of the disease processes the drugs are used to treat.[44]

The genomes of any two individuals are nearly 99.9% identical regardless of race.[44] Most variations in the human genome (polymorphisms) occur in drug-metabolizing enzyme genes. Others occur in the enzyme receptor genes and drug transporter genes.[45] Much of the observed variability in drug response has a basis in pharmacogenetic polymorphisms arising in genetically determined differences in drug absorption, disposition, metabolism, and excretion. The best-characterized pharmacogenetic polymorphisms are those in the cytochrome P-450 family of drug-metabolizing enzymes.[41]

Most drugs are lipophilic and must be metabolized to polar products for excretion. This involves hepatic enzymes and a sequence of steps dependent on the cytochrome P-450 system. Drugs are first metabolized by phase I enzymes (oxidation) and then phase II enzymes (conjugation that involves sulphation, glucuronidation, or acetlyation). Although the effects of polymorphism in phase II enzymes are often less pronounced, the effects of inherited variations in both phase I and II metabolism can be synergistic.[41]

Genetic polymorphisms occur in most if not all of the human cytochrome P-450 (CYP) isoenzymes, but functional polymorphisms reside in only four, which account for 40% of all drug metabolism (CYP2A6, CYP2C9, CYP2C19, and CYP2D6). Thus genetically controlled variations are common.[36] For example, CYP2D6 metabolizes up to 25% of all commonly prescribed drugs and is inactive in 6% of the Caucasian population.[41] Similarly, the CYP2C19 poor metabolizer phenotype occurs in 2% to5% of Caucasians and 3% to 23% of Asians and results in

high sensitivity to diazepam, propranolol, amitriptyline, and hexobarbital.[41]

Individuality in the expression in the P-450 isoenzymes may have a variety of consequences. These include toxic side effects due to impaired metabolism, no therapeutic effect due to ultrarapid metabolism, activation of toxic products, and failure of prodrug activation.[41]

Individual Drug Response/Genetics

Many variations of pharmacogenetic interest have been elucidated, and with the deciphering of the human genome, many innovative opportunities exist. Genetic variations can modify responses to drugs. Variations in target pathways and metabolic enzymes may render a drug ineffective for some, yet effective for others.

Recognition of genetic differences among patients has the potential to allow for individualized drug therapy. Further, with the recognition that certain genetic differences are associated with risk of disease, opportunities to identify these individuals and treat them early may improve efficacy and specificity of their treatment.[36]

There are marked ethnic differences that need to be taken into account when drugs subject to polymorphic metabolism are prescribed to patients from different ethnic backgrounds.[41] The variation in CYP2C19 is reflected in a significant dosing reduction for diazepam in Asians, for example.

Genetic variation may also alter pharmacotherapy responses by creating idiosyncratic effects. These are not caused by alterations in target proteins, pathways, or metabolism, but rather result from chance interactions between the medication and the individual's physiology.[44]

The identification of specific polymorphisms and the ability to screen for them opens up the possibility of rational, individualized treatment with ideal dosing, as well as minimization of side effects based on genetic constitution. Recognition of differences may also facilitate identification of good responders versus poor responders to therapy.[37]

SUMMARY

Pharmacokinetics is an integral part of modern anesthesia clinical practice. Anesthesia providers balance the administration of a number of drugs simultaneously to achieve the necessary drug actions that constitute anesthesia. A thorough understanding of the processes that govern drug kinetics allows for safe and effective practice and facilitates operating room efficiency. This knowledge also allows the clinician to anticipate and avoid potential problems and tailor each anesthetic to particular patient characteristics. Recent advances in pharmacokinetics and pharmacogenomics will further impact anesthesia care in years to come. Pharmacogenomics has made a significant impact on the direction of drug research and drug therapy. Diseases and drug therapies are complex processes that may challenge the predictive powers of pharmacogenetics. A systems approach may be needed to integrate overall pharmacotherapeutic effects with polymorphisms in multiple genes.[45,46]

REFERENCES

1. Holford NHG. Pharmacokinetics & pharmacodynamics: rational dosing & the time course of drug action. In: Katzung BG, ed. *Basic and Clinical Pharmacology*. 10th ed. New York: McGraw-Hill; 2007:34-49.
2. Buxton ILO. Pharmacokinetics and pharmacodynamics: the dynamics of drug absorption, distribution and elimination. In: Brunton LL et al, eds. *Goodman & Gilman's Pharmacological Basis of Therapeutics*. 11th ed. New York: McGraw-Hill; 2006:3-30.
3. Atkinson AJ. Compartmental analysis of drug distribution. In: Atkinson AJ et al, ed. *Principles of Clinical Pharmacology*. 2nd ed. San Diego: Elsevier; 2007:25-36.
4. Du Souich P et al. Plasma protein binding and pharmacological response. *Clin Pharmacokinet*. 1993;24:435-440.
5. Shargel L, Yu AB. *Applied Biopharmaceutics and Pharmacokinetics*. Stamford, CT: Appleton and Lange; 1999:29-45.
6. Gibiansky E et al. Aquavan injection, a water-soluble prodrug of propofol, as a bolus injection: a phase 1 dose-escalation comparison with Diprivan (part 1): pharmacokinetics. *Anesthesiology*. 2005;103(4):718-729.
7. Gibaldi M, Perrier D. Pharmacokinetics. In: *Drugs and the Pharmaceutical Sciences*. Vol 15. New York: Marcel Dekker; 1982:54-109, 451-457.
8. Meibohm B, Evans WE. Clinical pharmacodynamics and pharmacokinetics. In: Helms RA et al, eds. *Textbook of Therapeutics: Drug and Disease Management*. 8th ed. Philadelphia: Lippincott Williams & Wilkins; 2006:1-30.
9. Wu C-Y et al. Differentiation of absorption and first-pass gut and hepatic metabolism in humans: studies with cyclosporine. *Clin Pharmacol Ther*. 1995;58:492-497.
10. Hollenberg PF. Absorption, distribution, metabolism and elimination. In: Minneman KP, Wecker L, eds. *Brody's Human Pharmacology, Molecular to Clinical*. 4th ed. Philadelphia: Mosby; 2005:27-40.
11. Hudson RJ, Henthorn TK. Basic principles of clinical pharmacology. In: Barash PG et al, eds. *Clinical Anesthesia*. 5th ed. Philadelphia: Lippincott Williams & Wilkins; 2006:247-274.
12. Koup JR, Gibaldi M. Some comments on the evaluation of bioavailability data. *Drug Intell Clin Pharm*. 1980;14:327-330.
13. Kazama T et al. Comparison of predicted induction dose with predetermined physiologic characteristics of patients and with pharmacokinetic models incorporating those characteristics as covariates. *Anesthesiology*. 2003;98:229-305.
14. Guyton AC, Hall JE. *Textbook of Medical Physiology*. 11th ed. Philadelphia: Saunders; 2006.
15. Want H et al. Development of a new generation of propofol. *Curr Opin Anaesthesiol*. 2007;20(4):311-315.
16. Wagner JG. *Fundamentals of Clinical Pharmacokinetics*. Hamilton, IL: American Pharmaceutical Association; 1980.
17. *Basic Considerations of Drug Availability*. Weber State University Website (public-domain).http://faculty.weber.edu/ewalker/Medicinal_Chemistry/topics/Basic/1_basi~1.htm. Accessed February 26, 2008.
18. Nelson DL, Cox MM. *Lehninger Principles of Biochemistry*. 4th ed. New York: Freeman; 2005.
19. Shafer SL. Pharmacokinetic principles. In: Hemmings HC, Hopkins PM, eds. *Foundations of Anesthesia: Basic Sciences for Clinical Practice*. 2nd ed. St. Louis: Mosby; 2006:101-118.
20. Rowland M, Tozer TN. *Clinical Pharmacokinetics: Concepts and Applications*. 3rd ed. Baltimore: Lippincott Williams & Wilkins; 1995:33-62.
21. Smith CM, Reynard AM. *Textbook of Pharmacology*. Philadelphia: Saunders; 1992:57-86.
22. Boobis AR et al. Dissecting the function of P450. *Br J Clin Pharmacol*. 1996;42:81-89.
23. Gonzalez FJ, Korzekwa KR. Cytochromes P450 expression systems. *Annu Rev Pharmacol Toxicol*. 1995;35:269-390.
24. Lin JH, Lu AY. Interindividual variability in inhibition and induction of cytochrome P450 enzymes. *Annu Rev Pharmacol Toxicol*. 2001;41:535-567.
25. Raunio H et al. Expression of xenobiotic-metabolizing cytochrome P450s in human pulmonary tissues. *Arch Toxicol Suppl*. 1998;20:465-469.
26. Hughes MA et al. Context-sensitive half-life in multi-compartment pharmacokinetic models for intravenous anesthetic drugs. *Anesthesiology*. 1992;76:334-341.
27. Kapila A et al. Measured context-sensitive half-times of remifentanil and alfentanil. *Anesthesiology*. 1995;83:968-975.
28. Fisher DM. (Almost) everything you learned about pharmacokinetics was (somewhat) wrong! *Anesth Analg*. 1996;8:901-903.
29. Bailey JM. Context-sensitive half-times: what are they and how valuable are they in anesthesiology? *Clin Pharmacokinet*. 2002;41(11):793-799.
30. Pleym H et al. Gender differences in drug effects: implications for anesthesiologists. *Acta Anaesthesiol Scand*. 2003;47:241-259.
31. Gan TJ et al. Women emerge from general anesthesia with propofol/alfentanil/nitrous oxide faster than men. *Anesthesiology*. 1999;90(5):1283-1287.
32. Knibbe CA et al. Population pharmacokinetics and pharmacodynamic modeling of propofol for long-term sedation in critically ill patients: a comparison between propofol 6% and propofol 1%. *Clin Pharmacol Ther*. 2002;72:670-684.
33. Pere P et al. Pharmacokinetics of ropivacaine in uremic and nonuremic patients after axillary brachial plexus block. *Anesth Analg*. 2003;96:563-569.
34. Goyal P et al. Evaluation of induction doses of propofol: comparison between endstage renal disease and normal renal function patients. *Anaesth Intensive Care*. 2002;30:584-587.
35. Hijazi Y et al. Pharmacokinetics and haemodynamics of ketamine in intensive care patients with brain or spinal cord injury. *Br J Anaesth*. 2003;90:155-160.
36. Vesell ES. Advances in pharmacogenetics and pharmacogenomics. *J Clin Pharmacol*. 2000;40:930-938.
37. Mancinelli L et al. Pharmacogenomics: the promise of personalized medicine. *AAPS PharmSci*. 2000;2(1):1-13.
38. Munir P. Pharmacogenetics and pharmacogenomics. *Br J Clin Pharmacol*. 2001;52(4):345-347.
39. Garrod AE. The incidence of alcaptonuria: a study in chemical individuality. *Lancet*. 1902;ii:1616-1620.
40. Motulsky AG. Drug reactions, enzymes and biochemical genetics. *JAMA*. 1957;165:835-837.
41. Wolf RC, Smith G. Pharmacogenetics. *Br Med Bull*. 1999;55(2):366-386.
42. Kalow W. *Pharmacogenetics: Heredity and the Response to Drugs*. Philadelphia: Saunders; 1962.
43. Wolfgang S, Zunyan D. Pharmacogenetics/genomics and personalized medicine. *Hum Mol Genet*. 2005;14(Review Issue 2):R207-R214.
44. Ch'ng Y et al. Pharmacogenomics. In: Golan DE et al, eds. *Principles of Pharmacology*. Philadelphia: Lippincott Williams & Wilkins; 2005:803-809.
45. Nebert DW. Pharmacogenetics and pharmacogenomics: why is this relevant to clinical geneticists? *Clin Genet*. 1999;56:345-347.
46. Nebert DW, Vessel ES. Can personalized drug therapy be achieved? A closer look at pharmaco-metabonomics. *Trends Pharmacol Sci*. 2006;27(11):580-586.

CHAPTER 8

PHARMACOKINETICS OF INHALATION ANESTHETICS

John J. Nagelhout

The basic action of an anesthetic in the body is largely a function of the drug's chemical structure and the resulting interaction with a cellular receptor complex (Figure 8-1). A number of heterogeneous compounds exhibit anesthetic properties. The inorganic molecule nitrous oxide and halogenated ethers (e.g., isoflurane, desflurane, and sevoflurane) are all capable of binding to central nervous system and spinal cord neuronal membranes to produce reversible depression. A single specific anesthetic receptor has yet to be found. In fact, multiple sites of action probably exist; however, once a critical concentration of drug has entered the brain and spinal cord, loss of consciousness ensues.[1,2]

The administration of inhalation anesthetic gases plays a primary role in modern clinical anesthesia. In anesthesia's early years, administration of a gas constituted the entire anesthetic regimen. Now, one or two gas anesthetics are combined with a variety of intravenous drugs to produce an anesthetic state. These intravenous drugs include sedative induction agents, analgesics, neuromuscular blocking drugs, and local anesthetics. The use of this combination allows the anesthetist to use smaller and more easily manipulated doses of specific receptor agonists and antagonists. Used in the proper combination, the desired amount of anesthesia, analgesia, amnesia, and muscle relaxation can be achieved. Current practice dictates that the anesthetic technique allow for a quick and pleasant induction and recovery with maximum patient safety and efficient caseload management. A sound understanding of inhalation anesthetic pharmacokinetics is essential to safe practice.

PRIMARY FACTORS CONTROLLING UPTAKE, DISTRIBUTION, AND ELIMINATION OF ANESTHETICS

The basic task of anesthetic administration involves taking a drug supplied as a liquid, vaporizing it in an anesthesia machine, and delivering it to the patient's brain and other tissues via the lungs. Therefore the main factors that influence the ability to anesthetize a patient are technical or machine specific, drug related, respiratory, circulatory, and tissue related. The primary factors that influence absorption of the inhalation anesthetics are ventilation, uptake into the blood, cardiac output, the solubility of the anesthetic drug in the blood, and alveolar-to-venous blood partial-pressure difference. Other factors such as the concentration and second gas effects also play a role (Figure 8-2).[3]

A few assumptions are usually made. The level of anesthesia is related to the alveolar concentrations of anesthetic agents, which can be readily and continuously measured or inferred.

The concentration or partial pressure of anesthetic in the lungs is assumed to be the same as in the brain, because the drugs are highly lipid soluble and diffusible, and they quickly and easily reach equilibrium among the body compartments. For this reason, the dose of an individual drug is expressed in terms of the minimum alveolar concentration (MAC) necessary to produce anesthesia (lack of movement) on surgical stimulation.[4,5] The faster the lung (and therefore brain) concentration rises, the faster anesthesia is achieved. Conversely, the faster the lung (brain) concentration falls after discontinuation of the drug, the more quickly the patient emerges.[6]

Machine-Related Factors

Concepts regarding the anesthesia machine and its function are described in detail in Chapter 16. Two factors that may affect uptake early in anesthetic administration are drug solubility in the rubber and plastic machine parts and total machine liter flow of the gases chosen.

The rubber and plastic components of the machine, as well as the ventilator and absorbent, can retain small quantities of anesthetic gases. Theoretically, this could slow administration to the patient at the start of anesthetic delivery. The effect on uptake is minimal in actual clinical practice and essentially ceases after approximately 15 minutes of administration.[7] Nonetheless, sequestration of small amounts of gas in the apparatus has other implications, such as when anesthetizing patients with malignant hyperthermia. All gases except nitrous oxide are potent triggering agents for a hyperthermic episode. To avoid exposure resulting from residual trace amounts of gases, a thorough flush of the anesthesia machine with 100% oxygen at 10 L/min for at least 20 minutes, replacement of breathing circuits and the carbon dioxide canister, and draining, inactivation, or removal of vaporizers are advised when preparing for a patient who is susceptible to malignant hyperthermia.[8]

Low liter flows of oxygen and nitrous oxide carrier gas, although economical, deliver the anesthetic more slowly at the start of induction. Increasing liter flows for the first few minutes of the anesthetic minimizes this effect without unduly adding to cost.[9]

Drug-Related Factors
Blood/Gas Solubility

The blood/gas solubility coefficient of an anesthetic is an indicator of the speed of uptake and elimination.[10,11] It reflects the proportion of the anesthetic that will be soluble in the blood, "bind" to blood components, and not readily enter the tissues (blood phase) versus the fraction of the drug that will leave the blood and quickly diffuse into tissues (gas phase). The more soluble the drug (high blood/gas coefficient), the slower the brain and spinal cord uptake and therefore the slower the anesthesia achieved by the patient. Soluble drugs stay in the blood in greater proportion than less soluble agents; therefore, less of the drug is released to the tissues during the early, rapid-uptake phase of induction. For example, isoflurane has a blood/gas solubility coefficient of 1.4 or, expressed as a ratio, 1.4:1. Therefore 1.4 times as much stays in the blood as a nonreleasable fraction for every molecule that enters the tissues and produces anesthesia. Conversely, agents with low solubility properties (low blood/gas coefficient) leave the blood quickly and enter the tissues, producing a rapid anesthetic state. Desflurane, for example, has a low blood/gas coefficient of 0.42 or, expressed as a ratio, 0.42:1. Only 0.42 of a molecule stays in the blood for every 1 (greater than twice as much) that enters the brain. Anesthesia is achieved quickly. Blood/gas solubility coefficients for the inhalation anesthetic agents are listed in Table 8-1.[12] The rate of rise of an anesthetic in the alveoli relative to the concentration administered is graphically depicted by plotting the fraction in the alveoli over the fraction inspired (Figure 8-3).

As noted previously, the lower the blood/gas solubility, the faster the rise in lung concentration. The rate of rise of low solubility agents such as nitrous oxide and desflurane is greater than moderately soluble drugs such as isoflurane. Note that nitrous oxide exhibits a slightly faster rate of rise compared with desflurane, despite a higher blood/gas coefficient. This variation in the usual trend is a result of the concentration effect—that is, nitrous oxide is given at much higher concentrations (50% to 70%) than

desflurane (3% to 9%). Figure 8-4 depicts the effect of anesthetic blood solubility on uptake.

Ventilation Factors

As with all diffusible drugs, anesthetics move down a concentration gradient. Continuous inhalation administration of the agent into the lungs promotes subsequent diffusion into the blood and tissues as the anesthetic progresses. Anesthetic uptake slows throughout the surgical procedure.[13] The anesthetic is delivered, along with the necessary amount of

TABLE **8-1**	General Anesthetic Properties of Inhalation Agents		
Anesthetic	MAC (%)	Blood/Gas Partition Coefficient (at 37° C)	Oil/Gas Partition Coefficient (at 37° C)
Sevoflurane (Ultane)	2	0.6	50
Isoflurane (Forane)	1.15	1.4	99
Nitrous oxide	105	0.47	1.4
Desflurane (Suprane)	5.8	0.42	18.7

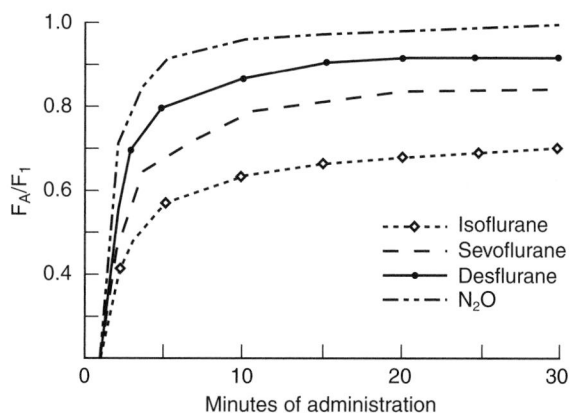

FIGURE **8-3** Rate of rise (F_A/F_1) of alveolar concentration of inhalation anesthetics over time. Low blood/gas anesthetics such as nitrous oxide and desflurane achieve a lung concentration much faster than high-solubility gases such as halothane. Note that nitrous oxide rises in the lungs more quickly than desflurane, in spite of a slightly higher blood/gas solubility. This is due to the concentration effect.

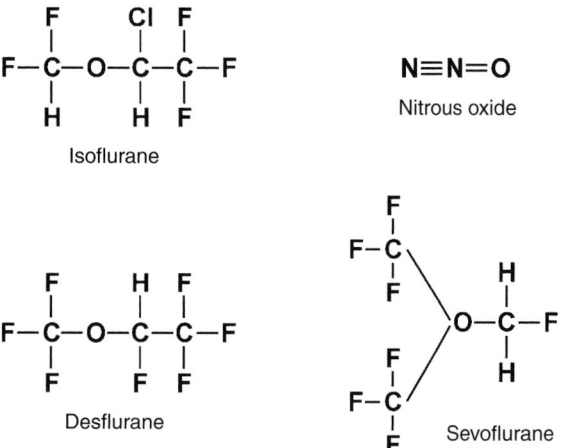

FIGURE **8-1** Chemical structure of anesthetic agents. Nitrous oxide is inorganic, and the rest are halogenated ethers.

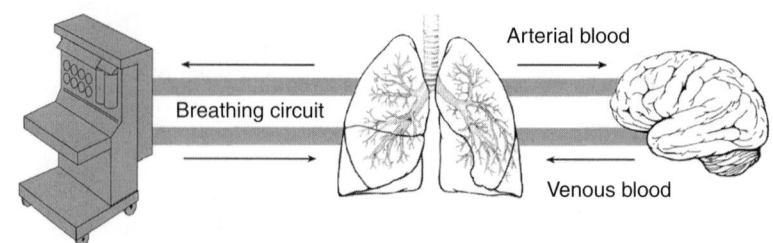

FIGURE **8-2** Transfer of an anesthetic gas from the machine through the lungs into the blood and tissues.

oxygen or an oxygen mix appropriate for the patient's condition. Supplemental nitrous oxide is commonly used. Basically, the faster and more deeply a patient breathes or is ventilated, the faster the patient loses consciousness at the start of anesthesia and emerges at the end.[11] This is often referred to as the *ventilation effect*.

Ventilation-perfusion deficits or poor lung function hinders inhalation drug administration.[14] Rapid-acting (low blood/gas solubility) agents are affected by these deficits to a greater extent than are slower-acting (high blood/gas solubility) drugs.[15] These decreases in speed can be partially compensated for by increasing the concentration of insoluble (fast) agents or increasing ventilation with soluble (slow) drugs.

Concentration or Dose

During the first minutes of gas administration, a higher concentration of the drug than necessary for maintenance, or a loading dose, is delivered to speed initial uptake. This is commonly referred to as *overpressuring* or the *concentration effect*.[16] Overpressuring during initial administration is a common clinical practice and is more effective the more soluble the anesthetic. Overpressuring can speed the effect of slow agents but has less of an effect on relatively fast agents. This practice follows the kinetic standard of using a loading dose to speed onset. After the first few minutes, the dose is decreased to normal maintenance levels.[17-19]

As noted previously, the dose of an anesthetic is expressed in terms of MAC—the relative concentration when the anesthetic is combined with all the other gases in the lungs. Induction and maintenance doses are given in Table 8-2.

Second-Gas Effect

Simultaneous administration of a relatively slow agent such as isoflurane and a faster drug such as nitrous oxide (in high concentrations) can speed the onset of the slower agent. This is known as the *second-gas effect*.[20] The uptake of the slower agent is increased by administering it with a high concentration of the faster anesthetic nitrous oxide. The faster the inherent speed of the second slower gas on its own, however, the less prominent the augmentation when given with nitrous oxide. For example, sevoflurane, which has a low blood solubility (blood/gas solubility coefficient 0.6) is rapidly taken up into tissues. Coadministration of sevoflurane with the slightly faster nitrous oxide produces only small and brief increases in uptake as compared with sevoflurane administration alone.[17-19,21] Some have questioned the validity of this concept.[22]

Tissue-Related Factors
Oil/Gas Solubility

The oil/gas solubility coefficient is an indicator of potency. The higher the solubility, the more potent the drug (see Table 8-1).[23,24] A high solubility coefficient reflects high lipid solubility. Because the anesthetic must traverse the blood-brain barrier and penetrate lipid cell membranes to produce its action, highly lipid-soluble drugs tend to be the most potent. Of current agents, isoflurane (oil/gas partition coefficient 99) is the most potent, and nitrous oxide (oil/gas partition coefficient 1.4) is the least potent. Remember that two factors are at play: how fast the drug is delivered to the tissues (blood/gas solubility) and how efficiently it can access and affect the sites of action (oil/gas solubility). Recent investigations suggest that polarity along with lipophilicity plays an important yet not fully understood role in the mechanism of inhalation anesthetics.[25,26]

Circulatory Factors

The cardiovascular system exerts two major influences on anesthetic uptake and distribution.[27] First, the majority of the blood leaving the lungs with anesthetic is normally distributed to the vital organs or high-blood-flow areas, commonly referred to as the *vessel-rich group* or *central compartment*. Organs such as the heart, liver, kidneys, and brain receive proportionately more anesthetic sooner than the muscle and fat areas (Table 8-3). The longer the anesthetic is given, the greater the saturation of all body compartments.

Second, during induction, increases in cardiac output slow onset. All anesthetics are affected; however, the more soluble the agent (higher blood/gas coefficient, and therefore slower),

TABLE **8-2**	Inhalation Anesthetic Doses*	
Anesthetic	**Induction (%)**	**Maintenance (%)**
Nitrous oxide	50-70	Same
Isoflurane (Forane)	1-4	0.5-2
Desflurane (Suprane)	3-9	2-6
Sevoflurane (Ultane)	4-8	1-4

Doses vary according to patient status, procedure, and types of medications coadministered.

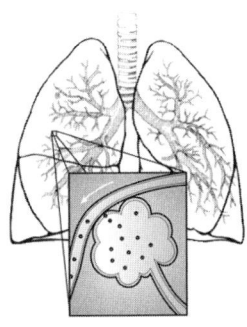
Low solubility

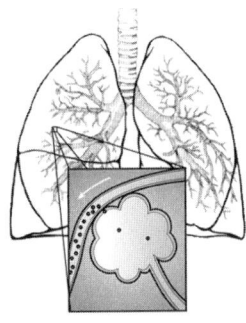
High solubility

FIGURE **8-4** Effect of anesthetic blood/gas solubility on uptake. *Left,* an anesthetic gas with a low blood/gas solubility is not taken into the blood; therefore, the alveolar (thus brain) concentration rises rapidly, and the patient achieves anesthesia quickly. *Right,* an anesthetic gas with a high blood/gas solubility is taken up and held in the blood, resulting in a slower rise in alveolar (thus brain) concentration and a slower onset of anesthesia.

TABLE 8-3	Tissue Compartments and Perfusion Comparisons			
Characteristic	Vessel Rich	Muscle	Fat	Vessel Poor
Body weight	10%	50%	20%	20%
Cardiac output	75%	19%	6%	0%
Perfusion	75 mL/min/100 g	3 mL/min/100 g	3 mL/min/100 g	0 mL/min/100 g

TABLE 8-4	Anesthetic Metabolism
Agent	Average Metabolism (%)
Sevoflurane	3-6
Nitrous oxide	<1
Isoflurane	<1
Desflurane	<0.1

the greater the effect. An increased cardiac output removes more anesthetic from the lungs, which slows the rise in lung and brain concentration.[28-30] This effect dissipates as the anesthetic proceeds.

Metabolism

Anesthetics are metabolized in the body to varying degrees (Table 8-4).[31] The effect on uptake, distribution, and elimination with modern anesthetics other than halothane is minimal. Possible toxic metabolite formation remains an important clinical issue.[32] Drug metabolism has historically been associated with various anesthetic-related toxicities. These include hepatotoxicity from halothane[33] and other agents and theoretically nephrotoxicity from sevoflurane, although these incidents are rare.[34-37] Nitrous oxide, desflurane, and isoflurane are the least metabolized and do not result in metabolism-related toxicity. Although sevoflurane is metabolized, no related clinically significant toxicity has been noted.

Emergence

After surgery, when the anesthetic is discontinued, the same principles that influence onset apply. The anesthetic leaves the tissues via the blood and exits the lungs with ventilation. Routine practice is to administer 100% oxygen to assist recovery. If nitrous oxide was given, 100% oxygen prevents diffusion hypoxia. Anesthetics redistribute out of the tissues in a more uniform manner compared with the way they distribute during onset. An equilibrium is approached among tissues during the anesthetic period, so recovery tends to be smoother than induction with respect to the excitatory stage responses. The longer an anesthetic is administered, the slower the patient emerges. Differences among anesthetics are small but significant and are seen during the final 20% of the elimination process.[35,38]

Diffusion Hypoxia

During emergence, when high concentrations of a rapid (insoluble) anesthetic such as nitrous oxide have been given, the drug exits the body quickly through the lungs and is replaced by less soluble nitrogen in air. This may result in a transient dilution of normal respiratory gases such as oxygen

and carbon dioxide. This phenomenon is referred to as *diffusion hypoxia*. Administration of 100% oxygen for several minutes when anesthesia is terminated entirely avoids this potential problem.

Diffusion of Nitrous Oxide into Closed Spaces

Nitrous oxide diffuses into air-containing cavities in the body during an anesthetic procedure. These air-containing spaces are normally rich in nitrogen, which is 34 times less soluble than nitrous oxide. If the space is expandable, it increases in volume. Examples of expandable air cavities include air embolism, pneumothorax, acute intestinal obstruction, intraocular air bubbles produced by sulfur hexafluoride gas injection, and pneumoperitoneum. Rigid air-containing spaces will undergo an increase in pressure. This includes tympanic membrane grafting after tympanomastoid procedures and intracranial air during diagnostic or surgical intracranial procedures. Nitrous oxide should be avoided in these situations. The endotracheal tube cuff, laryngeal mask airway, and balloon-tipped pulmonary artery catheters may expand during nitrous oxide anesthesia, and appropriate precautions and adjustments should be considered.[39-41]

Other Factors

The interaction of two agents with the carbon dioxide absorber in the breathing circuit should be noted, although this does not directly affect anesthetic kinetics.

Sevoflurane reacts with the carbon dioxide–absorbing granules in the anesthesia machine.[42-44] The reaction increases with heat and total gas flows less than 2 L/min.[45,46] Anesthetic administration duration naturally plays a role. The by-product, compound A, exhibits toxicity in animals.[47,48] To date, no clinical morbidity has been reported.

Carbon monoxide production has been reported after use of desflurane and sevoflurane and carbon dioxide granules such as sodalime, especially when they lose their moisture.[49,50] Toxin production is increased with dehydrated granules.[51] Proper machine maintenance decreases the likelihood of problems. A new type of granule, Amsorb, is available and is less reactive with inhalation anesthetics.[52,53]

PEDIATRICS

The uptake of anesthetic drugs is faster in children than in adults.[54,55] In other words, a child goes to sleep faster than an adult patient.[56] The child's higher alveolar ventilation per weight accounts for this effect.

Infants and children have a higher cardiac output per weight than adults. As noted previously, the higher the cardiac output, the slower the onset. This effect is minimized, however, by the increased cardiac output distributed to the vessel-rich group in children. The infant's lower muscle mass allows more of the agent to concentrate in the vital organs. This overall effect is to promote uptake to the brain.

TABLE 8-5	Inhalational Anesthetic Pharmacokinetic Concepts
Concept	**Comments**
Ventilation effect	The greater the alveolar ventilation, the faster the patient achieves anesthesia.
Concentration effect	The higher the concentration of anesthetic delivered, the faster anesthesia is achieved. This is also referred to as *overpressuring*. As with any drug, the larger the initial dose administered, the faster the onset of action.
Blood/gas solubility coefficient	The blood/gas solubility coefficient is the indicator of an anesthetic's speed of onset and emergence. The higher the coefficient, the slower the anesthetic. Conversely, the lower the coefficient, the faster the anesthetic.
Oil/gas solubility coefficient	The oil/gas solubility coefficient is the indicator of an anesthetic's potency. The higher the coefficient, the more potent the agent.
Second-gas effect	The second-gas effect is a phenomenon in which two anesthetics of varying onset speeds are administered together. A high concentration of a fast anesthetic such as nitrous oxide is administered with a slower second anesthetic gas. The slower gas achieves anesthetic levels more quickly than if it had been given alone.
Diffusion hypoxia	Diffusion hypoxia occurs when high concentrations of nitrous oxide are administered. At the end of the procedure when nitrous oxide is discontinued, it leaves the body very rapidly, causing a transient dilution of the oxygen and carbon dioxide in the lungs. Hypocarbia and hypoxia may occur. Administration of 100% oxygen for approximately 3-5 min when nitrous oxide is discontinued alleviates this problem.
Cardiac output effect	Increases in cardiac output decrease the speed of onset of all anesthetics. The more soluble anesthetics are affected to a much greater extent than the insoluble anesthetics.
Ventilation-perfusion abnormalities	Ventilation-perfusion abnormalities reduce the speed of onset of all anesthetics and affect the insoluble agents to a much greater degree than the soluble agents.
Pediatrics	Children achieve anesthesia more rapidly than adults because of a higher ventilatory rate and vessel-rich-group blood flow. This occurs despite the fact that the required dose and cardiac output are higher in children.
Obesity	Obesity has minimal clinical effects on anesthetic induction; however, emergence may be slower because of deposition of anesthetics in fat.

Finally, anesthetics appear to be less blood soluble (i.e., they work faster) in children than in adults. This effect varies with age and the agent.[57-59] The MAC or required dose of anesthetics is higher in children and decreases with increasing age.[5]

Recent data suggest that during recovery from anesthesia with some inhalation agents, especially sevoflurane and desflurane, emergence reactions and agitation may occur in infants, children, and young adults.[60,61] Recent evidence suggests that this phenomenon is not pharmacokinetic or related to rapidity of emergence.[62] Coadministration of fentanyl or dexmedetomidine reduces the incidence of emergence agitation.[63,64] Propofol and midazolam have no reducing effect.[65] A glossary of pharmacokinetic concepts is given in Table 8-5.

SUMMARY

A thorough understanding of the basic pharmacokinetic principles involved in administering anesthetic gases and the development of clinical skills in their use are the cornerstones of modern anesthesia practice. Adults are generally induced with one of the several available intravenous agents and maintained with a combination of inhalation and intravenous drugs. Better anesthesia machines and more sophisticated monitoring have greatly facilitated the quantification of clinical anesthetic levels and depth, contributing to the remarkable safety of modern anesthesia practice.

REFERENCES

1. Campagna JA et al. Mechanisms of action of inhaled anesthetics. *N Engl J Med.* 2003;348:2110-2124.
2. Sonner MJ et al. Inhaled anesthetics and immobility: mechanisms, mysteries, and minimum alveolar anesthetic concentration. *Anesth Analg.* 2003;97(3):718-740.
3. Eger EI II, Saidman LJ. Illustrations of inhaled anesthetic uptake, including intertissue diffusion to and from fat. *Anesth Analg.* 2005;100(4):1020-1033.
4. Eger EI II. Age, minimum alveolar anesthetic concentration, and minimum alveolar anesthetic concentration-awake. *Anesth Analg.* 2001;94(4):947-953.
5. Quasha AL et al. Determinations and application of MAC. *Anesthesiology.* 1980;53:314-334.
6. Yasuda N et al. Comparison of kinetics of sevoflurane and isoflurane in humans. *Anesth Analg.* 1991;72:316-324.
7. Eger EI II et al. Circuit absorption of halothane, isoflurane, and sevoflurane. *Anesth Analg.* 1998;86:1070-1074.
8. The Malignant Hyperthermia Association of the United States Website. Available at: http://www.mhaus.org/NonFB/Slideshow_eng/SlideShow_ENG_files/frame.htm. Accessed April 14, 2008.
9. Odin I, Feiss P. Low flow and economics of inhalational anaesthesia. *Best Pract Res Clin Anaesthesiol.* 2005;19(3):399-413.
10. Ekbom K et al. The effects of fresh gas flow on the amount of sevoflurane vaporized during 1 minimum alveolar concentration anaesthesia for day surgery: a clinical study. *Acta Anaesthesiol Scand.* 2007;51(3):290-293.

11. Lerou JG, Booij LH. Model-based administration of inhalation anaesthesia 2. Exploring the system model. *Br J Anaesth.* 2001;86(1):29-37.

12. Sakai EM et al. Inhalation anesthesiology and volatile liquid anesthetics: focus on isoflurane, desflurane, and sevoflurane. *Pharmacotherapy.* 2005;25(12):1773-1788.

13. Pal SK et al. Uptake of isoflurane during prolonged clinical anaesthesia. *Br J Anaesth.* 2001;86:645-649.

14. Eger EI II, Severinghause JW. Effect of uneven pulmonary distribution of blood and gas on induction with inhalation anesthetics. *Anesthesiology.* 1964;25:620-626.

15. Peyton PH et al. Effect of ventilation-perfusion in homogeneity and N_2O on oxygenation: physiological modeling of gas exchange. *J Appl Physiol.* 2001;91(1):17-25.

16. Eger EI II. The effect of inspired anesthetic concentration on the rate of rise of alveolar concentration. *Anesthesiology.* 1963;24:153-157.

17. Korman B, Maples WW. Concentration and second gas effects: can the accepted explanation be improved. *Br J Anaesth.* 1997;78:618-625.

18. Taheri S, Eger EI II. A demonstration of the concentration of second gas effects in humans anesthetized with nitrous oxide and desflurane. *Anesth Analg.* 1999;89:774-780.

19. Goldman LJ. Anesthetic uptake of sevoflurane and nitrous oxide during an inhaled induction in children. *Anesth Analg.* 2003;96:400-406.

20. Epstein RM et al. Influence of the concentration effect on the uptake of anesthetic mixtures: the second gas effect. *Anesthesiology.* 1964;25:364-371.

21. Hendrickx JF et al. Large volume N_2O uptake alone does not explain the second gas effect of N_2O on sevoflurane during constant inspired ventilation. *Br J Anaesth.* 2006;96(3):391-395.

22. Sun X et al. The "second gas effect" is not a valid concept. *Anesth Analg.* 1999;88:188-192.

23. Strum DP, Eger EI II. Partition coefficient of sevoflurane in human blood, saline and olive oil. *Anesth Analg.* 1987;66:654-666.

24. Eger EI II. Partition coefficient of I-653 in human blood, saline and olive oil. *Anesth Analg.* 1987;66:971-973.

25. Zhang Y et al. The anesthetic potencies of alkane thiols for rats: relevance to theories of narcosis. *Anesth Analg.* 2000;91:1294-1299.

26. Koblin DD et al. Polyhalogenated methyethyl ethers: solubilities and anesthetic properties. *Anesth Analg.* 1999;88:1161-1167.

27. Eger EI II. Uptake of inhaled anesthetics: the alveolar to inspired anesthetic difference. In: *Anesthetic Uptake and Action.* Baltimore: Williams & Wilkins; 1974:77.

28. Watt SJ et al. The relationship between anaesthetic uptake and cardiac output. *Anaesthesia.* 1996;51:24-28.

29. Kennedy RR, Baker AB. The effect of cardiac output changes on end-expired volatile anaesthetic concentrations—a theoretical study. *Anaesthesia.* 2001;56:11, 1034.

30. Hendrickx JF et al. Sevoflurane pharmacokinetics: effects of cardiac output. *Br J Anaesth.* 1998;81:495-501.

31. Carpenter RL et al. The extent of metabolism of inhaled anesthetics in humans. *Anesthesiology.* 1986;65:201-205.

32. Reichle FM, Conzen PF. Halogenated inhalational anaesthetics. *Best Pract Res Clin Anaesthesiol.* 2003;17:29-46.

33. Splinter W. Halothane: the end of an era? *Anesth Analg.* 2002;95:1471.

34. Kharasch ED et al. Clinical sevoflurane metabolism and disposition. *Anesthesiology.* 1995;82:1369-1377.

35. Kharash ED et al. Human kidney methoxyflurane and sevoflurane metabolism. *Anesthesiology.* 1995;82:689-699.

36. Brown BR. Shibboleths and jigsaw puzzles: the fluoride nephrotoxicity enigma [editorial]. *Anesthesiology.* 1995;82:607-608.

37. Malan GBA. Renal toxicity with sevoflurane: a storm in a teacup? *Drugs.* 2001;61:2155-2162.

38. Eger EI 2nd, Shafer SL. Tutorial: context-sensitive decrement times for inhaled anesthetics. *Anesth Analg.* 2005;101(3):688-696.

39. Ouellette RG. The effect of nitrous oxide on laryngeal mask cuff pressure. *AANA J.* 2000;68:411-414.

40. Algren JT et al. The effect of nitrous oxide diffusion on laryngeal mask airway cuff inflation in children. *Paediatr Anesth.* 1998;8(1):31-36.

41. Hohlrieder M et al. Middle ear pressure changes during anesthesia with or without nitrous oxide are similar among airway devices. *Anesth Analg.* 2006;102(1):319-321.

42. Anders MW. Formation and toxicity of anesthetic degradation products. *Annu Rev Pharmacol Toxicol.* 2005;45:147-176.

43. Ikeuchi Y et al. Quantification of the degradation products of sevoflurane using four brands of CO_2 absorbent in a standard anesthetic circuit. *J Anesth.* 2000;14(3):143-146.

44. Goldberg ME et al. Dose of compound A, not sevoflurane, determines changes in the biochemical markers of renal injury in healthy volunteers. *Anesth Analg.* 1999;88:437-445.

45. Bito H et al. Effects of low-flow sevoflurane anesthesia on renal function. *Anesthesiology.* 1999;86:1231-1237.

46. Cróinin DF, Shorten GD. Anesthesia and renal disease. *Curr Opin Anaesthesiol.* 2002;15(3):359-363.

47. Stabernack CR et al. Sevoflurane degradation by carbon dioxide absorbents may produce more than one nephrotoxic compound in rats. *Can J Anaesth.* 2003;50:249-252.

48. Eger EI II. Compound A: does it matter? *Can J Anaesth.* 2001;48:427-430.

49. Baum J et al. Carbon monoxide generation in carbon dioxide absorbents. *Anesth Analg.* 1995;81:144-146.

50. Stabernack CR et al. Absorbents differ enormously in their capacity to produce compound A and carbon monoxide. *Anesth Analg.* 2000;90(6):1428-1435.

51. Kharasch E et al. Comparison of Amsorb, sodalime, and Baralyme degradation of volatile anesthetics and formation of carbon monoxide and compound A in swine in vivo. *Anesthesiology.* 2002;96:173-182.

52. Mchaourab A et al. Lack of degradation of sevoflurane by a new carbon dioxide absorbent in humans. *Anesthesiology.* 2001;94:1007-1009.

53. Stabernack CR et al. Absorbents differ enormously in their capacity to produce compound A and carbon monoxide. *Anesth Analg.* 2000;90:1428-1435.

54. Salanitre E, Rackow H: The pulmonary exchange of nitrous oxide and halothane in infants and children. *Anesthesiology.* 1969;30:388-394.

55. Brondom BW et al. Uptake and distribution of halothane in infants: in vivo measurements and computer simulations. *Anesth Analg.* 1983;62:404-410.

56. Sarner JB et al. Clinical characteristics of sevoflurane in children: a comparison with halothane. *Anesthesiology.* 1995;82:38-46.

57. Eger EI II et al. The effect of age on the rate of increase of alveolar anesthetic concentration. *Anesthesiology.* 1971;35:365-372.

58. Lerman J et al. Effect of age on the solubility of volatile anesthetics in human tissues. *Anesthesiology.* 1986;65:307-311.

59. Malviya S, Lerman J. The blood-gas solubilities of sevoflurane, isoflurane, halothane, and serum constituent concentrations in neonates and adults. *Anesthesiology.* 1990;72:793-796.

60. Lerman J. Inhalation agents in pediatric anaesthesia—an update. *Curr Opin Anaesthesiol.* 2007;20(3):221-226.

61. Vlajkovic GP, Sindjelic RP. Emergence delirium in children: many questions, few answers. *Anesth Analg.* 2007;104(1):84-91.

62. Cohen IT et al. Rapid emergence does not explain agitation following sevoflurane anaesthesia in infants and children: a comparison with propofol. *Paediatr Anaesth.* 2003;1391:63-67.

63. Cohen IT et al. The effect of fentanyl on the emergence characteristics after desflurane or sevoflurane anesthesia in children. *Anesth Analg.* 2002;94:1178-1181.

64. Ibacache ME et al. Single-dose dexmedetomidine reduces agitation after sevoflurane anesthesia in children. *Anesth Analg.* 2004;98(1):60-63.

65. Cohen IT et al. Propofol or midazolam does not reduce the incidence of emergence agitation associated with desflurane anaesthesia in children undergoing adenotonsillectomy. *Paediatr Anaesth.* 2002;12:604-609.

INHALATION ANESTHETICS

Mark A. Kossick

Historically, major advances have been made in the development of inhalation anesthetics (Table 9-1). In 1800 the anesthetic property of nitrous oxide (N_2O) was first recognized by Humphry Davy. He achieved pain relief from a toothache while inhaling N_2O and later described the experience as one of merriment and exhilaration. Humphry Davy also predicted that N_2O could be used to advantage during surgical operations.[1] It is surprising to note that his 19th-century prediction not only came to pass but also remains true today. The predominant reason for this is the pharmacokinetic profile that N_2O possesses.

The present-day use of N_2O can be credited to Edmund Andrews, a professor of surgery in Chicago. In 1868 he declared that a safer anesthetic could result from combining oxygen (O_2) with N_2O.[2] Before that time N_2O was administered through a mouthpiece with a nose clamp to prevent the rebreathing of air.

One of the earliest "complete" anesthetic agents used was diethyl ether ($C_2H_5-O-C_2H_5$). The first ether anesthetic was administered in Georgia in March 1842 when C.W. Long anesthetized a patient for a minor operation.[3] However, the recognition of numerous unfavorable characteristics (excessive secretions with inhalation induction, laryngospasm, excessive depths of anesthesia) promoted its disappearance from clinical practice as newer agents were subsequently developed.

In the 1930s, research into potential anesthetic agents was based on the principle of a structure-activity relationship.[4] One of the earliest inhalation anesthetics developed in this manner was divinyl ether. Halothane was introduced into clinical practice in 1956 by Bryce-Smith and O'Brien in Oxford[5] and Johnstone in Manchester[6] and represented a significant advancement in inhalation anesthesia. Its sweet odor, nonflammability, and high potency offered clinical characteristics that were absent from the previous inhaled anesthetics. The search for newer and improved inhalation anesthetics persisted as concerns with hepatotoxicity and arrhythmogenicity of this alkane derivative began to be documented.

The two most recently released inhalation agents, sevoflurane (synthesized by Regan in the late 1960s) and desflurane (the 653rd compound of more than 700 synthesized by Terrell and colleagues between 1959 and 1966), have become accepted by many anesthesia providers as viable anesthetics for a diverse surgical population, based on their pharmacokinetic profile. What remains as a significant variable in determining the use of sevoflurane and desflurane among anesthesia providers is the cost (relative to isoflurane) versus clinical benefit to the patient. Although none of the inhalation anesthetic agents currently in use approaches the standards required of the ideal agent, some properties of an ideal anesthetic agent are listed in Box 9-1.

RELATIONSHIP OF CHEMICAL STRUCTURE AND AGENT CHARACTERISTICS

An understanding of the chemical structure of inhalation agents provides insight into their physical properties (e.g., flammability). However, the relationship between the pharmacologic characteristics (e.g., arrhythmogenic properties) and chemical structure of agents is not as predictable. This section reviews the structure-activity relationship of anesthetic vapors and their clinical relevance. Some selected physical and chemical properties are listed in Table 9-2.

All commonly used inhalation agents are ethers (R—O—R) or aliphatic hydrocarbons (straight-chained or branched nonaromatic hydrocarbons) with no more than four carbon atoms (Figure 9-1). The length of the anesthetic molecule is significant in that immobility (anesthetic effect) is attenuated or lost if carbon atom chain length exceeds a distance of four or five carbon atoms (5 angstroms [Å]).[7] The molecular shape of the agents is spherical or cylindrical with a length less than 1.5 times the diameter.[8]

Of primary importance to the development of volatile agents was the discovery of the impact of halogenation of organic compounds. Halogenation of hydrocarbons and ethers (the addition of fluorine [F], chlorine [Cl], bromine [Br], or iodine [I]) influences anesthetic potency, arrhythmogenic properties, flammability, and chemical stability (e.g., oxidation during storage and reactions with bases).

Anesthetic potency has been shown to increase when a halogen with a lower atomic mass unit (amu) is replaced by a heavier halogen (e.g., Br at 80 amu substituted for F at 19 amu).[9-11] Nonetheless, a ceiling effect exists with halogenation of anesthetic compounds. For example, adding F atoms to ether results in a continuum in which the ether becomes more potent, then acts as a strong convulsant, and finally changes to an inert compound with full fluorination.[12]

In general, the potency of volatile agents has also been found to correlate with the physical property of lipid solubility. A decline in potency (meaning an *increase* in the minimum alveolar concentration [MAC] of volatile agents) is associated with a proportional decrease in oil/gas partition coefficient values. Exceptions to this principle exist and demonstrate that the correlation between potency and lipid solubility is not perfect.

With regard to arrhythmogenic properties, increasing the number of halogen atoms within a volatile agent favors the genesis of cardiac dysrhythmias.[12] Nevertheless, alkanes that contain five halogens (e.g., halothane) are more prone to induce arrhythmias than ethers with six halogen atoms (e.g., isoflurane).[13] Ether molecules also contain oxygen, which reduces arrhythmogenic effects.

Flammability is reduced and chemical stability enhanced by substituting hydrogen atoms with halogens. The epitome of this relationship is demonstrated with desflurane, a compound that contains fluorine as its only halogen and thus strongly resists biodegradation; desflurane is metabolized one tenth as much as isoflurane.[14,15]

METABOLISM

As stated previously, the chemical structure of each inhalation agent determines the extent to which each volatile agent is

TABLE **9-1**	History of the Introduction of Inhalation Anesthetics
Anesthetic	**Year(s) Introduced**
N_2O	1840s
Ether	1840s
Chloroform	1840s
Cyclopropane	1930s
Fluroxene	1951
Halothane	1956
Methoxyflurane	1960
Enflurane	1973
Isoflurane	1981
Desflurane	1993
Sevoflurane	1995

BOX **9-1**

Properties of the Ideal Inhalation Anesthetic Agent

- It should have a pleasant odor, be nonirritating to the respiratory tract, and result in pleasant and rapid induction of anesthesia.
- It should possess a low blood/gas solubility, which permits rapid induction of and rapid recovery from anesthesia.
- It should be chemically stable in storage and should not interact with the material of the anesthetic machine and circuits or with soda lime.
- It should be neither flammable nor explosive.
- It should be capable of producing unconsciousness with analgesia and preferably some degree of muscle relaxation.
- It should be sufficiently potent to allow the use of high inspired-oxygen concentrations when necessary.
- It should not be metabolized in the body, should exert no systemic toxicity, and should not provoke allergic reactions.
- It should produce minimal and predictable depression of the cardiovascular and respiratory systems and should not interact with other drugs used commonly during anesthesia (e.g., pressor agents or catecholamines).
- It should be completely inert and eliminated completely and rapidly in an unchanged form via the lungs.
- It should be easy to administer using standard vaporizers.
- It should have a reasonable cost.
- It should not be epileptogenic or raise intracranial pressure.

Modified from Aitkenhead AR. Textbook of Anaesthesia. 5th ed. Edinburgh: Churchill Livingstone; 2007; and Bovill JG, Howie MB. Clinical Pharmacology for Anaesthetists. London: Saunders; 1999.

TABLE **9-2**	Select Properties of Volatile Anesthetics				
Property	**Halothane**	**Isoflurane**	**Desflurane**	**Sevoflurane**	**Nitrous Oxide**
MAC in O_2 30-60 yr at 37° C (EC_{50}; % atmosphere)	0.75	1.17	6.6	1.8	104
MAC in 60%-70% N_2O (%)	0.29	0.56	2.38	0.66	
MAC >65 yr (%)	0.64	1.0	5.17	1.45	
Blood/gas partition coefficient	2.5	1.46	0.42	0.65	0.46
Oil/gas partition coefficient	224	91	19	47	1.4
Specific gravity (g/mL)	1.87	1.50	1.47	1.50	NA
Boiling point (° C)	50	49	24	59	−88
Vapor pressure (mm Hg, 20° C)	243	238	669	157	Gas
Molecular weight (daltons)	197	184	168	200	44
Preservative	Thymol	None	None	None	None
Stability in CO_2 absorbers	Stable	Stable	Stable	No	Stable
Extent metabolized (%)	12-25	0.2	0.02	2-5	

Modified from Aitkenhead AR et al. Textbook of Anaesthesia. 5th ed. Edinburgh: Churchill Livingstone; 2007; and Hemmings H, Hopkins P. Foundation of Anesthesia Basic and Clinical Sciences. London: Mosby; 2000.
EC_{50}, Effective concentration in 50% of the population; MAC, minimum alveolar concentration.

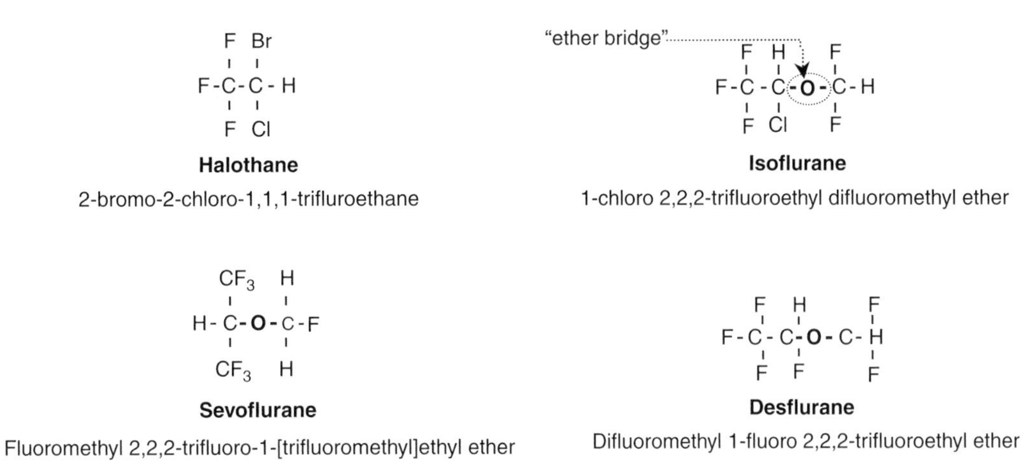

Halothane
2-bromo-2-chloro-1,1,1-trifluroethane

Isoflurane
1-chloro 2,2,2-trifluoroethyl difluoromethyl ether

Sevoflurane
Fluoromethyl 2,2,2-trifluoro-1-[trifluoromethyl]ethyl ether

Desflurane
Difluoromethyl 1-fluoro 2,2,2-trifluoroethyl ether

FIGURE **9-1**   Chemical structure of volatile agents. The "ether bridges" (R—O—R) are seen with sevoflurane, desflurane, and isoflurane. R refers to alkyl group. Halothane is a halogenated hydrocarbon.

metabolized. In general, increasing the number of fluorine atoms to an anesthetic molecule retards biodegradation (halothane has 3 and desflurane has 6). The current agents undergo metabolism at the following rates: sevoflurane 5% to 8% and isoflurane, desflurane, and nitrous oxide trace amounts.[16-21] Desflurane has been shown to resist biodegradation, even after 7.35 MAC-hours, as determined by peak mean urinary excretion rate of trifluoroacetic acid (TFA). This metabolite (TFA) is recognized as being a sensitive marker of desflurane metabolism.[22]

The biodegradation of all currently used volatile anesthetics is predominantly by way of hepatic metabolism through oxidation (phase I).[23] Halothane is unique in that it can also be metabolized by an alternative reductive pathway.[24] Sevoflurane has been used in the United States since 1995. Its biotransformation and lack of nephrotoxicity[25] are reviewed later in this chapter.

PHARMACODYNAMICS

Mechanisms of Action

The following properties of anesthetics must be taken into account when developing a theory that attempts to explain their mechanism of action:

1. Lipid solubility is directly proportional to potency (Meyer-Overton rule).[26,27]
2. Reversal of anesthetic effect can be achieved with the application of pressure, with some exceptions (species variation).[28]
3. No common chemical structure for the variety of compounds is capable of producing anesthesia.
4. The molecular and structural changes responsible for producing anesthesia must occur within seconds and be reversible.
5. A reduction in body temperature lowers anesthetic requirements.

In keeping with most of these prerequisites is the unitary hypothesis. This theory proposes that all inhalation anesthetics work via a similar (undefined) mechanism of action but not necessarily at the same site of action. One factor that supports this hypothesis is the Meyer-Overton correlation, which recognizes that the more lipid soluble the agent, the greater its potency (the lower its MAC value). This correlation suggests that anesthesia is produced by the volume of anesthetic

molecules present (dissolved) at the site, not by the type of volatile agent present. The additive effect observed among different anesthetics also supports the unitary hypothesis by suggesting independent sites of action[29]; nonetheless, disagreement remains regarding the validity of the unitary hypothesis.[30]

Research of the mechanism of action of volatile agents has caused some investigations to advocate for the redefining of the term *anesthesia*. A parsimonious view of inhalation anesthesia corresponds to compounds that produce amnesia and immobility in response to noxious stimuli. Amnesia in this context is defined as being unaware of one's environment or the inability to recall a previous episode of awareness. Any agent that produces both characteristics is termed a *full anesthetic*, and drugs that cause amnesia alone are termed *nonimmobilizers and nonanesthetics*.[31] The other traditional characteristics of an anesthetic state (analgesia, skeletal muscle relaxation) are viewed as "side effects" that are not essential to what defines anesthesia.[32] For clarification, this does not mean these side effects are of no concern to the anesthesia provider. Quite the contrary, adequate modulation of a patient's sympathetic response to painful stimuli can determine the success or failure of some anesthetics.

Research has permitted the description of the mechanism of action of inhaled anesthetics relative to distinct anatomic regions of the body and molecular changes. The spinal cord is known to mediate immobility to a painful stimulus via several mechanisms including (1) enhancing background potassium (K⁺) currents in tandem-pore-domain, weak inward-rectifying K^+ channels (TWIK)[33,34] and (2) reducing spontaneous action potential firing of spinal neurons via glycine receptors and γ-aminobutyric acid type A [GABA$_A$] receptors.[35] Investigators have also demonstrated nonimmobilizers with lipophilic characteristics (e.g., perfluoropentane) are able to produce amnesia but not immobility to noxious stimuli, which suggests two separate sites and mechanisms of anesthetic action for some drugs.[36] In contrast with other research, spinal *and* cerebral GABA$_A$ receptors (same receptor-clinical effect) were shown to contribute to volatile anesthetic's ability to produce immobility; therefore, the anesthetic effect of immobility is modulated at the spinal cord and supraspinal level.[37] In summary, research has validated the concept of a distinct anatomical division for the mechanism of action of volatile agents as being oversimplistic (and inaccurate); one example being the isolation of TWIK (a member of the tandem-pore-domain K channel family) in both the spinal cord and brain.[33] Clearly, supraspinal areas of the nervous system are recognized to mediate amnesia and immobility.[33,37-39]

Other specific anatomic sites where volatile anesthetics produce an effect include the reticular formation within the brainstem,[40] cerebral cortex,[41] and hippocampus.[42] Evidence of changes in cortical activity by volatile agents includes alterations in electroencephalogram (EEG) activity. All inhalation agents cause a dose-dependent change in the EEG—an initial increase in voltage (and decrease in frequency), then a peak, followed by a decline.[43,44] Deeper levels of anesthesia produce burst suppression and eventually a flat EEG.[45] Nonspecific generalized EEG changes may also persist for several days postoperatively.[46]

Increased or decreased neuronal excitability and enhanced or depressed inhibitory postsynaptic currents can occur, depending on which anesthetic agent or specific area within the CNS is manipulated. In addition to supraspinal effects, modulation of afferent and efferent impulses within the spinal cord has also occurred with volatile anesthetics.[47,48]

On a molecular level, researchers have found that the most likely site of action for volatile anesthetics involves interactions with membrane proteins in specific receptors (stereoselective) and not perturbation of lipid bilayers.[49-51] The primary receptor within the CNS believed to modulate anesthetic effects is the GABA receptor, specifically the subtype A.[38,39,52] This receptor is located abundantly in the CNS and is a ligand-gated chloride (Cl^-) ion channel.[53] Agonism of this receptor by full anesthetics (volatile agents) results in enhanced Cl^- conductance,[54] which leads to inhibitory actions on local neurons.[53] Ultimately, what is expressed is an extension of the amount of time the Cl^- channel remains open.[45] In contrast to full anesthetics, nonimmobilizers do not enhance the effect of GABA on these receptors. Neuronal nicotinic acetylcholine receptors (nAChRs) have also been shown to be highly sensitive to inhalational anesthetics and are believed to significantly influence several stages of anesthesia.[55]

An investigation by Kaech and colleagues revealed a new anesthetic site of action within the CNS; chloroform, diethyl ether, methoxyflurane, halothane, enflurane, and isoflurane were each shown (in clinically relevant concentrations) to block the morphologic plasticity of dendritic spines.[56] Prior research has demonstrated that dendritic spines can change shape in seconds.[57] This phenomenon occurs secondary to motile actin, which is abundant in the spines.[58] These volatile agents were found to strongly inhibit actin motility, which blocked changes in dendritic spine shape; the inhibition was fully reversed after removal of the agents. The dendritic spines serve as excitatory postsynaptic contact sites.[59] They are extremely abundant in the cerebral cortex (greater than 10^{13}) and are also located in large numbers in the cerebellum, basal ganglia, and olfactory bulb.[60] The details of how these rapid morphologic changes in dendritic spines contribute to an anesthetic state are unclear and merit further research.

The CNS effects of amnesia and loss of consciousness likely are produced separately from the immobility conceptualized in the theory of MAC.[61] The concept of MAC refers to the concentration required to prevent movement in response to a surgical situation. This is the result of an effect at the spinal cord level via glycine, 5-hydroxytriptamine$_{2A}$, sodium, and N-methyl-D-aspartate receptor action. Potassium, α-amino-3-hydroxy-5-methyl-4-isoxazolepropionic (AMPA) and kainate, GABA,

opioid, α$_2$-, 5HT$_3$, and acetylcholine receptors are likely not involved in producing immobility. They may be involved in varying degrees in the amnestic and anesthetic effects in the CNS.

MINIMUM ALVEOLAR CONCENTRATION

A useful means of comparing the potencies of inhalation agents is to use the concept of MAC, defined as the minimum alveolar concentration at equilibrium (expressed as a percentage of 1 atmosphere) in which 50% of subjects will not respond to a painful stimulus (i.e., initial surgical skin incision).[62] The response is defined as gross, *purposeful* movement of the head or extremities. The MAC values for the modern inhalation agents are listed in Table 9-3.[63-67]

The MAC of volatile agents can be affected by numerous factors, surprisingly even hair color.[68,69] With increasing age, the MAC of all inhaled anesthetics is reduced; in humans with mean age 18 to 30 years, the MAC of desflurane is 7.25%, in contrast to 6% in humans 30 to 55 years of age.[67] Infants represent an exception to the MAC age concept in that their anesthetic requirements exceed those of neonates. Box 9-2 lists variables shown to reduce and increase MAC.

Two other areas related to MAC are MAC-awake and MAC-BAR (block adrenergic response). *MAC-awake* is defined as the minimum alveolar concentration at which 50% of subjects will respond to the command "open your eyes." It has also been described as the anesthetic concentration that is between the end-tidal values that allow and prevent response to a command.[70] This end-tidal concentration is usually associated with a loss of recall and encompasses approximately one third of MAC values. MAC-awake can also be used in combination with MAC values to evaluate the potency of each agent with regard to amnestic properties. This is done by dividing MAC-awake by MAC (MAC-awake/MAC ratio). This parameter indicates that agents with ratios between 0.3 and 0.4 (e.g., desflurane, sevoflurane, isoflurane) are considered potent anesthetics. In contrast, N_2O, which has a ratio of 0.64, is considered a weak amnestic agent.

The MAC-BAR parameter represents the MAC necessary to block the adrenergic response (e.g., changes in plasma norepinephrine concentration, heart rate [HR], rate-pressure product, and mean arterial pressure) to skin incision. It can be expressed as a MAC-BAR$_{50}$ or MAC-BAR$_{95}$. The former is similar to AD$_{95}$

TABLE 9-3	Potencies of Volatile Anesthetics in Humans With and Without N_2O Expressed in MAC and MAPP Values*	
Anesthetic	**†MAC (MAPP)**	**In 60%-70% N_2O MAC (MAPP)**
Nitrous oxide	104 (798)	—
Desflurane	6.6 (50.16)	2.38 (18.08)
Sevoflurane	1.8 (13.68)	0.66 (5.01)
Isoflurane	1.17 (8.89)	0.56 (4.25)
Halothane	0.75 (5.7)	0.29 (2.20)

FIO$_2$, *Fraction of inspired oxygen*; MAC, *minimum alveolar concentration*; MAPP, *minimum alveolar partial pressure*; N_2O, *nitrous oxide*.
*MAC is expressed as volume percent of end-tidal gas at standard pressure. MAPP is calculated as MAC value times 760 mm Hg ÷ 100 (expressed in mm Hg).
†Age 30 to 60 years.

values, which represent the anesthetic dose that inhibits somatic evidence of light anesthesia in 95% of subjects in response to skin incision. Established MAC-BAR$_{50}$ values for volatile agents include (in 60% N_2O) 1.45 MAC (0.75% × 1.5 = 1.125%) for halothane,[71] and 1.3 MAC for both isoflurane and desflurane.[72] The MAC-BAR$_{50}$ for sevoflurane in 66% N_2O is 2.2.[73] The MAC-BAR$_{95}$ of halothane is 2.1 and 2.6 for enflurane.[71] It should be emphasized that MAC-BAR values exceed the requirements for ablation of skeletal muscle movement with surgical stimulation; therefore, blocking an adrenergic response requires a greater depth of anesthesia than preventing skeletal muscle movement. From a clinical standpoint, patients usually require anesthetic concentrations that exceed MAC by 20% to 30% (1.2 to 1.3 times MAC). At this alveolar concentration, somatic evidence of light anesthesia will commonly be abated, and fewer patients will respond adrenergically to the stresses of surgery.[74]

The concept of MAC has limitations when applied clinically to determine adequacy of anesthesia. It should be viewed as a general guide to the overall depth of anesthesia. One variable that restricts its application is the frequency at which surgical patients receive muscle relaxants, which attenuates the recognition of skeletal muscle movement in response to light planes of anesthesia. This results in the dependence of anesthesia providers on other traditional signs of anesthetic depth, such as changes in heart rate (HR), blood pressure, pupillary size, and sweating. Unfortunately, a light plane of anesthesia can exist even with a decreased blood pressure and a normal heart rate (e.g., patients with limited cardiac reserve). Pupillary changes can also be affected by opioids (miosis) and volatile agents (mydriasis) over time, even in the absence of surgical stimuli.[75] Also, the usefulness of a traditional clinical end-point as a guide to depth of anesthesia can change over time. For example, one investigator found that decreases in blood pressure served as an estimate of anesthetic depth during the first hour of an anesthetic, but after 5 hours they were unreliable—further declines in blood pressure did not occur even with increasing concentrations of halothane.[76] The challenge to the anesthesia provider is to estimate anesthetic depth based on a collation of variables (HR, blood pressure, synergistic and additive effects of anesthetic adjuvants, volume status, physiologic reserve, MAC, MAC-BAR, and MAC intubation values). The last variable (MAC intubation) is similar to MAC-BAR in that its values exceed the anesthetic requirements for surgical skin incision. Clearly, different stimuli require different end-tidal concentrations (brain anesthetic partial pressures) of volatile anesthetics.[77]

INFLUENCE OF INHALATION AGENTS ON ORGANS AND SYSTEMS

Central Nervous System

The volatile agents can adversely affect the care provided to patients with CNS pathology. Such effects include areas related to intracranial compliance, autoregulation of cerebral blood flow (CBF; e.g., cerebrovascular reactivity to carbon dioxide [CO_2]), cerebral metabolic rate, cerebrospinal fluid pressure (CSFP), and neurologic assessment.

Cerebral Metabolic Rate and Cerebral Blood Flow

In general, volatile agents decrease cerebral metabolic rate of O_2 consumption ($CMRO_2$) in a dose-dependent manner, whereas their effect on cerebral blood flow is variable; the latter has been reported by various researchers to be unchanged,[78] increased (dose-dependent and time-dependent manner),[79,80] or decreased.[81] When vascular resistance is decreased, CBF, cerebral blood volume (CBV), and CSFP increase. The order of potency for increasing CBF varies; it is affected by the dose of volatile anesthetic,[82] the administration of other drugs (e.g., propofol, N_2O),[83] the rate of change in end-tidal concentration of agent,[79] and the animal model used.[84] In other cases, differences in research findings lack a plausible explanation. A distinct picture of a homogeneous versus heterogeneous change in CBF, $CMRO_2$, and other

---

BOX 9-2

Relationship of Physiologic and Pharmacologic Factors to the MAC of Inhaled Anesthetics

Factors That Reduce MAC
Increase in age
Hypothermia
Administration of depressant medications (e.g., opioids, opioid agonist-antagonist analgesics, benzodiazepines, barbiturates, chlorpromazine, hydroxyzine)
α_2 Agonists
Acute ethanol consumption
Metabolic acidosis
Hypoxemia
Anemia (<4.3 mL O_2/dL blood)
Hypotension (MAP < 50 mm Hg)
Hyponatremia
Pregnancy
N_2O, ketamine, verapamil, lidocaine, clonidine, alpha-methyldopa, reserpine, chronic dextroamphetamine use, lithium, levodopa

Factors That Increase MAC
Decrease in age
Hyperthermia
Hyperthyroidism
Hypernatremia
Chronic alcohol consumption
Acute administration of dextroamphetamine
Monoamine oxidase inhibitors
Cocaine, levodopa

Factors with No Effect on MAC
Duration of anesthesia
Gender
Redheaded females
Hypocarbia and hypercarbia
Metabolic alkalosis
Hypertension
Administration of propranolol, isoproterenol, promethazine, naloxone, aminophylline, and neuromuscular blocking agents.

MAC, *Minimum alveolar concentration*; N_2O, *nitrous oxide*.

anesthetic effects of volatile agents has been noted[85] For example, halothane has been shown to globally increase CBF, whereas isoflurane's sphere of influence predominates in the subcortical regions and hindbrain structures.[86]

Uncoupling of Cerebral Blood Flow and Metabolism

When decreases in $CMRO_2$ are accompanied by increases in CBF, *uncoupling* is said to occur. As noted above, volatile anesthetics are capable of producing this effect. This paradoxical response (decreased $CMRO_2$ occurring in conjunction with increased CBF) seems not to occur with 1.0 MAC or less of halothane and isoflurane[87]; the magnitude of change is variable and dose dependent, meaning some flow-metabolism coupling mechanism is preserved.[88-90]

Nitrous oxide reduces cerebrovascular tone significantly. This effect is unmasked and enhanced when N_2O is combined with a volatile anesthetic (decreased autoregulation).[91] The mechanism for increased CBF may be related to a sympathoadrenal-stimulating effect of N_2O. The changes produced by N_2O in the $CMRO_2$ are the reverse of what takes place with volatile agents (i.e., increased $CMRO_2$),[92] although other investigators have reported no effect.[93] Nevertheless, a general impression is that N_2O probably increases $CMRO_2$ and CBF. The combination of elevated CBF and $CMRO_2$ still results in an uncoupling between flow and metabolism, because in goats the increase in $CMRO_2$ exceeds, albeit slightly, the elevation in CBF.[94] In summary, N_2O use in neurosurgical procedures is acceptable, as long as the anesthesia provider recognizes that its vasodilatory effects might adversely affect surgical outcome in patients with reduced intracranial compliance. Hyperventilation helps attenuate the increase in CBF that accompanies the use of N_2O.[95]

Cerebral Vasculature Responsiveness to CO_2

The normal physiologic response of the cerebral vasculature to CO_2 is to vasoconstrict in the presence of hypocapnia and vasodilate with hypercarbia. This reflex is effective in the acute setting when used during neurosurgical procedures to counteract drug-induced vasodilation and to reduce brain bulk within a closed compartment (cranial vault).[96] The usual goal for patients in which a reduction in intracranial volume is desired is a $Paco_2$ of 30 to 35 mm Hg with a duration of effectiveness being perhaps no more than 4 to 6 hours.[97]

Differences exist among the volatile agents in their ability to interfere with the cerebral vasculature's responsiveness to CO_2. Variables that affect the reported differences include the type of surgical procedure the patient is undergoing, associated pathophysiology, and the presence of any coexisting disease(s). For example, patients with hypertension given 1 MAC isoflurane with 67% N_2O have better control of CBF via manipulation of arterial CO_2 than those receiving 1 MAC sevoflurane with 67% N_2O.[98] Similar results have been reported by other investigators.[99] In contrast, CO_2 reactivity in insulin-dependent patients is equally impaired by 1 MAC isoflurane and 1 MAC sevoflurane, each given with 67% nitrous oxide.[100] Others have suggested that sevoflurane is less vasoactive than halothane, isoflurane, and desflurane and recommend it as a good alternative to propofol in patients with normal intracranial pressure.[101] It has also been reported to better preserve dynamic cerebral autoregulation than isoflurane when both are given at 1.5 MAC in combination with 100% O_2.[102] Desflurane administered to patients undergoing craniotomy for tumor resection with an air-O_2 mixture at 1.0 to 1.5 MAC has been shown to act similarly to isoflurane and maintain cerebrovascular reactivity to CO_2 and

cerebrospinal fluid pressure.[103-105] These research findings suggest that increases in CBF produced by isoflurane, desflurane,[104] and sevoflurane[106] can be effectively prevented by hyperventilation and using concentrations less than 1.5 MAC.

Electroencephalogram and Evoked Potentials

The volatile agents produce a dose-related suppression of EEG activity (initial increase [later a decline] in amplitude and decreased frequency) and at high concentrations produce electrical quiescence.[107] At deeper levels of anesthesia, the EEG may temporarily stop recording; at such time, burst suppression is said to have occurred. The effect of anesthetic agents on evoked potential is given in Chapter 29, Box 29-3.

For those procedures requiring monitoring of the integrity of the spinal cord or mapping of cortical regions of the brain, the anesthetist should be aware that inhalation agents can skew cortical somatosensory, motor, brainstem, auditory, and visual evoked potentials. Isoflurane, desflurane, sevoflurane, and N_2O produce a dose-dependent reduction in these evoked potentials, with visual evoked potentials being most sensitive and brainstem-evoked potentials most resistant.[97,107,108] Two evoked-potential variables commonly assessed are latency and amplitude. An increase in latency or decrease in amplitude of evoked potentials can reflect ischemia or be secondary to the volatile agent. Latency is the time between the initiation of a peripheral stimulus (e.g., electrical stimulation of the median nerve at the wrist) and onset of the evoked potential (e.g., cortical) recorded by scalp electrodes.

Isoflurane has been shown to interfere with the recording of cortical somatosensory evoked potentials (cSSEP) at light planes of anesthesia (0.5 MAC with 60% N_2O)[109] and desflurane and sevoflurane at 1.5 MAC (without N_2O).[97] Of these three agents, isoflurane produces the greatest reduction in cSSEP amplitude, whereas no difference exists among the volatile anesthetics' effect on latency.[110] The addition of N_2O to isoflurane, desflurane, and sevoflurane can also produce a significant reduction in the amplitude of cSSEPs.[111,112] It may be prudent to avoid the use of this agent in patients who have baseline low-amplitude evoked potentials.

Sevoflurane,[113,114] unlike desflurane[115] and isoflurane,[43] can predispose pediatric and adult patients to epileptic activity, even though sevoflurane[116-119] can suppress drug-induced convulsive activity in a manner similar to desflurane[120] and isoflurane.[118] Sevoflurane combined with N_2O has produced epileptiform EEG activity during inhalation induction with adults in a single-breath technique. A hyperdynamic response can accompany the EEG changes if concurrent hyperventilation occurs. The incidence of epileptiform EEG changes has been shown to nearly double in the presence of hypocapnia (100% versus 47%).[121] Similar results have been observed in children aged 2 to 12 years.[113] In contrast, intravenous induction with thiopental followed by anesthetic maintenance with 2% end-tidal sevoflurane in air does not produce seizurelike changes in the EEG in children.[114] Epileptiform activity has also been reported to occur during emergence from sevoflurane.[122]

Emergence and Neurologic Assessment in Adults

Although the objective of a smooth and rapid emergence from a general anesthetic is desirable for all surgical patients, it is especially meaningful for neurosurgical candidates. Delayed emergence in this specialty of anesthesia can have devastating consequences. A slow return of consciousness makes it difficult to perform the initial postoperative neurologic examination. It can also add to unnecessary therapeutic or diagnostic intervention and predispose the patient to respiratory complications.[123]

Because of this, the bias of some anesthesia providers is to administer total intravenous anesthetic (TIVA) techniques such as propofol with remifentanil for neurosurgical procedures involving supratentorial tumors. Some investigators report a more rapid awakening (after approximately 2 hours of anesthesia) from TIVA in non-neurosurgical patients compared with sevoflurane and desflurane combined with N_2O.[124] Recovery profiles for sevoflurane and desflurane indicate they are superior to isoflurane.[125,126] In side-by-side comparisons of desflurane and sevoflurane, desflurane permits for a more rapid awakening than sevoflurane in volunteers after 8 hours of exposure.[127] In contrast, sevoflurane allows for acute changes in vaporizer settings without evoking neurocirculatory excitation (significant increases in sympathetic nerve activity, norepinephrine concentrations, heart rate, and mean arterial blood pressure); of particular interest was the finding that desflurane's sympathomimetic response occurred in response to a controlled adjustment in vaporizer settings (i.e., changing from 6% to 9%)—that is, in the absence of overpressurization.[128] Sevoflurane may be preferred over desflurane if concentrations equal to or in excess of 1 MAC are used during neurologic surgery.[79] One study also found no difference in early postoperative recovery and cognitive function between a balanced sevoflurane-fentanyl technique versus propofol-remifentanil (TIVA) management in patients undergoing supratentorial intracranial surgery.[129] Further research is necessary to clarify whether the use of one volatile agent over another or TIVA technique influences neurosurgery outcome. In addition, questions remain regarding the potential neuroprotective effect of currently used inhalational agents. Current research suggests that anesthetics can provide long-term durable protection against ischemic injury that is mild to moderate in severity. Experimental data do not provide support for the premise that anesthetics reduce injury when the ischemic injury is severe.[130] Anesthetics consistently and meaningfully improve outcome from experimental cerebral ischemia, but only if present during the ischemic insult.[131] Not all research supports this clinical benefit.[132]

Emergence Phenomenon in Children

Sevoflurane and desflurane are associated with emergence agitation or delirium in children.[133] The emergence phenomenon is short-lived but troublesome, and the etiology is uncertain. A variety of factors have been suggested to play a potential role in emergence delirium (ED). Restless behavior upon emergence causes discomfort to the child, postanesthesia recovery nurses, and parents. Some suggested factors related to transient emergence agitation are noted in Box 9-3. These children may require analgesics or sedatives, which can delay discharge. Emergence delirium is self-limiting and devoid of apparent sequelae, as long as the child is protected from self-injury. Preventive measures include reducing preoperative anxiety and postoperative pain and providing a quiet, stress-free environment for postanesthesia recovery. Treatment may include small doses of midazolam, fentanyl, clonidine, or dexmedetomidine. Reuniting the child with the parents is also helpful.[134]

Cardiovascular System

All inhalation agents are capable of altering hemodynamics, the extent being related to various preoperative and intraoperative factors (e.g., American Society of Anesthesiologists physical status, coadministration of vasoactive drugs, opioids, barbiturates). This section reviews the influence of volatile agents on the cardiovascular system.

Systemic Hemodynamics

Isoflurane, desflurane, and sevoflurane all reduce mean arterial pressure (MAP) (Figure 9-2) and cardiac output (CO) and cardiac index (CI) in a dose-dependent fashion.[128,135-137] The mechanism by which each accomplishes this varies. For example, desflurane, sevoflurane, and isoflurane predominantly reduce MAP via a reduction in systemic vascular resistance (SVR), with the dose-response relationship being least with sevoflurane (Figure 9-3).[128,138] Halothane, by comparison, causes less disruption in inherent vascular tone and therefore predominantly reduces MAP by direct myocardial depression versus a reduction in preload.[139] Nitrous oxide activates the sympathetic nervous system and increases SVR,[140] which can also lead to an increase in central venous pressure (CVP) and arterial pressure. This sympathetic nervous system response appears to be intact during co-administration of volatile agents.[135]

From Vlajkovic GP, Sindjelic RP. Emergence delirium in children: many questions, few answers. Anesth Analg. 2007;104(1):84-91.

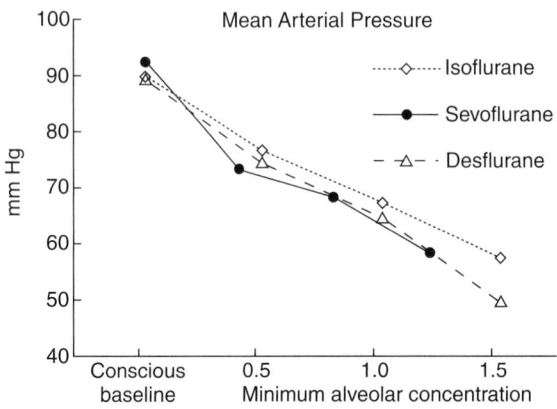

FIGURE **9-2** Mean arterial pressure response to the administration of isoflurane, sevoflurane, and desflurane in healthy volunteers. With increasing minimum alveolar anesthetic concentration, progressive decreases in blood pressure occurred with each of the volatile anesthetics. (*Adapted from Ebert TJ, Muzi M. Sympathetic hyperactivity during desflurane anesthesia in healthy volunteers: a comparison with isoflurane. Anesthesiology. 1993;79:444-453; and Ebert TJ et al. The neurocirculatory responses to sevoflurane anesthesia in humans: a comparison to desflurane. Anesthesiology. 1995;83:88-95.*)

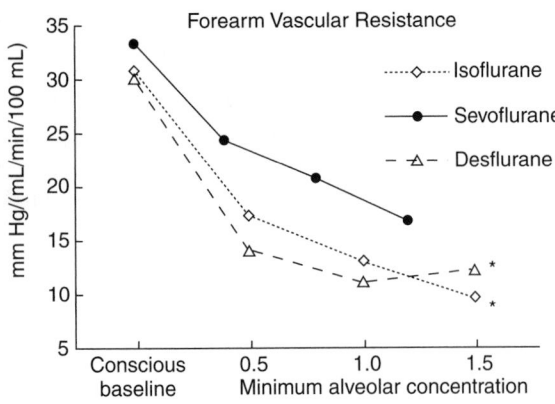

FIGURE **9-3** Forearm vascular resistance response to the administration of isoflurane, sevoflurane, and desflurane in healthy volunteers. In general, forearm vascular resistance was progressively decreased with increasing minimum alveolar anesthetic concentrations of each of the volatile anesthetics; however, this decline was less in the group receiving sevoflurane. (*Adapted from Ebert TJ, Muzi M. Sympathetic hyperactivity during desflurane anesthesia in healthy volunteers: a comparison with isoflurane. Anesthesiology. 1993;79:444-453; and Ebert TJ et al. The neurocirculatory responses to sevoflurane anesthesia in humans: a comparison to desflurane. Anesthesiology. 1995;83:88-95.*)

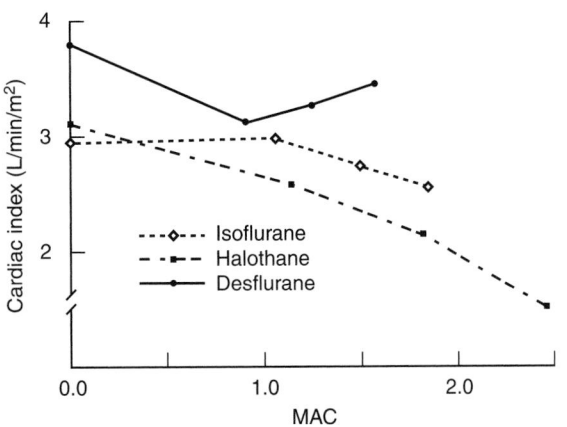

FIGURE **9-4** Cardiac index measured in healthy normocarbic volunteers during conscious state (0) MAC and during various steady-state MAC levels of halothane, isoflurane, and desflurane. (*Reprinted with permission from Warltier DC, as modified from Weiskopf et al. Cardiovascular and respiratory actions of desflurane: Is desflurane different from isoflurane? Anesth Analg. 1992;75:S23.*)

In general, N_2O used in combination with inhalation agents increases SVR and helps support arterial blood pressure.[141] In contrast, with opioids, the addition of N_2O augments cardiac depression instead of supporting it[142] because N_2O also produces a direct negative inotropic effect. This property can be unmasked in patients with decreased left ventricular function secondary to coronary artery disease or valvular heart defects.[143] Desflurane supports CI better than halothane at both low and high MAC levels (i.e., 1.66 MAC)[144] (Figure 9-4). With light levels of anesthesia, desflurane maintains the CI without

an accompanying elevation in HR. For deeper levels of anesthesia, the CI is probably supported by the associated rise in HR. Some investigators believe the favorable circulatory profile of desflurane, isoflurane, and sevoflurane results from their ability to attenuate the body's circulatory compensatory mechanisms in a dose-related manner.[128,145] In summary, there is no appreciable difference in the ether anesthetics' ability to produce dose-dependent depression in arterial pressure and cardiac output.[135-137,144]

Regarding the impact of the duration of anesthesia on hemodynamics, isoflurane, sevoflurane, and desflurane produce a similar response—that being as MAC-hours of anesthesia increase, CI and HR increase slightly.[135,144] The CI effect may be secondary to a continued reduction in SVR and increase in HR following prolonged exposure to each of the agents. Protracted anesthesia (8 hours) in healthy volunteers anesthetized with desflurane and sevoflurane leads to an increase in pupil size and HR independent of surgery.[75] These changes are not associated with increases in plasma catecholamines, blood pressure, or CO_2 production; therefore mydriasis and tachycardia as signs of anesthetic depth could be misleading at times.

Although anesthetic changes produced at the cellular level have already been discussed, it is sensible to briefly review the cellular effects of inhaled anesthetics on the aforementioned areas of the cardiovascular system. In vitro and in vivo studies have revealed that isoflurane, sevoflurane, and desflurane reduce intracellular free calcium (Ca^{2+}) concentrations in cardiac and vascular smooth muscle.[136,137] The mechanism for this is believed to be a reduction in Ca^{2+} influx through the sarcolemma and a depression of depolarization-activated Ca^{2+} release from the sarcoplasmic reticulum.[136,137,146] The end result is a depression in the contractile state of the myocardium, along with dilation of the peripheral vasculature. Other reported cellular effects of volatile agents include augmentation and attenuation of endothelium-derived relaxation factor, inhibition of acetylcholine-induced vascular relaxation,[147] and attenuation of sodium (Na^+)- Ca^{2+} exchange that leads to a reduction in the quantity of intracellular Ca^{2+}.[148] Future research is needed to clarify the effect of volatile agents in patients with cardiovascular dysfunction (hypertension, diabetes, geriatric patients) in which vascular responses can be altered. In these populations (compared to patients with normal physiology) the mechanisms for regulating vascular tone at the cellular level are altered.

Heart Rate

Volatile agents and N_2O induce changes in HR relative to the concentration of the anesthetic being used. Alterations in HR are a result of several variables: antagonism of SA node automaticity,[149] modulation of baroreceptor reflex activity,[150] and sympathetic nervous system activation via activation of tracheopulmonary and systemic receptors.[151]

Halothane and sevoflurane produce only minor alterations in HR, even when used in excess of 1 MAC,[152] although a rapid and large increase in the inspired concentration (i.e., from 0.5 MAC to 2.9 MAC) of sevoflurane (and isoflurane) may produce an increase in plasma epinephrine concentrations.[153] Isoflurane and desflurane can cause an increase in HR,[154] and when more than 1 MAC of desflurane is used (even without overpressurization), the dose-response relationship becomes more prominent, particularly when compared with sevoflurane (Figure 9-5).[128] Desflurane's steep dose-response to HR can potentially be problematic by diminishing the reliability of HR as a guide to anesthetic depth and by predisposing patients at risk for coronary

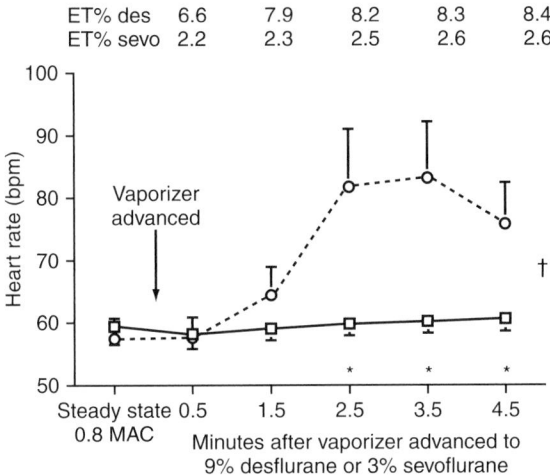

| ET% des | 6.6 | 7.9 | 8.2 | 8.3 | 8.4 |
| ET% sevo | 2.2 | 2.3 | 2.5 | 2.6 | 2.6 |

FIGURE **9-5** The effects of sevoflurane (*solid line with squares*) and desflurane (*dashed line with circles*) on heart rate in healthy young volunteers when the inspiratory concentration is rapidly increased from a steady-state value of 0.83 MAC to 1.25 MAC. (*Reprinted with permission from Ebert TJ. Neurocirculatory responses to sevoflurane in humans. Anesthesiology. 1995;83:88.*)

artery disease to myocardial ischemia secondary to an increased myocardial oxygen demand.

Research has shown pretreatment with fentanyl (1.5 or 4.5 mcg/kg) 5 minutes before an increase in end-tidal desflurane concentration from 4% to 8% modulates (not abolishes) an increase in HR by 61% and 70%, respectively.[155] In this same study, increase in MAP was attenuated by 31% and 46%. Another group of investigators found 5 mcg/kg of fentanyl followed by a continuous infusion of 2 mcg/kg/hr initiated 12 minutes before induction significantly blunted the HR and MAP response to a rapid increase in end-tidal desflurane concentration (5.4% to 11%).[156] The acute change in desflurane concentration occurred 20 minutes after intubation. Fentanyl's efficacy was also assessed 2 minutes after induction when desflurane was given in three incremental 1-minute steps (3.6%, 7.2%, 11%). Of interest was the finding that fentanyl was ineffective in diminishing the desflurane stimulatory effect during this induction period. Therefore the optimal use of fentanyl may be during steady-state periods of anesthesia when acute adjustments of desflurane are desired.

Esmolol (0.75 mg/kg) has been shown to attenuate HR response but not MAP and therefore may be less desirable than fentanyl.[155] Prior administration of intravenous lidocaine (1.5 mg/kg) has not been shown to be effective in modulating the sympathetic response associated with an acute change in desflurane end-tidal MAC value of 0.7 to 1.5.[157]

Coronary Blood Flow

The term *coronary steal* is defined as a reduction in perfusion of ischemic myocardium with simultaneous improvement of blood flow to nonischemic tissue. Simply stated, blood has been taken from the "poor" and given to the "rich" (a "reverse—Robin Hood" syndrome). In addition, this phenomenon has been demonstrated to occur more easily with "coronary steal–prone anatomy" (i.e., multivessel disease models).[158] Several articles have suggested that isoflurane and perhaps desflurane are capable

of producing a coronary steal with clinically relevant concentrations,[159] but other researchers have not found this to occur.[160,161] One investigator's results suggest that the use of 0.5% isoflurane in combination with 50% N_2O might be protective to the myocardium (i.e., improve the tolerance to pacing-induced myocardial ischemia).[162]

An important qualifier to isoflurane's ability to maldistribute coronary blood flow is the presence of hypotension; when normotension is maintained, a steal phenomenon is abated.[163] Reduced blood flow to ischemic myocardium can also be reversed if normotension is reestablished with phenylephrine administration.[164] To summarize the effects of isoflurane, desflurane, and sevoflurane on the coronary circulation, it can be stated that each produces vasodilation, with sevoflurane doing so the least.[159,165] In the presence of hypotension, a steal phenomenon can occur (as it can with inappropriate use of intravenous nitroglycerin or sodium nitroprusside), and this effect is reversible if normotension is reestablished. The magnitude of coronary vasodilation also is markedly less for isoflurane than that which occurs with dipyridamole[166] and the endogenous nucleoside, adenosine,[167] both of which produce coronary vasodilation even in the presence of normotension. Any of these three volatile anesthetics can be used in patients with a history of ischemic heart disease. If ECG monitoring demonstrates ST-segment or T-wave changes suggestive of myocardial ischemia (in the absence of abnormal hemodynamics), a change in primary anesthetic techniques may be warranted (e.g., substituting isoflurane for sevoflurane).[161]

As mentioned previously, volatile agents may produce a neuroprotective effect; similarly, the heart appears to benefit from isoflurane, sevoflurane, and desflurane inhaled anesthetics via initiating the phenomenon of preconditioning.[168] Anesthetic preconditioning (APC) results in a cascade of intracellular events that help protect the myocardium from ischemic and reperfusion insult, potentially limiting infarct size. The mechanism for this effect is multifactorial and includes such things as improving contractile function, preventing the down-regulation of major sarcoplasmic reticulum Ca^{2+} cycling proteins, thereby reducing calcium overload in the myocardial cells. The latter effect has been shown to be independent of potassium-sensitive adenosine triphosphate (K_{ATP}) channels[169] and confers 30% to 40% of the cardioprotective effect produced by inhalational anesthetics.[170] On the molecular level, sevoflurane has been found to produce in healthy male volunteers late preconditioning (24 to 48 hours after sevoflurane administration), as evidenced by altering gene expression in white blood cells (e.g., reduced pro-inflammatory L-selectin [CD62L] expression on granulocytes).[171] A potential application of APC, along with other cardioprotective substances such as insulin and adenosine, is administering preconditioning drugs during early coronary artery reperfusion, as is currently done with antiplatelet and antithrombotic therapies. Research has shown the administration of volatile agents during myocardial reperfusion activates a group of prosurvival kinases called the *Reperfusion Injury Salvage Kinase* (RISK) pathway. These prosurvival kinases produce potent cardioprotective effects.[172] The RISK pathway has also been found to be activated during ischemic preconditioning (a brief stimulus of myocardial ischemia/occlusion leading to cardioprotection).[172] Other factors that have been identified with preconditioning include protein kinase C activation of K_{ATP} channel opening, adenosine receptors (α_1 and α_2 subtypes), and inhibitory G proteins.[173-175] The recent American College of Cardiology/American Heart Association Guidelines on perioperative cardiac evaluation and care note that it can be beneficial to use volatile anesthetic agents during noncardiac surgery for the maintenance of general anesthesia in hemodynamically stable patients at risk for myocardial ischemia.[176] This is due to a protective effect on the myocardium associated with preconditioning.

It has been advocated that sulfonylurea oral hyperglycemic drugs be discontinued 24 to 48 hours prior to elective surgery, owing to their ability to close K_{ATP} channels.[25,177] Insulin is recommended as replacement therapy during this time period to abate the negative impact of hyperglycemia on preconditioning.[177]

Dysrhythmias

The dysrhythmic potential of inhalation agents has long been recognized. All of the agents, with the exception of isoflurane and probably desflurane, are conducive to the development of bradycardia and disturbances in atrioventricular (AV) nodal conduction (excluding second- or third-degree AV block). The mechanism for this is their ability to depress slow-response (sinoatrial and atrioventricular nodal tissue) and fast-response (atrial or ventricular musculature, Purkinje fibers) action potentials. When fibers become ischemic or injured, the volatile agents (particularly halothane) are prone to produce reentrant excitation.[178,179]

The ability of the volatile agents to reduce the quantity of catecholamines necessary to evoke dysrhythmias is commonly but inaccurately called "sensitization." It is more accurate to describe this phenomenon as an adverse drug interaction.[178] Researchers have determined the nasal and oral submucosal ED_{50} dosage of epinephrine for volatile agents to be 2.11 ± 0.15 mcg/kg for halothane and 6.72 ± 0.66 mcg/kg for isoflurane.[180] With these dosages, 50% of subjects developed three or more premature ventricular contractions or ventricular tachycardia during or immediately after a single injection of epinephrine (which required 3.5 to 11 minutes to complete). Variables that may influence epinephrine ED_{50} values are differences in systemic absorption, route of administration, existing plasma catecholamine levels, preexisting atrial or ventricular dysrhythmias, and the previous administration of induction agents (i.e., thiopental,[181,182] ketamine,[183,184] each of which increases the incidence of epinephrine-induced dysrhythmias). When these variables are taken into consideration it is not surprising that data regarding volatile agent "sensitization" are conflicting.[185] Regarding the two newest volatile agents, desflurane and sevoflurane, both appear to be similar to isoflurane in their epinephrine-arrhythmogenic potential.[186,187]

In general, it is reasonable to anticipate the fewest difficulties with dysrhythmias in physical status I and II patients if the submucosal epinephrine dose remains 7.0 mcg/kg or less with 1.0 to 1.3 MAC desflurane,[186] or 5.0 mcg/kg or less with 1.0 to 1.3 MAC sevoflurane or isoflurane.[187] Additional protection can be achieved by combining 0.5% lidocaine with epinephrine, the net effect being an increase in the minimum threshold dose of epinephrine.[180]

One other point is worth mentioning in relation to rhythm disturbances and inhalation agents: patients who are given a general anesthetic (primary opioid supplemented with a volatile anesthetic) and who are on amiodarone can have significant dysrhythmias intraoperatively or postoperatively (e.g., atropine-resistant bradycardia requiring isoproterenol infusions, atrioventricular sequential pacing). These significant rhythm disturbances can also result in death.[188] For clarification and emphasis, it should be understood that amiodarone and its major metabolite

are detectable in plasma for up to 9 months after discontinuation of therapy.[189]

Pulmonary Circulation

Pulmonary vascular resistance (PVR) is also affected by the volatile agents and N_2O. The effects of N_2O on PVR vary with age and preexisting levels of PVR. In adults with normal PVR, the addition of N_2O results in a small increase in PVR,[190] presumably due to an increase in sympathetic nervous system tone.[140] If a subject has preexisting pulmonary hypertension, the addition of N_2O results in larger increases in PVR,[190] which may become clinically significant. Volatile agents (including 0.8 or 1.2 MAC desflurane) decrease pulmonary artery pressure[135,144]; the opposite effect occurs when desflurane is administered at 1.6 MAC.[144]

The pulmonary vasculature also minimizes changes in alveolar-arterial oxygen tension gradient via hypoxic pulmonary vasoconstriction (HPV). This normal physiologic response to atelectasis or hypoxia is attenuated in vivo by halothane and isoflurane and markedly by N_2O.[191] All of the currently used volatile agents only marginally affect HPV.[192-194] Consistent with this finding, one group of researchers noted only minimal impairment in oxygenation (approximately 20% reduction in HPV at 1 MAC) in patients having one-lung ventilation performed during thoracotomy procedures. Desflurane and sevoflurane delivered at 1 MAC without N_2O have also been shown to only slightly affect arterial oxygenation in patients placed in a lateral position while undergoing esophagogastrectomy.[193,194]

Respiratory System

As seen with other systems of the body, the volatile agents exert a dose-response effect on the respiratory system, primarily tidal volume (TV). Responsiveness to CO_2 is depressed and the TV reduces as concentrations of the agents are increased. The compensatory mechanism for the diminished TV with halothane, isoflurane, sevoflurane, desflurane, and N_2O is an increase in respiratory rate (RR).[195-197] However, the increase in RR is not sufficient to prevent elevations in arterial CO_2 tension. Nevertheless, surgical stimulation is a variable that helps to overcome the respiratory-depressant effects of volatile agents.[198]

Emergence from an anesthetic can be associated with hypercarbia if minute volume (MV) is not adequately supported, owing to a volatile agent's capacity to depress the ventilatory response to $PaCO_2$ and PaO_2.[196,199-201] Hypercarbia also represents an increase in the apneic threshold (higher $PaCO_2$ values are required for spontaneous ventilation to occur). Patients should be closely monitored during emergence from an anesthetic and following adequate reversal of muscle relaxants to avoid acidemia or hypercarbia. During this phase of the anesthetic, significant end-tidal values of residual volatile anesthetic may persist, particularly if there was recent administration of an opioid (synergistic effect). It is important to recognize that impairment of the hypoxic ventilatory response by volatile agents is not abated with central nervous system arousal or acute pain[202]; even as little as 0.1 MAC of a volatile agent (excluding desflurane) can suppress ventilatory drive to hypoxia.[203] These research findings have implications for patients whose MVs are maintained via a hypoxic drive (e.g., emphysematous patients with depressed central chemoreceptors).

The smoothness of an inhalation induction is directly related to the ability of an inhalation agent to avoid provoking an irritant response. Halothane, N_2O, and sevoflurane are considered the standards by which other agents are measured because of the low incidence of breath holding, coughing, secretions, and laryngospasm encountered during inhalational induction.[204] In contrast, desflurane is considered a respiratory irritant when used for mask induction in concentrations greater than 6%[204,205]; therefore, it is generally not used to induce anesthesia in pediatric[206] and adult patients. One alternative method to incorporate desflurane in the pediatric population is to induce the child with sevoflurane, then change to desflurane for maintenance. Researchers have shown that reactive airway problems encountered during inhalational induction with desflurane are lost when this agent is used for anesthetic maintenance.[207] Lastly, the volatile agents have been shown to relax airway smooth muscle and produce bronchodilation. They have also been used in the treatment of refractory status asthmaticus.[208]

Kidneys

In general, autoregulation of the renal circulation remains intact during the administration of inhalation agents. Reductions in systolic blood pressure are accompanied by decreases in renal vascular resistance.[209] Nevertheless, compensatory reductions in renal vascular resistance can still lead to a decline in the glomerular filtration rate. This may contribute to the commonly observed intraoperative reduction in urinary output.

The potential for a volatile agent to produce renal damage is commonly assessed by the extent to which it elevates creatinine, blood urea nitrogen (BUN), and serum inorganic fluoride (F^-) concentrations.[210] With the older volatile agent methoxyflurane, a "toxic threshold" for peak serum concentration of F^- was established (50 µmol/L)[211]; at this value, vasopressin-resistant polyuric renal insufficiency occurs.[212]

Of the currently used inhalation agents, desflurane has been shown in both healthy and chronic renal disease patients[213] to alter indices of renal integrity the least, including no change in the renal function tests of urinary retinol-binding protein and N-acetyl-β-glucosaminidase (NAG).[214] The significance of this is that NAG is considered a sensitive indicator of drug-induced proximal tubular necrosis,[215,216] and retinol-binding protein has been shown to be a specific marker for indicating the presence of tubular damage of any cause.[217] Recent advancements in clinical markers for renal integrity have shown two new, perhaps better, biomarkers of tubular injury. Isoforms of glutathione-S-transferase (GST) include alpha GST, which is located exclusively in the proximal tubules, and pi GST, found only in the distal tubules.[218] In humans the urinary levels of each of these enzymes have been shown to increase after acute tubular necrosis and renal infarction.[219]

In contrast to studies involving desflurane (and isoflurane[220]), research with sevoflurane has generated concerns about compromised renal function. However, the current debate has settled on the degradation of sevoflurane by carbon dioxide absorbents. Most researchers now accept that serum inorganic fluoride (F^-) levels associated with sevoflurane administration do not represent a significant risk to patients, including those with compromised renal function.[221,222] Millions of sevoflurane anesthetics worldwide have failed to demonstrate any significant untoward renal outcomes in the general surgical population. Nevertheless, current FDA guidelines recommend sevoflurane be used with caution in patients with renal insufficiency (creatinine >1.5 mg/dL). In morbidly obese patients, researchers have found no appreciable difference in sevoflurane's biotransformation and subsequent fluoride levels, compared to nonobese patients.[223]

A concern still exists regarding sevoflurane's degradation within anesthesia circuits by soda lime,[224,225] with each having a chemical makeup of monovalent hydroxide bases (KOH and NaOH). These carbon dioxide absorbers break down all modern-day volatile agents.[226] The two by-products of sevoflurane's degradation that have been measured in a closed circuit are fluoromethyl-2,2-difluoro-1(trifluoromethyl)-vinyl ether (also known as compound A, an olefin) and fluoromethyl-2-methoxy-2,2-difluoro-1-(trifluoromethyl) ethyl ether (compound B).[227] The former is known to produce proximal corticomedullary tubular necrosis in rats.[228] Clinical studies involving low-flow (1 to 2 L/min) sevoflurane given over approximately 3 to 8 MAC-hours[229] in healthy patients[230] and in patients with stable renal insufficiency[229] were found to have no statistically significant changes in serum creatinine, blood urea nitrogen, urine protein, and glucose. It has also been reported that sevoflurane with desiccated soda lime can yield excessive temperatures that produce anesthesia machine fires and patient injuries,[231,232] the potential explanation being the by-product of hydrogen (3 moles) following the chemical reaction of sevoflurane with heated desiccated absorbent.[233]

In summary, it is widely recognized that the following variables do increase compound A content: low fresh gas flows, high concentrations of sevoflurane, and drying of soda lime CO_2 absorbant.[234,235] One way to eliminate compound A is to replace soda lime with Amsorb or DragerSorb Free.[236-238] These new CO_2 absorbents do not contain strong bases (sodium hydroxide [NaOH] or potassium hydroxide [KOH]), which are responsible for the degradation of sevoflurane to compound A, as well as the production of carbon monoxide from the breakdown of desflurane and isoflurane.[239,240] In the absence of Amsorb or DragerSorb Free carbon dioxide absorbents, current FDA dosing guidelines recommend sevoflurane exposure not exceed 2 MAC-hours at flow rates of 1 to less than 2 L/min. Fresh gas flow rates less than 1 L/min are not recommended.

Liver

All of the volatile anesthetics have been shown to decrease total hepatic blood flow, with halothane producing the greatest reduction.[25,241] By contrast, isoflurane, sevoflurane, and desflurane have been shown to increase or maintain hepatic artery blood flow, thereby limiting any accompanying attenuation in portal vein blood flow.[242-244] Hepatocyte hypoxia is of clinical concern, and its etiology can be multifactorial (e.g., volatile agents, surgical manipulation, enzyme induction). One significant outcome of liver hypoxia is increased reductive metabolism (which does not occur with the ether-based anesthetics) of halothane, which has been linked to "halothane hepatitis." This phenomenon has been investigated for nearly 45 years since the appearance of case reports in the literature of hepatic damage following halothane's use.[245] A better understanding of the pathophysiology of this phenomenon has improved diagnostic capabilities for volatile-agent hepatitis.[246,247]

Halothane-associated hepatitis is most common in the adult population (children are not immune to the response[248]) and is expressed as one of two clinical forms. The first is a mild hepatic reaction that occurs secondary to a direct hepatic effect or following reductive metabolism of halothane.[249] It is associated with low morbidity and moderately increased concentrations of elevated serum glutathione-S-transferase (GST) levels[246] or transient jaundice. It can occur shortly after the first exposure to a volatile agent, and the incidence may be as high as 20% to 50%.[250]

The second syndrome is characterized by fulminant hepatic failure with a high mortality rate. Multiple anesthetic exposures precede its onset, which has led researchers to theorize that an immune response evokes this syndrome (although not all research supports this theory).[251] Oxidative metabolism of halothane by hepatic cytochrome P-450 releases an unstable intermediate, trifluoroacetyl chloride (CF$_3$COCl). This substance binds to liver proteins to form trifluoroacetylated-protein (TFA-protein) neoantigens. Unfortunately, some patients form antibodies to TFA-protein neoantigens and on reexposure to halothane develop an immune response that is expressed as hepatic necrosis.[250,252-255] TFA-protein antibodies occur in up to 70% of patients with fulminant hepatic failure.[253,254] These antibodies do not appear in patients with normal liver function, patients with hepatic injury due to other causes, or in subjects who have previously received halothane but have not developed fulminant hepatic failure.

The predominant P-450 isoform responsible for the oxidation of halothane is cytochrome P-450 2E1. This may help explain why morbidly obese patients are prone to halothane hepatitis; the enzymatic activity of CYP-450 2E1 increases in this patient population.[256] In addition, the fatty liver infiltration observed in obese patients is associated with a greater quantity of CYP-450 2E1. Other risk factors identified for development of halothane hepatitis include fatty liver infiltration, having multiple anesthetics, and isoniazid and ethanol use.[257]

The overall incidence of the fulminant form of halothane hepatitis is reported to be 1:35,000 anesthetics.[258] In addition to the laboratory changes noted previously, the development of more specific serologic markers for detecting the presence of viral hepatitis C (including surrogate markers for recurrent hepatitis C [i.e., AST to platelet ratio index[259]]), D, and E has led to fewer false-positive diagnoses of halothane-associated hepatitis.[260-262]

Isoflurane and desflurane are similar to halothane in that each possesses a common metabolic pathway via cytochrome P-450 that eventually yields TFA-protein molecules.[247,250] However, because of differences in the rate of biodegradation, these volatile agents are probably less likely to produce hepatic injury than halothane. For example, isoflurane is metabolized 100-fold less than halothane, and as such it is estimated that fulminant hepatic failure caused by isoflurane may occur in 1:3,500,000 anesthetics.[247] Several case reports and clinical studies suggest that a potential immunologic mechanism (including cross-sensitization) may exist for the development of "isoflurane hepatitis,"[263] "sevoflurane hepatitis,"[264] and "desflurane hepatitis."[265] In one report, following isoflurane anesthesia the patient developed fulminant hepatic failure that led to death.[266]

Although desflurane is metabolized the least of all volatile anesthetics, it has also been associated with hepatotoxicity.[265] In one case report, a 65-year-old woman without a history of liver disease developed desflurane hepatitis 12 days postoperatively. The patient had a rash, nausea, polyarthralgias, marked elevations in liver transaminases, and jaundice. Serologic markers for hepatitis A, B, and C were negative. It was significant that the patient had undergone two prior halothane anesthetics lasting approximately 45 minutes each (death from a halothane anesthetic given 28 years after primary exposure has been documented[267]). The patient was discharged from the hospital 27 days after surgery, with continued improvement in liver function. This patient's exposure to halothane decades earlier combined with the ether-based anesthetic produced hepatic damage, probably secondary to "immunologic memory" and possible cross-sensitization.[265]

Sevoflurane is unique among the volatile anesthetics in that it is the only one that appears not to be biodegraded to TFA-protein molecules.[268] This step is a prerequisite to the formation of TFA-protein antibodies, so it is unlikely that sevoflurane will produce fulminant hepatic failure via an immunoallergic mechanism.[269] Nonetheless, there have been several case reports of hepatic injury associated with sevoflurane use,[264,270,271] including one that involved a child.[272]

In spite of the case reports listed, it is extremely rare for isoflurane, sevoflurane, and desflurane to produce clinically significant liver damage. Their molecular structure (increased fluorination) resists hepatic degradation, and their pharmacodynamic profile is associated with no changes or slight reductions in hepatic blood flow.[273-276]

In vitro research suggests that N$_2$O is metabolized minimally (0.004%) by intestinal microflora, yielding molecular nitrogen (N$_2$).[277] The limited metabolism does not necessarily mean that N$_2$O is an inert substance within the body. On the contrary, studies have demonstrated that chronic exposure to N$_2$O can lead to inactivation of the vitamin B$_{12}$ component of methionine synthetase,[278] which can disrupt deoxyribonucleic acid (DNA) synthesis.[279] For routine surgical cases this is generally not an issue, but caution should be exercised with patients who are pregnant, patients who receive a general anesthetic more than once a week, or patients who are debilitated and have problems with wound healing.[279,280]

In summary, the ether-based volatile agents have an extremely low risk for evoking hepatic injury. The discontinuation of halothane anesthesia in adults and pediatrics is warranted, particularly given the availability of sevoflurane for inhalational induction in children. Future research will help to further clarify the incidence and cellular mechanism by which isoflurane, sevoflurane, and desflurane evoke hepatic pathophysiologic processes. Nonetheless, with the knowledge that cross-sensitization and immunologic memory are factors to be considered in any patient who has received a prior halothane anesthetic, even decades before, vigilance by anesthesia providers is still required.

Neuromuscular System

All volatile agents produce a dose-dependent relaxation of skeletal muscle, as well as potentiation of the effects of depolarizing and nondepolarizing muscle relaxants.[281] The mechanism by which this occurs is multifactorial, involving reduced neural activity within the CNS and a presynaptic or postsynaptic effect at the neuromuscular junction.[47,282] Of the synaptic changes produced, the volatile agents predominantly affect the postjunctional membrane.[283]

With the exception of halothane, it is variable as to which volatile agent potentiates neuromuscular blocking agents the most.[284] Studies incorporating a broader methodology indicate that the greatest degree of potentiation of neuromuscular blockade occurs with sevoflurane, then isoflurane, and finally halothane.[285,286] Desflurane has been found by some investigators to potentiate the effects of neuromuscular blockers to the same extent as isoflurane[287] and sevoflurane. Similarly, other studies have shown that sevoflurane and isoflurane equally augment[288] and prolong[284] neuromuscular blockade produced by nondepolarizing muscle relaxants. In contrast, one investigation found that desflurane and sevoflurane enhanced the intensity of neuromuscular blockade with rocuronium, whereas isoflurane's effect was no different than that observed with a total intravenous anesthetic (TIVA).[281]

The discrepancies reported with interactions between volatile agents and muscle relaxants may be the result of differences in research methodology (e.g., type of muscle relaxant used in the study). For example, recovery of neuromuscular blockade after the use of cisatracurium and rocuronium is prolonged with sevoflurane but not isoflurane.[286,288] In contrast, the recovery profile for both volatile agents is the same after the use of vecuronium.[284]

Isoflurane[289] and N_2O[290] have been shown to potentiate the effects of succinylcholine. The former can accelerate the transition from a phase I to phase II block during an infusion of succinylcholine.[289] In general, nondepolarizing muscle relaxant dosages are decreased by approximately 25%[281,291] (sometimes as much as 50%)[286] of that required with TIVA when they are used in combination with a volatile agent. Of interest are two studies that found no difference in potentiation of nondepolarizing muscle relaxants and neuromuscular recovery profiles between an isoflurane/N_2O and TIVA technique.[286,288]

The volatile agents have also been shown to produce a time-dependent potentiation of nondepolarizing muscle relaxants (beginning in 5 to 10 minutes),[292] as well as a delayed recovery. For example, after 30 minutes of exposure to sevoflurane, recovery from vecuronium to 25% of baseline neuromuscular function is prolonged by 89%, and after 60 minutes, recovery exceeds 100%.[293] The inhalation agents have also been implicated in impairing reversal of nondepolarizing neuromuscular block.[294,295] For the reasons listed, anesthetists should carefully titrate muscle relaxants used in combination with inhalation anesthetics. Also, in select cases, a volatile anesthetic alone may produce adequate skeletal muscle relaxation without concurrent use of muscle relaxants.[296,297]

Malignant Hyperthermia

All of the volatile agents are capable of triggering malignant hyperthermia. These agents should not be used in malignant hyperthermia–susceptible patients. If a reaction occurs, it is treated instituting a hyperthermia protocol that includes intravenous dantrolene; the recommended dose is 2.5 mg/kg repeated every 5 minutes up to 10 mg/kg (although a dose of 29 mg/kg has been used).[298] Of interest is the observation that a delayed response (e.g., 6 hr) to malignant hyperthermia provoked by inhalation agents has been reported to occur with the use of nondepolarizing muscle relaxants and with desflurane if it is administered in the absence of succinylcholine.[299]

Nitrous oxide is considered at most a weak trigger of malignant hyperthermia in susceptible patients.[300-302] Overall, the clinical use of N_2O, in combination with many other agents (e.g., barbiturates, propofol, ketamine, etomidate, opiates, amide and ester anesthetics), is considered acceptable in patients susceptible to malignant hyperthermia.[298,303]

SUMMARY

Inhalation agents remain the most common class of drugs used to maintain a general anesthetic. The pharmacokinetic and pharmacodynamic profile of desflurane and sevoflurane facilitate meeting the anesthetic goals of an ever-increasing, same day–surgery population. Sevoflurane use continues to expand and is viewed by many anesthesia providers as a beneficial substitute/replacement for halothane—particularly given the potential for hepatic injury and prolonged immunologic memory. The ease of

TABLE 9-4	Effects of the Inhalation Anesthetics			
	Halothane	**Isoflurane**	**Desflurane**	**Sevoflurane**
Kinetics				
Alveolar equilibration	Slow	Moderate	Fast	Fast
Recovery	Slow	Moderate	Very fast	Fast
Liver				
Hepatotoxicity	Yes	No	No	No
Metabolism (%)	12-25	0.2	0.02	3-5
Musculoskeletal relaxation	Moderate	Significant	Significant	Significant
Cardiovascular System				
Heart rate	Reduced	Increased	Increased	Stable
Cardiac output	Reduced	Slightly reduced	Stable	Slightly reduced
SVR	Stable	Reduced	Reduced	Reduced
MAP	Reduced	Reduced	Reduced	Reduced
Coronary vasodilation	Minimal	Marked	Minimal	Moderate
Sensitization of myocardium	Yes	No	No	No
Respiratory System				
Respiratory irritation	No	Significant	Significant	No
Respiratory depression	Yes	Yes	Marked	Yes
Central Nervous System				
Seizure activity on EEG	No	No	No	No
Renal System				
Renal toxic metabolites	No	No	No	No

Modified from Aitkenhead AR et al, Textbook of Anaesthesia. 5th ed. Edinburgh: Churchill Livingstone; 2007.
EEG, Electroencephalogram; SVR, systemic vascular resistance; MAP, mean arterial pressure.

TABLE 9-5	Clinical Advantages and Disadvantages of Selected Inhalation Anesthetics	
Anesthetic	**Advantages**	**Disadvantages**
Nitrous oxide	Analgesia Rapid uptake and elimination Little cardiac or respiratory depression Nonpungent Allows less potent anesthetic to be administered	Expansion of closed air spaces Requires high concentrations Diffusion hypoxia Teratogenic
Halothane	Inexpensive Effective in low concentrations Excellent bronchodilator	Slow uptake and elimination Susceptible to biotransformation Idiosyncratic hepatic necrosis Catecholamine-induced ventricular ectopy Use is rapidly declining Impairs pulmonary macrophage activity and bronchial ciliary mucus transport Trigger for malignant hyperthermia
Isoflurane	Moderate muscle relaxation Decreases cerebral metabolic rate Minimal biotransformation No significant systemic toxicity Maintains cardiac output because of vasodilation Inexpensive	Pungent odor Airway irritant Fewer negative inotropic effects than halothane Trigger for malignant hyperthermia

Desflurane	Rapid uptake and elimination
	Stable molecules
	Minimal biotransformation
	No significant systemic toxicity
		Airway irritant
		Low boiling point
		Sympathetic stimulation
		Expensive
		Low boiling point and high saturation vapor
		  pressure
		Needs special electrically heated vaporizer
		Rapid increases in inspired concentration can lead
		  to reflex tachycardia and hypertension
		Trigger for malignant hyperthermia

Sevoflurane	Rapid uptake and elimination
	Nonpungent
	Excellent for inhalation induction
	Cardiovascular effects broadly comparable
	  to those of isoflurane
		Susceptible to biotransformation
		Reacts with soda lime
		Increases serum fluoride concentration
		Expensive
		3%-5% metabolized, but current evidence is that
		  it causes neither hepatic nor renal toxicity
		Trigger for malignant hyperthermia

administration of all ether-based volatile anesthetics, with or without N_2O, lends itself to common use among a diverse surgical population. Continued research will help guide anesthetists in the selection and application of a variety of inhalation anesthetic techniques. A summary of the systemic effects of the major inhalation anesthetics is given in Table 9-4. Some advantages and disadvantages of selected inhalation anesthetics are given in Table 9-5.

REFERENCES

1. Frost EA. A history of nitrous oxide. In: Eger EI II, ed. *Nitrous Oxide*. New York: Elsevier; 1985:1-22.
2. Andrews E. The oxygen mixture, a new anaesthetic combination. *Chicago Med Exam*. 1868;9:656-661.
3. Keys TE. *The History of Surgical Anesthesia*. New York: Krieger; 1978.
4. Calverley RK. Fluorinated anesthetics. 1. The early years 1932-1946. *Surv Anesthesiol*. 1986;30:170-173.
5. Bryce-Smith R, O'Brien HD. Fluothane: an non-explosive anaesthetic agent. *Br Med J*. 1956;2:969-972.
6. Johnstone M. The human cardiovascular response to fluothane anesthesia. *Br Med J*. 1956;28:392-410.
7. Eger EI II et al. Hypothesis: volatile anesthetics produce immobility by acting on two sites approximately five carbon atoms apart. *Anesth Analg*. 1999; 88(6):1395-1400.
8. Halsey MJ. A reassessment of the molecular structure-functional relationships of the inhaled general anaesthetics. *Br J Anaesth*. 1984;56(Suppl 1): 9S-25S.
9. Robbins JH. Preliminary studies of the anaesthetic activity of fluorinated hydrocarbons. *J Pharmacol Exp Ther*. 1946;86:197-204.

10. Larsen ER. Fluorine compounds in anesthesiology. In: Tarrant P, ed. *Fluorine Chemistry Reviews*. New York: Marcel Dekker; 1946:3.

11. Targ AG et al. Halogenation and anesthetic potency. *Anesth Analg.* 1989;68(5):599-602.

12. Rudo FG, Krantz JC Jr. Anaesthetic molecules. *Br J Anaesth.* 1974; 46(3):181-189.

13. Terrell RC. Physical and chemical properties of anaesthetic agents (with an appendix on the manufacture of isoflurane). *Br J Anaesth.* 1984; 56(Suppl 1):3S-7S.

14. Sutton TS et al. Fluoride metabolites after prolonged exposure of volunteers and patients to desflurane. *Anesth Analg.* 1991;73(2):180-185.

15. Holaday DA et al. Resistance of isoflurane to biotransformation in man. *Anesthesiology.* 1975;43(3):325-332.

16. Rehder K et al. Halothane biotransformation in man: a quantitative study. *Anesthesiology.* 1967;28(4):711-715.

17. Cascorbi HF et al. Differences in the biotransformation of halothane in man. *Anesthesiology.* 1970;32(2):119-123.

18. Carpenter RL et al. The extent of metabolism of inhaled anesthetics in humans. *Anesthesiology.* 1986;65(2):201-205.

19. Carpenter RL et al. Pharmacokinetics of inhaled anesthetics in humans: measurements during and after the simultaneous administration of enflurane, halothane, isoflurane, methoxyflurane, and nitrous oxide. *Anesth Analg.* 1986;65(6):575-582.

20. Shiraishi Y, Ikeda K. Uptake and biotransformation of sevoflurane in humans: a comparative study of sevoflurane with halothane, enflurane, and isoflurane. *J Clin Anesth.* 1990;2(6):381-386.

21. Yasuda N et al. Kinetics of desflurane, isoflurane, and halothane in humans. *Anesthesiology.* 1991;74(3):489-498.

22. Koblin DD. Characteristics and implications of desflurane metabolism and toxicity. *Anesth Analg.* 1992;75(4 Suppl):S10-S16.

23. Baden JM, Rice SA. Metabolism and toxicity of inhaled anesthetics. In: Miller RD, ed. *Anesthesia*. Vol 1. 5th ed. Philadelphia: Churchill Livingstone; 2000:147-173.

24. Spracklin DK et al. Human reductive halothane metabolism in vitro is catalyzed by cytochrome P450 2A6 and 3A4. *Drug Metab Dispos.* 1996; 24(9):976-983.

25. Ebert TJ. Inhalation anesthesia. In: Barash PG et al, eds. *Clinical Anesthesia*. 6th ed. Philadelphia: Lippincott Williams & Wilkins; 2006:384-420.

26. Meyer HH. Theorie der alkoholnarkose. *Arch Exp Pathol Pharmakol.* 1899;42: 109-118.

27. Overton CE. *Studien uber die Narkose, zugleich ein Beitrag zur allgemeinen Pharmakologie*. Jena, Ger: G Fischer; 1901.

28. Wann KT, Macdonald AG. Actions and interactions of high pressure and general anaesthetics. *Prog Neurobiol.* 1988;30(4):271-307.

29. DiFazio CA et al. Additive effects of anesthetics and theories of anesthesia. *Anesthesiology.* 1972;36(1):57-63.

30. Gelman S. A step toward consensus on general anesthesia. *Anesth Analg.* 1998;86(2):446.

31. Eger EI II et al. Hypothesis: inhaled anesthetics produce immobility and amnesia by different mechanisms at different sites. *Anesth Analg.* 1997; 84(4):915-918.

32. Eger EI II, Koblin DD. A step toward consensus on general anesthesia [letter; comment]. *Anesth Analg.* 1998;86:446.

33. Liu CP et al. Potent activation of the human tandem pore domain K channel TRESK with clinical concentrations of volatile anesthetics. *Anesth Analg.* 2004;99(6):1715-1722.

34. Cheng G, Kendig JJ. Enflurane decreases glutamate neurotransmission to spinal cord motor neurons by both pre- and postsynaptic actions. *Anesth Analg.* 2003;96(5):1354-1359.

35. Grasshoff CMD, Antkowiak BPD. Propofol and sevoflurane depress spinal neurons in vitro via different molecular targets. *Anesthesiology.* 2004; 101(5):1167-1176.

36. Kandel L et al. Nonanesthetics can suppress learning. *Anesth Analg.* 1996;82(2):321-326.

37. Zhang Y et al. Both cerebral GABA(A) receptors and spinal GABA(A) receptors modulate the capacity of isoflurane to produce immobility. *Anesth Analg.* 2001;92(6):1585-1589.

38. Salmi EMD et al. Sevoflurane and propofol increase 11C-flumazenil binding to gamma-aminobutyric acid A receptors in humans. *Anesth Analg.* 2004; 99(5):1420-1426.

39. Katayama SD et al. Increased [gamma]-aminobutyric acid levels in mouse brain induce loss of righting reflex, but not immobility, in response to noxious stimulation. *Anesth Analg.* 2007;104(6):1422-1429.

40. Ogawa T et al. The divergent actions of volatile anaesthetics on background neuronal activity and reactive capability in the central nervous system in cats. *Can J Anaesth.* 1992;39(8):862-872.

41. Angel A. Central neuronal pathways and the process of anaesthesia. *Br J Anaesth.* 1993;71(1):148-163.

42. Pearce RA. Volatile anaesthetic enhancement of paired-pulse depression investigated in the rat hippocampus in vitro. *J Physiol* (Lond). 1996; 492(Pt 3):823-840.

43. Rampil IJ et al. The electroencephalographic effects of desflurane in humans. *Anesthesiology.* 1991;74(3):434-439.

44. Watts AD et al. The effect of sevoflurane and isoflurane anesthesia on interictal spike activity among patients with refractory epilepsy. *Anesth Analg.* 1999;89(5):1275-1281.

45. Osawa M et al. Effects of sevoflurane on central nervous system electrical activity in cats. *Anesth Analg.* 1994;79(1):52-57.

46. Bruchiel KJ et al. Electroencephalographic abnormalities following halothane anesthesia. *Anesth Analg.* 1978;57(2):244-251.

47. Rampil IJ, King BS. Volatile anesthetics depress spinal motor neurons. *Anesthesiology.* 1996;85(1):129-134.

48. Zhou HH et al. Spinal cord motoneuron excitability during isoflurane and nitrous oxide anesthesia. *Anesthesiology.* 1997;86(2):302-307.

49. Franks NP, Lieb WR. Molecular and cellular mechanisms of general anaesthesia. *Nature.* 1994;367(6464):607-614.

50. Jenkins A et al. Effects of temperature and volatile anesthetics on GABA(A) receptors. *Anesthesiology.* 1999;90(2):484-491.

51. Campagna JA et al. Mechanisms of actions of inhaled anesthetics. *N Engl J Med.* 2003;348(21):2110-2125.

52. Solt K, Forman SA. Correlating the clinical actions and molecular mechanisms of general anesthetics. *Curr Opin Anaesthesiol.* 2007;20(4): 300-306.

53. Bloom FE. Neurotransmission and the central nervous system. In: Hardman JG, Limbird LE, eds. *Goodman & Gilman's Pharmacological Basis of Therapeutics*. 9th ed. New York: McGraw-Hill; 1996:267-293.

54. Quinlan JJ et al. Isoflurane's enhancement of chloride flux through rat brain gamma-aminobutyric acid type A receptors is stereoselective. *Anesthesiology.* 1995;83(3):611-615.

55. Yamashita MD et al. Isoflurane modulation of neuronal nicotinic acetylcholine receptors expressed in human embryonic kidney cells. *Anesthesiology.* 2005;102(1):76-84.

56. Kaech S et al. Volatile anesthetics block actin-based motility in dendritic spines. *Proc Natl Acad Sci U S A.* 1999;96(18):10433-10437.

57. Fischer M et al. Rapid actin-based plasticity in dendritic spines. *Neuron.* 1998;20(5):847-854.

58. Kaech S et al. Isoform specificity in the relationship of actin to dendritic spines. *J Neurosci.* 1997;17(24):9565-9572.

59. Shepherd GM. The dendritic spine: a multifunctional integrative unit. *J Neurophysiol.* 1996;75(6):2197-2210.

60. Shepherd GM, Koch C. *The Synaptic Organization of the Brain*. Oxford, England: Oxford Univ. Press; 1998.

61. Sonner JM et al. Inhaled anesthetics and immobility: mechanisms, mysteries, and minimum alveolar anesthetic concentration. *Anesth Analg.* 2003; 97(3):718-740.

62. Eger EI II et al. Minimum alveolar anesthetic concentration: a standard of anesthetic potency. *Anesthesiology.* 1965;26(6):756-763.

63. Saidman LJ et al. Minimum alveolar concentrations of methoxyflurane, halothane, ether and cyclopropane in man: correlation with theories of anesthesia. *Anesthesiology.* 1967;28(6):994-1002.

64. Stevens WD et al. Minimum alveolar concentrations (MAC) of isoflurane with and without nitrous oxide in patients of various ages. *Anesthesiology.* 1975;42(2):197-200.

65. Hornbein TF et al. The minimum alveolar concentration of nitrous oxide in man. *Anesth Analg.* 1982;61(7):553-556.

66. Katoh T, Ikeda K. The minimum alveolar concentration (MAC) of sevoflurane in humans. *Anesthesiology.* 1987;66(3):301-303.

67. Rampil IJ et al. Clinical characteristics of desflurane in surgical patients: minimum alveolar concentration. *Anesthesiology.* 1991;74(3):429-433.

68. Miller RD et al. The effects of alpha-methyldopa, reserpine, guanethidine, and iproniazid on minimum alveolar anesthetic requirement (MAC). *Anesthesiology.* 1968;29(6):1153-1158.

69. Liem EB et al. Anesthetic requirement is increased in redheads. *Anesthesiology.* 2004;101(2):279-283.

70. Stoelting RK et al. Minimum alveolar concentrations in man on awakening from methoxyflurane, halothane, ether and fluroxene anesthesia: MAC awake. *Anesthesiology.* 1970;33(1):5-9.

71. Roizen MF et al. Anesthetic doses blocking adrenergic (stress) and cardiovascular responses to incision–MAC BAR. *Anesthesiology.* 1981; 54(5):390-398.

72. Daniel M et al. Fentanyl augments the blockade of the sympathetic response to incision (MAC-BAR) produced by desflurane and isoflurane: desflurane and

isoflurane MAC-BAR without and with fentanyl. *Anesthesiology.* 1998;88(1):43-49.

73. Katoh T et al. The effect of fentanyl on sevoflurane requirements for somatic and sympathetic responses to surgical incision. *Anesthesiology.* 1999; 90(2):398-405.

74. de Jong RH, Eger EI. MAC expanded: AD50 and AD95 values of common inhalation anesthetics in man. *Anesthesiology.* 1975;42(4):384-389.

75. Tayefeh F et al. Time-dependent changes in heart rate and pupil size during desflurane or sevoflurane anesthesia. *Anesth Analg.* 1997;85(6):1362-1366.

76. Cullen DJ et al. Clinical signs of anesthesia. *Anesthesiology.* 1972;36(1):21-36.

77. Zbinden AM et al. Anesthetic depth defined using multiple noxious stimuli during isoflurane/oxygen anesthesia. II. Hemodynamic responses. *Anesthesiology.* 1994;80(2):261-267.

78. Kolbitsch C et al. Sevoflurane (0.4 MAC) does not influence cerebral compliance in healthy individuals. *J Neurosurg Anesthesiol.* 2000;12(4): 319-323.

79. Bedforth NM et al. Cerebral hemodynamic response to the introduction of desflurane: a comparison with sevoflurane [comment]. *Anesth Analg.* 2000;91(1):152-155.

80. Kolbitsch C et al. A subanesthetic concentration of sevoflurane increases regional cerebral blood flow and regional cerebral blood volume and decreases regional mean transit time and regional cerebrovascular resistance in volunteers. *Anesth Analg.* 2000;91(1):156-162.

81. Mielck F et al. Effects of one minimum alveolar anesthetic concentration sevoflurane on cerebral metabolism, blood flow, and CO_2 reactivity in cardiac patients. *Anesth Analg.* 1999;89(2):364-369.

82. Matta BF et al. Direct cerebrovasodilatory effects of halothane, isoflurane, and desflurane during propofol-induced isoelectric electroencephalogram in humans. *Anesthesiology.* 1995;83(5):980-985.

83. Strebel S et al. Dynamic and static cerebral autoregulation during isoflurane, desflurane, and propofol anesthesia. *Anesthesiology.* 1995;83(1):66-76.

84. Manohar M, Parks CM. Porcine systemic and regional organ blood flow during 1.0 and 1.5 minimum alveolar concentrations of sevoflurane anesthesia without and with 50% nitrous oxide. *J Pharmacol Exp Ther.* 1984; 231(3):640-648.

85. Heinke WA, Koelsch SB. The effects of anesthetics on brain activity and cognitive function. *Curr Opin Anaesthesiol.* 2005;18(6):625-631.

86. Hansen TD et al. Distribution of cerebral blood flow during halothane versus isoflurane anesthesia in rats. *Anesthesiology.* 1988;69(3):332-337.

87. Hansen TD et al. The role of cerebral metabolism in determining the local cerebral blood flow effects of volatile anesthetics: evidence for persistent flow-metabolism coupling. *J Cereb Blood Flow Metab.* 1989;9(3):323-328.

88. Lam AM et al. Change in cerebral blood flow velocity with onset of EEG silence during inhalation anesthesia in humans: evidence of flow-metabolism coupling? *J Cereb Blood Flow Metab.* 1995;15(4):714-717.

89. Heath KJ et al. The effects of sevoflurane on cerebral hemodynamics during propofol anesthesia. *Anesth Analg.* 1997;85(6):1284-1287.

90. Mielck F et al. Effects of 1 MAC desflurane on cerebral metabolism, blood flow and carbon dioxide reactivity in humans. *Br J Anaesth.* 1998;81(2):155-160.

91. Bedforth NM et al. The effects of sevoflurane and nitrous oxide on middle cerebral artery blood flow velocity and transient hyperemic response. *Anesth Analg.* 1999;89(1):170-174.

92. Nakanishi O et al. Inhibition of cerebral metabolic and circulatory responses to nitrous oxide by 6-hydroxydopamine in dogs. *Can J Anaesth.* 1997; 44(9):1008-1013.

93. Petersen-Felix S et al. Isoflurane minimum alveolar concentration decreases during anesthesia and surgery. *Anesthesiology.* 1993;79(5):959-965.

94. Pelligrino DA et al. Nitrous oxide markedly increases cerebral cortical metabolic rate and blood flow in the goat. *Anesthesiology.* 1984;60(5):405-412.

95. Algotsson L et al. Effects of nitrous oxide on cerebral haemodynamics and metabolism during isoflurane anaesthesia in man. *Acta Anaesthesiol Scand.* 1992;36(1):46-52.

96. Cho S et al. Effects of sevoflurane with and without nitrous oxide on human cerebral circulation. Transcranial Doppler study. *Anesthesiology.* 1996;85(4):755-760.

97. Bendo AA et al. Anesthesia for neurosurgery. In: Barash PG et al, eds. *Clinical Anesthesia.* 6th ed. Philadelphia: Lippincott Williams & Wilkins; 2006:746-789.

98. Kadoi Y et al. The comparative effects of sevoflurane vs. isoflurane on cerebrovascular carbon dioxide reactivity in patients with hypertension. *Acta Anaesthesiol Scand.* 2007;51(10):1382-1387.

99. Nishiyama T et al. Cerebrovascular carbon dioxide reactivity during general anesthesia: a comparison between sevoflurane and isoflurane. *Anesth Analg.* 1999;89(6):1437-1441.

100. Kadoi Y et al. The comparative effects of sevoflurane versus isoflurane on cerebrovascular carbon dioxide reactivity in patients with diabetes mellitus. *Anesth Analg.* 2006;103(1):168-172.

101. Engelhard K, Werner C. Inhalational or intravenous anesthetics for craniotomies? Pro inhalational. *Curr Opin Anaesthesiol.* 2006;19(5):504-508.

102. Summors AC et al. Dynamic cerebral autoregulation during sevoflurane anesthesia: a comparison with isoflurane. *Anesth Analg.* 1999;88(2):341-345.

103. Muzzi DA et al. The effect of desflurane and isoflurane on cerebrospinal fluid pressure in humans with supratentorial mass lesions. *Anesthesiology.* 1992;76(5):720-724.

104. Ornstein E et al. Desflurane and isoflurane have similar effects on cerebral blood flow in patients with intracranial mass lesions. *Anesthesiology.* 1993;79(3):498-502.

105. Kaye AM et al. The comparative effects of desflurane and isoflurane on lumbar cerebrospinal fluid pressure in patients undergoing craniotomy for supratentorial tumors. *Anesth Analg.* 2004;98(4):1127-1132.

106. Artru AA et al. Intracranial pressure, middle cerebral artery flow velocity, and plasma inorganic fluoride concentrations in neurosurgical patients receiving sevoflurane or isoflurane. *Anesth Analg.* 1997;85(3):587-592.

107. Banoub M et al. Pharmacologic and physiologic influences affecting sensory evoked potentials: implications for perioperative monitoring. *Anesthesiology.* 2003;99(3):716-737.

108. Vaughan DJ et al. Effects of different concentrations of sevoflurane and desflurane on subcortical somatosensory evoked responses in anaesthetized, non-stimulated patients. *Br J Anaesth.* 2001;86(1):59-62.

109. Peterson DO et al. Effects of halothane, enflurane, isoflurane, and nitrous oxide on somatosensory evoked potentials in humans. *Anesthesiology.* 1986;65(1):35-40.

110. Rehberg B et al. Concentration-dependent changes in the latency and amplitude of somatosensory-evoked potentials by desflurane, isoflurane and sevoflurane. *Anasthesiol Intensivmed Notfallmed Schmerzther.* 1998;33(7):425-429.

111. Schindler E et al. Changes in somatosensory evoked potentials after sevoflurane and isoflurane. A randomized phase III study. *Anaesthetist.* 1996;45(Suppl 1):S52-S56.

112. Schindler E et al. Modulation of somatosensory evoked potentials under various concentrations of desflurane with and without nitrous oxide. *J Neurosurg Anesthesiol.* 1998;10(4):218-223.

113. Vakkuri A et al. Sevoflurane mask induction of anaesthesia is associated with epileptiform EEG in children. *Acta Anaesthesiol Scand.* 2001;45(7):805-811.

114. Nieminen K et al. Sevoflurane anaesthesia in children after induction of anaesthesia with midazolam and thiopental does not cause epileptiform EEG. *Br J Anaesth.* 2002;89(6):853-856.

115. Voss LJ et al. Cerebral cortical effects of desflurane in sheep: comparison with isoflurane, sevoflurane and enflurane. *Acta Anaesthesiol Scand.* 2006;50(3):313-319.

116. Fukuda H et al. Sevoflurane is equivalent to isoflurane for attenuating bupivacaine-induced arrhythmias and seizures in rats. *Anesth Analg.* 1996;83(3):570-573.

117. Murao K et al. The anticonvulsant effects of volatile anesthetics on penicillin-induced status epilepticus in cats. *Anesth Analg.* 2000;90(1):142-147.

118. Murao K et al. The anticonvulsant effects of volatile anesthetics on lidocaine-induced seizures in cats. *Anesth Analg.* 2000;90(1):148-155.

119. Jaaskelainen SK et al. Sevoflurane is epileptogenic in healthy subjects at surgical levels of anesthesia. *Neurology.* 2003;61(8):1073-1078.

120. Fang Z et al. Convulsant activity of nonanesthetic gas combinations. *Anesth Analg.* 1997;84(3):634-640.

121. Yli-Hankala A et al. Epileptiform electroencephalogram during mask induction of anesthesia with sevoflurane. *Anesthesiology.* 1999;91(6):1596-1603.

122. Hilty CA, Drummond JC. Seizure-like activity on emergence from sevoflurane anesthesia. *Anesthesiology.* 2000;93(5):1357-1359.

123. Parr SM et al. Level of consciousness on arrival in the recovery room and the development of early respiratory morbidity. *Anaesth Intensive Care.* 1991;19(3):369-372.

124. Larsen B et al. Recovery of cognitive function after remifentanil-propofol anesthesia: a comparison with desflurane and sevoflurane anesthesia. *Anesth Analg.* 2000;90(1):168.

125. Smiley RM et al. Desflurane and isoflurane in surgical patients: comparison of emergence time. *Anesthesiology.* 1991;74(3):425-428.

126. Campbell C et al. A phase III, multicenter, open-label, randomized, comparative study evaluating the effect of sevoflurane versus isoflurane on the maintenance of anesthesia in adult ASA class I, II, and III inpatients. *J Clin Anesth.* 1996;8(7):557-563.

127. Eger EI II et al. Recovery and kinetic characteristics of desflurane and sevoflurane in volunteers after 8-h exposure, including kinetics of degradation products. *Anesthesiology.* 1997;87(3):517-526.

128. Ebert TJ et al. Neurocirculatory responses to sevoflurane in humans. A comparison to desflurane. *Anesthesiology.* 1995;83(1):88-95.

129. Magni GM et al. No difference in emergence time and early cognitive function between sevoflurane-fentanyl and propofol-remifentanil in patients

undergoing craniotomy for supratentorial intracranial surgery. *J Neurosurg Anesthesiol.* 2005;17(3):134-138.

130. Head BP, Patel P. Anesthetics and brain protection. *Curr Opin Anaesthesiol.* 2007;20(5):395-399.

131. Fukuda S, Warner DS. Cerebral protection. *Br J Anaesth.* 2007;99(1):10-17.

132. Koerner IP, Brambrink AM. Brain protection by anesthetic agents. *Curr Opin Anaesthesiol.* 2006;19(5):481-486.

133. Vlajkovic GP, Sindjelic RP. Emergence delirium in children: many questions, few answers. *Anesth Analg.* 2007;104(1):84-91.

134. Voepel-Lewis T et al. Nurses' diagnoses and treatment decisions regarding care of the agitated child. *J Perianesth Nurs.* 2005;20(4):239-248.

135. Malan TP Jr et al. Cardiovascular effects of sevoflurane compared with those of isoflurane in volunteers. *Anesthesiology.* 1995;83(5):918-928.

136. Akata TM. General anesthetics and vascular smooth muscle: direct actions of general anesthetics on cellular mechanisms regulating vascular tone. *Anesthesiology.* 2007;106(2):365-391.

137. Park WK et al. Myocardial depressant effects of desflurane: mechanical and electrophysiologic actions in vitro. *Anesthesiology.* 2007;106(5):956-966.

138. Lowe D et al. Influence of volatile anesthetics on left ventricular afterload in vivo. Differences between desflurane and sevoflurane. *Anesthesiology.* 1996;85(1):112-120.

139. Bahlman SH et al. The cardiovascular effects of halothane in man during spontaneous ventilation. *Anesthesiology.* 1972;36(5):494-502.

140. Ebert TJ. Differential effects of nitrous oxide on baroreflex control of heart rate and peripheral sympathetic nerve activity in humans. *Anesthesiology.* 1990;72(1):16-22.

141. Warltier DC et al. Recovery of contractile function of stunned myocardium in chronically instrumented dogs is enhanced by halothane or isoflurane. *Anesthesiology.* 1988;69(4):552-565.

142. Lunn JK et al. High dose fentanyl anesthesia for coronary artery surgery: plasma fentanyl concentrations and influence of nitrous oxide on cardiovascular responses. *Anesth Analg.* 1979;58(5):390-395.

143. Houltz E et al. The effects of nitrous oxide on left ventricular systolic and diastolic performance before and after cardiopulmonary bypass: evaluation by computer-assisted two-dimensional and Doppler echocardiography in patients undergoing coronary artery surgery. *Anesth Analg.* 1995;81(2):243-248.

144. Weiskopf RB et al. Cardiovascular actions of desflurane in normocarbic volunteers. *Anesth Analg.* 1991;73(2):143-156.

145. Ebert TJ et al. Desflurane-mediated sympathetic activation occurs in humans despite preventing hypotension and baroreceptor unloading. *Anesthesiology.* 1998;88(5):1227-1232.

146. Schotten U et al. Effect of volatile anesthetics on the force-frequency relation in human ventricular myocardium: the role of the sarcoplasmic reticulum calcium-release channel. *Anesthesiology.* 2001;95(5):1160-1168.

147. Muldoon SM et al. Attenuation of endothelium-mediated vasodilation by halothane. *Anesthesiology.* 1988;68(1):31-37.

148. Haworth RA, Goknur AB. Inhibition of sodium/calcium exchange and calcium channels of heart cells by volatile anesthetics. *Anesthesiology.* 1995;82(5):1255-1265.

149. Bosnjak ZJ, Kampine JP. Effects of halothane, enflurane, and isoflurane on the SA node. *Anesthesiology.* 1983;58(4):314-321.

150. Kotrly KJ et al. Baroreceptor reflex control of heart rate during isoflurane anesthesia in humans. *Anesthesiology.* 1984;60(3):173-179.

151. Weiskopf RB et al. Cardiovascular stimulation induced by rapid increases in desflurane concentration in humans results from activation of tracheopulmonary and systemic receptors. *Anesthesiology.* 1995;83(6):1173-1178.

152. Holaday DA, Smith FR. Clinical characteristics and biotransformation of sevoflurane in healthy human volunteers. *Anesthesiology.* 1981;54(2):100-106.

153. Wajima Z et al. Changes in hemodynamic variables and catecholamine levels after rapid increase in sevoflurane or isoflurane concentration with or without nitrous oxide under endotracheal intubation. *J Anesth.* 2000;14:175-179.

154. Weiskopf RB et al. Rapid increase in desflurane concentration is associated with greater transient cardiovascular stimulation than with rapid increase in isoflurane concentration in humans. *Anesthesiology.* 1994;80(5):1035-1045.

155. Weiskopf RB et al. Fentanyl, esmolol, and clonidine blunt the transient cardiovascular stimulation induced by desflurane in humans. *Anesthesiology.* 1994;81(6):1350-1355.

156. Pacentine GG et al. Effects of fentanyl on sympathetic activation associated with the administration of desflurane. *Anesthesiology.* 1995;82(4):823-831.

157. Gormley WP et al. Intravenous lidocaine does not attenuate the cardiovascular and catecholamine response to a rapid increase in desflurane concentration. *Anesth Analg.* 1996;82(2):358-361.

158. Gross GJ, Warltier DC. Coronary steal in four models of single or multiple vessel obstruction in dogs. *Am J Cardiol.* 1981;48(1):84-92.

159. Hirano M et al. A comparison of coronary hemodynamics during isoflurane and sevoflurane anesthesia in dogs. *Anesth Analg.* 1995;80(4):651-656.

160. Hartman JC et al. Influence of desflurane on regional distribution of coronary blood flow in a chronically instrumented canine model of multivessel coronary artery obstruction. *Anesth Analg.* 1991;72(3):289-299.

161. Kersten JR et al. Sevoflurane selectively increases coronary collateral blood flow independent of KATP channels in vivo. *Anesthesiology.* 1999;90(1):246-256.

162. Priebe HJ, Foex P. Isoflurane causes regional myocardial dysfunction in dogs with critical coronary artery stenosis. *Anesthesiology.* 1987;66(3):293-300.

163. Hartman JC et al. Alterations in collateral blood flow produced by isoflurane in a chronically instrumented canine model of multivessel coronary artery disease. *Anesthesiology.* 1991;74(1):120-133.

164. Wilton NC et al. Transmural redistribution of myocardial blood flow during isoflurane anesthesia and its effects on regional myocardial function in a canine model of fixed coronary stenosis. *Anesthesiology.* 1993;78(3):510-523.

165. Mignella R, Buffington CW. Inhaled anesthetics alter the determinants of coronary collateral blood flow in the dog. *Anesthesiology.* 1995;83(4):799-808.

166. Habazettl H et al. Left ventricular oxygen tensions in dogs during coronary vasodilation by enflurane, isoflurane and dipyramidole. *Anesth Analg.* 1989;68(3):286-294.

167. Hartman JC et al. Steal-prone coronary circulation in chronically instrumented dogs: isoflurane versus adenosine. *Anesthesiology.* 1991;74(4):744-756.

168. De Hert SG et al. Choice of primary anesthetic regimen can influence intensive care unit length of stay after coronary surgery with cardiopulmonary bypass. *Anesthesiology.* 2004;101(1):9-20.

169. An JMD et al. Myocardial protection by isoflurane preconditioning preserves Ca^{2+} cycling proteins independent of sarcolemmal and mitochondrial KATP channels. *Anesth Analg.* 2007;105(5):1207-1213.

170. Novalija E et al. Sevoflurane mimics ischemic preconditioning effects on coronary flow and nitric oxide release in isolated hearts. *Anesthesiology.* 1999;91(3):701.

171. Lucchinetti EP et al. Molecular evidence of late preconditioning after sevoflurane inhalation in healthy volunteers. *Anesth Analg.* 2007;105(3):629-640.

172. Hausenloy DJ, Yellon DM. Reperfusion injury salvage kinase signaling:: taking a RISK for cardioprotection. *Heart Fail Rev.* 2007;12(3-4):217-234.

173. Kevin LG et al. Anesthetic preconditioning: effects on latency to ischemic injury in isolated hearts. *Anesthesiology.* 2003;99(2):385-391.

174. Novalija E et al. Reactive oxygen species precede the [epsilon] isoform of protein kinase C in the anesthetic preconditioning signaling cascade. *Anesthesiology.* 2003;99(2):421-428.

175. Novalija E et al. Anesthetic preconditioning improves adenosine triphosphate synthesis and reduces reactive oxygen species formation in mitochondria after ischemia by a redox-dependent mechanism. *Anesthesiology.* 2003;98(5):1155-1163.

176. ACC/AHA 2007 guidelines on perioperative cardiovascular evaluation and care for noncardiac surgery: executive summary: a report of the American College of Cardiology/American Heart Association Task Force on Practice Guidelines (Writing Committee to Revise the 2002 Guidelines on Perioperative Cardiovascular Evaluation for Noncardiac Surgery). *Anesth Analg.* 2008;106(3):685-712.

177. Gu W et al. Modifying cardiovascular risk in diabetes mellitus. *Anesthesiology.* 2003;98(3):774-779.

178. Atlee JL. Causes for perioperative dysrhythmias. In Atlee JL, eds. *Perioperative Cardiac Dysrhythmias.* 2nd ed: Chicago: Year Book Med Pub; 1990:187-273.

179. Atlee JLd, Bosnjak ZJ. Mechanisms for cardiac dysrhythmias during anesthesia. *Anesthesiology.* 1990;72(2):347-374.

180. Johnston RR et al. A comparative interaction of epinephrine with enflurane, isoflurane, and halothane in man. *Anesth Analg.* 1976;55(5):709-712.

181. Atlee JLd, Malkinson CE. Potentiation by thiopental of halothane/epinephrine-induced arrhythmias in dogs. *Anesthesiology.* 1982;57(4):285-288.

182. Hayashi Y et al. Arrhythmogenic threshold of epinephrine during sevoflurane, enflurane, and isoflurane anesthesia in dogs. *Anesthesiology.* 1988;69(1):145-147.

183. Koehntop DE et al. Effects of pharmacologic alterations of adrenergic mechanisms by cocaine, tropolone, aminophylline, and ketamine on epinephrine-induced arrhythmias during halothane-nitrous oxide anesthesia. *Anesthesiology.* 1977;46(2):83-93.

184. Roberts FL et al. Effects of ketamine and etomidate on epinephrine-induced ventricular dysrhythmias in dogs anesthetized with halothane. *Anesthesiology.* 1984;61(3):A36.

185. Atlee JL, Roberts FL. Thiopental and epinephrine-induced dysrhythmias in dogs anesthetized with enflurane or isoflurane. *Anesth Analg.* 1986;65(5):437-443.

186. Moore MA et al. Arrhythmogenic doses of epinephrine are similar during desflurane or isoflurane anesthesia in humans. *Anesthesiology*. 1993; 79(5):943-947.

187. Navarro R et al. Humans anesthetized with sevoflurane or isoflurane have similar arrhythmic response to epinephrine. *Anesthesiology*. 1994;80(3): 545-549.

188. Liberman BA, Teasdale SJ. Anaesthesia and amiodarone. *Can Anaesth Soc J*. 1985;32(6):629-638.

189. Holt DW et al. Amiodarone pharmacokinetics. *Am Heart J*. 1983; 106(4 Pt 2):840-847.

190. Schulte-Sasse U et al. Pulmonary vascular responses to nitrous oxide in patients with normal and high pulmonary vascular resistance. *Anesthesiology*. 1982;57(1):9-13.

191. Lennon PF, Murray PA. Attenuated hypoxic pulmonary vasoconstriction during isoflurane anesthesia is abolished by cyclooxygenase inhibition in chronically instrumented dogs. *Anesthesiology*. 1996;84(2):404-414.

192. Pagel PS et al. Desflurane and isoflurane produce similar alterations in systemic and pulmonary hemodynamics and arterial oxygenation in patients undergoing one-lung ventilation during thoracotomy. *Anesth Analg*. 1998;87(4):800-807.

193. Wang JY et al. Comparison of the effects of sevoflurane and isoflurane on arterial oxygenation during one-lung ventilation. *Br J Anaesth*. 1998; 81(6):850-853.

194. Wang JY et al. A comparison of the effects of desflurane and isoflurane on arterial oxygenation during one-lung ventilation. *Anaesthesia*. 2000;55(2):167-173.

195. Fourcade HE et al. The ventilatory effects of forane, a new inhaled anesthetic. *Anesthesiology*. 1971;35(1):26-31.

196. Lockhart SH et al. Depression of ventilation by desflurane in humans. *Anesthesiology*. 1991;74(3):484-488.

197. Green WB Jr. The ventilatory effects of sevoflurane. *Anesth Analg*. 1995; 81(6 Suppl):S23-S26.

198. Eger EI et al. Surgical stimulation antagonizes the respiratory depression produced by forane. *Anesthesiology*. 1972;36(6):544-549.

199. Doi M, Ikeda K. Respiratory effects of sevoflurane. *Anesth Analg*. 1987;66(3):241-244.

200. Yacoub O et al. Depression of hypoxic ventilatory response by nitrous oxide. *Anesthesiology*. 1976;45(4):385-389.

201. Hirshman CA et al. Depression of hypoxic ventilatory response by halothane, enflurane and isoflurane in dogs. *Br J Anaesth*. 1977;49(10):957-963.

202. Sarton E et al. Acute pain and central nervous system arousal do not restore impaired hypoxic ventilatory response during sevoflurane sedation. *Anesthesiology*. 1996;85(2):295-303.

203. van den Elsen M et al. Influence of 0.1 minimum alveolar concentration of sevoflurane, desflurane and isoflurane on dynamic ventilatory response to hypercapnia in humans. *Br J Anaesth*. 1998;80(2):174-182.

204. TerRiet MF et al. Which is most pungent: isoflurane, sevoflurane or desflurane? *Br J Anaesth*. 2000;85(2):305-307.

205. Jones RM et al. Clinical impressions and cardiorespiratory effects of a new fluorinated inhalation anaesthetic, desflurane (I-653), in volunteers. *Br J Anaesth*. 1990;64(1):11-15.

206. Zwass MS et al. Induction and maintenance characteristics of anesthesia with desflurane and nitrous oxide in infants and children. *Anesthesiology*. 1992;76(3):373-378.

207. Ashworth J, Smith I. Comparison of desflurane with isoflurane or propofol in spontaneously breathing ambulatory patients. *Anesth Analg*. 1998;87(2): 312-318.

208. Mori N et al. Prolonged sevoflurane inhalation was not nephrotoxic in two patients with refractory status asthmaticus. *Anesth Analg*. 1996;83(1):189-191.

209. Crawford MW et al. Hemodynamic and organ blood flow responses to halothane and sevoflurane anesthesia during spontaneous ventilation. *Anesth Analg*. 1992;75(6):1000-1006.

210. Cousins MJ et al. The etiology of methoxyflurane nephrotoxicity. *J Pharmacol Exp Ther*. 1974;190(3):530-541.

211. Cousins MJ, Mazze RI. Methoxyflurane nephrotoxicity. A study of dose response in man. *JAMA*. 1973;225(13):1611-1616.

212. Crandell WB et al. Nephrotoxicity associated with methoxyflurane anesthesia. *Anesthesiology*. 1966;27(5):591-607.

213. Zaleski L et al. Desflurane versus isoflurane in patients with chronic hepatic and renal disease. *Anesth Analg*. 1993;76(2):353-356.

214. Jones RM et al. Biotransformation and hepato-renal function in volunteers after exposure to desflurane (I-653). *Br J Anaesth*. 1990;64(4):482-487.

215. Price RG. Urinary enzymes, nephrotoxicity and renal disease. *Toxicology*. 1982;23(2-3):99-134.

216. Price RG. Measurement of N-acetyl-beta-glucosaminidase and its isoenzymes in urine methods and clinical applications. *Eur J Clin Chem Clin Biochem*. 1992;30(10):693-705.

217. Bernard AM et al. Assessment of urinary retinol-binding protein as an index of proximal tubular injury. *Clin Chem*. 1987;33(6):775-779.

218. Sundberg AG et al. Immunohistochemical localization of alpha and pi class glutathione transferases in normal human tissues. *Pharmacol Toxicol*. 1993;72(4-5):321-331.

219. Sundberg A et al. Glutathione transferases in the urine: sensitive methods for detection of kidney damage induced by nephrotoxic agents in humans. *Environ Health Perspect*. 1994;102(Suppl 3):293-296.

220. Stevens WC et al. Comparative toxicity of isoflurane, halothane, fluroxene and diethyl ether in human volunteers. *Can Anaesth Soc J*. 1973;20(3):357-368.

221. Higuchi H et al. The effects of low-flow sevoflurane and isoflurane anesthesia on renal function in patients with stable moderate renal insufficiency. *Anesth Analg*. 2001;92(3):650-655.

222. Story DA et al. Changes in plasma creatinine concentration after cardiac anesthesia with isoflurane, propofol, or sevoflurane: a randomized clinical trial. *Anesthesiology*. 2001;95(4):842-848.

223. Frink EJ Jr et al. Clinical comparison of sevoflurane and isoflurane in healthy patients. *Anesth Analg*. 1992;74(2):241-245.

224. Liu J et al. Absorption and degradation of sevoflurane and isoflurane in a conventional anesthetic circuit. *Anesth Analg*. 1991;72(6):785-789.

225. Steffey EP et al. Dehydration of Baralyme increases compound A resulting from sevoflurane degradation in a standard anesthetic circuit used to anesthetize swine. *Anesth Analg*. 1997;85(6):1382-1386.

226. Kharasch ED. Putting the brakes on anesthetic breakdown. *Anesthesiology*. 1999;91(5):1192.

227. Hanaki C et al. Decomposition of sevoflurane by sodalime. *Hiroshima J Med Sci*. 1987;36(1):61-67.

228. Kharasch ED et al. Role of renal cysteine conjugate beta-lyase in the mechanism of compound A nephrotoxicity in rats. *Anesthesiology*. 1997; 86(1):160-171.

229. Conzen PF et al. Low-flow sevoflurane compared with low-flow isoflurane anesthesia in patients with stable renal insufficiency. *Anesthesiology*. 2002;97(3):578-584.

230. Ebert TJ et al. Absence of biochemical evidence for renal and hepatic dysfunction after 8 hours of 1.25 minimum alveolar concentration sevoflurane anesthesia in volunteers [comment]. *Anesthesiology*. 1998;88(3):601-610.

231. Castro BA et al. Explosion within an anesthesia machine: Baralyme(R), high fresh gas flows and sevoflurane concentration. *Anesthesiology*. 2004;101(2): 537-539.

232. Fatheree RS, Leighton BL. Acute respiratory distress syndrome after an exothermic Baralyme(R)-sevoflurane reaction. *Anesthesiology*. 2004;101(2): 531-533.

233. Dunning MB et al. Sevoflurane breakdown produces flammable concentrations of hydrogen. *Anesthesiology*. 2007;106(1):144-148.

234. Bito H, Ikeda K. Effect of total flow rate on the concentration of degradation products generated by reaction between sevoflurane and soda lime. *Br J Anaesth*. 1995;74(6):667-669.

235. Fang ZX et al. Factors affecting production of compound A from the interaction of sevoflurane with Baralyme and soda lime. *Anesth Analg*. 1996;82(4):775-781.

236. Kobayashi S et al. Compound A concentration in the circle absorber system during low-flow sevoflurane anesthesia: comparison of Dragersorb Free, Amsorb, and Sodasorb II. *J Clin Anesth*. 2003;15: 33.

237. Keijzer C et al. Compound A and carbon monoxide production from sevoflurane and seven different types of carbon dioxide absorbent in a patient model. *Acta Anaesthesiol Scand*. 2007;51(1):31-37.

238. Marini F et al. Compound A, formaldehyde and methanol concentrations during low-flow sevoflurane anaesthesia: comparison of three carbon dioxide absorbers. *Acta Anaesthesiol Scand*. 2007;51(5):625-632.

239. Yamakage M et al. Carbon dioxide absorbents containing potassium hydroxide produce much larger concentrations of compound A from sevoflurane in clinical practice [comment]. *Anesth Analg*. 2000;91(1):220-224.

240. Versichelen LF et al. Only carbon dioxide absorbents free of both NaOH and KOH do not generate compound A during in vitro closed-system sevoflurane: evaluation of five absorbents. *Anesthesiology*. 2001;95(3):750-755.

241. Gelman SM et al. Liver circulation and function during isoflurane and halothane anesthesia. *Anesthesiology*. 1984;61(6):726-730.

242. Merin RG et al. Comparison of the effects of isoflurane and desflurane on cardiovascular dynamics and regional blood flow in the chronically instrumented dog. *Anesthesiology*. 1991;74(3):568-574.

243. Frink EJ et al. Plasma inorganic fluoride with sevoflurane anesthesia: correlation with indices of hepatic and renal function. *Anesth Analg*. 1992;74(2):231-235.

244. Gatecel C et al. The postoperative effects of halothane versus isoflurane on hepatic artery and portal vein blood flow in humans. *Anesth Analg*. 2003;96(3):740-745.

245. Brody GL, Sweet RB. Halothane anesthesia as a possible cause of massive hepatic necrosis. *Anesthesiology*. 1963;24: 29.

246. Hussey AJ et al. Plasma glutathione S-transferase concentration as a measure of hepatocellular integrity following a single general anaesthetic with halothane, enflurane or isoflurane. *Br J Anaesth*. 1988;60(2):130-135.

247. Elliott RH, Strunin L. Hepatotoxicity of volatile anaesthetics. *Br J Anaesth*. 1993;70(3):339-348.

248. Kenna JG et al. Halothane hepatitis in children. *Br Med J (Clin Res Ed)*. 1987;294(6581):1209-1211.

249. Kharasch ED et al. Identification of the enzyme responsible for oxidative halothane metabolism: implications for prevention of halothane hepatitis. *Lancet*. 1996;347(9012):1367-1371.

250. Ray DC, Drummond GB. Halothane hepatitis. *Br J Anaesth*. 1991;67(1): 84-99.

251. Njoku DB et al. Autoantibodies associated with volatile anesthetic hepatitis found in the sera of a large cohort of pediatric anesthesiologists. *Anesth Analg*. 2002;94(2):243-249.

252. Neuberger J et al. Specific serological markers in the diagnosis of fulminant hepatic failure associated with halothane anaesthesia. *Br J Anaesth*. 1983;55(1):15-19.

253. Kenna JG et al. Specific antibodies to halothane-induced liver antigens in halothane-associated hepatitis. *Br J Anaesth*. 1987;59(10):1286-1290.

254. Hubbard AK et al. Halothane hepatitis patients generate an antibody response toward a covalently bound metabolite of halothane. *Anesthesiology*. 1988;68(5):791-796.

255. Njoku D et al. Biotransformation of halothane, enflurane, isoflurane, and desflurane to trifluoroacetylated liver proteins: association between protein acylation and hepatic injury. *Anesth Analg*. 1997;84(1):173-178.

256. O'Shea D et al. Effect of fasting and obesity in humans on the 6-hydroxylation of chlorzoxazone: a putative probe of CYP2E1 activity. *Clin Pharmacol Ther*. 1994;56(4):359-367.

257. Cousins MJ et al. Risk factors for halothane hepatitis. *Aust N Z J Surg*. 1989;59(1):5-14.

258. Bunker JP et al. *A Study of the Possible Association Between Halothane Anaesthesia and Post Operative Hepatic Necrosis*. Washington, DC: US Government Printing Office; 1969.

259. Toniutto P et al. Role of AST to platelet ratio index in the detection of liver fibrosis in patients with recurrent hepatitis C after liver transplantation. *J Gastroenterol Hepatol*. 2007;22(11):1904-1908.

260. Liaw YF. Diagnosis and onset of acute hepatitis delta virus infection. *Hepatology*. 1990;12(2):378-379.

261. Zuckerman AJ. Hepatitis C virus: a giant leap forward. *Hepatology*. 1990;11(2):320-322.

262. Zuckerman AJ. Hepatitis E virus. *Br Med J*. 1990;300(6738):1475-1476.

263. Scheider DM et al. Hepatic dysfunction after repeated isoflurane administration. *J Clin Gastroenterol*. 1993;17(2):168-170.

264. Ohmori H et al. A case of postoperative liver damage after isoflurane anesthesia followed by sevoflurane anesthesia. *J Jpn Soc Clin Anesth*. 1994;14: 68-71.

265. Martin JL et al. Hepatotoxicity after desflurane anesthesia. *Anesthesiology*. 1995;83(5):1125-1129.

266. Carrigan TW, Straughen WJ. A report of hepatic necrosis and death following isoflurane anesthesia. *Anesthesiology*. 1987;67(4):581-583.

267. Martin JL et al. Halothane hepatitis 28 years after primary exposure. *Anesth Analg*. 1992;74(4):605-608.

268. Green WB et al. Covalent binding of oxidative metabolites to hepatic protein not detectable after exposure to sevoflurane or desflurane. *Anesthesiology*. 1994;81:A437.

269. Kenna JG, Jones RM. The organ toxicity of inhaled anesthetics. *Anesth Analg*. 1995;81(6 Suppl):S51-S66.

270. Shichinohe Y et al. A case of postoperative hepatic injury after sevoflurane anesthesia. *Masui*. 1992;41(11):1802-1805.

271. Watanabe K et al. A case of suspected liver dysfunction induced by sevoflurane anesthesia. *Masui*. 1993;42(6):902-905.

272. Ogawa M et al. Drug induced hepatitis following sevoflurane anesthesia in a child. *Masui*. 1991;40(10):1542-1545.

273. Kanaya N et al. Comparison of the effects of sevoflurane, isoflurane and halothane on indocyanine green clearance. *Br J Anaesth*. 1995;74(2):164-167.

274. Hongo T. Sevoflurane reduced but isoflurane maintained hepatic blood flow during anesthesia in man. *J Anesth*. 1994;8: 55-59.

275. Schindler E et al. Blood supply to the liver in the human after 1 MAC desflurane in comparison with isoflurane and halothane. *Anasthesiol Intensivmed Notfallmed Schmerzther*. 1996;31(6):344-348.

276. O'Riordan J et al. Effects of desflurane and isoflurane on splanchnic microcirculation during major surgery. *Br J Anaesth*. 1997;78(1):95-96.

277. Hong K et al. Metabolism of nitrous oxide by human and rat intestinal contents. *Anesthesiology*. 1980;52(1):16-19.

278. Deacon R et al. Inactivation of methionine synthase by nitrous oxide. *Eur J Biochem*. 1980;104(2):419-423.

279. Nunn JF, Chanarin I. Nitrous oxide inactivates methionine synthetase. In: Eger EI II, ed. *Nitrous Oxide*. New York: Elsevier; 1985:216-228.

280. Nunn JF, O'Morain C. Nitrous oxide decreases motility of human neutrophils in vitro. *Anesthesiology*. 1982;56(1):45-48.

281. Wulf H et al. Neuromuscular blocking effects of rocuronium during desflurane, isoflurane, and sevoflurane anaesthesia. *Can J Anaesth*. 1998; 45(6):526-532.

282. Paul MM et al. Characterization of the interactions between volatile anesthetics and neuromuscular blockers at the muscle nicotinic acetylcholine receptor. *Anesth Analg*. 2002;95(2):362-367.

283. Waud BE, Waud DR. Comparison of the effects of general anesthetics on the end-plate of skeletal muscle. *Anesthesiology*. 1975;43(5):540-547.

284. Saitoh Y et al. Post-tetanic burst count and train-of-four during recovery from vecuronium-induced intense neuromuscular block under different types of anaesthesia. *Eur J Anaesthesiol*. 1998;15(5):524-528.

285. Taivainen T, Meretoja OA. The neuromuscular blocking effects of vecuronium during sevoflurane, halothane and balanced anaesthesia in children. *Anaesthesia*. 1995;50(12):1046-1049.

286. Lowry DW et al. Neuromuscular effects of rocuronium during sevoflurane, isoflurane, and intravenous anesthesia. *Anesth Analg*. 1998;87(4):936-940.

287. Kumar N et al. A comparison of the effects of isoflurane and desflurane on the neuromuscular effects of mivacurium. *Anaesthesia*. 1996;51(6):547-550.

288. Wulf H et al. Augmentation of the neuromuscular blocking effects of cisatracurium during desflurane, sevoflurane, isoflurane or total i.v. anaesthesia. *Br J Anaesth*. 1998;80(3):308-312.

289. Donati F, Bevan DR. Long-term succinylcholine infusion during isoflurane anesthesia. *Anesthesiology*. 1983;58(1):6-10.

290. Szalados JE et al. Nitrous oxide potentiates succinylcholine neuromuscular blockade in humans. *Anesth Analg*. 1991;72(1):18-21.

291. Bock M et al. Rocuronium potency and recovery characteristics during steady-state desflurane, sevoflurane, isoflurane or propofol anaesthesia. *Br J Anaesth*. 2000;84(1):43-47.

292. Kelly RE et al. Depression of neuromuscular function in a patient during desflurane anesthesia [see comments]. *Anesth Analg*. 1993;76(4):868-871.

293. Ahmed AA et al. Sevoflurane exposure time and the neuromuscular blocking effect of vecuronium. *Can J Anaesth*. 1999;46(5 Pt 1):429-432.

294. Morita T et al. Sevoflurane and isoflurane impair edrophonium reversal of vecuronium-induced neuromuscular block. *Can J Anaesth*. 1996;43(8): 799-805.

295. Morita T et al. Factors affecting neostigmine reversal of vecuronium block during sevoflurane anaesthesia. *Anaesthesia*. 1997;52(6):538-543.

296. Kiran U et al. Sevoflurane as a sole anaesthetic for thymectomy in myasthenia gravis. *Acta Anaesthesiol Scand*. 2000;44(3):351-353.

297. Baraka A. Anesthesia and critical care of thymectomy for myasthenia gravis. *Chest Surg Clin N Am*. 2001;11(2):337-361.

298. Gronert GA et al. Malignant hyperthermia. In: Miller RD, ed. *Miller's Anesthesia*. Vol 1. 6th ed. Philadelphia: Churchill Livingstone; 2005:1169-1190.

299. Papadimos TJ et al. A suspected case of delayed onset malignant hyperthermia with desflurane anesthesia. *Anesth Analg*. 2004;98(2):548-549.

300. Reed SB, Strobel GE. An in-vitro model of malignant hyperthermia: differential effects of inhalation anesthetics on caffeine-induced muscle contractures. *Anesthesiology*. 1978;48(4):254-259.

301. Gronert GA. Malignant hyperthermia. *Anesthesiology*. 1980;53(5):395-423.

302. Ellis FR et al. Malignant hyperpyrexia induced by nitrous oxide and treated with dexamethasone. *Br Med J*. 1974;4(5939):270-271.

303. Gronert GA, Milde JH. Hyperbaric nitrous oxide and malignant hyperpyrexia. *Br J Anaesth*. 1981;53(11):1238.

CHAPTER 10

INTRAVENOUS INDUCTION AGENTS

John J. Nagelhout

A single ideal intravenous anesthesia induction drug has yet to be developed; however, the variety of agents currently available can be exploited to select an appropriate drug for most all surgical and anesthetic requirements. Desirable properties for an induction agent include rapid and smooth onset and recovery, analgesia, minimal cardiac and respiratory depression, antiemetic actions, bronchodilation, lack of toxicity or histamine release, and advantageous pharmacokinetics and pharmaceutics. This chapter will discuss the advantages and limitations of the currently used intravenous anesthesia induction agents.

BARBITURATES

The first intravenous agents used for general anesthesia were the opioids, which were widely accepted for relief of the suffering patient. However, not until barbiturates were introduced in the 1930s was intravenous anesthesia taken seriously. Waters and Lundy introduced the thiobarbiturate thiopental in 1935. Despite the discovery of more than 2000 barbiturate agents since then, thiopental remains the barbiturate of choice for general anesthesia.

Chemical Structure

Barbituric acid is a cyclic compound formed from the condensation of urea and malonic acid. This compound has no intrinsic central nervous system (CNS) depressant activity by itself. Drugs that are derivatives of barbituric acid are categorized as *barbiturates* (Figure 10-1).

Various substitutions to the barbituric acid compound can create different pharmacologic actions. By replacing both hydrogen atoms at position 5 with *alkyl-* or *aryl-* groups, the pharmacologic action is as a sedative-hypnotic.

These derivatives of barbituric acid are known as *oxybarbiturates* or as the *true barbiturates*. Although insoluble in water, these compounds are soluble in nonpolar solvents such as chloroform and oil; this solubility is a common feature of organic CNS depressants. These drugs have a relatively slower onset of action and a prolonged duration. Alterations in molecular side-chain lengths affect potency; longer chains result in a higher potency. The structures of the barbiturates used in anesthesia are shown in Figure 10-2.

The replacement of the number 2 carbon atom of the barbituric acid molecule with a sulfur atom produces the

thiobarbiturates (thiopental). These compounds have a more rapid onset and a shorter duration of action than the oxybarbiturates.

The sulfurization of oxybarbiturates increases lipid solubility. Any structural change that increases the lipid solubility of barbiturates decreases the duration of action and the latency to onset of action. It also accelerates metabolic degradation, often increasing hypnotic potency.[1]

The ultra–short-acting barbiturate methohexital is produced by the methylation of the active barbiturate phenobarbital at C-1.

Methylation produces an agent that has a more rapid onset and a shorter duration but increased excitatory side effects. The addition of a methyl radical at C-5 confers some convulsant activity, such as involuntary muscular movement (Table 10-1).

Barbiturates are weak acids (the dissociation constant [pK_a] of thiopental is 7.6; of methohexital, 7.9) and are prepared as sodium salts. They are usually combined with 6% anhydrous sodium carbonate, which is used for preventing precipitation of the insoluble free acid form of the barbiturate by atmospheric carbon dioxide.[2] The solution produced has an alkalinity of 10.5 to 11. Barbiturates must be reconstituted before administration using aseptic technique with sterile water for injection, U.S. Pharmacopeia (USP) 0.09% sodium chloride injection or 5% dextrose injection. If lactated Ringer's solution or acidic solutions of drugs are used for reconstitution, the barbiturate precipitates out in the form of free acids. This moderate alkalinity also makes this solution incompatible with opioids, catecholamines, and muscle relaxants, all of which are acidic in solution. Intraarterial or extravascular infusion of this alkaline solution can cause severe tissue injury. One advantage of the alkalinity of barbiturates is the bacteriostatic property it confers. If properly reconstituted and refrigerated, it is stable at room temperature for 2 weeks.[2] Wong and associates[3] studied the risk of contamination in vials left out at room temperature for up to 25 days and found neither significant change in pH nor positive bacteriologic growth. Abbott Laboratories advises that thiopental be at room temperature for no longer than 24 hours after it is reconstituted. When reconstituted with sterile water, methohexital remains stable for 6 weeks.[4] The preparations of the induction drugs are listed in Table 10-2.

Pharmacokinetics

Stereoisomers

Barbiturates are enantiomeric. Many barbiturates have asymmetric side chains attached to the number 5 carbon atom of the barbiturate ring. They contain equal amounts of stereoisomers

The author would like to thank Mike and Nadine Fallacaro for their contributions to this chapter in previous editions.

and are marketed as racemic compounds. In thiopental, pentobarbital, and secobarbital, the L-isomers are the most potent. Methohexital has four stereoisomers that have varying degrees of activity. The β-L-stereoisomers are the most potent, but they create excessive motor activity. Methohexital is therefore a racemic mixture of the α-L-stereoisomers, which are the least potent and do not cause excessive motor activity.[5]

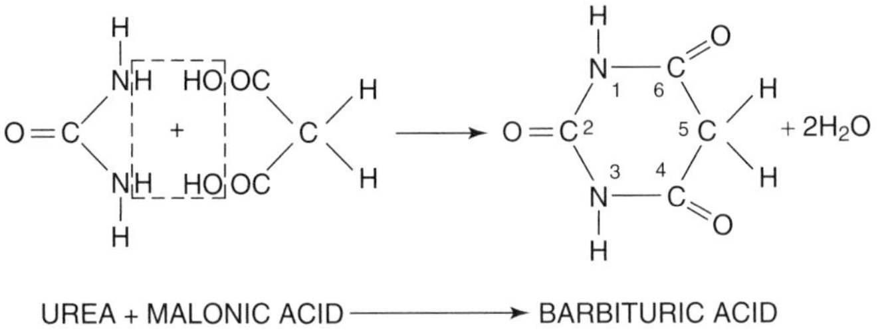
UREA + MALONIC ACID → BARBITURIC ACID
+ 2H₂O

FIGURE **10-1** Formation of barbituric acid.

TABLE **10-1** Chemical Modification of Barbiturates

	Placement	Substitute	Example
Oxybarbiturates	C-2	Oxygen	Pentobarbital, secobarbital, phenobarbital
Thiobarbiturates	C-2	Sulfur	Thiopental
Methylated oxybarbiturates	C-1	Methyl	Methohexital

- Thiomethylated and *N*-methylated drugs are ultra–short acting.
- Synthesized by condensation of urea and malonic acid to form barbituric acid ring (barbital).
- Metabolized via liver cytochrome enzymes by desulfuration (thiopental), producing the clinically active oxyanalogue pentobarbital, which contributes to the hangover effect. Oxidation of carbon-5 radicals and to a lesser extent ring hydrolysis also occur.
- Methohexital undergoes demethylation. Oxidation at carbon-5 and ring hydrolysis occur.

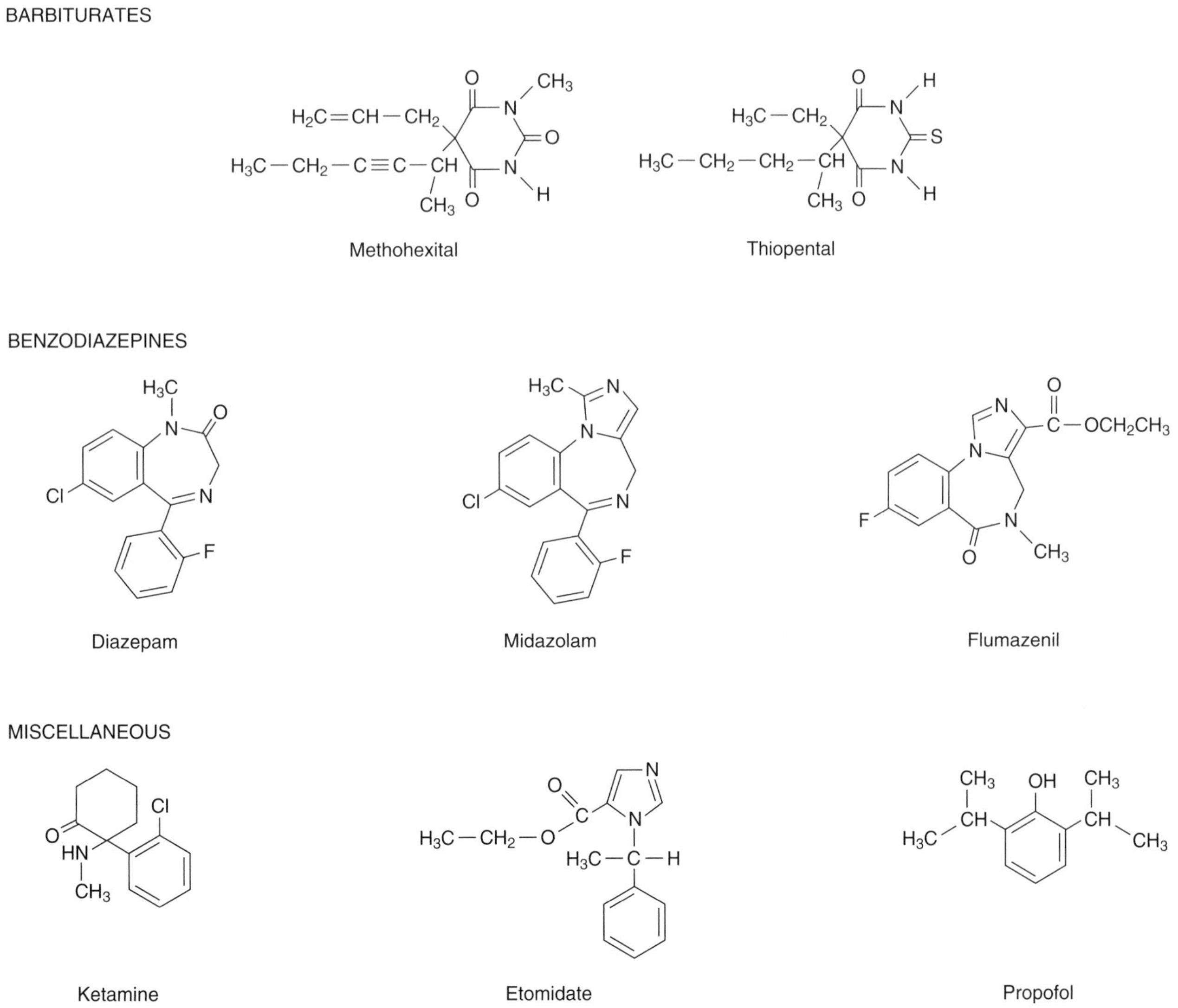
BARBITURATES
Methohexital
Thiopental
BENZODIAZEPINES
Diazepam
Midazolam
Flumazenil
MISCELLANEOUS
Ketamine
Etomidate
Propofol

FIGURE **10-2** Agents used for the induction of general anesthesia.

TABLE 10-2	Pharmaceutic Preparation of Intravenous Anesthetic Agents		
Class	**Drug Name**	**Available Solution**	**Pain on Injection***
Thiobarbiturates	Thiopental (Pentothal)	pK_a 7.5; sodium salts mixed with anhydrous sodium bicarbonate; pH 10.5-11	+++
N-methylated oxybarbiturate	Methohexital (Brevital)	pK_a 7.9; same as thiopental; pH 10-11	+
Benzodiazepines	Diazepam (Valium)	0.5% in 40% propylene glycol and 10% alcohol	+++
		0.5% emulsion formula; intralipid	+/−
	Lorazepam (Ativan)	0.4% in propylene glycol	+
	Midazolam (Versed)	0.5% buffered aqueous solution (pH 3.5)	0
Imidazoles	Etomidate (Amidate)	Water soluble at acidic pH, lipophilic at physiologic pH (pK_a 4.24); 0.2% solution in 30% propylene glycol (pH 5)	+++
Alkylphenol	Propofol (Diprivan)	1% solution in an aqueous emulsion containing 10% soybean oil, 2.25% glycerol, and 1.2% egg phosphatide, EDTA (pK_a 11); AstraZeneca	++
	Generic	Generic formulation from Baxter contains metabisulfate and a lower pH of 4.5-6.4 (use with caution in patients with allergies and asthma)	
	Generic	Generic formulation from Bedford contains benzyl alcohol; pH 7-8.5 (benzyl alcohol should be avoided in infants)	
	Aquavan	Water-soluble prodrug of propofol that undergoes hydrolysis by alkaline phosphatases to propofol	
Arylcyclohexylamines	Ketamine (Ketalar)	White crystalline salt 1% or 10% aqueous solution (pH 3.3-5.5; pK_a 7.5)	0

EDTA, *Disodium ethylenediaminetetraacetate.*
0, None; +, mild; ++, moderate; +++, marked.

Protein Binding

Barbiturates are reversibly bound to plasma proteins, most commonly to plasma albumin.[4] This binding has an effect on the pharmacologic actions of these drugs, because bound drugs are unable to cross biologic membranes. The greater the amount of free drug available, the greater the pharmacologic effect. Thiopental is approximately 80% protein bound, making it more highly protein bound than the oxybarbiturates.[1] The sulfur substitution may be responsible for the change in the affinity of the thiobarbiturate compound for protein.[6] Factors that change protein binding are listed in Table 10-3.

When competition with other drugs for protein binding sites occurs, the unbound fraction of thiopental is increased. Such competitive drugs include aspirin, indomethacin, naproxen, and warfarin. The greater the unbound fraction, or amount of free drug available, the shorter the duration of action as more rapid redistribution occurs.[7] Decreased plasma protein concentrations that occur in some patients (e.g., those with uremia or hepatic disease and those in the third trimester of pregnancy) may also cause an increase in circulating free-drug levels, but the clinical significance is questionable.

Physiologic pH favors the un-ionized fraction of thiopental. Its high lipid solubility accounts for its rapid movement across the blood-brain barrier and the quick onset of anesthesia it provides. Phenobarbital has much lower lipid solubility, a characteristic that accounts for its slower onset of action.

TABLE 10-3	Factors That Alter Protein Binding
Factors	**Percent Bound**
Decreased lipid solubility	Decreases binding
Increased pH ($\leq$8.0)	Increases binding
Increased drug concentration	Decreases binding
Increased protein concentration	Increases binding
Increased competition for binding sites with other drugs	Decreases binding

Barbiturate distribution depends on lipid solubility, protein binding, and degree of ionization. Of these, lipid solubility is the most important. Drugs that are highly lipid soluble cross cell membranes rapidly. There is a more rapid transfer into the CNS when the drug is more soluble. Solubility also accounts for transplacental drug transfer. Thiopental, being highly soluble, easily crosses the placental barrier.

Ionization

The 7.5 pK_a of thiopental is close to the physiologic pH of 7.4. Because formation of the nonionized pharmacologically active thiopental compound depends on the H^+ concentration, tissue pH exerts some control over the amount of active compound formed. Because the pK_a of thiopental is so close to physiologic pH, 61% of the compound exists in the nonionized state at a pH of 7.4. The pH is not uniform throughout the body; intracellular pH is more acidic than extracellular fluid pH, creating a difference in concentration of ionized and nonionized thiopental at either side of the membrane. Thiopental is an acid compound; therefore, acidosis increases the amount of nonionized thiopental in the extracellular fluid and allows greater diffusion across membranes into tissues.

The distribution, redistribution, and ultimate elimination of thiopental have been studied extensively in various physiologic and pharmacologic models. In the first decade of clinical use of thiopental, its short duration was attributed to rapid metabolism and elimination.[1] Brodie and associates[8] changed that theory by introducing the idea of redistribution into fat stores to account for the short duration of action. Price and colleagues, however, not convinced that adipose tissue uptake was rapid enough to account for this effect, looked to other tissue groups for an explanation of uptake that would terminate thiopental's drug action. These investigators found that the fat uptake of thiopental was too slow and that the relatively poorly perfused tissues, muscle, connective tissue, bone, and skin, in full, were responsible for depleting the brain of thiopental in the time considered.[9]

The role of metabolism in the short duration of effect of thiopental was reexamined with consideration given to the rapid decrease in plasma levels of barbiturates. After an intravenous injection of thiopental, its presence is restricted to the central blood volume, where its concentration is high. Distribution to the tissues is dependent on drug concentration in blood and cardiac output, which perfuses tissues and organs. The vessel-rich group of organs receives a major percentage of the cardiac output. The brain receives 20% of the cardiac output and achieves a peak plasma concentration of thiopental in one circulation time, accounting for the rapid onset of anesthesia after a bolus injection. In a three-compartment pharmacokinetic model, the brain is placed within or in immediate proximity to the central compartment.[10] After an intravenous injection, the first phase of distribution transports most of the injected drug to the vessel-rich group. Two phases begin shortly thereafter in which the drug is distributed to all other tissues, causing the drug blood levels to fall. A rapid phase of distribution begins with a redistribution of blood to the vessel-poor group, which is composed primarily of muscle tissues. This phase lasts 2 to 4 minutes, during which a patient would awaken from an initial bolus dose of thiopental. The second distribution phase is slow because of the equilibration of the drug concentration into peripheral compartments.[7] Although the capacity to store thiopental in fat is high, limited blood flow delays equilibration. The slow phase becomes predominant after four or five rapid distribution half-lives, or 12 to 17 minutes.

Distribution and redistribution of thiopental are largely dependent on cardiac output. Alterations in cardiac function and circulating blood volume may change some pharmacologic characteristics, including duration and therapeutic effect. Impaired cardiac function or hypovolemia decreases tissue perfusion to peripheral compartments; this phenomenon does not change the initial concentration of circulating drug in the central compartment after injection. Less hemodilution of the drug results in higher drug concentrations to the vessel-rich groups such as the CNS (causing anesthesia) and heart (causing cardiac depression).[5] Sympathetic stimulation from pain or increased

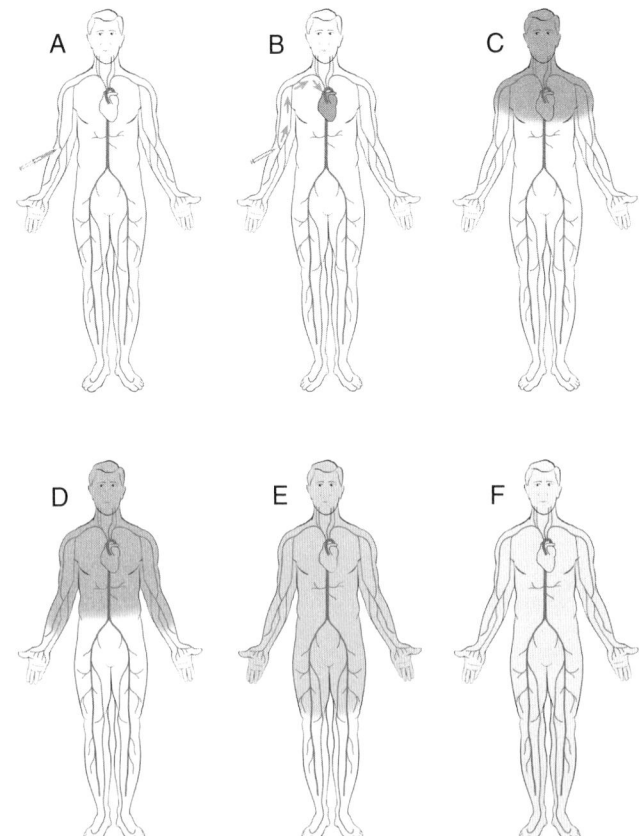

FIGURE **10-3**   Redistribution of intravenous drugs is shown. **A** and **B**, A drug is administered in the arm and follows the venous circulation to the heart. **C**, The high cardiac output and circulatory flow initially distribute the drug to the brain and upper body, and rapid central nervous system effects begin. **D**, **E**, and **F**, As time passes, usually minutes, the drug more evenly distributes throughout the body, lowering the initial high brain concentration, and the patient awakens.

anxiety increases cardiac output and speeds distribution to peripheral compartments from the brain, thereby decreasing the duration of the anesthesia.[11]

As tissue saturation of thiopental approaches equilibrium with the blood, termination of the drug action depends on the slow uptake of the drug into the vessel-poor group and on elimination. The phenomenon of redistribution is shown in Figure 10-3.

Metabolism

Investigators have looked for the rationale behind the rapid termination of the anesthetic effects of thiopental and methohexital. The role of hepatic metabolism has been extensively examined. The pharmacokinetics of the induction drugs is given in Table 10-4.

By use of a pharmacokinetic model with the brain concentration of thiopental as an approximation of the central compartment concentration, measurements were made 1 minute after intravenous bolus administration. Only 14% of the injected dose was lost through metabolism. This percentage correlated very well with a hepatic extraction ratio of 0.15. After 15 minutes, the amount of drug lost to metabolism was 18%, only a 4% change from the previous measurement. However, the CNS effects were greatly diminished, indicating that the redistribution of the central compartment, not hepatic metabolism, was

TABLE 10-4	Select Pharmacokinetic Values for Intravenous Anesthetic Agents				
Drug Name	Distribution Half-Life (min)	Elimination Half-Life (hr)	Clearance (mL/kg/min)	Volume of Distribution (L/kg)	Protein Binding (%)
Thiopental	2-4	10-12	3.5	2.5	80
Methohexital	5-6	2-4	10	2.3	85
Diazepam	10-15	20-50	0.3	0.8-1.3	98
Midazolam	7-15	2-4	7-11	1-1.7	94
Etomidate	2-4	2-5	22.5	2.5-4.5	75
Propofol	2-4	1-5	25	2-8	98
Ketamine	11-17	2-3	14.5	2.5-3.5	12

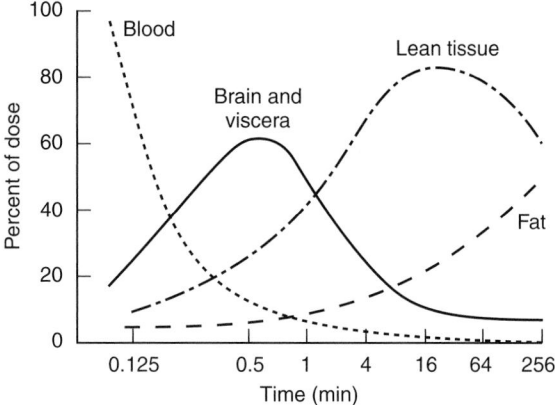

FIGURE 10-4 Pentothal kinetics. Note that thiopental rapidly enters the brain and other vital organs, with peak effects at 1 minute after bolus injection. The brain concentration then falls rapidly over the next 10 to 15 minutes as the drug redistributes more evenly throughout the body to muscle and fat.

responsible for awakening.[12] The pharmacokinetic movement of thiopental is given in Figure 10-4. Note that thiopental rapidly enters the brain and other vital organs with peak effects at 1 minute after bolus injection. The brain concentration then falls rapidly over the next 10 to 15 minutes as the drug redistributes more evenly throughout the body to muscle and fat.

In comparisons of methohexital and thiopental, the distribution kinetics are very similar, but the clearance-elimination half-times are different.[9] The hepatic extraction ratio for methohexital is three times greater than that for thiopental. Although hepatic metabolism has a much greater role in the termination of action of methohexital than of thiopental, the total difference in hepatic extraction after 30 minutes was not great enough to account for the much larger difference in clearance between the two agents.[13-14] Redistribution again is proved to be of much greater importance than hepatic metabolism in awakening from thiobarbiturate anesthesia.

The metabolism and elimination of barbiturates are almost entirely the result of hepatic biotransformation by microsomal enzymes and renal excretion. The role of the kidney in metabolism is small because thiobarbiturates are highly protein bound and thus are not freely filtered at the glomerulus. The lipid solubility of barbiturates allows them to be easily reabsorbed into the circulation via the renal tubules. Whereas oxybarbiturates

are metabolized by hepatocytes alone, other tissues (brain and kidney) are capable of metabolizing thiobarbiturates to a small extent.[12]

The most significant metabolic pathway involves the oxidation of the side-chain radicals at the C-5 position.[1,2] Omega oxidation produces thiopental carboxylic acid, which is not pharmacologically active. Thiobarbiturates can undergo desulfurization to the corresponding oxybarbiturate (pentobarbital), which does have pharmacologic activity, and breaks down further to inactive metabolites. The amount of pentobarbital produced has been studied in low- and high-dose administration techniques. After a 450- to 1275-mg intravenous bolus injection of thiopental, serum levels of pentobarbital at 15 minutes were found to be too low to produce pharmacologic effects.[14] Doses of thiopental for cerebral resuscitation (300-500 mg/kg given over 2 to 3 days) produced concentrations of pentobarbital that were pharmacologically active at approximately 10% of thiopental concentration.[15] In dosages used for achieving anesthesia for induction, the amount of pentobarbital produced is not significant.

Methohexital undergoes N-demethylation in addition to C-5 oxidation. Only minute amounts of active metabolites are generated.[1]

Barbiturates combine with cytochrome P-450 enzymes and compete for biotransformation with other substrates. In addition, they are responsible for the induction of the microsomal activity of these enzymes, probably by increasing their numbers rather than altering their properties.[1]

In a study of the effect of hepatic cirrhosis on thiopental metabolism, Pandele and colleagues[16] found that the pharmacokinetics were only slightly modified. Besides altered protein binding, hepatic blood flow and hepatic intrinsic clearance are decreased in the cirrhotic patient.[17] The decrease in hepatic blood flow is not a key factor because of thiopental's low hepatic extraction ratio. The liver's intrinsic abilities to metabolize drugs and influence protein binding are linked because only unbound drug is available for biotransformation. With the increase in free drug that occurs in hypoalbuminemic states, the rate of clearance should increase, but it remains unchanged. Although the findings of Pandele and co-workers[16] were statistically insignificant, they did show that the impairment of intrinsic metabolism of hepatocytes was decreased in liver disease. Redistribution still has a major influence on the duration of therapeutic effect.

Burch and Stanski[18] studied the effects of renal failure on thiopental pharmacokinetics. They determined that in

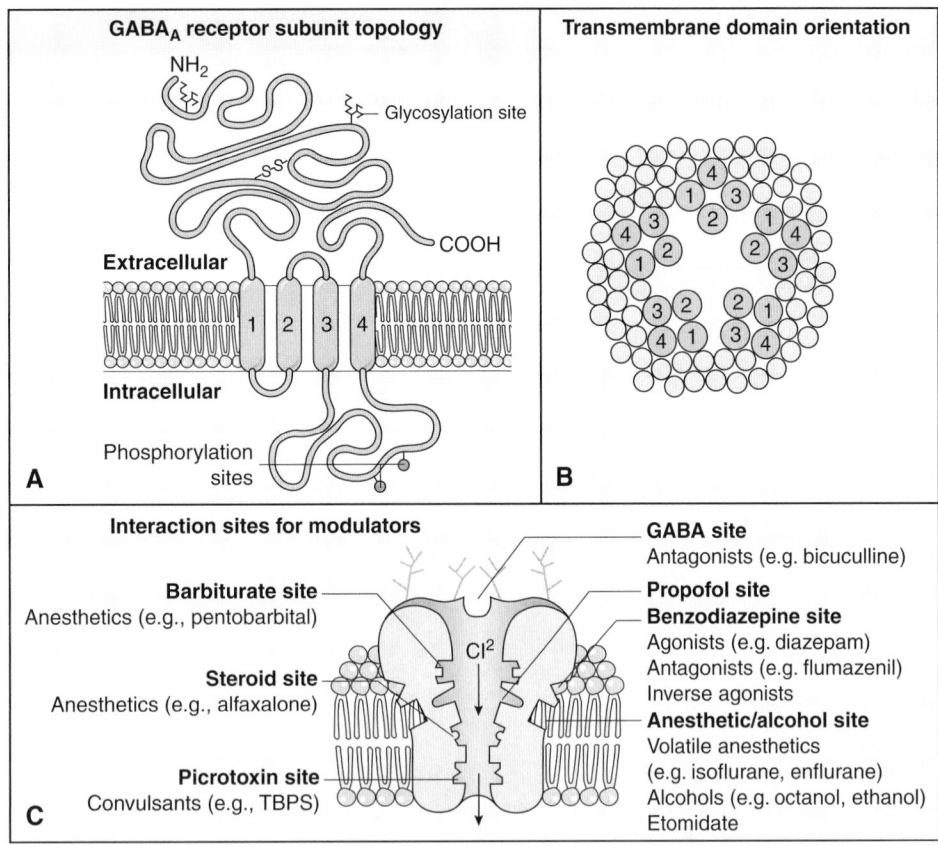

FIGURE **10-5**   The GABA$_A$ receptor. **A,** The generic GABA$_A$ receptor subunit has four hydrophobic transmembrane segments that are thought to form amphipathic α-helices. The N-terminal domain contains N-glycosylation sites and a conserved cysteine bridge; it forms the agonist-binding site. The large intracellular loop undergoes phosphorylation in several isoforms. **B,** Plane view of the transmembrane hydrophobic segments showing interactions to form a central ion-conducting pore lined by the second transmembrane domains. The hetero-oligomeric structure consists of five subunits, with each subunit contributing to the ion channel pore. **C,** The GABA$_A$ receptor gates an anion channel permeable to Cl$^-$ and HCO$_3$$^-$. The general anesthetics are distinguished from the benzodiazepines (which allosterically modulate GABA binding to potentiate GABA responses) by their ability to activate/gate the GABA$_A$ receptor channel directly. A separate site at the interface between the third and fourth transmembrane segments appears to interact with volatile anesthetics, alcohols, and etomidate, as demonstrated by site-directed mutagenesis studies. *(From Hemmings HC, Hopkins PM, eds.* Foundations of Anesthesia Basic and Clinical Sciences. *St Louis: Mosby; 2006.)*

chronic renal disease, the intrinsic hepatic metabolism and thiopental distribution remain essentially unchanged. Additionally, they found an increase in unbound drug (caused by altered protein binding) and therefore an increase in hepatic drug clearance. This increase in hepatic drug clearance was offset, however, by an increase in the volume of distribution attributed to increases in unbound drug available for distribution to the tissues. As a result, the elimination half-life is unchanged because differences in altered clearance and volume of distribution were approximately equal.[18] Injection of thiopental into an acidemic patient results in a higher proportion of un-ionized, unbound drug and therefore a more profound pharmacologic effect. Alterations in the blood-brain barrier that accompany uremia increase sensitivity to CNS depressants as well. A shorter titrated administration of thiopental and methohexital avoids the transient high concentration of these drugs that could cause CNS and cardiovascular depression.

Mechanism of Action

γ-Aminobutyric acid (GABA) is a major inhibitory transmitter in the CNS. The barbiturate mechanism of action is linked to postsynaptic enhancement of GABA-mediated inhibition.[19] The GABA$_A$ receptor, which is a ligand-gated ion channel receptor, is activated by the binding of the neurotransmitter GABA. This binding of GABA to the GABA$_A$ receptor initiates the movement of chloride (Cl$^-$) through ion channels into the cell. This results in hyperpolarization of postsynaptic cell membrane and the inhibition of neuronal cell excitation. A model has been developed that includes sites of action for GABA on the postsynaptic membrane, as well as sites of action for barbiturates and benzodiazepines. Propofol, etomidate, ethanol, and volatile anesthetics may also have binding sites on this receptor.[20] The GABA receptor and its function is described in Figure 10-5. The intravenous anesthetics mentioned earlier achieve hypnotic activity by binding to their distinctive sites on the

GABA$_A$ receptor. They may also have GABA-mimetic effects, allowing the influx of Cl$^-$ in the absence of GABA. Barbiturates increase the mean open time of GABA receptor channels by increasing the frequency with which longer openings occur, not by changing the duration of these channel openings.[21]

Thiopental

The two commonly used barbiturates in anesthesia are thiopental and methohexital. Thiopental is prepared as a 2.5% solution. The usual induction dose of these agents is 3 to 4 mg/kg. It produces few excitatory symptoms, has a rapid onset and a short duration, and is associated with some pain on injection. Patient age, size, physical condition, and current disease must be taken into consideration when a dose is chosen.

Methohexital

An ultra–short-acting barbiturate, methohexital is also primarily used for procedures outside the operating room such as electroconvulsive therapy (ECT), dental procedures, and cardioversion.[22] Its popularity is not as great as that of the thiobarbiturates because of actions such as excitatory movements (myoclonia) on induction, pain on injection, hiccough, and seizures.[22,23] Spontaneous muscle movements may be influenced by the total amount of drug given and the rapid rate of injection. The hepatic extraction ratio of methohexital is 0.5 (three times greater than that of thiopental). Therefore, hepatic blood flow is a major factor in methohexital clearance. The pharmacokinetics (distribution, redistribution, protein bonding, and lipid solubility) of thiopental and methohexital are similar. Although the hepatic clearance of methohexital is greater than that of thiopental, the difference is not as great as would be expected. Hence, redistribution is the most important determinant in the termination of effects for both drugs.[13]

Simulated driving tests showed mental impairment 8 hours after methohexital administration, even though clinical recovery with methohexital was more rapid than with thiopental.[24] The cardiovascular and respiratory effects of methohexital are also similar to those of thiopental.

Methohexital is 2.5 times more potent than the thiobarbiturates, and the incidence of pain on injection is 5%, compared with 1% to 2% with the thiobarbiturates.[22] Key points of barbiturate pharmacology are noted in Box 10-1.

Pharmacodynamics

Central Nervous System Effects. Thiopental has a firmly rooted place as an anesthetic induction agent because of its ability to promptly (within 15 to 30 seconds) and predictably induce a loss of consciousness. In recent years, however, propofol has become a much more popular induction agent because it is associated with less postanesthesia drowsiness. Thiopental's spectrum of CNS depressive effects ranges from sedation to dose-dependent unconsciousness. It is not useful in the maintenance of anesthesia, however, because it does not possess any intrinsic analgesic properties, and the sedative properties are prolonged with accumulation. On the contrary, it has been found to be antianalgesic or hyperalgesic, especially at low blood levels. Patients may exhibit a heightened response to pain at low doses (sedation) or at emergence.[25] In studies of somatic pain, the pain threshold to deep pain stimulus (tibial pressure) was decreased with thiopental.

Loss of consciousness occurs when the bolus of thiopental enters the cerebral circulation and crosses the blood-brain barrier. Factors that alter the onset of anesthesia are lipid solubility,

---

BOX 10-1

Key Points for Barbiturates Used in Anesthesia

- Use of thiopental has rapidly decreased in recent years, owing to the popularity of propofol.
- Barbiturates produce their action by binding to a specific site on the GABA$_A$ receptor.
- Barbiturates reduce cerebral blood flow (CBF), cerebral metabolic rate of oxygen consumption (CMRO$_2$), and intracranial pressure.
- Barbiturates are commonly used for their cerebral protective effects, but the benefits are controversial.
- Barbiturates exhibit a rapid onset and short duration but accumulate with repeat dosing. Their offset is due to redistribution.
- Barbiturates cause CNS and myocardial depression and vasodilation, leading to transient hypotension.
- Respiratory effects include transient respiratory depression or apnea, depending on dose. Bronchial tone is not directly affected; however, histamine release may occur.
- Porphyria is an absolute contraindication to the use of barbiturates.
- Standard induction doses of thiopental are 4 mg/kg, and methohexital 2 mg/kg.

---

protein binding, degree of ionization, plasma drug concentration, and cardiac output.

With regard to the evaluation of the effect of thiopental on the brain, the electroencephalograph (EEG) produces characteristic changes associated with dose-dependent stages of anesthesia. Stage 1 occurs as the patient loses consciousness and the EEG waveform displays a slight increase in amplitude and a slowing in frequency. Stage II EEG patterns show a marked slowing of the frequency of delta and theta waves and correspond to the loss of the corneal reflex and to amnesia. Stage III is marked by burst suppression, in which bursts of electrical activity are interspersed with periods of isoelectric waveforms. There is a lack of awareness to pain in stage III, and like stage II, stage III corresponds to surgical anesthesia. The isoelectric periods are more prolonged in stage IV, and a flat EEG is produced in stage V. Stages IV and V are induced for barbiturate coma.[26]

The complexity of the EEG and the different patterns produced by different agents have led investigators to seek alternative measures for evaluating pharmacodynamic information. The term *spectral-edge frequency* (see Chapter 19) refers to the frequency below which 95% of the EEG energy or power is located or the highest frequency at which significant EEG energy exists. The spectral-edge tracing for the thiopental effect on the brain would theoretically imitate the curve for the concentration of thiopental in the brain.[27]

Hudson and co-workers[28] used spectral-edge frequency and continuous infusions of thiopental to show that acute tolerance to thiopental does not exist as originally believed. The difference in study results was explained by thiopental concentration differences in the peripheral venous blood and brain circulation.[29] Energy production in the brain depends on glucose metabolism. In the presence of oxygen, glucose is metabolized through the glycolytic pathway, citric acid cycle, and oxidative phosphorylation to produce adenosine triphosphate (ATP) for the maintenance of cerebral energy requirements. Cerebral metabolism depends on ATP for ion transport across membranes, on molecular transport within neurons, and on cellular metabolism of carbohydrates, proteins, and lipids. Barbiturates have a pronounced effect on cerebral metabolism. A dose-dependent decrease occurs in cerebral metabolic rate of oxygen consumption (CMRO$_2$) and cerebral blood flow.[30] Under pentobarbital anesthesia, the CMRO$_2$ was decreased 30% when the reaction to painful stimuli was blocked.[31] In studies using large doses of thiopental in dogs, the CMRO$_2$ was decreased by 50% when the EEG was isoelectric. Any further increase in dosage was unable to alter the CMRO$_2$.[30] Pharmacologically decreasing cerebral function and causing a resultant decrease in CMRO$_2$ diminish the ATP requirements of the brain, thereby maintaining a supply-and-demand state that is favorable for electrophysiologic and cellular mechanics of brain cells. A parallel decrease in cerebral blood flow occurs with barbiturates. When CMRO$_2$ is decreased, cerebral blood flow and intracranial pressure are decreased. Barbiturates are used for brain protection before potential ischemic events. Collateral circulation to the ischemic areas is promoted by decreasing brain function and metabolic needs. The decreased cerebral blood flow in well-perfused tissue allows collateral circulation to the ischemic areas to increase, because the acidemic milieu favors vasodilation. Normal systemic blood pressure and cerebral perfusion pressure must be maintained.[32] The effects on cerebral metabolism and blood flow are useful in inducing anesthesia, especially in patients undergoing intraoperative somatosensory evoked potential (SSEP) recording.

Thiopental causes only minor alterations in SSEP; wave amplitude is maintained, allowing for SSEP monitoring.[33]

Thiopental administration decreases intraocular pressure.[34] Mechanisms thought to be responsible for this decrease include an increase in the outflow of aqueous humor, relaxation of extraocular muscles, and peripheral vasodilation.[35] Additionally, in doses used for anesthesia, thiopental has anticonvulsant properties and can abruptly stop seizures. CNS effects of the intravenous induction drugs are given in Table 10-5.

Cardiovascular Effects. Among the many factors that influence the cardiovascular effects seen with barbiturates are rate of administration and dose. Lower doses are associated with fewer cardiovascular effects.

The condition of the patient influences the patient's hemodynamic response. Patients who come to the operating room often experience high levels of psychologic and physiologic stress. Their drug profile may include use of antihypertensives, β-adrenergic–blocking agents, calcium channel–blocking agents, and antidepressants. These drugs alter the cardiovascular system compensatory mechanisms that respond to changes caused by induction agents.[36]

Barbiturates cause a dose-dependent depression of the cardiovascular system, resulting in a reduction in cardiac output.[37] One of the factors that decreases cardiac output is a decrease in the tone of systemic capacitance vessels that results in venous pooling.[38] With an increase in circulating volume in the periphery, decreases in venous return, left ventricular filling, and cardiac output occur. In addition, a direct negative inotropic effect occurs, with decreased myocardial contractility and sympathetic nervous system outflow that result in decreased sympathetic tone and vasodilation.[39] The systemic vascular resistance is either unchanged or mild vasodilation occurs. Baroreceptor reflexes are minimally depressed and respond to the change in cardiac output with an increase in heart rate. Barbiturates do not sensitize the myocardium to catecholamines and are not arrhythmogenic in the presence of normal oxygen and carbon dioxide balance.

Barbiturate induction agents should be used with caution or avoided in medically compromised patients. The hypovolemic patient may have a 69% reduction in cardiac output and a significant decrease in systemic blood pressure.[40] Patients unable to tolerate the tachycardia and associated increase in myocardial oxygen demand (e.g., those with coronary artery disease, pericardial tamponade, or congestive heart failure) should receive an alternative induction agent that has fewer cardiovascular depressant properties. The cardiac effects are compared in Table 10-6.

TABLE **10-5**	Central Nervous System Effects of Intravenous Anesthetics				
Agent	**CBF**	**CPP**	**CMRO$_2$**	**ICP**	**IOP**
Thiopental	↓↓	↓↓	↓↓	↓↓	↓
Methohexital	↓↓	↓↓	↓↓	↓↓	↓
Etomidate	↓↓	0	↓↓	↓↓	↓
Propofol	↓↓	↓↓	↓↓	↓↓	↓↓
Ketamine	↓↓	↑	↑	↑	↑
Midazolam	↑↓	↓	↓	↓	↓

CBF, *Cerebral blood flow;* CMRO$_2$, *cerebral metabolic rate of oxygen consumption;* CPP, *cerebral perfusion pressure;* ICP, *intracranial pressure;* IOP, *intraocular pressure.*
↓, *Decreases;* ↑, *increases;* 0, *no effect.*

TABLE **10-6**	Cardiac and Respiratory Effects of Intravenous Anesthetic Agents						
Drug Name	**Mean Arterial Pressure**	**Heart Rate**	**Cardiac Output**	**Venous Dilation**	**Systemic Vascular Resistance**	**Respiratory Depression**	**Bronchodilation**
Thiopental	−	+	−	++	−	−	0
Methohexital	−	++	−	+	−/+	−	0
Etomidate	0	0	0	0	0	0/−	0
Propofol	− −	−	−	++	− −	− −	0/+
Ketamine	++	++	+	0	+/−	0	++
Diazepam	0/−	−/+	0	+	−/0	0	0
Midazolam	0/−	−/+	0	+	−/0	0	0

−, *Mild decrease;* − −, *moderate decrease;* +, *mild increase;* ++, *moderate increase;* 0, *no effect.*

Respiratory Effects. Barbiturates can cause a dose-related, centrally mediated respiratory system depression. Dose, speed of injection, premedication, and concomitant use of other CNS depressants increase the degree of respiratory depression. The central origin of the respiratory effects has been determined from the inverse relationship between EEG depth and minute ventilation.[41] Peak respiratory depression occurs and dissipates rapidly, probably because of the pharmacokinetics of distribution and redistribution. Originally, thiopental was considered to be spasmogenic, and its use was thought to increase the risk for laryngospasm and bronchospasm. Actually, airway and laryngeal reflexes remain intact unless large doses are used. Stimulation of the airway at light levels of anesthesia would therefore explain the occurrence of laryngospasm. Comparative respiratory effects of the intravenous induction drugs are given in Table 10-6.

Considerations in the Elderly

Various studies have examined the effects of barbiturates on the elderly and the requirements of this population for a decreased dose for induction of anesthesia.[42] Using the EEG spectral-edge frequency effect versus time curve for each patient, investigators found that with increasing age, the dose of thiopental necessary to achieve anesthesia decreased 50% to 67%, the initial volume of distribution was decreased, and brain sensitivity was not a factor. A reevaluation by Stanski and Maitre showed that the initial volume of distribution was not age related and that EEG pharmacodynamics did not change with increased age. The rapid distribution phase is altered in the elderly population, resulting in a longer period of higher plasma concentrations of thiopental before redistribution. This longer time period allows an increased amount of thiopental to be available to the brain, often causing dramatic pharmacologic effects.[11]

Other Considerations

Thiobarbiturates cause a dose-dependent histamine release. Anaphylactic and anaphylactoid reactions have been reported.[43] Extravascular injection of thiopental in subcutaneous tissue can cause chemical irritation ranging from tenderness to venospasm and tissue necrosis.[25,44]

Intraarterial injection of thiopental causes immediate arteriospasm, vasoconstriction, and intense pain along the course of the artery. Blanching of the arms, hand, and fingers occurs and may result in gangrene if not immediately treated. Interventions include the following: (1) dilution of drug by injection of normal saline; (2) treatment of vasospasm with papaverine 40 to 80 mcg, procaine 1% 10 mL, or lidocaine injection into the artery; (3) administration of stellate ganglion or brachial plexus block to increase circulation; (4) heparinization (if not contraindicated); and (5) local infiltration of the area with phentolamine or topical application of nitroglycerin. Precautions when using the barbiturates are given in Box 10-2.

All barbiturates are able to rapidly cross the placenta into the fetal circulation. Rapid redistribution of thiopental in the mother during the time between dosing and delivery may account for the difference in the level of consciousness between the neonate and the mother.[45] Higher doses (8 mg/kg) were associated with higher maternal and fetal blood levels.[46]

Contraindications. Absolute contraindications to thiopental include a history of allergic reaction to barbiturates and acute intermittent porphyria or variegate porphyria. Acute exacerbations of this phenomenon do not occur with every exposure to a drug, but when they do occur, the mortality rate is as high as 10%. All symptoms are related to neurologic disturbances,

---

BOX 10-2

Precautions for Use of Intravenous Barbiturates

- Reduce dose and rate of injection in cardiovascularly compromised and hypovolemic patients.
- Solution has high pH (>10).
  - Avoid eye splash.
  - Extravascular injection is painful and can cause tissue damage.
  - Intraarterial thiopental causes arterial spasm thrombosis and distal limb ischemia:
    - Stop the injection but leave the needle in the artery.
    - Arterial injection of lidocaine (10 mL of 1%) provides analgesia and vasodilation.
    - A brachial plexus block has the same action for a more prolonged period.
    - Papaverine (70-80 mg in 20 mL of saline) is an effective vasodilator.
    - Topical nitroglycerin is also effective.
    - Anticoagulate with a heparin.
  - Methohexital does not result in thrombosis although it may be painful.
- Porphyria is an absolute contraindication to the use of barbiturates.

Modified from Bovill JG, Howie MB, eds: Clinical Pharmacology for Anaesthetists. *London: Saunders; 1999.*

---

especially the autonomic nervous system, and may include abdominal pain, nausea and vomiting, hypertension, tachycardia, seizures, and mood disturbances.[17] Other induction agents (ketamine and propofol) are available for use in affected patients.

NONBARBITURATE INTRAVENOUS ANESTHETICS

Etomidate

Etomidate (1-[1-phenylethyl]-1H-imidazole-5-carboxylic acid ethyl ester) is an intravenous induction agent whose CNS effects result in hypnosis. No intrinsic analgesic properties are associated with the use of this drug.[47] Etomidate has a cardiovascular stability and a wider margin of safety that appeared to challenge the long-standing role of thiopental as the induction agent of choice in intravenous anesthesia. Side effects such as pain on injection, myoclonia, and adrenocortical suppression, however, have limited wider acceptance of the drug. Etomidate is a carboxylated imidazole derivative that was synthesized in 1965 and introduced to European anesthesia practice in 1972.[48] Etomidate has two isomers, but the (+) isomer is the only one with hypnotic properties.[40] (See Figure 10-2 for the chemical structure of etomidate.)

Etomidate is currently supplied as a 2-mg/mL preparation; each milliliter contains 35% propylene glycol as a solvent and has a pH of 8.1. This formulation has been changed over the years in an effort to decrease the incidence of pain on injection and spontaneous muscle movements. It is also supplied as a lipid emulsion, Etomidate-Lipuro.[49] Previously used preparations included polyethylene glycol, aqueous ethanol, Cremophor EL, and an aqueous solution.[50]

Pharmacokinetics

Etomidate is rapidly metabolized in the liver by hepatic microsomal enzymes and plasma esterases. Ester hydrolysis is the primary mode of metabolism in the liver and plasma. Etomidate is hydrolyzed to form inactive carboxylic acid metabolites. Approximately 10% of the administered dose can be recovered in bile, 13% can be recovered in feces, and the remainder is eliminated by the kidney.[51]

The rapid distribution half-life of etomidate accounts for its extremely short duration of action (see Table 10-4). The drug is lipid soluble and has a volume of distribution that is several times greater than its body weight. Shortly after intravenous injection (within 1 minute), the brain concentration rises rapidly because of the drug's lipid solubility, and extensive redistribution to organs and tissues occurs.

The total body clearance of etomidate is rapid—five times greater than that of thiopental. The hepatic extraction ratio is 67%. The rapid distribution and clearance of etomidate make it especially useful in repeated doses and continuous infusions. Studies examining dose-response relationships have found a lack of accumulation with this compound.[47]

Awakening occurs 7 to 14 minutes after bolus administration. This attribute, combined with the cardiovascular stability of the drug, has led to extensive use of etomidate as a hypnotic-sedative infusion agent in critical care units. Etomidate is 76% protein bound, mostly to albumin. As with other intravenous anesthetics, variations in the amount of available plasma protein alter the amount of free drug available to exert pharmacologic actions. Disease states that produce alterations in plasma protein content should alert the anesthetist to decrease the administered dose.

The mechanism of action of etomidate involves GABA modulation. GABA antagonists can antagonize the effects of etomidate.[4] In clinical investigations of 2500 cases, Doenicke and co-workers[52] confirmed that no histamine is released by etomidate (see Figure 10-5).

Pharmacodynamics

Central Nervous System Effects. Etomidate produces a dose-dependent CNS depression within one arm-brain circulation. Its duration of action is also dose dependent,[47] with awakening occurring 5 to 10 minutes after a 0.2- to 0.4-mg/kg dose. The drug is devoid of analgesic properties because it is unable to block afferent pain stimulus to the thalamus.

Cerebral blood flow and cerebral metabolic rate of oxygen consumption are both decreased by etomidate.[53,54] In a study of fully alert patients without neurologic deficit or impaired consciousness, an etomidate induction was followed by an infusion of 2 to 3 mg/min. Cerebral blood flow decreased 34%, and cerebral metabolism was also reduced (mean decrease of 45%). Decreased oxygen consumption and the associated decrease in carbon dioxide production can cause cerebrovascular vasoconstriction, decreased cerebral blood flow, and decreased intracranial pressure. Also noted during this trial was the maintenance of cerebral blood vessel responsiveness to changes in carbon dioxide levels.[53]

In a study of patients with intracranial pathology, etomidate (0.2 mg/kg given intravenously) was shown to decrease intracranial pressure while maintaining cerebral perfusion pressure. Because of the cardiovascular stability of this drug, mean arterial pressure did not decrease below cerebral autoregulation values at which cerebral blood flow would become pressure dependent. Cerebral perfusion pressure was maintained adequately in all study subjects.[54]

The electroencephalographic changes that follow administration of etomidate are similar to those that follow administration of other intravenous induction anesthetics. When compared with thiopental, a lack of beta-wave activity was present during induction, along with a longer duration of stages III and IV.[55]

One negative characteristic of etomidate is its excitatory phenomenon of muscle movements and tremors.[55,56] Referred to as *myoclonia*, this phenomenon is defined as sudden, generalized, asynchronous muscle contractions.[57] Myoclonia can affect many muscle groups or a single muscle. The movements can be so severe that they resemble, and are often mistaken for, seizures. In EEG patterns monitored during etomidate anesthesia, no specific EEG disturbances occurred during or after myoclonic episodes.[55] The origin of these muscle movements is thought to be related to uneven drug distribution into the brainstem or deep cerebral structures and not to CNS stimulation.[33,55] Etomidate has been associated with epileptic seizures.[58] The incidence of myoclonia ranges between 10% and 60% and varies with the type and the amount of premedication given. Investigators associated the 35% incidence of myoclonic movement with painful stimuli (e.g., drug injection, mandibular lifting). Horrigan and colleagues[56] reported that premedication with fentanyl (100 mg) given intravenously 2 minutes before induction did not significantly decrease motor activity. However, other studies reported better outcomes with fentanyl and diazepam given before induction.[52,59] Etomidate is shown to decrease intraocular pressure. The use of etomidate in sensory evoked potential (SSEP) recording is avoided because the drug increases wave amplitudes recorded on the scalp. This alteration makes assessing neurologic function with SSEP difficult.[36]

Cardiovascular Effects. A major advantage of etomidate over propofol or thiopental is the hemodynamic stability of etomidate. Originally documented in animal studies,[60,61] these findings were later confirmed in humans. In studies of subjects who did not have cardiac disease but had compensated heart disease, changes in heart rate, pulmonary artery pressure, cardiac index, systemic vascular resistance, and arterial blood were not significant.[62] In one study of high-risk patients with significant cardiac disease, hemodynamic stability was maintained with induction doses of 0.3 mg/kg. Also, minimal changes in heart rate, blood pressure, central venous pressure, and intrapulmonary shunting have been demonstrated after etomidate administration.[63] Patients with aortic and mitral valve disease, however, are noted to have significant decreases in systemic blood pressure (17% to 19%), pulmonary artery pressure (11%), and pulmonary capillary wedge pressure (17%).[64] Slight decreases in blood pressure are thought to be caused by decreases in systemic vascular resistance. Myocardial oxygen supply and demand are kept constant by a balance of decreased myocardial blood flow and decreased oxygen consumption.[65] No reports have been made of cardiac dysrhythmias associated with etomidate administration. Both renal and hepatic blood flow are maintained by the stability of cardiac output (see Table 10-6). In summary, at equivalent anesthetic doses, propofol depresses cardiorespiratory function to the greatest degree, followed by thiopental; etomidate depresses it the least.

Respiratory Effects. Etomidate affects the respiratory system in a dose-dependent manner. Minute volume decreases, but respiratory rate increases. The respiratory depression seen with propofol or thiopental use is significantly greater than that seen with etomidate.[65] The ventilatory response to carbon dioxide is decreased, and etomidate administration may cause brief periods of apnea followed by a period of hyperventilation (see Table 10-6).[66]

Adrenocortical Effects. The pharmacokinetics of etomidate (rapid onset, short duration, lack of cumulative response, hemodynamic stability, lack of histamine release, and hypnosis) made it the agent of choice for sedation in critically ill patients. After 10 years of use in Europe, a study reported an increased mortality rate in critically ill patients who received etomidate infusions. This phenomenon was attributed to adrenocortical hypofunction, demonstrated by decreased levels of plasma cortisol.[67] After infusions of etomidate were discontinued, this decrease in adrenal hormone level lasted for 4 days.[68]

Multiple studies have shown adrenal hormone levels to be decreased for 5 to 8 hours after infusion or an induction dose (0.4 mg/kg).[68-74] These effects are caused by a reversible dose-dependent inhibition of adrenocortical enzymes. These enzymes are the cytochrome P-450–dependent mitochondrial enzymes and 11β-hydroxylase. To a lesser degree, 17α-hydroxylase is also affected. The result yields an increase in cortisol precursors but a decrease in cortisol, aldosterone, and corticosterone levels. This enzyme inhibition results in decreased ascorbic acid synthesis, which is necessary for steroid production.[75] These effects are caused by a reversible dose-dependent inhibition of the adrenalocortical enzyme 11β-hydroxylase.

The adrenocortical hypofunction that results from the administration of etomidate administered for the induction of anesthesia (Figure 10-6) is reversible.

Other Effects. Etomidate has been formulated in various solvents in an effort to decrease pain on injection and myoclonia. When etomidate was in a saline base, the incidence of burning and pain was 33% to 80%. After etomidate was reformulated with propylene glycol, no significant difference existed in painful

sensations between thiopental and etomidate (18% for both agents).[56] The effects of this reformulation on the incidence of myoclonia, however, have been negligible. Different studies have produced conflicting reports on patients' perception of pain on injection. Some of the variables identified as contributing to pain on injection include site and speed of injection, size of vessel used, and premedication (opioids, benzodiazepines, and lidocaine). One study showed that the use of propylene glycol slightly increased thrombophlebitis. The lipid emulsion formulation produces less pain on injection.[49] Unlike thiopental, no vascular injury occurs after intraarterial injection of etomidate. Nausea and vomiting are more common with etomidate (30% to 40%) than with thiopental (19% to 20%).[76,77] Opioids also increase the susceptibility to nausea and vomiting. Key points of etomidate pharmacology are given in Box 10-3.

Ketamine

In the search for the ideal induction agent, phencyclidine and its congeners were introduced into clinical practice. However, they were deemed unacceptable because they caused serious psychic disturbances, including hallucinations and delirium.[78,79] These agents produced a dissociative state of anesthesia, a concept described by Corssen and Domino,[80] in which the patient is in a catatonic state, feels separated from the environment, and has analgesia and amnesia. Continued research into the congeners of phencyclidine produced ketamine (Ketaject, Ketalar), which was found to be an acceptable drug for anesthesia. Ketamine produced profound analgesia and less severe psychic reactions when it was first introduced in clinical studies.[81]

The structural formula for ketamine is given in Figure 10-2. The chemical structure of ketamine is 2-(O-chlorophenyl)-2-(methylamino)cyclohexanone. It has a pK_a of 7.5, is partially water soluble, and is slightly acidic (pH 3.5 to 5.5). Pharmacologic preparations contain a preservative, Phemerol (benzethonium chloride), at a ratio of 1:10,000.

ADRENOCORTICOID SUPPRESSION BY ETOMIDATE

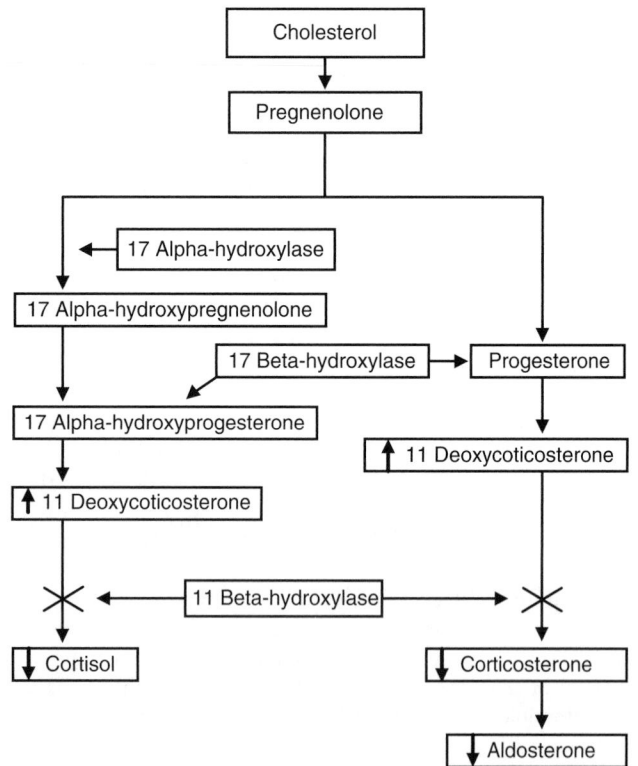

FIGURE **10-6** Adrenocorticoid suppression by etomidate. Etomidate produces prolonged inhibition of 11β-hydroxylase, which leads to reductions in cortisol and aldosterone.

BOX **10-3**

Key Points for Etomidate

- Etomidate is used in compromised patients when the use of the other intravenous anesthetics may be problematic.
- The major advantage of etomidate is minimal cardiorespiratory depression.
- Etomidate reduces intracranial pressure, cerebral blood flow, and $CMRO_2$.
- The mechanism of action of etomidate appears to be GABA-mimetic.
- Involuntary movements or myoclonia during onset is common.
- Etomidate frequently causes burning on injection.
- Etomidate inhibits the enzyme 11β-hydroxylase, which is essential in the production of both corticosteroids and mineralocorticoids. Clinically significant reductions in steroid production may occur with prolonged infusions.
- Etomidate increases postoperative nausea and vomiting.
- The induction dose is 0.2-0.3 mg/kg.

$CMRO_2$, *Cerebral metabolic rate of oxygen consumption.*

Chemical Structure

Ketamine is an optically active drug with a chiral center that exists as two optical isomers. A racemic mixture is available for use at this time, although investigators have looked at the different pharmacologic properties of the two stereoisomers. In studies of the S(+) isomer, the R(−) isomer, and the racemic mixture, many pharmacologic differences were found. The S(+) isomer was found to have less spontaneous motor activity; patients were calm and cooperative in the recovery room and had fewer complaints of pain and much lower levels of postoperative anxiety than with either the R(−) isomer or the racemic mixture. The R(−) isomer caused more instances of combativeness and delirium on emergence from anesthesia.[82]

Mechanisms of Action

The primary site of the analgesic action of ketamine is the thalamoneocortical system. Ketamine causes antagonism at N-methyl-D-aspartate amino acid (NMDA) receptors in the brain, resulting in a selective depressant effect on the medial thalamic nuclei that is responsible for blocking afferent signals of pain perception to the thalamus and cortex. The NMDA receptor is a ligand-gated ion channel where anions Ca^{2+} and Na^+ are voltage dependent. L-glutamate, an amino acid, is probably the most important excitatory neurotransmitter in the CNS. At the NMDA receptor, it causes the opening of the ion channel. A rapid influx of Na^+, Ca^{2+}, and K^+ results in the depolarization of the normally negative postsynaptic membrane that initiates the action potential. Ketamine is a noncompetitive antagonist at this receptor.[83,84] Afferent impulses are transmitted to cortical regions of the brain but are not interpreted, so responses to visual, auditory, and pain stimuli are inappropriate.[81] Although cortical association areas are depressed, the limbic system, which is thought to cause excitatory behavior, is simultaneously activated. The NMDA receptor is shown and described in Figure 10-7.

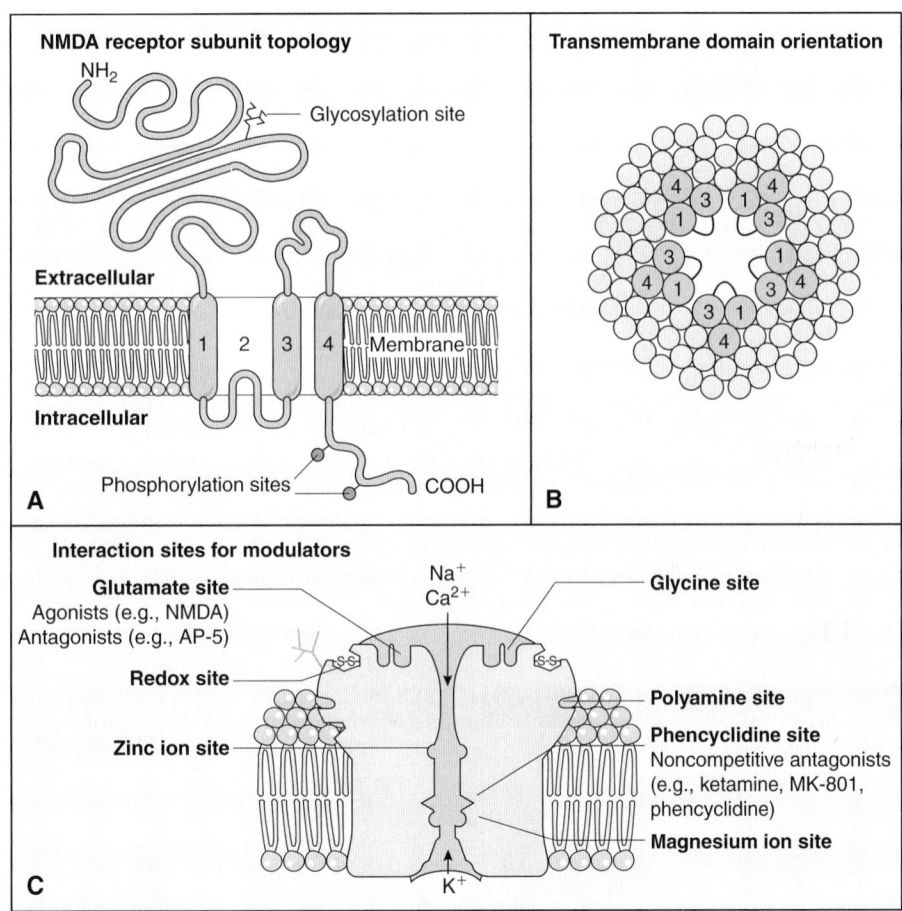

FIGURE **10-7** The N-methyl-D-aspartate amino acid (NMDA) receptor. **A,** The NMDA NRI receptor has three transmembrane segments and a fourth hydrophobic segment (*designated 2*) that loops into the membrane without traversing it. Mutation studies suggest that this loop is the putative channel-lining segment and that blockade by dizocilpine (MK-801), phencyclidine, and ketamine occurs through binding to a site that overlaps the Mg^{2+} site in the pore. The C-terminal domain undergoes phosphorylation, which regulates channel activity and mediates interactions with intracellular anchoring proteins. **B,** Transmembrane hydrophobic segments interact to form a central ion-conducting pore lined by the second hydrophobic segments. The stoichiometry of the hetero-oligomer is not known but may be four or five (as shown), by analogy with the homologous nicotinic cholinergic receptor. **C,** The NMDA receptor gates a cation channel that is permeable to Na^+, Ca^{2+}, and K^+ and is gated by Mg^{2+} in a voltage-dependent fashion. Agonists (glutamate, NMDA) and the coagonist glycine, required for full activation, bind to the extracellular domain. (*From Hemmings HC, Hopkins PM, eds.* Foundations of Anesthesia Basic and Clinical Sciences. *St Louis: Mosby; 2006.*)

The analgesia produced by ketamine has a spinal cord component. By injecting bradykinin intraarterially as a noxious stimuli, Nagasaka and co-workers[85] were able to demonstrate that ketamine blocked the stimulated excitatory activity of wide-dynamic-range neurons in the dorsal horn, thereby preventing transmission of noxious stimuli to the brain. Ketamine may also act as an agonist at opiate receptors.[86]

Neurotransmitter systems have been implicated in ketamine's mechanism of action. The use of acetylcholine was reduced in the caudate nucleus and hippocampus in rats during ketamine anesthesia, a finding that indicates that ketamine may induce electrophysiologic changes that reduce acetylcholine turnover. Physostigmine has been shown to reverse the sedative effect of ketamine but not its analgesic effect.[87]

Metabolism

Hepatic microsomal enzyme systems are responsible for the biotransformation of ketamine. The primary pathway for ketamine metabolism by the cytochrome P-450 system is demethylation to form the metabolite I, norketamine. Hydroxylation of norketamine occurs at one of two positions in the cyclohexone ring to form hydronorketamine metabolites I, II, and III. These metabolites form a glucuronide derivation via conjugation to produce a more water-soluble compound that is eliminated primarily via renal excretion. Thermal dehydration forms dehydroxynorketamine, a cyclohexene derivative (metabolite II).[40,88]

The pharmacologic activity of the metabolite norketamine is approximately 20% to 30% of ketamine's activity. The activity of the other metabolites is unknown.[89]

Pharmacokinetics

The distribution kinetics of ketamine follows a two-compartment model. Ketamine is able to cross the blood-brain barrier quickly to achieve rapid pharmacologic effect.[90] Peak plasma concentrations are reached within 5 minutes of intravenous injection, and termination of action occurs within 10 to 15 minutes. Ketamine is less protein bound than thiopental (12%), so more drug is immediately available for distribution to the CNS. Brain concentrations decrease rapidly as ketamine is redistributed from the central compartment to peripheral tissue compartments. Redistribution to low-blood-flow tissue compartments accounts

---

BOX 10-4

Recommendation Doses of Ketamine

Premedication
- A benzodiazepine such as midazolam is administered if patient status allows. An antisialagogue should be given to decrease secretions.

Induction of Anesthesia
- Ketamine 2-4 mg/kg IV, or 4-6 mg/kg IM

Maintenance of Anesthesia
- Ketamine 15-45 mcg/kg/min (1-3 mg/min) by continuous IV infusion

Sedation and Analgesia
- Ketamine 0.2-0.8 mg/kg IV (over 2-3 min) followed by a continuous ketamine infusion (5-120 mcg/kg/min) 10-20 mg may produce preemptive analgesia.

IM, *Intramuscular*; IV, *intravenous*.

---

for the termination of drug effect and return to consciousness. The slow elimination half-life of the drug is the result of hepatic metabolism and excretion. A large amount of ketamine remains in peripheral tissues as active drug and may be responsible for prolonged or cumulative effects.[91] Hepatic extraction of ketamine is high because the mean total body clearance is approximately the same as the hepatic blood flow.[92] Ketamine elimination is therefore dependent on hepatic blood flow. Pharmacokinetic values remain consistent with analgesic and anesthetic doses of ketamine, which implies that distribution of ketamine is not dose dependent (see Table 10-4).

Intramuscular Route. Given intramuscularly, ketamine reaches peak plasma concentrations within 22 minutes.[93] Dosages range from 4 to 6 mg/kg[83] to 5 to 10 mg/kg. The onset of anesthetic effects is seen within 2 to 3 minutes. Analgesic doses of ketamine (0.44 mg/kg) can be used for painful procedures without causing loss of consciousness and psychic disturbances.[40] After intramuscular administration, approximately 93% of the drug is bioavailable.[94] A consideration with the intramuscular route is the delayed onset of anesthesia. Box 10-4 gives complete dosing information.

Placental Transfer. Ketamine is highly lipid soluble and readily crosses the placenta into fetal tissue. When standard induction doses of 2 to 2.5 mg/kg were given to mothers, neonates were depressed on delivery.[95] Decreasing this dose to 0.2 to 1 mg/kg spared the newborn this CNS depression because of the rapid redistribution of the drug in the mother and the shunting of the drug past the fetal circulation.

Pharmacodynamics

Central Nervous System Effects. Ketamine produces a dissociative state of anesthesia, so called because the patient appears to be dissociated from the environment. The onset of anesthesia is slower than with propofol or thiopental and may make judgments regarding the onset of sleep and analgesia difficult. In the dissociative state, as originally described by Corssen,[40] the patient is cataleptic: the eyes remain open, the pupils are reactive to light, the corneal reflexes are intact, and horizontal nystagmus is present. Lacrimation and eye blinking continue, and salivary gland secretions are increased. Airway reflexes also remain intact (e.g., laryngeal reflex, pharyngeal reflex, coughing, sneezing, and swallowing). Skeletal muscle tone is increased, and occasional purposeless movements occur that are unrelated to painful stimuli.

Movement in response to painful stimuli is often required for judgments of adequate anesthesia. After administration of a single dose, full reorientation to person, place, and time takes place in 15 to 30 minutes, though wide variability in durations have been noted.[96] Ketamine is a profound analgesic that has a preference for skin, bones, and joints. Analgesia occurs with subdissociative doses[92] of ketamine, and this agent may be used for painful procedures without inducing a loss of consciousness. Analgesia is present after the anesthetic effects are terminated and correlates well with plasma levels of ketamine. Anesthetic levels are present with plasma levels of 640 to 1000 µg/mL, and analgesic levels are present with plasma ketamine concentrations of 100 to 150 µg/mL.[88]

Cerebral blood flow is increased 60% to 80% by ketamine and returns to normal within 20 to 30 minutes of administration. This increase in blood flow is attributed to the excitatory effects of ketamine; these effects increase the cerebral metabolic rate of oxygen consumption, which in turn increases central blood flow and cerebrospinal fluid pressure. This indirect effect of ketamine can be attenuated with hyperventilation; this finding indicates that the response of cerebral vessels to carbon dioxide is left intact with ketamine anesthesia.

On loss of consciousness and onset of analgesia, ketamine induces a transition from alpha to theta waves (slow waves with moderate to high amplitude) on the EEG. Alpha waves do not reappear until after consciousness returns and analgesia is lost.[81]

Ketamine anesthesia emergence is associated with psychic disturbances immediately on return of consciousness.[97] These emergence reactions are the result of visual, auditory, proprioceptive, and confusional illusions.[98] Descriptions of this phenomenon include vivid illusions, sensations of drunkenness, delirium, restlessness, altered states of consciousness, extracorporeal sensations, and combativeness.[82,98] The onset occurs with the first verbal contact and usually resolves with full return of orientation to person, place, and time.[37] The incidence of emergence reactions is approximately 12%.[99] Recurrent dreams have been reported to occur weeks after a ketamine anesthetic.[100] The benzodiazepines diazepam and midazolam were found to significantly decrease the incidence of these reactions. There has been a recent resurgence in the use of subanesthetic doses of ketamine for the treatment of acute and chronic pain. Low doses of ketamine are being used for sedation, postoperative pain relief, analgesia during regional or local anesthesia, and opioid-sparing effect.[99]

Cardiovascular Effects. Ketamine, unlike other intravenous anesthetics, acts as a circulatory stimulant, producing increases in systemic blood pressure, heart rate, cardiac output, and central venous pressure.[80,82,97] Systemic vascular resistance responded differently among patients undergoing cardiac catheterization and angiography (±25%), possibly because of patient variability in autonomic tone and disease states. Other studies have failed to show significant effects in systemic vascular resistance but have found evidence of an increase in pulmonary vascular resistance (42%), pulmonary artery pressure (47%), and right ventricular stroke work. These values persisted throughout the 12-minute measurement period, although they were somewhat decreased (pulmonary vascular resistance 42% at 3 to 5 minutes and 25% at 12 minutes; mean pulmonary arterial pressure 47% at 3 to 5 minutes and 23% at 12 minutes). In patients with congenital heart disease and increased pulmonary pressure and resistance, ketamine administration did not adversely affect myocardial function (ejection fractions remained constant).[101]

Ketamine administration causes an increase in myocardial contractility, thereby affecting the myocardial oxygen balance. This increase in myocardial oxygen consumption has not been shown to cause inadequate myocardial perfusion, because a concomitant rise in coronary artery perfusion occurs that is produced by a decrease in coronary artery vasodilation.[101]

Ketamine-induced activation of the sympathetic nervous system that results in endogenous catecholamine release is believed to be the mechanism for the cardiostimulatory properties experienced after administration of the drug. Injection of ketamine directly into the CNS via the carotid artery causes an immediate increase in blood pressure, heart rate, and cardiac output.[102] The positive inotropic effect of ketamine in vitro results from an inhibition of neuronal and extraneuronal uptake of norepinephrine. This norepinephrine then activates β-adrenergic receptors.[103] Studies have indicated that the negative inotropic effects of ketamine are the result of a decrease in the available calcium ions (Ca^{2+}) intracellularly, caused by an interference with Ca^{2+} delivery mechanisms (net transsarcolemmal Ca^{2+} influx).[104] When the positive inotropic effects of ketamine are blocked, the negative inotropic effects predominate

and may result in decreased blood pressure and cardiac output. This phenomenon may be seen clinically in the critically ill patient who, as a result of protracted illness, has decreased available catecholamine stores and limited ability to compensate. With an intact sympathetic nervous system, the positive inotropic effects dominate and counteract the negative inotropic effects. By decreasing sympathetic responses, some inhalation anesthetics are able to block the cardiovascular effects of ketamine to produce a decrease in systemic blood pressure and cardiac output.[105] The cardiovascular stimulation produced by ketamine may be deliberately decreased by the prior administration of benzodiazepines in patients in whom that response should be avoided.[97]

Ketamine has been used successfully in patients who are hemodynamically compromised because of shock, trauma, debilitation, or hypovolemia.

Changes in systemic blood pressure are dose related; systolic and diastolic blood pressures increase when larger doses of ketamine are administered (0.5 to 2.0 mg/kg). However, the heart rate response to different dosages reaches a plateau, with no significant change in rate occurring between doses of 0.5 and 2 mg/kg.

Ketamine has been used successfully for both pediatric and adult cardiac surgery patients with congenital and acquired disease processes.[101,106] The cardiac and respiratory actions of ketamine are summarized in Table 10-6.

Respiratory Effects. The effects of ketamine on the respiratory system are minor and of short duration. Respiratory depression, which is reflected in a decrease in tidal volume over respiratory rate, begins 2 to 3 minutes after parenteral administration.[81]

Significant respiratory depression, demonstrated by decreased oxygen constant and increased partial pressure of arterial carbon dioxide, follows rapid bolus intravenous injection and may last 5 to 10 minutes. The addition of other CNS depressants augments the respiratory depression produced by ketamine. With slow administration or infusion methods, arterial blood gases remain within normal limits, and the central response to carbon dioxide is maintained.[82]

Ketamine increases pulmonary compliance and decreases pulmonary resistance in patients with bronchospastic disease. In case reports, the effects of ketamine on resolving bronchospasm coincide with peak blood levels toward the end of the drug's distribution half-life, with recurrence of bronchospasm. Increased circulation catecholamine levels stimulated by ketamine, along with bronchial smooth muscle relaxation and vagolytic actions, are thought to be the reason for the bronchodilating effects of the drug. Tracheal, bronchial, and salivary muscle gland secretions are increased with ketamine, requiring the use of an antisialagogue. The muscle tone of the tongue and jaw is retained, and protective pharyngeal and laryngeal reflexes are left intact. Coughing, gagging, and swallowing remain in response to airway stimulation, although silent pulmonary aspiration has occurred in some patients.[83] (See Table 10-6.)

Intraocular Effects. Research into the effects of ketamine administration on intraocular pressure has yielded varied results. Some investigators have reported marked increases in intraocular pressure with ketamine administration, whereas others have concluded that no change in intraocular pressure occurs.[107] Measurement techniques and adjunctive anesthetics may have affected these results. Ketamine causes nystagmus, increased muscle tone, and muscle spasms, which may not be appropriate for ophthalmic procedures.[108] The common clinical effects of ketamine are given in Box 10-5.

BOX 10-5

Primary Clinical Characteristics and Effects of Ketamine

- Phencyclidine derivative
- Causes unconsciousness, amnesia referred to as *dissociative anesthesia*
- Increases cerebral metabolic rate, cerebral blood flow, intracranial pressure
- Causes nystagmus, increased intraocular pressure
- Moderate analgesic
- Increases blood pressure and pulse
- Potent bronchodilator
- Maintains respirations and airway reflexes (Note: A period of initial apnea may occur, especially with high doses and rapid administration.)
- Increases salivation and respiratory secretions
- Increases muscle tone
- Increases postoperative nausea and vomiting
- Associated with emergence delirium, nightmares, and hallucinations
- Requires caution in patients with hypertension, angina, congestive heart failure, increased intracranial pressure, increased intraocular pressure, psychiatric disease, airway problems

---

BOX 10-6

Clinical Uses of Ketamine

Induction of Anesthesia in High-Risk Patients
- Shock or cardiovascular instability
- Severe dehydration
- Bronchospasm
- Severe anemia
- One-lung anesthesia

Obstetric Patients
Induction of General Anesthesia
- Severe hypovolemia
- Acute hemorrhage
- Acute bronchospasm

Low Dose for Analgesia
- To supplement regional anesthetic techniques at the time of delivery or during the postpartum period

Adjunct to Local and Regional Anesthetic Techniques
- For sedation and analgesia during performance of nerve block procedures
- To supplement an inadequate block

Outpatient Surgery
- For brief diagnostic and therapeutic procedures
- To supplement local and regional block techniques

Use Outside the Operating Room
- In burn units (e.g., débridement, dressing changes)
- In emergency rooms (e.g., closed reduction)
- In intensive care units (e.g., sedation, painful procedures)
- In recovery rooms (e.g., postoperative sedation and analgesia)
- During x-ray examinations

Modified from Bowdle TA et al, eds: The Pharmacological Basis of Anesthesiology. *New York: Churchill Livingstone; 1994.*

Obstetric Use

Ketamine can be used in obstetrics for analgesia or anesthesia. As an induction agent, ketamine in doses of 0.5 to 1 mg/kg produces rapid anesthesia without compromising uterine tone, uterine blood flow, or neonatal status at delivery. For analgesia, 0.25 mg/kg of ketamine provides pain-related relief, airway stability, and a sustained maternal blood pressure and uninhibited uterine contractions. Use of doses reserved for surgical procedures (2 to 2.2 mg/kg) results, however, in a depressed neonate on delivery.[109,110] Clinical uses of ketamine are given in Box 10-6. Recommendations for using ketamine as a sedative, analgesic, or anesthetic during the postoperative period are listed in Box 10-4. Key points of ketamine pharmacology are given in Box 10-7.

Propofol
Chemical Structure

Propofol is a 2,6-diisopropyl phenol (see Figure 10-2). It is prepared in a milky-white emulsion of 10% soybean oil, 2.25% glycerol, and 1.2% purified egg lecithin. This unique vehicle has been reported to be especially favorable to bacterial contamination. The pH of Diprivan (propofol) is 7 to 8.5, and the pK_a is 11. The pH of the generic form of propofol is 4.5 to 6.4, and the pK_a is 11. Diprivan contains 0.005% disodium edetate, and the generic propofol contains 0.025% sodium metabisulfite to retard the growth of organisms. These preservatives may be effective in decreasing the risk of bacterial contamination. However, these formulations may still support bacterial growth. It is recommended that aseptic conditions be maintained and disinfection of the vial with 70% isopropyl alcohol be employed when syringes are prepared for use. Opened vials and syringes should be discarded if they are not used within 6 hours of preparation.[111]

New generic formulations are available with different preservatives and varying clinical considerations. An aqueous prodrug is also in phase 3 clinical trials.[112] The pharmaceutical preparations are given in Table 10-2.

Pharmacokinetics

Propofol exhibits a generally favorable kinetic profile, which is one of its main clinical benefits in comparison with other induction drugs.[113,114] (See Table 10-4.)

Rapid redistribution from the central to the peripheral compartments produces a quick initial decline in blood levels. This effect leads to a rapid reawakening after sedative and anesthetic doses. The characteristic of propofol that differentiates it from thiopental is its rapid metabolic clearance, which actually exceeds hepatic blood flow.[114] It was concluded by Veroli and colleagues[115] that extrahepatic routes of metabolism exist, because metabolites of propofol were found in the urine during the anhepatic phase of a liver transplantation. Residual drug undergoes hepatic elimination, and effects can be prolonged in patients with liver disease. The drug's kinetics are also influenced by age, with the elderly requiring lower doses.[116] Children require higher doses because they have an increased volume of distribution based on body weight. Their rate of clearance is also higher.[117] Accumulation can occur with prolonged infusion because of extensive tissue saturation.[118]

Mechanism of Action

Like other intravenous induction agents, propofol appears to exert its effect via an interaction with the inhibitory neurotransmitter GABA and the $GABA_A$ glycoprotein receptor complex.[119] Recent studies are also implicating the excitatory amino acid neurotransmitter glutamate and NMDA receptors in the anesthetic action of propofol but to a lesser extent. Other actions include a rapid, pleasant recovery and antiemetic and antipruritic effects.[120]

Other Pharmacologic Actions. It is recognized that propofol possesses mild antiemetic effects that are most prominent when given by continuous infusion.[121,122]

Patients experience varying degrees of pain on injection of propofol.[123] Different formulations have not changed this spontaneous complaint, and various techniques of administration have been used to minimize this problem. The addition of

---

BOX **10-7**

Key Points for Ketamine Anesthesia

- Site of action of ketamine appears to be the NMDA receptor, where it inhibits glutamate as a noncompetitive antagonist. Other actions are likely.
- Ketamine produces an anesthetic state referred to as *dissociative anesthesia*.
- Onset of effect is relatively slow compared to other induction drugs (2-5 min).
- Ketamine increases postoperative nausea and vomiting.
- Ketamine produces a rise in cerebral perfusion pressure by increased sympathetic outflow, which causes a rise in mean arterial pressure.
- Ketamine is a bronchodilator, preserves airway reflexes, and increases secretions.
- Emergence phenomena—including vivid dreams, floating sensations, and delirium—can occur after ketamine administration. They are more common in adults than children and are reduced by benzodiazepine or other sedative administration.
- Ketamine is an indirect sympathomimetic, releasing catecholamines. This action accounts for the cardiac stimulation and bronchodilation

NMDA, *N-methyl-D-aspartate*.

---

lidocaine to the emulsion has been used with good results. Lidocaine (1% or 2%) 0.1 or 0.2 mg/kg reduces the pain on injection.[124,125] A study using chilled propofol failed to reduce the incidence of pain.[124] The lidocaine may also be given before the administration of propofol. The use of larger veins for intravenous access in the antecubital fossa or forearm can decrease the incidence of pain on injection. The pain on infusion is not associated with an increased incidence of phlebitis. Intraarterial injection of propofol does not cause vascular injury. Newer formulations of propofol prodrug are being proposed to address this issue. The inherent slower onset as the drug is metabolized to active propofol will limit this benefit to the administration of infusions and not bolus dosing.[126,127] Figure 10-8 depicts the conversion of the prodrug of propofol by alkaline phosphatases to the active propofol molecule, releasing formaldehyde and phosphate.

Pharmacodynamics

Central Nervous System Effects. The use of propofol in neuroanesthesia, as well as in prolonged sedation in neurologic intensive care unit settings, has increased steadily since its introduction. Significant reductions in cerebral blood flow, $CMRO_2$, intracranial pressure, and cerebral perfusion pressure have been reported with the use of numerous administration techniques.[128] These effects result in part from the decreased mean arterial pressure and cerebral vasoconstriction produced by standard doses in a manner comparable to the effects of barbiturates and etomidate.[129] Craen and co-workers[130] have found that cerebral autoregulation and reactivity to changes in CO_2 were preserved with propofol.

EEG data produced a delta rhythm without evidence of epileptiform activity and burst suppression with higher doses.[131] Even with these findings, controversy exists over the use of propofol in the epileptic patient.[132] Three epileptic patients were reported to experience increased epileptiform activity on EEG after the administration of propofol 2 mg/kg.[133] Studies in epileptic patients showed a different response in that the EEG showed no increase in epileptogenic activity at any of the sites monitored.[134] It was also found that activation or extension of EEG activity was greater with thiopental than with propofol (although not statistically significant).[135] Propofol has been used successfully to manage status epilepticus.[136] Seizures induced by propofol may be spontaneous excitatory movements secondary to selective disinhibition of subcortical centers. Adequate dosage may prevent the occurrence of these movements. Myoclonia may occur on induction, but the incidence appears to be lower than that with etomidate, thiopental, and methohexital. Opisthotonos has also been associated with propofol. Intraocular pressure is decreased by propofol.[137]

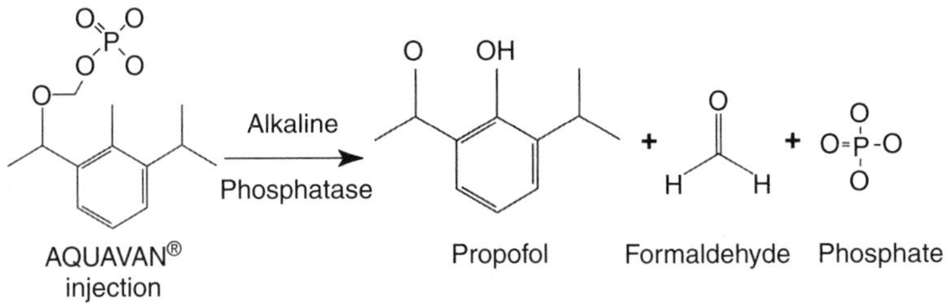

FIGURE **10-8** Conversion of the prodrug of propofol to the active propofol molecule by alkaline phosphatases.

The use of propofol for ECT has been somewhat controversial as a result of this drug's effects on seizure duration. Several studies have shown that propofol reduces the duration of the ECT-induced seizure when compared with barbiturates.[138,139] Evaluating the efficacy of ECT as an antidepressant was typically based on the duration of the seizure; a shortened seizure implied a less effective therapy. However, researchers have found that a reduction in seizure duration does not decrease the efficacy of the ECT, and that propofol is an appropriate agent for use in this procedure.[139,140] Some patients with a prolonged seizure response would benefit from the shorter seizure time caused by propofol. ECT is associated with cardiovascular changes (elevated blood pressure and heart rate) that may be prevented or modified with the use of propofol.[141]

Cardiovascular Effects. Propofol produces significant cardiac depression in the usual induction doses. The effects are more pronounced than those seen with equivalent doses of thiopental, midazolam, or etomidate. Predictors of hypotension when propofol is used for induction are age greater than 50 years old, ASA class 3-4, baseline mean arterial pressure less than 70, and coadministration of high doses of fentanyl.[70] As with most cardiac-depressing sedatives, the effect is the result of a combination of CNS, cardiac, and baroreceptor depression and systemic vasodilation. Decreased cardiac contractility and negative inotropy have been identified in animal studies on isolated papillary muscle. A decrease in dose or alternative agents should be considered in the elderly or cardiac-compromised patients. Propofol has been used successfully for cardiac anesthesia when combined with fentanyl in low-dose or infusion regimens.[142] (See Table 10-6.)

Respiratory Effects. Respiratory depression, more prominent than that seen with thiopental, has been reported with induction doses of propofol. Decreases in tidal volume are more prominent than decreases in respiratory rate, although apnea is common on initial administration of induction doses.[143]

Studies have shown propofol to have a minimal bronchodilating effect in asthmatic patients, nonasthmatic patients, and patients who smoke. After tracheal intubation, respiratory resistance was lower, and the incidence of wheezing was decreased, compared with the effects of etomidate, thiopental, and methohexital.[144,145]

The effect on airway reflexes by propofol is controversial. McKeating and co-workers[146] compared propofol with thiopental and found more satisfactory conditions for intubation with propofol than with thiopental. In a study of 90 patients, Kallar[147] confirmed that intubation without muscle relaxants could be done more successfully with propofol, compared with thiopental and methohexital.

Contraindications and Precautions. Few absolute contraindications exist for propofol other than cases in which a known hypersensitivity exists to propofol or its components.[148-150] The new generic formulation of propofol, which contains sodium metabisulfite, does issue a precaution to its use. The sulfite may cause allergic-type reactions such as anaphylactic symptoms and life-threatening or less severe asthmatic episodes in certain susceptible people. Sulfite sensitivity is more common in patients with asthma than in patients without asthma.[44] As noted, caution is advised in elderly, debilitated, and cardiac-compromised patients.

Uses

Propofol is widely used for the induction of anesthesia in doses of 0.5 to 2.5 mg/kg. Infusion rates of 25 to 200 mg/min are common for intraoperative sedation for a wide variety of surgical and diagnostic procedures. Higher rates of 100 to 200 mcg/kg/hr are required for hypnosis. Induction doses for children are higher (2.5 to 3.5 mg/kg) as a result of their larger central volume of distribution and more rapid rate of clearance. Use of propofol is especially popular in shorter procedures in an ambulatory setting and in monitored anesthesia care. Other uses include sedation for cardioversion, ECT, malignant hyperthermia, facilitation of laryngeal mask airway insertion, and obstetric anesthesia.[19,149]

Propofol Infusion Syndrome. Propofol has been used successfully in adult and pediatric intensive care units for prolonged sedation; however, a fatal syndrome has been proposed with long-term high-dose infusions of propofol.[151] This has not occurred in anesthesia, even with prolonged administration of relatively high doses, because it seems to require long duration infusions of increasing doses, as only encountered in critical care units.[152] Many of the patients have been children, but several cases in adults have been identified. The syndrome has occurred in patients with acute inflammatory disease with infection or sepsis or acute neurologic disease. One common denominator was the presence of impaired systemic microcirculation with tissue hypoperfusion and hypoxia. Propofol seemed to be a triggering agent when catecholamines and corticosteroids are also administered. Fatty acid metabolism and mitochondrial activity are impaired, creating an oxygen supply-and-demand mismatch that results in cardiac and peripheral muscle necrosis. Symptoms include severe metabolic acidosis, refractory cardiac failure, persistent bradycardia refractory to treatment, fever, lipemia, rhabdomyolysis, and possible renal failure.[153] Dosing recommendations include (1) initiation of sedation should begin at 5 mcg/kg/min (0.3 mg/kg/hr); (2) the infusion rate should be increased by increments of 5 to 10 mcg/kg/min (0.3 to 0.6 mg/kg/hr) until the desired level of sedation is achieved; and (3) a minimum period of 5 minutes between adjustments should be allowed for onset of peak drug effect. Most adult patients require maintenance rates of 5 to 50 mcg/kg/min (0.3 to 3 mg/kg/hr) or higher. Caution is advised for infusion doses of over 5 mg/hr for longer than 48 hours. Changes in dosing recommendations, especially in children, are likely.[154] Key points are listed in Box 10-8. Induction doses of the intravenous anesthetics are given in Table 10-7.

Recent Reformulations of Propofol. Propofol was initially manufactured as a preservative-free product. However, after initial introduction, reports of bacterial contamination of propofol emulsion started to appear, suggesting that some cases of postoperative infection might have been the result of the injection of contaminated product. The concern that the preservative-free product could easily be contaminated through handling led the original patent holder, AstraZeneca, to reformulate the preparation. Antimicrobial studies demonstrated that disodium ethylenediaminetetraacetic acid (EDTA) at a concentration of 0.005% successfully retards microbial growth and has no adverse effects on the physicochemical stability of the product.

At approximately the same time that the EDTA preparation of propofol was being formulated, another manufacturer was marketing a sulfite-containing product. This product, generic propofol injectable emulsion 1% (Baxter Pharmaceutical Products), contains sodium metabisulfite 0.25 mg/mL and is formulated in a slightly more acidic medium (pH 4.5 to 6.4) than the AstraZeneca product (pH 7 to 8.5). The release of these products has initiated a number of studies examining whether the new additives might have any effect on the stability of the emulsion product. It has been determined that both EDTA- and

CMRO$_2$, *Cerebral metabolic rate of oxygen consumption;* ICP, *intracranial pressure.*

TABLE **10-7**	Induction Doses of the Intravenous Anesthetics
Agent	**Dose (mg/kg)**
Thiopental	2-4
Methohexital	1-2
Etomidate	0.2-0.3
Propofol	1-2.5
Ketamine	0.1-0.2 (see Box 10-4)
Midazolam	0.1-0.2

sulfite-containing propofol products promote the formation of a propofol dimer. Although the propofol dimer was found in only trace amounts in the propofol-EDTA product (<0.015%), its concentration in the sulfite-propofol product was significantly higher (0.18%). In addition, reports have been made of yellow discoloration in sulfite-propofol products, which could result from increased dimer production. Of interest, both products are promoted by their respective manufacturers as being "preservative free," because the concentrations of both EDTA and sodium metabisulfite are below the USP minimum standard that would require other labeling.[155] Another generic product containing benzoyl alchohol is now available. (See Table 10-2.)

Allergy. Propofol has also been scrutinized because of its lecithin content. Lecithin (from the Greek *lekithos,* meaning "egg yolk") is a phospholipid compound composed of a range of phosphatidyl esters such as phosphatidyl choline, ethanolamine, and serine. These are combined with varying amounts of triglycerides and fatty acids. Lecithin was originally obtained from eggs, although now soybeans and other vegetables with high lecithin content are also useful sources. Apart from its use as an antioxidant synergist, lecithin has important surfactant properties and is used as an emulsifying agent.

It is questionable whether propofol injection, because of its lecithin content, should be avoided in patients with egg allergy. A case has been reported of possible anaphylaxis after propofol administration in a child with allergies to egg and peanut oil.[156] Hypersensitivity reactions to both soybean extract and lecithin have been demonstrated, but they have been reported only when the allergens have been inhaled or ingested. Furthermore, patients who are designated as having a so-called "egg allergy" generally demonstrate an IgE-mediated hypersensitivity to allergenic proteins found in egg whites and life-threatening reactions are rare.[157] The derivation and chemical structure of egg lecithin suggest that the risk associated with its administration to such individuals is very low. Current evidence suggests that egg-allergic patients are not more likely to develop anaphylaxis when exposed to propofol.[44,155]

BENZODIAZEPINES

Benzodiazepines are used in many clinical situations because of their multiple pharmacologic properties, including sedation, hypnosis, muscle relaxation, anxiolysis, anticonvulsant effects, and amnesia. They also are noted to have a low incidence of side effects. Benzodiazepines used clinically in the United States are listed in Table 10-8.

Although similar compounds were first synthesized in 1933, the first benzodiazepine synthesized was chlordiazepoxide (Librium) in 1955. It was not introduced into clinical practice until 1960, when it was found to have antianxiety and hypnotic effects. Diazepam was synthesized in 1959, and its metabolite, oxazepam (Serax), was synthesized in 1961. Lorazepam (Ativan) was derived from oxazepam in 1971.[158] The last benzodiazepine to be developed was midazolam (in 1976, by Fryer and Walser), which was the first of the benzodiazepine group to be formulated with anesthesia as its target clinical use.[4] The benzodiazepines available for clinical use have different potencies, pharmacokinetics, and intensities of clinical properties. Diazepam, lorazepam, and midazolam, which are available as intravenous preparations, are the most commonly used benzodiazepines in anesthesia practice.

Chemical Structure

The chemical structures of the benzodiazepines share some common features: (1) the benzodiazepine ring system; (2) the presence at positions 1 and 4 of two nitrogen atoms; (3) a phenyl group at position 5; and (4) an electronegative group at position 7 (see Figure 10-2).[158]

Midazolam has a unique chemical structure in comparison with the other benzodiazepines. The imidazole ring is responsible for its basic formulation, which permits the preparation of salts that are water soluble at a pH of 4.0. In a chemical reaction that depends on the environmental pH, the diazepine ring opens reversibly between positions 4 and 5. Midazolam is water soluble and does not require a lipoidal vehicle (such as propylene glycol) for parenteral use. Minimal if any side effects of venous irritation

TABLE 10-8	Benzodiazepines Used Clinically in the United States		
Generic Name	**Trade Name**	**Half-Life (hr)**	**Clinical Application**
Alprazolam	Xanax	12-15	Anxiolysis
Chlordiazepoxide	Librium	8-18	Treatment of alcohol withdrawal, etc.
Clonazepam	Klonopin	18.7-39	Treatment of epilepsy
Clorazepate	Tranxene	2.4	Treatment of epilepsy and alcohol withdrawal
Diazepam	Valium	36-50	Sedation; induction and maintenance of anesthesia
Estazolam		14	Treatment of insomnia
Flurazepam	Dalmane	2-3	Treatment of insomnia
Lorazepam	Ativan	10-22	Anxiolysis and sedation
Midazolam	Versed	1.7-2.6	Sedation; induction and maintenance of anesthesia
Oxazepam	Serax	3-21	Anxiolysis
Quazepam	Doral	25-41	Treatment of insomnia
Temazepam	Restoril	10-21	Treatment of insomnia
Triazolam	Halcion	2-3	Treatment of insomnia
Flumazenil	Romazicon	0.7-1.3	Reversal of benzodiazepine agonists

or phlebitis occur. Once in physiologic solution with a pH greater than 4.0, the diazepine ring closes, and midazolam becomes lipophilic, an effect that accounts for its rapid onset of action and the acceptance it has received as an alternative intravenous induction agent.[158]

In each milliliter of solution of diazepam, 0.4 mL of propylene glycol and 0.1 mL of ethyl alcohol are present as solvents, 0.015 mL of benzyl alcohol is present as a preservative, and sodium benzoate or benzoic acid in water is present as a buffer. Each milliliter contains 5 mg of diazepine, and the pH is 6.2 to 6.9.[159]

Each milliliter of lorazepam solution contains 0.18 mL of polyethylene glycol and 2% benzyl alcohol, a preservative. Lorazepam is available in solutions of 2 or 4 mg/mL.[159]

Injectable midazolam is compounded with 0.8% sodium chloride and 0.01% disodium edetate and 1% benzyl alcohol as a preservative. A pH of 3 is adjusted with hydrochloric acid and, if necessary, sodium hydroxide. Each milliliter of preparation contains 1 or 5 mg of midazolam.

Mechanisms of Action

In 1977, specific benzodiazepine receptors were identified in vivo. Benzodiazepine binding sites were found in great density in the olfactory bulb, cerebral cortex, cerebellum, and substantia nigra, with lesser concentrations in the lower brainstem and spinal cord. The clinical effects of benzodiazepines are a result of their occupation of the benzodiazepine receptors within a complex of receptors on the synaptic membrane of the effector neuron. This complex is a $GABA_A$ receptor complex that modulates GABA, the major inhibitory neurotransmitter in the CNS. This complex is composed of protein subunits that contain binding sites for benzodiazepines, GABA, the barbiturates, ethanol, and a chloride ion channel. When these sites are occupied, GABA receptor modulation increases the frequency of chloride channel opening, which results in postsynaptic membrane hyperpolarization, and neuronal transmission is inhibited.[160] A ceiling effect exists on the CNS depression produced by benzodiazepines and is a result of a limitation of the extent of modulation of GABA. Different receptor subtypes and concentration-dependent receptor occupancy may have a role in whether anxiolysis, sedation, or hypnosis occurs when a benzodiazepine is administered.

Three classes of ligands that bind to the benzodiazepine receptors have been identified: agonists, antagonists, and inverse agonists. Midazolam is a receptor agonist that has an increased binding affinity for GABA, resulting in the opening of the chloride channels. Antagonists (e.g., flumazenil) form reversible bonds with the agonist receptor but produce no agonist activity. Inverse agonists cause CNS stimulation by interfering with GABA transmission, which is inhibitory.[161]

The pharmacologic effects of agents depend on which receptors in the CNS are occupied. The brainstem or cortical receptors mediate sedation, the forebrain and hippocampus mediate amnesia, and the benzodiazepine receptors in the amygdala, hippocampus, and other limbic areas mediate anxiolytic properties. Like the other induction agents, except ketamine, the benzodiazepines exert their effect via the GABA receptor. (See Figure 10-5.)

Diazepam

In each milliliter of solution of diazepam, 0.4 mL of propylene glycol and 0.1 mL of ethyl alcohol are present as solvents, 0.015 mL of benzyl alcohol is present as a preservative, and sodium benzoate or benzoic acid in water is present as a buffer. Each milliliter contains 5 mg of diazepine, and the pH is 6.2 to 6.9.[159]

Pharmacokinetics

The elimination pharmacokinetics of benzodiazepines can be examined in both two- and three-compartment models Benzodiazepines have been classified according to their elimination half-lives. These classifications take into account the elimination half-lives of both the parent drug and the active metabolites it produces. Diazepam is long lasting, lorazepam has an intermediate duration, and midazolam is short lasting.[162]

Diazepam has a very slow distribution half-life, which limits its usefulness as an acceptable induction agent. Its inability to cause unconsciousness rapidly may be the result of its ability to produce profound CNS depression and renders it unacceptable.[162] Diazepam is extremely lipid soluble, a characteristic that promotes extensive distribution to the tissues. The volume of distribution is large, a characteristic of all benzodiazepines. Also characteristic is extensive protein binding, which can be affected by disease states that decrease plasma protein levels. The total body clearance of diazepam is only 0.24 to 0.53 mL/min/kg and is totally dependent on hepatic metabolism.

The hepatic extraction ratio of diazepam is very low, making it dependent on hepatic blood flow, protein binding, and hepatic metabolism. Cimetidine, a hepatic enzyme inhibitor, decreases the hepatic biotransformation of diazepam and prolongs its effects.[163] The pharmacologic effects seen with benzodiazepines are terminated primarily by redistribution of the drug out of the CNS. Oral diazepam has a 100% bioavailability, which reflects no first-pass removal of the drug by the liver. Intramuscular administration of similar doses, however, results in a plasma blood level of only 50% to 60% of that administered. Diazepam does not stay in solution after intramuscular injection. After the solvent dissolves, the diazepam precipitates, leaving less drug available for absorption. The preparation with propylene glycol also causes pain and irritation at the injection site.

Diazepam exhibits a near-linear relationship between elimination half-life and patient age.[164] Pharmacokinetics in the elderly are altered as a result of slowed drug absorption; increased percentage of adipose tissue in body mass; decreased plasma proteins, hepatic blood flow, and metabolism; and decreased cardiac output and circulation time. A prolonged circulation time allows for a slower onset and a higher plasma drug level that remains in the CNS longer before it redistributes; this phenomenon exaggerates the effects of the drug.[165]

Hepatic microsomal enzymes are responsible for the metabolism of diazepam. Diazepam is demethylated to dimethyl diazepam (nordiazepam), which is an active metabolite that, although less potent, is responsible for prolonged drug effect as a result of its slower metabolism. Diazepam can also be hydroxylated to 3-hydroxydiazepam, which is then demethylated to oxazepam, which is also pharmacologically active and commercially marketed. The termination of action of diazepam is caused by redistribution, and the distribution half-life is 30 to 66 minutes, much longer than that of other induction agents.

Pharmacodynamics

Central Nervous System Effects. Diazepam produces all the characteristic CNS depressant effects of the benzodiazepines, from sedation to anxiolysis and sleep. Diazepam produces anterograde but not retrograde amnesia; the amnesia is dose related. Benzodiazepines also possess anticonvulsant activity, and diazepam has been shown to be effective in the treatment of status epilepticus and sedative-hypnotic withdrawal syndromes. In vitro studies in animals have shown it to be effective in the prevention of seizures induced by local anesthetics. EEG changes include disappearance of the alpha rhythm and the onset of higher-frequency beta-rhythm activity.[166] (See Table 10-5.)

Respiratory Effects. Some respiratory depression occurs with diazepam, as evidenced by a decrease in minute ventilation and slope of the carbon dioxide response curve.[163] This response curve is not shifted to the right, as occurs with some other CNS depressants. Increased respiratory depression and apnea are possible when benzodiazepines are combined with other CNS depressants such as opioids.

Uses

Diazepam has been used successfully for preanesthesia medication and sedation during therapeutic or diagnostic procedures. Three main concerns with its use are pain on injection, thrombophlebitis, and duration of action. Dosages should be adjusted in elderly patients and in patients with hepatic or renal disease. Intravenous diazepam has been associated with patient dissatisfaction regarding pain and postoperative thrombophlebitis. The use of small veins and a rapid rate of injection can increase the high rate of these complications. The longer duration of action compared with that of midazolam explains the currently limited anesthetic use of diazepam.

Midazolam

Midazolam is an imidazobenzodiazepine similar to diazepam in potency but shorter acting. Its chemical structure differs from that of the classic benzodiazepines in that it has an imidazole ring that gives the drug basicity, which allows the preparation of the drug as a salt. This quality makes the drug soluble and stable in aqueous solutions. No solvents are necessary as a vehicle for injection, and the venous irritation produced by other benzodiazepines is therefore omitted. A methyl group exists at position 1; this group produces a very short duration of action because it is rapidly metabolized by hepatic oxidizing enzymes. The imidazole ring structure is altered by physiologic pH, and at a pH of less than 4 the ring is 80% to 85% in the closed ring form and 15% to 20% in the open form. When the pH is greater than 4, the ring structures are totally closed, and the drug becomes highly lipophilic, which results in a rapid onset of action.[158] The closed ring form has an increased affinity for hydrolysis by hepatic microsomal oxidative mechanisms, which contributes to the drug's short duration of action.

Absorption

Oral midazolam is rapidly absorbed and subject to first-pass hepatic extraction, which results in a systemic availability of less than 50% of the administered dose. The greater the dose, the larger the percent of active drug available.[167]

Intramuscular injection produces a bioavailability of between 80% and 100%. Peak plasma concentrations are reached within 45 minutes of intramuscular injection.[168]

Mechanisms of Action

The pharmacologic effects of midazolam include all actions common to benzodiazepines, such as anticonvulsant effects, hypnosis, amnesia, muscle relaxant effects, and anxiolysis. Midazolam has a higher affinity for benzodiazepine receptors in the CNS than diazepam. In animal studies, the anticonvulsant effects of midazolam were found to be equivalent to diazepam, although of shorter duration. Midazolam was also found to be a more effective sedative than diazepam but for a shorter duration.[169]

Pharmacokinetics

The rapid onset of this drug is a result of its high lipid solubility at physiologic pH and its ability to rapidly cross the blood-brain barrier. Midazolam is extensively protein bound (95% to 96%), which may contribute to clinically evident alterations in the effects of the drugs in patients with alterations in protein states.[170] Termination of action is dependent on a rapid redistribution of the drug. Midazolam may be described in a three-compartment model, with elimination occurring from the central compartment.

Metabolism of midazolam is via hydroxylation in the liver. It has a high hepatic extraction ratio (7 to 9 mL/min/kg) and a high clearance, resulting in the shortest elimination half-life of the benzodiazepines. The metabolites of midazolam are alpha-hydroxymidazolam (which has minimal potency), 4-hydroxymidazolam (which is similar in potency to alpha-hydroxymidazolam but is produced in very small amounts), and alpha-4-hydroxymidazolam (which is also produced in small amounts but is practically inactive). Combined, the metabolites do not contribute significantly to the pharmacologic effects of midazolam or its duration of action. All metabolites are excreted in the urine as glucuronide conjugates.[171]

In animal studies, three metabolites of midazolam were evaluated for pharmacologic activity. Alpha-hydroxymidazolam levels measured 30 minutes after administration in mice were one tenth to one fortieth as potent as those of midazolam. The metabolite 4-hydroxymidazolam had similar levels of potency, and alpha-4-hydroxymidazolam was practically inactive.

Pharmacodynamics

Cardiovascular Effects. Blood pressure was not significantly changed, and heart rate was only slightly increased in conscious dogs. Under barbiturate anesthesia, midazolam caused slight dose-related decreases in systolic and diastolic blood pressure. In humans, the use of midazolam is associated with a relatively stable cardiac profile.[170] When the drug was used for induction of anesthesia in healthy humans (0.15 mg/kg given intravenously over 15 seconds), systolic blood pressure was decreased 5%, diastolic blood pressure was decreased 10%, and heart rate was increased 18% (significance $P < 0.05$).[172] The decrease in arterial blood pressure is the result of a reduction in systemic vascular resistance.

Respiratory Effects. Midazolam, as well as all the other benzodiazepines, produces less respiratory depression in usual doses than older sedatives, such as the barbiturates or phenothiazines. As expected with any CNS depressant drug, however, respiratory depression may occur in the very young, elderly, or debilitated, as well as in patients receiving other respiratory depressant agents.[164]

Central Nervous System Effects. Amnesia is an important pharmacologic effect of midazolam. Intravenous administration produces anterograde amnesia in low doses. Amnesia occurs within 2 to 5 minutes of administration and remains for 20 to 30 minutes.[173] In one study, partial amnesia remained for 90 minutes in 40% of the patients studied.

Previous studies have shown that midazolam produces a decrease in cerebral blood flow and cerebral metabolic oxygen consumption without significant cardiovascular depression.[174]

Knudsen and co-workers[174] studied 30 patients with different serum concentrations of midazolam and the presence of nitrous oxide. They concluded that no drug response relationship existed between midazolam and cerebral blood flow or oxygen consumption. In this study, mean arterial pressure and arterial partial pressure of CO_2 were maintained at constant levels.

Uses

The popularity of midazolam in modern anesthesia is widespread. Its rapid onset and short duration and half-life make it ideal for use as a preoperative anxiolytic and a perioperative sedative drug.

Flumazenil

Flumazenil is the sole benzodiazepine antagonist available in the United States (see Figure 10-2). It is a competitive antagonist with a high affinity for the receptor site. It produces prompt and effective specific reversal of benzodiazepine agonist effects after anesthesia and overdose.[175,176] Actual available receptors for occupancy by flumazenil effect its pharmacologic action. Benzodiazepine affinity for the receptors and concentration of free benzodiazepines at the sites determine receptor occupancy of flumazenil. Its relatively short duration and half-life make the possibility of resedation clinically relevant, especially in overdose situations. A slow titration of 0.2-mg doses (2 mL) is given intravenously (up to 1 mg) until the desired level of consciousness is achieved. Doses rarely exceed 1 mg for the reversal of midazolam-induced sedation and 3 mg for suspected benzodiazepine overdose. Withdrawal reactions are possible in patients who are benzodiazepine dependent, and its use in these patients is contraindicated. Flumazenil does not reverse the actions of ethanol or barbiturates.[177] Side effects are rare, although mild anxiogenic effects have been reported.[178] Seizures have been reported in patients with suspected tricyclic and antidepressant overdose, and the use of flumazenil in these situations and in patients with a known history of seizures should be avoided.[179]

SUMMARY

The availability of a variety of unique intravenous drugs that contain the necessary properties for use in induction has allowed the clinician to tailor the induction to fit the needs of the patient and surgeon. This characteristic has made it much easier to care for an increasingly diverse and complex patient population. Intravenous anesthetics can be chosen with consideration for the health status of the patient, the type of procedure to be performed, and the patient's susceptibility to possible adverse effects to produce the remarkably safe techniques and excellent outcomes achieved today.

REFERENCES

1. Charney DS et al. Hypnotic and sedatives. In: Brunton LL et al, eds. *Goodman and Gilman's Pharmacologic Basis of Therapeutics.* New York: Macmillan; 2006:401-428.
2. Stoelting RK, Hillier SC. *Pharmacology and Physiology in Anesthetic Practice.* 4th ed. Philadelphia: Lippincott; 2006:127-139.
3. Wong CL et al. Reconstituted thiopentone retains its alkalinity without bacterial contamination for up to four weeks. *Can J Anaesth.* 1992;39:504-508.
4. Ghoneim MM et al. Binding of thiopental to plasma proteins. *Anesthesiology.* 1976;45:635-639.
5. Reves JG et al. Intravenous nonopioid anesthesia. In Miller RD, ed. *Anesthesia,* 6th ed. New York: Churchill Livingstone; 2005:317-378.
6. Eger EI II. *Anesthetic Uptake and Action.* Baltimore: Williams & Wilkins; 1974.
7. Stanski DR. Pharmacokinetics of barbiturates. In: Prys-Roberts C, Hug CC Jr, eds. *Pharmacokinetics of Anaesthesia.* Oxford: Blackwell Scientific; 1984: 86-93.
8. Brodie BB et al. The role of body fat in limiting the duration of thiopental. *J Pharmacol Exp Ther.* 1952;105:421-426.
9. Price HL et al. The uptake of thiopental by body tissues and its relation to the duration of narcosis. *Clin Pharmacol Ther.* 1960;1:16-22.
10. Nguyen KT et al. Pharmacokinetics of thiopental and pentobarbital enantiomers after intravenous administration of racemic thiopental. *Anesth Analg.* 1996;83:552-558.
11. Stanski DR, Maitre PO. Pharmacokinetics and pharmacodynamics of thiopental: the effect of age revisited. *Anesthesiology.* 1990;72:412-422.
12. Shanks CA et al. A pharmacokinetic-pharmacodynamic model for quantal responses with thiopental. *J Pharmacokinet Biopharm.* 1993;21:309-321.

13. Hudson RJ et al. Pharmacokinetics of methohexital and thiopental in surgical patients. *Anesthesiology*. 1983;59:215-219.

14. Jones DJ et al. Determination of (R)-(+)- and (S)-(−)-isomers of thiopentone in plasma by chiral high-performance liquid chromatography. *J Chromatogr*. 1996;675:174-179.

15. Abramson NS. Randomized clinical study of thiopental loading in comatose survivors of cardiac arrest. *N Engl J Med*. 1986;314:397-399.

16. Pandele G et al. Thiopental pharmacokinetics in patients with cirrhosis. *Anesthesiology*. 1983;59:123-126.

17. Diasio RB. Principles of drug therapy. In: Goldman L, Avsiello D, eds. *Cecil Textbook of Medicine*. 23rd ed. Philadelphia: Saunders; 2008:139-150.

18. Burch PG, Stanski DR. Thiopental pharmacokinetics in renal failure. *Anesthesiology*. 1981;55:A176.

19. Olsen RW et al. Barbiturate and benzodiazepine modulation of GABA receptor binding and function. *Life Sci*. 1986;39:1969-1976.

20. Perouansky MA, Hemmings HG. Intravenous anesthetic agents. In: Hemmings HC, Hopkins PM, eds. *Foundations of Anesthesia, Basic Sciences for Clinical Practice*. 2nd ed. Philadelphia: Mosby; 2006:295-310.

21. MacDonald RL et al. Barbiturates regulation of kinetic properties of the GABAA receptor channel of mouse spinal neurons in culture. *J Physiol*. 1989;417:483-500.

22. Chernin EL, Smiler B. The cost-effectiveness of methohexital versus propofol: the stability of reconstituted methohexital should eliminate waste. *Anesth Analg*. 1999;89:1064.

23. Todd MM et al. The hemodynamic consequences of high dose methohexital anesthesia in humans. *Anesthesiology*. 1984;61:495-501.

24. Korttila K et al. Recovery and simulated driving after intravenous anesthesia with thiopental, methohexital, propanidid, or alphadione. *Anesthesiology*. 1975;43:291-299.

25. Gentry WB, Henthorn TK. Barbiturates. In: White PF, ed. *Textbook of Intravenous Anesthesia*. Baltimore: Williams & Wilkins; 1997;65-76.

26. Ross AK, Glass PSA. Pharmacology and physiology of intravenous anesthesia. In: Miller RD, ed. *Atlas of Anesthesia*. Philadelphia: Churchill Livingstone; 1998.

27. Rampil ID et al. Spectral edge frequency: a correlate of anesthesia depth. *Anesthesiology*. 1980;53:S12.

28. Hudson RJ et al. A model for studying depth of anesthesia and acute tolerance to thiopental. *Anesthesiology*. 1980;59:301-308.

29. Barratt R et al. The influence of sampling site in the distribution phase kinetics of thiopentone. *Anaesth Intensive Care* 1984;56:1385-1391.

30. Michenfelder JG. The interdependency of cerebral function and metabolic effects following massive dose of thiopental in the dog. *Anesthesiology*. 1974;41:231-236.

31. Albrecht RF et al. Cerebral blood flow and metabolic changes from induction to onset of anesthesia with halothane or pentobarbital. *Anesthesiology*. 1977;47:252-256.

32. Asrup J et al. Minimal cerebral blood flow and metabolism during craniotomy: effect of thiopental loading. *Acta Anaesthesiol Scand*. 1984;28:478-481.

33. McPherson RW et al. Effects of thiopental, fentanyl and etomidate on upper extremity somatosensory evoked potentials in humans. *Anesthesiology*. 1986;65:584-589.

34. Joshi C, Bruce DL. Thiopental and succinylcholine: action in intraocular pressure. *Anesth Analg*. 1975;54:471-475.

35. Calla S et al. Comparison of the effects of etomidate and thiopental on intraocular pressure. *Br J Anaesth*. 1987;59:437-439.

36. Prys-Roberts C et al. Studies of anaesthesia in relation to hypertension. I. Cardiovascular responses of treated and untreated patients. *Br J Anaesth*. 1971;43:122-137.

37. Flickenger H et al. Effect of thiopental induction on cardiac output in man. *Anesth Analg*. 1961;40:693-700.

38. Eckstein JW et al. The effect of thiopental on peripheral venous tone. *Anesthesiology*. 1961;22:525-528.

39. Skorsted P et al. The effects of short-acting barbiturates on arterial pressure, preganglionic sympathetic activity and barostatic reflexes. *Anesthesiology*. 1970;33:10.

40. Corssen G. *Intravenous Anesthesia and Analgesia*. Philadelphia: Lea & Febiger; 1988.

41. Patrick RT, Faulconer A. Respiratory studies during anesthesia with ether and with pentothal sodium. *Anaesthesiology*. 1952;13:252.

42. Sedik H. Use of intravenous methohexital as a sedative in pediatric emergency departments. *Arch Pediatr Adolesc Med*. 2001;155:665-668.

43. Mertes PM et al. Anaphylactic and anaphylactoid reactions occurring during anesthesia in France in 1999-2000. *Anesthesiology*. 2003;99(3):536-545.

44. Chacko T, Ledford D. Peri-anesthetic anaphylaxis. *Immunol Allergy Clin North Am*. 2007;27:213-230.

45. Ebo DG et al. Anaphylaxis during anaesthesia: diagnostic approach. *Allergy*. 2007;62(5):471-487.

46. Kosaka Y et al. Intravenous thiobarbiturate anesthesia for cesarean section. *Anesthesiology*. 1969;31:489-506.

47. Kay B. A dose response relationship for etomidate with some observations on cumulation. *Br J Anaesth*. 1976;48:213-215.

48. Doenicke A. Etomidate: a new intravenous hypnotic. *Acta Anaesthesiol Belg*. 1974;25:307-315.

49. Nyman Y et al. Etomidate-Lipuro is associated with considerably less injection pain in children compared with propofol with added lidocaine. *Br J Anaesth*. 2006;97(4):536-539.

50. Giese JL, Stanley TH. Etomidate: a new intravenous anesthetic induction agent. *Pharmacotherapy*. 1983;3:251-258.

51. Thoheim MM, VanHamme MJ. Hydrolysis of etomidate. *Anesthesiology*. 1979;50:242-244.

52. Doenicke A et al. Histamine release with intravenous application of short-acting hypnotics. *Br J Anaesth*. 1973;45:1097-1104.

53. Renou AM et al. Cerebral blood flow and metabolism during etomidate anaesthesia in man. *Br J Anaesth*. 1978;50:1047-1050.

54. Moss E et al. Effect of etomidate on intracranial pressure and cerebral perfusion pressure. *Br J Anaesth*. 1979;51:347-352.

55. Ghoneim MM, Yamada T. Etomidate: a clinical and electroencephalographic comparison with thiopental. *Anesth Analg*. 1977;56:479-485.

56. Horrigan RW et al. Etomidate vs. thiopental with and without fentanyl: a comparative study of awakening in man. *Anesthesiology*. 1980;52:362-364.

57. Lang A. Other movement disorders. In: Goldman L, Ausiello D, eds. *Cecil Medicine*, 23rd ed. Philadelphia: Saunders; 2008:2734-2742.

58. Gancher S et al. Activation of epileptogenic activity by etomidate. *Anesthesia*. 1984;61:616-621.

59. Korttila K et al. Comparison of etomidate in combination with fentanyl or diazepam, with thiopentone as an induction agent for general anesthesia. *Br J Anaesth*. 1979;51:1151-1156.

60. Prakash O et al. Cardiovascular effects of etomidate with emphasis on regional myocardial blood flow and performance. *Br J Anaesth*. 1981;53:591-599.

61. Skovsted P, Sapthavichaikul S. The effects of etomidate on arterial pressure, pulse rate and preganglionic sympathetic activity in cats. *Can J Anaesth*. 1977;24:565-570.

62. Gooding JM, Corssen G. Effect of etomidate on the cardiovascular system. *Anesth Analg*. 1977;56:717-719.

63. Gooding JM et al. Cardiovascular and pulmonary responses following etomidate induction of anesthesia in patients with demonstrated cardiac disease. *Anesth Analg*. 1979;58:40-41.

64. Colvin MP et al. Cardiorespiratory change following induction of anaesthesia with etomidate in patients with demonstrated cardiovascular disease. *Br J Anaesth*. 1979;51:551-556.

65. Daehlin L, Gran L. Etomidate and thiopentone: a comparative study of their respiratory effects. *Curr Ther Res*. 1980;27:5.

66. Morgan M et al. Respiratory effects of etomidate. *Br J Anaesth*. 1977;49:233-236.

67. Ledingham IM, Watt I. Influence of sedation on mortality in critically ill multiple trauma patients. *Lancet*. 1983;1:1270.

68. Fragen RJ et al. Effects of etomidate on hormonal response to surgical stress. *Anesthesiology*. 1984;61:652-656.

69. Absalom A et al. Adrenocortical function in critically ill patients 24 h after a single dose of etomidate. *Anaesthesia*. 1999;54:861-867.

70. Reich DL et al. Predictors of hypotension after induction of general anesthesia. *Anesth Analg*. 2005;101(3):622-628.

71. Kamp R, Kress JP. Etomidate, sepsis, and adrenal function: not as bad as we thought? *Crit Care*. 2007;11(3):145.

72. Ostwald P, Doenicke AW. Etomidate revisited. *Curr Opin Anaesthesiol*. 1998;11(4):391-398.

73. Mohammad Z et al. The incidence of relative adrenal insufficiency in patients with septic shock after the administration of etomidate. *Crit Care*. 2006;10(4):R105.

74. Lundy JB et al. Acute adrenal insufficiency after a single dose of etomidate. *J Intensive Care Med*. 2007;22(2):111-117.

75. Boidin MP et al. The role of ascorbic acid in etomidate toxicity. *Eur J Anaesthesiol*. 1986;37:417-422.

76. Fragen RJ, Caldwell N. Comparison of the new formulation of etomidate with thiopental: side effects and awaking times. *Anesthesiology*. 1979; 50:242-244.

77. Giese JL et al. Etomidate versus thiopental for induction of anesthesia. *Anesth Analg*. 1985;64:871-876.

78. Lear E et al. Cyclohexamine (CI-400): a new intravenous agent. *Anesthesiology*. 1961;20:525.

79. Maddox VH. The historical development of phencyclidine. In: Domino EF, ed. *PCP (Phencyclidine). Historical and Current Perspectives*. Ann Arbor, MI: NPP Books; 1981:46-54.

80. Corssen G, Domino EF. Dissociated anesthesia: further pharmacologic studies and first clinical experience with the phencyclidine derivative. *Anesth Analg.* 1966;45:26-40.

81. Domino EF et al. Pharmacologic effects of CI-581, a new dissociated anesthetic in man. *Clin Pharmacol Ther.* 1965;6:279-291.

82. Schuttler J et al. Ketamine and its isomers. In: White PF, ed. *Textbook of Intravenous Anesthesia.* Baltimore: Williams & Wilkins; 1997:171-190.

83. Franks NP, Lieb WR. Molecular and cellular mechanisms of general anesthesia. *Nature.* 1994;367:607-614.

84. Leeson PD, Iverson LL. Perspective: the glycine site on the NMDA receptor—structure-activity relationships and therapeutic potential. *J Med Chem.* 1994;37:4053-4060.

85. Nagasaka H et al. The effect of ketamine on the excitation and inhibition of dorsal horn WDR neuronal activity induced by bradykinin injection into the femoral artery in cats after spinal cord transection. *Anesthesiology.* 1993;78:722-732.

86. Smith DJ et al. Ketamine interacts with opioid receptors as an agonist. *Anesthesiology.* 1980;53:55.

87. Toro-Matos A et al. Physostigmine antagonizes ketamine. *Anesth Analg.* 1980;59:764-767.

88. Kharasch ED, Labroo R. Metabolism of ketamine stereoisomers by human liver microsomes. *Anesthesiology.* 1992;77:1201-1207.

89. Ihmsen H et al. Stereoselective pharmacokinetics of ketamine: R(−)-ketamine inhibits the elimination of S(+)-ketamine. *Clin Pharmacol Ther.* 2001; 70:431-438.

90. Henthorn TK et al. Ketamine distribution described by a recirculatory pharmacokinetic model is not stereoselective. *Anesthesiology.* 1999;91:1733-1743.

91. Nimmo WS, Clements JA. Ketamine. In: Prys-Roberts C, Hug CC, eds. *Pharmacokinetics of Anaesthesia.* Oxford: Blackwell Scientific; 1984:235.

92. Roytblat L et al. Postoperative pain: the effect of low-dose ketamine in addition to general anesthesia. *Anesth Analg.* 1993;77:1161-1165.

93. Grant IS et al. Pharmacokinetics and analgesic effects of IM and oral ketamine. *Br J Anaesth.* 1981;53:805-810.

94. Stanski DR, Watkins DW, eds. *Drug Disposition in Anesthesia.* New York: Grune & Stratton; 1982.

95. Woolf CJ, Chong MS. Preemptive analgesia: treating postoperative pain by preventing the establishment of central sensitization. *Anesth Analg.* 1993;77:362-379.

96. Corssen G, Bjarnesen W. Recent advances in intravenous anesthesia. *AANA J.* 1966;34:416-427.

97. Zsigmond EK, Domino EF. Clinical pharmacology of ketamine. In: Domino EF, ed. *Status of Ketamine in Anesthesiology.* Ann Arbor, MI: NPP Books; 1990:27-76.

98. Engelhardt W. Recovery and Psychomimetic reactions following S-(+)-ketamine. *Anaesthetist.* 1997;46(Suppl 1):38-42.

99. Annetta MG et al. Ketamine: new indications for an old drug. *Curr Drug Targets.* 2005;6(7):789-794.

100. Gray C et al. Target controlled infusion of ketamine as analgesia for TIVA with propofol. *Can J Anaesth.* 1999;46:957-961.

101. Pedersen T et al. Effects of low dose ketamine and thiopentone on cardiac performance and myocardial oxygen balance in high risk patients. *Acta Anaesthesiol Scand.* 1982;26:235-239.

102. Ivankovich AD et al. Cardiovascular effects of centrally administered ketamine in goats. *Anesth Analg.* 1974;53:924-933.

103. Cook DJ et al. Mechanisms of the positive inotropic effect of ketamine in isolated ferret ventricular papillary muscle. *Anesthesiology.* 1991; 74:880-888.

104. Kongsayreepong S et al. Mechanisms of direct, negative inotropic effect of ketamine in isolated ferret and frog ventricular myocardium. *Anesthesiology.* 1993;80:313-322.

105. Bidwal AV et al. The effects of ketamine on cardiovascular dynamics during halothane and enflurane anesthesia. *Anesth Analg.* 1975;54:588-592.

106. Corssen G. Ketamine for high risk cardiac patients. *Anesthesiology.* 1972; 36:413.

107. Yoshikawa K, Marai Y. The effect of ketamine on intraocular pressure in children. *Anesth Analg.* 1971;50:199-202.

108. Ausinsch B et al. Ketamine and intraocular pressure in children. *Anesth Analg.* 1976;55:773-775.

109. Little B et al. Study of ketamine as an obstetrical agent. *Am J Obstet Gynecol.* 1972;113:247-260.

110. Sen S et al. The persisting analgesic effect of low-dose intravenous ketamine after spinal anaesthesia for caesarean section. *Eur J Anaesthesiol.* 2005; 22(7):518-523.

111. *Propofol.* St Louis: Mosby Drug Consult; 2007.

112. Baker MT, Naguib M. The challenges of formulation. *Anesthesiology.* 2005; 103(4):860-876.

113. Schuttler J, Ihmsen H. Population pharmacokinetics of propofol: a multicenter study. *Anesthesiology.* 2000;92:727-738.

114. Fechner J et al. Pharmacokinetics and clinical pharmacodynamics of the new propofol prodrug GPI 15715 in volunteers. *Anesthesiology.* 2003;99:303-313.

115. Veroli P et al. Extrahepatic metabolism of propofol in man during the anhepatic phase of orthotopic liver transplantation. *Br J Anaesth.* 1992; 68:183-186.

116. Dindee JW et al. Sensitivity to propofol in the elderly. *Anesthesia.* 1986; 41:482-485.

117. Hannollah RS. Induction dose of propofol in children. *Semin Anesth.* 1992; 11(Suppl 1):48-49.

118. Gan TJ. Pharmacokinetic and pharmacodynamic characteristics of medications used for modern sedation. *Clin Pharm.* 2006;45(6):855-869.

119. Solt K, Forman SA. Correlating the clinical actions and molecular mechanisms of general anesthetics. *Curr Opin Anaesthesiol.* 2007;20(4):300-306.

120. Irifune M et al. Propofol induced anesthesia in mice is mediated by γ-aminobutyric acid-A and excitatory amino acid receptors. *Anesth Analg.* 2003;97:424-429.

121. Mukherjee K et al. A comparison of total intravenous with balanced anaesthesia for middle ear surgery: effects on postoperative nausea and vomiting, pain, and conditions of surgery. *Anaesthesia.* 2003;58:176-180.

122. Pollard BJ et al. Anaesthetic agents in adult day case surgery. *Eur J Anaesthesiol.* 2003;20:1-9.

123. Cork RC, Scipione P. Appendix: patient perceptions of propofol versus thiopental-isoflurane for outpatient anesthesia. *Semin Anesth.* 1992; 11(Suppl 1):50-54.

124. Parmar AK, Koay CK. Pain on injection of propofol. A comparison of cold propofol with propofol mixed with lignocaine. *Anaesthesiology.* 1998;53:79-83.

125. Gehan G et al. Optimal dose of lignocaine for preventing pain on injection of propofol. *Br J Anaesth.* 1991;66:324-326.

126. Gibiansky E et al. Aquavan injection, a water-soluble prodrug of propofol, as a bolus injection: a phase I dose-escalation comparison with Diprivan (part 1): pharmacokinetics. *Anesthesiology.* 2005;103(4):718-729.

127. Struys MM et al. Aquavan injection, a water-soluble prodrug of propofol, as a bolus injection: a phase I dose-escalation comparison with Diprivan (part 2): pharmacodynamics and safety. *Anesthesiology.* 2005;103(4):730-743.

128. Herregods L et al. Effect of propofol on elevated intracranial pressure: preliminary results. *Anesthesia.* 1988;43:107-109.

129. Aikire MT et al. Cerebral metabolism during propofol anesthesia in humans studied with positron emission tomography. *Anesthesiology.* 1995;82:393-403.

130. Craen RA et al. Human cerebral autoregulation is maintained during propofol air/O₂ [abstract]. *Anesthesiology.* 1992;77:A220.

131. Mahla ME et al. Prolonged anesthesia with propofol or isoflurane: intraoperative electroencephalographic patterns and postoperative recovery. *Semin Anesth.* 1992;11(Suppl 1):31-32.

132. Collier C, Kelly K. Propofol and convulsions: the evidence mounts. *Anesth Intensive Care.* 1991;19:573-575.

133. Hodkinson BP et al. Propofol and the electroencephalogram. *Lancet.* 1987; 2:1518.

134. Samra SK et al. The effects of propofol sedation on seizures and intracranially recorded epileptiform activity in patients with partial epilepsy. *Anesthesiology.* 1995;82:843-851.

135. Hewitt PB et al. Effects of propofol on the electrocorticogram in epileptic patients undergoing cortical resection. *Br J Anaesth.* 1999;82:199-202.

136. MacKensie SJ et al. Propofol infusion for control of status epilepticus. *Anaesthesia.* 1990;45:1043-1045.

137. DeFriez CB, Wond HC. Seizures and opisthotonos after propofol anaesthesia. *Anesth Analg.* 1992;75:630-632.

138. Boey WK, Lai FO. Comparison of propofol and thiopentone as anaesthetic agents for electroconvulsive therapy. *Anaesthesia.* 1990;45:623-628.

139. McArtensson B et al. A comparison of propofol and methohexital as anesthetic agents for ECT: effects on seizure duration, therapeutic outcome, and memory. *Biol Psychiatry.* 1994;35:179-189.

140. Malsch E et al. Efficacy of electroconvulsive therapy (ECT) after propofol (P) or methohexital (M) anesthesia [abstract]. *Anesth Analg.* 1992;74:S192.

141. Malsch E et al. The effect of antihypertensive medication on the cardiovascular (CV) response to electroconvulsive therapy (ECT) after methohexital (M) or propofol (P) anesthesia [abstract]. *Anesthesiology.* 1992;77:A76.

142. Patrick MR et al. A comparison of the hemodynamic effects of propofol (Diprivan) and thiopentone in patients with coronary artery disease. *Postgrad Med J.* 1985;61(Suppl 3):23-27.

143. Goodman NW et al. Some ventilatory effects of propofol as a sole anesthetic agent. *Br J Anaesth.* 1987;59:1497-1503.

144. Eames WO et al. Comparison of effects of etomidate, propofol, and thiopental on respiratory resistance after tracheal intubation. *Anesthesiology.* 1996; 84:1307-1311.

145. Pizov R et al. Wheezing during induction of general anesthesia in patients with and without asthma: a randomized, blinded trial. *Anesthesiology.* 1995; 82:1111-1116.
146. McKeating K et al. The effects of thiopentone and propofol on upper airway integrity. *Anaesthesia.* 1988;43:638-640.
147. Kallar SK. Propofol allows intubation without relaxants [abstract]. *Anesthesiology.* 1992;73(A22):3A.
148. Smith I et al. Propofol: an update on its clinical use. *Anesthesiology.* 1994;81:1005-1043.
149. Nathan N, Odin I. Induction of anaesthesia: a guide to drug choice. *Drugs.* 2007;67(5):701-723.
150. Sneyd JR. Recent advances in intravenous anaesthesia. *Br J Anaesth.* 2004;93(5):725-736.
151. Wysowski DK, Pollock ML. Reports of death with use of propofol (Diprivan) for nonprocedural (long-term) sedation and literature review. *Anesthesiology.* 2006;105:1047-1051.
152. Ahlen K et al. The "propofol infusion syndrome": the facts, their interpretation and implications for patient care. *Eur J Anaesthesiol.* 2006; 23:990-998.
153. Crozier TA. The "propofol infusion syndrome"; myth or menace? *Eur J Anaesthesiol.* 2006;23:987-989.
154. Vasite B et al. The pathophysiology of propofol infusion syndrome: a simple name for a complex syndrome. *Intensive Care Med.* 2003;9:1417-1425.
155. MacPherson RD. Pharmaceutics for the anaesthetist. *Anaesthesia.* 2001; 56:965-979.
156. Hofer KN et al. Possible anaphylaxis after propofol in a child with food allergy. *Ann Pharmacother.* 2003;37(3):398-401.
157. Allen CW et al. Egg allergy: are all childhood food allergies the same? *Paediatr Child Health.* 2007;43(4):214-218.
158. Walser A et al. Quinazolines and 1,4 benzodiazepines. Synthesis and reactions of imidazo(1,5-a)(1,4)-benzodiazepines. *J Org Chem.* 1978;43:936.
159. Galloon S. Ketamine for obstetrical delivery. *Anesthesiology.* 1976;44: 522-544.
160. Goodchild CS. GABA receptors and benzodiazepines. *Br J Anaesth.* 1993;71:127-133.
161. Mohler H, Richards JG. The benzodiazepine receptor: a pharmacologic control element of brain function. *Eur J Anaesthesiol.* 1988;2(Suppl):15-24.
162. Greenblat DJ et al. Benzodiazepines: a summary of pharmacokinetic properties. *Br J Clin Pharmacol.* 1981;11:11-16.
163. Stanski DR, Watkins DW, eds. *Drug Disposition in Anesthesia.* New York: Grune & Stratton; 1982.
164. Roy-Bryne P, Crowley D, eds. *Benzodiazepines in Clinical Practice: Risk and Benefits.* Washington, DC: American Psychiatric; 1991.
165. Cote P et al. Systemic and coronary hemodynamic effects of diazepam in patients with normal and diseased coronary arteries. *Circulation.* 1974; 50:1210-1216.
166. Tomichek RL et al. Cardiovascular effects of diazepam-fentanyl anesthesia in patients with coronary artery disease. *Anesth Analg.* 1982;61:217-218.
167. Allonen H et al. Midazolam kinetics. *Clin Pharmacol Ther.* 1981;30:653-661.
168. *Versed [product information].* Nutley, NJ: Hoffmann-LaRoche; 1991.
169. Dundee JW et al. Midazolam: a review of its pharmacological properties and therapeutic use. *Drugs.* 1984;28:519-543.
170. Dundee JW et al. Variations in response to midazolam. *Br J Clin Pharmacol.* 1984;17:645-646.
171. Heizmann P et al. Pharmacokinetics and bioavailability of midazolam in man. *Br J Clin Pharmacol.* 1983;16:435-495.
172. Greenblatt DJ et al. Effect of age, gender, and obesity on midazolam kinetics. *Anesthesiology.* 1984;61:27-35.
173. Dundee JW, Wilson DB. Amnesia action of midazolam. *Anaesthesia.* 1980;35:459-461.
174. Knudsen L et al. The effects of midazolam on cerebral blood flow and oxygen consumption. *Anaesthesia.* 1990;45:1016-1019.
175. Nagelhout J et al. The effect of flumazenil on patient recovery and discharge following ambulatory surgery. *AANA J.* 1999;67:229-236.
176. Klotz V, Kanto J. Pharmacokinetics and clinical use of flumazenil. *Clin Pharmacokinet.* 1988;14:1-12.
177. Martens F et al. Clinical experience with the benzodiazepine antagonist flumazenil: suspected benzodiazepine or ethanol poisoning. *Clin Toxicol.* 1990;28:341-356.
178. Brogen RN, Goa KL. Flumazenil: a preliminary review of its benzodiazepine antagonist properties, intrinsic activity and therapeutic use. *Drugs.* 1988; 35:448-467.
179. Spivey WH. Flumazenil and seizures: analysis of 43 cases. *Clin Ther.* 1992; 14:292-305.

CHAPTER 11

LOCAL ANESTHETICS

John J. Nagelhout

Local anesthetics are drugs that reversibly block the conduction of electrical impulses along nerve fibers. Their ability to perform this function depends on various factors, including the microscopic and gross anatomy of the nerve being blocked and the physicochemical properties of the local anesthetics used. Anesthesia providers are primarily interested in the neural blocking effect this group of drugs has on the spinal cord, spinal nerve roots, and peripheral nerves.

Equally important in considering local anesthetics is the knowledge that absorption of these drugs into the circulation can produce significant systemic effects. The intrinsic potency and the fate of the drugs after absorption influence their ability to produce systemic effects and possible toxicity. Symptoms of toxicity can occur whether the drug is administered by local infiltration, intravenously, or regionally.

ANATOMY OF THE PERIPHERAL NERVE

The axon, an extension of a centrally located neuron, is the functional unit of peripheral nerves. A cell membrane, or axolemma, and intracellular contents, or axoplasm, are the major components of the axon. Schwann cells, whose functions are support and insulation, surround each axon. In unmyelinated nerves, single Schwann cells cover several axons. Conversely, in larger nerves the Schwann cell sheath covers only one axon and has several concentric layers of a liquid substance known as *myelin*.

Between Schwann cells are small segments of nerve that do not contain myelin. These areas, known as *nodes of Ranvier*, have limited diffusion barriers for drugs to penetrate and therefore may be the primary sites at which local anesthetics exert their action. In addition, these uncovered areas contain a large number of sodium (Na^+) channels; these channels are able to generate an action potential so intense that it can jump from node to node.[1] This phenomenon, known as *saltatory conduction*, significantly facilitates conduction speed along the axon.[2] Because of their better insulation, myelinated nerves are larger, conduct impulses faster, and are more difficult to block with local anesthetics than are unmyelinated nerves[3,4] (Figure 11-1).

Peripheral nerves have structures containing bundles of axons called *fasciculi*. Three layers of connective tissue—the endoneurium, perineurium, and epineurium—also are components of the peripheral nerve.[4,5] The endoneurium, which is a delicate connective tissue composed of longitudinally arranged collagen, surrounds and embeds the axons in the fasciculi. The perineurium,

which consists of layers of flattened, overlapping cells, binds a group of fascicles together. The epineurium, which surrounds the perineurium, is composed of areolar connective tissue that functionally holds the fascicles together to form the peripheral nerve.[5] These layers of connective tissue are important because they serve as barriers through which local anesthetics must diffuse if they are to exert their pharmacologic action (Figure 11-2).

NEURON ELECTROPHYSIOLOGY AND THE ACTION MECHANISM OF LOCAL ANESTHETICS

Electrophysiology

Measurement with an electrode placed in the axoplasm of a resting peripheral nerve demonstrates a negative membrane potential of -70 to -90 mV.[5,6] This voltage difference across the neuronal membrane at steady state is called the *resting membrane potential* (Figure 11-3). An ionic imbalance between the axoplasm and the extracellular fluid causes the electrical potential.[7,8] Several physiologic mechanisms create the ionic gradient; the primary one is an active, energy-dependent process executed by a sodium-potassium pump (Na^+-K^+ pump) located in the axolemma.[7,8]

Although the membrane is relatively permeable to the outward diffusion of K^+, an intracellular-to-extracellular K^+ ratio of 150:5 mmol, or 30:1, exists. An important contributor to this concentration difference is the impermeability of the membrane to other cotransported ions such as Na^+.[8] In addition, the movement of K^+ out of the neuron leaves an excess of intracellular negatively charged organic ions. The negative charge results in an electrostatic counterforce that limits K^+ movement out of the neuron.

Two opposing forces influence K^+ movement into and out of the neuron. First, a concentration gradient pushes K^+ outward. Second, an electrostatic gradient, created by the impermeability of the membrane to cations, tends to keep the K^+ in the cell. The net effect of these counterforces is modest movement of K^+ out of the cell, and this movement creates an intracellular negative charge. The Nernst equation expresses the charge created by the K^+ concentration gradient[9]:

Equation 11-1

$$\text{Membrane potential} = -58 \log \frac{(K^+ 30 \text{ inside})}{(K^+ \text{ outside})}$$

Determination of the resting membrane potential is not as simple as the Nernst equation for K^+ indicates, because Na^+ and chloride (Cl^-) ions have a minor role in establishing the intracellular resting potential.[6]

The author would like to thank Joe Williams for his contributions to this chapter in previous editions.

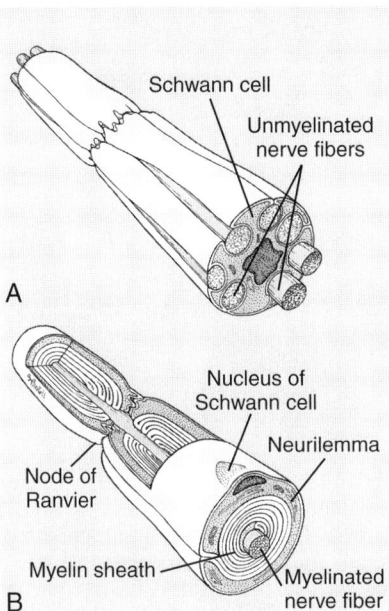

FIGURE **11-1**   **A,** Unmyelinated nerve fiber. **B,** Myelinated nerve fiber. Local anesthetics have better access to the axon at the node of Ranvier. (*From Thibodeau GA, Patton KT.* Anatomy & Physiology. *6th ed. St Louis: Mosby; 2007.*)

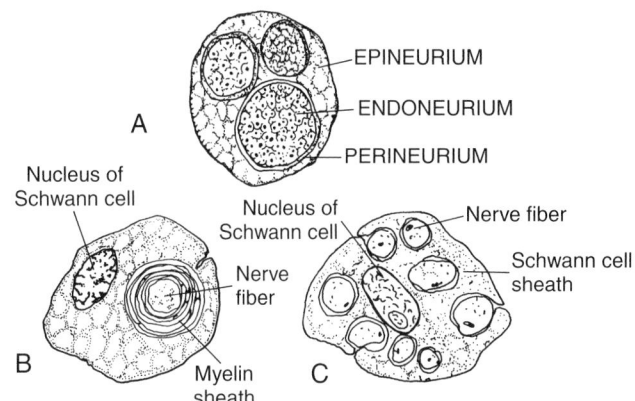

FIGURE **11-2**   Transverse sections of a peripheral nerve **(A)** showing the outermost epineurium; the inner perineurium, which collects nerve axons in fascicles; and the endoneurium, which surrounds each myelinated fiber **(B),** is encased in the multiple membranous wrappings of myelin formed by one Schwann cell, each of which stretches longitudinally over approximately 100 times the diameter of the axon. The narrow span of axon between these myelinated segments, the node of Ranvier, contains the ion channels that support action potentials. Nonmyelinated fibers **(C)** are enclosed in bundles of 5 to 10 axons by a chain of Schwann cells that tightly embrace each axon with but one layer of membrane. (*From Miller RD.* Miller's Anesthesia. *6th ed. Vol 1. Philadelphia: Churchill Livingstone; 2005.*)

When an electrical impulse is applied to a resting nerve, the membrane potential is reversed because of the intracellular movement of Na^+. This occurs because of the higher concentration of Na^+ outside the cell and the stimulation-induced increase in membrane permeability to this ion. The sudden influx of Na^+ that occurs in response to stimulation overrides the efflux of K^+ directed at maintaining the resting membrane potential. Once the process has reversed the membrane potential to 20 mV, an outward electrochemical gradient develops; this gradient resists the concentration-dependent, inward diffusion of Na^+.[5] This state of equilibrium causes the Na^+ channels to close. Shortly after Na^+ enters the cell, K^+ channels begin to open, and the ion rapidly diffuses out of the neuron, according to its concentration gradient. The active removal of intracellular Na^+ by the Na^+-K^+ pump and the passive diffusion of K^+ outward restore the resting membrane potential. During repolarization, three Na^+ ions leave the cell for each two K^+ ions that enter[10] (Figure 11-4).

The sequence of events that results in an action potential results from the passage of ions through pores, or "channels," located in the axolemma. These channels, which are composed of globular proteins, have transmural orientation to the phospholipid molecules that constitute the axolemma.[11] Although K^+ and calcium (Ca^{2+}) channels are important, the Na^+ channels are the most significant and best understood with respect to the initiation and propagation of the action potential.[12-14]

Mechanism of Action

Sodium channels have three functional states: resting (closed), open, and inactive. The resting state exists when the membrane

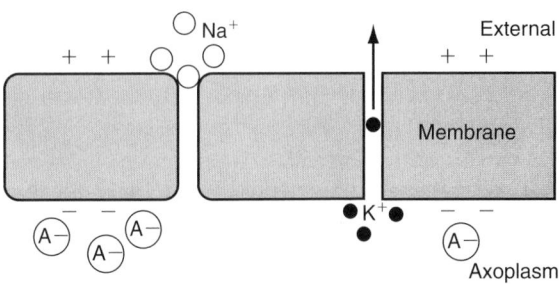

FIGURE **11-3**   In the polarized resting state, the membrane is permeable to the movement of potassium (K^+) out of the axon (*closed circles*) and impermeable to the influx of sodium (Na^+) into the cell (*open circles*). The selective movement of the positively charged cation K^+ out of the cell results in an intracellular negative charge. (*From de Jong RH.* Local Anesthesia. *St Louis: Mosby; 1994:29.*)

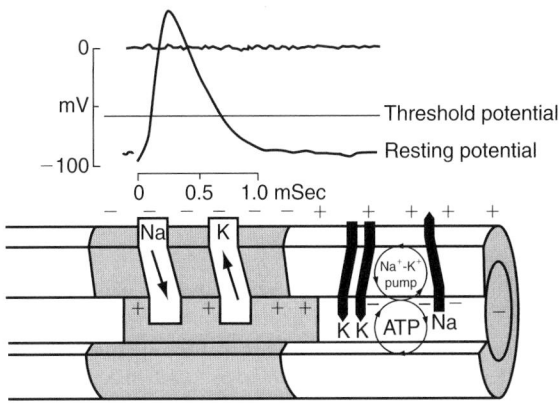

FIGURE **11-4**   Local anesthetic mechanism of action and clinical use. (*From Covino BG, Vassallo HG.* Local Anesthetics: Mechanism of Action and Clinical Use. *New York: Grune & Stratton; 1976:20.*)

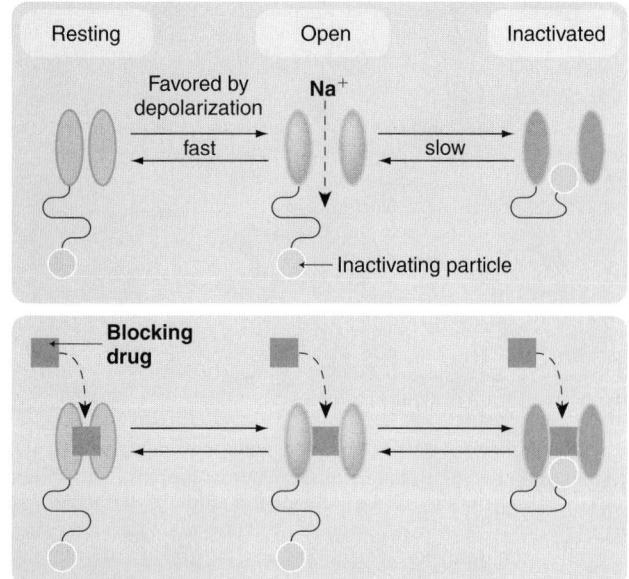

FIGURE **11-5** Resting, activated, and inactivated states of voltage-gated channels, exemplified by the sodium channel. Membrane depolarization causes a rapid transition from the resting (closed) state to the open state. The inactivating particle (part of the intracellular domain of the channel protein) is then able to block the channel. Blocking drugs (e.g., local anesthetics and antiepileptic drugs) often show preference for one of the three channel states, and thus affect the kinetic behavior of the channels, with implications for their clinical application. (*From Rang HP et al. Rang and Dale's Pharmacology. 6th ed. Edinburgh: Churchill Livingstone; 2007.*)

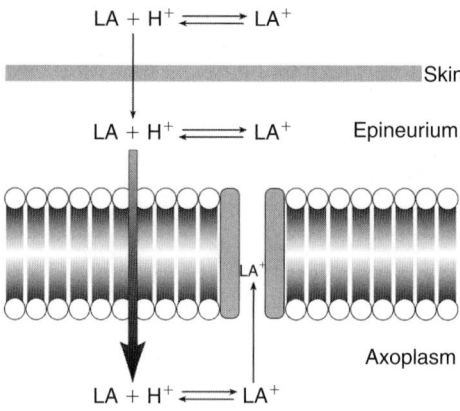

FIGURE **11-6** Schematic conceptualization of local anesthetic action. Equilibrium forms outside the nerve between the ionized and nonionized portions. The nonionized portion (*LA*), which is lipid soluble, enters the nerve. Once inside the axoplasm, the drug re-equilibrates, and the ionized fraction (*LA⁺*) attaches to the local anesthetic receptor on the inside of the sodium channel. *LA*, Nonionized form of the local anesthetic; *LA⁺*, ionized form.

polarizes to its resting potential. When a nerve is stimulated, reversal of the membrane potential occurs until the threshold potential is reached. When this happens, a conformational change in the proteins that compose the channel occurs; this results in the open state. An inactive state, characterized by the return of the Na^+ channel to an impermeable state, follows the open state. This state, which prevents initiation of an action potential, lasts until the restoration of the resting membrane potential.[12] At distal and central terminals, the inhibition of voltage-gated Ca^{2+} channels by local anesthetics will suppress neurogenic inflammation and the release of neurotransmitters. Actions on receptors that contribute to nociceptive transduction, such as TRPV1 (transient receptor potential vanilloid subfamily 1) and the bradykinin B2 receptor, provide an independent mode of analgesia. In the spinal cord, where local anesthetics are present during epidural or intrathecal anesthesia, inhibition by the anesthetics of inotropic receptors such as those for glutamate further interferes with neuronal transmission. Activation of spinal cord mitogen-activated protein (MAP) kinases, which are essential for the hyperalgesia following injury or incision and occur in both neurons and glia, is inhibited by spinal local anesthetics[13] (Figure 11-5).

Local anesthetics produce their effects by blocking Na^+ channels. The following four possible mechanisms of action have been suggested:

1. One theory postulates that local anesthetics produce their effect by displacing Ca^{2+} from the axolemma. According to this theory, Ca^{2+} controls Na^+ permeability in the axolemma.
2. Investigators have suggested that local anesthetics produce their effects by altering the membrane surface charge. Such changes

in charge could hyperpolarize the membrane or influence the process of repolarization.
3. Because local anesthetics are relatively lipophilic molecules, they could "dissolve" into the axolemma, resulting in membrane expansion. Such conformational changes in the membrane could result in distortion and closure of the Na^+ channel.
4. Although all of the aforementioned effects may influence the mechanism of action of local anesthetics, at present these theories do not have as much support in the literature as the specific receptor theory. The specific receptor theory states that local anesthetics block the propagation of the action potential by binding reversibly to specific receptors within or adjacent to the internal opening of the Na^+ channel.[2] Studies have indicated that these receptors, located on the intracellular side of the cell membrane, have a greater affinity for the charged or protonated form of the local anesthetics.[12,15] Consequently, local anesthetics must first penetrate the cell membrane before they produce their effects. This penetration is greatly facilitated if the drug is in the uncharged or un-ionized state.

Figure 11-6 shows the penetration of local anesthetic into a nerve.

Studies indicate that local anesthetics have a greater tendency to bind to receptors in the open or inactive state (phasic or frequency-dependent block). This finding is referred to as the *Modulated Receptor Hypothesis* of local anesthetic action. The open or inactive state may increase the affinity for binding, the physical access of the drug to the receptor, or both.[13,16] Because of this preference, local anesthetics are more likely to block rapidly firing nerves than nerves in which action potentials are less frequent. Compared with motor fibers, sensory fibers often fire at greater frequencies; hence, sensory blockade occurs before motor blockade with a given concentration of a local anesthetic.[7] This may be one of the factors that influence the "margin of safety," as discussed under the topic of differential block in the next section. The following is a summary of possible events that lead to neural blockade with the use of local anesthetics:

1. Local anesthetics gain access to the interior of the neuron. This occurs by the diffusion of neutral, uncharged molecules across the cell membrane.

2. Both charged and neutral molecules bind to the receptor located on the cytoplasm side of the Na^+ channel (however, the protonated moiety has a greater binding affinity than the neutral molecule).

3. Local anesthetics bind more readily to open or inactive channels than to resting channels. This type of binding prevents the channels from returning to the resting or repolarized state, which results in blockade.[11]

In addition, there have been some indications that the uncharged base form of a drug may produce an effect by interacting with the ion channel from within the lipid membrane. The receptor-membrane interface is probably the binding site for this type of interaction.[17] This site is probably responsible for the local anesthetic action of benzocaine, which exists only in the uncharged state. However, with most local anesthetics, this site of action is not thought to be as important as the interaction with the intraneuronal receptors.

Wynn has indicated that local anesthetics have actions other than those directly involved with the Na^+ channel in the axolemma. Wynn's research has focused on substance P, a pain transmitter located in the dorsal horn of the spinal cord. This polypeptide transmitter is released by neurons in the spinal cord and binds to adjacent receptors to produce pain and inflammation. This finding indicates that localanesthetics prevent binding of substance P to its spinal cord receptor, blocking nociceptive responses. Wynn suggests that this is not a factor when these agents are used for infiltration or nerve block, but it does suggest a more analgesic property of local anesthetics.[18] The prevention of substance-P binding may explain why local anesthetics administered by intravenous infusion are effective in the attenuation of postoperative pain.

Minimum Blocking Concentration and Differential Block

Important to local anesthetic action is the scientific concept related to minimum blocking concentration (C_{min}) and differential block. The C_{min} for local anesthetics can be defined as the lowest concentration of drug that is needed for blocking impulse propagation.[10] This parameter is analogous to minimum alveolar concentration (MAC), which is used for designating the potency of inhalation anesthetics. However, the determination of these values differs in that MAC is experimentally determined in vivo, whereas C_{min} is determined through in vitro in studies on isolated nerves. Experimentally, the C_{min} value can vary, depending on the temperature, pH, or Ca^{2+} concentration of the bathing solution.[19-21] Also important, C_{min} varies significantly with the type of nerve being studied.

In actual clinical use versus experiments on isolated nerves, the C_{min} for local anesthetics is significantly greater in vivo than in vitro.[22] This is because several factors can influence the amount of drug that comes into contact with neuronal tissue once the drug has been injected into tissue. These factors include drug movement away from the site of action, dilution, systemic absorption, and degradation.[22]

It has been observed clinically that nerves functionally have different sensitivity or rates of effect when exposed to local anesthetics. For example, loss of autonomic function occurs first, followed in sequence by perception of superficial pain, touch, and temperature, motor function, and proprioception.[10] This phenomenon is termed differential block. Seen clinically, an excellent example of differential block occurs with the use of bupivacaine. When administered epidurally for labor pain, this local anesthetic spares motor function while providing adequate analgesia.

Essential to the understanding of differential block is the concept that the diameter and myelination of nerve fibers may influence the sensitivity to local anesthetics. For simplicity, nerve fibers are separated into three groups—A, B, and C—on the basis of diameter.[23,24]

The A fibers are further divided into four subgroups known as alpha, beta, gamma, and delta fibers. The alpha fibers are the largest in diameter (15 to 20 µm) and the most heavily myelinated; they have the fastest conduction velocity of all the fibers, including B and C fibers.[10] Alpha fibers are responsible for motor functions and proprioception. The A beta and A gamma fibers have similar diameters (4 to 15 µm) and have conduction velocities second only to A alpha fibers. The A beta fibers provide motor function, touch, and pressure sensation; the A gamma fibers innervate muscle spindles and are responsible for reflexes.[10] The A delta fibers provide pain and temperature sensation. These fibers have a smaller diameter (3 to 4 µm) and slower conduction velocity than other A fibers. The beta, gamma, and delta fibers are all myelinated to a similar extent.[10]

B fibers have a similar diameter (4 µm) to A delta fibers; however, they exhibit slower conduction velocity and less myelination than the A fibers. These fibers constitute the preganglionic autonomic nerves. The C fibers, which conduct pain and temperature impulses, are the smallest of all fibers (1 to 2 µm) and have the slowest speed of conduction. These are the only fibers that are unmyelinated.[10]

It was first believed that nerve fiber diameter was the sole determinant of differential blockade.[25] This assumption came from the results of isolated in vitro studies performed only on myelinated nerves. Subsequent isolated studies on the small, unmyelinated C fibers revealed that they were more resistant to blockade than the larger A delta or B fibers.[10]

This apparent inconsistency can possibly be explained by the concept of conduction safety. This concept refers to the voltage change needed for the propagation of the action potential along the nerve. This voltage change is significantly greater than the action potential threshold and provides a safety factor for impulse conduction. Gissen and co-workers defined this safety factor as the "ratio between the magnitude of the action potential and the magnitude of the critical membrane potential." Research has indicated that the margin of safety for transmission is greater in small, slow fibers than in large, fast fibers.[26]

Lastly, differential block may be influenced by the rate of diffusion of local anesthetic molecules across multilayered lipoprotein membranes of the myelin sheath. For example, the clinical resistance to blockade observed in A fibers may be the result of a slower onset resulting from a greater diffusion barrier. As discussed in more detail later, diffusion can be influenced by such factors as the pK_a and the concentration of the local anesthetic, as well as the pH of the surrounding tissue and nerve fiber.[26]

As the preceding discussion indicates, the concept of differential block is more complex than originally proposed. Future research will probably indicate that an isolated mechanism does not explain this phenomenon, but rather several factors interact to produce the effect.

CHEMICAL STRUCTURE OF LOCAL ANESTHETICS

The local anesthetics used clinically for neural blockade are significantly similar in chemical structure. The molecules of these drugs have three characteristic segments: (1) an intermediate carbon group separates (2) an unsaturated (aromatic) ring

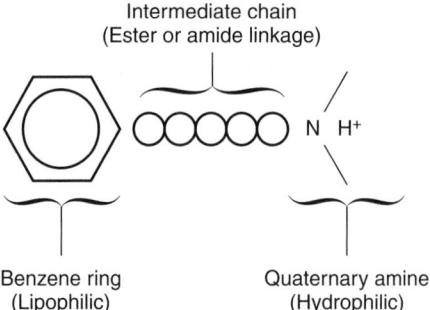

FIGURE **11-7** Core structure for local anesthetics, which includes a benzene ring and a quaternary amine separated by an intermediate carbon group. The bond between the benzene ring and the carbon group determines whether the drug is an amide or an ester. *(From Carpenter RL, Mackey DC. Local anesthetics. In: Barash GP et al, eds. Clinical Anesthesia. 2nd ed. Philadelphia: Lippincott Williams & Wilkins; 1989:510. Reprinted with permission.)*

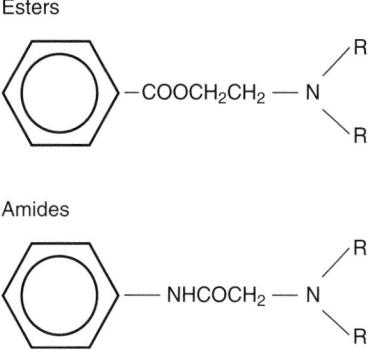

FIGURE **11-8** Representative chemical formula for ester and amide local anesthetic drugs.

system from (3) a tertiary amine (Figure 11-7). The aromatic ring provides lipophilic characteristics, whereas the quaternary amine gives hydrophilicity to the molecule. One reason the quaternary amine is hydrophilic is that this part of the molecule is partially charged at physiologic pH.

Chemically, local anesthetics do have one major difference in their core structure. Either an ester or an amide linkage binds the aromatic ring to the carbon group. This linkage is responsible for the classification of these drugs as either esters or amides. The type of linkage is important clinically because it has implications for metabolism and allergic potential (Figure 11-8). Box 11-1 classifies local anesthetics according to this bond. The chemical structures are important in determining these drugs' pharmacologic effects. Minor chemical alterations to drugs within these two "bond-related" groups can result in significant changes in drug potency, speed of onset, and duration of action[5,27] (Figure 11-9). These changes are discussed in detail as the specific pharmacologic factors associated with local anesthetics are noted.

PHARMACODYNAMICS AND PHARMACOKINETIC CONCEPTS

An important difference to note when describing the pharmacokinetics of local anesthetics is intuitive yet bears discussion.

BOX **11-1**

Ester and Amide Local Anesthetics

Esters	Amides
Procaine	Lidocaine
Chloroprocaine	Mepivacaine
Tetracaine	Prilocaine
Cocaine	Bupivacaine
	Levobupivacaine
	Ropivacaine
	Etidocaine
	Articaine

Unlike most medications, these agents are meant to remain localized in the area of injection or application. The higher the concentration (number of molecules) of drug injected that remain in the area of the nerve or nerves to be blocked, the faster the onset of action. If multiple nerves are being blocked a greater intensity may also be evident. Therefore, systemic absorption away from the deposition site results in the offset and termination of drug effect, rather than the onset as with most other drugs. Factors that affect absorption, such as the vascularity and blood flow of the injection area, lipid and protein binding, and addition of vasoconstrictors, greatly influence duration of action. The same local anesthetic dose and concentration injected in different areas of the body, with or without added epinephrine, can result in vastly different durations of action. Absorption also influences toxicity. The slower a local anesthetic is systemically absorbed, the less likely that high blood levels and therefore central nervous system (CNS) or cardiac toxicity will result. Drug metabolism and elimination more readily "keep up" with absorption, ensuring that toxic blood levels are avoided. A conceptual kinetic depiction of the fate of an injected local anesthetic is given in Figure 11-10.

Potency

There is a strong relationship between the lipid solubility of local anesthetics and their potency.[22,26,27] This finding is understandable, considering that the axolemma and myelin sheath are composed primarily of lipids[27,28]; therefore, lipid-soluble drugs can pass easily through the nerve membrane. Larger, more lipid-soluble local anesthetics are relatively water insoluble, highly protein bound in blood, and less readily washed out from nerves. They bind to Na^+ channels with a higher affinity than agents with lower lipid solubility. Increased lipid solubility correlates with increased protein binding, increased potency, longer duration of action and a higher tendency for severe cardiac toxicity.[27] It follows that fewer molecules or lower concentrations of these drugs are required for the production of blockade than if non–lipid-soluble anesthetics are used.[29] Changes in either the aromatic or amine moieties of the local anesthetic molecule can affect the lipid-water partition coefficient. In the amide series, for example, the addition of a butyl group to the amine end of mepivacaine leads to the formation of bupivacaine. Bupivacaine is 35-fold as lipid soluble and fourfold as potent as mepivacaine. In the case of the esters, the addition of a butyl group to the aromatic end of procaine produces tetracaine, which is considerably more lipid soluble and potent than procaine.[9]

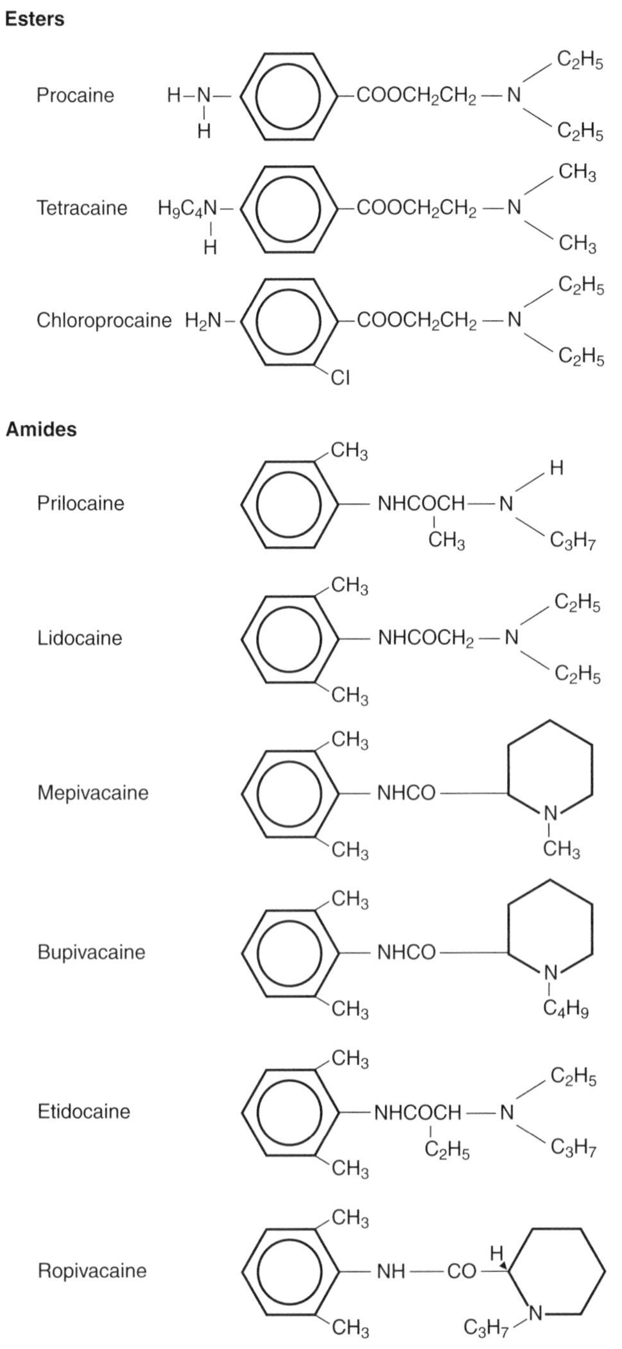

Esters

Procaine

Tetracaine

Chloroprocaine

Amides

Prilocaine

Lidocaine

Mepivacaine

Bupivacaine

Etidocaine

Ropivacaine

FIGURE **11-9** Chemical structure of the most commonly used local anesthetics. Note the chemical substitutions on the benzene ring and the amine end of the molecules. (*Modified with permission from Longnecker DE, Murphy FL. Introduction to Anesthesia. 9th ed. Philadelphia: Saunders; 1997:204.*)

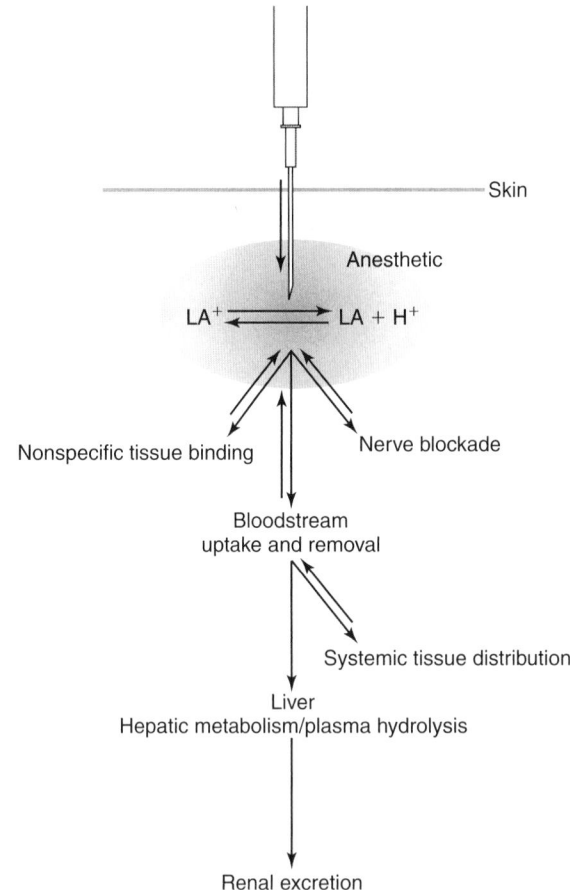

FIGURE **11-10** Representation of the fate of a local anesthetic injected into tissue.

similar potencies. This may be explained by the fact that lidocaine has greater vasodilating properties than prilocaine and therefore may be absorbed away more rapidly; this means that less drug is available for interaction with the neuron.[31]

Duration of Action

The duration of action of local anesthetics demonstrates a relationship to protein binding and lipid solubility.[9,27,32] In theory, drugs that have a high affinity for protein and lipids attach more firmly to these substances in the vicinity of the Na^+ channel receptor. This means that the drug remains in the channel for a longer time, producing prolonged conduction blockade[27] (Figure 11-11).

The addition of larger chemical radicals to the amide or aromatic end of the drugs results in greater protein binding. The duration is directly proportional to plasma protein binding, presumably because the local anesthetic receptor on the neural membrane is also composed of protein.[5,6,33] It has been posited that local anesthetics that have increased protein-binding properties (e.g., etidocaine 95%, ropivacaine 94%, bupivacaine 97%, levobupivacaine 97%) produce longer-duration anesthesia as a consequence of more efficient binding of the anesthetic to the Na^+ ion channel.[34] For example, bupivacaine and etidocaine are more than 90% bound to plasma protein; however, their homologues, mepivacaine and lidocaine, are only 65% to 75% bound, respectively.[32] The duration of action of bupivacaine and etidocaine is significantly longer than for mepivacaine or lidocaine.

Factors other than lipid solubility can affect potency. For example, the potency of local anesthetics as demonstrated in isolated in vitro studies is not always the same as that observed in vivo. The discrepancy between in vitro and in vivo findings may be the result of many factors, including the vascular and tissue distribution properties of the drug.[30] For example, the results of in vitro studies show that lidocaine is twice as potent as prilocaine; however, clinical use indicates that they have

The lipid solubility of these drugs was discussed earlier in this chapter.

As in the case of potency, the effect local anesthetics have on the vasculature at the injection site influences the duration of action. This is discussed in detail in the section on vasomotor action and absorption.

Onset of Action

As stated previously, local anesthetics must diffuse through the axolemma before they can interact with receptors. How readily they diffuse through the nerve membrane depends on their chemical structure, lipid solubility, and state of ionization. Of these, ionization is the most important, because the charged form of a drug does not penetrate membranes well.[28,30,33]

Local anesthetics are bases and therefore proton acceptors. As with all bases, a drug's pK_a is the pH at which 50% of the drug is in the charged form while the remaining half is uncharged. A basic drug becomes predominantly ionized if it is placed in an environment with a pH that is significantly less than its pK_a. Therefore drugs that have a greater pK_a are ionized to a greater extent at body pH than those with a lower pK_a. For example, if lidocaine (pK_a 7.74) is placed in plasma (pH 7.4), 65% of the drug is ionized and 35% remains un-ionized.

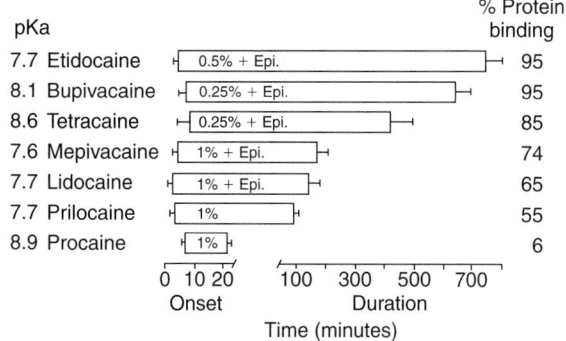

FIGURE **11-11**   The relationship between pK_a and onset of action, as well as protein binding and duration of action. (*From Covino BG. Clinical pharmacology of local anesthetic agents. In: Cousins MJ, Bridenbaugh PO, eds.* Neural Blockade. *Philadelphia: Lippincott Williams & Wilkins; 1988:115. Reprinted with permission.*)

Similarly, if tetracaine (pK_a 8.6) is placed in plasma, 95% of the drug becomes ionized and 5% remains un-ionized.[27]

Because their ionization is less, local anesthetics with lower pK_a (7.6 to 7.8), such as lidocaine, mepivacaine, prilocaine, and etidocaine, tend to have a more rapid onset of action than drugs with a greater pK_a (8.1 to 8.6), such as bupivacaine, tetracaine, and procaine. Chloroprocaine is one exception; it has a high pK_a and a rapid onset, probably because the clinical use of high concentrations of the drug attenuates the ionization effect.[27] In general, the onset of anesthesia slows with increasing local anesthetic lipid solubility. Some researchers downplay the role of pK_a on onset.[27]

These properties are beneficial in the classification of local anesthetics. The classification presented in Table 11-1 assists in the selection of the appropriate drug with respect to pharmacokinetic properties and toxicity.[35]

Vasomotor Action and Absorption

All local anesthetics except cocaine and ropivacaine produce relaxation of vascular smooth muscle.[31] The resultant vasodilation increases blood flow to the tissue, where the drug is deposited. This results in an increase in the drug's absorption, which limits its duration of action and increases the probability of toxic effects. It is interesting to note that ropivacaine is the only parenterally administered local anesthetic with vasoconstrictive properties.[2] This factor is related to its longer duration of action and lower toxicity when compared with other local anesthetics.[36] Cocaine also has vasoconstrictive properties because of its ability to block reuptake of norepinephrine. It is used only topically.

As indicated previously, not all local anesthetics have the same ability to produce vasodilation. For example, lidocaine is a more potent vasodilator than mepivacaine or prilocaine.[31] This may explain why lidocaine has a slightly shorter duration of action when compared with other drugs with an intermediate duration of action. Bupivacaine, etidocaine, and levobupivacaine have equal vasodilating properties and produce a longer duration of vasodilation when compared with intermediate-acting drugs.[31]

The speed of absorption and entry into the systemic circulation obviously has significant implications for toxicity. Absorption of drugs occurs most rapidly after intercostal blocks, followed by caudal-lumbar epidural, brachial plexus, sciatic-femoral, and

TABLE **11-1**	Classification of Local Anesthetics Based on Onset, Duration of Action, and Potency				
Characteristics	**Drug**	**Common Name**	**Relative Potency***	**Onset**	**Duration of Action (min)**
Low potency, short duration of action	Procaine	Novocain	1	Slow	60-90
	Chloroprocaine	Nesacaine	1	Fast	30-60
Intermediate potency, duration	Mepivacaine	Carbocaine	2	Fast	120-240
	Prilocaine	Citanest	2	Fast	120-240
	Lidocaine	Xylocaine	2	Fast	90-200
High potency, long duration	Tetracaine	Pontocaine	8	Slow	180-600
	Bupivacaine	Marcaine, Sensorcaine	9	Intermediate	180-600
	Etidocaine	Duranest	6	Fast	180-600
	Ropivacaine	Naropin	10	Slow	180-600
	Levobupivacaine	Chirocaine	9	Slow	180-600

Modified from Covino BG. Pharmacology of local anesthetics. Res Staff Physician. *June 1982. Modified with permission from Resident and Staff Physician (June 1982) by Romaine Pierson Publishers, Inc; and Mosby's Drug Consult. St Louis: Mosby; 2007.*
*On a milligram-for-milligram basis with procaine, 1 mg.

subcutaneous blocks. Table 11-2 shows the approximate peak plasma levels after lidocaine injection (400 mg) for intercostal versus brachial block.[8] These data indicate that toxicity probably occurs more frequently after intercostal block than after brachial plexus block if the dose administered is the same.

The total dose of local anesthetic, rather than the volume or concentration, linearly determines the peak plasma concentration.[37] For example, 400 mg of lidocaine yields the same peak plasma concentration regardless of whether 40 mL of a 1% or 80 mL of a 0.5%

Local anesthetic additives include α_1- and α_2-adrenergic agonists, opioids, sodium bicarbonate, ketorolac, and hyaluronidase. These are variously added to increase the safety, quality, intensity, duration, and rate of onset of anesthesia, as well as reduce blood loss. Epinephrine is added to constrict vessels and serve as a marker for intravascular injection. Alpha$_2$-adrenergic agonists have local anesthetic properties and alter pharmacodynamics.[27]

The addition of a vasoconstrictor (e.g., epinephrine) to local anesthetics can reduce the rate of vascular absorption. The availability of the drug is increased for neuronal uptake, resulting in a longer and more profound block. Of importance, the slower rate of absorption also attenuates the peak plasma concentration of the drug, thereby reducing systemic toxicity. The magnitude of this effect depends on the drug, dose, and concentration of both the local anesthetic and the vasoconstrictor, as well as the site of injection.[8] For example, addition of epinephrine to mepivacaine prolongs the time to maximum arterial plasma drug concentration in all situations; however, a 2% solution used for an intercostal block has the greatest effect.[38]

Epinephrine does not prolong the duration of blockade to the same extent with all local anesthetics. For example, it prolongs the duration for local infiltration, peripheral nerve block, and epidural anesthesia with procaine, mepivacaine, and lidocaine.[28,39-42] Recent research indicates that adding epinephrine to lidocaine solutions increases the intensity and duration of block.[42] The early increase in intensity is not matched with an increase in intraneural lidocaine content at these early times, although the prolonged duration of block by epinephrine appears to correspond to an enlarged lidocaine content in nerve at later times, as if a very slowly emptying "effector compartment" received a larger share of the dose. The increase in early analgesia without increased lidocaine content may be explained by a pharmacodynamic action of epinephrine that transiently enhances lidocaine's potency, but also by a pharmacokinetic effect that alters the distribution of the same net content of lidocaine within the nerve. In the case of prilocaine, bupivacaine, and etidocaine, infiltration and peripheral nerve blocks are prolonged with epinephrine, whereas no significant effect occurs with epidural anesthesia.[43] The rationale for this discrepancy might be that epidural fat significantly absorbs ropivacaine, bupivacaine, and etidocaine, owing to their lipid solubility. These drugs are released slowly from the fat depot, which could prolong the block.[41,43-45] This process overrides the effects of epinephrine on duration of action. In addition, the drug concentration can contribute to the differential effect seen with epinephrine. For example, epinephrine can prolong epidural blocks with 0.125% or 0.25% bupivacaine when used in patients in labor.[44,45] Conversely, epinephrine has less effect with the epidural administration of 0.5% or 0.75% bupivacaine.[46]

The addition of epinephrine does not attenuate the peak plasma level of all local anesthetics; for example, epinephrine significantly reduces the peak plasma concentration of lidocaine

TABLE 11-2	Peak Plasma Concentration of Lidocaine (400 mg) with Intercostal versus Brachial Plexus Block	
Site of Injection	**Peak Plasma Level**	
Intercostal	7 g/mL	
Brachial plexus	3 g/mL	

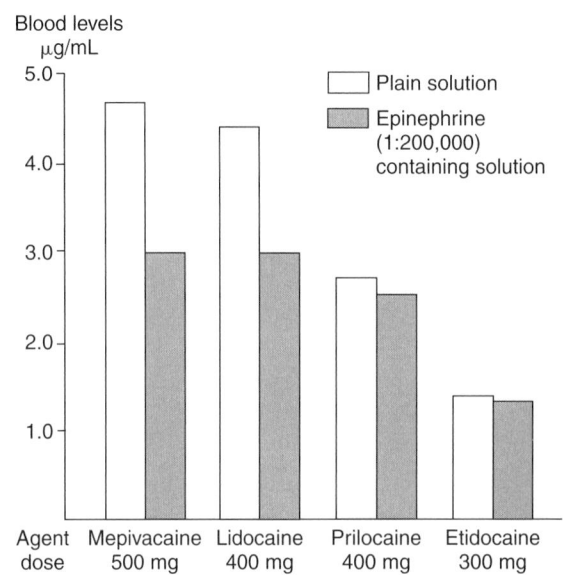

FIGURE **11-12** Peak plasma levels of local anesthetics injected into the epidural space with and without epinephrine. (*From Covino BG, Vassallo HG. Local Anesthetics: Mechanism of Action and Clinical Use. New York: Grune & Stratton; 1976:97.*)

and mepivacaine, regardless of the site of administration. On the other hand, epinephrine does not significantly affect the peak plasma level of prilocaine, bupivacaine, or etidocaine after epidural anesthesia. The lack of effect seen with prilocaine may be explained by its slower absorption and rapid tissue redistribution. In the case of bupivacaine and etidocaine, it may be explained by the significant lipid solubility and uptake of these drugs in epidural adipose tissue[26] (Figure 11-12).

Studies that have compared vasoconstrictors conclude that epinephrine is superior to drugs such as phenylephrine and norepinephrine in producing vasoconstriction with local anesthetics.[47,48] The usual concentration of epinephrine used for this purpose is 1:200,000 or 5 mcg/mL.

Miscellaneous Factors That Influence Onset and Duration

Local anesthetics are basic drugs. As discussed previously, they have both water- and lipid-soluble properties. Factors that raise the pH of their environment increase their lipid solubility, and, conversely, lower pH environments result in increased water solubility. These changes to pH result in altered proportions of lipid-water soluble fractions of the drugs, which may have clinical consequences. At times, the term used for this phenomenon is *ion trapping*. Ion trapping results from changes in pH in

BOX 11-2

Ion Trapping: Clinical Situations in Which Differences Between pK$_a$ and pH May Affect Patient Response

- In the event of local anesthetic overdose, associated respiratory depression may occur, resulting in hypoxia and acidosis. The acidosis resulting from hypoxia may increase the ionized fraction of local anesthetic within the cerebral circulation, thereby decreasing the ability of the anesthetic to cross the blood-brain barrier, leave the brain, and reenter the systemic circulation. This phenomenon may prolong and enhance the central nervous system toxicity of local anesthetics.
- Local anesthetic accumulation in the fetal circulation is enhanced by the fact that fetal pH is lower than maternal pH, which may result in high fetal levels of local anesthetics.
- Local anesthetics injected into acidotic, infected tissues are rendered ineffective because of the loss of lipid solubility. The lipid solubility of local anesthetics is diminished in an acidotic environment because of an increased concentration of the ionized, water-soluble form of the drug. The loss of lipid solubility prevents absorption into the nerve, thereby preventing access to the site of action.
- Carbonation of local anesthetics speeds the onset and intensity of action of neural blockade. Carbon dioxide readily diffuses into the nerve, lowering the pH within the nerve. The lipid-soluble form of local anesthetic, after passing through the neuronal membrane, receives protons from the intraneuronal environment and ionizes. An increase in the ionized fraction within the neuron produces a higher concentration of the active form of the anesthetic available at the sodium channel, the site of action.
- Commercially available local anesthetics are prepared in a slightly acidic formulation that improves the stability of the drug by increasing the concentration of the ionized, water-soluble form of the drug. Addition of sodium bicarbonate to the local anesthetic mixture increases the pH of the solution, thereby increasing the concentration of the un-ionized, lipid soluble form of the drug. Improving the lipid solubility of the local anesthetic improves diffusion of the local anesthetic through the neuronal membrane, leading to a more rapid onset of action.

relationship to the agent's pK$_a$. Instances in which ion trapping may have clinical consequences are noted in Box 11-2.

Local anesthetics have been carbonated to speed onset. In isolated nerve preparations, carbonation gives a more rapid onset and greater intensity of block.[49] Diffusion of carbon dioxide through the nerve membrane can lower the intracellular pH. When local anesthetics accompany this process, they become more ionized within the neuron; this results in an increase in the concentration of the drug in the protonated form at the intracellular binding site.

Controversy exists concerning whether carbonation improves onset time in the in vivo situation.[50] Separate double-blind studies of lidocaine and bupivacaine have failed to yield positive results.[51] This inconsistency may exist because the injected carbon dioxide is rapidly buffered in vivo, so intracellular pH is not greatly affected.[50,51]

The addition of sodium bicarbonate to local anesthetics may reduce the latency of onset and increase the duration of action.[52,53] In theory, this would increase the pH of the local anesthetic solution, resulting in the presence of more drug in the nonionized state. As stated previously, this form of the drug readily diffuses across the cell membranes and could decrease the latency of onset. Studies done with bupivacaine and lidocaine have indicated that this alteration does facilitate the onset and duration of action.[52,53]

The major limitation to the addition of bicarbonate is the precipitation that can occur in the local anesthetic solution. Table 11-3 indicates the propensity for precipitation, which depends significantly on the local anesthetic and whether the solution contains epinephrine. It also should be noted that the amount of bicarbonate that can be added without precipitation depends on whether the epinephrine is commercially or "freshly" mixed.[52] Manufacturers acidify local anesthetic solutions to increase solubility and stability (the free base is more susceptible to photodegradation and aldehyde formation), which results in a longer shelf-life. For example, the pH range of plain lidocaine is 6.5 to 6.8, compared with 3.5 to 4.5 for preparations that contain epinephrine. The lower pH is used with epinephrine because of the instability of this compound in alkaline solutions. Adjusting alkalization to prevent precipitation can be accomplished with the proposed mixing regimens for bicarbonate and local anesthetics shown in Table 11-3.[54]

Another benefit of alkalization is that it may result in less pain on injection. The mechanism of action for this effect could be more complex than just an increase in pH. It may be that the nociceptive nerve fibers may not be as sensitive to the un-ionized form of the drug. It also is possible that the un-ionized drug diffuses so rapidly through the tissue and axolemma that a sensory block occurs almost instantaneously.[55,56]

The addition of dextran to local anesthetics may increase their duration of action.[57,58] Studies indicate that this alteration does not consistently prolong the block. Animal studies demonstrate that dextran is effective if the pH of the solution is high (pH 8).[59]

The addition of hyaluronidase to local anesthetics facilitates the spread of the drugs in the tissue. This additive accomplishes the effect via the hydrolysis of hyaluronic acid, which is a polysaccharide that inhibits the diffusion of foreign substances within the interstitial tissue. Also, it has been suggested that hyaluronidase reduces hematoma size if a needle that is used with the regional technique punctures a major blood vessel. The addition of hyaluronidase can result in certain undesirable effects, such as the initiation of allergic reactions, a shortening of the duration of anesthetic action, and an increase in drug toxicity.[60] Nevertheless, some clinicians still use the drug with local anesthetics for certain regional techniques in an attempt to improve the success rate and onset of action.

Clinicians mix local anesthetics to obtain a more rapid onset and a longer duration of action. For example, a chloroprocaine and bupivacaine mixture might yield a rapid onset because of the former and a prolonged duration because of the latter. Studies exploring these combinations have yielded conflicting results.[61,62] This combination probably does yield a faster onset; however, the duration of action is shorter than that seen with only bupivacaine.[56]

TABLE 11-3	Sodium Bicarbonate and Local Anesthetic Mixtures		
Local Anesthetic	**Concentration(%)**	**HCO$_3^-$ (mL/20 mL)***	**pH after Addition of HCO$_3^-$**
2-Chloroprocaine	2	4	7.51
	3	4	7.43
Mepivacaine	1	4	7.26
	1.5	2	7
Etidocaine	1	0.015	5.90
	1 + epi[†]	0.100	5.73
	1 + epi[‡]	0.015	5.85
	1.5 + epi[†]	0.100	5.76
Bupivacaine	0.25	0.10	6.97
	0.5	0.05	6.62
	0.5 + epi[†]	0.30	6.37
	0.5 + epi	0.05	6.78
	0.75	0.05	6.56
	0.75 + epi	0.30	6.32
	0.75 + epi[‡]	0.05	6.58
Lidocaine	1	4	7.43
	1 + epi[†]	4	7.21
	1 + epi[‡]	4	7.37
	1.5	4	7.31
	1.5 + epi[†]	4	7.16
	1.5 + epi[‡]	4	7.35
	2	4	7.24
	2 + epi[†]	4	7.08
	2 + epi[‡]	4	7.26

Modified from Peterfreund RA et al. Adjustment of local anesthetic solutions with sodium bicarbonate: laboratory evaluations of alkalization and precipitation. Reg Anesth. 1989;14:265-270.
epi, Epinephrine.
*Data compiled for sodium bicarbonate 4% (weight/volume; 0.48 mEq/mL).
[†]Commercially added epinephrine, 1:200,000.
[‡]Freshly added epinephrine, 1:200,000.

Distribution

The absorption or injection of local anesthetics into the systemic circulation results in rapid distribution throughout the body. Distribution results in a rapid decrease in the plasma concentration, owing to the movement of drug into tissues that have the greatest perfusion. A secondary, slower disappearance follows; this reflects either distribution into tissues with a more limited blood supply, drug metabolism and excretion, or both of these processes. In a two-compartment model, distribution is known as the *alpha phase of plasma decay*, and the slower elimination component is referred to as the *beta phase of plasma decay*[63] (Figure 11-13). Some describe the pharmacokinetics of drugs, including local anesthetics, using a three-compartment model. In a three-compartment model, the distribution phase is subdivided into rapid (alpha) and slow (beta) phases. The elimination (gamma) phase remains conceptually similar to the usual two-compartment model.

Although local anesthetics are distributed throughout the body, their concentration varies in different tissues. Immediately after vascular uptake, more greatly perfused tissues, such as those of the lungs, receive more of these drugs than do less perfused tissues.[64] Once equilibration occurs, the local anesthetic leaves the highly perfused tissue and is deposited in tissue with less perfusion. Muscle tissue receives the greatest amount of local anesthetic from distribution. This is not because it has a greater affinity for these drugs, but rather because muscle acts as a depot, owing to its greater tissue mass.[9]

The distribution process varies significantly with different local anesthetics. For example, the disappearance rate of prilocaine is more rapid than that of mepivacaine or lidocaine. Of the longer-acting amides, etidocaine has a shorter distribution half-life than bupivacaine.[63] Ropivacaine also has shorter half-life than bupivacaine. Levobupivacaine appears to have a half-life similar to that of bupivacaine.[64-66] Distribution of the ester local anesthetics occurs as it does with the amides; however, their site and rate of metabolism tend to result in distribution having a lesser effect on plasma concentration.[67]

Metabolism

The metabolism of local anesthetics differs according to their chemical classification as either amides or esters. Ester hydrolysis is the primary metabolic route of ester local anesthetics. The hydrolysis occurs through the action of esterase in plasma, red

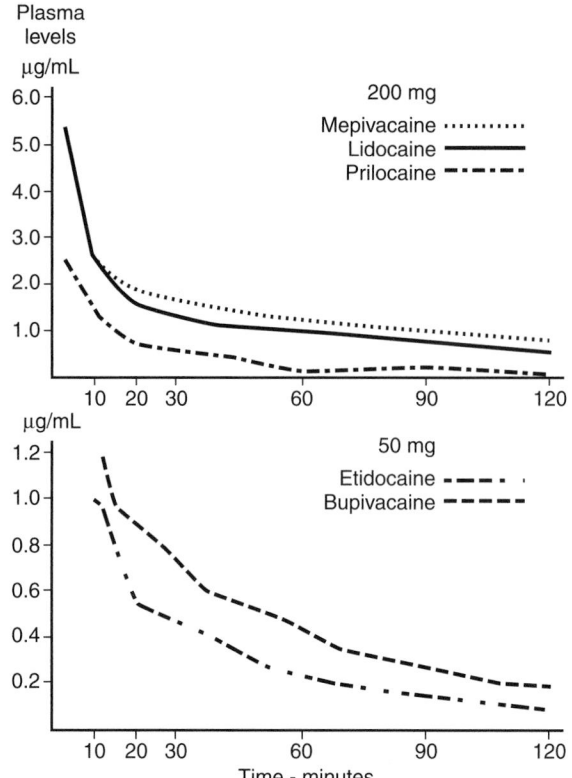

FIGURE **11-13** Plasma concentration curves of three intermediate-acting (*top*) and two long-acting (*bottom*) local anesthetics. Note that prilocaine and etidocaine (*dot-dashed lines*) are cleared more rapidly than the other local anesthetics in their respective groups. (*From Covino BG, Vassallo HG. Local Anesthetics: Mechanism of Action and Clinical Use. New York: Grune & Stratton; 1976.*)

TABLE **11-4**	Clearance Half-Life of Local Anesthetics	
Drug	**Clearance (L/min)**	**Half-Life (min)**
Chloroprocaine	—	0.3
Procaine	—	0.75
Tetracaine	—	—
Prilocaine	2.84	5
Lidocaine	0.95	9.6
Mepivacaine	0.78	7.2
Bupivacaine	0.47	28
Levobupivacaine	0.35	120
Ropivacaine	7.2	112
Etidocaine	1.22	19

blood cells, and the liver.[63,68-70] Primarily, plasma cholinesterase rapidly metabolizes the ester local anesthetics. Enzymatic hydrolysis in the plasma is rapid (half-life is 1 minute). An outcome of rapid hydrolysis is that toxic effects are short lived. Table 11-4 shows the clearance rates for select amide and ester local anesthetics.[71]

The plasma half-lives of procaine and chloroprocaine are shorter than 1 minute. The rapid rate of clearance of these drugs significantly reduces the incidence and severity of toxicity. Conversely, tetracaine is the most toxic ester and therefore is of limited clinical use. Saturated, inhibited, or genetically atypical plasma cholinesterase can significantly prolong the plasma half-life of ester local anesthetics.[70,72] For example, atypical plasma cholinesterase has been shown to significantly reduce the rate of procaine metabolism.[73] Drugs that are metabolized by plasma cholinesterase, such as succinylcholine, could also reduce the metabolism of ester local anesthetics.

In theory, patients who have liver disease severe enough to reduce plasma cholinesterase could be more prone to develop toxicity from ester local anesthetics. In fact, the plasma half-life of procaine is longer in patients with liver disease.[70] However, toxicity is unlikely in patients with liver disease who receive procaine and 2-chloroprocaine because of these drugs' intrinsic rate of metabolism and the esterase activity that is maintained in the erythrocytes.[68]

Metabolism of the amide local anesthetics occurs primarily in the liver. Metabolism is predominantly by microsomal cytochrome P-450.[74] The rate of hepatic metabolism—and

therefore clearance—is slowest for bupivacaine, followed in order by mepivacaine, lidocaine, etidocaine, and prilocaine.[75] This suggests that prilocaine, with intermediate potency, and etidocaine, with high potency, would be the least toxic drugs in their respective potency-related groups. It is obvious that clearance functions are independent of such factors as potency, lipid solubility, protein binding, and chemical structure. Table 11-5 presents pharmacokinetic data for the amide local anesthetics.[76]

Hepatic enzyme activity and blood flow are the primary factors that determine the rate of elimination of amide local anesthetics. The hepatic extraction ratio represents the activity level specific to the liver for metabolizing a drug. This ratio names the percentage of drug removed with each pass through the liver. The clearance of drugs that have higher hepatic extraction ratios, such as etidocaine, depends on adequate hepatic blood flow.[77] Hepatic enzyme activity is important when drugs with lower ratios, such as bupivacaine, are used[35,77] (see Figure 11-13). Table 11-6 indicates the extraction ratios for some amide local anesthetics.[71]

Consequently, pathologic conditions that influence hepatic function prolong the plasma half-life of these drugs by a reduction in hepatic blood flow, enzyme activity, or both. For example, lidocaine has a plasma half-life of 1.8 hours; however, in severe hepatic disease, its half-life is 4.9 hours. This probably results from both an enzymatic and a perfusion effect. A second example is found in congestive heart failure, which significantly reduces the rate of elimination of lidocaine because of a concomitant reduction in hepatic blood flow[78] (Table 11-7). These data indicate that reduced doses of amide local anesthetics should be used for patients with hepatic or circulatory dysfunction. Both of these pathologic states are common in the geriatric patient, necessitating the use of lower doses of anesthesia.

Only 1% to 5% of the injected dose of local anesthetic is accounted for by unchanged renal and hepatic excretion. However, the inactive, more water-soluble metabolites of local anesthetics appear in the urine. Although renal dysfunction affects the clearance far less than does hepatic failure, it can result in the accumulation of potentially toxic metabolites.[71]

The use of local anesthetics in pregnancy deserves some special pharmacokinetic and pharmacodynamic consideration. Clinical observations and studies both indicate that the spread and depth of spinal and epidural anesthesia are increased in pregnant women. Spread of neuraxial anesthesia increases during pregnancy due to decreases in thoracolumbar CSF volume and

TABLE 11-5	Pharmacokinetics of Amide Local Anesthetics				
Drug	Half-Life Alpha (min)	Half-Life Beta (min)	Half-Life Gamma (min)	V_{dss} (L)	Clearance (L)
Prilocaine	0.5	5	2	261	2.84
Lidocaine	1	9.6	1.6	91	0.95
Mepivacaine	0.7	7.2	1.9	84	0.75
Bupivacaine	2.7	28	3.5	72	0.47
Etidocaine	2.2	19	2.6	133	1.22
Ropivacaine	2.7	1.9	—	66.9	0.73

Modified from Longnecker DE, Murphy FL: Introduction to Anesthesia. 9th ed. Philadelphia: Saunders; 1997.
V_{dss}, Volume of distribution at steady state.

TABLE 11-6	Hepatic Extraction of Amide Local Anesthetics	
Drug		Hepatic Extraction Ratio
Lidocaine		0.68
Bupivacaine		0.37
Etidocaine		0.73

TABLE 11-7	Effect of Disease on Lidocaine Pharmacokinetics		
	Half-Life (hr)	V_{dss} (L/kg)	Clearance (mL/kg/min)
Normal	1.8	1.32	10
Renal disease	1.3	1.2	13.7
Heart failure	1.9	0.88	6.3
Liver disease	4.9	2.31	6

From Thompson PD et al. Lidocaine pharmacokinetics in advanced heart failure, liver disease, and renal failure in humans. Ann Intern Med. 1973;78:499.
V_{dss}, Volume of distribution at steady state.

increased neural susceptibility to local anesthetic. At first this was thought to be the result only of mechanical factors produced by a gravid uterus. For example, mechanical factors result in dilation of epidural veins, which leads to narrowing of the epidural and subarachnoid space, thereby reducing the dose requirement.[79] However, hormonal changes may explain some of this finding: there is a greater segmental spread of local anesthetics administered in the epidural during the first trimester of pregnancy.[80] A relationship appears to exist between the progesterone level in cerebrospinal fluid and the segmental spread of the drugs. Studies performed on isolated nerve taken from pregnant animals demonstrate more sensitivity to local anesthetic block than in nonpregnant animals.[81,82] Pregnancy appears to influence the potency of the local anesthetics.

TOXICITY OF LOCAL ANESTHETICS

Local anesthetics exert their action by inhibiting the passage of Na^+ ions through nerve membranes. Stabilized excitable tissue in the application region prevents normal function of afferent neurons. If the plasma concentration of these drugs becomes significantly elevated, this "stabilizing" property can lead to toxicity of the cardiovascular system and CNS. Toxic reactions to local anesthetics may be either local or systemic. Local reactions include pain, hematoma, abscess, ecchymosis, tissue necrosis, and neurotoxicity.[83] (Because tissue necrosis is often associated with the concomitant administration of epinephrine, the local anesthetic may not be the primary cause.) The most common causes of systemic local anesthetic toxicity are inadvertent intravascular injection and administration of an excessive dose.

Central Nervous System Toxicity

In one study, local anesthetics were infused into volunteers until they demonstrated symptoms of CNS toxicity.[84] This study demonstrated that although often similar, the patterns of CNS toxic effects varied among individuals. For example, some volunteers initially experienced tinnitus, whereas others became irrational. Despite individual variability, a sequence of symptoms was identified when all subjects were compared. Sequential symptoms are shown in Figure 11-14.

All of the symptoms noted in Figure 11-14 are the result of CNS effects, except for circumoral numbness, which is a result of extracellular extravasation of the drug in the tongue and mouth.[85] It has been noted that more of these symptoms are seen when plasma concentrations increase slowly. Conversely, a sudden increase in plasma concentration, as might occur with failure of an intravenous regional technique, may result in convulsion as the initial symptom.[84] Some patients manifest CNS depression as the initial symptom, especially if they have received a CNS depressant for sedation. For example, a CNS depressant such as midazolam, administered for anxiety associated with a regional technique, precludes the manifestation of the excitability component of the local-anesthetic reaction.

The effect of local anesthetics on the brain is depression of neuronal function. At first this may appear paradoxical, because many of the symptoms (e.g., muscle twitching and convulsion) indicate stimulation. The explanation lies in the fact that the local anesthetics selectively depress inhibitory functions in the cerebral cortex. Consequently, stimulatory activity results because facility neurons function are unopposed. If plasma levels increase significantly, both inhibitory and facility pathways are depressed and generalized CNS depression results.[86]

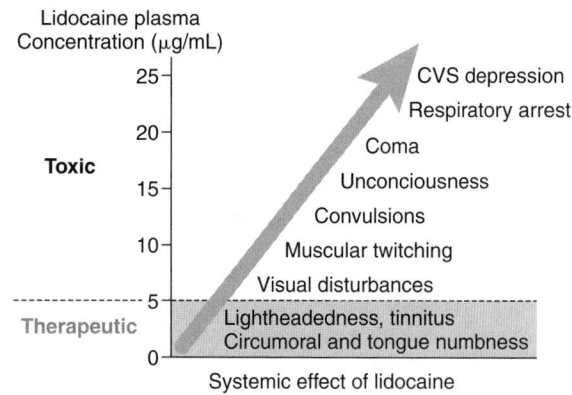

FIGURE **11-14**   Clinical signs after increased central nervous system concentration of lidocaine.

The potential for a local anesthetic to produce CNS toxicity relates to its potency. For example, animal studies have indicated that lidocaine 20 mg/kg results in convulsion. More potent drugs, such as etidocaine and bupivacaine, produced seizures at 8 and 5 mg/kg, respectively.[87] This results in a CNS toxicity ratio of 4:2:1, which correlates with the relative potency of these agents in establishing epidural anesthesia. Studies in human subjects have also demonstrated a similar correlation between potency and CNS toxicity.[86]

The acid-base status of animals and humans is important in the determination of CNS toxicity. For example, studies in cats have indicated that the convulsive threshold decreases by approximately 50% when carbon dioxide tension increases from 25 to 40 mm Hg to 45 to 81 mm Hg.[88] Both respiratory and metabolic acidosis increase the propensity for toxicity, whereas alkalosis reduces it. Several factors may be responsible for this effect. An elevation in carbon dioxide tension leads to cerebral vasodilation, which results in the delivery of more drug to the brain. Also, diffusion of carbon dioxide across the neuronal membrane causes a reduction in intracellular pH. This results in ionic trapping of the local anesthetic within the neurons. Finally, more free drug is available for diffusion into the CNS because of the reduction in plasma protein binding caused by acidosis.[89]

Some clinicians advocate having patients voluntarily hyperventilate while breathing oxygen when they first experience premonitory signs of CNS toxicity. Acute lowering of the intracerebral carbon dioxide tension may prevent seizure by raising the local anesthetic seizure threshold. However, if seizure should occur, the patient is less likely to develop hypoxia because of the denitrogenation that occurs when a high concentration of oxygen is breathed.[10]

Cardiovascular Toxicity

Studies have indicated (with some notable exceptions) that the cardiovascular system, when compared with the CNS, is more resistant to toxicity of local anesthetics. For example, in animals, the doses that cause significant cardiovascular depression are approximately threefold greater than those that produce convulsion.[90] Nevertheless, toxicity to the cardiovascular system does occur and is extremely important because it can result in grave clinical outcomes. As with the CNS, cardiovascular toxicity appears to be related to the anesthetic potency of the drugs.

Local anesthetics produce toxicity by influencing the heart and peripheral vascular system. The peripheral vascular effects of these drugs appear to be biphasic. At low concentrations, they produce vasoconstriction and an increase in systemic vascular resistance. As doses are increased, vasodilation occurs, resulting in significant hypotension.[91]

In the heart, these drugs influence electrophysiologic and contractile functions. An example of this is the prolongation of conduction time through the heart that occurs with the use of bupivacaine.[92] On electrocardiography, these effects result in an increase in the PR interval and in the duration of the QRS complex. As the dose of these drugs is increased, complete atrioventricular block, sinus bradycardia, or both can occur, possibly leading to cardiac arrest. Cardiac pacing, as indicated in the treatment of extreme bradycardia or cardiac arrest, may be difficult in this situation. By stabilizing nerve tissue, local anesthetics may elevate the pacing threshold.

In addition, because these drugs depress automaticity, extreme bradycardia is not well tolerated.[88] The effect of local anesthetics on conductivity, automaticity, and pacing potential is attributable to the blockade of Na^+ channels.[13,14]

Local anesthetics also depress contractility of the myocardium.[92] The mechanism for this depression is unknown; however, it is probably related to the blockade of Na^+ channels and the displacement of Ca^{2+} from the cardiac muscle.[93] The negative inotropic effect results in a depression in V_{max} (maximum velocity of shortening of cardiac muscle fibers), a reduction of cardiac output, and an elevation in left ventricular end-diastolic pressure and volume. As stated previously, a relationship exists between myocardial depression and the potency of a drug.[94] For example, tetracaine is 8 to 10 times more potent than procaine as a local anesthetic and as a myocardial depressant.[95,96]

The selectivity in the cardiovascular toxicity of local anesthetics is thought to be significant. For example, bupivacaine and etidocaine appear to produce toxicity at lower doses than a less potent drug such as lidocaine.[97,98] More important, the cardiovascular toxicity seen with the potent drugs is severe and recalcitrant to treatment and may occur prior to CNS toxicity.[99,100] Studies on isolated papillary muscles have demonstrated greater depression of Na^+ current by bupivacaine than by lidocaine. Also, the highly lipid-soluble bupivacaine dissociates from the channel more slowly than lidocaine.[101] Lastly, tachycardia, by a frequency-dependent effect, facilitates the binding of bupivacaine to Na^+ channels, thereby enhancing cardiac toxicity.[102]

This selectivity has special implications in the consideration of ventricular arrhythmias. Bupivacaine can produce severe and even fatal ventricular arrhythmias in patients; however, lidocaine, mepivacaine, and tetracaine rarely produce arrhythmias. The arrhythmogenic effect of bupivacaine is probably a result of the inhibition of both fast Na^+ and slow Ca^{2+} channels. Because this drug dissociates slowly from Na^+ channels, it is possible that it produces a persistent, slow conduction velocity, reentry pathways, and ventricular tachycardia, which lead to ventricular fibrillation.[101,102] Studies on the cardiotoxicity of ropivacaine and levobupivacaine suggest that they are much safer in this regard.[103,104] On comparison, ropivacaine is less cardiotoxic than levobupivacaine, which is less cardiotoxic than bupivacaine. With increased vigilance in clinical practice, the number of reported cases of bupivacaine toxicity has declined significantly in recent years.[105,106]

Several cases of cardiovascular toxicity in pregnant patients have been reported. These reports have led to the assumption that pregnancy possibly has a role in increasing sensitivity to the cardiovascular toxicity of local anesthetics. It has been noted that bupivacaine produces cardiovascular collapse at a lower plasma concentration in pregnant animals than in nonpregnant animals.[101,107] This difference possibly results from pregnancy-induced hormonal changes.[106] Neither pregnant animals nor humans have demonstrated this degree of toxicity in response to lidocaine or mepivacaine. It does not appear that this differential effect is the result of an increase in the myocardial uptake of bupivacaine.[108] Although the mechanism is unknown, case reports and animal studies have resulted in the recommendation that bupivacaine 0.75% not be used in obstetrics.

Hypercarbia, acidosis, and hypoxia potentiate the negative chronotropic and inotropic effects of lidocaine and bupivacaine in isolated myocardial tissue. This effect is most significant in the case of bupivacaine. Animal studies demonstrate that the use of bupivacaine in the presence of hypoxia and acidosis also increases the frequency of arrhythmias and death.[109] These facts emphasize the importance of good airway management during seizure activity resulting from the toxicity of local anesthetics.

Allergic Reactions

Local anesthetics can produce allergic, hypersensitive, and anaphylactic reactions, although the incidence of true allergy is very low. The use of ester local anesthetics is associated with a greater incidence of these reactions than the use of amides. This is likely because esters are derivatives of para-aminobenzoic acid, which is an allergenic compound.[110] Cross-reactivity among the ester-type local anesthetics is high; among the amide types, it is low but still possible. Although reports indicate that amide local anesthetics can produce allergic reactions, the incidence in this class is extremely low. Skin testing is possible but at times difficult to interpret.[106,111,112]

Intradermal experiments demonstrate the difference between amides and esters.[113] Both amides and esters were injected intradermally in patients with no history of allergic response to local anesthetics. Of these patients, 30% had skin reactions to esters, but no reactions to the amides were observed. None of these patients had systemic anaphylactic reactions. True immunologic reactions to local anesthetics are rare, encompassing less than 1% of all adverse reactions.[114] Cross-allergy between ester- and amide-type local anesthetics is rare.

Some commercially available amide local anesthetics are in solution with the preservative methylparaben. This substance, which has a chemical structure similar to that of para-aminobenzoic acid, can increase the incidence of allergic reactions with the amide local anesthetics.[115] Patients who are allergic to ester local anesthetics, whether determined through the patient's history or through intradermal skin testing, should be treated with a preservative-free amide local anesthetic to avoid a possible allergic reaction to the para-aminobenzoic acid metabolite of methylparaben.[114]

In clinical practice, adverse reactions after injection of local anesthetics are frequently observed. In most cases, they can be attributed to (1) toxic events (both cardiovascular and neurotoxic) related to the dose of the local anesthetic or vasoconstrictor (epinephrine) or accidental intravascular injections; (2) psychomotor reactions; and (3) reactions caused by preservatives or hidden allergens (e.g., the latex in surgical gloves).[114]

Methemoglobinemia

Methemoglobinemia is a disorder characterized by high concentrations of methemoglobin in the blood. Methemoglobin does not bind to oxygen, and tissue hypoxia can occur. The use of prilocaine can produce methemoglobinemia because of the metabolite o-toluidine, which oxidizes hemoglobin to methemoglobin. The tendency of prilocaine to produce methemoglobin is dose related. Significant methemoglobin does not result until the dose administered epidurally reaches 600 mg.[116] High concentrations of methemoglobin produce a brownish gray cyanosis, tachypnea, and metabolic acidosis. Severe methemoglobinemia causes signs and symptoms related to tissue hypoxia, headache, and irritability. Loss of consciousness may occur in 50% to 60% of cases.[117] Spontaneous reversal of methemoglobin occurs in 2 to 3 hours; however, the administration of methylene blue can result in immediate reversal. The formation of the usual clinical levels of methemoglobin is of little consequence in healthy patients; however, patients with severe anemia or heart failure cannot tolerate the reduction in oxygen-carrying capacity. Prilocaine should not be used in obstetrics because clinical doses can result in a 10% conversion of fetal hemoglobin to methemoglobin, leading to neonatal cyanosis. Benzocaine and benzocaine-containing mixtures such as Cetacaine, which are widely used for topical anesthesia, may also produce methemoglobinemia although the incidence is extremely low.[118,119] In a large-scale recent study of benzocaine use for transesophageal echocardiography, the incidence of methemoglobinemia was low (1 case per 1499) and had a good outcome if promptly recognized and treated. Clinical factors associated with the development of methemoglobinemia included sepsis, anemia, and hospitalization. Minimizing or avoiding the use of benzocaine in these patients is recommended.[118]

Local Tissue Toxicity

Chloroprocaine is the only local anesthetic that has produced prolonged sensory and motor deficits after epidural and subarachnoid administration.[120] Because of this, animal experiments were conducted to determine the effect of chloroprocaine on neural function.[121,122] It appeared that nerve damage is likely to result if chloroprocaine 3% is added to a solution of sodium bisulfite 0.2% at a pH of 3. However, chloroprocaine and sodium bisulfite at these concentrations did not produce damage if put into a solution with a pH of 7. Also, chloroprocaine 3% with a pH of 3 does not produce nerve damage if sodium bisulfite is omitted. Sodium bisulfite, without chloroprocaine and at a pH of 3, can produce nerve damage; however, other studies showed an actual protective effect of bisulfite.[120] In an animal model of neurotoxicity, researchers concluded clinical deficits associated with unintentional intrathecal injection of chloroprocaine likely resulted from a direct effect of the anesthetic, not the preservative. The data also suggested that bisulfite can reduce neurotoxic damage induced by intrathecal local anesthetic.[120-122] Even though the exact mechanism of neurotoxicity remains unresolved, clinically used preparations now omit sodium bisulfite because of this problem. A comparison of the common features of local anesthetic reactions are given in Table 11-8.

Prevention of Toxicity

Animal studies have demonstrated that pretreatment with benzodiazepines is effective in prevention of local anesthetic–induced CNS seizures.[123,124] Although this has been demonstrated in several species, the results are difficult to extrapolate to humans. Owing to ethical considerations, it is difficult to perform well-controlled clinical studies in humans, and without clinical studies it is impossible to determine the appropriate dose and

TABLE 11-8	Common Features of Local Anesthetic Reactions		
Cause	**Major Clinical Features**	**Comments**
Local Anesthetic Toxicity		
Intravascular injection relative overdose	Immediate convulsion or cardiac toxicity; in 5 to 15 minutes, onset of irritability progressing to convulsions	
Reaction to vasoconstrictor	Tachycardia, hypertension, headache	
Vasovagal reaction	Rapid onset bradycardia, hypotension, pallor, faintness	Apprehension
Allergy		
Immediate	Anaphylaxis (hypotension, bronchospasm, edema)	Allergy to amides is extremely rare
Delayed	Urticaria	Cross-allergy possible, e.g., with preservatives in local anesthetics and food

timing for administration. Nevertheless, the results of the animal studies tend to indicate that benzodiazepines are the drugs of choice, especially if sedation is needed for a regional technique. Administration of midazolam 5 to 10 minutes before the injection of the local anesthetic seems prudent.

The dose administered is important in determination of toxicity. There is much controversy and discussion involving the use of maximum doses of local anesthetics, with some clinicians calling for abandoning blanket maximum recommendations.[125] They should be replaced by recommended dose ranges for an intended purpose, for example, spinal, epidural, or continuous epidural infusion. The dose of local anesthetics that produces toxicity is difficult to predict because, as previously discussed, the site of injection, agent used, patient size, technical skill of the provider, and several other factors have a significant influence on the peak plasma level. Nevertheless, as shown in Table 11-9, manufacturers have issued recommended dose limits for single, nonvascular injections.[76] Some techniques for the recognition, prevention, and treatment of an accidental overdose of a local anesthetic are listed in Boxes 11-3 and 11-4.

Treatment of Systemic Toxicity

Treatment of adverse local anesthetic reactions depends on their nature and severity. The severity of toxic effects depends on the drug used and the amount administered. Drugs such as lidocaine, prilocaine, and chloroprocaine produce toxicity of limited duration because of short distribution times and elimination half-lives. A drug such as bupivacaine, ropivacaine, or levobupivacaine, which have longer half-lives, produces more protracted toxicity.

A primary concern when toxicity occurs is the treatment of CNS symptoms. During convulsions oxygen consumption increases and ventilation is significantly compromised; this situation can result in respiratory acidosis and hypoxemia. Therefore the assurance and maintenance of a patent airway and ventilation with oxygen are the initial actions taken.

If distribution allows the plasma concentration of the drug to rapidly fall below the convulsive threshold, airway management and ventilation with oxygen may be the only treatment needed. However, convulsions may be severe and protracted, making airway management difficult. The administration of anticonvulsant sedatives treats seizures in this situation. Care is taken to

use a minimal dose, because an excessive dose can potentiate cardiovascular and postconvulsive CNS depression. Propofol 0.5 to 1.0 mg/kg, midazolam 0.05 to 0.10 mg/kg, or thiopental 50 to 100 mg, is usually satisfactory. Also, use of a rapid-onset, short-acting muscle relaxant such as succinylcholine helps control the convulsive state. It should be noted that if this mode of treatment is used, the patient should undergo endotracheal intubation.

If hypotension occurs, conservative treatment includes the correction of hypoxia and acidosis. The patient's legs should be elevated and the intravenous infusion increased. Vasopressors are administered if hypotension is persistent and severe. Sympathomimetic drugs with alpha and beta effects can be used to treat hypotension resulting from local anesthetic–induced myocardial depression and vasodilatation. Ephedrine, 15 to 30 mg, is commonly used. Atropine, 0.4 mg, adequately treats bradycardia that may be present. In more severe cases, infusion of intravenous fluids and vasopressors such as phenylephrine 0.5 to 5 mcg/kg/min, norepinephrine 0.02 to 0.2 mcg/kg/min, or vasopressin 2 to 20 units IV may be necessary. If myocardial failure is present, epinephrine 1 to 15 mcg/kg IV bolus may be required. When toxicity progresses to cardiac arrest, it is reasonable to follow the guidelines for advanced cardiac life support.[27] Significant doses of atropine, dopamine, or epinephrine can be used to treat severe hypotension and bradycardia that might occur, especially in the case of bupivacaine toxicity.

Widening of the QRS complex usually precedes cardiovascular collapse. Cardiopulmonary resuscitation and cardioversion are used for treating ventricular tachycardia and fibrillation. The electrical energy needed for cardioversion may be greater than normal. With bupivacaine-induced cardiovascular collapse, resuscitation can be difficult and may require large doses of epinephrine, atropine, or both. The unique cardiotoxicity of bupivacaine has been well established, and all clinicians are aware of its special precautions for anesthetic use. With unresponsive bupivacaine cardiac toxicity, intravenous lipid or cardiopulmonary bypass may be considered. Recent experiments in animals and anecdotal clinical reports demonstrate the rapid ability of lipid infusion to resuscitate animals from bupivacaine overdosage. The mechanism is not yet clear. A growing number of case reports (available at http://www.lipidrescue.org/) provide evidence that lipid infusion may also be effective in humans.[126]

TABLE 11-9 | Manufacturers' Recommended Single-Injection Dose

Drug	Concentration (%)	Dose* (mg/kg)
Chloroprocaine	3	11 (14)
Lidocaine	1	4 (7)
Lidocaine	2	4 (7)
Mepivacaine	2	4 (7)
Prilocaine	3	7 (8.5)
Bupivacaine	0.75	2.5 (3.2)
Etidocaine	1	6 (8)
Etidocaine	2	(8)
Ropivacaine	0.75	3 (3.5)
Levobupivacaine	0.75	2.5 (3.2)

*Drug alone and (drug with epinephrine).

BOX 11-3

Techniques to Prevent Regional Block Toxicity

Patient Evaluation
- Identification of significant systemic disease, age, and surgical requirements to permit individualization of local anesthetic dose

Premedication
- A moderate dose of midazolam or other appropriate central nervous system depressant

Preparation

Resuscitative Drugs
- Midazolam, propofol or thiopental, succinylcholine, atropine, cardiac support drugs

Equipment
- Oxygen administration and suction equipment
- Airway management supplies, including airway, laryngoscope, and endotracheal tube and laryngeal mask airway
- Ensure adequate intravenous access is available before beginning procedure.
- Be aware of allergies to locals and preservatives.
- Physically separate neural blockade tray from any other drugs.

Prevention
- Personally check dose of local anesthetic and vasoconstrictor.
- Administer a test dose of 5%-10% of total dose.
- Aspirate frequently and discard bloody solutions.
- Monitor for cardiovascular signs such as increase in heart rate if epinephrine is used.
- Maintain constant verbal contact with patient and vigilance for premonitory signs of toxicity after time of peak plasma concentration.

BOX 11-4

Treatment of Acute Local Anesthetic Toxic Response

Airway
- Secure clear airway

Breathing
- Administer oxygen with face mask
- Encourage adequate ventilation, which prevents acidosis and ion trapping
- Use artificial ventilation, intubation as required

Circulation
- Increase intravenous fluids to treat hypotension
- Administer cardiovascular support drugs as required to treat blood pressure and heart rate changes
- Administer antiarrhythmic agents as required

Drugs
- Administer incremental doses of benzodiazepine, thiopental, or propofol as needed to prevent or treat seizure
- Administer muscle relaxant to secure airway
- Use cardiovascular support and resuscitation agents as required

Outcomes
- Local anesthetic toxicity may result in convulsions or abrupt respiratory and cardiac changes; however, with rapid and appropriate treatment long-term sequelae are rare

The regimens used in these cases consisted of bolus doses of lipid emulsion (20% Intralipid), 1.2 to 2 mL/kg, followed by continuous infusions of 0.25 to 0.5 mL/kg/min.

NEWER LOCAL ANESTHETIC COMPOUNDS

Ropivacaine

Researchers have attempted to identify drugs that have a long duration of action but do not have the cardiovascular toxicity of bupivacaine. Ropivacaine was designed to meet these specifications. Chemically, ropivacaine differs from bupivacaine in that it has a propyl group in place of the butyl group on the nitrogen atom in the piperidine ring. In addition, local anesthetics that have asymmetric carbon atoms can exist in either sinister (S−) or rectus (R−) stereoisomers. Bupivacaine exists as a racemic compound in that it has both S− and R− isomers. Conversely, ropivacaine exists only in the S− stereoisomer form. This difference between ropivacaine and bupivacaine has resulted in less cardiotoxicity.[127]

Isolated in vitro studies of ropivacaine have indicated that it is less potent than bupivacaine in its ability to block Na$^+$ channels. More important, this compound has a more rapid rate of reversal of Na$^+$ channel blockade than bupivacaine.[128,129] This may result in less toxicity.[103,130] As stated earlier in the section on cardiovascular toxicity, the slow dissociation of local anesthetics from Na$^+$ channels can result in the development of recalcitrant ventricular arrhythmias.

Ropivacaine and bupivacaine have been administered intravenously at equal doses in dog studies. These studies have demonstrated that ropivacaine produces less slowing in cardiac conduction velocity, less cardiovascular collapse, and less ventricular fibrillation than bupivacaine.[131-133] Conversely, studies in sheep have indicated that the mortality rate from ventricular fibrillation is the same for the two drugs.[134] Also important, studies in animals have shown that cardiac resuscitation is more successful after ropivacaine use when toxic doses of both drugs were administered by intravenous bolus.[135]

Clinical studies have indicated that the therapeutic profiles of both ropivacaine and bupivacaine are similar, but differences do exist. Ropivacaine has advantages over bupivacaine. It provides more differential block when given epidurally, allowing for a better separation between sensory and motor block. This feature can be used to its advantage in obstetrics and in postoperative epidural pain relief. It also exhibits less systemic toxicity than both racemic and levobupivacaine. Especially, its better cardiotoxic profile has been well documented and is an important advantage when using techniques with a potential for high plasma concentrations. Ropivacaine is less potent than bupivacaine and has a shorter duration of action.[136-138]

The elimination half-life of ropivacaine is less than that of bupivacaine.[127] A study in which the two drugs were infused at a rate of 10 mg/min demonstrated that 25% more ropivacaine was needed to produce minor symptoms. When the infusions were stopped, the toxic symptoms disappeared more rapidly in the subjects who had received ropivacaine. These findings seem to indicate that ropivacaine has a pharmacokinetic advantage over bupivacaine.[139] In summary, the most important aspect of the overall clinical profile of ropivacaine is reduced CNS and cardiac toxicity and less motor blockade, most likely because of a lower potency.[140]

Levobupivacaine

Levobupivacaine is the S− enantiomer of bupivacaine.[141-143] Levobupivacaine is clinically similar to bupivacaine and has a long duration of action. The advantage of levobupivacaine is a reduced CNS and cardiac toxicity profile compared with that of bupivacaine.[144]

In a study in human volunteers, levobupivacaine and ropivacaine appear to have similar CNS toxicity profiles. Because levobupivacaine is more potent then ropivacaine, the conclusion can be reached that levobupivacaine also has a higher therapeutic index.[145-147] Cost is a major factor in the decision regarding which long-acting agent to use. The type of block, the dose and concentration of local anesthetic required, and the realistic risk of bupivacaine toxicity compared with that associated with the new agents must be considered.[148]

Eutectic Mixture of Local Anesthetics

For years, researchers have sought to develop techniques and drugs that produce anesthesia on application to intact skin. As a result of their work, the eutectic mixture of local anesthetics (EMLA) was developed. EMLA is a mixture of lidocaine and prilocaine that when applied to skin, accumulates at the site of dermal pain receptors and nerve endings.

The clinical effectiveness of EMLA has been studied in the performance of venipuncture in children. A study of 41 ill children revealed that the application of EMLA for 45 minutes before the procedure resulted in lower pain scores than if no pretreatment was used. The effectiveness was not seen in situations classified as "difficult venipunctures." As might be expected, EMLA also was less effective in children younger than age 7 years than it was in older children.[149]

Pharmacokinetic studies indicate that satisfactory dermal analgesia is achieved 1 hour after application with an occlusive dressing; maximal analgesia occurs 2 to 3 hours after application.[150] When EMLA is applied to areas of abnormal skin (e.g., where psoriasis or eczema is present), absorption is faster, plasma levels are higher, and the duration of anesthesia is shorter. This results from an impairment of diffusion barriers and an increase in regional blood flow.[151] Systemic absorption of lidocaine and prilocaine is dependent on the duration and surface area of application. Blood levels of 5% and 2.8% of those needed to produce systemic toxicity are seen with use of lidocaine and prilocaine, respectively, when the drugs are applied in accordance with appropriate dosage recommendations.[152] Toxicity is more likely to occur in infants and small children than in adults. Also, toxicity can result if the emulsion is applied to broken or inflamed skin or to areas of 2000 cm² or greater or if it is left on for longer than recommended periods.[150]

The recommended dose of EMLA for minor dermal procedures such as venipuncture is 2.5 g; the dose is applied over a 20- to 25-cm² skin surface at least 60 minutes before the procedure. Analgesia does not occur until 15 minutes after application of the drug. For painful procedures, 2 g of EMLA per 10 cm² of skin surface area are applied and left in place for at least 2 hours.[151] EMLA should not be used in infants younger than age 12 months because EMLA contains prilocaine. Prilocaine can cause a dose-related increase in oxidation of hemoglobin to methemoglobin, which is especially problematic in neonates.[153] Studies have indicated that simultaneous use of EMLA and drugs that cause oxidation of hemoglobin (e.g., sulfonamides, benzocaine, aniline drugs, nitrites) also increases this risk.[150] Because of the rapid rate of absorption, the use of EMLA for mucous membrane anesthesia is not recommended.

Tetracaine, Epinephrine, and Cocaine

A common use of local anesthetics is to produce analgesia for the irrigating, débridement, and suturing of traumatic dermal lacerations. An ideal local anesthetic for this use would be painless, produce minimal systemic toxicity, maintain tissue viability, and not distort the wound margins.[154] In an attempt to produce some of these characteristics, three previously available agents—tetracaine, epinephrine, and cocaine (TAC)—were combined for use on traumatic lacerations. The relative concentration of each component is as follows: tetracaine 0.5%, epinephrine 1:200, cocaine 10%.[155] This combination has been as effective as infiltration of local anesthetics for the closure of certain types of laceration. Tetracaine and cocaine can produce excellent topical anesthesia, and cocaine and epinephrine result in vasoconstriction at the site of application. The vasoconstriction that results from the combination should slow the absorption of the local anesthetics, which should reduce toxicity and facilitate the quality and duration of anesthesia produced.

The clinical use of TAC has not been without problems. TAC is more expensive to administer than lidocaine when the latter is used for local infiltration. Because the combination contains cocaine, TAC must be treated as a Schedule II controlled substance.[156] Therefore it must be kept in a locked cabinet, and records of its use must be kept. This further increases the cost of administering the drug combination.

The drug combination in TAC can produce significant toxicity. Both cocaine and tetracaine can individually produce significant systemic toxicity. Cocaine can also increase the α-adrenergic response to epinephrine by blocking the reuptake of epinephrine into the peripheral adrenergic nerve terminal. The types of severe toxicity seen with TAC have been status epilepticus and death. It appears that complications are more likely to occur when TAC is administered topically to mucous membrane. The maximum recommended safe dose is 3 to 4 mL in adults and 0.05 mL/kg in children.[155] Because of toxicity seen with TAC, other non–cocaine-containing drug combinations have been used and demonstrated similar effectiveness.[156]

An over-the-counter anesthetic cream (ELA-Max) and gel (Topicaine) are also available. ELA-Max contains 4% lidocaine in a liposomal delivery system and is more than twice as fast as EMLA. Topicaine is a 4% microemulsion gel with an onset of approximately 1 hour and a duration of 1 hour after removal.

Sustained Release of Local Anesthetics

Pain can be easily alleviated with local anesthetics; however, their clinical usefulness is limited by their relatively short duration of action. Even long-acting local anesthetics, such as bupivacaine, etidocaine, ropivacaine, and levobupivacaine, are of limited use in relieving pain that lasts longer than between 2 and 12 hours.[157] To address this problem, indwelling catheters that provide continuous infusion of mixtures of local anesthetic and opiates are commonly used. Problems associated with the use of indwelling catheters are blockage or breakage, migration subdurally (after epidural insertion), and infection.

Because of the problems associated with indwelling catheters, researchers are investigating the use of liposomal microspheres for the slow release of local anesthetics. Liposomal microspheres consist of a phospholipid bilayer that encapsulates an aqueous core. Pharmacokinetically the liposomes act as a depot for local anesthetics and allow for the slow clearance of the drugs into the injected tissue. Liposomal microspheres impregnated with lidocaine and bupivacaine and injected into the epidural space have resulted in a prolonged duration of neural blockade. In addition, it appears that the administration of local anesthetics by this method results in lower plasma concentrations than those seen when the drugs are administered as regular preparations.[157] The lower plasma concentrations should certainly result in an attenuation of CNS and cardiac toxicity. It will be interesting to see if this new technology will have a significant impact on the clinical use of local anesthetics.

CLINICAL USE OF LOCAL ANESTHETICS

Specific regional anesthetic techniques and blocks are discussed in detail in Chapters 45-46.

Topical Anesthesia

The application of local anesthetics to the mucous membranes of the nose, mouth, tracheobronchial tree, esophagus, and genitourinary tract can produce satisfactory anesthesia. Local anesthetics used for this purpose are tetracaine (2%), lidocaine (2% to 10%), and cocaine (1% to 5%). Cocaine and lidocaine yield their maximum anesthetic effect in 2 to 5 minutes; the onset of tetracaine is slightly slower, at 3 to 8 minutes. The duration of action of tetracaine (30 to 60 minutes) is longer than that of lidocaine or cocaine (30 to 45 minutes).[158]

Absorption of local anesthetics from the mucous membrane is significant and therefore can result in systemic toxicity. Tetracaine has the most rapid rate of absorption, followed by cocaine and lidocaine, respectively. Peak plasma levels occur 5 minutes after the application of tetracaine or cocaine to the

pyriform fossae of the laryngopharynx.[158] The peak plasma level in this study was one third to one half that seen with intravenous bolus infusion. Lidocaine applied to the trachea manifests peak plasma levels in 15 to 20 minutes. However, high peak blood levels can occur after tracheal application of these drugs. This probably occurs because the drugs migrate to the distal airways and alveoli, where a large vascular surface is available for absorption. For example, absorption is faster if the drugs are instilled while the patient is in the erect position rather than in the supine position.[159]

Cocaine is a unique local anesthetic in that it produces vasoconstriction. This action facilitates nasal surgery because it results in shrinking of the mucosa. Cocaine produces vasoconstriction by blocking norepinephrine and epinephrine uptake into the adrenergic nerve ending. This uptake is responsible for the termination of the action of catecholamines. Epinephrine is usually injected shortly after the application of cocaine, setting the stage for a significant drug interaction. Because absorbed cocaine can block the uptake of epinephrine systemically, a toxic effect can result from the injection of epinephrine. This interaction can result in life-threatening ventricular arrhythmias. The possibility is even more significant if the patient is taking other adrenergic uptake blockers, such as tricyclic antidepressants, or catecholamine metabolism blockers, such as monoamine oxidase inhibitors.

Local Infiltration Anesthesia

Local infiltration involves the injection of local anesthetics into tissue to block diffuse nerve endings. Most local anesthetics are used for this purpose. The addition of epinephrine almost doubles the duration of action of all the local anesthetics; however, this effect is greater with the short- and intermediate-acting drugs. Also, epinephrine reduces the peak plasma concentration attained by the local anesthetics.

Epinephrine should not be injected around end arteries, such as are present in the fingers, toes, ear, nose, and penis. A large volume of 1:200,000 solution can be absorbed and result in significant adrenergic stimulation. Doses of 5 mcg/kg or less are usually safe but could be harmful to certain patients, such as those with ischemic heart disease or hypertension.

The local anesthetics most often used for infiltration are lidocaine (0.5% to 1%), procaine (0.5% to 1%), and bupivacaine (0.125% to 0.25%). The selection of the drug depends on the duration of anesthesia needed and on the tissue area to be blocked. For example, procaine is used for short procedures, whereas bupivacaine provides anesthesia for longer surgeries. If significant volumes are needed to block large areas, lidocaine and procaine are less likely to result in toxicity than bupivacaine. When injected without epinephrine, 4.5 mg/kg of lidocaine, 7 mg/kg of procaine, or 2.5 mg/kg of bupivacaine is the recommended maximum dose.[160] With the addition of epinephrine, these doses can be increased by one third.

The main disadvantage of local infiltration is that a large volume of local anesthetic must be used for blocking relatively small areas. Also, patients often object to the pain of injection, which may be attenuated by a slow rate of injection and by the alkalization of the local anesthetic. A single-blind study of 42 adult volunteers compared the effect that rate of administration versus buffering has on the pain associated with subcutaneous infiltration of local anesthetics. The findings indicated that the rate of injection had a greater effect on pain than did buffering; even with buffered drugs, rapid injection rates increased pain.[160]

Tumescent liposuction and anesthesia require infiltration of large volumes of crystalloids or "wetting" solution subcutaneously. Wetting solutions are used to facilitate fat suctioning, both for their local anesthesia effect and to decrease blood loss. These solutions commonly contain lidocaine 0.05% to 0.1% (0.5 to 1 mg/mL) and epinephrine 0.5 to 1.5 mg/L. Many surgeons also add sodium bicarbonate to increase absorption, speed onset, and decrease pain of infiltration. Steroids such as triamcinolone may also be added to decrease scarring and aid healing. Even though these are dilute solutions, large amounts of local anesthetic may be absorbed. Fortunately, the epinephrine slows absorption, and the peak plasma levels of lidocaine are within normal ranges. Intravenous fluid administration with these techniques should be limited. A reasonable goal is two times the volume of aspirate. Intravenous fluids and wetting solution are counted in the total fluids.[161,162]

Nerve Block Anesthesia

Injection of local anesthetics around peripheral nerves or plexuses can provide anesthesia for a large area, obviating the need for excessive doses or volumes.

Many clinicians classify nerve blocks as major or minor. *Minor nerve blocks* refer to anesthesia for individual nerves, such as the ulnar and median nerves at the elbow. *Major nerve blocks* produce anesthesia for two or more nerves that supply large areas. Analgesia of the brachial plexuses, which innervate the arms, is an excellent example of a major nerve block. This classification of nerve block is important because it influences many local anesthetic parameters.

Most local anesthetics manifest a rapid onset of action in all minor nerve blocks. This occurs because minor nerves are single nerves that have limited diffusion barriers for local anesthetics. The duration of action with these blocks is similar to those seen with local infiltration. Also, the addition of epinephrine prolongs the duration of block provided by all the drugs to an extent similar to that of local infiltration. The duration of block with epinephrine varies from 30 to 60 minutes with chloroprocaine to 240 to 480 minutes with bupivacaine.[163] Toxicity is usually not a problem because of the small volumes (5 to 20 mL) and concentrations required for minor nerve blocks. Chloroprocaine, lidocaine, and bupivacaine, which represent the three potency or duration groups, are usually selected for these blocks. The selection is dependent on the duration of the anesthesia required.

Major nerve blocks differ from minor nerve blocks in that (1) they usually require a higher concentration of local anesthetic and (2) their time of onset can vary significantly. For example, the onset time for major blocks with lidocaine or mepivacaine is 7 minutes; in contrast, with bupivacaine, 23 minutes is required.[164] Differences most likely exist because of the greater diffusion barriers of the larger nerves. As a result, latency of onset becomes dependent on the factors that influence diffusion of drug through tissues, such as the ionization state.

If an appropriate concentration is used, the duration of major nerve blocks is the same as or longer than that observed with minor nerve blocks. Epinephrine prolongs major blocks with all anesthetics; however, it has a smaller effect with local anesthetics that have a longer duration of action, such as bupivacaine, ropivacaine, etidocaine, and levobupivacaine. A significant variation exists in the duration of a brachial plexus block when compared with other conduction blocks. The long-acting agents can produce a brachial plexus block that lasts from 4 to 30 hours.[163]

Spinal Anesthesia

Spinal anesthesia is most commonly conducted with bupivacaine or tetracaine combined with analgesics such as fentanyl or sufentanil. Tetracaine is usually administered as a hyperbaric solution obtained by mixing 2 mL of 1% solution with 2 mL of 10% dextrose. Hypobaric solutions can be obtained by mixing the tetracaine with sterile water to yield a 0.1% solution. Isobaric solutions are acquired by mixing 20 mg of tetracaine crystals with cerebrospinal fluid. The use of the latter two formulations is indicated for specific surgical procedures. Tetracaine provides approximately 75 to 150 minutes of anesthesia; the duration can be increased by 50% with the addition of 0.2 to 0.3 mg of epinephrine.

The mixture of bupivacaine (0.75%) and dextrose 8.25% results in a hyperbaric solution. Bupivacaine is similar to tetracaine in that it is indicated for surgical procedures lasting 2 to 2.5 hours. However, some clinicians believe that bupivacaine may produce less hypotension and may better obliterate tourniquet pain in orthopedic procedures of the lower extremities.[164] It has largely replaced tetracaine as the most widely used spinal anesthetic drug. Epinephrine prolongs the duration of action of bupivacaine, as it does tetracaine.[165]

Transient neurologic symptoms (TNSs) have been reported after the use of lidocaine for spinal anesthesia, although many other agents have also been implicated.[166-168] Risk factors include lidocaine spinal anesthesia, lithotomy position, and outpatient procedures, especially knee arthroscopy. Avoidance of lidocaine in these situations is justified. Symptoms include a burning, aching, cramplike, and radiating pain in the anterior and posterior aspect of the thighs. Half of affected patients report that the pain radiates to the lower extremities, and lower back pain is common. Symptoms occur within 12 to 24 hours after surgery and resolve within several hours to 4 days. Treatment is supportive and should include nonsteroidal antiinflammatory agents. This transient syndrome is completely sensory in nature with no motor involvement and can therefore be differentiated from more serious abnormalities such as epidural hematoma, cauda equina syndrome, and nerve root damage. Many possible causes of TNS are theorized, including a specific local-anesthetic toxicity, needle trauma, and neural ischemia. It could also be secondary to sciatic stretching, patient positioning, pooling of local anesthetics administered via small-gauge, pencil-point needles, or to muscle spasm, myofascial trigger points, early mobilization, or irritation of the dorsal root ganglion.[169] The exact mechanism is unknown.

Epidural Anesthesia

Almost all local anesthetics can be used for epidural anesthesia. However, clinicians avoid tetracaine and procaine because of their long latency of onset. The intermediate-acting local anesthetics have a duration of 1 to 2 hours. The long-acting drugs produce anesthesia for 3 to 5 hours.[163] Epinephrine significantly prolongs the duration of the intermediate-acting agents but has little effect on the long-acting drugs. In addition, it has been postulated that clonidine might prolong the duration of action of local anesthetics by a mechanism similar to that observed with epinephrine. Studies show that clonidine reduces local blood flow, and the decrease in blood flow correlates with the injected dose. Higher doses were needed (300 mcg), and this reduction may be relevant only at the higher doses.[165] The onset is 5 to 15 minutes with all the drugs except bupivacaine, which has a longer onset of 10 to

20 minutes. Bupivacaine (0.25% and 0.5%) produces a good sensory block but has minimal effect on motor function. This makes it an ideal drug for obstetric anesthesia. Ropivacaine has been successfully used for epidural anesthesia; however, it is less potent than bupivacaine, which likely accounts for a reduced motor block.[103] Etidocaine (1% to 1.5%) produces adequate analgesia and a profound motor block; therefore, this drug is not used in obstetric anesthesia.

Prolonged Administration

It is common in clinical practice to administer local anesthetics by continuous infusion for several days after surgery or for weeks during treatment of chronic pain. It has been noted that administration of local anesthetics by continuous infusion can result in the attenuation of effectiveness. Also, it has been demonstrated that allowing pain to return between bolus epidural injections results in attenuation of intensity and duration of the block. Animal studies have indicated that the mechanism for the tolerance associated with local anesthetics probably has both a pharmacokinetic and pharmacodynamic component. For example, repeated injections of the sciatic nerve in rats result in a lower intraneural lidocaine content and a shorter duration of block (pharmacokinetic). Tachyphylaxis in rats is associated with hyperalgesia, indicating a pharmacodynamic component.[170,171]

SUMMARY

Local anesthetic techniques are becoming more commonplace in outpatient procedures, obstetrics, and pain services. The nurse anesthetist must thoroughly understand the pharmacologic properties of local anesthetics in order to administer and manage local, topical, and regional anesthesia appropriately. For example, this knowledge is important in the selection of a drug with an appropriate dose, concentration, time to onset, and duration of action for a selected regional technique.

Local anesthetics are drugs used for blocking the conduction of nerve impulses. They accomplish this primarily by blocking Na^+ channels on the cytoplasmic side of the axolemma. To do this, they must diffuse through tissue barriers. These include the supportive structures within the nerve trunk, such as the endoneurium, perineurium, and epineurium.

Different local anesthetics have similar chemical structures: they have an aromatic ring, an intermediate carbon chain, and an amine moiety. However, the structures differ with respect to the type of boundary that connects the aromatic ring to the carbon chain and because of substitutions on the amine and aromatic ends of the molecules. These structural differences can make a significant difference in the anesthetics' time to onset, duration, and potency, as well as the site used and rate of metabolism of these drugs. Therefore, the chemical structure is a primary determinant of which drug is selected in a given clinical situation.

Local anesthetics can be inadvertently injected intravascularly or can be absorbed systemically in quantities large enough to produce significant effects on the CNS and the cardiovascular system. In the CNS they produce depression that can result in seizures and coma. Cardiovascular toxicity may also be problematic. Manifestations of cardiovascular toxicity are myocardial depression, cardiac conduction abnormalities, and vasodilatation, which can result in cardiovascular collapse and cardiac arrest. Toxicity can be prevented through the avoidance of intravascular injection and the administration of appropriate doses. Less common forms of toxicity are allergic reactions, local tissue effects, and methemoglobinemia.

Local anesthetics can be used topically, as well as for local infiltration, nerve block, spinal anesthesia, and epidural anesthesia. Onset, duration, concentration, dose, and rate of absorption vary significantly with the site of anesthesia and the local anesthetic administered.

REFERENCES

1. Koster J. Passive membrane properties of the neuron. In: Kandel ER, ed: *Principles of Neural Sciences*. Norwalk, CT: Appleton & Lange; 1991:3.
2. Skidmore RA. Local anesthetics. *Dermatol Surg.* 1996;22:511-522.
3. Guyton AC, Hall JE. *Textbook of Medical Physiology*. 11th ed. Philadelphia: Saunders; 2006:57-70.
4. Jaffe RA, Rowe MA. Differential nerve block. Direct measurements on individual myelinated and unmyelinated dorsal root axons. *Anesthesiology.* 1996;84:1455-1464.
5. Wildsmith JAW. Peripheral nerve and local anesthetic drugs. *Br J Anaesth.* 1986;58:692-699.
6. Guyton AC, Hall JE. *Textbook of Medical Physiology*. 11th ed. Philadelphia: Saunders; 2006:61.
7. Stevens CE. The neuron. *Sci Am.* 1979;241:55.
8. Tetzlaff JE. *Clinical Pharmacology of Local Anesthetics*. Boston: Butterworth-Heinemann; 2000.
9. Guyton AC, Hall JE. *Textbook of Medical Physiology*. 11th ed. Philadelphia: Saunders; 2006:66.
10. de Jong RH. *Local Anesthesia*. Springfield, IL: Charles C Thomas; 1994;65-66, 82-84.
11. Singer SJ, Nicolson GL. The fluid mosaic model of the structure of cell membranes. *Science.* 1972;175:723.
12. Ragsdale DS et al:Common molecular determinants of local anesthetic, antiarrhythmic, and anticonvulsant block of voltage-gated Na^+ channels. *Proc Natl Acad Sci U S A.* 1996;93:9270-9275.
13. Yanagidate F, Strichartz GR. Local anesthetics. *Handb Exp Pharmacol.* 2007;177:95-127.
14. Power I, Kam P. *Principles of Physiology for the Anaesthetist*. London: Arnold; 2001:1-15.
15. Ragsdale DS et al: Molecular determinants of state-dependent block of Na^+ channels by local anesthetics. *Science.* 1997;265:1724-1728.
16. Carboni M et al. Slow sodium channel inactivation and use-dependent block modulated by the same domain IV S6 residue. *J Membr Biol.* 2005;207(2):107-117.
17. Fukuda K et al. Compound-specific Na^+ channel pore conformational changes induced by local anaesthetics. *J Physiol.* 2005;564(Pt 1):21-31.
18. Wynn RL. Recent research on mechanisms of local anesthetics. *Gen Dent.* 1995;4:316-318.
19. Franz DN, Perry RS. Mechanism for differential block among single myelinated and nonmyelinated axons by procaine. *J Physiol (London).* 1973;236:193.
20. Rosenburg PH, Heavner JE. Temperature dependent nerve blocking action of lidocaine and halothane. *Acta Anaesthesiol Scand.* 1980;24:324.
21. Bromage PR. *Epidural Anesthesia*. Philadelphia: Saunders; 1978:525.
22. Truant AP. Differential physical-chemical and neuropharmacologic properties of local anesthetic agents. *Anesth Analg.* 1959;38:478-484.
23. Gasser HS, Erlanger J. The role of fiber size in the establishment of nerve block by pressure or cocaine. *Am J Physiol.* 1929;88:581-591.
24. Collins WF et al. Relation of peripheral nerve fiber size and sensation in man. *Arch Neurol.* 1960;3:381-385.
25. Raymond SA, Gissen AJ. Mechanisms of differential nerve block. In: Strichartz GR, ed. *Local Anesthetics*. Berlin: Springer-Verlag; 1987:95.
26. Gissen A et al. Differential sensitivity of fast and slow fibers in mammalian nerve. II. Margin of safety for nerve transmission. *Anesth Analg.* 1982;61(7):561-569.
27. Given BG. Pharmacology of local anesthetic agents. *Br J Anaesth.* 1986;58:701.
28. Butterworth J. Local anesthetics, agents, additives, mechanisms and misconceptions. *ASA Annual Meeting Refresher Course Lectures*. Park Ridge, IL: American Society of Anesthesiologists; 2007:132.

29. Wildsmith JAW et al. Differential nerve blocking activity of amino-ester local anesthetics. *Br J Anaesth.* 1985;57:612.

30. Wildsmith JA et al. Differential nerve blockade: esters v. amines and the influence of pKₐ. *Br J Anaesth.* 1987;59:379-384.

31. Blair MR. Cardiovascular pharmacology of local anesthetics. *Br J Anaesth.* 1975;47(Suppl):247-252.

32. Tucker GT et al. Binding of amide-type local anesthetics in human plasma: relationships between binding, physiochemical properties, and anesthetic activity. *Anesthesiology.* 1970;33:287.

33. Ritchie JM et al. The active structure of local anesthetics. *J Pharmacol Exp Ther.* 1965;150:152.

34. Covino BG, Wildsmith JA. Clinical pharmacology of local anesthetic agents. In: Cousins MJ, Bridenbaugh PO, eds. *Neural Blockade in Clinical Anesthesia and Management of Pain.* Philadelphia: Lippincott-Raven; 1998:111-144.

35. Covino BG. Pharmacology of local anesthetic agents. *Br J Anaesth.* 1986;58:701-716.

36. Cederholm I et al. Local analgesic and vascular effects of intradermal ropivacaine and bupivacaine in various concentrations with and without addition of adrenaline in man. *Acta Anaesthesiol Scand.* 1994;38:322-327.

37. Scott DB et al. Factors affecting plasma level of lidocaine and prilocaine. *Br J Anaesth.* 1972;44:1040.

38. Cox B et al. Toxicity of local anaesthetics. *Best Pract Res Clin Anaesthesiol.* 2003;17:111-136.

39. Faccenda KA, Finucane BT. Complications of regional anaesthesia. Incidence and prevention. *Drug Saf.* 2001;24:413-442.

40. Tagariello V et al. Mepivacaine: update on an evergreen local anaesthetic. *Minerva Anestesiol.* 2001;67(Suppl 1):5-8.

41. Naguib M et al. Adverse effects and drug interactions associated with local and regional anaesthesia. *Drug Saf.* 1998;18:221-250.

42. Sinnott CJ et al. On the mechanism by which epinephrine potentiates lidocaine's peripheral nerve block. *Anesthesiology.* 2003;98(1):181-188.

43. Albert J, Tofstrom B. Bilateral ulnar blocks in the evaluation of local anaesthetic agents. *Acta Anaesthesiol Scand.* 1965;9:203.

44. Eisennach JC et al. Epinephrine enhanced analgesia produced by epidural bupivacaine during labor. *Anesth Analg.* 1987;66:467.

45. Sandler AN et al. Pharmacokinetics of three doses of epidural ropivacaine during hysterectomy and comparison with bupivacaine. *Can J Anaesth.* 1998;45:843-849.

46. Sinclair CJ, Scott DB. Comparison of bupivacaine and etidocaine in extradural blockade. *Br J Anaesth.* 1984;56:147.

47. Neal JM. Effects of epinephrine in local anesthetics on the central and peripheral nervous systems: neurotoxicity and neural blood flow. *Reg Anesth Pain Med.* 2003;28:124-134.

48. Chen TY et al. The clinical use of small-dose tetracaine spinal anesthesia for transurethral prostatectomy. *Anesth Analg.* 2001;92:1020-1023.

49. Bokesch PM et al. Dependence of lidocaine potency on pH and PCO₂. *Anesth Analg.* 1987;66:9.

50. Gosteli P et al. Effects of pH adjustment and carbonation of lidocaine during epidural anesthesia for foot or ankle surgery. *Anesth Analg.* 1995; 81:104-149.

51. Nickel PM et al. Comparison of hydrochloride and carbonated salts of lidocaine for epidural analgesia. *Reg Anesth.* 1986;11:66.

52. Chassard D et al. Alkalinization of local anesthetics: theoretically justified but clinically useless. *Can J Anaesth.* 1996;43:384-393.

53. Ramos G et al. Does alkalinization of 0.75% ropivacaine promote a lumbar peridural block of higher quality? *Reg Anesth Pain Med.* 2001;26:357-362.

54. Peterfreund RA et al. Adjustment of local anesthetic solutions with sodium bicarbonate: laboratory evaluations of alkalization and precipitation. *Reg Anesth.* 1989;14:265, 270.

55. Carvalho B et al. Local infiltration of epinephrine-containing lidocaine with bicarbonate reduces superficial bleeding and pain during labor epidural catheter insertion: a randomized trial. *Int J Obstet Anesth.* 2007;16(2): 116-121.

56. Christoph RA et al. Pain reduction in local anesthetic administration through pH buffering. *Ann Emerg Med.* 1988;17:117-120.

57. Navaratnarajah M, Davenport HT. The prolongation of local anaesthetic action with dextran. The effect of molecular weight. *Anesthesia.* 1985; 40:259-262.

58. Alkhawajah A, Farag H. The effect of dextran on the pharmacokinetics of lignocaine during epidural anaesthesia. *J Int Med Res.* 1992;20:127-135.

59. Rosenblatt RM, Fung DL. Optional ratio of bupivacaine and dextran for regional anesthesia. *Reg Anesth.* 1979;4:2.

60. Dempsey GA et al. Hyaluronidase and peribulbar block. *Br J Anaesth.* 1997;78:671-674.

61. Cunningham ML, Kaplan JA. A rapid onset long acting regional anesthesia technique. *Anesthesiology.* 1974;41:509.

62. Cohen SE, Thurlow A. Comparison of a chloroprocaine-bupivacaine mixture with chloroprocaine and bupivacaine used individually for obstetric epidural analgesia. *Anesthesiology.* 1979;51:288.

63. Reynolds F. Adverse effects of local anaesthetics. *Br J Anaesth.* 1987;59:78-95.

64. Sandler AN et al. Pharmacokinetics of three doses of epidural ropivacaine during hysterectomy and comparison with bupivacaine. *Can J Anaesth.* 1998;45:843-849.

65. Johnson RF et al. A comparison of the placental transfer of ropivacaine versus bupivacaine. *Anesth Analg.* 1999;89:703-708.

66. Santos AC et al. The placental transfer and fetal effects of levobupivacaine, racemic bupivacaine, and ropivacaine. *Anesthesiology.* 1999;90:6.

67. Lofstrom JB et al. Lung uptake of lidocaine. *Acta Anaesthesiol Scand.* 1978;70: 80.

68. Calvo R et al. Effects of disease and acetazolamide on procaine hydrolysis by red cell enzymes. *Clin Pharmacol Ther.* 1980;27:175.

69. Bowill JG, Howie MB. *Clinical Pharmacology for Anaesthetists.* London: Saunders; 1999:157-172.

70. Wildsmith JAW. Local anesthetics. In: Aitkenhead AR et al, eds. *Textbook of Anaesthesia.* 5th ed Edinburgh: Churchill Livingstone; 2007:52-63.

71. Arthur GR. Pharmacokinetics of local anesthetics. *Handb Exp Pharmacol.* 1987;81:165-186.

72. Smith AR et al. Grand mal seizures after 2-chloroprocaine epidural anesthesia in a patient with plasma cholinesterase deficiency. *Anesth Analg.* 1987; 66:677.

73. Davis L et al. Cholinesterase. Its significance in anaesthetic practice. *Anaesthesia.* 1997;52:244-260.

74. Simpson D et al. Ropivacaine: a review of its use in regional anaesthesia and acute pain management. *Drugs.* 2005;65(18):2675-2717.

75. Tucker GT et al. Hepatic clearance of local anesthetics in man. *J Pharmacokinet Biopharm.* 1977;5:111.

76. Longnecker DE, Murphy FL. *Introduction to Anesthesia.* Philadelphia: Saunders; 1992:204.

77. Jokinen MJ. The pharmacokinetics of ropivacaine in hepatic and renal insufficiency. *Best Pract Res Clin Anaesthesiol.* 2005;19(2):269-274.

78. Thompson PD et al. Lidocaine pharmacokinetics in advanced heart failure, liver disease and renal failure in humans. *Ann Intern Med.* 1973;78:499.

79. Nakayama M et al. Effects of volume and concentration of lidocaine on epidural anaesthesia in pregnant females. *Eur J Anaesthesiol.* 2002;19:808-811.

80. Fagraeus L et al. Spread of analgesia in early pregnancy. *Anesthesiology.* 1983;58:184.

81. Datta S et al. The effect of pregnancy on bupivacaine induced conduction blockade in the rabbit vagus nerve. *Anesth Analg.* 1987;66:123.

82. Datta S et al. Differential sensitivities of mammalian nerve fibers during pregnancy. *Anesth Analg.* 1983;62:1070.

83. McCaughey W. Adverse effects of local anesthetics. *Drug Saf.* 1992;77:74-78.

84. Mulroy MF. Systemic toxicity and cardiotoxicity from local anesthetics: incidence and preventive measures. *Reg Anesth Pain Med.* 2002;6(27): 556-561.

85. Scott DB. Toxic effects of local anaesthetic agents on central nervous system. *Br J Anaesth.* 1986;58:732.

86. Graf BM. The cardiotoxicity of local anesthetics: the place of ropivacaine. *Curr Top Med Chem.* 2001;1:207-214.

87. Liu PL et al. Comparative CNS toxicity of lidocaine, endocaine, bupivacaine and tetracaine in awake dogs following rapid IV administration. *Anesth Analg.* 1973;62:375.

88. Englesson S. The influence of acid-base changes on central nervous system toxicity of local anesthetic agents: an experimental study in cats. *Acta Anaesthesiol Scand.* 1974;18:79.

89. Covino BG. Clinical pharmacology of local anesthetic agents. In: Cousins MJ, Bridenbaugh PO, eds. *Neural Blockade in Clinical Anesthesia and Management of Pain.* Philadelphia: Lippincott; 1998:100-105.

90. Covina BG. Toxicity of local anesthetics. *Adv Anesth.* 1986;3:37.

91. Johns RA et al: Lidocaine constricts or dilates rat arterioles in a dose-dependent manner. *Anesthesiology.* 1985;62:141.

92. Gristwood RW. Cardiac and CNS toxicity of levobupivacaine: strengths of evidence for advantage over bupivacaine. *Drug Saf.* 2002;25:153-163.

93. Feldman HS et al. Direct chronotropic and inotropic effects of local anesthetic agents in isolated guinea pig atria. *Reg Anesth.* 1982;7:149.

94. Mather LE, Chang DH. Cardiotoxicity with modern local anaesthetics: is there a safer choice? *Drugs.* 2001;61:333-342.

95. Till R et al. Acute cardiovascular toxicity of procaine, chloroprocaine and tetracaine anesthetized ventilated dogs. *Reg Anesth.* 1982;7:14.

96. Mulroy MF. Systemic toxicity and cardiotoxicity from local anesthetics: incidence and preventive measures. *Reg Anesth Pain Med.* 2002;27:556-561.

97. Morishima HO et al: Is bupivacaine more cardiotoxic than lidocaine? *Anesthesiology.* 1983;59:A409.

98. Morishima HO et al: Etidocaine toxicity in the adult, newborn, and fetal sheep. *Anesthesiology.* 1981;58:342.

99. Davis ML, de Jong RH. Successful resuscitation following massive bupivacaine overdose. *Anesth Analg.* 1982;61:62-64.

100. Royse CF, Royse AG. The myocardial and vascular effects of bupivacaine, levobupivacaine, and ropivacaine using pressure volume loops. *Anesth Analg.* 2005;101(3):679-687.

101. Heavner JE. Cardiac toxicity of local anesthetics in the intact isolated heart model: a review. *Reg Anesth Pain Med.* 2002;27:545-555.

102. Graf BM. The cardiotoxicity of local anesthetics: the place of ropivacaine. *Curr Top Med Chem.* 2001;1:207-214.

103. Polley LS et al. Relative analgesic potencies of ropivacaine and bupivacaine for epidural analgesia in labor. *Anesthesiology.* 1999;90:944-950.

104. Chan VWS et al. Comparison of ropivacaine and lidocaine for intravenous regional anesthesia in volunteers. *Anesthesiology.* 1999;90:1602-1608.

105. Kopaz DJ, Allen HW. Accidental intravenous levobupivacaine. *Anesth Analg.* 1999;89:1027-1029.

106. Tetzlaff J. Local anesthesia: are the new agents any better? *Audio Digest Anesthesiol.* 2002;44:4.

107. Crandall JT, Kotelks DM. Cardiotoxicity of local anesthetics during pregnancy. *Anesth Analg.* 1985;61:60.

108. Morishima HO et al. Bupivacaine toxicity in pregnant and non-pregnant ewes. *Anesthesiology.* 1985;63:134.

109. Sage DJ et al. Influence of bupivacaine and lidocaine on isolated guinea pig atria in the presence of acidosis and hypoxia. *Anesth Analg.* 1984;63:1.

110. Malamed SF. Allergy and toxic reactions to local anesthetics. *Dent Today.* 2003;22:114-116, 118-121.

111. Finder RL, Moore PA. Adverse drug reactions to local anesthesia. *Dent Clin North Am.* 2002;46:747-757.

112. Boren E et al. A critical review of local anesthetics sensitivity. *Clin Rev Allergy Immunol.* 2007;32(1):119-128.

113. Phillips JF et al. Approach to patients with suspected hypersensitivity to local anesthetics. *Am J Med Sci.* 2007;334(3):190-196.

114. Eggleston ST, Lush LW. Understanding allergic reactions to local anesthetic. *Ann Pharmacother.* 1996;30:851-857.

115. Nagel JE et al. Paraben allergy. *JAMA.* 1977;237:1594.

116. Climic CR et al. Methaemoglobinemia in mothers and fetus following continuous epidural analgesia with prilocaine. *Br J Anesth.* 1967;30:195.

117. Law RMT et al. Measurement of methemoglobin after EMLA analgesia for newborn circumcision. *Biol Neonate.* 1996;70:213-217.

118. Kane GC et al. Benzocaine-induced methemoglobinemia based on the Mayo Clinic experience from 28,478 transesophageal echocardiograms: incidence, outcomes, and predisposing factors. *AMA Arch Intern Med.* 2007;167(18):1977-1982.

119. Gupta PM et al. Benzocaine-induced methemoglobinemia. *South Med J.* 2000;93(1):83-86.

120. Taniguchi M et al. Sodium bisulfite: scapegoat for chloroprocaine neurotoxicity? *Anesthesiology.* 2004;100(1):85-91.

121. Lambert DH, Strichartz GR. In defense of in vitro findings. *Anesthesiology.* 2004;101(5):1246-1247.

122. Baker MT. Chloroprocaine or sulfite toxicity? *Anesthesiology.* 2004;101(5):1247.

123. Feinstein MB et al. The antagonism of local anesthetic induced convulsions by the benzodiazepine derivative diazepam. *Arch Int Pharmacodyn Ther.* 1970;187:144-154.

124. Wesseling H et al. Effects of diazepam and pentobarbitone on convulsions induced by local anesthetics in mice. *Eur J Pharmacol.* 1971;1:150-154.

125. Heavner JE. Let's abandon blanket maximum recommended doses of local anesthetics. *Reg Anesth Pain Med.* 2004;29:564-575.

126. Rowlingson JC. Lipid rescue: a step forward in patient safety? Likely so! *Anesth Analg.* 2008;106:1333-1336.

127. Reynolds F. Ropivacaine. *Anesthesiology.* 1991;46:339.

128. Wang GK. Binding affinity and stereoselectivity of local anesthetics in single batrachotoxin-activated sodium channels. *J Gen Physiol.* 1990;96:105.

129. Bader AM et al. Comparison of bupivacaine- and ropivacaine-induced conduction blockade in the isolated rabbit vagus nerve. *Anesth Analg.* 1989;68:724.

130. Finucane BT. Ropivacaine cardiac toxicity—not as troublesome as bupivacaine. *Can J Anaesth.* 2005;52(5):449-453.

131. Ritz S et al. Cardiotoxicity of ropivacaine: a new amide local anesthetic. *Acta Anaesthesiol Scand.* 1989;33:93.

132. Hurley RJ et al. The effects of epinephrine on the anesthetic and hemodynamic properties of ropivacaine and bupivacaine after epidural administration in the dog. *Reg Anesth.* 1991;16:303.

133. Feldman HS et al. Comparative systemic toxicity of convulsant and supraconvulsant doses of ropivacaine, bupivacaine, and lidocaine in the conscious dog. *Anesth Analg.* 1989;69:794.

134. Rutten AJ et al. Hemodynamic and central effects of intravenous bolus doses of lidocaine, bupivacaine, and ropivacaine in sheep. *Anesth Analg.* 1989;69:291.

135. Feldman HS et al. Treatment of acute systemic toxicity after the rapid intravenous injection of ropivacaine and bupivacaine in the conscious dog. *Anesth Analg.* 1991;73:373.

136. Stienstra R. The place of ropivacaine in anesthesia. *Acta Anaesthesiol Belg.* 2003;54:141-148.

137. McClellan KJ, Faulds D. Ropivacaine: an update of its use in regional anaesthesia. *Drugs.* 2002;60:1065-1093.

138. Owen MD, Dean LS. Ropivacaine. *Expert Opin Pharmacother.* 2002;1:325-336.

139. Scott BD et al. Acute toxicity of ropivacaine compared with that of bupivacaine. *Anesth Analg.* 1989;69:563.

140. Pollock JE. Local anesthetic toxicity. *Audio Digest Anesthesiol.* 2003;45:11.

141. Gunter JB et al. Levobupivacaine for ilioinguinal/iliohypogastric nerve block in children. *Anesth Analg.* 1999;89:647-649.

142. McClellan KJ, Spencer CM. Levobupivacaine. *Drugs.* 1998;56:355-362.

143. Markham A, Faulds D. Ropivacaine: a review of its pharmacology and therapeutic use in regional anaesthesia. *Drugs.* 1996;52:429-449.

144. Foster RH, Markham A. Levobupivacaine: a review of its pharmacology and use as a local anaesthetic. *Drugs.* 2000;59(3):551-579.

145. Stewart J et al. The central system and cardiovascular effects of levobupivacaine and ropivacaine in healthy volunteers. *Anesth Analg.* 2003;97:412-416.

146. Lacassie HJ et al. The relative motor blocking potencies of epidural bupivacaine and ropivacaine in labor. *Anesth Analg.* 2002;95:204-208.

147. Polley LS et al. Relative analgesic potencies of ropivacaine and bupivacaine for epidural analgesia in labor: implications for therapeutics indexes. *Anesthesiology.* 1999;90:944-950.

148. Panni M, Segal S. New local anesthetics. Are they worth the cost? *Anesthesiol Clin North Am.* 2003;21:19-38.

149. Robieux I et al. Assessing pain and analgesia with a lidocaine/prilocaine emulsion in infants and toddlers during venipuncture. *J Pediatr.* 1991;118: 970.

150. EMLA *[package insert].* Westboro, MA: Astra Pharmaceutical Products; 1993.

151. Goede IA, Betcher DL. EMLA. *J Pediatr Oncol Nurs.* 1994;11:38.

152. Ohlsen C et al. An anesthetic lidocaine/prilocaine cream (EMLA) for epicutaneous applications tested for cutting split skin grafts. *Scand J Plast Reconstr Surg.* 1985;19:201.

153. Jokobson B, Nilsson A. Methemoglobinemia associated with a prilocaine/lidocaine cream and trimethoprim/sulfamethazole: a case report. *Acta Anaesthesiol Scand.* 1985;29:453.

154. Grant S, Hoffman RS. Use of tetracaine, epinephrine, and cocaine as a topical anesthetic in the emergency department. *Ann Emerg Med.* 1992; 21:987.

155. Strichartz GR, Berde CB. Local anesthetics. In: Miller RD, ed. *Anesthesia.* 6th ed. New York: Churchill Livingstone; 2005:573-604.

156. Smith G et al. New non–cocaine-containing topical anesthetics compared with tetracaine-adrenaline-cocaine during repair of lacerations. *Pediatrics.* 1997;100:825.

157. Jeffrey JM et al. Extended duration nerve blockade using large unilamellar vesicles that exhibit a proton gradient. *Anesthesiology.* 1996;85:635.

158. Astrom A, Persson NH. The toxicity of some local anesthetics after application on different mucous membranes and its relation to anesthetic action on the nasal mucosa of the rabbit. *J Pharmacol Exp Ther.* 1961;132:87.

159. Scarfone RJ et al. Pain of local anesthetics: rate of administration and buffering. *Ann Emerg Med.* 1998;31:36-40.

160. Campbell D, Adriani I. Absorption of local anesthetics. *JAMA.* 1958;168:873.

161. Liu SS, Joseph RS. Local anesthetics. In: Barash PG et al, eds. *Clinical Anesthesia.* 5th ed. Lippincott Williams & Wilkins; 2006:453-474.

162. Morell RC. What the anesthesiologist needs to know about tumescent anesthesia. *Audio Digest Anesthesiol.* 2002;44:10.

163. Liisanantti O et al. High-dose bupivacaine, levobupivacaine and ropivacaine in axillary brachial plexus block. *Acta Anaesthesiol Scand.* 2004;48(5): 601-606.

164. Concepcion MA et al. Tourniquet pain during spinal anesthesia: a comparison of plain solutions of tetracaine and bupivacaine. *Anesth Analg.* 1988; 67: 828.

165. Mazoit JX et al. Clonidine and or adrenaline decrease lidocaine plasma peak concentration after epidural injection. *Br J Clin Pharmacol.* 1996;42:242-245.

166. Phillip J et al. Transient neurologic symptoms after spinal anesthesia with lidocaine in obstetric patients. *Anesth Analg.* 2001;92:405-409.

167. Zaric D et al. Transient neurologic symptoms (TNS) following spinal anaesthesia with lidocaine versus other local anaesthetics. *Cochrane Database Syst Rev.* 2005;19(4):CD003006.

168. Sime AC. AANA *Journal* course: transient neurologic symptoms and spinal anesthesia. *AANA J.* 2000;68:163-168.

169. Pollock JE. Transient neurologic symptoms: etiology, risk factors, and management. *Reg Anesth Pain Med.* 2002;27:581-586.

170. Lee KC et al. Thermal hyperalgesia accelerates and MK-801 prevent the development of tachyphylaxis to rat sciatic nerve blockade. *Anesthesiology.* 1994;81:1284.

171. Choi R et al. Pharmacokinetic nature of tachyphylaxis to lidocaine: peripheral nerve blocks and infiltration anesthesia in rats. *Life Sci.* 1997; 61:177-184.

OPIOID AGONISTS AND ANTAGONISTS

Wanda O. Wilson

In the past, opium was used as a topical, intravenous, and inhaled analgesic. One of the earliest uses of opium is found in Greek literature dating from 300 BCE. Opium sponges, referred to as *soporific sponges*, were used for the control of pain as early as the 14th century. An attempt to administer opioids by the intravenous route was attributed to Elscholtz in 1665, approximately 200 years before the invention of the syringe and needle. The first attempt to administer an opium vapor by inhalation was documented in 1778. It was not until 1853, when the syringe and needle were introduced into clinical practice by Wood, that an accurate dose of opioid could be administered intravenously.

In 1803, Sertürner reported the isolation of a pure substance from opium that he named *morphine*, after Morpheus, the Greek god of dreams. Abuse of opium and isolated alkaloids led to the synthetic production of potent analgesics. Other opium alkaloids were soon discovered—codeine by Robiquet in 1832 and papaverine by Merck in 1848. The goal of synthetic manufacture of analgesics was the creation of potent analgesics that would have high specificity for receptors, were not addictive, and were free of side effects. Synthetic production led to the development of opioid agonists, partial agonists, agonists-antagonists, and antagonists.

OPIOIDS

Opioid is a term used to refer to a group of drugs, both naturally occurring and synthetically produced, that possess opium- or morphine-like properties. Opioids exert their effects by mimicking naturally occurring endogenous opioid peptides or endorphins. *Narcotic* is derived from the Greek word *narkōtikos*, "benumbing," and refers to potent morphine-like analgesics with the potential to produce stupor, insensibility, and dependence. The term *narcotic* is not useful in a pharmacologic or clinical discussion because of its legal connotations.

At least four systems of classification are used to describe opioids. The first divides the opioids into four categories: agonists, partial agonists, agonists-antagonists, and antagonists (Table 12-1). A second descriptive classification separates the opioids into classes according to their lipophilicity. Another system of categorization is based on the chemical derivation of the opioids and divides them into naturally occurring, semisynthetic, and synthetic compounds, with each group having subgroups (Box 12-1). A final, simple classification system describes the drugs as either weak or strong.

The term *opioid* is derived from the word *opium* (from *opos*, Greek for "sap"), an extract from the poppy plant *Papaver*

somniferum. The properties of opium are attributable to the 20 different isolated alkaloids, and the alkaloids are divided chemically into two types: phenanthrene (from which morphine and codeine are derived) and benzylisoquinoline (from which papaverine, a nonanalgesic drug, is derived). Modification of the morphine molecule with retention of the five-ring structure results in the semisynthetic drugs heroin and hydromorphone. When the furan ring is removed from morphine, the resulting four-ring synthetic opioid levorphanol is formed. The phenylpiperidines (e.g., meperidine, fentanyl) and the phenylheptylamines (e.g., methadone, propoxyphene) all have only two of the original five rings of the basic morphine molecular structure. A close relationship exists between the stereochemical structure and potency of opioids, with the *levo-* isomers being the most potent.[1] All opioids, despite the diverse molecular structures, share an N-methylpiperidine moiety, which seems to confer analgesic activity.[2] Figure 12-1 illustrates the structures of the commonly used opioids.

Opioid drugs produce pharmacologic activity by binding to opiate receptors primarily located in the central nervous system (CNS), supraspinal and spinal; however, evidence of sites outside the CNS, such as peripheral sites, has emerged.[3] Supraspinal analgesia occurs through activation of postsynaptic opioid receptors in the medulla and midbrain, which causes inhibition of neurons involved in pain pathways via increased flux of potassium ions. Spinal analgesia occurs by activation of presynaptic opioid receptors, which leads to decreased calcium influx and decreased release of neurotransmitters involved in nociception. Clinically, supraspinal and spinal opioid analgesic mechanisms are synergistic.[4] This explains why opioids such as fentanyl and sufentanil produce more profound analgesia when delivered epidurally than when delivered systemically, despite the similar blood concentrations measured with both routes of administration.[2,5]

Inflammatory hyperalgesic conditions appear to be especially amenable to peripheral opioid antinociceptive actions.[4] The mechanism of peripheral actions appears to be activation of opioid receptors located on primary afferent nerves.

Opiate Receptors

The discovery of opioid receptors can be traced back to the 1940s and 1950s, when pharmaceutical companies were involved in research in anticipation of the development of an effective nonaddictive analgesic. In 1973, the examination of vertebrate species led to the discovery of three opiate receptor classes that mediate analgesia.[3] Questions emerged as to why the receptors

TABLE 12-1	Opioid Agonists, Partial Agonists, Agonists-Antagonists, and Antagonists at Sites of Activity		
Opioid	Mu	Kappa	Delta
Morphine	Agonist	Agonist	Agonist
Meperidine	Agonist	Agonist	Agonist
Fentanyl	Agonist	Agonist	Agonist
Sufentanil	Agonist	Agonist	Agonist
Alfentanil	Agonist	Agonist	Agonist
Remifentanil	Agonist	Agonist	Agonist
Butorphanol	Antagonist	Partial agonist	Agonist
Nalbuphine	Antagonist	Partial agonist	Agonist
Naloxone	Antagonist	Antagonist	Antagonist
Naltrexone	Antagonist	Antagonist	Antagonist
Nalmefene	Antagonist	Antagonist	Antagonist

BOX 12-1

Classification of Opioids Based on Derivation of Drug

Naturally Occurring Opium Alkaloids
Phenanthrene derivatives
    Morphine
    Codeine
Benzylisoquinoline derivatives
Papaverine

Semisynthetic Derivatives of Opium Alkaloids
Morphine derivatives
    Oxymorphone
    Hydromorphone
    Heroin
Thebaine derivatives
    Buprenorphine
    Oxycodone

Synthetic Opioids
Morphinans
    Levorphanol
    Nalbuphine
Phenylheptylamines
    Methadone
    Propoxyphene
Phenylpiperidines
    Alfentanil
    Fentanyl
    Naloxone
    Naltrexone
    Meperidine
    Sufentanil
    Remifentanil

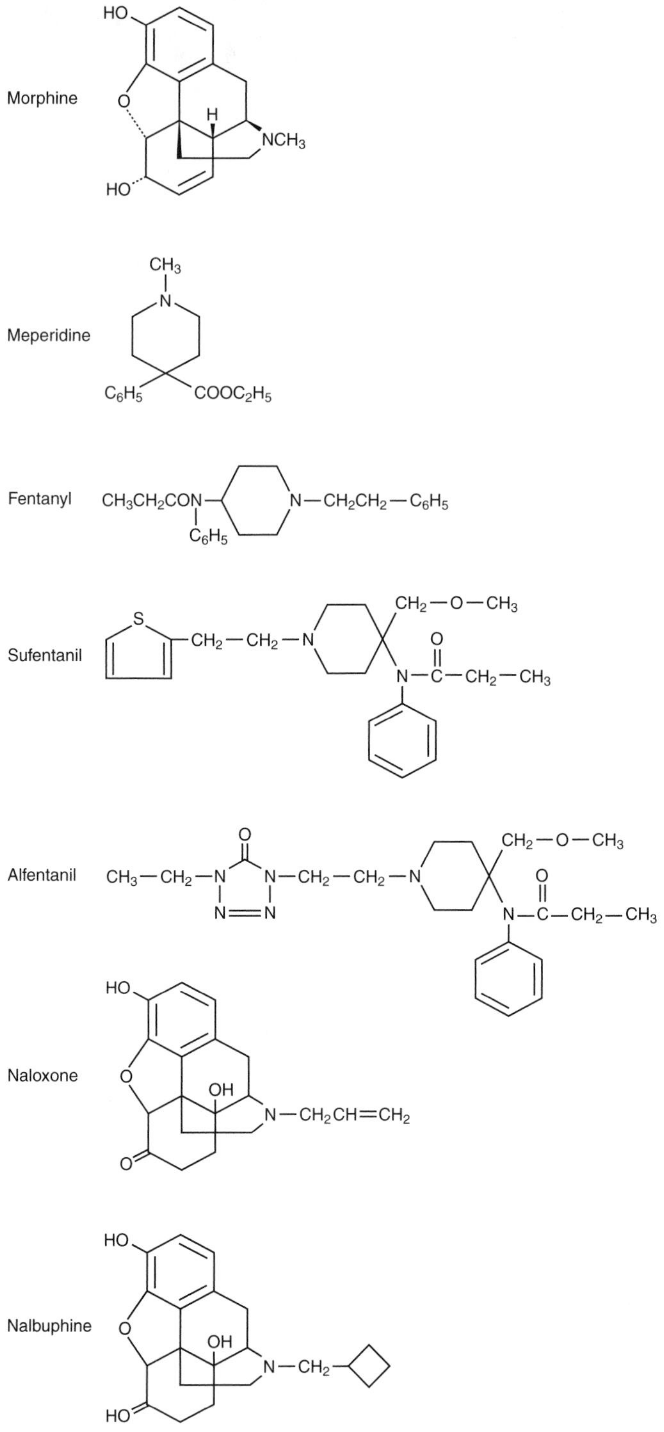

FIGURE 12-1 Selected opioid agonists and antagonists used as anesthesia adjunct drugs.

existed, and further research led to the hypothesis that the receptors possess endogenous functions.

After the discovery of opiate receptors in the early 1970s, the search began for endogenous substances that were their agonists. In 1975, three such agonists were identified: enkephalins,

endorphins, and dynorphins.[3] Each group is derived from a distinct precursor polypeptide and has a characteristic anatomic distribution. By the early 1980s, three precursor molecules to these agonists were identified and named after the active fragments: proenkephalin, proadrenocorticotropic hormone (ACTH)–endorphin (also called *proopiomelanocortin*), and prodynorphin.[2,3] Opioid peptides share the common amino-terminal sequence of Try-Gly-Gly-Phe-(Met or Leu), which has been labeled the *opioid motif* or *message* and is necessary for interaction at the receptor site. The peptide selectivity resides in the

TABLE **12-2** Characteristics of Opioid Receptor Subtypes*				
Effects	**Mu-1**	**Mu-2**	**Kappa Receptor**	**Delta Receptor**
Analgesia	Supraspinal	Spinal	Supraspinal, spinal	Supraspinal, spinal; modulates mu-receptor activity
Cardiovascular	Bradycardia	Bradycardia		
Respiratory		Depression	Possible depression	Depression
Central nervous system	Euphoria, sedation, prolactin release, hypothermia, catalepsy, indifference to environmental stimulus	Euphoria, dopamine turnover, possible growth hormone release	Sedation, dysphoria, psychomimetic reactions (hallucinations, delirium)	
Pupil	Miosis	Miosis	Miosis	
Gastrointestinal		Inhibition of peristalsis, nausea, vomiting		
Genitourinary	Urinary retention	Urinary retention	Diuresis (inhibition of vasopressin release)	Urinary retention
Pruritus		Yes		Yes
Physical dependence	Low abuse potential	Yes	Low abuse potential	Yes

Other opioid subtypes exist in animals, such as kappa-1, kappa-2, and kappa-3. Mu-1 and mu-2 agonists have not been developed for human use.

carboxy-terminal extension, providing the *address*.[2] In 1975, Hughes and Kosterlitz identified the first endogenous substance with opioid activity.

Martin and co-workers[6] were the first to provide evidence for opiate receptor subtypes (Table 12-2). Their findings provided evidence for the existence of three opiate receptors: mu, kappa, and sigma, named after their respective agonists—morphine, ketocyclazocine, and SK&F 10047. Each major opioid receptor has a unique anatomic distribution in the brain, spinal cord, and periphery.[7]

Stimulation of the mu receptor produces supraspinal analgesia, euphoria, and a decrease in ventilation. Studies of mu receptor subtypes revealed that the mu-1 subtype mediates analgesia and the mu-2 subtype mediates ventilatory depression, bradycardia, and dependence. Kappa stimulation produces spinal analgesia, sedation, and miosis. Currently, kappa-opioid drugs are being investigated for antiinflammatory actions that reduce disease severity of arthritis in a dose-dependent manner.[8] Sigma stimulation is responsible for an increase in ventilation, motor movement, and hallucinations. The delta receptor, discovered later, is responsible for spinal analgesia, responds to enkephalins, and serves to modulate activity of the mu receptors.[9] Evidence supports the existence of three kappa and two delta receptor subtypes.[3] Because sigma receptor stimulation produces effects so different from that of the opiate receptors, and its effects cannot be reversed by antagonists, the sigma receptor is no longer considered an opiate receptor.

At the cellular level, endogenous peptides and exogenous opioids produce effects by altering patterns of interneuronal communications. Receptor binding initiates a series of physiologic functions that result in cellular hyperpolarization and inhabitation of neurotransmitter release, effects mediated by second messengers.[9] All opioid receptors appear to be coupled to G-proteins[1] and inhibit the activity of adenylate cyclase. G-protein interactions affect ion channels. All three receptors decrease conductance of the voltage-gated calcium channels or open the potassium channels, resulting in decreased neuronal

TABLE **12-3** Endogenous Opioid Ligands	
Precursor	**Endogenous Peptide**
Proopiomelanocortin	β-Endorphin
Proenkephalin	Met-enkephalin Leu-enkephalin
Prodynorphin	Dynorphin A Dynorphin A(1-8) Dynorphin B α-neoendrophin β-neoendrophin
Pronociceptin/OFQ	Nociceptin
Proendomorphin*	Endomorphin-1 Endomorphin-2

Presumed to exist, awaiting discovery.

activity.[10] The endogenous ligands for opiod receptors are noted in Table 12-3.

Pharmacokinetics and Pharmacodynamics

Effects of opioids result from the combination of opioids with one or more receptors at specific tissue sites. The relationship between opioid dose and effects varies with pharmacokinetic and pharmacodynamic characteristics. *Pharmacokinetics* determines the relationship between drug dose and its concentration at receptor sites and refers to the study of plasma drug concentration versus time. *Pharmacodynamics* relates to the concentration of the drug at its site of action and the intensity of its effects. Changes in drug concentration over time in the blood, at the effect site and other sites, are determined by physiochemical properties of the drug, as well as biologic functions involved in the processes of absorption, redistribution, biotransformation, and elimination.

Clinically, opioids are administered parenterally, even though the drugs are well absorbed from the gastrointestinal (GI) tract.

TABLE 12-4		Physicochemical Characteristics and Pharmacokinetics						
Opioids	pK$_a$	Percent Nonionized	Protein Binding (%)	V$_c$ (L/kg)	V$_d$ (L/kg)	Clearance (mL/min/kg)	Elimination Half-Life (hr)	Partition Coefficient (Octanol/Water)
Morphine	7.9	23	35	0.23	2.8	15.5	1.7-3.3	1
Meperidine	8.5	7	70	0.6	2.6	22.7	3-5	21
Methadone	9.3	N/A	85	0.15	3.4	1.6	23	115
Fentanyl	8.4	8.5	84	0.85	4	13	2-4	820
Sufentanil	8	20	93	0.1	2	12	2-3	1750
Alfentanil	6.5	89	92	0.12	0.6	5	1-2	130
Remifentanil	7.26	58	93	0.1-0.2	0.39	41	0.1-0.3	N/A
Butorphanol	8.6	17	80	0.1	5	38.6	2.65	140
Nalbuphine	8.71	N/A	N/A	0.45	4.8	23.1	3.7	N/A

N/A, Not applicable; V$_c$, volume of distribution central compartment; V$_d$, volume of distribution.

Some opioids undergo extensive first-pass metabolism in the liver, greatly reducing their bioavailability and therapeutic efficacy after oral dosing. The early rapid decline in plasma concentration after the peak is the distribution phase, and the slower decline is the elimination phase. Orally administered morphine has limited absorption from the gastrointestinal tract. Drugs with greater lipophilicity are better absorbed through nasal and buccal mucosa and dermis.

Physiochemical properties of opioids influence both pharmacokinetics and pharmacodynamics. To reach effector sites in the CNS, opioids must cross biologic membranes from the blood to receptors on neural cell membranes. The ability of opioids to cross the blood-brain barrier depends on molecular size, ionization, lipid solubility, and protein binding. The physicochemical characteristics, pharmacokinetic variables, and partition coefficients (octanol and water as a measure of lipid solubility) for several of the commonly used opioid analgesics are summarized in Table 12-4. Pharmacokinetic parameters of opioids vary, in part, according to population and study differences. When the table is reviewed, it is most important to note how the opioids relate to one another. For example, the fact that fentanyl and morphine have similar elimination half-lives can explain how the drugs develop a similar duration of action when high doses of fentanyl are used.

Opioids are usually metabolized to more polar and less active or inactive compounds. Common mechanisms of metabolism include N-dealkylation, O-demethylation, glucuronidation, and hydrolysis. Some opioids, such as morphine, have active metabolites that can produce the therapeutic effects of the parent compound. Opioid metabolites and parent compounds are excreted primarily by the kidneys and secondarily by the biliary system and GI tract.

Pharmacogenetics

Opioids have a narrow therapeutic index, calling for a fine balance between optimizing pain control and sedative effects (without respiratory depression) and recognizing great variability from patient to patient in response and dose requirements. Genetic factors regulating their pharmacokinetics (metabolizing enzymes, transporters) and pharmacodynamics (receptors and signal transduction) contribute to this variability and to the possibility of adverse drug effects, toxicity, or therapeutic failure of pharmacotherapy. *Pharmacogenetics* describes genetically determined variability in the metabolism of drugs.

BOX 12-2

Factors Affecting Opioid Use

- Age
- Body weight
- Renal failure
- Hepatic failure
- Cardiopulmonary bypass
- Acid-base changes
- Hemorrhagic shock
- Genetic factors

Variation in DNA sequences explains some of the variability in metabolizing enzyme activities that contribute to alterations in drug cleavage and affect the response to drug therapy. Specific drug recommendations for opioids based on genotypes will be a future tool to guide clinicians. This development will lead to more patient-tailored drug therapy, resulting in fewer adverse drug reactions and higher efficacy of pharmacotherapy.[11]

The clinical use of opioids involves knowledge regarding patient characteristics, their perception, severity and likely duration of pain, lifestyle variables like smoking habits and alcohol intake, and opioid drug and dosing regimen selection.[12] Other factors affecting pharmacokinetics and pharmacodynamics of opioids include age, body weight, renal failure, hepatic failure, cardiopulmonary bypass, acid-base changes, and hemorrhagic shock (Box 12-2).

In adults, advancing age requires lower opioid doses for the treatment of postsurgical pain. Also, in relative similar patient groups, dosage requirements vary. Aubrun and colleagues reported that in more than 3000 patients, morphine dosage requirements for postoperative hip replacement therapy varied almost 40-fold.[13] Large variabilities have been reported in cancer patients receiving morphine via various routes.[12] Variability is contributed to by inherent pain sensitivity and factors, including pharmacogenetics influencing the clinical pharmacology of opioids.[14]

Clinical Effects of Opioids
Systemic Effects

Potency, speed of onset, and duration of action of the opioid analgesics are the most clinically relevant pharmacodynamic measures. The relative potencies of commonly used opioids,

TABLE **12-5**	Potencies of Opioids	
Drug	**Relative Potency, IM (mg)**	**Relative Potency, Oral (mg)**
Morphine	10	30
Meperidine	80	300
Methadone	10	12.5
Fentanyl	0.1	N/A
Butorphanol	2	N/A
Nalbuphine	12	N/A

IM, *Intramuscular*; N/A, *not applicable.*

BOX 12-3

Common Clinical Effects of Opioid Agonists

Acute	**Chronic**
Analgesia	Tolerance
Respiratory depression	Physical dependence
Sedation	Constipation
Euphoria	
Dysphoria	
Vasodilation	
Bradycardia	
Cough suppression	
Miosis	
Nausea and vomiting	
Skeletal muscle rigidity	
Smooth muscle spasm	
Constipation	
Urinary retention	
Biliary spasm	
Pruritus, rash	
Antishivering (meperidine only)	

---

based on acute administration, are listed in Table 12-5. However, apparent potencies can change over time and be a function of the route of administration. For example, morphine administered over a long period of time may seem to become more potent as a result of the gradual accumulation of active metabolites.[5] Tolerance usually predominates with any opioid drug and results in a diminishing effect with multiple dosing.

Probably of greatest importance in determining the speed of onset of analgesia of systemically administered analgesics is the gradient between blood and brain tissue. Although other factors (e.g., percent of free, nonionized drug in the blood and lipid solubility) appear to play a significant role in the drug entry rate into the CNS, empirically these factors do not correlate with drug onset. For example, alfentanil has a shorter time to onset of drug effect than either fentanyl or morphine. Fentanyl, however, is more than 7 times more lipid soluble than alfentanil, and morphine has 16 times more nonionized free drug available to the CNS for any given dose. Alfentanil's rapid onset is probably the result of its small volume of distribution and its low pK_a, allowing a rapid effect-site equilibrium.[4]

All the opioid agonists have similar clinical effects that vary in some degree from one drug to another. Sedation, respiratory depression, nausea, constipation, cough suppression, euphoria, dysphoria, and miosis are also known dose-dependent effects of the opioid agonists, in addition to analgesia. The commonly produced clinical effects of opioid agonists are given in Box 12-3. Morphine and related opioids affect the central nervous, renal, cardiovascular, GI, and endocrine systems.

CNS actions include analgesia, euphoria, respiratory depression, changes in temperature regulation, diuresis, miosis, and nausea. The effect of opioids on electroencephalographic and evoked-potential activity is minimal; therefore, neurophysiologic monitoring can be conducted during opioid anesthetic techniques. Analgesia results from the activity of morphine at several spinal and supraspinal sites within the CNS (Table 12-6). The analgesic effects of opioids come from their ability to (1) directly inhibit the ascending transmission of nociception information from the spinal cord dorsal horn and (2) activate pain control pathways that descend from the midbrain, via the rostral ventromedial medulla, to the spinal cord dorsal horn.[2]

Most opioids produce miosis by stimulating the autonomic segment of the nucleus of the oculomotor nerve. The respiratory depression produced by opioids is the result of direct depression of the respiratory centers and activation of the mu-2 receptors in

TABLE **12-6**	Opioid-Mediated Analgesia in the Central Nervous System
Central Nervous System Location	**Opioid Receptor**
Supraspinal	
Periaqueductal gray area	
Raphe nuclei	Mu = kappa > delta
Caudal linear	Kappa
Dorsal	Kappa > mu
Median	Mu > kappa
Magnus	Mu > kappa
Pallidus	Delta
Gigantocellular reticular	Mu = kappa = delta
Spinal	
Spinal cord	Mu = delta = kappa
Dorsal root ganglia	Mu = delta = kappa

the brainstem. Respiratory rate, minute volume, and tidal volume are decreased.

Opioids can act either as diuretics or as antidiuretics, depending on the opioid receptors stimulated. Opioids that are agonists at kappa receptors cause diuresis, whereas those that are agonists at mu receptors produce an antidiuretic effect. The increase in smooth muscle tone from opioid administration can result in urinary retention because of action on the urinary sphincter. However, with systemic opioids, the tone of the detrusor muscle may be enhanced, leading to urinary retention.[4] Urinary retention is a common side effect with intrathecal and epidural opioid administration.

Opioids have no major effects on nerve conduction at the neuromuscular junction or at the skeletal muscle membrane. A generalized hypertonus of skeletal muscle can be produced by large intravenous doses of most opioid agonists. Although morphine can produce rigidity, the problem is most often associated with fentanyl, alfentanil, sufentanil, and remifentanil. The difficulty is caused in part by loss of chest-wall compliance and by constriction of pharyngeal and laryngeal muscles. It is commonly referred to as *tight chest* or *truncal rigidity*. Opioid-induced muscle rigidity is thought to be mediated by mu receptors at supraspinal sites, including the nucleus raphe pontis and sites lateral to it in the hindbrain.[9] These effects are reduced or eliminated by an antagonist and by muscle relaxants.

The degree to which opioids affect the cardiovascular system depends on the specific opioid agent used. All opioids induce some degree of peripheral vasodilation and diminish the responses of baroreceptor reflexes. Much of the hypotension produced by morphine is attributed to histamine release, which is absent with meperidine, fentanyl, sufentanil, alfentanil, and remifentanil.[4] Histamine$_1$ antagonists only partially block the vasodilation that results from the administration of morphine. The antagonist naloxone effectively reverses morphine-induced vasodilation. The vasoconstriction response initiated by an increase in the partial pressure of carbon dioxide also is inhibited by morphine. At high doses, most opioids produce significant bradycardia via medullary vagal stimulation.[2] An exception is meperidine, which often causes tachycardia as a result of its having a structure similar to that of atropine or via a reflex response to hypotension.[4] Morphine may also cause tachycardia as a reflex to the hypotension that results from the histamine release.

Opioids have several effects on the GI tract in addition to the nausea produced via the CNS. The effects include constipation, nausea, and vomiting. Opioids decrease gastric motility, prolong gastric emptying, and potentially increase the incidence of esophageal reflux. Opioids directly stimulate the chemoreceptor trigger zone, causing nausea in some patients and both nausea and vomiting in others. The use of morphine decreases biliary, pancreatic, and intestinal secretions, leading to delayed digestion of food in the small intestine. Constipation is probably the result of decreased GI transit via mu-2 receptor action both within the brain and in the peripheral nerve plexus.[2]

Other GI effects from the administration of opioids include an increase in biliary duct pressure and sphincter of Oddi tone in a dose-dependent manner via opioid receptor–mediated mechanisms. Pentazocine has shown less biliary sphincter spasm than any of the other opioids.

Endocrinologic effects of opioids include the release of vasopressin and inhibition of the stress-induced release of corticotropin and gonadotropins from the pituitary. Release of thyrotropin from the adenohypophysis is also inhibited. Basal metabolic rate and temperature may also be decreased in patients receiving chronic opioids, although animal data indicate that acute administration either systemically or intrathecally can increase temperature.[2] Opioids slightly decrease body temperature by resetting the equilibrium point of temperature regulation in the hypothalamus.[2]

Neuraxial Effects

Opioids delivered by epidural or subarachnoid routes behave differently in onset, duration, and side effects than the same drugs given systemically. Pain that is unresponsive to systemic opioids may respond to the same drugs given centrally, reducing some side effects while increasing the incidence of others. Systemic opioids suppress nociception in lamina II and V cells of the dorsal horn of the spinal cord, leaving lamina IV and VI cells, which mediate non-nociceptive information relatively unaffected.[15]

Spinal administration of opioids is a selective and potent means of producing analgesia. Intrathecal administration allows injection of the opioids directly into the cerebrospinal fluid (CSF), a more efficient method of delivering the drug to the spinal cord opiate receptors. The analgesic response is the result of activity at spinal opiate receptors, especially kappa receptors in the substantia gelatinosa, lamina II of the dorsal horn.[15] Opioids can be given with local anesthetics intraoperatively at the initiation of spinal anesthesia or postoperatively for pain control.[16] Side effects with spinal administration are similar to those with systemic administration, except that pruritus and urinary retention occur with much greater frequency. Less lipid-soluble agents such as morphine and hydromorphone produce a delayed ventilatory depression, the result of migration of opioid via the CSF to the midbrain vestibular centers.

Respiratory depression is the most common serious complication associated with intrathecally and epidurally administered opioids. Two different levels of respiratory depression can occur after neuraxial morphine administration. An early phase observed soon after administration reflects rapid systemic absorption and is similar to parenteral dosing. A later, more insidious depression that occurs over a period of 8 to 12 hours has been related to rostral flow of CSF and delivery of morphine to the brainstem respiratory center.[17] Awareness of delayed respiratory depression has resulted in increased monitoring of patients and dose reduction, thereby greatly reducing the incidence of serious respiratory depression to that seen with patient-controlled analgesia (PCA) opioids.

Generalized pruritus has been observed with neuraxial morphine and to a lesser extent with other opioids. Mild itching, usually involving the face or chest, is common; however, the intensity of itching can become so annoying that it interferes with sleep. Pruritus is commonly seen with opioids such as fentanyl and sufentanil that do not release histamine. Pruritus can be treated with antihistamines or with opiate receptor antagonists. The incidence of postoperative nausea and vomiting increases for patients treated with neuraxial opioids. Nausea may result either from the rostral spread of the drug in the spinal fluid to the brainstem or vascular uptake and delivery to the vomiting center and chemoreceptor trigger zone in the area postrema of the medulla.

Urinary retention after spinal opioid analgesia has been related to inhibition of sacral parasympathetic outflow, which results in relaxation of the bladder detrusor muscle and an inability to relax the sphincter.[4]

Opioids with higher lipid solubilities (see Table 12-4) tend to be rapidly absorbed into the spinal tissues after central administration, resulting in a faster onset of action. However, higher lipid solubility is associated with a small area of distribution of the drug along the length of the spinal cord and therefore a more limited area of analgesia.[5,7] Higher lipid solubility is also associated with faster clearance of the drug out of the epidural and intrathecal space, resulting in a shorter duration of action and higher blood concentrations of the opioid.[15,17] Intraspinal opioids are advantageous in selective analgesia, which occurs in the absence of motor and sympathetic blockade.

Epidural anesthesia and analgesia have been successfully used in obstetric patients and surgical patients. Epidural doses of opioids, however, are much higher than doses of opioids for intrathecal use. Small portions of epidural opioids cross the dura, enter the CSF, and penetrate spinal tissue in amounts proportional to their lipid solubility. The remaining drug is absorbed by the vasculature, producing plasma levels comparable to those after intramuscular injections and providing supraspinal analgesia.[17] In fact, the doses of the more lipid-soluble agents approach those of systemic doses.

Opioid Techniques and Delivery

In clinical practice, opioids are used to relieve pain during monitored anesthesia care and regional anesthesia and as a component of balanced anesthesia, as well as an adjuvant in general anesthesia. The inclusion of opioids reduces pain and anxiety, decreases somatic and autonomic responses to airway manipulation, improves hemodynamic stability, lowers requirements for inhaled anesthetic agents, and provides postoperative analgesia.

Initially, the most common method of administering opioids in the practice of anesthesia was intermittent bolus injection, which produces wide swings in drug plasma concentration. Intermittent periods of deep and light anesthesia are produced. Continuous opioid infusion is a more common method of administration because plasma concentration can be maintained more accurately and consistently with continuous infusion than with intermittent bolus injection. Continuous infusion of opioids is associated with hemodynamic stability, reduces the total necessary dose of opioids, and decreases the need for opioid reversal agents.

Continuous intravenous administration involves the infusion of a loading dose that "fills" the volume of distribution, followed by continuous drug replacement that keeps the volume of distribution "filled" as the drug is eliminated.[18]

Equation 12-1

Loading dose (mcg/kg) = V_d (mL/kg) × C_p (mcg/mL)
Maintenance infusion (mcg/kg/min) = Cl (mL/kg/min)

where V_d is volume of distribution, C_p is plasma concentration, and Cl is drug clearance. See Table 12-4 for the V_d and Cl of various opioids.

The rate of continuous infusion does not remain constant, but rather is adjusted to meet the patient's needs and to control varying surgical stimuli. The volume of distribution is decreased for patients with hypovolemia and trauma and for geriatric patients. The anesthetist must exercise proper judgment when administering the maintenance dose, considering factors such as enzyme induction, hepatic failure, and adjunctive drug use. Table 12-7 provides dose ranges for continuous infusions.

Continuous intravenous infusion can be administered by gravity flow with a manual control device (e.g., Buretrol), an infusion pump, or a syringe pump. The least accurate method is the gravity flow device, the accuracy of which depends on counting the drops delivered. Most infusion pumps deliver medication in units of milliliters per hour. Syringe pumps are advantageous because they are programmed to administer drug in units of micrograms per kilogram per minute. Some advantages of continuous infusion techniques are listed in Box 12-4.

Anesthesia practitioners are exploring nonparenteral routes of opioid delivery. Fentanyl is the prototypic opioid for transdermal application. Transdermal administration of fentanyl does not require cooperation from the patient; also, first-phase hepatic metabolism is not a factor, and the route does not produce discomfort. Currently available formulations permit delivery of 25 to 100 mcg per hour for 24 to 72 hours. The transdermal fentanyl patch provides a relatively constant

TABLE 12-7	Infusion Rates*	
Opioid	Induction (mcg/kg)	Maintenance (mcg/kg/min)
Fentanyl	5.75	0.01-0.05
Sufentanil	1-10	0.025-0.15
Alfentanil	40-100	0.25-10
Remifentanil	5-20	0.05-0.10

Lower dose range with nitrous oxide and benzodiazepines; higher dose range with oxygen only.

BOX 12-4

Advantages of Continuous Opioid Infusion

- Hemodynamic stability
- Decreased side effects
- Reduced need for opioid-reversal agents
- Reduced use for vasopressor drugs
- Suppression of cortisol and vasopressin response to cardiopulmonary bypass
- Reduced total dosage of opioids
- Decreased recovery time

---

plasma concentration for 72 hours. It is not currently recommended for use in managing postoperative pain.

Oral transmucosal fentanyl citrate is used for providing analgesia in children. Fentanyl is dissolved in a sucrose solution and shaped into a lozenge. The transmucosal route is effective, owing to the characteristics of the oral mucosa. The oral mucosa is thinner than the skin and is supplied by numerous blood and lymphatic vessels. The opioid administered transmucosally is also absorbed directly into the systemic circulation without passing through the liver. Pruritus is a common side effect with transmucosal administration.

Nasal administration of sufentanil preoperatively in the pediatric patient has been studied. The children remained calm, and some experienced somewhat decreased ventilatory compliance. Recovery room time was not increased, and the highest incidence of nausea and vomiting occurred in the group that received the highest dose of sufentanil. Nasal butorphanol is currently available and is widely used in the management of migraine headaches.

Spinal and epidural opioid administration has been successfully used in obstetric patients, surgical patients, and patients with postoperative pain. Neuraxial administration of opioids is a selective and potent means of producing analgesia. Table 12-8 gives neuraxial opioid dosages,[15,17] and Table 12-9 compares dosages for other routes of opioid administration.[4,19]

CLASSIFICATION OF OPIOIDS

Agonists

Naturally Occurring Opioids

Morphine. Morphine, the prototype for opioid agonists, is the most abundant alkaloid in raw opium. The primary therapeutic use of morphine is the abatement of moderate to severe pain. Morphine can be administered via the intramuscular, intravenous, subcutaneous, oral, intrathecal, and epidural routes.

TABLE 12-8	Doses of Neuraxial Opioids*	
Opioid	**Single Dose**	**Infusion Rate**
Epidural		
Morphine	2-5 mg	0.1-1 mg/hr
Meperidine	25-50 mg	5-20 mg/hr
Methadone	5 mg	0.3-0.5 mg/hr
Fentanyl	50-100 mcg	25-100 mcg/hr
Sufentanil	25-50 mcg	10-50 mcg/hr
Butorphanol	2-4 mg	0.2-0.4 mg/hr
Subarachnoid		
Morphine	0.25-0.3 mg	
Meperidine	10 mg	
Fentanyl	10-20 mcg	
Sufentanil	5-10 mcg	

Doses adjusted for age and level of regional injection.

Effects of intravenous morphine on the time course of sedation and analgesia occur with sedation first, followed by analgesia.[20] Morphine-induced sedation, therefore, should not be considered as an indicator of appropriate analgesia. When given intrathecally, morphine has the longest duration of action of the specific opioids. Morphine is among the least lipophilic of the opioids, resulting in slow penetration of biologic membranes, less accumulation in lipid membranes or fatty tissues, and slower onset.

Morphine is glucuronidated in the liver at both the 3 position (which produces morphine-3-glucuronide, M3G) and the 6 position (which produces morphine-6-glucuronide, M6G), in a 2:1 ratio.[21] As a result of the active metabolite, M6G, morphine appears to produce a more prolonged effect, often excessive sedation, in the patient with renal failure. Within the CNS, M6G metabolite is 100 times more potent than the parent drug, whereas M3G metabolite is inactive.[21,22] The greater hydrophilicity of M6G than the parent drug normally impedes its passage into the CNS. However, after chronic administration or in patients with renal failure, M6G at a high blood level can enter the CNS by mass action.

Morphine produces a nonimmunologic release of histamine from tissue mast cells, resulting in local itching, redness, or hives near the site of intravenous injection or generalized flushing. When sufficient histamine is released, the patient may exhibit signs of decreased systemic vascular resistance, hypotension, and tachycardia. Localized histamine release after a morphine injection is not uncommon.

Codeine. Considered a weak opioid, codeine is generally not used for treatment of severe pain. Approximately 10% of the administered dose of codeine is O-demethylated to morphine, which accounts for most of its analgesic activity.[7] It has good antitussive activity, but on a weight basis, codeine is a less potent antitussive than morphine. Combinations of codeine with acetaminophen remain very popular as prescribed analgesics.

Semisynthetic Opioids

Hydromorphone. Derived from morphine in the 1920s, hydromorphone has a pharmacokinetic profile similar to that of morphine. Hydromorphone is absorbed from the oral, rectal,

and parenteral sites. Because of its lipid solubility, it is sometimes used instead of morphine for epidural or spinal administration when a wide area of analgesia is needed.[23] Studies performed on parenteral hydromorphone relative to morphine tend to demonstrate similar analgesia and side-effect profiles. Because of the lack of any known active metabolites, it is often recommended for patients with renal failure.[2]

Oxycodone. Since its approval for use in the treatment of pain, oxycodone has been studied in the setting of various pain conditions. Its relative potency in oral form is similar to that of oral codeine. Intravenous and oral oxycodone has differing potency results compared with morphine.

Synthetic Opioids

Methadone. Introduced in the 1940s, methadone is used primarily for relief of chronic pain, treatment of opioid abstinence syndromes, and treatment of heroin addiction. Supplied as a racemic mixture of two optical isomers, most of methadone's activity comes from the *l*-isomer. Unlike most opioids, it has a long half-life, allowing less frequent dosing.[24] Because its prolonged effect is the result of extensive protein binding (90%) with slow release and a lower intrinsic ability of the liver to metabolize it, methadone does not require a specific formulation. It also has the advantage of a high bioavailability and no active metabolites. Disadvantages include accumulation and a longer time to reach steady state than other opioids.

Meperidine. Meperidine, a mu-receptor agonist, exerts its pharmacologic action on the CNS and the neural elements in the bowels. It is structurally similar to atropine and has an atropine-like antispasmodic effect. After demethylation in the liver, meperidine is partially metabolized to normeperidine, which is half as analgesic as meperidine but lowers the seizure threshold and induces CNS excitability. Normeperidine's elimination half-life is significantly longer than that of meperidine. With accumulation of normeperidine, subjects may experience a CNS excitation characterized by tremors, muscle twitches, and seizures. Because of accumulation of normeperidine, limitations on its use should be considered in patients with renal failure and those with cancer who are receiving high doses of meperidine. Side effects may include dry mouth and blurring of vision.

Meperidine is effective in reducing shivering from diverse causes, including general and epidural anesthesia. It reduces or eliminates visible shivering, as well as the accompanying increase in oxygen consumption.[9] It produces local anesthesia when applied locally or intrathecally, but it can also cause significant local tissue irritation.[2]

Alfentanil. After bolus injection, alfentanil has a more rapid onset of action and shorter duration than fentanyl, even though it is less lipid soluble. The high nonionized fraction (90%) of alfentanil at physiologic pH and its small volume of distribution increase the amount of drug available for binding in the brain. Although alfentanil is effective epidurally, the duration of analgesia is short, and for this reason it has never achieved popularity. Alfentanil is metabolized in the liver by oxidative N-dealkylation and O-demethylation in the cytochrome P-450 system, and the inactive metabolites are excreted in the urine. Alfentanil has great patient-to-patient variability, as seen in the original studies, in which a high coefficient of variation was reported. Erythromycin has been shown to prolong the metabolism of alfentanil and interact with alfentanil to produce clinical symptoms of prolonged respiratory depression and sedation.

Fentanyl. A single administered dose of fentanyl has a short duration of action (approximately 20 to 40 minutes). It produces

TABLE **12-9**	Opioid Dose Comparisons				
Opioid	**Route**	**Onset**	**Peak**	**Duration of Action**	**Half-Life**
Morphine	PO	60 min	30-60 min	4-5 hr	Neonates 4.5-13 hr
	IM	30-60 min	30-60 min	4-5 hr	Adults 3-5 hr
	IV	20 min	30-60 min	4-5 hr	
	Epidural	60-90 min	30-60 min	8-24 hr	
Codeine	PO	30-60 min	60-90 min	4-6 hr	2.5-3.5 hr
	IM	10-30 min	30-60 min	4-6 hr	2.5-3.5 hr
Hydromorphone	IV	15-30 min	30-90 min	4-5 hr	1-3 hr
Oxycodone	PO	10-15 min	30-60 min	4-5 hr	3.2-4.5 hr
Methadone	PO	30-60 min	30-60 min	6-8 hr	15-30 hr
	IV	5-10 min	15-20 min	4-6 hr	15-30 hr
Meperidine	PO	10-15 min	30-60 min	2-4 hr	2.5-4 hr
	IM	10-15 min	30-60 min	2-4 hr	2.5-4 hr
	IV	5 min	30-60 min	2-4 hr	2.5-4 hr
Alfentanil	IV	Immediate	Immediate		1.5 hr
Fentanyl	Transmucosal	5-15 min	20-30 min	Related to blood levels	6.6 hr
	IM	7-15 min	20-30 min	1-2 hr	2-4 hr
	IV	2-5 min	20-30 min	0.5-1 hr	2-4 hr
	Epidural	20-30 min		2-3 hr	2-4 hr
Remifentanil	IV	1 min	1 min	5-10 min	9 min
Sufentanil	IV	1-3 min		Dose dependent	6 hr
Tramadol	PO	60 min	120 min	9 hr	2-3 hr
Buprenorphine	IM	10-30 min	60 min	6 hr	2-3 hr
	IV	10-30 min	60 min	6 hr	2.5-4 hr
Butorphanol	IM	10-15 min	30-60 min	3-4 hr	2.5-4 hr
	IV	Immediate	30-60 min	3-4 hr	2.6-2.8 hr
Dezocine	IM	15-30 min	60 min	4-6 hr	2.6-2.8 hr
	IV	15-30 min	60 min	4-6 hr	3.5-5 hr
Nalbuphine	IM		30 min		3.5-5 hr
	IV		1-3 min		2-3 hr
Pentazocine	PO	15-30 min		4-5 hr	2-3 hr
	IM	15-30 min		2-3 hr	2-3 hr
	IV	2-3 min		2-3 hr	Neonates 1.2-3 hr
Naloxone	IM	5 min	5-15 min	20-60 min	Adults 1-1.5 hr
	IV	2 min	5-15 min	20-60 min	10.8 hr
Nalmefene	IM	5-15 min	120 min	8 hr	10.8 hr
	IV	2 min	2-3 min	8 hr	6-10 hr
Naltrexone	PO	45-60 min	60 min	24-72 hr	

a profound dose-dependent analgesia, ventilatory depression, and sedation. The action of a single dose of fentanyl is terminated by redistribution. The high lipid solubility of fentanyl allows for rapid tissue uptake.[4] Fentanyl and its derivatives all undergo significant first-pass uptake in the lungs with temporary accumulation before release. When fentanyl is given in multiple doses or as a continuous infusion, the termination of action reflects elimination but not redistribution. Clearance of fentanyl is dependent on hepatic blood flow. Fentanyl is metabolized by *N*-dealkylation and hydroxylation to inactive metabolites that are eliminated in urine and bile. The delayed postoperative respiratory depression that can occur has been attributed to sequestering of

fentanyl in the gastric juice and muscles; the drug returns to the plasma and produces a secondary peak of action. Fentanyl elimination is prolonged in the elderly and the neonate.

Initially used intravenously during surgery, fentanyl later was administered for intrathecal, epidural, and postoperative PCA intravenous use. Fentanyl transdermal patches deliver 75 to 100 mcg/hr, resulting in peak plasma concentrations in approximately 18 hours because a subcutaneous depot of drug must be saturated before the drug is consistently absorbed into the bloodstream.[4] The dose remains stable during the presence of the patch. After removal, the decline in blood concentration follows an apparent 17-hour half-life; the true elimination half-life of fentanyl remains at approximately 3 hours, but continued absorption from the subcutaneous depot during elimination makes it appear longer.

Transmucosal fentanyl (Oralet) was initially developed in the form of a lollipop as an adjunct to pediatric anesthesia. A similar fentanyl product is available in higher strengths and is used for relief of breakthrough cancer pain. The pharmacokinetics of this form are dose related, with an apparent elimination half-life of approximately 6 hours. Not all opioids are absorbed sublingually. Hydromorphone, oxycodone, and heroin are minimally absorbed, whereas absorption for morphine is 18%; fentanyl, 51%; and methadone, 34%.[25]

Remifentanil. Remifentanil is a moderately lipophilic, piperidine-derived opioid with an ester link. The addition of the ester group allows the drug to be easily and rapidly metabolized by blood and tissue esterases. Kinetic studies indicate that the drug has a small volume of distribution (V_d 0.39 ± 0.25) and an elimination half-life of 8 to 20 minutes. It is metabolized by hydrolysis catalyzed by general esterase enzymes to a less active compound. It is not dependent on cholinesterase enzyme for metabolism and therefore is not influenced by quantitative or qualitative changes in cholinesterase. Succinylcholine metabolism does not influence remifentanil breakdown.

Because of the potential for respiratory depression and muscle rigidity, bolus dosing in the preoperative or postoperative care unit or during monitored anesthesia care is not recommended. Because of its unique metabolic pathway, remifentanil has brevity of action, a precise and rapid titratable effect because of rapid onset and offset, and noncumulative effects and results in rapid recovery after discontinuation of its administration by infusion. However, because of the rapidity of emergence from remifentanil anesthesia, it is important to develop and start a plan for alternative analgesic therapy in the postoperative period.[26]

The commercial preparation of remifentanil is a water-soluble, lyophilized powder that contains a free base and glycine as a vehicle to buffer the solution. Because of potential glycine neurotoxicity, remifentanil should not be administered epidurally or intrathecally.[2]

Sufentanil. Sufentanil is more tightly bound to receptors than fentanyl and has minimal nonspecific brain-tissue binding. Despite its high lipophilicity and potency, sufentanil has a shorter elimination half-life and duration of effect than fentanyl because of its high degree of plasma protein binding, lower volume of distribution, tighter binding to receptors, and minimal binding to brain tissue. Hepatic clearance of sufentanil approaches liver blood flow. Sufentanil metabolism involves O-demethylation and N-dealkylation, with minimal amounts being excreted unchanged in the urine.

The effects of age on the distribution and elimination of sufentanil are reflected in a decrease in the initial volume of distribution for the elderly. The reduced volume of distribution of sufentanil in elderly patients is associated with increased respiratory depression.

Tramadol. Tramadol is a synthetic codeine analog that is a weak mu opioid receptor agonist, with analgesic effects produced by inhibition of norepinephrine and serotonin neuronal reuptake as well as presynaptic stimulation of 5-hydroxytryptamine release.[4] Tramadol is a racemic mixture; the (+) enantiomer binds to the mu receptor and inhibits serotonin uptake, whereas the (−) enantiomer inhibits norepinephrine uptake and stimulates α_2-adrenergic receptors. It has an elimination half-life of 5 to 6 hours and is an effective analgesic for the treatment of mild to moderate pain. Tramadol can cause seizures and possibly

exacerbate them in patients with predisposing factors. Tramadol-induced analgesia is not entirely reversed by naloxone, but tramadol respiratory depression can be reversed. In overdose situations, most of the toxicity is related to monoamine uptake inhibition rather than to opioid effects.[2]

Partial Agonists and Agonists-Antagonists

Buprenorphine. Buprenorphine, a synthetic derivative, is a potent partial agonist opioid that binds mainly to the mu receptors.[27] Its slow dissociation from the receptor is a result of its long duration of action (approximately 8 hours). Its high affinity for the mu receptor accounts for the reduced ability of naloxone to reverse buprenorphine's effects. Clinically significant respiratory depression can occur with therapeutic doses. Buprenorphine exhibits a ceiling effect in which an increase in the dose does not increase respiratory depression; this is believed to result from the fact that the drug's antagonistic effects become more apparent at higher doses. It also has minimal effect on GI motility and smooth muscle sphincter tone. A transdermal system of buprenorphine was developed for treatment of moderate to severe cancer pain.[28] Administered transdermally, it provides analgesia and has a low incidence of adverse events.

Butorphanol. Butorphanol, a highly lipophilic opioid, acts as an agonist at the kappa and sigma receptors and as a weak antagonist at mu receptors. It is more potent than morphine in the production of analgesia. It produces respiratory depression, but its ceiling effect is below that of mu agonists. Intranasal butorphanol is used for the treatment of migraine headaches and postoperative pain. Butorphanol has also been studied for epidural use, although it tends to produce significant sedation. It has been shown to be effective in the treatment of postoperative shivering, but the mechanism of this effect is unknown.

Dezocine. Dezocine, an agonist-antagonist, demonstrates a greater anesthetic sparing effect than other agonist-antagonists. It demonstrates less affinity for sigma receptors, but it does have significant activity at kappa receptors and a high affinity for mu receptors.[2]

Nalbuphine. Nalbuphine has the ability to reverse respiratory depression that results from opioid use and to maintain analgesia. Nalbuphine acts as both an agonist and an antagonist at the opioid receptors. Nalbuphine's analgesic response is equal to that of morphine. Nalbuphine provides an agonist effect at the kappa and sigma receptors and an antagonist effect at the mu receptor. A ceiling effect for respiratory depression and difficulty with reversal with naloxone has been demonstrated with both nalbuphine and butorphanol.[9] Nalbuphine has been used to antagonize pruritus induced by epidural and intrathecal morphine. Nalbuphine effectively antagonizes fentanyl-induced respiratory depression, maintains analgesia, and does not produce adverse endocrinologic and circulatory changes.

During laparoscopic cholecystectomy, opioid use can cause spasms of the sphincter of Oddi, which complicates the interpretation of intraoperative cholangiography. In one case study, nalbuphine was effectively used to reverse a spasm produced by morphine at the time of contrast medium injection. Nalbuphine 10 mg intravenously released an occluded common bile duct around the sphincter of Oddi within 3 minutes.[2]

Pentazocine. Pentazocine has analgesic and weak antagonistic effects. It is considered to be a competitive antagonist at the mu receptor and an agonist at the kappa and sigma receptors. Although it does not reverse morphine-induced respiratory depression, it can precipitate withdrawal in morphine-dependent patients.

Antagonists

Naloxone. Naloxone, an oxymorphone derivative, is a pure opioid antagonist. Naloxone blocks the opioid receptor sites and reverses respiratory depression and opioid analgesia. The reversal of respiratory depression and analgesia occurs as a result of competitive antagonism at the mu, kappa, and delta receptors. The duration of action of naloxone is less than that of most opioid agonists, allowing the return of respiratory depression in some patients treated with naloxone. Naloxone is effective only when it is administered intravenously or intramuscularly.

Naloxone may antagonize intrinsic analgesic systems, as evidenced by its ability to blunt the placebo effect and inhibit the analgesia of electroacupuncture. Studies have demonstrated that naloxone's effect on reversing the effects of morphine is in fact titratable. Administration of low doses of naloxone can reverse the side effects of epidural opioids while preserving the analgesic effects. This effect is also possible by titrating the intravenous dose as seen in reversal of the side effects of intravenous morphine.

The effects of naloxone use range from discomfort to pulmonary edema to sudden death. Pulmonary edema after naloxone administration has been observed in patients with a documented history of cardiovascular disease. Prough and co-workers[29] reported two cases of acute onset of pulmonary edema in young male patients who received either 100 or 200 mcg of naloxone. The report discusses the ability of naloxone to inhibit endogenous pain suppression pathways and to allow unopposed noradrenergic transmission from medullary centers that can produce neurogenic pulmonary edema. Neurogenic pulmonary edema results from an increase in catecholamine levels in healthy patients, as well as in patients with a history of cardiovascular disease. Cautious titration of naloxone is of paramount importance in both cardiovascular patients and healthy patients. Andree[30] reported two cases of sudden death after naloxone administration. This study suggests that naloxone produces increases in blood catecholamine levels that predispose to ventricular fibrillation and subsequent cardiac arrest.

Nalmefene. Structurally similar to naloxone, nalmefene (Revex) is a long-acting parenteral opioid antagonist. It has an elimination half-life of approximately 10 hours (compared with naloxone's half-life of 1 hour) and duration of action of 8 hours when it is given in the usual doses.[31] The clinical effects of nalmefene are similar to those of naloxone.

Reversal of postoperative respiratory depression is accomplished with the administration of nalmefene 0.1 to 0.5 mcg/kg titrated at 2- to 5-minute intervals. In acute opioid overdose, it is recommended that 0.5 to 1.6 mcg be given intravenously. Administration of doses higher than 1.6 mcg does not elicit additional effects and is not recommended. As with all antagonists, slow titration of small doses may minimize side effects. As with naloxone, nalmefene should not be administered to opioid-dependent patients.[32]

Naltrexone. As a synthetic cogener of oxymorphone, naltrexone has antagonist and receptor-binding properties similar to those of naloxone but higher oral efficacy and longer duration of action. Its activity is the result of both the parent drug and its 6-beta metabolite. The parent and metabolite have half-lives of 6 and 13 hours, respectively.

Naltrexone has a duration of action of approximately 24 hours. Naltrexone is administered to patients addicted to opioids so that the euphoric effects of opioids can be prevented. When doses greater than 100 mg are administered to the opioid-addicted patient, plasma concentrations are reached within 2 hours, and the agent's half-life is approximately 10 hours. Naltrexone produces an active metabolite with a half-life even longer than that of naltrexone.[2] A major disadvantage associated with the use of naloxone and naltrexone is the potential for reversal of opioid analgesia.

CLINICAL USES OF OPIOIDS

Cardiovascular Considerations

Opioids have been shown to produce greater cardiovascular stability when compared with inhalation agents. An advantage of the use of fentanyl and its analogs during cardiac surgery is their lack of cardiovascular depression. Less depression of cardiac output and less decrease in systemic vascular resistance occur. A goal of managing cardiac patients is providing continuous cardiac protection. Opioids can provide the cardiac patient with a stable heart rate and blood pressure. Opioids blunt sympathetic stimulation and maintain perfusion pressure without producing cardiac depressant effects. The degree of myocardial impairment influences patient responses. Critically ill patients or patients with significant myocardial dysfunction appear to require lower doses of an opioid for anesthesia. Patients with poor left ventricular function may develop higher plasma and brain concentrations for a given loading dose or infusion rate of opioids than patients with good left ventricular function.

Before the 1970s, morphine was the drug of choice for patients who underwent open-heart procedures. Side effects associated with morphine anesthesia included venodilation, tachycardia, hypotension, and a high incidence of awareness. These side effects promoted the search for a more predictable opioid for use in such patients. In the late 1970s, fentanyl became the primary agent for patients who were to undergo open-heart surgery. Patients given fentanyl had a greater degree of cardiovascular stability than patients given morphine.[33] The bradycardia that occasionally occurs with the use of fentanyl can be countered with the administration of pancuronium bromide or treated with anticholinergics or sympathomimetics. Fentanyl does not produce the hypotension that can be seen with the use of morphine. Fentanyl rarely produces histamine release and has little effect on peripheral vascular resistance except in massive doses. The combination of benzodiazepines and fentanyl produces decreases in blood pressure, cardiac output, and stroke volume and an increase in central venous pressure. For patients dependent on catecholamines for blood pressure maintenance, fentanyl must be titrated slowly and in small doses so that arterial blood pressure remains constant. High-dose fentanyl, 15 to 50 mcg/kg, is used in cardiac anesthesia for producing cardiac stability. Because of the prolonged respiratory depression, postoperative ventilation is necessary for cardiac patients who have received high-dose fentanyl.

In the late 1970s, the opioid sufentanil was introduced into the practice of anesthesia. Sufentanil is 5 to 10 times more potent than fentanyl and has approximately the same or a slightly shorter duration of action. Sufentanil provides excellent cardiovascular stability for the cardiac patient. Sufentanil has a greater vasodilating effect than fentanyl does, and bradycardia and hypotension may occur when it is used as the induction agent. The vasodilating effects of sufentanil are not associated with histamine release. High-dose sufentanil for patients undergoing cardiac surgery is administered in the range of 8 to 30 mcg/kg. Considerations for postoperative ventilation are the same as for patients receiving high-dose fentanyl. Hemodilution, hypotension, altered regional blood flow, and hypothermia alter the pharmacokinetics of drugs during cardiac anesthesia.[33]

Remifentanil, with its fast decay in plasma concentration, even with high doses and long infusion times, ensures a rapid recovery from cardiac surgery. It allows rapid and precise control of analgesia during surgery. However, because of its rapid offset, the requirement for postoperative analgesia needs to be considered before the remifentanil infusion is discontinued at the end of surgery.

Obstetrics

Concerns attendant with the use of opioids in obstetrics are (1) the implications of respiratory depression in the mother, which results in acid-base imbalance in the fetus and possible hypoxia, and (2) the transfer of opioids across the placenta to the fetus. The plasma concentration of opioids available for placental transfer depends on the distribution of the opioids, on the metabolism and excretion of opioids and metabolites, on protein binding, and on the acid-base status of the mother.

Many different opioids have been used successfully in the obstetric setting. Opioids, whether administered intravenously, intramuscularly, epidurally, or intraspinally, are effective in obstetric patients during and after labor and delivery. Meperidine, administered both systemically and epidurally, has been shown safe and effective, as have fentanyl, sufentanil, and morphine when used for epidural analgesia during labor.[34] However, use of opioids without local anesthetics is likely to be effective in only the very early stages of labor; local anesthetics will ultimately need to be added.

Butorphanol and nalbuphine, synthetic agonist-antagonists, are used in obstetric practice for analgesia during labor. Because of its strong kappa-receptor activity, butorphanol can modulate visceral pain and be effective for the relief of labor pain. The major advantage attributed to these drugs is the ceiling effect for respiratory depression. Butorphanol systemically was found to be similar to intramuscular meperidine for labor analgesia.[35]

Nalbuphine is considered equipotent to morphine and is used in obstetric practice to reverse the itching associated with epidural morphine while maintaining the analgesia.[34] Major side effects associated with both nalbuphine and butorphanol are drowsiness and dizziness. They can cause psychomimetic effects in the obstetric patient and rarely cause a sinusoidal fetal heart pattern after administration.[35]

Pediatrics

Opioids have been widely used in recent years for infants and children as adjuncts to inhaled anesthetics, as the primary or major anesthetic component for balanced anesthesia techniques, and as analgesics for postoperative pain. Morphine, meperidine, methadone, fentanyl, sufentanil, alfentanil, and, more recently, remifentanil have been safely used in the pediatric population.[36] Dosage varies a great deal, depending on the age and size of the patient and the purpose and plan for anesthetic and postoperative management.

Pediatric patients are at increased risk for complications associated with anesthesia, and the younger the patient, the greater the risk. Failure to recognize and treat perioperative stress may account for the poor anesthesia outcomes in pediatric patients. Infants who undergo surgery experience stress as a result of catabolism and substrate mobilization. Critically ill neonates have a precarious metabolic balance and poor metabolic reserve, and they experience the metabolic cost of rapid growth. The added stress of surgery can be detrimental to the metabolic state of the neonate. Opioid-related suppression of the stress response in infants can improve these patients' postoperative course.

Fentanyl is the opioid most commonly used in the pediatric population. Its major advantage relates to its rapid onset and brief duration of action. It induces a very stable cardiovascular response. Excellent recovery characteristics and ventilatory function were provided when fentanyl, either 2 or 10 mcg/kg, was used for anesthesia in full-term infants who underwent hernia repair. It did not result in apnea and produced better pain control in comparison with other opioids; however, time to discharge was prolonged.

Effective analgesia can also be achieved in pediatric patients by injecting epidural (bolus or continuous infusion) and intrathecal opioids.[37] Control of respiratory depression, the major complication, requires careful dosing and monitoring. Other side effects, including pruritus, nausea, vomiting, and urinary retention, are often easily managed by administration of a small dose of naloxone.

Neurosurgery

Administration of opioids can increase CSF pressure if ventilation is not controlled and if the $PaCO_2$ is allowed to increase. Opioid premedication should therefore be used cautiously when elevated intracranial pressure is suspected. However, opioids are useful during induction of anesthesia in neurosurgical patients to blunt the stress of intubation. When ventilation is controlled, opioids have little effect on cerebral metabolic rate and blood flow.

Studies have been conducted on the use in neurosurgery of multiple opioids, including morphine, fentanyl, alfentanil, sufentanil, remifentanil, and meperidine. Results of these studies on opioids during intraoperative neurologic monitoring were similar for all types of evoked potentials. The effects of opioids on evoked responses are generally mild, causing small dose-dependent increases in latency and decreases in amplitude.[38] Effects are not clinically significant; they are maximal when the drug is peaking and then remain fairly stable.

Opioids, even in relatively high doses, can be used for patients who require intraoperative monitoring without compromising the ability to monitor neurologic function adequately.[38] Large intravenous bolus administration of opioids should be avoided at times of potential surgical compromise to neurologic function to prevent confusion regarding the interpretation of the measurements. Continuous infusions of opioids provide stable recordings, whereas bolus injections can affect both the evoked potentials and the wake-up test. Continuous infusions of remifentanil allow a rapid return to consciousness for neurologic examination if a wake-up test is needed during surgery.

Trauma

Opioids are commonly the agent of choice in the anesthetic management of trauma patients.[39] Opioid use provides cardiovascular stability for trauma patients, who are often in an unstable condition. Patients with major trauma have hypotension, hypovolemia, and hypothermia.

The selection of a specific opioid must be based on knowledge of its characteristics and the experience of the anesthesia provider. It is important to avoid the use of opioids that produce histamine release and hypotension. Histamine release after intravenous administration of equipotent doses of meperidine, morphine, fentanyl, and sufentanil for anesthesia induction must be considered. Morphine results in a great degree of histamine release. Patients receiving either meperidine, sufentanil, or fentanyl do not experience histamine release. The hemodynamic instability of trauma patients decreases opioid anesthetic requirements. The decreased anesthetic requirements that are the result of hemodynamic instability can result in surgical recall. The most distressing component of recall was pain. Less distressing components were voices and awareness of the experience of surgery.

Ambulatory Surgery

Because of patient preferences, improved technology, and financial considerations, more and more surgical procedures are being performed in an ambulatory setting. Choosing the ideal anesthetic for ambulatory surgery patients is difficult because of the variation in duration and stimulation among procedures.

Fentanyl, alfentanil, and remifentanil have all been used in the ambulatory setting. Comparison of the pharmacokinetics of these three opioids has shown that fentanyl is more lipid soluble and has a larger volume distribution, a longer elimination half-life, and a more basic pK_a. Alfentanil has a more acidic pK_a; therefore, the component of nonionized drug is larger, and this allows a more rapid onset of action. Because alfentanil has a shorter elimination half-life, it is excreted more rapidly than fentanyl but not as rapidly as remifentanil. Fentanyl and alfentanil can be administered as a single bolus or intermittent infusion in the ambulatory setting, but remifentanil can be administered only as an infusion. Fentanyl is a better choice for ambulatory surgery patients than nalbuphine, because nalbuphine is associated with a greater incidence of nausea, vomiting, unpleasant dreams, and hospital admission.

Pharmacokinetic differences between adults and children can influence opioid effect in outpatient pediatric surgery. The use of opioids in adults and children is an effective technique for inducing and maintaining analgesia in the ambulatory setting. Considerations with regard to opioid use in ambulatory surgical settings include drug ionization, elimination half-life, plasma clearance, and bolus versus infusion techniques.

Postoperative Pain Control

In the 1980s, several devices that enabled patients to control their postoperative pain were marketed. Patient-controlled analgesia (PCA) requires that patients be taught preoperatively about the equipment. PCA programming requires selection of the opioid, dosage, and a lockout interval measured in minutes. To decrease postoperative discomfort, the patient triggers the device, which then delivers a dose of the chosen opioid.

The incidence of respiratory depression is low with the use of PCA devices. The potential for operator, patient, and mechanical errors during PCA exists but has been reduced with the improvement of devices. Continuous infusion can be used to supplement PCA dosages, but it can increase side effects without an increase in analgesia.

The role of intrathecal and epidural opioids has been evolving since their first use in 1979. From intermittent boluses of epidural morphine only to combinations of other opioids with bupivacaine in continuous infusions or patient-controlled epidural analgesia, the safety and efficacy of this form of analgesia have been defined. However, with the introduction of ketorolac and the use of less invasive surgical approaches, fewer cases require the effect and cost of epidural analgesia.

SUMMARY

Opioids are a group of drugs that bind to receptor sites in the CNS, supraspinal and spinal, and at peripheral sites, producing morphine-like effects. Opioid analgesia results from the inhibition of nociceptive reflexes and the release of neurotransmitters. Because of their multiplicity of sites and mechanisms of action, opioids are a uniquely valued means for analgesia and anesthesia. Opioids can be used for preoperative medication, as induction agents, as maintenance anesthetics, and for treatment of postoperative pain. The newer methods of opioid delivery have been growing in popularity. Opioids provide the anesthesia practitioner with a multitude of delivery modalities. The introduction of other forms of delivery (e.g., inhalation) will further expand their role in perioperative pain management. Specific drug recommendations for opioids based on genotypes will be a future tool to better guide clinicians in developing patient-tailored drug therapy that will result in fewer adverse drug reactions and higher efficacy of pharmacotherapy.

REFERENCES

1. Kazuhiko F. Intravenous opioid anesthetics. In: Miller RD, ed. *Anesthesia*. 6th ed. Philadelphia: Churchill Livingstone; 2005:379-438.
2. Gutstein HB, Akil H. Opioid analgesics. In Brunton LL et al, eds. *Goodman and Gilman's Pharmacological Basis of Therapeutics*. 11th ed. New York: McGraw-Hill; 2006:547-590.
3. Synder SH, Pasternak GW. Historical review: opioid receptors. *Trends Pharmacol Sci*. 2006;547-590.
4. Stoelting RK, Hiller SC. *Pharmacology and Physiology in Anesthesia Practice*. Philadelphia: Lippincott-Raven; 2006.
5. Klepstad P et al. Start of oral morphine to cancer patients: effective serum morphine concentrations and contribution from morphine-6-glucuronide to the analgesia produced by morphine. *Eur J Clin Pharmacol*. 2000;55:713-719.
6. Martin WR et al. The effects of morphine and nalorphine-like drugs in non-dependent and morphine dependent chronic spinal dogs. *J Pharmacol Exp Ther*. 1976;197:517-532.
7. Inturrisi CE. Clinical pharmacology of opioids and pain. *Clin J Pain*. 2002;18:S3-S13.
8. Walker JS. Anti-inflammatory effects of opioids. *Adv Exp Med Biol*. 2003;521:148-160.
9. Coda BA. Opioids. In: Barash PG et al, eds. *Clinical Anesthesia*. 5th ed. Philadelphia: Lippincott Williams & Wilkins; 2006:353-383.
10. Stein C, Rosow CE. Analgesics: Receptor ligands and opiate narcotics. In: Evers AK, Maze M, eds. *Anesthetic Pharmacology: Physiologic Principles and Clinical Practice*. Philadelphia: Churchill Livingstone; 2004:457-489.
11. Stamer UM et al. Genetics and variability in opioid response. *Eur J Pain*. 2005;9:101-104.
12. Somogyi AA et al. Pharmacogenetics of opioids. *Clin Pharmacol Ther*. 2007;81:429-444.
13. Aubrun F et al. Relationships between measurement of pain using visual analog score and morphine requirements during postoperative intravenous morphine titration. *Anesthesiology*. 2003;98:1415-1421.
14. Samer CF et al. Individualizing analgesic prescription part 1: pharmacogenetics of opioid analgesics. *Personalized Med*. 2006;3:239-269.
15. Carr DB, Cousins MJ. Spinal route of analgesia: opioids and future options. In: Cousins M, Bridenbaugh P, eds. *Neural Blockade*. 3rd ed. Philadelphia: Lippincott-Raven; 1998:915-983.
16. Bernards CM. Understanding the physiology and pharmacology of epidural and intrathecal opioids. *Best Pract Res Clin Anaesthesiol*. 2002; 16:489-505.
17. Ayoub CM, Sinatra RS. Postoperative analgesia: epidural and spinal techniques. In: Chestnut DH, ed. *Obstetric Anesthesia Principles and Practice*. St Louis: Mosby; 2004:472-503.
18. Glass P et al. Intravenous drug delivery systems. In: Miller RD, ed. *Anesthesia*. 6th ed. Philadelphia: Churchill Livingstone; 2005:439-480.
19. Donnely AJ et al. *Anesthesiology and Critical Care Drug Handbook*. Hudson, TX: Lexi-Comp, Inc; 2006.
20. Paqueron X et al. Is morphine-induced sedation synonymous with analgesia during intravenous morphine titration? *Br J Anaesth*. 2002;89:697-701.
21. Smith MT. Neuroexcitatory effects of morphine and hydromorphone: evidence implicating the 3-glucuronide metabolites. *Clin Exp Pharmacol Physiol*. 2000;27:524-528.
22. Cann C et al. Unwanted effects of morphine-6-glucuronide and morphine. *Anaesthesia*. 2002;57:1200-1203.

23. Quigley C. Hydromorphone for acute and chronic pain. *Cochrane Database Syst Rev.* 2002;(1):CD003447.

24. Bruera E, Sweeney C. Methadone use in cancer patients with pain: a review. *J Palliat Med.* 2002;5:127-138.

25. Weinberg D et al. Sublingual absorption of selected opioid analgesics. *Clin Pharmacol Ther.* 1988;44:335-342.

26. Munoz HR et al. Effect of timing of morphine administration during remifentanil-based anaesthesia on early recovery from anaesthesia and postoperative pain. *Br J Anaesth.* 2002;88:814-818.

27. Tzschentke TM. Behavioral pharmacology of buprenorphine, with a focus on preclinical models of reward and addiction. *Psychopharmacology.* 2002;161:1-16.

28. Budd K. Buprenorphine and the transdermal system: the ideal match in pain management. *Int J Clin Pract Suppl.* 2003;133:9-14.

29. Prough DS et al. Acute pulmonary edema in healthy teenagers following conservative doses of intravenous naloxone. *Anesthesiology.* 1984;60:485-486.

30. Andree R. Sudden death following naloxone administration. *Anesth Analg.* 1980;59:782-784.

31. Glass P et al. Comparison of potency and duration of action of nalmefene and naloxone. *Anesth Analg.* 1994;78:536-541.

32. Henderson CA, Reynolds JE. Acute pulmonary edema in a young male after intravenous nalmefene. *Anesth Analg.* 1997;84:218-219.

33. Eaton MP, Bailey PC. Cardiovascular pharmacology of anesthetics. In: Estafanous FG et al, eds. *Cardiac Anesthesia Principles and Clinical Practice.* 2nd ed. Philadelphia: Lippincott; 2001:295-318.

34. Riley ET, Ross BK. Opioid techniques. In: Chestnut DH, ed. *Obstetric Anesthesia Principles and Practice.* St Louis: Mosby; 2004:349-368.

35. Wakefield ML. Systemic analgesia: parenteral and inhalational agents. In: Chestnut DH, ed. *Obstetric Anesthesia Principles and Practice.* St Louis: Mosby; 2004:311-323.

36. Ross AK et al. Pharmacokinetics of remifentanil in anesthetized pediatric patients undergoing elective surgery or diagnostic procedures. *Anesth Analg.* 2001;93:1393-1401.

37. Cote CJ. Pediatric anesthesia. In: Miller RD, ed. *Anesthesia,* 6th ed. Philadelphia: Churchill Livingstone; 2005:2367-2407.

38. Mahla ME et al. Neurologic monitoring. In: Miller RD, ed. *Anesthesia.* 6th ed. Philadelphia: Churchill Livingstone; 2005:1511-1550.

39. Alpen MA, Morse C. Managing the pain of traumatic injury. *Crit Care Nurs Clin North Am.* 2001;13:243-257.

NEUROMUSCULAR BLOCKING AGENTS, REVERSAL AGENTS, AND THEIR MONITORING

John J. Nagelhout

HISTORY

In the nineteenth century, Claude Bernard, a famous French physiologist and philosopher, carried out experiments with curare, then in use by the Amazonian Indians of South America.[1] He noted that animals the Indians hunted for food were paralyzed by arrows poisoned with curare and subsequently died of asphyxiation.[2] Bernard's experiments with the poison the Indians tipped their arrows with, formed the basis for our ideas of the neuromuscular junction, neuromuscular transmission, and neuromuscular pharmacology.[3] Indeed, curare had been used since 1857 as an anticonvulsant treatment in tetany and other types of spastic disorders.[4]

Laewen also described the use of curare in anesthetized humans in a German report in 1912.[3] For readers who are interested in historical aspects of this topic, a fascinating and more complete report of the earliest work of these and other researchers, beginning as early as the year 1548, is available in an outstanding review article by Bisset.[5]

In 1936, Dale and colleagues[6] found that acetylcholine (ACh) was the chemical neurotransmitter that activated the postjunctional muscle membrane receptors after excitation of the nerve terminal. This finding contradicted the once widely held theory that direct electrical transmission from the nerve to the muscle occurs.[6] This discovery provided the impetus for further research concerning pharmacologic agents that could either enhance the action of ACh or prevent it, thereby causing a temporary and reversible state of therapeutic paralysis.

Griffith and Johnson[7] of Montreal, Canada, are universally acknowledged as the persons responsible for the introduction of neuromuscular blockers into anesthetic practice. Their groundbreaking report laid the foundations for other studies that followed. Within a year of their study, Cullen[4] reported on the use of curare in 131 general anesthetic procedures. His only report of an adverse reaction dealt with a 44-year-old woman who experienced "complete paralysis and severe salivation," accompanied by muscular twitching.[4]

Despite initial successes with the neuromuscular blockers, an early study nearly doomed their use before they became widely accepted. Henry Beecher and Donald Todd, two physicians in the anesthesia department of Harvard Medical School, reviewed 599,548 anesthetic procedures administered at 10 institutions between 1948 and 1952. As part of this review, they examined the death rate in patients receiving *curares* (the term by which they described any neuromuscular blocking agent, including tubocurarine chloride, decamethonium bromide, succinylcholine chloride, gallamine triethiodide, and dimethyltubocurarine [*d*-tubocurarine] iodide). Beecher and Todd found that the overall death rate for persons treated with neuromuscular blockers was 1:370, compared with a death rate of 1:2100 in patients who did not receive these agents.[8]

After reviewing the conditions of the patients; the educational background and training of the practitioners who administered the anesthetic (e.g., physician, nurse anesthetist, or physician-in-training); the size of the institution; the sexes, races, and ages of the patients; and numerous other combinations of these factors, the investigators reached the following conclusions.

> [I]n our judgment the situation is one where neither experience of individual nor experience of institution appears to protect. This adds up to evidence that neither mistakes nor preventable error of any kind are involved in the main, but rather the inherent toxicity of the "curares" themselves.[8]

In the litigious environment of modern anesthetic practice, such a statement may have ended the administration of these agents. It would certainly have slowed their development. The positive attributes of the agents, however, were discussed later in the same paper, as Beecher and Todd added this caveat:

> Having presented the foregoing evidence and comment, one can ask what, then, is to be done about these agents? Are they to be banned as a practical solution of the problem? We believe not. These data strongly suggest that great caution in the use of muscle relaxants should be exercised, that the agents available at present be considered as on trial, and that they be employed only when there are clear advantages to be gained by their use, that they not be employed for trivial purposes or as a corrective for generally inadequate anesthesia.[8]

Beecher and Todd's admonition still echoes through the halls of anesthetic practice today. Although the safety and efficacy of neuromuscular blocking agents have markedly increased, the sage advice is still germane for the practitioner: Neuromuscular blocking agents, like all anesthetic agents, are best used where and when they are indicated. Nevertheless, as one leg of the anesthetic triad that includes analgesia, amnesia, and muscle relaxation, neuromuscular blockade has become an integral part of most modern anesthetic techniques. A broad spectrum of these

The author would like to thank Richard Haas, PhD, CRNA, for his contributions to this chapter in previous editions.

agents now exists, although no single agent has all of what would be the ideal properties. Their individual pharmacokinetic and pharmacodynamic attributes enable the anesthetist to tailor the use of the agent to the physiologic needs of the patient and the requirements of the surgeon.

MONITORING OF NEUROMUSCULAR BLOCKADE

Monitoring of neuromuscular blockade has become a standard during most anesthetics when a relaxant is administered. The response to a peripheral nerve stimulator (PNS) indirectly infers the relaxation of musculature. The PNS is an electrical device that delivers a series of shocks to the patient through electrodes applied to the skin near a nerve.[9] There are several methods for monitoring neuromuscular blockade intensity, including acceleromyography, electromyography, phonomyography, mechanomyography, and others. Visual and tactile response to evoked electrical stimulus is the most common. On activation of the PNS, various predictable muscle contraction patterns are visible in the presence and absence of neuromuscular blockers.

Depolarization and contraction of a muscle are caused by an action potential traveling along the course of a nerve. As the impulse reaches the motor endplate, ACh is released across the synaptic cleft. It subsequently travels toward the receptor sites on the muscle membrane, resulting in depolarization and subsequent contraction of the muscle.[2] The PNS elicits the same activity, which makes it useful for the monitoring of neuromuscular blockade.

The administration of neuromuscular blocking agents (NMBAs) places patients in a high-risk situation. Respiratory function is compromised. The monitoring of neuromuscular blockade is essential for proper dosing and provides the anesthetist a more accurate assessment of the patient. Inadequate doses of NMBAs may result in complications during surgical procedures because of unexpected patient movement. In contrast, overdosage may result in residual paralysis in the postoperative period, increased drug cost, and labor-intensive intervention (e.g., mechanical ventilation).

Contraction of the adductor muscle of the thumb via stimulation of the ulnar nerve is the preferred method of determining the level of neuromuscular blockade. Disposable electrodes are applied over the ulnar nerve. The distal electrode is placed over the proximal flexor crease of the wrist, and the other electrode is placed over and parallel to the carpi ulnaris tendon. On stimulation of these electrodes with the PNS, adduction of the thumb is visible.[9] Other monitoring sites include the first dorsal interosseous muscle in the hand, the abductor muscle of the little finger, the nerves of the foot, and the facial nerve, which stimulates the orbicular muscle around the eye or the orbicular muscle that contracts the lip.[10] The facial and ulnar nerves are the most commonly used sites (Figures 13-1 and 13-2).

Tests of Neuromuscular Function

The first (and simplest) type of stimulation is a single twitch at 0.1 to 1 Hz for 0.1 to 0.2 ms. These impulses can be delivered automatically every second, every 10 seconds, or manually, depending on the sophistication of the neurostimulating apparatus.[10] The second and most common means of stimulation is the train-of-four (TOF), which delivers four separate stimuli, each with a duration of less than 0.5 ms at a frequency of 2 Hz.[11] In the event that four twitches remain after NMBA administration, it is important to remember that the patient may be 0% to 70% blocked. As relaxation increases, the twitches in the TOF pattern progressively fade. The fourth twitch disappears first, which

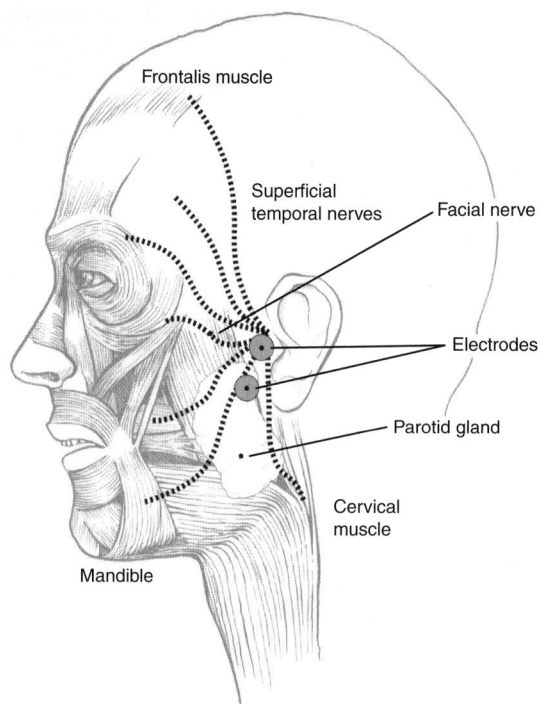

FIGURE **13-1**   Facial neuromuscular blockade testing.

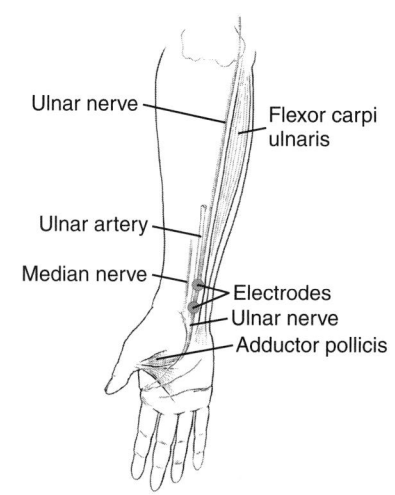

FIGURE **13-2**   Ulnar neuromuscular blockade testing.

represents a block of more than 80%. Disappearance of the third and second twitches indicates a 75% and 90% block, respectively.[9] Assessment of the TOF test is given in Figure 13-3.

Other types of stimulation that may be delivered are tetany, posttetanic count, and double-burst stimulation (DBS).[11] Tetanus may be used to determine whether "fade" occurs after the administration of nondepolarizing neuromuscular blockers.[12,13] It consists of continuous electrical stimulation for 5 seconds at 50 or 100 Hz. If fade is present, clinically significant block remains. The posttetanic count (PTC) mode releases a 50-Hz tetanic stimulation for 5 seconds, followed in 3 seconds by a series of single 1-Hz twitch stimulations.[14] The number of twitches inversely correlates with the time necessary for the

Train-of-four
suppression

Percent neuromuscular block

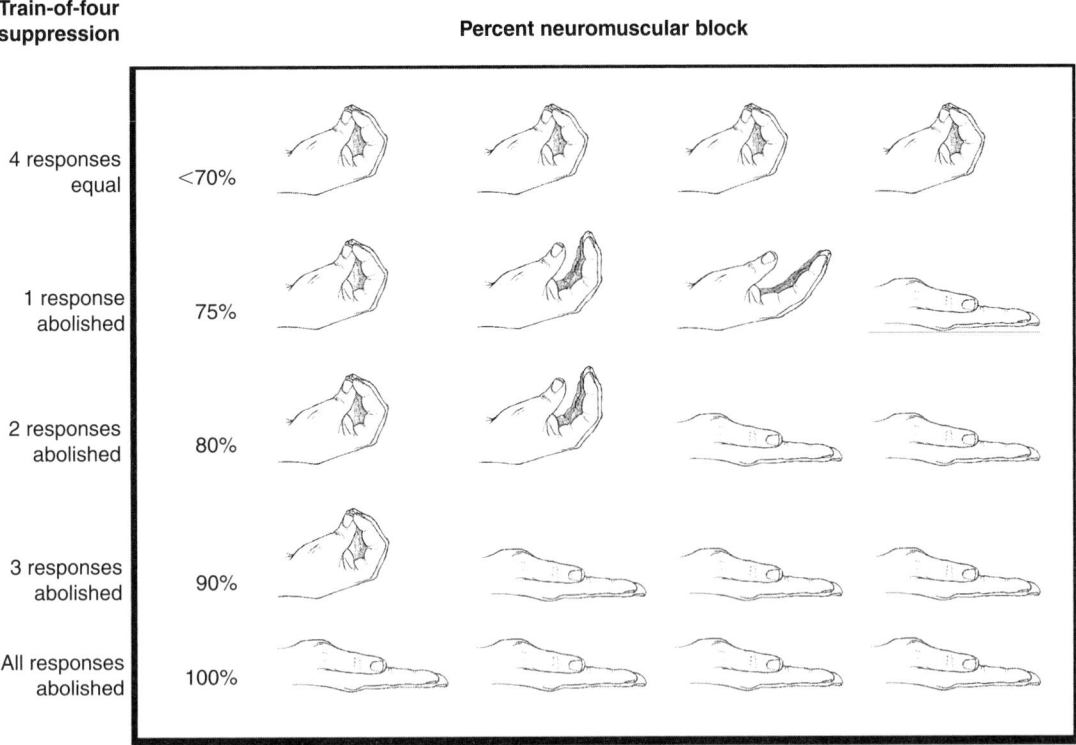

4 responses
equal   <70%

1 response
abolished   75%

2 responses
abolished   80%

3 responses
abolished   90%

All responses
abolished   100%

FIGURE **13-3**   Train-of-four test.

BOX **13-1**

Commonly Used Neuromuscular Terminology

- *Onset time:* time from drug administration to maximum effect
- *Clinical duration:* time from drug administration to 25% recovery of the twitch response
- *Total duration of action:* time from drug administration to 90% recovery of twitch response
- *Recovery index:* time from 25% to 75% recovery of the twitch response
- *Train-of-four ratio:* compares the fourth twitch of a TOF with the first twitch; when the fourth twitch is 90% of the first, recovery is indicated

return of the first twitch of a TOF stimulation; however, these values vary and should be investigated for each individual agent.[15,16] Double-burst stimulation is a means of administering two brief bursts of three impulses at 50 Hz, separated by a time period of 750 ms.[11] This is proposed to be a more accurate means of assessing nondepolarizing blockade, in part because of its ability to be detected by tactile sensation.[11,14] Neuromuscular monitoring terminology and tests are summarized in Box 13-1 and Tables 13-1 and 13-2. Some key points related to tests of neuromuscular transmission are given in Box 13-2.[17]

DEPOLARIZING AGENTS

Succinylcholine Chloride

Succinylcholine chloride (Anectine, Quelicin, and others) is very familiar to every clinical anesthetist, having been a standard for several decades of practice. Although its widespread use in clinical anesthesia represents the standard of care for a variety of situations, opinions regarding its use remain divided because of some of its untoward effects.

Stephen Thesleff at the Karolinska Institute in Stockholm was one of the pioneers who introduced the drug into clinical practice to induce neuromuscular paralysis in humans. Initial description of the neuromuscular blocking properties of succinylcholine is credited to Daniel Bovet. (Bovet was awarded the Nobel Prize for Physiology and Medicine in 1957 for his discovery of synthetic compounds that act on the vascular system and skeletal muscle.)[18] The first use of succinylcholine in the United States occurred in 1952. Foldes and co-workers[19] described this agent in the following manner:

> Compared to other muscle relaxants used in anesthesiology, succinylcholine possesses several advantages, the outstanding one, in our experience, being its easy controllability, which permitted almost instantaneous changes in degree of muscular relaxation. With succinylcholine, both increasing and decreasing muscular relaxation took less than a minute.[19]

The disadvantages of succinylcholine have been well recorded through years of clinical experience. It has no action in the ganglionic nicotinic receptors but may cause bradycardia by an action on cardiac cholinergic muscarinic receptors.[20,21] Prolonged neuromuscular blockade can result from excessive doses of succinylcholine in patients with atypical, inhibited, or deficient levels of plasma cholinesterases.[3,20]

Succinylcholine is the only remaining depolarizing muscle relaxant licensed for use in the United States. Remembering the composition of the drug is helpful in better understanding its effects and side effects. Succinylcholine results from the joining of two ACh molecules and is represented by the chemical formula $C_{14}H_{30}N_2O_4$. Although succinylcholine mimics the

TABLE 13-1	Neuromuscular Monitoring Modalities	
Monitoring Test	**Definition**	**Comments**
Single twitch	A single supramaximal electrical stimulus ranging from 0.1-1 Hz	Requires baseline before drug administration; generally used as qualitative rather than quantitative assessment
Train-of-four	A series of four twitches at 2 Hz every half-second for 2 seconds	Reflects blockade from 70%-100%; useful during onset, maintenance, and emergence
Tetanus	Generally consists of rapid delivery of a 30-, 50-, or 100-Hz stimulus for 5 seconds	Should be used sparingly for deep block assessment; painful; assess for presence of fade, indicating residual weakness
Posttetanic count	50-Hz tetanus for 5 seconds, a 3-second pause, then single twitches of 1 Hz	Used only when train-of-four or double-burst stimulation response is absent; count less than eight indicates a deep block, and prolonged recovery is likely
Double-burst stimulation	Two short bursts of 50-Hz tetanus separated by 0.75 second	Similar to train-of-four; useful during onset, maintenance, and emergence; may be easier to detect fade than with train-of-four; tactile evaluation

TABLE 13-2	Key Points Related to Tests of Neuromuscular Transmission and Reversal		
Test	**Acceptable Clinical Result to Suggest Normal Function**	**Approximate Percent of Receptors Occupied When Response Returns to Normal Value**	**Comments, Advantages, and Disadvantages**
Tidal volume	At least 5 mL/kg	80	Necessary, but insensitive as an indicator of neuromuscular function
Single twitch strength	Qualitatively as strong as baseline	75-80	Uncomfortable; need to know twitch strength before relaxant administration; insensitive as an indicator of recovery, but useful as a gauge of deep neuromuscular blockade
Train-of-four (TOF)	No palpable fade	70-75	Uncomfortable, but more sensitive as indicator of recovery than single twitch; used as a gauge of depth of block by counting the number of responses perceptible
Sustained tetanus at 50 Hz for 5 seconds	At least 20 mL/kg	70	Very uncomfortable, but a reliable indictor of adequate recovery
Vital capacity	At least 20 mL/kg	70	Requires patient cooperation, but is the goal for achievement of full clinical recovery
Double-burst stimulation	No palpable fade	60-70	Uncomfortable, but more sensitive than TOF as an indicator of peripheral function; no perceptible fade indicates TOF of at least recovery of 60%
Inspiratory force	At least −40 cm H_2O	50	Difficult to perform with endotracheal intubation, but a reliable gauge of normal diaphragmatic function
Head lift	Must be performed unaided with patient supine and sustained for 5 seconds	50	Requires patient cooperation, but remains the standard test of normal clinical function
Hand grip	Sustained at a level qualitatively similar to preinduction	50	Sustained strong grip, though also requires patient cooperation; is another good gauge of normal function
Sustained bite	Sustained jaw clench on tongue blade	50	Very reliable with patient cooperation; corresponds with TOF of 85%

Modified with permission from Miller RD, ed. Miller's Anesthesia. 6th ed. Philadelphia: Churchill Livingstone; 2005.

action of ACh by depolarizing the motor end plate, its degradation is distinct. In contrast with the degradation of ACh by acetylcholinesterase (AChE), succinylcholine is hydrolyzed by plasma cholinesterase (pseudocholinesterase). The popularity of this muscle relaxant is rooted in its unique ability to provide a quick onset and short duration of effect. A bolus of 0.5 to 1.5 mg/kg is the recommended dose for adequate adult paralysis and relaxation for intubation.[22] The dose of succinylcholine that provides the desired effect in 95% of the population (ED$_{95}$) is approximately 0.25 mg/kg.[23]

BOX **13-2**

General Guidelines for Successful Neuromuscular Monitoring

- During onset, paralysis begins with the eye muscles, followed by the extremities, trunk (from the neck muscles downward through the intercostals), abdominal muscles, and finally the diaphragm. Recovery returns in the opposite manner. Protective reflex muscles of the pharynx and upper esophagus recover later than the diaphragm, larynx, hands, or face.
- Monitoring of the facial nerve for determination of onset and readiness for intubation may be preferable to monitoring of the ulnar nerve.
- Monitoring of the offset and recovery from neuromuscular blockade is probably better at the ulnar nerve.
- Tactile evaluation of double-burst stimulation may be better to differentiate "fade" than train-of-four (TOF).
- When there is only one response to TOF stimulation, successful reversal may take as long as 30 minutes.
- At a TOF count of two or three responses, recovery may take up to 10 to 12 minutes after administration of long-acting relaxants and 4 to 5 minutes after intermediate-acting drugs.
- When the fourth response to TOF stimulation appears, adequate recovery can be achieved within 5 minutes of reversal with neostigmine or 2 to 3 minutes after use of edrophonium.
- When the fourth twitch of the TOF returns, the TOF ratio (TOFR) may be determined. Compare the size of the fourth twitch (T4) with the size of the first twitch (T1), using T4:T1 as a ratio. When the ratio reaches 0.9 or 90%, the patient has recovered significant muscle strength.

Pharmacokinetics

Onset. Succinylcholine has an extremely rapid onset and remains the gold standard against which other agents are compared. A typical intubating dose of 1 to 1.5 mg/kg results in a maximum suppression of muscle twitch and good to excellent intubating conditions within 1 to 1.5 minutes of administration.[23,24] Onset of action of succinylcholine at the larynx with administration of 1 mg/kg is 34 seconds.[25,26] The onset as measured at peripheral sites such as the adductor pollicis is slightly longer at 1 minute.[27] The rapid onset of succinylcholine is based on its action as an initial agonist at the nicotinic receptor, rather than as a competitive antagonist. Succinylcholine works by activating the muscle-type nicotinic cholinergic receptors, followed by desensitization.[21] This action results in the need for significantly less drug at the receptor site to produce neuromuscular block. In contrast, most NMBAs require 75% or more receptor occupancy for paralysis to result. Variable onset must be considered in patients with altered physiology. Patients with atypical plasma cholinesterase may exhibit prolonged onset after succinylcholine administration.[28] A summary of the dose, onset, and duration of the neuromuscular blocking drugs is given in Table 13-3.

Duration. The plasma half-life of succinylcholine is 2 to 4 minutes.[29] The clinical duration of succinylcholine (i.e., the length of time during which its clinical effects can be recognized) is 5 to 10 minutes, with full recovery evident at 12 to 15 minutes. Twitch recovery of 25%, as measured by the laryngeal adductor pressure responses, is 4.3 minutes, whereas 90% to 95% twitch recovery has been reported to occur in 8 minutes.[25] Other studies have yielded similar results, with researchers citing a range of duration of 7 to 12 minutes.[20,23]

Elimination. Succinylcholine is degraded via hydrolysis by plasma cholinesterases. These enzymes, although found in the plasma, are produced by the liver. Initially, hydrolysis results in the transformation of succinylcholine into succinylmonocholine and choline (Figure 13-4). Succinylmonocholine is further degraded by plasma cholinesterase into succinic acid and choline. Succinylcholine metabolism is so rapid that only 10% of the injected dose ever reaches the neuromuscular junction.[22] A summary of the elimination routes for the neuromuscular blocking drugs is given in Table 13-4.

Pharmacokinetic Summary. The onset of succinylcholine given in a dose of 1 to 1.5 mg/kg is 30 to 90 seconds. The clinical duration of succinylcholine is 8 to 15 minutes. It is degraded via the plasma cholinesterase into succinic acid and choline.

| TABLE **13-3** | Neuromuscular Blocking Agents: Dose, Onset, and Duration* |

Agent	ED$_{95}$ (mg/kg)	Intubating Dose (mg/kg)	Time to Onset	Duration of Action (min)
Succinylcholine (Anectine)	0.25	1-1.5	30-60 sec	Ultrashort, 5-15
Atracurium (Tracrium)	0.15	0.5	2-4 min	Intermediate, 30-60
Cisatracurium (Nimbex)	0.05	0.1	2-4 min	Intermediate, 30-60
Rocuronium (Zemuron)	0.3	0.6-1	1-1.5 min	Intermediate, 30-60
Vecuronium (Norcuron)	0.05	0.1	2-4 min	Intermediate, 30-60
Pancuronium (Pavulon)	0.05	0.08-1.8	2-4 min	Long, 60-90

ED$_{95}$, *Effective dose for 95% paralysis.*
All data for adult patients without significant disease.

Central Nervous System

Succinylcholine increases intracranial pressure (ICP), and therefore concern has always existed as to the appropriateness of its use in certain neurosurgical procedures and in patients with brain pathology and increased intracranial pressure.[25] Research conducted in animals shows a small and transient rise of 10 to 15

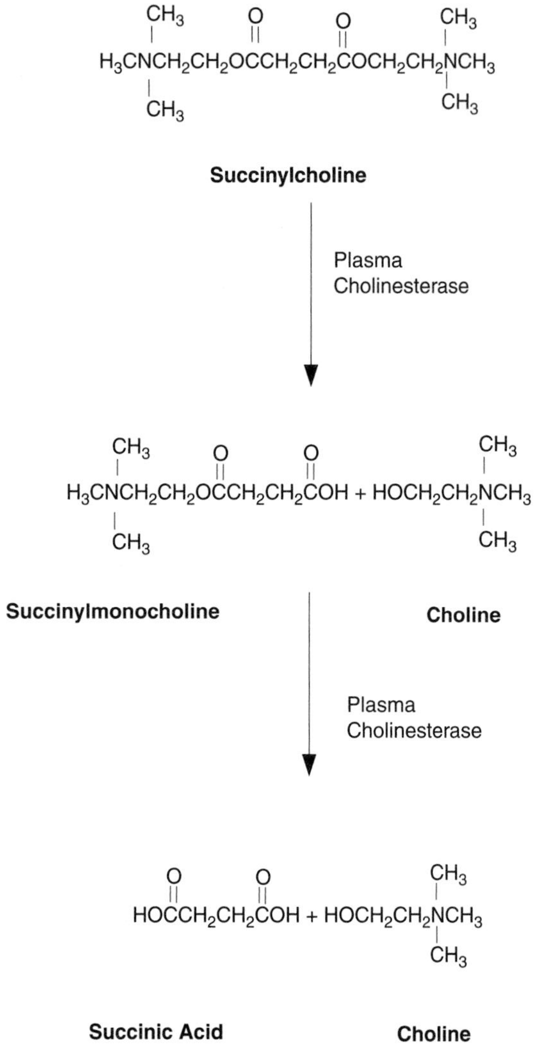

FIGURE 13-4 Metabolism of succinylcholine.

mm Hg for 5 to 8 minutes after administration.[29] The rise may be associated with an increased cerebral blood flow secondary to muscle spindle afferent activity and actions on peripheral neuromuscular junctions. The ICP effects are blocked by pretreatment with a small dose of nondepolarizing relaxant.[30] In clinical practice, the administration of succinylcholine is preceded by an anesthetic induction agent that lowers ICP, so there is little reason to avoid the use of succinylcholine in neurosurgery. This is especially true in emergency procedures requiring rapid airway control.

Cardiovascular System

Succinylcholine usually results in slight tachycardia; however, sudden abrupt bradycardia may result from repeat dosing in adults and any dose in children. Many types of arrhythmias have been reported. Another possible mechanism for the bradycardia associated with succinylcholine administration is thought to be related to its metabolite, succinylmonocholine, which causes stimulation of cholinergic receptors in the sinoatrial node.[31]

An intubating dose of succinylcholine increases serum potassium levels by 0.5 to 1 mEq/L.[29] Although this may not be significant in the normokalemic patient, it may be life threatening in patients with preexisting hyperkalemia.[32] Gronert presents a case that involved an 11-year-old girl who experienced cardiac arrest after receiving succinylcholine. Her cardiac arrest and eventual death were directly attributed to a high potassium release after the succinylcholine administration (10.2 mEq/L). The exaggerated potassium release after the succinylcholine administration in this case was determined to be related to a familial myopathy evidenced by extremely high patient levels of creatine kinase.[33] Succinylcholine administration and myopathy are discussed below.

Some clinicians believe that a second dose of succinylcholine indicated by any event should be preceded by intravenous (IV) atropine or glycopyrrolate for its anticholinergic effects; however, others do not.[32,34]

Hepatic System

Cholinesterase enzyme subtypes are produced in the liver. Pseudocholinesterase (PChE) degrades succinylcholine; therefore, certain types of liver damage may prolong the effects of the drug.[29] Ester compounds like succinylcholine are metabolized by adding water, the process referred to as *hydrolysis*. The basic reaction is ESTER + H_2O ↔ ACID + ALCOHOL. Three esterase enzymes that can act as catalysts for these hydrolysis reactions exist in the plasma: cholinesterase, paraoxonase, and albumin

TABLE 13-4	Neuromuscular Blockers: Elimination Mechanism	
Agent	Elimination Mechanism	Comments
Atracurium	Hofmann elimination; nonspecific esterases	Non–organ-dependent elimination produces consistent duration in patients with significant hepatic and renal disease, as well as the elderly
Cisatracurium	Hofmann elimination; nonspecific esterases	Similar to atracurium but without the histamine release
Rocuronium	Renal; hepatic	May be prolonged with hepatic and renal disease
Vecuronium	Renal (20%-30%); hepatic (40%-80%)	May be prolonged with hepatic disease
Pancuronium	Renal primarily; some hepatic	May be prolonged with renal disease
Succinylcholine	Plasma cholinesterase	Prolonged in patients with cholinesterase deficiency

esterase. Paraoxonase and albumin esterase are frequently referred to as *nonspecific esterases*. Red blood cells (RBCs) contain two esterase enzymes in their cytosol. One is referred to as *RBC esterase*, *esterase D*, or *S-formylglutathione*, and the other is AChE in small amounts.

Cholinesterase is a generic term used for a family of related enzymes that hydrolyze choline esters at a faster rate than other esters under optimal conditions. The major function of cholinesterase is to terminate the action of ACh at cholinergic nerve endings in synapses or in effector organs. Two types of cholinesterase exist in the human body, with several variations and a confusing set of names. One type of cholinesterase is AChE, also known as *true, specific, genuine,* and *type 1 cholinesterase*. This enzyme is found in erythrocytes, nerve endings, the lungs, the spleen, and the gray matter of the brain. It is a membrane-bound glycoprotein and exists in several molecular forms. The other subgroup, PChE, also known as *plasma, serum, benzoyl, false, butyryl, nonspecific,* and *type II cholinesterase*, exists in plasma and has more than 11 isoenzyme variants. PChE is also present in the liver, smooth muscle, intestines, pancreas, heart, and white matter of the brain.

Measurements of PChE activity can serve as a sensitive measure of the synthetic capacity of the liver. In the absence of known inhibitors, any decrease in activity reflects impaired synthesis of the enzyme. A moderate decrease (30% to 50%) is seen in acute hepatitis and long-standing chronic hepatitis, whereas a severe decrease (50% to 70%) is seen in advanced cirrhosis and in some carcinomas with metastases to the liver. Decreased levels of PChE are also found in patients with acute infections, pulmonary embolism, muscular dystrophy, myocardial infarction, pregnancy, and after surgical procedures. Essentially normal levels are noted in patients with chronic hepatitis, mild cirrhosis, or obstructive jaundice. Increased levels have been observed in cases of nephrotic syndrome, thyrotoxicosis, and hemochromatosis, in obese patients with diabetes, and in patients with anxiety and other psychiatric states. Patients generally develop neuromuscular symptoms at approximately 60% of normal activity, and serious neuromuscular effects are seen at approximately 20% of normal. Reference intervals are 2900 to 7100 units/L. Table 13-5 lists some common anesthesia-related drugs that undergo hydrolysis, with the enzyme catalyst involved.

TABLE **13-5**	Common Esterase-Dependent, Anesthesia-Related Drugs
Drug	**Enzyme**
Succinylcholine	Pseudocholinesterase
Ester local anesthetics: Cocaine Procaine Chloroprocaine Tetracaine	Pseudocholinesterase
Neostigmine	Pseudocholinesterase
Edrophonium	Pseudocholinesterase
Atracurium	Nonspecific esterases (plasma)
Cisatracurium	Nonspecific esterases (plasma)
Remifentanil	Nonspecific esterases (plasma)
Esmolol	RBC esterases

RBC, *Red blood cell.*

Genetic Variants and the Dibucaine Inhibition Test

Some patients exhibit genetic variations that cause a prolonged response and apnea when the patient is exposed to succinylcholine. Although such individuals may lead a normal life in every other respect, their atypical variants of cholinesterase are unable to hydrolyze certain drugs in the usual fashion. Low levels or even the absence of serum cholinesterase is indicative of atypical variants. The most frequent variations in the PChE gene are the atypical (A) and Kalow (K) variants.[35] An additional 58 mutations in the coding sequence have been reported; however, most are extremely rare.[36] In the usual clinical scenario, a patient completes surgery and is unable to breathe. If succinylcholine was used to facilitate intubation, differential diagnosis leads the anesthesia provider to conclude that a potential atypical pseudocholinesterase may be present. The patient is taken to the postanesthesia care unit, placed on a ventilator, sedated, and monitored until the succinylcholine wears off. The patient recovers and is subsequently discharged, but prior to discharge, a blood sample is taken to perform a dibucaine inhibition test to help determine (1) whether an atypical enzyme was present and (2) the cause of the prolonged apnea. The dibucaine number and enzyme activity are both determined. By treating the patient's serum with dibucaine and measuring the residual PChE activity compared with the PChE of an untreated sample, the metabolic sensitivity to succinylcholine can be measured. The patient is contacted post-discharge and counseled as appropriate, according to the findings.

Dibucaine is an amide local anesthetic that inhibits typical or usual PChE but not atypical. For example, the normal dibucaine number of 80 means that 80% of the PChE activity was inhibited by dibucaine. If a dibucaine number of 20 is obtained, the patient has atypical enzyme because dibucaine did not inhibit the patient's enzyme activity. If a patient experiences prolonged apnea following succinylcholine administration, it is imperative to differentiate between an atypical genetic variant of PChE or simply low levels of normal PChE enzyme. Possible interpretations of a dibucaine test are given in Box 13-3.

Patients with acute or chronic liver disease, organophosphate poisoning, or chronic renal disease, patients in the late stages of pregnancy, and patients undergoing estrogen therapy may have markedly decreased PChE activities but normal enzyme. PChE phenotype interpretation is based on the total PChE activity and the percent of inhibition caused by dibucaine. (Table 13-6).

Based on the method of denaturing high-performance liquid chromatography, a highly accurate detection approach for the most common variants has recently been reported. This new test offers a rapid and accurate screening method for the most common variants of cholinesterase.[35]

Renal System

Succinylcholine may be used in surgical patients with renal disease when preoperative potassium levels are normal. The use of succinylcholine in patients with elevated preoperative potassium levels is contraindicated.[37] Patients with renal failure and end-stage renal disease are frequently dialyzed prior to surgery, so as long as the serum potassium is within normal limits, succinylcholine may be safely used.[38]

Effects in Special Populations

Elderly Patients. The onset of succinylchoine may be slightly prolonged due to a slower circulation time, but the clinical relevance is minimal.[39] Reduced plasma cholinesterase levels in elderly men allow for a reduced dose of succinylcholine.[40]

Obese Patients. No contraindication to the use of succinyl-choline exists in obese patients. The utility of rapid-sequence induction in anesthetic management of the obese patient makes its use common.[41] The recommended dose of succinylcholine is 1.0 mg/kg, based on total body weight, to produce excellent intubating conditions.[42] In a 2003 study by Brodsky and Foster, succinylcholine was given to 14 morbidly obese patients (body mass indices ranging from 35.8 to 58) who underwent laparoscopic gastric bypass surgery. The authors administered doses ranging from 120 to 140 mg and successfully intubated all of the patients. Only 2 of the 14 patients complained of postoperative myalgia.[43]

Pediatrics. In children, succinylcholine is used only in emergency situations to secure an airway. Routine use in elective procedures was abandoned in the early 1990s, owing to several widely reported cases of severe hyperkalemia and rhabdomyolysis in what appeared to be healthy children. The cases involved routine procedures in children with undiagnosed Duchenne muscular dystrophy (DMD).[44-48] This is an X chromosome–linked disorder with onset of symptoms usually around 5 years of age. Patients exhibit a typical progression of weakness and atrophy that starts in the legs and pelvis, spreads to the shoulders and neck, and finally involves the upper extremities and respiratory muscles. Life expectancy is rarely more than 30 years; death is often a consequence of cardiac and respiratory diseases. Children with DMD frequently require orthopedic surgery for repair of scoliosis or contractures.[49]

BOX **13-3**

Dibucaine Inhibition Test Outcomes

1. Low dibucaine number + normal activity = atypical enzyme and prolonged apnea
2. Normal dibucaine number + low activity = normal enzyme with low levels present and prolonged apnea
3. Low dibucaine number + low activity = atypical enzyme with low levels present and prolonged apnea
4. Normal dibucaine number + normal activity = normal enzyme and amount (Another reason for the prolonged apnea must be investigated.)

The Food and Drug Administration, in conjunction with the anesthesia community, placed the following warning on the use of succinylcholine:

RISK OF CARDIAC ARREST FROM HYPER-KALEMIC RHABDOMYOLYSIS.

There have been rare reports of acute rhabdomyolysis with hyperkalemia followed by ventricular dysrhythmias, cardiac arrest and death after the administration of succinylcholine to apparently healthy children who were subsequently found to have undiagnosed skeletal muscle myopathy, most frequently Duchenne's muscular dystrophy.

This syndrome often presents as peaked T-waves and sudden cardiac arrest within minutes after the administration of the drug in healthy appearing children (usually, but not exclusively, males, and most frequently 8 years of age or younger). There have also been reports in adolescents.

Therefore, when a healthy appearing infant or child develops cardiac arrest soon after administration of succinylcholine not felt to be due to inadequate ventilation, oxygenation or anesthetic overdose, immediate treatment for hyperkalemia should be instituted. This should include administration of intravenous (IV) calcium, bicarbonate, and glucose with insulin, with hyperventilation. Due to the abrupt onset of this syndrome, routine resuscitative measures are likely to be unsuccessful. However, extraordinary and prolonged resuscitative efforts have resulted in successful resuscitation in some reported cases. In addition, in presence of signs of malignant hyperthermia, appropriate treatment should be instituted concurrently.

Since there may be no signs or symptoms to alert the practitioner to which patients are at risk, it is recommended that the use of succinylcholine in children should be reserved for emergency intubation or instances where immediate securing of the airway is necessary (e.g., laryngospasm, difficult airway, full stomach) or for intramuscular use when a suitable vein is inaccessible.

Because neither succinylcholine nor halothane is routinely used in children, the incidence of masseter spasm and malignant hyperthermia has decreased. Older studies have been reported in which jaw-opening ability and the presence or absence of masseter spasm, often considered a precursor of malignant hyperpyrexia, were studied. Research was conducted on 63 children anesthetized with halothane then relaxed with succinylcholine, pancuronium, or vecuronium. Although vecuronium and pancuronium did not cause problems with jaw opening, succinylcholine

---

TABLE **13-6**	Select Inherited Variants of Plasma Cholinesterase			
PChE Variant	**Genetic Label***	**Frequency (%)**	**Enzyme Activity**	**Duration of Succinylcholine**
Usual	Homozygote U	96	Normal	Normal; dibucaine number 70-80
—	Heterozygote U/A	3	Decreased	Slightly prolonged; dibucaine number 50-69
Atypical	Homozygote A	0.3	Decreased by 70% or more	Significantly prolonged; dibucaine number 16-30
Fluoride	Homozygote F	0.03	Decreased by 60%	Moderately prolonged
Silent	Homozygote S	0.04	No activity	Significantly prolonged

PChE, *Plasma cholinesterase.*

The gene controlling the synthesis of PChE is known to exist in at least four allelic forms. There are more than 25 different phenotypes, but most are extremely rare. The allelic forms are designated EU, EA, EF, and ES.

was associated with this problem, and some of the succinylcholine patients were difficult to intubate.[50] Masseter spasm was noted to be more frequent in children administered succinylcholine concomitantly with halothane, compared with children who received succinylcholine and thiopental.[51]

A random sample of 6500 anesthetic records (53% of 12,169 anesthetic procedures performed) was reviewed. Fifteen cases of masseter spasm were identified. In each case, the patient underwent halothane induction and was then given succinylcholine intravenously. Seven of the 15 cases of masseter spasm developed in children between ages 8 and 10 years.[52] Researchers noted an increased incidence of masseter spasm in children with strabismus who were anesthetized with halothane and received IV succinylcholine. Of 1468 halothane anesthetic procedures, 15 cases of masseter spasm were discovered, and of these 15 cases, 6 occurred in the 211 patients with strabismus.[53]

In current practice, masseter spasm, although rare, is seen in adults during anesthesia induction and often in emergency rooms or critical care units during emergency airway management.[54,55]

Other Factors
Common side effects of succinylcholine and contraindications for its use are noted in Table 13-7 and Box 13-4.

Intraocular Pressure. Intraocular pressure (IOP) is known to increase by 5 to 15 mm Hg for as much as 10 minutes after succinylcholine administration.[29,56] The average is about 10 mm Hg for approximately 6 minutes. The exact mechanism of this increase is unknown. Some feel that tonic contractions of the extraocular muscles via fasciculation may explain this IOP increase. It is now thought, however, that succinylcholine-induced IOP increase is a vascular event, with choroidal vascular dilation or a decrease in drainage secondary to elevated central venous pressure temporarily inhibiting the flow of aqueous humor through the canal of Schlemm.[56]

This rise in IOP with succinylcholine administration is significantly less than the IOP increase associated with coughing or bucking. Patients who receive succinylcholine and are intubated 1 minute after its administration had IOPs that were not significantly higher than baseline. There are no documented reports of the extrusion of globe contents following the use of succinylcholine in open-eye emergency procedures. A recent review has essentially refuted the issue of eye damage following succinylcholine administration in open-globe injuries. It appears as a theoretical but not a clinical concern. Securing the airway remains the primary issue.[29,56] A thorough discussion of the use of succinylcholine and eye injuries is found in Chapter 40.

Hyperkalemia. Succinylcholine administration results in a transient hyperkalemia. A 0.5- to 1-mEq/L increase in serum potassium levels within 3 minutes after administration is usual. The effects were reported as lasting fewer than 10 to 15 minutes.[37]

TABLE **13-7** Side Effects of Succinylcholine	
Side Effect	**Probable Cause**
Hyperkalemia	Normally, serum K^+ is increased by up to 0.5 mEq/L secondary to potassium leaking from the depolarized muscle; in up-regulated patients, levels may rise much higher.
Dysrhythmias	Tachycardia (usually mild) is the most common effect. Bradycardia secondary to hyperkalemia, especially with repeat doses, can occur. (Wide electrocardiographic complexes leading to cardiac arrest have been seen in children with Duchenne muscular dystrophy and other muscle disorders.)
Myalgia	Secondary to fasciculation, even though some patients complain of muscle pain without having shown visible evidence of fasciculation
Myoglobinemia	Rare complication after extensive fasciculation or in malignant hyperthermia
Elevated intragastric pressure	Secondary to transient contraction of abdominal muscles during fasciculation; however, elevations of intragastric pressure seen after succinylcholine are not clinically relevant; less significant than occur with CO_2 insufflation during laparoscopic procedures
Elevated intracranial pressure	Postulated to be secondary to fasciculation, increased central venous pressure; associated with increased cerebral blood flow secondary to muscle-spindle afferent activity and actions on peripheral neuromuscular junctions (ICP effects can be blocked by pretreatment with a small dose of nondepolarizing relaxant and the usual initial administration of an induction agent. May safely be used in neurosurgical procedures.)
Elevated intraocular pressure	Increases IOP within 1 minute and peaks at an increase of 9 mm Hg within 6 minutes after administration; increase is a vascular event, with choroidal vascular dilatation or a decrease in drainage secondary to elevated central venous pressure, temporarily inhibiting the flow of aqueous humor through the canal of Schlemm. Generally considered safe in ocular emergencies
Malignant hyperthermia	Associated with a genetic predisposition; mechanism by which succinylcholine triggers the syndrome is not understood
Masseter spasm	Seen in adults in anesthetic and emergency use; sometimes followed by malignant hyperthermia

Modified from Kirby RR et al, eds. Clinical Anesthesia Practice. 2nd ed. Philadelphia: Saunders; 2002; and Atlee JL. Complications in Anesthesia. 2nd ed. Philadelphia: Saunders; 2007.
CO_2, Carbon dioxide; ICP, intracranial pressure; IOP, intraocular pressure; K^+, potassium.

BOX **13-4**

Contraindications to the Use of Succinylcholine

Hyperkalemia
Burn patients with burns over 35% TBSA, third-degree burn
Severe muscle trauma
Neurologic injury (e.g., paraplegia, quadriplegia)
Hyperkalemia resulting from renal failure
Severe sepsis (e.g., abdominal)
Muscle wasting, prolonged immobilization, extensive muscle
    denervation
Malignant hyperthermia
Duchenne muscular dystrophy
Selected muscle disorders (see Table 13-8)
Should be used in children under 8 years old only in
    emergency situations; not for routine intubation
Genetic variants of pseudocholinesterase
Allergy

TBSA, *Total body surface area.*

BOX **13-5**

Pathologic Conditions* with Potential for Hyperkalemia with Succinylcholine

Upper or lower motor neuron defect
Prolonged chemical denervation (e.g., muscle relaxants,
    magnesium, clostridial toxins)
Direct muscle trauma, tumor, or inflammation
Thermal trauma
Disuse atrophy
Severe infection

All of these conditions have the potential to up-regulate (increase) acetylcholine receptors.[57]

A muscle receives signals to perform various functions from action potentials. As the action potential traverses the neuron, an influx of sodium and release of potassium occur. This mechanism of potassium release during normal muscle signaling is the same mechanism by which serum potassium increases because of the depolarization associated with receiving succinylcholine.[37]

Hyperkalemia may be profound in certain patients. In a recent review, Martyn and Richtsfeld noted that lethal hyperkalemic responses to succinylcholine continue to be reported, although the mechanisms have not been completely elucidated. In the normally innervated mature muscle, acetylcholine receptors (AChRs) are located only in the junctional area. But in certain pathologic states—including upper or lower motor denervation, infection, direct muscle trauma, muscle tumor, muscle inflammation, burn injury, immobilization, and prolonged chemical denervation by muscle relaxants, drugs, or toxins—there is an up-regulation (increase) of AChRs spreading throughout the muscle membrane. There is also an additional expression of two new isoforms of AChRs. The depolarization of these AChRs by succinylcholine and its metabolites leads to potassium efflux from the muscle and severe hyperkalemia. The nicotinic (neuronal) α7 acetylcholine receptors, which are also in muscle, are depolarized not only by acetylcholine and succinylcholine but by choline. Persistent choline stimulation may play a critical role in the hyperkalemic response to succinylcholine in patients with up-regulated AChRs.[57] Pathologic conditions with the potential for producing hyperkalemia associated with succinylcholine use are listed in Box 13-5.

Succinylcholine has been implicated in hyperkalemia after its administration to burn patients, so it is contraindicated in these patients.[58] Receptor up-regulation resulting from thermal trauma has been associated with several documented cases of cardiac arrest involving succinylcholine administration.[33] Indeed, plasma potassium levels as high as 15 mEq/L have been reported after the administration of succinylcholine, with this effect occurring 4 to 10 days after the burn and lasting for years after the burn.[59] The burn injury–related increase of AChRs is probably related to inflammation and local denervation of muscle. Major third-degree burns involving extensive

body surface area may up-regulate AChRs throughout the body because of the extent and direct inflammation and injury to muscle. Hyperkalemia after burn injury to a single limb (8% body surface area) has been observed, indicating that burn size alone is not the only contributing factor. It is generally reported that the administration of succinylcholine to a burn patient more than 24 hours after the burn is unsafe; however, others note that succinylcholine can be safely used with burn patients for several days after the burn, because receptor up-regulation does not begin until 24 to 48 hours after the burn.[60,61] Changes in responses to both succinylcholine and the nondepolarizing agents have been noted for years after a major burn injury. Immobilation due to contractures may play a role. Succinylcholine should never be used in these patients, regardless of the time post-burn.[56]

Treatment of succinylcholine-induced hyperkalemia involves the emergency administration of drugs that promote the cellular uptake of potassium; these include insulin with glucose, catecholamines, and sodium bicarbonate.

The use of various muscle relaxants in patients with muscle disorders is reviewed in Table 13-8.

Malignant Hyperthermia. Malignant hyperthermia (MH) is a pharmacogenetic skeletal muscle disorder triggered by volatile anesthetics and succinylcholine and stress. Succinylcholine is absolutely contraindicated in patients with known or suspected MH and their families. Mutations in the skeletal muscle ryanodine receptor gene may result in altered calcium release from sarcoplasmic reticulum stores, giving rise to MH. Patients who develop MH show signs such as muscle rigidity, rhabdomyolysis, increased carbon dioxide production, convulsions, metabolic acidosis, tachycardia, and a rapid increase in temperature.[62-64] A complete discussion of the physiologic and treatment aspects of MH can be found in Chapter 33.

Myalgias and Fasciculations. Postoperative muscle pain, particularly in the subcostal region, trunk, neck, upper abdominal muscles, and shoulders, is a common occurrence after succinylcholine administration.[65] A recent meta-analysis that included 52 randomized clinical trials found several interesting results.[66] The incidence of succinylcholine-induced myalgia is high, and symptoms sometimes last for several days. Small doses of nondepolarizing muscle relaxants, approximately 10% to 30% of the ED95, reduce the incidence of fasciculations and myalgia, although pretreatment side effects occur. Higher doses of succinylcholine decrease the risk of myalgia compared with lower doses, and opioids do not have any impact; however, there is

TABLE 13-8	Response of Neuromuscular Blocking Agents in Select Muscle Disorders	
Neuromuscular Disorder	**Succinylcholine**	**Nondepolarizing Neuromuscular Blocking Agents**
Multiple sclerosis	Contraindicated	Increased sensitivity; anesthetic stress may increase rate of relapse
Motor neuron disease (amyotrophic lateral sclerosis [ALS, Lou Gehrig disease])	Contraindicated	Increased sensitivity
Guillain-Barré syndrome	Contraindicated	Increased sensitivity; avoid agents with cardiac side effects
Charcot-Marie-Tooth disease	Contraindicated	Response to atracurium and mivacurium normal; all others, increased sensitivity
Muscular dystrophies	Contraindicated	Increased sensitivity
Myotonias	Contraindicated	Increased sensitivity; anticholinesterase agents may precipitate myotonia
Myasthenic syndromes	Resistant; prolonged duration of action may be present with plasmapheresis or anticholinesterase therapy	Extreme sensitivity
Mitochondrial myopathies	Contraindicated	Increased sensitivity
Hyperkalemic periodic paralysis	Contraindicated	Normal response
Hypokalemic periodic paralysis	Contraindicated	Normal response
Malignant hyperthermia	Contraindicated	Normal response
Myasthenia gravis	Resistant	Increased sensitivity
Huntington chorea	Increased sensitivity	Increased sensitivity
Up-regulation of acetylcholine receptors because of spinal cord trauma, stroke, or prolonged immobility	Contraindicated	Usually resistant, but depends on time since injury

Modified from Naguib M et al. Advances in neurobiology of the neuromuscular junction: implications for the anesthesiologist. Anesthesiology. 2002;96:202-231; and Malignant Hyperthermia Association of America, 11 East State Street, PO Box 1069, Sherburne, NY 13460; 2008.

less myalgia with thiopental compared with propofol. There is no clear relation between succinylcholine-related fasciculation and myalgia. Pretreatment with sodium channel blockers (i.e., lidocaine) or nonsteroidal antiinflammatory drugs (diclofenac and aspirin) may prevent myalgia. Myalgias are generally attributed to the occurrence of fasciculations resulting from repetitive firing of the motor nerve terminals, which causes uncoordinated muscle contractions. Patients who experience muscle pain most often are women and those persons who rarely participate in muscular activity. Conversely, patients at extremes of age, as well as pregnant patients, are least affected. Postoperative myalgias associated with succinylcholine increase in severity with early ambulation, which may consequently delay postoperative healing.[65]

Prevention is the key to avoiding postoperative muscle pain. Although not always effective, the incidence of myalgia is greatly reduced with nondepolarizer pretreatment. Use of no more than 10% of the ED$_{95}$ is safe and effective and will avoid most of the difficulties of the patient experiencing weakness prior to loss of consciousness. Effective and equivalent doses have been reported as 2 mg rocuronium, 1.5 mg atracurium, and 0.3 mg vecuronium.[67] Postulated mechanisms of action of various pretreatment agents are given in Table 13-9.

Phase II Block. Administration of large doses of succinylcholine results in an alteration in the characteristics of the block.[32] Succinycholine produces specific unique responses to nerve stimulation when compared with the nondepolarizing agents. These include a sustained response to tetanic stimulation, no fade with TOF or double-burst stimulation (DBS), and no posttetanic potentiation. Box 13-6 presents the characteristics of neuromuscular blockade. Large doses cause changes that resemble more of a nondepolarizing block, as evidenced by fade in response to tetanic stimuli, TOF and DBS, the appearance of posttetanic potentiation, and theoretically, antagonism with drugs such as neostigmine. This commonly is referred to as a *desensitization, dual,* or *phase II block.*

Tetanic fade is caused by an interaction with cholinergic presynaptic autoreceptors mediating acetylcholine release from the motor nerve end.[21,57] The finding that high doses of succinylcholine inhibited presynaptic $\alpha_3\beta_2$ AChRs (i.e., the compound behaved like a nondepolarizing relaxant) may help explain how high or repeated doses of succinylcholine result in a nondepolarizing type of block (phase II block) characterized by fade and posttetanic potentiation.[68] Development of a desensitization block is a historical discussion because doses exceeding 6 to 8 mg/kg are required, and high doses, as seen with succinylcholine infusions, are rarely used in current practice.

NONDEPOLARIZING AGENTS

The efficacy of the nondepolarizing relaxants is similar, so the choice of one drug over another is largely made on

TABLE 13-9	Postulated Mechanisms of Action of Pretreatment Agents	
Component in Mechanism of Postoperative Myalgia	**Pretreatment Agent**	**Postulated Mechanism of Action**
Neuromuscular junction	Nondepolarizing neuromuscular blockers	Prejunctional
	Phenytoin	Prejunctional
	Self-taming	Neuromuscular desensitization
Muscle fibers, stretch receptors	Stretching exercises	Desensitization of stretch receptors
	Vitamin C	Prevents damage to muscle fibers
Cell membrane, intracellular calcium mechanisms	Lidocaine	Cell membrane stabilization
	Calcium gluconate	Cell membrane stabilization
	Dantrolene	Interferes with intracellular calcium transfer
Fasciculations	Dose of succinylcholine	Synchronicity of muscle contractions
	Magnesium	Abolishes fasciculations
Muscle damage	Aspirin or nonsteroidal antiinflammatory drugs	Interrupt prostaglandin-mediated destructive cycle
	Chlorpromazine	Inhibits cellular phospholipases

Modified from Wong SF, Chung F. Succinylcholine-associated postoperative myalgia. Anaesthesia. 2000;55:144-152.

BOX 13-6

Characteristics of Neuromuscular Blockade

Depolarizing (Phase I) Block
- Muscle fasciculation precedes onset of neuromuscular blockade
- Sustained response to tetanic stimulation
- Absence of posttetanic potentiation, stimulation, or facilitation
- Lack of fade to tetanus, train-of-four, or double-burst stimulation
- Block antagonized by prior administration of nondepolarizer as pretreatment (approximately 20% more succinylcholine required)
- Block potentiated by anticholinesterase drugs

Nondepolarizing (Phase II) Block
- Absence of muscle fasciculation
- Appearance of tetanic fade and posttetanic potentiation, stimulation, or facilitation
- Train-of-four and double-burst fade
- Reversal with anticholinesterase drugs
- In rare cases may be produced by an overdose and desensitization with succinylcholine at doses >6 mg/kg

---

pharmacokinetic factors. Specific patient characteristics, type of surgical procedure, pharmacokinetics, and side-effect profile guide the selection of an individual relaxant for a given situation.

Rocuronium Bromide

The introduction of vecuronium and atracurium, both of which were marketed as intermediate-acting neuromuscular blocking agents (NMBAs) improved the flexibility of the clinician in matching the agent to the expected duration of surgery.[69] Slow onset, solution stability, and histamine release remained problems to be overcome.[70] Rocuronium (Zemuron) has been developed to partially fill this void. It combines a duration and cardiovascular profile comparable to those of vecuronium, with an onset that is only slightly longer than that of succinylcholine.[69-72]

A derivative of vecuronium, rocuronium bromide is chemically designated as 1-[17β-(acetyloxy)-3α-hydroxy-2β-(4-morpholinyl)-5α-androstan-16β-yl]-1-(2-propenyl) pyrrolidinium bromide, and it has one seventh to one eighth the potency of its derivative.[24,32,72] It is a monoquaternary structure that also shares its aminosteroid structure with pancuronium.[73] It has a molecular weight of 609.7 and a molecular formula of $C_{32}H_{53}BrN_2O_4$ (Figure 13-5). The pH of rocuronium is adjusted to 4, and the agent contains no preservative. It exists in a solution that is stable at room temperature for up to 30 days.[74] Each 1 mL of solution contains 10 mg of rocuronium bromide and 2 mg of sodium acetate.[72]

Results of clinical studies of both healthy children and healthy adults suggest an ED_{95} of approximately 0.3 mg/kg.[23] Its steady-state volume of distribution in healthy adults is 207 (14) mL/kg and is slightly smaller for children ages 4 to 8 years. Rocuronium is approximately 30% bound to human plasma proteins, somewhat less than other neuromuscular blockers.[72] Other researchers dispute these data. For example, Chaudhry and associates[75] found the agent in vitro to be 72% bound to plasma proteins. Even so, with regard to this characteristic, rocuronium compares very favorably with similar agents such as vecuronium, which is 91% bound.[72] This decreased plasma protein binding may lead to a more rapid onset because more unbound drug is readily available at the neuronal binding sites.[72,76,77]

Pharmacokinetics

Onset. Rocuronium is the drug of choice and is widely used as the NMBA for rapid sequence induction (RSI) when succinylcholine is contraindicated. A disadvantage of using rocuronium during RSI is its long duration of action.[31]

Administration of rocuronium with doses ranging from 0.6 to 1.2 mg/kg provides good to excellent intubating conditions

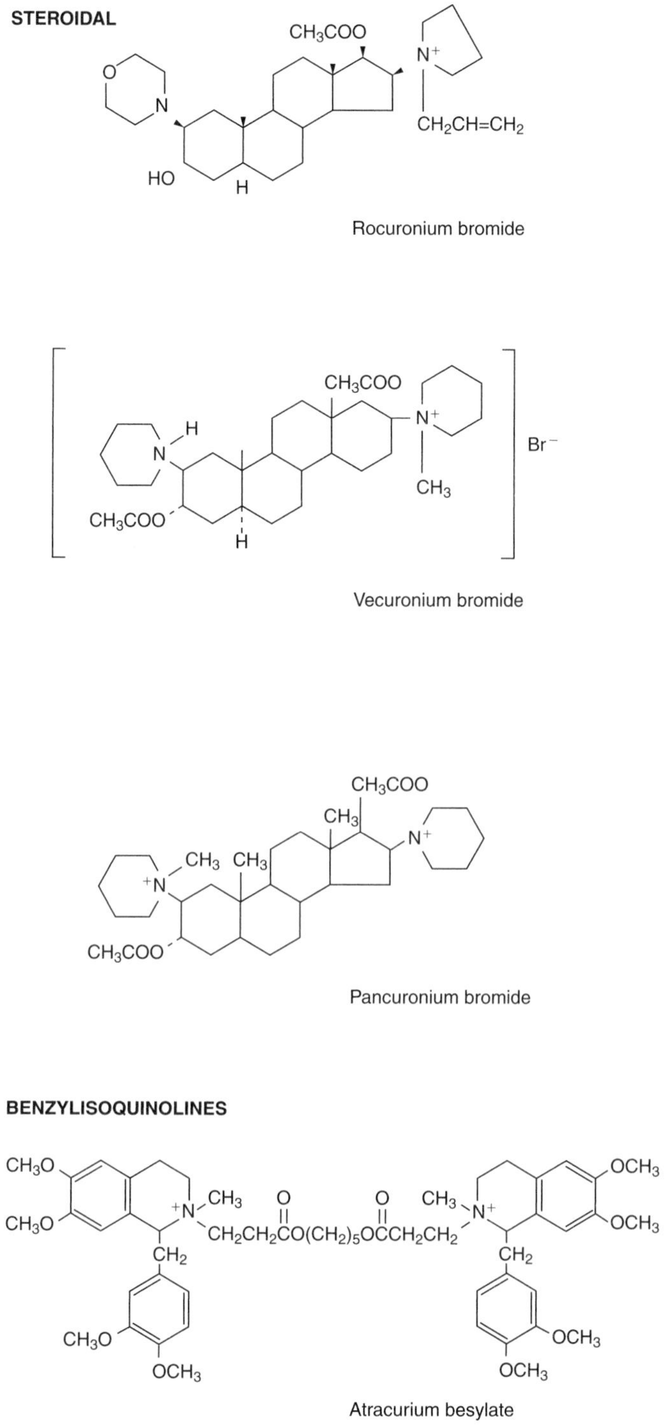

STEROIDAL

Rocuronium bromide

Vecuronium bromide

Pancuronium bromide

BENZYLISOQUINOLINES

Atracurium besylate

FIGURE **13-5** Chemical structures of nondepolarizing muscle relaxants.

within 45 to 90 seconds.[15,25,78] A 95% probability of successful intubation at 60 seconds was noted after a 1.04-mg/kg dose.[79,80] The onset of muscle relaxants is related to potency. The less potent an agent, the faster the onset. Rocuronium has an onset of action that is inversely proportional to its potency[71] and is less potent than other steroidal-based neuromuscular blockers.[76,81] This decreased potency together with the decrease in the amount of drug that is protein bound allow a larger mass

of drug at the prejunctional and postjunctional cholinoreceptors.[25,76] This large drug mass at the receptor site yields a faster onset.[72,75]

One method used clinically to accelerate the onset of rocuronium when administering it to intubate during RSI is referred to as *priming*. Priming involves giving 10% of the calculated intubating dose prior to inducing anesthesia. After a period of 1 to 3 minutes, the patient is anesthetized, and the remaining rocuronium is given. Giving a small portion of the relaxant dose in this manner speeds the onset by valuable seconds without undue stress to the patient.[82-84]

Duration. With regard to length of action, rocuronium is classified as intermediate in duration.[28] Its duration of action is similar to that of vecuronium, and its duration depends, like that of many other agents, on the dose administered.[24] An intubating dose of 0.6 to 1 mg/kg provides a clinical duration of 30 to 90 minutes.[24,25] The administration of 0.6 mg/kg resulted in 10% recovery of T1 within 27.2 (5.5) minutes, whereas 25%, 75%, and 90% recovery of T1 occurred in 31.1 (5.6) minutes, 39.3 (6.2) minutes, and 41.2 (6.1) minutes, respectively.[85] Recovery of the TOF ratio to 0.8 when rocuronium was administered with sevoflurane, isoflurane, and propofol occurred in 103 (30.7), 69(20.4), and 62(21.1) minutes, respectively.[86]

Elimination. Rocuronium undergoes both hepatic and renal elimination. The primary means of rocuronium elimination is deacetylation via the liver.[85-87] Renal excretion accounts for 35% of elimination.[32] Plasma levels of rocuronium follow a three-compartment open model. This results in extensive redistribution after IV injection. Therefore, before elimination occurs, serum levels of the drug are low enough to result in recovery.[23] The elimination half-life of rocuronium is 60 to 120 minutes. The elimination half-lives of the agent in children, normal adults, and elderly persons are 38.3 minutes, 56 minutes, and 137 minutes, respectively.[76,88]

Pharmacokinetic Summary. The onset of rocuronium is 45 to 90 seconds. The duration of rocuronium is 30 to 90 minutes. Elimination of the agent is via the liver and kidneys.

Atracurium Besylate

Atracurium (Tracrium) was developed as a result of a joint venture between the Department of Pharmaceutical Chemistry at the University of Strathclyde and Wellcome Research Laboratories.[89] The objective of the investigators was to develop an agent with the following characteristics:

1. Competitive bisquaternary neuromuscular blocker
2. Highly selective in action
3. Degradable without renal or hepatic intervention[89,90]

The resulting agent was a bisquaternary competitive neuromuscular blocker in the form of a besylate salt.[89-91] Atracurium besylate is designated as 2,2'-[1,5-pentanediylbis[oxy(3-oxo-3,1-propanediyl)]] bis[1-[(3,4-dimethoxyphenyl) methyl]-1,2,3,4-tetrahydro-6,7-dimethoxy-2-methylisoquinolinium] dibenzenesulfonate. It has a molecular weight of 1243.49 and a molecular formula of $C_{65}H_{82}N_2O_{18}S_2$ (see Figure 13-5).[80] The pH of atracurium is adjusted to 3.25 to 3.65, and the agent contains the preservative benzyl alcohol. Atracurium loses potency at the rate of 6% per year when it is refrigerated at 5° C. At room temperature, the agent degrades approximately 5% per month, and its recommended unrefrigerated shelf life is 14 days.[92] It was developed with an intermediate duration in mind, and it spontaneously degrades to inactive products. It is well absorbed intravenously, with an ED_{95} of 0.10 to 0.25 mg/kg.[91,93]

Atracurium is rapidly distributed throughout the extracellular space after IV injection and has a volume of distribution of 153 (13) mL/kg.[71] It is approximately 82% protein bound and does not distribute into the fat, because it is ionized.[94] Obese patients who received atracurium demonstrated no difference in recovery indices or recovery times when compared with control patients of normal weight because of the agent's lack of organ dependency for elimination.[95-97]

Pharmacokinetics

Onset. As expected, atracurium has an onset time that is inversely proportional to dosage, in the range of 1.2 to 2.8 minutes. When various doses of atracurium were given to 70 patients anesthetized with fentanyl, thiopental, and nitrous oxide–oxygen (N_2O-O_2) anesthesia, clinical effects were seen at doses of 0.3 to 0.6 mg/kg. Other investigators, however, have found the onset to be longer, in the range of 2.31 to 3.55 minutes.[98-100]

Duration. The duration of atracurium increases as its dose increases. Duration of maximum effect and duration to 95% recovery of peak contraction are reported in the range of 5.6 to 69.5 minutes.[98,101,102]

Elimination. The development of atracurium arose from the discovery of the plant *Leontice leontopetalum* and one of its components, designated *petaline*. This component was similar to tubocurarine and was observed to undergo an unexpectedly facile degradation in mild alkali by the well-known Hofmann elimination pathway, with loss of water and formation of a tertiary base.[93] Stenlake's pursuit of this research led to the development of atracurium, which does not rely on any organ system for its breakdown and elimination. Study of the clinical pharmacology of atracurium reveals that its molecules decompose by Hofmann elimination, as well as by nonspecific ester hydrolysis.[89,93,95,103]

Hofmann elimination is a temperature- and pH-dependent breakdown of the drug molecule. In the vial, atracurium is at room temperature in an acidic medium. When injected, the pH rises to blood pH of 7.4, and the temperature increases to body temperature. These increases in pH and temperature allow the Hofmann elimination to ensue. Atracurium degrades via Hofmann elimination (10% to 40%). In mild alkaline states, fission occurs at the quaternary nitrogen position, and laudanosine is subsequently released.[103,104] The agent then degrades further. After ester hydrolysis, it is catalyzed by nonspecific esterases into a quaternary alcohol and a quaternary acid.[73,89,103] These metabolites are excreted primarily in bile and urine.

Pharmacokinetic Summary. Onset time of atracurium is 1 to 3 minutes. The duration of atracurium is 20 to 60 minutes. It is degraded via Hofmann elimination and nonspecific ester hydrolysis, and its metabolites are subsequently excreted in bile and urine. The chemical structure of atracurium besylate is shown in Figure 13-5.

Cisatracurium Besylate

The most notable of the 10 stereoisomers of atracurium, cisatracurium besylate (Nimbex) has gained popularity in the clinical arena since the mid-1990s. It is a nondepolarizing muscle relaxant, three times more potent than atracurium but with a slower onset of action. The agent is available as a sterile, nonpyrogenic aqueous solution in 5-, 10-, and 20-mL vials. The pH is 3.25 to 3.65, and the concentration is 2 mg/mL (except in the 20-mL vial, in which the concentration is 10 mg/mL for convenience in the intensive care unit setting).[105] Advantages of cisatracurium include maintenance of cardiovascular stability and a lack of histamine release after injection.[106,107]

Pharmacokinetics

Onset. Cisatracurium is regarded as intermediate in its onset and duration of action. In adults the ED_{95} is 0.05 mg/kg during N_2O-O_2 opioid anesthesia.[108] It has been noted to be five times more potent than rocuronium, with a slower onset of action, longer duration, and slower spontaneous recovery.[109,110] An IV bolus of 0.1 mg/kg (twice the ED_{95}) produces desired levels of relaxation within 3.1 (1) minutes.[111] Doses of three to four times the ED_{95} (0.15 to 0.2 mg/kg) decrease the mean time of onset to 3.4 and 2.8 minutes, respectively.[112]

Duration. After doses of three to four times the ED_{95}, the average time for the first twitch in a TOF to recover to 25% of control is 65 minutes.[113] Further studies report that the duration of cisatracurium with an intubating dose of 0.25 mg/kg is 55 to 75 minutes. Full recovery at the aforementioned dose occurs in 75 to 100 minutes.[25] Additional sources report the duration as 55 to 61 minutes.[114]

Elimination. Cisatracurium, like atracurium, undergoes Hofmann elimination (which is pH and temperature dependent) in the plasma and tissues. Hofmann elimination accounts for 77% of total body clearance, and nonspecific esterases are responsible for 23% of total body clearance. Of the organ-dependent clearance, 16% occurs through renal pathways.[115] Studies have demonstrated a half-life of approximately 26 to 36 minutes, with an increase in the rate of degradation as pH increases.[116] As with atracurium, one of cisatracurium's metabolites is laudanosine. However, cisatracurium liberates one fifth as much laudanosine as atracurium.[117]

Pharmacokinetic Summary. The onset of cisatracurium is 2 to 4 minutes. The duration of cisatracurium is 40 to 75 minutes. The agent is degraded via Hofmann elimination and nonspecific ester hydrolysis, and its metabolites are partially excreted in urine.

Vecuronium Bromide

Vecuronium bromide (Norcuron) is a potent nondepolarizing neuromuscular blocker. Studies comparing vecuronium with pancuronium, its predecessor, found vecuronium to be 1.5 times more potent than its parent compound.[118,119] Both agents were developed by manipulation of the steroid nucleus. The molecule was successfully altered from bisquaternary pancuronium to a monoquaternary compound, creating an agent with a more rapid onset and a shorter duration. Vecuronium is more lipophilic than pancuronium, although it is still predominantly a hydrophilic compound. This change in its solubility is thought to be the cause of its differing pharmacokinetic profile.[91,120,121]

The chemical formula of vecuronium bromide is $C_{34}H_{57}BrN_2O_4$, and the drug has a molecular weight of 637.74 (see Figure 13-5). It is chemically designated as piperidinium 1-[(2β, 3α, 5α, 16β, 17β)-3, 17-bis(acetyloxy)-2-(1-piperidinyl) androstan-16-yl]-1-methyl bromide.[120]

Vecuronium is available as a 10- or 20-mg, sterile, nonpyrogenic powder for IV use only. Once reconstituted, the solution has a pH of 4 and is stable for 24 hours at 25° C.[120] Researchers' determinations of ED_{90} to ED_{95} of vecuronium are variable. An ED_{90} of 0.044 to 0.056 mg/kg was reported when vecuronium was administered with N_2O-O_2 and narcotic anesthesia.[89] Miller and associates constructed dose-response curves to derive the ED_{90}, which they found to be 0.023 to

0.044 mg/kg.[91] The agent has a steady-state volume of distribution of 0.21 to 0.27 L/kg.[121,122]

Pharmacokinetics

Onset. Vecuronium has an onset of action that is 1.5 times that of pancuronium, a proportion similar to that of its potency.[118,123] At a dose of twice the ED_{95}, 0.1 mg/kg, the maximum suppression of muscle twitch occurs within 3 minutes of administration.[99] The onset varies with the concurrent anesthetic administered and is inversely proportional to the dose.[9] With balanced anesthesia, a 0.1-mg/kg dose of vecuronium resulted in an onset of 3.1 minutes, whereas in patients receiving isoflurane, N_2O-O_2 anesthesia, the onset time decreased to 1.8 minutes.[98,121,124,125]

Duration. Duration of action varies with the type of anesthetic being administered and the dose of the agent. This phenomenon has been noted with other nondepolarizing agents, as well as with vecuronium.[125] Haines[98] reported a duration of 36.2 ± 6.4 minutes after a dose of 0.1 mg of vecuronium per kilogram was given patients undergoing balanced anesthesia. The time from 25% twitch recovery to 75% twitch recovery at a dose of 0.1 mg/kg was 11 to 12 minutes and the duration 30 to 45 minutes.

Elimination. Vecuronium is eliminated via hepatic and renal mechanisms. Vecuronium undergoes elimination via an orthodox three-compartment model. Because it is more lipophilic than other agents in its class, vecuronium does not depend solely on the kidneys for elimination. Only 20% to 30% of the administered dose is recovered unchanged in the urine within 24 hours.[88,91] A major portion of the dose, 40% to 80%, is taken up by the liver and excreted in bile.[123] Small amounts of its metabolites (3-hydroxy, 17-hydroxy, and 3,17-hydroxy) can be detected by thin-layer chromatography, but the amounts are minimal and have little if any neuromuscular blocking activity.[91] Reported elimination half-lives range from 51 to 90 minutes in healthy adults. Total clearances have been reported from 3 to 5.6 mL/kg/min.[6,119,126,127]

Pharmacokinetic Summary. The onset of vecuronium is 2 to 3 minutes. The duration of vecuronium is 30 to 45 minutes. It is eliminated by the kidneys (20% to 30%) and liver (40% to 80%).

Pancuronium Bromide

Pancuronium bromide was first synthesized for Organon in England in 1966. Researchers, especially Lewis and co-workers, were searching for an agent that was nondepolarizing, had a rapid onset, had an intermediate duration of action, was easily reversed, and had no significant unwanted side effects.[6] After clinical use by Baird and Reid in 1967 in Europe, the agent was introduced in the United States in 1972.[128,129]

Pancuronium bromide's chemical designation is 2β, 16β-dipiperidine-5α-androstane-3α, 17-β-diol diacetate dimethobromide (see Figure 13-5). It has a volume of distribution of 0.18 to 0.26 L/kg; is an odorless, white, crystalline powder; and has a melting point of 215° C.[6,88] Extensive testing revealed an effective dose of 0.02 to 0.05 mg/kg in mice, rats, rabbits, cats, and dogs.[6] Further research determined the ED_{95} of pancuronium to be 0.075 mg/kg in human beings.[130,131]

Pharmacokinetics

Onset. The mean time to depression of twitch to 5% of control values after a dose of twice the ED_{95} (0.14 mg/kg) is 4.4 (0.5) minutes.[132] At a dose of 1.5 ED_{95}, which is estimated as 0.08 mg/kg, an onset time to 90% blockade was 2.3 ± 0.3 minute.[133,134]

Duration. Pancuronium is a long-acting nondepolarizer that does not have the histamine-releasing effects of metocurine or d-tubocurarine.[129] Numerous authors have reported the duration of action of pancuronium since the development of the agent. In a comparative study with vecuronium, d-tubocurarine, and metocurine at an ED_{90} dose of 0.062 mg/kg, the mean duration of blockade was 109 minutes.[135]

Elimination. Pancuronium theoretically undergoes triphasic elimination via the kidney through glomerular filtration, and a small amount of the drug is also released in the bile.[88] Up to 24 hours after the injection of pancuronium, anywhere from 43% to 67% of unchanged drug may be found in the urine.[135]

Pharmacokinetic Summary. The onset of pancuronium is 2 to 3 minutes. The duration is 60 to 90 minutes. The majority of the agent undergoes renal elimination, but hepatic breakdown is also part of the degradation of this agent. A summary of the selected properties of the muscular blocking agents is given in Table 13-10.

Nondepolarizing Agents' Effect on Various Organ Systems

Central Nervous System

All muscle relaxants are quaternary ammonium compounds and therefore water soluble at physiologic pH. As such, they are unable to cross physiological barriers such as the blood-brain, placental, and gastric and therefore have no CNS effects. A minor, largely academic consideration has been noted: CNS stimulation has been seen in studies of animals after atracurium administration.[94] This CNS stimulation is primarily attributed to laudanosine, one of the metabolites produced from the breakdown of atracurium.[104] In one case report in which a patient received atracurium infusion for tetanus at a mean rate of 1.3 mg/kg/hr over a 71-day period, laudanosine concentrations were no more than 0.985 mcg/mL, and the patient incurred no CNS dysfunction.[136] With renal failure, laudanosine levels are roughly 3.5 times those of patients with normal renal function (1200 versus 4300 ng/mL).[137] Despite this level, no adverse CNS reactions have been found.[138,139] Cisatracurium, which is given in lower doses than atracurium because of its increased potency, is less likely to produce any significant change in metabolic levels and therefore has no significant CNS effects.[138]

Cardiovascular System

The NMBAs have no direct effect on cardiac muscle. Any cardiovascular changes that occur with the administration of a muscle relaxant are caused by indirect actions such as histamine release or effects on the autonomic nervous system. Of the current nondepolarizing relaxants, only atracurium and pancuronium exhibit any cardiac effects. Atracurium has been associated with increases in heart rate and decreases in blood pressure at doses of 0.5 mg/kg and greater because of histamine release.[140-143] Systolic and diastolic pressures significantly decrease, and cardiac output was significantly increased at 2, 5, and 10 minutes after a bolus dose. The increase in cardiac output is the result of a markedly decreased systemic vascular resistance. Nearly all of the hemodynamic changes associated with the administration of atracurium have been linked to the release of histamine.[128,144,145] Administration of cisatracurium does not result in histamine release.[15] The effects of stimulation of histamine receptors and the resulting effects are listed in Box 13-7.

Pancuronium produces tachycardia. Significant increases in heart rate 3 minutes after the administration of the agent were

TABLE **13-10**   Summary of Select Properties of Neuromuscular Blocking Agents

Classification	ED$_{95}$ (mg/kg)	Intubating Dose Usually 2-3× ED$_{95}$ (mg/kg)	Onset	Duration	Metabolism	Elimination		Automatic Ganglia Effect (SNS & PNS)	Cardiac Muscarinic Effect (Vagal Block)	Histamine Release	Resulting Cardiac Action
						Kidney (%)	Liver (%)				
Ultrashort											
Succinylcholine (Anectine, Quelicin)	0.3	1-1.5	30-60 sec	5-10 min	Plasma cholinesterase	<2	0	Stimulates	Stimulates and/or blocks	0 ?	Usually tachycardia, bradycardia with repeat doses
Intermediate											
Atracurium (Tracrium)	0.15	0.5	2-4 min	30-60 min	Hofmann elimination, nonspecific esterase hydrolysis	10-40 metabolites	0	0	0	yes	Hypotension, tachycardia, flushing
Cisatracurium (Nimbex)	0.05	0.1	2-4 min	30-60 min	Hofmann elimination, nonspecific esterase hydrolysis	Up to 77 metabolites	0	0	0	0	0
Rocuronium (Zemuron)	0.3	1	1-3 min	30-60 min	Hepatic and renal	10-30	70-90	0	0	0	0
Vecuronium (Norcuron)	0.05	0.1	2-4 min	30-60 min	Hepatic and renal	40-50	50-60	0	0	0	0
Long											
Pancuronium (Pavulon)	0.05	0.1	2-4 min	60-90 min	Hepatic 10%-20%	85	15	0	Blocks moderately	0	Slight vagolytic - tachycardia

---

BOX 13-7

Effects of Stimulation of Histamine Receptors by Neuromuscular Blockers

H_1 Receptors	H_2 Receptors
Increased capillary permeability	Increased gastric acid production
Bronchoconstriction	Systemic and cerebral vasodilation
Intestinal contraction	Positive inotropic effects
Negative dromotropic effects	Positive chronotropic effects

Atracurium releases modest amounts of histamine. Slight histamine release may occur with succinylcholine. The amount of histamine release is dependent on dose and speed of injection.

With endogenous histamine release, all receptor responses are elicited.

Prophylaxis against histamine release requires administration of both H_1- and H_2-receptor blockers.

H, Histamine.

BOX 13-8

Cardiac Effects of Neuromuscular Blocking Drugs

- Atracurium causes histamine release and may produce hypotension and tachycardia.
- Pancuronium is vagolytic and causes slight catecholamine release (indirect sympathomimetic), producing tachycardia.
- Succinylcholine usually results in slight tachycardia. Repeat dosing in adults and any dose in children may produce sudden, abrupt bradycardia. Many types of arrhythmias have been reported.

---

noted in patients with coronary artery disease who were scheduled for coronary artery bypass graft and who received a dose of 0.1 mg/kg, despite administration of narcotics.[144,146,147] Increases in heart rate are often accompanied by mild increases in mean arterial pressure. The tachycardia results from a vagolytic and an indirect sympathomimetic action. The other steroidal relaxants vecuronium and rocuronium have no significant cardiac effects at clinical doses. The cardiovascular effects of the neuromuscular blocking agents are summarized in Box 13-8.

Hepatic System

The steroidal relaxants rocuronium, vecuronium, and pancuronium are affected by changes in hepatic status. They are primarily eliminated by a combination of liver metabolism and biliary and renal excretion, and therefore their duration of action is prolonged in patients with hepatic disease. Vecuronium, which is metabolized in the liver, has been administered to patients with hepatic disease.[148-152] Lebrault and colleagues, for example, compared patients with cirrhosis who received 0.2 mg of vecuronium per kilogram with healthy control patients and found that elimination half-life was prolonged approximately 60%. This effect resulted in a time to return of 50% twitch height of 130 minutes in the cirrhotic group, compared with 62 minutes in healthy patients. Differences in clearance among alcoholic patients with liver disease are dose dependent and usually not significant.[148,152] Rocuronium and pancuronium have an increased volume of distribution and elimination times, resulting in significantly longer durations.[148-151] The duration of action of rocuronium, as well as the onset, is typically prolonged in patients with hepatic disease such as cirrhosis.[25] Patients with hepatic dysfunction demonstrate an elimination half-life that is increased to 173 minutes, compared with the normal 60 to 120 minutes.[23,88] This supports the finding that the route of plasma clearance of rocuronium is predominantly by hepatic uptake, through which much of the drug is excreted unchanged in bile.[76,153] Cautious dosing is

warranted, along with vigilant monitoring of neuromuscular function in these patients.[25]

An active desacetyl metabolite results from the breakdown of each of the steroidal relaxants. These metabolites exhibit relaxant activity and accumulate with prolonged use. Although this does not pose a problem perioperatively, prolonged paralysis and myopathies in patients with multiorgan failure in critical care units has been a problem with multi-day use. Practice guidelines for sustained neuromuscular blockade in critically ill adults and children have recently been published.[154,155]

Atracurium and cisatracurium are not affected by changes in liver function and are the agents of choice for use in patients with liver disease because of their unique method of metabolism, specifically their breakdown pathway via Hofmann elimination and nonesterase-dependent hydrolysis.[91] Cisatracurium is preferred for its lack of histamine release.[88] The pharmacokinetics of atracurium in patients with hepatic and renal disease were compared with those in nonimpaired control subjects. No differences in plasma elimination half-lives were noted.[130,156] The effect of atracurium infusions in patients with fulminant hepatic failure who were awaiting liver transplantation, as well as during liver transplantation, has been studied. Plasma clearances and half-lives were similar to those reported in healthy individuals, and no cumulative effects were noted.[139,157]

Renal System

The steroidal relaxants rocuronium, vecuronium, and pancuronium are affected by changes in renal status. Since all three drugs depend to varying degrees on renal and hepatic elimination, their duration of action is prolonged in patients with decreases in renal function. Pancuronium is largely (80% to 85%) dependent on renal elimination, which is markedly decreased in patients with chronic renal failure and therefore leads to the prolongation of neuromuscular blockade.[158] A small portion of rocuronium is excreted unchanged in the urine, resulting in a prolonged elimination half-life in patients with renal disease.[76,88,153] The onset time of rocuronium is not affected by renal failure.

Atracurium and cisatracurium are considered the agents of choice in patients with renal disease. Onset and duration are not affected by changes in renal function. Doses of three times the ED_{95} (0.15 mg/kg) of cisatracurium were given to 39 patients with decreased renal function, all of whom were induced with fentanyl and thiopental. Onset time, mean arterial blood pressure, heart rate, and time to recovery of 25% T1 were assessed, and there was no significant variation in the drug effects compared with patients with normal renal function.[159]

Effects in Special Populations

Elderly Patients. The onset times of the NMBAs are generally longer in the elderly due to slower circulation times and other kinetic changes associated with aging.[160] This is true for all relaxants. The dosing interval and duration of action of the steroidal relaxants rocuronium, vecuronium, and pancuronium are prolonged in the elderly due to decreased hepatic and renal clearance and an increased volume of distribution.[160-163] The duration of atracurium and cisatracurium is not affected by aging, making these the most predictable NMBAs in the elderly.

Obese Patients. The use of the NMBAs in obese patients raises some special clinical considerations. Obese patients require a rapid-sequence induction more frequently than nonobese patients, owing to their higher risk for gastroesophageal reflux and pulmonary aspiration. A difficult airway is more often encountered. It is especially important to ensure full reversal of the relaxant actions in this patient group because of the higher occurrence of breathing abnormalities and lung compromise. Sleep apnea syndrome and the associated anesthetic management must be considered.[164-167] The duration of action of the steroidal relaxants rocuronium, vecuronium, and pancuronium are all prolonged. This is likely due to a decrease in elimination.[25]

The kinetics of atracurium and cisatracurium are not significantly changed in obese patients, making these the most reliable agents. Cisatracurium is preferred for its lack of histamine release. Several authors recommend that to avoid overdosing, NMBAs should be dosed at ideal body weight plus 25%, rather than according to actual body weight.[168-171]

Pediatrics. When compared with adults, several differences exist among neonates, infants, and children in relation to their response to NMBAs. A more complete discussion of neonatal and pediatric pharmacology is given in Chapters 48 and 49. A few general observations can be made here. The neuromuscular junction is incomplete at delivery and continues to mature throughout infancy.[172] The sensitivity to any relaxant may change from birth through childhood. Neonates and infants have a higher volume of distribution and differences in redistribution, elimination, and metabolic rates, which vary with age. Infants appear to be more sensitive to nondepolarizing drugs than adults. The onset of action of the relaxants tends to be faster in children than adults. The duration of action of the intermediate NMBAs is longer in infants younger than 10 months of age than in children 1 to 5 years of age.[173] Recovery is faster in children than adults.[174]

Other Factors

Hypothermia. The importance of keeping the patient's core body temperature normothermic cannot be overstated. Hypothermic patients exhibit a prolonged duration of action to all muscle relaxants. Severe (but not mild) hypothermia makes it more difficult to antagonize a neuromuscular block.[175-177]

Allergy. The role of muscle relaxants in perioperative anaphylaxis is well established. An ongoing report from France notes that of 491 recent cases, the most common causes of anaphylaxis were NMBAs (n = 271, 55%), latex (n = 112, 22.3%), and antibiotics (n = 74, 14.7%). Succinylcholine (n = 102, 37.6%) and rocuronium (n = 71, 26.2%) were the most frequently incriminated NMBAs. Cross-reactivity between NMBAs was observed in 63.4% of cases of anaphylaxis to an NMBA.[178] Neuromuscular blocking agents carry two quaternary ammonium ions that are considered the main epitopes involved in anaphylaxis to these drugs.[179] Skin testing and follow-up guidelines have been published.[180] A complete discussion of anaphylaxis management and anesthesia is given in Chapter 42.

REVERSAL OF NEUROMUSCULAR BLOCKADE

Complete and effective reversal of the action of the muscle relaxants is one of the most important aspects of clinical practice. Incomplete relaxant reversal and the resulting difficulties continue to be an issue. This is due in part to the reversal agents and their indirect antidotal action. The use of nerve stimulators and our knowledge of relaxant pharmacology continue to evolve; however, a significant incidence of postoperative residual paralysis stubbornly remains.[181] Three anticholinesterase agents are available, although neostigmine is usually given. Edrophonium may be used when a faster onset is desired, but its efficacy is less than that of neostigmine. This lower effectiveness limits its use to situations in which significant recovery has already occurred. Pyridostigmine is largely historical. Fortunately, a new paradigm may be unfolding with the introduction of the selective relaxant binding agent (SRBA) sugammadex.[182]

Selective Relaxant Binding Agents—Sugammadex

Sugammadex is a modified gamma-cyclodextrin that works by forming very tight water-soluble complexes at a 1:1 ratio with steroidal neuromuscular blocking drugs. The concentration of free muscle relaxant falls rapidly, and muscle strength is reestablished. It is most effective reversing rocuronium, vecuronium, and pancuronium in that order. It does not affect the bezylisoquinolones atracurium and cisatracurium. Sugammadex is biologically inactive and appears to be safe and well tolerated. The most commonly reported adverse drug reactions included dry mouth, dysgeusia, nausea, vomiting, allergy, chills, and procedural hypertension. No anticholinesterase or anticholinergic drugs are needed.[183] In a dosing study, Sorgenfrei noted that sugammadex reversed 0.6 mg/kg rocuronium—induced neuromuscular block within 3 minutes at doses at or above 2 mg/kg. Sugammadex was safe and well tolerated, and no evidence of residual blockade was observed in any patient.[184] Reversal of a deep block was reported by de Boer and colleagues.[185] Sugammadex was administered just 5 minutes after administration of high-dose rocuronium 1.2 mg/kg. Increasing the dose of sugammadex up to 16 mg/kg reduced the mean recovery time to a TOF ratio of 0.9, from 122.1 minutes for spontaneous recovery to less than 2 minutes. A clear dose-response relation was seen. There were no apparent side effects. The mechanism by which sugammadex encapsulates rocuronium seems to be superior to currently used neuromuscular blockade reversal strategies in terms of speed, efficacy, and side effects. As the clinical use of sugammadex evolves, it is expected to produce significant benefits in current practice.[186-189] Sugammadex (Bridion) has been approved in Europe but not in the United States.

CHOLINESTERASE INHIBITORS

The mechanism of each of the cholinesterase inhibitors is primarily the result of its structural relationship and interaction with AChE, a protein with a molecular weight of approximately 320,000 and the capacity to hydrolyze an estimated 300,000 molecules of ACh per minute.[25,190,191]

Edrophonium, pyridostigmine, and neostigmine all contain an ionized center that actively combines either at the active center or at the site specifically removed from the active center of AChE. Edrophonium is a simple alcohol that contains a quaternary ammonium group.[191] It is considered a reversible inhibitor of cholinesterase because it electrostatically attaches to the anionic site of AChE and is stabilized by hydrogen binding at the esteratic site of the enzyme. Because a true chemical bond is not formed, ACh competes with edrophonium for the binding site of AChE, and therefore it has a shorter duration of action than those of compounds that form a bond.[192]

Neostigmine and pyridostigmine are carbamic acid esters of alcohols and contain a quaternary or tertiary ammonium group.[191] These agents form a carbamyl-ester complex at the esteratic site of cholinesterase.[25] This drug-enzyme complex then degrades in the same manner as the ACh-cholinesterase complex. The carbamate group is transferred to AChE, leaving it unable to hydrolyze ACh.[25,190]

The indirect-acting cholinesterase inhibitors exert their effect by inhibiting AChE, thereby increasing the concentration of endogenous ACh around the cholinoreceptors.[191] They act as alternative substrates for the enzyme. This provides a twofold mechanism in the reversal of neuromuscular blockade. First, increasing the concentration of ACh in the junctional cleft changes the agonist-antagonist ratio, thereby increasing the likelihood that the agonist will reoccupy the receptor site once occupied by the neuromuscular blocker, as well as occupying sites not previously engaged. Second, the life of the ACh within the cleft is increased. Because ACh is so rapidly hydrolyzed, it is seldom still available to occupy a receptor site when the antagonist spontaneously dissociates. The increased concentration of ACh prolongs the time it remains in the cleft, allowing time for the antagonist dissociation and the reactivation of the receptor site.[193] Evidence also suggests that these agents have direct influences on neuromuscular transmission independent of enzyme inhibition. These include at least three distinct although possibly interacting mechanisms, including a weak agonist action, the formation of desensitized receptor complex intermediates, and the alteration of the conductance properties of active channels.[194]

Although the result of inhibition of AChE is the same when edrophonium, neostigmine, or pyridostigmine is administered, the means by which these agents accomplish the task varies. Edrophonium binds reversibly with the negatively charged enzyme site by electrostatic attraction of its positively charged nitrogen. This effect prevents catalytic binding with ACh for the short time that edrophonium occupies the binding site. Although the duration of receptor site occupation is short for edrophonium, the duration of its effects is prolonged by the fact that once it leaves the receptor site, it finds another to occupy and continues with this process until eliminated.[193]

Enzymatic inactivation is accomplished by neostigmine and pyridostigmine. Electrostatic interaction between the ionized centers of drug and enzyme takes place initially as with edrophonium. This phenomenon then leads to a hydrolytic chemical reaction in which a shift in covalent bonds occurs, resulting in the formation of a carbamylated enzyme.[193] This methy-carbamyl AChE is much more stable and resistant to hydrolysis than the acetyl enzyme, resulting in an enzyme that is incapable of inactivating ACh.[190]

These differences in chemical deactivation of AChE result in differing pharmacokinetic profiles. Edrophonium, neostigmine, and pyridostigmine are all quaternary ammonium compounds that are poorly lipid soluble. At moderate doses, penetration through lipid barriers (e.g., gastrointestinal tract, placenta, and blood-brain barrier) is minimal if present at all.[25]

Edrophonium is the most rapid acting of these agents, with an onset time of 30 to 60 seconds after IV administration and a duration of 5 to 10 minutes. Intramuscular administration results in an onset of 2 to 10 minutes.[195] Renal excretion accounts for approximately 75% of the edrophonium eliminated, although in the absence of renal function, hepatic metabolism accounts for the inactivation of 30% of the injected dose; this amount undergoes conjugation to inactive edrophonium glucuronide.[25] The elimination half-life of edrophonium is 110 minutes in the healthy patient and 304 minutes in the anephric patient.[25,193] The volume of distribution is 1.1 and 0.7 L/kg in normal and anephric patients, respectively.[25]

Although similar in structure and mechanism of AChE deactivation, neostigmine is more potent than pyridostigmine and has a more rapid onset of action. After IV administration of neostigmine, onset occurs within 4 to 8 minutes. Duration of action is 0.5 to 2 hours, although other sources suggest durations from 60 minutes to 4 hours. Renal excretion accounts for roughly 50% of the neostigmine eliminated, primarily by glomerular filtration.[25,193] The remaining 50% of the neostigmine dose is hydrolyzed by plasma esterases and hepatic metabolism to 3-hydroxyphenyltrimethyl ammonium (3-OH PPM) and conjugated 3-OH PPM. These metabolites have approximately one tenth the activity of the parent compounds and are renally eliminated. The elimination half-life of neostigmine is 70 to 80 minutes, increasing to 181 to 183 minutes in anephric patients.[192,196] The volume of distribution of 0.7 L/kg in healthy patients increases to 0.8 L/kg in those with renal failure.[193]

Pyridostigmine is the cholinesterase inhibitor with the longest onset and duration, primarily because of slower hydrolization of the pyridostigmine-enzyme complex. Onset of action after IV administration is from 2 to 5 minutes. Duration of action has been reported to be from 90 minutes to 3 to 6 hours.[25,191] Pyridostigmine is 75% eliminated by the kidneys.[25,193] The remaining 25% is metabolized by the hepatic microsomal enzyme system to 3-hydroxy—methyl pyridinium, its major metabolite, and six other minor metabolites.[25] All of these metabolites are excreted in the urine. The elimination half-life and volume of distribution are 113 minutes and 1.1 L/kg, respectively. In patients with renal failure, the elimination half-life dramatically rises to 379 minutes, whereas the volume of distribution decreases slightly to 1 L/kg.[25,193]

Important evidence suggests that many patients are often inadequately reversed and exhibit clinically significant residual blockade in the postoperative period.[55,197,198] This phenomenon is frequently referred to as *recurarization*, although it is most likely unrecognized residual paralysis. Qualitative assessment of the signs of recovery are frequently misinterpreted by even the most experienced clinicians. Debaene and colleagues[198] noted that 45% of patients arrived in the recovery room with residual muscular block after intermediate-duration relaxant administration. Residual paralysis was evident even up to 2 hours after relaxant administration. This can have several important consequences, such as interference with pulmonary function, recovery of protective reflexes and protection of the airway, and a reduction of the ventilatory response to hypoxia. They suggest that all patients should receive reversal agents, regardless of the recovery status noted on clinical testing. A meta-analysis of 21 studies involving postoperative residual paralysis noted that the incidence of residual weakness was greater after the use of long- rather than intermediate-acting agents. Furthermore the use of

TABLE 13-11	Commonly Used Anticholinesterase and Anticholinergic Agents			
Agent	Dose Range	Onset (min)	Duration	Comments
Neostigmine	25-75 mcg/kg	5-15	45-90 min	Most commonly used reversal agent; may increase incidence of postoperative nausea and vomiting
Pyridostigmine	100-300 mcg/kg	10-20	60-120 min	Slow onset, long duration, and slow reversal
Edrophonium	500-1000 mcg/kg	5-10	30-60 min	Not recommended for deep block; rapid onset, short duration
Atropine	15 mcg/kg	1-2	1-2 hr	Should be combined with edrophonium because of more rapid onset
Glycopyrrolate	10-20 mcg/kg	2	2-4 hr	Less initial tachycardia than atropine; no central nervous system effects; most frequently used
Sugammadex	2-4 mg/kg	1-2	2-16 hr	Selective relaxant binding agent; up to 16mg/kg has been safely used

BOX 13-9

Common Clinical Signs of Recovery from Neuromuscular Blockers

Adequate tidal volume and rate
Respirations smooth and unlabored
Opens eyes widely on command; no diplopia
Sustained protrusion and purposeful movement of tongue
Effective swallowing and sustained bite
Able to sustain head or leg lift for at least 5 seconds
   (In small children, a strong knee-to-chest movement is
   equivalent.)
Strong, constant hand grip
Effective cough
Adequate vital capacity of at least 15 mL/kg
Adequate inspiratory force of at least 25 to 30 cm H_2O
   negative pressure
Sustained tetanic response to 50 Hz for 5 seconds
Train-of-four ratio >0.9 with no fade
No fade to double-burst stimulation

BOX 13-10

Considerations When Return of Muscle Function Is Incomplete

- As with any reversal agent, the ability to counteract a nondepolarizing blocking agent depends on the amount of spontaneous recovery before the administration of a reversal drug.
- Has enough time been allowed for the anticholinesterase to antagonize the block (at least 15 to 30 minutes)?
- Is the neuromuscular blockade too intense to be antagonized?
- Has an adequate dose of antagonist been given?
- Are the other anesthetics and adjunctive agents contributing to patient weakness?
- Has metabolism or excretion of the relaxant been reduced by a possibly unrecognized process?
- Have acid-base and electrolyte status, temperature, age, drug interactions, and other factors that may prolong relaxant action been contemplated?
- The safest approach when any question as to successful reversal remains is to provide proper sedation and controlled ventilation until adequate recovery is ensured.

neuromuscular monitoring did not affect the occurrence of residual weakness.[181]

The pharmacology of the reversal agents is summarized in Table 13-11. The common clinical signs of muscle recovery after administration of a muscle relaxant are listed in Box 13-9. Some considerations that apply when reversal is incomplete are noted in Box 13-10. Factors that may prolong paralysis are listed in Box 13-11.

ANTICHOLINERGICS

Atropine or glycopyrrolate is used in combination with neostigmine or edrophonium to prevent the parasympathomimetic side effects of the anticholinesterase drugs. If given alone,

neostigmine and the other anticholinesterase drugs would cause severe vagal effects due to the systemic buildup of acetylcholine. These would include bradycardia, hypotension, bronchoconstriction, hypersalivation, diarrhea, and an increase in postoperative nausea and vomiting. Glycopyrrolate is used more often because it produces less initial tachycardia and has no CNS effects. The antimuscarinic can be given first or the glycopyrrolate and neostigmine may be mixed in the same syringe.

Anticholinergic, antimuscarinic, and *parasympatholytic* are three common terms used to describe compounds that originate from

BOX **13-11**

Factors That May Prolong Paralysis

Pathophysiologic Causes
Acid maltase deficiency
Adrenocortical dysfunction
Acute intermittent porphyria
Amyotrophic lateral sclerosis
Anoxia and ischemia
Carcinomatous
  polyneuropathy
Cholinesterase deficiency or
  genetic variance
Compressive neuropathy
Critical illness polyneuropathy
Diphtheria
Eaton-Lambert syndrome
Guillain-Barré syndrome
Hypokalemia and
  hypocalcemia
Hypomagnesemia
Hypophosphatemia
Hypothermia
Motor neuron disease
Multiple sclerosis
Muscular dystrophy
Myasthenia gravis
Myotonic syndromes
Neurofibromatosis
Nonspecific nutritional
  deficiency
Poliomyelitis
Pyridoxine abuse
Polymyositis
Renal failure (variable
  prolongation)
Respiratory acidosis
Sepsis
Thiamine deficiency
Tick bite paralysis
Trauma
Vitamin E deficiency
Wound botulism

Pharmacologic Causes
Aminoglycoside toxicity
Penicillin toxicity
Steroid myopathy

Antihypertensives
Ganglionic blockers
Calcium channel blockers
β-blockers
Furosemide

Antidysrhythmics
Quinidine
Bretylium
Procainamide
Local anesthetics in
  large doses

Antibiotics
Aminoglycoside antibiotics
Polymyxin B
Clindamycin
Tetracycline

Miscellaneous Drugs
Cyclosporine
Steroids
Volatile anesthetics
Dantrolene
Magnesium
Lithium
Azathioprine
Organophosphate
  (poisoning)

Modified from Kirby RR et al, eds. Clinical Anesthesia Practice. *2nd ed. Philadelphia: Saunders; 2002.*

alkaloids of the belladonna plant. Each group name divides these compounds into subgroups that have a more similar mechanism of action. For the purposes of this section, all of the compounds are referred to as *antimuscarinics*. Atropine (*dl*-hyoscyamine) is the prototype of this group, and many of the currently available products are structural derivatives obtained both naturally and synthetically.[199] Atropine is found in the plant *Atropa belladonna*, or deadly nightshade, and in *Datura stramonium*, also known as *jimson weed*.[94] Preparations of these plants have been used by clinicians for centuries; belladonna was used as a poison during the time of the Roman Empire and in the Middle Ages. In 1867,

Bezold and Bloebaun began to study the cardiac effects of belladonna's vagal inhibition, and in 1931 Mein isolated atropine in the pure form.

Atropine and scopolamine are naturally occurring tertiary amines. Semisynthetic congeners of the belladonna alkaloids represented by glycopyrrolate are usually quaternary ammonium derivatives. These quaternary ammonium derivatives often have potent peripheral effects without CNS activity.

All the antimuscarinics are absorbed orally to some extent, although this route is often unpredictable. Intramuscular or IV administration is usually the route used. Scopolamine has the additional advantage of transdermal absorption. Atropine is well absorbed from the gastrointestinal tract by inhalation via endotracheal administration and by IV and intramuscular routes. Given orally, 90% of the dose is absorbed and reaches peak plasma levels within 1 hour. Intramuscular and IV administration results in peak plasma levels within 30 minutes and 2 to 4 minutes, respectively. Atropine is well distributed throughout the body. It crosses both the blood-brain barrier and the placental barrier. Both the kidneys and liver aid in the elimination of atropine. Although elimination is biphasic, the terminal half-life is 2 to 3 hours. Metabolism by the liver results in several metabolites: tropic acid, tropine, and glucuronide conjugates. Approximately 30% to 50% of a dose is excreted unchanged in the urine. Small amounts of atropine may also be eliminated in expired air as carbon dioxide and in feces.[199]

Glycopyrrolate is a quaternary ammonium compound whose ionization limits gastrointestinal absorption, blood-brain barrier, and placental penetration. After IV administration, glycopyrrolate has an onset of 1 minute. Intramuscular and subcutaneous administration results in an onset of 15 to 30 minutes. Vagal blockade can persist for 2 to 3 hours. Serum levels of glycopyrrolate decline quickly, and less than 10% of the drug remains in the serum after 5 minutes. Glycopyrrolate is excreted in feces and urine, primarily as unchanged drug. Small amounts are metabolized to inactive metabolites. Eighty-five percent of an IV dose is excreted in the urine within 48 hours.[94]

Atropine and glycopyrrolate are commonly administered to prevent the muscarinic effects of anticholinesterase inhibitors. Atropine induces its vagolytic effect more rapidly than glycopyrrolate. Atropine appears to be somewhat better suited for use with edrophonium, whereas the onset times of glycopyrrolate and neostigmine are more closely matched. When administered with edrophonium, the usual recommended dose of atropine is 7 mcg/kg.[94,200] With 0.5 to 2.5 mg of neostigmine, the recommended dose of atropine is 0.6 to 1.2 mg, and that of glycopyrrolate is 0.2 to 0.6 mg.[201] (See Chapter 14, Table 14-4 for a comparison of the anticholinergics.)

SUMMARY

Like every other agent used in the practice of anesthesia, neuromuscular blocking agents are useful tools in the hands of skilled clinicians. It should go without saying that these agents ought never to be administered without first appropriately sedating the patient. The exception is if the patient's condition is so marginal that even the most careful use of sedation could increase the chance for morbidity or death. The decision to use neuromuscular blockers in the absence of sedation should be made only after the most careful and thorough consideration. Prevention of movement should provide the surgeon with the optimum field on which life-saving skills can be practiced.

REFERENCES

1. Bloch H. Francois Magendie, Claude Bernard, and the interrelation of science, history, and philosophy. *South Med J.* 1989;82:1259-1261.
2. Rowlee SC. Monitoring neuromuscular blockade in the intensive care unit: the peripheral nerve stimulator. *Heart Lung.* 1999;28:352-362.
3. Lee C. Succinylcholine: its past, present and future. In: Katz RL, ed. *Muscle Relaxants: Basic and Clinical Aspects.* Orlando, FL: Grune & Stratton; 1985:69-70.
4. Cullen SC. The use of curare for the improvement of abdominal muscle relaxation during inhalational anesthesia: a report on one hundred and thirty-one cases. *Surgery.* 1943;14:261-266.
5. Bisset NG. War and hunting poisons of the new world. I. Notes on the early history of curare. *J Ethnopharmacol.* 1992;36:1-26.
6. Karis JH, Gissen AJ. Evaluation of the new neuromuscular blockers. *Anesthesiology.* 1971;35:149-157.
7. Griffith HR, Johnson GE. The use of curare in general anesthesia. *Anesthesiology.* 1942;3:418-420.
8. Beecher HK, Todd DP. A study of the deaths associated with anesthesia and surgery. *Ann Surg.* 1954;140:2-34.
9. Pena O et al. Agreement between muscle movement and peripheral nerve stimulation in critically ill pediatric patients receiving neuromuscular blocking agents. *Heart Lung.* 2000;29:309-318.
10. Silverman DG, Brull SJ. Monitoring neuromuscular block. *Anesthesiology.* 1994;12:237-260.
11. Bevan DR. Recovery from neuromuscular block and its assessment. *Anesth Analg.* 2000;90:S7-S13.
12. Wierda JM et al. The pharmacokinetics, urinary, and biliary excretion of pipecuronium bromide. *Eur J Anaesthesiol.* 1991;8:451-457.
13. Ornstein E et al. Pharmacokinetics and pharmacodynamics of pipecuronium bromide in elderly surgical patients. *Anesth Analg.* 1992;74:841-844.
14. Viby-Mogensen J. Neuromuscular monitoring. In: Miller RD, ed. *Anesthesia.* 6th ed. Philadelphia: Churchill Livingstone; 2005:1551-1570.
15. Donati F, Bevan DR. Muscle relaxants. In: Barash PG et al, eds. *Clinical Anesthesia.* 5th ed. Philadelphia: Lippincott Williams & Wilkins; 2006:421-452.
16. Rupp SM. Monitoring neuromuscular blockade: twitch monitoring. *Anesthesiol Clin North Am.* 1993;11:361-378.
17. Kervin MW. Residual neuromuscular blockade in the immediate postoperative period. *J Perianesth Nurs.* 2002;17:152-158.
18. Martyn J, Durieux ME. Succinylcholine: new insights into mechanisms of action of an old drug. *Anesthesiology.* 2006;104(4):633-634.
19. Foldes FF et al. Succinylcholine: a new approach to muscular relaxation in anesthesiology. *N Engl J Med.* 1952;247:596-600.
20. Flynn PB. Pharmacokinetics and pharmacodynamics of succinylcholine. *Anesthesiol Clin North Am.* 1993;11:309-324.
21. Jonsson M et al. Activation and inhibition of human muscular and neuronal nicotinic acetylcholine receptors by succinylcholine. *Anesthesiology.* 2006;104:724-733.
22. Leuwer M. Do we need muscular blockers in ambulatory anaesthesia? *Curr Opin Anaesthesiol.* 2000;13:625-629.
23. Donati F. Neuromuscular blocking drugs for the new millennium: current practice, future trends—comparative pharmacology of neuromuscular blocking drugs. *Anesth Analg.* 2000;90:S2-S6.
24. Mendez DR et al. Safety and efficacy of rocuronium for controlled intubation with paralytics in the pediatric emergency department. *Pediatr Emerg Care.* 2001;17:233-236.
25. White PF, Katzung BG. Skeletal muscle relaxants. In: Katzung BG, ed. *Basic and Clinical Pharmacology.* 10th ed. New York: McGraw-Hill; 2007:424-441.
26. Sluga M et al. Rocuronium versus succinylcholine for rapid sequence induction of anesthesia and endotracheal intubation: a prospective, randomized trial in emergent cases. *Anesth Analg.* 2005;101(5):1356-1361.
27. Heier T et al. Hemoglobin desaturation after succinylcholine-induced apnea: a study of the recovery of spontaneous ventilation in healthy volunteers. *Anesthesiology.* 2001;94:754-759.
28. Kopman AF et al. Molar potency is not predictive of the speed of onset of atracurium. *Anesth Analg.* 1999;89:1046.
29. Vachon CA et al. Succinylcholine and the open globe. Tracking the teaching. *Anesthesiology.* 2003;99:220-223.
30. Todd MM et al. Neuroanesthesia. In: Longnecker DE et al, eds. *Anesthesiology.* New York: McGraw-Hill; 2008:1099.
31. Morgan JE et al. *Clinical Anesthesiology.* 4th ed. New York: McGraw-Hill; 2006.
32. Calvey TN, Williams NE. Drugs acting on the neuromuscular junction. In: Calvey TN, Williams NE, eds. *Principles and Practice of Pharmacology for Anaesthetists.* 3rd ed. Cambridge: Blackwell Science; 1997:317-361.
33. Gronert GA. Cardiac arrest after succinylcholine. *Anesthesiology.* 2001; 94:523-529.
34. Calvey TN, Williams NE. *Principles and Practice of Pharmacology for Anaesthetists.* 3rd ed. Cambridge: Blackwell Science; 1997.
35. Levano S et al. Rapid and accurate detection of atypical and Kalow variants in the butyrylcholinesterase gene using denaturing high performance liquid chromatography. *Anesth Analg.* 2008 Jan;106(1):147-151.
36. Li B et al. Production of the butyrylcholinesterase knockout mouse. *J Mol Neurosci.* 2006;30(1-2):193-195.
37. Garwood S. Renal disease. In: Hines RL, Marschall KE eds. *Stoeltings Anesthesia and Co-Existing Disease.* 5th ed. Philadelphia: Churchill Livingstone; 2008:323-348.
38. Thapa S, Brull SJ. Succinylcholine-induced hyperkalemia in patients with renal failure: an old question revisited. *Anesth Analg.* 2000;91(1):237-241.
39. Cope TM, Hunter JM. Selecting neuromuscular-blocking drugs for elderly patients. *Drugs Aging.* 2003;20(2):125-140.
40. Seiber FE, Pauldine R. Anesthesia for the elderly. In: Miller RD, ed. *Anesthesia.* 6th ed. Philadelphia: Churchill Livingstone; 2005:2435-2450.
41. Freid EB. The rapid sequence induction revisited: obesity and sleep apnea syndrome. *Anesthesiol Clin North America.* 2005;23(3):551-564.
42. Lemmens HJ, Brodsky JB. The dose of succinylcholine in morbid obesity. *Anesth Analg.* 2006;102(2):438-442.
43. Brodsky JB, Foster PE. Succinylcholine and morbid obesity. *Obes Surg.* 2003;13:138-139.
44. Rosenberg H, Gronert G. Intractable cardiac arrest in children given succinylcholine [letter]. *Anesthesiology.* 1992;77:1054.
45. Al-Takrouri H et al. Hyperkalemic cardiac arrest following succinylcholine administration: the use of extracorporeal membrane oxygenation in an emergency situation. *J Clin Anesth.* 2004;16(6):449-451.
46. Huggins RM et al. Cardiac arrest from succinylcholine-induced hyperkalemia. *Am J Health Syst Pharm.* 2003;60(7):694-697.
47. Gronert GA. The dilemma of the undiagnosed hypotonic child. *Paediatr Anaesth.* 2007;17(8):809.
48. Hayes J et al. Duchenne muscular dystrophy: an old anesthesia problem revisited. *Paediatr Anaesth.* 2008;18(2):100-106.
49. Brambrink AM, Kirsch JR. Perioperative care of patients with neuromuscular disease and dysfunction. *Anesthesiol Clin.* 2007;25(3):483-510.
50. Van Der Speck AFL et al. The effects of succinylcholine on mouth opening. *Anesthesiology.* 1987;67:459-465.
51. Cook DR. Can succinylcholine be abandoned? *Anesth Analg.* 2000;90:S24-S28.
52. Schwartz L et al. Masseter spasm with anesthesia: incidence and implications. *Anesthesiology.* 1984;61:772-775.
53. Carroll JB. Increased incidence of masseter spasm in children with strabismus anesthetized with halothane and succinylcholine. *Anesthesiology.* 1987;67: 559-561.
54. Girard T, Ummenhofer W. Masseter spasm after succinylcholine administration. *J. Emerg Med.* 2007;33(1):75-76.
55. Gill M et al. Masseter spasm after succinylcholine administration. *J Emerg Med.* 2005;29(2):167-171.
56. Chidiac EJ, Raiskin AO. Succinylcholine and the open eye. *Opthalmol Clin North Am.* 2006;19(2):279-285.
57. Martyn JA, Richtsfeld M. Succinylcholine-induced hyperkalemia in acquired pathologic states: etiologic factors and molecular mechanisms. *Anesthesiology.* 2006;104(1):158-169.
58. Dutton RP, McCunn M. Anesthesia for trauma. In: Miller RD, ed. *Anesthesia.* 6th ed. Philadelphia: Churchill Livingstone; 2005:2451-2496.
59. Gronert GA, Theye RA. Pathophysiology of hyperkalemia induced by succinylcholine. *Anesthesiology.* 1975;43:89-99.
60. MacLennan N et al. Anesthesia for major thermal injury. *Anesthesiology.* 1998;89:749-770.
61. Gronert GA. Succinylcholine hyperkalemia after burns. *Anesthesiology.* 1999;91:320-322.
62. Galley HF et al. Pharmacogenetics and anesthesiologists. *Pharmacogenetics.* 2005;6(8):849-856.
63. Anderson AA et al. Identification and biochemical characterization of a novel ryanodine receptor gene mutation associated with malignant hyperthermia. *Anesthesiology.* 2008;108(2):208-215.
64. Ball C. Unraveling the mystery of malignant hyperthermia. *Anaesth Intensive Care.* 2007;35(Suppl 1):26-31.
65. Wong SF, Chung F. Succinylcholine-associated postoperative myalgia. *Anaesthesia.* 2000;55:144-152.
66. Schreiber J et al. Prevention of succinylcholine-induced fasciculation and myalgia. *Anesthesiology.* 2005;103:877-884.
67. Donati F. Dose inflation when using precurarization. *Anesthesiology.* 2006; 105(1):222-223.

68. Jonsson M et al. Distinct pharmacologic properties of neuromuscular blocking agents on human neuronal nicotinic acetylcholine receptors: a possible explanation for the train-of-four fade. *Anesthesiology*. 2006;105(3):521-533.

69. Foldes FF et al. The neuromuscular effects of ORG9426 in patients receiving balanced anesthesia. *Anesthesiology*. 1991;75:191-196.

70. Booij LH, Knape HT. The neuromuscular blocking effects of ORG 9426. *Anaesthesia*. 1991;46:341-343.

71. Lien CA. What is really new about the new relaxants? *Anesthesiol Clin North Am*. 1993;11:729-778.

72. *Rocuronium bromide for injection* [package insert]. West Orange, NJ: Organon; 2004.

73. Rose M, Fischer M. Rocuronium: high risk for anaphylaxis? *Br J Anaesth*. 2001;86:678-682.

74. Doobinin KA, Nakagawa TA. Emergency department use of neuromuscular blocking agents in children. *Pediatr Emerg Care*. 2000;16:441-447.

75. Chaudhry I et al. The protein binding effect of ORG9426 and its inhibitory effect on human cholinesterases. *Anesthesiology*. 1991;75:A786.

76. Mirakhur RJ. Newer neuromuscular blocking drugs. *Drugs*. 1992;44:182-199.

77. Szenohradszky J et al. Interaction of rocuronium (ORG 9426) and phenytoin in a patient undergoing cadaver renal transplantation: a possible pharmacokinetic mechanism? *Anesthesiology*. 1994;80:1167-1170.

78. Sieber TJ et al. Tracheal intubation with rocuronium using the "timing principle." *Anesth Analg*. 1998;86:1137-1140.

79. Kirkegaard-Nielsen H et al. Rapid tracheal intubation with rocuronium. *Anesthesiology*. 1999;91:131-136.

80. Perry J et al. Rocuronium versus succinylcholine for rapid sequence induction intubation. *Cochrane Database Syst Rev*. 2003;(1):CD002788.

81. Bartkowski RR et al. Rocuronium onset of action: a comparison with atracurium and vecuronium. *Anesth Analg*. 1993;77:574-578.

82. Leykin Y et al. Intubation conditions following rocuronium: influence of induction agent and priming. *Anaesth Intensive Care*. 2005;33(4):462-468.

83. Bock M et al. Priming with rocuronium accelerates neuromuscular block in children: a prospective randomized study. *Can J Anaesth*. 2007;54(7):538-543.

84. Schmidt J et al. A priming technique accelerates onset of neuromuscular blockade at the laryngeal adductor muscles. *Can J Anaesth*. 2005;52(1):50-54.

85. Wicks TC. The pharmacology of rocuronium bromide. *AANA J*. 1994;62:33-38.

86. Lowry DW et al. Neuromuscular effects of rocuronium during sevoflurane, isoflurane, and intravenous anesthesia. *Anesth Analg*. 1998;87:936-940.

87. Adejumo SW, Hunter JM. Muscle relaxants in the critically ill. *Curr Opin Crit Care*. 1999;5:263.

88. Ducharme J, Donati F. Pharmacokinetics and pharmacodynamics of steroidal muscle relaxants. *Anesthesiol Clin North Am*. 1993;11:283-307.

89. Torda TA. The "new" relaxants: a review of the clinical pharmacology of atracurium and vecuronium. *Anaesth Intensive Care*. 1987;15:72-82.

90. Payne JP. Atracurium. In: Katz RL, ed. *Muscle Relaxants: Basic and Clinical Aspects*. Orlando, FL: Grune & Stratton; 1985:87-101.

91. Miller RD et al. Clinical pharmacology of vecuronium and atracurium. *Anesthesiology*. 1984;61:444-453.

92. *Atracurium* [package insert]. Research Triangle Park, NC: Burroughs Wellcome; 1992.

93. Stenlake JB et al. Atracurium: conception and inception. *Anaesthesia*. 1983; 55:3S-10S.

94. Service AHF. Skeletal muscle relaxants. In: McEvoy GK, ed. *AHFS*. Bethesda, MD: American Society of Hospital Pharmacists; 1994:817.

95. Weinstein JA et al. Pharmacodynamics of vecuronium and atracurium in the obese surgical patient. *Anesth Analg*. 1988;67:1149-1153.

96. Papadimitriou L, Foustanos A. Continuous intravenous infusion of atracurium in idiopathic obesity [letter]. *Anaesthesia*. 1988;43:900.

97. Payne JP, Hughes R. Evaluation of atracurium in anaesthetized man. *Br J Anaesth*. 1981;53:45-54.

98. Haines M. A comparison of the onset time, duration of action, and fade characteristics of atracurium and vecuronium. *AANA J*. 1993;61:592-596.

99. Healy TE et al. Atracurium and vecuronium: effect of dose on the time of onset. *Br J Anaesth*. 1986;58:620-624.

100. Gramstad L et al. Comparative study of atracurium, vecuronium (ORG NC45) and pancuronium. *Br J Anaesth*. 1982;54:827-829.

101. Ward S et al. Pharmacokinetics of atracurium and its metabolites in patients with normal renal function and in patients in renal failure. *Br J Anaesth*. 1987;59:697-706.

102. Fahey MR et al. The pharmacokinetics and pharmacodynamics of atracurium in patients with and without renal failure. *Anesthesiology*. 1984;61:699-702.

103. Shea JHA. Atracurium: a review of a new non-depolarizing muscle relaxant. *AANA J*. 1984;52:299-302.

104. Hughes R, Chapple DJ. The pharmacology of atracurium: a new competitive neuromuscular blocking agent. *Br J Anaesth*. 1981;53:31-44.

105. *Nimbex Injection* [package insert]. Research Triangle Park, NC: Glaxo Wellcome; 1995.

106. Doenicke AW et al. Onset time, endotracheal intubating conditions, and plasma histamine after cisatracurium and vecuronium administration. *Anesth Analg*. 1998;87:434-438.

107. Konstadt SN et al. A two-center comparison of the cardiovascular effects of cis-atracurium (Nimbex) and vecuronium in patients with coronary artery disease. *Anesth Analg*. 1995;81:1010-1014.

108. Bryson HM, Faulds D. cis-Atracurium besylate. A review of its pharmacology and clinical potential in anaesthetic practice. *Drugs*. 1997;53:848-866.

109. Naguib M et al. Comparative clinical pharmacology of rocuronium, cisatracurium, and their combination. *Anesthesiology*. 1998;98:1116-1124.

110. Tran T et al. Pharmacokinetics and pharmacodynamics of cis-atracurium after a short infusion in patients under propofol anesthesia. *Anesth Analg*. 1998;87:1158-1163.

111. Mellinghoff H et al. A comparison of cis-atracurium and atracurium: onset of neuromuscular block after bolus injection and recovery after subsequent infusion. *Anesth Analg*. 1996;83:1072-1075.

112. Bluestein LS et al. Evaluation of cis-atracurium, a new neuromuscular blocking agent, for tracheal intubation. *Can J Anaesth*. 1996;43:925-931.

113. Savarese JJ et al. The clinical pharmacology of new benzylisoquinoline-diester compounds, with special consideration of cis-atracurium and mivacurium. *Anaesthetist*. 1997;46:840-849.

114. Donnelly AJ et al. *Anesthesiology and Critical Care Drug Handbook*. 5th ed. Hudson, OH: Lexi-Comp Corp; 2004.

115. Kisor DF et al. Importance of the organ-independent elimination of cis-atracurium. *Anesth Analg*. 1996;83:1065-1071.

116. Welch RM et al. The in vitro degradation of cis-atracurium, the R, cis-R'-isomer of atracurium, in human and rat plasma. *Clin Pharmacol Ther*. 1995;58:132-142.

117. Smith CE et al. A comparison of the infusion pharmacokinetics and pharmacodynamics of cis-atracurium, the 1R-cis-1R' isomer of atracurium, with atracurium besylate in healthy patients. *Anaesthesia*. 1997;52:833-841.

118. Savarese JJ et al. The cardiovascular effects of mivacurium chloride in patients receiving nitrous oxide-opiate-barbiturate anesthesia. *Anesthesiology*. 1989;70:386-394.

119. Fahey MR et al. Clinical pharmacology of ORG NC45 (Norcuron): a new nondepolarizing muscle relaxant. *Anesthesiology*. 1981;55:6-11.

120. Baird WLM, Savage DS. Vecuronium—the early years. *Anesthesiol Clin North Am*. 1985;3:347-360.

121. Shanks CA et al. Pharmacokinetics and pharmacodynamics of vecuronium administered by bolus and infusion during halothane or balanced anesthesia. *Clin Pharmacol Ther*. 1987;42:459-464.

122. Belmont MR. Pharmacodynamics and pharmacokinetics of benzylisoquinoline (curare-like) neuromuscular blocking drugs. *Anesthesiol Clin North Am*. 1993;11:251-281.

123. Cronnelly R et al. Pharmacokinetics and pharmacodynamics of vecuronium (ORG NC45) and pancuronium in anesthetized humans. *Anesthesiology*. 1983;58:405-408.

124. Gramstad L et al. Onset time and duration of action for atracurium, ORG NC45 and pancuronium. *Br J Anaesth*. 1982;54:827-830.

125. Rorvik K et al. Comparison of large dose of vecuronium with pancuronium for prolonged neuromuscular blockade. *Br J Anaesth*. 1988;61:180-185.

126. Fisher DM, Rosen JI. A pharmacokinetic explanation for increasing recovery time following larger or repeated doses of nondepolarizing muscle relaxants. *Anesthesiology*. 1986;65:286-291.

127. Sohn YJ et al. Pharmacokinetics of vecuronium in man. *Anesthesiology*. 1982;57:A256.

128. Hoskings MP et al. Combined H_1 and H_2 receptor blockade attenuates the cardiovascular effects of high dose atracurium for rapid sequence endotracheal intubation. *Anesth Analg*. 1988;67:1089-1092.

129. Rupp SM et al. Pharmacokinetics and pharmacodynamics of vecuronium in the elderly. *Anesthesiology*. 1983;59:A270.

130. Estafanous FG. Anesthetics and muscle relaxants in patients with heart disease: historical perspective. *J Cardiovasc Anesth*. 1990;6(suppl 4):3-13.

131. Lynam DP et al. The pharmacodynamics and pharmacokinetics of vecuronium in patients anesthetized with isoflurane with normal renal function or with renal failure. *Anesthesiology*. 1988;69:227-231.

132. Rathmell JP et al. Hemodynamic and pharmacological comparison of doxacurium and pipecuronium with pancuronium during induction of cardiac anesthesia: does the benefit justify the cost? *Anesth Analg*. 1993;76:513-519.

133. Murray DJ et al. Cardiovascular and neuromuscular effects of bwa938u: comparison with pancuronium. *Anesthesiology*. 1987;67:A367.

134. Lebowitz PW et al. Combination of pancuronium and metocurine: neuromuscular and hemodynamic advantages over pancuronium alone. *Anesth Analg*. 1981;60:12-17.

135. Booij LH et al. Comparative cardiovascular and neuromuscular effects of ORG NC45, d-tubocurarine and metocurine. *Anesthesiology*. 1979;51:S280.

136. Peat SJ et al. The prolonged use of atracurium in a patient with tetanus. *Anaesthesia.* 1988;43:962-963.

137. Parker CJR et al. Disposition of infusions of atracurium and its metabolite, laudanosine, in patients in renal and respiratory failure in an ITU. *Br J Anaesth.* 1994;61:531-540.

138. Buck ML, Reed MD. Use of nondepolarizing neuromuscular blocking agents in mechanically ventilated patients. *Clin Pharmacokinet.* 1991;10:32-48.

139. Bion JF et al. Atracurium infusions in patients with fulminant hepatic failure awaiting liver transplantation. *Intensive Care Med.* 1993;19:S94-S98.

140. Schramm W et al. The cerebral and cardiovascular effects of cisatracurium and atracurium in neurosurgical patients. *Anesth Analg.* 1998;86:123-127.

141. Modica P, Templehoff R. Effect of chronic anticonvulsant therapy on recovery from atracurium. *Anesth Analg.* 1989;68:S198.

142. Caldwell JE et al. The influence of renal failure on the pharmacokinetics and duration of action of pipecuronium bromide in patients anesthetized with halothane and nitrous oxide. *Anesthesiology.* 1989;70:7-12.

143. Savarese JJ, Kitz RJ. Does clinical anesthesia need new neuromuscular blockers? *Anesthesiology.* 1975;42:236-239.

144. Ferres CJ et al. Haemodynamic effects of vecuronium, pancuronium, and atracurium in patients with coronary artery disease. *Br J Anaesth.* 1987;59:305-311.

145. Gallo JA et al. Comparison of effects of atracurium and vecuronium in cardiac surgical patients. *Anesth Analg.* 1988;67:161-165.

146. Gravlee GP et al. Rapid administration of a narcotic and neuromuscular blocker: a hemodynamic comparison of fentanyl, sufentanil, pancuronium, and vecuronium. *Anesth Analg.* 1988;67:39-47.

147. Emmott RS et al. Cardiovascular effects of doxacurium, pancuronium, and vecuronium in anaesthetized patients presenting for coronary artery bypass surgery. *Br J Anaesth.* 1990;65:480-486.

148. Lebrault C et al. Pharmacokinetics and pharmacodynamics of vecuronium (ORG NC45) in patients with cirrhosis. *Anesthesiology.* 1985;62:601-605.

149. Fahey MR et al. Pharmacokinetics of ORG-NC45 (Norcuron) in patients with and without renal failure. *Br J Anaesth.* 1981;53:1049-1052.

150. Durant NN et al. The neuromuscular and autonomic blocking activities of pancuronium, Org NC45, and other pancuronium analogues in the cat. *J Pharm Pharmacol.* 1979;31:831-836.

151. Arden JR et al. Vecuronium in alcohol liver disease: a pharmacokinetic and pharmacodynamic analysis. *Anesthesiology.* 1988;68:771-776.

152. Garg RK. Anesthetic considerations in patients with hepatic failure. *Anesthesiol Clin.* 2005;46(4):45-64.

153. Cook DR. Pharmacokinetics of mivacurium in normal patients and in those with hepatic or renal failure. *Br J Anaesthesia.* 1992;69:580-585.

154. Playfor S et al. Consensus guidelines for sustained neuromuscular blockade in critically ill children. *Paediatr Anaesth.* 2007;17(9):881-887.

155. Murray MJ et al. Clinical practice guidelines for sustained neuromuscular blockade in the adult critically ill patient. *Crit Care Med.* 2002;30(1):142-156.

156. Ward S, Neill EAM. Pharmacokinetics of atracurium in acute hepatic failure (with acute renal failure). *Br J Anaesth.* 1987;55:1169-1172.

157. Farman JV et al. Atracurium infusion in liver transplantation. *Br J Anaesth.* 1986;58:96S-102S.

158. McLeod K et al. Pharmacokinetics of pancuronium in patients with normal and impaired renal function. *Br J Anaesth.* 1976;48:341-345.

159. Soukup J et al. *cis*-Atracurium in patients with compromised kidney function. Pharmacodynamic and intubation conditions under isoflurane-nitrous oxide anesthesia. *Anaesthetist.* 1998;47:669-676.

160. Lortat-Jacob B, Servin F. Pharmacology of intravenous drugs in elderly. In: Siebert F, ed. *Geriatric Anesthesia.* New York: McGraw-Hill; 2007:91-104.

161. Bata SJ et al. Neuromuscular effects and pharmacokinetics of mivacurium in elderly patients under isoflurane anesthesia. *Anesth Analg.* 1989;68:S18.

162. Matteo RS et al. Pharmacokinetics and pharmacodynamics of rocuronium (ORG9426) in elderly surgical patients. *Anesth Analg.* 1993;77:1193-1197.

163. Arain SR et al. Variability of duration of action of neuromuscular-blocking drugs in elderly patients. *Acta Anaesthesiol Scand.* 2005;49(3):312-315.

164. Freid EB. The rapid sequence induction revisited: obesity and sleep apnea syndrome. *Anesthesiol Clin North Am.* 2005;23(3):551-564.

165. Suzuki T et al. Neostigmine-induced reversal of vecuronium in normal weight, overweight and obese female patients. *Br J Anaesth.* 2006;97(2):160-163.

166. Lemmens HJ, Brodsky JB. The dose of succinylcholine in morbid obesity. *Anesth Analg.* 2006;102(2):438-442.

167. Ebert TJ et al. Perioperative consideration for patients with morbid obesity. *Int Anesthesiol Clin.* 2006;24(3):621-636.

168. Leykin Y et al. The pharmacodynamic effects of rocuronium when dosed according to real body weight or ideal body weight in morbidly obese patients. *Anesth Analg.* 2004;99(4):1086-1089.

169. Leykin Y et al. Anesthetic management of morbidly obese and super-morbidly obese patients undergoing bariatric operations: hospital course and outcomes. *Obes Surg.* 2006;16(12):1563-1569.

170. Leykin Y et al. The effects of cisatracurium on morbidly obese women. *Anesth Analg.* 2004;99(4):1090-1094.

171. Naguib M, Lien C. Pharmacology of muscle relaxants and their antagonists. In: Miller RD, ed. *Anesthesia.* 6th ed. Philadelphia: Churchill Livingstone; 2005:481-572.

172. Goudsouzian NG, Standaert FG. The infant and the myoneural junction. *Anesth Analg.* 1986;65(11):1208-1217.

173. Davis PJ et al. Pharmacology of pediatric anesthesia. In: Motoyama EK, Davis PJ, eds. *Smith's Anesthesia for Infants and Children.* 7th ed. Philadelphia: Mosby; 2006:177-238.

174. Baykara N et al. Predicting recovery from deep neuromuscular block by rocuronium in children and adults. *J Clin Anesth.* 2002;14(3):214-217.

175. Caldwell JE et al. Temperature-dependent pharmacokinetics and pharmacodynamics of vecuronium. *Anesthesiology.* 2000;92:84.

176. Heier T et al. The influence of mild hypothermia on the pharmacokinetics and time course of action of neostigmine in anesthetized volunteers. *Anesthesiology.* 2002;97(1):90-95.

177. Heier T, Caldwell JE. Impact of hypothermia on the response to neuromuscular blocking drugs. *Anesthesiology.* 2006;104(5):1070-1080.

178. Mertes PM, Laxenaire MC; GERAP. Anaphylactic and anaphylactoid reactions occurring during anaesthesia in France. Seventh epidemiologic survey (January 2001-December 2002). *Ann Fr Anesth Reanim.* 2004;23(12):1133-1143.

179. Mertes PM et al. Skin reactions to intradermal neuromuscular blocking agent injections: a randomized multicenter trail in healthy volunteers. *Anesthesiology.* 2007;107(2):245-252.

180. Mertes PM. Anaphylactic reactions during anaesthesia—let us treat the problem rather than debating its existence. *Acta Anaesthesiol Scand.* 2005;49:431-433.

181. Naguib M et al. Neuromuscular monitoring and postoperative residual curarisation: a meta-analysis. *Br J Anaesth.* 2007;98(3):302-316.

182. Miller RD. Sugammadex: an opportunity to change the practice of anesthesiology? *Anesth Analg.* 2007;104(3):477-478.

183. Nicholson WT et al. Sugammadex: a novel agent for the reversal of neuromuscular blockade. *Pharmacotherapy.* 2007;27(8):1181-1188.

184. Sorgenfrei IF et al. Reversal of rocuronium-induced neuromuscular block by the selective relaxant binding agent sugammadex: a dose-finding and safety study. *Anesthesiology.* 2006;104(4):667-674.

185. de Boer HD et al. Reversal of rocuronium-induced (1.2 mg/kg) profound neuromuscular block by sugammadex: a multicenter, dose-finding and safety study. *Anesthesiology.* 2007;107(2):239-244.

186. Kopman AF. Sugammadex: A revolutionary approach to neuromuscular antagonism. *Anesthesiology.* 2006;104:631-633.

187. Donati F. Sugammadex: an opportunity for more thinking or more cookbook medicine? *Can J Anaesth.* 2007;54(9):689-695.

188. Naguib M. Sugammadex: another milestone in clinical neuromuscular pharmacology. *Anesth Analg.* 2007;104(3):575-581.

189. de Boer HD et al. Non-steroidal neuromuscular blocking agents to re-establish paralysis after reversal of rocuronium-induced neuromuscular block with sugammadex. *Can J Anaesth.* 2008;55(2):125-126.

190. Service AHF. Parasympathomimetic agents. In: McEvoy GK, ed. *AHFS 94 drug information.* Bethesda, MD: American Society of Hospital Pharmacists; 1994:721-728.

191. Taylor P. Anticholinesterase agents. In: Brunton LL et al, eds. *Goodman and Gilman's Pharmacological Basis of Therapeutics.* 11th ed. New York: McGraw-Hill; 2006:201-216.

192. Sparr HJ et al. Comparison of intubating conditions after rapacuronium (ORG 9487) and succinylcholine following rapid sequence induction in adult patients. *Br J Anaesth.* 1999;82:537-541.

193. Haas RE et al. Cardiovascular effects of atropine and glycopyrrolate on anesthetized children. *AANA J.* 1987;55:529-538.

194. Naguib M et al. Advances in neurobiology of the neuromuscular junction: implications for the anesthesiologist. *Anesthesiology.* 2002;96:202-231.

195. Service AHF. Myasthenia gravis. In: McEvoy GK, eds. *AHFS 94 drug information.* Bethesda, MD: American Society of Hospital Pharmacists; 1994:1565-1567.

196. Goulden MR, Hunter JM. Rapacuronium (ORG 9487): do we have a replacement for succinylcholine? *Br J Anaesth.* 1999;82:489-492.

197. Eriksson LI. Evidence-based practice and neuromuscular monitoring. *Anesthesiology.* 2003;98:1037.

198. Debaene B et al. Residual paralysis in the PACU after a single intubating dose of nondepolarizing muscle relaxant with an intermediate duration of action. *Anesthesiology.* 2003;98:1042.

199. Pappano AJ. Cholinoreceptor blocking agents. In: Katzung BG, ed. *Basic and Clinical Pharmacology.* 10th ed. New York: McGraw-Hill; 2007:108-120.

200. Stoelting RK, Hillier SC. Anticholinesterase drugs and cholinergic agonists. *Pharmacology and Physiology in Anesthetic Practice.* 4th ed. Philadelphia: Lippincott Williams & Wilkins; 2006:251-265.

AUTONOMIC AND CARDIAC PHARMACOLOGY

John J. Nagelhout

Providing high-quality anesthetic care involves continuous monitoring of all the body's systems, with a special emphasis on the cardiovascular status of the patient. Complex anesthetic plans and invasive surgical intervention can produce profound stress on patients' cardiovascular balance and require careful manipulation of vital signs. The array of diagnostic tests, monitors, and drugs available makes a thorough understanding of autonomic and cardiac pharmacology essential. The anesthetist is able to plan preoperative interventions that make the anesthetic course flow smoothly. Intraoperative planning for the immediate and late postoperative periods is critical to avoiding untoward outcomes. The number and variety of medications in a patient's profile require a delicate balance between the anesthetic requirements and maintaining a successful continuum of therapy for the long-term needs of the patient. This chapter will present a broad overview of the many autonomic and cardiovascular medicines anesthetists may encounter during the perioperative period and their important anesthetic considerations.

AUTONOMIC DRUGS—SYMPATHOMIMETIC AMINES

The sympathomimetic amines include the three naturally occurring catecholamines epinephrine, norepinephrine, and dopamine and a number of synthetic agents such as phenylephrine and dobutamine. These drugs are used in a variety of situations, including the treatment of anesthesia-induced hypotension, bradycardia, anaphylaxis, shock, heart failure, and cardiac resuscitation.

The basic structure of the sympathomimetic amines is β-(3,4-dihydroxyphenyl)-ethylamine. This structure consists of a substituted benzene ring and an ethylamine side chain.[1] The effects elicited by this pharmacologic class are the result of the stimulation of β-adrenergic, α-adrenergic, and dopamine adrenergic receptors. The innervation of the effector organs by the autonomic system is outlined in Table 14-1.

The efficacy of a particular sympathomimetic amine depends on its concentration at the receptor site, its affinity for specific receptors, and the population of receptors available for binding. The effects of the common autonomic drugs are summarized in Table 14-2.

Epinephrine

Epinephrine, one of the naturally occurring catecholamines, is the final product in the chain of catecholamine synthesis. (See Chapter 34 for a complete description of catecholamine synthesis.) Although both epinephrine and norepinephrine have agonistic activity at both α- and β-receptors, norepinephrine has minimal β_1 activity in low doses, whereas epinephrine strongly stimulates both β_1- and β_2-receptors.

Epinephrine is useful not only in the treatment of anaphylaxis and cardiopulmonary resuscitation, but also its combination of α and β effects makes it an appropriate choice for the treatment of some shock states in which poor tissue oxygen delivery and hypotension are combined. In small doses, epinephrine may well be useful as a sympathomimetic agent in patients unresponsive to indirect-acting agents and in those in whom simultaneous β_1-and β_2-receptor stimulation may be helpful. With epinephrine, the dominance of α or β effects is dose related.

Epinephrine's β_1 effect produces marked positive inotropic (force of contraction), chronotropic (heart rate), and dromotropic (conduction velocity) actions. It should be noted that as heart rate, left ventricular stroke work, stroke volume, and cardiac output increase, so does myocardial oxygen consumption. In addition, the corresponding increased automaticity of all foci, including those that are ectopic, may lead to arrhythmia. Marked vigilance must be maintained in an effort to ensure that an imbalance of myocardial oxygen supply and demand does not occur. It should be recalled that the effects resulting from epinephrine administration are capable of both increasing myocardial demand and decreasing supply.

Beneficial effects of β_2 stimulation include bronchodilation, vasodilation, and stabilization of mast cells, with a resultant diminution of histamine release. Concurrently, α stimulation promotes a decrease in bronchial secretion. The net effect is a decrease in airway resistance with an improvement in oxygenation.

With low doses of epinephrine, β_2 stimulation in the peripheral vasculature promotes the redistribution of blood flow to skeletal muscle, thereby producing a decrease in systemic vascular resistance. As the dose of epinephrine is increased, the α effect predominates, with resultant vasoconstriction and an increase in systemic pressures. The systolic pressure is increased, whereas the diastolic pressure remains relatively unchanged, with a resultant increase in pulse pressure. It should be noted that if the coronary arteries are not obstructed, autoregulation increases oxygen delivery to meet the increased demand.[2] However, in the presence of a coronary artery lesion, oxygen delivery may be insufficient to meet demand, and myocardial ischemia results.[3]

The increased α effect that occurs with greater doses of epinephrine also results in renal and splanchnic vasoconstriction. Renal vascular resistance and ultimately renal blood flow are decreased. Beta stimulation leads to activation of the renin-angiotensin system and also to an increase in lipolysis, glycogenolysis, gluconeogenesis, ketone production, and lactate release by skeletal muscle.[4] Insulin secretion is inhibited by an overriding β_2 stimulation. Epinephrine-induced β_2 stimulation also can cause a

TABLE 14-1	Typical Autonomic Influences on Peripheral Effector Organs			
Organ System	**Sympathetic Effect**	**Adrenergic Receptor Type**	**Parasympathetic Effect**	**Cholinergic Receptor Type**
Eye				
Radial muscle, iris	Contraction (mydriasis)	α_1		
Sphincter muscle, iris			Contraction (miosis)	M_3, M_2
Ciliary muscle	Relaxation for far vision	β_2	Contraction for near vision (accommodation)	M_3, M_2
Heart				
Sinoatrial node	Increase in heart rate	β_1	Decrease in heart rate	M_2
Atria	Increase in contractility and conduction velocity	β_1	Decrease in contractility	M_2
Atrioventricular node	Increase in automaticity and conduction velocity	β_1	Decrease in conduction velocity; AV block	M_2
His-Purkinje system	Increase in automaticity and conduction velocity	β_1	Little effect	M_2
Ventricle	Increase in contractility, conduction velocity, automaticity	β_1	Slight decrease in contractility	M_2
Blood Vessels				
Arteries				
Coronary	Constriction; dilation	α; β_2	None	—
Skin and mucosa	Constriction	α_1; β_2	None	—
Skeletal muscle	Constriction; dilation	α_1; β_2	None	—
Cerebral	Constriction (slight)	α_1	None	—
Pulmonary	Constriction; dilation	α_1; β_2	None	—
Abdominal viscera	Constriction; dilation	α_1; β_2	None	—
Salivary glands	Constriction and reduced secretions	α_1; α_2	Dilation and increased secretions	M_3
Renal	Constriction +++; dilation	α_1, α_2; $\beta_1\ \beta_2$	None	—
Veins	Constriction; dilation	α_1, α_2; β_2	None	—
Lung				
Tracheal and bronchial smooth muscle	Relaxation	β_2	Contraction	M_2, M_3
GI Tract				
Motility and tone	Decrease	α_1, α_2; β_1, β_2	Increase	$M_2\ M_3$
Sphincters	Contraction	α_1	Relaxation	M_3, M_2
Secretion	Inhibition	α_2	Stimulation	M_3, M_2
Gallbladder and ducts	Relaxation	β_2	Contraction	M
Kidney				
Renin secretion	Increase	β_1	None	—
Urinary Bladder				
Detrusor	Relaxation	β_2	Contraction	M_3, M_2
Trigone and sphincter	Contraction	α_1	Relaxation	M_3, M_2
Uterus	Contraction (pregnant)	α_1	None	—
	Relaxation (pregnant and non-pregnant)	β_2		
Liver	Glycogenolysis and gluconeogenesis; increased blood sugar	α_1; β_2		
Pancreas				
Islets (β cells)	Decreased insulin secretion	α_2	None	—
	Increased insulin secretion	β_2	None	—
Adipocytes	Lipolysis	α_1; $\beta_1, \beta_2, \beta_3$	None	—

α, *Alpha receptor;* β, *beta receptor;* M, *muscarinic receptor.*

TABLE **14-2** Effects of Autonomic Drugs					
Organ Systems	**Alpha Agonists**	**Alpha Blocker**	**Beta Agonists**	**Beta Blocker**	**Cholinergic Agonists**	**Anticholinergic**
Eye	Mydriasis	Miosis (slight)	NCRE	↓ Intraocular pressure	Miosis, ↓ intraocular pressure	Mydriasis, cycloplegia, ↑ intraocular pressure
Heart						
Rate	Bradycardia (reflex)	Tachycardia (reflex)	Tachycardia	Bradycardia	Bradycardia	Tachycardia
Contractility	NCRE	Slight increase (reflex)	↑	→	↓ (slight)	↑ (slight)
Conduction velocity	NCRE	NCRE	↑	→	→	↑
Blood (vessels)	Vasoconstriction	Vasodilation	Vasodilation	Vasoconstriction	NCRE	NCRE
Lungs	NCRE	NCRE	Bronchodilation	Bronchoconstriction	Bronchoconstriction	Bronchodilation (slight)
GI Tract	↓ Motility and secretion	NCRE	↓ Motility and secretion	NCRE	↑ Motility and secretion	↓ Motility and secretion
Uterus	Contraction	NCRE	Relaxation	NCRE	NCRE	NCRE
Liver	↑ Blood sugar	NCRE	↑ Blood sugar	Hypoglycemia	NCRE	NCRE

↑, *Increase;* ↓, *decrease;* NCRE, *no clinically relevant effect.*

transient hyperkalemia as potassium follows glucose out of hepatic cells. This is followed by a longer hypokalemia as β_2 stimulation then forces this extracellular potassium into red blood cells.[5] Because of the mechanism of action of the drug, care must be exercised in treating hypotension with epinephrine in patients who are concomitantly receiving α-antagonists. Alpha-blocking drugs such as phentolamine block the peripheral vasoconstricting effects of the α-agonism usually associated with epinephrine. This leaves the peripheral β_2 effects, which cause vasodilation, virtually unopposed.

Norepinephrine

Norepinephrine is a potent vasopressor. Although it is not as potent as epinephrine in stimulating α-receptors in equal doses, it has little β_2 activity at low doses, and the end result is, for the most part, unopposed α stimulation. The chronotropic effect seen with β_1 stimulation is generally absent with norepinephrine in low doses because of the increase in systemic vascular resistance, which induces reflex vagal activity.

The aforementioned combination of adrenergic stimulation results in a decrease in vital organ flow; however, coronary artery perfusion may be increased because of the increase in diastolic pressure. Renal vascular resistance is increased, and urine output may fall. Simultaneous administration of dopamine has been recommended to correct the increase in renal vascular resistance seen with norepinephrine.[6] Fenoldopam may also have some benefit in increasing renal blood flow. An increase in preload may be seen because norepinephrine is a venoconstrictor.[7,8]

Norepinephrine is generally used in patients with adequate cardiac output but low systemic vascular resistance. In this group of patients, however, the underlying problem of peripheral tissue perfusion-oxygenation may be exacerbated by the intense norepinephrine-induced peripheral vasoconstriction, even if adequate blood pressure has been achieved.

Norepinephrine does have some generalized metabolic effects, such as a decrease in insulin production, but these metabolic effects are present to a lesser degree than those seen with epinephrine. Adverse effects are usually a result of the intense vasoconstriction associated with norepinephrine.

Dopamine

Dopamine is an endogenous central neurotransmitter that is derived from dopa in the chain of catecholamine synthesis. Pharmacologically, dopamine stimulates dopamine receptors, β-receptors, and α-receptors in a dose-dependent manner. Dopaminergic receptors are stimulated with low doses of less than 2 mcg/kg/min. At moderate doses of 2 to 5 mcg/kg/min, β effects are elicited, and α effects are seen with high infusion rates of greater than 10 mcg/kg/min. Dopamine also has an indirect sympathomimetic effect, eliciting the release of norepinephrine via β_1 stimulation.[9]

Dopamine is often the first inotropic agent chosen by the anesthetist presented with a patient in systemic shock. Some clinicians have found dopamine to have a poor response in cases of gram-negative sepsis because of a down-regulation in which the sensitivity of β-receptors is diminished.[10,11]

During surgery and anesthesia, dopamine is administered for its dopaminergic effect. The stimulation of dopamine receptors in the renal artery promotes an increase in renal blood flow and a resultant increase in glomerular filtration rate and urine output. Benefits, however, of so-called "renal" dopamine are in doubt, and many clinicians are abandoning the practice.[12,13]

Dopamine also inhibits aldosterone, resulting in an increase in sodium excretion and urine output.

Dopamine has been implicated in several cases of severe limb ischemia. If dopamine is administered through a peripheral line, increased vigilance in pediatric patients and in patients with any type of vascular disease such as diabetes, atherosclerosis, or Raynaud phenomenon is advised. The presence of an arterial line in the affected limb also increases the incidence of limb ischemia with concurrent dopamine infusion. Other metabolic and central nervous system effects, similar to those seen with epinephrine but less extensive, have been attributed to dopamine administration.

The monoamine oxidase enzymes metabolize dopamine; therefore, the effects of dopamine can be prolonged in patients receiving a monoamine oxidase inhibitor. Tricyclic antidepressants may also augment the activity of sympathomimetic drugs.

Isoproterenol

Isoproterenol is a synthetic catecholamine with the same underlying chemical structure as the endogenous catecholamines. It is a potent nonselective agonist of β_1- and β_2-receptors but has no agonistic activity at α-receptors or dopamine receptors. The uses of isoproterenol have been limited, and the drug is rarely used. In current practice, it is occasionally used in the treatment of bradycardia, heart block characterized by hemodynamic instability unresponsive to atropine, and in pediatrics for the management of status asthmaticus. Despite these two applications, other more selective drugs are frequently chosen for the treatment of these conditions.

The profound β_1 stimulation of isoproterenol results in both positive inotropic and chronotropic effects. In combination with the peripheral β_2-induced vasodilation and resultant drop in systemic vascular resistance, an increase in cardiac output is seen. However, the positive inotropic and chronotropic effects dramatically increase myocardial oxygen consumption, which may already be compromised by the β_2-induced peripheral vasodilation, causing a decrease in diastolic blood pressure and ultimately a decrease in coronary artery perfusion. Furthermore, the patient who is hypovolemic may become hypotensive as a result of the peripheral vasodilation.

Isoproterenol is also a potent bronchial dilator and pulmonary vasodilator. Initially this may cause a drop in arterial oxygen tension secondary to ventilation-perfusion mismatch if supplemental oxygen is not administered.

The detrimental effects of isoproterenol on the heart, such as excessive tachycardia, induction of myocardial ischemia, and arrhythmia production, are the major factors limiting its use to the treatment of significant heart block unresponsive to atropine. Other side effects are similar to those seen with epinephrine but occur to a lesser extent. One difference is that the profound β stimulation of the pancreatic islet cells increases insulin secretion and diminishes the degree of hyperglycemia.

Dobutamine

Dobutamine is a synthetic sympathomimetic amine. It is a modification of isoproterenol, but its use currently is much more widespread than that of isoproterenol. Dobutamine is a primarily a β_1-agonist with some β_2 effects.[14] Consequently, dobutamine displays a strong inotropic response with minimal chronotropy. It also produces a slight drop in systemic vascular resistance, owing to peripheral vasodilation. However, the resultant increase in cardiac output compensates for the decrease in systemic vascular resistance, and the blood pressure is increased or, at low doses, relatively unchanged. Pulmonary artery pressure decreases, and an increase in left ventricular stroke work index is observed.[15]

The positive inotropic effects, coupled with the lack of chronotropy and maintenance of normal blood pressure, have made this agent a frequent choice in the treatment of acute congestive heart failure (CHF). Patients who do not have heart failure but do have coronary artery disease may develop myocardial ischemia if given dobutamine.[16] In hypovolemic patients, the decrease in systemic vascular response can become exacerbated, with a resultant drop in blood pressure. This decrease in blood pressure may also be seen in patients with sepsis.

Dobutamine enhances conduction through the atrioventricular node, necessitating that caution be exercised in patients with atrial fibrillation. Dobutamine-induced arrhythmias do occur, but the incidence is considerably less than that seen with the other sympathomimetic amines. Another potential side effect of dobutamine of interest to the anesthetist is platelet inhibition; however, the clinical significance of this inhibition is negligible.

DIRECT-ACTING α-AGONISTS

α₁-Agonists
Phenylephrine
Phenylephrine (Neo-Synephrine) is the most commonly employed pure α-agonist. Phenylephrine has strong α-stimulating effects, with virtually no β stimulation. A sharp rise in blood pressure is seen after administration; this rise is primarily the result of a significant increase in peripheral resistance secondary to the α_1 stimulation.

A reflex bradycardia can be elicited secondary to baroreceptor stimulation, and the anesthetist should allow for the return of an adequate baseline heart rate before using one of these agents. An antimuscarinic also can be used selectively in the treatment of bradycardia. Intravenous (IV) bolus administration of phenylephrine is frequently used, but caution should be used because profound increases in blood pressure and decreases in heart rate can result. The onset of action of IV phenylephrine is immediate, with the duration of action ranging from 5 to 20 minutes. Because of its vasoconstricting effects, phenylephrine is frequently used topically for the prevention of nosebleeds during nasal intubation.

α₂-Agonists
Clonidine
Clonidine (Catapres) is presynaptic α_2-agonist. Clonidine decreases blood pressure by acting as an agonist at peripheral presynaptic α_2-receptors and central α_2-receptors. Stimulation of the peripheral presynaptic α_2-receptors causes inhibition of catecholamine release, with subsequent vasodilation. Stimulation of the central α_2-receptors, which is considered the main antihypertensive mechanism of action, results in diminished sympathetic outflow and a resultant decrease in circulating catecholamines and renin activity. Rebound hypertension, seen after abrupt discontinuation of clonidine use, is a major concern. The resultant increase in catecholamine levels manifests as tachycardia and hypertension. Continuing the medication throughout the perioperative period is the desired approach. Tapering the dose and discontinuation may occasionally be indicated. Patches may also be used during surgery to prevent withdrawal.

Clonidine is available in oral and transdermal forms. The transdermal form is frequently encountered and administered at a fixed rate for a period of 1 week. Use of clonidine as a premedicant has been advocated by some because of the sedative and

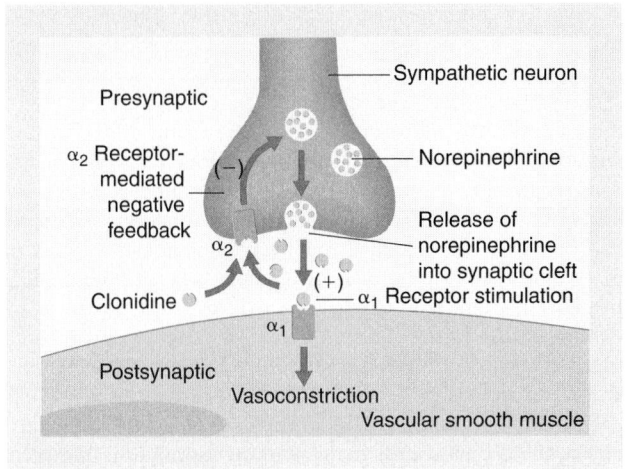

FIGURE **14-1** Presynaptic α_2 agonism. (*From Page C et al: Integrated Pharmacology. 2nd ed. Edinburgh: Mosby; 2002.*)

analgesic qualities of the agent.[17] Clonidine also is used as a catecholamine suppression test in the diagnosis of pheochromocytoma. A newer α_2-agonist, dexmedetomidine (Precedex), has been introduced for sedation in critical care. It is an IV infusion drug for short-term use.

Dexmedetomidine
Dexmedetomidine is an α_2-agonist that is marketed for short-term sedation in critical care. It is being used as an adjunct to anesthesia in a variety of situations.[18] Dexmedetomidine provides dose-dependent sedation, analgesia, sympatholysis and anxiolysis without significant respiratory depression. The side effects are predictable from the pharmacologic profile of α_2-adrenoceptor agonists and include hypotension, bradycardia, oversedation, and delayed recovery. It has been widely used to treat pediatric emergence delirium associated with general anesthesia. A prophylactic dose of 1 mcg/kg approximately 30 minutes prior to emergence is usually effective. Existing emergence delirium can be treated with a 0.125 mcg/kg bolus and repeated as needed to avoid oversedation.[19,20] Early promise is leading to many new perioperative applications.[21] The mechanism of presynaptic α_2 agonism is shown in Figure 14-1.

MIXED FUNCTION AGONISTS

Ephedrine
Ephedrine is a synthetic noncatecholamine sympathomimetic commonly used in anesthesia practice. It stimulates both α- and β-receptors directly, and it indirectly causes release of endogenous catecholamines, leading to multiple mechanisms of action. It has both central and peripheral actions. Ephedrine's effects are similar to those seen with epinephrine; however, they are lesser and not accompanied by a dramatic increase in serum glucose concentrations. The duration of action of ephedrine is also longer than that of epinephrine, owing to its lack of a basic catechol structure; this characteristic makes it resistant to metabolism by monoamine oxidase.

Ephedrine often is the first sympathomimetic chosen for alleviation of hypotension due to the cardiac-depressant effects of anesthetic agents or vasodilation resulting from spinal anesthesia. Intravenously administered ephedrine, in doses ranging from 10 to 25 mg, has an immediate onset and a duration of action of 1 to 1.5 hours. This drug should be used cautiously in patients with questionable coronary perfusion, because myocardial oxygen consumption may be more dramatically increased than is anticipated as a result of ephedrine's positive inotropic effect. In obstetrics, ephedrine has long been considered the drug of choice to address maternal hypotension following regional anesthesia, magnesium administration, or other causes. Newer data are questioning this long-standing practice, with phenylephrine being recommended over ephedrine.[22] As with any indirect-acting agent, tachyphylaxis may develop with subsequent dosing, because catecholamine stores become depleted. In addition, some authors believe that the tachyphylaxis seen with repeated dosing occurs because adrenergic receptors are still occupied; consequently, fewer receptors are available to bind with the drug.[23]

Ephedrine also may be administered by oral, intramuscular, or subcutaneous routes. Patients may receive long-term oral ephedrine for its bronchodilating effects secondary to β_2 stimulation.

SELECTIVE β_2-AGONISTS

The β_2-agonists include terbutaline (Brethine, Brethaire, Bricanyl), metaproterenol (Alupent, Metaprel), albuterol (Proventil, Ventolin), and salmeterol (Serevent). These "selective" β-agonists are effective in treating obstructive airway diseases such as asthma, chronic obstructive pulmonary disease, and acute bronchospasm.

The selectivity of these agents for β_2-receptors results in the desired response of bronchodilation and a lower incidence of the undesired β_1 responses of tachycardia and arrhythmia. As a result, these drugs have replaced epinephrine as the agent of choice for treatment of acute bronchospasm in anesthetic practice. All these agents are available in aerosol form, and it is widely accepted that aerosol delivery is as effective as subcutaneous or other means of administration. Drugs of this class also have an increased duration of action because of their noncatecholamine structure; this renders them resistant to methylation by catechol-O-methyltransferase.

Two puffs of nebulized or metered-dose inhaler–administered terbutaline, albuterol, or salmeterol 10 to 15 minutes before exercise have been shown to have similar efficacy in preventing exercise-induced asthma. However, salmeterol provides protection against bronchospasm for up to 12 hours, whereas terbutaline and albuterol have 2- to 2.5-hour durations of action.[24]

Chronic use of these agents can result in tachyphylaxis secondary to down-regulation (i.e., diminished quantity) of β-receptors. Increased hyperresponsiveness of the airway also has been suspected with chronic use of these agents. Salmeterol, the newest agent in this class, has been indicated for long-term use. Some investigators[25] have found it to be an effective β_2-agonist for long-term use because its effect is less diminished over time.[26] These drugs are frequently combined with a corticosteroid for chronic therapy.[27]

The β_2-agonists also are used for arresting premature labor. This is referred to as a *tocolytic effect*. Uterine relaxation is achieved through increases in the levels of cyclic adenosine monophosphate (cAMP); this decreases intracellular calcium levels and ultimately diminishes the level of actin-myosin coupling. Currently, terbutaline and ritodrine are used.

The parturient who receives a β_2-agonist usually shows some degree of both β_1 and β_2 stimulation. Common findings include tachycardia and increased cardiac output, along with a widened pulse pressure due to a lower diastolic pressure. Increased renin levels diminish the degree of urinary excretion of sodium and water, potentially increasing the risk of pulmonary edema if

fluids are not carefully titrated. Maternal hyperglycemia and hypokalemia also are seen. The total body potassium level is not altered, but an intracellular shift does occur. Ritodrine and terbutaline both freely cross the placenta. Contraindications to tocolytic therapy include fetal death or lethal abnormality, eclampsia, placental abruption, and proven chorioamnionitis. Relative contraindications are preeclampsia, severe chronic hypertension, renal disease, heart disease, fetal distress, and fetal growth retardation.[28] The effectiveness of tocolytic therapy was recently reviewed, with the following practice points: (1) β_2 agonists are effective in delaying delivery for 48 hours but have no effect on perinatal mortality. (2) There is no evidence to support the use of magnesium sulfate or the nitric oxide donors such as nitroglycerin. (3) Indomethacin is an effective tocolytic, but there are concerns about possible fetal and neonatal effects. (4) Nifedipine is an effective tocolytic with a low maternal side effect profile and positive effects on neonatal outcomes. (5) The oxytocin receptor antagonist atosiban is no better than other tocolytics in delaying or preventing preterm birth but has fewer maternal side effects.[29]

Nifedipine is recommended for initial tocolysis, given the oral route of administration, low frequency of side effects, and efficacy in reducing neonatal complications. Nifedipine can be used at any gestational age. For pregnancies of less than 32 weeks' gestation, a reasonable alternative to nifedipine is indomethacin or other COX inhibitors. These agents are more effective than the β-adrenergic receptor agonists in comparative studies. Indomethacin should be avoided in women with a platelet dysfunction or bleeding disorder, hepatic or renal dysfunction, gastrointestinal ulcerative disease, or aspirin-sensitive asthma. To avoid in utero closure or narrowing or neonatal patency of the ductus arteriosus, indomethacin and other COX inhibitors are not used in gestations of more than 32 weeks.[30] Doses of selected vasoactive drugs are listed in Table 14-3.

α-RECEPTOR ANTAGONISTS

The α-receptor antagonists are used for treatment of hypertension, benign prostatic hyperplasia, pheochromocytoma, Raynaud phenomenon, and ergot alkaloid toxicity.[31] Common side effects include orthostatic hypotension and baroreceptor-mediated reflex tachycardia, which may make their use in the treatment of hypertension somewhat difficult in the ambulatory patient. In addition, because of the significantly longer duration of action of the α-receptor antagonists, the direct vasodilators are considered more predictable in the treatment of emergent episodes of hypertension.

Phenoxybenzamine

Phenoxybenzamine (Dibenzyline) is a halo alkylamine with both α_1- and α_2-blocking activity. Its α-receptors are irreversibly bound by phenoxybenzamine, and its action is terminated only by metabolism of the drug and generation of additional α-receptors. Clinically this drug is used preoperatively in patients with pheochromocytoma for diminishing the response to endogenous catecholamines. The preoperative course is started 1 to 3 weeks before surgery, with the maximum oral dosage being 40 to 120 mg in two or three divided doses given daily. Phenoxybenzamine also prevents the sympathomimetic response expected from phenylephrine. The response to norepinephrine is limited to its β_1-agonist activity, and epinephrine may show "epi-reversal," which is an enhanced β_2 response with a worsening of hypotension and tachycardia. Nasal stuffiness has been frequently associated with phenoxybenzamine use.

TABLE **14-3**	Doses of Selected Vasoactive Drugs		
Drug	**Bolus Dose**	**Infusion Dose Rate**	**Comments**
Calcium chloride ($CaCl_2$) or gluconate	500-1000 mg (chloride)		Onset: <1 min Peak effect: <1 min Duration: 10-20 min
Dobutamine (Dobutrex)	500-2000 mg (gluconate)	2-20 mcg • kg^{-1} • min^{-1}	Onset: 1-2 min Peak effect: 1-10 min Duration: 10 min
Dopamine		1-2 mcg • kg^{-1} • min^{-1} (renal doses) 2-10 mcg • kg^{-1} • min^{-1} (cardiac doses) 10-20 mcg • kg^{-1} • min^{-1} (vasopressor doses)	Onset: 2-4 min Peak effect: 2-10 min Duration: <10 min
Ephedrine	5- to 10-mg incremental doses		Dilute to 5 or 10 mg • mL^{-1} Onset: <1 min Peak effect: 2-5 min Duration: 10-60 min
Epinephrine	10-100 mcg	0.01-0.03 mcg • kg^{-1} • min^{-1} (β doses) 0.03-0.15 mcg • kg^{-1} • min^{-1} (α and β doses) 0.15-0.3 mcg • kg^{-1} • min^{-1} (α doses)	Onset: <1 min Peak effect: 1-2 min Duration: 5-10 min
Fenoldopam		0.1-1.6 mg • kg • min	Onset: 4-5 min Peak effect: 7 min Duration: 15 min
Glucagon	1-5 mg over 2-5 min		
Isoproterenol (Isuprel)	1 mL over 1 min *after diluting* in 10 mL (= 0.02 mg • mL^{-1})	0.015-0.15 mcg • kg^{-1} • min^{-1}	Onset: <1 min Peak effect: 1 min Duration: 1-5 min
Milrinone (Primacor)	50 mcg • kg^{-1}	0.375-0.75 mcg • kg^{-1} • min^{-1}	
Nesiritide (Natrecor)		0.01 mcg • kg • min	Onset: 15 min Peak effect: 1 hr Duration: 60 min
Norepinephrine (Levophed)		0.01-0.2 mcg • kg^{-1} • min^{-1}	Onset: <1 min Peak effect: 1-2 min Duration: 2-10 min
Phentolamine	5 mg (50-100 mcg • kg^{-1}) Repeat as required	1-10 mcg • kg^{-1} • min^{-1}	Onset: 1-2 min Peak effect: 2 min Duration: 10-15 min
Phenylephrine (Neo-Synephrine)	40-100 mcg	0.15-0.75 mcg • kg^{-1} • min^{-1}	Onset: <1 min Peak effect: 1 min Duration: 15-20 min
Sodium nitroprusside (Nitropress)		0.1-10 mcg • kg^{-1} • min^{-1}	Onset: <1 min Peak effect: 1-2 min Duration: 1-10 min
Vasopressin (Pitressin)	10-20 units	0.1-1.0 units/min	Onset: 1-5 min Peak effect: 5 min Duration 10-30 min

Phentolamine

Phentolamine, an imidazole, is a competitive antagonist of α_1- and α_2-receptors. It has a rapid onset after IV administration and a much shorter duration of action when compared with phenoxybenzamine. It can be used for the short-term control of hypertension in patients with pheochromocytoma. The recommended dose is 1 to 5 mg by slow IV push. Phentolamine has also been used in the treatment of local infiltrations of vasoconstricting agents. Phentolamine (5 to 10 mg) can be mixed with 10 mL of normal saline and injected directly into the site of the infiltration.

Prazosin and Others

Prazosin (Minipress), doxazosin (Cardura), and terazosin (Hytrin) are selective α_1-antagonists used in the chronic treatment of hypertension. Their lack of α_2-blocking activity indicates that they have no effect on norepinephrine levels. Therefore, selectivity for α_1-receptors leaves the inhibitory action of α_2-receptors on norepinephrine release intact, and less norepinephrine-induced tachycardia results than when a nonselective α-antagonist is used. Prazosin induces vasodilation in both arterioles and veins. Peripheral vascular resistance and cardiac preload and afterload are diminished. The drugs are administered orally, and orthostatic hypotension can be a major side effect.

Droperidol

Droperidol (Inapsine), a butyrophenone, has been and continues to be used as an antiemetic and sedative agent in anesthesia practice. It also produces a minimal degree of α-adrenergic blockade and minimal reduction in blood pressure. Droperidol has proved to be useful clinically in the treatment of mild increases in blood pressure. Marked decreases in blood pressure in isolated patients may occur, especially in volume-depleted patients. The use of droperidol has decreased markedly as a result of the "black box" warning required by the U.S. Food and Drug Administration (FDA) as part of the package insert for this drug. Use of droperidol has been associated with prolongation of the corrected Q-T interval in certain patients, increasing the probability of the development of torsades de pointes, which has led to serious morbidity and death. There has been considerable debate regarding the relationship between the anesthetic administration of droperidol in very low doses as an antiemetic and the complications described.[32] Little doubt remains, however, that the potential for administrative and legal difficulties added to issues of patient safety have led to significant changes in the pattern of use of this drug.[33] A 12-lead electrocardiogram is required by the FDA prior to the use of droperidol. Off-labeled use of low doses as an antiemetic may still be useful. Evidence suggests that the serotonin type 3 receptor antagonists have a similar frequency of Q-T interval prolongation.[32] Fortunately, the FDA has recently agreed to revisit the issue of the cardiac effects of droperidol and the ominous restrictions placed on its use.

β-ADRENERGIC BLOCKING AGENTS

The β-blockers are one of the most widely prescribed classes of drugs. Common applications of these agents include the treatment of angina pectoris, hypertension, "fresh" myocardial infarctions, supraventricular tachycardias (including Wolff-Parkinson-White syndrome), and atrial fibrillation; the suppression of increased sympathetic activity (e.g., as occurs with intubation); the management of hypertrophic obstructive cardiomyopathies and CHF; the treatment of migraine headaches; and the preoperative preparation of hyperthyroid patients. Some authors also point out the effectiveness of β-blockers in the treatment of digitalis-induced arrhythmias and in the management of ventricular arrhythmias.[34] Substantial evidence supports the perioperative use of β-blockers in vascular and select general surgery patients to reduce cardiac perioperative mortality and ischemic complications by 15%.[27,35,36] The use of perioperative β-blockade in high-risk patients is discussed in Chapter 26.

The β-blockers are structurally related to isoproterenol. They bind β-receptors in a competitive manner and prevent the actions of catecholamines and other β-agonists. Because these agents are competitive antagonists, the law of mass action is applicable to their efficacy. If an agonist is present in sufficient concentration at the receptor, the blocking actions of the β-antagonists can be overcome.

The β-blockers are subdivided on the basis of their selectivity for cardiac β_1-receptors. Examples of cardioselective β_1-receptor antagonists include metoprolol (Lopressor), atenolol (Tenormin), acebutolol (Sectral), and esmolol (Brevibloc). Agents that block both β_1- and β_2-receptors include the prototype β-receptor antagonist propranolol (Inderal), as well as nadolol (Corgard), timolol (Blocadren), and pindolol (Visken). The degree of receptor selectivity is important because antagonism of β_1-receptors results in lowered heart rate, decreased myocardial contractility, and diminished atrioventricular conduction velocity; it also has beneficial effects with regard to decreasing myocardial oxygen consumption and the treatment of arrhythmias. However, antagonism of β_2-receptors can result in the unbeneficial effects of bronchoconstriction, hypoglycemia and peripheral vasoconstriction. It is important to note that as the dose of the selective β-blockers is increased, the degree of selectivity is diminished.

Some of the β-blockers act as partial agonists and as such possess intrinsic sympathomimetic activity. A partial agonist does not stimulate β-receptors to the extent that a full agonist does, and in the presence of a full agonist, the partial agonist acts as a competitive antagonist. It follows that β-blockers with intrinsic sympathomimetic activity (ISA) competitively antagonize the effects of a full agonist (e.g., endogenous catecholamines released during times of maximal sympathetic tone) down to the activity level of its partial agonist component. Intrinsic sympathomimetic activity minimizes the risk of bronchoconstriction in patients with reactive airway disease who require β-blockade. Pindolol, acebutolol, penbutolol, and carteolol are β-adrenergic blocking agents that possess intrinsic sympathomimetic activity.

Membrane-stabilizing activity is another property of some β-blockers. These agents diminish arrhythmogenicity by exerting a quinidine-like effect. However, membrane-stabilizing activity is seen only with high drug concentrations.[37] Propranolol and pindolol are two β-blockers with membrane-stabilizing activity. Bisoprolol has been shown to reduce the risk of myocardial infarction when administered before vascular surgery in high-risk patients.[38] Fifty-nine high-risk patients received 5 to 10 mg of bisoprolol versus placebo. A 3.4% mortality rate within 30 days occurred in the β-blocker–treated group versus 17% in the placebo group. Nebivolol (Bystolic) is a new cardioselective β-blocker approved for the treatment of hypertension. It is unique in that it has nitric oxide–mediated vasodilating properties.

Some potential problems with β-adrenergic blocking agents have already been mentioned. β-blockade can result in both

Beta Blockade Effects on Ischemic Heart

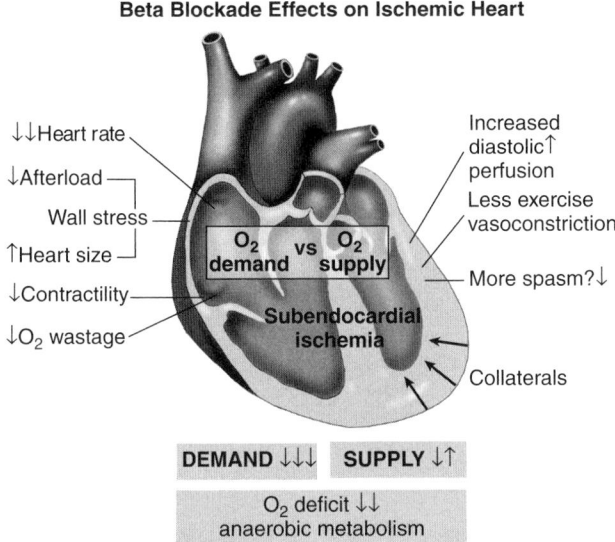

FIGURE **14-2** Effects of β-blocker aid the ischemic heart. (*Modified from Opie LH: Drugs for the Heart. 4th ed. Philadelphia: Saunders; 1995.*)

bronchospasm and the development of overt cardiac failure in some patients with high doses or IV administration. Other potential problems arise with β_2-receptor blockade in patients with peripheral vascular disease and Raynaud syndrome because of the possible potentiation of peripheral vasoconstriction. In diabetic patients, signs of hypoglycemia may be masked, and the patient's ability to increase serum glucose levels may be impaired. Serum potassium levels may also become elevated with β_2-blockade, because uptake into skeletal muscle is inhibited. In patients whose heart rate is controlled to maintain cardiac output, β-blockade may have a significant impact on blood pressure.

The β-receptors are considered to be "labile" receptors—that is, they are subject to significant up- and down-regulation. Chronic therapy with β-blockers can lead to up-regulation of β-receptors or an increase in the absolute number and activity of receptors. This phenomenon is suspected to be the underlying cause of the withdrawal syndrome seen with abrupt discontinuation of β-adrenergic antagonist use. This syndrome is characterized by increased sympathetic activity for up to 2 days. Obviously this means the patient receiving β-blockers should continue to receive them without interruption throughout the perioperative period. The effects of the β-blocking agents on the ischemic heart are summarized in Figure 14-2.

Propranolol, Metoprolol, and Esmolol

Three β-adrenergic blocking agents useful in the perioperative period are propranolol, metoprolol and esmolol. Propranolol may take up to 15 minutes to exert an effect. Its elimination half-life is approximately 4 hours, and its duration of action permits administration two to four times per day. The elimination of propranolol can be prolonged in patients with hepatic disease. Intravenous administration of propranolol is 1 to 5 mg, but most clinical practitioners start with 0.25 to 0.5 mg IV and titrate upward if needed. Esmolol has replaced propranolol in most instances of β-blocker application in anesthesia because of its rapid onset and short duration of action. Esmolol has an onset time of 2 minutes and an elimination half-life of

approximately 9 minutes. Its rapid onset and short half-life, as well as its duration of action of 10 to 15 minutes, make it easily and reliably titratable in acute-care situations. The recommended IV loading dose of esmolol is 500 mcg/kg; this is followed by an infusion of 100 to 300 mcg/kg/min. Most anesthesia practitioners start with a bolus of 10 to 15 mg and continue administration according to patient response. Esmolol is metabolized by nonspecific plasma esterases found in the cytosol of red blood cells. Metoprolol is frequently used following myocardial infarction or in some types of angina, once the patient is stable, to normalize vital signs. Administration of 5-mg doses intravenously at 5-minute intervals to a maximum dose of 15 mg is recommended.

Labetalol

Labetalol (Normodyne, Trandate) is classified as a nonselective β-blocker but is unique in that it also possesses an α-blocking component. It provides β-blockade along with α-blockade in a ratio of 7:1. Unlike the standard β-blocker, labetalol produces vasodilation secondary to its α-blocking properties. This action can be extremely beneficial in situations in which an acute rise in blood pressure could be devastating to the clinical outcome. The usual IV dose of labetalol is 0.25 mg/kg; this dose can be repeated every 10 minutes as indicated and followed by an infusion at a rate of 2 mg/min. In clinical practice, most practitioners use a bolus dose of labetalol (5-10 mg) and gauge follow-up administration on the basis of patient response. Labetalol can have a duration of action ranging from 2 to 18 hours, depending on dose. Because labetalol provides both β- and α-blockade, an adequate heart rate must be present before labetalol can be used in the acute management of hypertension. It should be noted that uterine blood flow is not affected in obstetric patients, even in the event of a dramatic decrease in systemic blood pressure.[39] Labetalol undergoes hepatic metabolism and renal elimination.[40] A new combined β- and α-blocker, carvedilol, has been introduced. It is available as an oral formulation for the treatment of hypertension and CHF.

CHOLINERGICS

Cholinergic agents mimic the actions of the neurotransmitter acetylcholine but have been developed to differ in terms of comparative nicotinic and muscarinic activity and duration of action. Acetylcholine (Miochol) has no clinical application, owing to its generalized enhancement of cholinergic effects throughout the body and its extremely short duration of action (approximately 1 ms), which is a result of its rapid metabolism by acetylcholinesterase.

Methacholine (Provocholine), carbachol (carbamylcholine chloride), and bethanechol (carbamylmethylcholine) are choline esters that have limited clinical applications. Methacholine can be used as an aerosol in the diagnosis of reactive airway disease, whereas carbachol, because of its significant muscarinic and nicotinic activity, is used only as a topical ophthalmic solution in the treatment of narrow-angle glaucoma and for inducing miosis during diagnostic testing and surgery. Bethanechol is theoretically useful in instances of ileus and urinary retention, such as in postvagotomy and postpartum patients, respectively. Bethanechol's relative lack of nicotinic activity makes it the most attractive of these three agents, and it is the agent most frequently encountered in clinical practice. Potential side effects of these agents include any cholinergic-induced response such as bradycardia, varying degrees of heart block, hypotension, bronchoconstriction, and an increase in gastric secretions.

ANTICHOLINERGICS

The anticholinergics are familiar agents in anesthesia practice and therefore are discussed only briefly. Atropine, scopolamine, and glycopyrrolate are the three anticholinergics used in anesthesia practice. These agents are competitive antagonists of acetylcholine at muscarinic receptors. A comparison of the basic properties of the anticholinergic agents is given in Table 14-4. Subtypes of muscarinic and nicotinic receptors are summarized in Table 14-5 and Table 14-6.

Atropine

Atropine, a belladonna alkaloid, is the prototype anticholinergic. The anesthetist can use atropine for its antisialagogue effects, for the prevention or treatment of bradycardia, and concurrently with anticholinesterase agents in the reversal of muscle relaxants for preventing the resultant bradycardia from anticholinesterase-induced acetylcholine buildup. The usual adult IV dose for increasing heart rate during anesthesia is 0.4 to 0.6 mg, with the time to onset being 1 to 2 minutes. Atropine is a tertiary amine; this allows it to cross the blood-brain barrier freely and may result in bradycardia when low doses are given. However, at usual clinical doses, significant central nervous system effects are rarely evident. Hepatic metabolism accounts for approximately half of a dose of atropine, with the remainder being eliminated unchanged in the urine. The elimination half-life of atropine is approximately 4 hours. Atropine should be avoided in patients with narrow-angle glaucoma, owing to its potential to increase intraocular pressure. Atropine poisoning or belladonna alkaloid toxicity manifests with extreme antimuscarinic effects, with potential progression to central nervous system depression and coma. The decades-old mnemonic "red as a beet, blind as a bat, dry as a bone, mad as a hatter, and hot as a hare" was devised to be an easy way to remember the signs and symptoms of belladonna overdose. These include flushing ("red as a beet"); extreme mydriasis ("blind as a bat"); lack of secretions and dry mouth ("dry as a bone"); confusion ("mad as a hatter"); and hyperthermia ("hot as a hare").

Scopolamine

Scopolamine (hyoscine) is another belladonna alkaloid with anticholinergic effects. Scopolamine is a tertiary amine. Compared

TABLE 14-4 Comparative Effects of Anticholinergic Drugs			
Effect	Atropine	Scopolamine	Glycopyrrolate
Sedation	+	+++	0
Antisialagogue	+	+++	++
Increase heart rate	+++	+	++
Relax smooth muscle	++	+	++
Mydriasis, cycloplegia	+	+++	0
Prevent motion-induced nausea	+	+++	0
Decrease gastric hydrogen ion secretion	+	+	+

TABLE 14-5 Properties of Muscarinic (M_1-M_5) Receptors					
	M_1	M_2	M_3	M_4	M_5
Location	CNS Stomach	Heart CNS	Glands GI, CNS	CNS Heart	CNS
Important clinical effects	Increased cognition and memory; gastric acid production	Bradycardia, smooth muscle contraction	Salivary secretions, bladder contraction	Promotes dopamine release	Promotes dopamine release, dilation of cerebral arteries

TABLE 14-6 Characteristics of Subtypes of Nicotinic Acetylcholine Receptors (nAChRs)		
Receptor Subtype	Main Synaptic Location	Membrane Response
Skeletal muscle (N_M)	Skeletal neuromuscular junction (postjunctional)	Excitatory; end-plate depolarization; skeletal muscle contraction
Peripheral neuronal (N_N)	Autonomic ganglia; adrenal medulla	Excitatory; depolarization; firing of postganglion neuron and secretion of catecholamines
Central nervous system (CNS)	CNS; pre- and postjunctional	Pre- and postsynaptic excitation Prejunctional control of transmitter release

with atropine, scopolamine has central nervous system effects that are much more pronounced at lower doses. Compared with atropine, it does not substantially increase heart rate. It can be used as a preoperative medication, with sedation and amnesia being a desirable effect. Scopolamine also is used to diminish the incidence of postoperative nausea and vomiting resulting from motion sickness. A scopolamine patch contains a total dose of 1.5 mg.

Glycopyrrolate

Glycopyrrolate (Robinul), a synthetic quaternary ammonium compound, has become the most frequently used anticholinergic in anesthesia practice. It has an excellent antisialagogue action,[41] with a longer duration of action than belladonna alkaloids. It prevents bradycardia without inducing significant levels of tachycardia. The quaternary ammonium structure of glycopyrrolate prevents it from crossing the blood-brain barrier to any significant degree; therefore, central nervous system effects are not seen. This property also makes it the agent of choice in obstetrics because it does not pass the placental barrier. Adult IV doses are generally 0.1 to 0.2 mg for antisialagogue activity and for the treatment of bradycardia. Onset of action is rapid, and the duration of action is up to 4 hours.

DIRECT VASODILATORS

Within this category, sodium nitroprusside, nitroglycerin, and hydralazine are the three drugs most commonly employed (Table 14-7). All three produce direct vasodilation. Sodium nitroprusside produces arterial and venous relaxation; nitroglycerin has a greater effect on venous than arterial relaxation; and hydralazine produces primarily arterial relaxation. The mechanism of action of all three agents is believed to be primarily an induced increase in the concentration of vascular nitric oxide, although that has not been confirmed with hydralazine.[42] The mechanism of action is described in Figure 14-3. The vasodilators nitroprusside and nitroglycerin are frequently used for controlled hypotension under anesthesia. Combined with the inhalation and intravenous anesthetics, they facilitate a reduction in blood loss and need for transfusions during a variety of surgical procedures.[43]

Nitrovasodilators
Sodium Nitroprusside

Sodium nitroprusside is frequently used for the emergent control of hypertension, for inducing hypotension to decrease blood loss during surgical procedures, and for the treatment of acute pulmonary edema. Its rapid onset (within seconds) and its short duration of action (1 to 3 minutes) make it unique among agents for the rapid control of blood pressure. Sodium nitroprusside reduces both afterload and preload, which results in a decrease in cardiac filling pressures and an increase in stroke volume and cardiac output. Left ventricular volumes are decreased, and diminished myocardial wall tension should contribute to a decrease in myocardial oxygen consumption.

Usually, sodium nitroprusside is started as an infusion at 0.5 mcg/kg/min and is titrated until a response occurs. An infusion rate of 3 mcg/kg/min is rarely exceeded, but young, normotensive patients may require up to 5 mcg/kg/min to achieve the desired response. A bolus dose of 1 to 2 mcg/kg has been found to be effective in blunting the hypertensive response to intubation.[44] Sodium nitroprusside is mixed with 5% dextrose in water, and the bottle and tubing are covered in a protective wrap; light causes the sodium nitroprusside to decompose. An infusion pump should

always be used with sodium nitroprusside because of its potency and the associated risk of cyanide toxicity.

Cyanide Toxicity. Sodium nitroprusside contains five cyanide ions within its chemical structure, and its metabolism by plasma hemoglobin causes the release of these cyanide ions. One cyanide ion binds methemoglobin to form cyanmethemoglobin, whereas the other four cyanide ions undergo rhodanese-catalyzed conversion to thiocyanate in the liver, with the thiocyanate undergoing renal elimination. This conversion to thiocyanate requires the cofactor thiosulfate B_{12}. Cyanide toxicity results when this metabolism is overwhelmed. Preventing cyanide toxicity from sodium nitroprusside begins with awareness of maximum doses and lengths of administration. In general, infusions of 8 to 10 mcg/kg/min for periods of 3 hours or longer should be avoided, and chronic administration should not exceed 0.5 mcg/kg/min. Clinically the development of metabolic acidosis, increased mixed venous oxygen content, tachycardia, and tachyphylaxis during sodium nitroprusside use are signs of cyanide toxicity.

Treatment of cyanide toxicity consists of discontinuing the sodium nitroprusside infusion, administering oxygen, and treating metabolic acidosis. Sodium nitrite 3%, 4 to 6 mg/kg, can be administered over 3 to 5 minutes to promote the production of methemoglobin so that excess cyanide ions can be bound. Sodium thiosulfate, 150 to 200 mg/kg over 15 minutes, can be administered every 2 hours as needed; vitamin B_{12} also can be administered. If available, hydroxycobalamin can be used. Methylene blue may also be useful.

Nitroglycerin

Nitroglycerin is used in the treatment of angina pectoris and ischemia under anesthesia and also can be used for lowering blood pressure. Nitroglycerin causes venodilation, with an increase in venous capacitance and a resultant decrease in preload.[45] This results in a lowering of cardiac filling pressures, a lessening of myocardial wall tension, and ultimately a decrease in myocardial oxygen requirements. Nitroglycerin's mechanism of action in the relief of angina is not a significant increase in coronary artery blood flow, which may actually be decreased during an infusion of nitroglycerin, but rather the aforementioned decrease in preload. Some of the larger coronary vessels may become dilated, with a resultant redirection and increase in blood flow to ischemic myocardium. At relatively high concentrations of nitroglycerin, arterial vasodilation also can occur.

Use of sublingual nitroglycerin (0.3-mg tablets), up to a total of three tablets, is the most efficient treatment for acute angina. Relief is generally achieved in 1 to 2 minutes and lasts up to 30 minutes. IV nitroglycerin also has an onset time of 1 to 2 minutes and a duration of action of up to 10 minutes. Nitroglycerin is extensively metabolized in the liver and has a half-life of only 3 minutes.[46] IV nitroglycerin is used for "unloading" of the heart in CHF and myocardial infarction. Nitroglycerin infusions are usually started at 5 to 10 mcg/min and titrated until effective. IV nitroglycerin can also be used for controlled hypotension but is not as potent in this regard as an infusion of sodium nitroprusside. Because nitroglycerin exerts its main effect on venous capacitance, any decrease in blood pressure is more volume dependent when compared with sodium nitroprusside–induced hypotension. Of note to the anesthesia provider is the ability of nitroglycerin to relax the smooth muscle of the biliary tract and provide relief from narcotic-induced biliary spasm. It also should be noted that nitroglycerin, as well as sodium nitroprusside, can cause mild cerebral steal in patients with cerebral injury, although the clinical significance

TABLE 14-7	Drugs Used in the Perioperative Management of Congestive Heart Failure				
Drug	Mechanism	Preload Reduction	Afterload Reduction	Usual Dose	
Renin-Angiotensin System Antagonists					
Captopril	Inhibition of renal systemic and tissue generation of angiotensin II by ACE; decreased metabolism of bradykinin	++	++	6.25-50 mg PO q8h	
Enalaprilat		++	++	2.5-10 mg PO q12h	
Quinapril		++	++	0.5-2.0 mg IV q12h	
Lisinopril		++	++	10-80 mg PO daily	
Ramipril		++	++	2.5-50 mg PO q12-24h	
Benazepril		++	++	10-40 mg in one or three doses	
Fosinopril		++	++	10-40 mg in one or two doses	
Moexipril		++	++	7.5-30 mg in one or two doses	
Perindopril		++	++	4-8 mg in one or two doses	
Trandolapril		++	++	1-4 mg in one dose	
Losartan	Blockade of angiotensin II (AT I) receptors	++	++	25-50 mg q12h	
Candesartan		++	++	8-32 mg in one dose	
Eprosartan		++	++	400-800 mg in one or two doses	
Irbesartan		++	++	150-300 mg in one dose	
Telmisartan		++	++	40-80 mg in one dose	
Valsartan		++	++	80-320 mg in one dose	
Direct Nitrovasodilators					
Nitroglycerin	Nitric oxide donors	+++	+	0.2-10 mcg/kg/min IV, 5-6 mg transdermal	
Isosorbide dinitrate		+++	+	10-60 mg qid	
Nitroprusside		+++	+++	0.1-3 mcg/kg/min IV	
		+++	+++		
Direct Vasodilator					
Hydralazine	Unclear	+	+++	10-100 PO q6h	
Calcium Channel Blocking Drug					
Amlodipine	Inhibition of L-type voltage-sensitive Ca^{2+} channels	+	+++	5-10 mg PO daily	
Phosphodiesterase Inhibitors					
Milrinone		++	++	50 mcg/kg, then 0.25-1 mcg/kg/min IV	
Sympathomimetics					
Dobutamine	Myocardial and vascular β-adrenergic agonist	+	++	2-20 mcg/kg/min	
Dopamine	Selective renal arterial vasodilation	−	−−	≤2 mcg/kg/min	
	Inotropic action	−	−	5-10 mcg/kg/min	
	β-receptor mediated				
	α-receptor mediated vasoconstriction	+	+	>15 mcg/kg/min	
Sympatholytics					
Prazosin (and other quinazoline derivatives)	α-Adrenergic receptor antagonist	++	++	1-5 mg PO q12h	
Labetalol	Combined β- and α-adrenergic blockade	+	+	12.5-50 mg PO bid	
Carvedilol		+	+	3.125-50 mg in two doses (titrate up every 2 wk)	
Bucindolol	Additional mechanisms	+	++	6.25-100 mg PO bid	

Modified from Treatment guidelines: drugs for treatment of heart failure. Med Lett. 2006;4(41):1-4.
ACE, Angiotensin-converting enzyme; bid, twice a day; IV, intravenous; PO, oral; qid, four times a day.

seems minimal.[47] Generally, 50 mg of nitroglycerin is mixed with 250 mL of dextrose 5% in water.[48] For extended coverage, nitroglycerin patches and ointments are also available (Table 14-8). A summary of antihypertensive agents dosing information is found in Table 14-9.

Hydralazine

Hydralazine causes direct relaxation of arterial smooth muscle. It can be administered intravenously for the control of hypertension in doses ranging from 2.5 to 20 mg. Tachycardia frequently accompanies the decrease in blood pressure. It is important to remember that the onset of action can occur from 2 to 20 minutes after administration; therefore; adequate time should be allowed before the initiation of repeat dosing so that profound decreases in blood pressure can be prevented. The elimination half-life in plasma is approximately 1 hour, but the duration of vasodilating action can be as long as 12 hours.[49-51] Hydralazine undergoes hepatic metabolism with renal excretion. Acetylation is partly responsible for the metabolism of hydralazine. Slow acetylators may be more prone to a drug-induced lupus syndrome that can result from high serum concentrations of hydralazine during chronic treatment.

CALCIUM ANTAGONISTS

The calcium antagonists have proved to be useful pharmacologic agents in the treatment of angina, hypertension, arrhythmias, peripheral vascular disease, esophageal spasm, and controlled hypotension and in blocking the stress response for intubation and skin incision.[52] The five calcium antagonists most likely to be encountered in clinical practice are of three chemical classes: nifedipine (Adalat, Procardia), nicardipine (Cardene), amlodipine (Norvasc), felodipine (Plendil), nisoldipine (Sular), and nimodipine (Nimotop) are 1,4-dihydropyridine derivatives; diltiazem (Cardizem) is a benzothiazepine derivative; and verapamil (Calan, Isoptin) is a phenylalkylamine derivative. In anesthesia practice, nicardipine for the control of blood pressure, nimodipine for treatment of cerebral vasospasm, and verapamil for the control of atrial tachyarrhythmias are the most commonly used calcium antagonists.

A discussion of the generalized mechanism of action of the calcium antagonists is necessary for a better understanding of their role. Depolarization of the sinoatrial and atrioventricular nodes is dependent on the inward flux of calcium during the phase 2 plateau of the cardiac action potential. Calcium antagonists "block" these channels, diminishing the inward flux of calcium and prolonging phase 2, and in this way exert a negative chronotropic effect on the heart. Ventricular pacemaker foci are dependent on the inward flux of sodium, which is minimally if at all affected by the calcium antagonists. It then follows that the calcium antagonists are effective in patients with atrial tachyarrhythmias but could be detrimental if used in patients with ventricular tachycardias. In clinical doses, verapamil exerts the greatest antiarrhythmic effect and has been found to be effective in treating atrial tachyarrhythmias (including Wolff-Parkinson-

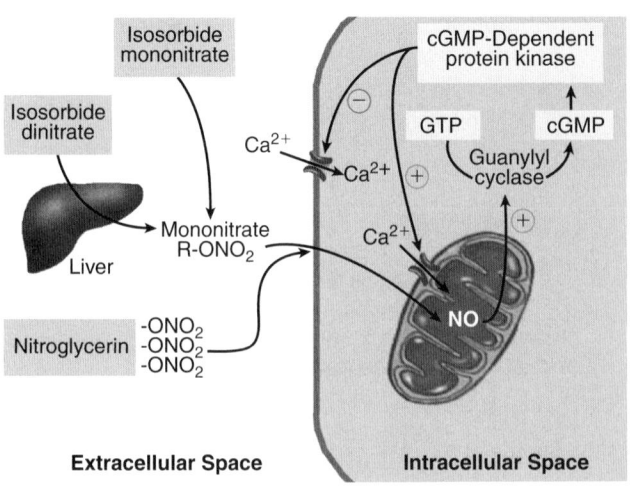

FIGURE 14-3 Mechanism of action of nitrates. (*Modified from Gori T, Parker JD: Nitrate tolerance: a unifying hypothesis. Circulation. 2002;106:2510; and Opie LH: Drugs for the Heart. 4th ed. Philadelphia: Saunders; 1995.*)

TABLE **14-8**	Pharmacologic Characteristics of Currently Available Nitrates			
Agent	**Dose**	**Dosing Interval**	**Onset of Action**	**Duration of Action**
Nitroglycerin				
Sublingual	0.15-0.6 mg	prn	1-5 min	10-30 min
Sublingual spray	0.4 mg/spray	prn	2-5 min	10-30 min
Buccal	1-3 mg	prn or q4-5h (while awake)	2-5 min	3-5 hr
Oral SR	2.6-13 mg	tid, qid	30-45 min	2-8 hr
Transdermal patches	2.5-15 mg/24 hr (1 patch)	daily (12 hr on/12 hr off)	30-60 min	8-14 hr
2% Ointment	0.5-2 in	q6h (daytime)	20-60 min	3-8 hr
Isosorbide Dinitrate				
Sublingual	2.5-10 mg	prn	3-15 min	1-2 hr
Chewable	5-10 mg	prn	3-15 min	1-2 hr
Oral	5-40 mg	bid, tid	15-30 min	3-6 hr
Oral SR	40 mg	daily	30-60 min	6-10 hr
Isosorbide Mononitrate				
Oral	10-20 mg	bid	30 min	6-8 hr
Oral SR	60 mg	daily	30 min	6-10 hr

bid, *Twice a day*; prn, *as needed*; qid, *four times a day*; tid, *three times a day.*

TABLE 14-9	Antihypertensive Drugs	
Drug	**Daily Adult Maintenance Dosage**	**Frequent or Severe Adverse Effects**
Angiotension-Converting Enzyme (ACE) Inhibitors		
Benazepril (Lotensin)	10-40 mg in one or two doses	Cough; hypotension, particularly with a diuretic or volume depletion; rash; acute renal failure with bilateral renal artery stenosis or stenosis of the artery to a solitary kidney; angioedema; hyperkalemia if also taking potassium supplements or potassium-sparing diuretics; loss of taste, usually not severe; blood dyscrasias and renal damage rare, except in patients with renal dysfunction; increased fetal mortality with second- and third-trimester exposure; may decrease excretion of lithium
Captopril (Capoten)	12.5-150 mg in two or three doses	
Enalapril (Vasotec)	2.5-40 mg in one or two doses	
Fosinopril (Monopril)	10-40 mg in one or two doses	
Lisinopril (Prinivil or Zestril)	5-40 mg in one dose	
Moexipril (Univasc)	7.5-30 mg in one or two doses	
Perindopril (Aceon)	4-8 mg in one or two doses	
Quinapril (Accupril)	5-80 mg in one or two doses	
Ramipril (Altace)	1.25-20 mg in one or two doses	
Trandolapril (Mavik)	1-4 mg in one dose	
Angiotensin-Receptor Antagonists		
Candesartan cilexetil (Atacand)	8-32 mg in one dose	Similar to ACE inhibitors but do not cause cough
Eprosartan (Teveten)	400-800 mg in one or two doses	
Irbesartan (Avapro)	150-300 mg in one dose	
Losartan (Cozaar)	25-100 mg in one or two doses	
Olmesartan (Benicar)	20-40 mg in one dose	
Telmisartan (Micardis)	40-80 mg in one dose	
Valsartan (Diovan)	80-320 mg in one dose	
β-Adrenergic Blocking Drugs		
Atenolol (Tenormin)	25-100 mg in one or two doses	Fatigue; depression; bradycardia; decreased exercise tolerance; congestive heart failure; aggravate peripheral arterial insufficiency; aggravate allergic reactions; bronchospasm; mask symptoms of and delay in recovery from hypoglycemia; Raynaud phenomenon; insomnia; vivid dreams or hallucinations; acute mental disorder; impotence; increased serum triglycerides
Betaxolol (Kerlone)	5-40 mg in one dose	
Bisoprolol (Zebeta)	5-20 mg in one dose	
Metoprolol (Lopressor, Toprol-XL)	50-200 mg in one or two doses	
Nadolol (Corgard)	50-400 mg in one dose	
Propranolol (Inderal)	20-240 mg in one dose	
Timolol (Blocadren)	40-240 mg in two doses	
	10-40 mg in two doses	
β-Adrenergic Blocking Drugs with Intrinsic Sympathomimetic Activity		
Acebutolol (Sectral)	200-1200 mg in one or two doses	Similar to other β-adrenergic blocking drugs but with less resting bradycardia and lipid changes; acebutolol has been associated with positive antinuclear antibody test and occasional drug-induced lupus
Carteolol (Cartrol)	2.5-10 mg in one dose	
Penbutolol (Levatol)	20 mg in one dose	
Pindolol (Visken)	10-60 mg in two doses	
α- and β-Blockers		
Carvedilol (Coreg)	12.5-50 mg in two doses	Similar to other β-adrenergic blocking drugs, but more orthostatic hypotension; no affect on serum lipids
β-Blocker Nitrovasodilator		
Nebivolol (Bystolic)	5-40 mg once	Vasodilator due to nitric oxide mediated action
Thiazide-Type Diuretics (Usually Once Daily)		
Chlorothiazide (Diuril)	125-500 mg	Hyperuricemia; hypokalemia; hypomagnesemia; hyperglycemia; hyponatremia; hypercholesterolemia; hypertriglyceridemia; pancreatitis; rashes and other allergic reactions; sexual dysfunction; photosensitivity reactions; may decrease excretion of lithium
Hydrochlorothiazide (Microzide)	12.5-50 mg	
Chlorthalidone (Hygroton)	12.5-50 mg	
Indapamide (Lozol)	1.25-5 mg	
Metolazone (Zaroxolyn)	1.25-5 mg	
Loop Diuretics		
Bumetanide (generic tablets)	0.5-2 mg in two or three doses	Dehydration; circulatory collapse; hypokalemia; hyponatremia; hypomagnesemia; hyperglycemia; metabolic alkalosis; hyperuricemia; blood dyscrasias; rashes; lipid changes as with thiazide-type diuretics
Ethacrynic acid (Edecrin)	25-100 mg in two or three doses	
Furosemide (Lasix)	20-320 mg in two or three doses	
Torsemide (Demadex)	5-20 mg in one or two doses	
Potassium-Sparing Diuretics		
Amiloride (Midamor)	5-10 mg in one or two doses	Hyperkalemia; GI disturbances; rash; headache

From Medical Letter Treatment Guidelines. Drugs for hypertension. Med Lett. 2005;3(4):39-48. With permission. Aliskiren (Tekturna) for hypertension. Med Lett. 2007;49(1258):29-31. Nebivolol (Bystolic) for hypertension. Med. Lett. 2008;50(1281):17-19.
AV, Atrioventricular; CNS, central nervous system; GI, gastrointestinal; HDL, high-density lipoprotein.

| TABLE **14-9** | Antihypertensive Drugs—cont'd |

Drug	Daily Adult Maintenance Dosage	Frequent or Severe Adverse Effects
Eplerenone (Inspra)	25-100 mg in one or two doses	Hyperkalemia; hypernatremia
Spironolactone (Aldactone)	12.5-100 mg in one or two doses	Hyperkalemia; hyponatremia; mastodynia; gynecomastia; menstrual abnormalities; GI disturbances; rash
Triamterene (Dyrenium)	50-150 mg in one or two doses	Hyperkalemia; GI disturbances; nephrolithiasis
Calcium Channel Blockers		
Diltiazem (Cardizem CD)	120-360 mg in two doses	Dizziness; headache; edema; constipation (especially verapamil); AV block; bradycardia; heart failure; lupus-like rash with diltiazem
(Dilacor)	120-480 mg in one dose	
(Diltia XT)	120-480 mg in one dose	
(Tiazac)	120-480 mg in one dose	
Verapamil (Calan)	120-480 mg in two or three doses	
(Calan SR)	120-480 mg in one or two doses	
(Isoptin SR)	120-480 mg in one or two doses	
(Verelan)	120-480 mg in one dose	
(Covera HS)	180-480 mg in one dose	
Dihydropyridines		
Amlodipine (Norvasc)	2.5-10 mg in one dose	Dizziness; headache; peripheral edema (more than with verapamil and diltiazem; more common in women); flushing; tachycardia; rash; gingival hyperplasia
Felodipine (Plendil)	2.5-10 mg in one dose	
Isradipine (DynaCirc, DynaCirc CR)	5-10 mg in two doses	
Nicardipine (Cardene, Cardene SR)	5-10 mg in one dose	
Nifedipine (Adalat CC, Procardia XL)	60-120 mg in three doses	
Nisoldipine (Sular)	60-120 mg in two doses	
	30-90 mg in one dose	
	30-90 mg in one dose	
	10-60 mg in one dose	
α-Adrenergic Blockers		
Prazosin (Minipress)	First day: 1 mg at bedtime	Syncope with first dose; dizziness and vertigo; headache; palpitations; fluid retention; drowsiness; weakness; anticholinergic effects; priapism
Terazosin (Hytrin)	Maintenance: 1-2 mg in two or three doses	Both similar to prazosin, but with less hypotension after first dose
Doxazosin (Cardura)	First day: 1 mg at bedtime	
	Maintenance: 1-20 mg in one dose	
	First day: 1 mg at bedtime	
	Maintenance: 1-6 mg in one dose	
Central α-Adrenergic Agonists		
Clonidine (Catapres)	0.1-0.6 mg in two or three doses	CNS reactions similar to methyldopa, but more sedation and dry mouth; bradycardia; heart block; rebound hypertension (less likely with patches); contact dermatitis from patches
(Catapres TTS)	One patch weekly (0.1-0.3 mg/day)	Similar to clonidine
Guanabenz (Wytensin)	4-64 mg in two doses	Similar to clonidine but milder
Guanfacine (Tenex)	1-3 mg in one dose	Drowsiness; sedation, fatigue; depression; dry mouth; heart block; autoimmune disorders, including colitis, hepatitis, hepatic necrosis; Coombs-positive hemolytic anemia; lupus-like syndrome; thrombocytopenia; red cell aplasia; impotence
Methyldopate (Aldomet)	250 mg-2g in 2-4 doses	
Direct Vasodilators		
Hydralazine (Apresoline)	40-200 mg in two to four doses	Tachycardia; aggravation of angina; headache; dizziness; fluid retention; nasal congestion; lupus-like syndrome; hepatitis
Minoxidil (Loniten)	2.5-40 mg in one or two doses	Tachycardia; aggravation of angina; marked fluid retention; pericardial effusion; hair growth on face and body
Peripheral Adrenergic Neuron Antagonists		
Guanadrel (Hylorel)	10-75 mg in two doses	Similar to guanethidine, but less diarrhea
Renin Inhibitor		
Aliskiren (Tekturna)	150-300 mg once daily	

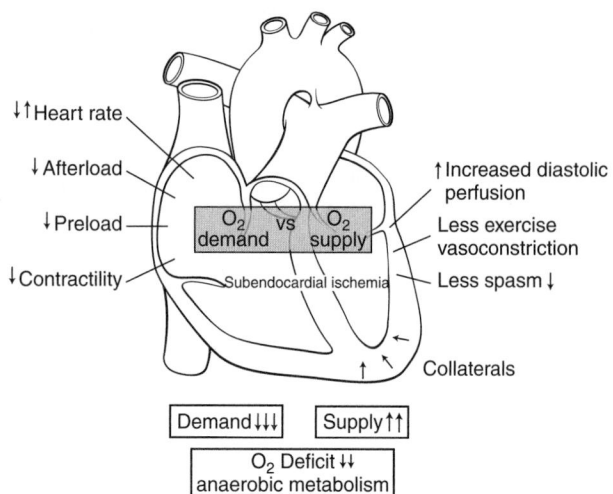

FIGURE **14-4**   Effects of calcium channel blockers on the ischemic heart.

White syndrome) and in controlling the ventricular response to atrial fibrillation and flutter. Verapamil is not indicated for the treatment of atrial fibrillation associated with Wolff-Parkinson-White syndrome, nor is it indicated for the treatment of "simple" atrial tachycardia, for which β-blockers may be a better choice.

Calcium antagonists also exert a negative inotropic effect on the heart, which can be beneficial in patients with angina. Cardiac contractility is dependent on the influx of calcium into cardiac cells. The calcium binds with the regulatory protein troponin, neutralizing troponin's inhibitory influence on the interaction between the structural proteins actin and myosin. The greater the degree of interaction between actin and myosin, the greater the degree of cardiac contraction. It follows that the calcium antagonists, by diminishing the influx of calcium into cardiac cells, diminish the degree of cardiac contractility. This negative inotropic effect then leads to a decrease in myocardial oxygen consumption. However, it should be noted that a significant decrease in cardiac contractility could prove to be detrimental in patients with CHF.

Calcium antagonists produce relaxation of vascular smooth muscle tone. Cytoplasmic calcium concentrations play an important role in the degree of vascular smooth muscle tension. Calcium antagonists, by diminishing the concentration of cytoplasmic calcium concentrations, induce vascular dilation or relaxation. Peripheral arteries are affected, with a resultant decrease in afterload and blood pressure, which contributes to an increase in cardiac output and a decrease in myocardial work and oxygen consumption. Coronary arteries also are affected, with an increase in coronary blood flow. The calcium antagonists have been found to be especially beneficial in the prevention of angina resulting from spasm of the coronary arteries, such as Prinzmetal angina.

Most calcium antagonists induce vascular smooth muscle relaxation, except for verapamil, which has virtually no effect. Nimodipine has been found to be beneficial in the prevention of cerebral vasospasm associated with acute subarachnoid hemorrhage.[53]

Verapamil, 2.5 to 10 mg intravenously (dose can be repeated every 30 minutes), can be given for the treatment of atrial tachyarrhythmias. The onset time is up to 10 minutes, and the duration of action ranges from 2 to 4 hours. Verapamil is metabolized hepatically, has an elimination half-life of 4 to 7 hours, and is renally eliminated. Verapamil has been largely replaced by adenosine as the first-line drug of choice in the emergent treatment of atrial tachyarrhythmias. Nicardipine is also useful as an IV preparation for the treatment of hypertension or controlled hypotension under anesthesia.[54-56] The effects of calcium channel blockers on the ischemic heart are summarized in Figure 14-4.

Varying degrees of atrioventricular block, myocardial depression, and hypotension are associated with the use of the calcium antagonists. An additive effect should be anticipated if the calcium antagonists are used with other cardiodepressant agents. In addition, verapamil and nifedipine can increase serum digoxin levels by up to 30%.[57] Calcium antagonists may also potentiate muscle relaxants, but this effect is minimal at clinically relevant doses.[58] It is interesting to note that hemodynamic but not electrophysiologic effects of the calcium antagonists can be reversed with the administration of calcium (Table 14-10).[59]

ANGIOTENSIN-CONVERTING ENZYME INHIBITORS

Angiotensin-converting enzyme (ACE) inhibitors have proved useful in the treatment of hypertension and CHF and in the management of the post–myocardial infarction patient.[60] These drugs exert their action by inhibiting the ACE peptidyl-dipeptidase. A brief description of the renin-angiotensin system is necessary for a full understanding of the actions of the ACE inhibitors (Figure 14-5).

Renin, a proteolytic protein, is released from the juxtaglomerular apparatus in response to diminished blood pressure. Renin is responsible for the conversion of angiotensinogen to the decapeptide angiotensin I. Angiotensin I is then converted to the octapeptide angiotensin II by peptidyl-dipeptidase, which is primarily located in the endothelial tissue of the lung. Angiotensin II is a potent vasopressor that also stimulates the release of endogenous norepinephrine and aldosterone. The end result is an increase in peripheral vasoconstriction, with an increase in blood pressure and a resultant decrease in cardiac output. The increased aldosterone level results in increased sodium and water reabsorption, with concomitant secretion of potassium. Ultimately, angiotensin II is converted to angiotensin III via the activities of aminopeptidase. Angiotensin III retains most of the potency of angiotensin II[61] and is ultimately degraded to peptide fragments through the actions of angiotensinase. Peptidyl-dipeptidase is also responsible for the metabolism of bradykinin, which has potent vasodilatory effects. Of interest, the majority of people with hypertension do not have high serum levels of renin, but the ACE inhibitors have been shown to be effective in all patients with hypertension.[62]

Common ACE inhibitors are listed in Table 14-9. Enalapril and lisinopril usually require administration only once per day. Enalapril is a prodrug, and it undergoes hepatic metabolism to its active form of enalaprilat. Enalaprilat is currently the only ACE inhibitor available for IV administration; it is available for use in perioperative hypertension but rarely used. All of these agents are renally eliminated, and their elimination half-lives can be expected to be prolonged in renally compromised patients. Potential problems with the ACE inhibitors include cough, angioedema, hyperkalemia, neutropenia, and proteinuria. Drug-induced renal failure also can be seen, especially in patients with renal artery stenosis, which is usually reversible with discontinuation of ACE inhibitor therapy. Interaction between the anesthetic agents and the ACE inhibitors has been suspected to

TABLE **14-10**	Drugs of Choice for Common Arrhythmias		
Arrhythmia	**Drug of Choice**	**Alternatives**	**Remarks**
Atrial fibrillation or flutter	*Rate control:* IV verapamil, diltiazem, β-blocker or digoxin	IV procainamide or ibutilide; dofetilide; single large oral dose of propafenone or flecainide	Amiodarone also may slow ventricular response, and conversion to normal rhythm can occur, but generally after delay of several hours
Acute management	*Conversion:* DC cardioversion		Ibutilide infusion may increase effectiveness of DC cardioversion
			Incidence of atrial fibrillation following cardiac surgery can be reduced by preoperative sotalol, amiodarone, or a β-blocker
Chronic treatment	*Rate control:* verapamil, diltiazem, a β-blocker, or digoxin	Quinidine, procainamide, disopyramide	Radiofrequency ablation may be effective in selected patients
	Maintenance of sinus rhythm: amiodarone, sotalol, flecainide, propafenone, or dofetilide		
Supraventricular tachycardias Acute management	IV adenosine, verapamil, or diltiazem	IV esmolol, another β-blocker, or digoxin for termination	Direct current cardioversion or atrial pacing may be effective for some patients; only rarely required
Long-term suppression	β-blockers, verapamil, diltiazem, flecainide, propafenone, amiodarone, sotalol, or digoxin	Quinidine, procainamide or disopyramide	Radiofrequency ablation can cure many patients
Premature ventricular complexes (PVCs) or nonsustained ventricular tachycardia	*Asymptomatic patients* without structural heart disease: no drug therapy indicated *Symptomatic patients:* β-blocker	Lidocaine IV for acute suppression under anesthesia	No evidence that prolonged suppression with drugs improves survival; for post-MI patients, treatment with a β-blocker has decreased mortality, treatment with flecainide or moricizine has increased it
Sustained ventricular tachycardia	Amiodarone	Procainamide, lidocaine	Long-term therapy ICD, amiodarone
Ventricular fibrillation	*Prevention of recurrence:* amiodarone	Procainamide, lidocaine	Long-term therapy ICD, amiodarone
Cardiac glycoside–induced ventricular tachyarrhythmias	Digoxin-immune Fab (digoxin antibody fragments—Digibind, DigiFab)		Self-limited if digoxin stopped; avoid direct current cardioversion, except for ventricular fibrillation or sustained ventricular tachycardia. A β-blocker or procainamide can make heart block worse.
Drug-induced torsades de pointes	IV magnesium sulfate	Cardiac pacing, isoproterenol	Causative agents should be discontinued; magnesium sulfate may be effective, even in absence of hypomagnesemia; potassium should be used to raise serum K to 4.5 to 5.0 mEq/L

Adapted from Medical Letter Treatment Guidelines. Drugs for cardiac arrhythmias. Med Lett. 2007;5(58):51-58.
ICD, *Implantable cardioverter/defibrillator;* IV, *intravenous;* MI, *myocardial infarction.*

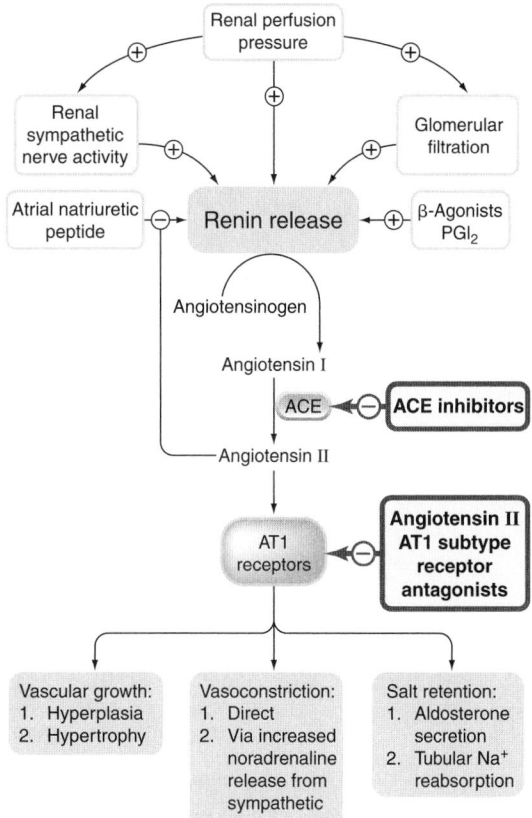

FIGURE **14-5** Renin-angiotensin system. Angiotensin-converting enzyme (ACE) inhibitors block the conversion of angiotensin I to angiotensin II. Angiotensin receptor blockers act as antagonists at the (AT1) receptors. (*From Rang HP et al. Rang and Dale's Pharmacology. 6th ed. Edinburgh: Churchill Livingstone; 2007.*)

lead to bradycardia and hypotension during the perioperative period.[63] The patient receiving an ACE inhibitor also is frequently being treated with a β-blocker and a diuretic. The interaction of these three pharmacologic classes should be considered. ACE inhibitors have been associated with adverse outcomes in obstetric patients and are contraindicated.

ANGIOTENSIN II RECEPTOR ANTAGONISTS

Several angiotensin receptor blockers (ARBs) have been introduced (see Table 14-9 and Figure 14-5). ARBs are receptor antagonists that interfere with binding at angiotensin II subtype 1 (AT_1) receptors; they are effective for lowering blood pressure without the cough and angioedema associated with ACE inhibitors. ACE inhibitors, but not ARBs, prevent formation of angiotensin II, but angiotensin II is also formed by other enzymes. ACE inhibitors also prevent the breakdown of bradykinin and substance P, which accumulate and are thought to cause the troublesome cough response. This blockade, which the angiotensin II receptor antagonists do not produce, may also contribute to the cardiac and renal protective effects of the ACE inhibitors.[64] Due to cost, the ARBs are usually reserved for patients who cannot tolerate an ACE inhibitor.[65]

CATECHOLAMINE-DEPLETING AGENTS

Catecholamine-depleting agents are rarely encountered in anesthesia practice, but the anesthetist should be familiar with their mechanism of action. The classic member of this group is reserpine. Reserpine blocks the uptake of catecholamines into storage vesicles within the presynaptic adrenergic neuron. This exposes the catecholamines to metabolism by monoamine oxidase in the axoplasm. This "catecholamine depletion" is responsible for reserpine's antihypertensive action.

TYROSINE HYDROXYLASE INHIBITORS

Metyrosine (Demser) is the only tyrosine hydroxylase inhibitor. Tyrosine hydroxylase is responsible for catalyzing the conversion of tyrosine to dopa and is considered the rate-limiting step in the synthesis of catecholamines. Inhibition of tyrosine hydroxylase results in a decrease in circulating catecholamine levels.

CATECHOL-*O*-METHYLTRANSFERASE INHIBITORS

Tolcapone (Tasmar) and entacapone (Comtan) have been introduced for the treatment of Parkinson disease as an adjunct to levodopa or carbidopa therapy. They are selective and reversible inhibitors of catechol-O-methyltransferase (COMT). They enhance the action of levodopa and produce less fluctuation in drug response. There are concerns that COMT inhibitors may interact with various cardiac drugs such as isoproterenol, dobutamine, and methyldopa, so a reduction in COMT inhibitor dose should be considered in patients receiving these drugs.[66]

PHOSPHODIESTERASE III INHIBITORS

The phosphodiesterase III (PDE III) inhibitors, also known as *nonglycoside noncatecholamines*, include amrinone (Inocor)[67] and the more potent milrinone (Primacor).[68-70] They differ structurally and functionally from the catecholamines (see Table 14-7) and are generally used as alternatives or adjuncts to the standard inotropes.

The PDE III inhibitors have several benefits over other inotropes currently in use. Their mechanism of action—the inhibition of intracellular phosphodiesterase III—allows for the buildup of cAMP and a subsequent increase in the uptake of intracellular calcium.[71] Adrenergic receptors are not used to achieve the inotropic effect. It follows that these drugs retain their inotropic effect even in the presence of β-blocking agents or the phenomenon of β-receptor down-regulation, situations frequently encountered in patients with heart failure. Therefore PDE III inhibitors may be used, by virtue of their alternative pathway, to augment the effect of direct-acting β-agonists such as dobutamine or dopamine.[72]

These agents act as vasodilators because of the differential mechanism of cAMP in the smooth muscle versus its actions in the myocardium. In the smooth muscle, cAMP causes an efflux of calcium, with a resultant relaxation of the muscle.[73] The clinical result is a decrease in both preload and afterload. Although this effect is desirable, caution must be exercised in treating the hypovolemic patient. This effect, along with the absence of an associated increase in heart rate, probably contributes to the absence of an increase in myocardial oxygen consumption seen in some patients with the use of these agents.[74]

Amrinone-induced thrombocytopenia has led to the drug rarely being used.

Milrinone acts to enhance diastolic function, increase cardiac output, and decrease pulmonary wedge pressure. It causes an increase in atrioventricular conduction when given within therapeutic dose ranges.[75] The increase in cAMP also increases the automaticity of cardiac cells and can lead to calcium overload at high levels.[76] These effects can be arrhythmogenic. Because increases in heart rate are rare with the use of either milrinone or amrinone but elimination is via the kidney, these drugs should be used with caution in patients in renal failure because of the potential for life-threatening arrhythmias.

Milrinone has demonstrated a 15-fold increase in inotropic potency compared with amrinone.[77,78] The current manufacturer's recommendation for the administration of milrinone is an IV loading dose of 50 mcg/kg, administered slowly over 10 minutes, followed by an infusion ranging from 0.375 to 0.75 mcg/kg/min, up to a total daily dose of 0.59 to 1.13 mg/kg.

CARDIAC GLYCOSIDES

Characterized by the digitalis preparations, the cardiac glycosides have been used to treat CHF for two centuries. The most common preparation now used is digoxin. The primary inotropic effect of digitalis is achieved by the binding to sodium-potassium adenosine triphosphatase (Na/K ATPase) in cardiac cells.[79,80] This allows the level of intracellular sodium to increase, which eventually results in an increase in the concentration of intracellular calcium. The increased intracellular calcium available to the sarcoplasmic reticulum is what causes the enhancement of myocardial contractility or inotropic effect. Electrophysiologically, enhancement of vagal tone, an indirect effect of digitalis, results in slowing of the heart rate. This combination results in an increase in both diastolic filling and ejection fraction. Central venous pressure, ventricular end-diastolic volume, and pulmonary artery pressure are all reduced.[81] Because of its direct and indirect vagal effects, digitalis also is frequently used to control the ventricular response to atrial fibrillation and other atrial tachyarrhythmias. The digitalis-induced enhancement of vagal tone leads to slowing of impulse conduction through the atrioventricular node and prolongation of the effective refractory period of the atrioventricular node.

Digitalis preparations have a narrow therapeutic index, great variability in action among patients, and several side effects. Hypokalemia greatly enhances the effects of digoxin, whereas hyperkalemia has the opposite effect.[82] A patient with hypokalemia whose digitalis level is within a therapeutic range may show toxic effects. Digoxin serum levels are also mediated by the P-glycoprotein transporter. All known arrhythmias have been attributed to digitalis preparations. Other signs and symptoms of digitalis toxicity include nausea, vomiting, diarrhea, headache, fatigue, and colored vision. Under anesthesia the first sign is usually an arrhythmia, frequently PVCs. Close monitoring of electrolytes should be performed in digoxin-treated patients receiving a preoperative bowel prep. Calcium administration is contraindicated in digoxin-treated patients; it may lead to cardiac arrest. Preoperatively the serum levels of potassium and digitalis must be closely monitored in patients receiving digitalis; additionally, electrocardiographic monitoring is required for the detection of arrhythmias.

OTHER AGENTS

Calcium

Calcium, through its interaction with actin and myosin, enhances myocardial contraction. Anesthetists usually use a bolus of calcium chloride (250 to 1000 mg) to improve cardiac output; calcium gluconate also is available. It is interesting to note that various studies have failed to show exogenous calcium to increase cardiac output significantly if the level of ionized calcium is normal or slightly depressed. However, exogenous calcium has been found to be beneficial if ionized calcium levels are significantly diminished (see Table 14-3 for doses).

Glucagon

Glucagon is an endogenous hormone produced by the α-cells of the pancreas and secreted in response to hypoglycemic states. It induces the release of catecholamines and has a direct inotropic effect. Exogenous glucagon can be administered as an inotrope in IV doses of 1 to 10 mg. Potential problems include tachycardia and hyperglycemia. In patients with inadequate glycogen stores, hypoglycemia may result from compensatory increases in serum insulin levels. Glucagon is not indicated for the maintenance of prolonged inotropy (see Table 14-3 for doses).

Some common mechanisms for drugs affecting the sympathetic nervous system are shown in Figure 14-6.

MANAGEMENT OF SPECIFIC DISEASES

In past decades, the treatment of cardiovascular diseases under anesthesia was difficult and limited. The lack of specific cardiac drugs and the limited selection of anesthetic agents warranted symptomatic therapy designed to facilitate surgery until the patient was in the recovery room. Currently, with the vast array of cardiac drugs, the improved sophistication of anesthetic management, and monitoring that provides extensive hemodynamic information, the anesthetist is able to treat patients in a manner that is appropriate for management of their diseases. Therapies can be chosen that fit into a patient's plan of care. The anesthetic process can safely and effectively continue the care management of the individual patient. To assist in predicting possible poor outcomes, the American College of Cardiology and the American Heart Association have classified the cardiovascular and surgical risks (Boxes 14-1 and 14-2). Evidence of effectiveness of various risk-reduction strategies is given in Table 14-11.

The drugs listed for therapy of the cardiovascular disorders that follow are presented not so much for their specific intraoperative use but as a means of continuing the patient's current drug profile. Patient treatment mirrors general nonoperative indications and considerations. Anesthetic techniques take into account the combined effects of cardiac drugs and anesthetic agents when administered together.

Congestive Heart Failure

In the United States, 4 to 5 million people have chronic CHF, with 400,000 to 700,000 new cases occurring each year. The incidence will undoubtedly increase as the population ages. Heart failure results in almost 1 million hospitalizations each year. It is the most common hospital discharge diagnosis in patients older than age 65 years. More than 300,000 patients die as a direct or an indirect consequence of heart failure each year, a sixfold increase during the past 40 years. It is the only major cardiovascular disorder that is increasing in prevalence, with an estimated annual cost of $40 billion. Once cardiac failure has been diagnosed, 5-year survival rates are typically 25% to 40%, similar to the survival rates for cancer.[83] The classification of heart failure is given in Box 14-3.

CHF represents a significant risk factor for general anesthesia. Mortality estimates range from 3% to as high as 30% in patients undergoing abdominal surgery.[84] In patients with CHF and renal failure undergoing emergency surgery, mortality rates as high as 76% have been reported.

CHF is a syndrome resulting from a cardiac malfunction that impairs the ability of the heart's left ventricle to eject blood and

Noradrenergic Varicosity

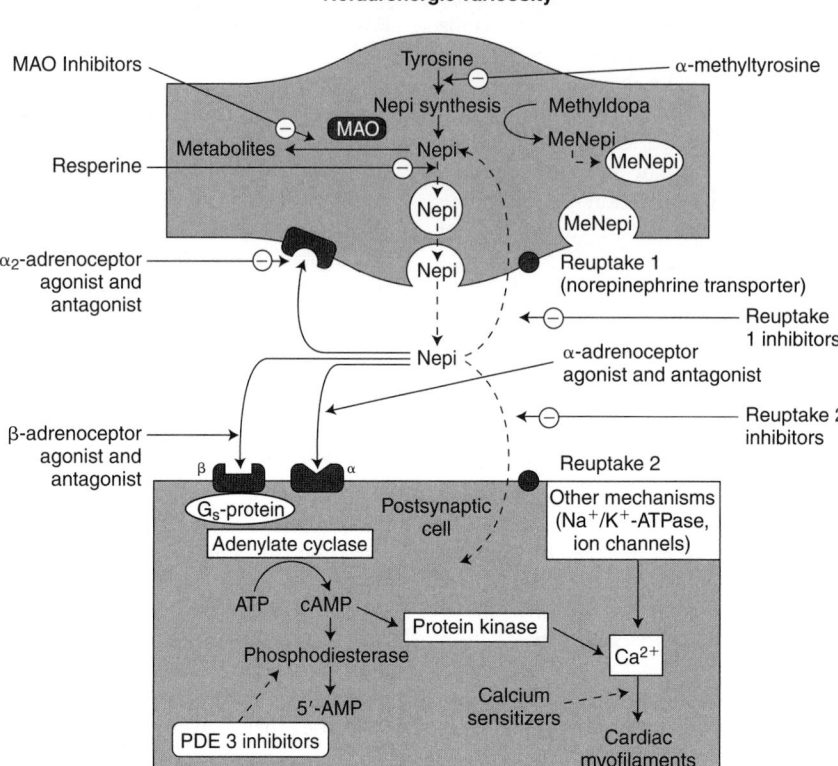

FIGURE **14-6**   Common mechanisms for drugs affecting the sympathetic nervous system.

meet the circulatory demands of the body. It is defined as a complex clinical syndrome that can result from any structural or functional cardiac disorder that interferes with the ability of the ventricle to fill with or eject blood. Alterations associated with CHF include impairment-induced complex changes in the structure of the ventricle called *ventricular remodeling*, along with hormonal and physiologic alterations.[85] The chamber dilates, hypertrophies, and becomes more spherical. Substantial evidence suggests that activation of the body's endogenous neurohormonal systems, such as the renin-angiotensin system, plays an important role in cardiac remodeling and the progression of heart failure. Treatment is complex and tailored to the patient's age, current disease state, and associated concurrent disorders. It usually involves a polypharmaceutical approach that includes[86] digoxin,[87] diuretics, ACE inhibitors,[88-92] β-blockers,[73-95] and spironolactone.[96] Neutral endopeptidase (NEP) inhibitors block the metabolism of atrial natriuretic factor and are being tried as adjuncts to other agents for heart failure. Candoxatril and ecadotril are two new NEP inhibitors. Recommendations for the management of CHF are given in Box 14-4.

In the perioperative period, anesthesia providers are faced with managing therapy for all degrees of severity of acute CHF. The goal can range from prevention of symptom progression to surviving the operation in life-threatening cases. When appropriate, regional nerve block techniques should be considered, but patients may have difficulty lying flat during surgery. No single general anesthetic technique has proven superior. Invasive arterial blood pressure monitoring and transesophageal echocardiography (TEE) are useful to guide intraoperative decision making and fluid management. TEE is especially useful in diagnosing whether hypotensive episodes are the result of

inadequate circulating blood volume, worsening ventricular function, or arterial vasoconstriction.

Drugs such as the inotropes, phosphodiesterase inhibitors, diuretics, and vasodilators are commonly used intraoperatively in acute episodes.[97] Some useful drugs for the treatment of heart failure during anesthesia are listed in Table 14-7.

Arrhythmias

The incidence of serious arrhythmias requiring intervention during general anesthesia is relatively low. A large multicenter study found that not counting simple tachycardia, bradycardia, or clinically minor rhythm disturbances, the frequency of serious arrhythmias was 1.6% in a series of more than 17,000 patients who underwent general anesthesia.[98] It is surprising that the incidence is not higher, because several contradictory factors are involved; most drugs given during anesthesia are cardiac depressants; therefore, they tend to be antiarrhythmic. However, patients with multiple drug profiles in combination with the anesthetics may experience drug interactions that lead to rhythm disturbances. Add to these pharmacologic factors the stresses of surgery and anesthesia, and a multitude of effects on cardiac rhythms may be expected.

In recent years, new pharmacologic and nonpharmacologic management approaches for cardiac arrhythmias have emerged. New drugs, implantable cardiac devices, and ablation therapy are available for managing these disorders. The use of antiarrhythmic drugs in the United States is declining because of major trials indicating an increasing mortality rate with clinical use. Proarrhythmic side effects and the use of nondrug therapies have also contributed to the decline. Some causes of intraoperative rhythm disturbances are listed in Box 14-5.

Clinical Predictors of Increased Perioperative Cardiovascular Risk

Major Risk Factors
Unstable coronary syndromes
- Acute or recent myocardial infarction with evidence of important ischemic risk by clinical symptoms or noninvasive study*
- Unstable or severe angina (Canadian class III or IV)

Decompensated heart failure
- New York Heart Association functional class IV; worsening or new onset heart failure

Significant arrhythmias
- High-grade atrioventricular block
- Mobitz II atrioventricular block
- Third-degree atrioventricular block
- Symptomatic ventricular arrhythmias
- Supraventricular arrhythmias, including atrial fibrillation with uncontrolled ventricular rate greater than 100 at rest
- Symptomatic bradycardia
- Newly recognized ventricular tachycardia

Severe valvular disease
- Severe aortic stenosis with mean pressure gradient greater than 40 mm Hg; aortic valve area less than 10 cm^2; or exhibiting symptoms
- Symptomatic mitral stenosis; progressive dyspnea on exertion, exertional presyncope or heart failure

Intermediate Risk Factors
Mild angina pectoris (Canadian class I or II)
Previous myocardial infarction identified by history or pathologic Q waves
Compensated or previous heart failure
Diabetes mellitus (particularly insulin dependent)
Renal insufficiency

Minor Risk Factors
Advanced age
Abnormal ECG (left ventricular hypertrophy, left bundle-branch block, ST-T abnormalities)
Rhythm other than sinus (e.g., atrial fibrillation)
Low functional capacity (e.g., inability to climb one flight of stairs with a bag of groceries)
History of stroke
Uncontrolled systemic hypertension

From ACC/AHA Guideline update for perioperative cardiovascular evaluation for noncardiac surgery—executive summary: a report of the American College of Cardiology/American Heart Association Task Force on Practice Guidelines (Committee to Update the 1996 Guidelines on Perioperative Cardiovascular Evaluation for Noncardiac Surgery). Circulation. 2002;105:10,1257-1267; and Fleischer LA et al. ACC/AHA 2007 guidelines on perioperative cardiovascular evaluation for noncardiac surgery—executive summary: a report of the American College of Cardiology/American Heart Association Task Force on Practice Guidelines. Circulation. 2007;116:418-499.
ECG, Electrocardiogram
The American College of Cardiology National Database Library defines recent myocardial infarction as having occurred more than 7 days previously, but less than or equal to 1 month (30 days); acute myocardial infarction is defined as having occurred within the last 7 days. May include "stable" angina inpatients who are unusually sedentary.

Cardiac Risk* Stratification for Noncardiac Surgical Procedures

High Risk (Reported Cardiac Risk Often Greater Than 5%)
- Emergent major operations, particularly in the elderly
- Aortic and other major vascular surgery
- Peripheral vascular surgery
- Anticipated prolonged surgical procedures associated with large fluid shifts or blood loss

Intermediate Risk (Reported Cardiac Risk Generally 1% to 5%)
- Carotid endarterectomy
- Head and neck surgery
- Intraperitoneal and intrathoracic surgery
- Orthopedic surgery
- Prostate surgery

Low Risk (Reported Cardiac Risk Generally Less Than 1%)†
- Endoscopic procedures
- Superficial procedures
- Cataract surgery
- Breast surgery
- Ambulatory surgery

*From ACC/AHA Guideline update for perioperative cardiovascular evaluation for noncardiac surgery—executive summary: a report of the American College of Cardiology/American Heart Association Task Force on Practice Guidelines (Committee to Update the 1996 Guidelines on Perioperative Cardiovascular Evaluation for Noncardiac Surgery). Circulation. 2002;105:10, 1257-1267; and Fleischer LA et al. ACC/AHA 2007 guidelines on perioperative cardiovascular evaluation for noncardiac surgery—executive summary: a report of the American College of Cardiology/American Heart Association Task Force on Practice Guidelines. Circulation 2007;116:418-499.
*Combined incidence of cardiac death and nonfatal myocardial infarction.
†These patients do not generally require further preoperative cardiac testing.*

The goal of drug therapy for arrhythmias during anesthesia should be to treat immediate hemodynamic problems and prevent progression of serious arrhythmias. Treatment is similar to that in the nonoperative setting, with the caveat that most therapies should be carefully titrated to avoid unexpected proarrhythmic or excessive hypotensive outcomes. Three cautionary statements should precede any discussion on the use of antiarrhythmic agents during anesthesia[99]:
- The cause of the arrhythmia should be explored before any treatment is instituted.
- Adequacy of ventilation, depth of anesthesia, acid-base balance, and fluid and electrolyte balance must be verified before appropriate therapy can be formulated.
- Multiple-drug administration, which constitutes modern anesthesia practice, may result in unexpected drug interactions. Analysis of complex arrhythmias with the commonly used three- or five-lead electrocardiograph system during a surgical procedure is less than ideal for proper diagnosis and treatment. Nonetheless,

TABLE 14-11	Perioperative Cardiac Risk-Reduction Strategies
Cardiac Risk-Reduction Strategies	**Effectiveness**
Perioperative Medical Therapy	
β-blockers	Strong evidence for effectiveness
Statins	Strong evidence for effectiveness
α_2-adrenergic blockers	Moderate effectiveness
Nitroglycerin/diltiazem	Not effective
Preoperative Coronary Revascularization	
Percutaneous revascularization	Conflicting results about effectiveness and increased risk of complications
Coronary artery bypass grafting	Moderate effectiveness
Perioperative Monitoring	
Pulmonary artery catheter	Conflicting results about effectiveness and increased risk of complications
Central venous catheter	Not effective
12-lead electrocardiography	Not effective
Transesophageal echocardiography	Not effective
Anesthetic Management	
Epidural anesthesia and analgesia	Not effective/moderate effectiveness
Intraoperative normothermia	Moderate effectiveness

Adapted from Kertai MD et al. *Predicting perioperative cardiac risk.* Prog Cardiovasc Dis. 2005;47(4):240-57.

BOX 14-3
New York Heart Association Functional Classification for Heart Failure

Class I
Patients with cardiac disease but without resulting limitation of physical activity. Ordinary physical activity does not cause undue fatigue, palpitation, dyspnea, or anginal pain.

Class II
Patients with cardiac disease resulting in slight limitation of physical activity. They are comfortable at rest. Ordinary physical activity results in fatigue, palpitation, dyspnea, or anginal pain.

Class III
Patients with cardiac disease resulting in marked limitation of physical activity. They are comfortable at rest. Less than ordinary activity causes fatigue, palpitation, dyspnea, or anginal pain.

Class IV
Patients with cardiac disease resulting in inability to carry out any physical activity without discomfort. Symptoms of heart failure or the anginal syndrome may be present even at rest. If any physical activity is undertaken, discomfort is increased.

Adapted from Helms RA et al, eds. *Textbook of Therapeutics: Drug and Disease Management. 8th ed. Philadelphia: Lippincott Williams & Wilkins; 2006.*

---

rhythm disturbances that compromise hemodynamic stability or may progress to more severe dysfunction must be addressed.

Classification of antiarrhythmic drugs is given in Table 14-12. The drugs of choice for the common arrhythmias are given in Table 14-10, and the dosages of the antiarrhythmic drugs are given in Table 14-13.

Hypertension

Hypertension is a major health problem in the United States; an estimated 50 million Americans have hypertension or should be monitored for elevated blood pressure.[100] The classification of hypertension has been revised and is given in Table 14-14. The optimal blood pressure is believed to be less than 120 systolic and less than 90 diastolic.[101,102] A new category, prehypertension, is included, and hypertension is classified as either stage 1 or 2. A number of drugs are available for the treatment of high blood pressure, including diuretics, β-blockers, calcium channel blockers, ACE inhibitors, and angiotensin receptor antagonists. Recommendations are that diuretics and β-blockers be first-line therapies in addition to combinations of other agents as warranted by patient characteristics and the concurrent presence of various target-organ disease states. Drugs available for the treatment of hypertension are listed in Table 14-9. Antihypertensive drugs that are safe for use during pregnancy are listed in Table 14-15.

Manipulation of the patient's blood pressure is an ongoing task during anesthesia. Many drugs are available to increase and decrease blood pressure when indicated. Improved monitoring and sophistication of anesthetic techniques has made control of blood pressure almost routine.

The problem of hypertension has varying significance in preoperative, intraoperative, and postoperative situations. Proper preoperative handling of patients with severe stage 2 hypertension sparks ongoing controversy. For a number of years, some practitioners thought it was better to postpone an operation to stabilize the patient's blood pressure, whereas others believed acute treatment was sufficient. Several studies have been done with somewhat conflicting results.[103,104] At present, what can be concluded is that blood pressure lability in the perioperative period is associated with postoperative morbidity.[105] Mild hypertension probably represents only a minor risk for anesthesia and surgery. Patients with more severe hypertensive episodes are at greater risk and will benefit from acute therapy combined with postoperative long-term follow-up. Hypertensive episodes during the perioperative period occur most often during emergence from anesthesia and may be associated with pain, airway stimulation, hypoxia-hypercarbia, hypothermia and shivering, bladder distention, withdrawal from preoperative medications, and intraoperative use of vasopressors. Drugs useful for the treatment of perioperative hypertension are listed in Table 14-16. Figure 14-7 summarizes the mechanism of arterial blood pressure regulation and the sites of action of antihypertensive drugs.

BOX **14-4**

Recommendations for the Management of Congestive Heart Failure

Prevention of Heart Failure
- Most patients with heart failure will be treated with "triple therapy" consisting of an angiotensin-converting enzyme (ACE) inhibitor, a β-blocker, and a diuretic, frequently an aldosterone antagonist. Occasionally digoxin is added or substituted for the aldosterone antagonist.
- Control of coronary risk factors, including hypertension, hyperlipidemia, and smoking
- In patients with a recent myocardial infarction (MI), reperfusion and neurohormonal antagonism with an ACE inhibitor and a β-blocker can reduce myocardial injury and the risk of subsequent events.
- In patients with asymptomatic left ventricular dysfunction, an ACE inhibitor and a β-blocker can produce complementary benefits.

General Measures
- Maintenance of fluid balance by salt restriction and daily monitoring of body weight
- Improved conditioning with encouragement of moderate exercise and avoidance of excessive bed rest
- Control of atrial fibrillation and anticoagulation in high-risk patients and revascularization in selected patients
- Avoidance of antiarrhythmic drugs, nonsteroidal antiinflammatory drugs, and most calcium channel blockers

Diuretics
- Diuretics should be prescribed for all patients with symptoms of heart failure who have a predisposition to fluid retention. These drugs should not be used alone, even if they are effective in controlling symptoms.
- The goal of diuretic therapy is to eliminate symptoms and physical signs of fluid retention, such as jugular venous distention and edema.
- Measurement of body weight is the best way of monitoring when to initiate or titrate a diuretic regimen.
- Diuretics may alter the efficacy of ACE inhibitors and β-blockers.

ACE Inhibitors
- All patients—not some, or most, but *all patients*—with heart failure resulting from left ventricular systolic dysfunction should receive an ACE inhibitor unless they are intolerant of the drug or have a contraindication to its use. Treatment should not be delayed until symptoms are severe or resistant to other drugs.
- Alleviation of symptoms may be delayed and disease progression modified, even if no symptomatic improvement occurs.
- Early side effects must not prevent long-term use.

β-Blockers
- All patients with stable New York Heart Association (NYHA) class II or III heart failure resulting from left ventricular systolic dysfunction should receive a β-blocker unless they are intolerant of the drug or have a contraindication to its use. Treatment should not be delayed until symptoms are severe or resistant to therapy.
- Alleviation of symptoms may be delayed and disease progression modified, even if no symptomatic improvement occurs.
- Early side effects must not prevent long-term use.

Digitalis
- Digitalis is recommended to improve symptoms of patients with heart failure resulting from left ventricular systolic dysfunction and should be used together with diuretics, ACE inhibitors, and β-blockers.
- Controversy exists about the proper dosing of digitalis, and it is unclear whether serum digoxin levels should be used to guide therapy.
- Digoxin is well tolerated, but there is some concern that the drug may be deleterious at levels within the therapeutic range.

Hydralazine-Nitrate Combinations
- Hydralazine-nitrate combinations should not be used in patients with no prior use of ACE inhibitors and should not be substituted for ACE inhibitors in patients who are tolerating ACE inhibitors without difficulty.
- Such combinations should be considered in patients who cannot tolerate ACE inhibitors because of hypotension or azotemia.
- Little evidence exists to support the use of nitrates alone or hydralazine alone in the treatment of heart failure.

Angiotensin and Aldosterone Antagonists
- Angiotensin receptor blockers should not be used in patients with no prior use of ACE inhibitors and should not be substituted for ACE inhibitors in patients who are tolerating ACE inhibitors.
- These agents should be considered only in those patients who are unable to tolerate ACE inhibitors because of cough or angioedema.

Calcium Antagonists
- Calcium antagonists should not be used for the treatment of heart failure.
- Most calcium antagonists should be avoided in heart failure, even when used for the treatment of angina or hypertension. There is persuasive evidence, however, that amlodipine does not adversely affect survival.
- Until further data are available, amlodipine should not be used to prolong survival in patients with a nonischemic cardiomyopathy.

Antiarrhythmic Drugs
- Class I antiarrhythmic agents should not be used, except for immediately life-threatening ventricular arrhythmias.
- Some class III agents, such as amiodarone, do not appear to increase the risk of death and are preferred over class I agents.
- Amiodarone is not recommended with ACE inhibitors and β-blockers.
- Electrolyte deficiencies may cause arrhythmias and alter the efficacy and safety of antiarrhythmic drugs.

Inotropic Infusions
- Use of intermittent infusions of positive inotropic agents at home, in the physician's office, or in a short-stay unit cannot be recommended, even in patients with advanced heart failure.
- Continuous outpatient infusions may be considered for improving the quality of life in the rare patient who cannot be weaned from inotropic therapy and in whom some relief of symptoms is worth the likelihood of an increased risk of death.

From Consensus recommendations for the management of chronic heart failure. On behalf of the membership of the advisory council to improve outcomes nationwide in heart failure. Am J Cardiol. 1999;83:1A-38A.

BOX **14-5**

Causes of Intraoperative Rhythm Disturbances

Structural Heart Disease
- Chronic coronary artery disease (infarction)
- Valvular and congenital heart disease
- Cardiomyopathies of diverse origins
- Sick sinus or long Q-T interval syndrome
- Wolff-Parkinson-White syndrome
- Hypertrophic, dilated, infiltrative, secondary to systemic disease (e.g., uremia, diabetes)

Transient Imbalance
- Stress: electrolyte or metabolic imbalance
- Laryngoscopy, hypoxia, hypercarbia
- Device malfunction, microshock
- Diagnostic or therapeutic intervention (pacemakers, cardioverter-defibrillators)
- Surgical stimulation
- Central vascular catheters

Adapted from Atlee JL. Perioperative dysrhythmias: diagnosis and management. Anesthesiology. 1997;86:1397-1424.

TABLE **14-12**   **Classification of Antiarrhythmic Drugs**

Class	Electrophysiologic Effect	Drug
I	Depression of phase 0 depolarization (block sodium channels)	
IA	Moderate depression and prolonged repolarization	Quinidine, procainamide, disopyramide
IB	Weak depression and shortened repolarization	Lidocaine, mexiletine, phenytoin, tocainide
IC	Strong depression with little effect on repolarization	Flecainide, propafenone, moricizine
II	β-Adrenergic blocking effects	Esmolol, propranolol, metoprolol, timolol, pindolol, atenolol, acebutolol, nadolol, carvedilol
III	Prolongs repolarization (blocks potassium channels)	Amiodarone, bretylium, sotalol, ibutilide, dofetilide
IV	Calcium channel blocking effects	Verapamil, diltiazem
Other		Adenosine, adenosine triphosphate, digoxin, atropine

Coronary Heart Disease

Coronary heart disease (CHD) is the most common cardiac disease encountered in the operating room. Approximately 12 million people in the United States have CHD. It is estimated that up to 208 deaths per 100,000 population result from significant coronary artery disease. The CHD death rate peaked in the mid-1960s and has declined in the general population over the past 35 years. This decline began in females in the 1950s and in males in the 1960s.[106]

High blood cholesterol is a major risk factor for CHD that can be modified. More than 50 million U.S. adults have blood cholesterol levels that require medical advice and treatment. More than 90 million adults have cholesterol levels that are higher than desirable. Experts recommend that all adults ages 20 years and older have their cholesterol levels checked at least once every 5 years to help them take action to prevent or lower their risk of CHD.[106]

The causes of coronary artery disease and management of patients with the disorder are discussed in detail in Chapters 24 and 25. The classification of angina pectoris is given in Table 14-17.

Pharmacotherapy includes nitrates, β-blockers, calcium channel blockers, aspirin, and "statin" drugs. Positive benefits have recently been noted for preoperative statin use.[107] Preoperative statin use was associated with reduced cardiac mortality after primary, elective coronary artery bypass grafting. Postoperative statin discontinuation was associated with increased in-hospital mortality. Recent evidence suggests that ACE inhibitors may also provide a reduction in mortality and infarction rates. The β-blockers and calcium channel blockers are listed in Table 14-9. The nitrates and the HMG-CoA reductase inhibitors ("statins") are listed in Tables 14-18 and 14-19, respectively.

PREOPERATIVE ADMINISTRATION OF CARDIAC DRUGS

Continuation of the patient's cardiac medications throughout the perioperative period is now considered routine practice. It is better to have the patient's disease state under proper control

than to discontinue any medications before surgery and risk having the patient in unstable condition. Withdrawal after abrupt discontinuation of β-blockers and clonidine is especially severe. This also includes aspirin, which adds little bleeding risk to surgical procedures. Based on recent clinical data, the risk of coronary thrombosis upon antiplatelet drug withdrawal is much higher than the risk of surgical bleeding when maintaining them. In secondary prevention, aspirin is a lifelong therapy and should never be stopped. Clopidogrel is mandatory for as long as coronary stents are not fully endothelialized (which takes 6 to 24 weeks, depending on the technique used) but might be required for a longer period.[108] A complete discussion of the anesthesia management of patients on antiplatelet drugs can be found in Chapter 35.

Some concern exists that the ACE inhibitors may precipitate significant hypotension during induction and that they should be withheld the morning of surgery.[109] Recent evidence suggests that patients who had withheld an ACE inhibitor for greater than 10 hours prior to induction exhibited less postinduction hypotension.[110] It is currently suggested that the ACE inhibitors be continued until the night before surgery but the morning dose be withheld.[111] Following anesthesia induction, hypotension refractory to fluids, ephedrine, or phenylephrine—although rare—may be successfully treated with the vasopressin analog terlipressin.[112] The same consideration for the angiotensin receptor blockers seems prudent.

New guidelines for antibiotic prophylaxis for the prevention of infective endocarditis were recently published. There are some significant changes, and the recommendations are much narrower. They are listed in Box 14-6, Table 14-20, and Table 14-21.

TABLE 14-13 Doses and Therapeutic Concentrations for Antiarrhythmic Agents

Drug	Usual Dosage Ranges				Time to Peak Plasma Concentration (Oral) (hr)	Elimination Half-Life (hr)	Bioavailability (%)	Major Route of Elimination
	Intravenous		Oral					
	Loading	Maintenance	Loading	Maintenance				
Quinidine	6-10 mg/kg at 0.3-0.5 mg/kg/min	NA	800-1000 mg	300-600 mg q6h	1.5-3.0	5-9	60-80	Liver
Procainamide	6-13 mg/kg at 0.2-0.5 mg/kg/min	2-6 mg/min	500-1000 mg	250-1000 mg q4-6h	1	3-5	70-85	Kidneys
Disopyramide	1-2 mg/kg over 15-45 min*	1 mg/kg/hr	N/A	100-300 mg q6-8h	1-2	8-9	80-90	Kidneys
Lidocaine	1-3 mg/kg at 20-50 mg/min	1-4 mg/min	N/A	N/A	N/A	1-2	N/A	Liver
Mexiletine	500 mg*	0.5-1.0 g/24 hr	400-600 mg	150-300 mg q8-12h	2-4	10-17	90	Liver
Acebutolol	N/A	N/A	200 mg bid, increase gradually to 600-1200 mg/day	NA	2-4	3-4	40	Liver
Flecainide	2 mg/kg*	100-200 mg q12h		50-200 mg q12h	3-4	20	95	Liver
Propafenone	1-2 mg/kg		600-900 mg	150-300 mg q8-12h	1-3	5-8	25-75	Liver
Esmolol	500 mcg/kg over 1 min, followed by 500 mcg/kg/min	100-300 mcg/kg/min	N/A	N/A	N/A	9 (min)	N/A	RBC esterases

From Libby P et al. Braunwald's Heart Disease. 8th ed. Philadelphia: Saunders; 2008; and Medical Letter Treatment Guidelines. Drugs for cardiac arrhythmias. Med Lett. 2007;5(58):51-58. Results presented may vary according to doses, disease state, and intravenous or oral administration.
*Intravenous use investigational.
N/A, Not applicable.

TABLE 14-13 Doses and Therapeutic Concentrations for Antiarrhythmic Agents—cont'd

| Drug | Usual Dosage Ranges | | | | Time to Peak Plasma Concentration (Oral) (hr) | Elimination Half-Life (hr) | Bioavailability (%) | Major Route of Elimination |
| | Intravenous | | Oral | | | | | |
	Loading	Maintenance	Loading	Maintenance				
Propranolol	0.25-0.5 mg q5min to ≤0.20 mg/kg	N/A	N/A	10-200 mg q6-8h	4	3-6	35-65	Liver
Amiodarone	15 mg/kg for 10 min, 1 mg/kg for 3 hr, 0.5 mg/kg thereafter	1 mg/min	800-1600 mg daily for 7-14 days	200-600 mg daily	3-7	56 days	50	Kidneys
Metoprolol	2.5-5 mg q 2-5 min (up to 15 mg)	N/A	50-200 mg/day divided q12-24h	N/A	1-2	3-7	50-70	Liver
Sotalol	10 mg over 1-2 min			80-320 mg q12h	2.5-4	12	90-100	Kidneys
Ibutilide	1 mg over 10 min	N/A	N/A	N/A	N/A	6	N/A	Kidneys
Dofetilide	2-5 mcg/kg infusion	N/A	N/A	0.1-0.5 mg q 12h		7-13	90	Kidneys
Diltiazem	10-25 mg over 2 min, may be repeated in 15 min	5-15 mg/hr	120-360 mg/day divided q6-24h	N/A	1-2	3-4.5	40	Kidneys
Verapamil	5-10 mg over 1-2 min	0.005 mg/kg/min		80-120 mg q6-8h	1-2	3-8	10-35	Liver
Adenosine	6-18 mg (rapidly)	N/A	N/A	N/A	N/A	1 (min)	N/A	Cellular uptake from plasma
Digoxin	0.5-1 mg	0.125-0.25 mg daily	0.5-1.0 mg	0.125-0.25 mg daily	2-6	36-48	60-80	Kidneys
Magnesium sulfate	2 g over 5-60 min	N/A	N/A	N/A	N/A	N/A	N/A	Kidneys

TABLE 14-14 Classification and Management of Blood Pressure for Adults

Blood Pressure Classification	Systolic Blood Pressure (mm Hg)	Diastolic Blood Pressure (mm Hg)
Normal	<120	and <80
Prehypertension	120-139	or 80-89
Stage 1 hypertension	140-159	or 90-99
Stage 2 hypertension	≤160	or ≤100

From Joint National Committee on Prevention, Detection and Treatment of High Blood Pressure. Seventh report of the National Committee on Detection, Evaluation and Treatment of High Blood Pressure (JNC-7) (NIH Publication No. 03-5233). Washington, DC: U.S. Department of Health and Human Services. National Institute of Health. National Heart, Lung and Blood Institute. National High Blood Pressure Education Program; May 2003.

TABLE 14-15 Antihypertensive Drugs Used in Pregnancy*

Suggested Drug	Comments
Central α-agonists	Methyldopa is the drug of choice
β-Blockers	Atenolol, metoprolol, and labetalol
Diuretics	Diuretics recommended for chronic hypertension if prescribed before gestation or if patients appear to be salt sensitive; diuretics not recommended in patients with preeclampsia
Direct vasodilators	Hydralazine is the parenteral drug of choice, based on its long history of safety and efficacy

From Joint National Committee on Prevention, Detection and Treatment of High Blood Pressure. Seventh report of the National Committee on Detection, Evaluation and Treatment of High Blood Pressure (JNC-7) (NIH Publication No. 03-5233). Washington, DC: U.S. Department of Health and Human Services. National Institute of Health. National Heart, Lung and Blood Institute. National High Blood Pressure Education Program; May 2003.
*ACE inhibitors and angiotensin II receptor blockers should not be used. Fetal abnormalities and death have been reported.

TABLE 14-16 Parenteral Drugs for Treatment of Severe Hypertension

Drug	Class	Route and Dose	Onset	Duration	Comments
Enalaprilat	Angiotensin-converting enzyme (ACE) inhibitor	IV: 1.25-5 mg q6h	15 min	6-12 hr	Variable, sometimes excessive response
Fenoldopam (Corlopam)	Dopamine-1 receptor agonist	IV infusion pump: 0.1-1.6 mcg/kg/min	4-5 min	<10 min	May cause reflex tachycardia; may increase intraocular pressure
Labetalol (Trandate Normodyne)	α- and β-adrenergic blocker	IV: 20 mg initially, then 40-80 mg q10min (300 mg max)	5 min or less	3-6 hr	Not for patients with bronchospasm, congestive heart failure, first-degree heart block, cardiogenic shock, or severe bradycardia
Nicardipine (Cardene IV)	Calcium channel blocker	IV: 5 mg/hr, increased by 2.5 mg/hr q15min up to 15 mg/hr	1-5 min	3-6 hr	May cause reflex tachycardia
Clevidipine (Cleviprex)	Calcium channel blocker	IV infusion: 1-2mg/hr initially; double the dose at 90-second intervals until desired results are achieved (16 mg/hr/max)	2-4 min	5-15 min	Rapidly degraded by tissue and blood esterases; contraindicated with allergy to soy or eggs; may cause reflex tachycardia
Nitroglycerin	Venous arteriolar vasodilator	IV infusion pump: 5-100 mcg/min	2-5 min	5-10 min	Headache, tachycardia can occur; tolerance may develop with prolonged use
Sodium nitroprusside	Arteriolar and venous vasodilator	IV infusion pump: 0.3-10 mcg/kg/min	Seconds	3-5 min	Thiocyanate or cyanide toxicity with prolonged or too rapid infusion
Esmolol	β-blocker	IV: 500 mcg/kg/min for 1 min Titration to effect Usually 50 mcg/kg/min	1-2 min	5-10 min	Cardioselective; however, use with caution in patients with asthma

From Medical Letter Treatment Guidelines. Cardiovascular drugs in the ICU. Med Lett. 2002;4:19-24; and Aggarwal M, Kahn IA. Hypertensive crises: hypertensive emergencies and urgencies. Cardiol Clin. 2006;24:135-146.

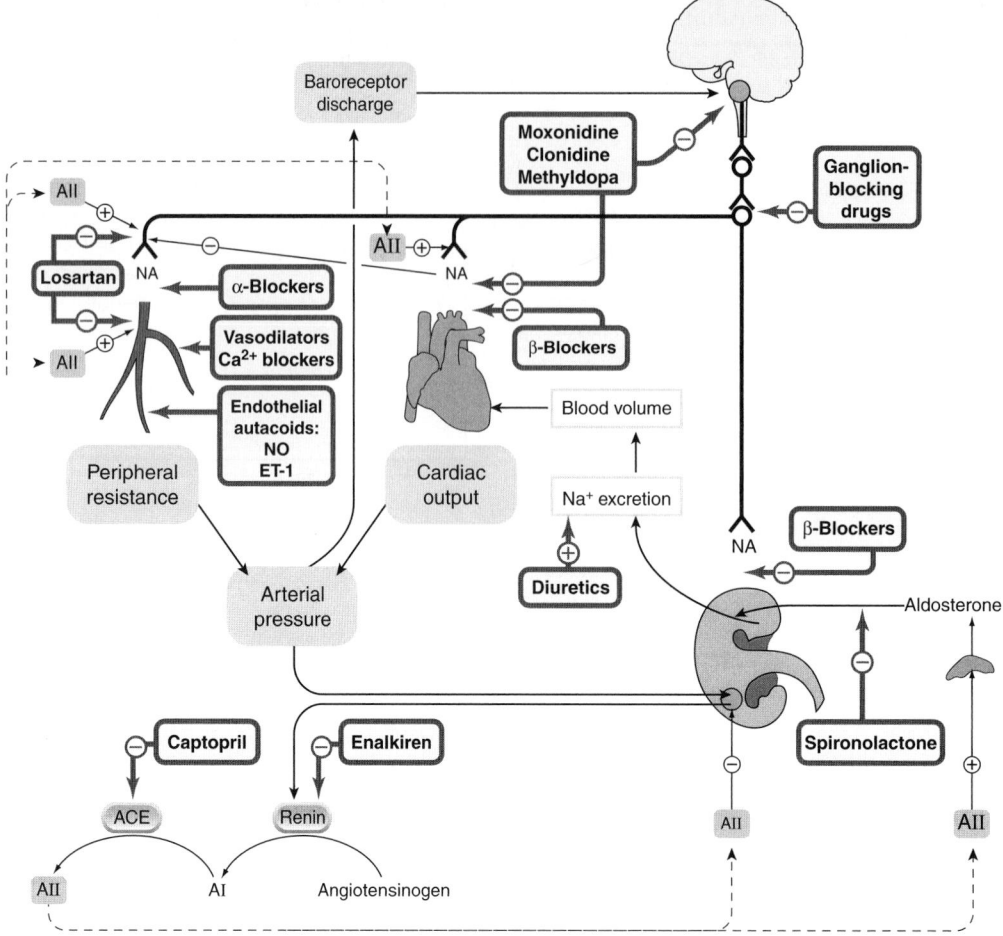

FIGURE **14-7**   Diagram showing the main mechanisms involved in arterial blood pressure regulation (*black lines*) and the sites of action of antihypertensive drugs (*boxes*). ACE, Angiotensin-converting enzyme; *AI*, angiotensin I; *AII*, angiotensin II; *NA*, noradrenaline; *NO*, nitric oxide; *ET-1*, endothelin-1. (*From Rang HP et al.* Rang and Dale's Pharmacology. *6th ed. Edinburgh: Churchill Livingstone; 2007.*)

TABLE **14-17**	Classification of Angina Pectoris
Class	**Canadian Cardiovascular Society Functional Classification**
I	No angina with ordinary physical activity (walking, climbing stairs) but may occur with strenuous, rapid, or prolonged exertion (work, recreation).
II	Early onset limitation of ordinary activity such as walking rapidly or > two blocks, climbing stairs rapidly or > one flight. Angina may be worse after meals, in cold temperatures, or with emotional stress.
III	Marked limitation of ordinary physical activity.
IV	Inability to carry out any physical activity without chest discomfort. Angina occurs during rest.

Adapted from Sangreddi V et al. Canadian Cardiovascular Society classification of effort angina: an angiographic correlation. Coron Artery Dis. 2004;15:11-114.

TABLE **14-18**	Drug Therapy for Angina
Drug	**Comments**
Nitrates	First-line therapy for acute attacks; mechanism is a decrease in oxygen demand via a reduction in preload and some beneficial redistribution in blood flow
β-Blockers	Cornerstone therapy for chronic prophylaxis; decrease cardiac demand via lower heart rate, blood pressure, and contractility
Calcium channel blockers	Especially effective in variant angina and in patients intolerant to β-blockers; reduce preload, afterload, and increase coronary flow
Aspirin	Inhibits platelet and endothelial cyclooxygenase; reduces coronary thrombosis; clopidogrel (Plavix) may be substituted in patients with contraindications to aspirin
Statins	HMG-CoA reductase inhibitors, commonly referred to as *statins*, reduce C-reactive protein, thrombogenicity, and adverse cardiac events

| TABLE **14-19** | HMG-CoA Reductase Inhibitors ("Statins") |

Drug	Initial Dosage	Maximum Dosage	Comments
Atorvastatin (Lipitor)	10 mg once	80 mg once	Statins are generally tolerated better than other lipid-lowering drugs. Mild transient gastrointestinal disturbances, muscle pain, rash, and headache have occurred. Some patients have reported sleep disturbances. An increase in liver enzymes and creatine phosphokinase may occur with significant myalgia and muscle weakness.
Fluvastatin (Lescol)	20 mg once	40 mg bid	
Lovastatin (Mevacor)	20 mg once	80 mg once	
Pravastatin (Pravachol)	40 mg once	80 mg once	
Rosuvastatin (Crestor)	10 mg once	40 mg once	
Simvastatin (Zocor)	20 mg once	80 mg once	

Adapted with permission from Medical Letter Treatment Guidelines. Drugs for lipids. Med Lett. 2008;6(66):9-16; and Mosby's Drug Consult. St Louis: Mosby; 2007.

BOX **14-6**

Indications for Antibiotic Prophylaxis for Prevention of Infective Endocarditis

Candidates for Antibiotic Prophylaxis
1. Prosthetic heart valve or prosthetic material used for cardiac valve repair
2. Previous endocarditis
3. Congenital heart disease
   a. Unrepaired cyanotic congenital heart disease, including palliative shunts and conduits
   b. During first 6 months after complete repair of heart defect with prosthetic material
   c. Incomplete repair with residual defects near prosthetic material which inhibits endothelialization
4. Heart transplant-associated valvulopathy

Procedures Requiring Antibiotic Prophylaxis
1. Any dental work involving gingival tissues or periapical region or peroration of the oral mucosa
2. Tonsillectomy & adenoidectomy
3. Bronchoscopy with incision
4. Empyema drainage
5. Gastrointestinal and genitourinary procedures on infected tissue
6. Procedures on infected skin or musculoskeletal tissue
7. Cardiac surgery to implant prosthetic valve/intracardiac device

From Wilson W et al. Prevention of infective endocarditis: guidelines from the American Heart Association. A guideline from the American Heart Association Rheumatic Fever, Endocarditis, and Kawasaki Disease Committee, Council on Cardiovascular Disease in the Young, and the Council on Clinical Cardiology, Council on Cardiovascular Surgery and Anesthesia, and the Quality of Care and Outcomes Research Interdisciplinary Working Group. Circulation. 2007;116(15):1736-1754.

| Table **14-20** | Regimens for Dental Procedures |

Situation		Regimen			
Allergy?	**Oral?**	**Agent**	**Adults**	**Children**
No penicillin allergy	Oral	Amoxicillin	2 g PO	50 mg/kg PO
No penicillin allergy	Nothing by mouth	Ampicillin or	2 g IM or IV	50 mg/kg IM or IV
		cefazolin*	1 g IM or IV	50 mg/kg IM or IV
Penicillin allergy	Oral	Cephalexin* or	2 g PO	50 mg/kg PO
		clindamycin or	600 mg PO	20 mg/kg PO
		azithromycin or	500 mg PO	15 mg/kg PO
		clarithromycin	500 mg PO	15 mg/kg PO
Penicillin allergy	Nothing by mouth	Cefazolin* or	1 g IM or IV	50 mg/kg IM or IV
		clindamycin	600 mg IM or IV	20 mg/kg IM or IV

Wilson W et al. Prevention of infective endocarditis: guidelines from the American Heart Association: a guideline from the American Heart Association Rheumatic Fever, Endocarditis, and Kawasaki Disease Committee, Council on Cardiovascular Disease in the Young, and the Council on Clinical Cardiology, Council on Cardiovascular Surgery and Anesthesia, and the Quality of Care and Outcomes Research Interdisciplinary Working Group. Circulation. 2007;116(15):1736-1754.
Single dose 30-60 minutes before dental procedure.

TABLE 14-21	Regimens for Non-Dental Procedures		
Procedure	**Criteria**	**Bacterial Targets**	**Antibiotic† for Empiric Coverage**
Respiratory tract procedures	Invasive procedure of respiratory tract to treat an established infection (drainage of an abscess or empyema)	*Streptococcus viridans* Suspected *Staphylococcus* aureus (MSSA) Suspected MRSA	Regimens in Table 14-20 active against *S. viridans* Nafcillin or cefazolin* or vancomycin Vancomycin
GI or GU tract procedures	GI or GU infection or currently receiving antibiotic therapy to prevent wound infection or sepsis associated with GI or GU procedure	Enterococci If infection is known to be caused by a strain of resistant enterococcus, consultation with an infectious disease expert is recommended.	Penicillin or ampicillin or vancomycin
Procedures on skin, skin structure, or musculoskeletal tissue	Infection of skin, skin structure, or musculoskeletal tissue	*Staphylococcus* β-hemolytic streptococci	Nafcillin or cefazolin* or vancomycin

Adapted with modification from Wilson W et al. Prevention of infective endocarditis: guidelines from the American Heart Association: a guideline from the American Heart Association Rheumatic Fever, Endocarditis, and Kawasaki Disease Committee, Council on Cardiovascular Disease in the Young and the Council on Clinical Cardiology, Council on Cardiovascular Surgery and Anesthesia, and the Quality of Care and Outcomes Research Interdisciplinary Working Group. Circulation. 2007;116(15):1736-1754.
MRSA, *Methicillin-resistant* Staphylococcus aureus; MSSA, *methicillin-sensitive* Staphylococcus aureus.
Cephalosporins should not be used in individuals with a history of anaphylaxis, angioedema, or urticaria with penicillins or ampicillin.
†*If antibiotic is inadvertently not administered before dental procedure, it may be administered up to 2 hours after.*

SUMMARY

Both advances in diagnostic and screening tests for heart disease and improvements in cardiac disease management continue to make impressive strides. Angioplasty is more effective and widely available, and electrophysiologic treatment of rhythm disorders is now considered routine. The number and diversity of cardiac medications we encounter in the perioperative period continues to grow in number and complexity. These advances require that anesthesia providers stay abreast of ever more complex clinical techniques but at the same time improve anesthesia quality and safety for our patients.

REFERENCES

1. Westfall TC, Westfall DP. Adrenergic agonists and antagonists. In: Brunton LL et al, eds. *Goodman and Gilman's Pharmacological Basis of Therapeutics.* 11th ed. New York: McGraw-Hill; 2006:237-296.
2. Nitenberg A, Antony I. Coronary vascular reserve in humans: a critical review of methods of evaluation and of interpretation of the results, *Eur Heart J.* 1995;16:7-21.
3. Vergroesen I et al. Coronary vasodilating drug effects on normal coronary blood flow regulation? *J Cardiothorac Vasc Anesth.* 1998;450-456.
4. Mersmann HJ. Species variation in mechanisms for modulation of growth by beta-adrenergic receptors, *J Nutr.* 1995;125:1777S-1782S.
5. Moss J, Glick D. The autonomic nervous system. In: Miller RD, ed. *Anesthesia.* 6th ed. New York: Churchill Livingstone; 2005:617-678.
6. Doggrell SA. The therapeutic potential of dopamine modulators on the cardiovascular and renal systems, *Expert Opin Investig Drugs.* 2002; 11:631-644.
7. Mannelli M et al. In vivo evidence that endogenous dopamine modulates sympathetic activity in man, *Hypertension.* 1999;34:398-402.
8. Brienza N et al. A comparison between fenoldopam and low-dose dopamine in early renal dysfunction of critically ill patients, *Crit Care Med.* 2006;34(3):707-714.
9. Abay MC et al. Current literature questions the routine use of low-dose dopamine, *AANA J.* 2007;75(1):57-63.
10. Matsuda N et al. Impairment of cardiac beta-adrenoceptor cellular signaling by decreased expression of G (s alpha) in septic rabbits, *Anesthesiology.* 2000; 93:1465-1473.
11. De Backer D et al. Effects of dopamine, norepinephrine, and epinephrine on the splanchnic circulation in septic shock: which is best? *Crit Care Med.* 2003;31:1659-1667.
12. Venkataraman R, Kellum JA. Prevention of acute renal failure, *Chest.* 2007;131(1):300-308.
13. Frost EA, Booij LH. Anesthesia in the patient for awake craniotomy, *Curr Opin Anaesthesiol.* 2007;20(4):331-335.
14. Chatterjee K, De Marco T. Role of nonglycosidic inotropic agents: indications, ethics, and limitations, *Med Clin North Am.* 2003;87:391-418.
15. MacLaren R et al. Use of vasopressors and inotropes in the pharmacotherapy of shock, In: Dipiro JT et al, eds. *Pharmacotherapy: A Pathophysiologic Approach.* 7th ed. New York: McGraw-Hill; 2008:417-440.
16. Wang CH et al. Dobutamine-induced hypotension is an independent predictor for mortality in patients with left ventricular dysfunction following myocardial infarction, *Int J Cardiol.* 1999;68:297-302.
17. Evers AS et al. General anesthetics. In: Brunton LL et al, eds: *Goodman and Gilman's Pharmacological Basis of Therapeutics.* 11th ed. New York: McGraw-Hill; 2006:341-368.
18. Gerlach AT, Dasta JF. Dexmedetomidine: an updated review, *Ann Pharmacother.* 2007;41(:2):245-252. Epub 2007 Feb 13.
19. Mayer J et al. Desflurane anesthesia after sevoflurane inhaled induction reduces severity of emergence agitation in children undergoing minor ear-nose-throat surgery compared with sevoflurane induction and maintenance, *Anesth Analg.* 2006;102(92):400-404.
20. Ibacache ME et al. Single-dose dexmedetomidine reduces agitation after sevoflurane anesthesia in children, *Anesth Analg.* 2004;98(1):60-63.
21. Shukry M, Kennedy K. Dexmedetomidine as a total intravenous anesthetic in infants, *Paediatr Anaesth.* 2007;17(6):581-583.
22. Ngan Kee WD, Khaw KS. Vasopressors in obstetrics: what should we be using? *Curr Opin Anaesthesiol.* 2006;19(3):238-243.
23. Stoelting RK, Hillier SC. Sympathomimetics. In: *Pharmacology and Physiology in Anesthetic Practice.* 4th ed. New York: Lippincott; 2006:292-310.
24. Bartow RA, Brogden RN. Formoterol. An update of its pharmacological properties and therapeutic efficacy in the management of asthma, *Drugs.* 1998;55:303-322.

25. Kumar VH et al. Effects of salmeterol on secretion of phosphatidylcholine by alveolar type II cells, *Life Sci.* 2000;66:1639-1646.

26. Kemp JP et al. A 1-year study of salmeterol powder on pulmonary function and hyperresponsiveness to methacholine, *J Allergy Clin Immunol.* 1999;104: 1189-1197.

27. Lundback B, Dahl R. Assessment of asthma control and its impact on optimal treatment strategy, *Allergy.* 2007;62(6):611-619.

28. Gal P, Ransom JL. Acute respiratory distress syndrome. In: Dipiro JT et al, eds: *Pharmacotherapy: A Pathophysiologic Approach.* 6th ed. New York: McGraw-Hill; 2005:557-576.

29. Giles W, Bisits A. The present and future of tocolysis, *Best Pract Res Clin Obstet Gynaecol.* 2007;21(5):857-868.

30. Simhan HN, Caritis SN. Prevention of preterm delivery, *N Engl J Med.* 2007;357:477-487.

31. *Mosby's Drug Consult 2007*[CD-ROM]. St Louis: Mosby; 2004.

32. Jackson CW et al. Evidence-based review of the black-box warning for droperidol, *Am J Health Syst Pharm.* 2007;64:1174-1186.

33. Arrhythmias from droperidol? *Med Lett.* 2002;44:53-54.

34. Sarkozy A, Dorian P. Advances in the acute pharmacologic management of cardiac arrhythmias, *Curr Cardiol Rep.* 2003;5:387-394.

35. Fleisher LA et al. ACC/AHA 2006 guideline update on perioperative cardiovascular evaluation for noncardiac surgery: focused update on perioperative beta-blocker therapy, *Anesth Analg.* 2007;104(1):15-26.

36. Fleisher LA. Perioperative β-blockade: how best to translate evidence into practice, *Int Anesth Res Soc.* 2007;104(1):1-3.

37. Miller JM, Zipes DG. Therapy for cardiac arrhythmias. In: Libby P et al, eds. *Braunwald's Heart Disease: A Textbook of Cardiovascular Medicine.* 8th ed. Philadelphia: Saunders; 2008:779-830.

38. Poldermans D. Bisoprolol reduces risk of cardiac death in high-risk vascular surgery patients, *N Engl J Med.* 1999;341:1789-1794, 1838-1840.

39. Henderson NL, Mason RC. Juxtaglomerular cell tumor in pregnancy, *Obstet Gynecol.* 2001;98(pt 2):943-945.

40. Jouppila P et al. Labetalol does not alter the placental and fetal blood flow or maternal prostanoids in preeclampsia, *Br J Obstet Gynaecol.* 1986;93:543-547.

41. Ali-Melkkila T et al. Pharmacokinetics and related pharmacodynamics of anticholinergic drugs, *Acta Anaesthiol Scand.* 1993;37:633-642.

42. Collard CL. Hypertension. Medication update, *South Med J.* 2001;94:1065-1070.

43. Degoute CS. Controlled hypotension: a guide to drug choice, *Drugs.* 2007;67(7):1053-1076.

44. Patterson KW et al. Inhaled nitric oxide potentiates actions of adenosine but not of sodium nitroprusside in experimental pulmonary hypertension, *Pharmacology.* 1999;58:246-251.

45. Hatsuoka S et al. Effect of L-arginine or nitroglycerine during deep hypothermic circulatory arrest in neonatal lambs, *Ann Thorac Surg.* 2003;75:197-203.

46. Kojda G et al. Nitric oxide inhibits vascular bioactivation of glyceryl trinitrate: a novel mechanism to explain preferential venodilation of organic nitrates, *Mol Pharmacol.* 1998;53:547-554.

47. Hlatky R et al. Role of nitric oxide in cerebral blood flow abnormalities after traumatic brain injury, *J Cereb Blood Flow Metab.* 2003;23:582-588.

48. Bauer JA et al. Vascular and hemodynamic differences between organic nitrates and nitrites, *J Pharmacol Exp Ther.* 1997;280:326-331.

49. Hoffman BB. Therapy of hypertension. In: Brunton LL et al, eds. *Goodman and Gilman's Pharmacological Basis of Therapeutics.* 11th ed. New York: McGraw-Hill; 2006:845-868.

50. Bang L et al. Hydralazine-induced vasodilation involves opening of high conductance Ca^{2+}-activated K^+ channels, *Eur J Pharmacol.* 1998;361:43-49.

51. Powers DR et al. Parenteral hydralazine revisited, *J Emerg Med.* 1998;16: 191-196.

52. Pepine CJ et al. Rationale and design of the International Verapamil SR/Trandolapril Study (INVEST): an Internet-based randomized trial in coronary artery disease patients with hypertension, *J Am Coll Cardiol.* 1998;32: 1228-1237.

53. Selman WR. Nimodipine in subarachnoid hemorrhage, *J Neurosurg.* 1999;91:520-521.

54. Epstein M. Role of a third generation calcium antagonist in the management of hypertension, *Drugs.* 1999;5:1-10.

55. Nishiyama T et al. Interactions between nicardipine and enflurane, isoflurane and sevoflurane, *Can J Anaesth.* 1997;44:1071-1076.

56. Cheung AT et al. Nicardipine intravenous bolus dosing for acutely decreasing arterial blood pressure during general anesthesia for cardiac operations: pharmacokinetics, pharmacodynamics, and associated effects on left ventricular function, *Anesth Analg.* 1999;89:1116-1123.

57. Nolte CW et al. Protection from digoxin-induced coronary vasoconstriction in patients with coronary artery disease by calcium antagonists, *Am J Cardiol.* 1999;8:440-442, A9.

58. Saitoh Y et al. Post-tetanic count and train-of-four response during neuromuscular block produced by vecuronium and infusion of nicardipine, *Br J Anaesth.* 1999;83:340-342.

59. Salhanick SD, Shannon MW. Management of calcium channel antagonist overdose, *Drug Saf.* 2003;26:65-79.

60. Nguyen T et al. Postinfarction survival and inducibility of ventricular arrhythmias in the spontaneously hypertensive rat: effects of ramipril and hydralazine, *Circulation.* 1998;98:2074-2080.

61. Jackson EK. Renin and angiotensin. In: Brunton LL et al, eds. *Goodman and Gilman's Pharmacological Basis of Therapeutics.* 11th ed. New York: McGraw-Hill; 2006:789-822.

62. Benowitz NL. Antihypertensive agents. In: Katzung BG. *Basic and Clinical Pharmacology.* 10th ed. New York: McGraw-Hill; 2007;159-182.

63. Brown NJ, Vaughan DE. Angiotensin-converting enzyme inhibitors, *Circulation.* 1998;97:1411-1420.

64. McMurray JJ. ACE inhibitors in cardiovascular disease—unbeatable? *N Engl J Med.* 2008;358(15):1615-1616.

65. Elliott WJ. Systemic hypertension, *Curr Probl Cardiol.* 2007;32(4):201-259.

66. Tolcapone: *Mosby's Drug Consult.* St Louis: Mosby; 2007.

67. Rathmell JP et al. A multicenter, randomized, blind comparison of amrinone with milrinone after elective cardiac surgery, *Anesth Analg.* 1998;86: 683-690.

68. Kikura M et al. The effect of milrinone on hemodynamics and left ventricular function after emergence from cardiopulmonary bypass, *Anesth Analg.* 1997;85:16-22.

69. Mehra MR et al. Safety and clinical utility of long-term intravenous milrinone in advanced heart failure, *Am J Cardiol.* 1997;80:61-64.

70. Leier CV, Binkley PF. Parenteral inotropic support for advanced congestive heart failure, *Prog Cardiovasc Dis.* 1998;41:207-224.

71. Van der Zypp A et al. The role of cyclic nucleotides and calcium in the relaxation produced by amrinone in rat aorta, *Gen Pharmacol.* 2000;34:245-253.

72. Okuno Y et al. Hemodynamic effects of amrinone combined with dopamine in patients undergoing living renal transplantation, *Masui.* 1997;46:87-94.

73. Matsuda F et al. Comparative effect of amrinone, aminophylline and diltiazem on rat airway smooth muscle, *Acta Anaesthesiol Scand.* 2000;44:763-766.

74. Ochiai Y et al. Effects of amrinone, a phosphodiesterase inhibitor, on right ventricular/arterial coupling immediately after cardiac operations, *J Thorac Cardiovasc Surg.* 1998;116:139-147.

75. Varriale P, Ramaprasad S. Short-term intravenous milrinone for severe congestive heart failure: the good, bad, and not so good, *Pharmacotherapy.* 1997;17:371-374.

76. Whitehurst VE et al. Reversal of propranolol blockade of adrenergic receptors and related toxicity with drugs that increase cyclic AMP, *Proc Soc Exp Biol Med.* 1999;221:382-385.

77. Lindsay CA et al. Pharmacokinetics and pharmacodynamics of milrinone lactate in pediatric patients with septic shock, *J Pediatr.* 1998;132:329-334.

78. Southworth MR. Treatment options for acute decompensated heart failure. *Am J Health Syst Pharm.* 2003;60:S7-S15.

79. Digitalis Investigation Group:The effect of digoxin on mortality and morbidity in patients with heart failure, *N Engl J Med.* 1997;336:525-533.

80. Hauptman PJ, Kelly RA. Digitalis, *Circulation.* 1999;99:1265-1270.

81. Campbell TJ, MacDonald PS. Digoxin in heart failure and cardiac arrhythmias, *Med J Aust.* 2003;179:98-102.

82. Dominiak P. Pharmacotherapeutic strategy in heart failure, *Clin Nephrol.* 2002;58:S2-S6.

83. Hunt SA et al. ACC/AHA guidelines for the evaluation and management of chronic heart failure in the adult, *Circulation.* 2001;104(24):2996-3007.

84. Aziz IN et al. Cardiac risk stratification in patients undergoing endoluminal graft repair of abdominal aortic aneurysm: a single-institution experience with 365 patients, *J Vasc Surg.* 2003;38:56-60.

85. Mann DL. Pathophysiology of heart failure. In: Libby P et al. *Braunwald's Heart Disease: A Textbook of Cardiovascular Medicine.* 8th ed. Philadelphia: Saunders; 2008:541-560.

86. Howard PA et al. Drug therapy recommendations from the 2005 ACC/AHA guidelines for treatment of chronic heart failure, *Ann Pharmacother.* 2006;40(9):1607-1617Epub 2006 Aug 8.

87. Dec GW. Management of acute decompensated heart failure, *Curr Probl Cardiol.* 2007;32(6):321-366.

88. Probstfield JL. How cost-effective are new preventive strategies for cardiovascular disease? *Am J Cardiol.* 2003;9:22G-27G.

89. Klein L et al. Pharmacologic therapy for patients with chronic heart failure and reduced systolic function: review of trials and practical considerations, *Am J Cardiol.* 2003;91:18F-40F.

90. Stojiljkovic L, Behnia R. Role of renin angiotensin system inhibitors in cardiovascular and renal protection: a lesson from clinical trials, *Curr Pharm Des.* 2007;13(13):1335-1345.

91. Sami M. Angiotensin-converting enzyme inhibitors and end-organ damage in heart failure, *Can J Cardiol.* 1999;15:19C-23C.

92. Manché A et al. Tolerance to ACE inhibitors after cardiac surgery, *Eur J Cardiothorac Surg.* 1999;15:55-60.

93. Krum H. Beta-blockers in heart failure. The "new wave" of clinical trials, *Drugs.* 1999;58:203-210.

94. Eichhorn EJ. Medical therapy of chronic heart failure. Role of ACE inhibitors and beta-blockers, *Cardiol Clin.* 1998;16:711-725.

95. McGavin JK, Keating GM. Bisoprolol: a review of its use in chronic heart failure, *Drugs.* 2002;62:2677-2696.

96. Follath F. Do diuretics differ in terms of clinical outcome in congestive heart failure? *Eur Heart J.* 1998;19(Suppl):P5-P8.

97. Groban L, Butterworth J. Perioperative management of chronic heart failure, *Anesth Analg.* 2006;103:557-575.

98. Forrest J et al. Multicenter study of general anesthesia. II, *Results. Anesthesiology.* 1990;72:262-268.

99. Bertrand M et al. Should the angiotensin II antagonists be discontinued before surgery? *Anesth Analg.* 2001;92(1):26-30.

100. Laird RD, Studenski SS. Management of hypertension for stroke prevention in older people, *Clin Geriatr Med.* 1999;15:663-684.

101. Joint National Committee on Prevention, Detection and Treatment of High Blood Pressure. Seventh Report of the National Committee on Detection, Evaluation and Treatment of High Blood Pressure (JNC-7) (NIH Publication No. 03-5233). Washington, DC: U.S. Department of Health and Human Services. National Institute of Health. National Heart, Lung and Blood Institute. National High Blood Pressure Education Program; May 2003.

102. Hansson L, HOT Study Group et al. Effects of intensive blood-pressure lowering and low-dose aspirin in patients with hypertension: principal results of the Hypertension Optimal Treatment (HOT) randomised trial. *Lancet.* 1998;351:1755-1762.

103. Prys-Roberts C et al. Studies of anesthesia in relation to hypertension. I. Cardiovascular responses of treated and untreated patients, *Br J Anaesth.* 1971;43:122.

104. Ali MJ et al. ACC/AHA guidelines as predictors of postoperative cardiac outcomes, *Can J Anaesth.* 2000;47:10-19.

105. Mangano DT et al. Association of perioperative stress myocardial ischemia with cardiac morbidity and mortality in men undergoing noncardiac surgery, *N Engl J Med.* 1990;323:1781.

106. Healthy People 2010. *Heart Disease and Stroke.* Hyattsville, MD: Centers for Disease Control and Prevention, National Center for Health Statistics; November 18, 2003.

107. Collard CD et al. Perioperative statin therapy is associated with reduced cardiac mortality after coronary artery bypass graft surgery, *Thorac Cardiovasc Surg.* 2006;132(2):392-400.

108. Chassot PG et al. Perioperative use of anti-platelet drugs, *Best Pract Res Clin Anaesthesiol.* 2007;21(2):241-256.

109. Bertrand M et al. Should the angiotensin II antagonists be discontinued before surgery? *Anesth Analg.* 2001;92(1):26-30.

110. Comfere T et al. Angiotensin system inhibitors in a general surgical population, *Anesth Analg.* 2005;100(3):636-644.

111. Schirmer U, Schürmann W. Preoperative administration of angiotensin-converting enzyme inhibitors, *Anaesthesist.* 2007;56(6):557-561.

112. Boccara G et al. Terlipressin versus norepinephrine to correct refractory arterial hypotension after general anesthesia in patients chronically treated with rennin-angiotensin system inhibitors, *Anesthesiology.* 2003;98(6):1338-1344.

CHAPTER 15

CHEMISTRY AND PHYSICS OF ANESTHESIA

Mark D. Welliver

The dynamics of much of anesthesia practice lie within the framework of chemical and physical science. Chemistry, the study of matter composition, properties, and behavior at the atomic and molecular level, and physics, the study of motion, matter, and energy interaction, are two foundations for nurse anesthetist practice. Chemistry and physics explain such actions as pressure, flow, diffusion, expansion, contraction and other processes that are intimately intertwined with the delivery of anesthetics. From the ancient philosophical beginnings of atomic theory and the proverbial falling apple of Newtonian physics (Sir Isaac Newton, 1642-1727) to current advances in quantum mechanics, discoveries have led to advances and application for anesthesiology. To understand these laws and theories is to understand the how and why of our practice, give us rationale for clinical interventions, and allow us the ability to manipulate dynamic processes to our patients' favor.

The dynamics of anesthesia herein are explained primarily by the atomic and kinetic molecular theories, Newtonian physics, thermodynamics, and the quantum mechanics of electromagnetic radiation. This chapter will provide a short, concise resource that focuses on the chemistry and physics of anesthesia.

GENERAL CHEMISTRY: MATTER AND ENERGY

The universe is composed of two main constituents, matter and energy. Energy is explored more thoroughly in the section on physics. Matter is the tangible composition of the universe that may be solid, liquid, gas, or plasma. Solids are defined as material that resists changes in shape and volume. Liquids are fluids that exhibit minimal to no compressibility and may change volume with changes in pressure and temperature. Gases are also fluids but are compressible and easily change volume with changes in pressure and temperature. Plasma is a mixture of ionized gas and free-floating electrons. It has been postulated that more than 99% of the universe's matter is plasma.

International System of Measurement

When studying and interacting with matter and energy, it is necessary to have a system of standardized units of measurement. The Systéme International (SI) is a set of standardized units of measure based on the metric scale. The SI uses 7 base quantities for measurement (Table 15-1) and 12 standard prefixes for naming units of measure to denote quantity (Table 15-2). Other units or combinations of units may be used in addition to those shown. Additionally, temperature and pressure affect the behavior of matter, and a standardized reference has been established for both. The standard temperature and pressure (STP) is 100.00 kilopascals at 273 kelvin.

Elements

Elements are matter that possess similar atoms containing the same protons. The periodic chart of the elements lists these elements according to their chemical characteristics.

TABLE 15-1	Systéme International Seven Base Quantities for Measurement	
SI Unit	**Symbol**	**Quantity**
meter	m	Length
kilogram	kg	Mass
second	s	Time
ampere	A	Electric current
kelvin	K	Temperature
candela	cd	Luminous intensity
mole	mol	Amount substance

TABLE 15-2	Systéme International Prefixes	
Name	**Symbol**	**Factor**
tera-	T	10^{12}
giga-	G	10^9
mega-	M	10^6
kilo-	k	10^3
hecto-	h	10^2
deca-	da	10^1
deci-	d	10^{-1}
centi-	c	10^{-2}
milli-	m	10^{-3}
micro-	µ	10^{-6}
nano-	n	10^{-9}
pico-	p	10^{-12}

1 H 1.008																	2 He 4.002
3 Li 6.941	4 Be 9.012											5 B 10.811	6 C 12.011	7 N 14.007	8 O 15.999	9 F 18.998	10 Ne 20.180
11 Na 22.990	12 Mg 24.305											13 Al 26.982	14 Si 28.086	15 P 30.974	16 S 32.066	17 Cl 35.452	18 Ar 39.948
19 K 39.098	20 Ca 40.078	21 Sc 44.956	22 Ti 47.867	23 V 50.942	24 Cr 51.996	25 Mn 54.931	26 Fe 55.845	27 Co 58.933	28 Ni 58.963	29 Cu 63.546	30 Zn 65.39	31 Ga 69.723	32 Ge 72.61	33 As 74.922	34 Se 78.96	35 Br 79.904	36 Kr 83.80
37 Rb 85.468	38 Sr 87.62	39 Y 88.906	40 Zr 91.224	41 Nb 92.906	42 Mo 95.94	43 Tc (98)	44 Ru 101.07	45 Rh 102.906	46 Pd 106.42	47 Ag 107.868	48 Cd 112.411	49 In 114.818	50 Sn 118.710	51 Sb 121.760	52 Te 127.60	53 I 126.904	54 Xe 131.29
55 Cs 132.905	56 Ba 137.327	57 La 138.905	72 Hf 178.49	73 Ta 180.948	74 W 183.84	75 Re 186.207	76 Os 190.23	77 Ir 192.217	78 Pt 195.08	79 Au 196.967	80 Hg 200.59	81 Tl 204.383	82 Pb 207.2	83 Bi 208.980	84 Po (209)	85 At (210)	86 Rn (222)
87 Fr (223)	88 Ra 226.025	89 Ac 227.028	104 Unq (261)	105 Unp (262)	106 Unh (263)	107 Uns (262)	108 Uno (265)	109 Une (266)	110 Uun (269)								

58 Ce 140.115	59 Pr 140.907	60 Nd 144.24	61 Pm (145)	62 Sm 150.36	63 Eu 151.965	64 Gd 157.25	65 Tb 158.925	66 Dy 162.50	67 Ho 164.930	68 Er 167.26	69 Tm 168.939	70 Yb 173.04	71 Lu 174.967
90 Th 232.038	91 Pa 231.036	92 U 238.029	93 Np 237.048	94 Pu (244)	95 Am (243)	96 Cm (247)	97 Bk (247)	98 Cf (251)	99 Es (252)	100 Fm (257)	101 Md (258)	102 No (259)	103 Lr (260)

FIGURE **15-1**   The Periodic Table. (*From Thibodeau GA, Patton KT. Anatomy & physiology. 6th ed. St Louis: Mosby; 2007.*)

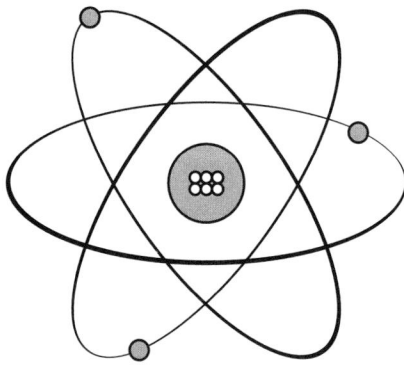

FIGURE **15-2**   Atomic structure showing nucleus containing protons and neutrons with orbiting electrons.

Vertical columns known as *groups* list elements with similar properties. Horizontal rows are known as *periods*. Atomic size progresses up across rows from left to right. Atomic weights are listed with each element on the chart (Figure 15-1).

ATOMIC STRUCTURE

Atomic theory has its origins in the philosophical musings of the ancient Greek philosopher Democritus, who described indivisible building blocks of matter referred to as "atomos."[1] The orbital theory of atomic structure was later put forth by Ernesto Rutherford (1871-1937) and improved upon by Neils Bohr (1885-1962), who described electron orbits in terms of energy levels and ability to emit quantized energy by stimulated emision. The atomic theory describes atoms as having a central core, the *nucleus*, with orbiting particles called *electrons* (Figure 15-2). The nucleus contains protons and neutrons. *Protons* have a positive charge and are larger than electrons. *Neutrons* are negatively charged and are similar in size to protons. The number of protons in an atom constitutes its *atomic number*. Electrons, much smaller than protons and neutrons, orbit around the nucleus and are negatively charged.

Electron Configuration

Atoms have electrons that orbit in shells around the nucleus. Each shell can contain only a set number of electrons. These shells have been designated K, L, M, N, O, P, Q. The corresponding maximal number of electrons that may occupy each shell is 2, 8, 18, 32, 32, 18, and 8. Electrons must fill lower shells before occupying higher shells. Quantum physics has refined the electron shell model by designating the K, L, M, N, O, P, Q shells with n-values 1, 2, 3, 4, 5, 6, and 7, which correspond with increasing energy levels. Electron shells are further divided into subshells with the designations s, p, d, f, and g. Subshells may hold only the following number of electrons: s(2), p(6), d(10), f(14), and g(18). Subshells are further subdivided into orbitals. Orbitals may only contain two electrons that spin in opposite directions. An s subshell has 1 orbital, a p subshell has 3 orbitals, a d subshell has 5 orbitals, and so forth. Electrons occupy lower energy level orbitals but may temporarily jump to higher level orbitals when they absorb energy. Electrons that jump to higher levels will emit their excess energy and return to their lower energy state. (See discussion on lasers later in this chapter.)

Angular Momentum/Spin

Nuclei and electrons have an angular momentum also known as *spin*. Atomic particles possess an intrinsic axis upon which they rotate (spin). Spin is analogous to the axis on which the earth rotates. The spin of an electron or proton is not directly measurable, but the uneven distribution of charge it produces is measurable. A magnetic moment is created and is essentially a minute electric current loop. (See discussion on magnetic resonance imaging later in this chapter.)

Ions

Ions are atoms that have gained or lost electrons from their natural composition. An atom that has gained an electron(s) is called an *anion*. Conversely, an atom that has lost an electron(s) is called a *cation*. Ions are important in chemical bonding and aqueous solubility. Mass number/atomic mass number is the amount of protons and neutrons in an atom. Isotopes of the same element have the same number of protons but different numbers of neutrons. Isotopes of the same element have differing mass numbers.

MOLECULAR BOND TYPES

Molecules are composed of two or more bonded atoms. Electrons in the outermost shell are called *valence electrons* and are involved in molecular bonding. Molecular bonding may occur by direct sharing of electrons or by thermodynamic interaction due to distribution of electron charge. Atoms with unpaired valence electrons are reactive and tend to form bonds that will fill their outer shell. Covalent and electrostatic are two general types of bonds. Atoms may bond to atoms of the same element (e.g., oxygen) or to different element atoms (e.g., water). Compounds are bonded atoms of differing elements.

Covalent Bonds

The physical sharing of electrons between atoms constitutes a *covalent bond*. The sharing of one pair of electrons is called a *single bond*, shairing two pairs of electrons is a *double bond*, and sharing three pairs of electrons is a *triple bond*. Often covalent bonds are stronger than electrostatic bonds. Covalent bonding may be between same or different atoms that share similar electronegativity.

Electrostatic Bonds

Electrostatic bonds are by attraction of electrons between atoms. Electrostatic bonding may be ion-to-ion interaction, ion-to-dipole interaction, or dipole-to-dipole interaction and follow the general rule of "opposites attract," with negative charges attracting positive charges.

Ion-Ion Bonding

Ion-to-ion bonds are the strongest of the electrostatic bonds. These bonds are not directional and occur anywhere along the outer electron shell of an atom. Molecules with ionic bonds have high melting and boiling points. Sodium chloride (table salt) is an example of ion-to-ion bonding (Figure 15-3).

Ion-Dipole Bonding

Ion-to-dipole bonds are weaker than ion-ion bonds, with only partial charges involved. Some molecules have structural arrangements that produce an uneven distribution of electrons. This uneven distribution of charges creates a dipole in which there is a more positive or more negative side to the molecule, although the molecule does not have a formal charge. An example of a molecule with an uneven charge distribution is water. The spatial arrangement of water's hydrogens toward one side of an oxygen atom causes that side to have a more positive character and the opposite side to have a more negative character. This dipole of water may bond to an ion of opposite charge. The ions of sodium and chlorine bond to water by ion-to-dipole interaction (Figure 15-4).

Dipole-Dipole Bonding

Water is an example of dipole-to-dipole molecular bonding. The spatial arrangement of water's hydrogens at a 105-degree angle to each other causes this molecule to be dipolar (Figure 15-5). The dipolar nature of water molecules allows them to form weak bonds with one another (Figure 15-6). The polar sides of water molecules also enable them to bond to ions and other polar molecules. For this reason, water is a convenient solvent for

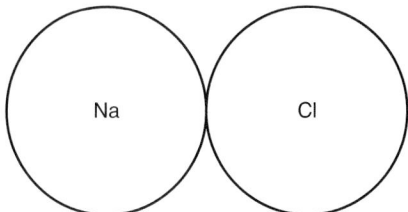

FIGURE **15-3** Ion-to-ion bond representation between sodium and chloride ions.

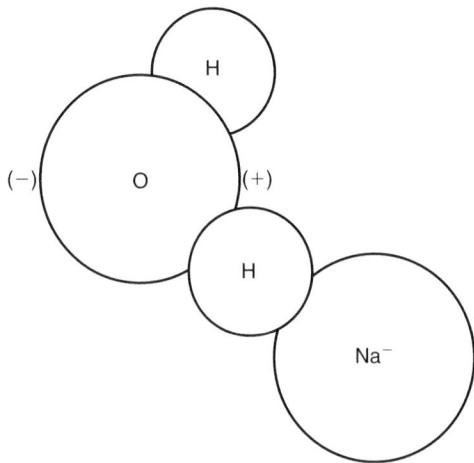

FIGURE **15-4** Ion-to-dipole bond representation between a water molecule and sodium ion.

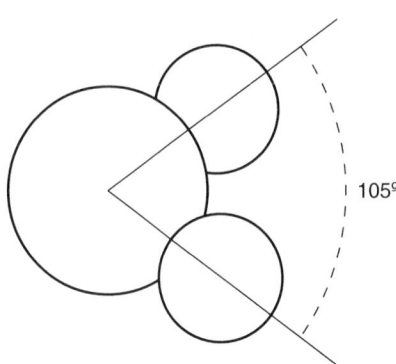

FIGURE **15-5** Hydrogen atoms bond angle in a water molecule.

many substances such as drugs. Surface tension of water is a physical characteristic that is caused by water's dipole-to-dipole intermolecular attractions.

Some molecules may have *induced dipoles* caused by momentary uneven spatial distribution of electrons. Induced dipoles are not permanent. These temporary dipoles may lead to weak bonding between nonpolar molecules. Oils represent nonpolar molecules that display induced dipole bonding, often called *London dispersion forces*. London dispersion forces are the weakest of all molecular bonds. Despite this weakness, London dispersion forces at very low temperatures allow oxygen and nitrogen to become liquids.

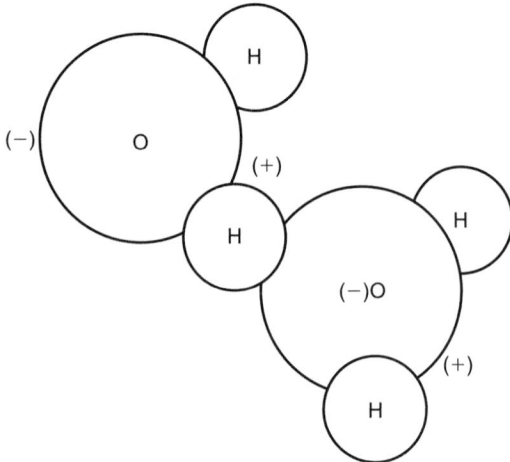

FIGURE **15-6**   Dipole-to-dipole bond representation between two water molecules.

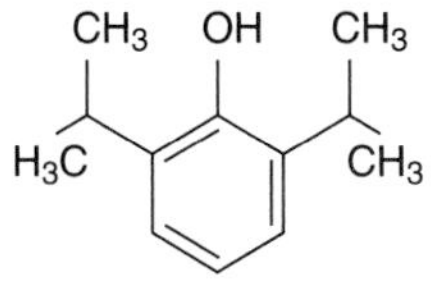

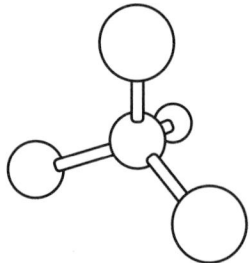

FIGURE **15-8**   VSEPR diagram of a tetrahedral-shaped molecule.

FIGURE **15-7**   Skeletal diagram of diisopropyl phenol molecule.

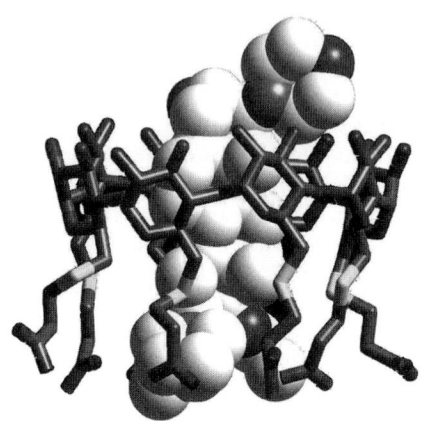

FIGURE **15-9**   Molecular model of sugammadex encapsulating a rocuronium molecule. *(Reproduced with permission. Angew Chem Int Ed. 2002;41(2):265. Copyright Wiley-VCH Verlag GmbH & Co. KGaA.)*

Molecular Bonding Representations

There are several ways to denote bonding and electron distribution. The Lewis structure (electron dot structure) shows the valence electrons as they bond among atoms. Lewis stuctures may show dots or lines to represent electrons. Again, only outer shell valence electrons are represented and not lower, fully filled shells. Skeletal diagrams are another frequently used method to represent molecular bonding. In organic chemistry, skeletal diagrams use lines to show atom bonding often omitting the letter C for carbon (Figure 15-7).

The Valence Shell Electron Pair Repulsion diagrams (VSEPR) are more descriptive Lewis structures based on the theory of the same name. These diagrams represent electron repulsions and the resultant approximation of the geometric distribution of atoms in covalently bonded molecules (Figure 15-8).

Molecular Modeling

Molecular models are detailed representations of molecules. Electrons are in constant "orbit" in an atom, and attempts have been made to graphically represent their space-occupying possible locations (Figure 15-9). Space-filling models reflect the "electron cloud" of specific atoms in a molecule. These models can appear as spherical, ball and stick, or ribbonlike representations of atoms and molecules that are affixed to one another. Molecular modeling is expanding our understanding not only of molecular geometries but also molecular behavior.[2]

Isomers

Isomers are molecules that have the same chemical formula but different structural formulas. The number and type of atoms and bonds are the same in isomers, but the arrangement of the atoms is different. Isomers may be *structural* or *stereoisomers*. Structural isomers have the same molecular formula, but their atoms are located in different places. Enflurane and isoflurane are examples of structural isomers. Structural isomers are truly different molecules with differing physical and chemical properties. Stereoisomers are molecules that that have a similar geometric arrangement of atoms but differ in their spatial position. Stereoisomers may be *enantiomers* or *diastereomers*. Enantiomers are mirror images of one another, cannot be superimposed, and possess similar chemical and physical properties. Enantiomers are optically active and can rotate polarized light in a clockwise fashion (prefix + or dextro) or counterclockwise fashion (prefix − or levo). Racemic chemical compositions contain 50% of the levo form isomer and 50% of the dextro form isomer. Diastereomers are not mirror images and may have differing physical and chemical properties.

BOND BREAKING

Bond energy is the amount of energy needed to make or break a bond. Energy is released when a bond is formed, and energy is consumed with breaking a bond. The energy released when a bond is formed is the same amount of energy needed to break that same chemical bond. Short bonds, such as covalent bonds, tend to possess greater bond energies than longer, electrostatic bonds. When molecular bonds are broken, new molecular bonds are often formed and energy is released. An example of this is adenosine triphosphate (ATP) conversion to adenosine diphosphate (ADP). Energy is actually consumed in the process of breaking an ATP bond. A greater amount of energy is released when the free phosphate forms new bonds with hydrogen.[3] Bond energies are measured as an enthalpy change.

Enthalpy

Enthalpy is the total amount of energy possessed by a system. A system can be on the atomic scale or the macroscopic scale. The enthalpy of a system is the total of all kinetic and potential energy. The stored, or potential, energy includes its height in relation to the force of gravity and the energy stored in the bonds of molecules and atoms and even subatomic particles. All movement, as well as stored energy, must be accounted for and summated to know the enthalpy of a system. Thus the total amount of energy contained within a system is increasingly difficult to quantify, especially with increasing complexity of a system. The difficulty in measuring all the energy in a particular system requires a simpler method to evaluate energy involved in chemical reactions. Therefore, *change of energy (ΔH)* rather total energy (enthalpy) of a system is measured.

ORGANIC COMPOUNDS

Organic chemistry is the study of carbon-containing molecules. Biological life on earth is based on carbon-containing compounds. Carbon is a unique atom that combines with many atoms in multiple arrangements, owing to its four valence electrons available for bonding. Carbon may make single, double, or triple covalent bonds with other atoms or molecules.

Hydrocarbons

Hydrocarbons are molecules composed entirely of carbon atoms with hydrogen atoms attached. These molecules are often found in straight chains, with or without branches. *Saturated hydrocarbons* are single-bonded carbon chains with all available carbon bonds attached to hydrogen. Hydrocarbons containing only single-bonded carbon atoms are called *alkanes*. The six-carbon hydrocarbon shown in Figure 15-10 is called a *hexane*. The *hex*-prefix denotes six carbons and the *-ane* suffix denotes an alkane with all single bonds.

Unsaturated hydrocarbons have one or more double or triple bonds between carbon atoms. Hydrocarbons containing double-bonded carbons are called *alkenes* and triple-bonded carbons are called *alkynes*. The six-carbon hydrocarbon containing a double bond is called *hexene* (Figure 15-11).

Cyclic hydrocarbons are carbon chains in a ring structure. They may contain multiple carbon atoms and may have single, double, or triple bonds. The cyclic hydrocarbons hexane and benzene (1,3,5 cyclohexatriene) are shown in Figure 15-12.

Saturated and unsaturated hydrocarbons that have hydrogens omitted are known as *alkyls*, are very reactive, and bond to functional groups. Cyclic hydrocarbons omitting a hydrogen on any carbon atom are called *aryls*, are reactive, and also bind with functional groups.

Functional Groups

Functional groups impart unique characteristics to molecules. There are many functional groups in organic chemistry, and several have importance in anesthesia.

Amines are derivatives of ammonia (NH_3) and have the general formula NR_3. Only one or two of the R groups may be hydrogen. All amines have a lone pair of electrons on the nitrogen.

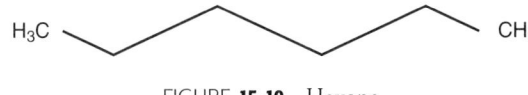

FIGURE **15-10**   Hexane.

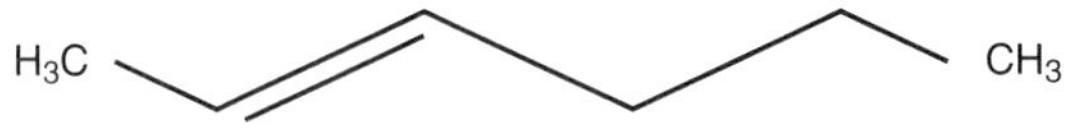

FIGURE **15-11**   Hexene.

FIGURE **15-12**   Hexane and benzene.

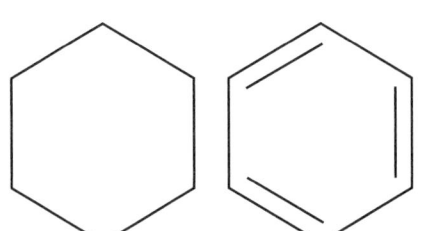

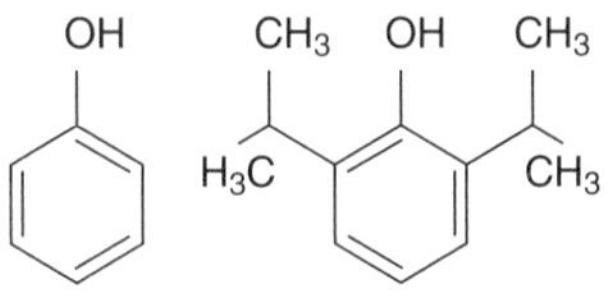

FIGURE **15-13**   Phenol and diisopropyl phenol molecules.

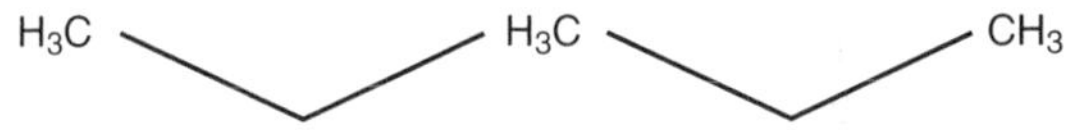

FIGURE **15-14**   Diethyl ether.

Alcohols have the general formula ROH, where *R* represents any alkyl group. The hydroxyl group (OH) of alcohols is highly polar and easily forms hydrogen bonds with other polar molecules. The polarity of the hydroxyl group allows alcohols to dissolve many other polar molecules.

Phenols are similar to alcohols in that they both have the general formula ROH. The *R* in phenols instead represents an aryl group (benzene). A simple phenol is polar due to the hydroxyl group, but more complex phenols such as propofol (diisopropyl phenol) are not water soluble (Figure 15-13).

Ethers have the general formula ROR′, where *R* and *R′* are alkyl groups attached by oxygen. Ethers are inert and do not react with oxidizing or reducing agents but are highly flammable. The outdated anesthetic agent diethyl ether clearly shows both alkyl groups bonded to oxygen (Figure 15-14). Halogen substitution on ethers alters anesthetic characteristics, such as blood solubility and potency, while lowering flammability.

Several functional groups contain a structural arrangement of carbon double bonded to oxygen. This is known as a carbonyl group and structurally identified as C=O. The carbonyl group is polar, with the oxygen being more electrically negative. This polar characteristic is imparted to functional groups that contain a carbonyl group. The carbonyl group, though not a functional group by itself, is a key component of the following functional groups: aldehydes, ketones, carboxylic acids, esters, and amides.

Aldehydes have the general formula RCHO.
Ketones have the general formula RCOR′.
Carboxylic acids have the general formula RCOOH.
Esters have the general formula RCOOR.
Amides have the general formulas $RCONH_2$, RCONHR, or $RCONR_2$.

SOLUBILTY

Solubility is the maximum amount of one substance (solute) that is able to dissolve into another (solvent). The factors that may affect solubility of solutes in solvents are the intermolecular interactions between the substances, temperature, and pressure.

Solids and Liquids

Solubility is enhanced by intermolecular interactions between substances that have similar electron configurations. "Like dissolves like" is often used to describe solubility. Salt (NaCl) in water is an example. The similar polarity of water and salt's constituent parts promote dissolving. Temperature also affects solubility. Energy is required to break the bonds of substances that are dissolving. Most often this is an endothermic reaction, which means it requires more energy than it produces. It consumes heat rather than produces heat. With endothermic reactions, solubility is increased with increased temperature; the additional energy (heat) drives greater dissolving. Most reactions of solids dissolving in liquids are endothermic. Occasionally the process may be exothermic, meaning energy is released in excess of the energy required to break the bonds of the solute. In this unique scenario, increases in temperature will decrease solubility. Pressure exerts little to no influence on solubility of solids and liquids.

Gases

Gas solubility in liquids is inversely related to temperature. As temperature increases, less gas is able to dissolve into a liquid. An increased temperature represents greater kinetic energy. Greater kinetic energy allows dissolved gas molecules to escape and prevents further dissolving. Lower temperature slows the kinetic energy of gas molecules, allowing them to dissolve into liquids. A clinical example of temperature affecting solubility is seen with the slower emergence of hypothermic patients receiving volatile-agent general anesthetics. The hypothermic patient retains anesthetic gases in the blood due to increased solubility related to temperature.[4] Gas solubility in a liquid is directly proportional to pressure and is described by Henry's law.[5]

Henry's Law

Henry's law (William Henry, 1775-1836) states "at constant temperature, the amount of gas dissolved in a liquid is directly proportional to the partial pressure of that gas at equilibrium above the gas-liquid interface." The formula is:

$$p = kc$$

where **p** is the partial pressure of the solute above the solution, **k** is Henry's constant, and **c** is the concentration of the solute in solution. Increasing the partial pressure of a gas above a liquid will increase the amount of gas that dissolves in the liquid. Increased delivery of oxygen (FIO_2) to patients to improve arterial

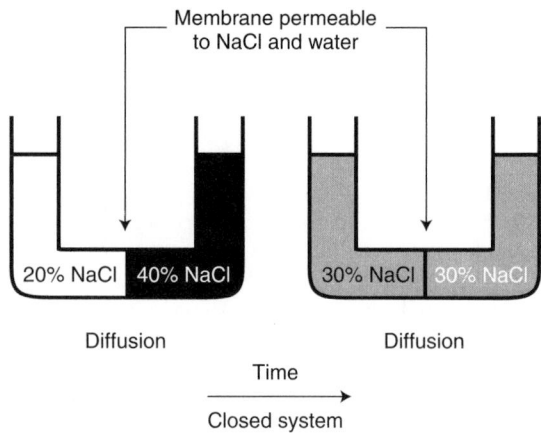

FIGURE **15-15**   Diffusion of water and NaCl.

oxygenation (PaO_2) and overpressurizing (high concentration) anesthetics reflect the direct relationship of pressure and solubility described by Henry's law. "Overpressurizing" is the process of significantly increasing a volatile anesthetic concentration (partial pressure) delivered to a patient to increase the alveolar concentration, and therefore the amount dissolved in the blood, to speed uptake.

DIFFUSION

Diffusion is the process of net movement of one type of molecule through space as a result of random motion intended to minimize a concentration gradient (Figure 15-15). This basic process occurs by Brownian (Robert Brown, 1773-1858) motion, which is driven by the inherent kinetic energy of the molecules.[6] Temperature is directly proportional to kinetic energy. Kinetic energy allows molecules to move freely in a fluid, and therefore mixtures of fluids tend to evenly distribute. The velocity at which a molecule may distribute is determined by its molecular weight. Every molecule at a given temperature will have the same kinetic energy, independent of its size, but its velocity may differ. From the formula for kinetic energy, $KE = (½)mv^2$, we can determine that if the mass of a molecule is changed, there must be an opposite change in velocity. Greater velocity correlates with faster diffusion. Thus, molecules with smaller mass will diffuse faster.

Graham's Law

Thomas Graham (1805-1869) determined that the rate of effusion (gas diffusion through an orifice) of a gas is inversely proportional to the square root of its molecular weight. The formula is:

$$r = 1/\sqrt{mw}$$

where **r** is the rate of diffusion, and **mw** is the molecular weight. Graham's law determines the faster diffusion of smaller molecules compared to larger molecules. Graham's law is helpful in understanding the effect of molecular weight on diffusion but is limited in fully describing all the factors influencing diffusion.

Diffusion Through Permeable and Semipermeable Membranes

Diffusion may occur through open space or through permeable membranes (tissues). If a fluid (gas or liquid) is permeable through a membrane, then the diffusion that occurs is dependent on five factors. These factors include concentration gradient,

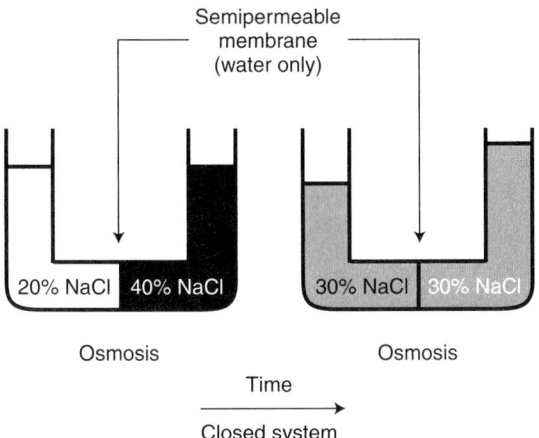

FIGURE **15-16** Osmosis of water through a semipermeable membrane.

tissue area, and fluid tissue solubility, which are all directly proportional to diffusion. Membrane thickness and molecular weight are factors that are inversely proportional to diffusion.

Osmosis

Osmosis is the movement of water across a semipermeable membrane to equilibrate a concentration gradient (Figure 15-16). Semipermeable membranes are permeable to water only and not to solute. *Osmotic pressure* is the force needed to stop osmosis from occurring. *Oncotic pressure* is the osmotic pressure caused by plasma proteins and electrolytes in capillaries. Oncotic pressure balances the hydrostatic pressure tendency to push water out of capillaries. Normal oncotic pressure is approximately 28 mm Hg. Our vascular system is a semipermeable membrane that responds to intravascular delivery of colloids by sequestering fluid.[7,8]

Diffusion in Anesthesia

Diffusion is a passive process driven by entropy (see Entropy in this chapter). The diffusion of oxygen and nitrous oxide represents both positive and negative consequences of this process. Nitrous oxide diffuses into air-filled cavities; therefore, delivery of nitrous oxide is contraindicated in patients with pneumothorax or where air-filled cavity expansion is undesirable.[9] Nitrous oxide expansion of endotracheal cuffs may cause tracheal mucosal damage.[10,11] Distention of bowel during nitrous oxide delivery also has been documented.[12,13] Apneic oxygenation is well known and exemplifies the beneficial process of diffusion.[14] An intubated patient who has previously been ventilated with 100% oxygen and remains connected to the ventilation circuit with 100% oxygen flow will maintain an acceptable Pao_2 if ventilation is ceased. The continual diffusion of oxygen into the blood is driven by a concentration gradient that continually diffuses oxygen into the alveoli via the ventilator circuit. The diffusion of gases across biological tissues is expressed by Fick's law.

Fick's Law

Fick's law for diffusion of a gas across a tissue plane is an encompassing law that accounts for molecular weight, concentration gradient, solubility, and membrane interactions. Fick's law states that diffusion of a gas across a semipermeable membrane is directly proportional to the partial pressure gradient, the membrane solubility of the gas, and the membrane area and is inversely proportional to the membrane thickness and molecular

weight of the gas. Specific application of the Fick equation for diffusion of respiratory gases is:

$$J = \alpha D / \Delta x (Pao_2 - Pcapo_2)$$

where **J** is diffusion flux, α is the solubility constant for oxygen, **D** is diffusivity, Δx is the membrane thickness, and ($Pao_2 -$ $Pcapo_2$) is the alveolar-capillary oxygen partial pressure difference. Fick's equation allows determination of pulmonary gas exchange.[15,16] The diffusion hypoxia that occurs after the delivery of nitrous oxide is discontinued, and low inspired oxygen is administered as explained by Fick's equation.[17]

NEWTONIAN PHYSICS

GRAVITY

All life on earth is well aware of gravity. From our first steps to our last, gravity affects every facet of our daily lives. It is a unidirectional force pulling objects down toward earth's center. Gravity appears to pull on heavy objects with greater force than lighter objects, but this is not necessarily true. Aristotle saw gravity this way and felt it was due to an object's desire to return to its natural position at rest on the earth. It took 2000 years to change that perspective. Gravity pulls on all objects with a force of 9.81m/sec/sec (32 ft/sec/sec). Sir Isaac Newton's law of gravity derived that, "Each particle of matter attracts every other particle with a force which is directly proportional to the product of their masses and inversely proportional to the square of the distance between them." The formula for gravity is:

Gravitational force = (G × m1 × m2)/(d²)

where **G** is the gravitational constant ($6.67 \times 10^{-11} Nm^2/kg^2$), **m1** and **m2** are the masses of the two objects for which you are calculating the force, and **d** is the distance between the centers of gravity of the two masses. Remember that mass and weight are not the same. Mass is the total of all matter in an object—the sum of all the electrons', protons', and neutrons' equal mass. Weight is the total effect of gravity pulling on all these electrons, protons, and neutrons of an object. An example often cited is that you may weigh 70 kilograms on earth due to the gravitational pull on all your atoms, but you would weigh less on the moon, which has less gravitational pull. Your mass or total amount of matter remains the same on earth or the moon.

Mass × force of gravity = weight

The earth attracts all other objects around it with a force of 9.81m/sec/sec, and those objects in turn attract the earth in relation to their mass and distance from the planet. The formula for gravitational acceleration is:

$$g = GM^e / r^2_e$$

where **g** is gravitational acceleration, **G** is the gravitational constant, M_e is the mass of earth, and r^2_e is the mean radius of earth. Earth's attraction for objects is proportional to mass for all objects at the same distance. One might want to say that larger-mass objects would accelerate or be pulled faster to earth, but objects also resist movement proportional to their mass (third law of motion). Gravity pulls on one atom of carbon with 9.81m/sec/sec force, and the carbon atom resists this pull with a force of *x*. Gravity pulls on two carbon atoms with a force of 9.81m/sec/sec on each atom for a total gravitational force of 9.81m/sec/sec × 2, or 19.62m/sec/sec. Two carbon atoms resist movement twice (2×) as much as one carbon atom, thus the net gravitational effect (falling) is the same. This is how greater-mass objects are pulled by gravity with the same force and fall at the same acceleration as lesser-mass objects.

This equal attraction on objects is often hidden in everyday life, owing to the effect of air molecules interacting with falling objects. Assuredly, all objects fall due to gravity at the same speed in a vacuum that is devoid of other molecules. Air molecules possess energy, move about, and interact with other matter. This causes friction. Greater friction equals greater force against the pull of gravity and slowing of a fall, but in a vacuum all objects fall equally at equal velocities.

NEWTON'S LAWS OF MOTION

Newton's first law (law of inertia): A body in motion tends to stay in motion unless acted upon by another force.

Newton's second law (law of acceleration): Acceleration of a body is in the direction of and proportional to the force (**F**), and that acceleration (**a**) is inverse to the mass (**m**) of the body, **F = ma**. If multiple forces exist, the direction and acceleration are proportional to the sum of all the forces. These are called *vectors*.

Newton's third law (law of reciprocal action): For every action, there is an equal and opposite reaction. It states that objects exert equal but opposite forces on one another.[18] Example: An apple on a desk pulls down with a gravitational force equal to the force that the table resists.

FORCE

Force is the amount of energy required to move an object. From the understanding that the force of gravity pulls equally on all objects proportional to mass, a standardization of force became possible. Because we know that gravity pulls (accelerates) all objects with a force of 9.81m/sec/sec, this force would also be 9.81m/sec/sec if applied to any given weight. The force of gravity applied to 1 kg weight creates a standard by which other forces may be compared quantified and measured. Thus the force required to accelerate a 1 kg weight 1 meter per second became known as the *newton*

The newton is the standard measure of force derived from the force of gravity.

$$\text{newton} = 1 \text{ meter/sec/sec}$$
$$= \frac{1}{9.81 \text{ kg weight or } 102 \text{ g weight}}$$
$$\text{gravity} = 9.81 \text{ meter/sec/sec}$$

One newton is equivalent to 1/9.81 kg weight or 102 g weight. Force is mass multiplied by acceleration. The formula for force is:

$$\text{F} = \text{ma}$$

where **F** is force, **m** is mass, and **a** is acceleration. Often in settings of small measures of force, the newton is too large. A dyne is 1000th newton. A dyne is the force required to move a 1-g weight 1 cm per second. Dynes are used in calculating systemic and pulmonary vascular resistance.[19,20]

Pulmonary vascular resistance (PVR) is the measure of the pulmonary vascular system's resistance to flow from the right ventricle. Normal PVR is 100 to 200 dyne sec/cm^5. Systemic vascular resistance (SVR) is the measure of the peripheral vascular system's resistance to flow that must be overcome for flow to occur. The left ventricle must therefore pump blood with a force greater than the resistance of the vascular system. The formula for calculating SVR is 80 × (MAP − CVP)/CO = SVR. Normal SVR is 900 to 1200 dyne sec/cm^5.

Another application of force measurement in anesthesia is the technology of accelerometry used to measure the degree of neuromuscular blockade.[21,22] Accelerometry uses a piezoelectric disk to generate an electric current in proportion to acceleration (see Piezoelectric Effect). An accelerometer measures the acceleration caused by the contraction of the adductor pollicis muscle after ulnar nerve stimulation. A comparison of baseline stimulated muscle twitches (forces) to twitches suppressed by neuromuscular blocking agents allows the quantification of the degree of neuromuscular blockade.[23] Accelerometers provide objective twitch data referenced to the patient's baseline twitch response.[24] Visual or tactile assessment of twitch heights is subjective and less reliable than accelerometry.[24,25]

Force is a basic phenomenon of physics that permeates the universe. Because all matter possess mass, and all mass has some degree of acceleration, force exists everywhere. All forces possess direction. The study of force direction is explored with vectors.

Vectors

Two basic types of values describe our physical world: *scalar* and *vector*. Scalar values are fully described by magnitude alone, they possess no motion, and they include mass, energy, and work. Vector values are fully described by magnitude and direction. Vectors express motion and are described by the mathematics of force, speed, velocity, acceleration, distance, and displacement. Vector diagrams are scaled representations of vectors, with an arrow starting at a given magnitude and pointing in the direction of the force summation.

An electrocardiogram (ECG) is an example of a type of vector diagram that allows us to calculate the predominant direction of electrical force in the myocardium. An ECG records electrical flow as an upward or downward deflection on graph paper. When the flow is toward the positive electrode, an upward deflection will record. When the flow is away from the positive electrode, a downward deflection will record. Twelve-lead ECGs are scaled graphs with multiple points of reference used to measure the force direction of the electrical conductance. As multiple points of reference are recorded, direction of electrical flow predominance may be made (vector summation). This is the principle behind determining axis deviation of the heart.

Axis deviation estimates the summation of forces that shift from the normal direction of electrical flow in the heart. Electrocardiogram vector diagrams are scaled clockwise from 0 degrees in the east position. The normal axis of electrical flow summation in the heart is between −30 degrees and +90 degrees. The axis determination steps that follow are based on identifying the positive (upward) deflections of the 12-lead electrocardiogram, which represents electrical flow toward the positive electrode. Because the normal axis of electrical flow is between −30 and +90 degrees, positive deflections in leads I and II would represent electrical flow in the normal direction. Negative deflections in lead I or lead II would reflect a deviation of normal axis and requires determination of the electrical flow vector. Vector deviations are described as *left*, *right*, or *right superior*. Several methods are available for quick determination of myocardial electrical axis deviation. Figure 15-17, Table 15-3, and Table 15-4 offer help in determining axis deviation.

PRESSURE

Pressure is defined as force over area, where **P** is pressure, **f** is force, and **a** is area.

$$\text{P} = \text{f/a}$$

Increasing the area in which a given force is applied will result in a lower pressure. The smaller the area the set force is applied, the

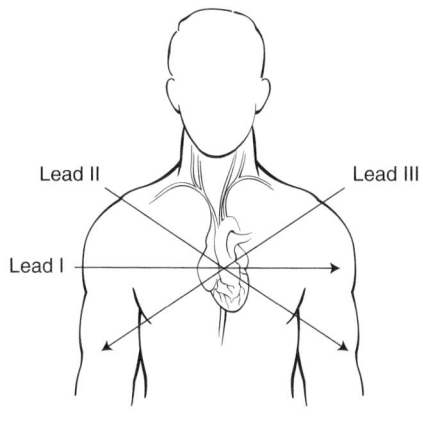

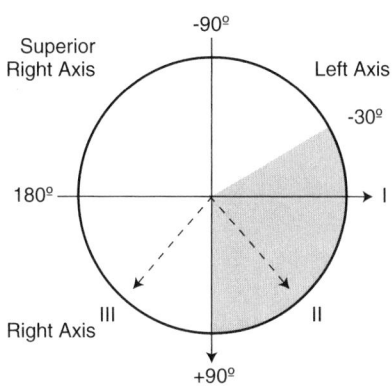

FIGURE **15-17** Electrocardiogram lead placement with vector direction and location of normal and abnormal axes.

Axis deviation vectors

TABLE **15-3**	Axis Deviation Determination Methods		
Vector Method		**Inspection Method**	**Grant Method**
I+, aVF+ = Normal axis		I+, III+ = Normal axis	I+, II+ = Normal axis
I−, aVF− = Superior right		I− = Right axis	I+, II− = Left axis
I−, aVF+ = Right axis		III−, II− = Left axis	I−, II+ = Right axis
I+, aVF− see lead II (if II+ = Normal; if II− = Left axis)			I−, II− = Superior right

TABLE **15-4**	Axis Deviations from Normal
Normal Axis	**−30 to +90 degrees**
Left axis deviation	−30 to −90 degrees
Right axis deviation	+90 to ±180 degrees
Superior right axis deviation	−90 to ±180 degrees

greater the pressure. The standard unit of measurement for pressure is the pascal (Pa). A pascal is the force of 1 newton (N) over 1 square meter.

$$Pa = \frac{1N}{1m^2}$$

A pascal equals 102 g weight acting over an area of 1 square meter. Remember, a newton equals 102 g weight. This is a very small unit of pressure. As the newton was fractionalized to the dyne for the purpose of establishing a more convenient unit of force measurement, the pascal was increased a thousand times to create the kilopascal (kPa) unit. A kilopascal is more convenient to use for measuring pressures. A kilopascal equals 1000 N or 102 kg acting over an area of 1 m^2.

$$Pa = 102 \text{ g/m}^2$$
$$kPa = 102 \text{ kg/m}^2$$

Syringes represent an example of the pressure generated by a force over a given area. Equal force (20 N) applied to the plungers of different syringes generates different pressures, depending on the area over which the force was applied. The force applied will cause greater pressure on injection with a tuberculin (TB) syringe (plunger area = 8.55×10^{-6} m^2) than with a larger 10-mL syringe (plunger area 2.14×10^{-4} m^2). As you increase the area to which a fixed force (20 N) is applied, the product of the equation, pressure (in atmospheres), becomes smaller.

$$P = f/a$$

TB syringe : $20N/8.55 \times 10^{-6}m^2 =$
2339.18 kPa, 17, 543.94 mm Hg, or 23.08 atm

10 mL syringe : $20N/3.42 \times 10^{-5}m^2 =$
584.79 kPa, 4, 386.28 mm Hg, or 5.77 atm

30 mL syringe : $20N/5.99 \times 10^{-5}m^2 =$
334.16 kPa, 2, 506.40 mm Hg, or 3.29 atm

These calculations show the extremely high pressures that can be generated by exerting a force over a small area. The tuberculin syringe generates more than 20 atmospheres of pressure and can rupture catheters if used to flush or dislodge blockages. Larger syringes are recommended for flushing or unclogging enteral feeding tubes because of the potential for generating high pressures with smaller syringes.[26-28]

Atmospheric Pressure

As previously discussed, gravity pulls on all objects, including the atoms and molecules of the atmosphere. Because these atoms and molecules have low mass, they have low gravitational pull but nonetheless are pulled toward Earth. The cumulative effect of gravity on atmospheric gases gives rise to atmospheric pressure. Atmospheric gases are less concentrated at altitude and more

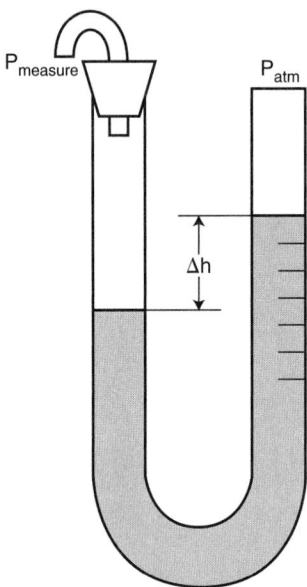

FIGURE **15-18** Manometer showing change in liquid column height (Δh) related to pressure applied.

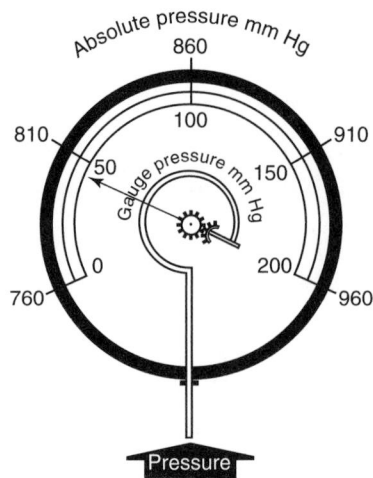

FIGURE **15-19** Bourdon gauge showing gauge pressure (*inside pressures*) referenced to absolute pressure (*outside pressures*).

concentrated at sea level. Atmospheric pressure is the column of gravitational force on gases over a given area. This can be measured and is equivalent at sea level to 100 kPa (or 14.7 lb per square inch, 1020 cm of H₂O, or 760 mm Hg—all equivalent to one another). *Standard pressure* in the SI is 100 kPa. Other units of pressure measurement include the following with their equivalents. It is best to memorize these:

> 1 torr = 1mm Hg
> 1 kPa = 10.2 cm H₂O = 7.5 mm Hg
> 1 atm = 760 mm Hg = 760 torr =
> 1 bar = 100 kPa = 1020 cm H₂ O = 14.7lb/inch₂

Pressure Measurement

The simplest method for determining pressure is the manometer. A manometer is a liquid-filled tube that is open to atmospheric pressure on one end and exposed to a pressure for measurement on the other end (Figure 15-18). A pressure greater than atmospheric pressure (760 mm Hg) will displace the column of liquid proportional to the pressure difference (Δh). Calibrating the column of liquid allows for quantification of the pressure.

A sphygmomanometer uses an inflatable cuff connected to a mercury-filled manometer to measure blood pressure. As the inflated cuff is slowly deflated, the arterial flow resumes, causing a pressure wave that is transmitted to a mercury column. The mercury column is calibrated to show the measured pressure in millimeters of mercury. A more recent advancement in blood pressure measurement is oscillometry. Oscillometry automates noninvasive blood pressure measurements by recording the oscillations in pressure caused by arterial pulsation.[29] As an inflated cuff is deflated, multiple measurements are made of these oscillations. Oscillations increase at systolic pressure and are maximal at the mean arterial pressure. Algorithmic computation of systolic and diastolic pressures is derived from the mean arterial pressure. Often these noninvasive automated blood pressure monitors use the piezoelectric principle to record the pressure oscillations and a microprocessor to derive the systolic and diastolic

measurements.[30] Invasive blood pressure monitors use a piezoelectric transducer that converts pressure waves into electrical signals. Blood pressure measurements are gauge pressures that are zeroed to atmospheric pressure.

Gauge and Absolute Pressure

Different pressure measurements may use different zero reference points. The zero reference point may be a complete vacuum devoid of all molecules and molecular collisions that impart pressure. This is true zero pressure and is the reference point used when measuring absolute pressure. Absolute pressure is atmospheric pressure plus gauge pressure. Gauge pressure is zero referenced at atmospheric pressure and reads zero at 760 mm Hg at sea level. Gauge pressure is absolute pressure minus atmospheric pressure.

Bourdon gauges are often used in anesthesia to measure high pressures, such as in gas cylinders, and are zero referenced to atmospheric pressure (Figure 15-19). Bourdon gauges contain a coiled tube that expands as pressure is applied. A linkage connects the coil to a rotating arm that records the pressure. The American Society for Testing Materials International mandates that the zero reading of Bourdon gauges lie between the 6 o'clock and 9 o'clock positions. Other methods of pressure measurement in anesthesia include manometers.

THERMODYNAMICS

The three laws of thermodynamics explain the relationship between heat and energy and their exchange during work processes:

1. *Law of conservation of energy.* Energy cannot be created or destroyed. The increase in the internal energy of a thermodynamic system is equal to the amount of heat energy added to the system minus the work done by the system on the surroundings.
2. *Energy moves toward greater entropy or randomness.* The entropy of an isolated system not in equilibrium will tend to increase over time, approaching a maximum value at equilibrium.
3. *Absolute zero (0° K or −273.15° C) is void of all energy.* Absolute zero is theoretical, because it has been impossible to achieve. As a system approaches absolute zero of temperature, all processes cease, and the entropy of a system approaches a minimum value.

ENERGY

Energy can be defined as the exertion of force (kinetic) or the capacity (potential) to do work. Energy can be expressed as mechanical work, chemical reactions, or heat. The unit of measurement for energy is the joule. A joule is the force of 1 newton that moves its point of application 1 meter in the direction of that force. Two types of energy are potential and kinetic. Potential energy is energy waiting to be used. It is energy that is stored and available to be converted into power. Potential energy is defined as mass (**m**) times gravity (**g**) times height (**h**).

$$PE = mgh$$

Kinetic energy is energy of movement. *Kinetic* means movement. *Kinetic energy* is defined as one half the product of mass times the velocity squared.

$$KE = (1/2)mv^2$$

ENTROPY

Entropy is the universe's trend to equilibrate all things. It is the process that allows everything from ice melting to gas expansion. Sleep and the induction of general anesthesia have been proposed to be entropic processes.[31-34] All of these processes involve the equilibration of energy. Even matter is a form of energy. Entropy is unidirectional; it is the movement of energy from high concentration to lower concentration. It moves because of a gradient. The difference in the gradient influences the speed of the flow. Greater difference usually equals greater flow, and always from higher concentration to lower concentration. All energy and matter tend to follow this rule. An example of this unidirectional action is ice added to lemonade. Ice does not make lemonade colder, lemonade makes ice warmer. Diffusion, which will be covered later, is also a process driven by entropy. Entropy ends when all energy is equally distributed. Entropy is the underlying process promoting spontaneous and elicited movement in our everyday lives and the universe in general. Essentially, entropy drives the universe. This process should be kept in mind when learning or reviewing any dynamic concepts of anesthesia.[35]

TEMPERATURE

Matter may change form with the addition of greater heat energy. An example we see every day is the melting of an ice cube into liquid water, and liquid water into vapor with the addition of greater heat energy. Liquid water, with the addition of heat energy, expands. This is due to the water molecules moving apart with greater kinetic energy that ultimately allows them to escape individually as a vapor. Another liquid, mercury, also expands with the addition of heat energy. When placed in the bottom of a closed glass cylinder, the expansion is limited to one direction in relation to the energy applied. This is a simple application of heat energy (kinetic energy) interacting with matter to allow analysis of the thermal state: a thermometer.

Temperature is the measurement of the thermal state of an object. Heat is thermal energy; temperature is the quantitative measurement of that energy. Several temperature scales exist: Fahrenheit, Celsius, and Kelvin (Figure 15-20). Gabriel Daniel Fahrenheit (1686-1736) is credited with inventing the mercury thermometer (1714) and devising the Fahrenheit temperature scale. The Celsius (Anders Celsius, 1701-1744) or centigrade scale is the primary scale used for everyday temperature measurements. The Kelvin scale (William Thompson Lord Kelvin, 1824-1907) was developed to better reflect

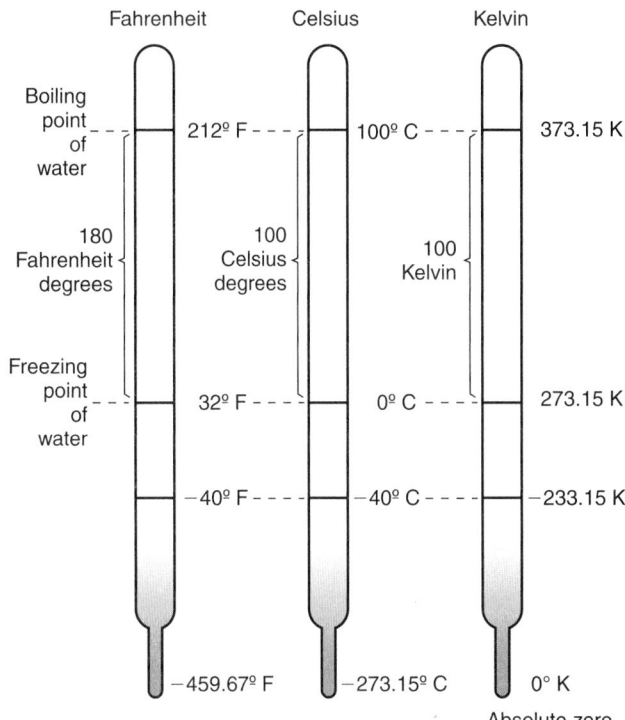

FIGURE **15-20** Temperature scales referenced to Kelvin.

mathematically the temperature/pressure relationship of gases and is used when calculating their behaviors. Water freezes at 273.15° K and boils at 373.15° K. Conversion among temperature scales is as follows:

> Celsius to Kelvin: °K = °C + 273
> Celsius to Fahrenheit: °F = 1.8 (°C) + 32
> Fahrenheit to Celsius: °C = (°F − 32)/1.8
> *Standard temperature* is 273.15 K (0° C)

Heat Loss

Heat and energy are the same. Heat loss (energy loss) of a system, as discussed previously, is unidirectional from higher concentration to lower concentration, from hotter to less hot. Even ice possesses heat (energy). Remember absolute zero, 0° K (−273.15° C or −459.67° F), is the absence of all energy and therefore absence of all heat. The human body is a system that contains energy. Much of this energy is in the form of heat. Our bodies continually exchange heat with the environment from high concentration to lower concentration. On a very hot day or in a very hot room, we could lead our bodies into hyperthermia. We will focus on heat loss in the cool operating room environment. Clothes, hair, skin, and fat insulate us from heat loss. Protective mechanisms exist that further lessen heat loss.

Vasoconstriction of peripheral vessels slows heat loss from our bodies. An example is the vasoconstriction seen in our limbs when exposed to a cold environment. The reverse thermoregulatory mechanism to promote heat loss is vasodilatation when exposed to a hotter environment. The directing of blood to or away from our periphery aids in the removal or conservation of our body's heat energy. This thermoregulatory mechanism is disrupted under anesthesia by vasodilating drugs, specifically volatile anesthetics. Volatile and regional anesthetics vasodilate vessels, including those in the periphery, causing greater blood flow to the surface of our bodies.

Core Temperature Redistribution

Core temperature redistribution is the process of increased heat loss from the body resulting from the vasodilating effects of volatile and regional anesthetics, which cause greater blood flow and therefore heat flow to the body's surface from the core.[36-38] A patient's core temperature can quickly drop by the vasodilating actions of anesthetics, with the greatest decrease in the first hour.[37] It is imperative that one be cognizant of this heat loss mechanism and take measures to decrease it.[39-41] Covering all exposed areas of a patient minus the surgical site, wrapping the head in blankets, and warming the operating room all decrease heat loss. The use of forced warm air devices is effective at decreasing heat loss in the operating room environment.[42-44]

Blood flow to our body's surface encourages heat loss by four primary processes. In decreasing order they are

1. Radiation
2. Convection
3. Conduction
4. Evaporation

Radiation

Radiation is the most significant mechanism of heat loss by our bodies, especially by patients under anesthesia. Radiation of the infrared electromagnetic wavelength transfers heat energy from our warm bodies to the less warm operating room environment (walls, ceiling, equipment, etc.). Electromagnetic radiation is pure energy. (See discussion on this later in the chapter.) Infrared radiation from our bodies is greatest in areas of highest blood flow. Our heads lose the greatest amount of heat due to the high percentage of blood flow. Blood carries body heat, and the greater amount of blood and heat transported to the head facilitates greater heat loss by radiation.

Convection

Convection is the process of creating air currents by heat. Our bodies transfer kinetic energy to air molecules on the surface of our skin. The heated air molecules then move about with greater kinetic energy, rise, and are replaced by colder (less kinetic energy) air molecules. Our bodies then transfer more kinetic energy to these molecules, they rise, and again are replaced by cooler air molecules. When thinking of convection, it helps to think in terms of *currents*.

Conduction

Conduction is the transfer of heat by physically touching a less warm object. Where two objects are in direct contact, heat exchange occurs from high concentration to lower concentration (entropy). An example would be holding a cold soda can. The sensation of cold is the direct loss of heat from your hand to the can. Cold is not transferred to your hand; heat is transferred to the can. A patient on a cold operating room table will conduct his or her heat to the less hot table wherever physical contact is present. This is not a significant process in adult patients, but for pediatric patients who have large body surface area to mass, it is quite significant. Use of warming blankets on operating room tables stops or reverses this heat transfer. Warming blankets may add heat energy to a patient, depending on the temperature and establishment of a thermal gradient.

Evaporation

Evaporation is not usually a large contributor to patient heat loss. Heat loss from evaporation includes moisture evaporated from the patient's skin, as well as exhaled water vapor. The process of evaporation, causing a phase change from liquid to gas, requires energy. The source of energy needed for this process comes from the surrounding environment of the evaporating substance. *Latent heat of vaporization* is the amount of heat energy per unit mass required to convert a liquid into the vapor phase. The energy withdrawn from the environment to convert one gram of water into vapor is 2500 joules, or approximately 600 calories. An example of this is the cooling off we feel after getting out of a swimming pool. The energy used to change the water into a vapor comes mostly from our bodies. Our body loses heat energy to this process, and we experience a state of lower thermal energy. Patients who have areas of their bodies surgically prepped with liquids (e.g., isopropyl alcohol, povidone-iodine, and chlorhexidine gluconate) experience heat loss by this method. The process of breathing also causes heat loss through exhaled water vapor. This is not usually a high heat loss method in adult patients, but may become significant in pediatric patients when using high carrier gas flow rates. Lower carrier gas flows, when appropriate, and use of in-line humidifying apparatus decrease the evaporation of pulmonary water content and limit heat loss by this mode. One should consider these interventions with all intubated general anesthetics to prevent not only heat loss but also the pulmonary drying effects of dehydrate carrier gases.

Heat loss from patients is primarily due to radiation of infrared electromagnetic radiation.[45] Convection is the second largest method of heat loss in anesthetized patients.[45,46] Conduction and evaporation cause heat loss to lesser extents but remain a concern. Prevention of heat loss is extremely important to decrease higher morbidity experienced by hypothermic patients.[47-49] As Figure 15-21 illustrates, the use of forced warm air devices, lower gas flow rates, humidification systems, warming the operating room, and covering and insulating patients all are effective methods to decrease patient heat loss.[43,50]

Vaporization. Vaporization is the process of converting liquids or solids into vapors. Evaporation is the specific process of vaporizing liquids. Vaporization requires energy. As stated previously, the latent heat of vaporization is the energy needed to transform a given amount of liquid into a gas and is measured in kilojoules (kJ). The temperature at which the bulk of a liquid at a given pressure converts to a vapor is the *boiling point*. The temperature of a liquid will not rise above its boiling point; instead, the energy is used to transform the liquid into gas. Heating a liquid to its boiling point increases the kinetic energy of the

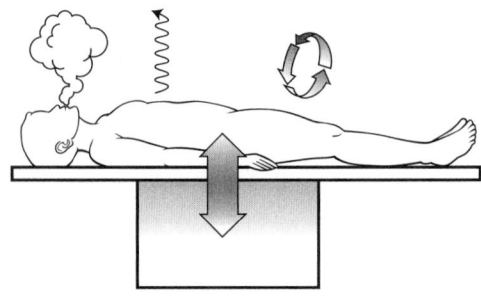

FIGURE **15-21** Heat loss mechanisms of radiation, convection, conduction, and evaporation in patients under anesthesia.

liquid's molecules. Further addition of heat energy, above the boiling point, is transferred to molecules so they may break away from the surface and become a gas. "The rate of vaporization depends only on the temperature, the vapor pressure of the liquid, and the partial pressure of the vapor above the evaporating liquid."[51] As gas molecules escape the liquid, they exert a pressure known as *vapor pressure*, measured in millimeters of mercury. Increasing heat will increase molecular kinetic energy, which will increase the rate of vaporization. In a closed container, equilibrium will be achieved between molecules in the gaseous phase and those in the liquid phase.

All liquids that have high vapor pressures at room temperatures are known as *volatile liquids*. Vapor pressure and boiling points are inversely related. Vapor pressures of the volatile anesthetics at STP are

- *Isoflurane:* 238 mm Hg
- *Sevoflurane:* 160 mm Hg
- *Desflurane:* 660 mm Hg

Vapor pressures are unique characteristics of liquids that depend solely on temperature. Different liquids exert different vapor pressures at a given temperature. Because different volatile anesthetics have differing vapor pressures, vaporizers must be calibrated for each specific agent. Placing the wrong agent into a vaporizer will cause a greater or lower delivered concentration than dialed. If a high-vapor-pressure volatile anesthetic agent is placed inside a vaporizer calibrated for a lower-vapor-pressure volatile anesthetic, the output of that vaporizer will be higher than indicated on the control dial. If a volatile anesthetic agent with a lower vapor pressure is placed inside a vaporizer calibrated for a higher-vapor-pressure anesthetic, the output of that vaporizer will be lower than indicated on the control dial.[52]

Absolute Zero

The preceding has covered the first and second laws of thermodynamics, with examples applied to the practice of anesthesia. With a unidirectional perspective and an understanding that energy can not be created nor destroyed, the third law becomes self-evident. Absolute zero is the theoretical state devoid of all energy. No matter how much energy is distributed, it will still be present. Entropy to its universal maximum distribution will possess energy, even though it would be very low. There is energy in the universe, and therefore it will always be present in some form and to some degree. The absolute absence of energy is therefore impossible. That does not prevent us from calculating the theoretical temperature that would be devoid of energy. The theoretical temperature of absolute zero is $-273°$ C ($0°$ K, $-460°$ F).

KINETIC MOLECULAR THEORY

Thermodynamics set the foundation for explaining the overall action of a system's energy. The kinetic molecular theory builds on Newtonian physics and thermodynamics and focuses on molecular movement (energy) and forces between these molecules. This theory explains how molecules behave as they follow the previously described laws of thermodynamics. Kinetic molecular theory was created to have a conceptual framework that encompassed the findings of Charles, Boyle, and Gay-Lussac and the *universal gas law* that unified their studies. A review of basic matter characteristics is as follows:

- *Matter* is composed of small particles called *molecules* and molecules are composed of atoms. Matter can take the form of solid, liquid, or gas.
- *Solids*—Molecules in a solid are held close together by intermolecular forces. They may move about slightly and vibrate.

- *Liquids*—Molecules in a liquid are held together by intermolecular forces and may slide or flow by one another.
- *Gases*—Molecules in a gas move linearly, and the attractive forces between molecules are less than their kinetic energy. They move almost completely free of one another.

The kinetic molecular theory, which best describes the action of gases, makes some generalized assumptions for simplicity:

1. Molecules have no volume.
2. Gas molecules exert no force on each other unless they collide.
3. Collisions of molecules with each other or the walls of the container do not decrease the energy of the system.
4. The molecules of a gas are in constant and random motion.
5. The temperature of a gas depends entirely on its average kinetic energy. The energy of a gas is entirely kinetic.

The kinetic molecular theory was created to explain the ideal gas law. Though the ideal gas law adequately explains the general behavior of gases, it does omit a gas molecule's small volume and intermolecular interactions. These flaws are further addressed in the section covering Van der Waal's equation.

GAS LAWS

The foundations for the kinetic molecular theory were based on the discoveries of three scientists, Jacques Charles (1746-1823), Robert Boyle (1627-1691), and Joseph Louis Gay-Lussac (1778-1850). They each studied isolated components of pressure, volume, and temperature to explore the relationship of these components. Charles studied the relationship of volume and temperature when pressure is maintained constant. He found that the volume-to-temperature relationship is directly proportional. This means that at a constant pressure, volume will increase as temperature increases and vice versa. Boyle studied the relationship of pressure and volume when temperature is maintained constant. Boyle found that the pressure-to-volume relationship is indirectly proportional. Thus at a constant temperature, pressure will increase as volume decreases and vice versa. Gay-Lussac studied the relationship of pressure and temperature when volume is maintained constant. Gay-Lussac found that the pressure-to-temperature relationship is directly proportional. As pressure increases, temperature will increase and vice versa. The gas laws allow us to calculate the behavior of gases when one of the three factors of pressure, volume, or temperature is maintained unchanged. The clinical significance of these laws is expressed by the ability to calculate the available liters of oxygen from a cylinder of any known pressure. This and other examples are available at the end of the chapter. Table 15-5 summarizes the laws and the interrelationship of pressure, volume, and temperature.

TABLE **15-5**	Gas Laws: Gas Properties and Relationships		
Property Constant	**Studied Properties**	**Property Relationship**	**Law**
Pressure	Temperature, volume	Directly proportional	Charles
Temperature	Pressure, volume	Indirectly proportional	Boyle
Volume	Pressure, temperature	Directly proportional	Gay-Lussac

Universal Gas Law

As the universal gas law unified the findings of Charles, Boyle, and Gay-Lussac, it also became known as the *unified gas law* or *ideal gas law*. The formula is:

$$PV = nrT$$

where at standard temperature, **P** is pressure, **V** is volume, **n** is the number of moles, **r** is the constant 0.0821 liter-atm/K/mole, and **T** is temperature. A *mole* is a gram molecular weight of a gas. Atomic, or molecular, weight is the addition of all atomic particles, protons, neutrons, and electrons in an atom or molecule. An example is a mole of helium. Helium has a molecular weight of 4. Placing "gram" after helium's atomic weight gives us a "mole" of helium. Four grams of helium is a mole of helium. This amount of gas establishes a standard reference for calculations.

Using the universal gas law, you can calculate the volume for which 1 mole of a gas will expand at any given temperature or pressure. In the example given, we will calculate the volume in liters that 1 mole of oxygen will expand to at 1 atmosphere pressure at standard temperature (0° C). Celsius is converted to Kelvin.

$$1 \text{ atm (x)} = 1 \text{ mole (0.0821 L atm/mol K)}(273K)$$
$$x = 22.4L$$

One mole of any gas at 0° C will expand to 22.4 liters volume.

As this is a conceptual text, it is easier to view the universal gas law as PV = T to focus on the relationship between pressure, volume, and temperature. It is easy to see mathematically how increasing or decreasing any value would affect the other values as described above. The universal gas law can be rearranged as follows:

$$PV = T \text{ or } \frac{T}{P} = V \text{ or } \frac{T}{V} = P$$

Increasing one value will increase or decrease the other values to maintain balance in the formula. The universal gas law allows understanding and quick determination of such things as: How much oxygen is available to be released from a partially full oxygen cylinder, and at what temperature will a full oxygen cylinder exceed its recommended pressure when heated?

Avogadro's Number

Amedeo Avogadro (1776-1856) was able to show that in a mole of any gas there are 6.023×10^{23} molecules. A mole of gas is equal to the molecular weight of the gas expressed in grams. A mole of helium would be 2 g, and 2 g of helium contain 6.023×10^{23} atoms. Similarly a mole of oxygen (O_2) would be 32 g and contain 6.023×10^{23} molecules of oxygen. Oxygen is a molecule composed of two oxygen atoms bonded together, and therefore the molecular weight of the diatomic oxygen molecule is 32, not 16.

Van der Waal's Forces

Unfortunately, the simplicity of the universal gas law is not 100% accurate in fully describing the interaction of gases with their environment. The universal gas law is also called the *ideal gas law* because it explains the behavior of gases if they were "ideal." An ideal gas would possess molecules that occupy no volume and never interact with other molecules. Gas molecules do have volume and occupy space, and therefore the volume they occupy must be taken into account when calculating a gas's expansion or contraction. The universal gas law does not account for gas molecule volume since Charles, Boyle, and Gay-Lussac did not account for this in their studies. (Remember, the universal gas law unified the work of Charles, Boyle, and Gay-Lussac.) An ideal gas also assumes no intermolecular forces. However,

molecules do interact with one another, and this behavior alters the net effect of kinetics as calculated by the universal gas law. Van der Waal's (Johannes Diderik van der Waal, 1837-1923) equation corrects the universal gas law and accounts for molecular volume and molecular interaction in a gas. Van der Waal's equation is:

$$(P + n^2a/V^2)(V/n - b) = RT$$

where **P** is the pressure of the fluid, **V** is the total volume of the container containing the fluid, **a** is a measure of the attraction between the particles, **b** is the volume excluded by a mole of particles, **n** is the number of moles, **R** is the gas constant, and **T** is the absolute temperature.

Because the deviations are not clinically significant, the universal gas law and molecular kinetic theory become immensely valuable in their simplicity to describe the behavior of gases.

Dalton's Law of Partial Pressures

Pressure in the kinetic molecular theory is purely the result of molecular collisions on the walls of a container. If there are more molecules in a container, there will be more collisions and thus greater pressure. Dalton's law (John Dalton, 1766-1844) states that the total pressure of a system is the additive pressures of each individual gas in a mixture. Multiple gases in a mixture each will exert a pressure in proportion to its percentage in the mixture. The total pressure is the summation of individual molecular collisions upon the walls of a container.

$$P_t = P_1 + P_2 + P_3 + P_4 + P_5 + ...$$

An example is the mixture of gases that compose medical air at atmospheric pressure:

79% Nitrogen: 0.79×760 mm Hg =
600.4 mm Hg partial pressure nitrogen
21% Oxygen: 0.21×760 mm Hg =
156.6 mm Hg partial pressure oxygen =
760 mm Hg total atmospheric pressure

Adiabatic Changes

Entropy in any system takes time. Rapid expansion or compression of gases may exceed the speed of energy equilibration with the surrounding environment. A rapid expansion or compression of a gas without equilibration of energy with the surrounding environment is called an *adiabatic* process and entails no increase or decrease in a system's energy.

Remember that the energy of a gas is almost entirely kinetic. Temperature is the measurement which quantifies the energy distribution among the molecules in a system. One could think of temperature measurement as a quantification of a system's kinetic energy per area. An example would be the experience of placing your hand into sunlight. The surface area of that sunlight measured is equal to the surface area of your hand. It is warm. Now place a magnifying glass of surface area equal to your hand into the sun and focus that same amount of sunlight energy onto a pinpoint area of your hand. Ouch! The same amount of energy experienced over less area is measured as a higher temperature. The temperature measurement is higher, but the system's energy total has not increased or decreased. The total sunlight energy hitting your hand is the same but distributed over different areas.

Energy Concentration Effect

Compressing a gas quickly will intensify the kinetic energy (molecular movement) such that the thermal measurement of the gas will be higher. This quick compression of the gas's area does not allow the system's energy to dissipate into the surrounding environment. Thus the temperature will quickly rise, proportional to the decreased volume. Although the temperature will be higher, the total energy of the system has not increased. A gas that is compressed quickly has little time to distribute any of its energy, so the thermal measurement becomes higher. This is the mechanism a diesel engine uses to ignite diesel fuel. Quick compression of fuel vapor intensifies the kinetic energy of the gas, with a corresponding increase in temperature, until the ignition temperature is achieved and spontaneous ignition occurs. This effect, though unlikely, could happen with a compressed gas cylinder that is quickly opened. The rapid reexpansion and recompression of gas as it rushes through the outlet channels of a cylinder could increase the temperature significantly. The high temperature generated could cause a burn or ignite any grease placed on the O-ring. Oil or grease is not recommended for use on any cylinder of compressed gas. Usually, rapid recompression in the cylinder stem is not a concern. It is possible and has occurred, but more likely the opposite will occur with rapid expansion of the gas as it leaves the cylinder.

Energy Dilution, Joule-Thompson Effect

The Joule-Thompson effect, named after James Prescott Joule, (1818-1889) and William Thompson Lord Kelvin, explains the cooling effect that occurs with adiabatic expansion of a gas. Rapid expansion of a gas causes the temperature measurement to decrease in the exact opposite process as explained previously. When we lower the pressure of a gas (increase its volume) quickly we lower the energy per area. The temperature measurement will be lower when the volume is rapidly expanded. The total energy of the gas has not changed, but the expression, or thermal measurement, is decreased related to the increased volume. The temperature may be so low that frosting may occur at the cylinder outlet. Potentially, one could suffer a freeze injury. So why does this not always occur? If done slowly, energy from the environment will move into the gas, and ambient temperature will equalize with the less kinetic energy per area of expanding gas. The second law of thermodynamics, entropy, explains the maintenance of temperature when opening a gas cylinder slowly. Opening a cylinder slowly, therefore, would not be an adiabatic process. The slow opening of a gas cylinder allows the expansion of gas to draw energy from the environment to maintain an equal distribution of energy, and we observe no changes in temperature of the gas.

FLUID FLOW

Basic Principles of Fluid Mechanics

Fluids are defined by their response to stress. Stress is the distribution of force per unit area. The stress, or force distribution, may be tangential, and thus designated a shear stress, or it may be perpendicular and designated as a normal force. Strain is the deformation caused by stress. Fluids continuously change shape (flow) when subjected to shear stress, and respond in one of two ways to perpendicular forces:

1. Resist compression (e.g., liquids)
2. Compressible and easily expandable (e.g., gases)

Both liquids and gases are fluids. Forces associated with fluids are gravity, pressure, and friction. Friction is resistance to flow from surface interaction and is proportional to viscosity. Viscosity is the physical property of a fluid that relates shear stress to rate of strain. Viscosity is the inherent property of a fluid that resists flow. Flow is the result of pressure forces in a fluid established by differences in pressure from one point to another, which creates a pressure gradient. All flow moves from higher pressure, or resistance, to lower. The following laws and principles apply to both compressible (gas) and incompressible (liquid) fluids. *Flow* is defined as the quantity of a fluid passing a point per unit of time, where **F** is the mean flow, **Q** is quantity, and **t** is time.

$$F = \frac{Q}{t}$$

Types of Flow

The three types of flow that occur through tubes and orifices are laminar, turbulent, and transitional. Laminar flow is a type of flow in which all molecules of a fluid travel in a parallel path within the tube. The molecules in the center of the tube encounter the least adhesive force of the walls of the tube and therefore move at a velocity twice that of the mean flow. Flow decreases approaching the walls and ceases at the wall. True laminar flow predominates in the smallest airways (terminal bronchioles). Transitional flow is a mixture of laminar flow along the walls of a tube with turbulent flow in the center. Turbulent flow is described as chaotic with irregular eddies throughout. Laminar, transitional, and turbulent airflow are illustrated in Figure 15-22.

Poiseuille's Law

Laminar flow is described mathematically by Poiseuille's law (Jean Louis Marie Poiseuille, 1797-1869). Poiseuille's law is:

$$F = (\pi r^4 \Delta P)/(8nl)$$

where **F** is flow, **π** is the constant *pie*, r^4 is radius to the fourth power, **ΔP** is the pressure gradient, **n** is viscosity of fluid, and **l** is the length of tube. According to Poiseuille's law, radius will have the most dramatic effect on flow. Doubling the radius will result in a 16-fold increase in flow. A tripling of the radius increases flow 81-fold. Therefore, flow through a 16-gauge (1.65 mm) intravenous catheter is much greater than through a 20-gauge (0.89mm). If the viscosity of a fluid is increased, flow decreases. Patients with polycythemia have decreased blood flow due to increased viscosity of blood. Increasing the length of a tube decreases the flow. If the length of tube is decreased by 50%, there will be a corresponding doubling of the flow. If the length of a tube is doubled, flow decreases by half.

Clinical application of Poiseuille's law in anesthesia is exemplified as follows. To improve flow when delivering a unit of

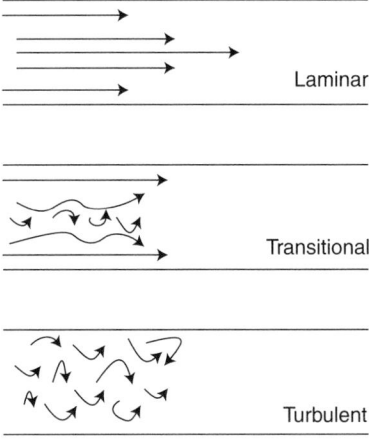

FIGURE **15-22** Three types of flow: laminar, transitional, and turbulent.

packed red blood cells, a large-diameter intravenous catheter (18 gauge or larger) is recommended, a pressure bag may be placed on the unit of packed red blood cells to increase the driving pressure (pressure gradient), and the packed red blood cells may be diluted with normal saline to lower viscosity.[53] These interventions are a direct manipulation of the factors associated with Poiseuille's law and significantly improve flow. Of all the changes that may be made, increasing the diameter of the intravenous catheter will have the most dramatic improvement of flow. Large-bore intravenous lines, such as an introducer central line, are best for rapid, large-volume infusion.

Mechanical ventilation of patients also reflects the factors associated with Poiseuille's law. The larger the endotracheal tube, the better flow of gas for ventilation. Delivery of β_2 receptor agonists, such as albuterol, has the effect of increasing the diameter of the bronchial tubes of the lungs to improve flow. Increasing the peak inspiratory pressure establishes a higher pressure gradient, which improves flow and delivered tidal volumes. Increases in the pressure gradient and flow velocity may initially improve flow but risks converting that flow to turbulent flow. Turbulent flow also may result when molecules of a fluid encounter rough, irregular walls or angles greater than 25 degrees. Turbulent flow often occurs in medium to large airways of the lung and predominates during periods of peak flow, coughing, and phonation. Orifice constrictions, such as glottic closure, cause laminar flow to become turbulent. Smaller bronchial tubes of the lung have slower velocities, and laminar flow is maintained. The presence of laminar, turbulent, or transitional flow is determined by Reynolds number.

Reynolds Number

Reynolds number (Osborne Reynolds, 1842-1912) is an index that incorporates the factors of Poiseuille's law with the addition of a fluid's density to determine whether a given flow will be laminar or turbulent. Reynolds number is directly proportional to the density of the fluid, linear velocity of the flow, and tube diameter; flow is inversely proportional to fluid viscosity. The equation is:

$$\text{Reynolds number} = \frac{vpd}{\eta}$$

where v is the linear velocity of fluid, p is density of fluid, d is diameter of tube, and η is viscosity. A calculated Reynolds number greater than 2000 will reflect a predominantly turbulent flow. Conversely, a Reynolds number less than 2000 will reflect predominantly laminar flow. Delivery of helium-oxygen mixtures to status asthmaticus patients, who are refractory to standard treatments, is based on the understanding of density's role in reestablishing laminar flow.[54] Helium, which has a significantly lower density (0.1786 g/L at STP) than nitrogen, (1.251 g/L at STP) improves flow by restoring laminar flow through the significantly narrowed airways of a severe asthma attack.

Bernoulli's Principle

Bernoulli's principle (Daniel Bernoulli, 1700-1782) describes the effect of fluid flow through a tube containing a constriction. As flow passes through a narrowing in a tube, the velocity of that flow increases and there is a corresponding decrease in pressure at the area of narrowing (Figure 15-23, A). This drop in pressure is explained by the conservation of energy law. For a steady flow of incompressible fluids, the sum of pressure, potential energy, and kinetic energy per unit of time must remain constant. The relationship of the pressure gradient to mass flow requires the

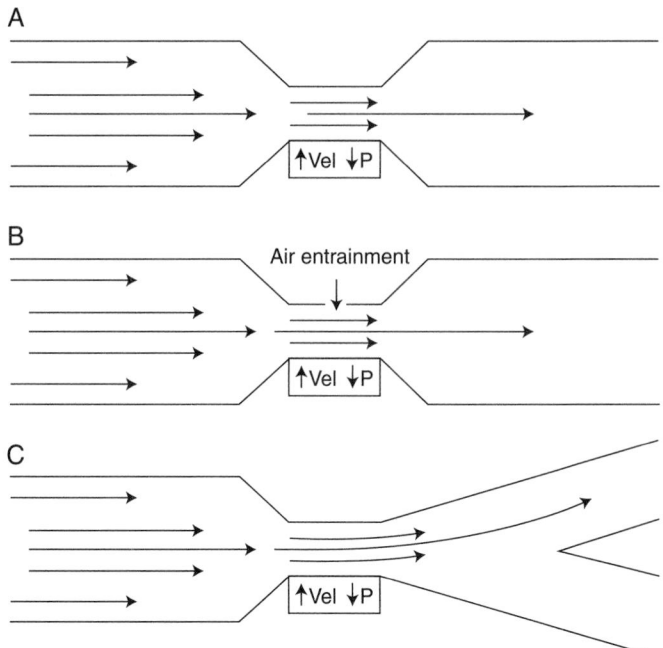

FIGURE **15-23**   **A,** Bernoulli principle; **B,** Venturi effect; **C,** Coanda effect. Vel, *Velocity*; P, *pressure*.

pressure to decrease when the velocity increases. The Bernoulli equation is:

$$p + {}^1/_2 \Delta V^2 + pgh = \text{constant}$$

where **p** is pressure,   is density, **V** is velocity, **g** is gravitational acceleration, and **h** is height. Bernoulli's equation is useful in determining flow through tubes that narrow, but it does not account for friction and assumes no changes in density or flow rate. The simplicity of this equation allows an explanation of the pressure velocity relationship if fluid flows across a constriction. The velocity of a fluid is the product of the flow rate divided by the area of flow.

$$\text{Velocity} = \frac{\text{Quantity of flow per unit of time}}{\text{area}}$$

If a given quantity of flow is 4 liters per minute over an area (tube) of 2 liters volume, the fluid velocity would be 2 liters per minute. If this flow meets a narrowing in its path which decreases the cross sectional area to 1 liter volume, the fluid velocity would increase to 4 liters per minute.

$$V1 = \frac{4 \text{ L/min}}{2 \text{ L/min}} = 2 \text{ L/min}$$

$$V2 = \frac{4 \text{ L/min}}{1 \text{ L/min}} = 4 \text{ L/min}$$

This shows the increase in velocity associated with a narrowing in a tube for a given fluid flow (assuming no changes in density or height), and the conservation of energy law dictates there must be a corresponding decrease in pressure.

Metered-dose inhalers (MDIs) use the Bernoulli principle to create a jet past a constriction that aerosolizes a drug in the expanding flow of gas. The necessity for large and sometimes cumbersome equipment is obviated by MDIs, which are able to consistently deliver aerosolized particles of medication into a fluid stream.[55] A more applicable example of the Bernoulli principle is the advantage taken of the pressure drop across the narrowing in a tube of fluid flow. The Venturi effect relies on the lower pressure at a constriction to entrain air or fluid into a fluid path.

Venturi Effect

The Venturi effect (Giovanni Battista Venturi, 1746-1822) utilizes the pressure drop across a narrowing in a tube. By placing an orifice at the narrowed region of flow, air is allowed to be entrained and enter the flow (see Figure 15-23, B). Air may be entrained into a flow of liquid, or a liquid may be entrained into the flow of a gas.[56] Jet ventilation uses this entrainment of air to augment lung ventilation volumes.[57-59] Nebulizers use the Venturi effect to deliver both humidification and medications such as albuterol.[60] Nebulizers effectively deliver medications into fluid paths, such as ventilator circuits, but have been replaced to a large extent by MDIs.

Coanda Effect

The Coanda effect (Henri Coanda, 1885-1972) explains the tendency of a fluid flow to follow a curved surface upon emerging from a constriction (see Figure 15-23, C). This may cause a preferential flow in one tube at a bifurcation just past a narrowing in a tube.[61] Beyond a narrowing in a tube, pressure will increase corresponding with a decrease in velocity of the fluid flow. If at a widening in a tube there is a division of flow with different angles, the return to a higher pressure will be at different points along the bifurcated tube. The bifurcated tube with the delayed reestablishment of higher pressure (and corresponding lower velocity) may preferentially attract a greater percentage of the total flow toward its path. The path with the greater flow will be at the expense of the other path. In situations in which the flow is blood in vessels or gas flow in the lungs, this diversion of flow could be consequential.[62-64]

Laplace's Law

Laplace's law (Pierre Simon Laplace, 1749-1827) describes the relationship of wall tension (**T**) to pressure (**P**) and radius(**r**) in cylinders and spheres.

- *Cylinders:* T = Pr
- *Spheres:* 2T = Pr

Tension is a stress force exerted over a given area. It is measured in newtons per centimeter (N/cm). In cylinders, wall tension is increased with increased radius; similarly, increasing pressure will increase wall tension.[65] Laplace's law shows why smaller-diameter capillaries do not burst during periods of hypertension and larger vessels or aneurysms may. An abdominal aorta maintains a mean arterial pressure along its length, including an aneurysm if present. Aneurysms, which have a greater radius than the rest of the aorta, have a corresponding greater tension and are more likely to rupture. Laplace's formula, when rearranged, reflects the direct relationship of tension to radius in both the aorta and an aortic aneurysm at a constant pressure.

$$P = \frac{T}{r}$$

Example 1—Cylinders: If the mean aortic pressure is 100 mm Hg with a normal radius of 2 cm and an aneurysm radius of 4 cm, the tension calculates as follows:

$$Pr = T$$

1. Normal aorta: 100 mm Hg (P) × 2.0 cm (r) = (T)
   1.33 N/cm² (100 mm Hg) × 2.0 cm = 2.66 N/cm
2. Aortic aneurysm: 100 mm Hg (P) × 4.0 cm (r) = (T)
   1.33 N/cm² (100 mm Hg) × 4.0 cm = 5.32N/cm

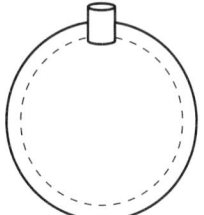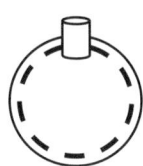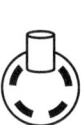

FIGURE **15-24** Increased surfactant concentration (*dashed line*) with decreasing alveolar size.

The aortic aneurysm in this example has twice the wall tension of the normal aorta. (Millimeters mercury were converted to newtons in formula). Any increases in blood pressure will increase the already high wall tensions of an aneurysm, and wall failure may result in dissection or rupture.[66]

In spheres, wall tension is increased twice as much, with increasing radius compared to cylinders. Applying Laplace's law to saccular aneurysms shows the relationship of increasing tension with increasing radius:

Example 2—Spheres: If the mean saccular aneurysm's pressures are 100 mm Hg, with one radius 0.5 cm and the other 1 cm, the tension for each calculates as follows:

$$Pr = 2T$$

1. Small saccular aneurysm:

100 mm Hg (P) × 0.5 cm (r) = (2T)
   1.33 N/cm² (100 mm Hg) × 0.5 cm =
   2 × 0.665 N/cm = 1.33 N/cm

2. Large saccular aneurysm:

100 mm Hg (P) × 1.0 cm (r) = (2T)
   1.33 N/cm² (100 mm Hg) × 1.0 cm =
   2 × 1.33 N/cm = 2.66 N/cm

Greater wall tension would be present in a large saccular aneurysm versus a small saccular aneurysm, and any increases in pressure would risk further increases in wall tension and rupture. Decreasing pressure will have the effect of decreasing wall tension across both cylinders and spheres and is the rationale for controlling blood pressure in patients with aneurysms.[67]

Laplace's law applied to a cardiac ventricle of increasing size explains the necessary inotropic response but eventual failure of contractility with increasing wall tension and pressure:

$$Pr = 2T$$
Increased pressure = increased wall tension
Increased radius = increased wall tension
Increased wall tension = increased contractility
(Frank-Starling curve)

Surfactant is a substance that lowers surface tension in alveoli to prevent the effects observed with Laplace's law. By lowering surface tension, the pressure in alveoli is lowered. Surfactant lowers surface tension more in smaller alveoli than in larger alveoli, owing to the effect of concentration when an alveolus contracts.[68] Greater surfactant concentration has greater surface tension–lowering ability. Surfactant therefore has the ability to equilibrate surface tension among different-sized alveoli and create stabilized alveolar pressures (Figure 15-24).

WAVES

Waves are a very important phenomenon in everyday life, as well as in anesthesia. Waves exist macroscopically, such as ocean waves and sound waves. They also exist within the atom and as light energy. Waves surround us and exist within us. To understand waves and wave action is to hold one key to understanding the basic ripple that permeates the universe. That basic ripple is energy. Waves are a periodic disturbance or motion. Waves are essentially the movement of energy. The "disturbance" is energy, and that is what is transported, or moved, along the wave front.

Wave Types

The two basic types of waves are transverse and longitudinal. *Transverse waves* are composed of up-and-down movement. In a transverse wave, the medium particles move perpendicular (up and down) to wave direction. *Electromagnetic radiation waves are transverse. Longitudinal waves* are composed of back-and-forth movement along the direction of the wave. In a longitudinal wave, the medium particles move forward parallel to the wave direction (propagation). There is no up-and-down motion in longitudinal waves. The wave energy causes only compression and decompression (rarefaction) to occur along its path. These are pressure fluctuations. *Sound waves are longitudinal.*

Wave characteristics:
- *Frequency*—Waves per second; measured in cycles per second called *hertz* (Hz)
- *Wave length*—Distance from one wave top (crest) to the next
- *Period or phase shift*—Describes how far the wave "slides"
- *Amplitude*—Height of wave
- *Speed*—Measured in meters per second
- *Wave part*—Crest is the wave top, trough is the wave bottom
- *Pressure waves*—Can be reflected, refracted, diffracted, or absorbed (interfered) by other waves
- *Reflection*—Waves reflect off of a medium in the same but opposite angle. The angle of incidence is the angle at which a wave strikes a medium.
- *Refraction*—Redirected in a new direction by contact with a new medium
- *Diffraction*—Spread or scattered; bending around an object
- *Absorption or interference*—Waves may interfere with other waves or be absorbed by matter. When waves interfere, amplitudes are additive. Constructive interference is when the **crest** of one wave passes through the **crest** of another wave or the **trough** of one wave passes through the **trough** of another wave, and the resultant wave is greater. Addition of two positive amplitudes or two negative amplitudes is a greater value or wave height. Destructive interference is when the *crest* of one wave passes through the *trough* of another wave. Amplitudes from one crest are added to the negative amplitudes from the other wave's trough, and the resultant wave is less.

Pressure Waves (Sound Waves)

Sound waves are pressure fluctuations that deviate from ambient pressure and are measured in pascals (Pa). Sound pressures are measured on a sound pressure level (SPL) that uses a logarithmic decibel scale to narrow the wide range (20 Hz to 20 kHz) of amplitudes audible to the human ear. Sound waves are longitudinal waves that propagate through matter (solid, liquid, gas) at varying speeds determined by the medium's elastic modulus (stiffness), density, and temperature. The speed of sound through air at 0° C is 740 miles per hour. In the absence of matter, there are no sound waves. Sound waves do not exist in a vacuum and only travel through matter.

Ultrasonography. Sound waves above the auditory limit of the human ear (20 kHz) are known as *ultrasound*. Ultrasonography uses ultrasound waves to construct a visual image of internal structures by examining the reflection of sound. Ultrasonography is useful for assisting simple procedures such as intravenous catheter insertion or for more invasive diagnostic assessment such as transesophageal echocardiograpghy.[69-73] Ultrasonography uses a signal generator that transmits sound waves through tissues and a transducer to record the time delay for the returning reflected sound waves. The speed of sound waves in tissues is unique and constant to specific tissue compositions, and therefore the time delay of the returning reflected sound waves allows calculation of the location of different internal structures. Not all sound waves are reflected back to the transducer; some sound waves will have been refracted in a new direction, diffracted in multiple directions, or interfered with by tissues that cause attenuation or conversion to heat and resultant dissipation. The fraction of the original signal that is reflected back to the transducer must be amplified and processed into a visual display. The introduction of ultrasonography has been made possible by piezoelectric crystals that act as both signal generators and signal transducers (see Piezoelectric Effect). The process of a burst of ultrasound pressure waves followed by measurement of the reflected waves is done many times a second, permitting real-time imaging of internal structures by computational analysis.

Piezoelectric Effect. Piezoelectric crystals are unique quartz, ceramic, or polymer compositions that contain a matrix of polarized molecules that (1) respond to electric current by changing shape and (2) respond to mechanical stresses by generating an electric current. Piezoelectric crystals derive their name from the Greek prefix *piezein*, which means "to press tight or squeeze." The shape change caused by an electric current creates a pressure fluctuation around the crystal; this is a pressure wave. If a piezoelectric crystal is subjected to an alternating electric current, it will vibrate, creating many pressure waves in quick succession. The rate at which the crystal vibrates is called its *resonant frequency.* When not responding to an electric current, piezoelectric crystals are at rest and respond to the mechanical stress of the pressure waves by creating a small electric current.

Doppler Effect. The Doppler effect (Christian Johann Doppler, 1803-1853) describes the change in frequency of a propagated wave from a moving object. The sound of a siren changes to a higher frequency as it approaches a listener and lowers in frequency as it departs. Listener 1 in the Doppler effect figure (Figure 15-25) will hear a sound emitted from a stationary object with a fixed frequency. Listener 2 will hear a sound emitted from a moving object with increasing frequency as the sound approaches and lessening frequency when it passes. This is due to the "stacking up" of the wave fronts emitted from an approaching object and the stretching of the wave fronts when it recedes.

The Doppler effect when applied to echocardiography allows the determination of blood flow direction and speed. As blood cells flow to or away from an ultrasound signal, reflected waves

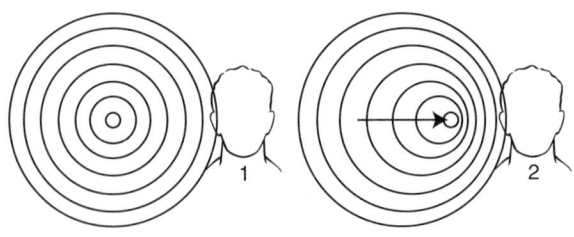

FIGURE **15-25** Doppler effect.

are either compressed or expanded. This change in frequency allows calculation of blood velocity:

$$v = \frac{\Delta f}{\cos\theta} \times \frac{c}{2f_t}$$

where velocity of blood is **v**, Δf is the difference in transmitted frequency and received frequency, f_t is the transmitted frequency, **c** is the speed of sound in blood, and θ is the angle of incidence between the ultrasound beam and blood. Spectral display presents Doppler ultrasound data in a time-velocity graph that allows greater assessment of hemodynamics on a beat-to-beat basis.

Electromagnetic Waves

The term *electromagnetic* succinctly expresses the dual nature of *electricity* and *magnetism*. The two are intimately intertwined. Where there is electric current, there are also magnetic waves. Where there are changing magnetic waves, there is also an electric current. Electromagnetic radiation is composed of two waves, electric and magnetic, oscillating in unison but perpendicular to one another. The whole electromagnetic wave propagation is perpendicular to these oscillating waves. Electromagnetic waves possess both electric and magnetic potential. Electromagnetic waves (electromagnetic radiation, EMR) are similar to pressure waves in that they both possess frequency and amplitude. Another similarity is that they may be reflected, refracted, diffracted, or absorbed. The unique wave properties of EMR include its composition, velocity, and independence of transport by matter. Electromagnetic radiation differs from pressure waves (sound waves) in their velocity. The speed of EMR in a vacuum is 3 $\times$ 10^8 m/sec (186,000 miles/sec), whereas sound cannot exist in a vacuum. The speed of EMR in air closely approaches 3 $\times$ 10^8 m/sec. The speed of sound in air is only 331 m/sec (740 miles/hr). Electromagnetic radiation and sound waves may travel through matter at varying speeds, but only electromagnetic radiation can propagate independently of matter. Sound waves only travel through matter and cannot exist in a vacuum, as shown in Figure 15-26 and Table 15-6.

Inverse Square Law

Waves represent a propagation of energy from a source. As energy moves away from its source, its strength decreases. Newton

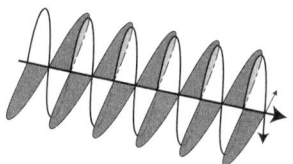

FIGURE **15-26** Electromagnetic wave showing electric wave oscillating perpendicular to magnetic wave.

TABLE **15-6**	Comparisons of EMR and Sound Wave Properties	
	EMR	**Sound Waves**
Speed	300,000,000 m/sec	344 m/sec
Wave type	Transverse	Longitudinal
Energy motion	Perpendicular to propagation	Parallel to propagation

EMR, *Electromagnetic radiation.*

showed that the strength of the emanating energy is inversely proportional to the square of its distance from its source. Newton originally calculated this for the force of gravity; however, it has application throughout physics.[74]

$$I1 = \frac{(d2)^2}{I2\,(d1)^2}$$

where **I1** equals intensity at the original distance, **I2** is the lower intensity at a new distance, **d1** is the distance from original source, and **d2** is the new distance from the source. This is represented by the inverse square law figure (Figure 15-27), where the *y* plane is twice the distance from the source than plane *x*. The energy intensity at **I2** is one fourth the intensity at **I1**. The inverse square law applies to pressure waves, electricity, light, and radiation, with the intensity of each decreasing with increasing distance from its source.

Magnetism

Magnets are unique matter that has charges aligned orderly. There are flows of magnetic currents, or field lines, in all magnets. To observe these invisible fields, place a magnet under a piece of paper and spread iron filings on top. The filings will line up along the magnetic fields. Magnetism is a force between electric currents. Flowing charged particles not only move energy along that current but also disrupt, or alter, the surrounding environment. This "altering" is not apparent unless one is looking. Hold a compass near a wire carrying an electric current. The needle will move and align itself along the flow of magnetism. Turn the wire, and the compass needle will turn. There is a force between the electric current and the compass needle (magnet). Magnetic fields are measured with a gauss meter in units of teslas. 10,000 gauss (G) equal one tesla (T). The earth's magnetic field strength is 0.00005 T (0.5 G). A small magnet's strength is 0.01 T (100 G). The magnet's strength in a magnetic resonance imaging machine is 1 to 3 T (10,000 to 30,000 G).

Magnetic Resonance Imaging

Magnetic resonance imaging (MRI) uses a strong, continuous magnetic field to uniformly realign the spin of protons within the hydrogen atoms of water. As the axes of protons are pulled into one of two possible positions of realignment, a radiofrequency pulse is delivered at resonant frequency to energize the protons. The protons will then reemit this energy. The radiofrequency pulses are delivered in thin "slices" that may be made in the sagittal, coronal, or axial planes. Computer-generated analysis of data produces very detailed representations of internal tissues. The magnetic field used is very strong, and specific safety considerations need to be addressed when delivering anesthesia care in an MRI suite.

MRI Safety. Because of the high strength of the magnetic field in and around an MRI scanner, special precautions must be observed. Any ferrous material will interact with the magnetic field, gaining kinetic energy and thermal heat. Movable ferrous objects will also be attracted to the MRI magnet and will be pulled into the magnetic field with great force. Patients and personnel are at potential risk for both thermal injuries from implanted ferrous objects and traumatic injury from ferrous objects violently pulled into the magnetic field. The American College of Radiology has designated four safety zones that surround an MRI scanner, with zone 4 representing the immediate area around the scanner. Zone 4 poses the greatest risk of injury and has the most stringent guidelines.[75] All ferrous materials such as pagers, phones, jewelry, identification badges, and pens must be removed before entering

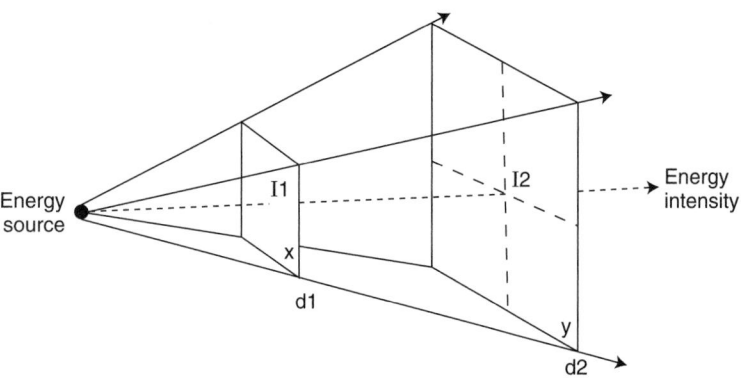

FIGURE **15-27** Inverse square law representation of decreasing intensity with increasing distance.

zone 4. Patient stretchers, oxygen tanks, IV poles, and any other ferrous objects must be kept outside zone 4. Specially designed stretchers and anesthesia machines are designated for zone 4 to prevent attraction to the magnet.

Implanted ferrous materials such as ferrous foreign bodies, prosthetics, stents, and pacemakers have been studied for MRI safety. Review of current literature for acceptability for scanning is recommended.[75-78] Many implanted devices can be safely scanned in an MRI, and any knowledge or concerns of potential ferrous interaction should be brought to the attention of the designated MRI personnel.[75]

Electricity

Electricity is the change in potential energy caused by the movement of electrons from an area of high concentration (high charge density) to an area of low concentration (low charge density). The fundamental unit of charge is *e*; it represents one electron's energy and is extremely small. Dealing with the energy of a single electron is difficult, so we use a quantized measurement called a *coulomb* (C): C $=1.60222210^{19}$ *e*.

Coulomb's Law

Coulomb's law (Charles-Augustin de Coulomb, 1736-1806) states that like charges repel each other, and opposite charges attract each other inversely to the square of their distance. In short, opposite charges will attract more when closer together, and like charges will repel more when closer together. The electrical potential energy unit is the *volt*. It represents electrical "pressure" or the gradient of charges that could potentially flow. Electric current (I) is the rate of flow of an electric charge through a *conductor*. In operating room electrical equipment, the conductor is usually copper wire. Copper is a good conductor, and therefore the resistance to flow is low. Insulators, also known as *dielectrics*, do not have electrons that are easily moved and therefore resist the flow of electricity. Current is measured in amperes. An *ampere* (A) is the flow of 1 coulomb per second, 1A = 1C/s. A *volt* is the SI unit for a joule per coulomb.

Ohm's Law

The potential flow of electric charge is proportional to actual current, after accounting for resistance. Resistance is calculated by Ohm's law (Georg Ohm, 1789-1854):

$$E = IR$$

where **E** represents volts (V) or potential energy, **I** is current, and **R** is resistance. Resistance is measured in ohms (Ω). Ohm's law measures resistance to electrical flow (Figure 15-28).

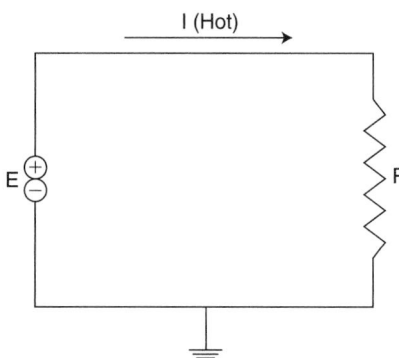

FIGURE **15-28** Basic electric circuit showing a live (hot) wire (*I* = *current*), a load (*R* = *resistance*), and a grounded neutral wire (*E* = *volts*).

Electrical Flow

The flow of electrons in electricity is from a surplus of electrons to a deficiency of electrons. Electricity must have a complete circuit for electrical flow to occur. A simple circuit is shown with a positive side (live, hot), a negative side (neutral), and a ground. The ground is a conductor that is connected to the earth (ground) and provides a low, resistive, alternate route for electricity to flow in the case of electrical surge. Electricity may be *direct current* (DC) or *alternating current* (AC). In DC circuits, the flow of electrons is always in one direction. In AC circuits, the flow of electrons reverses direction (alternates) at a set frequency, usually 60 Hz (United States) or 50 Hz (Europe) (1 Hz equals 1 cycle per second). Electricity is delivered by the power company as AC because its voltage can easily be maintained while traveling long distances to customers via the power grid. Operating room equipment and most residential and institutional electrical equipment operate on AC. A simple AC circuit is the same as a simple DC circuit, except resistance is more complex with AC circuits, and the positive side alternates between both wires. In AC circuits, resistance is called *impedance* and is the total of all forces that impede electrical flow. In addition to the inherent characteristics of the conductive material, capacitance and inductance contribute to AC impedance. *Capacitance* is the capacity to store charge. A capacitor is composed of two parallel conductive plates separated by an insulator. When a capacitor is exposed to a voltage source in an open circuit, one plate will store a positive charge, and the other will store a negative charge. Capacitors have useful application in electronic devices but have the ability to leak *stray capacitance*. There are no absolute insulators, and stray capacitance may create an unintended charge in the casing of electrical equipment. *Electromagnetic inductance* is the transfer of an electric current between circuits without physical contact, using induced magnetic waves. Any conductors carrying an electric current will also carry a magnetic field. In AC circuits, the charge is alternating and so too will the magnetic field change. This changing magnetic field may induce a small electric current in nearby conductive materials such as equipment metal casings, despite no physical contact between the circuit and the casing.

Electric Shock. Stray capacitance and inductance may contribute a low risk of shock because they are low current flows. Direct contact of exposed electrical wiring constitutes great risk of electric shock because of higher voltages. Current leakage from wires to equipment casing exposes patients and operating room personnel to the risk of shock by three mechanisms:

- Direct wire contact with metal casing due to insulation damage or faulty construction.
- Inductance due to the flowing alternating current's magnetic field, producing a small electrical flow in the surrounding metal casing despite no direct contact.
- Stray capacitance from the buildup of electrical potentials with an alternating current circuit despite no closed circuit electrical flow.[79]

If a patient or operating room personnel make contact with both a live wire and ground they may complete an electric circuit and receive a shock. For a shock to occur, a complete circuit must be made. This can happen if a person is standing on the earth and contacts the live wire in a circuit (Figure 15-29). Shocks may be macroshock or microshock. *Macroshock* refers to large amounts of current conducted through the patient's skin and other tissues. Injuries may be minor or severe, depending on amount of current and duration of exposure. Electric current seeks the path of least resistance and is often dissipated throughout the body tissues. The amount that reaches the heart is often insufficient to cause arrhythmias.

Conductive materials in a patient's body, though, may place that patient at greater risk by providing a low resistive path for electricity to flow to the heart. *Microshock* is the delivery of small amounts of current directly to the heart. The amount of current that may produce ventricular fibrillation has been found to be 50 microamperes or lower.[80,81] Table 15-7 gives a comparison of how different levels of microshock and macroshock affect the human body.

Electrical Safety. To decrease the risk of shock, operating room electrical systems are isolated from the main grounded electrical supply system. A *transformer* is used to isolate the electrical supply systems from one another. A transformer uses the principle of magnetic inductance to transfer electricity from one system to another system without having physical contact. This allows the operating room power supply to be ungrounded, preventing a circuit from being completed when a person contacts one live wire. However, if a person contacts both wires in a circuit, shock may occur as the path of electricity flows through the person from one line to the other. Operating room equipment casing (housing) is grounded to divert electrical flow in case of internal live wire contact with the metal housing.

If there is contact of the live wires to ground (fault), such as through touching the equipment casing, the system will become a grounded system. A second fault will enable a shock, because the newly grounded system will allow a completed circuit to pass through a person in the operating room that is grounded when

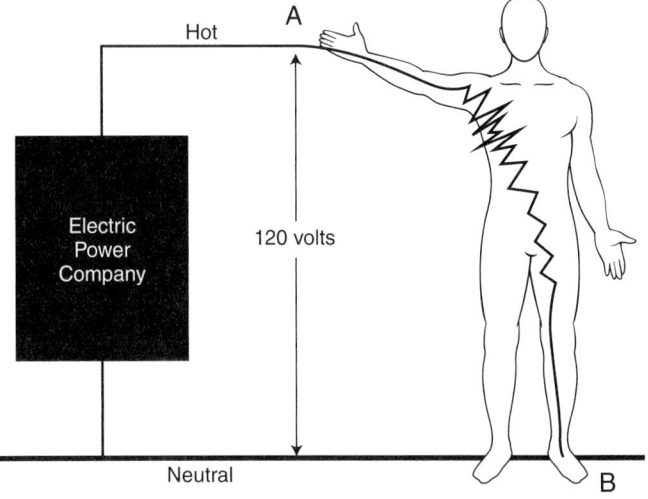

FIGURE **15-29** Electric shock. *A* is point of contact and *B* is connection to ground.

TABLE **15-7**	Effects of Macroshock and Microshock
Macroshock (mA)	**Effect**
1	Perception
5	Maximal harmless current
10-20	"Let-go" current
50	Loss of consciousness
100-300	Ventricular fibrillation
6000	Complete physiological damage
Microshock (μA)	**Effect**
20	Ventricular fibrillation in dogs
100	Ventricular fibrillation humans[53]

a live wire is contacted. To prevent a first fault from being unnoticed, a *line isolation monitor* is placed between the live wires and ground to measure their impedance to flow (Figure 15-30).[82] If a live wire has contact or high capacitance to ground, the line isolation monitor will alarm. Line isolation monitors are usually set to alarm at 2 to 5 mA potential leak. If a line isolation monitor alarms, the last equipment plugged in should be disconnected and inspected to verify it is the offending piece of equipment. Equipment that activates a line isolation monitor may still be operational but increase the potential risk of shock should a second fault occur, because it has converted the isolated power supply system to a grounded system. Line isolation monitor alarms may also be activated because of the cumulative effect of minor leakages of many pieces of properly functioning electrical equipment. This does not mean a risk is present. Newer systems alarm at 5 mA to account for this normal leakage.

Electrocautery

Electrocautery devices use high-frequency electric currents to cauterize, cut, and destroy tissue. These devices may be unipolar or bipolar. Bipolar electrocautery devices have two tips, one to

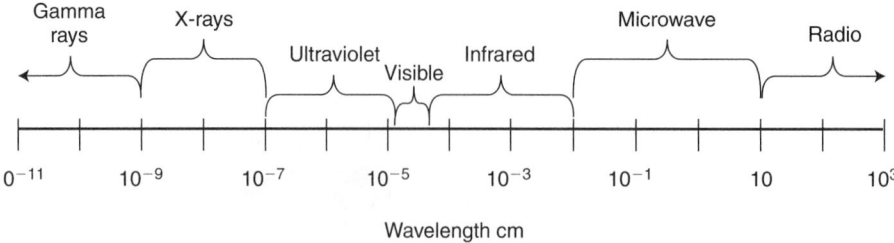

FIGURE **15-31** Electromagnetic radiation spectrum. Increasing energy associated with decreasing wavelength (increasing frequency) along the EMR spectrum is shown. Example: X-rays possess shorter wavelengths, greater energy, and greater ability to permeate matter than microwaves, which have longer wavelengths and lower energy.

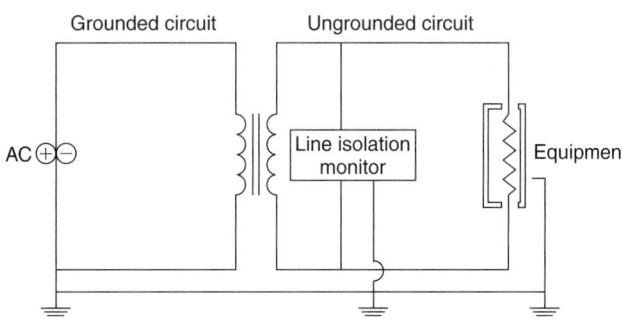

FIGURE **15-30** Ungrounded operating room electric circuit isolated from grounded hospital electrical system. Note electrical equipment casing and line isolation monitor are connected to ground, but the electric circuit is not.

supply the electric current and the other to return the current. Bipolar devices do not require a return electrode and are less likely to cause burn or injury apart from the local area of use. Unipolar devices have only one tip to deliver an electric current, and a large-surface-area return electrode with good conductive contact must be placed on the patient. The path of current flow from the unipolar device to the return electrode should not cross the patient's heart.

The high current flows used in electrocautery units may cause electromagnetic inductance, which in turn may cause artifact in other electrical equipment such as ECG monitors. Pacemakers may also sense the electromagnetic inductance as inherent electrical activity and not initiate a paced impulse. This would put the patient at risk for asystole if there is no inherent underlying heart rhythm.[83] Electrocautery interference has also been documented as initiating paced tachycardic rhythms.[84,85] Placing a pacemaker magnet over the patient's pacemaker resets it into a continuous, asynchronous mode. Not all pacemakers are reset into a continuous, asynchronous mode, and pacemaker interrogation to understand its settings and functions should be considered prior to surgery using electrocautery.

QUANTUM PHYSICS

ELECTROMAGNETIC RADIATION

Newtonian physics is helpful in describing the wavelike properties of EMR but is incomplete in its description. Originally it was assumed that EMR, like sound waves, was propagated through a medium. A "luminiferous ether" was thought to fill the universe

and was the suspected medium through which EMR traveled. The famous Michelson-Morley[86,87] experiment successfully disproved the existence of the "ether" but left open an explanation of how EMR propagates. Max Planck (1858-1947) later theorized EMR was *quantized*, meaning it was emitted only in discrete quantities of energy, and this revolutionized our perspective of the universe. Planck's constant expresses the quantized nature of EMR defined by energy, time, and frequency:

$$E = h\nu$$

where **E** represents energy, **h** is Planck's constant (6.626068 × 10^{-34} m^{2}kg/sec), and ν is frequency.[88] Albert Einstein introduced the photon concept of Planck's discrete energy quanta and together with others ushered in the study of quantum mechanics.[89,90] Quantum mechanics is a branch of physics that explores the subatomic dynamics of pure energy and the quasi-realm of energy/mass transition.

Electromagnetic radiation is now thought to travel as photons or packets of energy and can be observed as both a particle and a wave, depending on how scientists study and measure it. The dual nature of behaving as both a particle and a wave is unique to EMR.[91] EMR is called a *photon* when it exhibits particle-like behaviors. Despite its behavior, photons have no mass. They are pure energy. The energy of EMR is directly related to its frequency. Higher frequencies correspond to higher energies, and lower frequencies correspond to lower energies. The velocity of EMR in a vacuum remains constant and does not change related to frequency. The understanding of energy as a quantized event promoted numerous advances is physics, which ultimately found application in anesthesia. The perspective of EMR as photons allows us to better explain many dynamic interactions of EMR and matter. Figure 15-31 shows the EMR spectrum.

ELECTROMAGNETIC RADIATION/MATTER INTERACTION

Electromagnetic radiation exists independently of matter. Sound (pressure) waves do not exist without matter through which their energy is transmitted. Both may be reflected, refracted (scattered), diffracted (redirected), or absorbed (interfered) by matter (Figure 15-32). An example of the interaction of EMR with matter is visible light. Visible light is composed of a narrow band of EMR frequencies between 4.3 × 10^{14} and 7.5 × 10^{14} (400 to 700 nm). These frequencies of EMR are the only frequencies our eye receptors can detect. When we "see" a color, we see the reflected frequencies that correspond to that color. Visible light is composed of the colors red, orange, yellow, green, blue, indigo, and violet and were first described by Newton. Visualizing the color blue represents the reflected EMR frequencies between

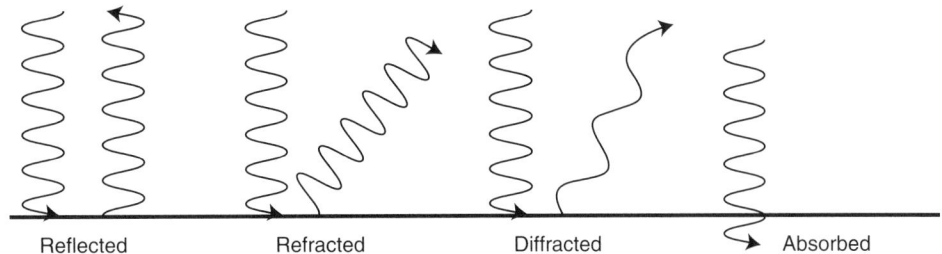

FIGURE **15-32** Electromagnetic radiation interactions with matter.

495 and 570 nanometers. The other visible light frequencies are not seen, because they have been absorbed and scattered by the material that appears blue. Materials that absorb EMR increase their vibration energy (kinetic energy), owing to their absorption of energy. We experience an example of this when wearing white or black clothing in sunlight. Black clothing absorbs many more frequencies of visible light and gains greater kinetic energy, which causes heat. White clothing appears white because of the high reflection of the visible light spectrum; it gains less kinetic energy and therefore less heat. The phenomenon of matter reflecting, scattering, and absorbing specific EMR frequencies has many applications in healthcare, anesthesia in particular.

Electromagnetic radiation may also be converted into other forms of energy such as electricity (gas discharge), heat (incandescence), and chemical energy (photoluminescence) but must obey the law of conservation of energy. When matter is exposed to EMR, it too may change form. The analysis of EMR's interaction with matter is the underlying principle of x-ray fluoroscopy, anesthetic gas measurement, pulse oximetry, and lasers.

RADIOGRAPHY

X-Rays

X-rays are able to pass through different organic materials to varying degrees and allow the "photographic" imaging of internal structures. Though x-ray and fluoroscopic imaging offer great medical benefit, they also possess potential for great harm. X-rays are ionizing radiation and lie in the higher energy frequencies of the electromagnetic radiation spectrum (see Figure 15-31). They possess high energy and have the ability to ionize atoms and molecules. X-rays can cause DNA damage and be mutagenic.[92] Proper protection is imperative for health care personnel when working near or with x-rays. Safety lies within the three factors of distance from source, barriers, and exposure time. The inverse square law explained how energy intensity significantly decreases with distance from its source.[93] X-rays obey this law, and the minimum recommended distance from an x-ray source is 6 feet. The greatest intensity of an x-ray is directly in front of the beam generator. Standing at least 6 feet away and behind or to the side of the beam direction lessens exposure. Although the energy intensity of x-rays decreases significantly with greater distance from the source, proper shielding is also important. Lead barriers are efficient absorbers of x-ray energy, and lead aprons and thyroid shields should be worn. X-ray technicians often wear badges that measure total exposure to x-rays over a period of time. Greater exposure to x-rays is associated with greater risks. Institutional policies establish guidelines of exposure limits. Unless practitioners are exposed to radiographic procedures frequently, the doses received usually fall well below established limits for maximal allowable exposure. Shielding and distance

---

BOX **15-1**

Organic and Inorganic Anesthetic Gas Analysis Technologies

Organic and Inorganic Anesthetic Gas Analysis
Infrared absorption analysis
Raman scattering
Mass spectrometry
Piezoelectric analysis
Interferometric refractometry
Gas-liquid chromatography

Oxygen Analysis
Electrogalvanic cell (fuel cell)
Polarographic electrode (Clark electrode)
Paramagnetic oxygen sensor
Fluorescence quenching
pH optode

Carbon Dioxide Analysis
Infrared absorption analysis
Severinghaus P_{CO_2} electrode
Fluorescence quenching
pH optode

---

from the x-ray source remain the two most important factors within the control of the practitioner.

GAS ANALYSIS

Gas analysis technologies use several methods to measure organic and inorganic gases. The methods described herein focus on the technologies prevalent in the field of anesthesia. The gas analysis technologies in Box 15-1 show the most common technologies for analysis of anesthetic gases, oxygen, and carbon dioxide.

Organic and Inorganic Anesthetic Gas Analysis
Infrared Absorption Analysis

Infrared absorption analysis uses each anesthetic gas's ability to absorb specific frequencies of EMR in the infrared spectrum. A sample of a gas or mixture of gases is subjected to a known range of infrared frequencies. The frequencies lost due to absorption are measured, and identification of the gas or gases may be made by the specific frequencies each gas absorbs. Anesthetic agents' infrared absorptions are unique but close in frequency. Newer infrared absorption analysis monitors are capable of identifying specific agents without preprogramming the specific agent. Concentration is determined by the amount of infrared absorption (Figure 15-33).

Raman Scattering Analysis

The interaction of electromagnetic radiation with matter is the underlying principle used with Raman scattering analysis of gases. Raman scattering passes a monochromatic laser beam through a gas mixture, causing an increased vibration frequency of the excited gas molecules (Figure 15-34). A laser is a high-intensity beam of a known specific EMR frequency (see laser discussion in this chapter). When this laser beam interacts with an anesthetic gas molecule, it may be absorbed, as previously described with infrared absorption analysis, or it may be scattered. Scattering is a frequency change (energy change) of the initial laser beam after it interacts with gas molecules. The laser frequency interacting with the molecules may be scattered at higher or lower frequencies. Each anesthetic gas scatters laser frequencies uniquely. Analysis and identification of a gas or gas mixture may be made by comparing the gas sample scattering spectrum to that of known gas-scattering spectrums. The scattered frequencies measured in this spectral analysis are represented as Stokes lines.

Raman scattering technology requires only that a gas molecule be polyatomic for identification. Raman scattering analysis can identify oxygen, carbon dioxide, nitrogen, nitrous oxide, and all volatile anesthetics, including mixtures of volatile anesthetics.[94]

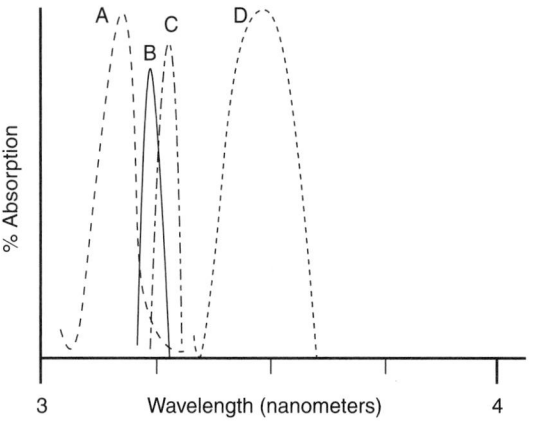

FIGURE **15-33** Individual anesthetic gas infrared absorption spectra (representation only, not actual).

Helium cannot be analyzed by Raman scattering. Raman scattering analyzers return the sample to the patient circuit and therefore do not need waste-gas scavenging. Raman scattering analyzers are small and portable but require calibration. They are less accurate with pediatric cases, which use high carrier gas flow rates and small tidal volumes.

Mass Spectrometry

Mass spectrometry historically has been the dominant technology for anesthetic gas analysis, though it has increasingly been replaced by more portable and efficient infrared absorption analysis and Raman scattering analysis technologies. Mass spectrometry ionizes gas molecules and passes them through a magnetic field. The gas molecules with the lowest mass-to-charge ratio are easily deflected by the magnetic field and collected by an ion detector (Figure 15-35). Ionized gas molecules with higher mass-to-charge ratios are deflected less by the magnetic field and detected by other ion detectors. Identification of a gas is based on the amount of deflection.

Piezoelectric Gas Analysis

Piezoelectric gas analysis incorporates both the piezoelectric effect and Henry's law.[95-97] A piezoelectric crystal will vibrate at a set frequency when an electric current is applied to it. A vibrating piezoelectric crystal coated with a liquid solution will alter its resonant frequency when exposed to a gas. As a gas dissolves into the liquid, in proportion to its concentration above the liquid gas interphase, the resonant frequency of the crystal is altered. The degree of frequency change is proportional to the concentration of gas that dissolves into the liquid. The amount of gas that dissolves into the piezoelectric crystal's liquid coating is directly related to the partial pressure of that gas. This is explained by Henry's law. A drawback of this technology is that it does not identify the specific anesthetic agent.[98]

Photoacoustic Gas Analyzer

The photoacoustic gas analyzer subjects a gas sample to a filtered, pulsating infrared light beam in a closed chamber. The pulsating beam causes the gas molecules to increase then decrease in temperature. The increase and decrease in temperature causes the chamber pressure to increase and decrease according to Gay-Lussac's law. Microphones along the chamber measure

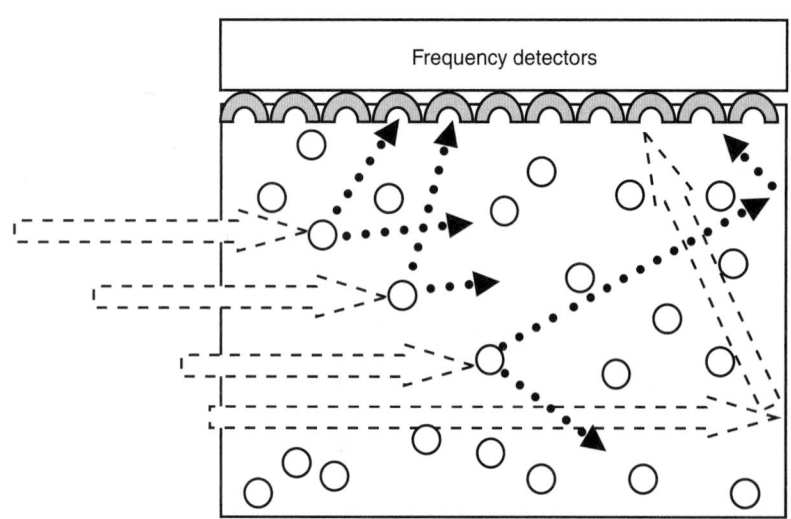

Gas sample chamber

FIGURE **15-34** Raman scattering gas analysis technology.

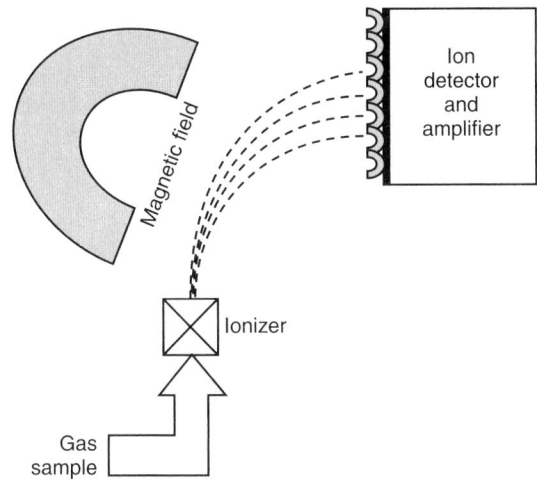

FIGURE **15-35**   Mass spectrometry gas analysis technology.

the pressure waves. A photoacoustic gas analyzer can measure anesthetic gases, mixtures of these gases, and carbon dioxide.[99] The units are small, portable, and accurate.

Oxygen Analysis

The primary role of oxygen in biological systems underscores the importance of identification and measurement of this gas when delivering anesthetics. Purposeful redundancy is used in oxygen measurement, often with more than one technology being used at a time. In the practice of anesthesia, oxygen content analysis is accomplished with several technologies. These technologies take advantage of oxygen's unique physicochemical properties and interaction with EMR. The most often used technologies pertaining to anesthesia practice are reviewed.

Electrogalvanic Cell (Fuel Cell) Electrochemical-Oxygen Analyzer

The electrogalvanic cell (Figure 15-36) is also called a *fuel cell* because the reaction that takes place creates its own electric current by consuming its "fuel." The electrogalvanic sensor has a membrane permeable to gases but not liquids. At the anode of the sensor, electrons are liberated in an oxidative reaction. This is shown with a lead anode:

$$2Pb \rightarrow 2(Pb^{+2}) + 4e^-$$

The meter measures the current produced by the electrons consumed in the reaction at the cathode (silver or gold):

$$O_2 + 4e^- \rightarrow 2O_2, 2O_2 + 2H_2O \rightarrow 4(OH)^-$$

The electron flow between the anode and cathode is directly proportional to the partial pressure of oxygen in the sample gas. Current flows in proportion to oxygen concentration.

Electrogalvanic cells have a limited life related to the concentration and duration of oxygen exposures. Because of this, some nurse anesthetists remove the oxygen sensor from the circle system if an anesthesia machine is left on and not in use for extended periods of time, such as overnight. Most anesthesia machines have minimal oxygen flow at all times, so removing the electrogalvanic cell from the flow of higher oxygen concentration will extend its duration of usefulness.

Polarographic Electrode (Clark Electrode)

The Clark polarographic oxygen electrode consists of a voltage source and a current meter connected to a platinum cathode and

a silver anode (Figure 15-37). The electrodes are immersed in a potassium chloride electrolyte cell. A membrane permeable to oxygen but not electrolytes covers one surface of the cell. A polarizing voltage is applied between the electrodes. At the anode, electrons are liberated by the oxidative reaction of silver with the chloride electrolyte:

$$4Ag \rightarrow 4Ag^+ + 4e^-, 4Ag^+ + Cl^- \rightarrow 4AgCl$$

The meter measures the current produced by the electrons consumed in the reaction at the cathode:

$$O_2 + 4e^- \rightarrow 2O_2, 2O_2 + 2H_2O \rightarrow 4(OH)^-$$

Current flows in proportion to oxygen concentration. If there is no current applied to these cells, there will be no consumption of the electrodes.[100]

Paramagnetic Oxygen Sensor: Magnetomechanical "Dumbbell Principle"

The paramagnetic oxygen sensor uses oxygen molecules' unique attraction into magnetic fields. Few other gases are attracted by magnetic fields. The paramagnetic oxygen sensor is constructed with two nitrogen-filled bulbs attached together by a stem; this resembles a dumbbell. This dumbbell-shaped apparatus is suspended parallel to a magnetic field in its "at-rest" state. Nitrogen is not attracted or repelled by magnetic fields. The introduction of oxygen into this sensor causes the dumbbell apparatus to be displaced out of the magnetic field as oxygen is attracted into the field (Figure 15-38). The amount of

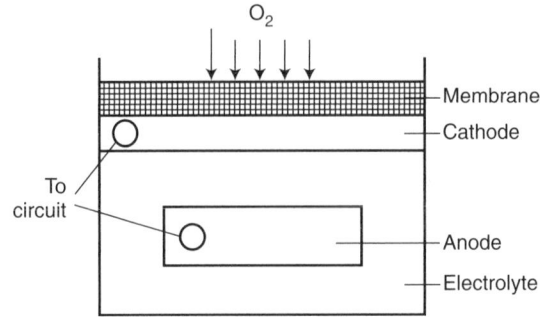

FIGURE **15-36**   Electrogalvanic fuel cell.

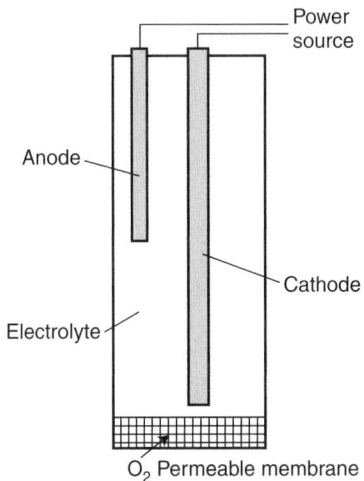

FIGURE **15-37**   Polarographic electrode.

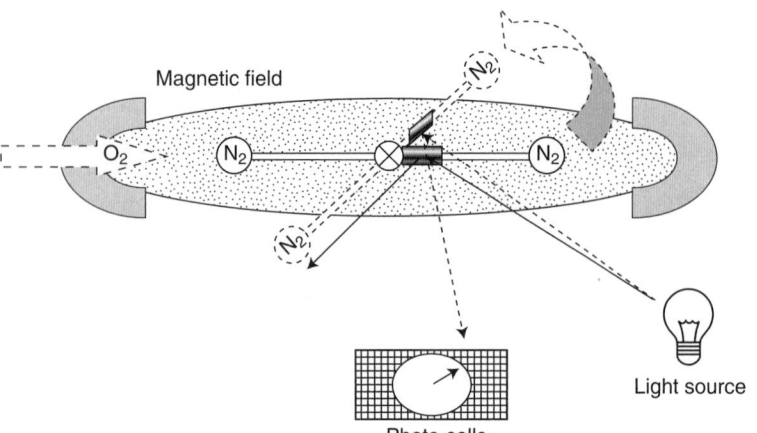

FIGURE **15-38**   Paramagnetic oxygen sensor.

displacement of the dumbbell apparatus is directly proportional to the concentration of oxygen. Originally these sensors measured the physical displacement of the dumbbell apparatus but were prone to artifact caused by vibration and external movement. These sensors now incorporate a small optical mirror that reflects a projected light beam. The light beam is reflected onto a photocell that generates a small voltage used to counteract the displacement of the dumbbell apparatus. Increased oxygen concentration increases the displacement of the dumbbell apparatus, which in turn directs a greater reflection of light onto the photocell. By using a generated electric current to counteract the dumbbell apparatus, displacement proportional to the oxygen concentration, external movement, and artifact are eliminated. These sensors are highly accurate, compact, and durable.

Fluorescence Quenching

Fluorescence is caused by a molecule emitting light (photons) in response to being energized. Certain molecules exhibit fluorescence in response to an electric current or exposure to EMR. These molecules are sometimes said to "glow in the dark." Neon lights are an example of noble gas fluorescence initiated by an electric current. Chemical fluorescence is seen in some sea life and in glow sticks. Both electrically and chemically initiated fluorescence is caused by energizing an electron to a higher energy level. The energized (excited) electron then returns to its lower energy level (resting state) by releasing a photon (spontaneous emission). The released photon is observed as light, with its color representing the emitted photon's frequency.[100]

Fluorescence quenching is a technology that uses oxygen's ability to suppress, or quench, certain molecules from fluorescing. When a fluorescent molecule is excited to a higher energy state, it will emit a photon. Oxygen, if present, will absorb this photon and prevent its release. The amount fluorescence is quenched is directly proportional to the concentration of oxygen present. By measuring the amount of emitted photons, analysis of oxygen concentration may be made (Figure 15-39).

Carbon Dioxide Analysis
Fluorescence Quenching

Fluorescence-quenching technology also may be used to measure carbon dioxide. Carbon dioxide is not the quencher of fluorescence; instead it causes a change in pH, liberating hydrogen ions, which react with a quenching agent or a fluorescent dye in the sensor. Fluorescence is altered by the protonation of these chemical components. The measured change in fluorescence is proportional to the concentration of carbon dioxide.

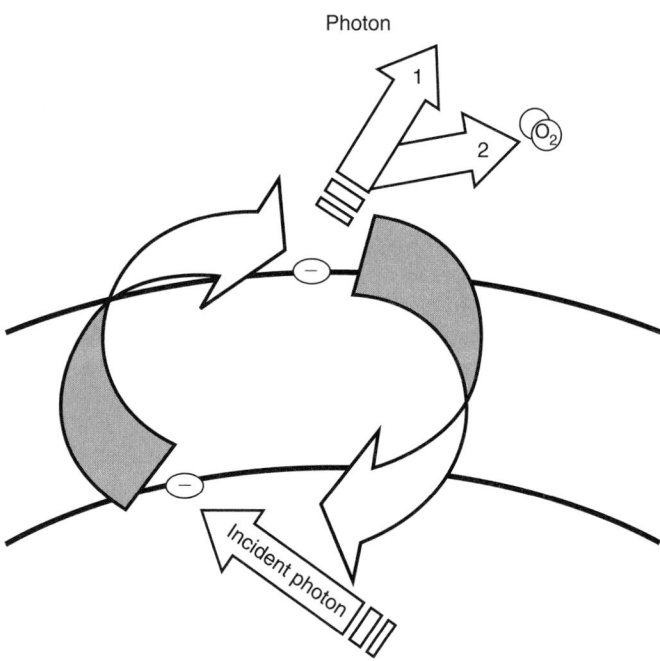

FIGURE **15-39**   Fluorescence-quenching principle. (*1*) Photon release as fluorescence. (*2*) Energy absorption by oxygen, which quenches fluorescence.

Colorimetric CO_2 Sensor

A dry-state sensor that uses a color change in the presence of carbon dioxide is often used to differentiate endotracheal intubation from esophageal intubation. These sensors use the fluorescence principle to indicate carbon dioxide in the gas phase. A paper is impregnated with a fluorescent dye that in the presence of carbon dioxide, will fluoresce or change color. A phase-transport agent facilitates the reaction to give an immediate color change (e.g., purple), indicating carbon dioxide. Colorimetric CO_2 sensors indicate the presence, but not the amount, of carbon dioxide.

Severinghaus P_{CO_2} Electrode

The Severinghaus P_{CO_2} electrode (Figure 15-40) is a frequently used method for analyzing carbon dioxide in anesthesia.[101] It uses a pH sensitive electrode immersed in a bicarbonate solution with a gas-permeable membrane. Carbon dioxide diffuses into the

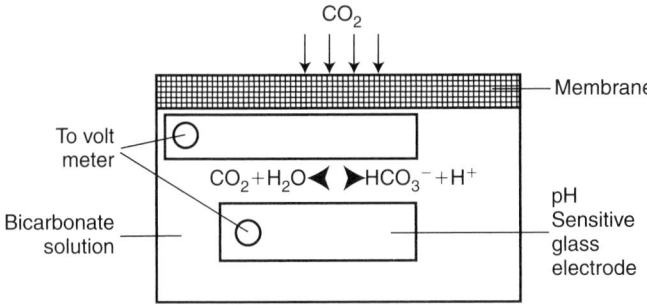

FIGURE **15-40**   Severinghaus Pco$_2$ electrode.

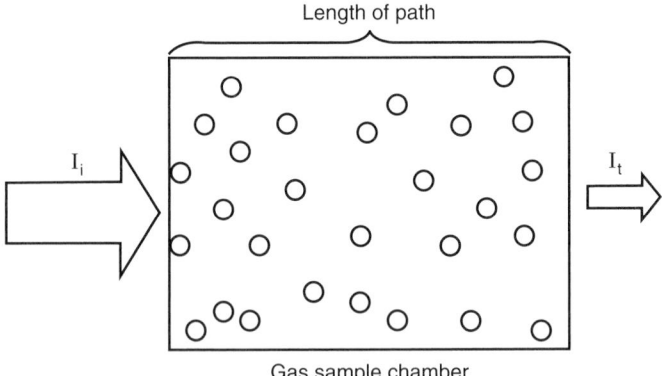

FIGURE **15-41**   Incident light intensity change when transmitted through a medium.

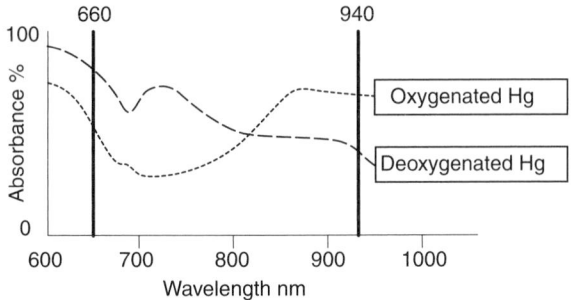

FIGURE **15-42**   Oxygenated hemoglobin and deoxygenated hemoglobin wavelength absorption spectra. The intersection where oxygenated and deoxygenated hemoglobin absorb the same frequency amount is the isobestic point.

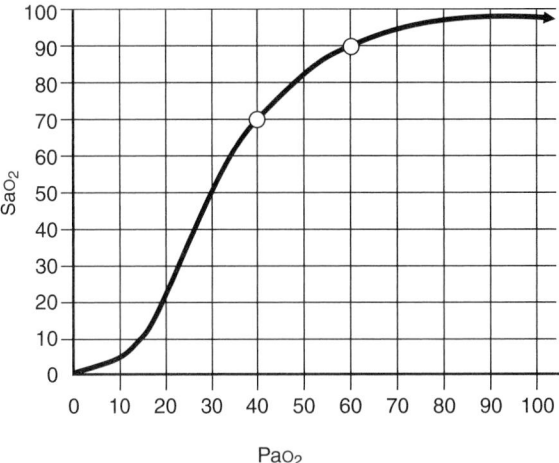

FIGURE **15-43**   Oxyhemoglobin dissociation curve.

frequencies that are absorbed by a pulsatile blood supply, a calculation may be made to determine the percentage of oxygenated and deoxygenated blood in that sample. The algorithm used to make these calculations is derived from the Beer-Lambert law (August Beer, 1825-1863, and Johann Heinrich Lambert, 1728-1777). This law is based primarily on the work of Lambert. Lambert's laws state the following: (1) The luminance of perpendicular light on a surface is proportional to the inverse square of the distance it travels from its source. (2) The luminance intensity of angled light is proportional to the cosine of the angle with the normal. (3) Luminance intensity decreases exponentially as the light travels through a medium. The Beer-Lambert law is:

$$It = Ii \times e^{-DC\alpha}$$

where **It** is the transmitted light, **Ii** is the incident light, $e^{-DC\alpha}$ is the distance through the medium, concentration, and absorption coefficient (Figure 15-41). Pulse oximetry applies the Beer-Lambert law to the absorption of two specific frequencies, infrared and visible red, by hemoglobin. Oxygenated hemoglobin absorbs the infrared frequency that corresponds to a wavelength of 940 nanometers, and deoxygenated hemoglobin absorbs the visible red wavelength of 660 nanometers (Figure 15-42). Analysis of the wavelength that is most absorbed corresponds to that form of hemoglobin. If the wavelength of 940 is absorbed, the hemoglobin present is the oxygenated form. Pulse oximeters display a percentage measurement of saturated hemoglobin. Pulse oximeters measure the amount of absorption of these two specific wavelengths many times a second.

Pulse oximetry is inexpensive, portable, and allows early detection of hemoglobin desaturation.[102-104] Probe placement may be on the digits, ears, nose, or even the forehead to detect a pulsatile arterial blood flow. The oxyhemoglobin saturation curve displays the oxygen saturation (SaO$_2$) relationship to PaO$_2$. Important points along this curve include the SaO$_2$ of 90%, which corresponds to the critically low PaO$_2$ of 60 mm Hg oxygen tension. The SaO$_2$ of 70% corresponds to a PaO$_2$ of 40 mm Hg oxygen tension (Figure 15-43) and is the saturation at which cyanosis becomes apparent.[105] Pulse oximetry is of great value and has become a standard of practice. Both a digital display and an auditory tone alert the nurse anesthetist to the patient's hemoglobin saturation.[106]

Disadvantages of pulse oximetry include the susceptibility of artifact from movement and ambient light sources, the risk of

sensor and is converted into free hydrogen ions, generating a current of electric charge. The current is proportional to CO$_2$ concentration.

PULSE OXIMETRY

Pulse oximetry uses the property of matter that absorbs certain frequencies but not other frequencies of EMR. Oxygenated and deoxygenated hemoglobin are uniquely different molecules and thus interact differently with EMR. By measuring specific

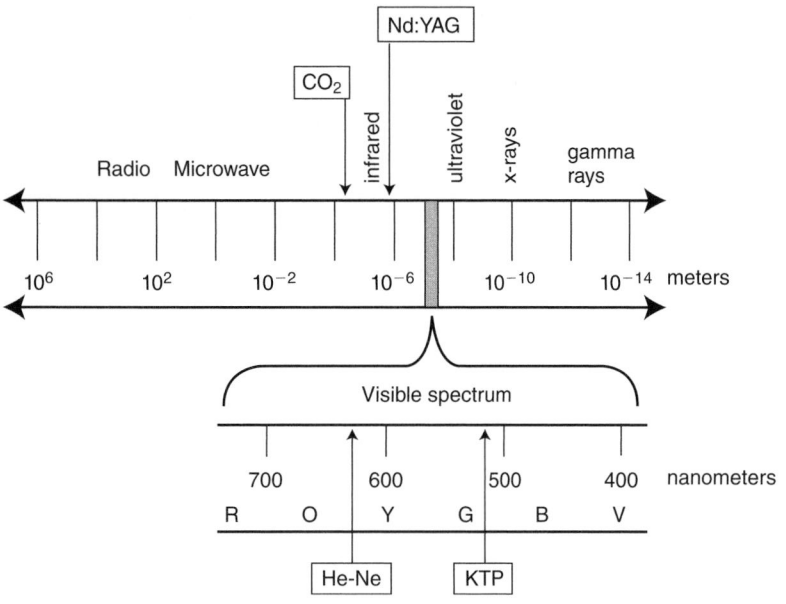

FIGURE **15-44** Common medical laser frequencies. *He-Ne*, Helium neon; *KTP*, potassium titanyl phosphate; *Nd:YAG*, neodymium-doped yttrium aluminum garnet.

TABLE 15-8	Medical Lasers and Uses		
Laser	**Wavelength**	**Tissue Penetration**	**Characteristics/Uses**
Helium neon	633 nm	none	Aiming beam for invisible lasers
CO_2	10,600 nm	<0.5 mm	Highly absorbed by water
			Good for superficial lesions
			Used in airway surgeries
Argon	488 nm	0.5-2.0 mm	Selectively absorbed by hemoglobin
	514 nm		Good for hemangiomas, moles
			Used also in eye and ear surgery
KTP	1060 nm	0.5-2.0 mm	Highly absorbed by hemoglobin
			Multiple uses
YAG lasers	1064-2940 nm	2-6 mm	Variable intensities
			Used to ablate and destroy tissues
			Multiple uses

CO_2, *Carbon dioxide*; KTP, *potassium titanyl phosphate*; YAG, *yttrium aluminum garnet*.

burns in poor perfusion states, and the limitation in detecting pulsatile blood flow in hypothermic or vasoconstricted patients. Additionally, some nail polish pigments interfere with accurate estimates of oxygen saturations. During high F_{IO_2} delivery, ventilation-perfusion abnormalities may be masked. A PaO_2 of 100 mm Hg and a PaO_2 of 500 mm Hg will both give the same pulse oximeter reading of 100%, regardless of the delivered oxygen. Lastly, pulse oximeters do not measure respiratory rate.[107-110]

LASERS

Lasers derive their name from the acronym **L**ight **A**mplification by **S**timulated **E**mission of **R**adiation. Certain atoms that have been energized by an incident photon may move an electron to a higher orbit, but that electron only stays there momentarily, releases a photon, and quickly returns to its resting energy level (see Fluorescence Quenching). This is called *spontaneous emission*. When many incident photons raise many electrons to higher energy levels, the *spontaneous emission* that occurs is chaotic, with photons radiating in multiple directions. However, if many atoms of a particular matter are continually energized by incident photons while their electrons are already in a higher energy state, then photons of the same frequency and direction will be emitted as the electrons are forced down to their natural resting state. This is called *stimulated emission* and is the basis of laser function. Continual energizing of certain atoms forces photons of the same frequency (monochromatic) and direction to be emitted in unison. Population inversion is the condition in which the majority of electrons in an atom are in the higher energy level rather than their natural resting state. The natural balance of resting electrons to energized electrons has been inverted. Population inversion is required to allow continual production of monochromatic, coherent, and unidirectional photons used in lasers. The intensity of lasers and the ability to direct the beam have many applications in medicine and present unique considerations for nurse anesthetists (Figure 15-44 and Table 15-8).

Laser Risks

Lasers have the ability to burn and ignite fires. The patient should have his or her eyes shielded with saline pads and laser goggles. Operating room personnel also should wear appropriate eye protection when lasers are in use.[111] The risk of fire is ever present with lasers. Three components are needed to produce a fire: fuel, oxygen, and an ignition source. Lasers are a potent ignition source. The nurse anesthetist should be aware of this risk during laser surgeries and be prepared to take rapid action. Drapes, dressings, and linens are a few of the combustible materials that may ignite during surgery.[112] Lasers should never be kept active when not in use. Lasers are often used for otorhinolaryngologic surgeries. Endotracheal tube fires can occur during these cases. Low inspired oxygen concentrations and nonflammable or shielded endotracheal tubes should be used.[113] Some authors recommend placing saline with methylene dye in the endotracheal tube cuff to dissipate heat and signal cuff rupture.[114] A source of saline to extinguish a potential fire should be immediately available. If an airway fire occurs, stop oxygen flow, stop ventilation, extubate the patient, extinguish the fire, mask ventilate, and reintubate the patient.[115] The patient will require airway assessment and medical treatment, including bronchoscopy, lavage, and steroids.

SUMMARY

The historical view of the universe as a machine following fixed specific rules often allowed for unequivocal laws to be discovered. For a time, the actions of the universe seemed destined to be unlocked and forever understood. Unfortunately or fortunately, this is not the case. The mechanistic view of the universe in Newtonian physics loses its ability to describe certain phenomena, and this underscores a significant limitation. Advances in our knowledge of quantum events may shed light on phenomena that remain elusive.[116]

Quantum physics has brought us new insight into the subatomic world and uncovered the limitations of classical physics in fully describing the actions and reactions of the universe. What Newtonian physics has done for the physical world, quantum physics holds for the nonphysical world, the world of pure energy and the quasi-world of energy/mass transition. Events in the quantum world are not determined by fixed, describable outcomes. Quantum events are described by probabilities. Phenomena that remain only partially understood in anesthesia may be clarified by discoveries in quantum study. Consciousness, awareness, and minimum alveolar concentrations (MACs) all are described in anesthesia as probabilities. Consciousness and awareness are not "on-off" phenomena. Delivery of anesthetics is sometimes measured not in fixed set doses but rather in ranges, MACs that provide a guideline of probability for a desired outcome. Though controversial, some have suggested that consciousness is a quantum event with understanding to be found in the study of quantum mechanics.[117-120] Newtonian physics and physical chemistry will remain valued sciences that well describe many processes in the field of anesthesia, but quantum study may someday bring new advances and applications to anesthesia. Safer, more effective anesthesia techniques and technologies may evolve out of quantum understanding, or the mere search itself may stimulate new developments. Regardless, the future is exciting. Chemistry and physics have and will continue to provide a conceptual and analytical framework from which we can derive understanding, establish clinical rationales, and direct the practice of safe and effective anesthetic management of patients under our care.

The author acknowledges and appreciates the University of North Florida Nurse Anesthetist Class of 2008 for assistance with referencing this chapter.

REFERENCES

1. van Melsen AG. From Atmos to Atom. The History of the Concept Atom. 1960. New York: Dover; 2004.
2. Trudell JR, Bertaccini E. Molecular modeling of specific and non-specific anaesthetic interactions. Br J Anaesth. 2002;89(1):32-40.
3. Gutierrez G. Sepsis, cellular energy metabolism, and tissue adenosine triphosphate concentration [editorial]. Crit Care Med. 2000;28(7):2664.
4. Zhou JX, Lui J. The effect of temperature on solubility of volatile anesthetics in human tissues. Anesth Analg. 2001;93:234-238.
5. Coburn CM, Eger EI II. The partial pressure of isoflurane or halothane does not affect their solubility in rabbit blood or brain or human brain: inhaled anesthetics do obey Henry's law. Anesth Analg. 1986;65:960-962.
6. Mezzasalama SA. The special theory of Brownian relativity: equivalence principle for dynamic and static random paths and uncertainty relation for diffusion. J Colloid Interface Sci. 2007;307(2):386-397. doi:10.1016./j.jcis.2006.11.042.
7. Cabrales P et al. Increased plasma viscosity sustains microcirculation after resuscitation from hemorrhagic shock and massive bleeding. Shock. 2005;23(6):549-555.
8. Persson J, Grande PO. Volume expansion of albumin, gelatin, hydroxyethyl starch, saline and erythrocytes after haemorrhage in the rat. Intensive Care Med. 2004;31(2):1432-1438.
9. Kaur S et al. Diffusion of nitrous oxide into the pleural cavity. Br J Anaesth. 2001;87(6):894-896.
10. Combes X et al. Intracuff pressure and tracheal morbidity: influence of filling cuff with saline during nitrous oxide anesthesia. Anesthesiology. 2001;95(5):1120-1124.
11. Atlas GM. A mathematical model of differential tracheal tube cuff pressure: effects of diffusion and temperature. J Clin Monit. 2005;19(6):415-425.
12. Akca O et al. Nitrous oxide increases the incidence of bowel distension in patients undergoing elective colon resection. Acta Anaesthesiol Scand. 2004;48(7):894-898.
13. Reinelt H et al. Diffusion of xenon and nitrous oxide into the bowel during mechanical ileus. Anesthesiology. 2002;96(2):512-513.
14. Frumen MJ et al. Apneic oxygenation in man. Anesthesiology. 1959;20:789-798.
15. Wu CC et al. Application of the mixed venous blood concentration equation in desflurane anesthesia. Acta Anaesthesiol Scand. 2006;50:536-541.
16. Ho WM et al. A real-time method for estimating the concentration of isoflurane in mixed venous blood by a derived Fick's equation. Anesth Analg. 2005;100:38-45.
17. Cheney FW. An early example of evidence-based medicine. Hypoxia due to nitrous oxide. Anesthesiology. 2007;106:186-188.
18. Pfister H. How about a magnet and a paper clip. Experiencing the interaction forces kinesthetically. The Physics Teacher. 2005;43:95-97.
19. Hoskote A et al. The effect of carbon dioxide on oxygenation and systemic, cerebral, and pulmonary vascular hemodynamics after the bidirectional superior cavopulmonary anastamosis. J Am Coll Cardiol. 2004;44(7):1501-1509. doi:10-1016/j.jacc.2004.06.061.
20. Ouzounian JG et al. Systemic vascular resistance index determined by thoracic electrical bioimpedance predicts the risk for maternal hypotension during regional anesthesia for cesarean section. Am J Obstet Gynecol. 1996;174(3):1019-1025.
21. Viby-Mogenson J. Measurement of acceleration: a new method of monitoring neuromuscular function. Acta Anaesthesiol Scand. 1988;32:450-458.
22. Eikerman M et al. Accelerometry of adductor pollicis muscle predicts recovery of respiratory function from neuromuscular blockade. Anesthesiology. 2003;98:1333-1337.
23. Ferreira TA et al. Fentanyl or remifentanil to potentiate a single dose of rocuronium in patients anesthetized with propofol with evaluation by accelerometry. Rev Esp Anestesiol Reanim. 2004;51(4):190-194.
24. Capron F et al. Tactile fade detection with hand or wrist stimulation using train-of-four, double-burst stimulation, 50-hertz tetanus, 100-hertz tetanus, and acceleromyography. Anesth Analg. 2006;102:1578-1584.

25. Kopman AF, Sinha N. Acceleromyography as a guide to anesthetic management: a case report. *J Clin Anesth.* 2003;15:145-148.
26. Lord LM. Restoring and maintaining patency of enteral feeding tubes. *Nutr Clin Pract.* 2003;18:422-426.
27. Mateo MA. Maintaining the patency of enteral feeding tubes. *Worldviews Evid Based Nurs.* 1993;1(1):72-78.
28. Reising DL, Neal RS. Enteral tube flushing: what you think are the best practices may not be. *Am J Nurs.* 2005;105(3):58-63.
29. Staessen JA et al. Modern approaches to blood pressure measurement. *Occup Environ Med.* 2000;57:510-520.
30. Von Montfrans GA. Oscillometric blood pressure measurement: Progress and problems. *Blood Press Monit.* 2001;6(6):287-290.
31. Dickson R et al. Thermodynamics of anesthetic/protein interactions temperature studies on firefly luciferase. *Biophys J.* 1993;1264-1271.
32. Sleigh JW et al. Cortical entropy changes with general anaesthesia: theory and experiment. *Physiol Meas.* 2004;25(4):921-934. doi:10.1088/0967-3334/25/4/011.
33. Steyn-Ross ML et al. Toward a theory of the general-anesthetic-induced phase transition of the cerebral cortex. I. A thermodynamics analogy. *Phys Rev E Stat Nonlin Soft Matter Phys.* 2001;64(1 Pt 1):011917. Epub 2001 Jul 27.
34. Brown LK. Entropy isn't what it used to be: applying thermodynamics to respiration in sleep. *Chest.* 2003;123:9-12.
35. Heimberg T, Jackson AD. The thermodynamics of general anesthesia. *Biophys J.* 2007;92(9):3159-3165. Epub 2007 Feb 9.
36. Arkilic CF et al. Temperature monitoring and management during neuraxial anesthesia: an observational study. *Anesth Analg.* 2000;91:662-666.
37. Matsukawa T et al. Heat flow and distribution during induction of general anesthesia. *Anesthesiology.* 1995;82(3):662-673.
38. Matsukawa T et al. Heat flow and distribution during epidural anesthesia. *Anesthesiology.* 1995;83(5):961-967.
39. Macario A, Dexter F. What are the most important risk factors for a patient's developing intraoperative hypothermia? *Anesth Analg.* 2002;94:215-220.
40. Winkler M et al. Aggressive warming reduces blood loss during hip arthroplasty. *Anesth Analg.* 2000;91:978-984.
41. Buggy DJ, Crossley AWA. Thermoregulation, mild perioperative hypothermia and post anaesthetic shivering. *Br J Anaesth.* 2000;84(5):615-628.
42. Negishi C et al. Resistive-heating and forced-air warming are comparably effective. *Anesth Analg.* 2003;96:1683-1687.
43. Ng SF et al. A comparative study of three warming interventions to determine the most effective in maintaining perioperative normothermia. *Anesth Analg.* 2003;96:171-176.
44. Bräuer A et al. Efficacy of forced-air warming systems with full body blankets. *Can J Anesth.* 2007;54:34-41.
45. Sessler DI. Perioperative heat balance. *Anesthesiology.* 2000;92(2):578.
46. Nilsson AL. Blood flow, temperature, and heat loss of skin exposed to local radiative and convective cooling. *J Invest Dermatol.* 1987;88(5):586-593.
47. Bush HL et al. Hypothermia during elective abdominal aortic aneurysm repair: the high price of avoidable morbidity. *J Vasc Surg.* 1995;21(3):392-400.
48. Insler SR et al. Association between postoperative hypothermia and adverse outcomes after coronary artery bypass surgery. *Ann Thorac Surg.* 2000;70:175-181.
49. Sessler DI. Complications and treatment of mild hypothermia. *Anesthesiology.* 2001;95(2):531-543.
50. Vanni S. Preoperative combined with intraoperative skin-surface warming avoids hypothermia caused by general anesthesia and surgery. *J Clin Anesth.* 2003;15(2):119-125.
51. Dosch MP. Anesthesia equipment. In: Nagelhout J, Zaglaniczny K, eds. *Nurse Anesthesia.* 3rd ed. St. Louis: Saunders; 2005:275.
52. Block F Jr, Schulte T. Observations of use of wrong agent in an anesthesia agent vaporizer. *J Clin Monit Comput.* 1999;15:57.
53. Boytim M. Chemistry and physics. In: Nagelhout J, Zaglaniczny K, eds. *Nurse Anesthesia.* 3rd ed. St Louis: Saunders; 2005:247-257.
54. Linck SL. Use of heliox for intraoperative bronchospasm: a case report. *AANA J.* 2007;75(3):189-192.
55. Mestitz H et al. Comparison of outpatient nebulized vs. metered dose inhaler terbutaline in chronic airflow obstruction. *Chest.* 1989;96:1237-1240.
56. Bossart PJ, Wolfe T. Venturi atomizers as potential sources of patient cross-infection. *Am J Infect Control.* 2003;31:441-444.
57. Patel A. The shared airway. *Curr Anesth Crit Care.* 2001;12(4):213-217.
58. Ihra A. On the use of Venturi's principle to describe entrainment during jet ventilation. *J Clin Anesth.* 2000;12(5):417-419.
59. Unzueta M et al. Endobronchial high frequency jet ventilation for endobronchial laser surgery: an alternative approach. *Anesth Analg.* 2003;96:298-300.
60. Hess DR. Nebulizers: principles and performance. *Respir Care.* 2000;45(6):609-622.
61. Chiang TP et al. Side wall effects on the structure of laminar flow over a plane-symmetric sudden expansion. *Computers & Fluids.* 2000;9:467-492.
62. Goubergrits L et al. Geometry of the human common carotid artery. A vessel cast study of 86 specimens. *Pathol Res Pract.* 2002;198(8):543-551.
63. Albert AA et al. Is there any impact of the shape of aortic end-hole cannula on stroke occurrence? Clinical evaluation of straight and bent-tip aortic cannulae. *Perfusion.* 2002;17:451-456.
64. Ussia GP et al. Images in cardiovascular medicine. Late device dislodgement after percutaneous closure of mitral prosthesis paravalvular leak with Amplatzer muscular ventricular septal defect occluder. *Circulation.* 2007;115(8):e208-210.
65. Slam KD et al. LaPlace's law revisited: cecal perforation as an unusual presentation of pancreatic carcinoma. *World J Surg Oncol.* 2007;5:14.
66. Wooley JG et al. Lethal aortic dissection in a 33-week parturient: a case report. *AANA J.* 2006;74(6):440-443.
67. Mayberg MR et al. Guidelines for the management of aneurismal subarachnoid hemorrhage: a statement for healthcare professionals from a special writing group of the Stroke Council, American Heart Association. *Circulation.* 1994;90:2592-2605.
68. Zuo YY, Possmayer F. How does pulmonary surfactant reduce surface tension to very low values? *J Appl Physiol.* 2007;102(5):1733-1734. Epub 2007 Feb 15.
69. Aponte H et al. The use of ultrasound for placement of intravenous catheters. *AANA J.* 2007;75(3):212-216.
70. Hopkins PM. Ultrasound guidance as gold standard in regional anesthesia [editorial]. *Br J Anaesth.* 2007;98(3):299-301.
71. Marhofer P, Frickey N. Ultrasonographic guidance in pediatric regional anesthesia part 1: theoretical background [electronic version]. *Pediatr Anesth.* 2006;16:1008-1018.
72. Mendelsohn AH et al. Strobokymographic and videostroboscopic analysis of vocal fold motion in unilateral superior laryngeal nerve paralysis. *Ann Otol Rhinol Laryngol.* 2007;116(2):85-91.
73. Willschke H et al. Epidural catheter placement in neonates: sonoanatomy and feasibility of ultrasonographic guidance in term and preterm neonates. *Reg Anesth Pain Med.* 2007;32(1):34-40.
74. Hoyle CD et al. Submillimeter test of the gravitational inverse-square law: a search for "large" extra dimensions. *Phys Rev Lett.* 2001;86:1418-1421.
75. Kanal E et al. American College of Radiology white paper on MR safety. *Am J Radiol.* 2002;178:1335-1347.
76. Shellock FG. Magnetic resonance safety update 2002: Implants and devices. *J Magn Reson Imaging.* 2002;16(5):485-496.
77. Gimbel JR et al. Safe performance of magnetic resonance imaging on five patients with permanent cardiac pacemakers. *Pacing Clin Electrophysiol.* 1996;19(6):913-919.
78. Yeung CJ et al. RF safety or wires in interventional MRI: using a safety index. *Magn Reson Med.* 2001;47(1):187-193.
79. Buczko GB, McKay WPS. Electrical safety in the operating room. *Can J Anaesth.* 1987;34(3):315-322.
80. Swerdlow CD et al. Cardiovascular collapse caused by electrocardiographically silent 60-Hz intracardiac leakage current: implications for electrical safety. *Circulation.* 1999;99:2559-2564.
81. Roy OZ. Summary of cardiac fibrillation thresholds for 60 Hz currents and voltages applied directly to the heart. *Med Biol Eng Comput.* 1980;18(5):657-659.
82. Johnston MJ. Isolated power systems [electronic version]. *IAEI.* Nov-Dec 2002. Available at: http://magazine.iaei.org/magazine/02_f/johnston.htm. Accessed July 2, 2007.
83. Bales JG et al. Electrocautery-induced asystole in a scoliosis patient with a pacemaker. *J Pediatr Orthop.* 2007;16(1):19-22.
84. Wong D. Electrocautery-induced tachycardia in a rate-responsive pacemaker. *Anesthesiology.* 2001;94(4):710-711.
85. Rozner M, Nishman R. Electrocautery-induced pacemaker tachycardia: Why does this error continue? [correspondence]. *Anesthesiology.* 2002;96(3):773-774.
86. Michelson AA, Morley EW. On the relative motion of Earth and the luminiferous ether. *Am J Sci.* 1887;34:333.
87. Shankland RS. Michelson-Morley experiment. *Am J Phys.* 1964;32(1):16-35.
88. Planck M. On the law of distribution of energy in the normal spectrum. *Ann Physik.* 1901;4:553-563.
89. Einstein A. On a heuristic viewpoint concerning the production and transformation of light. *Ann Physik.* 1905;17:132-148.
90. Clark RW. *Einstein: The Life and Times.* New York: Harper Collins; 1984.
91. Diner S et al. *The Wave-Particle Dualism: A Tribute to Louis de Broglie on His 90th Birthday.* New York: Springer; 1984.
92. Wagner LK et al. Potential biological effects following high x-ray dose interventional procedures. *J Vasc Interv Radiol.* 1994;5(1):71-84.

93. Tasbas BA et al. Which one is at risk in intraoperative fluoroscopy? Assistant surgeon or orthopaedic surgeon? *Arch Orthop Trauma Surg.* 2003;123(5): 1434-3916.

94. Westenskow DR et al. Clinical evaluation of a Raman scattering multiple gas analyzer for the operating room. *Anesthesiology.* 1989;70(2):350-355.

95. Kumar A. Biosensors based on piezoelectric crystal detectors: theory and application. *JOM-e.* 52(10);2000. Available at: http://www.tms.org/pubs/journals/JOM/0010/Kumar/Kumar-0010.html. Accessed May 6, 2007.

96. Westenkow DR, Silva FH. Laboratory evaluation of the vital signs (ICOR) piezoelectric anesthetic agent analyzer. *J Clin Monit.* 1991; 7(2):189-194.

97. Hayes JK et al. Monitoring anesthetic vapor concentrations using a piezoelectric detector: evaluation of the Engstrom EMMA. *Anesthesiology.* 1983;59(5):435-439.

98. Mohiuddin S, Block FE. What really happens when the wrong agent is poured into a modern vaporizer? *ASA Abstract A568.* Available at: www.asaabstracts.com/strands/asaabstracts/abstractList.htm?year=2000&index=7. Accessed May 6, 2007.

99. Walder B et al. Accuracy and cross-sensitivity of 10 different anesthetic gas monitors. *J Clin Monit.* 1993;9(5):364-373.

100. Shaw AD et al. Assessment of tissue oxygenation tension: comparison of dynamic fluorescence quenching and polarographic electrode technique. *Crit Care.* 2001;6(1):76-80.

101. Severinghaus JW. The invention and development of blood gas analysis apparatus. *Anesthesiology.* 2002;97(1):253-256.

102. Bohnhorst B et al. Pulse oximeters' reliability in detecting hypoxemia and bradycardia: comparison between a conventional and two new generation oximeters. *Crit Care Med.* 2000;28(5):1565-1568.

103. Sequin P et al. Evidence for the need of bedside accuracy of pulse oximetry in an intensive care unit. *Crit Care Med.* 2000;28(3):703-706.

104. Witting MD et al. The sensitivity of room-air pulse oximetry in the detection of hypercapnia. *Am J Emerg Med.* 2005;23:497-500.

105. Jubran A. Pulse oximetry. *Intensive Care Med.* 2004;30(11):2017-2020.

106. Giuliano KK, Liu LM. Knowledge of pulse oximetry among critical care nurses. *Dimens Crit Care Nurs.* 2006;25(1):44-49.

107. Barker SJ. "Motion-resistant" pulse oximetry: a comparison of new and old models. *Anesth Analg.* 2002;95:967-972.

108. Leonard P et al. Standard pulse oximeters can be used to monitor respiratory rate. *Emerg Med J.* 2003;20:524-525.

109. Rodden AM et al. Does fingernail polish affect pulse oximeter readings? *Intensive Crit Care Nurs.* 2007;23:51-55.

110. Netzer N et al. Overnight pulse oximetry for sleep-disordered breathing in adults. A review. *Chest.* 2001;120:625-633.

111. Anderson K. Safe use of lasers in the operating room: what perioperative nurses should know. *AORN J.* 2004;79:171-188.

112. Goldberg J. Brief laboratory report: surgical drape flammability. *AANA J.* 2006;75(5):352-354.

113. Barnes AM, Frantz RA. Do oxygen-enriched atmospheres exist beneath surgical drapes and contribute to fire hazard potential in the operating room? *AANA J.* 2000;68(2):153-161.

114. Morgan EG, Mikhail MS. *Clinical Anesthesiology.* 3rd ed. New York: McGraw-Hill; 2002.

115. Santos P et al. Airway ignition during CO_2 laser laryngeal surgery and high frequency jet ventilation. *Eur J Anaesthesiol.* 2000;17:204-207.

116. Hammeroff SR. The entwined mysteries of anesthesia and consciousness: is there a common underlying mechanism? *Anesthesiology.* 2006;105(2):400-412.

117. Hu H, Wu M. Spin-mediated consciousness theory: possible roles of neural membrane nuclear spin ensembles and paramagnetic oxygen. *Med Hypotheses.* 2004;63:633-646.

118. Woolfe NJ, Hameroff SR. A quantum approach to visual consciousness. *Trends Cogn Sci.* 2001;5(11):472-478.

119. Seife C. Cold numbers unmake the quantum mind. *Science.* 2004; 28(5454):791.

120. Hameroff S. Anesthesia, consciousness and hydrophobic pockets: a unitarian quantum hypothesis of anesthetic action. *Toxicol Lett.* 1998;100-101:31-39.

ANESTHESIA EQUIPMENT

Michael P. Dosch

"To a large extent, anesthesia machines are *inherently dangerous*. A machine that has the power to induce anesthesia necessarily has the power to cause death and serious injury. An anesthesia department may want to institute periodic training to make sure that everyone in the department is familiar with *all* of the machines in the hospital."[1] It would disturb any of us to read in the news about an adult without driver's training who attempted to drive a car and caused injury or death as a result. Shouldn't it be equally disturbing to learn that only a minority of anesthetists report that they check their gas machines before use?[2,3] Because anesthesia equipment malfunction is so rare, misuse and human error are much more of a threat to patient safety than outright malfunction.[4-7] However, when errors in the use of gas delivery equipment occur, the outcome is often mortality or serious morbidity.[4] Human error can be most effectively combated by a strong individual, department, and industry commitment (in the words of the mission of the Anesthesia Patient Safety Foundation) "to ensure that no patient is harmed by anesthesia."[8] The means of accomplishing this goal is primarily educational. We anesthetize patients with many different kinds of problems, for many different kinds of surgical and diagnostic procedures. But there is one thing that is present in every anesthetic: the anesthesia gas machine. It is the purpose of this chapter to provide timely, accurate, and patient-safety-focused information about this important and ubiquitous patient-safety technology.

As the previous generation of equipment passes out of use (Excel, Modulus, Narkomed 3), it is deemphasized in this edition to allow more focus on current anesthesia equipment systems. Additions to this chapter include the current status of the pre-use checklist for the anesthesia gas machine; protocols for troubleshooting (high and low pressure in the breathing circuit, oxygen pipeline failure); new modes of ventilation such as pressure support; carbon dioxide absorbent hazards; and the equipment implications of malignant hyperthermia. Differences between gas machines are presented here if understanding these differences is important to using the machine safely. Brief descriptions of new gas machines are presented (Aestiva, Aespire, Avance, Aisys, and ADU [GE Healthcare, Madison, Wisconsin]; Fabius GS, Narkomed 6000, and Apollo [Dräger Medical, Telford, Pennsylvania]; Anestar [Datascope, Mahwah, New Jersey]).

A major objective of this chapter is that readers will gain skill and safety in the use of the anesthesia gas machine. Therefore throughout the chapter, explicit directions on how to use the machine safely are presented; these directions are based on manufacturers' guidelines and on reports of pitfalls from the anesthesia literature. Because of the variety of machines currently in use, no direction in this chapter can be considered universally applicable. The directions given here must be adapted to individual practice settings only after study of the operator's manuals and appropriate local peer review.

Several factors make learning about gas machines difficult. Each model has unique aspects—even those from the same manufacturer. It is not always possible for the anesthetist to be available when department in-service education is conducted. Also, continuing education content may be too limited, or an opportunity to use new equipment soon after an educational session may not be available. Various pieces of new equipment are introduced frequently in the anesthesia work area. Although anesthesia equipment is designed to meet all legal and technical requirements, the designers of the equipment are not users. Some designs may be recognized as flawed only when the devices are used clinically. Instructional materials accompanying equipment often are inadequate. For example, no matter how well written, supplying one instruction manual per *machine* is inferior to supplying one instruction manual per *user*. The potential lack in equipment competency can be a safety problem.[9-11] Users may be legally obligated to know and follow manufacturers' instructions (operating manuals) and warnings, because these may contribute to the standard of care. Some courts have defined deviation from manufacturers' instructions as *prima facie* negligence.[12]

To make learning the content easier, this chapter views the machine from a systems approach. For example, all machines have systems to provide (and measure) gas composition, including life-sustaining gases (oxygen), anesthetizing gases, and metabolic by-products (carbon dioxide). When this capability of every gas machine is understood, one need only determine how a particular machine accomplishes this and how this function is checked before use to operate the machine safely (in this respect). Once all the systems—and their interplay—are understood, learning new equipment is easier. High-fidelity patient simulation is a novel approach that holds promise for both learning anesthesia equipment more efficiently and studying gas-machine hazards. Simulation has been used in several studies recently, which have allowed exploration of questions that could not be studied in the past because of risks to patients.[13,14]

ORGANIZATION OF THE ANESTHESIA GAS MACHINE

Presenting the anesthesia gas machine as a litany of components does not promote retention, much less aid in the development

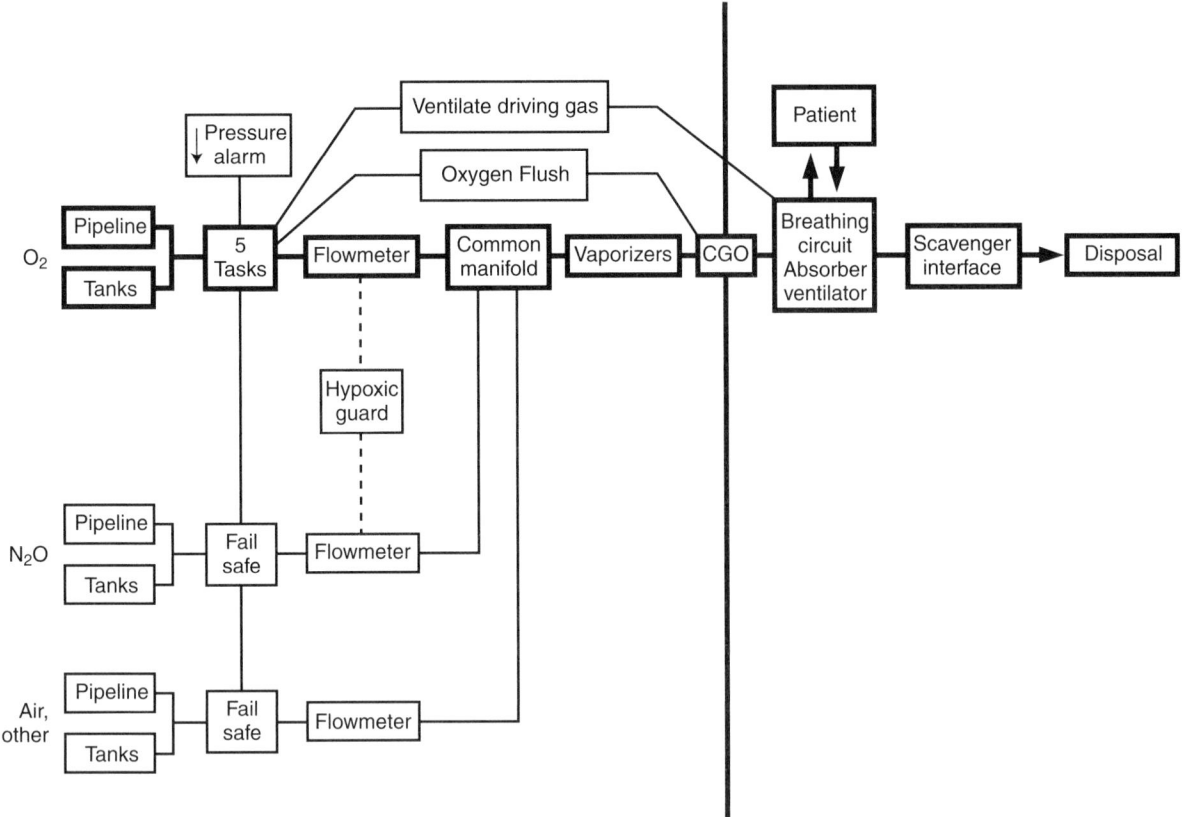

FIGURE **16-1** Supply, processing, delivery, and disposal (SPDD) model. CGO, Common gas outlet. (*Courtesy of Michael P. Dosch.*)

of a solid concept of the overall organization of the machine. An accurate concept of the overall organization should help one to understand the role of the individual components better, which should in turn promote correct use and thus patient safety. This section presents the *supply, processing, delivery, and disposal (SPDD) model.*

Supply, Processing, Delivery, and Disposal Model

The SPDD model is depicted in Figure 16-1 and Box 16-1. This model is comprehensive in that the path of gases can be followed from their arrival in the operating room to their disposal from it. Most anesthesia gas-machine components can be located easily within the overall scheme. Gas flows in the diagram proceed generally from left to right. The vertical bar separates components within the machine and proximal to the common gas outlet (left side), from external components downstream from the common gas outlet (right). The fact that nitrous oxide and air, unlike oxygen, have only one task in the machine is easy to appreciate. The five tasks of oxygen are easy to follow. Understanding the similarities and differences between the fail-safe and hypoxic guard systems is facilitated. The model makes clear that the scavenging system, rather than the patient, is the ultimate destination of gases. Oxygen is central to the figure, because it is the most essential gas delivered. The reader should note that not every component of the SPDD model in Box 16-1 is depicted graphically in Figure 16-1. The reader should make frequent reference to the model while reading this chapter.

The model organizes the information on the basis of how components are used, rather than on the pressures to which they are exposed. From the viewpoint of pressure that components are exposed to, components are classified as part of the high-, intermediate-, or low-pressure systems within (proximal to the common gas outlet) the gas machine (Box 16-2).

Introduction of new gas machines raises questions about the adequacy and safety of older equipment.[1,15] One can begin the determination of whether current equipment is obsolete by considering how closely it matches current safety standards.[16] Certain systems or components are required by the anesthesia workstation standard, which is a voluntary industry-group consensus standard (Box 16-3).

SUPPLY

The concept of supply is concerned with these questions. How do gases (and electrical power) come to the anesthesia gas machine? What are the likely faults and hazards?

Pipeline Supply

Configuration

Oxygen is produced by the fractional distillation of liquid air. It is delivered to facilities and stored as a liquid at a temperature of 184° C.[17] Various components convert the liquid oxygen to a gas and supply it to hospital pipelines at a pressure of 50 psi (344 kPa). In the operating room suite, main and partial-area shutoff valves are present to isolate sections with leaks, interrupt supply in case of fire, and allow repair work on subsections.

BOX 16-1

Components in Supply, Processing, Delivery, and Disposal (SPDD) Model

Supply
How do gases come to the anesthesia gas machine?
(Site: back of the machine)
Pipeline
Wall outlets
Connecting valves and hoses
Filters and check valves
Pressure gauges
Cylinders
Hanger yokes (yoke block)
Filters and check valves
Pressure gauge
Pressure regulators

Processing
How does the anesthesia gas machine prepare gases
before their delivery to the patient? (Site: within the
machine, proximal to common gas outlet)
Fail-safe (oxygen pressure-failure devices)
Flowmeters (main, auxiliary, common gas outlet, scavenging)
Oxygen flush
Low oxygen pressure alarms
Ventilator-driving gas
Proportioning systems (hypoxic guard)
Oxygen second-stage regulator (if present)
Vaporizers
Check valves distal to vaporizers (if present)
Common gas outlet

Delivery
How is the interaction of gases with the patient
controlled and monitored? (Site: breathing circuit)
Gas delivery hose connecting common gas outlet and
  breathing circuit
Breathing circuits
Nonrebreathing
Circle
Carbon dioxide absorption
Ventilators
Integral monitors
Oxygen analysis
Disconnect
Spirometry (volumes and flows), capnography, airway
  pressure
Ventilator alarms
Addition of positive end-expiratory pressure
Means of humidification

Disposal
How are gases disposed of? (Site: scavenger)
Scavenger systems
Interface—closed (active and passive) or open
Scavenger flowmeter

Wall outlets or hoses dropped from the operating room ceiling are finished with quick-connect couplers. These couplers are used so that the connection of gas-machine supply hoses to wall outlets does not require tools. However, the springs and rubber gaskets (O-rings) these couplers contain provide a connection that is less secure than a wrench-tightened connection; thus they are a common source of leaks.[18-20]

Systems processing nitrous oxide are similar in many respects. Nitrous oxide is delivered to the hospital in large (size H) cylinders, which are connected to a manifold. Regulators reduce the pressure so that nitrous oxide, like oxygen, is supplied to the pipelines at 50 psi.[17] Consequently, this is the normal working pressure of the anesthesia gas machine. Shutoff valves and wall outlets with quick-connect couplers are similar for nitrous oxide and oxygen. Delivery piping for both nitrous oxide and oxygen uses the diameter index safety system (DISS) to prevent misconnections. In this system, gas-piping connections are sized and threaded differently so that cross-connection is difficult, though not impossible (Figure 16-2).[18]

Supply hoses connect the pipeline inlets on the back of the machine to the wall outlets. At the pipeline inlet, a filter, check valve, and pressure gauge are present. The check valve ensures unidirectional flow so that a machine running on cylinder supplies, with the hoses disconnected at the wall outlet, does not leak (Figure 16-3). The filter is required by the current anesthesia workstation standard (ASTM-F1850) because it may help

BOX 16-2

Components in the High-, Intermediate-, and Low-Pressure Pneumatic Systems

High-Pressure System (Exposed to Cylinder Pressure)
Hanger yoke
Yoke block with check valves
Cylinder pressure gauge
Cylinder pressure regulators

Intermediate-Pressure System (Exposed to Pipeline Pressure—About 50 psi)
Pipeline inlets, check valves, and pressure gauges
Ventilator power inlet
Oxygen pressure-failure devices
Flowmeter valve
Oxygen second-stage regulator (if present)
Flush valve

Low-Pressure System (Distal to Flowmeter Needle Valve)
Flowmeter tubes
Vaporizers
Check valves (if present)
Common gas outlet

BOX **16-3**

Required Components of an Anesthesia Workstation

The current anesthesia gas machine (workstation) standard is **ASTM F1850** (a standard promulgated by the American Society for Testing and Materials. *Standard Specification for Particular Requirements for Anesthesia Workstations and Their Components [F1850-00].* Philadelphia; 2005). The comparable European standard is EN740. F1850 specifies what is needed for an anesthesia workstation. The components are typically built into new gas machines, or they may be added to older machines. Required components include:

Battery backup for 30 minutes
Alarms
- Grouped into high, medium, and low priority.
- High-priority alarms may not be silenced for more than 2 minutes.
- Certain alarms and monitors must be automatically enabled and functioning prior to use, either through turning the machine on or by following the pre-use checklist: breathing circuit pressure, oxygen concentration, exhaled volume or carbon dioxide (or both).
- A high-priority pressure alarm must sound if user-adjustable limits are exceeded, if continuing high pressure is sensed, or for negative pressure.
- Disconnect alarms may be based on low pressure, exhaled volume, or carbon dioxide.

Required monitors
- Exhaled volume
- Inspired oxygen, with a high-priority alarm within 30 seconds of oxygen falling below 18% (or a user-adjustable limit)
- Oxygen supply failure alarm
- A hypoxic guard system must protect against less than 21% inspired oxygen if nitrous oxide is in use.
- Anesthetic vapor concentration must be monitored.
- Pulse oximetry, blood pressure monitoring, and ECG are required.

Pressure in the breathing circuit is limited to 12.5 kPa (125 cm water).
The electrical supply cord must be nondetachable or resistant to detachment.

Cylinder supplies
- The machine must have at least one oxygen cylinder attached.
- The hanger yoke must be pin-indexed, have a clamping device that resists leaks, and contain a filter. It must have a check valve to prevent transfilling and a cylinder pressure gauge.
- There must be cylinder pressure regulators. The machine must use pipeline gas as long as pipeline pressure is greater than 345 kPa (50 psi).

Flowmeters:
- Single control for each gas
- Each flow control next to a flow indicator
- Uniquely shaped oxygen flow control knob
- Valve stops (or some other mechanism) are required such that excessive rotation will not damage the flowmeter.
- Oxygen flow indicator is to the right side of a flowmeter bank.
- Oxygen enters the common manifold downstream of other gases.
- An auxiliary oxygen flowmeter is strongly recommended.

An oxygen flush is present, capable of 35-75 L/min flow that does not proceed through any vaporizers.

Vaporizers
- Concentration-calibrated
- An interlock must be present.
- Liquid level indicated, designed to prevent overfilling
- "Should" use keyed-filler devices
- No discharge of liquid anesthetic occurs from the vaporizer, even at maximum fresh gas flow.

Only one common gas outlet at 22 mm outer diameter, 15-mm inner diameter, which is designed to prevent accidental disconnection

Pipeline gas supply
- Pipeline pressure gauge
- Inlets for at least oxygen and nitrous oxide
- DISS protected
- In-line filter
- Check valve

Checklist must be provided (it may be electronic or performed manually by the user).

A digital data interface must be provided.

---

prevent damage to the anesthesia gas machine from particulate matter present in the pipeline gas supply.[21]

Problems with Pipeline Supply

Some of the problems associated with pipeline use can be particularly dangerous because they are occult. Pressure loss, excess pressure, cross-connection of gas delivery pipelines, contamination, leaks, and theft of nitrous oxide (for recreational use) have been reported.[22] These problems are not all relegated to the past, and they have consequences for patient safety. There were 45 deaths related to pipeline problems in the United States from 1972 to 1993, and this number is probably an underestimate.[17] Two patients became hypoxemic during anesthesia due to

delivery to a hospital of nitrogen tanks with oxygen fittings in 1996.[23] Seven deaths related to piped medical gases were reported from 1997 to 2001.[24] Two patients became hypoxemic due to purging of oxygen lines with nitrogen in 2000.[25] A serious failure of the bulk liquid oxygen supply was noted in 2004, but no patients were harmed.[26] Complications can arise if oxygen analyzers fail or are misused.[2,11,27] Always trust an oxygen analyzer until you can prove it wrong.

Pipeline supplies of gas have been reported to contain particulate, gaseous, and bacterial matter; other contaminants; and water.[22,28-30] In 1993, the National Fire Protection Association (NFPA) adopted more stringent testing standards.[28] The Joint Commission has established standards that allow site visitors to

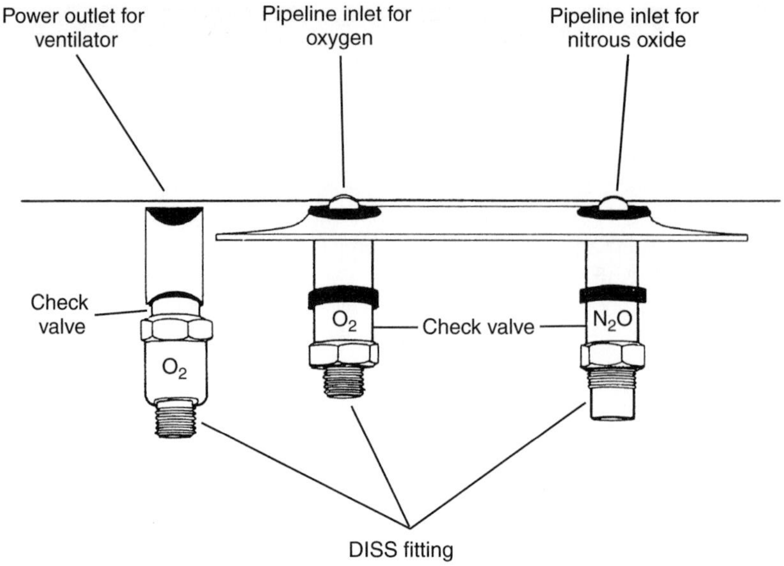

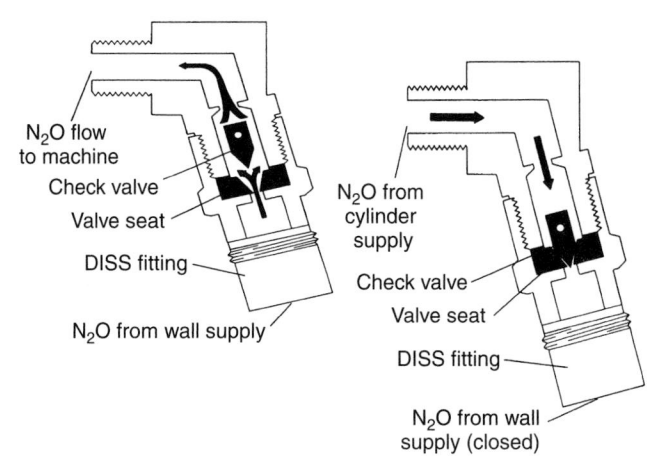

Power outlet for ventilator

Pipeline inlet for oxygen

Pipeline inlet for nitrous oxide

FIGURE **16-2** Diameter index safety system (DISS) for gas connections on the back of the anesthesia gas machine. (*From Bowie E, Huffman LM:* The Anesthesia Machine: Essentials for Understanding. *Madison, WI: Datex-Ohmeda; 1985.*)

Check valve

O₂

Check valve

N₂O

DISS fitting

FIGURE **16-3** Check valve in the nitrous oxide supply hose at the back of the anesthesia gas machine. (*From Bowie E, Huffman LM:* The Anesthesia Machine: Essentials for Understanding. *Madison, WI: Datex-Ohmeda; 1985.*)

N₂O flow to machine
Check valve
Valve seat
DISS fitting
N₂O from wall supply

N₂O from cylinder supply
Check valve
Valve seat
DISS fitting
N₂O from wall supply (closed)

randomly approach and question operating room and other hospital staff to ensure they are aware of the location and function of shutoff valves and alarms related to gas supplies in their area.[28]

Loss of Oxygen Pipeline Pressure

Loss of oxygen pipeline pressure is indicated by the pipeline pressure gauge. In addition, if pressure loss is profound, the oxygen low-pressure alarm sounds, and the fail-safe valves halt the delivery of all other gases. Some newer machines are designed to switch to air to drive the ventilator bellows with loss of oxygen pipeline pressure. With the new electronic alarms, operator response may be delayed because the electronic alarms lack the distinctive and familiar "whistle" of a pneumatic oxygen low-pressure alarm.[31] Two recent simulation studies point to the

need for change in the way we teach and respond to loss of oxygen pipeline pressure.[32,33] A minority of second- and fourth-year residents recognized oxygen supply and pressure alarms. They correctly did the following: opened the oxygen cylinder on the machine, recognized the oxygen cylinder was empty, changed it successfully, or recognized that bag-valve-mask (Ambu) ventilation would lead to patient awakening.[32] A group of volunteer specialist anesthetists (completed residency and in practice) managed a simulated oxygen pipeline failure equally poorly.[33] In their pre-use check, 70% failed to identify an empty oxygen cylinder, and only 25% checked for backup ventilation equipment (a bag-valve-mask) before induction. Most failed to conserve cylinder oxygen (by using low flows or turning off the mechanical ventilator), and all used untested

BOX **16-4**

Guideline for Oxygen Pipeline Supply Failure

Always check for the presence of a full E cylinder and an alternative means of ventilation (bag-valve-mask device) before using an anesthesia machine. If pipeline pressure fails or fraction of inspired oxygen drops, follow these steps:

1. Do not attempt to fix the oxygen analyzer—it must be trusted until it can be proved wrong.
2. Turn on backup oxygen cylinder on machine fully, and disconnect pipeline. Ensure measured fraction of inspired oxygen begins to rise. If the fraction of inspired O_2 does not increase (with fresh gas flow adequate to wash in the O_2 quickly), ventilate the patient by Ambu bag with room air.
3. Use low flows of oxygen. Maintain anesthesia with a volatile agent. Ensure Fio_2 and agent concentration are appropriate.
4. Turn off the ventilator and ventilate manually through the circle system.
5. Call for help if needed; calculate the time remaining for the current cylinder; call for additional oxygen cylinders, and install them on the machine if needed.
6. Find out how long the problem is expected to last; participate in the hospital disaster plan, which may require prioritizing oxygen for those patients who need it most.
7. Do not reconnect patient to pipeline gas until the gas supply is tested.
8. If unable to use the circle, ventilate with an oxygen source (freestanding cylinder) or with room air via a bag-valve-mask device, and institute total intravenous anesthesia.

pipeline supplies of oxygen when informed that pressure had been restored.[33] These responses could be categorized as unwise at least or unsafe at worst. In a third recent report, more than 700 anesthetics were claimed to be given over a 3-week period without any checks for a full E cylinder in reserve.[34]

Optimal management of loss of oxygen pipeline pressure has the following goals: maintenance of oxygenation, ventilation, and depth of anesthesia; and ensuring the safety of the oxygen supply.[33] Box 16-4 gives a suggested guideline for management.[26,32,33,35-38] The rationale is that with complete loss of oxygen pipeline pressure, the anesthetist should fully open the E cylinder of oxygen, disconnect the pipeline, and consider the use of low fresh gas flows and manual ventilation (to conserve the emergency cylinder supply of oxygen). If the E cylinder of oxygen is not opened fully, flow from it may end before the cylinder is empty. The pipeline is disconnected so that retrograde flow from within the machine to the pipeline is prevented. Retrograde flow occurs only if the pipeline inlet check valve fails simultaneously. Although this is unlikely, the author recommends disconnecting the hose at the quick-connect fitting for two reasons. First, it *must* be disconnected in the case of a cross-connection (which is more fully described later in the chapter), otherwise the contents of the oxygen cylinder will not flow. Remembering one strategy that is effective for two reasonably similar problems is easier than remembering two different strategies. Second, if the loss of pipeline pressure is

followed by the flow of contaminated contents from the oxygen pipeline, disconnecting when pipeline pressure is lost protects the patient from exposure to these contaminants.

Although excessive pipeline pressure will not trigger alarms in the machine, it should do so in the hospital physical plant or engineering department. Excessive pressure can damage respiratory apparatus or machinery of various types connected to the pipeline, including the anesthesia gas machine.

Cross-Connection of Gases

Cross-connection of gases can occur anywhere from the liquid oxygen supply and piping to the wall outlets, hoses, and internal circuitry of the anesthesia gas machine. Incidents of cross-connection continue to be reported. Fatalities in which cross-connection was a factor have been reported as recently as 2002.[39-41] These fatalities have been associated with the shipment in error to the hospital of liquid nitrogen instead of oxygen, liquid carbon dioxide rather than nitrous oxide, the unintentional cross-connection of oxygen and nitrous oxide pipelines during renovation of an operating room, and alteration of an oxygen flowmeter so that it would fit a nitrous oxide outlet in a cardiac catheterization laboratory. A common factor associated with patient injury has been failure to use an oxygen analyzer.

Although not all incidents involve patients connected to anesthesia gas machines, cross-connections continue to be reported in anesthetized patients. In 1997, a case was described in which the nitrogen hose from the gas machine was discovered to be fitted with a quick-connect coupler for air (at the end that would be plugged into the wall outlet).[23] This did not result in patient injury but would have allowed the delivery of 100% nitrogen had the machine been set to deliver air only. The consequences of this type of error in the oxygen wall-outlet hose could be disastrous. In 1995, it was reported in the United States that two patients became hypoxemic as a result of delivery of liquid nitrogen to the hospital in a tank with oxygen fittings.[42] These incidents underscore the importance of oxygen analysis, checking the oxygen analyzer before use, and proper response to oxygen-analyzer alarms.

In the event of a suspected crossover, one would see declining inspired oxygen concentration. The anesthetist must open the emergency cylinder oxygen supply, disconnect the pipeline, and consider the use of low fresh gas flows and manual ventilation. If the pipeline is not disconnected, the pipeline gas will continue to flow, rather than the cylinder oxygen supply. This is because the pressure distal to the cylinder regulator is set at 45 psi (310 kPa), compared with the typical pipeline pressure of 50 psi (344 kPa). Lower pressure is intentionally set on the cylinder regulator so that flow proceeds from the higher-pressure pipeline source if a cylinder is inadvertently left open after the machine has been checked.[43] This is analogous to the situation with an intravenous main line and a piggyback line: The one held higher is the one that will flow (greater hydrostatic pressure). In the case of cross-connection between oxygen and nitrous oxide pipelines, the contents of the oxygen pipeline (now nitrous oxide) continue to flow (because the pipeline pressure is 50 psi), whether or not the oxygen cylinder is open. Thus, regardless of the problem with the pipeline supply (lack of pressure or cross-connection), the cylinder *must* be opened; the author advocates disconnecting the pipeline in any instance of problems with the pipeline. If the pipeline is not disconnected and has pressure within it, the emergency supply of oxygen may not flow from the cylinder.

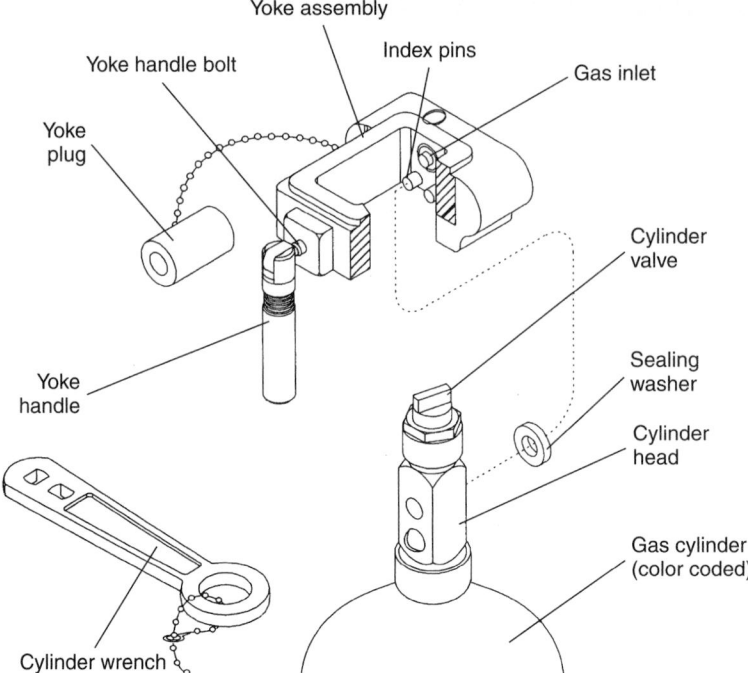

FIGURE **16-4** Pin index safety system, cylinder valve, and yoke. (*From Cicman J et al. Operating Principles of Narkomed Anesthesia Systems. Telford, PA: Dräger; 1993.*)

TABLE **16-1**	E Cylinder Characteristics			
Gas	**Color, United States (International)**	**Service Pressure psi (kPa x 10^{-2})**	**Capacity (L)**	**Pin Position**
Oxygen	Green (white)	1900 (131)	660	2-5
Nitrous oxide	Blue (blue)	745 (51)	1590	3-5
Air	Yellow (black and white)	1900 (131)	625	1-5

Data from Standard Specification for Particular Requirements for Anesthesia Workstations and Their Components [F1850-00]. *Philadelphia: American Society for Testing and Materials; 2000; and* NFPA 99: Health Care Facilities [Table C-12.5]. *Quincy, MA: National Fire Protection Association; 1990:184.*
Note that slightly different values may be found in different sources.

Cylinder Supply

Cylinders are present on the anesthesia machine as reserves for emergency use. Thus they should be open only when they are checked or when the pipeline supply is unavailable.[44] A fresh oxygen cylinder need not be obtained if at least one reserve cylinder on the machine has an adequate pressure, the amount of which would depend on the availability of pipeline supplies and additional backup oxygen cylinders. Cylinders are labeled, marked, and color coded (Table 16-1). Anesthetists who practice outside the United States must be aware that the color scheme may differ from country to country. Service pressure and cylinder contents are reported slightly differently in various sources.[45] *Pin position* refers to the pin index safety system (PISS) illustrated in Figures 16-4 and 16-5. In this system, each cylinder valve has a unique arrangement of pins that corresponds to its intended contents. The pin arrangement matches holes in the yoke, which is the point where cylinders are attached to the gas machine. The PISS is thus another means of preventing misconnections. The system can be defeated if the pins are missing, are removed, or if more than one washer is used. Anesthetists should check both pins and washers whenever cylinders are replaced. Furthermore, they should be aware that not all E cylinders are

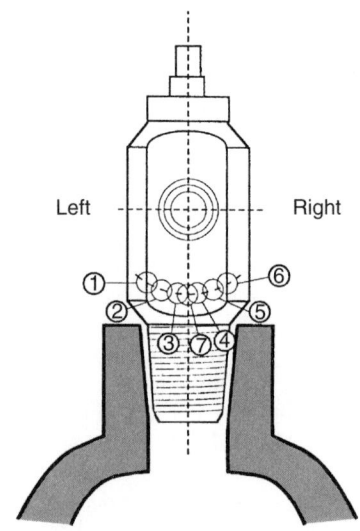

FIGURE **16-5** Pin index safety system: pin positions. (*Modified from Eichhorn JH, Ehrenwerth J: Medical Gases: Storage and Supply. In: Ehrenwerth J, Eisenkraft JB, eds. Anesthesia Equipment: Principles and Applications. St Louis: Mosby; 1993:1-26.*)

of precisely the right size to fit properly on the machine. Installation of a longer aluminum cylinder has prevented an anesthesia gas machine from rolling.[46]

The cylinder valve is the most fragile part of the cylinder, so it must be protected during transport. The cylinder valve consists of a body, the port where gas exits, a conical depression (opposite the port) for the securing screw, PISS pins, and safety relief devices. If a fire causes the temperature and pressure within the cylinder to increase, safety relief devices release cylinder contents in a controlled fashion, rather than explosively. Manufacturers use one or more of the following on cylinder valves: a frangible disk that bursts under pressure, a valve that opens at extreme

pressure, or a fusible plug made of Wood's metal (which melts at elevated temperatures).

The hanger yoke serves three functions: it orients cylinders, provides a gas-tight seal, and ensures unidirectional flow. It also contains a filter that is required by standard.[21] The check valve within the hanger yoke minimizes the likelihood of transfilling or of leakage to the atmosphere (if a yoke is empty). It also allows cylinders to be replaced during use. If two cylinders are open, transfilling occurs when gas flows from the cylinder with higher pressure into the cylinder with lower pressure, rather than proceeding toward the flowmeters. Transfilling is a potential fire hazard because filling a cylinder generates heat. The cylinder pressure gauge is a Bourdon-type gauge that indicates pressure within whichever of the cylinders for the same gas (if two are present and both open) has the higher pressure (Figure 16-6).

Immediately distal to the hanger yoke for each gas is a regulator (Figure 16-7). Two diaphragms move together, connected by a rod. The smaller of the two diaphragms opens or closes the high-pressure inlet (from the cylinder). Gas entering the regulator exerts pressure on the larger diaphragm, whose movement tends to close the inlet. Thus gas can enter the regulator only at a rate controlled by a feedback loop. The outlet pressure is adjustable with a screw and spring that bear on the inlet diaphragm. Thus the regulator converts the high (but variable) cylinder pressure to a constant downstream pressure (45 psi [310 kPa]), which is intentionally slightly less than pipeline pressure.[21,28,31] This is done to prevent silent depletion of cylinder contents. Pipeline pressure varies, depending on the load that is placed on it throughout the facility. If a cylinder is left open and pipeline pressure drops below 45 psi, gas will flow from the cylinder. No alarm will sound to warn the user of this condition.[22] Further, if the cylinder is left open after checking and the pipeline fails, the operator will not be alerted to the failure at the time it occurs, because gas will simply begin to flow from the cylinder, without alarms. If the mechanical ventilator is in use, a full E cylinder of oxygen may be depleted in as little

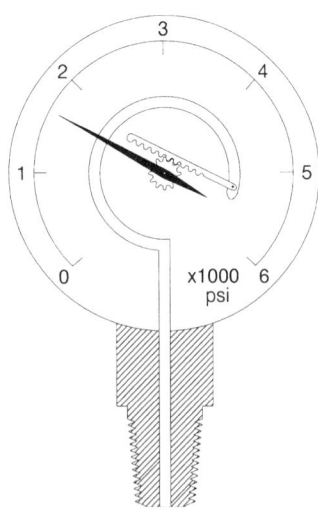

FIGURE **16-6** Bourdon-type pressure gauges are aneroid gauges used for measuring cylinder (and pipeline) pressure. (*From Cicman J et al. Operating Principles of Narkomed Anesthesia Systems. Telford, PA: Dräger; 1993.*)

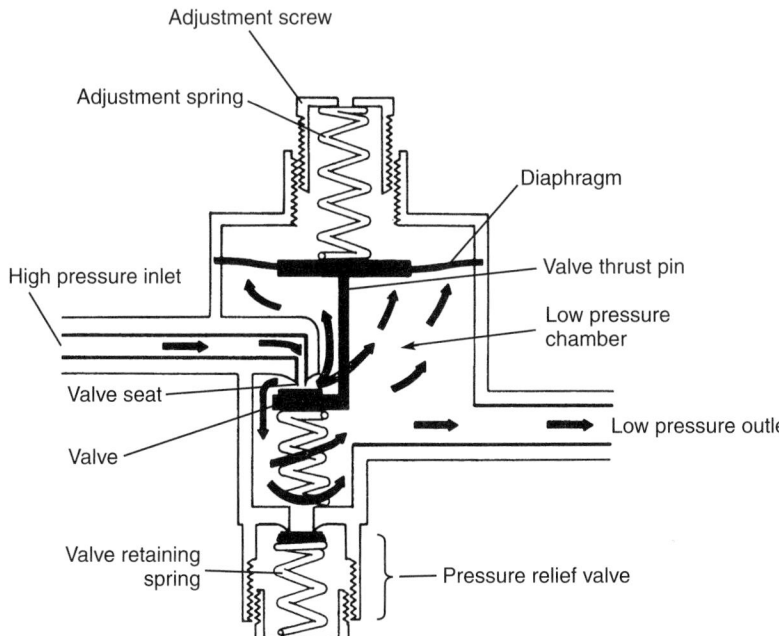

FIGURE **16-7** A schematic view of a cylinder regulator. (*From Bowie E, Huffman LM: The Anesthesia Machine: Essentials for Understanding. Madison, WI: Datex-Ohmeda; 1985.*)

BOX 16-5

Rules for Safe Handling of Cylinders

Never stand a cylinder upright without support; instead, lay it on its side.

Never leave empty cylinders on the machine.

Never leave the plastic cover on the port while installing the cylinder.

Never use more than one washer between a cylinder port and the yoke.

Never rely only on a cylinder's color for identification of its contents; read its labeling.

Never oil valves.

Never remove a cylinder from a yoke without filling the space with a yoke plug if available (see Figure 16-4), which is a backup strategy for guarding against check valve failure.

Always protect the cylinder valve when carrying a cylinder; it is the most fragile part.

---

as 1 hour, because the ventilator-driving gas often is oxygen.[35] The low oxygen supply failure alarm that rings subsequently announces the *end* of the emergency supply, instead of its beginning. This is the rationale for keeping cylinders closed after their pressure has been checked.

The U.S. Department of Transportation issues regulations for the manufacture, handling, transport, storage, and disposal of cylinders. These regulations have binding legal force. Industry advisory groups such as the Compressed Gas Association (CGA) and the National Fire Protection Association also have a role in setting cylinder standards. Cylinders are constructed of steel approximately one-quarter inch in thickness. Only nonferrous (aluminum) cylinders may be used in the magnetic resonance imaging (MRI) environment.[45] Fatalities have occurred when steel cylinders have affected patients in the MRI scanner.[47]

Anesthetists must be aware of the rules for the safe handling and use of cylinders.[22,48] Gas under pressure in cylinders has an enormous potential energy, which may be lethal if it is released in a rapid, uncontrolled fashion following damage to the cylinder valve. Selected rules for safe handling of cylinders are presented in Box 16-5.

When installing a cylinder, check the labels, crack the valve, check that both PISS pins are present, check that only one washer is present, place the cylinder in the hanger yoke, observe for the absence of an audible leak, and check for proper gauge pressure. The valve is "cracked" to remove dirt from the port. This is done by opening the valve briefly and carefully before the cylinder is placed on the machine. While cracking the valve, hold the cylinder securely, and do not point the port toward oneself or other personnel.

When relying on cylinder supplies in an emergency, one must be able to calculate how long an oxygen cylinder will last. The following relationship should be used:

$$\frac{\text{Capacity L}}{\text{Service Pressure psi}} = \frac{\text{Contents Remaining L}}{\text{Gauge Pressure psi}}$$

Remember to consider the oxygen flow rate set on the flowmeter when deciding how long the available liters will last.

As an example, if the oxygen flow is 2 L/min, and the cylinder's oxygen gauge pressure is 500 psi, how long will the cylinder last? From Table 16-1, we know that the service pressure is 1900 psi and that the capacity is 660 L. Substituting these values into the previous relationship, we obtain the following:

$$\frac{600\ \text{L}}{1900\ \text{psi}} = \frac{x\text{L}}{500\ \text{psi}}$$

$$x = 174\ \text{L}$$

Because 2 L of oxygen flow each minute, the cylinder will last approximately 86 minutes (174 L ÷ 2 L/min). This type of calculation is not applicable to compressed gases stored as liquids (nitrous oxide or carbon dioxide). It should be remembered that this calculation refers only to requirements at the flowmeters and assumes manual ventilation. Use of a mechanical ventilator consumes approximately a minute volume of driving gas each minute and thus should be avoided in situations in which oxygen supply is limited to cylinders only.

The contents of cylinders must meet the purity requirements for medical gases established by the United States Pharmacopeia (USP). The contents are also regulated in the United States by the U.S. Food and Drug Administration (FDA). Oxygen is used to power ventilators throughout the hospital because it is dry, readily available, and relatively inexpensive.

Nitrous oxide is stored as a liquid; therefore, the cylinder pressure of 745 psi ($51\ \text{kPa} \times 10^{-2}$) represents the vapor pressure of liquid nitrous oxide at room temperature. The nitrous oxide cylinder pressure gauge remains at 745 psi until the liquid is gone; at this point, the cylinder is more than threequarters empty. After this point, the nitrous oxide cylinder pressure swiftly declines with further use. Thus nitrous oxide cylinders should be changed if their pressure is less than 745 psi. Rapid removal (more than 4 L/min) from a cylinder may cause the formation of frost on its wall or freezing of the valve, owing to the loss of the latent heat of vaporization from the liquid nitrous oxide. Nitrous oxide is nonflammable, but it does support combustion.[22,45] Anesthesia personnel must be alert to the possibility of nitrous oxide abuse.[49]

Compressed air is not entirely dry. Its composition varies from sample to sample, but its major constituents are nitrogen (78%), oxygen (21%), and argon (nearly 1%). Carbon dioxide (0.03%) and other gases are present in trace amounts.

Electrical Power Supply

Electrical power is supplied to the gas machine through a single power cord, which can become dislodged. Because of this possibility, as well as the possibility of loss of main electrical power, new gas machines must be equipped with battery backup sufficient for at least 30 minutes of limited operation.[21] Which systems remain powered during this period is specific to each model, thus users must read the operator's manuals. For example, if you disconnect electrical power from the ADU (GE Healthcare) it loses patient monitors (electrocardiogram, noninvasive blood pressure, gas analysis, pulse oximetry, and other monitors displayed on the right screen), but fresh gas flow, volatile-agent delivery, and ventilation continue during the period that battery backup is used. Once battery power is lost, nitrous oxide and agent delivery are cut off.[50]

Convenience receptacles are usually found on the back of the machine so that monitors or other equipment can be plugged in. These convenience receptacles are protected by circuit breakers or fuses. It is a mistake to plug devices that convert electrical power into heat into these receptacles (air or water warming blankets, intravenous fluid warmers) for two reasons.[51] First, these devices draw a lot of amperage (relative to other electrical devices), so they are more likely to cause a circuit breaker to open. Second, the circuit breakers are in non-standard locations (so check for their location before your first case). If a circuit breaker opens, all devices that receive power there (such as monitors and in some configurations, the mechanical ventilator) may cease to function. If one is not familiar with the circuit-breaker location, valuable time may be lost while a search is conducted.

Loss of Main Electrical Power

Devices that typically *require* wall-outlet electrical power include mechanical ventilators, physiologic monitors, room and surgical-field illumination, digital flowmeter displays for electronic flowmeters, cardiopulmonary bypass pump/oxygenators, air warming blankets, gas/vapor blenders (Suprane Tec 6 [GE Healthcare]), and vaporizers with electronic controls (Aladin cassettes in the ADU).

Devices (or techniques) that typically *do not* rely on wall-outlet electrical power include spontaneous or manually assisted ventilation, mechanical flowmeters, scavenging, laryngoscope, flashlights, intravenous bolus or infusion, battery-operated peripheral nerve stimulators or intravenous infusion pumps, monitoring by the anesthetist using the five senses, and variable bypass vaporizers (Tec 7 [GE Healthcare]; Vapor 2000 [Dräger Medical).

Generally, hospitals have emergency generators that will supply operating-room electrical outlets in the event power is lost. But these backup generators are not completely reliable. A 90-minute interruption in power during cardiopulmonary bypass, complicated by almost immediate failure of the hospital generators, has been described.[52] One unanticipated hazard was injuries to personnel as they hurried in the dark to fetch lights and equipment.

With power failure in older gas machines, the principal problems were loss of room illumination and failure of mechanical ventilators and electronic patient monitoring. In general, new gas machines have battery backup sufficient for 30 minutes of operation—however, typically without patient monitors (electrocardiogram, pulse oximetry, gas analysis). Mechanical ventilation may or may not be powered by the backup battery (depending on the model). New flowmeters that are entirely electronic (Aisys and Avance [GE Healthcare])require a backup pneumatic/mechanical (needle-valve and flowtube) flowmeter.[15,53,54] Mechanical flowmeters with digital display of flows may have a backup glass flow tube that indicates total fresh gas flow (ADU[50] [GE Healthcare]; Fabius GS[55] [Dräger Medical]). New gas machines with mechanical needle valve flowmeters and variable bypass vaporizers (e.g., Fabius GS or Aestiva [GE Healthcare]) have an advantage during electrical power failure in that delivery of gases and agent can continue indefinitely.[44,55] However, in the event of generator failure, anesthesia would be limited to flashlight illumination and monitoring by the five senses. The Narkomed 6000 (Dräger Medical) provides gas and vapor delivery and integrated monitoring (oxygen, breathing circuit volume and pressure, gas analysis) for 30 minutes if main electrical power is lost.[56]

Because of the differences between models, it remains important to understand and anticipate how each particular anesthesia gas machine type responds when main electrical power is lost. This information must be reviewed in the operator's manual.

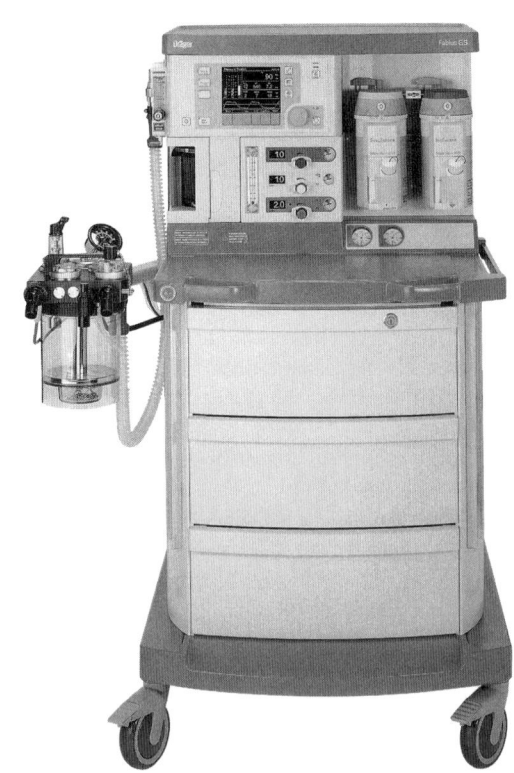

FIGURE **16-8** Fabius GS. (*Courtesy of Dräger Medical, Telford, PA.*)

PROCESSING

In this section, the various aspects of the anesthesia gas machine's preparation of gases before their delivery to the patient are discussed.

Manufacturers and Models

Manufacturers of anesthesia gas machines in the United States include Dräger Medical, GE Healthcare, and Datascope. Dräger Medical Inc. (Telford, Pennsylvania) is the manufacturer of the Narkomed series (6000 and 6400, GS, MRI, Mobile models), the Apollo, and the Fabius GS. GE Healthcare (Madison, Wisconsin) is the manufacturer of the Aestiva, Aestiva MRI, Avance, Aisys, Aespire, and ADU. Datascope (Montvale, New Jersey) manufactures the Anestar.

Gas machines not currently produced remain in widespread use. Currently produced models meet or exceed the specifications of the anesthesia workstation standard F1850. The differences among new gas machines are significant; thus what one learns on one may not transfer very well to a different model. The differences are pointed out in this chapter when they are relevant to clinical practice or to demonstrate by comparison how systems function. This section continues with an overview of several current gas machines.

Dräger Fabius GS

The Fabius GS (Figure 16-8) includes volume, pressure, flow, and inspired oxygen monitoring but not physiologic monitors or gas analysis. The thermal anemometry ("hot wire") flow sensor in the breathing circuit is unique to this machine and Anestar.[55]

The screen displays tidal and minute volume, respiratory rate, and a respiratory pressure waveform. The ventilator is piston driven; corrects tidal volume for compliance and leaks; and features manual, spontaneous, volume-controled ventilation (VCV); pressure-controlled ventilation (PCV); pressure-support ventilation (PSV); and synchronized intermittent mandatory ventilation (SIMV) with PSV.[57] Like all current machines, the mechanical ventilator is activated in one step. The machine uses a manual checklist with several electronic self-tests (system, leaks and compliance, flow sensor, oxygen sensor). With the Fabius GS (as with all the new models), users must review the operator's manual to check the machine correctly. The flowmeters are needle valves with electronic capture and display, with a common gas outlet glass flowmeter as backup. Variable-bypass vaporizers are used, and these may be removed without tools.

The Fabius GS breathing circuit is lower volume than older gas machines (2.8 L; of which 1.5 L is absorbent volume).[57] The absorber head is not warmed. Loose carbon dioxide absorbent granules or prefilled canisters may be used. There is an open scavenger interface. Fresh gas decoupling causes the manual breathing bag to fluctuate during the mechanical ventilator cycle, which serves as a further disconnect alarm.

In case of electrical power failure, there is a 45-minute battery reserve with fresh gas, vaporizers, integrated monitors, and ventilator operational. Because they are not part of the gas machine, patient monitors will not function. Several pneumatic functions remain after the battery is exhausted: vaporizers, hypoxic guard, adjustable pressure-limiting (APL or "popoff") valve, flowmeters, breathing pressure gauge, cylinder and pipeline pressure gauges, and common gas outlet flowmeter.

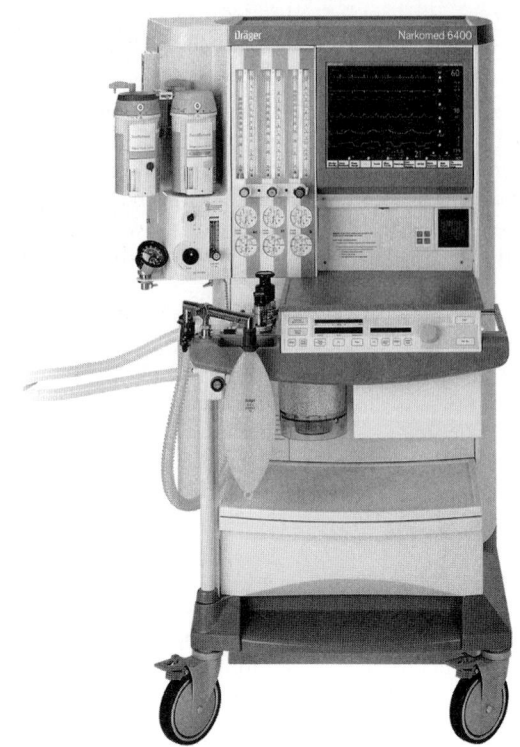

FIGURE **16-9** Dräger Narkomed 6000/6400. (*Courtesy of Dräger Medical, Telford, PA.*)

Dräger Narkomed 6000/6400

The Narkomed 6000 (Figure 16-9) includes volume, pressure, flow, and inspired oxygen monitoring. It also includes gas monitoring (infrared agent and carbon dioxide) and an ultrasonic flow sensor in the breathing circuit (unique to this machine). An integrated patient monitoring module is available as an option, so all parameters are displayed on the single touch screen.[56,58]

The 6000 includes a piston ventilator (Divan) with tidal volume corrected for leaks, patient and breathing circuit compliance, and fresh gas flow (by fresh gas decoupling). The ventilator is capable of manual, spontaneous, VCV, PCV, and SIMV modes. Like the Fabius GS, there is no "bag/vent" switch because changing ventilator mode is controlled electronically. Like most new model ventilators, it is accurate to very low tidal volume (range 10 to 1400 mL), which lessens the need for nonrebreathing circuits.

From a cold startup, there is a 1-minute power-on self-test, then a 5-minute ventilator self-test.[56] One can bypass the ventilator test for 10 days (or 10 times) only, after which the ventilator is unavailable until its self-test is performed. The machine checkout follows FDA guidelines,[59] but there are some differences. For example, the manufacturer recommends breathing through each circuit limb to test unidirectional valves and disconnecting the oxygen wall hose to check the oxygen pipeline pressure-failure device.

Flow meters are composed of needle valves and glass flowtubes, but electronic capture of fresh gas flows has been added in the 6400. Variable-bypass vaporizers are used, and these may be removed without tools. The breathing circuit is lower volume (1.5 L absorbent volume), and the absorber head is warmed. Only loose carbon dioxide–absorbent granules may be used. An open

scavenger interface or passive evacuation may be used. In case of power failure, there is a 30-minute battery reserve with fresh gas, vaporizers, monitors, and ventilator operational.

Dräger Apollo

The Dräger Apollo (Figure 16-10) includes volume, pressure, flow, and inspired oxygen monitoring. It also includes gas monitoring (agent and carbon dioxide) and spirometry.[15,60] The piston ventilator corrects tidal volume for leaks, compliance, and fresh gas flow (by fresh gas decoupling). The ventilator is capable of manual, spontaneous, VCV, pressure PCV, PSV, and SIMV modes. SIMV may be added to either volume or pressure modes. It is accurate to very low tidal volume (range 20 to 1400 mL). Mechanical needle valves govern fresh gas flow, which is electronically measured and displayed onscreen. A backup total flowtube is present. An electronic checklist assists the user in preuse checkout.[60] The scavenger interface is open.

GE Healthcare Aestiva

The Aestiva (Figure 16-11) has many traditional (mechanical/pneumatic) systems, but with an improved and capable ventilator. It includes volume, pressure, flow, and inspired oxygen monitoring. Gas analysis and patient physiologic monitors must be added (like most current machines except ADU, Aisys, Avance, and 6400).[15,61] The 7900 ventilator uses an oxygen-driven standing bellows capable of manual, spontaneous, VCV, PCV, PSV-Pro, which includes apnea backup,[62] and SIMV.

The flow sensors compensate tidal volume for compliance losses and leaks in the absorber head and bellows, so the ventilator is accurate to very low tidal volume. These variable orifice

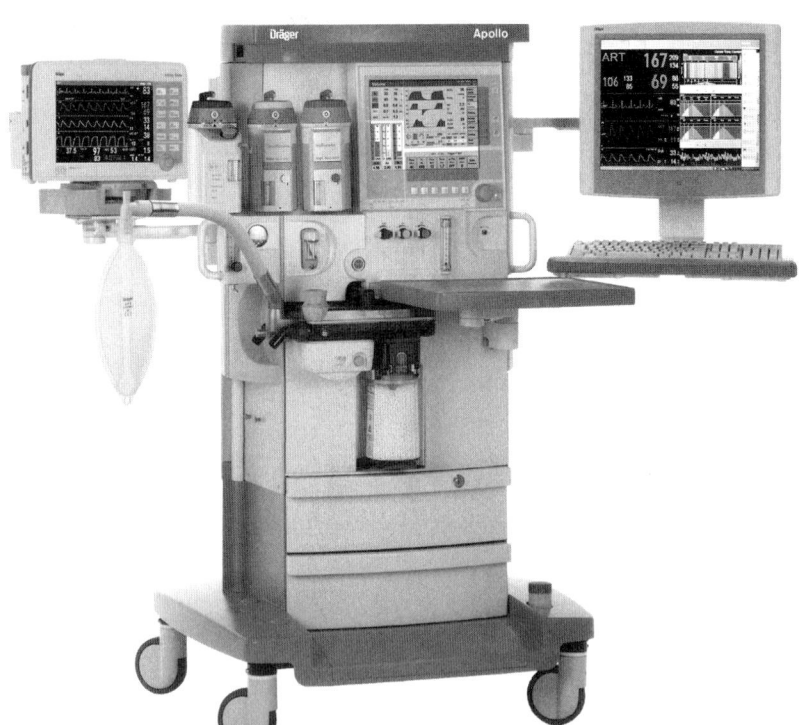

FIGURE **16-10** Dräger Apollo. (*Courtesy of Dräger Medical, Telford, PA.*)

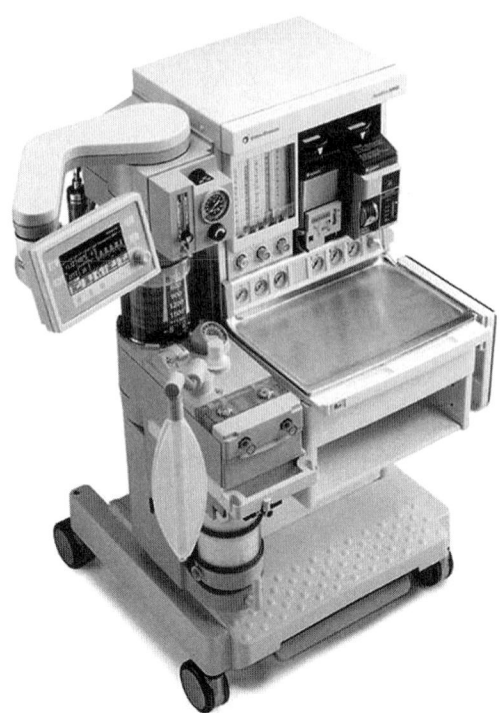

FIGURE **16-11** GE Healthcare Aestiva. (*Courtesy of GE Healthcare, Madison, WI.*)

flow sensors have shown some sensitivity to moisture in the breathing circuit in the past.[63] The "bag/vent" switch activates the mechanical ventilator in one step. The absorber head design allows for easier disassembly and cleaning than older models. The Aestiva uses a nonelectronic (FDA-style) checklist.

Flowmeters are traditional mechanical needle valves and glass flowtubes. There is no electronic capture of fresh gas flows. The oxygen sensor is the galvanic fuel cell type, and the hypoxic guard is mechanical (Link-25).[61] Variable-bypass vaporizers are used, and these may be removed without tools. The breathing circuit is relatively high volume (5.5 L, including dual canisters of 1.35 kg absorbent each).[64] Loose fill granules or prepackaged absorbent may be used. The machine is compatible with nonrebreathing circuits. The scavenger is available as a closed scavenger interface. There is a 30-minute battery reserve with fresh gas, vaporizers, and ventilator operational. The Aestiva is also available in a version compatible with the magnetic resonance imaging (MRI) suite.

GE Healthcare Aespire

The Aespire (Figure 16-12) is like the Aestiva in most of its systems but is more compact. The standing bellows, oxygen-driven ventilator offers tidal volume compensation. Volume control and pressure control are the two modes of ventilation available.[65]

GE Healthcare Aisys

The Aisys (along with Avance, ADU, and 6400) is a complete workstation in that physiologic monitors are included (electrocardiography, blood pressure, pulse oximetry).[54] The Aisys (Figure 16-13), introduced in 2005, uses the oxygen-driven, standing bellows 7900 Smartvent (like Aestiva) but offers more modes. Modes available include manual, spontaneous, VCV, PCV, pressure control with volume guarantee, PCV-VG, which is unique to Aisys and Avance, PSV-Pro with apnea backup, and SIMV with pressure support of the patient's spontaneous breaths (SIMV-PS) in either volume or pressure mode. Spirometry is included to help monitor and control ventilation. The ventilator can support a very wide range of tidal volumes, so there is no need for nonrebreathing circuits for children. Like most modern

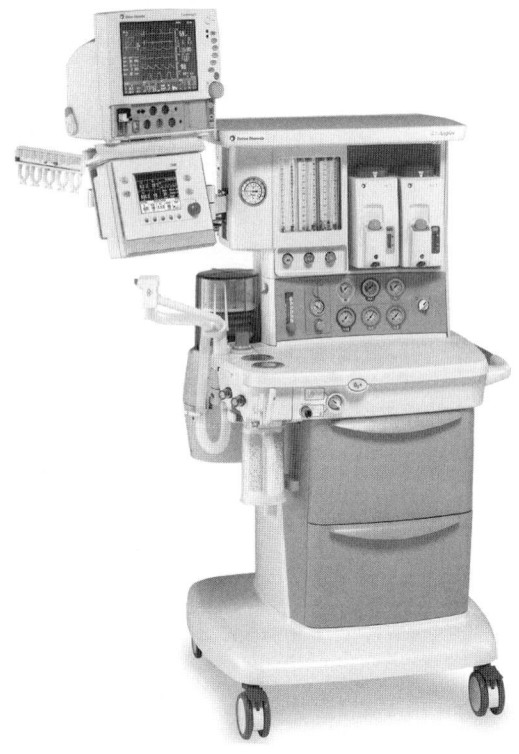

FIGURE **16-12**   GE Healthcare Aespire. (*Courtesy of GE Healthcare, Madison, WI.*)

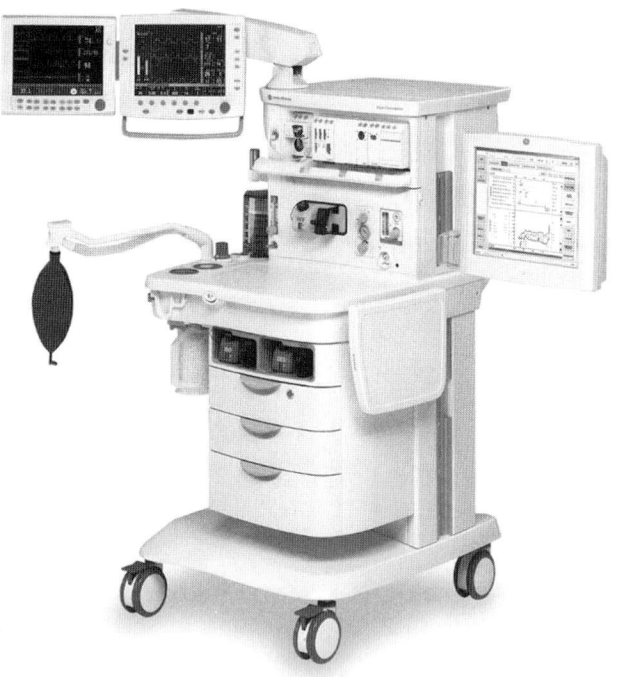

FIGURE **16-13**   GE Healthcare Aisys. (*Courtesy of GE Healthcare, Madison, WI.*)

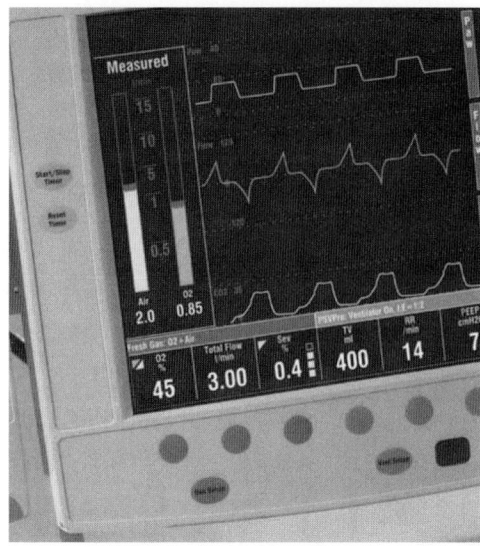

FIGURE **16-14**   Electronic control of inspired oxygen, carrier gas, and total fresh gas flow, Aisys. (*Courtesy of GE Healthcare, Madison, WI.*)

ventilators, the low circuit volume, freedom from leaks, and microprocessor control support the use of low-flow anesthesia. The fresh gas inlet enters the circle system distal to the inspiratory valve (like Avance and ADU), supporting fast response to changes in desired gas concentrations, even at low flows.

Aisys is similar to the ADU in that it uses Aladin cassette vaporizers, which are electronically controlled. There are no needle valves or glass flowtubes for fresh gas flow. It is similar to Avance—and unique in the North American market—in that it uses electronic control, measurement, and display of fresh gases (Figure 16-14). The user does not control the flow of each gas directly, as is usual, but instead selects the desired carrier gas (nitrous oxide or air), total fresh gas flow, and inspired oxygen concentration. In case of failure, there is a backup needle valve and total flow glass flowtube for display.[15,54]

GE Healthcare Avance

The Avance (Figure 16-15) is similar to the Aisys in most respects: electronic gas mixer with backup pneumatic control, modern and capable multi-mode 7900 ventilator, spirometry, and integrated physiologic monitoring. The pneumatic/mechanical Tec 6 and Tec 7 vaporizers included in the Avance are the primary difference between it and the Aisys.

GE Healthcare ADU

The ADU (Figure 16-16) includes all monitoring: volume, pressure, flow, inspired oxygen, gas analysis (agent and carbon dioxide), patient physiologic monitoring, and spirometry (flow-volume and pressure-volume respiratory loops). The ventilator is an oxygen-driven standing bellows, with tidal volume corrected for leaks, compliance, and fresh gas flow (via the D-Lite sensor at the Y-piece). It is accurate to very low tidal volumes and capable of manual, spontaneous, VCV, PCV, SIMV, and PSV. The "bag/vent" switch activates the mechanical ventilator in one step.[50]

The ADU uses an almost completely automated checklist routine that conforms to FDA recommendations. Since the D-Lite sensor is removed from the breathing circuit during checkout, one must perform a high-pressure check of the breathing circuit after reassembly.

The flowmeters are mechanical needle valves. Flow is captured and displayed electronically, with a glass common gas outlet flowmeter as an optional backup. The Aladin vaporizer cassettes may be tipped from the vertical during transport

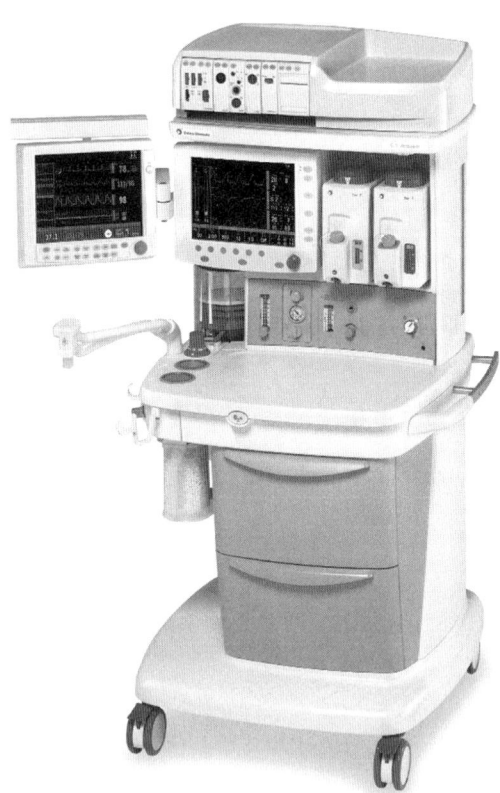

FIGURE **16-15** GE Healthcare Avance. (*Courtesy of GE Healthcare, Madison, WI.*)

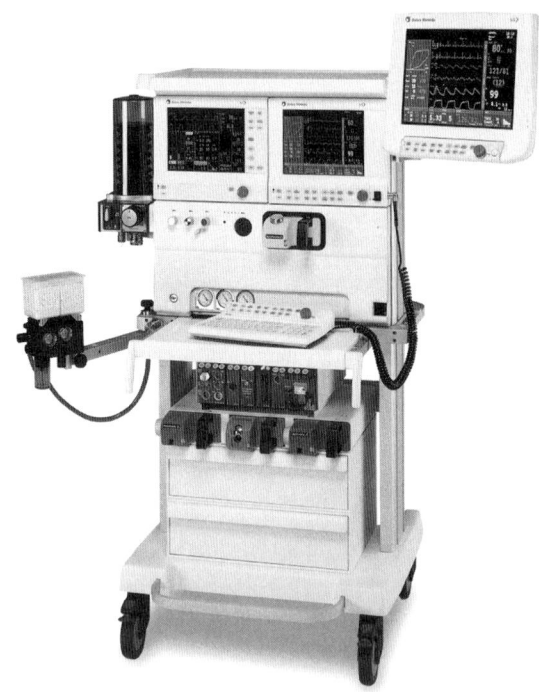

FIGURE **16-16** GE Healthcare Anesthesia Delivery Unit (ADU). Machine monitors are on the left screen (including video screen display of fresh gas flow); patient monitors are on the left (including electrocardiograph and blood pressure). (*Courtesy of GE Healthcare, Madison, WI.*)

without any risk because they are merely repositories for liquid anesthetic. The vaporizer's electronic mechanisms, which are within the gas machine, control the delivery of any agent chosen.

The breathing circuit is very low volume (the absorbent volume is only 750 mL). Only the manufacturer's carbon dioxide absorbent canisters may be used, which are single-use or refillable with loose granules. Certain disposables are only available from the manufacturer (spirometry tubing, D-Lite sensor, absorbent granule canisters). The machine is technically compatible with nonrebreathing circuits, but the need for them is questionable because the machine can ventilate patients who weigh as little as 3 kg. The scavenger interface is open. Scavenger suction adequacy is indicated on an optional glass flowmeter below the bellows. There is a 30-minute battery reserve with fresh gas, vaporizers, and ventilator operational. Patient monitoring (right screen) is lost unless main electrical power (or generator backup) is available. In this respect most gas machines, new or old, function similarly.

Datascope Anestar

The Anestar (Figure 16-17) includes volume, pressure, flow (hot-wire anemometer), and inspired oxygen monitoring (by galvanic fuel cell). Gas analysis and patient physiologic monitors must be added (like many other current machines).[66,67] The ventilator delivers tidal volumes of 40 to 1400 mL. The ventilator uses an oxygen-driven hanging bellows (unique to this machine). The ventilator is capable of manual, spontaneous, VCV, PCV, and PSV. Tidal volume is compensated for compliance, and fresh gas flow changes (by fresh gas decoupling). The breathing circuit is heated. Mechanical ventilation is activated in one step.

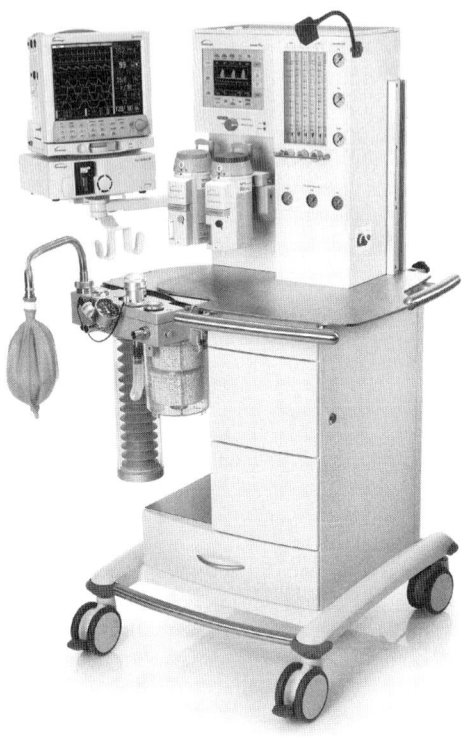

FIGURE **16-17** Anestar. (*Courtesy of Datascope, Mahwah, NJ.*)

Flowmeters are traditional mechanical needle valves and glass flowtubes. There is no electronic capture of fresh gas flows. Traditional variable-bypass vaporizers are used (Vapor 2000 [Dräger Medical]), and these may be removed without tools. The breathing circuit is relatively low volume (2.5 L, including one loose-fill canister for 1.6 kg of absorbent).[15,66]

Path of Gases Through the Machine

Oxygen, nitrous oxide, and air follow similar paths through the anesthesia gas machine (see Figure 16-1). Each passes from its supply point to a flowmeter. All gases (except oxygen and in newer models, air) pass through a fail-safe valve before proceeding to their flowmeters. This valve is held open by pressure in the oxygen circuitry within the anesthesia gas machine. After passing through their respective flowmeters, the gases are joined for the first time in a common manifold. Oxygen is always added to the common manifold downstream of other gases so that the chance of hypoxic breathing mixtures is lessened (e.g., in the event that a flowtube has cracked).[68] The combined gases enter any vaporizer that is turned on and then pass through the common gas outlet. A delivery hose with a locking connection conducts gases from the common gas outlet to the breathing circuit.

The breathing circuit and ventilator (if used) transport gases to and from the patient. An amount equal to the fresh gas flow per minute (minus patient uptake, plus gases excreted), leaves the breathing circuit and is conducted to the scavenger interface. From there, it is disposed of in the hospital ventilation or suction systems.

Five Tasks of Oxygen

Oxygen has five tasks in the anesthesia gas machine: It (1) proceeds to the fresh gas flowmeter, (2) powers the oxygen flush, (3) activates fail-safe mechanisms, (4) activates oxygen low-pressure alarms, and (5) compresses the bellows of mechanical ventilators (see Figure 16-1). The other gases supplied by the machine have only one pathway; they are transported via flowmeter and breathing circuit to anesthetize the patient (nitrous oxide) or sustain life (the oxygen component in the air flowmeter). Newer machines can switch to air as a driving gas for the ventilator bellows if oxygen pressure is lost.

Flowmeter

The first task of oxygen is proceeding through the flowmeter and on to the patient as a life-sustaining gas. Flowmeters have several components (Box 16-6). Control knobs are color and touch coded; thus the oxygen flow control knob is distinct in visual and tactile terms from the control knobs for the other gases (Figure 16-18).[69] The needle valve, which controls gas flow through the flowmeter, can be damaged if it is closed by excessive force. Valve stops (Figure 16-19) are usually incorporated to prevent damage. Note that there are no valve stops in the ADU needle valves. Flow increases when the knob is turned counterclockwise. All current gas machines use mechanical needle valves except Avance and Aisys, which use electronic controls for flow. On these machines, backup mechanical/pneumatic needle valves are present in case of electronic or electric failure.

Display of Fresh Gas Flow. An indicator float in a glass flowtube (Thorpe tube) is the classic way to capture and display fresh gas flow. Oxygen flow and concentration is calibrated to ±5% (or ±20 mL/min) accuracy at room temperature and 101.3 kPa.[53] Flowtubes are specific for each gas and cannot be interchanged. The flowtube is tapered to be narrower at its bottom.

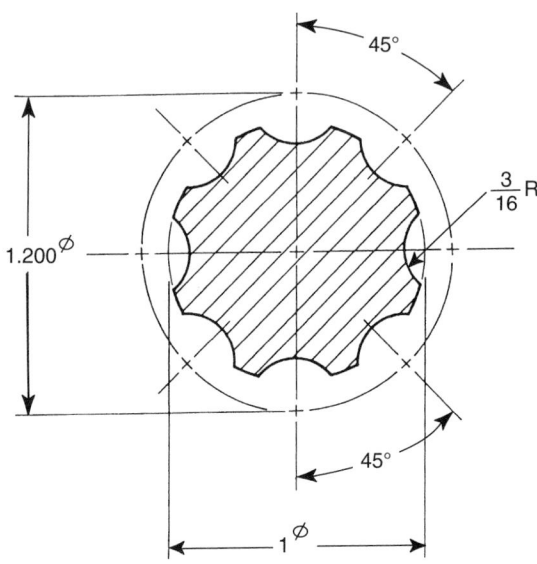

FIGURE **16-18** Oxygen knobs are touch coded to make them more distinct. *(From Schreiber P. Safety Guidelines for Anesthesia Systems. Telford, PA: Dräger; 1985.)*

Thus it may be referred to as a *variable orifice flowmeter* because the annular opening around the float is larger at higher flows. If a gas has two tubes, they are connected in series with a single control valve (Figure 16-20). It is standard in the United States (but not in the United Kingdom) for the oxygen flowtube to be placed to the right of other flowtubes. Flowmeters on the Fabius GS are unique in that they are arranged vertically, rather than side by side (Figure 16-21).[55,57] The flowtubes are the most fragile part of the machine. They are susceptible to breakage, leaks at their seals, and inaccuracy due to the presence of dirt or static electricity.[22]

Rather than using glass flowtube displays, many newer gas machines capture flows electronically by means of an anemometer or by a transducer and chamber of known volume. The chamber fills to a set pressure, and then the gas is allowed to proceed. The number of times this cycle occurs per minute can be converted to gas flow, which can be saved and sent to automated record keepers. These newer machines (for example ADU and Fabius GS) dispense with glass flowtubes, instead displaying fresh gas flows as colored bar graphs (with numeric data) on a computer screen. At the common gas outlet, both have a backup glass flowmeter, to measure total fresh gas flow continuously and in the event of screen or electrical power failure. The Narkomed 6400 uses regular glass flowtubes for display of flows but can capture flows electronically.

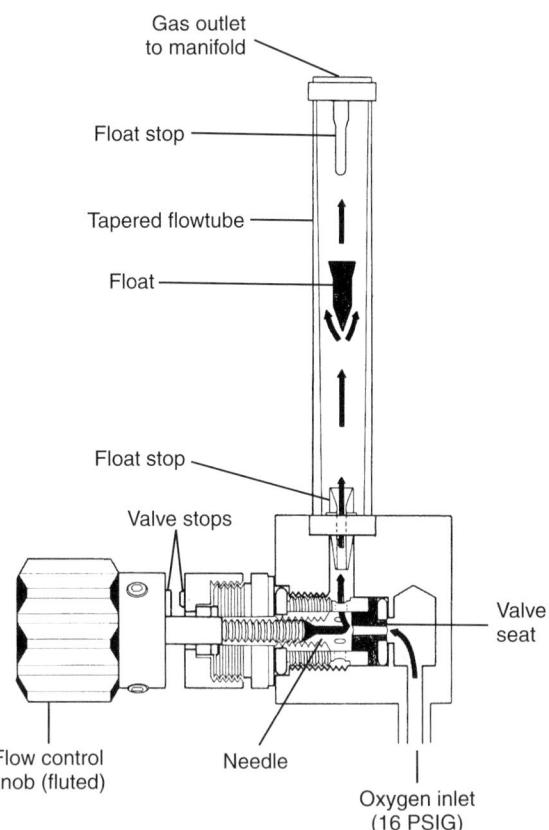

Gas outlet
to manifold

Float stop

Tapered flowtube

Float

Float stop

Valve stops

Valve
seat

Flow control
knob (fluted)

Needle

Oxygen inlet
(16 PSIG)

FIGURE **16-19** Flowmeter components. *(From Bowie E, Huffman LM: The Anesthesia Machine: Essentials for Understanding. Madison, WI: Datex-Ohmeda;1985.)*

Setting fresh gas flow on the Aisys and Avance is quite different. The flowmeter controls and display are all electronic. The display is numeric, with an optional bar-graph display. The user sets inspired oxygen concentration desired, the total fresh gas flow, and what carrier gas is desired (nitrous oxide or air) (see Figure 16-14).[53,54]

Care of Flowmeters. Flowmeters should be turned off before pipelines are connected, cylinders are opened, or the machine is turned on. If a flowtube is left open, the float will shoot to the top of a glass flowtube and may damage it. Flowmeters should be included in visual monitoring sweeps. Never adjust a flowmeter without looking at it. Read ball-type indicator floats in their center (Dräger) and plumb bob–type floats at the top (older Datex-Ohmeda). Remember to turn off flowmeters after each case and particularly at the end of the day. Failure to do so may contribute to premature drying of the carbon dioxide absorbent, which not only hastens its exhaustion but also has been implicated in the increase of the degradation of volatile agent, the generation of carbon monoxide in canisters, and canister fires.[70-74]

Other Flowmeters. Auxiliary oxygen flowmeters are an accessory currently offered on most models of gas machines. They are useful for attaching a nasal cannula or other supplemental oxygen delivery device. In the past, it was common to attach a nasal cannula to an adapter at the common gas outlet. The auxiliary oxygen flowmeter is advantageous because the breathing circuit and gas delivery hose (between the common gas outlet and breathing circuit) remain intact while supplemental oxygen is delivered to a spontaneously breathing patient. Thus if the anesthetist needs to switch from a nasal cannula to the circle breathing system during a case, he or she can accomplish this instantaneously and without the possibility of forgetting to

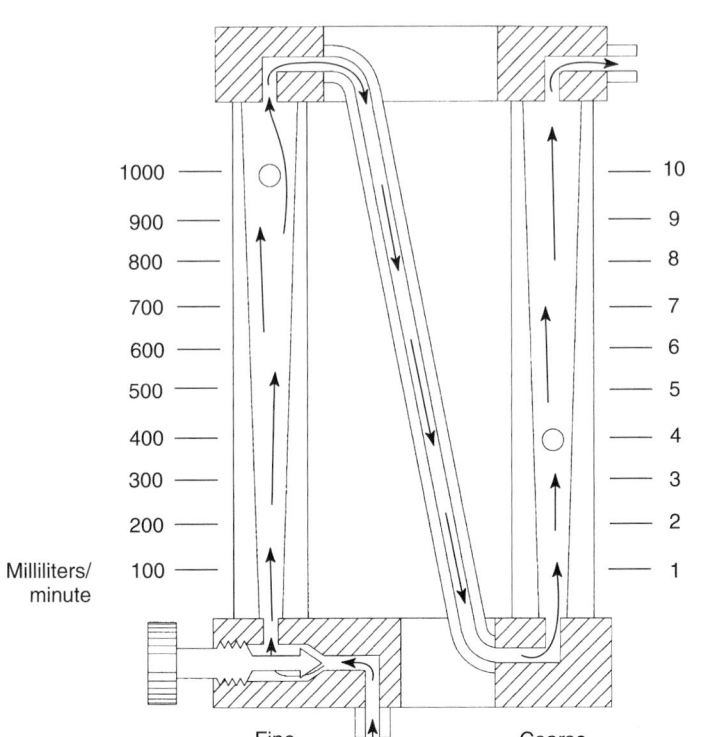

1000
900
800
700
600
500
400
300
200
100

10
9
8
7
6
5
4
3
2
1

Milliliters/
minute

Liters/
minute

Fine
flowtube

Coarse
flowtube

FIGURE **16-20** When two flowmeters are present for one gas, they are arranged in series. *(From Cicman J et al. Operating Principles of Narkomed Anesthesia Systems. Telford, PA: Dräger; 1993.)*

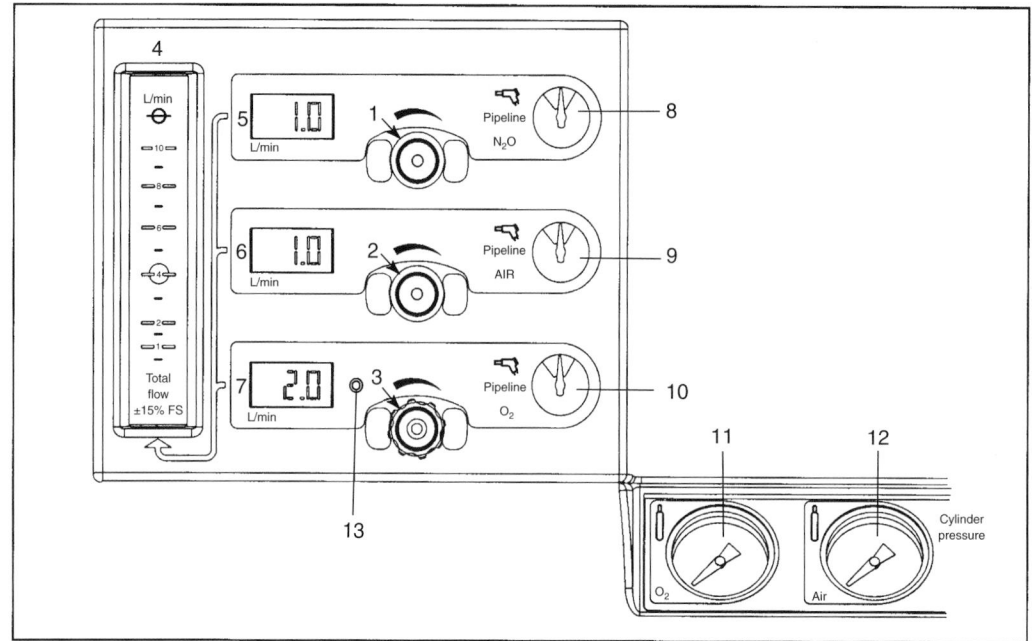

FIGURE **16-21**   Flowmeters on the Fabius GS are arranged vertically. The common gas outlet flowmeter is to the left (*marked 5*). Oxygen flowmeter is at the bottom of the bank, nitrous oxide at the top. To the left of each flow-control knob is a digital display of flow, to the right is the pipeline pressure gauge for each gas. Cylinder gauges are to the right. (*From* Fabius GS Operator's Instruction Manual. *Catalog No. 4117102-001. Telford, PA: Dräger; 2002.*)

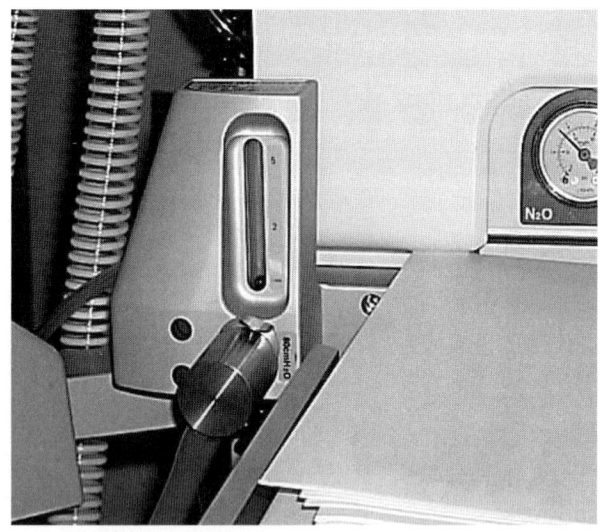

FIGURE **16-22**   The common gas outlet flowmeter on the ADU is located to the left of the writing surface. (*From* S/5 Anesthesia Delivery Unit User's Reference Manual. *Catalog No. 8502304. Madison, WI: Datex-Ohmeda; 2000.*)

reconfigure the breathing circuit properly. Another advantage is that an oxygen source is readily available for the Ambu bag if the patient needs to be ventilated manually for any reason during a case (for example, breathing circuit failure). One disadvantage is that the auxiliary flowmeter becomes unavailable if the pipeline supply has lost pressure or been contaminated;

this is because the auxiliary flowmeter is supplied by the same wall outlet and hose connection that supplies the main oxygen flowmeter. If users do not realize this, time could be wasted while they attempt to use this potential oxygen source.[75] Another disadvantage is that the fraction of inspired oxygen supplied cannot be varied with the auxiliary flowmeter. The chance of fire in sedated patients undergoing head and neck surgery can be lessened with reduced FiO_2, scavenging the oxygen, and tenting the drapes.[76]

Common gas outlet flowmeters (Figure 16-22) are used as a backup on gas machines that electronically capture and display flows on a computer screen. If offered as an option, they are strongly recommended; they are the only indication of oxygen flow if the computer display fails, or in a power-failure situation after battery backup is exhausted.

Scavenging flowmeters are used on most new machines that use scavenging interfaces. An indication that suction is adequate is mandatory with these systems to avoid exposure to waste anesthesia gases (see Disposal section). Unfortunately, the suction indicator may not be visible from the operator's normal position. On the Fabius GS, for example, it is on the back of the machine near the E cylinders.[55] It is behind and beneath the bellows block on the left side of the ADU (Figure 16-23).[50] Even though scavenging flowmeters are desirable, they may not be included with the basic package but only as an optional accessory (e.g., the ADU).

Oxygen Flush

The second task of oxygen in the processing area of the machine is to supply the oxygen flush valve. The flush valve is required by standard to deliver from 35 to 75 L/min.[21,77] The purpose of the flush valve is to quickly fill the breathing circuit with oxygen.

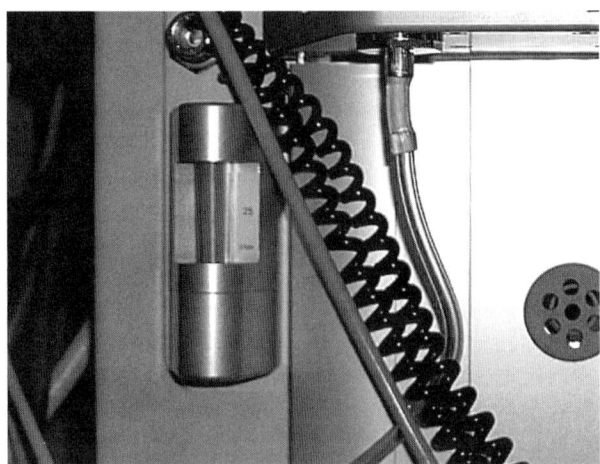

FIGURE **16-23** Scavenger suction flowmeter on ADU is located behind and beneath the bellows block on the left side of the machine.

The flush valve is often protected by a rim that lessens the chance of accidental activation of the flush. Should this occur, barotrauma can result. Users should avoid activating the flush while the ventilator is in use, particularly during the inspiratory phase; this is because the ventilator relief valve closes during this phase, preventing gas from exiting to the scavenger.[78] If flushing is necessary for filling the ventilator bellows, it may be done with caution, in short bursts, during the expiratory phase.

The oxygen flush line proceeds directly from the gas supply source to the common gas outlet (see Figure 16-1). Activating the flush bypasses the vaporizers and adds 100% oxygen to the breathing circuit. If partial pressures of nitrous oxide or volatile agent have already been established in the breathing circuit (during maintenance), excessive use of the oxygen flush tends to dilute these inhaled agents and may lessen the depth of anesthesia.

Fail-Safe Systems

If pipeline oxygen pressure fails, and other gases such as nitrous oxide keep flowing, the patient might receive a hypoxic gas mixture (less than 21% oxygen). Therefore, gas machines incorporate devices that halt the supply of nitrous oxide in the event of oxygen supply pressure failure. These are called *fail-safe systems*. It is required by standard that the set concentration of oxygen at the common gas outlet does not decline if the pipeline pressure decreases.[21] This requirement is satisfied by the presence of gatelike fail-safe valves in the internal supply line for nitrous oxide. The "gate" in each is held open by pressure in the oxygen line (Figure 16-24). Flow of nitrous oxide may be shut off with low oxygen pressure (Avance, Fabius GS) or proportionally decreased (Aestiva, ADU).[50,53,61,64,79] It is important to note that fail-safe systems do not analyze oxygen pipeline contents, so they would not be activated in a crossover, only if oxygen pipeline pressure is lost.

Fail-safe devices were once placed in air lines as well, with the rationale of leaving oxygen (however briefly) as the last gas flowing, even if oxygen pipeline pressure is lost. However, it is not possible to deliver a hypoxic mixture of air (and it is useful to drive ventilator bellows in case of oxygen pipeline pressure failure), so the trend is to place fail-safes in the nitrous oxide line only and rely on electronic proportioning systems to prevent hypoxic gas mixtures.

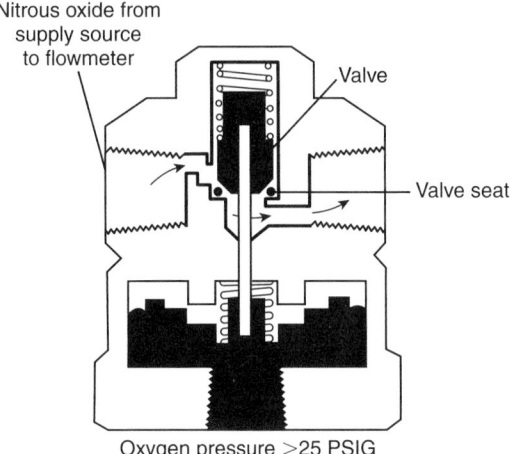

Oxygen pressure >25 PSIG

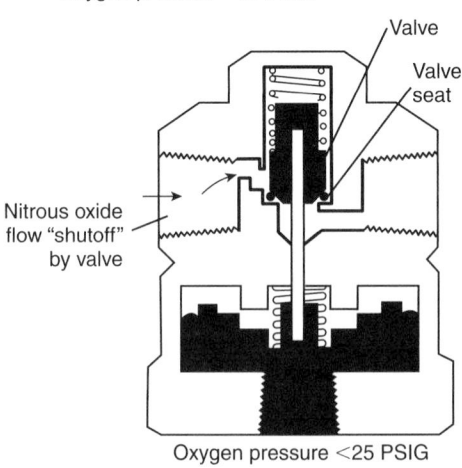

Oxygen pressure <25 PSIG

FIGURE **16-24** Pressure-sensor shutoff valve (fail-safe) in the nitrous oxide line. (*From Bowie E, Huffman LM: The Anesthesia Machine: Essentials for Understanding. Madison, WI: Datex-Ohmeda; 1985.*)

Low-Pressure Alarms

The fourth task of oxygen is powering the low-pressure alarms, which signal the operator when pressure is lost in the oxygen circuitry. The older oxygen supply failure alarm was a container with a whistle at its outlet that was pressurized by oxygen when the anesthesia gas machine was turned on. When pipeline pressure decreased to 28 psi, or when the machine was shut off, a characteristic and loud sound was heard as the container released its contents. Newer models lack this distinctive alarm, substituting a variety of visual and auditory alarms.[18,27,31] The proper response of the anesthetist to loss of pipeline pressure is discussed earlier in this chapter (see Supply section).

Ventilator Driving Gas

The fifth task of oxygen in many anesthesia gas machines is compression of the ventilator bellows. All GE Healthcare anesthesia ventilators use 100% oxygen as their driving gas.[64,79] The ADU may use either air or oxygen and will switch from oxygen to air automatically if oxygen pressure is lost.[50,79]

The older Dräger ventilators (AV-E, AV-2) used oxygen to drive a Venturi device, which augmented the driving gas with entrained room air.[80] Room air enters through a shiny (chrome or stainless steel) cylindrical muffler, which may be seen at the back of some Narkomed models. If this muffler becomes dirty, insufficient gas may enter; the lack can interfere with the ability of the ventilator to compress the bellows. If driving gas is prevented from exiting via the muffler, the bellows may remain compressed and barotrauma results.

Newer model piston ventilators use electric motors to compress the bellows and deliver tidal volume (Narkomed 6000/6400, Fabius GS, Apollo).[55-58,60] Thus ventilator delivery of tidal volume is unaffected by variation in oxygen pipeline pressure. Piston ventilators may operate for prolonged periods with only cylinder supplies of gases because they do not consume oxygen to drive the bellows.

Proportioning Systems (Hypoxic Guard)

All current anesthesia gas machines incorporate nitrous oxide–oxygen proportioning ("hypoxic guard") systems designed to prevent the delivery of hypoxic breathing mixtures. All link oxygen and nitrous oxide so that final breathing mixtures are at least 23% to 25% oxygen.* The ratio of nitrous oxide to oxygen is thus not more than 3:1.

An example of a pneumatic-mechanical proportioning system is the Link-25 (used on Aestiva and Aespire). In this system, the flowmeter control knobs for nitrous oxide and oxygen are linked by a chain; oxygen flow is increased automatically when nitrous

---

*References 53, 55-58, 60, 61, 64, 79

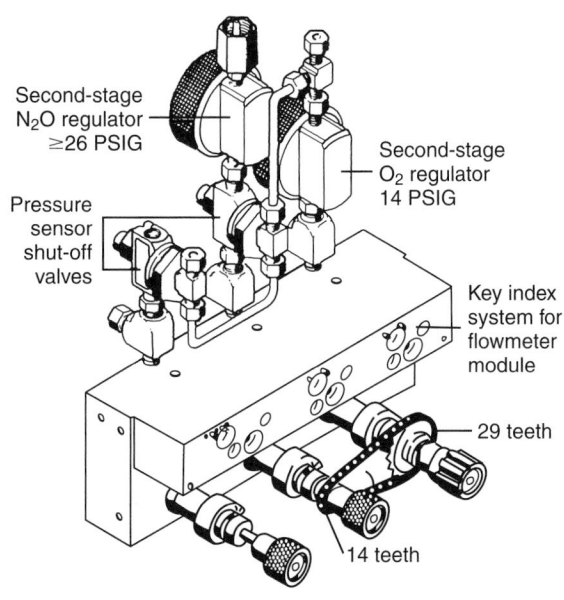

FIGURE 16-25 Link-25 proportioning system. (Courtesy of Datex-Ohmeda, Madison, WI.)

---

oxide flow is increased. The Link-25 system (Figure 16-25) also incorporates secondary regulators, so it has both pneumatic and mechanical components.

An alternative design is the electronic hypoxic guard system, the sensitive oxygen ratio controller (S-ORC; Apollo, Fabius, 6000).[60] This system also maintains at least 23% oxygen but does so by limiting nitrous oxide flow. Electronic alarms are incorporated, and the system includes a nitrous shutoff (so a fail-safe system is incorporated as well).

Hypoxic guard systems are not foolproof. Box 16-7 lists four situations in which a hypoxic breathing mixture can be delivered despite the use of these systems. Lack of oxygen in the oxygen pipeline may be detected with an oxygen analyzer. A system that is broken or defective[81] should be detected in the pre-use checklist, as should leaks downstream of the flowmeters. The most dangerous of these circumstances is the last, the administration of a third gas, especially that of an inert gas such as helium. It is not widely appreciated that the hypoxic guard systems link *only* nitrous oxide and oxygen. Perhaps because of the name, the assumption is made that *all* hypoxic breathing mixtures are prevented. These systems would *not* prevent the administration of a hypoxic mixture if a third inert gas (such as helium) is present on the gas machine. The proper use of a calibrated oxygen analyzer in each general anesthetic will always be of vital importance.

Many older Narkomed machines have a switch with two positions: "Nitrous Oxide–Oxygen" and "All Gases." In the Nitrous Oxide–Oxygen position, the hypoxic guard is active, and only these two gases may flow. In the All Gases position, the hypoxic guard and alarms are inactivated, and all gases (except nitrous oxide) may flow.[80]

Oxygen Analysis

Systems that warn of trouble with oxygen supply (supply failure alarms) or lessen the chances of hypoxemia (hypoxic guard system, fail-safe system) are based on *pressure* within the oxygen circuitry of the gas machine. They do *not* sample the oxygen lines to determine that *oxygen* is present. There is only one system that ensures that oxygen is present in the oxygen pipeline or cylinder: inspired oxygen analysis. Monitoring inspired oxygen is mandatory in every general anesthetic.[82]

Two types of sensors are in current use: electrochemical (galvanic fuel-cell; found in Aestiva, Aespire), and the paramagnetic analyzer (most others). The paramagnetic analyzer (Figure 16-26) has become more widely used because of its fast response, low cost, and extremely low maintenance requirements.[83]

BOX **16-7**

Circumstances Under Which Hypoxic Guard Systems Can Permit Formation of a Hypoxic Mixture

Wrong supply gas in oxygen pipeline or cylinder
Defective pneumatics or mechanics
Leaks downstream of flow control valves
Inert gas administration (e.g., a third gas such as helium)

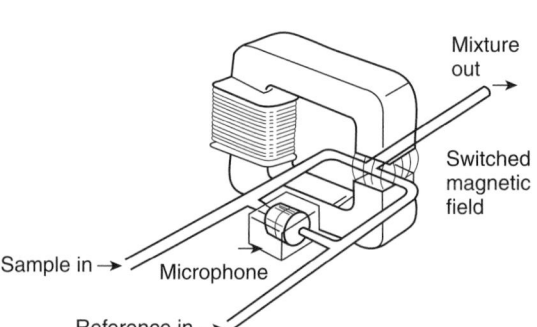

Figure **16-26** Paramagnetic oxygen analyzer. (Courtesy of Datex-Ohmeda, Madison, WI.)

A paramagnetic analyzer is often found in gas analysis (anesthetic agent and carbon dioxide) monitors.

Vaporizers

Underlying Physical Principles

A vapor is composed of molecules (in the gaseous phase) of a substance that is a liquid at room temperature and 1 atmosphere of pressure. Vaporization proceeds at a rate that depends on the physical characteristics of the vaporizing liquid and the temperature. Different liquids evaporate at different rates. Elevated temperature increases the rate of evaporation of any liquid, whereas decreased temperature slows the rate. As evaporation proceeds, the remaining liquid and its container cool because heat energy is carried from the liquid with the energetic, mobile, evaporating molecules. An example would be the cooling effect of evaporating perspiration or the chilling effect of evaporating gasoline or ether on the hand. In both cases, the molecules acquire the latent heat of vaporization from their surroundings. In the same way, one would expect an anesthetic vaporizer to cool as vaporization proceeds. This cooling limits the rate of further vaporization. To prevent this, materials such as copper are chosen for containing liquid anesthetics in current vaporizers. Copper has high thermal conductivity (transferring environmental heat easily to the liquid anesthetic) and high thermal capacity (acting as a thermal reservoir to help stabilize liquid anesthetic temperature).[22,84]

The rate of vaporization depends only on the temperature, the vapor pressure of the liquid, and the partial pressure of the vapor above the evaporating liquid—not on the ambient pressure of the remaining gases present. For example, water at constant temperature evaporates at the same rate into completely dry air whether it is at sea level, in a hyperbaric chamber, or at elevations far above sea level.

Classification and Design

Variable-Bypass. Table 16-2 presents a comparison of current variable-bypass vaporizers with heated-vapor types.[22,85-90] All vaporizers blend the combined flow of fresh gases from the flowmeters with sufficient vapor to form clinically useful concentrations. The problem is ensuring that the vapor concentration is appropriately limited. For example, a fully saturated isoflurane vapor consists of nearly 31% isoflurane (238 mm Hg [31 kPa], the saturated vapor pressure of isoflurane at 20° C divided by the

barometric pressure of 760 mm Hg [101 kPa]). To limit vapor output to a clinically useful concentration, only a small portion of the fresh gas flow is allowed to come into contact with the liquid and pick up anesthetic vapor.

The *splitting ratio* (gas entering the vaporizing chamber divided by total fresh gas flow) is automatically determined in a variable-bypass vaporizer by the internal resistance to flow; the operator merely has to set the control dial to the desired concentration (Figure 16-27). Setting the dial to a higher percentage increases the amount of flow sent through the vaporizing chamber. The small portion of the gas flow entering the vaporizing chamber ("carrier gas" or "chamber flow") flows over the liquid and picks up anesthetic vapor. Full saturation of the carrier gas is ensured by means of a series of wicks and baffles. This fully saturated (and thus known) concentration of carrier gas at the vaporizing chamber outlet is then diluted with the balance of the fresh gas that bypassed the vaporizing chamber ("bypass flow") to produce the desired final concentration at the vaporizer outlet.

A temperature-compensation device is built into variable-bypass vaporizers, so that more gas is directed into the vaporizing chamber as the vaporizer cools. Variable-bypass vaporizers are calibrated for concentration and are agent specific. Like the

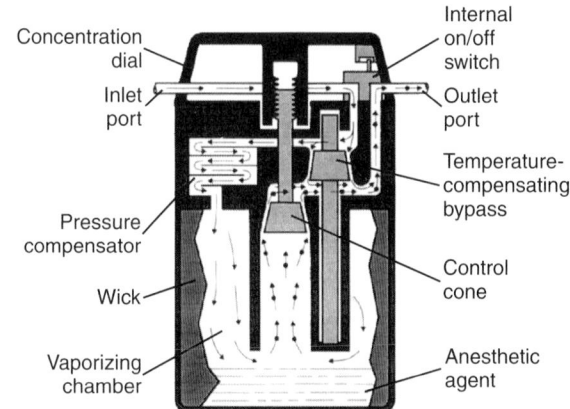

FIGURE **16-27** The Dräger Vapor 19 vaporizer. (*From Cicman J et al. Operating Principles of Narkomed Anesthesia Systems.* Telford, PA: Dräger; 1993.)

TABLE **16-2**	Classification of Vaporizers	
Characteristic	**Variable Bypass**	**Injector**
Example	Datex-Ohmeda Tec 4, 5, 7; ADU Aladin; Dräger Vapor 19, 2000	Datex-Ohmeda Tec 6 (Desflurane)
Splitting ratio (carrier gas flow)	Variable-bypass (vaporizer determines carrier gas split)	Dual-circuit (carrier gas is not split)
Method of vaporization	Flow-over	Gas/vapor blender (heat produces vapor, which is injected into fresh gas flow)
Temperature compensation	Automatic temperature compensation mechanism	Electrically heated to a constant temperature (39° C, thermostatically controlled)
Calibration	Calibrated, agent specific	Calibrated, agent specific
Position	Out of circuit	Out of circuit
Capacity	Tec 5, 300 mL; Tec 7, 225 mL; Vapor 19, 200 mL; Aladin, 250 mL	390 mL

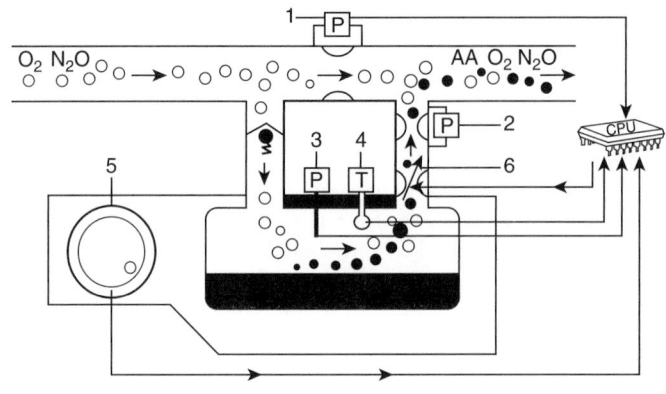

FIGURE **16-28** The ADU vaporizer. A microprocessor controls (6) and monitors (2) the vaporizer chamber flow, based on inputs of bypass flow (1), vaporizing chamber pressure (3), temperature (4), and the setting of the control dial (5). (*From S/5 Anesthesia Delivery Unit User's Reference Manual. Catalog No. 8502304. Madison, WI; Datex-Ohmeda; 2000*)

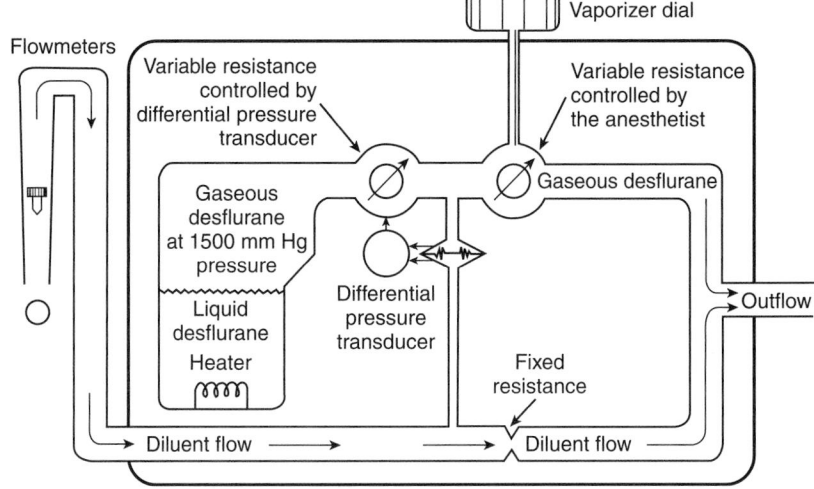

FIGURE **16-29** Principle of operation of the Datex-Ohmeda Tec 6 vaporizer. (*From The Datex-Ohmeda Tec 6 Vaporizer: For the Administration of Suprane (desflurane) [brochure with prescribing information]. Liberty Corner, NJ: Anaquest; 1992.*)

Tec 6, variable-bypass vaporizers are *out of circuit*, meaning they are out of the breathing circuit. Their capacities for liquid agent are listed in Table 16-2. Variable-bypass vaporizers in the ADU add microprocessor control, based on inputs from pressure or temperature sensors at various sites in the vaporizer (Figure 16-28).

Measured-Flow (Vernitrol). Anesthetists who practice in the military, or who use older equipment on mission trips outside of North America, may encounter *measured-flow* vaporizers. In a measured-flow vaporizer, the operator determines how much gas should be bubbled through the anesthetic liquid by means of a formula; this amount is then set on a second oxygen flowmeter, marked "Oxygen for Vernitrol." If the vaporizer cools, the operator must recalculate and set a new chamber gas flow; this is called *manual temperature compensation*. These devices can be used with multiple agents and are out of circuit. It is possible to use them safely, but their design is not as inherently safe as that of more modern types.[91] Measured-flow vaporizers are no longer manufactured in the United States, and factory service for them is no longer available. The military still trains anesthetists on the use of these vaporizers, and they may be seen overseas. They are not addressed in the current anesthesia gas machine standard.[21,91]

Tec 6 Injector. The Tec 6 vaporizer uses a completely different principle of operation as compared with variable-bypass types (Figure 16-29): it is a heated, dual-circuit vaporizer.[85,88,90,92-95] Fresh gas flow from the common manifold passes through the vaporizer in one circuit. This fresh gas never flows over or comes into contact with the liquid agent. Instead, an appropriate amount of vapor is added to the fresh gas flowing through the vaporizer. The second (vapor) circuit has two control points. One is the setting on the concentration control dial, the other is keyed to a transducer that is responsive to the amount of fresh gas flow. Thus more vapor is delivered from the vapor circuit if either the desired volume-percent setting or the fresh gas flow is increased. To maintain a known vapor pressure in the second circuit, the Tec 6 is heated to 39° C; this produces a vapor pressure of approximately 1500 mm Hg (200 kPa). Desflurane is near boiling at room temperature; if it were placed in a variable-bypass vaporizer, it would constitute nearly 100% of the output at first, and a hypoxic breathing mixture would result.[96]

The output of modern vaporizers may be influenced by extremes of fresh gas flow, extremes of temperature, or back pressure from the breathing circuit and ventilator. Current vaporizers function accurately over a wide range of settings at various

TABLE **16-3**	Accuracy of Current Vaporizers*					
Characteristic	**Datex-Ohmeda Tec 4**	**Datex-Ohmeda Tec 5**	**Datex-Ohmeda Tec 6**	**Datex-Ohmeda Tec 7**	**Dräger Vapor 19.3**	**Datex-Ohmeda Aladin (ADU)**
Fresh gas flow (L/min)	0.2-10	0.2-15	0.2-10	0.2-15	0.25-15	0.2-8
Temperature (° C)	20-35	17-35	18-30	18-35	15-35	18-25

The vaporizers listed function accurately within the ranges specified.

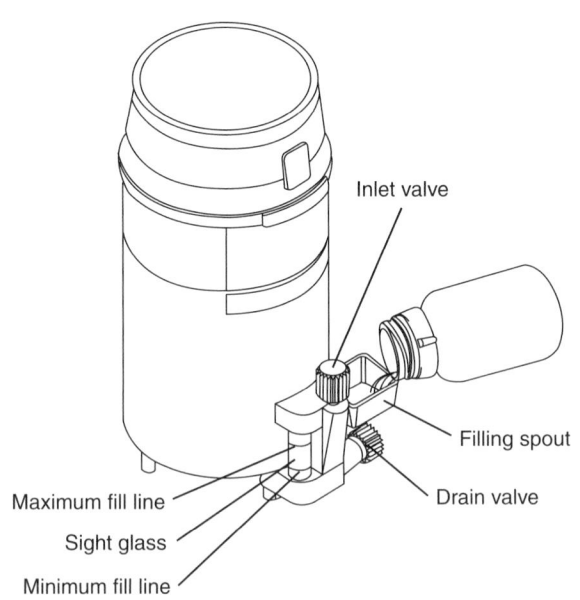

FIGURE **16-30** Filling a vaporizer with a funnel-type filling system. (*From* Narkomed 2C Anesthesia System—Setup and Installation Manual. *Telford, PA: Dräger; 1994.*)

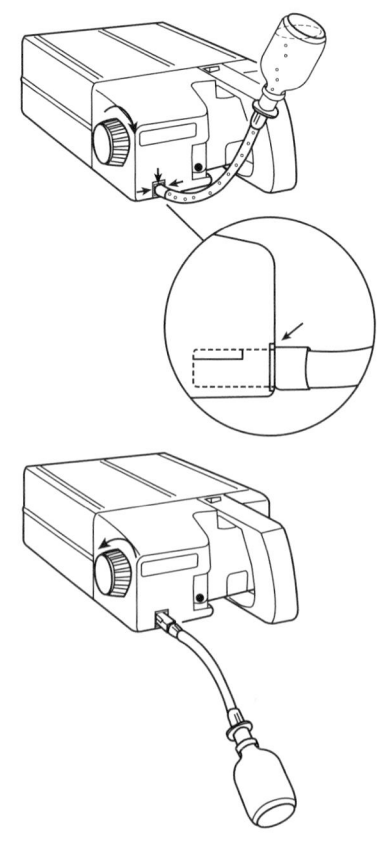

FIGURE **16-31** Filling a vaporizer with a keyed-filler system. (*From S/ 5 Anesthesia Delivery Unit User's Reference Manual. Catalog No. 8502304. Madison, WI: Datex-Ohmeda; 2000.*)

ambient temperatures and fresh gas flows (Table 16-3).[86-90,92,97] Furthermore, they are more resistant than previous models to the effects of intermittent back pressure (the so-called "pumping effect") that increases vaporizer output. This can be accomplished by incorporating unidirectional valves at the vaporizing chamber inlet or outlet, or distal to the vaporizer.

Using Vaporizers

Contemporary vaporizers are secured to the anesthesia machine in manifolds that hold two or three units. The operator is prevented from delivering more than one agent simultaneously by an interlock system. The interlock ensures that only one vaporizer is on, that gas enters only the one that is on, that all vaporizers are locked in so that leaks are decreased, and that trace vapor output is minimal when a vaporizer is off.[98]

Variable-bypass and Tec 6 vaporizers are all filled in a similar fashion. Funnel-type (Figure 16-30) and keyed-filler-type (Figure 16-31) systems are permitted by standard.[21] Keyed-filler types are preferred because their use lessens the chance that filling with the wrong agent will occur (although it is still possible).[99,100] The standard requires that overfilling be prevented in the normal operating position and that liquid level indicators be visible to the operator.[21,101] These indicators usually take the form of a sight glass with two etched lines corresponding to low and maximum liquid levels within the

vaporizer. To fill either the funnel-type or keyed-filler vaporizers, the anesthetist should turn the vaporizer off, check the anesthetic liquid (to ensure that the agent and the vaporizer match) and then pour it in. The vaporizer is full when the liquid level reaches the maximum line on the sight glass.[97,101] It is a misconception that while using the keyed-filler vaporizer, one should hold the bottle up until it stops bubbling. If the vaporizer is turned on, is not horizontal, or the keyed-filler device is not perfectly tight on the bottle, this method results in overfilling.[102] Overfilling may result in discharge of liquid anesthetic from the vaporizer outlet, which has caused patient injuries.[22] The Tec 6 uses a similar system, but the desflurane bottle has a permanently attached, non-interchangeable spout. The sight glass on the Tec 6 is a liquid crystal display that indicates when the level of liquid is low enough to allow the addition of a full bottle, and it shows when the sump is full. Although the Tec 6 vaporizer is unique in that it can be filled while in operation,[88] it is safe to turn it off momentarily to do so. All variable-bypass vaporizers *must* be shut off while they are being filled.[55,56,86,87,97,102]

Models

The Dräger Vapor 19 fits in a manifold with an interlock system. If a vaporizer is removed from the machine, a short-circuit block must be added for leaks to be prevented. The interlock continues to protect against simultaneous inhaled agent administration, regardless of which vaporizer is removed. There is no check valve between the vaporizer outlets and the common gas outlet in Dräger anesthesia gas machines. The Vapor 19 has a button that must be depressed before the control dial can be turned on. All contemporary vaporizers are designed to increase agent concentration as the dial is turned counterclockwise (as viewed from above).

The Dräger Vapor 2000 (Figure 16-32) is similar to the Vapor 19, except that is removable by hand. It has a unique "T" (transport) setting that allows the vaporizer to be tipped or transported.

The Datex-Ohmeda Tec 7 is a variable-bypass vaporizer similar to the older Tec 4 and 5. It is designed to require less frequent and less complicated service.

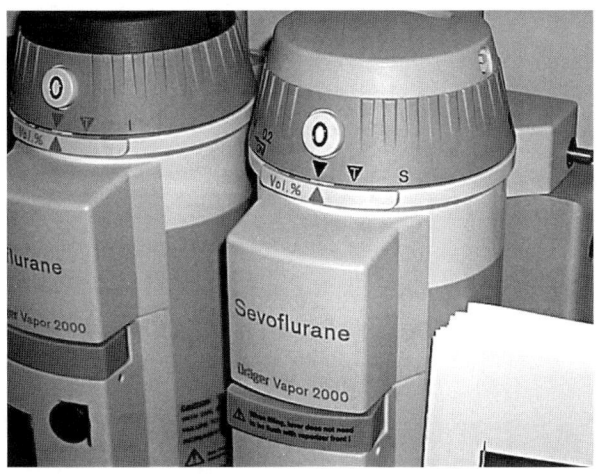

FIGURE **16-32** The Dräger Vapor 2000. Note the "T" (transport) setting to the right of "0."

Use of the Datex-Ohmeda Tec 6 vaporizer is unique, as could be suspected from its unique principle of operation. However, it is not difficult to use. Filling the Tec 6 has been described in general terms. The operator must check the desflurane bottle to ensure that it is the right agent, push it into the vaporizer firmly, and rotate it upward until the display indicates that the vaporizer is full. The operator then rotates the bottle downward and holds it for an instant (to allow any drops to drain back into it). Finally, he or she supports the bottle while withdrawing it from the vaporizer (Figure 16-33).[88]

The operator turns the Tec 6 vaporizer on by turning the concentration control dial to the "On" position while depressing the dial release located opposite the zero indicator (which is on the front of the dial). The vaporizer requires electric power and a warm-up period of approximately 10 minutes before it can be used.[88]

The Tec 6 has several visual indicators that are grouped in a status display (Figure 16-34).[88] These include a light that indicates "Operational" status, a "No Output" indicator light (and audible alarm), a "Low Agent" light (and audible alarm), a "Warm-Up" status light, and an "Alarm Battery Low" light. The No Output alarms are activated if the agent level is less than 20 mL, if the vaporizer is tilted more than 10 degrees from the vertical, if there is a power failure lasting longer than 10 seconds, or if an internal malfunction occurs. The cause of a No Output alarm may be sought if it occurs during a case; however, considering the rapid emergence that is characteristic with the use of desflurane, the operator should ensure the continued depth of anesthesia by switching to a different agent without undue delay.

Preoperative checkout for variable-bypass vaporizers is relatively straightforward. They are checked to determine whether they are turned off, whether they are full, whether the filling cap is tightly closed, and whether the interlock is functioning. Depending on the machine, they may need to be checked for leaks as well.[44] The Tec 6 requires a more extensive checkout. After performing the appropriate leak test of the machine low pressure system, the operator checks the amber Alarm Battery Low indicator and replaces the battery if necessary. Next, he or she turns the Tec 6 on to at least 1%, and disconnects its electrical plug. Within 15 seconds of disconnection, the No Output

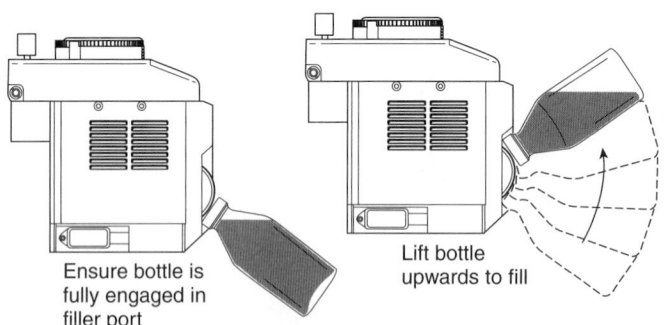

Ensure bottle is fully engaged in filler port

Lift bottle upwards to fill

FIGURE **16-33** Filling the Datex-Ohmeda Tec 6 vaporizer. (*From* Tec 6 Vaporizer: Operation and Maintenance Manual. *Madison, WI: Datex-Ohmeda; 1993.*)

light and alarm should activate. If they do not, the battery must be replaced and the vaporizer retested before use. If everything is functioning correctly, the operator reconnects the power and turns the dial to the "Off" position; he or she then presses the mute button for 4 seconds to test all alarms and the display. When the mute button is pressed, all lights and the alarm should activate.[88]

The Aladin (ADU) vaporizer uses one central electronic control mechanism for all agents.[50,90] Cassettes containing the volatile liquid anesthetic are inserted into a port connected to these control mechanisms, which recognizes the contents of the cassette and dispenses agent into the stream of fresh gas flow (Figure 16-35). The cassettes and control mechanisms are checked as part of the electronic equipment checklist daily. The ADU will not deliver volatile agent or nitrous oxide without main power or battery backup and adequate oxygen pressure.

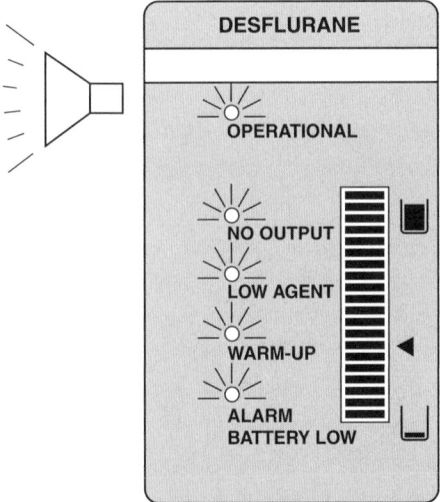

FIGURE **16-34** Display panel of the Datex-Ohmeda Tec 6 vaporizer. (*From Tec 6 Vaporizer: Operation and Maintenance Manual. Madison, WI: Datex-Ohmeda; 1993.*)

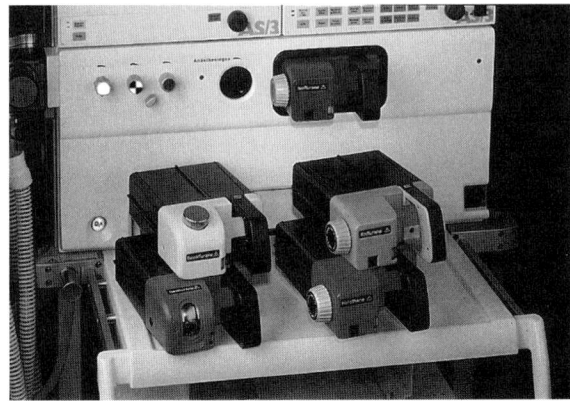

FIGURE **16-35** Datex-Ohmeda ADU vaporizer cassettes. The isoflurane cassette is plugged into the vaporizer port, and controls may be adjusted with the control wheel to the left of the port. (*Courtesy of Datex-Ohmeda, Tewksbury, MA.*)

Hazards of Contemporary Vaporizers

Many of the hazards historically associated with the use of vaporizers have been corrected by advances in design, but a few hazards remain (Box 16-8). Vaporizer contamination with incorrect agents continues to be noted.[99,100] Diligence during filling is not enough to prevent contamination. Departments should strongly consider replacing funnel-type with keyed-filler vaporizers in equipment purchases. If a vaporizer tips by more than 45 degrees from vertical, the operator's manual or a field service technician must be consulted. Tipping is hazardous because the entry of liquid agent into the control assembly at the top of the vaporizer can have unpredictable effects on its function. The vaporizer sump can be drained and gas run through it for a specified time and at a specified concentration before the vaporizer is returned to use. For the recommended corrective action for a particular make and model, the operator's manual must be consulted.

Overfilling may be prevented by following the manufacturer's guidelines for filling (e.g., fill only to the top etched line on the liquid level indicator glass, fill only when the vaporizer is off).[101] Managers should not conclude, in this era of cost constraints, that breath-by-breath agent analysis can substitute for regular preventive maintenance of vaporizers. Vaporizers go out of calibration and may then deliver too-high or too-low concentrations of agent.[103] Leaks are relatively common, often due to malposition of vaporizers on the back bar, accidental dislodgement, loss of gaskets, or mechanical damage,[104-107] and these leaks may not be detected with the standard checklist unless the negative pressure check is performed. Tec 6 vaporizers can also leak liquid while being filled if the desflurane bottle is missing the rubber O-ring near its tip.[108] This can be mistaken for a defective vaporizer. As vaporizers incorporate electronics, they are susceptible to electronic failure or unanticipated interactions of new designs with each other.[105,109,110] Recent case reports detail ADU vaporizers failing due to fresh gas unit failure and from copious emesis soaking the machine.[111,112]

New Agents and Low Flows

Low fresh gas flows should not be instituted too early when desflurane or sevoflurane is used. Induction at low flows would be extremely prolonged, creating the risk of awareness in the time interval between induction and onset of action of the volatile agent. Overpressure can be combined with low flows, but 18% of 2 L contains fewer desflurane molecules than 18% of 6 L, and it is the number of molecules presented to the brain per unit time that causes an increase in anesthetic tension within the brain.

Imagine a 1000-mL sink filled with water, with 100 mL/min inflow (of which 1 mL is methylene blue) and 100 mL/min outflow. The goal is turning the initially colorless water in the sink as blue as the inflow solution. Now, imagine the effect of increasing

BOX **16-8**

Hazards of Modern Vaporizers

Incorrect agent administration
Tipping
Overfilling with agent
Reliance on breath-by-breath gas analysis rather than
  preventive maintenance
Leaks
Electronic failures

the inflow to 500 mL/min (of which 5 mL is methylene blue) and increasing the outflow to 500 mL/min. Would the 1000 mL in the sink turn blue any faster in the second case? Of course, but not because the concentrations are different (both inflows are 1% methylene blue) but rather because the rate of inflow in the second example is a greater proportion of the capacity.

Wash-in is based on the concept of a time constant. One time constant (equal to capacity divided by flow) brings a system 63% of the way to equilibrium; two time constants to 86%; and three time constants to 95%. Thus, the first sink will reach 63% of equilibrium in 10 minutes (1000 mL ÷ 100-mL flow), whereas the second sink reaches this same state of equilibrium in only 2 minutes (1000 mL ÷ 500-mL flow). In the same way, the volume (capacity) of the functional residual capacity, hoses, and breathing circuit can be brought to equilibrium with the inflow more quickly as the rate of inflow increases. A rational approach for ensuring anesthesia that conserves volatile agents would include a nonrebreathing (semiopen) induction (fresh gas flow, 5 to 8 L/min) followed by a low-flow maintenance (fresh gas flow, 1 to 2 L/min). This approach helps conserve tracheal heat and humidity, gases, and agent. Emergence, like induction, must occur at higher, nonrebreathing flows; otherwise, it will be unacceptably prolonged.

DELIVERY

This section will discuss how the flow of gases to and from the patient is controlled and monitored.

Breathing Circuits
Fundamental Considerations

The purpose of all types of anesthesia breathing circuits is the delivery of oxygen and anesthetic and the elimination of carbon dioxide. Carbon dioxide is eliminated from the breathing circuit by washout with adequate fresh gas flow or by absorption in carbon dioxide absorbent granules.

Any breathing circuit creates some resistance to gas flow. Resistance in a circuit may be minimized by reducing the circuit's length and increasing its diameter, by avoiding the use of sharp bends, by eliminating valves, and by maintaining laminar flow. It is important to decrease resistance to flow, because added airway resistance is uncomfortable for the conscious patient. Furthermore, the unconscious or anesthetized patient challenged by the increased work of breathing may not be able to increase respiratory effort and may hypoventilate. The resistance of the anesthesia breathing circuit is low—typically less than that of an endotracheal tube.

Rebreathing of exhaled gases occurs with the use of anesthesia breathing circuits (as it does in space or submarine environments), but it is not found with other breathing circuits, such as those in the ventilators used in intensive care units. Rebreathing may be useful. Its advantages include cost reduction, an increase in tracheal warmth and humidity, and a decrease in the potential for exposure of operating room personnel to trace and waste gases (because of decreased rate of release of anesthetic gases into the environment). The degree of rebreathing in an anesthesia breathing circuit is increased as the fresh gas flow is decreased because there is relatively less fresh gas added to the circuit, and more of the next inhalation will be exhaled gas. Higher fresh gas flow is associated with less rebreathing in any type of circuit. The higher the fresh gas flow, the more quickly the composition of gas in the breathing circuit will resemble that at the common gas outlet (the dialed-in concentrations of agent, N_2O, and O_2).

Patients under anesthesia may rebreathe any component of their exhalations—nitrogen, O_2, CO_2, N_2O, and volatile agent. The effects of rebreathing each of these components differ. Rebreathing of exhaled oxygen has no ill effects. Rebreathing of exhaled nitrogen slows induction. Nitrogen that is not eliminated from the breathing circuit delays the establishment of the desired agent concentration; thus high fresh gas flows are appropriate during induction. In contrast, rebreathing of exhaled agent during maintenance is highly desirable for cost and environmental considerations. Rebreathing of CO_2 has the undesirable effect of producing respiratory acidosis, so it is best avoided. Because higher flows reduce the discrepancy between desired concentrations and the concentrations actually inspired, they are appropriate during emergence as well. At the end of an anesthetic, as the flow of volatile agent and N_2O is turned off, it would be undesirable for exhaled agent and N_2O to be rebreathed because this would delay emergence. So gas that is free of agent (and nitrous oxide) is supplied at high flow to create a favorable concentration gradient that speeds elimination of agents from the body.

Dead space is increased to some degree with the use of any respiratory equipment. The effect of an increase in mechanical (apparatus) dead space is that rebreathing of exhaled CO_2 is more likely. This is one reason that ventilator tidal volumes are set much larger than the volume of a spontaneous breath. To avoid hypercarbia in the face of an acute increase in dead space, a patient must increase minute ventilation (V_E). Conversely, because alveolar ventilation is the minute ventilation minus dead space ventilation ($V_A = V_E - V_D$), if the patient's minute ventilation is fixed, increasing dead space decreases alveolar ventilation and increases arterial CO_2 tension.[113] Dead space ends where the inspiratory and expiratory gas streams diverge. In a circle system, dead space ends at the Y-piece. Use of a face mask is associated with greater dead space than is the use of an endotracheal tube.

The anesthesia gas machine uses dry gases so that the problems of internal corrosion and bacterial colonization are avoided. However, provision of completely dry gases to the patient's airway can cause various problems. It is common for anesthesia providers to use various means of passively humidifying and heating inspired gases (with a heat and moisture exchanger and by using low fresh gas flows). Active humidification has become less common because it is less effective at preventing hypothermia than heated-air surface warming blankets, and because the added moisture can clog gas-analysis lines and soda lime granules or obstruct unidirectional valves.[114]

Anesthesia breathing circuits are unique among respiratory equipment in the degree to which they allow manipulation of the inspired concentration of a variety of components for therapeutic benefit. Each component of the breathing mixture follows its own concentration gradient as it is made to wash in or out of the breathing system, and then to wash in or out of the breathing system into the patient's lungs. In the lungs, gases flow down their concentration gradients, interchanging with pulmonary and blood gases. Understanding the pharmacokinetics of inhaled agent administration involves not only knowledge of respiratory physiology, but also familiarity with the "physiology" of the patient-machine system. For example, the concentration set on the dial differs from the concentrations in the breathing circuit, in the lungs, in the blood, and in the brain. Furthermore, these concentration differences are not constant but vary over time, depending on a number of patient- and machine-related factors. The concentration inspired most closely resembles that delivered

TABLE **16-4**			Classification of Breathing Circuits
Type	**Reservoir**	**Rebreathing**	**Example**
Open	No	No	Open drop, insufflation, nasal cannula
Semi-open	Yes	No	Circle at high fresh gas flow (more than minute ventilation); or a nonrebreathing circuit
Semi-closed	Yes	Yes (partial)	Circle at low fresh gas flow (less than minute ventilation)
Closed	Yes	Yes (complete)	Circle at extremely low fresh gas flow, with adjustable pressure-limiting valve closed

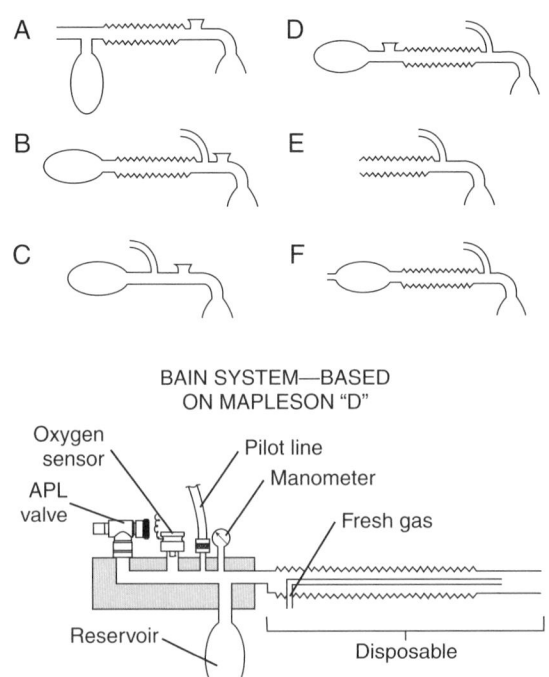

BAIN SYSTEM—BASED
ON MAPLESON "D"

FIGURE **16-36** Mapleson's classification of breathing systems. (*From Cicman J et al. Operating Principles of Narkomed Anesthesia Systems. Telford, PA: Dräger; 1993.*)

BOX **16-9**

Common Features of Nonrebreathing Systems

All lack unidirectional valves.
All lack soda lime carbon dioxide absorption.
Amount of rebreathing is highly dependent on fresh gas flow in all.
Amount of resistance is low in all (no unidirectional valves).

---

from the common gas outlet when rebreathing is minimal or absent (this is typical at high fresh gas flow). Of course, it is desirable that the alveolar concentration differ from the inspired concentration at times. At the start of the emergence phase, the inspired concentration of anesthetic is decreased so that anesthetic gas is washed out while ventilation is continued. Thus emergence is very different from merely "waking up," and is as much an active process as induction.

Classification of Breathing Circuits

Table 16-4 gives a classification of breathing circuits that is based on whether a reservoir (breathing bag) is present and on the degree to which rebreathing occurs.[115] Patients have access to the atmosphere only in open systems; this is not true in semi-open, semi-closed, or closed systems. A reservoir is present in these three types to provide for the moments during the inspiratory phase when flow in the trachea is greater than fresh gas flow. Both nonrebreathing (Mapleson, Bain) systems and the circle system, at fresh gas flows greater than minute ventilation, are semi-open.[116] If the fresh gas flow to the circle system is less than $\dot{V}_E$, some rebreathing must be occurring. In a closed

system, rebreathing is total. The adjustable pressure-limiting (APL or "popoff") valve is closed, and the supply of O_2, N_2O, and agent just matches the patient's uptake.[117]

Nonrebreathing Circuits. Mapleson published a classification of nonrebreathing circuits in 1954; this classification is still used today (Figure 16-36).[118] Rebreathing is prevented in systems like the Mapleson D because during the expiratory pause, fresh gas fills the corrugated limb, forcing the previously exhaled gas distally (toward the reservoir). If fresh gas flow is sufficient, no alveolar gas is rebreathed. The Mapleson F circuit is also referred to as the *Jackson-Rees modification of Ayre's T-piece.* The common features of nonrebreathing systems are listed in Box 16-9. These circuits offer very low resistance to breathing and can be used for patients of almost any age, from premature infants to adults. The fresh gas flow required to prevent rebreathing is two to three times minute ventilation.[22] This number can be calculated; however, in practice, many use a minimum fresh gas flow of 5 L/min.

The Bain system, shown at the bottom of the figure, often is referred to as a *modified Mapleson D circuit,* because the arrangement of its components (entry point of fresh gas, reservoir bag, and APL valve) is similar to that of the Mapleson D. However, in the Bain system the fresh gas hose is directed coaxially within the corrugated limb, and this configuration gives the inhaled gases greater heat and humidity. Unfortunately, unrecognized kinking or disconnection of this relatively hidden fresh gas hose converts the entire corrugated limb into dead space.[119] The resulting respiratory acidosis has been associated with arrhythmias.[120] Users of Bain systems must test the circuit for these problems before they use the system. Pethick's test and a similar test are available and should be used.[22]

The popularity of the nonrebreathing type of circuit has declined for several reasons. Many modern gas machines are not designed to accommodate them (e.g., Fabius GS or Narkomed 6000). It is more common to see a pediatric circle system used, which is characterized by smaller and less compliant corrugated limbs as compared with the adult circle system. The minimum weight of a child for which a pediatric circle would be suitable is approximately 10 to 20 kg. No one guideline applies to all situations because the decision on whether to use a pediatric circle system in any given child depends on familiarity, clinical judgment, and the anticipated duration of unassisted respiration. Pediatric circle systems do not place undue burdens (in terms of work of breathing) on spontaneously ventilating patients.[121] The pediatric circle system is low compliance; the work of breathing associated with it is reasonable; it requires less reconfiguration to set up; and it allows the use of lower fresh gas flows (the high fresh gas flow required in nonrebreathing circuits cools children and is more costly).[122] Modern ventilators are accurate to very low tidal volumes (10 to 20 mL), and modern monitoring such as capnography and spirometry allows a high degree of confidence that a child is being ventilated adequately with the pediatric circle. If a nonrebreathing circuit is used in the middle of a number of adult cases using the circle system, some disassembly and reassembly is required, accompanied by the possibility of error or misconnection. The small amount of resistance offered by the soda lime canisters and unidirectional valves of the circle system is deleterious only during spontaneous respiration, which is limited in duration in most general anesthesia for children. The advantages and disadvantages of nonrebreathing circuits are summarized in Box 16-10. Although they are useful, nonrebreathing circuits are associated with loss of heat from the patient and with greater use of volatile agents, owing to their requirement for relatively high fresh gas flow.

Circle System. The circle system is the breathing circuit most commonly used in the United States, because it prevents rebreathing of carbon dioxide while allowing rebreathing of all other gases. Gas flow during mechanical ventilator inspiration is shown in Figure 16-37, and during ventilator expiration in Figure 16-38.

A coaxial circle system is also available in which like the Bain, the inspiratory limb is contained within the expiratory (Figure 16-39). It is checked and used like any circle system. Like the Bain, the coaxial circle is less bulky and is thought to provide greater heat and humidity to inhaled gases.

Disadvantages include the potential for obstruction or lack of patency of either limb, which may cause respiratory acidosis or even mimic esophageal intubation.[119,123] This respiratory acidosis does not respond to increased minute ventilation—if exhaled gases are not forced through the absorbent granules, no amount of ventilation will cleanse carbon dioxide from the exhaled gases. The tests for inner tube patency that can be used for a Bain circuit are not readily adaptable to the coaxial circle system.

Gas enters the circle system from the common gas outlet by way of the fresh gas delivery hose, and it exits the circle via the APL valve (or the ventilator relief valve if mechanical ventilation is used) to the scavenger. The APL valve creates an adjustable leak during manual ventilation. If it is completely open and the bag is squeezed, all gas exits to the scavenger, because this is the path of least resistance. If the valve is completely closed, all gas ventilates the lungs. The setting of the APL is constantly adjusted during manual ventilation of the lungs so that a variable resistance sufficient to force gas to inflate the lungs is maintained. If gas cannot exit through the APL or ventilator relief valve, pressure will build within the system.[124]

Unidirectional valves enforce a pattern of gas flow by which exhalations are made to pass through the CO_2 absorbent granules (Figure 16-40). The valve leaflet (disk) is subject to damage, occlusion, foreign body contamination, and sticking with collected moisture or absorbent dust, particularly on the expiratory valve disk.[125-128] Daily performance of a preanesthesia checklist and regular maintenance should enable the operator to detect most of these problems. There are only two common reasons for an increase in inspired CO_2: absorbent granules have been exhausted, or unidirectional valves are faulty. Figure 16-41 shows that incompetence of an inspiratory or expiratory valve turns the entire corrugated limb into dead space.[129] This usually results in an increase in inspired and expired CO_2.

If inspired CO_2 of more than 1 to 3 mm Hg is detected on the capnograph (Figure 16-42 and Figure 16-43), the fresh gas flow should be increased to 5 to 8 L/min; this converts the system to a semi-open configuration in which rebreathing of exhaled gases is minimized. If this causes the inspired CO_2 to decrease substantially, the absorbent granules are exhausted and should be replaced at the end of the case. Some gas machines (ADU, others) with prepackaged granules or canisters allow granules to be changed during the case, although they are not meant to function for more than very brief periods without a canister attached. If elevated inspired CO_2 persists in spite of the higher fresh gas flow, the unidirectional valves are likely to be incompetent. The operator should remove the expiratory valve, inspect and dry it, and then reassemble it (while ventilating the patient with an Ambu bag).[22,127] Note that this may be more difficult in newer absorber heads (e.g., the ADU) as compared with older and will always be more difficult when the user has never performed it before. This argues for reading the operator's manual and practicing without a patient attached before the maneuver is attempted because failure to reassemble the valve quickly will result in hypoventilation and interruption in volatile anesthetic delivery. Perhaps the best recommendation is to bring a new gas machine into the room; any valve adjustment can take place outside the pressure of the clinical situation and will not distract the anesthetist from patient care.

It is mandatory to check unidirectional valves before use. There are a multitude of means proposed to check the

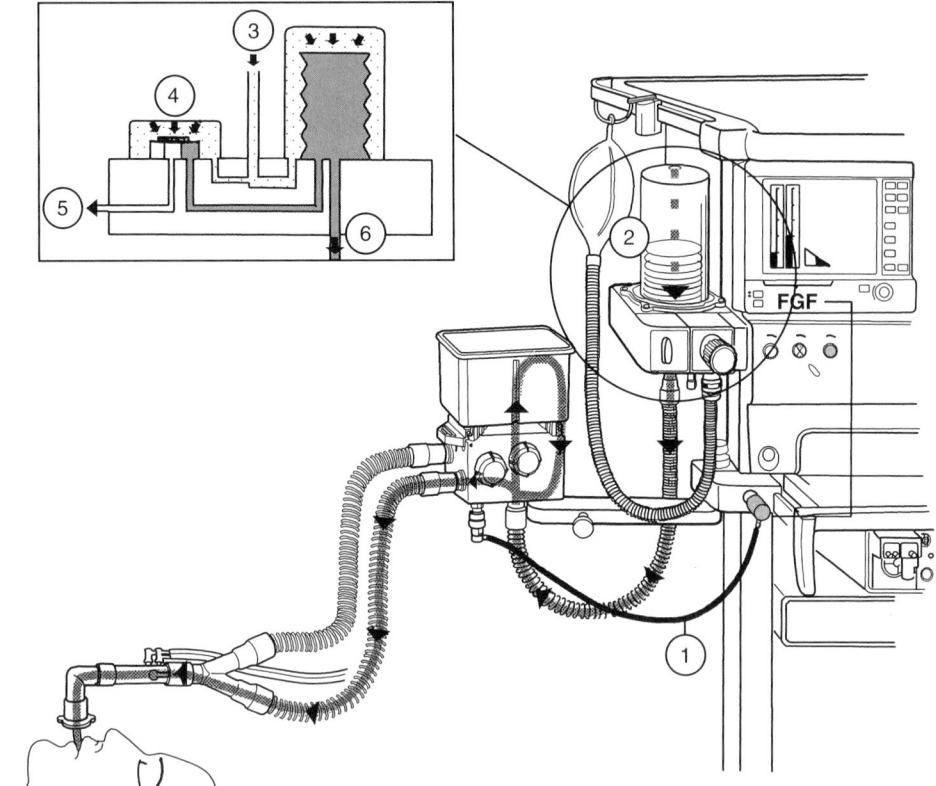

FIGURE **16-37** Gas flow in a circle system during mechanical ventilator inspiration. *(1)* Hose from common gas outlet to absorber head (which contains attachments for disposable breathing circuit hoses, inspiratory and expiratory unidirectional valves, and CO_2 absorbent granules). *(2)* Bellows block with Manual/Auto switch, APL valve, and manual breathing bag. *(3)* Ventilator driving gas. *(4)* Ventilator relief valve (pathway to scavenging, which is closed during inspiration). *(5)* Pathway for exhaled gas to scavenger interface. *(6)* Pathway for gas to patient. *(From S/5 Anesthesia Delivery Unit User's Reference Manual. Catalog No. 8502304. Madison, WI: Datex-Ohmeda; 2000.)*

unidirectional valves, which vary in ease of performance and complexity.* One suggested method with applicability to a variety of gas machines follows. The daily check of the unidirectional valves is done during the ventilator checkout. A reservoir bag is placed on the elbow fitting at the patient's end of the Y-piece, and mechanical ventilation of this "artificial lung" is begun. The user carefully observes that the valves lift and fall, and the bellows and artificial lung fluctuate in a to-and-fro fashion as expected during the appropriate phase of ventilation.[50] Breathing through the elbow or mask of a clean circuit (with a paper mask on) is an alternative method but presents problems of cross-contamination. Breathing through the circle has a second advantage; it checks for obstruction to expiration secondary to mold flash or plastic wrap emboli, problems that have resulted in mortality.[127,131-133] Dräger suggests a similar test but also breathing through each limb individually as follows.[55,56] If the inspiratory limb is detached and occluded with one's palm, the operator should be able to exhale, but *not* inhale, through the expiratory limb. Similarly, if the inspiratory limb is replaced and the expiratory limb detached and occluded, the operator should be able to inspire, but *not* expire, through the inspiratory

limb. This test may be more sensitive than the first test mentioned. If a preanesthesia check is performed daily, the capnograph is used properly, and the operator is aware of the steps that should be taken in the event of an increase in inspired CO_2, perhaps this more rigorous test need be performed only if unidirectional valve function is in doubt, particularly because it is problematic to perform the more rigorous test in a hygienic fashion.

Newer machines have electronic routines to check for leaks and compliance. This helps the ventilator accurately deliver the desired tidal volume. These checks must be repeated when the type of circuit is changed, for example, from adult to pediatric. Dräger does not recommend expandable breathing circuit hoses with the Narkomed 6000 because their volume and compliance may change after the leak and compliance testing is performed, which will degrade the accuracy of the delivered tidal volume.[56] With any newer gas machine, these hoses should be expanded before the leak and compliance test is initiated.

The advantages and disadvantages of the circle system are listed in Box 16-11. One advantage of at least partial rebreathing is relative constancy of inspired concentrations. In a completely nonrebreathing circuit, each breath is fresh gas, so depth can vary much more quickly. The use of lower flows also reduces the rate of release of anesthetic agents into the environment. The circle conserves respiratory tract humidity.

*References 55, 56, 80, 125, 127, 130.

Misconnections, although a potential disadvantage, occur much less frequently now than in the past because the diameter of breathing hoses (22 mm) has been standardized to be different from the diameter of scavenger hoses (19 or 30 mm).[21] Nevertheless, misconnections continue to be reported.[134,135] Maintenance of the circle system is detailed in the operator's manuals, that must be consulted before one disassembles and cleans the absorber head.

Several design changes in newer circle systems facilitate low-flow anesthesia. Low fresh gas flow is desirable to reduce pollution and cost of using volatile agents and nitrous oxide, preserve tracheal heat and moisture, delay the drying of carbon dioxide absorbent granules, and preserve patient body temperature. Factors that enhance the safety and efficiency of low flows in modern circle breathing systems and ventilators are shown in Box 16-12. A traditional-sized absorber head like the Aestiva is roughly twice the volume of many of the newer designs. Circles with smaller volume will have shorter time constants. The time constant equals capacity divided by flow, and measures how quickly a breathing system reaches equilibrium with a change in the inflow. In a circle system with lower volume, changes in dialed concentration of agent will be reflected more quickly in the inspired concentration at any flow rate, as compared to a higher volume circle system. In a nonrebreathing circuit, or a circle system at flows substantially higher than minute ventilation, each breath reflects the dialed concentration of agent because there is no rebreathing of exhaled gases in either. Thus a circle system with higher flows is suitable when rapid changes are desired, such as at induction and emergence.

There are, however, circumstances in which to avoid low flows (fresh gas flow 1 L/min).[136] Absolute contraindications include patients with smoke inhalation injury, malignant hyperthermia, or other conditions in which washout of potentially dangerous gases or a high oxygen uptake is expected. Any time equipment breakdown that would affect the safety of low flows occurs mid-case (i.e., inspired oxygen or anesthetic agent monitors or failure of soda lime granules), higher flows should be used. Relative contraindications include when using older equipment that is less leak proof; face mask anesthesia; and during rigid bronchoscopy or with uncuffed endotracheal tubes.[136]

Humidification and prevention of nosocomial infection are desirable with the use of any respiratory apparatus. Both of these goals may be addressed with breathing circuit filters that incorporate heat and moisture exchange with filtration (HMEF).[137] The use of low flows during maintenance results in an increase

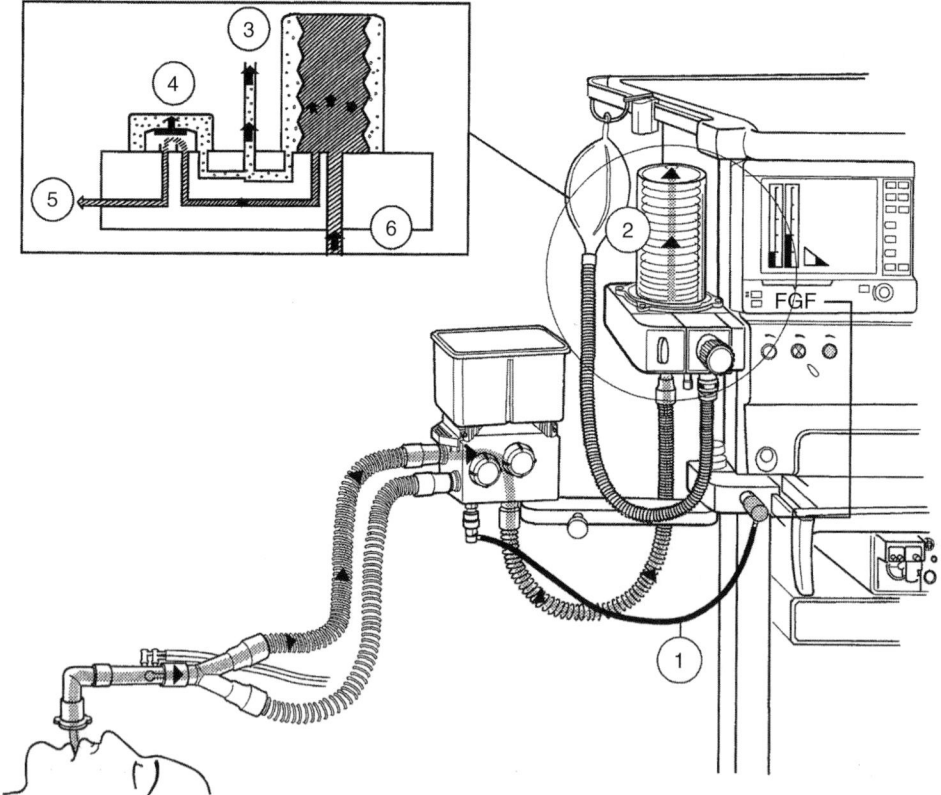

FIGURE **16-38** Gas flow in a circle system during mechanical ventilator expiration. The ventilator relief valve was held shut during inspiration. When the driving gas flow ceases, the patient's exhalation fills the bellows. Once the pressure within the bellows reaches +2 to 3 cm water, the ventilator relief valve opens, and any excess gas can exit to the scavenger. (*1*) Hose from common gas outlet to absorber head. (*2*) Bellows block (bellows refilling with patient's exhalation). (*3*) Ventilator driving gas pressure released as it leaves upper section of bellows. (*4*) Ventilator relief valve (pathway to scavenging, open during expiration). (*5*) Exhaled gas passing to scavenger interface. (*6*) Gas from patient. (*From S/5 Anesthesia Delivery Unit User's Reference Manual. Catalog No. 8502304. Madison, WI: Datex-Ohmeda; 2000.*)

in circuit humidity and a lower rate of use of volatile agents. Heat- and moisture-exchanging filters precipitate exhaled water vapor on their filter media. The next inhalation returns this water to the patient. These filters may slow the rate of heat loss from the patient because they decrease the rate of evaporation of water from the tracheal mucosa. They may also confer the benefit of bacterial and viral filtration.[138,139] Cleaning the bellows is necessary after anesthesia has been provided to a patient with a disease transmitted by air or oral secretions. To limit contamination of the machine, consider avoiding the mechanical ventilator, using bacterial/viral filters on the Y-piece or on each limb, and changing the soda lime after the case.

The Standards for Nurse Anesthesia Practice call on anesthetists to use safety precautions to minimize the risk of infection for the patient, the anesthetist, and other staff.[140,141] It is certain that anesthesia equipment (and providers) is contaminated with potential pathogens.[142] Furthermore, many of the surfaces of the anesthesia gas machine and monitors have been shown to be contaminated with blood—visible and occult.[143] It is therefore mandatory to ensure that departmental cleaning and sterilization programs are adequate, that "good housekeeping" during administration of anesthesia is practiced, and that universal precautions are observed. For equipment, the American Association of Nurse Anesthetists advocates a classification system and specific equipment recommendations that are published in their *Infection Control Guide*.[141] In addition, manufacturers include directions for cleaning and sterilizing equipment in their operation and maintenance manuals.

Electrically heated (active) humidifiers are no longer used. Problems associated with heated humidifiers included overhydration, underhydration, hypothermia, hyperthermia, melting of disposable breathing circuits, aspiration, interference with gas analysis accuracy (clogged lines or sensors) and infection.[144]

Carbon Dioxide Absorption

Carbon dioxide absorption makes rebreathing of exhalations possible. Thus it conserves agent, gases, and humidity, while preventing the respiratory acidosis that would result from the rebreathing of CO_2.

Gas flows set on the flowmeters determine the amount of rebreathing in the circle system. A circle system with fresh gas flows of 0.3 to 0.5 L/min provides near-total rebreathing and full reliance on absorbent for prevention of rebreathing of CO_2. At the other extreme, use of a circle system with fresh gas flows above minute ventilation (greater than 5 to 8 L/min for a traditional large, dual-canister absorber head) is associated with little if any reliance on absorbent granules because exhaled carbon dioxide is rapidly diluted and sent to the scavenger with such high fresh gas inflows.[116,145] This relationship can be confusing. When faced with exhausted granules, which cause an increase in expired (and inspired) CO_2, one may be tempted to increase V_E. This approach is ineffective if the absorbent has been exhausted (even though it is the obvious response for controlling hypercarbia from other causes), because the patient simply inspires more of a gas mixture containing CO_2. The correct response to hypercarbia associated with absorbent exhaustion is increasing fresh gas flow (then changing the absorbent at the end of the case).

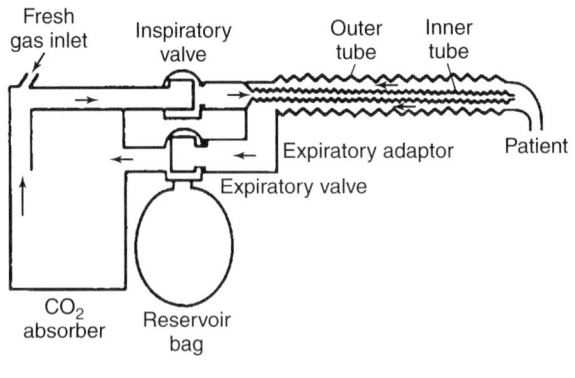

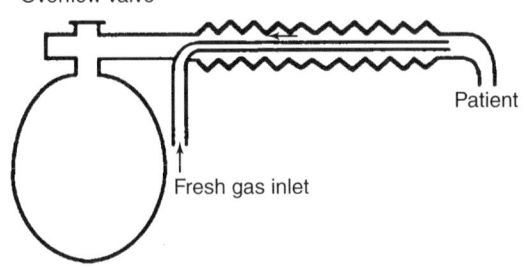

FIGURE **16-39** In the coaxial circle system (*top*), the inspiratory limb is contained within the expiratory limb, like the Bain (*bottom*).

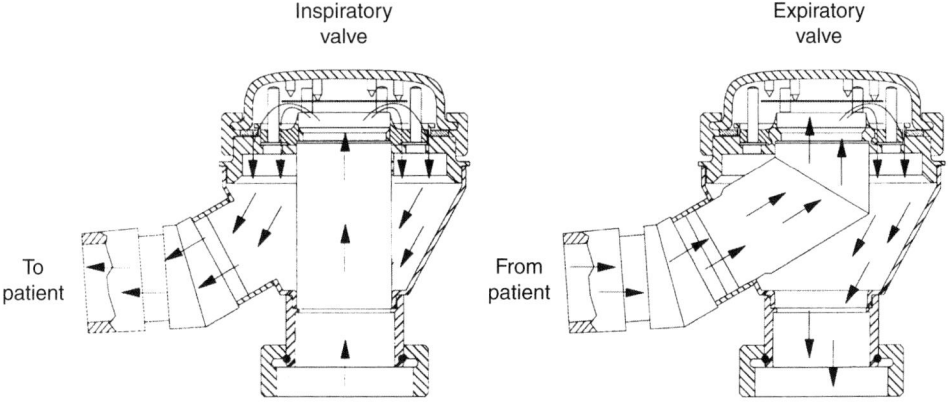

FIGURE **16-40** Gas flows in inspiratory and expiratory unidirectional valves. (*From Cicman J et al. Operating Principles of Narkomed Anesthesia Systems. Telford, PA: Dräger; 1993.*)

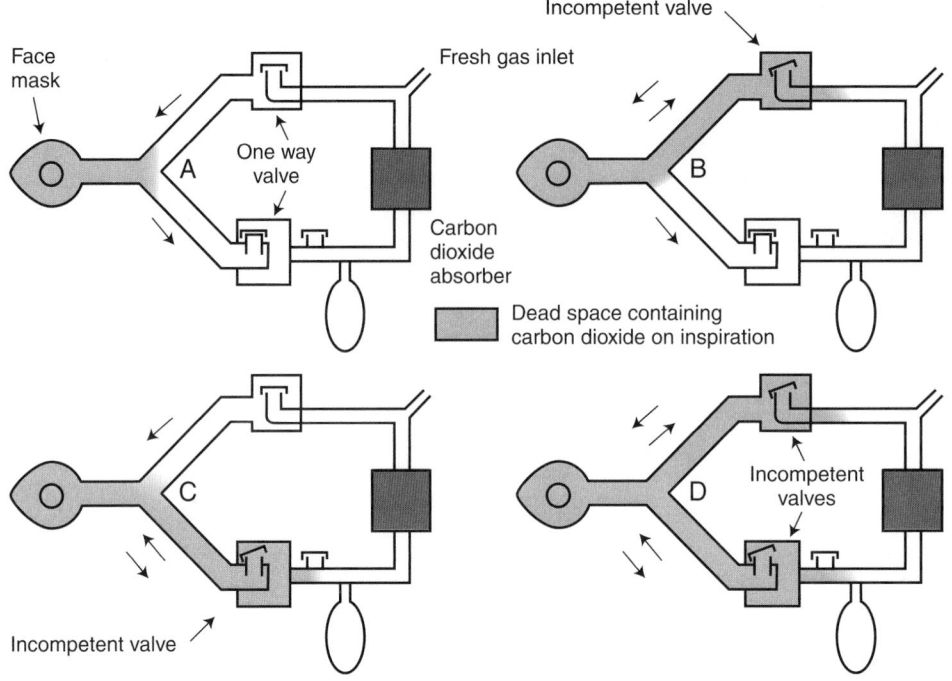

FIGURE **16-41**   Incompetence of a unidirectional valve. **A,** Normal function. Incompetence of an inspiratory valve **(B),** an expiratory valve **(C),** or of both unidirectional valves **(D)** creates dead space (*stippled area*) that extends through the entire ipsilateral corrugated breathing hose. (*Modified from Gravenstein JS et al.* Capnography in Clinical Practice. *Boston: Butterworth; 1989.*)

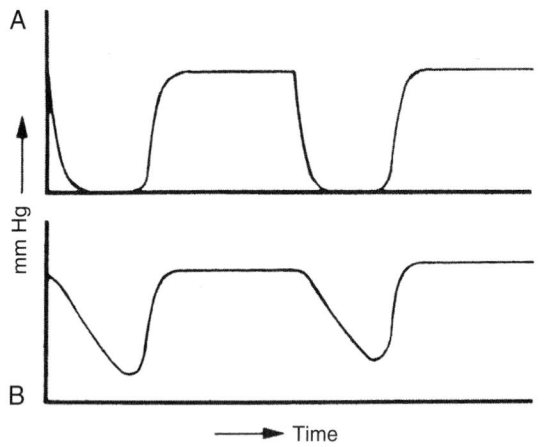

FIGURE **16-42**   Compared with a normal capnogram (A), a capnogram recorded when the inspiratory unidirectional valve is incompetent (B) shows increases in inhaled and exhaled carbon dioxide pressure and an abnormally prolonged downstroke. The prolonged downstroke during the inspiratory phase occurs because the patient inspires mixed alveolar and fresh gas from the inspiratory limb rather than fresh gas alone. (*Modified from Gravenstein JS et al.* Capnography in Clinical Practice. *Boston: Butterworth; 1989.*)

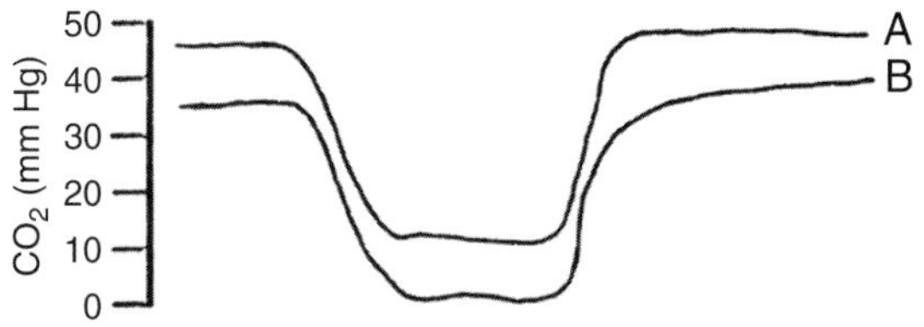

FIGURE **16-43**   Compared with a normal capnogram (A), a capnogram recorded with an incompetent expiratory unidirectional valve (B) shows increases in inspired and expired carbon dioxide concentration but no changes in morphology. (*Modified from Gravenstein JS et al.* Capnography in Clinical Practice. *Boston: Butterworth; 1989.*)

Chemistry

The chemistry of soda lime CO_2 absorption is shown in Box 16-13 (barium hydroxide lime is not shown because it has been withdrawn from the North American market by its manufacturer).[22,113] The ionic reactions take place in the aqueous medium on the surface of the granules. An appropriate water content (10% to 20%) is important for the speed and efficiency of the reactions. Dry granules become exhausted much more quickly than moist granules. Activators (NaOH, KOH) are added to increase the speed of the reaction. They combine with carbonate ions or CO_2 in a reversible reaction that produces water and energy. The absorption of 1 mole of CO_2 produces 13,000 kcal of heat energy.[113] Absorbents contain ethyl violet as an additive. The ethyl violet serves as an indicator of absorbent pH. Fresh CO_2 absorbent has a caustic alkaline pH because of the sodium hydroxide. As the reactions proceed, the pH becomes less alkaline. At a critical pH of 10.3, the ethyl violet changes from colorless to blue-purple.

Soda lime does not *regenerate* to any extent; in other words, it does not regain capacity to absorb CO_2 during periods when it is not in use. Its capacity is similar whether it is used continuously or intermittently. However, it does exhibit some *color reversion* (a change in appearance from blue-purple to white) during a rest period. The color of the absorbent at the beginning of the day may not reflect its remaining capacity because of this color reversion.[113] When a subsequent anesthetic is begun, the color of absorbent that had not seemed exhausted initially may quickly change to blue-purple. Therefore it is recommended that the user judge the degree of color change at the end of each case and change the canister before the next case if necessary.[113]

Soda Lime

The characteristics of soda lime and other selected absorbents are listed in Table 16-5.[73,146-148] The main constituent of all is calcium hydroxide. Hardeners (silica and kieselguhr) may be added to soda lime. Soda lime is manufactured to have a water content between 13% and 20% by weight. The size of all absorbent granules is 4 to 8 mesh, meaning they will pass through screens with 4 to 8 holes per linear inch. The selection of granule size involves a compromise between resistance to flow and absorption efficiency. Larger granules have less resistance to gas flow; however, they are also less efficient because their surface area is relatively small with respect to their mass. Fine granules or soda lime dust would have a great deal of resistance to gas flow, but their efficiency would be high because of their increased surface area.

Soda lime degrades most current volatile agents to some extent,[50,73] with sevoflurane degraded most and desflurane least. Degradation may produce compound A (sevoflurane), carbon monoxide (the ethyl methyl ethers), and other compounds. Degradation is favored by desiccated absorbent and the presence and quantity of strong bases (potassium hydroxide more than sodium hydroxide).[73,148-153] Sevoflurane may be degraded so much at low flows in desiccated barium hydroxide lime that it is impossible to attain 1 MAC in the breathing circuit, regardless of the dial setting.[154]

Sevoflurane is unstable in soda lime, producing compound A. Compound A is lethal at 130 to 340 ppm, and may cause renal injury at 25 to 50 ppm in rats. Compound A concentrations of 25 to 50 ppm are easily achievable in normal clinical practice. The incidence of toxic (hepatic or renal) or lethal effects in millions of humans are comparable to desflurane.[155] The product insert does not recommend sevoflurane at total fresh gas flows less than 1 to 2 L/min for more than 2 MAC-hours.[156] The production of compound A may be affected by the particular gas machine used.[152]

Carbon monoxide is produced by desflurane much more than isoflurane when these agents are in contact with absorbent granules. Halothane and sevoflurane produce little if any carbon monoxide. Production of carbon monoxide is greatest in dry absorbent, or with barium hydroxide lime as compared with soda lime. It is recommended that oxygen be turned off at the end of each case, absorbents changed regularly (particularly if fresh gas flow is left on over the weekend or overnight), and low flows used (this will tend to keep granules moist). Current recommendations for avoiding problems with carbon monoxide are summarized in Box 16-14.[70,147,154,157-159]

New Absorbents Lacking Strong Bases

The strong bases (the activators NaOH, and particularly KOH) have been convincingly implicated in the carbon monoxide problem with the ethyl methyl ethers and the generation of compound A by sevoflurane. Many absorbents available in

TABLE 16-5	Characteristics of Absorbents			
Component	**Sodasorb (WR Grace)**	**Medisorb (GE Medical)**	**Drägersorb 800 Plus (Dräger Medical)**	**Amsorb Plus (Armstrong Medical)**
$Ca(OH)_2$ %	50-100	70-80	75-83	>80
NaOH %	3.7	<3.5	1-3	0
KOH %	0	0	0	0
$CaCl_2$ % (humectant)	—	—	—	1
$CaSO_4$ and Polyvinylpyrrolidine % (hardener)	—	—	—	1
Water content %	15-17	16-20	~16	13-18
Size (mesh)	4-8	4-8	4-8	4-8
Indicator	Yes	Yes	Yes	Yes

Data from APSF Newsl. 2005;2:25-29; Anesth Analg. 2001;93:221-225; Anesthesiology. 2001;95:1205-1212; Anesth Analg 2000;91:220-224.
$Ca(OH)_2$, Calcium hydroxide; NaOH, sodium hydroxide; KOH, potassium hydroxide; $CaCl_2$, calcium chloride; $CaSO_4$, calcium sulfate. Numbers are approximations which may not sum to 100%.

BOX **16-14**

Recommendations on the Safe Use of Carbon Dioxide Absorbents

1. Use carbon dioxide absorbents with lower (or no) amounts of strong bases (particularly potassium hydroxide; KOH).
2. Create institutional, hospital, and/or departmental policies regarding steps to prevent desiccation of the carbon dioxide absorbent.
3. Turn off all gas flow when the machine is not in use.
4. Change the absorbent regularly—on Monday morning, for instance.
5. Change absorbent whenever the color change indicates exhaustion.
6. Change all absorbent, not just one canister in a two-canister system.
7. Change absorbent when uncertain of the state of hydration, such as if the fresh gas flow has been left on for an extensive or indeterminate time period.
8. If compact canisters are used, consider changing them more frequently.
9. Low flows also have a role in preserving humidity in absorbent granules. Use relatively low fresh gas flows for the majority of procedures, changing flows from high to low as soon as practical in any given case (after the patient has attained maintenance levels of volatile anesthetic).

North America lack KOH and may have reduced amounts of NaOH (see Table 16-5). Eliminating both activators (Amsorb Plus [Armstrong Medical Ltd., Coleraine Northern Ireland]) produces an absorbent that has similar physical characteristics and carbon dioxide absorption efficiency (the second is controversial) as compared with soda lime.[73,146,160] Lithium hydroxide is also an effective carbon dioxide absorbent.

Because of the controversial efficiency of absorbents that lack all strong bases, absorbents have been developed with reduced

NaOH and no KOH (see Table 16-5). The goal is to maintain efficiency while lessening the production of by-products. Dräger Medical makes an absorbent with decreased amounts of NaOH and no KOH: Drägersorb 800 Plus. GE Medical includes Medisorb, which lacks KOH, in the prefilled canisters for all their gas machines (i.e., ADU, Aestiva).

Using Carbon Dioxide Absorbents

Certain similarities are apparent with all absorbents. The resistance of filled canisters in a circle system is low (less than 1.5 cm H_2O at a flow rate of 100 L/min). Resistance of other breathing circuit components, particularly the endotracheal tube, is greater.[113] Inhaled dust is caustic and is an irritant, and its presence may lead to laryngospasm, bronchospasm, and pneumonia.[113] A trap for water and dust that prevents the passage of dust toward the patient may be incorporated distal to the granules in the circle systems; if present, it must be emptied periodically. In addition, when the breathing circuit is pressurized for check-out, the pressure should be released through the APL valve, rather than through the elbow at the patient's end. This technique not only prevents the propulsion of dust toward the patient but also is useful to check APL valve function.

Absorbent efficiency is decreased by channeling and the wall effect.[160,161] The amount of CO_2 absorbed varies throughout the canister. The inside edge of the canister is a low-resistance pathway. Exhaled gas follows this pathway or other low-resistance pathways through the canister, forming channels whose capacity to absorb CO_2 is exhausted before the capacity of the bulk of the absorbent is used. Thus the wall effect and channeling produce exhaustion of absorbent before its theoretic capacity has been reached. Efforts for preventing these two effects include shaking the canister before installation in the circle system to promote uniform packing throughout.[113]

Exhaustion and Replacement of Canisters

The clinical signs of absorbent exhaustion are shown in Box 16-15. Some of these signs (e.g., hyperventilation) may be masked in the anesthetized patient. In practice, capnography and indicator color change are primary indications of exhaustion. It is unwise to rely on color change or canister temperature

Clinical Signs of Carbon Dioxide Absorbent Exhaustion

Early

Increase in partial pressure of end-tidal carbon dioxide; may be accompanied by an increase in inspired carbon dioxide
Respiratory acidosis
Hyperventilation
Signs of sympathetic nervous system activation (flushed appearance, cardiac irregularities, sweating)
Increased bleeding at surgical site
Color of indicator

Late

Increase (and later a decrease) in heart rate and blood pressure
Dysrhythmia

General Steps for Changing Carbon Dioxide Absorbent Canisters

Protect eyes and skin with goggles and gloves.
Note purple color, date last changed, or both.
Loosen clamp or screw.
Remove and discard top canister.
Remove plastic wrap and seals from new canister.
Insert new canister on bottom and old bottom canister on top.
Retighten screw.
Check breathing circuit for leaks.

NOTE: *Do not change canister in the middle of a case; convert to semi-open with 5 L/min fresh gas flow.*

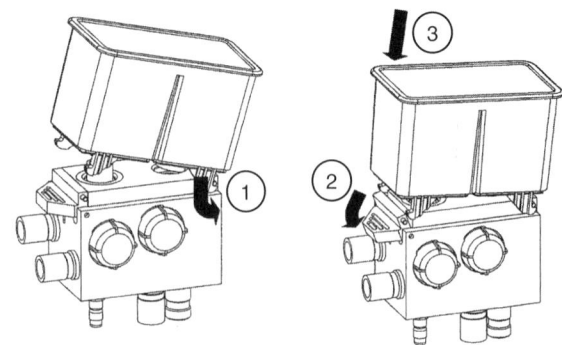

FIGURE **16-45** Changing carbon dioxide cassette in the ADU. (*From S/5 Anesthesia Delivery Unit User's Reference Manual. Catalog No. 8502304. Madison, WI: Datex-Ohmeda; 2000.*)

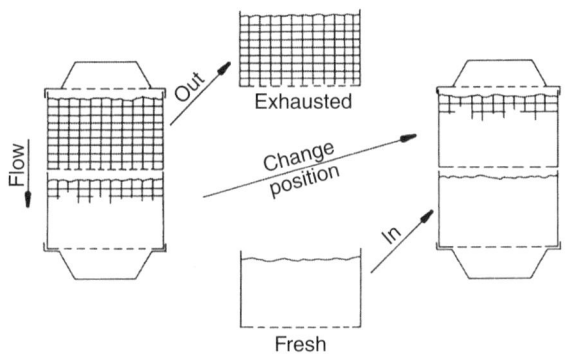

FIGURE **16-44** Changing carbon dioxide absorber canisters. (*From Schreiber P: Safety Guidelines for Anesthesia Systems. Telford, PA: North American Dräger; 1985.*)

alone as a measure of exhaustion.[162] The process of canister replacement for Aestiva-style absorbers is illustrated in Figure 16-44, and the steps for replacement are shown in Box 16-16. Canister replacement for the ADU is shown in Figure 16-45. Do *not* change Aestiva-style canisters or loose fill in the middle of a case. If the new canister is placed in its clear plastic holder upside down or if for any other reason the circuit cannot be reassembled promptly, resumption of ventilation might be delayed. If granules do become exhausted, a safer alternative strategy is to change fresh gas flow to one to two times the minute ventilation; this approach should ensure that expired CO_2 is reduced to acceptable levels. The granules can then be replaced after the case.

Each canister (top or bottom) in an Aestiva-style absorber contains approximately 1 to 1.3 kg of granules in a volume of 1400 to 1500 mL.[61,64,163] Each 100 g of granules can absorb as much as 15 L of CO_2 before the outlet concentration is 1% (7.6 mm Hg). This assumes that no channeling occurs. The average to maximum production of CO_2 by the anesthetized adult is 12 to 18 L/hr.[113] Therefore, when total rebreathing is occurring, the top canister might be expected to last approximately 8 to 10 hours. A much longer life is observed clinically for these large

canisters, principally because higher flows are used (typically in many clinical settings, 2 to 4 L/min of fresh gas flow). At these higher flows, both the dilution of exhaled CO_2 and the rate of washout of exhalations from the breathing circuit to the scavenger are greater. In one study in which fresh gas flows of 4 L/min were used, two canisters were used for 67 and 79 hours (anesthesia time) over 2.5 weeks without exhaustion, with a final minimum water content in some segments of 4% to 8.5%.[164] As lower flows become more common for economic and environmental reasons, and canisters become smaller, anesthetists will need to become more aware of the signs of absorbent exhaustion and realize that absorbent must be changed more frequently.[165]

The manufacturer of soda lime recommends that the absorbent be changed if it is left in the machine for longer than 48 hours.[113] This extremely cautious guideline is based on recognition of two problems that arise with extended use. First, the ethyl violet indicator present along the wall of the canister may be inactivated by gas flows or intense light. Second, dehydration of the granules occurs over time, particularly if higher gas flows or an excessive amount of flushing with O_2 is used. It is not uncommon for gases to be left flowing accidentally overnight or over the weekend. Dehydration of the granules reduces their efficiency. Dräger recommends that their loose-fill absorbent in

---

BOX 16-17

Classification of Modern Ventilators

Power Source
- Gas-driven bellows—compressed gas and electricity
- Piston ventilator—electricity only

Drive Mechanism
- Double-circuit (bellows compressed by driving gas) and pneumatically driven
  - Driving gas is 100% oxygen or compressed air (GE), or Venturi mix of oxygen and room air (older Dräger)
- Piston ventilators (bellows compressed by electric motor)

Cycling Mechanism
- Electronically time-cycled

Modes
- Manual/spontaneous
- Volume-controlled ventilation (VCV)

- Pressure-controlled ventilation (PCV)
- Synchronized intermittent mandatory ventilation (SIMV) in either volume or pressure mode, with or without pressure support of the patient's spontaneous breaths
- Pressure support ventilation (PSV)

Bellows Classification
- Gas-driven bellows
  - Most have ascending (standing) bellows (mnemonic: *ascend* and *descend* have *e*'s, so look at the bellows during expiration).
  - The Anestar has descending (hanging) bellows.
- Piston ventilators are driven by electric motors.

Data from 7800 Ventilator: Operation and Maintenance Manual Software Revision 4. Madison, WI: Datex-Ohmeda; 1993; 7000 Electronic Anesthesia Ventilator: Operation Maintenance. Madison, WI: Datex-Ohmeda; 1985; Andrews JJ. Understanding your anesthesia machine and ventilator. In: 1989 Review Course Lectures. Cleveland, OH: International Anesthesia Research Society; 1989; Cicman J et al. Operating Principles of Narkomed Anesthesia Systems. Telford, PA: Dräger; 1993.

---

the Fabius GS be changed if the machine has been idle for 48 hours, or at least each week on Monday.[55]

Ventilators

Classification and Theory of Operation—Gas-Driven Bellows

Modern ventilators using compressible bellows are multi-mode, double-circuit, electronically controlled, volume- or pressure-limited ventilators. Because they are electronically controlled, these ventilators do not operate without electrical power or a backup battery. Ventilators in current use may be classified with respect to a number of parameters (Box 16-17).* Figures 16-37 and 16-38 show gas flow in the breathing circuit with mechanical ventilation. Similar to the anesthetist's hand squeezing a breathing bag to assist the patient's respiration, the mechanical ventilator uses the force of compressed gas (air or O_2) as the driving mechanism to compress the bellows. The bellows contains the gas inspired and expired by the patient and separates it from the surrounding driving gas. Leaks in the bellows may cause dilution of gas within the bellows by driving gas or loss of agent and oxygen from within it.[166]

The potential buildup of volume and pressure within the breathing circuit (and in the patient's lungs) from the continual addition of fresh gas flow is prevented by a ventilator relief valve (also known as the *spill valve*, or *overflow valve*) that remains open during the expiratory phase (see insets in Figures 16-37 and 16-38). During the inspiratory phase, driving gas closes this relief valve, preventing gas within the bellows from exiting to the scavenger as the bellows are compressed. During early expiration, a weight within the ventilator relief valve holds the pathway to the scavenger closed until the bellows have filled. This creates 2 to 3 cm water of positive end-expiratory pressure (PEEP) within the breathing circuit. This small amount of PEEP is inherent to the design when standing-bellows mechanical ventilation is used.[44,50,166,167] Note that the "Bag/Vent" switch set to "Vent"

or "Auto" removes the reservoir bag and APL valve from the breathing circuit (not true for ventilators with fresh gas decoupling), so the APL valve can be open without causing a leak during mechanical ventilation.

Hanging Bellows

Ventilators generally have standing (ascending) bellows (except for the Anestar and the piston ventilators). To distinguish between ascending (standing) and descending (hanging) bellows, use the mnemonic, "Asc**e**nd and desc**e**nd contain *e*'s, so look at the bellows during **e**xpiration to distinguish them." Both standing and hanging bellows are safe in that both are capable of alerting the user to a disconnection, so long as appropriate monitoring is used.[168] Standing bellows are thought by some to have an advantage because they will not fill in the event of a disconnect, whereas hanging bellows may fill with room air even when completely disconnected from the patient.[167]

The hanging design may provide compactness and ease of sterilization of the entire breathing circuit. The Anestar incorporates disconnect alarms based on chemical (capnograph) and mechanical principles (pressure, volume, and flow sensors). Because this design uses fresh gas decoupling, the manual breathing bag is always in the circuit and fluctuates in volume while the mechanical ventilator is operating. Water may gather in the bellows (lessening tidal volume and creating an infection risk), but this tendency should be opposed by the heated absorber head of the Anestar.

Theory of Operation—Piston-Driven Ventilators

Piston ventilators use an electric motor to compress the gas in a rigid piston during the inspiratory phase. Thus they use no driving gas and may be used without depleting the oxygen cylinder in case of oxygen pipeline failure.[169] Piston ventilators, like gas-driven bellows designs, are safe and effective.

In the Narkomed 6000/6400 Divan ventilator, the piston is out of the operator's view, being placed horizontally under the writing surface. Although the piston can be viewed by lifting

---

*References 15, 18, 22, 44, 50, 53-56, 60-62, 64-66, 79.

the writing surface, their to-and-fro movement is not normally visible during mechanical ventilation. The anesthetist relies on pressure and capnography waveforms, plus the movement of the manual breathing bag, to guard against disconnects or other problems. The Fabius GS has a piston ventilator similar to the Divan, but the bellows travel vertically, and their movement is continuously visible through a window to the left of the flowmeter bank.

The piston ventilator has positive and negative pressure relief valves built in. If the pressure within the piston reaches 75 ± 5 cm H_2O, the positive pressure relief valve opens. If the pressure within the piston declines to -8 cm H_2O, the negative pressure relief valve opens, and room air is drawn into the piston, protecting the patient from negative end-expiratory pressure (NEEP).[55,57,60]

There are several advantages to a piston ventilator.[169] It is quiet. There is no PEEP (2 to 3 cm H_2O is mandatory on standing bellows ventilators because of the design of the ventilator spill valve). There is great precision in delivered tidal volume, owing to compliance and leak compensation, fresh gas decoupling, and the rigid piston design. There are fewer compliance losses with a piston, as compared with a flexible standing bellows compressed by driving gas. Measuring compliance and leaks with a transducer near the piston eliminates a bulky, costly sensor close to the patient's airway (such as the D-Lite sensor on the ADU). Electricity is the driving force for the piston, so if oxygen pipeline pressure fails or pipeline supplies are unavailable (as in an office-based setting), and one must rely on oxygen from the emergency cylinder, mechanical ventilation may continue (without exhausting the cylinder oxygen simply to drive the bellows, as in a gas-driven bellows). Piston ventilators (like gas-driven bellows) are capable of all modern ventilation modes.

The piston design also has some disadvantages. The familiar visible behavior of a standing bellows is lost during disconnects or when the patient is breathing over and above the ventilator settings. The piston is quiet, so that it may be harder to hear its regular cycling. The piston ventilator design cannot easily accommodate nonrebreathing circuits, although this is also true of traditional absorber heads like the Ohmeda GMS or newer ascending bellows ventilators like the ADU. The piston has the potential for NEEP and dilution of the patient's inspired gas with room air.

Typical Ventilator Alarms
Modern ventilators have safety alarms to protect the patient from a number of conditions (Box 16-18). One important safety feature of modern equipment is that apnea (disconnect) alarms are enabled with the first breath sensed.

Ventilator Modes and Settings
Besides increased accuracy because of compliance and leak compensation, the biggest improvement in current ventilators is their flexibility in modes of ventilation. Offering PCV allows more efficient and safe ventilation for certain types of patients. PSV is an important recent addition for patients who are spontaneously breathing, which is seen with much greater frequency with the adoption of the laryngeal mask airway. The improvement in accuracy afforded by modern ventilators means that switching of circuits (e.g., to a nonrebreather for small children) is not as necessary as formerly. This helps avoid potential misconnects.

Volume-Controlled Ventilation (VCV). All ventilators offer VCV. In this mode, the desired tidal volume V_T is set

---

> **BOX 16-18**
>
> #### Typical Ventilator Alarms
>
> Pressure
> High (isolated or continuing)
> Subatmospheric
> Volume—low tidal or minute volume
> Rate—high respiratory rate
> Reverse flow (may indicate incompetence of expiratory unidirectional valve in the breathing circuit)
> Apnea/disconnect alarms may be based on:
>   Chemical monitoring (lack of end-tidal carbon dioxide)
>   Mechanical monitoring:
>   Failure to reach normal inspiratory peak pressure, or
>   Failure to sense return of tidal volume
>   Spirometry
>   Failure of standing bellows to fill during exhalation
>   Failure of manual breathing bag to move and fill during mechanical ventilation (machines with fresh gas decoupling—the Anestar, Apollo, Fabius GS, Narkomed 6000)
>   Other—lack of breath sounds, visible chest movement

and delivered at a constant flow. The ventilator is volume limited, time cycled, and constant flow in VCV. Inspiration is terminated when the desired V_T is delivered or if an excessive pressure is reached (60 to 100 cm H_2O).[50,57,60,64] Patients under general anesthesia often have decreased functional residual capacity and compliance. Because volume is controlled, alveolar ventilation and arterial carbon dioxide can be maintained despite changes in pulmonary function.[170] The peak inspiratory pressure is uncontrolled and varies according to the patient's compliance and airway resistance.

V_T is adjusted to prevent atelectasis, and respiratory rate (RR) is adjusted to keep end-tidal carbon dioxide at the desired value. Peak inspiratory pressure (PIP) is monitored but not controlled. Typical initial settings for VCV in an adult are V_T 10 mL/kg, RR 6 to 12 breaths per minute, PEEP 0 cm H_2O, and inspiratory: expiratory (I:E) ratio 1:2.

Pressure-Controlled Ventilation (PCV). In PCV mode, the ventilator operates as pressure is limited and time cycled, with a decelerating flow pattern. Inspiratory pressure is controlled rather than volume (as with VCV).[171] Inspired volume varies with changes in compliance and airway resistance. The ventilator generates sufficient flow to attain the target pressure early in inspiration then maintains this set pressure throughout the inspiratory time. High flow is needed at first, and less flow is required to maintain this pressure. Target pressure is adjusted for the desired V_T; RR is adjusted to maintain a reasonable end-tidal carbon dioxide. V_T is monitored. PCV may result in an increased tidal volume at a lower PIP, especially if PIP had been high when employing VCV (for example, in laparoscopic abdominal or pelvic surgery). During PCV, if pulmonary compliance drops (i.e., pneumoperitoneum) or airway resistance increases (i.e., bronchospasm, kinked endotracheal tube), delivered V_T may drop substantially. Conversely, if pulmonary compliance improves (i.e., release of pneumoperitoneum, return to supine from steep Trendelenburg position) or airway resistance decreases, V_T may increase substantially.

There are several indications for PCV. Patients for whom high inspiratory pressure is particularly dangerous may benefit (laryngeal mask airway,[172] emphysema, neonates/infants). In patients with low compliance, PCV can often produce higher tidal volumes than VCV (pregnancy, laparoscopic surgery, morbid obesity, or adult respiratory distress syndrome). PCV can compensate for leaks (infants with uncuffed endotracheal tubes, laryngeal mask airway). PCV may provide effective ventilation and lower airway pressure during one-lung ventilation.[171,173]

Typical initial settings for PCV in an adult include pressure limit 20 cm H_2O, RR 6 to 12 breaths per minute, PEEP 0 cm H_2O, I:E ratio 1:2. PCV has also been implemented as PCV with Volume Guarantee (which adjusts pressure limit to prevent significant variation in delivered V_T)[53,54] and as SIMV in pressure mode.[60]

Synchronized Intermittent Mandatory Ventilation (SIMV). With the advent of the laryngeal mask airway (LMA) and the prevalence of short, ambulatory or office-based surgical procedures, spontaneous unassisted breathing has become much more common during general anesthesia. But it is difficult to maintain a light enough plane of anesthesia to permit spontaneous ventilation while retaining sufficient depth for surgery to proceed. If the patient is maintained in a plane of anesthesia that is too deep, respiratory acidosis will occur; too light, and bucking and awareness are risks. The traditional solution was to assist ventilation manually because VCV was all the mechanical ventilator could provide. Ventilation modes that could support a spontaneously breathing patient (provide normocapnia without bucking) include SIMV,[174] PSV,[175] continuous positive airway pressure (CPAP), and airway pressure release ventilation (APRV).[176]

Of these modes, SIMV and PSV are currently available. SIMV is like VCV in that it is volume-controlled ventilation, but the intermittent mandatory breaths are delivered in synchrony with, and triggered by, the patient's spontaneous efforts. Typical initial settings thus include not only volume and rate, but trigger window (percent) and sensitivity (Figure 16-46). Trigger window controls the amount of time during each expiratory cycle that the ventilator is sensitive to negative pressure generated by the patient's diaphragm. It also sensitivity controls how much negative pressure the patient needs to produce before a breath is triggered.

SIMV can be used for anything from full to partial ventilatory support. On new gas machines, pressure or volume modes of SIMV may be selected. The spontaneous breaths may be pressure supported (SIMV-PS).[57] When switching from SIMV to VCV, the I:E ratio does not reset to default values automatically, so this should be checked as part of the review of all settings when placing a subsequent patient on the mechanical ventilator. Typical settings for SIMV mirror those used for VCV (or PCV if a pressure control mode is chosen).

Pressure-Support Ventilation (PSV). PSV is like PCV in that it is a pressure-targeted ventilation mode—but with a RR of zero. It is like SIMV in that it is responsive to the patient's efforts, delivering a breath within a trigger window and as long as the patient's negative inspiratory pressure matches the sensitivity setting. Thus it is only useful for patients who are breathing spontaneously. There is no minimum minute ventilation, although some ventilators allow setting an apnea backup rate or delay.

PSV is useful to augment the V_T of a spontaneously ventilating patient during maintenance or emergence. The primary setting is the pressure support level, which for adults may be

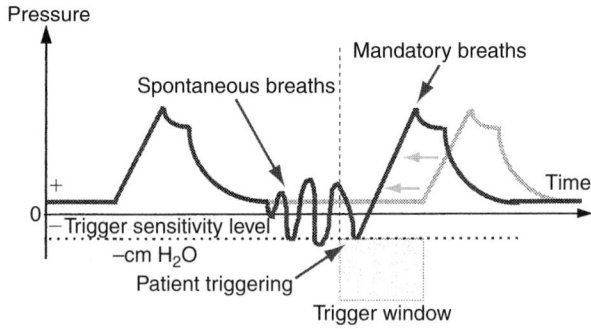

FIGURE **16-46** Trigger window and sensitivity may be set when choosing SIMV mode. (*From S/5 Anesthesia Delivery Unit User's Reference Manual.* Catalog No. 8502304. Madison, WI: Datex-Ohmeda; 2000.)

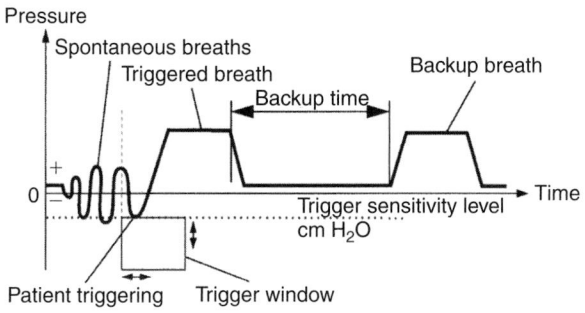

FIGURE **16-47** Trigger window and sensitivity settings for pressure support ventilation. (*From Datex-Ohmeda ADU Ventilation Supplement.* Document No. M1038740. Issue M1044700. Madison, WI: Datex-Ohmeda; 2005.)

started at 10 cm H_2O. Trigger window, sensitivity, maximum inspiratory flow, and apnea backup rate may also be set, depending on the particular ventilator (Figure 16-47).

Safety Features of Modern Ventilators

Flexibility. The appearance of pressure control ventilation is a major advantage, allowing more challenging patients to be ventilated efficiently, such as patients with ARDS or morbid obesity who are difficult with VCV mode. PCV also increases safety for patients in whom excessive pressure must be strictly avoided, such as neonates and infants, and emphysematous patients. Pressure support and SIMV are quite valuable in supporting the patient with spontaneous respirations. Perhaps the biggest hurdle in implementation for all new modes is the education of generations of providers who are only familiar with "plain vanilla" volume control mode.

Accuracy at Lower Tidal Volumes. Factors contributing to a discrepancy between set and delivered tidal volumes are especially acute in pediatrics and include the large compression volume of the circle system relative to the infant's lung volume, leaks around uncuffed endotracheal tubes, the augmentation of delivered tidal volume produced by fresh gas flow, and the difficulty of setting a small tidal volume using an adult bellows assembly.[15]

Modern ventilators have an unprecedented tidal volume range because of the greatly increased accuracy in tidal volume delivery achieved through electronic compliance and leak testing, and tidal volume that is compensated for these factors, as well as changes in fresh gas flow. They are able to ventilate smaller patients much more accurately than any previous anesthesia ventilator could. This has significantly lessened the need for nonrebreathing (Mapleson & Bain) circuits and made care safer, because anesthetists will no longer have to disassemble and reconfigure a nonrebreathing circuit for a child in the middle of several adult cases. However, it is mandatory to substitute pediatric circle disposable hoses for tidal volumes less than 200 mL with the Narkomed 6000 and the Fabius GS.[177] Smaller filters, a pediatric D-Lite sensor, and less compliant pediatric circle breathing systems must be used on the ADU for V_T less than 150 mL.[50] The lower limit of accuracy for tidal volume is 10 mL (for the Narkomed 6000), 20 mL (Fabius GS, Aestiva, ADU, Apollo, Avance, Aisys), or 40 mL (Anestar).* When sensors or disposable breathing circuit types are changed for a pediatric case, users must repeat the leak and compliance tests of the preanesthesia check so that maximum V_T accuracy is ensured. Likewise, these must be repeated when returning to the adult configuration.

Compliance and Leak Testing. Accuracy in delivered V_T comes with a price. An electronic leak and compliance test is part of the morning checklist, and it must be repeated every time the circuit is changed, particularly if changing to a circuit with a different configuration (adult circle to pediatric circle, or adult to long circuit). Users must familiarize themselves with whether vaporizers and other components are included in the leak and compliance test because these tests vary among gas machines.

The placement of the sensor used to compensate tidal volumes for compliance losses and leaks has some interesting consequences. The Aestiva flow sensors are placed between disposable corrugated breathing circuit limbs and the absorber head. Here they are able to compensate tidal volumes for fresh gas flow, compliance losses, and leaks internal to the machine and absorber head—but not in the breathing hoses. The D-Lite sensor (ADU) is placed at the Y-piece. In this position, it can compensate for all leaks and compliance losses out to the Y-piece (thus including the breathing circuit hoses). However, at this point it adds appreciable bulk and weight close to the patient's face. This may make mask ventilation more cumbersome. Further, a sensor closer to the patient is exposed to more exhaled moisture, but the impact can be lessened with a heat and moisture exchanger between patient and sensor. Unfortunately, this adds further bulk and weight. The Narkomed 6000, Apollo, and Fabius test compliance and leaks of all components to the Y-piece via a pressure transducer within the internal circuitry near the bellows. Here the sensor is relatively protected from moisture.

Fresh Gas Decoupling versus Tidal Volume Compensation. A final factor adding to modern ventilator accuracy is that they compensate delivered tidal volume for changes in fresh gas flow. In older ventilators, the delivered tidal volume is the sum of the volume delivered from the ventilator and the fresh gas flowing during the inspiratory phase, so delivered tidal volume may change as fresh gas flow is changed. For example, consider a patient with a fresh gas flow of 4 L/min, a respiratory rate of 10, an inspiratory to expiratory ratio of 1:2, and a tidal volume of 700 mL. During each minute, the ventilator spends a total of

20 seconds in inspiratory time and 40 seconds in expiratory time (1:2 ratio). During this 20 seconds, the fresh gas flow is 1320 mL (one third of 4000 mL/min fresh gas flow). So each of the 10 breaths of 700 mL is augmented by 132 mL of fresh gas flowing while the breath is being delivered, and the actual delivered tidal volume is 832 mL/breath (19% increase).

But what happens if we decrease the fresh gas flow? Assume the same parameters, but a fresh gas flow of 1000 mL/min. During each minute, the ventilator spends 20 seconds in inspiratory time and 40 seconds in expiratory time (1:2 ratio). During this 20 seconds, the fresh gas flow is 330 mL (1000 mL/min fresh gas flow times 1/3). So each of the 10 breaths of 700 mL is augmented by 33 mL of fresh gas flowing while the breath is being delivered, making the total delivered tidal volume 733 mL/breath. This means that changing fresh gas flow from 4000 mL/min to 1000 mL/min, *without changing ventilator settings*, has resulted in a 14% decrease in delivered tidal volume (832 to 733 mL). It would not be surprising if the end-tidal carbon dioxide rose as a result.

The situation is more acute with a traditional anesthesia ventilator used for a child. Assume a 10-kg patient with a fresh gas flow of 4 L/min, a respiratory rate of 20, inspiratory to expiratory ratio of 1:2, and a tidal volume of 100 mL. During each minute, the ventilator spends 20 seconds in inspiratory time and 40 seconds in expiratory time (1:2 ratio). During this 20 seconds, the fresh gas flow is 1320 mL (one third of 4000 mL/min fresh gas flow). So each of the 20 breaths of 100 mL is augmented by 66 mL of fresh gas flowing while the breath is being delivered, making the total delivered tidal volume 166 mL/breath. This is a 66% increase above what is set on the ventilator. Decreasing fresh gas flow from 4 to 1 L/min, again without changing ventilator settings, decreases minute ventilation from 3320 to 2333 mL (a 30% reduction).

There are two approaches to dealing with the problem. The Apollo, Anestar, Narkomed 6000 and Fabius GS use fresh gas decoupling (Figure 16-48). Fresh gas flow during inspiration is diverted to the manual breathing bag, which remains in circuit during mechanical ventilation and is not added to the delivered tidal volume. Thus fresh gas decoupling helps ensure that the set and delivered tidal volumes are equal. The action of the piston closes a decoupling valve, diverting fresh gas flow to the manual breathing bag during the inspiratory cycle. The visual appearance of the circuit during mechanical ventilation is unusual in that the manual breathing bag (normally quiescent) moves with each breath. Further, this manual breathing bag movement is opposite to the movement seen in a mechanical ventilator bellows, which empties during inspiration, and fills during expiration. With fresh gas decoupling, the bag inflates during inspiration (due to fresh gas flow) and deflates during expiration as the contents empty into the piston. With fresh gas decoupling, if there is a disconnect, the manual breathing bag rapidly deflates because the piston retraction draws gas from it.

The second approach is tidal volume compensation for fresh gas flow, which is used in the Aestiva and ADU (among others). The volume and flow sensors at the Y piece provide feedback that allows the ventilator to adjust the delivered tidal volume so that it matches the set tidal volume, in spite of changes in fresh gas flow.

Suitability for Low Flows. Low fresh gas flow is desirable to reduce pollution, reduce the cost of volatile agents and nitrous oxide, preserve tracheal heat and moisture, prevent soda lime granules from drying, and help preserve patient body temperature. Factors that enhance the safety and efficiency of low flow

---

*References 50, 57, 58, 60, 64, 66.

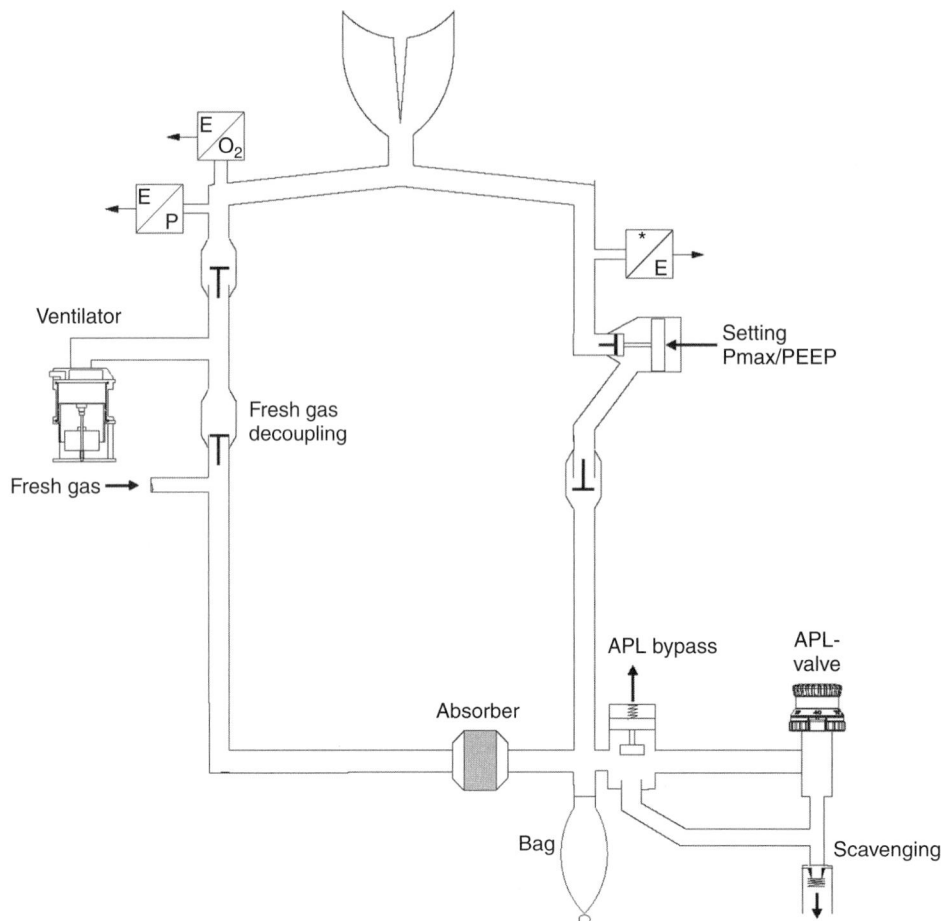

FIGURE **16-48** Circle breathing system with fresh gas decoupling unidirectional valve. (*From Fabius GS. Operator's Instruction Manual. Catalog No. 4117102-001. Telford, PA: Dräger; 2002.*)

anesthesia in modern ventilators are shown in Box 16-12. As you can see, a traditional-sized absorber head like the Aestiva is roughly twice the volume of some of the newer designs. All newer non-disposable portions of the breathing circuit are designed to be more leak-proof than earlier designs.

Electronic Selection of Positive End-Expiratory Pressure. Electronic selection of positive end-expiratory pressure (PEEP) is safer than previous approaches, which involved adding adapters to the breathing circuit. Add-on adapters came in different varieties, depending on how much PEEP was desired (e.g., 5 or 10 cm H_2O). They were intended to be placed between the expiratory limb of the breathing hoses and the expiratory unidirectional valve. They have been placed accidentally in the inspiratory limb, where they cause complete obstruction to flow in the breathing circuit.[178] Although it would seem easy to find this fault immediately, in the heat of the moment with a patient who is already hypoxemic, the clinician may become distracted and unable to focus effectively on the problem. This is an example of a clinical pearl: When a change in the patient's condition is noticed, think back to the last alteration made to the equipment (or to the last drug *thought* to be given), and determine whether it might have contributed to the change.

Current Ventilator Designs

GE Healthcare 7900 "SmartVent." The 7900 was designed to provide consistent delivered VT in spite of changes in fresh gas flow, small leaks, and absorber or bellows compliance losses.[179]

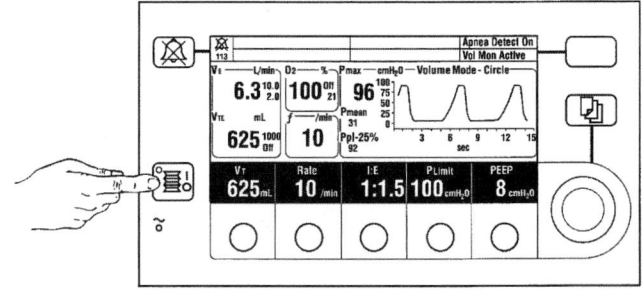

FIGURE **16-49** Display and control panel of the Datex-Ohmeda 7900 ventilator. (*From Ohmeda 7900 Ventilator Operation and Maintenance Manual. Madison, WI: GE Healthcare; 1997.*)

It uses variable-orifice flow sensors (proximal to the inspiratory and expiratory limbs) and pressure sensors to accomplish this. Compliance losses in the corrugated hoses are not corrected for, but these are a relatively small portion of compliance losses.[179] Available modes include manual/spontaneous, volume control, pressure control, pressure support, and SIMV (in either volume or pressure mode with pressure support). PEEP is integrated and electronically controlled. It is found on a variety of machines, including Aestiva, Aisys, and Avance. Typical controls are shown in Figure 16-49.

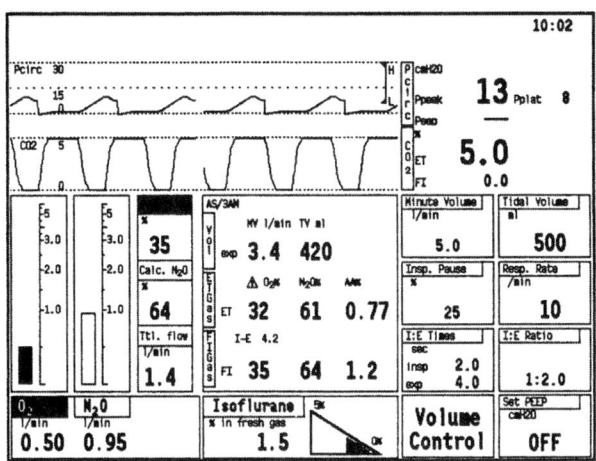

FIGURE **16-50** Machine monitors and ventilator controls are on the left display screen of the Datex-Ohmeda ADU. (*From Datex-Ohmeda AS/3 Anesthesia Delivery Unit User's Reference Manual. Tewksbury, MA: GE Healthcare; 1998.*)

GE Healthcare 7100. The 7100 model is similar to the 7900, except that the selection of modes is not as extensive. The 7100, like the 7900, features tidal volume compensation. It is found on the Aespire.

GE Healthcare ADU Ventilator. The design of the ADU ventilator and gas machine system has many innovative features.[50] The ventilator (like all modern designs) is activated by a single switch (setting the "Bag/Vent" switch to "Auto"). The ventilator can use either oxygen or air as a driving gas and will switch automatically to air if oxygen pipeline pressure is lost. Delivered VT is adjusted to compensate for changes in fresh gas flow and total (absorber head and corrugated limbs) breathing circuit compliance losses (through the D-Lite sensor at the elbow). Entering the patient's weight will suggest appropriate ventilator settings. Volume control, pressure control, pressure support, manual/spontaneous and synchronized intermittent mandatory ventilation (SIMV) modes are offered, along with integrated electronic PEEP. Flow-volume (resistance) or pressure-volume (compliance) loops may be displayed breath by breath. The controls are straightforward (Figure 16-50).

Users should exercise caution with regard to the displayed oxygen concentration. "Calc. O₂%," which is optionally displayed in the mid–lower left of the primary (left) machine status screen, is based on the flowmeter settings only, unlike the oxygen analysis results displayed in the lower center area. The danger arises in a crossover situation in which the pipeline oxygen supply is lost and replaced with another gas (e.g., nitrogen). In this emergency, two sections of the same display offer conflicting information. Because it is based on flowmeter settings, Calc. O₂% will indicate only the intended inspired oxygen concentration, not the actual. The oxygen analyzer display will simultaneously alarm, accurately showing a dangerous hypoxic mixture. Although the manual clearly warns of this problem, the design may confuse providers in this rare emergency situation, delaying the correct response, which might lead to patient injury.[50]

Dräger Divan Ventilator. The Divan ventilator is a piston ventilator found on the Narkomed 6000/6400.[56,58] It offers

pressure control, volume control, manual/spontaneous and SIMV modes. There is no mechanical Bag/Vent switch. Switching between modes is accomplished by electronic keypad. It corrects delivered tidal volume for compliance losses by measuring circuit compliance and fresh gas flow by fresh gas decoupling. Electronic PEEP is integrated. The absorber head is warmed. The Divan is limited to a pressure of 70 cm H₂O, so like most ventilators, it cannot ventilate patients in volume-controlled mode beyond this pressure (but it is possible and perhaps preferable to ventilate the ARDS patient with pressure-controlled mode). It is accurate to very low tidal volumes (range 10 to 1400 mL). Use pediatric circle system (low compliance) hoses for tidal volumes less than 200 mL, and remember to repeat the ventilator self-test when changing circuits.

Unlike most other anesthesia ventilators, there are no visible bellows on the Divan ventilator. It is unique among current models in having a horizontal piston, which is hidden within the writing surface of the gas machine. To provide a visible indication of lung inflation, fresh gas is diverted to the manual breathing bag, which inflates during mechanical ventilator inspiration and deflates during expiration. The piston design avoids negative end-expiratory pressure by entraining room air if pressure within the bellows is less than atmospheric pressure. The "Fresh gas low" error message warns of this condition.

Fabius GS Ventilator. The Fabius GS ventilator is another piston ventilator.[55,57] It offers pressure control, volume control, pressure support, SIMV/PS, and manual/spontaneous modes. There is no mechanical Bag/Vent switch. Switching between modes is accomplished by electronic keypad. It corrects delivered tidal volume for compliance losses by measuring circuit compliance and fresh gas flow by fresh gas decoupling. Electronic PEEP is integrated. One can view measured respiratory parameters or ventilator settings but not both simultaneously on the monitor screen. It is accurate to very low tidal volumes (range 20 to 1400 mL). Use pediatric circle system (low compliance) hoses for tidal volumes less than 200 mL, and remember to repeat the ventilator self-test when changing circuits.

The piston movement is visible in a window to the left of the flowmeter bank. Like the Divan, it provides a visible indication of lung inflation and potential disconnects in that fresh gas is diverted to the manual breathing bag, which inflates during mechanical ventilator inspiration and deflates during expiration. The piston design avoids negative end-expiratory pressure by entraining room air if pressure within the bellows is less than atmospheric pressure. The "Fresh gas low" error message warns of this condition.

Apollo Ventilator. The Apollo ventilator is a piston similar to the Fabius, except that spirometry is displayed. It is similar to the Narkomed 6000 in that the absorber head is heated. Modes are manual/spontaneous, volume and pressure control, pressure support, SIMV in either volume or pressure mode.[15,60]

Traditional Anesthesia Ventilators
The Datex-Ohmeda 7000 and 7800 and the Dräger AV-2 and AV-E ventilators were covered in previous editions of this text. Departments who still retain or use these ventilators should ensure that all personnel are familiar with them and can use them safely in an emergency.[1]

Critical Incidents Related to Ventilation
Disconnects and Other Causes of Low Pressure in the Breathing Circuit. Clinical experience with anesthesia ventilators and breathing circuits has identified several situations that

movement (both are recommended by standard).[82] Electronic monitors for disconnection include capnography and pressure-based and volume-based alarms (see Box 16-18).[37,168,188] Because electronic monitors may have alarms disabled either inadvertently or intentionally (because of artifacts and because of monitor failure), there is no substitute for the anesthetist's vigilance in remaining in touch with the patient through the five senses.

To manage inability to ventilate due to low pressure in the breathing circuit, first ensure ventilation is occurring by checking breath sounds. If not, and the circuit has obviously lost volume, check for leaks quickly (disconnect, suction in trachea, scavenger settings, incompetent ventilator relief valve), then try to ventilate manually using the anesthesia breathing circuit. If no volume loss is apparent, check settings of fresh gas flow, scavenger, and ventilator, as well as monitor artifact.[37] Do not interrupt ventilation for diagnosis of machine problems; proceed to manual ventilation with backup ventilation equipment (Ambu bag) without delay.[188]

Failure to Initiate or Resume Ventilation. Failure to initiate or resume ventilation may be less likely in the future because of the incorporation of modern monitoring in current gas machines. All possess common features that add to patient safety.[50,55,56] They have a centralized data and alarm display, as well as alarms prioritized to warnings, cautions, and advisories. They provide electronic pre-use checklists.[189] Furthermore, the apnea and disconnect alarms are typically placed on standby when the system's main power switch is activated, and their alarms are enabled once a breath is sensed. Therefore the anesthesia gas machine should alert the operator to a failure to turn on a mechanical ventilator after intubation or to a failure to resume ventilation after the ventilator is shut off either temporarily (in the middle of a case for radiography) or permanently (during emergence). If turning off a mechanical ventilator temporarily, it is safest to leave one's finger on the switch until it is time to resume ventilation.

The number of different alarm conditions programmed into a modern anesthesia gas machine with integrated monitoring is staggering. It is absolutely necessary to read the manuals and participate in training for machines of such complexity.[190] Although equipment has improved dramatically, some of the underlying causes of failure to ventilate and of barotrauma will likely remain problems for the foreseeable future (e.g., lack of knowledge or training and failure to use checklists).

Barotrauma and High Pressure in the Breathing Circuit. Although such problems as misconnections are less likely now than in the past because of improvements in design, other possible causes of failure to ventilate or barotrauma are still hazards: occlusion, bellows leaks, failure of gas supply, failure of the ventilator relief valve, and inadvertent application of suction to the airway.[124,191-197]

Unlike disconnects and other low-pressure breathing circuit problems, high pressure in the breathing circuit can evolve quickly and produce devastating consequences while allowing little time for diagnosis or correction. The causes of sustained high pressure in the breathing circuit are diverse. Obstruction to exhalation (but not inhalation) has been caused in recent times by direct connection of wall oxygen to a tracheal tube,[198] improper manufacture of a scavenger assembly,[199] failure to remove plastic wrap around a soda lime canister before installing it in the machine,[200,201] malfunctioning ventilator relief valve,[124] occlusion of the lumen of a breathing circuit extender adaptor by mold flash,[131,133] insertion of an occluded disposable PEEP

have led to critical incidents. Vigilance directed toward situations that have the potential to cause patient injury may contribute to the prevention of future occurrences (Box 16-19). Failure to ventilate caused by disconnection has been called the most common preventable equipment-related cause of mishaps.[22] The most common site for disconnection is between the breathing circuit and the endotracheal tube (at the Y-piece).[168] Disconnects can be partial or complete. Recent reported causes of low pressure (leak) conditions are many: absorbent granules changed between cases by ancillary personnel but improperly reassembled or even left open[180,181]; defective absorber canister[182]; failure of the Bag/Vent switch[183,184]; leaks in corrugated hoses[185]; incompetent ventilator relief valve[186]; leaks from a hot-wire anemometer sensor[187]; and ventilator failure due to moisture in flow sensors.[114]

Prevention of disconnects involves a thorough preanesthesia check of equipment, including testing the breathing circuit with a second breathing bag as an artificial lung (or breathing through the circuit). A primary monitor for disconnection is continuous auscultation of breath sounds with a precordial or esophageal stethoscope, as well as direct visual observation of chest valve into the breathing circuit,[131] and an occluded expiratory unidirectional valve.[128] Most of these obstructions would have easily been detected by a preinduction high-pressure check of the breathing circuit, with release of pressure through the APL valve, or simply by breathing through the circuit. Consequences included high PEEP, decreased venous return, cardiovascular collapse, pneumothorax, massive subcutaneous emphysema, or death.

The algorithm for responding to sustained high pressure in the breathing circuit is as follows.[37] Assess patient-related causes such as bronchospasm. Try manually ventilating the patient with the breathing circuit (in "Bag" mode). If the high pressure is relieved, it is likely that the ventilator relief valve is at fault; the ventilator is unusable until this valve is serviced. If circuit pressure is sustained during manual ventilation with the circuit, it is likely that the scavenger is obstructed or that its relief valves have failed. In either case, attempt to disconnect the scavenger gas collection tubing from the back of the APL if possible. If the tubing cannot be disconnected, disconnect the patient from the breathing circuit and continue ventilation by Ambu bag.[37]

Fire in the Breathing Circuit. Although rare, fires in the breathing circuit have been reported in vivo[72,74,202] and in vitro.[74,154,203] These events are often associated with first cases on Monday, sevoflurane, and desiccated barium hydroxide lime. The most important preventive actions include (1) turning off all gas flows and vaporizers between cases and at the end of the day and (2) ensuring that carbon dioxide absorbents are changed regularly.[72-74] The response to breathing circuit fires is the same as for airway fires.[74]

The Anesthesia Gas Machine and Malignant Hyperthermia. When an unexpected malignant hyperthermia (MH) crisis arises, one follows a protocol including (as far as equipment is concerned) withdrawal of triggering agents. This would include stopping the administration of volatile agents, hyperventilating with oxygen 100%, increasing fresh gas flow, and (if time and help are available and can be spared from other more important tasks such as mixing dantrolene) changing the disposable breathing circuit components and granules.[204] When preparing the gas machine for a patient who is known to be susceptible, one prepares the anesthesia machine by changing the breathing circuit and granules, disabling or removing the vaporizers, and flushing the machine at a rate of 10 L/min for 20 min.[204] Keep fresh gas flows high during maintenance.[205]

DISPOSAL

The final *D* of the SPDD model is concerned with a simple but vital question: How are gases disposed of?

Disposal of Gases in Scavenging Systems
Scavenging is the collection of waste anesthetic gases from the breathing circuit and ventilator and their removal from the operating room. An amount equal to the fresh gas flow must be scavenged each minute.[206-209] Otherwise, the breathing circuit and the patient's lungs will either gain or lose volume, resulting in barotrauma or failure to ventilate. The components of the scavenger are listed in Box 16-20.

A standard for exposure to waste anesthetic gases is published by the Occupational Safety and Health Administration (OSHA).[210] OSHA directs that no worker be exposed to more than 2 ppm halogenated agents (0.5 ppm if used with nitrous oxide) and no more than 25 ppm nitrous oxide, based on a time-weighted 8-hour average concentration. Levels in unscavenged anesthetizing locations may be as high as 7000 ppm

BOX **16-20**
Components of the Scavenger System

Gas collection assembly—at APL valve and ventilator relief valve
Transfer tubing—19 or 30 mm, sometimes color coded yellow
Scavenging interface (most important part)
- Closed Interface (all older models)
  - Communicates to atmosphere only through valves
  - If used with passive disposal system, must have positive pressure relief
  - Used with active (suction) disposal system; must have positive *and* negative pressure relief
- Open Interface (most new models)
  - No valves; open to atmosphere (both negative and positive pressure relief "built in")
  - Must be used *only* with active systems
  - Reservoir required
  Safety:
  - Safer than closed interface for the patient; no barotrauma
  - Less safe than closed interface for the caregiver (if used improperly)
Gas disposal tubing
Gas disposal assembly—active disposal (common) or passive disposal

(0.7%) N_2O and 85 ppm (0.008%) halothane.[19] The highest levels are found in the anesthetist's workstation and between the anesthesia gas machine and the wall.[18] Operating-room personnel (anesthesiologists, surgeons, and nurses) working in ear, nose, and throat operating rooms had measurable levels of exhaled sevoflurane higher than controls up to 18 hours after being on duty, although this study did not report what type of scavenging if any was employed.[211] The health effects of chronic exposure to volatile agents are unproved, though occupational exposure to nitrous oxide should definitely be avoided.[155]

Several variables determine the attainable reduction in waste anesthetic gases in the operating room, including the degree of room ventilation, the condition of anesthesia equipment, the effectiveness of the scavenger, and the anesthetic techniques of the user. However, with appropriate attention to these areas, trace gas levels within the operating room can meet OSHA requirements.[19]

The most important component of the scavenger system is the interface, because it protects the patient from excessive buildup of positive pressure and from exposure to suction. There are two types of interfaces: closed and open. The closed interface is found on older machines, though it is available as an option on new models.[212,213] A closed interface is useful where passive scavenging is used (no dedicated suction line for the scavenger, and waste gases flow passively along with room ventilation exhaust). A closed interface communicates with the atmosphere only through valves (Figure 16-51). A means for relief of positive pressure is mandatory for all closed interfaces. If the suction attached to the scavenger fails or if a hose distal to it becomes kinked, positive pressure relief valves operate before the pressure buildup within the scavenger is transmitted to the breathing

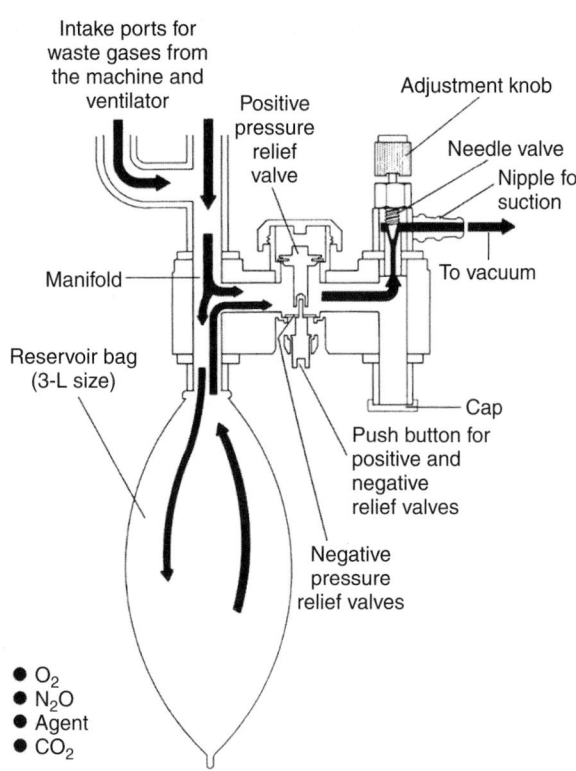

Intake ports for
waste gases from
the machine and
ventilator

Positive
pressure
relief
valve

Adjustment knob

Needle valve
Nipple for
suction

Manifold

To vacuum

Reservoir bag
(3-L size)

Cap

Push button for
positive and
negative
relief valves

Negative
pressure
relief valves

● O_2
● N_2O
● Agent
● CO_2

FIGURE **16-51**   Closed scavenger interface attached to suction. Note the reservoir, the positive and negative pressure relief valves, and the capped extra port. (*From Bowie E, Huffman LM:* The Anesthesia Machine: Essentials for Understanding. *Madison, WI: Datex-Ohmeda; 1985.*)

circuit and the lungs. In this case, the positive pressure relief valve opens and allows the release of waste gases into the operating-room air. If the closed interface is attached to suction, a negative pressure relief valve opens to draw in room air when suction is excessive, preventing the emptying of gas from the patient circuit. Suction should be adjusted as fresh gas flows change so that the scavenger reservoir bag is neither flat nor overdistended.[213]

Because the scavenger interface relief valves can fail,[214] an open scavenger interface is much more common on new machines. The open interface has large open holes or ports around the top. There are no valves to impede the flow of gases into or out of the reservoir, such as are found in closed-interface systems. Each patient exhalation is led to the bottom of the open interface reservoir, where a second tube withdraws it by suction before the next exhalation arrives. Use of the device with appropriate suction is critical to its proper function.[215] Yet because the device is so different from the closed interface, errors in its use have already been reported. In one report, 10 of 10 newly purchased machines equipped with open interfaces had the suction to the scavenger turned off, resulting in the release of all patient exhalations into the operating room.[214] This error in use may be related to the sounds produced by the two different interfaces. When a closed interface is leaking gas into the room through the positive pressure relief valve, one can hear a soft, intermittent hiss. The open interface, on the other hand, should hiss continuously when it has been properly adjusted.

The open interface affords patient safety advantages. With the open interface, there is no chance of relief valve failure, which can cause barotrauma or the application of suction to the

breathing circuit. The device is perhaps less safe for the operator who is unfamiliar with its use; however, the only danger of this ignorance is increased exposure to waste anesthetic gases. The smell of volatile agent during a case is abnormal, and its cause must be sought. The threshold for smelling volatile agents is variously stated as 5 to 300 ppm.[19,116,208,216] Thus, if any agent is smelled, the concentration is excessive (i.e., above that described in the OSHA standard).

Many factors in addition to the scavenger affect exposure to waste anesthetic gases. Guidelines for limiting exposure are listed in Box 16-21.[19,208,216-218] Some may be applied generally, whereas others are applicable only to selected practice settings.

RISK MANAGEMENT

Department-Level Aspects

Risk management is defined as a detection system designed to predict failures and ensure that precautions to prevent patient harm are taken.[116] Typical anesthesia risk management components include preoperative and postoperative rounds, avoiding indifferent treatment of patients, maintaining vigilance and high standards of care, peer review, continuing education, and the commitment to delivery of high-quality and humane patient care. In terms of equipment, risk management includes cleanliness, daily performance of equipment checklists, familiarity with equipment manuals, and appropriate maintenance.[116,219]

The Safe Medical Device Act of 1990 requires hospitals to report instances in which medical devices cause or contribute to death, serious illness, or serious injury.[220] All medical personnel who become aware of a problem with a device must remove the equipment from contact with patients and report the problem to their supervisors. The hospital risk manager then conducts an

BOX **16-21**

Means of Limiting Exposure to Waste Anesthetic Gases

Check the scavenger before use.
Perform regular preventive maintenance of room ventilation systems.
Perform regular preventive maintenance of all anesthesia equipment.
Conduct personnel monitoring and ambient trace gas monitoring.
Seek the source of the smell of anesthetics noted during a case.
Keep a good mask fit.
Avoid unscavengeable techniques (open drop, insufflation).
Prevent flow from breathing system into room air.
Turn on anesthetic gases only after mask is on the patient.
Turn off anesthetic gases before suctioning.
Wash out anesthetics into the scavenger at the end of the case.
Do not spill liquid agent.
Use cuffed endotracheal tubes.
Use low fresh gas flows.
Check the machine regularly for leaks.
Disconnect nitrous oxide at wall outlet at end of day.
Use total intravenous anesthesia.
Avoid use of nitrous oxide.

investigation and reports the results to the FDA within 10 working days. The most common barrier to investigation of a critical incident, and the degree to which anesthesia equipment may have contributed to it, is alteration of the equipment (i.e., it has been cleaned, disassembled, or tested).[221] In the case of patient injury in which equipment may be at fault, it is most helpful if equipment (including wastebaskets and syringes in the anesthesia work area) is sequestered "as is," pending a forensic evaluation conducted by the representatives of the hospital, the manufacturer, and perhaps the patient. Equipment logs should be kept for each anesthesia machine and include reports of maintenance, critical incidents, additions or alterations, pollution control, and vaporizer calibration. Preventive maintenance should be done at intervals specified by the manufacturer (usually two to four times per year) by qualified, factory-trained technicians.[116]

Individual Risk Management
The department-level risk management plan requires the active involvement of all department members. In addition to participation in the department-level activities noted earlier, individuals play a vital role in three further aspects: performance of the machine checklist before use, limiting equipment-related disease transmission, and reducing trace and waste gas exposure through alteration of work practices (the latter two were discussed earlier in this chapter).

Anesthesia Gas Machine Checklist
Reports of equipment problems surfacing in the 1980s prompted the professional societies and government to develop a

recommended anesthesia checklist.[222-225] Although equipment failures are rare, they are often the result of human error in the use of the equipment.[11,222] Failure to check anesthesia equipment adequately has been reported as a factor in up to 30% of critical incidents.[226,227] Users report that they often do not perform the FDA checklist, and many do not feel competent in their ability to perform it correctly.[3] When a checklist is performed, 30% of the gas machines in one study had serious faults discovered.[2] Checklists have been the focus of several studies of fault-detection ability[9,10,59,228-231] and much comment.[189,232-237] It is probable, but as yet unproved, that proper and consistent use of checklists will not only prevent critical incidents but also help teach and reinforce knowledge of the function and use of the anesthesia gas machine.[14] Performance of the pre-use anesthesia checkout is required by various standards.[238]

New developments in the pre-use anesthesia checkout are the abandonment of the 1990s FDA checklist and the proposal of a new checkout for anesthesia machines.[239] In view of the significant differences between models and variations in their self-test routines, no one set of procedures will cover all gas machines. This new checklist will be a statement of principles of what should be checked, rather than a procedures list. For example, the availability of backup ventilation equipment and backup oxygen supplies and the calibration of the oxygen analyzer and other monitors must be checked, regardless of which machine is used. But how these actions are performed varies from machine to machine. If they have not done so already, anesthesia departments will need to develop specific procedures and training for the machines they use, in consultation with manufacturers and the operator's instruction manuals.

The Aestiva is a system that must be manually checked—there are no electronic aspects to the checklist.[44] At the other extreme, some gas machines feature primarily electronic checklists. These electronic self-check routines, like that in the ADU, may help prevent errors and omissions in the preanesthesia checklist.[240] This checklist covers all essential functions, and it can detect leaks and measure breathing circuit compliance. The machine halts the checklist if leaks greater than 150 mL/min are detected.[50] If leaks are detected, check the tightness of all connections—respiratory and patient circuit tubing and bellows (bellows, bellows block, ventilator relief valve, and bellows chamber). Ensure that the Y-piece is properly occluded, gas flows are closed, and the gas sampling lines in the D-Lite sensor are not still connected to the circuit. The user performs a few manual tests at the end—suction, cylinder pressure, unidirectional valves, and gas analysis. Occupying a middle ground, the Fabius GS, Apollo, and Narkomed 6000/6400 have checklists that are partially electronic and partially manually performed by the user. All of these new machine checklists require that the circuit be occluded for compliance and leak testing, then reconfigured for use.

The anesthetist should ensure that a few activities are part of the preanesthesia checklist for any gas machine. To ensure that all breathing circuit connections are gas-tight, always perform a high-pressure check after the checklist is complete. Check that the oxygen analyzer reads 21% when exposed to room air, and the reading increases when the sensor is exposed to gas from the oxygen pipeline. Test the unidirectional valves with an artificial lung (or by breathing through the circuit) to ensure that the circuit is not obstructed by mold flash or plastic wrapping.[131,132] While checking for backup ventilation equipment (Ambu bag) and cylinder oxygen, walk around the machine, checking for suction and an extra circuit, the location of circuit breakers, the presence of a cylinder wrench and head strap, and whether gas analysis monitors are scavenged. If a manual high-pressure check and ventilator check are done, users should consider testing the ventilator and unidirectional valves before checking for leaks of the manual limb of the breathing system. In this way, the relatively common fault of beginning a case with the Bag/Vent switch in the Vent mode can be avoided. Because in some machines the vaporizers must be individually checked for leaks, it is possible that care of a patient could begin with the vaporizers inadvertently turned on. So the anesthetist must check that vaporizers are off at the end of the checklist.

Use of negative-pressure tests to check for leaks in the low pressure circuit within the gas machine remains unfamiliar to users. This is unfortunate. The negative-pressure test has been demonstrated to be the most effective test for leaks in the low-pressure system (that area within the machine distal to the flowmeters).[241] Leaks here may lead to hypoxic breathing mixtures or awareness under anesthesia.

There is no "minimum" test other than that suggested by the operator's instruction manuals. In administering an anesthetic for an emergency surgical procedure, one should always check the suction and high-pressure-test the breathing circuit. In addition, the breathing bag should be evaluated for fluctuations during preoxygenation. This evaluation ensures that the patient is breathing, the mask fit is good, oxygen is flowing, and the Bag/Vent switch is in the Bag mode. A situation in which any of these conditions is absent requires immediate attention.

SUMMARY

Compared with its forebears, the anesthesia gas machine available today is a system of tremendous capability, power, safety, and complexity. The machine is a result both of improvements in design and of the integration of physiologic monitors and machine function monitors. Use of an anesthesia gas machine was more straightforward in the past because all types of anesthesia machines contained simpler, similar elements. With the introduction of new designs, this is no longer the case. The days when a few "wizards" in an anesthesia department could specialize in equipment operation and maintenance and could instruct or troubleshoot for all of his or her co-workers have likewise passed. Equipment competency must be a part of everyone's toolkit of patient-care skills. It is hoped that through study of this chapter, current equipment will be more widely understood. In this manner, our future patients may "sleep" in safety, afforded the level of care that we all wish for ourselves and our loved ones.

REFERENCES

1. Blumenreich GA. Legal briefs: improving technology. *AANA J.* 1996; 64(3):213-216.
2. Kendell J, Barthram C. Revised checklist for anaesthetic machines. *Anaesthesia.* 1998;53:887-890.
3. Lampotang S et al. Anesthesia machine pre-use check survey—preliminary results [electronic version]. A1195. *ASA Abstracts 2005.* Available at: http://www.asaabstracts.com/strands/asaabstracts/abstract.htm;jsessionid=AD33DD5E71EE86C52238215FD321EF5D?year=2005&index=14&absnum=1619. Accessed June 30, 2008.
4. Caplan RA et al. Adverse anesthetic outcomes arising from gas delivery equipment: a closed claims analysis. *Anesthesiology.* 1997;87(4):741-748.
5. Cooper JB, Gaba D. No myth: Anesthesia is a model for addressing patient safety. *Anesthesiology.* 2002;97(6):1335-1336.
6. Fasting S, Gisvold SE. Equipment problems during anesthesia—are they a quality problem? *Br J Anaesth.* 2002;89(6):825-831.
7. Larson SL, Jordan L. Preventable adverse patient outcomes: a closed claims analysis of respiratory incidents. *AANA J.* 2001;69(5):386-392.
8. Anesthesia Patient Safety Foundation: *Welcome to APSF.org.* Web site. http://www.apsf.org/. 2007. Accessed June 30, 2008.
9. Larson ER et al. A prospective study on anesthesia machine fault identification. *Anesth Analg.* 2007;104:154-156.
10. Olympio MA et al. Instructional review improves performance of anesthesia apparatus checkout procedures. *Anesth Analg.* 1996;83:618-622.
11. Hellewell SA. Anaesthetic machine safety—the story continues. *Anaesthesia.* 2002;57:183-208.
12. Peters JD et al. Products liability [and] anesthesia mishaps. In: *Anesthesiology and the Law.* Ann Arbor, MI: Health Administration Press; 1983.
13. Dalley P et al. The use of high-fidelity human patient simulation and the introduction of new anesthesia delivery systems. *Anesth Analg.* 2004; 99(6):1737-1741.
14. Hart EM, Owen H. Errors and omissions in anesthesia: a pilot study using a pilot's checklist. *Anesth Analg.* 2005;101(1):246-250.
15. Olympio MA. Modern anesthesia machines: what you should know. *2005 Annual Meeting Refresher Course Lectures.* Park Ridge, IL: American Society of Anesthesiologists; 2005:501.
16. Dorsch JA: Guidelines published for determining anesthesia machine obsolescence [electronic version]. *APSF Newsl.* 2004;winter. Available at: http://www.apsf.org/resource_center/newsletter/2004/winter/05guidelines.htm. 2005. Accessed June 26, 2008.
17. Petty WC. AANA Journal Course: update for nurse anesthetists—medical gases, hospital pipelines, and medical gas cylinders: how safe are they? *AANA J.* 1995;63(4):307-324.
18. Bowie E, Huffman LM. *The anesthesia machine: essentials for understanding.* Madison, WI: Datex-Ohmeda; 1985.
19. Kole TE. Environmental and occupational hazards of the anesthesia workplace. *AANA J.* 1990;58:327-331.
20. ECRI: Waste anesthetic gas [and] minimizing anesthetic gas leakage. *Technol Anesth.* 1991;12:1-3.
21. American Society for Testing and Materials. *Standard specification for particular requirements for anesthesia workstations and their components [F1850-00].* Philadelphia: ASTM; 2005.
22. Dorsch JA, Dorsch SE. *Understanding anesthesia equipment.* 4th ed. Baltimore: Lippincott Williams & Wilkins; 1999.
23. Bernstein DB, Rosenberg AD. Intraoperative hypoxia from nitrogen tanks with oxygen fittings. *Anesth Analg.* 1997;84(1):225-227.
24. Council for Public Interest in Anesthesia. Piped medical gases cause deaths. *Qual Rev Anesth.* 2003;6:3.
25. Elizaga AM, Frerichs RL. Nitrogen purging of oxygen pipelines: an unusual cause of intraoperative hypoxia. *Anesth Analg.* 2000;91(1):242-243.
26. Schumacher SD et al. Bulk liquid oxygen supply failure. *Anesthesiology.* 2004;100(1):186-189.
27. Harris B, Weinger MB. An insidious failure of an oxygen analyzer. *Anesth Analg.* 2006;102(5):1468-1472.
28. Nagle TA. New standards focus on piped medical gas systems. *APSF Newsl.* 1993;8:42-43.
29. Moss E. Medical gas contamination: an unrecognized patient danger. *APSF Newsl.* 1994;9:20-22.
30. Moss E. Danger seen possible from contaminated medical gases. *APSF Newsl.* 1993;8:6-7.
31. Andrzejowski J, Freeman R. Oxygen failure alarms on modern anaesthetic machines. *Anaesthesia.* 2002;57:931-932.
32. Lorraway PG et al. Management of simulated oxygen supply failure: is there a gap in the curriculum? *Anesth Analg.* 2006;102(3):865-867.
33. Weller J et al. Anaesthetists' management of oxygen pipeline failure: room for improvement. *Anaesthesia.* 2007;62(2):122-126.
34. Serlin S. Check your tanks. *Anesth Analg.* 2004;98(3):871.
35. Taenzer AH et al. E-cylinder-powered mechanical ventilation may adversely impact anesthetic management and efficiency. *Anesth Analg.* 2002; 95(1):148-150.
36. University of Florida Department of Anesthesiology: Proposed hypoxic "O2" pipeline algorithm. 2002. Available at: http://vam.anest.ufl.edu/Hypoxicalgorithm.pdf. Accessed April 22, 2003.
37. Rieker M. Anesthesia machine perils and pitfalls: how well do you know your best friend? *Curr Rev Nurs Anesths.* 2005;28(7):81-92.
38. Council for Public Interest in Anesthesia. Oxygen pipeline failure: are you prepared? *Qual Rev Anesth.* 2007;10(3):3.
39. Morrell RC: Gas delivery mistakes continue to kill [electronic version]. *APSF Newsl.* 2002; spring. Available at: http://www.apsf.org/resource_center/newsletter/2002/spring/11gasdelivery.htm. Accessed June 30, 2008.

40. Sato T. Fatal pipeline accidents spur Japanese standards. *APSF Newsl.* 1991;6:14.
41. Holland R. Another "wrong gas" incident in Hong Kong. *APSF Newsl.* 1991;6:9.
42. Neubarth J. Another hazardous gas supply misconnection. *Anesth Analg.* 1995;80(1):206.
43. Lampotang S et al. *Anesthesia Patient Safety Foundation (APSF) Anesthesia Machine Workbook, Version 1.1a* [electronic version]. 2007. Available at: http://vam.anest.ufl.edu/members/workbook/apsf-workbook-english.html. Accessed June 30, 2008.
44. Datex-Ohmeda: *Aestiva 3000 Software Revision 3.X; Operation Manual Part 1.* Document No. 1006-0401-000 9/13/1999. Madison, WI: Datex-Ohmeda; 1999.
45. Eichhorn JH, Ehrenwerth J. Medical gases: storage and supply. In: Ehrenwerth J, Eisenkraft JB, eds. *Anesthesia Equipment: Principles and Applications.* St Louis: Mosby; 1993:1-26.
46. Andrews JJ, Johnston RV Jr. Not all E cylinders were created equal. *Anesth Analg.* 1992;75(1):154.
47. Miller JC. MRI Safety [electronic version]. *Radiology Rounds.* 2005; February. Available at: http://www.mghradrounds.org/index.php?src=gendocs&link=2005_february. 2005/2005. Accessed June 30, 2008.
48. Compressed Gas Association. *Handbook of Compressed Gases.* 3rd ed. Arlington, VA: Van Nostrand Reinhold; 1990.
49. Yudenfreund-Sujka SM. Nitrous oxide abuse presenting as premature exhaustion of Sodasorb. *Anesthesiology.* 1990;73:580.
50. Datex-Ohmeda. *S/5 Anesthesia Delivery Unit User's Reference Manual,* Catalog No. 8502304. Madison, WI: Datex-Ohmeda; 2000.
51. Chawla AV, Newton NI. Machine and monitoring failure from electrical overloading. *Anaesthesia.* 2002;57:1134-1135.
52. Troianos CA. Complete electrical failure during cardiopulmonary bypass. *Anesthesiology.* 1995;82:298-302.
53. GE Healthcare: *Avance.* Document AN-0105-04.06-EN-US. 2006. Available at: http://www.gehealthcare.com/usen/anesthesia/docs/an4583a.pdf. Accessed June 30, 2008.
54. GE Healthcare. *Aisys.* Document No. M1058500/1006. 2006. Available at: http://www.gehealthcare.com/usen/anesthesia/docs/AN4597-A%20US.pdf. Accessed June 30, 2008.
55. Dräger Medical Inc. *Fabius GS Operator's Instruction Manual.* Catalog No. 4117102-001. Telford, PA: Dräger; 2002.
56. Dräger Medical Inc. *Narkomed 6000 Anesthesia Machine Operator's Instruction Manual.* Catalog No. 4114915-006. Telford, PA: Dräger; 2000.
57. Dräger Medical Inc. *Fabius GS.* 2006. Web site. http://www.draeger.com/MT/internet/pdf/CareAreas/ORAnesthesia/or_fabiusgs_br_us.pdf. Accessed June 30, 2008.
58. Dräger Medical Inc. *Narkomed 6400.* 2002. Web site. http://www.draeger.com/MT/internet/pdf/CareAreas/ORAnesthesia/or_nar_br_us_64009049503.pdf. Accessed June 30, 2008.
59. Manley R, Cuddeford JD. An assessment of the effectiveness of the revised FDA checklist. *AANA J.* 1996;64(3):277-282.
60. Dräger Medical Inc: *Apollo Anesthesia Workstation.* 2006. Web site. http://www.draeger.com/MT/internet/pdf/CareAreas/ORAnesthesia/or_apollo_-br_us.pdf. Accessed June 30, 2008.
61. GE Healthcare. *Aestiva/5 Anesthesia Machine.* Document AN2594-K 7/05. 2005. Available at: http://www.gehealthcare.com/usen/anesthesia/docs/an2594j.pdf. Accessed June 30, 2008.
62. GE Healthcare. *Key differences between PSVPro and PSV on the ADU: Marketing Bulletin MB LSS 05 043.* Madison, WI: GE Healthcare; 2005.
63. Cantillo J et al. Ventilatory failures with the Datex-Ohmeda 7900 SmartVent. *Anesthesiology.* 2002;96):766-768.
64. Datex-Ohmeda. *Aestiva 3000 Software revision 3.X: Operation Manual Part 2.* Document No. 1006-0402-000 4/21/1999. Madison, WI: GE Healthcare; 1999.
65. GE Healthcare. *Aespire 7100:* DocumentAN3969-B11/05. Available at: http://www.gehealthcare.com/usen/anesthesia/docs/an3969a.pdf. Accessed June 30, 2008.
66. Datascope. *Anestar S Specifications.* 2004. Available at: http://www.proactmedical.com.au/resource/specsheet6.pdf. Accessed June 30, 2008.
67. Abramovich A. Descending bellows drives question. *APSF Newsl.* 2005; Summer:34-35.
68. Eger EII et al. Anesthetic flowmeter sequence: a cause for hypoxia. *Anesthesiology.* 1963;24:396.
69. Schreiber P. *Safety guidelines for anesthesia systems.* Telford, PA: Dräger; 1985.
70. Fang ZX, Eger EI. Source of toxic CO explained: CF_2 anesthetic + dry absorbent. *APSF Newsl.* 1994;9:25-30.
71. Berry PD et al. Severe carbon monoxide poisoning during desflurane anesthesia. *Anesthesiology.* 1999;90(2):613-616.
72. ECRI: Hazard report: Anesthesia carbon dioxide absorber fires. *Health Devices.* 2003; November:1-6.
73. Olympio MA. Carbon dioxide absorbent desiccation safety conference convened by Anesthetic Patient Safety Foundation. *APSF Newsl.* 2005; 20:25-29.
74. Olympio MA, Morrell RC. Canister fires become a hot safety concern [electronic version]. *APSF Newsl.* 2003;winter. Available at: http://www.apsf.org/newsletter/2003/winter/01fires.htm. Accessed April 6, 2004.
75. Haas RE. A simple technique to instantly convert from insufflation to positive-pressure ventilation (response). *AANA J.* 1992;60:526.
76. Pollock GS. AANA Journal Course: Update for nurse anesthetists—eliminating surgical fires: a team approach. *AANA J.* 2004;72:293-298.
77. Petty C. Understanding your machine: O2 flush valve key to safety. *APSF Newsl.* 1993;8:31.
78. ECRI. Hazard: barotrauma from anesthesia ventilators. *Technol Anesth.* 1988;9:1-2.
79. GE Healthcare. *ADU Plus Carestation Specifications.* Document No. AN3199-E 7/05. 2005. Available at: http://www.gehealthcare.com/usen/anesthesia/docs/AN3199_E_USSpec.pdf. Accessed June 30, 2008.
80. Dräger Medical Inc. *Narkomed 2C Anesthesia System—Setup and Installation Manual.* Telford, PA: Dräger; 1994.
81. Cheng CJ, Garewal DS. A failure of the chain-link mechanism on the Ohmeda Excel 210 anesthetic machine. *Anesth Analg.* 2001;92(4):913-914.
82. American Society of Anesthesiologists: *Standards for Basic Anesthetic Monitoring.* 2005. Available at: http://www.asahq.org/publicationsAndServices/standards/02.pdf. Accessed June 30, 2008.
83. Pekka M et al. *Patient Oxygen: Your Margin of Safety.* Document No. 896355/PG5/0199. Madison, WI: Datex-Ohmeda; 1999.
84. Davis PD, Kenny GNC. *Basic Physics and Measurement in Anaesthesia.* 5th ed. Edinburgh, United Kingdom: Butterworth Heinemann; 2003.
85. Anaquest: *The Datex-Ohmeda Tec 6 Vaporizer: for the Administration of Suprane (desflurane).* Liberty Corner, NJ: Anaquest; 1992.
86. Datex-Ohmeda. *Operators Manual: Tec 4 Continuous Flow Vaporizers.* Madison, WI: Datex-Ohmeda; 1986.
87. Datex-Ohmeda. *Tec 5 Continuous Flow Vaporizer: Operation and Maintenance Manual.* Madison, WI: Datex-Ohmeda; 1990.
88. Datex-Ohmeda. *Tec 6 Vaporizer: Operation and Maintenance Manual.* Madison, WI: Datex-Ohmeda; 1993.
89. GE Healthcare. *Tec 7 Vaporizer Specifications.* 2002. Available at: http://www.gehealthcare.com/usen/anesthesia/docs/AN3688.pdf. 2002. Accessed June 30, 2008.
90. Hendrickx JF et al. The ADU vaporizing unit: a new vaporizer. *Anesth Analg.* 2001;93:391-395.
91. Walter Reed Army Medical Center: *Ohmeda 885A Field Anesthesia Machine Use Tutor.* (Undated.) Available at: http://www.wramc.army.mil/Patients/healthcare/surgery/anesthesiology/Pages/introamachine.aspx. Accessed June 30, 2008.
92. Andrews JJ, Johnston RV. The new Tec 6 desflurane vaporizer. *Anesth Analg.* 1993;76:1338-1341.
93. Eger EI. *Desflurane (Suprane): a Compendium and Reference.* Rutherford, NJ: Healthpress; 1993.
94. Johnston RV et al. The effects of carrier gas composition on the performance of the Tec 6 desflurane vaporizer. *Anesth Analg.* 1994;79:548-552.
95. Miller D. The Tec 6 vaporizer: why desflurane needs to be heated. *AANA J.* 1994;62:527-531.
96. Andrews JJ et al. Consequences of misfilling isoflurane vaporizers with desflurane. *Anesth Analg.* 1994;78:S7.
97. Drägerwerk. *Dräger Vapor 19.n Anaesthetic Vaporizer: Instructions for Use.* Lübeck, Germany: Drägerwerk; 1991.
98. Petty C. Equipment safety: vaporizer exclusion or interlock systems. *APSF Newsl.* 1992;7:10.
99. Freeman RC, Siebert EM. Keyed vaporizer filling not infallible. *AANA J.* 2005;73:337-338.
100. Keresztury MF et al. A surprising twist: an unusual failure of a keyed filling device specific for a volatile inhaled anesthetic. *Anesth Analg.* 2006; 103:124-125.
101. Daniels D. Overfilling of vaporizers. *Anaesthesia.* 2002;57:288.
102. Mitton M. In response: tribulations with filling Tec 7 vaporizers. *Anesth Analg.* 2007;104:1604-1605.
103. Council for Public Interest in Anesthesia. Be vigilant: vaporizers can go out-of-calibration. *Qual Rev Anesth.* 2005;8:2.
104. Ghai B, Makkar JK. An unusual cause of faulty Tec 7 vaporizer. *Anesth Analg.* 2005;101:1890-1891.
105. Geffroy J-C et al. Massive inhalation of desflurane due to vaporizer dysfunction. *Anesthesiology.* 2005;103:1096-1098.

106. Chun NL. A potential circuit leak with Tec 5 vaporizers. *Anesthesiology.* 1997;87:1599.

107. Macleod DM, McEvoy L. Report of vaporizer malfunction. *Anaesthesia.* 2002;57:299-300.

108. Rupani G. Refilling a Tec 6 desflurane vaporizer. *Anesth Analg.* 2003;96:1534-1535.

109. Hendrickx JFA et al. Severe ADU desflurane vaporizing unit malfunction. *Anesthesiology.* 2003;99:1459.

110. Hercock T, Dawoojee D. Desflurane vaporizer: two hazardous incidents. *Anesth Analg.* 2006;103:1625.

111. Aziz E, Sanders GM. Failure of Datex AS/3 anaesthesia delivery unit. *Anaesthesia.* 2000;55:1214-1215.

112. Macartney NJD, Cohen J. Another case of anaesthetic machine failure. *Anaesthesia.* 2000;55:1215.

113. Grace WR. *The Sodasorb Manual of Carbon Dioxide Absorption.* Lexington, MA: WR Grace, Dewey and Almy Chemical; 1992.

114. Cantillo J et al. Ventilatory failures with the Datex-Ohmeda 7900 SmartVent. *Anesthesiology.* 2002;96:766-768.

115. Moyers J. A nomenclature for methods of inhalation anesthesia. *Anesthesiology.* 1953;14:609-611.

116. Petty C. *The Anesthesia Machine.* New York: Churchill Livingstone; 1987.

117. Forrester K. Cost savings associated with low flow anesthesia. *AANA J.* 1989;57:329-334.

118. Mapleson WW. The elimination of rebreathing in various semiclosed anaesthetic systems. *Br J Anaesth.* 1954;26:323-332.

119. Jellish WS et al. Hypercapnia related to a faulty adult co-axial breathing circuit. *Anesth Analg.* 2001;93(4):973-974.

120. Ghai B et al. Hypercarbia and arrhythmias resulting from faulty Bain circuit: a report of two cases. *Anesth Analg.* 2006;102(6):1903-1904.

121. Nakae Y et al. Comparison of the Jackson-Rees circuit, the pediatric circle, and the MERA F breathing system for pediatric anesthesia. *Anesth Analg.* 1996;83(3):488-492.

122. Fritz MR. Safety danger in cost cutting discussed at ASA. *APSF Newsl.* 1995;9:46.

123. Randhawa N et al. Coaxial breathing system outer tube occlusion: What goes in must come out. *Anaesthesia.* 2002;57(7):716-717.

124. Bourke DL, Tolentino D. Inadvertent positive end-expiratory pressure caused by a malfunctioning ventilator relief valve. *Anesth Analg.* 2003;97(2):492-493.

125. Dawood AM, Digger T. An apparently normal looking valve as a cause of rebreathing. *Anaesthesia.* 2002;57(9):929-930.

126. Kitagawa H et al. A new leak test for specifying malfunctions in the exhalation and inhalation check valve. *Anesth Analg.* 1994;78(3):611.

127. Aung SM et al. An unusual cause of carbon dioxide rebreathing in a circle absorber system. *Anesth Analg.* 1994;78(5):1027-1028.

128. Council for Public Interest in Anesthesia. Failed exhalation valve causes death. *Qual Rev Anesth.* 2004;6:3.

129. Gravenstein JS et al. *Capnography in Clinical Practice.* Boston: Butterworth; 1989.

130. Weigel WA, Murray WB. Detecting unidirectional valve incompetence by the modified pressure decline method. *Anesth Analg.* 2005;100(6):1723-1727.

131. ECRI. Hazard report: injuries—one fatal—highlight the need for pre-use testing of disposable breathing circuits. *Health Devices.* 2000;29:188-189.

132. Thorpe CM. Plastic in anaesthetic circuit. *Anaesthesia.* 2002;57(1):85-86.

133. Eckhout GV, Bhatia S. Another cause of difficulty in ventilating a patient. *J Clin Anesth.* 2003;15(2):137-139.

134. Khorasani A et al. Inadvertent misconnection of the scavenger hose: a cause for increased pressure in the breathing circuit. *Anesthesiology.* 2000;92(5):1501-1502.

135. Cróinín DF, Keogh J. Connector mix-up on an anaesthetic machine. *Anaesthesia.* 2002;57(11):1137-1138.

136. Baum JA. *Low Flow Anesthesia with Dräger Machines.* Lubeck, Germany: Dräger; 2004.

137. Yamashita K et al. Efficacy of a heat and moisture exchanger in inhalation anesthesia at two different flow rates. *J Anesth.* 2007;21(1):55-58.

138. Berry AJ, Nolte FS. An alternative strategy for infection control of anesthesia breathing circuits: a laboratory assessment of the Pall HME Filter. *Anesth Analg.* 1991;72(5):651-655.

139. Gunn N. *Pall Technical Report: Nosocomial Infection from Anesthetic and Ventilation Equipment.* Portsmouth, England: Pall Biomedical Products; 1991.

140. American Association of Nurse Anesthetists. *Scope and Standards for Nurse Anesthesia Practice.* 2005. Available at: http://www.aana.com/uploadedFiles/Resources/Practice_Documents/scope_stds_nap07_2007.pdf. Accessed June 30, 2008.

141. American Association of Nurse Anesthetists. *Infection Control Guide, Part III: Infection Control Procedures for Anesthesia Equipment.* 1997. Available at: http://www.aana.com/resources.aspx?ucNavMenu_TSMenuTargetID=51&ucNavMenu_TSMenuTargetType=4&ucNavMenu_TSMenuID=6&id=737. Accessed June 30, 2008.

142. Tessler MJ et al. Bacterial counts on the hands of anesthetists and anesthesia technicians. *Anesth Analg.* 1994;78(5):1030-1031.

143. Hall JR. Blood contamination of anesthesia equipment and monitoring equipment. *Anesth Analg.* 1994;78(6):1136-1139.

144. ECRI: An overview of heated humidifiers. *Technol Anesth.* 1994;15:1-4.

145. North American Dräger. *Absorber System: Operator's Instruction Manual.* Telford, PA: Dräger; 1988.

146. Higuchi H et al. The carbon dioxide absorption capacity of Amsorb is half that of soda lime. *Anesth Analg.* 2001;93(1):221-225.

147. Wissing H et al. Carbon monoxide production from desflurane, enflurane, halothane, isoflurane, and sevoflurane with dry soda lime. *Anesthesiology.* 2001;95(5):1205-1212.

148. Yamakage M et al. Carbon dioxide absorbents containing potassium hydroxide produce much larger concentrations of compound A from sevoflurane in clinical practice. *Anesth Analg.* 2000;91(1):220-224.

149. Versichelen LF et al. Only carbon dioxide absorbents free of both NaOH and KOH do not generate compound A during in vitro closed-system sevoflurane: evaluation of five absorbents. *Anesthesiology.* 2001;95(3):750-755.

150. McHaourab A et al. Lack of degradation of sevoflurane by a new carbon dioxide absorbent in humans. *Anesthesiology.* 2001;94(6):1007-1009.

151. Kharasch ED et al. Comparison of Amsorb, sodalime, and Baralyme degradation of volatile anesthetics and formation of carbon monoxide and compound A in swine in vivo. *Anesthesiology.* 2002;96(1):173-182.

152. Yamakage M et al. Production of compound A under low-flow anesthesia is affected by type of anesthetic machine. *Can J Anaesth.* 2001;48(5):435-438.

153. Bouche MP et al. No compound A formation with Superia during minimal-flow sevoflurane anesthesia: a comparison with Sofnolime. *Anesth Analg.* 2002;95(6):1680-1685.

154. Holak EJ et al. Carbon monoxide production from sevoflurane breakdown: Modeling of exposures under clinical conditions. *Anesth Analg.* 2003;96(3):757-764.

155. Eger EI et al. *The Pharmacology of Inhaled Anesthetics.* San Antonio, TX: Dannemiller Memorial Educational Foundation; 2002.

156. Abbott Laboratories: *Ultane (sevoflurane): Volatile Liquid for Inhalation.* 2006. Available at: http://www.rxabbott.com/pdf/ultanepi.pdf. Accessed June 30, 2008.

157. Lemmens HJ. Amsorb causes no less carbon monoxide formation than either "new" or "classic" sodalime. *Anesthesiology.* 2002;97(4):1038.

158. Knolle E et al. Small carbon monoxide formation in absorbents does not correlate with small carbon dioxide absorption. *Anesth Analg.* 2002;95(3):650-655.

159. Epstein RA. In my opinion: carbon monoxide: what should we do? *APSF Newsl.* 1995;9:39-41.

160. Cummings K 3rd. Carbon dioxide rebreathing due to unrecognized Amsorb Plus exhaustion. *Anesth Analg.* 2007;105(1):289.

161. Olympio MA. Channeling causes concern. *APSF Newsl.* Spring 2006; 21:14-15.

162. Pond D et al. Failure to detect CO_2-absorbent exhaustion: seeing and believing. *Anesthesiology.* 2000;92(4):1196-1198.

163. GE Healthcare: *Medisorb Medical Soda Lime.* Document No. M1072529/0306. 2006. Available at: http://www.gehealthcare.com/euen/anesthesia/docs/Medisorb_M1072529_eng.pdf. Accessed June 30, 2008.

164. Strum DP, Eger EI 2nd. The degradation, absorption, and solubility of volatile anesthetics in soda lime depend on water content. *Anesth Analg.* 1994;78(2):340-348.

165. Johnstone RE. CO_2 removal: a concern with new anesthesia machines. *Anesth Analg.* 2003;97(6):1852.

166. Lampotang S et al. The effect of a bellows leak in an Ohmeda 7810 ventilator on room contamination, inspired oxygen, airway pressure, and tidal volume. *Anesth Analg.* 2005;101(1):151-154.

167. Datex-Ohmeda. *Standing Bellows Technology.* Document No. ED2013-B. Madison, WI: Datex-Ohmeda; 1998.

168. Adams AP. Breathing system disconnections. *Br J Anaesth.* 1994; 73(1):46-54.

169. Dräger Medical Inc. *The Anesthesia Ventilator: Why Is the Piston Replacing the Bellows?* Document No. 90 49 447/01.04-1. Lubeck, Germany: Dräger; 2004.

170. Datex-Ohmeda. *Volume Control Ventilation.* Document No.ED2010-B. Madison, WI: Datex-Ohmeda; 1998.

171. Datex-Ohmeda. *Pressure Control Ventilation*. Document No. ED2011-B. Madison, WI: Datex-Ohmeda; 1998.

172. Brimacombe J et al. Pressure support ventilation versus continuous positive airway pressure with the laryngeal mask airway: a randomized crossover study of anesthetized adult patients. *Anesthesiology.* 2000;92(6): 1621-1623.

173. Marcy TW, Marini JJ. Control mode ventilation and assist/control ventilation. In: Stock MS, Perel A, eds. *Handbook of Mechanical Ventilatory Support*, 2nd ed. Baltimore, MD: Williams & Wilkins; 1997:89-110.

174. Datex-Ohmeda. *Synchronized Intermittent Mandatory Ventilation*. Document No. ED4130-B. Madison, WI: Datex-Ohmeda; 2002.

175. Datex-Ohmeda. *Pressure Support Ventilation: Impact on Anesthesia Practice*. Document No. ED4137-B/12 02 1. Madison, WI: Datex-Ohmeda; 2002.

176. Frawley PM, Habashi NM. Airway pressure release ventilation: theory and practice. *AACN Clin Issues.* 2001;12(2):234-246.

177. Feldman JM, Smith J. Compliance compensation of the Narkomed 6000 explained. *Anesthesiology.* 2001;94(3):543-544.

178. Cooper JB. Unidirectional PEEP valves can cause safety hazards. *APSF Newsl.* 1990;5:28.

179. Rothschiller JL et al. Evaluation of a new operating room ventilator with volume-controlled ventilation: The Ohmeda 7900. *Anesth Analg.* 1999; 88(1):39-42.

180. Ianchulev SA, Comunale ME. To do or not to do a preinduction check-up of the anesthesia machine. *Anesth Analg.* 2005;101(3):774-776.

181. Ezaru CS. Preinduction check-up of the anesthesia machine. *Anesth Analg.* 2006;102(5):1588-1589.

182. Kshatri AM, Kingsley CP. Defective carbon dioxide absorber as a cause for a leak in a breathing circuit. *Anesthesiology.* 1996;84(2):475-476.

183. Gravenstein D et al. Aestiva ventilation mode selector switch failures. *Anesth Analg.* 2007;104(4):860-862.

184. Gunter JB et al. Catastrophic failure of Aestiva 3000 absorber manifold. *Anesthesiology.* 2004;100(1):199-200.

185. Rossberg MI, Greenberg RS. Anesthesia respiratory circuit failure. *Anesthesiology.* 2002;97(3):762-763.

186. Wagner K, Loy J. A strange place to find a cable tie. *Anesth Analg.* 2006;102(2):655-656.

187. Bader SO et al. A novel leak from an unfamiliar component. *Anesth Analg.* 2006;102(3):975-976.

188. Raphael DT: The low-pressure alarm condition: safety considerations and the anesthesiologist's response [electronic version]. *APSF Newsl.* 1998;winter: Available at: http://www.apsf.org/resource_center/newsletter/1998/winter/07special.html. Accessed June 30, 2008.

189. Feldman JM et al. New electronic checklists aim at decreasing anesthetist errors. *APSF Newsl.* 1992;7:1-2.

190. Anesthesia Patient Safety Foundation. *Technology Training Initiative.* 2007. Available at: http://www.apsf.org/initiatives/technology_training.mspx. Accessed June 30, 2008.

191. Yassin K, Gibbons JJ. A hidden leak in the circle system. *Anesth Analg.* 1991;73(2):236.

192. Lee O, Sommer RM. Pressure monitoring hose causes leak in anesthesia breathing circuit. *Anesth Analg.* 1991;73(3):365.

193. Milliken RA, Bizzarri DV. An unusual cause of failure of anesthetic gas delivery to a patient circuit. *Anesth Analg.* 1984;63(11):1047-1048.

194. Johnstone R, Graf D. Bellows failure with Drager Anesthesia Ventilator. *Anesth Analg.* 1993;76(3):685-686.

195. Chaney MA. Delivery of excessive airway pressure to a patient by the anesthesia machine. *Anesth Analg.* 1993;76(5):1166-1167.

196. Sosis MB. Drager ventilator failure on changing the respiratory rate setting. *Anesth Analg.* 1993;76(2):453-454.

197. Ananthanarayan C, Fisher JA. Drager ventilator failure. *Anesth Analg.* 1993;77(3):638.

198. Singh S, Loeb RG. Fatal connection: death caused by direct connection of oxygen tubing into a tracheal tube connector. *Anesth Analg.* 2004;99(4): 1164-1165.

199. Berry JM, Blanks S. Misplaced valve poses potential hazard. *APSF Newsl.* 2004;19:8-9.

200. Wright T. Absorbent wrapper design questioned. *APSF Newsl.* 2006; 20:70-71.

201. Ransom ES, Norfleet EA. Obstruction due to retained carbon dioxide absorber canister wrapping. *Anesth Analg.* 1997;84:703.

202. Aso Kanno T et al. A combustive destruction of expiration valve in an anesthetic circuit. *Anesthesiology.* 2003;98(2):577-579.

203. Laster M et al. Fires from the interaction of anesthetics with desiccated absorbent. *Anesth Analg.* 2004;99:769-774.

204. Malignant Hyperthermia Association of the United States: *ABCs of Managing Malignant Hyperthermia*. 2006. Available at: http://medical.mhaus.org/index.cfm/fuseaction/OnlineBrochures.Display/BrochurePK/BCD9151D-3048-709E-5A445BC0808B4767.cfm. Accessed June 30, 2008.

205. Petroz GC, Lerman J. Preparation of the Siemens KION anesthetic machine for patients susceptible to malignant hyperthermia. *Anesthesiology.* 2002; 96(4):941-946.

206. Petty C. Scavenger is often a neglected safety device. *APSF Newsl.* 1992;7:28.

207. Huffman LM. Common problems in waste gas management. *AANA J.* 1991;59:109-112.

208. American Association of Nurse Anesthetists. *Management of Waste Anesthetic Gases*. Park Ridge, IL: AANA; 1992.

209. American Society of Anesthesiologists. *Waste Anesthetic Gases: Information for Management in Anesthetizing Areas and the Postanesthesia Care Unit (PACU)*. (Undated.) Available at: http://www.asahq.org/publicationsAndServices/wasteanes.pdf. Accessed June 30, 2008.

210. Occupational Safety and Health Administration: *Waste Anesthetic Gases*. Fact Sheet No. OSHA 91-38. 1991. Available at: http://www.osha.gov/pls/oshaweb/owadisp.show_document?p_id=128&p_table=FACT_SHEETS. Accessed June 30, 2008.

211. Summer G et al. Sevoflurane in exhaled air of operating room personnel. *Anesth Analg.* 2003;97(4):1070-1073.

212. North American Dräger. *Scavenger Interface for Suction Systems: Operator's Instruction Manual*. Telford, PA: Dräger; 1987.

213. Datex-Ohmeda. *Waste Gas Scavenging Interface Valve Assembly: Operation and Maintenance Manual*. Madison, WI: Datex-Ohmeda; 1991.

214. Connell GR, Mangar D. Is your scavenger system functional? *Anesth Analg.* 1992;75(6):1075.

215. Dräger Medical AG. *Anaesthetic Gas Scavenging System*. Document No. 90 29 327-GA 6913.305 de/en. Lubeck, Germany: Dräger; 2001.

216. Kole TE. Reduce, reuse, and recycle in the anesthesia workplace. *AANA J.* 1992;60:109-112.

217. Troyer GT. Controlling the legal liabilities of anesthetic gases. *Health Care Strateg Manage.* 1985;3:11-15.

218. Ward BG. Monitoring toxic substances: protecting your employees and your institution. *Health Care Strateg Manage.* 1985;3:16-17.

219. Karp D, Graham K. *Risk Management Guide for Certified Registered Nurse Anesthetists*. Park Ridge, IL: AANA; 1987.

220. Cooper JB. New law requires hospitals to report device-related injuries and deaths. *APSF Newsl.* 1991;6:13-17.

221. Huffman LM. Safe Medical Device Act: new law alters practice patterns. *Anesth Today.* 1992;3:7-11.

222. Spooner RB, Kirby RR. Equipment-related anesthetic incidents. *Int Anesthesiol Clin.* 1984;22(2):133-147.

223. Kumar V et al. An analysis of critical incidents in a teaching department for quality assurance. A survey of mishaps during anaesthesia. *Anaesthesia.* 1988;43(10):879-883.

224. Kumar V et al. A random survey of anesthesia machines and ancillary monitors in 45 hospitals. *Anesth Analg.* 1988;67(7):644-649.

225. Holley HS, Carroll JS. Anaesthesia equipment malfunction. *Anaesthesia.* 1985;40(1):62-65.

226. Craig J, Wilson ME. A survey of anaesthetic misadventures. *Anaesthesia.* 1981;36(10):933-936.

227. Cooper JB et al. An analysis of major errors and equipment failures in anesthesia management: considerations for prevention and detection. *Anesthesiology.* 1984;60(1):34-42.

228. Henry DW Jr. Examination of the efficacy of education concerning a standardized anesthesia machine checkout procedure upon the machine fault detection ability of anesthetists. *AANA J.* 1989;57(6):500-504.

229. Buffington CW et al. Detection of anesthesia machine faults. *Anesth Analg.* 1984;63(1):79-82.

230. Biddle C. Report of controlled prospective study of students vs. practicing CRNAs on performance of routine gas machine maintenance and fault-detection ability [letter]. *AANA J.* 1985;53:286-287.

231. March MG, Crowley JJ. An evaluation of anesthesiologists' present checkout methods and the validity of the FDA checklist. *Anesthesiology.* 1991; 75(5):724-729.

232. Lees DE. FDA preanesthesia checklist being evaluated, revised. *APSF Newsl.* 1991;6:25-27.

233. Chopra V et al. Checklists: aviation shows the way to safer anesthesia. *APSF Newsl.* 1991;6:26-29.

234. Witham-Wilson MJ. FDA pre-use equipment checklist spurred by accidents, studies. *APSF Newsl.* 1991;6:27.

235. Charlton JE. Checklists cited as contributing to safety. *APSF Newsl.* 1990;5:30-31.

236. Williams JR. What is the current status of the FDA checklist? *Nurse Anesth.* 1991;2:3-5.

237. Good ML. Comments sought on new FDA preanesthesia checklist. *APSF Newsl.* 1992;7:47-51.

238. Dean RJ. Reader seeks standards for equipment check. *APSF Newsl.* 2006;21:78-79.

239. Feldman JM: Efforts under way to revise the pre-use checkout recommendations [electronic version]. *ASA Newsletter.* 2005;October. Available at: http://www.asahq.org/Newsletters/2005/10-05/feldman10_05.html. Accessed June 30, 2008.

240. Blike G, Biddle C. Preanesthesia detection of equipment faults by anesthesia providers at an academic hospital: comparison of standard practice and a new electronic checklist. *AANA J.* 2000;68(6):497-505.

241. Myers JA et al. Comparison of tests for detecting leaks in the low-pressure system of anesthesia gas machines. *Anesth Analg.* 1997;84(1):179-184.

CHAPTER 17

CLINICAL MONITORING I: CARDIOVASCULAR SYSTEM

Mark A. Kossick

Monitoring of anatomic and physiologic variables during an anesthetic procedure enables anesthetists to enhance patient safety and meet established standards of care.[1] Many different monitors are commonly used to assist in the delivery of an anesthetic, and it is the responsibility of the anesthetist to assimilate data provided by monitors to make appropriate clinical judgments. Consequently, the application of critical thinking skills, thorough physical assessment, vigilance, and the appropriate selection and application of monitors are key requirements in the process of anesthesia monitoring.

Basic monitoring techniques include inspection, auscultation, and palpation. They provide essential subjective and objective data not available from technologic monitors and can alert the anesthetist to impending dangers in select patients. *Inspection* of the patient can provide information regarding the adequacy of oxygen delivery and carbon dioxide elimination, fluid requirements, and positioning and alignment of body structures. *Auscultation* is used to verify correct placement of airway devices such as the endotracheal tube and laryngeal mask airway, to assess arterial blood pressure, and to continually monitor heart sounds and air exchange through the pulmonary system. *Palpation* can aid the anesthetist in assessing the quality of the pulse and degree of skeletal muscle relaxation, as well as locating major vascular structures when placing central venous lines or performing anesthesia regional techniques.

Critical thinking skills are cardinal prerequisites for successful monitoring of a patient's anesthetic. In addition, it is well known that errors in anesthesia care are minimized when anesthetists remain alert and vigilant. This chapter reviews the more commonly used noninvasive and invasive cardiovascular monitors in anesthesia practice.

PULMONARY ARTERY CATHETERIZATION

One of the most significant advances made in critical care medicine was the introduction of the pulmonary artery catheter (PAC) by Swan and Ganz in 1970.[2] Their development of the flow-directed right-sided heart catheter allowed for direct bedside assessment of pulmonary artery (PA) pressures, indirect assessment of left ventricular (LV) filling pressures and right-sided cardiac outputs (CO), and calculation of pulmonary and systemic vascular resistances (SVRs), along with various cardiopulmonary indices. This section of the chapter reviews the interpretation of hemodynamic data obtained from a PAC, variables that can skew the data, and an extension of its use beyond the recording

of vascular pressures to include mixed venous oxygen saturation ($S\overline{V}O_2$), vascular resistance, and CO.

An important question related to the use of the PAC is-To what extent has morbidity and/or mortality been reduced when the PAC has been used to guide medical and nursing care? Practice guidelines for PAC use have been recommended and established by various professional societies through the critique of the literature.[3-5] Such recommendations reveal that the indications and potential benefit (or harm) of PAC use remains controversial.[6-12] Factors that may contribute to the discrepancies in research findings include differences in patient populations and limitations in research methodology, such as retrospective analysis, lack of randomization, and double-blind techniques, and variations in desired hemodynamic clinical end-points.[13-15] Another explanation for conflicting study results deals with competency levels in managing PAC data.[16,17] This explanation was supported by a multicenter study conducted by Iberti and co-workers in 1990.[16] These investigators developed a questionnaire that covered four main topic areas (insertion techniques, cardiac physiology, interpretation of waveforms along with pressure-volume relationships, and application of PAC data in patient treatment) related to PAC use. Examinees from the departments of medicine, surgery, and anesthesiology scored an average of 67% (range 19% to 100%). It is surprising to note that the attendings from all departments scored a mean value of 69%. Statistically, examinees had the most difficulty in interpreting hemodynamic variables (e.g., 47% of 496 respondents were unable to correctly determine the PA occlusive pressure [PAOP] from a clear tracing) and applying PAC data for proper patient treatment. Anesthesia providers who specialize in cardiovascular anesthesia have also been shown to have difficulty in interpreting one of the cardinal waveforms derived from PAC; 39% of cardiovascular anesthesiologists could not correctly interpret a PAOP waveform.[18] Results from these two studies suggest that the understanding of PAC data among patient care providers is extremely variable, and misinterpretation of PAC data may result in increased morbidity and mortality. It is likely that similar deficiencies in the application and interpretation of PAC data exists for nurses, knowing failing scores were noted on competency tests used to assess other areas of critical care.[19] Similarly, the 1988 prospective blinded study by Shoemaker and co-workers[20] supports the contention that PAC use per se does not improve patient outcome, but the way the physiologic information is interpreted and applied in patient care does. Such research findings have caused several groups to develop

FIGURE **17-1** Positive and negative waveforms of a CVP tracing. The third cardiac cycle in this figure does not produce a *c* wave.

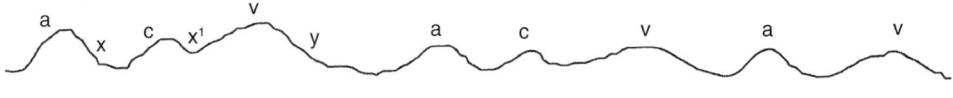

guidelines for the indications of a PAC, along with competency requirements for interpretation of data.[5,21]

Physiology and Morphology of Hemodynamic Waveforms

Essential to accurate interpretation of hemodynamic data derived from central venous lines is a solid foundation in what constitutes "normal" distances, pressures, and waveform morphology for central venous pressure (CVP), right ventricular (RV), PA, and PAOP recordings. Table 17-1 illustrates the approximate distances for reaching the junction of the venae cavae and the right atrium (RA) from various distal anatomic sites. Table 17-2 lists the anticipated distances for reaching various cardiac and pulmonary structures from the right internal jugular vein. Advancement of a catheter 10 cm beyond these distances without the production of a characteristic waveform could indicate coiling of the central line. If this problem arises with a PAC, the balloon should be deflated and the catheter withdrawn. If any resistance is met during withdrawal, a chest radiograph should be taken to rule out knotting or entanglement with the chordae tendineae.

Right Atrial Pressure Waveform

In addition to familiarity with proper distances, knowledge of normal intracardiac pressures, pulmonary pressures (Table 17-3), and waveform morphology facilitates accurate interpretation of PAC data and placement of central lines. For example, under normal circumstances, a CVP tracing will generate mean RA pressures in the range of 1 to 10 mm Hg. The fidelity of the transducing system determines if discernible *a*, *c*, and *v* waves will be displayed once the distal tip of a central line lies just above the junction of the venae cavae and the RA (Figure 17-1). The *a* wave is produced by contraction of the RA, the *c* wave by closure of the tricuspid valve, and the *v* wave by passive filling of the RA (which encompasses a portion of RV systole). The reason the *a* wave is commonly larger than the *c* wave is based on the position of the catheter relative to the physiologic event responsible for the pressure change. In essence, RA systole and the subsequent increase in atrial pressure is directly sensed by a catheter positioned just above (or inappropriately within) the RA, whereas RV systole (a more distal physiologic event relative to the position of a CVP catheter) indirectly increases RA pressure by closure of the tricuspid valve.

Right Ventricular Pressure Waveform

Further advancement of a PAC (approximately 10 cm) produces dramatic changes in the morphology of the hemodynamic waveform. As shown in Figure 17-2, a brisk upstroke (isovolumetric contraction and rapid ejection [RV systole]) and steep downslope (reduced ejection and isovolumetric relaxation [RV systole and diastole]) are viewed on an oscilloscope when a PAC is advanced through the right intraventricular cavity. A PAC with the distal balloon inflated should remain in the RV for as short a time as possible to reduce the incidence of ventricular ectopy, or the development of a conduction defect such as bundle branch block. Because it is undesirable to leave the tip of a central line in the RV, pressures generated during RV systole and RV diastole are assessed indirectly via the CVP port of a PAC and distal tip of the PAC. The former is used to estimate RV

TABLE **17-1**	Distance to the Junction of the Venae Cavae and Right Atrium from Various Distal Anatomic Sites	
Location		**Distance (cm)**
Subclavian		10
Right internal jugular vein		15
Left internal jugular vein		20
Femoral vein		40
Right median basilic vein		40
Left median basilic vein		50

TABLE **17-2**	Distance from the Right Internal Jugular Vein to Distal Cardiac and Pulmonary Structures	
Location or Structure		**Distance (cm)**
Junction venae cavae and right atrium		15
Right atrium		15-25
Right ventricle		25-35
Pulmonary artery		35-45
Pulmonary artery wedge position		40-50

TABLE **17-3**	Normal Intracardiac and Pulmonary Pressures	
Location	**Absolute Value (mm Hg)**	**Range (mm Hg)**
MRAP	5	1-10
RV	25/5*	15-30/0-8
PA S/D	25/10*	15-30/5-15
MPAP	15	10-20
PAOP	10	5-15
MLAP	8	4-12
LVEDP	8	4-12

LVEDP, *Left ventricular end-diastolic pressure;* MLAP, *mean left atrial pressure;* MPAP, *mean pulmonary artery pressure;* MRAP, *mean right atrial pressure;* PA, *pulmonary artery;* PAOP, *pulmonary artery occlusive pressure;* RV, *right ventricular;* S/D, *systolic/diastolic.*
*Values are systolic pressure/diastolic pressure.

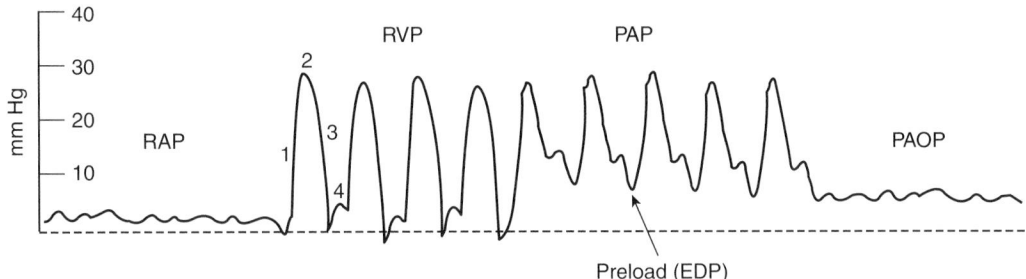

FIGURE **17-2** Pressure waveforms during positioning of a PAC. *EDP*, End-diastolic pressure; *PAOP*, pulmonary artery occlusive pressure; *PAP*, pulmonary artery pressure; *RAP*, right atrial pressure; *RVP*, right ventricular pressure. *1*, isovolumetric contraction (ascent of pressure waveform); *2*, rapid ejection; *3*, isovolumetric relaxation (mid-descent of pressure waveform); *4*, atrial systole (slight increase in pressure).

end-diastolic pressure (EDP) and the latter RV systolic pressure via the PA systolic recording. Thus RVEDP is used to estimate RVED volume (RVEDV), which approximates RV preload (and less accurately LV preload).

Pulmonary Artery Pressure Waveform
When a catheter enters the PA, the diastolic pressure is acutely increased with little change in systolic pressure. The upstroke of the PA tracing is produced by opening of the pulmonic valve, followed by RV ejection. The downstroke contains the dicrotic notch, which is produced by sudden closure of the pulmonic valve leaflets (the beginning of diastole).

Pulmonary Artery Occlusive Pressure Waveform
Final advancement of a PAC by 5 to 10 cm should produce a PAOP tracing. This waveform is similar to a CVP (the *a* wave is produced by left atrial [LA] systole, the *c* wave by closure of the mitral valve, and the *v* wave by filling of the LA, as well as upward displacement of the mitral valve during left ventricular [LV] systole), except that the pressure values are higher. In addition, it is less common to detect a *c* wave on a PAOP tracing, because retrograde transmission of LA pressure (produced by closure of the mitral valve) is significantly attenuated within the pulmonary circulation. The characteristic waveform morphologies of a PAOP tracing are shown in Figure 17-2.

Negative Waveforms
The descents that follow the *a*, *c*, and *v* waves of a CVP or PAOP tracing are labeled as *x*, *x¹*, and *y* (see Figure 17-1). The *x* descent corresponds to the start of atrial diastole (its terminal component [just before the upstroke of the *c* wave (or in its absence, the *v* wave)] with RVEDP and LVEDP), the *x¹* descent is produced by downward pulling of the septum during ventricular systole, and the *y* descent corresponds to opening of the tricuspid valve.

Correlation of Pressure Waveforms and the Electrocardiogram
The interpretation of hemodynamic waveforms can be facilitated by correlating their morphology and timeline with the electrocardiogram (ECG). The *a* wave of a CVP tracing, which is produced by atrial contraction, will follow electrical activation (depolarization) of the atria, and displayed as the P wave on the ECG. The *c* and *v* waves occur after the beginning of ventricular depolarization (QRS complex), or the *v* wave may

not appear until shortly after the T wave (Figures 17-3 and 17-4). When compared with the CVP tracing, the PAOP recording shows greater hysteresis between the waveforms of the ECG and the display of *a*, *c*, and *v* waves—meaning there is a greater distance between ECG activity and the subsequent pressure waveform. Identification of abnormal waveforms is greatly facilitated by the use of the ECG; for example, without an ECG recording, large positive waveforms on a PAOP tracing can be diagnosed as either cannon *a* waves or large *v* waves.

Distortion of Pressure Waveforms
Dysrhythmias can produce significant alterations in hemodynamic waveforms. Atrial fibrillation, junctional rhythms, and premature ventricular contractions (PVCs) can alter the shape of *a* waves. With atrial fibrillation, no synchronized atrial contraction occurs. In the CVP or PAOP tracing, this can lead to the loss of *a* waves or the appearance of small fibrillatory *a* waves. Complete atrioventricular block and some forms of junctional dysrhythmias cause the atria to contract against a closed tricuspid valve, which can produce large cannon *a* waves (Figure 17-5). Ventricular pacing can be associated with both the presence of cannon *a* waves and loss of *a* waves. The former occurs if a patient does not have an atrioventricular sequential pacemaker; the latter when ventricular pacing is used in the setting of asystole (neither atrial or ventricular depolarization is occurring). Valvular defects can also produce dramatic changes in the CVP and PAOP tracings, causing an increase in the amplitude of the *v* wave secondary to regurgitation (e.g., with mitral regurgitation, a portion

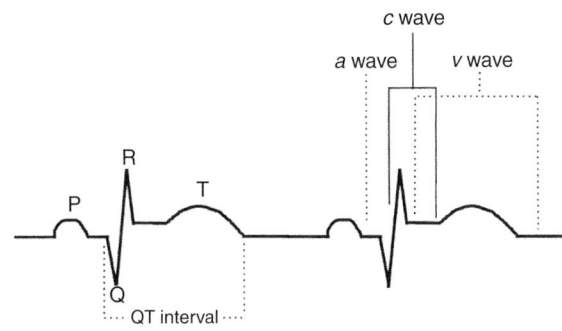

FIGURE **17-3** Temporal relationship between the electrocardiogram and hemodynamic waveforms.

FIGURE **17-4** Electrocardiographic recording with a concurrent central venous pressure tracing that shows the temporal relationship between atrial depolarization (P wave) and the production of an *a* wave, and the QRS complex and the *c* and *v* wave that follow.

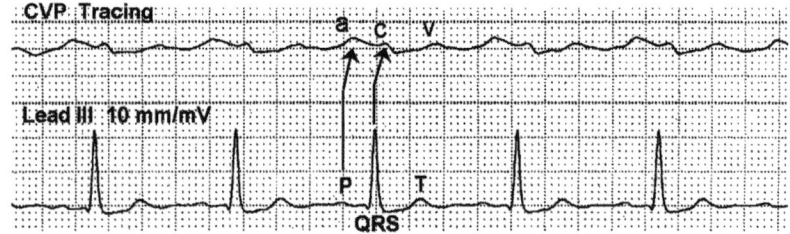

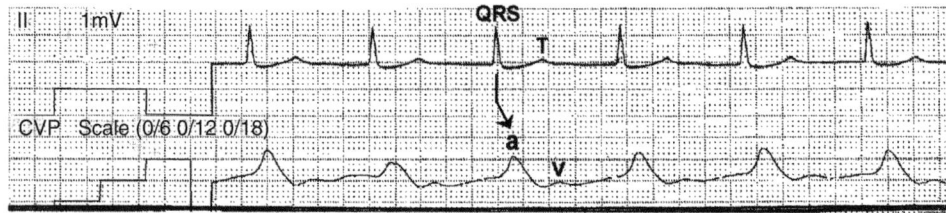

FIGURE **17-5** Electrocardiographic recording of a junctional rhythm (*top*) in which there is simultaneous retrograde atrial and antegrade ventricular depolarization (as evidenced by the lack of a P wave in each cardiac cycle). This results in the right atrium contracting against a closed tricuspid valve. As a consequence, the CVP tracing (*bottom*) has Cannon *a* waves. CVP, Central venous pressure.

of the stroke volume is ejected retrograde into the pulmonary circuit, owing to an incompetent mitral valve). Recognition of such abnormalities is critical for accurate recording of pressure measurements and proper placement of central lines. Significant tricuspid regurgitation can cause a CVP recording to mimic an RV tracing, and mitral regurgitation can cause a PAOP recording to appear as a PA tracing. Specifically, large *v* waves become superimposed on *a* waves. For the indistinguishable PA and PAOP recording, analysis of an $S\overline{V}O_2$ blood sample can assist in making a differential diagnosis. The saturation will be elevated (greater than 77%) if the catheter is in a wedged position, assuming the distal tip is not in a region of the lung that is atelectatic or has pneumonia; both of these factors would produce a false-negative result (normal or low $S\overline{V}O_2$). As a precautionary measure, a catheter suspected of being in a wedged position should not be flushed with the fluid contained in the pressurized transducing system. Although the overall incidence of PA rupture is low (0.064%),[22] flushing of a wedged catheter (as well as balloon overinflation) can result in vascular damage ranging from minor endobronchial hemorrhage to massive hemoptysis.

Significant tricuspid regurgitation and mitral regurgitation may also be associated with normal CVP and PAOP tracings.[23] These occur in patients with a low volume status and compliant atria. In addition, a poor correlation has been found between the size of the *v* wave and the degree of regurgitation. Also of interest is the finding that large *v* waves can be observed in the absence of significant regurgitation. This phenomenon can occur whenever an acute increase in preload occurs, which dynamically reduces atrial and pulmonary vascular compliance.[23]

Whenever large *v* waves are detected on a CVP or PAOP tracing, estimates of preload should be measured just before the upstroke of the v wave (or c wave when present). This point on the pressure recording equates with the EDP, the moment just before ventricular systole that ultimately produces the large *v* waves; the literature demonstrates alternative preload measurement points can be considered as well.[24,25] Box 17-1 indicates

---

BOX 17-1

Factors That Can Distort Central Venous Pressure and Pulmonary Artery Occlusive Pressure Tracings

Loss of *a* Waves or Only *v* Waves
- Atrial fibrillation
- Ventricular pacing in the setting of asystole

Giant *a* Waves—"Cannon" *a* Waves
- Junctional rhythms
- Complete AV block
- PVCs (simultaneous atrial and ventricular contraction)
- Ventricular pacing (asynchronous)
- Tricuspid or mitral stenosis
- Diastolic dysfunction
- Myocardial ischemia
- Ventricular hypertrophy

Large *v* Waves
- Tricuspid or mitral regurgitation
- Acute ↑ in intravascular volume

↑, *Increase;* AV, *atrioventricular;* PVCs, *premature ventricular contractions.*

---

how various rhythm disturbances, pacing, and valvular defects can distort the CVP tracing.

Implications of Abnormal Hemodynamic Values

The CVP serves as an estimate of right ventricular preload (RVEDP). Table 17-4 lists the causes of an elevated CVP. A low CVP correlates with hypovolemia of any cause. As stated previously, RV pressures can be assessed indirectly from the CVP and PA pressure (PAP) recordings. Right ventricular values can be elevated secondary to pulmonary hypertension,

TABLE **17-4**	Potential Causes of Elevated Central Venous Pressure, Pulmonary Artery Pressure, and Pulmonary Artery Occlusive Pressure	
CVP	**PAP**	**PAOP**
• RV failure	• LV failure	• LV failure
• Tricuspid stenosis or regurgitation	• Mitral stenosis or regurgitation	• Mitral stenosis or regurgitation
• Cardiac tamponade	• L-to-R shunt	• Cardiac tamponade
• Constrictive pericarditis	• ASD or VSD	• Constrictive pericarditis
• Volume overload	• Volume overload	• Volume overload
• Pulmonary HTN	• Pulmonary HTN	• Ischemia
• LV failure (chronic)	• "Catheter whip"	

ASD, *Atrial septal defect;* CVP, *central venous pressure;* HTN, *hypertension;* L, *left;* LV, *left ventricular;* PAOP, *pulmonary artery occlusive pressure;* PAP, *pulmonary artery pressure;* R, *right;* RV, *right ventricular;* VSD, *ventricular septal defect.*

TABLE **17-5**	Factors That Alter the Relationships Among Central Cardiovascular Pressures and Volumes
CVP ≠ PADP	• Change in RV compliance (e.g., PS) • Tricuspid valve disease
PADP ≠ PAOP	• Pulmonary HTN • MR or AR • Lung zone I or II • Tachycardia • ARDS • RBBB
PAOP ≠ MLAP	• Juxtacardiac pressure (e.g., PEEP) • Lung zone I or II • Mediastinal fibrosis • RBBB
MLAP ≠ LVEDP	• Juxtacardiac pressure (e.g., PEEP) • Mitral valve disease • Change in LV compliance (e.g., AS)
LVEDP ≠ LVEDV	• Juxtacardiac pressure (PEEP) • Ventricular interdependence • Change in LV compliance (e.g., ischemia)

AR, *Aortic regurgitation;* ARDS, *acute respiratory distress syndrome;* AS, *aortic stenosis;* CVP, *central venous pressure;* HTN, *hypertension;* LVEDP, *left ventricular end-diastolic pressure;* LVEDV, *left ventricular end-diastolic volume;* MLAP, *mean left atrial pressure;* MR, *mitral regurgitation;* PADP, *pulmonary artery diastolic pressure;* PAOP, *pulmonary artery occlusive pressure;* PEEP, *positive end-expiratory pressure;* PS, *pulmonic stenosis;* PVR, *pulmonary artery vascular resistance;* RBBB, *right bundle branch block;* RV, *right ventricular.*

ventricular septal defect, pulmonary stenosis, RV failure, constrictive pericarditis, or cardiac tamponade.

Like the RV waveform, the PA tracing occurs within the QT interval of the ECG. LVEDP can be estimated by measuring the pressure value that exists just before the upstroke of the PA waveform (see Figure 17-2). See Table 17-4 for a list of causes of an increase in the PAP. A false high value can also be produced by a phenomenon called *catheter whip,* which is exaggerated oscillation of the PA tracing. This can occur with excessive catheter coiling if the tip of the PA catheter is near the pulmonic valve; it also occurs in patients with dilated pulmonary arteries. The latter may occur if pulmonary hypertension exists.

One of the most valuable hemodynamic parameters is the PAOP recording. Like the CVP, it indirectly assesses ventricular function and therefore has distinct limitations. To ensure that accurate pressure recordings are documented, the mean or diastolic pressure should always be determined at end-expiration (whether the patient is spontaneously breathing or receiving positive pressure ventilation). This is usually the time when pleural pressures are approximately equal to atmospheric pressures (except when positive end-expiratory pressure [PEEP] is being used). The rationale for this timing relates to the fact that vascular pressure recordings are calibrated relative to atmospheric pressure. As stated previously, the correct area on the pressure recording to determine preload (e.g., LVEDP) is just before the upstroke of the *v* wave (or *c* wave if present). Causes of an elevated PAOP are listed in Table 17-4.

Variables That Influence Hemodynamic Measurements

Essential for proper management of hemodynamic parameters is the recognition of how numerous variables can skew recorded pressure values. The foundation for understanding PAC data begins with the recognition that absolute numbers are generally not as important as trends. In addition, most of the data obtained from a PAC allows for only *indirect* assessment of cardiovascular function and pulmonary indices. For example, PA diastolic pressure (PADP) approximates PAOP, which approximates LA

pressure, which approximates LVEDP, which provides an estimate of left ventricular end-diastolic volume (LVEDV). Table 17-5 lists clinical factors that can skew these pressure and volume relationships. Obviously, reliance on indirect pressure measurements mandates that the anesthetist understand how to interpret these data in light of such limitations. It should be assumed that for most patients who require a PAC or CVP that several, if not numerous, pathophysiologic states exist (e.g., cardiovascular disease, pulmonary dysfunction) that will skew the pressure-to-pressure and pressure-to-volume relationships.

Of the variables listed in Table 17-5, several require further discussion. Many of the factors listed can be viewed as disruptions or obstructions of the continuous column of blood that exists between the RA and LV. This is the case for valvular defects and pulmonary factors.

The goal for placement of a PAC is to have it reside in a West zone III[26] of the lung; this usually does occur, because the bulk of pulmonary blood flow lies within this region of the lung. In this position, the PAP is greater than the pulmonary venous pressure, which is greater than the alveolar pressure. This zone corresponds to a complete circuit or conduit that allows for direct communication between right-sided heart and pulmonary pressures with left-sided intraventricular pressures (see Figure 17-6). It is important to recall that each of the lung zones is physiologically—not anatomically—defined; thus a zone III can change into a zone II (PAP > alveolar pressure > pulmonary venous pressure) or zone I (alveolar pressure > PAP > pulmonary venous pressure).

Factors that contribute to the dynamic state of zone III include the application of PEEP (Figure 17-6), significant

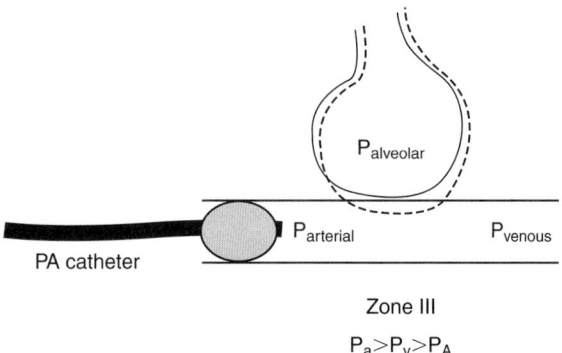

Zone III

$P_a > P_v > P_A$

FIGURE **17-6** Pulmonary artery catheter with balloon inflated (wedging) in a West lung zone III. In this zone, pulmonary pressures equilibrate during diastole because both arterial and venous pulmonary pressures are greater than alveolar pressures. The addition of positive end-expiratory pressure (*dashed-line alveolus*) or hypovolemia can convert a zone III to a zone I or II and lead to distended alveoli and inaccurate estimates of pressures distal to the invagination. P_a, Arterial pressure; P_A, alveolar pressure; P_v, venous pressure; PA, pulmonary artery.

diuresis, hemorrhage, and a change in patient position (e.g., supine to sitting). The influence of PEEP is contingent on the quantity applied, intravascular volume status, and pulmonary compliance. Normally, less than 50% of PEEP is transmitted to the microvasculature—even less if pulmonary compliance is poor (e.g., patients with adult respiratory distress syndrome).[25] In contrast, patients with decreased volume status (e.g., left atrial pressure less than 5 mm Hg) who receive PEEP as low as 7.5 cm H_2O can have collapse of the pulmonary capillaries, which distorts the PAOP.[24] A PAC located in zone I or II will produce marked variations in the PAOP waveform recording during the ventilatory cycle. In addition, *a* and *v* waves (cardiac influences) are lost, and the PAOP exceeds the PADP. This is in contrast to a PAOP recording produced by a catheter located in a true wedge position. The distinguishing criteria include the development of a characteristic waveform with balloon inflation and a PAOP reading less than or equal to the PADP. The latter criterion assumes that no valvular defect, which could also cause the mean PAOP to exceed the PADP, is present.

A rapid heart rate (HR) can also skew the relationship between PADP and the PAOP. Research has demonstrated that left-atrial-paced induced tachycardia (increased HR from 74 to 124 beats per minute) can produce an 11-mm Hg gradient between the PADP and LVEDP.[27] The increase in PADP and decrease in LVEDP result from the shortening of diastole, which reduces the amount of blood being transported from the pulmonary circulation to the LV.[27] Also, as HR increases, the left atrium begins to contract against a partially closed mitral valve.[28]

Another variable that significantly influences PAC data is a change in ventricular compliance. To illustrate this point, consider the fact that a high PAOP (or LVEDP) can exist in patients with an elevated preload with normal ventricular compliance, as well as in patients with a low preload with poor ventricular compliance. A patient with reduced ventricular compliance (e.g., myocardial ischemia, left ventricular hypertrophy, cardiac tamponade, ventricular interdependence) has a high PAOP or PADP that results in overestimation of LVEDV (Figure 17-7) and underestimation of LVEDP. In the setting of poor compliance,

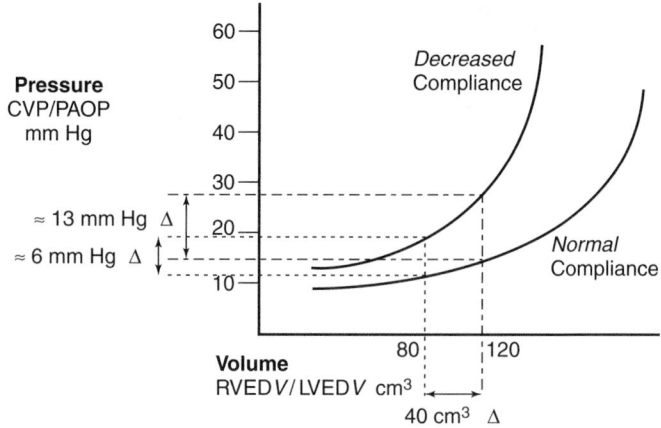

FIGURE **17-7** Effect of changes in ventricular compliance on CVP (which estimates RVEDP) and PAOP (which estimates LVEDP). The curve with *decreased compliance* distorts the relationship between pressure values and estimated ventricular volume. A preload of 80 cm³ in a compliant versus noncompliant ventricle generates a pressure difference of $\approx$ 6 mm Hg (*flat portion of each curve*). On the steeper portion of both curves, the relationship between volume and pressure is skewed even more dramatically. A preload of 120 cm³ generates a pressure difference of $\approx$ 13 mm Hg, which can ultimately lead to a gross overestimation of ventricular preload. Δ, Change; CVP, central venous pressure; LVEDP, left ventricular end-diastolic pressure; PAOP, pulmonary artery occlusive pressure; RVEDP, right ventricular end-diastolic pressure; RVEDV, right ventricular end-diastolic volume; LVEDV, left ventricular end-diastolic volume.

PAOP is not a reliable index for LVEDV.[29] In fact, it has been shown that during myocardial revascularization procedures, high PAOP values exist more than 50% of the time in conjunction with a low volume status (as determined by echocardiography), with patients responding favorably (despite a high PAOP) to an increase in intravascular volume.[30] As previously stated, one must be careful not to be misled by the wedge.[29]

To summarize, the PADP correlates poorly (by 5 mm Hg or more) with the PAOP under the following circumstances: when pulmonary vascular resistance (PVR) is elevated (e.g., chronic obstructive pulmonary disease, human papillomavirus, pulmonary embolus, adult respiratory distress syndrome, hypercarbia), when heart rates exceed 130 beats per minute, when severe mitral or aortic regurgitation is present, or when a lung zone III has changed to a zone II or I (e.g., in the presence of hypovolemia, PEEP). Increases in PVR and HR cause the PADP to exceed PAOP. Severe regurgitation and lung zone changes produce the opposite effect, with PADP being less than the PAOP; this may also hold true for right bundle branch block, based on one researcher's findings of how this conduction defect caused the PADP (in the setting of normal PVR) to be up to 7 mm Hg less than the mean left atrial pressure.[31] A review of the gross interpretation of CVP and PAOP values is presented in Table 17-6.

Other Hemodynamic Indexes

Some authors encourage the use of calculated indexes to optimize the care of critical care patients. These indexes include the pulmonary vascular resistance index (PVRI), systemic vascular resistance (SVR) index (SVRI), and cardiac index (CI). The potential advantages and limitations of each index will be reviewed.

The PVRI (PVR calculated with the CI instead of the CO) is equal to the difference in pressure across the pulmonary circuit

TABLE **17-6**	Potential Clinical Diagnosis via the Use of Hemodynamic Values: Interpretation of Pulmonary Artery Catheter Data		
CVP	**PADP**	**PAOP**	**Interpretation**
Low	Low	Low	Hypovolemia, transducer not at phlebostatic axis*
Normal or high	High	High	LV failure
High	Normal or low	Normal or low	RV failure, TR, or TS
High	High	Normal or low	Pulmonary embolism
High	High	Normal	Pulmonary HTN
High	High	High	Cardiac tamponade, ventricular interdependence, transducer not at phlebostatic axis*
Normal	Normal or high	High	LV myocardial ischemia or MR
Low	High	Normal	ARDS†

ARDS, Acute respiratory distress syndrome; CVP, central venous pressure; HTN, hypertension; LV, left ventricular; MR, mitral regurgitation; PADP, pulmonary artery diastolic pressure; PAOP, pulmonary artery occlusive pressure; RV, right ventricular; TR, tricuspid regurgitation; TS, tricuspid stenosis.

Phlebostatic axis is the fourth intercostal space, midanteroposterior level (not midaxillary line); for the right lateral decubitus position, fourth intercostal space midsternum; for the left lateral decubitus position, fourth intercostal space at the left parasternal border.

†*ARDS patients commonly require initial fluid administration for hemodynamic stability.*

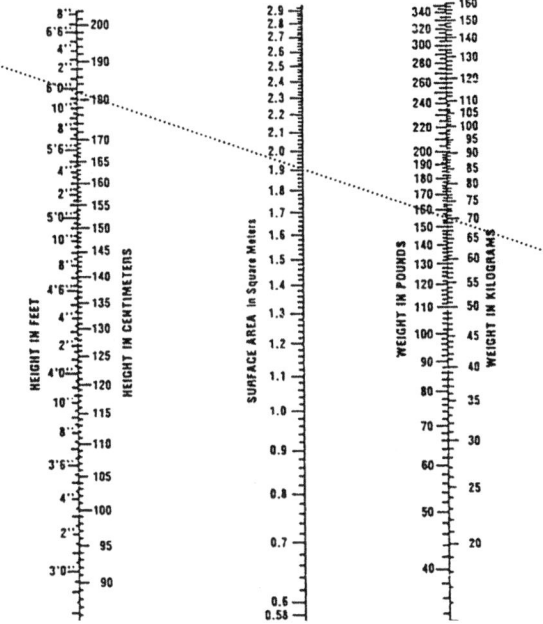

FIGURE **17-8**   Chart used to calculate body surface area. In this example, a height of 6 feet and a weight of 155 lb translate into a surface area of approximately 1.9 m².

(mean PAP − PAOP) divided by flow (CI) times 80. This formula is taken from Ohm's law (with the variables mathematically manipulated) for electric currents (R [Resistance] = V [Voltage] = I [Current]). A normal value is considered to be 45 to 225 dynes • sec/cm⁵ • m². Two limitations of extrapolating physiologic resistance from Ohm's law are that blood flow is pulsatile (not flowing continuously through a set of rigid pipes), and resistance is not uniform throughout the pulmonary circuit. The electrical counterpart describes resistance not in alternating currents, but direct currents.[32]

When PVR is used clinically, it is viewed as an *estimate* of RV afterload. *Afterload* is defined as systolic wall stress or the impedance the ventricle must overcome to eject its stroke volume. Vascular resistance is not synonymous with afterload but is used as an extension of the concept. Pulmonary vascular resistance, like SVR, can affect afterload, but neither formula accounts for changes in ventricular wall thickness or radius, which are components of afterload.

Systemic vascular resistance is commonly used to provide guidance in the use of vasoconstrictors (e.g., phenylephrine infusion) or afterload reduction (e.g., intravenous nitroglycerin or sodium nitroprusside). The limitations described previously for PVR also hold true for SVR, although perhaps to a lesser extent, because the systemic vasculature has lower compliance. Nevertheless, manipulation of SVRI to achieve normal or high values in shock syndromes (e.g., septic shock with low

blood pressure, low blood flow, and low SVRI) has been shown not to correlate with survival, and the development of a low SVRI in shock syndromes does not correlate well with death.[33] In general, the use of vasoconstrictors to support afterload should be deferred until maximization of preload or the use of positive inotropes has proved ineffective. Indiscriminate use of α-adrenergic agonists can worsen microcirculatory blood flow by exaggerating existing nonuniform vasoconstriction; this can lead to a further deterioration in cellular oxygen debt.[34] The SVRI is calculated as the difference between systemic input pressure (mean arterial pressure) minus the output pressure (right atrial pressure or CVP), divided by the CI times 80. The normal range is 1760 to 2600 dynes • sec/cm⁵ • m².

Determination of CO assists critical care specialists in providing rational hemodynamic therapy; evaluating the response to therapy; and determining the adequacy of tissue perfusion, which is linked to maintenance of arterial blood pressure, the delivery of oxygen, and removal of wastes. It also permits the calculation of other hemodynamic indices (e.g., PVR and SVR). A normal CO value should be qualified by taking into account age differences, metabolic activity (declines with anesthesia and increases with hyperthermia), and patient size.

This last factor may be adjusted for by converting a CO to a CI, which attempts to normalize CO for the large number of values found in the general population. However, CI adjusts only for the variables of height and weight. It does not address the lack of uniformity of predicted basal oxygen consumption and metabolic rates resulting from differences in sex and age.[35] In addition, the relationship between body surface area (BSA) and blood flow is indistinct.[35] CI is calculated by dividing CO by BSA. The plotting of height and weight on a body surface chart estimates the BSA in square meters (Figure 17-8). Commonly quoted "normal" values are 5 to 6 L/min for CO and 2.8 to 3.6 L/min • m² for CI.

The most commonly used technique for determining CO is thermodilution, whereby an analog computer calculates the CO by using the modified Stewart-Hamilton equation. This method was first used by Fegler in 1954.[36] It entails the injection of a known quantity of an indicator solution (most commonly 5% dextrose in water, although 0.9% normal saline has a similar density factor)[37] through the proximal port of a thermodilution PAC.[38]

The injected solution is considered a thermal indicator because it is cold relative to body temperature. It rapidly mixes with the incoming blood and is carried through the RV until it is detected by the thermistor near the end of the catheter in the PA. The computer plots a time-temperature curve, with the area under the curve being inversely proportional to the CO; therefore larger curves are not desired. Variables that can influence recorded values include the computation constant (which varies with catheter size, injectate volume, and temperature), temperature of the injectate (desired range of 0° to 24°C),[37,39] volume of injection,[37,39] speed of injection (should be done in 4 seconds or less),[37,40] and the timing of injection (it should be consistent, i.e., the same time during each respiratory cycle).[37,41,42] Iced injectates have not been shown to offer any significant advantage over room-temperature injectates.[37,39] In fact, cold indicator solutions injected rapidly into the right atrium have been shown to produce arrhythmias such as sinus bradycardia.[43,44] Research that has examined the impact of valvular or septal defects on thermodilution CO (TDCO) values has produced conflicting results.[45-47] A list of variables that can skew CO measurements is provided in Table 17-7.

The accuracy for TDCO (including when performed in patients in the lateral position) is ±10%, and the reliability is ±5%.[48,49] These values are lower in the pediatric population,[50] in patients who have low CO,[51] and for measurements taken in the operating room.[52] Anesthetists should be careful not to overinterpret small changes (e.g., 5% to 10%) and should never express values beyond one decimal point. The common practice of averaging three CO output values has also been shown to improve accuracy.[48]

A further advancement in CO technology has been achieved via the placement of thermal filaments within the right ventricular portion of the PAC and near the tip of the thermistor. With the former, a sophisticated computer algorithm permits for analysis of a thermal signal created by small quantities of heat being emitted from the PAC—a pulsed warm thermodilution technique. This heat signal is eventually transmitted by the blood to the distal thermistor, which permits for continuous cardiac output (CCO) assessment.[53] An adequate signal-to-noise ratio is necessary to produce accurate CCO measurements. Research has shown a low ratio (derived from a core body temperature >38.5° C) can result in inaccurate CCO values.[54] One advantage of a CCO catheter is the elimination of the time-consuming administration of a thermal injectate through the proximal port of the PAC. It also reduces the number of discrepancies in thermodilution CO values that can occur with inconsistent injectate administration relative to the respiratory cycle.

A significant drawback to the CCO device is the hysteresis in recording hemodynamic information. Although the monitor displays updated CO figures every 30 seconds, they nonetheless do not represent real-time data. Instead, the CCO values depict the average CO from the prior 3 to 6 minutes.[55] This can be a significant limitation in patients who develop acute hemodynamic changes occurring in response to hemorrhage and resuscitation.[56] In this setting, a standard bolus thermodilution technique is preferable. Manufacturers of CCO monitors have attempted to circumvent this limitation by developing "Fast-Filter" and "Urgent" modes to supplement the "Normal" mode of data processing.

One investigation found a significant decline in the precision of CO measurements when the Fast-Filter and Urgent modes were used.[57] The reliability and accuracy of the device with intensive care and surgical patients have been established with recordings taken in the supine position[54,58] and with the backrest elevated up to 45 degrees.[59] Nevertheless, some investigators have found the CCO technique to be less precise than iced-bolus thermodilution.[60,61] In spite of reports in the literature of a positive clinical outcome based on the use of CCO,[62] future studies will be required to establish whether CCO measurements (as well as other monitoring modalities such as Doppler techniques) reduce the length of hospitalization and improve morbidity and mortality rates.[63]

Mixed Venous Oxygen Saturation

Since its introduction in 1981, use of $S\overline{V}O_2$ as an estimate of systemic oxygen delivery has generated controversy. The purported usefulness of monitoring $S\overline{V}O_2$ is based on the knowledge that it is determined by pulmonary function, cardiac function, oxygen delivery, tissue perfusion, oxygen consumption, and hemoglobin concentration. During the course of an anesthetic procedure (excluding cases of major trauma or hemorrhagic shock), it is not unusual for pulmonary function, hemoglobin content, and oxygen consumption to remain relatively stable. Therefore proponents of $S\overline{V}O_2$ monitoring state that it is reasonable to assume that a decrease in $S\overline{V}O_2$ reflects a change in oxygen delivery, presumably via a reduction in CO. However, numerous studies have shown that in the intensive care unit, $S\overline{V}O_2$ values correlate poorly with CO,[64,65] causing some investigators to criticize its use. Nevertheless, other researchers have found changes in $S\overline{V}O_2$ to parallel changes in CO,[66,67] as well as reduce hospital morbidity and mortality.[68,69] In addition, $S\overline{V}O_2$ monitoring may serve as a prognostic indicator in patients with acute myocardial infarction.[70]

TABLE **17-7**	Variables That Influence Thermodilution CO Values	
Overestimates	**Underestimates**	**Unpredictable**
• Low injectate volume	• Excessive injectate volume	• Right-to-left ventricular septal defect
• Injectate that is too warm	• Injectate solutions that are too cold	• Left-to-right ventricular septal defect
• Thrombus on the thermistor of the PAC		• Tricuspid regurgitation
• Partially wedged PAC		

CO, *Cardiac output;* PAC, *pulmonary artery catheter.*

Continuous mixed venous oximetry is measured with the use of fiberoptic reflectance spectrophotometry through two fiberoptics housed in the PAC. One fiberoptic transmits light-emitting diodes (narrow wavebands of light) to the distal catheter. The extent of light absorption and reflection is a function of the quantity of oxyhemoglobin and deoxyhemoglobin present in the PA.[71] The receiving fiberoptic transports the reflected light to a microprocessor that interprets the signal and displays an $S\overline{V}O_2$ value; the normal range of $S\overline{V}O_2$ is 65% to 77%. Factors that increase $S\overline{V}O_2$ values include left-to-right shunts, hypothermia, sepsis, cyanide toxicity, a wedged PAC, and an increase in CO. $S\overline{V}O_2$ decreases with hyperthermia, shivering, seizures, reduced pulmonary transport of oxygen, hemorrhage, and decreased CO. Sustained low values (e.g., 50%) merit investigation followed by appropriate intervention(s).

It has also been demonstrated that some $S\overline{V}O_2$ monitoring systems adapt well to acute changes in hematocrit.[72] In addition, research with two-wavelength and three-wavelength $S\overline{V}O_2$ oximetry catheters has shown the systems to be comparable in accuracy.[73]

In conclusion, the cost-benefit ratio of using PACs that provide CCO or $S\overline{V}O_2$ measurements remains controversial.[5,55] The use of the PAC has the potential to promote health[11] or cause harm—the major determinant is the clinician's ability to interpret and apply data from this sophisticated diagnostic tool.[74] Therapeutic strategies should be guided by a knowledge of the patient's underlying pathophysiology.

AUTOMATED ST-SEGMENT MONITORING

Computerized real-time ST-segment analysis continues to be incorporated in operating rooms (ORs), intensive care units (ICUs), and postanesthesia care units (PACUs) across the country. Many factors support this trend, including the development of practice guidelines by professional societies that advocate such monitoring techniques in select patient populations[75] and the demographics of the general surgical population. Approximately one third of patients scheduled for noncardiac surgery have risk factors for coronary artery disease (CAD), and postoperative myocardial infarction is three times as frequent in patients with ischemia.[76,77] Research has shown prolonged stress-induced ischemia (i.e., ST-segment depression) to be the major cause for cardiac morbidity (myocardial infarction) after significant vascular surgery.[78] The overall incidence of perioperative ischemia in patients with CAD scheduled for cardiac or noncardiac surgery ranges from 20% to 80%.[79,80]

Because of its low cost, noninvasiveness, widespread availability, and designation as a standard of care for monitoring of all anesthetized patients,[1] the ECG remains a common and required diagnostic tool in the operating room. Compared with Holter monitors, ST-segment trending monitors have on average a sensitivity of 74% and specificity of 73% in detecting myocardial ischemia.[81] When used in high-risk cardiac patients to guide early treatment, they may reduce morbidity.[82]

Although universal standards for an "ECG ischemic threshold" do not exist, acceptable ECG criteria *suggestive* of myocardial injury include the following: (1) ≥1 mm horizontal ST-segment depression; (2) ≥1 mm upsloping or downsloping ST-segment depression measured 60 ms (1.5 mm) or 80 ms (2 mm) from the J point; and (3) ≥1 mm ST-segment elevation (Figure 17-9).[83-85] The J point is used in analyzing depressed ST-segments that are upsloped or downsloped. It is defined as the *junction* (hence J point) between the S wave and ST segment (Figure 17-10). The magnitude of ST-segment depression is determined by measuring a previously established horizontal distance (e.g., 60 ms) from the J point. For example, a vertical line is drawn at a distance of 60 ms from the J point, and the intersection

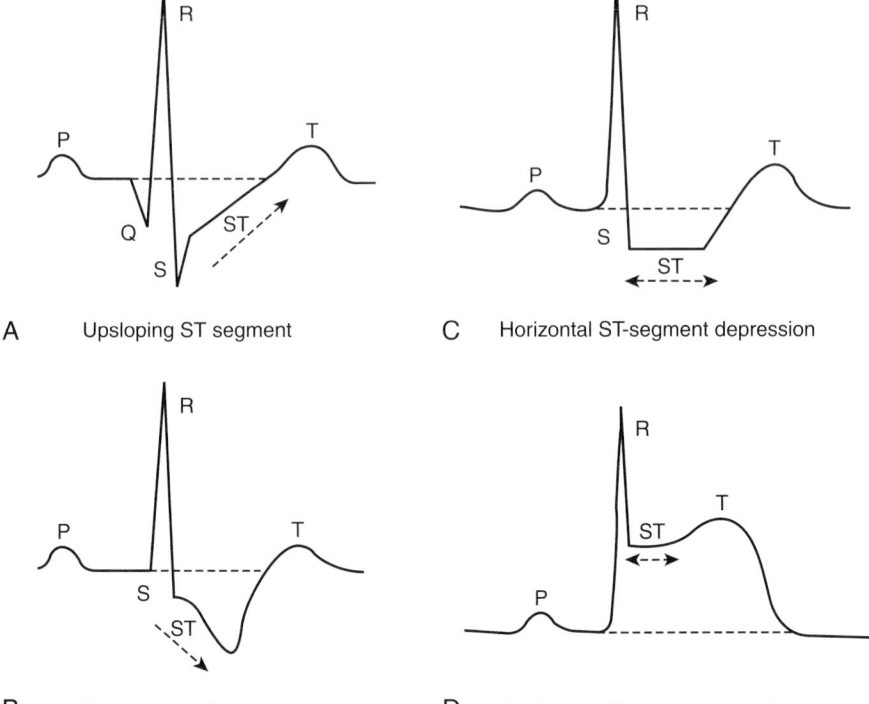

A   Upsloping ST segment

B   Downsloping ST segment

C   Horizontal ST-segment depression

D   Horizontal ST-segment elevation

FIGURE **17-9** Various forms of ST-segment deviation that may occur as a result of myocardial injury. Depression of the ST segment (**A, B, C**) correlates with subendocardial injury, ST-segment elevation (**D**) with transmural injury.

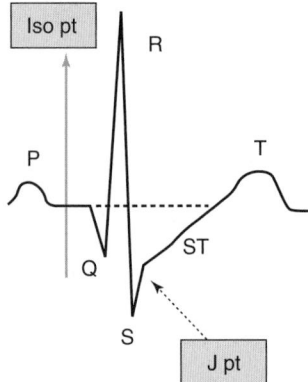

FIGURE **17-10** A single cardiac cycle demonstrating a depressed *ST* segment that is upsloping. The junction between the *S* wave and *ST* segment defines the *J point*. The *Iso point (vertical arrow)* intersects the *PR* segment. The *PR* segment is measured from the end of the *P* wave to the beginning of the *QRS* complex. (*Reprinted with permission from Kossick MA. Recognizing EKG evidence of ischemia, injury, and infarction. In:* EKG Interpretation: Simple, Thorough, Practical. *2nd ed. Park Ridge, IL: AANA Publishing; 1999:22.*)

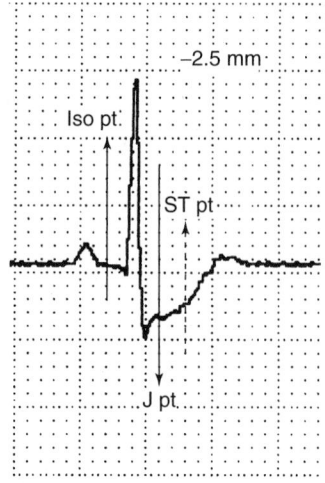

FIGURE **17-12** Correct placement of the *Iso, J,* and *ST* points. (*Reprinted with permission from Kossick MA. Recognizing EKG evidence of ischemia, injury, and infarction. In:* EKG Interpretation: Simple, Thorough, Practical. *2nd ed. Park Ridge, IL: AANA Publishing; 1999:20.*)

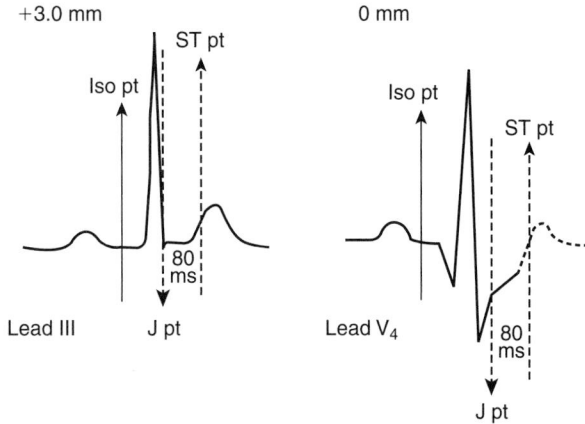

FIGURE **17-11** Two cardiac cycles from *lead III* and V$_4$ illustrating a shortened ST segment. Use of a J point + 80 ms value to measure ST-segment deviation in each lead results in the *ST point* intersecting the T wave, producing inaccurate ST-segment deviation values. For lead III the misplaced ST point produces a false positive and for lead V$_4$, a false negative. *pt*, Point. (*Reprinted with permission from Kossick MA. Recognizing EKG evidence of ischemia, injury, and infarction. In:* EKG Interpretation: Simple, Thorough, Practical. *3rd ed. Park Ridge, IL: AANA Publishing. In press.*)

of this line with the ST segment is noted. This point of intersection defines the degree of ST-segment deviation relative to the isoelectric line, which is referenced as the *Iso point* (i.e., intersects an extended PR segment [see dashed line in Figure 17-10]).

A 60-ms distance measured from the J point is preferred with rapid HRs because during tachyarrhythmias, a shortened ST segment can result from the T wave encroaching on the ST segment. The use of a J + 80-ms distance in this circumstance could actually lead to an ST point that intersects a T wave instead of the ST segment. Should this occur, the computer-derived ST-segment deviation value would reflect a *false*

significant shift in the ST segment, suggesting myocardial injury (false positive) or masking a significant ST-segment depression (false negative [Figure 17-11]).

Regarding the significance of the various forms of ST-segment depression, it is important to recall that a horizontal or down-sloping depressed ST segment has greater specificity (fewer false positives) than an upsloping depressed ST segment. Adding upsloping ST-segment changes to myocardial injury diagnostic criteria does improve overall sensitivity but at a sacrifice to specificity and positive predictive value.[86,87]

Setting the ST-Segment Parameters

Most manufacturers of automated ST-segment analysis monitors have sophisticated algorithms that allow fairly consistent and accurate placement of the ST measurement points, but no system is perfect. Anesthetists should periodically assess ST measurement points and change them as needed; responding to false trends could lead to iatrogenic injury. In fact, manufacturers have incorporated software that permits the health-care provider to override the monitor's placement of the ST measurement points. A common technique for setting ST measurement points involves adjustment of three variables: Iso point, J point, and ST point (Figure 17-12). Manipulation of a keypad on the ECG monitor permits the operator to scroll each of these "points" or vertical lines along a horizontal axis. Figures 17-13 and 17-14 illustrate the consequences when real-time ST-segment analysis software incorrectly places ST-segment measurement points (i.e., the display of inaccurate ST-segment deviation values). The application of an ST-segment deviation algorithm can reduce the occurrence of such mishaps and improve overall management of patients at risk for ischemic changes (Figure 17-15).

Other significant variables to account for when monitoring patients at risk for ischemic events include ECG electrode placement, ECG lead selection, gain setting, and frequency bandwidth. Each of these is briefly reviewed here.

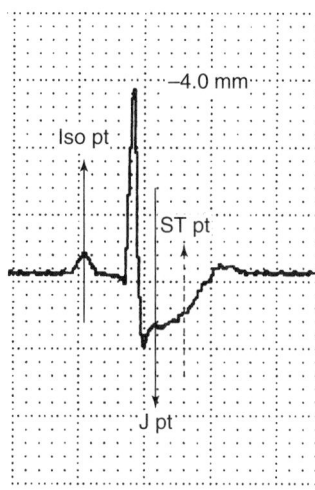

FIGURE **17-13** Iso point incorrectly placed on top of the P wave by an ECG monitor, producing an exaggerated ST-segment deviation value. (*Reprinted with permission from Kossick MA. Recognizing EKG evidence of ischemia, injury, and infarction. In: EKG Interpretation: Simple, Thorough, Practical. 2nd ed. Park Ridge, IL: AANA Publishing; 1999:21.*)

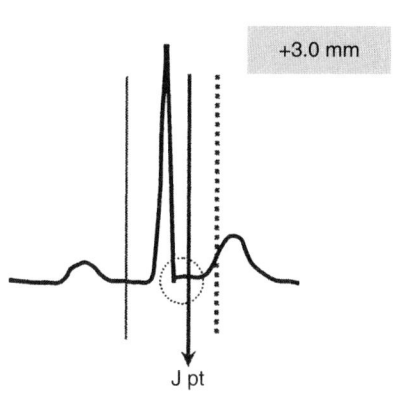

FIGURE **17-14** Incorrect placement of the J point leads to an ST point that intersects on the T wave. (*Reprinted with permission from Kossick MA. Recognizing EKG evidence of ischemia, injury, and infarction. In: EKG Interpretation: Simple, Thorough, Practical. 2nd ed. Park Ridge, IL: AANA Publishing; 1999:21.*)

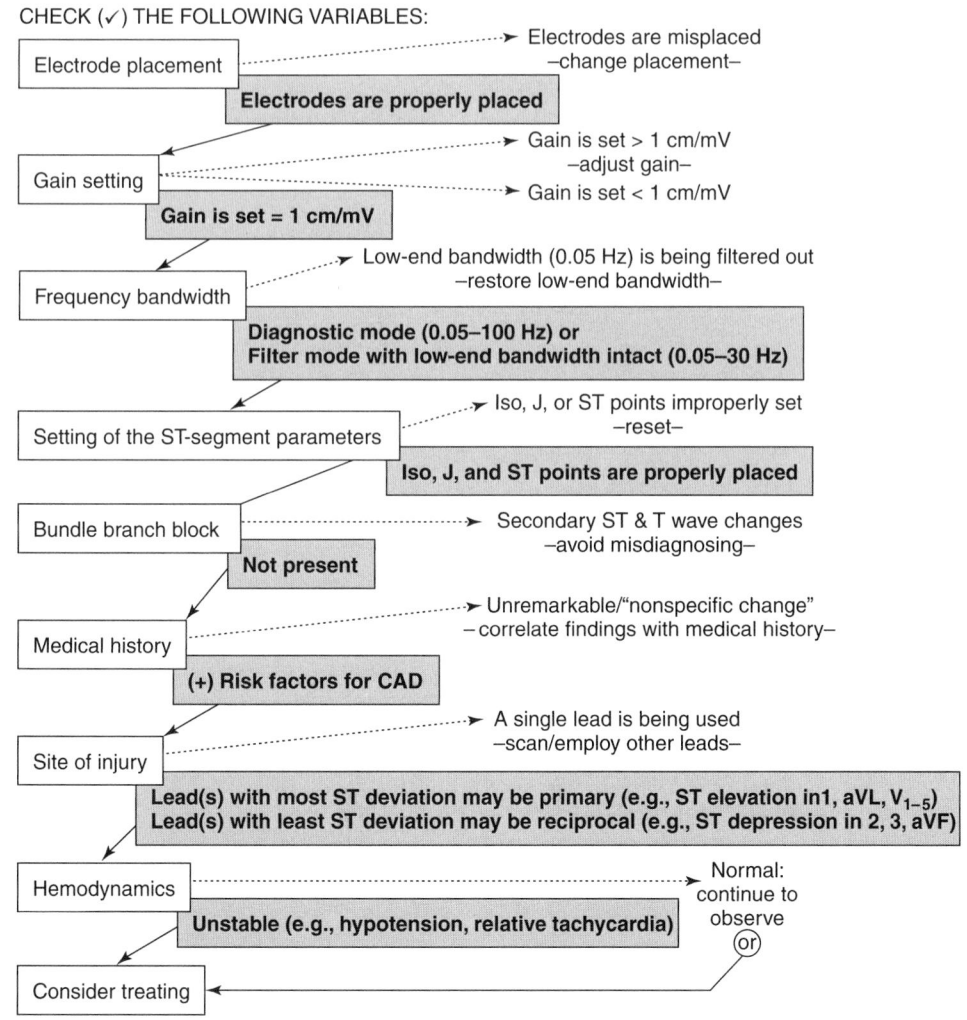

FIGURE **17-15** An ST-segment deviation assessment and treatment algorithm (threshold of 1 mm elevation or depression). (*Reprinted with permission from Kossick MA. Recognizing EKG evidence of ischemia, injury, and infarction. In: EKG Interpretation: Simple, Thorough, Practical. 2nd ed. Park Ridge, IL: AANA Publishing; 1999:16.*)

* Each of the above variables could produce a false positive or false negative

Electrocardiograph Electrode Placement

It is not uncommon to see ECG electrodes inaccurately placed on a patient in an attempt to "move an operating room schedule along." Many times in a physical status (PS) I or II patient, correct ECG electrode placement is a moot point. However, in patients with risk factors for CAD, such inattentiveness can lead to iatrogenic injury by producing deviated ST segments or flipped T waves that can be viewed as "real" problems. Proper placement of the limb lead and chest lead electrodes is described in Table 17-8. For emphasis, the precordial leads should be placed via palpation of the costae, not by gross visual estimation of an intercostal space (Figure 17-16). Understandably, some surgical procedures do not permit the use of optimal ECG lead selection and placement; ECG electrode(s) can interfere with skin preparation and surgical incision. Under these circumstances, a less than optimal ECG lead placement is acceptable.

Electrocardiographic Lead Selection

The decision regarding which ECG leads to monitor during the course of an anesthetic can be extremely important relative to the medical history of the patient. Improper selection can result in unrecognized myocardial ischemia, injury, or infarction. Research has validated that use of a single ECG lead for ischemic monitoring in patients with documented CAD is inadequate; monitoring with multiple leads enhances patient safety.[88] In patients at risk for ischemic events, this author recommends the maximum number of ECG leads be displayed (e.g., 3, 7, 12 [Derived 12-lead]) during the perioperative period to enhance continuous and comprehensive assessment of ST-segment and T-wave changes (Figures 17-17 and 17-18). Which lead(s) is/are best in detecting significant ST-segment changes remains somewhat controversial. First and foremost, if a preoperative 12-lead ECG has been done, "fingerprinting" of this tracing should serve as the primary guide for lead selection during the perioperative period. If the baseline 12-lead shows significant primary ST-segment changes in leads V3, V4 and V5, then this

TABLE **17-8**	Proper Placement of Electrocardiographic Electrodes for Monitoring Limb Leads and Chest Leads*
RA	Near the right shoulder directly beneath the clavicle
LA	Near the left shoulder directly beneath the clavicle
LL	Near the left iliac crest
RL	At any convenient location
V1	Fourth intercostal space right of the sternal border
V2	Fourth intercostal space left of the sternal border
V3	Equal distance between V2 and V4
V4	Midclavicular line at the fifth intercostal space
V5	Horizontal to V4 on the anterior axillary line
V6	Horizontal to V5 on the midaxillary line

LA, *Left arm electrocardiographic (ECG) electrode;* LL, *left leg ECG electrode;* RA, *right arm ECG electrode;* RL, *right leg ECG electrode.*
Placement of the LL electrode in a more superior location (e.g., near the left nipple) can affect the accuracy of ST-segment interpretation and dysrhythmia analysis.

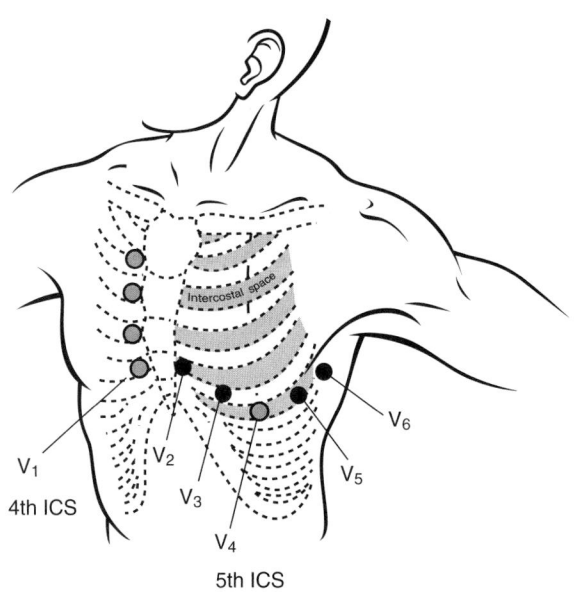

FIGURE **17-16** Precordial electrodes positioned across the ventrolateral aspect of the thorax. V$_1$ placement: 4th intercostal space (ICS) right of the sternum; V$_4$: 5th ICS, left midclavicular line. (*Reprinted with permission from Kossick MA. Basic Concepts. In: EKG Interpretation: Simple, Thorough, Practical. 3rd ed. Park Ridge, IL: AANA Publishing. In press.*)

FIGURE **17-17** Monitoring in 3 ECG leads during anesthetic administration captured significant ST-segment elevation. The greatest change in ST segments occurred in limb lead 3, followed by limb lead 2. Noteworthy was the failure of lead V5 to demonstrate any appreciable change in the ST segment. Postoperatively a cardiology consultation resulted in a diagnosis of Prinzmetal angina.

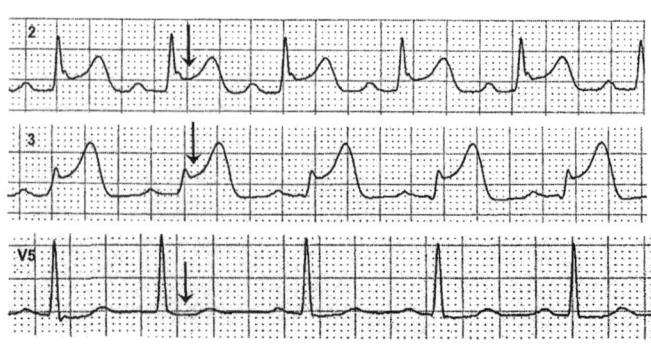

lead set should be prioritized for continuous display in the operating room. The ECG monitoring system will dictate what lead display options can be configured. For example, with Philips software and a five-cable ECG lead system, a derived 12-lead (EASI) can be continuously displayed (see Figure 17-18). With other manufacturers and a five-cable ECG lead system, a true V3 *or* V4, a modified chest lead V5 (e.g., central subclavicular 5 [CS5]), and a bipolar limb lead (e.g., lead II) can be configured for ECG monitoring (Figure 17-19).

In patients without a preoperative 12-lead or who have a baseline 12-lead that is essentially normal, the literature suggests leads V3, V4, and limb lead III be selected for continuous monitoring for ST-segment elevation.[88-90] Leads V3 and III are sensitive for detecting supply ischemia/transmural myocardial injury (as seen during angioplasty procedures). Lead II is recommended for assessment of narrow QRS complex rhythms, particularly if the P wave is significant for diagnostic criteria (e.g., atrial flutter, atrial fibrillation, junctional rhythms). If the anticipated change in ST segment is depression, which would correlate with subendocardial injury (demand and/or supply ischemia), then perhaps V5, limb lead II, and III may be best.[91-93]

However, some researchers with strong internal validity in their study have found V5 and II to be insensitive leads for detecting ST-segment changes.[94] The recommendation for V5 and limb lead II as preferred leads[92] has also been challenged by Landesberg and colleges in 2002. In their research, 185 consecutive patients undergoing vascular surgery were monitored by continuous 12-lead ST-trend analysis during the perioperative period and up to 72 hours postoperatively. Chest lead V3 was

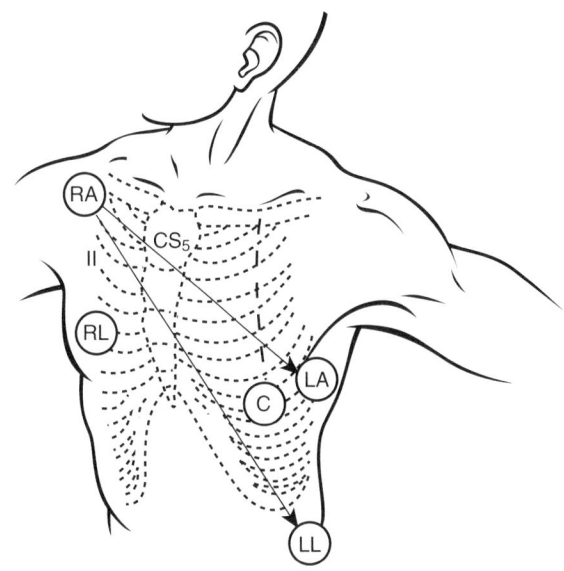

FIGURE **17-19** Perioperative ECG configured with a five-cable ECG system to continuously display limb lead II (right arm *[RA]* negative and left leg *[LL]* positive), true V4 chest lead *(C)*, and modified chest lead 5 (MCL5, i.e., central subclavicular 5 *[CS5]*). V4 electrode placement: left midclavicular line at 5th intercostal space (ICS). Lead selector switch set to display lead I, which causes the RA electrode to become negative and the left arm *(LA)* electrode (placed in the V5 position) to become positive. *(Reprinted with permission from Kossick MA. Basic Concepts. In: EKG Interpretation: Simple, Thorough, Practical. 3rd ed. Park Ridge, IL: AANA Publishing; In press.)*

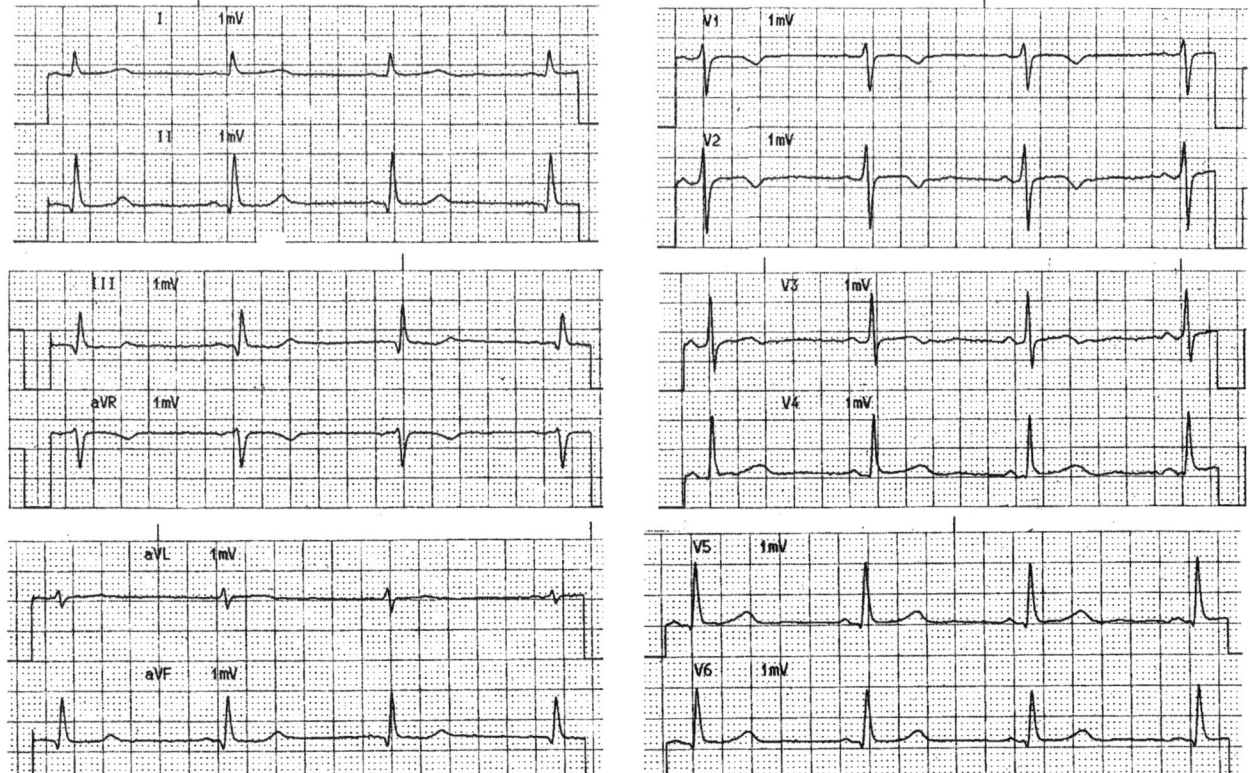

FIGURE **17-18** Derived 12-lead electrocardiogram (ECG [EASI]) recorded just prior to anesthetic induction in the operating room. The ECG monitor can be configured to continuously display all 12 leads for comprehensive assessment of ST segments and rhythm changes.

found to detect ischemia earliest and most frequently (86.8%). Lead V4 was the second most diagnostic lead (78.9%), and V5 was third (65.8%). With those patients sustaining a myocardial infarction, V4 was the most sensitive lead (83.3%), and V3 and V5 almost as sensitive (75%).[95] In this study, myocardial infarction was diagnosed if cardiac troponin I levels were greater than 3.1 ng/mL and were accompanied by symptoms of ischemia or the presence of ECG criteria (i.e., ST-segment elevation, ST-segment depression, or large Q waves). As reported by other researchers, monitoring in multiple leads improved sensitivity.[88,92,96] Of interest was the observation that 97% of ischemic events were expressed as ST-segment depression—not elevation—and ST shifts were considered significant if their duration of change exceeded 10 minutes.

Given this information, it is prudent for anesthesia providers to monitor and assess multiple ECG leads in the operating room. In the absence of an ST-segment fingerprint, this author advocates the following ECG lead combinations (for ST-segment elevation or depression) in patients with documented or identified significant risk factors for ischemic heart disease:

1. For a five-cable ECG recording system, the 3-lead set of V3, MCL$_4$, and MCL$_5$ or V3 or V4 combined with limb lead III and limb lead aVF.
2. For a three-cable ECG recording system, a two-lead set comprising MCL$_3$ and MCL$_{4\ or\ 5}$ or MCL$_{3\ or\ 4}$ combined with limb lead aVF.

Extended monitoring capabilities help to optimize detection of regionalized myocardial ischemia. Many times this entails nothing more than changing the lead selector switch to another ECG lead (e.g., III changed to aVF) or displaying a multilead ECG when indicated. The latter produces an ECG recording of all six limb leads and a single chest lead, permitting the anesthetist to more comprehensively assess ECG data, including dysrhythmias, the mean QRS axis (limb leads I and aVF), T-wave morphology, ST-segment changes, and QT intervals.

With the introduction into clinical practice of the derived 12-lead lead system (EASI), nurses and physicians have a convenient method to globally assess the overall well-being of the myocardium (see Figure 17-18). The 12-lead is derived from modified vectorcardiographic leads and requires the use of a five-cable ECG lead system.[97,98] To monitor with this system, the five ECG electrodes are placed in the following locations: LA electrode over the manubrium; chest (V) electrode over the lower body of the sternum; LL electrode left midaxillary, horizontal to the chest electrode; RA electrode right midaxillary, also horizontal to the chest electrode; and RL electrode in any convenient location. Current and past research suggests the derived 12-lead is comparable to the standard 12-lead for multiple cardiac diagnosis in adults and children (e.g., ST-segment changes, myocardial infarction, wide QRS-complex tachycardia, QT-interval measurements).[90,89-100] It is likely that patients at substantial risk for CAD would benefit from global ischemic monitoring via a derived 12-lead. This software option also eliminates any need to consider "preferred" ECG leads because all six limb leads and six chest leads can be viewed during an anesthetic.

In contrast to a derived 12-lead or five-cable ECG electrode system, a three-cable system offers challenges to anesthesia providers concerning potential errors with ECG lead configuration. The literature documents that health-care providers consistently struggle with modified chest lead configuration—even those who routinely monitor the ECG.[19] Modified chest leads offer an alternative to true chest leads when only a three-cable ECG recording system is available. Recently introduced into clinical practice is the modified chest lead MAC$_{1(L)}$ (modified augmented chest lead V1). This modified chest lead is configured using unipolar limb lead aVL and has been shown to have a diagnostic accuracy similar to true chest lead V1. The internal validity of this finding was based on His-bundle recordings, used as the gold standard for distinguishing between premature ventricular ectopy and premature aberrantly conducted beats.[101] The simplicity of this unique ECG lead has the potential to reduce modified chest lead configuration errors (e.g., through application of a unipolar lead system rather than a bipolar limb lead system to replicate a V1). To substantiate this theoretical advantage (e.g., ease of configuration of MAC$_{1(L)}$ versus modified chest lead V1 [MCL$_1$]), more research will be needed. Figure 17-20 illustrates the ECG configuration of MAC$_{1(L)}$, as well as the similarities in morphologic characteristics of single cardiac cycles recorded in V1 and MAC$_{1(L)}$.

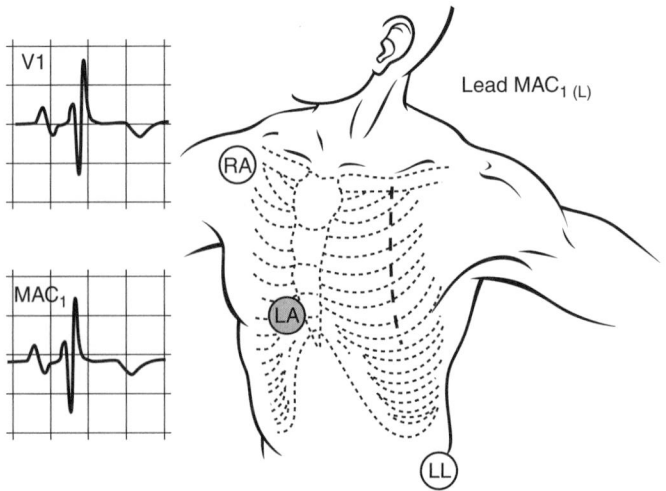

FIGURE **17-20** Modified augmented chest lead V1 (MAC$_1$ $_{[L]}$). It is configured by using unipolar limb lead a VL—which causes the left arm (LA) electrode to become positive—and placing the LA electrode in the V1 position. Remaining ECG electrodes are placed in their normal positions. The two single cardiac cycles shown illustrate the great similarity in cardiac-cycle morphology between V1 and MAC$_{1(L)}$. (*Modified and Reprinted with permission from Kossick MA. Evaluation of a new modified chest lead in diagnosing wide complex beats of unknown origin [dissertation]. Memphis, TN: University of Tennessee Health Science Center; 2003.*)

In summary, practitioners who limit ECG monitoring and assessment to a single lead or pair of leads *in patients with documented or recognized risk factors for ischemic heart disease* are potentially compromising patient safety by not using (when available) multiple-ECG-lead display configuration options. In such patients, the continuous display of three ECG leads (e.g., V4, MCL₅, and limb lead II with a five-cable ECG recording system (see Figure 17-19) or a derived 12-lead could be of clinical benefit. The literature substantiates myocardial ischemia (TW and/or ST-segment changes) can be regionalized and completely missed when viewing two or fewer ECG leads. Unarguably, critical assessment of all available patient data will help anesthetists exercise better judgment during an anesthetic and potentially improve anesthetic outcome.

Gain Setting and Frequency Bandwidth

Two other potential problems with continuous ST-segment monitoring relate to the amplitude at which the ECG monitor has been set and whether filtering of the electrical signal is excessive. When accurate visual assessment of ST segments is a priority during an anesthetic, the gain of the ECG monitor should be set at standardization (i.e., a 1 mV signal delivered by the ECG monitor produces a 10-mm calibration pulse). This gain setting fixes the ratio of the ST-segment and QRS-complex size so that a 1-mm ST-segment change is accurately assessed (e.g., potential myocardial injury). Failure to recognize the use of other gain settings can lead to overdiagnosis or underdiagnosis of myocardial injuries (ST-segment changes). Figure 17-21 illustrates how changes in gain settings and improper lead placement can confound ST-segment assessment.

The filtering capacity of the ECG monitor is yet another potential source of artifact. Research has demonstrated that filtering out the low end of the frequency bandwidth (e.g., 0.05 to 0.5 to produce a new bandwidth range of 0.5 to 40 Hz) of the monitor's electrical signal can lead to distortion of the ST segment (elevation or depression).[102,103] For this reason in many (but not all) cases, the *diagnostic mode* of an ECG monitor should be used when ST-segment analysis is a priority during an anesthetic.

Clearly, the sensitivity and specificity of computerized real-time ST-segment analysis software is dependent on the ability of the anesthetist to critically analyze the large number of factors that influence ST-segment values. Attentiveness to such variables as the patient's physical status, ECG lead placement and selection, type of electronic filtering used by the ECG monitor, and gain setting used can affect anesthetic outcome in patients at risk for myocardial ischemia or injury.

ARTERIAL PRESSURE MONITORING

As with ECG monitoring, professional societies have designated the routine assessment of arterial blood pressure (BP) to be essential for the safe conduct of any anesthetic; at minimum, BP should be recorded at least once every 5 minutes. This frequency of assessment should be increased for patients noted to have any systemic disease that limits physiologic reserve, such as coronary artery disease (CAD) or valvular heart defects (e.g., aortic stenosis). This author advocates BP assessment at 1-minute intervals during the induction period of most anesthetics, the rationale being that many commonly administered induction agents are associated with cardiac depressant effects. The concomitant

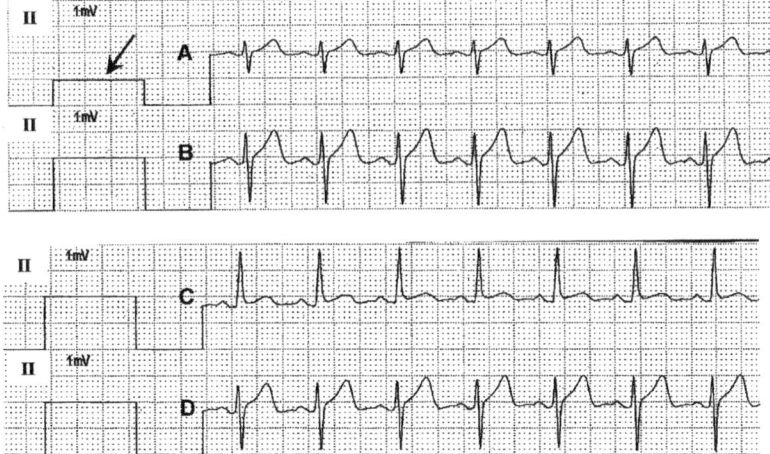

FIGURE **17-21** Series of electrocardiographic (ECG) recordings illustrating how the gain setting and incorrect ECG electrode placement can lead to misinterpretation of ST-segment changes. In strip A, the gain setting (*arrow*) on the ECG monitor has been set at half standardization (1 mV = 5 mm); it grossly gives the appearance of a minor ST-segment change. When concurrent strip B is compared with strip A, it becomes apparent that use of smaller gain settings can mask ST-segment deviation. Therefore if a 0.5-mm ST-segment deviation in ECG strip A were to occur, it would equate with a 1-mm change. A similar error in assessment of ST-segment changes can occur secondary to misplaced ECG electrodes. ECG strip recording C has all limb lead electrodes properly placed and displays an ST-segment elevation of approximately 0.8 mm. In contrast, ECG strip D mistakenly has the left leg electrode placed in the second intercostal space, midclavicular line, and therefore is not a literal lead II. The end result is an ST segment that is falsely elevated (in excess of 2 mm), suggesting inferior transmural myocardial injury. (*Reprinted with permission from Kossick MA. Recognizing EKG evidence of ischemia, injury, and infarction. In: EKG Interpretation: Simple, Thorough, Practical. 2nd ed. Park Ridge, IL: AANA Publishing; 1999:26-27.*)

disruption or gross activation of homeostatic reflexes can lead to substantive changes in hemodynamics—even in relatively healthy patients. It is also known that the hemodynamic response to many drugs used during induction of anesthesia can be unpredictable, owing to differences in pharmacokinetics and pharmacodynamics among patients.

BP monitoring can be accomplished through both noninvasive and invasive techniques. Each recording modality will be reviewed with an emphasis on clinical relevance. Other resources provide a comprehensive description of the theoretical underpinnings for the calculation of noninvasive and invasive arterial BP data. In today's modern OR environment, noninvasive blood pressure (NIBP) monitoring is most often recorded by automated BP cuffs that can be configured to measure systolic blood pressure (SBP), diastolic blood pressure (DBP), and mean arterial blood pressure (MAP) in a standard mode, stat mode, at varied frequencies of assessment, and adjusted for patient age and habitus. The literature recommends BP cuffs have a bladder dimension of approximately 40% of the circumference of the extremity.[104] Bladders not properly sized and cuffs not applied firmly to the extremity can lead to inaccurate recordings. For example, cuffs that are applied loosely to the extremity, positioned below the level of the heart, or too small can produce arterial blood pressure values that are falsely elevated.[105]

The physics associated with auscultation of BP relates to the audible discernment of Korotkoff sounds through a stethoscope. These sounds are produced by turbulent blood flow within an artery during cuff deflation. A second mechanism for BP assessment is via an oscillometric technique (Figure 17-22). NIBP devices have inflation and deflation cycles controlled by a microprocessor. During deflation of the cuff, oscillations are sampled over the span of several cardiac cycles. Any oscillations sensed by the pressure transducer are then processed numerically. If none are sensed, a stepwise reduction in cuff pressure followed by sustained measurement for oscillations occurs. This process repeats until SBP, DBP, and MAP are derived. MAP can also be estimated by taking the sum of the SBP and DBP—the latter multiplied by two, then dividing this figure by three. Example: a BP of 120/80 has a MAP of (120 + 80 + 80) ÷ 3 = 93 mm Hg). This formula accounts for diastole comprising approximately two thirds of a normal cardiac cycle.

Generally speaking, the benefits outweigh the risks of frequent NIBP recordings taken during an anesthetic. Nevertheless, injury and harm can occur with automatic NIBP measurements and may include damage to peripheral nerves (e.g., ulnar), development of a compartment syndrome, or interference with delivery of drugs through an intravenous (IV) line. For example, propofol sequestered in a forearm during BP-cuff inflation can cause intense pain. The latter can be avoided by routinely placing the BP cuff on the extremity without the peripheral IV. In circumstances in which the scheduled surgery involves an upper extremity, the BP cuff and IV can be placed on the contralateral arm (brachium or antebrachium), with the caveat that the NIBP be configured so BP measurements are recorded in the manual mode to prevent unexpected disruption of the delivery of IV induction drugs. Alternatively, a lower extremity (thigh or calf) can be used for BP measurements.

In morbidly obese patients, it is not unusual to have to relocate a BP cuff from the upper arm because of the cone shape of the extremity. An alternative BP monitoring site is the forearm. However, NIBP measurements taken in the forearm with the patient in supine or sitting position or the head of the bed

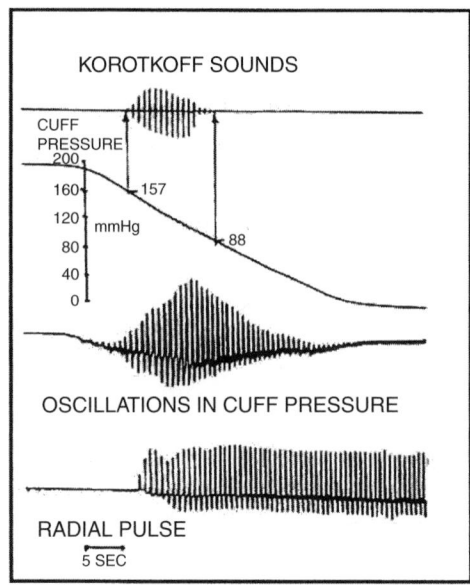

FIGURE **17-22**   Arterial blood pressure, comparing Korotkoff sounds, oscillations with a BP cuff, and radial artery palpation. Note correlation between onset of the first Korotkoff sound, onset of oscillations in the cuff pressure, and radial pulse wave. (*From Saidman LJ, Smith NT, eds.* Monitoring in Anesthesia. *New York: Wiley & Sons; 1978.*)

elevated 45 degrees can *overestimate* the more proximal brachial BP.[106,107] Formulas have been proposed to correct for such discrepancies. For example, in an obese patient with a diastolic forearm pressure of 80 mm Hg and arm circumference between 32 and 44 cm, the adjusted DBP would equal 72.4 mm Hg. This is derived from the following equation:

$$\text{Brachial DBP} = 25.2 + 0.59 \times \text{Forearm DBP}$$

This formula was proposed relative to 129 subjects with an average body mass index of 40 ± 7 kg/m²[106] Discrepancies in BP measurements have also been noted between upper and lower extremities and between arms. In study participants up to 16 years of age, SBP has been shown to be *greater* in the thigh and calf than in the arm. In contrast, DBP and MAP are *lower* in the calf and thigh than in the arm. [108] Patients most likely to exhibit inter-arm BP differences are those who are obese and have a higher HR and SBP.[109] Concerns about accuracy also arise when measuring BP noninvasively versus invasively. One group of investigators found NIBP taken in the upper arm in patients with septic shock to correlate poorly with arterial-line pressure measurements, specifically causing an overestimation of MAP with the noninvasive technique.[110]

It is apparent that in the demographics of the population of the United States, a substantive change has occurred in recent years in the number of adults and children who are classified as obese. Consistent with this change are the findings that mean mid-arm circumference has increased across the country, with the greatest increase occurring in 20- to 39-year-olds. This change should cause anesthesia providers to be more attentive to the daily task of selecting properly sized BP cuffs. In fact, research has shown that up to 39% of all hypertensive patients and 47% of self-reported diabetic patients should not have their BP measured with the standard adult-size cuff.[111] Inattentiveness to this basic

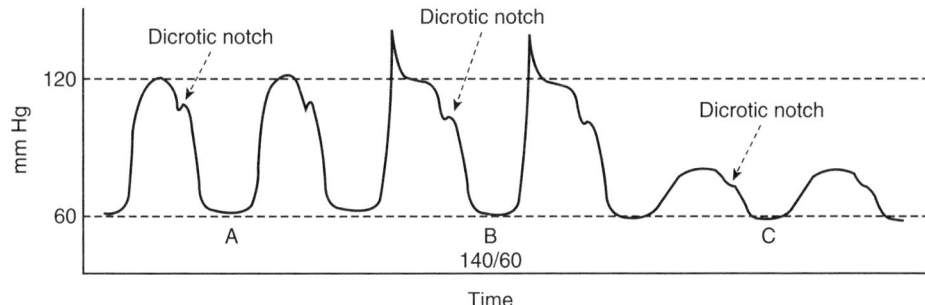

FIGURE **17-23** Radial arterial pressure waveforms. (A) normal morphology, (B) overshoot, (C) dampened. With waveform B, the overshoot should be ignored regarding the displayed systolic blood pressure.

and essential monitoring need could cause the anesthetist to process inaccurate hemodynamic data (e.g., overestimated BP recordings) and ultimately contribute to a poor surgical outcome.

Direct measurement of arterial BP is considered by many the gold standard for recording BP. Many anatomic locations can be used for direct BP measurement, with the most common being the radial artery. Other less commonly used arteries are the ulnar, brachial, axillary, femoral, and dorsalis pedis. Risks associated with placement of an intraarterial catheter include infection (localized and systemic), thrombus formation, hematoma, vasospasm, embolization, injury to adjacent nerves and veins, ischemia to extremities or digits, loss of a limb secondary to poor collateral circulation, iatrogenic injuries (air embolization, intraarterial injection of drugs meant to be administered intravenously), and acute blood loss due to an unexpected disruption of the transducing system (e.g., cracked or disconnected stopcock). A displaced transducer (no longer level with the phlebostatic axis) can cause an "increase" in arterial blood pressure if positioned substantially below the level of the heart. Assessment of an abnormal BP recording should include an understanding of problems inherent to a fluid-pressure monitoring system. To mitigate the ongoing risks of direct arterial BP monitoring, constant vigilance on the part of the anesthetist is paramount.

Monitoring BP directly offers several distinct advantages, including beat-to-beat assessment of BP, limited hysteresis in measured values, and easy access for arterial sampling of blood for any number of laboratory tests (e.g., arterial blood gases, serum electrolytes, glucose, hemoglobin levels). Indications for direct arterial BP monitoring include surgical procedures in which there is potential for acute and/or gross changes in hemodynamics. This would include operations such as repair of aortic aneurysms, carotid endarterectomy, and craniotomies. Even with lower risk surgical procedures, direct arterial BP monitoring may be indicated, particularly if preoperative BP is poorly controlled (labile). Patients with comorbidities may be at substantial risk for a stroke or heart attack during periods of acute stress (e.g., laryngoscopy or emergence from an anesthetic) if BP is not directly monitored.

Risks associated with placement of a radial artery catheter can be minimized if precautionary measures are taken. This would include positioning of the hand and wrist on an armboard. A roll should be placed beneath the wrist, and the fingers and thumb should be taped securely across the board. This position keeps the hand from interfering with manipulation and placement of the needle-catheter system; it also facilitates palpation of the radial artery. Commonly, a 20-gauge nontapered catheter is used (a 22-gauge is optional) to penetrate an area of skin that has been prepped with antiseptic solution and infiltrated with local anesthetic. The needle, bevel pointing upward, is directed

at a 45-degree angle toward the palpated pulse. If bone is encountered with the tip of the needle during advancement, the complete catheter system (catheter and needle) is slowly withdrawn while observing for the free flow of arterial blood; sometimes the artery can be pierced without a "flash back" (unintentional transfixion-withdrawal method). If during catheter withdrawal no blood is seen, the needle system is directed slightly laterally (in either direction) and readvanced. Once arterial blood is seen in the lumen of the catheter, the angle of the needle is reduced to approximately 30 degrees, then advanced slightly (a few millimeters). The catheter is subsequently threaded off the needle. "Fatigue" at a puncture site may occur, at which time a new artery may be chosen to cannulate or a "fresh set of hands" (perhaps another anesthesia provider or member of the surgical team) used to repeat the attempt at arterial puncture. After verifying correct placement of the catheter within the lumen of the artery (free flow of blood through the rigid tubing when vented to air), it is important to securely fasten the arterial catheter to the skin, preferably with suture and a sterile dressing applied on top of the puncture site.

The transducing system should be zeroed to atmospheric pressure (with the stopcock vented to air) and referenced at the level of the left atrium. In patients with poor vascular compliance, the arterial tracing can produce an "overshoot" or "ringing" phenomenon. If not recognized, BP recordings will overestimate SBP and MAP values. In contrast, a dampened waveform, which can develop with a flexed wrist or low pressure in the continuous-flush device, can lead to an underestimation of BP recordings (Figure 17-23). Direct arterial pressure measurements, although very accurate in many clinical circumstances, can still produce BP recordings that are significantly skewed and lead to inappropriate interventions (e.g., preload augmentation, indiscriminate use of vasoactive drugs).

TRANSESOPHAGEAL ECHOCARDIOGRAPHY MONITORING

Transesophageal echocardiography (TEE) has been established as a safe, noninvasive diagnostic tool for monitoring numerous cardiac parameters to guide medical and nursing care. Systolic wall motion abnormalities (SWMA), vascular aneurysms, calculation of ejection fraction, ventricular preload, and measuring blood flow within heart chambers and across valves are a few of the utilities of ultrasound imaging applied during TEE. Guidelines for indications and training proficiency have been advocated by medical professional societies.[112,113]

Sound waves used to define anatomic structures in the human body were first described by Dussik and colleagues in 1947. These investigators attempted to outline the cerebral ventricles by driving sound waves across the skull.[114] In 1971, C.D. Side and R.G. Gosling were the first to report the assessment of

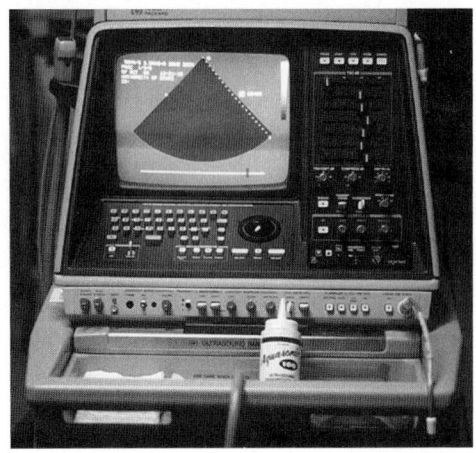

FIGURE **17-24**   Echograph machine.

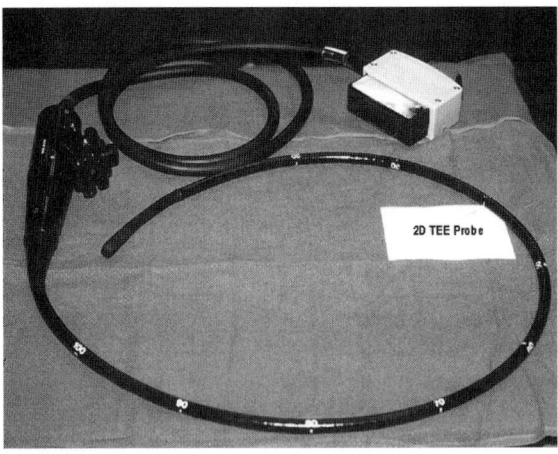

FIGURE **17-25**   A 170-cm transesophageal echocardiography probe with cm markings is displayed. Examination depth is approximately 35 to 40 cm from teeth. The positioning-holding mechanisms is located on control knobs, allowing for manipulation of the probe in the anterior, posterior, and lateral planes. *2D TEE,* Two-dimensional transesophageal echocardiography.

cardiac function via transesophageal techniques.[115] Thirty-six years later, substantial advancements in the medical application of ultrasound have occurred, leading in some circumstances to an improvement in surgical outcomes.[116] Fundamental to the interpretation of data obtained by TEE is an understanding of the physics of ultrasound. Ultrasound waves are inaudible to the human ear, having a frequency greater than 20,000 Hz. Piezoelectric crystals are known to produce ultrasound by vibrating when exposed to an electric current. The opposite also occurs, in that they produce voltage in response to an ultrasound echo or when pressed (mechanical stress) or released. The electric current produced has been shown to be of sufficient magnitude to temporarily illuminate a small bulb. Thus they function as both generators and receivers of ultrasound waves and electric currents.

Within the esophagus, ultrasound waves emitted by piezoelectric elements are absorbed, reflected, or scattered. When reflected by an organ (e.g., heart), the ultrasound echo produced is received by the piezoelectric elements housed within the TEE probe. These elements then generate an electrical impulse that is processed, amplified, and subsequently displayed as an image on the echograph machine (Figure 17-24). Manufacturers can place as many as 32 linearly arranged elements within a probe (Figure 17-25). The frequency of the piezoelectric crystals in TEE probes ranges from 3.7 to 7 MHz. This frequency range allows for greater detail in displayed images. Unfortunately, the tradeoff for clearer images is lower tissue penetration. Thus smaller frequency values (e.g., 2.5 MHz) are required in transthoracic echocardiographic (TTE) probes because of greater distances between elements and distal anatomic structures.

Clinically, three primary ultrasound imaging techniques are used: the M-mode, 2-dimensional (2-D) imaging, and the Doppler exam. The M-mode provides high picture resolution with 1000 images per second. It is commonly referenced as being unidimensional and produces a well-focused, narrow ultrasound beam. It is sometimes referred to as an *ice-pick view.* With the 2-D scan, the ultrasound beam is electronically steered across a target field. The intermittent pulses of ultrasound are produced by varying the firing sequence (phasing) of individual piezoelectric crystals. The monitor subsequently displays an image that is somewhat triangular or appears as a "slice" of pie. This produces excellent spatial orientation; however, at 30 images per second, the pictures are less well defined. The Doppler exam incorporates the concept of frequency shift, which was first described in 1842 by Austrian physicist Christian Doppler. The clinical application of this concept involves viewing red blood cells (RBCs) as moving reflectors of ultrasound. As ultrasound reflects off the moving RBCs, echos are produced, which are then recorded by the TEE transducer. With the flow of RBCs toward the TEE probe, the distance between the sound source and its reception is changing. This phenomenon is referred to as a *frequency shift.* It is analogous to the change in pitch of a train whistle as the locomotive approaches the station; sound waves are compressed, and the pitch increases (frequency shift). In contrast to RBCs, body fluids (plasma) only minimally reflect ultrasound. Spectral and color-flow Doppler exams performed with echographs incorporate this concept by assigning different colors to RBCs that move toward and away from the source of ultrasound. This permits easy visualization of retrograde flow of blood across incompetent heart valves, as may occur with mitral regurgitation (MR). For example, the retrograde flow of blood from the left ventricle into the left atria during MR is seen distinctly as a mosaic pattern of color. Doppler exams are recognized as being beneficial in determining the etiology of regurgitation and the adequacy of valve repair, as well as influencing surgical management, such as the use or nonuse of cardiopulmonary bypass.[116,117]

Fundamental elements of the TEE exam include positioning the TEE probe in the esophagus, either under sedation or after induction of the anesthetic (Figure 17-26). During the examination, cardiac anatomy can be assessed, myocardial ischemia diagnosed via the presence of SWMA, and blood flow through heart chambers and across valves seen. By convention, the posterior structures are displayed at the top of the screen (apex of the sector) and anterior structures at the bottom. The first image displayed in a standard exam is the short-axis view of the aortic valve. At a depth of approximately 35 to 40 cm from the teeth, the aortic valve leaflets and coronary arteries are seen.

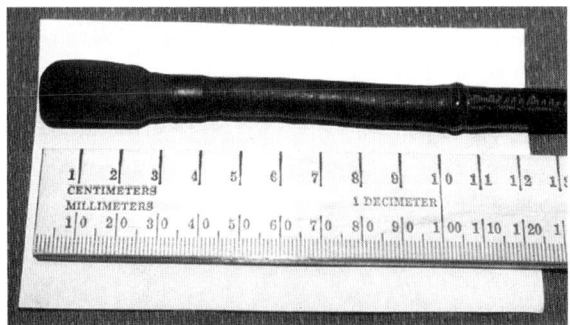

FIGURE **17-26** Transesophageal echocardiography probe. Distal tip contains thermistor and piezoelectric elements.

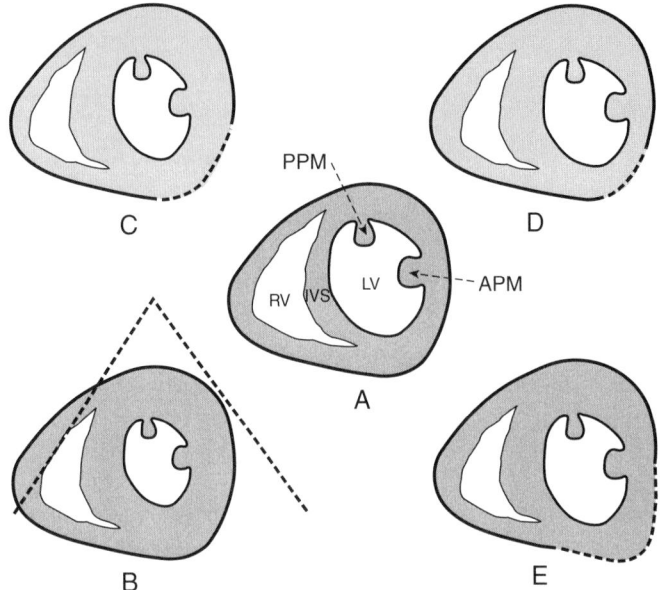

FIGURE **17-27** Midpapillary muscle level short-axis view of the heart (**A**) during diastole, (**B**) during systole with normal wall thickening and inward movement of endocardial surface, (**C**) systole with area of hypokinesia (decreased wall thickening), (**D**) systole with an area of akinesia (no change in wall thickness), and (**E**) systole with an area of dyskinesia (paradoxical movement). *APM,* Anterior papillary muscle; *IVS,* interventricular septum; *LV,* left ventricle; *PPM,* posterior papillary muscle *RV,* right ventricle.

Rotation and angulation of the probe can allow a long-axis view of the right and left atria, tricuspid and mitral valves, pulmonic and aortic valves, and right and left ventricles. This view is useful for assessing stenotic valves, identifying masses within the atria or ventricles, and observing the overall size of each heart chamber. A short-axis view of the left ventricle can be obtained with further advancement of the probe and angling of the tip. This position is also referred to as the *standard monitoring view,* which allows the echocardiographer to assess for SWMA. Normal ventricular wall motion (which is not entirely uniform) thickens during systole, and the endocardial surface moves inward. Approximately 87% of the normal stroke volume is derived from shortening in the short axis of the ventricle—with little contribution from the long axis.

Abnormal wall motion can be described by three terms: hypokinesia, akinesia, and dyskinesia. *Hypokinesia* represents contraction that is less vigorous than normal; wall thickening is decreased. *Akinesia* depicts the absence of wall motion and can be associated with myocardial infarction. *Dyskinesia* correlates with paradoxical movement (i.e., outward motion during systole) and is a hallmark of myocardial infarction and ventricular aneurysm (Figure 17-27). Not all wall motion abnormalities are diagnostic of an imbalance between myocardial oxygen supply and demand. Abnormal loading conditions, asynchronous ventricular depolarization (e.g., left bundle branch block), echo dropout due to haphazard reflection of ultrasound off myocardial walls in lateral fields of the sector arc, or improper use of the gain controls of the TEE probe can lead to an erroneous diagnosis of SWMA. Also, the duration of SWMA can persist well after coronary reperfusion has been restored (e.g., 6 hours), indicating a stunned myocardium.[118] In canine research, a 50% decline in coronary blood flow has been shown to serve as a threshold for hypokinesia. In contrast, a 75% reduction in coronary blood flow commonly produces ST-segment deviation. Thus there is greater hysteresis and less sensitivity with ischemia-induced ECG changes than with ischemia-induced SWMA.[94,119] This finding is consistent with classic research done by Tennant and Wiggers in 1935.[120]

To summarize, the best single view for routine monitoring for SWMA (myocardial ischemia) is the short axis at the midpapillary muscle level (see Figure 17-27), followed by the apical segment in the same axis. The midpapillary muscle level includes segments of the myocardium perfused by all three coronary arteries. This level is created by dividing the long axis of the left ventricle into three parts (i.e., basal, mid-, and apical regions). The mid-region extends from the tips to the bases of the papillary muscles. Interesting is the finding that the skills required of anesthesiologists, residents, and CRNAs (compared with trained observers) for recognizing gross SWMA can be acquired with little training; the study group successfully identified 95% of regional wall motion abnormalities.[121]

Newer imaging techniques introduced with TEE include contrast echocardiography, selected three-dimensional techniques, parametric imaging modes, and harmonic imaging modalities. Continued research with these echocardiographic diagnostic tools will help elucidate what patient populations may benefit most from their application. A recent investigation found real-time, three-dimensional (3-D) echocardiography in biplane mode to be a feasible way to estimate the area of the aortic valve orifice in patients with stenotic lesions.[122] Also of interest was porcine research that showed intracardiac transvenous echocardiography (ICE) to be superior to precordial Doppler and TEE techniques in diagnosing venous air embolism and retrieving as little as 0.05 to 1 mL of air.[123]

SUMMARY

With continued advancements in technology and improved clinical databases derived from research, future monitoring techniques offer much promise for improving anesthesia care. The development of specialized task forces comprising multiple professional societies also contributes substantively to professional practice. Understandably, anesthesia providers should continue to maintain a healthy skepticism of reported advancements in monitoring modalities. The decision to change practice routines should occur only after critiquing the reported merits of any research findings. Ultimately, this clinical paradigm will allow patients to benefit from medical and nursing care derived from evidence-based practice.

REFERENCES

1. American Association of Nurse Anesthetists. *Scope and Standards of Nurse Anesthesia Practice.* Park Ridge, IL: AANA; 2005. Available at: http://aana.com/uploadedFiles/Resources/Practice_Documents/scope_stds_nap07_2007.pdf.
2. Swan HJ et al. Catheterization of the heart in man with use of a flow-directed balloon-tipped catheter. *N Engl J Med.* 1970;283(9):447-451.
3. Naylor CD et al. Pulmonary artery catheterization: can there be an integrated strategy for guideline development and research promotion? [miscellaneous]. *JAMA.* 1993;269(18):2407-2411.
4. Bernard GR et al. Pulmonary artery catheterization and clinical outcomes: National Heart, Lung, and Blood Institute and Food and Drug Administration workshop report. *JAMA.* 2000;283(19):2568-2572.
5. American Society of Anesthesiologists. Practice guidelines for pulmonary artery catheterization: an updated report by the ASA Task Force on Pulmonary Artery Catheterization. *Anesthesiology.* 2003;99(4):988-1014.
6. Sandham JD et al. A randomized, controlled trial of the use of pulmonary-artery catheters in high-risk surgical patients [comment]. *N Engl J Med.* 2003;348(1):5-14.
7. de Jonge E et al. The value of the pulmonary-artery catheter: not ruled out, but not proven either. *Ned Tijdschr Geneeskd.* 2003;147(17):792-795.
8. Handa F et al. Reduction in the use of pulmonary artery catheter for cardiovascular surgery. *Masui.* 2003;52(4):420-423.
9. The Escape Investigators, *ESC. Evaluation study of congestive heart failure and pulmonary artery catheterization effectiveness: the ESCAPE trial. *JAMA.* 2005;294(13):1625-1633.
10. Smartt S. The pulmonary artery catheter: gold standard or redundant relic. *J Perianesth Nurs.* 2005;20(6):373-379.
11. Jeger RV et al. Hemodynamic parameters are prognostically important in cardiogenic shock but similar following early revascularization or initial medical stabilization: a report from the SHOCK trial. *Chest.* 2007;132(6):1794-1803.
12. Dellinger RP et al. Surviving sepsis campaign: international guidelines for management of severe sepsis and septic shock: 2008. *Crit Care Med.* 2008;36(1):296-327.
13. Rao TL et al. Reinfarction following anesthesia in patients with myocardial infarction. *Anesthesiology.* 1983;59(6):499-505.
14. Heyland DK et al. Maximizing oxygen delivery in critically ill patients: a methodologic appraisal of the evidence. *Crit Care Med.* 1996;24(3):517-524.
15. Leibowitz AB, Oropello JM. The pulmonary artery catheter in anesthesia practice in 2007: an historical overview with emphasis on the past 6 years. *Semin Cardiothorac Vasc Anesth.* 2007;11(3):162-176.
16. Iberti TJ et al. A multicenter study of physicians' knowledge of the pulmonary artery catheter. Pulmonary Artery Catheter Study Group. *JAMA.* 1990;264(22):2928-2932.
17. Gnaegi A et al. Intensive care physicians' insufficient knowledge of right-heart catheterization at the bedside: time to act? *Crit Care Med.* 1997;25(2):213-220.
18. Jacka MJ et al. Pulmonary artery occlusion pressure estimation: how confident are anesthesiologists? [comment]. *Crit Care Med.* 2002;30(6):1197-1203.
19. Drew BJ et al. Accuracy of bedside electrocardiographic monitoring: a report on current practices of critical care nurses. *Heart Lung.* 1991;20(6):597-607.
20. Shoemaker WC et al. Prospective trial of supranormal values of survivors as therapeutic goals in high-risk surgical patients. *Chest.* 1988;94(6):1176-1186.
21. American College of Physicians/American College of Cardiology/American Heart Association Task Force on Clinical Privileges in Cardiology. Clinical competence in hemodynamic monitoring. *J Am Coll Cardiol.* 1990;15:1460-1464.
22. Shah KB et al. A review of pulmonary artery catheterization in 6245 patients. *Anesthesiology.* 1984;61(3):271-275.
23. Pichard AD et al. Large v waves in the pulmonary capillary wedge pressure tracing without mitral regurgitation: the influence of the pressure/volume relationship on the v wave size. *Clin Cardiol.* 1983;6(11):534-541.
24. Nadeau S, Noble WH. Misinterpretation of pressure measurements from the pulmonary artery catheter. *Can Anaesth Soc J.* 1986;33(3 Pt 1):352-363.
25. Beique F, Ramsay JG. The pulmonary artery catheter: a new look. *Semin Anesth.* 1994;13:14-25.
26. West JB et al. Distribution of blood flow in isolated lung: relation to vascular and alveolar pressures. *J Appl Physiol.* 1964;19:713-724.
27. Enson Y et al. The influence of heart rate on pulmonary arterial-left ventricular pressure relationships at end-diastole. *Circulation.* 1977;56(4 Pt 1):533-539.
28. Mitchell JH et al. The transport function of the atrium: factors influencing the relation between mean left atrial pressure and left ventricular end diastolic pressure. *Am J Cardiol.* 1962;9:237-247.
29. Raper R, Sibbald WJ. Misled by the wedge? The Swan-Ganz catheter and left ventricular preload. *Chest.* 1986;89(3):427-434.
30. Douglas PS et al. Unreliability of hemodynamic indexes of left ventricular size during cardiac surgery. *Ann Thorac Surg.* 1987;44(1):31-34.
31. Herbert WH. Pulmonary artery and left heart end-diastolic pressure relations. *Br Heart J.* 1970;32(6):774-778.
32. McGregor M, Sniderman A. On pulmonary vascular resistance: the need for more precise definition. *Am J Cardiol.* 1985;55(1):217-221.
33. Shoemaker WC. Circulatory mechanisms of shock and their mediators. *Crit Care Med.* 1987;15(8):787-794.
34. Shoemaker WC. Diagnosis and treatment of the shock and circulatory dysfunction. In: Shoemaker WC et al, eds. *Textbook of Critical Care.* 4th ed. Philadelphia: Saunders; 2000:92-114.
35. Reeves JT et al. Cardiac output in normal resting man. *J Appl Physiol.* 1961;16:276-278.
36. Fegler G. Measurement of cardiac output in anesthetized animals by a thermodilution method. *Q J Exp Physiol.* 1954;39:153-164.
37. Hines R, Barash P. Pulmonary artery catherization. In: Blitt C, Hines R, eds. *Monitoring in Anesthesia and Critical Care Medicine.* 3rd ed. New York: Churchill Livingstone; 1995:231-259.
38. Forrester JS et al. Thermodilution cardiac output determination with a single flow-directed catheter. *Am Heart J.* 1972;83(3):306-311.
39. Pearl RG et al. Effect of injectate volume and temperature on thermodilution cardiac output determination. *Anesthesiology.* 1986;64(6):798-801.
40. Nelson LD, Houtchens BA. Automatic vs manual injections for thermodilution cardiac output determinations. *Crit Care Med.* 1982;10(3):190-192.
41. Synder JV, Powner DJ. Effects of mechanical ventilation on the measurement of cardiac output by thermodilution. *Crit Care Med.* 1982;10(10):677-682.
42. Stevens JH et al. Thermodilution cardiac output measurement. Effects of the respiratory cycle on its reproducibility. *JAMA.* 1985;253(15):2240-2242.
43. Weisel RD et al. Current concepts measurement of cardiac output by thermodilution. *N Engl J Med.* 1975;292(13):682-684.
44. Nishikawa T, Dohi S. Slowing of heart rate during cardiac output measurement by thermodilution. *Anesthesiology.* 1982;57(6):538-539.
45. Hamilton MA et al. Effect of tricuspid regurgitation on the reliability of the thermodilution cardiac output technique in congestive heart failure. *Am J Cardiol.* 1989;64(14):945-948.
46. Pearl RG, Siegel LC. Thermodilution cardiac output measurement with a large left-to-right shunt. *J Clin Monit.* 1991;7(2):146-153.
47. Heerdt PM et al. Inaccuracy of cardiac output by thermodilution during acute tricuspid regurgitation. *Ann Thorac Surg.* 1992;53(4):706-708.
48. Stetz CW et al. Reliability of the thermodilution method in the determination of cardiac output in clinical practice. *Am Rev Respir Dis.* 1982;126(6):1001-1004.
49. Spahn DR et al. Noninvasive versus invasive assessment of cardiac output after cardiac surgery: clinical validation. *J Cardiothorac Anesth.* 1990;4(1):46-59.
50. Maruschak GF et al. Overestimation of pediatric cardiac output by thermal indicator loss. *Circulation.* 1982;65(2):380-383.
51. Hillis LD et al. Analysis of factors affecting the variability of Fick versus indicator dilution measurements of cardiac output. *Am J Cardiol.* 1985;56(12):764-768.
52. Fischer AP et al. Analysis of errors in measurement of cardiac output by simultaneous dye and thermal dilution in cardiothoracic surgical patients. *Cardiovasc Res.* 1978;12(3):190-199.
53. Yelderman M. Continuous measurement of cardiac output with the use of stochastic system identification techniques. *J Clin Monit.* 1990;6(4):322-332.
54. Luchette FA et al. Effects of body temperature on accuracy of continuous cardiac output measurements. *J Invest Surg.* 2000;13(3):147-152.
55. Nelson LD. The new pulmonary artery catheters: continuous venous oximetry, right ventricular ejection fraction, and continuous cardiac output. *New Horiz.* 1997;5(3):251-258.
56. Poli de Figueiredo LF et al. Thermal filament continuous thermodilution cardiac output delayed response limits its value during acute hemodynamic instability. *J Trauma.* 1999;47(2):288-293.
57. Zollner C et al. Evaluation of a new continuous thermodilution cardiac output monitor in cardiac surgical patients: a prospective criterion standard study. *Crit Care Med.* 1999;27(2):293-298.
58. Yelderman ML et al. Continuous thermodilution cardiac output measurement in intensive care unit patients. *J Cardiothorac Vasc Anesth.* 1992;6(3):270-274.
59. Giuliano KK et al. Backrest angle and cardiac output measurement in critically ill patients. *Nurs Res.* 2003;52(4):242-248.

60. Schmid ER et al. Continuous thermodilution cardiac output: clinical validation against a reference technique of known accuracy. *Intensive Care Med.* 1999;25(2):166-172.

61. Zollner C et al. Continuous cardiac output measurements do not agree with conventional bolus thermodilution cardiac output determination. *Can J Anaesth.* 2001;48(11):1143-1147.

62. Forster MR, Ip-Yam PC. Pericardial injury following severe sepsis from faecal peritonitis—a case report on the use of continuous cardiac output monitoring. *Ann Acad Med Singapore.* 1998;27(6):857-859.

63. Cecconi M et al. Haemodynamic monitoring in acute heart failure. *Heart Fail Rev.* 2007;12(2):105-111.

64. Sommers MS et al. Mixed venous oxygen saturation and oxygen partial pressure as predictors of cardiac index after coronary artery bypass grafting. *Heart Lung.* 1993;22(2):112-120.

65. Steib A et al. Mixed venous oxygen saturation monitoring during liver transplantation. *Eur J Anaesthesiol.* 1993;10(4):267-271.

66. Powelson JA et al. Continuous monitoring of mixed venous oxygen saturation during aortic operations. *Crit Care Med.* 1992;20(3):332-336.

67. Krafft P et al. Mixed venous oxygen saturation in critically ill septic shock patients. The role of defined events. *Chest.* 1993;103(3):900-906.

68. Tweddell JS et al. Patients at risk for low systemic oxygen delivery after the Norwood procedure. *Ann Thorac Surg.* 2000;69(6):1893-1899.

69. Tweddell JS et al. Improved survival of patients undergoing palliation of hypoplastic left heart syndrome: lessons learned from 115 consecutive patients. *Circulation.* 2002;106(12 Suppl 1):182-189.

70. Sumimoto T et al. Mixed venous oxygen saturation as a guide to tissue oxygenation and prognosis in patients with acute myocardial infarction. *Am Heart J.* 1991;122(1 Pt 1):27-33.

71. Krouskop RW et al. Accuracy and clinical utility of an oxygen saturation catheter. *Crit Care Med.* 1983;11(9):744-749.

72. van Woerkens EC et al. Accuracy of a mixed venous saturation catheter during acutely induced changes in hematocrit in humans. *Crit Care Med.* 1991;19(8):1025-1029.

73. Bongard F et al. Simultaneous in vivo comparison of two- versus three-wavelength mixed venous (SVO_2) oximetry catheters. *J Clin Monit.* 1995;11(5):329-334.

74. Squara P et al. A computer program for interpreting pulmonary artery catheterization data: results of the European HEMODYN resident study. *Intensive Care Med.* 2003;29(5):735-741.

75. American College of Cardiology/American Heart Association Task Force on Practice Guidelines. 2007 Guidelines on perioperative cardiovascular evaluation and care for noncardiac surgery: a report of the ACC/AHA. *J Am Coll Cardiol.* 2007;50(17):e159-e241.

76. Slogoff S, Keats AS. Does perioperative myocardial ischemia lead to postoperative myocardial infarction? *Anesthesiology.* 1985;62(2):107-114.

77. Mangano DT et al. The Study of Perioperative Ischemia (SPI) Research Group. Perioperative myocardial ischemia in patients undergoing noncardiac surgery-I: incidence and severity during the 4-day perioperative period. *J Am Coll Cardiol.* 1991;17(4):843-850.

78. Landesberg G et al. Myocardial infarction after vascular surgery: the role of prolonged stress-induced, ST depression-type ischemia. *J Am Coll Cardiol.* 2001;37(7):1839-1845.

79. Coriat P et al. Clinical predictors of intraoperative myocardial ischemia in patients with coronary artery disease undergoing non-cardiac surgery. *Acta Anaesthesiol Scand.* 1982;26(4):287-290.

80. Sonntag H et al. Myocardial blood flow and oxygen consumption during high-dose fentanyl anesthesia in patients with coronary artery disease. *Anesthesiology.* 1982;56(6):417-422.

81. Leung JM et al. Automated electrocardiograph ST-segment trending monitors: accuracy in detecting myocardial ischemia. *Anesth Analg.* 1998;87(1):4-10.

82. Landesberg GM et al. Reduced postoperative myocardial infarction by prevention of prolonged ischemia on 12-lead ECG in vascular surgery. *ASA Annual Meeting Abstracts Clinical Circulation.* 2000;93(3A):A255.

83. Lehtinen R et al. Effect of ST segment measurement point on performance of exercise ECG analysis. *Int J Cardiol.* 1997;61(3):239-245.

84. Kossick MA. Recognizing EKG evidence of ischemia, injury, and infarction. In: *EKG Interpretation: Simple, Thorough, Practical.* 2nd ed. Park Ridge, IL: AANA Publishing; 1999:18-29.

85. Glancy DL, Patterson CM. Exercise electrocardiography. *J La State Med Soc.* 2003;155(1):26-35.

86. Ribisl PM et al. Comparison of computer ST criteria for diagnosis of severe coronary artery disease. *Am J Cardiol.* 1993;71(7):546-551.

87. Sansoy V et al. Significance of slow upsloping ST-segment depression on exercise stress testing. *Am J Cardiol.* 1997;79(6):709-712.

88. Mizutani M et al. ST monitoring for myocardial ischemia during and after coronary angioplasty. *Am J Cardiol.* 1990;66(4):389-393.

89. Bush HS et al. Twelve-lead electrocardiographic evaluation of ischemia during percutaneous transluminal coronary angioplasty and its correlation with acute reocclusion. *Am Heart J.* 1991;121(6 Pt 1):1591-1599.

90. Horacek BM et al. Optimal electrocardiographic leads for detecting acute myocardial ischemia. *J Electrocardiol.* 2001;34(Suppl):97-111.

91. Kaplan JA, King SB 3rd. The precordial electrocardiographic lead (V5) in patients who have coronary artery disease. *Anesthesiology.* 1976;45(5):570-574.

92. London MJ et al. Intraoperative myocardial ischemia: localization by continuous 12-lead electrocardiography. *Anesthesiology.* 1988;69(2):232-241.

93. Jain U. An electrocardiographic lead system for coronary artery bypass surgery. *J Clin Anesth.* 1996;8(1):19-24.

94. Smith JS et al. Intraoperative detection of myocardial ischemia in high-risk patients: electrocardiography versus two-dimensional transesophageal echocardiography. *Circulation.* 1985;72(5):1015-1021.

95. Landesberg GM et al. Perioperative myocardial ischemia and infarction: identification by continuous 12-lead electrocardiogram with online ST-segment monitoring. *Anesthesiology.* 2002;96(2):264-270.

96. Drew BJ. 12-lead ST-segment monitoring vs single-lead maximum ST-segment monitoring for detecting ongoing ischemia in patients with unstable coronary syndromes. *Am J Crit Care.* 1998;7(5):355-363.

97. Dower GE et al. Deriving the 12-lead electrocardiogram from four (EASI) electrodes. *J Electrocardiol.* 1988;21(Suppl):S182-S187.

98. Drew BJ et al. ST segment monitoring with a derived 12-lead electrocardiogram is superior to routine cardiac care unit monitoring. *Am J Crit Care.* 1996;5(3):198-206.

99. Pahlm O et al. Comparison of waveforms in conventional 12-lead ECGs and those derived from EASI leads in children. *J Electrocardiol.* 2003;36(1):25-31.

100. Martinez JP et al. Accuracy of QT measurement in the EASI-derived 12-lead ECG. Paper presented at: 28th Annual International Conference of the IEEE Engineering in Medicine and Biology Society; August 2006; New York, NY.

101. Kossick MA. *Evaluation of a new modified chest lead in diagnosing wide complex beats of unknown origin* [dissertation]. Memphis, TN: University of Tennessee Health Science Center; 2003.

102. Berson AS, Pipberger HV. The low-frequency response of electrocardiographs, a frequent source of recording errors. *Am Heart J.* 1966;71(6):779-789.

103. Slogoff S et al. Incidence of perioperative myocardial ischemia detected by different electrocardiographic systems. *Anesthesiology.* 1990;73(6):1074-1081.

104. O'Brien EI: Review: a century of confusion; which bladder for accurate blood pressure measurement? *J Hum Hypertens.* 1996;10(9):565-572.

105. Fonseca-Reyes S et al. Effect of standard cuff on blood pressure readings in patients with obese arms. How frequent are arms of a "large circumference"? *Blood Press Monit.* 2003;8(3):101-106.

106. Pierin AMG et al. Blood pressure measurement in obese patients: comparison between upper arm and forearm measurements. *Blood Press Monit.* 2004;9(3):101-105.

107. Schell K et al. Clinical comparison of automatic, noninvasive measurements of blood pressure in the forearm and upper arm with the patient supine or with the head of the bed raised 45 degrees: a follow-up study. *Am J Crit Care.* 2006;15:196-205.

108. Park MK et al. Oscillometric blood pressures in the arm, thigh, and calf in healthy children and those with aortic coarctation. *Pediatrics.* 1993;91(4):761-765.

109. Arnett DK et al. Interarm differences in seated systolic and diastolic blood pressure: the hypertension genetic epidemiology network study. *J Hypertens.* 2005;23(6):1141-1147.

110. Subramanian S et al. Correlation between noninvasive and invasive blood pressure measurements in early septic shock. *Chest.* 2006;130(4):150S.

111. Ostchega Y et al. US demographic trends in mid-arm circumference and recommended blood pressure cuffs: 1988-2002. *J Hum Hypertens.* 2005;19(11):885-891.

112. Cheitlin MD et al. American College of Cardiology/American Heart Association Task Force on Practice Guidelines. ACC/AHA/ASE 2003 Guideline update for the clinical application of echocardiography: summary article: a report of the ACC/AHA/ASE committee to update the 1997 guidelines for the clinical application of echocardiography. *J Am Soc Echocardiogr.* 2003;16(10):1091-1110.

113. American Society of Echocardiography, American College of Emergency Physicians, American Society of Nuclear Cardiology, Society for Cardiovascular Angiography and Interventions, Society of Cardiovascular Computed Tomography, and the Society for Cardiovascular Magnetic Resonance. Appropriateness criteria for transthoracic and transesophageal

echocardiography: a report of the American College of Cardiology Foundation Quality Strategic Directions Committee Appropriateness Criteria Working Group. *J Am Soc Echocardiogr.* 2007;20(7):787-805.

114. Dussik KT et al. Auf dem Wege zur Hyperphonographie des Gehirnes. *Wien Med Wochenschr.* 1947;97:425-429.

115. Side CD, Gosling RG. Non-surgical assessment of cardiac function. *Nature.* 1971;232(5309):335-336.

116. Minhaj M et al. The effect of routine intraoperative transesophageal echocardiography on surgical management. *J Cardiothorac Vasc Anesth.* 2007;21(6):800-804.

117. Douglas PS et al. 2007 appropriateness criteria for transthoracic and transesophageal echocardiography: a report of the American College of Cardiology Foundation Quality Strategic Directions Committee Appropriateness Criteria Working Group, American Society of Echocardiography, American College of Emergency Physicians, American Society of Nuclear Cardiology, Society for Cardiovascular Angiography and Interventions, Society of Cardiovascular Computed Tomography, and the Society for Cardiovascular Magnetic Resonance endorsed by the American College of Chest Physicians and the Society of Critical Care Medicine. *J Am Coll Cardiol.* 2007;50(2): 187-204.

118. Heyndrickx GR et al. Regional myocardial functional and electrophysiological alterations after brief coronary artery occlusion in conscious dogs. *J Clin Invest.* 1975;56(4):978-985.

119. Waters DD et al. Early changes in regional and global left ventricular function induced by graded reductions in regional coronary perfusion. *Am J Cardiol.* 1977;39(4):537-543.

120. Tennant R, Wiggers CJ. The effect of coronary occlusion on myocardial contraction. *Am J Physiol.* 1935;112:351-361.

121. Clements FM et al. How easily can we learn to recognize regional wall motion abnormalities with 2D-transesophageal echocardiography? Paper presented at Proceedings of the 8th Annual Meeting of the Society of Cardiovascular Anesthesiologists; 1986; Montreal, Quebec, Canada.

122. Blot-Souletie N et al. Comparison of accuracy of aortic valve area assessment in aortic stenosis by real time three-dimensional echocardiography in biplane mode versus two-dimensional transthoracic and transesophageal echocardiography. *Echocardiography.* 2007;24(10):1065-1072.

123. Schafer ST et al. Intracardiac transvenous echocardiography is superior to both precordial doppler and transesophageal echocardiography techniques for detecting venous air embolism and catheter-guided air aspiration. *Anesth Analg.* 2008;106(1):45-54.

CHAPTER 18

CLINICAL MONITORING II: RESPIRATORY AND METABOLIC SYSTEMS

Gregory Bozimowski

"EVERY BREATH YOU TAKE, EVERY MOVE YOU MAKE . . . I'LL BE WATCHING YOU"

(STING, 1983)[1]

It can be said that those haunting lyrics, when spoken in a nurse anesthesia context, are what provide the safety and reassurance for patients receiving anesthesia every day. Clinical monitoring in the perioperative setting is the process of observing physiologic responses to surgery and anesthesia. It is the essence of what the Certified Registered Nurse Anesthetist (CRNA) does to ensure an optimal, safe outcome. It is important to note that the modalities chosen to obtain physiologic feedback may or may not in and of themselves reduce the likelihood of patient morbidity and mortality. Literature provides rationale for the standardization of minimal monitoring requirements, and such standards are available to the anesthesia provider from both the American Association of Nurse Anesthetists (AANA) and the American Society of Anesthesiologists (ASA).[2] It then becomes a matter of the anesthetist's clinical judgment as to what modalities beyond those required by standards will provide useful information when added to the anesthetic plan of care.

It is crucial in a world of advancing technology that human vigilance is maintained. Human error is always possible and often associated with adverse outcomes. Monitoring alone cannot prevent adverse outcomes, but timely response by the anesthetist to any physiologic changes those monitors display can have a positive effect.[3] It cannot be emphasized enough that reliance on technology must never be allowed to lull the anesthetist into complacency. Though accuracy and reliability of monitors continually improve, the potential for machine malfunction and artifact is ever present. Despite the sophistication of current electronic monitors, timely human response to intraoperative events remains the key to predicting, avoiding, and managing untoward responses to anesthesia and surgery. The basic human senses of sight, hearing, touch, and even smell remain useful in clinical monitoring. The anesthetist must focus attention on the primary source of assessment data: the patient.

This chapter reviews current monitoring standards as outlined by the AANA. In addition, a practical systems approach to monitoring is presented as it relates to the avoidance of critical incidents. Respiratory monitoring will be reviewed as it relates to the ongoing assessment of airway, breathing, and circulation, using not only the human senses but also the technologic tools used by nurse anesthetists. The modalities to be discussed in this chapter include the precordial stethoscope, carbon dioxide detection devices, and pulse oximetry. Noninvasive blood pressure monitoring is discussed in general terms; advanced, invasive cardiovascular monitoring is discussed elsewhere in the text.

Thermoregulation is significantly altered under anesthesia, so temperature monitoring modalities are reviewed in this chapter. Finally, implications for the education of nurse anesthetists and the future of clinical monitoring are visited.

MONITORING STANDARDS

Monitoring standards have been published by anesthesia provider professional associations to recommend minimal standards in the provision and monitoring of care. Such standards are intended to provide assistance to anesthesia providers and health-care facilities in evaluating quality care and improving the safety of practice while educating the public regarding patient rights and expectations. Standard V of the AANA *Scope and Standards for Nurse Anesthesia Practice* outlines specific monitoring requirements necessary for compliance (Table 18-1)[4]. The standard acknowledges the importance of vigilant monitoring as the basis of safety in anesthesia practice. In addition, the standards point out that the CRNA must constantly be in attendance with the patient until the responsibility for care can be safely transferred to another qualified health-care provider. As with most position statements, they further point out that these are intended to be minimum requirements and should be exceeded as deemed necessary in the judgment of the anesthetist. In most cases, when certain monitoring modalities are not used, they must be at least immediately available. The AANA interpretation specifically indicates that alarm-limit parameters and audible warning systems should be used. A specific statement is made recommending the use of variable pitch alarms. The value of variable pitch technology commonly used in pulse oximetry equipment has been appreciated widely by nurse anesthetists for its ability to distinguish subtle changes in saturation, using the sense of hearing prior to visualizing the monitor. The ever-changing and developing technologies equipped with electronic capabilities warrant that these standards also allow for consideration of new monitoring modalities as they are introduced. It is important to note that the type of anesthetic given may influence the specific monitoring required but should not be a factor in considering the level of vigilance or accessibility of advanced monitoring and interventional equipment.

PRACTICAL APPROACH TO MONITORING

A systematic, evidence-based process shown to be effective in reducing anesthetic morbidity and mortality should be the goal when planning appropriate monitoring to be used. As monitoring

TABLE 18-1	Scope and Standards for Nurse Anesthesia Practice

Standard V

Monitor the Patient's Physiologic Condition as Appropriate for the Type of Anesthesia and Specific Patient Needs

Parameter	Modifier
Monitor ventilation continuously	Verify intubation of the trachea by auscultation, chest excursion, and confirmation of carbon dioxide in the expired gas. Continuously monitor end-tidal carbon dioxide during controlled or assisted ventilation, including any anesthesia or sedation technique requiring artificial airway support. Use spirometry and ventilatory pressure monitors as indicated.
Monitor oxygenation continuously	By clinical observation, pulse oximetry, and if indicated, arterial blood gas analysis.
Monitor cardiovascular status continuously	Via electrocardiogram and heart sounds. Record blood pressure and heart rate at least every 5 minutes.
Monitor body temperature continuously	On all pediatric patients receiving general anesthesia and when indicated, on all other patients.
Monitor neuromuscular function and status	When neuromuscular blocking agents are administered.
Monitor and assess the patient positioning	Assess and institute protective measures.

Adapted from the American Association of Nurse Anesthetists. Scope and Standards for Nurse Anesthesia Practice. June 2005. Available at: http://www.aana.com/uploadedFiles/Resources/Practice_Documents/scope_stds_nap07_2007.pdf

standards guide practice by prescribing minimums to be adhered to, other processes can be helpful in defining how monitoring should occur and which modalities should be used. In the spirit of learning from previous errors or untoward events, closed-claim studies can provide valuable insight into monitoring techniques and habits that could be useful in preventing future anesthesia mishaps. In a manner of speaking, clinical monitoring can be thought of as a means to avoid critical incidents.

The act of administering anesthesia results in a physiologic response that is dependent on the pharmacodynamics and pharmacokinetics of each substance. In addition, the insult of the surgical or diagnostic procedure performed results in physiologic alterations as well. As such, the anesthetist's observation of the human systems response is the monitoring of the pharmacology of the agents used and the physiology of the human system. As the science and process for quality assurance and improvement have evolved, much has been learned and written about the value of a systematic approach to the analysis of critical incidents and crisis management. The concepts used in quality assurance management are therefore easily applied to anesthesia monitoring because a primary function of the nurse anesthetist is to prevent or respond to critical incidents. In short, a systematic approach to clinical monitoring is the anesthetist's means of ensuring timely responses to physiologic changes presented by the patient. Many algorithms and protocols have been written to guide the practitioner through the monitoring process and ensure thorough, vigilant observation. One simple, systematic approach to crisis management is spelled out in the algorithm "COVER ABCD," the letters of which represent circulation and color, oxygen and oxygen analyzer, ventilation and vaporizer, endotracheal tube and elimination, review monitors and equipment, airway, breathing, circulation, and drugs[5] (Table 18-2). Perhaps without even having thought about it, the well-prepared anesthetist can attest to the enormous value of developing such a systematic approach to monitoring. The habit sometimes referred to as "sweeping" the anesthesia field to

visualize the patient, with the eyes following a path to the anesthesia machine via the airway and breathing circuit and progressing to the monitoring modalities used, has long been taught as a means of increasing vigilance and attention to detail.

Review of critical incidents has provided insight into how anesthetists can enhance safety and prevent mishaps through their use of monitors with alarms. Closed-claims review of various databases supports the notion that vigilance remains a key point, and respiratory events are of particular concern.[6] It has been suggested that in cases in which anesthesia is provided outside the operating room (e.g., a rapidly growing practice in which monitoring may not be as focused as in a standard anesthetizing area), the number and severity of liability claims may be increased.[7] The well-known mantra of the ABCs—observing the airway, breathing (respiration), and circulation—remains foremost and critical in anesthesia clinical monitoring. Monitoring drug effect completes the basic monitoring approach. Monitoring central nervous system responses also may be useful and is discussed in detail elsewhere in this text.

Airway Monitoring

Monitoring the airway includes observing ventilation and the adequacy of gas exchange from the upper to lower airways. Assessment of airway patency is performed in very subtle yet essential ways. The anesthetist must observe ventilatory movement of the chest and note the presence of any sign of airway obstruction, such as retractions or seesaw motion of the chest and abdomen. Seeing condensation in an airway device or clear mask can serve to indicate the presence of gas exchange. The sense of touch can be used to perceive subtle movement of air exchange, felt on the hand of the anesthetist. The sense of smell can be the first aid in detecting a disconnected circuit or airway device when volatile agents are being used. Listening for the presence of abnormal airway sounds such as stridor is crucial in noting airway obstruction. The precordial stethoscope is a valuable

TABLE **18-2**	Crisis Management Algorithm
Algorithm	**Descriptor**
C—Circulation, Color	Determine adequacy of circulation, check pulse, blood pressure, ECG. Note oxygenation through assessment and oximetry.
O—Oxygen, Oxygen analyzer	Check oxygen delivery system, hypoxic guard.
V—Ventilation, Vaporizer	Ventilate by hand to assess breathing circuit and airway patency, assess chest excursion and auscultation, assess ETCO2, check vaporizer function.
E—Endotracheal tube, Elimination	Systematic assessment of ETT if used, including patency, seal, etc. Eliminate the anesthetic machine as source of problem if indicated (ventilate with bag-valve-mask [BVM; Ambu] and oxygen tank).
R—Review monitors, Review equipment	Review all monitors in use, assure appropriate calibration and maintenance, review any and all equipment in contact with the patient.
A—Airway	Check patency of the unintubated airway, assess for laryngospasm, foreign body, etc.
B—Breathing	Assess pattern, rate, and depth of respirations. Examine, auscultate, and review ETCO2 and pulse oximeter monitors.
C—Circulation	Repeat assessment of circulation.
D—Drugs	Review drugs given, consider needed pharmacologic intervention, consider possibility of medication administration error.

Adapted from Runciman WB, Merry AF. Crises in clinical care: an approach to management. Qual Saf Health Care. 2005;14(3):156-163.
NOTE: *COVERABCD applies to a ventilated patient, whereas for a spontaneously breathing patient, the proper order should follow the algorithm AB-COVER_CD.*
ECG, *Electrocardiograph;* ETCO2, *end-tidal carbon dioxide;* ETT, *endotracheal tube.*

tool in auscultating the presence or absence of airway exchange during all phases of the anesthetic, regardless of the type administered. Ensuring adequacy of ventilation, whether an endotracheal tube or laryngeal mask airway is in use, must include verification of placement by assessing breath sounds and chest expansion, as well as verification of the presence of carbon dioxide (CO_2) in the expired gas.[8] Although failure to successfully intubate is problematic, failure to recognize an esophageal intubation is catastrophic.

Respiratory Monitoring: Ventilation

Monitoring respiratory parameters is aimed at evaluating both ventilation and oxygenation. Above all, the patient must be observed for adequate minute ventilation throughout the anesthetic course. At the most basic level, this is accomplished through visualization of chest excursion and auscultation of breath sounds. The value of the precordial or esophageal stethoscope is twofold: it provides continuous assurance that ventilation is occurring and can be used to detect changes in breath sounds. Assessing the respiratory rate and tidal volume (rate alone is not adequate to determine adequacy of ventilation) is crucial to ensuring adequacy of minute ventilation, as well as interpreting patient response to pharmacologic agents and surgical stimuli.

Skin color changes alone are not a reliable measure of whether ventilation and oxygenation are adequate; the CRNA should observe skin and nailbed color as part of the whole patient-assessment picture. Cyanosis is a late sign of anemia or hypoxia and can be difficult to assess accurately, given the variability of lighting during certain procedures. Besides physical assessment skills, monitoring the adequacy of ventilation must be done throughout the perioperative period, using multiple parameters. Several themes related to safety and vigilance in monitoring emerge when reviewing closed-claims studies for anesthesia incidents.

The most prominent of these themes is the value of certain specific monitors and their alarms. These include end-tidal carbon dioxide (ETCO2) measurement, pulse oximetry, oxygen (O_2) analyzers, and disconnect alarms. Of equal importance is the user's ability to ensure these are functioning properly *prior to* an anesthetic.[6]

Carbon Dioxide Monitoring

The measurement of arterial blood gases for CO_2 provides direct assessment of ventilation and metabolic status and may be indicated in certain cases. The means of measuring the carbon dioxide tension in the blood ($PaCO_2$) is based on the hydrogen ion concentration because CO_2 reacts with water to produce hydrogen ions through a reversible reaction. This reaction yields carbonic acid, which dissociates to yield hydrogen and bicarbonate ions,[9] as shown in equation 18-1.

Equation 18-1

$$CO_2 + H_2O \leftrightarrow H_2CO_3 \leftrightarrow H^+ + HCO_3^-$$

The production of carbonic acid also allows for the qualitative—and to a limited extent, quantitative—detection of the presence of CO_2 through the use of disposable ETCO2 detector devices. These colorimetric devices react to changes in pH and display it as a color change. They are widely used in emergency settings to verify proper placement of an endotracheal tube.[10] Although they are sensitive enough to detect CO_2 quickly, a minimum of six breaths has been suggested to avoid misinterpretation. False positives may result from the detection of CO_2 from air forced into the stomach during mask ventilation or the presence of carbonated beverages or antacids in the stomach.[11]

The anesthetist's choice of the means to measure CO_2 level must be based on the patient's condition, the type of anesthetic administered, and the complexity of the surgical procedure. The continuous electronic measurement of CO_2 in expired gas provides a practical, noninvasive, and accurate reflection of arterial blood CO_2 and is the most common means of monitoring CO_2 levels in the anesthesia setting. It is also a monitoring standard of care for the patient being ventilated or whose ventilations are being assisted. Accuracy of $ETCO_2$ as a reflection of arterial CO_2 has been well documented. End-tidal CO_2 is said to be approximately 2 to 5 torr lower than arterial CO_2 in patients who have no cardiac or pulmonary abnormalities.[11] This is the result of the normal alveolar-to-arterial pressure gradient that develops as a result of normal regional differences in ventilation and perfusion. *Capnometry* is a term that encompasses all means of measuring CO_2, whereas *capnography* refers to recording the measurement. The term *capnogram* is used to describe a continuous display of CO_2 during the phases of ventilation. The continuous measurement of $ETCO_2$ is accomplished through the use of infrared analysis. When a gas mixture containing more than one substance (e.g., an exhaled gas sample) is analyzed, a quantitative measurement can be made to determine the proportional contents. Each gas in the mixture absorbs infrared radiation at a different wavelength. The amount of CO_2 is measured by detecting its absorbance at specific wavelengths and filtering the absorbance related to other component gases. Older monitors had difficulty distinguishing between nitrous oxide and CO_2, but this fault is corrected in current models.[9]

Sampling of $ETCO_2$ can be accomplished through either a nondiverting (also known as *mainstream*) or diverting (also known as *sidestream*) monitor. A nondiverting monitor measures gas directly within the breathing system. Gas passes through a wide-chambered sensor that fits over a connector between the anesthesia circuit and mask adapter. The sensor is connected to the monitor by a cable. Nondiverting monitors offer several advantages. They have minimal sampling-time delays, use few disposable items, and do not require scavenging because gas is not removed from the system. Disadvantages include the inability to measure gases other than CO_2 and nitrous oxide, an increase in circuit deadspace by the adapter, and greater risk of interference by condensation and secretions. Also, because the sensor and cable are attached in proximity to the patient, the added weight may cause traction on the tube, increase the risk of circuit disconnect, and make sampling in a nonintubated patient difficult.

The other more commonly used CO_2 monitor type is the diverting monitor. The diverting monitor extracts gas from sample tubing attached near the patient end of the circuit and pumps it to the monitor. Disadvantages include the need for scavenging of sampled gases because they are removed from the circuit and some risk of contamination by condensation or secretions. Advantages of the diverting system include minimal increase in deadspace and versatility in gas analysis because the sample can also be sent to anesthetic agent monitors. In addition, the small, lightweight tubing can be adapted to sample awake, spontaneously breathing patients through the mouth, nares, or simple mask.[11]

It has become common to adapt the sampling line of a diverting $ETCO_2$ monitor to trace a capnogram in awake or sedated, spontaneously breathing patients receiving O_2 via simple mask or nasal cannula. Nasal cannula tubing already equipped with a sampling line is commercially available. It has been shown that sampling $ETCO_2$ in the spontaneously breathing patient's hypopharynx is reliable and accurate and that the exact position and use of supplemental O_2 flow will not affect reliability.[12]

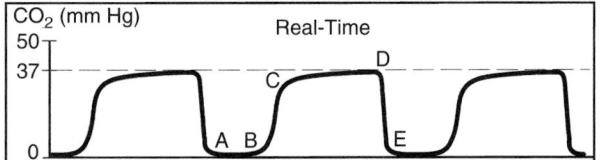

FIGURE **18-1** The four phases of a normal capnogram. *A-B* represents baseline; *B-C* represents expiratory upstroke; *C-D* represents expiratory plateau; *D* represents end-tidal concentration; and *D-E* represents descent to original baseline. (*Courtesy Novametrix Medical Systems, Wallingford, CT.*)

The use of $ETCO_2$ monitoring as a warning of hypoventilation or excess sedation has gained attention outside the anesthesia setting. $ETCO_2$ monitoring has been shown to be a more sensitive indicator of hypoventilation than clinical observation or pulse oximetry when used during sedation in the emergency department setting.[13] Other studies note the value of $ETCO_2$ monitoring during sedation as well and note the advantage over pulse oximetry alone in detecting hypoventilation in patients receiving supplemental O_2. It has been suggested that like pulse oximetry, $ETCO_2$ monitoring should be considered a standard of care for patients receiving sedation outside the operating room.[14]

End-Tidal Carbon Dioxide Capnography. Capnography can record CO_2 as a component of expired lung volume or as a measure of CO_2 alone throughout the phases of respiration plotted against time. Time capnography is most commonly used in the perioperative setting. Basic interpretation of the $ETCO_2$ capnogram is a necessary skill. The capnogram can differentiate between normal and abnormal patterns of ventilation that result from patient pathologies, anesthesia system problems, or unexpected patient responses during anesthesia.

The normal-time capnogram can be recorded at varying speeds. A fast speed setting of approximately 12.5 mm/second allows interpretation of individual respiratory components and short-term changes, whereas a slow speed of approximately 25 mm/minute displays long-term changes.[15] Although no standard descriptions exist for the components of the capnogram, it is typically described as encompassing four basic phases (Figure 18-1). These phases are often displayed in the literature in a classic waveform shape best recorded during mechanical ventilation in an intubated patient. It is important to note that the basic shape of the waveform will vary, depending on the mode of airway management used (endotracheal tube, laryngeal mask airway, simple mask, nasal cannula, etc.), as well as in comparison to the spontaneously breathing patient.

Although the shapes may vary, the represented phases apply universally. The first phase is the end of inspiration and very beginning of expiration. Gas sampled at this point identifies the baseline; it comes from the anatomic deadspace and contains no CO_2. This portion in a normal capnogram should approximate zero. The second phase is the expiratory upstroke. Gas sampled represents a mix of deadspace and alveolar gas and thus records measurable CO_2. This phase represents the rapid passing of initial expired gas through the upper airways. The third phase represents the plateau and records alveolar emptying of CO_2. In the normal pulmonary measurement, the plateau is very nearly flat. This phase represents the longest duration of the measurement. $ETCO_2$ is measured at the end of the plateau just prior to the beginning of phase four. The fourth phase is displayed as the rapid decrease in CO_2 concentration of sampled gas as a result of inspiration of air or O_2. This downstroke returns the recorded CO_2 measurement at or very near to zero.

Variations in the capnograph tracing can be very subtle and represent specific alterations in the ventilatory process. Some common deviations are worth noting. In the process of evaluating the capnogram, the anesthetist should note the respiratory rate, whether ventilation is spontaneous or mechanical, the value of measured end-expired CO_2, the shape of the recorded waveform, and the presence of additional respiratory efforts. Deviations from what is normally a close approximation of arterial CO_2 can occur. End-tidal CO_2 measurements may be inaccurate in the presence of significant ventilation and perfusion mismatching. When ventilation-to-perfusion ratio is large, the resultant increase in deadspace causes a low concentration of ET_{CO_2} overall.[16] In addition, small tidal volumes—reflecting inadequate alveolar ventilation—may produce ET_{CO_2} recordings that significantly underestimate arterial CO_2 levels. Some controversy exists as to the relative accuracy of capnography during laparoscopic procedures.[17]

Following esophageal intubation, an initial slight upstroke of CO_2 may be seen in those rare circumstances when CO_2 may be sampled from the stomach, as mentioned previously in reference to disposable ET_{CO_2} detector devices. These CO_2 measurements are the result of excess air blown into the stomach during over-zealous ventilation or a partially obstructed airway. Such a waveform will display for a very brief period and be followed by a measurement of zero. A waveform that fails to return to baseline during phases one and four indicates that rebreathing of CO_2 is occurring. This can be the result of inadequate fresh gas flow in the nonrebreathing system or a depleted or ineffective soda-lime absorber (Figure 18-2). Although this may be detected over time, it can be difficult to distinguish.

Sloping of the plateau phase represents a progressive prolongation of expiration. It is typically the result of either an obstruction of expired gas flow at some point along the airway or ventilation-perfusion mismatch (Figure 18-3). It also can be indicative of chronic obstructive lung disease because CO_2 is exhaled more slowly from diseased portions of the lungs (with more significant airway narrowing) than from areas with less severe narrowing. Plateau-phase sloping also can occur with kinking of the endotracheal tube (ETT) or any aspect of the circuit tubing. Changes in the waveform from baseline normal should always be evaluated to determine the cause and necessary interventions.

Regular, sawtooth waves within the expiratory phase at a rate equal to the heart rate are likely the result of cardiac oscillations (Figure 18-4). This is the result of the contraction of the heart and great vessels forcing gas in and out of the lungs and a common occurrence in pediatric patients, owing to the relative size of the heart to the thorax.

During mechanical ventilation in an anesthetized and/or paralyzed patient, spontaneous respiratory effort may be seen if anesthetic depth is insufficient to prevent rebreathing or when inadequate muscle relaxation is present. The resultant capnogram is often referred to as *curare cleft* (Figure 18-5). This irregular asynchronous waveform may occur within the mechanically ventilated wave or separate from it.

Transcutaneous Carbon Dioxide Monitoring. As previously stated, accurate analysis of CO_2 reflects adequacy of ventilation. Transcutaneous CO_2 monitoring does not provide immediate, breath by breath verification of endotracheal tube placement but is a reliable, noninvasive means of measurement. Transcutaneous CO_2 monitoring can be accomplished using the same technology commonly used for measuring oxygen

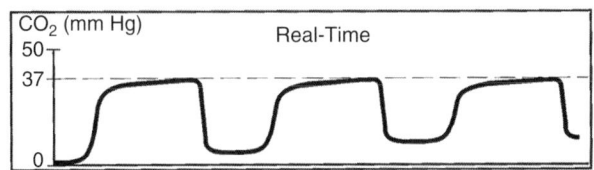

FIGURE **18-2**   Elevation of the baseline indicates rebreathing. (*Courtesy Novametrix Medical Systems, Wallingford, CT.*)

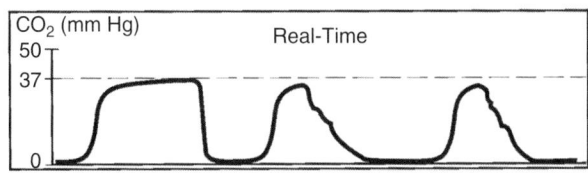

FIGURE **18-3**   Sloping plateau may indicate COPD. (*Courtesy Novametrix Medical Systems, Wallingford, CT.*)

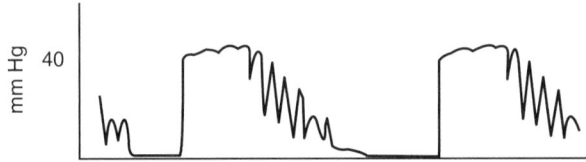

FIGURE **18-4**   Cardiac oscillations occur as a result of contractions of the heart and great vessels. (*From Miller RD. Miller's Anesthesia. 6th ed. Philadelphia: Churchill Livingstone; 2005.*)

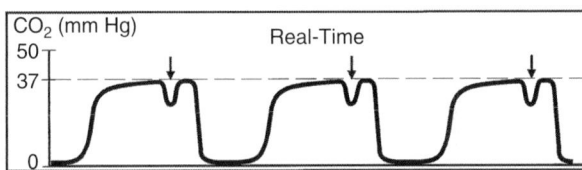

FIGURE **18-5**   Clefts displayed as a spontaneous inspiration asynchronous with controlled ventilation. (*Courtesy Novametrix Medical Systems, Wallingford, CT.*)

saturation through pulse oximetry. The electrode used provides a measurement of CO_2 through measurement of hydrogen ion (H^+) change. Transcutaneous CO_2 measurement is a noninvasive measure of Pa_{CO_2}. It can either estimate Pa_{CO_2} or determine trends in the measurement. Progress in the technical aspects of developing these monitors is beginning to be noted among researchers and clinicians.[18] Transcutaneous CO_2 monitors are not commonplace in the anesthesia setting but have gained notice for their value in analyzing CO_2 in circumstances in which ET_{CO_2} measurement may be inaccurate, as in the case of ventilation-perfusion mismatching. In such cases as severe obesity, which may affect ventilation-perfusion ratios as a result of reduced functional residual capacity, transcutaneous CO_2 monitoring may provide a more accurate estimate of arterial CO_2 than ET_{CO_2}.[19] Transcutaneous CO_2 measurement may prove beneficial during one-lung anesthesia for thoracic surgery, because it has been shown to provide a close correlation with arterial CO_2 An added benefit of transcutaneous CO_2 measurement may be seen in monitoring the awake patient at risk of hypoventilation in whom $ETCO_2$ monitoring is impractical.

Respiratory Monitoring: Oxygenation

To note that ensuring adequate O_2 delivery to the tissues is of paramount importance in the safe delivery of anesthesia is a statement of the obvious. Monitoring of oxygenation follows the continuum of O_2 delivery from the source to the patient until distribution within the body. The anesthetist must evaluate the adequacy of the gas machine's delivery of O_2 and the efficiency of its delivery to the alveoli during ventilation. The anesthetist must be aware that oxygenation monitoring by itself only constitutes a part of the whole picture when considering the respiratory process. Hypoventilation, hypercapnia, and impending respiratory arrest can occur despite adequate oxygenation, particularly during the administration of supplemental O_2.[20]

Like ventilation monitoring, the means to ensure oxygenation uses multiple senses and technologies. Monitoring oxygenation starts with O_2 delivery analysis and is covered in depth elsewhere in the text. It is crucial to note that ensuring delivery of O_2 from the source does not ensure adequate uptake and distribution of O_2 on the part of the patient.

To assess the major aspects of acid-base balance and respiratory function, including oxygenation, arterial blood gas analysis (ABG) is most helpful. Although frequent sampling and analysis of ABG is indicated in certain circumstances—dictated by the patient's physiologic status or surgical procedure—noninvasive, continuous monitoring of oxygenation through clinical observation and pulse oximetry is the standard of care[4] (see Table 18-1). Clinical observation parameters include an assessment of skin color and temperature, nailbed perfusion signs, assessment of depth and rate of respirations, auscultation of breath sounds, and assessment of upper airway patency.

Pulse Oximetry

The use of pulse oximetry has become commonplace in many health-care settings, both inside and outside critical care areas, and has proven valuable in detecting hypoxemia. Pulse oximetry measures heart rate and percent of arterial oxygen saturation (SpO_2) of hemoglobin (Hb) continuously and noninvasively. The technology involved in providing the transcutaneous measurement uses a spectrophotometer to determine SpO_2. Oxygenated Hb absorbs infrared light at a different wavelength than unoxygenated Hb. A light signal is emitted from one diode and transmitted through tissue, most commonly a finger, to an oppositely placed photosensitive diode that measures the amount of unabsorbed red light. Pulse oximeters can distinguish arterial from venous blood by measuring the change in transmitted light during pulsatile flow. The pulse oximeter converts the detected light to a plethysmographic signal that measures the drop in light intensity with each beat.[19,21,22]

Oxygen Saturation Physiology. To understand the measurement and significance of monitoring oxygen saturation via pulse oximetry, it is important to understand the physiology of oxygen transport and the factors that influence its binding to and release from Hb. This is expressed in equation 18-2.

Equation 18-2

$$Hb + O_2 \leftrightarrow HbO_2$$

The reversibility of the reaction allows for the release of O_2 to the tissues. Oxygen is transported throughout the body either

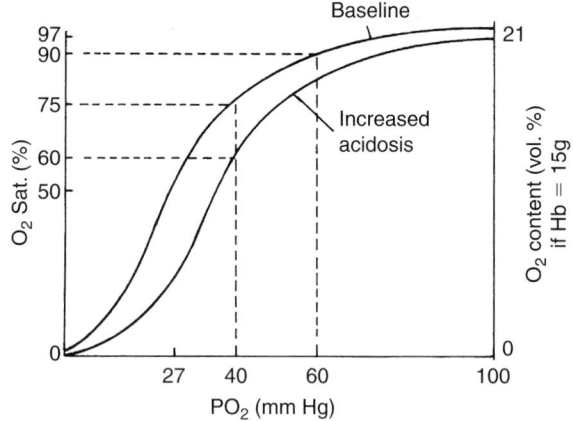

FIGURE **18-6** Oxyhemoglobin dissociation curve. (*From Roberts JR et al. Clinical Procedures in Emergency Medicine. 4th ed. Philadelphia: Saunders; 2004.*)

physically dissolved in the blood or chemically combined with Hb. The vast majority is carried bound to Hb. As a result, the oxygen-carrying capacity is mainly dependent on the amount of Hb. If varying concentrations of O_2 are added to a volume of blood, after allowing the mixture to equilibrate, the oxygen tension (PO_2) of the gas can be measured. Because it is known that 0.003 mL of O_2 will dissolve in 100 mL of blood at a PO_2 of 100 mm Hg, the remaining O_2 bound to Hb can be determined. In short, the PO_2 of the plasma determines the amount of O_2 that binds to Hb. Like oxygen-carrying capacity, this is expressed in mL per 100 mL of blood. The oxygen-carrying capacity of Hb, taking into account the existence of impure portions such as methemoglobin, is 1.34 mL/g of Hb. This means that if completely (100%) saturated, 1 g of Hb binds 1.34 mL of O_2. The formula for determining arterial oxygen content (CaO_2) is expressed in Equation 18-3:

Equation 18-3

$$CaO_2 = (0.003 \times PaO_2) + (1.34 \times Hb \times SaO_2)$$

For example, the CaO_2 for an individual whose Hb is 15, PaO_2 is 92, and SaO_2 is 98% can be calculated as follows:

$$CaO_2 = (0.003 \times 92) + (1.34 \times 15 \times 0.98)$$
$$CaO_2 = 0.28 + 19.7$$
$$CaO_2 = 19.98 \text{ mL } O_2/100 \text{ mL of blood}$$

The value of CaO_2 is crucial in calculating actual O_2 delivered, which is a product of oxygen content and cardiac output. It becomes obvious that adequate cardiac output does not ensure adequate delivery of O_2 to the tissues.

It is important to distinguish between terms used in discussing oxygenation. The proportion of Hb bound to O_2 is expressed as percent saturation and excludes that amount dissolved in the blood.[23,24] The relationship between oxygen tension and percent of oxygen saturation is illustrated in the oxyhemoglobin dissociation curve (Figure 18-6). It shows how the availability of O_2 (PO_2 in plasma) can affect the reversible reaction between O_2 and Hb. The curve demonstrates that the amount of O_2 carried by Hb (percent saturated) increases rapidly to a PO_2 of approximately 50 and slows thereafter, as displayed by a flattening of the curve.

TABLE 18-3	Factors Influencing the Oxyhemoglobin Dissociation Curve	
Curve Shift to the Right	**Curve Shift to the Left**	
Elevated CO_2	Decreased CO_2	
Elevated temperature	Decreased temperature	
Elevated levels of 2,3-DPG	Decreased levels of 2,3-DPG	
Decreased pH, acidosis (elevated H^+ ions)	Elevated pH, alkalosis (decreased H^+ ions)	

Adapted from Levitzky MG: Pulmonary Physiology. 7th ed. New York: McGraw-Hill; 2007.

As blood travels to the systemic capillaries, the oxygenated Hb releases O_2 to tissue with lower oxygen tension. In the 10 to 40 mm Hg range, the curve is very steep. This demonstrates that small decreases in P_{O_2} can result in significant dissociation of O_2 for use by the tissue. For example, at a P_{O_2} of 40 mm Hg, Hb is approximately 75% saturated with O_2, whereas at 20 mm Hg only 32% is saturated. This relationship can be altered by a variety of physiologic changes. The result is a shift in the curve either to the *right*, indicating a more ready release of O_2 from Hb at the tissue level, or to the *left*, indicating a greater attachment of O_2 to Hb, thereby decreasing release to tissues[23,25] (Table 18-3).

Clinical Use. Although many studies regarding the use of pulse oximetry show conflicting impact on outcome, it should be intuitive that early detection and warning of hypoxemia, followed by appropriate interventions, will improve care. Pederson and colleagues reviewed more than 21,000 perioperative patients and reported that the incidence of hypoxemia ranged from 1.5 to 3 times less in patients monitored with pulse oximetry.[26] Perhaps one of the greatest benefits of pulse oximetry is its simplicity. The pulse oximeter is calibrated by the manufacturer and needs little or no further maintenance. It is easy to apply, and ongoing product development has made the device quite portable and durable. Its efficiency in measuring oxygen saturation has been shown to be accurate within 2% when oxygen saturation is between 80% and 100% and approximately 5% when saturation falls below 80%.[3]

It is, however, essential that the anesthetist understand the optimal use and limitations of pulse oximetry. Pulse oximeters can use a variety of sensor types applied to the body. The finger probe is the most commonly used and is available as a reusable clip-on device or disposable stick-on probe. The finger probe is often used successfully on the toe as well, particularly in the pediatric population. One common problem with pulse oximeter monitoring is motion artifact.[27] To address this issue, monitors have been improved since their development, but motion artifact can still be problematic. Using alternative sites can be helpful or forehead, ear, or nose probes can be used with comparable accuracy and reliability.[11,28] The site of application of the pulse oximeter probe should be assessed at reasonable intervals during particularly long periods of use and changed as needed. Prolonged application of a clip-on probe could compromise perfusion. Another common problem associated with inaccurate measurement or sensor difficulties when pulse oximeter monitoring is in use is the vasoconstriction state that results from cold temperatures or inadequate circulation. It has been noted that during such circumstances, measurement may be improved by

using oximeter sites closer to the central circulation and away from the periphery, such as the forehead, nose, or ear.[28-30] Much discussion has surrounded whether the presence of nail polish affects pulse oximeter measurement. Some authors have noted that the presence of nail polish, particularly certain colors, will cause artifact and/or inaccurate measurements. More recent studies suggest that improved monitor sensitivity has virtually eliminated any effect nail polish might once have had on pulse oximetry readings.[31,32] A less commonly occurring but problematic issue is the presence of abnormal Hb. Methemoglobin absorbs light equally to oxyhemoglobin. As a result, pulse oximeter measurements falsely underestimate oxyhemoglobin concentrations when oxygen saturation is above 85% and overestimate oxyhemoglobin concentrations when oxygen saturation is below 85%. Likewise, abnormally high levels of carboxyhemoglobin can cause the oximeter to overestimate oxygen saturation. Sickle cell anemia and other rarer forms of anemia may also affect the accuracy of pulse oximeter measurements. Injectable dyes for diagnostic procedures, such as methylene blue or indigo carmine, will result in a significant but transient decrease in the measured oxygen saturation by pulse oximetry.[11] This is because the presence of the dye alters the absorption of infrared light. Technology available on some pulse oximeters enables the monitor to distinguish between normal Hb and carboxyhemoglobin or methemoglobin. In fact, oximetry principles in these monitors can quantitatively measure amounts of these variant forms of Hb.[33]

The versatility and accuracy of pulse oximeters have sparked their use for other diagnostic purposes such as assisting in the measurement of systolic blood pressure by inflating a cuff and noting the point at which the pulse oximeter waveform is obliterated. The pulse oximeter may be useful in assisting in the location of a vessel by occluding the anatomy proximal to the probe until that point is reached where the waveform is lost.[11] Because of their sensitivity to changes in vascular supply, pulse oximeters have been used to determine the presence of vascular disease, such as in diabetic patients.[34] Changes in sympathetic tone are perceived by pulse oximeter plethysmography. Vessels of the arm are subject to changes in autonomic tone, and pulse oximetry has demonstrated an ability to detect the subtle changes in blood flow that occur during regional anesthesia; indirectly, it can indicate degree of regional blockade. Research shows that circulation to the earlobe is not greatly affected by changes in sympathetic tone but rather by changes in pulse pressure. As a result, pulse oximetry measured at the earlobe may be a sensitive indicator of systemic circulation and possibly stroke volume.[29] The degree and sensitivity to which individual monitors perform under circumstances of hypothermia or circulatory changes may vary by manufacturer.[35]

The practice of closely monitoring respiration (ventilation and oxygenation) through the measurement of carbon dioxide and oxygen saturation during the anesthetic period has proved to be priceless in ensuring safe care. As technology has advanced to allow reliable, affordable, noninvasive measurement, this practice is being adopted in other settings. Combined sensors that measure both carbon dioxide and oxygen saturation are now available and may prove valuable in managing patients at risk for respiratory complications—during the postoperative period or whenever potent opiates are administered, for example.[20,36,37]

Circulation

In completing the systematic approach to patient monitoring, circulation follows breathing. As previously stated, pulse oximetry provides insight into both circulation and oxygenation. Monitoring electrocardiography and heart sounds continuously and blood pressure at frequent intervals is part of the standard of care (see Table 18-1). Adequacy of circulation can be estimated by heart rate in some circumstances. Anesthesia may result in expected decreases in blood pressure. During spinal anesthesia, the variability of heart rate may serve as a predictor of impending hypotension.[38] In certain circumstances and at the discretion of the anesthesia provider, continuous monitoring of arterial blood pressure may be indicated. This practice is, however, not without some risk (infection, embolization, thrombosis, hemorrhage or ischemia), so it behooves the anesthetist to be prudent prior to initiating invasive monitoring modalities.[39] Indications for invasive blood pressure monitoring are often centered on the type of surgery, such as cardiac, major vascular, major abdominal, thoracic or neurosurgery. Patient-centered factors also must be considered and include the presence of significant cardiovascular disease, shock, increased intracranial pressure, and multiple trauma.[3] For the remainder of patients and procedures, noninvasive intermittent blood pressure measurement has proved to be sufficient. Noninvasive, or indirect, measurement of blood pressure is achieved by the occlusion of the artery (typically the brachial) sufficient to obliterate the pulse, followed by the controlled release of the occluding pressure. The measurement of the pressure at which the pulse can first be sensed during release is the systolic pressure. As the pressure continues to be released, that measurement at which the pulse can no longer be sensed represents the diastolic pressure.

Various forms of blood pressure monitoring equipment have been used and improved upon over the years. The environmental impact of inadvertently leaked mercury forced the removal of the classic mercury sphygmomanometer in use for decades. The means of sensing the loss and return of the pulse may be simple auscultation by stethoscope, but automated blood pressure monitoring equipment uses the oscillometric technique to detect pulsatile movement.[9] Blood pressure monitors, whether freestanding or integrated into the anesthesia delivery system, typically display a mean arterial pressure as well and are equipped with high- and low-alarm limits. Automated blood pressure monitors, when adequately calibrated and maintained, will provide accurate measurements. Comparisons of the accuracy of noninvasive, invasive, or direct measurement are difficult because noninvasive methods provide intermittent measurement, and direct methods provide continuous readings. During periods of extreme high or low blood pressure, the degree of accuracy may be impaired. In addition, improper cuff fit may result in false readings. A cuff that is too small may overestimate pressure, and one that is too large may underestimate it. The site of indirect blood pressure measurement also will affect accuracy. The presence of peripheral vascular disease or vasoconstriction may result in lower measured pressures. Measurements taken at the arm, for example, will likely vary significantly from those taken in the calf.[11,40]

Although indirect, noninvasive blood pressure monitoring is typically harmless to the patient, the anesthetist must be aware of some potential problems and adverse effects. Motion artifact as a result of shivering or voluntary movement can prevent accurate measurement and cause prolonged inflation times. Inflation time also may be prolonged during extremes in blood pressure. Patient discomfort during prolonged or frequent measurement is a common issue. Patients may exhibit petechiae, bruising, or other skin damage secondary to excessive pressure. It is not uncommon for practitioners to use padding to prevent damage to underlying tissues. Certain patient risk factors such as advanced age, use of medications affecting coagulation, or preexisting skin defects should be noted and considered by the anesthetist.

Temperature Monitoring

The standards of care from both the AANA and the ASA support the notion that the ability to monitor patients' body temperature is essential.[4,8] Temperature monitoring alerts the anesthetist to hyperthermia and, as is more commonly the case, hypothermia. Despite clinical standards and the known physiology, hypothermia is an occurrence often underestimated in significance. It has been reported that approximately 70% of postoperative patients experience some degree of hypothermia.[41] Risks of hypothermia include wound infection and delayed healing, increased O_2 consumption through shivering, increased risk of cardiovascular incidents and myocardial infarction, and increased rate of sickling in sickle cell patients.[3,42] In addition, hypothermic patients have been shown to have a prolonged stay in the postanesthesia care unit, thus increasing the cost of care during the perioperative period.[41,43] It becomes apparent that appropriate and aggressive means of maintaining normothermia intraoperatively should be instituted, and a keystone to implementing these interventions is temperature monitoring. National quality-improvement initiatives supported by the Centers for Medicare and Medicaid Services have partnered with healthcare organizations to promote best practices aimed at improving surgical care. These initiatives have identified essential factors in preventing postoperative complications. Not the least of these identified areas of care is centered on maintenance of normothermia.[43] Understanding the potential causes of variations in core body temperature is valuable in appreciating the importance of temperature monitoring.

Thermoregulation

Normothermia can be defined as a core body temperature of 37° C. The human body regulates core temperature in a tightly controlled manner via the hypothalamus. Core temperature variations trigger autonomic response mechanisms to raise or lower the temperature as needed. These responses include vasoconstriction and shivering during hypothermia and vasodilation and sweating during hyperthermia. It is important to note that there is typically a variance between core and peripheral temperatures. This is key to appreciating the value of core versus peripheral temperature measurement.[41]

Hyperthermia or core temperatures exceeding 38° C can be seen intraoperatively. The genetic predisposition to drug-induced malignant hyperthermia is well documented. Other causes of fever, such as infection or hypermetabolic states, typically are not seen in patients electively brought to surgery. Certain recreational drugs such as amphetamine or cocaine can raise the body temperature through an increased rate of metabolism.[44] Drugs such as atropine can inhibit the sweating response, resulting in impaired regulatory response and a rise in the core temperature. In the anesthesia setting, these effects are typically overshadowed by the multiple factors in place that serve to lower core temperature.

Hypothermia, or core temperature below 36° C, occurs for multiple reasons. Upon entering many operating rooms, one cause of hypothermia becomes obvious to anyone, especially the patient: the low ambient temperature. Reports suggest that the greatest amount of heat loss occurs during the first hour in the perioperative setting and that patients in rooms at a temperature of 21° C will all develop hypothermia. Radiant heat loss, or that transfer of body heat into a cooler environment, accounts for the majority of heat loss in the patient undergoing surgery.

This is followed by evaporative loss from liquids on the skin, such as from cleansing or perspiration or through the expiration of warm, moist air. In addition, convective heat loss (through moving cool air) and conductive heat loss (through contact with a cooler object such as an operating room table) contribute. Redistribution of lower-temperature blood from the vasodilated, anesthetized periphery to the central compartment also accounts for significant heat loss.[41,45] Examples of ways to minimize heat loss are through the use of warming blankets, infusion of warmed intravenous fluids and irrigation solutions, and maintenance of reasonable room temperatures.

General and regional anesthesia inhibit thermoregulation and cause significant vasodilation such that temperature monitoring is warranted. During local anesthesia or sedation, temperature monitoring should be considered during circumstances in which the patient is at risk of hypothermia and should, at the very least, always be immediately available. It is important to note that normal core body temperature can vary among individuals, as well as within individuals at different points within their circadian rhythms.[44] Monitoring a patient's temperature is most beneficial when done continuously rather than intermittently and is most valuable when evaluated for trends.

Temperature Monitoring Modalities. The AANA and ASA practice standards allow for some discretion on the part of the anesthesia provider in deciding under what circumstances temperature monitoring should occur. The ASA states that body temperature monitoring should occur whenever significant changes in temperature are "intended, anticipated, or suspected." The AANA states that temperature should be monitored "on all pediatric patients receiving general anesthesia and when indicated, on all other patients."[4,8] To ensure monitoring is done and active warming strategies employed, it is essential that the anesthetist be well versed in the factors that place patients at risk for perioperative hypothermia. Some of these risk factors include high ASA status, lengthy or involved surgical procedures, combined epidural and general anesthesia, surgery of long duration, elderly patients, and those with lean body mass. Interestingly, another identified risk factor for hypothermia is failure to monitor temperature. Protective factors of increased body weight, higher preoperative temperature, and warmer rooms were noted to help maintain normothermia.[46,47]

Technology used for temperature monitoring often varies by site measured. Thermistor, thermocouple, and platinum-wire devices are frequently used with electronic monitors and have shown to be accurate and reliable. In addition, liquid crystal temperature monitors have been used for skin temperature monitoring. Although these are noninvasive and convenient, they lack specific accuracy both in measurement and in interpretation between readings by separate observers.[11]

How best to measure temperature arouses some debate. Skin temperature measurement is convenient and noninvasive; however, its accuracy as a reflection of core body temperature is unreliable. The anesthetist's sense of touch is not reliable for assessing the patient's temperature, but the sensation of being uncomfortable in a cold operating room can serve as an alert that the patient is most likely cold as well and would benefit from temperature monitoring and warming modalities. As far as choosing a site for monitoring, the Society for Critical Care Medicine's Fever Task Force concluded that the intravenous or bladder thermistor measures core temperature most accurately. They further state that electronic probe measurement orally or by rectum is also reliable.[48] Other useful and reliable measurements of core temperature include esophageal, tympanic membrane, and nasopharynx. Consistency in measurement site is identified by many authors as imperative in monitoring heat loss.

ADDITIONAL MONITORING ISSUES

Monitoring for Procedures Outside the Operating Room

As health-care delivery and technology have changed, so has the role of the anesthetist. One area of change is the location in which anesthesia is delivered. It has now become common for anesthesia departments to administer all forms of anesthesia in areas outside the traditional operating-room setting. Multiple factors could be anticipated to increase anesthesia risk outside an operating room. These include decreased availability of anesthesia personnel, less adjunct equipment, and unfamiliarity with supportive staff and settings. Procedures and settings often involve risk of allergic reactions to radiologic dyes, sharing of access to airway, and (in general) support staff with less experience with the anesthetized patient.

As anesthetists continue to work in areas outside the norm, there is a growing need for studies on morbidity and mortality as they relate to setting. A review of the ASA closed-claims database was done by Robbertze and colleagues to assess for trends and look for insight into how to best provide anesthesia safely in remote settings. Reviewers noted that anesthesia claims in these settings had a higher severity of injury and more often demonstrated that anesthesia was administered below the accepted standard level of care. The most common mechanism of injury was inadequate oxygenation or ventilation.[7] Close review of these cases emphasizes that monitoring standards during anesthesia administered outside the operating room must never be lower than what one would otherwise use. In fact, the circumstances may necessitate even closer vigilance. Frequent review and refinement of airway management skills is crucial for anesthesia providers caring for patients in these settings. Focused attention and pressure is being applied in many areas to recognize and prevent the dangerous effects of potent opioids and other sedative drugs given for pain and procedural sedation. Emphasis should be placed on ensuring adequate ventilation and oxygenation through close visualization, monitoring of ET_{CO_2}, and pulse oximetry.[20] Education, training, and certification are crucial for nonanesthesia nurses, physicians, or physician extenders involved in the administration of sedation in the absence of a nurse anesthetist or anesthesiologist. It behooves a health-care facility to have strict policies in place, and such policies should be reviewed by qualified anesthesia providers.

ANESTHESIA EDUCATION AND PATIENT MONITORING

As with all aspects of anesthesia education, teaching the art and science of clinical monitoring of the patient must be well thought out. Many educational programs and anesthesia departments use some form of simulation-based education as a supplement to clinical experience, and many more will likely join them. Simulation learning is designed to give additional interactive practice and can serve to review incidents; it has been shown to assist in the development of critical thinking skills. Research offers evidence that debriefing following the simulated event is of value.[49,50] Certainly the use of simulated clinical experience can assist in developing critical decision-making skills through repetition. It is worth noting that although the simulated experience can measure response, a certain lack of realism occurs because of the sense of anticipation of the soon-to-be-designed event. As a result, a level of "hypervigilance" can occur, masking the true habits of the learner.[51]

It is worth emphasizing that a part of vigilance in monitoring lies in developing habits that promote frequent, almost ritualistic patterns of assessment and visualization. Many students have a tendency to first focus on the electronic devices and forget the ongoing physical assessment of the patient. It is the role of the instructor to promote effective routines by explaining the underlying rationale, as well as by example. Another important part of learning how to closely monitor a patient is training the senses to notice changes in the clinical picture. Every anesthetist should be able to discern when the changing audible tones of the pulsatile measurement of the pulse oximeter monitor indicate decreasing oxygen saturation. One should rapidly recognize the subtle development of abnormal airway sounds heard through a precordial stethoscope. These are only several of the basic clinical skills essential to anesthesia practice, and the anesthesia student requires time, experience, and appropriate habits to hone them.

Beyond learning the use and interpretation of monitoring methods, the student must also learn to appreciate the potential artifacts that can occur during electronic measurement. Because artifacts can result in false alarms, there exists the potential to ignore important alarms if their validity is uncertain. The student and experienced provider must learn to assimilate all data to make the right interpretation.[52]

FUTURE OF CLINICAL MONITORING

As developments in science allow for improved accuracy, reliability, portability, and ease of use of monitoring devices, undoubtedly their applications will expand. This is a prediction that has been written many times for many years. Modalities such as cardiac output monitoring were once only estimated by invasive techniques but are now frequently monitored noninvasively. Closer monitoring of metabolic processes such as oxygen uptake or analysis of autonomic nervous system responses through noninvasive means will likely find a place in anesthesia settings as they develop.[53,54] The trend of moving toward electronic medical record keeping will affect the type of monitoring interfaces, as well as the documentation of measurements. Although the accuracy and usefulness of these systems are a source of debate, it is likely that their reliability will improve. Automated anesthesia record systems have proved valuable in ways that include avoiding and defending medical malpractice claims.[55]

Advancements in monitoring alarm systems and display capabilities also may prove valuable. Continuous auditory and integrated visual displays, including head-mounted screens, have been tested and shown to shorten time to response; however, they may bring with them detrimental effects to visual fields and increase noise levels in the operating room.[56,57]

Although the availability of devices and advancements in monitoring capabilities may be an ever-present reality, another harsh reality is the cost associated with obtaining and using them. As health-care delivery costs continue to increase, there will also be continued pressure to use these resources wisely. Outcome data are crucial to justifying the expense of keeping up with technology. Simply displaying patient-related data for the sake of defining physiologic or disease states without directly benefiting the patient will not justify the potential risk to the patient as well.[58]

The importance of the human factor in anesthesia delivery and monitoring does not appear to be replaceable any time soon. New devices may prove to be useful tools, but it is imperative for the anesthetist to remain vigilant and well informed as to their proper use and interpretation. Although studies may be published to demonstrate the capabilities of electronic devices, practitioners continue to fall back on the value of the human senses—as is the case with the simple precordial stethoscope in perceiving apnea or other events—and emphasize the importance of learning to use and interpret them appropriately.[59]

SUMMARY

Clinical monitoring is above all a human skill using all of the senses. The importance of maintaining adequate ventilation and oxygenation has been underscored in reviews of closed-claim studies, thereby emphasizing the need for vigilant, continuous monitoring of these parameters in the patient receiving anesthesia. Of all monitoring modalities, $ETCO_2$ and pulse oximetry have been shown to be of particular value. Hypothermia is an all-too-common occurrence under anesthesia, and management must center on prudent temperature monitoring. Clinical standards of care, as developed by the recognized professional anesthesia organizations, must be adhered to continually and reevaluated frequently. Outcome studies are warranted to justify the use of new monitoring modalities, and the potential benefits must outweigh the potential risks.

REFERENCES

1. Sting. Every breath you take [song]. On: The Police. *Synchronicity*. Los Angeles, CA: A&M Records; 1983. Available at: http://www.sting.com/discog/?v=so&a=1&id=130. Accessed May 30, 2008.
2. Brodsky JB. What intraoperative monitoring makes sense? *Chest.* 1999;115:101S-105S.
3. Buhre W, Rossaint R. Perioperative management and monitoring in anaesthesia. *Lancet.* 2003;362(9398):1839-1846.
4. American Association for Nurse Anesthetists. *Scope and Standards for Nurse Anesthesia Practice.* Available at: http://www.aana.com/resources.aspx?ucNavMenu_TSMenuTargetID=51&ucNavMenu_TSMenuTargetType=4&ucNavMenu_TSMenuID=6&id=783. Accessed June 19th, 2008.
5. Runciman WB, Merry AF. Crises in clinical care: an approach to management. *Qual Saf Health Care BMJ Journals.* Vol 14;2005:156-163.
6. Petty WC et al. A synthesis of the Australian Patient Safety Foundation Anesthesia Incident Monitoring Study, the American Society of Anesthesiologists Closed Claims Project, and the American Association of Nurse Anesthetists Closed Claims Study. *AANA J.* 2002;70(3):193-202.
7. Robbertze R et al. Closed claims review of anesthesia for procedures outside the operating room. *Curr Opin Anaesthesiol.* Aug 2006;19(4):436-442.
8. American Society of Anesthesiologists. *Standards for Basic Anesthetic Monitoring.* Available at: http://www.asahq.org/publicationsAndServices/standards/02.pdf. Accessed June 19th 2008.
9. Davis PD. *Basic Physics and Measurement in Anaesthesia.* 5th ed. Edinburgh: Butterworth-Heinemann; 2004.
10. Jain H. Use of disposable end tidal carbon dioxide detector device for checking endotracheal tube placement. *J Clin Diagn Res.* 2007;1(3):104-109.
11. Dorsch JA. *Understanding Anesthesia Equipment.* 5th ed. Baltimore: Lippincott Williams & Wilkins; 2007.
12. Oberg B. The effect of nasal oxygen flow and catheter position on the accuracy of end-tidal carbon dioxide measurements by a pharyngeal catheter in unintubated, spontaneously breathing subjects. *Anaesthesia.* 1995;50(8):695-698.
13. Burton JH et al. Does end-tidal carbon dioxide monitoring detect respiratory events prior to current sedation monitoring practices? *Acad Emerg Med.* 2006;13(5):500-504.
14. Lightdale JR et al. Microstream capnography improves patient monitoring during moderate sedation: a randomized, controlled trial. *Pediatrics.* 2006; 117(6):1170-1178.
15. Thompson JE, Jaffe MB. Capnographic waveforms in the mechanically ventilated patient. *Respir Care.* 2005;50(1):100-108; discussion 108-109.

16. Oshibuchi M et al. A comparative evaluation of transcutaneous and end-tidal measurements of CO_2 in thoracic anesthesia. *Anesth Analg.* 2003;97(3): 776-779.

17. Bhavani-Shankar K et al. Arterial to end-tidal carbon dioxide pressure difference during laparoscopic surgery in pregnancy. *Anesthesiology.* 2000; 93(2):370-373.

18. Chhajed PN et al. Cutaneous carbon dioxide monitoring in adults. *Curr Opin Anaesthesiol.* 2004;17(6):521-525.

19. Griffin J et al. Comparison of end-tidal and transcutaneous measures of carbon dioxide during general anaesthesia in severely obese adults. *Br J Anaesth.* 2003;91(4):498-501.

20. Weinger MB. Dangers of postoperative opioids. *APSF Newsletter.* 2006; 21(4):61-88.

21. Reuss JL, Siker D. The pulse in reflectance pulse oximetry: modeling and experimental studies. *J Clin Monit Comput.* 2004;18(4):289-299.

22. Clark AP et al. Pulse oximetry revisited: "But his O_2 sat was normal!" *Clin Nurse Spec.* 2006;20(6):268-272.

23. Levitzky MG. *Pulmonary Physiology.* 7th ed. New York: McGraw-Hill; 2007:142-148.

24. West J. *Respiratory Physiology. the Essentials.* 7th ed. Philadelphia: Lipincott Williams & Wilkins; 2005.

25. Leow MK. Configuration of the hemoglobin oxygen dissociation curve demystified: a basic mathematical proof for medical and biological sciences undergraduates. *Adv Physiol Educ.* 2007;31(2):198-201.

26. Pedersen T et al. Pulse oximetry for perioperative monitoring: systematic review of randomized, controlled trials. *Anesth Analg.* 2003;96(2):426-431.

27. Next-generation pulse oximetry. *Health Devices.* 2003;32(2):49-103.

28. Sugino S et al. Forehead is as sensitive as finger pulse oximetry during general anesthesia. *Can J Anaesth.* 2004;51(5):432-436.

29. Awad AA et al. Different responses of ear and finger pulse oximeter wave form to cold pressor test. *Anesth Analg.* 2001;92(6):1483-1486.

30. Awad AA et al. Analysis of the ear pulse oximeter waveform. *J Clin Monit Comput.* 2006;20(3):175-184.

31. Brand TM et al. Enamel nail polish does not interfere with pulse oximetry among normoxic volunteers. *J Clin Monit Comput.* 2002;17(2):93-96.

32. Rodden AM et al. Does fingernail polish affect pulse oximeter readings? *Intensive Crit Care Nurs.* 2007;23(1):51-55.

33. Barker SJ et al. Measurement of carboxyhemoglobin and methemoglobin by pulse oximetry: a human volunteer study. *Anesthesiology.* 2006;105(5):892-897.

34. Parameswaran GI et al. Pulse oximetry as a potential screening tool for lower extremity arterial disease in asymptomatic patients with diabetes mellitus. *Arch Intern Med.* 2005;165(4):442-446.

35. Nishiyama T. Pulse oximeters demonstrate different responses during hypothermia and changes in perfusion. *Can J Anaesth.* Feb 2006;53(2):136-138.

36. Bendjelid K et al. Transcutaneous Pco_2 monitoring in critically ill adults: clinical evaluation of a new sensor. *Crit Care Med.* 2005;33(10):2203-2206.

37. Rohling R, Biro P. Clinical investigation of a new combined pulse oximetry and carbon dioxide tension sensor in adult anaesthesia. *J Clin Monit Comput.* 1999;15(1):23-27.

38. Hanss R et al. Heart rate variability-guided prophylactic treatment of severe hypotension after subarachnoid block for elective cesarean delivery. *Anesthesiology.* 2006;104(4):635-643.

39. Cousins TR, O'Donnell JM. Arterial cannulation: a critical review. *AANA J.* 2004;72(4):267-271.

40. Zahn J et al. Comparison of noninvasive blood pressure measurements on the arm and calf during cesarean delivery. *J Clin Monit Comput.* 2000;16(8): 557-562.

41. Welch TC. AANA journal course. Update for nurse anesthetists. A common sense approach to hypothermia. *AANA J.* 2002;70(3):227-231.

42. Frank SM et al. Perioperative maintenance of normothermia reduces the incidence of morbid cardiac events. A randomized clinical trial. *JAMA.* 1997;277(14):1127-1134.

43. Wagner DV. Unplanned perioperative hypothermia. *AORN J.* 2006; 83(2):470, 473-476.

44. Henker R, Carlson KK. Fever: applying research to bedside practice. *AACN Adv Crit Care.* 2007;18(1):76-87.

45. Forstot RM. The etiology and management of inadvertent perioperative hypothermia. *J Clin Anesth.* 1995;7(8):657-674.

46. Kasai T et al. Preoperative risk factors of intraoperative hypothermia in major surgery under general anesthesia. *Anesth Analg.* 2002;95(5):1381-1383.

47. Kongsayreepong S et al. Predictor of core hypothermia and the surgical intensive care unit. *Anesth Analg.* 2003;96(3):826-833.

48. O'Grady NP et al. Practice guidelines for evaluating new fever in critically ill adult patients. Task Force of the Society of Critical Care Medicine and the Infectious Diseases Society of America. *Clin Infect Dis.* 1998;26(5):1042-1059.

49. Lasater K. High-fidelity simulation and the development of clinical judgment: students' experiences. *J Nurs Educ.* 2007;46(6):269-276.

50. Seropian MA. General concepts in full scale simulation: getting started. *Anesth Analg.* 2003;97(6):1695-1705.

51. Hotchkiss MA et al. Assessing the authenticity of the human simulation experience in anesthesiology. *AANA J.* 2002;70(6):470-473.

52. Takla G et al. The problem of artifacts in patient monitor data during surgery: a clinical and methodological review. *Anesth Analg.* 2006;103(5):1196-1204.

53. Stuart-Andrews C et al. Non-invasive metabolic monitoring of patients under anaesthesia by continuous indirect calorimetry—an in vivo trial of a new method. *Br J Anaesth.* 2007;98(1):45-52.

54. Avellanal M et al. Skin flowmetry: a new "depth of anesthesia" monitor? *Acta Anaesthesiol Scand.* 2006;50(6):771.

55. Feldman JM. Do anesthesia information systems increase malpractice exposure? Results of a survey. *Anesth Analg.* 2004;99(3):840-843.

56. Sanderson P. The multimodal world of medical monitoring displays. *Appl Ergon.* 2006;37(4):501-512.

57. Sanderson PM et al. Advanced patient monitoring displays: tools for continuous informing. *Anesth Analg.* 2005;101(1):161-168.

58. Young D, Griffiths J. Clinical trials of monitoring in anaesthesia, critical care and acute ward care: a review. *Br J Anaesth.* 2006;97(1):39-45.

59. Fisher QA. Can capnography substitute for auscultation in sedation cases? *Anesth Analg.* 2005;100(5):1546.

CHAPTER 19

CLINICAL MONITORING III: NEUROLOGIC SYSTEM

Gary D. Clark, Julie A. Stone, Nicholas C. Curdt

The practice of anesthesia requires constant vigilance and evaluation of the patient. Historically, early anesthetists like John Snow and Arthur Guedel proposed the use of clinical and neurologic signs to evaluate and determine the depth of anesthesia. Snow described the "five stages of narcotism" for chloroform anesthesia.[1] Guedel further refined these signs of anesthesia by developing a table of "clinical signs and stages of anesthesia" the patient passes through during anesthesia.[2] Guedel used neurologic signs like respiratory rate and rhythm, ocular movement, pupillary size, and reflexes to evaluate the depth of ether anesthesia.[1,2]

Today, the practice of anesthesia incorporates sophisticated technology for neurologic monitoring. The administration of a variety of drugs for anesthesia makes it impractical to depend solely on Snow's or Guedel's clinical signs for assessing anesthetic levels or neurologic function. Monitoring the neurologic status of a patient demands a thorough knowledge of the modern devices used and the skills to navigate a rapidly changing clinical environment. Essential for the nurse anesthetist are several goals for monitoring the neurologic system, including:

1. Possessing a thorough knowledge of the monitors and modalities available for neurologic monitoring
2. Selecting appropriate neurologic monitor(s) for data acquisition and patient management
3. Understanding the various pathologic and anesthetic effects on the electroencephalogram (EEG), somatosensory evoked potential (SSEP), motor evoked potential (MEP), and other neurologic monitors
4. Managing neurologic changes during periods of surgical stimulation
5. Recognizing data changes that reflect neurologic changes and ischemia
6. Being able to use numerical-processed EEG parameters or Bispectral Index (BIS) monitoring

The considerations for monitoring neurologic functions are given in Box 19-1.

The basic methods for assessing neurologic function are the raw electroencephalogram and the electromyogram (EMG). Recently, evoked potentials (EPs) have been added to the armamentarium for evaluating neurologic function. New strategies to improve neurologic outcome and reduce morbidity and mortality during anesthesia should include monitoring neurologic function. This chapter examines the monitors currently used, the methods for using these monitors in clinical

---

BOX **19-1**

Considerations for Monitoring Neurologic Function

Specialized Monitoring Methods for Neurologic Monitoring
EEG—electroencephalogram
SSEP—somatosensory evoked potentials
MEP—motor evoked potentials
VEP—visual evoked potentials
BAEP—brainstem auditory evoked potentials
BIS—Bispectral Index
PSI—patient state index
Transcranial Doppler
Near-infrared spectroscopy (NIRS)

Specialized Modalities for Neurologic Monitoring
Recognizing neurologic changes and ischemia
Understanding the effects of anesthesia on neurologic function and monitoring
Managing neurologic changes during the perianesthetic period

---

practice and managing the neurologic function of patients during the perianesthetic period.

ELECTROENCEPHALOGRAM

Normal EEG

The brain is an electrochemical organ generating electrical signals in a specific pattern. The electrical activity displayed through an EEG is sometimes called *electrical brainwaves*. Ebersol suggests that the EEG is actually a measurement of differences in electrical potentials in groups of neurons between brain regions rather than the brain emitting electrical waves.[3] Electrodes for the EEG are placed in a standardized sequential configuration (or montage) that examines known electrical potentials. This configuration was internationally standardized by Jasper in 1958 as the 10-20 system and is usually used to record the spontaneous EEG. With this system, 21 electrodes are placed on the surface of the scalp. The positions of the electrodes are determined by following three primary reference points: (1) the *nasal-frontal angle*, which is the depression at the top of the nose, (2) the level with the eyes; and (3) the *inion*, which is the bony lump at the base of the skull on the midline at the back of the head. These reference points allow the practitioner to measure the skull perimeters in the transverse and median planes. Electrode locations are determined by dividing these perimeters into 10% and 20% intervals.[3] Freeman suggested that the electrodes should be placed in areas that emit similar signals to concentrate and better record the electrical activity.[4] The 10-20 system montage for the placement of EEG leads is illustrated in Figure 19-1.

The electrical signals are first amplified then passed through a low filter that usually filters out electromyographic activity and a high filter that filters out the electrical resistance created by the tissues. There is currently no agreement on the exactness of how

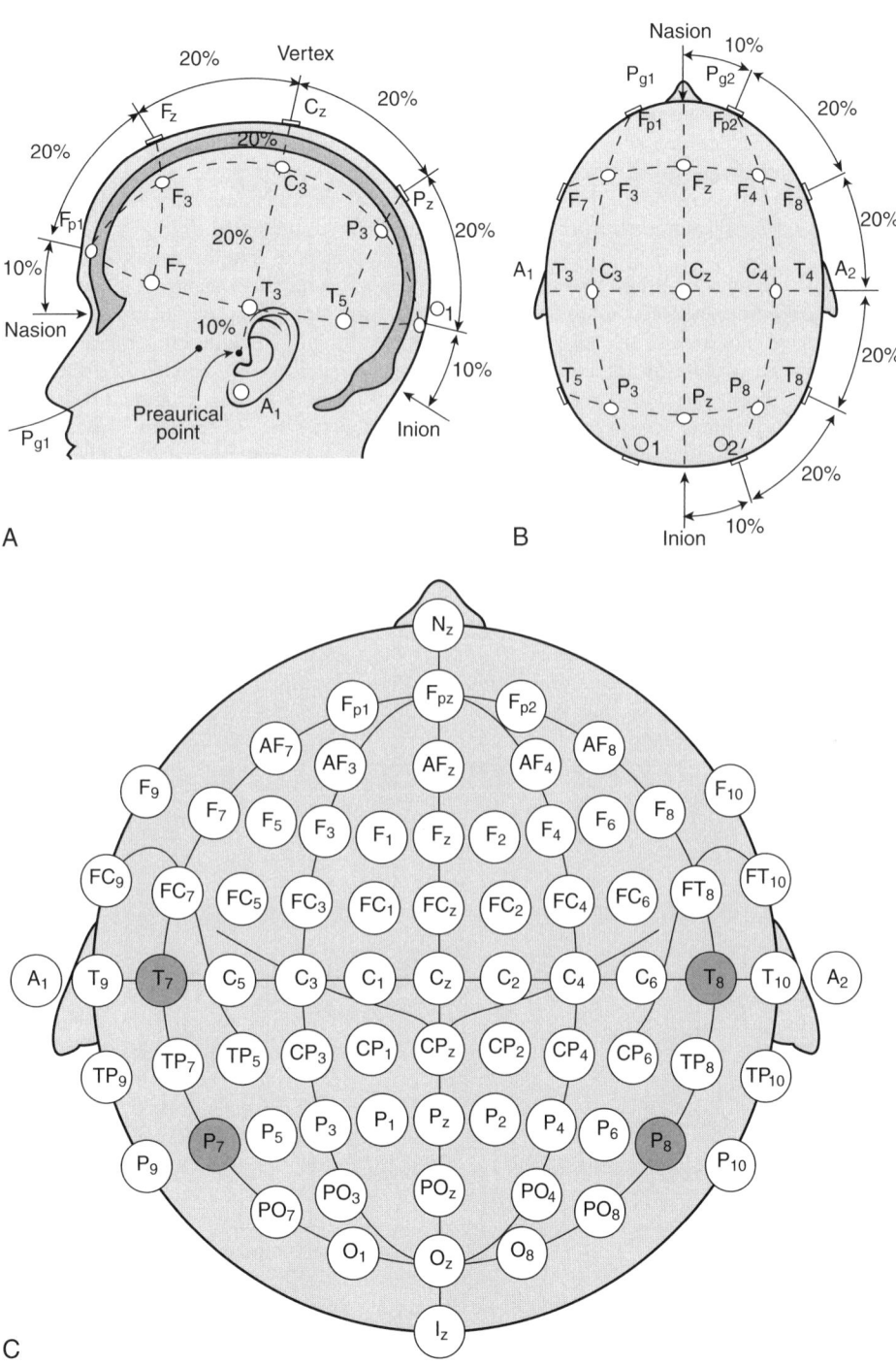

FIGURE **19-1** International 10-20 system seen from **(A)** left and **(B)** above the head. A = Ear lobe, C = central, *Pg* = nasopharyngeal, *P* = parietal, *F* = frontal, *Fp* = frontal polar, *O* = occipital. **(C)** International 10-20 system montage for EEG electrode placement. *(From Malmivuo J, Plonsey R. Bioelectromagnetism—Principles and Applications of Bioelectric and Biomagnetic Fields. New York: Oxford University Press; 1995.)*

the electrical brainwaves are categorized. Generally, the basic parameters of the EEG include frequency, amplitude, shape (amplitude and shape constitute morphology of the wave), and time of each of these electrical discharges. The waveforms are then arranged in the following manner. Four common types of brainwaves are noted on the EEG; they are alpha, beta, delta, and theta waves. There are also several variants or subgroups of waves noted during specific activities, which are only briefly described in this text. Some of these waveform variants are gamma, mu, and lambda waves. Gamma waves are typically seen with high-order activity like problem solving and analytical thinking. The amplitude of the mu wave is about one half that of the beta wave and is seen more frequently over the motor areas of the brain.[5-7] Lambda waves occur in the awake patient and are usually present when staring, reading, or looking at objects for long periods, as happens with videogames and TV.[8] Difficulty for the nurse anesthetist in assessing EEG patterns lies in distinguishing artifact and normal variations of the EEG from the four common types of known brainwaves.[9-11]

Brainwave frequencies, or the number of nonfiltered waves per second, range between 1 and 500 cycles per second or Hertz (Hz) in the adult. However, the electrical filters in the EEG are typically set to collect waves between 0.5 and 80 Hz and therefore allow for clearer interpretation of the signal. The signal emitted is reflective of the high-frequency electrical activity of the brain. This high-frequency signal of electrical activity is then divided further into several high-frequency waveforms. Additionally, the filtered amplitude usually ranges between 20 and 250 μV. The shape or morphology of the wave also aids in identification, although in a lesser capacity than the amplitude, frequency, and time, when the impedance is less than 3000 to 5000 ohms.[12] Alpha waves are higher in amplitude but slower in frequency at 9 to 14 Hz. Alpha waves are typically recorded over the posterior area of the head during awake, alert, but relaxed activities. Beta waves are low-amplitude waves that are generated rapidly at 15 to 40 Hz and recorded predominantly over the frontal portions of the head. Beta waves are usually seen with awake, anxious, active, business-thinking activities. Rhythmic variations of beta waves are sometimes seen and increased with the administration of benzodiazepines, propofol, and some pathologic abnormalities. These beta-wave variants can also be classified as *mu waves*. The delta wave has the greatest amplitude and the slowest frequency at 1 to 4 cycles per second. Delta waves are seen in a sleeping adult but are considered abnormal in an awake adult.[13] Lastly, theta waves are higher in amplitude than alpha and beta but lower than delta waves. The frequency of the theta wave is 4 to 8 Hz. All of these waves seen on the EEG are used in both raw data form and as a compressed spectrum of signals. In the normal EEG, the signals are usually symmetric. Although use of the EEG is supported in neurovascular procedures and assessing anesthetic levels during anesthesia, the interpretation is still highly dependent on the experience of the nurse anesthetist.[5-7]

Anesthetic Effects on EEG
Induction Agents
Induction doses of thiopental, etomidate, and propofol all cause similar effects on the EEG by increasing the frequency of beta waves and decreasing their amplitude. This beta-rhythm EEG activity correlates with the patient losing consciousness after drug administration; a dose-related depression is seen with anesthetic drugs.[14] As the concentration of these drugs is increased, barbiturate spindles, slow waves, and burst suppression with electronic silence intermittently occur, as seen in Figure 19-2.[15]

One difference noted with the administration of etomidate is that myoclonus, frequently seen with its use, is not reflected on EEG signals.[16] Coincidentally, the EEG frequency decreases as the serum levels of etomidate rise, thereby leading to burst suppression. Burst suppression can be achieved with all three of these induction agents in their higher dosage ranges. *Burst suppression* is an alternating high-frequency activity with 0.5- to several-second periods of electrical suppression. This type of electrical activity is unpredictable, and the duration constantly varies. Burst suppression is also typically seen with a decrease in cerebral circulation and oxygenation, as well as with hypothermia, particularly during cardiopulmonary bypass surgery. Many of these effects can be additive. Burst suppression EEG patterns remain somewhat controversial relative to cardiopulmonary bypass surgery. However, to reduce cerebral oxygen requirements and provide neuroprotective properties, burst suppression may be desirable during manipulation of brain tissues.[17-19] Burst suppression can be achieved during anesthesia using a variety of anesthetic agents. These agents include thiopental, etomidate, propofol, and the inhalation agents, which all provide varying levels of suppression of electrical activity with increasing depth; effects usually remain bilateral and uniform.[14,16,20] Unilateral burst suppression is usually indicative of ischemia or injury to the brain. Forethought should be given to the use of enflurane and sevoflurane in patients with known epileptiform EEG activity; the activity may be accentuated by these inhalation agents in their lower concentrations.[15,21,22]

PROCESSED EEG WAVEFORMS

The interpretation of a raw EEG can many times be difficult and depend on the quality of the waveform, lead placement, any artifact or electrical interference that might be present, and the skill level of the anesthesia provider in interpreting the waveforms. To further analyze the EEG, multiple methods are used, including compressed spectral array (CSA) and density spectral array (DSA). The CSA and DSA are obtained, calculated, and displayed by collecting, assessing, and providing a summary of each of the waves (alpha, beta, theta, delta) over a period of time. A mathematical description for the timeframe, using the amplitude and frequency of the waves, is accomplished by using a fast Fourier transform (FFT) algorithm. Applying an FFT is typically thought of as breaking down a signal into a variety of components and then reconstructing the useful information into an analysis of the complex signals. The cell phone, TV, and radio are examples of where this technology is best known. The Fourier analysis also results in a compressed view of EEG waveforms. The compressed data are presented in a two- or three-dimensional graph. Depending on the display used, these data appear as either a compressed spectral array (CSA) or a dot matrix called a *density spectral array* (DSA), as seen in Figure 19-3.[23]

The processed information collected and displayed for the CSA and DSA is analyzed for the waveform relationships using the amplitude and frequency and illustrated in two- or three-dimensional graphs. These relationships are expressed as the spectral edge frequency (SEF), median frequency (MF), and relative delta power (RDP). Most commonly, the SEF is used and represented by the EEG frequency and power activity, which falls below 90% (SEF90).[24,25] Figure 19-4 shows an EEG power spectrum demonstrating the SEF of waveforms within 90% of power and frequency. As frequency declines below a predetermined power, the spectral edge changes. In the presence of general anesthesia or injury, frequency and power decline, causing a change in the spectral edge. The modern EEG calculates the computerized spectral array, which is then used during anesthesia to determine the "depth of anesthesia" or unilateral injury, based on the processed results. The compressed spectral array (CSA) in Figure 19-5 shows the spectral edge shifted to the right, indicating lower power and frequency in brainwave activity. This pattern is typically found during deep sedation and sleep, and in Figure 19-5 is produced by the presence of 0.2%

isoflurane anesthesia, indicating the patient's brainwave activity is suppressed. General anesthesia produces a reduction in high-frequency waves and an increase in low-frequency amplitudes. In Figure 19-4, the spectral edge is positioned well to the left, indicating a higher power and frequency, suggesting that the patient is awake.[26-28]

Considerations for Inhalation Anesthetics and EEG Interpretation

Interpreting the EEG in the presence of anesthetic drugs can be confounding, since the different drug classes used for anesthesia may affect the EEG in different ways. Instead, generalized assumptions can be made from the interpretation of the EEG. There are two major reasons why EEG remains difficult to correlate with the course of the anesthetic and patient outcomes.

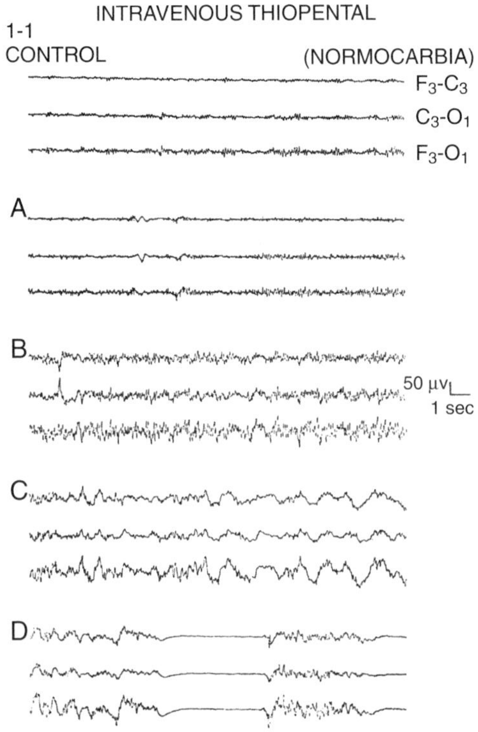

INTRAVENOUS THIOPENTAL

1-1
CONTROL   (NORMOCARBIA)

(traces labeled F₃-C₃, C₃-O₁, F₃-O₁)

A

B   50 µv
                                        1 sec

C

D

FIGURE **19-2** Progressive effects of intravenous thiopental on the EEG wave pattern in adults. **Control** and **A,** Normal rapid activity. **B,** Barbiturate spindles. **C,** Slow EEG waves. **D,** Burst suppressionz alternated with slow waves. (*From Clark DL, Rosner BS: Neurophysiologic effects of general anesthetics. Anesthesiology. 1973;38:564.*)

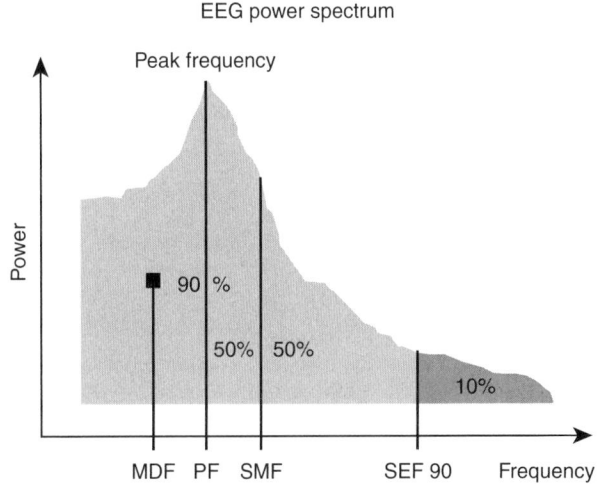

FIGURE **19-4** EEG power spectrum demonstrating the spectral edge frequencies of waveforms within 90% of power and frequency. (*Adapted from Rampil IJ. A primer for EEG signal processing in anesthesia. Anesthesiology. 89[4]:980-1002.*)

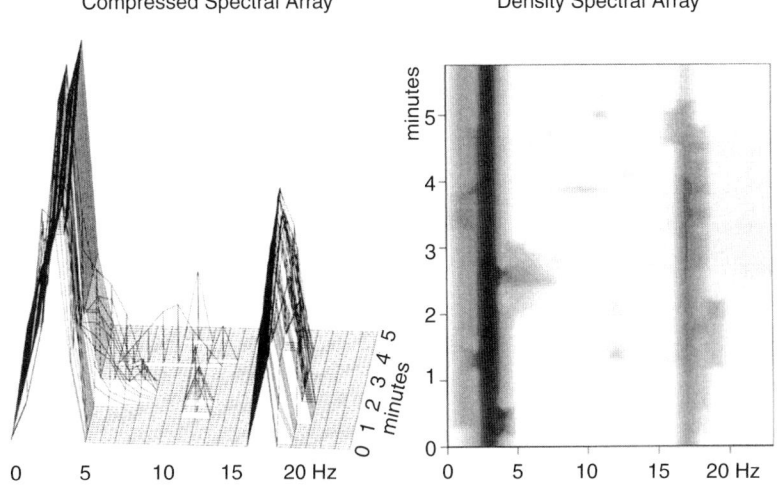

FIGURE **19-3** The compressed spectral array (CSA) histogram on the left is the compression and transformation of raw EEG waveform data and plotted over time. The density spectral array (DSA) on the right is created by converting each brainwave value as a shade of gray and then plotting them on the DSA graph. (*From Rampil IJ. A primer for EEG signal processing in anesthesia. Anesthesiology. 89[4]:980-1002.*)

The first major variable preventing exact correlation between the EEG and anesthetic depth is the combination of the many different drugs used to induce and maintain general anesthesia. Dose-related effects are seen with each general inhalation and intravenous anesthetic. The inhalation agents affect the frequency and amplitude of the EEG waveforms (Table 19-1).[28-31] Alpha waves seen primarily in the occipital and posterior lobes are increasingly abolished with inhalation anesthesia. Beta activity is usually seen in the frontal lobe and typically increases slightly with general anesthesia. The second major variable involves environmental factors and manipulation of the brain intraoperatively, adding to the complexity of interpretation.

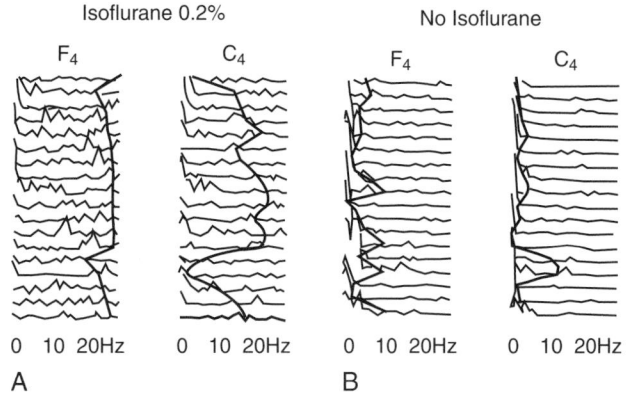

FIGURE 19-5 **A,** The solid line indicates a compressed spectral edge with the administration of isoflurane 0.2%. **B,** The solid line indicates the compressed spectral edge with no anesthesia. (*Adapted from Heyer EJ et al. Erroneous conclusion from processed electroencephalogram with changing anesthetic depth. Anesthesiology. 2000;92[2]:603.*)

Extensive research with bispectral analysis has sought to clarify EEG interpretation by analyzing the EEG electrical signals, processing them, and displaying the result as a final numerical value of 0 to 100. BIS measurement is effective in determining the level of anesthesia produced with inhalation agents but remains less predictable with pediatric patients and during regional and intravenous anesthesia.[32]

Processing Devices

Several devices on the market today use a combination of processed EEG signals to determine the "hypnotic" levels of anesthetics. The BIS machine (Aspect Medical Systems) uses a combination of bispectral analysis, power spectral analysis, and time domain analysis in combination with a mathematical algorithm that produces an index of the hypnotic state of the patient. The SEDLine, and the *PSA* (Hospira), monitor multiple parts of the brain to compute a proprietary measurement called the *patient state index*, or PSI. These devices are not intended to be used as stand-alone, depth-of-anesthesia monitors but rather in conjunction with traditional physiologic monitoring to guide the anesthesia practitioner in producing the safest anesthetic possible.

These devices do have their limitations. Most important is a time delay that is steadily being remedied by faster processors. The intraoperative gold standard is still the 16- to 32-channel analog EEG monitored by an experienced electroencephalographer. Studies still need to be done to evaluate whether systems with processing software using fewer channels are comparable to 16- to 32-analog EEG encephalography.

Near-Infrared Spectroscopy

Near-infrared spectroscopy (NIRS) is a relatively new method of analyzing brain hemodynamics, especially hemoglobin oxygenation and blood volumes, by using the near-infrared spectrum of electromagnetic waves from approximately 600 to

TABLE 19-1	Effects of Inhalation Anesthetics on EEG					
Inhalation Agent and Effect on EEG	Low-Dose Inhalation Anesthesia	Moderate-Dose Inhalation Anesthesia	High-Dose Inhalation Anesthesia	EEG Amplitude	Dose for Burst Suppression	[a]Blood/Gas and [b]Tissue (Brain)/ Blood Partition Coefficients
Desflurane	<Alpha waves >Beta waves	>Beta waves	Diffuse delta and theta	←Low dose →Anesthetic dose →High dose	>1.2 MAC	[a]0.45 [b]1.22
Isoflurane	<Alpha waves >Beta waves	>Beta waves	Diffuse delta and theta	←Low dose →Anesthetic dose →High dose	>1.5 MAC	[a]1.4 [b]1.57
Sevoflurane	<Alpha waves >Beta waves	>Beta waves	Diffuse delta and theta	←Low dose →Anesthetic dose →High dose	>1.2	[a]0.65 [b]1.69
Nitrous oxide (alone)	>Beta waves	>Beta waves	>beta waves	→Low dose →Anesthetic dose →High dose	Not seen with clinical concentrations	[a]0.46 [b]1.07

Data from Barter L et al. The effect of isoflurane and halothane on electroencephalographic activation elicited by repetitive noxious c-fiber stimulation. Neurosci Lett. 2005;382(3):242-247; Miller RD. Miller's Anesthesia. 6th ed. Philadelphia: Churchill Livingstone; 2005; Yasuda N et al, Solubility of I-653, sevoflurane, isoflurane and halothane in human tissues. Anesth Analg 1989;69(3): 370-373. Eger EI, Saidman LJ. Illustrations of inhaled anesthetic uptake, including intertissue diffusion to and from fat. Anesth Analg. 2005;100:1020-1033.

2500 nanometers (nm). Near-infrared spectroscopy can better penetrate deep into thick tissues, allowing noninvasive physiologic interpretation of oxygenation by evaluating, in real time, the transmission and absorption of infrared light in the hemoglobin in brain tissue. As each area of the brain is evaluated with NIRS, the local blood volume is also analyzed, thus determining flow to that area. Constant monitoring with NIRS allows the anesthetist to quickly determine regional volume and hemoglobin changes in the brain tissue. Not only is NIRS used to evaluate oxygenation and blood volume during anesthesia, it can also facilitate motor-function monitoring of patients, with strong clinical correlations. However, because NIRS devices differ, some caution in their use is encouraged.[33-35]

EVOKED POTENTIALS

EPs are electrical potentials that are measured in response to some type of stimulus. These stimuli can be changed or completely depressed with the administration of anesthesia. In the operating room, EPs are used to help alert surgeons and aid adjustments to surgical strategy, to confirm their decisions, and help them improve subsequent procedures and outcomes, therefore avoiding neurologic damage. This is all done to preserve or improve neurologic structures at risk and prevent irreversible damage. It is also sometimes effective in localizing anatomic structures. Auditory, visual, motor, and somatosensory stimuli are commonly used for clinical evoked-potential studies during surgical procedures. Attempting to preserve neural function with evoked potentials can be daunting. Once the basic science of measurement is understood, interpretation and diagnosis can be challenging, owing to harsh operating room environments. Injuries to neural structures can arise from heat (electrocautery), mechanical stress (retraction), ischemia (ligation and vessel damage), and loss of functional integrity (transection). Some if not most nerves encountered during surgical procedures lack perineurium, which protects against longitudinal retraction, and epineurium, which protects against retraction. The "elastic limit" of such nerves is around 20%, suggesting that stretching the nerve farther may produce irreversible damage to the nerve itself.[36] Evoked potentials also can be affected by hypothermia, hypotension, positioning, and anesthetic agents themselves. These systemic effects usually develop slowly and show more potential to be reversible defects rather than permanent.

It is important to remember that some injuries may be reversible, but early detection is the key to reducing more serious complications. Early detection must then be paired with good communication among the anesthesia provider, surgeon, and neurophysiologist. Adequate understanding of evoked potentials is essential if anesthesia providers are to have productive dialogue to guide care for the patient. There currently is no set standard for the amount of change in latency or amplitude that necessitates warning the surgeon. A rule of thumb offered by several sources states that a 50% decrease in amplitude or a 10% decrease in latency should exist before warning.[36] A better plan of care would be to ask the surgeon and neurophysiologist prior to surgery what they deem an acceptable amount of change in the evoked potential before warning.

One important question all anesthesia providers have is this: What are the best anesthetic agents to use for surgical procedures when using evoked potentials? A fine balance must be established between adequately anesthetizing patients while at the same time optimizing conditions that monitor neurologic structures and preserve them. Each different type of evoked potential has a unique interaction with the anesthetics delivered. However, there are some generic rules to help guide the nurse anesthetist. The first rule is that lipophilic agents that interfere with neuronal membrane conduction also interfere with subcortical conduction. Therefore these agents cause an increase in both interpeak latencies and control conduction time. The second rule is that anesthetic agents that interfere with EEG also interfere with EP. Changes occur because the component frequencies of the EP are the same as the EEG. Lastly, intravenous agents, at equipotent doses to inhalation agents, will have less effect than inhaled agents. However, when combinations of drugs are used for anesthesia, like those used in balanced anesthesia techniques, they too can have additive effects.

Somatosensory Evoked Potentials

Somatosensory evoked potentials (SSEPs) are used to monitor a number of neural structures along both the peripheral and central somatosensory pathways. Stimulation for SSEPs is created by stimulating peripheral nerves electrically. These stimulations can be induced through mechanical devices, but electrical stimulation gives a more robust response and may be better controlled. A supermaximal electrical stimulation is not required to elicit a response from the nerve. SSEPs are usually induced by stimulation of a peripheral nerve, which contains both a sensory and motor component combining to provide a mixed signal. Typically, the lower extremities can be monitored by stimulating the posterior tibial nerve located between the Achilles tendon and medial malleolus of the ankle. The upper extremities are monitored by placing the stimulus at the median nerve located between the tendons of the flexor carpi radialis and the palmaris longus. If these common sites cannot be accessed, two alternate sites are the common peroneal in the popliteal fossa (may be used for the lower extremity) and the ulnar nerve (either at the wrist or ulnar notch) for the upper extremities.

Recording electrodes used for SSEPs are placed at C2, C3, and C4, referencing to F2 of the montage for cortical SSEPs. An electrode placed over cervical spine C7 is used for subcortical SSEPs. For upper limb SSEP studies, electrodes are placed over Erb's point both ipsilateral and contralateral to the stimulus. Erb's point is located on the side of the neck 2 to 3 cm above the clavicle and in front of the transverse process of the sixth cervical vertebra. Pressure over this point elicits the Duchenne-Erb paralysis, and electrical stimulation over this area elicits various potentials measured in the arm. For lower limb studies, the electrode is placed at the iliac crest. Several different characteristics of SSEPs can be measured. Peak latencies are the easiest to measure and standardize, but like other characteristics, they can vary with age, tissue mass, electrical stimulus, and limb length. Spinal SSEP electrodes are placed over the spinal cord. SSEPs usually are *processed* signals, meaning they are processed as an average, with electrical filters to remove background noise, instead of providing real-time electrical waveforms. Interpretation of the compound action potential depends on the site of stimulus and distance to the recording electrodes.

Almost all anesthetic agents produce change in latency or amplitude, with the exception of ketamine, etomidate, and opiates.[37] Anesthesia and SSEPs provide a challenge for the anesthetist; the less anesthesia one administers, the better the SSEP monitoring results. Many researchers report that better monitoring conditions for SSEPs are obtained with narcotic-based anesthetics, less than 1 MAC total end-tidal inhaled concentration of inhalation agent, and nitrous oxide. If monitoring SSEPs alone, use of paralytic agents is acceptable, and potentials can be measured. However, in the absence of paralytics, motor responses can be elicited.

Although limited in their evaluation of neurologic diseases, the value of SSEPs in the clinical setting is valuable, and interest remains high.[38] because changes in SSEPs are sensitive to cerebral ischemia, they have multiple uses in vascular surgery. During carotid endarterectomy procedures, SSEPs can help determine the need for shunting intraoperatively. If changes are immediate, SSEPs can indicate high risk or neurologic injury during aortic cross-clamping. During cerebral aneurysm surgery, changes in SSEPs can possibly indicate occlusion of parental vessels, directing the positioning of important aneurismal vascular clips.

Brainstem Auditory Evoked Potentials

Brainstem auditory evoked potentials (BAEPs) are used to monitor the entire auditory pathway from the distal auditory nerve to the midbrain, inadvertently allowing monitoring of basic brainstem function. The stimulus used is typically a standard broadband repeating click. Repetition is generally around 10 Hz, and the intensity is around 65 to 70 decibels (dB) above the click-perception threshold. The stimulus is delivered via earphone. Because an external earphone is impractical, an earphone placed in the auditory canal, or "insert earphone," is used. For best results, care must be taken (1) to place the transducer after the head is positioned so as not to cause abrasive injury to the ear canal and (2) that the internal auditory canal is free of any built-up cerumen or fluid. Such things as fluid, saline, cerebrospinal fluid, and soap can dampen the sound and delay responses. Recording electrodes are determined by the type of evoked BAEPs performed on the patient. There are several common evoked responses used as BAEPs that will be discussed further.

Brainstem auditory evoked potentials have five main peaks represented by roman numerals (Figure 19-6). Peak I relates to the peripheral portion of the cochlear nerve inside the internal auditory canal. Peak II relates to the cochlear nucleus and the area where the eighth cranial nerve enters the brainstem. Peak III correlates to the area of the brainstem at the level of the cochlear nucleus and potentially the ipsilateral superior olivary nucleus. Peaks IV and V relate to the brainstem along the ascending auditory pathway between the cochlear nucleus and the inferior colliculi. Measured peaks must be compared with relative norms for age, sex, intensity, polarity, and repetition rate.

Brainstem auditory evoked potentials are clinically useful in that they are very resistant to alteration by anything other than structural pathology in the brainstem. This means that BAEPs are not significantly affected by barbiturates, benzodiazepines, ketamine, nitrous oxide, propofol, or muscle relaxants. There is one reported case of abolishment of the wave with the use of thiopental and lidocaine infusion.[39,40] However, inhalation agents can mildly affect BAEPs' latency and amplitude, and their effect is proportional to the dose of inhalation agent administered.[39]

A common effect on BAEP during anesthesia and in the operating room environment is hypothermia. Even mild hypothermia (patient temperature less than 35° C) has been associated with decreased latency and prolonged interpeak intervals during BAEP.[41] BAEPS can also be exaggerated, as demonstrated by an increase in latency with low P_{CO_2} seen during hyperventilation.[36]

The auditory nerve can be directly monitored during the surgical procedure by the surgeon. The monitoring electrode is placed on the nerve itself after surgical exposure and its response

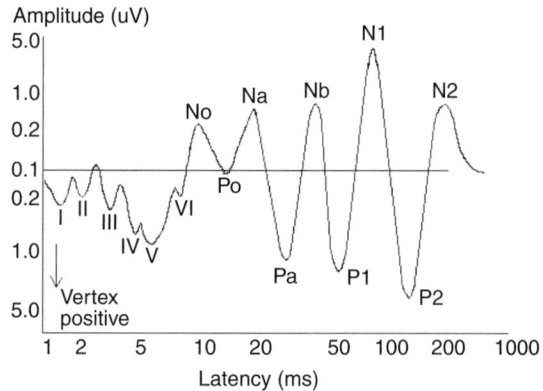

FIGURE **19-6** Auditory evoked potentials—common labeled potentials *(roman numerals)* that can be measured to assess different areas of the auditory and brainstem pathways. Peak I relates to the peripheral portion of the cochlear nerve inside the internal auditory canal. Peak II relates to the cochlear nucleus and the area where the 8th cranial nerve enters the brainstem. Peak III correlates to the area of the brainstem at the level of the cochlear nucleus and potentially the ipsilateral superior olivary nucleus. Peaks IV and V relate to the brainstem along the ascending auditory pathway between the cochlear nucleus and the inferior colliculi. Peak VI relates to the medial geniculate body and VII (not shown) relates to auditory radiations. *(Modified from Barlow HB, Mollon JD. The Senses. Cambridge, England: Cambridge University Press; 1982.)*

is measured as an *auditory nerve compound action potential* (AN-CAP). When the eighth nerve is involved, the AN-CAP is referred to as the *eighth nerve potential* (8NP). The AN-CAP, like the BAEP, can be used to determine auditory nerve insult or injury.

For auditory brainstem responses (ABRs), the noninverting (positive) electrode is placed at C2 or high on the forehead. The inverting (negative) electrode is typically placed on the mastoid or earlobe. However, if neither of these sites is practical, owing to surgical exposure, then the tragus of the ear may be used as an alternate site.

Electrocochleography (ECochG) is a specific test used to provide information about the cochlea and the distal section of the auditory nerve. It is typically used to evaluate and/or verify blood supply to the cochlea. The measure itself is called the *ECochG-CAP*. The inverting electrode is placed near the cochlea, tympanic membrane, or the cochlear promontory. The noninverting electrode is placed on the opposite ear.

Otoacoustic emissions (OAEs) are sometimes used, but this test is not an evoked potential. Because a stimulus is not used, there is only a recording device. No stimulus is required because the normal cochlea does not just receive sound but can produce low-intensity sounds called *OAEs*, produced specifically by the cochlea and most probably by the cochlear outer hair cells as they expand and contract. These sound transmissions can be recorded; they are typically used to assess auditory hair-cell function and not internal structure of the ear.

Motor Evoked Potentials and Electromyography

Motor evoked potentials (MEPs) are used to monitor the functional integrity of motor tracts, particularly in the corticospinal tract. Stimuli used for MEPs can be either electrical or magnetic.

Either the motor cortex or spinal cord can be used for sites of stimulation. Magnetic stimulation of the motor cortex can be accomplished using a rapidly changing magnetic field (compared with a constant field from MRI). Based on the Faraday law, electrical current is created in a nearby conductor, generating the stimulus. Although useful, magnetic stimulation is cumbersome in the operating room because of the interference of magnetic fields with other operating-room equipment, as well as the size and position of equipment during the procedure. Magnetic stimulation also generates intense heat that needs to dissipate to safe levels and can prolong procedures. Magnetic fields also produce a high-intensity noise, however brief, so ear protection is recommended. Contact with magnetic stimulation is contraindicated in patients with pacemakers, spinal or bladder stimulators, epilepsy, metallic foreign body, or previous craniotomy. Direct stimulation of the motor cortex may also be produced by cutaneous electrodes on the scalp or electrodes placed directly on the brain after surgical exposure. Electrical stimulation is more commonly used for spine cases.

Potentials are recorded as neurogenic potentials in the distal spinal cord or peripheral nerve. They also can be recorded as myogenic potentials of innervated muscle. While SSEP can assess the dorsal column (fasciculus cuneatus and gracilis) and the lateral sensory tract of the spinal cord, it also can make assumptions on changes in anterior motor tracts because the stimulation is a mixed nerve (motor and sensory) signal. However, because they are not directly measured, motor deficits have been seen in spinal cord cases in which SSEPs have been normal. In such cases, MEPs can be used in combination with SSEP to improve accuracy of monitoring.

Stimulation and monitoring of motor components of nerves are important in the operating room, but they require an active stimulus to produce an action potential. Electromyography (EMG) can be both passive and active. EMG has the capability to stimulate a motor nerve and monitor the known innervated muscle groups, as well as passively "listen" to all muscle groups. The ability to passively monitor nerves allows the surgeon to become more aware of what nerve is being stimulated with surgical manipulation.

EMG analysis of the facial nerve for related surgeries has been used and researched extensively. Other cranial nerves can and have been used for monitoring purposes as well. Monitoring needle electrodes are typically placed in the orbicularis oculi and the orbicularis oris muscles. To assess the cervicofacial and temporofacial divisions of the facial nerve as it divides from the posterior aspect of the parotid gland, both of these muscles require monitoring. Frequency and density of discharges elucidate the type of damage to the actual nerve. Simple benign contact with the nerve causes few random discharges. A response train is associated with more significant nerve irritation. Neurotonic discharges are associated with nerve irritation, as well as impending nerve damage. Elimination of environmental factors should be considered prior to diagnosing nerve damage. Trains of stimulation also can be caused by thermal changes (electrocautery or cold irrigation), drilling, traction, and/or nerve ischemia. The choice of anesthesia is essentially unrestricted, with the exception of avoiding paralytic agents. Additionally, the efficacy of partial paralysis has not been studied extensively.

Visual Evoked Potentials
Visual evoked potentials (VEPs) are used to monitor the function of the visual pathway, which comprises the retina to the occipital cortex and everything in between, including the optic nerve and optic chiasm. A visual stimulus is presented to the subject for

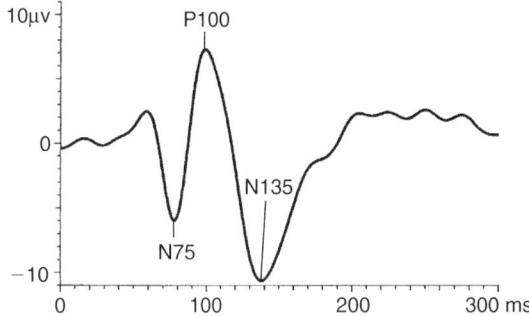

FIGURE **19-7** Pattern reversal visual evoked potentials. The three peaks that characterize the potential and are subsequently measured are denoted as N75, P100, and N135. (*Adapted from Odom J et al. Visual evoked potentials standard [2004]. Doc Ophthalmol. 2004;108:115-123.*)

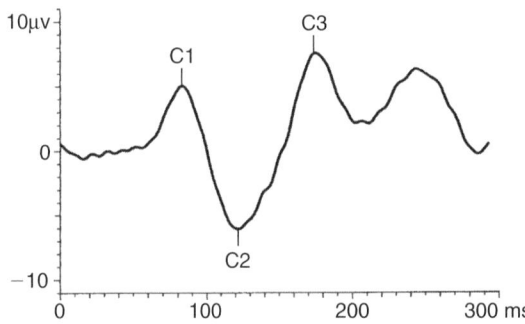

FIGURE **19-8** Pattern onset/offset visual evoked potential. The three peaks that characterize the potential and are subsequently measured are denoted as C1, C2, and C3. (*Adapted from Odom J et al. Visual evoked potentials standard [2004]. Doc Ophthalmol. 2004;108:115-123.*)

a selected number of times, and the cerebral responses are amplified, averaged by a computer, and displayed. The two major classes of VEP stimulation are patterned and unpatterned (luminance). Typically, awake tests consist of a pattern stimulus. The two most common pattern stimuli are pattern reversal and pattern onset/offset stimuli. Pattern reversal stimulus consists of black-and-white checks (checkerboard) that change phase (same luminescence) at a predetermined number of reversals per second (Figure 19-7). Pattern onset/offset stimulus consists of a black-and-white checkerboard that exchanges with a diffuse background with the same luminance (Figure 19-8).

Because such stimulation cannot be used in conjunction with anesthesia or even sedation, a stroboscopic flash (luminance) stimulus must be used in such cases. The flash VEP is created from a flash that has a predetermined strength against a dim background of certain luminance. Recording electrodes are fixed to the scalp and, as always, placed relative to bony landmarks. The active electrode is placed on the scalp over the visual cortex at Oz, with the reference electrode at Fz. The ground electrode can be placed at the forehead, vertex (Cz), mastoid, earlobe (A1 or A2), or linked earlobes.

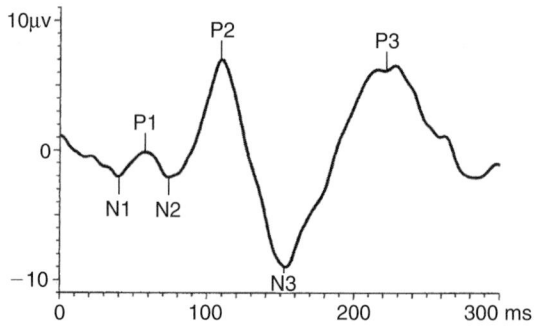

FIGURE **19-9**　Flash visual evoked potential. The three positive deflections that characterize the potential and are subsequently measured are denoted as *P1, P2,* and *P3.* The three negative deflections that characterize the potential and are subsequently measured are denoted as *N1, N2,* and *N3. (Adapted from Odom J et al. Visual evoked potentials standard [2004]. Doc Ophthalmol. 2004;108: 115-123.)*

Monocular stimulation is typically used to avoid masking of unilateral conduction abnormality. Care should be taken to ensure that no light enters the unstimulated eye. Close assessment must be made of the eyes preoperatively and should be noted in the record because they may affect recorded outcomes. Examples of such consideration include extreme pupil size or anisocoria (inequality of pupil diameter). Pupils do not need to be dilated for flash VEPs. Mydriatics and miotics should not be used with awake tests. It is also important to compare VEPs with appropriate age- and sex-related normal values.

The action potential of VEPs varies, depending on the type of stimulus used. Flash VEPs consist of a series of negative and positive waves, with the earliest detectable response occurring around 30 ms post-stimulus. For flash VEP, the N2 and P2 peaks are the most robust components, peaking around 90 and 120 ms, respectively (Figure 19-9). Unfortunately, flash VEPs are more variable between subjects than pattern responses. Some question the usefulness of intraoperative VEPs because in anesthetized patients, stable recording was either not obtainable or consistent across subjects.[42,43]

SUMMARY

The use of neurologic monitors does not guarantee prevention of neurologic injury. However, the use of neurologic monitors adds one more tool to aid the nurse anesthetist in patient assessment. Several factors contribute to intraoperative EEG changes, making the monitoring device more challenging to interpret. Some of these factors include hypothermia, hyperthermia, volatile and intravenous anesthetic agents, surgical intervention, previous neurologic injury, and excessive auditory and visual stimulation. Providing anesthesia for neurologic surgical procedures requires knowledge in both basic and advanced anesthesia techniques. The anesthetist should not only use all the usual techniques for safe anesthesia practice but also many times must apply these principles while being at a distance from the airway, particularly in cranial cases. Postoperative neurologic changes can occur, so continued monitoring is essential to reduce the incidence of preventable permanent changes. Cooperation and communication between the surgeon and the nurse anesthetist remain a vital key for safe neurologic monitoring and surgical outcomes.

REFERENCES

1. Snow J. *On Chloroform and Other Anaesthetics: Their Action and Administration.* London: John Churchill; 1858.
2. Lee JA. *A Synopsis of Anaesthesia.* 3rd ed. Baltimore: Williams and Wilkins; 1973.
3. Jasper HH. Report of the Committee on Methods of Clinical Examination in Electroencephalography. *Electroencephalogr Clin Neurophysiol.* 1958;10:370-371.
4. Freeman WJ. The electrical activity of a primary sensory cortex: analysis of EEG waves. *Int Rev Neurobiol.* 1963;5:53-119.
5. Blume W et al. Significance of EEG changes in carotid endarterectomy. *Stroke.* 1986;17:891.
6. Redekop G, Ferguson G. Correlation of contralateral stenosis and intraoperative electroencephalographic change with risk of stroke during carotid endarterectomy. *Neurosurgery.* 1992;30:191.
7. Sundt TM et al. Cerebral blood flow measurements and electroencephalograms during carotid endarterectomy 1974. *J Neurosurg.* 2007;107(4):887-897.
8. Chang B et al. *Atlas of Ambulatory EEG.* New York: Academic Press; 2005.
9. Hughes JR. *EEG in Clinical Practice.* 2nd ed. Newton, ME: Butterworth-Heinemann; 1994.
10. Malmivuo J, Plonsey R. *Bioelectromagnetism—Principles and Applications of Bioelectric and Biomagnetic Fields.* New York: Oxford University Press; 1995.
11. Sharbrough F et al. American Electroencephalographic Society guidelines for standard electrode position nomenclature. *J Clin Neurophysiol.* 1999; 8:200-202.
12. Schneider G. EEG and AEP monitoring during surgery. Paper presented at: 9th ESA Annual Meeting; April 2001; Gothenburg, Sweden. Available at Clinical Window. International Web Journal for Medical Professionals. www.clinicalwindow.net/cw_issue_05_article3.htm#. Accessed July 25, 2007.
13. Wang B et al. Effect of sedative and hypnotic doses of propofol on the EEG activity of patients with or without a history of seizure disorders. *J Neurosurg Anesthesiol.* 1997;9(4):335-340.
14. Schwilden H et al. Quantitation of the EEG and pharmacodynamic modelling of hypnotic drugs: etomidate as an example. *Eur J Anaesthesiol.* 1985;2:121.

15. Clark DL, Rosner BS. Neurophysiologic effects of general anesthetics. I. The electroencephalogram and sensory evoked responses in man. *Anesthesiology.* 1973;38:564-582.
16. Meinck HM et al. Neurophysiological effects of etomidate, a new short-acting hypnotic. *Electroencephalogr Clin Neurophysiol.* 1980;50:515.
17. Ghaly RF et al. Etomidate dose-response on somatosensory and transcranial magnetic induced spinal motor evoked potentials in primates. *Neurol Res.* 1999;21(8):714-720.
18. Cortínez LI et al. Performance of the cerebral state index during increasing levels of propofol anesthesia: a comparison with the bispectral index. *Anesth Analg.* 2007;104(3):605-610.
19. Roach GW et al. Multicenter Study of Perioperative Ischemia (McSPI) Research Group. Ineffectiveness of burst suppression therapy in mitigating perioperative cerebrovascular dysfunction. *Anesthesiology.* 1999;90(5):1255-1264.
20. Ravussin P, de Tribolet N. Total intravenous anesthesia with propofol for burst suppression in cerebral aneurysm surgery: preliminary report of 42 patients. *Neurosurgery.* 1993;32(2):236-240.
21. Jääskeläinen SK. Sevoflurane is epileptogenic in healthy subjects at surgical levels of anesthesia. *Neurology.* 2003;61:1073-1078.
22. Najjar S et al. Procedures in epilepsy patients. In: Ettinger AB, Devinsky O, eds. *Managing Epilepsy and Co-existing Disorders.* Boston: Butterworth-Heinemann; 2002:499-513.
23. Rampil IJ. A primer for EEG signal processing in anesthesia. *Anesthesiology.* 1998;89(4):980-1002.
24. Schwarz G et al. Specific problems in interpretation of absolute values of spectral edge frequency (SEF) in comparison to Bispectral Index (BIS) for assessing depth of anesthesia. *The Internet Journal of Neuromonitoring.* 2004;3(2)_Available at http://www.ispub.com/ostia/index.php?xmlFilePath=journals/ijnm/vol3n2/sef.xml Accessed July 14, 2008.
25. Heyer EJ et al. Erroneous conclusion from processed electroencephalogram with changing anesthetic depth. *Anesthesiology.* 2000;92(2):603-607.
26. Nieuwenhuijs D et al. Bispectral Index values and spectral edge frequency at different stages of physiologic sleep. *Anesth Analg.* 2002;94:125-129.

27. PhiTools. Software Tools and Services for Psychophysiology and Chronobiology. Website. http://www.phitools.com/pro_visualization.html. Updated February 14, 2008. Accessed July 20, 2007.

28. Barter L et al. The effect of isoflurane and halothane on electroencephalographic activation elicited by repetitive noxious c-fiber stimulation. *Neurosci Lett.* 2005;382(3):242-247.

29. Mahla ME et al. Neurologic monitoring. In: Miller RD, ed. *Anesthesia.* 6th ed. Philadelphia: Churchill Livingstone; 2005:1511-1550.

30. Yasuda N, et al. Solubility of I-653, sevoflurane, isoflurane and halothane in human tissues. *Anesth Analg.* 1989;69(3):370-373.

31. Eger EI, Saidman LJ. Illustrations of inhaled anesthetic uptake, including intertissue diffusion to and from fat. *Anesth Analg.* 2005;100:1020-1033.

32. Watcha MF. Investigations of the Bispectral Index monitor in pediatric anesthesia: first things first. *Anesth Analg.* 2001;92:805-807.

33. Bhambhani Y et al. Reliability of near-infrared spectroscopy measures of cerebral oxygenation & blood volume during handgrip exercise in brain injured patients. *J Rehabil Res Dev.* 2006;43(7):845-856.

34. Kenji Yoshitani K et al. A comparison of the INVOS 4100 and the NIRO 300 near-infrared spectrophotometers. *Anesth Analg.* 2002;94: 586-590.

35. Ali MS et al. Spatially resolved spectroscopy (NIRO-300) does not agree with jugular bulb oxygen saturation in patients undergoing warm bypass surgery. *Can J Anesth.* 2001;48:497-501.

36. Luders H. Surgical monitoring with auditory evoked potentials. *J Clin Neurophysiol.* 1988;5(3):261-285.

37. Banoub M et al. Pharmacologic and physiologic influences affecting sensory evoked potentials in humans. *Anesthesiology.* 2003;65:35.

38. Aminoff M, Jefferey M. *Electrodiagnosis in Clinical Neurology.* Philadelphia: Elsevier; 2005.

39. Nuwer MR. *Brainstem Auditory Monitoring and Related Techniques: Evoked Potential Monitoring in the Operating Room.* New York: Raven; 1986:158-161.

40. Garcia-Larrea L et al. Transient drug induced abolition of BAEPs in coma. *Neurology.* 1988;38(9):1487-1489.

41. Stockard JJ et al. Effects of hypothermia on human brainstem auditory response. *Ann Neurol.* 1978;3:368-370.

42. Weidemeyer H et al. Visual evoked potentials for intraoperative neurophysiologic monitoring using total intravenous anesthesia. *J Neurosurg Anesthesiol.* 2003;15(1):19-24.

43. Odom J et al. Visual evoked potentials standard (2004). *Doc Ophthalmol.* 2004;108:115-123.

PREOPERATIVE EVALUATION AND PREPARATION OF THE PATIENT

Rex A. Marley

A crucial element of the anesthesia provider's perioperative care of the patient includes a timely and thorough preoperative assessment. A fine-tuned approach to patient evaluation then enables appropriate interventions when required to properly prepare the patient for the upcoming anesthesia and surgery. For any patient scheduled to undergo anesthesia, preoperative evaluation is compulsory to help identify factors that increase the risk associated with anesthesia and the status of the patient relative to the proposed surgery. Essential goals of preoperative assessment and preparation of the patient include the following:

1. Optimize patient care, satisfaction, comfort, and convenience.
2. Minimize perioperative morbidity and mortality by accurately assessing factors that influence the risk of anesthesia or might alter the planned anesthetic technique.
3. Minimize surgical delays or preventable cancellations on the day of surgery.
4. Determine appropriate postoperative disposition of the patient (i.e., given the patient's status, whether the procedure is best performed on an ambulatory, inpatient, or intensive care basis).
5. Evaluate the patient's health status, determining which if any preoperative investigations and specialty consultations are required.
6. Formulate a plan for the most appropriate perianesthetic care and postoperative supportive patient care.
7. Communicate patient management issues effectively among care providers.
8. Ensure time-efficient and cost-effective patient evaluation.

During the preoperative visit, patient assessment begins with a thorough review of the patient's medical records and patient interview, followed by the physical examination. A comprehensive medical history and physical examination are the cornerstones of a systematic approach to continued patient preparation. Information gathered from this evaluative process guides further individualized assessment (e.g., obtaining diagnostic tests, specialist consultation). The extent of this preoperative workup depends on the existing medical condition of the patient, the proposed surgical procedure, and the type of anesthesia. Significant findings from this initial evaluation enable the anesthesia provider to make adjustments in the patient's care (i.e., initiate specific treatment modalities to optimize the patient's condition for the proposed surgery and anesthesia).

An evolving challenge confronting anesthesia providers in the current managed care environment is the provision of high-quality patient care at a discounted cost. Changes designed to decrease costs include patient screening techniques (e.g., the preanesthesia assessment clinic) and intense scrutiny regarding the appropriate requisitioning of preoperative diagnostic testing. Important strategies for achieving high-quality, cost-effective patient evaluation include the following[1]:

1. Educating the practitioner (e.g., regarding the cost of diagnostic tests) and thereby modifying practice patterns
2. Developing and implementing practice guidelines
3. Using clinical pathways (interdepartmental teamwork required)
4. Disseminating information regarding protocols, thereby avoiding duplication of services
5. Performing economic analyses of services, including cost effectiveness, and cost-benefit studies
6. Rendering efficient resource management
7. Providing for outcomes measurement

These concepts will become more familiar to practitioners as *economic-based management.*

PREANESTHESIA ASSESSMENT CLINIC

The preanesthesia assessment clinic has emerged as the most effective means of providing convenient "one-stop shopping" designed to (1) permit patient registration, (2) obtain a medical history and perform a physical examination, (3) promote patient teaching, (4) meet or schedule appointments with medical consultants, and (5) complete any required preoperative diagnostic testing. Successful preanesthesia assessment clinics have realized a reduction in patient anxiety, last-minute surgical cancellations, overall length of hospitalization after surgery, and diagnostic testing, as well as improvement in patient education and a shift from inpatient to outpatient surgery status.[2] The preanesthesia assessment clinic allows patients scheduled for elective surgery to be evaluated and their condition optimized sufficiently in advance of the surgery.

Timing of Patient Assessment

To allow ample time for necessary risk assessment, preoperative testing, and specialty consultations, ideal preoperative assessment for surgery and anesthesia should take place well in advance of the proposed surgery. Patients with complex medical conditions should be evaluated at least 1 week before the scheduled procedure. Because of the present economic realities, patients undergoing more complex procedures and those who have complicated

---

BOX 20-1

Conditions That Would Benefit from Early Preoperative Evaluation

General
Medical conditions inhibiting ability to engage in normal daily activity

Medical conditions necessitating continual assistance or monitoring at home within the past 6 months

Admission within the past 2 months for acute episodes or exacerbation of chronic condition

Use of medications (e.g., anticoagulants or monoamine oxidase inhibitors) for which modification of schedule or dosage might be required

Cardiocirculatory
History of angina, coronary artery disease, myocardial infarction, symptomatic arrhythmias

Poorly controlled hypertension (diastolic >110 mm Hg, systolic >160 mm Hg)

History of congestive heart failure

Respiratory
Asthma or chronic obstructive pulmonary disease that requires chronic medication; acute exacerbation and progression of these diseases within the past 6 months

History of major airway surgery, unusual airway anatomy, or upper or lower airway tumor or obstruction

History of chronic respiratory distress requiring home ventilatory assistance or monitoring

Endocrinologic
Diabetes treated with insulin or oral hypoglycemic agents (unable to control with diet alone)

Adrenal disorders

Active thyroid disease

Hepatic
Active hepatobiliary disease or compromise

Musculoskeletal
Kyphosis or scoliosis causing functional compromise

Temporomandibular joint disorder with restricted mobility

Cervical or thoracic spine injury

Oncologic
Patients receiving chemotherapy

Other oncologic process with significant physiologic residua or compromise

Gastrointestinal
Morbid obesity (>140% ideal body weight)

Hiatal hernia

Symptomatic gastroesophageal reflux

Modified from Barash PG, ed. ASA Refresher Courses in Anesthesiology. Philadelphia: Lippincott; 1996.

---

medical conditions (Box 20-1)[3] are frequently not admitted to the hospital before the day of surgery. Preoperative evaluation on the day of surgery can result in last-minute discoveries (e.g., of inappropriate fasting, suspected difficult airway, preexisting medical condition) that may result in surgical delay or cancellation. The timing of the preanesthesia assessment does not appear to influence outcome of anesthesia.[4] In one study, no difference in the cancellation rate for ambulatory patients was observed between groups seen within 24 hours and groups seen within 1 to 30 days of the scheduled surgery.[5]

CHART REVIEW

To provide the basis for and direction of the patient interview and physical assessment, the patient's past and current medical records should be reviewed preoperatively. Ideally the anesthesia provider will have the opportunity to review the patient's medical records before the interview with the patient or caregiver.

Past Medical Records

For a patient who has undergone surgery at the same institution in the past, previous anesthesia records should be retrieved and reviewed, especially if complications are suspected. If past medical records are not available, the patient must provide details of significant anesthetic experiences. If this information suggests that the patient has an unusual condition (e.g., atypical plasma cholinesterase, susceptibility to malignant hyperthermia), surgery

is delayed so that medical records can be obtained for review to provide further information that might affect patient care, or measures should be taken (e.g., avoidance of succinylcholine; provision of trigger-free anesthetic technique) to avoid consequences associated with the condition.

Patient Chart

A review of the current medical record includes verifying that the surgical consent is accurate and complete. The names of the patient and surgeon, the date, and the proposed procedure should be matched with those on the operating room schedule. Demographic or baseline data, such as the age, height, and weight of the patient, can often be obtained from the admitting record. Vital-sign trends and input-output totals are transcribed from graphic flow sheets, which may also contain pertinent data (e.g., daily blood glucose values for the diabetic patient).

Progress notes and consultation reports provide a valuable overview of the health history and physical status of the patient. Medical treatments, such as drug dosages and schedules, may be derived from these materials, but diagnostic test results should be obtained directly from their original sources. This retrieval of primary data prevents the possible misinterpretation of data that were transcribed incorrectly. Knowledge gleaned from a review of progress notes and consultative reports enables the anesthesia provider to formulate supplementary questioning, seek further specialist consultations, or obtain additional diagnostic testing as needed.

Baseline data concerning the patient, such as cultural diversity, coping mechanisms, or patient limitations (e.g., hearing impairment), can often be derived from nursing notes and can effectively guide the anesthesia provider in conducting a thorough preoperative interview. Increasingly the anesthetist must be able to appropriately interact with culturally diverse populations to properly evaluate and educate patients.

A preanesthesia questionnaire is included on the patient's chart (Figure 20-1). This questionnaire should be part of the admission paperwork to be completed by the patient or the patient's caregiver and consists of a concise checklist regarding the patient's health history and medical care. When properly completed and readily available on the chart, the preanesthesia questionnaire enables the anesthesia provider's visit with the patient to be accomplished more efficiently. Interview questions and physical assessment are appropriately directed to abnormal findings and areas of concern.

PATIENT INTERVIEW

The preoperative interview may be conducted in person or by telephone. The in-person patient interview is preferred, but for patients who are unable to visit the hospital setting (e.g., who live far from the hospital or have transportation constraints), an opportunity to participate in a telephone interview should be made available. Regardless of the location or approach used, the interview promotes a trusting relationship between the patient and anesthesia provider. When the interview is performed in a caring and unhurried manner, the patient's degree of trust and confidence in anesthesia care is enhanced. Furthermore, compliance with perioperative instructions is increased when the patient is treated with respect; an example of such respect is using the surname (Mr. Smith, Mrs. Jones) unless instructed differently by the patient.

The title of the anesthesia provider and his or her specific role in the patient's perioperative care should also be defined. The patient is entitled to know whether the interviewer is a Certified Registered Nurse Anesthetist, student registered nurse anesthetist, anesthesiologist, or medical resident in anesthesiology. The professional appearance and attitude of the anesthesia provider also can create a positive impression during the preoperative visit.

The environment of the preoperative interview should be staged to maximize the quality and effectiveness of the interaction. Adequate lighting enhances effective communication with the patient. Distractions such as an operating television set can be eliminated. The anesthesia provider should ensure that the time and location of the interview, whether it occurs in person or by telephone, are convenient and private for the patient. A return visit or call may be necessary if the patient is eating or receiving medical therapy.

Because the preoperative interview is a private interaction between the patient and the anesthesia provider, a tactful request that visitors remain outside the interview area, unless the patient wishes family members to be present, may be necessary. Otherwise, the patient may not volunteer confidential health information, such as a history of substance abuse or the sexual history. In certain situations, however, assistance from a family member or caregiver is required. The health history may be provided, for example, by the parent of a pediatric patient or by an interpreter for a patient with cognitive or language barriers.

The patient interview is designed to achieve specific objectives (Box 20-2). The interview process, along with patient education, yields beneficial consequences of reduced patient anxiety and increased patient satisfaction. A valuable step in preparing the patient or responsible caregivers (e.g., family members, legal guardian) for the scheduled surgery includes an educational process during which the staff counsels the patient concerning fundamental perioperative issues (Box 20-3). Reinforcing information to the patient verbally and in writing is essential to gaining patient compliance.[6] Coordinating the patient's visit to the preanesthesia assessment clinic to include educational time is ideal for the patient.

Patient History

The extent of a patient's health history depends partly on the amount of information available in the chart before surgery. If the surgeon has already documented a thorough medical history and physical examination, the interview can focus on confirming major findings and obtaining information that directly relates to the anesthetic management of the patient. The anesthesia provider must obtain and document a detailed health history, however, if one is unavailable in the chart during the preoperative visit.

The health history should be obtained in an organized and systematic way, as with the preanesthesia questionnaire, to minimize omission of important data. Open-ended and direct questions targeting each category of the checklist can be posed. With this approach, more detailed and graded responses are elicited from the patient. To avoid overwhelming or confusing a patient, questions are asked separately and formulated in comprehensible or layperson's terms.

Surgical History

The surgical history of a patient may be learned from the chart or preoperative interview. Most patients only vaguely recall surgical experiences, even from childhood operations. Information regarding complications related to previous operations, such as a peripheral nerve injury or uncontrolled blood loss, should be elicited to determine the need for further investigation.

Anesthetic History

Past anesthetic experiences are often not as easily defined as the surgical history. It is vitally important to determine the reaction of a patient to previously administered anesthetics. Adverse reactions to anesthetic agents and techniques (prolonged vomiting, difficult airway, malignant hyperthermia, postoperative delirium, anaphylaxis, and cardiopulmonary collapse) may have simply been an annoyance to the patient or could have been life threatening. Preoperative knowledge of these complications allows the anesthetic approach to be modified and the recurrence of the complication prevented. Causative factors are also thoroughly investigated in patients who note that a previous operation was aborted. Difficulties with airway management can alter the approach to endotracheal intubation, if indicated. Vague reports of fever and convulsions merit further investigation to rule out an episode of malignant hyperthermia.

Familial Anesthetic History. Numerous inherited diseases involving metabolic derangements may affect a patient's reaction to stress and certain drugs, including anesthetic agents. The patient is specifically asked whether any family member ever experienced an adverse reaction to anesthesia during surgery. Familial tendencies for diseases such as atypical plasma cholinesterase, malignant hyperthermia, porphyria, or glycogen storage diseases (e.g., glucose-6-phosphate dehydrogenase deficiency) are then investigated. A diagnosis should be established before the surgery proceeds, because adjustments in the anesthetic management of the patient may be required.

QUESTION	YES	NO	COMMENTS
Height: _____ (cm) Weight: _____ (kg)			
Current medications, including over-the-counter & herbal (dose, frequency):			
Allergies (include drugs, foods, & environmental items, e.g., latex):			
Previous surgeries/hospitalizations (list):			
Scheduled surgery/procedure:			
Anesthesia History			
Problems with anesthesia – self or blood relative?			
Respiratory			
Lung or breathing problems?			
Cough? If yes, do you bring up anything when you cough?			
Asthma? If yes, what is current treatment?			
Cold, flu, respiratory infection within the past 6 weeks?			
Diagnosed with sleep apnea? Do you snore?			
Ever required supplemental oxygen therapy?			
Abnormal chest x-ray?			
Smoke now or in past? If so, what type, how much, and for how many years?			
Exposed to passive smoke?			
Can you walk up two flights of stairs without getting short of breath?			
Do you have trouble walking one block?			
Cardiovascular			
Short of breath at night?			
Heart murmur?			
Heart attack, angina (with activity; at rest), or chest pain related to your heart?			
Irregular heartbeat or pacemaker?			
Congestive heart failure?			
Abnormal electrocardiogram?			
Problems with high blood pressure?			

FIGURE **20-1** Preanesthesia questionnaire.

Continued

QUESTION	YES	NO	COMMENTS
Renal			
Kidney, bladder, or urine problems?			
Hepatic			
Jaundiced, now or in past?			
Liver problems, e.g., hepatitis?			
Use alcohol? If so, how much, how often, and when did you last use alcohol?			
Gastrointestinal			
Acid reflux, hiatal hernia, ulcer, or heartburn?			
Recent diarrhea?			
Neurologic			
Stroke, seizures, episodes of unconsciousness or fainting, or other neurological problems?			
Numbness or weakness in an arm or leg?			
Frequent headaches?			
Eye problem or problems with your vision?			
Hearing problems?			
Endocrine			
Diabetes or high blood sugar?			
Thyroid problems?			
Steroids (e.g., prednisone) during the past year?			
Musculoskeletal			
Back or neck problems?			
Arthritis?			
Physical disabilities?			
Hematologic			
Bleed easily?			
Anticoagulants (blood thinners) within the past month?			
Ever been anemic?			
Evaluated for sickle cell anemia?			
Object to blood products under any circumstances?			

FIGURE **20-1**   **cont'd**

QUESTION	YES	NO	COMMENTS
Cancer			
Diagnosed with cancer?			
Received treatment for cancer?			
Obstetrical			
Could you be pregnant? If yes, how many weeks?			
Airway			
Chipped or loose teeth, dentures, caps, bridgework?			
Problems with opening your mouth? Temporomandibular joint (TMJ) problems?			
Difficult airway management with previous anesthesia?			
Psychosocial			
Ever had mental health treatment?			
Taken prescribed psychiatric medications?			
Used "street" or "recreational" drugs? If so, when did you last use?			
Birth & Developmental (pediatrics)			
Child's delivery premature or at term?			
Neonatal complications?			
History of low heart rate or periods of low or absent respirations?			
Sudden infant death syndrome (SIDS) in your family?			
Do you have any medical problems that have not been discussed?			

FIGURE **20-1   cont'd**

BOX 20-2

Objectives of the Preoperative Interview

- Ensure that the goals of preoperative assessment are met.
- Provide preoperative education to the patient and family.
- Obtain informed consent.
- Acquaint the patient and family with the surgical process (to reduce stress and increase familiarity).
- Evaluate the patient's social situation with respect to surgery (e.g., support network).
- Motivate the patient to comply with preventive care strategies (e.g., smoking cessation, improvement of cardiovascular fitness).

Modified from Cassidy J, Marley RA. Preoperative assessment of the ambulatory patient. J Perianesth Nurs. 1996;11:334-343.

Drug History

A preoperative drug history provides an excellent guide for the direction and depth of the patient interview and assessment. Drug dosages, schedules, and durations of treatment are reviewed and the patient questioned about the purpose and effectiveness of these medications. An interview with a patient receiving β-adrenergic blockers, for example, can focus in greater detail on the cardiovascular system. Patients on medications for hypertension or angina pectoris require further investigation and possibly specialty consultation if they have not been recently evaluated.

Adverse Drug Effects and Interactions. During the preoperative evaluation, current drug therapy must be carefully reviewed for side effects and potential interactions with anesthetic agents. Table 20-1 lists selected drugs and their potential anesthetic interactions.[7-12] One drug-management strategy is to discontinue

Patient Education Objectives

- Promote interactive communication between patient and care provider.
- Encourage patient participation in making decisions about perioperative care.
- Maximize and enhance patient self-care skills and participation in continuing care during the postoperative phase.
- Increase the patient's ability to cope with his or her health status.
- Increase patient compliance with perioperative care.
- Provide individualized preoperative instructions regarding the following:
  Where and when laboratory tests, consultations, and diagnostic procedures will be completed
  Appropriate time at which the patient should cease ingestion of food and drink
  Personal considerations (e.g., comfortable clothes to wear; no jewelry or makeup; what personal items to bring; leave valuables at home; bring favorite toy, comforter, or book)
  Postoperative considerations and instructions (e.g., anticipated recovery course, discharge instructions, how to deal with complications)
  Person to contact if the patient's physical conditions changes (e.g., upper respiratory tract infection, cancellation)
- Detail the process of arrival and registration on arrival to the surgical facility (i.e., time and location of arrival).
- Review advance directive information as required by law in some states.
- Explain the surgical facility policies to the patient and family.

Modified from Cassidy J, Marley RA. Preoperative assessment of the ambulatory patient. J Perianesth Nurs. 1996;11:334-343.

particular drugs preoperatively in the hope of reducing the potential for adverse interactions. The therapeutic benefits of these drugs are weighed against the risks of abrupt discontinuation. Abrupt discontinuation of long-standing medication may lead to the development of undesirable withdrawal symptoms.[10] With occasional exceptions, the majority of medications are continued preoperatively. Should a decision be made to withhold a particular drug before surgery, sufficient time should be allowed for metabolic clearance (ideally three to five half-lives).[7]

Drug Allergies. A patient's drug history should include information regarding allergic reactions to certain foods and medications. Prior allergic responses are investigated so they can be differentiated from adverse drug reactions. Use of certain antibiotics and opioids may be avoided because of gastrointestinal side effects. These do not represent a true allergic response, however. A distinction between allergic reactions and adverse effects is crucial, because an allergy to a drug is an absolute contraindication to its use. Medications within the same classification of a drug allergy should be avoided, and heightened awareness of a potential allergic reaction is required during the perioperative period.

Latex Sensitivity. Patient sensitivity to latex products has recently been identified as a frequent basis of allergic reaction. Up to 20% of intraoperative anaphylactic reactions have been attributed to latex sensitivity.[13] The preoperative questioning of patients should include inquiry regarding specific latex sensitivity or allergy. Patients at increased risk for latex sensitivity should be cared for in a no-latex setting and scheduled as the first case of the day to reduce the likelihood of aeroallergen latex exposure. The diagnosis of latex allergy is based on the findings of the history and physical examination and if necessary, in vivo (skin-prick test is the most sensitive) and in vitro testing. Preoperative testing is indicated only when there is a family history of reactions or when patients report experiencing symptoms such as a rash, swelling, or wheezing when exposed to latex.[14] Patients at high risk for latex sensitivity include those with a history of the following[13]:

- Chronic exposure to latex-based products (e.g., workers in the natural rubber industry)
- Spina bifida, urologic reconstructive surgery
- Repeated surgical procedures (more than nine)
- Intolerance to latex-based products (e.g., balloons, rubber gloves, condoms, dental dams, rubber urethral catheters)
- Allergy to food and tropical fruits (e.g., banana, avocado, mango, peach, passion fruit, kiwi, celery, chestnut)
- Intraoperative anaphylaxis of uncertain cause
- Working in health care, especially with a history of atopy or hand eczema

Social History

The addictive nature of tobacco and alcohol, as well as illegal drugs, exerts a detrimental influence on several aspects of life in the United States.

- More than 9% of persons 12 years of age or older were classified with substance dependence or abuse in 2005.[15]
- Nearly one quarter of all deaths (75,000 annually)[16] in the United States are caused by addictive substances.[17]
- The economic burden of addiction (e.g., health-care expenditures, missed work, crime) is estimated at more than $400 billion annually.[17]

Certain drugs, despite their social or recreational application, may be associated with adverse and life-threatening consequences with long- or short-term use or overdose. The social history provides an excellent opportunity to explore the extent of self-medication. Open-ended questions, posed in a professional and nonjudgmental manner, are most likely to elicit detailed information from the patient. At this time, the patient can also be educated about the adverse consequences of substance abuse, especially as such substances affect anesthetic care.

Tobacco Use. Many patients arrive for anesthesia and surgery with a history of tobacco smoking. In the United States, some disturbing statistics are associated with this form of substance abuse.

- One in five deaths in the United States is related to smoking. Cigarette smoking is the leading cause of preventable premature death in the United States (approximately 438,000 premature deaths annually).[18]
- Of adults in the United States, 23% smoke.[19] In 2006 in the United States, 46 million adults were smokers.[20]
- Teen smoking rates increased by nearly one third from 1991 to 1997.[21] Currently, 23% of high school students in the United States smoke cigarettes.[22]

TABLE **20-1**	Potential Drug Interactions Affecting Perianesthesia Care		
Perianesthesia Concern			
Drug Category	**Intraoperative Concerns**	**Management**	**Discontinuation Issues**
Drugs Affecting the Cardiovascular System			
Angiotensin-converting enzyme (ACE) inhibitors	Hypotension with or without bradycardia; intolerance to hypovolemia	Optimize hydration; moderate doses of vasopressor	Brief interruption is well tolerated; continuation may improve regional blood flow and oxygen delivery and preserve renal function; consider withholding in patients taking amiodarone, on multiple (three or more) antihypertensives, or in whom even a brief period of hypotension is unacceptable; omit AM dose on day of surgery
β-adrenergic blockers	Discontinuation may increase perioperative cardiovascular morbidity and development of withdrawal symptoms (increased nervousness, tachycardia, headache, nausea, exacerbation of myocardial ischemia or sudden death)	Optimize hydration	Beta-adrenergic blockers should be continued in patients undergoing surgery who are receiving β-blockers to treat angina, symptomatic arrhythmias, or hypertension
Calcium channel blockers	Decrease systemic vascular resistance and blood pressure via peripheral vasodilation; exhibit a negative inotropic effect by slowing sinus automaticity & arterioventricular conductivity; demonstrate a negative chronotropic effect by slowing the sinoatrial & arteriovenous (AV) nodes & prolonging AV nodal conduction	Optimize hydration; phenylephrine as needed to maintain atrial pressure	Continue chronic calcium channel blocker therapy preoperatively in patients with normal or slightly impaired heart function; exercise caution in patients with left ventricular dysfunction (ejection fraction <40%)
Diuretics	Hypokalemia; hypovolemia	Monitor potassium levels preoperatively; maintain hydration	Patients rarely become symptomatic if morning dose withheld; patients appreciate lack of urinary urgency while awaiting surgery; it might be desirable to continue in patients for whom diuretics are part of treatment for chronic renal failure
Antiarrhythmics	Cardiac depression; prolonged neuromuscular blockade; amiodarone— hypotension and atropine-resistant bradycardia requiring ventricular pacing	Monitor serum drug levels as needed; amiodarone—large doses of vasopressors or inotropes and pacemaker capability	Discontinuation rarely recommended, because usually not prescribed for benign arrhythmias; amiodarone—impractical to discontinue because half-life is 58 days; withhold concurrent medications (e.g., ACE inhibitors)
Drugs Affecting Hemostasis			
Antiplatelet drugs and nonsteroidal antiinflammatory drugs (NSAIDs)	Impaired platelet function; altered renal function; gastrointestinal bleeding		Antiplatelet drugs, e.g., aspirin, clopidogrel, ticlopidine, should be discontinued 7-10 days prior to high-risk surgery; unless surgery puts

Data from Doak GJ. Discontinuing drugs before surgery. Can J Anaesth. 1997;44:R112-R117; Pass SE, Simpson RW. Discontinuation and reinstitution of medications during the perioperative period. Am J Health Syst Pharm. 2004;61:899-912; Schirmer U, Schurmann W. Preoperative administration of angiotensin-converting enzyme inhibitors. Anaesthesist. 2007;56:557-561; Baillard C. Preoperative management of chronic medications. Ann Fr Anesth Reanim. 2005;24:1360-1374; Huyse FJ et al. Psychotropic drugs and the perioperative period: a proposal for a guideline in elective surgery. Psychosomatics. 2006;47:8-22; Fleisher LA et al. ACC/AHA 2006 guideline update on perioperative cardiovascular evaluation for noncardiac surgery: focused update on perioperative beta-blocker therapy. Anesth Analg. 2007;104:15-26.
IV, Intravenous; PT, prothrombin time; PTT, partial thromboplastin time.

Continued

| TABLE **20-1** | Potential Drug Interactions Affecting Perianesthesia Care—cont'd |

Perianesthesia Concern

Drug Category	Intraoperative Concerns	Management	Discontinuation Issues
Antiplatelet drugs and nonsteroidal antiinflammatory drugs (NSAIDs)—cont'd			patient at particular risk for increased or catastrophic bleeding or impaired renal function, it is reasonable to continue NSAIDs up to morning of surgery; if desirable to discontinue NSAIDs preoperatively, short-acting NSAIDs should be withheld for at least 1 day, longer-acting agents for 2-3 days
Anticoagulants (heparin, Coumadin, low-molecular-weight heparins [LMWH])	Increased hemorrhage	May reverse heparin with IV protamine; may reverse Coumadin with vitamin K or fresh frozen plasma	Heparin—discontinue IV 6 hr before surgery and check PTT; Coumadin—discontinue 3-5 days (5 days if INR <1.5 is required) before surgery and check INR or PT; LMWH—discontinue 12 hr before surgery
Fibrinolytic drugs (streptokinase, urokinase, tissue plasminogen activator)	Hemorrhage	Antifibrinolytic agent (aprotinin) may be indicated	Discontinuation usually not an option when administered for treatment of life-threatening conditions (e.g., acute myocardial infarction, massive pulmonary embolus)
Hypoglycemic Agents			
Insulin	Hyperglycemia; hypoglycemia	Monitor serum glucose; use insulin-supplementation protocol	Morning dose either withheld or reduced and adjustments in therapy based on periodic serum glucose determinations
Oral hypoglycemic agents	Hyperglycemia; hypoglycemia	Monitor serum glucose; avoid dehydration	Withhold oral hypoglycemic agents beginning on day of surgery
Drugs Affecting the Central Nervous System			
Monoamine oxidase inhibitors	Hypertension secondary to indirect-acting sympathomimetic drugs causing release of norepinephrine; excitatory state (from meperidine) or depressive phenomena secondary to opioid administration	Avoid known triggering agents such as meperidine, pentazocine, dextromethorphan, and indirect-acting sympathomimetic agents (e.g., ephedrine)	Older, nonselective, irreversible monoamine oxidase inhibitors—discontinue for 2 wk with risk of serious psychiatric consequences or provide MAOI-safe anesthesia if drugs continued; newer, reversible inhibitors of monoamine oxidase A—have short half-life; therefore, discontinue drug on morning of surgery; consider changing irreversible MAOIs to a reversible MAOI in the weeks prior to surgery, then only discontinuing reversible MAOI on morning of surgery
Tricyclic antidepressants	α-adrenergic blocking activity & potential to block norepinephrine uptake may lead to cardiac arrhythmias or hypotension; lowers seizure threshold	Norepinephrine should be considered the vasopressor of choice for related hypotension	Discontinue gradually over 2 wk before surgery; obtain baseline ECG; if continued, take precautions to reduce the significance of adverse events
Lithium	T-wave smoothing, ventricular arrhythmias, myocarditis; sinus dysfunction can lead to extreme atropine-resistant sinus bradycardia; dehydration will lead to increases in lithium blood levels	Optimize hydration	Discontinue 72 hours before surgery

- Smokers die 14 years earlier than nonsmokers.[23]
- Exposure to secondhand smoke causes 3000 deaths a year from lung cancer and 46,000 deaths from coronary heart disease; 430 newborns a year die from sudden infant death syndrome attributed to secondhand smoke.[24]

The inhaled components of tobacco smoke lead to multiple pathophysiologic changes within the body. Nicotine and carbon monoxide are just two of the more than 6000 noxious components that have been identified in tobacco smoke.[25] Nicotine, a toxic alkaloid, produces ganglionic stimulant effects and is the tobacco component that affects the cardiovascular system.[26] Acute side effects of nicotine include increased heart rate, blood pressure, myocardial contraction, myocardial oxygen consumption, myocardial excitement, and peripheral vascular resistance. Net effects of nicotine's cardiovascular influence include impaired coronary blood flow and an adverse myocardial oxygen supply/demand ratio.[27] Carbon monoxide readily occupies the oxygen-binding sites of hemoglobin (approximately 250 to 300 times greater affinity for hemoglobin than oxygen).[28] Oxygen transport to the tissues and resultant oxygen use is thereby drastically reduced. In the heavy smoker, carboxyhemoglobin may be as high as 15%, which effectively reduces the patient's oxyhemoglobin percentage accordingly. The adverse effects of nicotine on the cardiovascular system and carbon monoxide on oxygen-carrying capacity are short lived (half-life of nicotine is 40 to 60 minutes[29,30]; half-life of carbon monoxide if room air is breathed is 130 to 190 minutes).[31,32] Patients should be instructed to stop smoking at least 12 hours before surgery. *Short-term (e.g., 12 hours) preoperative abstinence from tobacco smoke reduces the deleterious effects of nicotine and carbon monoxide on cardiopulmonary function.*[33] Smoking cessation for even 1 night before surgery reduces heart rate, blood pressure, and circulating catecholamine levels[34] and allows carboxyhemoglobin values to return to normal levels.[35]

Patients who smoke have a higher incidence (a nearly sixfold increase[36]) of postoperative pulmonary complications (pneumonia and atelectasis).[37] Whereas short-term preoperative smoking cessation may be beneficial in reducing postoperative pulmonary complications—and should be encouraged—longer periods of smoking cessation (8 weeks or longer) result in a marked improvement in pulmonary mechanics (e.g., enhanced ciliary function, decreased mucous secretion and small airway obstruction, and enhanced immune function).[38] Patients who stopped smoking less than 2 months before surgery had nearly four times the pulmonary complications (e.g., purulent sputum, secretion retention, bronchospasm, pleural effusion, pneumothorax, segmental pulmonary collapse, pneumonia) of those who abstained from smoking for longer than 2 months.[39] However, even short-term smoking cessation is effective in reducing postoperative complications when compared with patients who continued to smoke up until the time of surgery.[38] Patients who smoke should be advised to quit even immediately prior to surgery, without fear of worsening pulmonary outcomes or increasing psychologic stress as a result of acute abstinence.[40] Effective interventions, including behavioral support and pharmacotherapy, should be made available to smokers considering abstinence at this time.[41]

The influence of environmental tobacco smoke (also known as *secondhand* or *passive smoke*) on children has been found to produce disturbing respiratory consequences, including increased reactive airway disease,[42] abnormal results of pulmonary function tests,[43,44] and increased respiratory tract infections.[45] The perioperative complications in children exposed to smoke include laryngospasm, coughing on induction or emergence, breath holding, and postoperative oxyhemoglobin desaturation.[46,47]

Alcohol Intake. An estimated 14 million Americans are dependent on alcohol, with 105,000 deaths annually attributed to alcohol abuse.[48] Perioperative complications such as arrhythmias, infection, and alcohol withdrawal syndrome, are increased two- to fivefold in chronic excessive alcohol users.[49] Information regarding the type and amount of alcohol regularly consumed and the frequency of consumption is important in the evaluation for anesthesia and surgery. Often an accurate assessment of a patient's alcohol intake may be difficult to obtain. The Alcohol Use Disorders Identification Test (AUDIT), a self-reporting questionnaire designed to identify problem drinkers, can be incorporated into the preoperative interview of suspected problem drinkers.[50] A less confrontational and a reliable approach to evaluating a patient's potential for an alcohol problem uses the mnemonic CAGE, which refers to the following four questions[51]:

- Do you feel you should **c**ut down on your alcohol consumption?
- Have people **a**nnoyed you by criticizing your drinking habits?
- Have you felt **g**uilty about your drinking?
- Have you ever had a drink first thing in the morning to steady your nerves or get rid of a hangover (**e**ye-opener)?

A patient reporting more than two positive responses is at high risk for alcoholism and an increased likelihood of experiencing withdrawal symptoms.[52] Both AUDIT and CAGE have been shown to be effective in identifying the abusive alcohol consumer.[53]

In the heavy drinker, it is important to determine whether the patient has experienced seizures, abrupt withdrawal syndrome, or delirium tremens as a consequence of alcohol abuse. Clinical signs suggestive of alcohol withdrawal include increased hand tremors, autonomic hyperactivity (e.g., sweating, tachycardia, systolic hypertension), insomnia, anxiety, restlessness, nausea or vomiting, transient hallucinations (visual, tactile, or auditory), psychomotor agitation, and grand mal seizures.[52]

Chronic alcohol abuse results in the development of tolerance, physical dependence, and multisystem organ dysfunction. Tolerance to alcohol is evidenced by a resistance or cross-tolerance to other central nervous system (CNS) depressants. For example, the anesthetic requirement of hypnotics, opioids, and inhalation agents is increased in the chronic alcoholic; however, exaggerated responses to anesthetic agents are likely during periods of acute intoxication or advanced alcoholism. This effect is attributed to the additive depressant effects of alcohol and anesthetic agents. Enzymatic function and plasma albumin concentrations may also be reduced in patients with alcoholic hepatic insufficiency. As a result, greater circulating concentrations of unbound intravenous agents (e.g., thiopental) may result in an exaggerated and prolonged drug effect.[54] This enhanced drug response has not been shown to occur with propofol in patients with moderate liver cirrhosis.[55]

An insidious progression of multisystem organ dysfunction is also characteristic of long-term alcohol abuse. Numerous illnesses are attributable to the toxic adverse effects of advanced alcoholism on overall health and nutrition. Predictably, postoperative morbidity and mortality rates are increased in alcoholic patients as a result of poor wound healing, infection, bleeding, and further hepatic deterioration.[56]

Illicit Drug Use. Use of illicit drugs (e.g., cocaine, cannabis, "crack," lysergic acid diethylamide-25 [LSD], amphetamines) is a significant health-care issue in the United States. The most popular recreational drugs continue to be cocaine and marijuana. Approximately 20 million Americans used illicit drugs monthly in 2006.[57] Americans use 80% of all opioids available in the world.[58] The use of these substances increases the risk for adverse consequences and drug interactions during anesthesia. An accurate illicit drug history is often difficult to obtain because of the patient's fear of legal reprisal or refusal to believe a drug problem exists. During the physical examination, the anesthesia provider should look for signs that indicate illicit drug use by the patient. A diagnosis of recent or continuing drug abuse should be suspected in patients exhibiting the following on physical examination[59]:

- Evidence of drug injection (e.g., track marks or scarring), thrombotic veins, phlebitis, tattoos (may be used to mask the sites), ablation of venous return leading to unilateral edema of the nondominant hand, subcutaneous skin abscesses
- Ophthalmologic changes, such as pupillary constriction from opioid use, pupillary dilation with amphetamine use, nystagmus from phencyclidine (PCP) use
- Lymphadenopathy secondary to nonspecific activation of the immune system as a result of repeated injections of impurities
- Malnourishment as a result of amphetamine abuse (opioid users tend to be well nourished)
- Poor dental care and bruxism (involuntary grinding and clenching of teeth) from amphetamine use
- Nasal perforation from cocaine abuse

Primary concerns for the anesthesia provider are the likelihood of the patient exhibiting acute abuse or possible withdrawal syndrome.[60] Signs and symptoms of acute abuse of the more common substances are listed in Box 20-4.[59,60] Elective surgery should be delayed or canceled in patients suspected of being under the influence of an illicit drug until further patient evaluation can be performed. Suspicion of acute substance abuse should be followed up with a urine screen for drug identification. Abstinence syndrome typically exhibits increased sympathetic and parasympathetic responses resulting in hypertension, tachycardia, abdominal cramping and diarrhea, tremors, anxiety, irritability, lacrimation, mydriasis, algid sweat, and yawning.[61]

Synthetic Androgens. Anabolic steroids are self-administered in an attempt to increase strength and muscle mass but can result in hepatic and endocrine system dysfunction. Risks associated with long-term androgen steroid supplementation include impaired liver function, hepatic adenocarcinoma, peliosis hepatis, myocardial infarction (MI), atherosclerosis, hypercoagulopathy, stroke, hypertension, dyslipidemia, and psychiatric and behavioral disturbances in susceptible patients.[62] The hepatotoxic effects have important implications for the anesthetic management of a chronic steroid abuser, particularly with agents metabolized by the liver, and such patients should undergo preoperative liver function testing.

Herbal Dietary Supplements. Patients should be questioned regarding their use of nonprescription medications to determine the herb's name, the duration of herbal therapy, and the dose taken. If patients are in doubt as to the herbal medications they are taking, they should be encouraged to bring in the herbal products with them to their preoperative workup. Certain herbal products are known to influence blood clotting, affect blood glucose levels, produce CNS stimulation or depression, or interact with psychotropic drugs (Table 20-2).[63,64]

PATIENT EVALUATION: OVERVIEW OF SYSTEMS

Upper Airway
Assessment of the airway should be performed preoperatively in every patient, regardless of the plan of anesthetic management.

BOX **20-4**

Signs and Symptoms of Acute Substance Abuse

Cannabis (Marijuana or Hashish)
Tachycardia, labile blood pressure, headache
Euphoria, dysphoria, depression, occasional anxiety and panic reactions, psychosis (rare)
Poor memory and decreased motivation with chronic use

Cocaine and Amphetamines
Tachycardia, labile blood pressure, hypertension, myocardial ischemia, arrhythmias, pulmonary edema
Excitement, delirium, hallucinations to psychosis
Euphoria, feeling of excitation, well-being, and enhanced physical strength & mental capacity
Hyperreflexia, tremors, convulsions, mydriasis, sweating, hyperpyrexia, exhaustion, coma with overdose

Hallucinogens: LSD, PCP
Sympathomimetic and weak analgesic effects
Altered perception and judgment; high doses may progress to toxic psychosis
PCP produces dissociative anesthesia with increasing doses

Opioids
Respiratory depression, hypotension, bradycardia, constipation
Euphoria (most marked with heroin)
Pinpoint pupils with overdose; decreased level of consciousness to coma

From Cheng DCH. The drug addicted patient. Can J Anaesth. 1997;44:R101-R106; Cavaliere F et al. Anesthesiologic preoperative evaluation of drug addicted patient. Minerva Anestesiol. 2005;71:367-371. LSD, Lysergic acid diethylamide-25; PCP, phencyclidine.

It is important to evaluate the patient before anesthesia to identify those patients at risk for difficult airway management. The initial physical examination of the patient includes careful inspection of the teeth, inside of the mouth, mandibular space, and neck in a sequential fashion to determine predictors of airway management difficulties (Table 20-3).[65] Certain body structural features, metabolic disease states, and congenital or acquired structural anomalies are associated with difficult airway management (Box 20-5).[66] The combination of subtle or minor physical anomalies may result in a difficult tracheal intubation, even when each factor individually is not expected to pose a problem.

Tests for Prediction of Difficult Intubation
Several screening tests for predicting difficult endotracheal intubation are recommended as part of the preoperative patient evaluation. No single test should be relied on exclusively when the airway is evaluated; a combination of evaluative criteria should be used to increase the predictive value for difficult intubation.

Mallampati Classification. A popular technique for airway assessment is the modified Mallampati airway classification, which entails examination of tongue size relative to the oral cavity.[67] During the assessment for the Mallampati classification, the patient is seated upright with the head in neutral alignment, while the examiner sits opposite the patient at eye level. The patient is asked to open the mouth as wide as possible and

TABLE 20-2 Clinically Important Effects and Perioperative Concerns of Selected Herbal Medicines and Recommendations for Discontinuation of Use Before Surgery

Herb: Common Name(s)	Relevant Pharmacologic Effects	Perioperative Concerns	Preoperative Discontinuation
Echinacea: purple coneflower root	Activation of cell-mediated immunity	Allergic reactions; decreased effectiveness of immunosuppressive actions of corticosteroids & cyclosporine; potential for immunosuppression with long-term use; inhibition of hepatic microsomal enzymes may precipitate toxicity of drugs metabolized by the liver, e.g., phenytoin, rifampin, phenobarbital	No data
Ephedra: ma huang	Increased heart rate & blood pressure through direct & indirect sympathomimetic effects	Risk of myocardial ischemia & stroke from tachycardia & hypertension; ventricular arrhythmias with halothane; long-term use depletes endogenous catecholamines & may cause intraoperative hemodynamic instability (control hypotension with direct vasoconstrictor, e.g., phenylephrine); life-threatening interaction with monoamine oxidase inhibitors	At least 24 hours before surgery
Garlic: ajo, *Alium sativum*	Inhibition of platelet aggregation (may be irreversible); increased fibrinolysis; equivocal antihypertensive activity	Potential to increase risk of bleeding, especially when combined with other medications that inhibit platelet aggregation	At least 7 days before surgery
Ginkgo: duck foot tree, maidenhair tree, silver apricot	Inhibition of platelet-activating factor	Potential to increase risk of bleeding, especially when combined with other medications that inhibit platelet aggregation	At least 36 hours before surgery
Ginseng: American ginseng, Asian ginseng, Chinese ginseng, Korean ginseng	Lowers blood glucose; inhibition of platelet aggregation (may be irreversible); increased PT-PTT in animals; many other diverse effects	Hypoglycemia; potential to increase risk of bleeding; potential to decrease anticoagulation effect of warfarin	At least 7 days before surgery
Kava: awa, intoxicating pepper, kawa	Sedation, anxiolysis	Potential to increase sedative effect of anesthetics; potential for addiction, tolerance, & withdrawal after abstinence unstudied	At least 24 hours before surgery
St John's wort: amber, goat week, hardhay, *Hypericum*, klamatheweed	Inhibition of neurotransmitter reuptake, monoamine oxidase inhibition is unlikely	Induction of cytochrome P-450 enzymes, affecting cyclosporine, warfarin, steroids, protease inhibitors, & possibly benzodiazepines, calcium channel blockers, & many other drugs; decreased serum digoxin levels	At least 5 days before surgery
Valerian: all heal, garden heliotrope, vandal root	Sedation	Potential to increase sedative effect of anesthetics; benzodiazepine-like acute withdrawal; potential to increase anesthetic requirements with long-term use	No data

Modified from Ang-Lee MK et al. *Herbal medicines and perioperative care.* JAMA. 2001;286:208-216; Kaye AD et al. *Perioperative anesthesia clinical considerations of alternative medicines.* Anesthesiol Clin North America. 2004;22:125-139.

TABLE 20-3	Components of the Preoperative Airway Physical Examination
Airway Examination Component	**Cautionary Findings**
Length of upper incisors	Relatively long
Relation of maxillary and mandibular incisors during normal jaw closure	Prominent "overbite" (maxillary incisors anterior to mandibular incisors)
Relation of maxillary & mandibular incisors during voluntary protrusion of the jaw	Patient mandibular incisors anterior to (in front of) maxillary incisors
Interincisor distance	<3 cm
Visibility of uvula	Not visible when tongue is protruded with patient in sitting position (e.g., Mallampati class >II)
Shape of palate	Highly arched or very narrow
Compliance of mandibular space	Stiff, indurated, occupied by mass, not resilient
Thyromental distance	Less than three ordinary fingerbreadths
Length of neck	Short
Thickness of neck	Thick
Range of motion of head and neck	Patient cannot touch tip of chin to chest or cannot extend neck

From American Society of Anesthesiologists Task Force on Management of the Difficult Airway. Practice guidelines for management of the difficult airway: an updated report by the American Society of Anesthesiologists Task Force on Management of the Difficult Airway. Anesthesiology. 2003;98:1269-1277.

maximally extrude the tongue. The patient is encouraged not to phonate during this maneuver because phonation may inappropriately elevate the soft palate. The airway is then classified based on the structures visible on direct examination of the oropharynx (Figure 20-2).[67] Endotracheal intubation is generally easy in a patient with a Mallampati class I airway and can be expected to be difficult in a patient with a Mallampati class III or IV airway. Mallampati airway classification has been criticized as not being a reliable or sensitive predictor of difficult intubating conditions.[68] Because of the unusually high incidence of false-positive and false-negative findings associated with the system, it should not be used as the only means of screening for the difficult airway.

Thyromental Distance. Thyromental distance can be quantified to enable prediction of difficulties with laryngoscopy. Thyromental distance represents the straight distance, with the neck fully extended and the mouth closed, between the prominence of the thyroid cartilage and the bony point of the lower mandibular border. In adults, a thyromental distance of less than 7 cm, which is approximately three adult fingerbreadths, is associated with difficult endotracheal intubation[69] because the pharyngeal and laryngeal axes may not properly align, and difficult laryngoscopy can be anticipated.[69]

Interincisor Distance. The degree of mouth opening, largely a function of the temporomandibular joint, is a vital component of airway assessment. Limited temporomandibular joint movement is a well-recognized contributor to difficult endotracheal intubation. An adult should be able to open the mouth at least 4 cm, allowing two large fingers to be placed between the upper and lower incisors. An interincisor gap of less than two fingerbreadths is associated with difficulty in endotracheal intubation.[70] Some patients who are able to open their mouths sufficiently while awake experience limitations in temporomandibular joint mobility after anesthesia is induced. This limited movement renders the visualization of laryngeal structures difficult. In this situation, forward protrusion of the mandible can be attempted for opening the mouth adequately to allow direct laryngoscopy.[71]

Head and Neck Movement (Atlantooccipital Function). Moderate flexion of the neck on the chest and full extension of the atlantooccipital joint aligns the oral, pharyngeal, and laryngeal axes into the McGill, or "sniff," position. In this position, less tongue obscures the laryngeal view during laryngoscopy. Limitations to atlantooccipital joint extension, which are frequently attributed to cervical arthritis or a small C-1 gap, enhance the convexity of the neck and push the larynx anteriorly. This situation can impair laryngoscopy and render endotracheal intubation difficult.

Mandibular Mobility. Have the patient demonstrate the ability to move the jaw forward and bite their upper lip. Being able to protrude the mandible in front of the central incisors indicates relative ease for maneuvering the laryngoscope.

Dentition

The incidence of perianesthetic dental injury in patients undergoing general anesthesia involving endotracheal intubation approximates 1:2100 and is associated with patients who have preexisting poor dentition and characteristics linked with difficult laryngoscopy and intubation (e.g., limited neck motion, previous head and neck surgery, craniofacial abnormalities, history of previous difficult tracheal intubation).[72] Because dental injuries are the most common reason for anesthesia-related medicolegal claims[73] (accounting for one third of all claims in the United States),[74] a preanesthesia inspection of the teeth should be performed and documented for each patient. Otherwise, fractured or missing teeth may be falsely attributed to damage occurring during airway instrumentation. The patient with protuberant or loose maxillary incisors should also be informed of the increased risk of tooth injury or loss with laryngoscopy. An informed consent to proceed with the anesthetic plan, despite this dental risk, must then be documented. If the patient is properly informed of the likelihood of dental damage, the anesthesia provider may not be held liable should dental injury occur.[75]

The location and condition of crowns, braces, and other significant dental work are also noted. Prosthetic devices such as partial plates and dentures are removed before surgery, unless they significantly improve the mask fit. An extremely loose tooth may be extracted before laryngoscopy to prevent its aspiration during anesthesia.

Musculoskeletal System
Obesity

Evaluation of the musculoskeletal system usually begins with a general assessment of the size and stature of the patient. Baseline height and weight information can be obtained from the admission data or by direct questioning of the patient during the health

BOX 20-5

Conditions Associated with Difficult Airway Management

Head
Mass defects (e.g., encephalocele, soft-tissue sarcoma)
Macrocephaly (e.g., severe hydrocephaly, Dandy Walker
  syndrome, mucopolysaccharidoses [Hurler syndrome])
Interference with airway access (e.g., thoracopagus conjoined
  twins, stereotactic frame)

Facial Anomalies
Maxillary and mandibular deformities
Maxillary hypoplasia (e.g., Apert syndrome, Crouzon disease)
Mandibular hypoplasia, microgenia, micrognathia (e.g., Pierre
  Robin syndrome, Treacher Collins syndrome, Goldenhar
  syndrome, cri du chat syndrome, Nager syndrome)
Mandibular hyperplasia (e.g., cherubism)
Temporomandibular joint anomalies
Reduced mobility (e.g., arthrogryposis multiplex, diabetes, Dutch-
  Kentucky syndrome, Hecht-Beals syndrome),
  ankylosis (inflammatory, congenital, traumatic, infectious)

Thoracoabdominal
Morbid obesity, sleep apnea syndrome, Prader-Willi syndrome
Kyphoscoliosis
Prominent chest or large breasts
Full-term or near-term pregnancy

Mouth and Tongue Anomalies
Microstomia
Congenital anomalies (e.g., Freeman-Sheldon [whistling face]
  syndrome)
Acquired anomalies (e.g., burn)
Stomatitis (e.g., noma)
Tongue disease
Macroglossia
Congenital (e.g., Beckwith-Wiedemann syndrome, Down
  syndrome, congenital hypothyroidism, Pompe disease)
Swelling (e.g., burns, trauma, Ludwig angina)
Tumors (e.g., hemangiomas, lymphangioma)
Protruding upper incisors (e.g., Cockayne syndrome)
Foreign body

Nasal Pathology
Choanal atresia
Tumors (e.g., encephaloceles, gliomas, foreign body)

Palate Pathology
Arch and cleft defects
Soft-palate swelling and hematomas

Pharynx
Adenoid and tonsillar disease
Hypertrophy
Tumors and abscesses

Lingual tonsils
Pharyngeal wall pathology
Retropharyngeal and parapharyngeal abscesses
Inflammatory disease (e.g., epidermolysis bullosa, erythema
  multiforme bullosum)
Scarring (e.g., Behçet syndrome)

Laryngeal Pathology
Supraglottic
Laryngomalacia
Supraglottis (epiglottitis)
Glottic
Congenital lesions (vocal cord paralysis, laryngeal web, cyst,
  laryngocele)
Papillomatosis
Granuloma formation
Foreign body
Subglottic
Congenital stenosis
Infectious (croup)
Inflammatory (edema, traumatic stenosis)

Tracheal and Bronchial Tree Pathology
Tracheomalacia (e.g., Larsen syndrome)
Croup
Bacterial tracheitis
Mediastinal masses
Vascular malformation
Foreign body aspiration
Other (e.g., tracheal stenosis, webbing, fistula, diverticulum)

Neck
Mass lesions
Lymphatic malformation, hemangioma, teratoma, goiter, abscess
Skin contracture (postburn, inflammatory [scleroderma,
  epidermolysis bullosa, erythema multiforme bullosum])
Webbed (e.g., Turner syndrome)

Spine
Limited cervical spine mobility
Congenital (e.g., Klippel-Feil syndrome)
Acquired (e.g., surgical [fusion], trauma [vertebral fracture],
  inflammatory [ankylosing spondylitis])
Cervical spine instability
Congenital (e.g., Down syndrome, Larsen syndrome, Möbius
  syndrome, Morquio syndrome)
Acquired (e.g., trauma [subluxation, fracture], inflammatory
  [rheumatoid arthritis])

Modified from Riazi J, ed. Anesthesiology Clinics of North America: The Difficult Pediatric Airway. *Philadelphia: 1998; Saunders.*

history interview. Body weight is then compared with normal values for a given height in relation to the patient's age and gender. Ideal body weight, for example, can be determined for men and women (see Box 20-6). The actual weight of the patient is compared with the calculated ideal body weight. Body weight that is 20% in excess of the ideal body weight at a particular height constitutes obesity. A body weight that is twice the ideal body weight is deemed morbidly obese.

A more scientific approach to describing weight in relation to height uses the measure of body mass index (BMI).

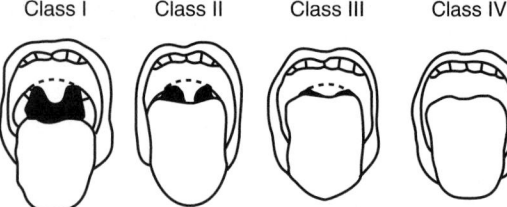

Class I   Class II   Class III   Class IV

FIGURE **20-2** Modified Mallampati classification of pharyngeal structures. *Class I*, Soft palate, tonsillar fauces, tonsillar pillars, and uvula visualized. *Class II*, Soft palate, tonsillar fauces, and uvula visualized. *Class III*, Soft palate and base of uvula visualized. *Class IV*, Soft palate not visualized. (*From Samsoon GL, Young JR. Difficult tracheal intubation: a retrospective study. Anaesthesia. 1987;42:487-490.*)

BOX **20-6**

Calculation of Ideal Body Weight and Body Mass Index

Ideal Body Weight (IBW)
IBW (male) = 105 lb + 6 lb for each inch >5 ft
IBW (female) = 100 lb + 5 lb for each inch >5 ft

To Calculate Body Mass Index (BMI):
BMI = Weight in kg/(height in meters)^2
  Example 1:
    70 kg/1.7 m^2 = 70 kg/2.89 m = 24 kg/m^2
  Example 2:
    125 kg/1.7 m^2 = 125 kg/2.89 m = 43 kg/m^2

BOX **20-7**

Obesity-Related Comorbidities

Cardiovascular
Hypertension
Coronary heart disease
Hypertrophic cardiomyopathy
Peripheral vascular disease
Thromboembolic disease
Stroke

Dermatologic
Dermatitis
Cellulitis
Panniculitis
Hirsutism (presence of excess body and facial hair)

Endocrine
Dyslipidemia (e.g., high total cholesterol, low levels of high density lipoprotein [HDL] cholesterol, or hypertriglyceridemia)
Liver dysfunction
Type 2 diabetes
Gout

Gastrointestinal
Gallbladder disease (cholelithiasis)
Hiatal hernia, heartburn
Gastroesophageal reflux disease (GERD)

Genitourinary
Complications of pregnancy
Menstrual irregularities
Stress incontinence

Malignancies
Some cancers (e.g., endometrial, uterine cervical, ovarian, breast, prostate, esophagus, liver, pancreas, kidney, gallbladder, & colorectal)

Maternal
Pregnancy-induced hypertension (PIH)
Induced labor, prolonged labor, difficult delivery
Increased primary cesarean section rate (>50%)
Increased perinatal mortality
Pulmonary embolism
Wound infection
Maternal death

Musculoskeletal
Osteoarthritis
Degenerative joint disease

Psychologic
Depression
Anxiety disorders

Pulmonary
Chronic obstructive pulmonary disease (COPD)
Restrictive pulmonary disease
Reactive airway disease
Obstructive sleep apnea
Pulmonary hypertension

From Marley RA et al. Perianesthesia respiratory care of the bariatric patient. J Perianesth Nurs. 2005;20:404-431.

Box 20-6 presents the formula for calculating BMI and incorporates it into examples for an average and an overweight individual of the same height. The adult patient weight classification based on BMI is: overweight, 25 to 29.9 kg/m^2; moderate obesity, 30 to 34.9 kg/m^2; severe obesity, 35 to 39.9 kg/m^2; and morbidly obese, greater than or equal to 40 kg/m^2.[76]

Two thirds of the adult population in the United States are overweight or obese.[77] Obese patients are at risk of illness from a multitude of conditions (Box 20-7) that require detailed workup.[76]

Appropriate diagnostic testing prior to bariatric surgery has been proposed (Box 20-8).[78] Much of this testing centers around the likelihood of patients presenting for bariatric surgery with preexisting metabolic complications or nutritional deficiencies.

The morbidly obese patient is at greater risk for cardiopulmonary aberrations and abnormal airway issues, and the preoperative assessment should reflect careful attention to these concerns.[76] Patients should receive cardiac assessment in accordance with the American Heart Association guidelines.[79] Asymptomatic patients should be screened for coronary disease if they have an abnormal baseline electrocardiogram; a history of coronary artery disease/valvular disease; or are more than 50 years of age with at least two of the following: metabolic syndrome, diabetes, hypertension, smoking, dyslipidemia, or family history of coronary disease.[80]

Obstructive sleep apnea is a breathing disorder distinguished by periodic, partial, or complete obstruction of the upper airway during sleep.[81] Particular attention is given to a history of snoring, apneic episodes, frequent arousals during sleep (vocalization, shifting position, extremity movements), morning headaches, and daytime somnolence. The physical examination would include airway evaluation, nasopharyngeal characteristics, neck circumference, tonsil size, and tongue volume.[81] If the findings of the history and physical examination are suggestive of obstructive sleep apnea, a decision in consultation with the surgeon should be made regarding obtaining a preoperative sleep study. Polysomnography is the best test for establishing a diagnosis of obstructive sleep apnea. If the diagnosis of obstructive sleep apnea is confirmed, the patient will be evaluated to determine optimal levels of continuous positive airway pressure (CPAP) therapy. Patients already receiving CPAP therapy will be asked to bring their cleaned home CPAP units to the hospital for postoperative application as needed. If the hospital is to provide the CPAP device, the patient needs to be queried as to the type of interface device the patient uses, pressure settings, and whether supplemental oxygen is required.

Particular attention is given to airway evaluation to determine the likelihood of difficult endotracheal intubation. Patients who are obese or have short, thick necks or obstructive sleep apnea have a higher incidence of difficult or failed endotracheal intubation (1:20) than the general population (1:2200).[76] If a problem is anticipated and an awake or fiberoptic tracheal intubation

is planned, proper patient preparation, which includes a drying agent and proper upper airway anesthesia, should be planned.

The patient should be questioned about the use of antiobesity drugs such as amphetamines, nonamphetamine Schedule IV appetite suppressants, and antidepressants (e.g., fluoxetine, sertraline).

Ankylosing Spondylitis and Rheumatoid Arthritis

Disorders of the musculoskeletal system include degenerative disk disease (osteoarthritis), ankylosing spondylitis, and rheumatoid arthritis. The chronic pain and inflammation of spinal or extraspinal joints associated with these diseases limit the degree of patient mobility. Tolerance for positions required during surgery and regional anesthesia techniques should therefore be ascertained preoperatively. Aspirin, nonsteroidal antiinflammatory drugs, and corticosteroids may be included in pharmacologic regimens for such patients. A thorough family history and previous dental, obstetric, surgical, traumatic injury, transfusion, and drug histories should be elicited from patients taking these drugs to evaluate the propensity for bleeding. A history suggestive of a bleeding disorder (e.g., excessive bruising or prolonged bleeding) should lead to a patient work-up that may include measurement of international normalized ratio (INR), platelet count, prothrombin time, and activated partial thromboplastin time.[82]

If the dosage and duration of corticosteroid therapy are considerable in patients with a musculoskeletal disorder, perioperative supplementation also may be necessary to avoid hemodynamic instability. Patients considered at risk for adrenal insufficiency include those who received the hydrocortisone equivalent of more than 20 to 30 mg daily for longer than 2 weeks during the previous year and those who are receiving replacement corticosteroid treatment for adrenal insufficiency.[83] Patients with proven or suspected adrenal insufficiency or suppression should receive adequate perioperative steroid coverage (Table 20-4).[84-86]

Although less common than osteoarthritis, ankylosing spondylitis and rheumatoid arthritis have greater implications for anesthetic management. Systemic manifestations are extensive during the advanced stages of both disorders. Patients frequently have pain, inflammation, and limited mobility in affected joints, such as those in the back and hands. Extreme ankylosis and joint deformity often make peripheral venous access and intraoperative positioning a challenge. On physical examination, limited range of motion of the temporomandibular joint and cervical spine can make tracheal intubation more difficult.[87] In rheumatoid arthritis, this limitation is compounded by restrictions in vocal cord movement or tracheal stenosis caused by cricoarytenoid arthritis. These changes may be evidenced by preoperative hoarseness, stridor, painful speech, or dysphagia. Restrictive lung disease, polychondritis, pleural and pericardial effusions, and cardiac conduction abnormalities may be present during advanced stages of ankylosing spondylitis or rheumatoid arthritis.[88,89]

Neurologic System

Preoperative evaluation of the neurologic system includes the determination of CNS or peripheral nervous system dysfunction. An initial neurologic examination consisting of the following should be performed[90]:

- *Musculoskeletal (motor) system:* observe the patient's gait, ability to perform toe-and-heel walk, ability to maintain the arms held forward; evaluate the patient's grip strength
- *Sensory system:* physical distinction of vibration, pain, and light touch on the patient's hands, feet, and limbs

TABLE 20-4	Steroid Supplementation Regimen		
Patients currently taking steroids	<10 mg prednisolone per day	Assume normal hormonal response	Additional steroid cover not required
	>10 mg prednisolone per day	Minor surgery (inguinal hernia repair, colonoscopy)	25 mg hydrocortisone at induction
		Moderate surgery (open cholecystectomy, hemicolectomy)	Usual preoperative steroids plus 25 mg hydrocortisone at induction plus 100 mg/day for 24 hr; taper rapidly to usual dose over next 1-2 days
		Major surgery (major cardiothoracic surgery, Whipple procedure, liver resection)	Usual preoperative steroids plus 25 mg hydrocortisone at induction plus 100 mg/day for 48-72 hr; taper rapidly to usual dose over next 1-2 days
	High-dose immunosuppression	Give usual immunosuppressive doses during perioperative period	
Patients who have stopped taking steroids	<3 mo	Treat as if on steroids	
	>3 mo	No perioperative steroids necessary	

Data from Nicholson G et al. Perioperative steroid supplementation. Anaesthesia. 1998;53:1091-1104; Mieure KD et al. Supplemental glucocorticoid therapy. Orthopedics. 2007;30:116-119; Connery LE, Coursin DG. Assessment and therapy of selected endocrine disorders. Anesthesiol Clin North America. 2004;22:93-123.

- *Muscle reflexes:* deep, superficial, and pathologic
- *Cranial nerve abnormalities:* obtained by patient medical history and observation
- *Mental status and speech pattern:* appearance, mood, thought processes, cognitive function

Knowledge of clinical manifestations of neurologic disease is essential for the preoperative evaluation of patients with CNS or peripheral nervous system disorders. Signs and symptoms of increasing intracranial pressure and cerebral ischemia, for example, may include papilledema; unilateral mydriasis; headaches, made worse by coughing; nausea and vomiting; slurred speech, disorientation, and altered levels of consciousness; flaccid hemiplegia or hemiparesis; abducens or oculomotor palsy; neck rigidity; and respiratory disturbances. Hypertension, with corresponding decreases in heart rate, represents a physiologic attempt to enhance cerebral perfusion when intracranial pressure is high. The appearance of Q waves, deep and inverted T waves, prolonged QT intervals, and ST-segment elevations on the electrocardiogram (ECG) may reflect hypothalamic ischemia and sympathetic overactivity. These abnormalities are most often attributed to vasospasm after a subarachnoid hemorrhage, but myocardial ischemia should be ruled out before surgery.[91] Fever and leukocytosis also can follow a subarachnoid hemorrhage as a result of meningeal irritation by subarachnoid blood. The progression of neurologic dysfunction to coma, obtundation, and decerebrate rigidity worsens the overall prognosis of the patient with an intracranial mass or hemorrhage. This prognosis mirrors that of a patient who has sustained an acute head injury. The patient with an initial Glasgow Coma Scale (Table 20-5)[92] score of less than 8 is considered comatose. Patients with a score of 8 or less usually require tracheal intubation and mechanical hyperventilation.[93]

Diagnostic reports should be reviewed so that the extent of neurologic and coexisting disease can be determined.

TABLE 20-5	Glasgow Coma Scale
Response	**Score**
Eyes Open	
Spontaneously	4
To speech	3
To pain	2
Never	1
Best Motor Response	
Obeys commands	6
Localizes pain	5
Withdraws (flexion)	4
Abnormal flexion (decortication)	3
Extensor response (decerebration)	2
None	1
Best Verbal Response	
Oriented	5
Confused conversation	4
Inappropriate words	3
Incomprehensible sounds	2
None	1
Range of Scores	3-15

Modified from Teasdale G, Jennett B. Assessment of coma and impaired consciousness. A practical scale. Lancet. 1974;2:81-84.

These reports include the results of electromyography, conduction velocity studies, electroencephalography, computed tomography (CT), magnetic resonance imaging (MRI), and cerebral arteriography studies. Consultation with a neurologist and obtaining preoperative electromyography, for example, are recommended for patients with complaints of extremity weakness, pain, or paresthesia. This screening is especially important in patients at greater risk for peripheral neuropathy (e.g., patients with long-standing diabetes, patients with uremia, chronic alcoholics with nutritional deficits). Documentation of symptoms and reports of abnormal preoperative neurologic findings is important in these patients. Preoperative CT that reveals a 0.5-cm midline shift of the brain is significant and can confirm suspicions of intracranial hypertension. The size and location of an intracerebral aneurysm are represented on cerebral arteriography. This information can facilitate the prediction of the surgical approach and guide the evaluation of neurologic involvement. The degree of collateral circulation in the patient with cerebrovascular occlusive disease can be determined from arteriographic films. In a patient with vertebral artery involvement, for example, extremes in head flexion, extension, and rotation are avoided. Because of the associated risks of perioperative myocardial ischemia and infarction in patients undergoing a carotid endarterectomy procedure, a thorough cardiac evaluation by a cardiologist, including 12-lead ECG and stress testing, is advised.[94]

Information gained from the preoperative evaluation of neurologic function can enlighten the management of a patient with a CNS or peripheral nervous system disorder. For example, sedatives are avoided in patients with intracranial hypertension, especially when an altered level of consciousness accompanies it. Affected patients may be extremely sensitive to the CNS-depressant effects of such drugs as opioids.

Doses, schedules, and adverse effects of therapeutic regimens should also be considered before surgery. Serum concentrations of anticonvulsants such as phenytoin and phenobarbital are measured to determine whether levels are therapeutic. A complete blood cell count is obtained for patients receiving prolonged phenytoin therapy because of the risk of agranulocytosis associated with this drug. As with anticonvulsant therapy, corticosteroid therapy is continued perioperatively in patients with a CNS tumor. Although the exact mechanism of the beneficial effects of corticosteroids is unknown, it is theorized to involve the reduction of cerebrospinal fluid production or cerebral edema as a result of capillary membrane stabilization. Blood glucose levels are also determined for the patient treated with either dexamethasone or methylprednisolone, because hyperglycemia frequently accompanies the use of these drugs. Heightened risks of pulmonary infection and gastrointestinal irritation are unlikely in the patient undergoing perioperative therapy.[95]

Cardiovascular System

Evaluation of the cardiovascular system includes the determination of (1) preexisting cardiac disease (e.g., hypertension, ischemic heart disease, valvular dysfunction, cardiac arrhythmias, and cardiac conduction abnormalities, with or without evidence of ventricular failure); (2) disease severity, stability, and prior treatment; (3) comorbidity (e.g., diabetes mellitus, peripheral vascular disease, chronic pulmonary disease); and (4) the type of surgery to be performed (major abdominal, orthopedic, and vascular procedures are associated with high risk). The prevalence and adverse consequences of cardiovascular disease make it a prime consideration in the overview of systems. Major cardiovascular risk factors that correlate with increased perioperative morbidity and mortality have been described by an American College of Cardiology and American Heart Association (ACC/AHA) Task Force (Box 20-9).[96,97]

A standard means of categorizing the degree of cardiovascular disability is the New York Heart Association classification (Table 20-6).[98] When the patient interview is conducted, specific inquiry should be made regarding the presence of dyspnea, chest pain, fatigability, syncope, palpitation, and the factors that predispose to angina. Whenever a patient has signs of cardiovascular disease, referral to a cardiologist is indicated if a recent workup has not been conducted.

Hypertension

Hypertension, defined as a systolic blood pressure greater than 140 mm Hg or a diastolic pressure greater than 90 mm Hg,[99] is the most common circulatory derangement to affect humans (approximately 60 million in the United States) and is a major risk factor for coronary artery disease[100] and increased perioperative mortality.[101] All too often, patients undergoing surgery have uncontrolled stage 3 hypertension (systolic blood pressure greater than 180 mm Hg, diastolic pressure greater than 110 mm Hg, or both). This problem can be attributed to the lack or inadequacy of medical treatment or to patient noncompliance. In such a situation, elective surgery may be postponed for further patient assessment and normalization of the preoperative blood pressure. Consultation with an internist can be pursued for the medical evaluation and treatment of the patient with uncontrolled or newly diagnosed hypertension. These recommendations are aimed at reducing the occurrence of perioperative hemodynamic instability and consequently the incidence of myocardial ischemia. Both complications are more likely to occur when hypertension is not effectively treated before surgery.[102-104] With the goal of reducing perioperative risk, delaying surgery is justified in hypertensive patients with target-organ damage (or suspected) such as ischemic heart disease, heart failure, renal, and cerebrovascular diseases, whose:

- conditions can be improved by such postponement to the extent that the perioperative risk would be considerably decreased; or whose
- care may be influenced by further preoperative examination.[105]

Delaying elective surgery in mild to moderate hypertension only for the purpose of blood pressure control may not reduce perioperative risk.[105] A systolic blood pressure below 180 mm Hg and diastolic blood pressure below 110 mm Hg is not an independent risk factor for perioperative cardiovascular complications.[97]

The practitioner taking the medical history should focus on identifying comorbid diseases, such as diabetes mellitus, and social risk factors (i.e., tobacco use, alcohol or caffeine consumption, illicit drug use [especially cocaine or amphetamines]). What medications the patient takes to manage hypertension should be established. In general, the substances used affect the central and peripheral components of the sympathetic nervous system by altering the synthesis, release, biotransformation, or end-organ action of norepinephrine. Because the circulatory-depressant effects of general anesthesia may be additive, the combination of antihypertensive drugs and anesthetics is of concern. Complaints of syncope and dizziness also are investigated. These symptoms may be the clinical manifestations of cerebrovascular insufficiency, although a diagnosis of drug-induced orthostatic hypotension should be considered preoperatively. This diagnosis can be confirmed by measuring a significant decrease in the blood pressure as the patient rises from the supine position. The lack of hemodynamic compensatory

BOX 20-9

Active Cardiac Conditions for Which the Patient Should Undergo Evaluation and Treatment Before Noncardiac Surgery

Major Risk Factors
Unstable coronary syndromes
  Acute or recent myocardial infarction* with evidence of important ischemic risk by clinical symptoms or noninvasive study
  Unstable or severe† angina (Canadian class III or IV)‡
Decompensated congestive heart failure
Significant arrhythmias
  High-grade atrioventricular block, Mobitz II atrioventricular block, third-degree atrioventricular heart block
  Symptomatic ventricular arrhythmias in the presence of underlying heart disease
  Supraventricular arrhythmias (including atrial fibrillation) with uncontrolled ventricular rate (heart rate greater than 100 beats/minute at rest)
  Symptomatic bradycardia
  Newly recognized ventricular tachycardia
Severe valvular disease
  Severe aortic stenosis (mean pressure gradient greater than 40 mm Hg, aortic valve area less than 1 cm², or symptomatic)

Symptomatic mitral stenosis (progressive dyspnea on exertion, exertional presyncope, or heart failure)

Intermediate Risk Factors
Mild angina pectoris (Canadian class I or II)
Prior myocardial infarction identified by history or pathologic Q waves
Compensated or prior congestive heart failure
Diabetes mellitus (particularly insulin-dependent)
Renal insufficiency

Minor Risk Factors
Advanced age
Abnormal electrocardiograph (left ventricular hypertrophy, left bundle branch block, ST-T abnormalities)
Rhythm other than sinus (e.g., atrial fibrillation)
Low functional capacity (e.g., inability to climb one flight of stairs with a bag of groceries)
History of stroke
Uncontrolled systemic hypertension

From Fleisher LA et al. ACC/AHA 2006 guideline update on perioperative cardiovascular evaluation for noncardiac surgery: focused update on perioperative beta-blocker therapy. Anesth Analg. 2007;104:15-26; Fleisher LA et al. ACC/AHA 2007 guidelines on perioperative cardiovascular evaluation and care for noncardiac surgery. Circulation. 2007;116:1971-199.
*The American College of Cardiology National Database Library defines recent myocardial infarction as having occurred more than 7 days but less than or equal to 30 days previously; acute myocardial infarction is within 7 days.
†May include "stable" angina in patients who are unusually sedentary.
‡Campeau L. Grading of angina pectoris. Circulation. 1976;54:522-523.

responses that normally accompany positional changes may then predict their absence during anesthesia and surgery.

The physical examination of the patient includes the following[106]:

- *Overall appearance:* truncal obesity with purpura and striae suggestive of Cushing disease
- *Vital signs:* measurement of blood pressure in both arms.
- *Funduscopic examination:* hypertensive retinopathy
- *Neck:* carotid bruits, distended veins, or enlarged thyroid gland
- *Heart:* abnormal rhythm or size, murmurs, or heart sounds
- *Lungs:* rales or bronchospasm
- *Abdomen:* bruits, masses, enlarged kidneys, or abnormal aortic pulsation
- *Extremities:* delayed or absent femoral pulses secondary to aortic coarctation; evidence of atherosclerosis, peripheral edema
- *Neurologic evaluation:* see the discussion of the neurologic system earlier in this chapter

Ischemic Heart Disease

Myocardial ischemia occurs secondary to insufficient oxygen and nutrient supply (increased demand, reduced blood supply, or both) to meet the metabolic requirements of the myocardial cells. Nearly one third of the estimated 30 million patients undergoing surgery annually in the United States is at high risk for coronary artery disease or factors for cardiovascular disease.[107]

Risk factors for ischemic heart disease include advanced age, smoking, diabetes mellitus, hypertension, pulmonary disease, previous MI, left ventricular wall motion dysfunction, and peripheral vascular disease.[108] The preoperative evaluation of a patient with known or suspected ischemic heart disease is aimed at determining the severity, progression, and functional limitations imposed by cardiovascular disease. Myocardial ischemia, cardiac arrhythmias, and left ventricular dysfunction are usually precipitating factors for patient symptomatology. Complaints of undue fatigue, angina pectoris, palpitations, syncope, or dyspnea should be thoroughly investigated. A 12-lead ECG is reviewed for evidence of myocardial ischemia or infarction, cardiac arrhythmias or conduction abnormalities, and ventricular hypertrophy. Signs and symptoms of myocardial ischemia may not be apparent at rest, however. Therefore the response of the patient to various activities, such as walking a certain distance or climbing several stairs, must be determined (see Table 20-6).

Anginal symptoms can also be classified according to the stability of precipitating factors, the frequency of the events, and the duration of pain. Stable angina (characterized as substernal discomfort brought on by exertion, relieved by rest or nitroglycerin or both in less than 15 minutes, and having a typical radiation to the shoulder, jaw, or the inner aspect of the arm)[98] poses no greater threat of MI perioperatively than the absence of anginal symptoms.[109] Unstable angina is defined as newly developed

TABLE **20-6**	New York Heart Association Functional Classification of Cardiovascular Disability
Classification	**Cardiovascular Status**
Class I	*Patients with cardiac disease.* No functional limitations to physical activity, such as walking or climbing stairs. Ordinary physical activity is not associated with undue fatigue, palpitations, dyspnea, or anginal pain.
Class II	*Patients with cardiac disease who are comfortable at rest.* Slight functional limitations to physical activity, such as walking or climbing stairs rapidly, or during emotional stress. Patients are comfortable at rest. Ordinary physical activity results in fatigue, palpitation, dyspnea, or anginal pain.
Class III	*Patients with cardiac disease resulting in marked limitations to physical activity.* Patients are comfortable at rest. Less than ordinary physical activity causes fatigue, palpitations, dyspnea, or anginal pain.
Class IV	*Patients with cardiac disease resulting in inability to carry on any physical activity without discomfort.* Symptoms of cardiac insufficiency or anginal syndrome may be present even at rest. If any physical activity is undertaken, discomfort is increased.

Modified from Kaplan JA, ed. Cardiac Anesthesia. 4th ed. Philadelphia: Saunders; 1999.

TABLE **20-7**	New Clinical Classifications of Myocardial Infarction
Classification	**Description**
1	Spontaneous MI related to ischemia due to a primary coronary event, such as plaque erosion and/or rupture, fissuring, or dissection.
2	MI secondary to ischemia due to an imbalance of O_2 supply and demand, as from coronary spasm or embolism, anemia, arrhythmias, hypertension, or hypotension
3	Sudden unexpected cardiac death, including cardiac arrest, often with symptoms suggesting ischemia with new ST-segment elevation, new left bundle branch block, or pathologic or angiographic evidence of fresh coronary thrombus—in the absence of reliable biomarker findings
4a	MI associated with PCI
4b	MI associated with documented in-stent thrombosis
5	MI associated with CABG surgery

From Thygesen K et al. Joint ESC/ACCF/AHA/WHF Task Force for the Redefinition of Myocardial Infarction. Universal definition of myocardial infarction. J Am Coll Cardiol. 2007;50(22):2173-2195.
MI, Myocardial infarction; PCI, percutaneous coronary intervention; CABG, coronary artery bypass graft.

angina occurring within the past 2 months; angina that has progressively worsened, that occurs with increased frequency, intensity, or duration, that is less responsive to medicine, or that occurs when the patient is at rest; or angina that lasts longer than 30 minutes, exhibiting transient ST- or T-wave changes without development of Q waves or diagnostic elevation of enzymes.[98] *Unstable angina is associated with the highest risk for perioperative MI.*[110] In the patient with unstable angina, elective surgery is canceled until the cardiovascular status of the patient has been thoroughly evaluated and optimized. Advanced diagnostic techniques such as coronary angiography and exercise ECG may be used for determination of the extent and functional impairment of ischemic heart disease.

The overall risk of MI after general anesthesia is between 0.1% and 0.7% in the population at large. In patients known to have had an MI in the remote past (more than 6 months previously), the risk of perioperative reinfarction increases to approximately 6%. If MI occurred 3 to 6 months previously, the risk of reinfarction is 15%; within 3 months previously, 30%. If reinfarction occurs, the mortality rate is approximately 50%. The highest at-risk period appears to be within 30 days after an acute MI; therefore the ACC/AHA guidelines recommend waiting at least 4 to 6 weeks after an MI before a patient

undergoes elective surgery.[97] Patients who have survived coronary revascularization and are asymptomatic are at lower risk of reinfarction when undergoing noncardiac surgery.[97] The new clinical classification of myocardial infarction is noted in Table 20-7.

Left Ventricular Dysfunction

Active left ventricular failure is the prominent cardiovascular risk factor for patients undergoing noncardiac surgery.[111] Patients with ischemic cardiomyopathy are at even greater risk for perioperative MI and ventricular dysfunction.[112] Heart failure is defined by the presence of any of the following: history of congestive heart failure, pulmonary edema, or paroxysmal nocturnal dyspnea; physical examination showing bilateral rales or S_3 gallop; or chest X-ray showing pulmonary vascular redistribution.[97] Prominent signs include moist rales in the lungs, often associated with tachypnea. These extraneous sounds may be confined to the bases, with mild degrees of left ventricular failure, or they may be generalized throughout the lungs, with acute pulmonary edema. As a result of sympathetic nervous system stimulation, resting tachycardia may also be present. A third heart sound (S_3) or ventricular gallop, jugular vein distention, and peripheral edema are significant. In the presence of congestive heart failure as confirmed by a chest radiograph, elective surgery should be postponed until optimal ventricular performance can be achieved.

Patients exhibiting dyspnea of unknown origin or current or prior heart failure with worsening dyspnea or other relevant change in clinical status should undergo preoperative evaluation of left ventricular function if an assessment has not been performed within the previous 12 months.[97] Tests of resting left ventricular function include radionuclide angiography, echocardiography, and contrast ventriculography. A left ventricular ejection fraction of less than 35% as determined by echocardiography is associated with greater incidence of postoperative heart failure and death.[113]

Valvular Heart Disease

Basic lesions of valvular heart disease may involve stenosis, incompetence, or both. In adults, aortic and mitral valve lesions are more common than those involving the tricuspid or pulmonic valve. Despite decreasing incidence, rheumatic heart disease is still the most common cause of adult valvular disease. Degenerative disorders (sclerosis, fibrosis) and congenital diseases are less common causes. With stenosis, the chamber proximal to the obstruction must increase the work of maintaining a stroke volume; this eventually results in hypertrophy. Normal valves can episodically accommodate up to seven times the normal cardiac output—for example, in intense physical exercise in the normally active patient. Valvular stenosis usually is chronic and severe before cardiac output decreases. In valvular incompetence, the chambers both proximal and distal to the lesions are involved, because regurgitant flow during one phase of the cardiac cycle is added to forward flow during subsequent systole. Because lesions are almost never entirely unitary, in stenosis some regurgitation is common, and vice versa. It is important to identify the type of valvular lesion before surgery. Evaluation of the clinical symptoms and cardiac catheterization data regarding valve area and gradients, combined with assessment of data from any surgical history (e.g., correction of congenital heart lesions), is an important component of the preoperative evaluation of patients with valvular heart disease.

Severe aortic stenosis poses the greatest patient risk for noncardiac surgery,[97] especially when the cross-sectional area of the aortic valve is less than 1 cm^2. Severe aortic stenosis is associated with a 14-fold greater incidence of perioperative sudden death.[114] For patients in whom aortic stenosis is symptomatic, elective noncardiac surgery should be postponed until after cardiac surgical consultation.[97] Chapter 24 describes the perioperative care of patients with valvular heart disease.

Arrhythmias

Patients with cardiac arrhythmias must have an adequate preoperative evaluation to ascertain the nature of the arrhythmia, associated underlying heart disease, and type of antiarrhythmic therapy. Whether symptoms of palpitations or dizziness have been relieved may be a sign of successful therapy or continuing problems. Other cardiac symptoms such as dyspnea, angina, or syncope may suggest worsening of associated cardiac disease. Treatment of the underlying disease preoperatively may aid in control of arrhythmia in the perioperative period. All patients with a history of symptomatic arrhythmias should undergo electrocardiography with rhythm strip before surgery. Other preoperative laboratory evaluations should include measurement of potassium and magnesium levels, determination of antiarrhythmic drug levels (if possible), and chest radiography (in the presence of structural cardiac disease).

Ventricular arrhythmias are classified into three categories: benign ventricular arrhythmias (unifocal premature ventricular contractions); potentially malignant ventricular arrhythmias (patient has known organic heart disease and is on antiarrhythmic therapy); and malignant ventricular arrhythmias (patient has

organic heart disease, hemodynamic compromise, and possibly a family history of sudden death).[115] Few data are available to help correlate the risk of arrhythmias and perioperative risk.[98] In the absence of cardiac disease, benign ventricular arrhythmias do not carry a significantly increased surgical risk.[116] In patients with severe coronary artery disease, recent MI, or peripheral vascular disease, arrhythmias may increase perioperative risk.[117,118]

Pacemaker

Anesthesia providers must be familiar with the different types of pacemakers or implanted defibrillators, the indications for insertion, the evaluation of pacemaker function, and the perioperative management of patients with these devices (Box 20-10). Too often, the presence of a permanent pacemaker is merely noted. Direct examination with a programmer remains the only trustworthy method for evaluating battery status, lead performance, and adequacy of current settings.[119] Pacemakers can mask the toxicity of antiarrhythmic drugs, electrolyte disorders, and myocardial ischemia and irritability. In general, the ECG should be examined for pacemaker malfunction, as evidenced by unexpected pauses. If the patient's heart rate is slower than the pacing rate, pacing spikes should appear on the ECG. To determine whether these pacing impulses are associated with myocardial contractions, the clinician should palpate a peripheral pulse. Evaluation of a pacemaker becomes more difficult when the patient's heart rate is faster than the pacing rate. A Valsalva maneuver slows the patient's rate so that pacing impulses appear on the ECG. Generally, because sensing is lost before pacing, the pacemaker is probably functioning normally if (1) it has been in place for fewer than 2 years, (2) chest radiography demonstrates that leads are intact, and (3) impulses do not appear on the ECG.[120] Chest radiography should provide information on electrode placement, the presence of electrode fracture, and even battery depletion.[121]

If each pacing impulse is not associated with a pulse or if the symptoms that led to pacemaker implantation have returned, cardiology consultation should be considered.[120] Anesthesia providers sometimes must decide whether a transvenous, temporary pacing wire should be inserted preoperatively. Persistent bradycardia not responsive to intravenous administration of atropine or exercise is one indication. Bifascicular block in a patient with a history of syncope suggests underlying, unrecognized complete heart block. Such patients can benefit from the availability of transvenous pacing.

It also must be determined whether exercising the muscles adjacent to the generator causes dizziness. The presence of this symptom, indicating that myopotentials may be inhibiting the pacemaker, implies that muscle fasciculations caused by succinylcholine and shivering should be avoided.

Diagnostic Testing to Assess Cardiovascular Disease

Multiple tests are available to define the presence of cardiac disease. Preoperative cardiac testing should not be performed unless the results are likely to influence patient management. The ACC/AHA guidelines include an algorithm for determining the appropriateness of preoperative testing (Figure 20-3).[97]

Exercise stress testing is designed to increase myocardial work and permit measurement of myocardial response to the increased workload. The exercise stress test not only is a standardized means of obtaining a functional history of angina but also provides excellent documentation of how ischemia manifests its effects on the cardiovascular system. By examining the stress test report, one can learn the extremes of blood pressure and

BOX **20-10**

Perioperative Guidelines for the Patient with a Cardiac Generator

Preoperative Key Points

- Have the pacemaker or defibrillator interrogated by a competent authority shortly before the anesthetic.
- Obtain a copy of this interrogation. Ensure that the device will pace the heart with appropriate safety margins.
- Consider replacing any device near its elective replacement period in a patient scheduled to undergo either a major surgery or surgery within 25 cm of the generator.
- Determine the patient's underlying rhythm/rate to evaluate the need for backup pacing support.
- Identify the magnet rate and rhythm if a magnet mode is present and magnet use is planned.
- Program minute ventilation rate responsiveness "Off," if present.
- Program all rate enhancements "Off."
- Consider increasing the pacing rate to optimize oxygen delivery to tissues for major cases.
- Disable antitachycardia therapy if the device is a defibrillator.

Intraoperative Key Points

- Monitor cardiac rhythm/peripheral pulse with pulse oximeter or arterial waveform.
- Disable the "artifact filter" on the ECG monitor.
- Avoid use of monopolar electrosurgery.
- Use bipolar ESU if possible; if not possible, then pure cut (monopolar ESU) is better than "blend" or "coag."
- Position the ESU current return pad in such a way that it will prevent electricity from crossing the generator-heart circuit, even if the pad must be placed on the distal forearm and the wire covered with sterile drape.
- If the ESU causes ventricular oversensing, pacer quiescence, or tachycardia, limit the period(s) of asystole or reprogram the device.

Postoperative Key Points

- Have the device interrogated by a competent authority postoperatively. Some rate enhancements can be reinitiated, and optimum heart rate and pacing parameters should be determined. The ICD patient must be monitored until the antitachycardia therapy is restored.

From Rozner MA. The patient with a cardiac pacemaker or implanted defibrillator and management during anaesthesia. Curr Opin Anaesthesiol. 2007;20:261-268.

heart rate the patient can tolerate while awake (although exactly how these correlate with the anesthetized state is a matter of debate), the location of ischemic leads, and whether arrhythmias are associated with ischemia. Significant coronary disease is likely if ST-segment depression is greater than 0.2 mV, if ST depression occurs early in the test, if little increase in blood pressure or heart rate occurs at the time of ST depression, or if hypotension occurs. Hypotension is considered an ominous finding and usually prompts cardiac catheterization. Perioperative risk is considered low if exercise stress testing does not produce signs of myocardial ischemia at a reasonable workload (greater than 85% of predicted maximum heart rate).[122] Although it is useful in diagnosing coronary artery disease, its value as a preoperative test has been questioned.[112] Patients who are able to tolerate a good exercise stress workload, even those with stable angina, are unlikely to have myocardial dysfunction.[123]

Pharmacologic stress testing can be performed in patients unable to exercise or in those who take digoxin. Two pharmacologic techniques, which incorporate either echocardiography or radionuclide scintigraphy, are used: (1) dipyridamole or adenosine, both of which cause a coronary steal phenomenon by redistributing coronary blood flow without direct negative inotropic effects, and (2) dobutamine for inotropic stress testing.[124]

Cardiac catheterization provides definitive information about the distribution and severity of coronary artery disease and may be indicated for patients with New York Heart Association class III or IV criteria who are undergoing high-risk surgical procedures.[122] Significant stenosis means narrowing of a major coronary artery by more than 70% or narrowing of the left main coronary artery by more than 50%. It is important to look beyond the coronary anatomy and concentrate on other findings that can guide perioperative decision making. Three readily identifiable findings that indicate poor ventricular function are a cardiac index of less than 2.2 L/m^2, a left ventricular end-diastolic pressure of greater than 18 mm Hg, and an ejection fraction of less than 40%.[125] Taking note of ischemia-induced dysfunction of the papillary muscles can help in avoiding later confusion about the configuration of the pulmonary wedge pressure waveform and the significance of intraoperative changes in wedge pressure. Wall motion abnormalities should be noted. Areas of akinesis (no movement during systole) usually represent nonviable regions of myocardium and are relatively fixed deficits. In contrast, areas of hypokinesis (reduced contraction during systole) may represent ischemic but nonetheless viable regions of myocardium. This should alert anesthesia providers to a potentially dynamic situation in which alterations in the balance of myocardial oxygen supply and demand can either improve or worsen regional ischemia and associated contractility.

Respiratory System

A detailed evaluation of the respiratory system is crucial because of the relative frequency of and complications associated with respiratory disease. From an epidemiologic perspective, some form of lung disease is present in nearly 25% of the adult population. The most common problems are chronic obstructive pulmonary diseases (COPDs), such as chronic bronchitis, emphysema, and asthma, which are major predictors for postoperative pulmonary disorders.[126] In their acute or chronic forms, the lung diseases are second only to coronary artery disease

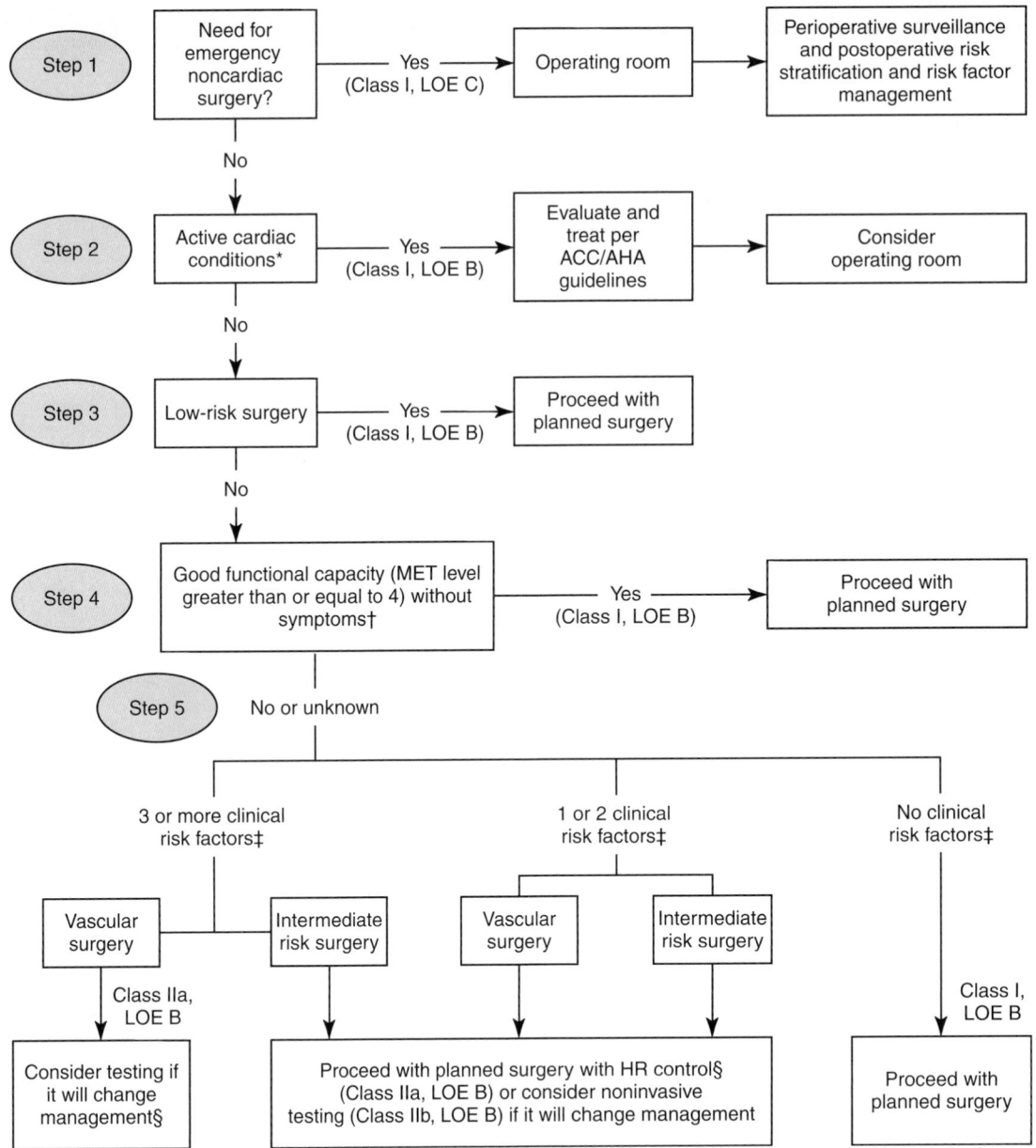

FIGURE **20-3** Cardiac evaluation and care algorithm for noncardiac surgery, based on active clinical conditions, known cardiovascular disease, or cardiac risk factors for patients 50 years of age or older. *See Box 20-9 for active clinical conditions. ‡Clinical risk factors include ischemic heart disease, compensated or prior HF, diabetes mellitus, renal insufficiency, and cerebrovascular disease. §Consider perioperative beta blockade for populations in which this has been shown to reduce cardiac morbidity/mortality. ACC/AHA, American College of Cardiology/American Heart Association; *HR*, heart rate; *LOE*, level of evidence; *MET*, metabolic equivalent. (*From Fleisher LA et al. ACC/AHA 2007 guidelines on perioperative cardiovascular evaluation and care for noncardiac surgery. Circulation. 2007;116:1971-1996.*)

as a cause of death. Patients with COPD are twice as likely to have postoperative pulmonary complications.[127] Risk factors associated with increased postoperative respiratory morbidity and mortality rates include preoperative sepsis, emergency operations, age (older than 60 years), history of smoking, comorbid diseases (e.g., cardiovascular disease, congestive heart failure, diabetes, American Society of Anesthesiologists [ASA] physical status class III or greater), chronic bronchitis, obesity (as little as 20% overweight), type of surgery (abdominal, thoracic), prolonged duration of anesthesia (3 to 4 hours or longer) and elevated creatinine.[127,128] The surgical site (aortic and thoracic surgeries) has been found to be the most important risk factor for the development of postoperative pulmonary complications.[129]

Emphysema and Chronic Bronchitis

The preparation of a patient with two forms of COPD—emphysema and chronic bronchitis—depends largely on the severity of the respiratory disease, as reflected by the preoperative history, physical examination, and diagnostic testing. Elective surgery is postponed when severe dyspnea, wheezing, pulmonary congestion, or hypercarbia ($PaCO_2$ greater than 50 mm Hg) is evident. The risk of postoperative respiratory failure in such circumstances is drastically increased. Consultation with a pulmonologist may be necessary for further evaluation and optimization of the respiratory status of the patient before anesthesia and surgery. Interventions to improve the pulmonary status of the patient with chronic bronchitis are the primary focus before surgery. Prophylactic measures that may reduce pulmonary risk are cited in Box 20-11.[130-132] Specific antibiotic therapy is initiated in patients with thick, purulent sputum and pulmonary infiltrates on the chest radiograph. Administration of prophylactic antibiotics to "sterilize" the sputum is not recommended, because secondary resistant infections may develop and complicate the perioperative management of the patient. To enhance the mobilization and clearance of pulmonary secretions, chest physiotherapy and adequate hydration can be instituted. Instruction on incentive spirometric techniques to lessen the incidence of postoperative atelectasis is crucial in these patients.

The most reliable way to reduce the incidence of perioperative pulmonary complications is to have patients stop smoking cigarettes. Eight weeks after smoking cessation, the pulmonary complication rate correlates with that of nonsmokers.[39] This intervention may not be feasible when initial meetings with the patient occur within days or hours of the scheduled procedure.

Several diagnostic tests are used for clinically differentiating bronchitis and emphysema in patients in the advanced stages of COPD. Arterial blood gases, for example, may document the presence of preoperative hypoxemia or hypercarbia. An abnormally low partial pressure of arterial oxygen (PaO_2) value (less than 60 mm Hg), with or without partial pressure of arterial carbon dioxide ($PaCO_2$) retention, often reflects a state of chronic bronchitis. Over time, the patient develops cor pulmonale because of the adverse effects of chronic hypoxia on pulmonary vasculature. The chest radiograph may suggest a diagnosis of COPD if slight abnormalities on the chest radiograph, including emphysemic bullae and pulmonary hyperlucency (which reflect vascular deficiencies in the lung periphery) are apparent. Diaphragmatic flattening and a vertical orientation of the cardiac silhouette also are characteristic. Chronic bronchitis, on the other hand, is rarely recognized through chest radiography unless secondary infections are present.

In addition to their role in categorizing patients with COPD, pulmonary function tests are occasionally used as diagnostic adjuncts for confirming the severity of airflow obstruction and its reversibility with bronchodilator therapy. In both chronic bronchitis and pulmonary emphysema, a decrease of the forced exhaled volume in 1 second (FEV_1) occurs in comparison with the forced vital capacity (FVC). FEV_1/FVC ratios of less than 80% indicate the presence of an obstructive process. Individual values of pulmonary function test results may be misleading. The FEV_1, for example, may already be low if the vital capacity is also decreased or the patient is uncooperative with the spirometric tests.

Numerous studies have found preoperative pulmonary function studies to be poor indicators of postoperative pulmonary

---

BOX **20-11**

Therapeutic Maneuvers to Decrease Risk of Pulmonary Complications

Preoperative
Instruction in respiratory maneuvers
Smoking cessation
Antibiotic treatment of pulmonary infection
Antibiotic treatment of chronic bronchitis
Expectorants
Psychologic preparation
Bronchodilator therapy for asthmatics
Maintenance of good nutrition
Chest physiotherapy
Weight reduction

Postoperative
Adequate pain control with minimization of postoperative opioid analgesia
Maximal inspiration maneuvers, incentive spirometry, chest physiotherapy
Mobilization of secretions
Early mobilization of elderly patients
Cough encouragement
Heparin prophylaxis in selected cases

Data from Mohr DN, Lavender RC. Preoperative pulmonary evaluation. Identifying patients at increased risk for complications. Postgrad Med. 1996;100:241-256; Marienau MES, Buck CF. Preoperative evaluation of the pulmonary patient undergoing nonpulmonary surgery. J Perianesth Nurs. 1998;13:340-348; Wang JS. Pulmonary function tests in preoperative pulmonary evaluation. Resp Med. 2004;98:598-605.

---

complications.[133-135] All patients scheduled to undergo lung resection should have spirometric assessment preoperatively to estimate postoperative FEV_1 and suitability for resection.[127] It is not necessary to routinely obtain spirometric data prior to high-risk noncardiothoracic surgery. The value of pulmonary function testing prior to noncardiothoracic surgery is unproven and should be reserved for symptomatic patients suspected of having COPD.[136]

Asthma

Unlike other COPDs, asthma is characterized by reversible airflow obstruction. Inflammation of the airways is the hallmark of asthma. Distal bronchoconstriction results from airway hyperreactivity to stimuli that have little or no effect on normal airways. Precipitating factors include allergens, exercise, upper respiratory tract infections (URTIs), emotional stressors, and unidentified triggers.[130] Pertinent data obtained from the medical history are detailed in Box 20-12.[137,138]

Information gleaned from these questions will help establish the nature and stability of the disease process. Patients with a history of coexistent cardiovascular disease, copious sputum production, previous perioperative complications from asthma, recurrent nocturnal awakenings from asthma, frequent or continuous systemic corticosteroid requirement, or a recent hospitalization or emergency visit for asthma are considered to be at greater risk for perioperative aggravation of their asthma.

BOX **20-12**

Pertinent Data Obtained from the Medical History

Asthma Control and Current Therapy

- The frequency of asthmatic attacks
- The time interval since the last attack
- Recent asthma exacerbation? How long since the patient was last hospitalized or treated in the emergency department for an asthmatic attack?
- Increased use of inhaled short-acting β-agonists? Use per week?
- Current or past use of inhaled corticosteroids?
- Most recent course of oral corticosteroids?
- What works best for treating an acute asthmatic event?

Asthma History and Complicating Conditions or Factors

- Recent upper respiratory tract infection or sinus infection?
- Recent pneumonia? Was this documented on chest radiograph?
- What triggers an asthmatic attack?
- The severity of attacks (Was endotracheal intubation or intensive care unit admission required?)
- History of pulmonary complications with prior surgical procedures?
- History of long-term corticosteroid use or corticosteroid-dependent asthma?

Modified from Zaglaniczny K, Aker J, eds. Clinical Guide to Pediatric Anesthesia. *Philadelphia: Saunders; 1999; Tirumalasetty J, Grammer LC. Asthma, surgery, and general anesthesia: a review.* J Asthma. *2006;43:251-254.*

Asthma should be under optimal medical management before a patient undergoes elective surgery and anesthesia. If the patient has a persistent cough, wheezing, or tachypnea on the day surgery is scheduled, it is best to reschedule surgery to allow for additional treatment of the asthma.

The need for diagnostic testing is based on the clinician's assessment of the severity of the disease and magnitude of the operative procedure. An ECG is indicated if right ventricular hypertrophy is presumed, typically implying long-standing insufficient therapy. A chest radiograph is considered only if the patient is suspected of having an acute infiltrative process (e.g., pneumonia, pneumothorax in an acute exacerbation) or if a recent change in the patient's physical status is suggestive of a worsening pulmonary condition.[139] Arterial blood gases are usually indicated only when signs of chronic respiratory insufficiency (e.g., hypoxia, hypercarbia) are suspected or in patients with acute asthma who require emergency surgery. If age appropriate, spirometric evaluation consisting of a peak expiratory flow rate should be performed the morning of surgery if active disease is suspected. The results should be compared with the patient's best value in recent weeks. Findings will be:

- Normal: 80% to 100% of baseline
- Moderate exacerbation: 50% to 80% of baseline
- Severe episode indicating the need for delay of surgery and more intensive therapy: less than 50% of baseline

Peak expiratory flow is of limited use in assessing asthma preoperatively, because other symptoms or clinical signs of poor asthma control are usually present.[139]

Early preoperative patient assessment promotes optimizing pharmacotherapy in the days prior to the scheduled surgery (Table 20-8).[140] Patient medications should be continued up to and on the day of surgery. Prophylactic β-adrenergic metered-dose inhalers should be used on the morning of surgery and accompany the patient to the operating room. Oral medications (e.g., theophylline) may be taken with a sip (1 to 2 oz) of water up to 1 to 2 hours before surgery. Therapeutic serum theophylline levels, 10 to 20 mcg/mL, should be confirmed if theophylline is used. Supplemental stress doses of corticosteroids may be appropriate if the patient has recently taken corticosteroids. Antianxiety premedication should be considered; psychologic triggers such as anxiety are common.

Ensure adequate hydration (e.g., minimize the fasting interval) to reduce airway desiccation and improve mobilization of secretions. If signs and symptoms of infection are present, surgery may be postponed while antibiotic therapy, based on sputum Gram stain and cultures, is initiated.

Upper Respiratory Tract Infection

Children with URTIs, particularly those younger than 1 year, have an increased risk (twofold to sevenfold increase) of respiratory-related adverse events intraoperatively and postoperatively (e.g., bronchospasm, laryngospasm, hypoxemia, atelectasis, croup, stridor). Signs and symptoms of URTI include sore throat; inflamed and reddened nasopharyngeal and oropharyngeal mucosa; sneezing; rhinorrhea (clear secretions) or mucopurulent nasal secretions; nasal congestion, including watery eyes; malaise; bulging, tender eardrums with associated inflammation; nonproductive cough; fever of 37.5° to 38.5° C (greater than 38° C associated with lower respiratory tract involvement); laryngitis or tonsillitis; viral ulcers in the oropharynx; and white blood cell count greater than 12,000 cells/mm³ with a left shift. Positive chest findings such as pulmonary congestion and rales are usually associated with lower respiratory tract involvement.

Each case should be reviewed individually. The decision to operate frequently depends on the urgency of the surgery, the duration and complexity of the surgery, and the need for instrumentation of the airway (Figure 20-4).[141] Children with uncomplicated URTIs may undergo elective procedures without significantly increasing anesthesia complications.[142] It is important to obtain a specific history to distinguish a chronic state from an acute, superimposed infectious process, which has predictive value for morbidity. Parents will be the best resource for establishing baseline conditions. If the parents state that the child typically has a cold or chronic runny nose (clear rhinorrhea) and is in his or her optimal state (afebrile, without respiratory distress), short elective procedures may be considered. If the child has a productive cough from lower respiratory tract involvement or an infectious-appearing runny nose, elective surgery should be postponed. However, it may be necessary to schedule children who have chronic URTIs for procedures such as myringotomy with ventilation tube placement or tonsillectomies, because URTIs are commonly associated with these conditions. Exercise caution with children younger than 5 years (consider postponing the procedure for children less than age 1) because risks are increased. If the child is older than 1 year with a resolving URTI, it is reasonable to proceed with minor procedures not requiring endotracheal intubation (intubation with URTI increases risk 11-fold).

TABLE 20-8	Guidelines for Preoperative Asthma Pharmacotherapy
Clinical Characteristics of Asthma	**Corresponding Preoperative Pharmacologic Therapy**
No asthma symptoms	No additional asthma therapy preoperatively
Not on any asthma medications	
No flares in asthma symptoms over past year	
Spirometry does not show significant obstruction	
On bronchodilators only	Initiate therapy with inhaled corticosteroid, beclomethasone 320 mcg per day or equivalent dose, 1 week before surgery
No history of oral corticosteroid use	
Spirometry is not below baseline	If spirometry is below baseline or patient is having flare of symptoms, consider adding prednisone 0.5 mg/kg for 5 days before surgery
Already on inhaled corticosteroid	Continue treatment with inhaled corticosteroid
Spirometry at or below baseline	Treat with prednisone 0.5 mg/kg for 5 days before surgery
	Treat with hydrocortisone 100 mg IV every 8 hours the morning before surgery and postoperatively until stable
Patient is already on oral steroids	Increase dose of oral steroids for 5 days before surgery
	Treat with hydrocortisone 100 mg IV every 8 hours the morning before surgery and postoperatively until stable

From Tirumalasetty J, Grammer LC. Asthma, surgery, and general anesthesia: a review. J Asthma. 2006;43:251-254.

Infectious nasopharyngitis (without lower respiratory tract involvement) requires postponing the surgery for 2 weeks after peak symptoms.[143] If the child exhibits signs and symptoms of lower respiratory tract involvement, it is prudent to postpone an elective surgical procedure for 4 to 6 weeks, the time necessary to minimize airway hyperactivity.

Laboratory testing may consist of a complete blood count, including differential. The value of obtaining a preoperative white blood cell count has been questioned because it is of little value and rarely is a factor in determining whether to proceed with the surgery.[144] Nasal or throat cultures may be obtained if signs of an infectious process are observed. A chest radiograph is not warranted, especially if chest sounds are clear. Pulmonary function tests and arterial blood gas analysis rarely offer any useful information.

Gastrointestinal System

Evaluation of the gastrointestinal system includes preoperative determination of the presence of nausea and vomiting, diarrhea, occult or overt gastrointestinal bleeding, abdominal or referred pain, abdominal distention, palpable masses, dysphagia, or gastric hyperacidity, with or without reflux. The fluid and electrolyte status of the patient is reviewed, especially when gastrointestinal symptoms are associated with weight loss or malabsorption. Active bleeding requires preoperative hemoglobin concentration measurement. The hematocrit value may be falsely elevated as a result of hemoconcentration in patients with acute or chronic bleeding. Radiographic and CT scans of the abdomen are reviewed for evidence of obstruction or masses. The presence of peptic ulcer disease or esophageal hiatal hernia is also ascertained. For affected patients, prophylactic measures to reduce the risk of aspiration and its adverse pulmonary sequelae (e.g., aspiration pneumonitis) are instituted before surgery.

Hepatobiliary System

Preoperative evaluation of the hepatobiliary system includes screening for the presence of acute or chronic liver parenchymal disease, such as hepatitis or cirrhosis, or cholestatic liver disease. Because of the tremendous reserve of the liver, progression of hepatic disease is often insidious. Signs and symptoms may be inapparent or vague until physiologic functions of the hepatobiliary system (Box 20-13) are markedly affected. Liver function tests are also limited in their ability to reflect the acuity and extent of hepatobiliary disease.[145] Considerable damage to the liver may be evident before laboratory test results are altered.

During the early stages of hepatitis or cirrhosis, the clinical presentation ranges from one in which the patient is asymptomatic with normal liver function tests to one in which the patient has malaise, weight loss, abdominal discomfort, and mild jaundice with mild elevations in bilirubin levels. In cases of unexplained jaundice or elevated transaminase levels, suspicions of hepatobiliary dysfunction should be thoroughly investigated by a preoperative consultation with a gastroenterologist. Elective surgery is postponed until a definitive diagnosis and treatment are established and indicators of active inflammation (e.g., transaminase levels, cellular infiltration on liver biopsy, etc.) have subsided. Further decompensation of hepatic function may follow anesthesia and surgery, notably after intraabdominal procedures. Figure 20-5 offers an algorithm for the preoperative assessment of the patient with known or suspected liver disease.[146]

Progression of hepatobiliary disease to overt hepatic failure may be evidenced by gross abnormalities of liver function test results, including coagulopathies; extreme jaundice with or without cyanosis; generalized tremors and increased deep tendon reflexes; ascites, spider nevi, and hepatosplenomegaly; hepatorenal failure; and signs of hepatic encephalopathy.[147]

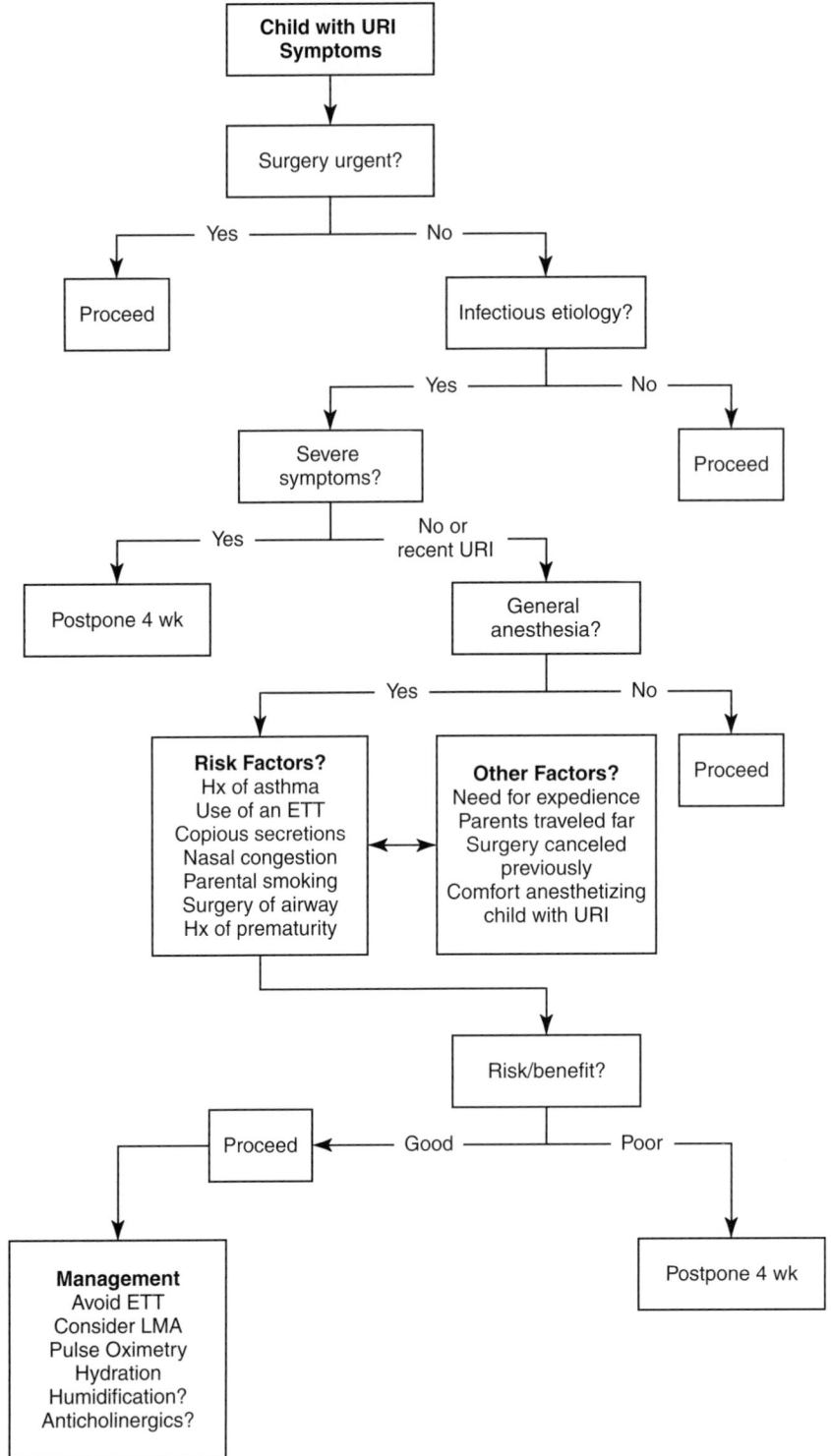

FIGURE **20-4** Suggested algorithm for the assessment and anesthetic management of the child with an upper respiratory infection. *Hx*, History; *ETT*, endotracheal tube; *LMA*, laryngeal mask airway; *URI*, upper respiratory infection. (*From Tait AR, Malviya S. Anesthesia for the child with an upper respiratory tract infection: still a dilemma? Anesth Analg. 2005;100:59-65.*)

Elective surgery is avoided at this time because surgery on a patient with hepatic failure is associated with an extremely high incidence of morbidity and mortality. Anesthesia may be required, however, for a patient who requires a palliative or emergent procedure. Placement of a portocaval shunt and the surgical control of hemorrhage from esophageal varices are common procedures, given the growing number of patients with advanced liver disease. Anesthetic management is supportive in such situations and focused on minimizing the risk of further hepatobiliary deterioration. Administration of

BOX **20-13**

Physiologic Functions of the Hepatobiliary System

Bilirubin Formation and Excretion
Conjugation of free bilirubin and secretion into bile

Carbohydrate Metabolism
Glycogenesis
Gluconeogenesis
Glycogenolysis

Fat Metabolism
Lipogenesis
Lipolysis

Protein Metabolism
Formation of proteins, such as albumin, prothrombin, transferrin, and glycoprotein
Synthesis of plasma cholinesterase
Deamination of proteins, such as hormones, into ammonia and urea

Hormone Metabolism Drug Detoxification
Conversion of lipophilic drugs into inactive hydrophilic substances
Hydrolysis of ester linkages by plasma cholinesterase

Vitamin Storage
Storage of fat-soluble vitamins A, D, E, and K
Storage of anti–pernicious anemia factor, vitamin B_{12}

Synthesis of Coagulation Factors and Inhibitors
Synthesis of most clotting factors, including prothrombin, fibrinogen, factors V, VII, IX, and X
Synthesis of antithrombin
Mast-cell production of heparin

Phagocytosis
Filtration and destruction of bacteria and debris in blood circulating through hepatic sinusoids by Kupffer cells

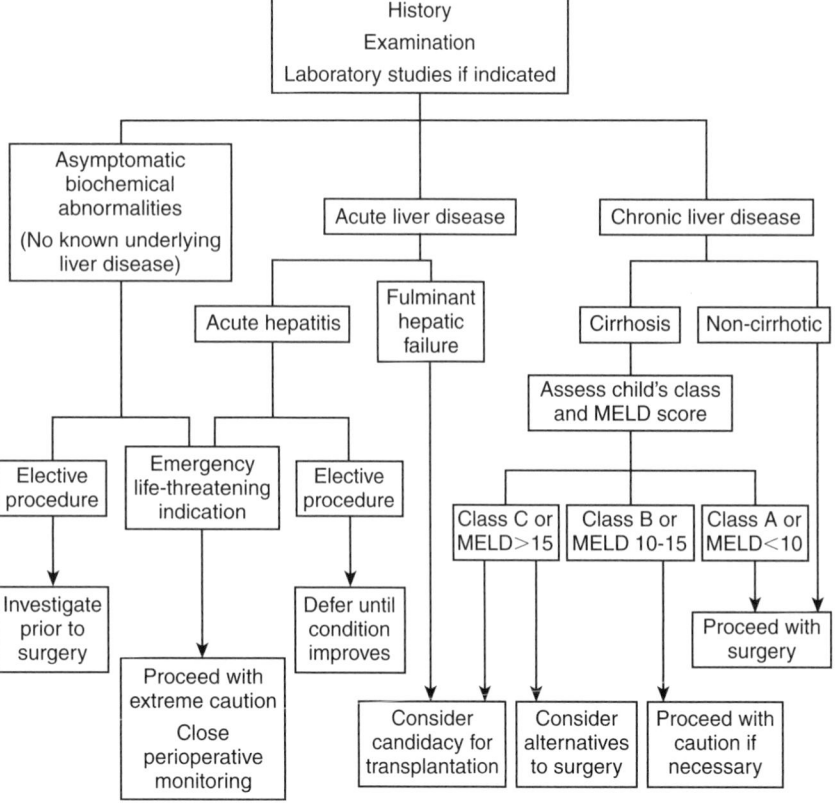

FIGURE **20-5** Suggested algorithm for assessing the patient with known or suspected liver disease. The MELD (Model for End-stage Liver Disease) scoring system to objectively assess liver disease severity. (*From Keegan MT, Plevak DJ. Preoperative assessment of the patient with liver disease.* Am J Gastroenterol. *2005;100:2116-2127.*)

phytonadione (AquaMEPHYTON) and transfusion of fresh frozen plasma and cryoprecipitate may be required for the correction of preoperative coagulopathies. Sedative premedicants are avoided in the disoriented or somnolent patient in whom hepatic encephalopathy has been diagnosed. Because of the rapid development of hypoglycemia, the patient's blood glucose level is checked preoperatively. The acid-base balance, electrolyte status, and extent of hepatorenal reserve may be determined by arterial blood gas analysis, serum multiphasic profiles, and liver function tests.[147]

The interpretation of liver function tests should be approached cautiously. Differential diagnosis of parenchymal versus cholestatic liver disease is limited by the insensitivity and nonspecificity of current lab analysis, especially serum transaminase and alkaline phosphatase levels.[148] Aspartate transaminase (AST) or serum glutamic oxaloacetic transaminase (SGOT); alanine transaminase (ALT) or serum glutamic pyruvic transaminase (SGPT); and lactate dehydrogenase (LDH) are commonly measured hepatocellular enzymes also distributed throughout cells of the lungs, heart, kidneys, and skeletal muscles. Increases in their serum concentrations are therefore not always indicative of hepatobiliary disease. Greater specificity can be derived from isoenzyme-5 fractions of the enzymes, such as LDH.[149]

In cases of biliary obstruction or irritation, alkaline phosphatase enzymes may be released from the cells of bile ducts. Increases in serum concentrations of these enzymes also help differentiate hepatic dysfunction caused by parenchymal disease from that caused by cholestasis. The interpretation of these results is again limited by the presence of extrahepatic stores of alkaline phosphatase. In this situation, cholestatic liver disease can be confirmed by high serum levels of conjugated (direct) bilirubin.[150] Causative factors are then determined from discussions with a gastroenterologist and the results of ultrasound, CT, and endoscopic retrograde cholangiopancreatographic scans.

When acute parenchymal injury is evident, prolongation of prothrombin time offers the most rapid and reliable hallmark of liver dysfunction and is shown to have prognostic significance. It reflects the inability of the acutely damaged liver to synthesize clotting factors. Although the production of albumin is also affected, its plasma half-life exceeds that of prothrombin. Hypoalbuminemia may then be inapparent for days after an acute hepatocellular insult.[151]

Once a functional impairment of the liver has been established, the cause is investigated as part of the preoperative evaluation. Cirrhosis and hepatitis, for example, are frequently associated with long-standing alcohol abuse. The increasing consumption of alcohol in the United States parallels the rising incidence of liver disease. Exposure to hepatotoxic agents in the workplace, such as carbon tetrachloride or vinyl chloride, should be ruled out. Hepatotoxic drugs may then be discontinued or avoided before surgery. These drugs commonly include acetaminophen and other nonsteroidal antiinflammatory drugs, aspirin, methyldopa, isoniazid, and rifampin.[152,153] Finally, a diagnosis of infectious hepatitis should be pursued in patients with hepatobiliary disease of unknown cause and in patients considered to be at high risk, which includes those with a history of hemodialysis, multiple blood transfusions, or intravenous drug abuse. Because of the virulent nature of the hepatitis viruses, care of an infected patient also poses an occupational hazard for anesthesia providers.[154] Maximum precautions must be consistently exercised, and vaccination with the hepatitis B virus, as recommended by the Centers for Disease Control and Prevention, should be performed.[155]

Renal System

Evaluation of the kidneys and urinary tract includes preoperative determination of the patient's volume status and presence of polyuria; urinary incontinence or retention; microscopic or frank hematuria; recurrent infections in the form of glomerulonephritis, pyelonephritis, or cystitis; dysuria; and oliguria or anuria. Fluid balance is calculated from the patient's intake and output during the hospital stay. Preoperative dehydration may be evident, for example, in a patient receiving long-term diuretic therapy. Polyuria, when not attributed to diuretics, may reflect glycosuria or, rarely, inadequate secretion of antidiuretic hormone (diabetes insipidus). Urinary retention and other signs of

TABLE **20-9**	Common Renal Function Tests
Test	**Reference Range**
Urea nitrogen	5-25 mg/dL
Creatinine	0.5-1.5 mg/dL
Sodium	133-147 mmol/L
Potassium	3.2-5.2 mmol/L
Chloride	94-110 mmol/L
CO_2	22-32 mmol/L
Uric acid	2.5-7.5 mg/dL
Calcium	8.5-10.5 mg/dL
Phosphorus	2.2-4.2 mg/dL
Urinalysis, routine	
Color	Straw-amber
Appearance	Clear-hazy
Protein	0 mg/dL
Blood	Negative
Glucose	0 mg/dL
Ketones	0 mg/dL
pH	4.5-8
Specific gravity	1.002-1.030
Bilirubin	Negative
Urinalysis, micro	
Red blood cells	0-3/high-power field
White blood cells	0-5/high-power field
Casts	0-2/low-power field

Modified from Malhotra V, ed. Anesthesia for Renal and Genitourinary Surgery. New York: McGraw-Hill; 1996.

neurogenic bladder may be caused by a spinal cord injury or long-standing diabetes mellitus. Frequent catheterizations are often necessary in such situations, increasing the patient's risk for developing chronic urinary tract infections. Preoperative urinalysis and culture are therefore required so infection can be ruled out. Treatment and resolution should be accomplished before elective surgery is performed, especially for procedures involving the placement of a prosthetic graft for a mitral valve or total hip replacement. Problems with intraoperative bladder catheterization can be anticipated in patients with dysuria or voiding difficulties. In older men, these problems are frequently attributed to chronic prostatism. Untreated prostatic hypertrophy, as well as renal calculi and congenital malformations of the ureters, results in obstructed urinary outflow. Over time these conditions may lead to a state of chronic renal insufficiency or failure.

Any suspicion of renal dysfunction should be investigated before surgery. Unfortunately, clinical evidence of renal insufficiency may not be apparent until at least 70% of nephrons are nonfunctional. Accurate diagnosis of renal insufficiency is further limited by the insensitivity of laboratory tests (Table 20-9).[156] Blood urea nitrogen (BUN) concentrations, for example, do not accurately reflect glomerular filtration rate (GFR). Although urea is freely filtered at the glomerulus, it is reabsorbed to a large and variable extent through the tubules. BUN levels are also affected by the amount of protein ingested in the gastrointestinal tract and the amount of urea metabolized by the liver, as well as by the catabolic state of the patient. Because tubular reabsorption of creatinine does not occur, creatinine levels correlate more with the rate of glomerular filtration than do BUN concentrations. The serum levels of creatinine, a by-product of skeletal muscle metabolism, can reflect the muscle mass and catabolic state of each patient. This characteristic limits its precision in determining the magnitude of nephron loss. Normal serum creatinine levels may be higher, for example, in a muscular man than in a woman. Conversely, serum creatinine levels can remain within the normal range in the elderly patient, despite a progressive decline in glomerular function,[157] because of the decrease in muscle mass associated with aging.

The most accurate reflection of renal reserve or GFR is creatinine clearance, which reflects the ability of glomeruli to excrete creatinine into the urine at a given blood concentration. The drawbacks of this assessment lie in the cost and time required for the collection of urine samples. As a general principle, urine is collected over a 24-hour period and the creatinine clearance rate is measured by the following equation:

Equation 20-1

$$GFR \ (mL/min) = UV \div P$$

where U is the urinary concentration of creatinine (mg/dL), V is the volume of urine (mL/min), and P is the plasma concentration of creatinine (mg/dL).

Accurate measures of GFR also can be calculated from a 2-hour specimen.[158] Creatinine clearance or GFR values between 50 and 80 mL/min are indicative of mild renal dysfunction. Renal failure is otherwise evident when creatinine clearance levels decrease to less than 10 mL/min.

Practically all surgical patients with chronic renal failure are undergoing dialysis, usually hemodialysis performed at the hospital or renal facility. Others undergo continuous ambulatory peritoneal dialysis. The goal of dialysis therapy is to maintain a reasonable degree of homeostasis, although BUN and creatinine concentrations remain abnormal. The preoperative evaluation and preparation of the patient with chronic renal failure should therefore focus on fluid and electrolyte balance, as well as on the extent of concomitant diseases. Estimates of volume status are derived from the amount of weight gained between periods of dialysis. Fluid overload may also be evidenced by jugular vein distention, peripheral and periorbital edema, and bibasilar rales.

Preoperative measurement of serum potassium concentration is recommended within 6 to 8 hours of surgery, regardless of whether dialysis is performed, because unexpected hyperkalemia, with its adverse cardiac effects, is known to occur rapidly. In cases in which the serum potassium level exceeds 5.5 mEq/L and congestive heart failure is apparent, elective surgery should be delayed until after dialysis. When postponement is not feasible, as with emergency surgery to relieve a pericardial effusion or procedures to revise a hemodialysis shunt, measures to reduce the serum potassium concentration are then instituted. In the presence of tall, tented T waves on the ECG, these measures may include the infusion of a dextrose-insulin solution.

Although hemoglobin ranges from 5 to 8 mg/dL are not unusual in patients with chronic renal failure, a hemoglobin level should also be obtained as part of the preoperative evaluation. Chronic anemia is predominantly caused by decreases in renal erythropoietin production and enhanced fragility of red blood cells in the presence of uremia. It is further exacerbated by blood loss experienced with hemodialysis and chronic gastrointestinal bleeding. When extreme fatigue and pallor, limited exercise tolerance, and persistent tachycardia are evident before major surgery, the transfusion of packed red blood cells may be necessary. Because repeat transfusion and immunosuppression therapy are often required during the course of chronic renal failure, the patient is at greater risk for being infected with the hepatitis virus, human immunodeficiency virus (HIV), or both. Coagulopathies are also suspected. The most likely cause is a decrease in platelet adhesiveness secondary to the chronic state of metabolic acidemia. Hemodialysis can be effectively used for the correction of prolonged bleeding times before surgery in this situation.

Throughout the perioperative period, most therapeutic regimens for patients with chronic renal failure can be continued, including the administration of antihypertensives, digitalis preparations, corticosteroids, and insulin.[159] Requirements for preoperative sedation may be less than anticipated, and medications with prolonged durations, such as diazepam, are avoided.[160] Peripheral arteriovenous shunts should be assessed for patency and infection. Measurement of noninvasive blood pressures and application of intravenous lines are avoided in the limb of the graft. Administration of gastrointestinal preparations (e.g., antacids and gastrokinetic agents) and drainage of peritoneal dialysate, aimed at reducing the risks of regurgitation and pulmonary aspiration, are instituted when preparing the patient with chronic renal failure for anesthesia and surgery.

Endocrine System

Endocrine diseases of concern in the preoperative evaluation include diabetes mellitus, thyroid gland disorders, and adrenocortical dysfunctions. End-organ effects of each of these diseases increase perioperative risk substantially. For example, morbidity and mortality rates are 5 to 10 times greater in diabetic patients with renal and autonomic nervous system involvement.[161]

Diabetes

Diabetes mellitus is the most common of endocrine disorders, affecting more than 20.8 million people—7% of the population—in the United States.[162] Thirty-eight percent of people ages 65 years or older report having diabetes. It represents a dysfunction in glucose metabolism caused by impaired synthesis, secretion, or use of insulin.

Most patients with diabetes (90% to 95%) are not dependent on exogenous insulin for the regulation of blood glucose levels. As shown in Table 20-10, the patient with non–insulin-dependent, or type 2, diabetes often benefits from diet modification, weight control, and exercise alone. An oral hypoglycemic agent (Table 20-11) may also be added to the patient's therapeutic regimen.[163] The remaining 5% to 10% of patients with diabetes are dependent on insulin preparations listed on Table 20-12 and are therefore classified as having insulin-dependent, or type 1, diabetes mellitus.[164,165] These patients are susceptible to periods of hyperglycemia and ketoacidosis. As a result of microvascular changes, they are also prone to the development of severe end-organ complications, including diabetic retinopathy and cataract formation, somatic and autonomic insufficiency (orthostatic hypotension, bradycardia, gastroparesis), and nephropathy. Because of acquired abnormalities in the macrovasculature, patients with type 2 diabetes are more likely to have hypertension, coronary artery disease (which frequently is asymptomatic), and peripheral vascular disease. Death in the majority of patients with diabetes is secondary to complications of atherosclerosis (MI, stroke).[166]

The aim of an evaluation of a patient with diabetes, notably one with type 1 diabetes mellitus, is ascertaining the degree of preoperative blood glucose control and the presence of major organ system dysfunction. Renal and cardiovascular complications of diabetes substantially heighten perioperative morbidity and mortality. Particular attention should be paid to:

- Diabetes—type of disease, method of home monitoring and usual metabolic control
- Drugs—antidiabetic medication, medication for associated diseases

- Cardiovascular disease—including an assessment of exercise tolerance
- Renal disease
- Neuropathy—peripheral and autonomic, in particular gastric paresis
- Airway—diabetics with stiff joint syndrome (due to glycosylation) often have limited mobility of the upper cervical spine and are more likely to have a poor view on direct laryngoscopy, and they may therefore present difficulties with tracheal intubation.[167]

Early preoperative evaluation and workup of diabetic patients are important. This is especially true in patients who are noncompliant, patients whose blood glucose level is poorly controlled, and patients with newly diagnosed diabetes, because modifications in their care may be necessary before surgery. Early assessment of a patient allows for consultation with a medical internist to optimize the patient's preoperative condition before anesthesia and surgery. Elective surgery is also postponed in cases of extreme hyperglycemia and ketoacidosis. Aggressive fluid, electrolyte, and insulin therapy are initiated, and the cause of ketoacidosis must be investigated before surgery.

Consultation with a cardiologist may also help a practitioner evaluate and improve the preoperative cardiac status of a patient with diabetes, especially if the patient is undergoing a procedure associated with a greater risk of perioperative myocardial ischemia, such as a carotid endarterectomy or an abdominal aortic aneurysm resection. Because of the high incidence of ischemic heart disease in this population, exercise stress testing and a 12-lead ECG may be performed. Orthostatic hypotension, resting tachycardia, and lack of respiratory variability in cardiac rhythm may reflect autonomic neuropathy (20% to 40%). Abnormalities in autonomic function may also result in bladder atrophy and delayed gastric emptying times in nearly 50% of diabetic patients.[168] A gastrokinetic agent, such as metoclopramide, should be administered before surgery to reduce the incidence of regurgitation and pulmonary aspiration during general anesthesia.

TABLE 20-10   Distinguishing Features of Diabetes Mellitus

	Type 1	Type 2
Previous name	Insulin-dependent diabetes	Non–insulin-dependent diabetes
Age of onset	Childhood	Middle age or elderly
Timing of onset	Abrupt	Gradual
Predisposing factors	Genetic	Obesity, pregnancy, drugs
Prevalence	0.2%-0.3%	2%-4%
Insulin requirement	Always	Infrequent
Ketoacidosis	Common	Rare
Systemic complications	Frequent	Frequent

Modified from Inzucchi SE, Sherwin RS. Diabetes mellitus. In: Goldman L, Ausiello D, eds. Cecil Textbook of Medicine. 23rd ed. Philadelphia: Saunders; 2008; Barash GP et al, eds. Clinical Anesthesia, 2nd ed. Philadelphia: Lippincott; 1992.

TABLE 20-11   Oral Hypoglycemic Therapy

Drug Class	Drug Name	Onset	Duration of Action
First-generation sulfonylureas	Tolbutamide	1 hr	12 hr
	Acetohexamide	3 hr	24 hr
	Tolazamide	4 hr	16 hr
	Chlorpropamide	2 hr	24 hr
Second-generation sulfonylureas	Glyburide	30 min	24 hr
	Glipizide	IR 30 min	IR 24 hr
		ER 2-4 hr	ER 24 hr
	Glimepiride	2-3 hr	24 hr
Biguanides	Metformin	1-3 hr	17 hr
Thiazolidinediones	Rosiglitazone	1-3 hr	4 hr
	Pioglitazone	2 hr	N/A
Glinides	Repaglinide	30-90 min	4 hr
Alpha-glucosidase inhibitor	Acarbose	2 hr	4 hr
	Miglitol	1 hr	4 hr

From Schwartz AJ, ed. ASA Refresher Courses in Anesthesiology. Philadelphia: Lippincott; 2001.
ER, *Extended release;* IR, *immediate release;* N/A, *not available.*

TABLE **20-12**	Insulin Preparations and Guidelines			
Insulin Type	**Onset**	**Peak (hr)**	**Duration (hr)**	**Comments**
Very Rapid				
Lispro; Aspart	IV immediate; subQ 5-15 min	subQ 0.5-1.5	subQ 3-4	Usually administered immediately prior to a meal; use subQ or via an insulin pump, but not recommended for continuous infusion
Short-Acting				
Regular	IV immediate; subQ 30-60 min	subQ 2-3	subQ 3-6	Usually administered 30-60 min before meals; most common in continuous IV infusions
Intermediate-Acting				
NPH	subQ 2-4 hr	subQ 6-10	subQ 10-16	Often combined with regular insulin
Lente	subQ 3-4 hr	subQ 6-12	subQ 12-18	
Long-Acting				
Ultralente	subQ 6-10 hr	subQ 10-16	subQ 18-20	Perioperative use uncommon
Glargine	subQ 4 hr	Minimal peak activity	subQ 24	May be administered as usual to provide basal insulin levels during surgery
Combinations				
75/25 (75% protamine lispro, 25% insulin lispro)	subQ 30-60 min	Dual	10-14	
70/30 (70% NPH, 30% regular)	subQ 30-60 min	Dual	10-16	Usually given before breakfast
50/50 (50% NPH, 50% regular)	subQ 30-60 min	Dual	10-16	Usually given before dinner

From Connery LE, Coursin DB. Assessment and therapy of selected endocrine disorders. Anesthesiology Clin North America. 2004;22:93-123; Powers AC. Diabetes mellitus. In: Fauci AS et al, eds. Harrison's Principles of Internal Medicine. 17th ed. New York: McGraw-Hill; 2008:2275-2304.
IV, Intravenous; subQ, subcutaneous.

It is best to schedule surgery as early in the day as possible to minimize the fasting period. Just before surgery, diabetic patients who require insulin or oral hypoglycemic agents should have blood glucose checked. Depending on the type and length of surgery and the lability of diabetes, serum glucose levels are checked intraoperatively and in the postanesthesia care unit at 2- to 4-hour intervals. The goal of perioperative insulin therapy is to maintain the serum glucose level less than 180 mg/dL while avoiding hypoglycemia.[169] Several different regimens are available for the treatment of diabetic patients undergoing surgery and anesthesia. Consultation with the physician responsible for managing the diabetes is helpful in determining an acceptable range of serum glucose and when and what type of insulin therapy may be appropriate. Patients taking oral hypoglycemic agents should withhold the short half-life agents (e.g., repaglinide and acarbose) on the day of surgery and withhold the longer-lasting agents (e.g., chlorpropamide and glimepiride) for up to 48 hours. Fasting patients who are receiving insulin should have intravenous access established with a crystalloid solution containing 5% glucose. Insulin may then be administered to the patient intravenously (bolus or continuous infusion) or subcutaneously. The intravenous technique of administering regular insulin offers the advantage of providing a more predictable serum drug level and metabolic control. The intravenous route still has the risk of making the patient hyperglycemic or hypoglycemic if the glucose or insulin infusions become unbalanced. The tighter the control of glucose levels, the more frequent the glucose monitoring. The subcutaneous route of insulin administration has been criticized

as being too unpredictable in its absorption, especially perioperatively, with alterations in blood pressure and cutaneous blood flow.[170] In the patient with type I diabetes, a common approach, especially for brief procedures, is to subcutaneously administer a fraction (often one third to one half) of the patient's usual morning dose of intermediate- or long-acting insulin. For patients with either insulin-dependent or non–insulin-dependent diabetes, the most important goal of perioperative management is the prevention of hyperglycemia and especially hypoglycemia, as well as their adverse consequences, during surgical stress.

Thyroid Gland Disorders
Although disorders of the thyroid gland are relatively uncommon, the anesthesia provider may still encounter patients with hyperthyroidism or hypothyroidism who require surgery. Most have undergone adequate medical therapy before anesthesia and surgery are performed. Nevertheless, the anesthesia provider should be aware of the clinical manifestations of thyroid gland dysfunctions (Table 20-13).[86,171]

Hyperthyroidism. Hyperthyroidism is caused by an excess secretion of thyroid hormones, 3,5,3'-triiodothyronine (T_3) and tetraiodothyronine (thyroxine or T_4). It is evident in such conditions as Graves disease, toxic goiter (multinodular, single), thyroid carcinoma, and pituitary tumors that oversecrete thyroid-stimulating hormone (TSH). Signs and symptoms reflect a hypermetabolic state with sympathetic overactivity resulting from the primary effects of thyroid hormones on the adenylate cyclase system.[171]

TABLE 20-13	Clinical Features of Thyroid Gland Disorders	
	Hyperthyroidism	**Hypothyroidism**
General	Heat intolerance, weight loss, tremor, sweating, warm, moist skin	Cold intolerance, thinning hair, arthralgia, alopecia, "strawberries and cream" complexion, gruff voice
Cardiovascular	Tachycardia, cardiac arrhythmias, wide pulse pressure, elevated systolic blood pressure, decreased diastolic blood pressure, increased left ventricular contractility & ejection fraction, atrial fibrillation & heart failure in elderly	Bradycardia, cardiomegaly, cardiac failure, increased peripheral resistance, pericardial effusions
Respiratory	Dyspnea	Hypoventilation, sleep apnea
Gastrointestinal	Diarrhea, nausea, vomiting	Decreased gastrointestinal motility, constipation
Neurologic	Anxiety, irritability, hyperactive reflexes, insomnia; depression, withdrawal, and apathy in elderly	Fatigue, lethargy, slow mental function, hypoactive reflexes, myxedema coma
Musculoskeletal	Goiter, weight loss, proximal myopathy, bone resorption	Goiter, lethargy, large tongue, amyloidosis, peripheral neuropathy, muscle stiffness
Ophthalmic	Exophthalmos, lid lag, lid retraction, reduced blinking	
Renal		Impaired free water clearance
Hematologic	Hypercalcemia, thrombocytopenia, mild anemia	Anemia, coagulopathy

Modified from Connery LE, Coursin DB. Assessment and therapy of selected endocrine disorders. Anesthesiol Clin North America. 2004;22:93-123; Barash PG et al, eds. Clinical Anesthesia. 5th ed. Philadelphia: Lippincott Williams & Wilkins; 2006.

The preoperative preparation of the hyperthyroid patient is aimed at attaining a euthyroid state. This may be accomplished through administration of antithyroid drugs such as methimazole or propylthiouracil for 6 to 8 weeks followed by iodine for 7 to 14 days.[171] Not only does propylthiouracil decrease the overall synthesis of thyroxine, it lessens its conversion into the more potent T_3. Reversible agranulocytosis is infrequently seen with long-term therapy.[172] A complete blood cell and platelet count should be determined preoperatively. Beta-antagonist drugs, such as propranolol and esmolol, are also useful adjuncts in the management of hyperthyroidism. They ameliorate signs of sympathetic nervous system overstimulation such as tachycardia, diaphoresis, and tremors.

All drugs used to manage hyperthyroidism, including propylthiouracil and propranolol, should be continued perioperatively, and elective surgery is postponed until the patient is rendered euthyroid. If emergency surgery cannot be delayed for a patient with symptomatic hyperthyroidism, a continuous infusion of esmolol (100 to 300 mcg/kg/min) may be initiated to control unwanted tachycardia.[173] Higher doses of preoperative anxiolytics and sedatives, such as benzodiazepines, may also be required. Anticholinergics are avoided because of their interference with normal heat-regulating mechanisms and their potentiation of tachyarrhythmias.

Hypothyroidism. Hypothyroidism represents several conditions, such as chronic thyroiditis or Hashimoto disease, in which tissues are exposed to decreased circulating concentrations of T_3 and T_4. The cause of hypothyroidism may be primary, resulting from the destruction or hypofunction of the thyroid gland, or secondary, resulting from insufficient TSH production. The diagnosis of hypothyroidism is confirmed by decreased serum concentrations of T_3 and T_4, with or without secondary increases in TSH levels.[174]

The treatment of hypothyroidism consists of administration of T_4, levothyroxine sodium (Synthroid) replacement therapy, with the restoration of intravascular volume and electrolyte status. Elective surgery need not be delayed for patients with mild to moderate hypothyroidism. No difference in perioperative outcome has been noted between untreated hypothyroid patients and patients who are euthyroid.[86]

Adrenocortical Disorders. Disorders of the adrenal cortex, ranging from hyperadrenocorticism to hypoadrenocorticism, are the result of primary disease of the adrenal cortex or pituitary gland, ectopic production of adrenocortical hormones by malignant tissue, or most commonly treatment with exogenous corticosteroids. Steroids are commonly used to treat bronchial asthma, autoimmune diseases, and connective tissue disorders such as rheumatoid arthritis. Their high-dose administration for prolonged periods or their excess levels in circulating glucocorticoid hormones characteristically results in a syndrome referred to as *Cushing syndrome*. This syndrome is clinically manifested as hypertension and hypovolemia, truncal obesity with an accumulation of interscapular fat ("buffalo hump"), abdominal and gluteal striae, plethoric facial appearance ("moon facies"), easy bruising, osteoporosis, personality changes, and menstrual irregularities and hirsutism. Hyperaldosteronism—an excess of mineralocorticoid hormones—may be manifested as hypertension in association with marked hypokalemia (plasma potassium [K] less than 3 mmol/L). Its major alterations involve sodium and water retention, potassium depletion, and metabolic alkalosis.

Adrenocortical insufficiency may be of a primary origin (Addison disease) or caused by the secondary inhibition of adrenocortical function by prolonged exogenous steroid therapy. Clinical signs are less obvious than those of Cushing disease and include skin hyperpigmentation, weight loss, muscle wasting, hypotension, intravascular volume depletion, hypoglycemia, hyponatremia, and hyperkalemia.[175]

The preoperative preparation of a patient with adrenocortical dysfunction includes the correction of fluid and electrolyte disturbances and the treatment of coexisting disorders, such as hypertension and diabetes mellitus. Glucocorticoid or mineralocorticoid replacement therapy is also continued perioperatively. Exogenous corticosteroids should be provided for patients who have been treated with steroids for more than 1 month within the previous year (see Table 20-4).[84] For patients currently receiving high-dose steroid therapy, such as those with chronic hypoadrenocorticism or Addison disease, further supplementation of the daily maintenance doses is required. This recommendation is based on concerns that additional cortisol may not be released from the adrenal cortex as a result of its primary hypofunction or secondary suppression in response to surgical stress. Cardiovascular collapse may then ensue during major surgical procedures.

DIAGNOSTIC TESTING

Appropriate laboratory evaluations and diagnostic procedures should be obtained and the results considered to determine the patient's surgical and anesthetic risk, as well as the need for appropriate health-care modifications. The controversy lies in which tests are necessary and appropriate for specific settings. The rationale for performing "routine" tests has been under intense scrutiny, primarily because of recent and ongoing changes in health-care economics. A protocol that delineates the indications for testing should be established by each surgical facility and approved by the medical staff. When protocols are followed for ordering preoperative laboratory tests, the total number of tests performed has been reduced 50% to 60%, and the appropriateness of the tests has improved.[176] A necessary step in the implementation process for preoperative testing guidelines is the education of the medical staff. Centralizing the test-ordering process, such as in the preoperative assessment clinic, makes standardization and compliance more attainable.

Routine Diagnostic Testing

It has been traditional practice, even within the past decade, to order a "battery" of routine evaluative tests before a patient undergoes surgery and anesthesia. Routine ordering of preoperative diagnostic tests remains a common practice in many institutions. Until the early 1990s, the rationale for obtaining preoperative diagnostic tests was rarely questioned. Tests were frequently ordered for a variety of reasons but were often unrelated to findings based specifically on the patient's history and physical examination. Reasons cited for ordering the standard battery of preoperative tests included the following[177-179]:

- To follow customary practice at an institution
- To adhere to institutional or legislative mandates that dictate the tests be performed
- To further evaluate and determine the progress of a known disease or condition, because preexisting medical conditions have a greater risk for intraoperative and postoperative complications
- To detect asymptomatic yet modifiable conditions that could alter anesthetic and surgical care
- To detect asymptomatic but unmodifiable conditions that could alter anesthetic and surgical risk

- To screen for conditions unrelated to the planned surgery
- To acquire baseline results that might be useful in the perioperative period
- To protect against medicolegal involvement

When considering the value of preoperative tests, the following must be considered:

1. The diagnostic procedure should be cost effective—that is, the costs saved from knowing the results exceed the expense of performing the test.
2. The diagnostic procedure should have a positive benefit-risk ratio—that is, the benefit derived from conducting the test outweighs the harm that might ensue from a false-positive result.
3. Test results are available for interpretation and recuperative intervention before surgery.
4. Test results will yield information that could not be obtained from the history and physical examination.
5. Abnormal test results in an asymptomatic patient would influence the patient care, the surgery, or the anesthesia management.

Without any clinical sign, the likelihood of observing a significant anomaly is very small for diagnostic procedures such as ECG,[178] chest radiography,[178,180,181] or laboratory tests.[178,182] Asymptomatic disease is rarely of clinical concern in perioperative surgical care. In addition, unexpected abnormal findings from preoperative testing tend not to affect the upcoming surgery.[183] When a battery of routine preoperative tests are conducted, abnormal test results potentially alter patient care only 0.22% to 0.56% of the time.[178,182] A consistent conclusion of most studies is that routine preoperative laboratory screening is not cost-effective or predictive of postoperative complications[177,184] and is unnecessary when an extensive history and physical examination do not suggest any patient abnormalities.[185,186]

Limitations to Routine Preoperative Diagnostic Testing

Studies estimate that at least 10% of the more than $30 billion spent on laboratory testing annually in the United States goes to preparing patients for surgery.[187] Although added health-care costs are the most apparent limitation to performing the routine battery of preoperative tests, additional factors can negatively affect the patient and care providers. The indiscriminant ordering of tests for diagnostic evaluation increases the likelihood that at least one test will be abnormal in a healthy patient.[179] False-positive, or even false-negative, test results can lead to additional medical evaluation and the potential for increased morbidity. Abnormal laboratory tests for continuous data are defined in probabilistic terms and assume a normal patient population distribution.[178,179] The end points of the bell-shaped distribution curve are arbitrarily set at 2.5%; therefore, 5% of test results in normal patients are reported as abnormal. False-positive test results may lead to additional follow-up tests, which can place the patient at risk of increased morbidity.[188] Abnormal test results that were not further pursued and lack of documentation of the rationale for not investigating abnormal test results have increased the medicolegal risk for physicians.[189]

Timing of Diagnostic Testing

In general, diagnostic testing results are deemed current within 6 months of the scheduled surgery if the test results are normal and if the patient's current health status indicates no change has occurred since the test was performed.[190] However, specific tests require more current data analysis. A serum potassium level should be obtained within 7 days of surgery for patients receiving diuretics or digitalis, and blood glucose level determinations should be obtained on the day of surgery for patients with diabetes controlled by medication. An electrocardiogram, when indicated, within 30 days prior to elective surgery is considered adequate for patients with stable disease.[97] Chest radiographs taken within 6 months are generally acceptable if the patient's pulmonary condition is stable.[191]

Indications for Diagnostic Testing

A continuing point of controversy relates to disagreement about which tests are appropriate for specific patients, surgeries, and conditions. Difference of opinion exists among and within medical specialties regarding which tests are appropriate. Suggested guidelines for ordering various diagnostic tests based on results of the patient's history and physical examination have been offered for ordering diagnostic procedures (Box 20-14) and laboratory tests (Box 20-15).

Pregnancy Testing

Routine preoperative pregnancy testing in women of childbearing age remains controversial. If a patient is uncertain of her status or if the physical examination or medical history suggests the possibility of pregnancy (e.g., because of information regarding sexually active status, time of last menstrual period, presence or absence of birth control methods), a preoperative pregnancy test should be performed.[1] Issues to address when deciding whether to test include the following:

- Policies of the hospital or health-care facility based on medical staff bylaws. The medical facility should have established guidelines that delineate when testing for pregnancy is appropriate.
- Patients should be advised of the fetal risk (e.g., spontaneous abortion) should anesthesia be performed during pregnancy. The incidence of congenital abnormalities is no greater in pregnant women who undergo surgery, however, than it is in those with a surgery-free pregnancy.[192] Despite this finding, patients are advised to postpone elective surgery until well after the first trimester, when fetal organogenesis is complete.
- Patients should be privately questioned about the possibility of pregnancy. Female staff should interview adolescent patients in the absence of family members.

Chest Radiography

A preoperative chest radiograph is of minimal predictive importance and is not cost effective as a screening test for postoperative respiratory problems, so it is not to be recommended without specific indications from the medical history and physical examination.[193,194] The risk of performing a routine preoperative chest radiograph in asymptomatic patients less than 75 years of age is greater than the benefit.[189]

Electrocardiography

Many medical facilities continue to use an age-specific criterion for acquiring a preoperative ECG, regardless of indications—or lack of indications—based on the patient's medical history and physical examination. The recommended minimum age for routinely conducting a baseline ECG has gradually increased to 50 years or older.[1,3,195-197] Inquiry has even been raised regarding the appropriateness of an age-only basis for preoperative ECG testing.[198]

The value of obtaining a routine preoperative 12-lead ECG in asymptomatic, low-risk patients has been questioned.[199,200] This rethinking of indications for when to order a preoperative ECG has been challenged for the following reasons:

- It has not been shown to be cost-effective.[183,201,202]
- It is a poor predictor of perioperative complications.[200,202,203]
- It is of limited value in detection of ischemia in asymptomatic individuals.[204,205]
- Abnormal preoperative ECGs rarely lead to alteration in patient care.[183,201,206]
- No evidence supports the value of a "baseline" ECG.[195,199,200]

FASTING CONSIDERATIONS

Part of the anesthesia provider's role in patient preparation involves establishing an appropriate fasting interval for the patient. This requires knowledge of risk factors for pulmonary aspiration of gastric contents weighed against the consequences of prolonged fasting. The risk of perioperative pulmonary

BOX **20-15**

Indications for Laboratory Testing

Complete Blood Count
Hematologic disorder
Vascular procedure
Chemotherapy
Unknown sickle cell syndrome status

Hemoglobin and Hematocrit
Age <6 mo (<1 yr if born prematurely)
Hematologic malignancy
Recent radiation or chemotherapy
Renal disease
Anticoagulant therapy
Procedure with moderate to high blood loss potential
Coexisting systemic disorders (e.g., cystic fibrosis, prematurity,
   severe malnutrition, renal failure, liver disease, congenital
   heart disease)

White Blood Cell Count
Leukemia and lymphomas
Recent radiation or chemotherapy
Suspected infection that would lead to cancellation of surgery
Aplastic anemia
Hypersplenism
Autoimmune collagen vascular disease

Blood Glucose Level
Diabetes mellitus
Current corticosteroid use
History of hypoglycemia
Adrenal disease
Cystic fibrosis

Serum Chemistry
Renal disease
Adrenal or thyroid disease
Chemotherapy
Pituitary or hypothalamic disease
Body fluid loss or shifts (e.g., dehydration, bowel prep)
Central nervous system disease

Potassium
Digoxin therapy
Diuretic therapy

Creatinine and Blood Urea
Nitrogen
Cardiovascular disease (e.g., hypertension)
Renal disease
Adrenal disease
Diabetes mellitus
Diuretic therapy
Digoxin therapy
Body fluid loss or shifts (e.g., dehydration, bowel prep)
Procedure requiring radiocontrast

Liver Function Tests
Hepatic disease
Exposure to hepatitis
Therapy with hepatotoxic agents

Coagulation Studies
INR, Prothrombin Time, and Partial Thromboplastin Time
   Leukemia
   Hepatic disease
   Bleeding disorder
   Anticoagulant therapy
   Severe malnutrition or malabsorption
Platelet Count and Bleeding Time
   Bleeding disorder
   Abnormal hemorrhage, purpura, history of easy bruising

Urinalysis
Not indicated as a routine screening test

Pregnancy Test
Possibility of pregnancy

Medication Levels
Monitor for medications (e.g., theophylline, phenytoin,
   digoxin, carbamazepine) if patient exhibits signs
   of ineffective therapy, potential drug side effects,
   or poor drug compliance or has recently changed
   medication therapy without documentation of the
   drug level

aspiration of gastric contents that results in morbidity or mortality is relatively low, so the recommendations for withholding oral feeding before elective surgery have recently become much more liberal. When studies were conducted challenging the traditional fasting times (7 hours or greater) for clear liquids, the results appeared to show that a reduced fasting interval does not increase the risk of pulmonary aspiration in normal, healthy individuals.[207]

The traditional policy of fasting after midnight fails to address three variables that influence gastric emptying for surgery: the time of the scheduled surgery, the time at which the patient retired for the night, and the variability in gastric emptying for solids and fluids among individuals. Prolonged fasting, especially in children, can be highly distressing in addition to causing physiologic alterations. Periods of long preoperative fasting have been shown to contribute to the following:

- Dehydration[208]
- Hypoglycemia (in smaller children)[209]
- Hypovolemia
- Increased irritability[209]
- Enhanced preoperative anxiety[210]
- Reduced compliance with preoperative fasting orders[208]
- Thirst[211] and related discomforts (e.g., hunger, headache, unhappiness)

BOX 20-16

Conditions That Increase the Risk of Regurgitation and Pulmonary Aspiration During Anesthesia

- Age extremes (<1 yr or >70 yr)
- Anxiety
- Ascites
- Collagen vascular disease (e.g., scleroderma)
- Depression
- Esophageal surgery
- Exogenous medications (e.g., opioids, premedication)
- Failed intubation or difficult airway history
- Gastroesophageal junction dysfunction (e.g., hiatal hernia)
- Mechanical obstruction (e.g., pyloric stenosis, duodenal ulcer)
- Metabolic disorders (e.g., hypothyroidism, chronic diabetes, hepatic failure, hyperglycemia, obesity, renal failure, uremia)
- Neurologic sequelae (e.g., those of developmental delays, head injury, hypotonia, seizures)
- Pain
- Pregnancy
- Prematurity with respiratory problems
- Smoking
- Type and composition of gastric contents (e.g., solid foods and milk products)

BOX 20-17

Fasting Guidelines for Healthy Patients (All Ages) Undergoing Elective Surgery

- No chewing gum (nicotine gum allowed with patient counseling) or candy after midnight (foreign body aspiration concern)
- Clear liquids up to 2 hr before surgery*
- Breast milk until 4 hr before surgery
- No infant formula, nonhuman milk,† or light meal‡ for at least 6 hr before surgery
- Prescribed medications (e.g., premedication) administered with a sip of water or prescribed liquid mixture (up to 150 mL for adult; up to 75 mL for children) up to 1 hr before anesthesia

*Consider the possibility that the case may proceed earlier than scheduled.
†Because nonhuman milk is similar to solids in gastric emptying time, the amount ingested must be considered when determining an appropriate fasting period.
‡A light meal typically consists of toast and clear liquids. Meals that include fried or fatty foods or meat may prolong gastric emptying time. Both the amount and type of foods ingested must be considered when determining an appropriate fasting period.

Pulmonary Aspiration Risk

Recent ingestion of food and liquid before surgery does contribute to an increased risk of pulmonary aspiration. Solid foods must be digested to a bolus diameter of less than 2 mm before the food can pass through the pylorus.[212] This process normally takes several hours for solids, whereas liquids pass through the pylorus in 1 to 2 hours. Historically, patients have been required to fast for extended periods in an attempt to ensure an empty stomach. However, sustained fasting does not guarantee that the stomach will be empty at the time of surgery.[213]

Part of the preoperative evaluation process identifies patients who are at risk for aspirating gastric contents into the lungs and developing aspiration pneumonitis. Factors associated with an increased risk of pulmonary aspiration of gastric contents are listed in Box 20-16.[214-225]

Fasting Interval

When the fasting interval is minimized, patients (especially children) are reported to be less irritable, less thirsty, and less hungry; to have fewer headaches; to be more comfortable; and generally to tolerate the preoperative phase better than patients who have fasted for longer periods of time. Modest amounts of clear liquids taken orally 2 hours[226-228] to 3 hours[229,230] preoperatively, when compared with a conventional fasting interval of "7 to 8 hours" or "after midnight," are acceptable and have been shown to lower residual gastric volume (stimulation of the gastric emptying reflex) and raise gastric pH in a majority of patients. Acceptable clear fluids (e.g., water, apple juice, black coffee, black tea, clear juice drinks, clear Jell-O, clear broth, ice, Popsicles, Pedialyte) may be given to healthy, unpremedicated

patients. In light of these recent findings, recommended fasting guidelines for otherwise healthy individuals have been liberalized (Box 20-17).[225,231]

AMERICAN SOCIETY OF ANESTHESIOLOGISTS PHYSICAL STATUS CLASSIFICATION SYSTEM

With the conclusion of the preanesthesia assessment, assignment of an ASA physical status classification is made for each patient. The classification ideally represents a reflection of the patient's preoperative status and is not an estimate of anesthetic risk. For greater accuracy to be attained from its interpretation, the ASA status should also remain independent of the proposed surgical procedure.[232-235]

Advent and Purpose

In 1940, the ASA developed a system "to classify the physical condition of a patient requiring anesthesia and surgery." This six-category classification was then revised by the ASA in 1961 to the current system of five categories (Table 20-14).[236] The purpose of the ASA classification, then and now, is to provide a consistent means of communication to anesthesia staff, within and among institutions, about the physical status of a patient.[236] Furthermore, it allows for a standardized interpretation of anesthesia outcome based on one criterion.

Despite rough correlations between patient physical status and postoperative outcome, the ASA classification system does not represent an estimate of anesthesia risk.[232-235] Although a patient in poor physical health is known to be at greater risk for negative outcome, this does not account for other factors that influence perioperative morbidity and mortality. These factors include the duration and involvement of the surgical procedure, the degree of

TABLE **20-14**	American Society of Anesthesiologists Physical Status Classification
Classification	**Physical Status**
ASA Class I	No organic, physiologic, biochemical, or psychiatric disturbance *Example:* Healthy patient
ASA Class II	Mild to moderate systemic disturbance *Examples:* Heart disease that slightly limits physical activity, essential hypertension, diabetes mellitus, chronic bronchitis, anemia, morbid obesity, age extremes
ASA Class III	Severe systemic disturbance that limits activity *Examples:* Heart or chronic pulmonary disease that limits activity, poorly controlled essential hypertension, diabetes mellitus with vascular complications, angina pectoris, history of previous myocardial infarction
ASA Class IV	Severe systemic disturbance that is life threatening *Examples:* Congestive heart failure; persistent angina pectoris; advanced pulmonary, renal, or hepatic dysfunction
ASA Class V	Moribund patient undergoing surgery as a resuscitative effort, despite a minimal chance for survival *Example:* Uncontrolled hemorrhage from a ruptured abdominal artery aneurysm
ASA Class E	Emergency surgery is required *Example:* An otherwise healthy 30-year-old woman who requires a dilation and curettage for moderate but persistent hemorrhage is classified as ASA IE

Modified from American Society of Anesthesiologists. New classification of physical status. Anesthesiology. 1963;24:111.
ASA, American Society of Anesthesiologists.

perioperative monitoring, and unfortunate circumstances, such as human error or equipment failure.

Definition

The current ASA classification system ranges from class I through V, with E denoting an emergent procedure. At some institutions, a classification of ASA status VI also may be assigned to postmortem patients undergoing organ procurement procedures. By definition, a patient classified as ASA status I is a healthy individual except for the condition that has necessitated surgery. A healthy young woman about to undergo an emergency dilation and curettage for vaginal bleeding, for example, is classified as ASA status IE. At the other end of the spectrum, a 74-year-old man with hypertension, uncontrolled diabetes, and unstable angina who is scheduled for a coronary artery bypass graft procedure is classified as ASA status IV.[236]

Limitations of the Current System

Despite the numerous benefits of the ASA classification system, it has its shortcomings. Namely, the current system is not explicit enough in its categorization to account for every patient, and this can result in patient misclassification.[237] If the physical status classification system is used for statistical or reimbursement purposes within a department, overclassification is often the consequence. Overclassification of a patient also occurs when the proposed surgical procedure is incorporated

into the assignment of ASA physical status. This improper classification, or overclassification, of patient status thereby limits the degree of accuracy attained from its original interpretation. As a result, correlations between preoperative status and postoperative outcome are skewed. Despite the shortcomings of the system, ASA physical status continues to be assigned to each patient as a summary of the preoperative evaluation.

PREVENTING OPERATIVE ERRORS

The Joint Commission has endorsed a universal protocol for eliminating wrong site, wrong procedure, wrong patient surgeries. It has been endorsed by more than 40 of the leading medical, nursing, and health-care leadership organizations. The guidelines will be used in all hospitals, ambulatory care surgery centers, and office-based surgery sites, as shown in Box 20-18.

SUMMARY

An important feature of patient care is a timely and thorough preoperative assessment to identify factors that increase the risk of anesthesia and surgery. The preoperative evaluation and preparation of the patient involve integration of information obtained from the patient interview, chart review, physical examination, and interpretation of the results of necessary diagnostic tests. The anesthesia provider can then assimilate the assessment data and devise and implement the most appropriate anesthetic plan for the patient.

BOX 20-18

Guidelines for Implementing the Universal Protocol for Preventing Wrong Site, Wrong Procedure, and Wrong Person Surgery

The following guidelines provide detailed implementation requirements, exemptions, and adaptations for special situations.

Preoperative Verification Process

Verification of the correct person, procedure, and site should occur (as applicable):

- At the time the surgery or procedure is scheduled
- At the time of admission or entry in the facility
- Any time the responsibility for care of the patient is transferred to another caregiver
- With the patient involved, awake, and aware if possible
- Before the patient leaves the preoperative area or enters the procedure/surgical room

Before the start of the procedure, a preoperative verification checklist may be helpful to ensure availability and review of the following:

- Relevant documentation (e.g., history and physical, consent)
- Relevant images, properly labeled and displayed
- Any required implants and special equipment

Marking the Operative Site

- Make the mark at or near the incision site. Do NOT mark any nonoperative site(s) unless necessary for some other aspect of care.
- The mark must be unambiguous (e.g., use initials or "YES" or a line representing the proposed incision; consider that "X" may be ambiguous).
- The mark must be positioned to be visible after the patient is prepped and draped.
- The mark must be made using a marker that is sufficiently permanent to remain visible after completion of the skin prep. Adhesive site markers should not be used as the sole means of marking the site.
- The method of marking and type of mark should be consistent throughout the organization.
- At a minimum, mark all cases involving laterality, multiple structures (fingers, toes, lesions), or multiple levels (spine). NOTE: In general spinal region, special intraoperative radiographic techniques are used for marking the exact vertebral level.
- The person performing the procedure should do the site marking.
- Marking must take place with the patient involved, awake, and aware if possible.
- Final verification of the site mark must occur during the time-out.
- A defined procedure must be in place for patients who refuse site markings.

Exemptions

- Single-organ cases (e.g., cesarean section, cardiac surgery)
- Intervention cases for which the catheter or instrument insertion site is not predetermined (e.g., cardiac catheterization)
- Teeth—BUT indicate operative tooth name(s) on documentation OR mark the operative tooth (teeth) on the dental radiographs or dental diagram
- Premature infants, for whom the mark may cause a permanent tattoo

Time-Out Immediately Before Starting the Procedure

Must be conducted in the location where the procedure will be done, just before starting the procedure. It must involve the entire operative team, use active communication, be briefly documented (the type and amount of documentation) and must, at the least, include:

- Correct patient identity
- Correct side and site
- Agreement on the procedure to be done
- Correct patient position
- Availability of correct implants and any special equipment or special requirements.

The organization should have processes and systems in place for reconciling differences in staff responses during the time-out.

Procedures for Non–Operating Room (OR) Setting, Including Bedside Procedures

- Site marking must be done for any procedure that involves laterality, multiple structures, or levels (even if the procedure takes place outside an OR).
- Verification, site marking, and time-out procedures should be as consistent as possible throughout the organization, including the OR and other locations where invasive procedures are done.
- Exception: Cases in which the individual doing the procedure is in continuous attendance with the patient from the time of decision to do the procedure and consent from the patient to the execution of the procedure may be exempted from the site-marking requirement. The requirement for a time-out final verification still applies.

Modified from The Joint Commission. Guidelines for Implementing the Universal Protocol to Prevent Wrong Site Surgery. *Chicago: Dec 2, 2003. Available at* http://www.jointcommission.org/NR/rdonlyres/4CF3955D-CD1F-4230-86C5-D04485CAFBEA/0/16G_final.pdf. *Accessed November 18, 2008.*

REFERENCES

1. Fischer SP. Cost-effective preoperative evaluation and testing. *Chest.* 1999;115(Suppl):96S-100S.
2. Lew E et al. Outpatient preanaesthesia evaluation clinics. *Singapore Med J.* 2004;45:509-516.
3. Pasternak LR. Preanesthesia evaluation of the surgical patient. In: Barash PG, ed. *ASA Refresher Courses in Anesthesiology.* Philadelphia: Lippincott; 1996:205-219.
4. Solca M. Evidence-based preoperative evaluation. *Best Pract Res Clin Anaesthesiol.* 2006;20:231-236.
5. Pollard JB, Olson L. Early outpatient preoperative anesthesia assessment: does it help to reduce operating room cancellations? *Anesth Analg.* 1999; 89:502-505.
6. Malins AF. Do they do as they are instructed? A review of outpatient anaesthesia. *Anaesthesia.* 1978;33:832-835.
7. Doak GJ. Discontinuing drugs before surgery. *Can J Anaesth.* 1997; 44:R112-R117.
8. Schirmer U, Schurmann W. Preoperative administration of angiotensin-converting enzyme inhibitors. *Anaesthetist.* 2007;56:557-561.
9. Baillard C. Preoperative management of chronic medications. *Ann Fr Anesth Reanim.* 2005;24:1360-1374.
10. Pass SE, Simpson RW. Discontinuation and reinstitution of medications during the perioperative period. *Am J Health Syst Pharm.* 2004;61:899-912.
11. Huyse FJ et al. Psychotropic drugs and the perioperative period: a proposal for a guideline in elective surgery. *Psychosomatics.* 2006;47:8-22.
12. Fleisher LA et al. ACC/AHA 2006 guideline update on perioperative cardiovascular evaluation for noncardiac surgery: focused update on perioperative beta-blocker therapy. *Anesth Analg.* 2007;104:15-26.
13. Hepner DL, Castells MC. Anaphylaxis during the perioperative period. *Anesth Analg.* 2003;97:1381-1395.
14. Demaegd J et al. Latex allergy: a challenge for anaesthetists. *Acta Anaesth Belg.* 2006;57:127-135.
15. Substance Abuse and Mental Health Services Administration. *Results from the 2005 National Survey on Drug Use and Health: National Findings* (Office of Applied Studies, NSDUH Series H-30, DHHS Publication No. SMA 06-4149). Rockville, MD: U.S. Dept. of Health and Human Services; 2006.
16. Coleman P. Overview of substance abuse. *Prim Care.* 1993;20:1-18.
17. McGinnis JM, Foege WH. Mortality and morbidity attributable to use of addictive substances in the United States. *Proc Assoc Am Physicians.* 1999;111:109-118.
18. Centers for Disease Control and Prevention. Annual smoking: attributable mortality, years of potential life lost, and economic costs—United States, 1995-1999. *MMWR Morb Mortal Wkly Rep.* 2002;51:300-303.
19. Centers for Disease Control and Prevention. Tobacco use among adults—United States, 2005. *MMWR Morb Mortal Wkly Rep.* 2006;55: 1145-1148.
20. Centers for Disease Control and Prevention. Cigarette smoking among adults—United States, 2002. *MMWR Morb Mortal Wkly Rep.* 2004;53: 427-431.
21. Centers for Disease Control and Prevention. Cigarette use among high school students—United States, 1991-2003. *MMWR Morb Mortal Wkly Rep.* 2004;53:499-502.
22. Centers for Disease Control and Prevention. Cigarette use among high school students—United States, 1991-2005. *MMWR Morb Mortal Wkly Rep.* 2006;55:724-726.
23. Centers for Disease Control and Prevention. Annual smoking: attributable mortality, years of potential life lost, and productivity losses—United States, 1997-2001. *MMWR Morb Mortal Wkly Rep.* 2005;54:625-628.
24. U.S. Department of Health and Human Services. *The Health Consequences of Involuntary Exposure to Tobacco Smoke: A Report of the Surgeon General* (USDHHS Publication No. O2NLM: WA754H43252006). Atlanta GA: U.S. Department of Health and Human Services, Centers for Disease Control and Prevention, Coordinating Center for Health Promotion, National Center for Chronic Disease Prevention and Health Promotion, Office on Smoking and Health; 2006.
25. O'Rourke JM et al. The effects of exposure to environmental tobacco smoke on pulmonary function in children. *Ped Anesth.* 2006;16:560-567.
26. Comroe JH Jr. The pharmacological actions of nicotine. *Ann N Y Acad Sci.* 1960;90:48-51.
27. Nicod PJ et al. Acute systemic and coronary hemodynamic and serologic responses to cigarette smoking in long-term smokers with atherosclerotic coronary artery disease. *J Am Coll Cardiol.* 1984;4:964-971.
28. Nunn JE. Oxygen. *Nunn's Applied Respiratory Physiology.* 4th ed. Boston: Butterworth-Heinemann; 1993:247-305.
29. Kyerematen GA et al. Pharmacokinetics of nicotine and 12 metabolites in the rat. Application of a new radiometric high performance liquid chromatography assay. *Drug Metab Dispos.* 1988;16:125-129.
30. Duan MJ, et al. Disposition kinetics and metabolism of nicotine-1'-N' oxide in rabbits. *Drug Metab Dispos.* 1991;19:667-672.
31. Sasaki T. On half-clearance time of carbon monoxide hemoglobin in blood during hyperbaric oxygen therapy (OHP). *Bull Tokyo Med Dent Univ.* 1975;22:63-77.
32. Wagner JA, Horvath SM, Dahms TE. Carbon monoxide elimination. *Respir Physiol.* 1975;23:41-47, 1975.
33. Moller AM, Pedersen T. The effect of tobacco smoking on risks in connection with anesthesia and surgery. Development of complications and the preventive effect of smoking cessation. *Ugeskr Laeger.* 1999;161:4273-4276.
34. Pearch AC, Jones RM. Smoking and anesthesia: preoperative abstinence and perioperative morbidity. *Anesthesiology.* 1984;61:576-584.
35. Kambam JR et al. Effect of short-term smoking halt on carboxyhemoglobin levels and P50 values. *Anesth Analg.* 1986;65:1186-1188.
36. Bluman LG et al. Preoperative smoking habits and postoperative pulmonary complications. *Chest.* 1998;113:883-889.
37. Moores LK. Smoking and postoperative pulmonary complications. An evidence-based review of the recent literature. *Clin Chest Med.* 2000;21:139-146.
38. Theadom A, Cropley M. Effects of preoperative smoking cessation on the incidence and risk of intraoperative and postoperative complications in adult smokers: a systematic review. *Tob Control.* 2006;15:352-358.
39. Warner MA et al. Role of preoperative cessation of smoking and other factors in postoperative pulmonary complications: a blinded prospective study of coronary artery bypass patients. *Mayo Clin Proc.* 1989;64:609-616.
40. Warner DO. Helping surgical patients quit smoking: why, when, and how. *Anesth Analg.* 2005;101:481-487.
41. Moller A, Villebro N. Interventions for preoperative smoking cessation [electronic version]. *Cochrane Database Syst Rev.* 2005;3:CD002294. PMID: 16034875. DOI:10.1002/14651858.
42. Chilmonczyk BA et al. Association between exposure to environmental tobacco smoke and exacerbation of asthma in children. *N Engl J Med.* 1993;328:1665-1669.
43. Eisner MD et al. Secondhand smoke exposure, pulmonary function, and cardiovascular mortality. *Ann Epidemiol.* 2007;17:364-373.
44. O'Rourke JM et al. The effects of exposure to environmental tobacco smoke on pulmonary function in children undergoing anesthesia for minor surgery. *Ped Anesth.* 2006;16:560-567.
45. Forastiere F et al. Effects of environment and passive smoking on the respiratory health of children. *Int J Epidemiol.* 1992;21:66-73.
46. Skolnick ET et al. Exposure to environmental tobacco smoke and the risk of adverse respiratory events in children receiving general anesthesia. *Anesthesiology.* 1998;88:1144-1153.
47. Lyons B et al. The effect of passive smoking on the incidence of airway complications in children undergoing general anaesthesia. *Anaesthesia.* 1996;51:324-326.
48. Stahre MA et al. Alcohol-attributable deaths and years of potential life lost—United States, 2001. *MMWR Morb Mortal Wkly Rep.* 2004;53:866-870.
49. Shourie S et al. Pre-operative screening for excessive alcohol consumption among patients scheduled for elective surgery. *Drug Alcohol Rev.* 2007; 26:119-125.
50. Babor TF et al. *AUDIT. The Alcohol Use Disorders Identification Test: Guidelines for Use in Primary Care.* World Health Organization: 2001; Geneva.
51. Kitchens JM. Does this patient have an alcohol problem? *JAMA.* 1994;272:1782-1787.
52. Lohr RH. Treatment of alcohol withdrawal in hospitalized patients. *Mayo Clin Proc.* 1995;70:777-782.
53. Bradley KA et al. AUDIT-C as a brief screen for alcohol misuse in primary care. *Alcohol Clin Exp Res.* 2007;31:1208-1217.
54. Pandele G et al. Thiopental pharmacokinetics in patients with cirrhosis. *Anesthesiology.* 1983;59:123-126.
55. Costela JL et al. Serum protein binding of propofol in patients with renal failure or hepatic cirrhosis. *Acta Anaesthesiol Scand.* 1996;40:741-745.
56. Gordon AJ et al. Identification and treatment of alcohol use disorders in the perioperative period. *Postgrad Med.* 2006;119:46-55.
57. Substance Abuse and Mental Health Services Administration. *Results from the 2006 National Survey on Drug Use and Health: National Findings* (Office of Applied Studies, NSDUH Series H-32, DHHS Publication No. SMA 07-4293). Rockville, MD: U.S. Department of Health and Human Services; 2007.

58. Manchikanti L. National drug control policy and prescription drug abuse: facts and fallacies. *Pain Physician.* 2007;10:399-424.

59. Cheng DCH. The drug addicted patient. *Can J Anaesth.* 1997;44:R101-R106.

60. Cavaliere F et al. Anesthesiologic preoperative evaluation of drug addicted patient. *Minerva Anestesiol.* 2005;71:367-371.

61. Mitra S, Sinatra RS. Perioperative management of acute pain in the opioid-dependent patient. *Anesthesiology.* 2004;101:212-227.

62. Kam PC, Yarrow M. Anabolic steroid abuse: physiological and anaesthetic considerations. *Anaesthesia.* 2005;60:685-692.

63. Ang-Lee MK et al. Herbal medicines and perioperative care. *JAMA.* 2001;286:208-216.

64. Kaye AD et al. Perioperative anesthesia clinical considerations of alternative medicines. *Anesthesiol Clin North America.* 2004;22:125-139.

65. American Society of Anesthesiologists Task Force on Management of the Difficult Airway. Practice guidelines for management of the difficult airway: an updated report by the American Society of Anesthesiologists Task Force on Management of the Difficult Airway. *Anesthesiology.* 2003;98:1269-1277.

66. Gregory GA, Riazi J. Classification and assessment of the difficult pediatric airway. In: Riazi J, ed. *Anesthesiology Clinics of North America: The Difficult Pediatric Airway.* Philadelphia: Saunders; 1998:729-741.

67. Samsoon GL, Young JR. Difficult tracheal intubation: a retrospective study. *Anaesthesia.* 1987;42:487-490.

68. Lee A et al. A systematic review (meta-analysis) of the accuracy of the Mallampati tests to predict the difficult airway. *Anesth Analg.* 2006;102:1867-1878.

69. Frerk CM. Predicting difficult intubation. *Anaesthesia.* 1991;46:1005-1008.

70. Block C, Brechnew VL. Unusual problems in airway management. II. The influence of the temporomandibular joint, the mandible, and associated structures on endotracheal intubation. *Anesth Analg.* 1971;50:114-123.

71. Wilson ME et al. Predicting difficult intubation. *Br J Anaesth.* 1988;61:211-216.

72. Newland MC et al. Dental injury associated with anesthesia: a report of 161,687 anesthetics given over 14 years. *J Clin Anesth.* 2007;19:339-345.

73. Cass NM. Medicolegal claims against anaesthetists: a 20 year study. *Anaesth Intensive Care.* 2004;32:47-58.

74. Chadwick RG, Lindsay SM. Dental injuries during general anaesthesia: can the dentist help the anaesthetist? *Dent Update.* 1998;25:76-78.

75. Blumenreich GA. Res ipsa loquitur: dental damage during anesthesia. *AANA J.* 1997;65:33-36.

76. Marley RA et al. Perianesthesia respiratory care of the bariatric patient. *J Perianesth Nurs.* 2005;20:404-431.

77. Ogden CL et al. Prevalence of overweight and obesity in the United States, 1999-2004. *JAMA.* 2006;295:1549-1555.

78. Collazo-Clavell ML et al. Assessment and preparation of patients for bariatric surgery. *Mayo Clin Proc.* 2006;81:S11-S17.

79. Fleisher LA et al. ACC/AHA 2007 guideline on perioperative cardiovascular evaluation and care for noncardiac surgery: executive summary. *Anesth Analg.* 2008;106(3):685-712.

80. Kuruba R et al. Preoperative assessment and perioperative care of patients undergoing bariatric surgery. *Med Clin N Am.* 2007;91:339-351.

81. Gross JB et al. Practice guidelines for the perioperative management of patients with obstructive sleep apnea: a report by the American Society of Anesthesiologists Task Force on Perioperative Management of Patients with Obstructive Sleep Apnea. *Anesthesiology.* 2006;104:1081-1093.

82. Peterson P et al. The preoperative bleeding time test lacks clinical benefit: College of American Pathologists' and American Society of Clinical Pathologists' position article. *Arch Surg.* 1998;133:134-139.

83. MacKenzie CR, Sharrock NE. Perioperative medical considerations in patients with rheumatoid arthritis. *Rheum Dis Clin North Am.* 1998;24:1-17.

84. Nicholson G et al. Perioperative steroid supplementation. *Anaesthesia.* 1998;53:1091-1104.

85. Mieure KD et al. Supplemental glucocorticoid therapy. *Orthopedics.* 2007;30:116-119.

86. Connery LE, Coursin DG. Assessment and therapy of selected endocrine disorders. *Anesthesiol Clin North America.* 2004;22:93-123.

87. Lai HY et al. The use of the GlideScope for tracheal intubation in patients with ankylosing spondylitis. *Br J Anaesth.* 2006;97:419-422.

88. Tanoue LT. Pulmonary manifestations of rheumatoid arthritis. In: Matthay RA, ed. *Clinics in Chest Medicine. Thoracic Manifestations of the Systemic Autoimmune Diseases.* Philadelphia: Saunders; 1998:667-685.

89. Lee-Chiong TL Jr. Pulmonary manifestations of ankylosing spondylitis and relapsing polychondritis. In: Matthay RA, ed. *Clinics in Chest Medicine. Thoracic Manifestations of the Systemic Autoimmune Diseases.* Philadelphia: Saunders; 1998:747-757.

90. Fischer SP. Preoperative evaluation of the adult neurosurgical patient. In: Jaffe RA, Giffard RG, eds. *International Anesthesiology Clinics. Topics in Neuroanesthesia.* Boston: Little, Brown; 1996:21-32.

91. Manno EM. Subarachnoid hemorrhage. *Neurol Clin.* 2004;22:347-366.

92. Teasdale G, Jennett B. Assessment of coma and impaired consciousness. A practical scale. *Lancet.* 1974;2:81-84.

93. Moppett IK. Traumatic brain injury: assessment, resuscitation and early management. *Br J Anaesth.* 2007;99:18-31.

94. Henke PK. Improving quality of care in vascular surgery: the tools are available now. *Am J Surg.* 2005;190:333-337.

95. Bruewer M et al. Preoperative steroid administration: effect on morbidity among patients undergoing intestinal bowel resection for Crohn's disease. *World J Surg.* 2003;27:1306-1310.

96. Vernick W, Fleisher LA. Risk stratification. *Best Pract Res Clin Anesthesiol.* 2008;22(1):1-21.

97. Fleisher LA et al. ACC/AHA 2007 guidelines on perioperative cardiovascular evaluation and care for noncardiac surgery. *Circulation.* 2007;116:1971-1999.

98. Horak J, Fleisher LA. Assembly of cardiac risk and cardiology consultation: examining, imaging, optimizing, and recommending. In: Kaplan JA, ed. *Cardiac Anesthesia.* 5th ed. Philadelphia: Saunders; 2006:283-298.

99. The Joint National Committee on Prevention, Detection, Evaluation, and Treatment of High Blood Pressure. The seventh report of the Joint National Committee on Prevention, Detection, Evaluation, and Treatment of High Blood Pressure: the JNC 7 report. *JAMA.* 2003;289:2560-2572.

100. Elliott WJ, Black HR. Prehypertension. *Nat Clin Pract Cardiovasc Med.* 2007;4:538-548.

101. Aronson S, Fontes ML. Hypertension: a new look at an old problem. *Curr Opin Anaesthesiol.* 2006;19:59-64.

102. Howell SJ et al. Risk factors for cardiovascular death after elective surgery under general anaesthesia. *Br J Anaesth.* 1998;80:14-19.

103. Kim HS et al. Abnormal cardiac autonomic activity and complexity in newly diagnosed and untreated hypertensive patients after general anesthesia. *Clin Exp Hypertens.* 1999;21:1357-1372.

104. Howell SJ et al. Predictors of postoperative myocardial ischaemia. The role of intercurrent arterial hypertension and other cardiovascular risk factors. *Anaesthesia.* 1997;52:107-111.

105. Hanada S et al. Hypertension and anesthesia. *Curr Opin Anaesthesiol.* 2006;19:315-319.

106. Murray MJ. Perioperative hypertension: evaluation and management. *ASA 40th Annual Refresher Course: Lecture 221.* Park Ridge, IL: American Society of Anesthesiologists; 1989.

107. Maddox TM. Preoperative cardiovascular evaluation for noncardiac surgery. *Mt Sinai J Med.* 2005;72:185-192.

108. Eagle KA et al. Long-term survival in patients with coronary artery disease: importance of peripheral vascular disease. The Coronary Artery Surgery Study (CASS) Investigators. *J Am Coll Cardiol.* 1994;23:1091-1095.

109. Goldman L et al. Multifactorial index of cardiac risk in noncardiac surgical procedures. *N Engl J Med.* 1977;297:845-850.

110. Shah K et al. Angina and other risk factors in patients with cardiac diseases undergoing noncardiac operations. *Anesth Analg.* 1990;70:240-247.

111. Detsky AS et al. Cardiac assessment for patients undergoing noncardiac surgery. A multifactorial clinical risk index. *Arch Intern Med.* 1986;146:2131-2134.

112. Fleisher LA, Lehmann HP. Preoperative cardiac evaluation and perioperative monitoring for noncardiac vascular surgery. *JAMA.* 1995;274(24):1671-1672.

113. Kertai MD et al. A meta-analysis comparing the prognostic accuracy of six diagnostic tests for predicting perioperative cardiac risk in patients undergoing major vascular surgery. *Heart.* 2003;89:1327-1334.

114. Goldman L. Multifactorial index of cardiac risk in noncardiac surgery: ten-year status report. *J Cardiothorac Anesth.* 1987;1:237-244.

115. Royster R. Anesthesia and cardiac dysrhythmias. *40th Annual Refresher Course: Lecture 221.* Park Ridge, IL: American Society of Anesthesiologists; 1989.

116. Belzberg H, Rivkind AI. Preoperative cardiac preparation. *Chest.* 1999;115:82S-95S.

117. Schulze RA Jr et al. Sudden death in the year following myocardial infarction. Relation to ventricular premature contractions in the last hospital phase and left ventricular ejection fraction. *Am J Med.* 1977;62:192-199.

118. Cooperman M et al. Cardiovascular risk factors in patients with peripheral vascular disease. *Surgery.* 1978;84:505-509.

119. Rozner MA. The patient with a cardiac pacemaker or implanted defibrillator and management during anaesthesia. *Curr Opin Anaesthesiol.* 2007;20:261-268.

120. Vijayakumar E. Anesthetic considerations in patients with cardiac arrhythmias, pacemakers, and AICDs. *Int Anesthesiol Clin.* 2001;39:21-42.

121. Hata TM, Moyers JR. Preoperative evaluation and management. In: Barash PG et al, eds. *Clinical Anesthesia.* 5th ed. Philadelphia: Lippincott Williams & Wilkins; 2006:475-501.

122. Almany SL et al. Preoperative cardiac evaluation. Assessing risk before noncardiac surgery. *Postgrad Med.* 1995;98:171-182.

123. Flood C, Fleisher LA. Preparation of the cardiac patient for noncardiac surgery. *Am Fam Physician.* 2007 Mar 1;75(5):656-665.

124. Hultman J. Pre-anaesthetic evaluation and management of patients with cardiovascular disease. *Acta Anaesthesiol Scand.* 1996;40:996-1003.

125. Caplan R. Preoperative evaluation of the patient with ischemic heart disease. *40th Annual Refresher Course: Lecture 221.* Park Ridge, IL: American Society of Anesthesiologists; 1989.

126. Williams-Russo P et al. Predicting postoperative pulmonary complications. Is it a real problem? *Arch Intern Med.* 1992;152:1209-1213.

127. Smetana GW. Preoperative pulmonary evaluation: identifying and reducing risks for pulmonary complications. *Cleve Clin J Med.* 2006;73:S36-S41.

128. Johnson RG et al. Multivariable predictors of postoperative respiratory failure after general and vascular surgery: results from the patient safety in surgery study. *J Am Coll Surg.* 2007;204:1188-1198.

129. Arozullah AM et al. Development and validation of a multifactorial risk index for predicting postoperative pneumonia after major noncardiac surgery. *Ann Intern Med.* 2001;135:847-857.

130. Marienau MES, Buck CF. Preoperative evaluation of the pulmonary patient undergoing nonpulmonary surgery. *J Perianesth Nurs.* 1998;13:340-348.

131. Mohr DN, Lavender RC. Preoperative pulmonary evaluation. Identifying patients at increased risk for complications. *Postgrad Med.* 1996;100:241-256.

132. Wang JS. Pulmonary function tests in preoperative pulmonary evaluation. *Respir Med.* 2004;98:598-605.

133. De Nino LA et al. Preoperative spirometry and laparotomy. Blowing away dollars. *Chest.* 1997;111:1536-1541.

134. Kocabas A et al. Value of preoperative spirometry to predict postoperative pulmonary complications. *Respir Med.* 1996;90:25-33.

135. Lawrence VA et al. Risk of pulmonary complications after elective abdominal surgery. *Chest.* 1996;110:744-750.

136. Qaseem A et al. Risk assessment for and strategies to reduce perioperative pulmonary complications for patients undergoing noncardiothoracic surgery: a guideline from the American College of Physicians. *Ann Intern Med.* 2006;144:575-580.

137. Marley RA. Preoperative preparation for the pediatric patient. In: Zaglaniczny K, Aker J, eds. *Clinical Guide to Pediatric Anesthesia.* Philadelphia: Saunders; 1999:29-45.

138. Tirumalasetty J, Grammer LC. Asthma, surgery, and general anesthesia: a review. *J Asthma.* 2006;43:251-254.

139. Doherty GM et al. Anesthesia and the child with asthma. *Ped Anesth.* 2005;15:446-454.

140. Tirumalasetty J, Grammer LC. Asthma, surgery, and general anesthesia: a review. *J Asthma.* 2006;43:251-254.

141. Tait AR, Malviya S. Anesthesia for the child with an upper respiratory tract infection: still a dilemma? *Anesth Analg.* 2005;100:59-65.

142. Serafini G et al. Upper respiratory tract infections and pediatric anesthesia. *Minerva Anestesiol.* 2003;69:457-459.

143. Elwood T, Bailey K. The pediatric patient and upper respiratory infections. *Best Pract Res Clin Anaesthesiol.* 2005;19:35-46.

144. Tait AR, Malviya S. Anesthesia for the child with an upper respiratory tract infection. *Curr Rev Nurs Anesth.* 1999;21:170-175.

145. Schemel WH. Unexpected hepatic dysfunction found by multiple laboratory screening. *Anesth Analg.* 1976;55:810-812.

146. Keegan MT, Plevak DJ. Preoperative assessment of the patient with liver disease. *Am J Gastroenterol.* 2005;100:2116-2127.

147. Ward ME et al. Acute liver failure. Experience in a special unit. *Anaesthesia.* 1977;32:228-239.

148. Gitnick G. Assessment of liver function. *Surg Clin North Am.* 1981;61:197-207.

149. Viegas O, Stoelting RK. LDH5 changes after cholecystectomy or hysterectomy in patients receiving halothane, enflurane, or fentanyl. *Anesthesiology.* 1979;51:556-558.

150. Marschall KE. Diseases of the liver and biliary tract. In: Stoelting RK, Dierdorf SF, eds. *Anesthesia and Co-existing Disease.* 5th ed. Philadelphia: Churchill Livingstone; 2008:259-278.

151. O'Grady JG et al. Early prognostic indicators in acute liver failure and application to selection for orthotopic liver transplantation. *Gastroenterology.* 1988;94:A578.

152. Tucker RA. Drugs and liver disease: a tabular compilation of drugs and the histopathological changes that can occur in the liver. *Drug Intell Clin Pharm.* 1982;16:569-580.

153. Kaplowitz N et al. Drug-induced hepatotoxicity. *Ann Intern Med.* 1986;104:826-839.

154. Browne RA, Chernesky MA. Infectious diseases and the anaesthetist. *Can J Anaesth.* 1988;35:655-665.

155. Centers for Disease Control and Prevention. Protection against viral hepatitis. Recommendations of the Immunization Practices Advisory Committee (ACIP). *MMWR Morb Mortal Wkly Rep.* 1990;39:1-26.

156. Miller ED Jr. Understanding renal function and its preoperative evaluation. In: Malhotra V, ed. *Anesthesia for Renal and Genitourinary Surgery.* New York: McGraw-Hill; 1996:9.

157. Beck LH. Changes in renal function with aging. *Clin Geriatr Med.* 1998;14:199-209.

158. Sladen RN et al. Two-hour versus 22-hour creatinine clearance in critically ill patients. *Anesthesiology.* 1987;67:1013-1016.

159. Weir PH, Chung FF. Anaesthesia for patients with chronic renal disease. *Can Anaesth Soc J.* 1984;31:468-481.

160. Garwood S. Renal disease. In: Stoelting RK, Dierdorf SF, eds. *Anesthesia and Co-existing Disease.* 5th ed. Philadelphia: Churchill Livingstone; 2008:323-348.

161. Roizen MF. Preoperative evaluation. In: Miller RD, ed. *Miller's Anesthesia.* 6th ed. Philadelphia: Churchill Livingstone; 2005:927-997.

162. Centers for Disease Control and Prevention. *National Diabetes Fact Sheet: General Information and National Estimates on Diabetes in the United States, 2005.* Atlanta, GA: U.S. Department of Health and Human Services, Centers for Disease Control and Prevention; 2005.

163. Angelini G et al. Perioperative care of the diabetic patient. In: Schwartz AJ, ed. *ASA Refresher Courses in Anesthesiology.* Philadelphia: Lippincott; 2001:1-9.

164. Connery LE, Coursin DB. Assessment and therapy of selected endocrine disorders. *Anesthesiol Clin North America.* 2004;22:93-123.

165. Powers AC. Diabetes mellitus. In: Fauci AS et al, eds. *Harrison's Principles of Internal Medicine.* 17th ed. New York: McGraw-Hill; 2008:2275-2304.

166. Beckman JA et al. Diabetes and atherosclerosis: epidemiology, pathophysiology, and management. *JAMA.* 2002;287:2570-2581.

167. Robertshaw HJ, Hall GM. Diabetes mellitus: anaesthetic management. *Anaesthesia.* 2006;61:1187-1190.

168. Syed AA et al. Current perspectives on the management of gastroparesis. *J Postgrad Med.* 2005;51:54-60.

169. Smiley DD, Umpierrez GE. Perioperative glucose control in the diabetic or nondiabetic patient. *South Med J.* 2006;99:580-589.

170. Marks JB. Perioperative management of diabetes. *Am Fam Physician.* 2003;67:93-100.

171. Schwartz JJ, Rosenbaum SH. Anesthesia and the endocrine system. In: Barash PG et al, eds. *Clinical Anesthesia.* 5th ed. Philadelphia: Lippincott Williams & Wilkins; 2006:1129-1151.

172. Andersohn F et al. Systematic review: agranulocytosis induced by nonchemotherapy drugs. *Ann Intern Med.* 2007;146:657-665.

173. Duggal J et al. Utility of esmolol in thyroid crisis. *Can J Clin Pharmacol.* 2006;13:292-295.

174. Devdhar M et al. Hypothyroidism. *Endocrinol Metab Clin North Am.* 2007;36:595-615.

175. Nieman LK, Chanco Turner ML. Addison's disease. *Clin Dermatol.* 2006;24:276-280.

176. Finegan BA et al. Selective ordering of preoperative investigations by anesthesiologists reduces the number and cost of tests. *Can J Anaesth.* 2005;52:575-580.

177. Velanovich V. Preoperative laboratory screening based on age, gender, and concomitant medical diseases. *Surgery.* 1994;115:56-61.

178. Perez A et al. Value of routine preoperative tests: a multicentre study in four general hospitals. *Br J Anaesth.* 1995;74:250-256.

179. Macpherson DS. Preoperative laboratory testing: should any tests be "routine" before surgery? *Med Clin North Am.* 1993;77:289-308.

180. Archer C et al. Value of routine preoperative chest x-rays: a meta-analysis. *Can J Anaesth.* 1993;40:1022-1027.

181. Charpak Y et al. Prospective assessment of a protocol for selective ordering of preoperative chest x-rays. *Can J Anaesth.* 1988;35:259-264.

182. Kaplan EB et al. The usefulness of preoperative laboratory screening. *JAMA.* 1985;253:3576-3581.

183. Johnson H et al. Are routine laboratory screening tests necessary to evaluate ambulatory surgical patients? *Surgery.* 1988;104:639-645.

184. Ransom SB et al. Cost-effectiveness of routine blood type and screen testing before elective laparoscopy. *Obstet Gynecol.* 1995;86:346-348.

185. van Klei WA et al. Role of history and physical examination in preoperative evaluation. *Eur J Anaesthesiol.* 2003;20:612-618.

186. Smetana GW, Macpherson DS. The case against routine preoperative laboratory testing. *Med Clin North Am.* 2003;87:7-40.

187. Pasternak LR. Preoperative laboratory testing: general issues and considerations. *Anesthesiology Clin North America.* 2004;22:13-25.

188. Roizen MF. Cost-effective preoperative laboratory testing. JAMA. 1994;271:319-320.

189. Roizen MF, Cohn S. Preoperative evaluation for elective surgery: what tests are needed? In: Stoelting et al, eds. Advances in Anesthesia. St Louis: Mosby; 1993:25-47.

190. Pasternak LR et al. Practice advisory for preanesthesia evaluation: a report by the American Society of Anesthesiologists Task Force on Preanesthesia Evaluation. Anesthesiology. 2002;96:485-496.

191. Calderini E et al. Indications to chest radiograph in preoperative adult assessment: recommendations of the SIAARTI-SIRM commission. Minerva Anestesiol. 2004;70:443-451.

192. Duncan PG et al. Fetal risk of anesthesia and surgery during pregnancy. Anesthesiology. 1986;64:790-794.

193. Archer C et al. Value of routine preoperative chest x-rays: a meta-analysis. Can J Anaesth. 1993;40:1022-1027.

194. Bouillot JL et al. Are routine preoperative chest radiographs useful in general surgery? A prospective multicentre study in 3959 patients. Eur J Surg. 1996;162:597-604.

195. Callaghan LC et al. Utilisation of the preoperative ECG. Anaesthesia. 1995;50:488-490.

196. Wagner JD, Moore DL. Preoperative laboratory testing for the oral and maxillofacial surgery patient. J Oral Maxillofac Surg. 1991;49:177-182.

197. Haug RH, Reifeis RL. A prospective evaluation of the value of preoperative laboratory testing for office anesthesia and sedation. J Oral Maxillofac Surg. 1999;57:16-20.

198. Gloyna DF et al. The incidence of an abnormal ECG in the surgical patient: is a positive history predictive? Anesthesiology. 1998;89:A1349.

199. Munro J et al. Routine preoperative testing: a systematic review of the evidence. Health Technol Assess. 1997;1:1-62.

200. Tait AR et al. Evaluation of the efficacy of routine preoperative electrocardiograms. J Cardiothorac Vasc Anesth. 1997;11:752-755.

201. Turnbull JM, Buck C. The value of preoperative screening investigations in otherwise healthy individuals. Arch Intern Med. 1987;147:1101-1105.

202. Gold BS et al. The utility of preoperative electrocardiograms in the ambulatory surgical patient. Arch Intern Med. 1992;152:301-305.

203. Murdoch CJ et al. The pre-operative ECG in day surgery: a habit? Anaesthesia. 1999;54:907-908.

204. Orkin FK, Gold B. Selection. In: Wetchler BV, ed. Anesthesia for Ambulatory Surgery. 2nd ed. Philadelphia: Lippincott; 1991:81-129.

205. Margolis JR et al. Clinical features of unrecognized myocardial infarction—silent and symptomatic. Eighteen year follow-up: the Framingham study. Am J Cardiol. 1973;32:1-7.

206. Golub R et al. Efficacy of preadmission testing in ambulatory surgical patients. Am J Surg. 1992;163:565-570.

207. Stuart PC. The evidence behind modern fasting guidelines. Best Pract Res Clin Anaesthesiol. 2006;20:457-469.

208. Hannallah R. Clear liquids before surgery offer ASCs more flexibility. Same Day Surg. 1991;15:105-108.

209. Dose VA, White PF. Effects of fluid therapy on serum glucose levels in fasted outpatients. Anesthesiology. 1987;66:223-226.

210. Sutherland AD et al. Effects of preoperative fasting on morbidity and gastric contents in patients undergoing day-stay surgery. Br J Anaesth. 1986;58:876-878.

211. Splinter WM et al. The effect of preoperative apple juice on gastric contents, thirst, and hunger in children. Can J Anaesth. 1989;36:55-58.

212. Minami H, McCallum RW. The physiology and pathophysiology of gastric emptying in humans. Gastroenterology. 1984;86:1592-1610.

213. Farrow-Gillespie A et al. Effect of the fasting interval on gastric fluid pH and volume in children. Anesth Analg. 1988;67:S59.

214. Cote CJ. Aspiration: an overrated risk in elective patients. In: Stoelting RK, ed. Advances in Anesthesia. St Louis: Mosby; 1992:1-26.

215. Yogendran S, Chung FF. How long should we fast our patients? Soc Ambul Anesth Newsl. 1992;7:10.

216. Simpson KH, Stakes AF. Effect of anxiety on gastric emptying in preoperative patients. Br J Anaesth. 1987;59:540-544.

217. Borland LM et al. Pulmonary aspiration in pediatric patients during general anesthesia: incidence and outcome. J Clin Anesth. 1998;10:95-102.

218. Nimmo WS. Drugs, diseases and altered gastric emptying. Clin Pharmacokinet. 1976;1:189-203.

219. Morgan M. Anaesthetic contribution to maternal mortality. Br J Anaesth. 1987;59:842-855.

220. Morrison JE Jr, Lockhart CH. Preoperative fasting and medication in children. Anesthesiol Clin North America. 1991;9:731-743.

221. Cote CJ. Changing concepts in preoperative medication and "NPO" status of the pediatric patient. ASA 1992 Annual Refresher Course Lecture. Philadelphia: Lippincott; 1992:132.

222. Hinder RA, Kelly KA. Canine gastric emptying of solids and liquids. Am J Physiol. 1977;233:E335-E340.

223. Warner ME. Risks and outcomes of perioperative pulmonary aspiration. J Perianesth Nurs. 1997;12:352-357.

224. Nagelhout JJ. Aspiration prophylaxis: is it time for changes in our practice? AANA J. 2003;71:299-303.

225. Soreide E et al. Pre-operative fasting guidelines: an update. Acta Anaesthesiol Scand. 2005;49:1041-1047.

226. Read MS, Vaughan RS. Allowing preoperative patients to drink: effects on patients' safety and comfort of unlimited oral water until 2 hours before anaesthesia. Acta Anaesthesiol Scand. 1991;35:591-595.

227. Shevde K, Trivedi N. Effects of clear liquids on gastric volume and pH in healthy volunteers. Anesth Analg. 1991;72:528-531.

228. Splinter WM, Schaefer JD. Unlimited clear fluid ingestion two hours before surgery in children does not affect volume or pH of stomach contents. Anaesth Intensive Care. 1990;18:522-526.

229. Maltby JR et al. Gastric fluid volume and pH in elective patients following unrestricted oral fluid until three hours before surgery. Can J Anaesth. 1991;38:425-429.

230. Splinter WM, Schaefer JD. Ingestion of clear fluids is safe for adolescents up to 3 h before anaesthesia. Br J Anaesth. 1991;66:48-52.

231. Warner MA et al. Practice guidelines for preoperative fasting and the use of pharmacologic agents to reduce the risk of pulmonary aspiration: application to healthy patients undergoing elective procedures. Anesthesiology. 1999;90:896-905.

232. Keats AS. The ASA classification of physical status—a recapitulation. Anesthesiology. 1978;49:233-236.

233. Keenan RL, Boyan CP. Cardiac arrest due to anesthesia. A study of incidence and causes. JAMA. 1985;253:2373-2377.

234. Marx GF et al. Computer analysis of postanesthesia deaths. Anesthesiology. 1973;39:54-58.

235. Vacanti CJ et al. A statistical analysis of the relationship of physical status to postoperative mortality in 68,388 cases. Anesth Analg. 1970;49:564-566.

236. American Society of Anesthesiologists. New classification of physical status. Anesthesiology. 1963;24:111.

237. Owens WD et al. ASA physical status classifications: a study of consistency of ratings. Anesthesiology. 1978;49:239-243.

CHAPTER

21

FLUIDS, ELECTROLYTES, AND BLOOD COMPONENT THERAPY

Edward Waters, Anne Kiyomi Nishinaga

In the clinical practice of anesthesia, an important priority in patients experiencing the stresses of surgery and anesthesia is maintenance of homeostasis. Maintaining a physiologic balance of body fluids in both volume and composition is critical to maintaining overall homeostasis. The following discussion focuses on factors of fluid and electrolyte management and transfusion therapy that are of greatest consequence to patients in the perioperative period.

FLUID COMPARTMENTS

A prerequisite to understanding clinical fluid management is an appreciation of the role of fluids in the human body and the distribution of fluids and electrolytes among the fluid compartments. The body is in large part composed of fluid, ranging between 46% and 80%, depending on the age and gender of the individual and the body's composition of fat relative to muscle. Compared with muscle, fat contains less fluid as a percentage of weight (Table 21-1).

Total body water is partitioned into two principal compartments: the intracellular fluid (ICF) and the extracellular fluid (ECF). The extracellular compartment is further subdivided into intravascular fluid (IVF) and interstitial fluid (ISF) spaces. The fluid compartments are divided by water-permeable membranes[1]; the intracellular space is separated from the extracellular space by the cell membrane, and the extracellular space is divided into intravascular and interstitial spaces by the capillary membrane.

The ICF compartment contains approximately two thirds of the body's total fluid volume[2] and is characterized by high concentrations of potassium, phosphate, and magnesium. The adenosine triphosphatase (ATPase)–driven sodium-potassium pump (Na-K-ATPase pump) located in the cell membrane maintains the high concentration of potassium found in ICF[3] (Figure 21-1 and Table 21-2). The Na-K-ATPase pump exchanges three sodium ions for two potassium ions and offsets the tendency for sodium to diffuse into the intracellular space.

The ECF compartment contains approximately one third of the body's fluid volume[2] and contains high concentrations of sodium and chloride compared with the ICF compartment. The IVF (also known as *plasma*) space contains approximately one quarter of the ECF volume and has essentially the same composition and concentration of electrolytes as the ISF. The presence in the IVF of relatively high concentrations of osmotically active plasma proteins, of which albumin is most important, is a

significant difference distinguishing ISF from IVF.[4] The capillary membrane is relatively impermeable to the plasma proteins contained within the vascular space, unless a disease state such as trauma or sepsis alters the capillary permeability.

The properties of the membranes that separate the fluid compartments, as well as the relative concentration of osmotically active substances within each compartment, are the factors primarily responsible for the movement of fluid (water and electrolytes) among compartments in the body. Because the intravascular space is the fluid compartment accessible to the clinician and the chief focus of fluid therapy, it is useful to understand the motion of fluid from the IVF space to the ISF space across the capillary membrane. Four forces known commonly as *Starling forces* determine the motion of fluids across the capillary membrane. The four forces that govern fluid dynamics in the microcirculation are capillary pressure, ISF pressure, ISF colloid osmotic pressure, and plasma colloid osmotic pressure.[2]

The plasma colloid osmotic pressure is significant to the anesthetist because this force is determined primarily by plasma protein concentration and serves to maintain the circulating fluid volume within the intravascular space. Plasma protein concentrations can be increased or decreased, depending on the types and volumes of intravenous (IV) fluids the clinician administers.

INFLUENCES OF SURGERY AND ANESTHESIA ON FLUID BALANCE

Illness, surgery, and anesthetics can profoundly alter the fluid and electrolyte balance of patients during the perioperative period.

Preoperatively, patients can become volume depleted and experience alterations of electrolyte balance due to several processes. Burns, vomiting, diarrhea, fever, and gastric suction can lead to hypovolemia before surgery.[5] If a large volume of fluid is lost from the gastrointestinal (GI) tract, careful evaluation of electrolytes and appropriate replacement is indicated.[4] Quite often, preoperative hypovolemia is at least in part an iatrogenic phenomenon secondary to bowel preparation and preoperative fasting. Unless surgery is of the greatest urgency, to reduce the risk of hypotension and complications resulting from electrolyte imbalances, preoperative fluid deficits and electrolyte abnormalities should be corrected before anesthetic induction.[6]

During the intraoperative period, the effects of surgery and anesthesia combine to challenge fluid and electrolyte homeostasis. Surgery can lead to hemorrhage and a need to replace fluids or blood. Surgery can also lead to evaporative loss; loss from exposed viscera is composed entirely of water (without electrolytes) and is most appropriately replaced with free water (water available for dissolving substances). Manipulation of tissues during surgery can lead to "third spacing," which is the redistribution of fluid from the intravascular space to the interstitial space. Replacement of fluid lost from the intravascular space in the phenomenon of third spacing is best carried out by balanced

TABLE 21-1	Approximate Values of Total Body Fluid as Percentage of Body Weight in Relation to Age and Sex
Age	**Total Body Fluid (% of Body Weight)**
Full-term newborn	70-80
1 year	64
Puberty to 39 years	Men: 60 / Women: 52
40-60 years	Men: 55 / Women: 47
>60 years	Men: 52 / Women: 46

From Metheney N. Fluid and Electrolyte Balance: Nursing Considerations. 4th ed. Philadelphia: Lippincott; 2000:4.

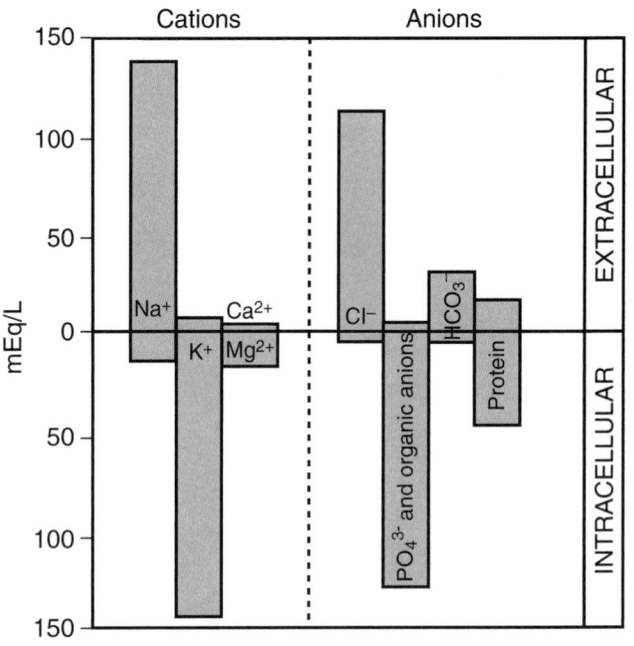

FIGURE 21-1 Major cations and anions of the intracellular and extracellular fluids. (From Guyton AC, Hall JE. Textbook of Medical Physiology. 11th ed. Philadelphia: Saunders; 2006:294.)

TABLE 21-2	Osmolar Substances in Extracellular and Intracellular Fluids		
	Plasma (mOsm/L H₂O)	Interstitial Fluid (mOsm/L H₂O)	Intracellular Fluid (mOsm/L H₂O)
Na^+	142	139	14
K^+	4.2	4	140
Ca^{2+}	1.3	1.2	0
Mg^{2+}	0.8	0.7	20
Cl^-	108	108	4
HCO_3^-	24	28.3	10
$HPO_4^-, H_2PO_4^-$	2	2	11
SO_4^{2-}	0.5	0.5	1
Phosphocreatine	—	—	45
Carnosine	—	—	14
Amino acids	2	2	8
Creatine	0.2	0.2	9
Lactate	1.2	1.2	1.5
Adenosine triphosphate	—	—	5
Hexose monophosphate	—	—	3.7
Glucose	5.6	5.6	—
Protein	1.2	0.2	4
Urea	4	4	4
Others	4.8	3.9	10
Total mOsm/L	301.8	300.8	301.2
Corrected osmolar activity (mOsm/L)	282	281	281
Total osmotic pressure at 37° C (mm Hg)	5443	5423	5423

From Guyton AC, Hall JE. Textbook of Medical Physiology. 11th ed. Philadelphia: Saunders; 2006:294.

salt solutions that have an electrolyte composition similar to ECF.[1,6] Absorption of electrolyte-free irrigation solutions during transurethral prostate surgery or endometrial ablation can result in a life-threatening hyposmolar state that must be addressed appropriately by the clinician.[7]

Anesthesia in and of itself can lead to derangements of fluid balance in surgical patients. The vasodilatory effects of both regional and general anesthesia can result in a relative hypovolemia, which may lead to hypotension on induction. General anesthesia increases the release of antidiuretic hormone, causing increased retention of water,[1,8] which can predispose the patient to hyponatremia.[9] Mechanical ventilation can increase evaporative loss of water and decrease the release of atrial natriuretic peptide, leading to renal conservation of sodium.[1]

The effects of surgery on fluid balance can persist into the postoperative period. Third-spaced fluids are typically mobilized (returned to the intravascular space) on the third postoperative day. The increased circulating volume may be poorly tolerated by patients with marginal renal or cardiovascular performance and can result in heart failure or pulmonary edema.[4,10]

FLUID VOLUME DISORDERS

Fluid volume disorders, particularly hypovolemia, are often encountered in patients undergoing surgery. Discussion of disorders of concentration and volume of body fluids is facilitated by careful consideration of the concepts of osmolarity, osmolality, and tonicity. Osmolarity is an expression of the number of osmoles of solute in a liter of solution, whereas osmolality expresses the number of osmoles of solute in a kilogram of solvent. Because of the dilute nature of body fluids, the difference between osmolarity and osmolality is minimal. Tonicity, a concept related to osmolarity and osmolality, describes how a solution affects cell volume. Isotonic solutions have an effective osmolality close to that of body fluids (approximately 285 mOsm/L)[3]; therefore, cells placed in an isotonic solution are not expected to swell or shrink.

Volume depletion, or *hypovolemia*, refers to the loss of ECF and is not to be confused with *dehydration*, which refers to a concentration disorder in which insufficient water is present relative to sodium levels.[3] Hypovolemia can result from an absolute loss of fluid from the body or a relative loss of bodily fluids in which water is redistributed within the body, leading to a reduced circulating volume. Causes of absolute fluid loss include loss of fluid from the GI tract, polyuria, and diaphoresis. Decreased intake of fluids is a common cause of absolute fluid deficit in surgical patients because of intolerance to oral fluids and prolonged preoperative fasting. Relative fluid losses can be caused by conditions such as burns and third-space losses resulting from surgery. It should be noted that patient weight does not decrease in cases of relative fluid loss.

Because most cases of hypovolemia are caused by the loss of ECF, replacement with isotonic crystalloids (which have a composition similar to ECF) is appropriate.[3] Determining the appropriate volume of fluids to administer for maintenance and replacement needs is discussed later; however, in certain circumstances such as oliguria or hemodynamic instability, a fluid bolus (also known as *fluid challenge*) may be warranted (Table 21-3). Estimated fluid and blood requirements based on the clinical presentation of a patient have been described by the American College of Surgeons (Table 21-4).

Hypervolemia is an excess of fluid volume in an isotonic concentration. Hypervolemia is not usually encountered in surgical patients but can be seen if diseases such as congestive heart

TABLE 21-3	Fluid Challenge Guideline Chart	
Baseline Values		
PAWP* (mm Hg)	**Challenge Volume**	**CVP* (mm Hg)**
<12	200 mL/10 min or 20 mL/min	<8
12-16	100 mL/10 min or 10 mL/min	8-13
>16-18	50 mL/10 min or 5 mL/min	>13

- Reprofile at the end of 10 minutes of fluid challenge.
- Discontinue challenge if PAWP increases >7 mm Hg or CVP increases >4 mm Hg.
- Repeat challenge if PAWP increases <3 mm Hg or CVP increases <2 mm Hg.
- Observe patient for 10 minutes and reprofile if PAWP increases >3 mm Hg but <7 mm Hg, or CVP increases >2 mm Hg or <4 mm Hg.

Adapted from Lichtenthal, PR. Quick Guide to Cardiopulmonary Care. Irvine, CA: Edwards Lifesciences; 2002:60.
CVP, Central venous pressure; PAWP, pulmonary artery wedge pressure.
**References differ on CVP and PAWP range.*

failure, renal failure, or cirrhosis of the liver are present. Iatrogenic causes of fluid overload include administration of steroids and excessive IV administration of isotonic fluids. Excessive consumption of sodium in the diet or in medications can lead to retention of water and hypervolemia. Treatment of hypervolemia may include sodium restriction, diuretics, and in cases of renal failure, hemodialysis or ultrafiltration.

DISORDERS OF SODIUM BALANCE

Disorders of sodium balance may be encountered in anesthetic care and are of great clinical significance. Sodium is the most abundant electrolyte in the ECF; along with its accompanying chloride anion (NaCl), it is responsible for most of the osmotic activity of the ECF. The physiologic significance of sodium can be appreciated when one considers that gain or loss of sodium is accompanied by a gain or loss of water.[3] Because sodium concentration in the ECF is much higher than in the intracellular space (as a result of the action of the Na-K-ATPase pump in the cell membrane), alteration of sodium levels in the extracellular space greatly affects the osmotic relationship between intracellular and extracellular spaces, leading to movement of water across the cell membrane.

The clinical importance of sodium disorders is due largely to the influence of sodium on the water content in brain cells. The blood-brain barrier, unlike peripheral capillary beds, has only limited permeability to ionic solutes. The result of the limited permeability in the blood-brain barrier is prevention of equilibration of osmotically active ionic solutes between intravascular and interstitial spaces. This lack of permeability to sodium (and consequent failure to equilibrate osmotically active solutes between the intravascular and interstitial spaces) changes the osmotic gradients between fluid compartments, leading to the precedence of sodium over plasma proteins as the most important osmotically active substance influencing the water content of the brain tissues.[10,11]

TABLE 21-4	Advanced Trauma Life Support Estimates of Fluid and Blood Requirements in a 70-kg Man			
	Initial Presentations			
	Class I	**Class II**	**Class III**	**Class IV**
Blood loss (mL)	<750	750-1500	1500-2000	≥2000
Blood loss (% of blood volume)	<15	15-30	30-40	≥40
Pulse rate (bpm)	<100	>100	>120	≥140
Blood pressure	Normal	Normal	Decreased	Decreased
Pulse pressure (mm Hg)	Normal or increased	Decreased	Decreased	Decreased
Capillary blanch test	Normal	Positive	Positive	Positive
Respiratory rate	14-20	20-30	30-40	>35
Urine output (mL/hr)	30 or more	20-30	5-15	Negligible
CNS-mental status	Slightly anxious	Mildly anxious	Anxious and confused	Confused and lethargic
Fluid replacement	Crystalloid	Crystalloid	Crystalloid + blood	Crystalloid + blood

From Lichtenthal PR. Quick Guide to Cardiopulmonary Care. Irvine, CA: Edwards Lifesciences; 2002:59.
bpm, *Beats per minute;* CNS, *central nervous system.*

BOX 21-1

Hyponatremia (Serum Sodium <135 mEq/L)

Causative Factors and Classification
Isotonic Hyponatremia (Pseudohyponatremia)
Serum osmolality 280-285
Causes: Hyperlipidemia, hyperproteinemia, infusion of isotonic nonelectrolytic substances (glucose, mannitol glycine)

Hypertonic Hyponatremia
Serum osmolality >285
Causes: Hyperglycemia, infusion of hypertonic nonelectrolytic substances

Hypotonic Hyponatremia
Serum osmolality <280
Hypovolemic hypotonic hyponatremia
Causes: Diuretics, salt-losing nephropathy, ketonuria, third spacing, adrenal insufficiency, vomiting, diarrhea, third spacing of fluids
Isovolemic hypotonic hyponatremia
Causes: SIADH, renal failure, hypothyroidism, drugs, water intoxication, drugs

Hypervolemic hypotonic hyponatremia
Causes: Nephrotic syndrome, cirrhosis, congestive heart failure

Clinical Manifestations
Neurologic Manifestations
Seizure
Coma
Agitation
Confusion
Headache
Confusion
Cerebral edema

Gastrointestinal Manifestations
Anorexia
Nausea and vomiting

Muscular Manifestations
Cramps
Weakness

From Metheney N. Fluid and Electrolyte Balance: Nursing Considerations. *4th ed. Philadelphia: Lippincott; 2000:58-89; Ferri FF. Practical Guide to the Care of the Medical Patient. 5th ed. St Louis: Mosby; 2001:594-601; Barash PG et al. Handbook of Clinical Anesthesia. 5th ed. Philadelphia: Lippincott; 2005:95-96.*
ADH, *Antidiuretic hormone;* SIADH, *syndrome of inappropriate secretion of antidiuretic hormone;* U_Na, *urinary sodium.*

Because sodium imbalances reflect impaired concentration between water and sodium, evaluation of sodium imbalance should take into consideration both the volume of the solvent (water) and the amount of solute (sodium) present in the solution. Likewise, treatment of sodium imbalances can involve restriction or expansion of water volume and enhanced elimination or supplementation of sodium.

Hyponatremia may have multiple causes (Box 21-1). Of particular interest to anesthetists is hyponatremia resulting from

inappropriate secretion of antidiuretic hormone (SIADH), which is discussed in Chapter 34. Water intoxication resulting from the absorption of electrolyte-free irrigation solution during procedures such as transurethral resection of the prostate and endometrial ablation are discussed in Chapter 30. Water intoxication and SIADH lead to hyponatremia from an excess of water, not loss of sodium.[1,12]

Hyponatremia results in a condition in which the intracellular environment is hyperosmolar relative to the ECF, leading to an

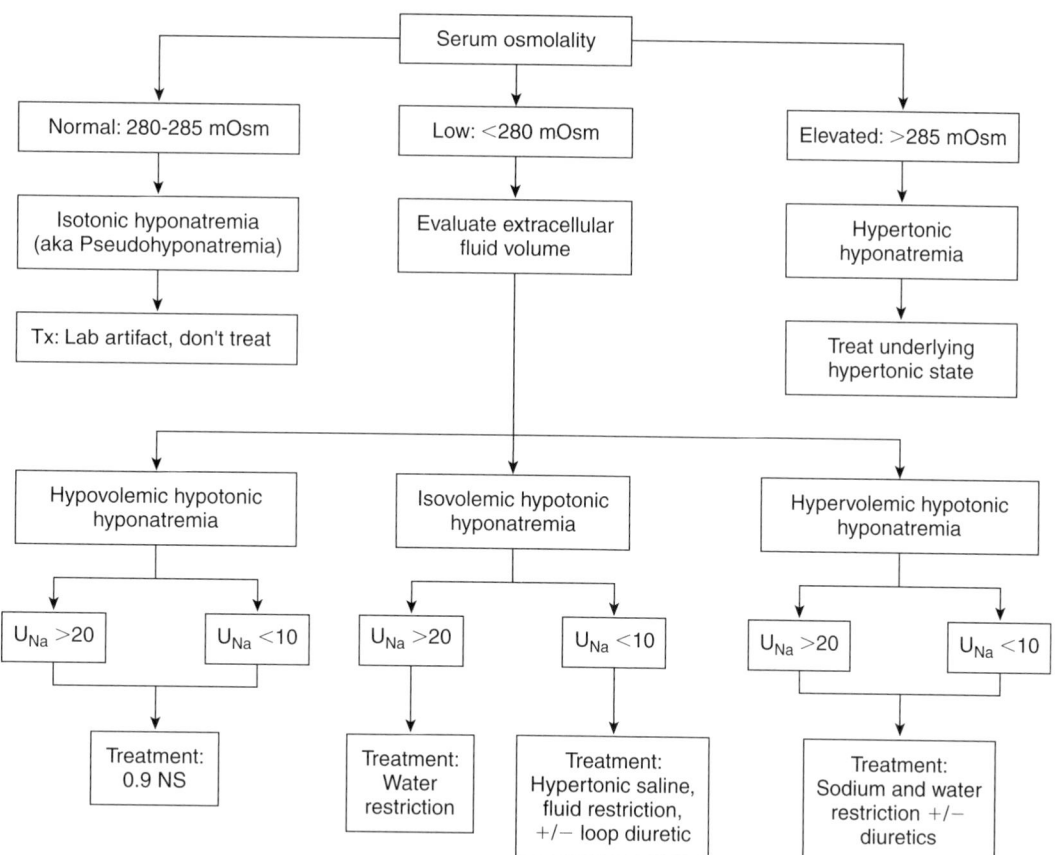

FIGURE **21-2** Treatment of hyponatremia. *Tx,* Treatment; U_{Na}, urinary sodium; NS, normal saline. (*Modified from Ferri FF: Practical Guide to the Care of the Medical Patient. 5th ed. St Louis: Mosby; 2001.*)

influx of water into the intracellular space. One of the most significant consequences of hyponatremia is cerebral edema. Because the brain is contained within the fixed confines of the skull, cerebral edema is poorly tolerated.[13] Compensatory mechanisms can forestall the development of symptomatic cerebral edema for a period of time.[14] Brain cells can maintain osmotic equilibrium by extruding intracellular solutes, thereby reducing intracellular osmolality.[9,13] However, if the extrusion of solute by brain cells is inadequate to compensate for the hyposmolar influence of the ECF, an intracellular influx of water may lead to symptomatic cerebral edema.[13]

Clinical studies have demonstrated that compared with men or postmenopausal women, menstruant women are at increased risk of brain damage resulting from hyponatremia.[3,13] It is believed that estrogen and progesterone inhibit the efficiency of the Na-K-ATPase pump, which is essential to the extrusion of intracellular solutes to maintain osmotic equilibrium in hyponatremia; female sex hormones may facilitate movement of water into the brain through the mediation of ADH.[13]

Some controversy exists as to how aggressively hyponatremia should be treated (Figure 21-2). In chronically hyponatremic patients, rapid correction of serum sodium can lead to the neurologic disorder known as *myelinolysis*. Myelinolysis, originally known as *central pontine myelinolysis*, can lead to disorders of the upper neurons, spastic quadriparesis, pseudobulbar palsy, mental disorders, and in some cases death.[14] Patients at particular risk for myelinolysis are those who have been hyponatremic for more than 48 hours[9,14] and individuals who have had orthotopic

liver transplantation or a history of alcohol abuse.[14] Optimal treatment of hyponatremia must balance the risks of cerebral edema against the risks of myelinolysis.[12]

The risk of myelinolysis can be reduced by correcting serum sodium levels in a deliberate manner. It has been suggested that serum sodium concentrations should be increased by no more than 1 to 2 mEq/L/hr. In symptomatic patients, this is accomplished by infusing 3% saline at a rate of 1 to 2 mL/kg/hr. Once the patient is clinically stable, sodium administration should be slowed to raise serum sodium not more than 10 to 15 mmol/L in 24 hours.[9,12,14]

Hypernatremia can result from several causes (Figure 21-3 and Box 21-2) but is usually the result of impaired water intake.[12] Inadequate administration of free water to hospitalized patients can lead to an iatrogenic hypernatremia. Debilitated, mentally impaired, and intubated individuals are at particular risk for developing hypernatremia.[4,12] In cases of slow-onset hypernatremia, the brain can adapt by conserving intracellular solutes, which allows maintenance of normal intracellular volume. Rapidly occurring hypernatremia can be accompanied by rapid shrinking of the brain and concomitant traction on intracranial veins and venous sinuses, leading to intracranial hemorrhage.[7]

As with hyponatremia, overly aggressive treatment of chronic hypernatremia can lead to unwanted effects. In the case of hypernatremia, rapid correction of serum sodium with solutions containing large amounts of free water may lead to cerebral edema.[7]

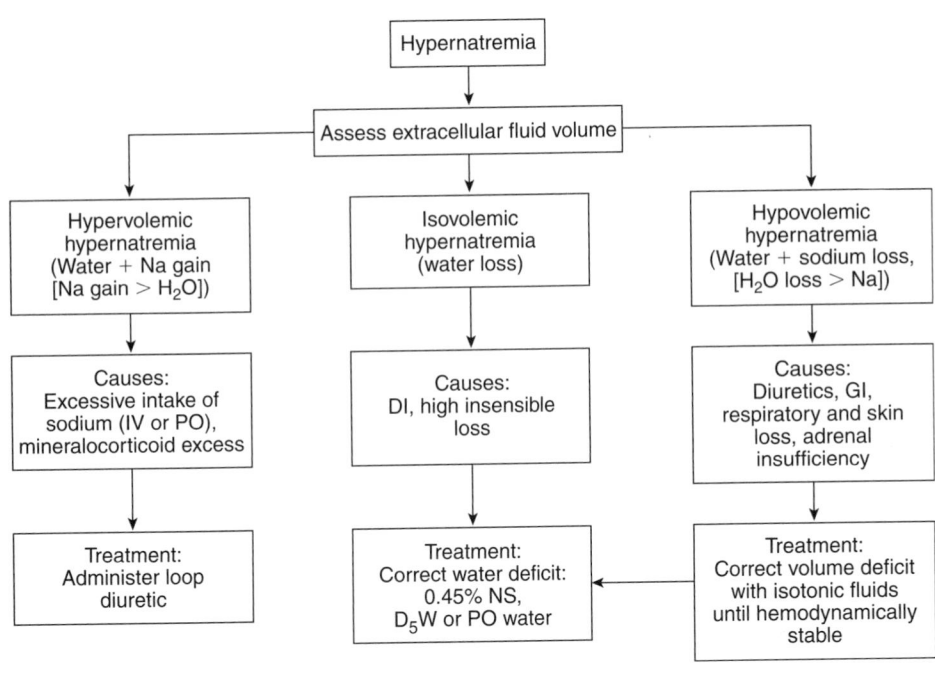

FIGURE 21-3 Hypernatremia (serum sodium [Na] >145 mEq/L). *PO, Oral; NS, normal saline. (Modified from Ferri FF. Practical Guide to the Care of the Medical Patient. 5th ed. St Louis: Mosby; 2001; Morgan GE et al. Clinical Anesthesiology. 3rd ed. New York: Lange Medical; 2002.)*

BOX 21-2

Clinical Manifestations of Hypernatremia (Serum Sodium >145 mEq/L)

Neurologic Manifestations
Thirst
Weakness
Seizure
Coma
Intracranial bleeding
Disorientation
Hallucinations
Irritability

Cardiovascular Manifestations
Hypovolemia

Renal Manifestations
Polyuria or oliguria
Renal insufficiency

Modified from Metheney N. Fluid and Electrolyte Balance: Nursing Considerations. 4th ed. Philadelphia: Lippincott; 2000:58-59; Ferri FF. Practical Guide to the Care of the Medical Patient. 5th ed. St Louis: Mosby; 2001:594-601; Barash PG et al. Handbook of Clinical Anesthesia. 5th ed. Philadelphia: Lippincott; 2005.

BOX 21-3

Estimation of Water Deficit

1. Solve for current total body water (TBW):

$$\text{(Normal TBW [weight} \times \text{fluid as \% TBW])(Target Na}^+) = \text{(Current TBW)(Current Na}^+)$$

2. Solve for deficit:

$$\text{Water deficit} = \text{Normal TBW} - \text{Current TBW}$$

From Morgan GE et al. Clinical Anesthesiology. 4th ed. New York: Lange Medical; 2006:671.

Correction of hypernatremia is carried out by replacement of the water deficit, which can be calculated by the formula shown in Box 21-3. If the hypernatremia is acute (i.e., less than 24 hours' duration), water deficits can be replaced relatively rapidly with hypotonic solutions. If chronic hypernatremia accompanied by volume depletion is present, the volume disorder is corrected first with isotonic crystalloids. Once the circulating volume has been restored, hypotonic solutions are used to correct the water deficit. Correction of chronic hypernatremia, like treatment of chronic hyponatremia, calls for prudence. Plasma sodium should be decreased by 1 to 2 mEq/hr until the patient is clinically stable, and correction of serum sodium to normal levels should gradually progress over the subsequent 24 hours.[12]

DISORDERS OF POTASSIUM BALANCE

Potassium is the principal electrolyte of the ICF, where 98% of the body's supply of potassium is located. The difference between intracellular and extracellular potassium concentration is in large part responsible for the resting membrane potential of the cell.[15] Potassium exists in a dynamic balance between the intracellular and extracellular compartments. Abnormal serum potassium levels may be the result of disturbances in the balance between intracellular and extracellular distribution of potassium or an abnormality in the total body store of potassium. Evaluation and treatment of disorders of potassium homeostasis should

BOX **21-4**

Hypokalemia (Serum Potassium <3.5 mEq/L)

Causative Factors
Redistribution
  Alkalosis
  Insulin administration
  β-Agonists

Increased Renal Excretion
  Multiple drug use, especially potassium-losing
    diuretics, penicillin, aminoglycosides, corticosteroids
  Hyperaldosteronism
  Renal tubular acidosis
  Magnesium deficiency

Gastrointestinal Loss
  Diarrhea
  Gastric suctioning
  Villous adenoma
  Fistulas

Inadequate Intake
  Anorexia
  Alcoholism
  Debilitation

Clinical Manifestations
Cardiovascular Manifestations
  ST-segment depression
  Widened QRS complex
  Flattened T waves
  Ventricular ectopy

Neuromuscular Manifestations
  Weakness
  Decreased reflexes
  Confusion

Renal Manifestations
  Polyuria
  Concentrating defect

Metabolic Manifestations
  Glucose intolerance
  Potentiation of hypercalcemia and hypomagnesemia

From Metheney N. Fluid and Electrolyte Balance: Nursing Considerations. 4th ed. Philadelphia: Lippincott; 2000:90-109; Ferri FF. Practical Guide to the Care of the Medical Patient. 5th ed. St Louis: Mosby; 2001:601-606; Barash PG et al. Handbook of Clinical Anesthesia. 5th ed. Philadelphia: Lippincott; 2005.

address factors that can shift potassium into the cell and total body levels of potassium. The symptoms associated with disorders of potassium homeostasis are largely a reflection of disorders of resting membrane potential. Clinically this is seen most clearly in the dysrhythmias associated with abnormal potassium levels (Box 21-4).

Hypokalemia, defined as plasma potassium of less than 3.5 mEq/L, can result from an absolute deficiency caused by GI loss, renal loss, or from a poor intake of potassium (see Box 21-4). Redistribution of potassium from the extracellular to the intracellular compartment can also lead to hypokalemia. β-Adrenergic stimulation, insulin, and alkalosis all promote movement of potassium into the intracellular space.[16]

Treatment of hypokalemia depends on the severity of the symptoms accompanying the potassium deficit. In the face of malignant dysrhythmias, aggressive IV administration of potassium is warranted.[15] IV replacement of potassium should be accomplished with the patient under continuous ECG monitoring. Rates of IV administration as fast as 40 mEq/hr have been reported,[16] although a maximum rate of 10 to 20 mEq/hr is usually recommended to avoid an iatrogenic hyperkalemia.[4,7]

Once serious symptoms of hypokalemia such as respiratory muscle weakness or dysrhythmia have ceased, IV replacement can be discontinued in favor of oral supplementation.[16] It is recommended that IV potassium be replaced as a chloride, because the hypochloride state makes it difficult for the kidney to conserve potassium.[4] Furthermore, potassium chloride should be mixed in a dextrose-free solution to prevent stimulation of insulin, leading to increased redistribution of potassium to the intracellular space.[7]

Some clinicians have questioned whether surgery should be canceled because of low serum potassium. In a study of 447 patients scheduled for cardiovascular surgery, Hirsch and co-workers used continuous electrocardiographic monitoring to evaluate the preoperative and intraoperative incidence of ectopy. They found no significant difference in frequent or complex ventricular ectopy among patients with normal serum potassium and those with mild to severe hypokalemia. The authors concluded that cancellation of surgery based on low serum potassium was not warranted.[17]

Hyperkalemia is less common than hypokalemia; if renal causes are excluded, the incidence is quite uncommon.[16] In addition to impaired renal excretion of potassium, causes of hyperkalemia include a high intake of potassium and a shift of potassium from the intracellular to the extracellular space. Movement of potassium from the intracellular to the extracellular compartment can result from lysis of cells, as well as from acidemia and the administration of β-adrenergic blockers, which inhibit the Na-K-ATPase pump and disrupt movement of potassium into the cell (Box 21-5).

Treatment of hyperkalemia should be preceded by exclusion of pseudohyperkalemia, which is a laboratory artifact. Pseudohyperkalemia results from hemolysis of the blood sample, leukocytosis, thrombosis, or prolonged fist clenching during blood drawing. Treatment of hyperkalemia is based on the severity of the patient's presenting signs and symptoms (Figure 21-4).

BOX **21-5**

Hyperkalemia (Serum Potassium >5.0 mEq/L)

Causative Factors
Redistribution
  Acidosis
  Hypertonicity
  Hemolysis
  Tissue necrosis
  Rhabdomyolysis

Decreased Renal Excretion
  Renal insufficiency and failure
  Potassium-sparing diuretics
  Hypoaldosteronism
  Drugs (e.g., NSAIDs, β-blockers, ACE inhibitors)

Excessive Potassium Intake
  IV or PO supplementation
  Excessive use of salt substitutes
  Rapid transfusion of banked blood

Clinical Manifestations
Cardiovascular Manifestations
  Tall, peaked T waves
  Widened QRS complex
  Ventricular dysrhythmias
  Cardiac arrest

Neuromuscular Manifestations
  Muscle weakness
  Confusion
  Paresthesias

From Metheney N. Fluid and Electrolyte Balance: Nursing Considerations. 4th ed. Philadelphia: Lippincott; 2000:90-109; Ferri FF. Practical Guide to the Care of the Medical Patient. 5th ed. St Louis: Mosby; 2001:606-613; Barash PG et al. Handbook of Clinical Anesthesia. 5th ed. Philadelphia: Lippincott; 2005.
ACE, Angiotensin-converting enzyme; IV, intravenous; NSAIDs, nonsteroidal antiinflammatory drugs; PO, orally.

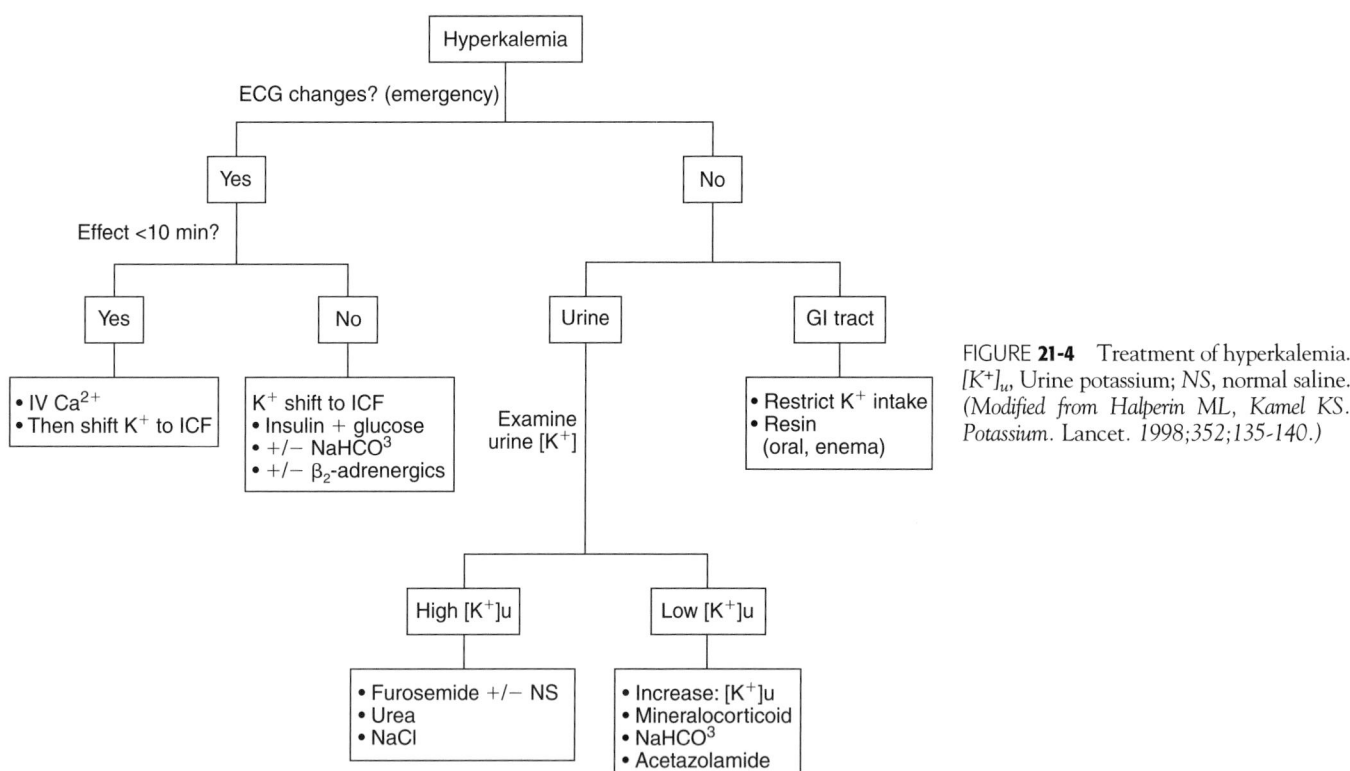

FIGURE **21-4**   Treatment of hyperkalemia. $[K^+]_u$, Urine potassium; *NS*, normal saline. *(Modified from Halperin ML, Kamel KS. Potassium. Lancet. 1998;352;135-140.)*

DISORDERS OF CALCIUM BALANCE

Calcium is a divalent cation, 99% of which is found in bones. Calcium has an important structural function, but perhaps most important to anesthetists is its role as a second messenger that couples cell membrane receptors to cellular responses. The action of calcium as a second messenger is critical to functions such as muscle contractions and release of hormones and neurotransmitters.[2,18] In addition to the second messenger function, calcium plays an important role in coagulation of blood and in muscle function.

BOX 21-6

Hypocalcemia (Serum Calcium <8.9 mg/dL, Ionized Calcium <4.6 mg/dL)

Causative Factors
Hypoparathyroidism (can be surgically induced)
Pseudohypoparathyroidism
Malabsorption
Acute pancreatitis
Malignancy
Alkalosis
Hyperphosphatemia
Rhabdomyolysis
Chronic renal insufficiency
Hypomagnesemia

Clinical Manifestations
Cardiovascular Manifestations
Dysrhythmia
Prolonged QT interval
T-wave inversion
Hypotension
Decreased myocardial contractility

Neuromuscular Manifestations
Cramps
Muscle weakness
Chvostek sign
Trousseau sign
Seizure
Numbness
Tingling

Pulmonary Manifestations
Laryngospasm
Bronchospasm
Hypoventilation

From Metheney N. Fluid and Electrolyte Balance: Nursing Considerations. 4th ed. Philadelphia: Lippincott; 2000:111-129; Barash PG et al. Handbook of Clinical Anesthesia. 5th ed. Philadelphia: Lippincott; 2005.

BOX 21-7

Hypercalcemia (Serum Calcium >10.5 mg/dL, Ionized Calcium >5.6 mg/dL)

Causative Factors
Hyperparathyroidism
Malignancy
Thiazide diuretics
Thyrotoxicosis
Renal failure
Excessive intake of calcium supplements

Clinical Manifestations
Cardiovascular Manifestations
Hypertension
Heart block
Shortened QT interval
Dysrhythmia

Neuromuscular Manifestations
Muscle weakness
Decreased deep tendon reflexes
Sedation

Renal Manifestations
Hypercalcuria
Polyuria

Gastrointestinal Manifestations
Anorexia
Pancreatitis

Modified from Metheney N. Fluid and Electrolyte Balance: Nursing Considerations. 4th ed. Philadelphia: Lippincott; 2000:111-129; Barash PG et al. Handbook of Clinical Anesthesia. 5th ed. Philadelphia: Lippincott; 2005.

Although most of the body's calcium is found in the bones, a small percentage is freely exchangeable with the ECF. Calcium in the ECF is found in three distinct fractions. Ionized calcium accounts for 50% of the calcium in the ECF and is the physiologically active portion of circulating calcium.[1] The remainder of the circulating calcium is bound either to anions (10%) or plasma proteins, primarily albumin (40%).[19] Changes in pH alter the extracellular distribution of calcium, with acidemia decreasing the protein-bound fraction and increasing the ionized fraction.[4]

Because the ionized fraction of calcium is the most clinically significant form, and total serum calcium levels are largely dependent on albumin levels, direct measurement of ionized calcium is the preferred method in critically ill patients.[3] Mathematical formulas to "correct" total calcium measurement for albumin concentration are available but have been characterized as inaccurate.[4,19]

Hypocalcemia has numerous causes (Box 21-6). In the intraoperative period, the most likely causes of hypocalcemia are hyperventilation and massive transfusion of citrated blood. Hyperventilation leads to an increased pH and an increased protein-bound fraction of calcium. Massive transfusion of citrated blood is discussed later in this chapter.

Treatment of acute hypocalcemia involves the infusion of calcium salts. Calcium chloride is the most bioavailable parenteral preparation of calcium and results in the most rapid correction of hypocalcemia; however, it is more irritating to the vein than calcium gluconate.[19] One technique for treatment of hypocalcemia calls for administration of 10 mL of 10% calcium gluconate (93 mg of elemental calcium) over 10 minutes, followed by an infusion of 0.3 to 2 mg/kg/hr of elemental calcium.[4]

Hypercalcemia typically results from a situation in which the movement of calcium from the bone to the ECF exceeds the ability of the kidney to excrete calcium (Box 21-7). Primary hyperparathyroidism accounts for more than half of all cases of hypercalcemia, with malignancy being the second most common cause.[19] Treatment of hypercalcemia involves volume expansion with normal saline (NS) (severely hypercalcemic patients are typically hypovolemic), which in and of itself increases renal excretion of calcium. Addition of a loop diuretic further

---

BOX **21-8**

Hypomagnesemia (Serum Magnesium <1.7 mg/dL)

Causative Factors
Inadequate Intake
  Total parenteral nutrition without supplementation
  Starvation
  Chronic alcoholism

Increased Gastrointestinal Losses
  Diarrhea
  Fistulas
  Nasogastric suctioning
  Vomiting

Increased Renal Losses
  Diuretics
  Aminoglycosides

Changes in Distribution
  Pancreatitis
  Insulin
  Glucose
  Catecholamines

Clinical Manifestations
Cardiovascular Manifestations
  Coronary vasospasm
  Dysrhythmia
  Ventricular fibrillation
  Congestive heart failure
  QT and PR prolongation
  QRS widening

Neuromuscular Manifestations
  Weakness
  Chvostek sign
  Trousseau sign

Miscellaneous Manifestations
  Hypocalcemia
  Hypokalemia
  Nausea
  Anorexia

Modified from Metheney N. Fluid and Electrolyte Balance: Nursing Considerations. 4th ed. Philadelphia: Lippincott; 2000:131-144; Ferri FF. Practical Guide to the Care of the Medical Patient. 5th ed. St Louis: Mosby; 2001:608-609; Barash PG et al. Handbook of Clinical Anesthesia. 5th ed. Philadelphia: Lippincott; 2005.

---

enhances the renal excretion of calcium. Bisphosphonates, mithramycin, calcitonin, glucocorticoids, and phosphate salts also have been used in the treatment of hypercalcemia.[3]

DISORDERS OF MAGNESIUM BALANCE

Magnesium is the second most abundant intracellular cation, second only to potassium. The physiologic importance of magnesium lies in its role as a cofactor in more than 300 enzymatic reactions, including those involving energy metabolism and the function of the Na-K-ATPase pump.[18]

Hypomagnesemia is common in hospitalized patients, especially critically ill patients.[1,7] Magnesium deficiency is usually the result of increased renal or GI loss or poor intake of the electrolyte[3] (Box 21-8). Thirty percent of alcoholics admitted to the hospital are hypomagnesemic because of poor dietary intake.[7] Severe hypomagnesemia can be treated with administration of 1 to 2 g of magnesium sulfate over 5 minutes while the ECG is monitored, followed by administration of 1 to 2 g/hr of magnesium sulfate.[3]

Hypermagnesemia is most commonly the result of iatrogenesis (Box 21-9). Hypermagnesemia can result from the treatment of preeclampsia, preterm labor, ischemic heart disease, and cardiac dysrhythmias.[20] The symptoms of hypermagnesemia tend to reflect depression of the peripheral and central nervous systems and are dose related. Because magnesium potentiates the action of nondepolarizing neuromuscular relaxants, their use should be carefully monitored in patients with hypermagnesemia.[1] Treatment of hypermagnesemia involves discontinuing the administration of magnesium; in urgent situations such as bradycardia, heart block, and respiratory depression, calcium should be used as an antagonist.[7,21]

BOX **21-9**

Hypermagnesemia (Serum Magnesium >2.5 mg/dL)

Causative Factors
  Renal failure
  Excessive magnesium administration
  Adrenal insufficiency

Clinical Manifestations
Serum Magnesium Levels
  3-5 = Flushing, nausea and vomiting
  4-7 = Drowsiness, decreased deep tendon reflexes, weakness
  5-10 = Hypotension, bradycardia
  7-10 = Loss of patellar reflex
  10 = Respiratory depression
  10-15 = Respiratory paralysis, coma
  15-20 = Cardiac arrest

Modified from Metheney N. Fluid and Electrolyte Balance: Nursing Considerations. 4th ed. Philadelphia: Lippincott; 2000:131-144; Ferri FF. Practical Guide to the Care of the Medical Patient. 5th ed. St Louis: Mosby; 2001:609; Barash PG et al. Handbook of Clinical Anesthesia. 5th ed. Philadelphia: Lippincott; 2005.

PARENTERAL FLUIDS

Intravenous fluids are the primary means by which the anesthetist addresses a patient's need for fluid and electrolytes. Parenteral fluid therapy serves three principal purposes: provision of maintenance fluids, replacement of fluids lost as a result of surgery and anesthesia, and correction of electrolyte disturbances.[3] In anesthesia practice, IV fluids fall into two main categories: crystalloids (Table 21-5) and colloids.

Crystalloid solutions, which consist of fluids and electrolytes, are the most commonly used fluids in the surgical setting. Balanced salt solutions are crystalloids formulated to consist of an electrolyte concentration similar to ECF.[1] Two balanced salt solutions commonly administered to patients undergoing surgery include NS (also known as *0.9% normal saline* or *0.9% NS*) and lactated Ringer's (LR) solution.

Isotonic solutions such as NS and LR are commonly used to correct the hypovolemia resulting from surgery and anesthesia because the bulk of fluid lost is isotonic. Excessive volumes of NS have been associated with hyperchloremic metabolic acidosis.[22] A study by Scheingraber and colleagues revealed that a significant acidosis was noted when NS but not LR was administered at a rate of 35 mL/kg/hr over a 2-hour period during the perioperative period.[23] Although large-volume administration of LR may not result in acidosis, metabolic alkalosis may result when lactate is metabolized into bicarbonate by the liver[6]; furthermore, the potassium in LR can accumulate in patients with renal failure.

Hypertonic saline solutions (3% or 5% NaCl), or saline solutions containing Na concentrations exceeding 154 mEq/L, have been used as low-volume solutions for fluid resuscitation. Because of its hyperosmolar characteristics, hypertonic saline draws water from the interstitium into the vascular space. However, hypertonic saline carries with it a risk of unwanted hyperchloremia, hypernatremia, and cellular dehydration, as well as a limited intravascular duration. In the past, the principal role for hypertonic saline was the treatment of hyponatremia.[1] Current research suggests that hypertonic saline solutions can be effective in treating hemorrhagic shock, particularly in patients with traumatic brain injury (TBI).[24] Hypertonic saline has been shown to increase blood pressure, increase cardiac output, and decrease intracranial pressure (ICP).[25]

Dextrose is often added to crystalloid parenteral solutions for a variety of reasons. Dextrose 5% in water (D5W) is mildly hypotonic and is often used to provide free water that is available to the body once the dextrose has been metabolized. Dextrose also can be used as a metabolic substrate but is not usually administered intraoperatively because of the risk of hyperglycemia. Intraoperative dextrose administration is warranted in patients such as neonates, who have limited glycogen stores,[26] and diabetic patients who have received insulin and are at risk of hypoglycemia and protein catabolism.[1]

Colloids are solutions containing osmotically active substances of high molecular weight that do not easily cross the capillary membrane and therefore draw fluid into the intravascular space and expand circulating volume.[3] Colloids can be manufactured from human blood or synthesized from nonanimal substances.

Normal human serum albumin is manufactured from pooled donor plasma and is available in 5% and 25% (commonly called *salt-poor albumin*) solutions. Albumin 5% replaces plasma loss in a 1:1 ratio and remains in the vascular space for a prolonged time because of the presence of high-molecular-weight protein molecules. Albumin 25% can expand intravascular volume up to five times the volume infused, owing to its high osmotic pressure. Albumin 25% is well suited for use in patients with excessive ECF who need intravascular expansion.[1] Colloids formulated from human blood have at least a theoretic risk of disease transmission via pathogens such as prions,[27] and availability can be limited by donor supply.[28]

Synthetic colloids include dextran, gelatins, and hetastarch. Gelatins are generally not available for use in North America.[28] Dextrans are polysaccharides that are useful for volume expansion but are also associated with anticoagulation, which limits their application to settings such as vascular surgery, in which prevention of thrombosis is desired. Dextran is also associated with risk of anaphylaxis.[3]

Hetastarch is a synthetic colloid made from plant starch. It has fluid expansion properties similar to those of albumin[3] but is far less expensive than albumin. Use of hetastarch 6% in saline has been limited by its effect on coagulation. It can produce a dilutional dysfunction of coagulation like other colloids and crystalloids. Hetastarch also directly inhibits clot formation by movement into fibrin clots.[1] Because of the effect of this colloid on coagulation, it is generally not administered in volumes exceeding 20 mL/kg. Another formulation of hetastarch, Hextend, is a solution containing 6% hetastarch with balanced electrolytes, a lactate buffer, and physiologic glucose. A study by Gan and colleagues evaluated hetastarch in saline versus the hetastarch in the buffered solution and found that patients with the newer formulation could receive the colloid in volumes exceeding 20 mL/kg without coagulopathy.[28]

Estimation of intraoperative fluid requirements is an imperfect science and is based on an understanding of patient fluid needs as well as the dynamics of fluid compartments. Fluid therapy in surgical patients should include administration of fluids to compensate for preoperative fluid deficit, maintenance fluids to compensate for evaporative losses and provide solute for excretion of waste,[26] and fluids to replace surgical fluid losses (e.g., third-space loss and blood loss).

Hourly maintenance fluid requirements are estimated according to the 4-2-1-formula (Table 21-6). A shortcut for estimating hourly maintenance fluid requirements in patients who weigh more than 20 kg is to add weight in kilograms to 40 to arrive at an hourly infusion volume in milliliters. Fluid deficit is estimated by multiplying the hourly maintenance requirement by the number of hours the patient has been without oral or parenteral fluids. Calculation of the fluid deficit also should account for fluids lost through preoperative events such as nasogastric suctioning and bowel preparation.

Surgical fluid loss consists of blood loss, evaporative loss resulting from an open wound, and third-space losses resulting from fluid redistribution. Estimation of third-space loss is based on the degree of tissue trauma expected during the surgical procedure (Table 21-7) and can be substantial (e.g., as in major abdominal surgery). Estimation of blood loss is discussed in the section on transfusion therapy; blood volume loss can be replaced by crystalloids in a 3:1 or 4:1 ratio of crystalloid to blood. The 3:1 or 4:1 ratio has come into question because of the understanding that as crystalloids are infused, plasma osmotic pressure decreases, which leads to an increased loss of fluid from the intravascular to the interstitial space. This has led some authors to suggest replacement ratios of 7:1 or even 10:1 in certain circumstances.[29] Replacement of blood with crystalloid or colloid solutions replaces volume only and does not replace lost oxygen-carrying capacity or coagulation factors.

The rate at which fluids are administered intraoperatively is determined after summation of fluid requirements for surgical loss, deficit, and maintenance. Typically, maintenance and replacement fluids are administered to meet the hourly needs of the patient, and the deficit is replaced within the first 3 hours after induction. In clinical practice, induction of anesthesia frequently requires a fluid bolus to maintain blood pressure and

TABLE 21-5   Composition of Crystalloid Solutions

Solution	Tonicity (mOsm/L)	Na⁺ (mEq/L)	Cl⁻ (mEq/L)	K⁺ (mEq/L)	Ca²⁺ (mEq/L)	Mg²⁺ (mEq/L)	Glucose (g/L)	Lactate (mEq/L)	HCO₃⁻ (mEq/L)	Acetate (mEq/L)	Gluconate (mEq/L)
5% Dextrose in water (D₅W)	Hypotonic (253)	—	—	—	—	—	50	—	—	—	—
Normal saline (NS)	Isotonic (308)	154	154	—	—	—	—	—	—	—	—
D₅ ¼ NS	Isotonic (355)	38.5	38.5	—	—	—	50	—	—	—	—
D₅ ½ NS	Hypertonic (432)	77	77	—	—	—	50	—	—	—	—
D₅ NS	Hypertonic (586)	154	154	—	—	—	50	—	—	—	—
Lactated Ringer's injection (LR)	Isotonic (273)	130	109	4	3	—	—	28	—	—	—
D₅ LR	Hypertonic (525)	130	109	4	3	—	50	28	—	—	—
½ NS	Hypotonic (154)	77	77	—	—	—	—	—	—	—	—
3% S	Hypertonic (1026)	513	513	—	—	—	—	—	—	—	—
5% S	Hypertonic (1710)	855	855	—	—	—	—	—	—	—	—
7.5% NaHCO₃	Hypertonic (1786)	893	—	—	—	—	—	—	893	—	—
Plasmalyte	Isotonic (294)	140	98	5	—	3	—	—	—	27	23

Modified from Morgan GE et al. Clinical Anesthesiology. 4th ed. New York: Lange Medical; 2006:693.

TABLE **21-6**	Estimating Maintenance Fluid Requirements
Weight	**Rate**
For the first 10 kg	4 mL/kg/hr
For the next 10-20 kg	Add 2 mL/kg/hr
For each kg above 20 kg	Add 1 mL/kg/hr
Example: What are the maintenance fluid requirements of a 25-kg child?	
Answer: 40 + 20 + 5 = 65 mL/hr	

From Morgan GE et al. Clinical Anesthesiology. 6th ed. New York: Lange Medical; 2006:695.

TABLE **21-7**	Redistribution and Evaporative Surgical Fluid Losses
Degree of Tissue Trauma	**Additional Fluid Requirements**
Minimal (e.g., in herniorrhaphy)	0-2 mL/kg
Moderate (e.g., in cholecystectomy)	2-4 mL/kg
Severe (e.g., in bowel resection)	4-8 mL/kg

From Morgan GE et al. Clinical Anesthesiology. 4th ed. New York: Lange Medical; 2006:697.

often results in an initial infusion of IV fluids that exceeds what might be suggested by calculations.

The subject of much discussion, selection of IV fluid for therapy is based in large part on the purpose of the fluid. Maintenance needs are ideally met by fluids such as 5% dextrose and ¼% NS (D_5-¼ NS), which provide free water to facilitate excretion of waste and replace evaporative loss.[26] IV therapy in the operating room is principally focused on replacement of fluids lost during surgery and uses balanced salt solutions such as NS or LR. Replacement needs can also be met by colloid solutions such as hetastarch.

The relative merits of LR versus NS as a replacement solution for trauma resuscitation were explored in an animal model by Healey and colleagues. They found that in cases of moderate hemorrhage, NS and LR were both acceptable solutions. However, in cases of massive hemorrhage, LR was found to be superior to NS because of an absence of hyperchloremic metabolic acidosis.[30]

Whether crystalloids or colloids are superior as replacement fluids has been debated for decades. The relative merits and disadvantages of each fluid are well known (Table 21-8). There is a definite lack of consensus in the literature regarding the superiority of a particular type of intravenous fluid. Literature is available to support both sides of the debate. It is noteworthy, however, that a review of existing randomized controlled trials published in 2007 concluded that crystalloids and colloids were equally effective[31] The debate not only includes the colloid versus crystalloid controversy but also extends to compare colloids and their relative merits. According to one source, albumin is easily replaced by synthetic colloid.[32] Another study published the same year discussed the merits of albumin in fluid resuscitation.[33] An additional facet to this ongoing debate is the possiblity that colloids may decrease postoperative complications such as nausea, vomiting, severe pain, periorbital edema and double vision.[34]

TABLE **21-8**	Advantages and Disadvantages of Crystalloid and Colloid Solutions for Fluid Resuscitation	
Crystalloid	**Colloid**	
Advantages		
Inexpensive	Causes sustained increase in plasma volume	
Promotes urinary flow	Requires smaller volume for resuscitation	
Restores third-space loss	Causes less peripheral edema	
Used for extracellular fluid replacement	Tends to remain intravascular after repletion	
Used for initial resuscitation	Causes more rapid resuscitation	
	Useful in conditions of altered vascular permeability	
Disadvantages		
Dilutes plasma proteins	Expensive	
Causes reduction of capillary osmotic pressure	Can cause coagulopathy (dextran > hetastarch > Hextend)	
Causes peripheral edema	Can cause anaphylactic reaction (dextran)	
Has transient effect	Decreases Ca^{2+} (albumin)	
Has potential for pulmonary edema	Can cause renal failure (dextran) Can cause osmotic diuresis Can cause impaired immune response (albumin)	

BLOOD COMPONENT THERAPY

For the purpose of volume replacement, perioperative blood loss can be replaced with crystalloids and/or colloids, but if hemorrhagic losses are significant, transfusion therapy involving the administration of blood or blood components may be necessary to restore oxygen transport and hemostasis. Decisions regarding transfusion therapy must take into account several factors, including perioperative blood loss, the clinical condition of the patient, and patient blood type.

Estimation of blood volume and blood loss and calculation of allowable blood loss are important factors to consider when making decisions about blood component therapy. Estimating blood volume takes into account patient age, gender, and weight and is summarized in Table 21-9.

Once blood volume has been estimated, a clinician can, by a simple calculation, determine the volume of blood loss that would decrease hematocrit to a target value. The formula for maximum allowable blood loss (MABL) is as follows:

Equation 21-1

$$MABL = \frac{EBV \times (\text{Starting hct} - \text{Target hct})}{\text{Starting hct}}$$

where *EBV* is estimated blood volume and *hct* is hematocrit.

Unfortunately, estimation of intraoperative blood loss is fraught with error because of a lack of practical objective measures. Intraoperative measurement of hematocrit can often be useful as a reflection of the ratio of formed elements to plasma

TABLE 21-9	Average Blood Volumes
Age	**Blood Volume**
Neonates	
Premature	95 mL/kg
Full-term	85 mL/kg
Infants	80 mL/kg
Adults	
Men	75 mL/kg
Women	67 mL/kg

From Morgan GE et al. Clinical Anesthesiology. 4th ed. New York: Lange Medical; 2006:696.

TABLE 21-10	Relationship Among Blood Groups, Antigens, Antibodies, and Blood Compatibility		
Blood Group	**Antigen on Red Blood Cell**	**Antibodies in Serum**	**Blood Group Compatibility**
A	A	Anti-B	A, O
B	B	Anti-A	B, O
AB	A and B	—	AB, A, B, O
O	—	Anti-A and anti-B	O only
Rh-positive	D	—	Rh-positive and Rh-negative
Rh-negative	—	Anti-D if sensitized	Rh-negative

but does not measure blood loss.[35] Intraoperative administration of replacement fluids can produce lowered hemograms[36]; furthermore, rapid hemorrhage is not immediately reflected in changes in hemoglobin and hematocrit *values*. Measuring net suction volume (amount of fluid suctioned minus amount of irrigant) and counting or weighing sponges are common methods used to determine the volume of blood lost during surgery. A study by Orth and co-workers examined the accuracy of conventional, subjective techniques for estimation of blood loss by comparing the results of conventional techniques to those derived from an objective technique (sodium fluorescein dye). The investigators found a significant difference between subjective and objective techniques; in general, blood loss was underestimated by an average of approximately 300 mL when subjective techniques were used.[37]

In addition to estimating blood loss, patient response to intraoperative hemorrhage should be taken into consideration when making decisions regarding transfusion therapy. Tachycardia and decreased mixed venous oxygen saturation are suggestive of anemia, especially in the setting of intraoperative hemorrhage. A useful metric in decision making for transfusion therapy involves the measurement of systemic oxygen delivery (DO_2), which integrates cardiac index, oxyhemoglobin saturation, and hemoglobin concentration to produce a global measure of DO_2, rather than one isolated parameter such as hemoglobin. Survival in high-risk patients is associated with a DO_2 greater than or equal to 600 mL O_2/min/m^2.[10,37]

A further prerequisite of blood component therapy is establishing blood compatibility. Because of the presence of antigens in red blood cell (RBC) membranes and circulating antibodies, a blood recipient can receive red cells only from a compatible donor (Table 21-10). Two blood groups deserve special attention. Individuals with group AB blood possess both A and B antigens on their RBCs and lack anti-A and anti-B antibodies; therefore, such individuals can receive blood from any ABO group and are known as *universal recipients*. Individuals with type O blood are known as *universal donors* because their RBCs are devoid of any of the ABO antibodies.

The most important tests of blood compatibility are those used to determine ABO and Rh (also known as *type D*) blood groupings; transfusion of ABO- or Rh-incompatible blood can result in serious hemolysis. Patients at risk for needing transfusion (as well as banked blood for transfusion) are "typed" to determine ABO and Rh status. To further reduce the risk of a transfusion reaction, patients and banked blood are screened for clinically significant antibodies other than ABO and D. The ultimate test of blood compatibility is a type and crossmatch, during which donor blood and recipient blood are mixed together in what is essentially a trial transfusion. In contemporary clinical practice, patients are often prepared for surgery with only a type and screen, which predicts compatible transfusions 99.94% of the time. The addition of crossmatching increases the possibility of a compatible transfusion only one hundredth of 1%.[38]

In an emergency situation in which a patient's blood group is unknown, uncrossmatched type O, Rh-negative blood can be given. However, if two or more units of O-negative whole blood have been given, the patient may not be able to receive transfusions of his or her own type (A, B, or AB) because of the risk of hemolysis.[38]

Currently in the United States, most donor blood is fractionated into its component parts (i.e., RBCs, plasma, and platelets). Because of fractionation, blood component therapy can be targeted to a specific patient need (e.g., diminished oxygen-carrying capacity). In addition, storage of blood as components rather than as whole blood has distinct advantages[39]; however, banked blood does undergo undesirable changes during storage (Box 21-10). The deleterious effect of storage on RBCs in particular has been well known for some time and has been referred to as "the storage lesion." The clinical effects of the functional and morphologic changes observed in banked blood are not fully understood at present and are the subject of intense investigation.[40] A recent observational study of almost 6000 cardiac surgery patients found an association between transfusion of blood stored longer than 14 days and increased postoperative morbidity and mortality when compared with patients receiving blood stored for less than 14 days.[41]

Deciding when to administer blood components is an important clinical judgment that should be based on sound evidence, not custom. In recent years, critical attention has been directed to transfusion practices because of concerns regarding the expense, availability, and risks of transfusions. In 1996 and 2006, the American Society of Anesthesiologists (ASA) convened task forces on blood component therapy to develop guidelines to help inform clinicians of the best practices in transfusion therapy.[36,42]

A single threshold for transfusion, a so-called *transfusion trigger*, has been the subject of much discussion and study. The literature, based largely on clinical experience with Jehovah's Witnesses, records the survival of patients with hemoglobin values as low as 1.8 g/dL, although significant mortality is associated with hemoglobin values of less than 5 g/dL.[27] During anemic episodes, oxygen delivery to the tissues can be improved

BOX **21-10**

Changes in Banked Blood

- Depletion of 2,3-diphosphoglycerate (DPG)
- Depletion of ATP (adenosine triphosphate)
- Oxidative damage
- Increased adhesion to human vascular endothelium
- Acidosis
- Altered morphology of red blood cells (change in shape, decreased flexibility)
- Accumulation of microaggregates
- Hyperkalemia (as high as 17.2 mEq/L)
- Absence of viable platelets (after 2 days of refrigerated storage)
- Absence of factors V and VIII

From Corazza ML, Hranchook AM. Massive blood transfusion. AANA J. 2000;68:311-314; Tinmouth A et al. ABLE Investigators Canadian Critical Care Trials Group. Clinical consequences of red cell storage in the critically ill. Transfusion. 2006;46:2014-2027.

by increased cardiac output and improved microvascular blood flow resulting from the decreased viscosity of diluted blood.[43] The current consensus is that no single transfusion threshold exists and that decisions regarding RBC transfusions should be based on the specific clinical situation.

In practice, packed RBCs (PRBCs) are the component of choice for improving oxygen-carrying capacity. PRBC infusions are generally administered in a ratio of 1 mL for each 2 mL of blood loss (along with crystalloids or colloids for volume). A commonly used rule of thumb states that each unit of PRBCs increases hemoglobin 1 g/dL and hematocrit 2% to 3%.[35]

The ASA Task Force concluded that transfusion is "rarely" indicated in patients with hemoglobin greater than or equal to 10 g/dL and "almost always" indicated when hemoglobin is less than 6 g/dL.[36] Transfusing patients with a hemoglobin level of 6 to 10 g/dL is based on specific clinical factors. Factors that affect the selection of a transfusion threshold in individual patients include consideration of cardiopulmonary reserve, experienced and expected blood loss, O_2 consumption (reflected in indices such as arterial oxygen saturation and mixed venous oxygen saturation), and the presence or absence of atherosclerotic disease.[27,36,42]

Outcomes in patients whose transfusions were guided by restrictive transfusion triggers have been studied. The Cochrane Injuries Group conducted a systematic review of 10 studies examining restrictive transfusion triggers and concluded that in patients without cardiovascular disease, renal failure, or hematologic disorders, withholding transfusions in those with hemoglobin as low as 7g/dL was a justifiable practice.[44] A compelling study by Hebert and colleagues randomized 838 critically ill patients to receive transfusions at a threshold of either 7 or 10 g/dL of hemoglobin (Hb). Hebert found that the more restrictive transfusion threshold was at least as effective and in some subsets superior to the more liberal transfusion threshold.[45] A later study by Hebert and colleagues[46] suggested that a restrictive transfusion threshold (7 to 9 g/dL Hb) may be appropriate and safe in critically ill, hemodynamically stable cardiac patients. The author did warn against applying this restrictive transfusion trigger to patients experiencing acute myocardial infarction or unstable angina. A metaanalysis examining restrictive transfusion triggers cited a 42% reduction in the probability of a patient receiving a transfusion when restrictive standards were applied.[47]

Massive transfusion of RBCs, variously defined as (1) replacement of estimated blood volume within 24 hours or (2) 50% of blood volume within 3 hours or less or (3) transfusion of more than 10 units of whole blood,[48] presents special concerns to anesthetists. Replacement of lost blood volume by PRBCs, often accompanied by crystalloids and colloids, does not provide coagulation factors and can lead to a dilutional coagulopathy or dilutional thrombocytopenia. Banked blood is commonly anticoagulated by a solution containing sodium citrate, which binds calcium, thereby preventing coagulation. Very rapid infusion of blood can reduce the level of ionized calcium.[38] This phenomenon, sometimes referred to as *citrate intoxication*, presents as acute hypocalcemia. Fortunately, normothermic patients with normal kidney and liver function can metabolize the amount of citrate present in 20 units of banked blood per hour and are not likely to display citrate intoxication.[4]

Fresh frozen plasma (FFP) contains all coagulation factors[49] and is administered to provide coagulation factors that may be inadequate because of dilution or dysfunctions of coagulation. Indications for administration of FFP include reversal of the effects of warfarin, correction of known coagulopathy, correction of microvascular bleeding in the presence of elevated prothrombin time or partial thromboplastin time, and correction of microvascular bleeding in patients suspected of dilutional coagulopathy. For the reversal of warfarin, FFP is usually administered in doses of 5 to 8 mL/kg; 10 to 15 mL/kg is the guideline for all other purposes.[36,42,49]

Platelets are essential for adequate hemostasis and may need to be transfused because of thrombocytopenia or abnormal function.[39] Platelets are available as platelet concentrates separated from one unit of whole blood or as apheresis platelets, which originate from a single donor and are the equivalent of approximately six platelet concentrates.[50] Transfusion of platelets is usually indicated when the count is less than $50 \times 10^3/\mu L$ but not more than $100 \times 10^3/\mu L$. Platelet transfusions in patients with platelet counts of $50 \times 10^3/\mu L$ to $100 \times 10^3/\mu L$ are indicated when the patient displays microvascular bleeding or if the patient is at risk for platelet dysfunction or continued bleeding. The usual dose of platelets is one platelet concentrate per 10 kg of body weight; transfusion raises the platelet count for 6 to 7 days.[36,39,42]

A less frequently used blood component, cryoprecipitate, contains factor VIII, von Willebrand factor, and fibrinogen.[39] Cryoprecipitate is recommended for treatment of patients with von Willebrand disease and in patients with probable or documented deficits in fibrinogen (e.g., fibrinogen <80 to 100 mg/dL).[36,42]

Benefits of transfusion include increased oxygen-carrying capacity and improved coagulation. Unfortunately, transfusion of blood and blood products is not without risk. Infectious and noninfectious complications are possible, and the risk of complications is increased by massive transfusion, as well as by transfusion of blood that has been stored for a prolonged period.

Some of the most common serious complications of blood transfusion are due to incompatibility. In a survey of hematologists in the United Kingdom and Ireland (the Serious Hazards Of Transfusion [SHOT] initiative), reports of transfusion reactions over a 2-year period in the late 1990s were carefully examined. Clinicians participating in the SHOT initiative reported 366 cases of serious transfusion reactions, 191 of which were "wrong blood to patient" incidents.[51] The result of transfusion to an incompatible recipient is an immune reaction, with the risk of intravascular hemolysis because of an interaction between the circulating antibodies of the recipient and the RBCs of the donor.

Approximately half of all deaths from acute hemolytic reactions are caused by ABO-incompatible transfusions resulting from procedural or administrative error.[52] Volumes of donor blood as small as 10 mL may lead to hemolytic reactions that may result in death for 20% to 60% of patients.[38] The clinical picture is complicated by the fact that general anesthesia may obscure the symptoms associated with a hemolytic reaction.[36]

Incorrect transfusions in the SHOT study were typically the result of procedural errors that led to the misidentification of patients. In five cases the erroneous transfusion was the result of six errors; in one case seven errors preceded the incorrect transfusion. Almost 10% of the cases involved patients without identity wristbands.[51]

Other life-threatening complications seen in the context of transfusion include transfusion-associated graft-versus-host disease and transfusion-related acute lung injury (TRALI). Transfusion-associated graft-verses-host disease results when donor lymphocytes incorporate themselves into the tissues of the recipient, leading the recipient's immune system to attack the embedded recipient tissues. Rash, leukopenia, and thrombocytopenia occur, with sepsis and death usually ensuing.[38]

Since 2003, TRALI has been recognized by the U.S. Food and Drug Administration as the leading cause of transfusion-related death in the United States and is believed to occur as frequently as once in every 432 units of platelets or as infrequently as once in every 7900 units of FFP.[53,54] It is likely that TRALI is underreported because the syndrome may be confused with other forms of acute lung injury (ALI) and was without a clear definition until 2005. TRALI has been defined as ALI occurring within 6 hours of transfusion in individuals who were previously free of ALI and without other risk factors for ALI.[53]

The etiology of TRALI has not been fully explained, but two theories have been proposed to describe the syndrome. One explanation proposes that antibodies in donor plasma activate recipient neutrophils, leading to pulmonary capillary leakage. An alternative explanation puts forward a two-event model in which a physiologic stressor such as sepsis leads to sequestration of neutrophils in the lungs, then the transfusion of biologically active mediators (the second event) leads to activation of the neutrophils and capillary leakage. Treatment of TRALI is supportive and should include notifying the blood bank that a transfusion reaction suspected to be TRALI has occurred.[53,54]

Several undesirable effects of transfusions have been linked to the presence of leukocytes in allogenic blood. Homologous transfusions, which invariably contain some leukocytes, have been implicated in immunosuppression of recipients, leading to unexpectedly early recurrences of cancer and higher than expected rates of postoperative infection—a condition known as transfusion-related immunomodulation (TRIM).[36,39,52]

Nonhemolytic transfusion reactions are relatively common, occurring in 1% to 5% of all transfusions, and are associated with symptoms such as fever, chills, and urticaria. Like hemolytic reactions, these reactions are difficult to detect during general anesthesia.[36] Although not usually life threatening, febrile nonhemolytic and allergic reactions can cause concern and may lead to interruption of the transfusion.[38,55]

Leukoreduction, the use of filters to reduce the level of WBCs, is one technique used to reduce the incidence of certain adverse events related to transfusion. Leukoreduction has proved to be effective in reducing the incidence of nonhemolytic transfusion reactions and is likely to be effective in the reduction of TRIM. The effects of universal leukoreduction have been so promising (Box 21-11) that several nations, including Canada and France,

---

BOX 21-11

Clinical Benefits of Leukoreduction

A. Proved clinical relevance:
1. Reduced frequency and severity of NHFTRs
2. Reduced risk of CMV transmission
3. Reduced risk of HLA alloimmunization and platelet refractionness

B. Likely clinically relevant:
4. Reduced infectious risk associated with immunomodulation (TRIM)
5. Reduced organ dysfunction and mortality
6. Reduced direct risk of transfusion-transmission bacteria

C. Unproved clinical relevance:
7. Avoidance of vCJD transmission
8. Avoidance of HTLV I/II, EBV, etc.
9. Reduced risk of GVHD

From Blajchman MA. *The Clinical benefits for the leukoreduction of blood products.* J Trauma. 2006;60(6 Suppl):S83-90.
CMV, *Cytomegalovirus*; EBV, *Epstein-Barr virus*; GVHD, *graft-versus-host disease*; HLA, *human leukocyte antigen*; HTLV, *human T-lymphotrophic virus*; NHFTRs, *nonhemolytic febrile transfusion reactions*; TRIM, *transfusion-related immunomodulation*; vCJD, *variant Creutzfeldt-Jakob disease.*

---

have mandated universal leukoreducion for their nations' blood supply.[56]

Despite enhanced safety of the blood supply, infectious complications remain a real, although perhaps overemphasized, possibility (Table 21-11).[51,57,58] The current rates of transmission of viral illness by transfusion are so low that mathematical models are now used to estimate risk.[52] Even with improved testing, transmission of viral disease can still occur during a period of time commonly called the *window period*, during which the donor blood is infectious, but screening tests used by blood banks are insensitive. Polymerase chain reaction (PCR) assays have improved testing for antibodies and shortened the window period to approximately 11 days for HIV and 8 to 10 days for HCV.[59] Although hepatitis and HIV continue to be the subjects of considerable attention, other newly emerging (in the United States) viral diseases threaten the safety of the blood supply. West Nile virus is one example of a newly recognized transfusion-related illness. Fortunately, rapidly developed testing procedures for the virus have greatly reduced the risk of transmission by transfusion.[60]

One of the most recently identified transfusion-related diseases is variant Creutzfeldt-Jakob disease (vCJD). Theories suggest that this disease is contracted by blood donors through the ingestion of beef from cattle infected with bovine spongiform encephalopathy (BSE). The infectious agent responsible for BSE—believed to be an abnormal prion protein—can be passed from blood donor to transfusion recipient and become manifest in the recipient as vCJD, leading to degeneration of the central nervous system. Fortunately, vCJD remains a rare disease, with the majority of cases confined to the United Kingdom. Measures to protect the integrity of the blood supply include careful donor screening and leukodepletion.[61]

Bacterial contamination of blood remains a risk and increases with the length of time the blood is stored.[52] Contamination of platelets is of particular concern. Platelets are stored for a maximum of 5 days[62] at room temperature and carry a risk of bacterial contamination of 1 in 12,000.[52]

TABLE 21-11	Risks and Side Effects of Allogenic RBC Transfusion
Type of Risk	**Incidence (per Unit Transfused)**
Infections	
Viruses	
Human immunodeficiency virus (HIV)	1:1,468,000 – 1:4,700,000
Hepatitis B virus (HBV)	1:31,000 – 1:205,000
Hepatitis C virus (HCV)	1:1,935,000 – 1:3,100,000
Bacteria	
All	1:28,000 – 1:143,000
Parasites	
Malaria	1:4,000,000
Prions	
New variant Creutzfeldt-Jakob disease	Possible
Immunologic Reactions	
Hemolytic transfusion reactions	
Acute hemolytic TR	1:13,000
Delayed hemolytic TR	1:9000
Alloimmunization	1:1600
Immunosuppression	1:1
Transfusion-related acute lung injury	1:70,000
Mistransfusion	
All RBC mistransfusions	1:14,000 – 1:18,000

From Spahn DR, Kocian R. Artificial O_2 carriers: status in 2005. Curr Pharm Des. 2005;11:4099-4114.
RBC, Red blood cell.

Concerns regarding cost, availability, and complications associated with blood and blood products have led to strategies to reduce the risk of intraoperative blood loss, such as careful preoperative evaluation of the patient focusing on conditions that place the patient at increased risk of hemorrhage. In the surgical setting, these factors generally include medications that affect coagulation (e.g., wafarin, clopidogrel) and inherited and acquired defects of coagulation. An important tool to reduce the risk of significant intraoperative blood loss is the preoperative administration of agents to promote coagulation or reverse anticoagulants. The ASA transfusion practice guidelines recommend judicious preoperative administration of reversal agents such as vitamin K, prothrombin-complex concentrate, recombinant factor VII, and FFP. Antifibrinolytic agents should be considered in cases in which large amounts of blood loss are anticipated. This may lead to the administration of agents such as tranexamic acid G.[42,63]

In the event that blood transfusion becomes unavoidable, alternatives to blood transfusion from anonymous donors have been developed in the hope of reducing patient risk. One option involves the use of directed donors. Donor-directed blood transfusions are homologous blood transfusions from a donor selected by the recipient and believed by some to decrease the risk of transmission of disease. Studies comparing the safety of donor-directed blood with blood from anonymous donors,

however, fail to demonstrate any advantage to using donor-directed blood.[35,50]

A widely used alternative to allogenic blood transfusion is the use of autologous transfusion. Autologous transfusion techniques can be divided into three main categories: intraoperative and postoperative blood salvage, preoperative blood donation, and acute normovolemic hemodilution.[64]

Intraoperative red-blood-cell salvage involves the aspiration of blood shed into the surgical field into a specialized apparatus that concentrates the RBCs and washes the shed blood to remove debris, after which the RBCs are reinfused. Cell salvage may be used in surgical cases in which significant blood loss is likely, as well as in cases of unexpected massive blood loss (Table 21-12). Generally accepted contraindications to cell salvage include surgery involving wounds contaminated by bacteria, bowel contents, amniotic fluid, or malignant cells, as shown in Box 21-12.[65] Cell-washing devices can provide a volume equivalent to 10 units of blood per hour for transfusion in cases of massive blood loss.[66]

Preoperative blood donation consists of the collection and storage of a potential recipient's own blood for possible reinfusion of the blood at a later date, the intraoperative period. Although this procedure may eliminate certain risks associated with transfusions, some risks remain, and other risks arise (Box 21-13).[64] The process of autologous preoperative blood donation and transfusion carries with it the risks of preoperative anemia and resultant myocardial ischemia, the risk of bacterial contamination, and the risk of clerical error leading to the administration of the wrong blood.[38] In addition to these patient risks, approximately half of autologously donated blood is discarded,[66] which contributes to waste.

Acute normovolemic hemodilution is a transfusion alternative involving the removal of whole blood from a patient immediately before or after the initiation of anesthesia and surgery and replacing volume with crystalloid or colloid solutions. Blood lost during surgery will have a low hematocrit. Reinfusion of the whole blood (with a normal hematocrit) is initiated when intraoperative loss of blood has stopped, or earlier if the patient's condition warrants it. Advocates of acute normovolemic hemodilution suggest that hemodilution, compared with autologous donation, eliminates the expense of testing, the risks of bacterial contamination, and opportunity for wrong unit transfusion because the whole blood remains in the operating room.[66]

The search for a "blood substitute" has evolved over time into efforts to develop "oxygen therapeutics," which involves the use of technology to increase the oxygen-carrying capacity of the circulating volume.[67] Main areas of concentration in this field include the development of cell-free hemoglobin solutions to carry oxygen and perfluorochemicals to carry dissolved oxygen in a manner similar to that of plasma.[57,63,66-68]

SUMMARY

Surgery and anesthesia challenge the body's ability to maintain the dynamic balance of fluids and electrolytes necessary for proper function. Skillful management of fluids and electrolytes in the perioperative period is one of the most challenging and important tasks of the anesthetist and requires knowledge of both basic sciences and clinical research.

A subject intimately related to fluid and electrolyte management is transfusion therapy. An expanding body of evidence addressing transfusion therapy is better informing the clinician, who must evaluate risks versus benefits in the process of clinical decision making.

TABLE **21-12**	General Indications for Cell Salvage	
Specialty	**Surgical Procedure**	**Comments**
Cardiac	Valve replacement Redo bypass grafting	
Orthopedics	Major spine Bilateral knee replacement Revision hip replacement	
Urology	Radical retropubic prostatectomy Cystectomy Nephrectomy	Individualized by surgeon Limited to patients with prior radiation therapy When tumor involves major vessels
Neurosurgery	Giant basilar aneurysm	
Vascular	Thoracoabdominal aortic aneurysm repair Abdominal aortic aneurysm repair	Should be individualized by patient characteristics and surgeon
Liver transplant		
Other	Jehovah's Witnesses Unexpected massive blood loss RBC antibodies	When accepted by patient

From Waters JH. *Indications and contraindications of cell salvage*. Transfusion. 2004;44(12 Suppl):40S-44S.

BOX **21-12**

Contraindications to Cell Salvage

Pharmacologic Agents
- Clotting agents (Avitene, Surgical, Gelfoam, etc.)
- Irrigating solutions (Betadine, antibiotics meant for topical use)
- Methylmethacrylate

Contaminants
- Urine
- Bone chips
- Fat
- Bowel contents
- Infection
- Amniotic fluid

Malignancy

Hematologic Disorders
- Sickle cell disease
- Thalassemia

Miscellaneous
- Carbon monoxide (electrocautery smoke)
- Catecholamine (pheochromocytoma)
- Oxymetazoline (Afrin)

From Waters JH. *Indications and contraindications of cell salvage.* Transfusion. 2004;44(12 Suppl):40S-44S.

BOX **21-13**

Autologous Blood Donation

Advantages
1. Prevents transfusion-transmitted disease
2. Prevents red-cell alloimmunization
3. Supplements the blood supply
4. Provides compatible blood for patients with alloantibodies
5. Prevents some adverse transfusion reactions
6. Provides reassurance to patients concerned about blood risks

Disadvantages
1. Does not affect risk of bacterial contamination
2. Does not affect risk of ABO incompatibility error
3. More costly than allogeneic blood
4. Results in wastage of blood not transfused
5. Increased incidence of adverse reactions to autologous donation
6. Subjects patient to perioperative anemia and increased likelihood of transfusion

From Goodnough LT. *Autologous blood donation*. Anesthesiol Clin North America. 2005;23:263-270.

REFERENCES

1. Kaye AD, Kucera IJ. Fluid and electrolyte physiology. In: Miller RD, ed. *Anesthesia*. 6th ed. Philadelphia: Churchill Livingstone; 20051763-1798.
2. Guyton AC, Hall JE. The microcirculation and the lymphatic system: capillary fluid exchange, interstitial fluid and lymph flow. In: *Textbook of Medical Physiology*. 11th ed. Philadelphia: Saunders; 2006:181-193.
3. Metheney N. *Fluid and Electrolyte Balance: Nursing Considerations*. 4th ed. Philadelphia: Lippincott; 2000.
4. Prough DS et al. Acid-base, fluids, and electrolytes. In: Barash PG et al, eds. *Clinical Anesthesia*. 5th ed. Philadelphia: Lippincott Williams & Wilkins; 2005:175-207.

5. Kreimeier U. Pathophysiology of fluid imbalance. *Crit Care*. 2000; 4(Suppl 2):S3-S7.

6. Rosenthal MH. Intraoperative fluid management—what and how much? *Chest*. 1999;115(Suppl 5):106S-112S.

7. Kapoor M, Chan G. Fluid and electrolyte abnormalities. *Crit Care Clin*. 2001;7:503-529.

8. Gold MS. Perioperative fluid management. *Crit Care Clin*. 1992;8:409-421.

9. Kumar S, Berl T. Sodium. *Lancet*. 1998;352:220-228.

10. Prough DS, Svens C. Current concepts in perioperative fluid management. *Anesth Analg*. 2001;92(suppl):70-77.

11. Zornow MH et al. The acute cerebral effects of changes in plasma osmolality and oncotic pressure. *Anesthesiology*. 1987;67:936-941.

12. Fried F, Palevsky PM. Hyponatremia and hypernatremia. *Med Clin North Am*. 1997;81:585-609.

13. Fraser CL, Arieff AI. Epidemiology, pathophysiology, and management of hyponatremic encephalopathy. *Am J Med*. 1997;102:67-77.

14. Laureno R, Karp BI. Myelinolysis after correction of hyponatremia. *Ann Intern Med*. 1997;126:57-62.

15. Halperin ML, Kamel KS. Potassium. *Lancet*. 1998;352:135-140.

16. Mandal AK. Hypokalemia and hyperkalemia. *Med Clin North Am*. 1997;81:611-639.

17. Hirsch IA et al. The overstated risk of preoperative hypokalemia. *Anesth Analg*. 1988;67:131-136.

18. Malloch A, Bodenham AR. Regulation of blood volume and electrolytes. In: Hemmings HC, Hopkins PM, eds. *Foundations of Anesthesia: Basic and Clinical Sciences*. London: Mosby; 2000:571-581.

19. Bushinsky DA, Monk RD. Electrolyte quintet: Calcium. *Lancet*. 1998;352: 306-311.

20. Weisinger JR, Bellonin-Font E. Magnesium and phosphorus. *Lancet*. 1998;325:391-396.

21. Tolksdorf W. Electrolyte disorders relevant to anesthesia. *Acta Anaesthesiol Scand Suppl*. 1997;111:328-329.

22. Prough DS, Bidani A. Hyperchloremic metabolic acidosis is a predictable consequence of intraoperative infusion of 0.9% saline. *Anesthesiology*. 1999;90:1247-1249.

23. Scheingraber S et al. Rapid saline infusion produces hyperchloremic acidosis in patients undergoing gynecological surgery. *Anesthesiology*. 1999;90: 1265-1270.

24. Prough D. Fluid management in head injury. *53rd Annual Refresher Course Lectures, Clinical Updates and Basic Science Reviews Program*. Park Ridge, IL: American Society of Anesthesiologists; 2002.

25. Kaakinen T et al. Hypertonic saline dextran improves outcome after hypothermic circulatory arrest: a study in a surviving porcine model. *Ann Thorac Surg*. 2006;81:183-190.

26. Culpepper TL. AANA *Journal* course; update for nurse anesthetists—intraoperative fluid management for the pediatric surgical patient. *AANA J*. 2000;68:531-538.

27. Goldhill D, Boralessa H. Anaemic and red cell transfusion in the critically ill. *Anaesthesia*. 2002;57:527-529.

28. Gan TJ et al. Hextend Study Group. Hextend, a physiologically balanced plasma expander for large volume use in major surgery: a randomized phase III clinical trial. *Anesth Analg*. 1999;88:992-998.

29. Rizoli SB. Crystalloids and colloids in trauma resuscitation: a brief overview of the current debate. *J Trauma*. 2003;54(Suppl 5):S82-S88.

30. Healey MA et al. Lactated Ringer's is superior to normal saline in a model of massive hemorrhage and resuscitation. *J Trauma*. 1998;45:894-899.

31. Perel P, Roberts I. Colloids versus crystalloids for fluid resuscitation in critically ill patients. *Cochrane Database Syst Rev*. 2007;4:CD000567.

32. Boldt J. Fluid choice for resuscitation of the trauma patient: a review of the physiological, pharmacological, and clinical evidence. *Can J Anaesth*. 2004;51:500-513.

33. Vincent JL et al. Morbidity in hospitalized patients receiving human albumin: a meta-analysis of randomized, controlled trials. *Crit Care Med*. 2004;32: 2029-2038.

34. Moretti EW et al. Intraoperative colloid administration reduces postoperative nausea and vomiting and improves postoperative outcomes compared with crystalloid administration. *Anesth Analg*. 2003;96:611-617.

35. Morgan GE et al. Fluid management and transfusion. In: *Clinical Anesthesiology*. 4th ed. New York: Lange Medical; 2006:690-707.

36. American Society of Anesthesiologists Task Force on Blood Component Therapy. Practice guidelines for blood component therapy. *Anesthesiology*. 1996;84:732-747.

37. Orth VH et al. First clinical implications of perioperative red cell volume measurement with a nonradioactive marker (sodium fluorescein). *Anesth Analg*. 1998;87:1234-1238.

38. Miller RD. Transfusion therapy. In: *Anesthesia*. 6th ed. Philadelphia: Churchill Livingstone; 2005:1799-1830.

39. Carrico CJ et al. Transfusion, autotransfusion and blood substitutes. In: Mattox KL et al, eds. *Trauma*. 4th ed. New York: McGraw-Hill; 2000.

40. Tinmouth A et al. ABLE Investigators, Canadian Critical Care Trials Group. Clinical consequences of red cell storage in the critically ill. *Transfusion*. 2006;46:2014-2027.

41. Koch CG et al. Duration of red-cell storage and complications after cardiac surgery. *N Engl J Med*. 2008;358:1229-1239.

42. American Society of Anesthesiologists Task Force on Perioperative Blood Transfusion and Adjuvant Therapies. Practice guidelines for perioperative blood transfusion and adjuvant therapies: an updated report by the American Society of Anesthesiologists Task Force on Perioperative Blood Transfusion and Adjuvant Therapies. *Anesthesiology*. 2006;105:198-208.

43. Leone BJ, Spahn DR. Anemia, hemodilution, and oxygen delivery. *Anesth Analg*. 1992;75:651-653.

44. Hill SR et al. Transfusion thresholds and other strategies for guiding allogenic red blood cell transfusion. *Cochrane Database Syst Rev*. 2003;3.

45. Hebert PC et al. Transfusion Requirements in Critical Care Investigators, Canadian Critical Care Trials Group. A multicenter, randomized, controlled clinical trial of transfusion requirements in critical care. *N Engl J Med*. 1999;340:409-417.

46. Hébert PC et al. Is a low transfusion threshold safe in critically ill patients with cardiovascular diseases? *Crit Care Med*. 2001;29:227-234.

47. Carson JL et al. Transfusion triggers: a systematic review of the literature. *Transfus Med Rev*. 2002;16:187-199.

48. Corazza ML, Hranchook AM. Massive blood transfusion. *AANA J*. 2000;68:311-314.

49. Manino PL. Transition practicing in critical care. In: *The ICU Book*. 3rd ed. Philadelphia: Lippincott Williams & Wilkins; 2007:659-681.

50. Menitore JE. Blood transfusion. In: Stein JH, ed. *Internal Medicine*. 5th ed. St Louis: Mosby; 1998:572-576.

51. Williamson LM et al. Serious hazards of transfusion (SHOT) initiative; analysis of the first two annual reports. *BMJ*. 1999;319:16-19.

52. Goodnough LT et al. Transfusion medicine. First of two parts—blood transfusion. *N Engl J Med*. 1999;340:438-447.

53. Barrett NA, Kam PC. Transfusion-related acute lung injury: a literature review. *Anaesthesia*. 2006;61:777-785.

54. Toy P et al. Transfusion-related acute lung injury: definition and review. *Crit Care Med*. 2005;33:721-726.

55. Perrotta PL, Synder EL. Non-infectious complications of transfusion therapy. *Blood Rev*. 2001;15:69-83.

56. Blajchman MA. The clinical benefits of the leukoreduction of blood products. *J Trauma*. 2006;60(6 Suppl):S83-90.

57. Spahn DR, Kocian R. Artificial O_2 carriers: status in 2005. *Curr Pharm Des*. 2005;11:4099-4114.

58. Boraless H et al. A survey of physicians' attitudes to transfusion practice in critically ill patients in the UK. *Anesthesia*. 2002;57:584-588.

59. Busch MP et al. Current and emerging infectious risks of blood transfusions. *JAMA*. 2003;289:959-962.

60. Goodnough LT. Risks of blood transfusion. *Anesthesiol Clin North America*. 2005;23:241-252.

61. Anstee DJ. Prion protein and the red cell. *Curr Opin Hematol*. 2007;14: 210-214.

62. Snyder EL, Rinder HM. Platelet storage—time to come in from the cold? *N Engl J Med*. 2003;2032-2033.

63. Henkel-Honke T, Oleck M. Artificial oxygen carriers: a current review. *AANA J*. 2007;75:205-211.

64. Goodnough LT. Autologous blood donation. *Anesthesiol Clin North America*. 2005;23:263-270.

65. Waters JH. Indications and contraindications of cell salvage. *Transfusion*. 2004;44(12 Suppl):40S-4S.

66. Goodnough LT et al. Transfusion medicine—blood conservation—second of two parts. *N Engl J Med*. 1999;340:525-533.

67. Wahr JA. Clinical potential of blood substitutes or oxygen therapeutics during cardiac surgery. *Anesthesiol Clin North America*. 2003;21:553-568.

68. Kim HW, Greenburg AG. Artificial oxygen carriers as red blood cell substitutes: a selected review and current status. *Artif Organs*. 2004;28:813-828.

CHAPTER 22

POSITIONING FOR ANESTHESIA AND SURGERY

Elizabeth Monti Seibert

The act of positioning a patient for surgery is a group endeavor that requires teamwork, timing, communication, and knowledge of measures to protect the patient. CRNAs are intimately involved in coordinating and directing patient positioning and continually monitoring and assessing the subsequent effects on the patient's physiologic status. To prevent patient injury, nurse anesthetists must be knowledgeable about possible hazards associated with various surgical positions.

Surgical positions are associated with numerous potential complications that can be detrimental to a patient's short- and long-term outcomes. Although the potential for various complications is generally well known, the precise incidence and cause of position-related injuries are often difficult to determine. Because the frequency of these events is low, contributing causes are frequently multifactorial,[1,2] and uniform reporting mechanisms do not exist. Position-related injuries are probably underreported in the scientific literature. Fear of litigation or damage to one's professional reputation may prevent anesthesia providers from reporting such events. However, case reports, closed-claims studies, and retrospective analyses of databases can provide insight into position-related injuries and shed light on precipitating causes and outcomes.

CLOSED-CLAIMS STUDIES

Studies of closed malpractice claims from professional liability insurance companies provide a rich source of data about position-related complications. Both the American Association of Nurse Anesthetists Foundation (AANA-F) and the American Society of Anesthesiologists (ASA) have conducted such studies. The ASA Closed Claims Project (ASA CCP) was initiated in 1985. Since then, this ongoing project has collected data on 7348 anesthesia-related claims filed with more than 35 liability insurance carriers.[3,4] Because the ASA CCP involves primarily anesthesiologists, the AANA-F conducted a similar study to examine outcomes of care provided by CRNAs. The AANA-F database covers 223 cases that occurred between 1989 and 1997 and is derived from records of the primary insurer of CRNAs at that time.[5,6] Dental claims are excluded from both the AANA-F and ASA CCP studies.

In 1999, the ASA CCP contained 4183 cases. An analysis of these cases revealed that death (32%), nerve injuries (16%), and brain damage (12%) were the major causes of liability.[1] Nerve damage included injuries to both the peripheral nervous system and spinal cord but not to the brain. Nerves most commonly affected were the ulnar (28%), brachial plexus (20%), lumbosacral nerve root (16%), and spinal cord (13%). Injuries to all other

nerves accounted for only 8% of the nerve damage claims. Although claims for nerve injury have remained constant over time, claims for ulnar nerve injury have decreased while those from spinal cord injury have increased.[1]

Specific causative factors could not be identified in the majority of claims in the ASA CCP. When the association of anesthetic technique with nerve injury was examined, regional anesthesia was more frequently associated with nerve-injury claims—particularly of the spinal cord and lumbosacral nerve root—than general anesthesia. However, 85% of ulnar nerve injuries were associated with general anesthesia. The quality of anesthesia care was judged as appropriate in 66% of all nerve injury claims, as compared with 42% of non–nerve-damage cases. However, care was deemed appropriate in only 46% of spinal cord damage claims. Other factors associated with nerve damage included positioning and positioning devices, intraoperative trauma, and paresthesias during regional block performance.[1]

The AANA-F closed-claims study compared 151 claims (68%) in which a CRNA was judged to have contributed to the adverse outcome (CRNA-related) with 72 claims (32%) in which the CRNA was judged not to have contributed to the adverse event (non–CRNA related).[6] Death (32%), nerve injury (18%), brain injury (12%), and eye injury were the primary outcomes of CRNA-related claims. No significant difference in the type of outcome was found between CRNA-related claims and non–CRNA-related claims. Reviewers evaluated the appropriateness of care and found care inappropriate in 52% of CRNA-related cases, appropriate for 30%, and impossible to assess in the remaining cases.

A subsequent analysis was conducted of 44 cases of nerve injury in the AANA-F database.[7] The distribution of nerve injuries was as follows: brachial plexus (15 [34%]), ulnar nerve (7 [16%]), radial nerve (5 [11%]), peroneal nerve (4 [9%]), spinal cord (4 [9%]), and lumbosacral nerves (3 [7%]). A variety of other nerves accounted for the remaining injuries. In the majority of claims filed, documentation of the patient's position and the use of protective padding was inadequate, preventing investigators from identifying possible causative factors. However, a higher percentage of nerve injuries were associated with inadequate positioning, preexisting patient conditions, general anesthesia, extremes of body habitus, and procedures lasting longer than 2 hours.

The AANA-F and ASA CCP studies highlight the importance of following standards of care and properly documenting perianesthetic activities. Standards for nurse anesthesia practice identify thorough, complete, and accurate documentation as an expectation of nurse anesthesia practice.[8] In the event of a malpractice claim, thorough documentation assists reviewers in determining the quality of care provided.

Quality of care was judged as inappropriate in 34% of nerve injury claims from the ASA CCP and 52% of all cases in the AANA-F study.[1,6] In both studies, monetary awards were higher in those cases resulting in more severe outcomes and when anesthesia care was determined to be less than appropriate. Although some suggest that position-related nerve injuries are largely preventable,[9] the ASA analysis of nerve injury claims revealed that payouts were frequently made even when anesthesia care was judged appropriate.[1] This suggests that current knowledge of methods for preventing nerve injury is inadequate and that further research into mechanisms of nerve injury is needed.

Several limitations are inherent in closed-claims studies. First, the purpose of data collected by professional liability insurance companies is to investigate malpractice claims, not to improve patient safety. Not all anesthesia-related injuries result in a liability claim. Therefore, data from closed-claims studies are not a random or even representative sample, because only those cases in which a claim was filed and subsequently closed are included. Second, the incidence of various outcomes cannot be described because the total number of cases performed by insured providers is unknown.[6] For these two reasons, closed-claims data are not suitable for calculation of risk. However, analysis of closed-claims data can identify issues confronting practitioners and suggest methods for improving practice or making changes in systems.[6,10]

Other factors limit the conclusions that can be drawn from closed-claims data. Many cases that might be included in the database are eliminated because of inadequate documentation. In addition, closed-claim studies and quality assurance data categorize claims by type of injury rather than cause. Inadequate documentation and inability to determine the role played by various factors can limit the ability of reviewers to determine the cause of injury.[1] Finally, reviewers' knowledge of patient outcomes may bias their opinions on the quality of care provided.[5]

PATHOPHYSIOLOGY OF NERVE INJURY

Transection, compression, stretch, and kinking are the primary mechanisms responsible for nerve injuies.[11,12] Nerves may be transected by surgical maneuvers or by trauma. Compression can happen when a nerve is forced against a bony prominence or a hard surface such as an armboard or operating table. In the lateral position, for example, the weight of the superior leg pushes against the dependent extremity and may compress the common peroneal nerve in the dependent leg against the operating table. Stretch or traction injuries occur where nerves such as the sciatic nerve or brachial plexus have a long course across many structures. Like telephone wires, peripheral nerves have some laxity that allows a limited amount of elongation. However, excessive elongation or stretch may cause conduction changes, axonal disruption, or interruption of the nerve's vascular supply.[13-16] Use of neuromuscular blocking agents during general anesthesia may increase joint mobility and allow greater than normal degrees of stretch. Kinking injuries happen when a peripheral nerve is pinched between two immovable structures. For example, the femoral nerve can be kinked under the inguinal ligament when the thighs are flexed on the abdomen, as in the exaggerated lithotomy position.

A common component of all peripheral nerve injuries is ischemia. Intraneural blood flow may be compromised by stretch, compression, or disruption of the nerve tissue itself.[17]

Other causes include occlusion of major vessels, emboli, tissue edema, or inhibition of perfusion at the capillary level. For example, pressure applied over a body surface may limit venous capillary outflow, causing a rise in venous capillary pressure and a decrease in the hydrostatic pressure gradient between interstitial tissues and the capillary.[18] Ultimately, tissue edema occurs as fluid is sequestered in the cells and interstitial space. As venous capillary pressure rises, the arterial-venous pressure gradient is reduced, decreasing flow to tissues along the capillary. As venous and tissue pressures continue to rise, arterial inflow is eventually obstructed and ischemia results. Low mean arterial blood pressure may augment the development of ischemic conditions.

Tissue metabolism continues even in the absence of blood flow. When ischemia ensues, adenosine triphosphate (ATP) production is decreased, causing failure of the transmembrane sodium-potassium pump and accumulation of sodium within the cell. The resulting osmotic pressure gradient favors the movement of water into the cells. Intracellular volume is increased, and tissue edema occurs.[19] A vicious cycle of ischemia results as tissue pressures increase, preventing the movement of fluid and nutrients from the capillaries into the cells.

The susceptibility of peripheral nerves to ischemia may be partially due to their anatomic structure (Figure 22-1). Like a telephone cable constructed from hundreds of smaller wires, peripheral nerves are composed of bundles of nerve fibers (fascicles) and their vascular supply encased in protective connective-tissue coverings. Each nerve fiber is composed of one or more axons sheathed by Schwann cells (neurolemma) that are either myelinated or unmyelinated. The axons and neurolemma are covered by a loose connective tissue called the *endoneurium*. The *perineurium* is a tough connective tissue that binds the fascicles into identifiable structures. The *epineurium* consists of two layers: an inner epineurium that supports the fascicles and an outer epineurium that covers the external surface of the nerve.[16,20] The quantity of these protective tissues varies between nerves and even along the same nerve. The entire nerve trunk is covered by a loose layer of connective tissue that allows it to slide across joints and other tissues.[16]

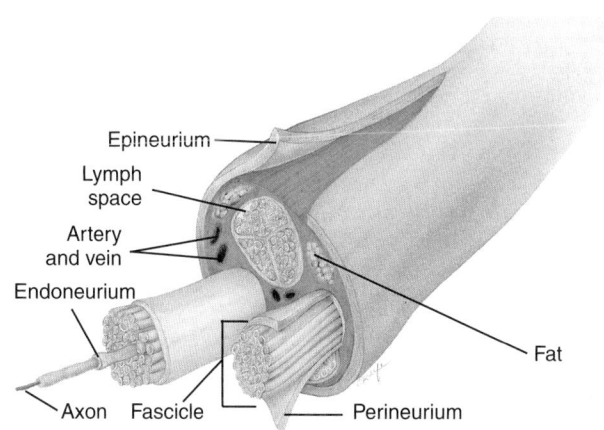

FIGURE **22-1** Cross-section of a peripheral nerve trunk showing its components. (*From Thibodeau GA, Patton KT. Anatomy & Physiology. 6th ed. St Louis: Mosby; 2007.*)

Peripheral nerves have an extensive microvascular supply. Blood vessels in the epineurium run parallel to the nerve and form numerous anastomoses with the perineurium. Collateral connections between the perineurium and the endoneurial capillaries run obliquely between the layers and thus may be more susceptible to compression by increases in tissue pressure.[16] In addition, the endoneurial space lacks lymphatic vessels, so edema and fluid accumulation in this region may obstruct the microcirculation.[16]

PERIOPERATIVE FACTORS CONTRIBUTING TO NERVE INJURIES

Postoperative peripheral nerve injuries are frequently attributed to incorrect surgical positioning; however, current evidence indicates that multiple factors are involved in postoperative peripheral neuropathies.[1,2,11,21] Perioperative factors that contribute to the development of nerve injuries include ancillary positioning devices, prolonged surgical procedures, and anesthetic technique. Patient-related factors include gender, age, body habitus, and preexisting medical conditions. However, the precise mechanism of nerve injury is often unclear, suggesting that further investigation is needed to identify causative factors.[1,2,22]

Positioning Devices

Controlled studies of complications related to specific positioning devices are largely nonexistent. Isolated case reports provide much of the evidence that is known about nerve injuries attributable to improper use of positioning devices. Ancillary positioning devices, such as straps used to restrain the patient or an extremity, may cause pressure and temporary injury if excessively tightened. For example, the lateral femoral cutaneous nerve in the thigh is susceptible to injury by tight table straps or the leg-holding device used for knee arthroscopy.[23] Common peroneal nerve injury has been attributed to the use of crutch-type stirrups. Brachial plexus injury has been caused by a damaged armboard falling off the operating room (OR) table[24] or the use of shoulder braces with steep Trendelenburg.[1] Compression injury of the radial nerve has been reported following the intraoperative use of tourniquets and blood pressure cuffs and by compression between the humerus and a firm surface, such as a positioning device.[25,26] Improper placement of an axillary roll may cause compartment syndrome and compression of neural and vascular structures.[27]

Length of Procedure

Prolonged surgical procedures contribute to postoperative positioning complications. Postoperative visual loss, nerve injuries, and compartment syndrome have been associated with a variety of procedures and positions where the common denominator was a duration of more than 4 hours.[28-31] Rhabdomyolysis and acute renal failure also have been reported following lengthy procedures.[32,33] One possible explanation is that during long procedures, the weight of the body causes external compression of dependent tissues and states of low perfusion.[33] The longer this situation persists, the higher the potential for development of edema and ischemic injury.

Anesthetic Techniques

Anesthetic techniques may contribute to the development of position-related injuries.[1] Patients receiving general anesthesia cannot move in response to painful stimuli generated by uncomfortable body positions. The constraints of the procedure or surgeon may limit movement even when patients are sedated.

Muscle relaxation due to neuromuscular blocking drugs or volatile anesthetics may contribute to stretch injuries by allowing increased mobility of joints.[17] For example, limited elbow extension from tight biceps muscles can be overcome by neuromuscular blockade, allowing the arms to be extended flat and subsequently stretching the median nerve.[17,34] The hypotensive effects of general anesthetics may lower perfusion pressures below acceptable levels in patients who are hypertensive or have other comorbidities. The use of hypotensive techniques to reduce blood loss should be balanced against the risk of possible complications resulting from decreased perfusion pressures, particularly during prolonged procedures and in the sitting, lithotomy, and Trendelenburg positions, where gravity affects blood flow.

Although neuraxial and peripheral nerve blocks are associated with both permanent and temporary nerve injuries, the majority of injuries are not related to positioning but to block technique, hematoma formation, and needle trauma.[35] However, recognition of compartment syndrome may be delayed when providers attribute the patient's symptoms to the residual effects of regional blocks and local anesthetics.[36,37] Anesthetists must have a high index of suspicion when return of function is delayed beyond what is expected for a particular technique or local anesthetic and when patients complain of severe pain in the presence of a seemingly adequate block.

PATIENT-RELATED FACTORS CONTRIBUTING TO NERVE INJURIES

Body Habitus

Extremes of body habitus are correlated with an increased incidence of positioning complications.[30,32,33] Individuals who are underweight may develop decubiti or nerve damage due to lack of adequate adipose tissue over bony prominences.[30,38] For example, thin patients may be at higher risk for sciatic nerve damage when the opposite buttock is elevated,[11] and thinner women (body mass index [BMI] <22) are more likely to develop ulnar neuropathy.[34,39] Individuals with a muscular physique may also be at increased risk for compartment syndrome and ulnar nerve injury.

Obesity increases morbidity from positioning because large tissue masses place increased pressure on dependent body parts; in addition, adipose tissue is poorly perfused. For example, in the lateral position, a heavy superior extremity may interfere with perfusion by exerting substantial pressure on the inferior extremity. Obesity also may compromise ventilation by restricting chest and abdominal excursion, particularly in the supine, lithotomy, and Trendelenburg positions. In the lithotomy position, extreme flexion of heavy thighs onto the abdomen also can limit ventilation.

Preexisting Conditions

Preexisting conditions appear to be associated with an increased risk of developing postoperative position-related injuries (Box 22-1). Hypertension, diabetes mellitus, peripheral vascular disease, peripheral neuropathies, and alcoholism can exacerbate the physiologic effects of various positions. Nerve injury and preexisting neuropathies are more common in patients with diabetes,[11] and diabetes is the most common metabolic cause of spontaneous isolated femoral neuropathy.[40] A history of smoking within 1 month of the surgical procedure has been identified as a risk factor for nerve injury, as well as for delayed healing.[30,41] Individuals with subclinical ulnar nerve entrapment, which may not be apparent to the patient or anesthetist, are also at risk for nerve injuries.[42,43]

PERIOPERATIVE NEUROPATHIES

Ulnar Neuropathy

Ulnar neuropathy is one of the most frequently reported injuries following surgery and anesthesia, with a reported incidence ranging from 0.04% to 0.5%.[42,44,45] Ulnar neuropathy is a

---

<table>
<tr><td style="background:black; color:white">BOX **22-1**</td></tr>
</table>

Factors Associated with Position-Related Injuries

Positioning Devices
  Table straps
  Leg holders and stirrups
  Axillary roll
  Bolsters
  Fracture table post
  Shoulder braces
  Positioning frames
  Headrests
  Ether screen

Length of Procedure
  Longer than 4-5 hr

Body Habitus
  Obesity
  Malnutrition
  Bulky musculature

Preexisting Pathophysiology
  Anemia
  Diabetes mellitus
  Peripheral vascular disease
  Liver disease
  Peripheral neuropathies
  Alcoholism
  Limited joint mobility
  Smoking

Anesthetic Technique
  General anesthesia
  Hypotensive techniques
  Neuromuscular blockade

---

well-known complication of cardiac surgery, with a prevalence as high as 38%.[46] The ASA and AANA-F closed-claims studies found that the ulnar nerve was the first (28%) and second (16%) most commonly injured nerve.[1,6]

The ulnar nerve traverses the length of the upper extremity from its origins as a branch of the medial cord of the brachial plexus to its terminal branches in the hand. In the upper arm, the ulnar nerve passes along the anterior aspect of the medial head of the triceps muscle and posterior into the groove between the medial epicondyle of the humerus and the olecranon (Figure 22-2).[47] In this region, the nerve is sheathed in the cubital tunnel before exiting and passing between the two heads of the flexor carpi ulnaris.[38] The cubital tunnel retinaculum (CTR) forms the roof of the cubital tunnel (Figure 22-3), a potential area for nerve compression because fibrous tissue and the elbow capsule form a semirigid canal that changes shape with flexion and extension of the forearm.[47] When the elbow is flexed, the distance between the olecranon and medial epicondyle increases, stretching the CTR, decreasing the size of the tunnel, and increasing pressure on the nerve.[12]

Surgical positioning, age, preexisting diseases, and mechanical factors such as tourniquets and blood pressure cuffs have all been proposed as contributing to ulnar nerve injuries. However, ulnar neuropathy is more frequently associated with male gender,[39,42,45] the presence of a preexisting asymptomatic neuropathy,[42] prolonged hospital stays,[42,45] and extremes of body habitus.[34,45] Median sternotomy and sternal retraction are also proposed as a cause of ulnar nerve injury following cardiac surgery.[48] A subclinical ulnar neuropathy that is exacerbated by perioperative events is proposed to exist in patients that develop postoperative ulnar nerve injury without obvious predisposing factors.[42,48] Additionally, in some individuals the nerve is congenitally hypermobile and easily slides anteriorly when the elbow is flexed. As a result, the nerve may become inflamed from constant friction.[47]

The incidence of ulnar neuropathy is higher in men—particularly those older than age 50—than in women.[1,39,44,45] Gender-related anatomic variations are hypothesized to explain this difference. The coronoid process is larger in men compared with women, and men have less subcutaneous tissue over the ulnar nerve in this region.[17,38] Also, the cubital tunnel may be narrower in men who have more well-developed forearm musculature,[11] making the nerve in this region more susceptible to compression and potential ischemia. However, women with a

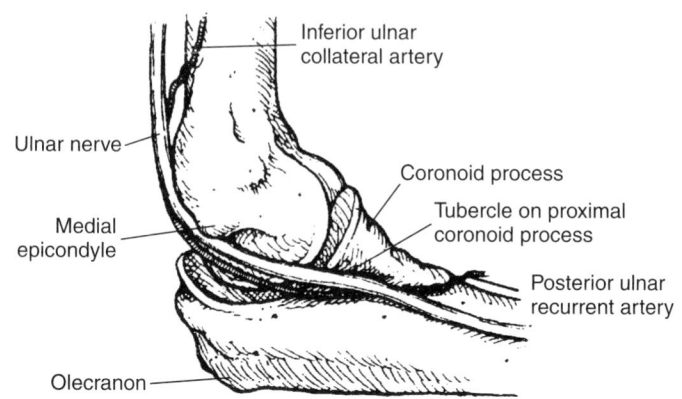

FIGURE **22-2** Ulnar nerve at the elbow. (*From Prielipp RC et al. Ulnar nerve injury and perioperative arm positioning. Anesthesiol Clin North America. 2002;20[3]:589-603.*)

low BMI (<22) are more likely to develop ulnar neuropathy than men of similar weight.[34,39]

Although postoperative ulnar neuropathy is often blamed on intraoperative positioning, other perioperative factors may be involved. The prevalence of ulnar neuropathy is similar in medical and surgical patients, and prolonged hospital stays are significantly related to the development of ulnar neuropathy.[44,45,49] Bedrest is suspected as contributing to ulnar neuropathy, because the initial presentation is often delayed 24 or more hours.[44,45,49] Medical patients and those with longer hospital stays are likely to spend considerable time in bed lying in the supine position with their hands folded on the chest or abdomen or sitting in chairs with the elbows resting on the armrest. When the elbow is flexed, the cubital tunnel is narrowed and can compress the ulnar nerve. Pain, abdominal and thoracic incisions, and orthopedic procedures may also cause surgical patients to lie immobile or in the supine position for long periods. In addition, clasping the hands on the abdomen causes supination of the hands and rotation of the humerus, allowing the ulnar nerve in the postcondylar groove to be compressed against the bed.[49]

Recommendations for positioning to prevent ulnar nerve injury in anesthetized patients include the use of padding, placing the arms in a supinated position, and abducting the arms less than 90 degrees if armboards are used.[47,50] Although padding the elbow is suggested as potentially helpful in preventing ulnar neuropathies,[50] no evidence supports the benefit of padding, and injuries have occurred despite the prophylactic use of padding. If the arms are secured on armboards, the forearm should be supinated (palm up), because pronation (palm down) increases pressure over the ulnar nerve.[51] Anatomic changes in the cubital tunnel with flexion and extension suggest that excessive flexion of the elbow should be avoided when the patient is in the lateral position or if the arms are secured across the chest. Although patients who are sedated may feel more comfortable with their elbows flexed, sedated patients should have their arms positioned in the same manner as anesthetized patients.

BRACHIAL PLEXUS INJURIES

The brachial plexus arises from the nerve roots of C5-T1, which subsequently merge to form the superior, middle, and inferior trunks (Figure 22-4). The trunks split into divisions as they pass over the first rib and posterior to the clavicle.[52] After passing into the infraclavicular region, the divisions separate into cords in the axilla and then subdivide into the terminal branches. The brachial plexus is susceptible to stretch injuries for two reasons. First, the plexus is relatively fixed between its origins at the vertebral foramina and its terminal branches.[53] Second, the clavicle, first rib, and humeral head may compress or stretch the plexus as it passes these structures.

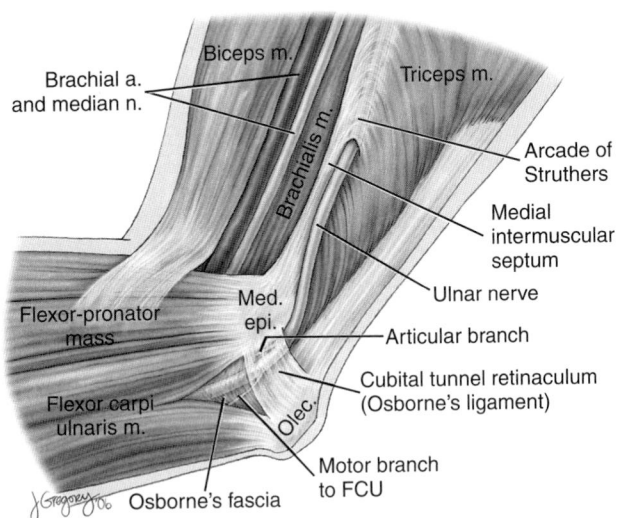

FIGURE **22-3**   Anatomy of the ulnar nerve in the cubital tunnel. Flexion of the elbow stretches the cubital tunnel retinaculum between the olecranon and medial epicondyle and may compress the ulnar nerve in the cubital tunnel. *a*, Artery; *FCU*, flexor carpi ulnaris; *Med epi*, medial epicondyle; *m*, muscle; *n*, nerve; *olec*, olecranon. (*From Polatsch DB et al. Ulnar nerve anatomy. Hand Clin. 2007;23[3]:283.*)

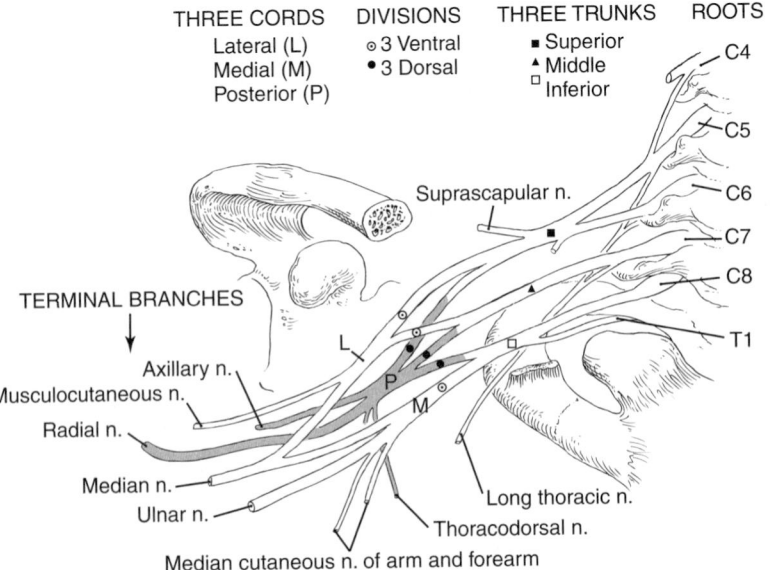

FIGURE **22-4**   Derivation of the brachial plexus from the cervical spine. *n*, Nerve.

The brachial plexus is vulnerable to injuries in almost every surgical position, particularly if the arms are abducted, the shoulders are depressed, or the head is rotated (Figure 22-5). When the patient is supine, abduction of the arms greater than 90 degrees stretches the plexus around the humeral head. Turning the head to the side with the arms abducted can cause stretching and compression of the contralateral brachial plexus beneath the clavicle.[54,55] Even tucking the arms next to the body is not without risk if the head is turned laterally and the shoulders are depressed. When the patient is prone, inadequate support of the shoulders allows them to sag anteriorly, causing traction on the plexus. Also in the prone position, extending the arms over the head (superman position) may compress the plexus between the clavicle and first rib.

In the lateral decubitus position, brachial plexus injury is most commonly the result of excessive stretching, usually because of arm abduction greater than 90 degrees, external rotation, extension and lateral flexion of the head, and posterior shoulder displacement.[11] In the lateral position, the humeral head of the dependent arm can also compress the plexus against the thorax, requiring the use of a pad or roll placed just below the axilla.[56] Injuries to the brachial plexus and the musculocutaneous and ulnar nerves have occurred with shoulder arthroscopies in which the lateral decubitus position was used, and traction was applied to the arm to improve joint visualization[23]; manual traction may be preferable to mechanical. If the nondependent arm is suspended on an arm holder with traction, abduction of 45 to 60 degrees should be maintained and less than 10 pounds of traction applied.[57]

Brachial plexus injuries are also associated with positioning devices. Injuries have been caused by a damaged armboard falling off the OR table and the use of shoulder braces with steep Trendelenburg.[1,24,58] Improper placement of shoulder braces close to the base of the neck or along the midpoint of the clavicle can compress neurovascular structures and cause brachial plexus neuropathy. If used, shoulder braces are properly placed at the distal end of the clavicle.

Sternal retraction during cardiac surgery has been implicated as a cause of brachial plexus injury that presents as a postoperative ulnar neuropathy. Spreading of the sternal retractor causes the clavicle to move posteriorly and the first rib to rotate upward, pinching the plexus between the two (Figure 22-6).[48] Dissection of the internal mammary artery requires wider, asymmetric chest retraction to allow adequate visualization and may predispose to brachial plexus neuropathy.[53,59] Rib fractures also occur with sternal retraction, and fracture of the first rib and associated hematoma formation may contribute to brachial plexus injury. To prevent brachial plexus injury during cardiac surgical procedures, caudad placement of the sternal retractor and avoidance of excessive and prolonged asymmetric chest wall retraction are recommended.[48]

SPINAL CORD INJURY

Quadriplegia and paraplegia are well-known complications of aortic vasular and thoracic procedures where there is potential for interupting the blood supply of the spinal cord. Although rare, hemiparesis and quadriplegia are also associated with surgical procedures performed in the sitting and prone positions.[60-63] Midcervical flexion myelopathy with temporary or permanent quadriplegia may occur when the head is flexed on the neck in the sitting or prone positions. When the head is flexed, the spinal cord moves anteriorly and may be compressed against the posterior vertebral body.[61] Ischemia may result from a combination of compression and stretch, because the spinal cord lengthens with flexion. Like a rubber band, the cord becomes thinner as it stretches, and the caliber of the vessels supplying the cord can be reduced.[61] Increased vertebral venous pressure is also proposed as leading to postoperative spinal cord injury. The absence of valves between the central venous and epidural venous systems allows direct transmission of increased abdominal or intrathoracic pressure to the vertebral venous systems.[64] Congestion in the veins draining the spinal cord, coupled with hypotension, may result in decreased spinal cord perfusion and the onset of new neurologic deficits.[63]

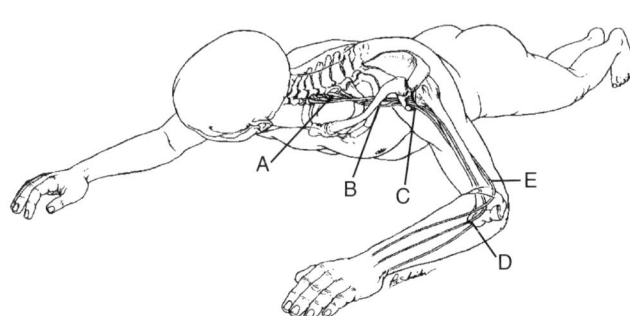

FIGURE **22-5** Sources of potential injury to the brachial plexus and its peripheral components in a pronated patient. **A,** Head position stretching the plexus. **B,** Clavicle trapping the neurovascular bundle against the first rib with the patient's arms at sides, and cephalad end of chest roll compressing the clavicle. **C,** Head of humerus thrust into the neurovascular bundle with nonrelaxation of arm and axilla. **D,** Compression of ulnar nerve at the elbow. **E,** Area of vulnerability of the radial nerve to lateral compression above the elbow. (*From Martin JT, ed. Positioning in Anesthesia and Surgery. 2nd ed. Philadelphia: Saunders; 1987.*)

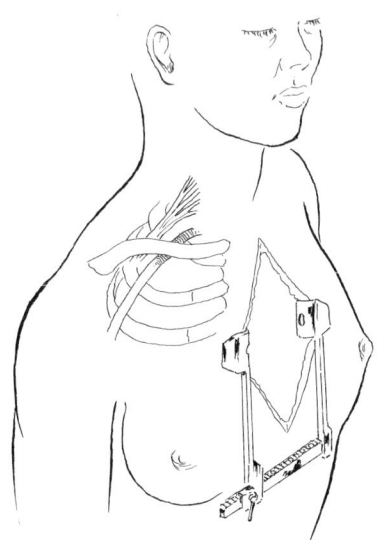

FIGURE **22-6** Opening the sternal retractor pinches the medial cord of the brachial plexus between the middle third of the clavicle and the fixed first rib. (*Modified from Casscells CD et al. Ulnar neuropathy after median sternotomy. Clin Orthop. 1993;291:263.*)

Somatosensory evoked potentials (SSEPs) have been suggested as useful in identifying position-related changes in spinal cord function.[65] However, new neurologic defects have emerged postoperatively despite normal intraoperative SSEP readings.[60,66] Hyperflexion of the head on the neck in any position may be avoided by allowing a minimum of two fingerbreadths between the sternum and mandible.

POSTOPERATIVE VISUAL LOSS

Postoperative visual loss (POVL) is a rare but devastating complication of nonophthalmic surgery. It may occur in one or both eyes and refers to a variety of visual defects ranging from decreased visual acuity to total blindness. The incidence of visual loss after surgery and anesthesia is estimated at 0.0008% to 0.2% and varies with the type of procedure.[67-70] The prevalence of POVL is higher following certain surgical procedures, ranging from 0.113% following cardiac surgery to 1:3526 following prone spinal surgeries.[68,70] Its incidence appears to be increasing over the last decade.

The optic nerves are extensions of the brain, with the retina containing cell bodies that supply axons to the optic nerves and brain. The optic nerve extends from the globe to the optic chiasm and is divided into four sections: intraocular, intraorbital, intracannalicular, and intracranial (Figure 22-7).[71] The anterior or intraocular optic nerve is that portion of the nerve within the globe. It includes the optic disc and is about 1 mm long and 1.5 × 1 mm in diameter. Nerve fibers and blood vessels of the anterior optic nerve pass through holes in a sievelike structure called the *lamina cribrosa*.[72] The posterior or intraorbital optic nerve, that section of the nerve posterior to the lamina cribrosa (outside the globe) yet still within the orbit, is approximately 25 mm long. Like the brain, the optic nerve is sheathed by the meninges. Beneath the dura, which reaches to the globe, lie the arachnoid, subarachnoid space, and pia.

The retina and optic nerves are supplied by the central retinal artery and long and short posterior ciliary arteries that arise from the internal carotid artery (Figure 22-8).[72] The central retinal artery supplies the retina; the anterior optic nerve and choroid are supplied by the choriocapillaris, which emanates from the long and short posterior ciliary arteries. The posterior optic nerve is supplied by pial vessels that branch off the ophthalmic artery.[73] Blood flow is lower in the posterior optic nerves because the pial vessels are end-arteries and lack autoregulation.[74,75] There is considerable interindividual variation in the ophthalmic blood supply.[72,73,76]

The optic nerves may be susceptible to hypoperfusion. The central retinal and posterior ciliary arteries are end-arteries and lack anastomoses with other arteries.[77] Thus the structures supplied by these vessels are in a "watershed" region, meaning that the region receives a dual blood supply from the most distal branches of two arteries. Watershed areas are reportedly vulnerable to ischemia if a portion of the blood supply is interrupted.[73,78] Finally, the ocular circulation lacks autonomic innervation; however, autoregulation does occur in the ophthalmic and central retinal arteries.[72] The limits of autoregulation in the ocular circulation are unknown. Preexisting diseases such as diabetes and hypertension that disrupt autoregulatory mechanisms may contribute to ischemic episodes during periods of hypotension.[79]

Causes of Postoperative Visual Loss

The visual pathways reach from their origins in the retinal ganglion cells to the primary visual cortex in the occipital lobes. Visual loss may result from a variety of lesions along these pathways, including trauma, tumors, stroke, and ischemia. However, visual loss following nonophthalmic surgery is generally attributable to five causes: ischemic optic neuropathy (ION), central retinal artery occlusion (CRAO), central retinal vein occlusion, cortical blindness, and glycine toxicity.[72] In the ASA POVL registry, ION and CRAO accounted for 81% of all cases, with ION accounting for 89% of POVL following prone spinal procedures.[74]

As the name implies, ION is the result of ischemia in a portion of the optic nerve. Anterior ION (AION) affects the portion of the optic nerve within the globe and is further subdivided into arteritic and nonarteritic forms. Temporal arteritis is the usual cause of the arteritic variant, with all other causes classified as nonarteritic AION.[72] Posterior ION affects the optic nerve posterior to the globe.

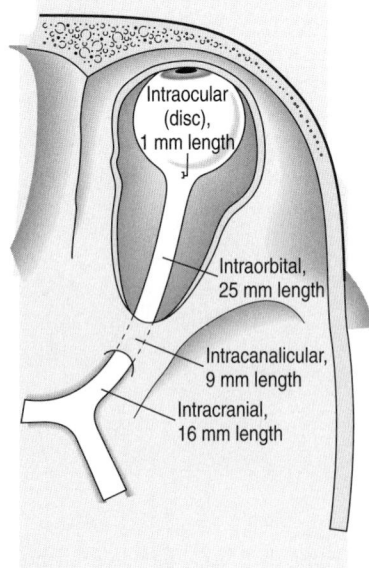

FIGURE **22-7** The four portions of the optic nerve. (*From Yanoff M et al, eds. Ophthalmology. 2nd ed. St Louis: Mosby; 2004.*)

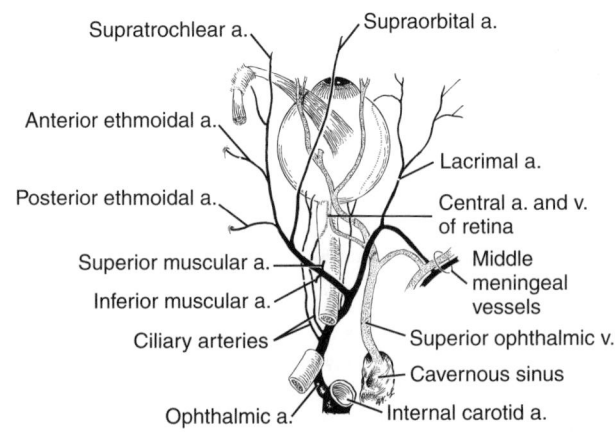

FIGURE **22-8** Superior view of the orbital arteries and veins. *a*, Artery, *v*, vein.

A variety of patient factors are associated with postoperative ION, including male gender and the presence of coexisting diseases such as hypertension, vascular disease, obesity, and diabetes.[74,79] However, postoperative ION is as likely to occur in healthy patients as those who have coexisting diseases.[74,78] Intraoperative factors related to ION include spinal surgery, the prone position, prolonged surgical procedures, large blood loss, low hematocrit, and systolic blood pressure less than 100 mm Hg.[74,75,79] However, ION has occurred in the absence of any of these factors.[78]

The most common causes of ION are decreased perfusion and increased intraocular pressure.[78] Just as cerebral perfusion pressure equals mean arterial pressure (MAP) minus intracranial pressure, ocular perfusion pressure (OPP) is the difference between MAP and intraocular pressure (IOP).[72,76] Intraoperative and anesthetic events that decrease MAP and thus reduce OPP include general anesthetics, hypotension, hemorrhage, and hypovolemia. Venous pressure and the ratio of aqueous humor production to absorption affect IOP. An increase in venous pressure may impede aqueous humor outflow into the venous system, causing a rise in IOP.[76] As IOP approaches MAP, OPP will decrease. During surgery, ocular venous pressure can be increased by a head-down tilt, increased abdominal and right atrial pressure, and obstruction of jugular venous return.[73] Unlike CRAO, ION does not seem to be associated with pressure on the globe, because ION has occurred in patients whose heads were secured with pin-type headrests.[74]

CRAO is a less common cause of POVL than ION. In 93 cases of POVL following prone spinal surgery, only 10 cases were attributed to CRAO.[74] The central retinal artery is one of the first branches of the internal carotid artery (Figure 22-9), and nourishes the internal layer of the retina. Emboli from the ipsilateral carotid can migrate to the central retinal artery and cause unilateral blindness. Perioperative factors associated with CRAO are cardiopulmonary bypass, hypotension, and increased extraocular pressure. Some recovery of vision is possible if blood flow is restored within 4 hours. Although many treatments are recommended for CRAO, few have proven efficacy.[76]

General risk factors for central retinal vein obstruction syndrome include hypertension, cardiovascular disease, increased body mass index, open angle glaucoma, and sickle cell anemia.[72] Because external pressure on the globe may cause central retinal vein obstruction,[72] when the patient is placed prone for procedures on the head and neck, some suggest the use of 3-pin headrests that securely immobilize the head rather than the horseshoe headrest. Although the 3-pin headrest avoids the potential for external ocular compression, POVL from ION has occurred despite the use of the pin-type headrest.[74]

Visual changes due to central retinal vein obstruction can be subtle or marked, but in either situation the prognosis for recovery of vision is poor.[72] No definitive treatment is available for central retinal vein obstruction.

Cortical blindness is the result of ischemia or trauma and a subsequent infarction of the visual pathways in the parietal or occipital lobes.[77] Operative causes of cortical blindness include air and particulate emboli, cardiopulmonary bypass, and hypoperfusion due to hemorrhage or hypotension. No specific treatment is available for cortical blindness. Vision may improve over time.[72]

Glycine toxicity is a rare syndrome that occurs in patients with a deficiency of L-arginine, the enzyme needed to metabolize ammonia.[80] Ammonia is a by-product of the metabolism of glycine, a nonessential amino acid, to glycolytic acid and ammonia. Temporary vision loss occurs in these patients as a consequence of high blood ammonia levels. Vision returns to normal as blood ammonia levels decrease.

Much remains to be learned about POVL. Although factors such as hypertension, vascular disease, obesity, and smoking have been associated with POVL, specific methods for identifying at-risk patients are not available, and reasons why POVL occurs in patients without obvious risk factors are unknown. Patients at high risk of developing POVL include those undergoing lengthy spinal procedures in the prone position (>6.5 hours), especially if surgery is accompanied by significant blood loss. During the preoperative interview, high-risk patients should be informed of the small risk of POVL. Presently there are no intraoperative monitoring methods that might detect the onset of POVL. Although periodic intraoperative monitoring of hemoglobin or hematocrit is suggested, safe lower limits for hematocrit are unknown. Deliberate hypotensive techniques to prevent blood loss during spine surgery should be avoided in individuals with chronic hypertension or other factors that place them at risk for POVL. Avoidance of direct pressure over the eye is recommended to avoid CRAO. The prone patient's head should be placed in a neutral position (avoid excessive flexion) and level with or slightly elevated above the heart (10-degree head-up tilt) when possible. If an exceptionally long procedure is anticipated, the anesthetist should discuss the possibility of staging the procedure with the surgeon.[50]

The ASA has established a Postoperative Visual Loss Registry to study the phenomenum. The registry, accessible on the Internet, is a venue where anesthesia providers can submit voluntary, anonymous reports of nonophthalmic visual loss cases.

OTHER POSITION-RELATED INJURIES

Position-related injuries run the gamut from minor skin abrasions and backache to events with serious morbidity (Table 22-1). Complications of these injuries can lead to tissue necrosis, infection, renal failure, paralysis, loss of limbs, and even loss of life. Although most individuals recover from minor position-related injuries without sequelae, more serious injuries may prolong a patient's hospital stay and recovery, cause psychological trauma, and perhaps even result in permanent disability. Anesthetists must not minimize the physical, psychological, social, and financial impact of transient injuries that resolve over hours, days, or months. Permanent, disabling injuries are even more devastating to patients and providers.

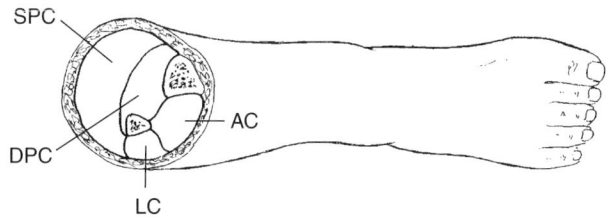

FIGURE **22-9** Compartments of the lower leg. *AC,* Anterior compartment; *DPC,* deep posterior compartment; *LC,* lateral compartment; *SPC,* superficial posterior compartment. *(Modified from Matsen FA III. Compartmental Syndromes. New York: Grune & Stratton; 1980:82.)*

Compartment Syndrome

Compartment syndrome is a potentially life-threatening complication that causes damage to neural and vascular

TABLE **22-1**	Potential Position-Related Injuries
System	**Potential Injury**
Head, eyes, ears, nose, and throat	Blindness Corneal abrasion Facial edema Vocal cord edema
Cardiovascular	Vascular occlusion Deep vein thrombosis Ischemic injuries
Respiratory	Atelectasis Endobronchial intubation
Neurologic	Peripheral neuropathy Quadriplegia Decreased cerebral blood flow Increased intracranial pressure
Genitourinary	Myoglobinuria Acute renal failure
Musculoskeletal	Amputation Backache Compartment syndrome Rhabdomyolysis
Integumentary	Abrasion Alopecia Decubiti

structures from swelling of tissues within a muscular compartment.[81] Prolonged surgical procedures, operative positions, elevation of the extremities, intraoperative hypotension, increasing age, and extremes of body habitus are reported to contribute to the development of compartment syndrome in surgical patients.[36,82-84] Compartment syndrome can be precipitated by intraoperative hypotension in conjunction with leg elevation that causes low-flow states; blood pressure decreases by 0.75 mm Hg per centimeter change in height.[85] Pneumatic compression boots and fluid extravasation into tissues have been linked to the syndrome.[82,86]

Unless the syndrome is promptly diagnosed and treated, permanent neuromuscular damage will occur.[81,84] Fasciotomy is generally considered the definitive treatment because less aggressive therapies will not release the constricted compartments. If untreated, the syndrome progresses to tissue necrosis with myoglobinuria and acute renal failure (crush syndrome).[36] Amputation and even death can occur.[36,84]

Compartment syndrome is the result of increased pressures and decreased tissue perfusion in muscles with tight fascial borders (see Figure 22-9). Just as increased intracranial pressure reduces cerebral blood flow, increased compartmental pressure compromises arteriolar supply and results in ischemia with subsequent muscle and nerve infarction. Although compartment syndrome occurs most often in the extremities, abdominal compartment syndrome also occurs following tight wound closures.[81] Because tissue swelling typically occurs when blood flow returns following a period of ischemia, the syndrome has also been dubbed a "reperfusion injury."[87,88]

Trauma, embolic phenomena, tumors, and vascular insufficiency are common causes of compartment syndrome.

Other predisposing perioperative factors include tight wound closures, expanding hematomas, prolonged surgical procedures, and external compression. A higher incidence has been reported in patients undergoing surgery in the lithotomy and lateral decubitus positions.[36,83,84,89,90] Although anesthetic technique has not been implicated as causing compartment syndrome, general and regional anesthesia can contribute to intraoperative hypotension and impaired blood flow. Controversy exists over whether regional anesthesia contributes to delayed diagnosis of the syndrome.[84,91-93]

Venous Air Embolism
Venous air embolism (VAE) is a well-known consequence of surgery performed in the sitting position. However, VAE may occur in any position where a negative pressure gradient exists between the right atrium and the veins at the operative site.[94-97] The precise incidence of VAE is unknown but is variously estimated at between 1% and 76%.[97-102] Differences in estimates result from variations in the sensitivity of monitoring devices used and the type of surgical procedure.[85,98,100,102,103] Complications of VAE are proportional to both the rapidity and volume of air entrainment and range from no effect for minimal amounts of air to hypotension, arrhythmias, cardiac arrest, and death with larger volumes.[97,100,102-104] Air that enters the right side of the heart can limit gas exchange in the lungs as it displaces blood in the pulmonary vasculature.

Paradoxical air embolism (PAE) can occur in the patient with a patent foramen ovale (PFO) or when right atrial pressures are higher than left atrial pressures. Studies in vivo and in cadavers indicate that the incidence of PFO can be as high as 35% in the general population.[102,103,105] In the patient with PFO, air can enter the systemic circulation when right atrial pressure is greater than left atrial pressure, a reversal of the normal pressure gradient. Very small amounts of air in the arterial system can result in severe cardiovascular and neurologic complications. Positive end-expiratory pressure (PEEP) and other conditions that elevate right atrial pressure can also predispose to PAE.[85,106]

Because VAE and PAE are results of surgical intervention and carry the potential for serious consequences, much attention has been placed on identifying individuals at risk for these complications. Preoperative transesophageal echocardiograph (TEE) with contrast is the gold standard for detection of PFO in patients scheduled for surgery in the sitting position.[100,103] The cost of TEE is thought to be justified because it is a low-risk, semiinvasive procedure and the sequelae of PAE are severe. However, the low incidence of VAE and PAE in some types of procedures may not justify the expense.[107] In addition, PFO can be present and PAE can occur despite negative preoperative TEE.[102] Because echocardiography is uncomfortable for patients and has rare but serious complications, transcranial Doppler studies are recommended as an alternative, noninvasive approach for detection of PFO.[103,105]

In addition to the use of standard anesthetic monitoring techniques, patients who are susceptible to VAE should be monitored with devices that detect VAE and allow aspiration of entrained air. TEE, Doppler ultrasonography, capnography, and pulmonary artery catheterization vary in their ability to detect VAE. TEE is the most sensitive monitor for VAE detection, having the ability to identify emboli less than 0.2 mL/kg, but it is not specific for gas emboli.[100,102,108] Although TEE is the gold standard for VAE detection and can be used to position right atrial catheters, disadvantages are that it requires specialized training, considerable time, and experience to use and may not provide a continuous monitor of cardiovascular events.

The precordial Doppler is often used to monitor for VAE when patients are in the sitting position. The probe is placed over the third to sixth intercostal spaces to the right of the sternum. The Doppler is equally as sensitive as TEE and less expensive and cumbersome, but it does not have the advantage of localizing entrained air within the cardiac chambers.[97,100,108] The device is sensitive to electrical interference from other operating room equipment, and its effectiveness can be reduced by auditory fatigue in the anesthetist. False positives can be generated by rapid infusion of fluid or flushing transducers. Most frequently used for sitting cases, Doppler devices have not traditionally been advocated for management of VAE during procedures performed in the prone position. Positioning of the Doppler probe is difficult in the prone position and requires adequate padding to prevent excessive pressure on the chest wall.

Both TEE and Doppler detect changes resulting from VAE at smaller air volumes than either capnography or measurement of PAP.[85,108,109] Because VAE increases dead space and contains nitrogen, capnography reveals a drop in end-tidal CO_2 and the presence of end-tidal nitrogen. The esophageal stethoscope, ECG, and pulse oximeter can also be used to detect changes caused by VAE. A "mill-wheel murmur" is a characteristic of VAE that can be heard through the esophageal stethoscope.[85,109] However, most anesthesia providers are unfamiliar with the rumbling sound of a mill wheel. Air in the coronary arteries can cause ischemic electrocardiographic changes, and air in the pulmonary vessels can result in an increase in PAP and hypoxia. These signs occur later than changes detected by TEE, Doppler, or capnography and are indicative of PAE or large emboli.

Entrained air emboli are removed from the circulation by aspiration through a multiorifice central venous catheter. For patients undergoing surgery in the sitting position, the catheter is placed in the right atrium at the junction of the superior vena cava.[85] However, patients who are prone should have the CVP catheter positioned at the junction of the inferior vena cava (IVC) and right atrium because air emboli from spinal surgery enter the venous circulation through the lumbar epidural veins and IVC. The risks of central venous catheter placement, the potential for VAE, and the cardiopulmonary risks of the position must be weighed against the benefits of fluid volume management and air recovery with a CVP catheter.

At one time or another, intravascular volume expansion, PEEP, leg wraps, and the antigravity suit (G-suit) have been advocated to reduce the negative incision-to-heart pressure gradient and the incidence of VAE. The G-suit was ineffective in preventing VAE, and hypervolemia and PEEP are no longer recommended as means of reducing the chance of VAE.[85] PEEP has been suggested to decrease VAE by increasing right atrial pressure and decreasing venous return from cerebral and intrathoracic veins.[104] However, studies of canine cerebral venous pressures in the sitting position found no change in cerebral venous pressure when PEEP of up to 20 cm H_2O was applied.[106] A similar incidence of VAE was found in patients who received controlled ventilation without PEEP and those who received PEEP of 10 cm H_2O.[110] Valves located at the thoracic inlet of the jugular veins prevent retrograde blood flow when intrathoracic pressures are increased.[106] Significant levels of PEEP may actually increase the incision-heart pressure gradient by decreasing atrial pressures.[102] PEEP can also worsen right-to-left shunts in patients with PFO and cause systemic VAE. The release of PEEP has been demonstrated to cause a recurrence of VAE in patients who had intraoperative episodes of intracardiac air.[104]

Airway Complications of Surgical Positions

Anesthetized patients in various surgical postures are vulnerable to endotracheal tube displacement, airway edema, and passive regurgitation. The endotracheal tube may become dislodged, kinked, or disconnected when the patient is moved or turned. Inadvertent one-lung ventilation may occur when the head is flexed upon the neck or when the patient is in a steep head-down position. With flexion, the endotracheal tube moves downward and can accidentally enter the right mainstem bronchus.[111] In the head-down position, pressure of the abdominal contents against the diaphragm may cause a similar occurrence.[112] The endotracheal tube can become kinked with extreme degrees of flexion or may compress the arytenoids and epiglottis, resulting in postoperative supraglottic edema. Use of a wire-reinforced tube is recommended when extreme flexion is anticipated.

Extensive edema of the face, tongue, and oropharyngeal structures has been reported after procedures in the prone, sitting, and head-down positions.[113-115] In the prone and head-down positions, gravitational forces or increases in hydrostatic pressures may restrict venous return from the head and neck. Undue flexion of the head on the neck may also obstruct jugular venous return and may be compounded by excessive fluid administration. Oral airways, endotracheal tubes, and esophageal stethoscopes may compress the base of the tongue and limit lymphatic drainage.[114] Macroglossia or upper airway edema may necessitate leaving the patient intubated following surgery until the edema subsides.[115]

The risk of aspiration is assumed to increase with the Trendelenburg position because gastric pressure is increased, and secretions can accumulate in the oropharynx and nasopharynx. However, studies of awake, non-fasted subjects in the supine, head-up, and head-down postions have found no significant differences in reflux between the positions.[116,117] The potential for reflux depends on the difference between intragastric pressure and lower esophageal sphincter (LES) pressure. Therefore, the risk of reflux may be higher during laparoscopy or in obese patients in the head-down position because intragastric pressure may be higher than LES pressure in these situations. The minimum airway pressure necessary to inflate the stomach is approximately 25 cm H_2O.[117]

SURGICAL POSITIONING

The Supine Position (Dorsal Recumbent)

The supine position is most frequently used for surgical procedures on the abdomen, head, neck, extremities, and chest, owing to the favorable exposure it allows. When positioning the patient supine, the head should be maintained in a neutral position on a small pad, pillow, or donut. If the patient has severe arthritis or decreased mobility of the head and neck, the head is best placed in the position preferred by the patient before induction. During prolonged procedures, the head should be repositioned at intervals and the occiput massaged to prevent alopecia due to prolonged pressure. Gel-type donuts may more evenly distribute pressure. However, the head should not be turned laterally when the arms are abducted on armboards because brachial plexus stretch can occur.[12]

A small support such as a folded sheet or bag of IV fluid may be placed under the lumbar spine to prevent postoperative back pain due to abolition of the normal lumbosacral curve. Awake individuals typically cross their ankles to alleviate lumbosacral strain in the supine position. The legs must be uncrossed once the patient is anesthetized because the pressure from the superior extremity may damage the superficial peroneal nerve in the

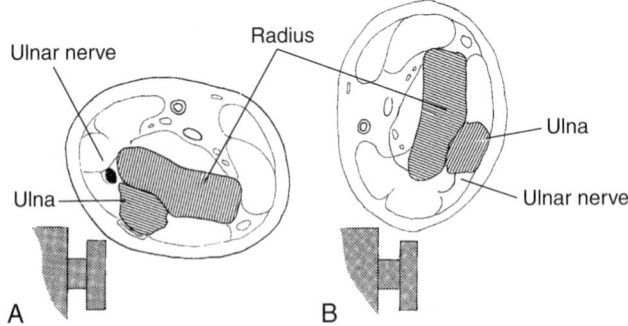

FIGURE **22-10**   Cross-sections of the right upper extremity viewed distally at the level of the ulnar groove, with the patient lying supine on the operating table. **A,** With the patient's hand supinated, the ulnar groove is at the posteromedial aspect of the elbow, and the ulnar nerve is vulnerable to pressure from the equipment rail of the table if the elbow slips out of the restraint. **B,** Pronating the patient's hand rotates the ulnar groove outward, protecting the ulnar nerve. (*From Dornette WH. Compression neuropathies: medical aspects and legal implications.* Int Anesth Clin. 1986;24:215.)

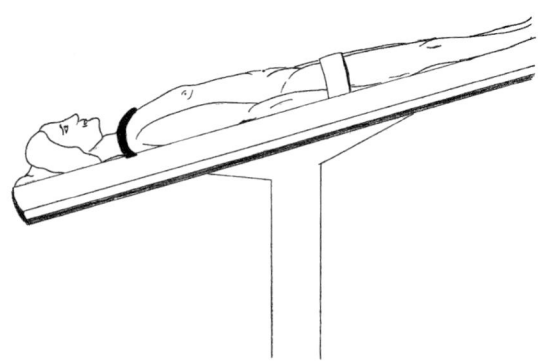

FIGURE **22-11**   In a supine patient, pronating the forearm places the ulnar nerve in contact with supporting surfaces. Placing the forearm with the palm up (supination) rotates the ulnar nerve away from compressive surfaces. (*From Rothrock JC.* Alexander's Care of the Patient in Surgery. *13th ed. St Louis: Mosby; 2007:139.*)

dependent leg and the sural nerve in the superior leg. Placing the table in a slight "lounge chair" position and the patient with hips and knees flexed and the trunk slightly elevated increases patient comfort. If prolonged surgery is anticipated, the heels should be elevated off the mattress to prevent pressure sores; however, using too large a support to elevate the heels can cause hyperextension of the knees and pain postoperatively. Gel pads or mattresses more evenly distribute the patient's body weight and prevent reddened areas following lengthy procedures.

The arms can be placed in several positions. One or both arms may be tucked at the sides or abducted on padded armboards that are level with the top of the table. If the arms are tucked, the elbow must not be allowed to hang over the edge of the operating table, or ulnar nerve damage may occur (Figure 22-10). When tucked, the hands should be parallel to the legs and trunk. Compression of the fingers and hands may result if the arms are pronated with the hands placed under the buttocks. If the arms are secured on armboards, the forearm should be supinated; pronation may result in compression of the ulnar nerve against the armboard (Figure 22-11)[118] The arms should be abducted less than 90 degrees, and the head should be maintained in a neutral position to avoid brachial plexus injuries.

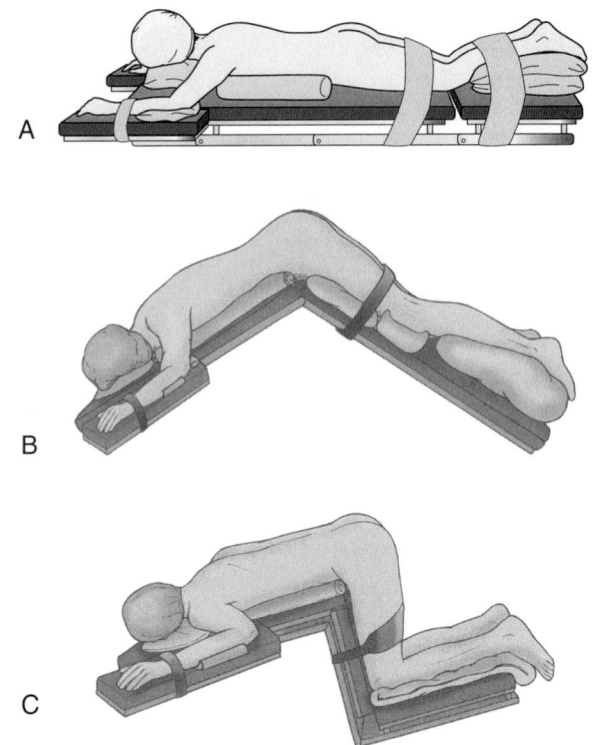

FIGURE **22-12**   Variations of the prone position. **A,** Classic prone position with the torso supported on chest rolls. **B,** Jackknife position. **C,** Knee-chest position. (**A** *from Phillips N:* Berry & Kohn's Operating Room Technique. *11th ed. St Louis: Mosby; 2007:509;* **B** *and* **C** *from Rothrock JC.* Alexander's Care of the Patient in Surgery. *13th ed. St Louis: Mosby; 2007:155.*)

The Prone Position

The prone position provides optimal exposure for a variety of procedures performed on the spine. The prone position has also been advocated for intracranial procedures, owing to the decreased risk of venous air embolism compared with the sitting position. Many modifications of the prone position exist (Figure 22-12). Anesthetists must become familiar with the various methods of securing the patient in the prone position and recognize the potential hazards of each variation or device.

In the prone position, the torso is typically supported on a frame or with rolls that extend from the shoulders to the iliac crests. Alternatively, supports can be placed crosswise at the pelvis and shoulders. The lower legs are supported with pillows, and the upper extremities may be tucked at the sides or supported on armboards with the arms flexed at the shoulders and elbows. Care must be taken to pad pressure points at elbows, knees, ankles, and genitalia. Breasts must be positioned to limit pressure on the nipples.

When a prone approach is planned, the patient is anethetized on a guerney and then log-rolled onto the frame or rolls while good body alignment is maintained. Some anesthetists disconnect all monitors and vascular access lines before turning to prevent tangling or inadvertent detachment; others do not. However, thoughtful planning of monitor placement allows turning without removal of monitors during this critical period and avoids delays. Typically the patient is disconnected from the breathing circuit to avoid accidental extubation. The anesthetist should control the airway, head, and neck, as well as coordinate the turn.

Head, neck, shoulder, and arm mobility must be assessed preoperatively; arm placement can be limited by ankylosis of shoulder or elbow joints. Depending on the surgeon's preference, the arms may be tucked parallel to the sides with a draw sheet or supported on armboards. If tucked, the arms should be pronated and the elbows padded in the event the arm slips over the edge of the table. Plastic or metal arm "sleds," with sufficient padding, can be used to protect the arms and vascular access sites from compression by the bodies of the surgical team. If the arms are not tucked at the sides, they should be carefully rotated into position. The preferred arm placement is flexed, slightly abducted, and with the forearms and hands lower than the shoulders and adequately supported. The arms should rest at a comfortable height on the armboards and should not support the weight of the shoulders. Padding should be placed under the shoulders to prevent sagging of the shoulders and stretching of the brachial plexus. Although anesthetists commonly place padding between the elbow and armboard to prevent ulnar nerve damage, postoperative ulnar neuropathy has occurred despite this practice. Care must be taken to avoid pressure against the medial aspect of the upper arm by positioning devices or the operating room table, because radial nerve damage may occur.

Particular care must be taken to maintain alignment of the head and neck in the prone position. The head should be supported in a neutral position with a head-holding device. Hyperextension or lateral rotation of the neck should be avoided, since either may compromise spinal cord blood flow, especially in elderly individuals with narrowing of the spinal canal due to osteoarthritis. Also, stretch injuries of the brachial plexus may occur with lateral head rotation.

A primary goal of positioning the prone patient is to avoid pressure over the abdomen, which can impede venous return, increase venous pressures, and interfere with ventilation by inhibiting movement of the diaphragm.[119,120] Valves are not present in the intervertebral veins that drain the vertebral and spinal cord venous plexuses into the lumbar veins. External abdominal pressure is transmitted to the vena cava and communicated to the lumbar epidural veins (Figure 22-13).[74,121] Positioning devices that allow the abdomen to hang freely are associated with greater decreases in inferior vena cava pressures than those that compress the abdomen and therefore prevent engorgement of spinal venous plexuses. Engorged epidural veins are fragile and easily traumatized, and the ensuing blood loss will decrease surgical exposure and contribute to hypotension.

Meticulous attention must be paid to protection of the eyes, because corneal abrasions and POVL are complications of the prone position.[74] Several devices including 3-point skull fixation, the horseshoe headrest, and foam cushions allow the head to be placed in a neutral position while the eyes are kept free of pressure. However, the head may slip or rotate on the horseshoe headrest, allowing pressure to be applied over the globe and placing the patient at risk of central retinal artery thrombosis. Although 3-point skull fixation is often recommended for securing the head and protecting the eyes in the prone position, POVL has occurred despite the use of this device.[85]

The Lithotomy Position

The lithotomy position is used for surgical procedures that require access to any perineal structure. In the typical lithotomy position, the legs are held in flexion and abduction above the level of the

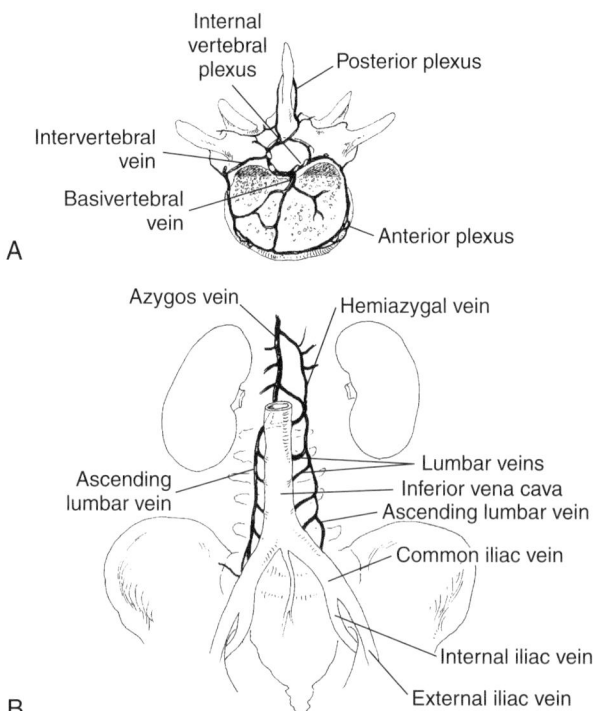

FIGURE **22-13** Venous drainage of the lumbar epidural space. **A,** Internal and external venous plexuses communicate with the intervertebral veins, posterior branches of the lumbar veins. **B,** The lumbar veins anastomose with the iliac veins, vena cava, or azygos veins. (*Modified from Williams PL et al, eds. Gray's Anatomy. 37th ed. London: Churchill Livingstone; 1989:809-811.*)

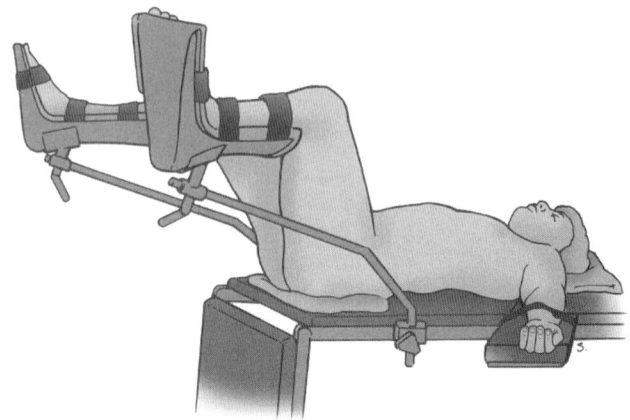

FIGURE **22-14** Legs are supported by leg cradles in the Lloyd-Davies variation of the lithotomy position. (*From Rothrock JC. Alexander's Care of the Patient in Surgery. 13th ed. St Louis: Mosby; 2007:151.*)

torso by a leg-holding device (Figure 22-14). The position is termed *low, standard, high,* or *exaggerated lithotomy*, depending on the distance the legs are elevated above the torso (Figure 22-15). In low lithotomy position, the legs are almost level with the torso, whereas in exaggerated lithotomy position, the legs are suspended with boots or stirrups so that the feet are well above the body. A hemilithotomy position, with one leg elevated, is used for some orthopedic procedures.

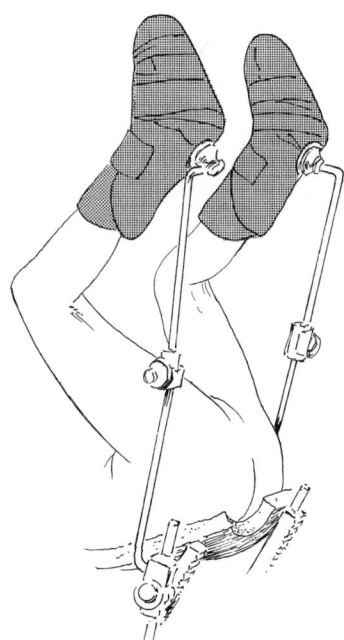

FIGURE **22-15**   Exaggerated lithotomy position. Hips and lower back are elevated, and legs are suspended in boot-type stirrups. (*Modified from Angermeier KW, Jordan GH. Complications of the exaggerated lithotomy position: a review of 177 cases. J Urol. 1994;151:867.*)

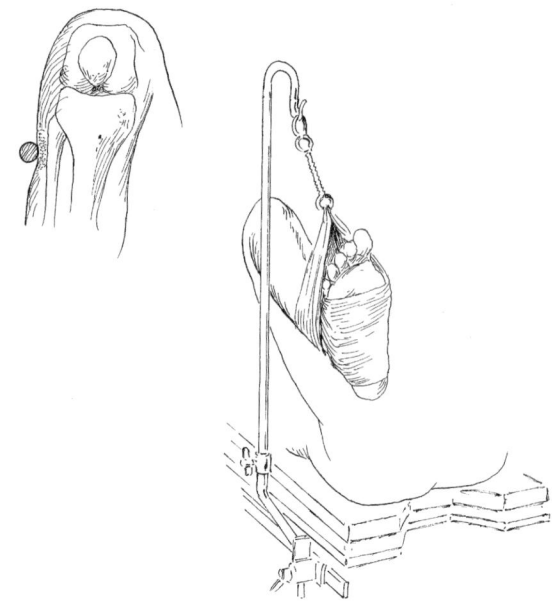

FIGURE **22-16**   Compression of the common peroneal nerve by the upright post of the leg holder. (*From Smith BE. Unusual patients: obstetrics. In: Martin JT, ed. Positioning in Anesthesia and Surgery. 2nd ed. Philadelphia: Saunders; 1987:275.*)

The arms are usually positioned as for the supine position, either tucked at the sides or abducted on armboards. In the hemilithotomy position, one arm may be secured across the chest. The same cautions for positioning the upper extremity apply as in the supine position. Additionally, care must be taken to avoid injury to the fingers if the arms are tucked at the sides and the hands extend over the edge of the table, where they may be trapped when the foot section is raised.

Many neurologic and vascular complications occur in the lithotomy position because of the position of the leg and hip. Both legs should be elevated and flexed at the hip simultaneously when they are placed in a leg-holding device; raising the legs separately can cause hip dislocation or postoperative back and hip pain. Acute abduction and external rotation of the hips can also cause femoral nerve or lumbosacral plexus stretch injuries. Flexion of the hips more than 90 degrees in the lithotomy position can cause kinking or compression of femoral neurovascular structures under the tight inguinal ligament, with subsequent arterial or venous occlusion and nerve palsy.[122,123] Extreme flexion of the knee can obstruct the popliteal vein and impede venous outflow from the extremity. Leg holders that support the leg under the knee can also compromise vascular structures in the popliteal space.

The peroneal nerve is susceptible to injury at the knee because of its superficial course and fixation against the fibular head posteriorly and inferiorly (Figure 22-16). Peroneal nerve injury is frequently associated with the lithotomy position, regardless of the type of leg-holding device used.[28,30] Depending on the type of leg holder used, the nerve can be injured by compression against the upright bar or against the supporting cradle of the leg holder. Care must be taken to adequately pad any points of potential compression.

The Lateral Decubitus Position

The lateral decubitus position is often used for surgeries involving the thorax and kidneys when the supine position cannot provide sufficient lateral or posterior-lateral exposure. The lateral position is also useful for procedures that require access to the lateral or posterior spine or cranium. Orthopedic procedures involving the hips, shoulders, or upper or lower extremities can require this position for better access to the surgical site. When a nephrectomy is performed using a lateral approach, exposure of the kidney can be facilitated by elevating the kidney rest beneath the dependent iliac crest and flexing the operating table so that the operative flank is higher than the upper torso or legs (Figure 22-17).[124]

Initially the patient is placed supine for induction of anesthesia and intubation. If a beanbag is used to support the torso, it is placed flat on the operating table prior to the patient's arrival in the OR. Before the patient is positioned, the endotracheal tube, breathing circuit, intravenous and monitoring lines, and any other devices should be secured so that none are beneath the body after the turn. The anesthetist should control the airway, head, and neck, as well as coordinate the turn.

Particular attention should be paid to body alignment in the lateral position. The shoulders, hips, head, and legs are maintained in the same plane and turned simultaneously to avoid stress and twisting of the torso and spine. The head and neck remain aligned with the spine in a neutral position. The head should be supported on pillows, donuts, or unwrinkled, folded blankets and not allowed to hang, tilt laterally, hyperflex, or hyperextend (see Figure 22-17A). Extreme neck angulation places the patient at risk for occlusion of the vertebral or carotid arteries, compromise of perfusion to the head, impairment of jugular venous drainage, and increased intracranial pressure.

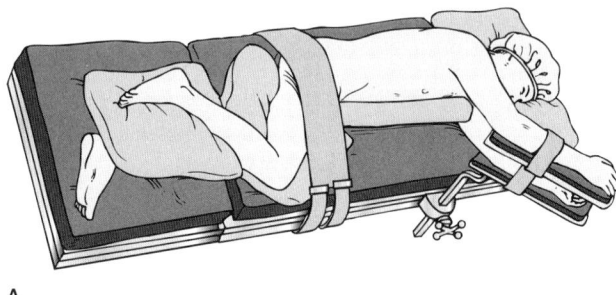

A

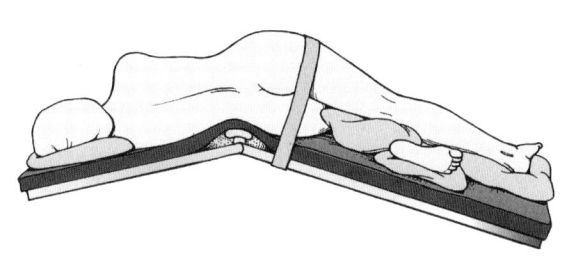

B

FIGURE **22-17 A,** Standard right lateral decubitus position. **B,** Flexed lateral position with the kidney rest properly elevated under the iliac crest. *(From Phillips N: Berry & Kohn's Operating Room Technique. 11th ed. St Louis: Mosby; 2007:511.)*

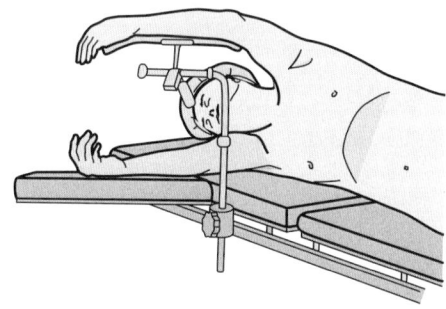

FIGURE **22-18** Proper placement of an armboard with elevated arm positioner. *(From Phillips N: Berry & Kohn's Operating Room Technique. 11th ed. St Louis: Mosby; 2007:502.)*

Angulation of the head and neck also places tension on the brachial plexus, which can cause postoperative neuropathies.[56] The anesthetist should make sure the dependent eye and ear are free of pressure. A gel donut is useful for keeping the dependent ear suspended and pressure free.

Padding and pillows are required at bony prominences and between extremities to prevent nerve compression, to pad cutaneous pressure points, and to promote venous drainage.[56] Once the patient is in the lateral position, flexing the knee and hip of the dependent leg stabilizes the patient. The nondependent leg remains straight and is supported by a pillow placed between the lower extremities. Positioning the legs in this manner prevents bony prominences of the legs from resting on each other and reduces compression of the inferior leg by the superior extremity (see Figure 22-17A). Padding should be placed along the lateral aspect of the dependent leg, extending from the knee to the heel to protect the peroneal nerve from external pressure against the table or beanbag.[11,50]

The dependent arm is positioned on a padded armboard perpendicular to the torso and flexed less than 90 degrees at the elbow.[11,50] The nondependent arm is placed to avoid interference with surgical exposure—usually parallel to the dependent arm and level with the shoulder. It can be supported with a well-cushioned arm-holding device or with pillows or blankets between the arms. Caution must be taken with the use of folded blankets or pillows because they can obstruct the anesthetist's view of the inferior arm. Perfusion to the upper extremities, especially the dependent arm, should be periodically assessed by palpating the radial artery and checking capillary refill.

The dependent shoulder and upper extremity are susceptible to compression in the lateral position. An axillary support is placed under the dependent side of the thorax, slightly caudad to but not directly in the axilla, to decompress the shoulder,

axillary vessels, and brachial plexus of the dependent arm.[87,125] Because of the risk of brachial plexus stretch and injury, posterior displacement of the shoulder should not occur.[125]

Ancillary positioning devices such as beanbags, pillows, sandbags, braces, and adhesive tape aid in securing the patient and preventing rotation of the trunk. If tape or straps are used to stabilize the torso, they should be placed just caudal to the axilla to reduce the risk of brachial plexus injury.[56] Placement across the ribs can impair ventilation. Soft tissue injury may occur if straps or tape is overly tight.

Meticulous care must be taken to prevent nerve injury when positioning the patient in the lateral decubitus position. Compression and stretching of nerves are the usual causes of injury. The most common sites of injury are the brachial plexus and the ulnar and peroneal nerves.[11] If an arm-holding device is used to support the nondependent arm, the radial nerve can be injured by compression against an edge of an improperly placed armboard (Figure 22-18).[126] Padding the elbows is suggested to prevent ulnar nerve compression in the cubital tunnel.[50] Damage to the dependent eye also can occur in lateral decubitus position if the eye is not adequately protected. Permanent blindness can result from retinal artery thrombosis secondary to pressure on the eye when the head is improperly placed on a headrest or pillow.[56] Intraoperative hypotension can further reduce retinal artery perfusion pressure and potentiate ischemia from compression.

Rhabdomyolysis has been reported after use of the lateral decubitus position.[127,128] Prolonged operating time, hypotension, and pressure of the operating table against gluteal and flank muscles have been described as contributory factors. The anesthetist, as well as the entire operating team, should ensure that the operating table is well padded and that positioning devices are properly placed. Furthermore, prolonged or excessive hypotension should be avoided to ensure adequate tissue perfusion.

The Sitting Position

The term *sitting position* commonly refers to any position in which the torso is elevated from the supine position and is higher than the legs. Depending on the surgical procedure, the amount of elevation of the head above the heart can vary greatly. A true sitting position in which the torso is elevated at 90 degrees to the legs is rarely used. The modified sitting position, in which the torso is elevated 45 degrees, the head is flexed, and the legs are elevated and flexed at heart level, is probably most familiar to anesthetists. This position is variously described as the *lounging, lawn chair,* or *beach chair* position.

The sitting position offers advantages to the surgeon and anesthetist.[1] Although its use is reportedly decreasing in popularity, some neurosurgeons favor the sitting position for posterior fossa and cervical spine procedures because it allows excellent visualization of intracranial structures and facilitates drainage of blood and cerebral spinal fluid from the wound. Plastic surgeons favor the sitting position for mammoplasty and breast reconstruction because the breasts are viewed in the natural, upright position. During shoulder arthroplasty and arthroscopy, the sitting position reduces brachial plexus stretch and aids surgical exposure and manipulation of the arm and shoulder.[129] Access to the airway and monitoring devices is easier for the anesthetist with the sitting position.

Placement of the patient in the sitting position involves flexion of the operating room table, elevation of the backrest and legs, and head-down rotation. The degree of torso elevation desired determines the amount of operating table manipulation required. For neurosurgical procedures, a 3-pin head holder is generally used to secure the head. The device provides better head stabilization compared with horseshoe-type headrests and avoids eye compression, but jugular venous obstruction can occur if the head is excessively flexed on the neck. At least two finger-breadths of space should be allowed between the neck and mandible. Care must be taken when fixing the head in the 3-point head holder because sharp skull pins can lacerate or perforate ears and eyelids. Additionally, incorrect placement of the head holder and direct contact of its metal bars with the nose or skin can cause pressure necrosis.

A horseshoe headrest is often used to support the head for shoulder procedures performed in the sitting position. Straps or adhesive tape secure the head to the headrest. The anesthetist should be aware that vigorous surgical manipulation of the arm and shoulder can move the patient's body toward the operative side of the table. If the head is firmly secured to the headrest, excessive traction or stretch can be placed on the neck and brachial plexus. If the restraining straps are loose, the head can become partially or completely dislodged from the headrest, introducing the potential for cervical spine injury. Accidental extubation can occur if the endotracheal tube is secured by a supporting device and the head is displaced. Profound hypotension and bradycardia from activation of the Bezold-Jarisch reflex occurs frequently when shoulder surgery is performed in the sitting position under an interscalene block.[129]

Serious complications associated with the sitting position are among the reasons that the position is falling out of favor. VAE is the most feared complication, but pneumocephalus, quadriplegia, and peripheral nerve injuries are also possible. Pneumocephalus is a frequent occurrence after neurosurgical procedures performed using the sitting or supine positions and is typically a benign condition.[130-132] Gravity is the most important factor in the development of pneumocephalus. Opening of the dura, drainage of cerebrospinal fluid, and surgical decompression allow relaxation of the brain and entrance of air, which rises to the top of the cranial vault. Contributing factors are those that decrease brain volume, such as the use of diuretics, hypocarbia, the presence of intraventricular shunts, and gross hydrocephalus.[132,133] Tension pneumocephalus, on the other hand, rarely occurs, but its advent requires immediate intervention to prevent rapid deterioration of the patient. The onset of tension pneumocephalus manifests as restlessness, deterioration of consciousness, convulsions, or other changes in neurologic status.[132,133] Definitive diagnosis is made by the presence of air on computed tomographic scan. Prompt evacuation of the air collection through twist drill holes is indicated.[130,131]

Trendelenburg Position

Use of the Trendelenburg (head-down) or reverse Trendelenburg (head-up) position often augments surgical exposure. The Trendelenburg position was first described in the 1860s but was used before then.[134] The position used today bears little resemblance to the original, which entailed suspension of the patient's legs over the shoulders of an assistant to improve exposure of the pelvic organs. Today the term *Trendelenburg* refers to any position in which the head is lower than the rest of the body; *reverse Trendelenburg* indicates a head-up tilt. Typically, Trendelenburg and reverse Trendelenburg are used to supplement the primary surgical position and improve exposure. Physiologic alterations vary greatly depending on the degree of tilt and the primary position.

Various complications, many transient, have been observed as outcomes of the Trendelenburg position. Many are the result of devices designed to prevent the patient from sliding when in a steep Trendelenburg or reverse Trendelenburg position. Wristlets used to restrain the patient can cause traction on the arm and stretch of the brachial plexus. Improperly positioned shoulder braces can also injure the brachial plexus. Placement of the shoulder brace in a position that is either too lateral or too medial can result in depression of underlying bony structures and compression or stretching of the plexus.[1,58,135] Shoulder braces should be avoided if at all possible. The arms are vulnerable to injury in the Trendelenburg position, particularly if they are positioned on armboards and inadequately restrained. The arms can slip off, hyperextend, and abduct above the level of the shoulder, stretching the plexus. Suspension of the patient by ankle restraints can cause sore knees or hips. When too tight, table straps used to prevent the patient from sliding in the reverse Trendelenburg position have resulted in lower-extremity neuropathies.[136] Use of a foot board is preferable to the overzealous tightening of the table strap if the use of a steep reverse Trendelenburg position is anticipated.

PHYSIOLOGIC EFFECTS OF SURGICAL POSITIONS

Humans normally assume an upright posture. As a result, gravity plays a significant role in the functioning of the cardiovascular and respiratory systems. Position changes in conscious human beings are accompanied by numerous compensatory mechanisms to maintain a stable heart rate, cardiac output, and blood pressure. Administration of general or central neuraxial anesthesia significantly depresses or attenuates these responses. Therefore hemodynamic and ventilatory changes often accompany position alterations in adequately anesthetized patients.

Hemodynamic Effects of Surgical Positions

Cardiac output and blood pressure are generally decreased under general anesthesia in response to myocardial depression and vasodilation induced by volatile anesthetics. As a result, blood pools in dependent body areas, reducing preload and decreasing stroke volume. Administration of neuromuscular blocking agents also contributes to decreased venous return because normal muscle tone is abolished. Additionally, opioids and volatile agents slow the heart rate, further decreasing cardiac output and blood pressure. In healthy patients, MAP is maintained by compensatory increases in heart rate and systemic vascular resistance (SVR), but elderly patients and those with preexisting diseases can be less adaptive. Compensatory mechanisms to increase heart rate when hypotension occurs are blunted by general anesthetics, rendering cardiac output and blood pressure more susceptible to gravitational forces.

Hemodynamic changes are usually minimal in the supine and lateral positions.[137,138] However, cardiac output and blood pressure are often decreased in the sitting, prone, and flexed lateral positions, where the lower extremities are dependent.[56,137] Although CVP is increased in the prone position, left ventricular volume is reduced, probably due to decreased venous return and increased intrathoracic pressure.[139] Cardiac index may be decreased[140,141] or unchanged[140] in the prone position compared with the supine; the effect may be frame dependent.[141] In the lateral decubitus position with the kidney rest elevated, hypotension is likely because the legs are dependent, venous return is reduced by extreme flexion, and the kidney rest may compress the great vessels.[56,137] Conversely, blood pressure may appear normal or higher in the lithotomy position, in which elevation of the legs above the trunk provides an autotransfusion of 100 to 250 mL per leg.

Mean arterial pressure increases or decreases by 0.75 mm Hg for each centimeter change in height between the heart and a body region.[89,142] Therefore regions elevated above the heart in the head-up, sitting, and lithotomy positions may be at risk for hypoperfusion and ischemia, particularly if hypotension occurs. The decrease in hemodynamic parameters depends on the degree of elevation of the torso. Hemodynamic changes are minimal if the patient is placed in a 45-degree, head-up sitting position, but cardiac output decreases 20% if the patient is raised to 90 degrees, because venous blood pools in the extremities. When the patient is in the seated position, as compared with supine, cardiac index (CI), CVP, and pulmonary artery wedge pressure decrease significantly, and SVR increases.[110,143] In procedures in which the head is elevated and cerebral perfusion is a concern, invasive arterial blood pressure monitoring should be instituted, with the transducer placed at the level of the circle of Willis.[85]

Positioning devices and mechanical ventilation may contribute to decreased cardiac output and hypotension. In the lateral decubitus position, elevation of the kidney rest under the flank may cause vena cava compression. When the patient is in the lateral decubitus position, the kidney rest should lie under the dependent iliac crest.[137] Extreme flexion of the hips in some variations of the prone or lithotomy positions may occlude the femoral vessels and contribute to decreased venous return. Large tidal volumes and PEEP may generate high intrathoracic pressures, with a subsequent reduction in atrial filling and cardiac output.

A variety of methods have been suggested for attenuating the hemodynamic changes associated with surgical positioning. Slow assumption of the surgical position is assumed to allow the cardiovascular system time to compensate for position-induced hemodynamic alterations. Because hemodynamic changes may be influenced by anesthetic technique, using a nitrous-narcotic technique or a lighter level of anesthesia (less than 0.5 minimum alveolar concentration) or gradually attaining a deeper level of anesthesia may attenuate position-induced hypotension.[56] Intravascular volume loading before positioning can reduce or eliminate hypotension.[137,141] However, volume replacement must be done judiciously because excessive fluid administration can lead to volume overload in susceptible individuals when the patient is returned to supine position, or when the vasodilatory effects of general anesthetics are terminated.[56] The use of leg wraps, hip flexion, and G-suits to reduce hypotension in the sitting position has fallen out of favor.

The Trendelenburg position is often used to treat hypotension, because it is assumed to increase venous return and MAP. When placed in a head-down position, normotensive individuals compensate for increases in CVP and PAP with vasodilation and a decrease in heart rate from stimulation of baroreceptor reflexes. However, hypotensive individuals may not respond in the same manner. Investigators have demonstrated variable effects of the Trendelenburg position on cardiovascular parameters. Changes in intrathoracic blood volume of 2% to 3% in unanesthetized normovolemic individuals are reported with the Trendelenburg position.[144,145] CVP, mean PAP, and pulmonary artery occlusion pressure can be increased in the head-down position, but this increase may not reflect changes in CI, stroke volume, or MAP.[145-147] Others have shown no increase in MAP, an increase in SVR, and a decrease in CI in hypotensive patients placed in Trendelenburg.[148]

Hypovolemia can be unrecognized in the lithotomy and Trendelenburg positions, because MAP can appear normal despite volume deficit. Volume replacement can be assessed as adequate until acute hypotension occurs when the patient is returned to the horizontal position. An additive effect can occur if the Trendelenburg position is used to supplement the lithotomy position.

Patients with comorbidities may be susceptible to the detrimental effects of various positions. The combination of the lithotomy position and a head-down tilt can have a detrimental effect on myocardial function in patients with coronary artery disease, because CVP, pulmonary artery pressure (PAP), and pulmonary capillary wedge pressure (PCWP) are increased, whereas cardiac output is decreased.[149] The Trendelenburg position may increase myocardial work by increasing central blood volume, cardiac output, and stroke volume. Individuals with very poor cardiac function can have decreased cardiac output if the increased central blood volume moves them to a worse position on the Frank-Starling curve. The lower extremities of individuals with peripheral vascular disease may be at risk of ischemia in the lithotomy and Trendelenburg positions because a relative state of hypoperfusion exists when the lower extremities are elevated above the heart.

The prone and Trendelenburg positions may increase venous pressure in the head, with resultant swelling of facial, pharyngeal, and orbital structures. Intracranial pressure can be elevated when the head is dependent, because venous pressures are transmitted to the head and intracranial structures through the valveless jugular system. Cerebral blood flow can be decreased when inflow is limited by venous congestion in intracranial structures. POVL may result from an increase in ocular venous pressures and concomitant decrease in ocular perfusion pressure. Facial chemosis, macroglossia, and airway edema are reported following the prone and head-down positions.[113,115] A 10-degree head-up tilt may prevent the development of facial edema.

Respiratory Effects of Surgical Positions

During spontaneous respiration in awake patients, contraction of the diaphragm and intercostal muscles causes expansion of the thoracic cavity in both an anterior-posterior and lateral direction. Downward displacement of the diaphragm generates a negative intrathoracic pressure and allows lung expansion as gas flows inward. Lung elastance and chest-wall compliance affect the amount of pressure necessary to expand the alveoli for a given change in volume. Gravitational factors affect the distribution of ventilation and perfusion within the lung, as well as the shape of the thoracic cavity and movement of the diaphragm and abdominal contents.

Postural changes may significantly alter compliance, lung volumes, and the distribution of ventilation and pulmonary blood flow. Positioning devices may cause mechanical interference with movement of the belly wall and abdominal contents, the chest wall, or the diaphragm.[150] Therefore anesthetic-induced depression of ventilation may be worsened by the majority of surgical positions. Individuals with preexisting diseases that alter respiratory function may be more susceptible to the deleterious ventilatory effects of surgical positions.

Gravity plays an important role in position-related ventilatory changes. On a vertical gradient, dependent regions of the lung are heavier than nondependent regions, owing to the effects of gravity. In essence, the lung is deformed by gravity. The volume and weight of dependent lung tissue will vary depending on the position adopted. For example, although overall lung density is not different between the supine and prone positions, lung density is significantly increased in dependent regions and decreased in nondependent regions in both positions.[151] Increases in lung density are accompanied by concomitant decreases in perfusion in that region.

Effective respiratory gas exchange depends on a balance of ventilation and perfusion throughout the lungs. Traditionally, gravitational effects on gas and blood flow are thought to result in differences in ventilation and perfusion in different lung segments. In both awake and anesthetized patients, gravitational forces are theorized to create a gradient that favors perfusion in dependent portions of the lungs and ventilation in nondependent regions.[152,153] However, new imaging techniques have identified a concentric pattern of blood flow in the lungs, with central regions receiving a greater proportion of flow than the periphery.[154] The mechanism for this gradient has not been identified, but the diameters and branching patterns of pulmonary vessels and the distance blood must flow to reach a site are possible factors. Nongravitational factors such as cardiac output, pleural pressures, and lung volumes are also thought to play a factor in regional lung perfusion.[152,154]

Positional changes result in redistribution of ventilation and perfusion that are least in the sitting position and greatest in the prone and lateral positions. In the prone position, changes in ventilation-perfusion ($\dot{V}/\dot{Q}$) ratios have been postulated as the cause of improved oxygenation.[152] More lung volume is present posteriorly than anteriorly, where anterior mediastinal structures occupy significant space; as a consequence, posterior lung segments are better ventilated. Ventilation is more uniform and $\dot{V}/\dot{Q}$ matching is better in the prone position than in the supine position.[153] In the lateral decubitus position, ventilation and perfusion are greater in the dependent lung than in the nondependent lung in awake, spontaneously breathing patients.

Improvements in functional residual capacity (FRC), lung compliance, and oxygenation are also reported in obese patients in the prone position.[155] In the lithotomy position, ventilation and perfusion ratios are unchanged in normal individuals receiving epidural anesthesia, but obese individuals and patients under general anesthesia demonstrate reductions in ventilation-perfusion ratios and lung aeration.[156]

$\dot{V}/\dot{Q}$ mismatching in the lateral decubitus position affects oxygenation, especially with procedures requiring one-lung ventilation. Hypoxic pulmonary vasoconstriction in the unventilated lung further redistributes blood flow to the dependent lung to improve ventilation.[154] Patients are susceptible to atelectasis in the lateral position, because closing volumes occur above FRC,

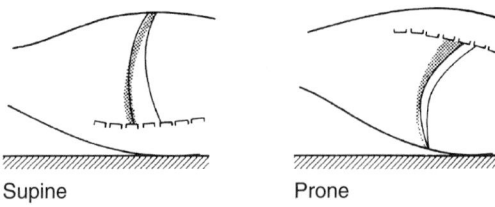

FIGURE **22-19** Position of the diaphragm in supine and prone subjects. *Solid lines* represent end-expiratory and end-inspiratory diaphragm positions during spontaneous breathing while the patient is awake. *Stippled areas* represent diaphragm excursions during mechanical ventilation for anesthesia paralysis. (*Modified from Krayer S et al. Position and motion of the human diaphragm during anesthesia-paralysis.* Anesthesiology. 1989;70:895.)

with closing occurring earlier in the dependent than in the nondependent lung. Tidal volumes of 10 to 12 mL/kg and an F_{IO_2} of 0.5 or higher have been suggested to compensate for $\dot{V}/\dot{Q}$ mismatch in the lateral position; however, excessive tidal volumes can cause barotrauma, decrease hypoxic vasoconstriction, and reduce oxygenation in patients in the lateral position.[154] Tidal volumes of 5 to 7 mL/kg and higher respiratory rates cause smaller declines in oxygenation.[154] Although PEEP applied to both lungs can increase ventilation to the dependent lung, controversy exists regarding whether PEEP selectively applied to the dependent lung increases or decreases ventilation to that lung. Application of 2 to 5 cm H_2O of continuous positive airway pressure (CPAP) to the dependent lung can significantly improve oxygenation during one-lung ventilation.[154]

Changes in the elastance and resistance of the diaphragm and abdomen occur when shifting between positions. These changes have little effect on movement of the chest wall in healthy individuals but may have an effect in persons with conditions that predispose to abnormalities of lung function.[157] Lung and chest-wall compliance in sitting and supine patients is not different, because increases in thoracic compliance are paralleled by reductions in the abdominal compartment. Expansion of the rib cage is not limited by the supine position; however, the elastic recoil of the chest wall and its anterior-posterior diameter are decreased in the anesthetized state. The rib cage contributes less to ventilation in the prone position than in the sitting position because of limitations in anterior chest expansion.[158] In the prone position, diaphragmatic excursion can be limited by the abdominal viscera if the abdomen is compressed by the weight of the body or positioning devices (Figure 22-19). If the abdomen hangs free, gravity allows the abdominal contents to shift anteriorly, reducing interference with diaphragmatic movement.[159] In the anesthetized patient who is in the lateral position, induction of anesthesia allows the the abdominal contents to shift cephalad, moving the hemidiaphragm of the dependent lung upward, thereby decreasing ventilation in the dependent lung and reducing its compliance. In the nondependent lung of the anesthetized patient, ventilation is greater and compliance increased because the caudal shift of the upper hemidiaphragm allows unrestricted lung excursion. The lithotomy position has little effect on the compliance of the respiratory system in healthy, conscious volunteers.[150] However, extreme flexion of the thighs on the belly in the exaggerated lithotomy position compresses the abdomen, shifts the abdominal viscera cephalad, and limits diaphragmatic movement. As a result, compliance and tidal volume are reduced, and airway pressures and dead space–to–tidal volume ratios are increased.[160] This effect may be amplified in obese individuals.

Pulmonary mechanics may be inhibited by positioning devices. Pneumoperitoneum combined with a head-down tilt and devices that restrict chest expansion such as tight straps or tape can decrease chest-wall compliance. Studies suggest that in the prone position, the degree to which pulmonary mechanics are altered depends on the positioning device used, not on body habitus.[159] The Jackson table resulted in the smallest change in pulmonary compliance and peak airway pressures when compared with the Wilson frame and chest rolls. The investigators hypothesized that the Jackson table allows the abdomen to hang freely, permitting better diaphragmatic excursion and lower intraabdominal and intrathoracic pressures.[159]

Lung capacities are decreased with most position changes. In the supine position, FRC and total lung capacity are significantly decreased compared with the sitting position.[157] A cephalad shift of the dependent diaphragm caused by pressure of the abdominal viscera has been proposed for this reduction (see Figure 22-19).[150] Conflicting evidence exists regarding the effect of the prone position on FRC. Some investigators have found a decrease in FRC compared with the sitting position, although less so than the supine position,[158] whereas others have found an increase in FRC.[152,161] Theories posit that better matching of ventilation and perfusion, rather than changes in lung volumes or capacities, cause improvements in oxygenation in the prone position.[150]

In the lateral position, the mediastinum shifts toward the dependent lung, decreasing FRC in that lung and increasing it in the nondependent lung.[154] Vital capacity and tidal volume are reduced in awake, anesthetized individuals in the lateral position. Vital capacity in an awake, spontaneously breathing patient is reduced by 10%; elevation of the kidney rest produces an additional 5% reduction.[56] Similar reductions in tidal volume occur in anesthetized, mechanically ventilated patients.

Ventilatory changes associated with the lithotomy position are dependent on the extent to which the legs are flexed on the abdomen and the concomitant use of the head-down position. In the normal lithotomy position without Trendelenburg, changes in FRC are similar to those associated with the supine position, and the diaphragm does not shift farther cephalad.[156] However, adding Trendelenburg position to lithotomy can cause an additional decrease in FRC. In spontaneously breathing individuals, the lithotomy position can restrict diaphragmatic movement and tidal volume.

The effect of the sitting position on the respiratory system varies, depending on the relationship among the chest, abdomen, and lower extremities. The sitting position is more favorable for ventilation and has less effect on lung volumes than other positions. The more the torso is elevated, the smaller the effect on lung mechanics. Forced vital capacity and FRC are within normal parameters in the seated position.[158] The abdominal contents shift caudally and anteriorly, causing less interference with diaphragmatic movement and allowing greater expansion of dependent lung regions.[150] Compared with the supine position, in which the abdominal muscles are used for breathing, in the sitting position, the rib cage contributes more to ventilation.[158]

Respiratory benefits of the sitting position are attenuated when the sitting position is modified to minimize cardiovascular effects. Flexion of the lower extremities at the hip and elevation of the legs causes abdominal contents to shift cephalad against the diaphragm. The sitting position then more closely resembles the supine position, limiting diaphragmatic excursion and decreasing FRC and closing volumes.[85] External compression devices (G-suit) to prevent VAE can compound this effect.

The Trendelenburg position exacerbates the deleterious ventilatory effects of the various positions. The diaphragm is displaced cephalad, and its excursion is limited by shifting of the abdominal contents, decreasing the FRC progressively as the degree of Trendelenburg increases. Movement of the mediastinum toward the head moves the carina closer to the endotracheal tube and can result in preferential ventilation of one lung if the tube moves into the right mainstem bronchus.[111,162] This complication also occurs in the reverse Trendelenburg position during laparoscopic procedures, in which the diaphragm is displaced in a cephalad direction by pressurized gas.[112,162]

SUMMARY

Surgical positioning disturbs normal cardiovascular and respiratory physiology. These positional changes can be augmented by anesthetic techniques, patient pathophysiology, and body habitus. The implications of physiologic changes associated with each position should be considered when the procedure is planned, when positioning is initiated, and when the patient is returned to the supine posture. Anesthetists must recognize and anticipate both the publicized complications and the potential for damage inherent in each surgical position. Prevention is the best method for decreasing both the incidence of position-related injuries and the associated physical, psychological, and economic costs to the patient.

REFERENCES

1. Cheney FW et al. Nerve injury associated with anesthesia: a clinical closed claims analysis. *Anesthesiology.* 1999;90(4):1062-1069.
2. Warner MA et al. Ulnar neuropathy in surgical patients. *Anesthesiology.* 1999;90(1):54-59.
3. Cheney FW et al. Trends in anesthesia-related death and brain damage. *Anesthesiology.* 2006;105:1081-1086.
4. American Society of Anesthesiologists. Closed Claims Project. *Overview.* Available at: http://depts.washington.edu/asaccp/ASA/index.shtml. Accessed July 10, 2008.
5. MacRae MG. Closed claims studies in anesthesia: a literature review and implications for practice. *AANA J.* 2007;75(4):267-275.
6. Jordan LM et al. Data-driven practice improvement: the AANA Foundation Closed Malpractice Claims Study. *AANA J.* 2001;69(4):301-311.
7. Fritzlen T et al. The AANA Foundation Closed Malpractice Claims Study on nerve injuries during anesthesia care. *AANA J.* 2003;71(5):347-352.
8. American Association of Nurse Anesthetists. *Scope and Standards for Nurse Anesthesia Practice.* Available at: http://www.aana.com. Accessed Jure 2, 2008.
9. Winfree CJ, Kline DG. Intraoperative positioning nerve injuries. *Surg Neurol.* 2005;63(1):5-18.
10. Murff HJ et al. Detecting adverse events for patient safety research: a review of current methodologies. *J Biomed Inform.* 2003;36:131-143.
11. Sawyer RJ et al. Peripheral nerve injuries associated with anaesthesia. *Anaesthesia.* 2000;55:980-991.
12. Prielipp RC et al. Ulnar nerve injury and perioperative arm positioning. *Anesthesiol Clin North America.* 2002;20(3):589-603.
13. Wall EJ et al. Experimental stretch neuropathy. Changes in nerve conduction under tension. *J Bone Joint Surg Br.* 1992;74(1):126-129.
14. Tanoue M et al. Acute stretching of peripheral nerves inhibits retrograde axonal transport. *J Hand Surgery [Br].* 1996;21(3):358-363.

15. Brown R et al. Effects of acute graded strain on efferent conduction properties in the rabbit tibial nerve. *Clin Orthop Relat Res*. 1993;296:288-294.

16. Rempel D et al. Pathophysiology of nerve compression syndromes: response of peripheral nerves to loading. *J Bone Joint Surg Am*. 1999;81(11):1600-1610.

17. Warner MA. Perioperative neuropathies. *Mayo Clin Proc*. 1998;73:567-574.

18. Huether SE. The cellular environment: fluids and electrolytes, acids and bases. In: McCance KL, Huether SE, eds. *Pathophysiology: The Biologic Basis for Disease in Adults and Children*. 4th ed. St Louis: Mosby; 2002:85-113.

19. McCance KL, Grey TC. Altered cellular and tissue biology. In: McCance KL, Huether SE, eds. *Pathophysiology: The Biologic Basis for Disease in Adults and Children*. 4th ed. St Louis: Mosby; 2002:43-84.

20. Moore KL, Dalley AF. *Clinically Oriented Anatomy*. 5th ed. Philadelphia: Lippincott Williams & Wilkins; 1999.

21. Schinsky MF et al. Nerve injury after primary total knee arthroplasty. *J Arthroplasty*. 2001;16(8):1048-1054.

22. Angermeier KW, Jordan GH. Complications of the exaggerated lithotomy position: a review of 177 cases. *J Urol*. 1994;151:866-868.

23. Rodeo SA et al. Neurological complications due to arthroscopy. *J Bone Joint Surg Am*. 1993;75(6):917-926.

24. Wong DH, Ward MG. A preventable cause of brachial plexus injury. *Anesthesiology*. 2003;98(3):798.

25. Lundborg G, Dahlin LB. The pathophysiology of nerve compression. *Hand Clin*. 1992;8(2):225-227.

26. Lowe J et al. Current approach to radial nerve paralysis. *Plast Reconstr Surg*. 2000;110:1099-1112.

27. Martin JT. Compartment syndromes: concepts and perspectives for the anesthesiologist. *Anesth Analg*. 1992;75:275-283.

28. Jacobs D et al. Unusual complication after pelvic surgery: unilateral lower limb crush syndrome and bilateral common peroneal nerve paralysis. *Acta Anaesthesiol Belg*. 1994;43:139-143.

29. Fowl RJ et al. Neurovascular lower extremity complications of the lithotomy position. *Ann Vasc Surg*. 1992;6:357-361.

30. Warner MA et al. Lower-extremity motor neuropathy associated with surgery performed on patients in a lithotomy position. *Anesthesiology*. 1994;81:6-12.

31. Lee LA, Lam AM. Unilateral blindness after prone lumbar spine surgery. *Anesthesiology*. 2001;95(3):793-795.

32. Guzzi LM et al. Rhabdomyolysis, acute renal failure, and the exaggerated lithotomy position. *Anesth Analg*. 1993;77:635-637.

33. Ali H et al. Acute renal failure due to rhabdomyolysis associated with the extreme lithotomy position. *Am J Kidney Dis*. 1993;22(6):865-869.

34. Landau ME et al. Effect of body mass index on ulnar nerve conduction velocity, ulnar neuropathy at the elbow, and carpal tunnel syndrome. *Muscle Nerve*. 2005;32(3):360-363.

35. Lee LA et al. Injuries associated with regional anesthesia in the 1980s and 1990s. *Anesthesiology*. 2004;202(1):143-152.

36. Goldsmith AL, McCallum MI. Compartment syndrome as a complication of the prolonged use of the Lloyd-Davies position. *Anaesthesia*. 1996;51(11):1048-1052.

37. Thonse R et al. Differences in attitudes to analgesia in post-operative limb surgery put patients at risk of compartment syndrome. *Injury*. 2004;35(3):290-295.

38. Contreras MG et al. Anatomy of the ulnar nerve at the elbow: potential relationship of acute ulnar neuropathy to gender differences. *Clin Anat*. 1998;11(6):372-378.

39. Richardson JK et al. Gender, body mass and age as risk factors for ulnar mononeuropathy at the elbow. *Muscle Nerve*. 2001;24(4):551-554.

40. Sharma K et al. Incidence of acute femoral neuropathy following renal transplantation. *Arch Neurol*. 2002;59:541-545.

41. Warner DO. Tobacco dependence in surgical patients. *Curr Opin Anaesthesiol*. 2007;20(3):279-283.

42. Alvine FG, Schurrer ME. Postoperative ulnar nerve palsy. *J Bone Joint Surg Am*. 1987;69(2):255-259.

43. Stoelting RK. Postoperative ulnar nerve palsy—is it a preventable complication? *Anesth Analg*. 1993;76:7-9.

44. Warner MA et al. Ulnar neuropathy in surgical patients. *Anesthesiology*. 1999;90(1):54-59.

45. Warner MA et al. Ulnar neuropathy: incidence, outcome, and risk factors in sedated or anesthetized patients. *Anesthesiology*. 1994;81:1332-1340.

46. Unlu Y et al. Brachial plexus injury following median sternotomy. *Interact Cardiovasc Thorac Surg*. 2007;6(2):235-237.

47. Polatsch DB et al. Ulnar nerve anatomy. *Hand Clin*. 2007;23(3):283-289.

48. Casscells CD et al. Ulnar neuropathy after median sternotomy. *Clin Orthop*. 1993;291:259-265.

49. Warner MA et al. Ulnar neuropathy in medical patients. *Anesthesiology*. 2000;92(2):613-615.

50. American Society of Anesthesiologists. Practice advisory for the prevention of perioperative peripheral neuropathies: a report by the ASA Task Force on Prevention of Perioperative Peripheral Neuropathies. *Anesthesiology*. 2000;92(4):1168-1182.

51. Prielipp RC et al. Ulnar nerve pressure: influence of arm position and relationship to somatosensory evoked potentials. *Anesthesiology*. 1999;91(2):345-354.

52. Moore KL, Agur AMR. *Essential Clinical Anatomy*. Baltimore: Lippincott Williams & Wilkins; 2002.

53. Sharma AD et al. Peripheral nerve injuries during cardiac surgery: risk factors, diagnosis, prognosis, and prevention. *Anesth Analg*. 2000;91(6):1358-1369.

54. Bhardwaj D, Peng P. An uncommon mechanism of brachial plexus injury. A case report. *Can J Anaesth*. 1999;46(2):173-175.

55. Coppieters MW et al. Positioning in anesthesiology: toward a better understanding of stretch-induced perioperative neuropathies. *Anesthesiology*. 2002;97:75-81.

56. Lawson NW, Meyer DJ. Lateral positions. In: Martin JT, Warner MA, eds. *Positioning in Anesthesia and Surgery*. Philadelphia: Saunders; 1997:127-152.

57. Rao AG et al. Shoulder arthroscopy: principles and practice. *Phys Med Rehabil Clin N Am*. 2004;15(3):627-642.

58. Kent CD, Cheney FW. A case of bilateral brachial plexus palsy due to shoulder braces. *J Clin Anesth*. 2007;19(6):482.

59. Jellish WS et al. Somatosensory evoked potential monitoring used to compare the effect of three asymmetric sternal retractors on brachial plexus function. *Anesth Analg*. 1999;88(2):292-297.

60. Bhardwaj A et al. Neurologic deficits after cervical laminectomy in the prone position. *J Neurosurg Anesthesiol*. 2001;13:314-319.

61. Haisa T, Kondo T. Midcervical flexion myelopathy after posterior fossa surgery in the sitting position: case report. *Neurosurgery*. 1996;38(4):819-821.

62. Rau C-S et al. Quadriplegia in a patient who underwent posterior fossa surgery in the prone position. *J Neurosurg*. 2002;96(1 Suppl):101-103.

63. Morandi X et al. Extensive spinal cord infarction after posterior fossa surgery in the sitting position: case report. *Neurosurgery*. 2004;54(6):1512-1515.

64. Lee RR et al. Dynamic physiologic changes in lumbar CSF volume quantitatively measured by three-dimensional fast spin-echo MRI. *Spine*. 2001;26(10):1172-1178.

65. Deinsberger W et al. Somatosensory evoked potential monitoring during positioning of the patient for posterior fossa surgery in the semisitting position. *Neurosurgery*. 1998;43(1):36-40.

66. Wenger M et al. Post-traumatic cervical kyphosis with surgical correction complicated by temporary anterior spinal artery syndrome. *J Clin Neurosci*. 2005;12(2):193-196.

67. Warner ME et al. The frequency of perioperative vision loss. *Anesth Analg*. 2001;93(6):1417-1421.

68. Kalyani SD et al. Incidence of and risk factors for perioperative optic neuropathy after cardiac surgery. *Ann Thorac Surg*. 2004;78(1):34-37.

69. Chang SH, Miller NR. The incidence of vision loss due to perioperative ischemic optic neuropathy associated with spine surgery: the Johns Hopkins Hospital experience. *Spine*. 2005;30(11):1299-1302.

70. Stevens WR et al. Ophthalmic complications after spinal surgery. *Spine*. 1997;22(12):1319-1324.

71. Sadun AA. Anatomy and physiology. In: Yanoff M et al, eds. *Ophthalmology*. 2nd ed. St Louis: Mosby; 2004.

72. Williams EL. Postoperative blindness. *Anesthesiol Clin North America*. 2002;20(3):605-622.

73. Buono LM, Foroozan R. Perioperative posterior ischemic optic neuropathy: review of the literature. *Surv Ophthalmol*. 2005;50(1):15-26.

74. Lee LA et al. The American Society of Anesthesiologists Postoperative Visual Loss Registry: analysis of 93 spine surgery cases with postoperative visual loss. *Anesthesiology*. 2006;105(4):652-659.

75. Kamming D, Clarke S. Postoperative visual loss following prone spinal surgery. *Br J Anaesth*. 2005;95(2):257-260.

76. Hayreh SS, Zimmerman MB. Central retinal artery occlusion: visual outcome. *Am J Ophthalmol*. 2005;140(3):376-391.

77. Williams EL et al. Postoperative ischemic optic neuropathy. *Anesth Analg*. 1995;80(5):1018-1029.

78. Abraham M et al. Unilateral visual loss after cervical spine surgery. *J Neurosurg Anesthesiol*. 2003;15(4):319-322.

79. Dunker S et al. Perioperative risk factors for posterior ischemic optic neuropathy. *J Am Coll Surg*. 2002;194(6):705-710.

80. Levin H, Ben-David B. Transient blindness during hysteroscopy: a rare complication. *Anesth Analg*. 1995;81:880-881.

81. Tiwari A et al. Acute compartment syndromes. *Br J Surg*. 2002;89(4):397-412.

82. Verdolin MH et al. Bilateral lower extremity compartment syndromes following prolonged surgery in the low lithotomy position with compression stockings. *Anesthesiology*. 2000;92:1189-1191.

83. Tuckey J. Bilateral compartment syndrome complicating prolonged lithotomy position. *Br J Anaesth.* 1996;77:546-549.
84. Warner ME et al. Compartment syndrome in surgical patients. *Anesthesiology.* 2001;94:705-708.
85. Porter JM et al. The sitting position in neurosurgery: a critical appraisal. *Br J Anaesth.* 1999;82(1):117-128.
86. Kaper BP et al. Compartment syndrome after arthroscopic surgery of the knee: a report of two cases managed nonoperatively. *Am J Sports Med.* 1997;25:123-125.
87. Azar FM. Traumatic disorders. In: Canale ST, ed. *Campbell's Operative Orthopedics.* 10th ed. St Louis: Mosby; 2003.
88. Tuncer R, Zorludemir U. Lower limb compartment syndrome following urethroplasty. *Brit J Urol.* 1997;79:646.
89. Meyer RS et al. Intramuscular and blood pressures in legs positioned in the hemilithotomy position: clarification of risk factors for well-leg acute compartment syndrome. *J Bone Joint Surg Am.* 2002;84(10):1829-1835.
90. Venkatesh R et al. Compartment syndrome. *Brit J Urology.* 1996;78:964-965.
91. Kumar V et al. Gluteal compartment syndrome following joint arthroplasty under epidural anaesthesia: a report of 4 cases. *J Orthop Surg (Hong Kong).* 2007;15(1):113-117.
92. Davis ET et al. The use of regional anaesthesia in patients at risk of acute compartment syndrome. *Injury.* 2006;37(2):128-133.
93. Turnbull D, Mills GH. Compartment syndrome associated with the Lloyd Davies position: three case reports and review of the literature. *Anaesthesia.* 2001;56:980-987.
94. Jolliffe MP et al. Venous air embolism during radical perineal prostatectomy. *J Clin Anesth.* 1996;8(8):659-661.
95. McDouall SF, Shlugman D. Fatal venous air embolism during lumbar surgery: the tip of an iceberg? *Eur J Anaesthesiol.* 2007;24(9):803-805.
96. Brown J et al. Cardiac arrest during surgery and ventilation in the prone position: a case report and systematic review. *Resuscitation.* 2001;50(2):233-238.
97. Duke DA et al. Venous air embolism in sitting and supine patients undergoing vestibular Schwannoma resection. *Neurosurgery.* 1998;42(6):1282-1286.
98. Rath GP et al. Complications related to positioning in posterior fossa craniectomy. *J Clin Neurosci.* 2007;14(6):520-525.
99. Bithal PK et al. Comparative incidence of venous air embolism and associated hypotension in adults and children operated for neurosurgery in the sitting position. *Eur J Anaesthesiol.* 2004;21(7):517-522.
100. Girard F et al. Incidences of venous air embolism and patent foramen ovale among patients undergoing selective peripheral denervation in the sitting position. *Neurosurgery.* 2003;53:316-319.
101. Lobato EB et al. Venous air embolism and selective denervation for torticollis. *Anesth Analg.* 1997;84(3):551-553.
102. Papadopoulos G et al. Venous and paradoxical air embolism in the sitting position. A prospective study with transoesophageal echocardiography. *Acta Neurochir (Wien).* 1994;126(2-4):140-143.
103. Stendel R et al. Transcranial Doppler ultrasonography as a screening technique for detection of a patent foramen ovale before surgery in the sitting position. *Anesthesiology.* 2000;93:971-975.
104. Schmitt HJ, Hemmerling TM. Venous air emboli occur during release of positive end-expiratory pressure and repositioning after sitting position surgery. *Anesth Analg.* 2002;94(2):400-403.
105. Engelhardt M et al. Neurosurgical operations with the patient in sitting position: analysis of risk factors using transcranial Doppler sonography. *Br J Anaesth.* 2006;96(4):467-472.
106. Toung TJK et al. Effects of positive end-expiratory pressure ventilation on cerebral venous pressure with head elevation in dogs. *J Appl Physiol.* 2000;88(2):655-661.
107. Cucchiara RF, Bechtle PS. Comment on "Incidences of venous air embolism and patent foramen ovale among patients undergoing selective peripheral denervation in the sitting position." *Neurosurgery.* 2003;53:320.
108. Schafer ST et al. Intracardiac transvenous echocardiography is superior to both precordial Doppler and transesophageal echocardiography techniques for detecting venous air embolism and catheter-guided air aspiration. *Anesth Analg.* 2008;106(1):45-54.
109. Albin MS et al. Venous air embolism during lumbar laminectomy in the prone position: report of three cases. *Anesth Analg.* 1991;73:346-349.
110. Giebler R et al. Effect of positive end-expiratory pressure on the incidence of venous air embolism and on the cardiovascular response to the sitting position during neurosurgery. *Br J Anaesth.* 1998;80(1):30-35.
111. Yap SJ et al. Alterations in endotracheal tube position during general anaesthesia. *Anaesth Intensive Care.* 1994;22:586-588.
112. Lobato EB et al. Pneumoperitoneum as a risk factor for endobronchial intubation during laparoscopic gynecologic surgery. *Anesth Analg.* 1998;86(2):301-303.
113. Pivalizza EG et al. Massive macroglossia after posterior fossa surgery in the prone position. *J Neurosurg Anesthesiol.* 1998;10(1):34-36.
114. Kotil K et al. Postoperative massive macroglossia in Klippel-Feil syndrome after posterior occipitocervical fixation surgery in the sitting position. *J Spinal Disord Tech.* 2006;19(3):226-229.
115. Sinha A et al. Oropharyngeal swelling and macroglossia after cervical spine surgery in the prone position. *J Neurosurg Anesthesiol.* 2001;13(3):237-239.
116. Heijke SA et al. The effect of the Trendelenburg position on lower esophageal sphincter tone. *Anaesthesia.* 1991;46:185-187.
117. Jeske HC et al. The influence of postural changes on gastroesophageal reflux and barrier pressure in nonfasting individuals. *Anesth Analg.* 2005;101(2):597-600.
118. Lee T-C et al. Effect of patient position and hypotensive anesthesia on inferior vena caval pressure. *Spine.* 1998;23:941-947.
119. Park CK. The effect of patient positioning on intraabdominal pressure and blood loss in spinal surgery. *Anesth Analg.* 2000;91:552-557.
120. Chaynes P et al. Microsurgical anatomy of the internal vertebral venous plexuses. *Surg Radiol Anat.* 1998;20:47-51.
121. Roth S et al. Eye injuries after nonocular surgery. *Anesthesiology.* 1996;85:1020-1027.
122. Al Hakim M, Katirji MB. Femoral mononeuropathy induced by the lithotomy position: a report of 5 cases with a review of the literature. *Muscle Nerve.* 1993;16:891-895.
123. Hsieh L-F et al. Bilateral femoral neuropathy after vaginal hysterectomy. *Arch Phys Med Rehabil.* 1998;79(8):1018-1021.
124. Matin S, Novick A. Renal dysfunction associated with staged bilateral partial nephrectomy: the importance of operative positioning. *J Urol.* 2001;165:880-881.
125. Della Valle A et al. Inflatable pillows as axillary support devices during surgery performed in the lateral decubitus position during epidural anesthesia. *Anesth Analg.* 2001;93:1338-1343.
126. Tuncali BE et al. Radial nerve injury after general anaesthesia in the lateral decubitus position. *Anaesthesia.* 2005;60(6):602-604.
127. Mathes D et al. Rhabdomyolysis and myonecrosis in a patient in the lateral decubitus position. *Anesthesiology.* 1996;84(3):727-729.
128. Irvine J et al. Rhabdomyolysis following laparoscopic radical nephrectomy: a case to heighten awareness. *Nephrology (Carlton).* 2006;11(4):282-284.
129. D'Alessio JG et al. Activation of the Bezold-Jarisch reflex in the sitting position for shoulder arthroscopy using interscalene block. *Anesth Analg.* 1995;80:1158-1162.
130. Hernandez-Palazon J et al. Anesthetic technique and development of pneumocephalus after posterior fossa surgery in the sitting position. *Neurocirugia.* 2003;14:216-221.
131. Satapathy GC, Dash HH. Tension pneumocephalus after neurosurgery in the supine position. *Br J Anaesth.* 2000;84:115-117.
132. Prabhakar H et al. Tension pneumocephalus after craniotomy in supine position. *J Neurosurg Anesthesiol.* 2003;1:278-281.
133. Suri A et al. Posterior fossa tension pneumocephalus. *Childs Nerv Syst.* 2000;16:196-199.
134. Wilcox S, Vandam LD. Alas, poor Trendelenburg and his position! A critique of its uses and effectiveness. *Anesth Analg.* 1988;67(6):574-578.
135. Phong SV, Koh LK. Anaesthesia for robotic-assisted radical prostatectomy: considerations for laparoscopy in the Trendelenburg position. *Anaesth Intensive Care.* 2007;35(2):281-285.
136. Johnston RV et al. Lower extremity neuropathy after laparoscopic cholecystectomy. *Anesthesiology.* 1992;77:835.
137. Yokoyama M et al. Haemodynamic effects of the lateral decubitus position and the kidney rest lateral decubitus position during anaesthesia. *Br J Anaesth.* 2000;84(6):753-757.
138. Fahy BG et al. Transesophageal echocardiographic detection of gas embolism and cardiac valvular dysfunction during laparoscopic nephrectomy. *Anesth Analg.* 1999;88:500-504.
139. Toyota S, Amaki Y. Hemodynamic evaluation of the prone position by transesophageal echocardiography. *J Clin Anesth.* 1998;10(1):32-35.
140. Sudheer PS et al. Haemodynamic effects of the prone position: a comparison of propofol total intravenous and inhalation anaesthesia. *Anaesthesia.* 2006;61(2):138-141.
141. Dharmavaram S et al. Effect of prone positioning systems on hemodynamic and cardiac function during lumbar spine surgery: an echocardiographic study. *Spine.* 2006;31(12):1388-1393.
142. Halliwill JR et al. Effect of various lithotomy positions on lower-extremity blood pressure. *Anesthesiology.* 1998;89(6):1373-1376.
143. Buhre W et al. Effects of the sitting position on the distribution of blood volume in patients undergoing neurosurgical procedures. *Br J Anaesth.* 2000;84:354-357.

144. Bivins HG et al. Blood volume distribution in the Trendelenburg position. *Ann Emerg Med.* 1985;14(7):641-643.

145. Hofer CK et al. Changes in intrathoracic blood volume associated with pneumoperitoneum and positioning. *Acta Anaesthesiol Scand.* 2002;46: 303-308.

146. Reuter DA et al. Trendelenburg positioning after cardiac surgery: effects on intrathoracic blood volume index and cardiac performance. *Eur J Anaesthesiol.* 2003;20(1):17-20.

147. Sibbald WJ et al. The Trendelenburg position: hemodynamic effects in hypotensive and normotensive patients. *Crit Care Med.* 1979;7(5):218-224.

148. Sing RF et al. Trendelenburg position and oxygen transport in hypovolemic adults. *Ann Emerg Med.* 1994;23:564-567.

149. Hirvonen EA et al. Hemodynamic changes due to Trendelenburg positioning and pneumoperitoneum during laparoscopic hysterectomy. *Acta Anaesthesiol Scand.* 1995;39(7):949-955.

150. Barnas GM et al. Effect of posture on lung and regional chest wall mechanics. *Anesthesiology.* 1993;78(2):251-259.

151. Prisk GK et al. Pulmonary perfusion in the prone and supine postures in the normal human lung. *J Appl Physiol.* 2007;103(3):883-894.

152. Mure M, Lindahl SGE. Prone position improves gas exchange—but how? *Acta Anaesthesiol Scand.* 2001;45:150-159.

153. Mure M et al. Regional ventilation-perfusion is more uniform in the prone position. *J Appl Physiol.* 2000;88:1076-1083.

154. Dunn PF. Physiology of the lateral decubitus position and one-lung ventilation. *Int Anesthesiol Clin.* 2000;38(1):25-53.

155. Pelosi P et al. Prone positioning improves pulmonary function in obese patients during general anesthesia. *Anesth Analg.* 1996;83:578-583.

156. Reber A et al. Lung aeration and pulmonary gas exchange during lumbar epidural anaesthesia and in the lithotomy position in elderly patients. *Anaesthesia.* 1998;53(9):854-861.

157. Krayer S et al. Position and motion of the human diaphragm during anesthesia-paralysis. *Anesthesiology.* 1989;70:891-898.

158. Lumb AB, Nunn JF. Respiratory function and ribcage contribution to ventilation in body positions commonly used during anesthesia. *Anesth Analg.* 1991;73:422-426.

159. Palmon SC et al. The effect of the prone position on pulmonary mechanics is frame-dependent. *Anesth Analg.* 1998;87:1175-1180.

160. Choi SJ et al. The effects of the exaggerated lithotomy position for radical perineal prostatectomy on respiratory mechanics. *Anaesthesia.* 2006; 61(5):439-443.

161. Pelosi P et al. The prone positioning during general anesthesia minimally affects respiratory mechanics while improving functional residual capacity and increasing oxygen tension. *Anesth Analg.* 1995;80:955-960.

162. Kim JH et al. Tracheal shortening during laparoscopic gynecologic surgery. *Acta Anaesthesiol Scand.* 2007;51(2):235-238.

CHAPTER 23

AIRWAY MANAGEMENT

Anthony Chipas, Wayne E. Ellis

Nurse anesthetists are responsible for managing the airway in a wide variety of settings. The best preparation for managing the difficult airway is being excellent at the management of routine airways. Patients are not harmed from inadequate intubation but rather inadequate ventilation. *Difficult ventilation* has been defined as the inability of a trained anesthetist to maintain the oxygen saturation at greater than 90% using a face mask for ventilation and 100% inspired oxygen, provided that the pre-ventilation oxygen saturation level was within normal range.[1] It is imperative that anesthesia providers perfect their technique by obtaining the requisite knowledge and management skills associated with routine and alternative airway management procedures. Techniques range from simple mask management to advanced skills such as fiberoptic intubation and cricothyrotomy.

Outcomes related to airway management have focused on injury to the airway and management of the difficult airway. In a review of 266 closed claims related to airway injury, 87 involved the larynx, with the most common lesions being vocal cord paralysis, granulomas, arytenoid dislocation, and hematomas. Of laryngeal injuries, 80% were associated with a routine (not "difficult") tracheal intubation, and only 17 were associated with a difficult intubation. Airway injuries placed fourth (6%) behind three other major types of outcomes: death (32%), spinal cord or peripheral nerve damage (16%), and brain damage (12%). Outcomes related to difficult airway claims included death (46%), brain damage (11%), airway injury (34%), and aspiration (7%).[2] The Difficult Airway Algorithm, introduced in 1992, established a structure for the management of expected and unexpected difficult airways.[3] These practice guidelines have improved the assessment and management of potentially difficult airways. Recent advances in equipment, technology, and monitoring have significantly improved airway management options and outcomes. This chapter describes the anatomy and physiology, patient assessment, anesthetic considerations, and techniques related to airway management.

ANATOMY AND PHYSIOLOGY OF THE AIRWAY

The airway is divided into two sections: upper and lower. Various anatomists divide the upper from the lower airway at the cricoid cartilage. The upper airway includes the nose, mouth, pharynx, hypopharynx, and larynx. The lower airway consists of the trachea, bronchi, bronchioles, terminal bronchioles, respiratory bronchioles, and alveoli. This section reviews primary structures, innervation, blood supply, and normal and abnormal function of the upper airway structures.

Developmental Anatomy
Upper Respiratory Tract
Unlike the structures of the lower respiratory tract, the upper respiratory tract arises from bony structures of the head. Endochondral bone is preformed in cartilage. The bones form initially from the optic, olfactory, and otic capsules. These merge with the midline cartilaginous structures to form the embryologic vestiges of the ethmoid, sphenoid, the petrous portion of the temporal bone, and the base of the occipital bone. Direct ossification of membranous tissue known as the *mesenchyme* occurs during early embryologic development to form membranous bone. The membranous bones include the temporal, parietal, frontal, and portions of the occipital bones and the pharyngeal arches. The pharyngeal arches are complex structures also known as the *branchial arches* that extend anterior to posterior. Development of these structures begins at day 22 (week 4 following fertilization).[4]

Embryologically, there are six arches that develop from five structures. Arches one through four and six go on to develop the airway structures, and the fifth arch disappears with fetal development. The arches all contain a covering of tissue that will eventually become the nerves, muscles, and cartilage of the airway. These will become the tissues of the oropharynx, middle ear, the hyoid bone, and the laryngeal cartilages. Arch one becomes the jaws; arch two becomes the facial structures and the ears; arch three becomes the hyoid bone and structures of the upper pharynx; arches four and six become the structures of the larynx and the lower pharynx; and arch five disappears. The tongue is formed from the mesoderm of multiple arches. The anterior two thirds of the tongue is developed from the first arch. The mesoderm of the third and fourth arches comprises the posterior third of the tongue. There are identified spaces between the arches that are known externally as *clefts* and internally as *pouches*. The cleft between the first two arches becomes the external auditory meatus. The internal pouch between the first and second arches forms the majority of the tympanic cavity and the eustachian tubes. The other clefts disappear as the fetus develops. The pouches contribute to the development of the glandular structures of the head and neck. The palatine tonsils arise from pouch two; the inferior parathyroid glands and the thymus come from pouch three; the superior parathyroid glands arise from pouch four, and the ultimobranchial structures arise from the inferior portion of pouch four.[4]

Nose. The nose and mouth are the external openings to the respiratory tree. The large surface area of the nasal mucosa warms and humidifies inspired air but also provides almost two thirds of the resistance to breathing. The nose is the primary passage by which air enters the lungs. Because of the surface area over the turbinates and the sinuses, the nasal passages are well suited for the task of humidification of air and primary filtration. As air passes through the nose, it meets the turbinates, which cause directional changes in the airflow. Branches of three arteries—the maxillary (sphenopalatine), ophthalmic, and facial (septal)—provide a rich supply of blood to the nasal mucosa. The innervation of the nose is from the nasopalatine and ethmoidal branches of the facial nerve. These nerves also supply the nasopharynx, nasal septum, and palate. Sensory-nerve supply to the nasal mucosa is from the ophthalmic and maxillary divisions of the trigeminal nerve. Parasympathetic innervation arises from the seventh cranial nerve and pterygopalatine ganglion. Sympathetic innervation is derived from the superior cervical ganglion. Sympathetic stimulation results in vasoconstriction and shrinkage of the nasal tissue. Depression of the sympathetic nervous system, as occurs with general anesthesia, may cause engorgement of the nasal tissues, increasing the likelihood of bleeding with manipulation from nasal airways or endotracheal tubes.

Mouth. The oral cavity is separated from the nasal passages by the hard and soft palates. The hard palate is stationary and remains positionally unchanged. The soft palate covers the posterior third to half of the oral cavity. The palate rises during eating to prevent food and liquids from passing from the mouth into the nose and thereby decreases the chance of aspiration. With age, obesity, and other conditions, this structure may stretch and become more movable. When an individual is asleep or paralyzed, as with general anesthesia, this structure can fall back against the nasal passages, blocking air movement and causing symptoms of sleep apnea. The tongue is a large muscular organ that fills most of the oral cavity and is involved in the tasting and ingestion of food. It relaxes when the individual is either asleep or paralyzed, which increases the potential for airway obstruction. The passage from the oral cavity into the oropharynx is "guarded" by the uvula. This pendulous piece of tissue extends from the posterior edge of the middle of the soft palate into the oral cavity. If swollen, enlarged, or injured, it can be a cause of airway obstruction. The tonsils are walnut-shaped structures that sit on both sides of the posterior opening of the oral cavity. They are partially buried in the soft tissue at the base of the tongue and are protected by the anterior and posterior tonsillar pillars.

Pharynx. The pharynx is divided into three compartments—the nasopharynx, oropharynx, and hypopharynx (laryngopharynx)—and extends from the base of the skull to the level of the cricoid cartilage. The nasopharynx lies anterior to C1 and is bound superiorly by the base of the skull and inferiorly by the soft palate. The openings to the auditory (eustachian) tubes and the adenoids are found in the nasopharynx. Sensory innervation of the mucosa is derived from the maxillary nerve. The oropharynx lies at the C2 to C3 level and is bound superiorly by the soft palate and inferiorly by the epiglottis. It opens into the mouth anteriorly through the anterior and posterior tonsillar pillars. The hypopharynx lies posterior to the larynx and is bound by the superior border of the epiglottis and the inferior border of the cricoid cartilage at the C5 to C6 level. The upper esophageal sphincter lies at the lower edge of the hypopharynx and arises from the cricopharyngeus muscle. This muscle acts as a barrier to regurgitation in the conscious patient.

Numerous nerves supply motor and sensory fibers to the airway. The glossopharyngeal, vagus, and spinal accessory

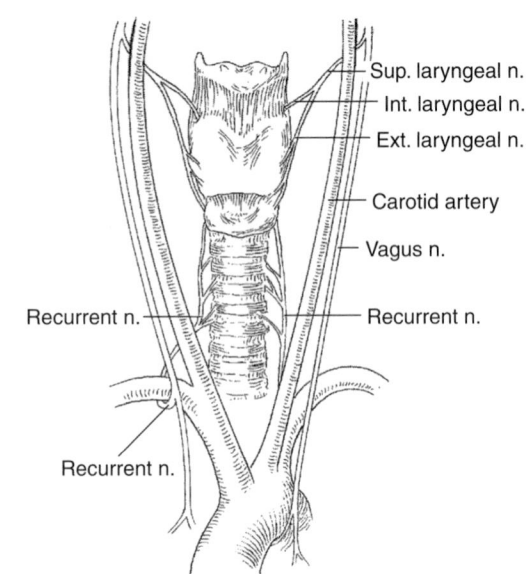

FIGURE **23-1** Anatomy of the superior laryngeal and recurrent laryngeal nerves. *n.*, Nerve.

nerves share nuclei in the medulla and innervate all the muscles of the pharynx, larynx, and soft palate. Afferent (sensory) stimuli elicited when the posterior wall of the pharynx is touched are carried by the glossopharyngeal nerve to the medulla, where they synapse with nuclei of the vagus nerve and the cranial portion of the spinal accessory nerve. The efferent response returns primarily through the vagus nerve, resulting in the gag reflex as the muscles of the pharynx elevate and constrict.

Two branches of the vagus nerve innervate the hypopharynx: the superior laryngeal nerve and the recurrent laryngeal nerve (RLN) (Figure 23-1). The superior laryngeal nerve divides into the internal and external branches. The internal branch of the superior laryngeal nerve provides sensory input to the hypopharynx above the vocal folds (cords). The external branch provides motor function to the cricothyroid muscle of the larynx.

The RLN provides sensory innervation to the subglottic area and the trachea. The recurrent layngeal nerve is so named because it recurs (loops around) another structure. The right recurrent laryngeal nerve recurs around the brachiocephalic (innominate) artery, and the left recurrent laryngeal nerve loops around the aorta. Traction on either of these structures during thoracic surgery can cause injury to the RLN, causing hoarseness or stridor. The motor component of the RLN provides motor function to all the muscles of the larynx except the cricothyroid muscle.

The superior laryngeal nerve and the RLN may be damaged by surgery, neoplasms, and neck trauma. Dissecting aortic arch aneurysms and mitral stenosis place traction on the RLN, causing hoarseness. Unilateral injury to the RLN usually results in hoarseness but does not compromise respiratory status. The vocal cords compensate by shifting the midline toward the uninjured side. In the acute phase of bilateral injury to the RLN, unopposed tension and adduction of the vocal cords result in stridor, which may deteriorate into severe respiratory distress and possibly death. Patients with chronic injury develop compensatory mechanisms that allow for normal respiration and gruff or husky speech. Injury to the superior laryngeal nerve does not usually cause respiratory distress.

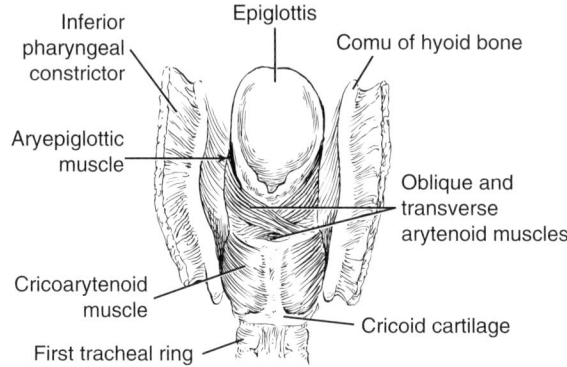

FIGURE **23-2** Larynx.

TABLE **23-1**	Intrinsic Muscles of the Larynx
Muscle	**Action**
Posterior cricoarytenoid	Separates the vocal cords (abducts) and opens the glottis
Lateral cricoarytenoid	Closes the glottis (adducts)
Arytenoids	Closes the glottis, especially posterior
Cricothyroid	Produces tension and elongates the vocal cords
Thyroarytenoid	Shortens and relaxes the vocal cords

TABLE **23-2**	Extrinsic Muscles of the Larynx
Muscle	**Action**
Sternohyoid	Draws hyoid bone inferiorly
Sternothyroid	Draws thyroid cartilage caudad
Thyrohyoid	Pulls hyoid bone inferiorly
Omohyoid	Pulls hyoid bone caudad

Larynx. The larynx begins with the epiglottis and extends to the cricoid cartilage. It is composed of three single cartilages, three paired cartilages, and intrinsic and extrinsic muscles connected by ligaments and membranes (Figure 23-2). These structures function intricately together to protect the airway from aspiration, provide airflow between the hypopharynx and trachea, provide cough and gag reflexes, and produce phonation. The larynx begins between the third and fourth cervical vertebrae and ends (in the adult) at the cricothyroid muscle at the level of the sixth cervical vertebra. The anterior and lateral larynx is formed by the thyroid cartilage. This cartilage fuses anteriorly and is identified by the thyroid notch. Posteriorly, the thyroid cartilage rises toward the hyoid bone at the base of the tongue as the posterior horns, or cornu. The thyroid cartilage is connected to the hyoid bone by the thyrohyoid fascia and muscle. The posterior border of the larynx is formed by the posterior portion of the cricoid cartilage. Internal to the larynx are the articulating cartilages, the arytenoids, and the epiglottis. The epiglottis is a single cartilage that is leaflike in shape. It sits above the glottic opening and closes during swallowing. The space between the epiglottis and the base of the tongue is known as the *superior vallecula*. Applying upward force on this area results in "lifting" or pulling of the epiglottis away from the glottic opening. This tissue is very delicate in the infant and child, and pressures exerted to lift the epiglottis can result in damage to the tissues of the vallecula, bleeding, edema, and airway obstruction. The inferior vallecula is between the inferior edge of the epiglottis and the true vocal cords.

The intrinsic muscles of the larynx control the tension of the vocal cords and the opening and closing of the glottis (Table 23-1). The extrinsic muscles connect the larynx with the hyoid bone and other neighboring structures (Table 23-2). Their primary function is to adjust the position of the trachea and other structures during phonation, breathing, and swallowing.

Branching from the external carotid, the superior thyroid artery gives rise to the superior laryngeal artery. This artery supplies the supraglottic region of the larynx. The infraglottic region is supplied by the inferior laryngeal artery, a terminal branch of the inferior thyroid artery.

Lower Respiratory Tract

As the fetus develops, the respiratory system evolves in complex developmental interactions between the endodermal-derived epithelium and the mesoderm. Both contribute to lung development. The lungs and airways develop through a process of five stages.

These include the embryonic, pseudoglandular, canalicular, terminal sac phases, and maturation.[5]

During the embryonic phase, the endodermal respiratory diverticulum (laryngotracheal groove) develops. This occurs during the fourth through the seventh week. The laryngotracheal groove develops from the ventral surface of the foregut. During this period, fibroblast growth factor (FGF-10) causes stimulation and proliferation of cells that will eventually express fibroblast homologous factor (FHF). As the laryngotracheal groove grows and develops, it becomes the primitive lung bud. By day 28, it has grown caudally to the splanchnic mesoderm. It divides into the right and left bronchial buds. This then progresses through the development and expression of the epithelial lining of the lower respiratory system. Cartilage, muscle, and connective tissue arise from the same tissues that form the smooth muscle of the blood vessels. The bronchopulmonary segments appear by the 42nd day.

During the pseudoglandular stage, there is rapid growth and proliferation of the peripheral airways. This occurs during the 6th through the 16th week. Repeated branching of the distal ends of the epithelial tubes results in 16 or more generations of the bronchial tubes and the development of the terminal bronchioles. The airways are filled with liquid at this time. The cellular structure is more characterized by tall columnar epithelium.

The next phase of development is known as the *canalicular stage*. This occurs most frequently during the 16th and the 26th week. At this time, the airways widen and lengthen. The proliferation of this space will eventually become the large volume of air space in the expanded lung after birth. Terminal and respiratory bronchioles and terminal saccules develop. Cuboidal cells of the terminal sacs differentiate into alveolar type-II cells. Secretion of surfactant begins at this time. Type II alveolar cells that are adjacent to a vessel flatten and differentiate into

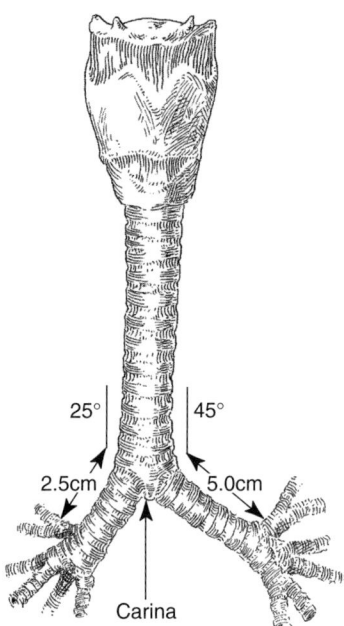

FIGURE **23-3**   Trachea.

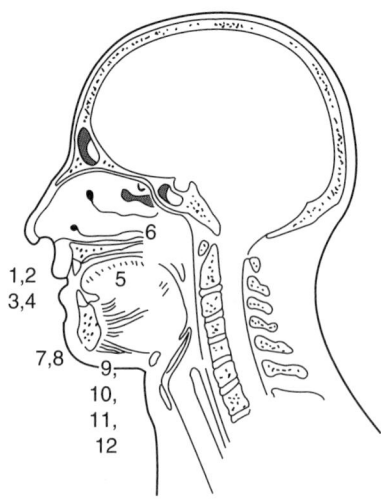

FIGURE **23-4**   Airway assessment—12 identification points.

type I cells. As the type II and type I cells develop, vascularization appears. The vascularization is associated with the development of the respiratory bronchioles and the alveoli necessary for air exchange following birth. Along with other growth factors, vascular endothelial growth factor (VEGF) participates in the formation of blood vessels that will surround the alveoli. At the end of this phase, air exchange is possible although inefficient.

The terminal sac phase occurs during the 24th through the 36th week. Branching of the respiratory bud continues, and further development of the terminal buds is expressed as primitive alveoli. Capillaries begin to develop and proliferate around the terminal buds and proliferate at the same time as the primitive alveoli develop. Cells further differentiate throughout this period, and by the 26th week, a primitive blood-gas barrier has developed.

By the 36th week, mature alveoli are seen. This requires FGF and platelet-derived growth factor (PDGF). Development of alveoli will continue for approximately 3 years after birth. A change in the relative relationship of parenchyma to total lung volume contributes to lung growth until the second year of life. From the third year of life until adulthood, lung growth continues.[5]

Trachea. The trachea originates at the inferior border of the cricoid cartilage and extends to the carina (Figure 23-3). It is approximately 10 to 20 cm long in adults. The cricoid cartilage is the only cartilage of the trachea that is a complete ring. The remainder of the trachea is composed of 16 to 20 C-shaped cartilaginous rings. The posterior side of the trachea lacks cartilage, thereby accommodating the esophagus during the act of swallowing. The cartilaginous rings and plates continue until the bronchi reach 0.6 to 0.8 mm in size. At this point the cartilage disappears, and the bronchi are termed *bronchioles*. The function of the bronchi is to provide humidification and warming of inspired air as it passes to the alveoli.

The angle of bifurcation of the right mainstem bronchus is approximately 25 to 30 degrees. The bifurcation to the right

upper lobe is approximately 2.5 cm from the carina. The angle of the left mainstem bronchus is 45 degrees. The left mainstem bronchus is approximately 5 cm long before it bifurcates into the left superior and inferior lobe bronchi.

The tracheobronchial trees receive sympathetic innervation from the first through fifth thoracic ganglia. Parasympathetic innervation is derived from branches of the vagus nerve. The carina is richly innervated, making it sensitive to sensory stimulation.

Diaphragm

The diaphragm arises from four structures: (1) septum transversum, (2) dorsal esophageal mesentery, (3) the pleuroperitoneal folds, and (4) the body-wall mesoderm. The diaphragm develops in the cephalic region and descends into the position between the abdominal and pleural cavity contents as the embryo develops. The nerve supply for the diaphragm arises from the cords of the third, fourth, and fifth cervical nerves and travels with the descending diaphragmatic structure as the phrenic nerve. Owing to this process of descent, the phrenic nerves lie within the pericardium as the fetus matures and after birth. Because of the development of the diaphragm in the cephalic position and the merging of four structures, drugs that impair fetal development can result in many potential congenital deformities, including diaphragmatic hernia.[5]

AIRWAY ASSESSMENT

The best way to prevent anesthesia disasters, especially with airway management, is to be prepared, informed, and vigilant. A thorough and systematic airway assessment and physical examination should be performed in the preoperative period. "Examination of the airway to predict difficulties with face mask ventilation and intubation is an essential component of the preoperative assessment of patients who are scheduled for surgery."[6] This statement agrees with Standards I and III of the Standards of the American Association of Nurse Anesthetists. Standard I states that the practitioner shall "perform a thorough and complete preanesthesia assessment," allowing the practitioner to "formulate a patient-specific plan for anesthesia care" (Standard III). This assessment (Figure 23-4) includes a 12-point evaluation of the airway and surrounding tissues, including multiple patient physical characteristics to identify potential airway

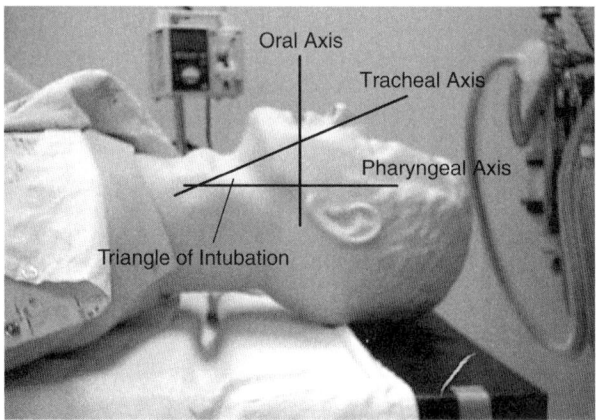

FIGURE **23-5** Triangle of intubation—flat.

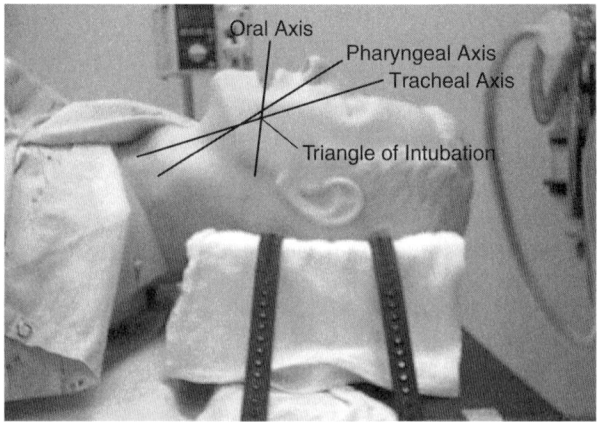

FIGURE **23-6** Triangle of intubation—sniffing.

problems that might help identify a difficult airway. Known physical characteristics associated with difficult intubation include obesity, head and neck movement, jaw movement, receding mandible, buck teeth, Mallampati scores, maxillary incisor characteristics, male sex, age 40 to 59, decreased mouth opening, short thyromental distance, and short neck.[7] Evaluation of the airway requires the practitioner to use the senses of sight, hearing, touch, and (unfortunately sometimes) smell. Proper assessment of the airway can facilitate proper positioning of the head into the sniffing position and make the "triangle of intubation" smaller, allowing for successful intubation (Figures 23-5 and 23-6).

Criteria that can be assessed (Table 23-3) to identify potentially difficult airways include interincisor distance (width of mouth), thyromental distance (length of jaw), head and neck extension, Mallampati classification (tongue to oropharyngeal ratio), body weight, and a history of difficult airway. Evaluation of the length of the upper incisors, visibility of the uvula, shape of the palate, compliance of the mandibular space, and length and thickness of the neck provide further assessment.[3] The most prominent factors predictive of a difficult airway are obesity, decreased head and neck movement, decreased jaw movement, receding mandible, and buck teeth.[7] In determining the probability of a difficult airway, no ideal method exists that is highly

sensitive and specific with minimal false-positive or false-negative reports.[8-11] In an attempt to standardize the physical examination, it is recommended that all tests be completed with the patient in the sitting position with the head in full extension, mouth opened wide, tongue extruded, and phonation elicited. The history should focus on prior airway management problems, acute or chronic diseases, and syndromes associated with difficult airways (Table 23-4).

During the airway physical examination, findings that may indicate a difficult airway are integrated into the proposed airway management. Normally the interincisor distance should be at least 4 cm; less than 3 cm indicates a potential problem. If the mouth is narrow, it may be difficult to get the 2-cm flange of the laryngoscope blade and the endotracheal tube (ETT) into the mouth while maintaining good visualization of the cords. The thyromental distance is measured from the thyroid notch to the inner border of the mandible when the patient's head is extended. A thyromental distance less than 6 cm or three ordinary fingerbreadths is associated with a higher incidence of difficult intubation. The full range of flexion-extension of the neck varies from 90 to 165 degrees, decreasing approximately 20% between ages 16 and 75 years. The atlantooccipital joint is capable of extending up to 35 degrees and provides the highest degree of mobility in the neck. When extension is reduced to 23 degrees, visualization may become difficult.[12] Patients should be able to touch the tip of the chin to the chest.

The Mallampati classification is an indirect method of relating the size of the base of the tongue to the oral cavity (Table 23-5, Figure 23-7). It is based on the theory that the tongue is the single largest obstacle to directly visualizing the glottis.[13] The incidence of grades III and IV laryngoscopic views varies throughout the literature. Variability in observation, years of experience, and definitions of airway categories result in differences in reporting statistics. Approximately 15% to 18% of patients have a grade III view, requiring multiple intubation attempts. Approximately 1% to 4% have a grade IV view, and approximately 0.0001% to 0.02% fit into the "cannot intubate, cannot ventilate" category.[14] Difficult direct laryngoscopy occurs in 1.5% to 8.5% of general anesthetic procedures, and difficult intubation occurs with a similar incidence. Failed intubation occurs in 0.13% to 0.3% of general anesthetic procedures.[15]

An alternative method of airway assessment termed the *Lemon method* uses five categories for assessment and can be stratified to determine difficulty of intubation (Table 23-6). In a study performed by Reed and colleagues, they found that the higher the Lemon assessment score, the greater the chance of a difficult airway. The Lemon method did not, however, predict all difficult intubations, even at lower scores.[16]

By applying an assessment scale, Reed and colleagues quantified the possibility of a difficult airway[16] (Table 23-7). Like the Lemon method, it did not identify all difficult airways but seemed to provide practitioners additional information to allow them time to prepare. The scale ranges from 0 to 9 points, with higher scores equating to the possibility of more difficult airways.

TRACHEAL INTUBATION

The mainstay of traditional airway management is tracheal intubation. For the administration of anesthesia and for emergency airway conditions, intubation of the trachea can be performed by means of a variety of techniques and equipment. Competency with various intubation techniques and equipment is primarily related to the skill and expertise of the provider. The challenge of a can't intubate/can't ventilate situation can arise, requiring the

TABLE 23-3	Airway Assessment		
Assessment Item	**Acceptable End-Point**	**Implication**	**Airway Axis**
Length of upper incisor	Qualitative/short incisors	Long incisors → blade enters mouth in a cephalad direction	Oral
Maxillary teeth anterior to mandibular teeth	No overriding of maxillary teeth (overbite)	Overriding → blade enters mouth in a cephalad direction	Oral
Protrusion of mandibular teeth anterior to maxillary teeth	Anterior protrusion of mandibular teeth relative to maxillary (underbite)	Test TMJ; limits adequate mouth opening	Oral
Intercisor distance	> 3 cm	2-cm flange on blade can insert between teeth	Oral
Oropharyngeal class (see Table 23-5)	= Class II	Tongue small in relation to size of oropharyngeal cavity	Oral
Narrowness of palate	Should not appear narrow or highly arched	Narrow palate decreases oropharyngeal volume (↓ room blade & ETT)	Pharyngeal
Mandibular space length (thyromental)—head in a neutral position	= 5 cm or 3 ordinary fingerbreadths	Larynx relative posterior to other upper airway structures	Pharyngeal
Mandibular space compliance	Qualitative palpation normal softness	Scope retracts tongue; if mandibular space not compliant, tongue obstructs	Pharyngeal
Length of neck	Qualitative index not available	Short neck decreases ability to align upper airway axes	Pharyngeal/tracheal
Thickness of neck	40 cm neck = 5% chance difficult airway ↑1.3% per 1 cm ↑ neck size 60 cm neck = 35%	Thick neck decreases ability to align upper airway axes	Pharyngeal/tracheal
Range of motion (head and neck)	Neck flexed on chest 35 degrees + head extension on neck 80 degrees = sniffing position	Sniffing position aligns oral, pharyngeal, and laryngeal axes to create favorable line of sight	Pharyngeal/tracheal
Identification of cricothyroid membrane	Proper identification and if necessary marking cricothyroid membrane	Finding insertion point for subglottic airway intervention prior to its being needed is lifesaving	Tracheal

TMJ, *Temporomandibular joint;* ETT, *endotracheal tube.*

prompt initiation of various airway management strategies. Tracheal intubation is recommended in the following situations: compromise or inaccessibility of the patient's airway; long surgical procedures; surgical procedures involving the head, neck, abdomen, or chest; need for controlled positive pressure ventilation; inability to maintain airway with a mask or airway device; disease process involving the airway; risk of aspiration from a full stomach; and pregnancy.

Proper positioning of the head is essential to facilitate success with mask ventilation and tracheal intubation. The use of the "sniffing position" requires the head to be flexed forward 35 degrees and extended 80 degrees. This position allows for better alignment of the oral, pharyngeal, and tracheal axis and promotes optimal conditions (see Figures 23-5 and 23-6). Techniques for routine laryngoscopy and intubation are detailed in basic anesthesia texts.

With the patient under general anesthesia, if the first attempt is unsuccessful, the patient should be evaluated for adequate muscle relaxation and repositioned. The type and length of the laryngoscope blade may need to be changed. Use of optimal external laryngeal pressure during laryngoscopy may improve the view of the vocal cords. This is accomplished by applying pressure in a posterior-cephalad direction sequentially over the thyroid, hyoid, and cricoid cartilages with the free hand during laryngoscopy. An assistant, when available, may help with the cricoid pressure. Subsequent intubation attempts should adhere to practice guidelines, with prompt consideration of waking up the patient.

Management of the Difficult Airway

The Difficult Airway Algorithm established in 1991 by the American Society of Anesthesiologists (ASA) gave anesthesia

TABLE 23-4	Acute and Chronic Diseases and Syndromes Associated with Difficult Airways
Category	**Diseases and Syndromes**
Congenital	Pierre Robin, Treacher Collins, Down, choanal atresia
Physical	Large, protruding teeth; thick neck; spinal malformations ("humpback," scoliosis); large tongue; micrognathia; maxillary overbite
Traumatic	Oral or airway burns, facial trauma, head and neck injuries, mandibular fracture, dislocation of the temporal mandibular joint
Chronic diseases	Rheumatoid or degenerative arthritis, diabetes mellitus, obesity, supraglottic tumors, acromegaly
Acute disorders	Peritonsillar or retropharyngeal abscess, epiglottitis, postoperative airway bleeding, Ludwig angina

TABLE 23-5	Mallampati Airway Classification	
Classification	**Description**	**Ease of Intubation**
1	Soft palate, fauces, uvula, and anterior and posterior tonsillar pillars seen	Easy
2	Same as 1, except tonsillar pillars hidden by tongue	Possibly difficult
3	Only base of uvula seen	Probably difficult
4	Even uvula not visualized	Very difficult

From Mallampati SR et al. Clinical signs to predict difficult tracheal intubation. Can Anaesth Soc J. 1985;32(4):429-434.

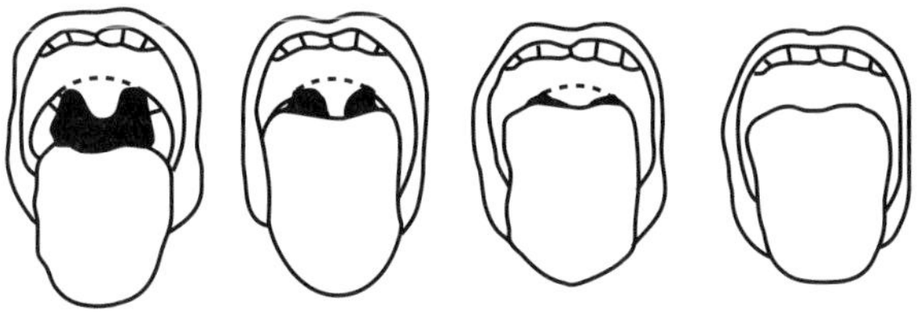

FIGURE 23-7 Modified Mallampati classification of pharyngeal structures. *Class I,* Soft palate, tonsillar fauces, tonsillar pillars, and uvula visualized. *Class II,* Soft palate, tonsillar fauces, and uvula visualized. *Class III,* Soft palate and base of uvula visualized. *Class IV,* Soft palate not visualized. (*From Samsoon GL, Young JR. Difficult tracheal intubation: a retrospective study. Anaesthesia. 1987;42:487-490.*)

TABLE 23-6	LEMON Law Airway Assessment
Criteria for Assessment	
Look Externally	Look at patient characteristics known to cause difficult laryngoscopy, intubation, and ventilation
Evaluate 3-3-2 (Head extended)	3 fingerbreadths between incisors, 3 fingerbreadths between tip of the chin and hyoid bone, and 2 fingerbreadths between hyoid bone and thyroid notch
Mallampati score	Hypopharynx should be visualized adequately; Mallampati class I or II
Obstruction	Any conditions that can cause obstruction? Listen to respiration; inspiratory wheeze signifies upper airway obstruction, expiratory wheeze signifies lower airway or thoracic obstruction
Neck mobility	Assess by having patient place chin on chest then extend head backward as far as possible; patients in hard collars have limited movement, therefore harder to intubate

Modified from Wilson ME et al. Predicting difficult intubation. Br J Anaesth. 1988;61:211-216.

TABLE 23-7	LEMON Airway Assessment Scores
Airway Assessment Score	**Points**
Number of positive unfavorable "look" criteria	0-4 points
Mouth opens less than 3 fingerbreadths	1 point
Hyomental distance less than 3 fingerbreadths	1 point
Thyrohyoid distance less than 2 fingerbreadths	1 point
Presence of an obstructed airway	1 point
Presence of poor neck mobility	1 point
Total maximum score = 9; minimum score = 0	

Modified from Wilson ME et al. Predicting difficult intubation. Br J Anaesth. 1988;61:211-216.

practitioners the first standardized approach to managing the anticipated or unanticipated difficult airway (Figure 23-8). The practice guidelines were updated in 2003 to reflect current management strategies.[4] The airway algorithm provides guidelines for dealing with difficult face mask ventilation, difficult laryngoscopy, difficult tracheal intubation, and failed intubation. Assessment of the airway and use of the Difficult Airway Algorithm provide the practitioner with four end-points: (1) intubation awake or asleep, (2) intubation emergent or nonemergent, (3) approach supraglottic or subglottic, and (4) airway access surgical or nonsurgical. Each of these end-points (Table 23-8) entails

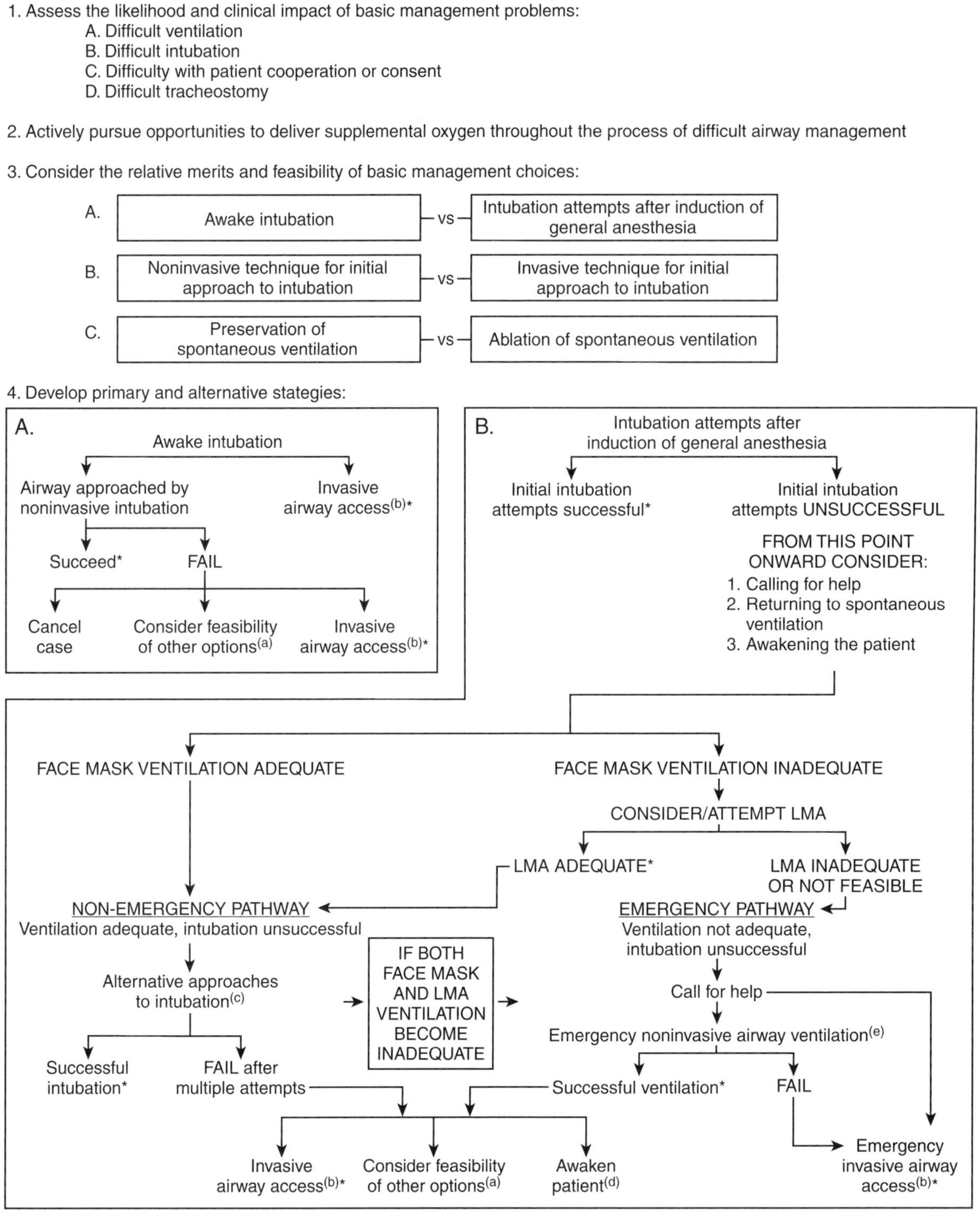

1. Assess the likelihood and clinical impact of basic management problems:
   A. Difficult ventilation
   B. Difficult intubation
   C. Difficulty with patient cooperation or consent
   D. Difficult tracheostomy

2. Actively pursue opportunities to deliver supplemental oxygen throughout the process of difficult airway management

3. Consider the relative merits and feasibility of basic management choices:

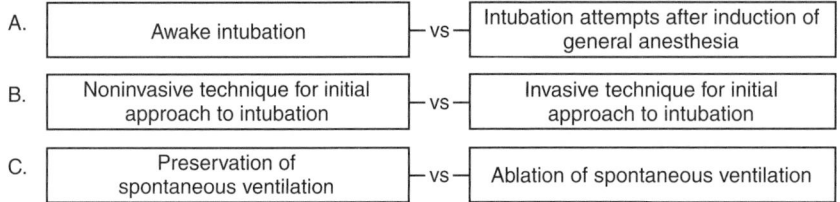

A. | Awake intubation | — vs — | Intubation attempts after induction of general anesthesia |

B. | Noninvasive technique for initial approach to intubation | — vs — | Invasive technique for initial approach to intubation |

C. | Preservation of spontaneous ventilation | — vs — | Ablation of spontaneous ventilation |

4. Develop primary and alternative stategies:

A.

Awake intubation

- Airway approached by noninvasive intubation
- Invasive airway access[(b)]*

Airway approached by noninvasive intubation →
- Succeed*
- FAIL

Succeed* →
- Cancel case

FAIL →
- Consider feasibility of other options[(a)]
- Invasive airway access[(b)]*

B.

Intubation attempts after induction of general anesthesia

- Initial intubation attempts successful*
- Initial intubation attempts UNSUCCESSFUL

FROM THIS POINT ONWARD CONSIDER:
1. Calling for help
2. Returning to spontaneous ventilation
3. Awakening the patient

FACE MASK VENTILATION ADEQUATE

FACE MASK VENTILATION INADEQUATE

CONSIDER/ATTEMPT LMA
- LMA ADEQUATE*
- LMA INADEQUATE OR NOT FEASIBLE

NON-EMERGENCY PATHWAY
Ventilation adequate, intubation unsuccessful

EMERGENCY PATHWAY
Ventilation not adequate, intubation unsuccessful

Alternative approaches to intubation[(c)]
- Successful intubation*
- FAIL after multiple attempts

IF BOTH FACE MASK AND LMA VENTILATION BECOME INADEQUATE

Call for help
Emergency noninvasive airway ventilation[(e)]
- Successful ventilation*
- FAIL

- Invasive airway access[(b)]*
- Consider feasibility of other options[(a)]
- Awaken patient[(d)]

Emergency invasive airway access[(b)]*

*Confirm ventilation, tracheal intubation, or LMA placement with exhaled CO_2

a. Other options include (but are not limited to) surgery utilizing face mask or LMA anesthesia, local anesthesia infiltration, or regional nerve blockade. Pursuit of these options usually implies that mask ventilation will not be problematic. Therefore, these options may be of limited value if this step in the algorithm has been reached via the Emergency Pathway.
b. Invasive airway access includes surgical or percutaneous tracheostomy or cricothyrotomy.
c. Alternative noninvasive approaches to difficult intubation include (but are not limited to) use of different laryngoscope blades, LMA as an intubation conduit (with or without fiberoptic guidance), fiberoptic intubation, intubating stylet or tube changer, light wand, retrograde intubation, and blind oral or nasal intubation.
d. Consider re-preparation of the patient for awake intubation or canceling surgery.
e. Options for emergency noninvasive airway ventilation include (but are not limited to) rigid bronchoscope, esophageal-tracheal Combitube ventilation, or transtracheal jet ventilation.

FIGURE **23-8** The American Society of Anesthesiologists (ASA) Difficult Airway Algorithm. (*From ASA Task Force on Management of the Difficult Airway. Practice guidelines for management of the difficult airway: an updated report. Anesthesiology. 2003;98:1269-1277.*)

TABLE **23-8**	Appropriate Airway Equipment for Techniques							
	Awake	**Asleep**	**Emergent**	**Nonemergent**	**Supraglottic**	**Subglottic**	**Surgical Airway**	**Nonsurgical Airway**
Airtrach	X*	X	X	X	X			X
Bronchoscope fiberoptic	X*	X		X	X			X
Bullard scope	X*	X		X	X			X
Cobra PLA	X*	X	X	X	X			X
Combitube	X*	X	X	X	X			X
Eschmann stylet	X*	X	X	X	X			X
Fastrach	X*	X	X	X	X			X
GlideScope	X*	X	X	X	X			X
KING LT/LTS-D	X*	X		X	X			X
ILA (Mercury)	X*	X	X	X	X			X
Laryngoscope	X*	X	X	X	X			X
Lighted stylet	X*	X	X	X	X			X
LMA, ProSeal, C-Trach	X*	X	X	X	X			X
Mask management	X	X	X	X	X			X
Shikani Optical Stylet	X*	X	X	X	X			X
SLIPA	X*	X	X	X	X			X
Upsher scope	X*	X	X	X	X			X
Retrograde wire	X	X					X	X
Cricothyrotomy	X	X	X			X	X	
Transtracheal jet	X	X	X			X	X	

SLIPA, Streamlined liner of the pharynx airway.
*Requires airway blocks.

specific airway equipment and techniques to facilitate ventilation. An organized plan should be initiated when a difficult airway is encountered. A *difficult airway* is defined as any intubation that takes a skilled anesthetist more than three attempts or greater than 10 minutes.[3] All departments have a dedicated difficult airway cart or box that must be readily available and well stocked (Box 23-1). This cart should be checked on a routine basis to ensure that all materials are available and all devices are working. Team members should know their responsibilities and be ready to react calmly.

Devices and techniques used for difficult intubation and ventilation may include different laryngoscope blades, a fiberoptic scope, light wand, Bullard scope, laryngeal mask airway (LMA), intubating stylet, retrograde intubation kit, Eschmann stylet, transtracheal jet ventilation (TTJV), and Combitube. A commercial kit is available for retrograde intubation, or the practitioner can choose to insert either a "J-wire" or #2 Mersiline suture via a cricothyrotomy and pass the device into the oropharynx. Adjunct airway equipment should be routinely used in nonemergent or practice situations to increase familiarity with the equipment and facilitate ease of use in emergent situations.

Failure to acknowledge that the patient cannot be intubated or ventilated and reluctance to accept the fact that the ETT is in the esophagus contribute to adverse outcomes. These include brain injury, death, cardiopulmonary arrest, unnecessary tracheotomy, airway trauma, and damage to teeth.[3] Continued attempts at intubation and exertion of unnecessary force can cause bleeding and edema of the mucous membranes. Ventilation can become progressively more difficult, leading to morbidity from hypoxemia and hypercarbia.

The patient with a potentially difficult airway should be optimally positioned. Pillows and blankets should be built up under the head and shoulders to afford the optimal "sniffing" position. This also provides more space for introduction of the laryngoscope blade into the mouth. Locating and marking the cricoid cartilage or cricothyroid ligament enables the assistant applying cricoid pressure to easily find the correct position and identify landmarks should a surgical airway be needed.

With the difficult airway, preoxygenation (actually denitrogenation) is an essential component to delay arterial desaturation during subsequent apnea. It increases the oxygen content and eliminates much of the nitrogen (79% of room air) from the functional residual capacity (FRC). Without preoxygenation (denitrogenation), the oxygen reserve in the FRC will last approximately 2.5 minutes in a can't ventilate/can't intubate situation. With good preoxygenation, the FRC has enough oxygen to last almost 12 minutes. Adequate preoxygenation should include having the patient breathe at normal tidal volumes for 3 to 5 minutes with a fresh gas flow of no less than 5 L and a tight mask fit. The respiratory bag should move with each inspiration/expiration, and there should be a good end-tidal CO_2 waveform.[13] This is easily accomplished by applying the face mask as soon as the patient arrives in the operating room, before the application of other monitors. If time is limited, "fast-track" preoxygenation, in which the patient takes four vital capacity breaths in 30 seconds, can be used before induction of anesthesia. This does not completely denitrogenate the blood but is useful in the emergent situation.[7]

Alternative anesthetic management options exist if a difficult airway is anticipated, including use of monitored anesthesia care

BOX 23-1

Components of a Difficult Airway Cart

Airways—oral and nasal—various sizes
  Tongue blades
  Flexible stylets
  Endotracheal tubes—cuffed and uncuffed—2.5, 3.0, 3.5, 4.0,
    4.5, 5.0, 5.5, 6.0, 7.0, 8.0 (two of each size)
  Miller laryngoscope blades—sizes 0, 1, 2, 3, 4
  Macintosh laryngoscope blades—sizes 2, 3, 4
  Laryngoscope handles—regular and stubby
  Extra laryngoscope batteries and bulbs
  Magill forceps
  Syringes—3, 5, 10, and 20 mL (three or four of each size)
  Angiocatheters—14, 16, 18, 20 gauge (three each)
  Xylocaine jelly 2%
  Surgilube
  Salem sump—16 and 18 French
  Suction catheters—10, 12, 14 French
  Nebulizer
  Atomizer
  Oxygen mask
  Nasal cannula
  Oxygen with 15 L/min regulator

Alternate airway devices
  Laryngeal mask airways—sizes 3, 4, 5
  Intubating laryngeal mask airway
  Combitube
  Lighted stylet (Trachlite) (two)
  Eschmann stylet
  Tube exchanger—small, medium, large
  Ventilating stylet
  Needle cricothyrotomy set
  Retrograde intubation set
  Melker percutaneous dilational cricothyrotomy set
Transtracheal jet ventilator
Ambu bag
Bullard or Upsher scope
Intubating bronchoscope
  Tongue clamp
  Light source
  Endoscopy mask
  Ovassapian intubating airway
Lidocaine—4% topical, 2% for injection

(MAC) and regional anesthesia. The selection of MAC or regional anesthesia does not obviate the need to plan for management of the difficult airway. Failure of the regional block or complications resulting from placement may require emergent intubation under less than desirable conditions. It is not recommended that regional anesthesia be used for conditions in which the patient is unwilling to cooperate, the surgery cannot be quickly terminated, or access to the airway is lost.

The essence of the ASA Difficult Airway Algorithm is this:
1. Plan ahead. Be ready for anything.
2. If you are suspicious of airway trouble, intubate awake.
3. If you get into trouble and can still ventilate the patient, wake him or her up.
4. When making intubation choices, do what you do BEST.[17]

Awake Intubation

Awake intubation is the cornerstone on which the Difficult Airway Algorithm is based. Awake intubation should be planned any time a difficult intubation is anticipated. In many situations, an oral or nasal intubation while the patient is awake is the preferred method of intubating the trachea. Examples of such situations include patients with anticipated difficult airway, unstable neck fractures, halo devices, small or limited oral openings, and intubation of awake patients in the critical care setting. With proper patient preparation and a sufficiently anesthetized airway, an awake intubation can be accomplished quickly and with minimal discomfort to the patient.

Patient Preparation

For maximum cooperation to be elicited from the patient, the procedure must be clearly explained and consent obtained. It is difficult if not impossible to proceed if the patient is uncooperative or unwilling to participate. Depending on the situation and the patient's condition, judicious use of anxiolytics and

narcotics may be considered. Administration of antisialagogues to dry secretions can also maximize the view of the laryngeal structures. The risk of aspiration must always be considered when the airway reflexes have been anesthetized. Initiation of aspiration prophylaxis protocols may be warranted.

The most widely used local anesthetic for anesthetizing the airway is lidocaine in various forms and concentrations. Cocaine 4%, benzocaine 20%, and tetracaine are also effective anesthetics. Peak serum lidocaine levels are highest 30 minutes after instillation. Use of lidocaine within the recommended dosage keeps serum lidocaine levels well within the acceptable range.[18,19] Vasoconstrictors are commonly used to decrease bleeding associated with nasal intubation. Cocaine 4% or solutions containing oxymetazoline 0.05% should be used before insertion of local anesthetic gels into the nares.

The nares and nasopharynx are easily anesthetized by insertion of 5 mL of lidocaine viscous down each naris. The solution "melts" and drips down the back of throat. The nares and oral pharynx may also be anesthetized by adding 2% lidocaine to either a hand-held nebulizer or a nebulizer attached to a face mask. As the patient breathes through the nose and mouth, small droplets of local anesthetic are deposited on the mucous membranes. This method also is effective for anesthetization of subglottic tissue.

Anesthetization of the mouth and oral pharynx helps decrease the gag reflex and coughing associated with awake intubations. Benzocaine spray is a topical anesthetic with a quick onset and short duration. Flavored sprays may increase salivation. A lidocaine lollipop can be made by coating the tip of a tongue blade with lidocaine ointment and then placing it on the back of the tongue to provide anesthesia to the oropharynx. Another method is to have the patient swish and gargle for 2 minutes with 2% lidocaine viscous.

Anesthetizing the vocal cords may be accomplished by instilling local anesthetic directly onto the cords or through transtracheal blocks. After the nares have been anesthetized, a nasal airway or ETT is passed and positioned in close approximation to the vocal cords. The patient is instructed to take a deep breath. On inspiration, 5 mL of 2% lidocaine is inserted down the lumen of the nasal airway. This causes the patient to cough, indicating that local anesthetic was deposited on the vocal cords. If a fiberoptic scope is to be used, local anesthetic may be administered through the injection port onto the vocal cords under direct visualization.

AIRWAY BLOCKS

Superior Laryngeal Nerve Block
The superior laryngeal nerve block is easily performed and provides a dense block of the supraglottic region. To perform the block, the practitioner locates the hyoid bone and displaces it toward the side that is being injected (Figure 23-9). This stabilizes the bone and eases identification of structures and injection of the local anesthetic. The inferior border of the cornu is palpated, and the needle is inserted perpendicular to the skin, approximately 0.25 inch caudad and 0.25 inch medially. This approximates the site at which the superior laryngeal nerve pierces the thyrohyoid membrane. Just below the subcutaneous tissue, the tip of the needle may be felt to "bounce" on the thyrohyoid membrane; 1 to 2 mL of local anesthetic is deposited above this membrane, then the membrane is "popped through," and 2 mL of local anesthetic is deposited just below the membrane. Aspiration is performed before injection of the local anesthetic. If air is obtained, the needle has been placed too deep and is in the pharynx. The tip of the needle is withdrawn and repositioned. The block is repeated on the other side.

Transtracheal Block
The transtracheal block is accomplished by injecting local anesthetic through the cricothyroid membrane (Figure 23-10). To administer the block, the practitioner attaches a 23-gauge needle or a 24-gauge angiocatheter to a syringe containing 5 mL of 2% lidocaine. While aspiration is constantly performed, the needle is advanced in a caudad direction through the cricothyroid membrane. When air bubbles up through the solution, the tip of the needle is in the tracheal lumen.

The patient usually coughs when this occurs. The patient is then instructed to take a deep breath. On inspiration, the local anesthetic is injected into the tracheal lumen. This causes the patient to cough, spraying the local anesthetic onto the vocal cords. Care must be taken to stabilize the needle so as not to tear the

tracheal mucosa when the patient coughs. Use of the softer angiocatheter may decrease trauma.

Glossopharyngeal Block
The lingual branch of the glossopharyngeal nerve supplies sensory innervation to the back of the tongue (Figure 23-11). To block the lingual branch, the practitioner has the patient open his or her mouth and displaces the tongue to the opposite side with a tongue blade; this forms a gutter. Where the gutter meets the base of the palatoglossal arch, a 26-gauge spinal needle is inserted approximately ¼ inch. If air is obtained on aspiration, the needle has been placed too deeply. If blood is obtained, the needle must be withdrawn and repositioned more medially. One to 2 mL of 2% lidocaine is injected, and the block is repeated on the other side.

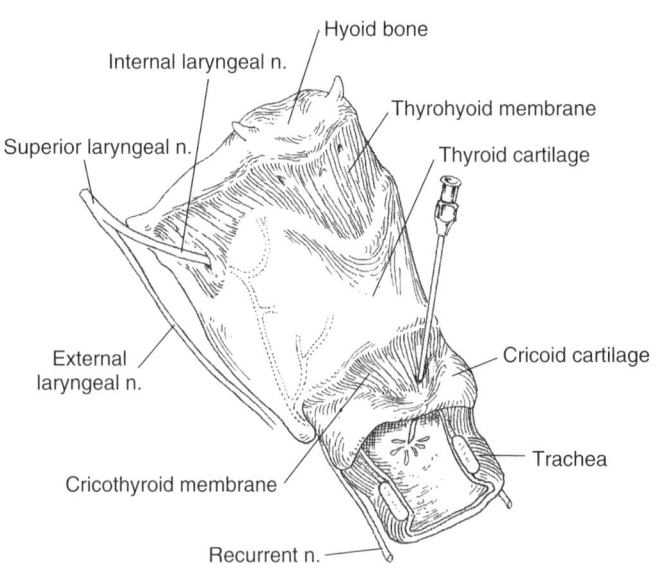

FIGURE **23-10** Transtracheal injection. *n.*, Nerve.

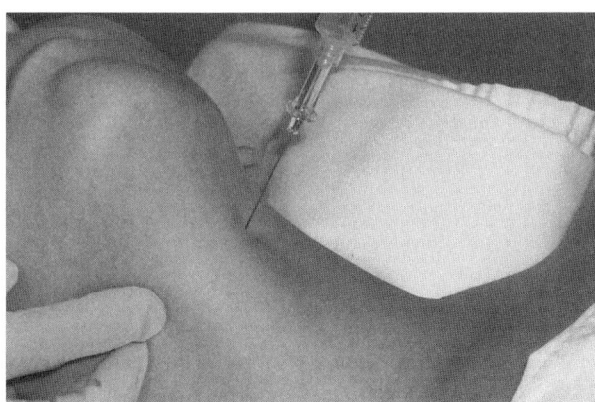

FIGURE **23-9** Superior laryngeal nerve block.

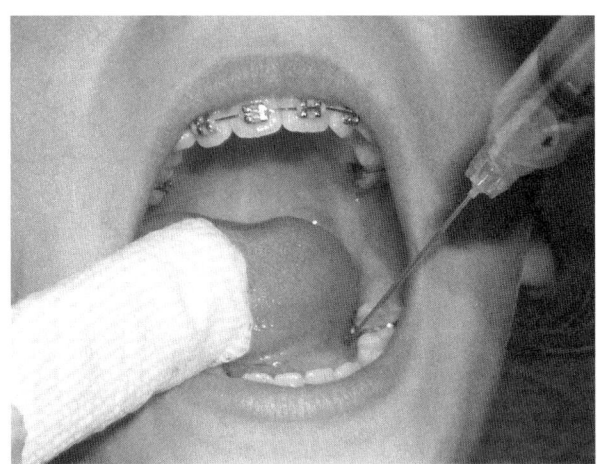

FIGURE **23-11** Glossopharyngeal nerve block.

CRICOID PRESSURE

Any time a patient is suspected of having a full stomach, such as in a trauma, diabetic patient, pregnant patient or any other emergency situation, use of cricoid pressure is considered the standard of care in the anesthesia community. Debate and controversy exist regarding the effectiveness of routine use of cricoid pressure in actual practice. Sellick described cricoid pressure as the posterior displacement of the cricoid cartilage against the cervical vertebrae with the patient in a 20-degree head-up position.[20] The most recent recommendation is that as long as the procedure is performed properly and does not impede effective airway management, cricoid pressure as a requirement for rapid sequence induction may be beneficial.[21]

This procedure occludes the esophagus, thereby preventing aspiration of gastric contents and insufflation of the stomach during positive pressure ventilation. However, errors are commonly made when cricoid pressure is applied.[22,23] Inadequate force applied at the wrong anatomic position and improper timing contribute to the decreased effectiveness of cricoid pressure and put the patient at increased risk for aspiration. Cricoid pressure is properly applied with the thumb and first finger placed on either side of the cricoid cartilage. Proper application then calls for **b**ackward, **u**pward, **r**ightward **p**ressure (BURP) until the fingers blanch. Because the esophagus is to the right side of the airway in approximately 75% of patients, displacement of the cricoid cartilage to the patient's right side should occlude the esophagus. Application of cricoid pressure can also cause flexion of the neck and may distort or deviate the trachea from midline. If pressure is applied too forcefully, difficulty in ventilation and ETT passage may be encountered.

The upper and lower esophageal sphincters serve as barriers to aspiration when the patient is awake. On loss of consciousness, the upper esophageal sphincter relaxes and allows for passive flow of gastric contents into the hypopharynx. Use of neuromuscular blockers further exacerbates relaxation of the upper esophageal sphincter. If aspiration is to be prevented, cricoid pressure must be applied before loss of consciousness. The recommended pressure to be exerted before loss of consciousness is 20 N, or approximately 2 kg of pressure. On loss of consciousness the pressure exerted must be increased to 44 N, or approximately 4 kg of pressure.[23] Required pressures are independent of age and sex. Also, the force applied declines steadily after 30 seconds. In the management of a difficult airway, recovery from induction drugs and neuromuscular blockers may take a significant length of time, during which the maintenance of adequate cricoid pressure is necessary. Care must be taken in the proper application of cricoid pressure because if done incorrectly, it can worsen the laryngoscopic view by as much as 30%.[14]

To add to the risk of aspiration, lower esophageal pressure is also affected by the force of cricoid pressure. Mechanoreceptors in the esophagus are stimulated by the pressure of a bolus of food. Cricoid pressure mimics this pressure, decreasing lower esophageal pressure by 9 to 12 mm Hg.[24] Insufflation of air into the stomach during forceful mask ventilation and use of succinylcholine increase intragastric pressures, increasing the risk that the gastric contents will be expelled into the esophagus.

Assistants who apply cricoid pressure should be instructed in noncritical situations regarding the required force of application and location of correct anatomic landmarks. As stated previously, inappropriately applied pressure can result in difficulty ventilating the patient or inserting the ETT, as well as displacement of the esophagus lateral to the larynx with no compression of the esophagus. The assistant holding cricoid pressure must be instructed to not release pressure until placement of the ETT is verified and the tube secured in place.

When a difficult airway is anticipated, the cricoid cartilage can be marked before induction of anesthesia. Marking the cricothyroid ligament may be of additional value if a surgical airway must be established.

ADJUNCT AIRWAY EQUIPMENT AND TECHNIQUES

Over the past decades, alternative airway devices and techniques have been developed and implemented for use in airway management. The devices include the LMA, ETT guides, lighted stylets, rigid laryngoscopes, indirect rigid fiberoptic laryngoscopes, and supraglottic ventilatory devices. Special airway techniques include flexible fiberoptic intubation. Supraglottic airway ventilation devices include both airway masks and tubes.

Supraglottic Laryngeal Masks
Laryngeal Mask Airway
Since its introduction, the LMA has been used extensively in the administration of anesthesia. Its development has been hailed as one of the most significant advances in airway management since the ETT.[25] The LMA is a valuable airway tool in managing the difficult airway. The literature contains anecdotal reports of the successful use of the LMA for establishing an airway and providing a conduit for intubation of the trachea.[25-27]

The LMA was used extensively in Europe, primarily in England, before its introduction in the United States. Several variations of the LMA exist, including the classic and ProSeal devices. In daily clinical use, this airway can be used in place of mask ventilation. It is inserted blindly into the posterior pharynx until resistance is felt. At that point the LMA is positioned in the hypopharynx below the base of the tongue and above the epiglottis. If the appropriately sized LMA is selected, the resistance denotes placement of the LMA's tip in the hypopharynx, and the black line on the tubing will be even with the upper lip. The cuff is then inflated, sealing the airway over the larynx. The esophageal opening at the base of the hypopharynx has no seal. If the cuff is overinflated, it can actually open the upper esophageal sphincter. The ProSeal LMA is designed with a second posterior cuff that inflates, closing the hypopharynx. The LMA is designed with a second tube so that a gastric tube can be inserted into the esophagus without passing through the hypopharynx.

Familiarity with the LMA, its ease and speed of insertion, and its high likelihood of success in difficult airway situations make it an extremely valuable rescue device. One of the concerns with the LMA is the possibility of aspiration during insertion or when the LMA is in place. The LMA devices do not prevent inflation of the stomach, regurgitation, or aspiration if the inflation pressure is too high. If ventilation is accomplished using positive pressure greater than 20 torr within the airway, the stomach may become inflated. The device can also be malpositioned or the cuff overinflated, resulting in failure to ventilate the patient. Both malpositioning of the airway and overinflation of the cuff result in additional pressure to the side walls of the pharynx and pressure on the posterior wall of the larynx. When this pressure is generated, the epiglottis can be folded back against the glottic opening, sealing the airway. Pathology at or below laryngeal level may make the LMA ineffective as a supraglottic device. In obstetric anesthesia, the LMA is used when tracheal intubation has failed and ventilation with face mask is difficult or impossible. Attempted use of the LMA should precede a cricothyroidotomy.

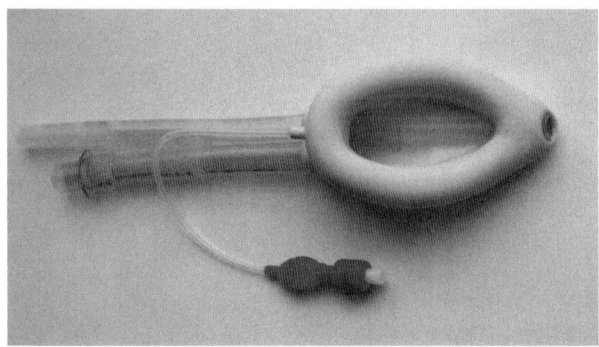

FIGURE **23-12** ProSeal LMA. (*Courtesy of LMA North America.*)

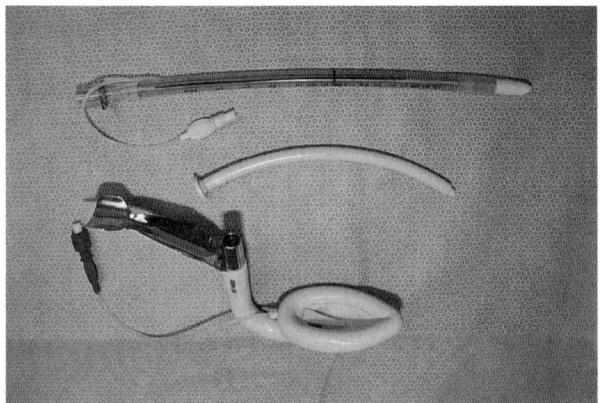

FIGURE **23-13** Fastrach.

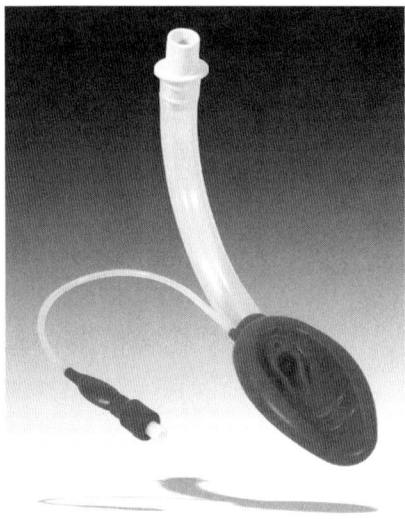

FIGURE **23-14** Intubating laryngeal airway. (*Courtesy of Mercury Medical.*)

The ProSeal LMA (Figure 23-12) allows the practitioner to pass a nasogastric tube through a side lumen to decompress the stomach or allow for removal of passive gastric contents. It differs from the traditional LMA in another important characteristic in that it provides a seal against the posterior wall of the pharynx, allowing positive inspiratory pressures of up to 30 psi. The ProSeal LMA can be used with a ventilator.

Other supraglottic laryngeal masks have been introduced, including the Ambu laryngeal mask, which combines an anatomic curve and a built-in bite block.

Fastrach
The Fastrach (Figure 23-13) is a new model of the LMA specifically designed to improve blind endotracheal intubation through a laryngeal mask.[27-29] It has been used successfully in the can't intubate/can't ventilate scenario, as well as in situations in which difficult intubation is anticipated. The design of the Fastrach allows for reasonable control of the airway throughout the intubation process, first with the laryngeal mask, then with endotracheal intubation. Most practitioners are familiar with the insertion of the LMA and adapt readily to insertion of the Fastrach. As with all adjunct airway equipment, the Fastrach should be used in routine cases to ensure familiarity with the technique before its use is attempted in an emergent situation or with a difficult airway.

An adaptation of the Fastrach is the C-Trach intubation device. This device adds a video screen to the standard Fastrach. The C-Trach allows the anesthetist to visualize the ETT passing through the vocal cords, confirming proper placement of the tube.

Intubating Laryngeal Airways (Cookgas ILA) and air-Q
Physician inventor Daniel Cook developed an oval-shaped supraglottic intubating airway that allows the anesthetist to maintain ventilation through the airway device or intubate with a standard ETT. The Cookgas ILA (Figure 23-14) comes with a removable stylet to stabilize the ETT while the laryngeal mask is removed. As with most devices, the ILA is able to be re-autoclaved only 40 times. A companion product, the air-Q, is disposable. The stylet with the ILA cannot be autoclaved but can be sterilized with liquids up to 10 times. The ILA and air-Q come in varying sizes, and both are usable on patients from 20 to 100 kg.

Supraglottic Tubes
Several supraglottic tubes have been developed over the past several years. These devices are placed blindly through the mouth and into the esophagus. The tube has a distal balloon to occlude the esophagus, as well as a larger proximal balloon to occlude the posterior oropharynx. Between the two balloons is a ventilation port at approximately the level of the trachea. These devices are meant for both rescue and routine management.

Combitube
The Combitube (Figure 23-15) is a double-lumen airway device that is inserted blindly into the hypopharynx. Irrespective of where the tip is placed, the lungs may be ventilated.[30] The usual placement of the tip is into the esophagus. This blind insertion is easily accomplished, and the patient's head can be kept in the neutral position. With the cuffs of both lumens inflated, the Combitube may offer some protection from aspiration. The Combitube is a supraglottic device, and pathology at or below the laryngeal level may make the Combitube ineffective. The esophageal lumen offers a way to further decompress the stomach. To successfully insert the Combitube, cricoid pressure must be released. Reported complications include esophageal rupture. In 2002, King Systems introduced the King LT, a minimally invasive airway device similar to the Combitube. This device is inserted in a manner similar to insertion of the Combitube but has only one ventilation port.

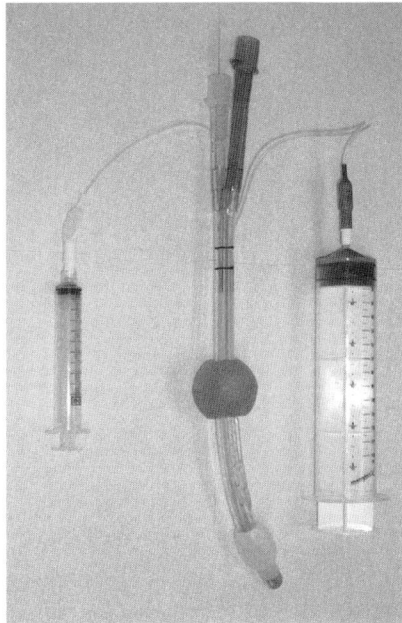

FIGURE **23-15** Combitube.

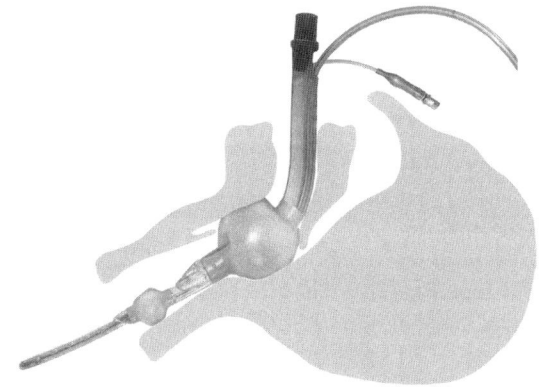

FIGURE **23-16** KING LTS-D. (*Courtesy of King Systems.*)

KING LT/LTS-D

The KING LT is a reusable supraglottic airway created as an alternative to tracheal intubation or mask ventilation. The KING LT is designed for positive pressure ventilation, as well as for spontaneously breathing patients, thereby allowing maximum versatility as an airway management tool.

The KING LT consistently achieves a ventilatory seal of 30 cm H_2O or higher. It is easy to insert and results in minimal airway trauma. The KING LT is 100% latex free and can be autoclaved up to 50 cycles or is available in a disposable model. The LT model has a single opening for ventilation. The LTS-D (Figure 23-16) has a second port that an 18-French nasogastric tube can be inserted through.

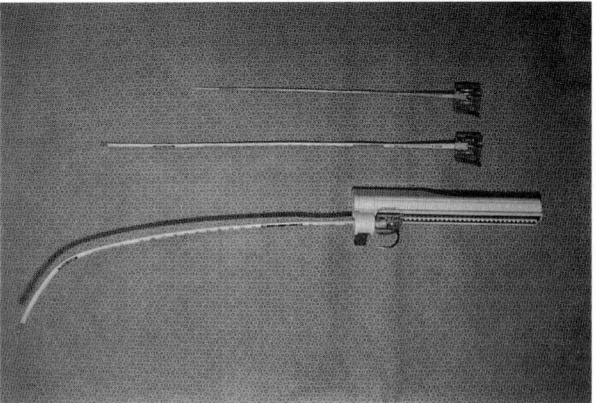

FIGURE **23-17** Trachlite.

Stylets
Trachlite

The Trachlite (Figure 23-17) is a recent adaptation of the light wand or lighted stylet that uses transillumination of the neck to accomplish endotracheal intubation.[31] Because the placement of the glottic opening is anterior to the esophagus, as the light source enters the trachea, a well-defined, circumscribed glow is noticed below the thyroid prominence and can be readily seen on the anterior neck. Placement of the light wand in the esophagus results in much more diffuse transillumination of the neck without this circumscribed glow. The Trachlite has a bright light source that does not require low ambient light for optimum performance. In addition, it has a retractable stylet that increases the success rate for intubation.

The success rate of the Trachlite is similar to that of conventional direct laryngoscopy. It is less affected by anterior placement of the larynx, is less stimulating than conventional laryngoscopy, and is associated with a lower incidence of sore throat. It can be used in both the anticipated and the unanticipated difficult airway in which conventional laryngoscopy has failed. Intubation of the trachea can be accomplished with a small oral opening and minimal neck manipulation.

Because the Trachlite is inserted blindly using transillumination, risk of injury or failure is increased when the device is used in patients with any upper airway anomaly, such as foreign body, tumor, polyps, or soft-tissue injuries. If these anomalies exist, other airway adjuncts should be used. In addition, it may be more difficult to accurately place the Trachlite in patients with short, thick necks or redundant soft tissue.

Eschmann Stylet (Gum Elastic Bougie)

The Eschmann stylet (Figure 23-18) is a flexible stylet with a bent tip that can be useful when the glottic opening is difficult to visualize. The stylet is placed into the glottic opening. An ETT is inserted over the stylet and slid into place in the trachea. Confirmation of proper placement of the Eschmann stylet is made by feeling the stylet bounce along the tracheal rings as it is advanced.

Scopes

Scopes allow for the visual placement of ETTs under less than optimal circumstances. Scopes can be either rigid or flexible.

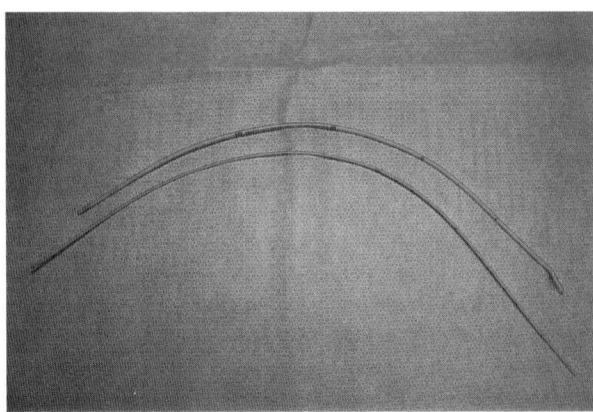

FIGURE **23-18** Eschmann stylet.

Fiberoptic Laryngoscope (Bronchoscope)

The fiberoptic bronchoscope can be used to evaluate the airway, ease intubation of the patient with a difficult airway, check placement of ETTs, change ETTs, and perform pulmonary toilet and post-extubation evaluations.[32] The flexible fiberoptic laryngoscope consists of multiple strands of tiny glass fibers that carry light. These fibers are bound together inside a rubberized coating that allows for flexibility. Within the scope are working channels that can act as suction ports or be used to instill local anesthetic or carry oxygen. The handle contains an eyepiece for viewing and a lever for controlling the distal end of the scope through one plane. The second plane is navigated by turning the scope. Light is supplied by an external light source or most recently by battery.

Limitations of the fiberoptic laryngoscope include the following:

- The scope can become fogged, especially if it is cold. Soaking the scope in warm saline before use may help prevent this.
- Limitation of view can result when multiple fiberoptic strands are broken or damaged. The scope should never be banged or dropped and should always be stored flat in a protective case or cart.
- Vision can be obstructed by secretions or blood. This can be prevented with the instillation of 10 to 15 L of oxygen per minute through one of the side channels.

The fiberoptic bronchoscope can be used for oral or nasal intubation, with the patient either awake or asleep. For awake intubation, instillation of local anesthesia or nerve blocks should be accomplished as previously described. With oral intubations, a bite block should be used to prevent damage to the fibers caused by the patient's biting the scope.

When the fiberoptic bronchoscope is prepared for use, a cart should be dedicated to the equipment. The light source and extension cord should be securely mounted to the cart, along with any outlet adapters required, suction devices, and oxygen delivery systems. Oral airways, irrigation catheters, and suction catheters or devices, as well as other equipment used in the management of the airway, should be placed on the cart and labeled. Practitioners should use the equipment frequently to ensure that they are comfortable with it and to verify that the devices are functionally ready for use.

A Yankauer suction device must be available and set up whenever the fiberoptic bronchoscope is used. Medications used in airway management should be readily available. These include local anesthetics, resuscitation drugs, induction agents, and muscle relaxants. If the equipment is to be used outside of the operating room, the appropriate monitors should be on the cart as well. This cart can become the central location for all emergency airway devices, including the TTJV and LMAs.

Debate and controversy exist regarding the administration of drying agents and sedation. Atropine or glycopyrrolate may be administered 5 to 20 minutes before the procedure. Administration of light sedation (midazolam 0.04 mg/kg) may help reduce the patient's stress and provide for a more relaxed environment for the practitioner. Some practitioners routinely administer narcotics as an adjunct to midazolam, although this practice must be a cautious choice whenever control of the airway is in doubt. The most widely used sedation-analgesia technique seems to be administration of fentanyl and midazolam, carefully titrated in small bolus doses. A short-acting and easily titratable opioid such as remifentanil is an alternative choice for the intensely stimulating, but usually brief, airway manipulation during fiberoptic nasotracheal intubation.[33]

The fiberoptic scope is first inserted through the ETT and is then inserted through either the mouth or the nose and advanced to the posterior pharynx. Care must be taken to keep the tube and scope in the midline while the tip is advanced toward the epiglottis. Instillation of oxygen through the suction port not only aids in the oxygenation of the patient but also helps keep the optics clear. The anesthetist can manipulate the scope in two planes by rotating the lever on the right side of the handle back and forth and by rotating the scope laterally. The tip of the scope is slipped through the epiglottis and advanced until the tracheal rings come into view. The ETT is slipped downward, with the scope used as a stylet, and then through the cords. Care must be taken to ensure that the tube does not damage the rubber coating of the scope.

One way to gain experience with the device is to use it routinely to secure the airway in controlled intubation procedures in class I and II airway patients. After the induction of anesthesia and the securing of the airway, the evaluation of the airway and tube placement can be accomplished using the fiberoptic bronchoscope. Use of the fiberoptic bronchoscope to observe airway landmarks in the pharynx and the epiglottis can help the practitioner become acquainted with the anatomy. Additionally, intubation mannequins made by Laerdal and Ambu can be used to practice intubation techniques with this equipment.

Suctioning is almost impossible through the suction port. A more advantageous use of this channel is to provide the patient with supplemental oxygen. A 2- to 4-L flow through this port provides the patient with up to 26% oxygen insufflation and keeps debris from collecting on or near the port and lens. Another use of this port can be the administration of local anesthesia through an epidural catheter threaded down the port.

The fiberoptic bronchoscope is contraindicated in patients with epiglottitis, laryngotracheitis, or bacterial tracheitis. The manipulation of the fiberoptic bronchoscope through the glottis may cause enough stimulation to convert a partial obstruction into a total obstruction of the airway. Caution should be strictly exercised in patients with airway burns because of the restricted size and the hyperirritability of the airway. Special care should be used in patients who have been irradiated. Radiation can cause fibrosis and loss of mucus-producing glands, so drying of the airway can be extensive with the use of either glycopyrrolate or atropine. The use of the fiberoptic bronchoscope is very limited in airway trauma. The presence of blood and mucus in the airway obscures the lens and makes visualization impossible. If significant soft-tissue trauma is present, edema of the tissues can prevent adequate visualization of the larynx and trachea.

Additionally, all personnel who will be using the device should be trained in its care and cleaning. The fibers in the bronchoscope are very fragile. Bending, curling, or any other type of kinking of the scope will break the fibers. Cleaning is very important. All of the channels, suction and injection, must be cleaned thoroughly after each use. This requires flushing with warm saline immediately after use. Manufacturers will indicate which detergent and sterilizing solution they recommend. Instructions regarding solution, dilution, soak times, and rinsing must be closely followed to ensure the integrity of the equipment. After external washing is performed, a small bottle brush is used to clean the channels. This brush is usually supplied with the device, but it is wise to buy several extras. Flushing with warm water after cleaning is mandatory.

Shikani Optical Stylet

The Shikani Optical Stylet (SOS) (Figure 23-19) is a malleable, semirigid, intubating fiberoptic stylet for use in adults and children. It features a battery-operated light source with a high-resolution eyepiece on the handle to which the stylet is attached. The SOS also has the ability to insufflate oxygen into the pharynx via the ETT that is placed over the stylet prior to intubation. The malleable distal end allows configuration for varying the intubation angles that may be encountered in different patients; this can be particularly useful for patients with a rigid or unstable cervical spine. The SOS can be used alone or in conjunction with direct laryngoscopy or as a conventional light wand.[34]

GlideScope

The GlideScope (Figure 23-20), which is similar to a Macintosh blade, slides into the vallecula, allowing for visualization of the cords. The advantage of the GlideScope is that it includes a fiber bundle built into the one-piece blade and handle. This fiber bundle not only allows for light to illuminate the cords but also for a camera for external visualization of the airway on a small monitor. According to Sun and Warriner, "It provided a laryngoscopic view equal to or better than that of direct laryngoscopy"[35] without manipulation of the head into a sniffing position.

Airtraq Optical Laryngoscope

The Airtraq (Figure 23-21) optical laryngoscope is designed to provide a view of the glottic opening, also without manipulating the neck into a sniffing position. This potentially makes the Airtraq important in situations in which manipulation of the head would be dangerous to the patient, such as an unstable cervical fracture, temporomandibular joint (TMJ) immobility, burns, and trauma. The blade of the Airtraq has two channels. The first channel has a lighted, heated lens, and the second channel is for passage of any style ETT up to an 8.5 mm. The Airtraq has a unique system that turns on an antifogging system when the LED light is on for at least 30 seconds. There is an optional video camera that clips on to the viewfinder. The Airtraq is available in two sizes, regular and small. In simulated difficult laryngoscopy scenarios, the Airtraq was more successful in achieving tracheal intubation, required less time to intubate successfully, caused less dental trauma, and was considered by the anesthetists to be easier to use.[36]

The ETT is placed into the side channel until the tip is at the end of the channel. The LED light is turned on for at least 30 seconds prior to placing it into the mouth to allow the

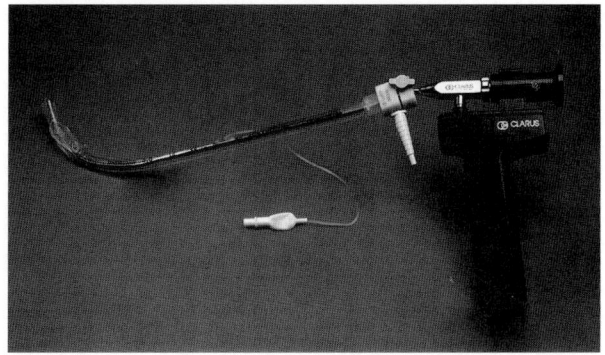

FIGURE **23-19**   Shikani Optical Stylet. (*From Marx JA et al*: Rosen's Emergency Medicine. *6th ed. St Louis: Mosby; 2006:22.*)

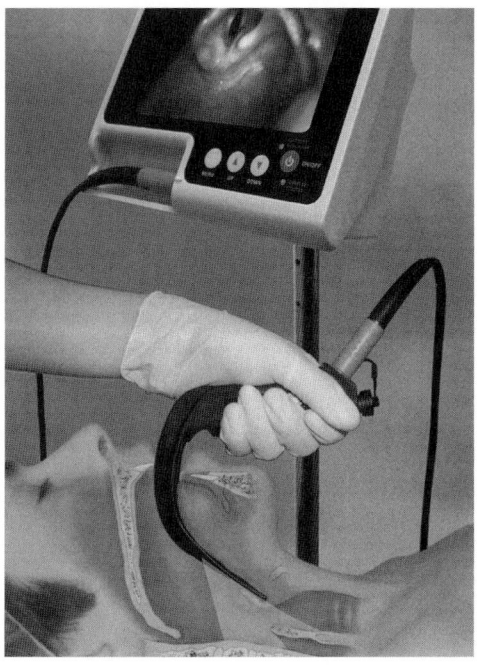

FIGURE **23-20**   GlideScope in airway. (*Courtesy of Verathon Medical.*)

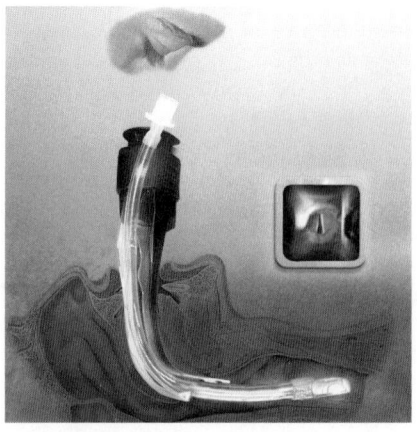

FIGURE **23-21**   Airtraq visualization. (*Courtesy of Prodol Meditec.*)

antifogging system to be activated. The battery will allow enough power for the LED light to stay on for 90 minutes. The tip of the Airtraq is placed in the vallecula in a manner similar to the MacIntosh. Once in place, the scope is lifted vertically, allowing the epiglottis to flip up onto the blade and the cords to be visualized. Once the cords are visualized, the ETT is advanced through, securing the airway. If the practitioner has difficulty visualizing the cords or advancing the ETT through the cords, the scope should be withdrawn slightly.

Bullard Scope, Upsher Scope, and McGrath Scope

Maharaj and colleagues describe the Bullard laryngoscope as "an indirect fiberoptic laryngoscope with a rigid anatomically shaped blade with fiberoptic bundles."[36] The anatomic curve of the blade allows for visualization and intubation of the airway without aligning the oral, pharyngeal, and tracheal axes. The scope serves as a channel for insufflation of oxygen while intubating, as well as a detachable stylet to position the ETT along the right side of the flat blade.

The Bullard scope can be used on either an awake or an anesthetized patient, and because it does not require the sniffing position, it is ideal for patients with limited range of motion of the neck, such as those in cervical collars. Optimal use of the Bullard scope takes place with the patient in a neutral head position. The scope is advanced along the hard palate and when in the vertical position, it is lifted slightly. This position should allow the optimal view of the larynx. While observing through the scope, the ETT is slid off the attached stylet through the cords.

Mercury Medical Corporation's Upsher scope was developed as a device that uses the traditional laryngoscope handle but takes advantage of the provider's skills with the curved blade when accomplishing endoscopy. The device is a single piece, unlike the Bullard scope, but the view through the lens is the same, and the device can be connected to an external camera and television screen. The Upsher scope serves the same purposes and has the same advantages as the Bullard scope in relation to moving the neck. Unlike the Bullard's wide, flat blade, the Upsher has a curved channel to accommodate passage of the ETT. With both of these scopes, the ETT should pass wherever the scope is looking. The most common difficulty is hanging up on the arytenoids. This problem can usually be solved with either gentle cricoid pressure or lifting slightly with the blade.

LMA America introduced a scope in 2007 called the *McGrath* (Figure 23-22). It provides a small view of the camera similar to the intubating scopes, with the familiarity of the Macintosh blade. The tip of the blade is clear plastic and disposable.

Subglottic Interventions

With the advent of the intubating laryngeal mask airway (iLMA) and other effective airway rescue devices, there has been less need for the practitioner to be overly concerned with subglottic airway interventions. But as good as the iLMA and other devices are, they may not rescue the patient in all can't ventilate/can't intubate airway situations. It is then that the anesthesia provider must be familiar with emergency subglottic airway techniques such as transtracheal jet ventilation and cricothyrotomy.

Transtracheal Jet Ventilation

In the can't intubate/can't ventilate scenario, a means to deliver oxygen must be made available if hypoxemia and other adverse outcomes are to be avoided. This can be accomplished quickly and easily with TTJV[37-40] (Figure 23-23), a technique used to provide oxygenation using high-pressure delivery systems and used widely in anesthesia practice for surgical procedures on the airway. A large-bore intravenous (IV) catheter is inserted through the cricothyroid membrane in a caudad direction (Figure 23-24). The lungs are ventilated using a high-pressure oxygen source and a regulating valve to control oxygen flow through noncompliant tubing attached to the IV catheter. As high-flow oxygen is introduced for 1 second through the catheter, air is also entrained (Venturi effect) through the upper airway. At a delivered pressure of 50 psi, a 20-gauge catheter delivers approximately 400 mL of oxygen per second, a 16-gauge catheter delivers 500 mL of oxygen per second, and a 14-gauge catheter delivers 1600 mL of oxygen per second.[41] High-pressure oxygen is delivered reliably through central wall outlets and high-flow (50 to 100 psi) tank regulators. Most jet ventilators have a regulator to allow for a decrease in the inspiratory pressure; in most instances, 25 psi is a sufficient inspiratory pressure. A 1-second inspiration at 25 psi with a rate of 20 breaths per minute (1 second inspiration/2 second expiration) delivers a 285-mL tidal volume or 5.7 L/min ventilation. Expiration is

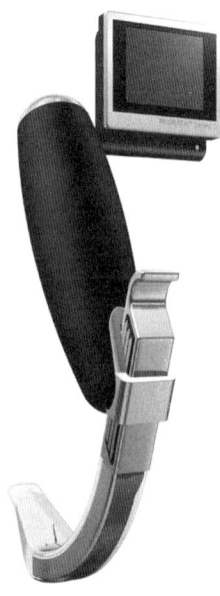

FIGURE **23-22** McGrath scope. (*Courtesy of LMA North America.*)

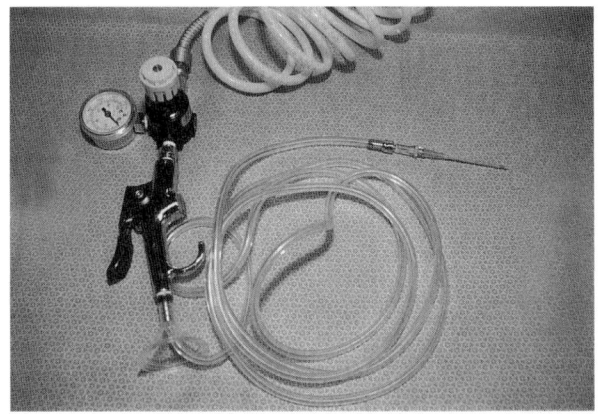

FIGURE **23-23** Transtracheal jet ventilation.

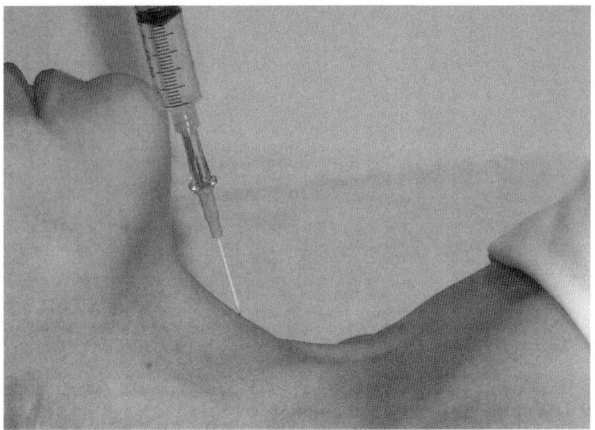

FIGURE **23-24**   Insertion of needle for transtracheal jet ventilation.

through the normal airway, with a normal elastic contraction of 15 psi.[42,43] If the inspiratory cycles are too rapid, there tends to be air trapping in the lungs and incomplete elimination of carbon dioxide. Use of corrugated tubing or other compliant tubing decreases the minute volume delivered. Multiple devices are available for use in the operating room, including the Cook Emergency Cricothyrotomy Kit.

Complications associated with the use of TTJV include barotrauma, tissue emphysema, and exhalation difficulties. Exhalation occurs passively through the upper airway. Obstructions to passive exhalation or excessively large tidal volumes result in hyperinflation. Placement of bilateral nasal airways or an oral airway facilitates exhalation. Use of an in-line pressure gauge and inspiration to expiration ratios of 1:2 or 1:3 decrease the incidence of barotrauma. Bilateral breath sounds should be confirmed frequently to rule out pneumothorax and subcarinal placement or dislodgement of the catheter.

Retrograde Intubation

This procedure is performed by inserting a 14- to 18-gauge IV catheter or a Cook needle through the cricothyroid membrane and directing it cephalad. A wire or suture is inserted through the needle and passed cephalad until it can be visualized in the posterior pharynx and then passed through the mouth or nose. The distal end of the wire is secured with a clamp to prevent the wire from being pulled into the trachea prematurely. An ETT can be directed over the wire and passed into the trachea. As the tube enters the larynx, tension is increased on the wire or suture. When this occurs, the distal wire is cut at the level of the skin and permitted to pass into the trachea. The tube is passed into the trachea, placement confirmed, and the tube secured in place. This is not an emergent process and often can be completed by a skilled practitioner in 5 to 7 minutes.

Percutaneous Dilational Cricothyrotomy

Percutaneous dilational cricothyrotomy is the emergency method of ventilation for patients in a can't ventilate/can't intubate situation. A skilled anesthesia provider can insert a tube through the cricothyroid membrane and ventilate the patient in approximately 70 seconds, as opposed to the 4 to 5 minutes required for a surgical tracheostomy. According to Melker and Orlando, "Emergency cricothyrotomy has largely replaced emergency tracheostomy in an ED setting because of its simplicity, rapidity and minimal morbidity."[44] Indications for cricothyrotomy include

(1) can't ventilate/can't intubate situations, (2) traumatic injuries that make intubation through the nose or mouth difficult or hazardous, and (3) need for a definitive airway for neck or facial surgery.

Contraindications for cricothyrotomy are rare but include preexisting laryngeal diseases such as cancer or chronic inflammation, distortion of neck anatomy, bleeding diathesis and history of coagulopathy, and children younger than 6 years of age.[44]

"Needle-puncture" cricothyrotomy allows emergency oxygenation through insertion of a 14-gauge IV catheter placed through the cricothyroid membrane. Oxygen can be instilled by attaching the barrel of a 3-mL syringe to the proximal end of the IV catheter and connecting this to an oxygen supply via the connector from a 7-mm ETT. The oxygen flow must be provided through TTJV or other high-pressure system. A needle cricothyrotomy can provide a patient with oxygenation for 30 minutes while a tracheotomy or other rescue airway intervention is performed.

The most common method of intervention through the cricothyroid membrane is easy to perform with a commercially prepared tray such as the Melker Cricothyrotomy Set (Figure 23-25) by Cook Critical Care or alternative sets such as the Quicktrach or Pertrach cricothyrotomy sets, with the Melker set being the most common.

The Melker set contains all of the necessary equipment to perform a percutaneous dilational cricothyrotomy. The set includes an airway catheter with dilator, scalpel, syringe, introducer needle and catheter introducer needle, stiff guide wire, and tie tapes for securing the airway catheter once it is placed in the neck.

Although putting a needle and knife blade into a patient's neck can be daunting, placing the airway catheter is relatively simple. The steps are:

1. Place the patient's head in a neutral position.
2. Open the proper tray and place it in a position that is comfortable for the person inserting the device. Insert the dilator into the airway catheter.
3. Palpate the cricothyroid membrane, and using the introducer needle with the syringe attached, enter the neck in a caudad direction while aspirating on the syringe. Once air is aspirated, thread the catheter off of the needle, attach the syringe to the catheter, and again aspirate air (Figure 23-26).
4. Insert the flexible end of the guide wire through the catheter until it is approximately 2 inches beyond the tip of the catheter (Figure 23-27).
5. Using the enclosed scalpel, incise the neck with a single insertion along the guide wire (Figure 23-28).
6. Thread the airway catheter/dilator over the exposed guide wire and advance, applying steady pressure by pushing on the dilator. Once there is loss of resistance, usually preceded by a "pop" as the catheter penetrates the cricothyroid membrane, advance the airway catheter off of the dilator until it rests firmly against the neck. Remove the dilator (Figure 23-29).
7. Using suture or the tape ties, secure the airway catheter into the neck, and ventilate (Figure 23-30).

Tracheotomy

An additional technique for securing the airway in a patient with airway problems is the tracheotomy. This surgical intervention is not a procedure performed by an anesthetist. Patients with facial and neck trauma, for example, are cases in which a difficult airway might be anticipated, so a surgical consultation should be requested as part of the patient assessment and anesthesia plan. The standard tracheotomy is performed at the level of

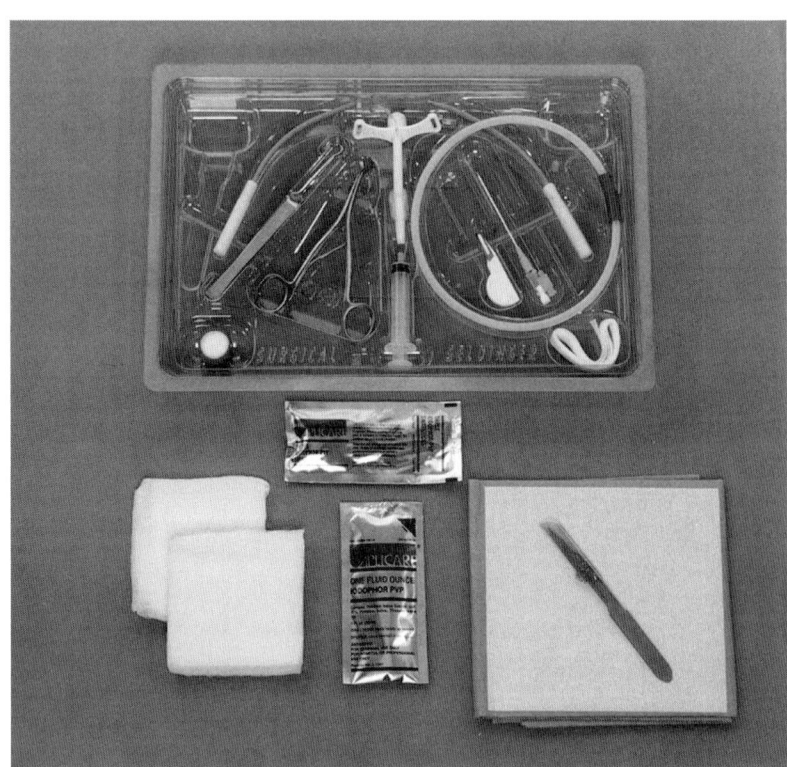

FIGURE **23-25** Melker Cricothyrotomy Set. (*Courtesy of Cook Critical Care.*)

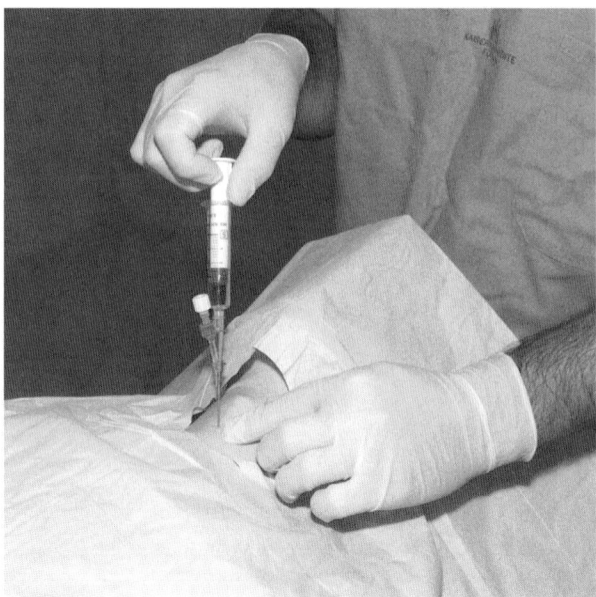

FIGURE **23-26** Needle inserted in caudad direction aspirating air.

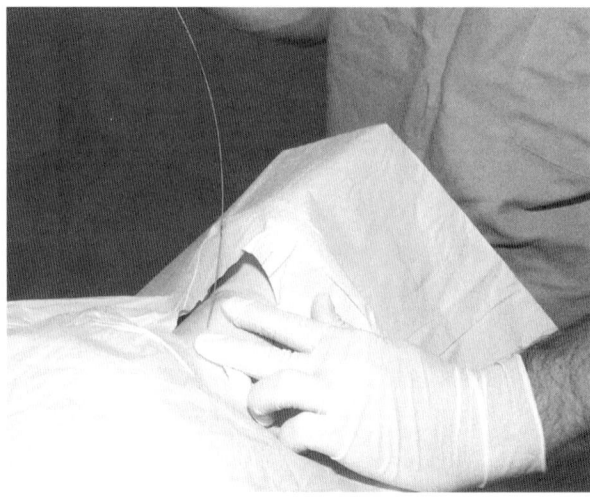

FIGURE **23-27** Guide wire threaded through catheter in neck.

the fourth to sixth tracheal ring, below the isthmus of the thyroid gland. This procedure can take up to 30 minutes. If a need to perform a tracheotomy exists, the airway should be secured first or the procedure performed with the patient under a local anesthetic.

Extubation

Extubating the trachea at the completion of surgery depends on a number of factors, including the type of airway anatomy encountered during induction, the type of surgery, and the potential for bleeding or severe airway edema. Criteria for extubation provide guidelines for safe removal of the ETT. The same care taken to secure the airway should be exercised when control of the airway is returned to the patient. Extubation may occur when the patient is in a deep plane of anesthesia, awakening, or fully awake. Extubation criteria commonly used in patients undergoing general anesthesia with neuromuscular blockers include an adequate tidal volume and rate; ability to open the eyes widely on command with no diplopia; demonstration of sustained protrusion and purposeful movement of the tongue; ability to swallow effectively; completion of sustained head or leg lift for at least 5 seconds (in small children a strong knee-to-chest movement is equivalent); demonstration of a strong, constant hand grip; presence of effective cough; adequate vital capacity of at least 15 mL/kg; and inspiratory force of at least 25 to 30 cm H_2O

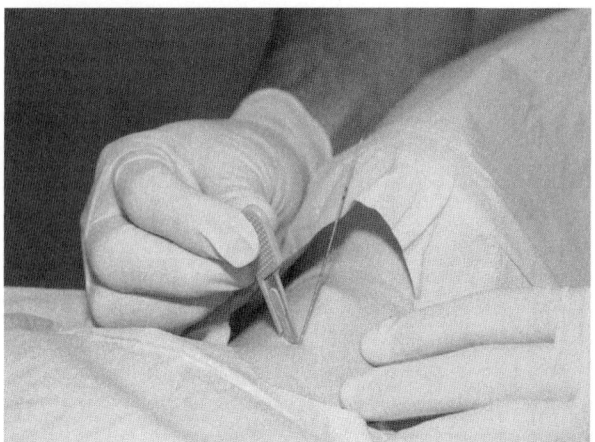

FIGURE **23-28** Neck incised with scalpel along guide wire.

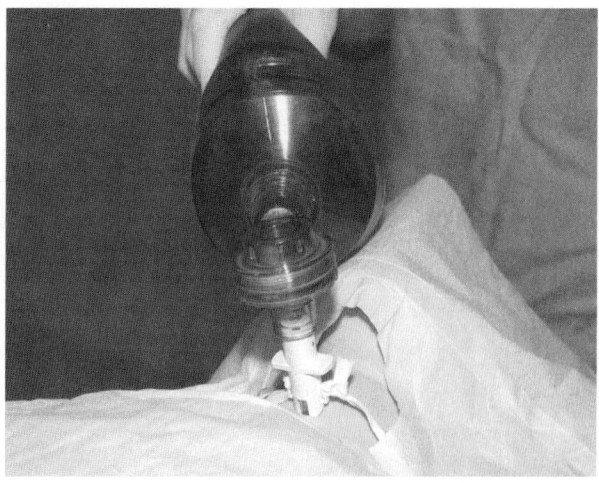

FIGURE **23-30** Dilator and guide wire removed, allowing ventilation.

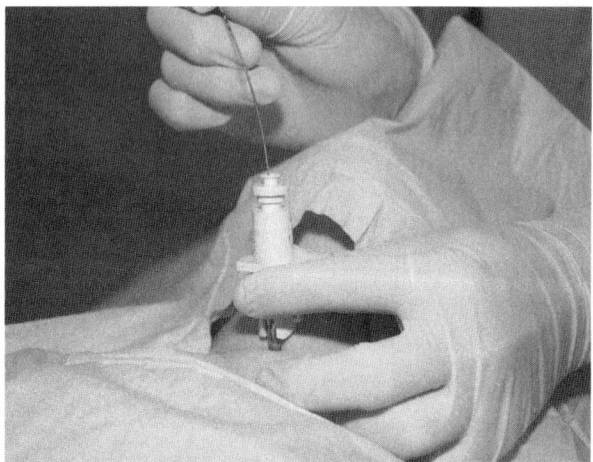

FIGURE **23-29** Airway catheter/dilator threaded over guide wire.

TABLE **23-9**	Causes of Injury and Complications of Intubation
Cause of Injury	**Complications of Intubation**
Physical	
Tubeinduced	Nasal mucosal damage; turbinate fractures; dissection of posterior pharyngeal wall; sore throat; hoarseness; granulomas; tracheal mucosa damage leading to scarring and strictures; endobronchial intubation; pressure injuries to recurrent laryngeal, laryngeal, or hypoglossal nerves
Laryngoscopy	Hypertension, tachycardia, bradycardia, dental trauma, spinal cord trauma, aspiration, corneal abrasion
Mechanical	
Obstruction resulting from kinking, dried secretions	Negative-pressure pulmonary edema, hypoxia, hypercarbia
Disconnect	Hypoxia, hypercarbia
Airway fire	Airway burns, pulmonary edema

negative pressure. The neuromuscular monitor must also identify a sustained tetanic response to 50 Hz for 5 seconds, train-of-four ratio greater than 0.90 with no fade, and no fade to double-burst stimulation.

The patient who was difficult to ventilate or intubate should be fully awake, able to follow commands, and have all protective reflexes present before extubation. Guidelines for extubating patients with a difficult airway are noted in the ASA Difficult Airway Algorithm.[3] One of the suggestions is the use of a device over which the ETT is removed, such as a fiberoptic broncho-scope, a jet stylet, or a gum-elastic bougie. Because these devices may not be suitable in very small infants, the use of a guide wire from the Cook Airway Exchange Catheter (CAEC; Cook, Inc., Bloomington, Indiana) has been described. This guide wire is 0.018 inch and permits the use of the 8-French CAEC, over which a 3.0 ETT can be passed. This technique of leaving a device in the trachea in the patient with a difficult airway has proved useful in a number of reports.

COMPLICATIONS OF TRACHEAL INTUBATION

Airway Mishaps

Complications from intubation can occur at any point during management of the airway (Table 23-9). Intubation attempts during light anesthesia, numerous attempts at intubation, or prolonged intubations are only a few of the reasons complications occur.[45] Gentle manipulation of the airway, adequate preparation, and vigilance are all required to decrease the incidence and severity of complications. Laryngeal swelling can be caused by placement of an ETT that significantly contributes to the increment of laryngeal resistance. Laryngeal resistance increases because of anatomic narrowing of the laryngeal aperture (anatomic mechanisms) or imbalance between the abductor and adductor of the vocal cords (neural mechanisms). The increased laryngeal resistance may not manifest clinical symptoms in subjects with normal preoperative laryngeal function.

However, the results should be taken seriously, prompting routine airway management procedures with ETTs, particularly in patients with preoperative laryngeal narrowing and small children who may have no clinical symptoms preoperatively.

Esophageal Intubation

Unrecognized esophageal intubation can lead to catastrophic complications from hypoxia. Signs of an esophageal intubation include absence of breath sounds over the lung fields, a gurgling over the epigastrium with progressive distention of the abdomen, and lack of sustained end-tidal CO_2 on the capnogram. Signs of hypoxemia may not readily appear if the patient was adequately preoxygenated. Once an esophageal intubation has been recognized and corrected, the stomach should be decompressed to decrease the risk of aspiration.

Endobronchial Intubation

When the ETT is placed too deeply, it may migrate into a mainstem bronchus. In adults, endobronchial intubation most commonly occurs in the right mainstem bronchus. The distance to the right upper lobe is short, and a right mainstem intubation may also occlude the right upper lobe.

Signs of an endobronchial intubation include increased peak inspiratory pressures, uneven chest excursion, decreased breath sounds on the unventilated side, a drop in the end-tidal CO_2 concentration, tachycardia, and hypoxemia. If endobronchial intubation is suspected, the balloon on the ETT should be deflated and withdrawn until bilateral breath sounds are heard. The fiberoptic scope may be used to confirm placement of the tube.

Risks of Intubation

Trauma to the structures of the upper and lower airway and the neck can occur during placement of the ETT.[45] Careful positioning, proper depth of anesthesia, and gentle manipulation of the airway limit the incidence of injury.

The ETT is often a cause of injury. The larger the diameter of the tube and the longer it is left in place, the greater the incidence of injury. Most susceptible to injury are the arytenoids, the posterior half of the vocal cords, and the posterior tracheal wall (Figure 23-31). The natural curve of the ETT rests on these structures and can cause desquamation, inflammation, and ulceration of the tissue. Formation of scar tissue over areas of ulceration may lead to tracheal stenosis. Granuloma formation

on scar tissue most often occurs on the posterior wall of the trachea (Figure 23-32). The most common injuries are:

- Injuries to lips, gums, and soft tissues of the oral cavity caused by insertion of the laryngoscope.
- Dental trauma from the laryngoscope, causing teeth to be chipped, broken, or loosened. All possible attempts should be made to find the missing fragments so they are not aspirated. If not all fragments are found, radiographs of the chest and abdomen must be taken to check for aspiration.
- Nasal intubation can result in nosebleed. This can be prevented by progressive dilation of the nasal passage with progressively larger, well-lubricated nasal airways. Use of a vasodilator such as Neo-Synephrine or Afrin is recommended.
- Puncture or tearing of the trachea can result when a stylet is used. The tip should never protrude beyond the end of the ETT or through the Murphy's eye.

Nasal intubation carries the additional risks of turbinate fractures, hemorrhage, laceration of the nasal mucosa, and dissection of the adenoids. Prolonged intubation may contribute to infection of the paranasal sinuses.

Endotracheal Tube Obstruction

The ETT can become obstructed by foreign materials or mechanically obstructed by the patient. The obstruction can be partial or complete. Obstruction may be more troublesome with spontaneous ventilation because positive-pressure ventilation overcomes some of the increased resistance. This obstruction, especially in young, healthy patients, can lead to negative pressure pulmonary edema (NPPE), caused by the movement of fluid from the interstitial space of the lung into the plural cavity. Treatment includes administration of diuretics and positive pressure ventilation.

Some of the possible causes of obstruction include:

1. *Biting*. A partially anesthetized patient may react to the presence of an ETT by biting down. This action may partially or totally occlude the ETT. This can be prevented by insertion of an oral airway or bite block.
2. *Kinking*. Kinks are one of the most common causes of ETT obstruction and may occur anywhere along the length of the tube. The tube may be kinked because of the patient's position or because increased weight distal to the patient causes the tube to kink at the patient's mouth. If the anesthetist does not have immediate access to the airway because of surgical positioning, use of an armored or reinforced ETT should be considered.

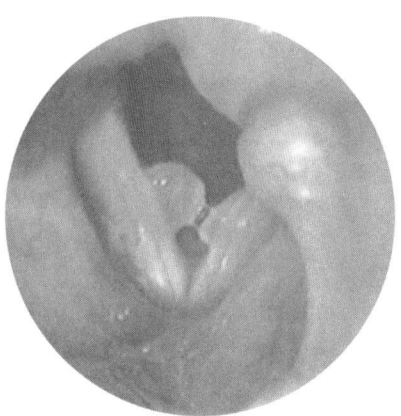

FIGURE **23-31** Fiberoptic view of vocal cord polyps.

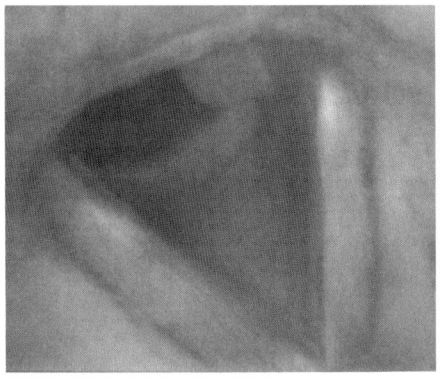

FIGURE **23-32** Fiberoptic view of granuloma.

3. *Foreign materials.* As the ETT passes through the pharynx, any number of substances can be picked up and cause obstruction. These substances include mucus, blood, pus, and tissue.

Endotracheal Tube Ignition

With the use of lasers becoming common in laryngeal surgery, the possibility of tracheal tube fires has increased. Direct penetration of the tube (combustible material) with the laser (ignition source) in the presence of an oxygen-rich environment (O_2 greater than 21%) (Oxidizer) involves all of the three components required for fire. Special ETTs, avoidance of nitrous oxide, and use of lower oxygen concentrations are recommended.

Sore Throat

Sore throat is the most common postoperative anesthesia complaint. It usually is transient and not severe. Factors contributing to a sore throat include ETT size, difficulty with the intubation, use of a nasogastric tube, female gender, and a history of smoking. The use of local anesthetic lubricants has not been shown to be effective in prevention and may in fact increase the incidence of a sore throat. The best prevention is a careful, gentle technique when inserting the ETT and the placement of as few tubes as possible through the pharynx.

Laryngospasm

Forceful, involuntary spasm of the laryngeal musculature occurs through sensory stimulation of the superior laryngeal nerve and afferent responses from the RLN. Laryngospasm can be caused by either secretions or stimulation of the larynx while the patient is in a light plane of anesthesia. In the awakening patient, it can be lessened by extubation when the patient is either in a deeper plane of anesthesia or fully awake. Extubation should occur during a full-tidal-volume breath as the patient exhales, so that any secretions are projected out of the airway.

Laryngospasm consists of two phases—a "shutter" mechanism that results in partial airway obstruction, followed by a "ball-valve" mechanism in which complete obstruction occurs.[46] The shutter mechanism reflects adduction of the vocal cords, whereas the ball-valve mechanism entails constriction of the false vocal cords and supraglottic soft tissue. Treatment of a partial or shutter laryngospasm includes the administration of gentle positive-pressure ventilation with 100% oxygen (10 to 20 cm H_2O pressure). Care must be taken not to force air into the esophagus or stomach, causing gastric distention. If the condition persists, administration of lidocaine or succinylcholine 0.1 mg/kg IV may be necessary. The treatment of a full or ball-valve laryngospasm requires an intubating dose of succinylcholine (1 to 2 mg/kg IV or 4 mg/kg administered intramuscularly).

Croup

Croup can be caused by post-intubation edema around the glottic and subglottic regions. Croup is more common in children than in adults because children have smaller airways. This condition is often associated with multiple intubation attempts, a large ETT without an air leak, or exaggerated movement of the patient's head. Croup usually occurs within 3 hours of extubation. Symptoms include respiratory stridor and a barking cough. Treatment is aimed at reducing swelling via inhalation of cool, moist oxygen and inhalation of racemic epinephrine (0.5 mL of a 2.25% solution in 2.5 mL of normal saline). Dexamethasone 0.1 to 0.5 mg/kg may also be helpful.

DIFFICULT AIRWAY IN OBSTETRIC ANESTHESIA

Case Presentation

A healthy primigravida has developed sustained fetal bradycardia. The decision is made to proceed with an emergency cesarean section. Anesthesia is induced with sodium thiopental and succinylcholine. The laryngoscopic view is grade III, and a blind attempt at intubation is made. It is immediately apparent that the ETT is in the esophagus. The tube is removed, the head is repositioned, and a second attempt is made, resulting in another esophageal intubation. Mask ventilation has become increasingly difficult, and the SaO_2 is 80 and falling. What is the next step?

Defining the Problem

This case demonstrates the challenges of providing obstetric anesthesia care. Maternal mortality in the United States has remained approximately 7.5 maternal deaths per 100,000 live births over the last 15 years.[47] Anesthesia-related problems are the sixth leading cause of maternal mortality. General anesthesia carries a higher risk than regional anesthesia in obstetric patients, primarily because airway management is more difficult in obstetric patients. Airway problems are by far the most common cause of anesthesia-related death. The incidence of failed intubation in obstetric patients is 1:280, whereas the incidence of failed intubation in the general operating room population is 1:2230.[48] The primary causes of maternal death are related to aspiration, complications from failed or difficult intubations, local anesthetic toxicity, and high regional blocks.

The Obstetric Airway

Because of the dynamic nature of obstetrics, a thorough airway examination should be performed on every parturient who requests anesthesia services. A stable patient may quickly deteriorate and require emergent interventions. Obstetric patients have classic changes of the airway. By virtue of their age they are likely to have full dentition. Edema of the airway structures and soft tissues may limit visualization and access to the laryngeal opening. In addition to weight gain, breast tissue is enlarged and engorged and may interfere with the introduction of the laryngoscope into the patient's mouth or with the practitioner's vision during laryngoscopy. The gravid uterus pushes up against the diaphragm, making full diaphragmatic excursion difficult and decreasing the FRC of the lungs. Oxygen consumption is increased by approximately 20% during pregnancy. During active labor, it is increased an additional 23%. These factors contribute to rapid desaturation once oxygen delivery is interrupted, as it is during laryngoscopy.

Aspiration Syndrome

Hormonal changes during pregnancy delay emptying of the stomach and increase gastric volume and acid content. It is estimated that 45% of pregnant patients at term have reflux corresponding to moderate to severe heartburn. A gravid uterus can increase intragastric pressures up to 17 cm H_2O. Multiple gestations, polyhydramnios, and obesity can increase intragastric pressures up to 40 cm H_2O. Medications commonly used in anesthesia, such as narcotics, benzodiazepines, and anticholinergics, decrease the lower esophageal sphincter tone, further increasing aspiration risk.

After a failed intubation attempt, intermittent mask ventilation is necessary to provide oxygenation. Positive pressure ventilation may result in gastric insufflation, further increasing intragastric pressure. Peak airway pressures less than 15 cm H_2O rarely cause gastric insufflation. As higher pressures are required for ventilation (greater than 25 cm H$_2$O), gastric insufflation occurs. Cricoid pressure (Sellick maneuver) is used universally to decrease the incidence of passive regurgitation and to prevent gastric insufflation. Application of appropriate cricoid pressure allows the use of peak airway pressures up to approximately 45 cm H$_2$O.

Aspiration Prophylaxis

Aspiration remains a significant cause of morbidity and mortality in obstetrics. Interventions should be taken to prevent the occurrence of this potentially catastrophic complication. Whenever possible, regional anesthesia should be considered for cesarean delivery. Methods to reduce the acidity and volume of gastric contents may reduce maternal morbidity should aspiration occur. The administration of nonparticulate antacids such as sodium citrate in a 30-mL dose 10 to 20 minutes before induction of anesthesia effectively raises gastric pH. A histamine-blocking agent (e.g., ranitidine) administered preoperatively either orally or IV is effective in raising gastric pH. Metoclopramide (10 mg) accelerates gastric emptying. Although the onset of action after IV administration occurs within minutes, sufficient time must be given for gastric emptying to be complete. In a synthesis of the data from several large-scale clinical studies and revised practice recommendations, revisions in the standard practices with regard to aspiration prophylaxis were noted.[49] These included the following:

- The use of gastric fluid volume of greater than 0.4 mL/kg (25 mL/70 kg) and pH less than 2.5 should be abandoned as surrogate end-points for aspiration risk.
- Cricoid pressure as a requirement for rapid sequence induction may be beneficial as long as it is performed properly and does not impede effective airway management.
- Patients should be ventilated during a rapid sequence induction. There is no evidence that smooth, controlled light ventilation increases the incidence of aspiration. Prolonged periods of apnea should be abandoned.

SUMMARY

Airway management is a critical component of anesthesia practice. Knowledge of anatomy, equipment, and techniques is paramount if safe airway management is to be provided. Adherence to established standards and protocols including the Difficult Airway Algorithm could minimize complications. Competence and skill with a variety of airway management techniques will facilitate the appropriate management when a difficult airway situation occurs.

REFERENCES

1. Reynolds SF, Heffner J. Airway management of the critically ill patient: rapid-sequence intubation. *Chest*. 2005;124(4):1397-1412.
2. Miller CG. Management of the difficult intubation in closed malpractice claims [electronic version]. *ASA Newsl*. 2000;64:1-6. Available at: http://www.asahq.org/Newsletters/2000/06_management0600.html. Accessed Feb. 17, 2008.
3. American Society of Anesthesiologists. Practice guidelines for management of the difficult airway: an updated report by the ASA Task Force on Management of the Difficult Airway. *Anesthesiology*. 2003;98:1269-1277.
4. German RZ, Palmer JB. Anatomy and development of oral cavity and pharynx. *GI Motility online*. 16 May 2006. Available at http://www.nature.com/gimo/contents/pt1/full/gimo5.html. doi:10.1038/gimo5.
5. Lerner KL, Lerner BW. Respiratory system, embryological development. In: *World of Anatomy and Physiology*. Detroit: Thompson Gale; 2002.
6. Reed MJ et al. Can an airway assessment score predict difficulty at intubation in the emergency department? *J Emerg Med*. 2005;22:99-102.
7. Wilson ME et al. Predicting difficult intubation. *Br J Anaesth*. 1988;61: 211-216.
8. Yamamoto K et al. Predicting difficult intubation with indirect laryngoscopy. *Anesthesiology*. 1997;86:316-321.
9. Khan ZH et al. A comparison of the upper lip bite test with the Mallampati classification in predicting difficult airway in endotracheal intubation: a prospective double blind study. *Anesth Analg*. 2003;96:595-599.
10. Karkouti K et al. Predicting difficult intubation: a multivariate analysis. *Can J Anaesth*. 2000;47:730-739.
11. Karkouti K et al. Inter-observer reliability of ten tests used for predicting difficult tracheal intubation. *Can J Anaesth*. 1996;43:554-559.
12. Frerk CM et al. Difficult intubation: thyromental distance and the atlanto-occipital gap. *Anaesthesia*. 1996;51:738-740.
13. Mallampati SR et al. A clinical sign to predict difficult tracheal intubation: a prospective study. *Can J Anaesth*. 1985;32:429-434.
14. Domino KB et al. Airway injury during anesthesia: a closed claims analysis. *Anesthesiology*. 1999;91:1703-1711.
15. Crosby ET et al. The unanticipated difficult airway with recommendations for management. *Can J Anaesth*. 1998;45:757-776.
16. Reed MJ et al. Can an airway assessment score predict difficulty at intubation in the emergency department? *Emerg Med J*. 2005;22(2):99-102.
17. Hagberg CA, Benumof J. The American Society of Anesthesiologists' management of the difficult airway algorithm and explanation-analysis of the algorithm. In: Hagberg CA, ed. *Benumof's Airway Management*. 2nd ed. Philadelphia: Mosby; 2007:236-254.
18. Parkes SB et al. Plasma lignocaine concentration following nebulization for awake intubation. *Anaesth Intensive Care*. 1997;25:369-371.

19. Milman N et al. Serum concentrations of lignocaine and its metabolite mono-ethylglycinexylidide during fiber-optic bronchoscopy in local anaesthesia. *Respir Med*. 1998;92:40-43.
20. Sellick BA. Cricoid pressure to control regurgitation of stomach contents during induction of anesthesia. *Lancet*. 1961;2:404-406.
21. Herman NL et al. Cricoid pressure: teaching the recommended pressure. *Anesth Analg*. 1996;83:859-863.
22. Tournadre JP et al. Cricoid cartilage pressure decreases lower esophageal sphincter tone. *Anesthesiology*. 1997;86:7-9.
23. Lichtwarck-Aschoff M et al. Good short-term agreement between measured and calculated tracheal pressure. *Br J Anaesth*. 2003;91:239-248.
24. Asai T, Morris S. Cricoid pressure impedes placement of the laryngeal mask airway. *Br J Anaesth*. 1995;74:521-525.
25. Tanaka A et al. Laryngeal resistance before and after minor surgery: endotracheal tube versus laryngeal mask airway. *Anesthesiology*. 2003;99:252.
26. Cook TM et al. Randomized comparison of laryngeal tube with classic laryngeal mask airway for anaesthesia with controlled ventilation. *Br J Anaesth*. 2003;91:373-378.
27. Joo H, Rose K. Fastrach—a new intubating laryngeal mask airway: successful use in patients with difficult airways. *Can J Anaesth*. 1998;45:253-256.
28. Ferson DZ et al. Use of the intubating LMA-Fastrach in 254 patients with difficult to manage airways. *Anesthesiology*. 2001;95:1175-1181.
29. Fukutome T et al. Tracheal intubation through the intubating laryngeal mask airway (LMA Fastrach) in patients with difficult airways. *Anaesth Intensive Care*. 1998;26:387-391.
30. Blostein PA et al. Failed rapid sequence intubation in trauma patients: esophageal tracheal Combitube is a useful adjunct. *J Trauma*. 1998;44: 534-537.
31. Sdrales L, Benumof JL. Prevention of kinking of a percutaneous transtracheal intravenous catheter. *Anesthesiology*. 1995;82:288-291.
32. Liem EB et al. New options for airway management: intubating fiberoptic stylets. *Br J Anaesth*. 2003;91:408-418.
33. Machata AM et al. Awake nasotracheal fiberoptic intubation: patient comfort, intubating conditions, and hemodynamic stability during conscious sedation with remifentanil. *Anesth Analg*. 2003;97:904-908.
34. Jansen AH, Johnston G. The Shikani Optical Stylet: a useful adjunct to airway management in a neonate with popliteal pterygium syndrome. *Paediatr Anaesth*. 2008;18(2):188-90.
35. Sun DA, Warriner CB. The GlideScope Video Laryngoscope: randomized clinical trial in 200 patients. *Br J Anaesth*. 2005;94(3):381-384.
36. Maharaj CH et al. Retention of tracheal intubation skills by novice personnel: a comparison of the Airtraq and Macintosh laryngoscopes. *Anesthesia*. 2007;62(3):272-278.

37. Petty WC. Establish the airway; use percutaneous high-pressure transtracheal jet ventilation in an emergency [letter]. *AANA J.* 1993;61:349.

38. Somerson SJ, Sicilia MR. AANA *Journal* course: update for nurse anesthetists—beyond the laryngoscope; advanced techniques for difficult airway management. *AANA J.* 1993;61:64-71.

39. Biro P, Moe KS. Emergency transtracheal jet ventilation in high-grade airway obstruction [letter]. *J Clin Anesth.* 1997;9:604-607.

40. Smith RB et al. Percutaneous transtracheal jet ventilation [letter]. *J Clin Anesth.* 1996;8:689-690.

41. Gaughan SD et al. A comparison in a lung model of low and high flow regulators for transtracheal jet ventilation. *Anesthesiology.* 1992;77:189-199.

42. Ho AM. A simple anesthesia machine driven transtracheal jet ventilation system. *Anesth Analg.* 1994;78:405-406.

43. Gaughan SD et al. Can an anesthesia machine flush valve provide for effective jet ventilation? *Anesth Analg.* 1993;76:800-808.

44. Melker R, Orlando G. Percutaneous dilational cricothyrotomy and tracheostomy. In: Benumof JL, ed. *Airway Management: Principles of Practice.* St Louis: Mosby; 1996:484-511.

45. Weber S. Traumatic complications of airway management. *Anesthesiol Clin North America.* 2002;20:265-274.

46. Landsman IS. Mechanism and treatment of laryngospasm. *Anesthesiol Clin North America.* 2002;20:67-73.

47. Hawkins JL. Maternal mortality: anesthetic implications. *Int Anesthesiol Clin.* 2002;40:1-11.

48. Ross BK. ASA closed claims in obstetrics: lessons learned. *Anesthesiol Clin North America.* 2003;21:183-197.

49. Nagelhout JJ. AANA *Journal* course update for nurse anesthetists. Aspiration prophylaxis: is it time for some changes in our practice? *AANA J.* 2003;71:299-303.

CARDIOVASCULAR ANATOMY, PHYSIOLOGY, PATHOPHYSIOLOGY, AND ANESTHESIA MANAGEMENT

Sass Elisha

CARDIOVASCULAR SYSTEM

Knowledge of anatomy and physiology of the cardiovascular system is essential to anesthesia practice. Every anesthetic agent has either a direct or an indirect effect on the cardiovascular system. Therefore whether the nurse anesthetist is concerned about a sympathectomy and a decrease in blood pressure during neuraxial blockade or about myocardial depression during inhalation anesthesia, a thorough understanding of these effects and their implications with regard to human physiology is vital if competent anesthesia care is to be provided.

The cardiovascular system is composed of the heart and the vasculature that carries blood to provide nutrients to all cells in the body. In addition, the cardiovascular system transports substances such as hormones and electrolytes from one part of the body to another.

At the center of this network is the heart. The heart pumps unoxygenated blood to the lungs and then supplies oxygenated blood to all parts of the body. This chapter describes the anatomic and physiologic characteristics, as well as pathophysiologic changes, associated with the cardiovascular system.

Heart

Gross Anatomy

The heart is bound anteriorly by the sternum and the costal cartilages of the third, fourth, and fifth ribs and inferiorly by the diaphragm. It is positioned with the apex projecting anteriorly and inferiorly toward the left fifth intercostal space at the midclavicular line. At this location, the pulsation from the cardiac apex may be palpated. This is known as the *point of maximal impulse*. The first heart sound (S_1) is best auscultated in this area. A third (S_3) or fourth (S_4) heart sound, if present, can also be heard in this location. Heart sounds are generated from the vibrations caused by the closure of the semilunar and atrioventricular (AV) valves.[1]

Cardiac Silhouette

The superior aspect of the cardiac silhouette is formed by the transverse and ascending aortas. The right lateral border is composed of the right atrium (RA), and the mass of the right ventricle (RV) constitutes most of the inferior border. The left ventricle (LV) comprises the majority of the apex and the lower left lateral border. The left atrial appendage lies superior to the

LV and to one side of the pulmonary artery. This appendage may be seen radiographically between the LV and the pulmonary outflow tract. The heart is rotated on its base such that the anterior surface is almost entirely made up of the RV. The base of the heart is the most superior portion of the cardiac silhouette.

Pericardium

The heart is situated within the mediastinum and surrounded by a fibrous, double-walled sac called the *pericardium*,[2] which envelops the heart and the roots of the great vessels. It consists of a visceral portion, which is in intimate contact with the outer surface of the heart (epicardium), and an outer parietal portion, which is adherent to the fibrous pericardium (Figure 24-1).

The fibrous pericardium is pierced superiorly by the aorta, the pulmonary trunk, and the superior vena cava. The base of the fibrous pericardium is fused with the central tendon of the diaphragm. The visceral pericardium and parietal pericardium are separated by a thin potential space known as the *pericardial cavity*. This space normally contains approximately 10 to 25 mL of serous fluid, which provides lubrication for the free movement of the heart within the mediastinum. In disease states, the pericardial space can fill with blood, compress the heart, and decrease cardiac output (CO). In acute cardiac tamponade, the volume rapidly increases, producing myocardial dysfunction. In contrast, in chronic cardiac tamponade, the degree of pressure exerted on the heart increases slowly because the pericardial sac stretches to accommodate the blood that accumulates over time. However, the pressure may eventually increase as much as 10-fold before symptoms of cardiac tamponade occur.[3]

The pericardium receives its arterial blood supply from the branches of the internal thoracic arteries and through the bronchial, esophageal, and superior phrenic arteries. Venous drainage from the pericardium occurs through the azygos system and the pericardiophrenic veins, which anastomose with the internal thoracic veins. Nervous innervation to the pericardium is derived from the vagus nerve, the phrenic nerves, and the sympathetic trunks.

Surface Anatomy

The atria are separated from the ventricles by the coronary sulcus (AV sulcus), as seen in Figure 24-2, A. The right coronary artery travels within this sulcus. The circumflex artery arises from the left coronary artery and travels in the coronary sulcus until it branches posteriorly. The RV and LV are separated by the interventricular sulci, which descend from the coronary sulcus to the apex. The interventricular sulci are composed of an anterior interventricular sulcus and a posterior interventricular sulcus. The anterior interventricular sulcus contains the left anterior descending (LAD) artery, which courses over the interventricular septum and continues in the posterior interventricular sulcus.

The crux of the heart is the place at which the coronary and the posterior interventricular sulci meet. Internally, it is where the atrial and ventricular septa meet (Figure 24-2, *B*). This anatomic crux is important in determining coronary artery dominance.

Cardiac Skeleton

Essential to a discussion of the chambers of the heart is a description of the fibrous skeleton, the annulus fibrosus (Figure 24-3). Tough fibrous rings surround the AV valves and act as points of attachment for the valves. Two additional fibrous annuli develop in relation to the bases of the aorta and the pulmonary trunk. The aortic fibrous annulus is connected to the pulmonary annulus by a fibrous band called the *tendon of the conus*. The aortic annulus is connected to the AV annuli by the small left fibrous trigone and the larger right fibrous trigone, also called the *central*

fibrous body. The four annuli and their interconnections constitute the fibrous cardiac skeleton.

The annulus fibrosus is the fixation point for the cardiac musculature and plays an important role in the structure, function, and efficiency of the heart. The annulus acts as an insulator to prevent aberrant electrical conduction from the atria to the ventricles so that AV conduction moves through one pathway only: the AV node to the bundle of His. This element increases the electromechanical efficiency of the heart and helps prevent dysrhythmias.

Chambers of the Heart

Right Atrium. The atria act as the priming chambers for the ventricles. As such, the RA acts as a reservoir for the RV and has unique anatomic characteristics. It has a muscle wall thickness of approximately 2 μm.

The RA receives blood from several sources: the superior vena cava, the inferior vena cava, and the coronary sinus (Figure 24-4). The RA consists of two parts: an anterior, thin-walled trabeculated portion and a posterior, smooth-walled portion called the *sinus venarum*. The sinus venarum receives blood from the venae cavae and the coronary sinus. The auricle projects to the left from the root of the superior vena cava and overlaps the root of the ascending aorta.

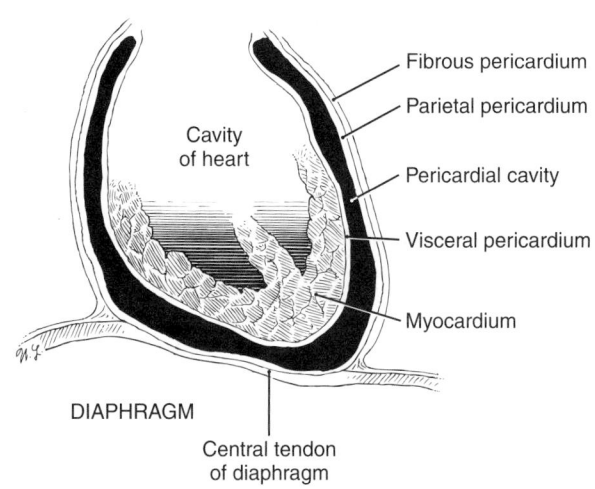

FIGURE **24-1**   The pericardium.

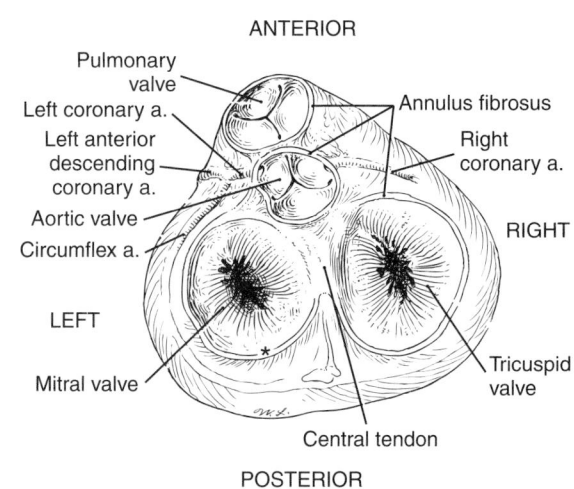

FIGURE **24-3**   The annulus fibrosus. *a.*, Artery.

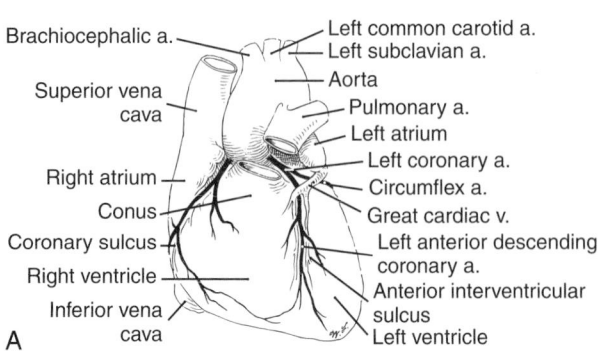

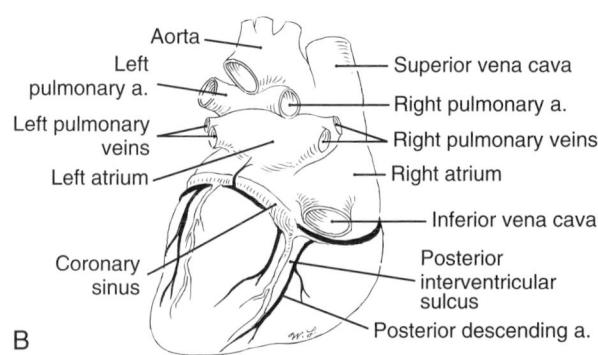

FIGURE **24-2**   **A,** Surface anatomy of the heart (anterior view). **B,** Surface anatomy of the heart (posterior view). *a.*, Artery; *v.*, vein.

The superior vena cava returns blood to the RA from the upper body. The inferior vena cava returns blood to the RA from the lower body. The entrance of the inferior vena cava into the RA is protected by a rudimentary valve called the *eustachian valve*.[4]

The entrance from the coronary sinus into the RA is located between the AV orifice and the valve of the inferior vena cava. This opening is protected in part by a rudimentary valve of the coronary sinus called the *thebesian valve*.[5] Other distinguishing structures in the RA include the interatrial septum and the fossa ovalis cordis, which is the remnant of the fetal foramen ovale within the septum.

Right Ventricle. The RV ejects blood into the pulmonary arteries for oxygenation and removal of carbon dioxide by the lungs. The RV communicates with the RA through the AV orifice, which is guarded by the tricuspid valve. The RV also communicates with the pulmonary outflow tract through the pulmonary orifice, which is guarded by the pulmonic valve (see Figure 24-4).

The walls of the RV are much thicker (4 to 5 mm) than those of the RA because of the increased pressures required to generate forward blood flow into the pulmonary circulation. The superior portion of the RV as it approaches the pulmonary orifice has a conical appearance and is called the conus arteriosus or infundibulum.[6]

The inner wall of the conus is smooth, but the remainder of the right ventricular wall has a rough appearance because of the presence of several irregular muscular bundles called the *papillary muscles* and the *trabeculae carneae*. One of the trabeculae carneae (the moderator band) crosses the cavity of the ventricles and carries the right branch of the AV bundle. The papillary muscles have attachments to the ventricular walls and to the chordae tendineae. The chordae tendineae are attached to the cusps of the tricuspid valve; together with the papillary muscles, they help prevent eversion of the tricuspid valve into the RA during ventricular systole.[7]

Left Atrium. The left atrium (LA) acts as a reservoir for oxygenated blood from the pulmonary veins and also as a pump during ventricular diastole. It provides a 20% to 30% increase in left ventricular end-diastolic volume (LVEDV), which is known as the *atrial kick*. A person who has normal myocardial performance does not rely on this increase in ventricular filling to achieve adequate CO. However, in certain cardiovascular or respiratory pathologic conditions, compromised patients rely on this atrial kick to maintain an adequate CO. The LA is located superiorly and posteriorly to the other cardiac chambers. The walls of the LA are slightly thicker (3 μm) than those of the RA. The LA connects to the LV through the left AV orifice, which contains the mitral valve. The atrial septum is smooth but may contain a central depression that corresponds to the location of the fossa ovalis cordis.

Left Ventricle. The apex of the LV is positioned within the mediastinum in an anterior and inferior orientation. The LV receives blood from the LA and ejects it into the aorta. Left ventricular wall thickness is approximately 8 to 15 mm, or two to three times the thickness of the RV. This additional muscle mass is required to overcome the systemic vascular resistance (SVR), or afterload, to maintain CO.

The ventricular septum separates the right and left ventricular cavities.[8] The upper third of the septum is smooth endocardium. The remaining two thirds of the septum and the rest of the ventricular wall are covered with trabeculae carneae.

Two large papillary muscles are present within the LV. The anterior papillary muscle attaches to the anterior part of the left ventricular wall, and the posterior papillary muscle arises from the posterior aspect of the inferior wall. The chordae tendineae of each muscle are attached to the cusps of the mitral valve and prevent eversion of the valve during ventricular systole.

Myocardium

Cardiac musculature comprises three distinct layers: an outer epicardium, a middle muscular myocardium, and an inner endocardium. The epicardium is composed of mesothelium, connective tissue, and fat. The middle muscular myocardium consists of two muscle layers—a superficial and a deep layer. These layers are arranged in a spiral fashion and appear on cross-section to run at right angles to each other. It has been postulated that the superficial and deep layers of the myocardium are not two separate layers but one tortuous and continuous layer. The arrangement of the muscle layers provides strength during contraction of the myocardium and efficient propulsion of blood toward the semilunar valves. The endocardium consists of endothelium and a layer of connective tissue.

Valves

The cardiac valves increase the heart's efficiency by ensuring a one-way flow of blood through the circuit. They open and close in response to pressure gradients that exist above or below the valves. These valves may be categorized as AV or semilunar in configuration.

One of the most accurate ways to determine the presence of valvular pathology is by calculating valve area. The standard method for determining valve area is by cardiac catheterization. A cardiologist is able to determine valve gradients using the Gorlin formula or its correction, which can provide information regarding the degree of pathology that exists.[9]

Equation 24-1

$$\text{Valve area} = \frac{\text{Flow across valve}}{K \times \sqrt{\text{Mean transvalvular gradient}}}$$

Where valve area is expressed in cm^2, blood flow across the mitral valve is expressed in mL/s, K is a hydraulic pressure constant, and mean transvalvular gradient is expressed in mm Hg.

Echocardiography is a noninvasive method of determining valve area and is used in the diagnosis of valvular heart disease.

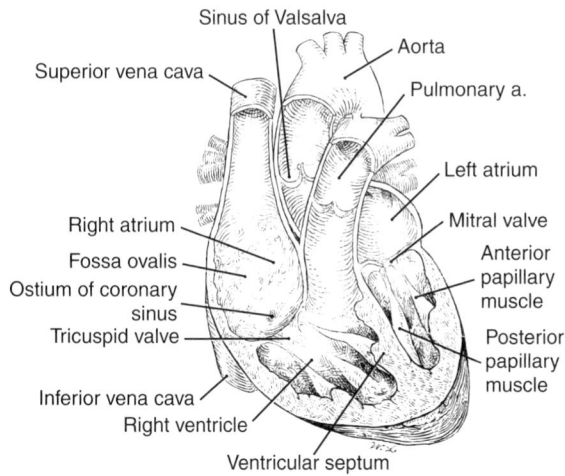

Sinus of Valsalva
Aorta
Superior vena cava
Pulmonary a.
Left atrium
Mitral valve
Right atrium
Anterior papillary muscle
Fossa ovalis
Ostium of coronary sinus
Posterior papillary muscle
Tricuspid valve
Inferior vena cava
Right ventricle
Ventricular septum

FIGURE **24-4** Internal anatomy of the heart chambers. *a.,* Artery.

The use of echocardiography will be discussed later in this chapter.

Atrioventricular Valves

Tricuspid Valve. The tricuspid valve is situated within the right AV orifice, which lies between the RA and the RV. The tricuspid leaflets are thinner and more translucent than the mitral valve and more easily separated into well-defined leaflets. Three leaflets of unequal size exist: the anterior, septal, and posterior leaflets. The leaflets are attached to the chordae tendineae, which are attached to the papillary muscles.[10] The normal tricuspid valve area is approximately 7 cm². Symptoms of tricuspid insufficiency occur when the valve area is less than 1.5 cm².

Mitral Valve. The mitral valve is situated in the left AV orifice between the LA and the LV. Two major leaflets, the anteromedial leaflet and the posterolateral leaflet, are connected by commissural tissue. The normal mitral valve area is 4 to 6 cm². When the surface area of the valve is decreased by half, clinical symptoms may appear. Like the tricuspid valve, the mitral valve has papillary muscles and chordae tendineae attached to the leaflets to prevent eversion of the valve during ventricular systole.[11]

Semilunar Valves. The configuration of the aortic and pulmonary valves is similar. The cusps of the aortic valve are slightly thicker because it is subjected to greater pressures, which are created by left ventricular ejection. The semilunar valves are situated within the outflow tracts of their corresponding ventricles. Each valve is composed of three cusps. Above the aortic valve is a dilation known as the *sinus of Valsalva*, which allows the valve to open efficiently without occluding the ostia or openings that communicate with the coronary arteries. Eddy currents form behind the valve leaflets and prevent contact between the valve leaflets and the walls of the aorta. The normal valve area of the aortic valve is 2.5 to 3.5 cm². Reduction of the valve area by one third to one half is associated with an increase in the symptoms caused by aortic stenosis.

Coronary Circulation

The heart is an aerobic organ that depends on a constant supply of oxygen to meet its high metabolic demand. It requires an elaborate arterial and venous network to ensure that myocytes are adequately supplied with oxygen. The arterial system consists of epicardial and subendocardial vessels. The epicardial vessels are located superficially and most commonly become obstructed at areas of bifurcation where the blood flow is turbulent rather than laminar. Significant obstruction (50% reduction in luminal diameter) can result in myocardial ischemia or infarction as a result of increased resistance to flow across the stenotic areas.

Coronary Arteries. The ostia of the two coronary arteries are located behind the aortic cusps near the superior part of the sinus of Valsalva. The ostium of the left coronary artery is superior and posterior to the right coronary ostium. The coronary arteries act as end arteries, and each supplies blood to its respective capillary bed[12] (Figure 24-5).

Left Main Coronary Artery. The left main coronary artery travels anteriorly, inferiorly, and leftward from the left coronary sinus to emerge from behind the pulmonary trunk. Within 2 to 10 µm of its emergence, the left main coronary artery divides into two or more branches of near-equal diameter. The branches include the LAD artery, the left circumflex coronary artery, and possibly the diagonal branch.

Left Anterior Descending Coronary Artery. The LAD is a continuation of the left main coronary artery. The branches of this vessel include the first diagonal branch, the first septal

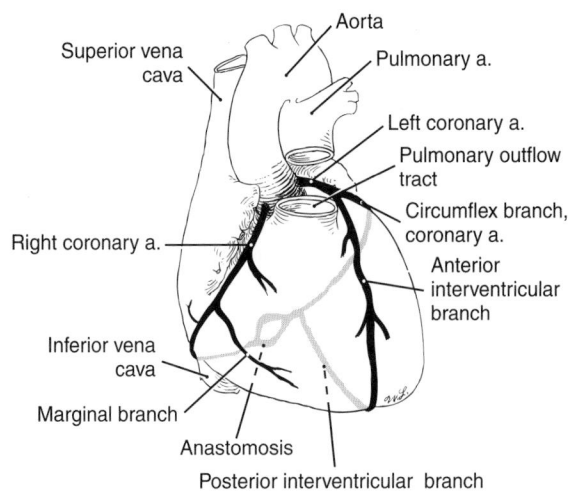

FIGURE **24-5**   The coronary arterial circulation. *a.*, Artery.

perforator, the right ventricular branches (not always observed), other septal perforators, and other diagonal branches. The LAD provides blood flow to the anterior two thirds of the interventricular septum, the right and left bundle branches, the anterior and posterior papillary muscles of the mitral valve, and the anterior lateral and apical walls of the LV. The LAD also provides collateral circulation to the anterior wall of the RV.

Left Circumflex Coronary Artery. The left circumflex artery arises from the left main coronary artery at an obtuse angle and is directed posteriorly as it travels around the left side of the heart within the left AV sulcus. Branches are variable and may include the sinus node artery (40% to 50% of the population), the left atrial circumflex artery, the anterolateral marginal artery, the distal circumflex artery, one or more posterolateral marginal arteries, and the posterior descending artery (10% to 15% of the population). The circumflex artery supplies blood to the left atrial wall, the posterior and lateral LV, the anterolateral papillary muscle, the AV node in 10% of the population, and the sinoatrial (SA) node in 40% to 45% of the population.

Right Coronary Artery. The right coronary artery supplies blood to the SA and AV nodes, the RA and RV, the posterior third of the interventricular septum, the posterior fascicle of the left bundle branch, and the interatrial septum. In approximately 90% of the population, the right coronary artery leaves the right coronary sinus and descends in the right AV groove. At the crux, the right coronary artery courses inferiorly in the posterior AV groove and terminates as a left ventricular branch.

The branches of the right coronary artery include the conus artery, the sinus node artery (50% to 60% of the population), several anterior right ventricular branches, the right atrial branches, the acute marginal branch, the AV node artery (90% of the population), the proximal bundle branches, the posterior descending artery, and the terminal branches to the LA and LV.

Coronary Artery Dominance. Dominance of one coronary artery is determined by the coronary artery that crosses the crux and provides blood flow to the posterior descending artery. The dominant coronary artery in 50% of the general population is the right coronary. In addition, 10% to 15% of the general population are left coronary dominant, and 35% to 40% of the general population have mixed right and left dominance.

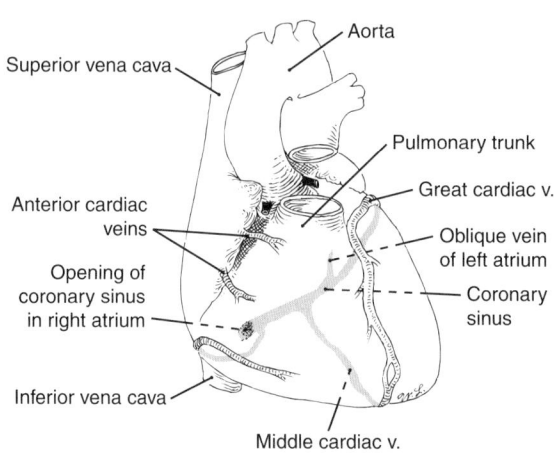

FIGURE **24-6** The coronary venous system. *v.*, Vein.

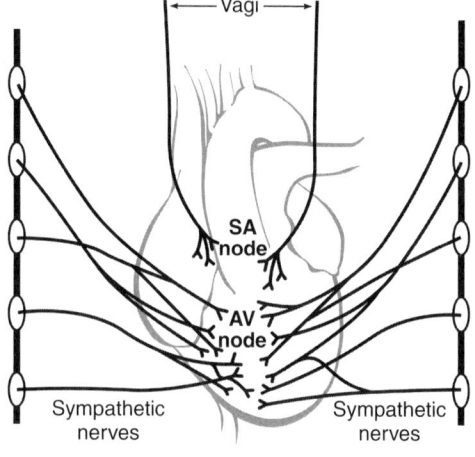

FIGURE **24-7** Distribution of sympathetic and parasympathetic innervation to the heart.

Venous Drainage. An extensive venous system exists in the heart. The three major systems include the coronary sinus, the anterior cardiac veins, and the thebesian veins (Figure 24-6).

The coronary sinus is located in the posterior AV groove near the crux. It collects approximately 85% of the blood from the LV, and for this reason it is catheterized when metabolic studies of the LV are performed. It may also be cannulated during cardiopulmonary bypass to deliver cardioplegia. The coronary sinus receives blood from the great, middle, and small cardiac veins; the posterior left ventricular veins; and the left atrial vein of Marshall.

Two to four anterior cardiac veins drain the anterior right ventricular wall. These veins may enter the RA directly, or they may empty into the coronary sinus.

The thebesian veins traverse the myocardium and drain into the various chambers, especially the RA, the RV, and to a lesser extent the LV. The thebesian veins may carry up to 40% of the blood that is returned to the RA.

Cardiac Innervation

The autonomic nervous system is divided into the sympathetic and parasympathetic nervous systems. Efferent impulses are transmitted from the brainstem and hypothalamus to numerous body systems, including the heart. The neurologic innervation to the heart originates from the autonomic nervous system, as well as from sensory fibers. The myocardium also has a specialized conduction system that is discussed in this chapter.

Increased sympathetic nervous system tone increases heart rate (chronotropic), force of myocardial contraction (inotropic), and rate of sinus node discharge (dromotropic). Sympathetic nervous system activation results in the mobilization of myocardial fat free acids and glycogen for energy use by the myocardial cells. The preganglionic sympathetic nervous system fibers originate from the cells in the intermediolateral columns of the higher thoracic segments of the spinal cord and synapse at the first through the fourth or fifth thoracic paravertebral ganglia. These spinal cord segments are known as the *cardioaccelerator fibers*. The postganglionic fibers then travel as the superior, middle, and inferior cardiac nerves and the thoracic visceral nerves. These fibers form an epicardial plexus and are distributed over the entire ventricular myocardium. There is greater distribution of sympathetic nerves to the ventricles, resulting in

increased ventricular contractility, as is shown in Figure 24-7. Catecholamines released during sympathetic stimulation bind with adrenergic receptors on the heart (primarily B_1) and change the biochemical properties within the myocyte. This process is discussed later in this chapter.

Some of these postganglionic sympathetic fibers also join with the postganglionic parasympathetic fibers from the cardiac plexus and primarily innervate the SA and AV nodes and the atrial myocardium. Suppression or blockade of this thoracic portion of the spinal cord by regional anesthesia causes bradycardia and hypotension as a result of the blockade of these sympathetic ganglia parasympathetic nervous system predominance.

The preganglionic parasympathetic fibers originate in the dorsal motor nucleus of the medulla. Short postganglionic fibers primarily innervate the SA and AV nodes and the atrial muscle fibers (see Figure 24-7). For this reason, increased parasympathetic tone decreases heart rate (HR). The function of the parasympathetic nervous system is primarily to slow the HR and secondarily to decrease contractility. In fact, maximal vagal (parasympathetic) stimulation reduces contractility by only 30%, whereas maximal sympathetic stimulation increases contractility by 100%. Acetylcholine is the neurotransmitter of the parasympathetic nervous system. Acetylcholine binds to muscarinic receptors on the heart and decreases the rate of sinus node discharge and slows conduction velocity through the AV node. The physiologic effects of parasympathetic nervous system stimulation occur because of increased permeability of cardiac muscle cell membranes to potassium, resulting in hyperpolarization. As a result, SA and AV node cells are less excitable.

Sensory innervation to the heart originates in the nerve endings in the walls of the heart, the coronary artery adventitia, and the pericardium. These nerve endings synapse with ascending fibers in the posterior gray columns of the spinal cord, where the fibers synapse with second-order neurons. From these neurons, the fibers ascend in the ventral spinothalamic tract and terminate in the posteroventral nucleus of the thalamus.

Cardiac Conduction System

Within the myocardium lies the specialized conduction system whose purpose is to automatically initiate and coordinate the cardiac rhythm. The cells of this system differ from the other

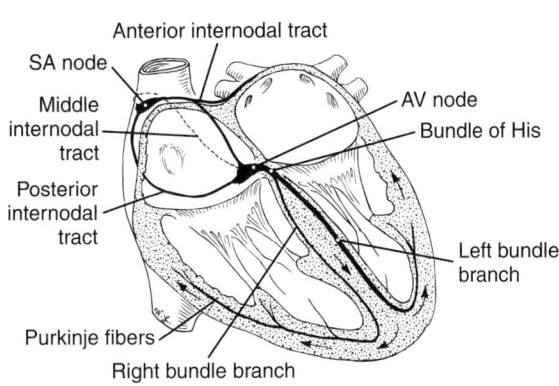

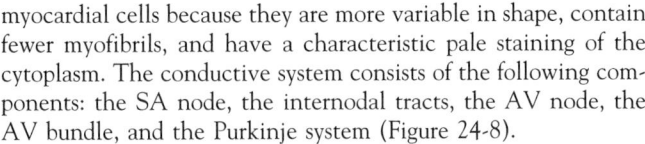

FIGURE **24-8**   The cardiac conduction system. AV, Atrioventricular; SA, sinoatrial.

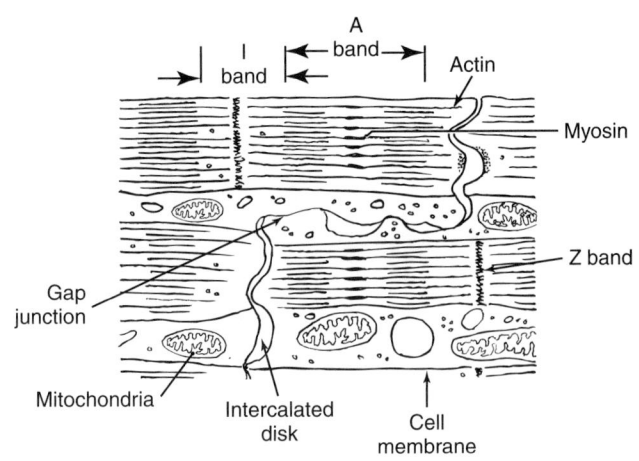

FIGURE **24-9**   The myocardial sarcomere.

myocardial cells because they are more variable in shape, contain fewer myofibrils, and have a characteristic pale staining of the cytoplasm. The conductive system consists of the following components: the SA node, the internodal tracts, the AV node, the AV bundle, and the Purkinje system (Figure 24-8).

Sinoatrial Node. The SA node (the Keith-Flack node) is a small mass of specialized cells and collagenous tissue located along the epicardial surface at the junction of the superior vena cava and the RA. It has a prominent central artery that is a branch of the right coronary artery. The SA node is derived from the junction of the right horn of the sinus venosus and the primitive atrium. The SA node consists of two cell types: P cells (pacemaker cells), which are pale and ovoid with large round nuclei, and intermediate or transitional cells, which are elongated. These transitional cells are intermediate between ovoid and ordinary cells. They conduct impulses within and away from the SA node.

Internodal Tracts. The internodal tracts are located within the atria and are the preferential conduction pathways between the SA and the AV nodes. They are composed of a combination of closely packed parallel myocardial fibers and large pale-staining cells with a perinuclear clear zone. They have large nuclei and sparse myofibrils that resemble the Purkinje cells. Like the SA node, the internodal tracts contain P cells and transitional cells.

Three major internodal tracts exist: the anterior, middle, and posterior internodal tracts. The anterior internodal tract, or Bachmann bundle, sends fibers to the LA and then travels down through the atrial septum to the AV node. The middle internodal tract, or Wenckebach tract, curves behind the superior vena cava before descending to the AV node. Finally, the posterior internodal tract, or Thorel tract, continues along the terminal crest to enter the atrial septum and then passes to the AV node.

Atrioventricular Node. The AV node is located beneath the endocardium on the right side of the atrial septum, anterior to the opening of the coronary sinus. The AV node is supplied by an abundance of nerve endings, as well as vagal (ganglionic) cells. The AV node causes a delay in the transmission of action potentials. This delay may be attributed to several factors, such as the size of the AV nodal cells (smaller than the surrounding atrial cells), a decreased distribution of gap junctions between cells, a resting membrane potential that is *more negative*

than the normal resting membrane potentials of the surrounding cells, and the paucity of gap junctions. Greater resistance to the transmission of an action potential exists within the AV node.

Atrioventricular Bundle. The AV bundle (bundle of His) extends from the lower end of the AV node and enters the posterior part of the ventricle and the Purkinje system. This AV bundle is the preferential channel for conduction of the action potential from the atria to the ventricles.

Purkinje System. The Purkinje system consists of the bundle branch system and its terminal branches. The left bundle branch extends outward under the endocardium and forms several fascicles, which innervate various parts of the LV. The anterior fascicle innervates the anterolateral wall of the LV and the anterior papillary muscle. The posterior fascicle innervates the lateral and posterior ventricular wall and the posterior papillary muscle. The anterior and posterior fascicles join to form the septal fascicle, which innervates the lower ventricular septum and the apical wall of the LV.

The right bundle branch travels under the endocardium along the right side of the ventricular septum to the base of the anterior papillary muscle.

Structural and Regulatory Proteins. The myocardium has characteristics of both skeletal and smooth muscle. Like smooth muscle, cardiac muscle fibers are interconnected (syncytial), which allows for an action potential to rapidly spread to adjacent cells. Because of this characteristic of cardiac muscle fibers, action potential propagation and muscle contraction occur as an "all-or-none" response.

The myocardial cell is similar to skeletal muscle in that it is composed of sarcomeres (Figure 24-9). These sarcomeres contain all the microfilaments and structures that are consistent with the skeletal muscle sarcomere. The sarcomere stretches from Z line to Z line. The A bands consist of the actin filaments, which contain a bilayer filament of F-actin and tropomyosin. Along the actin filament, many active sites exist that can attach to the head of the myosin molecule. A troponin complex is necessary to inhibit actin and myosin from interacting and initiating muscle contraction. The other microfilament in the cardiac muscle is the myosin molecule. This molecule is made up of two major parts: a light meromyosin chain and a heavy meromyosin chain. The heavy meromyosin chain consists of two hinged ends and a head that plays a role in the "ratchet theory" of muscle contraction (Figure 24-10).[1]

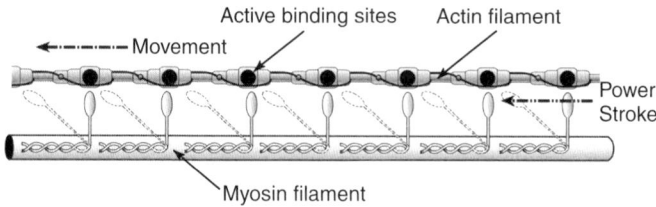

FIGURE **24-10** Interaction between actin and myosin that initiates cardiac muscle contraction.

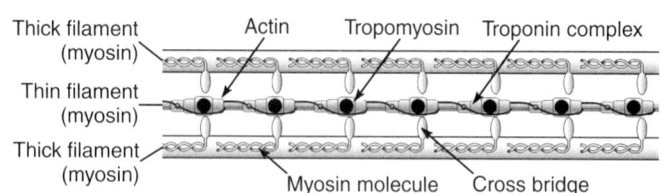

FIGURE **24-11** Arrangement of actin and myosin in cardiac muscle.

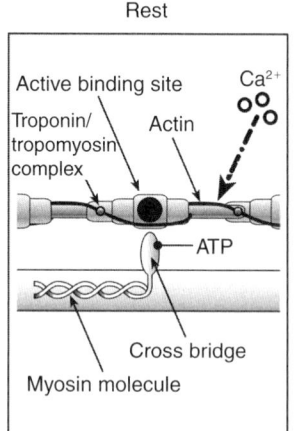 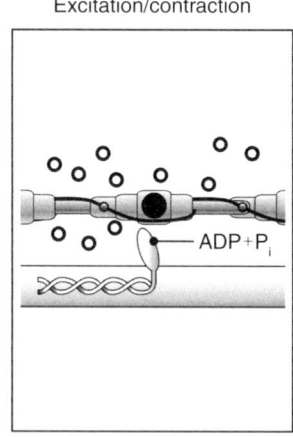 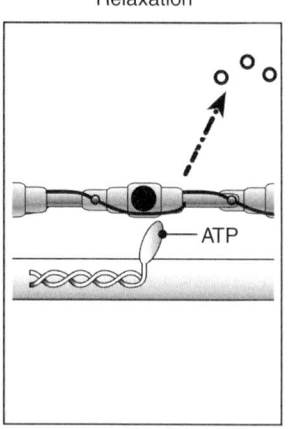

FIGURE **24-12** Phases of cardiac muscle contraction.

During sympathetic nervous system stimulation, catecholamines (primarily epinephrine and norepinephrine) are released from the central nervous system and the adrenal medulla. Increased cardiac conduction velocity, increased force of contraction, and increased heart rate are primarily mediated by beta$_1$ (β_1)-adrenergic receptors. When catecholamine hormones interact with β_1 receptors, they stimulate G protein activation. Adenyl cyclase activity increases and catalyzes the formation of cyclic adenosine monophosphate (cAMP). Specific protein kinase is formed, and phosphorylation occurs, increasing myocardial cell permeability to calcium and sodium. Threshold potential is reached, and depolarization occurs, which increases the concentration of calcium from the sarcoplasmic reticulum and the transverse tubular system. Calcium interacts with the troponin tropomyosin complex to initiate cardiac contraction. The force of myocardial contraction is dependent on the quantity of calcium present in the cardiac cell.

Evidence indicates that the troponin-tropomyosin complex inhibits the binding of the heads of the myosin filaments with the active sites on the actin molecule (Figure 24-11). During the initiation of contraction, calcium is released from the sarcoplasmic reticulum. Calcium binds to the troponin-tropomyosin complex and causes a conformational change so that the active binding sites on the actin filaments become exposed. The myosin cross bridges bind to the active filament and move along the actin filament by alternately attaching and detaching from the active sites, thereby causing shortening of the Z lines (Figure 24-12). This is known as the *sliding filament theory*. When the actin filaments and myosin cross bridges intermingle, muscle contraction occurs. Inhibition of calcium influx into the cardiac muscle cells is the proposed mechanism whereby the inhaled anesthetic agents cause depression of myocardial contractility.

Cellular energy or adenosine triphosphate (ATP) is required for this process, known as *excitation-contraction coupling*, to occur, as shown in For muscle contraction to cease, calcium reuptake into the sarcoplasmic reticulum occurs as a result of active transport. The troponin tropomyosin complex reinhibits the interaction between actin and myosin. That this process occurs constantly and within milliseconds is the primary reason for the heart's high metabolic demands (Figure 24-13). With a limited supply of oxygen and substrate (primarily fatty acids), such as with patients with coronary artery disease or an increased energy demand caused by tachycardia from sympathetic nervous system stimulation, myocardial dysfunction and infarction can occur.

Similar length-force relationships exist within the myocardium and in skeletal muscle. The resting sarcomere length at which the muscle cell is most efficient is 2 to 2.4 μm. At greater lengths, the interdigitation of the actin and myosin is compromised, and at shorter lengths the sarcomere is unable to generate an efficient contraction.

Clinically this concept is demonstrated by the ideal filling pressure of the LV necessary to achieve adequate CO. Filling pressures are used to reflect the filling volumes of the ventricles and (indirectly) the amount of stretch on the ventricular muscle at rest. Filling pressures are measured by the use of the pulmonary capillary wedge pressure (PCWP) or the pulmonary artery diastolic pressure. It has been demonstrated that at excessively high filling pressures (as in congestive heart failure) and at excessively low filling pressures (as in hypovolemia) the CO can be compromised as a result of either excessive or inadequate stretch of the left ventricular myocardium. The greater the degree of stretch of myocardial muscle fibers, the greater the number of actin filaments and myosin cross bridges that are more completely approximated. This will result in an increase in the force of cardiac contraction, as shown in Figure 24-14. This concept is the basis for the Frank-Starling law of the heart, which is discussed later in this chapter.

Differences Between Skeletal and Cardiac Muscle Cells. Several differences exist between myocardial muscle cells and skeletal muscle cells (see Figure 24-9). At the junctions between the fibers in the myocardial muscle mass, many branching, interconnected fibers are intercalated disks and gap junctions, or nexi. Areas of low resistance facilitate the conduction of the action potential from one myocardial cell to another.

The myocardial sarcomeres also contain higher concentrations of mitochondria than do other types of muscle cells. The cardiac cells are aerobic and cannot tolerate oxygen deficiency. Skeletal muscles can function both aerobically and anaerobically.

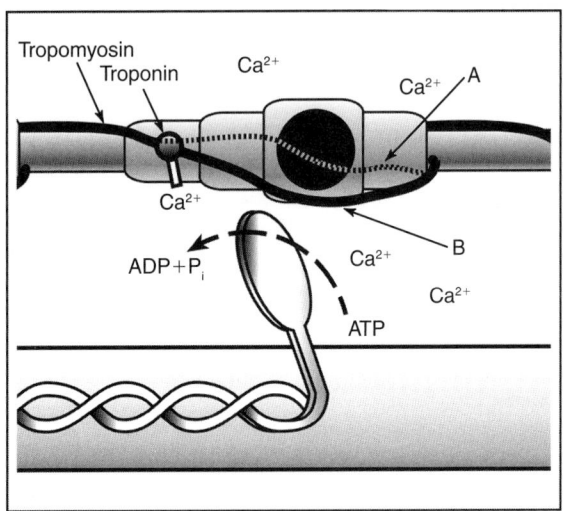

FIGURE **24-13** Letter A (dotted line) indicates that the troponin tropomyosin complex blocks the active binding site and inhibits contraction. Letter B (solid line) indicates that when calcium interacts with troponin, there is a conformational change. The troponin tropomyosin is displaced, and interaction between actin and myosin initiates muscle contraction. Note that ATP is used during the binding, the power stroke, and the unbinding process.

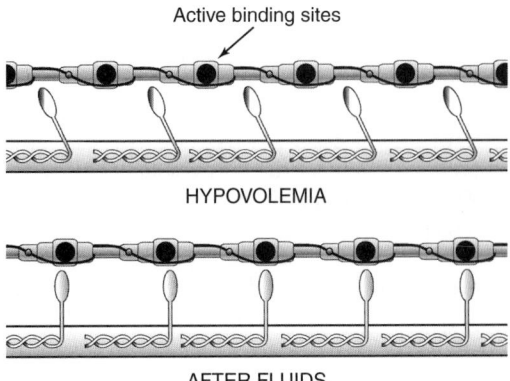

FIGURE **24-14** Greater alignment of actin binding sites and myosin cross bridges causes increased myocardial contractility.

The myocardial sarcomere system has a rich capillary supply (one capillary per fiber) that allows for efficient diffusion and perfusion. The T-tubular system and the sarcoplasmic reticulum are extensive within the cardiac sarcomere. This situation allows for the rapid release and reabsorption of calcium from the cells. It also serves to highlight the important role extracellular calcium plays in the contractile process of the myocardial cell.

Generation of Membrane Potentials

Resting Membrane Potentials. The myocardial sarcomere is not merely a contractile entity. It also possesses properties common to neural tissue, such as the generation of a resting membrane potential, the ability to generate an action potential, and the conduction of the action potential from one sarcomere to the next.

The resting cell membrane is relatively permeable to potassium and relatively impermeable to both sodium and calcium. The resting membrane potential is caused by a chemical force, an electrostatic counterforce, and the sodium-potassium active transport pump.

The chemical force relies on the potential difference in ion concentration between one side of the cell membrane and the other. The ions primarily responsible for this force are sodium, potassium, and calcium.[13] The electrostatic counterforce results from the negative potential generated by the ion difference of the interior of the cell. This force can pull ions into the cell, especially potassium.

The sodium-potassium pump requires an energy source (active transport) and involves the magnesium-dependent enzyme adenosine triphosphatase located in the cell membrane. Three molecules of sodium are pumped out of the cell into the extracellular fluid for every two molecules of potassium pumped into the intracellular fluid.

Calculation of the equilibrium potential (E_m, measured in millivolts) has been accomplished by examining the concentration of an ion inside the cell versus outside the cell (see the Nernst equation that follows). Table 24-1 lists the equilibrium potentials of the most physiologically important ions. The ion most responsible for the resting membrane potential is potassium.

Equation 24-2

$$E_m = (-RT/FZ) \times \log[K]_i/[K]_o$$

where R is a gas constant, T is temperature in Kelvin, F is Faraday's constant, $[K]_i$ is the intracellular concentration of potassium, and $[K]_o$ is the extracellular concentration of potassium.

TABLE **24-1**	Equilibrium Potential of Various Ions		
Ion	Intracellular Concentration (mmol)	Extracellular Plasma Concentration (mmol)	Equilibrium Potential E_m (mV)
Na$^+$	10	145	60
K$^+$	135	4	−94
Cl$^-$	4	114	−97
Ca^{2+}	10^{-4}	2	132

If a temperature of 310° K is assumed for a living human, the Nernst equation reduces to the following in a human heart:

Equation 24-3

$$E_m = (-61.5/Z) \times \log[K]_i/[K]_o$$

The Nernst potential is useful only in discussions of a single ion. The membrane potentials are generated because the cell membrane is permeable to several different ions. Three factors affect the calculation of the effect of these different ions on the resting membrane potential: the electric charge of each ion, the permeability of the membrane to each ion, and the concentration gradient across the membrane. The following equation, the Goldman-Hodgkin-Katz equation, is a modification of the Nernst equation that accounts for these factors.

Equation 24-4

$$EMF = 61.5 \times \log ([Na]_i P_{Na} + [K]_i P_K + [Cl]_o P_{Cl})/$$

$$([Na]_o P_{Na}[K]_o P_K[Cl]_i P_{Cl})$$

where $[K]_i$ is the intracellular ion concentration of potassium, $[K]_o$ is the extracellular ion concentration of potassium, and P_K is the membrane permeability of potassium.

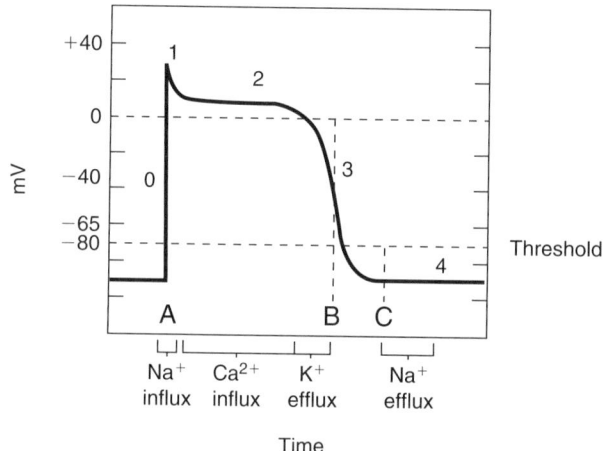

FIGURE **24-15** The ventricular muscle action potential. *A* to *B*, Absolute refractory period; *B* to *C*, relative refractory period; *0*, depolarization; *1*, overshoot; *2*, plateau; *3*, repolarization (rapid); *4*, repolarization (complete).

Ventricular Muscle Fiber Action Potential

Gate Theory. Several electrostatic gates have been elucidated for the various ions. These gates open (activated) and close (inactivated), depending on the electrical potential of the cell membrane. An electrostatic gate exists for each of the major cardiac ions (sodium, potassium, calcium, and chloride).

Phases of the Action Potential. The action potentials of the various parts of the conduction system vary according to their locations and functions.[14] The action potential of the ventricular muscle fiber is separated into five phases (Figure 24-15). Phase 0, or upstroke, is represented by depolarization and involves the fast sodium channels. The fast sodium channel activation gates (M gates) open between −70 and −65 mV (threshold potential). At 0 mV, both the activation and the inactivation gates (H gates) are open. The rapid upstroke velocity of phase 0 gives a relative indication of the conductivity of the myocardial cell. Local anesthetics like lidocaine have an inhibitory effect on phase 0 by decreasing the influx of sodium. Table 24-2 describes the phases and events of a cardiac action potential.

At *phase 1*, or early rapid repolarization (+2 to +30 mV), the sodium gates close, the rapid influx of sodium stops, and the slower influx of calcium begins. Also, potassium gates open and potassium moves out of the interior of the cell into the extracellular fluid.

One of the characteristics of the action potential unique to ventricular muscle is *phase 2*, or the plateau phase. The plateau phase exists because the slow calcium channels open at −30 to −40 mV and allow an influx of calcium. This inward calcium flux delays repolarization and prolongs the absolute refractory period. Toward the end of phase 2, a decreased permeability to potassium occurs that accounts for a small outward leakage of potassium balanced by the calcium and sodium influx that maintains a membrane potential near 0 mV. Calcium channel blockers exert their pharmacologic effect during phase 2. The physiologic effects include decreased contractility, decreased heart rate, and decreased cardiac conduction velocity.[15]

The terminal repolarization phase, *phase 3*, is initiated as the slow calcium channels become inactivated, and this phenomenon is sustained by an accelerated potassium efflux. These events return the transmembrane potential to its resting membrane value.

The sodium-potassium pump, which is dependent of ATP, reestablishes the proper intracellular-to-extracellular ionic concentrations during *phase 4* (diastolic repolarization phase). Phase 4 lasts from the completion of repolarization to the next

TABLE **24-2**	Cardiac Action Potential		
Phase	**Name**	**Cation Movement**	**Effect**
0	Upstroke	Na^+ ECF to ICF	Sodium channels open Potassium permeability decreased
1	Initial repolarization	K^+ ICF to ECF	Sodium channels close Potassium channels open
2	Plateau	Ca^{2+} ECF to ICF	Calcium channels open
3	Final repolarization	K^+ ICF to ECF	Calcium channels close Potassium channels open
4	Resting potential	K^+ ICF to ECF Na^+/Ca^{2+} ECF to ICF	Resting membrane permeability restored, sodium and potassium leak to ICF to increase threshold potential

ECF, Extracellular fluid; ICF, intracellular fluid.

action potential. Lidocaine lengthens the duration of phase 4 by decreasing the cardiac cell membrane's permeability to potassium ion, thereby decreasing the efflux of potassium and delaying the onset of the resting membrane potential.[15]

The cardiac glycoside digoxin inhibits the sodium-potassium ATP-dependent pump, decreasing sodium efflux into the extracellular fluid. As a result, higher concentrations of calcium remain in the cardiac cell, and this effect is believed to be responsible for the increased inotropic effect. [15]

Refractory Periods. The extended duration of the action potential of the myocardial cell protects it against premature excitation. This period of quiescence is known as the *refractory period* and can be divided into absolute and relative periods. The refractory periods are a result of the properties of the sodium channels during the action potential.

The term *effective or absolute refractory period* is used to describe the time during which a conducted action potential may not be evoked, even if an active response is elicited by a stimulus at the cellular level. This period lasts from phase 0 to the middle of phase 3, when the membrane potential drops below −60 mV. The relative refractory period is the time during the action potential when a second stimulus can result only in an action potential with decreased amplitude, upstroke velocity, and conduction velocity. The relative refractory period extends from this middle part of the phase 3 range to the beginning of phase 4, when the membrane potential is from −60 to −90 mV. This information can be clinically related to synchronized cardioversion. The shock will not be delivered during the T wave on the electrocardiogram, which represents ventricular repolarization. The relative refractory period occurs during the T wave, and electricity delivered to the chest during this time can cause electrical disorganization in cardiac cells, resulting in ventricular tachycardia or ventricular fibrillation.

Sinoatrial Node Action Potential. The myocardium has among its characteristics contractility, automaticity, and conductivity. Each of the various myocardial masses has its own intrinsic automaticity and rate of action-potential initiation. The SA node is the primary pacemaker of the heart and has several unique characteristics (Figure 24-16). As a result of its higher resting membrane potentials, the SA node membrane is more permeable to sodium than other atrial myocardial cells. This "leakiness" gradually raises the membrane potential closer to threshold potential (−55 to −60 mV), at which point an action potential may be initiated. Therefore the action potential originating within the SA node differs from the action potential generated within the ventricular muscle mass. For this reason, the SA node is the primary pacemaker of the heart.

The SA node and the other automatic cells exhibit only phase 4, phase 0, and phase 3 of the action potential. Because rapid depolarization does not occur, the phase 1 or phase 2 (plateau phase) does not occur.

If the SA node fails, the area of the heart with the next highest intrinsic rate, the AV node, replaces the SA node as the pacemaker of the heart. The intrinsic firing rate of the AV node is 40 to 60 beats per minute. If both the SA and the AV nodes fail, the ventricular cells take over and become automatic, firing at a rate of 15 to 30 beats per minute.

Physiology of the Heart

Cardiac Cycle. To understand the cardiac cycle, one must have a firm understanding of the basics of the anatomy of the heart and the pressures and volumes generated within the various chambers during the cardiac cycle. An appreciation for the valves and their positions during the phases of the cycle is essential (Figure 24-17). Additionally, notice that the electrocardiogram impulse generation precedes the mechanical action of the heart. This delay between the electrical impulse and the mechanical event occurs because time is needed for the wave of depolarization to spread across the myocardium before contraction can begin. In relation to the electrocardiogram, the P wave represents atrial systole, the QRS complex signifies ventricular systole, and the T wave represents ventricular repolarization.

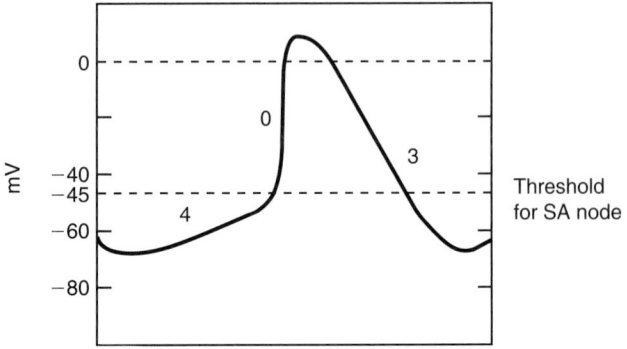

FIGURE **24-16** The sinoatrial nodal action potential.

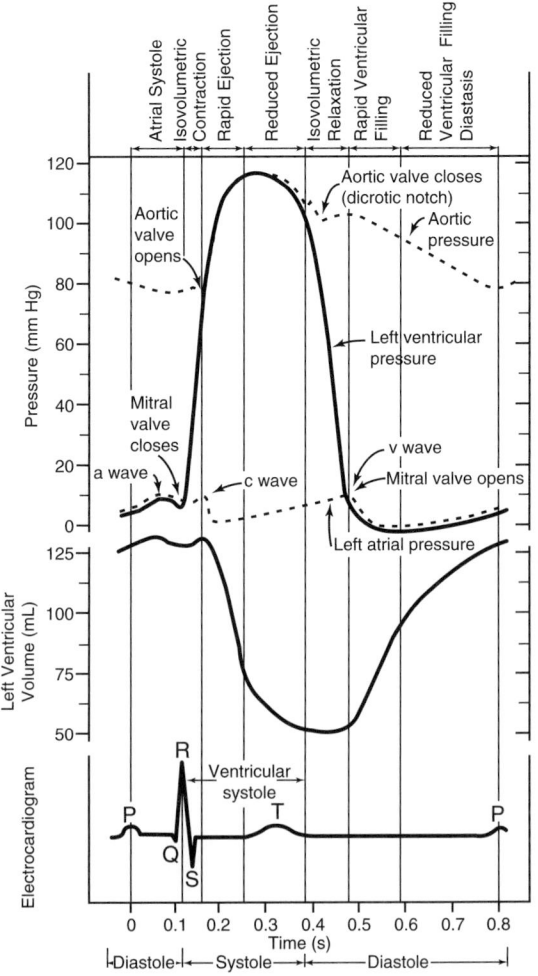

FIGURE **24-17** The cardiac cycle.

The cardiac cycle extends from one ventricular contraction to the next. It may be divided into two main phases—systole and diastole. Usually the cardiac cycle is described in relation to the left side of the heart. However, similar conclusions about the function of the right side of the heart may be drawn in the absence of cardiopulmonary pathology.

Diastole. During ventricular systole, the atria fill with blood returning from the venous system to the right side of the heart and from the pulmonary circulation to the left side of the heart. The first phase of diastole is the period of isovolumetric relaxation. The ventricular muscle mass relaxes, and the aortic and mitral valves are closed as long as the ventricular pressure remains higher than the atrial pressure. The true filling phase is divided into three periods: (1) rapid inflow, or diastasis, (2) reduced inflow, and (3) atrial systole. Once the ventricular pressure drops below atrial pressure, the mitral valve opens, and the period of rapid inflow to passively fill the ventricle begins. The second period of diastole is diastasis, in which minimal changes occur in volume and in pressure.

Atrial systole provides another period of rapid filling that is commonly referred to as the *atrial kick*. This phenomenon increases ventricular filling by 20% to 30%.

In patients who have severe mitral stenosis, the atrial kick may be responsible for up to 40% of the ventricular filling. During periods of strenuous exercise or in patients with many pathologic conditions such as shock or congestive heart failure, the additional ventricular filling is critical to maintaining CO.

Systole. After atrial systole, the isovolumetric phase, or isovolumetric contraction, which is the phase at the beginning of ventricular contraction, occurs. The myocardial fibers shorten, and pressure is generated within the ventricle but only enough to close the mitral valve. Therefore during this period, an increase in left ventricular pressure occurs without a change in ventricular diastolic volume. Isovolumetric contraction begins with closure of the mitral valve and lasts until opening of the mitral valve.

Systolic ejection begins with the opening of the aortic valve and occurs when the ventricular pressure exceeds the aortic pressure. This phase of the cardiac cycle is divided into two periods, with the period of rapid ejection taking the first third of systole and the period of reduced ejection taking the last two thirds of systole. During rapid ejection, ventricular systolic pressures reach their maximum, and the largest amount of volume is ejected. Therefore systole is composed of isovolumetric contraction, rapid ejection, and reduced ejection. The dicrotic notch or incisura on the arterial pressure tracing occurs within the period of isovolumetric relaxation. This segment represents retrograde blood flow back into the LV before aortic valve closure. Three waveform segments are present on the left atrial pressure tracing: the *a* wave, *c* wave, and *v* wave. The specific waveforms correspond to their position within the cardiac cycle. The *a* wave represents atrial systole as it ends just before mitral valve closure. The *c* wave represents ventricular contraction and is produced by bulging of the mitral valve caused by increasing left ventricular pressure. The *v* wave represents increased pressure in the LA caused by blood return from the pulmonary artery before mitral valve opening.

Physiology of Coronary Circulation. The anatomy of the coronary circulation has already been discussed. A description of the physiologic determinants of coronary blood flow follows.

Coronary Blood Flow. As in all hemodynamics, flow equals change in the pressure divided by resistance of the system.

Alterations of the radius of a vessel change the flow to the fourth power of the radius. This phenomenon is an extension of Poiseuille's law, which determines the flow of a fluid through a tube.

At rest, approximately 4% to 5% of the CO, or 225 mL/min of blood, passes through the coronary vasculature. Phasic changes have been documented during coronary blood flow. A greater amount of coronary flow in the LV occurs during diastole. During systole, left coronary artery blood flow ceases to the subendocardium due to compression of the subendocardial vessels by the myocardium; flow through the epicardial vessels is not affected during systole to this extent. The flow to the left coronary artery is greatest during diastole as a result of the decreased resistance to flow from decreased myofibril tension that occurs as the intracavitary pressure decreases (Figure 24-18).

Control of Coronary Circulation and Oxygen Supply and Demand. Coronary blood flow is regulated by intrinsic and extrinsic factors that affect coronary artery tone. Intrinsic factors include the anatomic arrangement and perfusion pressure of the coronary vessels. Extrinsic factors include compressive factors within the myocardium, as well as metabolic, neural, and humoral factors. Blood flow through the coronary circulation is primarily controlled by the factors that determine oxygen demand and oxygen supply. Myocardial oxygen supply is determined by arterial blood content, diastolic blood pressure, diastolic time as determined by HR, oxygen extraction, and coronary blood flow. Myocardial oxygen demand is determined by preload, afterload, contractility, and HR (Figure 24-19).

The factors that increase myocardial oxygen consumption ($m\dot{V}O_2$) are listed in Table 24-3. Notice in Figure 24-19 that heart rate appears on both the supply (diastolic time) side and

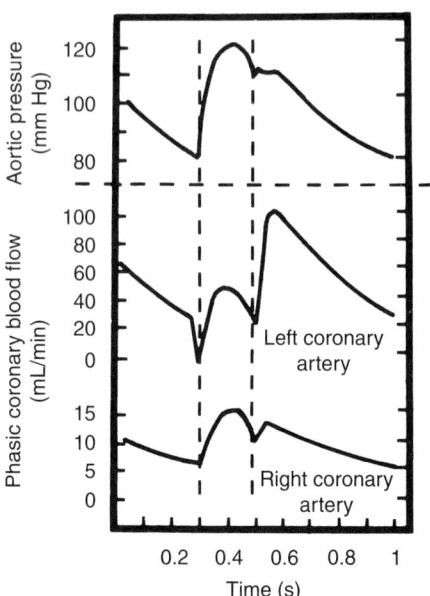

FIGURE **24-18** Blood flow in the left and right coronary arteries. The right ventricle is perfused throughout the cardiac cycle. Flow to the left ventricle is largely confined to diastole. (*From O'Brien ER, Nathan HJ. Coronary physiology and atherosclerosis. In: Kaplan JA. Kaplan's Cardiac Anesthesia. 5th ed. Philadelphia: Saunders; 2006:97.*)

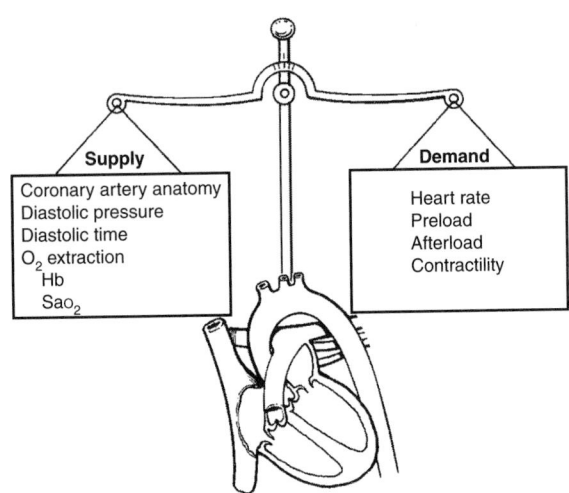

BOX 24-1

Normal Physiologic Parameters

Heart size	230-280 g (female)
	280-340 g (male)
Coronary blood flow	225-250 mL/min or 4%-7%
	total cardiac output
Myocardial O_2 consumption	65%-70% extraction
	8-10 mL O_2/100 g per min
Normal autoregulation	50-120 mm Hg (MAP)
Coronary filling	80%-90% during diastole

MAP, *Mean arterial pressure.*

FIGURE **24-19**   The heart's oxygen supply and demand must be balanced by the anesthetist, who should increase the former and reduce the latter. *Hb,* Hemoglobin; *SaO_2,* arterial oxygen saturation.

TABLE **24-3**	Components and Effects on Myocardial Oxygen Consumption
A 50% Increase in:	**Resultant Increase in m$\dot{V}O_2$**
Heart rate	50%
Pressure work	50%
Contractility	45%
Wall stress	25%
Volume work	4%

Modified from Opie LH. Mechanisms of cardiac contraction and relaxation. In: Libby P et al, eds. Braunwald's Heart Disease: A Textbook of Cardiovascular Medicine. 8th ed. 2008:509-540.
m$\dot{V}O_2$, *Myocardial oxygen consumption.*

demand side of the balance. Increasing heart rate not only increases demand but also decreases diastolic time, which is when 80% to 90% of coronary filling and myocardial perfusion occurs. Increased heart rate is the most important factor that negatively affects m$\dot{V}O_2$. Doubling the heart rate doubles (m$\dot{V}O_2$).[16] This phenomenon most dramatically affects patients with coronary artery disease, because the supply of blood is compromised and may not be able to meet the oxygen demands caused by tachycardia. As a result, myocardial dysfunction or infarction can occur. By slowing HR and decreasing contractility, β-blocking medications increase supply and decrease demand, protecting the heart from ischemia.[17]

Because at rest the myocardium extracts 65% to 70% of the available oxygen, the only way to increase oxygen delivery to the myocardium is by increasing blood flow. During periods of increased myocardial oxygen demands, flow through the coronary arteries can increase by three to four times. Several vasodilator substances have been identified and are released from the myocardium in response to decreased oxygen delivery or

concentration. Among these substances are adenosine, adenosine phosphate compounds, potassium ions, hydrogen ions, carbon dioxide, bradykinin, and prostaglandin. Many authors believe that adenosine is the primary substance responsible for coronary vasodilation.

The normal physiologic parameters of the heart are given in Box 24-1. The determinants of m$\dot{V}O_2$ include myocardial contractility, myocardial wall tension (preload), HR, and mean arterial pressure (MAP; afterload). Oxygen extraction is determined by measurement of the difference between the oxygen tension in the pulmonary arterial blood and that in the coronary sinus.

Oxygen supply relies on the blood oxygen content (see following equation), which is affected by both the oxygen carried on the hemoglobin (Hb) molecule (1.34 mL of oxygen per gram of Hb) and to a lesser extent the oxygen dissolved in the plasma (0.003 mL of oxygen per milliliter of plasma).

Equation 24-5

$$O_2 \text{ content (mL } O_2/\text{mL plasma)} = (Pa_{O_2} \times 0.003) + (\text{Hb content} \times \text{Hb-}O_2 \text{ saturation \%})$$

Other factors that have an influence on coronary circulation include the direct and indirect effects of the sympathetic nervous system and the effect of certain substrates of cardiac metabolism.

Autoregulation. Under normal physiologic conditions, the coronary circulation, like other tissue beds in the body, exhibits *autoregulation,* which is the ability to maintain coronary blood flow through a range of MAPs by dilating or constricting. Coronary blood flow is maintained at a constant rate through a MAP range of 50 to 120 mm Hg. When arterial blood pressure is less than or exceeds these pressure limits, coronary blood flow becomes pressure dependent. Therefore during hypotension, when the coronary arteries are maximally dilated, coronary blood flow is determined by the MAP minus the right atrial pressure.

A method for directly estimating coronary perfusion pressure (CPP) can be calculated by subtracting left ventricular end-diastolic pressure (LVEDP) from diastolic pressure (DBP)—that is, CPP = DBP − LVEDP. Because under normal conditions LVEDP (10 mmHg) is significantly less than DBP (80 mmHg), the major determinant of CPP is DBP.

Coronary vascular reserve is the difference between the maximal flow and the autoregulated flow. The closer these two values, the lower the coronary reserve of the patient. Factors that increase myocardial oxygen demand and limit supply decrease coronary reserve flow and can result in myocardial dysfunction.

The concept of "coronary steal" has emerged, especially in reference to the use of agents such as nitroglycerin and isoflurane. If vasodilator treatment is used in a patient who has both an ischemic area of the heart that is supplying a stenotic vessel with collateral flow and another area that has an intact autoregulated vessel, only the autoregulated vessel dilates further and has the ability to increase its flow. Constant maximal coronary artery dilation exists in an area where stenosis is present. Therefore, only the areas of the heart with intact autoregulation respond to vasodilators and receive preferential flow over the stenotic area. The existence of this phenomenon is questionable. Agnew and colleagues have determined that as long as adequate CPP is maintained, coronary steal and myocardial ischemia caused by isoflurane do not occur.[18,19] A second factor that could result in this phenomenon is coronary steal–prone anatomy. This has been defined as complete occlusion of one coronary artery and at least 50% occlusion of a second coronary artery that supplies collateral blood flow to the area in which the complete occlusion exists.[18] In addition, recent evidence suggests that isoflurane produces myocardial protection during periods of ischemia in humans by decreasing the formation of free radicals, preserving myocardial ATP stores, and inhibiting increased intracellular calcium.[19,20] Presently it has not been established whether sevoflurane and desflurane can cause coronary steal.

Cardiac Output. Cardiac output is the amount of blood ejected from the LV during 1 minute. Comparing various CO values among several patients requires a method for calculating output in relation to the size of the patient. The CO is measured in liters per minute. Cardiac output is indexed, because a CO of 3.5 L/min may be adequate for a patient who is 5 feet tall and weighs 95 lb, but it is less than optimal for a patient who is 6 feet 7 inches tall and weighs 300 lb. The average CO is 5 L/min, and the average cardiac index (CI) is 2.5 L/min or more per square meter of body surface area (BSA). The formula for this relationship is CI = CO/BSA.

The primary determinants of CO are stroke volume (SV) and HR. CO is derived by using the equation CO = HR × SV. The SV is the amount of blood ejected from the LV with each beat. The average SV is approximately 70 mL. If the average HR is 70 to 80 beats per minute, a CO of 5 L/min results.

Several key factors affect the SV, including preload, afterload, and myocardial contractility. Preload is the effective tension of the blood on the ventricle or the wall tension at the end of diastole. Preload can either be passive (the flow of blood from the atria to the ventricles during diastole) or active (the volume contributed by the atrial kick). With increased preload, there is an associated increase in contractility. This phenomenon is known as the *Frank-Starling law* of the heart, which states that the greater the wall tension (preload), the greater the compensatory increase in myocardial contractility. This mechanism allows the heart to immediately compensate for increased preload and avoid overdistention of the cardiac chambers by increasing SV, which facilitates chamber emptying. However, there is a point at which progressive increases in preload no longer increase contractility but can contribute to decreased myocardial performance. Increased preload increases myocardial oxygen demand. Clinically, preload can be estimated by using the PCWP and the pulmonary artery diastolic pressure. In patients with normal mitral valve and ventricular muscle function, either of these measures provides an estimate of the preload or LVEDP and volume.

Cardiac output can be determined indirectly by applying the Fick principle (see Equation 24-6). Assuming normal respiratory function, CO is equal to the amount of oxygen absorbed by the lungs divided by the arteriovenous oxygen difference.

Equation 24-6

CO (L/min) =

$$\frac{\text{Oxygen absorbed per minute by the lungs (mL/min)}}{\text{Arteriovenous oxygen difference (mL of blood)}}$$

Right-sided heart pressures (central venous pressure) that are obtained clinically can be estimates of left ventricular volumes in patients with good left ventricular function.[21]

Afterload is the wall tension the myocardium needs to overcome to eject the SV. It is the pressure within the LV during peak systole. Factors affecting the afterload of the LV include the ventricular chamber and the vasculature. The shape, size, and wall thickness of the ventricle play an important role in afterload. The vascular component of the afterload includes SVR and MAP because these variables relate to the vascular compliance of the aorta. Thus increases in blood pressure increase afterload.

Afterload is most often estimated clinically by determining the SVR. The SVR may be calculated once the CO and the difference between the MAP and the central venous pressure (CVP) are known (see equation). The normal SVR is 800 to 1500 dyn.s/cm⁵.

Equation 24-7

$$SVR = (MAP \times CVP)/CO \times 80$$

The problem with equating afterload with SVR is that ventricular wall tension, which is an integral part of the afterload, is not considered.

Contractility of the myocardium is the state of inotropy that is independent of either preload or afterload. It may be altered by many cardiovascular disease states. Factors such as rate of pressure changes over time (dP/dt), force-velocity or Starling ventricular function curves, pressure-volume loops, ejection fraction (EF), and velocity of circumferential fiber shortening have all been used to estimate contractility.

Left ventricular dP/dt measurements require a high-fidelity recording system, and for this reason these measures are not readily available in the clinical setting. A wide range of normal values exists (800 to 1700 mm Hg/sec), making patient-to-patient comparisons difficult. Assessment of the acute change in contractility of a single patient over time is still the common method of using this measurement.

Ventricular function curves[22] (Figure 24-20) define the relationship between the left ventricular filling pressure (left ventricular diastolic pressure, left atrial pressure, PCWP) and the left ventricular stroke work index (LVSWI), which is calculated by use of the following equation:

Equation 24-8

LVSWI (in g/m² per beat) = 0.0136 × SVI × (MAP − PCWP)

where SVI = CI/HR.

Each left ventricular function curve has a steep upstroke that has a plateau at higher filling pressures. To apply the Frank-Starling mechanism to Figure 24-20, notice in the "normal" and "hyperdynamic" curves that as pressure (horizontal axis) increases, so does LV output (vertical axis). However, at the top of these curves, there is a plateau where increasing the filling pressures no longer increases performance and can then decrease

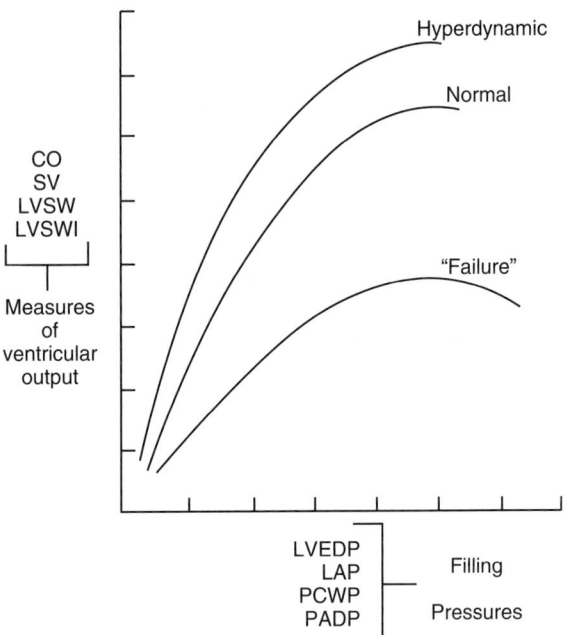

FIGURE **24-20**   The ventricular function curve. CO, Cardiac output; *LAP*, left atrial pressure; *LVEDP*, left ventricular end-diastolic pressure; *LVSW*, left ventricular stroke work; *LVSWI*, left ventricular stroke work index; *PADP*, pulmonary artery diastolic pressure; *PCWP*, pulmonary capillary wedge pressure; *SV*, stroke volume.

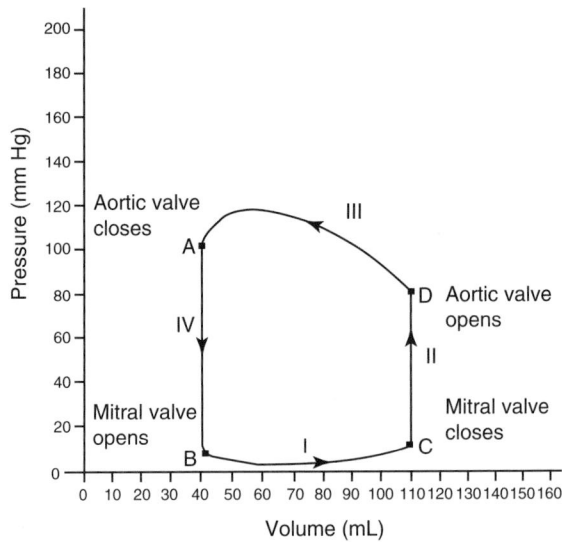

FIGURE **24-21**   Phases of the left ventricular (LV) pressure-volume loop, which is a continuous cycle divided into four phases. Phase **I** represents diastolic filling. Left ventricular filling begins at point B and ends at point C. Note the increase in volume of 70 mL and the upward movement of the curve at point C, representing a slightly increased pressure in response to the increased volume. Point C or mitral valve closure represents end-diastolic volume (EDV). Phase **II** represents isovolumetric contraction. Note there is a significant increase in pressure but no change in volume. Cardiac muscle fibers are shortening and increasing the pressure on the LV volume until point D, where the LV pressure exceeds aortic pressure. Phase **III** represents systolic ejection. Note the decrease in LV volume throughout LV systolic ejection. Phase **IV** represents isovolumetric relaxation. At point **A** the aortic pressure exceeds LV pressure, and the aortic valve closes. Point A represents end-systolic volume (ESV). The LV relaxes, and the pressure decreases significantly. At maximal LV relaxation, the mitral valve opens and the process starts again.

ventricular output. Symptoms may be elicited by either high or low filling pressures. On the "failure" curve, with compromised cardiac function, increases in filling pressures do not dramatically increase myocardial performance and can lead to cardiogenic shock. The clinical determination of LVSWI is worthwhile because it contains many of the factors that contribute to CO, and it gives measures of both systolic and diastolic performance.

Left ventricular pressure-volume loops have been mentioned before as indexes of the cardiac cycle. They may also be used as tools to determine myocardial performance. Left ventricular pressure-volume loops simultaneously measure chamber pressures and the resultant volumes (Figure 24-21). Movement from left to right on the horizontal axis represents increased volume. Movement from right to left on the horizontal axis represents decreased volume. Movement up and down on the vertical axis represents increases and decreases in pressure, respectively. The distinct phases of the left ventricular pressure-volume loop are represented in Figure 24-22.

The interior of the curve (distance between the two vertical lines of the LV pressure-volume loop) is representative of SV. In this diagram, SV is calculated by subtracting end-systolic volume from end-diastolic volume, or EDV (110 mL) − ESV (40 mL). Thus in this example, stroke volume is 70 mL. Ejection fraction can then be estimated using the following equations:

Equation 24-9

$$EF = (EDV \times ESV)/ EDV \times 100$$

or

Equation 24-10

$$EF = (SV/EDV) \times 100$$

The EF is the percentage of the end-diastolic volume ejected during systole, as seen in Figure 24-23. The normal EF is 60%

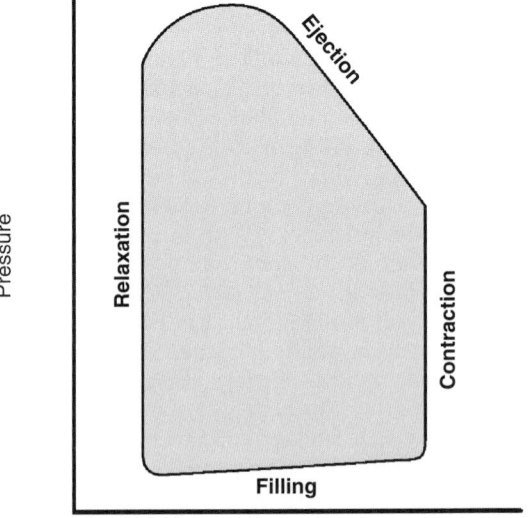

Volume
Left Ventricular Pressure-Volume Loop

FIGURE **24-22**   Phases of the cardiac cycle represented by a left ventricular pressure-volume loop.

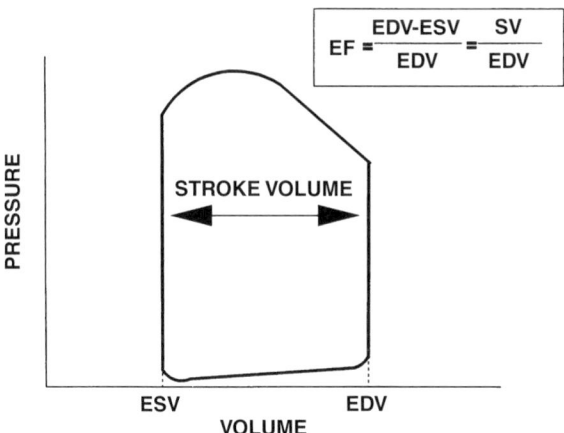

FIGURE **24-23** Pressure-volume diagram indicating end-diastolic volume (EDV), end-systolic volume (ESV), stroke volume (SV), and the equation for ejection fraction (EF). (*From Johnson B et al. Cardiac physiology. In: Kaplan JA: Kaplan's Cardiac Anesthesia. 5th ed. Philadelphia: Saunders; 2006:73.*)

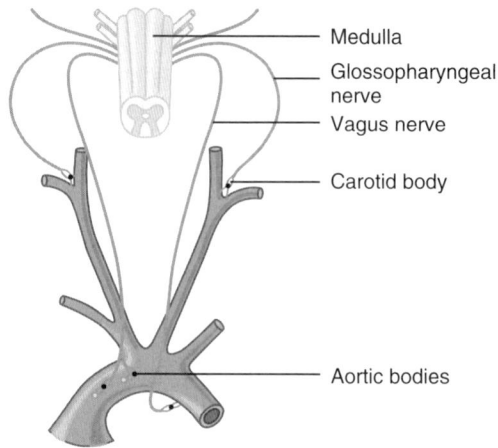

FIGURE **24-25** Afferent and efferent neural pathways from carotid and aortic baroreceptors. (*From Guyton AC, Hall JE. Medical Physiology. 11th ed. Philadelphia: Saunders; 2006:518.*)

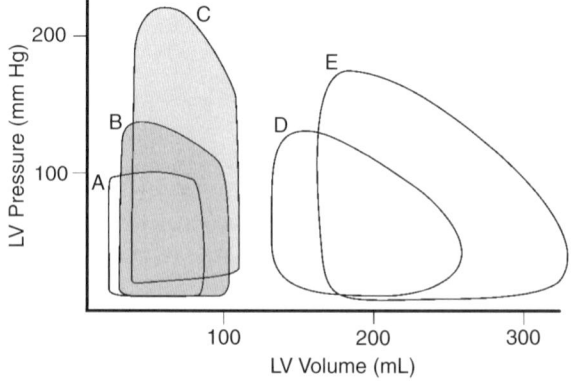

FIGURE **24-24** Pathologic left ventricular pressure-volume loops. A, mitral stenosis; B, normal curve; C, aortic stenosis; D, mitral regurgitation; E, aortic regurgitation.

to 70%. An EF of less than 40% is associated with significant left ventricular impairment.

Deviations from the normal left ventricular pressure-volume loops occur as a result of many causes. Factors that alter the normal loop include increases and decreases in LV preload, LV afterload, and LV contractility. These factors can be acute and transient, such as during the administration of vasoactive medications, or chronic as a result of myocardial compensation caused by valvular heart disease. In Figure 24-24, these changes are consistent with valvular heart disease. A discussion of these pathologic curves will occur later in this chapter.

A clinically useful tool is two-dimensional transesophageal echocardiography (TEE). When this technology is appropriately used, real-time movement of all four chambers of the heart, as well as that of the valves, may be visualized.

Transesophageal echocardiography can be used to detect valvular function and blood flows in both regurgitant and stenotic lesions. It is also useful in determining areas of hypokinesis, dyskinesis, or akinesis caused by myocardial infarction, ischemia,

or injury. It can be useful in determining myocardial contractility, and it is a more direct measure of intraventricular volume status than pulmonary artery catheter pressure measures. Transesophageal echocardiography has also proved useful in directing fluid and pharmacologic therapy in patients who have undergone coronary bypass and other surgical procedures. Ventricular dysfunction or reperfusion injury, as well as the presence of intraventricular air, can be determined with TEE. This diagnostic tool is the gold standard for assessing intraoperative myocardial performance. The practical problems associated with the clinical use of TEE entail acquiring the skills necessary for accurate interpretation of the visual data, the possibility of esophageal rupture, and the cost associated with its use.

CARDIOVASCULAR REFLEXES

Cardiac Output Regulation. A direct interplay exists between CO and venous return. As long as neither the contractility nor the HR is compromised, maintenance of a constant return of blood flow to the heart ensures an adequate CO. The body's regulation of CO depends on its ability to regulate HR and contractility of the myocardium, as well as constriction and distention of the vascular tree.

Many of the factors that affect CO also affect the MAP and are addressed in the section on regulation of MAP. Some of the more common reflexes that can alter the CO are described in this section or in the section on regulation of MAP.

Valsalva Maneuver. The Valsalva maneuver occurs as a result of forced expiration against a closed glottis. The reflex is mediated through the baroreceptors located near the bifurcation of the internal and external carotid arteries (carotid sinus) and the aortic arch. The afferent pathway is through the Hering nerve and either the glossopharyngeal nerve (carotid sinus) or the vagus nerve (aortic arch), as shown in Figure 24-25. Stimulation of either of these areas inhibits the vasomotor center in the medulla. The response inhibits the sympathetic nervous system and stimulates the parasympathetic nervous system, producing a decrease in HR, a decrease in myocardial contractility, and vasodilation, resulting in a decrease in blood pressure. The Valsalva maneuver also increases intrathoracic pressure, which decreases venous return and thereby decreases CO.

Baroreceptor Reflex. The baroreceptors respond to fluctuations in arterial blood pressure. Afferent and efferent impulse transmission travels along the same pathway as the Valsalva maneuver. Decreases in arterial blood pressure are sensed by the baroreceptors, increasing sympathetic tone, which results in increased myocardial performance and vasoconstriction. Acute hypertension causes the opposite cardiovascular response. A more in-depth explanation of the baroreceptor response and its role in short- and long-term blood pressure control is presented later in this chapter. The baroreceptor response is inhibited by volatile anesthetic agents in a dose-dependent manner and results in decreased ability of the baroreceptors to respond to blood pressure changes when these agents are used.

Oculocardiac Reflex. Traction on the extraocular muscles (especially the medial rectus), conjunctiva, or orbital structures causes hypotension and a reflex slowing of the HR, as well as arrhythmias. The oculocardiac reflex may also be elicited during retrobulbar block, ocular trauma, or pressure on the tissue that remains after enucleation. The afferent path of the reflex is mediated by the long and short ciliary nerves to the ciliary ganglion of the oculomotor nerve and then the ophthalmic division of the trigeminal nerve (cranial nerve V) to the gasserian ganglion. The efferent branch of the reflex is mediated by the vagus nerve (cranial nerve X). This reflex may be blunted by the use of retrobulbar block or the release of the offending stimulus. The resulting vagal response to the heart can be inhibited by an anticholinergic agent (atropine or glycopyrrolate).

Celiac Reflex. The celiac reflex is elicited by traction on the mesentery or the gallbladder or stimulation of the vagus nerve in other areas of the body, such as the thorax and abdominal cavity. Stimulation of this reflex causes bradycardia, apnea, and hypotension. Clinically, the celiac reflex can be initiated indirectly as a result of a pneumoperitoneum. As with the oculocardiac reflex, the celiac reflex is frequently resolved by stopping the initiating stimulus.

Bainbridge Reflex (Atrial Stretch Reflex). The Bainbridge reflex is elicited as a result of an increased volume of blood in the heart, which causes sympathetic nervous system stimulation. Stretch receptors are located in the right atrium, junction of the vena cava, and pulmonary veins. The sinoatrial node is also involved in this process and can increase heart rate by 10% to 15%. This reflex helps to prevent sequestration of blood in veins, atria, and pulmonary circulation. Antidiuretic hormone secretion from the posterior pituitary gland is decreased, resulting in decreased circulating blood volume. Atrial natriuretic peptide is increased, which also promotes diuresis.

Cushing Reflex. This physiologic response to CNS ischemia caused by increased intracranial pressure is called the Cushing reflex. It is triggered as a result of an elevation of intracranial pressure to a value greater than the MAP, thereby decreasing cerebral perfusion and cerebral-causing ischemia. An intense response from the vasomotor center is initiated, resulting in intense vasoconstriction. These compensatory physiologic changes attempt to restore adequate cerebral perfusion. However, if cerebral ischemia is not relieved, cerebral infarction results. When the vasomotor area becomes ischemic as a result of hypotension (MAP <50 mm Hg), maximal stimulation of the vasomotor center occurs. The Cushing triad is a late sign of high and sustained intracranial pressure prior to cerebral herniation. The signs include hypertension, bradycardia, and respiratory irregularity.

Chemoreceptor Reflex. The central chemoreceptors are located beneath the ventral surface of the medulla and are directly stimulated primarily by increased hydrogen ion concentration. The peripheral chemoreceptors are located at the bifurcation of the internal and external carotid arteries (carotid body) and within the aortic arch (aortic body) and are primarily stimulated by decreased arterial oxygen concentration. The response elicited from hypoxia, hypercarbia, and acidosis is increased minute ventilation and increased sympathetic nervous system stimulation, resulting in increased blood pressure. Like the baroreceptor reflex, the chemoreceptor response is inhibited by the volatile anesthetic agents in a dose-dependent manner. Thus if residual volatile agent is present during the emergence from anesthesia, the threshold for breathing will be increased. Table 24-4 provides a summary of the cardiovascular reflexes.

VASCULAR SYSTEM

Anatomy

Vascular Anatomy

The vascular circulation is divided into the pulmonary circulation and the peripheral systemic circulation (Figure 24-26). Several functional parts of this vascular system exist.

Arteries

Arteries transport blood to the tissues under high pressure. Arteries have an average diameter of 4 mm and a wall thickness of 1 mm. They have a thick layer of elastic tissue, smooth muscle, and fibrous tissue. Arteries are able to maintain the flow of blood because of their large internal diameter.

Arterioles

Arterioles are the last small branches of the arterial system, and they act as control valves for the release of blood into the capillary beds. Arterioles have an average diameter of 30 μm and a wall thickness of 20 μm. Like arteries, arterioles have a thick layer of elastic tissue, smooth muscle, and fibrous tissue. Constriction of the arterioles, compared with that of other structures within the vascular system, causes the greatest increase in SVR. Because of this contribution, arterioles exhibit the greatest pressure drop in the vascular system across the length of their vessels.

Capillaries

The exchange of fluids, nutrients, electrolytes, hormones, and other substances occurs between the blood and the interstitial fluids in the capillaries. Capillaries have an average diameter of 8 μm and a wall thickness of 1 μm. The walls of capillaries are only one cell thick and have no elastic tissue, smooth muscle, or fibrous tissue. The capillary cell membrane is semipermeable to water and other small molecules.

Venules

Venules collect blood from capillaries and gradually coalesce into progressively larger veins. Venules have an average diameter of 20 μm and a wall thickness of approximately 0.5 mm. They do not have an elastic or smooth muscle layer but have a thin fibrous layer.

Veins

Veins act as conduits for the transport of blood back to the heart. They also act as a large reservoir because they are very distensible. They have an average diameter of 30 mm and a wall thickness of 1.5 mm. The venous system contains approximately 60% of the blood volume, as opposed to the 20% contained within the arteries (Figure 24-27). The elastic

TABLE **24-4**	Cardiac Reflexes	
Reflex	**Stimulus**	**Response**
Baroreceptor reflex	Hypertension resulting in baroreceptor stimulation. Carotid baroreceptors send afferent response via Hering and glossopharyngeal nerves (CN IX). Aortic baroreceptors send afferent response via the vagus nerve (CN X).*	Decreased heart rate, decreased contractility, peripheral vasodilation from efferent response via the vagus nerve (CN X)
Valsalva maneuver	Forced expiration against a closed glottis mediated via baroreceptors; see baroreceptor reflex for neural pathways	Decreased heart rate, decreased contractility, peripheral vasodilation from efferent response via the vagus nerve (CN X)
Cushing reflex	Increased intracranial pressure resulting in cerebral ischemia	Sympathetic nervous stimulation resulting in increased blood pressure
Chemoreceptor reflex	Decreased oxygen saturation, increased carbon dioxide, increased hydrogen ion concentration. Peripheral chemoreceptors located in the carotid body and aortic arch; see baroreceptor reflex for neural pathways.	Increased respiratory drive, increased blood pressure
Atrial stretch reflex (Bainbridge reflex)	Hypervolemia, increased venous return causes stimulation of atrial stretch receptors	Increased heart rate, decreased blood pressure, decreased systemic vascular resistance, diuresis
Oculocardiac reflex	Traction on the extraocular muscles (especially medial rectus) or pressure on the globe causes an afferent response via the trigeminal nerve (CN V) and results in an efferent vagal response via the vagus nerve (CN X).	Bradycardia, hypotension, and arrhythmias
Celiac reflex	Traction or pressure on structures within abdominal and thoracic cavity causes vagal nerve stimulation	Bradycardia, hypotension, and apnea

CN, *Cranial nerve.*
Efferent response increases parasympathetic tone via the vagus and sympathetic nerves.

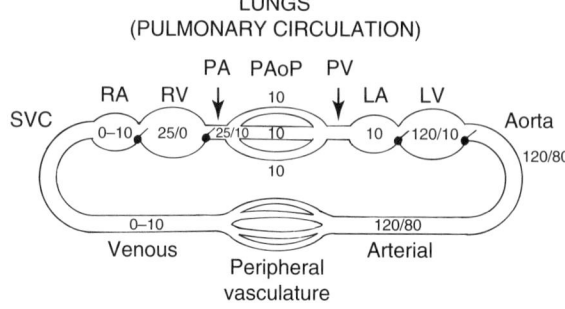

FIGURE **24-26** The vascular circuit *LA*, left atrium; *LV*, left ventricle; *PA*, pulmonary artery; *PAOP*, pulmonary artery occlusion pressure; *RA*, right atrium; *RV*, right ventricle; *SVC*, superior vena cava.

tissue and the fibrous tissue layers are similar in size to those of the arterioles, but the smooth muscle layer in the veins is smaller than that in the other large vessels.

Arterial Circulation

Knowledge of the anatomy of the arterial circulation is an important part of anesthesia practice. Such information is essential for obtaining intraarterial access, assessing HR and pulse quality, understanding the anatomic relationships for the purpose of regional blocks, and understanding the physiologic implications of blood flow in shock states.

Microscopic Anatomy of the Arterial Circulation. Arteries are classically divided into two types: conducting, or elastic, arteries and distributing, or muscular, arteries. Conducting arteries include the major arteries, such as the aorta, and their major branches, such as the brachial, radial, and ulnar arteries. The walls of the arteries are thicker than the walls of veins and consist of three major layers: the tunica intima, the tunica media, and the tunica adventitia.

Thoracic Aorta. The thoracic aorta is divided into three sections: the ascending aorta is the portion that leaves the LV; the transverse aorta, or arch, is the portion that levels off; and the descending aorta is the portion that descends into the thorax. After the thoracic aorta penetrates the diaphragm, the vessel is called the abdominal aorta (Figure 24-28).

The first branches of the ascending aorta are the right and left coronary arteries. From this point, three major branches of the thoracic aorta exist: the brachiocephalic (innominate) artery, the left common carotid artery, and the left subclavian artery.

The brachiocephalic artery branches and becomes the right common carotid artery and the right subclavian artery. The left and right common carotid arteries branch into internal and external carotid arteries. The external carotid arteries supply blood to the face and neck, and the major branches are the superior thyroid artery, the lingual artery, the facial artery, the posterior auricular artery, the maxillary artery, the transverse facial artery, the middle temporal artery, and the superficial temporal artery (Figure 24-29).

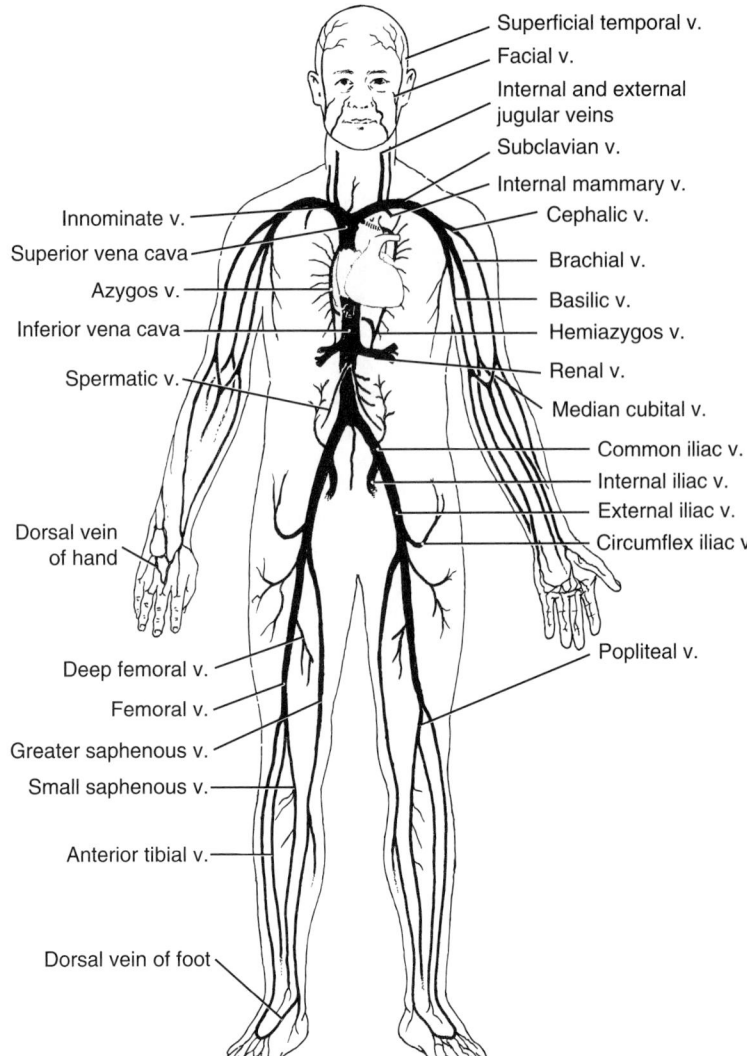

FIGURE **24-27**   The venous system. *v.*, Vein.

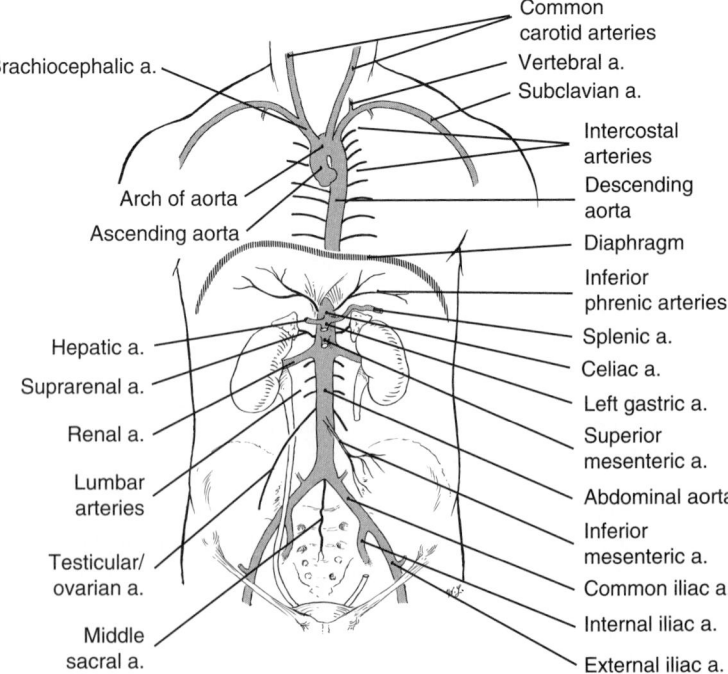

FIGURE **24-28**   Thoracic aorta and abdominal aorta and their branches. *a.*, Artery.

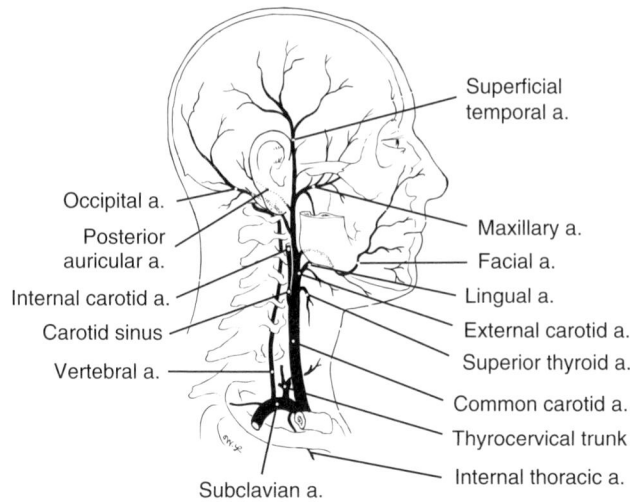

FIGURE **24-29** Arterial supply to the face. *a.*, Artery.

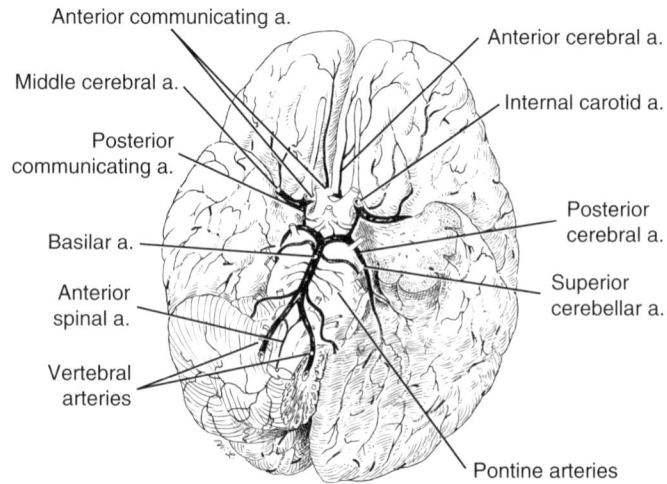

FIGURE **24-30** The circle of Willis. *a.*, Artery.

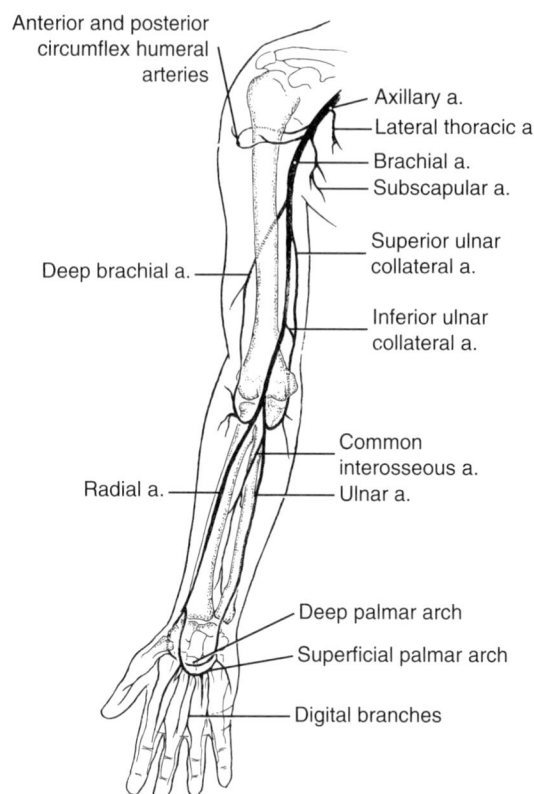

FIGURE **24-31** Arterial supply to the upper extremity. *a.*, Artery.

The internal carotid arteries supply blood to the brain via the circle of Willis and to the eyes via the ophthalmic arteries (Figure 24-30). The circle of Willis also receives a major part of its blood supply from the vertebral branches of the subclavian artery.

Upper Extremity Arteries. The subclavian arteries branch before entering the upper arm. These branches include the vertebral arteries, as noted earlier; the thyrocervical trunk, which supplies blood to the thyroid gland as well as other structures in the neck; the internal thoracic artery, which supplies blood to the anterior chest; and the costocervical trunk, which supplies blood to the first two intercostal spaces and the muscles of the neck.

The subclavian artery continues at the border of the first rib as the axillary artery (Figure 24-31). Branches from the axillary artery supply blood to the axillary region and include the highest thoracic artery, the thoracoacromial artery, the lateral thoracic artery, the subscapular artery, and the anterior and posterior circumflex humeral arteries.

The brachial artery begins at the terminal end of the axillary artery at the inferior border of the teres major muscle.

The artery continues until the neck of the radius, where it ends by dividing into the radial and ulnar arteries. The radial artery forms the deep palmar arch, and the ulnar artery supplies blood to the superficial palmar arch.

Descending Thoracic Aorta. The descending thoracic aorta passes caudad through the posterior mediastinum on the left side and at the level of the twelfth thoracic vertebra passes through the aortic opening in the diaphragm and becomes the abdominal aorta. Branches of the descending thoracic aorta include the lower nine posterior intercostal arteries, the subcostal arteries, the pericardial arteries, the esophageal arteries, and the bronchial arteries.

Abdominal Aorta. As the thoracic aorta passes through the aortic hiatus of the diaphragm, it becomes the abdominal aorta. The first branches of the abdominal aorta are the inferior phrenic arteries, which supply blood to the underside of the diaphragm and the adrenal glands (see Figure 24-28).

The next major branch of the abdominal aorta is the celiac trunk, which supplies blood to many of the organs in the upper abdomen. Its branches include the splenic artery, the left gastric artery, the gastroduodenal artery, and the hepatic artery. The cystic artery, which supplies blood to the gallbladder, is a branch of the hepatic artery.

Below the celiac trunk of the aorta lies the superior mesenteric artery, which arises at the level of L1. This artery supplies blood to the jejunum, the ileum, and the transverse colon by means of an anastomosis with the middle colic artery. The jejunal and ileal branches unite to form the arterial arcades of the colon.

Below the superior mesenteric artery are the right and left renal arteries. The right renal artery branches to the right adrenal

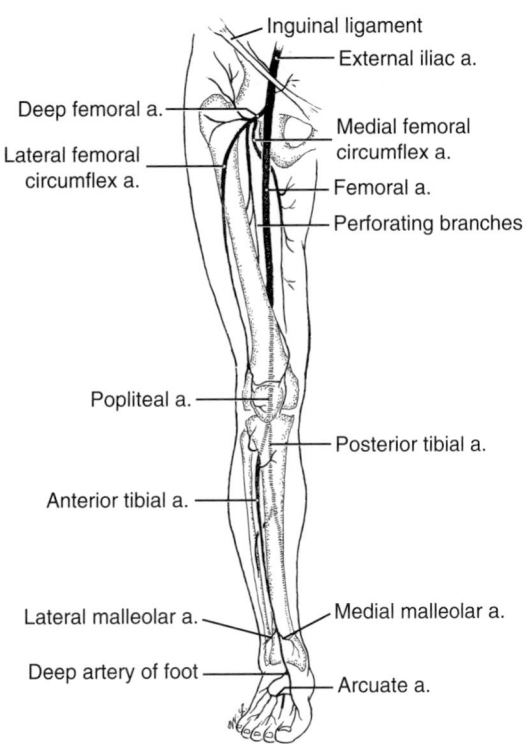

FIGURE **24-32** Arterial supply to the lower extremity. *a.*, Artery.

gland, where it is called the *middle suprarenal artery*. Below the renal arteries are the testicular or ovarian arteries.

Below the level of the renal arteries lies the inferior mesenteric artery. This artery has branches to the transverse colon, the descending colon, and the sigmoid colon and rectum.

Iliac Arteries. The abdominal aorta terminates at the common iliac arteries in the pelvis. These arteries divide into internal and external iliac arteries. The internal iliac arteries supply blood to structures within the pelvis, whereas the external iliac arteries supply blood to the legs.

Lower Extremities. The external iliac continues as the femoral artery and the deep femoral artery (Figure 24-32). The femoral artery becomes the popliteal artery behind the knee and then divides into the anterior and posterior tibial arteries. The anterior tibial artery continues as the dorsal artery of the foot. The posterior tibial artery continues and supplies blood to the plantar arches. Clinically, the dorsal artery of the foot is not only an important landmark for the assessment of lower extremity circulation but can also be used for arterial cannulation if the radial artery is not available.

Venous Circulation

An understanding of the anatomy of the venous system is essential in the practice of anesthesia, not only for vascular access but also for identification of significant landmarks for the location of nerve bundles for nerve blocks. Evaluation of venous distention is an important assessment tool for fluid overload and cardiovascular dynamics.

Head and Neck. In the head and neck, venous drainage returns to the heart via the internal and external jugular veins. The drainage from the brain comes from the sagittal, transverse, and sigmoid sinuses. These sinuses drain into the internal jugular vein, whereas the more superficial structures of the face and head drain into the external jugular vein.

Upper Extremities. Superficial veins of the upper extremities include those that drain into the axillary vein, the cephalic vein laterally, and the basilica vein medially. The axillary vein drains into the subclavian vein on the right and then into the right brachiocephalic vein. The left subclavian vein drains into the left brachiocephalic vein. The right and left brachiocephalic veins empty into the superior vena cava and account for the venous drainage that occurs from the upper extremities. Pressure and occlusion of the superior vena cava from a mass can result in a decrease in venous drainage, causing superior vena cava syndrome.

Thorax. Venous drainage of the chest comes from the branches of the superior and inferior vena cava and the azygos and hemiazygos systems. These systems are an important alternative blood return route if a major obstruction of the inferior vena cava occurs. These vessels include the intercostal vessels, the bronchial veins, and the pericardial veins.

Abdomen, Pelvis, and Lower Extremities. The deep femoral and femoral veins receive superficial and deep venous drainage from the legs and join to form the external iliac veins. The internal iliac veins drain blood from the pelvis. The common iliac vessels receive blood from the internal and external iliac veins and drain into the inferior vena cava. In this region, the common iliac vessels are joined by branches from the abdomen and the hepatic portal system.

Microcirculation

The function of the microcirculation is to control the delivery of nutrients to the capillary tissue beds, remove waste products, maintain ionic concentrations, and transport hormones to the tissues.

Anatomy. In general, a main nutrient artery enters an organ, where it branches six to eight times until the vessels are small enough to be called *arterioles* (<20 μm in diameter). Arterioles then branch two to five times and reach diameters of 5 to 9 μm, small enough to supply blood to the capillary bed.

In the capillary bed, the blood enters through an arteriole that has a muscular coat. Arterioles are connected to metarterioles, which have many interconnections to the true capillaries and whose branches are protected by precapillary sphincters. These sphincters can control blood flow through the capillary bed.

The capillary wall is a unicellular layer of endothelium surrounded by a basement membrane. The total wall thickness is 0.5 μm, and the diameter of the capillaries is 4 to 9 μm. In the capillary membrane, intercellular clefts allow the diffusion of water-soluble ions and small solutes. Plasmalemma vesicles exist and form channels in the cell membrane.

The diffusion of substances through the cell membrane is determined by several factors: lipid solubility, water solubility, size of the molecule, and concentration difference from one side of the membrane to the other.[1]

Movement of fluid volume from the plasma and the interstitial fluid is determined by four factors: capillary pressure, interstitial fluid pressure, plasma colloid osmotic pressure, and interstitial fluid colloid osmotic pressure. Excess fluid from the interstitial space is transported through the lymphatic system, which plays an important role in the prevention of pulmonary edema formation when pulmonary artery pressures are elevated.

Local Control of Capillary Blood Flow. Blood flow to the various capillary beds is regulated by local tissue metabolic requirements. Therefore capillary blood flow may be controlled by the delivery of oxygen and other nutrients, the removal of end products of metabolism, or the maintenance of ionic balance of pH in the tissues.

Two major theories that regulate capillary blood flow include the vasodilator theory and the oxygen-demand theory. According to these theories, the vessels dilate to increase the blood flow as a result of either hypoxemia or release of a vasodilator substance in response to hypoxemia. Some of the vasodilator substances that have been suggested are adenosine, carbon dioxide, lactic acid, adenosine phosphate compounds, histamine, potassium ions, and hydrogen ions. These theories indicate that an active microcirculatory process exists that responds to tissue metabolic needs.

Certain tissue capillary beds do not function as explained by the vasodilator and the oxygen-demand theories of microcirculatory blood flow. Blood flow to the skin is dependent on external temperature and dissipation of body heat, whereas blood flow to the kidneys is dependent on the amount of fluid and sodium that needs to be excreted.

Autoregulation is another process demonstrated by certain organ tissues; it keeps blood flow through the capillary bed constant, despite the normal changes in MAP. Autoregulation has been demonstrated in such tissues as the brain, the kidney, and the coronary circulation. Autoregulation keeps the blood flow to an organ constant by vasodilation or vasoconstriction as occurs in response to fluctuations in MAP.

A substance that causes secondary vasodilation of the large arteries in response to increased flow has been isolated and is called the *endothelium-derived relaxing factor*,[23] more commonly referred to as *nitric oxide*. This factor is synthesized by the endothelial lining of the arterioles and the small arteries. Shear stress on the walls of the vessels accelerates the release of this substance and allows larger vessels to dilate when blood flow to the tissues increases.

Growth of Collateral Circulation

Microcirculation is a good example of vascular growth that can occur to provide collateral circulation. The growth of new vessels results in part from angiogenesis and the release of angiogenic factors. These substances are released from ischemic tissues, rapidly growing tissues, and tissues with high metabolic rates.

Several angiogenic factors have been identified, including endothelial cell growth factor,[24] fibroblast growth factor,[25] and angiogen.[26] These factors act by the dissolution of the basement membrane of the endothelial cells, followed by the rapid dissolution of new endothelial cells that stream out of the vessels into cords. The cells in these cords divide and then gradually fold over into a tube. The tubes then connect with other tubes to form a vascular network.

Vascular flow is dependent on neurologic as well as hormonal regulation. Some vasoconstrictor hormones include epinephrine and norepinephrine from the central nervous system (CNS) and the adrenal medulla, angiotensin from the adrenal cortex, and vasopressin from the posterior pituitary. Some vasodilator substances include bradykinin, serotonin, histamine, and the prostaglandins. Various other ionic and chemical factors can produce vasoconstriction and vasodilation as well and have an effect on the flow of blood that is delivered to tissues.

Blood Pressure

Pressure, Flow, and Resistance Interrelationships

Ohm's Law. Ohm's law correlates the flow of electricity (current), the applied electrical pressure (voltage), and the resistance to this flow (resistance). A modification of this law is used

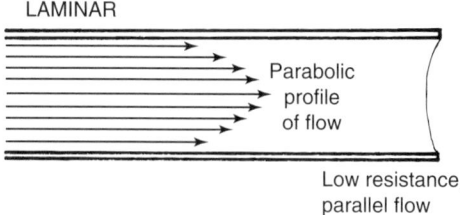

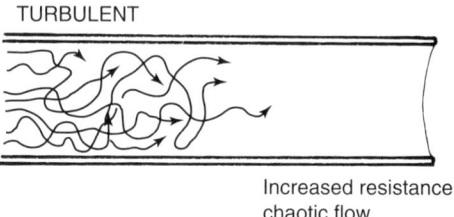

FIGURE **24-33** Laminar and turbulent flow.

in medicine to describe the flow of a fluid (blood) through a tube (blood vessel), even though the vessels are dynamic rather than static. Ohm's law and fluid flow are described by the following equation:

Equation 24-11

$$Q = (P_1 \times P_2)/R$$

where the flow through a cylinder (Q) is equal to the change in pressure from one end of the tube to the other ($P_1 \times P_2$) divided by the resistance (R) of the tube. Therefore either a decrease in resistance or an increase in pressure change across the tube increases the flow of fluid through the tube.

Blood Flow. Blood flow is the quantity of blood that passes a given point in a given amount of time. Clinically, CO may be inserted into the equation as blood flow. Two types of flow exist: laminar and turbulent (Figure 24-33).

Laminar flow has a parabolic profile that illustrates the parallel movement of molecules. Conversely, turbulent flow is described as a whirlpool and does not move as easily, thereby increasing resistance to flow. Reynolds number (Re) is a means of determining the type of flow in a tube and uses the diameter of the blood vessel (d) and the velocity (v), density (ρ), and viscosity (n) of the fluid to determine whether turbulence occurs.

The formula for calculating Reynolds number includes the velocity of blood flow in centimeters per second multiplied by the diameter of the tube in centimeters, multiplied by the density of the fluid in grams per cubic centimeter, divided by the viscosity (see equation). A Reynolds number below 200 indicates laminar flow. A Reynolds number of 200 to 400 indicates that turbulence occurs at bends in the tube, and a Reynolds number above 2000 indicates turbulent flow, even in straight, smooth vessels.

Equation 24-12

$$Re = (v \times d \times \rho)/n$$

Reynolds number demonstrates that in large vessels with high velocities, such as the aorta and large arteries, turbulent flow occurs even in the straight portions of these vessels.

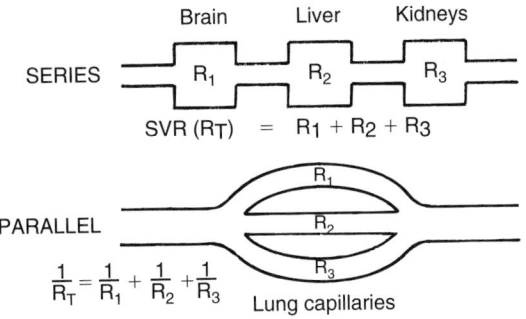

FIGURE 24-34 Resistance in series and parallel systems. *R*, Resistance; *SVR*, systemic vascular resistance. *R_T*, total resistance.

Poiseuille's Law. Poiseuille's law (see equation) describes the amount of fluid flowing through a tube (Q) in relation to the pressure drop across the tube ($P_1 - P_2$), the radius of the tube (r), the length of the tube (l), and the viscosity of the fluid (n):

Equation 24-13

$$Q = ([P_1 - P_2] \, r^4)/(8 \times n \times 1)$$

One of the most important factors in determining fluid flow is the radius of the vessel.

Clinical applications of Poiseuille's law include selection of intravenous catheter size and endotracheal tube size and determination of vascular distention and constriction in response to pharmacologic agents.

Resistance. Resistance is the impediment to blood flow in a blood vessel. Clinically it cannot be measured directly but is calculated from measures of blood flow (CO) and pressure differences in the vessels.

The units of measure most commonly used in the clinical area are centimeter-gram-second units. The normal SVR is 800 to 1500 dyne/sec per centimeter^{-5}, and the normal pulmonary vascular resistance is approximately one tenth of that number, or between 50 and 150 dyne/sec per centimeter^{-5}.

Resistance of Systems. Resistance is calculated for two major systems (Figure 24-34). In a series system, such as the systemic vasculature, the total resistance (R_T) is equal to the sum of the resistances for the individual tissue beds within the system (see equation):

Equation 24-14

$$R_T = R_1 + R_2 + R_3 + \ldots R_n$$

In a parallel system, such as a capillary bed, the total resistance is less than any of the individual resistances (see equation). Therefore the blood flow through a capillary bed such as the pulmonary capillaries is less than the resistance through any of the individual capillaries of the pulmonary system.

Equation 24-15

$$1/R_T = 1/R_1 + 1/R_2 + 1/R_3 + \ldots 1/R_n$$

Regulation of Mean Arterial Blood Pressure

Regulation of arterial blood pressure is an important function in maintaining the homeostasis of the patient receiving anesthesia. Mean arterial pressure is an important indicator of the perfusion of the tissue beds.

Blood pressure regulation can be categorized as either short term or long term. The choice of category depends on the onset of action, the duration of action, and the intensity of action to return the MAP to normal values.

Short-Term Regulation. The short-term blood pressure regulators are those that respond to rapid changes in MAP and attempt to rapidly (within 30 minutes) return the MAP back to normal range. These reflexes rely on an intact autonomic nervous system, and this interaction is responsible for the rapid onset of action of these blood pressure regulators. The reflexes include the baroreceptor response, the chemoreceptor response, atrial stretch reflex, and CNS ischemic mechanism. All of these reflexes are initiated rapidly in response to acute changes in MAP.

It is important to understand the role of the cardiovascular (vasomotor) center that is located in the medulla and pons. This center regulates four basic actions: vasoconstriction, vasodilation, cardiac excitation, and cardiac inhibition. These areas activate the sympathetic and parasympathetic nervous systems in response to certain stimuli. Under normal conditions, the vasomotor center maintains peripheral vascular tone.

Baroreceptors are located in the internal carotid arteries and the aortic arch and are called the *carotid and aortic sinuses*. They are spray-type nerve endings that increase impulse production when they are stretched. Impulses from the baroreceptors affect the inhibitory centers of the vasomotor center. At MAP of less than 60 mm Hg, the baroreceptors do not transmit impulses. However, as the MAP increases to between 60 and 180 mm Hg, impulses sent to the inhibitory area of the vasomotor center incrementally increase. The baroreceptors are most efficient in responding to rapid changes in blood pressure. They are not as efficient in long-term blood pressure regulation, because they adapt to the higher pressures, in effect by being reset. Therefore, the baroreceptors act as a buffer system to prevent extreme short-term swings in blood pressure. Two clinically significant examples of stimulation of the baroreceptor reflex during surgery include carotid sinus manipulation during carotid endarterectomy and aortic baroreceptor stimulation from pressure exerted on the aortic arch during mediastinoscopy.

Chemoreceptors are chemosensitive cells located within the carotid and aortic bodies. These are known as the *peripheral chemoreceptors*. Each area is supplied by a small nutrient artery and thereby maintains constant contact with the internal environment. Chemoreceptors send impulses to excite the vasomotor center, primarily in response to decreases in PaO₂. Chemoreceptors play a greater role in respiratory system regulation than in blood pressure regulation.

Low-pressure receptors, or stretch receptors, are located in many areas of the vasculature, especially within the atria and pulmonary arterial tree. They act in conjunction with the baroreceptors to buffer changes in the blood pressure caused by changes in volume status.

The *atrial stretch reflex* is initiated by input from low-pressure receptors. Stretching of the atria caused by an increase in volume results in a dilation of the peripheral arterioles, which decreases SVR, MAP, and CO. Furthermore, hypervolemia causes the release of the atrial natriuretic factor by the atria as a result of increased stretch.[27] This factor causes a reflex dilation of afferent arterioles in the kidney, a phenomenon that increases the glomerular filtration rate and decreases the secretion of antidiuretic hormone via signals to the hypothalamus. The combination of these events causes an increase in urine formation and an attempt to change the MAP by decreasing vascular volume.

The CNS ischemic mechanisms are another rapidly acting blood pressure control system. When hypotension exists, this reflex is initiated in an attempt to restore the MAP to adequate levels for CNS perfusion and especially for perfusion to the vasomotor center. The reflex is most intensely initiated when MAP is less than 20 mm Hg and results in one of the most powerful sympathetic vasoconstrictor responses within the human body.[1] The stimulation persists for approximately 10 minutes, by which time either the ischemia has been relieved or the vasomotor center has infarcted, and the stimulation ceases.

Several hormones are instrumental in the short-term regulation of MAP. The onset of action is not as rapid as that of neural control mechanisms, but activation occurs within a short time of stimulation. Norepinephrine and epinephrine are released from the central nervous system and the adrenal medulla during times of sympathetic stimulation and cause vasoconstriction.

Angiotensin I is converted to angiotensin II in the lungs by angiotensin-converting enzyme. This substance is one of the most potent vasoconstrictive substances secreted by the body. It takes approximately 20 minutes to become fully activated. Angiotensin II also plays a role in the secretion of aldosterone from the adrenal cortex. Aldosterone has a role in the long-term regulation of MAP.

The antidiuretic hormone vasopressin has both short-term and long-term effects on blood pressure control. The short-term effect of antidiuretic hormone causes potent and direct vasoconstriction. The long-term control effects of antidiuretic hormone decrease urine output from the kidneys.

Two short-term systems for maintenance of blood pressure that could be classified as intermediate mechanisms are the capillary fluid shift and the stress-relaxation mechanism. Both of these mechanisms depend on an intact vascular system.

The capillary fluid shift is a simple mechanism. As the hydrostatic pressure (MAP) increases within the capillaries, a larger movement of fluid occurs across the capillary membrane as increased pressure. This phenomenon lowers the fluid volume within the vasculature and results in a decrease in MAP.

The stress-relaxation mechanism is an example of the ability of the vasculature to compensate for hypervolemia and hypovolemia as a result of alterations of smooth muscle tone within the vasculature. When the fluid volume increases, tension on the blood vessels results in dilation of the vasculature to compensate for increased volume. Conversely, as the blood volume decreases, the vessels constrict to compensate for the decreased volume in order to maintain MAP.

Long-Term Regulation. Long-term regulation of MAP includes mechanisms that eventually regulate blood volume to within normal range. The renal body fluid system is one of the major long-term regulators of MAP. Renal homeostasis of blood pressure occurs as the kidneys preferentially excrete sodium and water to maintain a normal fluid balance.

It is important to understand the concept of fluid balance and its effect on arterial blood pressure. A chronic increase in blood volume leads to increases in mean filling pressure, venous return, CO, and SVR. The combination of an increased CO and an increased SVR can increase the arterial blood pressure by more than 30%. This causes an increase in myocardial oxygen demand.

Several factors govern the effectiveness of the renal body fluid system, including the renin-angiotensin system, aldosterone secretion, and the nervous system. As fluid intake and blood pressure increase, the secretion of renin by the kidneys decreases. This decreased renin secretion causes a reduced secretion of aldosterone as a result of the decreased production of angiotensin

II, which is a potent vasoconstrictor. A decrease in sympathetic nervous system response to the kidney also occurs. The net effect is an increased renal output of sodium and water.

Physiology of the Venous System
In the past, the venous system has been described as simply the return conduit for the arterial system. The venous system was not thought to play a very active role in the maintenance of circulation and CO. The modern view gives the venous system an integral role in support of the circulation.[28]

The venous system's ability to accommodate large volume changes helps to buffer the intravascular volume during periods of hypervolemia or hypovolemia and thereby helps to maintain CO. In addition, the venous system is well innervated by the autonomic nervous system and therefore has the ability to respond to the wide variations in intravascular volume that occur over the course of long surgical procedures and during times of intensive fluid resuscitation.

Knowledge of the anatomy and physiology of the cardiovascular system is essential for the safe practice of anesthesia. This section has discussed issues of concern to the anesthesia provider and has provided reference material for the integration of that knowledge into clinical practice.

HYPERTENSION
Extent, Definition, and Etiology
The pathophysiologic cardiovascular condition that is most commonly encountered in patients who require surgery is hypertension. Hypertension affects approximately 60 million people in the United States, and the frequency at which it occurs increases with age. Nearly two thirds of people over the age of 65 years have hypertension. It is vital for the anesthesia provider to understand the pathophysiology of the condition and its relation to the cardiovascular system and other body systems. Only then can a comprehensive anesthesia plan be constructed.

Patients frequently do not exhibit signs or symptoms associated with hypertension. Chronic uncontrolled hypertension affects specific target organs, including the heart, brain, and kidney. Hypertension accelerates and exacerbates the onset of atherosclerotic changes in the arterial vessels of the target organs. It is a primary risk factor for the development of coronary artery disease. Hypertension is a significant cause of congestive heart failure and cardiomyopathy because of increased afterload from chronic vasoconstriction. Because hypertension increases the likelihood of the development of atherosclerosis, it has been implicated as a causative factor responsible for the development of stroke and renal failure.[29]

Hypertension is classified on the basis of its causes. Essential (primary) hypertension, which has no identifiable cause, accounts for 95% of all cases of the disease, and its diagnosis is determined on the basis of exclusion. Remedial (secondary) hypertension has an identifiable and potentially curable cause. Sources of secondary hypertension include pheochromocytoma, coarctation of the aorta, renal artery stenosis, primary renal diseases (e.g., pyelonephritis, glomerulonephritis), primary aldosteronism (Conn disease), and hyperadrenocorticism (Cushing disease).

Guidelines regarding blood pressure values that constitute hypertension have been published by the National Institutes of Health (NIH). The classification of hypertension is listed in Table 24-5. To determine accurate blood pressure measurements, two readings taken 5 minutes apart with the patient in the sitting

TABLE 24-5	Classification of Blood Pressure for Adults Age 18 Years and Older			
Category	Systolic (mm Hg)		Diastolic (mm Hg)	
Normal	<120	And	<80	
Prehypertension	120-139	Or	80-89	
Hypertension, stage 1	140-159	Or	90-99	
Hypertension, stage 2	≥160	Or	≥100	

From National Institutes of Health, National Heart, Lung and Blood Institute, National High Blood Pressure Education Program. Seventh Report of the Joint National Committee on Prevention, Detection, Evaluation and Treatment of High Blood Pressure (NIH Publication No. 03-5233:3). Washington, DC: U.S. Government Printing Office; 2003.

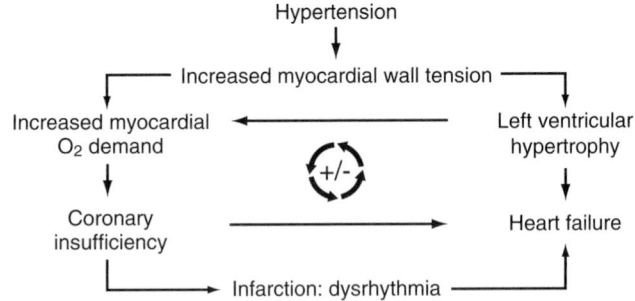

FIGURE 24-35   Schematic representation of the relationship between hypertension and heart failure. (*Modified from Wallace MC, Haddadin AS. Systemic and pulmonary hypertension. In: Hines RA, Marschall KE, eds. Stoelting's Anesthesia and Co-Existing Disease. 5th ed. Philadelphia: Churchill Livingstone; 2008:89.*)

position are necessary. The risk of cardiovascular disease doubles with each increment of 20/10 mm Hg above 115/75 mm Hg. The NIH has coined the term *prehypertension* to refer to those patients who would benefit from lifestyle modifications that decrease the likelihood of developing the pathophysiologic changes associated with hypertension.[30] It is estimated that the implementation of antihypertensive therapy is associated with a 25% decrease in cardiovascular complications and a 38% decrease in stroke.[31] If lifestyle modifications are unsuccessful in decreasing blood pressure to acceptable levels, then antihypertensive therapy should be prescribed.[32] In many instances, patients may have developed advanced atherosclerotic vascular disease or target-organ dysfunction before the start of treatment for hypertension.[33,34]

Pathophysiology

Systemic blood pressure is regulated by interactive feedback mechanisms involving the sympathoadrenal axis and baroreceptors in the heart and great vessels. It is accepted that some degree of sympathetic dysfunction is responsible for essential hypertension. Dysfunction of the sympathetic nervous system leads to a state of chronic vasoconstriction. In an attempt to maintain normal intravascular volume, the renal juxtaglomerular apparatus secretes renin. All the vascular and hormonal effects of renin are caused by its conversion of angiotensin I to angiotensin II. Angiotensin II is the major stimulus for the secretion of aldosterone by the adrenal cortex.

Anesthesia Management for the Patient with Hypertension
Preoperative Evaluation

The most important issues to be addressed in the preoperative evaluation of the hypertensive patient are the identification and the adequacy of treatment. A number of otherwise healthy patients scheduled for elective procedures are determined to have hypertension, even though they had no prior need for medical treatment. The goal of antihypertensive therapy is to maintain normotension on a consistent basis. Effective antihypertensive therapy that renders the patient normotensive on a routine basis may not necessarily prevent episodes of perioperative hypertension. However, patients whose condition is optimized before surgery have a more stable perioperative course and a lower incidence of cardiovascular system–related morbidity. Although not ideal, if perioperative diastolic blood pressure

is maintained below 110 mm Hg, the risk of perioperative cardiac morbidity does not increase significantly.[29,35]

It is imperative for anesthesia providers to have an adequate understanding of the pharmacology and side effects of the drugs used for treating hypertension. For a complete discussion of antihypertensive drugs, see Chapter 14. Some of the drugs used to treat hypertension block or depress homeostatic sympathetic reflexes. The depression of these reflexes may prevent homeostatic compensatory mechanisms from functioning at normal levels during the course of anesthesia. Subsequently, compensatory mechanisms (tachycardia and vasoconstriction) associated with blood loss may be diminished or may not occur. Patients treated with antihypertensive medication do not lose their responsiveness to vasoactive drugs but instead may respond to these substances in an exaggerated manner. Even with depression of the sympathetic reflexes, no predominance of the parasympathetic system occurs.

The clinician should carefully obtain a thorough history of the cardiovascular system to elicit any symptoms of ischemic cardiovascular disease. Hypertension is a major risk factor for coronary artery disease. Any symptoms related to coronary artery disease should be further investigated. In addition to being a risk factor for coronary artery disease, hypertension directly affects myocardial function. The chronic increase in myocardial wall tension caused by long-standing hypertension results in left ventricular hypertrophy (LVH; Figure 24-35). Ventricular diastolic dysfunction occurs before the development of hypertrophy. This diastolic dysfunction is not clinically apparent, and the patient may appear to have normal cardiac function except under stressful physiologic conditions. A delayed rate of passive ventricular filling is evidence of ventricular diastolic dysfunction. The rate of ventricular filling from atrial contraction becomes predominant in the hypertensive patient. This represents the inverse of normal ventricular filling patterns. Other information and results from preoperative tests that will help the nurse anesthetist to evaluate and create an individualized anesthetic plan for patients with cardiac dysfunction includes determining exercise tolerance, ECG, Doppler ultrasound, stress test, and cardiac catheterization results.

Left ventricular hypertrophy is a consequence of chronic hypertension and increased afterload that results in an enlargement of myocardial mass. This compensatory process increases myocardial oxygen demand. Hypertrophy that occurs in response to chronic increases in intracardiac pressure is termed *concentric hypertrophy.* Ventricular hypertrophy also may produce subendocardial ischemia at perfusion pressures that would normally be adequate in a healthy ventricle. Concomitant development of coronary artery disease coupled with increased myocardial oxygen demand hastens and exacerbates the development of ischemic symptoms. As a rule, all patients with chronic hypertension should be suspected of having some degree of coronary artery disease.

Hypertensive cardiomyopathy and systolic ventricular dysfunction are the direct result of the pathophysiologic changes associated with chronic hypertension. This hypertensive cardiomyopathy manifests as a decrease in both EF and SV. Increasing diastolic dysfunction results in ventricular dilation in conjunction with systolic dysfunction. The subsequent replacement of myocardial cells with fibrous tissue results in a cardiomyopathy.[4]

Long-standing hypertension that has remained either untreated or inadequately controlled has adverse consequences on brain and kidney function, and patients with long-standing disease have a higher incidence of strokes than do patients whose blood pressure has been controlled.[4] Inadequate control of hypertension can lead to alterations in cerebrovascular and coronary artery autoregulation. For example, normal physiologic coronary artery autoregulation occurs at a MAP between 50 and 120 mm Hg. However, a patient with chronic hypertension and coronary artery disease may develop ischemic changes at a MAP of 50 mm Hg or greater. The cerebral and coronary autoregulation curves are shifted to the right in patients with chronic hypertension, necessitating higher perfusion pressures to ensure adequate organ blood flow. Therefore, cerebral and myocardial ischemia may occur with significant decreases in MAP in patients with hypertension and coronary artery disease. This phenomenon makes patients with uncontrolled hypertension more susceptible to cardiac and cerebral ischemia, compared with normotensive individuals.[34] Chronic untreated hypertension can cause nephrosclerosis, which can impair renal function. Nephrosclerosis can produce proteinuria and a gradual decrease in renal function. Early treatment of hypertension results in little change in renal function and spares the kidneys. Signs of target organ involvement must be investigated in the hypertensive patient who is to undergo anesthesia.

Anesthesia Management

An individualized anesthetic plan must be created by taking into account the type and extent of cardiac pathophysiology, other disease states, and the surgical procedure. To maintain a stable intraoperative course, administration of antihypertensive medications should be continued on schedule until the time of surgery. All oral medications can be given with one or two sips of water without increased risk of aspiration.[33] It should be noted that acute hypertensive rebound can occur with abrupt cessation of antihypertensive medications. Tachycardia, hypertension, angina, and myocardial infarction can result from interruption of therapy with β-blockers and calcium channel–blocking agents. These drugs should be discontinued with caution and only after utmost discretionary review of the patient's physiologic status.

Determining whether to proceed with elective surgery in a patient in whom hypertension is untreated or poorly controlled remains controversial. However, evidence suggests that patients with diastolic blood pressures greater than 110 mm Hg have a significantly increased risk of perioperative cardiac morbidity.[34] This caveat may be modified in patients with hypertension in whom diastolic blood pressures greater than 110 mm Hg occur

frequently, despite aggressive antihypertensive drug therapy (e.g., patients with end-stage renal disease).

To attenuate sympathetic responsiveness, preoperative sedation may be indicated for patients with hypertension. Establishing control of the blood pressure before induction should result in a more stable hemodynamic course during the induction, maintenance, and emergence from anesthesia. A fluid bolus and incremental titration of anesthetic induction agents may help decrease the degree and duration of hypotension.

Induction of Anesthesia

Patients with hypertension may react in an exaggerated manner to induction agents and the stimulation associated with laryngoscopy and tracheal intubation. This response is highly variable and may result in hypertension or hypotension. It is dependent on the individual's physiology, degree of stimulation, adequacy of preoperative antihypertensive therapy, and amount and type of induction agents administered. Hypertensive patients are hypovolemic, either as a result of renal-compensatory mechanisms, extreme vasoconstriction, or pharmacologic therapy (diuretics). Increased vasoconstriction as a consequence of hypertension results in volume contraction and a greater susceptibility to hypotension from the vasodilating and cardiac-depressant effects of anesthetic agents. Of the anesthetic induction agents, etomidate, propofol, or sodium pentothal can be used in patients with hypertension. Etomidate offers an advantage in patients with cardiac pathology, as compared to propofol or sodium pentothal because it preserves stroke volume and cardiac output.[15] Due to the sympathomimetic response that occurs with the administration of induction doses of ketamine, this drug should be not be used routinely for patients with cardiovascular disease.

The stimuli of laryngoscopy and tracheal intubation can result in an exaggerated hypertensive response, despite postinduction hypotension. An existing hypertensive state is further compounded by intense stimulation caused by airway manipulation. Suppressing the exaggerated hypertensive response to intubation requires that a greater depth of anesthesia be achieved. However, the depth of anesthesia at induction necessary to suppress this response may produce a more profound hypotensive state. Administration of adjunct medications before induction (e.g., β-blockers or arterial dilators) can reduce the hyperdynamic sympathetic response to tracheal intubation. Hypotensive episodes can be treated with fluid administration, decrease in anesthetic depth, and administration of vasoconstrictors. Numerous strategies have been suggested for the management of this hyperdynamic response. Akhtar demonstrated that the pressor response to laryngoscopy and intubation could be significantly reduced by laryngotracheal or intravenous administration of lidocaine.[36] They also proposed that reducing the duration of airway manipulation to 15 seconds or less may be helpful. Use of a β-blocker before induction has been shown to reduce the hyperdynamic sympathetic responses, as may the administration of sodium nitroprusside before laryngoscopy.[33] Administration of fentanyl (2 to 3 mcg/kg) just before induction also helps attenuate the pressor response.

With regard to suppression of marked hemodynamic responses, a smooth induction followed by a rapid and atraumatic intubation is imperative. Maintaining an adequate depth of anesthesia at induction that produces extreme hypotension may be more detrimental to both coronary and cerebral perfusion than the hypertensive response it was intended to prevent. Because the hypertensive patient is frequently hypovolemic as compared with the normotensive patient, adequate hydration before induction may help prevent postinduction hypotension.[29,33]

Most intravenous induction agents are appropriate for the hypertensive patient. The propensity for these agents to cause vasodilation in a comparatively hypovolemic patient is a concern. In light of this, a combination of low doses of more than one agent in addition to titration of medications may prove a better choice than a full dose of a single agent. In emergency cases in which rapidly securing the airway is of paramount importance, the choice of agents may be limited, and hyperdynamic pressor responses become a secondary issue.

Maintenance of Anesthesia

The goal of anesthetic management for the hypertensive patient undergoing general anesthesia is to maintain blood pressure stability within 20% of the normal mean pressure. Intraoperative events that cause wide fluctuations in blood pressure should be anticipated and treated immediately. The most common event precipitating intraoperative hypertension is the painful stimulus of surgery. This induces increased sympathetic tone via a neurohormonal reflex and represents the stress-induced response of surgical stimulation. Volatile and opioid agents given alone and in combination have the ability to attenuate this response.[2,33,34] Altering the depth of anesthesia to suppress maximal surgical stimulation may not be adequate for achieving rapid and complete control of hypertensive responses. The adjunct use of drugs such as β-antagonists, nitroprusside, angiotensin-converting enzyme inhibitors (e.g., enalapril), α_2-agonists (e.g., clonidine), calcium-channel blockers (e.g., nifedipine), and α_1-blockers (e.g., droperidol) may be necessary for achieving control. These drugs offer the advantage of continued control of hypertensive response in the immediate postanesthesia recovery period. Box 24-2 lists hemodynamic goals for patients with coronary artery disease.

The onset of profound hypotension during anesthesia maintenance should be immediately recognized, diagnosed, and treated. Prolonged severe hypotension has predictive significance in perioperative cardiac morbidity.[35] Treatment of hypotension may require reduction of the amount of volatile agent used and infusion of adequate volume. Should these measures prove inadequate or untimely, a rapid-acting vasopressor such as phenylephrine or ephedrine may be administered as a temporizing measure until the cause of the hypotension can be diagnosed. It is important to realize that hypertensive patients may have exaggerated responses to vasopressor agents. The goal of intraoperative anesthesia management is maintenance of hemodynamic stability, which includes anticipation of intraoperative events that may affect cardiovascular stability and thereby prevent extreme fluctuations in blood pressure.

BOX **24-2**

Hemodynamic Goals for Management of Coronary Artery Disease

Preload	Decrease/Maintain
Afterload	Maintain
Contractility	Decrease/Maintain
Heart rate	Slow
Heart rhythm	Normal sinus rhythm

Postoperative Considerations in the Hypertensive Patient

Termination of anesthesia results in hyperdynamic, hypertensive responses, even in patients with well-controlled hypertension. Intraoperative control of blood pressure should continue into the immediate postoperative period. Initiation of adjunct administration of antihypertensive medications should be anticipated early in the postoperative period. Adequate control of pain represents a primary antihypertensive consideration. The hypertensive patient is more susceptible to perioperative cardiac morbidity than the normotensive patient during the postoperative period. Adequate control of blood pressure in the postoperative period reduces the incidence of cardiovascular complications.[29,37] Mangano and associates studied the effects of atenolol administered to patients who had confirmed coronary artery disease or were at risk for its development. Atenolol was administered preoperatively, postoperatively, and throughout the hospital stay. The results in the atenolol study group showed a 65% reduction in mortality caused by adverse cardiac events. In addition, patients in the atenolol study group had a 67% decrease in mortality within 1 year of surgery and a 48% decrease in mortality in the 2 years after surgery.[17]

Pericardial Disease

In reviewing the anesthetic management of patients with pericardial disease, this section focuses on the pathophysiology, clinical presentation, and anesthetic implications of three primary disease processes: acute pericarditis, constrictive pericarditis, and cardiac tamponade.

The pericardium surrounds the heart and anchors it to its anatomic position, concomitantly reducing contact between it and surrounding structures. It consists of an inner visceral layer, which envelops the surface of the heart, and an outer parietal layer. The pericardial space between these layers usually contains 20 to 25 mL of clear fluid, that under normal circumstances can accommodate gradual volume fluctuations. Rapid accumulation of pericardial fluid in the pericardial space can result in cardiac tamponade and cardiovascular collapse.[38]

Acute Pericarditis

Acute inflammation of the pericardium is caused by a number of disorders.[38] The most common cause of acute pericarditis is viral infection. Postmyocardial infarction syndrome (Dressler syndrome), postcardiotomy, metastatic disease, irradiation, tuberculosis, and rheumatoid arthritis represent the remaining primary predisposing conditions that contribute to the development of this process.[39]

Pathophysiology. It is common for a serofibrinous inflammatory reaction associated with a small intrapericardial exudative effusion to evolve. This may result in adherence of the two layers of the pericardium. The sequelae are largely dependent on the severity of the reaction, as well as on the specific cause. Most often when the condition is left untreated or undiagnosed, complete resolution is the end result. Infrequently, however, extended organization of fibrinous exudate within the pericardial sac may lead to encasement of the heart by dense fibrous connective tissue (chronic constrictive pericarditis) or to the accumulation of a large amount of pericardial fluid and consequent cardiac tamponade, usually when fluid levels exceed 1 L. Constrictive pericarditis and cardiac tamponade result in impaired diastolic filling and subsequent diminution of CO.[38,39]

Clinical Presentation. The principal symptom associated with acute pericarditis is chest pain with sudden onset.

Although similar in nature to that experienced during myocardial infarction, this pain is differentiated by the inclusion of a pleural component, which includes increased discomfort associated with postural changes and relief on sitting or leaning forward. Other signs that are characteristic of acute pericarditis include fever with a pericardial friction rub, absence of elevation of cardiac enzymes levels, and diffuse ST-segment elevation in two or three limb leads and in most of the precordial leads. Echocardiography is another reliable method for diagnosing pericarditis and pericardial effusion.

Anesthetic Management. Acute pericarditis in the absence of an associated pericardial effusion or scarring does not alter cardiac function. Specific considerations for anesthetic management are directed toward the underlying illness.

Chronic Constrictive Pericarditis

Chronic constrictive pericarditis results from pericardial thickening and fibrosis. In the past, tuberculosis was the most common cause of pericardial constriction. Currently the most common causes are idiopathic and include complications following cardiac surgery, neoplasia, uremia, radiation therapy, and rheumatoid arthritis.[39,40]

Pathophysiology. Stiff, fibrous tissue encircles the heart and limits its ability to expand during diastole. The fundamental hemodynamic abnormality in chronic constrictive pericarditis is abnormal diastolic filling. Reduced myocardial compliance impairs filling of both ventricles. Consequently filling pressures increase, and as a result, pulmonary and peripheral congestion occurs. SV and CO can also be decreased. Equilibration of pulmonary artery diastolic pressure, PCWP, and right atrial pressure commonly occurs. Initially, ventricular systolic function is normal. However, over time the underlying myocardial tissue may atrophy, and systolic function may decrease.

Clinical Presentation. Clinical features representative of chronic constrictive pericarditis include gradually increasing fatigue and dyspnea. Typical signs of increasing venous pressure and congestion are engorgement of neck veins, hepatomegaly, ascites, and peripheral edema. In approximately 50% of patients, the fibrous enclosure becomes calcified and is visible on a chest radiograph.[33] The electrocardiogram may reveal diffuse low-voltage QRS complexes, T-wave inversion, and notched P waves. As many as 25% of patients have atrial dysrhythmias because of the involvement of atrial conduction pathways. Diagnosis is confirmed by demonstration of pericardial thickening with echocardiography or computed tomography.

The treatment used for patients with hemodynamically significant constrictive pericarditis is pericardiotomy. Unfortunately, the surgical removal of adherent pericardium may precipitate malignant cardiac dysrhythmias and massive bleeding. Consequently, pericardiotomy is associated with relatively high perioperative morbidity and mortality rates, ranging from 6% to 19%.[41,42]

Anesthetic Management. Large-bore intravenous lines must be established preoperatively because of the potential for sudden, rapid hemorrhage. A cardiopulmonary bypass circuit should be readily available. Invasive hemodynamic monitoring is essential. Arterial catheterization allows beat-to-beat blood pressure monitoring and assists in the evaluation of significant cardiac dysrhythmia. A pulmonary artery catheter is useful because it permits measurement of filling pressures on both the right and left sides of the heart, as well as determination of CO.

The anesthetic agents chosen for management of patients with constrictive pericarditis should preserve myocardial contractility, HR, preload, and afterload. Among these parameters, HR is of greatest concern. Cardiac output is dependent on HR in patients with constrictive pericarditis. As a consequence of limited ventricular diastolic filling, bradycardia is poorly tolerated and reflects a decrease in SV that can lead to hypotension. Using anesthetic medications that preserve HR and myocardial contractility, such as pancuronium or ketamine, is hemodynamically advantageous. Inhalation agents that cause myocardial depression should be used with caution. The use of opioids and etomidate, benzodiazepines, and nitrous oxide for the induction and maintenance of anesthesia is suitable in this setting. The clinician should be aware that vigorous positive-pressure ventilation may cause a decrease in venous return to the heart and result in a further decrease in CO.[43]

Immediate hemodynamic improvement may not occur after removal of the constricting tissue. Consistently low CO after pericardiectomy may be secondary to diffuse atrophy of myocardial muscle fibers or myocardial damage from the underlying disease. Intensive postoperative care with inotropic support and awareness of the potential for dysrhythmia or bleeding are integral components of the anesthetic management plan.

Cardiac Tamponade

Cardiac tamponade is a syndrome caused by the impairment of diastolic filling of the heart because of continal increases in intrapericardial pressure.[44] Slow accumulation of fluid in the pericardial space can cause minute increases in intrapericardial pressure. This occurs as a result of the pericardium's ability to stretch to accommodate this increase in volume. If the pericardial fluid accumulates rapidly, the presence of a few hundred milliliters may cause a significant increase in intrapericardial pressure that may result in cardiovascular collapse. Cardiac tamponade is the cause of cardiac compressive shock that can result in inadequate peripheral perfusion, acidosis, and death (Figure 24-36).

Classification of the causes of cardiac tamponade includes (1) trauma, including sharp or blunt trauma to the chest and dissecting aortic aneurysms; (2) causes associated with cardiac surgery; (3) malignancy within the mediastinum; and (4) expansion of pericardial effusions after any form of pericarditis.[45]

Pathophysiology. Normal intrapericardial pressure is subatmospheric. Accumulation of pericardial fluid leads to an increase in intrapericardial pressure. As a result, diastolic expansion of the ventricles decreases. As in constrictive pericarditis, poor ventricular filling develops and leads to peripheral congestion and a decrease in SV and CO. The decrease in SV stimulates compensatory mechanisms for maintaining CO (tachycardia, vasoconstriction, and an increase in venous pressure). If these mechanisms fail, cardiac collapse can occur.[46] The left ventricular pressure-volume loop associated with cardiac tamponade represents decreased LV volume and decreased SV due to compression (Figure 24-37).

Clinical Presentation. In addition to obvious indications of cardiac distress, specific signs of cardiac tamponade include the Beck triad: hypotension, jugular venous distention, and distant muffled heart sounds.[47] Another common finding is pulsus paradoxus, an exaggerated (i.e., >10 mm Hg) decrease in systolic blood pressure that normally occurs with inspiration. Other conditions that may result in pulsus paradoxus are chronic obstructive pulmonary disease, obesity, and congestive heart failure. Jugular venous distention that occurs because of decreased forward blood flow through the heart may also be present.

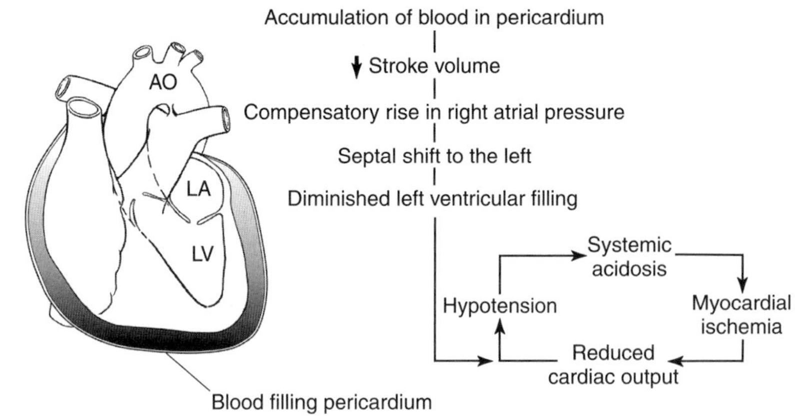

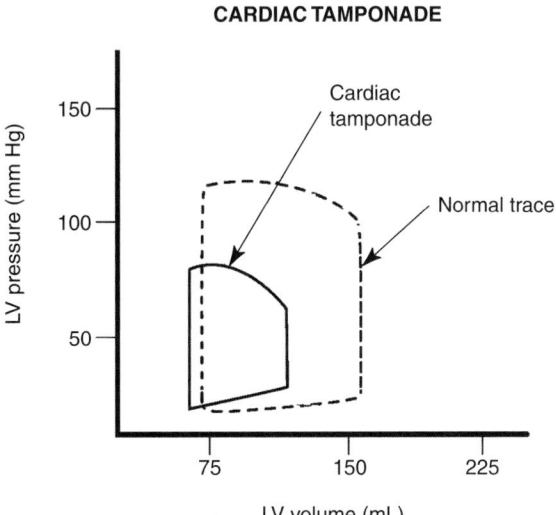

FIGURE **24-36** Pathophysiology associated with cardiac tamponade.

Accumulation of blood in pericardium
↓ Stroke volume
Compensatory rise in right atrial pressure
Septal shift to the left
Diminished left ventricular filling

Hypotension → Systemic acidosis → Myocardial ischemia → Reduced cardiac output

Blood filling pericardium

CARDIAC TAMPONADE

FIGURE **24-37** Left ventricular pressure-volume loop associated with cardiac tamponade.

In cardiac tamponade, chest radiography may show enlargement of the cardiac silhouette. The electrocardiogram usually demonstrates a decrease in voltage across all leads or electrical alterations of either the P wave or the QRS complex.[48] Echocardiography is the most sensitive, noninvasive method for detection of pericardial effusion and exclusion of tamponade. Use of a pulmonary artery catheter may reveal equilibration of right and left atrial pressures and right ventricular end-diastolic filling pressures at approximately 20 mm Hg.[49]

The definitive treatment for cardiac tamponade is pericardiocentesis, performed either percutaneously by needle decompression, through a subxiphoid incision, or via video-assisted thorascopic surgery and creation of a pericardial window. In contrast to patients with constrictive pericarditis, in patients with cardiac tamponade, immediate hemodynamic improvement occurs once the pericardium is opened. However, despite this fact, pulmonary edema, acute right and left ventricular dysfunction, and circulatory collapse can occur.[42]

Anesthetic Management. Preoperatively the patient's clinical status should be optimized. This includes expansion of intravascular fluid volume, use of positive inotropic agents, and correction of acidosis. The degree to which these measures are

instituted depends on the hemodynamic state of the patient. Severely compromised patients require immediate medical therapy, and therefore emergency pericardiocentesis is indicated. Invasive hemodynamic monitoring should be established before the procedure. Intraarterial and central venous pressure catheters are required for frequent drawing of blood, continuous blood pressure monitoring, and assessment of intravascular fluid status.

Local infiltration anesthesia is the technique of choice for operative correction of cardiac tamponade.[50] Many reports exist of severe hypotension and cardiac arrest after induction of general anesthesia in patients with tamponade.[51,52] The potential for decompensation associated with the use of general anesthetics is attributed to direct myocardial depression and vasodilation in patients with established impairment of cardiac filling. The use of positive-pressure ventilation in such patients may result in a decrease of venous return to the heart and can further decrease CO.[53] After percutaneous pericardiocentesis and the improvement of hemodynamic status, induction of general anesthesia and initiation of positive-pressure ventilation are sufficient for further surgical exploration.

When it is not possible to relieve intrapericardial pressure that causes cardiac tamponade before the induction of anesthesia, the same anesthetic principles that are applied to the anesthetic management of patients with constrictive pericarditis should be used, including the use of anesthetic agents that preserve myocardial contractility, HR, preload, and afterload. Because of the sympathomimetic effects of ketamine, this drug has been advocated for the induction and maintenance of anesthesia.[4,50] However, many combinations of anesthetic agents that preserve the previously mentioned determinants of CO have been used safely.[43,50,52]

Postoperative continuous monitoring of blood pressure, central venous pressure, and chest-tube drainage is necessary. Possible complications after pericardiocentesis include the reaccumulation of pericardial fluid, coronary laceration, cardiac puncture, and pneumothorax. Box 24-3 lists hemodynamic goals for patients with cardiac tamponade.

Acquired Valvular Heart Disease
The cardiac valves are membranous leaflets that separate the chambers of the heart. When open, they allow blood flow between the chambers and great vessels, and when closed, they prevent regurgitant blood flow between the chambers or backflow from the great vessels. A valve orifice of normal size presents a small degree of flow obstruction and thereby creates a

BOX **24-3**

Hemodynamic Goals for Management of Cardiac Tamponade

Preload	Maintain or increase
Afterload	Maintain
Contractility	Maintain or increase
Heart rate	Maintain
Heart rhythm	Normal sinus rhythm
Treatment	Pericardiocentesis, pericardial window

2. *Status of left ventricular loading*
   Left ventricle (LV) overload from mitral or aortic regurgitation (AR)
   Pressure overloading from aortic stenosis
   Volume underloading from mitral stenosis
3. *Acute versus chronic evolution of the dysfunction*
   Acute lesions have severe and precipitous hemodynamic consequences.
4. *Cardiac rhythm and its effects on ventricular diastolic filling time*
5. *Left ventricular function*
   Poor left ventricular function places the patient at higher risk for perioperative cardiac morbidity.
6. *Secondary effects on the pulmonary vasculature and right ventricular function*
   Secondary pulmonary hypertension from valvular lesions can significantly affect right ventricular function.
7. *Heart rate*
   Changes in HR (either bradycardia or tachycardia) can significantly alter the hemodynamic manifestations of a specific valvular lesion.
   Bradycardia occurring with regurgitant lesions can result in a significant increase in the regurgitant fraction.
   Tachycardia is detrimental in patients with stenotic lesions because it shortens the time of ejection and increases myocardial oxygen demand.[27-30,33,34]
8. *Perioperative anticoagulation as discussed in Chapter 35*
9. *Perioperative antibiotic therapy as discussed in Chapter 14*

Clinical Symptomatology. The most frequent clinical symptoms and signs of valvular dysfunction are congestive heart failure, dysrhythmias, syncope, and angina pectoris. Symptoms commonly associated with congestive heart failure include dyspnea, orthopnea, and fatigue. The severity of left ventricular dysfunction can be related to the patient's activity level before the onset of cardiac symptoms.[35]

Patient Evaluation: Compensatory Mechanisms. In order to maintain cardiac function despite progressive valvular dysfunction, sympathetic activity increases as a compensatory mechanism. A decrease in sympathetic tone that occurs during anesthesia can cause severe myocardial dysfunction. Evaluation of the patient should include recognition of sympathetic compensatory mechanisms and management strategies to maintain hemodynamic stability. Despite maximum medical therapy, patients with severe valvular dysfunction may remain in congestive heart failure.

The evaluation should also focus on associated organ dysfunction. Cardiac output that is decreased by chronic myocardial failure can cause significant major organ dysfunction, including renal and hepatic insufficiency, as well as poor cerebral perfusion, which can produce an altered level of consciousness, restlessness, agitation, and lethargy.

Diagnostic Modalities. The most valuable diagnostic modalities used to evaluate valvular heart disease include electrocardiography, chest radiography, color flow Doppler imaging, echocardiography, and cardiac catheterization of both the right and left chambers of the heart. Electrocardiography can be used for evaluation of ventricular hypertrophy, atrial enlargement, axis deviation and—most important—determining cardiac rhythm. Chest radiography demonstrates the size of the cardiac silhouette and signs of pulmonary vascular congestion. Color flow Doppler imaging can be used to determine the valvular area, transvalvular gradients, degree of regurgitation, and flow velocity and direction and can measure cardiac function. Cardiac catheterization can

hemodynamically insignificant gradient. Primary dysfunction of the mitral and aortic valves represents the most common and most severe hemodynamic derangement. Acquired primary dysfunction of the tricuspid or pulmonic valves is extremely rare and therefore is not addressed in this chapter.

Valvular disease is classified according to the type of lesion that exists—stenosis, insufficiency, or mixed lesions. Valvular stenosis is a narrowing of the valvular orifice, which restricts flow through the orifice when the valve is open. This situation creates an increase in flow resistance and increases turbulent blood flow. Valvular insufficiency results in regurgitation secondary to incomplete or partial valve closure, which allows blood to flow back through the valve into the previous chamber. In patients with mixed lesions (stenosis with insufficiency or insufficiency with stenosis), one type of dysfunction is considered dominant over the other on the basis of the severity of clinical symptoms.

Valvular dysfunction is classified as either primary or secondary. In primary valvular dysfunction, the valve leaflets or the anchoring and supporting structures are damaged or do not function properly. In secondary valvular dysfunction, the valve is not directly damaged. However, normal valve function is altered secondary to another pathophysiologic entity. Causes of this type of manifestation include ventricular dilation, which produces mitral insufficiency; retrograde aortic dissection, which creates aortic insufficiency (AI); and papillary muscle infarction, which causes mitral insufficiency.[54,55]

Cardiac Output. The primary components of CO are preload, afterload, contractility, LV compliance, and HR.[55-57] Blood flow may increase due to an increase in HR or an increase in SV. Because blood viscosity decreases with decreasing hematocrit and increasing flow rate, normovolemic anemia reduces cardiac afterload, thereby facilitating the augmentation of CO. This sequence of events occurs so long as intravascular volume is maintained and cardiac reserve is ample. The amount of afterload present determines the degree of tension cardiac fibers must develop before systolic ejection can occur.[58]

Evaluation of the Patient. Evaluation of the patient with valvular heart disease should focus on the pathophysiologic derangements and their effects on cardiac function. The systematic evaluation of primary valvular dysfunction should include the following:

1. *Category of valvular dysfunction*
   Stenosis (progressive narrowing of the valve orifice)
   Insufficiency (incomplete valve closure that causes backflow through the valve)
   Mixed (regurgitant and stenotic dysfunction)

be used directly to measure transvalvular gradients, estimate the degree of regurgitation, visualize the coronary arteries, and determine intracardiac pressures.[59-63]

MITRAL STENOSIS

Pathophysiology

In mitral stenosis, the mitral valve orifice becomes progressively narrowed. The normal mitral valve area is 4 to 6 cm². This narrowing reduces flow from the LA into the LV during diastole. The narrowing of the mitral valve orifice has two significant hemodynamic consequences. First, a gradient develops across the valve orifice. This change represents a compensatory response directed at maintaining adequate flow. Second, as the cross-sectional area of the orifice decreases and the gradient increases, flow is restricted and left ventricular volume is decreased. The clinical symptomatology of severe mitral stenosis results in pulmonary congestion and decreased CO. Pulmonary congestion occurs as a result of increases in left atrial pressure. Decreased SV is caused by decreased left ventricular volume. Left ventricular filling is dependent on the length of diastole, the gradient between the LA and LV, and the surface area of the mitral valve. As the valve area narrows to 1.5 to 2.5 cm², patients frequently develop increased heart rate and cardiac output.[64] At a mitral valve area of less than 1 cm², the prolonged diastolic filling time and elevated mean left atrial pressure are incapable of maintaining normal LVEDV, and decreases in left ventricular volume occur, resulting in symptoms that occur at rest.[55] Atrial systole accounts for 20% to 30% of LVEDV. Because mitral stenosis presents a fixed resistance to ventricular inflow, most of the pressure generated during atrial systole is used to overcome the resistance caused by the stenotic valve rather than for producing forward flow. As the HR increases to greater than 90 beats per minute and diastolic time intervals are shortened, LVEDV is decreased. This is demonstrated by the Gorlin equation, where mitral valve flow (MVF) is estimated utilizing equation 24-16.

Equation 24-16

$$\text{MVF} = \frac{\text{Cardiac output}}{\text{Diastolic filling time} \times \text{heart rate}}$$

Any subsequent increase in flow rate or decrease in diastolic filling time reflects an increase in the pressure gradient between the LA and the LV. As the diastolic time interval shortens, the pressure gradient increases by the square of the increase in flow rate. Therefore, any marked increase in HR can result in an increase in left atrial pressure, which can precipitate a rise in pulmonary artery pressures and ultimately leads to pulmonary edema.[65]

Left atrial hypertrophy and distention are consequences of elevated left atrial pressures. This distention of the LA can lead to atrial dysrhythmias, most commonly atrial fibrillation. The atrial systolic "kick" is lost during atrial fibrillation; this implies that diastolic filling can be maintained only by a further increase in left atrial pressure. Mean left atrial pressure is limited by the development of pulmonary congestion at pressures greater than 25 mm Hg. Elevation of left atrial pressures to greater than 25 mm Hg leads to pulmonary congestion and eventually pulmonary edema. In patients with chronic mitral stenosis, pulmonary hypertension develops because of continuous elevations in left atrial pressure (Figure 24-38).

Pulmonary Vascular Changes in Right Ventricular Function

The pulmonary vasculature and eventually the RV are adversely affected by the chronic elevation of left atrial pressure that occurs with mitral stenosis. As mitral stenosis progresses, chronic elevation of left atrial pressure causes increased blood volume in the pulmonary vascular circuit. This can cause perivascular edema, and changes in pulmonary vascular resistance may ensue. These changes in pulmonary vascular resistance result in an increase in RV afterload. As a compensatory response, right ventricular hypertrophy occurs; however, because the RV is not capable of generating high pressures, it eventually begins to fail.[55-57] As the disease progresses, overt signs of biventricular failure such as low CO with poor systemic perfusion become evident. Peripheral edema, hepatic congestion, and marked venous distention are signs of right ventricular failure. The deterioration of right ventricular function decreases adequate left ventricular filling and therefore causes further deterioration in CO (Figure 24-39).

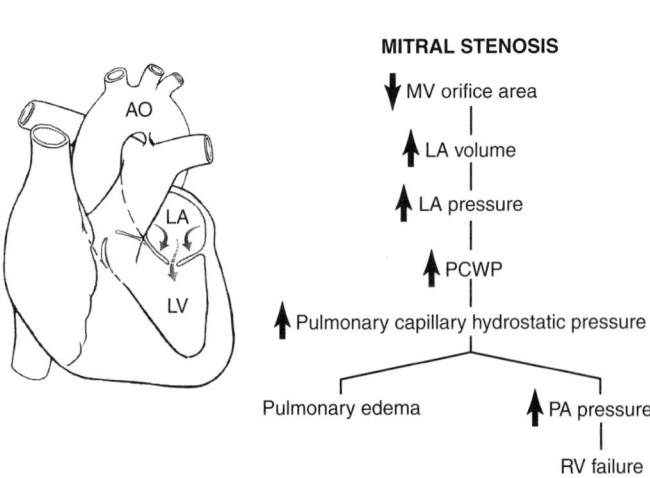

FIGURE **24-38** Pathophysiology associated with mitral stenosis.

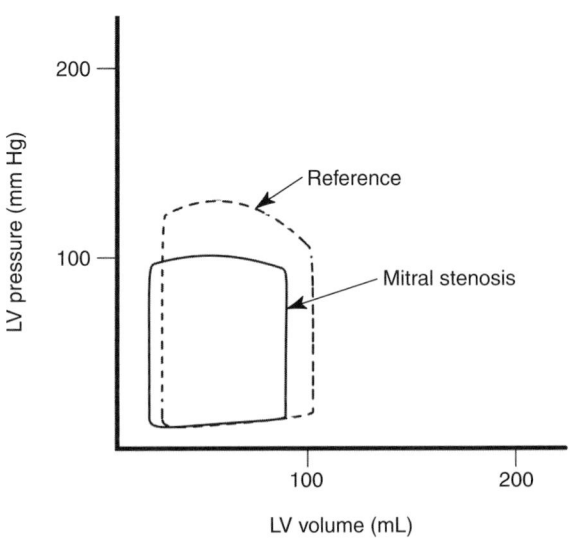

FIGURE **24-39** Left ventricular pressure-volume loop associated with mitral stenosis.

Anesthetic Considerations

Any anesthetic technique should be based on a thorough understanding of the pathophysiology of mitral stenosis, as well as the cardiovascular effects of the anesthetic agents employed. The following goals should be achieved in the anesthetic management of the patient with mitral stenosis:

1. Maintenance of sinus rhythm at low normal heart rate
2. LVEDV adequate to maintain adequate CO without increasing pulmonary congestion
3. Avoidance of extreme decreases in myocardial contractility
4. Reduction in both right ventricular and left ventricular afterload may improve hemodynamics; this must be done in a controlled manner and with careful monitoring. The extent of the surgical procedure and the degree and severity of mitral stenosis determine the level of monitoring necessary.
5. Cardioversion for hemodynamically compromising atrial tachyarrhythmias
6. Hypotension treated with small doses of phenylephrine

The LVEDV is normal in approximately 85% of patients with mitral stenosis. An increased LVEDV in patients with mitral stenosis should alert the anesthesia provider to the presence of mitral or aortic insufficiency or primary coronary artery disease. Most patients with moderate mitral stenosis also have low to normal SV and therefore may have a normal EF. Approximately 33% of patients with mitral stenosis have an EF below normal (normal, 0.67 ± 0.08).[56] When the mitral valve is narrowed to less than 1 cm^2 (severe mitral stenosis), a mean left atrial pressure of 25 mm Hg is necessary for maintaining even an adequate resting CO. Owing to the abnormal transvalvular gradient, the pulmonary capillary wedge pressure (PCWP) overestimates LVEDP. On the PCWP, a prominent *a wave* and a decreased y *descent* are present in patients with mitral stenosis.

MITRAL REGURGITATION AND INSUFFICIENCY
Pathophysiology

During ventricular systole, the mitral valve is closed, preventing blood flow from the LV back into the LA. However, if for any reason the two leaflets of the mitral valve are not in opposition to each other, a portion of systolic ventricular flow regurgitates back through this incompetent (insufficient) valve. Therefore, the LV has a double outlet for systolic ejection. Ejection into the aorta is a high-impedance outlet, and regurgitation through the mitral valve back into the LA is a low-impedance outlet. This condition is termed *mitral regurgitation* (MR) or *mitral insufficiency*.

The degree of regurgitation (quantitatively), called the *regurgitant fraction*, is determined by four factors:

1. Size of the regurgitant valve orifice (surface area measured in square centimeters)
2. The pressure gradient between the LA and the LV
   - Inotropic state of the LV (peak systolic pressure)
   - Compliance of the LA and pulmonary veins
3. Time available for regurgitation (systole); systolic interval determines length of time during which regurgitation can occur; length of systolic time interval is inversely proportional to HR
4. Aortic outflow impedance SVR; regurgitant fraction can be significantly influenced by changes in impedance to aortic blood flow

The major pathophysiologic derangement associated with MR is volume overload of the LV. This occurs because the regurgitant fraction (retrograde blood flow ejected into the LA during ventricular systole) delivers an increased diastolic volume to the LV. This increase in LVEDV results in ventricular dilation.[44,55,65] Acute MR and chronic MR have substantially different pathophysiologic manifestations. The primary determinant of these pathophysiologic adaptations is left atrial compliance. If acute MR is caused by papillary muscle rupture, the mortality rate approaches 75% within 24 hours and 95% within 48 hours.[66] Chronic MR produces a dilated, compliant LA, whereas the longstanding and gradual elevation of left atrial pressure results in left atrial dilation. This consequently facilitates containment of relatively large end-diastolic volumes while reflecting relatively low increases in LA pressures (Figure 24-40). With chronic MR, hypertrophic changes occur in response to a continual increased left ventricular volume by increasing the left ventricular chamber size. This type of hypertrophic change is called *eccentric hypertrophy*.

In contrast, in acute MR the LA is small and noncompliant, but over time eccentric hypertrophic changes occur to compensate for progressive increases in volume (Figure 24-41). In this situation, a small regurgitant volume bolus can generate deflections or *v* waves that appear in the PCWP tracing. This *v* wave appears as a result of a systolic jet (ejection) back through the incompetent mitral valve. The pressure wave produced by this jet is transmitted upstream into the pulmonary artery and designated as a *pathologic v wave*. The time delay for this pressure wave to be transmitted results in its appearance at the time interval in which the normal *v* wave (passive atrial filling) occurs.[55] The height of the *v* wave in MR does not represent a measurement of regurgitant volume but rather of left atrial compliance in relationship to

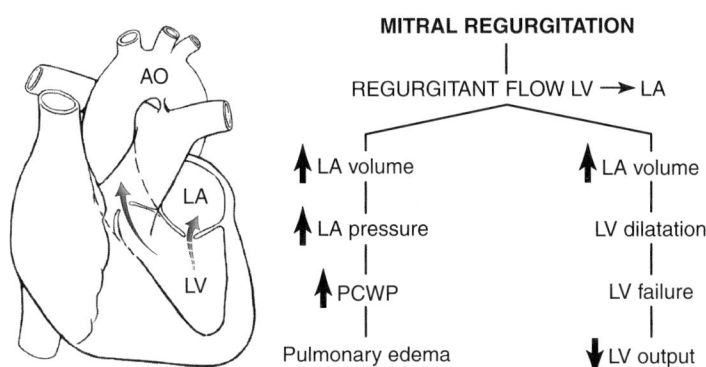

MITRAL REGURGITATION
|
REGURGITANT FLOW LV → LA

↑ LA volume   ↑ LA volume

↑ LA pressure   LV dilatation

↑ PCWP   LV failure

Pulmonary edema   ↓ LV output

FIGURE **24-40** Pathophysiology associated with mitral regurgitation.

the regurgitated volume. The hypertrophic LA accommodates a larger regurgitant volume, which results in small increases in pressure. The dilated and compliant LA allows the pulmonary vascular circuit to be buffered from the excessive left atrial volume. However, chronic MR causes pulmonary venous congestion, which creates pulmonary vascular reactive changes that eventually result in pulmonary artery hypertension. Distention of the LA may lead to atrial fibrillation, a common arrhythmia associated with MR.

Pulmonary Vasculature and Right Ventricular Function

In acute MR, the pulmonary circuit is exposed to immediate and marked elevation of left atrial pressure because of a small and noncompliant LA. Pulmonary vascular congestion is precipitous and results in almost immediate development of pulmonary edema. An acute rise in left atrial pressure and congestion of the pulmonary circuit creates an increased right ventricular workload. This immediate increase in right ventricular afterload results in ventricular dilation and consequently may lead to right ventricular failure. In chronic MR, elevation of baseline pulmonary pressures is much more gradual, occurring over a prolonged period. This allows secondary pulmonary artery hypertension via intimal fibroelastosis generated by chronic perivascular edema. If the patient has coexisting mitral stenosis, pulmonary vascular resistance and right ventricular pressures may be excessively elevated.[44,55,65]

Effects of Afterload Reductions

The path of least resistance for blood flow during left ventricular systole is retrograde into the LA. Reduction of SVR via arterial vasodilation reduces impedance to systolic outflow into the aorta and increases forward flow. Conversely, increases in SVR have marked effects on the reduction in forward flow and the increase in the regurgitant fraction. A 20% increase in MAP raises LA pressure by 50% and reflects a 120% increase in regurgitant flow concurrent with a 16% decrease in forward flow.[55]

Anesthetic Considerations

An otherwise healthy patient with stable and controlled MR undergoing an ambulatory or uncomplicated surgical procedure has a minimal increase in risk of adverse hemodynamic fluctuations. Patients with cardiovascular disease who undergo major vascular, intrathoracic, intraabdominal, neurosurgical, orthopedic, or emergency procedures may have a 25% to 50% higher mortality risk than patients without the disease process. Controversy exists regarding whether the duration of surgery correlates with perioperative cardiac morbidity.[35,54,55]

Preoperative assessment is essential for evaluating the degree of cardiac compensation (Table 24-6). Anesthetic management of the patient with MR should focus on these hemodynamic goals: decreasing regurgitant blood flow to enhance CO by decreasing afterload, maintaining or increasing preload, and maintaining cardiac contractility. Bradycardia or dysrhythmias that cause a loss of atrial kick can result in pulmonary congestion, left atrial and left ventricular overload, and a significant decrease in CO.[54-56]

Another anesthetic consideration of MR includes decreasing SVR or afterload. Cautiously lowering SVR via an arterial vasodilator such as sodium nitroprusside improves forward flow. However, extreme reductions in blood pressure, and especially diastolic pressure, can lead to decreased coronary artery blood flow and decreased CO.

Selection of the anesthetic technique should take into consideration the adverse effects associated with changes in HR and SVR. General anesthesia is the technique of choice in patients with MR. Regional anesthesia (spinal or epidural) is not contraindicated; however, the potential for profound and precipitous decreases in blood pressure via sympathetic blockade should be considered. Induction of general anesthesia can be safely achieved with any of the presently available agents. Hemodynamic goals include avoiding bradycardia and significant increases in afterload. The use of muscle relaxants does not present a significant risk as long as the resulting changes in HR do not cause severe bradycardia. The vagolytic properties of pancuronium may help to maintain HR. Maintenance of anesthesia can be accomplished with nitrous oxide and a volatile agent. Any changes in vascular resistance induced by nitrous

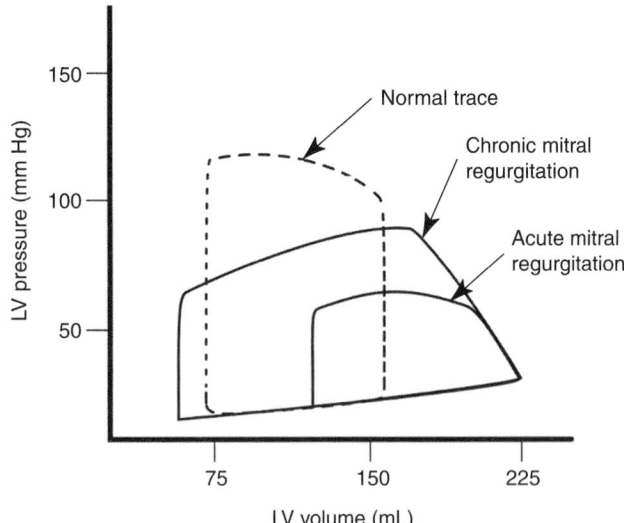

MITRAL REGURGITATION

FIGURE **24-41** Left ventricular (LV) pressure-volume loop associated with mitral regurgitation. The large volume and stroke volume associated with chronic mitral regurgitation occurs because of LV hypertrophy. Notice that during the isovolumetric contraction phase, LV volume decreases as a result of the incompetent mitral valve.

TABLE **24-6**	Hemodynamic Goals for Management of Mitral Valve Lesions	
Parameter	**Mitral Regurgitation (Insufficiency)**	**Mitral Stenosis**
Heart rate	Increase	Decrease to normal
Rhythm	Maintain normal sinus rhythm	Maintain normal sinus rhythm
Afterload	Decrease	Maintain normal
Pulmonary vascular resistance	Avoid increases	Avoid increases
Preload	Normal to increased	Normal to increased

oxide are frequently offset by pulmonary vasodilatation produced by the volatile agent. No volatile agent has been proved to be superior in patients with MR. Isoflurane may be an ideal choice because of its significant vasodilatory effects, causing an increased HR. Because all volatile agents induce a dose-dependent decrease in myocardial contractility, their use may be detrimental in patients with severe ventricular dysfunction. In this instance, the use of a high-dose opioid technique may provide for a more effective hemodynamic profile. Anesthetic management should focus on avoiding bradycardia or increases in SVR.[55] See Table 24-6 for anesthetic goals for management of mitral lesions.

AORTIC STENOSIS

Etiology and Pathophysiology

The most common causes of aortic stenosis include a congenital defect resulting in a bicuspid aortic valve (especially in males) and the sequelae of rheumatic valvular heart disease. Isolated aortic valvular dysfunction in patients with rheumatic heart disease is rare. Commonly, rheumatic valvular disease is associated with mitral valve involvement. Whatever the cause, the pathophysiology remains the same and results in the need for increased left ventricular systolic pressure to overcome the left ventricular outflow tract obstruction caused by a narrowed aortic valve orifice (Figure 24-42). During auscultation, a low-frequency, systolic ejection murmur is characteristic of aortic stenosis.[67]

An understanding of the flow rates through a normal aortic valve orifice is needed for gaining an appreciation of ventricular pressure overload. A normal aortic valve area of 2.5 to 3.5 cm^2 and SV of approximately 80 mL result in a flow rate of 250 mL/min during the interval of ventricular systole (80 mL/sec × 0.32 sec − systolic time interval). The flow rate through a normal orifice results in a minimal gradient (2 to 4 mm Hg). The normal left ventricular systolic pressure of 100 to 130 mm Hg is sufficient to generate flow rates of 250 to 300 mL/sec. To ensure normal flow rates and therefore CO through the narrowed orifice, the velocity of systolic ejection must increase. For systolic ejection to be increased, ventricular systolic pressure increases dramatically, depending on the degree of valvular pathology. The LV must compensate for gradually increasing mechanical impedance to ejection. This results in LVH, which allows the heart to generate high ventricular systolic pressure and overcome impedance to ejection. The elevation of systolic ejection pressure produces a gradient between the left ventricular cavity and the aorta. The valve area must be constricted by at least 50% before the gradient becomes significant to the point that symptoms occur at rest. An aortic valve area of less than 1 cm^2 produces a clinical triad of symptoms that include angina (even in the absence of significant coronary artery disease), syncope, and congestive heart failure.[65] An aortic valve area of less than 1 cm^2 represents severe aortic stenosis and should be a cause of concern in planning anesthetic management because of the associated increase in perioperative cardiac morbidity.[35] An aortic valve area less than 0.7 cm^2 is associated with sudden death.[68] For adequate assessment of the degree of valvular stenosis, both the flow rate across the valve and the pressure gradient should be evaluated, either by cardiac catheterization or echocardiography.[62,63]

Left Ventricular Function

Left ventricular concentric hypertrophy is the compensatory change associated with aortic stenosis. It results in several hemodynamic adaptations that are unique to aortic stenosis and present a challenge and a dilemma with regard to anesthesia management. The consequence of LVH in aortic stenosis is a decrease in ventricular compliance, hypertrophic remodeling, and an eventual decrease in the intrinsic contractility of the myocardium.[69] The reduction in ventricular compliance affects normal hemodynamics as follows:

I. Higher filling pressures are needed to produce the same amount of ventricular work.

II. To achieve adequate left ventricular filling, normal sinus rhythm must be maintained to ensure adequate LVEDV from the atrial kick.

III. Concentric ventricular hypertrophy causes alterations in myocardial oxygen balance.

  A. Myocardial oxygen consumption is increased.

    1. Myocardial mass is increased.

    2. Pressure generation (isovolumetric contraction) uses more energy than left ventricular ejection; a high intracavitary pressure must be generated to maintain CO.

    3. The ejection phase is prolonged.

  B. Myocardial oxygen supply is decreased.

    1. CPP is decreased as a result of an increase in LVEDP.

    2. Systolic coronary flow is absent because left ventricular systolic pressure exceeds aortic systolic pressure.

    3. Prolonged systolic ejection reduces the coronary perfusion interval.

    4. Subendocardial capillaries are compressed by hypertrophic myocardium.[44,54,55]

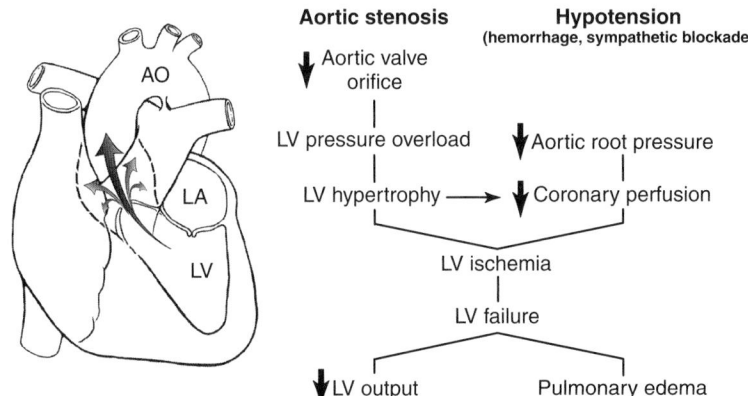

AORTIC STENOSIS

FIGURE **24-42** Pathophysiology associated with aortic stenosis.

Pulmonary Circuit and Right Ventricular Responses

To maintain CO in the presence of a noncompliant and hypertrophic LV, left atrial pressures increase to accommodate left ventricular filling (Figure 24-43). Left atrial pressures of greater than 18 mm Hg can cause an increase in pulmonary artery pressure, resulting in passive pulmonary venous congestion. Eventually, pulmonary fibroelastosis occurs, causing pulmonary artery hypertension. If the ventricular EF is decreased to less than 40% in association with aortic stenosis, CO can be maintained only with increases in left atrial pressures. These pressures increase to 25 to 30 mm Hg, which results in increased mean pulmonary artery pressure. Elevated mean pulmonary artery pressure increases pulmonary vascular resistance, which can cause right ventricular failure. Decreasing left ventricular preload in association with significant aortic stenosis can result in decreases in CO.

Anesthetic Considerations

The goals of anesthesia management include maintaining hemodynamic stability without causing significant alterations in compensatory mechanisms. Anesthetic management of patients with aortic stenosis should focus on the following hemodynamic factors:

1. Maintain normal sinus rhythm and HR 70 to 80 beats per minute
2. Enssure sufficient preload (LVEDV) to maintain CO
3. Enssure adequate coronary perfusion by maintaining diastolic blood pressure levels
4. Avoid myocardial depression, especially with poor LV function
5. Maintain or allow slight increase in afterload

General anesthesia is the preferred technique for major surgical procedures involving patients with aortic stenosis because of the ability to manipulate hemodynamic parameters, especially diastolic blood pressure. Central neural blockade (spinal or epidural) must be used with extreme caution, because precipitous reductions in blood pressure associated with a sympathectomy decrease SVR.[67] Epidural anesthesia offers the advantage of a slower onset of vasodilation. Depending on the degree of compromise, the heart may not be able to compensate for moderate to severe systemic vasodilation. Therefore, lower dermatome level blocks

decrease the degree of systemic vasodilation and maintain afterload. Successful cardiopulmonary resuscitation is virtually impossible because of the mechanical left ventricular outflow obstruction associated with this type of valvular pathology. The pressure necessary to overcome outflow obstruction and produce adequate coronary artery perfusion and CO cannot be generated with closed-chest compressions. Furthermore, short periods of hypotension may lead to a decrease in coronary perfusion and should be treated with volume and phenylephrine.[70] Because of the increased oxygen demands of the LV, irreversible myocardial ischemia and cardiovascular collapse can occur if hypotension is not promptly and aggressively treated.

Intraoperative control of HR and rhythm is a major goal of the anesthetic management of patients with aortic stenosis. Tachycardia can be detrimental because it decreases diastolic filling time, resulting in a reduction of left ventricular preload. The reduced time interval for coronary artery perfusion reduces oxygen supply to the myocardium. In patients with HRs of greater than 110 beats per minute, systolic ejection time and CO are decreased.[55,56] Bradycardia (fewer than 60 beats per minute) is detrimental in aortic stenosis. Prolonged diastolic filling time, which occurs as a result of bradycardia, causes ventricular distention, which can further decrease CPP, especially to the subendocardium.[44,54,55]

Monitoring and Premedication

It is prudent to titrate preoperative sedatives while vital signs can be continuously monitored. In addition to standard intraoperative monitoring, complete invasive monitoring may be required for patients with aortic stenosis, even for routine procedures. Any significant change in basic hemodynamic variables (i.e., HR, heart rhythm, LVEDV, CPP) can rapidly cause irreversible myocardial deterioration. It is imperative that these variables be monitored closely and appropriate interventions be performed to prevent adverse hemodynamic consequences. The complexity of hemodynamic monitoring modalities is dependent on the physical status of the patient, the severity of aortic stenosis, the extent of the surgical procedure, and the ability of the anesthesia provider to use and interpret hemodynamic values.

The use of intraarterial monitoring for direct beat-to-beat blood pressure assessment allows the anesthesia provider to rapidly treat undesirable hemodynamic changes. Pulmonary artery catheterization provides the ability to monitor all the hemodynamic parameters necessary for diagnosing and treating adverse hemodynamic events. Absolute criteria for intraoperative invasive monitoring for patients with aortic stenosis are controversial. However, clinical judgment, experience, and the ability to appropriately use the pulmonary artery catheter must be considered before implementation.[68,71]

Maintenance of Anesthesia

Commonly used induction agents can be used so long as caution to avoid profound hypotension is exercised. Tracheal intubation can be performed with any of the available muscle relaxants, but caution must be exercised to avoid histamine release, which can dramatically increase HR. Anesthetic maintenance can be accomplished with the use of a volatile agent in conjunction with nitrous oxide, opiates, or both. The adverse cardiovascular effects of the volatile agents must be considered before these drugs are used. Higher concentrations of inhaled agent result in greater degrees of myocardial depression and vasodilation. Volatile agents must be used with extreme caution, because the

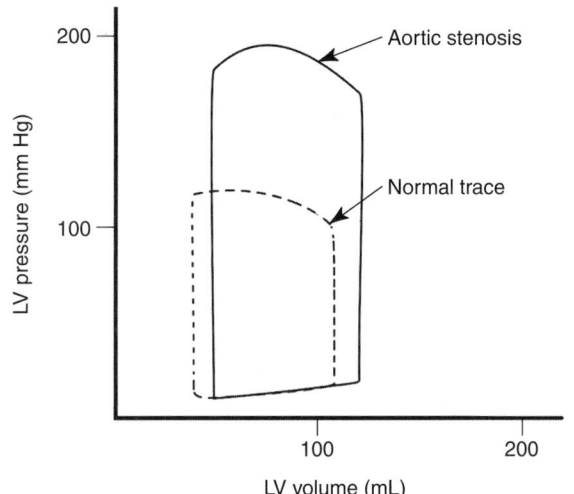

FIGURE **24-43** Left ventricular pressure-volume loop associated with aortic stenosis.

myocardial depressant effect can be deleterious in patients with impaired ventricular function. The use of high-dose opioid-based agents (fentanyl, 50 to 100 mcg/kg; sufentanil, 5 to 30 mcg/kg) is an alternative anesthetic approach that may help achieve cardiovascular stability by not causing a significant amount of myocardial depression. Finally, a combination of inhaled agents and narcotics has been used safely to provide anesthesia for patients with aortic stenosis. Whatever the anesthetic technique chosen for patients with aortic stenosis, immediate and aggressive treatment of adverse changes that occur in HR and rhythm, SVR, blood pressure, and LVEDV is paramount if successful anesthetic outcomes are to be achieved.[68,71]

AORTIC INSUFFICIENCY

AI, also known as *aortic regurgitation*, can be classified as acute or chronic and as primary or secondary, depending on the cause. Primary *chronic* AI is caused by rheumatic valvular disease and almost always involves the mitral valve to some degree. Primary *acute* AI usually is caused by infective endocarditis, which is caused by direct damage to the valve cusps. Acute secondary (functional) AI results from aortic root dissection caused either by trauma or aneurysm and results in a mechanical and functional impairment of functional aortic valve closure.

Pathophysiology

The major hemodynamic aberration related to AI occurs during diastole. A portion of the blood volume ejected from the LV into the aorta regurgitates back into the ventricle because of incomplete closure of the aortic valve. Aortic insufficiency causes volume overload of the LV. Chronic ventricular overload causes eccentric ventricular hypertrophy and chamber dilation (Figure 24-44). The degree of regurgitation depends on three factors: the diastolic time available for regurgitation to occur, the diastolic pressure gradient between the aorta and the LV, and the degree of incompetence of the aortic valve.[65,68]

Diastolic time and diastolic pressure can be manipulated during the course of anesthesia so that the amount of regurgitant flow is decreased and the amount of forward flow is increased. An HR of 90 to 110 beats per minute and decreases in diastolic time interval occur and thereby reduce the time available for regurgitation. Reducing SVR reduces aortic diastolic pressure and decreases the gradient between the aorta and the LV. Unique pathophysiologic adaptations differentiate chronic AI

from the acute form. In chronic AI, the LV has had time to compensate for the increased volume. In time, LV hypertrophy allows the LV to tolerate significant increases in volume without dramatic decreases in EF.[44,55] In situations in which the onset of AI is acute, the LV has inadequate time to adapt to volume overload, which renders compensatory mechanisms ineffective (Figure 24-45). Frequently left ventricular failure, pulmonary edema, and cardiovascular collapse occur. Left ventricular end-diastolic pressure rises precipitously in acute AI because of the inability of the LV to alter its compliance.

Patients with chronic AI can remain asymptomatic for long periods. Except during times of stress, the clinical symptoms associated with chronic AI are usually not incapacitating. End-stage AI is characterized by myocardial failure with decreased CO and precipitous elevation of LVEDV with evidence of pulmonary congestion. As long as ventricular hypertrophy and dilation do not affect the mitral valve, the pulmonary circulation is not affected by the pathophysiologic changes associated with AI. Increased myocardial oxygen consumption occurs because of the development of eccentric hypertrophy. The decrease in aortic diastolic pressure that results from AI reduces coronary flow and can cause subendocardial ischemia. In acute AI, a precipitous increase in LVEDP with a decrease in aortic diastolic pressure can severely compromise coronary blood flow and result in acute myocardial ischemia. The RV and pulmonary vascular circuit usually are spared in chronic AI until secondary (functional) MR occurs. This results in dilation of the mitral valve annulus. A gradual increase in LA pressure and pulmonary artery pressure caused by functional MR eventually causes pulmonary hypertension; right ventricular failure can occur if pulmonary hypertension becomes severe. In acute AI, functional MR is poorly tolerated, owing to a noncompliant LA. This situation leads to immediate pulmonary vascular congestion and pulmonary edema. Patients with asymptomatic AI have a 0.2% annual mortality rate as compared with symptomatic patients, who have a greater than 10% mortality rate per year.[72] Therefore, when evidence suggests that increases in left ventricular

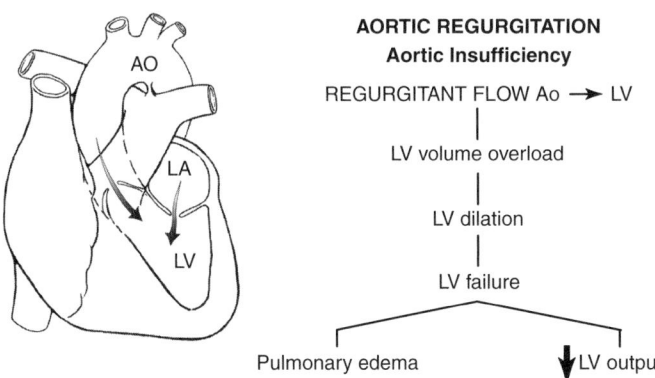

FIGURE **24-44** Pathophysiology associated with aortic regurgitation. AO, Aorta; *LA*, left atrium; *LV*, left ventricle.

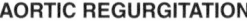
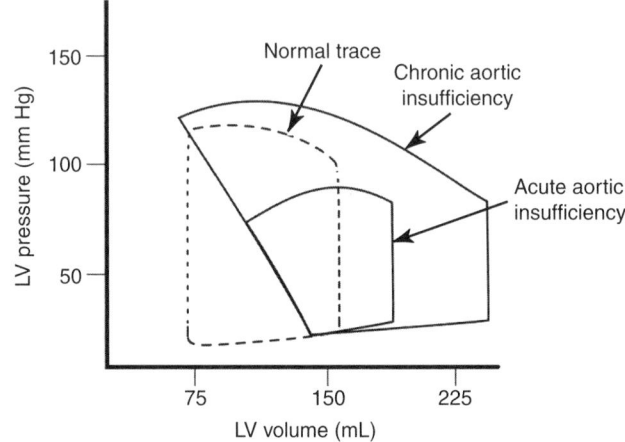

FIGURE **24-45** Left ventricular (LV) pressure-volume loop associated with aortic insufficiency. Increased LV pressure, volume, and stroke volume are associated with chronic aortic insufficiency and reflective of LV hypertrophy. Notice that during the relaxation phase, as isovolumetric relaxation occurs, LV volume increases as a result of the incompetent aortic valve.

volume result in left ventricular dysfunction, aortic valve replacement is recommended.

Anesthesia Management

The goals for anesthesia management are to increase forward flow and decrease the degree of regurgitation and therefore should focus on the following hemodynamic factors:

1. Heart rate should be maintained slightly higher than normal (80 to 110 beats per minute).
2. Afterload (especially diastolic pressure) should be decreased.
3. Avoid myocardial depression.[54]
4. Maintain NSR.
5. Maintain/increase preload.

Central neural blockade is an appropriate anesthetic choice, depending on the invasiveness of the surgical procedure. Reduction in SVR resulting from sympathetic blockade may reduce the degree of regurgitation. The potential for immediate and uncontrolled hypotension during spinal anesthesia is a concern. However, spinal and epidural anesthesia has been used successfully for patients with AI. Induction of general anesthesia can be accomplished with any of the available intravenous agents. Tracheal intubation can be achieved with the use of available nondepolarizing muscle relaxants. As mentioned in the anesthetic management for patients with mitral regurgitation, the vagolytic properties associated with pancuronium are desirable and may offset the vagotonic effects of narcotics. Succinylcholine may be used, but its potential to cause bradycardia (although rarely) must be considered. Maintenance of anesthesia can be achieved with nitrous oxide and a volatile agent. Isoflurane, with its ability to increase HR and decrease SVR, produces little myocardial depression, and therefore its use is preferred over use of other volatile agents. If significant ventricular dysfunction exists, an opioid-based anesthetic technique may be preferable.[26,52,53]

Monitoring and Premedication

Unless end-stage AR or significant preoperative ventricular dysfunction exists, aggressive invasive monitoring is not warranted. However, if the surgical procedure is extensive or if vasodilators or inotropes are being used, then an arterial line and a pulmonary artery catheter should be used for assessing the results and efficacy of these therapeutic agents. Premedication should be tailored to the patient's clinical condition. In elderly or debilitated patients, a conservative amount of premedication in a monitored environment should be titrated until effective.

Appropriate anesthetic management of the patient with valvular heart disease requires a basic knowledge of cardiac physiology and the pathophysiologic changes that occur with valvular dysfunction. The cardiovascular effects of all the agents, techniques, and adjunct pharmacologic agents used during anesthesia must be integrated into the anesthetic plan. A thorough understanding of the use of invasive monitoring along with other sophisticated diagnostic modalities enables the clinician to continuously monitor hemodynamic parameters. Contemporary anesthesia practice has allowed patients with severe valvular dysfunction to undergo surgical procedures that would not have been performed a decade ago.[68] Table 24-7 lists anesthetic goals for management of aortic lesions.

HYPERTROPHIC CARDIOMYOPATHY

Cardiomyopathy is a compensatory enlargement of the heart. Hypertrophic cardiomyopathy, a genetically transmitted disorder, is a form of myocardial dysfunction that can cause coronary

TABLE **24-7**	Hemodynamic Goals for Management of Aortic Lesions	
Parameter	**Aortic Regurgitation (Insufficiency)**	**Aortic Stenosis**
Heart rate	Moderate increase	Normal to slow
Heart rhythm	Normal sinus rhythm	Normal sinus rhythm
Afterload	Decrease	Maintain to slight increase
Pulmonary vascular resistance	Maintain	Maintain
Preload	Normal to increased	Increased

artery disease, valvular dysfunction, ventricular remodeling, and hypertension. The incidence in the adult population is approximately 1 in 500 persons.[73] Obstructive hypertrophic cardiomyopathy has previously been referred to as *idiopathic hypertrophic subaortic stenosis.* Currently the preferred term is *hypertrophic cardiomyopathy with or without left ventricular outflow obstruction.*[74]

The myocardial defect associated with hypertrophic cardiomyopathy is related to the contractile mechanism. An increase in the density of calcium channels appears to lead to myocardial hypertrophy. Asymmetric hypertrophy of the interventricular septum of the LV occurs. The asymmetric hypertrophy of the intraventricular septum causes a left outflow tract obstruction, and the hemodynamic consequences are similar to those that are characteristic of aortic stenosis. Hypertrophic cardiomyopathy is the most common cause of sudden death in the pediatric and young adult populations.[75]

Pathophysiology

Myocardial hypertrophy is the pathophysiologic abnormality that precipitates the hemodynamic derangements associated with hypertrophic cardiomyopathy and is caused by left ventricular outflow obstruction. Left ventricular myocytes are hypertrophic and chaotically arranged. Coronary arterial walls are narrowed because of the presence of collagen. If the entire myocardium is involved, a disproportionate hypertrophy of the intraventricular septum exists. The contraction of the hypertrophied septum bulging into the subaortic area of the left ventricular outflow tract creates a dynamic gradient. The left ventricular outflow tract is bounded anteriorly by the intraventricular septum and posteriorly by the anterior leaflet of the mitral valve. The rapid acceleration of blood traveling through the narrowed outflow tract creates a Venturi effect, which pulls the anterior mitral valve leaflet into the outflow tract. A LV outflow tract obstruction is present in approximately two thirds of patients with hypertrophic cardiomyopathy.[76] The systolic anterior motion of the anterior mitral valve leaflet further obstructs left ventricular outflow. The valve leaflet may even contact the septum and further compromise left ventricular outflow.[67]

The pathophysiologic abnormalities related to hypertrophic cardiomyopathy include the presence of systolic and diastolic dysfunction. A loss of diastolic compliance results in an abnormally elevated LVEDP in the presence of low-normal

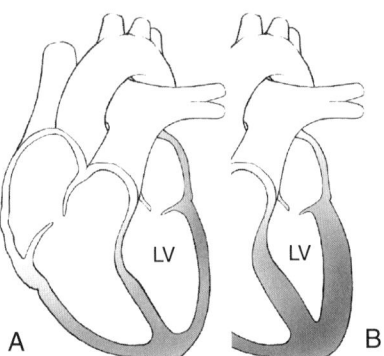

FIGURE **24-46** **A,** Normal left ventricular outflow tract. **B,** Hypertrophic cardiomyopathy with an enlarged interventricular septum and decreased left ventricular chamber size. A further decrease of left ventricular outflow is caused by migration of the anterior mitral leaflet toward the septum.

BOX **24-4**

Hemodynamic Goals for Management of Hypertrophic Cardiomyopathy

Preload	Increase
Afterload	Increase
Contractility	Decrease
Heart rate	Maintain
Heart rhythm	Normal sinus rhythm

end-diastolic volume. Loss of left ventricular diastolic compliance requires a greater contribution of volume from atrial contraction. As a result, congestive heart failure may ensue as left atrial pressures continue to increase.[68] Because as much as 75% of left ventricular preload comes from the LA, maintenance of normal sinus rhythm is vital. The increase in LVEDP, which results from a noncompliant LV, decreases CPP to the hypertrophic LV. Altered coronary perfusion decreases myocardial blood supply, and the presence of left ventricular hypertrophy increases myocardial oxygen demand. Thickening of the internal lumen of the coronary arteries decreases myocardial perfusion, leading to ischemia.[76]

Hypertrophic cardiomyopathy with obstruction is characterized by its dynamic nature. Three basic hemodynamic parameters can affect the degree of outflow obstruction. Manipulation of these parameters can exacerbate or ameliorate the hemodynamic consequences of outflow obstruction. These three parameters include preload, afterload, and contractility.[33] Increasing myocardial contractility in patients with dilated cardiomyopathy exacerbates the obstruction by increasing septal wall contraction and decreasing CO. Increased blood flow velocity causes a greater degree of systolic anterior motion of the mitral valve's anterior leaflet, creating further obstruction. Decreased preload changes left ventricular geometry and thereby brings the anterior leaflet of the mitral valve into closer proximity to the hypertrophied septum. Increases in left ventricular contractility cause the LV to empty more completely and increase the degree of septal contractility, which results in a greater degree of obstruction.[74]

In hypertrophic cardiomyopathy with obstruction, conditions that impair ventricular function under normal physiologic conditions improve cardiac function. This implies that factors that normally impair contractility (e.g., myocardial depression, increased end-diastolic volume, and increased SVR) improve forward flow and diminish the degree of obstruction. Figure 24-46 illustrates the pathology related to hypertrophic cardiomyopathy.

Anesthetic Considerations

Anesthetic management should focus on strategies that alleviate and do not increase left ventricular outflow obstruction. It is imperative that adequate or slightly elevated left ventricular volume be maintained. Measures that decrease venous return and interfere with adequate ventricular preload should be avoided. Factors that increase myocardial contractility should be avoided. Inadequate depth of anesthesia that causes sympathetic nervous system stimulation may be detrimental. In the event that hypotension occurs, adequate perfusion pressure should be maintained by increasing preload with fluid administration and increasing SVR with phenylephrine.

Pharmacologic therapy used to treat hypertrophic cardiomyopathy (including β-blockers and calcium channel blockers) should be continued until the time of surgery.[15] β-Blockers may be administered intraoperatively to reduce HR and contractility. Dysrhythmias must be avoided and immediately treated if they occur; the atrial contribution to left ventricular volume is necessary to achieve CO.[71,74] Box 24-4 lists hemodynamic goals for patients with hypertrophic cardiomyopathy.

Anesthetic management must focus on increasing left ventricular preload, decreasing myocardial contractility, controlling HR, and maintaining or increasing afterload. Regional anesthesia is not contraindicated in patients with dilated cardiomyopathy. Decreases in blood pressure must be treated immediately. Hypovolemia must be avoided and expeditiously treated if it occurs. Deep general anesthesia with a volatile agent is preferred in patients with hypertrophic cardiomyopathy and obstruction.

The potential for hemodynamic deterioration because of increasing subaortic obstruction along with secondary MR necessitates aggressive hemodynamic monitoring. Invasive monitoring via a pulmonary artery catheter allows for maintenance of adequate LVEDV. Because of reduced diastolic compliance associated with hypertrophic cardiomyopathy, PCWP does not correlate directly with LVEDV. The PCWP should be maintained at approximately 18 to 25 mm Hg. If hemodynamic status deteriorates and exacerbation of outflow obstruction is suspected, β-blocking drugs (propranolol or esmolol) should be administered. In addition, vasoconstrictors such as phenylephrine should be used to increase SVR.[33]

MITRAL VALVE PROLAPSE

Description and Etiology

The incidence of mitral valve prolapse, which was thought to be present in 5% to 15% of the U.S. population, is presently estimated at 1.6% to 2.4% of adults.[77] A familial predisposition exists, and women are three times more likely than men to develop mitral valve prolapse. Other conditions frequently associated with mitral valve prolapse include pectus excavatum and kyphoscoliosis. Symptoms are general and include weakness, dizziness, syncope, atypical chest pain, and palpitations. Atrial and ventricular dysrhythmias are common findings in asymptomatic patients. A diagnosis of mitral valve prolapse is confirmed

BOX 24-5

Hemodynamic Goals for Management of Mitral Valve Prolapse

Preload	Maintain or increase
Afterload	Maintain
Contractility	Maintain
Heart rate	Maintain
Heart rhythm	Normal sinus rhythm

through echocardiography. Most patients with this condition remain undiagnosed. Despite its benign nature, mitral valve prolapse can produce potentially life-threatening complications. Premature ventricular contractions are the most common dysrhythmia associated with mitral valve prolapse. Prolonged periods of ventricular tachycardia occur in approximately 21% of patients with mitral valve prolapse. Mitral valve prolapse is also the most common cause of isolated MR. Supraventricular tachyarrhythmias and bradycardia associated with AV block may occur. Medical therapy for mitral valve prolapse consists primarily of the use of β-blocking drugs, which are thought to inhibit an autonomic imbalance that exists in women with mitral valve prolapse. Additionally, β-blocking drugs may increase end-diastolic volume and thereby decrease the degree of prolapse. The majority of patients with mitral valve prolapse do not require medical or pharmacologic management, which reflects the asymptomatic nature of this relatively common valvular abnormality (Box 24-5).[33,71]

Pathophysiology and Unique Problems

The pathophysiologic changes that occur in mitral valve prolapse primarily affect the cusps and the chordae tendineae. Involved is a myxomatous degeneration of the valve cusps that replaces normal fibrous tissue. Also, this myxomatous degeneration affects the chordae tendineae and causes them to become pliable and elongated. The valve leaflets become supple and redundant, as the valve everts into the LA during systole.[78]

Mitral valve prolapse is undiagnosed in the majority of patients. A manifestation that commonly occurs in healthy patients who are receiving anesthesia is an unexpected dysrhythmia (e.g., premature ventricular contractions), many of which resolve spontaneously. Lidocaine does not always terminate the premature ventricular contractions in mitral valve prolapse. β-Blockers are the best choice for control of arrhythmias in patients with mitral valve prolapse. Hemodynamic events and certain positions tend to exacerbate the degree of mitral valve

prolapse and dysrhythmias. Hemodynamic changes that cause a decrease in ventricular preload and increase the incidence of eversion of the mitral valve are caused by increased myocardial contractility, decreased SVR, head-up or sitting positions, use of drugs that decrease ventricular preload (e.g., nitroglycerin and sodium nitroprusside), and hypovolemia.

Pharmacology

Preoperative anxiety stimulates the sympathetic nervous system and can increase the degree of mitral valve prolapse and concomitant dysrhythmias. Decreasing anxiety can reduce the sympathetically mediated responses and improve the hemodynamic profile characteristic of mitral valve prolapse. Anticholinergics can cause tachycardia and should therefore be omitted from the preoperative regimen.

Anesthetic Management

No contraindication to providing regional anesthesia exists, although SVR should be maintained slightly above normal, even in the presence of sympathetic blockade. General anesthesia is an appropriate choice and may be preferred in many instances. Whichever technique is chosen, it is important that preload be maintained. Induction of anesthesia can be accomplished with any of the available intravenous agents. Ketamine, with its ability to stimulate the sympathetic nervous system, should not be used in patients with mitral valve prolapse. Use of a volatile agent alone or in combination with opioids is appropriate for maintenance of anesthesia. Muscle relaxants that have a stable cardiovascular profile can be used. Because of the vagolytic effects of pancuronium, tachycardia and stimulation of the sympathetic nervous system can occur. These cardiovascular effects can be minimized if the drug is administered slowly.[78] Antibiotic prophylaxis is recommended for patients with mitral valve prolapse because of the potential for endocarditis. Currently the American Heart Association has guidelines for antibiotic prophylaxis in surgical patients with valvular disease. All patients who have valvular dysfunction or prosthetic valves are candidates for antibiotic prophylaxis.[27,60] These guidelines are provided in Chapter 14.

SUMMARY

As the population continues to age, the prevalence of cardiovascular disease will increase to reflect the progressive nature of this disease state. Anesthesia providers are able to safely manage extremely critical patients for the full spectrum of surgical needs. A thorough knowledge of cardiac physiology and function is imperative so that high-quality anesthesia care may continue to be administered. Improved patient outcomes are consistently being achieved as better assessment, monitoring, and anesthesia management techniques are discovered.

REFERENCES

1. Guyton AC. Textbook of Medical Physiology. 11th ed. Philadelphia: Saunders; 2006:213-269.
2. Freeman GL. The effects of the pericardium on function of normal and enlarged hearts. Cardiol Clin. 1990;8:579-586.
3. Shabetai R. Acute pericarditis. Cardiol Clin. 1990;8:639-644.
4. Powell EDU, Mullaney JM. The Chiari network and the valve of the inferior vena cava. Br Heart J. 1960;22:579-584.
5. Hellerstein HK, Orbison TL. Anatomic variations of the orifice of the human coronary sinus. Circulation. 1951;3:514-523.
6. Dell'Italia LJ. The right ventricle: anatomy, physiology and clinical importance. Curr Probl Cardiol. 1991;26:658-720.
7. Farb A et al. Anatomy and pathology of the right ventricle (including acquired tricuspid and pulmonic valve disease). Cardiol Clin. 1992;10:1-21.
8. Rosenquist GC, Sweeny LJ. The membranous ventricular septum in the normal heart. Johns Hopkins Med J. 1974;135:9-16.
9. Cannon SR et al. Hydraulic estimation of stenotic orifice area: a correction of the Gorlin formula. Circulation. 1985;71:1170.
10. Shah PM. Tricuspid valve, pulmonary valve and multivalvular disease. In: Fuster V et al, eds. Hurst's the Heart. 12th ed. New York: McGraw-Hill; 2008:1770-1782.
11. Rahimtoola SH et al. Mitral valve stenosis. In: Fuster V et al, eds. Hurst's the Heart. 12th ed, New York: McGraw-Hill; 2008:1757-1769.
12. Goldbert AH, Warltier DC. The coronary circulation: implications for anesthesiologists. Semin Anesth. 1990;9:232-244.

13. Wostczak JA. Basic cellular electrophysiology of the heart. In: Thys DM, Kaplan JA, eds. *The ECG in Anesthesia and Critical Care.* New York: Churchill Livingstone; 1987:109.

14. Little RC, Little WC. *Physiology of the Heart and Circulation.* 4th ed. Chicago: Yearbook Medical; 1989:53.

15. Stoelting RK, Simon SC. *Pharmacology and Physiology in Anesthetic Practice.* 4th ed. Philadelphia: Lippincott Williams & Wilkins; 2006:165, 312, 378,387.

16. Canty JM. Coronary blood flow and myocardial ischemia. In: Libby P et al. *Braunwald's Heart Disease.* 8th ed. Philadelphia: Saunders; 2005:1167-1194.

17. Mangano DT et al. Effect of atenolol on mortality and cardiac morbidity after noncardiac surgery. *N Engl J Med.* 1996;23:1713-1720.

18. Agnew NM et al. Isoflurane and coronary heart disease. *Anaesthesia.* 2002;57:338-347.

19. Teo A, Koh KF. Isoflurane and coronary steal. *Anaesthesia.* 2003;58:95-96.

20. Roscoe AK et al. Isoflurane, but not halothane, induces protection of human myocardium via adenosine A1 receptors and adenosine triphosphate sensitive potassium channels. *Anesthesiology.* 2000;92:1692-1701.

21. Tuman KJ et al. Pitfalls in interpretation of pulmonary artery catheter data. *J Cardiothorac Anesthesiol.* 1989;3:625-641.

22. Sarnoff SJ. Myocardial contractility as described by ventricular function curves: observations on Starling's law of the heart. *Physiol Rev.* 1955;35:107.

23. Johns RA. Endothelium-derived relaxing factor: basic review and clinical implications. *J Cardiothorac Vasc Anesth.* 1991;5:69.

24. Hoover GA. Endothelial cell growth factors in atherogenesis. *CMAJ.* 1990;143:1035.

25. Schelling ME. FGF medication of coronary angiogenesis. *Ann N Y Acad Sci.* 1991;638:467-469.

26. Klagsbrun M. Angiogenic factors: regulators of blood supply-side biology. FGF, endothelial cell growth factors and angiogenesis: a keystone symposium. *New Biol.* 1991;3:745-749.

27. deBold AJ. Atrial natriuretic factor: a hormone produced by the heart. *Science.* 1985;230:767.

28. Rothe CF. Physiology of venous return. *Arch Intern Med.* 1986;146:977.

29. Zweiten PA, Wetzel HB. Antihypertensive drug treatment in the perioperative period. *J Cardiothorac Vasc Anesth.* 1993;7:213-226.

30. National Institutes of Health, National Heart, Lung and Blood Institute, National High Blood Pressure Education Program. *Seventh Report of the Joint National Committee on Prevention, Detection, Evaluation and Treatment of High Blood Pressure (NIH Publication No. 03-5233).* Washington, DC: US Government Printing Office; 2003.

31. Wallis EJ et al. Cardiovascular and coronary risk estimation in hypertensive management. *Heart.* 2002;88:306-312.

32. Hopkins TJ. US guidelines say blood pressure of 120/80 mm Hg is not "normal." *BMJ.* 2003;326:1104.

33. Wallace MC, Haddadin AS. Systemic and pulmonary hypertension. In: Hines RA, Marschall KE, eds. *Stoelting's Anesthesia and Co-Existing Disease.* 5th ed, Philadelphia: Churchill Livingstone; 2008:87-102.

34. Chaney MA et al. Cardiac anesthesia. In: Longnecker DE et al, ed. *Anesthesiology.* New York: McGraw-Hill; 2008:1140-1174.

35. Mangano DT. Perioperative cardiac morbidity. *Anesthesiology.* 1990;72:151-165.

36. Akhtar S. Ischemic heart disease. In: Hines RA, Marschall KE, eds. *Stoelting's Anesthesia and Co-Existing Disease.* 5th ed. Philadelphia: Churchill Livingstone; 2008:1-27.

37. Frohlich ED et al. The heart of hypertension. *N Engl J Med.* 1992;327:998-1008.

38. Agner RC, Gallis HA. Pericarditis: differential diagnostic considerations. *Arch Intern Med.* 1979;139:401-412.

39. Robertson R. Constrictive pericarditis with particular reference to etiology. *Circulation.* 1982;65:525.

40. Spodick DH. Pericarditis, pericardial effusion, cardiac tamponade, and constriction. *Crit Care Clin.* 1989;5:455-476.

41. Seifert FC et al. Surgical treatment of constrictive pericarditis: analysis of outcome diagnostic error. *Circulation.* 1985;72:264-273.

42. Hoit BD. Management of effusion and constrictive pericardial disease. *Circulation.* 2002;105:2939-2942.

43. Konchigeri HN, Levitsky S. Anesthetic considerations for pericardectomy in uremic pericardial effusion. *Anesth Analg.* 1976;55:378-382.

44. Guyton AC. Cardiac tamponade. *Textbook of Medical Physiology.* 11th ed, Philadelphia: Saunders; 2006:238.

45. Williams C, Soutter L. Pericardial tamponade. *Arch Intern Med.* 1954;94:571.

46. Shabetai R et al. The hemodynamics of cardiac tamponade and constrictive pericarditis. *Am J Cardiol.* 1970;26:480-489.

47. Beck CA. Two cardiac compression triads. *JAMA.* 1935;104:715.

48. Lake CL. Anesthesia and pericardial disease. *Anesth Analg.* 1983;62:431-443.

49. Weeks KR et al. Bedside hemodynamic monitoring: its value in the diagnosis of tamponade complicating cardiac surgery. *J Thorac Cardiovasc Surg.* 1976;71:250-252.

50. Stanley TH, Weidauer HE. Anesthesia for the patient with cardiac tamponade. *Anesth Analg.* 1973;52:110-114.

51. Cyna AM et al. Hypotension due to unexpected pericardial tamponade. *Anaesthesia.* 1990;45:140-142.

52. Murray BR, Robertson DS. Anaesthesia for mitral valvotomy complicated by hypotension due to pericardial effusion. *Br J Anaesth.* 1964;36:256-258.

53. Guntheroth WG, Morgan BC. Effect of respiration on venous return and stroke volume in cardiac tamponade. *Circ Res.* 1967;20:381-390.

54. Mastropietro C. Anesthesia for cardiac and peripheral vascular surgery. In: Waugaman WR et al, eds. *Principles and Practice of Nurse Anesthesia.* Norwalk, CT: Appleton & Lange; 1992:705.

55. Swartz AJ, Maddi R. Anesthesia for cardiac surgery. In: Liu PL, ed. *Principles and Procedures in Anesthesiology.* Philadelphia: Lippincott; 1992:339.

56. Wray-Roth DL et al. Anesthesia for cardiac surgery. In: Barash PG et al, eds. *Clinical Anesthesia.* 5th ed. Philadelphia: Lippincott; 2006:886-932.

57. Lake CL. Cardiovascular anatomy and physiology. In: Barash PG et al, eds. *Clinical Anesthesia.* 5th ed. Philadelphia: Lippincott; 2006:856-885.

58. Mohrman DE, Heller LJ. *Cardiovascular Physiology.* 3rd ed, New York: McGraw-Hill; 1991:175.

59. Thrush DN et al. Blood pressure after cardiopulmonary bypass: which technique is accurate? *J Cardiothorac Vasc Anesth.* 1994;8:269-272.

60. Church JA et al. Incidence of cerebral air embolism during left atrial catheter insertion in cardiopulmonary bypass patients. *Anesthesiology.* 1993;79:52.

61. Edwards Critical Care Division. *Invasive Hemodynamic Monitoring: Physiologic Principles and Clinical Applications.* Santa Ana, CA: Baxter Healthcare; 1989:1.

62. Kato M et al. Does transesophageal echocardiography improve postoperative outcome in patients undergoing coronary artery bypass surgery? *J Cardiothorac Vasc Anesth.* 1993;7:285-289.

63. Sutton DC, Calahan MK. Transesophageal echocardiography is routine in anesthesia for cardiac surgery. *J Cardiothorac Vasc Anesth.* 1993;7:357-360.

64. Cook DJ et al. Valvular heart disease: replacement and repair. In: Kaplan JA, ed. *Kaplan's Cardiac anesthesia.* 5th ed, Philadelphia: Saunders; 2006:675.

65. Jackson MJ, Thomas SJ. Valvular heart disease. In: Kaplan JA, ed. *Kaplan's Cardiac Anesthesia.* 5th ed, Philadelphia: Saunders; 2006:645-690.

66. Iung B. Management of ischemic mitral regurgitation. *Heart.* 2003;89:459-464.

67. Wallace A. Cardiovascular disease. In: Stoelting RK, Miller RD. *Basics of Anesthesia.* 5th ed. Philadelphia: Churchill Livingstone; 2007:365-392.

68. Wilson WC, Benumof JL. Anesthesia for cardiac surgery procedures. In: Miller RD, ed. *Miller's Anesthesia.* 6th ed, New York: Churchill Livingstone; 2006:1962.

69. Zile MR, Gaasch WH. Heart failure in aortic stenosis—improving diagnosis and treatment. *N Engl J Med.* 2003;348:1735-1736.

70. Christ M et al. Preoperative and perioperative care for patients with suspected or established aortic stenosis facing noncardiac surgery. *Chest.* 2005; 128(4):2944-2953.

71. Mark JB, Slaughter TF. Cardiovascular monitoring. In: Miller RD, ed. *Miller's Anesthesia.* 6th ed, New York: Churchill Livingstone; 2006:1328.

72. Hicks GL, Massey TH. Update on indications for surgery in aortic insufficiency. *Curr Opin Cardiol.* 2002;17:172-178.

73. Maron BJ. Hypertophic cardiomyopathy. *Am J Med.* 2004;116:63-65.

74. Popescu WM. Heart failure and cardiomyopathies. In: Hines RL et al, eds. *Anesthesia and Co-existing Disease.* 5th ed. Philadelphia: Saunders; 2008:103-124.

75. Maron B. Hypertrophic cardiomyopathy: a systematic review. *JAMA.* 2002;287:1308-1320.

76. Poliac LC et al. Hypertrophic cardiomyopathy. *Anesthesiology.* 2006 Jan ;104(1): 183-192. Review.

77. Pellerin D et al. Degenerative mitral valve disease with emphasis on mitral valve prolapse. *Heart.* 2002;88:20-28.

78. Oliver WC, Nuttall GA. Uncommon cardiac diseases. In: Kaplan JA, ed. *Kaplan's Cardiac Anesthesia.* 5th ed, Philadelphia: Saunders; 2006:775.

CHAPTER 25

ANESTHESIA FOR CARDIAC SURGERY

Charlene V. Brouillette

Care of the patient with cardiac compromise is a complex undertaking and requires knowledge of basic cardiac physiology, mechanics of circulation, requirements of myocardial oxygen supply and demand, and the basics of pharmacologic and hemodynamic management. Preoperative evaluation and preparation of the patient are important facets of the anesthetic plan of care. Intraoperatively, anesthetic maintenance is often achieved in collaboration with the perfusionist during bypass procedures and in conjunction with the minute-to-minute needs of the surgeon during off-pump procedures. Postoperative management begins at cessation of the pump run on bypass procedures and with completion of anastomoses during off-pump cases. Postoperative care includes temperature management and prevention and control of coagulopathies, as well as regulation of hemodynamic stability and pain management.

The first recorded open-cardiac procedure was performed on April 15, 1952. Dr. R. E. Gross of Children's Hospital in Boston was able to close an atrial septal defect under direct visualization. In October of that year in Detroit, Dr. Dodril used right-sided heart bypass to perform an open pulmonary valvotomy. In May of 1953 in Philadelphia, Dr. Gibbon used a heart-lung machine to close an atrial septal defect. Also in 1953, the Mayo Clinic was the site of the first series of open-heart surgeries using a heart-lung machine.[1] This was a prototype for the coronary artery bypass grafting procedures familiar to practitioners today.

Coronary artery disease is the predominant cause of death in patients in the fourth and fifth decades and the most common cause of *premature* death in men aged 35 to 45 years. Annually approximately 1.5 million individuals endure some level of myocardial insult. The most recent data show that there are more than 1,285,000 inpatient angioplasty procedures, 427,000 inpatient bypass procedures, 1,471,000 inpatient diagnostic cardiac catheterizations, 68,000 inpatient implantable defibrillators, and 170,000 inpatient pacemaker procedures performed in the United States.[2]

CORONARY ARTERY DISEASE

The coronary arteries arise from the aorta. Coronary artery perfusion pressure is mainly determined by aortic diastolic pressure and left ventricular[3] end-diastolic pressure. Coronary artery disease alters coronary blood flow, decreases coronary reserve, and increases the incidence of coronary artery vasospasm. Risk factors associated with the progression of coronary artery disease include age, gender, genetic predisposition, obesity, hyperlipidemia, hypertension, stress, diabetes mellitus, and smoking. Exacerbating the effects of coronary artery disease are combinations of peripheral vascular disease, carotid disease, and a compromised pulmonary system.

Atherosclerosis is a disease process in which fatty lesions are deposited on the intimal layer of the arteries. These fatty deposits are called *atheromatous plaques* and begin as crystals of cholesterol that adhere to the intima and smooth muscle layer of the arteries. This disease rarely involves small arteries and should not be confused with arteriosclerosis, which is considered relatively benign. The cholesterol crystals develop and form a larger matrix that stimulates fibrous tissue and smooth muscle growth to create additional layers on which larger plaques grow. Eventually the plaques mature and develop into obstructive lesions or contribute to the formation of fibroblasts, which eventually deposit dense connective tissue, resulting in sclerosis (fibrosis). Atheromatous plaque and the resulting sclerotic lesions lead to loss of arterial distensibility and tissue degeneration and ulceration of the arterial wall. Inherent in this process are thrombi, which form and embolize, causing blood flow obstruction and distal tissue ischemia.[4]

Patients with atherosclerotic coronary disease become symptomatic when 75% of the coronary vessel is occluded, resulting in a decrease in coronary blood flow. Ischemia depresses myocardial function and causes severe chest pain referred to as *angina pectoris*. In addition to pain, cells are subject to increased irritability and become increasingly vulnerable to fibrillation, alterations in the conduction pathways, and thrombus formation.

EFFECTS OF CARDIOPULMONARY BYPASS

Pulmonary System

Cardiopulmonary bypass (CBP) can precipitate morphologic changes known as *pump lung*. This acute lung injury can result in diffuse congestion, edema in the alveolar and interstitial regions, and hemorrhagic atelectasis. One theory regarding this phenomenon is that microemboli of protein aggregates, disintegrated platelets, damaged fibrin, and fat particles contribute to the development of pump lung. Acute lung injury can also be caused by complement activation, inflammatory response, hemodilution, lung hypoxia, and elevated pulmonary artery (PA) pressure. Hypothermia and topical cooling contribute to instances of phrenic nerve dysfunction that can play a role in alterations in pulmonary function.[5] CPB has a negative influence on ventilation-perfusion parameters. Gas distribution occurs preferentially to nondependent areas of the lung, thereby producing hypoventilation of dependent lung sections, which can result in postoperative atelectasis.

Various approaches for prevention of atelectasis have been proposed and studied (e.g., delivery of positive-pressure ventilation, intermittent sighs, or static inflation [continuous positive airway pressure (CPAP)] during CPB), but none has demonstrated a definitive or reliable effect. It is recommended that a reduction of microemboli proliferation (using blood filtration), prevention of pulmonary vascular distention, and hemodilution along with steroids and vasodilator prostaglandins may preclude the onset of this problem.

Central Nervous System

The predominant postoperative neurologic complication after open-heart surgical procedures on CPB is stroke. The word *stroke* refers to a sudden onset of focal deficit of the central nervous system (CNS) that lasts more than 24 hours. Up to 50% of patients demonstrate postoperative neurophysiologic dysfunction in the postoperative period after CPB.[6] Cerebrovascular sequelae indicators include visual impairment, hemiparesis, aphasia, and sensory impairment. Other neurologic deficits include abnormal reflexes, loss of the sensation of vibration, impaired locomotion, and impaired visual acuity associated with retinal lesions or infarction. The incidence of cerebrovascular insult is related to age, valvular repair or replacement, the extent of aortic calcification, and preexisting cerebrovascular disease. The presence of preoperative cerebrovascular disease indicates the need to maintain higher perfusion pressures during CPB. A recent history of stroke should be considered a contraindication for anticoagulation therapy necessary in CPB-dependent procedures.

The CNS is sensitive to hypoxemia and is at risk when cerebral hypoperfusion occurs. At a mean arterial pressure (MAP) between 50 and 150 mm Hg (autoregulatory plateau), cerebral blood flow (CBF) is maintained at approximately 50 mL/100 g/min because of changes in cerebrovascular tone. Maintenance of adequate CBF may decrease the incidence of arterial hypoperfusion, which could result in stroke.[7] Cerebral autoregulation is dependent on CBF and MAP and is established at a lower plateau with hypothermia. Global ischemia is possible with rapid hypoperfusion of collaterals, lost autoregulation in profound hypothermia, or circulatory arrest of longer than 1 minute.[8]

Changes in arterial blood pressure and blood flow may be precipitated as a result of hypothermic responses, hypocarbia, venous congestion arising from superior vena caval obstruction, or emboli. Sources of emboli include aortic atheroma from the aortic clamp, intraventricular thrombi, valve calcification, air during open-chamber procedures, aortic cannulation, bubble oxygenators, nitrous oxide administered before bypass, or factors associated with a long pump run (CPB). Pump runs longer than 90 minutes are considered an independent risk factor, in which the risk of cognitive dysfunction is greatly increased.[9] Avoidance of nitrous oxide decreases the possibility of remobilization. The use of nitrous oxide can increase the size of gaseous emboli.

Hyperglycemia may intensify global and focal insults to the CNS. Strict glucose control is essential because evidence suggests that hyperglycemic states increase the magnitude and extent of neurologic injury that ensues during ischemia.[10] Solutions containing glucose are to be avoided, and patients who are diabetic must be monitored closely to maintain tight control of glucose status. Although it may be necessary to institute insulin therapy to manage hyperglycemia in some patients, insulin resistance develops during CPB in part because of increased endogenous

---

BOX 25-1

Cerebral Protection Techniques Used During Cardiopulmonary Bypass

Maintain mean arterial pressure >50 mm Hg after start of rewarming
Maintain euglycemia
Maintain mild hypothermia (nasopharyngeal temperature <37° C at rewarming)
Perform pharmacologic metabolic suppression:

Thiopental	Lidocaine
Propofol	β-blockers
Calcium channel blockers	Ketamine
Volatile anesthetics	

Emboli reduction
Acid-base management

---

catecholamines, which increase the incidence of refractory hyperglycemia.

Cerebral protection techniques include metabolic suppression with hypothermia, administration of medications such as thiopental or propofol, and the use of calcium channel blockers to reduce the incidence of vasospasm.[7] In addition, deep hypothermic circulatory arrest can be used for arch reconstruction and for treatment of giant aneurysms. This technique necessitates core and external cooling to temperatures of 15° to 20° C, selective cerebral perfusion, pH management, and intermittent or low-flow perfusion (as in pediatric hearts for aortic arch procedures). Brain protection by the volatile anesthetics has been recently reported.[11-13] Data indicate that the inhalation anesthetics can provide long-term durable protection against mild to moderate but not severe ischemic brain injury. Mechanisms reponsible for brain preconditing are complex and may involve changes in murine thymoma viral oncogene homolog (Akt gene) expression, adenosine triphosphate (ATP)-sensitive potassium channels, and nitric oxide. Cerebral protection techniques during cardiopulmonary bypass are listed in Box 25-1.

Neurocognitive function has been studied post-bypass for many years. Disagreement exists as to the extent (if any) decline occurs. Decline in cognitive function has been attributed to the use of cardiopulmonary bypass, cerebral microemboli and hypoperfusion, inflammation, cerebral hyperthermia and edema, blood-brain barrier dysfunction, and genetic influences. Recent data suggest none of these are the case.[14-17]

Gastrointestinal Tract

GI tract morbidity in the postoperative CPB patient is a significant complication of bypass procedures. Predictive factors include previous cerebrovascular accident (CVA), chronic obstructive pulmonary disease (COPD), type II heparin-induced thrombocytopenia (HIT-II), atrial fibrillation, prior myocardial infarction, renal insufficiency, hypertension, and the use of intraaortic balloon counterpulsation.[18-20] Valve surgery, concomitant valve and coronary bypass surgery, deep sternal infection, prolonged ventilation, and low ejection fraction

(<30%) also contributed to postoperative gastrointestinal complications.[21] The most common catastrophic GI complication is mesenteric ischemia, which is often fatal. This ischemia may result from atheroembolization, heparin-induced thrombocytopenia, or hypoperfusion.[18-20] Minimizing risk factors when possible may reduce associated morbidity and mortality.

Renal Function

Impairment of renal function is not uncommon in patients undergoing surgical procedures requiring CPB. Studies have demonstrated that renal dysfunction of varying degrees is related to length of time on bypass (longer than 3 hours), cardiac output (CO), infection, type of procedure (valve surgery has higher incidence of renal dysfunction), excessive blood loss, diabetes, increased use of vasopressors, perioperative myocardial infarction (MI), use of intraaortic balloon pump (IABP), and massive transfusion.[22] Independent risk factors for postoperative renal failure include use of IABP, deep hypothermic circulatory arrest, low CO syndrome, advanced age, and low urinary output during the pump run. CPB by itself is a less problematic risk factor.[18,23-26]

Serum creatinine levels are accepted predictors of morbidity. Normal creatinine is 1.8 mg/100 mL or less; values ranging from 1.9 to 5 mg/100 mL are considered abnormal. A creatinine level in excess of 5 mg/100 mL indicates renal failure, and the patient requires dialysis. Preoperative serum creatinine levels are directly proportional to predicted mortality rate and postoperative renal failure; they are inversely related to the preoperative cardiac index (CI).

Hypothermia during CPB depresses renal tubular function; however, hemodilution, administration of mannitol (CPB prime), and maintenance of glomerular filtration rate result in adequate urinary output. The standard for measurement of perfusion is a urinary output of at least 1 mL/kg/hr.[22] Perfusion pressure is a primary determinant of urinary output during CPB. Hypothermia does not seem to have a great influence on urinary output during bypass. Studies have shown no difference in urinary output (renal function) among cases in which hypothermic versus normothermic CPB is used.[27]

Nondiabetic hyperglycemia during CPB is largely the result of increased glucose reabsorption by the kidneys. Even small amounts of glucose introduced during CPB have been shown to precipitate hyperglycemia. This is problematic because hyperglycemia is detrimental to the brain, as well as the renal tubules.

Catecholamines rise progressively during CPB. The release and circulation of vasopressin (antidiuretic hormone; ADH) are thought to occur in response to low atrial pressures, hypotension, and nonpulsatile flow. Reduction in urinary output may be the result of renal vasoconstriction stimulated by high levels of vasopressin. Hemodilution has a significant effect in counteracting the effects of vasopressin by increasing perfusion to the outer cortex of the kidney, thereby stimulating renal plasma flow and the clearance of free water and potassium.

Urinary output is the single most important intraoperative monitor of the renal system during coronary artery bypass grafting (CABG) procedures using CPB. Anuria is not uncommon during CPB, and approximately one third of patients may experience acute renal failure. It is thought that the nonpulsatile flow of the extracorporeal circuit interferes with autoregulation of renal blood flow. Maintenance of good urinary flow (0.5 to 1 mL/kg/hr) during the pump run ensures that free water can be eliminated. Evaluation of electrolyte status is recommended before and after termination of CPB. Levels of cations such as potassium and calcium may have to be adjusted postoperatively.

Hypothermia

Hypothermia is an integral aspect of CPB and has a profound effect on enzyme systems and the coagulation cascade. Activated clotting time (ACT), prothrombin time (PT), and partial thromboplastin time (PTT) are prolonged, and platelets become nonfunctional as the body temperature is lowered to approximately 28° C. Cellular potassium uptake is increased and may result in hypokalemia.

The beneficial aspects of hypothermia include a reduced basal metabolic rate, improved myocardial protection, tissue and organ preservation, and reduced oxygen consumption. The metabolic requirement for O_2 is reduced by 50% for each 7° C drop in core body temperature. However, it may not be possible to convert heartbeat to normal sinus rhythm until the rewarming core temperature is 34° C.

ANESTHESIA CONSIDERATIONS

The goals of anesthetic management for coronary revascularization are directed toward (1) producing analgesia, amnesia, and muscle relaxation; (2) abolishing autonomic reflexes; (3) maintaining physiologic homeostasis; and (4) providing myocardial and cerebral protection. The avenues available to accomplish these goals include an effective preoperative evaluation, administration of modest doses of sedation and pain medication before any attempt at line placement is made, and use of O_2 in the preoperative setting. Administration of a balanced anesthetic with opioid, inhalation agents, sedative-hypnotics, and muscle relaxant provides a stable hemodynamic state for the difficult cardiovascular patient. The inhalation agents offer the additional advantage of anesthetic preconditioning that is cardioprotective. Anesthetic preconditioning is fully discussed in Chapter 9.

Preoperative Assessment

A thorough preoperative assessment of the patient who will undergo cardiac surgery should include comprehensive review of systems, airway status, and laboratory data; physical examination; review of surgical history; and review of current medications (Figure 25-1). Actual reports of diagnostic procedures such as cardiac catheterization, echocardiogram, and Doppler studies should be reviewed by the anesthesia care provider.

Airway assessment in cardiac patients is necessary because such patients are unable to compensate for a reduced oxygen supply. Often patients who undergo cardiac revascularization procedures are oxygen compromised because of body habitus, pulmonary disease, age, and general physical condition. These patients cannot tolerate decreases in oxygen supply. Careful evaluation and preparation for airway management is very important.

Myocardial Ischemia

Prevention of myocardial ischemia in patients undergoing myocardial revascularization procedures is paramount if the procedures are to be successful. Ischemia can be precipitated by hemodynamic alterations, which can occur at any time during the perioperative period. Alterations such as tachycardia, hypertension, hypotension, and ventricular distention can cause myocardial ischemia. Treatment of ischemia is directed at stabilizing hemodynamic parameters. A patient who is subjected to perioperative ischemia is three times more likely to suffer an MI.[28]

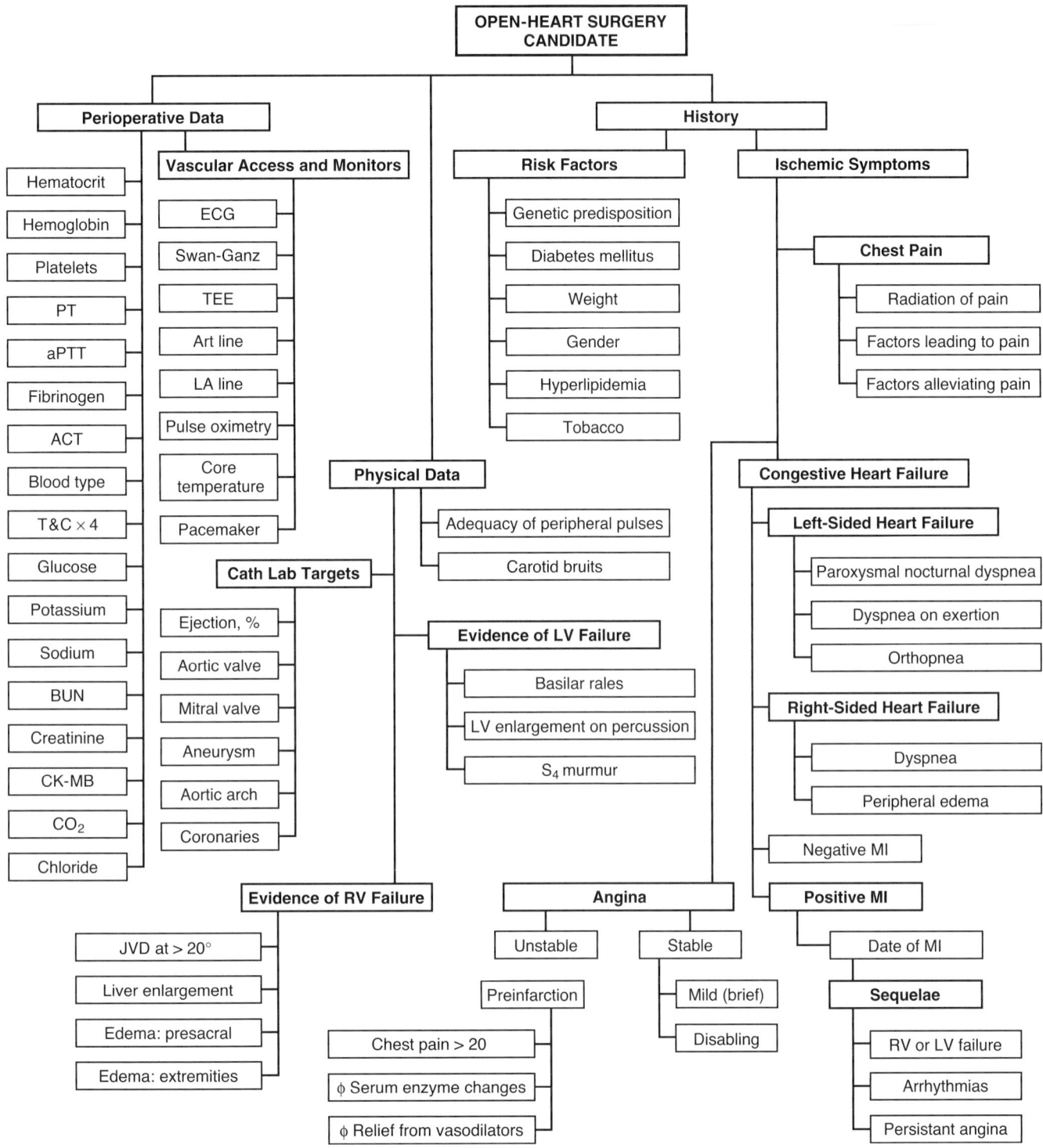

FIGURE **25-1** Preoperative assessment of patients with myocardial ischemia. *ACT,* Activated coagulation time; *aPTT,* activated partial thromboplastin time; *BUN,* blood urea nitrogen; *CK-MB,* creatinine phosphokinase myocardial band; *ECG,* electrocardiography; *JVD,* jugular venous distention; *LA,* left atrial; *LV,* left ventricular; *MI,* myocardial infarction; *PT,* prothrombin time; *RV,* right ventricular; *T&C,* type and cross-match; *TEE,* transesophageal echocardiography.

Perioperative hypertension may be responsible for myocardial ischemia, ventricular failure, intracerebral hemorrhage, pulmonary edema, or aortic dissection. Continuation of antihypertensive therapy is recommended during the preoperative preparation of cardiac patients. Patients should be instructed to take any antihypertensive or cardiac medications until the day of surgery. Providing sedation during the invasive placement and induction lessens the possibility of hypertension from sympathetic stimulation.

Intraoperative events that are known to precipitate ischemia are listed in Box 25-2. The goal of anesthetic management is to

TABLE 25-1	Normal Intracardiac Pressures	
	Notation	**Range (mm Hg)**
Central venous pressure	CVP	0-8
Right atrial pressure	RAP	0-8
Right ventricular end-systolic pressure	RVESP	15-25
Right ventricular end-diastolic pressure	RVEDP	0-8
Pulmonary artery pressure (systolic)	PAP systolic	15-25
Pulmonary artery pressure (diastolic)	PAP diastolic	8-15
Pulmonary artery pressure (mean)	PAP	10-20
Pulmonary capillary wedge pressure (PCWP); pulmonary artery occlusion pressure	PAOP (PCWP)	6-12

reduce or obtund responses to these stimuli to reduce exposure to ischemia. Treatment of ischemia is based on four modes of support: oxygen administration, stabilization of hemodynamic parameters, inotropic support, and mechanical support when indicated.[29]

Coexisting Disease States

Preoperative risk factors include age, cigarette smoking (which contributes to development of atherosclerosis), peripheral vascular and cerebral vascular disease, hypertension, angina, congestive heart failure (CHF), previous MI, and diabetes mellitus.

Angina pectoris is classified by degree of severity, based on factors promoting the onset, duration, and response to symptomatic treatment with vasodilator therapy (nitroglycerin). Angina is defined as *stable* if there has been no change in frequency, precipitating event, or duration for the previous 2 months. *Unstable angina* (crescendo angina) is defined as angina of new onset that lasts longer than 30 minutes and is associated with ST- or T-segment changes. Unstable angina often does not respond to rest or medication.[30,31]

Previous cardiac surgery results in an increase in blood loss because of reoperation through adhesions from a previous sternotomy. Anticipation of excessive blood loss may indicate the use of antihyperfibrinolytic agents and implementation of a cell-saver device. The sternotomy is a cause for significant concern because scar tissue formation may have led to anatomic distortion or superficial attachment of the pericardium to the anterior chest wall, which presents a potential hazard for laceration of the myocardium or great vessels. It may become necessary for the anesthesia care provider to heparinize the patient earlier than anticipated to allow for percutaneous femoral artery cannulation for bypass. Blood products and heparin bolus must be immediately available should this extremely emergent situation occur.

Because of the frequent need for PA catheterization or central venous pressure (CVP) monitoring, prior surgery that has distorted the vascular and anatomic features of the neck and upper thorax must be noted. Of particular importance is a history of radical neck dissection, subclavian bypass procedures, ligation of the internal jugular vein, or carotid artery surgery, which should be evaluated for effect on intubation and line placement.

For cardiac surgery involving recent or concomitant endarterectomy of carotid artery lesions, reinstitution of normal perfusion pressure may result in edema and hemorrhage. The inability of capillary beds to vasoconstrict and regulate flow leads some areas of the brain to exhibit a mismatch of CBF to metabolic ratio.[32] Cerebral perfusion is dependent on autoregulation to maintain constant blood flow regardless of changes in perfusion pressure or CO. Chronic hypoperfusion related to carotid stenosis may lead to maximal dilation of the cerebral vessels, compromising compensatory mechanisms normally available for tolerance of low-pressure or low-flow states.[23] In cases in which this condition remains uncorrected before cardiac surgery, systemic arterial pressure must be maintained at a level that ensures adequate cerebral perfusion.

Hemodynamic Status

Evaluation of cardiovascular status includes a discussion with the patient regarding his or her functional status. One method of qualifying the functional status is to determine by interview which activities of daily living the patient is able to perform. If a patient is unable to climb one flight of stairs without difficulty, then the anesthesia care provider can plan for a patient with reduced ability to handle the hemodynamic changes inherent to induction and maintenance of anesthesia.

Cardiac catheterization may be used for diagnostic assessment, electrophysiologic evaluation, or direct intervention in patients in cardiogenic shock. The catheterization report provides significant information regarding patient cardiac performance. The catheterization evaluation provides information about pressures and oxygen saturations of the four chambers of the heart, PA pressure, systemic pressure, body surface area, CI (liters per minute per square meter), stroke index (milliliters per beat per square meter), left ventricular ejection fraction (EF), degree of stenosis in coronary vessels, and coronary dominance (Table 25-1).

TABLE **25-2**	Cardiac Formulas		
Parameter	**Notation**	**Formula**	**Normal Range**
Stroke volume	SV	$SV = CO \div HR$	60-90 mL/beat
Stroke index	SI	$SI = SV \div BSA$	40-60 mL/beat/m^2
Cardiac output	CO	$CO = SV \times HR$	5-6 L/min
Cardiac index	CI	$CI = CO \div BSA$	2.5-4 L/min/m^2
Mean arterial pressure	MAP	MAP = diastolic pressure + ⅓ pulse pressure	80-120 mm Hg
Systemic vascular resistance	SVR	$SVR = (MAP - CVP) \div (CO \times 80)$	700-1400 dyne/sec/cm^5
Pulmonary vascular resistance	PVR	$PVR = (PAP - PCWP) \div (CO \times 80)$	50-300 dyne/sec/cm^5
Left ventricular stroke work index	LVSWI	$LVSWI = 0.0136 \times (MAP - PCWP) \times SI$	40-60 g • m/beat/m^2
Coronary perfusion pressure	CPP	$CPP = DIA\ BP - LVEDP$	50 mm Hg
Ejection fraction	EF	$EF = (EDV - ESV) \div EDV$	55%-70%
Rate-pressure product	RPP	$RPP = SYS\ BP \times rate$	>15,000
Triple index	TI	$TI = SYS\ BP \times rate \times PCWP$	>180,000

BSA, *Body surface area*; DIA BP, *diastolic blood pressure*; EDV, *end-diastolic volume*; ESV, *end-systolic volume*; HR, *heart rate*; LVEDP, *left ventricular end-diastolic pressure*; PCWP, *pulmonary capillary wedge pressure*; SI, *stroke index*; SYS BP, *systolic blood pressure*.

EF is the end-diastolic volume (EDV) minus the end-systolic volume (ESV), divided by the EDV:

Equation 25-1

$$EF = (EDV - ESV)/EDV$$

Tables 25-2 and 25-3 summarize cardiac formulas that are useful in clinical practice. An EF of 50% or greater in a patient with normal valve function is acceptable. If the patient has mitral regurgitation, an EF of 50% to 55% is considered to indicate left ventricular dysfunction. An EF of less than 50% reflects a moderate reduction of ventricular function. Poor cardiac function relates to an EF below 30% and may stem from ventricular hypokinesis, akinesis, or dyskinesis. Echocardiography is used to evaluate ventricular function by measuring wall motion during systole. It can permit a qualitative and quantitative assessment and reflects the four types of abnormal wall function described previously.[33] Single photon emission computed tomography (SPECT) scan is another diagnostic tool used in the preparation of patients for cardiac surgery. It is a noninvasive procedure that makes use of a radionuclide tracer to provide a three-dimensional picture of heart structures and function. It is capable of producing a measurement of rate and volume of blood flow, size and location of blockages or narrowing of vessels, and more accurate diagnosis of heart disease in women.[34]

Right Ventricular Function

Patients with right coronary artery disease may be susceptible to right ventricular ischemia and infarction when right ventricular distention or increased afterload results in diminished cardiac performance and reduced right coronary perfusion pressure. The interrelationships among aortic end-diastolic pressure, afterload volume, coronary perfusion pressure, and pulmonary vascular resistance play a significant role in the management of right-sided cardiac performance. Assessment of these variables before treatment is essential if compromise of function is to be avoided.

Common treatment for systemic hypotension before initiation of CPB incorporates the use of phenylephrine, an α_1-adrenergic agonist. The primary indication for use is hypotension induced by

TABLE **25-3**	Hemodilution	
Circulating Blood Volume		
Patient	**Estimated Red Blood Cell Count**	
Male	80 mL/kg	
Female	65 mL/kg	
Pediatric	85-105 mL/kg	
Hemodilutional Hematocrit		
	Notation	**Formula**
Estimated red blood cell count	ERBC	Determined by age and gender
Circulating blood volume	CBV	ERBC × weight (kg)
Red blood cell volume	RBCV	CBV × Hct
Total circulating volume	TCV	CBV + prime volume
Dilutional hematocrit	Dilutional Hct	RBCV ÷ TCV

a reduction in systemic vascular resistance (SVR) as opposed to compromised CO. The perceived advantage of the use of phenylephrine is its effect of increasing coronary perfusion pressure with minimal chronotropic side effects.[35]

Pulmonary Function

Risk factors of note for the pulmonary system include a history of cigarette smoking, dyspnea, and wheezing. Patients with chronic obstructive pulmonary disease and dyspnea or wheezing have two to six times more pulmonary complications in the postoperative phase of cardiac surgery. A recent respiratory infection predisposes to postoperative atelectasis and pneumonia.[36]

Diabetes Mellitus

Patients with diabetes mellitus are at increased risk intraoperatively and postoperatively because of the potential threat of silent ischemia and MI. These patients have both peripheral and autonomic neuropathies. With autonomic neuropathy, they are at an increased risk of aspiration and sudden death. Patients on NPH insulin have the added risk of allergic reaction to protamine, necessitating the possibility that heparin may have to be metabolized instead of being reversed. Investigational substances may be available in the future to safely reverse heparin in these allergic patients. Heparinase I has been introduced as an alternative to protamine. It is a carbohydrate-modifying enzyme that cleaves heparin at specific sites that are important for anticoagulation. This agent fractionates heparin into small inactive fragments with no apparent adverse hemodynamic changes.[37]

Laboratory Data

Laboratory examinations for patients with ischemic heart disease involving two or more associated risk factors (e.g., diabetes, obesity, family history, smoking) should include complete blood count; electrolytes, cardiac enzymes (including enzyme fraction for creatinine phosphokinase), serum creatinine, cholesterol; and coagulation screening profile.[38]

Coagulation function studies include platelet count (PT) and partial thromboplastin time (PTT). Activated clotting time (ACT) is used to monitor patients receiving heparin therapy, and PT and international normalized ratio (INR) are used to monitor patients receiving warfarin products.[39] Platelet inhibitors are often part of the drug regimens of patients who need cardiac surgery. These agents are associated with the risk of excess bleeding. However, no evidence suggests that surgery is contraindicated in this situation. It is recommended that 24 to 48 hours should elapse before surgery is performed after these drugs are discontinued. The platelet inhibitors (glycoprotein IIb/IIIa receptor inhibitors) in use at this time include abciximab (ReoPro), eptifibatide (Integrilin), and tirofiban (Aggrastat).[40] It should be emphasized that long-term heparin therapy results in prolonged bleeding times and may affect calculations of loading doses of heparin required for CPB.[41] Other issues related to the cause and treatment of adverse bleeding are discussed later in this chapter.

Long-Term Use of Medications

Patients on chronic therapy should continue their medications up to the time of surgery. This is especially important for their cardiac drugs.

It is recommended that antidysrhythmics be continued until the day of surgery except for disopyramide and flecainide, which should be discontinued except in the presence of the most life-threatening dysrhythmias. Disopyramide has been noted to cause difficulty in termination of CPB.

Antidepressants provide no advantage if continued up to the day of surgery and may interact negatively with sympathomimetics. However, as noted previously, it is important to give sedation and anxiolysis to these patients during the preoperative phase.

ANESTHESIA MONITORING

Electrocardiography and Noninvasive Blood Pressure

Leads II and V_5 can help in the diagnosis of dysrhythmias, ischemia, conduction defects, and electrolyte disturbances. None of the standard leads can detect posterior-wall ischemia. The noninvasive blood pressure cuff must be placed on the same side as the arterial line to allow for correlation of blood pressure. This is a backup monitor.

Radial Arterial Line

Sternal retraction may play a role in distorting the radial artery waveform. The right radial artery is usually selected in cases in which the left internal mammary artery is dissected for anastomosis and because radial arterial line monitoring may show a false low number because of compression of the subclavian artery at the retractor. The brachial artery is contraindicated because it is an end artery of the arm. Some authors evaluate results of an Allen test, because it screens for patients with inadequate palmar collateral flow from the ulnar artery. Reduced collateral flow is a relative contraindication to the use of a radial artery catheter.

Other Arterial Line Sites

Use of the brachial artery for monitoring is most commonly dismissed because it provides the bulk of circulation for the lower arm and is considered an end artery. The femoral artery is superficial and offers access to the central arterial tree. It also provides appropriate access should an IABP placement be necessary. However, if the femoral artery is used, it should be noted that an alternative site may become necessary if use of IABP is instituted. The dorsalis pedis arteries may have a more distorted wave form and are not recommended for patients with aortoiliac or peripheral vascular disease. The axillary artery is not commonly cannulated because of an increased risk of cerebral air embolus and because it has a tendency to bleed more easily. The ulnar artery can be cannulated for monitoring, but an Allen test of the ulnar artery is necessary before placement, and the risk of problems with placement on the same extremity as a radial attempt must be taken into consideration. The complications inherent to arterial line placement include ischemia, thrombosis, infection, and bleeding.

Central Venous Pressure

Use of the of the right internal jugular (IJ) vein is recommended because cannulation of the left IJ vein increases the risk of laceration of the left brachiocephalic vein. Relative contraindications to right IJ cannulation include carotid disease, recent cannulation (increases the risk of thrombosis), contralateral diaphragmatic dysfunction, thyromegaly, and prior major neck surgery. Central venous pressure lines may be used for monitoring, to provide a central line for fluid and drugs, and in situations in which a PA catheter is not used.[42,43]

Pulmonary Artery Catheter

The PA catheter was historically used for all CABG procedures, but it is associated with complications (Box 25-3) and now has a more narrow range of uses. It is indicated for use in high-risk patients with an EF of less than 40%.[43] (Table 25-4).

Inflation of the positioned balloon occludes the PA pressure and reflects left chamber pressures of the heart. This catheter also allows simultaneous monitoring of central venous pressure and pulmonary arterial blood temperature. The thermistor on the PA catheter allows calculation of derived parameters such as CO via

---

BOX **25-3**

Complications of Pulmonary Artery Catheters

- Tachyarrhythmias
- Right bundle branch block
- Complete heart block
- Cardiac perforation
- Pulmonary infarction and prolonged wedge times
- Pulmonary artery rupture
- Endocarditis
- Knotting of catheter
- Pulmonic valve insufficiency

TABLE **25-4**	Pulmonary Artery Catheter Insertion Sites	
Location	**Distance to Vena Cava–Right Atrium Junction (cm)**	
Internal jugular vein	15-20	
Superior vena cava	10-15	
Femoral vein	30	
Right antecubital fossa	40	
Left antecubital fossa	50	

Modified from Headley JM. Invasive Hemodynamic Monitoring: Physiological Principles and Clinical Applications. Irvine, CA: Baxter Healthcare; 1989.

---

the thermodilution method, SVR, CI, and stroke volume (SV). This hemodynamic tool is used to monitor demand factors such as preload, afterload, heart rate, and contractility.

During systole with the balloon deflated, the catheter transduces right ventricular systolic pressure. During diastole with the balloon deflated, the catheter transduces PA diastolic pressure, which also represents left atrial pressure. During ventricular diastole with the balloon inflated, the pulmonary catheter is said to be *wedged* and reflects left ventricular filling pressure. During ventricular systole with the balloon wedged, the catheter reflects left atrial filling pressure.[44] Types of PA catheters include the venous infusion port (with a third port for administration of intravenous [IV] solutions), pacing PA catheter, mixed venous saturation catheters, EF catheters, and PA catheters capable of measuring continuous CO, which is valuable during off-pump cardiac procedures.

Transesophageal Echocardiography

Transesophageal echocardiography (TEE) allows continuous monitoring of the chambers of the heart, ascending and descending aorta, valvular function, chamber filling, and wall contractility and motion. Detection of gaseous or particulate emboli, identification of intracardiac shunting, diagnosis of aortic dissection, evaluation of saphenous vein graft flow, and confirmation of left ventricular dimension (filling) during weaning are other potential applications for this monitoring method. TEE may predict or suggest myocardial ischemia as defined by regional wall motion abnormalities, valve replacement procedures, cardiac aneurysms, intracardiac tumors, aortic dissection, and repair of complex congenital lesions.[45]

Relative contraindications to the use of TEE include dysphagia, mediastinal radiation, upper GI surgery or bleeding, esophageal stricture, tumor, varices, and recent chest trauma. In conjunction with the increased use of TEE, certain complications have been reported to occur during open-heart surgery. Cardiac arrhythmias, bronchospasm, and esophageal laceration are rare. The Society of Cardiovascular Anesthesiologists has published guidelines for the perioperative use of TEE.[46,47]

Monitoring Core Temperature

Accurate monitoring of core temperature is essential in controlling target hypothermia, as well as reestablishing normothermia. The most accurate indicator of core temperature is at the thermistor of the PA catheter. Brain temperature is reflected in nasopharyngeal measurement, but a lag time occurs on rewarming. The probe should be inserted before heparinization to a depth of 7 to 10 cm through the nares. Tympanic temperature may also lag behind brain rewarmed temperature and is no better for monitoring this parameter. Bladder or rectal temperature measurement is today considered inaccurate when renal and splanchnic blood flow is decreased.[46] Brain temperature should not drop below 20° C; profound hypothermia (15° to 20° C) appears to cause a loss of cerebral autoregulation.[8]

Cerebral Monitoring

In addition to the monitoring of brain temperature, electrophysiologic monitoring is often used. EEG is not an effective method for monitoring subtle changes, but any asymmetric EEG activity is considered a problem. Bispectral analysis (BIS) monitoring *may* correlate with the depth of anesthesia, but it is actually a derived parameter to assess the degree of wakefulness. BIS does not measure brain function or the adequacy of oxygenation of the brain.[48,49]

Somatosensory and motor evoked potentials are useful measures for monitoring neurologic functions.

Monitoring glucose is important in cerebral preservation because hyperglycemia increases the extent and degree of any ischemia that may occur. Glucose is considered an independent risk factor for aggravation of ischemia. Hyperglycemia prevents the increase of adenosine (responsible for cerebrovasodilatation), thereby preventing the brain from protecting itself from ischemic damage.[50] Modalities and the function they measure are noted in Table 25-5.

PERFUSION PRINCIPLES

The goal of CPB is to provide a motionless heart in a bloodless field while the vital organs continue to be adequately oxygenated. The CPB pump provides respiration (oxygenation and elimination of CO_2), circulation (maintenance of perfusion pressure), and regulation of temperature (hypothermia to preserve myocardium). Initiation of CPB subjects the circulating blood of the patient to significant physiologic and physical changes. Anesthetic and perfusion management must address the effect of low-flow indices, reduced metabolic requirements, changing viscosity of the patient's circulating volume, and postoperative inflammatory response. Multiple factors interact to create a substantially new environment for physiologic homeostasis. Hemodynamic abnormalities that occur during CPB include endothelial dysfunction ("total body systemic inflammatory response"), which causes symptoms similar to those in patients

TABLE **25-5**	Multimodality Neuromonitoring for Cardiac Surgery
Modality	**Function**
Electroencephalography	Cortical synaptic activity
Middle latency auditory evoked potentials	Subcortical-cortical activity
Brainstem auditory evoked potentials	Brainstem synaptic activity
Transcranial Doppler	Blood flow change and emboli
Cerebral oximetry	Cortical oxygen balance

From Edmonds HL: Central nervous system monitoring. In: Kaplan JA et al. eds. Kaplan's Cardiac Anesthesia. 5th ed. Philadelphia: Saunders; 2006.

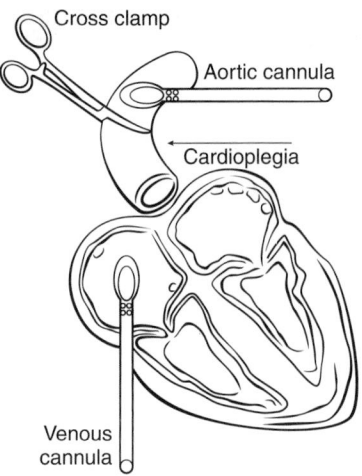

FIGURE **25-2**   Cannulation sites in the heart.

with sepsis or trauma.[51,52] Other abnormalities include persistent heparin effect, platelet dysfunction or loss, coagulopathy, fibrinolysis, and hypothermia.

Rapid recirculation of the total blood volume during CPB subjects blood and tissue components to a foreign environment that invites cellular trauma. The patient experiences tremendous alterations in core temperature, hematocrit (in the form of hemodilution), the coagulation cascade, and perfusion pressures (nonpulsatile perfusion). Clinical and experimental evidence indicates that CPB significantly alters the plasma and cellular constituents of blood, affecting both platelet count and function. As a result of excessive hemodilution, the platelet count decreases rapidly to 50% of the preoperative level but usually remains above 100,000 per microliter. Bleeding time is greatly prolonged, and platelet aggregation and function are impaired. Reductions occur in the plasma concentrations of coagulation factors II, V, VII, IX, X, and XII and are attributed to hemodilution.[53]

Extracorporeal Circuit

The CPB (pump) circuit consists of separate disposable components bioengineered to interface with perfusion pumps, fluid-based thermoregulating systems, air-oxygen blenders, anesthetic vaporizers, pressure transducers, temperature monitors, and in-line oxygen and blood gas analyzers. The pump components include venous cannulas from the right atrium or vena cava, which are usually fenestrated at the tip and reinforced. Venous tubing includes the venous return for the blood drained to the machine from the left ventricle. The venous drainage to the venous reservoir depends on gravity, patient intravascular volume, and the position of and resistance from the venous cannula. The table height can affect venous drainage to the pump. Drainage collects in the venous reservoir, where air bubbles are removed and drainage from other reservoirs is mixed together. If a low volume is allowed here, air can be entrained into the arterial circulation.[54] Blood suctioned from the heart, pericardium, and pleural spaces drains to the cardiotomy reservoir.

The pump's oxygenator can be of the bubble type or the membrane type. Bubble-type oxygenators are implicated in gas embolisms because of incomplete removal of bubbles. Membrane oxygenators made of artificial polypropylene remove CO_2 independently of oxygenation. Membrane oxygenators have a higher resistance to flow and are placed after the pump. A heat

exchanger cools or rewarms blood and is located in the venous reservoir or oxygenator.[53] An arterial cannula returns oxygenated blood from the pump to the patient. Blood pressure is usually reduced at the time of arterial cannulation so that blood does not spray from this high-pressure site.

The CPB circuit pushes blood forward and returns blood under pressure to the patient by means of either rollers (most common) or a centrifugal (vortex) pump. The roller-type pump can deliver blood to the body at a constant rate or in a pulsatile fashion. The centrifugal pump is affected by pressure downstream and will stop if air is present in the pump. The cannulation sites in the heart are noted in (Figure 25-2).

Various safety mechanisms are included to alert the operator of low venous operating reserve, high arterial line pressures, disconnection from air supply, and introduction of air embolus into the arterial line. As an extension of the extracorporeal circuit, the cardioplegia delivery system provides and maintains hypothermic and pharmacologic arrest of the heart during revascularization. Ultrafiltration and red blood cell–sequestering devices may be incorporated into the circuit to counteract hemodilution by removing excess volume through dialysis or centrifugal separation of fluid and plasma components from the circulating blood volume.

Prime

A significant factor is the amount of crystalloid solution required to prime the tubing, reservoir, filters, and oxygenator. Establishing an air-free circuit is essential for unimpaired fluid volume transport and preventing air embolism. Most circuits require at least 2000 mL of a solution such as Normosol, Plasma-Lyte A, or Isolyte S, with pH and electrolytes closely matching the composition of whole blood. Added to this base solution are heparin, sodium bicarbonate, mannitol, hetastarch, albumin, and possibly corticosteroids or antihyperfibrinolytic agents. The additions can result in priming volumes in excess of 2000 mL; when transfused to the patient at the onset of CPB, this can cause a hemodilutional bolus of 30% to 50% of the patient's circulating blood volume (see Table 25-3).

Vascular Transport

The heart and lungs are isolated and bypassed from systemic blood flow. This function is accomplished by right atrial or vena caval cannulation with subsequent diversion of venous blood that is returning to the heart. The venoatrial cannulas are connected to polyvinyl chloride (PVC) tubing that extends from the surgical field to the venous reservoir situated at a level well below the patient's heart to facilitate gravity exsanguination. Blood from the reservoir is propelled by roller or centrifugal pump to the oxygenator, where it becomes arterialized by interfacing with a membrane oxygenator. A heat exchanger mounted on the oxygenator provides for control of blood temperature. Oxygenated blood passes through an arterial filter and an in-line arterial gas monitoring device.

Aortic cannula placement is distal to the sinus of Valsalva and proximal to the brachiocephalic (innominate) artery. The arterial line pressure of the extracorporeal circulation (ECC) depends on flow and resistance but usually is maintained below 300 mm Hg.[54]

Myocardial Protection Techniques

Injury to the myocardium is a complex occurrence and may result from numerous physiologic events. Tachycardia, hypertension or hypotension, and ventricular distention can all play a role in the events that produce an oxygen supply/demand imbalance. Contractile function deteriorates rapidly after the initial insult of ischemia. Rapid cardioplegia-induced cardiac arrest, decompression of the ventricles, and hypothermia are the underlying techniques used to ensure myocardial protection during CPB. The duration of aortic cross-clamping time, collateral coronary blood supply, frequency of cardioplegia delivery, and composition of cardioplegia are factors that influence the extent of reperfusion injury.[55] Intermittent doses of cold crystalloid cardioplegia help maintain cardiac arrest, hypothermia, and pH; counteract edema; wash out metabolite; and provide oxygen and substrate for aerobic metabolism.

Administration of inhalation anesthetics has been shown to produce protection against myocardial ischemia and reperfusion injury.[56-59] This phenomenon is termed *anesthetic-induced preconditioning* (APC) and derives from positive effects on mitochondria, potassium ATP channels, reactive oxygen species, calcium overload, and inflammation. Anesthetic-induced preconditioning reduces myocardial necrosis and improves postoperative cardiac performance.

Cardioplegia

Cardioplegia is a potassium solution administered into the coronary circulation to provide diastolic arrest. It is composed of potassium (15 to 30 mEq/L), calcium to prevent ischemic contracture (stone heart), albumin or mannitol for osmolarity correction, and glucose or simple amino acids as a metabolic substrate. The cardioplegia delivers oxygen and nutrients, removes waste products, and cools or rewarms the heart. It is administered in an anterograde manner into the aortic root, from which it distributes to the coronaries and into the myocardium. It may also be administered in a retrograde fashion into the coronary sinus, from which it distributes through veins, venules, and capillaries of the myocardium.

The cardioplegia composition is blood or crystalloid based. Blood-based cardioplegia is oxygenated blood that is diluted with fluid at a 4:1 ratio. It has a hematocrit of 16% to 18% and is given at 4° to 14° C. Crystalloid-based solutions do not contain hemoglobin; therefore they deliver dissolved O_2 only. Because of this, crystalloid solutions can be used only with myocardial hypothermic techniques. Intracellular cardioplegia has a low sodium content to produce loss of membrane potential by eliminating the sodium gradient across the membrane. Extracellular solutions produce diastolic arrest by depolarization of the membrane with high potassium concentrations.[60]

COAGULATION

Coagulation Cascade
Intrinsic Pathway

The coagulation cascade is initiated when blood becomes traumatized by exposure to a foreign surface. In the initiation of CPB, contact with the PVC tubing used in the extracorporeal circuit, the squeezing mechanism of the roller head pump, and various filtering devices can cause lysis of the blood cells. This leads to activation of factor XII (Hageman factor), also known as the *contact factor.*[61]

Activated factor XII is a proteolytic enzyme that stimulates the production of factor XI. This reaction is mediated by high-molecular-weight kininogen and is accelerated by prekallikrein. Platelets are damaged because of adherence to collagen or secondary to damage associated with the extracorporeal circulation. Platelet disruption mediates the release of platelet phospholipids containing platelet factor III, which is a lipoprotein that plays a role in subsequent clotting reactions. Activated factor XI, factor VIII, and platelet factor III interact to activate factor X, which initiates the common pathway for both intrinsic and extrinsic coagulation mechanisms. An acute deficiency in either factor VII (hemophilia) or platelets (thrombocytopenia) results in a clotting deficiency.

Activated factor X combines with factor V and platelet or tissue phospholipids to form a complex called *prothrombin activator,* which cleaves prothrombin to form thrombin. This process and subsequent processes are mediated by the presence of calcium ions. Thrombin facilitates the conversion of fibrinogen to a fibrin monomer that polymerizes into long fibrin threads to form the reticulum of the clot. Clot is composed of a meshwork of fibrin threads extending in all directions, entrapping blood cells, platelets, and plasma. The fibrin threads adhere to damaged surfaces of blood vessels (or a foreign surface) and prevent further blood loss.[61]

Extrinsic Pathway

The extrinsic mechanism for coagulation is activated when blood comes into contact with traumatized vascular wall or extravascular tissues. Traumatized tissue releases a complex of factors called *tissue thromboplastin.* Of particular interest are the phospholipids (derived from tissue membranes) and a lipoprotein complex containing a glycoprotein that functions as a proteolytic enzyme. This lipoprotein complex of tissue thromboplastin interacts with factor VII and, in the presence of tissue phospholipids and calcium ions, converts factor X to its activated form. Activated factor X complexes with either the tissue phospholipids released from tissue thromboplastin or the tissue phospholipids released from platelets and, in combination with factor V, forms a new complex called *prothrombin activator.* Within seconds, prothrombin activator splits prothrombin to form thrombin, and the clotting process begins.[61]

Common Pathway

The end-point of activity for both the extrinsic and intrinsic coagulation pathways is the activation of factor X. Reactions beyond this point are common to both pathways and involve the combining of activated factor X with procoagulants (factor II, factor V, calcium ions, and platelet phospholipids) to form a prothrombinase complex. This complex catalyzes the conversion of circulating prothrombin to thrombin, which in turn converts circulating fibrinogen to insoluble fibrin. The coagulation process is terminated by the stabilization of fibrin via the activation of factor XIII.[62]

Blood Components

Fibrinogen

Fibrinogen is a high-molecular-weight protein present in the plasma in quantities of 100 to 700 mg/dL. In the presence of calcium ions it becomes the precursor for fibrin threads, the foundation of the blood clot. For replacement therapy, a target value of 150 mg/dL may be achieved with the administration of blood products such as cryoprecipitate or fresh frozen plasma (FFP).[63,64]

Fresh Frozen Plasma

FFP contains the same concentrations of plasma proteins present in the donor's plasma. Therefore, fibrinogen and all other factors are not concentrated. When some deficiency of a factor is present, a considerable amount of FFP is required to raise levels back to normal. Fibrinogen is accepted as the protein most critical in the coagulation cascade. Considering the fact that each unit of FFP is approximately 250 mL and that the patient's circulating blood volume averages 5000 mL or greater, the FFP usually is diluted in the patient's own plasma and has little effect in raising overall plasma fibrinogen concentrations.[65,66]

Platelets

The normal platelet concentration in blood is 150,000 to 300,000 platelets per microliter. Changes in platelet count and function can be associated with CPB. The circulating platelet count declines to approximately 50% of prebypass levels, partially as a result of hemodilution, adhesion to the surface of the oxygenator and bypass circuit, sequestration to the spleen, and platelet aggregation.[61] Platelet count rarely drops below 100,000 per microliter, but this decrease in count does explain the bleeding abnormalities found after CPB. Platelet dysfunction may be due to hypothermia, trauma-induced activation, fibrinolysis, or drug-related causes. Heparin, nitrates, phosphodiesterase inhibitors, and protamine can all affect platelet function. Platelet function cannot be appropriately assessed on the basis of count alone. The properties required for adhesion and aggregation may be diminished or nonexistent in platelets that have been subjected to ECC.

Anticoagulation

Initiation of CPB requires systemic heparinization to establish a safe level of anticoagulation. The currently accepted regimen is 300 units of heparin per kilogram of patient weight. The heparin dose is usually calculated to maintain an ACT of 400 seconds (the normal range is 130 seconds or less). Heparin is a catalyst and binds with circulating antithrombin (AT III) and potentiates its natural anticoagulant properties. Heparin is administered intravenously through the central venous port. Its peak effect occurs within 2 minutes, and verification is based on the ACT, which should be established 5 to 10 minutes after administration. Special circumstances such as long-term heparinization, antithrombin III deficiency, heparin-induced thrombocytopenia, and excessive hemodilution may cause "heparin resistance," which alters the algorithm for calculating the loading dose. The surgeon, anesthesia provider, and perfusion teams should consider these circumstances.

Management of a patient with heparin-associated thrombocytopenia and thrombosis (HATT or HIT) presents a particular challenge. HIT is evident after exposure to heparin, because the platelet count suddenly falls. The onset can be as soon as 2 days or as long as 5 days after institution of heparin therapy. Surgery should be postponed if at all possible, and heparin must be eliminated from the patient's medication regimen until the platelets are normal and do not aggregate in response to heparin. A polysulfated glycosaminoglycan (danaparoid) as well as a thrombin inhibitor (hirudin) have been used safely for CPB.[61]

Heparin should be a part of the resuscitation protocol for cardiac surgery patients. If the patient undergoes cardiac arrest during the induction or prebypass phase of the case, heparin can be given and the patient placed on bypass as a resuscitative measure.

Anticoagulation is imperative for CPB used during cardiac surgery. It is vital in all patients that the ACT be at least 350 before CPB is performed.

Coagulation Tests

Treatment for coagulopathy depends on the cause. A review of tests for assessing functions of coagulation is included as a guide to management.

Activated Clotting Time

ACT is a standardized measurement of the patient's procoagulation or anticoagulation level. The unit of measurement is the time (in seconds) required for an ACT counter to detect the formation of blood clot in a 2- to 3-mL sample of whole blood. Normal ACT levels range from 100 to 130 seconds. Because this test is a crude measure of clotting, CPB requires anticoagulation levels of 400 seconds or more. Patients may show significant variability in the reaction as a result of different rates of metabolism of heparin. Hypothermia and hemodilution are factors associated with CPB that directly affect the ACT. Hypothermia has the most profound effect in terms of prolonging intraoperative values.[60]

Whole Blood Heparin Concentration

The whole blood heparin concentration method of assessing anticoagulation is usually followed by use of an automated protamine titration (Medtronic HemoTec). However, the amount of heparin necessary for this technique is increased, and any benefit may be at the expense of greater platelet activation, which could confound platelet dysfunction after CPB.[61]

Other Anticoagulation Monitors

Because ACT and heparin concentration testing is less than perfect, other tests are being investigated. Activated PTT (aPTT) and thrombin time are too sensitive to be useful in CPB monitoring.

Thromboelastogram

The thromboelastogram assesses clot function from the time of initial activation and clot formation through the acceleration phase, clot-strengthening phase, and retraction phase to eventual lysis. It grossly examines the entire life cycle of a clot but does not isolate the subsegments of procoagulant precursors and their individual contributions to clot dynamics. It is capable of indicating abnormalities in formation and lysis of clots. Its primary function is to examine clot strength. This coagulation test is finding utility in the diagnosis of fibrinolysis for liver transplants.[61]

PROPHYLAXIS AND TREATMENT OF COAGULOPATHY

Patients for CABG procedures on CPB receive an antifibrinolytic. Antifibrinolytics are hemostatic agents usually given as an IV loading dose and then by continuous infusion. First-time patients are treated with aminocaproic acid. Patients undergoing subsequent surgeries, those with renal failure, those at high risk of bleeding, and Jehovah's Witnesses may require alternative antifibrinolytics.

∈-Aminocaproic Acid and Tranexamic Acid

Aminocaproic acid (Amicar) was initially proposed for the treatment of fibrinolysis associated with prostate and cardiac surgery. Tranexamic acid is considered to be more potent than aminocaproic acid. The loading dose of aminocaproic acid is 100 to 150 mg/kg, followed by an infusion dose of 10 to 15 mg/kg/hr. The dose of tranexamic acid is 10 to 15 mg/kg loading, with an infusion of 1 to 1.5 mg/kg/hr. The drug has renal excretion and a plasma half-life of approximately 80 minutes. These drugs have proved effective in reducing bleeding after bypass.[61]

Aprotinin

Aprotinin (Trasylol) is a serine inhibitor extracted from the bovine lung and has demonstrated efficacy in reducing blood loss in cardiac surgery. Safety concerns regarding the use of aprotinin have recently been raised, and its use has been suspended in the United States. Increased rates of thrombotic and renal morbidity, as well as increased mortality have been noted.[67-70] Aminocaproic acid and tranexamic acid are safer alternatives.

Desmopressin

Desmopressin acetate (DDAVP) is a synthetic analog of vasopressin that releases a variety of hemostatically active substances from the vascular endothelium. It is administered in doses of 0.3 mcg/kg intravenously, intranasally, or subcutaneously. It has a half-life of 55 minutes (with clinical effects lasting from 5 to 6 hours) and results in an approximately fourfold increase in circulating levels of factor VIII, prostacycline, tissue plasminogen activator, and von Willebrand factor. The overall effect of desmopressin is hemostatic. DDAVP has also been used to treat uremia, cirrhosis, platelet disorders, and mild or moderate cases of hemophilia A (von Willebrand disease). Current evidence does not support the broad administration of DDAVP to cardiac surgical patients as prophylaxis for bleeding.[61]

PHARMACOLOGIC APPROACHES TO BLOOD PRESSURE CONTROL

Blood pressure control during the perioperative phase may be accomplished with the use of pharmacologic agents independently or in combination. Vasodilators such as hydralazine, nitroglycerin, and nitroprusside are useful for controlling blood pressure and improving peripheral blood flow.

α-Adrenergic agonists (e.g., clonidine) reduce stress-mediated neurohumoral responses to induction and CPB. They decrease heart rate and blood pressure and have sedative and antinociceptive characteristics, which may reduce opioid requirements without respiratory depression. They can be used independently or in conjunction with IV induction agents and opioids; they help to reduce the amount of agent required.

Careful use of β-blockers can decrease heart rate, contractility, and blood pressure, which works to reduce oxygen use. These drugs increase the duration of diastole to allow for a more complete oxygenation of the left ventricle. They act synergistically with nitroglycerin and blunt tachycardia and decrease ischemia of the myocardium. They have the ability to reduce

catecholamine-induced ventricular arrhythmias. The disadvantage associated with β-blockers is that they may precipitate bradyarrhythmias, heart block, or bronchospasm. β–Blockers available in IV form for use during cardiac surgery include esmolol, labetalol, metoprolol, and propranolol. Reversal of the effects of β-blockers can be achieved through use of β-agonists (isoproterenol) and cardiac pacing (unless emergent CPB initiation is possible).

Vasodilator therapy includes direct vasodilators (hydralazine, nitroglycerin, or nitroprusside), α- and β-adrenergic blockers (labetalol), angiotensin-converting enzyme (ACE) inhibitors (enalaprilat IV), central α-agonists (clonidine), or calcium channel blockers (nicardipine IV, verapamil, or diltiazem). The drug therapy is to be selected individually for each patient and situation and administered judiciously for the desired effect.

Vasopressor therapy includes agents with selective direct effects (phenylephrine), α_1-agonist mixed agents (dopamine, ephedrine, epinephrine, noradrenaline), or vasopressin (direct peripheral vasoconstriction with no β-adrenergic effects).[71,72] Other drugs include the positive inotropic drugs (e.g., dobutamine, dopamine, and milrinone).[57] Calcium reverses hypotension associated with the use of halogenated agents, calcium channel blockers, hypocalcemia, β-blockers, and CPB. When administered intravenously by central line, it can increase blood pressure, as well as reverse the negative cardiac effects of hyperkalemia.[73]

PREOPERATIVE PERIOD

Considerations during the preoperative period include sedation and monitoring of the patient while placement of appropriate invasive monitoring lines ensues. All equipment should be available and invasive lines inserted before the patient is taken to the operating room. Invasive monitors are useful during induction and should be placed before induction except in emergency situations like ruptured aneurysms, cardiac tamponade, or ventricle rupture.

Premedication should provide anxiolysis, amnesia, and some degree of pain relief for the insertion of invasive lines. Midazolam (0.05 to 0.1 mg/kg) IV titrated or lorazepam (15 to 20 mcg/kg) titrated with either fentanyl (10- to 20-mcg increments IV) or sufentanil (5- to 10-mcg increments) until effective work well in compensated patients. For patients who are poorly compensated, a titrated low dose of lorazepam or midazolam is sufficient.[74] Oxygen should be administered to these medicated patients during line placement and until preoxygenation for induction ensues.

Extensive preparation and setup are required for heart surgery. Each institution has specific setup guidelines with regard to medication and equipment needs. It is advisable that patients be intubated with an endotracheal tube that is as large as possible, because they may remain intubated and mechanically ventilated for several hours after surgery in some situations.

Induction

Hemodynamic alterations occur at induction of anesthesia. The induction plan should take into consideration left ventricular function. No single technique has been demonstrated as superior with regard to the prevention of postoperative MI by intraoperative ischemia. It is important to control heart rate because this parameter is most likely to produce myocardial ischemia.[74] Prevention of myocardial ischemia is a primary concern. Two factors associated with myocardial ischemia are inadequate oxygen supply to the myocardium from localized coronary lesions and excessive oxygen demand due to the increased hemodynamic workload associated with increased heart rate and blood pressure or adrenergic stimulation. On induction, myocardial ischemia can be detected through the electrocardiogram (ECG), TEE, or PA wedge pressure readings.

Methods for diminishing the incidence of ischemia include therapeutic interventions such as preoxygenation before induction, reduction of wall tension with nitroglycerin, control of heart rate with β-adrenergic blocking agents, reduction of the work of the myocardium through control of myocardial depression with increased anesthetic levels, and maintenance of coronary perfusion pressure through the use of a non-chronotropic agent such as phenylephrine. Many cardiac patients have low circulating blood volume because of hypertensive vasoconstriction. A reduced plasma volume may necessitate fluid loading or prophylactic treatment with pressors such as phenylephrine before induction. Hypovolemia should be anticipated and can be monitored by observation of blood pressure alterations and CVP.

High or low CO has a significant effect on the pharmacokinetics of anesthetic agents. The anesthetic ideally should not interfere with heart rate or metabolic demand for oxygen. Patients with disease of the left main coronary artery are more susceptible to insult during induction. Hemodynamic changes in these patients precipitate extension of already present ischemic effects. A slow, methodic, balanced technique with combinations of midazolam, fentanyl or sufentanil, etomidate, thiopental, or propofol and a nondepolarizing muscle relaxant reduces

hemodynamic changes and meets the goals of diminishing workload on the myocardium. Typical opioid maintenance doses are shown in Table 25-6.

INTRAOPERATIVE PERIOD

Incision to Bypass

After induction, the skin incision and sternal split constitute two very stimulating steps in the process of preparation for CPB. A patient in whom anesthesia is adequate will show minimal response to these steps, thereby reducing the need for additional adjuncts (Table 25-7). A continuous opioid infusion with "background" volatile agent or continuous infusion of propofol may help to maintain blood pressure and ensure amnesia, as well as provide a smooth transition toward CPB.

During sternotomy, for approximately 15 to 20 seconds, the lungs must be deflated to prevent laceration or puncture. In most cases, the left internal mammary artery is dissected and mobilized for anastomosis to the left anterior descending artery. This requires placement of an internal mammary artery retractor on the left side of the operating table. When there is a left radial arterial line, careful attention to wrist positioning ensures that the arterial waveform is not damped. When only saphenous vein grafts are to be harvested, the pace of the operation may increase significantly, and cannulation of the aorta and right atrium may occur earlier.

Once the internal mammary and saphenous grafts are mobilized or harvested, the patient requires heparinization before cannulation of the aorta and right atrium. Bolus administration

TABLE **25-6**	Common Opioid Doses for Maintenance During Cardiopulmonary Bypass		
	Loading Dose	**Infusion Rate**	**Additional Bolus**
Sufentanil	0.5-2 mcg/kg	0.5-1.5 mcg/kg/hr	2.5-10 mcg
Fentanyl	4-20 mcg/kg	2-10 mcg/kg/hr	25-100 mcg
Remifentanil	1-2 mcg/kg	0.1-1 mcg/kg/min	0.1-1 mcg/kg

TABLE **25-7**	Sample Adjunct Drugs for Cardiac Procedures	
Type of Drug	**Drug Name**	**Method of Administration**
Prepared		
Vasopressor	Phenylephrine	Titrate 50-100 mcg
Vasodilator	Nitroglycerin *or* Nitroprusside	Titrate as infusion or bolus Titrate as infusion
Available		
β-blocker	Esmolol	Titrate as bolus or infusion
Inotrope	Milrinone, epinephrine, dopamine, dobutamine	Titrate as infusion; usually facility or surgeon specific
Calcium chloride		Infusion or bolus
Vagolytic (anticholinergic)	Atropine	Bolus
Antiarrhythmic	Lidocaine, adenosine, diltiazem or verapamil, procainamide, amiodarone, magnesium	Titrate

of heparin is administered in a central line and *may* decrease arterial pressure 10% to 20%. Anticoagulation is measured with ACT approximately 3 to 5 minutes after heparin administration. The ACT should be approximately 400 seconds before it is safe to institute CPB.

Aortic cannulation is associated with a hypertensive response, probably because of direct stimulation of sympathetic nerves in the aortic arch. Reduction of MAP assists aortic cannulation and prevents laceration of the aorta. As a result of manipulation of the heart during cannula placement, venous cannulation (right atrium) may lead to fluctuations in arterial pressure. Right atrial cannulation drains the superior and inferior venae cavae; ventricular tachyarrhythmias may occur, and CO and blood pressure may decrease. If additional cannulation of the coronary sinus for retrograde cardioplegia delivery is required, severe hypotension may ensue and necessitate administration of volume by the perfusionist via the aortic cannula. Once the patient has been placed on extracorporeal support and adequate perfusion flow and pressure have been achieved, most surgeons prefer to stop ventilation to deflate the lungs and optimize surgical conditions. Some surgeons prefer to continue ventilation until the myocardium is motionless. CPB should not commence unless all the parameters for institution of bypass have been addressed by the anesthesia care provider (Box 25-4).

Initiation of Bypass

Multiple events occur simultaneously and can cause a significant drop in blood pressure at the initiation of CPB. Hemodilution decreases blood viscosity and dilutes catecholamines in the plasma, contributing to the drop in pressure. Rapid cooling of

---

BOX 25-4

Preparation for Bypass: Pre-Bypass Checklist

1. Anticoagulation
   a. Heparin administered
   b. Desired level of anticoagulation achieved
2. Arterial cannulation
   a. Absence of bubbles in arterial line
   b. Evidence of dissection or malposition?
3. Venous cannulation
   a. Evidence of superior vena cava obstruction?
   b. Evidence of inferior vena cava obstruction?
4. Pulmonary artery catheter (if used) pulled back
5. Are all monitoring/access catheters functional?
6. Transesophageal echocardiograph (if used)
   a. In "freeze" mode
   b. Scope in neutral/unlocked position
7. Supplemental medications
   a. Neuromuscular blockers
   b. Anesthetics, analgesics, amnestics
8. Inspection of head and neck
   a. Color
   b. Symmetry
   c. Venous drainage
   d. Pupils

From Mora-Mangona CT et al. Cardiopulmonary bypass and the anesthesiologist. In: Kaplan JA et al, eds. Kaplan's Cardiac Anesthesia. 5th ed. Philadelphia: Saunders; 2006.

---

the patient occurs to a target temperature of 28° C. When the target temperature is reached or spontaneous hypothermic fibrillation of the heart occurs, the aorta is cross-clamped. At times the myocardial arrest may require retrograde administration of cardioplegia via the coronary sinus.

Cerebral and renal protection are important during CPB. Techniques of cerebral protection include metabolic suppression, which can be accomplished with hypothermia, burst suppression, use of calcium channel blockers to reduce the incidence of vasospasm, and decrease in intraoperative bleeding attained through use of antifibrinolytics. The perfusionist also plays a central role in providing cerebral protection. As core temperature is lowered, the pH rises, placing the patient in an alkalotic state. The alpha-stat system represents alkalotic management of cerebral perfusion, but pH-stat relies on hypercarbia to manage CBF. The essential difference is that alpha-stat management represents CBF that is not dependent on MAP and does not mandate the addition of exogenous CO_2 to maintain pH in the normal range.

Renal protection is best maintained by preserving renal blood flow and monitoring urine production. Risk factors for renal dysfunction after CPB include prolonged bypass time (>3 hours) and low CO. Osmotic diuretics, low-dose dopamine, and fenoldopam are used during CPB in patients at risk for developing acute renal failure. Prevention of renal insufficiency postoperatively includes control of hypertension, control of hyperglycemia, reduction of "pump" time, maintenance of fluids, and the use of medications that promote urinary output.[75] Urinary output is considered satisfactory if it measures 1 mL/kg/hr during CPB.

Bypass

During bypass, anesthesia is maintained with an opioid drip, as described in Table 25-6, as well as the addition of volatile agent on the perfusion circuit. Controversy exists regarding an acceptable mean blood pressure (BP) range during CPB. Keep in mind that CBF is autoregulated, as is flow to other organs. Because of hypothermia, the lower limit of autoregulation is further decreased. This fact coupled with the presence of high perfusion pressures can result in an increase in the possibility of emboli and bleeding on the surgical field; the use of 50 to 70 mm Hg is promoted as a practical norm in most facilities.[75-77]

ACT is checked every 20 to 30 minutes by the perfusionist and maintained at greater than 400 seconds with the addition of heparin to the pump as necessary. Because of hemodilution, the hematocrit frequently falls to approximately 20 g/dL, which is an acceptable level in most patients. Hypokalemia can be problematic, so the perfusionist checks electrolytes frequently during the pump run. Fluids are kept to a minimum during the bypass phase, and the perfusionist often makes adjustments. Open communication among the perfusionist, surgeon, and anesthesia care provider are crucial during CPB so that coagulation, pressure maintenance, and adjustment of electrolyte imbalances are carefully regulated. A checklist for bypass is noted in Box 25-5.

DISCONTINUING CARDIOPULMONARY BYPASS

Weaning from Bypass

When a patient is weaned from CPB, considerations should include the ventricular function of the heart before bypass and the length of time the aorta was cross-clamped. If the ventricle was in good condition before bypass and the cross-clamp time was less than 60 minutes, the initiation of inotropes is probably not

Checklist for Bypass Procedure

1. Assess arterial inflow.
   Is arterial perfusate oxygenated?
   Is direction of arterial inflow appropriate?
   Evidence of arterial dissection?
   Patient's arterial pressure persistently low?
   Inflow line pressure high?
   Pump/oxygenator reservoir level falling?
   Evidence of atrial cannula malposition?
   Patient's arterial pressure persistently high or low?
   Unilateral facial swelling, discoloration?
2. Assess venous outflow.
   Is blood draining to the pump/oxygenator's venous reservoir?
   Evidence of SVC obstruction?
   Facial venous engorgement or congestion, CVP elevated?
3. Is bypass complete?
   High CVP/low PA pressure?
   Impaired venous drainage?
   Low CVP/high PA pressure?
   Large bronchial venous blood flow?
   Aortic insufficiency?
   Arterial and PA pressure nonpulsatile?
   Desired pump flow established?
4. Discontinue drug and fluid administration.
5. Discontinue ventilation and inhalation drugs to patient's lungs.

From Mora-Mangona CT et al. Cardiopulmonary bypass and the anesthesiologist. In: Kaplan JA et al, eds. Kaplan's Cardiac Anesthesia. 5th ed. Philadelphia: Saunders; 2006.
CVP, *Central venous pressure;* PA, *pulmonary artery;* SVC, *Superior vena cava.*

Preparation for Separation-from-Bypass Checklist

1. Air clearance maneuvers completed
2. Rewarming completed
   a. Nasopharyngeal temperature 36° to 37° C
   b. Rectal/bladder temperature $\geq$35° C but $\leq$37° C
3. Address issue of adequacy of anesthesia and muscle relaxation
4. Obtain stable cardiac rate and rhythm (use pacing if necessary)
5. Pump flow and systemic arterial pressure
   a. Pump flow to maintain mixed venous saturation $\leq$ 70%
   b. Systemic pressure restored to normothermic levels
6. Metabolic parameters
   a. Arterial pH, Po_2, Pco_2 within normal limits
   b. Hct: 20% to 25%
   c. K^+: 4 to 5 mEq/L
   d. *Possibly* ionized calcium
7. Are all monitoring/access catheters functional?
   a. Transducer re-zeroed
   b. TEE (if used) out of freeze mode
8. Respiratory management
   a. Atelectasis cleared/lungs reexpanded
   b. Evidence of pneumothorax?
   c. Residual fluid in thoracic cavities drained
   d. Ventilation reinstituted

From Mora-Mangona CT et al. Cardiopulmonary bypass and the anesthesiologist. In: Kaplan JA et al, eds. Kaplan's Cardiac Anesthesia. 5th ed. Philadelphia: Saunders; 2006.
Hct, *Hematocrit;* TEE, *transesophageal echocardiography.*

Protamine Reversal of Heparin

- 10 mg protamine reverses 1000 units heparin
- 10 mg protamine = 1 mL of protamine
- 1 mL of protamine reverses 30 mL heparin (an average initial dose)
- *Protamine reversal is 1:1 ratio with heparin dose.*

necessary. Otherwise, an inotrope should be chosen in consultation with the surgeon. Additional parameters that should be verified include patient temperature, heart rhythm, monitor status, and adequacy of perfusion. During weaning, the perfusionist partially occludes the venous line to increase right atrial pressure, blood flows into the right ventricle and out through the PA, and pressures become pulsatile (Box 25-6).

The rate of rewarming must be limited to 1° C per 3 to 5 minutes to prevent formation of gaseous emboli in the circulatory system or the ECC. Rewarming begins slightly before removal of the aortic cross-clamp, when the last distal anastomosis begins in multiple graft procedures, or when the valve sutures have been placed during valve replacement procedures. The temperature gradient between arterial and venous blood should be maintained below 10° C, and the time frame for rewarming is usually 30 minutes.[78]

Many tasks are required at this time. Laboratory values including arterial blood gases, electrolytes, and hematocrit should be obtained. Patient ventilation is reinstituted. An infusion of calcium chloride (1 g/100 mL 5% dextrose in water [D_5W]) is administered via a central line. After most of the calcium chloride has been given, a small test dose of protamine, usually 10 mg, is administered to test for an unexpected reaction before infusion. If the patient remains stable, protamine administration is initiated slowly over approximately 20 minutes to avoid hypotension. Protamine is given in a calculated dose that is approximately a 1:1 ratio of the initial heparin dose (Box 25-7). When one third of the dose of protamine has been given, notify the perfusionist to stop collecting blood via suction from the operative field because this would clot the pump. Small increments of phenylephrine may be administered to maintain blood pressure within desired ranges. The surgeon can restart bypass throughout the weaning process as necessary.

Communication is vital during the weaning process. The possibility always exists that the patient will have to be returned to bypass. Notify the surgeon when the protamine has been completely administered, and recheck the ACT. Recheck CO and pressures to establish postoperative baselines.

When bypass is completely discontinued, check ACT values and institute treatment if they are elevated. Bypass may have to be reinstituted if severe hypotension, excessive bleeding, or a persistently low CO is present. If the protamine is completely administered and a return to bypass is required, heparin (300 units/kg) may be readministered. At times an IABP may be required.

In anticipation of the increased metabolic uptake associated with this phase of the operation, administration of amnestic agents and muscle relaxants to maintain appropriate anesthetic levels should be instituted. When the aortic cross-clamp is removed, reperfusion to the myocardium allows the heart to rewarm and flushes residual cardioplegic solution and accumulated metabolic by-products out of the coronary vessels. Hypotension should be anticipated. Plasma levels of atrial natriuretic factor have been shown to decrease with the onset of aortic cross-clamping and either decrease or increase significantly when the cross-clamp is removed. Studies have demonstrated that this factor increases glomerular filtration, inhibits renin release, reduces aldosterone concentrations, and antagonizes endogenous vasoconstrictors, resulting in a reduction in blood pressure.[79]

Sweating during the rewarming phase of CPB represents a normal thermoregulatory response that can be associated with cutaneous dilation caused by elevated skin temperatures. Anesthetic agents depress vasoconstriction and shivering while increasing the propensity for sweating. Postoperative shivering should be avoided to prevent increased oxygen demand and carbon dioxide production.

Protamine Administration

Protamine sulfate is the drug of choice for heparin reversal. It inactivates heparin by binding with it to form an inert salt. At the conclusion of CPB, the residual amount of heparin is assessed and appropriately neutralized. Protamine is initiated after a test dose of 1 mg in 100 mL over 10 minutes before heparinization. It binds and inhibits the anticoagulation effects to circulating heparin. Adverse cardiopulmonary responses to protamine have been observed. Suggested risk factors include valvular heart disease (mitral), preexisting pulmonary hypertension, infusion rates greater than 5 mg/min, diabetes with prior exposure to NPH insulin, and vasectomy. Adverse reactions to protamine include histamine-releasing reactions, true anaphylaxis mediated by a specific antiprotamine antibody, or reactions in which release of thromboxane leads to pulmonary vasoconstriction or bronchoconstriction. In the presence of increased risk factors, heparinase I may be given.[80] In a small study by Heres and colleagues, heparinase I was found to result in no adverse hemodynamic changes when given to patients after heparinization for CPB in coronary artery surgery.[37]

MANAGEMENT OF COMPLICATIONS OF CARDIAC BYPASS

Separation from Cardiopulmonary Bypass

Preexisting ventricular dysfunction or myocardial insult associated with CPB complicates the process of weaning the patient from extracorporeal support. Separation from bypass presents a tremendous challenge in providing appropriate pharmacologic and mechanical support sufficient for the recovery of ventricular function. The major pharmacologic interventions include the use of both inotropic and vasodilator treatment of systolic or diastolic dysfunction.

Regardless of the therapeutic technique used, the focus on basic hemodynamic and physiologic goals should be maintained when one selects an anesthetic regimen for termination of bypass.

Tachycardia and arrhythmias must be prevented, arterial blood pressure maintained, and myocardial contractility promoted while constraints on oxygen demand are maintained. The ideal regimen for pharmacologic therapy includes drugs that have rapid onset and termination, have a neutralizing effect on ischemia, and are nontoxic to the myocardium.

A primary therapeutic consideration for patients not previously in atrial fibrillation is to establish an atrioventricular sequence. Altered ventricular compliance necessitates optimal loading conditions for nondynamic ventricles. Patients who are dependent on atrial kick for ventricular filling experience a serious compromise in CO in the presence of atrial fibrillation or supraventricular tachycardia. Impaired diastolic function may be managed by treating hypertension and decreasing ventricular load with vasodilator therapy. Nitric oxide–based drugs (nitroglycerin, sodium nitroprusside) are commonly used agents that promote vasodilation, counteract the vasoconstrictive effects of circulating catecholamines, and reduce ventricular distention by relieving myocardial wall tension. The aim of administration of vasodilators is treatment of specific hemodynamic conditions such as increased arterial blood pressure, left atrial pressure, pulmonary capillary wedge pressure, and rising central venous pressure. The intent is to optimize ventricular loading conditions and, in combination with inotropic support, provide adequate CO while minimizing demand on the revascularized myocardium.

Catecholamines have variable effects on heart rate, rhythm, and metabolism. Milrinone, epinephrine, norepinephrine, dopamine, and isoproterenol are selected based on targeted functions. Recent evidence suggests that administration of dobutamine to improve low cardiac output states following cardiac surgery and bypass is associated with adverse postoperative outcomes.[81,82] Dopamine increases pulmonary vascular resistance, PA pressure, and left ventricular filling pressures.

Calcium may be beneficial on termination of CPB and should be administered just before weaning, when ionized calcium levels are deficient and inotropic assistance is required. Phosphodiesterase inhibitors such as milrinone may be helpful in providing prophylactic inotropic support in anticipation of ventricular failure. In conjunction with decreased left ventricular wall tension, milrinone promotes cardiac function without increasing myocardial oxygen demand. Milrinone is similar to dobutamine in its effects on myocardial contractility, myocardial oxygen consumption rate, SVR, and pulmonary vascular resistance; however, patients are less susceptible to biochemical changes in neurohumoral regulation that may reduce the efficacy of β-agonists.[73]

Blood from the pump is sequestered into the cell-saver device and concentrated to be returned to the patient via IV infusion after separation from CPB. This will assist in bolstering the blood pressure without the administration of large amounts of crystalloid or pressors. In addition, colloid may be included to decrease the incidence of hypotension. Monitoring devices should be recalibrated before separation from the CPB, and the lungs should be expanded and mechanical ventilation instituted before weaning. This is done to assess the possibility of atelectasis, pneumothorax, and hydrothorax.

Pacing

Fibrillation of the myocardium typically occurs on rewarming, with a gradual progression to normal sinus rhythm. If defibrillation does not occur spontaneously, antiarrhythmic therapy, electrical cardioversion, or both are used. Heart rate and rhythm may be controlled through the use of atrial, ventricular,

TABLE 25-8	Pacemaker Codes and Functions			
I Chamber Paced	**II Chamber Sensed**	**III Response Mode**	**IV Program Function**	**V Special Function**
A = Atrial	Atrium	I = Inhibited	P = Program	B = Bursts
V = Ventricular	Ventricle	T = Triggered	M = Multiprogram	N = Norm Rate
D = Dual Chamber	Both	D = Dual	C = Communicating	S = Scanning
		O = None		E = External
		R = Reverse		
Assigned Function				
DDD	Atrial and ventricular sensing and pacing			
VDD	Programmable AV interval: senses both chambers, paces ventricle			
DVI	Programmable AV interval: senses R wave, paces atrium			
VVT	Programmable escape interval: senses ventricle, paces ventricle			
VVI	Inhibited output from sensed ventricle: demand ventricular pacing			
VOO	Asynchronous ventricular pacing			
AAT	Programmable escape interval: senses atrium, paces atrium			
AAI	Inhibited output from sensed atrium: demand atrial pacing			
AOO	Asynchronous atrial pacing			

AV, *Atrioventricular.*

atrioventricular (AV) sequential, or overdrive pacing in addition to necessary antiarrhythmic drugs. Epicardial electrode placement on the wall of the atrium is routine for cardiac surgery. Pacemakers allow for rapid adjustment of decreased CO when the conduction pathway is damaged or highly irritable.

Atrial contraction determines CO by controlling the volume of blood ejected into the ventricle. Atrial volume, ventricular volume and compliance, and the pattern of atrial contraction influence ventricular filling. If ventricular pacing is used alone, CO may decrease due to loss of the atrial "kick," but AV pacing alters the AV interval in relation to the PR interval, thereby improving CO.[83,84] Table 25-8 explains types of pacemakers.

Left Ventricular Dysfunction

Left ventricular dysfunction may be indicated by a rise in PA pressure in conjunction with depressed systemic arterial blood pressure. The causes of left ventricular failure can be varied and may include preoperative markers such as a diminished left ventricular EF and left ventricular hypokinesis or akinesis. TEE is an invaluable tool for confirming and isolating hypodynamic ventricular wall motion. If depressed contractility results from lack of appropriate inotropic and pharmacologic support, this should be remedied immediately. In some cases, the myocardium may be "stunned" and require the additional support of reengaging CPB, resting the heart, and examining the anastomoses for leaks and the grafts for air emboli or kinking. In the event cardiac depression remains unresolved or worsens, a mechanical assist device such as an IABP may be percutaneously introduced to provide diastolic augmentation and decreased afterload.

Right Ventricular Dysfunction

An inflammatory-mediated response from the ECC or acute anaphylactic reaction caused by protamine sulfate or blood product transfusion may lead to increased pulmonary vascular resistance, resulting in depressed right ventricular function. Pharmacologic intervention to reduce pulmonary vasoconstriction includes nitric oxide–based vasodilators and β_2-adrenergic agonists. In cases in which conventional treatment fails, intervention may also include the use of prostaglandin E_1. Left atrial injection of norepinephrine has been demonstrated to increase systemic pressures while avoiding first-pass effects on the pulmonary vascular system. When right ventricular failure is unrelated to pulmonary vascular resistance, phosphodiesterase inhibitors may be beneficial for resolving the condition without the vasodilatory effects of prostaglandins.[73]

Failure to Wean

The quality of surgical correction and the quality of myocardial preservation are important determinants of the success in weaning from CPB. Failure to wean can be attributed to multiple factors, including heart block or ventricular dysfunction resulting from hyperkalemia, interruption of coronary flow (because of air, fat, or particulate emboli), extended CPB and aortic cross-clamp times, and arrhythmias associated with reperfusion injury.

Failure to wean on the primary attempt may lead to significant damage or distention of the heart. Systemic hypotension may promote metabolic acidosis and organ damage or failure. Additional inotropic support may be required for returning to bypass under these conditions and may necessitate additional administration of blood products to compensate for excessive hemodilution.[85] If return to CPB becomes imperative, an additional heparin bolus may be needed. These situations are always emergent and require extreme caution in ensuring that the patient is being ventilated and adequately anticoagulated and that anatomic reconnection to ECC is achieved before bypass is reengaged. Preparations should include an avenue for mechanical support (e.g., IABP, ventricular assist device), should the need arise.

Intraaortic Balloon Pump

In the event of left ventricular failure or myocardial hypokinesia due to CPB or ischemic insult, insertion of an intraaortic balloon may be necessary to provide diastolic counterpulsation for the patient. The intraaortic balloon is a distensible polyurethane catheter that is percutaneously inserted through the femoral artery using the Seldinger technique for large-diameter catheter placement. The tip of the catheter allows aortic pressure monitoring and is threaded to the descending thoracic aorta with the tip at the distal aortic arch. The balloon (size 34, 40, or 50 mL) is inflated with helium or carbon dioxide gas. Balloon deflation can be triggered by the R wave of the electrocardiograph or by the arterial pressure waveform, atrial pacing mode, AV sequential pacing mode, or internal asynchronous timing (not recommended).[86]

Inflation of the intraaortic balloon is timed to occur during diastole, forcing blood into the coronary arteries and periphery. It deflates during systole to promote ventricular ejection. Diastolic augmentation is achieved during inflation and results in increased coronary perfusion pressure, as well as increased flow to the great vessels arising from the aorta. In most instances, this diastolic augmentation results in pressures greater than the patient's systolic pressure. Afterload reduction results when the balloon is rapidly deflated before ventricular ejection, reducing ventricular wall tension and therefore myocardial oxygen demand.

Ventricular Assist Devices

The placement of a ventricular assist device is an option when termination of bypass cannot be tolerated by the patient, and no other options to ensure survival exist. This effort in most cases represents a bridge to cardiac transplantation or allows for additional resting time to promote recovery of severely compromised cardiac contractile function. Most institutions have established protocols and criteria for considering a patient as a candidate for this device. Age, pulmonary function, and organ system viability are factors in the selection process.

CPB is reinstituted to prepare the circuit and cannulation sites for transfer from the ECC to a centrifugal assist device. Cannulation depends on which ventricle requires support and represents a mechanically assisted atrial-aortic shunt of blood flow to circumvent the impaired ventricle.[54] This is a simple circuit with no oxygenator or heating element component, so during the transfer from the ECC to the mechanical assist device, the patient must be ventilated. Appropriate pharmacologic support is essential.

EXTUBATION

The current trend is toward early extubation of the postoperative cardiac surgical patient. Controversy surrounds the efficacy of extubation within 2 to 4 hours of closure. However, "fast-tracking," a term used to describe early extubation and discharge from the intensive care unit, has become popular as a cost-effective technique associated with this major surgical procedure. The patient population for fast-track cardiac anesthesia must be a "less sick" group to prevent precipitation of hypertensive episodes and increased postoperative myocardial ischemia. Ideally, the fast-track candidate is less than 70 years of age, has normal ventricular and valvular function and an uncomplicated surgery, and is free of renal, neurologic, and coagulation disorders in the immediate postoperative period.

The selection of agents for fast-tracking starts in the preinduction phase with agents that have a short duration of action. Lower doses of opioids are supplemented with low-dose inhalation agents and propofol infusions. α-Agonists are used as adjuncts because of their ability to blunt neurohumoral stress responses. Postoperative analgesia can be accomplished with the use of low-dose morphine, nonsteroidal antiinflammatory drugs, patient-controlled analgesia, and thoracic epidurals with short acting opioids.[87]

Extubation criteria include a warm patient, low-dose or no inotropic drugs or vasoactive drips, no balloon pump, and bleeding less than 100 mL/hr.[88-90] The patient must be awake, pain free, and hemodynamically stable and must meet all conventional criteria for extubation. Regardless of the anesthetic technique used, the key to optimizing patient recovery is postoperative pain management, which facilitates early mobility and nutritional intake.[91,92]

UNIQUE SITUATIONS IN CARDIAC ANESTHESIA

Automatic Internal Cardioverter Defibrillator

Automatic implantable cardioverter defibrillators are surgically implanted to prevent sudden cardiac death from malignant ventricular tachyarrhythmias. These are self-contained diagnostic devices that continuously monitor the patient's heart rate and electrocardiographic activity. They sense potentially lethal ventricular arrhythmias and treat them with electrical discharges. Whereas pacemakers use low-energy impulses measured in microjoules, these defibrillators release an electrical discharge of approximately 30 joules after sensing periods of fibrillation lasting approximately 20 seconds. Most devices can now be programmed to reconfirm ventricular tachycardia or ventricular fibrillation after charging to prevent inappropriate shock therapy.[93]

Patients considered for implantation are those who have had minimal success with standard antiarrhythmic drug therapy. The majority of patients have severe coronary artery disease with reduced left ventricular function, ischemic cardiomyopathy, or idiopathic cardiomyopathy.

Anesthetic management is best handled by general anesthesia because of the testing necessary to properly place and program this device. Prolonged periods of asystole are at times encountered and can cause cerebral and myocardial ischemia. Vasoactive drugs are helpful for blood pressure stabilization. If ventricular tachycardia occurs before clinical induction, lidocaine treatment should be avoided—it may result in the inability to induce ventricular tachycardia on demand during testing.

Minimal monitoring includes ECG leads II and V_5 along with an arterial line. Although some institutions suggest IV sedation for these patients, the stress associated with testing and the amount of sedation necessary for the procedure suggest that general anesthesia with a controlled airway would be a better choice. Patients undergoing extracorporeal shock wave lithotripsy are a special problem, in that the automatic implantable cardioverter defibrillator (AICD) may discharge. The shock waves themselves are capable of damaging the pacemaker components. To reduce the risk of life-threatening arrhythmias, the shock waves are synchronized to the R wave of the ECG. In situations in which the AICD is involved, the manufacturer should be contacted to determine whether it is better to reprogram the device or use a magnet.[94]

Deep Hypothermic Circulatory Arrest

Hypothermic circulatory arrest is indicated for aortic arch lesions and in infants and children with small hearts. Exposure is improved when no multiple cannulas exist and no blood is present in the operative field. The margin of safe time for circulatory arrest under these conditions is unknown. The primary objective of this process is cerebral and major organ preservation. A gradient of no more than 10° C is allowed between the patient and the perfusate at initial institution of bypass for cooling. Core cooling is gradual, with a target temperature of 18° to 20° C.

Anesthetic considerations include prevention of prebypass respiratory alkalosis. During the circulatory arrest time frame, the perfusate is maintained at 28° C while CPB is off. At the time of rewarming, phentolamine is administered in the pump, and phenylephrine is administered to the patient to maintain perfusion pressure at 30 to 50 mm Hg. The maximum acceptable temperature for deep hypothermia circulatory arrest is below 22° C.[95-97]

Cardiac Tamponade

Cardiac tamponade is a rare but potentially lethal consequence of open-heart surgery. For the cardiac surgical patient, it is usually related to a leaking anastomosis that requires surgical reexploration. It can also occur as a result of infection, uremia, trauma, CHF, rheumatoid arthritis, and anticoagulant therapy. Clinical diagnosis of this condition is made on the basis of decreasing systolic blood pressure accompanied by pulsus paradoxus, jugular venous distention, tachycardia, and an enlarged cardiac silhouette.

Pericardial effusion can lead to cardiac tamponade after open-heart bypass. This condition can be relieved using either percutaneous pericardiocentesis or subxiphoid pericardiotomy. Percutaneous pericardiocentesis in conjunction with two-dimensional echocardiography has been demonstrated to be successful in preventing cardiac puncture. Patients require only local anesthetic and are placed in the supine position with the head slightly raised.[98]

MINIMALLY INVASIVE CORONARY ARTERY BYPASS TECHNIQUES

Port-Access Coronary Artery Bypass Grafting

To minimize postoperative pain and speed recovery, some cardiovascular surgeons have used a port-access method of coronary artery bypass (PACAB). In these procedures, multiple ports are placed in the chest wall for video surgery in addition to performance of a minithorocotomy in some patients. PACABs take advantage of the nonbeating heart on CPB. The Heartport system necessitates the femoral artery approach and uses an endoaortic balloon occlusion for instillation of cardioplegia. One-lung ventilation is necessary during the IMA dissection, and monitoring is extensive. The heart is not viewed directly; rather, it is viewed through echocardiography, video (endoscopy), and fluoroscopy. This makes the procedure somewhat cumbersome and tedious for the surgeon.

Anesthetic techniques include all monitors and considerations for CPB, as well as the need for one-lung ventilation. Patients benefit from this port-access technique because they experience less postoperative pain, a reduced ICU stay, an accelerated recovery time, improved postoperative pulmonary function, and a reduced need for inpatient cardiac rehabilitation.[99] Aortic atherosclerotic disease is a contraindication. Heartport has a long bypass run for single-vessel CABG, which maximizes the risk of stroke, even though the sternotomy is eliminated.

Procedures that benefit from port access include multivessel CABG, mitral valve procedures, aortic valve replacements, and some congenital heart defect procedures. Some concern remains about aortic dissection, stroke, and embolism because the surgeon does not have direct access to the surgical field and cannot directly suction air from the heart. Patient selection is an important factor in safety of the procedure.

Minimally Invasive Direct Coronary Artery Bypass

Minimally invasive direct coronary artery bypass (MIDCAB) follows the basics of conventional CABG procedures but does not require CPB, cardioplegia, or a large incision. Through a small incision (10 to 12 cm) and under direct vision, the graft is anastomosed while the heart is still beating. This procedure is beneficial to the patient because of the smaller incision, the absence of CPB and its inherent complications, and the reduced need for blood transfusions. Disadvantages include that it is limited to use for only one or two arteries and that one-lung ventilation often is requested by the surgeon. Because the heart continues to beat, the anastomoses are difficult to suture, and significant ischemia may occur, precipitating hemodynamic compromise of the patient. At times, urgent conversion to coronary bypass is necessary, and the perfusionist and equipment for this must be immediately available.[100] Anesthetic management is closely related to that for off-pump coronary artery bypass procedures with normal sternotomies.

Off-Pump Coronary Artery Bypass

Surgical techniques in this area, along with advances in equipment, allow multivessel procedures with median sternotomy to be performed. Because CPB is not used, hearts of patients undergoing off-pump coronary artery bypass (OPCAB) are normothermic, and maintenance of coronary perfusion and hemodynamic stability are absolutely necessary. Communication between the surgeon and the anesthesia care provider is of paramount importance. The anesthesia provider is a crucial member of the team who should be as observant of the surgical field as the surgeon. Unlike CPB cases, during OPCAB procedures, the grafting phase requires involvement and vigilance on the part of the anesthesia provider.

The hearts of patients undergoing OPCAB are anesthetized with the intent of "early" extubation. A modified fast-track approach that avoids ischemia while facilitating early extubation is desirable. The choice of an anesthetic must take into consideration that a slow heart rate facilitates the surgical procedures and reduces myocardial oxygen demand. A narcotic oxygen muscle relaxant technique facilitates minute-to-minute control of hemodynamics. Maintenance of the systolic pressure promotes hemodynamic stability when the heart position is changed during exposure of the different vessels. It is recommended that the systolic pressure be maintained above 100 mm Hg.[101] Prudent volume loading and positioning of the patient in the Trendelenburg position with a right rotation promote recovery of blood pressure when retraction is used in exposure of the posterior pericardium.

Extensive invasive monitoring is indicated, along with a large-bore peripheral IV and a right IJ triple-lumen catheter capable of handling continuous thermodilution CO and transvenous pacing. Multiple central ports must be available for continuous infusion of various vasoactive medications. Temperature monitoring is vital. It is necessary to maintain fluids and any other drips or instillations at warm temperatures, to use a forced-air warming device on the head and neck, and to maintain a warm room temperature.[102] If the grafts are completely arterial, as is often the case in OPCAB procedures, the possibility of placing a forced-air warmer on the patient's lower extremities should be investigated.

The muscle relaxant chosen should be one without histamine-releasing effects. Some anesthesia care providers insist that a neuromuscular blocker like pancuronium, which independently causes tachycardia, should be avoided.[103] However, when potent

TABLE **25-9** Monitoring Approaches for OPCAB and MIDCAB			
Monitor	**Advantages**	**Disadvantages**	**Comment**
ECG	Universal Simple Inexpensive Recognized criteria	Insensitive Position dependent (lead and heart) Incision dependent Loss of V4-5 (MIDCAB)	Best if multi-lead Should be calibrated ST-segment treading helpful

Central venous pressure	Simple
	Inexpensive
		Insensitive for LV dysfunction
		No cardiac output
			Important for drug infusions
			Affected by position of heart
			  and patient
			Use of "introducer" allows
			  rapid insertion of PAC

Pulmonary artery catheter	LV filling pressure
	Cardiac output
	Options may be helpful
	  (Svo₂, CCO, pacing)
		Expensive
		Insensitive for acute regional
		  dysfunction
		Postoperative nuisance
			Controversial monitor
			May prolong ICU stay with
			  "abnormal numbers"

Transesophageal echocardiography	Gold standard for acute
	  ischemia
	Verify restoration of function
	Guide surgical cannula
	  placement
		Expensive
		User dependent
		Distracting
		May not have good view
		  of heart
			Requires expertise
			May give false sense of security

Cardiac output (bioimpedance, aortic flow, CO₂ rebreathing)	Less invasive than PAC
	Can give beat-to-beat flow
		Expensive
		No measure of LV filling
		May be user dependent
			Bioimpedance questionable
			  with open chest
			Cannot get readings
			  on all patients

From Hensley FA et al, eds. A Practical Approach to Cardiac Anesthesia. 4th ed. Philadelphia: Lippincott Williams & Wilkins, 2008.
CCO, *Continuous cardiac output;* ICU, *intensive care unit;* LV, *left ventricular;* MIDCAB, *minimally invasive direct coronary artery bypass grafting;* OPCAB, *off-pump coronary artery bypass grafting;* PAC, *pulmonary artery catheter;* Svo₂, *mixed venous oxygen saturation.*

narcotics such as sufentanil are used, the bradycardia produced by the opiate drug may offset the tachycardia produced by pancuronium. A target heart rate of not greater than 70 beats per minute can be achieved with the addition of an esmolol drip. Because surgical manipulation itself precipitates arrhythmias, antiarrhythmic medications (lidocaine, magnesium, or amiodarone)[104] for treatment of these problems must be readily available. In addition to drugs, it is appropriate to let the surgeon know what effect surgical manipulations have on the myocardium and to ask the surgeon to stop temporarily, if possible, when the situation warrants it. If bradycardia becomes a problem, treatment with medications or epicardial or transvenous pacing may be necessary.

The use of antifibrinolytics is controversial; some surgeons are concerned about graft thrombosis associated with the use of these agents.[103] Anticoagulant therapy is facility specific but usually directed at a target ACT of 300 seconds and incomplete reversal. When protamine is given, it is usually at a reduced dose to achieve an anticoagulation level 25% to 50% above the control ACT. When instilling protamine, check the ACT one third and two thirds of the way through the dose to avoid overshooting the target ACT. In off-pump procedures, the coagulation system is normal because it has not been exposed to the ECC and its effects; therefore, the possibility of pulmonary embolus, graft clotting, and the like exists just as in other major vascular procedures.

For OPCAB patients to be extubated, they must be warm, awake, and pain free and receiving no or low-dose inotropes and vasoactive drugs; no balloon pump must be in use; bleeding must be less than 100 mL/hr; and patients must be hemodynamically stable and meet conventional metabolic and mechanical criteria for extubation. Some monitoring approaches for OPCAB and MIDCAB are given in Table 25-9.

ABLATION PROCEDURES

MAZE and Mini-MAZE Procedures

The MAZE procedure is offered to patients at high risk for stroke who have undergone unsuccessful attempts at chemical treatment of atrial fibrillation. It is an "open-heart" cardiac surgery procedure intended to eliminate atrial fibrillation (AF). The name refers to the series of incisions arranged in a maze-like pattern in the atria. The Cox maze III procedure is now considered to be the gold standard for effective surgical cure of AF. It may be performed concomitant with mitral valve repair (MVR) or replacement for patients who also have mitral valve disease. The MAZE procedure was introduced in 1987[105] and is performed using pulmonary vein isolation and a number of incisions in the right and left atria. These incisions, or cryoablations, ultimately form scar tissue that mechanically interrupts transmission of impulses that trigger atrial fibrillation.[106,107] MAZE procedures necessitate a sternotomy and CPB. All monitoring and medications used for CPB are also required. In addition to the lesions made in the atria, the left atrial appendage is often removed because it is thought to be a culprit in blood flow stasis, increasing the possibility of stroke should it remain.[108]

The term *mini-MAZE* is still sometimes used to describe an open-heart procedure requiring CPB, but it more commonly refers to minimally invasive, epicardial procedures not entailing CPB. A mini-MAZE procedure is performed using thoracoscopy on a beating heart, so no CPB is required. "Keyhole" incisions are used for the mini-MAZE. The patient is placed in lateral position, and routine monitoring with the addition of an arterial line and one-lung ventilation (OLV) are adjuncts of this procedure.

Pulmonary Vein Isolation and Catheter Ablation for Persistent Atrial Fibrillation

Surgical management of rate-related cardiac rhythm anomalies has historically been achieved with catheter ablation of the offending right atrial conduction pathways. For conditions such as Wolff-Parkinson-White syndrome, right atrial flutter, or supraventricular tachycardia, catheter ablation to permanently block impulses has been performed by groin catheterization, much like cardiac angiograms.[109]

Research on the contributing triggers for atrial fibrillation has illuminated the possibility that pulmonary vein isolation and ablation of offending fibers is an alternative when chemical means fail.[105] Beginning in 2000, catheter ablation for atrial fibrillation has been performed with patients under general anesthesia.[110] Groin catheterization continuing with a catheter puncture across the atrial septal wall and advancement of the catheter into the left atrium is performed.[109] A lesion is created with the catheter tip and a specified energy. The lesion then prevents transmission of offending impulses that trigger atrial fibrillation.

Catheter ablation under general anesthesia necessitates an endotracheal tube, an arterial line, and resuscitative drugs. Multiple arrhythmias and blood pressure swings may be evident during this procedure but are often short lived and resolve spontaneously with little if any intervention on the part of the anesthesia provider.

PEDIATRIC APPROACHES

A limited discussion of pediatric cardiac anesthesia is presented here because of the extent of information required to apply appropriate anesthetic techniques for the many types of anomalies present in pediatric patients. An entire career can be (and usually is) devoted to pediatric cardiac anesthesia. Basic information follows.

Pediatric physiology stipulates revised anesthetic approaches that take into consideration the fetal circulatory system, neonatal response to stress, and developmental alterations in anatomy and hemodynamics. Besides requiring the clinician to have excellent professional judgment, pediatric cardiac anesthesia is an anesthetic challenge. Pathophysiology such as coronary artery disease and life-threatening arrhythmias are not common problems in pediatric patients.[110] Congenital anomalies are.

Maturation of the fetal circulatory system may be incomplete in some newborns. In most circumstances, the ductus arteriosus spontaneously closes within 15 hours to 4 days after birth, and the foramen ovale closes within 1 month. A patent ductus arteriosus or incomplete closure of the foramen ovale may result in arteriovenous shunting that calls for surgical repair.

Neonates are less susceptible to anesthetic techniques traditionally applied to adults for increasing SV and myocardial contractility; CO in neonates is more dependent on heart rate than it is on SV. Parasympathetic tone is greater than sympathetic tone in neonates, making them more prone to bradycardia after stimulation of the parasympathetic nervous system.[110] Infants with congenital heart disease are more susceptible to cerebral insult or injury than adults. Depending on the type of malformation, a cardiac defect may represent a 10% morbidity from cerebral injury.

Principles of Intracardiac Shunts

In the presence of a congenital defect of the cardiac septum or great vessels in which a communication is present between the left and right cardiac structures, blood flow is diverted from the area of greater resistance to the chamber or vessel of lower resistance. As a result, part of the blood that characteristically flows from the right side of the cardiac structure through the pulmonary system may be shunted back to the venous side of the heart because of greater left heart pressures. This condition is referred to as a *left-to-right shunt* and is most commonly associated with a congenital lesion such as an atrial septal defect or a ventricular septal defect. If left unresolved, the left-to-right shunt results in right atrial enlargement as a compensatory mechanism for the increased volume and workload associated with the shunt. Pathologic changes occur in the pulmonary system because of this increase in blood flow and are eventually reflected as an extension of the muscle layer into peripheral vessels, resulting in medial hypertrophy of the lung. The subsequent development of pulmonary hypertension ultimately results in right ventricular hypertrophy, which in time elevates right cardiac pressures to a point at which the shunt is reversed (right-to-left). When outflow-tract resistance exceeds SVR, the result is reduced pulmonary blood flow, a condition commonly referred to as *Eisenmenger syndrome*.[111]

Anesthetic Considerations

Because more than 40 cardiac malformations are known and may manifest as isolated or combined lesions, the anesthesia care provider should tailor the therapeutic approach to the physiologic consequences associated with the specific condition. Cardiac defects are classified according to their effect in precipitating CHF, cyanosis, or a combination of the two. The key points for anesthetic assessment center on the net effect of the intracardiac or extracardiac shunts, the status of ventricular function, pulmonary vascular compliance and flow, and whether an obstructive lesion is involved.[110]

Cyanosis in newborns represents inadequate pulmonary blood flow due to right ventricular outflow tract obstruction, intracardiac right-to-left shunting, a common ventricle, or transposition of the pulmonary and aortic arteries. In severe cases, pulmonary blood flow may be diminished to less than 50% of the CO. This condition is immediately treated with a continuous infusion of prostaglandin to prevent closure of the ductus arteriosus. Cyanotic lesions result in polycythemia, a condition that may lead to dehydration, thrombosis, and elevations in pulmonary vascular resistance and SVR resulting from increased blood viscosity.[111] Survival of these patients is contingent on the existence of a systemic-to-pulmonary shunt and usually requires palliative surgery to create a temporary shunt. This allows the newborn time to develop sufficiently for future corrective cardiac surgery.

In the newborn, CHF may result from a combination of lesions that contribute to increased pulmonary flow with concomitant outflow-tract obstruction. These patients have left-to-right shunts through an existing atrial or ventricular septal defect or patent ductus arteriosus. Aortic coarctation, endocardial defects, transposition of the great vessels, anomalous pulmonary venous return, truncus arteriosus, and formation of a single ventricle are congenital defects that may lead to the development of CHF. Initial surgery is most often directed toward the correction of the pathology that caused the development of CHF; this allows postponing the eventual repair of other coexisting malformations.

Premedication depends on the type of lesion and symptoms. Infants who are cyanotic, dyspneic, or less than 6 months old should not be premedicated before surgery. For pediatric patients undergoing corrective surgery for congenital lesions, induction should not be focused simply on preventing hemodynamic or circulatory deterioration. Rather, it should be directed at improving circulatory performance and oxygen transport. If CO is not depressed, the decreased oxygen consumption associated with general anesthesia should result in overall improvement in mixed venous oxygen saturation. This improvement should be reflected in increased arterial saturations as a result of intracardiac shunting.

In neonates or infants with complex lesions, high-dose opiate anesthetic agents may be useful, owing to the ability of these agents to maintain cardiovascular stability. Continued use of opioids during the operation offers additional benefit by reducing the stress response associated with CPB, decreasing ventricular arrhythmias after bypass, and allowing hemodynamic stabilization during and after CPB. Volatile anesthetic agents may be less suitable because of the myocardial depression associated with their use. The myocardium of infants less than 2 years of age is immature and potentially more sensitive to these negative inotropic effects. Increases in pulmonary vascular resistance (PVR) may exacerbate cyanosis and must be avoided. Conditions that may increase pulmonary vascular resistance include light anesthesia, positive end-expiratory pressure, hypoxia, hypercarbia, acidosis, and hypothermia.[110]

When an intracardiac shunt is present, the anesthetic technique used should minimize decreases in SVR to prevent an increase in right-to-left shunting. Pretreatment with a vasoconstrictor such as phenylephrine or methoxamine may offset the reduction of SVR associated with induction. The administration of ketamine at a dose of 1 to 2 mcg/kg has been shown to have no significant effect on systemic or pulmonary vascular resistance in children and therefore causes no major fluctuations with regard to their shunts.[110] This ability to maintain systemic blood pressure makes ketamine a suitable choice for induction of anesthesia in pediatric patients with right-to-left shunts.[112]

SUMMARY

Anesthesia management for the cardiac patient continues to change as new surgical modalities enter clinical practice. More thorough risk assessment and monitoring throughout the perioperative period has improved outcomes and patient satisfaction. Angioplasty is now the treatment of choice for many situations in which surgery was once the only alternative. This has changed the profile of the typical patient presenting for cardiac surgery and required significant adjustments in how we conceptualize their care. This chapter updates some of those changes. Among the many areas of clinical anesthesia, management for cardiac surgery is the most varied and hospital specific. The general concepts presented here may be adapted to each clinician's unique need.

REFERENCES

1. Hessel EA II. History of cardiac surgery and anesthesia. In: Estefanous FG. *Cardiac Anesthesia Principles and Clinical Practice.* Philadelphia: Lippincott Williams & Wilkins; 2001:4.
2. American Heart Association. *Heart Disease and Stroke Statistics—2007 Update.* Dallas: American Heart Association; 2007:12.
3. Norton JM. Toward consistent definitions for preload and afterload. *Adv Physiol Educ.* 2001;25:53-61.
4. Hoit BD, Walsh RA. Normal physiology of the cardiovascular system. In: Fuster V et al, eds. *Hurst's the Heart.* 12th ed. New York: McGraw-Hill; 2008:83-109.
5. Maccherini M et al. Warm heart surgery eliminates diaphragmatic paralysis. *J Cardiac Surg.* 1995;10:257.
6. Roach GW et al. Multicenter Study of Perioperative Ischemia (McSPI) Research Group. Ineffectiveness of burst suppression therapy in mitigating perioperative cerebrovascular dysfunction. *Anesthesiology.* 1999; 90:1255-1264.
7. Arrowsmith JE et al. Central nervous system complications of cardiac surgery. *Br J Anaesth.* 2000;84(3):378-393.
8. Murkin JM et al. Cognitive dysfunction after ventricular fibrillation during implantable cardioverter/defibrillator procedures is related to duration of the reperfusion interval. *Anesth Analg.* 1997;84:1186-1192.
9. Arrowsmith JE et al. Central nervous system complications of cardiac surgery. *Br J Anaesth.* 2000;84:378-383.
10. Murkin JM. Intraoperative tight glucose control improves outcome in cardiovascular surgery: pro. *J Cardiothorac Vasc Anesth.* 2000;14:475-478.
11. Kitano H et al. Inhalational anesthetics as neuroprotectants or chemical preconditioning agents in ischemic brain. *J Cereb Blood Flow Metab.* 2007;27(6):1108-1128.
12. Head BP, Patel P. Anesthetics and brain protection. *Curr Opin Anaesthesiol.* 2007;20(5):395-399.
13. Koerner IP, Brambrink AM. Brain protection by anesthetic agents. *Curr Opin Anaesthesiol.* 2006;19(5):481-486.
14. Selnes OA et al. Cognition 6 years after surgical or medical therapy for coronary artery disease. *Ann Neurol.* 2008;63(5):581-590.
15. Sweet JJ et al. Absence of cognitive decline one year after coronary bypass surgery: comparison to nonsurgical and healthy controls. *Ann Thorac Surg.* 2008;85(5):1571-1578.
16. Newman MF et al. Longitudinal assessment of neurocognitive function after coronary artery bypass surgery. *N Engl J Med.* 2001;344(6):395-402.
17. Selnes OA et al. Neurocognitive outcomes 3 years after coronary artery bypass graft surgery: a controlled study. *Ann Thorac Surg.* 2007;84(6):1885-1896.
18. Yilmaz AT et al. Gastrointestinal complications after cardiac surgery. *Eur J Cardiothorac Surg.* 1996;10:763-767.
19. Mangi AA et al. Gastrointestinal complications in patients undergoing heart operations: an analysis of 8709 consecutive cardiac surgical patients. *Ann Surg.* 2005;241(6)895-901.
20. Bolcal C et al. Gastrointestinal complications after cardiopulmonary bypass: sixteen years of experience. *Can J Gastroenterol.* 2005;19(10):613-617.
21. Huddy SP et al. Gastrointestinal complications in 4473 patients who underwent cardiopulmonary bypass surgery. *Br J Surg.* 1991;78:293-296.
22. Mangano CM et al. The Multicenter Study of Perioperative Ischemia Research Group. Renal dysfunction after myocardial revascularization: risk factors, adverse outcomes, and hospital resource utilization. *Ann Intern Med.* 1998;128:194-203.
23. Picca S et al. Risks of acute renal failure after cardiopulmonary bypass surgery in children: a retrospective 10-year case control study. *Nephrol Dial Transplant.* 1995;10:630.
24. Brown JR et al. Multivariable prediction of renal insufficiency developing after cardiac surgery. *Circulation.* 2007;116(11 Suppl):I139-143.
25. Swaminathan M et al. Trends in acute renal failure associated with coronary artery bypass graft surgery in the United States. *Crit Care Med.* 2007;35(10):2286-2291.
26. Bove T et al. The incidence and risk of acute renal failure after cardiac surgery. *J Cardiothorac Vasc Anesth.* 2004;18(4):442-445.
27. Regragui IA et al. Cardiopulmonary bypass perfusion temperature does not influence perioperative renal function. *Ann Thorac Surg.* 1995;60:160.
28. Okum G, Horrow JC. Anesthetic management for myocardial revascularization. In: Hensley FA et al, eds. *A Practical Approach to Cardiac Anesthesia.* 4th ed. Philadelphia: Lippincott Williams & Wilkins; 2008:289-315.
29. Reich DL et al. Intraoperative hemodynamic predictors of mortality, stroke, and myocardial infarction after coronary artery bypass surgery. *Anesth Analg.* 1999;89:814-822.
30. Noronha B et al. Optimal medical management of angina. *Curr Cardiol Rep.* 2003;5:259-265.
31. Suematsu Y et al. Strategies for CABG patients with carotid artery disease and perioperative neurological complications. *Heart Vessels.* 2000;15:129-134.
32. Joshi S et al. Cerebral and spinal cord blood flow. In: Cottrell JE, Smith DS. *Anesthesia and Neurosurgery.* 4th ed. St Louis: Mosby; 2001:36.

33. Mantha S et al. Relative effectiveness of four preoperative tests for predicting adverse cardiac outcomes after vascular surgery: a meta-analysis. *Anesth Analg.* 1994;79:422-433.

34. Soman P et al. The prognostic value of a normal Tc-99m Sestamibi SPECT study in suspected coronary artery disease. *J Nucl Cardiol.* 1999; 6:252-256.

35. Riedel BJ. Ischemic injury and its prevention. On right ventricular function in patients undergoing myocardial revascularization. *J Cardiothorac Vasc Anesth.* 1995;9:2-8.

36. Martin DE, Chambers CE. The cardiac surgical patient. In: Hensley FA et al, eds. *A Practical Approach to Cardiac Anesthesia.* 4th ed. Philadelphia: Lippincott Williams &Wilkins; 2008:3-32.

37. Heres EK et al. A dose-determining trial of heparinase I (Neutralase) for heparin neutralization in coronary artery surgery. *Anesth Analg.* 2001; 93:1446-1452.

38. Merin RG. Preoperative preparation of the patient with myocardial ischemia. *Anesthesiol Clin North America.* 1999;9:555-563.

39. Whit GC. Approach to the bleeding patient. In: Colman RW et al, eds. *Hemostasis and Thrombosis.* Philadelphia: Lippincott; 1994.

40. Crouch MA et al. Glycoprotein IIb/IIIa receptor inhibitors in percutaneous coronary intervention and acute coronary syndrome. *Ann Pharmacother.* 2003;37:860-875.

41. Hirsh J, Fuster V. American Heart Association guide to anticoagulant therapy. Part 1, heparin. *Circulation.* 1994;89:1449-1468.

42. Grock H et al. Monitoring intravascular volumes for postoperative volume therapy. *Eur J Anaesthesiol.* 2003;19:288-294.

43. Godje O et al. Central venous pressure, pulmonary capillary wedge pressure and intrathoracic blood volumes as preload indicators in cardiac surgery patients. *Eur J Cardiothorac Surg.* 1998;13:533-539;539-540 [discussion].

44. Baxter Healthcare Corporation, Edwards Critical Care Division. *Invasive Hemodynamic Monitoring: Physiologic Principles and Clinical Applications.* Santa Ana, CA: Baxter Healthcare; 1989:1.

45. Shanewise JS. Transesophageal echocardiography. In: Hensley FA et al, eds. *A Practical Approach to Cardiac Anesthesia.* 4th ed. Philadelphia: Lippincott Williams & Wilkins; 2008:142-163.

46. American Society of Anesthesiologists and the Society of Cardiovascular Anesthesiologists Task Force on Transesophageal Echocardiography. Practice guidelines for perioperative transesophageal echocardiography. *Anesthesiology.* 1996;84:986-1006.

47. Shanewise JS et al. ASE/SCA guidelines for performing a comprehensive intraoperative multi-plane transesophageal echocardiography examination: recommendations of the American Society of Echocardiography Council for Intraoperative Echocardiography and the Society of Cardiovascular Anesthesiologists Task Force for Certification in Perioperative Transesophageal Echocardiography. *Anesth Analg.* 1999;89(4):870-884.

48. Lehmann A et al. Bispectral index-guided anesthesia in patients undergoing aortocoronary bypass grafting. *Anesth Analg.* 2003;96:336-343.

49. Heck M et al. Electroencephalogram bispectral index predicts hemodynamic and arousal reactions during induction of anesthesia in patients undergoing cardiac surgery. *J Cardiothorac Vasc Anesth.* 2000;14:693-697.

50. Newfield P, Cottrell JE. *Handbook of Neuroanesthesia.* 4th ed. Philadelphia: Lippincott Williams & Wilkins; 2007:55-72.

51. Hall RI et al. The systemic inflammatory response to cardiopulmonary bypass: pathophysiologic, therapeutic and pharmacologic considerations. *Anesth Analg.* 1997;85:766-782.

52. Asimakopoulas G. Systemic inflammation and cardiac surgery: an update. *Perfusion.* 2001;16:353-360.

53. Michelsen LG. Cardiopulmonary bypass. In: Kirby RR et al, eds. *Clinical Anesthesia Practice.* 2nd ed. Philadelphia: Saunders; 2002:329-350.

54. Brodie JE, Johnson BB. *The Manual of Clinical Perfusion.* Augusta, GA: Glendale Medical Corporation; 1994.

55. Buckberg GD. Recent progress in myocardial protection during cardiac operations. *Cardiac Surgery.* 2nd ed. Philadelphia: FA Davis; 1987:291.

56. Meco M et al. Desflurane preconditioning in coronary artery bypass graft surgery: a double-blinded, randomized and placebo-controlled study. *Eur J Cardiothorac Surg.* 2007;32(2):319-325.

57. Suleiman MS et al. Inflammatory response and cardioprotection during open-heart surgery: the importance of anaesthetics. *Br J Pharmacol.* 2008;153:21-33.

58. Stadnicka A et al. Volatile anesthetics-induced cardiac preconditioning. *J Anesth.* 2007;21(2):212-219.

59. Pratt PF II et al. Cardioprotection by volatile anesthetics: new applications for old drugs. *Curr Opin Anaesthesiol.* 2006;19(4):397-403.

60. Rinder CS et al. Platelet activation and aggregation during cardiopulmonary bypass. *Anesthesiology.* 1991;75:388-393.

61. Shore-Lesserson L et al. Coagulation management during and after cardiopulmonary bypass. In: Hensley FA et al, eds. *A Practical Approach to Cardiac Anesthesia.* 4th ed. Philadelphia: Lippincott Williams & Wilkins; 2008:348-373.

62. Guyton AC. *Hemostasis and blood coagulation.* In: *Textbook of Medical Physiology.* 11th ed. Philadelphia: Saunders; 2006:457-467.

63. Hunt BJ et al. Activation of coagulation and fibrinolysis during cardiothoracic operations. *Ann Thorac Surg.* 1998;65:712-718.

64. Tanaka K et al. Alterations in coagulation and fibrinolysis associated with cardiopulmonary bypass during open heart surgery. *J Cardiothorac Anesth.* 1989;3:181-188.

65. Wilhelmi M et al. Coronary artery bypass grafting surgery without the routine application of blood products: is it feasible? *Eur J Cardiothorac Surg.* 2001;19:657-661.

66. Kasper SM et al. Failure of autologous fresh frozen plasma to reduce blood loss and transfusion requirements in coronary artery bypass surgery. *Anesthesiology.* 2001;95:81-86;6A [discussion].

67. Ray WA, Stein CM. The aprotinin story—is BART the final chapter? *N Engl J Med.* 2008;358(22):2398-2400.

68. Sodha NR et al. Is there still a role for aprotinin in cardiac surgery? *Drug Saf.* 2007;30(9):731-740.

69. Mangano DT et al. The risk associated with aprotinin in cardiac surgery. *N Engl J Med.* 2006;354(4):353-65.

70. Mangano DT et al. Mortality associated with aprotinin during 5 years following coronary artery bypass graft surgery. *JAMA* 2007;297(5):471-479.

71. Chugh SS et al. Pressor with promise. *Using vasopressin in cardiac arrest.* 1997;96:2453-2454.

72. The American Heart Association in collaboration with the International Liaison Committee on Resuscitation (ILCOR). Guidelines 2000 for cardiopulmonary resuscitation and emergency cardiovascular care. Part 6: advanced cardiovascular life support, section 6: Pharmacology II: agents to optimize cardiac output and blood pressure. *Circulation.* 2000;102:I129-I135.

73. Balser JR et al. Cardiovascular drugs. In: Hensley FA et al, eds. *A Practical Approach to Cardiac Anesthesia.* 4th ed. Philadelphia: Lippincott Williams & Wilkins; 2008:33-103.

74. London MJ et al. Anesthesia for myocardial revascularization. In: Kaplan JA. *Cardiac Anesthesia.* 5th ed. Philadelphia: Saunders; 2006:585-644.

75. Michelsen LG. Cardiopulmonary bypass. In: Kirby RR et al, eds. *Clinical Anesthesia Practice.* 2nd ed. Philadelphia: Saunders; 2002:342.

76. Gold J et al. Improvement of outcomes after coronary artery bypass: a randomized trial comparing intraoperative high versus low mean arterial pressure. *J Thorac Cardiovasc Surg.* 1995;110:1302.

77. Cartwright CR, Mangano CM. Con: during cardiopulmonary bypass for elective coronary artery bypass grafting, perfusion pressure should not routinely be greater than 70 mm Hg. *J Cardiothorac Vasc Anesth.* 1998;12:36.

78. Thomas SJ, Davis RF. Termination of cardiopulmonary bypass. In: Gravlee GP et al, eds. *Cardiopulmonary Bypass. Principles and Practice.* 2nd ed. Baltimore: Lippincott Williams & Wilkins; 2000:613-632.

79. Morgan GE et al. *Cardiovascular physiology and anesthesia.* In: *Clinical Anesthesiology.* 4th ed. New York: McGraw-Hill; 2006:413-440.

80. Strong M et al. Efficacy and pharmacokinetics of neutralase in CABG. *Int Anesth Res Soc.* 1998;86:28SCA.

81. Butterworth J. Dobutamine: too dangerous for "routine" administration? *Anesthesiology.* 2008;108(6):973-974.

82. Fellahi JL et al. Perioperative use of dobutamine in cardiac surgery and adverse cardiac outcome: propensity-adjusted analyses. *Anesthesiology.* 2008;108(6):979-987.

83. Atlee JL, Bernstein AD. Cardiac rhythm management devices. Part I, indications, device selection and function. *Anesthesiology.* 2001;95:1265-1280.

84. Atlee JL, Bernstein AD. Cardiac rhythm management devices. Part II. Perioperative management. *Anesthesiology.* 2001;95:1492-1506.

85. Kikura M et al. The effect of milrinone on hemodynamics and left ventricular function after emergence from cardiopulmonary bypass. *Anesth Analg.* 1997;85:16.

86. Sun BCV et al. Devices for cardiac support and replacement. In: Hensley FA et al, eds. *A Practical Approach to Cardiac Anesthesia.* 4th ed. Philadelphia: Lippincott Williams & Wilkins; 2008:587-603.

87. Scott NB et al. A prospective randomized study of the potential benefits of thoracic epidural anesthesia and analgesia in patients undergoing coronary artery bypass grafting. *Anesth Analg.* 2001;93:528-535.

88. Leslie K, Sessler D. The implications of hypothermia for early extubation following cardiac surgery. *J Cardiothorac Vasc Anesth.* 1998;12(Suppl 2):30-34.

89. Montes F et al. The lack of benefit of tracheal extubation in the operating room after coronary artery bypass surgery. *Anesth Analg.* 2000;91:776-780.

90. Cheng D et al. Early tracheal extubation after coronary artery bypass graft surgery reduces costs and improves resources use. *Anesthesiology.* 1996;85:1300-1310.

91. Hardy JF. Cardiac anesthesia: perspective 1990s. *Can J Anaesth.* 1993;9:1115-1119.

92. Cheng D. Fast-track cardiac surgery: economic implications in postoperative care. *J Cardiothorac Vasc Anesth.* 1998;12:72-79.

93. Trankina MF. Automatic implantable cardioverter-defibrillator. In: Fause RJ et al, eds. *Anesthesiology Review.* 3rd ed. New York: Churchill Livingstone; 2002.

94. Vijayakumar E. Anesthetic considerations in patients with cardiac arrhythmias, pacemakers, and AICDs. *Int Anesthesiol Clin.* 2001;39:21-42.

95. Hennein HA. *Cardiopulmonary Bypass/Deep Hypothermia Circulatory Arrest.* PediHeart Organization's Practitioner Website 1998. Available at: http://anes01.wustl.edu/all-net/english/cardpage/operate/bypass/cpb-19.htm. Accessed May 5, 2003.

96. Caldarone CA, Abonassaly C. *Hypothermic Circulatory Arrest and Cardiopulmonary Bypass.* E-medicine 2002. Available at: http://www.emedicine.com/ped/topic2813.htm. Accessed April 2, 2003.

97. Kuimral E et al. Neurologic complications with deep hypothermic circulatory arrest. *Tex Heart Inst J.* 2001;28:83-88.

98. Spodick DH. Acute cardiac tamponade. *N Engl J Med.* 2003;349(7):684-690.

99. Ribakove GH et al. Port-access minimally invasive CABG: techniques and results. *J Card Surg.* 2000;15(4):296-302.

100. Ganapathy S. Anaesthesia for minimally invasive cardiac surgery. *Best Pract Res Clin Anaesthesiol.* 2002;16:63-80.

101. Chassot PG et al. Off-pump coronary artery bypass surgery: physiology and anaesthetic management. *Br J Anaesth.* 2004;92(3):400-413.

102. Shanewise JS, Ramsay JG. Off-pump coronary surgery: how do the anesthetic considerations differ? *Anesthesiol Clin North America.* 2003;21:613-623.

103. Barnes RD. Off-pump coronary artery bypass and minimally invasive direct coronary artery bypass. In: Faust RJ et al, eds. *Anesthesiology Review.* 3rd ed. New York: Churchill Livingstone; 2002.

104. Huss MG, Wasnick JD. Magnesium and off-pump coronary artery bypass. *J Cardiac Thorac Vasc Anesth.* 1999;13:374-375.

105. Gillinov Am, Saltman AE. Surgical approaches for atrial fibrillation. *Med Clin North Am.* 2008;92(1):203-215.

106. Department of Cardiothoracic Surgery, University of Southern California Keck School of Medicine: MAZE *Procedure for Treatment of Atrial Fibrillation.* Available at: www.CTS.USC.edu/mazeprocedure.html. Accessed July 17, 2008.

107. Nakajima H et al. The effect of cryo-maze procedure on early and intermediate term outcome in mitral valve disease: case matched study. *Circulation.* 2002;106[Suppl I]:I46-I50.

108. Gillinov AM. Advances in surgical treatment of atrial fibrillation. *Stroke.* 2007;38(Suppl 2):618-623.

109. Thomas SP. Operative and percutaneous procedures for cure of atrial fibrillation [electronic version]. *Heart Lung Circulation.* 2007;16(3):229-233 doi:10.1016/j.hlc.2007.03.008.

110. Stratford MA. Cardiovascular physiology in infants and children. In: Motayama EK, Davis PJ, eds. *Smith's Anesthesia for Infants and Children.* 7th ed. Philadelphia: Mosby; 2006:7-108.

111. Bell C, Kain ZN. *The Pediatric Anesthesia Handbook.* 2nd ed. St Louis: Mosby; 1997:540.

112. Reid RW et al. Anesthesia for children having heart surgery. In: Cote CJ et al. *A Practice of Anesthesia for Infants and Children.* 3rd ed. Philadelphia: Saunders; 2001:397.

ANESTHESIA FOR VASCULAR SURGERY

Sass Elisha

PERIPHERAL VASCULAR DISEASE

Atherosclerosis is the most common cause of occlusive disease in the arteries of the lower extremities. This degenerative process involves the formation of atheromatous plaques that may obstruct the vessel lumen and thereby cause a reduction in distal blood flow. The pathophysiologic processes that affect the arteries include plaque formation, which obstructs the lumen (stenosis); thrombosis, which results in acute ischemia; embolism from microthrombi or atheromatous debris, which decreases distal blood flow; and weakening of the arterial wall with aneurysm formation. The most common risk factors associated with atherosclerosis appear in Box 26-1. Cigarette smoking and diabetes mellitus are major risk factors in the pathogenesis of atherosclerosis in the peripheral vascular system. Typical symptoms of peripheral occlusive disease include claudication, skin ulcerations, gangrene, and impotence.[1] The extent of disability is primarily influenced by the development of collateral blood flow. Initially, collateral blood flow sufficiently meets tissue oxygen demands. As the disease process progresses, supply is unable to meet demand, and limb ischemia becomes symptomatic, requiring therapeutic intervention. The mortality rates associated with peripheral vascular disease are 30% at 5 years and 70% at 10 years.[2] There has been an interest in the relationship between inflammation and the development of atherosclerosis. Platelet interaction with leukocytes and other cells that modulate the immune response play a major role in the development of atherosclerosis.[3,4] Researchers have discovered heritable genetic factors that predispose patients to developing vascular disease.[5]

Treatment for peripheral occlusive disease may range from pharmacologic therapy to surgery. Surgical therapy includes transluminal angioplasty, endarterectomy, thrombectomies, endovascular stenting and arterial bypass procedures. Some common surgical maneuvers used for bypassing occlusive lesions are aortofemoral, axillofemoral, femorofemoral, and femoropopliteal bypass techniques. Bypass techniques may be classified as *inflow* or *outflow* procedures, depending on the level of the obstruction, with the dividing axis being at the level of the groin. Temporary occlusion of the operative artery is mandatory when bypass procedures are used. The response to aortic cross-clamping in patients with aortoiliac occlusive disease is of less magnitude than in patients with aneurysmal disease. The development of collateral circulation provides alternative vascular blood flow that occurs in patients with occlusive disease.[6,7]

Preoperative Evaluation

The atherosclerotic process in occlusive disease is not limited to the peripheral arterial beds and should be expected to be present in the coronary, cerebral, and renal arteries. More than half the mortality associated with peripheral vascular disease results from adverse cardiac events.[8] Szilagyi and co-workers[9] reported that 60% of late deaths that followed reconstructive operations for aortoiliac occlusive disease in 1647 patients were the result of atherosclerotic heart disease. The identification and management of cardiac pathology, which often occurs in this patient population, must be managed aggressively to optimize cardiac functioning and decrease morbidity and mortality from cardiac causes. For a complete discussion of a preoperative cardiac evaluation, refer to Chapter 20.

Owing to the advantages of β-blockade on factors that affect myocardial oxygen supply and demand, their use is recommended in patients at high risk for myocardial ischemia and infarction.[10] For patients having abdominal aortic aneurysm repairs, there was a 10-fold decrease in cardiac morbidity.[11] β-Blockade should be instituted days to weeks before surgery and titrated to a target heart rate between 50 and 60 beats per minute.[12] Vascular surgery patients with limited heart rate variability after β-blocking therapy exhibit less cardiac ischemia and troponin values postoperatively and have a decreased mortality from all causes 2 years postoperatively.[13]

The presence of concurrent pulmonary, renal, neurologic, and endocrine dysfunction should be identified, and measures should be taken to improve organ function prior to surgery. Preoperatively, the greater number of comorbidities that exist, the greater risk of morbidity and mortality during the perioperative period.

Monitoring

The extent of perioperative monitoring should be based on the presence of coexisting disease processes. Clearly the detection of myocardial ischemia should be a primary objective in patients with vascular disease. Methods for assessing cardiac function include monitoring pulmonary artery pressure and transesophageal echocardiography. The effectiveness of pulmonary artery catheters (PAC) to improve patient outcomes has been controversial for years. The authors of three randomized controlled trials sought to answer this question. The studies included patients with severe cardiac conditions from a variety of causes. It was unanimously determined that PAC monitoring had no effect on mortality or length of stay. Additionally, there were higher rates of pulmonary embolism, pulmonary infarction, and hemorrhage in the PAC group.[14-16] The recommendation by Eagle and colleagues[12] state that the routine use of PACs is not warranted.

Due to the global nature of atherosclerotic disease, the anesthetist should assume some degree of systemic cardiovascular disease in patients with peripheral vascular disease.[9] Patients with hypertension and/or angiopathy rely on increased mean arterial pressures to perfuse their vital organs. Thus cerebral and coronary autoregulation occurs at higher than normal

pressures. Direct intraarterial blood pressure monitoring allows for near–real-time determination of blood pressure values and is warranted because of dramatic fluctuations that can occur during anesthesia.

Anesthetic Selection

The anesthetic technique chosen for vascular surgery depends on the type of surgical procedure to be performed and the presence of coexisting disease. In certain instances, infiltration of local anesthetic and intravenous sedation may be sufficient, whereas other situations may require the use of general anesthesia. Regional anesthesia for surgery on the lower extremities may decrease the overall morbidity and mortality associated with this patient population. In a review of 912 patients who underwent peripheral vascular reconstruction, Baron and associates[17] documented the safety of a continuous epidural anesthetic technique for patients who had received heparin; these investigators identified specific advantages of this technique. Similarly, Raggi and co-workers[18] documented favorable consequences of the use of epidural anesthesia during vascular surgery in 85 patients (Box 26-2). Specific anesthetic techniques and their contribution to postoperative complications remain controversial. For example, Underwood and associates[19] reported a higher frequency of cardiac complications in patients who underwent peripheral vascular surgery while receiving epidural anesthesia; however, all patients studied were over 69 years of age. Presently, there is a lack of randomized controlled trials and no conclusive scientific evidence suggesting superiority of a specific type of anesthetic technique.

Postoperative Considerations

Postoperative pain management is an important issue related to peripheral vascular surgery. Most clinicians agree that

---

BOX 26-1

Risk Factors Related to the Development of Atherosclerotic Lesions

- Hypercholesterolemia
- Elevated triglycerides
- Cigarette smoking
- Hypertension
- Diabetes mellitus
- Obesity
- Genetic predisposition
- Sex (male>female)
- Impaired long-term glucose regulation
- Homocysteine
- C-reactive protein

From Fruchart JC et al. New risk factors for atherosclerosis and patient assessment. Circulation. 2004;109(23Suppl 1):15-19.

BOX 26-2

Benefits of the Epidural Technique in Vascular Surgery

Endocrine
Inhibits surgical stress response
Inhibits adrenaline and cortisol release
Inhibits hyperglycemia
Inhibits lymphopenia and granulocytosis
Causes nitrogen sparing
Blocks sympathetic tone

Cardiovascular
Decreases myocardial oxygen demand and afterload
Decreases myocardial infarct size (experimental model)
Increases endocardial perfusion at ischemic zone
Causes fewer sympathetic blood pressure swings
Causes less blood loss
Requires less general anesthesia depressant medication
Redistributes blood to lower extremities

Pulmonary
Decreases FVC, FEV_1, and PEFR
Requires less shunting oxygen consumption
Improves atrioventricular oxygen differentiation
Causes fewer pulmonary infections
Causes fewer thromboembolisms

Renal
Increases blood flow in the renal cortex
Causes less renovascular constriction

Geriatric
Causes less cardiorespiratory trespass
Improves postoperative mental status

Miscellaneous
Allows earlier extubation, ambulation, and discharge
Achieves greater postoperative pain control

Modified from Raggi R et al. Continuous epidural anesthesia and postoperative epidural narcotics in vascular surgery. Am J Surg. 1987;154:192-197. FEV_1, Forced expiratory volume in 1 second; FVC, forced vital capacity; PEFR, peak expiratory flow rate.

postoperative administration of narcotics not only provides patient comfort but also contributes to cardiac stability. The use of epidural opioid and local anesthetics in patients recovering from vascular surgery is an important component of postoperative care because pain can greatly enhance sympathetic nervous system stimulation. Despite a decrease in discomfort during the postoperative course, these patients must be monitored in an appropriate surgical unit that is capable of detecting possible adverse events, such as myocardial infarction or respiratory depression, which could be attributed to the administration of epidural opioids and local anesthetics. Presently there are insufficient data to confirm that adequate analgesic techniques decrease morbidity and mortality from postoperative complications.[20]

ABDOMINAL AORTIC ANEURYSMS

Incidence

The incidence of abdominal aortic aneurysm (AAA) has increased since the 1970s[21] and has risen over the last 5 decades from 12.2 to 36.2 per 100,000 surgical procedures.[22] This increase may partially be the result of the detection of asymptomatic aneurysms by noninvasive diagnostic modalities, such as computed tomography (CT), magnetic resonance imaging (MRI), and ultrasonography. The occurrence of AAAs has increased because of the increased age of the general population and the vascular changes that occur as a result of aging.[21] Aortic aneurysms can be identified in approximately 1% to 4% of the population older than 50 years and in approximately 5% of the population older than 60 years.[23-25] Aneurysms are more common in men than in women and in caucasians than in African Americans.[21,24,26,27]

Risk Factors

Atherosclerosis is thought to be the primary cause of AAAs in more than 90% of patients.[27] However, this traditional theory has been challenged by some who speculate that aneurysmal development may result from proteolysis of elastin and collagen within the vessel wall and that atherosclerosis may be an incidental finding in the pathogenesis of aneurysm development.[21,28] Hypertension is present in 60% of patients with aneurysmal lesions.[27] In cigarette smokers, the incidence of AAAs increases eightfold.[21,27,29] Although investigators have demonstrated a correlation between aneurysms and these factors, aneurysms can also be observed in normotensive nonsmokers. Perhaps it may be more judicious to suggest that hypertension and cigarette smoking increase the potential for the development of aneurysms.[21] Genetics may also contribute to the predisposition for aneurysmal development.[28,30] Obesity, although not an independent risk factor, may mask the signs and symptoms of an AAA until complications arise.[26,27]

Mortality

Mortality rates for elective abdominal aortic aneurysmectomies have decreased since the 1970s. The present mortality rate ranges from 1% to 11%, although it is most commonly estimated at 5%. This is compared with mortality rates of 18% to 30% in the 1950s.[26,27,30-34] Advanced detection capabilities, earlier surgical intervention, extensive preoperative preparation, refined surgical techniques, better hemodynamic monitoring, improved anesthetic techniques, and aggressive postoperative management have all contributed to this improvement in surgical outcomes. Data suggest that risk of rupture is very low for AAAs less than 4 cm in diameter, but the risk dramatically increases for AAAs with a 5-cm or greater diameter. Surgical intervention is recommended for AAAs 5.5 cm or greater in diameter.[35]

Unfortunately, mortality rates for undetected or untreated ruptured aortic aneurysms have not followed the trend of those for surgical intervention. Estimates of mortality resulting from ruptured AAAs vary from 35% to 94%.[23,26,36-38] The 5-year mortality rate for individuals with untreated AAAs is 81%, and the 10-year mortality rate is 100%.[32] Early detection and elective surgical intervention can be lifesaving.

Diagnosis

Frequently, asymptomatic aneurysms are detected incidentally during routine examination or abdominal radiography. Smaller aneurysms are often undetected on routine physical examination. Diagnostic techniques, such as ultrasonography, CT scan, and MRI, may identify vascular abnormalities in these patients. Such noninvasive techniques not only reveal the presence of aneurysms but also provide information about aneurysm size, vessel wall integrity, and adjacent anatomic definition.[39] Invasive techniques, including contrast-enhanced CT scan, contrast angiography, and digital subtraction angiography, can provide additional information and more detailed representations of arterial anatomy. Digital subtraction angiography is the best method of evaluating suprarenal aneurysms because it provides superior definition of the aneurysmal relationship to the renal arteries.[40]

ABDOMINAL AORTIC RECONSTRUCTION

Patient Selection

As a result of recent advances in surgical and anesthetic techniques, the mortality associated with elective repair of AAAs is fairly low compared with nonsurgical management. Most patients with abdominal aneurysms, including octogenarians, are considered surgical candidates. Although advancing age contributes to an increased incidence of morbidity and mortality, age alone is not a contraindication to elective aneurysmectomy.[41] Mortality in patients who undergo elective aortic reconstruction has been reported to be 5.6% for patients younger than 75 years and 11.3% for those older than 75 years.[42] However, physiologic age is more indicative of increased surgical risk than chronologic age. Contraindications to elective repair include intractable angina pectoris, recent myocardial infarction, severe pulmonary dysfunction, and chronic renal insufficiency.[6] Patients with stable CAD and coronary artery stenosis of greater than 70% who require nonemergent AAA repair do not benefit from revascularization if β-blockade has been established.[43] Table 26-1 lists characteristics that define high-risk patients; however, in most cases the presence of an AAA warrants surgical intervention.[32]

The dimensions of an aneurysm can change over time. Abdominal aortic aneurysms grow approximately 4 mm/yr.[28] Aneurysmal vessel dimensions correspond to the law of Laplace:

Equation 26-1

$$T = P \times r$$

where T = wall tension, P = transmural pressure, and r = vessel radius.

As the radius of a vessel increases, the wall tension increases. Therefore, the larger the aneurysm, the more likely the risk of spontaneous rupture. As stated, aneurysms measuring more than 4 to 5 cm in diameter generally require surgical intervention,[26] but aneurysms measuring less than 4 to 5 cm should not be considered benign. An aneurysm has the potential to rupture regardless of its size. On postmortem examination, Darling and associates[44] reported that 18% of ruptured aneurysms were less than 5 cm in diameter.

Patient Preparation

Preoperative fluid loading and restoration of intravascular volume are perhaps the most important techniques used to enhance cardiac function during abdominal aortic aneurysmectomies. Reliable venous access must be secured if volume replacement is to be accomplished. Large-bore intravenous lines and central lines can be used to infuse fluids or blood. Massive hemorrhage is an ever-present threat, therefore the availability of blood and blood products should be ensured. Provisions for rapid transfusion and intraoperative blood salvage should be confirmed.

Routine Monitoring

Standard monitoring methods include electrocardiography (with display of lead II for detection of dysrhythmias and the precordial V_5 lead for analysis of ischemic ST-segment changes), pulse oximetry, and capnography. An esophageal stethoscope allows for continuous auscultation of heart and breath sounds, as well as temperature determination. Placement of an indwelling urinary catheter is necessary for continuous measurement of urinary output and renal function. Neuromuscular function is also routinely monitored.

Invasive Monitoring

Maintaining cardiac function is crucial for a successful surgical outcome; cardiac function should be closely monitored during abdominal aortic reconstruction. Invasive blood pressure monitoring permits beat-to-beat analysis of the blood pressure, immediate identification of hemodynamic alterations related to aortic clamping, and access for blood sampling.

Pulmonary artery catheters can be used in abdominal aortic reconstruction for monitoring left-sided filling pressures as a guide for fluid replacement. Correlations between central venous pressure and PAOP have been demonstrated in both coronary revascularization[45] and aortic surgery.[46] This correlation is predictable only in patients with adequate ventricular function (ejection fraction 0.5).[45] Pulmonary artery catheterization not only provides clinical indices that reflect intravascular volume

but also facilitates calculations of stroke volume, cardiac index, and left ventricular stroke work index. Myocardial ischemia can be detected by analysis of pulmonary artery catheter tracings. Some pulmonary artery catheters allow for measurement of mixed venous oxygen saturation. However, information obtained from pulmonary artery catheters has been shown to have low sensitivity and low specificity in detecting myocardial ischemia when compared with electrocardiographic and transesophageal echocardiography. The results from two randomized controlled studies comparing pulmonary artery catheter monitoring versus central venous pressure monitoring showed no difference in cardiac morbidity.[47,48]

By detecting changes in ventricular wall motion, two-dimensional transesophageal echocardiography provides a sensitive method for assessing regional myocardial perfusion. Thys and associates[49] reported a positive correlation between hemodynamic indices obtained by invasive monitoring and those derived by two-dimensional echocardiography. Wall motion abnormalities also occur much sooner than electrocardiographic changes during periods of reduced coronary blood flow.[50] Myocardial ischemia poses the greatest risk of mortality after abdominal aortic reconstruction. Intraoperative monitoring may enable earlier detection and intervention during ischemic cardiac events.

Aortic Cross-Clamping

Abdominal aortic reconstruction may be one of the most challenging situations for the anesthetist. Patients with AAAs tend to be elderly and have varying degrees of coexisting disease. In addition to the risks associated with any major surgical procedure, these patients also experience physiologic changes that are specific to abdominal aortic aneurysmectomies. Perhaps the most dramatic physiologic change occurs with the application of an aortic cross-clamp. Temporary aortic occlusion produces various hemodynamic and metabolic alterations.

Hemodynamic Alterations

The hemodynamic effects of aortic cross-clamping depend on the application site along the aorta, the patient's preoperative cardiac reserve, and the patient's intravascular volume. The most common site for cross-clamping is infrarenal, because most aneurysms appear below the level of the renal arteries. Less common sites of aneurysm development are the juxtarenal and suprarenal areas.

During aortic cross-clamping, *hypertension* occurs *above* the cross-clamp and *hypotension* occurs *below* the cross-clamp. Organs proximal to the aortic occlusion may experience a redistribution of blood volume.[51] There is an absence of blood flow distal to the clamp in the pelvis and lower extremities.[6] Increases in afterload cause myocardial wall tension to increase. Mean arterial pressure (MAP) and systemic vascular resistance (SVR) also increase. Cardiac output may decrease or remain unchanged. Pulmonary artery occlusion pressure (PAOP) may increase or display no change. Table 26-2 summarizes the cardiac function observed during aortic cross-clamping and release, as measured by radionuclide angiography. Table 26-3 lists the percentages of change in cardiovascular indexes at different levels of aortic occlusion.

Patients with adequate cardiac reserve commonly adjust to sudden increases in afterload without the occurrence of adverse cardiac events. However, patients with ischemic heart disease or ventricular dysfunction are unable to fully compensate, as a result of the hemodynamic alterations. The increased wall stress

TABLE **26-1**	Criteria for High Risk in Abdominal Aortic Aneurysm Repair
Parameter	**Criterion**
Age	>85 yr
Pulmonary	Home oxygen, Pao_2 <50 mm Hg, FEV_1 <1 L/s
Renal	Serum creatinine level (>3 mg/dL)
Cardiac	Class III-IV angina Resting LVEF <30% Recent congestive heart failure Complex ventricular ectopy Large left ventricular aneurysm Severe valvular disease Recurrent congestive failure or angina after CABG Severe, noncorrectable CAD

Modified from Pairolero PC. Repair of abdominal aortic aneurysms in high-risk patients. Surg Clin North Am. *1989;69:765-774.*
CABG, *Coronary artery bypass grafting;* CAD, *coronary artery disease;* FEV_1, *forced expiratory volume in 1 second;* LVEF, *left ventricular ejection fraction;* Pao_2, *partial pressure of arterial oxygen.*

attributed to aortic cross-clamp application may contribute to decreased global ventricular function and myocardial ischemia. Clinically, these patients experience increases in PAOP in response to aortic cross-clamping. Aggressive pharmacologic intervention is required for restoration of cardiac function during this time.

Metabolic Alterations

After the application of an aortic cross-clamp, the lack of blood flow to distal structures makes these tissues prone to developing hypoxia. In response to hypoxia, metabolites such as lactate accumulate. Gelman and co-workers[52] demonstrated that the reduction in cardiac output during aortic cross-clamping might be partly the result of metabolic alterations, such as decreased oxygen consumption. Gold and co-workers[53] found that plasma catecholamine levels increase significantly during application of the aortic cross-clamp. Both epinephrine and norepinephrine stimulate myocardial β_1-receptors that can increase heart rate and myocardial oxygen demand.

The release of arachidonic acid derivatives may also contribute to the cardiac instability observed during aortic cross-clamping. Thromboxane A_2 synthesis, which is accelerated by the application of an aortic cross-clamp, may be responsible for the decrease in myocardial contractility and cardiac output that occurs. Numerous studies have attempted to determine if cyclooxygenase inhibition caused by the administration of aspirin or ibuprofen before elective aneurysmectomies can preserve myocardial function. Pretreatment with ibuprofen has been shown to have positive results; however, its effectiveness in stabilizing cardiac function remains unclear.[54,55]

Traction on the mesentery is a surgical maneuver used for exposing the aorta. Gottlieb and associates[56] and Seltzer and colleagues[57] described the mesenteric traction syndrome associated with this procedure. Decreases in blood pressure and SVR, tachycardia, increased cardiac output, and facial flushing are common responses to mesenteric traction. Although the cause of this syndrome is unknown, it has been associated with high concentrations of 6-ketoprostaglandin F_1, the stable metabolite of prostacyclin at the time of mesenteric traction.[56] The 6-ketoprostaglandin F_1 levels and hemodynamic stability return to preclamp values as reperfusion occurs. Pretreatment with cyclooxygenase inhibitors may reduce the incidence of mesenteric traction syndrome, although the effectiveness of these agents remains unclear.

The neuroendocrine response to major surgical stress is believed to be mediated by cytokines such as interleukin (IL)-1B, IL-6, and tumor necrosis factor, as well as plasma catecholamines and cortisol.[58] These mediators are thought to be responsible for triggering the inflammatory response that results in increased body temperature, leukocytosis, tachycardia, tachypnea, and fluid sequestration. Norman and Fink[59] demonstrated that patients who had an exaggerated plasma stress mediator release had longer operative and cross-clamp times and required a greater number of blood transfusions (see Table 26-3).

Effects on Regional Circulation

Structures distal to the aortic clamp are underperfused during aortic cross-clamping. Renal insufficiency and renal failure have been reported to occur after abdominal aortic reconstruction. Suprarenal and juxtarenal cross-clamping may be associated

TABLE 26-2	Responses of 26 Patients Undergoing Abdominal Aortic Aneurysm Resection with Aortic Occlusion	
	Response	
Parameter	Application of Clamp	Release of Clamp
LVEF	↓(0.56-0.48)	↑(0.51-0.58)
EDV	↑(171-225 mL)	↓(205-187 mL)
ESV	↑(85-127 mL)	↓(105-94 mL)
MAP	↑(82-91 mm Hg)	↓(84-69 mm Hg)
ESWS	↑(53-67 10^3 dyne/cm^2)	↓(67-46 10^3 dyne/cm^2)

Modified from Harpole DH et al. Right and left ventricular performance during and after abdominal aortic aneurysm repair. Ann Surg. 1989;209:356-362.
↑, Increased; ↓, decreased; EDV, end-diastolic volume; ESV, end-systolic volume; ESWS, end-systolic wall stress; LVEF, left ventricular ejection fraction; MAP, mean arterial pressure.

TABLE 26-3	Change in Cardiovascular Variables at Different Levels of Aortic Occlusion as Assessed by Two-Dimensional Transesophageal Echocardiography		
	Change After Occlusion at Different Levels (Percent Increase or Decrease)		
Variable	Infrarenal	Suprarenal Infraceliac	Supraceliac
Mean arterial pressure	↑ 2	↑ 5	↑ 54
Pulmonary artery occlusion pressure	0	↑ 10	↑ 38
End-diastolic area	↑ 9	↑ 2	↑ 28
End-systolic area	↑ 11	↑ 10	↑ 69
Ejection fraction	↓ 3	↓ 10	↓ 38
Number of Patients Affected			
Patients with wall motion abnormality	0	33	92
New myocardial infarction	0	0	8

Modified from Roizen MF et al. Monitoring with two-dimensional transesophageal echocardiography: comparison of myocardial function in patients undergoing supraceliac, suprarenal-infraceliac, or infrarenal aortic occlusion. J Vasc Surg. 1984;1:300-305.

with a higher incidence of altered renal dynamics; however, reductions in renal blood flow can occur with any level of clamp application. Infrarenal aortic cross-clamping is associated with a 38% decrease in renal blood flow and a 75% increase in renal vascular resistance.[6] These effects may lead to acute renal failure, which is fatal in 50% to 90% of patients who have undergone aneurysmectomies.[60] Preoperative evaluation of renal function is one of the most significant predictors of postoperative renal dysfunction. Therefore, a complete evaluation of renal function is required in the preoperative period.

Spinal cord damage is associated with aortic occlusion. Interruption of blood flow to the greater radicular artery (artery of Adamkiewicz) in the absence of collateral blood flow has been identified as a causative factor in paraplegia. The incidence of neurologic complications increases as the aortic cross-clamp is positioned in a higher or more proximal area. Somatosensory evoked potential (SSEP) monitoring has been advocated as a method of identifying spinal cord ischemia. However, SSEP monitoring reflects dorsal (sensory) spinal cord function and does not provide information regarding the integrity of the anterior (motor) spinal cord.[6] Motor evoked potential (MEP) monitoring is capable of determining anterior cord function. This monitoring modality relies on intact neuromuscular functioning for analysis, which limits its use in abdominal aortic aneurysmectomies because neuromuscular blocking drugs are routinely used. Alternative methods for reliable evaluation of spinal cord ischemia are still under investigation.[61]

Ischemic colon injury is a well-documented complication associated with abdominal aortic resections. Ischemia of the colon is most frequently attributed to manipulation of the inferior mesenteric artery, which supplies the primary blood supply to the left colon. This vessel is often sacrificed during surgery, and blood flow to the descending and sigmoid colon depends on the presence and adequacy of the collateral vessels. Mucosal ischemia occurs in 10% of patients who undergo AAA repair. In less than 1% of these patients, infarction of the left colon necessitates surgical intervention.[60]

Aortic Cross-Clamp Release

While the aorta is occluded, metabolites that are liberated as a result of anaerobic metabolism, such as serum lactate, accumulate below the aortic cross-clamp and induce vasodilation and vasomotor paralysis. As the cross-clamp is released, SVR decreases, and blood is sequestered into previously dilated veins, which decreases venous return. Reactive hyperemia causes transient vasodilation secondary to the presence of tissue hypoxia, release of adenine nucleotides,[60] and liberation of an unnamed vasodepressor substance that acts as a myocardial depressant and peripheral vasodilator. This combination of events results in decreased preload and afterload. The hemodynamic instability that may ensue after the release of an aortic cross-clamp is called *declamping shock syndrome.*[62] Evidence demonstrates that venous endothelin (ET)-1 may be partially responsible for the hemodynamic alterations that accompany declamping shock syndrome. Venous ET-1 has a positive inotropic effect on the heart and a vasoconstricting and vasodilating action on blood vessels. Fukuda and colleagues[63] found that venous ET-1 is released in response to tissue ischemia, which is associated with the release of the aortic cross-clamp. Table 26-4 summarizes the most frequently observed hemodynamic responses to aortic declamping.

The magnitude of the response to unclamping the aorta may be manipulated. Although SVR and MAP decrease, intravascular

volume may influence the direction and magnitude of change in cardiac output. Restoration of circulating blood volume is paramount in providing circulatory stability before release of the aortic clamp.[7,60,62-64] The site and duration of cross-clamp application, as well as the gradual release of the clamp, influence the magnitude of circulatory instability. For this reason, it is vital that communication between the anesthetist and the surgical team occurs. Partial release of the aortic cross-clamp over time frequently results in less severe hypotension.

Surgical Approach

The standard approach for elective abdominal aortic reconstruction is the transperitoneal incision. The advantages of this route include exposure of infrarenal and iliac vessels, ability to inspect intraabdominal organs, and rapid closure.[65] Unfavorable consequences associated with this approach include increased fluid losses, prolonged ileus, postoperative incisional pain, and pulmonary complications.

The retroperitoneal approach has gained popularity as an alternative to the standard route. Its advantages include excellent exposure (especially for juxtarenal and suprarenal aneurysms), decreased fluid losses, less incisional pain, and fewer postoperative pulmonary and intestinal complications. After implantation with a synthetic graft, the aortic adventitia is closed (Figure 26-1). In addition, the retroperitoneal approach does not elicit mesenteric traction syndrome.[65] The reported limitations of this approach are unfamiliarity of surgeons with this technique, poor right distal renal artery exposure, and inability to inspect the integrity of the abdominal contents. Table 26-5 compares the standard and retroperitoneal surgical approaches.

Management of Fluid and Blood Loss

Extreme loss of extracellular fluid and blood should be expected with abdominal aortic aneurysmectomies. Evaporative losses and third spacing occur, with the magnitude of loss depending on the surgical approach, the duration of the surgery, and the experience of the surgeon. Most blood loss occurs because of back bleeding from the lumbar and inferior mesenteric arteries after the vessels have been clamped and the aneurysm is opened.[60,66] The use of heparin also contributes to blood loss. Excessive bleeding, however, can occur at any point during surgery, and blood replacement is commonly administered during abdominal aortic resections.

Owing to the heightened awareness of transfusion-related morbidity, the use of autologous blood has generated increasing interest. Presently, three options are available for administering autologous transfusions: preoperative deposit, intraoperative phlebotomy and hemodilution, and intraoperative blood salvage. Preoperative deposit is becoming more feasible because

TABLE **26-4**	Hemodynamic Consequences of Aortic Declamping
Clinical Indexes	**Responses to Clamp Release**
Mean arterial pressure	Decrease
Systemic vascular resistance	Decrease
Cardiac output	No change or increase
Pulmonary artery occlusion pressure	Decrease

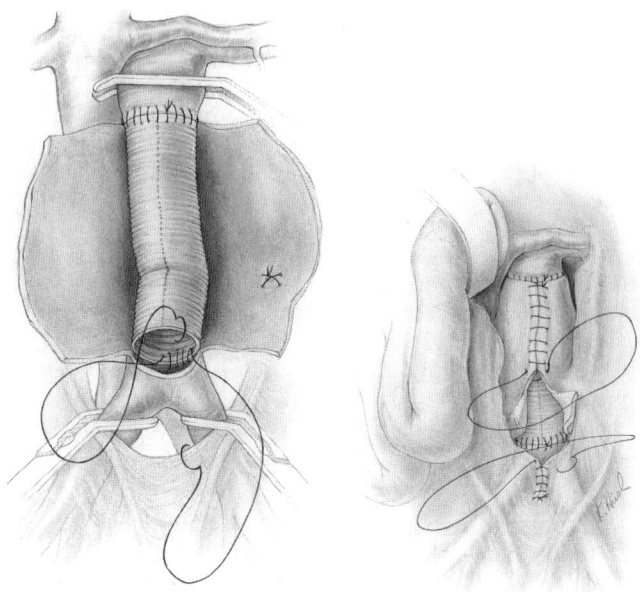

FIGURE **26-1** Dacron graft used to repair aneurysm. (*From Zarins CK, Fewertz BL. Atlas of Vascular Surgery. 2nd ed. Philadelphia: Churchill Livingstone; 2005.*)

TABLE **26-5**	Comparison of Transperitoneal and Retroperitoneal Approaches	
Transperitoneal	**Retroperitoneal**	
Advantages		
Familiarity	Exposure for juxtarenal and suprarenal aneurysms	
Access to infrarenal aorta and iliac vessels	Decreased fluid loss	
Visualization of intraabdominal viscera	Improved postoperative respiratory function	
Rapid opening and closure	Better-tolerated incisional pain avoids formation of intraabdominal adhesions	
Versatility	Mesenteric traction syndrome, non-elicited	
Disadvantages		
Increased fluid losses	Inaccessibility to distal right renal artery complications	
Less postoperative ileus		
More frequent postoperative respiratory complications		
Increased postoperative incisional pain		

Modified from Sicard GA et al. Retroperitoneal versus transperitoneal approach of repair of abdominal aortic aneurysms. Surg Clin North Am. 1989;69:795-806.

asymptomatic aneurysms are being detected with greater frequency. Ideally, patients donate their own blood to minimize the intraoperative use of homologous blood products and the subsequent risk of transfusion-related viruses. Autotransfusion systems may be used for replacing intraoperative blood loss. In a study at the Mayo Clinic in which intraoperative autologous red-cell salvage was used, 75% less banked blood was transfused. In a prospective study of 100 patents who underwent elective abdominal aortic resections, 80% of the patients received only their own blood.[66]

Presence of Concurrent Disease
Preoperative Management
The presence of underlying coronary artery disease (CAD) in patients with vascular disease has been well documented. Reports suggest that CAD exists in more than 50% of patients who require abdominal aortic reconstruction and is the single most significant risk factor influencing long-term survivability.[7,8,22,67,68] Myocardial infarctions are responsible for 40% to 70% of all fatalities that occur after aneurysm reconstruction.[6,7,31,68] In the presence of such threatening mortality rates, the extent of CAD and the subsequent functional limitations must be clearly defined and cardiac function optimized preoperatively before elective aortic vascular reconstruction is performed.

Preoperative cardiac evaluation begins with the identification of risk factors that may contribute to adverse cardiac events and subsequent death. When preoperative CAD exists, an increased incidence of postoperative adverse cardiac complications has been demonstrated.[69] Goldman[70] described the cardiac risk index, which is used to predict the likelihood of adverse cardiac complications and death in patients undergoing noncardiac surgery. In the cardiac risk index, advanced age, cardiac history, aberrations on physical examination, electrocardiographic

abnormalities, and previous surgical procedures are identifiable factors that contribute to cardiac complications. Cooperman and associates[71] used similar risk factors, that include angina, congestive heart failure dysrhythmias, myocardial infarction, cerebrovascular accidents, and abnormal electrocardiograph findings to derive an equation for computing the possibility of cardiac complications in patients undergoing vascular surgery. Although the reliability of multivariate risk factor analysis in the prediction of adverse cardiac events has been disputed, these systems are applicable to all patients and can serve as the initial evaluation of cardiac risk for patients undergoing elective aneurysmectomies.

Initially, controversy existed regarding which diagnostic modality should be used in the evaluation of patients undergoing elective vascular surgery. Patients with unremarkable medical histories and normal physical examinations, exercise testing, electrocardiography, and laboratory studies have a decreased surgical risk. Some centers advocated the use of routine coronary angiography in all candidates for elective aortic revascularization.[72] Currently, investigators advocate the use of coronary angiography in selected patients who have positive findings on the initial cardiac evaluation.[7,22,67]

Patients with symptomatic CAD require more extensive cardiac evaluation. Dipyridamole thallium testing is perhaps one of the most reliable methods for evaluating the extent of myocardial dysfunction associated with CAD and for predicting coronary events after vascular surgery.[6,23,31,73] In addition to its sensitivity in detecting myocardial dysfunction, dipyridamole thallium testing does not rely on exercise for detection of areas of myocardial hypoperfusion. Techniques capable of evaluating left ventricular performance, such as echocardiography, are of some value in predicting adverse cardiac events. Ambulatory electrocardiographic monitoring has also been very successful in the identification of postoperative cardiac complications.[74] Finally, coronary angiography provides the most reliable definition of coronary anatomy and the extent of CAD.

The end-point of any method of preoperative cardiac evaluation for aneurysmectomy is identification of functional cardiac limitations. Depending on the degree of cardiac dysfunction, preoperative optimization of cardiac function may range from simple pharmacologic manipulation to surgical intervention. Some centers advocate the use of cardiac revascularization for reversible CAD before AAA repair is performed and demonstrate reduced mortality rates for elective aneurysmectomies.[8,32,72] On the other hand, the risk associated with cardiac revascularization and the potential for aneurysmal rupture add credibility to approaches that proceed to aneurysmectomies in patients with reversible CAD.[11] Percutaneous transluminal coronary angioplasty may provide an alternative method of restoring oxygen supply to the myocardium; however, the advantages of this technique have not been established. Figure 26-2 is an algorithm for the evaluation and treatment of CAD for patients with AAAs.

Hypertension, chronic obstructive pulmonary disease, diabetes mellitus, renal impairment, and carotid artery disease are frequently observed in patients with AAAs. Table 26-6 lists the frequency rates of coexisting disease in patients who require AAA repair. Each of these disease entities deserves attention in the preoperative period. Measures must be taken to optimize organ function because each of these disease states contributes to postoperative complications. Preoperative renal dysfunction deserves special consideration because aortic cross-clamping produces alterations in renal dynamics. The degree of preoperative renal insufficiency contributes to the extent of any postoperative renal damage.[6]

Intraoperative Management
Anesthetic Selection
Many anesthetic techniques are available for abdominal aortic resections. Although each technique has its advantages and disadvantages, a superior technique has not been identified. Anesthetic selection should be based on the following objectives: providing optimum analgesia and amnesia, facilitating relaxation, maintaining hemodynamic stability, preserving renal blood flow, and minimizing morbidity and mortality.

Inhalation Agents. Circulatory stability is desirable for patients undergoing AAA reconstruction, especially for those with CAD. All inhalation anesthetics may depress the myocardium and cause hemodynamic instability. Therefore, high concentrations of inhalation agents in patients with moderate to severe decreased ejection fraction should not be used. Because the degree of myocardial depression is dose dependent, it is acceptable to administer inhalation agents at a dose of less than or equal to 1 MAC. Potential organ toxicity and lack of postoperative analgesia may be additional limitations to the use of these agents. Beneficial effects attributed to inhalation agents include the ability to alter autonomic responses, reversibility, rapid emergence, and potentially earlier extubation.

Narcotic Technique. A balanced technique using a combination of high-dose narcotics with nitrous oxide can be used as the anesthetic for major vascular surgery. The cardiovascular

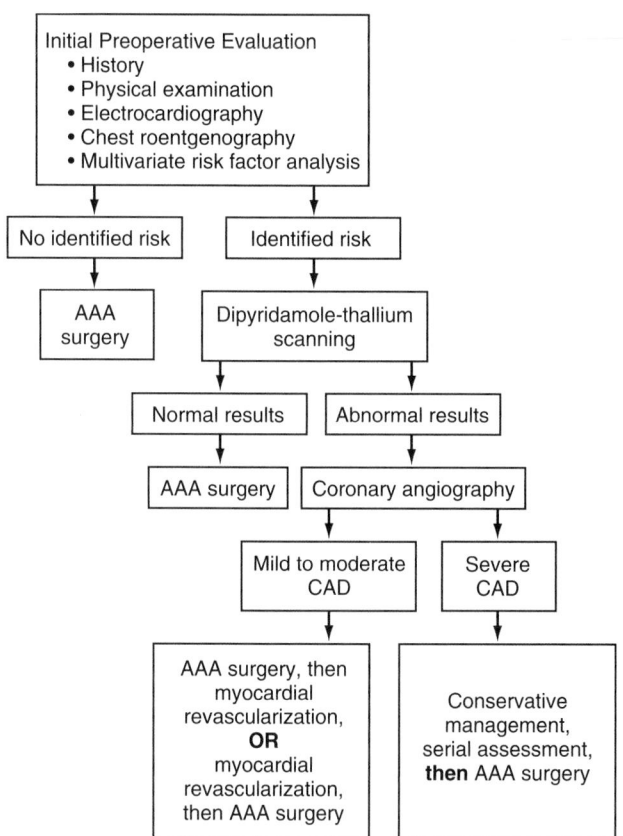

FIGURE **26-2** Algorithm for patient management and surgical selection for abdominal aortic aneurysm (AAA) resection. *CAD*, Coronary artery disease.

TABLE **26-6**	Occurrence of Coexisting Disease in Abdominal Aortic Resections
Disease	**Percent of Patients**
Hypertension	50-60
Heart disease	40-50
Chronic obstructive pulmonary disease	25-50
Diabetes mellitus	9-12
Renal impairment	5-17
Carotid artery disease	6-16

Data from Graor RA. Preoperative evaluation and management of coronary and carotid artery occlusive disease in patients with abdominal aortic aneurysms. Surg Clin North Am. 1989;69:737-743; Cunningham AJ. Anesthesia for abdominal aortic surgery. I: a review. Can J Anaesth. 1989;36:426-444.

stability provided by opioids has been well documented, and this feature is especially attractive for patients with ischemic heart disease and ventricular dysfunction. Provision of intense analgesia for the initial postoperative period after major abdominal vascular surgery (via the administration of neuraxial opioid) does not alter the combined incidence of major cardiovascular, respiratory, and renal complications.[75]

Regional Anesthesia. The use of epidural anesthesia for abdominal aneurysmectomies has gained renewed interest.

Hessel[64] and Yeager and co-workers[76] identified several benefits of epidural use, including decreased preload and afterload, preserved myocardial oxygenation, reduced stress response, excellent muscle relaxation, decreased incidence of postoperative thromboembolism, and increased graft flow to the lower extremities. However, Underwood and associates[19] reported more postoperative complications in the epidural group than in the general anesthetic group in 66 elderly patients who underwent vascular surgery. Hypotension may also be a significant unfavorable result of an epidural technique. In fact, this technique requires the administration of approximately 1600 to 2000 mL more intravenous fluid than is usual with general anesthetic.[64] The controversy regarding hematoma formation after heparinization during epidural techniques is still noteworthy. Rao and El-Etr[77] investigated the neurologic consequences of 3164 epidural anesthetics and 847 subarachnoid blocks; only 20 patients experienced neurologic complications, all of which were self-limiting and resolved with time, demonstrating that the simultaneous use of epidural anesthesia and low-dose heparinization rarely produces complications.

Postoperative pain control is vital for maintaining hemodynamic stability and alleviating patient suffering. Epidural narcotics have been shown to decrease pain after major surgery.[78] Because of the high incidence of CAD in patients presenting for abdominal aortic reconstruction, severe postoperative pain can result in increased heart rate and blood pressure, which may contribute to cardiac-related morbidity and mortality. Pain relief may decrease respiratory splinting and decrease the likelihood of hypoxemia.[79]

Combination Techniques. Combining anesthetic techniques for major vascular surgery is more popular than using them alone; the advantages of each technique contribute to a smoother anesthetic. A balanced technique supplemented by low-dose inhalation agents maintains cardiovascular hemodynamics and controls momentary autonomic responses to surgical stimulation. Similarly, epidural anesthesia combined with light general anesthesia provides the benefits of epidural anesthesia plus the ability to provide amnesia and controlled ventilation.

A combined spinal and epidural anesthetic has been used successfully for infrarenal abdominal aortic aneurysmectomy using an endovascular approach. Aadahl and associates[80] found that a lumbar epidural catheter at L2-L3 followed by a spinal block at L3-L4 using isobaric bupivacaine provided excellent muscle relaxation and hemodynamic stability during surgery. These patients were able to ambulate after the first postoperative day.

In summary, all the aforementioned anesthetic techniques can be used safely and can demonstrate positive outcomes. Even more important than anesthetic selection is the clinical management of each patient. Observation, accurate interpretation, and immediate intervention during the anesthetic process reduce morbidity and mortality to a much larger extent than does selection of the superior anesthetic technique.

Fluid Management

Maintaining intravascular volume may be an extreme challenge during abdominal aortic resections. Controversy exists regarding whether the administration of crystalloids or colloids affects the overall incidence of morbidity and mortality. Crystalloids may be used for replacing basal and third-space losses at an approximate rate of 10 mL/kg/hr.[64] Blood losses initially can be replaced with crystalloids at a ratio of 3:1. The combination of crystalloid and colloid administration is also acceptable. Regardless of the choice of fluid, volume replacement must be dictated by physiologic

parameters. Fluid replacement should be sufficient for the maintenance of normal cardiac filling pressures, cardiac output, and urine output of 1 mL/kg/hr.[7] Patients with limited cardiac reserve can develop congestive heart failure if hypervolemia occurs.

Hemodynamic Alterations

Hemodynamic changes are likely to occur throughout the anesthesia process. Adequate preoperative sedation should be given before placement of invasive monitoring equipment. Momentary fluctuations in heart rate and blood pressure should be anticipated during induction and intubation. Preoperative replacement of fluid deficits prevents exaggerated responses to vasodilating induction agents. For patients with adequate left ventricular function, hemodynamic stability can be preserved with a "slow" induction using opioids and β-adrenergic blocking agents. Etomidate has minimal myocardial depressant effects and may be most suitable for patients with limited cardiac reserve. The response to mesenteric traction (discussed previously) is also associated with momentary hemodynamic changes.

Application of the aortic cross-clamp produces various hemodynamic responses. Patients without underlying ischemic heart disease usually demonstrate slight changes in PAOP when the aorta is occluded, requiring minimal intervention. However, patients with a history of CAD may experience an increase in PAOP and a decrease in cardiac output, indicating left ventricular decompensation. Although several different pharmacologic agents may be used, nitroglycerin appears to be the drug of choice because of its primary pharmacologic effect of decreasing preload and thereby decreasing myocardial oxygen demand.[7,64] Inotropic agents, such as dopamine and dobutamine, may improve cardiac output, whereas pharmacologic agents that decrease afterload, such as sodium nitroprusside and isoflurane, may decrease SVR. The more proximal the application of the aortic cross-clamp, the greater the magnitude and severity of these responses. Vasoactive medications must be readily available throughout the surgery.

When the aortic cross-clamp is released, declamping shock syndrome may occur. Severe hypotension and reduction in cardiac output may ensue. These conditions can be prevented by volume loading and raising the central venous pressure 3 to 5 mm Hg[7] or raising the PAOP 3 to 4 mm Hg[7,55,64] just before the clamp is released. If severe acidosis is present, sodium bicarbonate may be administered.[64] Increasing minute ventilation may be useful for the control of acidosis.

Renal Preservation

The incidence of acute renal failure after infrarenal cross-clamping is 5%, and this value increases to 13% after suprarenal cross-clamping. Mortality is four to five times greater in patients who develop acute renal failure postoperatively. Alterations in renal dynamics during intrarenal cross-clamping may continue up to 1 hour after the clamp is released. Such alterations can be profound and extend into the postoperative period. Mechanisms for preserving renal function during aortic cross-clamping include improving renal and glomerular blood flow. Maintenance of cardiac output and intravascular volume is vital. Prevention of hypovolemia is the best prophylaxis against renal failure.[7] Administration of mannitol 20 to 30 minutes before aortic clamping may help preserve renal function, owing to mannitol's hydroxyl free-radical scavenging properties.[6,64] Further intervention includes intravenous administration of low-dose dopamine at 3 to 5 mcg/kg/min, fenoldopam, and loop diuretics.[64,81] Renal-dose dopamine has not proved to decrease the risk of postoperative renal dysfunction.[82]

Postoperative Considerations

Cardiac, respiratory, and renal failure are the most common complications observed postoperatively in patients recovering from abdominal aortic reconstruction. Cardiovascular function must be closely monitored in the intensive care unit (ICU) for at least 24 hours after surgery. Maintaining adequate blood pressure, intravascular fluid volume, and myocardial oxygenation is paramount during this period. Myocardial infarction frequently contributes to postoperative morbidity and mortality; serial cardiac enzyme analysis may be justified. Pharmacologic agents used in the treatment of hypertension must also be available.

Most patients require ventilatory assistance during the postoperative period. Vigilant monitoring of respiratory function is mandatory, especially when epidural catheters are used for postoperative analgesia. Yeager and colleagues[76] demonstrated fewer postoperative complications and improved pain control when epidural analgesia was provided postoperatively.

Finally, renal function must be continuously evaluated in the postoperative phase. Urine output should be maintained at 1 mL/kg/hr. To improve urine output, administration of fluid, maintenance of physiologic hemodynamics, and concurrent administration of pharmacologic agents should be considered.

Juxtarenal and Suprarenal Aortic Aneurysms

Although most AAAs occur below the level of the renal arteries, 2% extend proximally and involve the renal or visceral arteries.[24,25] Juxtarenal aneurysms are located at the level of the renal arteries, but they spare the renal artery orifice. More proximal suprarenal aneurysms include at least one of the renal arteries and may involve visceral vessels. The effects of aortic cross-clamping for juxtarenal or suprarenal aneurysms are similar to those for infrarenal aortic occlusions; however, the magnitude of hemodynamic alterations increases as the aorta is clamped more proximally.

Preoperative preparation includes a thorough evaluation of coexisting disease, with an emphasis on cardiac function. As the aorta is clamped more proximally, left ventricular afterload increases; consequently, myocardial ischemia is more likely to occur.[26] Diligent cardiac monitoring is necessary, and direct intraarterial blood pressure assessment, cardiac filling pressure monitoring, and transesophageal echocardiography are advocated to detect cardiac dysfunction and allow for immediate pharmacologic intervention.

Renal failure, although possible during infrarenal aortic cross-clamping, occurs more frequently due to suprarenal aortic occlusion. Maintaining adequate intravascular volume and administering osmotic and loop diuretics may minimize renal ischemia and dysfunction. If the ischemic episode persists for longer than 45 minutes, renal cooling is suggested. Renal cooling consists of flushing the kidney with an iced electrolyte perfusate that contains heparin and glucose.[25,60]

Paraplegia is possible when the blood supply to the spinal cord is interrupted by aortic cross-clamping at or above the level of the diaphragm. Increasing the MAP or decreasing cerebrospinal fluid (CSF) pressure may be used as a means to increase spinal cord perfusion pressure.[7,24,25] Box 26-3 summarizes the complications that may result from juxtarenal or suprarenal aortic occlusion.

Ruptured Abdominal Aortic Aneurysm

A high mortality rate of up to 94% is associated with a ruptured AAA.[26,27,37] A wide range of morbidity rates has been reported. One explanation for the discrepancies may be the parameters used for the definition of "rupture." Centers that have reported lower mortality rates may not be truly assessing rupture as intraperitoneal hemorrhage. Rutherford and McCroskey[38] attempted to identify mortality rates related to hemodynamic status. Their findings are presented in Table 26-7. This information further demonstrates the need for earlier detection of aneurysms and aggressive surgical intervention.

The most common symptoms of ruptured AAAs are abdominal discomfort with a pulsatile mass, back pain, decreased peripheral pulses, and hypotension.[36,38,83] Hypotension and a history of cardiac disease are two factors associated with the poorest prognosis.[23,37] Patients with these symptoms should be immediately transferred to the operating room for surgical exploration. When hypotension is absent, more time is available for a comprehensive CT scan to search for other causes of abdominal discomfort. Figure 26-3 provides a plan for the evaluation and treatment of the patient with a symptomatic but unruptured aneurysm.

Once the patient arrives in the operative suite, a brief preoperative evaluation, establishing venous access, and provisions

---

BOX 26-3

Potential Complications of Juxtarenal or Suprarenal Aortic Occlusion

- Renal failure
- Hemorrhage
- Distal arterial occlusion
- Infarction
- Pulmonary or cardiac dysfunction
- Impotence
- Paraplegia
- Thrombosis
- Pseudoaneurysm formation
- Aortoenteric fistula

From Hollier LH, Moore WM. Surgical management of juxtarenal and suprarenal aortic aneurysms. Acta Chir Scand. *1990;555(Suppl): 117-122.*

TABLE **26-7**	Mortality Rates for Ruptured Aortic Aneurysms Related to Hemodynamic Status at Time of Presentation
Hemodynamic Status	**Mortality Rate (%)**
Normal blood pressure	20
Hypotensive, but responding to resuscitation	40
Hypotensive, incompletely responding to resuscitation	60
Hypotension recurs with induction (unstable), incompletely responding to resuscitation	60
Hypotension recurs with induction (unstable), no urinary output	80

Data from Rutherford RB, McCroskey BL. Ruptured abdominal aortic aneurysms. Surg Clin North Am. *1989;69:859-868.*

for fluid and blood product administration can be completed. Induction of anesthesia should follow the principles of trauma anesthesia. Hemodynamic stability must be the primary objective, and anesthetic induction and maintenance agents must be selected on a case-by-case basis.

Cardiovascular resuscitation is the anesthetist's primary focus until blood loss from the proximal aorta is controlled by surgical intervention. Fluid resuscitation can begin with crystalloids, and blood products can be administered as they become available. Intraoperative blood salvage provisions should be secured. If large amounts of blood products are given, coagulation studies and ionized calcium values should be calculated. The use of fresh frozen plasma has been shown to decrease the total transfusion requirements and the incidence of coagulopathies.[23] The ability to administer platelets may also be necessary.

After initial fluid resuscitation has been performed and hemodynamic stability has been ensured, direct arterial blood pressure monitoring must be instituted. A central venous or pulmonary artery catheter may be inserted. The hemodynamic effects of aortic cross-clamping and release are similar to those for elective surgery; however, responses may be extreme, especially if hypotension exists when the clamp is released. Measures for ensuring the adequacy of renal circulation, such as administering mannitol, should be incorporated. Because mannitol is an osmotic diuretic, decreased vascular volume resulting in hypotension can occur. Because most patients require large amounts of fluid and blood replacement, postoperative mechanical ventilation is recommended.

THORACIC AORTIC ANEURYSMS

The mortality associated with thoracic aneurysms is well established. Patients with aortic dissections have only a 3-month survival if they do not undergo surgical repair, because the incidence of rupture is high.[84] Aneurysms have been described in the literature for hundreds of years, but not until 1951 did the development of the arterial prosthesis lead to successful bypass options.[85] The refinement of synthetic grafts, surgical and perfusion techniques, and intraoperative management has contributed to improved surgical outcomes. Today the early mortality rate is thought to be less than 10%, demonstrating that elective surgical intervention is an acceptable means of treating thoracic aortic aneurysms.[86,87]

Classification

Aneurysms of the thoracic aorta may be classified with respect to type, shape, and location. Typically, aneurysms involving all three layers of the arterial wall—tunica adventitia, tunica media, and tunica intima—are considered to be *true aneurysms*. In comparison, aneurysms that solely involve the adventitia are termed *false aneurysms*. The shape of the lesion can also serve as a means of characterizing aneurysms. Fusiform aneurysms have a spindle shape and result in dilation of the aorta. Saccular aneurysms are spherical dilations and are generally limited to only one segment of the vessel wall. Aortic dissection is the result of a spontaneous tear within the intima that permits the flow of blood through a false passage along the longitudinal axis of the aorta. Aneurysms can also be classified according to their location within the aortic arch (Figure 26-4). In addition, thoracoabdominal aneurysms can be classified into four types on the basis of their location, as illustrated in Figure 26-5.

Etiology

Atherosclerosis is the most common cause of aneurysmal pathology. Atherosclerotic lesions occur most often in the descending and distal thoracic aorta and are most often classified as fusiform. Less common causes include the histologic contributions of cystic medial necrosis observed in patients with Marfan syndrome, infective and inflammatory processes within the vessel wall, and Takayasu arteritis.[88,89] Finally, aneurysms that were once related to syphilitic aortitis are now rarely observed, as a result

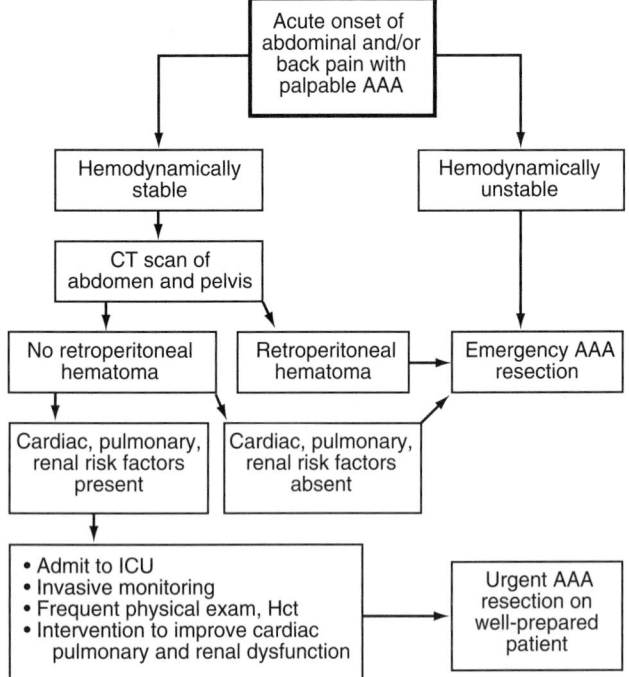

FIGURE **26-3** Algorithm for the management of the patient with an unruptured symptomatic abdominal aortic aneurysm (AAA). *CT*, Computed tomography; *Hct*, hematocrit; *ICU*, intensive care unit. (*From Sullivan CA et al. Clinical management of symptomatic but unruptured abdominal aortic aneurysm. J Vasc Surg. 1990;11:799-802.*)

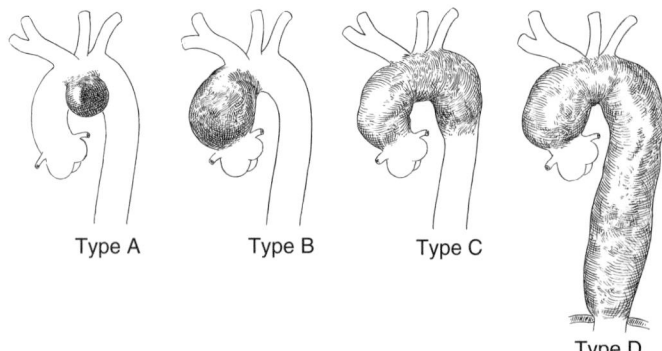

FIGURE **26-4** Cooley classification of aortic arch aneurysms. *Type A,* Saccular transverse arch. *Type B,* Fusiform ascending aorta and proximal arch. *Type C,* Fusiform aneurysm extending into the proximal aorta. *Type D,* Fusiform aneurysm involving the entire aorta.

of the advent of early diagnosis and treatment of syphilis. The various causes of arterial aneurysms are classified in Box 26-4.

Diagnosis

The symptomatology of thoracic aneurysms is often related to the site of the lesion and its compression on adjacent structures. Pain, stridor, and cough may result from compression of thoracic structures. Symptoms related to aortic insufficiency may be observed in aneurysms of the ascending aorta. An upper mediastinal mass may be an incidental finding on conventional chest radiography in an asymptomatic patient. Further investigation with noninvasive methods (e.g., CT scan, MRI) can describe the configuration and location of the aneurysm. Invasive aortography, although associated with a higher risk of complications, provides the most information because it allows evaluation of the coronary vessels and branches of the aortic arch.

Treatment

As previously described, a high mortality rate is associated with rupture of thoracic aneurysms. Crawford and DeNatale[90] investigated the survival of 94 patients who did not undergo surgery for thoracoabdominal aneurysms. The investigators reported that only 24% of the patients survived 2 years after detection of the lesion, and 50% of the deaths were the result of aortic rupture. Therefore early detection and surgical intervention have made a significant contribution to long-term survival.

Surgical approach and mode of resection vary according to the location of the lesion within the thoracic aorta. Resection of the ascending aorta and graft replacement necessitate the use of cardiopulmonary bypass. The aortic valve may also require replacement. Surgical resection of lesions in the transverse arch compromises cerebral perfusion, although various bypass techniques combined with profound hypothermia and circulatory arrest have been used.[91] Aneurysms of the descending aorta may be resected by application of an aortic cross-clamp. However, perfusion to distal organs can be compromised during this procedure.

AORTIC DISSECTION

As mentioned previously, aortic dissection is characterized by a spontaneous tear of the vessel wall intima, permitting the passage of blood along a false lumen. Although the cause of the dissection is unclear, lesions that were thought to be related to cystic necrotic processes may actually be caused by variations in wall integrity. Hypertension is the most common factor that contributes to the progression of the lesion. Manipulation of the ascending aorta during cardiac surgery may be associated with aortic dissection.[92] The symptoms of aortic dissection are the result of interruption of blood supply to vital organs. The most serious complication is aneurysm rupture. Diagnosis can be accomplished by the previously mentioned noninvasive techniques; however, aortography appears to be most reliable. Simon and associates[93] evaluated the efficacy of transesophageal echocardiography as a diagnostic tool for the detection and analysis of aortic dissections in 32 patients. The authors concluded that this bedside modality allows for the reliable, expedient diagnosis and

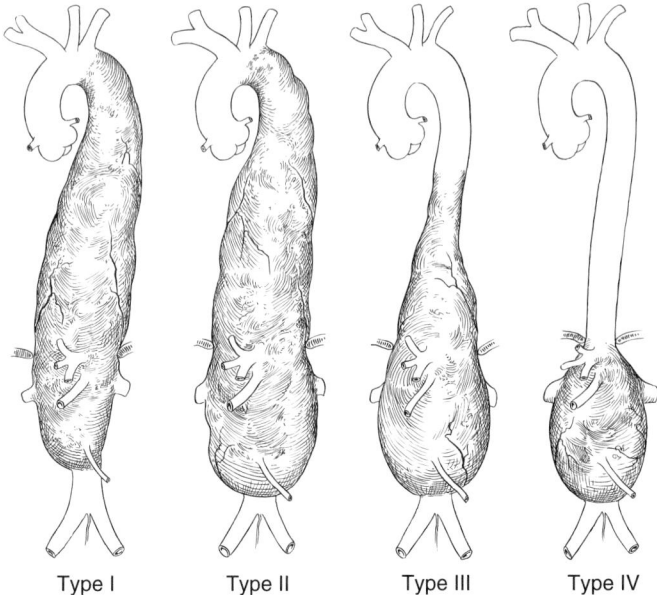

Type I   Type II   Type III   Type IV

FIGURE **26-5** Classification of thoracoabdominal aneurysms. *Type I*, Begins distal to the subclavian artery and extends to involve visceral artery orifices. *Type II*, Involves most of the descending aorta and most or all of the abdominal aorta. *Type III*, Involves the distal descending thoracic aorta and varying segments of the abdominal aorta. *Type IV*, Involves most or all of the abdominal aorta, including segments of visceral vessel origins.

BOX 26-4

Classification of Arterial Aneurysms by Cause

Congenital (Developmental)
Ehlers-Danlos syndrome
Marfan syndrome

Mechanical (Hemodynamic)
Poststenotic
Arteriovenous fistula associated
Traumatic
Blunt or penetrating trauma

Inflammatory (Noninfectious)
Takayasu disease
Behçet disease
Kawasaki disease
Microvascular disorder (e.g., polyarteritis)
Periarterial inflammatory disease (e.g., pancreatitis)

Infectious
Bacterial
Fungal
Spirochetal

Degenerative
Nonspecific (commonly considered arteriosclerotic), dysplastic

Anastomosis
Postarteriotomy

Modified from Johnston KW et al. Subcommittee on Reporting Standards for Arterial Aneurysms, Ad Hoc Committee on Reporting Standards, Society for Vascular Surgery and North American Chapter of International Society for Cardiovascular Surgery. Suggested standards for reporting on arterial aneurysms. J Vasc Surg. 1992;13:452-458.

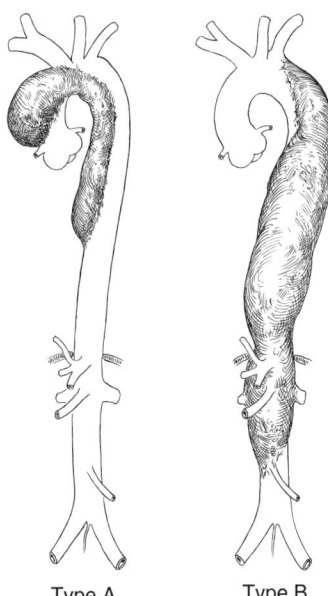

FIGURE **26-6** Types of aortic dissection. *Type A* involves the ascending aorta and may extend into the aortic arch. *Type B* starts at the proximal descending aorta and extends distally.

TABLE **26-8**	Risk Factors Identified in 101 Patients Undergoing Thoracoabdominal Aneurysm Repair	
Risk Factors		**Incidence (%)**
Smoking history		90
Coronary artery disease		67
Chronic lung disease		42
Renal insufficiency		38
Strokes or transient ischemic attacks		12
Diabetes mellitus		6

Modified from Hollier LH, Moore WM. Avoidance of renal and neurologic complications following thoracoabdominal aortic aneurysm repair. Acta Chir Scand. 1990;55(suppl):129-135.

TABLE **26-9**	Early Causes of Death in 54 Patients After Thoracoabdominal Aneurysm Repair	
Cause		**Incidence (%)**
Cardiac		44
Renal		37
Pulmonary		18
Sepsis		19
Stroke		9
Hemorrhage		9
Pulmonary embolus		7
Gastrointestinal bleeding		7

Modified from Hollier LH et al. Thoracoabdominal aortic aneurysm repair: analysis of postoperative morbidity. Arch Surg. 1988;123:871-875.

classification of thoracic lesions, thereby allowing urgent surgical intervention.

Treatment of dissecting aortic lesions depends on their location within the thoracic aorta (Figure 26-6). Type A lesions have the highest incidence of rupture and require immediate surgical intervention. Type B lesions may initially be managed medically, with the administration of arterial dilating and β-adrenergic blocking agents. However, some authors suggest that surgical intervention contributes to an improved long-term survival rate.[75] Studies by investigators using the newer techniques have shown a survival rate of 94% to 95% for repair of dissecting aortic aneurysm.[75,94]

In summary, surgical resection of thoracic aortic lesions enhances long-term survival. Refinement of surgical techniques and improvement in perfusion technology have reduced mortality rates to less than 10%. The surgical method used is dependent on the location of the aortic lesion. Anesthesia for aneurysms of the ascending and transverse aorta requires cardiopulmonary bypass.

DESCENDING THORACIC AND THORACOABDOMINAL ANEURYSMS

Preoperative Assessment

Patients who undergo major vascular surgery are frequently elderly and have varying degrees of concurrent disease. The incidence of thoracic aortic aneurysm is increasing, and the 5-year survival rate after diagnosis without intervention is 9% to 13%.[35] Crawford and colleagues[91] described the frequency with which atherosclerotic occlusive disease, heart disease, chronic obstructive pulmonary disease, hypertension, and renal insufficiency occurred in 605 patients who had thoracic aortic aneurysms. In this study, advancing age, atherosclerotic heart disease, chronic obstructive pulmonary disease, renal artery occlusive disease, and renal insufficiency were associated with diseases that most often contributed to early death. Hollier and Moore[95] identified risk factors associated with thoracoabdominal aneurysms in a smaller group consisting of 101 patients. Risk factors identified for patients undergoing thoracoabdominal aneurysmectomies are listed in Table 26-8.

The importance of a thorough preoperative evaluation cannot be overemphasized in this patient population. Special attention should be directed toward cardiac, renal, and neurologic function. Although most fatalities related to thoracic aortic surgery are cardiac in origin, renal and neurologic dysfunction contribute to poor surgical outcomes.[87] Table 26-9 lists the causes of early death after thoracoabdominal aneurysm repair. Preoperative renal dysfunction is directly related to postoperative renal failure and is thought to be one of the strongest contributors to renal deterioration after surgery.[87,95] Neurologic function should be carefully assessed in the preoperative phase. Because paraplegia is one of the most devastating consequences of thoracic aortic surgery, any alteration in lower-extremity function should be noted. Hoarseness related to compression of the recurrent laryngeal nerve should be assessed and documented. The left recurrent laryngeal nerve is most susceptible to damage because of its close proximity to the aortic arch. Bilateral recurrent laryngeal nerve compression or damage can result in respiratory compromise.

Intraoperative Management
Monitoring

Intraoperative monitoring devices used for thoracoabdominal aneurysm resection are the same as those used for abdominal aneurysmectomies. Direct intraarterial blood pressure and pulmonary artery pressure monitoring is mandatory. If the aneurysm involves the thoracic region or the distal aortic arch, right radial arterial line monitoring is preferred because left subclavian arterial blood flow may be compromised during surgery. Use of two-dimensional transesophageal echocardiography is suggested for cardiac monitoring in patients with myocardial dysfunction. An indwelling urinary catheter is used for assessing renal function. To facilitate exposing the descending thoracic aorta, a double-lumen endotracheal tube is inserted to allow for one-lung ventilation. As a result, careful monitoring of oxygenation is mandatory. Pulmonary artery catheters equipped with fiberoptics are useful for measuring mixed venous oxygen. Routine use of pulse oximetry may be limited if the left subclavian artery is manipulated; therefore, the right hand, the ear, or the nasal passages should be used for monitoring oxygen saturation. Finally, a lumbar intrathecal catheter is inserted to access CSF. Somatosensory evoked potentials or MEPs may be used to detect neurologic dysfunction; however, their clinical usefulness remains uncertain.[95-98]

Aortic Cross-Clamping

Simple aortic cross-clamping and graft replacement is an acceptable method for surgical repair of descending thoracic or thoracoabdominal aortic aneurysms.[87] Application of a simple cross-clamp has eliminated the need for shunts and extracorporeal circulation. However, the consequences of this maneuver include myocardial compromise and occlusion of blood flow to distal structures. The hemodynamic alterations produced by the application of an aortic clamp have previously been discussed. Similar responses are observed during proximal aortic occlusion; however, the magnitude of these responses is extreme. When the aorta is occluded, afterload and therefore myocardial workload increase. As a result, increases occur in left ventricular end-diastolic pressure, left ventricular stroke work index, and myocardial oxygen consumption.[86,99-101] When oxygen demands are not accompanied by an increase in oxygen supply, ischemia results, and myocardial failure can occur. Although methods have been instituted to decrease myocardial afterload (e.g., partial bypass and shunts), the use of sodium nitroprusside appears to be the most effective means of decreasing afterload during cross-clamp application.[86,99] To decrease preload during aortic occlusion, administration of nitroglycerin may be required.[99]

Hemodynamic Alterations

The hemodynamic consequences of releasing the aortic cross-clamp are similar to those of abdominal aortic occlusion, but they are of greater magnitude. Metabolites that have accumulated during aortic cross-clamping are released into circulation. The combination of reactive hyperemia and sequestration of blood volume within hypoperfused areas can lead to severe hypotension. Guided by left-sided filling pressures, restoration of blood volume before the gradual release of the clamp can minimize hemodynamic alterations. Increasing ventilation and administering sodium bicarbonate may control carbon dioxide increases at the time of declamping.

Spinal Cord Ischemia

Neurologic dysfunction is a serious complication of thoracic aortic reconstruction. The incidence of paraplegia is reported

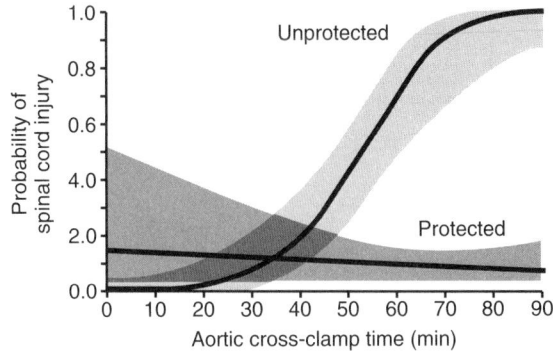

FIGURE 26-7 Relationship between probability of spinal cord injury and length of aortic occlusion. Note that risk of spinal cord injury increases substantially after 45 minutes of aortic occlusion for patients without protection of distal circulation. No such relationship between probability of spinal cord injury and length of aortic occlusion was noted for patients with protection of distal circulation. Shaded areas indicate the 70% confidence limits. (*From Jex RK et al. Early and late results after repair of dissections of the descending thoracic aorta.* J Vasc Surg. *1986;3:226-267.*)

to be approximately 20% after elective surgery and as high as 40% after surgery for dissecting and ruptured aneurysms.[95,100,101] Neurologic deficits are the result of hypoperfusion to the spinal cord during thoracic aortic reconstruction. The artery of Adamkiewicz, also known as the *greater radicular artery*, originates from an intercostal branch between T8 and L2 and provides the majority of blood flow to the anterior spinal artery. The anterior spinal artery perfuses the ventral aspect of the spinal cord, which is responsible for motor control.[95] Although attempts have been made to reimplant the intercostal branches that contribute blood flow to the spinal cord, these efforts do not always decrease the incidence of paraplegia.[95,102] The duration of aortic occlusion also contributes to spinal cord ischemia (Figure 26-7). Jex and co-workers[103] suggest that damage to the spinal cord can occur in as little as 34 minutes of unprotected aortic occlusion.

Several techniques have been described in an attempt to decrease the incidence of neurologic dysfunction after thoracic aortic surgery. However, few techniques have proved to decrease spinal cord ischemia. Systemic hypothermia and selective cooling of the spinal cord may lengthen ischemic time intervals; however, the clinical benefits of these methods are unclear.[99,104] The use of various bypass mechanisms and distal shunts may minimize the length of aortic occlusion time, but the risks associated with implementing these techniques could be greater than the potential benefits.

One method that has been successful is CSF drainage. McCullough and associates[101] reported a decrease in the incidence of paraplegia when CSF was drained before the thoracic aorta was cross-clamped in animal models. CSF drainage involves manipulation of spinal cord perfusion pressure during aortic clamping. *Spinal cord perfusion pressure* can be defined as the arterial pressure minus the CSF pressure. During aortic clamping, CSF pressure increases while arterial pressure decreases distal to the clamp. The spinal cord perfusion pressure can therefore be manipulated by altering arterial blood pressure and draining CSF through the intrathecal catheter.[103,104] Hollier and Moore[95] reported no cases of paraplegia in more than 50 patients who

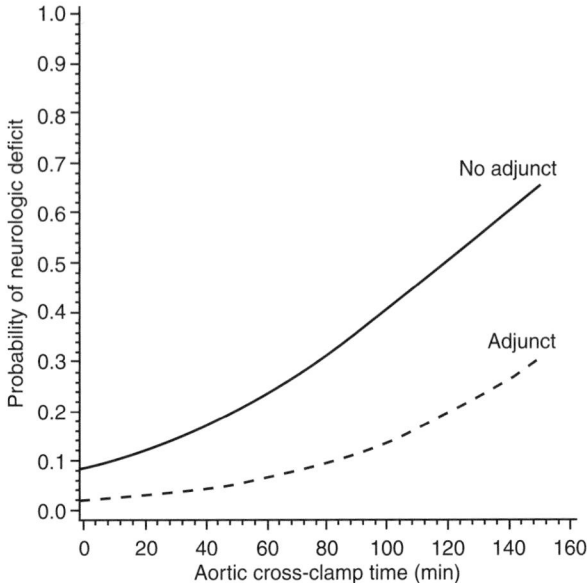

FIGURE **26-8** The probability of neurologic deficit increases with clamp time and is markedly higher in patients undergoing thoracoabdominal aortic aneurysm surgery without adjuncts. Adjuncts include distal aortic perfusion and cerebrospinal fluid drainage. (*From Rutherford RB et al. Vascular Surgery, 6th ed. Philadelphia: Saunders; 2005*)

From Hollier LH, Moore WM. Avoidance of renal and neurologic complications following thoracoabdominal aortic aneurysm repair. Acta Chir Scand. 1990;555(suppl):129-135.

underwent thoracic or thoracoabdominal aneurysm repairs in which CSF drainage was used.

Several studies have attempted to identify metabolic markers that are predictors of spinal cord ischemia. Drenger and colleagues[105] found that during and after thoracic aortic occlusion, a dramatic increase occurs in CSF lactate levels. Patients who became paraplegic had higher CSF lactate levels compared with those who were neurologically intact postoperatively. Van Dongen and colleagues[106] observed that S-100 protein, which is only found in glial and Schwann cells, is released during acute damage to the central nervous system. Increases in S-100 protein concentration occurred after aortic cross-clamping, despite normal SSEP and MEP monitoring values.

Methods for detecting spinal cord ischemia were previously discussed. The intraoperative use of SSEPs and MEPs can provide early identification of neurologic dysfunction, but these monitoring modalities do not ensure spinal cord integrity. Factors that contribute to the development of neurologic deficit include level of aortic clamp application, ischemic time, embolization or thrombosis of a critical intercostal artery, failure to revascularize intercostal arteries, and urgency of surgical intervention.[86,87] Neurologic dysfunction has also been reported to occur in the postoperative phase. Delayed paraplegia may be the result of reperfusion injury, although the exact mechanism of injury has not been proved.[86,101,107] Figure 26-8 shows the probability of neurologic deficits associated with aortic cross-clamp time with and without adjunctive measures.

Renal Dysfunction

The incidence of renal dysfunction after thoracoabdominal aortic resection is estimated to be between 30% and 50%. The possibility of permanent renal failure requiring hemodialysis is estimated to be between 2% and 12%.[95] The cause of renal insufficiency is ischemia related to aortic occlusion. Crawford and colleagues[91] identified preoperative renal dysfunction as one of the most significant factors that contributes to postoperative renal failure. These investigators also showed that renal artery perfusion with cold lactate solution demonstrated no apparent benefit with regard to renal function. Intraoperative hypotension has been identified as an independent predictor of postoperative renal dysfunction.[86] Maintenance of intravascular volume and stable circulatory status appears to be the most reliable method of minimizing renal dysfunction. Preoperatively, volume status should be corrected with non–glucose-containing crystalloid solutions. Intraoperative volume replacement should be guided by invasive monitoring. Pharmacologic adjuncts to produce diuresis, such as mannitol and furosemide, should be given approximately 20 to 30 minutes before clamp application.[99] Low-dose dopamine is also advocated as a means of increasing renal perfusion.

In summary, neurologic and renal dysfunction are devastating consequences of thoracic and thoracoabdominal aortic resections. A complete preoperative evaluation, identification of risk, optimization of organ function, and use of the suggested methods to minimize the consequences of ischemia all contribute to optimal surgical outcomes. Additional complications of thoracoabdominal aortic reconstruction are listed in Box 26-5.

Anesthetic Management

The principles of perioperative management of thoracic or thoracoabdominal aneurysms are similar to those previously discussed for abdominal aortic aneurysmectomies. Anesthetic selection should be based on the presence of concomitant disease processes, with the objective of maintaining cardiovascular stability and minimizing morbidity and mortality. Intraoperative monitoring should focus on detection of myocardial, neurologic, and renal ischemia. The hemodynamic consequences of aortic cross-clamping should be attenuated by the use of pharmacologic adjuncts. Restoration of circulating blood volume, as guided by left-sided filling pressure, minimizes the hemodynamic alterations caused by the release of the aortic clamp.

Unique to thoracic aortic surgery is the use of one-lung ventilation. To detect potential inadequacies in ventilation and oxygenation with this approach, the highest degree of vigilance must be used. Extreme blood loss should be anticipated. Venous access and blood product availability should be confirmed during the preoperative phase. Methods of minimizing the use of homologous blood products (e.g., perioperative blood salvage) can be used. Coagulopathy is a constant threat with the administration of blood products. Close monitoring of coagulation parameters and administration of fresh frozen plasma, platelets, or specific coagulation factors can minimize the incidence and severity of coagulopathies.

Postoperative Considerations

After surgery is completed, if a double-lumen endotracheal tube was used, it should be replaced with a standard endotracheal tube to provide a secure airway because postoperative ventilatory assistance is usually required. Anatomic landmarks may have become edematous during surgery, causing difficulty with reintubation. Under these circumstances, the double-lumen endotracheal tube may be left in place. Replacement, guided by fiberoptic evaluation, can proceed in the postoperative period after the airway edema has dissipated.

Close observation of circulatory and pulmonary status is warranted in the postoperative phase. Hemodynamic control is vital to maintaining perfusion to vital organs without creating excessive demands on the heart or the aortic graft. Administration of dopamine may be continued during this time. Careful monitoring of respiratory status aided by arterial blood gas analysis is important. Epidural analgesia using local anesthetics, narcotics, or both can be administered for pain relief.

ENDOVASCULAR AORTIC ANEURYSM REPAIR

In 1991, the first endovascular stent was performed to repair an infrarenal aortic aneurysm. The development of this technique has created a less invasive approach to aortic aneurysm repair. Studies suggest that severe cardiac and respiratory pathology make as many as 30% of patients with aortic aneurysms poor surgical candidates.[108] Endovascular aortic aneurysm repair (EVAR) was initially intended for patients with severe coexisting disease, but its popularity has increased as the success of the procedure has improved. It is estimated that 20,000 EVAR procedures a year now take place in the United States, accounting for 36% of aortic aneurysm repairs.[109] Schermerhorn and colleagues suggested that the patient population who may benefit most from EVAR are high-risk patients.[110]

The largest source of data is EUROSTAR (EUROpean collaborators on Stent/graft Techniques for aortic Aneurysm Repair), a registry that provides insight on the potential advantages and shortcomings of EVAR. The registry contains data on 5466 patients treated over 6 years in 135 European medical centers. The patient population included patients with infrarenal aortic aneurysms. Results suggest that the larger the diameter of

the AAA (greater than 5.5 cm), the greater the 30-day mortality rate. Cumulatively, the 30-day operative mortality was 2.5%. There were no statistically significant differences in the AAA-related death rate at 1 year comparing EVAR with open surgical treatment (98.2% versus 98.6%).[111] Five years after EVAR, the patient survival rate was 76%. There was a low incidence of intraoperative AAA rupture with EVAR, occurring in only 32 patients. The cumulative rate of rupture was estimated to be approximately 1% per year. *Endoleak* (defined as persistent blood flow and pressure ["endotension"] between the endovascular graft and the aortic aneurysm), graft migration, and kinking were determined to be significant risk factors for late open conversion. The overall risk of late failure was approximately 3% per year.[110,112]

The results comparing EVAR with traditional open AAA repair for abdominal aortic aneurysm assessing short-term success are promising. There are currently two large randomized controlled studies comparing the effects of EVAR to open AAA repair. These include the Endovascular Aneurysm Repair Trial 1 (EVAR 1), and the Dutch Randomized Endovascular Aneurysm Management (DREAM). A national audit of the effectiveness of EVAR by the Canadian Institute for Health Information database provides information that supports the endovascular technique.

The purpose of the EVAR 1 trial was to determine which surgical intervention—endovascular or open aneurysmectomy—was superior in patients who were deemed fit for open AAA repair. Patients were randomized to either the EVAR group (n = 543) or the open AAA repair group (n = 539). The 30-day mortality rate was 1.7% in the EVAR group versus 4.7% in the open AAA repair group. Secondary interventions were more common in the EVAR group (9.8% versus 5.8%).[113] However, there was no significant difference between the groups with respect to 2-year survival.

The DREAM study was a multicenter randomized controlled trial comparing short-term results (30 days) of conventional and endovascular repair of AAAs in 345 patients whose aneurysms were a minimum of 5 cm in diameter. For the open repair group, the operative mortality was 4.6%, and severe complications occurred in 9.8% of patients. In the EVAR group, operative mortality was 1.2%, and severe complications occurred in 4.7% of patients. The conclusion was that EVAR was superior to open repair in this patient population. However, it was also determined that 2-year moderate and severe adverse patient events were nearly identical for both groups. The researchers stated that long-term follow-up studies were needed to determine whether the advantages of EVAR would be sustained.[114]

The Canadian National Audit included results from 1996 patients with nonruptured AAAs. A comparison of EVAR (n = 178) versus open aneurysm repair (n = 1818) was completed. The findings indicated that in-hospital mortality was 0.6% and mean length of stay (LOS) was 5.8 days for EVAR, whereas in-hospital mortality for open procedures was 4.6% and LOS 11.9 days. The conclusion was that EVAR was presently being underused in Canada.[115]

Endovascular aortic aneurysm repair is also being used to treat patients with thoracic aortic aneurysms. The mortality rate for EVAR for elective descending thoracic aneurysm repairs range from 3.5 to 12.5%, as compared to an open approach, where mortality is approximately 10%.[116] Reports also show that EVAR has a low incidence (0 to 6%) of spinal cord ischemia and paraplegia.[117] Potential explanations for the absence of spinal cord complications are (1) no thoracic aortic cross-clamping and (2) no prolonged periods of extreme hypotension. Perioperative hypotension (MAP <70 mm Hg) was a significant predictor of spinal cord ischemia in patients having EVAR for thoracic aneurysm repair.[118] Endograft therapy has also been used with success and may eventually become the treatment of choice for thoracic aneurysm repair in patients older than 75 years of age.[119]

The mortality rate for patients with a ruptured AAA who are alive when diagnosed in emergency departments is 40% to 70%.[120] Since the 1950s, mortality from ruptured AAAs has only decreased 3.5% per decade.[121] The EVAR approach has been used successfully to repair ruptured AAAs, but the number of patients treated and the quality of randomized controlled data on this subject are limited. However, 30-day mortality rates were 10% to 45%.[122] Medical centers that consider EVAR for ruptured AAA repair must have emergent CT imaging capabilities, trained endovascular teams, adequate endovascular supplies available, and a surgical suite.

From the data presented above, it would appear that EVAR is clearly advantageous to the traditional open AAA repair. However, there are questions about the procedure that have yet to be answered, most importantly, Is there a long-term survival benefit to EVAR? As described in EVAR 1, reinterventions due to endoleak were required in three times as many patients who had EVAR. Of these, 7% of endoleaks were discovered within 1 month of implantation and another 13% occurred within 4 years postoperatively.[124] Problems with graft migration and durability are the primary determinants of this complication. However, the majority of this data was collected while physicians were implanting first- and second-generation endografts. Newer generation endografts and superior surgical techniques may decrease this adverse effect in the future. A comparison of outcomes evaluating EVAR and open AAA repair in nearly 23,000 patients was reported.[123] The conclusion was that EVAR was associated with lower short-term morbidity and mortality. Three-year survival rates were similar for both surgical approaches. Further randomized controlled studies must be done on the long-term effects of EVAR.

Procedure

Endovascular aortic aneurysm repair involves deployment of an endovascular stent graft within the aortic lumen. The graft restricts blood flow to the portion or the aorta where the aneurysm exists. This procedure can be performed for patients who have descending thoracic aortic aneurysms or AAAs. Cannulation of both femoral arteries is performed. As seen in

Figure 26-9, a guide wire is threaded through the iliac artery to the level of the aneurysm. Next, a sheath is inserted over the guide wire and positioned at the aneurysm location through use of fluoroscopy. The proximal end of the sheath must extend beyond the aneurysm. Once the sheath is deployed, radial force or fixation mechanisms such as hooks or barbs on the stent become embedded into the aortic wall to prevent stent migration (Figure 26-10).

The procedure frequently takes place in an interventional radiology suite. Compared with the conventional surgical method, advantages of the endovascular approach include improved hemodynamic stability, decreased incidence of embolic events, decreased blood loss, reduced stress response, decreased incidence of renal dysfunction, and decreased postoperative discomfort.[125,126] Systemic anticoagulation with heparin, 50 to 100 units/kg, is administered prior to catheter manipulation.[127] A first-generation cephalosporin is recommended at the beginning of surgery. The anesthetic techniques that can be used for EVAR include general anesthesia neuroaxial blockade or local anesthesia with sedation.[128] There is presently a lack of data suggesting that one anesthetic technique is superior for patients having EVAR. Verhoeven and colleagues determined that local anesthesia with sedation, as compared to general anesthesia, was associated with a decrease in nonfatal cardiac morbidity, respiratory complications, renal failure, and overall mortality.[129,130] Further studies are needed to determine if an ideal anesthetic technique exists. The goals for intraoperative management for EVAR include maintaining hemodynamic stability, providing analgesia and anxiolysis, and being prepared to rapidly convert to an open procedure.

With infrarenal or suprarenal EVAR, creatinine clearance values decreased by 10% in the first year.[131] However, proximal endovascular graft migration can occur, causing renal artery occlusion and postoperative renal failure.[132] Further randomized controlled trials are needed to substantiate these results. Plasma catecholamine concentrations and mediators of the systemic immune response were decreased in patients who underwent the endovascular approach as compared with patients who underwent conventional repair.[133,134] Pearson and colleagues determined that plasma cortisol release was lower in patients having EVAR than in traditional open AAA repair. The EVAR group also developed significantly less sepsis and systemic immune response syndrome.[135] Complications that can arise from the EVAR approach include endograft thrombosis, migration or

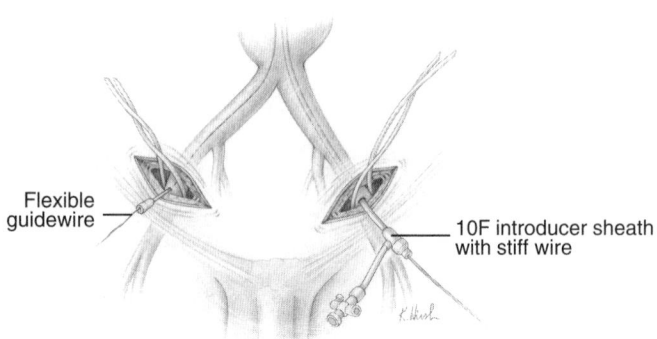

Flexible guidewire

10F introducer sheath with stiff wire

FIGURE **26-9**　Femoral cutdown and insertion of introducer sheath. (*From Zarins CK, Fewertz BL. Atlas of Vascular Surgery. 2nd ed. Philadelphia: Churchill Livingstone; 2005.*)

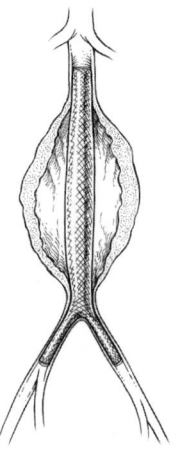

FIGURE **26-10**　Aortic endovascular graft.

rupture, graft infection, iliac artery rupture, and lower extremity ischemia.[136] Fatal cerebral embolism resulting in sudden respiratory arrest has occurred during EVAR.[137] Box 26-6 lists potential complications associated with EVAR.

Endovascular graft design and durability continue to improve. Graft devices are either unibody (comes in one piece) or modular (comes in multiple pieces). The endograft fabric is either woven polyester (Dacron) or polytetrafluoroethylene. There is no significant difference in biologic response when comparing these two materials.[138] The graft skeleton is constructed of stainless steel, nitinol, or Elgiloy (Figure 26-11). Nitinol stents are popular because they exhibit minimal shortening after deployment. There is considerable interest and research involving drug eluting stents. Drugs being tested are immunomodulators, antiinflammatories, and antiproliferative drugs. Researchers have shown in initial clinical trials that restenosis rates are improved with the newer-generation endovascular stents.[139,140]

Endoleak, shown in Figure 26-12 and noted earlier as persistent blood flow and pressure (endotension) between the endovascular graft and the aortic aneurysm, is a serious complication of this procedure. Types of endoleaks are listed in Table 26-10. Endoleak diagnosed by postoperative CT scan has been reported to occur in 15% to 52% of patients.[141] Most are type II, and 70%

BOX 26-6

Potential Complications Associated with EVAR

Graft and Deployment Complications
 Failed deployment
 Microembolization
 Migration/occlusion of major branch arteries
  (i.e., renal, mesenteric)
 Aortic perforation/aneurysm rupture
 Aortic dissection
 Hematoma formation
 Endoleak
 Stenosis/kink/thrombosis
 Graft tear
 Damage to access arteries (femoral → iliac)
 Infection

Radiologic Implications
 Radiation exposure
 Allergy to contrast dye
 Renal insufficiency from contrast dye

Systemic Complications
 Cardiac morbidity/mortality
 Pulmonary insufficiency
 Renal insufficiency
 Postimplant syndrome

EVAR, *Endovascular aneurysm repair.*

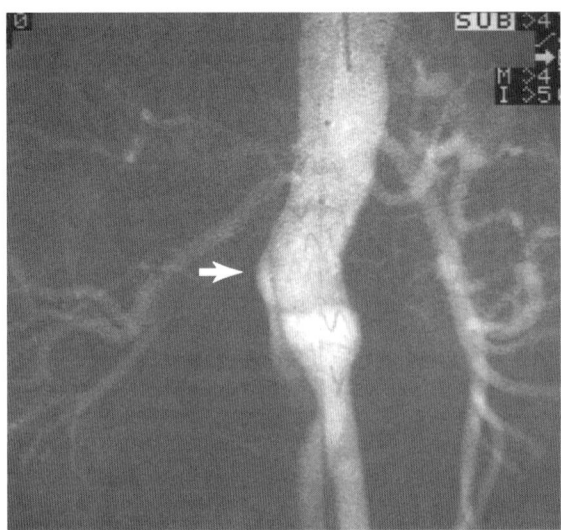

FIGURE **26-12** Proximal endoleak after stent graft treatment (*arrow*). (*From Rutherford RB et al. Vascular Surgery. 6th ed. Vol 2. Philadelphia: Saunders; 2005.*)

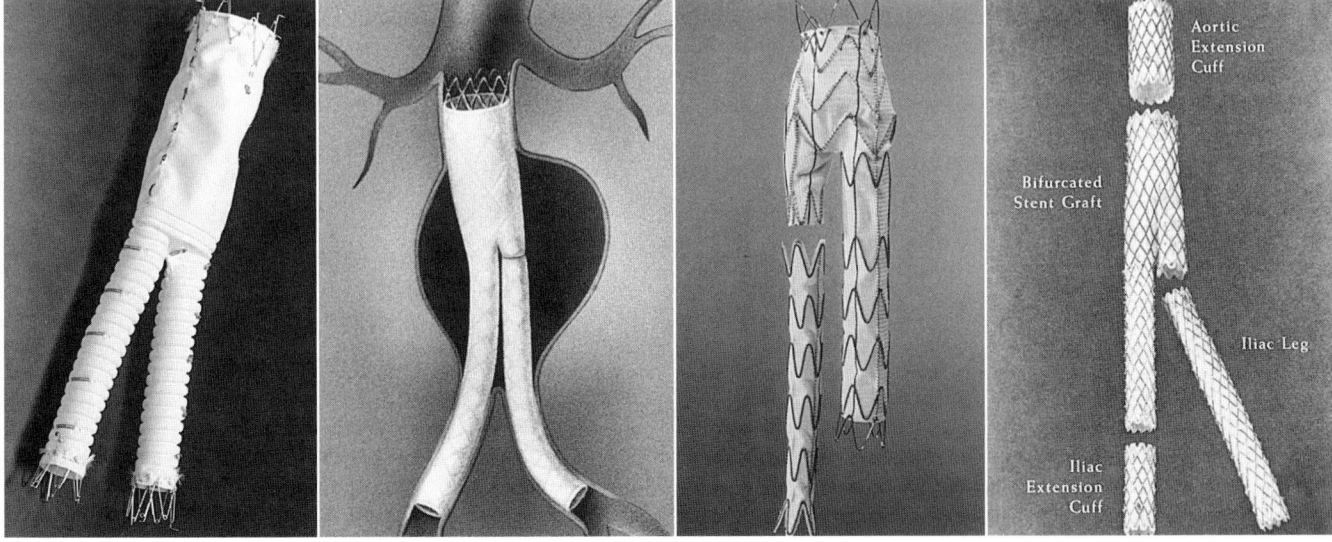

FIGURE **26-11** Various types of endovascular grafts. (*From Rutherford RB et al. Vascular Surgery. 6th ed. Vol 1. Philadelphia: Saunders; 2005.*)

spontaneously close within the first month after implantation.[142] Type II endoleaks are caused by collateral retrograde perfusion. Type I and type III endoleaks are caused by device-related problems. The most frequent intervention used to correct these complications include implantation of a second endograft or open repair.[143] Long-term results of endovascular aortic aneurysm repair have demonstrated that this procedure yields good results, but the overall durability of conventional surgical techniques is superior.[144]

Postoperative follow-up care for patients who have undergone EVAR is vital because long-term outcomes have not been quantitatively established. Physical examination and contrast-enhanced CT scan are recommended at 1, 6, 12 and 18 months postoperatively and then annually.[145] Additionally, abdominal x-rays should be obtained on a regular basis. Lifelong radiographic evaluation and surveillance is necessary to monitor aneurysm size, graft migration, and endoleak. Intensive follow-up care, the need for reinterventions, and the cost of the endograft make EVAR more expensive than open repair.[146]

In the future, minimally invasive aortic aneurysm surgery will continue to be used. Improvements in surgical techniques, imaging, and graft devices will allow a greater number of patients to experience the technical and physiologic advantages of EVAR.

CEREBROVASCULAR INSUFFICIENCY AND CAROTID ENDARTERECTOMY

Carotid endarterectomy is the second most common vascular operation performed in the United States per year (the first being coronary revascularization). Cerebrovascular accidents, or strokes, are the third leading cause of death in the United States and account for a yearly cost of 14 billion dollars in medical expenses and lost productivity.[147,148] Most strokes are caused by

cerebral ischemia. In carotid atherosclerotic disease, subintimal fatty plaques can increase in size over time and incrementally occlude the vascular lumen, which results in decreased cerebral blood flow. The plaque may rupture and release fibrin, calcium, cholesterol and inflammatory cells. This phenomenon can lead to abrupt occlusion of the lumen from thrombosis due to platelet activation, or an embolus may form and decrease cerebral blood flow distal to the carotid artery. In each scenario, an abrupt decrease in cerebral blood flow (CBF) leads to transient ischemic attacks (TIAs) or strokes. Note the anatomic details of the surgical site as seen in Figure 26-13.

More than half of all strokes are preceded by a TIA. The Framingham study reported that the risk of a stroke was 30% 2 years after a TIA and approximately 55% 12 years after a TIA had occurred.[149] It is this increased risk of stroke associated with TIA that provides the rationale for use of carotid endarterectomy (CEA), the surgical procedure in which the internal carotid artery is incised and the plaque within the carotid arterial lumen removed to improve cerebral blood flow.

Indications

Since 1954, specific indications for and expected outcomes of CEA have been the subject of heated debate. Ischemic stroke accounts for approximately 80% of first-time strokes and is primarily caused by atheromatous plaques. The initial indication for CEA was symptomatic stenosis but not complete occlusive carotid disease. This presentation occurs in most patients who undergo carotid surgery. Some centers have extended the indications to include evolved ("nondense"), nonhemorrhagic strokes and asymptomatic severe stenosis or lesser stenosis associated with contralateral occlusive disease.[147] The North American Symptomatic CEA Trial concluded that CEA for patients with recent hemispheric TIAs and high-grade stenosis (70% to 99%) had a risk reduction of 65% for the development of an ipsilateral stroke 2 years after surgery, compared with patients whose condition was medically managed.[150] The Executive Committee for Asymptomatic Carotid Atherosclerosis Study

TABLE **26-10**	Classification of Types of Endoleak	
Classification	**Description**	**Treatment**
Type I endoleak	• Attachment site leaks • Perigraft channel	• Proximal or distal graft extension • Embolization • Secondary endograft • Open repair
Type II endoleak	• Branch leaks (i.e., lumbar artery, renal artery, internal iliac artery, inferior mesenteric artery	• Conservative • Laparoscopic clip application
Type III endoleak	• Graft defect (fabric tear, modular disconnection)	• Secondary endograft • Open repair
Type IV endoleak	• Graft wall fabric porosity/suture holes	• Observation
Endotension	• Systemic pressure in aneurysm sac despite no evidence of endoleak	• Secondary endograft • Open repair

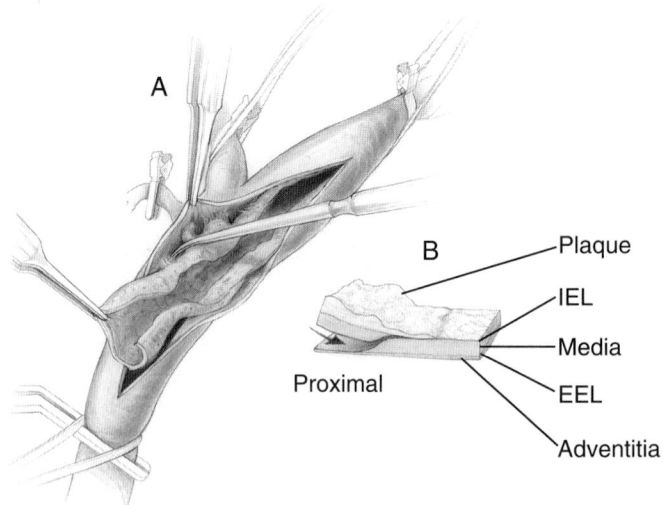

FIGURE **26-13** **A,** Removal of plaque from carotid artery; **B,** Formulation of plaque on the intima of carotid artery. (*From Zarins CK, Fewertz BL. Atlas of Vascular Surgery. 2nd ed. Philadelphia: Churchill Livingstone; 2005.*)

demonstrated that asymptomatic patients with carotid artery stenosis of at least 60% who underwent CEA had a 53% lower 5-year risk of ipsilateral stroke than patients who were treated medically.[151]

Morbidity and Mortality

The surgical outcomes reported for CEA remain inconclusive because of differences in patient populations and varying degrees of surgical expertise. Other variables that cannot be stratified in studies but may affect outcome include the state of collateral flow through the circle of Willis, the presence of concurrent atherosclerotic disease in the cerebral vasculature, the size and morphology of the offending plaque, the specific presenting symptoms, and the presence of concurrent cardiovascular disease.[152] If this information is obtained, the recommended acceptable perioperative stroke rates should be limited to less than 3% in asymptomatic patients, less than 5% in symptomatic patients, and 10% or less in patients with recurrent disease or existing strokes.[153] Morbidity rates related to CEA have been reported to be at or below these recommended limits.[153,154] The perioperative myocardial infarction rate of 2% to 5% illustrates the global nature of atherosclerotic disease and represents the greatest contribution to overall morbidity. The perioperative mortality rate for CEA is approximately 0.5% to 2.5%,[155,156] and the long-term postoperative stroke incidence ranges from 1% to 3% per year.[147,157]

Patient Selection

Criteria for the best candidates for carotid artery surgery remain unclear. The risks associated with having surgery and the possibility of a stroke must be measured against the risks associated with not having surgery and undergoing medical management. As mentioned previously, the Framingham study identified the incidence of stroke after TIAs and demonstrated an increased risk of stroke in untreated disease. In a study of 561 patients who underwent CEA during a 10-year period, Sieber and associates[158] attempted to identify the preoperative and intraoperative risk factors associated with stroke. Preoperative neurologic dysfunction was found to be the most significant factor for predicting postoperative stroke incidence (4%). Several conditions that can increase the risk of perioperative complications include severe preoperative hypertension, CEA performed in preparation for coronary artery bypass, angina, internal carotid artery stenosis near the carotid siphon, age older than 75 years, and diabetes mellitus.[159] Box 26-7 identifies various factors that contribute to morbidity during CEA. Because CEA is performed prophylactically, it would seem prudent that patient selection be based on the risks associated with the neurologic and myocardial ischemia of surgery, as opposed to risks associated with the neurologic sequelae of nonsurgical management.

Diagnosis

The neurologic symptoms of cerebral vascular dysfunction such as TIAs and strokes are most frequently related to decreased CBF. Asymptomatic carotid bruits may be a sign of the possibility of carotid artery disease. Amaurosis fugax or monocular blindness occurs in 25% of patients with high-grade carotid artery stenosis. This syndrome is believed to be caused by microthrombi that travel into the internal carotid artery and that decrease the blood supply of the optic nerve via the ophthalmic artery. Duplex ultrasonography, a noninvasive diagnostic modality that combines ultrasound and Doppler analysis, is currently one of the most sensitive noninvasive techniques capable of evaluating extracranial occlusive disease.[147] Arteriography may be performed if surgery is being contemplated and can provide anatomic details of arterial vessels. In patients with a neurologic deficit, in whom an alternative diagnosis may be discovered, CT scan or MRI may be useful.

Preoperative Assessment

The presence of concurrent CAD and carotid stenosis is well documented. Although stroke is a devastating consequence of CEA, myocardial infarction contributes more frequently to poor surgical outcomes than stroke. Callow and Mackey[153] reported on myocardial infarction as a cause of late mortality in 49% of patients who underwent CEA. The stroke-related fatality was 15%. The prevalence of cardiac disease and related risk factors is summarized in Table 26-11.

Hertzer and co-workers[72] performed coronary angiography in 1000 patients who underwent elective peripheral reconstruction as a means of identifying the presence of CAD. In this report the authors identified severe correctable CAD in 26% of the 195 patients with cerebrovascular disease. Although coronary angiography may not be justified in all patients undergoing CEA, a systematic approach to the identification of CAD and its subsequent risks should be performed before elective surgery (Figure 26-14).

Patients with no significant medical history, normal physical examination, and normal electrocardiography should proceed directly to surgery; these patients have low surgical risks. When abnormal cardiac information is obtained, further evaluation should be performed. Radionuclide imaging is highly sensitive in diagnosing CAD. Redistribution demonstrated on dipyridamole-thallium imaging is very suggestive of increased risk of adverse cardiac events. In these patients, coronary angiography is suggested as a means of quantifying CAD and selecting an appropriate therapeutic intervention.

BOX 26-7

Factors Contributing to Morbidity During Carotid Endarterectomy

- History of stroke or infarction on computed tomographic scan
- Early operation after stroke
- Significant medical problems
- Age
- Contralateral carotid artery disease
- Progressing stroke
- Hypercapnia
- Bilateral surgery
- Ulcerative lesion
- Low stump pressures
- Hemodynamic failure or hypoperfusion
- Surgery without intraoperative monitoring
- Surgery with shunt
- Surgery without shunt
- Vein patch closure
- Primary closure

Modified from Schroder T. How to predict which patient with carotid atherosclerosis is "high risk." Acta Chir Scand. 1990;555(suppl):209-222.

TABLE 26-11	Prevalence of Cardiac Disease and Associated Risk Factors in 614 Patients Undergoing Carotid Endarterectomy (CEA)	
Risk Factor		**Incidence (%)**
Cigarette smoking		62
Hypertension		62
Abnormal electrocardiographic results		34
Prior myocardial infarction		24
Angina		21
Diabetes mellitus		20
Hyperlipidemia		12

Modified from MacKey MC et al. Cardiac risk in patients undergoing CEA: impact on perioperative and long-term mortality. J Vasc Surg. 1990;11:226-234.

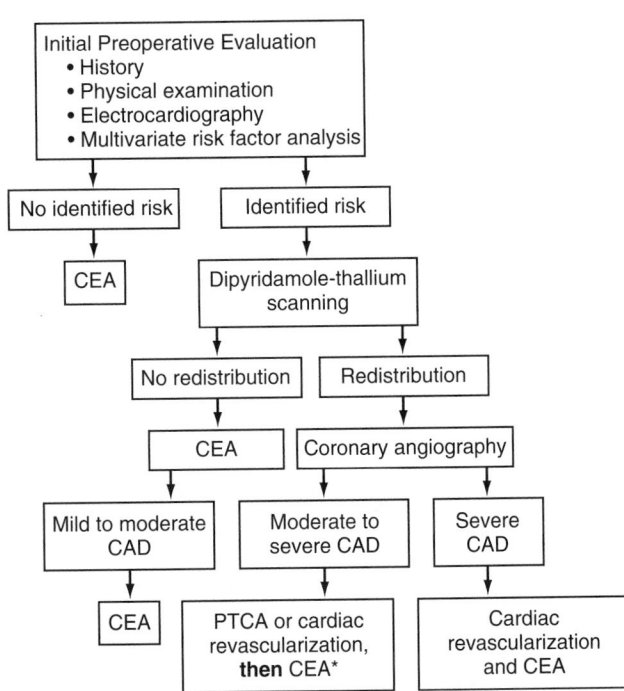

FIGURE **26-14** Algorithm for the management and the surgical selection of patients with concurrent carotid artery disease (CAD). Asterisk indicates that some may suggest reversing the order of these events. CEA, Carotid endarterectomy; PTCA, percutaneous transluminal coronary angioplasty.

The progression of surgical intervention when CAD is present with carotid artery disease is controversial. Most agree that in cases of mild CAD, patients may undergo CEA with a low degree of risk. However, in cases of moderate to severe CAD, the direction of surgical intervention is unclear. One option is the simultaneous performance of CEA and coronary revascularization. The safety of combined procedures has been addressed in the literature. Although some authors dispute the benefit of concomitant coronary and cerebral revascularization, most seem

to advocate this combination in a select group of individuals within the population who have severe CAD and significant carotid artery occlusion.[160,161] A combined CEA and coronary artery bypass surgery (CABG) has been suggested to decrease operative mortality rate and does not appear to put the patient at increased surgical risk.[162,163] However, Brown and associates[164] state that there is a high overall mortality rate of 17.7% when CABG and CEA are performed as a combined procedure. It is doubtful that strict conclusions will soon be drawn regarding the appropriate surgical management of concomitant CAD and carotid artery disease. Until more specific information is available, decisions should be guided by the individual's symptoms, the associated risk factors, and the center's experience.

Intraoperative Considerations
Cerebral Physiology
Cerebral blood flow (CBF) can remain relatively constant at different cerebral perfusion pressures as a result of cerebrovascular autoregulation. Cerebral perfusion pressure can be expressed as the difference between MAP and intracranial pressure. During CEA, intracranial pressure is usually not elevated; therefore MAP plays the predominant role in determining cerebral perfusion pressure. When MAP is maintained between 60 and 160 mm Hg, CBF remains constant. However, the adverse effects of chronic systemic hypertension shifts the patient's cerebral autoregulatory curve to the right, and therefore a higher than normal MAP may be required to ensure adequate cerebral perfusion. Cerebral blood flow is also influenced by arterial carbon dioxide and oxygen levels, as well as by inhalation agents.

Normal CBF is approximately 50 mL/100 g/min. Neuronal function is generally maintained at levels greater than 25 mL/100 g/min. Levels less than this critical value jeopardize cellular function. Decreased perfusion and ischemia can be reflected in changes in consciousness. Cellular death occurs at levels less than 6 mL/100 g/min, as evidenced by flattening seen on an electroencephalogram.

Carotid occlusive disease jeopardizes the cerebral perfusion pressure in the ipsilateral artery. Ischemia leads to the disruption of autoregulation and compensatory vasodilation, and thus blood flow becomes pressure dependent. During CEA the anesthetic goals must focus on improvement and protection of CBF and diligent monitoring of brain function.

Cerebral Monitoring
In addition to standard monitoring, direct intraarterial pressure is continuously assessed to evaluate near–real-time values. During the administration of anesthetic agents, blood pressure fluctuation commonly occurs in patients who have a history of hypertension. Owing to the high incidence of CAD and neurovascular disease in this patient population, prompt treatment of blood pressure values below 20% of the preoperative mean arterial pressure value is imperative. Pulmonary artery catheterization is not warranted in most individuals unless the presence of concurrent cardiac disease justifies its use. Carbon dioxide has a potent effect on cerebrovascular tone. Both hypocapnia and hypercapnia directly affect CBF; therefore, maintenance of normocapnia is paramount.

During repair, the carotid artery cross-clamp is applied. Various monitoring techniques have been proposed for assessing the adequacy of CBF during this maneuver. A summary of cerebral monitoring techniques is presented in Box 26-8. Each of these monitoring modalities has limitations; the most sensitive and specific measure of adequate cerebral blood flow is an awake patient. Electroencephalographic monitoring constitutes the gold standard in identifying neurologic deficits related to carotid artery cross-clamping.[165] Electroencephalogram has demonstrated reliability in monitoring cortical electrical function.[166] Loss of β-wave activity, loss of amplitude, and emergence of slow-wave activity all are indicative of neurologic dysfunction.

Carotid stump pressure has been used as a means of assessing collateral flow.[167] After the carotid cross-clamp is placed, distal pressure in the operative internal carotid artery is measured. A carotid stump pressure of less than 40 to 50 mm Hg reflects neurologic hypoperfusion and is a criterion for shunt placement. However, there is no correlation between stump pressures and electroencephalographic changes.[154] In a study by Harada and associates,[168] a carotid stump pressure of less than 50 mm Hg had a positive predictive value for only 36% of patients who exhibited ischemic EEG changes during carotid artery cross-clamping.

Regional CBF can be measured by the inhalation or direct administration of radioactive xenon 133 (^{133}Xe). In the operating room, intraarterial carotid injections of xenon 108 (^{108}Xe) are more feasible than inhalation, and the reliability of the injection technique has been well demonstrated. Intravenous methods have been recently proposed as a new means of measuring regional CBF for patients undergoing general anesthesia. Young and colleagues[169] demonstrated a positive correlation between intracarotid and intravenous ^{133}Xe methods in determining regional CBF.

The use of SSEP monitoring can be used to identify inadequate CBF during cross-clamping. Lam and co-workers[165] compared the efficacy of SSEP monitoring and electroencephalography (EEG) and concluded that these two monitoring techniques were similar. SSEP monitoring is a feasible alternative to conventional EEG for predicting neurologic deficits; however, false-positive results can occur. In addition, SSEPs are a measure of the integrity of the dorsal or sensory portion of the spinal cord. Therefore, a motor deficit can occur despite a normal SSEP waveform. Additionally, there are no values for decreased amplitude and increased latency that correlate with cerebral ischemia.

Transcranial Doppler velocity monitoring has been used as a method of detecting adverse cerebral events during CEA. McDowell and associates[170] used intraoperative transcranial Doppler monitoring during 238 carotid endarterectomies. They concluded that this method was more reliable than EEG for assessing interior integrity of the cerebral hemispheres.

The use of cerebral oximetry to determine the adequacy of cerebral perfusion is controversial. The critical oxygen saturation below which neurologic compromise will occur has not been quantified. This monitoring technique yields only a 33% positive predictive value. Box 26-8 outlines the cerebral monitoring modalities during general anesthesia for CEA.

Cerebral Protection
The major objective during carotid artery revascularization is to maintain CBF and decrease cerebral ischemia. Prevention of cerebral ischemia can be accomplished in one of two ways: by increasing collateral flow (placement of intraluminal shunt) or by decreasing cerebral metabolic requirements (pharmacologic adjunct).

Temporary Shunt Placement. Because 80% of cerebral blood flow is supplied via the carotid arteries, when the operative carotid artery is clamped, CBF is compromised. Therefore maintenance of CPP is dependent on collateral blood flow for adequate cerebral perfusion. The EEG changes associated with cerebral ischemia can be reversed when an intraluminal shunt is inserted.

> ### BOX **26-8**
> ### Cerebral Monitoring Modalities During General Anesthesia for CEA
>
> Electroencephalogram (EEG): assesses cortical electrical function
> Somatosensory evoked potential (SSEP): assesses sensory evoked potentials
> Carotid stump pressure (CSP): assesses perfusion pressure in the operative carotid artery
> Transcranial Doppler (TCD): assesses blood flow velocity in the middle cerebral artery
> Cerebral oximetry: assesses cerebral regional oxygen saturation
> Intraarterial xenon injection: assesses arterial xenon concentrations

CEA, *Carotid endarterectomy.*

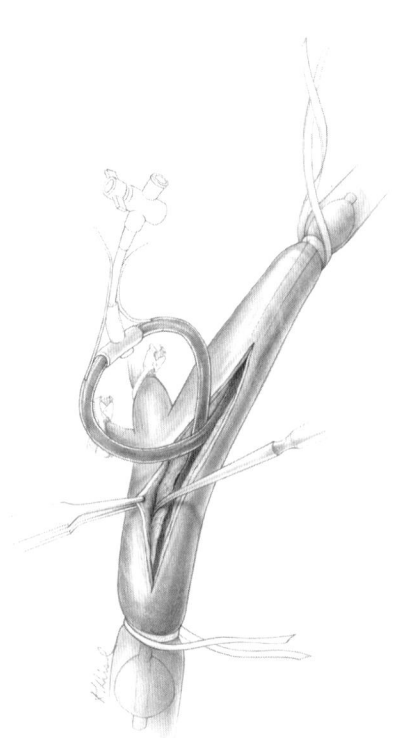

FIGURE **26-15** Shunting during carotid endarterectomy. (*From Zarins CK, Fewertz BL.* Atlas of Vascular Surgery. *2nd ed. Philadelphia: Churchill Livingstone; 2005.*)

The shunt acts as a temporary conduit that allows for arterial blood flow during the time the surgeon is dissecting plaque from the intima of the carotid artery (Figure 26-15). Although some surgeons routinely insert shunts prior to plaque removal, others do not use shunts or use shunts only in a select group of patients. Studies have demonstrated successful surgical outcomes when CEA was performed without the use of intraoperative shunting.[158,166] Schroder[157] reported a 5% incidence of stroke in patients who underwent CEA. In this group of

561 patients, neither the use of a shunt or cross-clamp nor administration of glucose was identified as a primary determinant of stroke severity.[158] The application of a shunt imposes the risk of embolic complications and intimal dissections.[159] Cerebral ischemic events are most often the result of embolic complications.[156] It has been suggested that 65% to 95% of neurologic deficits that occur as a result of CEA are related to thromboembolic events unrelated to the carotid artery cross-clamping.[171] Therefore surgeons more frequently reserve the use of shunts for patients with impaired contralateral cerebral circulation or an unstable neurologic history. However, Hankey and colleagues[172] state that inconclusive evidence exists, as reported by randomized controlled trials comparing routine or selective shunting and the overall mortality rate. The need for shunt placement can be based on information obtained using intraoperative monitoring techniques that determine CBF. Stump pressures and EEG measurements are the intraoperative monitoring modalities that can be used to determine the need for shunt placement.

Cerebral Metabolism

Barbiturates and propofol have the capability of decreasing cerebral metabolism to 40% below normal values.[104] During transient focal ischemia, barbiturates and propofol decrease the cerebral metabolic rate of oxygen consumption, which results in cerebral protection. The disadvantages of administering barbiturates and propofol during CEA surgery include myocardial depression and delayed emergence. The surgeon may request that one of these cerebral depressants be administered before the carotid artery is cross-clamped.

Hypothermia is also associated with decreases in cerebral metabolic rates and oxygen consumption. A decrease in core temperature of 1° C decreases $CMRO_2$ by 7%. When core temperature has been reduced to 12° C to 20° C, the safe duration of ischemia is 30 to 60 minutes.[104] Hypothermic techniques were initially advocated; however, the risks associated with these techniques outweigh the clinical usefulness. Mild hypothermia (33° C to 35°C) has also been a topic of interest. Mild hypothermia was not shown to improve neurologic outcomes during surgery for intracranial aneurysm. [173] More information regarding the use of hypothermia and its effectiveness are needed.

Blood Pressure Control

The presence of hypertension in patients with cerebrovascular disease is well known. Therefore, one of the most challenging aspects of care associated with anesthesia for CEA is blood pressure control. Patients with cerebral insufficiency are vulnerable to perioperative blood pressure instability. Hypotension occurs in 10% to 50% of patients who undergo CEA and is believed to be the result of carotid sinus baroreceptor stimulation. Conversely, 10% to 66% of patients experience hypertension, which is attributed to surgical manipulation of the carotid sinus.[174] Preoperative blood pressure control, volume status, and depth of anesthesia can also contribute to intraoperative hemodynamic instability.

Blood pressure control must begin in the preoperative phase. Mangano and associates[175] studied the effects of atenolol administered to patients who had confirmed or were at risk for CAD. Atenolol was administered preoperatively, postoperatively, and throughout patients' hospital stays. Overall the atenolol study group had a 65% reduction in mortality secondary to adverse cardiac events. In addition, patients in the atenolol study group had a 67% decrease in mortality within 1 year of surgery and a 48% decrease in mortality 2 years after surgery. All patients should continue taking their antihypertensive medications until the time of surgery. Additional pharmacologic adjuncts may be required in the preoperative period, especially during the insertion of intravenous and intraarterial catheters, in order to reduce increases in heart rate and blood pressure. The induction of anesthesia, the initial incision, the dissection, the manipulation of the carotid sinus, and the emergence from anesthesia are all events that precipitate blood pressure fluctuations. The use of pharmacologic adjuncts, such as short-acting β-adrenergic blockers, may stabilize blood pressure during induction and emergence. Continuous intravenous use of nitroglycerin or sodium nitroprusside should be available to treat hypertension. Patients with chronic hypertension are predisposed to dramatic decreases in blood pressure after the induction of general anesthesia. This condition must be treated promptly and can be successfully managed by providing intravenous fluids or administering a vasoconstrictor such as phenylephrine hydrochloride. Hypotension and bradycardia, which result from carotid sinus baroreceptor manipulation, can be inhibited by infiltration with local anesthetic. Although this maneuver is a fairly common practice during CEA, one series demonstrated no benefit from the prophylactic administration of local anesthetic to the carotid sinus nerve. These investigators suggested that this technique might be detrimental because it can cause hypertension.[174]

Anesthetic Management

The anesthetic objectives for vascular surgery are similar to those for any type of elective procedure: to provide analgesia and amnesia, to facilitate surgical intervention, and to minimize operative morbidity and mortality. Goals that are specific to CEA include maintaining cerebral and myocardial perfusion and oxygenation, minimizing the stress response, and facilitating a smooth and rapid emergence. However, it may be difficult to maintain the integrity of one system without adversely affecting the other. For example, raising the arterial blood pressure to augment cerebral perfusion can increase myocardial oxygen demand, which may lead to ischemia. In addition, significantly decreasing blood pressure can lead to cerebral hypoperfusion. Therefore, the anesthetic goal is to optimize perfusion to the brain, minimize myocardial workload, ensure cardiovascular stability, and allow for rapid emergence. An understanding of the physiology of the cerebrovascular system is important for optional anesthetic management. Figure 26-16 illustrates the anatomy of structures in this region. This knowledge enables the selection of appropriate monitoring and anesthetic techniques that will protect and improve cerebral and myocardial perfusion.

Anesthetic Selection

In an attempt to decrease the incidence of perioperative stroke during CEA, individual anesthetic techniques have been investigated. Many authors have reported the advantages and disadvantages of both general and regional anesthesia; however, no consensus indicates that a particular technique is more effective in decreasing overall perioperative morbidity and mortality. There are insufficient data from randomized controlled trials on the subject to suggest which technique yields superior results.[176] Authors of nonrandomized studies have shown that regional is associated with improved postoperative outcomes such as lower mortality, lower perioperative stroke rate, less intraoperative hemodynamic variability, fewer major adverse cardiac events, including myocardial infarction 30 days postendarterectomy, 10% decreased rate of unnecessary shunting, and decreased

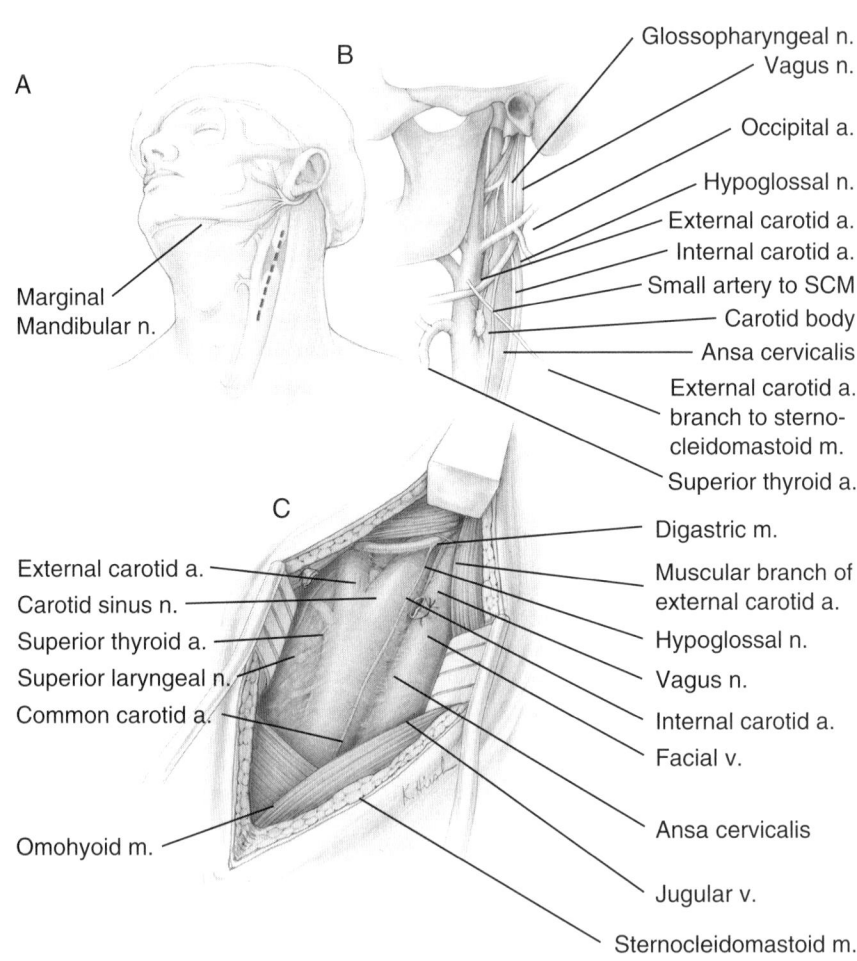

A

B

Glossopharyngeal n.

Vagus n.

Occipital a.

Hypoglossal n.

External carotid a.

Internal carotid a.

Small artery to SCM

Carotid body

Ansa cervicalis

External carotid a. branch to sterno-cleidomastoid m.

Superior thyroid a.

Marginal Mandibular n.

C

External carotid a.

Carotid sinus n.

Superior thyroid a.

Superior laryngeal n.

Common carotid a.

Omohyoid m.

Digastric m.

Muscular branch of external carotid a.

Hypoglossal n.

Vagus n.

Internal carotid a.

Facial v.

Ansa cervicalis

Jugular v.

Sternocleidomastoid m.

FIGURE 26-16   Carotid endarterectomy. **A,** Incision site. **B** and **C,** Anatomic structures presented at the carotid surgical site *a.,* Artery; *n.,* nerve; *v.,* vein. (*From Zarins CK, Fewertz BL. Atlas of Vascular Surgery. 2nd ed. Philadelphia: Churchill Livingstone; 2005.*)

length of hospital stay.[177-181] Therefore, anesthetic selection must be based on the anesthetist's familiarity and competence with a specific technique, as well as the patient's condition and the surgeon's preference.

Regional Anesthesia. A regional anesthetic technique during CEA can be accomplished by local infiltration or by superficial and deep cervical plexus block. Perhaps the greatest advantage of regional anesthesia is the anesthetist's ability to directly assess neurologic function in an awake individual. Assessing level of consciousness is the most effective method of assessing the adequacy of cerebral blood flow and detecting cerebral ischemia. In fact, assessment of consciousness in the awake patient may be more sensitive than conventional EEG in detecting cerebral ischemia. Corson and colleagues[182] reviewed data from 399 patients who underwent CEA in which general and regional techniques were used. The authors concluded that perioperative strokes occurred less frequently when a regional anesthetic was provided, especially in high-risk patients. McCarthy and colleagues[183] compared middle cerebral artery blood flow velocity using transcranial Doppler monitoring in patients undergoing CEA with either local or general anesthesia. It was determined that preservation of cerebral circulation was better maintained in patients who received local anesthesia. In addition, 67% of the general anesthesia group and 15% of the local anesthesia group received shunts. However, despite these seemingly physiologic advantages, no differences occurred in outcomes between the local and general anesthesia groups. The use of regional anesthesia has been associated with shorter operative times, less frequent

cardiopulmonary complications, and shorter postoperative hospitalization. In addition, there is a significant decrease of up to 20% in routine carotid artery shunting.[184-188]

The limiting factor for use of a regional technique is patient acceptance. Because these individuals are awake, preoperative patient education is essential, and their cooperation during surgery is vital. Anxiety, fear, and apprehension can initiate sympathetic stimulation, and as a result, extreme hemodynamic responses can occur. Deep sedation, which can be required in an apprehensive patient, may confound the neurologic assessment, negating the advantages of a regional technique. Additionally, hypercarbia can result from hypoventilation, and dysphoria is most likely to occur. Furthermore, converting to a general anesthetic technique once surgery has begun can be problematic. If adequate cerebral perfusion is compromised, symptoms include dizziness, contralateral weakness, decreased mentation, and loss of consciousness. In the event this scenario occurs, immediate shunt placement is warranted. Emergent airway management may be necessary.

General Anesthesia. Although the use of regional anesthesia has numerous advantages, general anesthesia is commonly used during CEA. Perhaps the greatest benefit of this technique is that it counters the most cited disadvantage of regional anesthesia: lack of patient cooperation. General anesthesia promotes a motionless field during surgery. In addition, inhalation agents may provide hemodynamic stability and may have beneficial effects on cerebral circulation.[189] By decreasing cerebral and cardiac metabolism, the inhalation agents provide a degree of protection against ischemia, an effect called *anesthetic preconditioning.*[190-192]

Comparison of inhaled agents with narcotic-based techniques yields no scientific evidence to suggest that patient outcome is improved. In studies of inhalation agents, the critical regional CBF (the blood level below which electroencephalographic signs of ischemia occur) during isoflurane anesthesia was less than when other volatile anesthetics were used.[189,193] Isoflurane also contributed to fewer adverse cardiac events when compared with enflurane and halothane in 2223 patients who underwent CEA at the Mayo Clinic.[194] The effects of sufentanil on cerebral hemodynamics were similar to those of isoflurane.[195] Remifentanil can be used; its rapid metabolism improves neurologic recovery. The inhalation agents may alter the monitoring methods used for detecting cerebral ischemia, such as EEG and SSEP monitoring. In these cases, general anesthetic techniques may require modification, and direct communication is required between the anesthetist and the surgical team. The use of nitrous oxide during CEA can potentially increase the incidence of a clinically significant pneumocephalus. During shunt placement and carotid artery cross-clamp release, microbubbles can be entrained into carotid artery blood flow. When carotid artery cross-clamping without shunting occurs, MAP valves should approximate or be slightly above preoperative levels to help ensure adequate cerebral perfusion through the contralateral carotid artery. For this reason, if nitrous oxide is used, some believe it should be discontinued before removal of the carotid artery cross-clamp.[196]

In summary, there is no scientific consensus supporting the idea that one anesthetic technique is superior in terms of decreasing perioperative morbidity and mortality. Palmer[197] investigated the type of anesthetic technique used and the associated morbidity and mortality in more than 200 patients. He concluded that no significant differences existed among all possible techniques. Furthermore, he recommended that the choice of anesthetic technique be governed by the preferences of the surgeon and the operative team. However, anesthetic agents that allow for a rapid assessment of neurologic function at the completion of surgery should be selected.

Postoperative Considerations

Perhaps the most common problem experienced in the postoperative period is hypertension. Although the specific cause remains unclear, postoperative hypertension may be related to events or conditions that alter cerebral autoregulation, such as use of halogenated hydrocarbons, diabetes mellitus, and cerebral hypoperfusion. Hypertension in the postoperative period occurs in 29% to 69% of patients undergoing CEA.[198] A systolic blood pressure greater than 180 mm Hg is associated with an increased incidence of TIA, stroke, or myocardial infarction.[159] Those patients with systolic blood pressures of 145 mm Hg or less had fewer postoperative complications.[150]

Although an uncommon complication, carotid artery hemorrhage can occur in the postoperative phase. Hemorrhage is a devastating event that requires immediate surgical intervention. Initial manifestations of hemorrhage may be those of upper airway obstruction, which may make reintubation difficult or impossible because of tracheal deviation. Emergency management of a patient with airway compromise as a result of carotid artery hemorrhage includes immediate evacuation of the hematoma. In addition, recurrent laryngeal nerve damage can occur and routinely manifests as inspiratory stridor. Respiratory insufficiency can be problematic for patients who have

---

BOX 26-9

Postoperative Complications After Carotid Endarterectomy

- Hemodynamic instability
- Myocardial ischemia/infarction
- Stroke
- Respiratory insufficiency
- Recurrent/superior laryngeal nerve damage
- Hematoma
- Carotid body dysfunction
- Tension pneumothorax

---

preexisting respiratory conditions. Tension pneumothorax can also occur, because the apices of the lungs extend above the clavicles toward the surgical site. Treatment includes immediate needle decompression. Damage to the carotid body can lead to a blunting of the chemoreceptor reflex, and therefore supplemental oxygen should be administered. Lastly, cerebral hyperperfusion syndrome (CHS) may result from increased blood flow to the brain as a result of loss of cerebral vascular autoregulation. The mechanism of action causing this phenomenon is unknown; however, it is hypothesized that CHS may occur as a result of chronic cerebral ischemia. Signs and symptoms of CHS include severe headache, visual disturbances, altered level of consciousness, and seizures. CHS may occur more often in patients who have had a contralateral CEA within the last 3 months and undergo a second CEA for occlusion on the ipsilateral side.[199]

The incidence of postoperative stroke after CEA was discussed previously. Unfortunately, even after successful revascularization of the carotid artery, occlusion can recur at a rate of 3% per year.[156] Although symptoms are present in only a small percentage of patients (3% to 5%), the incidence of recurrent carotid stenosis may be much larger than that reported, because asymptomatic cases may be overlooked.[200] As many as 25% of patients experience a neurocognitive decline up to 1 month after surgery. Patients who are predisposed are those with diabetes mellitus and advanced age.[201] The exact mechanism responsible for the cognitive dysfunction has not been scientifically identified. Postoperative complications of CEA are listed in Box 26-9.

Owing to the anatomic location and potential neurologic complications after CEA, postemergence neurologic integrity should be assessed. In addition to neurocognitive functioning, clinical assessment of cranial nerve function should be performed (Table 26-12).

CAROTID ARTERY STENTING

A less invasive surgical approach for treatment of carotid artery stenosis is carotid artery angioplasty and stenting. The safety and efficacy of carotid artery stenting (CAS) have been in question. Early stents were not equipped with distal protection devices, and a high number of patients developed CVAs as a result of embolization. Several randomized controlled trials have been published on the subject.

Controversy exists regarding the degree of success that this procedure affords as an alternative to CEA. The current incidence of stroke after CEA is approximately 2%. In a study of 100 patients undergoing CAS, Stankovic and associates[202] concluded that this procedure is a safe, effective, and reliable method of treating carotid artery disease. However, other researchers

TABLE 26-12	Cranial Nerve Assessment for the CEA Patient	
Cranial Nerve	**Function**	**Abnormal Response**
VII (facial)	Muscles of facial expression, saliva secretion	Inability to smile symmetrically; contralateral asymmetry indicates possible stroke; nerve injury on ipsalateral side
IX (glossopharyngeal)	Swallowing, pharyngeal muscle	Difficulty swallowing with ipsilateral Horner syndrome (ptosis, miosis, exophthalmos, reduced sweating)
X (vagus) → superior and recurrent laryngeal nerves	Laryngeal muscles movement	Minor swallowing problems, fatigued voice; vocal cord paralysis, hoarseness, inadequate gag reflex; may test speech by having the patient say "EEE"
X1 spinal accessory	Shoulder muscles	Ipsalateral weakness in neck and shoulder with shrugging
XII (hypoglossal)*	Muscles of tongue	Stick tongue out, move tongue side to side; tongue droops to ipsalateral side, difficulty with speech and chewing, high-pitched sounds, hoarseness

From Heffine MS. Care of the vascular surgical patient. In: Drain CB, Odom-Forren J, eds. Perianesthesia Nursing: A Critical Care Approach. 5th ed. St Louis: Saunders; 2009.
CEA, Carotid endarterectomy.
*This nerve traverses the internal carotid artery.

have stated that this procedure is associated with an increased stroke rate, poor durability of carotid angioplasty and stenting as evidenced by restenosis, and increased procedural costs.[203,204] The long-term results of CAS appear to be comparable to CEA in terms of preventing stroke, freedom from new neurologic events, and patency rates.[205]

The first large multicenter randomized controlled trial comparing CEA versus CAS was the Stenting and Angioplasty with Protection Patients at High Risk for Endarterectomy (SAPPHIRE trial). The rate of event-free survival at 1 year postsurgery was 88% for the CAS group and 79.9% for the CEA group. The stroke rate after 1 year was lower in the CAS group as compared with the CEA group—6.2% versus 7.9%, respectively. As for cardiac morbidity, the rate of MI for CAS versus CEA was 1.9% versus 6.6% 30 days postoperatively. Overall cardiac morbidity was 3% for CAS and 6.2% for CEA. The conclusion from SAPPHIRE was that CAS does not yield inferior outcomes as compared with CEA. However, the study methodology was criticized for several reasons. Nearly 60% of the patients were excluded from the trial because they were identified as too high risk. Therefore, the patients enrolled in the study were not particularly high risk. Also, 20% of the patients in each group were having CEA for restenosis, which increases surgical risk.[206,207]

The Endarterectomy versus Angioplasty with Symptomatic Severe Carotid Stenosis (EVA3S) trial was designed to compare the outcomes from CAS versus CEA. The study population were patients with symptomatic carotid stenosis of at least 60%. The study was stopped early because of a high incidence of stroke and death—9.6% compared with 3.9% for CEA 30 days after surgery. The conclusion was that CEA was superior to CAS for this patient population when considering risk of stroke at 30 days and 6 months postoperatively.[208] Another randomized controlled trial, the stent-protected angioplasty versus carotid endarterectomy (SPACE), yielded high but similar statistics for 30-day stroke death rates—CAS 6.8% and CEA 6.3%[209]

The goal of the Carotid Revascularization versus Stenting Trial (CREST), a randomized controlled trial was to determine which procedure, CAS or CEA, was more effective in preventing stroke and death. Inclusion criteria were patients who were symptomatic and had greater than 50% carotid artery stenosis and those who were asymptomatic with greater than 60% carotid

artery stenosis. The preliminary results from the first stage of the trial, which included 1000 patients, are encouraging and compare favorably with CEA. Death or stroke rates from any cause during the 30 days postprocedure include 3% for asymptomatic patients less than 80 years of age and 2.7% for symptomatic patients less than 80 years of age.[210] Initial indications were that CAS was associated with an increased incidence of stroke in octogenarians. However, it has now been determined the incidence of stroke resulting from CAS is similar to the CEA results for all age groups.[211] The CREST trial remains in progress.

The first Italian Concensus on Carotid Stenting (ICCS) recommends that further studies are needed to provide more evidence regarding the safety and efficacy of CAS. The authors believe that a cerebral embolic protective device should be used for CAS procedures. Carotid artery stenting should be used instead of CEA in the presence of specific patient factors and severe vascular or cardiac comorbidities, listed in Box 26-10.[212]

Prior to the CAS procedure, patients receive an aortic arch, carotid, and cerebral angiogram or a high-resolution MRI. This allows the physicians to evaluate the individual anatomy and angiopathology of the aortic arch, brachiocephalic artery (for right carotid artery stent), or left common carotid artery. Determination of the type of sheaths, stents, and cerebral embolic protection device can then be planned. Femoral artery access is obtained, then a sheath is threaded through the aortic arch and into the operative carotid artery. The guide wire/embolic protection device is advanced through the sheath and positioned across the stenotic region. An embolic protection device sequesters emboli during angioplasty and stenting to avoid distal occlusion in cerebral arteries (Figure 26-17). In elderly patients, adjunctive distal embolic protection lowers the risk of intraoperative and postoperative adverse events.[213] Angioplasty with a 5-mm balloon dilates the carotid artery, then the stent is deployed. The guide wire/device wire is removed after agiographic confirmation that carotid artery dissection or occlusion has not occurred. Figure 26-18 shows carotid artery patency after angioplasty and stent placement.

Anesthetic Considerations

The anethesia routinely used for CAS is local anesthesia at the femoral insertion site and minimal sedation. Fluroscopy will be used throughout the surgery, so it is important that all operating room personnel are protected with lead shielding. Anticoagulation is initiated with a heparin bolus, 50 to 100 units/kg, to maintain ACT greater than 250 seconds.[214] Balloon inflation in the internal carotid artery can stimulate the baroreceptor response, resulting in prolonged bradycardia and hypotension. Glycopyrrolate or atropine can be given prior to inflation to offset this vagal response.

Complications associated with CAS are listed in Box 26-11. The most common complication is stroke caused by thromboembolism. Interventions for a patient with an acute stroke include airway and hemodynamic management. Currently, the only treatment approved for acute ischemic stroke is intravenous recombinant tissue plasminogen activator (rt-PA). Mechanical devices such as snares and ballons are being developed so that the physician will be able to physically remove a thromboembolic material and restore blood flow.

Patients typically remain in the postanesthesia care unit for 30 minutes after carotid stent placement and then are transferred to a monitored floor. A carotid duplex scan is performed prior to discharge, and then routinely obtained at 6 weeks, 6 months, 1 year, and then yearly. Patients will remain on aspirin therapy for anticoagulation for life.[215]

PERIOPERATIVE COST CONTAINMENT

During the past few decades, a dramatic change in the way surgical care is delivered has taken place. For patients undergoing CEA, efforts to curtail hospital costs have led to changes in preoperative evaluations and anesthetic techniques and reductions in the length of stay.

In a patient without atypical neurologic symptoms, contrast arteriography, which was once the standard technique for evaluating the degree of carotid artery stenosis, usually does not provide any more information than carotid duplex scanning.[216] As discussed previously, a significant cost savings is associated with the use of regional anesthesia. The dramatic cost difference is the result of decreased ICU use, decreased length of stay, and reduced costs for pharmacologic agents.[217] A CEA protocol in which patients are discharged 1 day postoperatively has been evaluated. In a prospective study by Friedman and colleagues,[218] 72 patients were evaluated preoperatively on an outpatient basis, and hospital admission took place on the day of surgery. General anesthesia was administered to all patients in the study group. A total of 66 (88%) patients were discharged on the first postoperative day.

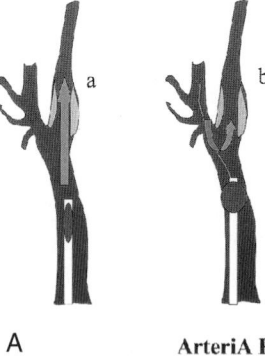
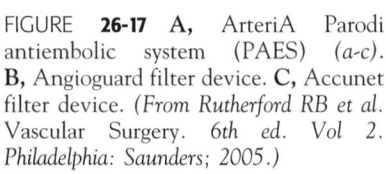
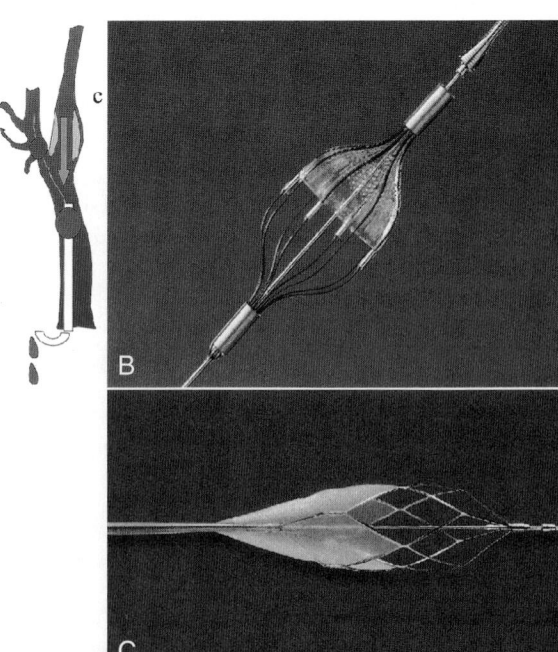

FIGURE **26-17 A,** ArteriA Parodi antiembolic system (PAES) *(a-c).* **B,** Angioguard filter device. **C,** Accunet filter device. *(From Rutherford RB et al. Vascular Surgery. 6th ed. Vol 2. Philadelphia: Saunders; 2005.)*

ArteriA PAES

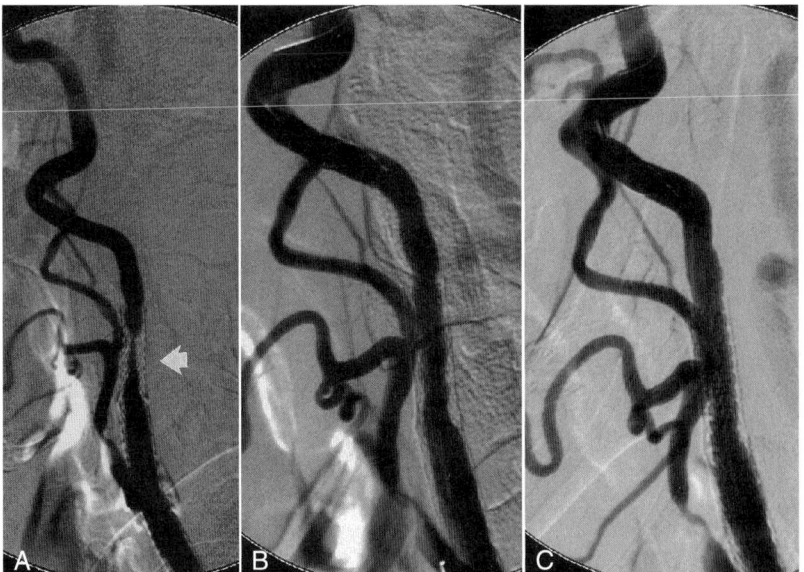

FIGURE **26-18** **A,** High-grade restenosis of internal carotid artery (*arrowhead*) 11 months after carotid angioplasty/stenting with Wallstent. **B,** After angioplasty alone. **C,** After placement of nitinol stent. Note filter protection device in distal internal carotid. (*From Rutherford RB et al. Vascular Surgery. 6th ed. Vol 2. Philadelphia: Saunders; 2005.*)

BOX **26-11**

Complications Associated with Carotid Artery Stenting

- Stroke
- Myocardial ischemia/infarction
- Bradycardia
- Hypotension
- Deformation of expandable stent
- Stent thrombosis
- Horner syndrome
- Cerebral hyperperfusion syndrome
- Carotid artery dissection
- Hemorrhage resulting from anticoagulation

The average length of stay was 1.13 days, and no complications were attributed to early discharge.

When complications are prevented and favorable surgical outcomes are demonstrated, health-care economics may be improved. Use of a regional technique during CEA has been associated with economic savings.[180] Godin and colleagues[219] examined hospital costs in a comparison of general versus regional techniques and determined that regional anesthesia was more cost-effective than regional anesthesia.

It has been suggested that carotid artery angioplasty and stenting is more cost effective than CEA; however, CEA is more cost-effective than CAS. The greater costs associated with the CAS procedure are related to a higher rate of stroke and the high costs of stents and neuroprotection devices.[220]

SUMMARY

The treatment of vascular disease is one of the fastest changing areas of medicine. Minimally invasive vascular surgical techniques are being introduced that are revolutionizing the options available for treatment. Many highly invasive surgical techniques are now being performed as interventional radiologic procedures. Anesthetic management for vascular procedures is far different from just a few years ago and requires that we adapt to ever-new treatment strategies. As practice evolves, we will be better able to assess growing evidence that suggests the superiority of these procedures in decreasing patient morbidity, mortality, and convalescence.

REFERENCES

1. Zarins CK, Graham HM. Aorta and arterial disease of the lower extremity. In: Miller TA, ed. *Physiologic Basis of Modern Surgical Care.* St Louis: Mosby; 1988:837.
2. Panetta TF, Veith FJ. Aortoiliac occlusive disease. In: Cameron JL, ed. *Current Surgical Therapy.* 4th ed. St Louis: Mosby; 1992.
3. Daub K et al. The evil atherosclerosis: adherent platelets induce foam cell formation. *Semin Thromb Hemost.* 2007;32(2):173-178.
4. May AE et al. Platelet leukocyte interactions in inflammation and atherothrombosis. *Semin Thromb Hemost.* 2007;32(2):123-127.
5. Brenner D et al. Cytokine polymorphisms associated with carotid intima thickness in stroke patients. *Stroke.* 2006;37(7):1691-1696.
6. Cunningham AJ. Anesthesia for abdominal aortic surgery. I. A review. *Can J Anaesth.* 1989;36:426-444.
7. Stenseth R. Advances in anesthesiological management of aortic surgery. *Acta Chir Scand.* 1990;155:123-128.
8. DeBakey ME, Lawrie GM. Combined coronary artery and peripheral vascular disease: recognition and treatment. *J Vasc Surg.* 1984;1:605-607.
9. Szilagyi DE et al. A thirty-year survey of the reconstructive surgical treatment of aortoiliac occlusive disease. *J Vasc Surg.* 1986;3:421-435.
10. Lindenauer PK et al. Perioperative beta-blocker therapy and mortality after major noncardiac surgery. *N Engl J Med.* 2005;353:346-361.
11. Olaf S et al. Pro beta-blockers are indicated for patients at risk for cardiac complications undergoing noncardiac surgery. *Anesth Analg.* 2007;104(1):8-10.
12. Eagle KA et al. ACC/AHA guideline update for perioperative cardiovascular evaluation for noncardiac surgery—executive summary. *J Am Coll Cardiol.* 2002;39(3):543-632.
13. Polderman D et al. High dose beta blockers and tight heart rate control reduce myocardial ischemia and troponin T release in vascular surgery patients. *Circulation.* 2006;114:344-349.
14. Harvey S et al. Assessment of the clinical effectiveness of pulmonary artery catheters in management of patients in intensive care (PAC-Man): a randomized controlled trial. *Lancet.* 2005;366:472-477.
15. Sandham JD et al. A randomized controlled trial of the use of pulmonary artery catheters in high risk surgical patients. *N Engl J Med.* 2003;348(1):5-14.

16. Shah MR et al. Impact of the pulmonary artery catheter in critically ill patients: meta analysis of randomized controlled trials. *JAMA.* 2005; 294(13):1664-1670.

17. Baron HC et al. Continuous epidural analgesia in the heparinized vascular surgical patient: a retrospective review of 912 patients. *J Vasc Surg.* 1987;6:144-146.

18. Raggi R et al. Continuous epidural anesthesia and postoperative epidural narcotics in vascular surgery. *Am J Surg.* 1987;154:192-197.

19. Underwood PS et al. A comparison of epidural versus general anesthesia for elderly patients undergoing peripheral vascularization. *Anesthesiology.* 1988;6:A105.

20. Liu SS, Wu CL. Effect of postoperative analgesia on major postoperative complications: a systematic update of the evidence. *Anesth Analg.* 2007;104(3):689-702.

21. Reilly JN, Tilson MD. Incidence and etiology of abdominal aortic aneurysms. *Surg Clin North Am.* 1989;69:705-711.

22. Hall SW. Endovascular repair of abdominal aortic aneurysms. *AORN J.* 2003;77(3):630-648.

23. Lambert ME et al. Ruptured abdominal aortic aneurysms. *J Cardiovasc Surg.* 1986;27:256-261.

24. Hollier LH, Moore WM. Surgical management of juxtarenal and suprarenal aortic aneurysms. *Acta Chir Scand.* 1990;555:117-122.

25. Budden J, Hollier LH. Management of aneurysms that involve the juxtarenal or suprarenal aorta. *Surg Clin North Am.* 1989;69:837-844.

26. Quill DS et al. Ultrasonic screening for the detection of abdominal aortic aneurysms. *Surg Clin North Am.* 1989;69:713-720.

27. Thurmond AS, Semler HJ. Abdominal aortic aneurysm: incidence in a population at risk. *J Cardiovasc Surg.* 1986;27:457-459.

28. Dobrin PB. Pathophysiology and pathogenesis of aortic aneurysms. *Surg Clin North Am.* 1989;69:687-703.

29. Brady AR et al. Risk factors for postoperative death following elective surgical repair of abdominal aortic aneurysm: results from the UK Small Aneurysm Trial. On behalf of the UK Small Aneurysm Trial participants. *Br J Surg.* 2000;87(6):742-743.

30. Webster MW et al. Abdominal aortic aneurysm: results of a family study. *J Vasc Surg.* 1991;13:366-372.

31. Graor RA. Preoperative evaluation and management of coronary and carotid artery occlusive disease in patients with abdominal aortic aneurysms. *Surg Clin North Am.* 1989;69:737-743.

32. Pairolero PC. Repair of abdominal aortic aneurysms in high-risk patients. *Surg Clin North Am.* 1989;69:755-763.

33. Johansen K. Treatment options for aneurysms in high-risk patients. *Surg Clin North Am.* 1989;69:765-774.

34. Hertzer NR et al. The risk of vascular surgery in a metropolitan community. *J Vasc Surg.* 1984;9:13-19.

35. Faxon DP et al. Atherosclerotic vascular disease conference: executive summary: atherosclerotic vascular disease conference proceeding for healthcare professionals from a special writing group of the American Heart Association. *Circulation.* 2004;109(21):2595-2604.

36. Sullivan CA et al. Clinical management of symptomatic but unruptured abdominal aortic aneurysm. *J Vasc Surg.* 1990;11:799-802.

37. Wakefield TW et al. Abdominal aortic aneurysm rupture: statistical analysis of factors affecting outcome of surgical treatment. *Surgery.* 1982;91:586-595.

38. Rutherford RB, McCroskey BL. Ruptured abdominal aortic aneurysms. *Surg Clin North Am.* 1989;69:859-868.

39. Bandyk DF. Preoperative imaging of aortic aneurysms: conventional and digital subtraction angiography, computed tomography scanning, and magnetic resonance. *Surg Clin North Am.* 1989;69:721-735.

40. Vowden P et al. A comparison of three imaging techniques in the assessment of an abdominal aortic aneurysm. *J Cardiovasc Surg.* 1989;30:891-896.

41. Glock Y et al. Abdominal aortic aneurysmectomy in octogenarian patients. *J Cardiovasc Surg.* 1990;31:71-76.

42. Plecha FR et al. The early results of vascular surgery in patients 75 years of age and older: an analysis of 3259 cases. *J Vasc Surg.* 1985;2:769-774.

43. McFalls EO et al. Coronary revascularization before elective major vascular surgery. *N Engl J Med.* 2004;27:2795-2804.

44. Darling RC et al. Autopsy study of unoperated abdominal aortic aneurysms: the case for early resection. *Circulation.* 1977;56:161-164.

45. Mangano DT. Monitoring pulmonary arterial pressure in coronary artery disease. *Anesthesiology.* 1980;53:364-370.

46. Rice CL et al. Central venous pressure or pulmonary capillary wedge pressure as the determinant of fluid replacement in aortic surgery. *Surgery.* 1978; 84:437-440.

47. Isaacson IJ et al. The value of pulmonary artery and central venous monitoring in patients undergoing abdominal aortic reconstructive surgery: a comparison study of two selected randomized groups. *J Vasc Surg.* 1990;12:754-760.

48. Joyce WP et al. The role of central hemodynamic monitoring in abdominal aortic surgery: a prospective randomized trial. *Eur J Vasc Surg.* 1990; 4:633-636.

49. Thys DM et al. A comparison of hemodynamic indices derived by invasive monitoring and two-dimensional echocardiography. *Anesthesiology.* 1987; 67:630-634.

50. Clements FM, deBruijn NP. Perioperative evaluation of regional wall motion by transesophageal two-dimensional echocardiography. *Anesth Analg.* 1987;66:249-261.

51. Gelman S et al. Blood volume redistribution during cross-clamping of the descending aorta. *Anesth Analg.* 1994;78:219-224.

52. Gelman S et al. The reason for cardiac output reduction after aortic cross-clamping. *Am J Surg.* 1988;155:578-586.

53. Gold MS et al. The effect of lumbar epidural and general anesthesia on plasma catecholamines and hemodynamics during abdominal aortic aneurysm repair. *Anesth Analg.* 1994;78:225-230.

54. Huval WV et al. Determinants of cardiovascular stability during abdominal aortic aneurysmectomy (AAA). *Ann Surg.* 1984;199:216-222.

55. Galt SW et al. The effect of ibuprofen on cardiac performance during abdominal aortic cross-clamping. *J Vasc Surg.* 1991;13:876-883.

56. Gottlieb A et al. The role of prostacyclin in the mesenteric traction syndrome during anesthesia for abdominal aortic reconstructive surgery. *Ann Surg.* 1989;209:363-367.

57. Seltzer JL et al. The hemodynamic response to traction on the abdominal mesentery. *Anesthesiology.* 1985;63:96-99.

58. Naito Y et al. Responses of adrenocorticotropic hormone, cortisol, and cytokines during and after upper abdominal surgery. *Anesthesiology.* 1992; 77:426-431.

59. Norman JG, Fink GW. The effects of epidural anesthesia on the neuroendocrine response to major surgical stress: a randomized prospective trial. *Am Surg.* 1997;63:75-80.

60. Hermreck AS. Prevention and management of surgical complications during repair of abdominal aortic aneurysms. *Surg Clin North Am.* 1989; 69:869-894.

61. Mongan PD et al. Spinal evoked potentials are predictive in a porcine model of aortic occlusion. *Anesth Analg.* 1994;78:257-266.

62. Damask MC et al. Abdominal aortic cross-clamping: metabolic and hemodynamic consequences. *Arch Surg.* 1984;119:1332-1337.

63. Fukuda S et al. Relationship between tissue ischemia and venous endothelin-1 during abdominal aortic aneurysm surgery. *J Cardiothorac Vasc Anesth.* 1995; 9:510-514.

64. Hessel EA. Intraoperative management of abdominal aortic aneurysms: the anesthesiologist's viewpoint. *Surg Clin North Am.* 1989;69:775-793.

65. Sicard GA et al. Retroperitoneal versus transperitoneal approach of repair of abdominal aortic aneurysms. *Surg Clin North Am.* 1989;69:795-806.

66. Hallett JW. Minimizing the use of homologous blood products during repair of abdominal aortic aneurysms. *Surg Clin North Am.* 1989;69:817-826.

67. Roger VL et al. Influence of coronary artery disease on morbidity and mortality after abdominal aortic aneurysmectomy: a population-based study, 1971-1987. *J Am Coll Cardiol.* 1989;14:1245-1252.

68. Pasternack PF et al. The value of radionuclide angiography as a predictor of perioperative myocardial infarction in patients undergoing abdominal aortic aneurysm resection. *J Vasc Surg.* 1984;1:320-325.

69. Mangano DT, et al. Association of perioperative myocardial ischemia with cardiac morbidity and mortality in men undergoing noncardiac surgery. *N Engl J Med.* 1990;323:1781-1787.

70. Goldman L. Multifactorial index of cardiac risk in noncardiac surgery: ten-year status report. *J Cardiothorac Anesth.* 1987;1:237-244.

71. Cooperman M et al. Cardiovascular risk factors in patients with peripheral vascular disease. *Surgery.* 1978;84:505-509.

72. Hertzer NR et al. Coronary artery disease in peripheral vascular patients: a classification of 1000 coronary angiograms and results of surgical management. *Ann Surg.* 1984;199:223-233.

73. Pohost GM. Dipyridamole thallium test: is it useful for predicting coronary events after vascular surgery? *Circulation.* 1991;84:931-932.

74. Raby KE et al. Correlation between preoperative ischemia and major cardiac events after peripheral vascular surgery. *N Engl J Med.* 1989; 321:1296-1300.

75. Fleron MH et al. A comparison of intrathecal opioid and intravenous analgesia for the incidence of cardiovascular, respiratory, and renal complications after abdominal aortic surgery. *Anesth Analg.* 2003;97:2-12.

76. Yeager MP et al. Epidural anesthesia and analgesia in high-risk surgical patients. *Anesthesiology.* 1987;66:729-736.

77. Rao TL, El-Etr AA. Anticoagulation following placement of epidural and subarachnoid catheters: an evaluation of neurological sequelae. *Anesthesiology.* 1981;55:618-620.

78. Gold MS et al. Comparison of lumbar and thoracic epidural narcotics for postoperative analgesia in patients undergoing abdominal aortic aneurysm repair. *J Cardiothorac Vasc Anesth.* 1997;11:137-140.

79. Major CP II et al. Postoperative pulmonary complications and morbidity after abdominal aneurysmectomy: a comparison of postoperative epidural versus parenteral epidural analgesia. *Am Surg.* 1996;62:45-51.

80. Aadahl P et al. Regional anesthesia for endovascular treatment of abdominal aortic aneurysms. *J Endovasc Surg.* 1997;4:56-61.

81. Miller Q et al. The effects of intraoperative fenoldopam on renal blood flow and tubular function following suprarenal aortic cross clamping. *Ann Vasc Surg.* 2003;17:656-662.

82. Girbes ARJ et al. Lack of specific renal and hemodynamic effects of different doses of dopamine and infrarenal aortic surgery. *Br J Anaesth.* 1996;77:753-755.

83. Bower TC et al. Unusual manifestations of abdominal aortic aneurysms. *Surg Clin North Am.* 1989;69:745-754.

84. Crawford ES et al. Aortic dissection and dissecting aortic aneurysms. *Ann Surg.* 1988;208:254-273.

85. Piotrowski JJ et al. Selection of grafts currently available for repair of abdominal aortic aneurysms. *Surg Clin North Am.* 1989;69:827-836.

86. Hollier LH et al. Thoracoabdominal aortic aneurysm repair: analysis of postoperative morbidity. *Arch Surg.* 1988;123:871-875.

87. Coselli JS et al. Thoracoabdominal aortic aneurysm repair: review and update of current strategies. *Ann Thorac Surg.* 2002;74:S1881-S1884.

88. Johnston KW et al. Subcommittee on Reporting Standards for Arterial Aneurysms, Ad Hoc Committee on Reporting Standards, Society for Vascular Surgery, and North American Chapter of International Society for Cardiovascular Surgery. Suggested standards for reporting on arterial aneurysms. *J Vasc Surg.* 1991;13:452-458.

89. Bickerstaff LK et al. Thoracic aortic aneurysms: a population-based study. *Surgery.* 1982;92:1103-1108.

90. Crawford ES, DeNatale RW. Thoracoabdominal aortic aneurysms: observations regarding the natural course of the disease. *J Vasc Surg.* 1986;3(4):578-582.

91. Crawford ES et al. Surgical treatment of aneurysm and/or dissection of the ascending aorta, transverse aortic arch, and ascending aorta and transverse aortic arch: factors influencing survival in 717 patients. *J Thorac Cardiovasc Surg.* 1989;98:659-673.

92. Murphy DA et al. Recognition and management of ascending aortic dissection complicating cardiac surgical operations. *J Thorac Cardiovasc Surg.* 1983;85:247-256.

93. Simon P et al. Transesophageal echocardiography in the emergency surgical management of patients with aortic dissection. *J Thorac Cardiovasc Surg.* 1992;103:1113-1117.

94. Svensson LG et al. Dissection of the aorta and dissecting aortic aneurysms: improved early and long-term surgical results. *Circulation.* 1990;82:24-38.

95. Hollier LH, Moore WM. Avoidance of renal and neurologic complications following thoracoabdominal aortic aneurysm repair. *Acta Chir Scand.* 1990;555(suppl):129-135.

96. Svensson LG et al. Influence of preservation or perfusion of intraoperatively identified spinal cord blood supply on spinal motor evoked potentials and paraplegia after aortic surgery. *J Vasc Surg.* 1991;13:355-365.

97. Laschinger JC et al. Direct noninvasive monitoring of spinal cord motor function during thoracic aortic occlusion: use of motor evoked potentials. *J Vasc Surg.* 1988;7:161-171.

98. Grubbs PE Jr et al. Somatosensory evoked potentials and spinal cord perfusion pressure are significant predictors of postoperative neurologic dysfunction. *Surgery.* 1988;104:216-223.

99. Stenseth R, Myhre HO. Anesthesia in surgery for aneurysm of the descending thoracic or thoracoabdominal aorta. *Acta Chir Scand.* 1988;154:147-150.

100. Coles JG et al. Intraoperative management of thoracic aortic aneurysm: experimental evaluation of perfusion cooling of the spinal cord. *J Thorac Cardiovasc Surg.* 1983;85:292-299.

101. McCullough JL et al. Paraplegia after thoracic aortic occlusion: influence of cerebrospinal fluid drainage. *J Vasc Surg.* 1988;7:153-160.

102. Naslund TC, Hollier LH. Thoracoabdominal aneurysm. In: Cameron JL, ed. *Current Surgical Therapy.* 4th ed. St Louis: Mosby; 1992:676.

103. Jex RK et al. Early and late results following repair of dissections of the descending thoracic aorta. *J Vasc Surg.* 1986;3:226-237.

104. Hollier LH. Protecting the brain and spinal cord. *J Vasc Surg.* 1987;5:524-528.

105. Drenger D et al. Changes in cerebrospinal fluid pressure and lactate concentrations during thoracoabdominal aortic aneurysm surgery. *Anesthesiology.* 1997;86:41-47.

106. van Dongen EP et al. Normal serum concentrations of S-100 protein and changes in cerebrospinal fluid concentrations of S-100 protein during and after thoracoabdominal aortic aneurysm surgery: is S-100 protein a biochemical marker of clinical value in detecting spinal cord ischemia? *J Vasc Surg.* 1998;27:344-346.

107. Naslund TC et al. Protecting the ischemic spinal cord during aortic clamping: the influence of anesthetics and hypothermia. *Ann Surg.* 1992;215:409-415.

108. Magee TR et al. A prosepective survey of patients presenting with abdominal aortic aneurysm. *Eur J Vasc Endovasc Surg.* 1997;13:403-406.

109. Katzen BT et al. Endovascular repair of abdominal aortic aneurysms. *Circulation.* 2005;112(11):1663-1675.

110. Schermerhorn ML et al. Life expectancy after endovascular versus open abdominal aortic aneurysm repair: results of a decision analysis model on the basis of data from EUROSTAR. *J Vasc Surg.* 2002;36:1112-1120.

111. Brewster D et al. Long-term outcomes after endovascular abdominal aortic aneurysm repair: the first decade. *Ann Surg.* 2006;244(3):426-438.

112. Harris P et al. Incidence and risk factors of late rupture, conversion, and death after endovascular repair of infrarenal aortic aneurysms: the EUROSTAR experience. *J Vasc Surg.* 2000;32(4):739-749.

113. Lifeline registry of EVAR Publications Committee. *J Vasc Surg.* 2005;42(1):1-10.

114. Prissen M et al. A randomized trial comparing conventional and endovascular repair of abdominal aortic aneurysms. *N Engl J Med.* 2004;351:1607-1618.

115. Forbes TT et al. National audit to the recent utilization of endovascular abdominal aortic aneurysm repair in Canada. *J Vasc Surg.* 2005;42(3):410-414.

116. Orend KH et al. Endovascular treatment in diseases of the descending thoracic aorta: six-year results of a single center. *J Vasc Surg.* 2003;37:91-99.

117. Cambria PR et al. Evolving experience with thoracic aortic stent graft repair. *J Vasc Surg.* 2002;35:1129-1136.

118. Chiesa R et al. Spinal cord ischemia after elective stent graft repair of the thoracic aorta. *J Vasc Surg.* 2005;42(1):11-17.

119. Kern JA et al. Thoracic aortic endografting is the treatment of choice for elderly patients with thoracic aortic disease. *Ann Surg.* 2006;243(6):815-823.

120. Lawrence PF et al. The epidemiology of surgically repaired aneurysms in the United States. *J Vasc Surg.* 1999;30:632-640.

121. Brown MJ et al. A meta-analysis of 50 years of ruptured abdominal aortic aneurysm repair. *Br J Surg.* 2002;89:714-717, 730.

122. Gerasimidis T et al. Endovascular management of ruptured abdominal aortic aneurysms: 6-year experience from a Greek center. *J Vasc Surg.* 2005;42(4):615-623.

123. Schermerhorn ML et al. Endovascular vs. open repair of abdominal aortic aneurysms in the Medicare population. *N Engl J Med.* 2008;358(5):464-474.

124. Van Marrewijk C et al. Significance of endoleaks after endovascular repair after abdominal aortic aneurysm. *J Vasc Surg.* 2002;35:461-473.

125. Carpenter JP et al. Durability of benefits of endovascular versus conventional abdominal aortic aneurysm repair. *J Vasc Surg.* 2002;35:222-228.

126. Boyle JR et al. Endovascular AAA repair attenuates the inflammatory and renal responses associated with conventional surgery. *J Endovasc Ther.* 2000;7(5):359-71.

127. Ayerdi J, Hodgson KJ. Fundamental techniques in endovascular surgery. In: Rutherford RB. *Vascular Surgery.* 6th ed. Philadelphia: Saunders; 2005:747-748.

128. Buth J et al. Outcome of endovascular abdominal aortic aneurysm repair in patients with conditions considered unfit for an open procedure. *J Vasc Surg.* 2002;35:211-221.

129. Verhoeven EL et al. Local anesthesia for endovascular abdominal aortic aneurysm repair. *J Vasc Surg.* 2005;42(3):402e1-402e9.

130. Henretta JP et al. Feasibility of endovascular repair of abdominal aortic aneurysms with local anesthesia with intravenous sedation. *J Vasc Surg.* 1999;29(5):793-798.

131. Alsac JM et al. The impact of aortic endografts on renal function. *J Vasc Surg.* 2005;41(6):926-930.

132. Katzen B et al. Retrograde migration of an abdominal aortic aneurysm endograft leading to postoperative renal failure. *J Vasc Surg.* 2005;42(2):784-787.

133. Thompson JP et al. Cardiovascular and catecholamine responses during endovascular and conventional abdominal aortic aneurysm repair. *J Vasc Surg.* 1999;17:326-333.

134. Sweeny KJ et al. Endovascular approach to abdominal aortic aneurysms limits the postoperative systemic immune response. *Eur J Vasc Surg.* 2002;23:303-308.

135. Pearson S et al. Endovascular repair of abdominal aortic aneurysm reduces intraoperative cortisol and perioperative morbidity. *J Vasc Surg.* 2005;41(6):919-925.

136. Fairman RM et al. Endovascular repair of aortic aneurysms: critical events and adjunctive procedures. *J Vasc Surg.* 2001;33:1226-1232.

137. Zaugg M et al. Sudden respiratory arrest resulting from brainstem embolism in a patient undergoing endovascular abdominal aortic aneurysm repair. *Anesth Analg.* 2001;92(2):335-337.

138. Gerasimidis T et al. Impact of endograft material on the inflammatory response after elective endovascular abdominal aortic aneurysm repair. *Angiology.* 2005;56(6):743-753.

139. Grube E et al. TAXUS 1: six- and twelve-month results from a randomized, double-blinded trial on a slow-release paclitaxel eluting stent for cardiac lesions. *Circulation.* 2003;107:38-42.

140. Morice MC et al. A randomized comparison of a sirolimus-eluting stent with a standard stent for coronary revascularization. *N Engl J Med.* 2002;346:1773-1780.

141. Brewster DC. Presidential address: what would you do if it was your father? reflections of endovascular abdominal aortic aneurysm. *J Vasc Surg.* 2001;33:1139-1147.

142. Buth J, Harris P. Endovascular treatment of aortic aneurysms. In: Rutherford RB, ed. *Vascular Surgery.* 6th ed. Philadelphia: Saunders; 2005:1452-1475.

143. Buth J, Laheij RJ. Early complications and endoleaks after endovascular abdominal aortic aneurysm repair: report of a multicenter study. *J Vasc Surg.* 2000;31:134-146.

144. Dattilo JB et al. Clinical failures of endovascular abdominal aortic aneurysm repair: incidence, causes and management. *J Vasc Surg.* 2002;35:1137-1144.

145. Chaikoff EL et al. Ad Hoc Committee for Standardization Reporting Practices in Vascular Surgery, Society of Vascular Surgery/American Association of Vascular Surgery. Reporting standards for endovascular aortic aneurysm repair. *J Vasc Surg.* 2002;35:1048-1060.

146. Haytner CL et al. Follow-up costs increase the cost disparity between endovascular and open abdominal aortic aneurysm repair. *J Vasc Surg.* 2005;42(5):912-918.

147. Mackey WC. Extracranial cerebral vascular disease. In: Cameron JL, ed. *Current Surgical Therapy.* 4th ed. St Louis: Mosby; 1992:684.

148. Warlow C. Surgical versus medical treatment for symptomatic carotid atherosclerosis. *Acta Chir Scand.* 1990;555(Suppl):223-224.

149. Wolf PA et al. Transient ischemic attacks and the risk of stroke: the Framingham study. *Circulation.* 1979;60:98.

150. Massachusetts Medical Society. Beneficial effect of CEA in symptomatic patients with high-grade carotid stenosis. *N Engl J Med.* 1991;325:445-453.

151. Executive Committee for the Asymptomatic Carotid Atherosclerosis (ACAS) Study. Endarterectomy for asymptomatic carotid artery stenosis. *JAMA.* 1995;273:1421-1428.

152. Wheeler HB. Presidential address: common sense and CEA. *J Vasc Surg.* 1990;11:735-744.

153. Callow AD, Mackey WC. Optimum results of the surgical treatment of carotid territory ischemia. *Circulation.* 1991;83(Suppl 1):190-195.

154. Callow AD, Mackey WC. Long-term follow-up of surgically managed carotid bifurcation atherosclerosis. *Ann Surg.* 1989;210:308-315.

155. Hsia DC et al. Epidemiology of carotid endarterectomies among Medicare beneficiaries. *J Vasc Surg.* 1992;16:201-208.

156. Ackroyd N et al. CEA long-term follow-up with specific reference to recurrent stenosis: contralateral progression, mortality and recurrent neurological episodes. *J Cardiovasc Surg.* 1986;27:418-425.

157. Schroder T. How to predict which patient with carotid atherosclerosis is "high risk.". *Acta Chir Scand.* 1990;555(Suppl):209-222.

158. Sieber FE et al. Preoperative risks predict neurological outcome of CEA-related strokes. *Neurosurgery.* 1992;30:847-854.

159. Young B et al. ACAS Investigators. Asymptomatic Carotid Atherosclerosis Study. An analysis of perioperative surgical mortality and morbidity in the asymptomatic carotid atherosclerosis patient. *Stroke.* 1996;27:2216-2224.

160. Cambria RP et al. Simultaneous carotid and coronary disease: safety of the combined approach. *J Vasc Surg.* 1989;9:56-64.

161. Perler BA et al. Should we perform CEA synchronously with cardiac surgical procedures? *J Vasc Surg.* 1988;8:402-409.

162. Chang BB et al. CEA can be safely performed with acceptable mortality and morbidity in patients requiring coronary artery bypass grafts. *Am J Surg.* 1994;168:94-96.

163. Riotta JJ et al. Modeling stroke risk after coronary artery bypass and combined coronary artery bypass graft and CEA. *Stroke.* 2003;34:1212-1217.

164. Brown KR et al. Multistate population-based outcomes of combined CEA and coronary artery bypass graft. *J Vasc Surg.* 2003;37:32-39.

165. Lam AM et al. Monitoring electrophysiologic function during CEA: a comparison of somatosensory evoked potentials and conventional electroencephalogram. *Anesthesiology.* 1991;75:15-21.

166. Redekop G, Ferguson G. Correlation of contralateral stenosis and intraoperative electroencephalogram change with risk of stroke during CEA. *Neurosurgery.* 1992;30:191-194.

167. Dared M. CEA: anesthesia and monitoring. *Acta Anaesthesiol Belg.* 1988;39(Suppl 2):271-273.

168. Harada RN et al. Stump pressure, electroencephalographic changes, and the contralateral carotid artery: another look at selective shunting. *Am J Surg.* 1995;170:148-153.

169. Young WL et al. Intraoperative 133Xe cerebral blood flow measurements by intravenous versus intracarotid methods. *Anesthesiology.* 1990;73:637-643.

170. McDowell HA Jr et al. CEA monitored with transcranial Doppler. *Ann Surg.* 1992;215:514-519.

171. Wilke HJ et al. CEA: perioperative and anesthetic considerations. *J Cardiothorac Vasc Anesth.* 1996;10:928-949.

172. Hankey GJ et al. Routine or selective carotid artery shunting for CEA. *Stroke.* 2003;34:824-825.

173. Todd MM et al. Mild intraoperative hypothermia during surgery for intracranial aneurysm. *N Engl J Med.* 2005;352:135-145.

174. Elliott BM et al. Intraoperative local anesthetic injection of the carotid sinus nerve: a prospective, randomized study. *Am J Surg.* 1986;152:695-699.

175. Mangano DT et al. Effect of atenolol on mortality and cardiac morbidity after noncardiac surgery. *N Engl J Med.* 1996;23:1713-1720.

176. Rerkasem K et al. Local versus general anesthetic for carotid endarterectomy. *J Vasc Surg.* 2005;36:169-170.

177. Sternbach Y et al. Hemodynamic benefits of regional anesthesia for carotid endarterectomy. *J Vasc Surg.* 2002;35(2):333-339.

178. Mehta M, Veith FJ. Regarding "Hemodynamic benefits of regional anesthesia for carotid endarterectomy." *J Vasc Surg.* 2003;37(5):1134-1135.

179. Mofidi R et al. Regional versus general anesthesia for carotid endarterectomy: impact of change in practice. *Surgeon.* 2006;4(3):158-162.

180. Meitzner MC et al. A literature review on anesthetic practice for carotid endarterectomy surgery based on cost, hemodynamic stability and neurologic status. *AANA J.* 2007;75(3):193-196.

181. Watts K et al. The impact of anesthetic modality on the outcome of carotid endarterectomy. *Am J Surg.* 2004;188:741-747.

182. Corson JD et al. The influence of anesthetic choice on CEA outcome. *Arch Surg.* 1987;122:807-812.

183. McCarthy RJ et al. Physiological advantages of cerebral blood flow during CEA under local anesthesia: a randomized trial. *Eur J Vasc Surg.* 2002;24:215-221.

184. Allen BT et al. The influence of anesthetic technique on perioperative complications after CEA. *J Vasc Surg.* 1994;19:834-842.

185. Mashiah M et al. Carotid surgery under local anesthesia in the elderly. *J Am Geriatr Soc.* 1988;36:545-547.

186. Zuccarello M et al. Morbidity and mortality of CEA under local anesthesia: a retrospective study. *Neurosurgery.* 1988;23:445-450.

187. Slutzki S et al. CEA under local anesthesia supplemented with neuroleptic analgesia. *Surg Gynecol Obstet.* 1990;170:141-144.

188. Knighton JD, Stoneham M. Carotid endarterectomy: a survey of UK anaesthetic practice. *Anaesthesia.* 2000;55(5):481-495.

189. Messick JM Jr et al. Correlation of regional cerebral blood flow (rCBF) with EEG changes during isoflurane anesthesia for CEA: critical rCBF. *Anesthesiology.* 1987;66:344-349.

190. De Hert SG et al. Cardioprotection with volatile anesthetics: mechanisms and clinical implications. *Anesth Analg.* 2005;100(6):1584-1593.

191. Nasu I et al. The dose-dependent effects of isoflurane on outcome from severe forebrain ischemia in the rat. *Anesth Analg.* 2006;103(2):413-418.

192. Feng J et al. Infarct-remodeled myocardium is receptive to protection by isoflurane preconditioning: role of protein B/AKT signaling. *Anesthesiology.* 2006;104(5):1004-1014.

193. Michenfelder JD et al. Isoflurane when compared to enflurane and halothane decreases the frequency of cerebral ischemia during CEA. *Anesthesiology.* 1987;67:336-340.

194. Cucchiara RF et al. Myocardial infarction in CEA patients anesthetized with halothane, enflurane or isoflurane. *Anesthesiology.* 1988;69:783-784.

195. Young WL et al. A comparison of the cerebral hemodynamic effects of sufentanil and isoflurane in humans undergoing CEA. *Anesthesiology.* 1989;71:863-869.

196. Herrick IA, Gelb AW. Occlusive cerebrovascular disease: anesthetic considerations. In: Cottrell JE, Smith DS, eds. *Anesthesia and Neurosurgery.* St Louis: Mosby; 2001.

197. Palmer M. Comparison of regional and general anesthesia for CEA. *Am J Surg.* 1989;157:329-333.

198. Skydell JL et al. Incidence and mechanism of post-CEA hypertension. *Arch Surg.* 1987;122:1153-1155.

199. Ascher E et al. Cerebral hyperperfusion syndrome after CEA: predictive factors and hemodynamic changes. *J Vasc Surg.* 2003;37:769-777.

200. Edwards WH Jr et al. Recurrent carotid artery stenosis: resection with autogenous vein replacement. *Ann Surg.* 1989;209:662-668.

201. Mocco J et al. Predictors of neurocognitive decline and carotid endarterectomy. *Neurosurgery.* 2006;58(5):844-850.

202. Stankovic G et al. Carotid artery stenting in the first 100 consecutive patients: results and follow up. *Heart.* 2002;88:381-386.
203. Leger AR et al. Poor durability of carotid angioplasty and stenting for treatment of recurrent artery stenosis after CEA: an institutional experience. *J Vasc Surg.* 2001;33:1008-1014.
204. Kilaru S et al. Is carotid angioplasty and stenting more cost effective than CEA? *J Vasc Surg.* 2003;37:331-339.
205. Bergeron P et al. Long-term results of carotid stenting are competitive with surgery. *J Vasc Surg.* 2005;41(2):213-221.
206. Yadav JS et al. Protected carotid artery stenting versus endarterectomy in high risk patients. *N Engl J Med.* 2004;351:1493-1501.
207. Roffi M, Yadav S. Carotid stenting. *Circulation.* 2006;114(1):1-4.
208. Mas JL et al. Endarterectomy versus stenting in patients with symptomatic severe carotid artery stenosis. *N Engl J Med.* 2006;355:1660-1671.
209. Ringleb PA et al. Thirty-day results from the SPACE trial of stent-protected angioplasty versus carotid endarterectomy in symptomatic patients: a randomized non-inferiority trial. *Lancet.* 2006;368:1239-1247.
210. Lal BK, Hobson RW. Treatment of carotid artery disease: stenting or surgery. *Curr Neurol Neurosci Rep.* 2007;7(1):49-53.
211. Longo GM et al. Carotid artery stenting in octogenarians: is it too risky? *Ann Vasc Surg.* 2005;19(6):812-816.
212. Cremonesi A et al. Carotid artery stenting: first consensus document of the ICCC-SPREAD Joint Committee. *Stroke.* 2006;37(9):2400-2409.
213. Villalobos HJ et al. Advancements in carotid stenting leading to reductions in perioperative morbidity among patients 80 years and older. *Neurosurgery.* 2006;58(2):233-240.
214. Sullivan TJ, Cloft H. Carotid angioplasty and stenting. In: Rutherford RB. *Vascular Surgery.* 6th ed. Philadelphia: Saunders; 2005:2006-2030.
215. Chaturvedi S, Yadav JS. The role of antiplatelet therapy in carotid stenting for ischemic stroke prevention. *Stroke.* 2006;37(6):1572-1577.
216. Kraiss LW et al. Short-stay CEA is safe and cost-effective. *Am J Surg.* 1995;169:512-515.
217. Ricotta JJ, Hargadon T. Cost-management strategies for CEA. *Am J Surg.* 1998;176:188-192.
218. Friedman SG, Tortolani AJ. Reduced length of stay following CEA under general anesthesia. *Am J Surg.* 1995;170:235-236.
219. Godin MS et al. Cost effectiveness of regional anesthesia in CEA. *Am Surg.* 1989;55:656-659.
220. Kilaru S et al. Is carotid angioplasty and stenting more cost effective than carotid endarterectomy. *J Vasc Surg.* 2003;37(2):331-339.

CHAPTER 27

RESPIRATORY ANATOMY, PHYSIOLOGY, PATHOPHYSIOLOGY, AND ANESTHESIA MANAGEMENT

Michael Rieker

Knowledge of the respiratory system is essential to the practice of anesthesia. Anesthetists are known as the airway experts, but we are also expected to possess an excellent command of the entire respiratory system. This is not surprising, considering that we administer oxygen to the majority of our patients, administer inhaled anesthetics down a cascade of concentration gradients through the lungs, provide artificial ventilation for many patients under general anesthesia, and monitor and interpret blood gas analysis, capnography, and oximetry in our patients. Indeed, the visual hallmark of an anesthetist is frequently a stethoscope earpiece pinned to the scrub top; a device that places each patient breath at the forefront of our consciousness.

Besides the basic functions of the respiratory system to extract oxygen (O_2) from the atmosphere and deliver it to the blood while excreting carbon dioxide (CO_2), the respiratory system functions in acid-base balance, phonation, pulmonary defense, and metabolism (synthesis and breakdown of bioactive materials). These functions will be discussed in this chapter.

ANATOMY OF THE RESPIRATORY SYSTEM

Knowledge of airway anatomy is not only necessary for understanding respiratory physiology but also essential for anesthesiology practice. The airway consists of the nose, mouth, pharynx, larynx, trachea, and lower airways.

The components of the respiratory system are the conducting airways, the lungs, the portions of the central nervous system responsible for control of the muscles of ventilation, and the chest wall and thoracic muscles responsible for ventilation.

Nose

Inhaled air enters the body through the nose or mouth. Air passing through the nose is filtered, heated to body temperature, and humidified. The external nose is only a small part of the nasal air passageway, the major portion of which lies directly behind and includes three scroll-shaped turbinate bones, also called the *nasal conchae*.

The cartilage around the entrance to the nostrils that can flare during heavy breathing is called the *alar cartilage* or *ala nasae* ("nasal wings"). Each nostril opening (anterior naris) leads directly into the vestibule, which is the forwardly expanded portion of the nasal cavity. The vestibule is lined with cutaneous epithelium. In its lower half, it has sebaceous glands and coarse hairs, sometimes referred to as *vibrissae*. The floor of the nose is at a level higher than the opening of the nostril; therefore, during nasal intubation, the apex of the nose should be elevated superiorly with gentle pressure while the tube is inserted parallel to the roof of the mouth. The tube should not be directed upward into the turbinates but rather along the floor of the nose formed by the superior aspect of the palatine bone, which below forms the hard palate of the mouth. Prolonged nasotracheal intubation is associated with obstruction of the nasal sinuses, sinus infection, and fever. Intranasal infections can produce intracranial infection via vascular connections, as discussed later in this section.

The anterior portion of the external nose, the vestibule, expands above and behind into triangular spaces, or fossae. The fossae are separated from each other by the nasal septum, which also separates the two nostrils. The septum is formed by the ethmoid and vomer bones superiorly and the vomeronasal and nasal septal cartilages inferiorly. The nasal fossae usually communicate freely with the paranasal air sinuses (frontal, ethmoid, maxillary, and sphenoid). They open into the nasopharynx by the posterior nares (also known as *choanae*) and are bordered medially by the nasal septum and laterally by three turbinates arranged one above the other. Choanal atresia is a birth defect that results in the obstruction of the airway of the obligate nose-breathing newborn.

The conchae are scroll-shaped prominences projecting from the lateral walls and have their free margins directed downward and inward. The spaces these conchae overlie and partly shut off from the nasal cavity are the superior, middle, and inferior meatus (which contain the openings to the paranasal sinuses).[1] The superior concha is by far the smallest of the three, and the middle concha extends forward much farther than the superior. The inferior concha, which lies along the lower part of the lateral wall of the nasal cavity, is in the pathway of airflow in the nose. It is the one most commonly injured during nasal intubation. It extends to within approximately 2 cm of the middle of the anterior naris, and its posterior tip lies approximately 1 cm in front of the pharyngeal orifice of the eustachian tube. Eustachian drainage can become obstructed when the inferior concha or adenoid tonsils become inflamed. Such obstruction can lead to middle ear pathology.

The nasal cavities are lined with mucous membranes that are continuous with those of the pharynx. The mucosa can be divided into respiratory and olfactory areas because it not only lines the tracts followed by respired air but also covers the cells that act as the receptors for smell. The olfactory epithelium occupies the apical third of the nasal cavity. This epithelium contains afferent fibers from the olfactory nerves (cranial nerve I) that communicate through the cribriform plate of the ethmoid bone to the adjacent olfactory bulb intracranially. Signals then progress to the other parts of the rhinencephalon. The respiratory mucosa lines the lower two thirds of the nose and consists of pseudostratified ciliated columnar epithelium interspersed with goblet cells that produce mucus. Although the morphology of cells changes progressively toward the terminal bronchioles, this general arrangement of stratified ciliated epithelium with goblet cells persists through the majority of the air passages of the respiratory system. The direction of motion of the cilia is toward the exterior of the nasal cavity, and the amount of mucus produced can often be copious. The principal arterial supply of the nasal fossae comes from the ophthalmic arteries through the anterior and posterior ethmoid branches and from the internal maxillary artery through the sphenopalatine arteries. Because of the location of the interior maxillary artery, it is sometimes ligated for the treatment of persistent nosebleed. The veins accompany the arteries; the ethmoid veins open into the superior sagittal sinus, and the nasal veins drain into the ophthalmic veins and then into the cavernous sinuses. Infections in the nose can result in meningitis because of this venous communication between the intracranial and intranasal circulation. The sensory nerves from the upper respiratory tract come from the ophthalmic nerve and the maxillary nerve (both are branches of cranial V). Lymphatic drainage from the cavities of the nose is via the deep cervical lymph nodes adjacent to the internal jugular vein.

Owing to the presence of the vibrissae, the mucus-producing epithelium, and the rich arterial supply, the nose carries out important functions, including the filtration, humidification, and heating of inspired air. As long as the incoming air is not extremely cold, the nose can warm the inspired air to nearly body temperature and moisten the air to nearly 100% relative humidity. The heating and humidifying functions of the nose are affected by general anesthesia. The inspiration of cold, dry gas often dries the nasal and pharyngeal passageways, causing sore throat even if no manipulation of the airway takes place. The hairs at the entrance to the nostrils are of minor importance to filtration because they remove only large particles. Much more important is the removal of particles by turbulent precipitation. Air passing through the nasal passageways hits many obstructions: the septum, the turbinates, and the pharyngeal wall. When the inspired air is forced to change direction, the inhaled particles cannot change course as rapidly, and they become embedded in the sticky mucus-covered surfaces of these processes. The particles trapped in the mucus are moved by the cilia either to the nostril or posteriorly to the pharynx to be either expectorated or swallowed. This nasal mechanism for removing particles from the air is so effective that almost no particle greater than approximately 6 mm in size is allowed to enter the trachea.[2]

Pharynx

The pharynx is a wide muscular tube that is a part of both the respiratory tract and the alimentary tract. Its upper border is the base of the skull, and it extends to the level of the C6 vertebra, where it becomes continuous with the esophagus. At this level, ingested foreign bodies, such as coins, are frequently lodged. The pharynx is lined by a musculomembranous coat and divided into three parts: the nasopharynx, which extends from the posterior nares (choanae) to the end of the soft palate; the oropharynx, which is bounded superiorly by the soft palate and anteriorly by the tonsillar pillars and oral cavity and extends inferiorly to the tip of the epiglottis; and the laryngopharynx, which extends from the tip of the epiglottis to the level of C6, or the beginning of the esophagus.

TABLE 27-1	The Nine Cartilages of the Larynx		
Unpaired Cartilages		**Paired Cartilages**	
Number	**Name**	**Number**	**Name**
1	Epiglottic	4 and 5	Arytenoids
2	Thyroid	6 and 7	Corniculates
3	Cricoid	8 and 9	Cuneiforms

The pharyngeal region includes the tonsils, which are composed of three aggregations of lymphoid tissue; the palatine tonsils (major tonsils), which lie in the tonsillar fossae at the boundary of the oral cavity and oropharynx; the lingual tonsils, which extend across the tongue from the base of each palatine tonsil; and the pharyngeal tonsils (adenoids), which lie on the lateral walls of the nasopharynx. The lymphoid tissue of the tonsils forms the Waldeyer tonsillar ring, which acts as a first line of defense against bacterial invasion of the nasal and buccal passages. If inflamed, the pharyngeal tonsils may obstruct air flow through the choanae and are sometimes removed by an adenoidectomy. Likewise, chronic tonsillitis may lead to removal of the palatine tonsils by tonsillectomy.

Blood supply to the entire mouth and pharyngeal region is from branches of the external carotid artery. Venous drainage is via the facial vein and the external jugular vein. The nerve supply to the inner mouth is from cranial nerves VII, IX, X, and XII. The lymphatic circulation is abundant, draining into the cervical lymph nodes located under and anterior to the sternocleidomastoid muscle (this configuration accounts for lumps in the neck that accompany a sore throat).

Larynx

The adult larynx extends from vertebrae C3 to C6 and is a protective structure that prevents aspiration during swallowing; vocalization evolved secondarily. The larynx consists of one bone, nine pieces of cartilage (Table 27-1), ligaments, muscles, and membranes.

The hyoid bone is the chief support for the larynx and is the only bone that does not form a joint with another bone. Its anterior aspect can be easily palpated, and its location is sometimes used as a measure of airway assessment for laryngoscopy. The thyroid cartilage and the cricoid cartilage make up the principal part of the framework of the larynx, whereas the epiglottis guards its entrance.

Laryngeal Cartilages

The epiglottic cartilage lies closest to the root of the tongue and is vertical to the opening of the larynx. It is attached to the body of the thyroid cartilage by the thyroepiglottic ligament just above the vocal cords and to the base of the tongue by the glossoepiglottic folds. The furrow between the glossoepiglottic fold and the base of the tongue is called the *vallecula epiglottica* and serves as the situation point for the tip of a curved laryngoscope blade. The epiglottis serves to protect the larynx from foreign body entry. During swallowing or laryngospasm, elevation of the larynx and closure of the epiglottis effectively "seal off" the trachea.

The thyroid cartilage is the largest cartilage of the larynx, formed by two quadrangular plates or laminae fused near the midline anteriorly. It has great strength and affords a great deal of protection to the larynx. The thyroid cartilage forms the

Adam's apple. Being larger and covered with less subcutaneous fat, the thyroid cartilage is more prominent in adult males.

The cricoid cartilage is palpable just below the thyroid gland, and its level corresponds to the beginning of the trachea and the esophagus. It is the only true ring of cartilage encircling the airway. Anteriorly, the cricoid cartilage lies below the thyroid cartilage, with the cricothyroid membrane intervening. The cricoid is the most inferior of the nine laryngeal cartilages. The arytenoid cartilages articulate on the superior posterior aspect of the cricoid cartilage, which is slanted forward. The paired arytenoid cartilages are attached to the posterior ends of the vocal cords. The paired corniculate (median) and cuneiform (more lateral) cartilages are embedded in the aryepiglottic folds and give support to these structures. These cartilages cause the two bumps seen in the aryepiglottic folds, which are mistakenly called the "arytenoids" when visualized during difficult intubation.

In adults, the narrowest portion of the laryngeal cavity is the area between the vocal cords; in children younger than 10 years, the narrowest part is just below the cords at the cricoid cartilage. This anatomic difference is of clinical significance: when small children are intubated, a tube may pass through the cords but will be unable to pass through the cricoid ring.[3] Likewise, because the complete circle of the cricoid cartilage can form a seal around the endotracheal tube; an uncuffed endotracheal tube may be used in children less than 8 to 10 years of age. In adults the space between the vocal cords (glottis) is smaller than the inside of the cricoid cartilage; therefore a cuffed tube is necessary to form a seal that allows for positive-pressure ventilation.

Membranes of the Larynx

The thyrohyoid membrane suspends the larynx from the hyoid bone. The conus elasticus, or cricothyroid membrane, lies between the cricoid and the thyroid cartilages. The easiest and most rapid laryngotomy can be performed through this membrane. Cricothyrotomy is recommended for the emergency establishment of an airway when both endotracheal intubation and mask ventilation are unsuccessful. The so-called "transtracheal block" also can be performed through the cricothyroid membrane.

Interior of Larynx

The cavity of the larynx is divided into three compartments by the false vocal cords and the true vocal cords. The supraglottic area, also called the *vestibule*, extends from above the false cords to the tip of the epiglottis. On each side of the vestibule is located a pharyngeal sinus (the pyriform sinus). This recess or sinus is

important because it is likely to be a place at which foreign bodies that enter the pharynx become lodged. The second compartment of the larynx is the area between the false cords and the true cords known as the *laryngeal ventricles*. The third area is the infraglottic region below the true cords and above the beginning of the trachea. The rima glottidis (glottic slit) is the space between the true cords.

Movements of the Vocal Cords

The true vocal cords are fibromembranous folds attached anteriorly to the thyroid cartilage and posteriorly to the arytenoids. The focal points of movement are the arytenoid cartilages, which rotate and slide up and down on the sloping cricoid cartilage. The muscles controlling laryngeal movement (Box 27-1) are most conveniently thought of as pairs having opposing actions. The laryngeal inlet is closed by the aryepiglottic muscle and opened by the thyroepiglottic muscle. The glottic slit is dilated by the posterior cricoarytenoid muscles and closed by the interarytenoid muscles assisted by the lateral cricoarytenoid muscles. The cricothyroid muscles lengthen the true vocal cords, and the thyroarytenoid muscles shorten them. Both sets of muscles can alter the tension on the vocal cords and are important for determining the pitch of the voice[4] (Figure 27-1).

Nerve Supply to the Larynx

Both the superior and inferior laryngeal nerves are branches of cranial nerve X (the vagus nerve). The superior laryngeal nerve

---

BOX 27-1

Intrinsic Muscles of the Larynx

Laryngeal Inlet
　Closed by the aryepiglottic muscle
　Opened by the thyroepiglottic muscle

Glottic Slit
　Open the posterior cricoarytenoid muscles
　Closed by the interarytenoid muscle and the lateral
　　cricoarytenoid muscles

True Vocal Cords
　Lengthened by the cricothyroid muscles
　Shortened by thyroarytenoid muscles

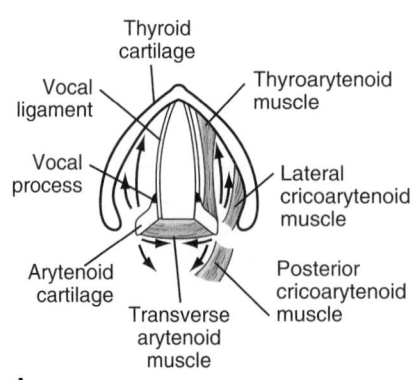
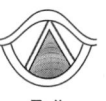

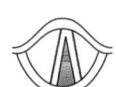
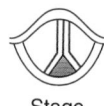
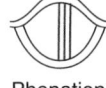

FIGURE **27-1** **A**, Anatomy of the throat. **B**, Laryngeal function in phonation showing the positions of the vocal folds during different types of phonation. (*Modified from Greene MC: The Voice and Its Disorders. 4th ed. Philadelphia: JB Lippincott; 1980.*)

A

B

arises from the ganglion nodosum of the vagus and divides into two branches, the internal and external. The external segment gives a branch to the inferior constrictor muscle of the pharynx and also to the cricothyroid muscles. These muscles change the position of the cricoid and thyroid cartilages and in doing so lengthen or increase the tension of the vocal cords. If these muscles are paralyzed, the voice becomes weak, rough, and easily fatigued. Voice hoarseness, particularly of recent onset, should be investigated in the preoperative evaluation as a potential indicator or vocal cord palsy or airway obstruction. The internal branch of the superior laryngeal nerve enters the larynx and then the thyrohyoid membrane and is distributed to the mucous membranes of the larynx and epiglottis. It provides sensation from the laryngeal side of the epiglottis down to the true cords (the tongue side of the epiglottis is innervated by the glossopharyngeal nerve). The internal branch also innervates the interarytenoid muscles, which are important in phonation.

The inferior (or recurrent) laryngeal nerves arise from the two vagus nerves at different levels. The left nerve descends with the vagus and then loops around the arch of the aorta to come back up to the neck. The right nerve travels with the vagus nerve as far as the subclavian artery; it loops around this artery and then comes back up the neck. The recurrent laryngeal nerve supplies sensation to the larynx below the level of the vocal cords and innervates all the muscles of the larynx except the cricothyroid and part of the interarytenoid muscles. Damage to the recurrent laryngeal nerve(s) during surgery on the neck or from airway devices or anesthetic blocks can lead to unilateral or bilateral vocal cord paralysis with hoarseness or dyspnea, respectively.[5,6] Blood supply to the larynx is provided by the superior thyroid artery (a branch of the external carotid artery) and the inferior thyroid artery (a branch of the thyrocervical trunk, which arises from the subclavian artery).[7]

Trachea

The trachea is lined by pseudostratified ciliated columnar epithelium, and it extends from the inferior larynx to the carina, where it bifurcates into the two mainstem bronchi. In adults of normal size, the distances are fairly constant: the distance from the incisors to the larynx is approximately 13 cm, as is that from the larynx to the carina. Therefore, the distance from the incisors to the carina is approximately 26 cm (note the distance marks on endotracheal tubes). The blood supply to the trachea is through the inferior thyroid artery, which comes from the thyrocervical branch of the subclavian artery. Some perfusion is also received from the superior thyroid, bronchial, and internal thoracic arteries. Blood is drained by the inferior thyroid veins. Sensory innervation of the trachea is via the vagus nerve for both parasympathetic and nociceptive stimuli.

The trachea has a diameter of approximately 2.5 cm and is supported by incomplete rings of cartilage that open posteriorly and prevent tracheal collapse under the negative pressure generated during spontaneous respiration. The trachea extends down to the level of T4-T5, where the carina is located. This posterior T4-T5 level corresponds anteriorly to the angle of Louis on the sternum, which is the articulation of the second rib. The trachea is not a "fixed" structure—that is, it moves with head or neck movement. If a patient flexes the neck, the trachea moves upward; as a result, the endotracheal tube moves downward and endobronchial intubation may result. During extension of the head and neck, the trachea moves downward, the endotracheal tube moves upward, and extubation can occur. The apparent movement of the endotracheal tube in relation to head

flexion may seem paradoxical, and can be remembered by the mnemonic "the hose follows the nose." Neck rotation to the left or right tends to cause tracheal elevation and risk of endobronchial intubation.

Bronchi

At the carina, the trachea divides into the right and left bronchi. The cellular structure begins to change at this point from columnar to cuboidal epithelium, and the cartilaginous rings thin into plates once the bronchi penetrate the lungs. From the carina, the bronchi branch off at slightly different angles. The right bronchus takes a less acute angle from the trachea, about 25 degrees, while the left bronchus takes off at 45 degrees. Also, the right mainstem bronchus is wider and shorter (2 cm) than the left one (4 cm).[8] Because the right bronchus is more nearly vertical than the left, the tendency is much greater for endotracheal tubes, suction catheters, or aspirated foreign materials to enter the right side after passing the carina. Additionally, the beveled tip of an endotracheal tube makes right-sided intubation more likely. The side hole (Murphy's eye) near the end of the endotracheal tube allows the delivery of gas if the beveled tip of the tube is closely opposed to the similarly angled right main bronchus.

Each mainstem bronchus divides into lobar bronchi (three on the right; two on the left), that lead to the major lung lobes. The right mainstem bronchus ends only 2 to 2.5 cm from the carina before giving rise to the right upper lobe (RUL) bronchus. This bronchus exits almost 90 degrees posteriorly, which, in addition to the shallow takeoff of the right main bronchus, promotes aspirated material flow to the RUL, following gravity in the supine position. After the RUL takeoff, the main bronchus then continues for 3 cm as the *bronchus intermedius* before giving rise to the right middle lobe bronchus and the right lower lobe bronchus. The left main bronchus is 4 cm long and terminates by bifurcating into the left upper lobe bronchus and the left lower lobe bronchus. The left upper lobe bronchus divides into halves, an upper half and a lower half (the lingular branch).

Each successive division of the airways is referred to as a *generation*, with the mainstem bronchi representing the first generation, the lobar bronchi representing the second, and so on. The lobar bronchi divide into the third generation of airways, called *segmental bronchi*, which deliver ventilation to the various bronchopulmonary segments of the lung. There are 10 bronchopulmonary segments in each lung, but on the left, the apical and posterior segments and the anterior basal and medial basal segment pairs each arise from a single bronchial branch (Box 27-2). Therefore, there are only eight third-generation bronchi on the left. Segments whose names contain the word *basal* are located adjacent to the diaphragm. The bronchopulmonary segments create distinct units. The segments are separated by connective tissue, so gas-exchange properties or pathology tend to be isolated to a segment. A bronchopulmonary segment can also be excised as a unit.

Each subsegmental bronchus divides several times, giving rise to many bronchioles. With succeeding generations and multiplication of the number of airways, the total cross-sectional area becomes very large, and the airflow velocity decreases. There are 20 to 25 total generations before the alveoli. By the seventh generation, the diameter of bronchioles is about 2 mm, and beyond this point, they are referred to as *small airways*. When the diameter has decreased to 1 mm they are referred to as *terminal bronchioles*. The terminal bronchioles are the last structures perfused by the bronchial circulation and are the end of the conducting airways (anatomic deadspace, as discussed later).

BOX 27-2

Lung Lobes and Segments

I. Right lung
   A. Right upper lobe (3 segments)
      1. Apical
      2. Anterior
      3. Posterior
   B. Right middle lobe (2 segments)
      1. Medial
      2. Lateral
   C. Right lower lobe (5 segments)
      1. Superior
      2. Anterior basal
      3. Posterior basal
      4. Lateral basal
      5. Medial basal
II. Left lung
   A. Left upper lobe (4 segments)
      1. Apical posterior
      2. Anterior
      3. Superior lingular
      4. Inferior lingular
   B. Left lower lobe (4 segments)
      1. Superior
      2. Anteromedial basal
      3. Posterior basal
      4. Lateral basal

BOX 27-3

Characteristics of Progressive Airway Divisions

With each succeeding generation:
- Number of airways ↑
- Cross sectional area ↑
- Airflow velocity ↓
- Cartilage ↓
- Mucous glands absent in bronchioles
- Goblet cells ↓
- Muscular layer ↑
- Ciliated cells ↓ & give way to cuboidal, then to squamous

In the latter generations, the cross-sectional area of the airway has expanded so much that the velocity of airflow becomes very slow, and gas moves largely by diffusion rather than by bulk flow.

With succeeding generations, the histology of the airways changes, in a progression characterized by thinning of the walls, to transition to the gas-exchanging morphology of the *respiratory zone* (Box 27-3). The terminal bronchioles divide into the respiratory bronchioles that are perfused by the pulmonary circulation and are the first place in the airway at which exchange of gas with the blood occurs. These airways are characterized by occasional outpouching of alveoli, or air sacs. The respiratory bronchioles divide into several alveolar ducts that lead to circular spaces called *atria*. Each atrium opens into two to five alveolar sacs, which are spaces lined by alveoli. The terminal airways are very small, and their walls are no longer tented open by cartilage but rather by connection with the adjacent matrix of pulmonary parenchyma in which they are situated. For this reason, they are prone to closure from compression of the pulmonary tissue during respiration or if emphysema, for example, expands the volume of adjacent air spaces and compresses the airways. The lung volume at which small airways tend to close is called the *closing volume*. In obesity and COPD, the closing volume increases into the range of normal tidal breathing such that some airways close before the intended tidal volume has been expired. Small pores in the alveoli, known as the *pores of Kohn*, serve to allow collateral gas flow between alveoli and provide a mechanism of relief from gas stagnation from airway closure.

Respiratory Zone

The respiratory bronchioles and alveolar ducts, sacs, and alveoli comprise the *respiratory zone*, the area where gas exchange takes place. All parts of the airway prior (nose to terminal bronchioles) conduct gas without exchanging gas with the blood and are referred to as the *conducting zone*. Some refer to the respiratory bronchioles and alveolar ducts where limited gas exchange takes place as the *transitional zone* because this zone not only functions to conduct gas but also participates in some gas exchange. The alveoli are the air sacs that are tightly packed and closely approximated with pulmonary capillaries. The typical maximum number of approximately 300 million alveoli is reached by age 9. The alveoli are characterized by very thin walls composed of squamous epithelium. There are three types of cells that form the alveoli: type I pneumocytes, which are the structural cells; type II pneumocytes, which produce surfactant to reduce alveolar collapse from surface tension; and type III pneumocytes, which are macrophages.

Pulmonary Hila and Coverings

The nerve supply to the bronchi and lungs arises chiefly from the sympathetic nerves and the vagus nerve (which supplies sensory and parasympathetic innervation). All conduits to the lung pass through the hilum, which is the connection of the mediastinum to the pedicle of each lung. The structures included in each hilum include the mainstem bronchus, pulmonary artery and vein, bronchial arteries and veins (which drain into the azygous system), lymphatics, lymph nodes, pulmonary nerve plexuses, and pulmonary ligament. All of this is surrounded by connective tissue. The serous membrane covering the lung is called the *pleura*. The parietal pleura lines the chest wall, mediastinum, and diaphragm, and at the hilum is then reflected back to cover the lungs as the visceral pleura. Between these two layers is a potential space called the *pleural cavity*. The touching surfaces of the two layers of pleura are kept slippery by a small amount of serous fluid. Certain conditions can result in occupation of the pleural space by liquids or gas (Table 27-2) and may affect ventilation and lung expansion. Infected intrapleural blood can clot and organize to form a fibrothorax, which must be peeled from the surface of the lung (in a procedure called *lung decortication*) so the lung can reexpand.

Mediastinum

The mediastinum is the region between the two pleural sacs. It lies roughly in the center of the thoracic cavity but is slightly

TABLE 27-2 Conditions That Affect the Pleural Space

Material in Pleural Space	Medical Name
Air	Pneumothorax
Air under pressure	Tension pneumothorax
Blood	Hemothorax
Serous fluid	Pleural effusion
Pus	Empyema or pyothorax
Organized blood clot	Fibrothorax
Lymph	Chylothorax

TABLE 27-3 Divisions of the Mediastinum

Subdivision	Location	Contents
Superior	Above level of the sternal angle, extending superior to the thoracic inlet	Thymus, esophagus, trachea, great vessels
Anterior	Between sternum and pericardium	Thymus
Posterior	Between vertebral column and posterior pericardium	Esophagus, thoracic aorta, thoracic duct
Middle	Between anterior and posterior divisions, bounded laterally by the parietal pleura	Heart, distal trachea, mainstem bronchi, and great vessel trunks

of the pleura may produce characteristic pain patterns: the costal pleura creates localized pain, the diaphragmatic pleura creates diffuse pain, and areas supplied by the phrenic nerve may radiate pain to the neck or back. Posterior to the mediastinum, the pleura doubles up and descends downward as the "pulmonary ligament."

If communication is created across the pleura, accumulation of air in the pleural space is referred to as *pneumothorax*. In a closed chest (e.g., a pulmonary bleb ruptures, creating a communication to the pleural space) a tension pneumothorax develops as inspired air accumulates in the pleural space and is not expelled. With an opening through both pleura (such as with open chest trauma) the external wound may create a simple pneumothorax, which does not tend to cause high intrathoracic pressures. In either type of pneumothorax, the elastic recoil of the lung tends to favor lung collapse once the negative pressure of the pleural space is disrupted by the breach.[9,10] (See Figure 28-9 in Chapter 28.)

MECHANICS OF BREATHING

Contraction of the muscles of inspiration lowers intrathoracic pressure and causes the volume of the thoracic cavity to increase. Boyle's law explains that the increase in volume creates a reduction in pressure, which causes air to enter from the atmosphere. Spontaneous respiration therefore involves passive movement of gas, as opposed to positive-pressure ventilation, which requires generation of positive pressure in the upper airway to overcome intrathoracic pressure and expand the lungs.

The diaphragm and external intercostals are the muscles that contract during normal breathing (eupnea). While the diaphragm increases the superior-inferior dimension of the chest, the external intercostals increase the anterior-posterior diameter by elevating the ribs and sternum. Each half of the diaphragm is innervated by a branch of the phrenic nerve, which arises from the third, fourth, and fifth cervical spinal nerve roots. This anatomy gives rise to the mnemonic "C-3, 4, and 5 keep the diaphragm alive." The diaphragm is almost solely responsible for quiet respiration, and loss of the function of intercostal muscles (by a thoracic spinal cord injury or high spinal or epidural block) usually does not impair respiration. However, if coupled with paralysis of the phrenic nerve and resulting paralysis of a hemidiaphragm (such as may occur with interscalene blocks), dyspnea may result. Spinal cord injuries above the level of C-5 usually lead to dependence on mechanical ventilation.

Normally, eupneic expiration results from passive recoil of the chest wall and does not require muscular contraction, although the internal intercostal muscles may be used to augment exhalation. During forced exhalation (e.g., with coughing and the clearing of secretions), the abdominal muscles—that is, the rectus abdominis, the transversus abdominis, and the external and internal oblique muscles of the abdomen—are used. For forced inhalation, the intercostal muscles play a more prominent role, and accessory breathing muscles in the neck are also used. The diaphragm descends approximately 1 to 2 cm during eupneic breathing, but this excursion can increase to as much as 10 cm during forceful breathing. During forceful inspiration, the sternocleidomastoid and scalene muscles contract in conjunction with the diaphragm and intercostals.

The muscles of ventilation are attached to the cartilaginous and bony components (ribs, sternum, and vertebrae) of the chest. Conditions that impede chest excursion, such as thoracic kyphosis, may require reduction to further increase the chest diameter. The two domes of the diaphragm separate the thoracic and

displaced to the left by the presence of the heart. Therefore the left lung represents 45% of the total lung capacity (TLC), whereas the right lung represents 55%. Perforation of the larynx, trachea, pharynx, or esophagus, which sometimes occurs during esophagoscopy, bronchoscopy, or traumatic intubation, can produce mediastinitis, a life-threatening infection of an area containing the trachea, esophagus, and major blood vessels and heart. The mediastinum is divided into four divisions separated by the pericardium (Table 27-3). Common procedures involving the mediastinum include coronary artery bypass, cardiac valve replacement, aortic aneurysm repair, thymectomy for myasthenia gravis, resection of tumors, and mediastinoscopy for diagnosis and staging of cancer.

Pleura

The pleura is a serous membrane that lines the thoracic wall and lungs. The parietal pleura is attached to the chest wall, diaphragm, and mediastinum but is then reflected back to cover the lungs and afterward referred to as the *visceral pleura*. These two layers are closely opposed, with only a capillary-thin layer of pleural fluid between them in a potential space known as the *pleural space*. The parietal pleura is very sensitive to pain, and conditions that cause accumulation of pleural fluid or friction between the layers can be very uncomfortable. Different areas abdominal cavities and function separately, such that injury to a phrenic nerve results in paralysis in the diaphragm only on that side. The central tendon on the underside of the diaphragm provides a site of rigidity, allowing the diaphragm to tense and flatten without pulling against an external insertion point, as with other muscles. The central tendon includes an orifice for passage of the inferior vena cava. The esophagus passes through the esophageal hiatus in the diaphragm. When the diaphragm contracts during spontaneous inspiration, it flattens and moves the abdominal contents downward, raising intraabdominal pressure while lowering intrathoracic pressure. Pressure within the alveoli becomes slightly negative with respect to atmospheric pressure, and gas flows inward through the conducting airways to expand the lungs. When the diaphragm is paralyzed, it cannot contract; therefore, it moves upward from its normal position, owing to the effects of intraabdominal pressure and negative intrapleural pressure. When the normal diaphragm contracts (moving downward), the paralyzed diaphragm moves upward, and when the normal diaphragm relaxes (moving upward), the paralyzed diaphragm moves downward, resulting in paradoxical movements.

The diaphragm descends approximately 1 to 2 cm during eupneic breathing and as much as 10 cm during forceful breathing. For air to move into the alveoli, alveolar pressure must be less than atmospheric pressure. This can be achieved either through an increase in atmospheric pressure (as in positive-pressure ventilation) or a reduction in alveolar pressure, as during spontaneous ventilation (negative-pressure breathing). During anesthesia, respiratory therapy, and cardiopulmonary resuscitation, the air or gas mixtures are delivered to the alveoli by means of an increase of the pressures at the nose and mouth or endotracheal tube to greater than alveolar pressure (positive-pressure ventilation).[9]

Lung Compliance

Lung compliance (CL) is defined as the change in volume divided by the change in pressure (V/P). For a certain change in pressure, a more compliant lung has a greater change in volume than a less compliant one. Figure 27-2 shows pressure-volume relationships for a lung. As with many concepts in respiratory physiology, the reader must make the jump from considering the application to a single alveolus (which aids in understanding), to conceptualizing the overall average state in the pulmonary system, which often involves many regional conditions along a continuum of conditions. In considering lung compliance, the curve in Figure 27-2 represents the contribution of alveoli that are almost collapsed at the beginning of inspiration, alveoli that are distended, and alveoli that exist at various intermediate volumes.

Static compliance is the pressure-volume relationship for a lung when the air is not moving. Static compliance is decreased by conditions that make the lung difficult to inflate, such as fibrosis, obesity, vascular engorgement, edema, ARDS, and external compression (e.g., that caused by tight dressings or a surgeon's leaning on the chest). Static compliance is increased by emphysema, which destroys the elastic tissue of the lung. This makes the emphysematous lung easier to inflate. The problem with emphysema is not inflation but rather deflation, because the loss of elastic tissue results in airway collapse as the lung deflates, which causes gas trapping. It is important to note that compliance changes as lung volume changes. In other words, compliance is volume dependent. Figure 27-2 shows that the lung is less compliant both at very high lung volumes and at very low lung volumes. Alveoli require greater pressure changes to be inflated and deflated when they are almost empty or almost full,

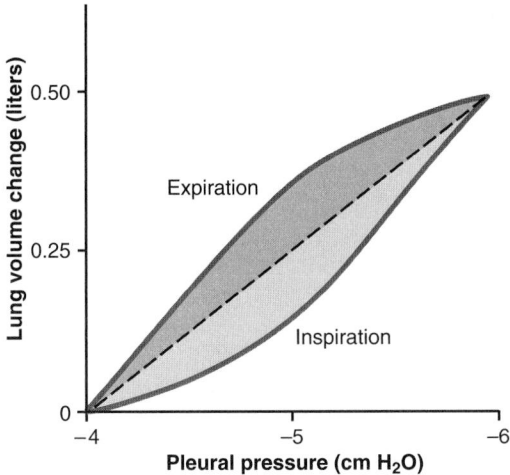

FIGURE **27-2** Compliance curve of the lungs. (*From Guyton AC, Hall JE. Textbook of Medical Physiology. 11th ed. Philadelphia: Saunders; 2006:473.*)

respectively. When an alveolus is collapsed, a great increase in pressure is necessary for inflation to begin. Observe in Figure 27-2 that the slope of the inspiratory curve is less at both low volumes and very high volumes. At low volumes, it takes more energy (more negative pressure, i.e., less compliant) to begin to expand the lungs. At high volumes, the alveoli are almost at capacity, and further changes in pressure result in less change in volume (less volume per given pressure = less compliant). As you follow the curve along the expiratory side, notice that an initial increase in pressure (with slower volume change) as the chest wall relaxes is followed by a smooth reduction in volume back to the resting level. Lung compliance results from the interplay of various factors that tend to either expand the lungs or restrict lung expansion. Much of the energy required to expand the lungs, particularly at low volumes, is created by surface tension in the fluid lining of the alveoli, which tends to attract the alveoli toward a smaller volume. Perhaps counterintuitively, a lung filled with fluid (and therefore does not have an air/fluid interface and the resulting surface tension) has a very high compliance—it requires much less energy to expand. Although not a high-fidelity measurement, you can calculate static effective compliance easily by inserting the values for lung volume versus pressure using the following equation:

Equation 27-1

$$\text{Static effective compliance} = \frac{\text{tidal volume}}{(\text{plateau pressure} - \text{PEEP})}$$

Plateau pressure is the pressure observed if you retard exhalation momentarily when the lungs are at end-inspiration. An inspiratory pause on the ventilator is an easy way to observe the plateau pressure. After subtracting the added pressure of PEEP, the plateau pressure is then divided into the measured tidal volume of that breath, producing a measure of lung compliance. A static compliance of 60 to 100 mL/cm H_2O is considered normal.

Dynamic compliance is the compliance of the lung while the air is moving. Here the forces involved in static compliance are added to the effects of airway resistance. Airway obstruction (e.g., that caused by bronchospasm or the presence of foreign bodies in the airway) can greatly decrease dynamic compliance.[10] Dynamic compliance is calculated as the tidal volume divided by (peak inspiratory pressure − PEEP). Many modern anesthesia ventilators can now calculate and trend compliance through tracing of pressure-volume curves.

Lung Elastic Recoil

The forces that cause elastic recoil of the lung are responsible for emptying the lung during exhalation and have a large role in determination of lung compliance. In addition to actual elastic fibers, the surface tension of the liquid film that lines the alveoli causes elastic recoil of the lung. Surface tension occurs at a gas/ liquid interface and is generated by the cohesive forces among the molecules of the liquid. Surface tension is what causes water to bead and form droplets.

If the alveolar interface were lined with water, surface tension would be high, making the lung harder to inflate. Laplace's law (P = T/r) states that if surface tension (T) is constant, pressure (P) would increase as radius (r) decreases. This does not occur in the lungs, because as alveolar radius decreases, surface tension also decreases, so that pressure remains the same. This occurs because of a substance secreted by alveolar type II cells and known as *pulmonary surfactant*, which consists mainly of the phospholipid dipalmitoyl lecithin. Pulmonary surfactant lowers the surface tension of the alveolar lining and decreases the work of breathing.

Another reason the alveoli do not obey Laplace's law is because surfactant preferentially lowers the surface tension in the small alveoli, thereby stabilizing the alveolar unit. Without surfactant, alveoli would all have the same surface tension, and the pressure in small alveoli would be much greater than in larger ones. This would cause small alveoli to empty into larger alveoli, resulting in the eventual collapse of the smaller alveoli and impairment of gas exchange. Also in relation to the application of Laplace's law to alveoli, there is controversy over whether alveoli should be treated as spherical (and thus subject to the law) or not. Geometricians postulate that closely packed alveoli would not maintain the shape of spheres, but rather of polyhedrons because their sides would be flattened against each other. In this case, connective tissue and elastic forces may play an important role in preventing alveolar closure.

Regardless of the shape of alveoli, it is clear that surfactant is crucial for reducing surface tension and preventing alveolar collapse. In the fetus, surfactant is not produced until approximately 28 to 32 weeks of gestation and does not reach mature levels until approximately 35 weeks' gestation. This is the prevalent cause of respiratory distress syndrome (RDS) in premature infants. Formation of surfactant can be hastened by the administration of glucocorticoids (particularly a steroid that crosses the placenta, such as betamethasone) to the parturient mother when premature delivery is threatened or imminent. The direct administration of synthetic surfactant to the airways of premature newborns has also greatly reduced the incidence of this RDS. Amniocentesis is sometimes performed to determine whether mature surfactant levels are present in the premature fetus. The ratio of lecithin to sphingomyelin (the L/S ratio) indicates the amount of mature surfactant (dipalmitoyl lecithin) in proportion to the amount of surfactant precursor (sphingomyelin).

Although the elastic forces of the lung tend to favor lung collapse, the chest wall is constantly under tension to expand. This is why normal inspiration requires very little energy. At the end of eupneic exhalation, the outward recoil of the chest wall is balanced by the inward elastic recoil of the lung. This is called the *resting end-expiratory point*. The opposing forces of the lungs and chest wall produce the negative intrapleural pressure in the pleural space.

The difference between intraalveolar pressure and pleural pressure is called the *transpulmonary pressure*. Under normal circumstances, the pleural pressure is always slightly negative. However, the transpulmonary pressure fluctuates as the intraalveolar pressure oscillates between slightly negative during inspiration to slightly positive during expiration, returning to zero whenever airflow is stopped at end-inspiration or end-expiration.

Resistance to Breathing

In addition to the static elastic recoil of the lung and chest wall, frictional resistance of lung tissues and chest wall (inertia), as well as resistance to airflow, opposes inflation of the lung.

Certain characteristics of airflow affect its ability to pass through conducting airways. Laminar flow is an orderly movement, where molecules are moving along a generally straight path. In laminar flow, the gas in the center of the tube moves faster than that closer to the wall because frictional resistance slows molecules near the vessel wall. Laminar flow is characterized by lower pressure than turbulent flow. During turbulent flow, resistance greatly increases because molecules move in various directions. The rheologic calculation of Reynolds number predicts when flow of a fluid (or gas) will be laminar or turbulent. Reynolds number (Re) is calculated as follows:

Equation 27-2

$$Re = \rho \ v \ d/\eta$$

where v = velocity of fluid flow, d = diameter of the vessel, ρ = density of the fluid, and η = viscosity of the fluid. This version of the formula would apply to flow through a tube (such as the airways). In open systems, *length* is substituted for diameter. When the inertial forces of density, velocity of flow, and diameter increase, Reynolds number increases. Increasing viscosity of the fluid reduces the product. Products up to 2000 predict laminar flow, above 4000 predicts turbulent flow, and a transitional area exists when results are between those numbers.

True laminar flow occurs in smaller airways, where the diameter is small and linear velocity is very low. (Linear velocity is inversely proportional to cross-sectional area for any flow rate.) Throughout the airways, both laminar and turbulent flow occur. Turbulence caused by sudden branching of the airways produces the breath sounds heard on auscultation. Resistance to laminar flow follows Poiseuille's law (R = $8\eta l/r^4$, where η equals viscosity). Resistance (R) to laminar airflow is directly proportional to the length (l) of the tube and inversely proportional to the fourth power of the radius (r). Therefore doubling the radius of the tube decreases resistance 16(2^4) times. Normally, about 40% of the total airway resistance resides in the upper airways (nasal cavity, pharynx, and larynx). Although resistance to airflow is greatest in individual small airways, the net total resistance to airflow of the small airways is very low because they represent a huge number of parallel pathways. Under normal circumstances, the greatest resistance to airflow resides in medium-sized bronchi, whose smooth muscle tone greatly affects airway resistance.

The clinical application of these laws resides in strategies to reduce airflow resistance. Bronchodilators will reduce resistance to laminar airflow by increasing the radius of the pathway, as predicted by Poiseuille. Selection of an endotracheal tube size may confer greater or lesser resistance, based on the length and (much more significantly) the internal diameter of the tube.

TABLE 27-4	Glossary for Static Lung Volumes and Capacities		
Measurement	**Symbol**	**Definition**	**Capacity (mL)**
Volumes			
Residual volume	RV	Volume of air remaining in the lungs after maximum expiration	1200
Expiratory reserve volume	ERV	Maximum volume of air expired from the resting end-expiratory level	1100
Tidal volume	V_T	Volume of air inspired or expired with each breath during quiet breathing	500
Inspiratory reserve volume	IRV	Maximum volume of air inspired from the resting end-inspiratory level	3000
Capacities			
Inspiratory capacity	$IC = IRV + V_T$	Maximum volume of air inspired from the end-expiratory level (the sum of IRV and TV)	3500
Vital capacity	$VC = IRV + V_T + ERV$	Maximum volume of air expired from the maximum inspiratory level	4500
Functional residual capacity	$FRC = RV + ERV$	Volume of air remaining in the lungs at the end expiratory level (the sum of RV and ERV)	2300
Total lung capacity	$TLC = IRV + V_T + ERV + RV$	Volume of air in the lungs after maximum inspiration (the sum of all volume compartments)	5800

As the Reynolds number equation tells us, greater airflow velocity (high I:E ratio) will favor turbulent flow and higher airway pressures. At the same time, lower density will favor laminar flow and reduce resistance when flow is turbulent, the conceptual basis for combining helium with oxygen ("heliox") to improve pulmonary gas distribution in obstructive lung disease.[11]

The autonomic nervous system affects the tone of the bronchial smooth muscle. The sympathetic nervous system, as well as sympathomimetic drugs (e.g., norepinephrine, epinephrine, and isoproterenol), produce bronchodilation. The parasympathetic nerves and parasympathomimetic drugs (e.g., acetylcholine) cause bronchoconstriction. Parasympatholytic drugs (e.g., atropine and ipratropium) therefore cause bronchodilation. Irritation of the airway by foreign bodies or inhaled irritants causes reflex bronchoconstriction. During lung inflation, increasing lung volumes exert retractive forces on the airways, resulting in a reduction in airway resistance. During forced expiration, dynamic compression of the airways increases airway resistance and may even cause airway collapse (most likely in small airways with no cartilaginous support).

The amount of O_2 consumed by the ventilatory muscles during eupneic breathing is usually less than 5% of the total body O_2 uptake. This percentage can greatly increase during exercise or with lung disease. For this reason, controlled ventilation is sometimes used in very ill patients to increase the availability of O_2 for other body functions.

The two major categories of lung disease are obstructive and restrictive. Pulmonary function tests reveal increased airway resistance in patients with obstructive lung disease (e.g., asthma, emphysema, and bronchitis). Airway obstruction can cause gas trapping (e.g., emphysematous blebs or early airway closure during expiration), which in turn can result in a barrel chest and increased lung volume. The time necessary for exhalation is increased in obstructive lung disease. Using higher I:E ratios during mechanical ventilation can allow for more expiratory time and reduce air trapping. In the spontaneously breathing person, normally approximately 80% of the vital capacity can be exhaled in 1 second. This is measured as the *forced expired volume in 1 second*, or FEV_1. In severe obstructive lung disease, expiratory flow rates are greatly decreased. Although obstructive lung disease restricts airflow through the airways, it is different from restrictive lung disease (as in pulmonary fibrosis, scoliosis, and obesity), which decreases lung compliance and lung volumes. Unfortunately, a patient can have both obstructive and restrictive disease simultaneously.[12]

Lung Volumes

The following discussion of lung volumes gives the parameters of a normal 70-kg male. Table 27-4 gives an overview of related terms and normal values. The amount of air that enters and leaves the body with each eupneic breath contains approximately 500 mL of air and is called the *tidal volume* (V_T). The *minute volume* (MV) equals the respiratory rate multiplied by V_T. The MV will be indirectly proportional to the arterial CO_2 tension. However, not the entire amount of minute ventilation ($\dot{V}_E$) participates in gas exchange. The amount of alveolar ventilation in a minute equals V_T minus the volume of the conducting airways (anatomic deadspace, which is approximately 2 mL per kg of body weight) multiplied by the ventilatory rate. The residual volume (RV) is the volume of gas left in the lung after a maximal exhalation (1.5 L). The RV cannot be removed from the lungs voluntarily and is important because it is a component of the functional residual capacity, which represents alveolar gas used for oxygenation of the blood, even between breaths or in periods

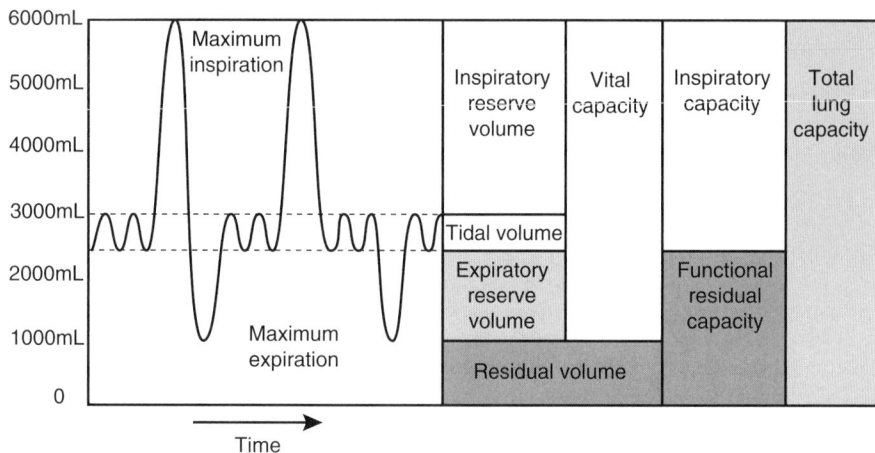

FIGURE **27-3** Lung volumes and capacities. (*From Applegate EJ. The Anatomy and Physiology Learning System. 3rd ed. Philadelphia: Saunders; 2006:294.*)

of apnea. The expiratory reserve volume is the volume of gas expelled from the lungs during a maximal forced exhalation, starting at the end of a normal tidal exhalation. The inspiratory reserve volume is the volume of gas inhaled into the lungs during a maximal forced inhalation, starting at the end of a normal tidal inspiration (2.5 L).

The sum of the four basic lung volumes is the TLC. Several types of lung capacity measures exist, each of which is the sum of two or more lung volumes. TLC is the volume of air in the lungs after a maximal inspiratory effort (approximately 6 L in a 70-kg adult). The vital capacity is the amount of air that can be forcibly exhaled from the lungs after a maximal inspiratory effort (approximately 4.5 L). The functional residual capacity (FRC) is the volume of gas contained in the lungs after normal quiet expiration. It is the sum of the RV and expiratory reserve volume (approximately 3 L). The inspiratory capacity is the volume of air inhaled into the lungs during a maximal inspiratory effort that begins at FRC (approximately 3 L). Figure 27-3 gives a graphic representation of lung volumes.

Closing volume is that phase of expiration that occurs as nitrogen-rich alveoli at the lung apexes continue to empty after closure of the small airways in the base of the lungs (which are exposed to greater intrapleural pressures and have less alveolar elastic recoil traction). The closing volume increases from approximately 30% of the TLC at age 20 years to approximately 55% at age 70 years. The closing volume may exceed the FRC in elderly people, which suggests that they may have airway closure and poorly ventilated or unventilated alveoli during normal tidal volumes, which would contribute to intrapulmonary shunt.[12]

Respiratory Pressure

During normal inspiration, intraalveolar pressure becomes slightly negative with respect to atmospheric pressure (normally by less than 1 mm Hg); this causes air to flow inward. During expiration, intraalveolar pressure increases to 1 mm Hg above atmospheric pressure, and air flows outward. Therefore very little pressure is applied during eupneic ventilation. During maximal expiration with a closed glottis (such as during coughing), intraalveolar pressure may be greater than 100 mm Hg, whereas during maximal inspiration it may be reduced to as low as −90 mm Hg. Even a newborn can attain an intraalveolar pressure from −40 to −60 mm Hg during the first few breaths of life.

Dead Space

The volume of the conducting airways is called the *anatomic dead space* and normally equals approximately 2 mL per kg of body weight. The conducting airways create dead space because their relatively thick walls do not allow the gas they contain to be exchanged with the gas contained in the blood. Alveoli that are ventilated but not perfused are known as *alveolar dead space* and contribute nothing to gas exchange with the blood. The sum of the anatomic dead space plus the alveolar dead space is the physiologic volume of dead space (V_{DS}). This is calculated with the Bohr equation:

Equation 27-3

$$\% \, V_{DS} = (Pa_{CO_2} - Pe_{CO_2})/Pa_{CO_2}$$

where Pa_{CO_2} is the arterial partial pressure of CO_2 as determined from arterial blood gas (ABG) measurement, and Pe_{CO_2} is the P_{CO_2} of mixed expired gas as determined with a CO_2 meter. Certain pathologic conditions, such as pulmonary embolus, increase the alveolar dead space and can abruptly decrease the end-tidal CO_2 levels monitored with capnography.

Distal to the anatomic dead space, the lung has 14 million alveolar ducts from which arise approximately 300 million alveoli perfused by 280 billion pulmonary capillaries. The average alveolar diameter is approximately 250 μm; therefore the total surface area available for gas exchange is 60 to 80 m².[13]

Regional Distribution of Alveolar Ventilation

In the normal upright lung, the alveoli at the bottom of the lung increase their volume more with each inspiration and decrease their volume more with each expiration during eupnea (from FRC) than do those alveoli at the top. This is because at FRC the dependent alveoli are more compliant. If lung volumes were decreased, upper alveoli would be more compliant and receive more ventilation, and the dependent alveoli would be emptier or even collapsed. Review of the compliance curve (see Figure 27-2) reveals that alveoli become less compliant at higher volumes (e.g., in upper alveoli at high lung volume) and also at lower volumes (e.g., in independent alveoli at low lung volumes).

Alveolar Oxygen and Carbon Dioxide Levels

The levels of O_2 and CO_2 in alveolar gas are determined by several factors. These include the amount of alveolar ventilation, the inspired concentrations of O_2 and CO_2, the flow of mixed venous blood to the lungs, and the body's consumption of O_2 and production of CO_2. Each breath brings approximately 350 mL of fresh air (21% of which is O_2) into the alveoli, which already contain approximately 3 L of gas (the FRC). Each exhalation removes approximately 350 mL of gas consisting of 5% to 6% CO_2. Every minute, approximately 250 mL of O_2 diffuses from the alveoli into the pulmonary capillary blood, whereas approximately 200 mL of CO_2 diffuses from the pulmonary capillary blood into the alveoli. The ratio of the amount of CO_2 produced to the quantity of O_2 consumed is called the *respiratory quotient* (RQ = 200 mL CO_2 produced divided by 250 mL O_2 consumed = 0.8).

Approximately 21% of dry atmospheric air is O_2; therefore, at the standard barometric pressure of 760 mm Hg, P_{O_2}atm equals 0.21×760 mm Hg, or 160 mm Hg. Only 0.04% of atmospheric air is CO_2, so P_{CO_2}atm = 0.3 mm Hg. As the inspired air passes through the upper airways, it is heated to body temperature and humidified to a relative humidity of nearly 100%. The partial pressure of water vapor at body temperature is a fairly constant 47 mm Hg. The P_{O_2} of inspired air (P_{IO_2}) saturated with water vapor at standard atmospheric pressure = $0.21 \times (760$ mm Hg − 47 mm Hg), or 149 mm Hg.

The inspired gas mixes with the gas already in the alveoli (FRC) and rapidly equilibrates with the pulmonary capillary blood. The alveolar P_{O_2} (P_{AO_2}) can be calculated with the alveolar air equation:

Equation 27-4

$$P_{AO_2} = P_{IO_2} - (P_{ACO_2}/RQ)$$

Thus during the breathing of atmospheric air, when P_{ACO_2} is 40 mm Hg and the RQ is 0.8, then P_{AO_2} = $(0.21 \times [760$ mm Hg − 47 mm Hg]) − 40 mm Hg/0.8 = 99 mm Hg. Therefore, using the alveolar air equation, one can calculate the P_{AO_2} if the atmospheric pressure, inspired O_2 concentration, and P_{ACO_2} (which is approximately equal both to the end-tidal P_{CO_2} and the arterial P_{CO_2} [P_{aCO_2}]) are known, because water vapor pressure and RQ are fairly constant. If the inspired O_2 concentration differs from that of room air, then that fraction replaces the 0.21.

The alveolar air equation works because the RQ represents the ratio of the amount of O_2 removed to the quantity of CO_2 delivered to the alveoli by the pulmonary capillary blood flow. P_{AO_2} is less than P_{IO_2} because the CO_2 is delivered to the alveoli by the pulmonary blood flow at the same time that O_2 is taken up from the alveoli. Therefore P_{ACO_2} divided by the RQ approximates the amount of O_2 that was removed from the alveoli by the pulmonary capillary blood flow.

Effects of Alveolar Ventilation on Carbon Dioxide and Oxygen

Within certain limits P_{ACO_2} is inversely proportional to alveolar ventilation. If alveolar ventilation is doubled, then P_{ACO_2} and P_{aCO_2} are reduced by half (if CO_2 production remains unchanged).

As alveolar ventilation increases, P_{AO_2} also increases slightly. However, doubling alveolar ventilation does not double P_{AO_2}; according to the alveolar air equation, reduction of the P_{ACO_2} raises the P_{AO_2}, bringing P_{AO_2} closer to the P_{IO_2}.

PULMONARY BLOOD FLOW

The lungs have a dual blood supply: (1) the bronchial arteries (usually one on the right and two on the left), and (2) the pulmonary arteries, which bring unoxygenated blood to the lungs from the right ventricle. The bronchial arteries arise from the descending aorta and carry approximately 2% of the cardiac output to nourish the nonrespiratory tissues: lung parenchyma, bronchi, nerves, pulmonary vessels, and visceral pleura. Bronchial arteries do not participate in fresh gas exchange with the alveoli. The branches of the bronchial arteries accompany the bronchial divisions as far as the respiratory bronchioles. The bronchial veins return deoxygenated blood from the first part of the bronchi and drain into the azygos, hemiazygos, or posterior intercostal veins. The remainder of the deoxygenated blood is returned by the pulmonary veins.

The pulmonary circulation provides blood flow to the structures distal to the terminal bronchioles, including distal nonrespiratory tissues, and the respiratory units. The pulmonary artery arises from the right ventricle and branches into the right and left pulmonary arteries, which further branch to accompany the bronchi. Although the pulmonary artery carries the entire cardiac output of the right ventricle, its walls are less muscular and more distensible that those of the aorta, and the pulmonary artery pressure is considerably less than the pressure in the aorta. The pulmonary arteries rapidly subdivide into terminal branches, which have thinner walls, much less smooth muscle, and greater internal diameters than corresponding branches of the systemic arterial tree. Pulmonary vessels are also much shorter than systemic vessels (and, according to Poiseuille's law, a decrease in length decreases resistance). Subsequently, pulmonary vascular resistance is very low, being approximately one eighth of systemic vascular resistance. Pulmonary vascular resistance is fairly evenly distributed among the arteries, capillaries, and veins, whereas most of the resistance in the systemic circulation is in the muscular arteries. Although pulmonary venous resistance is very low, it can decrease further when blood flow increases. This is because of passive changes in resistance caused by recruitment and distensibility of the pulmonary vessels. *Recruitment* is the opening to perfusion of pulmonary vessels that were previously not perfused. *Distensibility* is an increase in diameter of a pulmonary vessel that is already being perfused, and it results from the vessel's compliance. The sympathetic nervous system has some influence on pulmonary vascular resistance, as do certain substances circulating in the pulmonary blood. Pulmonary vascular resistance is increased by norepinephrine, serotonin, histamine, hypoxia, and hypercapnia, and it is decreased by acetylcholine and isoproterenol.

The respiratory units are the site of gas exchange between alveolar air and the pulmonary capillary blood. After participating in gas exchange in the respiratory zone, pulmonary arteriolar blood is returned to the heart by way of the pulmonary veins. The pulmonary vessels also anastomose with the bronchial vessels at the junction of the terminal and respiratory bronchioles. Therefore, the pulmonary veins carry oxygenated blood from the respiratory units and deoxygenated blood from the visceral pleura and distal bronchi. The venous bronchopulmonary anastomoses are significant in their contribution to the normal anatomic shunt (the addition of unoxygenated blood to the left chambers of the heart). Evidence of this crossover is seen when a patient is on complete bypass during cardiac surgery: blood enters the left atrium, even though all blood is shunted from the right ventricle by the venous cannula. This is because blood flow continues through the bronchial vessels, which anastomose with the pulmonary veins, which in turn ultimately drain into the left atrium—one reason why a ventricular drain may be inserted during the surgery to prevent overdistention of the heart. Five pulmonary veins ultimately return blood to the left heart.

Pulmonary Blood Flow Influences

Although pulmonary vessels have less muscular content than systemic arteries, the low pressure of the system makes pulmonary blood flow very sensitive to small changes in arterial tone. Unlike the systemic circulation, where hemodynamic influences are more global, pulmonary blood flow is more commonly regulated locally by changes in oxygen and carbon dioxide tension. In contrast to the systemic circulation, high oxygen tension and hypocapnia vasodilates pulmonary vessels (which helps those vessels pick up more oxygen), whereas hypercarbia and acidosis cause vasoconstriction. In the strongest influence to pulmonary local regulation, blood flow to hypoxic or atelectatic alveoli is actively diverted at a precapillary site by a process known as *hypoxic pulmonary vasoconstriction*. This decreases blood flow away from focal diseased areas of the lung and improves matching of ventilation and perfusion. See Chapter 28 for a more complete discussion of hypoxic pulmonary vasoconstriction.

Distribution of Pulmonary Blood Flow

In the normal upright lung, a greater portion of the blood flow goes to the bottom (dependent) portion because of the effects of hydrostatic pressure and greater distention of dependent pulmonary vessels. The variation in blood flow to the different regions of the lung allows the lung to be divided into zones (Figure 27-4). In the upper parts of the lung, alveolar pressure can be greater than pulmonary artery pressure (PAP), so that no blood flow occurs in this region. This is called *zone 1* and is alveolar dead space because the region is ventilated but not perfused. Normally,

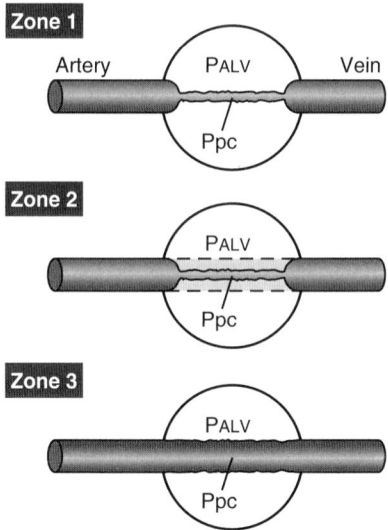

FIGURE **27-4** Alveolar and capillary mechanics in three lung zones. *Zone 1*, Gravity induces low perfusion pressure in capillary and larger resting volume of alveoli, owing to traction from parenchyma below. Alveolar air pressure is greater than capillary pressure, causing high $\dot{V}/\dot{Q}$, dead-space effect. *Zone 2*, Systolic capillary pressure rises higher than alveolar air pressure, but diastolic capillary pressure falls below alveolar air pressure. Blood flow is intermittent. *Zone 3*, Capillary pressure is highest because of hydrostatic gradient. Alveoli are relatively compressed by weight of parenchyma above and therefore have highest compliance. Ventilation and perfusion best matched. (*From Guyton AC, Hall JE. Textbook of Medical Physiology. 11th ed. Philadelphia: Saunders; 2006:486.*) *PALV,* Alveolar pressure; *Ppc,* pulmonary capillary pressure.

zone 1 exists only in a very small margin of lung area around the apical border during spontaneous ventilation, but the use of high airway pressures during mechanical ventilation can expand this zone.

The bottom portion of the lung, where both pulmonary artery and venous pressures exceed alveolar pressure, is known as *zone 3*. This zone represents continuous blood flow, and it is in this zone (dependent portion of the lung) that the tip of a pulmonary artery catheter should lie, for example, to ensure continuous communication with the left heart. The middle portion of the lung, where there is a variable relationship between vascular and alveolar pressure, is *zone 2*. Fluctuating increases in alveolar pressure can variably occlude capillary flow in this zone.

It should be noted that the prevalence of different zones is not as evenly distributed as diagrams would suggest. Nor are the zones necessarily "stacked" according to gravity. There is some evidence that regional perfusion zones may even be situated concentrically, independent of gravity, with the greatest blood flow in the center of the lungs.[14]

Pulmonary Edema

The normal distance for diffusion from the alveolar air space into the pulmonary capillary blood cells is less than 1 micron. The gas must traverse the surfactant layer, the flat alveolar type I cells, the interstitial space, the endothelial cells that make up the wall of the pulmonary capillary, a minute amount of plasma, and then finally the membrane of the red blood cell. The pulmonary system is designed to allow free passage of gases across this series of structures, collectively called the *respiratory membrane*. However, that inherent "leakiness" does predispose this area to unintended movement of fluid.

There is a fine balance between the plasma colloid oncotic pressure, which tends to hold fluid in the pulmonary capillaries, and the capillary hydrostatic pressure, interstitial fluid colloid oncotic pressure, and negative interstitial fluid pressure, which all tend to favor fluid movement into the interstitial space. In normal circumstances, the net of these forces favors movement into the interstitium, helping to divert fluid from accumulating in the alveoli from the adjacent "leaky" capillaries.[15] Although the interstitium has a large compliance for removing accumulating transudated fluid, derangements in the factors above can lead to fluid accumulation in the interstitium or alveoli and disrupt gas exchange.

Pulmonary vascular congestion causes increased capillary leakage into the interstitium, which can increase the distance for gas diffusion. If the capillary leak overcomes the compliance of the interstitial space, the fluid may then begin to pass into the alveoli. Pulmonary edema affects oxygenation more than CO_2 excretion because CO_2 is 20 times more diffusible than O_2. Many conditions can result in pulmonary edema. The high capillary pressures associated with heart failure or the excessive administration of intravenous fluids can increase lung water content. The size of the pulmonary capillary pores can be increased by sepsis, smoke inhalation, and other toxic conditions. Brain trauma can produce an intense sympathetic discharge, resulting in neurogenic pulmonary edema. A condition that occasionally occurs during emergence from anesthesia is postobstructive pulmonary edema also referred to as *negative-pressure pulmonary edema*. After extubation, the patient experiences laryngospasm and then attempts forceful inhalation against the closed glottis. The drastic decrease in intrathoracic pressure pulls fluid from the pulmonary capillaries. Postobstructive pulmonary edema probably occurs more frequently than is generally recognized.

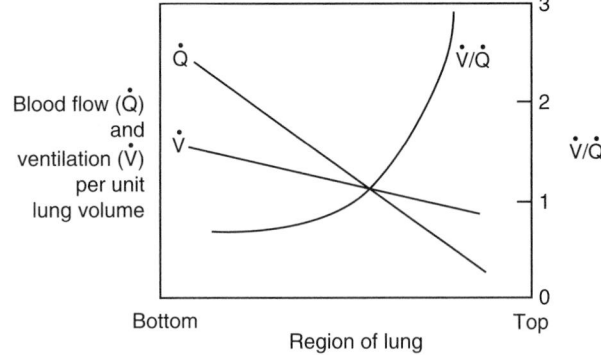

FIGURE **27-5** Ventilation-perfusion relationships.

The onset is rapid and relatively easy to treat. The symptoms resolve rapidly; in most cases patients are discharged within 24 hours. Treatment includes general supportive measures, oxygen, maintenance of a patent airway, a mask with continuous positive airway pressure (CPAP), and aggressive fluid therapy to restore depleted intravascular volume. Rarely are diuretics necessary, at least during initial treatment. The three mainstays of treatment remain normalization of ventilation and oxygenation, reduction of lung congestion and fluid, and treatment of the precipitating condition (Box 27-4).

Ventilation-Perfusion Relationships in the Lung

Normally, ventilation ($\dot{V}$) is approximately 4 L/min, whereas pulmonary blood flow ($\dot{Q}$) is approximately 5 L/min. Therefore, the ventilation-perfusion ratio ($\dot{V}/\dot{Q}$) for the whole lung is 0.8. However, $\dot{V}$ and $\dot{Q}$ must be matched at the alveolar-capillary level for gas exchange to occur in the lung.

Dependent portions of the lung receive relatively more blood flow than nondependent portions because of the effects of gravity. Additionally, ventilation goes to the more compliant portions of the lung. Normally at FRC, the dependent regions of the lung are more compliant, and the alveoli of the nondependent portions are more inflated ("tented open") and less compliant. Therefore, relatively more ventilation and perfusion go to the dependent portions, and this results in optimal gas exchange.

Although distribution of ventilation normally decreases going from dependent to nondependent regions of the lung, the accompanying decrease in perfusion is even greater; therefore the ratio, $\dot{V}/\dot{Q}$, increases as measured progressively from dependent to nondependent lung areas (Figure 27-5). Also, $\dot{V}/\dot{Q}$ varies: in alveoli that are ventilated but not perfused, $\dot{Q}$ equals 0, so $\dot{V}/\dot{Q}$ equals infinity (i.e., dead space); in alveoli that are perfused but not ventilated, $\dot{V}$ equals 0, so $\dot{V}/\dot{Q}$ equals 0 (i.e., a shunt). Similarly, alveoli that are ventilated but poorly perfused are described as "deadspace-like," whereas alveoli that are perfused but poorly ventilated are termed *shuntlike*; the latter contribute to the $\dot{V}/\dot{Q}$ mismatch of the lung. Shuntlike alveoli (low $\dot{V}/\dot{Q}$) have relatively low P_{O_2} and high P_{CO_2} when compared with deadspace-like alveoli (high $\dot{V}/\dot{Q}$), which have relatively high P_{O_2} and low P_{CO_2}.

$\dot{V}/\dot{Q}$ mismatch can result from a number of causes. A pulmonary embolus of thrombus, air, or other material that passes through the pulmonary artery to obstruct blood flow through the pulmonary capillaries creates alveolar dead space. Likewise, very high airway pressure can produce alveoli that are ventilated but not perfused. Furthermore, very low cardiac output (CO) results in low pulmonary blood flow and therefore in dead space. This is reflected by a low end-tidal CO_2 pressure on capnography and a wide gradient between the end-tidal and the arterial Pa_{CO_2}.

Total pulmonary venous admixture (unoxygenated blood delivered to the left chambers of the heart) is the sum of the shunt and shuntlike states. It can be calculated with the shunt equation, which is discussed below. Bronchopulmonary anastomoses are a cause of normal anatomic shunt, along with thebesian veins, which drain into the left side of the heart and usually account for less than 2% of the CO. Airway obstruction, alveolar collapse (atelectasis), and alveolar filling processes, such as pneumonia, also produce shunt.

Some diagnostic studies can definitively identify ventilation/perfusion abnormalities. A lung scan after a single breath of xenon 133 (^{133}Xe) gas or aerosolized technetium-99m can be used to determine the location of poorly ventilated areas in the lung, whereas IV injection of dissolved radioisotope reveals areas of the lung that are poorly perfused. Together, these comprise a ventilation-perfusion scan. Pulmonary angiography (radiography with injection of IV contrast dye) of the pulmonary vasculature can be used to demonstrate whether any pulmonary blood vessels are obstructed, such as in pulmonary embolism.[4]

Effects of General Anesthesia on Respiratory Physiology

General anesthesia affects the matching of ventilation and perfusion in several ways. Changing position from upright to supine and induction of general anesthesia produce a significant decrease in the FRC (see Chapter 28). With positive-pressure ventilation, the distribution of ventilation becomes more uniform throughout the lung, so both the dependent and nondependent alveoli receive about the same amount of ventilation. This leads to a wider scatter of ventilation and perfusion because there is relatively more ventilation of underperfused alveoli. General anesthesia usually also causes a significant decrease in the CO, which is exacerbated by positive-pressure ventilation, especially if it is accompanied by positive end-expiratory pressure (PEEP). This may promote an extension of zone 1 areas, although this theoretic effect is probably overstated. Atelectasis is a common finding with general anesthesia and is likely the main cause of the 10% shunt commonly observed in patients under anesthesia.[15]

Although hypoxic pulmonary vasoconstriction is partially effective in diverting blood flow away from poorly ventilated, unventilated, or atelectatic lung regions, most inhaled anesthetics (as well as potent vasodilators, such as nitroprusside and nitroglycerin) decrease the effectiveness of hypoxic pulmonary vasoconstriction, whereas most intravenous anesthetics do not. The inhibition of hypoxic pulmonary vasoconstriction contributes to the decrease in PaO_2 and the increase in the alveolar-arterial PO_2 difference usually seen with inhaled general anesthetic agents.

Although general anesthesia, particularly when administered in combination with muscle relaxants, tends to increase chest-wall compliance, the decrease in FRC actually produces a large decrease in the compliance of the respiratory system. Laryngoscopy and endotracheal intubation can increase airway resistance by stimulating airway irritant receptors, thereby decreasing dynamic compliance. However, most inhaled anesthetics (except for nitrous oxide [N_2O]) act as bronchodilators. Also, general anesthesia depresses the ventilatory response to CO_2, metabolic acidosis, and hypoxia (as discussed later in this chapter).[16,17]

Oxygen and Carbon Dioxide Exchange

As blood flows through the lungs, the mean pulmonary transit time is approximately 4 to 5 seconds, with the blood spending approximately 0.75 second in the pulmonary capillaries. However in the normal lung, it takes only one-third of this, or 0.25 second, for equilibration to occur between the alveolar air and the pulmonary capillary blood. During exercise, CO may be so greatly increased that the time a blood cell spends in a pulmonary capillary can be reduced to 0.25 second. This decreased time available for diffusion has a much greater effect on exchange of O_2 than on that of CO_2 because CO_2 diffuses approximately 20-fold more rapidly than O_2 does. *Diffusivity* is defined as the solubility divided by the square root of the molecular weight. CO_2 is a slightly heavier molecule than O_2, but it is 24-fold as soluble in body fluids as O_2.[4]

Oxygen Transport

The blood carries O_2 in two ways: (1) O_2 can be physically dissolved in the blood, and (2) O_2 can be chemically bound to hemoglobin (Hb) in the red blood cells. Normally all but a minute portion of the O_2 carried is bound to Hb. Without Hb, the cardiovascular system could not transport sufficient O_2 to meet the metabolic demands of the tissues. The ratio of the volume of the blood cells to the total volume of blood (expressed as a percentage) is called the *hematocrit*.

There is 0.003 mL of O_2 per every 1 mm Hg partial pressure of PO_2 dissolved in 100 mL of whole blood. Therefore, with a PaO_2 of 100 mm Hg, only 0.3 mL of O_2 is transported physically dissolved in 100 mL of blood. Hb rapidly and reversibly combines with O_2, allowing the O_2 to be released to the tissues. Each gram of Hb can combine with approximately 1.34 mL of O_2; therefore, if the level of Hb is 10 g/100 mL, then at 100% saturation, 13.4 mL of O_2 is bound to Hb per 100 mL of blood. Note that an Hb level of 10 g/100 mL of blood corresponds to a hematocrit of 30%—the hematocrit is approximately equal to Hb level multiplied by 3.

The normal hematocrit for a man is approximately 45% (Hb 15 g/dL) and for a woman is approximately 39% (Hb 13 g/dL). Centrifugation of the blood in a capillary tube separates the cells from the plasma. A thin layer called the *buffy coat* separates the plasma and the red blood cells (erythrocytes). This thin layer

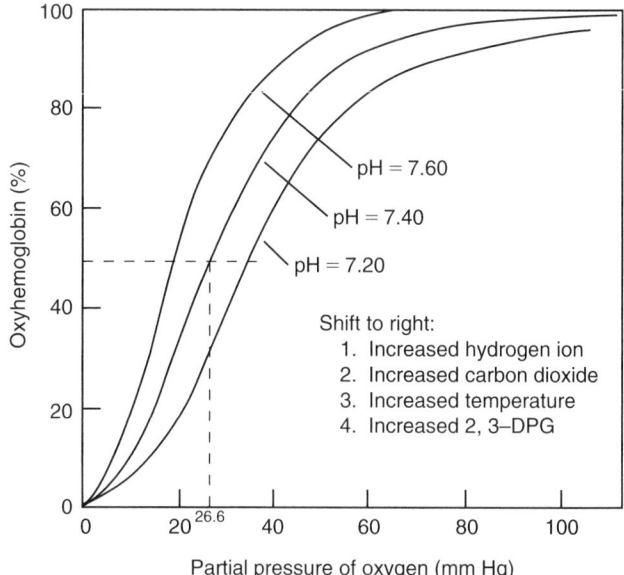

FIGURE **27-6** Oxyhemoglobin dissociation curve at various pH levels. *Dotted line* indicates P_{50}, the measure used to quantify any shift in the curve. The normal P_{50} is 26.6 mm Hg.

(approximately 1% of the volume of the blood) consists of white blood cells and platelets.[4]

Oxyhemoglobin Dissociation Curve

The relationship between the PO_2 of the plasma and the percent Hb saturation is represented by the oxyhemoglobin (HbO_2) dissociation curve (Figure 27-6). This relationship between PO_2 and HbO_2 is not linear; rather, it is described by an S-shaped curve that is steep at lower PO_2 values and nearly flat when the PO_2 is greater than 70 mm Hg. As the PO_2 of the plasma increases, the amount of O_2 bound to the Hb also increases, but not in a linear manner. This is because each of the four Hb subunits combines with O_2, and each combination facilitates the next. Similarly, when the O_2 is being unloaded at the peripheral tissues, each dissociation facilitates the next. Therefore, this S-shaped curve is extremely important physiologically. Interaction between O_2 and Hb is also influenced by the pH, PCO_2, temperature, and 2,3-diphosphoglycerate (a metabolite of glucose hydrolysis) levels.

The changing affinity of Hb for O_2 facilitates loading at the pulmonary capillaries and unloading of the O_2 at the peripheral tissues. The S-shaped HbO_2 dissociation curve is displaced to the left of the normal curve by hypocapnia, a decrease in temperature, alkalosis, and a decrease in 2,3-diphosphoglycerate levels, resulting in an increased affinity of the Hb for O_2 (a higher saturation for a given PO_2). When exposed to increased temperature, hypercapnia, acidosis, and elevated 2,3-diphosphoglycerate levels, the affinity of Hb for O_2 decreases. This results in a shift of the HbO_2 dissociation curve to the right, and therefore the O_2 is given up to the tissues. Note that the conditions that favor the release of O_2 from the Hb to the tissues are likely to be associated with increased tissue metabolism, which would increase the tissues' O_2 demand. The influence of pH and PCO_2 on the HbO_2 dissociation curve is referred as the *Bohr effect*. The position of the oxyhemoglobin curve can be quantified by the P_{50}. The P_{50} is the PaO_2 at which 50% of the Hb is saturated.

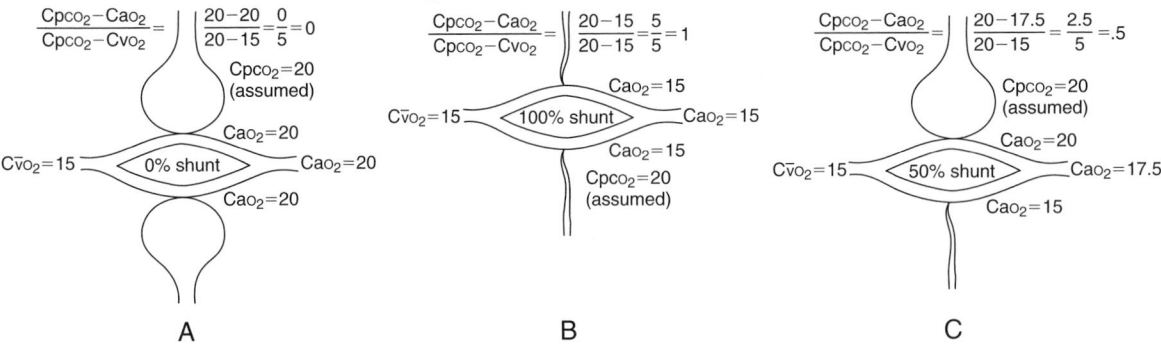

FIGURE **27-7** Calculation of the shunt fraction for various theoretic conditions. **A,** No shunt; **B,** complete shunt; **C,** 50% shunt.

Under normal conditions, adult human blood has a P_{50} of 26 to 27 mm Hg. If the HbO_2 dissociation curve shifts to the right, the P_{50} increases; if it shifts to the left, the P_{50} decreases.

Other factors that affect O_2 transport include carbon monoxide poisoning and methemoglobinemia. Carbon monoxide binds to Hb (forming carboxyhemoglobin) with 240 times the affinity of O_2. The carbon monoxide binds with Hb at the site that O_2 would occupy, making the carboxyhemoglobin unable to transport O_2. Without a multiple-channel oximeter, carboxyhemoglobin provides a misleadingly high reading because it interprets the hemoglobin as being "saturated," without distinguishing the inability of the Hb to unload its cargo.

Methemoglobin is Hb with its iron in the ferric state (Fe^{3+}) instead of the normal ferrous state (Fe^{2+}). In the ferric state, the Hb iron atoms do not combine with O_2. Methemoglobinemia can be caused by nitrate poisoning (nitroglycerin overdose) or toxic reactions to oxidant drugs, such as the local anesthetic prilocaine. Methemoglobinemia is treated with O_2 therapy and methylene blue at a dose of 1 to 2 mg/kg intravenously over 5 minutes.[4]

Oxygen Content Calculations

Values for the amount of O_2 in arterial blood are yielded by the O_2 content equation:

Equation 27-5

$$Ca_{O_2} = (0.003 \times Pa_{O_2}) +$$
$$(1.34 \times Hb \times \% \text{ arterial Hb saturation})$$

where Ca_{O_2} is the arterial O_2 content, and Pa_{O_2} and percent of Hb saturation are obtained from ABG analysis. Ca_{O_2} is normally approximately 20 mL of O_2 per 100 mL of arterial blood (when Hb is 15 g/dL and Pa_{O_2} is 90 mm Hg).

The amount of O_2 in mixed venous blood is calculated with the following equation:

Equation 27-6

$$C\bar{v}_{O_2} = (0.003 \times P\bar{v}_{O_2}) +$$
$$(1.34 \times Hb \times \% \text{ mixed venous Hb saturation})$$

where $C\bar{v}_{O_2}$ is the mixed venous O_2 content, and $P\bar{v}_{O_2}$ and percent of Hb saturation are obtained from mixed venous blood gas analysis of blood drawn from the distal lumen of a pulmonary artery catheter (the only site in the body with truly mixed venous blood). $C\bar{v}_{O_2}$ is normally about 15 mL of O_2 per 100 mL of mixed venous blood when Hb is 15 g/dL and $P\bar{v}_{O_2}$ is 40 mm Hg.

Subtraction of $C\bar{v}_{O_2}$ from Ca_{O_2} yields the arteriovenous O_2 content difference. This difference is useful in determining the relationship between O_2 delivery to the body's tissues and the tissues' O_2 demand. Normally the difference is approximately 5 mL/dL of blood. A difference greater than 5 mL/dL of blood can be associated with low CO because the blood takes longer to traverse the capillaries in the tissues; therefore, more O_2 is extracted. A difference of less than 5 mL/dL of blood can be associated with systemic arteriovenous shunts, which allow blood to bypass the tissue capillaries; such shunts occur during hyperdynamic sepsis.

The amount of O_2 in pulmonary capillary blood is calculated with the following equation:

Equation 27-7

$$Cpc_{O_2} = (0.003 \times Ppc_{O_2}) +$$
$$(1.34 \times Hb \times \% \text{ pulmonary capillary Hb saturation})$$

where Cpc_{O_2} is the pulmonary capillary O_2 content. Ppc_{O_2} (partial pressure of oxygen in the pulmonary capillary) is derived from the alveolar air equation described earlier in this chapter; the assumption is made that pulmonary capillary blood equilibrates completely with the partial pressure of oxygen in the alveolar air. The pulmonary capillary oxygen saturation cannot be measured, but is estimated by plotting the Ppc_{O_2} on the oxyhemoglobin dissociation curve and determining the corresponding hemoglobin saturation. Cpc_{O_2} is normally approximately 21 mL of O_2 per 100 mL of pulmonary capillary blood (when Hb is 15 g/dL and Ppc_{O_2} is 99 mm Hg).

The Ca_{O_2}, $C\bar{v}_{O_2}$, and Cpc_{O_2} are used in the shunt equation:

Equation 27-8

$$\dot{Q}S/\dot{Q}T = (Cpc_{O_2} - Ca_{O_2})/(Cpc_{O_2} - C\bar{v}_{O_2})$$

In this equation, $\dot{Q}S$ is the shunt blood flow, $\dot{Q}T$ is the total blood flow (CO), Cpc_{O_2} is the pulmonary capillary O_2 content, Ca_{O_2} is the arterial O_2 content, and $C\bar{v}_{O_2}$ is the mixed venous O_2 content.[17] The shunt equation estimates the fraction of cardiac output that perfuses alveoli that are absolutely nonventilated. In actuality, the shunt calculation represents the sum effects of countless lung units of varying ($\dot{V}/\dot{Q}$) relationships throughout the lung; however, the calculation is useful to monitor trends in oxygenation, help diagnose the cause of observed hypoxemia, and guide alveolar recruitment maneuvers, such as PEEP. The proof of this equation is illustrated in Figure 27-7 and lies in the assumption that if there is no shunt (Figure 27-7, *A*), all arterial blood would have been fully oxygenated in the alveolar capillaries.

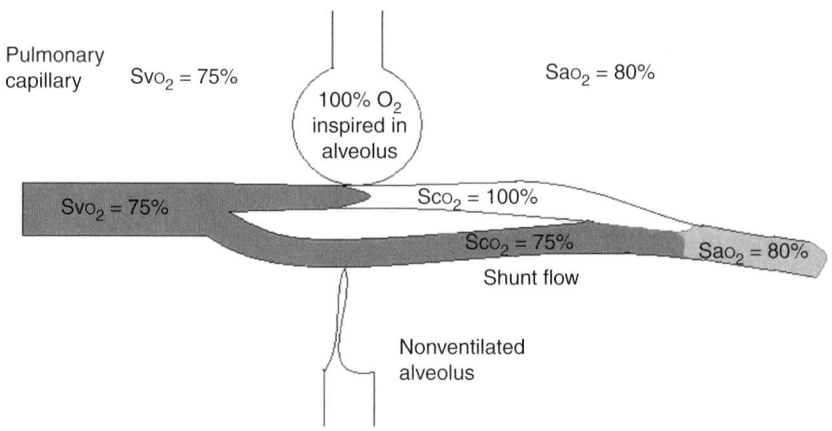

FIGURE **27-8** True shunt; unresponsiveness to supplemental oxygen. Sa_{O_2}, arterial oxygen saturation; Sc_{O_2}, capillary oxygen saturation; $S\overline{v}_{O_2}$, venous oxygen saturation.

Therefore, ($Cpc_{O_2} = Ca_{O_2}$), and the numerator of the equation would be zero, thus so would its quotient. On the other hand, with a theoretic 100% shunt (Figure 27-7, *B*), no blood would become oxygenated and thus ($C\overline{v}_{O_2} = Ca_{O_2}$); the difference of each from Cpc_{O_2} would be the same, and the number divided by itself would equal 1.0, denoting 100% shunt. Figure 27-7, *C* illustrates a theoretic 50% shunt, where the Ca_{O_2} equilibrates between the Cpc_{O_2} and the $C\overline{v}_{O_2}$, so its difference from the Cpc_{O_2} is twice that from the $C\overline{v}_{O_2}$, denoting a 0.5 shunt fraction.

One characteristic of the existence of a significant shunt proportion is hypoxemia unresponsive to supplemental oxygen administration. When blood is passing through the lungs unoxygenated, no increase in FI_{O_2} delivered to other regions can overcome the hypoxemia (Figure 27-8). This is because under normal circumstances, those normal lung regions are already achieving 100% saturation of the hemoglobin. Therefore they cannot overcompensate for the venous admixture contributed by the shunt areas. In assessing hypoxemia, once hypoventilation and low inspired oxygen are ruled out, improvement in Pa_{O_2} in response to supplemental oxygen favors $\dot{V}/\dot{Q}$ mismatch, as opposed to true shunt or possibly a diffusion disorder (the latter of which can be identified through a test of diffusing capacity of carbon monoxide [D_{LCO}]).

Transport of Carbon Dioxide

The blood carries CO_2 in three forms: (1) in physical solution, (2) chemically combined with the amino acids of blood proteins, and (3) as bicarbonate ions. Approximately 5% to 10% of the total CO_2 transported in the blood is carried in physical solution. Chemical combination of CO_2 with the terminal amine groups of blood proteins forms carbamino compounds. The reaction occurs rapidly and does not require enzymes. Carbamino compounds constitute another 5% to 10% of the blood's total CO_2 content. The remaining 80% to 90% of the CO_2 in the blood is carried as bicarbonate. In the presence of carbonic anhydrase, CO_2 combines with water to form carbonic acid. The carbonic acid can dissociate into a bicarbonate ion and H^+ according to the following chemical reaction:

Equation 27-9

$$CO_2 + H_2O \xrightarrow{\text{carbonic anhydrase}} H_2CO_3 \rightarrow H^+ + HCO_3^-$$

When HCO_3^- leaves the blood cells, chloride ions enter to maintain electrical neutrality (the so-called "chloride shift").[18]

Carbon Dioxide Dissociation Curve

As expected, decreases in the Pco_2 of the blood correspond to a decrease in the total CO_2 content of the blood. This is because of corresponding decreases in the levels of bicarbonate and carbamino compounds. When the Pco_2 falls, the amount of the total CO_2 decrease is affected by the presence of O_2 in the blood. When blood contains mainly oxygenated hemoglobin, the CO_2 dissociation curve shifts to the right, reducing the blood's capacity to hold CO_2. When the blood contains mostly deoxyhemoglobin, the curve shifts to the left, increasing the capacity to carry CO_2. This effect is known as the *Haldane effect*, and it allows the blood to load more CO_2 at the tissues, where more deoxyhemoglobin is present, and to unload CO_2 at the lung, where more Hb_{O_2} is present.

The fact that deoxyhemoglobin is a weaker acid than Hb_{O_2} accounts for the Bohr and Haldane effects. Deoxyhemoglobin more readily accepts the H^+ produced by the dissociation of carbonic acid. This permits more CO_2 to be carried in the form of bicarbonate ions (Haldane effect). Conversely, the association of H^+ with the amino acids of Hb lowers the affinity of Hb for O_2, shifting the Hb_{O_2} dissociation curve to the right at low pH or high Pco_2 (Bohr effect).[19]

ACID-BASE BALANCE

The respiratory system has an important role in maintaining a normal pH balance in the body. It works along with the kidneys and the buffer systems to balance the acids and bases of the blood and other body tissues, allowing them to function normally. Hydrogen ions interact with negatively charged regions of other molecules, such as proteins, altering their structural conformation and in doing so altering their behavior. As previously mentioned, pH affects the Hb_{O_2} dissociation curve and the activity of enzymes, thereby changing metabolic functions in all body tissues. Severe metabolic acidosis that results from prolonged cardiopulmonary arrest must be treated with sodium bicarbonate because protein-receptor sensitivity and other enzymatic functions must be restored before epinephrine can be effective in resuscitation.

Metabolism of substances ingested as food produces mainly acidic metabolic waste products. Under normal conditions, a tremendous amount of the acid produced daily can be removed from the body by the respiratory system as exhaled CO_2. The acidic products are known as *volatile acids* because they can be converted into carbonic acid gas that is exhaled at a rate of approximately 24,000 mEq/day. A much smaller amount of nonvolatile or fixed

Physiologic State	pH	Paco₂ (mm Hg)	HCO₃⁻ (mEq/L)	Examples
Normal	7.40 ± 0.05	40 ± 5	25 ± 1	
Uncompensated respiratory acidosis	↓↓	↑↑	↑	Acute hyperventilation (such as during neurosurgery)
Uncompensated respiratory alkalosis	↑↑	↓↓	↓	Acute hypoventilation (such as during an asthma attack)
Uncompensated metabolic acidosis	↓↓	↔	↓↓	Metabolic acidosis with controlled mechanical ventilation (respiratory compensations not possible)
Uncompensated metabolic alkalosis	↑↑	↔	↑↑	Metabolic alkalosis with controlled mechanical ventilation
Compensated respiratory acidosis	↓	↑↑	↑↑	Chronic hypoventilation (as in chronic obstructive pulmonary disease)
Compensated respiratory alkalosis	↑	↓↓	↓↓	Chronic hyperventilation (as in chronic increased intracranial pressure)
Compensated metabolic acidosis	↓	↓↓	↓↓	Renal failure or diabetic ketoacidosis
Compensated metabolic alkalosis	↑	↑↑	↑↑	Long-term hypokalemia or bicarbonate ingestion
Mixed respiratory and metabolic acidosis	↓↓↓	↑↑	↓↓	Respiratory and circulatory arrest
Mixed respiratory and metabolic alkalosis	↑↑↑	↓↓	↑↑	"Over-resuscitation" (hyperventilation and excess bicarbonate administration)

TABLE 27-5 Acid-Base States

acids also is produced during normal metabolic breakdown of food at the rate of approximately 50 mEq/day; these acids are primarily removed by the kidneys.

In addition to the efforts of the respiratory system and kidneys to regulate pH levels, buffers in the human body maintain pH in the physiologic range. The buffers consist mainly of bicarbonate, phosphate, and proteins. A buffer is a mixture of substances that usually consists of a weak acid and its conjugate base. When a strong acid or base is added to a buffer system, the changes in H⁺ concentration are much smaller than those that would occur if the same amount of acid or base were added to pure water or another nonbuffered solution.[20]

Interpretation of Arterial Blood Gases

Analysis of ABGs can provide useful information concerning the relationship of acid production and acid removal by the lungs and kidneys. Acid-base disturbances can be categorized into four major groups: respiratory acidosis, metabolic acidosis, respiratory alkalosis, and metabolic alkalosis.

Although it may seem that a great number of acid-base states are possible, actually only 11 conditions exist (Table 27-5). Blood gases in a normal individual have a pH in the range of 7.35 to 7.45, Paco₂ ranges from 35 to 45 mm Hg, and bicarbonate concentration is approximately 25 mEq/L.

Acidosis

Any process that leads to an elevation in Paco₂ tends to lower the arterial pH, resulting in respiratory acidosis. An acute change in Paco₂ of 10 mm Hg is associated with a change in pH of 0.08

units. An increase in Paco₂ with a normal bicarbonate level is termed *uncompensated respiratory acidosis.*

Metabolic acidosis should more properly be referred to as *non-respiratory acidosis* because it does not always involve alterations in metabolism. Causes of this condition include ingestion (poisoning), infusion, production of a fixed acid (lactic acidosis), and decreased excretion of acid by the kidneys. A base change of 10 mEq/L is associated with a pH change of 0.15 unit (in the absence of a change in Paco₂). Therefore, if the bicarbonate level increases by 10 mEq/L, then the pH also increases by 0.15 unit. A decrease in bicarbonate level when the Pco₂ remains at approximately 40 mm Hg is termed *uncompensated metabolic acidosis.* The combination of respiratory acidosis and metabolic acidosis is termed *mixed acidosis* and can produce a drastically decreased arterial pH.[21]

Alkalosis

When alveolar ventilation exceeds that necessary to keep up with CO₂ production in the body, both Paco₂ and Paco₂ decrease to below 35 mm Hg. This hyperventilation results in respiratory alkalosis. A decrease in Paco₂ in the presence of a normal bicarbonate level is termed *uncompensated respiratory alkalosis.* The relationship between alveolar ventilation and CO₂ production that results in hyperventilation can occur because of an increase in alveolar ventilation or a decrease in CO₂ production, as occurs with hypothyroidism or hypothermia, if alveolar ventilation is maintained at normal levels.

Metabolic alkalosis occurs when fixed acid loss is increased or when the intake of bases is abnormally high. Above-normal increases in the bicarbonate level when the P_{CO_2} is maintained at approximately 40 mm Hg is termed *uncompensated metabolic alkalosis*. The combination of respiratory alkalosis and metabolic alkalosis produces mixed alkalosis, in which the arterial pH is markedly elevated.

Compensatory Mechanisms

The respiratory system can rapidly compensate for metabolic acidosis or alkalosis by altering alveolar ventilation. It normally occurs because changes in blood H^+ concentrations affect the chemoreceptors, which in turn increases or decreases alveolar ventilation, altering Pa_{CO_2} within minutes. The kidneys can compensate for respiratory acidosis and metabolic acidosis of nonrenal origin by excreting fixed acid and retaining bicarbonate. Conversely, the kidneys compensate for respiratory alkalosis or metabolic alkalosis of nonrenal origin by decreasing H^+ excretion and decreasing retention of bicarbonate. Renal compensatory mechanisms act more slowly than do respiratory mechanisms and may take several days. When evaluating blood gas analyses, *compensated acidosis* involves finding the pH below 7.4 but within the normal range (above 7.35). Conversely, *compensated alkalosis* is characterized by a pH above 7.4 but within the normal range (below 7.45). In spite of observing a compensatory change in CO_2 or bicarbonate, an acid-base disorder is considered *uncompensated* if that mechanism has not been able to bring the pH back into a normal range.

TREATMENT OF BLOOD GAS ABNORMALITIES

For the patient being mechanically ventilated, respiratory acidosis and respiratory alkalosis can be treated with a simple increase or decrease in the amount of alveolar ventilation. Respiratory acidosis should not be treated with sodium bicarbonate, because through the reversible reaction in Equation 27-9, the bicarbonate dissociates into more CO_2, worsening the acidosis. To restore a stable spontaneous circulation, mild to moderate metabolic acidosis can be treated with hyperventilation and correction of shock. Certain types of severe metabolic acidosis (pH <7.20) may be treated with sodium bicarbonate. The total body bicarbonate deficit equals the base deficit (in mEq/L) that is obtained from the blood gas values: the patient's bicarbonate level is subtracted from the normal bicarbonate level; the difference is multiplied by the patient's weight (in kilograms) and then by 0.3 (which is equal to the extracellular fluid compartment and the volume of distribution for bicarbonate). Complete correction of the base deficit is not indicated; only half of the calculated dose of bicarbonate is used. Severe lactic acidosis is treated with bicarbonate, but the acidosis associated with renal failure is better treated with dialysis. The hyperosmolarity and high sodium content of bicarbonate are usually contraindicated for renal failure patients. Manipulation of the blood's volume and electrolyte composition is used in the treatment of certain types of metabolic acidosis or alkalosis.

Hypoxemia is treated with an increase in the inspired O_2 concentration (F_{IO_2}), PEEP, and correction of atelectasis (e.g., with bronchoscopy for the removal of foreign bodies in the airway). As previously mentioned, increasing alveolar ventilation usually has only a modest effect on Pa_{O_2}.

CONTROL OF BREATHING

The respiratory centers in the brainstem control breathing by automatically generating a cycle of inspiration and expiration (Figure 27-9). This spontaneously generated cycle can be modified by reflexes or by higher centers in the brain. The respiratory

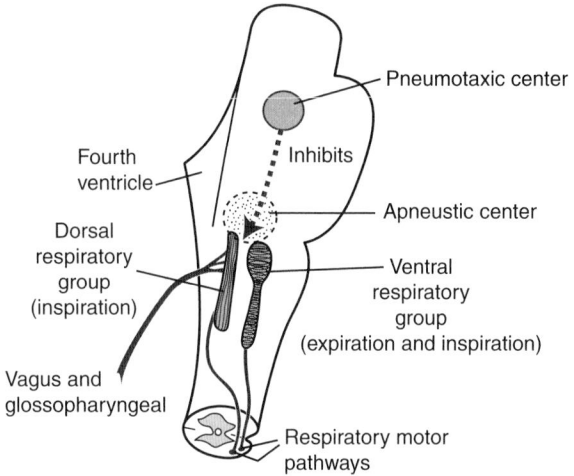

FIGURE **27-9**   Organization of the respiratory center. (*From Guyton AC, Hall JE. Textbook of Medical Physiology. 11th ed. Philadelphia: Saunders; 2006:515.*)

centers affect the nerves of the spinal cord, which innervate the muscles of respiration (the cervical branches of the spinal nerves C3, C4, and C5 form the phrenic nerves, which innervate the diaphragm). The spontaneous respiratory rhythm is generated by the medullary respiratory center, which is found in the reticular formation of the medulla under the floor of the fourth ventricle. The pons, which is the portion of the brainstem immediately above the medulla, contains the apneustic center (in the lower pons) and the pneumotaxic center (in the upper pons), both of which modify the output of the medullary respiratory center.

The activity of the brainstem's breathing centers is modulated by information received from afferent spinal nerves and higher brain centers, as occurs in voluntary control of breathing. Additionally, a great number of sensors in the lungs, cardiovascular system, muscles, tendons, skin, and viscera can affect the control of breathing by eliciting reflex changes. Stimulation of stretch receptors in the lungs can elicit three respiratory reflexes: the Hering-Breuer inflation reflex, the Hering-Breuer deflation reflex, and the paradoxical reflex of Head. The Hering-Breuer inflation reflex may help prevent overdistention of the alveoli at high lung volumes by inhibiting large V_Ts and may decrease the frequency of the inspiratory efforts by causing a transient apnea. The Hering-Breuer deflation reflex may be responsible for the increased ventilation elicited when the lungs are deflated abnormally, such as in pneumothorax, or it may have a role in the periodic spontaneous deep breaths (sighs) that help to prevent atelectasis. The paradoxical reflex of Head results during partial block of the phrenic nerves, such that lung inflation results in further deep inspiration instead of the apnea expected when the vagus nerve is fully functional. This reflex may be involved in generating the first breath of the newborn baby. Chemical or mechanical irritation of the airways may elicit a reflex cough or sneeze, hyperpnea, bronchoconstriction, and increased blood pressure. The vagus nerve provides afferent pathways for all of the airway's irritant receptors, except for the nasal mucosa receptors, which send information centrally by means of the trigeminal and olfactory tracts. Pulmonary embolism (PE) typically causes rapid, shallow breathing, whereas pulmonary vascular congestion causes hyperpnea. The vascular receptors that initiate these responses are named *J receptors* (for "juxtapulmonary capillary").

Stimulation of receptors in the muscles, tendons, and joints can also increase ventilation during exercise. Elevated blood pressure stimulates the arterial (carotid and aortic) baroreceptors, resulting in apnea and bronchodilation. Somatic pain tends to cause hyperpnea, whereas visceral pain usually causes apnea or decreased ventilation. Stimulation of the arterial chemoreceptors by decreased Po_2, increased Pco_2, or low pH tends to increase lung inflation and cause hyperpnea, bronchoconstriction, and an increase in blood pressure.[22] Table 27-6 summarizes the respiratory control reflexes.

Chemical Control of Breathing

The arterial and cerebrospinal fluid partial pressures of CO_2 are probably the most important inputs to the brainstem centers for establishing the ventilatory rate and V_T. Hypoxemia potentiates the ventilatory response to CO_2. Its effect is that for any particular $Paco_2$, ventilatory response becomes greater as the Pao_2 decreases. Narcotics and anesthetic drugs (Figure 27-10) may profoundly depress the ventilatory response to CO_2. Chronic obstructive lung disease (COLD) also depresses the ventilatory response to hypercapnia, so the hypoxic drive may be solely responsible for maintaining spontaneous breathing in these patients, and administering high Fio_2 may halt their spontaneous ventilatory efforts. Metabolic acidosis shifts the CO_2 curve to the left, so that for any particular Pco_2, ventilation is increased during metabolic acidosis.

A depressed or abnormal response to CO_2 during sleep may be involved in central sleep apnea (characterized by pauses of 2 minutes' duration between breaths). Central sleep apnea, which possibly is caused by a defect in the chemoreceptors or brainstem respiratory controller, may be an important contributor to sudden infant death syndrome.

Increased $Paco_2$ and decreased Pao_2 and arterial pH stimulate the arterial (peripheral) chemoreceptors, with the carotid bodies apparently exerting a much greater influence on the medullary respiratory centers than the aortic bodies. The afferent nerve from the carotid body is the Hering nerve, a branch of the glossopharyngeal nerve. The afferent pathway from the aortic body is the vagus nerve. The central chemoreceptors are in contact with cerebrospinal fluid but are not directly exposed to arterial blood (because of the blood-brain barrier). CO_2 is rapidly diffusible through the blood-brain barrier; therefore, changes in $Paco_2$ are rapidly transmitted to the cerebrospinal fluid, taking less than 2 minutes. Hydrogen ions and bicarbonate ions are slowly diffusible through the blood-brain barrier, so changes in arterial pH that do not result from changes in Pco_2 take considerably longer to affect the cerebrospinal fluid. The central chemoreceptors are located just beneath the surface of the medulla. They are not stimulated by hypoxia; their activity may even be suppressed by it. Although the central chemoreceptors are almost solely responsible for determining the resting ventilatory level and long-term response to and maintenance of blood CO_2 levels, the peripheral chemoreceptors may be more important in short-term responses to CO_2.[23]

CHRONIC OBSTRUCTIVE PULMONARY DISEASE

The American Thoracic Society defines chronic obstructive pulmonary disease (COPD) as a "disorder characterized by abnormal tests of expiratory flow that does not change markedly over periods of several months of observation."[23,24] The terminology can be confusing, because asthma, chronic bronchitis, and emphysema are all common obstructive diseases characterized by decreased airflow through the tracheobronchial tree and small airways.

The terms *chronic obstructive pulmonary disease* and *chronic obstructive lung disease* are widely used as synonyms for the combination of chronic bronchitis and emphysema. Because of the prevalence of cigarette smoking, the combination of these two entities is encountered much more commonly than either of the two in its "pure" form. As a rule the combination of chronic bronchitis and emphysema is seen in those who smoke heavily, and the disease process takes 30 years or longer to manifest.

Definition

The term *chronic bronchitis* refers to "the condition of subjects with chronic or recurrent excess [mucous] secretion into the bronchial tree." In this definition, *chronic* means "occurring on most days for at least 3 months of the year for at least 2 successive years."[24] A critical element is the presence of airway obstruction of expiratory airflow. A glossary of static lung volumes and capacities is presented in Table 27-4.

Emphysema is defined as "a condition of the lung characterized by abnormal permanent enlargement of the air spaces distal to the terminal bronchiole, accompanied by destruction of their walls and without obvious fibrosis."[23] Destroyed alveolar tissue is largely incapable of regeneration, and therefore the changes that occur in emphysema are irreversible.[25] Classification of COPD and suggested therapies for each stage are given in Table 27-7. Differential diagnosis of COPD compared with other common lung disorders is noted in Table 27-8 and Table 27-9.

Incidence and Outcome

COPD affects an estimated 15 to 20 million Americans and is the fifth leading cause of death in the United States, accounting for approximately 60,000 deaths each year. Chronic bronchitis and emphysema are the most common causes of COPD.[26]

The social and economic impacts of COPD are enormous. Patients in advanced stages of obstructive lung diseases are unable to work and frequently cannot participate in activities of daily living. Even in milder cases, activities often are restricted. The prognosis for patients with chronic bronchitis is poor, with death often occurring within 5 years after the first episode of acute respiratory failure.[27] *Acute respiratory failure* is defined as a functional disturbance of physiologic mechanisms characterized by a significant reduction in a patient's partial pressure of arterial O_2 (Pao_2) from his or her usual baseline or by an increase in the partial pressure of arterial CO_2 ($Paco_2$) with concomitant acidosis.[28] In the subset of patients with severe COPD and acute respiratory failure who require tracheal intubation, the presence of pulmonary infiltrates on chest radiography has been associated with diminished likelihood for survival.[29,30]

Etiology and Pathophysiology

The principal factor that predisposes a patient to the development of COPD is cigarette smoking.[29,31] Environmental pollution appears to have some role, but its effects are minor compared with those of cigarette smoking. The dominant feature of the natural history of COPD is progressive airflow obstruction, as reflected by a decrease in forced expiratory volume in 1 second (FEV_1). Three causes of decreases in FEV_1 are as follows: (1) a decrease in the intrinsic size of bronchial lumina; (2) an increase in the collapsibility of bronchial walls (this cause is the most difficult to quantify); and (3) a decrease in elastic recoil of the lungs.[27]

TABLE **27-6**	Reflex Mechanism of Respiratory Control			
Stimulus	**Reflex**	**Receptor**	**Afferent Pathway**	**Effects**
Lung inflation	Hering-Breuer inflation reflex	Stretch receptors within smooth muscles of large and small airways	Vagus	Respiratory—cessation of inspiratory effort, apnea, or decreased breathing frequency; bronchodilation Cardiovascular—increased heart rate; slight vasoconstriction
Lung deflation	Hering-Breuer deflation reflex	Possibly J receptors, irritant receptors in lungs, or stretch receptors in airway	Vagus	Respiratory—hyperpnea
Lung inflation	Paradoxical reflex of Head	Stretch receptors in lungs	Vagus	Respiratory—inspiration
Negative pressure in upper airway	Pharyngeal dilator reflex	Receptors in nose, mouth, upper airways		Respiratory—contraction of pharyngeal dilator muscles
Mechanical or chemical irritation of airways	Cough	Receptors in upper airways, tracheobronchial tree	Vagus	Respiratory—cough; bronchoconstriction
	Sneeze	Receptors in nasal mucosa	Trigeminal, olfactory	Respiratory—sneeze; bronchoconstriction
				Cardiovascular—increased blood pressure
Face immersion	Diving reflex	Receptors in nasal mucosa and face	Trigeminal	Respiratory—apnea
				Cardiovascular—decreased heart rate; vasoconstriction
Pulmonary embolism		J receptors in pulmonary vessels	Vagus	Respiratory—apnea or tachypnea
Pulmonary vascular congestion		J receptors in pulmonary vessels	Vagus	Respiratory—tachypnea, possible sensation of dyspnea
Specific chemicals in the pulmonary circulation	Pulmonary chemoreflex	J receptors in pulmonary vessels	Vagus	Respiratory—apnea or tachypnea; bronchoconstriction
Low Pa_{O_2}, high Pa_{CO_2}; low pH	Arterial chemoreceptor reflex	Carotid bodies, aortic bodies	Glossopharyngeal, vagus	Respiratory—hyperpnea; bronchoconstriction, dilation of upper airway Cardiovascular—decreased heart rate, vasodilation, etc.
Increased systemic arterial blood pressure	Arterial baroreceptor reflex	Carotid and aortic arch stretch receptors	Glossopharyngeal, vagus	Respiratory—apnea, bronchodilation Cardiovascular—decreased heart rate, vasodilation, etc.
Increased systemic arterial blood pressure		Muscle spindles, tendon, organs, proprioceptors	Various spinal pathways	Respiratory—provide respiratory controller with feedback about work of breathing; stimulation of proprioceptors in joints causes hyperpnea
Somatic pain		Pain receptors	Various spinal pathways	Respiratory—hyperpnea Cardiovascular—increased heart rate, vasoconstriction, etc.

Modified from Levitzky MG. Pulmonary Physiology. 7th ed. New York: McGraw-Hill; 2007:197-198.

Emphysema may develop in some patients because of an imbalance between protease and antiprotease activities in the lungs. α_1-Antitrypsin deficiency results in the unopposed degradation of pulmonary interstitial elastin fibers by the enzyme elastase and in the early development of emphysema.[32]

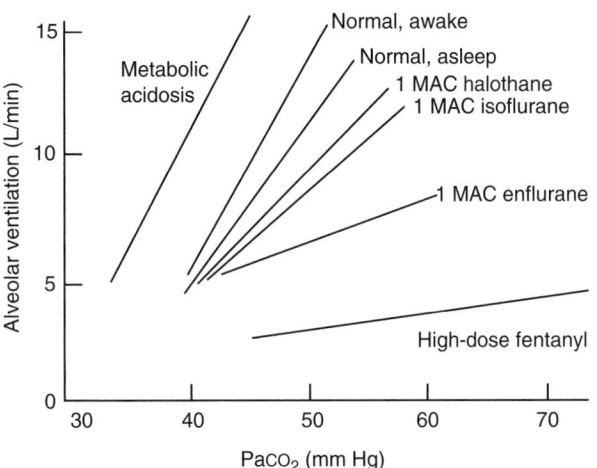

FIGURE **27-10** Carbon dioxide response curve. MAC, Minimum alveolar concentration.

Bullae, a form of emphysema, are air-containing spaces greater than 1 cm in diameter that result from the destruction and dilation of air spaces distal to terminal bronchioles. Their walls consist of attenuated and compressed parenchyma, are confined by connective tissue septa of the lung, and are deep to the internal elastic layer of the visceral pleura.[33]

Blebs are collections of air within the pleura. Because blebs do not involve the acinus, they are not a form of emphysema. If the definition of blebs included the presence of collections of air in the interstitium, as well as in the pleura, interstitial emphysema could be referred to more appropriately as *multiple blebs*. Pulmonary interstitial emphysema occasionally is seen in adults as a complication of assisted ventilation or if air from other sites has dissected backward into the lung.[33]

Distinct morphologic changes can be found in the airways of patients exposed to an ongoing inflammatory challenge. In chronic bronchitis, a proliferation of the compound tracheobronchial mucous glands occurs in the subepithelial layers of the airway wall. Excessive airway mucus and thickened airway walls cause a narrowing of the functional airflow channel. Approximately 25% of patients with COPD also have enhanced airway reactivity. In these patients, an increased amount of airway muscle is noted; this increase also may contribute to airway narrowing.[34]

The defense system of a patient with COPD is disrupted by the excessive production of mucus and by paralysis of the mucociliary transport system, which leads to microbial colonization. However, the presence of microbial organisms in the airway secretions of patients with chronic bronchitis is common and

TABLE **27-7**	Therapy at Each Stage of Chronic Obstructive Pulmonary Disease		
Stage	**Characteristics**	**Recommended Treatment**	
All		Avoidance of risk factors; influenza vaccination	
0: At risk	Chronic symptoms (cough, sputum); exposure to risk factors; normal spirometry		
I: Mild COPD	FEV_1/FVC <70%; FEV_1 ≥80% predicted; with or without symptoms	Short-acting bronchodilator when needed	
II: Moderate COPD	IIA: FEV_1/FVC ≥70%; 50% ≤FEV_1 <80% predicted; with or without symptoms	Regular treatment with one or more bronchodilators; rehabilitation	Inhaled glucocorticosteroids if significant symptoms and lung function response
	IIB: FEV_1/FVC <70%; 30% ≤FEV_1 >50% predicted; with or without symptoms	Regular treatment with one or more bronchodilators; rehabilitation	Inhaled glucocorticosteroids if significant symptoms and lung function response or if repeated exacerbations
III: Severe COPD	FEV_1/FVC <70%; FEV_1 <30% of predicted or presence of respiratory failure or right heart failure	Regular treatment with one or more bronchodilators; inhaled glucocorticosteroids if significant symptoms and lung function response or if repeated exacerbations; treatment of complications; rehabilitation; long-term oxygen therapy if respiratory failure; consider surgical treatments	

From Rable KF et al. Global strategy for the diagnosis, management, and prevention of chronic obstructive pulmonary disease. Am J Respir Crit Care Med. 2007;176:532-555.
COPD, *Chronic obstructive pulmonary disease;* FEV_1, *forced expiratory volume in 1 second;* FVC, *forced vital capacity.*

does not necessarily imply the presence of active infection.[34] Changes in lung functioning include:

1. Destruction of lung connective tissue, which normally provides elastic pull on the outsides of bronchi and bronchioles, reduces the tethering of airways of the pulmonary interstitium, leads to premature collapse of the airways from external pressure, and increases the unevenness of distribution of inspired air to different regions of the lungs. Consequently, the exchange of CO_2 and O_2 between the blood and alveolar air is impeded. Compensation for lower diffusion of gases is partly achieved via collateral ventilation by diffusion across alveolar walls.[35]

TABLE **27-8**	Differential Diagnosis of Chronic Obstructive Pulmonary Disease
Diagnosis	**Suggestive Features***
COPD	Onset in midlife; symptoms slowly progressive; long-term smoking history; dyspnea during exercise; largely irreversible airflow limitation
Asthma	Onset early in life (often childhood); symptoms vary from day to day; symptoms occur at night or in early morning; allergy, rhinitis, or eczema also present; family history of asthma; largely reversible airflow limitation
Congestive heart failure	Fine basilar crackles on auscultation; chest radiograph shows dilated heart, pulmonary edema; pulmonary function tests indicate volume restriction, not airflow limitation
Bronchiectasis	Large volumes of purulent sputum; commonly associated with bacterial infection; coarse crackles or clubbing on auscultation; chest radiograph or CT scan shows bronchial dilation, bronchial wall thickening
Tuberculosis	Onset at all ages; chest radiograph shows lung infiltrate or nodular lesions; microbiologic confirmation; high local prevalence of tuberculosis
Obliterative bronchiolitis	Onset at younger age, in nonsmokers; may have history of rheumatoid arthritis or fume exposure; CT scan taken on expiration shows hypodense areas
Diffuse panbronchiolitis	Most patients are male and nonsmokers; almost all have chronic sinusitis; chest radiograph and HRCT scan show diffuse small centrilobular nodular opacities and hyperinflation

From Rable KF et al. Global strategy for the diagnosis, management, and prevention of chronic obstructive pulmonary disease. Am J Respir Crit Care Med. 2007;176:532-555.
COPD, Chronic obstructive pulmonary disease; CT, computed tomography; HRCT, high-resolution computed tomography.
*These features tend to be characteristic of the respective diseases but do not occur in every case. For example, a person who has never smoked can develop COPD (especially in developing countries, where other risk factors may be more important than cigarette smoking); asthma can develop in adult and even elderly patients.

2. Injury and inflammation of the bronchial tubes and alveoli increase the resistance to airflow during both inspiration and expiration. More forceful breaths or quicker breaths are needed for maintaining even normal levels of ventilation.[36]

3. Lung compliance increases with the tissue damage, and the airways' narrowing and greater collapsibility impede the ability of the ventilatory muscles to empty the lung completely. Hyperinflation results, raising the resting end-expiratory position of the lungs. Because the lung is more expanded, the inspiratory muscles operate from a shorter initial length and produce less force when foreshortened.

4. The more horizontally placed diaphragm is less able to lift the rib cage. The diaphragm may contract ineffectively, such that the abdomen moves inward rather than outward with each inspiration.[37]

5. Because of the increased demands for work output placed on the respiratory muscles, the energy requirement of these muscles escalates. A greater proportion of the CO goes to these muscles. If hypoxemia is present and increased ventilation is required (e.g., as in exercise), the energy supply of the muscles may become inadequate, and respiratory muscle fatigue ultimately is produced.[38]

6. The expansion of the lung and thorax also misaligns the intercostal muscles and accessory respiratory muscles. To compensate, patients may assume special postures, such as leaning forward.[39]

7. Inflammation allows noxious agents in the air to reach the more deeply located tissues in the lung and gain access to blood vessels, macrophages, mast cells, and nerves in the lung. Airway irritation increases; as a result, asthmatic episodes occur because the introduction of noxious agents causes the release of spasmogenic agents from tissue cells and nerve endings.[39]

General Characteristics

The ability of compensatory mechanisms to preserve ventilation and ABG tensions varies. Ventilation usually is very well protected, even more than is gas exchange. CO_2 is 20 times more soluble than O_2 and therefore is more diffusible.[40] Also, if hypercapnia should occur, pulmonary ventilation is stimulated. Minute ventilation ($\dot{V}_E$) in COPD generally is normal to above normal. Usually, Pa_{CO_2} does not increase beyond normal levels in COPD until FEV_1 is less than 1 L. In comparison, Pa_{O_2} is not appreciably restored by an increase in depth of breathing, and even slight variations in $\dot{V}/\dot{Q}$ ratios in the lung adversely affect oxygenation.[30,41] O_2 delivery (D_{O_2}) to the tissues is preserved as much as possible by an increase in CO, a greater extraction of O_2 from the blood, polycythemia, or some combination of these three factors. Consequently, respiratory muscle work is greater than normal, and O_2 use by the muscles is increased.[42]

Associated Conditions
Cigarette Smoking

Cigarette smoking has been firmly established as the primary environmental risk factor associated with emphysema and bronchitis.[31] Its pathogenic mechanism is not known. The unchecked protease hypothesis holds that emphysema is caused by damage to elastic fibers because of an imbalance between elastase and antielastase in the lung.[43] Also, evidence that oxidants have a role in lung damage is increasing. The lungs of cigarette smokers are subject to an enhanced oxidant burden. Oxidants are highly reactive electron acceptors capable of removing electrons from a variety of molecules. The process of oxidation may reversibly or irreversibly damage compounds of all chemical classes, including nucleic acids, proteins and free amino acids, lipids and lipoproteins, and carbohydrates. In this regard, oxidants can damage cells and extracellular matrix components critical for normal lung function. Cigarette smoke and activated lung phagocytes generate an increase in the level of oxidants.[44] Additionally, excess sputum production and hyperplasia of the mucous glands of the trachea and large bronchi are linked to cigarette smoking.[30,44]

Chronic hyperinflation results in diaphragmatic shortening and a decrease in the length of each sarcomere. Over time the decrease in the number of sarcomeres impairs diaphragmatic contraction and contractile force.[45,46]

Peripheral Circulation in Chronic Obstructive Pulmonary Disease

COPD can change the determinants of systemic venous return by altering the mechanical characteristics of either the heart or lungs. When a patient adapts a forced expiratory breathing pattern (e.g., during exercise), very positive pressure swings occur during expiration. The positive swings cyclically decrease systemic venous return, leading to an exaggeration of respiratory variation in arterial blood pressure or to pulsus paradoxus.[47] Pulsus paradoxus is present in two thirds of patients with severe COPD, and its severity correlates with the degree of airflow obstruction.[48,49] Increases in lung volume may directly impede systemic venous return through compression of the vena cava or heart. Normally, inspiration augments systemic venous return because of a decrease in right atrial pressure.[48]

Patients with COPD often have an increase in CO mediated by an increase in catecholamine levels and by a redistribution of blood flow and volume from the high-capacitance splanchnic regions to the lower-capacitance cardiac, cerebral, and muscle regions.[48]

A characteristic enhanced heart rate response also has been identified. Four parameters of airway obstruction (forced vital capacity [FVC], the ratio of FEV_1 to FVC [% FEV_1], the ratio of RV to TLC [RV/TLC], and % RV) have been correlated with the heart rate response to hypoxia. This increased response appears to be the result of an unknown mechanism of diseased lung tissue.[50]

Fluid Retention in Chronic Obstructive Pulmonary Disease

It appears that patients with hypoxic and hypercapnic respiratory failure from emphysema or chronic bronchitis, or from both, have impaired renal function, with reduced renal plasma flow and decreases in glomerular filtration.[51]

Note that cardiac responses to chronic and acute pressure increases are not the same. Chronic pressure overload causes right ventricular hypertrophy, whereas acute pressure changes cause right ventricular dilation.

Clinical Features and Diagnosis

The clinical presentation of COPD varies markedly, and crippling changes for one person may be a minor incapacity for another. Chronic productive cough and progressive exercise limitation are the hallmarks of COPD. Spirometric evaluation in accordance with the standards of the American Thoracic Society establishes the diagnosis of COPD and is categorized by stage in Table 27-7.

Diagnostic Testing

Pulmonary Function Tests. It is desirable to perform spirometry in all patients with unexplained dyspnea and in those in whom COPD is suspected. A decrease in FEV_1/FVC on spirometry is characteristic of expiratory airflow obstruction. FEV_1 is typically less than 80% of FVC in the presence of COPD (Figure 27-11). Measurement of the FEV_1 alone may be misleading because this value may be low if the vital capacity (VC) also is low or if the patient is uncooperative. Likewise, a low FEV_1 combined with a low FEV_1/FVC is indicative of restrictive disease. Measurement of lung volumes in obstructive disease demonstrates an increased RV and often an increased FRC. Slowing of expiratory flow and gas trapping behind prematurely closed airways is responsible for the increase in RV.[52] The advantage of increased RV and FRC in the patient with significant COPD is enlargement of airway diameter, with greater radial support and elastic recoil for exhalation (compared with a patient with a smaller airway diameter, not with one who has a healthy airway and preservation of lung connective tissue). The cost to the patient is the need for greater work in breathing, owing to higher lung volumes.

Sputum examination may be helpful for guiding antimicrobial therapy during exacerbations.

Arterial Blood Gas Analysis. ABG analysis, which is often performed in patients with advanced COPD, helps in the categorization of patients as either "pink puffers" (PaO_2 >60 mm Hg, $PaCO_2$ normal) or "blue bloaters" (PaO_2 <60 mm Hg, $PaCO_2$ >45 mm Hg, and presence of cor pulmonale). Pink puffers usually have severe emphysema, whereas blue bloaters are more likely to have chronic bronchitis.[23] Cyanosis reflects the concentration of deoxygenated Hb (not the percentage of deoxygenated Hb) but not the amount of oxygenated Hb, because the dark blue color of

FIGURE **27-11** Schematic diagram of the forced expiratory volume in 1 second (FEV_1) and forced vital capacity (FVC). The total volume of air exhaled in the first second should be equivalent to at least 80% of the FVC (A). In the presence of obstructive airway disease, the FEV_1 is less than 80% of the FVC (B). (Modified from Stoelting RK, Miller RD. Chronic pulmonary disease. In: Stoelting RK, Miller RD, eds. Basics of Anesthesia. 2nd ed. New York: Churchill Livingstone;1989:288.)

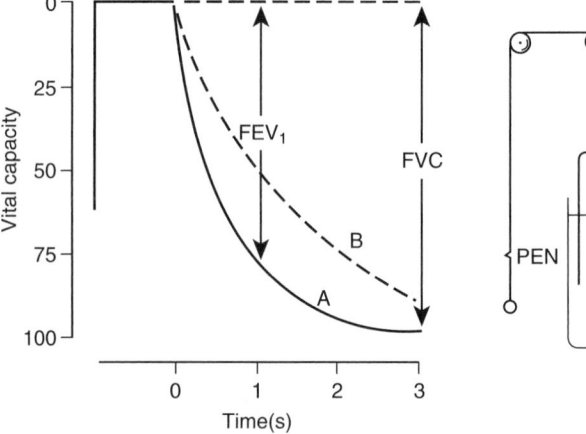
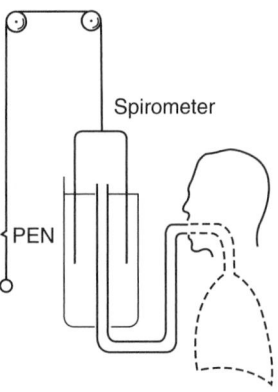

deoxygenated blood masks the red color of oxygenated blood. Cyanosis is present if the arterial blood contains more than 5 g of deoxygenated Hb per deciliter of blood.[53]

Pulmonary artery hypertension that leads to cor pulmonale is a likely development in bronchitic patients with arterial hypoxemia and hypercarbia. Conversely, loss of pulmonary capillaries from the destruction of alveoli in emphysema is manifested by a decrease in the diffusing capacity of carbon monoxide (D_{LCO}). Pulmonary vasoconstriction also is a late consequence, because arterial hypoxemia is not prominent in emphysema until the disease's very advanced stages (Table 27-10).[27]

TABLE 27-9	Clinical Hallmarks: Predominant Bronchitis versus Predominant Emphysema	
	Blue Bloater, Predominant Bronchitis	**Pink Puffer, Predominant Emphysema**
General appearance	Overweight; dusky; warm extremities	Thin, often emaciated; pursed-lip breathing; anxious; prominent use of accessory muscles; normal to cool extremities
Age (yr)	40-55	50-75
Onset	Cough	Dyspnea
Cyanosis	Marked	Slight to none
Cough	More evident than dyspnea	Less evident than dyspnea
Sputum	Copious	Scanty
Upper respiratory infections	Common	Occasional
Breath sounds	Moderately diminished	Markedly diminished
Cor pulmonale and right-sided heart failure	Common	Only during bouts of respiratory infection, and terminally
Radiographic features	Normal diaphragm position; cardiomegaly; lungs normal or with increased bronchovascular markings	Small pendulous heart; low, flat diaphragm; areas of increased radiolucency
Course	Ambulatory but constantly on verge of right-sided heart failure and coma	Incapacitation of breathlessness punctuated by life-threatening bouts of upper respiratory infections; prolonged course culminating in right-sided heart failure and coma

Modified from Fishman AP, ed. Update: Pulmonary Diseases and Disorders. 2nd ed. New York: McGraw-Hill; 1988:1165.

TABLE 27-10	Functional Hallmarks: Predominant Bronchitis versus Predominant Emphysema	
	Blue Bloater, Predominant Bronchitis	**Pink Puffer, Predominant Emphysema**
FEV_1/FC	Reduced	Reduced
FRC	Mildly increased	Markedly increased
TLC	Normal to slight increase	Considerably increased
RV	Moderately increased	Markedly increased
Lung compliance	Normal or high	Normal or low
Recoil pressure	Normal or high	Low
MVV	Moderately decreased	Markedly decreased
Airway resistance	Increased	Normal to slightly increased
D_{LCO}	Normal or low	Low
Arterial Pao_2	Moderate to severe decrease	Mildly to moderately reduced
Arterial hypercapnia	Often present	Present during an acute respiratory infection
Hematocrit	Generally high; may reach 70%	Normal or slightly high; uncommon exceeds 55%
Pulmonary arterial pressure	Generally increased	Normal or slightly increased

From Fishman AP, ed. Pulmonary Diseases and Disorders. 3rd ed New York: McGraw-Hill; 2002:106.
D_{LCO}, *Diffusing capacity of carbon monoxide;* FEV_1, *forced expiratory volume in 1 second;* FRC, *functional residual capacity;* MVV, *maximum voluntary ventilation;* Pao_2, *partial pressure of arterial oxygen;* RV, *residual volume;* TLC, *total lung capacity;* VC, *vital capacity.*

Chest Radiography and Computed Tomography. Radiographic abnormalities may be minimal, even in the presence of advanced COPD.[52] Hyperlucency of the lungs (caused by arterial vascular deficiency in the lung periphery) and hyperinflation (flattening of the diaphragm with loss of the silhouette) suggest the diagnosis of emphysema.[54] If bullae also are present, the diagnosis of emphysema is virtually certain; however, only a small percentage of patients who have emphysema have bullae. Chronic bronchitis can be detected only on chest radiography. Computed tomography (CT) can delineate the pulmonary parenchyma much better than standard chest radiography. CT may also be used to quantitate the amount of air trapping.

Preoperative Evaluation

The surgical site and the preoperative status of the patient are critical factors in determining the incidence of postoperative complications. Multiple factors are predictive of postoperative respiratory difficulties, but no preoperative pulmonary function test establishes absolute contraindications to surgery. The preoperative evaluation of patients with COPD should determine the severity of the disease and identify treatments for reducing inflammation, improving secretion clearance, treating underlying infection, and increasing airway caliber that can ensure the best surgical outcome. Supplemental administration of O_2 usually is recommended if the PaO_2 is less than 60 mm Hg, if the hematocrit is greater than 55%, or if evidence of cor pulmonale is present.[23]

The causes of acute exacerbations of COPD are multiple and may be explained only partially by airway infection or inflammation. Multiple contributing factors, including bronchitis, underlying airway hyperresponsiveness, inhalation of noxious agents, mucous plugging, pneumonitis, cardiovascular disease, congestive heart failure (CHF), and generalized systemic inflammation, must be considered.[30] Signs of COPD may be subtle.[55] The clinician must assess for increased respiratory effort, altered breathing patterns, abnormal breath sounds, and a productive cough.[56] A consensus statement by the American Thoracic Society defines dyspnea as "a term used to characterize a subjective experience of breathing discomfort that is comprised of qualitatively distinct sensations that vary in intensity. The experience derives from interactions among multiple physiological, psychological, social and environmental factors, and may induce secondary physiological and behavioral responses."[57,58] In evaluating a patient for dyspnea, a visual analogue scale is commonly used (Figure 27-12).

Visual analogue scale for dyspnea

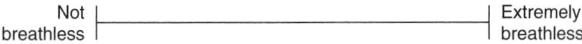

FIGURE **27-12** Visual analogue scales, such as the horizontal one shown here, can be used for measuring dyspnea during an activity (e.g., exercise testing) or in response to questions. Such scales may be depicted vertically as well. On request, the subject marks a point on the line in response to a question (e.g., "How short of breath are you right now?"). The score is determined by the length of the line from "not breathless" to the point marked by the patient. The scales are usually 10 cm long to facilitate scoring, and electronic scales may be used to allow online scoring (e.g., during exercise testing). Instructions about what is meant by the terms used to describe a sensation (e.g., "extremely breathless") must be clear and must be presented in a uniform fashion to provide meaningful results. (*From Murray JF, Nadel JA. Textbook of Respiratory Medicine. 4th ed. Philadelphia: Saunders; 2005:819*)

A history or the presence of atopy (predisposition to allergies), childhood respiratory impairment, high serum immunoglobulin E (IgE) levels, and eosinophilia is suggestive of asthmatic bronchitis, which is generally more responsive to treatment than is smoking-induced COPD. The clinician should perform ABG analysis or pulse oximetry (or both) for those patients with FEV_1 less than 1.5 L and should document the changes that occur with O_2 treatment. Pulmonary function tests should be repeated after bronchodilator or steroid treatment (or both) so that airway disease reversibility can be evaluated. Although β-agonists are the mainstay of treatment, increasing emphasis on the inflammatory component of reactive airway disease has resulted in an increase in the use of steroids.[55]

Conditions that predispose a patient to infectious complications include dehydration, decreased ability to cough, immobility, decreased level of consciousness, microatelectasis and macroatelectasis, decreased mucociliary clearance of inhaled particles and microbial organisms, pain, analgesia, and supplemental O_2 therapy. Optimal control of airway inflammation may require a course of broad-spectrum antimicrobial therapy preoperatively. A patient with an acute exacerbation of chronic bronchitis may have fatigue, chest tightness, increased cough, and dyspnea.[34]

The patient may observe a change in sputum volume, color, or consistency. Viruses are frequently causative organisms in acute exacerbations of chronic bronchitis and may be responsible for 25% to 50% of acute infections. In contrast to bacteria, viruses do not colonize the airways; when identified, they signify an active infective process.[34] Acute infection is associated with epithelial desquamation and correlates with airway hyperreactivity that may persist for 3 to 6 weeks after the resolution of symptoms.[58] The clinician should consider performing pulmonary function tests. They are useful for confirming the presence, severity, and reversibility of airflow obstruction and for monitoring the progression of the disease. Surgery is not likely to be withheld on the basis of a decrease in ventilatory capacity, because patients with FEV_1 in the low range of 0.3 to 1 L often undergo surgery and anesthesia successfully.[59,60] It should be recognized that decreased pulmonary function as reflected by FEV_1 correlates with coronary artery disease and increased total mortality; the reason for this relationship has yet to be determined. Measures to improve respiratory skeletal muscle strength include good nutrition and balanced fluid and electrolyte intake. Bronchodilators should be used if the patient exhibits some degree of airway obstruction (coughing may temporarily increase in frequency as greater quantities of sputum are removed). Some commonly used bronchodilators are listed in Table 27-11.

An increased plasma concentration of bicarbonate in the presence of a low or normal $PaCO_2$ suggests that acute hyperventilation is masking chronic CO_2 retention. If the $PaCO_2$ has been chronically elevated, it is important that the hypercarbia not be corrected too quickly. Sudden decreases in $PaCO_2$ can result in alkalemia because the kidneys cannot instantly excrete the excess bicarbonate.

Patients arriving for surgery who are already undergoing mechanical ventilation may require a ventilator that is more powerful than that on the anesthesia machine. High airway pressures (i.e., those >60 cm H_2O) create impedance to the high compressible volume of the anesthesia circuit, preventing adequate ventilation. Finally, the patient with COPD who arrives for an emergency operation presents a further challenge because of an increased risk for mortality.[55] The anesthetist must attempt to provide optimal care despite less than optimal conditions.

TABLE 27-11 Drugs for COPD

Drug	Formulation	Delivery Device	Adult Dosage
Short-Acting Beta₂ Agonists			
Albuterol generic Proventil (Schering-Plough)	90 mcg base/inhalation	MDI	2 inhalations q4-6h PRN
Albuterol sulfate			
ProAir HFA (Teva) *Proventil HFA* (Schering-Plough) *Ventolin HFA* (GSK) generic	90 mcg base/inhalation	MDI	2 inhalations q4-6h PRN
single-dose vials multi-dose vials	2.5 mg base/3 mL 2.5 mg base/0.5 mL	Nebulizer	2.5 mg q6-8h PRN
AccuNeb (Dey) single-dose vials	0.63 or 1.25 mg base/3 mL		
Levalbuterol tartrate			
Xopenex (Sepracor)	0.31, 0.63 1.25 mg/3 mL	Nebulizer	0.63-1.25 mg tid q6-8h
Xopenex HFA	45 mcg/inhalation	MDI	2 inhalations q4-6h PRN
Pirbuterol			
Maxair Autohaler (Graceway/3M)	200 mcg/inhalation	MDI	2 inhalations q4-6h PRN
Short-Acting Anticholinergic			
Ipratropium			
Atrovent HFA (Boehringer Ingelheim) generic	17 mcg/inhalation 250 mcg/mL	MDI Nebulizer	2 inhalations qid PRN 500 mcg qid PRN
Short-Acting Beta₂ Agonists/Short-Acting Anticholinergic Combination			
Albuterol sulfate/ipratropium			
Combivent (Boehringer Ingelheim)	90 mcg albuterol base/18 mcg ipratropium/inhalation	MDI	2 inhalations qid PRN
DuoNeb (Dey)	2.5 mg albuterol base/0.5 mg ipratropium/3 mL	Nebulizer	2.5 mg/0.5 mg qid PRN (max 6 doses/day)
Long-Acting Beta₂-Agonists			
Salmeterol—*Serevent Diskus (GSK)*	50 mcg/blister	DPI	50 mcg bid
Formoterol—*Foradil Aerolizer* (Schering-Plough)	12 mcg/capsule	DPI	12 mcg bid
Perforomoist (Dey)	20 mcg/2 mL	Nebulizer	20 mcg bid
Arformoterol—*Brovana* (Sepracor)	15 mcg/2 mL	Nebulizer	15 mcg bid
Long-Acting Anticholinergic			
Tiotropium—*Spiriva HandiHaler* (Boehringer Ingelheim)	18 mcg/capsule	DPI	8 mcg once/day
Corticosteroid/Long-Acting Beta₂ Agonist Combinations			
Fluticasone/salmeterol—*Advair Diskus (GSK)* Advair HFA (GSK)	100, 250, 500 mcg/50 mcg/ blister 45, 115, 230 mcg/21 mcg inhalation	DPI MDI	1 inhalation bid 2 inhalations bid
Budesonide/formoterol—*Symbicort* (AstraZeneca)	80, 160 mcg/4.5 mcg/ inhalation	MDI	2 inhalations bid
Theophylline			
Average generic	450 mg ER* tabs; 100, 125, 200, 300 mg ER* caps	—	300-600 mg/day
Theo-24† (UCB Pharma)	100, 200, 300, 400 mg ER* caps		
Theochron (Forest)	100, 200, 300, 450 mg ER* tabs		
Uniphyl (Purdue Pharma)	400, 600 mg ER* tabs		400-600 mg/day

Modified from *Drugs for chronic obstructive pulmonary disease. Treat Guidel Med Lett.* 2007;5(63):95-100.
DPI, *Dry powder inhaler;* ER, *extended-release;* HFA, *hydrofluoroalkane (propellant);* MDI, *metered-dose inhaler.*
Extended-release formulations may not be interchangeable.
†*If Theo-24 is taken with food, the entire 24-hour dose is released in a 4-hour period.*

Continued

TABLE **27-11**	Drugs for COPD—cont'd		
Drug	**Formulation**	**Delivery Device**	**Adult Dosage**
Corticosteroids			
Beclomethasone dipropionate QVAR HFA (Ivax)	40, 80 mcg/inhalation	MDI	40-320 mcg bid
Budesonide			
Pulmicort Flexhaler (AstraZeneca)	90, 180 mcg/inhalation	DPI	60-720 mcg bid
Pulmicort Turbuhaler	200 mcg/inhalation	DPI	200-800 mcg bid
Pulmicort Respules	0.25, 0.5 mg/2 mL	Nebulizer	250-500 mcg 1×/day or bid or 1.0 mg 1×/day
Flunisolide			
AeroBid (Forest)	250 mcg/inhalation	MDI	500-1000 mcg bid
Aerospan HFA (Forest)	80 mcg/inhalation	MDI	160-320 mcg bid
Fluticasone propionate			
Flovent Diskus (GSK)	50, 100, 250 mcg/blister	DPI	100-500 mcg bid
Flovent HFA (GSK)	44, 110, 220 mcg/inhalation	MDI	88-440 mcg bid
Mometasone furoate			
Asmanex Twisthaler (Schering-Plough)	220 mcg/inhalation	DPI	20-440 mcg 1×/day or bid (max 880 mcg/day)
Triamcinolone acetonide			
Azmacort (Kos)	75 mcg/inhalation	MDI	150 mcg tid-qid or 300 mcg bid
Corticosteroid/Long-Acting Beta₂-Agonist Combinations			
Fluticasone/salmeterol			
Advair Diskus (GSK)	100, 250, 500 mcg/50 mcg/blister	DPI	1 inhalation bid
Advair HFA (GSK)	45, 115, 230 mcg/21 mcg/inhalation	MDI	2 inhalations bid
Budesonide/formoterol			
Symbicort (FHA) (AstraZeneca)	80, 160 mcg/4.5 mcg/inhalation	MDI	2 inhalations bid

Anesthesia Management

The presence of COPD does not dictate the use of specific drugs or techniques for the management of anesthesia. It is crucial to realize that COPD patients are susceptible to the development of acute respiratory failure during the postoperative period. Therefore, continued intubation of the trachea and mechanical ventilation of the lungs may be necessary, particularly after thoracic and upper abdominal surgery. Postoperative ventilation is more likely to be needed in those patients with low PaO_2 and dyspnea at rest.

Regional Anesthesia

Regional anesthesia is useful if sedation is not needed, and it may be safer than general anesthesia. Anesthetists must avoid complacency if they use regional rather than general anesthesia, monitoring for potential adverse side effects (pneumothorax, impaired muscle function). Regional anesthetic techniques that produce sensory anesthesia above T6 are not recommended. The potential for decreasing expiratory reserve volume, impairing cough effort, and creating anxiety-provoking weakness is too great.[61]

General Anesthesia

General anesthesia often is provided with a volatile anesthetic (for facilitating bronchodilation) and humidification (for preventing the drying of secretions). However, there is some

evidence that volatile anesthetics (as opposed to intravenous agents) reduce the function of cilia in the respiratory tract.[62] Maintaining adequate anesthesia in patients with significant lung disease presents a challenge. General anesthesia is often associated with an increase in the alveolar-arterial difference in PO_2 ($PAO_2 - PaO_2$). Causes include a fairly consistent 20% decrease in FRC when neuromuscular relaxants are used, as well as airway closure, for which signs will lessen. Atelectasis normally occurs following induction of general anesthesia and has been found to worsen with muscle paralysis and prolonged surgical duration.[63] It is interesting to note that patients with chronic hyperinflation appear to be less likely to develop atelectasis than subjects with healthy lungs, possibly because of airway closure before alveolar collapse or because of resistance to early alveolar collapse from long-standing lung hyperinflation, which prevents prompt formation of atelectasis.[64] Reducing absorptive atelectasis by administering oxygen at less than 100% and providing intermittent vital capacity maneuvers to recruit atelectatic alveoli will help improve oxygenation during pulmonary surgery.[63]

If N_2O is used, bullae may enlarge and rupture; therefore, their presence is a contraindication to its use.[65] The anesthetist should provide adequate hydration to prevent excessive drying of secretions. The major limitation to gas movement in tissues is

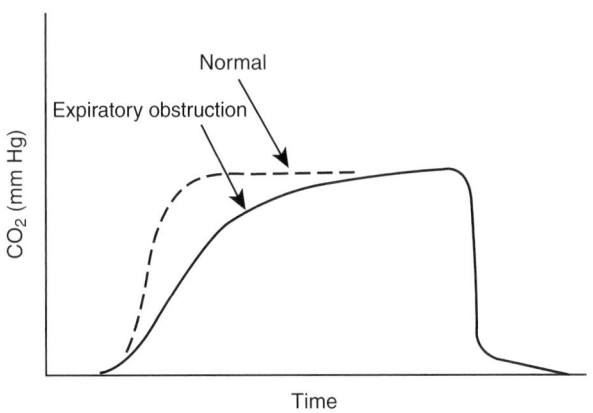

FIGURE **27-13** Capnograph of a patient with expiratory airway obstruction. (*Modified from Morgan GE, Mikhail MS. Anesthesia for patients with respiratory disease. In: Morgan GE, Mikhail MS, eds. Clinical Anesthesiology. 4th ed. Norwalk, CT: Appleton & Lange; 2006:575.*)

diffusion through tissue water. Impairment of gas exchange worsens during anesthesia.[66,67] Patients with COPD have slower diffusion and therefore may have longer induction and emergence times. The anesthetist should have the patient produce sighs during anesthesia; this has been found to improve the $PaO_2 - PaO_2$ significantly, ultimately improving oxygenation.[67] The capnograph should be monitored for expiratory airflow obstruction (Figure 27-13). Patients generally require an increased V_T. Gas exchange is very dependent on V_T in some who require an increase in V_T for the improvement of gas exchange at the periphery of the lobule. This response varies among patients.[68]

Positive End-Expiratory Pressure

Severe airflow obstruction prevents full lung decompression at end-expiration. As a result, inspiration begins at volumes at which the respiratory system exhibits positive recoil pressure, or auto or intrinsic PEEP (PEEPi).[69,70] Patients must generate pressure sufficient to overcome PEEPi before inspiratory flow can start.[70] In the past, external PEEP (PEEPe) was generally not used in patients with COPD because hypoxemia often is improved with increases in the fraction of inspired O_2 (FiO$_2$) and because the risk of barotrauma resulting from further hyperinflation was deemed too great. However, more recent studies suggest that a PEEPe that is less than the PEEPi in the presence of expiratory flow limitation may assist patients in overcoming the inspiratory mechanical load of PEEPi, ultimately decreasing the work of breathing and eliminating or decreasing atelectatic areas.[70,71] Patients whose peak cycling pressures remain essentially unaffected by PEEPe experience the greatest improvement and the least hazard.[72] In the operating room, the clinician can best diagnose PEEPi by assessing whether exhalation is still taking place when the next inhalation starts.[55]

Clinical judgment must dictate the judicious use of PEEPe because the results of PEEPe are largely unpredictable.[69] PEEPe that is less than 85% of PEEPi has been found helpful, whereas PEEPe greater than 85% of PEEPi can cause further hyperinflation and may compromise hemodynamics and gas exchange. When PEEPe is added, it should be titrated in 2.5- to 5-cm H_2O increments while peak cycling pressures are closely monitored. The inspiratory/expiratory ratio is adjusted so that expiration is prolonged, and the decrease in PEEPi is facilitated.[70]

Postoperative Care

Postoperative care of patients with COPD is directed at minimizing the incidence and severity of pulmonary complications, because such patients are at increased risk for the development of acute respiratory failure.[56] Postoperative pulmonary complications are most often characterized by atelectasis followed by pneumonia and decreases in PaO_2.[55] These patients require close monitoring; worsening $\dot{V}/\dot{Q}$ mismatch after extubation may not be detected by ABG analysis, possibly because of changes in breathing pattern and cardiovascular function. In fact, minute ventilation may not change, but often respiratory rate increases, and V_T decreases after the termination of mechanical ventilation.[72] The choice of drugs or techniques for producing anesthesia does not seem to predictably alter the incidence of postoperative pulmonary infections. Whether a relationship exists between the duration of anesthesia and the incidence of postoperative pulmonary complications is not clear.

To increase FRC and improve oxygenation via $\dot{V}/\dot{Q}$ matching, ambulation should be encouraged. Incentive spirometry with maintenance of peak inflation for 3 to 5 seconds reexpands collapsed alveoli.[58] Expiratory maneuvers (e.g., floating balls on an expiratory spirometer) generate pleural pressures that exceed airway pressures and can cause alveolar collapse.[56,73]

ASTHMA

Definition

The National Asthma Education and Prevention Program Expert Panel Report 3 (EPR-3) defines asthma as a chronic inflammatory disorder of the airways in which many cells and cellular elements play a role: in particular, mast cells, eosinophils, neutrophils (especially in sudden onset, fatal exacerbations, occupational asthma, and patients who smoke), T lymphocytes, macrophages, and epithelial cells. In susceptible individuals, this inflammation causes recurrent episodes of coughing (particularly at night or in the early morning), wheezing, breathlessness, and chest tightness. These episodes are usually associated with widespread but variable airflow obstruction that is often reversible either spontaneously or with treatment.[74]

Various subtypes of asthma exist. The most important consideration is identifying exacerbating factors whenever possible. A well-known system classifies asthmas as either extrinsic or intrinsic. Although this system is conceptually helpful, its two groups are not mutually exclusive. Extrinsic asthma (or allergic asthma) most commonly affects children and young adults and involves infectious, environmental, psychologic, or physical factors, whereas intrinsic asthma (or idiosyncratic asthma) usually develops in middle age without specifically identifiable attack-provoking stimuli. The term *atopy*, which refers to a hereditary, IgE-mediated, clinical hypersensitive state, is often used when extrinsic asthma is described.

Incidence and Outcome

Up to 22 million persons in the United States have asthma. It is the most common chronic disease of childhood, affecting an estimated 6 million children. The burden of asthma affects the patients, their families, and society in terms of lost work and school, lessened quality of life, and avoidable emergency department (ED) visits, hospitalizations, and deaths.[74]

Pathogenesis and Pathophysiology

Our contemporary understanding of asthma is that it is not a single entity, but rather a heterogeneous clinical syndrome characterized by episodes in which airways are hyperresponsive interspersed with symptom-free periods.[75] Bronchoconstriction is a factor long associated with the asthmatic symptom complex, but asthma is much more than bronchoconstriction. Airway inflammation and a nonspecific hyperirritability of the tracheobronchial tree are now recognized as being central to the pathogenesis of even mild cases of asthma. Permanent changes in airway anatomy, referred to as *airway remodeling*, magnify the inflammatory response.[75,76]

Allergic asthma (atopic or immunologic disease) is triggered by antigens that provoke a T-lymphocyte–generated, IgE-mediated immune response.[77] It is often associated with a personal or familial history of allergic disease.

In susceptible patients, exposure to even minute amounts of an offending agent can cause activation of lymphocytes and cytokine release, setting into motion an immune-mediated inflammatory response. Endobronchial biopsy specimens, even from asymptomatic patients, frequently show an active inflammatory process. Eosinophils, mast cells, neutrophils, and macrophages are prominent features in asthmatic airways, and their activation and degranulation fuel the proinflammatory cascade.

Potent biochemical mediators released from proinflammatory and airway epithelial cells promote vasoconstriction, increased smooth muscle tone, enhanced mucus secretion, submucosal edema, increased vascular permeability, and inflammatory cell chemotaxis. Leukotrienes have been identified as especially potent spasmogenic and proinflammatory substances. Released molecules that are toxic to the airway epithelium cause patchy desquamation, exposing cholinergic nerve endings and compounding the bronchoconstrictive and hyperresponsive response.

The asthmatic diathesis creates airways that are inflamed, edematous, and hypersensitive to irritant stimuli, and the degree of airway hyperresponsiveness and bronchoconstriction appears to parallel the extent of inflammation.[78-80] When airway reactivity is high, asthmatic symptoms are generally more severe and unrelenting, and the amount of therapy required to control the episode is greater.[75]

The mechanisms underlying idiosyncratic asthma (nonimmunologic disease) are less clearly defined. Nonimmunologic asthma occurs in patients with no history of allergy and normal serum IgE. These patients typically develop asthmatic symptoms in response to some provocative or noxious stimulus such as cold air, airway instrumentation or irritation, climate changes, or an upper respiratory illness. Recent upper respiratory infection may precipitate bronchospasm in any patient, but the risk is higher in patients with a history of asthma. The increased bronchomotor tone associated with viral respiratory infections may persist for as long as 5 weeks.[80] Nonasthmatic children with an upper respiratory infection are two to seven times more likely to experience an adverse event perioperatively and are more prone to postoperative desaturation.[81] Asthmatic children can be considered to be at a similar if not greater risk. Enhanced parasympathetic nervous system tone can contribute to the airflow obstruction.

Immune mechanisms appear to be causally related or contributory to the development of asthma in more than 50% of cases, but many patients with asthma have disease mechanisms from both categories. Asthma that has its onset in childhood tends to have a strong allergic component, whereas asthma that arises in adults tends to be nonallergic or to have a mixed cause.[75,82] As a general rule, nonallergic mechanisms are more prevalent in the perioperative period.[83] It is of significance that the clinical features of idiosyncratic asthma are essentially indistinguishable from the immune-mediated response.

IgE-mediated asthma occurs after initial antigen exposure has resulted in IgE antibody formation. On reexposure, in the presence of IgE, mast cells release multiple mediators. These mediators directly constrict small and large airways, increase capillary permeability, stimulate vasoconstriction, and increase mucous gland secretion, which contributes to mucous plugging (Figure 27-14).

The mechanism of exercise-induced bronchospasm (EIB) is unknown. One popular theory suggests that a high minute ventilation ($\dot{V}_E$) and the low temperature or low H_2O content of inspired gas (which requires greater heat and water transfer from the mucosal surface to the inspired gas) generates a bronchoconstrictive response. Another theory proposes that the evaporation of water from respiratory mucosa and the resultant increase in the osmolarity of the surface-lining fluid induces the degranulation of mast cells. A third theory suggests that reactive hyperemia of the bronchial mucosa occurs with rewarming, resulting in airway narrowing.[84] Regardless of the mechanism,

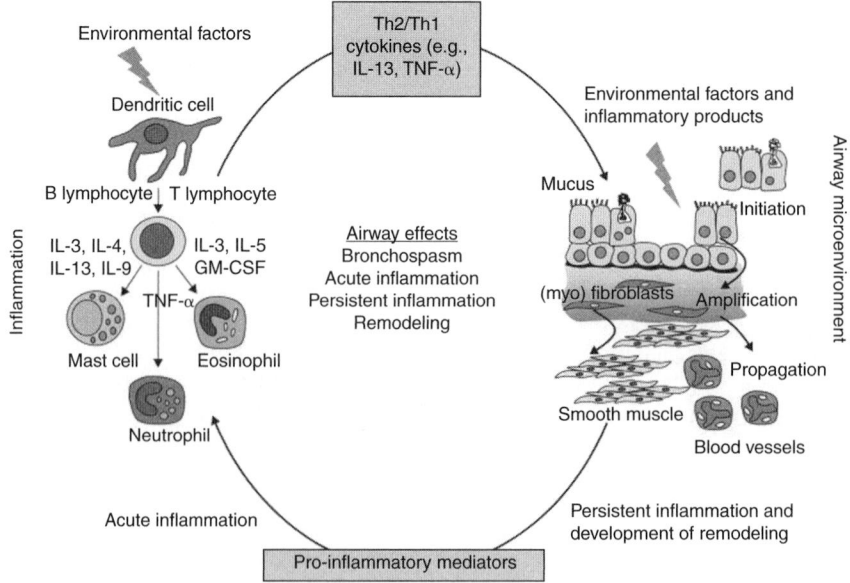

FIGURE **27-14** Factors limiting air flow in acute and persistent asthma. *GM-CSF,* Granulocyte-macrophage colony-stimulating factor; *IgE,* immunoglobulin E; *IL-3,* interleukin 3 (and similar); *TNF-α,* tumor necrosis factor-alpha. (*Modified and reprinted from Holgate ST, Polosa R. The mechanisms, diagnosis, and management of severe asthma in adults. Lancet. 2006;368: 780-793.*)

most symptoms last less than 1 hour and are usually quickly reversed with administration of β_2-adrenergic receptor agonists.[85]

Occupational asthma develops when irritants directly stimulate vagal nerve endings in the airway epithelium. Infection-induced asthma with acute inflammation of the bronchi may be caused by viral, bacterial, or mycoplasmal infections. Aspirin-induced asthma occurs when, in some predisposed persons, cyclooxygenase promotes an increase in leukotriene levels via the arachidonic acid pathway, thereby triggering the asthma attack. This peculiar response can also occur with the use of other nonsteroidal antiinflammatory agents. The aspirin-induced asthma variant is not IgE mediated or allergic in nature. It is clinically associated with nasal polyps.

Clinical Features and Diagnosis

Airflow limitation is caused by a variety of changes in the airway, all influenced by airway inflammation[74]:

- Bronchoconstriction—bronchial smooth muscle contraction that quickly narrows the airways in response to exposure to a variety of stimuli, including allergens or irritants
- Airway hyperresponsiveness—an exaggerated bronchoconstrictor response to stimuli

- Airway edema—As the disease becomes more persistent and inflammation becomes more progressive, edema, mucus hypersecretion, and formation of inspissated mucus plugs further limit airflow.

Key hallmarks of asthma include[74,78]:

- Recurrent wheezing
- Dyspnea (may parallel the severity of expiratory airflow obstruction)
- Cough (productive or nonproductive; frequently at night or early morning)
- Recurrent labored respirations with accessory muscle use
- Tachypnea (a respiratory rate >30 breaths per minute and a heart rate of 120 suggests severe bronchospasm)
- Recurrent chest tightness
- Prolonged expiratory phase of respiration
- Fatigue
- Symptoms occur or worsen with exercise, viral infection, environmental allergens or irritants, changes in weather, stress, or menstrual cycles.

Clinical classification of asthma is noted in Table 27-12 and Figure 27-15. Typical attacks are short-lived, lasting minutes to hours. Between attacks the asthmatic patient may be entirely

TABLE 27-12	Clinical Asthma Classification and Associated Pharmacotherapy	
	Clinical Characteristics Before Therapy	**Pharmacologic Treatment***
Step 1—Intermittent asthma	Signs and symptoms occur less than twice per week Patients generally asymptomatic with normal peak flows between exacerbations Exacerbations brief, although intensity may vary Nighttime symptoms occur twice per month or less frequently FEV_1 or PEFR $\geq$80% of predicted value FEV_1/FVC normal	Short-acting bronchodilator, as needed: inhaled β_2-agonists are the first-line selection
Step 2—Mild persistent asthma	Signs and symptoms occur more than twice per week but less than once per day Exacerbations may affect activity Nighttime symptoms occur more than three to four times per month FEV_1 or PEFR $\geq$80% of predicted value. FEV_1/FVC normal	Long-term antiinflammatory medication: inhaled corticosteroid (low dose) Cromolyn or nedocromil, particularly in children Sustained-release theophylline is an alternative Zafirlukast or zileuton may be considered for patients $\geq$12 years old
Step 3—Moderate persistent asthma	Daily symptoms Daily use of short-acting β_2-agonist Exacerbations that affect activity occur at least twice a week and may last for days Nighttime symptoms occur more than once per week but not nightly FEV_1 or PEFR 60% of 80% of predicted value. FEV_1/FVC reduced 5%	Long-term control medications: medium-dose inhaled corticosteroids or low- to medium-dose inhaled corticosteroids plus long-acting bronchodilator (inhaled or oral β_2-agonist, sustained-release theophylline), especially for treatment of nocturnal symptoms
Step 4—Severe persistent asthma	Continuous signs and symptoms, frequently exacerbated Often nightly symptoms Extremely limited physical activity FEV_1 or PEFR $\leq$60% of predicted value. FEV_1/FVC reduced >5%	High-dose inhaled corticosteroids Long-acting bronchodilators, as indicated in Step 3 Systemic corticosteroids (e.g., prednisone)

Modified from National Asthma Education and Prevention Program, Expert Panel Report 3. Guidelines for the diagnosis and management of asthma—summary report 2007. J Allergy Clin Immunol. 2007;120(Suppl 5):S94-138; Kaiser Permanente Care Management Program. Asthma: Successful Practice Guidelines. Pasadena, CA: Kaiser Permanente; 2003:1-14.
FEV_1, Forced expiratory volume in 1 second; FEV_1/FVC, forced expiratory volume in 1 second/forced vital capacity; PEFR, peak expiratory flow rate.
*For all severity steps, β_2-agonists are used for quick relief of acute symptoms.

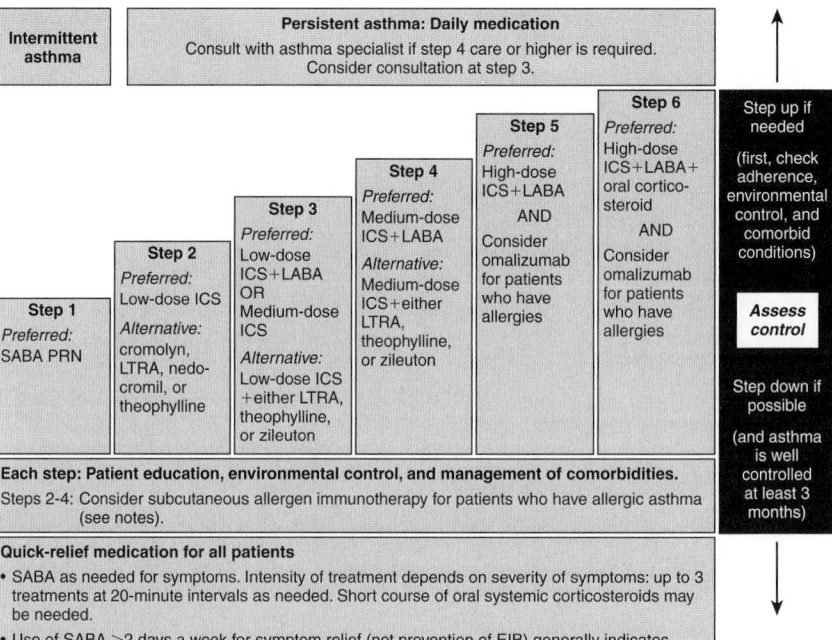

| Intermittent asthma | **Persistent asthma: Daily medication**
Consult with asthma specialist if step 4 care or higher is required.
Consider consultation at step 3. |

						Step 6 *Preferred:* High-dose ICS+LABA+ oral cortico- steroid AND Consider omalizumab for patients who have allergies
					Step 5 *Preferred:* High-dose ICS+LABA AND Consider omalizumab for patients who have allergies	
				Step 4 *Preferred:* Medium-dose ICS+LABA *Alternative:* Medium-dose ICS+either LTRA, theophylline, or zileuton		
			Step 3 *Preferred:* Low-dose ICS+LABA OR Medium-dose ICS *Alternative:* Low-dose ICS +either LTRA, theophylline, or zileuton			
		Step 2 *Preferred:* Low-dose ICS *Alternative:* cromolyn, LTRA, nedo- cromil, or theophylline				
	Step 1 *Preferred:* SABA PRN					

Step up if needed

(first, check adherence, environmental control, and comorbid conditions)

Assess control

Step down if possible

(and asthma is well controlled at least 3 months)

Each step: Patient education, environmental control, and management of comorbidities.
Steps 2-4: Consider subcutaneous allergen immunotherapy for patients who have allergic asthma (see notes).

Quick-relief medication for all patients
- SABA as needed for symptoms. Intensity of treatment depends on severity of symptoms: up to 3 treatments at 20-minute intervals as needed. Short course of oral systemic corticosteroids may be needed.
- Use of SABA >2 days a week for symptom relief (not prevention of EIB) generally indicates inadequate control and the need to step up treatment.

FIGURE **27-15** Stepwise approach to treating asthma in adults. (*Modified from Urbano FL. Review of the NAEPP 2007 expert panel report [EPR-3] on asthma diagnosis and treatment guidelines.* J Manag Care Pharm. 2008:Jan-Feb;14[1]:41-49.)

SABA=short acting β_2 agonist; ICS=inhaled corticosteroid; LABA=long acting β_2 agonist; LTRA=leukotriene receptor antagonist; PRN=as needed

Notes:
- The stepwise approach is meant to assist, not replace, the clinical decisionmaking required to meet individual patient needs. Steps vary with age.
- If alternative treatment is used and response is inadequate, discontinue it and use the preferred treatment before stepping up.
- Zileuton is a less desirable alternative because of limited studies as adjunctive therapy and the need to monitor liver function. Theophylline requires monitoring of serum concentration levels.
- In step 6, before oral corticosteroids are introduced, a trial of high-dose ICS+LABA+LTRA, theophylline, or zileuton may be considered, although this approach has not been studied in clinical trials.
- Step 1, 2, and 3 preferred therapies are based on Evidence A; step 3 alternative therapy is based on Evidence A for LTRA, Evidence B for theophylline, and Evidence D for zileuton. Step 4 preferred therapy is based on Evidence B, and alternative therapy is based on Evidence B for LTRA and theophylline and Evidence D for zileuton. Step 5 preferred therapy is based on Evidence B. Step 6 preferred therapy is based on (EPR-2 1997) and Evidence B for omalizumab.
- Immunotherapy for steps 2-4 is based on Evidence B for house dust mites, animal danders, and pollens; evidence is weak or lacking for molds and cockroaches. Evidence is strongest for immunotherapy with single allergens. The role of allergy in asthma is greater in children than in adults.
- Clinicians who administer immunotherapy or omalizumab should be prepared and equipped to identify and treat anaphylaxis that may occur.
- Alphabetical order is used when more than 1 treatment option is listed within either preferred or alternative therapy.

symptom free; however, underlying airway remodeling is still evident.[76,77] Severe obstruction persisting for days or weeks is known as *status asthmaticus*. Use of accessory muscles of respiration and the increased work of breathing associated with a protracted asthmatic episode can result in respiratory muscle fatigue and respiratory failure.

During exacerbations, pulmonary function tests may reflect acute expiratory airflow obstruction ($\downarrow$ forced expiratory flow [$FEF_{25\%-75\%}$; $\downarrow$ FEV_1/FVC). Viscid mucous secretion may compound the airway narrowing and produce airway collapse.[85]

The asthmatic episode produces not only airflow obstruction, but also gas exchange abnormalities. The resulting low $\dot{V}/\dot{Q}$ state produces arterial O_2 desaturation.[86] Hypoxemia is common, but in most patients with acute bronchospasm, CO_2 elimination is relatively well preserved until $\dot{V}/\dot{Q}$ abnormalities are severe. An increased arterial CO_2 tension may indicate impending respiratory failure in the acutely ill asthmatic patient. Chronic asthma may eventually lead to irreversible lung destruction, loss of lung elasticity, pulmonary hypertension (PH), and lung hyperinflation.

Diagnostic Testing

Pulmonary Function Tests. Lung function testing routinely should be performed in asthmatic patients. Pulmonary function tests allow the clinician to assess the degree of impairment and the reversibility of airway limitation (see Table 27-12). Spirometry is based on a VC or FVC maneuver, with volume recorded as a function of time. The FVC maneuver requires total patient effort; a lack of effort may produce faulty results.[87]

The FVC is divided into several time intervals, of which the FEV_1 is the most reproducible. Patients with increased airway resistance exhibit decreased FEV_1 and FEV_1/FVC ratios. Normal FEV_1 varies with age. FEV_1 is extremely useful and reliable, and the technique for its determination is noninvasive and easy to perform.[87]

Respiratory activity represented by the midportion of the FVC curve is the most effort independent and the most sensitive indicator of small airway disease. This parameter is the $FEF_{25\%-75\%}$. The normal $FEF_{25\%-75\%}$ of 4 to 5 L/sec may decrease markedly in pulmonary disease, with early changes evident sooner in patients with obstructive disease than in those with restrictive disease. The value of $FEF_{25\%-75\%}$ is computed electronically.[88]

RV, FRC, and TLC all increase because of an increase in volume of the gas trapped beyond closed airways, and lung deflation is less because of airway obstruction. Comparison of current and prior pulmonary function test results is useful. Tolerance of activities is used for classifying the degree of dyspnea.[89] The patient in remission may have negative results on all parameters of pulmonary function and may be tested with a cholinergic agonist for bronchial provocation. A typical abnormality is an increase in the FEV_1 of more than 15% in response to a bronchodilator. Episodes of severe airway obstruction may not respond to bronchodilator treatment, and cessation of wheezing may occur with the worsening of obstruction (i.e., the "ominously silent chest"). Although the diagnosis of asthma does not require the measurement of lung volumes, knowledge of these volumes is helpful in assessing the severity of the disease.

Arterial Blood Gas Analysis. Increased diffusibility of CO_2 (compared with that of O_2) in combination with an often increased respiratory rate generally produces ABG analysis results that reflect the presence of respiratory alkalosis. Even slight hypercapnia may indicate severe air trapping and potential impending respiratory failure.

Chest Radiography. Because nearly 75% of asthma patients have a normal chest radiograph, chest radiography is not helpful in diagnosing or determining the severity of asthma. Hyperinflation with flattening of the diaphragm may be evident. Chest radiography is more helpful in detection of complications.

Electrocardiography. Changes evident on electrocardiography, such as ST-segment changes, right ventricular strain, and right axis deviation, usually manifest only in severe attacks and generally are of little significance with regard to the asthmatic condition.

Sputum Analysis. Eosinophilia, which is common in asthmatic patients, may be manifested as the production of grossly purulent sputum. Microscopic evaluation may reveal Curschmann spirals and Charcot-Leyden crystals, rather than polymorphic neutrophils associated with infection.

Serum Values. Eosinophilia (defined as more than 275 eosinophils per cubic millimeter of blood) is common in asthmatic patients with active IgE-mediated bronchial asthma, but its presence does not serve to differentiate extrinsic from intrinsic asthma. Asymptomatic patients with asthma generally have a total blood eosinophil count that is less than $50/mm^3$, with an increasing count often signaling the acceleration of bronchial asthma even before such patients experience symptoms. Determination of an increased eosinophil value in the absence of signs and symptoms of asthma requires that a differential analysis be undertaken. Tests for detection of IgE antibodies are performed only if an identifiable and avoidable substance is suspected. In this instance, consultation with a physician skilled in testing for allergic disease may be indicated.

Anesthetized Patients

In anesthetized patients, prominent manifestations of the asthmatic episode are wheezing, mucous hypersecretion, high inspiratory pressures, a blunted expiratory CO_2 waveform, and hypoxemia.

Mechanical ventilation and positive airway pressure are associated with a higher incidence of air trapping and lung hyperinflation, and the associated barotrauma can result in a pneumothorax.[86] Additionally, alveolar overdistention may lead to decreased venous return and diminution of CO. The combination of impaired ventilation and hypoxia can precipitate increased pulmonary vascular resistance, enhanced right ventricular afterload, and finally hemodynamic collapse.

The onset of an asthmatic episode may occur abruptly in surgical patients. Airway manipulation, acute exposure to allergens, or the stress of surgery can provoke wheezing in a patient who was previously asymptomatic. The lability of the disease makes assiduous observation crucial.

Wheezing often suggests potentially reversible bronchoconstriction, but the extent or degree of wheezing is a notoriously poor indicator of the degree of airway obstruction.[90] In addition, care must be taken to differentiate wheezing of asthmatic origin from other causes of wheezing, such as pneumothorax, endotracheal tube obstruction, endobronchial intubation, anaphylaxis, pulmonary edema, and pulmonary aspiration.[91,92]

Anesthesia Management

Several important anesthetic considerations and risk-reduction strategies have been reported. The EPR-3 recommends that to reduce the risk of complications during surgery:[74]

- Before surgery, review the level of asthma control, medication use (especially oral systemic corticosteroids within the past 6 months), and pulmonary function.
- Provide medications before surgery to improve lung function if lung function is not well controlled. A short course of oral systemic corticosteroids may be necessary.
- For patients receiving oral systemic corticosteroids during the 6 months before surgery, and for selected patients on long-term high-dose inhaled corticosteroids (ICS), give 100 mg hydrocortisone every 8 hours intravenously during the surgical period, and reduce the dose rapidly within 24 hours after surgery.

Preoperative Evaluation

A careful preoperative history and physical examination are essential to discerning the current disease status and medication profile. Frequent nocturnal awakenings due to respiratory difficulty, recent increases in medication use, and signs of viral infection may signal an increased likelihood of intraoperative difficulties.[93-95] Elective procedures in patients who are exhibiting significant respiratory symptoms should be postponed, and the condition of such patients should be normalized as much as possible.[95]

The predictive value of routine pulmonary function testing remains controversial.[94-98] FEV and peak expiratory flow rate, which can be measured with inexpensive hand-held devices, may be helpful in assessing current respiratory status. Values that fall 30% to 50% below expected baseline values indicate a moderate episode of bronchoconstriction. Values below 50% of normal indicate a severe episode.[93]

Pretreatment with systemic corticosteroids has been advocated in asthma patients undergoing surgical procedures. Kabalin and co-workers[99] studied the administration of corticosteroids in asthmatic surgical patients. Of the 89 subjects in the study, 86 had no postoperative wheezing when given either prednisone or hydrocortisone preoperatively. Complications of steroid therapy such as delayed wound healing, infection, or adrenocortical insufficiency were not noted. Ensuring that a patient who is currently receiving inhaled or systemic steroids receives them immediately before surgery is a prudent course.

Routine preoperative medications should be given to allay anxiety. The anticholinergics atropine and glycopyrrolate exhibit mild bronchodilating effects. As noted earlier, asthmatics experience an increased parasympathetic tone, and these agents are most effective as prophylactic drugs given 20 to 30 minutes preoperatively, rather than for acute therapy.[100] Caution must be exercised when administering narcotics to patients whose

TABLE 27-13	Drug Therapy for Asthma	
Drug Group	**Specific Agent**	**Dose**
Antiinflammatory drugs, corticosteroids, mast cell–inhibiting agents	Hydrocortisone, intravenous	4-mg/kg bolus followed by infusion of 0.5 mg/kg/hr
	Methylprednisolone, intravenous	0.8 mg/kg bolus followed by infusion of 0.1 mg/kg/hr
	Beclomethasone dipropionate (QVAR)	40 mcg/puff; 2-8 puffs twice per day
	Budesonide (Pulmicort)	1-2 inhalations twice per day
	Flunisolide (AeroBid) (MDI)	250 mcg/puff; 2-4 puffs twice per day
	Fluticasone propionate (Flovent)	44 mcg/puff; 2-4 puffs twice per day
	Triamcinolone (Azmacort)	75 mcg/puff; 2 puffs 3-4 times per day or 4 puffs twice per day
	Ciclesonide (Alvesco)	80 mcg/puff; 1-4 puffs twice per day
	Mometasone (Asmanex)	110 mg/puff; 2-4 puffs per day or 2 puffs twice per day
	Cromolyn sodium (generic)	10 mg/mL; 20 mg 3 or 4 times per day
Bronchodilators, beta2-selective adrenergic drugs	Albuterol (generic)	90 mcg/puff; 2 puffs every 4-6 hr (nebulized solution, 1.25-5 mg every 4-8 hr)
	Salmeterol (Serevent Diskus)	50 mcg/blister; 50 mcg every 12 hr
	Pirbuterol (Maxair)	200 mcg/puff; 2 puffs every 4-6 hr
	Terbutaline (Brethine, Bricanyl) subcutaneous	0.25 mg (may repeat once after 15-30 min; maximum dose, 0.5 mg in 4 hr)
	Levalbuterol (Xopenex)	0.63-1.25 mg every 6-8 hr nebulized as needed
	Formoterol (Foradil Aerolizer)	12 mcg/puff; 12 mcg twice per day
Antimuscarinic	Ipratropium bromide (Atrovent)	17 mcg/puff; 2 puffs 4 times per day maximum, 12 puffs in 24 hr
Methylxanthine	Theophylline (Theo-Dur and others)	Extended-release capsules or tablets, 300-600 mg/day Intravenous: 5-6 mg/kg loading; 0.9-1 maintenance via slow infusion
Leukotriene modifiers	Montelukast (Singulair)	10 mg once per day
	Zafirlukast (Accolate)	20 mg twice per day
	Zileuton (Zyflo)	1200 mg twice per day
Anti-IgE antibody	Omalizumab (Xolair)	150-300 mg every 4 wk or 225-375 mg every 2 wk subcutaneous injection

Data from Drugs for asthma. Treat Guidel Med Lett. 2008;6(76):83-90; Mosby's Drug Consult 2007.

respiratory difficulties are evident or when using narcotics associated with histamine release, such as morphine. Fentanyl and the other phenylpiperidine analogs commonly used in anesthesia have been widely used and are safe.[94,100,101] The use of histamine-2 (H_2)-receptor blocking agents such as cimetidine and ranitidine to reduce gastric volume and acidity should be avoided.[81,100] Bronchospasm after their use has been reported, possibly resulting from loss of inhibitory feedback control via presynaptic H_2 autoreceptor blockade, resulting in increased histamine release. Usual drug therapy for asthma is listed in Table 27-13. Some suggested risk-reduction strategies for use in the perioperative period are listed in Box 27-5.

Intraoperative Management
Despite a lack of definitive controlled clinical studies, regional anesthetic techniques are generally felt to be safer than general anesthesia.[102,103] Spinal or epidural levels to the midthoracic area or higher, however, decrease FRC, expiratory reserve volume, and the ability to cough and should be avoided.

All of the common induction drugs—propofol, thiopental, etomidate, and ketamine—have been used successfully in asthmatic patients, but some differences exist. Ketamine is the only induction drug with bronchodilating properties, which makes it the agent of choice in patients with active asthmatic symptoms who require emergency surgery. Thiopental may cause histamine release in a small percentage of patients. Pizov and colleagues[104] compared thiopental, thiamylal, methohexital, and propofol in a double-blind randomized study in patients with and without asthma. None of the asthmatic patients who received propofol exhibited wheezing 2 and 5 minutes after intubation. Wheezing after intubation occurred in 26% to 45% of the patients who received one of the three barbiturates. These authors suggested that propofol is advantageous for routine induction in asthmatic patients.

The potent inhalation agents produce bronchial relaxation and have all been successfully used in asthmatic patients after administration of an intravenous induction drug. Isoflurane and desflurane, however, are both mild respiratory irritants, which

BOX 27-5

Risk Reduction Strategies for Anesthetization of Patients with Asthma

Preoperative
- Encourage cessation of cigarette smoking for at least 8 weeks.
- Aggressively treat airflow obstruction.
- Administer antibiotics and delay surgery if respiratory infection is present.
- Begin patient education regarding lung-expansion maneuvers.

Intraoperative
- Limit duration of surgery to less than 3 hours.
- Use regional anesthesia when possible.
- Avoid the use of long-acting neuromuscular blocking agents.
- Use laparoscopic procedures when possible.
- Substitute less ambitious procedure for upper abdominal or thoracic surgery when possible.

Postoperative
- Encourage deep-breathing exercises or incentive spirometry.
- Use continuous positive airway pressure.
- Use intercostal nerve blocks and local anesthesia infiltration of incisional area for pain when appropriate.

Modified from Smetana GW. Current concepts: preoperative pulmonary evaluation. N Engl J Med. 1999;340:937-944; Hurford WE. The bronchospastic patient. Int Anesthesiol Clin. 2000;38:77-89.

may be a consideration during emergence. It is common practice to blunt this effect with the administration of opiates. Sevoflurane has been shown to be effective for inhalation induction in children.[105,106] Other anesthesia-related medications that should be avoided in asthmatic patients include atracurium, because of histamine release, and esmolol and labetalol, which as β-receptor blockers produce bronchoconstriction. Many practitioners avoid long-acting muscle relaxants and the associated possibility of residual muscle weakness in patients with asthma. Ketorolac and other nonsteroidal antiinflammatory agents should be avoided in patients with aspirin-intolerant asthma.[107]

If an episode of bronchospasm occurs during anesthesia, the following steps are recommended: (1) deepen the level of anesthesia with a volatile agent, ketamine, propofol, lidocaine, or a combination that rapidly increases anesthetic depth; (2) administer 100% O_2; (3) administer a β_2-agonist—up to 10 puffs may be needed; (4) in severe cases, administer epinephrine intravenously or subcutaneously; (5) administer intravenous corticosteroids—hydrocortisone 2 to 4 mg/kg; (6) consider intravenous aminophylline if long-term postoperative mechanical ventilation is planned. Theophylline has little efficacy for the treatment of acute bronchoconstrictive episodes.[108]

A strategy for mechanical ventilation that avoids lung hyperinflation and barotrauma while allowing for longer expiratory times should be chosen. A reduction in $\dot{V}_E$, by limiting inspiratory times and prolonging expiratory times, and moderate permissive hypercapnia have been suggested.[109-111]

Emergence

The primary issue during emergence is when to extubate. Some authors suggest deep extubation to avoid the mechanical stimulation from the endotracheal tube on awakening. Others fear that the loss of a secure airway before patient awakening may present a greater difficulty than the presence of the endotracheal tube. Either way, a judgment must be made as to when to extubate the patient, with the understanding that the earliest possible time is advantageous for prevention of mechanical bronchial stimulation. Administration of lidocaine and opiates may help diminish airway sensitivity.

The use of anticholinesterase reversal agents has also been an area of concern. The anticholinesterase should be administered in the minimum adequate dose. To ensure a more complete anticholinergic effect, a small increase in the coadministered dose of atropine or glycopyrrolate is suggested.

Asthma and the Pregnant Surgical Patient

The EPR-3 report recommends the following general strategies when caring for the pregnant patient.[74] Maintaining asthma control during pregnancy is important for the health and well-being of both mother and baby. Maintaining lung function is important to ensuring oxygen supply to the fetus. Uncontrolled asthma increases the risk of perinatal mortality, preeclampsia, preterm birth, and low-birth-weight infants. It is safer for pregnant women to be treated with asthma medications than to have asthma symptoms and exacerbations.

- Monitor the level of asthma control and lung function during prenatal visits. The course of asthma improves in one third of women and worsens for one third of women during pregnancy. Monthly evaluations of asthma will allow the opportunity to step up therapy if necessary and to step down therapy if possible.
- Albuterol is the preferred short-acting β-agonist (SABA). The most data related to safety during human pregnancy are available for albuterol.
- Inhaled corticosteroids are the preferred long-term control medication. Budesonide is the preferred ICS, because more data are available on using budesonide in pregnant women than are available on other ICSs, and the data are reassuring. However, no data indicate that the other ICS preparations are unsafe during pregnancy.

Maintaining proper maternal oxygenation is essential to the health of the fetus. Some anesthetic considerations for the pregnant asthmatic patient are given in Box 27-6.[112-114]

PULMONARY HYPERTENSION

Definition

Pulmonary arterial hypertension (PAH) usually represents an advanced stage of a large number of cardiovascular diseases.[115] The mortality rate associated with PAH is high. The condition exists if the mean level of PAP increases by 5 to 10 mm Hg or if pulmonary artery systolic pressure exceeds 30 mm Hg and mean PAP exceeds 20 mm Hg.[116,117]

Incidence and Outcome

PAH may be (1) primary or idiopathic (unexplained) or (2) secondary to an associated condition. In young adults, the female-to-male incidence of primary PAH (PPH) is 4:1; this incidence is similar to that in older groups of men and women. PPH is a rare disorder, and its true incidence is unknown; however, it is found on autopsy in 1% of patients in whom cor pulmonale had been diagnosed.[117]

BOX 27-6

Anesthetic Considerations in the Pregnant Asthmatic Patient

Avoid nonemergency surgery until after delivery.
Postpone semiemergent surgery until after the first trimester.
Administer higher than normal oxygen concentrations.
Use antacids but not histamine₂-receptor blockers for gastric preparation.
Use uterine displacement, generous fluid replacement, compression stockings, or leg elevation to minimize hypotension.
If a vasopressor is necessary, use ephedrine.
Avoid nitrous oxide.
Shield the fetus from radiographic exposure when possible.
Use inhaled but not parenteral β₂-receptor agonists.
Use fetal monitoring and ultrasound when feasible.

Modified from Karlet M, Nagelhout J. Asthma: an anesthetic update. AANA J. 2001;69:317-324.

Etiology

PAH may be caused by many associated conditions. Pulmonary venous hypertension due to left atrial outflow obstruction or pulmonary venous occlusive disease is a common one. Others involve pulmonary arterial hypertension caused by hyperdynamic circulation (e.g., secondary to burns or sepsis), vasoconstriction, viscosity, obstruction, and reactive vascular disease.[117]

PPH is characterized by a rapidly progressive course with a 79% mortality rate within 5 years of clinical diagnosis.[118] The degree of increase in pressure in the pulmonary circulation has an important influence on the patient's life expectancy.[119] Resistant PAH has long been identified as a major cause of early death.[120] Prognosis is largely determined by right ventricular integrity.[121]

Pathophysiology

The normal pulmonary circulation is mostly passive, of low resistance, and highly distensible.[116] PAH is characterized by an increase in vascular tone and the growth and proliferation of pulmonary vascular smooth muscle. Initial reversible vasoconstriction may progress to muscle hypertrophy and irreversible degeneration.[117]

Pulmonary vasoconstriction appears to occur in some (but not all) patients with PAH. Some speculate that the disease progresses from vasoconstriction to fixed obstruction of the pulmonary vascular bed. Pathologic changes associated with a fixed resistance are the presence of intimal sclerosis, plexiform (resembling a plexus or network) lesions, and the obliteration of as many as 90% or more of the small vessels within the lung.[122] Other reported abnormalities include impairment of endothelium-dependent vasodilation.[123]

Clinical Features and Diagnosis

PAH may be either acute or chronic. In almost all patients with PAH, dyspnea and exercise intolerance usually are the first complaints.[121,124] Patients also may have angina. PAH associated with chest pain was reported as early as 1891; however, whether PAH actually causes anginal chest pain is uncertain. Many cases of this combination have been reported, suggesting that PAH

may be associated with chest pain and electrocardiographic changes typical of myocardial infarction, even in the absence of coronary artery disease. Some clinicians propose that the source of the chest pain is (1) an increase in right ventricular myocardial O₂ demand secondary to an increase in wall stress, or (2) a decrease in coronary blood flow because of a decrease in flow in the arteries supplying the right ventricle during systole.[125]

Right atrial hypertrophy or right ventricular hypertrophy (or both) may be evident on ECG. Chest radiography may demonstrate an enlarged pulmonary artery.[126] Cardiac catheterization combined with pulmonary angiography is most informative in assessment of PAH, cardiac reserve, and the effects of pulmonary vasodilator therapy.[117] Vasodilator therapy is attempted when a vasoconstrictor component is identified. Vasodilator challenge may be performed with cardiac catheterization using a rapid and effective pulmonary vasodilator such as nitroglycerin, isoproterenol, nifedipine, prostaglandin E₁, prostacyclin, prostaglandin E₂, hydralazine, nitroprusside, or adenosine for evaluation of the reversibility of PAH.[120] Frequently, open-lung biopsy is performed for assessment of the histopathologic composition of small pulmonary arteries.[127] Noninvasive evaluation includes Doppler echocardiography for measurement of the velocity of tricuspid regurgitation (which correlates well with invasive PAP measurements) and pulmonic peak flow velocity.[128,129]

Anesthesia Management

Attempts to alleviate pulmonary hypertensive disease states have had varied success.[130] Vasodilator agents are used most commonly and may be helpful in patients with reversible vasoconstriction (Table 27-14). Possible beneficial effects of pulmonary arterial dilation are preservation of lung function, prevention of right ventricle deterioration, and (it is hoped) improved survival.

The principal objectives during anesthesia in patients with PAH are preventing increases in PAH and avoiding major hemodynamic changes.[124] Considerations that apply to the care of patients with cor pulmonale also apply to those with PAH. Information regarding PAH and intravenous induction agents is lacking; however, most agents either have little effect on pulmonary vascular resistance (PVR) or decrease it.[117] Ketamine, which causes an increase in PVR, may be the exception.[130]

COR PULMONALE

Definition

The term *cor pulmonale* or *pulmonary heart disease* refers to patients exhibiting PAH resulting in progressive right ventricular hypertrophy, dilation, and eventual cardiac decompensation. This arises from disorders that affect ventilatory drive or musculoskeletal respiratory mechanics; pulmonary airway, infiltrative, fibrotic, or vascular diseases; and diseases that are primarily cardiac but affect the pulmonary circulation and the lungs (Box 27-7).

Incidence and Outcome

In individuals older than 50 years of age, cor pulmonale is the third most common cardiac disorder (after ischemic heart disease and hypertensive cardiac disease). The male-to-female ratio of incidence of the disease is 5:1; 10% to 30% of patients admitted to the hospital with coronary heart failure exhibit cor pulmonale.[131]

Prognosis is determined by the pulmonary disease responsible for the increased PVR. In patients with COPD in whom PaO₂ can be maintained at near-normal levels, the prognosis is favorable. However, cor pulmonale associated with hypoxic lung disease is

| TABLE **27-14** | Drug Treatment Options for Patients with Pulmonary Hypertension |

Drug or Drug Class	Rationale	Potentially Responsive Types of Pulmonary Hypertension	Limitations
Anticoagulants	Reduce risk of pulmonary thromboembolism	Primary PH and PH secondary to acute pulmonary thromboembolism, chronic pulmonary thromboembolism, and anorectic drugs	For primary hypertension, concomitant vasodilator treatment also required
Vasodilators			
Calcium antagonists	Inhibit influx of calcium into smooth muscle cells with elevated vasomotor tone; preferentially act on pulmonary vasculature	Primary PH and PH secondary to connective tissue vascular disease and COPD	Initial treatment in specialized centers recommended to avoid severe adverse outcomes such as negative inotropic effects
Epoprostenol (Flolan)—prostacyclin	May replace deficiencies in endogenous prostacyclin; also inhibits smooth muscle proliferation and platelet aggregation	Primary, persistent PH of the neonate and PH secondary to ARDS, crises after heart surgery in infants, and connective tissue disease in adults	Peripheral adverse effects occur when administered by continuous IV infusion
Nitric oxide	Interferes with endogenous vasoconstrictor mechanisms	Primary, persistent PH of the neonate and PH secondary to corrective cardiac surgery in children, lung or lung-heart transplant surgery in adults, and COPD	Potential adverse effects include increased bleeding times, negative inotropic effects, and formation of potentially toxic products (e.g., nitrogen dioxide, methemoglobin)
Alprostadil (prostaglandin E_1)	Interferes with endogenous vasoconstrictor mechanisms	Secondary to ARDS	Impaired pulmonary metabolism may result in systemic hypotension
Bosentan (Tracleer)	Oral endothelin receptor antagonist	Severe PH	Hepatotoxicity
Treprostinil (Remodulin)	Prostacyclin analog	Primary PH; classes II-IV	Given by continuous infusion via wearable infusion pump; peripheral edema, nasal congestion, and serious birth defects may occur
Ambrisentan (Letairis)	Selective endothelin type A (ET_A) receptor antagonist	Treatment of symptomatic patients (WHO class II or III) with pulmonary arterial hypertension (PAH)	
Sildenafil (Revatio)	Inhibits phosphodiesterase type 5	Treatment for PAH along with anticoagulant and a diuretic	Headaches, dyspepsia, and transient color vision
Iloprost (Ventavis)	Synthetic analog of prostacyclin PGI2	Treatment of PAH in patients with NYHA class III or IV symptoms	Requires inhalation administration 6-9 times a day
Inhibitors of Vasoconstriction			
α-Adrenoceptor antagonists	Inhibits formation of the vasoconstrictor angiotensin II	Persistent PH of the neonate (especially preterm infants) and PH secondary to COPD	Can cause severe systemic adverse effects
ACE inhibitors	Inhibit formation of the vasoconstrictor angiotensin II	Secondary to connective tissue disease, effects of high altitude, and congestive heart failure	Prolonged treatment required to obtain an effect

Modified from Treprostinil (Remodulin) for pulmonary arterial hypertension. Med Lett. 2002;44(1139):80-82; Sildenafil (Revatio) for pulmonary arterial hypertension. Med Lett. 2005; 47(1215/1216):65-66,165-167; Ambrisentan (Letairis) for pulmonary arterial hypertension. Med Lett. 2007;49(1272):87-90.
ACE, *Angiotensin-converting enzyme;* ARDS, *acute respiratory distress syndrome;* COPD, *chronic obstructive pulmonary disease;* IV, *intravenous;* PH, *pulmonary hypertension.*

BOX 27-7

Classification of Pulmonary Hypertension

1. Pulmonary Arterial Hypertension (PAH)
Idiopathic PAH
Familial PAH
PAH related to:
  Connective tissue disease
  Human immunodeficiency virus infection
  Portal hypertension
  Drug/toxins
  Congential heart disease
  Persistent pulmonary hypertension of the newborn
PAH with venular/capillary involvement (pulmonary
  venoocclusive disease, pulmonary capillary
  hemangiomatosis

2. Pulmonary Hypertension with Left Heart Disease
Arterial or ventricular
Valvular

3. Pulmonary Hypertension with Lung Disease/Hypoxemia
Chronic obstructive pulmonary disease
Interstitial lung disease
Sleep-disordered breathing
Developmental abnormalities

4. Pulmonary Hypertension Due to Chronic Thrombotic and/or Embolic Disease
Thromboembolic obstruction of proximal pulmonary arteries
Thromboembolic obstruction of distal pulmonary arteries
Nonthrombotic pulmonary emboli

5. Miscellaneous

Modified from Murray JF, Nadel JA. Textbook of Respiratory Medicine. 4th ed. Philadelphia: Saunders; 2005:1545.

---

associated with a 70% rate of mortality within 5 years after onset of associated peripheral edema.[132] Prognosis is poor for those patients in whom cor pulmonale is the result of gradual obstruction of pulmonary vessels by intrinsic pulmonary vascular disease or pulmonary fibrosis. These anatomic changes cause irreversible alterations in the pulmonary vasculature, resulting in fixed elevations of PVR.

Etiology

COPD is associated with the functional loss of pulmonary capillaries and subsequent arterial hypoxemia; these events initiate pulmonary vasoconstriction, which is the leading cause of chronic cor pulmonale. The World Health Organization has proposed a classification of conditions associated with cor pulmonale. Diseases associated with hypoxic pulmonary vasoconstriction include:

- COPD
- Bronchiectasis
- Chronic mountain sickness
- Cystic fibrosis
- Idiopathic alveolar hypoventilation
- Obesity-related hypoventilation syndrome

- Neuromuscular disease
- Kyphoscoliosis
- Pleuropulmonary fibrosis
- Upper airway obstruction

Diseases that produce obstruction or obliteration of the pulmonary vasculature include:

- PE
- Pulmonary fibrosis
- Pulmonary lymphangitic carcinomatosis
- Idiopathic PAH
- Progressive systemic sclerosis
- Sarcoidosis
- Intravenous drug abuse
- Pulmonary vasculitis
- Pulmonary venoocclusive disease[133]

Pathophysiology

Sustained pulmonary vasoconstriction produces hypertrophy of the smooth muscle in the tunica media and an irreversible increase in PVR.[134] In the presence of chronically elevated pulmonary capillary pressure, the lungs are increasingly resistant to pulmonary edema because lymph vessels expand, and their ability to carry fluid away from the interstitial spaces increases. The lymphatic pumping action creates a suction effect, which results in a negative pleural pressure.[135] The rate at which right ventricular dysfunction develops depends on the magnitude of pressure increase in the pulmonary circulation and on the rapidity with which this increase occurs. For example, PE may result in right ventricular failure in the presence of a mean PAP as low as 30 mm Hg. By contrast, when PAH occurs gradually, as it does in COPD, right ventricular compensation occurs; CHF rarely occurs before mean PAP exceeds 50 mm Hg.

The normal pulmonary circulation can accommodate a maximal right ventricular output with minimal increase in pulmonary pressure via distention of existing vessels or recruitment of unused vessels. However, patients with COPD have larger than normal increases in PAP when executing maneuvers that increase pulmonary blood flow (e.g., exercise, even if resting hemodynamic status is normal).[136] In COPD, derangements in intrapulmonary gas exchange are the major factors involved in the hemodynamic changes. Namely, alveolar hypoxia appears to locally mediate the vasoconstriction of precapillary pulmonary vessels. Acidosis and hypercarbia potentiate this effect.[137]

The compensatory mechanism for pressure overload on the right ventricle involves enhancement of contractility and an increase in preload, which result in an increase in right ventricular end-diastolic volume.[138] In response to chronic pressure overload imposed by the PAH, right ventricular hypertrophy occurs (chronic leads to hypertrophy). Preterminally, a bout of intolerable hypoxia often exaggerates the PAH and imposes an acutely rising afterload on the right ventricle, which accommodates by dilating (acute leads to dilation). Although acute hypercapnia does not directly affect pulmonary circulation, it does cause and potentiate PAH if it causes acidosis.[137] Acute hypercapnia stimulates ventilation, dilates cerebral vessels, and elicits central nervous system disturbances.[139]

Right ventricular hypertrophy is characterized by increased firmness of the myocardium and increased thickness of its wall, most prominently in the pulmonary outflow tract. The papillary muscles and the trabeculae carneae may be twice as thick as normal. The thickness of individual muscle fibers is also greater than normal and may approximate that of left ventricular myofibers.

Clinical Features and Diagnosis

Clinical manifestations of cor pulmonale often are nonspecific and obscured by coexisting COPD. Right-sided heart catheterization usually is required for diagnosis. Cardiac catheterization combined with pulmonary angiography provides the most definitive information on the degree of PAH, cardiac reserve, and the effects of pulmonary vasodilator treatment.[134]

Symptoms of cor pulmonale are retrosternal pain, cough, dyspnea on exertion, weakness, fatigue, early exhaustion, and hemoptysis.[134] Occasionally hoarseness secondary to left recurrent laryngeal nerve compression by the enlarged pulmonary artery is present. Syncope on effort may occur, reflecting the inability of the right ventricular stroke volume to increase in the presence of a fixed elevation of PVR.

Physical signs of cor pulmonale include the following:
- Elevation of jugular venous pressure
- Cardiac heave or thrust along the left sternal border and S_3 gallop
- Presence of an S_4 secondary to significant right ventricular hypertrophy
- A widely split S_2
- Possible murmur of pulmonic and tricuspid insufficiency
- Hepatomegaly, ascites, and lower-extremity edema (late signs)

Diagnostic Testing

Electrocardiography. Right atrial displacement, right ventricular hypertrophy, right atrial hypertrophy, and right atrial enlargement may be observed. Patients may develop concomitant supraventricular tachycardic arrhythmias (i.e., tachycardic atrial fibrillation, sinus tachycardia, and paroxysmal atrial tachycardia).

Chest Radiography. On chest radiography, enlargement of the pulmonary arteries is observed, followed by right ventricular hypertrophy.

Doppler Echocardiography. Enlargement, dilation, or thickening of the right ventricle, with or without tricuspid valve regurgitation, and a pulmonary artery systolic pressure estimated to be increased all suggest that at least acute or possibly chronic PAH is present.

Treatment

The three major drug classes for treatment of PAH are prostanoids, endothelin receptor antagonists and phosphodiesterase inhibitors. The goals of treatment are decreasing the workload of the right ventricle, reducing PVR, preventing increases in PAP, and avoiding major hemodynamic changes. Improvement of gas exchange is the primary focus of treatment in COPD patients with cor pulmonale.[134,140] Treatment includes supplemental administration of O_2 to maintain a PaO_2 of greater than 60 mm Hg or an arterial O_2 saturation of greater than 90%. O_2 is the only vasodilator with a selective effect on pulmonary vessels that is not associated with a risk of worsening hypoxemia.[141]

Heart-Lung Transplantation

A heart-lung transplantation may ultimately be needed when cor pulmonale progresses despite the provision of maximal medical therapy.

In general, preoperative preparation of the patient with cor pulmonale includes the following:
- Elimination and control of acute or chronic pulmonary infections
- Reversal of bronchospasm
- Improvement in clearance of secretions

- Expansion of collapsed or poorly ventilated alveoli
- Hydration
- Correction of any electrolyte imbalance

Anesthesia Management

Regional anesthesia technique may be appropriate as long as a high sensory level of anesthesia is not required, because any decrease in systemic vascular resistance in the presence of a fixed PVR may produce undesirable degrees of systemic hypotension.[131]

General Anesthesia

Volatile agents decrease PVR. Studies have demonstrated that PAP is decreased by isoflurane. N_2O has been shown to increase PVR in patients with PPH. Intravenous agents, with the exception of ketamine, appear to have little effect on PVR.[142] During all stages of anesthesia, manipulations that increase PAP must be avoided. Five key principles should be followed:
- Keep the patient well oxygenated
- Avoid acidosis
- Avoid the use of exogenous and endogenous vasoconstrictors
- Avoid presenting stimuli that increase sympathetic tone
- Avoid hypothermia[134]

PULMONARY EMBOLISM

Definition

PE is the impaction of a dislodged thrombus into the pulmonary vascular bed.

Incidence and Outcome

A major source of morbidity and mortality, PE claims the lives of more than 50,000 patients in the United States annually. It is the third most common cause of cardiovascular death after myocardial infarction and stroke. PEs originate from deep vein thrombosis (DVT) of the iliofemoral vessels in approximately 90% of patients, and the clinical course depends on the size of the clot. Evidence suggests that at least 5 million episodes of DVT occur annually in the United States, with approximately 10% leading to PE. Of those resulting in PE, approximately 10% are fatal.[143]

Etiology

PE is considered by some to be a clinical manifestation of DVT rather than a separate entity. As noted previously, most emboli (90%) arise in the proximal deep veins of the lower extremities, with the remainder originating from pelvic veins. DVT at proximal sites is more likely to cause symptoms. Three major factors promote the formation of venous thrombi: stasis of blood flow, venous injury, and hypercoagulation states. Other, less common causes of PE include air, tumor, bone, fat, catheter fragments, and amniotic fluid. Fillers used in illicit drug preparations by intravenous drug abusers also may cause PE. Of particular concern to anesthesia providers are air emboli caused by the opening of venous structures during surgery or by disconnected intravenous lines.

Most pulmonary emboli resolve within 8 to 21 days of the initial presentation; 10% to 20% are estimated to develop into unresolved emboli, and 0.5% to 4% lead to the development of chronic PAH. Chronically unresolved emboli that lodge in major pulmonary arteries may become incorporated into the vascular walls and obstruct blood flow. Patients with such emboli are surgical candidates, representing approximately 1000 cases in the United States each year.[143]

TABLE 27-15	The Virchow Triad: Clinical States Predisposing to Venous Thrombosis
Stasis	Immobility
	Bed rest
	Anesthesia
	Congestive heart failure or cor pulmonale
	Prior venous thrombosis
Hypercoagulability	Malignancy
	Anticardiolipin antibody
	Nephrotic syndrome
	Essential thrombocytosis
	Estrogen therapy
	Heparin-induced thrombocytopenia
	Inflammatory bowel disease
	Paroxysmal nocturnal hemoglobinuria
	Disseminated intravascular coagulation
	Protein C and S deficiencies
	Antithrombin III deficiency
Vessel wall injury	Trauma
	Surgery

Modified from Fedullo PF, Yung Gl. Pulmonary thromboembolic disease. In: Fishman AP et al, eds. Fishman's Pulmonary Diseases and Disorders. *New York: McGraw-Hill; 2008:1425.*

Pathophysiology

Once a thrombus has formed, it rarely remains static. It can be dissolved through fibrinolysis, become "organized" into a vessel wall, or be released into the circulation. Because thrombi are most friable early in their development, it is then that the greatest risk for embolism exists.

Once the fragment has been released from its site of formation, it can be rapidly swept into one of the pulmonary arteries. It may pass through the vasculature completely, break up, and block several smaller pulmonary vessels; or if the thrombus is sufficiently large, it may impact against one or both pulmonary arteries and cause pulmonary collapse, massive infarction, and ultimately cardiac arrest.[144] Emboli are most often seen in the lower lung lobes, which receive the greatest amount of blood flow. Fortunately, these lower lung lobes also tend to receive the least ventilation, so much of the $\dot{V}/\dot{Q}$ ratio is preserved in patients with small to moderate-sized emboli.

Within the pulmonary capillaries, hemorrhage is frequently seen distal to the site of the embolism. The alveolar structures in this area can remain viable for a period of time.[144] However, if the clot does not dissolve or if it is not quickly squeezed through the vasculature, the alveolar structure will be permanently damaged. Bronchial circulation limits this consequence of pulmonary infarction, and substantial damage is unusual unless an embolus completely blocks a large artery or preexisting lung disease is present.[145] In fact, less than 10% of emboli actually cause any type of infarction.[146] The three components of the Virchow triad—stasis, hypercoagulability, and vessel-wall injury—lead to venous thrombosis (Table 27-15).

Pulmonary Function

Pulmonary Circulation. Normally the pulmonary circulation has a very large reserve capacity. However, when PAPs increase, previously unfilled capillaries are recruited, and distention occurs. This allows for obstruction of at least half of the pulmonary circulation before a substantial increase in PAP becomes manifest.[144]

Occlusion of approximately 70% of the pulmonary vascular bed results in PAH with subsequent right ventricular failure, increased end-diastolic pressures, and development of arrhythmias and possibly of tricuspid valve incompetence.[145] Pulmonary edema may follow.[144,147] Acute pulmonary edema may develop when hyperperfusion from intact circulation to the perfused lung results in extravasation of fluid into the alveoli. If the clot breaks up and passes quickly or if the affected area is minimal, the PAPs gradually decrease with embolus resolution by fibrinolysis or transformation onto the vessel wall as a scar.[145]

Mechanism. When a pulmonary artery is occluded, ventilation distal to the obstruction is decreased. This is a result of the direct effect of alveolar P_{CO_2} (P_{ACO_2}) on the smooth muscle of the local small airways, which is bronchoconstriction. The reduction of airflow to the unperfused lung reduces the amount of wasted ventilation. This mechanism is very short lived, with distribution of ventilation returning to normal within several hours.[144,146] The elastic properties of the embolized region may change some hours after the event; localized atelectasis is believed to result from a loss of pulmonary surfactant, the rapid turnover of which requires adequate blood flow.[146]

Gas Exchange. An embolus can have a significant effect on gas exchange. Moderate hypoxemia without CO_2 retention is often seen after PE as both physiologic shunt and dead space increase. In spontaneously breathing patients, P_{ACO_2} is maintained at the normal level after PE by increasing the respiratory rate. The resultant increase in ventilation may be substantial because of the large physiologic dead space. The anesthetized patient obviously cannot increase his or her ventilation; as a result, the P_{ACO_2} builds up, and O_2 saturation decreases more quickly.[146,148]

The difference between P_{ACO_2} and end-tidal P_{CO_2} (P_{ETCO_2}) is a very useful indicator in PE.[144] The mixed P_{ACO_2} tends to be low because of the high $\dot{V}/\dot{Q}$ ratio in the embolized region; because little uneven ventilation occurs with this disease, the P_{ETCO_2} is an accurate and immediate indicator of the status of alveolar blood gas exchange. In anesthetized patients, the P_{ACO_2} continues to increase more quickly because of this increase in shunt without ventilatory compensation.[145] If the embolus does not completely occlude the vessel, the discrepancy between P_{ETCO_2} and P_{ACO_2} may not be as great.[144]

Clinical Features and Diagnosis

The patient's clinical presentation depends largely on the size of the embolus. Signs and symptoms of PE vary, and the differential diagnosis according to size of emboli may be difficult (Box 27-8). Dyspnea of sudden onset appears to be the only common historic complaint. Hypoxia is a constant feature of PE, possibly owing to intrapulmonary shunting. Several clinical features can be associated with emboli of varying sizes.

Small emboli frequently go unrecognized; uncommonly, however, multiple small emboli can produce extensive obstruction of the pulmonary capillary bed, possibly causing PAH and cardiac failure. Generally, however, small thromboemboli are incorporated into the arterial wall and have little effect on either parenchyma or the circulation. Patients may complain of dyspnea

---

BOX 27-8

Differential Diagnosis of Acute Pulmonary Embolism

Myocardial infarction (unstable angina)
Pericarditis
Heart failure
Pneumonia, bronchitis, chronic obstructive pulmonary disease
  exacerbation
Asthma
Chronic obstructive pulmonary disease
Pneumothorax
Pleurodynia
Pleuritis from collagen vascular disease
Thoracic herpes zoster (shingles)

Rib fracture pneumothorax
Primary or metastatic intrathoracic cancer
Infradiaphragmatic processes (e.g., acute cholecystitis, splenic
  infarction)
Hyperventilation syndrome
Cardiomyopathy
Primary pulmonary hypertension
Intrathoracic cancer
Costochondritis, musculoskeletal pain
Anxiety

From Tapson VF. Pulmonary embolism. In: Goldman L, Ausiello D, eds. Cecil's Textbook of Medicine. 2nd ed. Philadelphia: Saunders; 2008:689; Goldhaber SZ. Pulmonary embolism. In: Libby P et al, eds. Braunwald's Heart Disease: A Textbook of Cardiovascular Medicine. 8th ed. Philadelphia: Saunders; 2008:1879.

on exertion that may lead to syncope; sometimes, a right ventricular "heave" or a split-second heart sound can be detected on examination. For patients with chronic embolization, medical therapy with anticoagulant, thrombolytic, or vasodilating drugs does not alter the prognosis.

Patients with medium-sized emboli may present with pleuritic pain accompanied by dyspnea, a slight fever, and a productive cough that yields blood-streaked sputum. These patients usually are tachycardic. A small pleural effusion can develop and mimic the appearance of pneumonia.

Massive emboli can produce sudden cardiac collapse. Preceding symptoms range from pallor, shock, and central chest pain to sudden loss of consciousness. In patients with cardiac collapse, the pulse becomes rapid and weak, blood pressure decreases, neck veins become engorged, and cardiogenic shock may be present or impending. Also, a decrease in P_{ETCO_2} and an increase in P_{aCO_2} occur, with the difference between the values for these two indexes increasing as conditions worsen. If a pulmonary artery catheter is in place, PAPs are observed to increase rapidly; also, the ECG may begin to show right ventricular strain. The prognosis for these patients is very poor. The most common clinical signs are noted in Table 27-16.[144]

Diagnostic Testing

Few of the common preoperative tests indicate the presence of PE. A number of imaging and laboratory tests are now available for diagnosis (Table 27-17). Echocardiographic and electrocardiographic signs are noted in Box 27-9. In the patient with PE, ABG analysis generally reveals hypoxemia and increased differences between P_{ACO_2} and P_{aCO_2}, which result from ventilation of unperfused alveoli.[148] Massive PE is associated with severe hypoxemia and hypocapnia. An initial difference between P_{ACO_2} and P_{ETCO_2} is common early during the embolic event.[146] Some common conditions associated with an increased risk for deep vein thrombosis are given in Box 27-10.

Treatment

Aggressive efforts at prevention have been successful in reducing the incidence of DVT in surgical patients. Treatment mainly is aimed at preventing further embolism and providing ventilatory support (Table 27-18).[149] Use of graded compression stockings, intermittent pneumatic compression, administration of various

TABLE 27-16	Common Signs and Symptoms of Pulmonary Embolism
Sign or Symptom	
Dyspnea	
Tachypnea	
Tachycardia	
Hypotension	
Cyanosis	
Neck vein distention	
Chest pain	
Cough	
Syncope	
Hemoptysis	

Modified from Goldhaber SZ. Deep vein thrombosis and pulmonary thromboembolism. In: Fauci AS et al, eds. Harrison's Principles of Internal Medicine. 17th ed. New York: McGraw-Hill; 2008:1651-1657.

anticoagulants and thrombolytics, and ambulation are typical measures for preventing embolus formation. It must be remembered that PE is a mechanical disease caused by acute pulmonary obstruction in a previously healthy patient.

Treatment requires rapid intervention before vital signs are affected by hypoxia and mechanical failure of the heart. Guidelines for treatment of PE are summarized in Box 27-11.

Surgery

Surgical intervention often is indicated for patients who are unresponsive to other measures. Procedures that used to be the mainstay of this intervention, such as ligation of the inferior vena cava, are now rarely performed. Currently, the most common surgical procedure for patients with PE is placement of an umbrella filter, which traps thromboemboli. It is estimated that 30,000 to 40,000 patients receive such filters annually in the United States. Indications for vena cava filters are listed in Box 27-12. The filter is placed in the inferior vena cava under fluoroscopic guidance, usually below the renal veins at the level

TABLE 27-17	Diagnostic Tests for Suspected Pulmonary Embolism
Test	**Comments**
Oxygen saturation	Nonspecific but can raise suspicion if there is a sudden, otherwise unexplained decrement.
D-dimer	An excellent "rule out" test if normal, especially if accompanied by low clinical suspicion.
Electrocardiogram	May be normal, especially in younger, previously healthy individuals. May provide alternative diagnosis, such as myocardial infarction or pericarditis.
Lung scanning	Usually does not definitively diagnose or exclude PE. Being replaced by chest CT except for patients with anaphylaxis to contrast agent, renal insufficiency, or pregnancy.
Chest CT	Most accurate diagnostic imaging test for PE. May be problematic if CT result and clinical decision rule score are discordant.
Pulmonary angiography	Invasive, costly, uncomfortable. Has ceded to chest CT its designation as "diagnostic gold standard."
Echocardiography	Best used as a prognostic test in patients with established PE, rather than as a diagnostic test. Many patients with larger PE will have normal echocardiograms.
Venous ultrasonograph	Excellent for diagnosing acute symptomatic proximal DVT, but a negative test does not rule out PE, because a recent leg DVT may have embolized completely. Calf vein imaging is operator dependent.
Magnetic resonance imaging	Reliable only for imaging large, proximal pulmonary arteries.

From Goldhaber SZ. Pulmonary embolism. In: Libby P et al. Braunwald's Heart Disease. 8th ed. Philadelphia: Saunders; 2008:1871.

of the L2 to L3. Suprarenal placement is required when a thrombus directly involves the renal veins or has propagated above the level of the renal veins.

The presence of an infrarenal filter in a pregnant woman may place her and her fetus at risk because of the possibility that the filter will come into contact with the gravid uterus. Suprarenal placement prevents this risk.

Thromboendarterectomy is the treatment of choice for chronic large vessel thromboembolic PAH.[150] Desired results include decreased PVR, improved CO, restoration of exercise tolerance, and resolution of hypoxemia. Improvements in RV function and hemodynamics may be prompt, whereas improvements in gas exchange occur over weeks to months. Although the role of pulmonary embolectomy remains controversial, in the few patients who do not benefit from optimal medical therapy, it remains an acceptable procedure.[151]

BOX 27-9

Electrocardiographic and Echocardiographic Signs of Pulmonary Embolism

- Incomplete or complete right bundle branch block
- S in lead I and $aV_L > 1.5$ mm
- Transition zone shift to V_5
- Qs in leads III and aV_F but not in lead II
- QRS axis >90 degrees or indeterminate axis
- Low limb-lead voltage
- T-wave inversion in leads III and aV_F or in leads V_1-V_4
- Direct visualization of thrombus (rare)
- Right ventricular dilation
- Right ventricular hypokinesis (with sparing of the apex)
- Abnormal interventricular septal motion
- Tricuspid valve regurgitation
- Pulmonary artery dilatation
- Lack of decreased inspiratory collapse of inferior vena cava

Modified from Sreeram N et al. Value of the 12-lead electrocardiogram at hospital admission in the diagnosis of pulmonary embolism. Am J Cardiol. 1994;73:298.

BOX 27-10

Conditions Associated with Increased Risk for Deep Vein Thrombosis

Advancing age
Obesity
Previous venous thromboembolism
Surgery
Trauma
Active cancer
Acute medical illnesses—e.g., acute myocardial infarction, heart failure, respiratory failure, infection
Inflammatory bowel disease
Antiphospholipid syndrome
Dyslipoproteinemia
Nephrotic syndrome
Paroxysmal nocturnal hemoglobinuria
Myeloproliferative diseases
Behçet syndrome
Varicose veins
Superficial vein thrombosis
Congenital venous malformation
Long-distance travel
Prolonged bed rest
Immobilization
Limb paresis
Chronic care facility stay
Pregnancy/puerperium
Oral contraceptives
Hormone replacement therapy
Heparin-induced thrombocytopenia
Other drugs
Chemotherapy
Tamoxifen
Thalidomide
Antipsychotics
Central venous catheter
Vena cava filter
Intravenous drug abuse

TABLE **27-18** Prevention of Venous Thromboembolism	
Condition	**Strategy**
Total hip or knee replacement; hip or pelvis fracture	Warfarin (Coumadin) (target INR 2-2.5) × 4-6 weeks LMWH/subQ (e.g., enoxaparin 1 mg/kg subQ twice daily or fondaparinux 2.5 mg subQ (except for total knee replacement)) IPC ± warfarin
Gynecologic cancer surgery	Warfarin (Coumadin) (target INR 2-2.5) IPC Unfractionated heparin, 5000 units q8h ± IPC Dalteparin (Fragmin) 2500 units once daily ± IPC Enoxaparin 40 mg subQ once daily
Urologic surgery	Warfarin (Coumadin) (target INR 2-2.5) ± IPC
Thoracic surgery	IPC *plus* unfractionated heparin, 5000 units q8h
High-risk general surgery (e.g., prior VTE, current cancer, or obesity)	IPC *or* GCS *plus* unfractionated heparin, 5000 units q8h
General, gynecologic, or urologic surgery (without prior VTE) for noncancerous conditions	GCS *plus* unfractionated heparin 5000 units q12h Dalteparin 2500 units subQ once daily Enoxaparin 40 mg subQ once daily IPC alone
Neurosurgery, eye surgery, or other surgery when prophylactic anticoagulation is contraindicated	GCS ± IPC
Medical conditions	GCS ± heparin, 5000 units q12h IPC alone Enoxaparin (Lovenox) 40 mg subQ once daily
Orthopedic surgery	Enoxaparin 30 mg twice daily Enoxaparin 40 mg once daily* Dalteparin 5000 units once daily* Warfarin (target INR = 2-3) GCS plus IPC
General surgery	Enoxaparin 40 mg daily Dalteparin 2500 or 5000 units once daily GCS plus IPC
Pregnancy	Enoxaparin 40 mg daily Dalteparin 5000 units daily
Medical patients	Enoxaparin 40 mg daily GCS plus IPC
Long-haul air travel	LMWH for high risk patients

Modified from Goldhaber SZ. *Deep vein thrombosis and pulmonary thromboembolism. In: Fauci AS et al, eds. Harrison's Principles of Internal Medicine. 17th ed. New York: McGraw-Hill; 2008:1651-1657; Goldhaber SZ. Pulmonary embolism. In: Libby P et al, eds. Braunwald's Heart Disease: A Textbook of Cardiovascular Medicine. 8th ed. Philadelphia: Saunders; 2008:1879.*
GCS, *Graduated compression stockings;* INR, *international normalized ratio;* IPC, *intermittent pneumatic compression;* LMHW, *low-molecular weight heparin;* subQ, *subcutaneous;* VTE, *venous thromboembolism.*
**Approved only for total hip replacement prophylaxis.*

Anesthesia Management

Anesthesia for patients at risk for PE is aimed at supporting vital-organ function and minimizing anesthetic-induced myocardial depression. The use of a high FiO₂ aids in prevention of pulmonary vasoconstriction, and monitoring PAP helps the anesthesia provider optimize right-sided heart function and assess the effects of anesthetic management on PVR.[147] Many anesthesia providers choose not to place pulmonary artery catheters because of concerns about the possibility that these catheters dislodge clots in the right side of the heart.

Intravenous fluid infusion must be adjusted so that right ventricular stroke volume is optimized in the presence of marked increase in afterload. A continuous catecholamine infusion may be needed to enhance cardiac contractility.

Induction is often performed with etomidate or ketamine (for maintenance of hemodynamic stability), but ketamine must be titrated judiciously because it may increase PVR.[146]

The use of N_2O is generally believed to be acceptable. However, this may not be possible with the use of a high FiO₂.[146] Use of N_2O should be discontinued if PVR increases. Obviously the use of N_2O is contraindicated in patients with venous air embolism.[145] Patients with moderate to severe PE often are experiencing acute right-sided heart failure. Cardiac function can be optimized by the use of minimally depressing cardiac agents such as narcotics.[147]

Persistent, severe hypotension, such as that accompanying a massive PE, may necessitate the use of a cardiotonic agent. The goal is preservation of perfusion to the brain and heart until

BOX 27-11

Guidelines for the Treatment of Pulmonary Embolism

1. Treat DVT or PE with therapeutic levels of unfractionated intravenous heparin, adjusted subcutaneous heparin, or low-molecular-weight heparin for at least 5 days and overlap with oral anticoagulation for at least 4 to 5 days. Consider a longer course of heparin (approximately 10 days) for massive PE or severe iliofemoral DVT. Enoxaparin, tinzaparin, or fondaparinux may also be used depending on renal function and indications.
2. For most patients, heparin and oral anticoagulation can be started together and heparin discontinued on day 5 or 6 if the INR has been therapeutic for 2 consecutive days.
3. Patients with reversible or time-limited risk factors can be treated for at least 3 months. Patients with a first episode of idiopathic DVT should be treated indefinitely. Approved regimen is warfarin, target INR of 2.0 to 3.0 for 6 months, followed by low-intensity warfarin, target INR of 1.5 to 2.0.
4. The use of thrombolytic agents continues to be highly individualized, and clinicians should have some latitude in using these agents. Patients with hemodynamically unstable PE or massive iliofemoral thrombosis are the best candidates.
5. Inferior vena caval filter placement is recommended when there is a contraindication to or failure of anticoagulation, for chronic recurrent embolism with pulmonary hypertension, and with concurrent performance of surgical pulmonary embolectomy or pulmonary endarterectomy.

Modified from Goldhaber SZ. Deep vein thrombosis and pulmonary thromboembolism. In: Fauci AS et al, eds. Harrison's Principles of Internal Medicine. 17th ed. New York: McGraw-Hill; 2008:1651-1657.
DVT, *Deep vein thrombosis;* INR, *international normalized ratio;* PTE, *pulmonary thromboembolism.*

BOX 27-12

Indications for Inferior Vena Caval Filters

Active Bleeding That Precludes Anticoagulation
Active bleeding that might cause exsanguination (e.g., gastrointestinal)
Feared bleeding that might be catastrophic (e.g., postoperative craniotomy)
Ongoing complications of anticoagulation (e.g., heparin-associated thrombocytopenia)
Planned intensive cancer chemotherapy (with anticipated pancytopenia or thrombocytopenia)

Recurrent Venous Thrombosis Despite Intensive Anticoagulation
Extensive or progressive venous thrombosis
In conjunction with catheter-based or surgical pulmonary embolectomy
Severe pulmonary hypertension or cor pulmonale
Temporary high risk such as bariatric surgery in a patient with a history of PE

Modified from Goldhaber SZ. Deep vein thrombosis and pulmonary thromboembolism. In: Fauci AS et al, eds. Harrison's Principles of Internal Medicine. 17th ed. New York: McGraw-Hill; 2008:1651-1657.
PE, *Pulmonary embolism.*

established by intubation if the patient is not already intubated. Second, delivery of the anesthetic agent must be discontinued, and administration of a 100% FIO_2 initiated.[147] Next, the circulatory system should be supported with the infusion of intravenous fluids or blood (or both) as needed, and the use of sympathomimetics (e.g., dobutamine or dopamine) initiated if necessary. Dysrhythmias should be treated with intravenous administration of lidocaine, and the patient should receive PEEP for optimization of O_2 transport across the alveolar membrane.[145]

Pulmonary embolectomy may be necessary. Severe hemodynamic difficulty should be anticipated and resuscitative efforts continued. Patients with PE are extremely sensitive to any anesthetic agent and are likely to require femoral bypass under local anesthesia with partial cardiopulmonary bypass before induction. Again, it is critical to have heparin ready to infuse into a central line (if available). Although separation from bypass is beyond the scope of this chapter (see Chapter 25), the anesthetist must realize that difficulties may be encountered. Depending on the insult to the right ventricle, pulmonary vasodilation and catecholamine infusions may be indicated. Simultaneous left atrial and right atrial pressure monitoring is helpful.

Patients with PE present particular management challenges in their postoperative course, including reperfusion edema, persistent hypoxemia, pericardial effusion, psychiatric disorders, and pulmonary blood flow steal. The areas of the lung to which pulmonary artery flow has been restored are subject to development of reperfusion pulmonary edema, presumably as a manifestation of oxidant- and protease-mediated acute lung injury. Other possible causes are extracorporeal circulation, anticoagulation, and an increase in perfusion pressure in a previously obstructed pulmonary artery. Complications include immediate pulmonary hemorrhage and respiratory disturbance, and death may occur.[152] This syndrome may develop 3 to 5 days after surgery.[153] Olman and associates have observed that after pulmonary

cardiopulmonary bypass is started and surgical removal of the clot attempted.[147] As always, heparin should be readily available; when needed, it should be administered into a central line while blood aspiration is verified before and after injection. Reports of operative mortality during pulmonary embolectomy range from 11% to 55%, with much higher rates among patients experiencing cardiac arrest.[152]

Detection of Pulmonary Embolism During Anesthesia
In the intubated patient under general anesthesia, combinations of symptoms may occur. A decreasing $PETCO_2$ and tachycardia usually are the first symptoms seen in PE.[147,148] These can be followed by a decrease in SaO_2 and the generation of ABG values that indicate unexplained arterial hypoxemia. Increased PAP and central venous pressure (CVP) can be seen in combination with a decrease in systolic and diastolic blood pressures.[148] Bronchospasm may occur.[145] Finally, ECG changes that indicate right axis deviation, incomplete or complete right bundle branch block, or peaked T waves may be observed in the presence or absence of an accompanying systolic ejection murmur.[144,148]

Intraoperative Management
Several measures can be taken to support the anesthetized patient with suspected PE. First and most important, an airway must be

thromboendarterectomy for relief of chronic thromboembolic PAH, perfusion lung scans frequently reveal new perfusion defects in segments served by undissected pulmonary arteries. This phenomenon has been labeled *pulmonary blood flow steal* and is believed to be caused by postoperative redistribution of regional PVR and not by rethrombosis or embolism.[154]

RESTRICTIVE PULMONARY DISEASES

Definition

Restrictive pulmonary disease is defined as any condition that interferes with normal lung expansion during inspiration. Typically, it includes disorders that increase the inward elastic recoil of the lungs or chest wall (Table 27-19). Consequently, the alteration in pulmonary dynamics results in decreases in lung volumes and capacities and in lung or chest-wall compliance. Some restrictive diseases produce ventilation abnormalities and $\dot{V}/\dot{Q}$ mismatching, whereas others lead to impairment of diffusion. FEV_1 and FVC are both decreased, owing to a reduction in TLC or a decrease in chest-wall compliance or muscle strength However, the FEV_1/FVC ratio is normal or elevated.

Impairment-producing restrictive pulmonary diseases can be classified as (1) acute intrinsic, (2) chronic intrinsic, or (3) chronic extrinsic. Acute intrinsic disorders are primarily caused by the abnormal movement of intravascular fluid into the interstitium of the lung and alveoli secondary to the increase in pulmonary vascular pressures occurring with left ventricular failure, fluid overload, or an increase in pulmonary capillary permeability. Examples of acute intrinsic disorders include pulmonary edema, aspiration pneumonia, and acute respiratory distress syndrome (ARDS). Chronic intrinsic diseases are characterized by pulmonary fibrosis. Conditions that produce fibrosis of the lung include idiopathic pulmonary fibrosis (IPF), radiation injury, cytotoxic and noncytotoxic drug exposure, O_2 toxicity, autoimmune diseases, and sarcoidosis. Chronic extrinsic diseases can be defined as disorders that inhibit the normal lung excursion. They include flail chest, pneumothorax, atelectasis, and pleural effusions. They also include conditions that interfere with chest-wall expansion, such as ascites, obesity, pregnancy, and skeletal and neuromuscular disorders.

The pulmonary system and its functions are directly manipulated by the administration of anesthesia. The effect of intraoperative pulmonary insult or preexisting pulmonary disease on respiratory function during anesthesia and the postoperative period is predictable: greater degrees of pulmonary impairment lead to marked alterations in intraoperative respiratory status and higher rates of occurrence of postoperative pulmonary complications. This section illustrates the pathophysiologic changes involved in these clinical disorders and discusses their clinical presentation, diagnosis, treatment, and anesthetic implications.

Pulmonary Edema

Pulmonary edema is not itself an independent disease entity, but rather the result of a variety of disease processes. Simply stated, pulmonary edema is the accumulation of excess fluid in the interstitial and air-filled spaces of the lung. The mechanisms responsible for its development include an increase in hydrostatic pressure within the pulmonary capillary system, an increase in the permeability of the alveolocapillary membrane, and a decrease in intravascular colloid oncotic pressure.[155]

Before one can understand the etiology and pathophysiology of pulmonary edema, the Starling forces and Starling's law of transcapillary fluid exchange must be clearly understood. The pulmonary capillary endothelium is thought to be

TABLE **27-19**	Common Causes of Restrictive Lung Disease	
Cause	**Example**
Interstitium	
Interstitial fibrosis, infiltration	Asbestosis
Pulmonary edema	Left ventricular failure
Pleura	
Pleural disease	Fibrothorax
Thoracic Cage and Abdomen	
Neuromuscular disease	Poliomyelitis
Skeletal abnormalities	Severe kyphoscoliosis
Marked obesity	Gross obesity

Modified from Taichman DB, Fishman AP. Approach to the patient with respiratory symptoms. In: Fishman AP et al, eds. Fishman's Pulmonary Diseases and Disorders. 4th ed. New York: McGraw-Hill; 2008:400.

semipermeable. Pulmonary interstitial fluid pressures, both hydrostatic (Pif) and osmotic (πif), along with the hydrostatic pressure in the pulmonary capillaries (Pc) and the osmotic pressure of the plasma (πp), are the primary determinants that balance fluid exchange across this semipermeable barrier.[156] These factors, which ultimately determine the amount of fluid that actually leaves the pulmonary vascular space, are incorporated into what is known as the *Starling equation*. A simplified version of this equation is as follows:

Equation 27-10

$$\dot{Q} = k[(Pc - Pif) - (\pi p - \pi if)]$$

where $\dot{Q}$ is the total amount of fluid that traverses the endothelial membrane and k is the fluid filtration coefficient, which describes quantitatively the permeability of the membrane.[155,156]

The Pc, the force favoring fluid movement out of the vessel wall, is in direct opposition to the Pif. The Pif, when positive, tends to force fluid inward through the capillary membrane; when it is negative, it tends to force fluid outward.[41] The πp and Pif also oppose each other, with the πif keeping fluid within the capillary and the πif pulling it outward into the interstitium. Overall, the balance of forces shown in the Starling equation favors fluid filtration into the interstitial space. Fluid filtered out into the alveolar interstitial space does not enter the alveoli, because under normal conditions the alveolar epithelium is composed of very tight junctions that prevent fluid and protein from entering the alveolar air spaces. The fluid moves to the extravascular interstitial space, where the lymphatics remove all of the filtered fluid and return it to the systemic circulation.[157]

Pulmonary edema can occur if any variable in the Starling equation is altered in the direction favoring increased fluid filtration. High pressure (Pc) and increased permeability (k) are the two most important components of the Starling equation that are altered in states of pulmonary edema. Because of this, pulmonary edema is classified as being either cardiogenic (high pressure, hydrostatic) or noncardiogenic (permeability is increased).

Cardiogenic pulmonary edema occurs whenever the Pc is increased. Increased Pc is the most common form of pulmonary edema. Cardiogenic pulmonary edema is initiated by some type of left-sided heart incompetence or failure. The term *left ventricular failure* implies that a decrease has occurred in left ventricular contractility, which ultimately leads to a reduction in both stroke volume and CO. Incomplete left ventricular emptying elevates left ventricular end-diastolic volume, which in turn elevates left ventricular end-diastolic pressure. Increased left ventricular end-diastolic pressure is "reflected back," causing elevation of the left atrial, pulmonary venous, and pulmonary capillary pressures. When pulmonary capillary pressure reaches levels of 20 to 25 mm Hg (normal range, 10 to 16 mm Hg), the rate of fluid transudation often exceeds lymphatic drainage capacity, and alveolar flooding occurs.

Coronary artery disease, hypertension, cardiomyopathies, mitral regurgitation, and mitral stenosis are a few of the cardiac conditions that may increase pulmonary intravascular hydrostatic pressure (Pc) and predispose a patient to the development of pulmonary edema. Although an elevated left ventricular end-diastolic pressure is the major cause of an increase in Pc, and therefore pulmonary edema, it is important to realize that several noncardiac problems also may increase Pc. These include pulmonary venoocclusive disease, fibrosing mediastinitis, head trauma, cerebrovascular accident, exposure to high altitudes, and overhydration.

Noncardiogenic pulmonary edema is associated with an increase in endothelial permeability caused by an insult that disrupts the barrier function of the blood-tissue interface. Unlike cardiogenic pulmonary edema, in which the capillary endothelium remains intact and no leakage of protein is noted, noncardiogenic pulmonary edema is associated with leakage of both fluid and protein from the vascular space.[156] Because this respiratory membrane disruption cannot be easily or directly measured, noncardiogenic pulmonary edema is said to exist when suspicious chest radiographic evidence coexists with insufficient hemodynamic basis. The presence of a pulmonary wedge pressure less than 12 mm Hg and the absence of a significant history of cardiac disease generally suffice for exclusion of a hemodynamic mechanism.[155]

Although a multitude of disorders are associated with noncardiogenic pulmonary edema, the most commonly encountered cause is systemic sepsis that leads to ARDS. Other clinical conditions associated with noncardiogenic pulmonary edema include the aspiration syndromes, inhalation of toxic fumes and gases, and the embolization phenomena. (See also Box 27-15 on page 613.)

Pulmonary edema is nearly always associated with some type of preexisting disease state or insult. If a patient with pulmonary edema has a history of CHF, hypertension, or ischemic heart disease, the presence of cardiogenic pulmonary edema can be assumed. In addition to systemic sepsis, anaphylaxis, pancreatitis, disseminated intravascular coagulation, trauma, multiple transfusions, and near-drowning can all result in noncardiogenic pulmonary edema.

Neurogenic Pulmonary Edema

Neurogenic pulmonary edema begins with a massive outpouring of sympathetic nervous system stimulation triggered by central nervous system insult. This centrally mediated central nervous system overactivity typically occurs in the hypothalamic area.[158] Excessive sympathetic activation induces remarkable hemodynamic alterations—primarily systemic and pulmonary vasoconstriction. The left ventricle fails because of the inordinate pressure work imposed by the systemic hypertension, and pulmonary blood volume increases because of the functional imbalance between the failing left ventricle and the normal right ventricle.[156] Although this sequence seems to parallel

that of hemodynamic pulmonary edema, a permeability component exists, as evidenced by the high protein concentration found in the pulmonary secretions of affected patients.

Uremic Pulmonary Edema

Uremic pulmonary edema is seen in those patients with renal insufficiency or failure. Overhydration and expansion of the circulating blood volume lead to increases in pulmonary capillary pressures. Again, a "leaky" component exists because of the metabolic abnormalities associated with uremia. Reducing the circulating blood volume of these patients via hemodialysis promotes resolution of this type of pulmonary edema.[156]

High Altitude–Related Pulmonary Edema

High altitude–related pulmonary edema can occur in the absence of left ventricular failure whenever an individual overexerts before acclimating to a high altitude. The pathogenesis of this form of pulmonary edema is unclear, but it may be the result of intense hypoxic pulmonary arterial vasoconstriction or massive sympathetic discharge triggered by cerebral hypoxia.[157]

Pulmonary Edema due to Upper Airway Obstruction

Pulmonary edema due to upper airway obstruction results from prolonged, forced inspiratory effort against an obstructed upper airway. The most common cause of this type of pulmonary edema in adults is laryngospasm after extubation and general anesthesia. In children, pulmonary edema after obstruction caused by croup, epiglottitis, and laryngospasm also is well documented. Vigorous inspiration against obstruction creates high negative intrathoracic, transpleural, and alveolar pressures, enlarging the pulmonary vascular volume and subsequently the interstitial fluid volume. The capacity of the lymphatics becomes overwhelmed, and interstitial fluid transudes into the pulmonary alveoli. Hypoxia causes a massive sympathetic discharge that results in systemic vasoconstriction and a translocation of fluid from the systemic circulation to the already expanding pulmonary vascular and interstitial spaces. Hypoxia also increases pulmonary capillary pressures. Because hypoxia alters myocardial activity, left atrial function and left ventricular function are reduced.

During obstruction, vigorous inspiratory efforts are unsuccessful because of the airway obstruction. Unsuccessful expiration produces an increase in intrathoracic and alveolar pressures. Intrinsic PEEP also is produced during this stage. Relief of the obstruction results in cessation of intrinsic PEEP.

The consequence of these events is the sudden massive transudation of fluid from the pulmonary interstitium into the alveoli, which results in pulmonary edema. The malignity of pulmonary edema is determined by the extent of prior alveolar and capillary damage and the immensity of hemodynamic and cardiovascular alterations.

Not all of those who experience an acute airway obstruction develop pulmonary edema, and no specific risk factors for its occurrence have been identified. Factors that may predispose to its formation after obstruction include youth, male gender, long periods of obstruction, overzealous perioperative fluid administration, and the presence of preexisting cardiac and pulmonary disease.

Treatment includes prompt recognition of the condition, securing a patent airway, supportive therapy with oxygenation, and administering diuretics. Although the onset of pulmonary edema after laryngospasm usually is immediate, cases have been reported of the occurrence of pulmonary edema several hours after laryngospasm. Therefore, it is recommended that patients who develop laryngospasm be observed postoperatively longer than the typical 60 to 90 minutes. The diagnosis of pulmonary edema and its differentiation into cardiogenic and noncardiac categories necessitates taking a detailed medical history and performing a physical examination, chest radiography, and ABG analysis.

Physical examination reveals increased respiratory effort. As water accumulates, the lungs become heavy and noncompliant, and a decrease in FRC occurs. This increase in the volume of extravascular lung fluid provides a potent stimulus for surrounding interstitial stretch receptors (J-receptors), the activation of which results in tachypnea. Tachypnea is not relieved by the administration of O_2 and the return of PaO_2 to normal. Intercostal retractions and use of accessory muscles are apparent on physical examination. Signs of sympathetic stress stimulation, such as hypertension, diaphoresis, and tachycardia, often are noted. The expectoration of pink, frothy sputum signals that alveoli have been flooded.[158]

The detection of basilar crackles on auscultation is the traditional hallmark of early pulmonary edema. In reality, by the time these crackles become audible, excess water has already flooded the alveoli and overflowed into the terminal bronchioles.[154] It is in the bronchioles, not in the alveoli, that the crackles of pulmonary edema are generated. The earliest and most often disregarded clinical sign is rapid, shallow breathing.

In cardiogenic pulmonary edema, heart size may be increased. High CVPs, an S_3 or S_4 gallop, and jugular venous distention often are observed.[155] Chest radiography is still the most reliable and expedient tool for early detection of pulmonary edema. In cardiogenic pulmonary edema, the cardiac silhouette may appear abnormal or enlarged; in noncardiogenic pulmonary edema, it can be enlarged or remain normal. Interstitial edema can be observed before the alveoli flood and the onset of clinical signs occurs. Pleural effusions are common, and a "whited-out" or "butterfly" appearance may be noted.[156]

ABG analysis reveals hypoxemia secondary to $\dot{V}/\dot{Q}$ abnormalities. When right-to-left shunting is great, the PaO_2 can be affected by any change in the central venous O_2 content. Increases in O_2 consumption or decreases in CO further reduce the PaO_2. The $PaCO_2$ may be low, normal, or elevated. The initial hypocarbia is related to tachypnea and high MVs; at later stages, hypercarbia is frequently secondary to muscle fatigue and exhaustion. Changes in pH usually reflect changes in $PaCO_2$, but metabolic or lactic acidosis or both may occur from tissue O_2 deficiency, low CO, or sepsis.

Anesthesia Management

Pulmonary edema is considered a medical emergency, and immediate intervention is required for treatment of the underlying disease, support of other failing organ systems, and optimization of O_2 delivery.[155] O_2 should be administered either by nasal cannula, face mask, or endotracheal tube. If oxygenation does not improve with the administration of high FIO_2, positive-pressure ventilation with either PEEP or CPAP must be initiated. Institution of positive-pressure mechanical ventilation in patients with acute pulmonary edema usually results in a prompt increase in oxygenation and, in some cases, in CO. Improvement occurs because of superior inflation and $\dot{V}/\dot{Q}$ matching. Amelioration of left ventricular function (CO) may occur secondary to four possible mechanisms: (1) improvement in arterial oxygenation and therefore improvement of myocardial O_2 supply; (2) reduction in the extreme pleural pressure swings present with spontaneous ventilation and hence reduction in afterload on the left

ventricle; (3) decrease in the workload of the failing heart because of a reduction in work of breathing (and therefore a reduction in O_2 requirement) effected by a mechanical ventilator; and (4) decrease in preload (and a subsequent reduction in venous return) occurring secondary to the use of positive-pressure ventilation.

Pharmacologic therapy includes the use of vasodilators, inotropes, steroids, and diuretics. For more than 50 years, morphine sulfate has been used in the treatment of cardiogenic pulmonary edema because of its venodilatory and preload-reducing properties.[158] Nitroprusside is a very effective preload and afterload reducer. By reducing systemic blood pressure, nitroprusside decreases the afterload on the left ventricle; this may result in better cardiac function, with a subsequent lowering of left atrial pressures. Inotropic agents such as dopamine or dobutamine improve myocardial contractility and lower cardiac filling pressures. In patients with chronic CHF and pulmonary congestion, digitalis augments contractility and promotes decreases in left atrial and ventricular filling pressures. (The use of steroids is discussed later in this chapter in the section on ARDS.)

Fluid balance is managed with both fluid restriction and diuresis. This therapy helps achieve a "negative" fluid balance in hydrostatic pulmonary edema, in which Pc is high. Even in permeability pulmonary edema, in which Pc is thought to be low, any decrease in the hydrostatic pressure further reduces the net movement of pulmonary microvascular fluid outward.[155] Potent diuretics such as furosemide not only lower left atrial filling pressure by decreasing systemic venous tone but also induce diuresis of the expanded extravascular volume.

The type of fluid, whether crystalloid or colloid, that should be used in the presence of pulmonary edema remains controversial. Regardless of type used, it is generally agreed that administration should proceed slowly.

ASPIRATION PNEUMONITIS

Definition

Aspiration is a rare yet serious complication of general anesthesia. Much effort is expended to prevent this untoward occurrence and minimize sequelae if it does occur. It can occur at any time during the course of anesthesia administration, and if it is severe, a multitude of serious complications may follow. Pneumonitis adds an average of 15 hospital days' stay and $22,000 to the course of care of a patient who suffers this complication.[159]

Aspiration pneumonitis was described by Curtis Mendelson in 1946 after he observed a number of deaths among obstetric patients.[160] Mendelson's laboratory investigations led him to the conclusion that two entirely separate clinical aspiration disorders existed. One followed the aspiration of solid food and produced a picture of laryngeal or bronchial obstruction, whereas the other resulted from direct acid injury to the lung and produced the "asthmalike" syndrome that now carries his name.[161] By definition, pulmonary aspiration has two components. First, gastric contents escape from the stomach into the pharynx, and, second, they enter the lungs. This results from preexisting disease, airway manipulation, and the inevitable compromise in protective reflexes that accompany the anesthetized state. Aspirates are commonly categorized as contaminated, acidic, alkaline, particulate, and nonparticulate. Less than half of all aspirations lead to pneumonia. Pneumonia occurs most often in patients with aspiration of infected material or who are immunocompromised. Ingestion of highly acidic or particulate aspirate may cause severe respiratory damage without an infectious component. Patients who initially show no signs of infection, however, may develop pneumonia over time because of the severity of the lung injury and prolonged respiratory support.[162]

Incidence and Outcome

Although the incidence of regurgitation is estimated to be frequent (as high as 15%, according to some authors), pulmonary aspiration complicates only about 1 out of 3000 anesthetics. This incidence is roughly doubled for cesarean section surgery[163] and emergency surgery.[164] Fortunately, the majority of aspiration incidents require little or no treatment. Warner and colleagues[165] from the Mayo Clinic reviewed 215,488 general anesthetics and studied the outcomes of aspiration pneumonitis. They determined that approximately 60% of episodes were asymptomatic, 15% were symptomatic but required only conservative treatment, 20% required mechanical ventilation, and 5% of episodes led to death (Figure 27-16). The overall mortality was 1 in 71,829 anesthetic procedures. Several of their findings were interesting. Complications developed in equal percentages among those who received and those who did not receive pharmacologic acid aspiration prophylaxis. Patients who aspirated but did not develop symptoms within 2 hours could be discharged. If signs or symptoms did not emerge in that time frame, they would not occur subsequently. Not surprisingly, the largest number of aspirations occur during induction and intubation or on emergence within 5 minutes of extubation. They found no serious morbidity from pulmonary aspiration in nearly 120,000 elective procedures in ASA class I or II.

In a later study, the same group reported on the incidence of aspiration in infants and children.[166] Although pediatric patients are often reported as having a higher incidence of aspiration than adults,[164] these researchers found no increase in the incidence among young patients. They noted 24 aspirations in a series of 63,180 general anesthetic procedures. Fifteen of the 24 children did not develop symptoms within 2 hours, and no treatment was required. Five children required respiratory support, three for more than 48 hours. No deaths occurred. Common risk factors for aspiration are given in Box 27-13.

The Anesthetic Incidence Monitoring Study database in New Zealand noted 133 cases of aspiration out of 5000 reported anesthesia incidents.[167] Five deaths occurred. Aspiration was confirmed by clinical signs or radiography. Predisposing factors included abdominal pathology, obesity, diabetes, neurologic deficit, lithotomy position, difficult intubation, reflux disease, hiatal hernia, and inadequate anesthesia leading to straining and bucking.

In an interesting study, researchers looked at general anesthesia by mask in obstetric patients who required surgery immediately after vaginal delivery.[168] Procedures included placental

extraction; repair of vaginal, cervical, and perineal tears; and uterine manipulation. This database in Israel involved 1705 anesthetic procedures with only one case of mild pneumonitis.

Etiology

Although vomiting and gastroesophageal reflux are common clinical events, aspiration usually occurs only when normal protective reflexes (swallowing, coughing, gagging) fail.[165] Three broad categories of failure include (1) depression of reflex protection, (2) alteration in anatomic structures, and (3) iatrogenic disorder. Reflex responses to aspiration are automatically blunted with depression of consciousness. The most common setting for depression of reflex protection occurs during anesthesia induction and emergence.[165]

Three aspiration syndromes have been identified: (1) chemical pneumonitis (Mendelson syndrome); (2) mechanical obstruction; and (3) bacterial infection. Because acute chemical pneumonitis poses the greatest difficulty to anesthesia providers, the pathophysiology, presentation, and anesthetic implications of Mendelson syndrome are discussed.

The triphasic sequence of (1) immediate respiratory distress combined with bronchospasm, cyanosis, tachycardia, and dyspnea followed by (2) partial recovery and (3) a final phase of gradual return of function is characteristic of Mendelson syndrome.[169] This acute chemical pneumonitis is caused by the irritative action of hydrochloric acid, alkaline aspirates, or particulate materials, which are damaging to the lungs.

The etiology of aspiration pneumonia often is characterized according to the pH, volume, and type of gastric material aspirated. It has long been felt that gastric fluid volume (GFV)

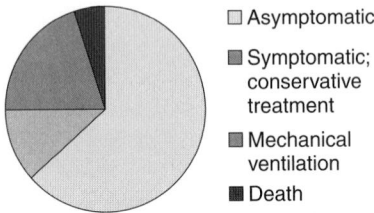

FIGURE **27-16** Sequelae of aspiration pneumonitis. (*Modified from Warner MA et al. Clinical significance of pulmonary aspiration during the perioperative period. Anesthesiology. 1993;78[1]:56-62.*)

greater than 0.4 mL/kg (25 mL/70 kg) and a pH less than 2.5 are significant indicators of risk for aspiration sequelae. In 1974, Roberts and Shirley[170] published a classic article advocating these arbitrarily defined surrogate end-points in patients undergoing cesarean section. These markers became widely accepted in clinical practice, and efforts to reach these levels preoperatively in many patient groups included insertion of nasogastric tubes, as well as multidrug pharmacologic intervention. Unfortunately, the experiment by Roberts and Shirley by far lacked adequate scientific design to derive recommendations on assessing risk or administering prophylaxis to patients to reduce aspiration. Questions have therefore been raised as to the validity of the data behind these recommendations, with the suggestion that a reappraisal is in order.[169] GFVs greater than 0.4 mL/kg are more common, even in fasting individuals, than the overall incidence of aspiration would suggest, if this were a major risk factor for aspiration. In a recent report comparing gastric content differences in healthy obese versus lean patients, GFV greater than 25 mL and pH less than 2.5 were noted in 26.6% of obese and 42% of lean patients.[171] These data suggest that healthy obese patients do not exhibit delayed gastric emptying and that many patients routinely fall into the arbitrary range of GFV greater than 25 mL and pH less than 2.5 without experiencing aspiration. Although the volume *aspirated* correlates with the severity of pulmonary damage, there is less correlation between the volume in the stomach and the risk of pneumonitis.

Acidity plays a role in aspiration-induced lung damage; however, preoperative pharmacologic manipulation of gastric pH has not been proven to be clinically effective.[165,166,172] It is time to shift the focus away from GFV and pH and toward patient characteristics, patient condition, and anesthetic practices that place the patient at risk of pulmonary aspiration. Attention to the presence of factors listed in Box 27-13 and in particular to the presence of *multiple* factors from that list will prove more fruitful to the anesthetist's ability to predict aspiration risk than will over-attention to the questionable and nonspecific factors of gastric fluid volume and gastric pH.

Pathophysiology

The pathophysiology of aspiration pneumonitis is typically characterized by four stages: (1) The aspirated substance causes immediate damage to the lung parenchyma, resulting in tissue necrosis. (2) Atelectasis results within minutes, owing to a parasympathetic response that leads to airway closure and a decrease in lung compliance. (3) One to two hours after the injury, there is an intense inflammatory reaction characterized by pulmonary edema and hemorrhage. Inflammatory cytokines, including interleukin-8 and tumor necrosis factor-alpha released by alveolar macrophages, play a central role. Neutrophils also play a key role in this phase by releasing oxygen radicals and proteases. (4) By 24 hours after the insult, secondary injuries result from fibrin deposits and necrosis of alveolar cells.

When aspiration is severe, damage to the entire alveolocapillary barrier, including the basement membranes and capillary endothelial cells, may occur. It is important to note that physical damage is done to the lung endothelium instantly on contact with caustic aspirate. Therefore, there is no benefit in performing bronchoscopy or deep tracheal suctioning with the intent of halting the damage. Unless the patient has aspirated a particulate substance that can be retrieved, deep suctioning following aspiration will probably cause more irritation than any benefit from reversing the process. Suctioning the mouth and pharynx to prevent further aspiration is helpful.

Hypoxia occurs secondary to a shunting effect due to atelectasis. Initially $PaCO_2$ tends to be low because of hyperventilation from hypoxic drive and because of the mechanical and irritative stimuli to the large airways and parenchyma. Hypercarbia associated with hypoventilation is a negative prognostic sign. Because atelectasis is common, PEEP is commonly a useful treatment modality for patients who require mechanical ventilation. Damage to the lung parenchyma causes an increase in the permeability of the pulmonary blood vessels followed by a profound capillary leak syndrome. This capillary leak produces flooding of the interstitium and alveolar spaces with a protein-rich fluid (permeability pulmonary edema). Mucus rapidly buffers the acidic fluid entering the lungs. Despite this, initial contact with highly acidic material has still been shown to increase the vascular permeability in a very predictable fashion. In addition to the inactivation of surfactant by the gastric aspirate itself, the loss of protein through the impaired capillary wall can cause changes in surfactant production and in turn can contribute to a loss of lung compliance. Hemodynamic changes may include hypotension and reduction in CO from hypoxemia-induced myocardial ischemia, pulmonary hypertension, and acidosis.

In the inflammatory stage, there is a release of various phagocyte-derived substances such as reactive oxygen metabolites, nitric oxide, and proteases. This stage is characterized by neutrophil infiltration, which has been found to be an important negative factor in the eventual outcome following aspiration. Recent research has demonstrated that inhibition of alveolar macrophages will decrease the levels of inflammatory mediators and neutrophil recruitment to the area of injury.[173] Direct inhibition of neutrophils with neutrophil aggregation inhibitors, such as pentoxifylline and lidocaine, also improve outcomes of pneumonitis.[174,175]

Clinical Features and Diagnosis

Arterial hypoxemia, the hallmark sign of aspiration pneumonitis, is frequently the first sign of aspiration. Because the majority of aspiration incidents are asymptomatic or mildly symptomatic, unexplained hypoxemia occurring in otherwise healthy patients postoperatively may frequently be a vague sign of silent aspiration. Other signs to alert the anesthetist to the possibility of aspiration include tachypnea, dyspnea, tachycardia, hypertension, and cyanosis.

Diagnosis may be difficult to establish unless the aspiration is witnessed or gastric contents are visualized directly in the airway or suctioned from an endotracheal tube. ABG analysis and chest radiography are needed for evaluation. Infiltrates in perihilar and basilar regions along with pulmonary edema are the most common findings on radiography. Table 27-20 outlines classifications and therapy of aspiration pneumonia. Differential diagnosis of these signs should include allergic bronchospasm, endotracheal tube displacement or obstruction, pneumothorax, and pulmonary embolism.

Anesthetic Management
Preoperative Management

When dealing with aspiration, "an ounce of prevention is worth a pound of cure." Avoiding the use of general anesthesia is the most effective means of preventing aspiration. However, regional and local sedation anesthesia is unrealistic for many procedures and in certain patient populations. When the use of general anesthesia is unavoidable, taking the following steps may help minimize the risk of aspiration, or at least limit its consequences.

TABLE 27-20	Classification of Aspiration Pneumonia		
Inoculum	**Pulmonary Sequelae**	**Clinical Features**	**Therapy**
Acid breathing	Chemical pneumonitis	Acute dyspnea, tachypnea; tachycardia; cyanosis, bronchospasm, fever Sputum: pink, frothy Radiographic: infiltrates in one or both lower lobes Hypoxemia	Positive-pressure Intravenous fluids Tracheal suction
Oropharyngeal bacteria	Bacterial infection	Usually insidious onset Cough, fever, purulent sputum Radiographic: infiltrate in dependent pulmonary segment or lobe ± cavitation	Antibiotics
Inert fluids positive-breathing with isoproterenol	Mechanical obstruction Reflex airway closure	Acute dyspnea, cyanosis ± apnea Pulmonary edema	Tracheal suction Intermittent pressure oxygen and matter
Particulate	Mechanical obstruction	Dependent on level of obstruction, ranging from acute apnea and rapid death to irritating chronic cough ± recurrent superimposed infections particulate matter	Extraction of matter Antibiotics for infection

From Fishman JA. *Aspiration, empyema, lung abscesses and anaerobic infections.* In: Fishman AP et al, eds. *Fishman's Pulmonary Diseases and Disorders.* 4th ed. New York: McGraw-Hill; 2008:2150.

Nil per os (NPO) policy has been a mainstay of prophylaxis against aspiration, by aiming to reduce patients' intragastric volume by the time they undergo anesthesia. The suggestion by Roberts and Shirley that a gastric fluid volume greater than 0.4 mL/kg would predispose to aspiration gave credence to this approach. Following this concept, practitioners have instructed patients to refrain from oral intake for 8, 12, and sometimes as much as 16 hours (e.g., afternoon-scheduled surgeries, for which the patient is told to remain "NPO after midnight"). However, these long NPO periods are unnecessarily long to ensure stomach emptying of most no-fat or low-fat foods, and the prolonged NPO periods contribute more to patient discomfort, dehydration, and insulin resistance than to ensuring an empty stomach.[176] It has become evident that clear liquids leave the stomach within 2 hours of ingestion, but gastric acid secretion continues, even in the absence of food intake. Therefore, in the absence of prokinetic stimulation by oral intake, a fasting patient may have a higher gastric volume and acidity than one who was allowed clear fluids closer to the time of surgery. The effects of gastrin and cholecystokinin on stimulating gastric emptying in response to clear liquid ingestion are greater than the effect of the migrating motor complex in emptying the stomach in the absence of food or liquid intake. Contemporary understanding of this concept has led to revision of blanket NPO guidelines in favor of food-specific guidelines, particularly a much more liberal approach to clear liquid ingestion preoperatively (Figure 27-17).

Pharmacologic prophylaxis for aspiration has been common practice for many years. Reliance on this approach arose from the belief that large volumes of acidic gastric contents, if aspirated, caused lung damage and increased the risk of serious morbidity and mortality. Agents such as gastrokinetics, histamine blockers, anticholinergics, antacids, proton pump inhibitors, and antiemetics are all used alone or in various combinations to raise gastric pH and lower volume. Recent evidence questioning the

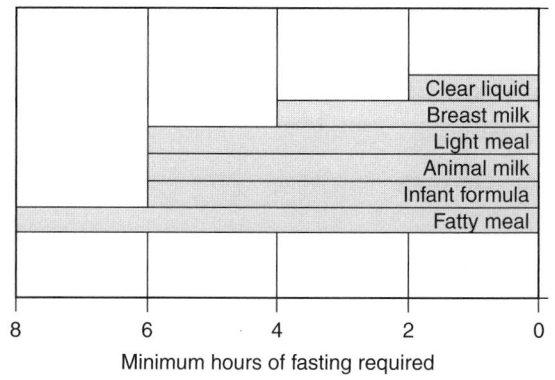

Preoperative fasting guidelines for various foods

FIGURE **27-17** Preoperative fasting guidelines. (*Modified from American Society of Anesthesiologists Task Force on Preoperative Fasting. Practice guidelines for preoperative fasting and the use of pharmacologic agents to reduce the risk of pulmonary aspiration: application to healthy patients undergoing elective surgery. Anesthesiology. 1999;90:896-905.*)

benefit of this practice of routinely administering such agents to healthy patients without an increased aspiration risk has led to new practice guidelines. A task force appointed by the ASA has reviewed data with an evidence-based approach to the current fasting guidelines and drug prophylaxis (Table 27-21).[177] Evidence does not support the practice of routine preoperative administration of these gastric-related agents. Some combinations of these agents even cancel out each others' intended effects. For example, metoclopramide raises barrier pressure (which opposes gastric regurgitation) by increasing the tone of the lower esophageal sphincter. However, anticholinergics used to reduce gastric secretion lower the tone of the lower esophageal sphincter and are therefore decreasing lower esophageal sphincter

TABLE 27-21	Drug Prophylaxis for Anesthesia	
Medication Type	**Common Examples**	**Recommendation**
Gastrointestinal stimulants	Metoclopramide	No routine use*
Gastric acid secretion blockers	Cimetidine Famotidine Omeprazole Lansoprazole	No routine use*
Antacids	Sodium citrate Sodium bicarbonate Magnesium trisilicate	No routine use*
Antiemetics	Droperidol Ondansetron	No routine use*
Anticholinergics	Atropine Scopolamine Glycopyrrolate	No use†
Combinations of the medications above		No routine use*

Modified from American Society of Anesthesiologists. Practice guidelines for preoperative fasting and the use of pharmacologic agents to reduce the risk of pulmonary aspiration: application to healthy patients undergoing elective surgery. Anesthesiology. 1999;90:896-905.
The routine preoperative use of these medications to decrease aspiration risk in patients with no apparent increased risk is not recommended.
†*The use of anticholinergics to decrease aspiration risk is not recommended.*

pressure (LESP). Metoclopramide stimulates gastric emptying and acts as an antiemetic. When this agent is used in combination with the H_2-receptor blockers or antacids, the resultant reduction in gastric volume and acidity may be helpful in reducing aspiration risk. Although not recommended for routine use, the administration of pharmacologic prophylactic agents is indicated for patients at specific risk of aspiration.

Clear, nonparticulate antacids such as sodium citrate or sodium citrate with citric acid ("bicitra") have been shown to be clinically effective in increasing the pH of gastric contents. Desired onset of action occurs within 15 minutes, and duration of action is 1 to 3 hours. Although citrate preparations may last up to 6 to 7 hours, some patients will also experience a rebound increase in gastric acid production, so if surgery is delayed more than 1 hour after citrate administration, it may be prudent to repeat the dose.[178]

Intravenous administration of the H_2-receptor blockers cimetidine, ranitidine, and famotidine 45 to 60 minutes before surgery can raise gastric pH. Of the H_2 blockers, famotidine provides the best profile of duration of action and low incidence of side effects.[179] Although the H_2 blockers reduce gastrin-induced acid production, they are less effective against vagal or muscarinic influence. In contrast, proton pump inhibitors irreversibly bind to H+/K+ ATPase, blocking the final pathway for acid production. They are therefore more effective in reducing acid production, but for maximal effectiveness, they must be administered as a dose the night before surgery and then repeated preoperatively. In emergency cases or where the prior-night dose was not performed, H_2-receptor blockers may provide a better option for single-dose therapy.

Although cricoid pressure has long been considered a foundation of management of aspiration risk, the effectiveness of this technique has recently been called into question.[180] Confounding findings include that in a significant number of patients, the esophagus is not aligned directly posteriorly to the trachea, so there are numerous reports of aspiration despite application of cricoid pressure. Other suggestions are that cricoid pressure is inconsistently applied, or cricoid pressure itself will reduce LESP, thereby increasing the gradient for gastric regurgitation. This LESP reduction appears to be a reflex mechanism in response to cricoid pressure and can be blunted by remifentanil.[181] Other nonpharmacologic mechanisms such as elevating the patient's head may offer limited benefit. In a small study of non-obese, awake, non-fasted patients, Jeske and colleagues found no difference in gastric regurgitation, regardless of 20-degree head elevation or depression.[182]

Intraoperative Management

If intubation is not expected to be difficult, a rapid-sequence induction (rather than awake endotracheal intubation) is indicated in the patient with aspiration risk. There is little evidence that "modified" rapid sequence technique (which allows for gentle mask ventilation) would worsen aspiration incidence, and this approach may be preferable in patients at risk for rapid oxygen desaturation. Because difficult intubation itself is a risk factor for aspiration, there should be a low threshold for performing awake intubation in a patient with aspiration risk who may also pose airway challenges. Endotracheal intubation is considered the optimal approach for airway isolation, but regurgitated material can seep around the ETT cuff, particularly if it is not lubricated.[183,184] Preventive measures in the anesthetic plan include ensuring that the patient is fully awake before extubation and manifesting protective reflexes, residual neuromuscular blockade is minimized to the extent possible, the degree of narcosis does not impair the level of consciousness postoperatively, and that the stomach has been evacuated.

If vomiting or aspiration occurs during induction, immediate treatment includes tilting of the patient's head downward or to the side, rapid suctioning of the mouth and pharynx, and intubation. As noted above, there is little benefit in performing tracheal or bronchial suctioning in most cases, and bronchoscopy should be reserved for those patients suspected of having aspirated solid material. If aspiration is severe, surgery may be postponed. ABG analysis should be performed for determination of the extent of hypoxemia. Early application of PEEP is recommended for improving pulmonary function and combating atelectasis.[169]

Oxygenation should be supported with supplemental oxygen only to the minimum extent necessary. The damage to pulmonary parenchyma from caustic aspiration predisposes the tissue to oxygen toxicity. Indiscriminate administration of oxygen may worsen tissue damage.[185] For pharmacologic treatment of aspiration pneumonitis, the use of steroids is controversial. Long considered a mainstay of treatment, steroid therapy is associated with more rapid resolution of radiologic evidence of pneumonitis but also with longer ICU stays for pneumonitis patients. Lidocaine 1.5 mg/kg as a neutrophil aggregation inhibitor may be useful in improving long-term outcome following aspiration.[186] Although most aspirations are of sterile material (such as typical gastric acid), leukocytosis, fever, and infiltrate on x-ray are common findings in aspiration pneumonitis. The clinical findings resemble but do not indicate bacterial colonization (i.e., pneumonia). For this reason, the routine use of antibiotics is not recommended.[177] Antibiotics are indicated only if the fever does not resolve within 48 hours, or there is risk for bacterial colonization (e.g., a patient on high-pH gastric tube feedings) or protected-sample bronchial or blood cultures indicate infection. Box 27-14 gives standard treatment protocol for aspiration pneumonitis.

The common time course of symptoms following aspiration has been characterized. Warner and colleagues[165] noted that the condition of the patient at 2 hours following the aspiration was prognostic of their eventual course. Patients could be discharged if they did not manifest significant symptoms within 2 hours of the incident. Their criteria were as follows: (1) patients did not develop symptoms that included a new cough or a wheeze; (2) no decrease in SpO2 of greater than or equal to 10% of preoperative levels occurred while the patient was breathing room air; (3) patients did not exhibit an A-a gradient of greater than or equal to 300 mm Hg; and (4) no radiographic evidence of pulmonary aspiration was present.

ACUTE RESPIRATORY DISTRESS SYNDROME

Definition

The term *acute respiratory failure* is often used synonymously with *acute* (formerly *adult*) *respiratory distress syndrome* (ARDS).

Although ARDS may be caused by or associated with a variety of clinical conditions, most patients with this disease demonstrate similar clinical and pathologic features, regardless of the cause of lung injury. Common features include (1) a history of a preceding noxious event that served as a trigger for the subsequent development of ARDS; (2) an interval from hours to days of relatively normal lung function after the insult; and (3) the rapid onset and progression over several hours of dyspnea, severe hypoxia, diffuse bilateral pulmonary infiltration, and stiffening and noncompliance of the lungs.[187] The consensus definition is given in Table 27-22.

Incidence and Outcome

Risk factors for the development of ARDS appear to be additive. Taylor reported the incidence of occurrence to be 25% with the presence of one risk factor, 42% with the presence of two, and 85% with the presence of three.[188] The mortality rate for ARDS remains high, ranging from 50% to 70%.[189] However, the mortality rate often exceeds 90% when gram-negative septic shock precedes ARDS development.[190]

Etiology

Events and risk factors associated with the development of ARDS include (1) shock (septic, cardiogenic, or hypovolemic); (2) trauma; (3) pulmonary infection (e.g., with *Pneumocystis jiroveci* or *Escherichia coli*); (4) disease states that result in the release of inflammatory mediators (e.g., extrapulmonary infections, disseminated intravascular coagulation, anaphylaxis, coronary bypass grafting, and transfusion reactions); (5) exposure to various agents (e.g., narcotics, barbiturates, and O_2); (6) diseases of the central nervous system; (7) aspiration (e.g., of gastric contents or as in drowning); and (8) metabolic events (e.g., pancreatitis and uremia) (Box 27-15).[187]

Pathophysiology

As with pulmonary edema and aspiration pneumonitis, the pathophysiology of ARDS is centered around severe damage and inflammation to the alveolocapillary membrane. Irrespective of the cause of acute respiratory failure, the lungs' structural response to injury and subsequent repair occurs in a similar fashion.[188] Although the exact mechanisms of this response and repair remain unclear, research has focused on the release of cytokines and membrane-bound phospholipids from the capillary endothelium and the activation of leukocytes and macrophages (via the complement system) within the lungs.[189]

Phospholipids are converted into prostaglandins and leukotrienes by the enzymes cyclooxygenase and lipoxygenase, respectively. It is believed that prostaglandin metabolites mediate pulmonary vasoconstriction, alter vascular reactivity (i.e., decrease hypoxic pulmonary vasoconstriction), and cause airway constriction.[191]

In addition, microembolus formation is a common manifestation of ARDS. Complement system activation and the release of thromboplastin from soft-tissue injury can trigger the coagulation cascade. Microemboli contribute to the severity of lung injury and are often found during autopsy.[192]

Clinical Features and Diagnosis

The clinical presentation of ARDS resembles that of pulmonary edema and aspiration pneumonitis. Patients are dyspneic, hypoxic, and hypovolemic and often require intubation and mechanical ventilation. Findings on histologic examination are similar to those of aspiration pneumonitis, with the exception

TABLE **27-22**	American-European Consensus Conference on ARDS: Recommended Criteria for Acute Lung Injury and Acute Respiratory Distress Syndrome				
Criteria	**Timing**	**Oxygenation**	**Chest Radiography**	**P Wedge**	
Acute lung injury	Acute onset	Pa_{O_2}/F_{IO_2} <300 mm Hg (regardless of PEEP level)	Bilateral infiltrates	<18 mm Hg or no clinical evidence of left atrial hypertension	
Acute respiratory distress syndrome	Acute onset	Pa_{O_2}/F_{IO_2} <200 mm Hg (regardless of PEEP level)	Bilateral infiltrates	<18 mm Hg or no clinical evidence of left atrial hypertension	

From Bernard GR et al. The American-European Consensus Conference on ARDS: definitions, mechanisms, relevant outcomes, and clinical trial coordination. Am J Respir Crit Care Med. 1994;149:818-824.
F_{IO_2}, *Fraction of inspired oxygen;* Pa_{O_2}, *partial pressure of oxygen in arterial blood; PEEP, positive end-expiratory pressure; P wedge, pulmonary capillary wedge pressure.*

BOX **27-15**

Clinical Disorders Associated with Acute Respiratory Distress Syndrome

Sepsis Trauma
Fat emboli
Lung contusion
Nonthoracic trauma

Liquid Aspiration
Gastric contents
Fresh and salt water (drowning)
Hydrocarbon fluids

Drug Associated
Heroin
Methadone
Propoxyphene
Barbiturates
Colchicine
Ethchlorvynol
Aspirin
Hydrochlorothiazide

Inhaled Toxins
Smoke
Oxygen (high concentration)
Corrosive chemicals (NO_2, Cl_2, NH_3, phosgene)

Shock from Any Cause
Hematologic disorders
Massive blood transfusion
Disseminated intravascular coagulation

Metabolic
Acute pancreatitis
Uremia

Miscellaneous
Lymphangiography
Reexpansion pulmonary edema
Increased intracranial pressure
After cardiopulmonary bypass
Eclampsia
Air emboli
Amniotic fluid embolism
Ascent to high altitude

Primary Pneumonias
Viral
Bacterial
Mycobacteria
Tuberculosis
Fungal
Pneumocystis jiroveci

From Ware LB, Matthay MA. Pulmonary edema and acute lung injury. In: George RB et al, eds. Chest Medicine: Essentials of Pulmonary and Critical Care Medicine. 5th ed. Philadelphia: Lippincott Williams & Wilkins; 2005:555.

---

that fibrosis of lung is more pronounced. Recovery of lung function is unpredictable. Milder cases resolve quickly, whereas others progress to fibrosis and death.

Treatment
Because lung infections (e.g., *P. jiroveci* pneumonia) mimic ARDS, antibiotic therapy often is initiated before the cause of respiratory failure is known. Maintaining tissue oxygenation and replacing lost intravascular fluids are the main goals of therapy. Preserving end-organ perfusion is of utmost importance. Treatment is supportive and includes correction of hypoxia,

preload and afterload reduction, and inotropic support as indicated.

Anesthetic Management
Anesthetic preparation includes evaluation of the patient's respiratory, cardiac, and renal status. Ventilator settings should be noted and special attention devoted to peak inspiratory pressures and PEEP levels. If the anesthesia ventilator cannot accommodate these settings, then arrangements must be made to bring the patient's ventilator into the operating room. The nature of lung sounds and amount of secretions should be noted.

The presence of excess secretions should alert the anesthetist to the potential risk of airway obstruction. The degree of barotrauma from prolonged mechanical ventilation with high levels of PEEP can be assessed by the presence of chest tubes and subcutaneous emphysema secondary to pneumothorax. The effectiveness of therapy with bronchodilators should be assessed, because the use of these drugs may be initiated preoperatively and continued intraoperatively if effective. An arterial line should be placed preoperatively and ABG analysis performed. If possible, lactic acid values should be determined.

Volume status should be evaluated closely because patients with ARDS often are hypovolemic. Invasive monitoring via central venous lines and pulmonary artery catheters often is available, and cardiac filling pressures along with CO values should be assessed. Patients requiring inotropic support may arrive for surgery with infusions of dopamine or dobutamine. For all procedures, renal function should be monitored with a bladder catheter. Antibiotic therapy should be continued intraoperatively, and continuation of steroid preparations should be considered if patients were receiving these medications preoperatively.

Because patients with ARDS often are hemodynamically unstable, judicious titration of anesthetic agents and adjunct agents is necessary. Owing to the multisystemic involvement characteristic of ARDS, drug metabolism and elimination should be carefully considered.

Transport should be carefully planned so that complications are minimized and safe arrival in the intensive care unit is ensured. Patients should undergo pulse oximetry, ECG, and blood pressure transport monitoring (by arterial line or noninvasively) before departure from the operating room. Breath sounds should be continually assessed with a precordial stethoscope. A full tank of O_2 and PEEP adapter valves should be available for transport. The potential need for emergency medications and a defibrillator should be considered. If the patient's ventilator needs to be returned to the intensive care unit, plans should be made so that it arrives there before the patient does. Finally, if possible, another member of the anesthesia team should accompany the patient during transport. Pulmonary dysfunction is the most common cause of postoperative complications after the administration of general anesthesia. To minimize pulmonary derangement, the anesthesia provider must identify those patients who are at risk for the development of pulmonary impairment and must have a thorough understanding of the preexisting lung dysfunction. Some common modes of positive pressure ventilation are shown in Table 27-23.

NONCYTOTOXIC AND CYTOTOXIC DRUG-INDUCED PULMONARY DISEASE

Currently, more than 100 pharmacologic agents are known to produce adverse effects on the lung parenchyma, the pleura, and the airway. Drug-induced pulmonary injury occurs in several

TABLE 27-23	Modes of Positive Pressure Ventilation	
Mode	**Description**	**Advantages and Disadvantages**
Controlled mechanical ventilation (CMV)	Ventilator f, inspiratory time, V_T (and therefore V_E) preset	May be used with sedation or paralysis; ventilator cannot respond to ventilatory needs
Assisted mechanical ventilation (AMV) or assisted-control mechanical ventilation	Ventilator V_T and inspiratory time preset, but patient can increase f (and therefore V_E)	Ventilator may respond to ventilatory needs; ventilator may undertrigger or overtrigger, depending on sensitivity
Intermittent mandatory ventilation (IMV)	Ventilator delivers preset V_T, f, and inspiratory time, but patient also may breathe spontaneously	May decrease asynchronous breathing and sedation requirements; ventilator cannot respond to ventilatory needs
Synchronized intermittent mandatory ventilation (SIMV)	Same as IMV, but ventilator breaths delivered only after patient finishes inspiration	Same as IMV, and patient not overinflated by receiving spontaneous and ventilator breaths at same time
High-frequency ventilation (HFV)	Ventilator f is increased and, V_T may be smaller than V_{DS}	May reduce peak airway pressure; may cause auto-PEEP
Pressure-support ventilation (PSV)	Patient breathes at own f; V_T determined by inspiratory pressure and CRS	Increased comfort and decreased work of breathing; ventilator cannot respond to ventilatory needs
Pressure-control ventilation (PCV)	Ventilator peak pressure, f, and respiratory time preset	Peak inspiratory pressures may be decreased; hypoventilation may occur
Inverse ratio ventilation (IRV)	Inspiratory time exceeds expiratory time to facilitate inspiration	May improve gas exchange by increasing time spent in inspiration; may cause auto-PEEP
Airway pressure release ventilation (APRV)	Patient receives CPAP at high and low levels to stimulate V_T	May improve oxygenation at lower airway pressure; hypoventilation may occur
Proportional assist ventilation (PAV)	Patient determines own f, V_T, pressures, and flows	May amplify spontaneous breathing; depends entirely on patient's respiratory drive

Modified from Goldman L, Ausiello D, eds. Cecil Textbook of Medicine. 22nd ed. Philadelphia: Saunders; 2004:604.
CPAP, *Continuous positive airway pressure;* CRS, *respiratory system compliance;* f, *respiratory rate;* PEEP, *positive end-expiratory pressure;* V_{DS}, *volume of dead space;* V_E, *minute ventilation;* V_T, *tidal volume.*

hundred thousand people each year in the United States. Knowledge of doses and the potential adverse effects of the prescribed medications may prevent or minimize drug-induced damage.

Mechanism

The mechanism of drug-induced pulmonary injury is not well defined. It has been shown that cytotoxic drugs used in the treatment of cancer cause pulmonary insult by a combination of the direct toxic effects of a drug or its metabolite and of their indirect effects—that is, the enhancement of inflammation or immune processes. The clinical features produced by different cytotoxic agents are similar, but chronic pneumonitis and fibrosis are the most commonly associated clinical syndromes. Box 27-16 lists various chemotherapeutic agents that may produce pulmonary toxicity. The pathogenesis of pulmonary toxicity is uncertain but has been found to include disruption of the endothelial cells and changes in calcium homeostasis that lead to toxic injury. The mechanisms of drug-induced pulmonary injury associated with noncytotoxic drugs are less well defined but may involve changes in pulmonary homeostasis. Noncytotoxic agents can induce the development of numerous clinical syndromes. Several commonly implicated agents are discussed in the following sections.

Noncytotoxic Drug-Induced Pulmonary Disease
Drugs Used in Treatment

Amiodarone. Amiodarone (Cordarone) is a potent and effective agent used primarily in the long-term management of refractory, life-threatening arrhythmias—predominantly ventricular tachycardia and fibrillation. Despite its therapeutic benefits, it is considered to be the drug of last resort because of the numerous

adverse effects with which it is associated—in particular, severe pulmonary toxicity.[193] Acute administration is common during life-support protocols for arrhythmias. Toxicity is rare when given acutely.

Pulmonary complications associated with amiodarone therapy are reported to occur in no patients to 61% of patients and are associated with an estimated mortality rate of 1% to 33%; however, patients with pulmonary complications usually have concomitant cardiac disease. Amiodarone has been found to accumulate in the lung. Kachel and associates have shown that α-tocopherol, a naturally existing antioxidant, offers protection against the effects of amiodarone.[194] According to Dusman and associates, clinical diagnosis of amiodarone-induced pulmonary toxicity is based on the presence of two or more of the following signs and symptoms:

1. New onset of pulmonary symptoms such as dyspnea, cough, or pleuritic chest pain
2. Detection of new chest radiographic abnormalities such as an interstitial or alveolar infiltrate
3. A decrease in D_{LCO} of 20% from the pretreatment value; if no pretreatment values are available, then a value equal to less than 80% of the predicted value
4. Abnormal gallium-67 uptake by the lungs
5. Characteristic histologic changes of lung tissue obtained by bronchoscopic or open-lung biopsy[195]

Two syndromes of amiodarone-induced pulmonary toxicity are recognized. The more common syndrome is characterized by an insidious onset with nonproductive cough, dyspnea, weight loss, and occasional fever. Hypoxemia is common. Chest radiographs demonstrate parenchymal infiltrates with a predominant diffuse interstitial pattern that may progress to fibrosis. Pleural thickening and effusions also have been reported.

BOX 27-16

Classification of Drug-Induced and Related Pulmonary Diseases by Type of Medication

Chemotherapeutic		Analgesic	Intravenous
Cytotoxic	Gemcitabine	**Analgesic**	**Intravenous**
Azathioprine inhibitors	Methotrexate*	Heroin*	Blood*
Bleomycin*	Procarbazine*	Methadone*	Ethanolamide Maolate
Busulfan		Naloxone*	(sodium morrhuate)*
Chlorambucil	**Antibiotic**	Placidyl*	Ethiodized oil
Cyclophosphamide	Amphotericin B*	Propoxyphene*	(lymphangiogram)
Etoposide	Nitrofurantoin	Salicylates*	Talc
Interleukin-2	Acute*		
Melphalan	Chronic	**Cardiovascular**	**Miscellaneous**
Mitomycin C*	Sulfasalazine	Amiodarone*	Appetite suppressants
Nitrosamines		Angiotensin-converting enzyme	Bromocriptine
Procarbazine	**Antiinflammatory**	Anticoagulants	Dantrolene
Tumor necrosis factor	Acetylsalicylic acid*	β-Blockers*	Hydrochlorothiazide*
Vinblastine	Gold	Dipyridamole	Methysergide
Zinostatin	Interferons	Flecainide	Tocolytic agents*
	Leukotriene antagonists	Protamine*	Tricyclics*
Noncytotoxic	Methotrexate	Tocainide	l-Tryptophan
Bleomycin*	Nonsteroidal		Radiation
Cytosine arabinoside*	antiinflammatory agents	**Inhalant**	Systemic lupus erythematosus
	Penicillamine	Aspirated oil	(drug induced)
		Oxygen	Complement-mediated
			leukostasis*

Modified from Murray JF, Nadel JA. Textbook of Respiratory Medicine. 4th ed. Philadelphia: Saunders; 2005:1889.
*Typically manifests as acute or subacute respiratory insufficiency.

Onset usually occurs after 2 months and with a dose of 400 mg/day or greater.[193] Case reports have shown favorable responses with and without the use of corticosteroids.[196]

The second syndrome has a more acute or explosive onset and accounts for 25% to 33% of cases. Presenting signs include rapidly progressive dyspnea, high fever, and hypoxemia. Chest radiographs show a predominant alveolar pattern with a patchy distribution that often involves the peripheral areas of the lung. The acute form is associated with a higher mortality rate than the insidious form, and prompt recognition and treatment are essential for a favorable recovery.

Pulmonary function tests performed at the onset of pulmonary toxicity reveal abnormalities typical of restrictive lung disease. Findings include a decrease in FVC and TLC, an elevation in FEV_1/FVC, and diffusion abnormalities.[195]

Therapeutic options are limited. Drug withdrawal is mandatory. Resolution is gradual because the drug's half-life is approximately 40 to 70 days; therefore, serum and tissue levels of amiodarone are measurable long after discontinuation of therapy. Radiographic clearing occurs within 2 months. However, as signs and symptoms of pulmonary toxicity abate, so does the therapeutic benefit. The underlying arrhythmia commonly returns during the same period. At times, reduction of the dose may be successful in decreasing toxicity while control of the dysrhythmia is maintained. This strategy may be the only option. The impression that corticosteroids are efficacious in this syndrome is unsubstantiated.

Gold. The administration of gold salts is common in the treatment of rheumatoid arthritis. Unfortunately, their use has been implicated in the development of hypersensitivity lung disease, interstitial pneumonitis, and pulmonary fibrosis.[197] The incidence of pulmonary insult occurs in fewer than 1% of patients who receive gold therapy. Several possible mechanisms of injury have been proposed, but none has been proved. Symptoms may occur as early as 6 hours to 1 month after administration of the last dose of gold salts, and they usually are seen within 4 months after the initiation of therapy. Rarely the presentation may be acute and characterized by fever, wheezing, and cough. More commonly it is insidious and manifested by progressive dyspnea and nonproductive cough. Fever and eosinophilia are present in 40% and 33% of patients, respectively.[196] Although chest radiography demonstrates the presence of an interstitial process, this process may predominate in the upper lung zones. Pulmonary function abnormalities show a restrictive ventilatory defect and impairment of diffusion. Discontinuation of therapy with gold salts after their causal role has been suspected is the most important treatment measure. Corticosteroids have been used with equivocal results.

Cytotoxic Drug-Induced Pulmonary Disease

Three clinical syndromes are associated with cytotoxic drug-induced pulmonary injury: (1) chronic pneumonitis and fibrosis, (2) acute hypersensitivity lung disease, and (3) noncardiogenic pulmonary edema.[193] These syndromes may coexist.

Chronic Pneumonitis and Fibrosis

Interstitial pneumonitis and fibrosis is the most frequently encountered pattern in drug-induced pulmonary injury. The mechanism of injury is a direct cytotoxic effect of a drug or its metabolites on the endothelial, interstitial, or alveolar epithelial cells. On lung parenchyma, the cytotoxic effect elicits an inflammatory response characterized by the proliferation of macrophages, lymphocytes, and other inflammatory cells. This inflammatory response leads to the deposition of fibrin within the alveoli, which produces interstitial inflammation and fibrosis.

Interstitial pneumonitis can be classified as acute, subacute, or chronic; the chronic form is the most frequently encountered. Common manifestations of these subgroups include dyspnea, dry cough, low-grade fever, fatigue, and malaise that develop over several weeks to months. Chest radiography demonstrates diffuse interstitial infiltrates. Bleomycin is the causative agent most frequently implicated in interstitial pneumonitis. Treatment includes discontinuation of the offending agent with or without institution of corticosteroid therapy; prognosis is variable.

Syndrome of Hypersensitivity Lung Disease

Hypersensitivity lung disease has been associated with the cytotoxic agents bleomycin, methotrexate, L-asparaginase, and procarbazine. Common pulmonary manifestations include a nonproductive cough, dyspnea, and chest pain. The systemic allergic response is manifested as fever, urticaria, arthralgias, hypotension, and eosinophilia. Chest radiography may reveal pneumonitis, pleuritis, and pleural effusion. Suspicion of a hypersensitivity drug reaction should be followed by prompt withdrawal of the agent. Corticosteroid use may or may not be indicated, and prognosis is generally favorable.

Noncardiogenic Pulmonary Edema

The development of noncardiogenic pulmonary edema is an acute but rare phenomenon that occurs after the administration of some antineoplastic agents. Cytotoxic drugs that contribute to its development include methotrexate, cytosine arabinoside (cytarabine), and cyclophosphamide. One major difference between the noncardiogenic pulmonary edema caused by cytotoxic agents and that produced by noncytotoxic ones is prognosis. The latter form usually is fully reversible on discontinuation of the offending agent. Patients with cytotoxic pulmonary insult have a variable prognosis, and survivors may show residual pulmonary dysfunction.

Numerous pharmacologic agents used in the treatment of cancer have been implicated in the development of toxic pulmonary side effects. The agents most commonly implicated in pulmonary insult include bleomycin, busulfan, carmustine, and methotrexate. Pulmonary toxicity in the use of antineoplastic agents is defined as the development of clinical signs and symptoms of pulmonary distress that were not present during the pretreatment studies. The prevalence of diffuse pulmonary infiltration occurring as a result of drug toxicity is reported to be as high as 20%.

Agents Implicated in Pulmonary Insult

Bleomycin. Bleomycin, an antitumor antibiotic, is the most common chemotherapeutically induced potentiator of pulmonary injury. It is used primarily in the treatment of lymphomas, testicular tumors, and squamous cell carcinomas of the head and neck. Despite the benefits of bleomycin therapy, the development of pulmonary toxicity is the limiting factor of its use.[198]

The most common adverse effect of bleomycin is the development of interstitial fibrosis. The incidence of pulmonary fibrosis is approximately 20%, with a 1% mortality rate. Anesthesia-related problems occur postoperatively and are associated with exposure to high O_2 concentrations. Those factors associated with an increased risk for bleomycin-related pulmonary toxicity include the following:

1. Therapy with a cumulative dose greater than 450 to 500 mg; however, cases of pulmonary toxicity occurring with doses of 100 mg have been well documented
2. Prior or concomitant irradiation to the thorax, which increases the incidence of toxicity to 35% to 55% and the mortality rate to more than 50%
3. Age greater than 70 years
4. Smoking, which increases the release of hydrogen peroxide and other reactive oxidative metabolites into the surrounding lung tissue, potentiating impairment of respiratory function
5. Treatment with multiple antineoplastic agents, especially cyclophosphamide
6. Hyperoxia and retention of carbon monoxide

Because bleomycin is predominantly excreted via the kidneys, impairment of renal function impedes the rate of elimination and may contribute to injury.

Concentration of bleomycin is preferentially in the skin, causing ulcerations. In the lungs it produces interstitial fibrosis. The cause o the adverse pulmonary effects induced by bleomycin is thought to be the generation of reactive oxidative metabolites. Pulmonary damage appears in two clinical syndromes: acute and chronic. The acute pattern is rare and occurs with lower doses of bleomycin.[199] The chronic form is more common; its severity is related to dose, and it develops within weeks to months of the initiation of therapy. Approximately 15% of patients who receive a cumulative dose greater than 450 mg develop clinical pulmonary dysfunction.[193]

Symptoms of toxicity initially include a dry hacking cough and dyspnea on exertion. Progression of lung disease is associated with dyspnea at rest, tachypnea, fever, and cyanosis. Changes on chest radiography usually occur later and manifest as bibasilar reticular infiltrates that may progress to frank consolidation.

Several investigators have suggested that patients undergoing general anesthesia who have a concurrent history of bleomycin therapy should receive the lowest possible O_2 concentrations that allow maintenance of adequate Po_2.[200,201] They also have suggested that excessive administration of crystalloid solutions be avoided, but data that demonstrate the superiority of colloid solution administration in these patients are unavailable. Treatment is supportive therapy and discontinuation of bleomycin treatment. The use of steroids has been effective in some patients. Prognosis for these patients is poor.[199]

Anesthetic Management of Bleomycin-Treated Patients. Although universally accepted guidelines for the management of bleomycin-treated patient undergoing general anesthesia are lacking, the following suggestions have been made:

1. O_2 saturation should be monitored continuously and ABG analysis performed intermittently.
2. Immediately before anesthesia, 100% O_2 should be administered for 1 to 4 minutes.
3. After induction, a target Pao_2 should be chosen and the Fio_2 maintained at the lowest level that allows adequate oxygenation.
4. The use of PEEP should be considered.
5. Crystalloid solutions should be administered carefully and the use of colloid solutions considered if large fluid volumes are required.
6. The patient should be informed of the possible need for postoperative ventilation.
7. Postoperatively the Fio_2 should be kept at the lowest possible setting that maintains the target Pao_2.

The choice of anesthetic technique varies, but as with all surgical procedures, careful evaluation and management are essential. There are no reports suggesting the superiority of regional anesthesia in patients treated with bleomycin.

Methotrexate. Methotrexate is an analog of folic acid that inhibits cellular reproduction by causing an acute intracellular deficiency of folate coenzymes. Methotrexate is used in the treatment of malignant and benign conditions, including leukemia, osteogenic sarcoma, choriocarcinoma, polymyositis, psoriasis, and connective tissue disorders (particularly rheumatoid arthritis). Regardless of the route of administration, pulmonary toxicity has been reported to occur with all forms of delivery, with an incidence of 7.6%. Clinically, the onset of pulmonary dysfunction may be chronic, but more commonly it is acute. Several cases of acute noncardiogenic pulmonary edema have been reported after intrathecal administration. The majority of reported methotrexate-induced pulmonary reactions occur in children with acute lymphocytic leukemia. The syndrome often develops over 7 to 14 days and is characterized by fever, dry cough, dyspnea, hypoxemia, and bilateral pulmonary infiltrates. Improvement may begin 10 to14 days after onset.

No precipitating factors—including age, total dose, duration of therapy, and underlying disease—have been conclusively implicated. In addition, no injury has been reported in individuals receiving less than 20 mg of methotrexate per week.[200]

The mechanism of pulmonary injury in humans is consistent with a hypersensitivity response and includes the presence of fever, eosinophilia, and occasionally granuloma and multinucleated giant cells in histopathologic specimens. Cytologic examination of bronchoalveolar lavage specimens reveals a lymphocytic alveolitis with a disproportionately high ratio of helper T lymphocytes to suppressor T lymphocytes, which suggests the presence of an immunologic disorder.[201]

As with injury by most agents that have toxic effects, the earlier the response is identified, the more likely it is that the damage will resolve fully. Treatment consists of the withdrawal of methotrexate. Corticosteroid use may be advantageous in severe cases.[200,201] Despite a mortality rate of 1%, the majority of patients return to their pretreatment status.

PULMONARY OXYGEN TOXICITY

Etiology

The administration of O_2 for the treatment of hypoxemia is a common practice. As with all prescribed drugs, the risks of the adverse effects of O_2 administration must be considered, despite its beneficial effects. The prolonged use of high concentrations of O_2 (greater than 50% for longer than 24 hours) is potentially toxic and may result in irreversible lung damage.[199] Injury to the lung affects the upper airways mildly; the predominant damage occurs in the lower respiratory tract, particularly in the alveolar structures.[200,202] The rate of development of O_2 toxicity is directly related to the partial pressure of inspired O_2.[201]

Normobaric hyperoxia can result in four clinical syndromes: (1) acute tracheobronchitis, (2) absorption atelectasis, (3) acute alveolar lung injury (ARDS), and (4) bronchopulmonary dysplasia.[201] When nitrogen is replaced with O_2, absorption atelectasis occurs in the alveoli that are poorly ventilated. The loss of the so-called "nitrogen splint" promotes alveolar collapse.

Pathophysiology

The pathogenesis of pulmonary O_2 toxicity is linked to the excessive production of free O_2 radicals. Free radicals are molecules that contain one or more unpaired electrons.[201] Free radicals are highly reactive metabolites of O_2 (e.g., superoxide anion, hydrogen peroxide, and hydroxyl radical) that overwhelm antioxidant systems, including cellular enzymatic defenses (superoxide dismutase, catalase, glutathione peroxidase) and nonenzymatic scavengers (α-tocopherol acetate). Free radicals exert their toxic effect on cell and organelle membranes; they interfere with vital cellular functions, causing inactivation of enzymes and transport proteins, membrane lipid peroxidation, and inhibition of cell growth and division.[203]

Five common risk factors have been described in the development of O_2 toxicity. First is an increased propensity for toxicity with use of increasing concentrations. This cumulative dose effect also has been noted with the use of the antineoplastic agents bleomycin, busulfan, and carmustine. The second risk factor is age. As an individual ages, a decrease in the antioxidant defense system may occur. Bleomycin and methotrexate administration in the elderly augments the risk of pulmonary toxicity. The third risk factor is previous or concurrent radiotherapy to the thorax. The production of superoxides secondary to gamma irradiation is believed to cause a synergistic reaction with bleomycin, busulfan, and mitomycin. The fourth factor is O_2 therapy concurrent with the use of various chemotherapeutic agents. Cytotoxic chemicals such as bleomycin, cyclophosphamide, and mitomycin either alter antioxidant defense mechanisms or generate oxidants, causing further pulmonary insult. The fifth factor is use of a combination chemotherapy regimen. Agents associated with an increased likelihood of lung damage include carmustine, mitomycin, cyclophosphamide, bleomycin, and methotrexate.

Pulmonary injury induced by hyperoxia has two phases: exudative and proliferative.[203] The exudative or acute phase is characterized by injury to alveolar type I cells and capillary endothelial cells; this injury increases the permeability of membranes to water, electrolytes, and proteins. Progression of damage causes interstitial and alveolar edema and alveolar hemorrhage, which are consistent with noncardiogenic pulmonary edema. These events of pulmonary insult usually occur within 24 to 72 hours, depending on the concentration and duration of hyperoxia. The proliferative or chronic phase is characterized by hyperplasia of alveolar type II cells, deposition of collagen and elastin in the interstitium, and the formation of hyaline membrane. Eventually, interstitial fibrosis develops.

Clinical Features and Diagnosis

The earliest manifestations are related to the effects on the tracheobronchial mucosa (Table 27-24). Symptoms may occur after 6 hours of O_2 exposure and include substernal chest pain that is prominent with inspiration, tachypnea, and a nonproductive cough. By 24 hours, paresthesia, anorexia, nausea, and headache occur. Physiologic changes include a decrease in tracheal mucous velocity, VC, pulmonary compliance, and diffusing capacity and increased $PAO_2 - PaO_2$. Some individuals develop signs of mild airway obstruction. Chest radiography demonstrates an alveolar and interstitial pattern. Respiratory failure and death ensue if O_2 poisoning persists.

Management

Both hyperoxia and hypoxemia have undesirable effects. Therefore, deciding whether to administer O_2 requires mature clinical judgment. The goal is to deliver the lowest level of FIO_2 needed for maintaining adequate arterial O_2 saturation (generally, a PaO_2 of >90 mm Hg, as determined by ABG analysis).

TABLE 27-24	Sequence of Pulmonary Changes During Hyperoxic Exposure in Humans	
O_2 at 1 atm	**Exposure Duration**	**Manifestation**
100%	>12 hr	Decreased tracheobronchial clearance; decreased forced vital capacity; cough; chest pain
	>24 hr	Altered endothelial function
	>36 hr	Increased alveolar-arterial oxygen gradient; decreased carbon monoxide diffusing capacity
	>48 hr	Increasing alveolar permeability; pulmonary edema; surfactant inactivation
	>60 hr	Acute respiratory distress syndrome
60%	7 days	Mild chest discomfort without changes in lung mechanics; possible changes in morphometry
24%-28%	Months	Subclinical pathologic changes; no clinical toxicity documented

From Beers ME. Oxygen therapy and pulmonary oxygen toxicity. In: Fishman AP, ed. Fishman's Pulmonary Disease and Disorders. New York: McGraw-Hill; 2008:2627.

Measures such as PEEP should be used for decreasing the need for high FIO_2. Corticosteroid therapy reduces antioxidant enzyme activity and may be useful during the exudative phase.

AUTOIMMUNE DISORDERS

Autoimmune diseases, connective tissue diseases, collagenosis, and rheumatologic diseases are terms used interchangeably in clinical medicine. These entities are frequently characterized by multiple-organ involvement and inflammation. On the whole, these disorders have unknown causes; however, the inflammatory process is immunologically mediated, as evidenced by the presence of autoantibodies, rheumatoid factor, and immune complexes, as well as by elevation of the sedimentation rate and the observation of certain clinical characteristics. Pulmonary manifestations are common and often assume a major role in the disease process. Characteristic restrictive lung changes may result if pulmonary impairment is sufficiently severe. Box 27-17 lists pulmonary manifestations of various collagen vascular diseases.

Sarcoidosis

Sarcoidosis is a multisystemic disorder characterized by the presence of noncaseating epithelioid-cell granulomata. It is described as an intense interaction of activated lymphocytes and macrophages that results in tissue injury. The disease most frequently involves the lungs, reticuloendothelial system, skin, eyes, and myocardium. The prevalence of disease in the United States is 10 to 40 persons per 100,000, with blacks being more commonly

BOX 27-17

Pulmonary Manifestations of Some Collagen Vascular Diseases

Rheumatoid Arthritis
Pleural disease (effusions)
Diffuse interstitial pneumonitis
Necrobiotic nodules
Caplan syndrome
Pulmonary hypertension (arteritis)
Apical fibrobullous disease
Bronchiolitis obliterans with and without organizing pneumonia
Cricoarytenoid arthritis

Systemic Lupus Erythematosus
Pleural disease (pleuritis, effusions)
Atelectasis
Acute lupus pneumonitis
Diffuse interstitial lung disease
Pulmonary hemorrhage
Respiratory muscle dysfunction

Progressive Systemic Sclerosis
Diffuse interstitial fibrosis
Pulmonary vascular disease
Aspiration pneumonia
Chest-wall restrictions secondary to thoracic skin sclerosis
Pleural disease

Polymyositis—Dermatomyositis
Interstitial pneumonitis
Aspiration pneumonia
Respiratory myositis
Pulmonary hypertension
Bronchiolitis obliterans organizing pneumonia

Mixed Connective Tissue Disease
Diffuse interstitial lung disease
Pulmonary hypertension (vasculitis)
Pleural disease
Diaphragmatic muscle dysfunction

Sjögren Syndrome
Respiratory mucosal dryness
Pleurisy
Chronic airway disease
Lymphocytic interstitial pneumonia
Pseudolymphoma
Lymphoma
Amyloid
Pulmonary hypertension (vasculitis)

damage. Pulmonary involvement is primarily in regions rich in lymphatic vessels, such as the subpleural, perivascular, and peribronchial areas. Frequently, adjacent nonspecific inflammatory changes as well as alveolitis with cellular infiltrates are noted.[205]

Parenchymal infiltration and fibrosis result in a decrease in lung compliance, impairment of diffusing capacity, and a reduction in lung volumes. Many patients exhibit a reduced FEV_1/FVC and increased airway resistance. $\dot{V}/\dot{Q}$ imbalance and an increase in Pao_2 occur in response to a nonuniform decrease in lung compliance. An obstructive pattern resulting from endobronchial disease or peribronchial fibrosis may occur simultaneously. Cor pulmonale may develop in the presence of severe pulmonary fibrosis. Clinical presentation is varied and may be categorized as asymptomatic (occurring in 20% of individuals investigated and based on the detection of abnormality of chest radiography) or symptomatic (characterized by nonspecific features ranging from fever, fatigue, anorexia, weight loss, chills, and night sweats to dyspnea and blindness).

The lung is the most commonly affected organ, with pulmonary involvement occurring in more than 90% of individuals with sarcoidosis. Respiratory symptoms are those typical of interstitial involvement and include dyspnea, dry cough, and retrosternal chest pain (35% to 50% of patients). Less common symptoms include wheezing, hemoptysis, pleural effusion, and clubbing of the fingers. Sarcoidosis is one of the few chest diseases that concurrently involve lymph nodes in the lung (hilar) and the mediastinum.[206] On radiography, intrathoracic involvement has been classified into three categories. Stage I is characterized by bilateral, symmetric, hilar adenopathy; stage II by hilar adenopathy and diffuse pulmonary changes; and stage III by diffuse pulmonary infiltrates without adenopathy. Stage I is associated with the most favorable prognosis, and stage III with the worst.

The distribution of extrathoracic involvement is as follows: peripheral lymphatic, 50% to 75%; skin, 25% to 70%; liver, 60% to 80%; eye, 25%; spleen, 20% to 30%; bone, 1% to 35%; salivary glands, 5%; heart, 5%; nervous system, 5%. Laryngeal involvement occurs in 1% to 5% of patients and may make insertion of an adult-sized tracheal tube difficult.[207] In patients with diffuse pulmonary involvement, a transbronchial approach that includes fiberoptic bronchoscopy is the procedure of choice.[206]

The diagnosis of sarcoidosis is typically based on the presence of a combination of clinical, radiographic, and histologic criteria, as follows: (1) a compatible clinical or radiologic picture; (2) the presence of noncaseating granulomas; and (3) negative results on bacterial and fungal studies of biopsied tissue and sputum. The overall prognosis in sarcoidosis is good. The acute onset usually is followed by a self-limiting course of approximately 2 years' duration with spontaneous resolution; sarcoidosis of insidious onset may be followed by progressive disease characterized by pulmonary fibrosis.[208] Approximately 15% to 20% of cases remain active or recur. Treatment with corticosteroids is frequently used and produces relief of symptoms, clinical remissions, and suppression of inflammation and granuloma formation. Conversely, because spontaneous and permanent remissions occur in 50% of patients, the use of corticosteroids in these individuals is controversial. Pulmonary disease is the most frequent indication for corticosteroid therapy in systemic disease.[209] Other treatment options include the use of antiinflammatory agents, antimalarials, radiation therapy, and immune system–modulating drugs.[210]

The mortality rate for patients with sarcoidosis after 5 years is approximately 4% to 10% and is attributed to respiratory failure,

affected than whites (12:1 ratio). In whites the distribution among men and women is equal; in blacks, however, the female-to-male ratio is 2:1. The disease predominantly occurs in those aged 20 to 40 years.[204] The cause of sarcoidosis is unclear; no organic or inorganic causative agent has been consistently found. The route of transmission also is uncertain.

Most sarcoid granulomata resolve spontaneously, leaving no scar. Others persist for a longer duration, with little or no fibrosis, and still others become hyalinized, fibrotic areas that cause tissue azotemia from renal injury caused by chronic hypercalciuria, cardiac arrest resulting from myocardial involvement, and massive hemoptysis due to colonization of bullae by *Aspergillus fumigatus*.

FLAIL CHEST

Flail chest, a condition that results from chest trauma and multiple rib fractures, is reported to occur in 5% of patients who sustain thoracic injury (Figure 27-18).[211] The hallmark of flail chest is paradoxical movement of the chest wall at the site of the fracture. During inspiration, the chest wall is drawn inward, owing to the negative intrathoracic pressure; its outward movement during expiration occurs when the intrathoracic pressure increases above atmospheric pressure (Figure 27-19). Inefficient lung inflation caused by rib fracture and paradoxical breathing limits alveolar ventilation and may progress to hypoventilation,

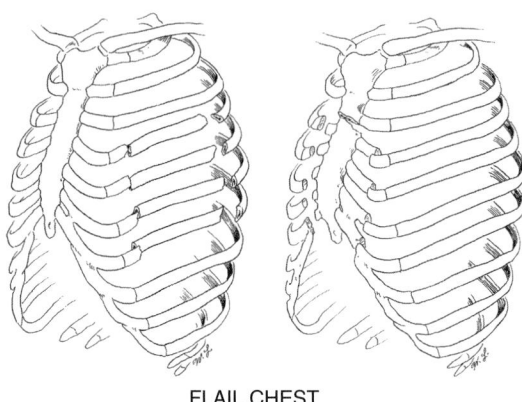

FLAIL CHEST

FIGURE **27-18** Fracture of several adjacent ribs in two places with lateral flail or central flail segments. (*Redrawn from Eckstein M et al. Thorax. In: Marx JA et al, eds. Rosen's Emergency Medicine: Concepts and Clinical Practice. 6th ed. St Louis: Mosby; 2006:457.*)

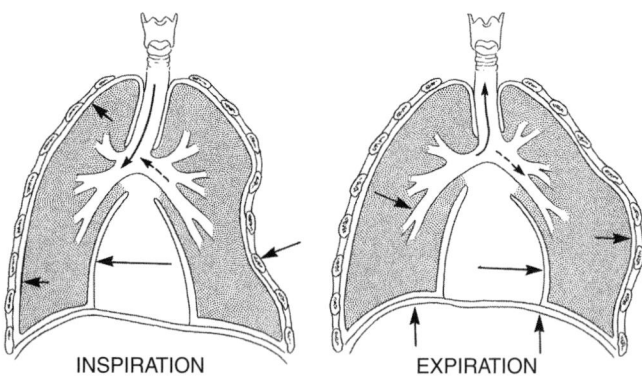

INSPIRATION   EXPIRATION

FIGURE **27-19** Flail chest: Paradoxical respiration. On inspiration, flail section sinks in as chest expands, impairing ability to produce negative intrapleural pressure to draw in air. Mediastinum shifts to uninjured side. On expiration, flail segment bulges outward, impairing ability to exhale. Mediastinum shifts to injured side. Air may shift uselessly from side to side in severe flail chest (*broken arrows*). (*Redrawn from Eckstein M et al. Thorax. In: Marx JA et al, eds. Rosen's Emergency Medicine: Concepts and Clinical Practice. 5th ed. St Louis: Mosby; 2002:389.*)

hypercapnia, and progressive alveolar collapse.[212] Treatment includes pain control with measures such as intercostal nerve block with a local anesthetic or insertion of an epidural catheter with a local anesthetic or a narcotic; incentive spirometry to reduce the risk of atelectasis; and in severe cases, tracheal intubation with mechanical ventilation and PEEP (Box 27-18). Ventilator settings are adjusted so that wide swings in pleural pressure are decreased or avoided. Surgical fixation of the rib cage may be indicated in some patients. The mortality rate is directly related to the underlying and associated injuries and is reported to be between 8% and 35%.[211]

PNEUMOTHORAX

Pneumothorax can be subdivided into three categories, depending on whether air has direct access to the pleural cavity.

Simple Pneumothorax

In simple pneumothorax, no communication exists with the atmosphere (Figure 27-20). Additionally, no shift of the mediastinum or hemidiaphragm results from the accumulation of air in the intrapleural space. The severity of pneumothorax is graded on the basis of the degree of collapse: collapse of 15% or less is small; collapse of 15% to 60% is moderate; and collapse of greater than 60% is large. Treatment of a simple pneumothorax is determined by the size and cause of injury and may include catheter aspiration or tube thoracostomy; close observation of the patient with simple pneumothorax is essential.

Communicating Pneumothorax

In communicating pneumothorax, air in the pleural cavity exchanges with atmospheric air through a defect in the chest wall (Figure 27-21). Because the exchange of air may often be heard through the site of injury, this entity is commonly known as a "sucking chest wound." Communicating pneumothorax represents a severe ventilatory disturbance because the affected lung collapses on inspiration and expands slightly on expiration. The exchange of air in and out of the wound results in a large functional dead space and a decrease in the efficacy of ventilation.

The wound should be covered with an occlusive dressing immediately. Development of tension pneumothorax is possible (see next section). The injury should never be packed during inspiration, because the negative pressure could suck the dressing into the chest cavity. Treatment measures include administration

---

BOX 27-18

Indications for Treatment of Flail Chest with Mechanical Ventilation

Respiratory Failure Manifested by One or More of the Following Criteria:
Clinical signs of respiratory fatigue
Respiratory rate >35/min or <8 min
Pa_{O_2} <60 mm Hg at Fi_{O_2} ≥0.5
Pa_{CO_2} <55 mm Hg at Fi_{O_2} ≥0.5
Alveolar-arterial oxygen gradient >450
Clinical evidence of severe shock
Associated severe head injury with lack of airway control or need to ventilate
Severe associated injury necessitating surgery

of supplemental O_2, tube thoracostomy, and intubation; mechanical ventilation may be indicated.

Tension Pneumothorax

Tension pneumothorax develops when air progressively accumulates under pressure within the pleural cavity (Figure 27-22). If the pressure becomes too great, the mediastinum shifts to the opposite hemithorax, and this causes compression of the contralateral lung and great vessels. Subsequently venous return is decreased, and air enters the pleural space but cannot exit. Respiratory and cardiac disturbances ensue, exhibited by a decrease in CO, a decrease in blood pressure, an increase in CVP, and a shunting of blood to nonventilated areas. The hallmark signs of tension pneumothorax are hypotension, hypoxemia, tachycardia, increased CVP, and increased airway pressure. Other findings include absence of breath sounds on the affected side, asymmetric chest wall movement, tracheal shift, displacement of the cardiac impulse, and hyperresonance to percussion in the affected hemithorax. Also, the patient may exhibit extreme anxiety.

Tension pneumothorax is potentially lethal; therefore, immediate treatment is essential. Decompression of the chest can be performed with the insertion of a 16- or 18-gauge angiocatheter into the second or third interspace anteriorly or the fourth or fifth interspace laterally. A rush of air is heard when decompression occurs. The angiocatheter must be covered if the sucking of more air into the pleura is to be prevented.

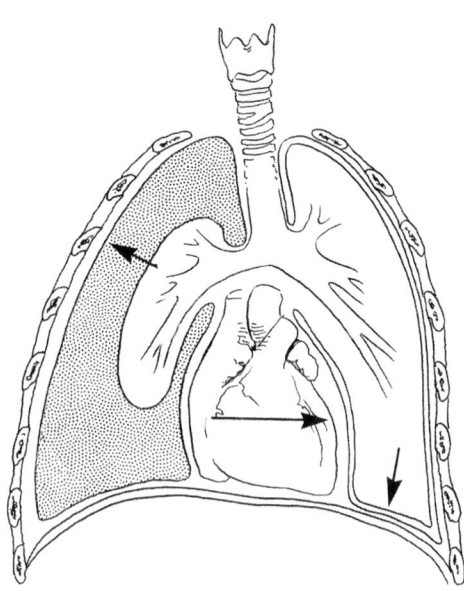

FIGURE **27-20** Closed pneumothorax. Simple pneumothorax is present in the right lung, with air in the pleural cavity and collapse of right lung. (*Redrawn from Eckstein M et al. Thorax. In: Marx JA et al, eds. Rosen's Emergency Medicine: Concepts and Clinical Practice. 6th ed. St Louis: Mosby; 2006:461.*)

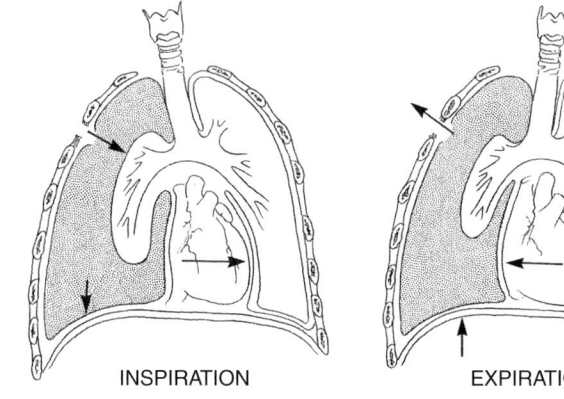

INSPIRATION   EXPIRATION

FIGURE **27-21** Communicating pneumothorax. The right lung has collapsed, and air is present in the pleural cavity, with communication to the outside through the defect in the chest wall. In sucking chest wounds, lung volume is greater with expiration. (*Redrawn from Eckstein M et al. Thorax. In: Marx JA et al, eds. Rosen's Emergency Medicine: Concepts and Clinical Practice. 6th ed. St Louis: Mosby; 2006:462.*)

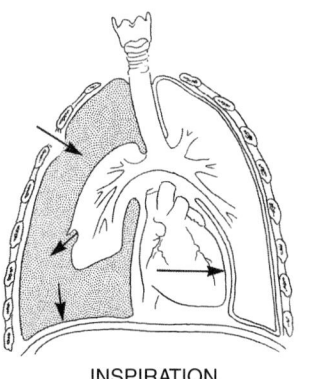
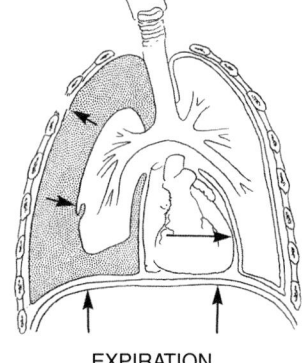

INSPIRATION   EXPIRATION

FIGURE **27-22** Tension pneumothorax. Shown are right pneumothorax under tension, total collapse of right lung, and shift of mediastinal structures to left. (*Redrawn from Eckstein M et al. Thoracic trauma. In: Marx JA et al, eds. Rosen's Emergency Medicine: Concepts and Clinical Practice. 6th ed. St Louis: Mosby; 2006:463.*)

Hemothorax

A hemothorax is the accumulation of blood in the pleural cavity. It usually is a result of trauma (Figure 27-23), but other causes include the rupture of small blood vessels in the presence of inflammation, pneumonia, tuberculosis, or erosion by tumors.

The treatment of hemothorax consists of airway management as necessary, restoration of circulating blood volume, and evacuation of the accumulated blood. Thoracostomy may be indicated if the initial bleeding rate is greater than 20 mL/kg/hr. If bleeding subsides but its rate remains greater than 7 mL/kg/hr, if chest radiograph worsens, or if hypotension persists after initial blood replacement and decompression, thoracostomy is indicated.

Pathogenesis

Different presentations may be distinguished, according to the mechanism of injury.

Spontaneous. Hemothorax usually is caused by rupture of alveoli near the pleural surface of the lung after a forceful sneeze or cough. This mechanism is most common in individuals with a long narrow chest and in those with emphysema.

Traumatic. Hemothorax, pneumothorax, and flail chest may occur after blunt chest trauma; however, they most frequently occur after rib fracture. Hemopneumothorax also may occur with penetrating injury.

Iatrogenic. Hemothorax, pneumothorax, and flail chest may occur after any of the following:

1. Subclavian central line insertion (incidence 2% to 16%)
2. Supraclavicular block to the brachial plexus (incidence 1%; hemothorax, pneumothorax, and flail chest can be complications of interscalene block but are rare with intercostal block)
3. Barotrauma (resulting from overdistention of the alveoli by PEEP; abrupt deterioration of Pa_{O_2} and cardiovascular function during PEEP administration should arouse suspicion of pulmonary barotrauma, especially pneumothorax)
4. Exposure to high airway pressures (e.g., during mechanical ventilation)
5. Other surgical procedures (e.g., mediastinoscopy, radical neck dissection, mastectomy, or nephrectomy)

Nitrous Oxide and Pneumothorax

The blood-gas partition coefficient of N_2O (0.47) is 34 times greater than that of nitrogen (0.014). This differential solubility

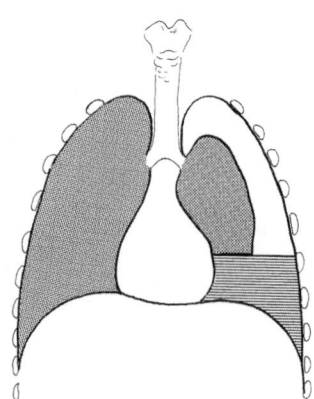

FIGURE **27-23** Hemopneumothorax. Note that the fluid level produces a straight line as opposed to a meniscus when pneumothorax is present with the pleural fluid. (*From Roberts RR, Hedges JR, eds. Clinical Procedures in Emergency Medicine. 2nd ed. Philadelphia: Saunders; 1991:129.*)

means than N_2O can leave the blood to enter an air-filled cavity 34 times more rapidly than nitrogen can leave the cavity and enter the blood. As a result, the volume or pressure of the air-filled cavity surrounded by a compliant wall increases. An often-cited study determined that 75% N_2O doubles the volume of a pneumothorax in 10 minutes.[213] N_2O is acceptable for use if the chest tube is patent and functioning. A closed pneumothorax is a contraindication to the administration of N_2O. Decreased pulmonary compliance (increased pulmonary inspiratory pressure) during administration of anesthesia to patients with a history of chest trauma may reflect the expansion of an unrecognized pneumothorax.

ATELECTASIS

Definition

Atelectasis is an abnormal condition characterized by a collapse of pulmonary tissue that prevents the respiratory exchange of CO_2 and O_2. Atelectasis can involve a small localized area or an entire lung. Atelectasis is common with all general anesthetics. It commonly develops within the first few minutes of induction of anesthesia, regardless of the mode of ventilation used, and persists for hours to days following anesthesia, depending on the extent and location of surgery.[214] Atelectasis commonly forms adjacent to the diaphragm in dependent lung regions. Compression of lung tissue, absence of diaphragmatic-induced negative pressure, impaired surfactant, and absorption of oxygen from nitrogen-free alveoli are common causes of atelectasis. Affecting 90% of patients under general anesthesia, atelectasis and airway closure are responsible for the vast majority of gas exchange impairment observed under anesthesia.[215]

Etiology and Pathophysiology

Atelectasis results from a blockage or obstruction of many small bronchi or of a major bronchus. The loss of diaphragmatic tone and function during general anesthesia is a major contributing factor to atelectasis, which characteristically develops within minutes following anesthesia induction. As small airways close due to maldistribution of ventilation under positive-pressure breathing, or due to the cephalad migration of abdominal contents, the gas within the affected alveoli is absorbed, and there is no further ventilation to reopen those alveoli. The higher the concentration of oxygen administered, the greater this effect, because nitrogen or nitrous oxide will not demonstrate ongoing movement from alveoli to blood and will therefore remain in the alveoli and act to stabilize their volume, even in the absence of continued ventilation. Reduction in the F_{IO_2} can help reduce the degree of atelectasis (as measured by the shunt fraction).[216]

Incidence and Outcome

Atelectasis occurs almost universally under general anesthesia and is the most common cause of postoperative respiratory dysfunction. Postoperatively, it occurs most frequently after thoracic and upper abdominal procedures, with rates of incidence reaching 80%. In lower-risk surgeries, postoperative atelectasis most often is subclinical and resolves spontaneously within 24 to 48 hours. No recent data support that atelectasis predisposes one to the development of pneumonia.

Treatment

Historically, practitioners have used large tidal volumes (10 to 15 mL/kg) to combat atelectasis intraoperatively. However, more contemporary data show that ventilator-induced lung injury (VILI) is in part caused by high ventilating volumes, even in the presence of moderate peak inspiratory pressures (so-called "volu-trauma," as opposed to barotrauma). To reduce the deleterious effect of high volumes, smaller tidal volumes of 6 to 10 mL/kg may be more beneficial for mechanical ventilation, particularly in cases of respiratory distress syndrome. There is evidence that this reduction in tidal volume does not worsen the degree of atelectasis.[217] Instead, PEEP and various maneuvers to reopen ("recruit") and maintain alveoli have been proposed to reduce atelectasis.[218] Most common of these are vital capacity maneuvers, where the lungs are intermittently expanded to vital capacity or 30 cm H_2O and held in that state for around 10 seconds. Such recruitment maneuvers are most effective when combined with other strategies such as reduction in FIO_2 or "open-lung" ventilation approaches.

Open-lung ventilation describes myriad approaches to providing mechanical ventilation with the goal of preventing atelectasis. Pressure-control inverse ratio ventilation (PC-IRV) and more recently airway pressure release ventilation (APRV) are approaches designed to maintain a higher mean lung volume and thereby reduce airway closure and atelectasis. Airway pressure release ventilation is analogous to CPAP, with intermittent release phases that allow the lung volume to drop briefly. APRV has an advantage over more "controlled" ventilation modes (such as PC-IRV) in that it is useful in spontaneously-breathing patients to reduce neuromuscular blockade, preserve respiratory effort and protective reflexes, and cause less patient-ventilator dysynchrony.[219]

Standard postoperative measures for improving pulmonary function include incentive spirometry, deep breathing, intermittent positive-pressure breathing, and administration of CPAP, with the last of these offering the greatest superiority by increasing FRC.

PLEURAL EFFUSION

Pleural effusion is the abnormal accumulation of fluid in the pleural space. It usually is an indication of disorders or disease complications in the surrounding structures. Possible causes of effusion are (1) blockage of lymphatic drainage from the pleural cavity; (2) cardiac failure, which causes an increase in pulmonary capillary pressures and eventual movement of fluid into the pleural cavity; (3) reductions in plasma colloid osmotic pressure; and (4) infection or any other inflammatory process of the pleural membranes that alters capillary membrane permeability.

Treatment modalities include tube thoracostomy, thoracentesis, and pleurodesis. Pleurodesis is a procedure used to prevent the reaccumulation of pleural fluid. Inflammation is produced with injection of a sclerosing agent, usually tetracycline, into the chest tube; adhesion formation and fusion of the pleural membranes result.

SKELETAL DISORDERS

The primary pathophysiology of skeletal disorders is an alteration in the structure of the thorax that diminishes chest-wall excursion. Disorders commonly producing this restriction of breathing include sternal deformities, kyphoscoliosis, and ankylosing spondylitis (AS).

Pectus Deformities
Pectus Excavatum
Pectus excavatum, also referred to as *funnel chest*, is the most common chest wall deformity, occurring in 1 in 400 children.[220] It is a congenital anomaly characterized by depression of the sternum (usually above the xiphisternal junction) and symmetric

or asymmetric prominence of the ribs on either side. The etiology of pectus excavatum is unknown, but it is thought that excessive diaphragmatic traction on the lower sternum or displacement of the heart into the left hemithorax is largely responsible.[221] Family history of some type of anterior thoracic deformity is present in 37% of patients. If uncorrected, the disease usually worsens at adolescence. Self-limiting deformities are either gone or vastly improved by the age of 3 years.[222]

Clinically the majority of patients are asymptomatic unless pectus excavatum is extreme. Patients with pectus excavatum have reduced chest cavities and TLC compared with normal subjects; however, pulmonary function often is normal except in severe cases, in which VC, TLC, and maximum breathing capacity may be diminished. The indications for repair of pectus excavatum are the subject of controversy. Conflicting data have been presented regarding whether the repair of pectus excavatum is performed only for cosmetic purposes or whether it actually improves cardiorespiratory function and exercise tolerance.[223] Some clinicians suggest that pectus excavatum should be corrected in childhood—ideally when patients are between the ages of 4 and 6 years—to relieve the structural compromise of the chest, to allow normal growth of the thorax, to prevent pulmonary and cardiac dysfunction in teens and adults, and to improve cosmetic appearance.[224] Others have found that surgery does not significantly improve pulmonary function and that exercise tolerance and cardiorespiratory function during exercise do not benefit significantly from surgical correction.[225] Patients with Marfan syndrome have a high incidence of chest-wall deformities. They usually are seen in their most severe form and often are accompanied by scoliosis. Other musculoskeletal diseases that may be present in patients with pectus excavatum are listed in Table 27-25. Congenital heart disease, mitral valve prolapse, and asthma also occur more frequently in patients with pectum excavatum. Electrocardiographic abnormalities are common and attributable to the abnormal chest-wall configuration and to the displacement and rotation of the heart into the left thoracic cavity. A systolic ejection murmur of grades II to III or IV frequently is identified.

Pectus Carinatum
Pectus carinatum is characterized by a longitudinal protrusion of the sternum. It is the second most common chest deformity, occurring in 1 or 2 persons per 1000. A familial tendency exists, and the disorder is more frequent in males than in females (4:1). The pathogenesis is unclear, and the disorder may be congenital or acquired. The development of pectus carinatum is thought to result from the overgrowth of the costal cartilages, which results in displacement of the sternum. The development of pectus carinatum has also been associated with severe childhood asthma and rickets.[226] The physiologic effects are probably related to the restriction of thoracic excursion. Patients with pectus carinatum have an increased incidence of congenital heart disease, including ventricular septal defect, patent ductus arteriosus, atrial-septal defects, and mitral valve abnormalities.[227]

Three classifications of pectus carinatum exist. Type I—pigeon breast or keel chest—consists of symmetric protrusion of the sternum and costal cartilages. Type II—pouter pigeon breast or Currarino-Silverman syndrome—is characterized by protrusion of the manubrium of the first two sternal cartilages, backward arching of the sternal body, and anterior displacement of the xiphoid process. Type III—lateral pectus carinatum—is manifested by unilateral protrusion of the anterior chest wall.[228]

TABLE 27-25	Musculoskeletal Abnormalities Identified in 133 of 704 Cases of Pectus Excavatum	
Abnormality		**Number of Cases**
Scoliosis		107
Kyphosis		4
Myopathy		3
Poland syndrome		3
Marfan syndrome		2
Pierre Robin syndrome		2
Prune-belly syndrome		2
Neurofibromatosis		3
Cerebral palsy		4
Tuberous sclerosis		1
Congenital diaphragmatic hernia		2

From Shields TW. General Thoracic Surgery. Philadelphia: Lea & Febiger; 1994.

Surgery is the only effective treatment for pectus carinatum and is performed to alleviate possible cardiopulmonary dysfunction and to prevent progressive postural deformities, as well as for cosmetic reasons.

Kyphoscoliosis
Definition
Kyphosis is a deformity marked by an accentuated posterior curvature. Scoliosis is a lateral curvature of the spine. Kyphoscoliosis results when kyphosis and scoliosis occur concomitantly, causing a lateral bending and rotation of the vertebral column. Scoliosis alone, despite its severity, does not cause sensory or motor impairment. In contrast, kyphosis and kyphoscoliosis may induce cord damage because of the sharp angulation of the spine. Respiratory dysfunction is associated with scoliosis, significant kyphosis, and severe kyphoscoliosis.

Incidence and Outcome
Scoliosis is the most common spinal deformity, with an incidence of 4 persons per 1000.[229] The etiologic classification of scoliosis falls into five categories: idiopathic, congenital, neuropathic (e.g., poliomyelitis, cerebral palsy, syringomyelia, and Friedreich ataxia), myopathic (e.g., muscular dystrophy and amyotonia), and traumatic. Idiopathic scoliosis is the most common deformity, accounting for 80% of all cases. On the basis of the time of onset, idiopathic scoliosis is divided into the following two categories: (1) the rare infantile form (male-to-female ratio, 6:4); and (2) the common adolescent form (male-to-female ratio, 1:9). The children in the adolescent group are born with a straight spine; however, at some point during the growth period, the spine begins to bend and deform, with deformation progressively worsening until growth ends. However, conflicting studies by Collis and Ponseti have demonstrated that curvatures tend to progress throughout life rather than to stop progressing at the end of growth.[230] In general, curves associated with adolescent idiopathic scoliosis are convex and deviated to the right, whereas those related to other disease may be deviated to the left. The

presence of cervical scoliosis should alert anesthesia personnel to potential difficulties in airway management. Any significant curvature involving the thoracic spine may alter lung function. Unless deformity is severe, patients with kyphosis are able to maintain normal pulmonary function. In contrast, even mild forms of scoliosis can result in impaired ventilatory function.

A long-term study of pulmonary function tests performed 20 years apart in patients with unfused scoliosis (nonoperated) demonstrated that respiratory failure occurred in patients with a VC less than 45% of that predicted during initial testing who had an angle of curvature greater than 110 degrees. Results also showed that the initial VC was the strongest predictor of the development of respiratory failure (magnitude of the scoliotic angle was the second strongest indicator).[231]

Severe thoracic deformity may result in respiratory alterations during sleep. Several types of breathing abnormalities have been documented, including obstructive apnea and hypopnea. The lowest HbO_2 saturations occurred during rapid-eye-movement sleep.[232]

Respiratory mechanics in anesthetized young patients with kyphoscoliosis are characterized by an increase in mean total respiratory elastance, chest wall elastance, and respiratory flow resistance during corrective spinal surgery for kyphoscoliosis that may have resulted from rib cage trauma and changes in airway caliber, with microatelectasis and uneven distribution of mechanical properties within the lung. Spinal correction results in immediate and short-term deterioration of respiratory mechanics in anesthetized patients.[233]

Clinical Features and Diagnosis
Diminution of pulmonary function occurs with curvatures of greater than 60 degrees, and pulmonary symptoms develop with curvatures greater than 70 degrees (as measured by the Cobb technique; Figure 27-24). Curvatures greater than 100 degrees may be associated with significant gas exchange impairment.[234] In general, the greater the curvature, the greater the loss of pulmonary function. Because of this, mechanical ventilation becomes inefficient; this inefficiency is the major factor causing respiratory embarrassment.[235] At the time of diagnosis, it is often possible to document a reduction in lung capacity. The characteristic deformity seen in scoliosis causes one hemithorax to become relatively smaller than the other.

Skeletal chest wall deformity in kyphoscoliosis leads to a reduction in lung volumes and the pulmonary vascular bed.[236] Ventilatory failure associated with severe kyphoscoliosis produces a lung size that is 30% to 65% of normal. As the patient ages, the chest wall becomes less compliant; this increases the work of breathing and leads to hypoventilation and respiratory muscle weakness.

The main features of lung mechanics in the patient with early-stage scoliosis are reduced lung volumes (VC, TLC, FRC, and RV) and reduced chest wall compliance; in the late stages of disease, $\dot{V}/\dot{Q}$ mismatching with hypoxemia (attributed to alveolar hypoventilation because of a decrease in V_T), increased PAP, hypercapnia, abnormal response to CO_2 stimulation, increased work of breathing, and cor pulmonale occur and eventually lead to cardiorespiratory failure.[236] Reduction in VC to 60% to 80% of the predicted value is a typical finding.[234] FEV_1/FVC is normal unless other pulmonary diseases are present. Although normocarbia prevails for most of the clinical course, an elevated $Paco_2$ signifies the onset of respiratory failure. The severity of hypercapnia most closely correlates with the patient's age and inspiratory muscle strength.

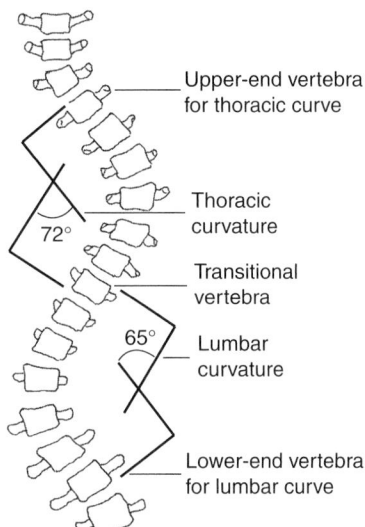

FIGURE **27-24** Cobb method of measuring scoliosis curves. First, the "end vertebrae" of the curve are identified. These are the vertebrae that have the maximum tilting toward the curve to be measured. Then, horizontal lines are drawn at the superior border of the superior end vertebra and at the inferior border of the inferior end vertebra. Then, perpendicular lines are erected from each of the horizontal lines. The angle between the intersecting perpendicular lines is the angle of curvature. *(From Prakash UB. Pulmonary manifestations in systemic diseases. In: Baum GL, Wolinsky E, eds. Textbook of Pulmonary Diseases. Vol 2. 5th ed. Boston: Little, Brown; 1993:1692.)*

Associated Conditions

Scoliosis may be associated with several cardiovascular abnormalities, of which mitral valve prolapse is the most common. If mitral regurgitation is present, antibiotic prophylaxis is indicated before surgical manipulation. Other common changes include an increase in PVR and ensuing PAH, which leads to the development of right ventricular hypertrophy. Several contributing factors are thought to be responsible for the development of increased PVR. First, arterial hypoxemia results in pulmonary vasoconstriction. Second, changes in the pulmonary arterioles consequent to the increased pulmonic pressure may cause narrowing and result in irreversible PH. Third, a compressed chest wall may increase vascular resistance in affected areas. Fourth, development of scoliosis at an early age inhibits growth of the pulmonary vascular bed. Alveolar multiplication is nearly complete by 2 years of age but continues until the age of 8 years. During the first few years, lung growth occurs primarily by enlargement of existing alveoli. Olgiati and co-workers have supported this argument by showing that a decrease in diffusion capacity results from partial failure of alveolar enlargement because of the thoracic deformity rather than any atrophy of the alveoli or pulmonary vasculature.[233]

Treatment

The management of scoliosis may include (1) observation of the problem without active medical treatment, (2) treatment by nonoperative methods that include the use of braces or electronic stimulators, and (3) operative methods such as anterior or posterior spinal fusion and instrumentation, such as Harrington rod insertion.[237] The largest studies by Nachemson and Nilsonne have shown that the mortality rate among persons with untreated scoliosis is twice that of the normal population, and the rate for those with thoracic curvatures alone was fourfold that of the normal population.[238,239] Patients with congenital thoracic scoliosis are particularly at risk for cor pulmonale.[239]

Anesthetic Management

Preoperative Evaluation. Preoperatively a thorough review of systems is essential. The severity of scoliosis and any underlying conditions must be noted. Any reversible pulmonary involvement such as pneumonia should be corrected before elective surgery. Laboratory data should include complete blood count; prothrombin time; partial thromboplastin time; values for electrolytes, blood urea nitrogen, and creatinine; ECG; chest radiography; and routine pulmonary function test values. ABG analysis may be indicated if the results of the pulmonary function tests reflect significant impairment or if the surgical procedure dictates its need. Because these procedures can potentially involve large blood losses, young, healthy, asymptomatic patients may donate autologous blood. Blood typing and cross-match also are required.

When sedatives are used in the preoperative area, care must be taken to ensure that respiratory status is not depressed. The need for intraoperative monitoring is dictated by the type of surgery and the physical status of the patient. No specific anesthetic techniques have been shown to be superior in patients with scoliosis, but N_2O may increase PVR by direct vasoconstrictive effects on the pulmonary vasculature. It has been suggested that scoliosis is associated with an increased incidence of malignant hyperthemia.[240] Ventilation should be adjusted so that adequate arterial oxygenation and normocarbia are maintained.

Patients undergoing surgery for correction of the spinal curvature should be informed preoperatively of the possible need for the "wake-up" test; once the patient is able to move both feet on request, and surgical correction has been achieved, anesthesia can be quickly reinstituted. The use of somatosensory evoked potentials may require an alteration in anesthetic technique. All anesthetic agents depress somatosensory evoked potentials to a varying degree. Administration of volatile anesthetics should not exceed a minimum alveolar concentration of 1. An N_2O–continuous infusion opioid technique often is preferred.

Communication between the technician and anesthetist is essential.

Intraoperative Management. Considerable fluid and blood loss may occur during surgery. The surgeon may request the institution of deliberate hypotension. Deliberate hypotension can be produced with the use of one or more of the following: potent inhalation anesthetics; vasodilators (e.g., sodium nitroprusside, nitroglycerin) or β-adrenergic blocking agents (e.g., propranolol and esmolol). The risks and potential benefits should be weighed against the effects of deliberate hypotension. The mean arterial blood pressure should be maintained at no lower than 60 to 65 mm Hg. Cell-saver blood is often used. Interventions for prevention of hypothermia, such as use of a hot-air warming blanket or heated humidifiers, should be used. Careful positioning is essential.

Postoperative Care. The decision whether to use mechanical ventilation postoperatively is based on the severity of scoliosis and intraoperative events. Most patients with mild to moderate pulmonary dysfunction are able to undergo safe extubation in the operating room. Those with severe deformity should be weaned slowly.

Ankylosing Spondylitis

Definition

Ankylosing spondylitis (AS), also known as *rheumatoid spondylitis* and *Marie-Strumpell disease*, is a chronic inflammatory disorder that primarily affects the spine and sacroiliac joints and produces fusion of the spinal vertebrae and the costovertebral joints.

Etiology and Incidence

The cause of AS remains unclear. However, it is strongly associated with the histocompatibility antigen HLA-B27, the presence of which is detected in more than 90% of Caucasians with the disease.[241,242] It is a disease of adults younger than 40 years, and it demonstrates a predilection for males (male-to-female ratio, 9:1). The disease is rare in non-Caucasians.

Clinical Features and Diagnosis

AS is diagnosed on the basis of clinical criteria that include (1) chronic low back pain with limitation of spinal motion (<4 cm as measured by the Schober test), (2) radiographic evidence of bilateral sacroiliitis, and (3) limitation of chest wall expansion (<2.5-cm increase in chest circumference measured at the fourth intercostal space). Extraskeletal manifestations of this disease include iritis, cardiovascular involvement (cardiac conduction defects, aortitis, and aortic insufficiency in 20% of individuals), peripheral arthritis, fever, anemia, fatigue, weight loss, and fibrocavitary (fibrobullous) disease of the apexes of the lungs. The most limiting factors associated with the disease are pain, stiffness, and fatigue.

Complications

Pulmonary complications are reported to occur in 2% to 70% of patients with AS, although one large review of 2080 AS patients found the frequency to be less than 2%.[243] Apical fibrosis is the most commonly occurring abnormality, followed by aspergilloma and pleural effusion with nonspecific pleuritis. In apical fibrosis, the pulmonary lesion begins with apical pleural thickening and patchy consolidation of one or both apexes and often progresses to dense bilateral fibrosis and air space enlargement. Patients with apical fibrosis usually have advanced AS.

Stewart and colleagues suggest that impaired thoracic-cage excursion caused by AS results in a greater impairment of apical ventilation and that this may be one factor in the pathogenesis of apical fibrosis.[244]

The most common thoracic complication is fixation of the thoracic cage as a result of costovertebral ankylosis, which can lead to pulmonary dysfunction.[242] In patients with this complication, motion of the thoracic cage is restricted due to fusion of the costovertebral joints; this restriction leads to a decrease in thoracic excursion. Respiratory function typically demonstrates a restrictive pattern with mild diminution of TLC, VC, and D_{LCO} and normal or slightly increased RV and FRC. Pulmonary compliance, diffusion capacity, and ABG values usually are normal.[241] Despite having abnormal pulmonary function, the majority of patients with AS are able to perform normal physical activities without pulmonary symptoms. It has been suggested that patients who exercise regularly and thus improve cardiovascular fitness could maintain a satisfactory work capacity.[245]

Bone ankylosis may occur in the numerous joints around the thorax (the thoracic vertebrae and the costovertebral, costotransverse, sternoclavicular, and sternomanubrial joints), resulting in limitation of chest-wall movement. Patients with AS rarely complain of respiratory symptoms or functional impairment unless they have coexisting cardiovascular or respiratory disease. Progressive kyphosis is equivalent to progressive rigidity of the thorax. Increased diaphragmatic function compensates for decreased thoracic motion, allowing lung function to be well preserved. Patients with advanced disease may have an entirely diaphragmatic respiration.[245] Regional lung ventilation in patients with AS is normal unless they have preexisting apical fibrosis.

Cervical spondylosis affects levels C5 to C6 and C6 to C7 most often, and less frequently C4 to C5, C7 to T1, and C3 to C4. The degenerative changes may result in nerve root entrapment by foraminal encroachment. The phrenic nerve, which innervates the diaphragm, is supplied primarily by the C4 nerve root, and to a lesser extent, by the C3 and C5 nerve roots. A case of hemidiaphragmatic paralysis secondary to C4 nerve root compression has been reported.

Cricoarytenoid involvement may exist and can lead to respiratory dysfunction and upper airway obstruction. Cricoarytenoid dysfunction can manifest as a hoarse, weak voice. Respiratory failure from cricoarytenoid ankylosis has necessitated therapeutic tracheostomy. In all reported cases, laryngeal symptoms were present before cricoarytenoid arthritis caused airway compromise. A case of acute respiratory failure and cor pulmonale resulting from cricoarytenoid arthritis has also been reported in a patient with AS.

Treatment

Medical therapy for adult patients with AS is supportive and preventive. Most patients with AS are asymptomatic. Depending on the severity of disease involvement, management may consist of the use of corticosteroids and nonsteroidal antiinflammatory agents. Patients should refrain from smoking tobacco.

Anesthetic Management

Patients with AS have specific anesthetic requirements.[245] Management of the upper airway is the priority because of the potential for obstruction. Cervical spine involvement may result in limitation of movement. The ankylosed neck is more susceptible to hyperextension injury, and cervical fracture may occur.

Intubation awake with or without the use of a fiberoptic bronchoscope is indicated. In rare situations, tracheostomy must be performed with the patient under local anesthesia before anesthesia can be induced. A regional anesthetic technique may not be feasible because of skeletal involvement that precludes access or because of neurologic complications such as spinal cord compression, cauda equina syndrome, focal epilepsy, vertebrobasilar insufficiency, and peripheral nerve lesions. Patients with cardiovascular system involvement may require antibiotic coverage, treatment of heart failure, or insertion of a temporary pacemaker before surgery. Restriction of chest expansion and rarely pulmonary fibrosis necessitate performance of a thorough preoperative assessment and immediate postoperative mechanical ventilation. Careful attention to positioning is essential.

SUMMARY

To conduct an accurate patient assessment and manage relevant pathophysiology, knowledge of the anatomy and physiology of the respiratory system is imperative for the anesthetist. Anatomical idiosyncrasies (such as the shorter, straighter, right mainstem bronchus), physiologic derangements from anesthesia (such as the atelectasis and ventilation-perfusion mismatch that occur), perianesthetic complications (such as aspiration pneumonitis), preexisting illness (such as COPD), and iatrogenic illness (such as pulmonary toxicity from chemotherapeutic agents) are all concerns for the anesthetist in caring for the pulmonary system.

REFERENCES

1. Krohner RG, Ramanathan S. Functional anatomy of the airway in Hagberg CA. In: *Benumof's Airway Management.* 2nd ed. Philadelphia: Mosby; 2007.
2. Ellis H, Feldman S. *Anatomy for Anaesthetists.* London: Blackwell; 1988:7.
3. Whitten C. *Anyone Can Intubate.* San Diego: KW Publications; 1997:12.
4. Guyton AC, Hall JE. *Textbook of Medical Physiology.* 11th ed. Philadelphia: Saunders; 2006:481-482.
5. Endo K et al. Bilateral vocal cord paralysis caused by laryngeal mask airway. *Am J Otolaryngol.* 2007;28(2):126-129.
6. Weiss A et al. Acute respiratory failure after deep cervical plexus block for carotid endarterectomy as a result of bilateral recurrent laryngeal nerve paralysis. *Acta Anaesthesiol Scand.* 2005;49(5):715-719.
7. Gal TJ. Airway management. In: Miller RD *Anesthesia.* 6th ed. New York: Churchill Livingstone; 2005:1616-1652.
8. Simoff M et al. *Thoracic Endoscopy: Advances in Interventional Pulmonology.* Malden, MA: Wiley-Blackwell; 2006.
9. Ackerman U. *Essentials of Human Physiology.* St Louis: Mosby; 1999:53.
10. Levitzky MG. *Pulmonary Physiology.* 7th ed. New York: McGraw-Hill; 2007:21.
11. O'Donnell DE. Pathophysiology of dyspnea in chronic obstructive pulmonary disease: a roundtable. *Proc Am Thorac Soc.* 2007;4(2):145.
12. Lumb AB. *Nunn's Applied Respiratory Physiology.* 6th ed. Philadelphia: Butterworth-Heinemann; 2005:39-50.
13. Ochs M, Weible ER. Functional design of the human lung for gas exchange. In: Fishman AP, ed. *Fishman's Pulmonary Disease and Disorders.* New York: McGraw-Hill; 2008:23-70.
14. Hakim TS et al. Gravity-independent inequality in pulmonary blood flow in humans. *J Appl Physiol.* 1987;63(3):1114-1121.
15. Lumb AB. *Nunn's Applied Respiratory Physiology.* 6th ed. Philadelphia: Butterworth-Heinemann; 2005:387-390.
16. Murray JF. *The Normal Lung.* 2nd ed. Philadelphia: Saunders; 1986.
17. West JB. *Pulmonary Pathophysiology.* 7th ed. Baltimore: Lippincott Williams & Wilkins; 2008:153-170.
18. Gal TJ. Anatomy & physiology of the respiratory system and the pulmonary circulation. In: Kaplan JA, ed. *Thoracic Anesthesia.* 3rd ed. New York: Churchill Livingstone; 2003:57-70.
19. West JB. *Pulmonary Physiology and Pathophysiology.* 2nd ed. Philadelphia: Lippincott Williams Wilkins; 2007:10.
20. West JB. *Respiratory Physiology—the Essentials.* 7th ed. Baltimore: Lippincott Williams & Wilkins; 2005:83-89.
21. Rose BD. *Clinical Physiology of Acid-Base and Electrolyte Disorders.* 4th ed. New York: McGraw-Hill; 1994:261.
22. Levitzky MG et al. *Introductions to Respiratory Care.* Philadelphia: Saunders; 1990.
23. Celli BR. ATS standards for the optimal management of chronic obstructive pulmonary disease. *Respirology.* 1997;2(Suppl 1):S1-4.
24. American Thoracic Society. Standards for the diagnosis and care of patients with chronic obstructive pulmonary disease (COPD) and asthma. *Am Rev Respir Dis.* 1987;136:225-243.
25. Ciba Guest Symposium Report. Terminology, definitions, and classification of chronic pulmonary emphysema and related conditions. *Thorax.* 1959; 14:286-299.
26. Senior RM, Atkinson JJ. Chronic obstructive pulmonary disease: epidemiology, pathophysiology, and pathogenesis. In: Fishman AP, ed. *Fishman's Pulmonary Disease and Disorders.* New York: McGraw-Hill; 2008:707-728.
27. Pauwels RA et al. Global strategy for the diagnosis, management, and prevention of chronic obstructive pulmonary disease. *Am J Respir Crit Care Med.* 2001;163:1256-1276.
28. Wright JL, Churg A. Pathologic features of chronic obstructive pulmonary disease: diagnostic criteria and differential diagnosis. In: Fishman AP, ed. *Fishman's Pulmonary Disease and Disorders.* New York: McGraw-Hill; 2008:693-706.
29. Sherman CB et al. Acute exacerbations in COPD patients. In: Cherniak NS, ed. *Chronic Obstructive Pulmonary Disease.* Philadelphia: Saunders; 1991:449.
30. American Thoracic Society. Standards for the diagnosis and care of patients with chronic obstructive pulmonary disease. *Am J Respir Crit Care Med.* 1995;152:S77-120.
31. Rieves RD et al. Severe COPD and acute respiratory failure: correlates for survival at the time of tracheal intubation. *Chest.* 1993;104:854-860.
32. US Public Health Service. *The Health Consequences of Smoking. A Report of the Surgeon General (US Department of Health, Education, and Welfare Publication No. HSM 72-7516).* Washington, DC: US Government Printing Office; 1972.
33. Carrell RW et al. Structure and variation of human α-1-antitrypsin. *Nature.* 1982;298:329-334.
34. Murphy DM, Fishman AP. Bullous disease of the lung. In: Fishman AP, ed. *Fishman's Pulmonary Disease and Disorders.* New York: McGraw-Hill; 2008:913-930.
35. Drain CB. Anesthesia care of the patient with reactive airways disease. *CRNA.* 1996;7:207-212.
36. Luijendijk SCM et al. Collateral ventilation by diffusion across the alveolar walls and the exchange of inert gases in the lung. *Eur Respir J.* 1991;4:1228-1236.
37. Cherniack NS, Milic-Emili J. Mechanical aspects of loaded breathing. In: Roussos C, Macklem PT, eds. *Thorax.* New York: Marcel Dekker; 1985:751.
38. Bellemare F, Grassino A. Force reserve of the diaphragm in patients with chronic obstructive pulmonary disease. *J Appl Physiol.* 1983;55:8-15.
39. Jardim J et al. The failing inspiratory muscles under normoxic and hypoxic conditions. *Am Rev Respir Dis.* 1981;124:274-279.
40. Kim CS et al. Airway responsiveness to inhaled and intravenous carbachol in sheep: effect of airway mucus. *J Appl Physiol.* 1988;65:2744-2751.
41. Guyton AC. Physical principles of gaseous exchange: diffusion of oxygen and carbon dioxide through the respiratory membrane. In: Guyton AC, Hall JE, eds. *Textbook of Medical Physiology.* 10th ed. Philadelphia: Saunders; 2006:491-501.
42. Burrows B et al. Patterns of cardiovascular dysfunction in chronic obstructive lung disease. *N Engl J Med.* 1972;286:912-917.
43. Rochester DF. Effects of COPD on the respiratory muscles. In: Cherniak NS, ed. *Chronic Obstructive Pulmonary Disease.* Philadelphia: Saunders; 1991:1135.
44. Shapiro SD. The pathogenesis of emphysema: the elastase/antielastase hypothesis 30 years later. *Proc Assoc Am Physicians.* 1995;107(3):346-352.
45. Hoidal JR et al. Oxidative damage and COPD. In: Cherniak NS, ed. *Chronic Obstructive Pulmonary Disease.* Philadelphia: Saunders; 1991:45.
46. Thurlbeck WM. Chronic airflow obstruction: correlation of structure and function. In: Petty T, ed. *Chronic Obstructive Pulmonary Disease.* 2nd ed. New York: Marcel Dekker; 1985:1985.

47. Cherniak NS. Control of breathing in COPD. In: Cherniak NS, ed. *Chronic Obstructive Pulmonary Disease*. Philadelphia: Saunders; 1991:118.

48. Natarajan TK et al. Immediate effect of expiratory loading on left ventricular stroke volume. *Circulation*. 1987;75:139-145.

49. Bilgi C et al. Relation between pulsus paradoxus and pulmonary function in patients with chronic airway obstruction. *CMAJ*. 1977;117:1389-1392.

50. Wise RA. COPD and the peripheral circulation. In: Cherniak NS, ed. *Chronic Obstructive Pulmonary Disease*. Philadelphia: Saunders; 1991:168.

51. Miyamoto K et al. Augmented heart rate response to hypoxia in patients with chronic obstructive pulmonary disease. *Am Rev Respir Dis*. 1992;145:1384-1388.

52. Kilburn KH. Fluid retention associated with pulmonary insufficiency and respiratory failure. In: Cherniak NS, ed. *Chronic Obstructive Pulmonary Disease*. Philadelphia: Saunders; 1991:187.

53. Fraser RG, Pare JA. Pulmonary emphysema. *Diagn Dis Chest*. 1979;3:11.

54. Guyton AC. Respiratory insufficiency-pathophysiology, diagnosis, oxygen therapy. In: Guyton AC, Hall JE, eds. *Textbook of Medical Physiology*. 11th ed. Philadelphia: Saunders; 2006:524-532.

55. Flenley DC. The diagnosis of emphysema. In: Cherniak NS, ed. *Chronic Obstructive Pulmonary Disease*. Philadelphia: Saunders; 1991:352.

56. Bishop MJ. The patient with respiratory disease: evaluation, preparation and timing of surgery. *ASA Annu Refresher Course Lect*. 1992;246:1-7.

57. Gass GD, Olsen GN. Preoperative pulmonary function testing to predict postoperative morbidity and mortality. *Chest*. 1986;89:127-135.

58. American Thoracic Society: Dyspnea. Mechanisms, assessment, and management: a consensus statement. *Am J Respir Crit Care Med*. 1999;159:321-340.

59. Hirshman CA, Bergman NA. Factors influencing intrapulmonary calibre during anesthesia. *Br J Anaesth*. 1990;65:30-42.

60. Nunn JF et al. Respiratory criteria for fitness for surgery and anesthesia. *Anesthesia*. 1988;43:543-551.

61. Fowkes FGR et al. Epidemiology in anesthesia III: mortality risk in patients with coexisting physical disease. *Br J Anaesth*. 1982;54:819-825.

62. Ledowski T et al. Bronchial mucus transport velocity in patients receiving propofol and remifentanil versus sevoflurane and remifentanil anesthesia. *Anesth Analg*. 2006;102(5):1427-1430.

63. Hedenstierna G, Edmark L. The effects of anesthesia and muscle paralysis on the respiratory system. *Intensive Care Med*. 2005;31(10):1327-1335.

64. Hedenstierna G. Gas exchange during anesthesia. *Br J Anaesth*. 1990;64:507-514.

65. Gunnarsson L et al. Chronic obstructive pulmonary disease and anesthesia: formation of atelectasis and gas exchange impairment. *Eur Respir J*. 1991;4:1106-1116.

66. Slinger P. Anesthesia for lung resection. *J Anaesth*. 1990;37:Sxv-Sxxiv.

67. Rehder K et al. Ventilation-perfusion relationship in young healthy awake and anesthetized-paralyzed man. *J Appl Physiol*. 1979;47:745-753.

68. Wagner PD et al. Ventilation-perfusion inequality in chronic obstructive pulmonary disease. *J Clin Invest*. 1977;59:203-216.

69. Bates DV. The lung in transition between health and disease. In: Macklem PT, Permutt S, eds. *Lung Biology in Health and Disease*. Vol 12. New York: Marcel Dekker; 1979.

70. Pepe PE, Marini JJ. Occult positive end-expiratory pressure in mechanically ventilated patients with airflow obstruction: the auto-PEEP effect. *Am Rev Respir Dis*. 1982;126:166-170.

71. Coursin DB et al. Pulmonary disorders. In: Cheng EY, Kay J, eds. *Manual of Anesthesia and the Medically Compromised Patient*. Philadelphia: Lippincott; 1990.

72. Rossi A et al. Measurement of static compliance of the total respiratory system in patients with acute respiratory failure during mechanical ventilation: the effect of intrinsic positive end-expiratory pressure. *Am Rev Respir Dis*. 1985;131:672-677.

73. Torres A et al. Ventilation-perfusion mismatching in chronic obstructive pulmonary disease during ventilator weaning. *Am Rev Respir Dis*. 1989;140:1246-1250.

74. National Asthma Education and Prevention Program, Expert Panel Report 3. Guidelines for the diagnosis and management of asthma–summary report 2007. *J Allergy Clin Immunol*. 2007;120(5 Suppl):S94-138.

75. Barnes PJ. Asthma. In: Fauci AS, ed. *Harrison's Principles of Internal Medicine*. 17th ed. New York: McGraw Hill; 2008:1596-1606.

76. Laitnen LA et al. Airway mucosal inflammation even in patients with newly diagnosed asthma. *Am Rev Respir Dis*. 1993;147:697-704.

77. Beach JR. Immunologic versus toxicologic mechanisms in airway responses. *Occup Med*. 2000;15:455-470.

78. Bigby TD, Wasserman SI. Asthma. In: Stein JH, ed. *Internal Medicine*. 5th ed. St Louis: Mosby; 1998:1185-1193.

79. Gibson PG et al. Airway mast cells and eosinophils correlate with clinical severity and airway hyperresponsiveness in corticosteroid-treated asthma. *J Allergy Clin Immunol*. 2000;105:752-759.

80. Hall WJ et al. Pulmonary mechanics after uncomplicated influenza A infection. *Am Rev Respir Dis*. 1976;113:141.

81. Moudgil GC. The patient with reactive airways disease. *Can J Anaesth*. 1997;44:R77-R83.

82. Boulet LP et al. Bronchial subepithelial fibrosis correlates with airway responsiveness to methacholine. *Chest*. 1997;112:45-52.

83. Geer RT. Pulmonary complications of anesthesia. In: Longnecker DE, et al, eds. *Principles and Practice of Anesthesiology*. St Louis: Mosby; 1998:232-241.

84. Argyros GJ et al. Water loss without heat flux in exercise-induced bronchospasm. *Am Rev Respir Dis*. 1993;147:1419-1424.

85. McFadden ER. Asthma. In: Kassper DL et al. *Harrison's Principles of Internal Medicine*. 16th ed. New York: McGraw-Hill; 2005:1508-1517.

86. Dietzel DP, Ciullo JV. Spontaneous pneumothorax after shoulder arthroscopy: a report of four cases. *Arthroscopy*. 1996;12:99-102.

87. Cherniack RM. Pulmonary function testing. In: Mitchell RS, et al, eds. *Synopsis of Clinical Pulmonary Disease*. 4th ed. St Louis: Mosby; 1988.

88. Macklem PT. Tests of lung mechanics. *N Engl J Med*. 1975;293:339.

89. Roizen MF. Preoperative evaluation. In: Miller RD, ed. *Anesthesia*. 6th ed. New York: Churchill Livingstone; 2005:927-998.

90. Roizen MF, Fleisher LA. Anesthetic implications of concurrent diseases. In: Miller ED. *Anesthesia*. New York: 6th ed. Churchill Livingstone; 2005:1017-1150.

91. Kurup V. Respiratory disease. In: Hines RL, Maraschall KE. *Stoelting's Anesthesia and Co-Existing Disease*. 5th ed. Philadelphia: Churchill Livingstone; 2008:161-198.

92. Hepner DL. Sudden bronchospasm on intubation: Latex anaphylaxis? *J Clin Anesth*. 2000;12:162-166.

93. Innes AL et al. Chronic pulmonary disease. In: Stoelting RK, Miller RD, eds. *Basics of Anesthesia*. 5th ed. Philadelphia: Churchill Livingstone; 2007:406-424.

94. Hurford WE. The bronchospastic patient. *Int Anesthesiol Clin*. 2000;38:77-89.

95. Wong DH et al. Factors associated with postoperative pulmonary complications in patients with severe chronic obstructive pulmonary disease. *Anesth Analg*. 1995;80:276-284.

96. Smetana GW. Current concepts: preoperative pulmonary evaluation. *N Engl J Med*. 1999;340:937-944.

97. Gass GD, Olsen GN. Preoperative pulmonary function testing to predict postoperative morbidity and mortality. *Chest*. 1986;89:127-135.

98. Kocabas A et al. Value of preoperative spirometry to predict postoperative pulmonary complications. *Respir Med*. 1996;90:25-33.

99. Kabalin CS et al. Low complication rate of corticosteroid-treated asthmatics undergoing surgical procedures. *Arch Intern Med*. 1995;155:1379-1384.

100. Gal TJ. Bronchial hyperresponsiveness and anesthesia: physiologic and therapeutic perspectives. *Anesth Analg*. 1994;78:559-573.

101. Karlet M, Nagelhout J. Asthma: an anesthetic update. Part 3, *AANA J*. 2001;69:317-324.

102. Christopherson R et al. Perioperative morbidity in patients randomized to epidural or general anesthesia for lower extremity vascular surgery. *Anesthesiology*. 1993;79:422-434.

103. Yeager MP et al. Epidural anesthesia and analgesia in high-risk surgical patients. *Anesthesiology*. 1987;66:729-736.

104. Pizov R et al. Wheezing during induction of general anesthesia in patients with and without asthma. A randomized, blinded trial. *Anesthesiology*. 1995;82:1111-1116.

105. Habre W et al. Respiratory mechanics during sevoflurane anesthesia in children with and without asthma. *Anesth Analg*. 1999;89:1177-1181.

106. Rooke GA et al. The effect of isoflurane, halothane, sevoflurane and thiopental/nitrous oxide on respiratory system resistance after tracheal intubation. *Anesthesiology*. 1997;86:1294-1299.

107. Blake K. Asthma. In: Herfindal ET, Gourley DR, eds. *Textbook of Therapeutics*. Philadelphia: Williams & Wilkins; 2000:727-764.

108. Treatment Guidelines from the Medical Letter. Drugs for asthma. *Med Lett*. 2005;3:22-38.

109. Levy BD et al. Medical and ventilatory management of status asthmaticus. *Intensive Care Med*. 1998;24:105-117.

110. Jain S et al. Ventilation of patients with asthma and obstructive lung disease. *Crit Care Clin*. 1998;14:685-705.

111. Corbridge TC, Hall JB. The assessment and management of adults with status asthmaticus. *Am J Respir Crit Care Med*. 1995;5:1296-1316.

112. Rosen MA. Management of anesthesia for the pregnant surgical patient. *Anesthesiology*. 1999;91:1159-1161.

113. Koren G et al. Drug therapy: drugs in pregnancy. *N Engl J Med*. 1998;338:1128-1137.

114. Urbano FL. Review of the NAEPP 2007 expert panel report (EPR-3) on asthma diagnosis and treatment guidelines. *J Manag Care Pharm.* 2008; 14(1):41-49.

115. Takaoka S et al. Current therapies for pulmonary arterial hypertension. *Semin Cardiothorac Vasc Anesth.* 2007;11(2):137-148.

116. Taichmann DB, Fishman AP. Pulmonary hypertension and cor pulmonale. In: Fishman AP, ed. *Fishman's Pulmonary Disease and Disorders.* New York: McGraw-Hill; 2008:1359-1422.

117. Armstrong P. Thoracic epidural anesthesia and primary pulmonary hypertension. *Anesthesia.* 1992;47:496-499.

118. Rostagno C et al. Pulmonary hypertension associated with long-standing thrombocytosis. *Chest.* 1991;99:1303-1305.

119. Gassner A et al. Differential therapy with calcium channel antagonists in pulmonary hypertension secondary to COPD: hemodynamic effects of nifedipine, diltiazem, and verapamil. *Chest.* 1990;98:829-834.

120. Costard-Jackle A, Fowler MB. Influence of preoperative pulmonary artery pressure on mortality after heart transplantation: testing of potential reversibility of pulmonary hypertension with nitroprusside is useful in defining a high-risk group. *J Am Coll Cardiol.* 1992;19:48-54.

121. Galie N et al. Evaluation of pulmonary arterial hypertension. *Curr Opin Cardiol.* 2004;19(6):575-581.

122. Reeves JT et al. The case for treatment of selected patients with primary pulmonary hypertension. *Am Rev Respir Dis.* 1986;134:342-346.

123. Uren NG et al. Response of the pulmonary circulation to acetylcholine, calcitonin gene-related peptide, substance P and oral nicardipine in patients with primary pulmonary hypertension. *J Am Coll Cardiol.* 1992;19:834-841.

124. Levine DJ. Diagnosis and management of pulmonary arterial hypertension: implications for respiratory care. *Respir Care.* 2006;51(4):368-381.

125. Morrison DA et al. Relief of right ventricular angina and increased exercise capacity with long-term oxygen therapy. *Chest.* 1991;100:534-539.

126. Speich R et al. Primary pulmonary hypertension in HIV infection. *Chest.* 1991;100:1268-1271.

127. Moser KM, Bloor CM. Pulmonary vascular lesions occurring in patients with chronic major vessel thromboembolic pulmonary hypertension. *Chest.* 1993;103:685-692.

128. Abramson SV et al. Pulmonary hypertension predicts mortality and morbidity in patients with dilated cardiomyopathy. *Ann Intern Med.* 1992; 116:888-895.

129. Eysmann SB et al. Echo/Doppler and hemodynamic correlates of vasodilator responsiveness in primary pulmonary hypertension. *Chest.* 1991;99: 1066-1071.

130. Hickey PR et al. Pulmonary and systemic hemodynamic responses to ketamine in infants with normal and elevated pulmonary vascular resistance. *Anesthesiology.* 1985;62:287-293.

131. Popescu WM. Heart failure and cardiomyopathies. In: Hines RL, Maraschall KE. *Stoelting's Anesthesia and Co-Existing Disease.* 5th ed. Philadelphia: Churchill Livingstone; 2008:103-124.

132. Morgan JM et al. Hypoxic pulmonary vasoconstriction in systemic sclerosis and primary pulmonary hypertension. *Chest.* 1991;99:551-556.

133. Weir EK, Reeves JT. *Pulmonary Hypertension.* Mount Kisco, NY: Futura; 1984:292.

134. Armstrong P. Thoracic epidural anaesthesia and primary pulmonary hypertension. *Anaesthesia.* 1992;47:496-499.

135. Guyton AC, Hall JE. Pulmonary circulation; pulmonary edema; pleural fluid. In: Guyton AC, Hall JE, eds. *Textbook of Medical Physiology.* 11th ed. Philadelphia: Saunders; 2006:483-489.

136. Burrows B et al. Patterns of cardiovascular dysfunction in chronic obstructive lung disease. *N Engl J Med.* 1972;286:912-918.

137. Enson Y et al. The influence of hydrogen ion concentration and hypoxia on the pulmonary circulation. *J Clin Invest.* 1964;43:1146.

138. Salvaterra CG et al. Is the early diagnosis of pulmonary hypertension possible, useful, and cost-effective? In: Weir EK et al, eds. *The Diagnosis and Treatment of Pulmonary Hypertension.* Mount Kisco, NY: Futura; 1992.

139. Grippi MA. Respiratory failure: an overview. In: Fishman AP, ed. *Fishman's Pulmonary Disease and Disorders.* New York: McGraw-Hill; 2008:2509-2522.

140. Mann DL. Heart failure and cor pulmonale. In: Fauci AS et al, eds. *Harrison's Principles of Internal Medicine.* 17th ed. New York: McGraw-Hill; 2008:1596-1606.

141. Cooper CB, Howard P. An analysis of sequential physiologic changes in hypoxic cor pulmonale during long-term oxygen therapy. *Chest.* 1991;100:76-80.

142. Bovill JG et al. Opioid analgesics in anesthesia: with special reference to their use in cardiovascular anesthesia. *Anesthesiology.* 1984;61:731-755.

143. Berqvist D, Lindblad B. A 30-year survey of pulmonary embolism verified at autopsy: an analysis of 1274 surgical patients. *Br J Surg.* 1985;72:105-108.

144. West JB. Vascular diseases. In: West JB, ed. *Pulmonary Pathophysiology: the Essentials.* 7th ed. Baltimore: Lippincott Williams & Wilkins; 2008: 99-120.

145. Eger EI. Uptake and distribution. In: Miller RD, ed. *Anesthesia.* 6th ed. New York: Churchill Livingstone; 2005:131-154.

146. Donegan J. *Manual of Anesthesia for Emergency Surgery.* New York: Churchill Livingstone; 1987.

147. Cartagen R et al. Respiratory diseases. In: Fleisher LA. *Anesthesia and Uncommon Diseases.* 5th ed. Philadelphia: Saunders; 2006:127-151.

148. Treggiari MM, Dunn S. Anesthesia and critical care medicine. In: Barash PG et al, eds. *Clinical Anesthesia.* 5th ed. Philadelphia: Lippincott Williams & Wilkins; 2006:1473-1498.

149. Carlbom DJ, Davidson BL. Pulmonary embolism in the critically ill. *Chest.* 2007;132(1):313-324.

150. Weichman K, Ansell JE. Inferior vena cava filters in venous thromboembolism. *Prog Cardiovasc Dis.* 2006;49(2):98-105.

151. Arcelus JI et al. The management and outcome of acute venous thromboembolism: a prospective registry including 4011 patients. *J Vasc Surg.* 2003;38:916-922.

152. Buchalter SE et al. Surgical management of chronic pulmonary thromboembolic disease. *Clin Chest Med.* 1992;13:17-22.

153. Daily PO et al. Risk factors for pulmonary thromboendarterectomy. *J Thorac Cardiovasc Surg.* 1990;99:670-678.

154. Olman MA et al. Pulmonary vascular steal in chronic thromboembolic pulmonary hypertension. *Chest.* 1990;98:1430-1434.

155. Perel A. Pulmonary edema. In: Civetta JM, et al, eds. *Critical Care.* Philadelphia: Lippincott; 1988:1043.

156. Matthay MA. Acute respiratory distress syndrome: pathogenesis. In: Fishman AP, ed. *Fishman's Pulmonary Disease and Disorders.* New York: McGraw-Hill; 2008:2523-2534.

157. Stoelting RK et al. Restrictive lung disease. *Anesthesia and Coexisting Disease.* 4th ed. New York: Churchill Livingstone; 2002:205-216.

158. Matthay MA, Matthay RA. Pulmonary edema: cardiogenic and noncardiogenic. In: George RB et al, eds. *Chest Medicine: Essentials of Pulmonary and Critical Care Medicine.* 2nd ed. Baltimore: Williams & Wilkins; 1990:439.

159. Kozlow JH et al. Epidemiology and impact of aspiration pneumonia in patients undergoing surgery in Maryland, 1999-2000. *Crit Care Med.* 2003;31(7):1930-1937.

160. Mendelson CL. The aspiration of stomach contents into the lungs during obstetric anesthesia. *Am J Obstet Gynecol.* 1946;52:191-205.

161. Goodwin SR. Aspiration syndromes. In: Civetta JM et al, eds. *Critical Care.* Philadelphia: Lippincott; 1988:1081.

162. Cassiere HA. Aspiration pneumonia: current concepts and approach to management. *Medscape J Med.* 1998;2:1-11.

163. Kalinowski CP, Kirsch JR. Strategies for prophylaxis and treatment for aspiration. Best practice & research. *Clin Anesth.* 2004;18(4):719-737.

164. Janda M et al. Management of pulmonary aspiration. Best practice & research. *Clin Anesth.* 2006;20(3):409-427.

165. Warner MA et al. Clinical significance of pulmonary aspiration during the perioperative period. *Anesthesiology.* 1993;78:56-62.

166. Warner MA et al. Perioperative pulmonary aspiration in infants and children. *Anesthesiology.* 1999;90:66-71.

167. Kluger MT, Short TG. Aspiration during anaesthesia: a review of 133 cases from the Australian Anaesthetic Incident Monitoring Study (AIMS). *Anaesthesia.* 1999;54:19-26.

168. Ezri T et al. Peripartum general anaesthesia without tracheal intubation: incidence of aspiration pneumonia. *Anaesthesia.* 2000;5:421-426.

169. Schreiner MS. Gastric fluid volume: is it really a risk factor for pulmonary aspiration? *Anesth Analg.* 1998;87:874-876.

170. Roberts RB, Shirley MA. Reducing the risk of acid aspiration during cesarean section. *Anesth Analg.* 1974;53:6:859-868.

171. Harter RL et al. A comparison of the volume and pH of gastric contents of obese and lean surgical patients. *Anesth Analg.* 1998;86:147-152.

172. Sakai T et al. The incidence and outcome of perioperative pulmonary aspiration in a university hospital: a 4-year retrospective analysis. *Anesth Analg.* 2006;103(4):941-947.

173. Beck-Schimmer B et al. Pulmonary aspiration: new therapeutic approaches in the experimental model. *Anesthesia.* 2005;103(3):556-566.

174. Pawlik MT et al. Early treatment with pentoxifylline reduces lung injury induced by acid aspiration in rats. *Chest.* 2005;127:613-621.

175. Azuma Y et al. Comparison of inhibitory effects of local anesthetics on immune functions of neutrophils. *Int J Immunopharmacol.* 2000; 22(10):789-796.

176. Soop M et al. Preoperative oral carbohydrate treatment attenuates immediate postoperative insulin resistance. *Am J Physiol Endocrinol Metab.* 2001;280:E576-0583.

177. American Society of Anesthesiologists. Practice guidelines for preoperative fasting and the use of pharmacologic agents to reduce the risk of pulmonary aspiration: application to healthy patients undergoing elective surgery. *Anesthesiology.* 1999;90:896-905.

178. Hauptfleisch JJ, Payne KA. An oral sodium citrate-citric acid non-particulate buffer in humans. *Br J Anaesth.* 1999;77:642-644.

179. Armstrong L, Bohenek W. Evaluation of histamine2-receptor-antagonists (H2-antagonists): switch to famotidine at the University of Chicago Hospitals. *U Chicago Med Center Topics in Drug Ther.* 1996;38(10).

180. Priebe H. Cricoid pressure? An alternative view. *Semin Anesth Periop Med Pain.* 2005;(24):120-126.

181. Thorn K et al. The effects of cricoid pressure, remifentanil, and propofol on esophageal motility and the lower esophageal sphincter. *Anesth Analg.* 2005;100(4):1200-1203.

182. Jeske HC et al. The influence of postural changes on gastroesophageal reflux and barrier pressure in nonfasting individuals. *Anesth Analg.* 2005;101:597-600.

183. Blunt MC et al. Gel lubrication of the tracheal tube cuff reduces pulmonary aspiration. *Anesthesiology.* 2001;95:377-381.

184. Sanjay PS et al. The effect of gel lubrication on cuff leakage of double lumen tubes during thoracic surgery. *Anesthesiology.* 2006;61(2):133-137.

185. Knight PR et al. Acid aspiration increases sensitivity to increased ambient oxygen concentrations. *Am J Physiol.* 2000;278(6):L1240-1247.

186. Nishina K et al. *Anesthesiology.* 1988;88(5):1300-1309.

187. Smith RM, Spragg RG. Adult respiratory distress syndrome. In: Bordow RA, Moser KM, eds. *Manual of Clinical Problems in Pulmonary Medicine.* 3rd ed. Boston: Little, Brown; 1991:263.

188. Taylor RW. The adult respiratory distress syndrome. In: Kirby RR, Taylor RW, eds. *Respiratory Failure.* Chicago: Year Book; 1986:208.

189. Epstein PE. Acute respiratory failure in the surgical patient. In: Fishman AP, ed. *Manual of Pulmonary Diseases and Disorders.* 3rd ed. New York: McGraw-Hill; 2002:1034-1043.

190. Ranieri VM et al. Mechanical ventilation as a mediator of multisystem organ failure in acute respiratory distress syndrome. *JAMA.* 2000;284:43-44.

191. Morgan GE, Mikhail MS. Anesthesia for patients with respiratory disease. *Clinical Anesthesiology.* 4th ed. East Norwalk, CT: Appleton & Lange; 2006:571-584.

192. Brown M. ICU: critical care. In: Barash PG et al, eds. *Clinical Anesthesia.* 4th ed. Philadelphia: Lippincott; 2001:1463-1484.

193. Fishman JA. Approach to the patient with pulmonary infection. In: Fishman AP, ed. *Fishman's Pulmonary Disease and Disorders.* New York: McGraw-Hill; 2008:1981-2016.

194. Kachel DL et al. Amiodarone-induced injury of human pulmonary artery endothelial cells: protection by α-tocopherol. *J Pharmacol Exp Ther.* 1990;254:1107-1112.

195. Dusman RE et al. Clinical features of amiodarone-induced pulmonary toxicity. *Circulation.* 1990;82:51-59.

196. Suarez LD et al. Subacute pneumopathy during amiodarone therapy. *Chest.* 1983;83:566-568.

197. Cooper JA et al. Drug-induced pulmonary disease: part 2. Noncytotoxic drugs. *Am Rev Respir Dis.* 1986;133:488-505.

198. Kawai K, Akaza H. Bleomycin-induced pulmonary toxicity in chemotherapy for testicular cancer. *Expert Opin Drug Saf.* 2003;2(6):587-596.

199. Bowden DH. Unraveling pulmonary fibrosis: the bleomycin model [editorial]. *Lab Invest.* 1984;50:487-488.

200. Weiss RB, Muggia FM. Cytotoxic drug-induced pulmonary disease: update 1980. *Am J Med.* 1980;68:259-266.

201. Beers ME. Oxygen therapy and pulmonary oxygen toxicity. In: Fishman AP, ed. *Fishman's Pulmonary Disease and Disorders.* New York: McGraw-Hill; 2008:2613-2630.

202. Clark JM, Lambertsen CJ. Pulmonary oxygen toxicity: a review. *Pharmacol Rev.* 1971;23:37-133.

203. Muzaffar A, Demeter SL. Drug-induced pulmonary disease. In: Baum GL, Wolinsky E, eds. *Textbook of Pulmonary Diseases.* Vol 1. 5th ed. Boston: Little, Brown; 1993:775.

204. Donat SM, Levy DA. Bleomycin associated pulmonary toxicity: is perioperative oxygen restriction necessary? *J Urol.* 1998;160:1347-1352.

205. Auger WR. Pulmonary oxygen toxicity. In: Bordow RA, Moser KM, eds. *Manual of Clinical Problems in Pulmonary Medicine with Annotated Key References.* 3rd ed. Boston: Little, Brown; 1991:282.

206. Cooper JA et al. Drug-induced pulmonary disease: part 1. Cytotoxic drugs. *Am Rev Respir Dis.* 1986;133:321-340.

207. Sharma OP. Sarcoidosis. In: Kelley WN, ed. *Textbook of Internal Medicine.* 2nd ed. Philadelphia: Lippincott; 1993:1742.

208. Moller DR. Systemic sarcoidosis. In: Fishman AP, ed. *Fishman's Pulmonary Disease and Disorders.* New York: McGraw-Hill; 2008:1125-1142.

209. Reynolds HY, Matthay RA. Diffuse interstitial and alveolar inflammatory diseases. In: George RB, et al, eds. *Chest Medicine: Essentials of Pulmonary and Critical Care Medicine.* 2nd ed. Baltimore: Williams & Wilkins; 1990:231.

210. Wills MH, Harris MM. An unusual airway complication with sarcoidosis. *Anesthesiology.* 1987;66:554-555.

211. Cheitlin MD, Trunkey DD. Chest trauma. In: Saunders CE, Ho MT, eds. *Emergency Diagnosis and Treatment.* 4th ed. East Norwalk, CT: Appleton & Lange; 1992:266.

212. Campbell L, Gropper M. Critical care medicine. In: Stoelting RK, Miller RD, eds. *Basics of Anesthesia.* 5th ed. New York: Churchill Livingstone; 2007:595-607.

213. Eger EI II, Saidman LJ. Hazards of nitrous oxide anesthesia in bowel obstruction and pneumothorax. *Anesthesiology.* 1965;26:61-66.

214. Aker J. Atelectasis during the perioperative period: etiology, contributing factors, and patient outcome. *Curr Rev Nurse Anesth.* 2007;23(29):271-277.

215. Hedenstierna G. Airway closure, atelectasis and gas exchange during anaesthesia. *Minerva Anestesiol.* 2002;68(5):332-336.

216. Rothen H et al. Atelectasis and pulmonary shunting during the induction of general anesthesia—can they be avoided? *Acta Anaesthesiol Scand.* 1996;40:524-529.

217. Cai H et al. Effect of low tidal volume ventilation on atelectasis in patients during general anesthesia: a computed tomographic scan. *J Clin Anesth.* 2007;19(2):125-129.

218. Hager D et al. Tidal volume reduction in patients with acute lung injury when plateau pressures are not high. *Am J Resp Crit Care Med.* 2005;172:1241-1245.

219. Habashi N. Other approaches to open-lung ventilation: airway pressure release ventilation. *Crit Care Med.* 2005;33(3):S228-S240.

220. Sugarbaker DJ, Lukanich JM. Chest wall and pleura. *Sabiston Textbook of Surgery: the Biological Basis of Modern Surgical Practice.* 18th ed. Philadelphia: Saunders; 2008:1655-1676.

221. Prakash UB. Skeletal diseases. In: Baum GL, Wolinsky E, eds. *Textbook of Pulmonary Diseases.* Vol 2. 5th ed. Boston: Little, Brown; 1993:1691.

222. Welch KJ, Shamberger RC. Chest wall deformities. In: Shields TW, ed. *General Thoracic Surgery.* 3rd ed. Philadelphia: Lea & Febiger; 1989:515.

223. Castile RG et al. Symptomatic pectus deformities of the chest. *Am Rev Respir Dis.* 1982;126:564-568.

224. Haller JA Jr et al. Evolving management of pectus excavatum based on a single institutional experience of 664 patients. *Ann Surg.* 1989;209:578-582.

225. Wynn SR et al. Exercise cardiorespiratory function in adolescents with pectus excavatum: observations before and after operation. *J Thorac Cardiovasc Surg.* 1990;99:41-47.

226. Dudley FR, Findley LJ. Neuromuscular and skeletal disease. In: Murray J, ed. *Pulmonary Complications of Systemic Disease.* New York: Marcel Dekker; 1992:333.

227. Chidambaram B, Mehta AV. Currarino-Silverman syndrome (pectus carinatum type 2 deformity) and mitral valve disease. *Chest.* 1992;102:780-782.

228. Robicsek F et al. Pectus carinatum. *J Thorac Cardiovasc Surg.* 1979;78:52-61.

229. Prakash UB. Pulmonary manifestations in systemic diseases. In: Baum GL, Wolinsky E, eds. *Textbook of Pulmonary Diseases.* Vol 2. 5th ed. Boston: Little, Brown; 1993:1691.

230. Collis DK, Ponseti IV. Long-term follow-up of patients with idiopathic scoliosis not treated surgically. *J Bone Joint Surg.* 1969;51A:425-445.

231. Pehrsson K et al. Lung function in adult idiopathic scoliosis: a 20-year follow up. *Thorax.* 1991;46:474-478.

232. Guilleminault C et al. Severe kyphoscoliosis, breathing, and sleep: the "Quasimodo" syndrome during sleep. *Chest.* 1981;79:626-630.

233. Baydur A et al. Respiratory mechanics in anesthetized young patients with kyphoscoliosis: immediate and delayed effects of corrective spinal surgery. *Chest.* 1990;97:1157-1164.

234. Zayas V. Scoliosis. In: Yao FS, Artusio JF, eds. *Anesthesiology: Problem-Oriented Patient Management.* 6th ed. Philadelphia: Lippincott; 2008:1155-1178.

235. Jones RS et al. Mechanical inefficiency of the thoracic cage in scoliosis. *Thorax.* 1981;36:456-461.

236. Boffa P et al. Lung developmental abnormalities in severe scoliosis. *Thorax.* 1984;39:681-682.

237. Winter R et al. Scoliosis, kyphosis, and lordosis. In: Youmans JR, ed. *Neurosurgical Surgery.* Vol 4. 3rd ed. Philadelphia: Saunders; 1990.

238. Nachemson A. A long-term follow-up study of nontreated scoliosis. *Acta Orthop Scand.* 1968;39:466-576.

239. Nilsonne U, Lundgren KD. Long-term prognosis in idiopathic scoliosis. *Acta Orthop Scand*. 1968;39:456-465.

240. Kafer ER. Respiratory and cardiovascular functions in scoliosis and the principles of anesthetic management. *Anesthesiology*. 1980;52:339-351.

241. Cosgrove GP, Schwarz MI. Pulmonary manifestations of the collagen-vascular diseases. In: Fishman AP, ed. *Fishman's Pulmonary Disease and Disorders*. New York: McGraw-Hill; 2008:1193-1212.

242. King TE. Connective tissue disease. In: Schwarz MI, King TE, eds. *Interstitial Lung Diseases*. 2nd ed. St Louis: Mosby; 1993:271.

243. Rosenow FC III et al. Pleuropulmonary manifestations of ankylosing spondylitis. *Mayo Clin Proc*. 1977;52:641-649.

244. Stewart RM et al. Regional lung function in ankylosing spondylitis. *Thorax*. 1986;31:433-437.

245. Fisher LR et al. Relation between chest expansion, pulmonary function, and exercise tolerance in patients with ankylosing spondylitis. *Ann Rheum Dis*. 1990;49:921-925.

ANESTHESIA FOR THORACIC SURGERY

Michael Rieker

Thoracic anesthesia has evolved as a specialty since the development of bronchial blockers and double-lumen endobronchial tubes. The anesthetist can safely and selectively ventilate one lung to create a quiet field for the surgeon. Patients undergoing thoracic surgery have varying degrees of respiratory disease and may experience profound changes in ventilation and blood flow through the lungs, so a thorough understanding of this complex physiology is vital.

PREOPERATIVE PREPARATION

Resection of affected lung tissue in bronchogenic carcinoma offers a better prognosis than radiation and chemotherapy. The prognosis without surgery is poor, even if detected in early stages; if detected upon presentation of symptoms, mean survival is only 13 months without surgical intervention.[1] Because most pulmonary patients have many risk factors for respiratory disease, evaluating respiratory function and predicting postresection function are crucial to anticipating the patient's intraoperative and postoperative care.[2]

Preoperative assessment of patients in need of pulmonary resection surgery should address two questions. First, does the risk of potential postoperative complications preclude performing the surgery? Second, will postoperative pulmonary function be sufficient to allow reasonable quality of life? Spirometry parameters (forced expiratory volume in first second [FEV_1] and forced vital capacity [FVC]) decline approximately 10% following lobectomy and approximately 33% following pneumonectomy.[3] However, in spite of these compromises usually superimposed on preexisting lung disease, mortality from unresected carcinomas is sufficiently high that the risks of postoperative complications would have to be extraordinarily high before they would preclude the operation.

Fear of creating pulmonary insufficiency by lung resection is an important concern, and numerous studies have been designed to determine the lowest limit of pulmonary function that will allow surgery to be safely performed. Research findings are limited in their ability to predict particular complications, though. Studies performed to predict postoperative pulmonary complications after lung resection demonstrate that patients develop both pulmonary and cardiac complications such as arrhythmias, myocardial infarction, pulmonary embolism, pneumonia, and empyema. These complications influence the duration of mechanical ventilation and outcome; however, none of these complications can be predicted by preoperative studies of pulmonary function. No consensus exists with regard to what should be included in a preoperative

evaluation for risk of complications following lung resection. See Box 28-1 and discussion in this chapter for commonly used preoperative criteria for lung resection.

Changes in surgical techniques, especially the use of video-assisted thoracoscopy, have markedly decreased the incidence of postoperative pulmonary complications and will necessitate a reevaluation of the testing required for preoperative assessment.[4] For smaller lung resections, minimal preoperative evaluations of cardiac disease, gas exchange, and oxygenation may suffice. Given the large physiologic changes that occur after pneumonectomy, complete pulmonary function testing, as well as cardiac testing, may still be reasonable in these patients.

Lung resection surgeries are now being performed on more patients who have end-stage chronic obstructive pulmonary disease (COPD), morbid obesity, or who are of advanced age.[5-7] Evidence shows that these patients can be treated safely, but further data are necessary to determine which preoperative tests are useful in predicting outcome and which tests are cost-effective.

Preoperative Evaluation

History and Physical Examination

Cancer patients who undergo lung resection typically have a history of multiple risk factors and signs of respiratory disease. Risk factors include cigarette smoking, air pollution, and industrial chemical exposure. Patients must be evaluated for exertional dyspnea, productive cough, hemoptysis, cyanosis, poor exercise tolerance, and chest pain. Difficulty breathing in the supine position can result from COPD or compression of the airway by a mediastinal mass. Lung cancer patients should be assessed for mass and metabolic effects, metastasis, and medications (Table 28-1).

A history of COPD is common. The chest radiograph of the patient with COPD shows hyperinflation, increased anteroposterior diameter, and increased vascular markings. Increased pulmonary vascular resistance (PVR) resulting from compression of the vascular bed increases the likelihood of right ventricular failure. The patient should be evaluated for ischemic and valvular heart disease. A high index of suspicion should be maintained for hormonal abnormalities, because some tumors secrete endocrine-like substances such as adrenocorticotropic hormone, antidiuretic hormone, serotonin, parathyroid hormones, and insulin, causing a variety of metabolic abnormalities (Table 28-2). Nutritional status, commonly compromised in patients with cancer, is also important to note because hypoalbuminemia and malnutrition are associated with increased postoperative complications such as pneumonia.[8] Box 28-2 lists important elements of the preoperative evaluation.

BOX **28-1**

Summary of Preoperative Factors That Predict Postoperative Complications

Factors That Characterize Low-Risk Patients
FEV_1 >2 L or 80% of predicted
PPO FEV_1 at least 80% of predicted normal value
$\dot{V}O_2$max >20 mL/kg/min
Ability to climb 5 flights of stairs

Factors That Characterize High-Risk Patients
FEV_1 <2 L or <40% of predicted
PPO FEV_1 <40% of predicted normal value
D_{LCO} <40% of predicted
Predicted postoperative product <1650
$\dot{V}O_2$max <10 mL/kg/min
Inability to climb 1 flight of stairs
Oxygen desaturation >4% during exercise

TABLE **28-2**	Initial Preanesthetic Assessment for Thoracic Surgery
Patient Type	**Assessments**
All patients	Assess exercise tolerance, estimate PPO FEV_1%*, discuss postoperative analgesia, consider discontinuation of smoking
Patients with PPO FEV_1 < 40%	D_{LCO}, $\dot{V}/\dot{Q}$ scan, $\dot{V}O_2$max
Patients with cancer	Consider the "4 Ms": mass effects, metabolic effects, metastases, medications
Patients with COPD	Arterial blood gas analysis, physiotherapy, bronchodilators
Patients with increased renal risk	Measure creatinine and blood urea nitrogen

Modified from Slinger PP, Johnston MR. Preoperative assessment and management. In: Kaplan JA, Slinger PD, eds. Thoracic Anesthesia. 3rd ed. Philadelphia: Churchill Livingstone; 2003.
COPD, *Chronic obstructive pulmonary disease;* D_{LCO}, *diffusing capacity for carbon monoxide;* FEV_1, *forced expiratory volume in 1 second;* PPO, *predicted postoperative;* $\dot{V}O_2$max, *maximum oxygen consumption;* $\dot{V}/\dot{Q}$, *ventilation perfusion ratio.*
*PPO FEV_1% = Preoperative FEV_1% × (1% functioning lung tissue removed/100). For values >40%, postoperative complications are rare; for values between 30% and 40%, postoperative problems are possible; for values <30%, postoperative ventilation is likely to be required.

TABLE **28-1**	Anesthetic Considerations in Lung Cancer Patients: "The 4 Ms"
Mass effects	Obstructive pneumonia, lung abscess, superior vena cava syndrome, tracheobronchial distortion, Pancoast syndrome, recurrent laryngeal nerve or phrenic nerve paresis, chest wall or mediastinal extension
Metabolic effects	Lambert-Eaton syndrome, hypercalcemia, hyponatremia, Cushing syndrome
Metastases	Particularly to brain, bone, liver, and adrenals
Medications	Chemotherapy-induced lung changes

Modified from Slinger PP, Johnston MR. Preoperative assessment and management. In: Kaplan JA, Slinger PD, eds. Thoracic Anesthesia. 3rd ed. Philadelphia: Churchill Livingstone; 2003.

Diagnostic Data

Chest Radiograph. Anteroposterior and lateral projections show hyperinflation and increased vascular markings in patients with COPD. Bullae of emphysema may be present. Infection or pleural effusions may be noted preoperatively and treated to improve the postoperative course.

The locations of masses can be identified. In some patients it can be ascertained whether lesions compress mediastinal structures, cause tracheal shift, or invade the airway. This information is important to predict whether intubation will be difficult, whether induction of anesthesia could cause collapse of the airway, or whether surgical dissection may be difficult or bloody.[9]

Electrocardiogram. Pulmonary disease can cause right ventricular hypertrophy and strain. In such a case, the electrocardiogram (ECG) shows low-voltage QRS waves and poor R-wave

progression over the precordial leads. Right ventricular hypertrophy causes an R/S ratio greater than 1 in lead V_1, along with a shift toward right-axis deviation.[10] Right atrial hypertrophy causes the initial component of a biphasic P wave in lead V_1 to be larger than the second component.[11] Increased PVR and right ventricular strain could preclude pneumonectomy because of the added resistance produced by clamping the vasculature of one lung.

Arterial Blood Gases. Measurement of preoperative room air arterial blood gases is useful in guiding the weaning of O_2 and ventilation postoperatively. Carbon dioxide (CO_2) retention with an arterial partial pressure ($PaCO_2$) greater than 45 mm Hg is an indicator of poor ventilatory function. However, hypercapnia is not a reliable predictor of increased risk of perioperative pulmonary complications.[12,13] Preoperative hypoxemia (SpO_2 < 90%) and particularly desaturation during exercise are predictive of increased complications following thoracic surgery.[14]

Pulmonary Function Tests. Multiple studies have been done to identify which preoperative pulmonary function tests are good indicators of postoperative complications. Indicators suggested to predict complications include a forced vital capacity (FVC) less than 50% of the predicted value, a forced expiratory volume in 1 second (FEV_1) less than 2 L, FEV_1/FVC less than 50%, and a lung carbon monoxide diffusing capacity (D_{LCO}) less than 50% of the predicted value. Assessment of spirometry should be based upon values obtained post-bronchodilator therapy, because these would represent the patient's potential lung function once optimized on medications.

While a static metric (such as FEV_1 <2 L) to predict postoperative pulmonary complications is easy to assess, a standard

Preoperative Evaluation of Patients for Pulmonary Surgery

1. Advanced age alone should not be considered a contraindication for lung resection surgery.
2. Patients should undergo cardiologic evaluation.
   - Unstable angina, MI within 6 weeks, or significant arrhythmias predict high risk of cardiac complications.
3. Prior to lung resection, spirometry should be performed.
   - FEV_1 >80% of predicted or >2 L indicates minimal risk; further testing is not indicated.
   - FEV_1 <40% of predicted indicates high risk for complications or death.
4. With evidence of interstitial lung disease or dyspnea,
   - D_{LCO} should be measured.
   - D_{LCO} <60% predicts increased complications; <40% = high risk.
5. If FEV_1 or D_{LCO} <80% of predicted, postoperative lung function should be estimated.
6. If preop or predicted postop FEV_1 or D_{LCO} are <40% of predicted normal, exercise testing should be performed.
   - A $\dot{V}O_2$max (>/< 15 mL/kg/min) will dispute or confirm the risk conferred by the low FEV_1.
   - Inability to climb one flight of stairs, $\dot{V}O_2$max <10 mL/kg/min or desaturation >4% during exercise indicates high risk for complications/mortality.
7. Lung volume reduction surgery may be associated with improved outcomes beyond what preoperative measurements would suggest.

From Beckles A et al. The physiologic evaluation of patients with lung cancer being considered for resectional surgery. Chest. 2003;123:105S-114S; British Thoracic Society. BTS guidelines on the selection of patients with lung cancer for surgery. Thorax 2001;56:89-108.

value does not account for the patient's age, gender, or height. A more reliable approach is to assess predicted postoperative (PPO) function tests. The PPO FEV_1 is calculated by multiplying the current FEV_1 by the fraction of functioning lung or the fraction of lung segments that will remain after surgery.[15] Predicted postoperative FEV_1 has been found to be an important parameter, serving as an independent predictor of complications.[16] Numerous studies demonstrate consistently that a PPO FEV_1 at least 40% of predicted is a good criterion for safe lung resection.[17] Patients with a preoperative FEV_1 less than 35% of predicted are considered at high risk for postoperative complications. However, Linden and colleagues reported a series of 100 thoracic surgery patients with FEV_1 less than 35% who demonstrated a low rate of mortality and ventilator dependence but who did demonstrate prolonged duration of hospitalization and air leak.[18]

Ventilation-Perfusion Tests. When the preoperative lung function tests indicate that the patient is at increased risk for perioperative complications, split lung function tests of ventilation and perfusion are valuable in the prediction of postresection lung function.[19] Removal of a diseased portion of lung may not decrease overall lung function. Ventilation can be measured by having the patient inhale one vital capacity breath of a radioisotope and measuring isotope counts with multiple scanners placed over the chest wall. Radioisotope injected intravenously and imaged shows the distribution of perfusion to all areas of the lung. After determining function in various areas of the lung, calculations can then estimate postresection function by multiplying current function by the fraction of functioning lung that will remain postoperatively. Although sound in principle, radionuclide studies have been found to suffer imprecision in the range of 20% in their ability to accurately predict pulmonary function postoperatively.[20]

Calculations based on segmental lung regions may help predict outcomes for patients undergoing lung volume reduction surgery. This procedure of removing emphysematous portions of lung to improve overall lung function has proved efficacious and particularly beneficial in allowing resection of cancerous lung tissue from patients in whom overall lung function studies would have contraindicated surgery. Lung volume reduction surgery is most useful in patients with heterogeneous emphysema (particularly when the emphysematous lobe is also the one containing the tumor), where removal of a lung segment or lobe will result in better pulmonary function overall.[15] Incidentally, this effect is appreciated more often with upper rather than lower lobectomy, in which patients with a low preoperative FEV_1 tend to demonstrate improvement in the FEV_1 following upper lobectomy.[21]

Diffusion Capacity. Diffusion capacity of the lung tests the lung's ability to allow transport of gas across the alveolar-capillary membrane. Because it is difficult to measure the diffusing capacity of oxygen, carbon monoxide (CO) is used, in which the patient inhales a small amount of CO, holds the breath for 10 seconds, exhales, and the amount of CO in the exhaled breath is measured. After subtracting the amount of CO that should be expired with dead space air, the amount exhaled provides an indicator of the diffusion of gases in the lung. A carbon monoxide diffusing capacity of the lungs (D_{LCO}) less than 60% of predicted has been associated with increased complications and mortality following pulmonary surgery.[22,23] However, D_{LCO} has also been found to have good specificity but low sensitivity as an independent measurement. The product of the predicted values for D_{LCO} and FEV_1 may provide better reliability than single measures. This measurement, called the *predicted postoperative product*, was found by Pierce to be less than 1650 in 75% of those who died.[24] Maximal oxygen consumption ($\dot{V}O_2$max) during exercise testing is also assessed as a strong predictor of outcomes.[25,26] A $\dot{V}O_2$max less than 10 mL/kg/min (or 50% of predicted) is associated with increased mortality, whereas a $\dot{V}O_2$max greater than 20 mL/kg/min is a favorable finding.[17] In a study of 125 pulmonary resection patients, Brutsche found maximal oxygen uptake to be a highly predictive independent indicator of postoperative complications.[27] A $\dot{V}O_2$max greater than 20 mL/kg/min suggests little risk of complications, but values less than 15 mL/kg/min can be interpreted as representing increased risk, and values less than 10 mL/kg/min indicate a high risk of death following surgery.[15] These values may be roughly estimated by evaluating the patient's physical ability, in which the ability to climb five flights of stairs suggests $\dot{V}O_2$max greater than 20 mL/kg/min, and the inability to climb one flight of stairs suggests $\dot{V}O_2$max less than 10 mL/kg/min.[28]

Patient Optimization

Aggressive treatment of acute or reversible components of respiratory disease greatly decreases the risk of postoperative complications. Treatable preoperative conditions include infections, excess bronchial secretions, bronchospasm, dehydration,

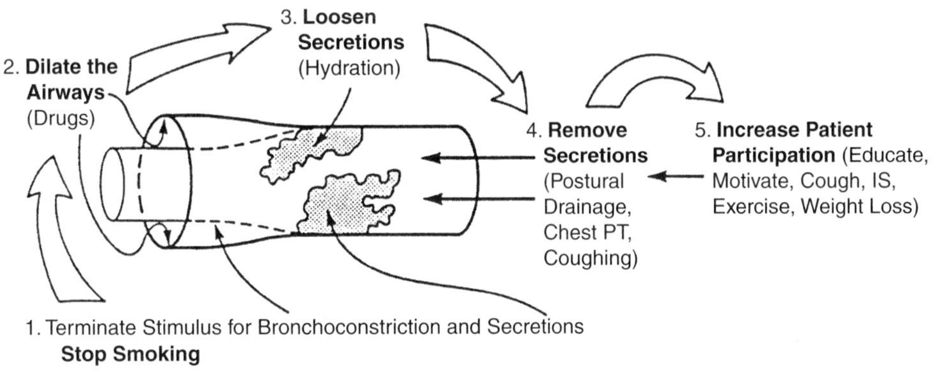

FIGURE **28-1**   A full, aggressive preoperative respiratory preparation regimen entails a five-pronged attack. *(1)* Require the patient to stop smoking. *(2)* Dilate the airways. *(3)* Loosen secretions. *(4)* Remove secretions. *(5)* Increase patient participation. *IS,* Incentive spirometry; *PT,* chest physiotherapy. *(From Wilson WC, Benumof JL. Anesthesia for thoracic surgery. In: Miller RD, ed. Miller's Anesthesia. 6th ed. Philadelphia: Churchill Livingstone; 2005.)*

electrolyte imbalance, cigarette smoking, alcohol abuse, and malnutrition (Figure 28-1).

Although smoking cessation may reduce postoperative complications,[29] the timing of this intervention is important. Transient increases in mucus production may *increase* complications in patients who have surgery within 2 months of stopping smoking.[30] Owing to the urgent nature of treating pulmonary carcinoma, delaying surgery to allow for an adequate period of smoking cessation is an impractical goal.

Monitoring

The purpose of monitoring during thoracic surgery is the quick recognition of sudden and severe changes in ventilation and hemodynamics that can accompany positioning, one-lung ventilation (OLV), and surgical manipulation of the airway and thoracic structures. All patients require continuous monitoring of the ECG. Monitoring a combination of leads II and V_5 will help detect more than 85% of ischemia.[2] Esophageal stethoscopes, temperature monitoring, and pulse oximetry are routine. An airway pressure monitor helps detect changes in airway compliance and assists in identifying the proper placement of double-lumen tubes (DLTs). Capnography is useful for determining whether ventilation is adequate when one lung is deflated.

Arterial Pressure Monitoring

Arterial blood pressure monitoring instantly identifies acute hypotension with surgical manipulation. It also allows for frequent sampling of arterial blood for gas analysis. For thoracotomies, the arterial cannula is generally placed in the dependent arm, where it is more easily stabilized. For mediastinoscopy, an arterial line placed in the right arm detects compression of the innominate artery and helps prevent a decrease in cerebral blood flow. Alternately, a pulse oximeter probe placed on a digit of the right hand also detects compression of the innominate artery and can be compared to an arterial pressure waveform on the left to differentiate general from regional hypoperfusion.

Central Venous Pressure Monitoring

Central venous pressure (CVP) monitoring is not required for routine thoracotomies but may be indicated if the patient's volume status is unclear or if large fluid shifts are anticipated.

In complex cases, a CVP line may help manage fluid status. Increased filling pressures (CVP or pulmonary capillary wedge) have been associated with greater lung injury and prolonged mechanical ventilation following complex pulmonary surgery.[31] In addition, a CVP can provide large-bore access for rapid infusion and an access site should transvenous pacing or pulmonary artery pressure monitoring become necessary.

The CVP line can be inserted via the external or internal jugular veins or the subclavian veins. An external jugular line is more easily kinked in the lateral position. One should remain alert to the possibility of pneumothorax with the insertion of central lines. A pneumothorax on the ventilated side can lead to severe hypoxemia during OLV. If a subclavian puncture is planned, the insertion site should be on the same side as the planned thoracotomy.

Pulmonary Artery Pressure Monitoring

Although pulmonary artery pressure monitoring is not helpful in predicting postoperative complications,[16] monitoring pulmonary artery pressure may be considered in the presence of a history of severe cardiovascular disease, valvular heart disease, or significant pulmonary hypertension. It may also be useful in preventing fluid overload, which may worsen postoperative pulmonary function. However, the anesthetist must be cautious in interpreting values because in these circumstances, the normal correlation of right and left ventricular pressures may be disturbed. Pulmonary artery pressure monitoring is intended to provide estimation of left ventricular pressures and facilitate the improvement of cardiac performance with fluids and cardiovascular drugs. In spite of its past popularity, pulmonary artery catheterization has not been demonstrated to improve patient outcomes in either cardiac or noncardiac surgery.[32] There have even been suggestions that right heart catheterization may *promote* cardiac complications.[33] The use of pulmonary artery catheters has specific limitations during OLV. Lung pathology or hypoxic pulmonary vasoconstriction may alter the resistance in pulmonary vessels and reduce the correlation between pulmonary artery occlusion pressure and left ventricular pressure.[34] More than 90% of pulmonary artery catheters float into the right lung.[35] During right thoracotomy, then, the catheter will likely be in the nondependent, collapsed lung and give a false low reading for cardiac output. Finally, care must be taken to ensure that a pulmonary artery catheter is not situated in a vessel that will be clamped during the course of lung resection.

LATERAL DECUBITUS POSITION

The most frequent position chosen for surgical exposure during thoracotomy is the lateral decubitus position. A roll is placed beneath the torso just caudal to the axilla to prevent compression of the neurovascular bundle and forward rotation of the humeral head. It is important to note that this commonly called "axillary roll" is better considered an "axillary *support* roll," because positioning it *in* the axilla may cause neurovascular compression. Hyperabduction of the arms is prevented to keep the brachial plexus from stretching against the humeral head. Arms can be separately padded and extended forward with armboards. Strategies for supporting the nondependent arm may include a pillow between the arms, a padded Mayo stand (which provides good access to intravenous or arterial lines in the dependent arm), or specially made double armboards. Pulse oximetry or frequent palpation of the radial pulse ensures the integrity of circulation to the hand.[36]

The head is supported on pillows to maintain alignment of the head and neck with the spine. Lateral flexion of the neck can cause compression of the jugular veins or vertebral arteries, compromising cerebral circulation. The dependent ear can be compressed by the weight of the head. Careful padding or use of a foam doughnut relieves this pressure, but care must be taken to prevent corneal abrasion and retinal ischemia by avoiding pressure on the eyes.

Other pressure points of concern in the lateral position include the peroneal nerve in the area of the fibular head of the dependent leg and the femoral head of the nondependent leg if a stabilizing strap is placed over the patient. Please refer to Chapter 22 for more information about proper positioning.

Physiology of the Lateral Decubitus Position

Positional changes and changes in chest-wall integrity produce significant alterations in ventilation and perfusion of the lungs during thoracic surgery.

Upright Position

The distribution of perfusion in the lungs depends on gravity in relation to the level of the heart and on pressures transmitted through alveoli. In a spontaneously breathing, upright patient, blood perfusion increases linearly from the apex to the base of the lung (Figure 28-2). Flow reaches very low rates in the apex and is greatest at the base.

Owing to downward traction from gravity, pleural pressure is most negative at the apex of the lung, and this keeps alveoli distended (Figure 28-3). Dependent alveoli are less distended and therefore more compliant (can expand by a greater volume for a given pressure change because they are starting at a lower resting volume). Therefore, most of a tidal breath is distributed to the dependent alveoli (Figure 28-4). The higher ventilation matches the higher perfusion in the dependent lung, making gas exchange efficient.[37]

Awake Lateral Position

Less vertical distance is present to cause differences in the intrapleural pressure and blood pressure gradients in the lateral position (Figure 28-5). Abdominal contents displace the diaphragm in a cephalad direction on the dependent side. Starting from a higher position in the thorax, the dependent hemidiaphragm can

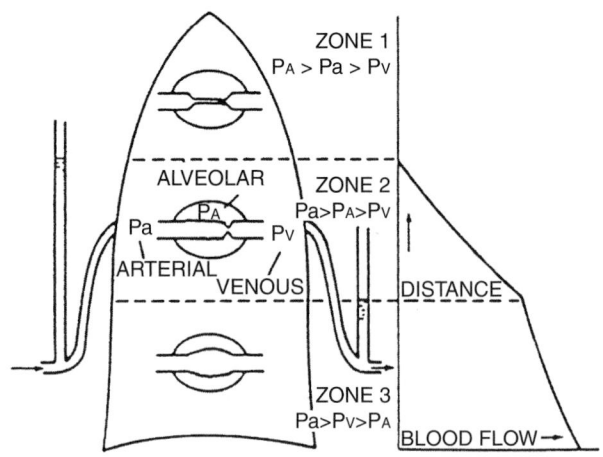

FIGURE **28-2**   The lung is divided into three zones according to the relative magnitudes of the pulmonary arterial, venous, and alveolar pressures (Pa, Pv, and Pa, respectively). In *zone 1*, alveolar exceeds arterial pressure, so the collapsible vessels are held closed and there is no flow. In *zone 2*, arterial exceeds alveolar pressure, but alveolar exceeds venous pressure. Under these conditions, a constriction occurs at the downstream end of each collapsible vessel, and the pressure inside the vessel at this point is equal to alveolar pressure, so the pressure gradient causing flow is arterial-alveolar. This gradient increases linearly with distance down the lung, and therefore so does blood flow. In *zone 3*, venous exceeds alveolar pressure, and the collapsible vessels are held open. Now the pressure gradient causing flow is arteriovenous, and this is constant down the zone. (*From West JB. Explanation of the uneven distribution of blood flow in the lung, based on the pressures affecting capillaries. In: West JB. Respiratory Physiology: The Essentials. 7th ed. Philadelphia: Lippincott Williams & Wilkins; 2005.*)

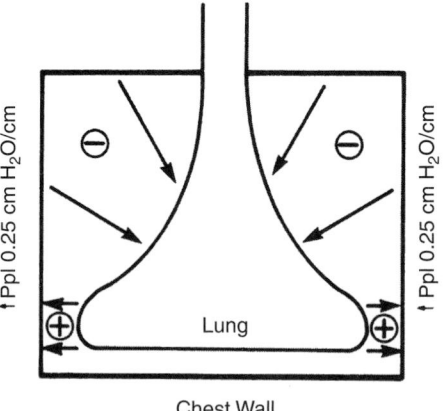

FIGURE **28-3**   Schematic diagram of the lung within the chest wall, showing the tendency of the lung to assume a globular shape because of its viscoelastic nature. The tendency of the top of the lung to collapse inward creates a relatively negative pressure at the apex, and the tendency of the bottom of the lung to spread outward creates a relatively positive pressure at the base. Therefore pleural pressure (Ppl) increases by 0.25 cm H_2O per centimeter of lung dependency. (*From Triantafillou AN et al. Physiology of the lateral decubitus position, the open chest, and one-lung ventilation. In: Kaplan JA, Slinger PD, eds. Thoracic Anesthesia. 3rd ed. Philadelphia: Churchill Livingstone; 2003.*)

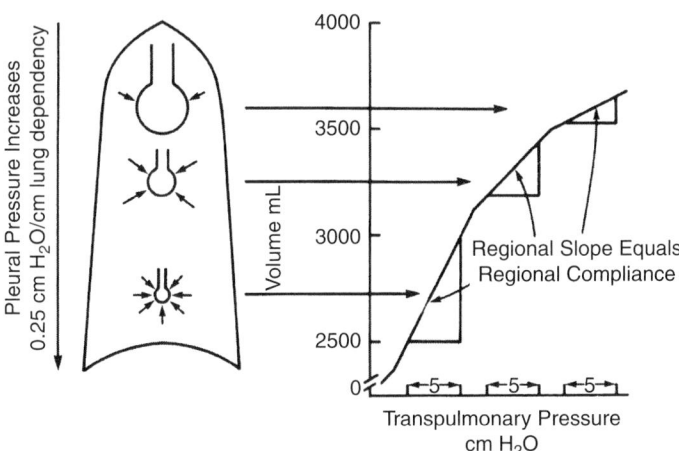

FIGURE **28-4**   Pleural pressure increases 0.25 cm H_2O every centimeter down the lung. The increase in pleural pressure causes a fourfold decrease in alveolar volume. Small alveoli are on the flat portion of the compliance curve and therefore receive the largest share of the tidal volume. Over the normal tidal volume range (lung volume increases by 500 mL from 2500 mL [normal functional residual capacity] to 3000 mL), the pressure-volume relationship is linear. (*From Triantafillou AN et al. Physiology of the lateral decubitus position, the open chest, and one-lung ventilation. In: Kaplan JA, Slinger PD, eds. Thoracic Anesthesia. 3rd ed. Philadelphia: Churchill Livingstone; 2003.*)

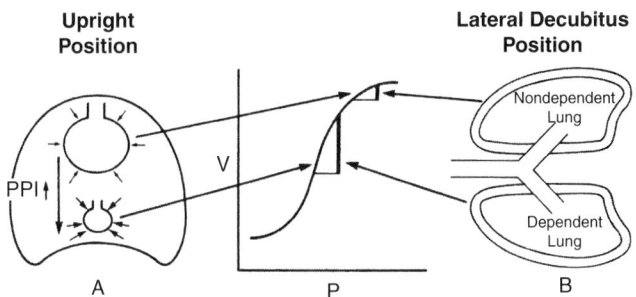

FIGURE **28-6**   In the lateral decubitus position, the dependent lung receives the majority of tidal ventilation. **A,** Pleural pressure (*Ppl*) in the awake, upright patient is most positive in the dependent portion of the lung, and alveoli in this region are the most compressed and have the lowest volume. Ppl is least positive (most negative) at the apex of the lung; alveoli in this region are least compressed and have the highest volume. When these regional differences in alveolar volume are translated into a regional transpulmonary pressure-alveolar volume curve, the small, dependent alveoli are on a steep portion of the curve, and the large, nondependent alveoli are on a flat portion of the curve. In this diagram, regional slope equals regional compliance. For a given and equal change in transpulmonary pressure, the dependent part of the lung receives a much larger share of the tidal volume than the nondependent lung. **B,** In the lateral decubitus position, gravity also causes pleural pressure gradients and affects the distribution of ventilation similarly. The dependent lung lies on a relatively steep portion of the pressure-volume curve, and the nondependent lung lies on a relatively flat portion. P, Transpulmonary pressure; V, alveolar volume. (*From Triantafillou AN et al. Physiology of the lateral decubitus position, the open chest, and one-lung ventilation. In: Kaplan JA, Slinger PD, eds. Thoracic Anesthesia. 3rd ed. Philadelphia: Churchill Livingstone; 2003.*)

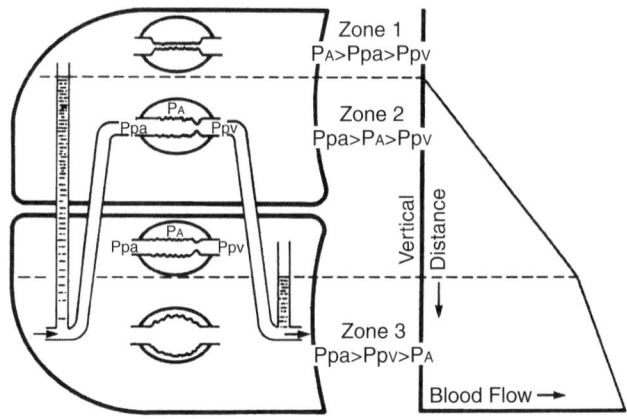

FIGURE **28-5**   Schematic representation of the effects of gravity on the distribution of pulmonary ventilation and blood flow in the lateral decubitus position. The vertical gradient in the lateral decubitus position is less than in the upright position; consequently blood flow in zones 2 and 3 is less. Nevertheless, pulmonary blood flow increases with lung dependency and is greater in the dependent lung than in the nondependent lung. PA, Alveolar pressure; *Ppa,* pulmonary arterial pressure; *Ppv,* pulmonary venous pressure. (*From Triantafillou AN et al. Physiology of the lateral decubitus position, the open chest, and one-lung ventilation. In: Kaplan JA, Slinger PD, eds. Thoracic Anesthesia. 3rd ed. Philadelphia: Churchill Livingstone; 2003.*)

ventilation and perfusion in the dependent lung is unchanged, and gas exchange remains efficient.

Anesthetized Lateral Position, Chest Closed, with Spontaneous Ventilation

A change in the distribution of ventilation is seen with the induction of anesthesia, even when spontaneous respiration is maintained. Functional residual capacity (FRC) decreases almost immediately with the induction of anesthesia. The weight of the mediastinum and the cephalad displacement of the diaphragm by abdominal contents further decrease FRC in the dependent lung and reduce the proportion of the favorable zone 3 area. Lower volumes in each lung shift their place on the compliance curve. The lungs are less compliant when they are either at a very high volume (distended alveoli) or a very low volume (atelectasis). In the anesthetized patient, the nondependent lung moves from a flat, noncompliant portion of the compliance curve to a more compliant position. Although anesthesia results in a net loss of FRC, the relative proportion of FRC in the nondependent lung increases in contrast to the dependent lung.[38] As the dependent lung loses FRC, its volume becomes so low as to decrease its compliance. It shifts to a less compliant, flatter portion of the curve (Figure 28-7). Ventilation is therefore preferentially distributed to the nondependent lung, while gravity-dependent blood flow preferentially goes to the dependent lung, resulting in a mismatch of ventilation and perfusion.

contract further. During inspiration, therefore, contraction of the diaphragm causes more of the tidal volume (VT) to fill the dependent lung. Because perfusion is dependent on gravity, perfusion in the lateral position is also greatest in the dependent lung (Figure 28-6). Overall, the relationship of greater

**Closed Chest, Lateral Decubitus Position
Distribution of Ventilation**

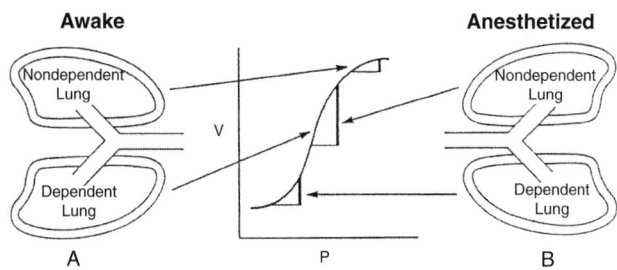

FIGURE **28-7** Schematic diagram showing **A,** distribution of ventilation in the awake patient in lateral decubitus position and **B,** distribution of ventilation in the anesthetized patient in lateral decubitus position. Induction of anesthesia has caused a loss of lung volume in both lungs, with the nondependent lung moving from a flat, noncompliant portion of the pressure-volume curve to a steep, compliant portion. The anesthetized patient in lateral decubitus position has the majority of tidal ventilation in the nondependent lung (where there is the least perfusion) and the minority of tidal ventilation in the dependent lung (where there is the greatest perfusion). *P,* Transpulmonary pressure; *V,* alveolar volume. *(From Triantafillou AN et al. Physiology of the lateral decubitus position, the open chest, and one-lung ventilation. In: Kaplan JA, Slinger PD, eds. Thoracic Anesthesia. 3rd ed. Philadelphia: Churchill Livingstone; 2003.)*

**Progressive Cephalad Displacement
of the Diaphragm**

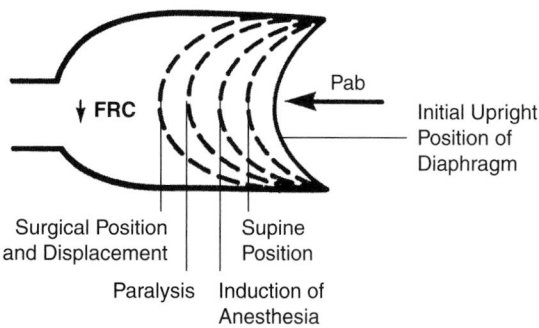

FIGURE **28-8** Anesthesia and surgery may cause a progressive cephalad displacement of the diaphragm. The sequence of events involves assumption of the supine position, induction of anesthesia, causation of paralysis, assumption of several surgical positions, and displacement by retractors and packs. The cephalad displacement of the diaphragm results in decreased functional residual capacity (FRC). *Pab,* Pressure of the abdominal contents. *(From Benumof JL. Anesthesia for Thoracic Surgery. 2nd ed. Philadelphia: Saunders; 1995.)*

Anesthetized, Paralyzed, Mechanically Ventilated Patient

Under mechanical ventilation, the diaphragm no longer contributes to ventilation of the lower lung, and FRC further declines as the compression from abdominal viscera is no longer counteracted by the force of the contracting diaphragm (Figure 28-8). With the initiation of mechanical ventilation and the deletion of effect of the contracting diaphragm, ventilation further shifts to follow the path of least resistance, favoring the nondependent lung. The ventilation-perfusion relationship further deteriorates. The addition of positive end-expiratory pressure (PEEP) to

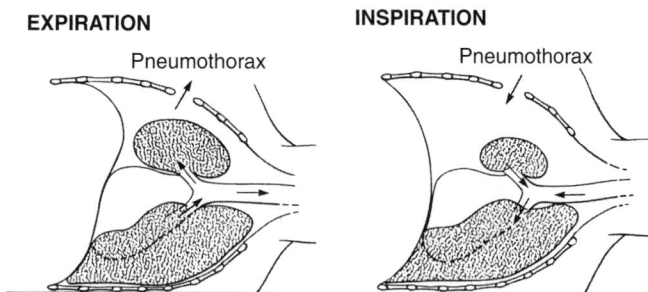

FIGURE **28-9** Paradoxical respiration in the spontaneously breathing patient lying on the side. *(From Tarhan S, Moffitt EA. Principles of thoracic anesthesia. Surg Clin North Am. 1973;53:813.)*

mechanical ventilation may help restore FRC and improve the ventilation-perfusion ratio.

Anesthetized Open-Chest Patient

The open chest greatly reduces resistance to gas flow in the nondependent lung by detaching the lung from its pleural connection with the chest wall. This causes further loss of ventilation to the dependent lung, in preference for the nondependent lung. The mediastinum also further shifts downward because of loss of negative intrapleural pressure in the nondependent lung, which helped to distend it. Ventilation to the dependent lung is decreased in proportion to the displacement of the lung by the mediastinal structures. Compression of the great vessels may cause a decrease in cardiac output and circulatory compromise. Any spontaneous respiration becomes very inefficient as paradoxical movement of air occurs on inspiration from the open-chest lung into the dependent lung, which has the greater negative intrapleural pressure. On expiration, gas exits the dependent lung and enters both the trachea and the open-chest lung, causing the lung to expand (Figure 28-9). Paradoxical respiration compromises fresh gas exchange in the dependent lung as part of the VT moves to and fro between the lungs.[39] Positive-pressure ventilation diminishes the effects of mediastinal shift and paradoxical respiration. However, during mechanical ventilation, the open chest provides no resistance, and the greatly increased compliance of that lung allows a higher proportion of ventilation to go to the nondependent lung, the least perfused area of the thorax. The less ventilated, better-perfused, dependent lung contributes to physiologic shunt, as blood flows through atelectatic areas without acquiring oxygen. Although the prevalence of different zones is not as evenly distributed as diagrams would suggest, the lateral, anesthetized, paralyzed, open-chest patient does exhibit the epitome of significant regional areas of disparity between ventilation and perfusion.

ONE-LUNG VENTILATION

Indications for Lung Separation

The ability to provide distinct ventilation to the separate lungs facilitates pulmonary surgery by providing a quiet surgical field. This is particularly helpful in the case of thoracoscopic surgery, in which visualization and the ability to manipulate the operative lung are limited. Thoracic surgeons will commonly consider lung separation an absolute requirement for pulmonary surgery. However, surgery can be performed on a lung that is being ventilated, and thoracic surgery alone is not an absolute indication for OLV. In fact, in the case of pediatric patients, gentle

Indications for Separation of the Two Lungs (Double-Lumen Tube Intubation) or One-Lung Ventilation

I. Absolute
   A. Isolation of one lung from the other to avoid spillage or contamination
      1. Infection
      2. Massive hemorrhage
   B. Control of the distribution of ventilation
      1. Bronchopleural fistula
      2. Bronchopleural cutaneous fistula
      3. Surgical opening of a major conducting airway
      4. Giant unilateral lung cyst or bulla
      5. Tracheobronchial tree disruption
      6. Life-threatening hypoxemia related to unilateral lung disease
   C. Unilateral bronchopulmonary lavage
      1. Pulmonary alveolar proteinosis
II. Relative
   A. Surgical exposure—high priority
      1. Thoracic aortic aneurysm
      2. Pneumonectomy
      3. Thoracoscopy
      4. Upper lobectomy
      5. Mediastinal exposure
   B. Surgical exposure—medium (lower) priority
      1. Middle and lower lobectomies and subsegmental resections
      2. Esophageal resection
      3. Procedures on the thoracic spine
   C. Postcardiopulmonary bypass pulmonary edema/hemorrhage after removal of totally occluding unilateral chronic pulmonary emboli
   D. Severe hypoxemia related to unilateral lung disease

From Sheinbaum R et al. Separation of the two lungs (double-lumen tubes, bronchial blockers, and endobronchial single-lumen tubes). In: Hagberg CA, ed. Benumof's Airway Management. 2nd ed. Philadelphia: Mosby; 2007.

TABLE **28-3**	Types of Double-Lumen Tubes	
Name	**Bronchus Intubated**	**Carinal Hook**
Carlens	Left	Yes
White	Right	Yes
Robertshaw	Right or left	No

the right upper lobe orifice. However, in an emergent situation, use of a single-lumen tube advanced blindly down the right bronchus or placed into the left bronchus aided by a bronchoscope can be life saving.

Bronchial blockers were developed in the mid-1930s. These generally consist of catheters with an inflatable balloon that blocks the bronchus. A separate ETT is then placed into the trachea. Bronchial blockers are very useful in patients in whom securing the airway is anticipated to be difficult. These devices are also appropriate for patients already intubated, when changing to another tube would be too dangerous. They can also be advanced down a nasally intubated patient or used for pediatric video-assisted thoracoscopy procedures.[41] Current options for stand-alone bronchial blockers include the 8F Fogarty embolectomy catheter and the Wire-Guided Endobronchial blocker (WEB). These blockers are inserted through a conventional ETT and guided into the appropriate bronchus with the aid of a bronchoscope.[42] The use of bronchial blockers has declined because of the risk of slippage and obstruction of the trachea. With the bronchial blocker approach, although insertion of the tube is less challenging than placing a DLT, correct positioning of the bronchial blocking device is more challenging and definitely requires use of a bronchoscope. Given that each approach (DLT vs. bronchial blocker) has relative merits, neither can be recommended as a clearly superior method of lung separation for thoracic surgery.[43]

The Univent tube was developed in Japan in the 1980s. It consists of an integrated ETT with a second lumen for a deployable bronchial blocker. After intubation of the trachea has been performed, the blocker is advanced into the bronchus with the aid of the fiberoptic bronchoscope. This tube is as easy to pass into the trachea as a single-lumen tube. Postlaryngectomy patients can also benefit from this tube because it is easily advanced through the stoma. The Univent tube is available in sizes from 6 to 9 mm internal diameter (although, accounting for the blocker channel, the outer diameter is greater than that of a corresponding-sized ETT). Because its shape and size are more similar to conventional ETTs, the Univent may be a good alternative to a DLT in patients with difficult airways.

DLTs consist of two bonded catheters, each with its own lumen; one lumen is used for ventilating the trachea and the other for ventilating the bronchus. Several types of DLTs have been used in thoracic surgery (Table 28-3). The Carlens tube is a left-sided DLT with a carinal hook to aid in stabilizing the tube. Insertion is difficult, and the hook can cause vocal cord damage. A White tube is a right-sided DLT with a carinal hook.

The Robertshaw DLT was developed in 1962. This tube is available as a right- or left-sided DLT without a carinal hook. Disposable polyvinyl chloride tubes are available in French (F) sizes 26, 28, 35, 37, 39, and 41. These correspond to internal lumen diameters ranging from 3.4 mm to 5 mm.[44] Although the presence of dual lumens limits the internal diameter of

dual-lung ventilation is indicated and appropriate in either the presence of airway concerns that preclude use of a lung-separating tube or the inability to maintain oxygenation with OLV. Certain situations, such as infectious contamination of one lung, are absolute indications for OLV, but most common thoracic surgeries actually create *relative* indications for lung separation in that they can safely be accomplished without it. Indications for lung separation are noted in Box 28-3.

Methods of Lung Separation

Several devices have been developed to enable isolation of one lung and ventilation of the other. The single-lumen endobronchial tube was developed in 1931 to isolate an infected lung.[40] Mimicking this simple approach by advancing a 7.5-mm, 32-cm endotracheal tube (ETT) over a fiberoptic scope into one bronchus may still be used in some circumstances. A disadvantage to use of a single-lumen tube for OLV is that the ability to ventilate or suction the other lung is lost. Another disadvantage is that use of a single-lumen tube in the right lung would probably occlude each, the external diameter of a DLT is very large. The 37F DLT has an outer diameter equivalent to that of a standard 11-mm ID ETT. For this reason, DLTs are not used for small children; the external diameter of the 26F DLT is 7.5 mm.[45] Sizing of DLTs is determined by patient height, usually leading to use of 35F to 37F tubes in females, and 39F to 41F tubes in males.[38]

When a right-sided DLT is placed, even slight movements in the tube's position can dislodge the bronchial lumen into the trachea or cause obstruction of the right upper lobe by the bronchial cuff. This happens because the distance from the carinal bifurcation to the beginning of the right upper lobe is 2.5 cm or less, as compared with a 4-5 cm left mainstem bronchus (Figure 28-10).

Modifications have been made in right-sided tubes to allow ventilation through a slot in the endobronchial cuff. It is thought that a greater margin of safety is associated with the use of a left-sided DLT for all right and left thoracotomies unless a left-sided tube is contraindicated. Contraindications to the use of DLTs include internal lesions of the trachea or main bronchi, compression of the trachea or main bronchi by an external mass, or the presence of a descending thoracic aortic aneurysm, which can compress or erode the left main bronchus. In these circumstances, it may be possible to use a DLT with the bronchial lumen on the unaffected side. An increased risk of aspiration may exist with the use of a DLT because it takes longer to place and to verify its placement, compared with a single-lumen tube. Another contraindication is a difficult airway in which direct laryngoscopy is impossible. Intubation with the large DLT can pose a challenge, even in patients with a normal airway; insertion in those with poor airway anatomy may require a creative approach.[46]

The use of a DLT may be precluded in a critically ill patient who arrives with a single-lumen tube if it is judged that the patient cannot tolerate a short period of extubation.[2] In that case, manual ventilation can be used to coordinate lung movement with surgical requirements. In patients too small to accommodate standard double-lumen tubes, a regular ETT may be used, with intentional endobronchial intubation during the period when lung separation is required. Owing to anatomic characteristics, it is easier to achieve right-sided ventilation with this method; however, the risk of occlusion of the right upper lobe is also high. Jet ventilation is another strategy that may be useful for ventilating the pediatric patient undergoing lung surgery. The combination of pneumothorax and the low mean airway pressures generated by jet ventilation should allow adequate deflation of the operative lung.[47] Recommendations for placement of the various lung separation devices are given in Table 28-4. For the practitioner with limited thoracic anesthesia experience, the failure rate for correct placement of a lung separation device is not different between the various equipment options available.[48]

Placement of Double-Lumen Tubes

The DLT has two curves along its length to aid in its placement. A stylet aids placement through the larynx. Some practitioners prefer the MacIntosh blade for intubation because it offers greater clearance for the tube and may decrease the chance of balloon rupture from the teeth.[49] For laryngoscopy, the lubricated DLT is advanced with the distal curve concave anteriorly until the vocal cords are passed. The stylet is usually removed at this point.

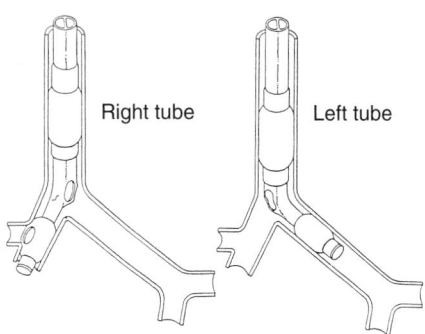

FIGURE **28-10** Correct position of a right- and left-sided double-lumen tube. (*From Morgan GE et al. Anesthesia for thoracic surgery. In: Clinical Anesthesiology. 4th ed. New York: McGraw-Hill; 2006.*)

TABLE **28-4**	Summary of Lung Separation Devices and Recommendations for Placement		
Device	**Indication**	**Tube Size**	**Placement and Confirmation**
Left-sided DLT	Majority of elective left or right thoracic surgical procedures	Determined by measurements of tracheal width from chest radiograph	Fiberoptic bronchoscopy
Right-sided DLT	Distorted left bronchus anatomy; left pneumonectomy		Fiberoptic bronchoscopy with guided technique
Fogarty occlusion catheter	Critically ill patient; small bronchus; difficult airway; nasotracheal intubation	Standard endotracheal tube at least 6 mm in diameter	Fiberoptic bronchoscopy
Univent blockers	Selective lobar blockade; difficult airway requiring lung separation		Fiberoptic bronchoscopy
WEB blockers	Critically ill patients; selective lobar blockade; difficult airway; nasotracheal intubation requiring lung separation	Standard endotracheal tube at least 8 mm in diameter	Fiberoptic bronchoscopy with guided technique

From Campos JH. Lung separation techniques. In: Kaplan JA, Slinger PD, eds. Thoracic Anesthesia. 3rd ed. Philadelphia: Churchill Livingstone; 2003.
DLT, *Double-lumen endotracheal tube;* WEB, *wire-guided endobronchial blocker.*

The tube is then rotated 90 degrees toward the bronchus to be intubated and advanced to around a 27-cm depth in females or 29 cm in males, or until resistance is met.[50] Because of concern about the rigid tube causing mucosal damage, usually the stylet is removed after the tube has passed the glottis. However, one study found that the success of initial placement was significantly improved by keeping the stylet in place until the tube was fully situated in the bronchus. This technique was not associated with increased tissue trauma.[51]

The tracheal cuff requires 5 to 10 mL of air, and the bronchial cuff requires 1 to 2 mL of air. Overinflation of the bronchial cuff can cause its lumen to be narrowed or occluded and increases the risk of tearing the bronchus. Unlike most tracheal high-volume, low-pressure cuffs, the bronchial cuff holds a small volume and can produce high pressures on the endobronchial mucosa. For that reason, the bronchial cuff should be deflated during the procedure once OLV is no longer needed. After the tube is situated in the bronchus, adapters are attached to the two lumens for interface with the anesthesia circuit. Auscultation of breath sounds is a simple though not highly reliable method of determining the position of a double-lumen tube. (Box 28-4). Figure 28-11 outlines auscultation findings with various tube malpositions.

Flexible fiberoptic bronchoscopy is essential to verify placement of the DLT (Figure 28-12 and Box 28-5). Fiberoptic bronchoscopy has revealed a 38% to 83% incidence of malpositioning of DLTs that were judged by auscultation to be properly placed.[44,51] Some particular advantages of fiberoptic inspection of the DLT over auscultation are guidance during initial placement, ability to visualize correct depth of the bronchial cuff, and visualization of proper positioning of the right upper lobe port (if present). Placement of the tube should again be verified by bronchoscopy after the patient is positioned laterally because the DLT will commonly withdraw from the bronchus by 1 cm.[52]

A fiberoptic bronchoscope of 4.9 mm external diameter can be lubricated and passed through an endobronchial tube of size 37F or larger. A fiberoptic bronchoscope of 3.6 mm can pass through a 35F tube.[53]

Double-Lumen Tube Malpositions

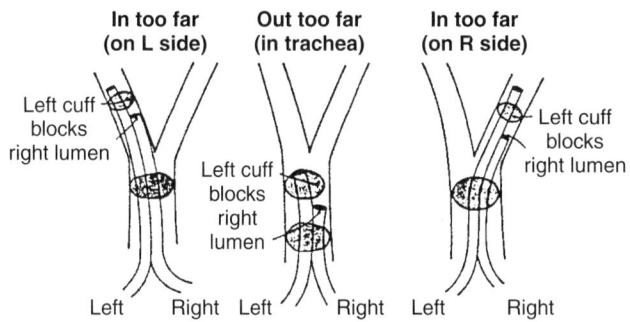

Procedure	Breath Sounds Heard		
	In too far (on left side)	Out too far (in trachea)	In too far (on right side)
Clamp right lumen both cuffs inflated	Left	Left and right	Right
Clamp left lumen both cuffs inflated	None or very ↓↓	None or very ↓↓	None or very ↓↓
Clamp left lumen deflate left cuff	Left	Left and right	Right

FIGURE **28-11** Three malpositions of the endobronchial tube and expected auscultatory findings with each. (*From Benumof JL. Anesthesia for Thoracic Surgery. 2nd ed. Philadelphia: Saunders; 1995.*)

BOX 28-4

Auscultation of Breath Sounds After Placement of a Double-Lumen Tube

1. Inflate the tracheal cuff.
2. Verify bilaterally equal breath sounds. If breath sounds are present on only one side, both lumens are in the same bronchus. Deflate the cuff and withdraw the tube 1 to 2 cm at a time until breath sounds are equal bilaterally.
3. Inflate the endobronchial cuff.
4. Clamp the endobronchial lumen and open its lumen cap proximal to the clamp.
5. Verify breath sounds in the correct lung and the absence of breath sounds in the opposite lung.
6. Verify that breath sounds are equal at the apex of the lung and at the lateral lung. If the apex is diminished, withdraw the tube until upper lung sounds return.
7. Verify the absence of air leakage through the opposite lumen cap.
8. Unclamp the endobronchial lumen and verify bilateral breath sounds.
9. Clamp the tracheal lumen and open its cap.
10. Verify breath sounds on the side opposite the lung with the endobronchial lumen and the absence of breath sounds on the other.
11. When absolute lung separation is needed, as in bronchopulmonary lavage, connecting a clamped lumen to an underwater drainage system will show air bubbles if a leak is present.

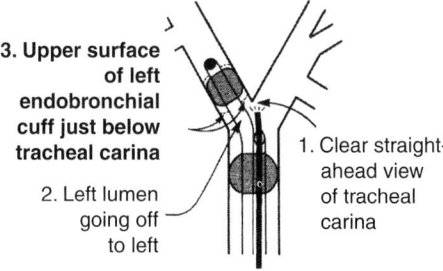

FIGURE **28-12** The fiberoptic bronchoscope is placed down the right lumen to determine precise left-sided double-lumen tube position. The endoscopist should see a clear straight-ahead view of the tracheal carina (*1*), the left lumen going off into the left mainstem bronchus (*2*), and most important, the upper surface of the left endobronchial cuff just below the tracheal carina (*3*). (*From Benumof JL. Anesthesia for Thoracic Surgery. 2nd ed. Philadelphia: Saunders; 1995.*)

BOX **28-5**

Fiberoptic Bronchoscopy to Verify Placement of a Double-Lumen Tube

1. Insert the scope through the tracheal lumen. Visualize the carina distally. (Confirm that the tracheal orifice is within the trachea and not a bronchus, or that the tube is not displaced proximally such that the bronchial cuff fills the trachea.)
2. Visualize the endobronchial (blue) cuff 1 to 2 mm beyond the carina. Ensure that the cuff is not too proximal or overinflated such as to herniate across the carina and obstruct the contralateral bronchus.
3. Insert the scope through the bronchial lumen. Visualize that the tip of the bronchial lumen is unobstructed. For left-sided tubes, visualize the LUL bronchus distal to the tube tip. For right-sided tubes with a RUL ventilation port, visualize that the RUL bronchus is aligned with the ventilation port.

RUL, Right upper lobe (of lung).

Complications of Double-Lumen Tubes

Placement of DLTs carries the same risks as laryngoscopy and intubation with ETTs. In addition, there exists a risk of hypoxemia with malpositioning of the tube. Figure 28-13 demonstrates some variations of DLT malposition. Part A demonstrates ideal placement of a right-sided tube, with the fenestrated bronchial cuff situated adjacent to the RUL takeoff. If insertion is too shallow (as in the right-sided tube shown in part B), the bronchial cuff may herniated over the carina or frankly obstruct tracheal flow. This situation would allow ventilation only through the bronchial lumen, and depending on how shallow the tube is, would ventilate one or both lungs. A DLT inserted too far could seat the tracheal lumen in a bronchus, but the resistance in the distal bronchus would make this malposition difficult if using an appropriate-sized tube. More likely would be to insert a right-sided tube slightly too far such as to exclude the RUL by having the bronchial cuff beyond the bronchus, as in Figure 28-13, C. Figure 28-13, D demonstrates proper positioning of a left-sided DLT. Because of the longer distance to the LUL bronchus, the threat of obstructing that lobe with the DLT is slight.

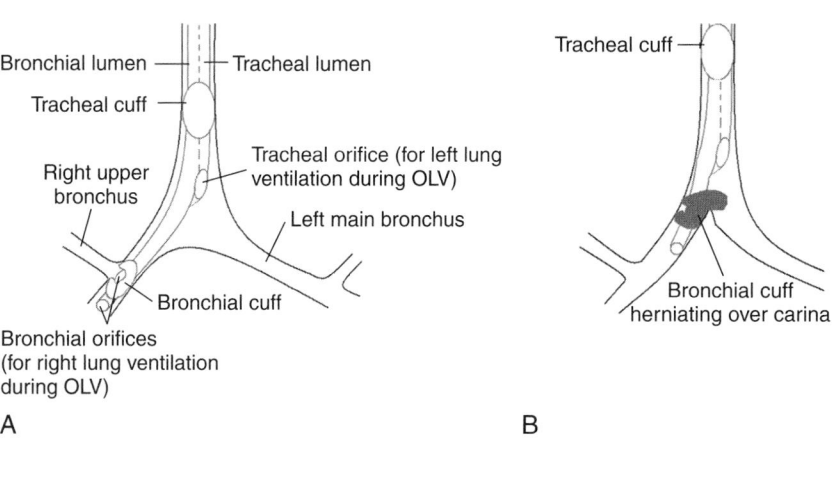

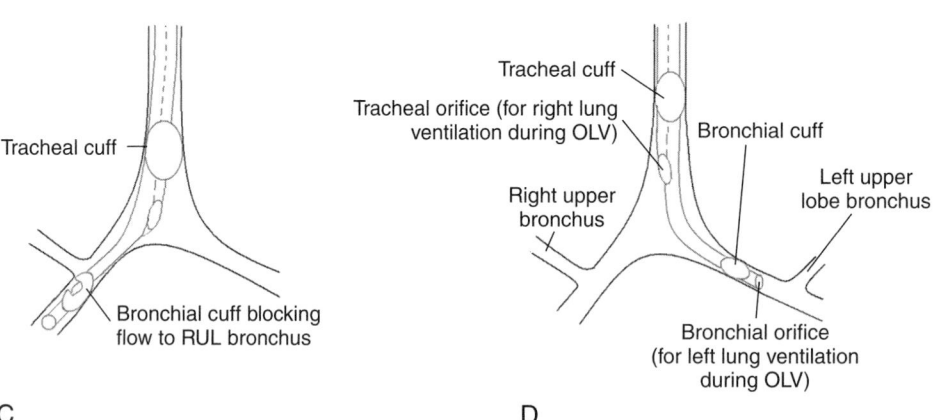

FIGURE **28-13** Positioning variations of the double-lumen endobronchial tube. **A,** Correct positioning of a right-sided DLT for lung separation, including alignment of the right upper lobe fenestration adjacent to the right upper lobe bronchus. **B,** A right-sided DLT at an inadequate depth, allowing for bronchial cuff herniation over the carina, possibly obstructing ventilation of the left lung. (The same could happen with a left-sided tube inserted too shallowly.) **C,** A right-sided DLT inserted too far, excluding the right upper lobe from ventilation. **D,** A left-sided DLT properly inserted. Note the distance to the left upper lobe and lack of potential for obstruction by the bronchial cuff of the DLT.

Blood Flow Distribution: Two Lung Ventilation

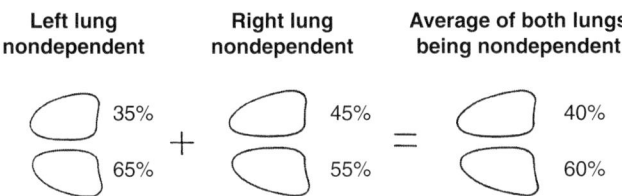

FIGURE **28-14** When the left lung is the nondependent lung, the distribution of blood flow between the nondependent and dependent lungs is 35%:65%. When the right lung is the nondependent lung, blood flow distribution between the nondependent and dependent lungs is 45%:55%. Average one-lung ventilation blood flow distribution is a nondependent-to-dependent ratio of 40%:60%. *(From Benumof JL. Anesthesia for Thoracic Surgery. 2nd ed. Philadelphia: Saunders; 1995.)*

Rupture of a thoracic aneurysm is possible with a left DLT if the aneurysm compresses the left mainstem bronchus. Damage to the vocal cords or arytenoid cartilages is possible from a carinal hook. A carinal hook can also break off, requiring retrieval with a bronchoscope. Bronchial rupture, which was thought to be caused by overinflation of the bronchial cuff, has been reported.[54,55] An incident was reported in which pulmonary artery exsanguination occurred on extubation after a Carlen DLT had been inadvertently sutured to the artery through the wall of the trachea.[56] Owing to the possibility of its being inserted too deeply, a DLT can also cause the entire tidal volume to be delivered to a single lung lobe, creating the potential for barotrauma. The larger size of the DLT is probably also responsible for the slightly increased incidence of hoarseness and vocal cord lesions observed in patients following DLT, versus using a bronchial blocker for lung separation.[57] Vocal cord paralysis can represent a life-threatening complication of DLT placement.[58]

Physiology of One-Lung Ventilation
During two-lung ventilation, blood flow to the dependent lung averages approximately 60% (Figure 28-14). When one lung is allowed to deflate and OLV is started, any blood flow to the deflated lung becomes shunt flow, causing the PaO_2 to decrease. Without autoregulation of pulmonary blood flow, a 40% shunt would be anticipated. The lungs have a compensatory mechanism of increasing vascular resistance in hypoxic areas of the lungs, and this diverts some blood flow to areas of better ventilation and oxygenation. This mechanism, present in most mammals, is termed *hypoxic pulmonary vasoconstriction* (HPV). HPV is a reflex intrapulmonary feedback mechanism in inhomogeneous lungs to improve gas exchange and arterial oxygenation. Whereas hypoxemia causes vasodilation in the general circulation, it has the opposite effect on pulmonary arteries. HPV is a unique mechanism, suited specifically to match pulmonary blood flow with well-oxygenated areas of lung.

The cellular mechanism for HPV involves a redox-based oxygen sensor in smooth muscle cells of the pulmonary arteries (probably focused on the electron transport chain of the mitochondria of these cells). Hypoxemia reduces production of activated oxygen species (AOS) such as H_2O_2. These AOS act as second messengers from the oxygen sensors, and reduction in their outflow leads to inhibition of voltage-dependent potassium channels. The result is influx of extracellular calcium,

BOX **28-6**

Characteristics of Hypoxic Pulmonary Vasoconstriction

1. A local reaction occurring in hypoxic areas of lung. May be very localized due to regional atelectasis or OLV, or affect both lungs entirely in hypoxic situations.
2. Opposite to systemic reaction, causes vaso*constriction* in response to hypoxia in all but very proximal pulmonary arteries.
3. Onset and resolution are very fast following changes in tissue PO_2.
4. Triggered by alveolar hypoxia, not arterial hypoxemia.
5. May be inhibited by calcium channel blockade (verapamil, volatile anesthetics) or vasodilators (nitrates). Augmented by chemoreceptor agonists (almitrine)

Data from Archer SL et al. Differential distribution of electrophysiologically distinct myocytes in conduit and resistance arteries determines their response to nitric oxide and hypoxia. Circ Res. 1996;78:431-442; Archer S, Michelakis E. The mechanism(s) of hypoxic pulmonary vasoconstriction: potassium channels, redox O_2 sensors, and controversies. News Physiol Sci. 2002;17:131-137; Nagendran J et al. An anesthesiologist's guide to hypoxic pulmonary vasoconstriction: implications for managing single-lung anesthesia and atelectasis. Curr Opin Anaesthesiol. 2006;19(1):34-43.

Conversion of Two-Lung to One-Lung Ventilation: Blood Flow Distributions

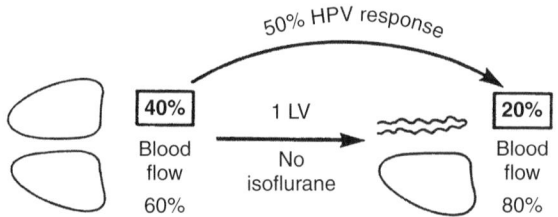

FIGURE **28-15** Two-lung ventilation nondependent/dependent lung blood flow ratio is 40%:60%. When two-lung ventilation is converted to one-lung ventilation (*1 LV*), the hypoxic pulmonary vasoconstriction (*HPV*) response decreases the blood flow to the nondependent lung by 50%, and the nondependent/dependent lung blood flow ratio becomes 20%:80%. *(From Benumof JL. Anesthesia for Thoracic Surgery. 2nd ed. Philadelphia: Saunders; 1995.)*

which causes vasoconstriction.[59] Box 28-6 lists the characteristics of HPV.

HPV during OLV is effective in decreasing the cardiac output to the nonventilated lung to 20% to 25% (Figure 28-15).[60] Shunt flow changes from 10% during two-lung ventilation to 27% during OLV. This increase in shunt decreases the mean PaO_2 from greater than 400 mm Hg during two-lung ventilation to slightly less than 200 mm Hg during OLV when the fraction of inspired O_2 (FIO_2) is 1.[48] Hypoxic pulmonary vasoconstriction can decrease the shunt fraction during OLV by 50%.[61]

HPV occurs whether the lung is rendered hypoxic by atelectasis or by ventilation with a hypoxic mixture. HPV improves arterial oxygenation when the amount of hypoxic lung is between 20% and 80%, which is the condition during OLV.[60] When less than 20% of the lung is hypoxic, the total amount of shunt is not significant. When more than 80% of the lung is hypoxic, HPV increases PVR, but the amount of well-perfused lung is not sufficient to accept shunt flow to maintain arterial oxygenation. This increase in PVR increases the work of the right side of the heart and can cause right ventricular strain and failure.[48]

Because HPV is effective in decreasing shunt flow, avoidance of drugs or events that inhibit the mechanism is important. Alveolar and intravascular volume derangements can inhibit the effect of HPV. Hypervolemia or high cardiac output may override HPV by recruiting constricted vessels.[62] Conversely, hypovolemia may trigger adrenergic vasoconstriction, reducing flow to well-ventilated portions of lung.[63] Overdistention of alveoli may also reduce perfusion to well-ventilated lung areas by creating the "zone 1" ventilation-perfusion scenario. For these reasons, normal fluid volume should be maintained during OLV; moderate tidal volumes (6 mL/kg) should be used, and excessive PEEP should be avoided.[38] Hypocapnia, alkalosis, and acidosis decrease HPV. Hypothermia causes pulmonary vasoconstriction and can shunt blood away from the ventilated lung.[2]

Inhalation agents have been studied extensively to determine their effect on HPV. Inhaled anesthetics have been reported to inhibit HPV in a variety of in vitro experimental preparations. In studies in which animal lungs were isolated from the body, inhalation agents have been found to decrease the vasoconstrictor response to hypoxic lung segments. However, when the same agents are used in intact specimens, human and animal, no change or very little change is seen in PaO_2, shunt flow, or regional blood flow. In patients, HPV can be expected to remain intact if volatile agents are administered at less than 1.5 minimum alveolar concentration (MAC).[64,65] Autoregulatory mechanisms (e.g., baroreceptor reflexes, humoral influences, and changes in cardiac output) probably account for the difference in inhibition of HPV between in vitro and intact in vivo specimens.[66]

The influence of various intravenous agents on HPV has also been investigated. In vitro and in vivo studies have revealed no change in HPV with fentanyl, pentazocine, ketamine, droperidol, diazepam, thiopental, or pentobarbital.[67] When propofol was administered after the institution of OLV, no change in venous admixture or PaO_2 was found.[68] However, many vasodilating drugs inhibit HPV, including nitroglycerin, nitroprusside, dobutamine, some calcium channel blockers (e.g., nifedipine nicardipine, and verapamil), and some β_2-agonists, such as isoproterenol.[38] Vasoconstrictive drugs, including dopamine, epinephrine, and phenylephrine, may preferentially constrict normally oxygenated pulmonary vessels and reestablish the shunt flow, in opposition to the effect of HPV.[60] Box 28-7 lists factors that reduce the effectiveness of HPV.

Anesthetic Management During One-Lung Ventilation
Choice of Anesthetic
Side effects of general anesthesia from a variety of mechanisms create concern for intraoperative and postoperative pulmonary function. They include impairment of hypoxic pulmonary vasoconstriction, disruption of ventilation/perfusion matching, neural and pain-induced hypoventilation, postoperative residual curarization, and atelectasis. Few studies have been able to demonstrate clear differences in patient outcomes based on anesthetic technique alone; however, some factors have emerged as important in the pulmonary surgical patient.

> ### BOX 28-7
>
> **Factors That Reduce Effectiveness of Hypoxic Pulmonary Vasoconstriction**
>
> Shunt fraction <20% or >80%
> Hypervolemia
> Hypovolemia
> Excessive tidal volume or PEEP
> Hypocapnia
> Acidosis
> Hypothermia
> Volatile agents >1.5 MAC
> Vasoactive medications

On the basis of the discussion of HPV, clinical doses of potent inhalation agents do not significantly alter the mechanism of HPV. Inhalation agents offer several benefits in thoracic surgery. They allow the use of a high FIO_2 to help prevent hypoxemia during OLV. They produce bronchodilatory effects and decrease airway irritability in patients to be subjected to direct manipulation of lung tissue. In contrast, the dose of narcotics required to obtund airway reflexes could depress ventilation and necessitate postoperative ventilation. Inhalation agents are rapidly eliminated at the end of surgery and allow for early extubation. For these reasons, inhalation agents are usually chosen as the primary anesthetics during thoracic surgery.

To prevent hypoxia and any significant increase in PVR, nitrous oxide is generally avoided in favor of 100% O_2. Nitrous oxide increases PVR in cardiac patients whose baseline PVR is within normal limits, from a mean of 112 to 130 dyne $\cdot$ sec$^{-1} \cdot$ cm^{-5}. Nitrous oxide raises PVR much more markedly in patients whose PVR is already elevated from mitral valve stenosis, from a mean of 357 to 530 dyne $\cdot$ sec$^{-1} \cdot$ cm^{-5}.[34] This is cause for even greater clinical concern with concurrent right ventricular dysfunction. Nitrous oxide should also be avoided in patients with bullous or emphysematous lungs, because it may increase the volume of trapped airspace.

The choice of specific opioids or hypnotics will not influence pulmonary outcomes, but there is concern related to the choice of muscle relaxants used. Postoperative residual curarization is a common occurrence with both intermediate and long-acting relaxants and is present regardless of the use of neuromuscular monitoring or reversal.[69] However, the incidence of residual relaxation associated with the use of long-acting relaxants (e.g., pancuronium) is significantly higher, and complications from it are more frequent compared with the use of intermediate-acting relaxants.[70] Muscle weakness may follow surgeries of long duration, even with adequate tests of neuromuscular recovery.[71] Therefore the use of shorter-acting, fast-offset relaxants and conservative monitoring, dosing, and reversal practices are indicated in the pulmonary surgical patient.

The Role of Regional Anesthesia
When compared with general anesthesia, regional anesthesia may be beneficial in reducing atelectasis, pneumonia, respiratory failure, and other pulmonary complications.[72] Unfortunately, regional anesthesia without general is impractical for the open-lung case. Some data do suggest that regional anesthesia may

reduce pulmonary complications when used instead of systemic opioids for postoperative analgesia; however, other studies offer conflicting evidence.[73]

Management of One-Lung Ventilation

The primary goal during OLV is maintaining adequate arterial oxygenation while providing a surgical field favorable for visualization and manipulation of the operative lung. Two-lung ventilation should be maintained as long as possible and the time of OLV minimized. In the past, large V_{TS} of 10 mL/kg (range 8 to 15 mL/kg) were recommended to prevent atelectasis in the dependent lung and maintain an adequate FRC. Recent data suggest that most patients during OLV develop "auto-PEEP" and have an increased FRC.[74,75] The use of a large V_T in that case may lead to volutrauma of the lung. Besides the direct physical effect, higher V_{TS} are also associated with increases in inflammatory mediators and in alveolar fibrin deposition and other markers of procoagulant effect, which characterize acute lung injury.[76,77] Understanding the detrimental effects of high tidal volumes has led to the more contemporary approach of using more physiologic volumes (e.g., 6 mL/kg), adding PEEP to those patients without auto-PEEP, and limiting plateau inspiratory pressures to less than 25 cm H_2O.[76-79] With this approach, patients will maintain adequate or even improved oxygenation (as compared with using higher V_T) and minimal elevations in $PaCO_2$.[38] In any case, the effect of hypercapnia (consider the use of "permissive hypercapnia" as a strategy in treating severe lung injury) is far less detrimental than the potential volutrauma from excessive ventilation.[80]

An appropriate air-O_2 mixture, at times as high as an FIO_2 of 1, is necessary to maximize the PaO_2. However, after ascertaining that oxygenation will be stable after 30 minutes of OLV, the FIO_2 should be reduced to lessen the effects of absorptive atelectasis. The respiratory rate can be adjusted to maintain an adequate $PaCO_2$. Although a high FIO_2 should induce vasodilation in the dependent lung, improving blood flow, hypocapnia would cause vasoconstriction and should be avoided. The relationship between $PaCO_2$ and end-tidal CO_2 is not altered by OLV. Should hypoxemia occur during OLV, the anesthetist should assess for physiologic causes or tube malpositioning. Physiologic causes may include bronchospasm, decreased cardiac output, hypoventilation, low FIO_2, or pneumothorax of the dependent lung. Tube malpositioning implies that movement of the DLT may have excluded a portion of dependent lung, usually the upper lobe. If physiologic causes have been ruled out and adequate lung separation and ventilation have been determined, one or more of the following interventions will help improve PaO_2. First, continuous positive airway pressure (CPAP) to the nondependent, nonventilated lung is almost 100% efficacious in increasing PaO_2. This can be accomplished with a compact breathing system, such as a Mapleson C with a manometer for pressure determination, attached to the lumen of the deflated lung. Alternatively, some DLTs can be purchased, which include such a CPAP device with each tube. Application of CPAP should help to oxygenate the persistent blood flow through the nondependent lung, but too much pressure will cause the lung to inflate, reducing surgical exposure. The lowest level of effective CPAP (start at 2 cm H_2O) should be sought. A CPAP device that incorporates a reservoir bag is also useful for providing intermittent ventilation to the operative lung, should that intervention become necessary. Providing gentle ventilation with a separate system will minimize the diminution of surgical exposure, as opposed to ventilating the lung with the same vigor as that required for the dependent lung.

Shunt flow through the operative lung is not the only cause of hypoxemia during OLV; atelectasis and reduced FRC in the dependent lung may also be significant factors. If CPAP to the nondependent lung does not improve oxygenation, PEEP applied to the dependent, ventilated lung acts to increase PaO_2 by recruiting collapsed airways, increasing compliance of the lung, and increasing FRC. Under different conditions, PEEP can exert pressure on small pulmonary vessels, causing more shunt to the unventilated lung and decreasing PaO_2.[81] Excessive PEEP may also detrimentally reduce cardiac output. Combined with a fast respiratory rate and/or high, PEEP may impair adequate exhalation, leading to a net volume increase through auto-PEEP and the potential for volu-trauma to the dependent lung. The actual end-expiratory pressure should be monitored during OLV to ensure that it does not significantly exceed the intended level of PEEP. Some authors have advocated using calculations of dead space to determine the optimal level of PEEP. Although the intention of PEEP is to recruit collapsed alveoli, overdistention of alveoli with excessive PEEP may increase the areas of zone 1 effect (alveolar pressure exceeding capillary pressure) and create more dead space ventilation.[82,83]

Other methods of improving oxygenation during OLV include combining PEEP and CPAP to the respective lungs, and intermittent reinflation of the nondependent lung. In a 1992 study by Lewis and colleagues, a PaO_2 of less than 80 mm Hg developed in 28.5% of patients during OLV with an FIO_2 of 1.[48] In 37% of these instances, hypoxia was transient and responded to suctioning, brief lung reinflation, DLT repositioning, V_T adjustment, or temporary reinflation of the operative lung. In the remaining 63% of these patients, some combination of PEEP and CPAP was required. When PEEP alone was added, PaO_2 rose above 80 mm Hg in only 40% of cases. CPAP was used alone in six patients and raised the PaO_2 above 80 mm Hg in all patients. PEEP plus CPAP raised the PaO_2 to higher than 80 mm Hg in all but one patient.[48] The use of different modes of ventilation, such as pressure-control, may provide a different distribution of ventilation and improve oxygenation as well.[84] Emerging in this area are innovative ventilatory approaches such as high-frequency jet ventilation to the operative lung and jet ventilation selectively to nonoperative *lobes* of the operative lung via a bronchial blocker with an insufflation port.[85,86]

In the failure of CPAP and PEEP, early ligation of the pulmonary artery in pneumonectomy patients may be used to improve oxygenation. If the pulmonary artery is planned to be ligated during the procedure, clamping it will immediately stop all significant flow through the lung contributing to the shunt. If it becomes impossible to maintain adequate oxygenation with OLV in spite of CPAP and PEEP, manual two-lung ventilation can be used, with pauses in ventilation coordinated with the surgeon's activities to facilitate exposure, suturing of the lung, or other needs. Communication with the surgical team is vital throughout the procedure, especially during the evaluation and correction of hypoxia.

At the conclusion of the resection, the surgeon will commonly ask that the operative lung be reinflated using large tidal volumes so that air leaks may be detected. At this time, the lung separator (DLT clamp, bronchial blocker) should be discontinued and the lung inflated with slow breaths, achieving a peak inspiratory pressure of 30 to 40 cm H_2O.[38] Reexpansion of the lung can be observed while performing this maneuver, which also helps to reverse atelectasis in the lungs. Following lung reexpansion, the bronchial cuff should be deflated on the DLT to both reduce pressure on the bronchial mucosa and obviate any detrimental effects of slight tube malpositioning. Deflated, the cuff does not pose the threat of herniating over the carina, obstructing the RUL takeoff.

ANALGESIA FOR THORACIC SURGERY

Thoracotomy is known as one of the most painful operations, and postoperative pain can be very protracted (as in post-thoracotomy pain syndrome) and lead to complications such as pneumonia and atelectasis.[87] Pain immediately after thoracic surgery causes splinting, decreased respiratory effort, hypoxemia, and respiratory acidosis. Aggressive management of pain is aimed at seeking a balance between comfort and respiratory depression in patients with decreased lung function. Residual pain exists in half of thoracotomy patients after 1 year and in one third of patients after 4 years.[88]

Several options can be considered in the management of postoperative pain. Patients can titrate intravenous patient-controlled analgesia to obtain a more constant level of analgesia than that provided by intermittent intramuscular injections, but the benefits of avoiding systemic opioids have made regional anesthesia emerge as a superior method of pain control.

Thoracic epidural analgesia is considered one of the most effective methods for treating postoperative pain.[89] An epidural catheter may be placed preoperatively (T6 to T8) and infused with epidural opioids or dilute solutions of local anesthetics to provide analgesia. The efficacy of epidural analgesia may be improved with adjunctive interventions, such as IV administration of the *N*-methyl-D-aspartate (NMDA)-blocker, ketamine.[90] Although epidural administration is found to provide excellent anesthesia and analgesia, evidence of improved postoperative outcomes or reduced pulmonary complications is not clear.[91]

As an alternative regional anesthesia technique, intercostal (paravertebral) nerve blocks can be placed at the level of the incision plus one or two intercostal interspaces above and below. This technique provides good short-term pain relief and reduces opioid requirements.[92] Rapid intravascular absorption of the local anesthetic is possible in this highly vascular area, so caution must be taken to avoid systemic toxicity.

Cryoanalgesia is performed by applying a cryoprobe cooled to $-60°$ C to nerves in intercostal spaces two to three spaces above and below the incision, disrupting nerve activity. This modality gained popularity because of its lasting duration. Onset of analgesia may be delayed for 24 hours, but the effect lasts for 1 to 3 months. However, studies have found conflicting conclusions about the benefit of cryoanalgesia and its efficacy in reducing the incidence of post-thoracotomy pain syndrome.[93] Other options for analgesia include local anesthesia instilled into the intrapleural space. Insertion of an intrapleural catheter (i.e., a single-lumen CVP catheter) is easily accomplished by the surgeon prior to closing the chest.

COMPLICATIONS AFTER THORACOTOMY

Significant factors associated with acute lung injury (ALI) after pulmonary resection include right pneumonectomy, intraoperative overhydration with high vascular volume, high intraoperative airway pressure during OLV, and preoperative alcohol abuse. Other factors that have been suggested are female gender, poor postoperative predicted lung function, trauma, infection, chemotherapy, mediastinal lymphatic damage, transfusion and administration of fresh frozen plasma, serum cytokines, O_2 toxicity, prolonged OLV greater than 100 minutes, and an increased postoperative urine output.[76,94] Fortunately, the incidence of postoperative pneumonia and

atelectasis is declining. Minimizing pulmonary intravascular pressures by intraoperative fluid restriction is advocated to decrease postoperative complications. Surgical requirements for proper hydration and tissue perfusion must be balanced with the desire to prevent high postoperative intravascular pressures and possible pulmonary edema. Avoidance of fluid overload is especially important to avoid respiratory dysfunction and pulmonary injury postoperatively.[22,75]

Several preoperative patient comorbidities such as chronic alcoholism and respiratory diseases are associated with increased susceptibility to ALI because they reduce lung defense mechanisms, restrict capillary volume, and enhance the inflammatory response against injurious agents. During and after surgery, the effects of lung hyperinflation, surgical trauma, ischemia, and reperfusion induce the release of inflammatory mediators and a combination of insults at the alveolar-endothelial barrier. The result is lung edema and eventual organ dysfunction. In addition, stretching of capillaries by overzealous fluid administration (or impaired pulmonary venous return) may cause stress failure within microvessels, which further aggravates permeability disturbances.[79,95]

Implementation of risk-reduction strategies for the occurrence of ALI, particularly in patients undergoing pneumonectomy and in those with underlying lung diseases, is important. Such strategies may include withdrawal of alcohol for a safe period of abstinence and correction of nutritional deficits before elective surgery; intraoperative application of pressure-controlled ventilation with small Vts and with air-O_2 mixtures to prevent barotrauma, volutrauma, and oxidative damages; limitation of fluid intake for the first 24 to 48 hours after surgery while maintaining tight control of hemodynamics; and monitoring to assess cardiac preload, intrathoracic blood volume, and pulmonary artery pressure (e.g., stroke volume or pressure variation, transpulmonary thermo-dye dilution technique, and echocardiography) that allow early detection of pulmonary hypertension and interstitial lung edema. These conditions can be treated with diuretics, inhaled nitric oxide, and noninvasive positive pressure ventilatory techniques.[79]

Low cardiac output in the early postoperative period can be caused by several factors, including blood loss, herniation of the heart through a pericardial defect, right-sided heart failure, and dysrhythmias. Generally, blood entering the pleural space drains into chest tubes at a rate of less than 500 mL per day. Chest tube drainage greater than 200 mL per hour necessitates surgical reexploration. An obstructed chest tube can conceal bleeding in a hemothorax. Hypotension, unexplained tachycardia, and decreasing hematocrit are other signs of bleeding.

Loss of pulmonary vasculature with lung resection can result in increased PVR and right-sided heart failure. Reduction in cardiac ejection fraction is greater following pneumonectomy than following lobectomy. One study noted that the ejection fraction following lobectomy patients changed from 40% to 36%, compared with a change from 41% to 29% in pneumonectomy patients.[96] Conditions that increase the likelihood of right-sided heart failure include postoperative pneumonia, hypercarbia, and acidosis. Vasodilating agents such as nitroglycerin, sodium nitroprusside, calcium channel blockers, and hydralazine have been used to dilate the pulmonary vasculature to decrease PVR. Amrinone or dobutamine can be administered if an inotrope is also needed.[97]

Dysrhythmias are relatively common after thoracotomy because of hypoxemia, vagal irritation, atrial inflammation, pre-existing cardiac disease, pulmonary hypertension, or right atrial or ventricular dilation. In a review of 236 pneumonectomy patients, 22% experienced cardiac dysrhythmias, most commonly atrial fibrillation, supraventricular tachycardia, and atrial flutter.[98] Atrial fibrillation occurs in 20% of patients following lung cancer resection and may herald other serious complications.[99] Morbidity and mortality rates in patients with supraventricular tachydysrhythmias are high, with 20% of the total associated with hypotension and 25% associated with death within 30 days postoperatively, despite institution of aggressive treatment. No correlation between the incidence of dysrhythmias and preoperative pulmonary function or age was found. The incidence of dysrhythmias in association with intrapericardial dissection and pulmonary edema was higher than expected. Administration of more than 2000 mL of fluids intraoperatively may increase the risk of pulmonary infiltration and the incidence of dysrhythmias.[98]

Administration of a β-blocking agent can help prevent atrial dysrhythmias. Jakobsen and co-workers administered 100 mg of oral metoprolol preoperatively and daily postoperatively. The incidence of atrial tachycardia lasting longer than 30 seconds was 6.7% compared with 40% in the placebo group.[100] Digitalis, adenosine, calcium channel blockers, and β-blockers are useful to treat supraventricular tachydysrhythmias. Cardioversion may become necessary if a patient is hemodynamically unstable.

The increased PVR and right-sided heart pressures after lung resection can cause a right-to-left shunt through a patent foramen ovale. Treatment is aimed at correction of hypoxemia, acidosis, and hypercarbia; use of pulmonary vasodilators; and treatment of infection to lower right-sided pressures and functionally close the defect.

Respiratory complications in the early postoperative period include atelectasis, pneumonia, respiratory failure, bronchopleural or bronchocutaneous fistula, pneumothorax, torsion of remaining lobes necessitating surgical correction, and pulmonary edema resulting from high fluid administration. Aggressive respiratory care to prevent deterioration and allow weaning from ventilation is vital. Blood, blood clots, or thick secretions can cause airway obstruction. Tracheal suction or bronchoscopy may be needed to clear the lungs.

Disruption of the bronchial stump repair creates a communication between the bronchus and the pleural space. The escape of gas causes massive bubbling in the chest tube drainage system if it is patent or a potential tension pneumothorax with mediastinal shift if the chest tube is occluded. A large portion of the V_T can be lost to this low-resistance pathway, compromising gas exchange. Any fluid present in the pleural space can enter the defect and contaminate the healthy lung.[39] A small leak may heal with conservative medical management, including placement of a chest tube and ventilatory support if needed. High-frequency ventilation has been used with varying results to allow the defect to heal. Surgical interventions to close the defect include endoscopic application of sealing agents, closure with vascular tissue or muscle flaps, and further lung resection.[101]

If the leak from the bronchopleural fistula is so large that it interferes with adequate ventilation, the placement of a DLT facilitates ventilation of the healthy lung and prevents further contamination. Until the DLT is placed, the patient should be positioned so that the lung with the fistula is dependent, and the patient should maintain spontaneous respiration. The endobronchial lumen should be in the healthy lung before positive-pressure ventilation is begun.[39]

BOX 28-8

Common Tumors of the Anterior Mediastinum: "The 4 Ts"

Thymoma
Thyroid
Teratoma
"Terrible" lymphoma

Thoracic duct injury is possible during a left thoracotomy or the placement of left-sided central lines. A chylothorax may occur in either thorax after removal of lymph nodes during thoracotomies. Creamy chyle may be noted in the chest tube drainage or may be suspected weeks later with weight loss and recurrent sepsis. Thoracic duct injury necessitates ligation of the duct or pleuroperitoneal shunting.[102]

Nerve injuries that may follow thoracic surgery include damage to the phrenic nerve as it passes through the mediastinum and damage to the left recurrent laryngeal nerve, which is vulnerable during dissection of aortopulmonary lymph nodes and mediastinal procedures.[103] Spinal cord injury is a possibility if an intercostal artery supplying a major radicular artery is injured or if an epidural hematoma is created by surgical dissection between the pleura and the epidural space.

MEDIASTINAL MASSES

Masses in the mediastinum can compress vital structures and cause changes in cardiac output, obstruction to airflow, atelectasis, or central nervous system changes. Masses can include benign or cancerous tumors, thymomas, substernal thyroid masses, vascular aneurysms, lymphomas, and neuromas (Box 28-8). Surgical procedures for diagnosis or treatment of these masses may include thoracotomy, thoracoscopy, and mediastinoscopy.

Tumors within the anterior mediastinum can cause compression of the trachea or bronchi, increasing resistance to airflow. Changes in airway dynamics with supine positioning, induction of anesthesia, and positive-pressure ventilation can cause collapse of the airway with total obstruction to flow. General anesthesia can therefore be very dangerous in these patients. Manipulation of tissue intraoperatively, edema, and bleeding into masses can increase their size and effects on airways or vasculature. As a result, total airway obstruction can occur at any phase of anesthesia: positioning, induction, intubation, emergence, or recovery. Positive-pressure ventilation may be impossible, even with a properly placed ETT, if the mass encroaches on the airway distal to the ETT. Localization of the mass by computed tomography or bronchoscopy may facilitate placement of the ETT distal to the mass. Maintenance of spontaneous ventilation retains normal airway-distending pressure gradients and can maintain airway patency when positive pressure will not.[104,105] Maintenance of spontaneous ventilation is the goal when managing these patients.

Signs and symptoms of respiratory tract compression should be sought preoperatively. Many mediastinal masses are asymptomatic, or characterized by vague signs such as dyspnea, cough, hoarseness, or chest pain. Wheezing may represent airflow past a mechanical obstruction rather than bronchospasm. Shortness of breath at rest or with exertion and coughing are other symptoms. Symptoms may be positional, worsening in the supine or other

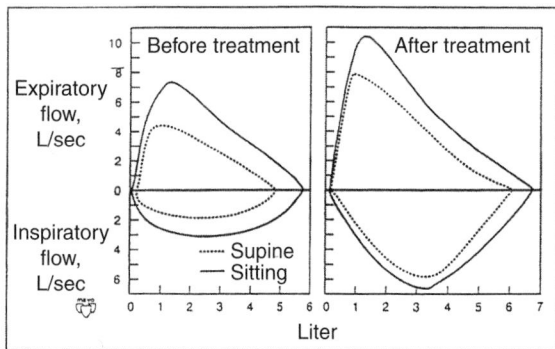

FIGURE **28-16** Flow-volume curves obtained in supine and upright positions before (*left*) and 4 weeks after (*right*) two courses of chemotherapy in a patient with mediastinal Hodgkin lymphoma. (*From Prakash UB et al. Mediastinal mass and tracheal obstruction during general anesthesia.* Mayo Clin Proc. 1988;63:1004-1011. By permission of the Mayo Foundation.)

BOX **28-9**

Symptoms of Mediastinal Mass

Sweats
Syncope
Orthopnea
Hoarseness
Inability to lie flat
Chest pain or fullness
Superior vena cava obstruction
Cough (especially when supine)

Data from Slinger P, Karsli C. Management of the patient with a large anterior mediastinal mass: recurring myths. Curr Opin Anaesthesiol. 2007;20(1):1-3.

---

position. A chest radiograph may show airway compression or deviation. Computed tomography, transesophageal echocardiography, and magnetic resonance imaging may further delineate the size and effects of masses. Subclinical airway obstruction may be revealed by flow-volume loops, which demonstrate changes in flow rates at different lung volumes. Decreased maximal inspiratory or expiratory flow rate alerts the anesthetist to increased risk of obstruction perioperatively. Comparison of flow rates obtained with the patient in the upright and supine positions can reveal whether the supine position will exacerbate obstruction intraoperatively (Figure 28-16 and Box 28-9).[106] However, the reader is cautioned that flow-volume loops do not demonstrate a high correlation to the degree or severity of airway compression.[107]

If any sign of respiratory obstruction is present, surgery for the biopsy of masses should be performed with the patient under local anesthesia whenever possible. Radiation to decrease mass bulk in radiosensitive tumors is recommended before surgery to reduce the risk of airway obstruction.[108]

In the case of mediastinal masses, awake fiberoptic bronchoscopy and intubation enables the anesthetist to evaluate the large airways for obstruction and place the ETT beyond the obstruction while maintaining spontaneous ventilation. The effect of positional changes can be checked with the bronchoscope.[109]

Spontaneous ventilation should be maintained as long as possible or throughout the procedure if feasible. The ability to effectively provide positive-pressure ventilation should be guaranteed prior to administering muscle relaxants. The use of a helium-O_2 mixture can improve airflow during partial obstruction. The use of this low-density gas decreases turbulence past a stenotic area, improving flow and decreasing the work of breathing.[110]

Previously, anesthetic management recommendations included having cardiopulmonary bypass on standby during induction of general anesthesia in patients with mediastinal masses. However, considering the time required for cannulation and full implementation of bypass, this approach may not confer the intended "escape plan" if the airway is suddenly lost. Instead, in high-risk patients, cannulation of the femoral vessels should be performed *prior to* induction of anesthesia if there is a high risk of airway loss.[111] Emergency strategies that may become necessary in the case of airway compromise include repositioning or awakening the patient, rigid bronchoscopy to establish a patent airway beyond the obstruction, or (in the case of life-threatening compromise) sternotomy with manual decompression of the mass off of the airway.[111]

Mediastinal masses can cause compression of great vessels or cardiac chambers. Compression of the pulmonary artery is rare because it is a higher-pressure vessel than the pulmonary vein and somewhat protected by the aortic arch. Compression of this vessel, however, can lead to sudden hypoxemia, hypotension, or cardiac arrest.[112] Patients with any cardiac or great vessel involvement should receive only local anesthesia whenever possible, remain in the sitting position, and maintain spontaneous respirations.[113] If general anesthesia is required, prior establishment of the means for extracorporeal ventilation should be established.

Superior vena cava syndrome is venous engorgement of the upper body caused by compression of the superior vena cava by a mass. It leads to the following signs and symptoms: dilation of collateral veins of the upper part of the thorax and neck; edema and rubor of the face, neck, and upper torso and airway; edema of the conjunctiva with or without proptosis; shortness of breath, headache, visual distortion, or altered mentation.[106] Placement of intravenous lines in the lower extremities is preferred; insertion in sites above the superior vena cava could delay the drug effect as a result of slow distribution. Fluids should be administered with caution because large volumes can worsen symptoms.

Mediastinoscopy

Mediastinoscopy involves passing a scope into the mediastinum via an incision above the suprasternal notch. The scope is passed anterior to the trachea in close proximity to the left common carotid artery, the left subclavian artery, the innominate artery, the innominate veins, the vagus nerve, the left recurrent laryngeal nerve, the thoracic duct, the superior vena cava, and the aortic arch. Complications of mediastinoscopy include pneumothorax, hemorrhage resulting from tearing of major vessels, arrhythmias, bronchospasm resulting from manipulation of the airway, laceration of the esophagus, and chylothorax secondary to laceration of the thoracic duct.[113-115] Large-bore intravenous access should be in place, and banked blood should be immediately available in the event of a tear in a major blood vessel. Air embolism is also a risk if a venous tear occurs. Arrhythmias such as bradycardia are possible with manipulation of the aorta or trachea during blunt dissection.

The mediastinoscope can place pressure on the innominate artery as it passes through the upper thorax, causing a decrease in

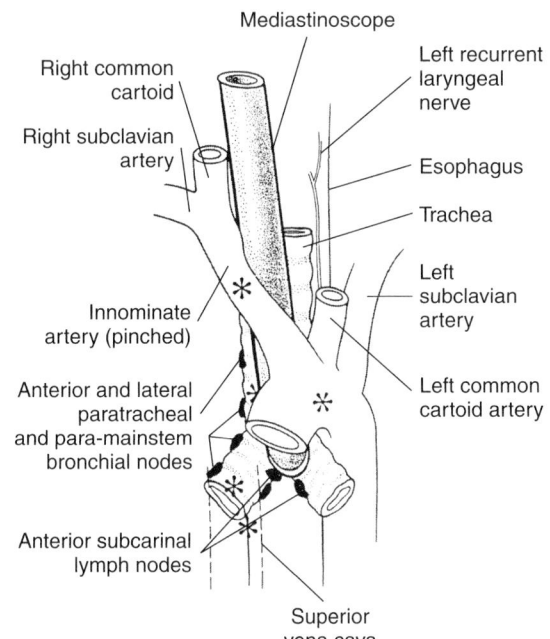

Mediastinoscope

Right common cartoid

Right subclavian artery

Left recurrent laryngeal nerve

Esophagus

Trachea

Left subclavian artery

Innominate artery (pinched)

Anterior and lateral paratracheal and para-mainstem bronchial nodes

Left common cartoid artery

Anterior subcarinal lymph nodes

Superior vena cava

FIGURE **28-17** Placement of a mediastinoscope into the superior mediastinum. The mediastinoscope passes in front of the trachea but behind the thoracic aorta. Anatomic structures that can be compressed by the mediastinoscope (*asterisks*), leading to major complications, are the thoracic aorta (rupture, reflex bradycardia), innominate artery (decreased right carotid and right subclavian flow), trachea (inability to ventilate), and vena cava (risk of hemorrhage with superior vena cava syndrome). (*From Benumof JL. Anesthesia for Thoracic Surgery. 2nd ed. Philadelphia: Saunders; 1995.*)

blood flow to the right common carotid artery and the right vertebral artery and a decrease in subclavian flow to the right arm (Figure 28-17).[116] The decrease in cerebral flow could be deleterious, especially if the patient has a history of cerebrovascular disease. Monitoring perfusion to the right arm with a pulse oximeter or radial artery catheter can detect decreased flow to the right arm and signal concurrent loss of flow to the brain via the innominate artery. Repositioning of the mediastinoscope is required to reestablish flow to the brain. A noninvasive blood pressure cuff placed on the left arm enables continued monitoring of systemic blood pressure during periods of innominate artery compression.

Thoracoscopy

Advances in videoscopic technology have led to the increased use of thoracoscopy. The uses of the thoracoscope and anesthetic techniques are still being expanded and refined. The procedure used most commonly involves placing the patient in the lateral decubitus position. A trocar is introduced at the fourth to fifth or fifth to sixth intercostal space to allow passage of the thoracoscope. Additional trocars and cannulas can be passed to insert suction, cautery, or other instruments.[117] Drainage and examination of the pleural space, débridement of an empyema, removal of foreign bodies, instillation of chemotherapeutic agents into the pleural space, pleurodesis with physical abrasion or talc, stapling of blebs, diagnostic biopsies and staging, and evaluation of bronchopleural fistulas are some of the procedures possible with thoracoscopy.[118-120]

Thoracoscopy has been performed under epidural anesthesia alone, and this technique is associated with the typical advantages of regional over general anesthesia.[121] However, general anesthesia with a double-lumen endobronchial tube offers several advantages for thoracoscopy. The airway is secured before lateral positioning. This avoids the need to change to general anesthesia under less than optimal conditions, should regional anesthesia or sedation techniques fail.[117] It allows for deflation of the lung before the introduction of the trocar. CPAP and PEEP can be applied as needed to improve oxygenation. Controlled ventilation helps prevent paradoxical respiration and mediastinal shift, and the lung can be actively reinflated at the end of the procedure.[122] Regardless of the anesthetic used, the anesthetist should always be prepared for a switch to an open thoracotomy in the event the surgeon encounters complications or cannot complete the procedure by thoracoscopy.

An arterial line is generally placed for thoracoscopy, except in selected healthy patients. Patients for thoracic procedures are generally at risk for cardiopulmonary morbidity. As a result of the ventilation-perfusion mismatch that may accompany OLV, the anesthetic plan should account for the potential need for rapidly obtaining arterial blood gas samples.

Thoracoscopic sympathectomy for hyperhydrosis is an outpatient procedure. A DLT is preferred over a bronchial blocker, because the procedure is bilateral. Positioning the DLT once at the beginning of the case so that each lung can be deflated one at time is much easier than repositioning a bronchial blocker into the opposite bronchus once one side has been completed. The patient is in the supine position, and no chest tubes are inserted. Air and O_2 are preferred carrier gases.

Pain after a thoracoscopy is generally more easily managed than after an open thoracotomy. The incision length is smaller, and spreading of the ribs is avoided. Adequate pain relief is commonly obtained with the use of oral analgesics or nonsteroidal antiinflammatory drugs. More extensive procedures such as decortication or pleurodesis often require parenteral narcotics. Intercostal block may also be used to treat pain from manipulation of the thoracoscope in the camera port.[122]

BULLAE

Bullae are air-filled spaces of lung tissue resulting from the destruction of alveolar tissues and consolidation of alveoli into large pockets. They offer low resistance to inspiration and tend to increase in size with positive-pressure ventilation. A valvelike mechanism may be present that causes air trapping on expiration. Enlarging bullae compress normal lung tissue and vasculature to the point of causing hypoxemia, polycythemia, and cor pulmonale. Overdistended bullae can rupture and cause pneumothorax or tension pneumothorax with cardiopulmonary collapse, requiring insertion of a chest tube. A chest tube may show a large, continuous air leak, and ventilation may be difficult.[123]

A DLT is indicated when a thoracotomy is planned to resect bullous tissue. This allows for separate ventilation of each lung and the ability to use adequate VTs on the healthy lung without risking further rupture of bullae. In the event of a pneumothorax, the unaffected lung can be ventilated while a chest tube is placed or the incision is made. When the surgery is nearing completion, each lung can be separately checked for air leaks.

During general anesthesia for bullous disease, to reduce the risk of rupture of bullae, spontaneous ventilation is desirable until the chest is opened. Patients with severe cardiopulmonary disease may not be able to ventilate adequately under general anesthesia, however, and positive-pressure ventilation may be required. Small V_Ts, high respiratory rates, and high F_{IO_2} can be delivered by gentle manual ventilation to keep airway pressures below 10 to 20 cm H_2O.[123] An alternative to positive-pressure ventilation is high-frequency jet ventilation, used to decrease the chance of barotrauma. Normandale[124] describes jet ventilation with settings of a respiratory rate of 250 per minute, a volume of driving gas of 18 L/min, and inspiratory time of 3% of the total respiratory cycle with an F_{IO_2} of 0.8.

Nitrous oxide should be avoided in bullous disease because it rapidly enlarges the air-filled spaces. The choice of other anesthetic agents depends on the patient's cardiopulmonary status and the anesthetist's desire to maintain spontaneous ventilation. Hasenbon and Gielen described a combination general-epidural technique using epidural bupivacaine with epinephrine and a light general anesthetic. Bupivacaine 0.25% with epinephrine 1:200,000, 8 mL, resulted in an anesthetic block of T2 to T10. After induction with intravenous anesthetics, the vocal cords were anesthetized with 10% lidocaine topically, and a DLT was placed. Spontaneous ventilation was maintained, occasionally with manual assistance. The catheter was then used for postoperative epidural analgesia.[125]

After excision of the bulla, normal lung tissue rapidly expands, and compliance and gas exchange rapidly improve. Care must still be taken with positive-pressure ventilation if some unresectable bullae remain.

SUMMARY

Anesthetizing a patient for thoracic surgery requires intricate coordination of multiple factors. The patient may have cardiac or respiratory diseases, masses, bullae, and other problems that complicate anesthetic management. Knowledge of respiratory physiology, pathophysiology, and the physiology of OLV is vital to safe and effective practice. Special equipment such as double lumen ETTs and fiberoptic bronchoscopes must be understood. A thorough understanding of the properties of anesthetic drugs is necessary so that the most beneficial combination of agents can be selected to manage the patient's anesthesia. Contemporary literature suggests that using general anesthesia with the ability to provide high F_{IO_2} be balanced by the concern for absorption of oxygen worsening atelectasis. Lung separation may be achieved by double lumen tubes or bronchial blockers. Each has its own advantages, but neither is clearly preferable over the other in every case. Fiberoptic bronchoscopy should be used to ensure proper placement of airway devices for lung separation. Ventilation management calls for modest tidal volumes with the judicious use of PEEP and intermittent lung expansion maneuvers to minimize intraoperative and postoperative hypoxemia. For hypoxemia caused by shunting during OLV, intermittent expansion of one or both lungs, CPAP applied to the operative lung, or PEEP applied to the nondependent lung should be used. Judicious fluid management is an important component of reducing postoperative lung injury. Regional anesthesia is a useful adjunct for postoperative pain control.

REFERENCES

1. Sobue T et al. The Japanese Lung Cancer Screening Research Group. Survival for clinical stage I lung cancer not surgically treated. Comparison between screen-detected and symptom-detected cases. *Cancer.* 1992;69:685-692.
2. Weiss SJ, Ochroch EA. Thoracic anesthesia. In: Longnecker DE, et al, eds. *Anesthesiology.* New York: McGraw-Hill; 2008:1213-1283.
3. Bollinger CT et al. Pulmonary function and exercise capacity after lung resection. *Eur Respir J.* 1996;9:415-421.
4. Tassi G, Marchetti G. Minithoracoscopy: a less invasive approach to thoracoscopy. *Chest.* 2003;124:1975-1977.
5. Lohser J et al. Anesthesia for thoracic surgery in morbidly obese patients. *Curr Opin Anaesthesiol.* 2007;20(1):10-14.
6. Castillo MD, Heerdt PM. Pulmonary resection in the elderly. *Curr Opin Anaesthesiol.* 2007;20(1):4-9.
7. Bolliger CT et al. Preoperative assessment for lung cancer surgery. *Curr Opin Pulm Med.* 2005;11(4):301-306.
8. Lawrence VA et al. Strategies to reduce postoperative pulmonary complications after noncardiothoracic surgery: systematic review for the American College of Physicians. *Ann Int Med.* 2006;144(8):596-608.
9. Cohen E et al. Anesthesia for thoracic surgery. In: Barash PG, et al, eds. *Clinical Anesthesia.* 5th ed. Philadelphia: Lippincott; 2006:813-852.
10. Marriot HJL. Chamber enlargement. *Practical Electrocardiography.* Baltimore: Williams & Wilkins; 1988:50-62.
11. Dubin D. Hypertrophy. In: *Rapid Interpretation of EKGs.* 6th ed. Tampa, FL: Cover; 2000:243-258.
12. Kearney DJ et al. Assessment of operative risk in patients undergoing lung resection: importance of predicted pulmonary function. *Chest.* 1994;105:753-759.
13. Harpole DH et al. Prospective analysis of pneumonectomy: risk factors for major morbidity and cardiac dysrhythmias. *Ann Thorac Surg.* 1996;61:977-982.
14. Ninan M et al. Standardized exercise oximetry predicts postpneumonectomy outcome. *Ann Thorac Surg.* 1997;64:328-333.
15. Beckles A et al. The physiologic evaluation of patients with lung cancer being considered for resectional surgery. *Chest.* 2003;123:105S-114S.
16. Ribas J et al. Invasive exercise testing in the evaluation of patients at high risk for lung resection. *Eur Respir J.* 1998;12:1429-1435.
17. Mazzone PJ, Arroliga AC. Lung cancer: preoperative pulmonary evaluation of the lung resection candidate. *Am J Med.* 2005;118(6):578-583.
18. Linden PA et al. Lung resection in patients with preoperative FEV_1 < 35% predicted. *Chest.* 2005;127(6):1984-1990.
19. Chetta A et al. Respiratory effects of surgery and pulmonary function testing in the preoperative evaluation. *Acta Biomed.* 2006;77(2):69-74.
20. Giordano A et al. Perfusion lung scintigraphy for the prediction of postlobectomy residual pulmonary function. *Chest.* 1997;111:1542-1547.
21. Kushibe K et al. Assessment of pulmonary function after lobectomy for lung cancer—upper lobectomy might have the same effect as lung volume reduction surgery. *Eur J Cardiovasc Surg.* 2006;29(6):886-90.
22. Bousamra M et al. Early and late morbidity in patients undergoing pulmonary resection with low diffusion capacity. *Ann Thorac Surg.* 1996;62:968-975.
23. Ferguson MK et al. Optimizing selection of patients for major lung resection. *J Thorac Cardiovasc Surg.* 1995;109:275-283.
24. Pierce R et al. Preoperative risk evaluation for lung cancer resection predicted postoperative product as a predictor of surgical mortality. *Am J Respir Crit Care Med.* 1994;150:947-955.
25. Sue DY et al. Diffusing capacity for carbon monoxide as a predictor of gas exchange during exercise. *N Engl J Med.* 1987;316:1301-1306.
26. British Thoracic Society. BTS guidelines on the selection of patients with lung cancer for surgery. *Thorax.* 2001;56:89-108.
27. Brutsche MH et al. Exercise capacity and extent of resection as predictors of surgical risk in lung cancer. *Eur Resp J.* 2000;15(5):828-832.
28. Pollock M et al. Estimation of ventilatory reserve by stair climbing. *Chest.* 1993;104:1378-1383.
29. Moller AM et al. Effect of preoperative smoking intervention on postoperative complications: a randomized clinical trial. *Lancet.* 2002;359:114-117.
30. Bluman LG et al. Preoperative smoking habits and postoperative pulmonary complications. *Chest.* 1998;113:883-889.
31. Pilcher DV et al. High central venous pressure is associated with prolonged mechanical ventilation and increased mortality after lung transplantation. *J Thorac Cardiovasc Surg.* 2005;129(4):912-918.
32. Sandham J et al. A randomized, controlled trial of the use of pulmonary-artery catheters in high-risk surgical patients. *N Engl J Med.* 2003;348:5-14.
33. Polanczyk CA et al. Right heart catheterization and cardiac complications in patients undergoing noncardiac surgery: an observational study. *JAMA.* 2001;286:309-314.
34. Ganter CG et al. Pulmonary capillary pressure. A review. *Minerva Anestesiol.* 2006;72(1-2):21-36.
35. Bowdle TA. Complications of invasive monitoring. *Anesthesiol Clin North America.* 2002;20:571-588.
36. Lawson NW, Meyer J. Lateral decubitus positions. In: Martin JT, Warner MA, eds. *Positioning in Anesthesia and Surgery.* 3rd ed. Philadelphia: Saunders; 1997:124-145.

37. West J. Ventilation-perfusion relationships. In: *Respiratory Physiology: The Essentials.* 7th ed. Baltimore: Williams & Wilkins; 2005:55-74.

38. Dunn PF. Physiology of the lateral decubitus position and one-lung ventilation. *Int Anesth Clin.* 2000;38(1):25.

39. Benumof JL. Special respiratory physiology of the lateral decubitus position, the open chest and one lung anesthesia. *Anesthesia for Thoracic Surgery.* 2nd ed, Philadelphia: Saunders; 1995:123-151.

40. Gale JW, Waters RM. Closed endobronchial anesthesia in thoracic surgery. *J Thorac Surg.* 1931;1:432-437.

41. Takahashi M et al. Selective lobar-bronchial blocking for pediatric video-assisted thoracic surgery. *Anesthesiology.* 2001;94:170-172.

42. Campos JH. Which device should be considered the best for lung isolation: double-lumen endotracheal tube versus bronchial blockers. *Curr Opin Anaesthesiol.* 2007;20(1):27-31.

43. Teleflex Medical. *Endobronchial Tubes.* Available at: http://www.myrusch.com/images/rusch/docs/A25C.pdf. Accessed November 24, 2007.

44. Campos JH. Lung isolation techniques. *Anesthesiol Clin North America.* 2001;19(3):455-474.

45. Satya-Krishna R, Popat M. Insertion of the double lumen tube in the difficult airway. *Anaesthesia.* 2006;61(9):896-898.

46. Hubner BL et al. Jet ventilation for anterior paediatric scoliosis surgery. *Paediatr Anaesth.* 2002;12(8):724-728.

47. Campos JH et al. Devices for lung isolation used by anesthesiologists with limited thoracic experience: comparison of double-lumen endotracheal tube, Univent torque control blocker, and Arndt wire-guided endobronchial blocker. *Anesthesiology.* 2006;104(2):261-266.

48. Lewis JW et al. The utility of a double-lumen tube for one-lung ventilation in a variety of noncardiac thoracic surgical procedures. *J Cardiothorac Vasc Anesth.* 1992;6:705-710.

49. Hurford WE, Alfille PH. A quality improvement study of the placement and complications of double-lumen endobronchial tubes. *J Cardiothorac Vasc Anesth.* 1993;7:517-520.

50. Lieberman D et al. Placement of left double-lumen-endobronchial tubes with or without stylet. *Can J Anaesth.* 1996;43:238-242.

51. Klein U et al. Role of fiberoptic bronchoscopy in conjunction with the use of double-lumen tubes for thoracic anesthesia. *Anesthesiology.* 1998;88:346-350.

52. Desiderio DP et al. The effects of endobronchial cuff inflation on double-lumen endobronchial tube movement after lateral decubitus positioning. *J Cardiothorac Vasc Anesth.* 1997;11:595-598.

53. Berchard D, Wetstein L. Assessment of exercise oxygen consumption as preoperative criterion for lung resection. *Ann Thorac Surg.* 1987;44:344-349.

54. Gilbert TB et al. Bronchial rupture by a double-lumen endobronchial tube during staging thoracoscopy. *Anesth Analg.* 1999;88:1252-1253.

55. Yuceyar L et al. Bronchial rupture with a left-sided polyvinylchloride double-lumen tube. *Acta Anaesthesiol Scand.* 2003;47:622-625.

56. Dryden GE. Circulatory collapse after pneumonectomy (an unusual complication from the use of a Carlen catheter): case report. *Anesth Analg.* 1977;56:451-452.

57. Knoll H et al. Airway injuries after one-lung ventilation: a comparison between double-lumen tube and endobronchial blocker: a randomized, prospective, controlled trial. *Anesthesiology.* 2006;105(3):471-477.

58. Sagawa M et al. Bilateral vocal cord paralysis after lung cancer surgery with a double-lumen endotracheal tube: a life-threatening complication. *J Cardiothorac Vasc Anesth.* 2006;20(2):225-226.

59. Archer S, Michelakis E. The mechanism(s) of hypoxic pulmonary vasoconstriction: potassium channels, redox O_2 sensors, and controversies. *News Physiol Sci.* 2002;17:131-137.

60. Benumof JL. One-lung ventilation and hypoxic pulmonary vasoconstriction: implications for anesthetic management. *Anesth Analg.* 1985;64:821-833.

61. Benumof JL. Isoflurane anesthesia and arterial oxygenation during one-lung ventilation. *Anesthesiology.* 1986;64:419-422.

62. Benumof JL, Wahrenbrock EA. Blunted hypoxic pulmonary vasoconstriction by increased lung vascular pressures. *J Appl Physiol.* 1975;38:846-850.

63. Colley PS et al. Mechanism of change in pulmonary shunt flow with hemorrhage. *J Appl Physiol.* 1977;42:196-201.

64. Hillier SC et al. Hypoxic vasoconstriction in pulmonary arterioles and venules. *J Appl Physiol.* 1997;82:1084-1090.

65. Carlsson AJ et al. Hypoxia-induced pulmonary vasoconstriction in the human lung. The effect of isoflurane anesthesia. *Anesthesiology.* 1987;66:312-316.

66. Eisenkraft J. Effects of anesthetics on the pulmonary circulation. *Br J Anaesth.* 1990;65:63-78.

67. Schulte-Sasse U et al. Pulmonary vascular responses to nitrous oxide in patients with normal and high pulmonary vascular resistance. *Anesthesiology.* 1982;57:9-13.

68. Van Keer L et al. Propofol does not inhibit hypoxic pulmonary vasoconstriction in humans. *J Clin Anesth.* 1989;1:284-288.

69. Cammu G et al. Postoperative residual paralysis in outpatients versus inpatients. *Anesth Analg.* 2006;102:426-429.

70. Berg H et al. Residual neuromuscular block is a risk factor for postoperative pulmonary complications. A prospective, randomized, and blinded study of postoperative pulmonary complications after atracurium, vecuronium and pancuronium. *Acta Anaesthesiol Scand.* 1997;41:1095-1103.

71. Eikermann M et al. Impaired neuromuscular transmission after recovery of the train-of-four ratio. *Acta Anaesthesiol Scand.* 2007;51(2):226-234.

72. Rodgers A et al. Reduction of postoperative mortality and morbidity with epidural or spinal anaesthesia: results from overview of randomized trials. *BMJ.* 2000;321:1493.

73. Ballantyne JC et al. The comparative effects of postoperative analgesic therapies on pulmonary outcome: cumulative meta-analysis of randomized, controlled trials. *Anesth Analg.* 1998;86:598-612.

74. Slinger P et al. Relation of the static compliance curve and positive end-expiratory pressure to oxygenation during one-lung ventilation. *Anesthesiology.* 2001;95:1096-1102.

75. Slinger PD, Johnston MR. Preoperative assessment and management. In: Kaplan JA, Slinger PD, eds. *Thoracic Anesthesia.* 3rd ed. Philadelphia: Churchill Livingstone; 2003:1-23.

76. Senturk M. New concepts of the management of one-lung ventilation. *Curr Opin Anaesthesiol.* 2006;19(1):1-4.

77. Choi G et al. Mechanical ventilation with lower tidal volumes and positive end-expiratory pressure prevents alveolar coagulation in patients without lung injury. *Anesthesiology.* 2006;105(4):689-695.

78. Slinger PD. Acute lung injury after pulmonary resection: more pieces of the puzzle. *Anesth Analg.* 2003;97:1555-1557.

79. Licker M et al. Risk factors for acute lung injury after thoracic surgery for lung cancer. *Anesth Analg.* 2003;97:1558-1565.

80. Amato MB et al. Effect of a protective-ventilation strategy on mortality in the acute respiratory distress syndrome. *N Engl J Med.* 1998;338:347-354.

81. Cohen E et al. Positive end-expiratory pressure during one-lung ventilation improves oxygenation in patients with low arterial oxygen tensions. *J Cardiothorac Vasc Anesth.* 1996;10:578-582.

82. Hedenstierna G, Sandhagen B. Assessing dead space. A meaningful variable? *Minerva Anestesiol.* 2006;72(6):521-528.

83. Blanch L et al. Volumetric capnography in the mechanically ventilated patient. *Minerva Anestesiol.* 2006;72(6):577-585.

84. Tugrul M et al. Comparison of volume controlled with pressure controlled ventilation during one-lung anaesthesia. *Br J Anaesth.* 1997;79:306-310.

85. Ng JM. Hypoxemia during one-lung ventilation: jet ventilation of the middle and lower lobes during right upper lobe sleeve resection. *Anesth Analg.* 2005;101(5):1554-1555.

86. Abe K et al. Effect of high-frequency jet ventilation on oxygenation during one-lung ventilation in patients undergoing thoracic aneurysm surgery. *J Anesth.* 2006;20(1):1-5.

87. Sabanathan S et al. Alterations in respiratory mechanics following thoracotomy. *J Royal Coll Surg Edinburgh.* 1990;35:144-50.

88. Tippana E et al. Post-thoracotomy pain after thoracic epidural analgesia: a prospective follow-up study. *Acta Anaethesiol Scand.* 2003;47:433-438.

89. Richardson J, et al. Post-thoracotomy spirometric lung function. the effect of analgesia. *J Cardiovasc Surg.* 1999;40:445-446.

90. Suzuki M et al. Low-dose intravenous ketamine potentiates epidural analgesia after thoracotomy. *Anesthesiology.* 2006;105(1):111-119.

91. Tziavrangos E, Schug SA. Regional anaesthesia and perioperative outcome. *Curr Opin Anaesthesiol.* 2006;19(5):521-525.

92. Kaya FN et al. Preoperative multiple-injection thoracic paravertebral blocks reduce postoperative pain and analgesic requirements after video-assisted thoracic surgery. *J Cardiothorac Vasc Anesth.* 2006;20(5):639-643.

93. Yang MK. The effects of cryoanalgesia combined with thoracic epidural analgesia in patients undergoing thoracotomy. *Anaesthesia.* 2004;59(11):1073.

94. Gothard J. Lung injury after thoracic surgery and one-lung ventilation. *Curr Opin Anaesthesiol.* 2006;19(1):5-10.

95. Losher J. Evidence based management of one lung ventilation. *Anesthesiology Clin.* 26;2008:241-272.

96. Boldt J et al. Cardiorespiratory changes in patients undergoing pulmonary resection using different anesthetic management techniques. *J Cardiothorac Vasc Anesth.* 1996;10:854-859.

97. Pate P et al. Preoperative assessment of the high-risk patient for lung resection. *Ann Thorac Surg.* 1996;61:1494-1500.

98. Krowka MJ et al. Cardiac dysrhythmias following pneumonectomy: clinical correlates and prognostic significance. *Chest.* 1987;91:490-495.

99. Roselli EE et al. Atrial fibrillation complicating lung cancer resection. *J Thorac Cardiovasc Surg.* 2005;130(2):438-444.

100. Jakobsen CJ et al. Perioperative metoprolol reduces the frequency of atrial fibrillation after thoracotomy for lung resection. *J Cardiothorac Vasc Anesth.* 1997;11:746-751.

101. Baumann MH, Sahn SA. Medical management and therapy of bronchopleural fistulas in the mechanically ventilated patient. *Chest.* 1990;97:721-728.

102. Milsom JW et al. Chylothorax: an assessment of surgical management. *J Thorac Cardiovasc Surg.* 1985;89:221-227.

103. Gallagher C et al. Thoracotomy: postoperative complications. *Probl Anesth.* 1990;4:393-415.

104. Gothard JWW. Anesthetic considerations for patients with anterior mediastinal masses. *Anesthesiol Clin.* 2008;26:305-314.

105. Rendina EA et al. Biopsy of anterior mediastinal masses under local anesthesia. *Ann Thorac Surg.* 2002;74:1720-1722, 1722-1723 [discussion].

106. Pullerits J, Holzman R. Anaesthesia for patients with mediastinal masses. *Can J Anaesth.* 1989;36:681-688.

107. Torchio R et al. Orthopnea and tidal expiratory flow limitation in patients with euthyroid goiter. *Chest.* 2003;124:133-140.

108. Piro AJ et al. Mediastinal Hodgkin's disease: a possible danger for intubation anaesthesia. *Int J Radiat Oncol Biol Phys.* 1976;1:415-419.

109. Prakash UBS et al. Mediastinal mass and tracheal obstruction during general anesthesia. *Mayo Clin Proc.* 1988;63:1004-1011.

110. Mizrahi S et al. Major airway obstruction relieved by helium/oxygen breathing. *Crit Care Med.* 1986;14:986-987.

111. Slinger P, Karsli C. Management of the patient with a large anterior mediastinal mass: recurring myths. *Curr Opin Anaesthesiol.* 2007;20(1):1-3.

112. Levin H et al. Cardiac arrest in a child with a mediastinal mass. *Anesth Analg.* 1985;64:1129-1130.

113. Keon TP. Death on induction of anesthesia for cervical node biopsy. *Anesthesiology.* 1981;55:471-472.

114. Goh MH et al. Anterior mediastinal masses: an anaesthetic challenge. *Anaesthesia.* 1999;54:670-674.

115. Hung JJ et al. Major hemorrhage and subsequent cardiac tamponade during mediastinoscopy. *J Thorac Cardiovasc Surg.* 2007;133(1):269-270.

116. Plummer S et al. Anaesthesia for telescopic procedures in the thorax. *Br J Anaesth.* 1998;80:223-234.

117. Fair J. Anesthesia for thoracoscopy: an overview. *AANA J.* 1994;62:133-138.

118. Conacher ID. Anaesthesia for thoracoscopic surgery. *Best Pract Res Clin Anaesthesiol.* 2002;16:53-62.

119. Allen MS et al. Video-assisted thoracic surgical procedures: the Mayo experience. *Mayo Clin Proc.* 1996;71:351-359.

120. Berrisford RG, Page RD. Video-assisted thoracic surgery for spontaneous pneumothorax. *Thorax.* 1996;51:523-528.

121. Pompeo E et al. The role of awake video-assisted thoracoscopic surgery in spontaneous pneumothorax. *J Thorac Cardiovasc Surg.* 2007;133(3):786-790.

122. Horswell JL. Anesthetic techniques for thoracoscopy. *Ann Thorac Surg.* 1993;56:624-629.

123. Cohen E et al. Case 1,1990. A 59-year-old, oxygen-dependent man with severe giant bullous emphysema is admitted for pulmonary angiography and pulmonary bulla resection. *J Cardiothorac Vasc Anesth.* 1990;4:119-129.

124. Normandale JP. Bullous cystic lung disease. *Anaesthesia.* 1985;40:1182-1185.

125. Hasenbon MA, Gielen MJ. Anesthesia for bullectomy: a technique with spontaneous ventilation and extradural blockade. *Anaesthesia.* 1985;40:977-980.

CHAPTER 29

NEUROANATOMY, NEUROPHYSIOLOGY, AND NEUROANESTHESIA

C. Wayne Hamm, John Maye

This chapter will review the organization of the central nervous system (CNS). Specific neurophysiologic concepts that are essential for the anesthesia provider will also be presented. These concepts include electrophysiology, cerebral blood supply, role of neurotransmitters, and the effects of selected anesthetic agents on cerebral physiology. This chapter will also provide recommendations for the management of specific neurosurgical procedures.

ORGANIZATION OF THE CENTRAL NERVOUS SYSTEM

Cells of the Central and Peripheral Nervous Systems

The central nervous system (CNS) includes the brain and spinal cord. The peripheral nervous system (PNS) includes the cranial and spinal nerves and their receptors and is divided into the somatic and autonomic nervous systems. The somatic nervous system contains sensory neurons for the control of skin, muscles, and joints. The autonomic nervous system, which consists of the sympathetic, parasympathetic, and enteric subdivisions, is responsible for involuntary innervation of various organ systems.

The CNS is derived from two primary cell types: neurons and neuroglial (or glial) cells. The neuron is the basic functional cell of the CNS and consists of a cell body (perikaryon) and specialized cytoplasmic processes, dendrites, and a single axon (Figure 29-1). A single axon emerges from the cell body at the axon hillock. The axon may branch to form collateral nerves at a point distal to the neuron cell body. Axon diameters range from 0.2 to 20 μm. Most of the axons in the brain are only a few millimeters long, although the axons that run from the spinal cord may be as long as 1 m. Stimulation of the dendrites produces antegrade impulse conduction (toward the neuron cell body) with subsequent conduction away from the neuron cell body by way of the axon.

Neuron cell bodies vary in size and shape and are classified as unipolar, bipolar, pseudounipolar, or multipolar. Unipolar neurons are found only in lower invertebrates. Bipolar neurons are found in the retina, ear, and olfactory mucosa. Pseudounipolar neurons have one cytoplasmic process that exits the cell and divides into two branches, one serving as the dendrite, the other as the axon. Pseudounipolar neurons are present in the dorsal root ganglia and cranial ganglion cells, enabling sensory impulses to travel from the dendrite directly to the axon without passing through the cell body. Multipolar neurons have multiple dendritic processes but only one axon and constitute the majority of the CNS neurons.

The gray matter of the CNS is composed of neuron cell bodies in the CNS, and the white matter is composed of myelinated axons. Regions of concentrated cell bodies within the peripheral nervous system form the cranial, spinal, and autonomic ganglia.

Neurons may be classified according to their specific function: motor neurons, sensory neurons, or interneurons. Motor neurons are multipolar and innervate and control effector tissues such as muscles and glands. Sensory neurons are pseudounipolar and receive exteroceptive, interoceptive, or proprioceptive input. Interneurons are pseudounipolar and connect adjacent neurons.

The neuron is bounded by a bilaminar lipoprotein membrane derived from phospholipid molecules arranged with their fatty acid chains facing one another, producing an inner hydrophobic membrane. The membrane surface in contact with the extracellular fluid contains polar hydrophilic groups of phospholipid molecules. The neuronal membrane contains integral membrane proteins, which form ionic pumps, ion channels, enzymes (e.g., adenylate cyclase), receptor proteins, and structural proteins.

The neuron contains a number of common cellular organelles including a well-developed nucleus, mitochondria (distributed throughout the cell body), and cytoplasmic processes. Ribosomes, endoplasmic reticulum, lysosomes, and Golgi complexes are also found. Neurotubules and neurofilaments extend through the cytoplasm from the dendrites to the axon terminal; they provide structural support and a pathway for intracellular transport of neurotransmitters.

The second major cell type found within the CNS is the neuroglial, or glial, cell (Table 29-1). Four types of glial cells are found within the CNS: astrocytes, oligodendrocytes, microglial cells, and ependymal cells. Most neoplasms of the CNS arise from glial cells (astrocytes). Glial cells are smaller, outnumber neuronal cells, and lack dendritic and axonal processes. Although they do not participate in neuronal signaling, glial cells are essential for neuronal function. The role of neuroglia includes the maintenance of a proper ionic environment, the modulation of nerve cell electrical conduction, control of reuptake of neurotransmitters, and repair after neuronal injury.

The astrocyte is the predominant glial cell. Astrocytes provide structural neuronal support, group and pair neurons and nerve terminals, regulate the metabolic environment, and are active in repair after neuronal injury.

Two distinct types of astrocytes exist: fibrous astrocytes, found in the white matter, and protoplasmic astrocytes, concentrated in the gray matter. Astrocytes have multiple processes that radiate from the cell, producing a star-shaped appearance. Some of these processes (astrocytic feet) terminate on the surfaces of blood vessels within the CNS (perivascular feet). The contact of the cerebral endothelium by astrocytes has been proposed to be essential in the development of the blood-brain barrier.[1]

Oligodendrocytes have fewer branches than astrocytes (*oligo*, "few"; *dendro*, "branches"). Oligodendrocytes form the myelin sheath of axons in the brain and spinal cord and are capable of myelinating more than one axon. However, oligodendrocytes are incapable of division and fail to regenerate after injury.

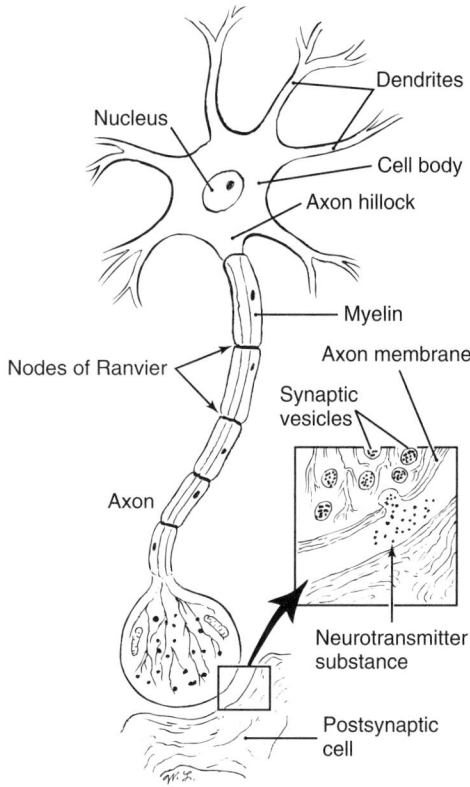

FIGURE **29-1** Neuron and chemical synapse.

The velocity of nerve impulse conduction in an unmyelinated axon increases with the square root of the diameter of the axon. Accordingly, a doubling of impulse conduction requires that the axon be doubled in size. One could only imagine the size of the peripheral nervous system without the presence of myelin. Myelin is essential to increase the velocity of impulse conduction and minimize the size of the axon.

Myelin is formed in the vertebral peripheral nervous system by modified glial cells termed *Schwann cells*.[2] Unlike the oligodendrocyte, the Schwann cell myelinates only one axon, surrounding the axon and forming successive layers of plasma membrane. The resultant thickness is variable in different axons. The junction between adjacent Schwann cells is devoid of myelin at 1-mm intervals along the length of the axon. This nonmyelinated portion of the axon, the node of Ranvier, is the site of electrical impulse propagation. Impulses in myelinated axons travel from one node of Ranvier to another (saltatory conduction), bypassing the area between the nodes and increasing the velocity of conduction (see Figure 29-1). Wallerian degeneration results in the distal degeneration of the axon after peripheral nerve injury. Proximal axon degeneration may also occur. Within 1 week of the initial injury, Schwann cells proliferate to form a tube into the area of degeneration, forming a scaffold to direct axon regeneration. Myelin regeneration precedes axon regeneration, with the myelin eventually reaching its previous thickness.

Microglial cells are the smallest neuroglial cells and are scattered throughout the CNS. They are transported throughout the CNS to sites of neuronal injury or degeneration, where they proliferate and develop into large macrophages that phagocytize neuronal debris.

Ependymal cells line the roof of the third and fourth ventricles of the brain and the central spinal canal. Ependymal cells form the cuboidal epithelium (choroid plexus), which secretes cerebrospinal fluid (CSF).

Blood-Brain Barrier

The injection of an intravenous dye causes most of the body tissues and internal organs to be stained, yet the brain and spinal cord remain unblemished. This finding led to the discovery of the blood-brain barrier, which effectively isolates the brain and spinal cord extracellular compartment from the intravascular compartment.

The endothelial cells of the CNS form tight junctions between adjacent cells, preventing the transport of polar substances from the intravascular to the cerebral extracellular fluid compartment. CNS endothelial cells lack transport mechanisms, so little intracellular transport takes place. A number of midline brain structures receive neurosecretory products from the blood and therefore lack a blood-brain barrier. These structures, the circumventricular organs, include the area postrema, pituitary gland, pineal gland, choroid plexus, and portions of the hypothalamus.

The blood-brain barrier is incompletely developed in the newborn. The high vascular content of bile pigments in jaundiced newborns may enter the basal ganglia, producing kernicterus. Blood-brain barrier disruption can be caused by traumatic head injury, subarachnoid or intracerebral hemorrhage, or cerebral ischemia. The development of mass lesions may also produce blood-brain barrier disruption. Osmotically active substances may penetrate the brain or spinal cord after blood-brain barrier disruption. Intentional intracarotid injection of a hyperosmolar solution shrinks the endothelial cells, opens tight junctions, and disrupts the blood-brain barrier. This technique allows the

TABLE **29-1**	Glial Cells
Type	**Major Functions**
Astrocytes	Support (for neurons) Metabolic and nutritive functions
Ependymal cells	Probable role in cerebrospinal fluid production
Microglia	Phagocytosis
Oligodendrocytes	Insulation (form myelin sheath in the brain and spinal cord)
Schwann cells	Insulation (form myelin sheath in the peripheral nerves)

delivery of chemotherapeutic drugs through the blood-brain barrier for the treatment of neural malignancy.[3]

ANATOMY OF THE CENTRAL NERVOUS SYSTEM

Cerebral Structures

The cerebral hemispheres are the most intricately developed and largest regions of the brain (Figure 29-2). They contain the cerebral cortex, hippocampal formation, amygdala, and basal ganglia. The cerebral cortex consists of the outer 3-mm layer of the cerebral hemispheres. The surface of the cerebral cortex is convoluted, increasing the surface area of the cerebral hemispheres. Elevated convolutions called *gyri* are separated by shallow grooves called *sulci* and by deeper grooves called *fissures*.

The medial longitudinal fissure divides the cerebral hemispheres into right and left halves. The lateral fissure of Sylvius and the central sulcus of Rolando divide each hemisphere into four lobes, which are named for the cranial bones that overlie each area. The frontal lobe, essential for motor control, and the parietal lobe, essential for the senses of pain and touch, are separated by the central sulcus. Voluntary muscle activity is controlled by the motor cortex located in the precentral gyrus, or the Brodmann areas (Figure 29-3). The sensations of touch, pain, and limb position, as well as the sensory perception of grasped objects, are controlled by the somatic sensory cortex located in the postcentral gyrus of the parietal lobe. The temporal lobe, which contains the auditory cortex, is separated from the frontal and parietal lobes by the sylvian fissure. The occipital lobe lies posterior to the parietooccipital sulcus. Here the visual

cortex lies within the walls of the calcarine fissure on the medial brain surface.

The corpus callosum lies deep in the longitudinal fissure and contains commissural fibers that interconnect the cerebral hemispheres. These fibers arise from neurons in one hemisphere and synapse with neurons in the corresponding area of the adjacent hemisphere. The remaining major structures of the cerebral hemispheres include the basal ganglia, the amygdala, and the hippocampal formation. The basal ganglia are involved in the control of movement. The amygdala functions in the regulation of emotional behavior, response to pain, and appetite and is essential in forming the response to stressors. The hippocampal formation is essential for memory formation and learning.

The diencephalon is located in the midline between the two cerebral hemispheres and contains two important structures—the thalamus and the hypothalamus. The oval-shaped thalamus integrates and transmits sensory information to various cortical areas of the cerebral hemispheres via separate thalamic nuclei. The hypothalamus is composed of several nuclei, including the mammillary bodies. The hypothalamus is the master neurohumoral organ.

The midbrain, pons, and medulla form the brainstem. The brainstem contains the reticular activating system, which functions to maintain consciousness, arousal, and alertness. The pons is anterior to the cerebellum, separated by the fourth ventricle, connecting the medulla oblongata and the midbrain (Figure 29-4). The pons contains ascending and descending fiber tracts and the nuclei of the trigeminal nerve (cranial nerve V) and the facial nerve (cranial nerve VII). The medulla extends from the pons to the foramen magnum, where it becomes continuous with the spinal cord (see Figure 29-4). In addition to ascending and descending fiber tracts, the medulla contains respiratory and cardiovascular control centers and the vestibulocochlear nerve (cranial nerve VIII), the glossopharyngeal nerve (cranial nerve IX), the vagus nerve (cranial nerve X), the spinal accessory nerve (cranial nerve XI), and the hypoglossal nerve (cranial nerve XII) nuclei.[4]

The cerebellum is convoluted in appearance and lies below the occipital lobe of the cerebral cortex and posterior to the pons and medulla. Structurally it resembles the cerebral cortex, containing an outer layer of gray matter and an inner core of white matter with several nuclei embedded within. The cerebellum can be divided into three functional areas. The flocculonodular lobe (archeocerebellum) is active in the maintenance of equilibrium, and the paleocerebellum (anterior lobe and part of vermis) regulates muscle tone. The neocerebellum (posterior lobe plus most of the vermis) is the largest subdivision of the cerebellum and is essential in coordinating voluntary muscle activity. The cerebellum integrates information received from other areas of the CNS and the peripheral nervous system. Information from the cerebellum is transmitted to the cerebral cortex and to lower motor neurons involved in the maintenance of muscle tone, equilibrium, and voluntary muscle activity.[4]

Meninges

The brain and spinal cord are enveloped by three meningeal layers: the dura mater, the arachnoid mater, and the pia mater (Figure 29-5). The dura mater, the thickest of the meningeal layers, overlies the cerebral hemispheres and brainstem and is functionally separated into an outer periosteal layer (adherent to the inner cranium) and an inner meningeal layer. The dura mater forms a fold, the falx cerebri, that functionally separates the cerebral hemispheres. A similar fold, the tentorium cerebelli,

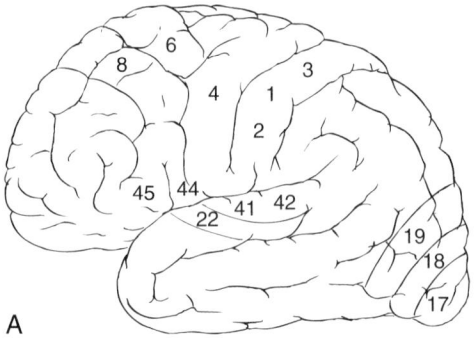

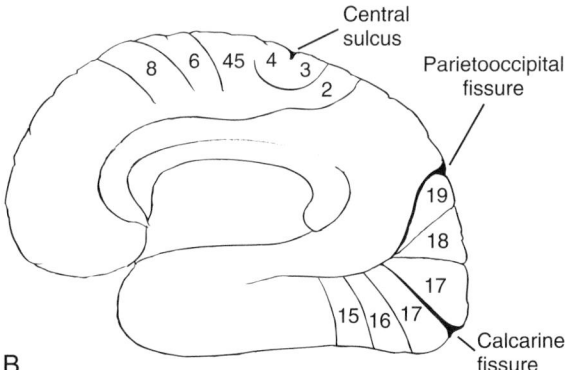

FIGURE **29-2** Cerebral cortex. **A,** Gyri, sulci, and fissures of the surface of the brain. **B,** Some functional areas of the cerebral cortex. (*Modified from Guyton AC. Basic Neuroscience: Anatomy and Physiology. Philadelphia: Saunders; 1991:12.*)

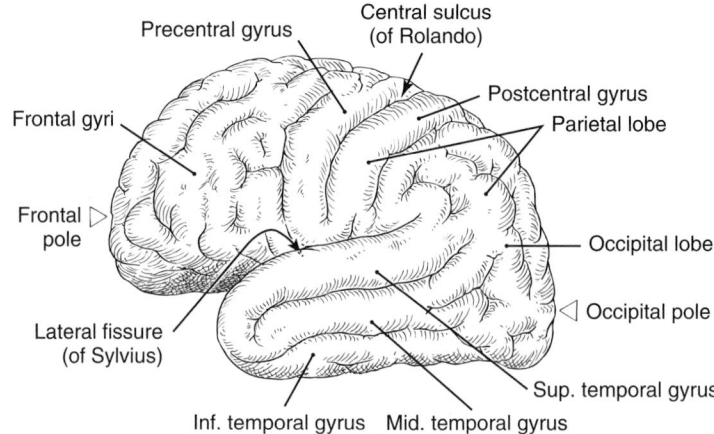

FIGURE **29-3** Brodmann areas of the cerebral cortex. *(Modified from Carpenter MD. Core Text of Neuroanatomy. Baltimore: Williams & Wilkins; 1991:286.)*

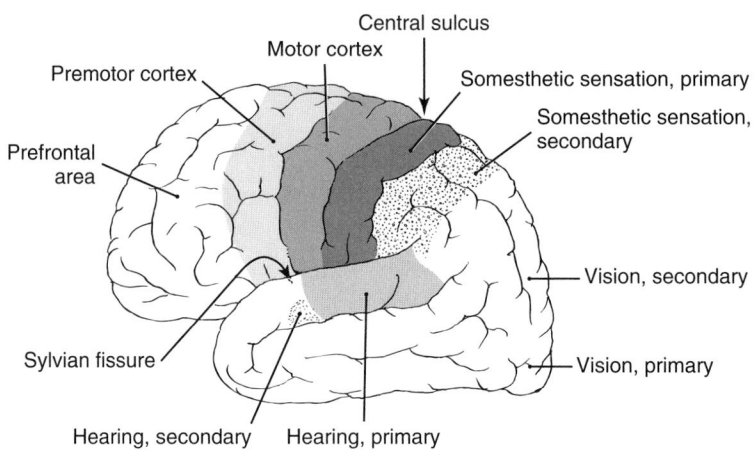

FIGURE **29-4** The pons and medulla and the origin of the cranial nerves.

separates the occipital lobe and the cerebellum. The dura mater of the spinal cord is continuous with the meningeal layer of the cranial dura mater and the perineurium of the peripheral nerves. Innervation of the dura mater is provided by the first three cervical roots and the trigeminal nerve. During awake

craniotomy, the patient may complain of pain "behind the eye" when traction is applied to the dura.

The arachnoid mater is a thin, avascular membrane joining the dura mater. The subdural space, a potential space between the dura mater and the arachnoid mater, is of clinical importance.

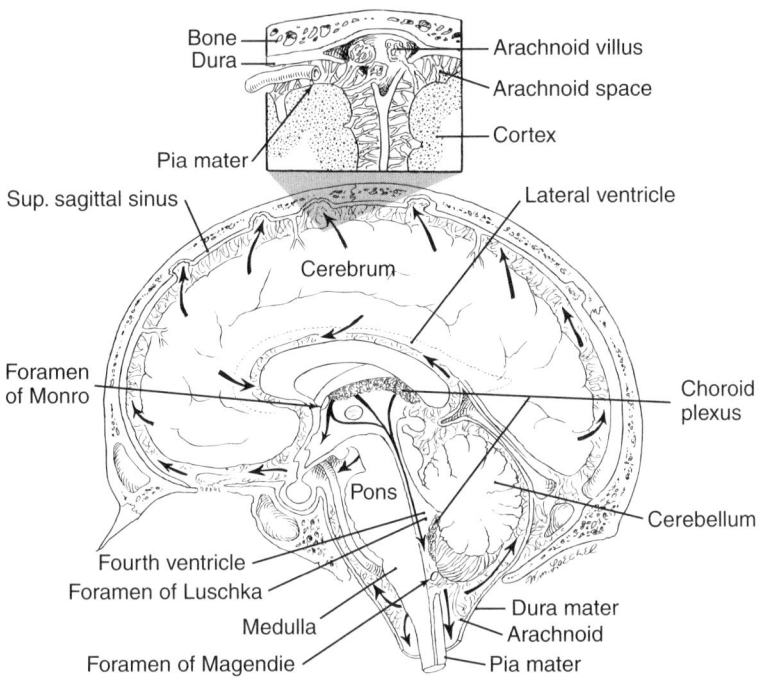

FIGURE **29-5** Meninges and the flow of cerebrospinal fluid through the ventricular system.

The unintentional injection of local anesthetic during spinal anesthesia into the subdural space produces patchy, asymmetric block. In addition, injury to a blood vessel in the subdural space can create bleeding (subdural hematoma), requiring surgical intervention.

The pia mater is a thin avascular membrane adherent to the brain and spinal cord. The subarachnoid space lies between the arachnoid mater and the pia mater. In the spinal cord, the subarachnoid space extends to the S2 to S3 level and is filled with CSF. In addition, the vasculature that overlies the CNS is located within the subarachnoid space. Injury to the vascular structures may produce subarachnoid hemorrhage and hematoma.

The epidural space is located outside the dura but inside the spinal canal. The epidural space contains a venous plexus and epidural fat that provides protection of the neural structures. The distance from the skin to the epidural space may be as little as 3 cm or as large as 8 cm.

Cerebrospinal Fluid

CSF is contained within the ventricles of the brain, the cisterns surrounding the brain, and the subarachnoid space of the brain and spinal cord (see Figure 29-5). The total volume of cranial and spinal CSF in the adult is approximately 150 mL. The specific gravity is 1.002 to 1.009, and the pH is 7.32. CSF bathes the brain and spinal cord, cushioning these delicate structures, and controls and maintains the extracellular milieu for neurons and glial cells.

CSF is secreted by the ependymal cells of the choroid plexus within the ventricular system at a rate of approximately 30 mL/hr. Although CSF is isotonic with plasma, it is not a plasma filtrate. CSF concentrations of potassium, calcium, bicarbonate, and glucose are lower than their respective plasma concentrations, and concentrations of sodium, chloride, and magnesium are higher. The entire CSF volume is replaced every 3 to 4 hours. Normal CSF pressure is between 5 and

15 mm Hg. CSF flows from the lateral ventricles of the cerebral hemispheres through the foramen of Monro into the third ventricle, through the aqueduct of Sylvius in the midbrain, into the fourth ventricle. CSF enters the subarachnoid space through the medial foramen of Magendie and the paired lateral foramina of Luschka, openings in the roof of the fourth ventricle.

The cisterna magna, located between the medulla and the cerebellum, is formed from the separation of the arachnoid mater from the pia mater and is filled with CSF. Two additional cisterns exist, the cisterna pontis and the cisterna basalis. CSF drains into the venous blood via the superior sagittal sinus and is absorbed by arachnoid granulations.

Spinal Cord

The spinal cord extends from the medulla at the foramen magnum to the filum terminale, a threadlike connective tissue structure that attaches to the first segment of the coccyx. Thirty-one pairs of spinal nerves carry motor and sensory information: 8 cervical, 12 thoracic, 5 lumbar, 5 sacral, and 1 coccygeal. The first pair of cervical nerves exits the spinal cord between the base of the skull and the first cervical vertebra (atlas), and the remaining 30 pairs exit between adjacent vertebrae. All of the exiting spinal nerves are covered with pia mater. Because the spinal cord is approximately 25 cm shorter than the vertebral canal in adults, the lumbar and sacral nerves have relatively long roots (the cauda equina). The spinal cord fills the canal in utero, but the canal elongates at a greater rate than does the neural tissue as the child ages, forming the cauda equina.

The spinal cord is divided into dorsal, lateral, and ventral regions by the entering dorsal sensory root fibers and the outgoing ventral motor root fibers. Neuron cell bodies and unmyelinated fibers lie in the H-shaped central gray region of the cord, surrounded by fiber tracts that form the white matter. Although it does not have a uniform appearance, this general arrangement continues throughout the entire spinal cord.

The spinal gray matter is divided into the ventral and dorsal gray commissures. The ventral projections of gray matter are called the *gray horns* or *columns*; the posterior projections are called the *posterior gray horns* or *columns*. Intermediolateral gray horns or columns are found between T1 and L2. The gray matter has been subdivided into 10 (I through X) laminae of Rexed. Rexed laminae I through VI are located in the dorsal (posterior) horn and contain cell bodies that receive sensory information from the periphery. Projections from the laminae form afferent tracts. A large number of interneurons are found in laminae V, VI, and X. Laminae VII, VIII, and IX make up the ventral (anterior) horn and contain motor neurons and interneurons involved in motor functions. The gray matter is enlarged in two areas of the spinal cord, C5 to C7 and L3 to S2. The cervical enlargement contains neuron cell bodies that innervate the upper extremities; the lumbosacral enlargement contains neuron cell bodies that innervate the lower extremities.

The tracts or fascicles that make up the white matter are highly organized, similar to the organization of the cerebral cortex and other areas of the brain. The dorsal white matter is composed almost exclusively of ascending sensory fiber tracts. The lateral and ventral white matter contains descending motor tracts. Commonly, fiber tracts at some level in the spinal cord or brain decussate, or cross over to the other side. As in the brain, spinal cord fiber tracts can be projection tracts connecting the spinal cord and brain, or they can be association (intersegmental, fasciculi proprii) tracts that originate and terminate entirely within the spinal cord. The association tracts play an important role in spinal reflexes.[4-7]

Shortly after leaving the spinal cord, the meningeal coverings of the peripheral nerves merge with the connective tissue layers that cover the peripheral nerve. The outermost covering of the peripheral nerve is called the *epineurium*. The bundles or fascicles of axons in each nerve are covered by the perineurium, and each axon in a fascicle is surrounded by the endoneurium.

Peripheral nerves may be classified according to their diameter. Generally, the larger the diameter, the faster the conduction velocity; therefore A alpha fibers, the fibers with the largest diameters, have the fastest conduction velocity, and C fibers, which have the smallest diameter, have the slowest conduction velocity. Between the two extremes lie A beta, A gamma, A delta, and B fibers, in decreasing order of size and conduction velocity. The degree of myelination affects the conduction velocity of the nerves.

PERIPHERAL NERVOUS SYSTEM

The peripheral nervous system is divided into the somatic and autonomic nervous systems (Figure 29-6). The somatic system contains sensory neurons for the control of skin, muscles, and joints. Somatic motor fibers arise from motor neurons in the ventral horn, their axons exiting the spinal cord via the ventral root. A few centimeters after leaving the spinal cord, the somatic motor fibers join with incoming sensory fibers carrying information from afferent receptors (muscles, skin, tendons, and joints) to form a mixed nerve. As a mixed nerve approaches its site of innervation, the motor and sensory fibers separate.

Cranial nerves emerge from the cranium. Cranial nerves provide sensory and motor innervation for the head and neck. The sensory cranial nerves include the olfactory nerve (cranial nerve I), optic nerve (cranial nerve II), and vestibulocochlear nerve (cranial nerve VIII); the motor cranial nerves include the oculomotor, trochlear, abducens, spinal accessory, and hypoglossal nerves; and the four mixed cranial nerves with both sensory and motor function are the trigeminal nerve (cranial nerve V), facial nerve (cranial nerve VII), glossopharyngeal nerve (cranial nerve IX), and vagus nerve (cranial nerve X). Table 29-2 lists cranial and peripheral nerve fiber types, locations, and functions.

The autonomic nervous system controls involuntary visceral functions and is composed of three subdivisions: the sympathetic, parasympathetic, and enteric nervous systems. The sympathetic nervous system (SNS) and the parasympathetic nervous system (PNS) are functionally antagonistic.[5,8] The SNS and PNS originate within the CNS and require two efferent neurons—a preganglionic neuron originating within the CNS and a postganglionic neuron terminating within the effector organ (smooth muscle, cardiac muscle, or sweat gland). Autonomic fibers originating in the brain arise from cell bodies located in the brainstem. PNS fibers supplying the lower gastrointestinal tract and genitourinary systems arise from the sacral portion of the spinal cord.

Sympathetic Nervous System

Preganglionic neurons of the SNS originate in the intermediolateral gray horn of the spinal cord between the first thoracic (T1) and second or third lumbar vertebra (L2 or L3). The myelinated preganglionic axons (preganglionic fibers of the preganglionic neurons) exit the spinal cord via the anterior (ventral) nerve root. These processes leave the spinal cord by way of a small trunk, the white rami communicans. A series of paired paravertebral ganglia is ranged bilaterally along the spinal cord (Figure 29-7). All of the paired segmental paravertebral ganglia are connected, forming the sympathetic trunks. These ganglia may contain the cell body of the second efferent neuron (postganglionic neuron). The preganglionic fibers of the preganglionic neuron enter the white rami communicans and may synapse with the second efferent neuron located within the ganglion. The postganglionic fiber of the postganglionic neuron may either exit the gray ramus to enter a spinal nerve or may extend through a connection between the paravertebral ganglion and one of the three (celiac, superior, or inferior) mesenteric ganglia. The postganglionic fibers then synapse with the smooth muscle of the digestive tract and other abdominal organs. SNS preganglionic axons secrete acetylcholine at their ganglionic synapses, and postganglionic fibers secrete norepinephrine.

Usually one paravertebral ganglion is present for each spinal nerve, except in the cervical area, where they fuse to form two or three ganglia. On entering the sympathetic chain the preganglionic fiber may synapse at the entry level or travel up or down the ganglionic chain before forming a synapse. Some preganglionic axons pass through the sympathetic chain without synapsing and after leaving the chain form a distinct nerve (e.g., splanchnic nerve) before synapsing in prevertebral ganglia, such as the superior or inferior mesenteric ganglia. Some preganglionic axons in the sympathetic trunk synapse with several postganglionic neurons located in several chain ganglia. This arrangement explains the manner in which a central SNS discharge spreads over several segments. After synapsing in the sympathetic chain, the postganglionic axons, which are unmyelinated, enter the spinal nerve through the gray ramus communicans and travel to the periphery.

The cervical ganglia are divided into superior, medial, and inferior cervical ganglia. The inferior cervical ganglion fuses with the first thoracic ganglion to form the stellate ganglion. Stimulation of SNS fibers from the superior cervical ganglion

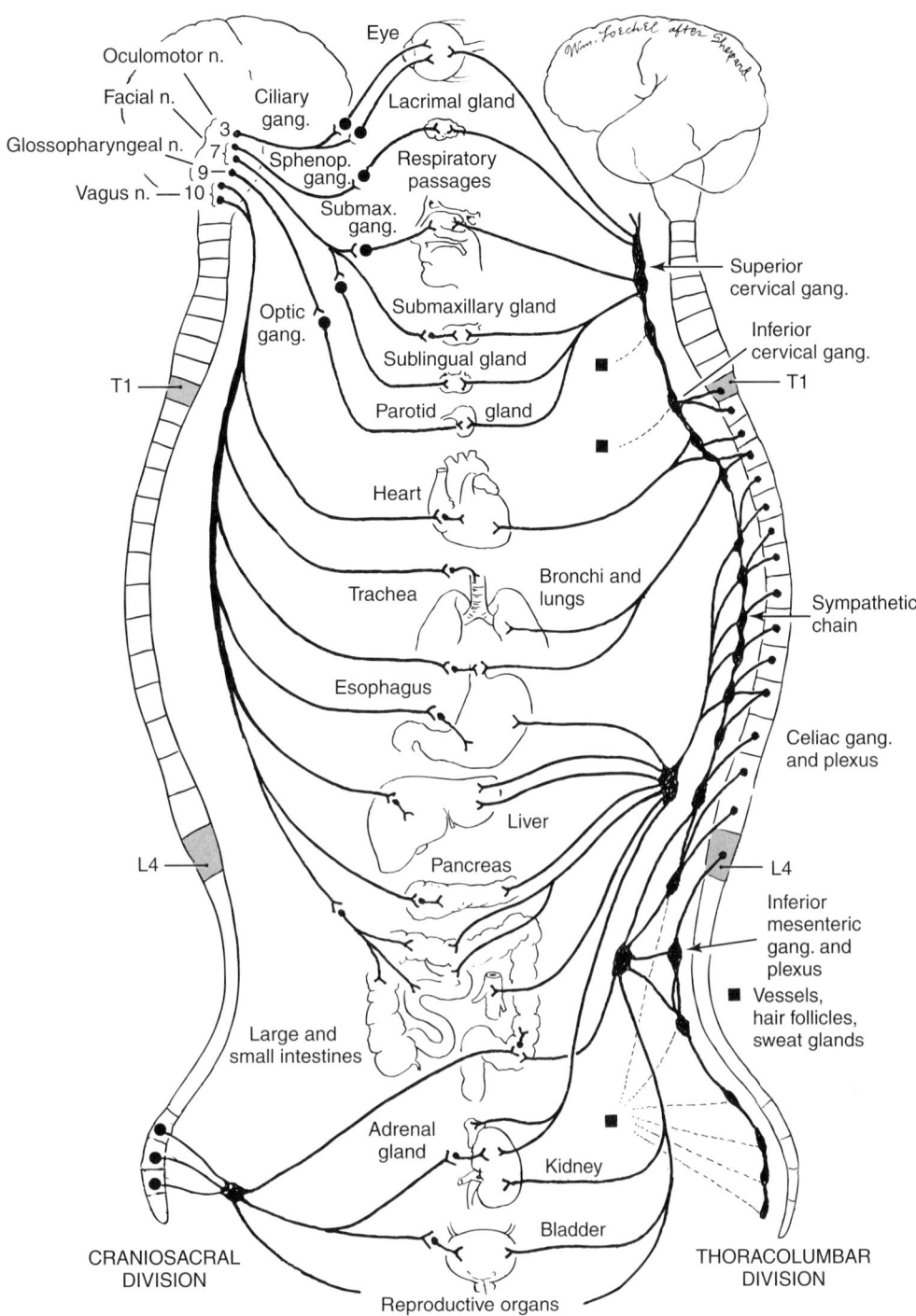

FIGURE **29-6** Both divisions of the autonomic nervous system. *gang.*, Ganglion; *n.*, nerve.

produces contraction of the radial muscle of the iris (mydriasis), relaxation of the ciliary muscle of the eye, and constriction of the blood vessels of the head (see Figure 29-6). Destruction of the superior cervical ganglion, central SNS damage, or injury to other cervical paravertebral ganglia produces Horner syndrome, clinically distinguished by miosis, anhydrosis (absence of sweating), and ptosis on the affected side. Ptosis is incomplete because the primary innervation to the levator palpebrae superioris muscle of the eyelid is through the oculomotor nerve, and only a few SNS fibers innervate this muscle.

Postganglionic fibers from the upper thoracic chain ganglia (stellate to T4 to T5) innervate the heart and lungs. β-Receptor stimulation produces an increased heart rate (positive chronotropic effect), an increase in conduction (positive dromotropic effect), and an increase in myocardial contractility (positive inotropic effect). Myocardial α-receptor stimulation produces coronary vasoconstriction. The resultant pulmonary effects also depend on the receptor type that is stimulated; bronchial dilation follows β$_2$-receptor stimulation, and mild bronchoconstriction follows α-receptor stimulation.

TABLE **29-2**	Cranial and Peripheral Nerves	
Fiber Type	**Location**	**Information Conveyed**
General somatic afferent	CN V, CN VII, CN IX, CN X, all spinal nerves	Pain, touch, temperature, pressure, and proprioception from muscles, tendons, and joint capsules
General visceral afferent	CN V, CN VII, CN IX, CN X, all spinal nerves	Conscious pain sensations
Special somatic afferent	CN II, CN VIII	Sight, hearing
Special visceral afferent	CN I, CN IX, CN X, CN VII (intermediate branch)	Olfaction, taste
Special visceral efferent	CN V, CN VII, CN IX, CN X, CN XI	Mastication, facial expressions
General somatic efferent	CN III, CN IV, CN VI, CN VII, all spinal nerves	Voluntary muscles (trunk and extremities), extrinsic muscles of eye, muscles of the tongue
General visceral efferent	CN III, CN VII, CN IX, CN X, spinal nerves T1 through L2 or L3, S2, S3, S4	Smooth muscle, cardiac muscle, some glands

CN, *Cranial nerve.*

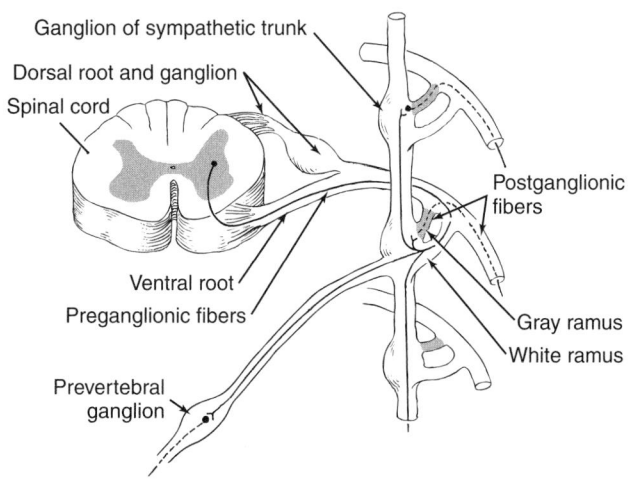

FIGURE **29-7**   Sympathetic ganglion.

The SNS fibers supplying abdominal and pelvic viscera (T5 through L3) pass through the chain ganglia forming the greater and lesser splanchnic nerves, which subsequently terminate in preterminal ganglia. Postganglionic fibers from the prevertebral ganglia, such as the superior and inferior mesenteric ganglia, travel to the abdominal and pelvic viscera. Stimulation of these SNS fibers activates liver glycogenolysis and gluconeogenesis, decreases secretions from pancreatic acinar cells and β-cells, initiates lipolysis, decreases the tone and motility of the gastrointestinal tract, contracts gastrointestinal sphincters, relaxes urinary smooth muscle, and increases renin secretion from the kidney.

Parasympathetic Nervous System

The efferent neurons of the parasympathetic subdivision are located in the gray matter of the midbrain and medulla. The preganglionic fibers exit the brain via cranial nerves II, VII, IX,

and X. The remainder of the cell bodies of the first efferent neurons arise from the lateral horn of the sacral portion of the spinal cord (S2 through S5). Acetylcholine is secreted by both parasympathetic preganglionic and postganglionic fibers (see Figure 29-6).

The second efferent neuron (postganglionic neuron) of the parasympathetic subdivision may be located in a small ganglion adjacent to the innervated organ or within the organ itself. Preganglionic axons travel with the vagus to ganglia located near the organ they innervate. The postganglionic axons innervate the bronchioles, heart, coronary arteries, stomach, and large intestine up to the left colic flexure. PNS postganglionic fibers to the descending colon and the genitourinary systems are supplied by parasympathetic fibers from sacral segments of the spinal cord. Most of the parasympathetic preganglionic fibers originate at the S3 and S4 segments. Shortly after exiting the spinal cord with the spinal nerves, the preganglionic fibers form the pelvic nerves (nervi erigentes), which synapse in ganglia in close proximity to the innervated organ.

VASCULATURE OF THE CENTRAL NERVOUS SYSTEM

The brain and spinal cord are dependent on an uninterrupted blood supply to deliver the essential fuels, oxygen, and glucose (Figure 29-8). The brain receives 15% of the cardiac output, or approximately 50 mL/100 g/min. The brain's blood supply originates from two arterial circulations that receive blood from two distinct systemic arteries: the anterior circulation receives blood from the carotid arteries, and the posterior circulation receives blood from the vertebral arteries. These arterial systems communicate through arterial anastomoses that form the circle of Willis. The paired anterior, middle, and posterior cerebral arteries originate from the circle of Willis. Although these arterial communications exist, under normal conditions, little mixing of blood flow occurs. Intraarterial contrast studies demonstrate that the carotid artery supplies the ipsilateral cerebral hemisphere, and the vertebrobasilar system supplies the structures of the posterior fossa.

The internal carotid arteries enter the skull through the foramen lacerum and bifurcate near the lateral border of the

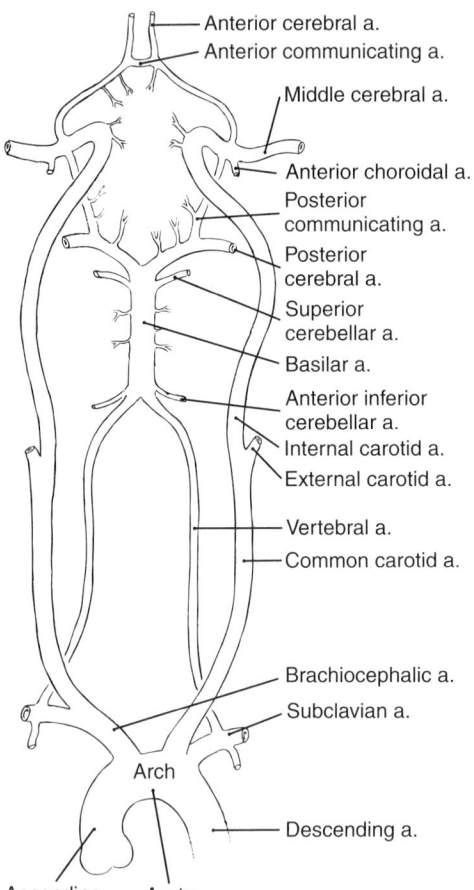

- Anterior cerebral a.
- Anterior communicating a.
- Middle cerebral a.
- Anterior choroidal a.
- Posterior communicating a.
- Posterior cerebral a.
- Superior cerebellar a.
- Basilar a.
- Anterior inferior cerebellar a.
- Internal carotid a.
- External carotid a.
- Vertebral a.
- Common carotid a.
- Brachiocephalic a.
- Subclavian a.
- Arch
- Descending a.
- Ascending   Aorta

FIGURE **29-8** Cerebral vasculature. *a.*, Artery.

optic chiasm, forming the anterior and middle cerebral arteries. The anterior cerebral arteries supply the medial surface of the cerebral hemispheres, and the middle cerebral arteries supply the lateral surface of the hemispheres. The striate arteries, which are branches of the middle cerebral arteries, supply the internal capsule and its motor tracts. Cerebrovascular accidents commonly involve the striate arteries. Communicating arteries provide connections between the two anterior cerebral arteries of each hemisphere (anterior communicating arteries) and between the middle and posterior cerebral arteries (posterior communicating arteries).

The vertebral arteries, branches of the subclavian artery, enter the cranium through the foramen magnum and join to form the basilar artery in the vicinity of the pons. Branches of the vertebral and basilar arteries supply a wide area, including the cervical region of the spinal cord, the brainstem, the cerebellum, the vestibular apparatus and cochlea of the inner ear, parts of the diencephalon, and the occipital and temporal lobes of the cerebral hemispheres.

Venous blood exits the brain via two separate systems. The blood from the cerebral and cerebellar cortex flows through veins on the surface and empties into overlying dural venous sinuses. Venous blood from the basal portions of the brain empties into the great vein of Galen and the straight sinus. These sinuses empty into the internal jugular veins. The superficial veins of the scalp are linked to the dural sinuses by the emissary veins.[4,5]

Like the brain, the spinal cord receives blood from two arterial sources: the anterior and posterior spinal arteries, which are branches of the vertebral artery, and the radicular arteries, which are branches of segmental vessels (cervical, intercostal, and lumbar). The spinal cord blood supply is not continuous along its length, and although each spinal cord segment is perfused, blood is delivered preferentially by one of the supply sources. The cervical cord is supplied by the vertebral and radicular arteries, and the thoracic and lumbar cord is supplied by the radicular arteries arising from this respective region (intercostal and lumbar). Of particular importance is the radicular artery, the artery of Adamkiewicz, which enters the cord at approximately T7 and supplies the lumbosacral segment. Spinal cord segments that receive blood from one source are particularly prone to ischemic injury if this blood supply is interrupted. Interruption of the blood flow from the artery of Adamkiewicz results in paraplegia.

ELECTROPHYSIOLOGY

The physiologic basis for the propagation of a nerve impulse lies in the structural nature of the axolemma, the differential concentration of electrolytes within the axolemma and extracellular space, and the semipermeability of the axolemma to these specific ions. The resting nerve cell has a potential difference, or voltage, created by the asymmetric distribution of sodium and potassium ions. Sodium ions are 10-fold richer in the extracellular medium, and potassium ions are 10-fold richer in the intracellular medium. The resting membrane potential is created through the excess positive charges on the extracellular surface and excess negative charges on the interior of the cell membrane. The nerve cell is said to be *polarized* in the resting state.

In the resting state, the cell membrane permeability to sodium ions is low, so little movement of extracellular sodium ions to the cell interior occurs. Although larger than sodium ions, potassium ions are freely permeable through the axolemma, and their movement creates a net deficit of positive ions within the interior of the axolemma. This ionic asymmetry is maintained by the sodium-potassium adenosine triphosphate (ATP) pump. The distribution of ions outside the cell produces a negative resting membrane potential of approximately −60 to −90 mV.

Nerve impulses are transmitted through action potentials that are generated with membrane alterations in permeability of the axolemma to sodium and potassium ions. Depolarization occurs when a stimulus of sufficient intensity (threshold potential) increases membrane permeability to sodium ions, facilitating the passage of a greater number of sodium ions into the cell interior than potassium ions to the cell exterior. The lowering of the voltage difference of the axolemma occurs as a result of "gating," or the opening or closing of integral membrane proteins. Gating occurs in response to voltage differences across the axolemma (voltage-gated channel) or after the binding of a specific molecule to a receptor or channel protein (chemically gated channel, e.g., the binding of acetylcholine to the neuromuscular junction). Sodium channels open when the threshold potential is reached, facilitating a rapid influx of sodium into the axolemma interior and producing depolarization (Figure 29-9). The initial flow of sodium ions results in the opening of additional sodium channels. The action potential develops as the cell interior undergoes a transition from negative to positive. At the peak of depolarization, the electrical potential is 30 to 40 mV higher than the cell exterior, and sodium channels close. The action potential develops as a result of the change from the resting potential of −60 to −90 mV to a peak of 30 to 50 mV at the

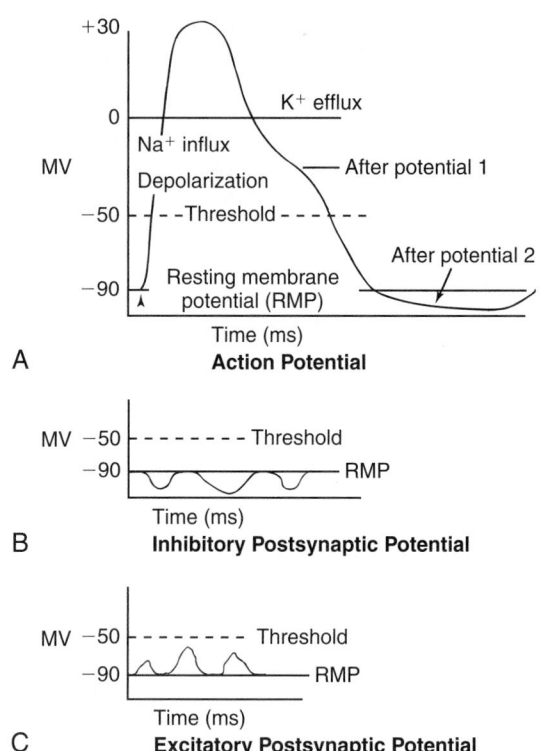

+30

0

MV

−50

−90

K⁺ efflux

Na⁺ influx

Depolarization

After potential 1

- -Threshold - - - - - -

Resting membrane
potential (RMP)

After potential 2

Time (ms)

A　**Action Potential**

MV −50 − − − − − − − Threshold

−90

RMP

Time (ms)

B　**Inhibitory Postsynaptic Potential**

MV −50 − − − − − − − Threshold

−90

RMP

Time (ms)

C　**Excitatory Postsynaptic Potential**

FIGURE **29-9**　**A,** Phases of the action potential (AP) and major ionic movements during the AP. **B** and **C,** Subthreshold changes in the resting membrane potential.

completion of depolarization. The action potential cannot occur without the delivery of a stimulus, or critical threshold potential. For myelinated mammalian nerves, the threshold potential is 20 to 30 mV less than the resting potential. This threshold potential can be modified by a variety of factors, including pH, partial pressure of oxygen (Po_2), and partial pressure of carbon dioxide (Pco_2). Alkalosis increases neuronal excitability, and hypoxemia and acidosis depress neuronal excitability.

After depolarization, cell repolarization is initiated with the closing of sodium channels and the opening of potassium channels, allowing the flow of potassium ions to the exterior of the axolemma to return the axon to the resting potential of −60 to −90 mV. The sodium pump is active in reestablishing this ionic asymmetry. During repolarization, the axon is refractory, or unable to respond to an additional stimulus, no matter how strong (it will not respond to an action potential). In the later phases of repolarization, the axolemma is in a state of ready refractoriness, that is, depolarization can be initiated only by a stimulus with an intensity greater than that which produced the original depolarization.

Chemical, mechanical, and electrical stimulation may elicit an action potential. Mechanical stimulation via pinching or crushing increases the membrane's permeability to sodium ions. The resulting change in ion permeability determines whether the postsynaptic neuron is either excited or inhibited.

Tissues whose sodium channels are not completely closed at rest (cardiac and smooth muscle) have a constant leak of sodium inside the cell, and excitation occurs by electrical stimulation to produce an action potential. Because these tissues repetitively discharge, they are described as having *rhythmicity*. The usual

resting membrane potential of cells displaying rhythmicity is −60 to −70 mV. After stimulation, a wave of depolarization is transmitted to the axon terminal. At electrical synapses, the wave of depolarization crosses the 2-nm synaptic space and spreads to the postsynaptic cell (neuron or muscle cell).

Synaptic Transmission

After depolarization, the flow of information is transmitted to adjacent neurons at specialized membrane sites called *synapses* (see Figure 29-1). Synapses are present on dendrites and axons. Synapses may be present on axon terminals of specific neurons in contact with endocrine glands (e.g., salivary glands) or skeletal muscle. The neuron sending the information is the presynaptic neuron, and the receiving neuron is the postsynaptic neuron. Separating the presynaptic and postsynaptic neurons is a small intracellular space (the synaptic cleft). The majority of synaptic transmission occurs in the direction from the presynaptic to the postsynaptic neuron, but retrograde nerve impulse conduction is known to occur and modulates the strength of synaptic connections.

Synaptic transmission may be electrically or chemically mediated. Electrically mediated synapses are large compared with chemically mediated synapses. Electrical synapses have direct cytoplasmic continuity and no synaptic delay. Electrical synapses are excitatory in nature and are located in the CNS, peripherally in smooth muscle, and in cardiac muscle. Synaptic delays (delayed synaptic transmission) occur in chemically mediated transmission because of the transit time of the chemical mediator (specific neurotransmitter) from the presynaptic terminal to the postsynaptic membrane.

The majority of CNS neurons have chemically mediated synapses. The presynaptic neuron releases a neurotransmitter, a low-molecular-weight compound that diffuses across the synaptic cleft and binds to specific receptors on the postsynaptic membrane. Depolarization stimulates the uptake of calcium by the nerve terminal, fusing intracellular vesicles that contain the neurotransmitter to the presynaptic membrane. The neurotransmitters are subsequently released into the synaptic cleft. The neurotransmitter diffuses across the synaptic cleft, interacting with a specific postsynaptic receptor. Neurotransmitters that increase the permeability of the axolemma to sodium ions are excitatory (e.g., acetylcholine, glutamate); neuroinhibitory neurotransmitters (e.g., γ-aminobutyric acid [GABA], glycine) hyperpolarize the membrane by increasing the permeability to chloride ions. The neurotransmitter serotonin excites some neurons and inhibits others. The attachment of the neurotransmitter to the postsynaptic receptor can produce either an immediate (fraction of millisecond) or a delayed (from a few milliseconds up to seconds) effect on the postsynaptic membrane. The delayed transmission involves second messengers, such as cyclic adenosine monophosphate and cyclic guanosine monophosphate, which are activated when the neurotransmitter attaches to the postsynaptic membrane.

NEUROTRANSMITTERS

Neurotransmitters are molecules contained within the presynaptic neuron that are discharged in a calcium-dependent manner after presynaptic depolarization and interact with specific receptors on the postsynaptic membrane. More than 100 molecules meet these criteria. Acetylcholine is an excitatory neurotransmitter that interacts with both nicotinic and muscarinic receptors. Additional neurotransmitters include biogenic amines (epinephrine, norepinephrine, dopamine, serotonin,

TABLE **29-3**	Common Neurotransmitters
Class	**Neurotransmitter**
Monoamines	Epinephrine
	Norepinephrine
	Dopamine
	5-Hydroxytryptamine (serotonin)
Amino acids	γ-Aminobutyric acid
	Glycine
	Glutamate
Peptides	Hypothalamic-releasing hormones (thyrotropin-releasing hormone, somatostatin)
	Posterior pituitary hormones (vasopressin, oxytocin)
	Substance P
	Opioids (β-endorphin, enkephalins, dynorphin)
	Insulin
	Glucagon
	Neurokinin A
	Endomorphin
	Orexin
Other	Acetylcholine
	Nitric oxide

histamine), amino acids (aspartate, glycine, GABA, glutamate), neuropeptides (substance P, the opioids, several hormones), and the second messenger nitric oxide (Table 29-3).

The synthesis of neurotransmitters occurs within the presynaptic neuron terminal. The neuron regulates the synthesis, packaging, release, and degradation of the synthesized neurotransmitter. The enzymes essential for neuron transmitter synthesis are obtained by axonal transport and taken into the nerve terminal by transport proteins. The synthesized neurotransmitter is then packaged into synaptic vesicles by membrane transport proteins.

Acetylcholine

Acetylcholine is an excitatory neurotransmitter with a widespread distribution. It is the predominant neurotransmitter within the CNS, at the neuromuscular junction, within all autonomic nervous system preganglionic fibers and postganglionic parasympathetic fibers, and within postganglionic sympathetic fibers innervating sweat glands. Acetylcholine is synthesized in the presynaptic nerve terminal from acetic acid, coenzyme A, and choline in the presence of the enzymes acetyl kinase and choline acetylase. This enzyme is also referred to as *choline acetyl transferase*. Acetylcholine is packaged in vesicles and stored in the presynaptic terminal. Calcium uptake into the presynaptic terminal is required for acetylcholine release, and magnesium (Mg^{2+}) and manganese (Mn^{2+}) block the uptake of Ca^{2+} and the subsequent release of acetylcholine. Acetylcholine interacts with the postsynaptic receptor for a few milliseconds before being hydrolyzed by acetylcholinesterase to acetic acid and choline. Both the acetic acid and the choline are taken up by the presynaptic nerve terminal and recycled.

Cholinergic receptors are classified as either nicotinic or muscarinic. Nicotinic receptors are found in autonomic ganglia and at the neuromuscular junction. Muscarinic receptors are found on smooth muscle, cardiac muscle, and sweat glands. Acetylcholine is the neurotransmitter at cranial nerve nuclei and ventral horn motor neurons of the spinal cord, including various collateral nerves to Renshaw cells (interneurons). Acetylcholine may be interactive in neuronal circuits involved with pain reception. Acetylcholine may also act as a sensory transmitter in thermal receptors and taste bud endings.

Biogenic Amines

The biogenic amines include epinephrine, norepinephrine, dopamine, serotonin, and histamine. The catecholamines epinephrine, norepinephrine, and dopamine are synthesized in a series of hydroxylation, decarboxylation, and methylation reactions from the amino acids phenylalanine and tyrosine. The adrenal medulla secretes both epinephrine (75%) and norepinephrine (25%). Postganglionic adrenergic neurons secrete norepinephrine; norepinephrine and dopamine are probably neurotransmitters within the CNS. Amacrine cells of the retina and some neurons of the intrinsic nervous system of the intestine secrete dopamine. As with acetylcholine, the release of norepinephrine, epinephrine, and dopamine is calcium dependent. One notable difference from acetylcholine is that norepinephrine and dopamine act by means of second messengers (slow synaptic transmission), whereas most of the actions of acetylcholine are directly on ion channels (fast synaptic transmission). The duration of effect of catecholamines is regulated by presynaptic reuptake. Enzymatic breakdown of catecholamines by monoamine oxidase and catechol-o-methyltransferase within the liver is primarily responsible for terminating their effects.

Dopamine is an inhibitory neurotransmitter and the predominant biogenic amine within the CNS. Dopamine is concentrated within the basal ganglia. Dopamine's inhibitory effects occur through action on adenylate cyclase, which is dopamine sensitive.

Norepinephrine is concentrated in the reticular activating system and the hypothalamus. Norepinephrine acts as an inhibitory neurotransmitter, inhibiting impulses to the cerebral cortex.

Serotonin is an inhibitory neurotransmitter that influences behavior and mood. Histamine is also an inhibitory neurotransmitter concentrated within the hypothalamus and the reticular activating system. Histamine requires the second messenger cyclic adenosine monophosphate to mediate its inhibitory effects.

Amino Acids

Glutamate is the primary excitatory transmitter found within the cerebral cortex, the hippocampus, and the substantia gelatinosa of the spinal cord.[9] Glutamate plays a formidable role in learning and memory (perhaps interactive in memory formation during awareness during anesthesia) and the appreciation of pain. Glutamate has also been implicated in excitotoxic neuronal injury after ischemic or traumatic brain injury.

Glutamate is formed from the deamination of glutamine supplied by the Krebs cycle. Glutamate may activate either an inotropic or a metabotropic amino acid receptor. N-methyl-D-aspartate (NMDA) receptors are ligand-gated inotropic receptors that produce a conformational change in the receptor, opening a sodium channel, which results in the depolarization of the postsynaptic membrane. The metabotropic receptor is an integral transmembrane receptor that regulates intracellular second messenger systems.

GABA is the major inhibitory neurotransmitter found in the CNS. It is concentrated in the basal ganglia, cerebral cortex, cerebellum, and spinal cord. Activation of the GABA receptor opens neuronal membrane chloride channels, producing hyperpolarization (the hyperpolarized neuron is resistant to excitation). GABA is important in antagonizing the excitatory effects of amino acid neurotransmitters.

Glycine is the primary inhibitory neurotransmitter in the spinal cord. In the past, glycine irrigation was employed during transurethral resection of the prostate. Postoperative visual impairment after the intravascular absorption of glycine suggests that glycine may act as an inhibitory neurotransmitter within the retina.

Neuropeptides

Neuropeptides are either excitatory or inhibitory. Common neuropeptides include the opioids, substance P, and many pituitary and pancreatic islet hormones.

Substance P is an excitatory neurotransmitter found in the striatum and substantia nigra of the basal ganglia, hypothalamus, brainstem (raphe nuclei), and dorsal root ganglia of the spinal cord. Substance P is released by pain-fiber terminals that synapse with the substantia gelatinosa of the spinal cord.

The opioid neuropeptides include β-endorphin, enkephalins, dynorphins and endomorphins. They act at opiate receptors distributed throughout the brain and spinal cord. Three classes of opiate receptors have been identified—delta, kappa, and mu. Dynorphin is a potent agonist at kappa receptors, and the enkephalins are agonists at delta and mu receptors. Opiate alkaloids like morphine interact with mu receptors. Morphine-like agents block slow pain pathways, raise the pain threshold, and modify the response to pain. Other effects, such as miosis and respiratory depression, result from the actions of these agents on opiate receptors located in the parts of the brain that control these functions.[2,7,10]

SENSORY PATHWAYS

Sensory or afferent pathways transmit pain, temperature, pressure, touch, vibratory sense, and proprioceptive information to the CNS. Sensory pathways also include the special senses of vision, taste, hearing, smell, and equilibrium.

Receptors for pain and temperature are located in the epidermis and the dermis; those for pressure, touch, vibratory sense, and proprioception are located in the dermis. Receptors can be classified as (1) exteroceptors, which are located near the surface of skin and oral mucosa, and (2) proprioceptors, which are located in deeper skin layers, joint capsules, ligaments, tendons, muscles, and periosteum. Several types of receptors exist. Pacinian corpuscles are receptors for vibration and pressure. Free nerve endings, Ruffini corpuscles, muscle spindles, and Golgi tendon organs are involved in movement sense. The receptors for light (or crude) touch sensations include Merkel disks, Meissner corpuscles, and the nerve plexuses surrounding some hair roots. Fibers travel from these receptors to a ganglion, where they synapse with first-order neurons, the fibers of which continue to the CNS. Fibers from receptors in the trunk and extremities travel to the dorsal root ganglion, where they synapse with first-order neurons. Most of the sensory fibers from the head, excluding those from the special sense organs (hearing, equilibrium, vision, taste, and smell), synapse in first-order neurons located in the semilunar or trigeminal ganglion.[7,8]

Pain and Temperature Pathways

Pain and temperature fibers from the head synapse in the trigeminal ganglion and enter the pons, forming the trigeminal nerve (cranial nerve V) (Figure 29-10). These fibers subsequently synapse with second-order neurons in the nucleus of the descending

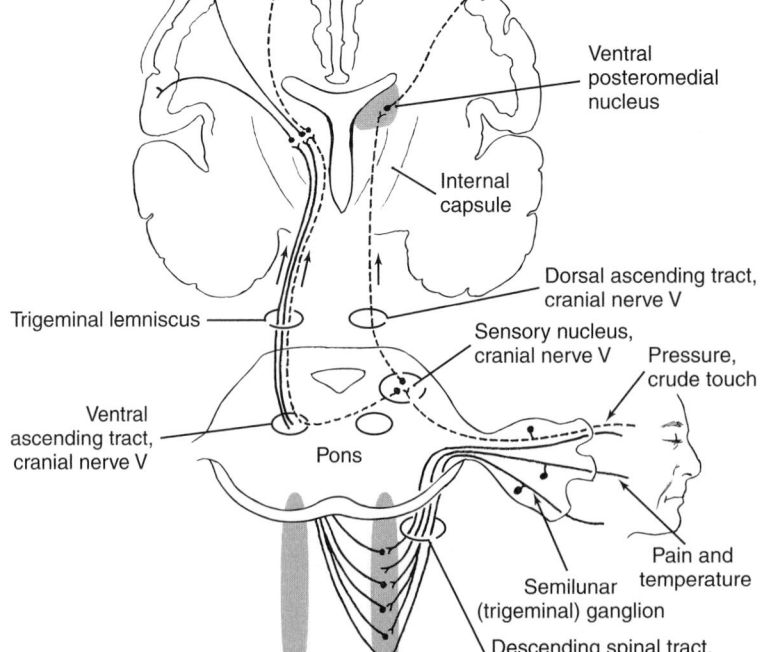

FIGURE **29-10** Sensory pathways from the head and neck. (*Modified from Liebman M. Neuroanatomy Made Easy and Understandable. Gaithersburg, MD: Aspen; 1991:19. Copyright 1991, Michael Liebman.*)

tract of cranial nerve V. The second-order axons cross to the ventrolateral side and ascend as the ventral trigeminal tract to the ventral posteromedial nucleus of the thalamus, where they synapse with third-order neurons. From the ventral posteromedial thalamic nucleus, third-order axons ascend in the internal capsule and end in the postcentral gyrus of the cerebral cortex, which is the primary somatic sensory area of the brain. Pain and temperature receptors in the skin of the trunk and extremities send fibers to the dorsal root ganglion, where they synapse with first-order neurons (Figure 29-11). The first-order axons enter the dorsal horn gray matter of the spinal cord and synapse with second-order neurons. Axons from the second-order neurons decussate (cross) in the ventral white commissure and enter the lateral white columns before ascending as the lateral spinothalamic tract to the ventral posterolateral thalamic nucleus, where they synapse with third-order neurons. Axons from the third-order neurons travel in the posterior limb of the internal capsule and ultimately synapse in the postcentral gyrus, where sensations of pain, temperature, touch, and pressure are interpreted, and responses to the sensations are initiated.

Some pain and temperature fibers in the dorsal horn give off branches that synapse with internuncial (messenger) neurons. The internuncial neurons have axons that synapse with motor neurons in the ventral horn, which are not necessarily at the same level of the spinal cord. The axons can cross over and travel up or down the spinal cord before synapsing. These circuits are part of the reflex response to pain, which results in a rapid, automatic response to nociceptive stimuli.

The afferent fibers from each dorsal root ganglion come from a relatively limited area of the skin termed a *cutaneous dermatome.* Some overlap exists, so if a spinal nerve that supplies a certain dermatome is severed, pain and temperature sensations from that dermatome are supplied by adjacent dermatome fibers. For example, if T6 is severed, T5 and T7 sensory neurons carry pain and temperature sensations from the skin area supplied by T6. Axons entering the dorsal horn from the dorsal root ganglion send branches to one spinal segment above and one segment below in the dorsolateral column of Lissauer.[2,6,8,11]

Pressure and Crude Touch

Pressure and crude (light) touch fibers from the head synapse with first-order neurons in the trigeminal ganglion. From the trigeminal ganglion, first-order axons travel to the pons, where they synapse with second-order neurons in the sensory nucleus of cranial nerve V (see Figure 29-11). From the sensory nucleus of cranial nerve V, second-order axons form the dorsal trigeminal tract, which has both crossed and uncrossed fibers. The second-order fibers terminate in the ventral posteromedial nucleus of the thalamus. Third-order axons from the ventral posteromedial nucleus subsequently terminate in the postcentral gyrus of the cerebral cortex.

After leaving the dorsal root ganglion, crude touch and pressure fibers from the extremities and trunk enter the dorsal white column on the ipsilateral side and bifurcate (Figure 29-12). One branch immediately enters the dorsal gray horn and synapses with second-order neurons. The other branch ascends for up to 10 spinal segments before synapsing with the second-order neurons in the dorsal horn. Second-order axons from both branches cross over and enter the ventral white column, forming the ventral spinothalamic tract, which ascends to the thalamus and synapses with third-order neurons in the ventral posterolateral nucleus. Tertiary axons travel through the internal capsule to the postcentral gyrus.

Owing to the branching arrangement of the first-order fibers from the trunk and extremities, injuries to the spinal cord rarely result in the total loss of these two sensations. Each cerebral cortex receives both crossed and uncrossed pressure and light-touch fibers from the face; as a result, damage to the postcentral gyrus on one side does not result in loss of pressure and crude touch sensations to the face, even though these sensations are lost on the trunk and extremities of the contralateral side.[2,7,8,11]

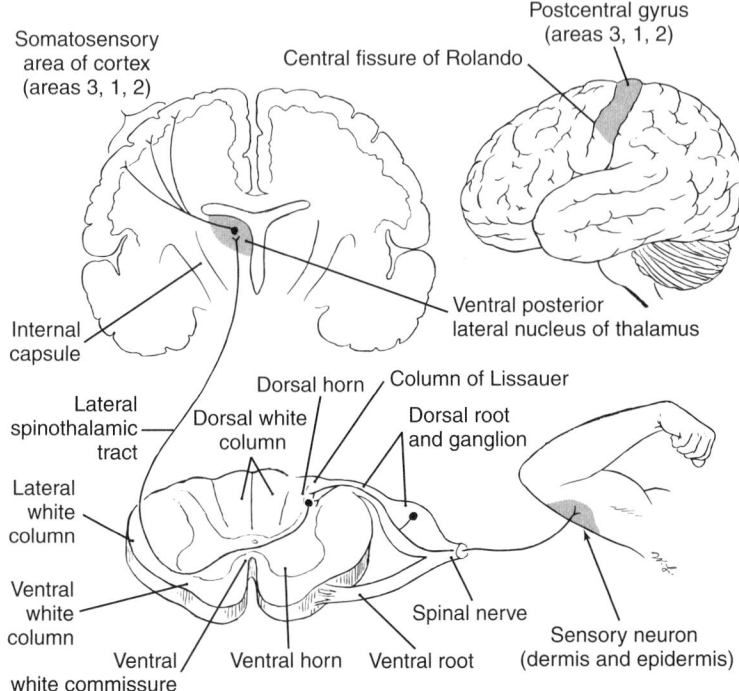

FIGURE **29-11** Pain and temperature pathways from the trunk and extremities. (*Modified from Liebman M. Neuroanatomy Made Easy and Understandable. Gaithersburg, MD: Aspen; 1991:11. Copyright 1991, Michael Liebman.*)

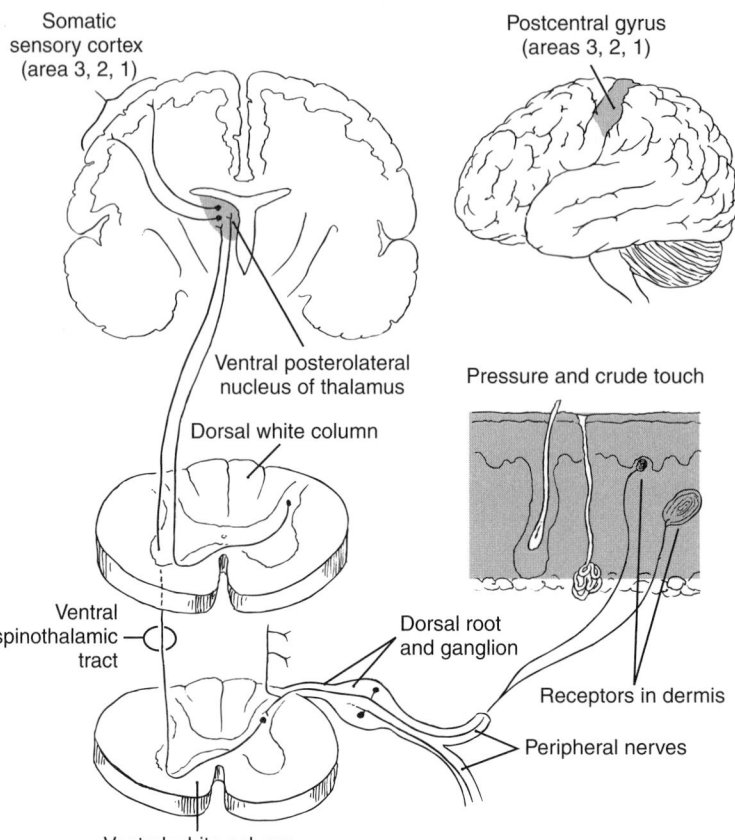

FIGURE **29-12** Crude touch and pressure sensations from the extremities and trunk. (*Modified from Liebman M. Neuroanatomy Made Easy and Understandable. Gaithersburg, MD: Aspen; 1991:14. Copyright 1991, Michael Liebman.*)

Vibratory Sense, Proprioception, and Discriminatory Touch

Proprioceptive fibers from muscles of the face involved in facial expression and mastication synapse in cell bodies located in the mesencephalic nucleus of the midbrain. Little is known about the rest of the pathway.

Fibers from the trunk and extremities carrying proprioceptive, vibratory, and discriminatory (fine) touch sensations synapse with neuron cell bodies in the dorsal root ganglion. From the dorsal root ganglion, first-order axons enter the dorsal white column and ascend to the medulla (Figure 29-13). The fibers are somatotopically organized in the white columns. Axons from the lumbar and sacral parts of the spinal cord travel medially in the fasciculus gracilis, and fibers from the cervical and thoracic areas of the cord are located laterally in the fasciculus cuneatus of the dorsal white column of the spinal cord. Each fasciculus terminates in its respective medullary nucleus; for example, the fasciculus gracilis terminates in the nucleus gracilis. Second-order axons decussate after leaving their medullary nucleus and form a bundle termed the *medial lemniscus*, which terminates in the ventral posterolateral thalamic nucleus. Third-order fibers from the ventral posterolateral nucleus terminate in the postcentral gyrus.[2,7,8,11]

Pupillary light and accommodation reflexes are mediated through the Edinger-Westphal nucleus and cranial nerve III. Pupillary dilation is produced by postganglionic sympathetic fibers from the superior cervical ganglion that travel with branches of the internal carotid artery to the radial muscle of the iris.[2,7,8,11]

MOTOR PATHWAYS

Motor, or efferent, pathways transmit information from the brain to the voluntary muscles of the body, to smooth and cardiac muscles, and to some glands. The corticospinal tracts supply the voluntary muscles of the trunk and extremities; nine cranial nerves supply the voluntary muscles of the head and neck. Autonomic preganglionic fibers arise in the brain and spinal cord and transmit efferent signals to smooth muscle, cardiac muscle, and some glands (lacrimal, bronchial).

Corticospinal Tract

The corticospinal tract originates in large, upper motor neurons located in the precentral gyrus of the frontal lobe (Figure 29-14). These neurons are arranged in a specific manner. Neurons supplying voluntary muscles of the head are found in the precentral gyrus near the lateral fissure of Sylvius, and those innervating the legs and feet are found in an area of the gyrus near the median longitudinal fissure. All parts of the body are represented in the gyrus. However, areas that perform complex movements (such as the hands when writing, typing, or playing the piano) have a larger area in the gyrus than other parts of the body not involved in intricate movements. Many of the upper motor neurons are pyramid shaped.

Axons travel from the pyramidal cells through the internal capsule, the major pathway for ascending and descending fibers between the cortex and other sites in the CNS. The internal capsule has three parts: the anterior limb, the posterior limb, and the genu, which lies between the anterior and posterior limbs. Fibers in the internal capsule are highly organized.

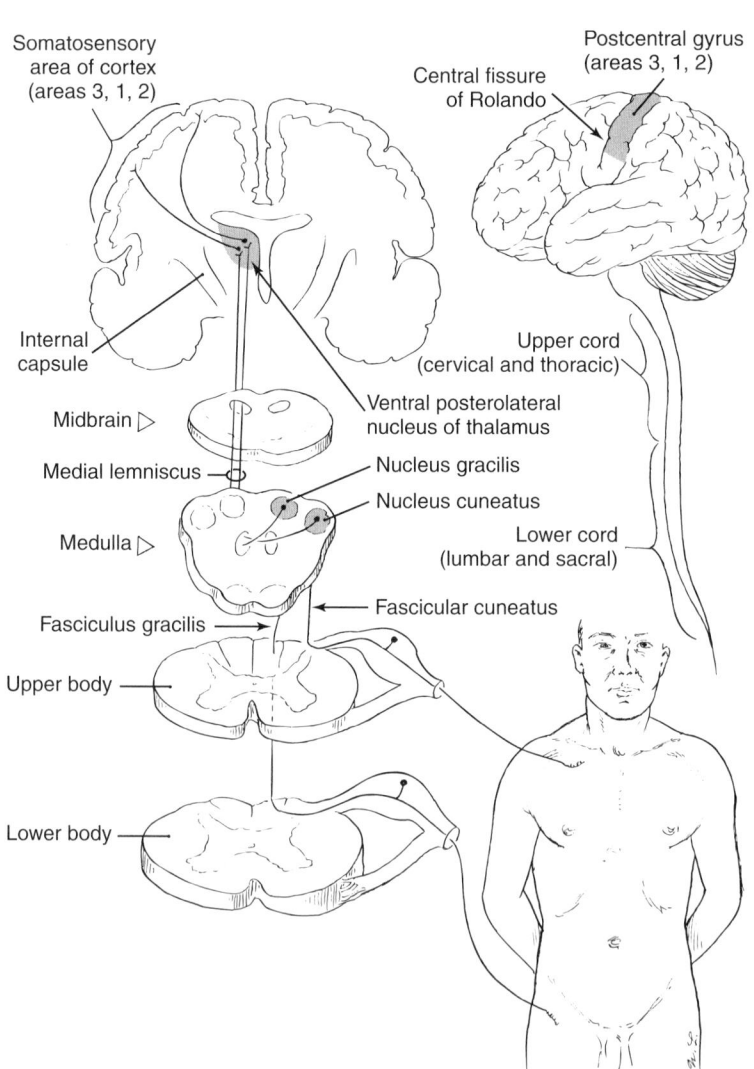

FIGURE **29-13** Proprioceptive, fine touch, and vibratory sensations from the extremities and trunk. (*Modified from Liebman M. Neuroanatomy Made Easy and Understandable. Gaithersburg, MD: Aspen; 1991:16. Copyright 1991, Michael Liebman.*)

Motor fibers to all parts of the body except the face are located in the anterior limb and part of the posterior limb. Fibers supplying the face are located in the genu. From the internal capsule, the axons travel through the midbrain (basis pedunculi) to the medulla, where approximately 90% of the fibers decussate, forming the pyramids of the medulla. The corticospinal tract is frequently called the *pyramidal tract,* either because of the shape of the upper motor neurons or because of the site at which the fibers decussate in the medulla. The fibers that cross over form the lateral corticospinal tract. Axons from the lateral corticospinal tract continue their descent to the spinal cord. At each level of the cord, some fibers leave the lateral corticospinal tract and enter the ventral horn gray matter, where they synapse with lower motor neurons. The fibers that do not decussate (approximately 10%) in the medulla continue to the spinal cord as the ventral corticospinal tract. The ventral corticospinal tracts cross over before synapsing with lower motor neurons in the gray matter. Axons from the lower motor neurons travel in the spinal nerves to innervate voluntary muscle.

A few corticospinal tract neurons are located anterior to the precentral gyrus. Axons from these neurons have an inhibitory effect on the lower motor neurons because they prevent them from discharging excessively. Damage to these suppressor fibers can stimulate the lower motor neurons either to overfire,

resulting in hyperreflexia, or to discharge simultaneously, causing spasticity. Damage to the corticospinal tract anywhere along its route to the spinal cord can cause upper motor neuron paralysis. If the injury occurs above the decussation in the medulla, the paralysis is on the opposite side of the body. Paralysis occurs on the same side of the body if the damage occurs below the medulla. With upper motor neuron paralysis, reflexes are intact, but suppressor-fiber activity is impeded. As a result, hyperreflexia is present, and the upper motor neuron paralysis is spastic. Damage to lower motor neuron cell bodies in the ventral horn or ventral root fibers produces lower motor neuron paralysis, a flaccid type of paralysis. Cerebral palsy and amyotrophic lateral sclerosis are diseases that affect the corticospinal tracts.

Motor Innervation to the Head

Upper motor neurons whose axons supply the voluntary muscles of the head are found in the precentral gyrus next to the lateral fissure of Sylvius. The cell bodies, whose axons supply the extrinsic muscles of the eye, are located in the middle frontal gyrus. Axons from both areas form the corticobulbar tracts, which travel through the genu of the internal capsule to the brainstem, where they synapse with neurons located in nuclei spread throughout the brainstem. Axons from these neurons form many of the cranial nerves.

Axons originating from neurons located in the midbrain form the oculomotor and trochlear nerves (Figure 29-15). The oculomotor nerve innervates most of the external muscles of the eye (inferior oblique and the inferior, medial, and superior rectus muscles), along with the levator palpebrae superioris muscle, which raises the upper eyelid. The trochlear nerve innervates the external oblique muscle of the eye. Three other groups of nuclei have neurons whose axons form the trigeminal, abducens, and facial nerves. The trigeminal nerve innervates part of the soft palate and all of the muscles of mastication. The abducens innervates the lateral rectus muscle of the eye, and the facial nerves supply all the muscles involved in facial expression.

Axons from neurons located in medullary nuclei form the glossopharyngeal, vagal, accessory, and hypoglossal nerves. Both the glossopharyngeal and vagal nerves arise from the ambiguous nucleus. The glossopharyngeal nerve supplies the stylopharyngeal muscle of the pharynx, and the vagal nerve innervates the muscles of the throat involved in swallowing and phonation. All of the tongue muscles are supplied by the hypoglossal nerve. The accessory nerve innervates the trapezius and sternocleidomastoid muscles of the neck. With the exception of the facial and hypoglossal nerves, the remaining nerves receive information from both the right and the left corticobulbar tracts. The nuclei of facial nerve fibers to the upper part of the face receive axons from the left and right corticobulbar tracts; the facial nerve nuclei whose fibers supply the lower part of the face receive fibers only from the contralateral corticobulbar tract. The nuclei from the origin of the hypoglossal nerves receive innervation from only the contralateral corticobulbar tract.[2,7,8,11]

Subcortical Motor Areas

Several motor areas in the brain are outside the cerebral cortex. For the most part, these are relatively primitive motor areas that have a modulating influence on motor function. Included in the subcortical motor areas are the basal ganglia, the nucleus of Luys, the red nucleus (nucleus ruber), the substantia nigra, and the reticular formation.

The basal ganglia lie deep within the cerebral hemispheres at the level of the internal capsule. They are composed of three nuclei: the globus pallidus, the putamen, and the caudate, which are collectively termed the *corpus striata*. The globus pallidus and the putamen are sometimes termed the *lentiform nucleus*. The globus pallidus makes up the paleostriatum, and the other two nuclei are part of the neostriatum.

The globus pallidus receives input from the motor cortex and from the other basal ganglia; it sends fibers to the subcortical motor areas. The globus pallidus is connected to the thalamus by two tracts, the ansa lenticularis and the lenticular fasciculus, which merge as they enter the thalamus to form the thalamic fasciculus. The thalamus forms a feedback process by sending fibers to the caudate nucleus and motor cortex. In this way, the motor activity of the basal ganglia can be influenced by the motor cortex without the presence of direct connections between the two structures. Dopamine, an important neurotransmitter in the basal ganglia, is produced in the substantia nigra of the midbrain and then travels by axonal transport to the caudate nucleus and the putamen.

The subthalamic nucleus of Luys is located in the diencephalon and is connected to other subcortical motor areas. Lesions in this nucleus result in a suppression of motor activity.

Three motor areas are located in the midbrain: the red nucleus, the substantia nigra, and the reticular formation. The red nucleus is located at the level of the corpora quadrigemina and gives rise to the crossed rubrospinal tract. When stimulated, this tract excites alpha and gamma flexor motor neurons and inhibits extensor motor neurons. The reticular formation consists of a diffuse collection of neurons found throughout the brainstem and into the diencephalon. Two major tracts arise from the reticular formation. One tract is the uncrossed medial reticulospinal tract, which excites alpha and gamma extensor motor neurons and inhibits flexor motor neurons when stimulated. The second tract is the lateral reticulospinal tract, which contains crossed

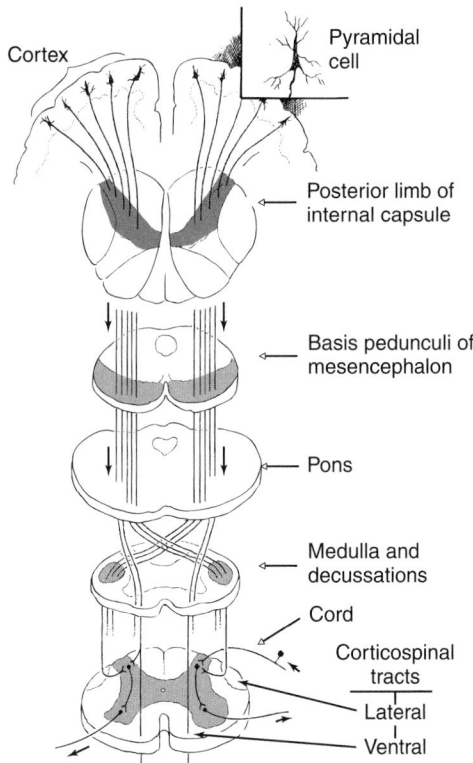

FIGURE **29-14**   Corticospinal tracts. (*Modified from Guyton AC.* Basic Neuroscience: Anatomy and Physiology. *Philadelphia: Saunders; 1991:212.*)

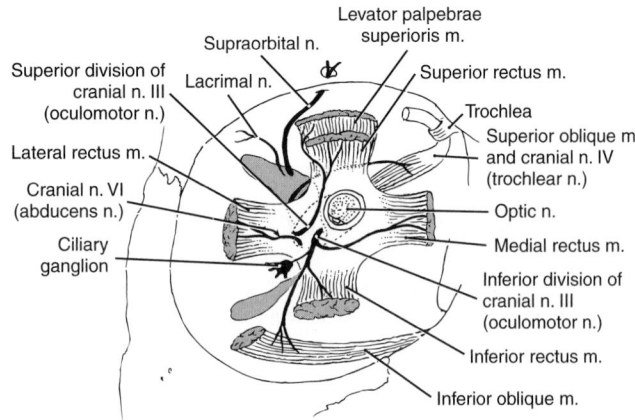

FIGURE **29-15**   Frontal view of the posterior orbit with its motor nerves and the extraocular muscles. *n.,* Nerve; *m.,* muscle.

and uncrossed fibers and activates alpha and gamma flexor motor neurons and inhibits extensor motor neurons when stimulated.

Lesions in the subcortical motor areas produce diseases characterized by disturbed muscle tone and dyskinesia (abnormal involuntary movements). In Parkinson disease, the globus pallidus and substantia nigra are affected. Huntington chorea involves atrophy of the caudate nucleus and putamen, as well as degeneration of cortical neurons. Other diseases that involve subcortical motor nuclei include athetosis, dystonia, ballismus, and Sydenham chorea.

NEUROANESTHESIA

Neuroanesthesia must take into account the unique set of circumstances each individual case represents. Comorbidities, pathology to be addressed, positioning, side of surgery, surgical approach, and procedure to be applied are all factors that must be clearly understood and fully addressed to administer a successful neuroanesthetic. Compounding the complexity is the constantly changing landscape of neurosurgical procedures, both cranial and spine. Providing competent neuroanesthesia in this environment demands thorough preparation and a degree of communication between surgeon and anesthesia not seen in other anesthesia environments.

This chapter will not assign specific anesthetics to specific procedures. That determination can only be made by thoughtful placement of each patient within the matrix of considerations discussed above. What follows will give a broad overview of the effects of anesthetic agents on cerebral blood flow (CBF), cerebral metabolic rate for oxygen (CMRO$_2$), and intracranial pressure (ICP). The remainder of this chapter provides a general discussion of the preoperative, intraoperative, and immediate postoperative care associated with common intracranial surgical procedures.

Effects of Anesthetic Agents on Cerebral Physiology

CBF, cerebral blood volume (CBV), ICP, CMRO$_2$ and cerebral compliance all must be considered in concert with pharmacologic principles in the design of a neurosurgical anesthetic regimen (Table 29-4).

Inhalation Agents

All anesthetic agents influence ICP by decreasing cerebrovascular resistance through cerebrovascular dilation and by dose-dependent impairment of autoregulation, producing increases in ICP and CBV and a decrease in CMRO$_2$. The changes in ICP are generally greater in patients who have an underlying increase in ICP.[12,13] The potent inhalational agents decrease mean arterial pressure (MAP) and increase ICP, reducing cerebral perfusion pressure (CPP).[14-16] Halothane produces the greatest increases in CBF and ICP, followed by isoflurane, sevoflurane, and desflurane. Additional increases in ICP after halothane administration in patients with increased ICP may be attenuated with hyperventilation for at least 10 minutes before halothane administration; however, this may not be successful if ICP is markedly increased.[12,17-19]

CBF in humans is unaltered with isoflurane-inspired concentrations of 0.6 to 1.1 minimum alveolar concentration (MAC); however, 1.6 MAC isoflurane doubles CBF. Animal studies have shown that isoflurane may enhance the carbon dioxide (CO$_2$) reactivity of the cerebral vessels. Cerebral autoregulation is impaired with concentrations exceeding 1 MAC.[20,21] CMRO$_2$ is depressed to a greater extent with isoflurane than with halothane, and progressive metabolic depression occurs with concentrations of isoflurane greater than 1 MAC until the electroencephalograph (EEG) becomes isoelectric at approximately 2.5 MAC.[22,23] These properties suggest that clinically relevant doses may provide a neuroprotective effect against

TABLE 29-4	Effects of Anesthetics on Cerebral Dynamics			
Drug	**Cerebral Blood Flow**	**CMRO$_2$**	**Intracranial Pressure**	**Cerebral Perfusion Pressure**
Inhalation				
Nitrous oxide	↑	↑↓	0	↓
Halothane	↑↑	↓	↑	↓
Sevoflurane	↑	↓	↑	↓
Isoflurane	↑	↓	↑	↓
Desflurane	↑	↓	↑	↓
Intravenous				
Barbiturates	↓↓	↓↓	↓↓	0/↓
Etomidate	↓↓	↓↓	↓	0
Propofol	↓	↓	↓	↓
Ketamine	↑	↑	↑↑	↓
Benzodiazepines	↓	↓	↓	0/↓
Morphine	0/↓	0/↓	↓	↑↓
Fentanyl	0/↓	0/↓	↓	0/↓
Alfentanil	0/↓	0/↓	↓	↓
Sufentanil	0/↓	0/↓	↓	↓
Remifentanil	0/↓	0/↓	↓	↓

From Aker J. Neuroanesthesia. In: Zaglaniczny K, Aker J, eds. Clinical Guide to Pediatric Anesthesia. Philadelphia: Saunders; 1999:176.
CMRO$_2$, Cerebral metabolic rate of oxygen.

ischemic insults, as demonstrated in human studies of critical regional CBF during carotid clamping.[24] Although strong experimental data support a neuroprotective potential of several anesthetic agents, specifically isoflurane and xenon, consistent long-term protection by either agent has not been demonstrated. Unfortunately, there is a lack of clinical studies to support the use of any one anesthetic agent over the others. Mechanisms of neuroprotection by anesthetic agents appear to involve suppression of excitatory neurotransmission and potentiation of inhibitory activity, which may contribute to the reduction of excitotoxic injury. Activation of intracellular signaling cascades that lead to altered expression of protective genes may also be involved.[25] The high concentrations of isoflurane necessary for abolishing cortical activity have no toxic effect on cerebral metabolic pathways; in contrast, high concentrations of halothane induce cerebral acidosis.[23,26] The majority of human studies show that inspired concentrations of isoflurane of less than 1% have minimal effect on ICP and that any increase in ICP is attenuated by hyperventilation. An exception to this generalization is that some patients with malignant brain tumors may show increases in ICP despite prior hyperventilation, particularly if computed tomography shows a midline shift.[27-29]

Desflurane is unique among the potent inhalation agents in that its low blood/gas solubility facilitates a rapid emergence, which may be useful for immediate postoperative neurologic evaluation. Desflurane has effects on EEG, CBF, and $CMRO_2$ similar to those of isoflurane. Young[30] and Ornstein and co-workers[31] compared the effects of desflurane and isoflurane on CBF at two concentrations, 1 MAC and 1.5 MAC, in an air-oxygen mixture during hypocapnia and reported no difference between isoflurane and desflurane at the two different MAC levels. Holmström and Akeson reported desflurane was associated with more CBF than isoflurane at the same depth of anesthesia.[32] However, the results of ICP studies are not as definitive. Muzzi and colleagues[33] reported that desflurane 1 MAC in an air-oxygen mixture with an arterial CO_2 tension ($PaCO_2$) of 26 mm Hg resulted in sustained increases in ICP until the dura was incised. The physiologic effects of sevoflurane are similar to those of other inhalation anesthetics, but some consider sevoflurane less vasoactive than isoflurane or desflurane.[34]

In summary, all potent inhalational agents are known to increase CBF, CBV and ICP. Hyperventilation attenuates these dose-dependent increases in ICP.

Nitrous oxide (N_2O) is more soluble than nitrogen and expands closed-gas spaces. This has relevance in patients with pneumocephalus.[35] Some practitioners abandon N_2O before closure of the dura to attenuate the development of iatrogenic pneumocephalus.

N_2O is a potent cerebral vasodilator and can produce increases in both CBF and ICP (after cerebral vasodilation) near or greater than those produced by the volatile anesthetic agents themselves. Concomitant hyperventilation or the administration of one of several intravenous anesthetics (barbiturates, propofol, benzodiazepines, opioids) can reduce the increases in CBF and $CMRO_2$ during N_2O administration. However, the combination of N_2O and volatile anesthetics behaves much differently. Administering a volatile anesthetic in low doses (below 1 MAC) may decrease CBF and $CMRO_2$. The addition of 50% N_2O with less than 1 MAC of the volatile anesthetic produces increases in both CBF and $CMRO_2$. The cerebral vasodilation produced by N_2O is greater when increasing doses (greater than 1 MAC) of the volatile anesthetic are administered. N_2O may increase CBF by 100% or more at approximately 0.5 MAC.

Even when it is added to a background of 1 MAC halothane, a threefold increase in CBF is noted. N_2O appears to produce nonuniform changes in CBF, increasing flow in anterior regions and decreasing flow in posterior brain regions. N_2O is not thought to affect CBV or CSF dynamics.[36]

Many neuroanesthesiologists have advocated that N_2O should no longer be administered in neurosurgical patients. But vast clinical experience of N_2O in thousands of neurosurgical patients, with little documentation of adverse neurologic events, argues against N_2O as having major neurotoxic effects during limited exposure. Typically, only very small amounts of N_2O are broken down in the body, but when used on long cases (over 12 hours), substantial accumulation of metabolic breakdown products may occur. These metabolites have been associated with megaloblastic anemia, leukopenia, impaired fetal development, and a depressed immune system. Circumstances in which the practitioner should consider eliminating N_2O are listed in Box 29-1.

Intravenous Agents

Barbiturates are beneficial neuroanesthetic agents because of their ability to decrease $CMRO_2$. This occurs as a result of a reduction in CNS neuronal activity that in turn leads to a coupled reduction in CBF and ICP. However, barbiturates decrease CBF only in normal regions. Because of vasomotor paralysis, vessels within injured or ischemic zones fail to react and remain maximally dilated. The result is the shunting of blood from normal to ischemic areas (termed *inverse steal*). CSF production and absorption are not affected. However, a dose-dependent depression of the CNS does occur. This depression is reflected as progressively slowing EEG activity.[36] A reduction in the metabolic requirement for EEG permits this energy to be used for neuronal basal metabolic needs. When the EEG is isoelectric, neuronal energy consumption is decreased approximately 50%.

Additional benefits of barbiturate administration include the reduction of free-radical formation (which may prevent further injury in ischemic zones, reduced ATP depletion, and provision of effective anticonvulsant activity) and a decrease in cytotoxic cerebral edema, often seen after incomplete ischemia. Barbiturates may be clinically useful for the control of ICP in patients with head injury when standard therapy is ineffective.[15,36,37]

Propofol is a popular induction and maintenance agent for neurosurgical patients. The cerebral effects are similar to those found after barbiturate administration, with a dose-dependent

---

BOX 29-1

Considerations for Eliminating Nitrous Oxide

Nitrous oxide should be eliminated:
- In the presence of intracranial air (recent craniotomy, craniofacial trauma)
- When signal quality during intraoperative evoked potential monitoring is inadequate
- When the patient has clinical evidence of moderate to severe increases in ICP
- When a "tight-brain" is clinically appreciated during the intraoperative period
- When a case longer than 8 hours is anticipated

ICP, Intracranial pressure.

reduction in CBF and $CMRO_2$ producing an isoelectric EEG. CPP may decrease because of reductions in blood pressure after bolus induction doses; however, the reduction in CBF appears to be independent of systemic hemodynamic changes.[38] Reductions in systemic blood pressure produce corresponding reductions in CPP. Very high doses (beyond those required to produce an isoelectric EEG) may produce an increase in CBF (direct cerebral vasodilatation).

Etomidate, like the barbiturates, has similar cerebrovascular and metabolic effects, reducing $CMRO_2$, CBF, and ICP in normal brains and in situations of reduced intracranial compliance. Etomidate has a rapid elimination, allowing a more prompt postoperative neurologic evaluation. In addition to the indirect effect of reduced cerebral metabolism on blood flow, etomidate has a direct vasoconstriction effect. Unlike barbiturates, etomidate does not produce clinically significant cardiovascular depression, resulting in an unchanged or mildly increased CPP.[39-41] Major disadvantages include a high incidence of nonpurposeful movements, thrombophlebitis, nausea, vomiting, and suppression of the adrenocortical response to stress.[41,42] Small doses of etomidate may elicit seizure activity in patients with an underlying seizure disorder. Renal toxicity may develop from the accumulation of propylene glycol after continuous intravenous infusions.

Dexmedetomidine is a new intravenous drug gaining popularity in neuroanesthesia and neurocritical care practice. This α_2-adrenergic receptor agonist offers a unique "cooperative sedation," anxiolysis, and analgesia with no respiratory depression.[43] Systemic administration of dexmedetomidine decreases CBF directly via α_2-mediated constriction of cerebral blood vessels and indirectly via its effect on the intrinsic neural pathway modulating vascular smooth muscle. Reduction in CBF without a concomitant decrease in $CMRO_2$ has raised concerns that dexmedetomidine may limit adequate cerebral oxygenation of brain tissue in patients with already compromised cerebral circulation.[44] Dexmedetomidine in isoflurane-anesthetized dogs is associated with a profound decrease in CBF and cardiac output in the presence of an unaltered $CMRO_2$. Despite the large reduction in the $CBF/CMRO_2$ ratio, there was no evidence of global cerebral ischemia.[45]

The greatest utilization of dexmedetomidine outside the neurosurgical intensive care environment is in the awake craniotomy.

Opioid-based anesthetic techniques are popular for neurosurgical procedures because they provide a steady hemodynamic course and predictable emergence. The synthetic opioids produce dose-related reductions in CBF (decrease to 25 mL/100 g/min and $CMRO_2$ (40% to 50%).[46-49] Later investigations in patients after acute head injury or those undergoing supratentorial craniotomy noted increases in ICP and decreases in CPP after administration of induction doses of fentanyl, sufentanil, and alfentanil.[50] These opioid-induced changes in ICP have been suggested to occur secondarily to an autoregulatory response to decreases in MAP.[51]

Fentanyl decreases the resistance to CSF absorption and results in a 10% reduction in CBV.[35,42,46] Sufentanil is 5 to 10 times more potent than fentanyl and has the highest therapeutic index of the clinically used opiates. Of the synthetic opiates, alfentanil produces the greatest decreases in MAP and CPP.[35,42,47] Remifentanil is the latest available compound of the 4-anilidopiperidine derivatives. It is characterized by an ultrashort duration of action and a metabolism independent of both hepatic and renal functions. Its main drawback is a lack

of residual analgesia and the risk of postoperative hyperalgesia.[52] Meperidine should probably be avoided in the neurosurgical patient, because its metabolite, normeperidine, is a well-known convulsant.

Judiciously titrated doses of naloxone reverse opioid-induced respiratory depression and normalize both CBF and $CMRO_2$. The abrupt reversal of opioid-induced respiratory depression should be avoided in neurosurgical patients. Naloxone administered in this fashion is associated with hypertension, cardiac dysrhythmias, pulmonary edema, and intracranial hemorrhage.[53,54]

The benzodiazepines—midazolam, diazepam, and lorazepam—are useful anesthetic adjuncts used for their anxiolytic, anticonvulsant, and amnestic effects. Benzodiazepines produce a dose-dependent decrease in $CMRO_2$ and reductions in CBF; however, their effects on ICP are minimal.

Flumazenil, the benzodiazepine-specific antagonist, has no effect on cerebral dynamics when administered alone. High-dose midazolam anesthetic in the canine was associated with rebound increases in CBF and ICP to values greater than baseline when abrupt reversal was accomplished with flumazenil.[55] Flumazenil may produce seizures when large doses are administered.

Ketamine has limited usefulness in neuroanesthesia. The dissociative mechanism of action and resultant stormy emergence from anesthesia are undesirable after neurosurgical procedures. The primary advantage of ketamine is the stable hemodynamic course in the face of hypovolemia that may occur in the head-injured patient with multisystem trauma. Ketamine is known to produce untoward alterations in cerebral physiology, increasing CBF by 60% to 80% and elevating ICP. Ketamine also increases the resistance to CSF reabsorption, which over time may increase ICP beyond that produced by increases in CBF alone. Cerebral metabolic rate is unchanged, but regional differences may exist.[35] A renewed interest in ketamine has been prompted because of its noncompetitive antagonism of the glutamine NMDA receptor. Similar compounds have been demonstrated to afford some degree of neuroprotection. Some studies now suggest that ketamine can be used safely in neurologically impaired patients under conditions of controlled ventilation, coadministration of a γ-aminobutyric acid receptor agonist, and avoidance of N_2O.[56] Yet, for most neuroanesthesia practitioners, ketamine continues to be an unpopular drug for neuroanesthesia.

Nondepolarizing neuromuscular relaxants do not appear to have clinically significant direct effects on CBF or $CMRO_2$, provided MAP is not altered after administration.[57] The depolarizing agent succinylcholine in select circumstances may produce elevations in ICP, CBF, and $CMRO_2$.

Upper motor neuron disease may alter the peripheral nerve–stimulating response of nondepolarizing neuromuscular relaxants. Generally, the twitch response shows relative resistance to muscle relaxants on the hemiparetic or hemiplegic side, compared with the unaffected side or respiratory muscles.[58,59] Decreased sensitivity to nondepolarizing muscle relaxants is most exaggerated in the first 3 weeks of upper motor neuron disease. Therefore, monitoring neuromuscular blockade is preferentially performed on the unaffected side. Patients on chronic anticonvulsant therapy may be more resistant to long-acting nondepolarizing muscle relaxants.[60] Patients receiving chronic phenytoin therapy have an increased dosage requirement and reduced duration of action for the nondepolarizing neuromuscular relaxants, with the exception of atracurium and cisatracurium.

Succinylcholine increases ICP through an increase in muscle-spindle activity and increased cerebral stimulation with coupled increases in CBF.[42] Despite the use of thiopental with hyperventilation during induction, greater increases in ICP have been noted with succinylcholine than with pancuronium. Succinylcholine is contraindicated in patients with neurologic or denervated muscle because of the potential for life-threatening hyperkalemia.[35,41] Succinylcholine should be avoided in patients with cerebrovascular accident, upper and lower motor neuron lesions, coma, encephalitis, and closed head injury and after severe burns and prolonged bed rest.

The availability of suitable nondepolarizing alternatives such as rocuronium (1 mg/kg intubating dose) facilitates endotracheal intubation within 60 to 90 seconds and avoids the known complications attendant on the administration of succinylcholine.

Antihypertensives

β-Adrenergic antagonists have great utility for the control of the inotropic and chronotropic effects of sympathetic stimulation that attend laryngoscopy, endotracheal intubation, and endotracheal extubation. Esmolol is a rapid-onset, short-acting selective β$_1$-adrenergic receptor antagonist. Administration of 0.5 to 1 mg/kg 2 minutes before laryngoscopy and endotracheal intubation attenuates the predictable increases in heart rate and blood pressure. Its effects on ICP are thought to be negligible. Labetalol is a selective α$_1$-adrenergic antagonist and nonselective β$_1$- and β$_2$-adrenergic antagonist (ratio of β-blockade to α-blockade is 7:1 for intravenous preparation). Labetalol spares presynaptic α$_2$-receptors; consequently, released norepinephrine produces further inhibition of catecholamine release via a negative feedback from the stimulation of β$_2$-receptors. Labetalol administration in a canine model with and without intracranial hypertension failed to alter ICP, despite reductions in MAP of up to 38%.[61] Esmolol may be preferred for the control of emergence hypertension after intracranial procedures. In one study, patients treated with labetalol as compared with esmolol experienced a higher incidence of bradycardia in the immediate postoperative period.[62]

The smooth muscle relaxants sodium nitroprusside and nitroglycerin produce increases in CBV and ICP. Sodium nitroprusside is a direct-acting cerebrovasodilator, increasing CBV after dilation of cerebral capacitance vessels.[57,63] Deliberate hyperventilation and the administration of a barbiturate may attenuate the cerebrovasodilation. Most contemporary neuroanesthesiologists consider nitroglycerin and sodium nitroprusside to be potent dilators of capacitance vessels and unsafe in patients with abnormal elastance. If a patient is on a tenuous portion of the pressure-volume curve, the dramatic rise in CBV caused by nitroglycerin or nitroprusside use would be catastrophic, resulting in spatial exhaustion and intracranial hypertension.[64]

The calcium channel blocking agents not only have been used for the control of blood pressure during the perioperative period but also have been studied for their potential cerebral protectant effects. Nimodipine is commonly used to prevent vasospasm after neurologic trauma or hemorrhage.

Nicardipine inhibits calcium ion from entering the "slow channels" or select voltage-sensitive areas of vascular smooth muscle and myocardium during depolarization, producing a relaxation of coronary vascular smooth muscle and coronary vasodilatation. Nicardipine also increases myocardial oxygen delivery in patients with vasospastic angina. Cerebral vasospasm and delayed cerebral ischemia remain common complications of aneurysm subarachnoid hemorrhage (SAH), and yet therapies for cerebral vasospasm are limited. Despite a large number of clinical trials, only calcium antagonists have strong evidence supporting their effectiveness.[65] Nicardipine prolonged-release implants reduce the incidence of cerebral vasospasm and delayed ischemic deficits and improve clinical outcome after severe subarachnoid hemorrhage.[66] Nicardipine has been compared to esmolol in controlling the hemodynamic response to emergence. Although esmolol 1.5 mg/kg IV was more effective than nicardipine 0.03 mg/kg IV for attenuating the HR response to extubation, nicardipine was more effective in controlling the blood pressure response.[67]

INTRACRANIAL PRESSURE

In its simplest definition, *intracranial pressure* refers to the supratentorial CSF pressure. The supratentorial pressure may be measured within the lateral ventricle or within the subarachnoid space over the convexity of the cerebral cortex. CSF pressure may vary markedly in different areas within the cranium, and similarly, CSF pressure in the cranial subarachnoid space may differ from that in the spinal subarachnoid space. In individuals free of neurologic pathology in the recumbent position, the CSF pressure measured at the lumbar cistern accurately reflects ICP. However, many factors, including the assumption of the upright position, can alter the relationship between cranial and spinal CSF pressures. In addition, in the presence of intracranial mass lesions, infratentorial CSF pressure (as measured in the cisterna magna or lumbar cistern) often decreases, whereas supratentorial pressure increases. Therefore, the measurement of supratentorial CSF pressure is a useful clinical concept.[15,68]

Determinants of Intracranial Pressure

The brain is enclosed within a rigid container, and because the brain is not compressible, any increase in total intracranial volume produces an accompanying increase in ICP (Monro-Kelly doctrine). Increased ICP may have a detrimental effect on the well-being of the brain. The intracranial contents consist of the brain (12%), intracellular water (78%), CSF (approximately 75 mL), and blood (approximately 50 mL), for a combined volume of approximately 1200 to 1500 mL.[69] The brain is surrounded by the dura mater and rigidly encased in the bone of the calvaria and skull base. In the strictest sense, the intracranial space, volume, and pressure are defined by the limits of the encasing bone. However, should the skull become disrupted, the remaining intracranial contents may be subject to the potential for abnormal pressure accumulation because of the restrictions imposed by an intact dura mater. The same dural restrictions also may contribute to regional ICP gradients in patients with intracranial mass lesions and an intact cranial vault.[70] Intracranial hypertension may lead to global reductions in CPP (CPP = MAP − ICP) from compression-induced ischemia or may produce shifting of intracranial contents, resulting in compression of the brain against the falx, the tentorium, or the foramen magnum.

The ICP is approximately 5 to 15 mm Hg in adults; lower values are recorded in children and infants. This pressure is determined by the relationship between the volume allowed by the structures that limit intracranial volume and the actual volume of the intracranial space. Because of the normal elastance of the intracranial contents, individuals without intracranial pathology maintain normal ICP despite transient increases that develop with coughing or during a Valsalva maneuver. Small increases in the intracranial volume do not produce abrupt increases in ICP. This normal elastance exists because the limits of the intracranial contents have not been reached. Once a growing

ICP Compliance Curve

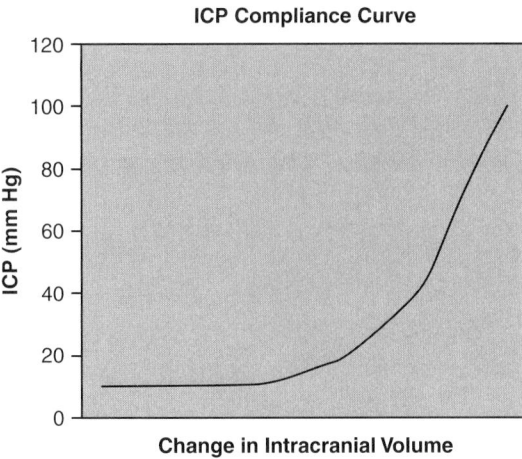

FIGURE **29-16** Intracranial pressure-volume curve. (*From Kofke WA, Stiefel M. Monitoring and intraoperative management of elevated intracranial pressure and decompressive craniectomy. Anesthesiol Clin. 2007;25[3]:580.*)

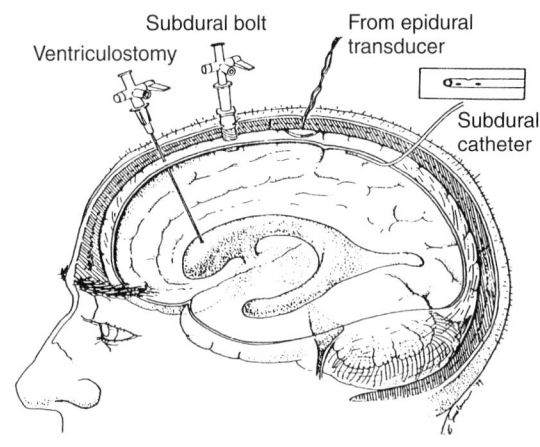

FIGURE **29-17** Representation of sites for placement of intracranial pressure monitors. (*From Shapiro HM. Neurosurgical anesthesia and intracranial hypertension. In: Miller RD, ed. Anesthesia. 3rd ed. New York: Churchill Livingstone; 1991:1749.*)

mass, blood or tumor, has increased intracranial volume to its limit, dramatic increases in ICP may occur.[71] This relationship is depicted in Figure 29-16. Although this ICP-volume curve is commonly used to explain these relationships, Todd and colleagues[72] suggest that the x-axis be relabeled as the "volume of the growing mass," because this axis does not really represent total intracranial volume. The initial portion of the curve in Figure 29-16 is relatively flat because the total intracranial volume does not change with early periods of bleeding or tumor growth. This portion of the curve reflects the phenomenon of spatial compensation. As the mass (blood or tumor) increases, the volume of the intracranial compartments must decrease to maintain normal ICP. In most cases, the CSF compartment decreases; that is, CSF is absorbed by the arachnoid granulations or shunted to the spinal subarachnoid space to compensate for the increasing intracranial volume. Compensation is exhausted when the CSF compartment cannot decrease further in size and total intracranial volume increases, accounting for the increase in ICP. In summary, an increase in total intracranial volume increases ICP.

Measurement of Intracranial Pressure

ICP monitoring is facilitated by ventriculostomy, subdural bolt, epidural transducer, or subdural fiberoptic catheter placed in a supratentorial location (Figure 29-17). Access to the subarachnoid space facilitates the removal of CSF for assistance in the control of increased ICP.[73,74]

Intracranial Hypertension

Intracranial hypertension occurs with a sustained increase in ICP above 15 to 20 mm Hg. Intracranial hypertension develops with expanding tissue or fluid mass, interference with normal CSF absorption, excessive CBF, or systemic disturbances promoting brain edema. Often, multiple factors are responsible for the development of intracranial hypertension. For example, tumors in the posterior fossa usually produce some degree of brain edema and readily obstruct CSF flow by compressing the fourth ventricle.[75]

Although many patients with intracranial hypertension are initially asymptomatic, all eventually develop characteristic signs and symptoms, including headache, nausea, vomiting,

papilledema, focal neurologic deficits, altered ventilatory function, decreasing consciousness, seizures, and coma. When ICP exceeds 30 mm Hg, CBF progressively decreases, and a vicious cycle is established: ischemia produces brain edema, which in turn increases ICP, and further precipitates ischemia. If this cycle remains unchecked, progressive neurologic damage or catastrophic herniation may result.[15,75,76]

Cerebrospinal Fluid Drainage. Intracranial hypertension may be reduced by a surgical CSF diversion. The long-term effectiveness of this therapeutic alternative depends on the cause of the increased ICP. When brain edema produces elevation of ICP, CSF drainage may provide only transient abatement of intracranial hypertension. If external drainage is continued in this circumstance, ventricular collapse can occur and prevent further venting of CSF. Successful chronic control of high ICP caused by hydrocephalus can be achieved with implanted CSF shunts.[50]

Intracranial Pressure Reduction

Box 29-2 lists the major methods for the treatment of elevated ICP. Selective application of these methods often results in ICP reduction accompanied by clinical improvement. A patent airway, adequate oxygenation, and hyperventilation provide the foundation for neuroresuscitative care in acute intracranial hypertensive states. Frequently, overlap occurs among causes of increased ICP, and this may necessitate simultaneous application of a number of different therapeutic modalities.[50]

Hyperventilation

Lowering Pa_{CO_2} increases cerebrovascular resistance, reducing CBV and ICP. The exact mechanism by which CO_2 exerts its effect on cerebral vessels is not completely understood. The prevailing theory is that changes in CO_2 produce alterations in the pH of the CSF surrounding the arterioles. This alteration occurs because CO_2 crosses the blood-brain barrier freely, whereas bicarbonate crosses more slowly. Therefore, decreases in Pa_{CO_2} increase pH in the CSF and arteriolar walls. Because bicarbonate ions cross the blood-brain more slowly, changes in CSF pH and CBF that result from alterations in Pa_{CO_2} last only a few hours. After this time, CBF returns to prehyperventilation values, despite continuing hypocapnia or hypercapnia.[68]

BOX 29-2

Methods for the Treatment of Elevated Intracranial Pressure

- Apply hyperventilation on demand ($Paco_2$ 30 to 35 mm Hg)
- Administer diuretics (osmotic mannitol 0.25-1 g/kg^{-1} IV) (may repeat if serum osmolarity <320 mOsm • 1^{-1} and patient is euvolemic) or furosemide
- Perform cerebrospinal fluid drainage (if available)
- Avoid overhydration; target normovolemia
- Elevate patient's head; position to improve cerebral venous return; avoid neck-vein compression
- Insert intracranial pressure monitor; Sjo_2, $AVDo_2$, and CBF monitoring recommended
- Optimize hemodynamics: mean arterial pressure, central venous pressure, pulmonary capillary wedge pressure, heart rate, and cerebral perfusion pressure; consider antihypertensive therapy as needed
- Administer corticosteroids (dexamethasone)
- Surgical decompression; consider decompressive craniectomy if hematoma is present
- Cerebral vasoconstriction (thiopental, propofol)
- Consider mild hypothermia

$AVDo_2$, *Arteriovenous difference in oxygen content*; CBF, *cerebral blood flow*; IV, *intravenous*; $Paco_2$, *partial pressure of arterial carbon dioxide*; Sjo_2, *jugular bulb oxyhemoglobin saturation*.

In cooperative patients, voluntary hyperventilation is encouraged just before induction of anesthesia. When this is not possible, airway control is obtained as early as possible after anesthetic induction, and hyperventilation is rapidly initiated. In emergency neuroresuscitative care, hyperventilation is the first step when acute decompensation occurs.[50] In previously normocapnic patients, acute hyperventilation to a $Paco_2$ range of approximately 30 mm Hg probably provides maximum intracranial decompression with minimal risk of cerebral ischemia.

Surgical Decompression

Surgical decompression may be used for uncontrollable increases in ICP. Internal decompression involves the excision of brain tissue, reduction in ICP, and reduction of the potential for brainstem displacement or herniation. External decompression involves excision of the skull overlying the site of either an epidural or a subdural hematoma. Decompressive surgery is generally considered to be a last resort in patients with persistent, intractable increases in ICP.[41]

Hypothermia

Hypothermia may assist in uncontrollable increases in ICP by decreasing $CMRO_2$ 7% for each degree centigrade decrease in core body temperature.[77]

Pharmacologic Manipulation of Intracranial Pressure
Diuretics

Loop diuretics (furosemide, bumetanide, ethacrynic acid) produce a general diuresis, decrease the rate of CSF production, and decrease cerebral edema. Osmotic diuretics are effective in decreasing the water content of the brain. Mannitol is the most widely used osmotic diuretic for acute control of intracranial hypertension. Rapid administration of mannitol may produce vasodilation, increases in CBF, a transient rise in ICP, and a transient increase in circulating blood volume. Increases in circulating blood volume may prove to be detrimental to patients with underlying cardiac dysfunction. Prior administration of intravenous furosemide may minimize these potential complications. Decreases in ICP begin shortly after mannitol administration and may continue for up to 6 hours. The typically prescribed dose of mannitol is 0.25 to 1 g/kg. Continued use of mannitol may produce hyperosmolality and electrolyte imbalance, which may be attenuated with concurrent administration of a loop diuretic.[78]

Hypertonic saline has an osmotic effect on the brain because of its high tonicity and ability to effectively remain outside the blood-brain barrier. Numerous animal studies have suggested that fluid resuscitation with hypertonic saline bolus after hemorrhagic shock prevents the ICP increase that follows resuscitation with standard fluids. There may be a minimal benefit in restoring CBF, which is thought to be mitigated through local effects of hypertonic saline on cerebral microvasculature. In animal models with cerebral injury, the maximum benefit is observed in animals with focal injury associated with vasogenic edema (cryogenic injury). The ICP reduction is seen for approximately 2 hours and may be maintained for longer periods by using a continuous infusion of hypertonic saline. The ICP reduction is thought to be caused by a reduction in water content in areas of the brain with intact blood-brain barrier, such as the nonlesioned hemisphere and cerebellum. Most comparisons with mannitol suggest almost equal efficacy in reducing ICP, but there is a suggestion that mannitol may have a longer duration of action. To date, human studies reporting on the use of hypertonic saline in treating cerebral edema and elevated ICP include case reports, case series, and small controlled trials. Results from studies directly comparing hypertonic saline with standard treatment in regard to safety and efficacy are inconclusive. However, the low frequency of side effects and a definite reduction of ICP observed with use of hypertonic saline in these studies are very promising. Systemic effects include transient volume expansion, natriuresis, hemodilution, immunomodulation, and improved pulmonary gas exchange. Adverse effects include electrolyte abnormalities, cardiac failure, bleeding diathesis, and phlebitis. Although unproven, a potential for central pontine myelinosis and rebound intracranial hypertension exists with uncontrolled administration.[79]

Corticosteroids

Glucocorticoids penetrate the blood-brain barrier and decrease edema associated with mass lesions. In the absence of mass lesions, glucocorticoid administration may produce pseudotumor cerebri (increased ICP) and papilledema. Additional complications ascribed to the continuous use of steroids in neurosurgical patients include hyperglycemia, glucosuria, gastrointestinal bleeding, electrolyte abnormalities, and an increase in the incidence of infection. Evidence remains contradictory regarding the efficacy of high-dose steroids for head injury.[80,81] Recent data suggest steroids are not indicated and may be harmful in the treatment of intracranial hypertension resulting from traumatic brain injury.[82] Steroids, even when clinically efficacious, require hours for their ICP decompression effects to become apparent.[50]

Barbiturates

A bolus injection of 1.5 to 5 mg of thiopental per kilogram has been shown to be effective in reducing ICP. Although the CPP in most patients increases because the magnitude of the decrease in ICP exceeds the magnitude of the decrease in MAP, close monitoring of both pressures is indicated. In situations in which either hypotension or hypovolemia is present, lidocaine, 1.5 mg/kg, may be useful in reducing ICP while maintaining MAP. Failure of intracranial hypertension to respond to barbiturates usually indicates a poor prognosis.

Barbiturate coma, hypothermia, or decompressive craniectomy should be considered for intracranial hypertension refractory to initial medical management. Steroids are not indicated and may be harmful in the treatment of intracranial hypertension resulting from traumatic brain injury.[14]

Barbiturate coma is used to capture refractory ICP, though not on a routine basis. Barbiturates will lower ICP by lowering CBF, and this is brought about by lowering the $CMRO_2$ and also to some degree by inducing hypotension, which at times may be very difficult to treat.[83] Because of this, they are almost always used in conjunction with intravenous pressor agents in the intensive care setting and can be titrated to ICP effect or to EEG depiction of burst suppression. The cerebral metabolic rate cannot be lowered further after burst suppression is achieved by barbiturates; theoretically, ICP will be at its lowest barbiturate-induced level when burst suppression is achieved.[84] Patients may be kept in burst suppression–induced barbiturate coma for hours to days.

NEUROPHYSIOLOGIC MONITORING

Great use is made of neurophysiologic brain monitoring. It is important to confer with the surgeon prior to surgery to determine which neurophysiologic monitoring is to be used and to plan the anesthetic in a manner that optimizes the results of the required monitoring.

Although not universally adopted, the growing body of literature provides strong evidence of the clinical utility of neurophysiologic monitoring in a variety of cerebrovascular surgical and endovascular procedures. The Therapeutics and Technology Subcommittee of the American Academy of Neurology and Fisher and colleagues concluded that the following are useful and noninvestigational: (1) EEG, compressed spectral array, and somatosensory evoked potentials (SSEPs) in carotid endarterectomies and brain surgeries that potentially compromise cerebral blood flow; (2) brainstem auditory evoked response and cranial-nerve monitoring in surgeries performed in the region of the brainstem or inner ear; and (3) somatosensory evoked monitoring performed for surgical procedures potentially involving ischemia or mechanical trauma of the spinal cord. The committee concluded that although promising, motor evoked potentials and visual evoked potentials remain investigational. Before intraoperative monitoring can become standard practice, further research investigations, especially in the area of outcomes research and cost-effectiveness, will be required.[85]

Electroencephalography

The EEG recorded from the scalp is a summation of the excitatory and inhibitory postsynaptic potentials produced in the pyramidal layer of the cerebral cortex. EEG activity requires about 50% of the total oxygen consumed by the brain; the remaining 50% is needed to maintain cellular integrity. When oxygen delivery is compromised, slowing of EEG activity ensues.

Changes in EEG frequency and amplitude may be caused by administration of anesthetic drugs and changes in anesthetic depth. Low doses of potent inhalation agents with N_2O produce an active EEG. Steady-state anesthesia, regardless of the agent

used, usually produces a stable EEG pattern. It is worth noting that deep levels of anesthesia and cerebral ischemia produce similar EEG changes. In both cases, fast activity is replaced by slower, larger EEG waveforms. Boluses of anesthetic drugs may produce large EEG changes indistinguishable from those seen during ischemia. The EEG provides information about the overall electrical functioning of the cerebral cortex but not much about the subcortical brain, spinal cord, or cranial and peripheral nerves.[86]

Somatosensory Evoked Potentials

An evoked potential differs from the EEG mainly in two ways: (1) The EEG is a random, continuous signal that arises from the ongoing activity of the outer layers of the cortex, and an evoked potential is the brain's response to a repetitive stimulus along a specific nerve pathway. (2) EEG signals range from 10 to 200 millivolts (mV). Evoked potentials are smaller in amplitude (1, 5, 20 microvolts), requiring precise electrode positioning and special techniques (signal averaging) to extract the specific response from the underlying EEG "noise." The technique of signal averaging has been further developed in computer processing. The technique now used applies a stimulus repeatedly—preferably at randomized intervals—and records the evoked response over the corresponding area of the brain, averaging out mathematically the change over the number of stimuli.[87]

SSEP can be used for detecting localized injury to specific areas of the neural axis by assessing cortically generated waves, or it can serve as a nonspecific indicator of the adequacy of cerebral oxygen delivery.[86]

Although anesthetics alter the generation and transmission of SSEP, suppression of muscle artifact by neuromuscular blocking drugs and the ability to use much higher stimulus intensity in the anesthetized patient allow rapid production of waves that are reproducible, although they differ from those found in the awake patient. Early components of SSEP are generally resistant to anesthetic depression. Etomidate and ketamine both increase the amplitude of scalp-recorded waves by 200% to 600%. Volatile anesthetics and N_2O depress the SSEP waveform in a dose-dependent manner. Avoiding changes in inhaled gas concentration and bolus injection of hypnotic drugs during periods of risk minimizes difficulties in determining whether waveform changes are due to surgical manipulation.[88]

Hypothermia increases SSEP latency. Latency increases about 3 milliseconds with every decrease in temperature of 2° C to 3° C. This amount of change is suggestive of neural injury. Hyperthermia suppresses SSEP amplitude, with the amplitude being only 15% of that at normothermia.[88-91]

Reproducible, very-short-latency waves of the trigeminal system are produced by stimulation of the lip at 2 to 4 Hz (512 stimuli). This modality of evoked potential is abnormal in patients with posterior fossa masses in the region of cranial nerve V or in symptomatic hydrocephalus.[92] This modality of evoked potential monitoring may be useful in patients with large posterior fossa tumors that cause severe cranial nerve VIII dysfunction and make brainstem auditory evoked response (BAER) monitoring impossible.[88]

BAER assesses only brainstem function, although long-latency cortical waves can be assessed to evaluate cortical function. BAER has been used extensively in patients at risk of brain injury during intracranial surgery, despite the extremely small amount of neural tissue assessed and the resistance of BAER to oxygen deprivation when compared with other neural monitors such as the EEG or SSEP waves.[88,93]

Compared with SSEPs, intraoperative factors other than surgical brain damage are relatively unlikely to seriously alter the BAER. BAER waveforms are resistant to both intravenous and inhalational drugs.[88] Fentanyl in large doses does not alter BAER.[88,94] Propofol (2 mg/kg, followed by an infusion) increases the latency of waves I, III, and V without a change in the amplitudes, but it completely suppresses middle-latency auditory waves.[88,95] N_2O produces a linear decrease in BAER amplitude from 10% to 40%[88,96]; N_2O at doses of 33% reduces the wave amplitude without altering latency.[88,97,98]

BAER waves are easily identifiable at more frequently used levels of hypothermia (29° C), although latencies are delayed by about 33%.[99] BAER latency is inversely related to temperature over the range of 36° C to 42° C, with a decrease in amplitude as temperature increases.[88,100]

BAER appears to be a sensitive monitor to the auditory apparatus in response to direct injury.[88] The auditory apparatus includes the cochlear hair cells, spiral ganglion, eighth cranial nerve, cochlear nuclei, superior olivary complex, lateral lemnisci, inferior colliculus, and medial geniculate thalamic nuclei.[86] Some have recommended BAER monitoring be undertaken in all patients at risk of brainstem injury, even if the primary disease causes hearing on the affected side to decrease below the functional level.[88] Some also consider BAER clinically useful and probably approaching standard of care for microvascular decompression procedures and acoustic tumor surgery.[86]

Aggressive intraoperative monitoring does not guarantee prevention of neurologic injury, because all parts of the brain are not assessed using currently available monitoring.[88] Except when the entire brainstem is at risk, there will likely be a high incidence of cases in which BAERs are unaffected intraoperatively, yet significant impairment in motor function or consciousness occurs postoperatively.[86]

Electromyography (EMG) monitoring is frequently used for facial nerve monitoring. Generally, two types of EMG activity are monitored. The first involves active stimulation of the nerve for localization and the second, spontaneous EMG activity initiated by irritation or manipulation of the nerve. It has been noted that in the presence of light anesthesia, spontaneous EMG activity caused by slight movements may become apparent and mimic neuronal irritation.[86]

The effects of muscle relaxants on EMG monitoring have not been adequately studied.[86,88] The degree of neuromuscular blockade should be maintained at a light level until response of the respective muscles (orbicularis oris and orbicularis oculi) is verified.[88] Chronically injured facial nerves may show greater sensitivity to the effects of neuromuscular blockade, suggesting lower levels of neuromuscular blockade be used.[101] Some do not paralyze patients during the time EMG monitoring is used. Facial nerve monitoring is considered the standard of care for acoustic tumor surgery and during other surgery that risks facial nerve function.[86]

The motor component of cranial nerves III, IV, X, XI, and XII also can be monitored using EMG.[86,102,103] Whereas some consider the use of EMG monitoring of cranial nerves other than VII not widespread or universally accepted,[86] recent interest in skull-base surgery has spurred EMG monitoring for lower cranial nerve preservation. Some recent evidence suggests EMG monitoring proved to be a safe tool for the intraoperative identification and localization of the lower cranial nerves, contributing to their anatomic and functional preservation. The predictive value of standard neurophysiologic parameters for functional outcome, however, is limited.[104]

There is great interest in intraoperative use of motor evoked potentials (MEPs) because of the theoretic limitations of SSEPs in monitoring motor function.[86] MEPs assess function of the motor cortex and descending tracts. The peripheral response of the MEP is recorded by measuring the compound muscle action potential.[88] The motor cortex is stimulated by electrical or magnetic stimulation. Both volatile anesthetics and neuromuscular blocking drugs obtund these responses.[88,105,106]

Some authors have concluded that MEPs produced by either transcranial magnetic or electrical stimulation using single stimuli cannot be recorded during general anesthesia using virtually any commonly used anesthetic drug.[86,107-112] But averaging of multiple stimuli may allow monitoring during anesthesia. Several studies, both in animals and humans, report that neuromuscular blockade resulting in a 70% or less reduction in the height of the response to ulnar nerve stimulation is compatible with MEP monitoring.[86,112] A combination of N_2O-narcotic anesthetic and a stable level of neuromuscular blockade, such as that provided by an infusion of neuromuscular blocking agent, has been advocated to provide a stable response.[88] Some authors recommend that N_2O be kept to less than 50% or not used if monitoring of MEPs is vital to safe spinal surgery.[108,113] Total intravenous anesthesia using infusions of etomidate or propofol in combination with a narcotic allow stable MEP recordings. Total intravenous anesthesia with ketamine has also been recognized as compatible with stable MEP readings.[86,114]

MEP responses produced by electrical stimulation of the spinal cord are resistant to the effects of anesthesia and require no special anesthetic considerations other than the need for muscle relaxants to prevent gross movements.[86]

ANESTHETIC CONSIDERATIONS FOR SPECIFIC PROCEDURES

Supratentorial Surgery

Intracranial masses may be congenital, neoplastic (benign, malignant, or metastatic), infectious (abscess or cyst), or vascular (hematoma or malformation). Most but not all anesthetics can be used safely in patients with cerebral lesions. Important considerations are the effects of the agent on ICP, CPP, CBF $CMRO_2$, promptness of return of consciousness, drug-related protection from cerebral ischemia or edema, blood pressure control, and compatibility with neurophysiologic monitoring techniques.[115]

Most craniotomy surgery in the United States today is probably performed following a thiopental/propofol induction of anesthesia with intubation of the trachea after a nondepolarizing relaxant. Maintaining anesthesia is commonly accomplished with a volatile agent (usually isoflurane) and a narcotic, such as fentanyl, sufentanil, or alfentanil, in various combinations during hypocarbia to $PaCO_2$ levels of 28 to 33 mm Hg.[115]

Preoperative Evaluation

The clinical signs of a supratentorial mass include seizures, hemiplegia, and aphasia. The clinical signs of infratentorial masses include cerebellar dysfunction (ataxia, nystagmus, dysarthria) and brainstem compression (cranial nerve palsies, altered consciousness, abnormal respiration). When ICP increases, frank signs of intracranial hypertension can also develop.[75]

Preanesthetic evaluation should attempt to establish the presence or absence of intracranial hypertension. Computed tomography or MRI data should be reviewed for evidence of brain edema, midline shift greater than 0.5 cm, and ventricular size. A neurologic assessment should evaluate the current mental status and any existing deficits. Anticonvulsant therapy and medications prescribed for control of ICP (corticosteroids, diuretics) should be reviewed. Laboratory evaluation should rule out corticosteroid-induced hyperglycemia and electrolyte disturbances that may develop secondary to diuretic therapy. For anticonvulsants, amount, time of last dose, and blood levels should be noted.

The decision regarding the amount and timing of the premedication administration should be made only after a thorough patient evaluation. Benzodiazepines produce respiratory depression and hypercapnia. Premedication should be omitted in patients with a large mass lesion, a midline shift, and abnormal ventricular size. Opioids are universally avoided in the preoperative period. If premedication is desired in those patients deemed appropriate, careful titration of intravenous midazolam may begin once the patient has been delivered to the preoperative holding area. In an attempt to help control ICP in patients with mass lesions, the head of the bed should be elevated 15 to 30 degrees during transport to the preoperative holding area and the operating room. Due diligence to all existing hospital recommendations for prophylactic antibiotics given at the appropriate time and in the appropriate amount should be performed.

Intraoperative Monitoring

Routine monitors for supratentorial procedures include continuous electrocardiography, cuff measurement of blood pressure, precordial stethoscope, monitoring of the fraction of inspired oxygen, pulse oximetry, temperature, peripheral nerve

stimulation, end-tidal CO_2 ($ETCO_2$) monitoring, and indwelling urinary catheterization. For patients with ischemic heart disease, use of a modified V_5 ECG lead is recommended. An arterial line placed either before or immediately after anesthetic induction provides for uninterrupted blood pressure monitoring and easy access for blood sampling for laboratory analysis. SSEPs may be assessed. The effect of various anesthetics on SSEPs is given in Table 29-5. Methods for cerebral oxygenation monitoring are listed in Table 29-6.

Fluid Management

Tissues within the CNS are subject to water movement governed by the blood-brain barrier. The pore size in the blood-brain barrier is only one tenth that of the periphery, at 0.7 to 0.9 nm.[116] There is a fundamental difference between capillaries within the CNS and the peripheral capillaries. The blood-brain barrier remains impermeable to both ions and proteins. The number of ions represents a greater magnitude in determining the net movement of water than the number of plasma proteins. There can be little doubt that osmolarity is the primary determinant of water movement across the intact blood-brain barrier.[117,118]

Preoperative fluid deficits and intraoperative blood and fluid losses must be adequately replaced during neurosurgical procedures. Judicious fluid administration minimizes the occurrence of cerebral edema and increased ICP, reduced CPP, and worsened cerebral ischemia. In most neurosurgical patients, fluids that contain sodium in a concentration similar to that of serum (e.g., lactated Ringer's solution or 0.9% saline) are administered in a volume sufficient for maintaining peripheral perfusion but avoiding hypervolemia (0.5 to 1 mL/kg/hr). Traditionally, less fluid is given than would be administered for nonneurologic surgery, although new recommendations indicate that patients should be kept isovolemic, isotonic, and isooncotic.[119-122] No single intravenous solution is best suited for the neurosurgical patient at risk for intracranial hypertension, but the use of isoosmolar crystalloids is widely accepted and can be justified on a scientific basis.[118]

Emerging evidence questions the rationale for routine administration of glucose. Hyperglycemia induces marked cerebrovascular changes during both ischemia and reperfusion.[123] Multiple studies have demonstrated that hyperglycemia before and during an episode of global cerebral ischemia will exacerbate the neurologic injury.[124]

Some argue that the hyperglycemia-enhanced ischemic injury is due to a rise in lactate production and concomitant tissue acidosis.[125-127] Another theory suggests that hyperglycemia enhances ischemic injury by attenuating an increase in

TABLE **29-5**	Effects of Anesthetics on Somatosensory Evoked Potentials	
Drug	**Latency**	**Amplitude**
Isoflurane	↑	↓
Sevoflurane	↑	↓
Halothane	↑	↓
Nitrous oxide	↑	↓
Desflurane	↑	↓
Thiopental	↑	↓
Fentanyl	Slight ↑	Slight ↓
Propofol	↑	No change
Ketamine	↑	↑
Etomidate	↑	↑

TABLE **29-6**	Cerebral Oxygenation Monitoring	
Monitor	**Abbreviations**	**Comments**
Jugular venous bulb oxygen saturation	$SjvO_2$	Lack of a gold standard for comparison; invasive; monitors global not regional ischemia and hypoxia
Transcranial cerebral oximetry	rSO_2	Lack of definition of brain tissue being monitored; trend monitor; patients act as their own control; technology rapidly changing
Cerebral oxygen tension monitors	$PbtO_2$	Highly invasive; reserved for severe head injuries; cerebral perfusion pressure must be at least 60 mm Hg

Modified from Smyth PR, Samra S. Monitors of cerebral oxygenation. Anesthesiol Clin. 2002;20:3-7.

adenosine.[125,128,129] Yet another theory suggests that hyperglycemia significantly worsens the degree of acute blood-brain barrier disruption that occurs during ischemia.[125,130] It is also thought that hyperglycemia is associated with a significantly reduced CBF and increased heterogeneity of regional CBF during the postischemic period.[125,131-134]

Animal studies report that during complete cerebral ischemia, hyperglycemia or the use of glucose-containing solutions is associated with a significantly greater neurologic or histopathologic injury and even an increased death rate when the periischemic blood glucose levels are only moderately increased or are similar to control levels.[125,127,135,136] Treatment with insulin, even after the ischemic insult, has been shown to attenuate this neurologic injury and death rate.[125,136,137]

Current critical care studies underscore the necessity of controlling blood glucose levels. Use of insulin protocols in critically ill patients improves blood glucose control and reduces morbidity and mortality in this population. Insulin protocols to control glucose levels should be implemented with the goal of achieving normoglycemia, regardless of the history of diabetes.[138] Frequent assessment of blood glucose levels and aggressive insulin treatment are recommended.[128]

Fluid therapy is most challenging during prolonged surgical procedures or in the surgical management of multiple traumas. If tissue trauma is severe or if hemorrhage has been prolonged, patients develop a marked reduction in functional extracellular volume as a result of the internal redistribution of fluids (third-space losses). Although the extent of tissue manipulation in most routine neurosurgical procedures is small, third-space fluid losses during prolonged surgery and in patients with severe associated systemic trauma can be sufficient to decrease intravascular volume, reduce peripheral perfusion, and impair renal function. The sequestered extracellular fluid can be cautiously replaced with lactated Ringer's solution or with 0.9% saline. In the absence of diuretic therapy, a urinary output of 0.5 to 1 mL/kg/hr suggests adequate replacement, as do hemodynamic stability and cardiac filling pressures within the normal range. Although some clinicians prefer to use colloid-containing solutions in neurosurgical patients, such solutions appear to exert negligible effects on brain water and ICP.[119,120]

Anesthetic Induction and Maintenance

Although induction of anesthesia for patients undergoing craniotomy can be performed with various agents, a smooth and gentle induction of general anesthesia is more important than the drug combination used. No evidence indicates that one technique or set of drugs is better than another. A reasonable induction sequence would combine preoxygenation, thiopental (2 to 4 mg/kg) or propofol (1 to 2 mg/kg), and a nondepolarizing muscle relaxant. No evidence suggests that any of the induction agents (midazolam, etomidate, propofol, and methohexital) is superior to thiopental. The hemodynamic response to intubation may be blunted with the administration of fentanyl (10 to 15 mcg/kg total dose) or lidocaine (1.5 mg/kg) administered 3 minutes before laryngoscopy. The dose of these induction agents may need to be adjusted according to the patient's age and physical status. Whatever agents are selected, the induction should be accomplished without the development of sudden hypertension or hypotension.

The head typically is elevated from 15 to 30 degrees to facilitate venous and CSF drainage. The head may also be turned to the side to facilitate exposure. Excessive neck flexion may impede jugular venous drainage and increase ICP. Because of the flexion-extension-rotation of the head in combination with head fixation in a pinion headrest, the use of an armored or reinforced endotracheal tube (ETT) is recommended to avoid kinking of the tube once positioning is accomplished. The ETT follows the position of the chin. With extension of the neck, the chin and ETT move cephalad; with neck flexion, the chin and ETT move caudad. The anesthesia circuit connections must be firmly secured by simultaneously pushing and twisting to seat the plastic connectors. The risk of unrecognized disconnections may be increased because the operating table is usually turned 90 to 180 degrees away from the anesthetist, and both the patient and the breathing circuit are almost completely covered by surgical drapes.[75]

Maintenance of anesthesia may be accomplished with an oxygen-air-opioid technique, a selected potent inhalation agent, or oxygen-air and a continuous infusion of propofol. After endotracheal intubation, mechanical hyperventilation is begun, decreasing $ETCO_2$ to 25 to 30 mm Hg, confirmed through arterial blood gas analysis. The patient should be covered with blankets or a forced-air warming blanket to maintain core body temperature.

An opioid-based anesthetic technique with air in oxygen with low-dose (less than 1%) isoflurane is a popular choice. Incremental administration of fentanyl, sufentanil, alfentanil, or an infusion of remifentanil is acceptable. Sufentanil as a 0.5 to 1 mcg/kg loading dose, followed by either incremental boluses (not to exceed 0.5 mcg/kg/hr) or an intravenous infusion of 0.25 to 0.5 mcg/kg/hr in combination with less than 1% isoflurane in oxygen may be used. Sufentanil administration should be discontinued approximately 45 minutes before the end of surgery to ensure that the patient awakens promptly. The primary advantage of remifentanil is rapid awakening. If the patient experiences hypertension or tachycardia near the end of surgery, the practitioner should consider giving either labetalol or esmolol, not additional opioids.[139]

A volatile agent (isoflurane, desflurane, or sevoflurane) with little or no opioid supplementation can also be used for maintenance of anesthesia. If isoflurane is used, the concentration should remain less than 1%. Hyperventilation in combination with less than 1% isoflurane generally results in stable intracranial dynamics.[139]

N_2O may be used in an anesthetic regimen if it is deemed desirable. However, if the patient is suspected to have a pneumocephalus or the potential for air embolism exists, N_2O use is contraindicated. N_2O expands both the pneumocephalus and the air embolus. A tension pneumocephalus acts like an expanding mass lesion. A large air embolus can cause cardiovascular collapse.[139]

Hyperventilation is an important adjunct to any neuroanesthetic technique. Hypocapnia decreases ICP before opening of the dura and attenuates the vasodilatation produced by the volatile anesthetic agents. Optimal hyperventilation during surgery would yield a $PaCO_2$ of 25 to 30 mm Hg. Diuretics, when indicated, may be timed just before or after the cranial vault is opened to facilitate surgical exposure.

Skeletal muscle relaxation prevents patient movement at inappropriate times. It may decrease ICP by relaxing the chest wall, decreasing intrathoracic pressure, and facilitating venous drainage. In choosing an agent for muscle relaxation, the length of the procedure and the effect of the drug on ICP should be considered.[139]

Emergence

Arguably, in no other anesthetic situation is careful attention to appropriate planning for the emergence from anesthesia as important as in neurosurgical brain tumor surgery. Sudden emergence from anesthesia can result in uncontrolled hypertension. Delirium with coughing and straining on the endotracheal tube should be avoided. In a patient with a compromised blood-brain barrier, this stormy emergence can produce devastating consequences. Late emergence from anesthesia can result in a confusing diagnostic picture with possible intracranial hematoma, acute hydrocephalus, or other diagnoses masked by the residual anesthesia.[124]

The goal for emergence is control. A controlled emergence focuses on regulation of blood pressure, ICP, and CBF. Controlled emergence also accounts for the preexisting pathophysiology, the surgical trauma, the length of the procedure, and appropriate management of the airway.[124]

Emergence from anesthesia begins when the surgical pathology has been addressed. Collaboration with the surgeon is essential. After the surgeon grants approval, the following strategy can be implemented for emergence. Prior to closing the dura, the appropriate levels of postoperative blood pressure can be determined. The $Paco_2$ should be allowed to return to a normal level. Blood pressure can then be raised to 120% of the normal baseline level prior to closing of the dura. Hypertension is considered a frequent occurrence of the postoperative period.[140-142] Tachycardia associated with hypertension "invariably" results from emergence excitement.[143] By raising the blood pressure and the $Paco_2$ prior to dural closure, the ability of the brain to withstand such challenges can be directly assessed by the surgeon.[124]

Once the dura has been closed, the blood pressure is maintained at baseline levels throughout the remainder of the closure.

There is strong support for the notion that sympatholytic drugs should be used to decrease blood pressure during emergence.[144] Studies have shown that during the first hour after craniotomy for supratentorial lesions, the arteriovenous oxygen content difference is low, suggesting a state of cerebral luxury perfusion.[145,146] This event coincides with a high level of mean arterial blood pressure. Accordingly, it is supposed that this correlation is caused by changes in the mean blood pressure and impaired autoregulation. This may be deleterious, because it enhances blood-brain barrier leakage, provoking edema and hemorrhage.

A relationship between hypertension and postoperative hematoma formation exists.[147] The parameters for these events for each individual patient are unknown. Normal autoregulation of CBF maintains adequate perfusion at mean blood pressures ranging from 50 to 150 torr,[148] but the effects on autoregulation of combinations of anesthetic agents over a prolonged case and under varying temperatures are unknown.[124] Labile hypertension and unstable blood pressure during the perisurgical period may contribute to intracerebral hemorrhage remote from the site of the initial neurosurgical procedure.[149] Given the evidence, and without the need to volume expand and maintain the patient in a hyperdynamic manner, it would seem prudent to institute some form of blood pressure control to provide the most controlled emergence possible.

Judicious titration of short-acting antihypertensives (esmolol, labetalol) has great clinical utility in controlling blood pressure during emergence. When access to the patient is regained, the use of anesthetic gases is discontinued, and the muscle relaxant is reversed. Intravenous lidocaine (1.5 mg/kg) can be given just before suctioning for cough suppression before extubation. Rapid awakening facilitates immediate neurologic assessment and can

generally be expected after a pure opioid-N_2O technique. Delayed awakening may result from residual opioid or remaining end-tidal concentrations of potent inhalation agent. After extubation, the patient is transported to the intensive care unit postoperatively for continued monitoring of neurologic function.[144]

Awake Craniotomy

In a small percentage of patients—those in whom a seizure focus may be suppressed during general anesthesia or may be adjacent to an area of eloquent cortical function—awake craniotomy may be necessary.[150] Sources feel awake craniotomy is the most reliable method to ensure neurologic integrity in cerebral gliomas that infiltrate or come close to the eloquent areas of the brain. Awake craniotomy allows for localization of eloquent cortical areas by electrical stimulation and of epileptic foci through cortical recordings. Continuous monitoring of the functional integrity of the brain in awake patients is inherently protective while surgical removal of the gliomatous tissue is performed.[151] Anesthetic techniques may vary, depending on whether the procedure is for tumor removal or seizure treatment.

Patient Selection

To minimize the risk of intraoperative complications, contraindications for awake craniotomy include developmental delay, lack of maturity, an exaggerated or unacceptable response to pain, a significant communication barrier, and a failure to obtain patient consent. Only those patients with the ability to clearly understand risks and benefits and who, in the opinion of the neurosurgeon and the neuroanesthesiologist, will cooperate during surgery should be considered as candidates for an awake craniotomy.[150] Seizure management should be optimized with acceptable levels of antiepileptic medications verified.

Patient Teaching

The single most important element in the successful awake craniotomy is a highly motivated, well-informed patient. Each step of the procedure is discussed with the patient and family. Special emphasis is paid to prolonged surgical procedure, positioning, head immobility, pain anxiety, monitoring, noise, seizure management, and any individual considerations.

Anesthesia Induction and Maintenance

Upon arrival to the holding area, an intravenous line is established. Preanesthesia medications are administered; they may include antibiotics, steroids, antiemetic prophylaxis, and anticonvulsants as indicated.

In the operating room suite, application of noninvasive monitoring is completed. Last-minute questions are addressed, and the patient is induced with propofol. Some sources use either dexmedetomidine singly or in combination with propofol.[152] After satisfactory general anesthesia is established, a laryngeal mask airway (LMA) is placed, with patient ventilation controlled using a continuous propofol infusion. Invasive monitoring is established (arterial line, central line, urinary catheter). The scalp is anesthetized with 0.5% bupivacaine and the head placed in a pinion head holder. The patient is carefully positioned with all bony surfaces padded and the patient carefully secured to the table to minimize a sense of falling when the table is moved during the awake phase of the surgery. Frameless stereotaxis registration is accomplished. Depending on the preoperative radiographic edema findings, hypertonic saline or mannitol is given. During the draping, an area is constructed around the patient's face such that the face may be clearly seen and accessed.

Clinical Situations Contributing to the Occurrence of Venous Air Embolism

- Patient positioning (seated, prone, steep Trendelenburg)
- Transfusion therapy
- Intravenous therapy
- Central venous catheterization
- Hepatic surgical procedures
- Urologic surgical procedures
- Posterior spinal procedures
- Epidural or caudal catheter insertion
- Bone marrow harvesting
- Laparoscopy
- Radical pelvic surgery

A light is introduced under the drapes to keep the patient from darkness. During the scalp opening, spontaneous ventilation is established. Prior to the bone flap removal, the LMA is removed and verbal contact established.

Awake Phase

All sedation is stopped. All issues regarding patient comfort and concerns are addressed prior to the incision of the dura. Conversation with the patient is confined to the surgeon and one member of the anesthesia team. Stimulation of eloquent areas is carried out with results noted. Any seizures are controlled with propofol, or cold saline is available if needed.[153] Following the stimulation and mapping, volumetric surgical removal of the tumor or seizure focus is accomplished with interval monitoring. Upon completion of the surgical removal and requisite monitoring, propofol sedation may be restarted and titrated to patient preference. Sedation is discontinued upon conclusion of surgery.

The most common complications associated with awake craniotomy are pain, seizures, nausea, and confusion.[154,155]

Posterior Fossa Surgery

Neuropathology within the posterior fossa may impair control of the airway, respiratory function, cardiovascular function, autonomic function, and consciousness. The major motor and sensory pathways, the primary cardiovascular and respiratory centers, the reticular activating system, and the nuclei of the lower cranial nerves are all concentrated in the brainstem. All these structures are contained in a tight space with little room for edema, tumor, or blood.

Venous Air Embolus

In addition to the previously mentioned monitoring modalities, monitoring during posterior fossa surgery requires consideration of patient position and the potential for venous air embolus (VAE). Clinical situations that contribute to the occurrence of VAE are listed in Box 29-3. Air may also be entrained from the cranial pin sites of the Mayfield head holder and from improperly connected vascular lines (arterial, central, and intravenous).

The occurrence of VAE depends on the development of a negative pressure gradient between the operative site and the right side of the heart. As the gradient between the cerebral

veins and the right atrium increases, the potential for air entry increases. The estimated incidence of VAE during neurosurgical procedures ranges from 5% to 50%, with an increased incidence in the sitting position.[156,157]

The physiologic consequences of VAE depend on both the volume and the rate of air entrainment. In the canine model, large cumulative doses of air produce sudden cardiac arrest and death; smaller cumulative doses produce less profound physiologic consequences, including increased pulmonary artery and central venous pressure, decreased cardiac output with accompanying hypotension, progressive hypotension, and dysrhythmias.[158] Despite the potentially devastating effects of VAE, a retrospective review of neurosurgery patients who had appropriate monitoring for the detection of VAE found that VAE contributed to patient morbidity or mortality in only six instances (0.4%).[159-161]

Paradoxical Air Embolism

Paradoxical air embolism (PAE) develops with the entry of air into the systemic circulation. Individuals with an existing anatomic connection between the right and left sides of the heart (atrial or ventricular septal defect, probe-patent foramen ovale) are at risk. A patent foramen ovale may exist in 30% to 35% of the population.[162] If right-sided heart pressures exceed left-sided pressures (a situation that may occur in fluid-restricted neurosurgical patients), systemic air may embolize and enter the arterial circulation through a probe-patent foramen ovale.

Patients who require the sitting position should be carefully evaluated with echocardiograms if the history suggests the presence of an intracardiac defect (presence of heart murmur) or probe-patent foramen ovale. The presence of a probe-patent foramen ovale may be elicited with the injection of contrast material before, during, and after the patient produces a Valsalva maneuver. If the condition is identified, the surgical procedure should be accomplished in an alternative position.

Detection of Venous Air Embolus

The entrainment of air into the vascular system is usually of little consequence, because the lungs serve as effective blood filters.[163] Small bubbles of air are absorbed into the blood or enter the alveoli, where they are eliminated. However, the efficient filtering capacity of the lung may be breached by a large bolus of air or after the administration of a pulmonary vasodilator (e.g., aminophylline), either of which acts to widen the venous-arterial barrier. Air enters the venous circulation as small bubbles that pass through the right side of the heart, entering the pulmonary arterioles. A reflexive sympathetic pulmonary vasoconstriction is produced after the release of endothelial mediators, which are ultimately responsible for the clinical manifestations (pulmonary hypertension, hypoxemia, CO_2 retention, increased dead-space ventilation, and decreased $ETCO_2$). The continued entry of air produces an airlock within the right ventricle, producing right ventricular failure and decreased cardiac output. Altered ventilation-perfusion relationships parallel the hemodynamic changes. Obstructed pulmonary blood flow increases dead-space ventilation, resulting in decreased $ETCO_2$. The entry of a large volume of air in the alveoli may be detected by the sudden appearance of end-tidal nitrogen.

The selection of appropriate monitoring for the detection of VAE is based on the various sensitivities of the available monitoring modalities (Figure 29-18). Precordial Doppler monitoring can detect air entrainment at rates as small as 0.0021 mL/kg/min.[164] The Doppler probe is affixed over the right side of the heart along the right sternal border between

HIGH SENSITIVITY - **LOW SENSITIVITY**

Transesophageal Echocardiography

Doppler

End-tidal CO_2

Pulmonary Artery Catheter

Cardiac Output

Central Venous Pressure

ECG Changes

Blood Pressure

Precordial Stethoscope

SMALL VAE VOLUME - **LARGE VAE VOLUME**

FIGURE **29-18** Sensitivity of venous air embolus (VAE) detection devices. *(From Aker JG. Clinical dilemmas in neuroanesthesia. CRNA. 1995;6:13.)*

the third and sixth intercostal spaces. Proper positioning over the right atrium is confirmed if a change in Doppler signal is elicited when a 10-mL bolus of saline is injected rapidly into a previously placed right central venous catheter.[164-166] Placement of a right atrial catheter affords the means for diagnosis and recovery of intravenous air and also reflects cardiac preload. When a right atrial catheter is placed, it is recommended that either radiographic confirmation or ECG confirmation of proper placement of the catheter tip be obtained.[16] Advantages and disadvantages of selected monitors for detection of VAE are noted in Table 29-7.

Capnography complements the capabilities of the Doppler device, because small, hemodynamically insignificant air emboli detected with the Doppler device can be differentiated from emboli that may produce arterial hypotension.

Transesophageal echocardiography (TEE) is the most sensitive method of air embolism detection, but it is also the most expensive. With TEE, it is possible to observe both cardiac contractility and air bubbles as they pass through the heart.[167] TEE is also capable of detecting PAE in the heart. The detection of a "mill-wheel" murmur via precordial or esophageal stethoscope is a late sign of air entrainment.

Treatment of Venous Air Embolus

Detection of VAE should prompt certain crucial steps (Box 29-4). The surgeon should be notified, and N_2O should be immediately discontinued, 100% oxygen delivered, and the right atrial catheter aspirated.[168] The surgeon should flood the surgical field with irrigation or pack the area with saline-soaked sponges. A Valsalva maneuver or bilateral compression of the jugular veins for 5 to 10 seconds increases the cerebral venous pressure and induced bleeding. The addition of positive end-expiratory pressure also slows air entry. However, 10 to 15 cm H_2O may be required to effectively elevate venous pressure when the head is elevated. The head should be lowered to decrease air entrainment. This may be accomplished by placing the operating table in Trendelenburg position. If air entrainment continues, the

anesthetist should ask for an assistant. A second pair of hands allows simultaneous jugular vein compression and central catheter aspiration.[169,170]

Supportive therapy is required for hemodynamic compromise. Administration of ephedrine, 10 to 20 mg intravenously, and an intravenous fluid bolus improves the blood pressure. If these measures do not restore blood pressure, additional vasopressors (epinephrine) may be required.

Anesthetic agent and technique may influence the rate of air entrainment and the resulting physiologic consequences. The anesthetist should recall the role N_2O may play in the patient at risk for VAE, because N_2O is known to increase the volume of embolized air. Munson and Merrick[168] demonstrated that the expansion of an intravascular air bubble is proportional to the delivered concentration of N_2O. A 50% concentration doubles the initial air-bubble volume, and a 70% concentration quadruples the air-bubble volume.

General endotracheal anesthesia with controlled ventilation is thought to be protective in patients experiencing VAE. Durant and colleagues demonstrated the appearance of a respiratory "gasp" with the onset of VAE in dogs that were spontaneously ventilating. This reflexive gasp may worsen VAE because additional air is entrained into the venous system with the gasping respiration.[171]

Surgical Positioning

Although most posterior fossa explorations may be performed with the patient in either the lateral or prone position, the sitting position (Figure 29-19) is occasionally preferred because the enhanced CSF and venous drainage facilitates surgical exposure. The use of this position, however, has declined dramatically because of the potential for serious complications.[172] The patient is semirecumbent in the standard sitting position with the back elevated to 60 degrees and the legs elevated (with the knees flexed) to the level of the heart. The latter is important for preventing venous pooling and reducing the risk of venous thrombosis. The head is fixed in a three-point head holder

TABLE 29-7	Monitors for Detection of Venous Air Embolism		
Monitor	**Advantages**	**Disadvantages**
Precordial Doppler	Noninvasive Most sensitive noninvasive monitor Earliest detector (before air enters pulmonary circulation)	Nonquantitative May be difficult to place in obese patients, patients with chest wall deformity, or patients in the prone or lateral position False negative result if air does not pass beneath ultrasonic beam (approximately 10% of cases) Useless during electrocautery IV mannitol may mimic intravascular air
Pulmonary artery (PA) catheter	Quantitative slightly more sensitive than $ETCO_2$ Widely available Placed with minimum difficulty in experienced hands Can detect right-atrial pressure more easily than pulmonary capillary wedge pressure	Small lumen, less air aspiration than with right-atrial catheter Placement for optimal air aspiration may not allow pulmonary capillary wedge pressure measurement Nonspecific for air
Capnography ($ETCO_2$)	Noninvasive Sensitive Quantitative Widely available	Nonspecific for air Less sensitive than Doppler, PA catheter Accuracy affected by tachypnea, low cardiac output, chronic obstructive pulmonary disease
End-tidal nitrogen (ETN_2)	Specific for air Detects air earlier than ($ETCO_2$)	May not detect subclinical air embolism May indicate air clearance from pulmonary circulation prematurely Accuracy affected by hypotension
Transesophageal echocardiography (TEE)	Most sensitive detector of air Can detect air in left side of heart and aorta	Invasive, cumbersome Expensive Monitor must be observed continuously Not quantitative May interfere with Doppler

Modified from Smith DS, Osborne I. Posterior fossa: anesthetic considerations. In: Cottrell JE, Smith DS. Anesthesia and Neurosurgery. 4th ed. St Louis: Mosby; 2001:343.
$ETCO_2$, *End-tidal carbon dioxide;* IV, *intravenous.*

BOX 29-4

Therapy for Venous Air Embolism

- Notify surgeon on detection (flood surgical field with saline and wax bone edges).
- Discontinue nitrous oxide administration. Administer 100% oxygen.
- Perform a Valsalva maneuver or compression of jugular veins.
- Aspirate air from atrial catheter.
- Support blood pressure with volume and vasopressors.
- Reposition patient in left lateral decubitus position with a 15-degree head-down tilt if blood pressure continues to decrease.
- Modify the anesthetic as needed to optimize hemodynamics.

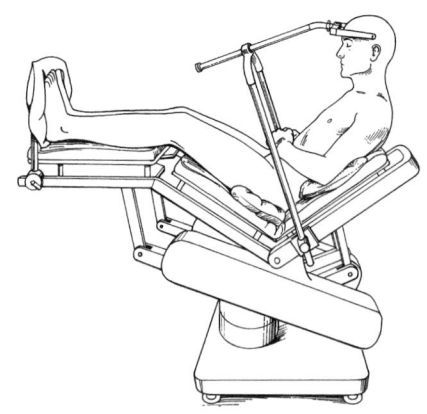

FIGURE **29-19** Representation of a patient properly positioned for seated posterior fossa operation with the knees at heart level and the neck not hyperflexed. (*From Phillips NF. Berry & Kohn's Operating Room Technique. 11th ed. St Louis: Mosby; 2007:794.*)

with the neck in flexion, and the arms remain at the sides with the hands resting on the lap.[75]

Careful positioning is essential to prevent iatrogenic injury. Pressure points such as the elbows, ischial spines, and forehead must be protected with foam padding. Excessive neck flexion has been associated with swelling of the upper airway (venous obstruction) and, rarely, quadriplegia resulting from compression of the cervical spinal cord and decreased cervical cord perfusion when the neck is elevated above the heart. Preexisting cervical spinal stenosis probably predisposes to the latter injury.[75]

Anesthetic Induction, Maintenance, and Emergence

Increased ICP, although common in patients with supratentorial lesions, is less common in patients with posterior fossa lesions. Obstructive hydrocephalus is more typical because CSF outflow is occluded at the level of the aqueduct of Sylvius or fourth ventricle. This can be readily identified preoperatively by magnetic resonance imaging or computed tomography and may be corrected before definitive surgical intervention with the placement of a ventricular catheter. Premedication is contraindicated in patients with obstructive hydrocephalus.

Induction should be slow and deliberate to avoid changes in cerebral perfusion and increased ICP. Because the head is generally flexed and fixed in this position, a wire-reinforced ETT may prevent intraoperative kinking. These tubes may become permanently kinked if the patient is lightly anesthetized and bites the tube. Intravenous fluid administration during posterior fossa surgery should be limited to the infusion of deficit and maintenance quantities of a balanced salt solution. Major volume resuscitation can be accomplished with the infusion of blood, colloid, or crystalloid solutions.

Emergence from anesthesia should be as smooth and gentle as possible. The intraoperative use of opioids facilitates a smooth emergence without significant coughing and bucking. The administration of lidocaine 1.5 mg/kg intravenously decreases the airway irritation of the ETT.[169]

The decision to remove the ETT should be made after the anesthetic course and surgical procedure are reviewed. Intraoperative air embolism may be followed by the development of pulmonary edema. Although this condition is self-limiting, continued mechanical ventilation is the treatment of choice. Consideration must also be given to the possibility of cranial nerve damage during the operative procedure. Provided the patient is safely extubated, continued vigilant observation is essential because airway compromise may develop after injury to cranial nerves IX, X, and XI (Box 29-5).

BOX **29-5**

Postoperative Considerations with Posterior Fossa Surgery

- Central apnea
- Impaired swallowing
- Hypertension
- Cardiac dysrhythmias
- Delayed awakening (brainstem compression)

From Barash PG et al, eds. Handbook of Clinical Anesthesia. *3rd ed. Philadelphia: Lippincott; 1997:392.*

Pituitary Surgery

Approximately 10% of intracranial neoplasms are found in the pituitary gland and come to clinical attention because of their mass effects or the hypersecretion of pituitary hormones. These tumors are rarely metastatic and produce local symptoms via bone invasion, hydrocephalus, and compression of a cranial nerve (most often the optic nerve). Frontotemporal headache and bitemporal hemianopsia are the most common nonendocrine symptoms of enlarging pituitary lesions. Nonsecreting pituitary tumors account for approximately 20% to 50% of lesions in this area and are classified as *chromophobe adenomas*.[172]

Tumors that secrete excess growth hormone produce acromegaly. Increased growth hormone increases the size of the skeleton, particularly the bones and soft tissues of the hands, feet, and face. The enlarged facial structures may increase the likelihood of difficult intubation. Excess growth hormone may also contribute to the development of coronary artery disease, hypertension, and cardiomyopathy. Hyperglycemia is also a common finding, reflecting a growth hormone–induced glucose intolerance.[173]

Surgical Approach

Medical and surgical therapies exist for both functional and nonfunctional pituitary tumors. Transsphenoidal surgery (Figure 29-20) offers several advantages over the intracranial approach. Statistically, morbidity and mortality rates are reduced because of a decrease in blood loss and less manipulation of brain tissue. In addition, the risk of inducing panhypopituitarism and the incidence of permanent diabetes insipidus are both reduced. For patients with large tumors (>10 mm), tumors of uncertain type, and tumors that have substantial extrasellar (beyond the sella turcica) extension, the transsphenoidal approach is inadequate, and a bifrontal intracranial approach is required for successful removal.[173] Current trends are moving toward endoscopic approaches to the pituitary tumor. Less invasive approaches, such as the transnasal approach combined with endoscopic resection of tumor, have been performed. The endoscopic technique entails less morbidity and a shorter hospital stay than the traditional approach.[174]

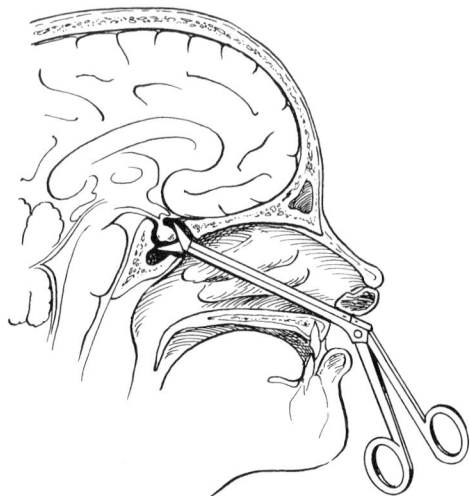

FIGURE **29-20** Transsphenoidal approach to the pituitary gland. *(From Black J, Hawks J.* Medical-Surgical Nursing: Clinical Management for Positive Outcomes. *8th ed. Philadelphia: Saunders; 2009:1829.)*

Preoperative Evaluation

Patients undergo transsphenoidal operations for the treatment of hypersecreting pituitary tumors. Clinical symptoms of pituitary tumors include amenorrhea, galactorrhea, Cushing disease, and acromegaly.

Each preoperative condition has its own constellation of systemic disorders and accompanying effects on intracranial dynamics that must be considered when an anesthetic technique is selected. Pituitary tumors can damage decussating optic fibers, producing blindness in the temporal half of the visual field of both eyes (bitemporal heteronymous hemianopsia). Occasionally, an aneurysm of one of the internal carotid arteries may produce nasal hemianopsia on the affected side. Patients who have Cushing disease may also be affected by hypertension, diabetes, osteoporosis, obesity, and friability of skin and connective tissue. Patients who have acromegaly may have hypertension, cardiomyopathy, diabetes, and osteoporosis, as well as cartilaginous and soft-tissue hypertrophy of the larynx and enlargement of the tongue, complicating intubation of the trachea. Patients who have panhypopituitarism may exhibit hypothyroidism, requiring preoperative thyroid supplementation.

The transsphenoidal approach usually necessitates the head and back to be elevated 10 to 20 degrees. The patient's head is supported by a three-point pin head holder and centered within a C-arm fluoroscopy unit for radiographic control during surgery. The patient's arms are placed at the sides and padded so that injury to the ulnar nerves is avoided. The patient's airway is shared with the surgeon; therefore, great attention must be directed to the proper securing of the ETT and anesthesia circuit to prevent unintended extubation and anesthesia-circuit disconnect. Hyperventilation is avoided after anesthetic induction, because reductions in ICP result in retraction of the pituitary into the sella, making surgical access difficult. The anesthetist should also consider the potential for massive hemorrhage, because the carotid arteries lie adjacent to the suprasellar area and may be inadvertently injured.

When the resection involves the suprasellar area, postoperative endocrine dysfunction may occur, namely diabetes insipidus. Diabetes insipidus that occurs after most transsphenoidal procedures is usually self-limited and resolves within a week to 10 days.[173] Although the onset is usually on the first or second postoperative day, diabetes insipidus may develop during the perioperative period or in the immediate recovery period. Intraoperative diagnosis is made with the sudden onset of diuresis. The diagnosis may be confirmed with concurrent urine and serum osmolalities. If diabetes insipidus persists or if it becomes difficult to match urinary losses, the patient may receive aqueous vasopressin (Pitressin) or desmopressin (DDAVP). Intravenous DDAVP is longer acting and is not associated with the coronary vasoconstriction that follows administration of aqueous vasopressin.

Anesthetic Induction, Maintenance, and Emergence

After anesthetic induction and intubation, the ETT is typically moved to the left corner of the patient's mouth and secured to the chin with adhesive and tape. A right-angled ETT may be effective because such tubes are pre-bent and curve along the mandible when exiting the mouth. The esophageal stethoscope and temperature probe are inserted and secured on the lower left as well, leaving the upper lip totally exposed. An orogastric tube is placed, aspirated, and then put to gravity drainage during the procedure. The oropharynx is then packed with moist cotton gauze. The eyes are first taped closed and then covered with cotton-padded adhesive patches to prevent corneal abrasion and seepage of cleansing solution and blood into the eyes.

Thiopental, propofol, an opioid (either fentanyl, sufentanil, alfentanil, or remifentanil), and a neuromuscular relaxant (either succinylcholine or a nondepolarizing neuromuscular relaxant for intubation, followed by a selected nondepolarizing agent), with a combination of air and oxygen is a commonly used anesthetic combination for this procedure. Isoflurane may be added in low concentrations for blood pressure control; alternatively, it may be used as the primary anesthetic drug. Halothane is contraindicated because of its potential for inducing ventricular dysrythmia after infiltration of the oral and nasal mucosa with epinephrine-containing local anesthetics and the application of cocaine-soaked pledgets.[175]

The topical use of cocaine and the oral and nasal submucosal injection of local anesthetic solutions containing epinephrine help constrict gingival and mucosal vessels and dissect the nasal mucosa away from the cartilaginous septum. Epinephrine use may produce hypertension or dysrhythmias or both. Cocaine interferes with the intraneuronal uptake of catecholamine and can augment both the hypertensive and dysrhythmogenic properties of epinephrine. The use of epinephrine is relatively safe if (1) halothane is avoided, (2) ventilation is adequate, (3) epinephrine is given in combination with lidocaine instead of saline, (4) epinephrine concentrations of 1:100,000 to 1:200,000 are used, and (5) total dose does not exceed 10 mL of 1:100,000 solution in 10 minutes for a 70-kg adult. A total dose of 200 mg of cocaine should not be exceeded. Persistent dysrhythmias may require treatment with lidocaine or possibly a β-blocker. Hypertension may be controlled with an increased concentration of the selected inhalation agent or with small intravenous doses of hydralazine, labetalol, or esmolol.[175,176]

In some cases, it may be necessary to insert a catheter into the lumbar subarachnoid space to facilitate the injection of preservative-free saline to delineate the suprasellar margins or for prevention of CSF leak postoperatively. If air is injected, N_2O must be discontinued from the anesthetic mixture because of rapid diffusion into the air present in the closed cranial vault.[176]

Emergence from anesthesia should be conducted as described for the previously discussed procedures. Intravenous lidocaine, 1.5 mg/kg given approximately 3 minutes before suctioning and extubation, decreases coughing, straining, and hypertension. Postoperatively, patients should be responsive to commands in the recovery room. Steroid therapy is continued throughout this period and tapered over time, if appropriate.

Cerebrovascular Surgery

Cerebral Aneurysms

Cerebral aneurysms are abnormal, localized dilations of the intracranial arteries. They are classified as berry or saccular, mycotic, traumatic, fusiform, neoplastic, or atherosclerotic. Rupture of a saccular aneurysm is a leading cause of subarachnoid hemorrhage (SAH).[177]

Approximately 5 million people in North America have cerebral aneurysms, with approximately 30,000 new cases of SAH occurring annually. The peak age for rupture of a cerebral aneurysm is 55 to 60 years. A slight female predilection also exists, with aneurysmal rupture occurring in three women for every two men.[178]

More than a third of patients with SAH die or develop significant and lasting neurologic disabilities before they receive any treatment. A small bleed occurs in approximately 50% of patients and is often tragically ignored or misdiagnosed.

TABLE **29-8**	Location and Occurrence of Cerebral Aneurysms
Location	**Occurrence (%)**
Internal carotid	38
Anterior cerebral system	36
Anterior communicating junction	30
Internal carotid at posterior communicating junction	25
Middle cerebral system	21
Vertebrobasilar system	5

From Frost AEM. Management of neurosurgical anesthesia: aneurysms. Curr Rev Clin Anesth. 1991;11:125-132. Used with permission of Current Reviews.

TABLE **29-9**	Hunt's Classification of Patients with Intracranial Aneurysms According to Surgical Risk	
Grade	**Perioperative Criterion**	**Mortality Rate (%)**
I	Asymptomatic or minimal headache and slight nuchal rigidity	0-5
II	Moderate to severe headache, nuchal rigidity, no neurologic deficit, possible cranial nerve palsy	2-10
III	Drowsiness, confusion, or mild focal deficit	10-15
IV	Stupor, moderate to severe hemiparesis, possibly early decerebrate rigidity and vegetative disturbances	60-70
V	Deep coma, decerebrate rigidity, moribund appearance	70-100

From Hunt WE, Hess RM. Surgical risk as related to time of intervention in the repair of intracranial aneurysms. J Neurosurg. 1968;28:14.

Even in patients who receive prompt care, only half remain functional survivors; the remainder die or develop serious neurologic deficits.[179]

Aneurysms may arise at any point in the circle of Willis. The most common locations for the occurrence of aneurysms are shown in Table 29-8. Most aneurysms are broad based and located in the middle cerebral system. Traumatic aneurysms develop as a result of direct trauma to an artery, with injury to the wall.

Mirror aneurysms of the internal carotid system are common, and other combinations of locations occur. The site of the bleeding aneurysm is best located by computed tomography studies, evidence of vasospasm in the immediate vicinity, and lobulation of the aneurysm wall on angiographic studies.[177]

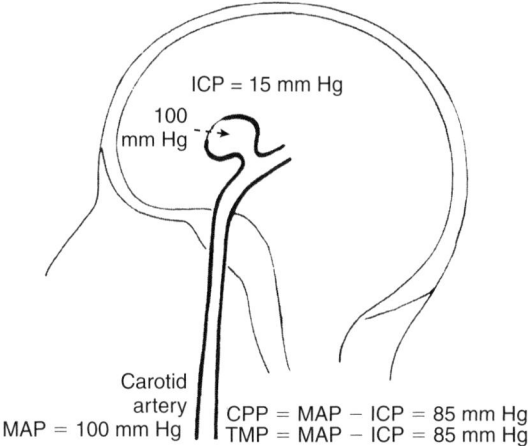

FIGURE **29-21** Transmural pressure (TMP) of the aneurysm. TMP is the same as the cerebral perfusion pressure (CPP) and is equal to the difference between mean arterial pressure (MAP) and intracranial pressure (ICP). *(From Newfield P, Cottrell JE, eds. Neuroanesthesia: Handbook of Clinical and Physiologic Essentials. 2nd ed. Boston: Little, Brown; 1991:195.)*

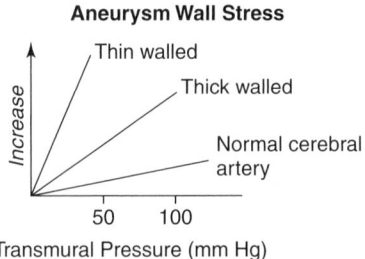

FIGURE **29-22** Aneurysm wall stress. Wall tension divided by wall thickness equals aneurysm wall stress. The relationship between transmural pressure and wall stress is linear: the thinner the wall, the greater the wall stress at any given pressure. *(From Newfield P, Cottrell JE, eds. Neuroanesthesia: Handbook of Clinical and Physiologic Essentials. 2nd ed. Boston: Little, Brown; 1991:195.)*

Diagnosis of Subarachnoid Hemorrhage

SAH produces an abrupt, intense headache in 85% of patients, and transient loss of consciousness may be seen in up to 45% of patients. Nausea and vomiting, photophobia, fever, meningismus, and focal neurologic deficits are not uncommon. The severity of a SAH can be graded clinically with the use of classifications developed by either Botterell or Hunt (Table 29-9). Although surgical mortality rates vary somewhat among institutions, patients with a neurologic grade I SAH generally undergo surgical clipping with a low mortality rate (less than 5%), whereas grade V patients generally do not survive.[179]

General Considerations

Hypertension often accompanies acute SAH and is postulated to develop secondary to autonomic hyperactivity, which may increase transmural pressure in the aneurysmal sac. *Transmural pressure* is defined as the differential pressure between MAP and ICP and represents the stress applied to the aneurysm's wall (Figures 29-21 and 29-22).[179]

Increases in blood pressure directly increase the transmural pressure and the likelihood of bleeding; conversely, reductions in blood pressure reduce transmural pressure. Caution should be exercised when purposefully reducing transmural pressure because cerebral autoregulation may be impaired after SAH, and a reduction in blood pressure may induce or aggravate cerebral ischemia, particularly if vasospasm is present. To balance these opposing concerns, many neurosurgeons attempt to maintain systolic blood pressure between 120 and 150 mm Hg before clipping the aneurysm.[179]

ECG changes are common after SAH and have been reported to occur in 50% to 80% of patients. The most common changes involve the T wave or the ST segment, but other changes such as the presence of a U wave, QTc interval prolongation and dysrhythmias may be present. Whether such changes in the ECG represent myocardial injury has long been debated. In the majority of patients, these changes do not appear to be associated with adverse neurologic or cardiac outcomes.[178,179]

Rebleeding from a previously ruptured aneurysm is a life-threatening complication. The incidence of rebleeding is approximately 50% in the first days after SAH, and rebleeding is associated with an 80% mortality rate.[180] The chance of rebleeding from an unsecured aneurysm declines over time; by 6 months, the risk stabilizes at approximately 3% per year. Approaches used to decrease the risk of rebleeding include early surgical clipping, the use of antifibrinolytic agents, and blood pressure control.[179,181]

Vasospasm

Vasospasm is reactive narrowing of cerebral arteries after SAH. Although arterial narrowing may be detected with angiography in 60% of patients, only half of these patients develop clinical symptoms. The accompanying neurologic deterioration, arising from impaired cerebral perfusion, ischemia, and secondary infarction of the brain, peaks between the fourth and ninth day after SAH and resolves over the next 2 to 3 weeks.[181]

Vasospasm and the ensuing delayed ischemic deficit are thought to result from several factors. First, direct trauma to vessels or mechanical distortion or displacement from the hemorrhage itself produces localized, short-lived spasm. Second, spasmogenic substances, such as oxyhemoglobin, may be present in the subarachnoid blood; the effects of these substances may be mediated by free radicals. Because of their high serotonin content, platelets are also spasmogenic.[182] Third, prostaglandins synthesized by platelets and brain tissue as a response to injury are known to produce prolonged arterial constriction when given intrathecally to laboratory animals. Fourth, mediators of the inflammatory response (eicosanoids, circulating immune complexes, complement activators) may have a role in vasospasm.[183]

Successful treatment of vasospasm depends on maintaining adequate CPP. This is accomplished by expanding intravascular volume (which augments blood pressure and cardiac output), avoiding hyponatremia, and preserving relative hemodilution (hematocrit approximately 32%).[183] Because of the risk of rebleeding, both hypertension and hypervolemia are used with caution in the period preceding surgical correction. Deliberate intraoperative hypotensive techniques are common. Postoperative hypertension is not treated aggressively and at times is encouraged.

Pharmacologic vasodilation of spastic vessels has been ineffective because vasospasm involves a structural alteration in the vessel wall rather than just a spastic contracture or failure of relaxation of the smooth muscle cells in the media of the vessels. Nimodipine and nicardipine, calcium channel blockers, are currently in wide use for preventing delayed neurologic deficit after SAH. They diminish the level of myoplastic calcium in smooth muscle cells and impede the entry of extracellular calcium necessary for the contraction of smooth muscle.[184-186] Recent literature supports a role for magnesium in possible vasospasm prophylaxis.[187,188]

Timing of Surgery

The presence or absence of vasospasm on angiographic studies has frequently determined the timing of aneurysmal surgery. Current neurosurgical practice suggests that a good outcome is achieved with early operation (within 24 to 48 hours) in patients who are neurologically intact (grades I or II), regardless of whether vasospasm has been demonstrated. Such emergency intervention decreases the likelihood of rebleeding. Only 53% of grade III patients achieve a good outcome after early surgery; this indicates that the gross neurologic condition preoperatively is the best prognostic indicator of intact survival.[177,180] In the first few days after hemorrhage, the brain is swollen, soft, hyperemic, and prone to contusion and laceration. Impaired autoregulation may decrease cerebral tolerance to brain retraction. Although removal of a subarachnoid clot probably decreases the incidence and severity of delayed arterial narrowing, clearly, operative management may be hazardous. In more severely injured patients (grades III through V), surgery is often delayed in anticipation of resolution of vasospasm and improvement in neurologic status.[177,189]

Endovascular coiling has been used increasingly as an alternative to neurosurgical clipping for treating SAH secondary to aneurysm rupture.[190] This has led some authors to conclude that endovascular obliteration by means of platinum spirals (coiling) is the preferred mode of treatment.[191] But coiling is not without its problems, as noted in the increased rate of recanalization. The most recent study on unruptured aneurysms treated with endovascular coiling concludes that compared with microvascular clipping, the rate of recanalization of unruptured intracranial aneurysms is higher after endovascular obliteration. With regard to ruptured intracranial aneurysms, the international subarachnoid aneurysm trial of neurosurgical clipping versus endovascular coiling in 2143 patients with ruptured intracranial aneurysms concluded that in patients with ruptured intracranial aneurysms suitable for both treatments, endovascular coiling is more likely to result in independent survival at 1 year than neurosurgical clipping; the survival benefit continues for at least 7 years. The risk of late rebleeding is low but is more common after endovascular coiling than after neurosurgical clipping.[192,193]

Preoperative Evaluation

The baseline neurologic status must be ascertained. The level of consciousness may vary from perfect alertness to deep coma and is an important prognostic factor for the postoperative state. Evidence of increased ICP should be elicited preoperatively so it can be managed appropriately. Focal motor and sensory signs may indicate intracerebral extension of SAH, vasospasm, or cerebral edema.[179]

Pulmonary complications, such as pneumonia, neurogenic pulmonary edema, and atelectasis, are not uncommon and are potentially treatable. Patients often have an increased risk of aspiration because of their depressed level of consciousness, and measures should be taken to reduce gastric acidity and volume preoperatively. The use of prophylactic hypervolemia also increases the likelihood of pulmonary edema.[179]

The hemodynamic status of the patient should be assessed, with particular attention paid to the relationship between neurologic deterioration and blood pressure changes. Continuous arterial blood pressure monitoring is essential. Serious dysrhythmias or evidence of ventricular dysfunction should be diagnosed preoperatively so appropriate monitoring and management can be instituted.[194]

The syndrome of inappropriate antidiuretic hormone and diabetes insipidus can occur in patients with subarachnoid hemorrhage.

The presence of blood in the subarachnoid space may produce a $1°$ C to $2°$ C elevation of body temperature. Temperature elevation increases cerebral oxygen requirements and therefore should be treated to prevent an increase of cerebral ischemia.[179,181]

Preoperative sedation is rarely necessary in these patients. Depression of ventilation associated with opioids, barbiturates, and benzodiazepines may result in hypercapnia, with resultant increases in CBF and ICP. Additionally, the reduced level of consciousness preoperatively and postoperatively may make clinical assessment difficult. Preoperative anxiety is not a problem in patients with a depressed level of consciousness (grades III through V), so sedation is not required. In awake patients, a reassuring preoperative visit usually allays anxiety. If preoperative sedation is considered necessary, the best choice is probably a small dose of a benzodiazepine (midazolam), with continued observation after its administration.

Anesthetic Induction, Maintenance, and Emergence

Maintaining adequate intravascular volume requires two large-bore intravenous cannulas. Intraoperative monitoring includes continuous ECG (V_5), arterial pressure monitoring, peripheral nerve stimulator, central venous pressure monitoring, EEG, ETCO$_2$ monitoring, pulse oximetry, and monitoring of temperature and fluid balance.[195]

The anesthetic induction should be slow and deliberate. The anesthetic depth should be sufficient to avoid the hypertensive responses that accompany laryngoscopy and endotracheal intubation. Anesthesia is induced with titrated doses of either thiopental or propofol. The addition of an opioid (5 to 10 mcg/kg of fentanyl or 1 to 2 mcg/kg of sufentanil) and intravenous lidocaine (1.5 mg/kg) further blunts the patient's response to the sympathetic stimulation of laryngoscopy and intubation. An additional dose of opioid or thiopental is required for the placement of the three-point pin head holder. Prior injection of local anesthetic minimizes the associated sympathetic stimulation. Epinephrine should not be included with the local anesthetic because delayed absorption (up to 30 minutes after injection) may produce significant increases in blood pressure. Isoflurane may be introduced after hyperventilation before laryngoscopy to increase the depth of anesthesia. Ventilation is controlled with administration of 100% oxygen to achieve a Paco$_2$ of 35 to 40 mm Hg with normal intracranial compliance. Mild hyperventilation (Paco$_2$ of 25 to 30) is instituted when intracranial compliance is impaired.[179]

Succinylcholine produces moderate increases in ICP.[196-198] Elevation of serum potassium sufficient to produce lethal dysrhythmias has been reported in comatose, nonparetic, head-injured patients and in patients after SAH who received succinylcholine. Alternatively, intubation can be accomplished with 1 mg/kg of rocuronium.

The patient is placed in one of several positions, depending on the site of the aneurysm. Aneurysms that arise from the anterior part of the circle of Willis require that the patient be supine for a frontotemporal approach. The lateral position for a temporal approach is required for aneurysms that arise from the posterior aspect of the basilar artery. Aneurysms that arise from the vertebral artery or from the lower basilar artery require a sitting or prone position for a suboccipital approach. Aneurysms that arise from the anterior communicating artery are usually approached from the right and those from the middle cerebral and posterior communicating arteries are approached from the side on which the aneurysm is located.[199]

Anesthesia is maintained with air and oxygen or N$_2$O in oxygen, with incremental titrated dosages of an opioid (fentanyl, alfentanil, or sufentanil) or an infusion of remifentanil and a muscle relaxant. Isoflurane may also be added in inspired concentrations not to exceed 1%. Patients who have intracranial aneurysms require precise intraoperative control of blood pressure to prevent rebleeding and counteract vasospasm.[200] In addition, controlled hypotension is commonly used intraoperatively to make aneurysms softer and more pliable at the time of clipping, as well as to minimize blood loss should aneurysmal rupture occur at this time.[178] Sodium nitroprusside and an inhalation anesthetic agent are the drugs most widely used for induction or hypotension.[200]

The safe limit of controlled hypotension has not been definitively established. Because autoregulation is maintained to a MAP of 50 to 60 mm Hg, some argue that this limit should not be exceeded. In addition, because patients with poor-grade aneurysms may not have intact autoregulation, some argue that a lower limit of 60 mm Hg should be adopted. Limits of autoregulation are shifted to higher pressures in patients with preexisting hypertension, so decreases in MAP should probably be limited to no more than 40% of preoperative values.[179]

Rather than induce hypotension to facilitate clip ligation of the neck of the aneurysm, many neurosurgeons now routinely use temporary proximal occlusion of the parent vessel.[201]

The use of mild intraoperative hypothermia has been advocated for cerebral protection during periods of temporary occlusion.[202] Deliberate mild hypothermia was first used in 1955 as an intraoperative technique to ameliorate new neurologic deficits following cerebral aneurysm clipping. Subsequently, it was also used following neonatal asphyxia, head trauma, and cardiac arrest. The Intraoperative Hypothermia for Aneurysm Surgery Trial (IHAST II) was a randomized control trial designed to evaluate the effectiveness of mild hypothermia in decreasing neurologic deficits following aneurysm surgery. Intraoperative hypothermia did not improve the neurologic outcome after craniotomy among good-grade patients with aneurysmal subarachnoid hemorrhage.[203]

At the conclusion of the anesthetic procedure, patients with good-grade aneurysms may be extubated in the operating room, although care must be exercised so that coughing, straining, hypercarbia, and hypertension are avoided. Propofol, lidocaine, or small doses of fentanyl may be used for short-term anesthesia as the procedure is being finished and for reducing the hemodynamic responses to extubation. Although the residual depressant effects of opioids may be reversed with judicious titrated dosages of naloxone, larger doses of naloxone can be hazardous in that they may cause sudden, violent awakening of the patient and marked increases in systemic blood pressure. Endotracheal tubes should be retained in patients with poor-grade aneurysms and in those who have had intraoperative complications; these patients will probably require postoperative ventilation.[181]

Postoperative Care

Postoperative care is directed at the prevention of vasospasm via the maintenance of intravascular volume expansion and moderate hypertension (MAP of 80 to 120 mm Hg). Changes in the level of consciousness and development of focal neurologic deficits are usually early signs of vasospasm. These clinical signs should be aggressively managed with hypertension, hypervolemia, and hemodilution. Dopamine may be used for blood pressure support. Computed tomography should be used for ruling out other causes of neurologic deterioration, including rebleeding, infarction, and hydrocephalus.[181]

Aneurysmal Rupture

Intraoperative aneurysmal rupture can be catastrophic. An abrupt increase in blood pressure during or after induction of anesthesia may indicate that an aneurysm has bled. The use of 100 to 200 mg of thiopental or 0.5 to 1 mcg/kg of sodium nitroprusside decreases the transmural pressure of the aneurysm, although hypotension can be detrimental at this juncture. Intraoperative aneurysmal rupture necessitates maintaining the MAP between 40 and 50 mm Hg or lower to facilitate surgical control of the neck of the aneurysm or the parent vessel. Alternatively, one or both carotid arteries may be compressed for up to 3 minutes to produce a bloodless field. Blood that is lost should be continuously replaced with blood, blood products, or colloid solution so that intravascular volume is maintained.[181]

Although barbiturates have been used for protection against focal cerebral ischemia, their efficacy has not been demonstrated in this clinical situation. Some practitioners advocate the administration of thiopental (3 to 5 mg/kg) before temporary clipping.[204]

Arteriovenous Malformation

Arteriovenous malformations are congenital intracerebral networks in which arteries flow directly into veins. Patients with these malformations generally are younger than those with aneurysms. They may have bleeding or seizures or less commonly ischemia resulting from "steal" from normal areas or occurring with high-output congestive heart failure. The anesthetic problems parallel those associated with patients undergoing aneurysm surgery. Notably, arteriovenous malformations do not autoregulate their blood flow. The operation is likely to be longer and bloodier than that of aneurysm clipping. Surgery may be preceded by an attempt at embolization by the neuroradiologist to diminish the risk of surgery. The neurologic examination should be repeated after embolization to document new deficits that otherwise might be attributed to anesthesia and surgery.

Head Trauma

Head injuries are a contributory factor in up to 50% of deaths resulting from trauma. Most patients with head trauma are young, and many (10% to 40%) have associated intraabdominal injuries, long-bone fractures, or both. The significance of a head injury is dependent not only on the extent of the irreversible neuronal damage at the time of injury but also on the occurrence of any secondary insults. Additional insults include systemic factors such as hypoxemia, hypercapnia, and hypotension; the formation and expansion of an epidural, subdural, or intracerebral hematoma; and sustained intracranial hypertension (Box 29-6). Studies suggest that sustained increases in ICP of approximately 60 mm Hg

---

BOX 29-6

Peripheral Sequelae of Head Trauma

Cardiopulmonary
Abnormal breathing patterns
Airway obstruction
Hypoxia
Shock
Adult respiratory distress syndrome
Neurogenic pulmonary edema
Electrocardiographic changes
Hematologic
Disseminated intravascular coagulation
Endocrinologic
Diabetes insipidus
Syndrome of inappropriate antidiuretic hormone
Skeletal
Cervical spine injury
Maxillofacial injuries

Modified from Newfield P, Cottrell JE, eds. Neuroanesthesia: Handbook of Clinical and Physiologic Essentials. *2nd ed. Boston: Little, Brown; 1991:301.*

---

result in irreversible brain edema. Surgical and anesthetic management of these patients is directed at preventing secondary insults.[75] Types of cerebral hematomas are illustrated in Figure 29-23.

Preoperative Management

Emergency therapy for head injury should begin before hospital admission, because a large proportion of deaths occur in the prehospital phase. Therapy is based on prevention of secondary brain injury resulting from hypoxia, hypercapnia, hypotension, and expanding intracranial masses.

Airway Management

Measures to ensure airway patency, adequacy of ventilation and oxygenation, and the correction of systemic hypotension should be instituted simultaneously with neurologic evaluation. Airway obstruction and hypoventilation are common. Up to 70% of head-injured patients have concurrent hypoxemia, which may be complicated by pulmonary contusion, fat emboli, or neurogenic pulmonary edema. All patients must be assumed to have a cervical spine injury (10% incidence) until disproved by radiography. Axial traction to maintain the head in a neutral position should be used during airway instrumentation. Fiberoptic intubation may be preferred for airway management in some cases. Patients with obvious hypoventilation, absence of the gag reflex, or a persistent total score below 7 on the Glasgow Coma Scale (Table 29-10) require tracheal intubation and hyperventilation. A modified coma scale for infants is given in Table 29-11 and outlines response patterns seen after neurologic injuries. All other patients should be carefully observed for deterioration. Table 29-12 summarizes respiratory patterns seen with various neurologic injuries. The Glasgow Coma Scale score generally correlates well with the severity of injury and outcome.[75]

When intubation is indicated, the oral route provides the most efficient means of safely securing the airway. Whenever possible, a modified, rapid-sequence endotracheal intubation

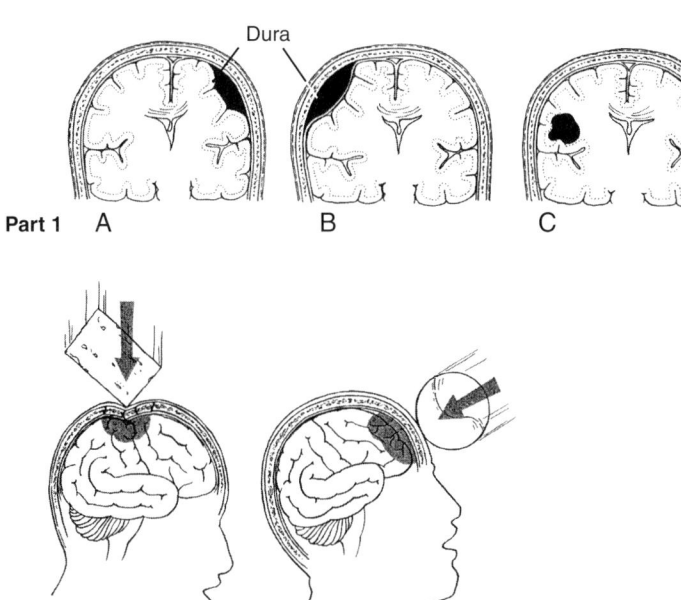

FIGURE **29-23** **Part 1:** Types of hematomas. **A,** Subdural hematoma. **B,** Epidural hematoma. **C,** Intracerebral hematoma. **Part 2:** Mechanisms of head injury. **A,** Direct injury resulting in depressed skull fracture and compression injury. **B,** Blow to skull resulting in tearing of blood vessels. Shaded areas represent cerebral contusion. *(Part 1 from Clochesy J et al. Critical Care Nursing. 2nd ed. Philadelphia: Saunders; 1996; Part 2 from Luckman J, Sorensen KC. Medical-Surgical Nursing: A Psychophysiologic Approach. 3rd ed. Philadelphia: Saunders; 1987.)*

TABLE **29-10**	Glasgow Coma Scale Scoring System
Parameter	**Score**
Eye Opening	
Spontaneously	4
To command	3
To pain	2
No response	1
Motor Response	
Obeys verbal command	6
Localizes pain	5
Flexion withdrawal	4
Decorticate rigidity	3
Decerebrate rigidity	2
No response	1
Verbal Response	
Oriented and converses	5
Disoriented and converses	4
Inappropriate words	3
Incomprehensible words	2
No response	1

TABLE **29-11**	Modified Coma Scale for Infants
Response	**Score**
Eye Opening	
Spontaneous	4
To speech	3
To pain	2
None	1
Verbal Response	
Coos, babbles	5
Irritable cries	4
Cries to pain	3
Moans to pain	2
None	1
Motor Response	
Normal spontaneous movement	6
Withdraws to touch	5
Withdraws to pain	4
Abnormal flexion	3
Abnormal extension	2
None	1

should be performed; that is, it should be preceded by a period of 100% oxygen administration and hyperventilation supplemented by continuous cricoid pressure.[205-207] Nasal intubation should be avoided in the presence of suspected basilar skull fracture, bleeding diathesis, suspected upper-airway foreign body, or severe facial fractures.[205] If a difficult intubation is anticipated,

awake intubation, fiberoptic techniques, or tracheostomy may be necessary.

Cardiovascular Assessment
Multisystem trauma frequently accompanies head injury. Hypotension results from intravascular loss from associated injuries.

688 UNIT V INTRAOPERATIVE MANAGEMENT

TABLE 29-12 Respiratory Patterns

Pattern	Description	Location of Injury and Other Causes
Cheyne-Stokes respiration	Regular increase in the rate and depth of breathing that peaks and is followed by a decreasing rate and depth of breathing, which progresses to apnea; then the cycle repeats itself	Bilateral dysfunction of cerebral hemispheres Midbrain and upper pons
Central neurogenic hyperventilation	Deep, rapid, and regular pattern of breathing	Low midbrain and upper pons Increased intracranial pressure with head trauma
Apneusis breathing	A pause at full inspiration occurs; may see prolonged inspiratory pause alternating with prolonged expiratory pause	Mid and low pons Hypoglycemia, anoxia, and meningitis
Cluster breathing	Periodic breathing with frequent apneic episodes	Low pons and high medulla
Ataxic breathing	Irregular breathing with shallow, deep respirations and irregular apneic episodes; usually slow	Medulla

From Drain CB. Care of the neurosurgical patient. In Drain CB, Odom-Forren J. eds. Perianesthesia Nursing. 5th ed. St Louis: Saunders; 2009:574.

These injuries must be identified and treated early in the resuscitative period. Fluid resuscitation is facilitated by the administration of isotonic fluid, either normal saline or lactated Ringer's solution, or colloids if blood is not readily available. Glucose in water should not be used because it decreases serum osmolarity and can aggravate cerebral swelling. The ideal replacement fluid, of course, is blood. Because the cerebral vessels are already dilated from hypotension, rapid restoration of the normal arterial pressure precipitates brain swelling. It is extremely valuable to insert an ICP monitor during resuscitation for the monitoring of both systemic arterial pressure and ICP.[205] Dysrhythmias and ECG abnormalities in the T wave, U wave, ST segment, and QT interval are common after head injuries but are not necessarily associated with cardiac injury.[75]

Coagulopathies

Chronic Subdural Hematoma. Bridging veins run between the dura and the surface of the brain. A subdural hematoma develops when these veins tear and leak blood, usually as the result of a head injury. A collection of blood then forms over the surface of the brain. In a chronic subdural collection, the problem is not discovered immediately, and blood leaks from the veins slowly over time. A subdural hematoma is more common in the elderly because normal brain shrinkage occurs with aging that stretches and weakens the bridging veins. Thus these veins are more likely to break in the elderly, even after a minor head injury. Rarely, a subdural hematoma can occur spontaneously. Risks include head injury, old age, chronic use of aspirin or antiinflammatory drugs such as ibuprofen, anticoagulant medication, chronic heavy alcohol use, or many diseases associated with blood-clotting problems.[208]

A recent study of 713 emergency referrals documented over 90 days evaluated the effect of antithrombotic therapy on neurosurgical emergency referral. Of the 713 patients, 174 (24.4%) were discovered to have intracranial or spinal hemorrhage, and 75 (43.1%) of these were on antithrombotic therapy. Seventeen of the 75 (22.6%) had no documented indication for antithrombotic therapy (all of these were on aspirin therapy), and 9 of the 29 on warfarin (31%) had an INR in excess of 3.5 on presentation.[209]

The key elements in dealing with coagulation abnormalities in patients presenting for emergent/urgent neurosurgery are (1) identify the coagulopathy, (2) implement a plan that allows for optimum coagulation status given the comorbidities of the patient, and (3) time the period of optimum coagulation to coincide with the conclusion of surgery and the immediate postoperative period.

The coincidence of coagulopathy and chronic subdural hematoma requires correction of coagulation to facilitate surgery.[210] Forty-two percent of 114 patients presenting for drainage of chronic subdural hematoma were found to have coagulation disorders prior to surgery. Addressing coagulopathies in the geriatric population is a situation best addressed by a multidisciplinary approach. The primary problem in this population has to do with limited vascular space that may not be able to accommodate the volume of blood products necessary for reversal in an urgent/emergent fashion. For example, studies suggest that 10 to 17 mL/kg of fresh frozen plasma is necessary to reverse coumadin toxicity.[211] This may not be a reasonable option in the face of imminent surgery. The Mayo Clinic asked seven experts on clinical stroke, neurologic intensive care, and hematology to address three scenarios for dealing with reversal of warfarin in patients with intracranial hemorrhage. All experts agreed that anticoagulation should be urgently reversed, but how to achieve it varied from the use of prothrombin complex concentrates only (three experts), to recombinant factor VIIa only (two experts), to recombinant factor VIIa along with fresh frozen plasma (one expert), to prothrombin complex concentrates and fresh frozen plasma (one expert).[212] Although a universally accepted treatment remains to be identified, the options available provide anesthesia providers with a number of options for treating warfarin toxicity that limit the fluid loads associated with fresh frozen plasma.

The broadening use of recombinant factor VIIa in treating active or impending bleeding in brain injury has led some to conclude that the compartmentalized mode of action of recombinant factor VIIa, along with its good safety profile and Intracerebral Hemorrhage Trial results, provide encouraging data to justify its off-label use in selected patients in the presence of any coagulopathy.[213]

Reversal of clopidogrel, aspirin, or aspirin plus clopidogrel may be addressed by platelet administration. Alternatively, recombinant factor VIIa has been shown to reverse the inhibitory effects of aspirin or aspirin plus clopidogrel and could be useful for bleeding complications or when acute surgery is needed during treatment with these antiplatelet drugs.[214]

Severe brain injury initiates the outpouring of tissue thromboplastin and activation of the complement system, causing disseminated intravascular coagulopathy and fibrinolysis and precipitating the development of adult respiratory distress syndrome. Early recognition of abnormal prothrombin and partial thromboplastin times is crucial. Prompt therapy with fresh frozen plasma, cryoprecipitate, whole blood, and if necessary, platelets may abort the development of disseminated intravascular coagulopathy.[207,208]

Increased Intracranial Pressure

The clinical appreciation of elevated ICP is difficult in unconscious patients. Therefore, initial therapy is directed toward lowering ICP or at least toward preventing further increases in ICP. Simple maneuvers such as using a head-up tilt of 15 to 20 degrees to keep the head in the midline position and not rotated to either side (to ensure jugular vein patency), avoiding overhydration, maintaining normovolemia, and maintaining normal (rather than increased) arterial pressure all help control ICP.[206]

In patients in whom intracranial hypertension is suspected, whether from an epidural or subdural hematoma or from diffuse brain swelling, emergency treatment directed at reducing ICP is the rational course. Ideally, a definitive study for identifying the cause of clinical deterioration is performed before therapy. The first and most rapidly effective therapy is hyperventilation. In a patient with multiple trauma and reduced blood volume, care must be taken during controlled ventilation to avoid increasing the intrathoracic pressure, decreasing venous return, and producing secondary hypotension. Corticosteroids (dexamethasone or methylprednisolone) are of little benefit in trauma, and these drugs must not be relied on to lower the ICP rapidly.[215]

Although mannitol effectively lowers the ICP minutes after administration, its use remains controversial. The drug is indicated, however, when either elevated ICP or a mass and herniation are responsible for the patient's deteriorating state. The risk of increasing the size of a hematoma is negligible compared with the disastrous effects of untreated progressive uncal herniation. If decompression of transtentorial herniation is delayed, secondary hemorrhage into the brainstem can occur and cause irreversible neurologic deficit. Once mannitol is given and the ICP is reduced, the specific intracranial disorder must be identified as soon as possible if a recurrence of the patient's deterioration is to be prevented.[215]

Animal and human studies have demonstrated that hypertonic saline has clinically desirable physiological effects on CBF, ICP, and inflammatory responses in models of neurotrauma.[216] Some studies suggest that 23.4% hypertonic saline is a safe and effective treatment for elevated ICP in patients after traumatic brain injury.[217,218]

Mannitol therapy for raised ICP may have a beneficial effect on mortality when compared wtih pentobarbital treatment but a detrimental effect on mortality when compared with hypertonic saline in treating increased ICP in head-injury patients.[219]

Neurodiagnostic Evaluation

The choice between operative and medical management of head trauma is based on radiographic and clinical findings. Patients should be stabilized before any computed tomography or angiographic studies are performed. Critically ill patients should be closely monitored during such studies. Restless or uncooperative patients may require general anesthesia if these diagnostic examinations are to be accomplished. Sedation without control of the airway should be avoided because of the risk of further increases in ICP from hypercapnia or hypoxemia. In the event of neurologic deterioration before completion of these studies, intravenous administration of mannitol should be considered.[75] Reductions of Paco$_2$ levels may, by decreasing CBF, allow better angiographic studies. The introduction of computed tomography and MRI has greatly facilitated neuroradiologic diagnosis. Serial computed tomography is an aid in predicting the outcome of patients with severe head injury. New findings after the initial study are associated with poorer outcomes.[220]

Intraoperative Management

Operative treatment is reserved for depressed skull fracture, depressed fractures associated with underlying brain injury, and evacuation of epidural, subdural, and some intracerebral hematomas.[221]

Monitoring during anesthesia is generally similar to that for other mass lesions associated with intracranial hypertension. Intraarterial and central venous (or pulmonary artery) pressure monitoring should be established if it is not already present, but it should not delay surgical decompression in a rapidly deteriorating patient.[75,208] Monitors for cerebral oxygenation are noted in Box 29-4.

Anesthetic Induction, Maintenance, and Emergence

Intubation must be accomplished as expeditiously as possible with the use of small, incremental doses of thiopental, rocuronium (assuming the airway can be instrumented), lidocaine, and labetalol (as needed for the treatment of systemic hypertension), with concurrent cricoid pressure. Hyperkalemia may be induced with succinylcholine in a patient with closed-head injury without paresis; therefore, use of this drug should be avoided.[222] Intracranial damage is usually associated with hypertension. The true state of hydration may be realized for the first time after induction, when catastrophic hypotension may occur if fluid replacement is inadequate or barbiturate dosage is excessive.

Ventilation should be controlled. A Paco$_2$ of 25 to 30 mm Hg promotes brain relaxation for surgical exposure without producing ischemia from hypocapnic vasoconstriction. A higher Paco$_2$ (30 to 35 mm Hg) is recommended for patients who require burr holes for evacuation of chronic subdural hematomas, particularly after decompression, because a slack brain may encourage recurrence.[221]

If the patient is unconscious in the absence of a drug overdose, the ICP is probably elevated. In this case, a barbiturate and an opioid in combination with oxygen (or air in oxygen) and a muscle relaxant are appropriate. A similar technique is indicated in the patient whose computed tomography scan demonstrates obliteration of basal cisterns, dilation of the fourth or lateral ventricles, or a midline shift of 10 mm.[221]

Although hyperventilation attenuates the increase in ICP when inhalation anesthetics are used, in patients with head injury, cerebral vasoconstriction in response to hypocapnia is not a dependable indicator. The introduction of inhalation agents in such patients may increase ICP and exacerbate the formation of edema. The administration of inhalation anesthetics in low inspired concentrations may have a role in the treatment of intraoperative hypertension.[221]

Patients who have chronic subdural hematoma and are alert and responsive may have burr holes placed for evacuation of accumulated blood under local anesthesia with sedation. Depressed skull fractures may also be elevated while the patient is awake and under local anesthesia with sedation. This technique must be used cautiously when the patient placed in the three-point pin head holder has a full stomach.[221]

Fluid replacement should be with glucose-free solutions. Hypovolemia results in systemic hypotension, an unstable anesthetic course, and (by decreasing cerebral oxygen delivery) increased cerebral vasodilatation. Rheologic conditions are optimal at hematocrit levels of 30% to 32%.[207]

The decision of whether to extubate the trachea at the conclusion of the surgical procedure depends on the severity of the injury, the presence of concomitant abdominal or thoracic injuries, preexisting illnesses, and the preoperative level of consciousness. A recent study noted that up to 54.5% of patients had an adverse event after surgery.[222] Occurrence of nausea, vomiting, and respiratory and cardiac problems was significantly more likely than in patients undergoing routine surgical procedures. Young patients who are conscious preoperatively may be extubated after the removal of a localized lesion, whereas patients with diffuse brain injury should remain intubated. Moreover, persistent intracranial hypertension requires continued paralysis, sedation, hyperventilation, and possibly a pentobarbital infusion postoperatively.[75]

SUMMARY

Anesthesia management of the neurosurgical patient continues to be one of the most challenging clinical issues encountered by the nurse anesthetist. Advances in surgical approaches to tumors, vascular lesions, and trauma necessitate constant reappraisal of the important role of anesthesia care in improving a patient's long-term outcome. Intraoperative monitoring modalities new to neurosurgical procedures remain to be definitively evaluated. Interventional radiologic approaches are now a primary therapy for several neurologic disorders, and anesthesia management presents many new challenges in caring for these patients. As clinical practice evolves, it is both exciting and satisfying to meet the demands of this area of anesthesia practice.

REFERENCES

1. Marieb E, Hoehn K. The central nervous system. In: *Human Anatomy & Physiology*. 7th ed. San Francisco: Pearson, Benjamin Cummings; 2007:430-463.
2. Snell RS. Nerve fibers and peripheral nerves. In: *Clinical Neuroanatomy for Medical Students*. Philadelphia: Lippincott-Raven; 1997:90-92.
3. Rapoport SI et al. Testing of a hypothesis for osmotic opening of the blood-brain barrier. *Am J Physiol*. 1972;223:323-331.
4. Sugarman RA. Neurological system. In: McCance KL, Heuther SE, eds. In: *Pathophysiology: The Biological Basis for Disease in Adults and Children*. 5th ed. St Louis: Mosby; 2006:411-482.
5. Marieb E, Hoehn K. The spinal cord. In: *Human Anatomy & Physiology*. 7th ed. San Francisco: Pearson, Benjamin Cummings; 2007:470-480.
6. Stoelting RK, Hillier SC. Central nervous system. In: *Pharmacology & Physiology in Anesthetic Practice*. 4th ed. Philadelphia: Lippincott Williams & Wilkins; 2006:663-667.
7. Guyton AC, Hall JE. Motor functions of the spinal cord: the cord reflexes. In: *Textbook of Medical Physiology*. 11th ed. Philadelphia: Saunders; 2006:673-684.
8. Marieb E, Hoehn K. The autonomic nervous system. In: *Human Anatomy & Physiology*. 7th ed. San Francisco: Pearson, Benjamin Cummings; 2007:532-554.
9. Hudspith MJ. Glutamate: a role in normal brain function, anesthesia, analgesia and CNS injury. *Br J Anaesth*. 1997;78:731-747.
10. Gustein HB, Akil H. Opioid analgesics. In: Brunton LL et al, eds. *Goodman & Gilman's the Pharmacological Basis of Therapeutics*. 11th ed. New York: McGraw-Hill; 2006:547-590.
11. Wilson DR et al. Chronic and interventional pain management. In: Cucchiara RF et al, eds. *Clinical Neuroanesthesia*. New York: Churchill Livingstone; 1998:623-642.
12. Jennett WB et al. Effect of anaesthesia on intracranial pressure in patients with space-occupying lesions. *Lancet*. 1969;1:61-64.
13. Sloan TB. Anesthetics and the brain. *Anesthesiol Clin North America*. 2002;20:265-292.
14. Albin MS. Anesthesia for neurosurgical procedures. In: Grossman RG, Hamilton WJ, eds. *Principles of Neurosurgery*. New York: Raven; 1991:1-17.
15. Baker AJ. Management of the severely head injured patient. *Can J Anaesth*. 1999;46:R35-R45.
16. Steen PA. Inhalational versus intravenous anesthesia: cerebral effects. *Acta Anaesthiol Scand*. 1982;75:32-35.
17. Fitch W, McDowal DG. Effect of halothane on intracranial pressure gradients in the presence of intracranial space-occupying lesions. *Br J Anaesth*. 1971;43:904-911.
18. Adams RW et al. Halothane, hypocapnia, and cerebrospinal fluid pressure in neurosurgery. *Anesthesiology*. 1972;37:510-517.
19. McGrath BJ, Matjasko MJ. Anesthesia and head trauma. *New Horiz*. 1995;3:523-533.
20. Drummond JC, Todd MM. The response of the feline cerebral circulation to $PaCO_2$ during anesthesia with isoflurane and halothane and during sedation with nitrous oxide. *Anesthesiology*. 1985;62:268-273.

21. Van Aken H et al. Cardiovascular and cerebrovascular effects of isoflurane-induced hypotension in the baboon. *Anesth Analg*. 1986;65:565-574.
22. Todd MM, Drummond JC. A comparison of the cerebrovascular and metabolic effects of halothane and isoflurane in the cat. *Anesthesiology*. 1984;60:274-282.
23. Oshima T et al. Effects of sevoflurane on cerebral blood flow and cerebral metabolic rate of oxygen in human beings: a comparison with isoflurane. *Eur J Anaesthesiol*. 2003;20:543-547.
24. Michenfelder JD et al. Isoflurane when compared to enflurane and halothane decreases frequency of cerebral ischemia during carotid endarterectomy. *Anesthesiology*. 1987;67:336-340.
25. Koerner IP, Brambrink AM. Brain protection by anesthetic agents. *Curr Opin Anaesthesiol*. 2006;19(5):481-486.
26. Michenfelder JD, Theye RA. In vivo toxic effects of halothane on canine cerebral metabolic pathways. *Am J Physiol*. 1975;229:1050-1055.
27. Adams RW et al. Isoflurane and cerebrospinal fluid pressure in neurosurgical patients. *Anesthesiology*. 1981;54:97-99.
28. Campkin TV. Isoflurane and cranial extradural pressure. *Br J Anaesth*. 1984;56:1083-1087.
29. Sponheim S et al. Effects of 5.0 and 1.0 MAC isoflurane, sevoflurane and desflurane on intracranial and cerebral perfusion pressures in children. *Acta Anaesthesiol Scand*. 2003;47:932-938.
30. Young WL. Effects of desflurane on the central nervous system. *Anesth Analg*. 1992;75:s32-s37.
31. Ornstein E et al. Desflurane and isoflurane have similar effects on cerebral blood flow in patients with intracranial mass lesions. *Anesthesiology*. 1993;79:498-502.
32. Holmström A, Akeson J. Desflurane induces more cerebral vasodilation than isoflurane at the same A-line autoregressive index level. *Acta Anaesthesiol Scand*. 2005;49(6):754-758.
33. Muzzi DA et al. The effect of desflurane and isoflurane on cerebrospinal fluid pressure in humans with supratentorial mass lesions. *Anesthesiology*. 1992;76:720-724.
34. Engelhard K, Werner C. Inhalational or intravenous anaesthetics for craniotomies? Pro inhalational. *Curr Opin Anaesthesiol*. 2006;19(5):504-508.
35. Boos DL, Stirt JA. Pharmacology. In: Sperry RJ et al, eds. *Manual of Neuroanesthesia*. Philadelphia: Decker; 1989:37-66.
36. Smith AL, Marque JJ. Anesthetics and cerebral edema. *Anesthesiology*. 1976;45:64-72.
37. Baughman VL. Brain protection during neurosurgery. *Anesthesiol Clin North America*. 2002;20;(vi):315-327.
38. Ramani R et al. A dose-response study of the influence of propofol on cerebral blood flow, metabolism, and the electroencephalogram of the rabbit. *Neurosurg Anesthesiol*. 1992;4:110-119.
39. Moss E et al. Effect of etomidate on intracranial pressure and cerebral perfusion pressure. *Br J Anaesth*. 1979;51:347-352.
40. Milde LN et al. Cerebral functional, metabolic, and hemodynamic effects of etomidate in dogs. *Anesthesiology*. 1985;65:371-377.

41. Alves S, Yermal S. Assessment of the neurological systems of the adult. In: Waugaman WR et al, eds. *Principles and Practice of Nurse Anesthesia.* 3rd ed. Norwalk, CT: Appleton & Lange; 1999:224-226.

42. Bendo AA et al. Anesthesia for neurosurgery. In: Barash PG et al, eds. *Clinical Anesthesia.* 5th ed. Philadelphia: Lippincott Williams & Wilkins; 2006:746-789.

43. Bekker A, Sturaitis MK. Dexmedetomidine for neurological surgery. *Neurosurgery.* 2005;57(1 Suppl):1-10.

44. Bekker A et al. Dexmedetomidine does not increase the incidence of intracarotid shunting in patients undergoing awake carotid endarterectomy. *Anesth Analg.* 2006;103(4):955-958.

45. Zornow MH et al. Dexmedetomidine, an alpha 2-adrenergic agonist, decreases cerebral blood flow in the isoflurane-anesthetized dog. *Anesth Analg.* 1990;30(6):624-630.

46. Keykhah MM et al. Influence of sufentanil on cerebral metabolism and circulation in the rat. *Anesthesiology.* 1985;63:274-277.

47. McPherson RW et al. Effects of alfentanil on cerebral vascular reactivity in dogs. *Br J Anaesth.* 1985;57:1232-1238.

48. Ostapkovich ND et al. Cerebral blood flow and CO_2 reactivity is similar during remifentanil/N_2O and fentanyl/N_2O anesthesia. *Anesthesiology.* 1998;89:358-363.

49. Paris A et al. The effect of remifentanil on cerebral blood flow velocity. *Anesth Analg.* 1998;87:569-573.

50. Drummond JC, Patel PM. Neurosurgical anesthesia. In: Miller RD, ed. *Anesthesia.* 6th ed. New York: Churchill Livingstone; 2005:2127-2174.

51. Vesely R et al. The cerebrovascular effects of curare and histamine in the rat. *Anesthesiology.* 1987;66:519-523.

52. Viviand X, Garnier F. Opioid anesthetics (sufentanil and remifentanil) in neuro-anesthesia. *Ann Fr. Anesth Reanim.* 2004;23(4):383-388.

53. Prough DS et al. Acute pulmonary edema in healthy teenagers following conservative doses of intravenous naloxone. *Anesthesiology.* 1984;60:485-486.

54. Estilo AE, Cottrell JE. Naloxone, hypertension and ruptured cerebral aneurysm. *Anesthesiology.* 1981;54:352.

55. Fleisher JE et al. Cerebral effects of high-dose midazolam and subsequent reversal with Ro 15-1788 in dogs. *Anesthesiology.* 1988;68:234-242.

56. Himmelseher S, Durieux ME. Revising a dogma: ketamine for patients with neurological injury? *Anesth Analg.* 2005;101(2):524-534.

57. Stirt JA et al. Vecuronium: effect on intracranial pressure and hemodynamics in neurosurgical patients. *Anesthesiology.* 1987;67:570-573.

58. Shayevitz JR, Matteo RS. Decreased sensitivity to metocurine in patients with upper motor neuron disease. *Anesth Analg.* 1985;64:767-772.

59. Iwasaki H et al. Response differences of paretic and healthy extremities to pancuronium and neostigmine in hemiplegic patients. *Anesth Analg.* 1985;64:864-866.

60. Hans P, Bonhomme V. Muscle relaxants in neurosurgical anaesthesia: a critical appraisal. *Eur J Anaesthesiol.* 2003;20:600-605.

61. Van Akne H et al. Effect of labetalol on intracranial pressure in dogs with and without intracranial hypertension. *Acta Anaesthesiol Scand.* 1982;26:615-619.

62. Muzzi DA et al. Labetalol and esmolol in the control of hypertension after intracranial surgery. *Anesth Analg.* 1990;70:68-71.

63. Griswold WR et al. Nitroprusside-induced intracranial hypertension. *JAMA.* 1981;246:2679-2680.

64. Sulek CA. Intracranial pressure. In: Cucchiara RF et al, eds. *Clinical Neuroanesthesia.* 2nd ed. New York: Churchill Livingstone; 1998:104.

65. Weyer GW et al. Evidence-based cerebral vasospasm management. *Neurosurg Focus.* 2006;21(3):E8.

66. Barth M et al. Effect of nicardipine prolonged-release implants on cerebral vasospasm and clinical outcome after severe aneurismal subarachnoid hemorrhage: a prospective, randomized, double-blind phase IIa study. *Stroke.* 2007;38(2):330-336.

67. Kovac AL, Masiongale A. Comparison of nicardipine versus esmolol in attenuating the hemodynamic responses to anesthesia emergence and extubation. *J Cardiothorac Vasc Anesth.* 2007;21(1):45-50.

68. Kass IS. Physiology and metabolism of the brain and spinal cord. In: Newfield P, Cottrell JE, eds. *Handbook of Neuroanesthesia.* 4th ed. Philadelphia: Lippincott Williams & Wilkins; 2007:3-22.

69. Lanier WL, Weglinski MR. Intracranial pressure. In: Cucchiara RF, Michenfelder JD, eds. *Clinical Neuroanesthesia.* New York: Churchill Livingstone; 1990:77-115.

70. Weaver DD et al. Differential intracranial pressure in patients with unilateral mass lesions. *J Neurosurg.* 1982;56:660-665.

71. Miller JD et al. Induced changes of cerebrospinal fluid volume. *Arch Neurol.* 1973;28:265-269.

72. Todd MM et al. Neuroanesthesia. In: Longnecker D et al, eds. *Anesthesiology.* New York: McGraw-Hill; 2008:1081-1139.

73. Jenkinson JL. Neuroanesthesia. In: Nimmo WS, Smith G, eds. *Anaesthesia.* Oxford: Blackwell Scientific; 1989:576-593.

74. Pavlin EG. Emergency anaesthesia and trauma. In: Nimmo WS, Smith G, eds. *Anaesthesia.* Oxford: Blackwell Scientific; 1989:687-692.

75. Morgan GE, Mikhail MS. Anesthesia for neurosurgery. In: *Clinical Anesthesiology.* 4th ed. New York: McGraw-Hill; 2006:631-646.

76. Miller JD, Sullivan HG. Severe intracranial hypertension. *Int Anesthesiol Clin.* 1989;17:19-75.

77. Cottrell JE et al. Furosemide- and mannitol-induced changes in intracranial pressure and serum osmolality and electrolytes. *Anesthesiology.* 1977;47:28-30.

78. Todd MM, Cutkomp J, Brian JE. Influence of mannitol and furosemide, alone and in combination, on brain water content after fluid percussion injury. *Anesthesiology.* 2006;105(6):1176-1181.

79. Qureshi A, Suarez J. Use of hypertonic saline solutions in treatment of cerebral edema and intracranial hypertension. *Crit Care Med.* 2000; 28(9):3301-3313.

80. Kobrine AL, Kempe LG. Studies in head injury: part II. Effect of dexamethasone on traumatic brain swelling. *Surg Neurol.* 1973;1:38.

81. Braakman R et al. Megadose steroids in severe head injury: results of a prospective double-blind clinical trial. *J Neurosurg.* 1983;58:326-330.

82. Rangel-Castillo L, Robertson CS. Management of intracranial hypertension. *Crit Care Clin.* 2006;22(4):713-732.

83. Kassell NF et al. Alterations in cerebral blood flow, oxygen metabolism, and electrical activity produced by high-dose thiopental. *Neurosurg.* 1980;7:598.

84. Atkinson JLD, Faust RJ. Central nervous system trauma. In: Cucchiara RF et al, eds. *Clinical Neuroanesthesia.* 2nd ed. New York: Churchill Livingstone; 1998:549-550.

85. Lopez JR. The use of evoked potentials in intraoperative neurophysiologic monitoring. *Phys Med Rehabil Clin N Am.* 2004;15(1):63-84.

86. Mahla ME. Neurological monitoring. In: Cucchiara RF et al, eds. *Clinical Neuroanesthesia.* 2nd ed. New York: Churchill Livingstone; 1998:129-135.

87. Freye E. Cerebral monitoring in the operating room and the intensive care unit - an introductory for the clinician and a guide for the novice wanting to open a window to the brain. Part II: Sensory-evoked potentials (SSEP, AEP, VEP). *J Clin Monit Comput.* 2005;19(1-2):77-168.

88. McPherson RW, Sloan TB. Evoked potentials. In: Cottrell JE, Smith DS, eds. *Anesthesia and Neurosurgery.* 4th ed. St Louis: Mosby; 2001:183-200.

89. Dubois M et al. Somatosensory evoked potential during whole body hyperthermia in humans. *Electroencephalogr Clin Neurophysiol.* 1981; 52:157-162.

90. Stejskal L et al. Somatosensory evoked potentials in deep hypothermia. *Appl Neurophysiol.* 1980;43(1-2):1-7.

91. Van Rheinek-Leyssius AT et al. Influence of moderate hypothermia on posterior tibial nerve. *Anesth Analg.* 1986;65:475-480.

92. Soustiel JF et al. Short latency trigeminal evoked potentials: normative data and clinical correlations. *Electrocephalogr Clin Neurophysiol.* 1991; 80:119-125.

93. Sohmer H, et al. Multi-modality evoked potentials in hypoxemia. *Electroencephalogr Clin Neurophysiol.* 1986;64:328-333.

94. Samra SK et al. Fentanyl anesthesia and human brainstem auditory evoked potentials. *Anesthesiology.* 1984;61:261-265.

95. Chassard D et al. Auditory evoked potentials during propofol anaesthesia in man. *Br J Anaesth.* 1989;62:522-526.

96. Houston GH et al. Effects of nitrous oxide on auditory cortical evoked potentials and subjective thresholds. *Br J Anaesth.* 1988;61:606-610.

97. Fenwick P et al. Contingent negative variation and evoked potential amplitude as a function of inspired nitrous oxide concentration. *Electroencephalogr Clin Neurophysiol.* 1979;47:473-482.

98. Harkins SW et al. Effects of nitrous oxide inhalation on brain potentials evoked by auditory and noxious dental stimulation. *Prog Neuropsychopharmacol Biol Psychiatry.* 1982;6(2):167-174.

99. Markland ON et al. Monitoring of multimodality evoked potentials during open-heart surgery under hypothermia. *Electroencephalogr Clin Neurophysiol.* 1984;59(6):432-440.

100. Gold S et al. Effects of body temperature elevation on auditory nerve brainstem evoked responses and EEGs in rats. *Electroencephalogr Clin Neurophysiol.* 1985;60(2):146-153.

101. Blair A et al. Effect of neuromuscular blockade on facial nerve monitoring. *Am J Otology.* 1994;15(2):161-167.

102. Schaefer SD. Laryngeal electromyography. *Otolaryngol Clin North Am.* 1991;24(6):1053-1057.

103. Sterkers JM et al. Preservation of facial, cochlear, and other nerve functions in acoustic neuroma treatment. *Otolaryngol Head Neck Surg.* 1994;110(2):146-155.

104. Schlake HP et al. Intraoperative electromyographic monitoring of the lower cranial nerves (LCN IX-XII) in skull base surgery. *Clin Neurol Neurosurg.* 2001;103(2):72-82.

105. Jellinek D et al. Noninvasive intraoperative monitoring of motor evoked potentials under propofol anaesthesia: effects of spinal surgery on the amplitude and latency of motor evoked potentials. *Neurosurgery.* 1991;29(4):551-557.

106. Taniguchi M et al. Effects of 4 IV anesthetic agents on motor evoked potentials elicited by magnetic transcranial stimulation. *Neurosurgery.* 1992;31(2):298-305.

107. Zetner J et al. Influence of halothane, enflurane, and isoflurane on motor evoked potentials. *Neurosurgery.* 1992;31(2):298-305.

108. Jellinek D et al. Effects of nitrous oxide on motor evoked potentials recorded from skeletal muscle in patients under anesthesia with intravenously administered propofol. *Neurosurgery.* 1991;29(4):558-562.

109. Ghaly RF et al. The effect of etomidate on motor evoked potentials induced by transcranial magnetic stimulation in the monkey. *Neurosurgery.* 1990;27(6):936-942.

110. Zentner J et al. Influence of anesthetics—nitrous oxide in particular—on electromyographic response evoked by transcranial electrical stimulation of the cortex. *Neurosurgery.* 1989;24(2):253-256.

111. Kalkman CJ et al. Effects of propofol, etomidate, midazolam, and fentanyl on motor evoked responses to transcranial electrical or magnetic stimulation in humans. *Anesthesiology.* 1992;76:502-509.

112. Kalkman CJ et al. Intraoperative monitoring of tibialis anterior muscle motor evoked responses to transcranial electrical stimulation during partial neuromuscular blockade. *Anesth Analg.* 1993;75:584.

113. Zentner J et al. Influence of nitrous oxide on motor evoked potentials. *Spine.* 1997;22(9):1002-1006.

114. Frei FJ et al. Intraoperative monitoring of motor-evoked potentials in children undergoing spinal surgery. *Spine.* 2007;32(8):911-917.

115. Black S, Cucchiara RF. Tumor surgery. In: Cucchiara RF et al, eds. *Clinical Neuroanesthesia.* 2nd ed. Edinburgh: Churchill Livingstone; 1994:343-365.

116. Alphin RS, Gravenstein N. Fluid management of the neurosurgical patient. In: Cucchiara RF et al, eds. *Clinical Neuroanesthesia.* 2nd ed. Edinburgh: Churchill Livingstone; 1998:229-246.

117. Zornow MH, Scheller MS. Intraoperative fluid management during craniotomy. In: Cottrell JE, Smith DS, eds. *Anesthesia and Neurosurgery.* 4th ed. St Louis: Mosby; 2001:237-250.

118. Zornow MH et al. The acute cerebral effects of changes in plasma osmolality and oncotic pressure. *Anesthesiology.* 1987;67:936-941.

119. Mears SL, Sperry RJ. Fluid management. In: Sperry RJ et al, eds. *Manual of Neuroanesthesia.* Philadelphia: Decker; 1989:107-118.

120. Tommasino C. Fluid management. In: Newfield P, Cottrell JE, eds. *Handbook of Neuroanesthesia.* 4th ed. New York: Lippincott Williams & Wilkins; 2007:379-395.

121. Prough DS et al. Effects of hypertonic saline versus lactated Ringer's solution on cerebral oxygen transport during resuscitation from hemorrhagic shock. *J Neurosurg.* 1986;64:627-632.

122. Tommasino C. Fluids and the neurosurgical patient. *Anesthesiol Clin North America.* 2002;20:329-346.

123. Kawai N et al. Hyperglycemia and the vascular effects of cerebral ischemia. *Stroke.* 1997;28:149-154.

124. Hamm CW. Neuroanesthesia considerations in skull base surgery. In: Robertson JT et al, eds. *Cranial Base Surgery.* London: Churchill Livingstone; 2000:99-130.

125. Milde LN. Cerebral protection. In: Cucchiara RF et al, eds. *Clinical Neuroanesthesia.* 2nd ed. Edinburgh: Churchill Livingstone; 1998:177-228.

126. Kraig RP, Chesler M. Astrocytic acidosis in hyperglycemia and complete ischemia. *J Cereb Blood Flow Metab.* 1990;10(1):104-114.

127. Pulsinelli WA et al. Moderate hyperglycemia augments ischemic brain damage: a neuropathologic study in the rat. *Neurology.* 1982;32(11):1239-1246.

128. Hsu SS et al. Influence of hyperglycemia on cerebral adenosine production during ischemia and reperfusion. *Am J Physiol.* 1991;262 (2 pt 2):H398-H403.

129. Phillis JW et al. The effect of hyperglycemia on extracellular levels of adenosine in the hypoxic rat cerebral cortex. *Brain Res.* 1990;524(2):336-338.

130. Dietrich WD et al. Moderate hyperglycemia worsens acute blood-brain barrier injury after forebrain ischemia in rats. *Stroke.* 1993;24(1):111-116.

131. Ginsberg MD et al. Deleterious effect of glucose pretreatment on recovery from diffuse cerebral ischemia in the cat. I. Local cerebral blood flow and glucose utilization. *Stroke.* 1980;11(4):347-354.

132. Duckrow RB et al. Regional cerebral blood flow decreased during chronic and acute hyperglycemia. *Stroke.* 1987;18(1):52-58.

133. Harik SI, LaManna JC. Vascular perfusion and blood-brain glucose transport in acute and chronic hyperglycemia. *J Neurochem.* 1988;51(6):1924-1925.

134. Kagstrom E et al. Recirculation in the rat brain following incomplete ischemia. *J Cereb Blood Flow Metab.* 1983;3(2):183-192.

135. Siemkowicz D, Hansen AJ. Clinical restitution following cerebral ischemia in hypo-, normo- and hyperglycemic rats. *Acta Neurol Scand.* 1978;58(1):1-8.

136. D'Alecy LG et al. Dextrose containing intravenous fluid impairs outcome and increases death after eight minutes of cardiac arrest and resuscitation in dogs. *Surgery.* 1986;100(3):505-511.

137. Strong AJ et al. Protection of respiration of a crude mitrochondrial preparation in cerebral ischaemia by control of blood glucose. *J Neurol Neurosurg Psychiatry.* 1985;48:450.

138. Zimmerman CR et al. An infusion protocol in critically ill cardiothoracic surgery patients. *Ann Pharmacother.* 2004;38(7-8):1243-1251.

139. Ravussin PA, Wilder-Smith O. General anaesthesia for supratentorial neurosurgery. *CNS Drugs.* 2001;15:527-535.

140. Bedford R et al. Supratentorial masses: anesthetic considerations. In: Cottrell JE, Smith DS, eds. *Anesthesia and Neurosurgery.* 4th ed. St Louis: Mosby; 2001:319-334.

141. Muzzi DA et al. Labetalol and esmolol in the control of hypertension after intracranial surgery. *Anesth Analg.* 1990;70(1):68-71.

142. Miner ME, Allen SJ. Cardiovascular effects of severe head injury. In: Frost EAM, ed. *Clinical Anesthesia in Neurosurgery.* 2nd ed. Boston: Butterworth-Heinemann; 1991:439-444.

143. Helmy A et al. Traumatic brain injury: intensive care management. *Br J Anaesth.* 2007;99(1):32-42.

144. Kofke WA et al. Neurological intensive care. In: Albin MS, ed. *Textbook of Neuroanesthesia with Neurosurgical and Neuroscience Perspectives.* New York: McGraw-Hill; 1997:1247-1348.

145. Engberg M et al. The cerebral arterio-venous oxygen content difference during halothane and neurolept anesthesia in patients subjected to craniotomy. *Acta Anaesthesiol Scand.* 1989;33:642-646.

146. Asmussen J et al. Peri- and postoperative changes in the arterio-venous oxygen content difference in patients subjected to craniotomy for cerebral tumors. *Acta Neurochir Wien.* 1989;101:9-17.

147. Kalfa IH, Little JR. Postoperative hemorrhage: a survey of 4992 intracranial procedures. *Neurosurgery.* 1988;23(3):343-347.

148. Cucchiari RF et al. Anesthesia and intensive care management of patients with brain tumors. In: Kaye AH, Laws ER Jr, eds. *Brain Tumors.* Edinburgh: Churchill Livingstone; 1995:263-292.

149. Waga S et al. Intracerebral hemorrhage remote from the site of the initial neurosurgical procedure. *Neurosurgery.* 1983;13(6):662-665.

150. Roper SN, Alphin RS. Epilepsy surgery. In: Cucchiara RF et al, eds. *Clinical Neuroanesthesia.* 2nd ed. Edinburgh: Churchill Livingstone; 1998:367-388.

151. Jaaskelainen J, Randell T. Awake craniotomy in glioma surgery. *Acta Neurochir Suppl.* 2003;88:31-35.

152. Souter MJ et al. Dexmedetomidine sedation during awake craniotomy for seizure resection: effects on electrocorticography. *J Neurosurg Anesthesiol.* 2007;19(1):38-44.

153. Karkar KM et al. Focal cooling suppresses spontaneous epileptiform activity without changing the cortical motor threshold. *Epilepsia.* 2002;43(8):932-935.

154. Sajpaul R. Awake craniotomy: controversies, indications and techniques in the surgical treatment of temporal lobe epilepsy. *Can J Neurolog Sci.* 2000;27(Suppl 1):S55-S63.

155. Signorelli F et al. The value of cortical stimulation applied to the surgery of malignant gliomas in language areas. *Can J Neurolog Sci.* 2001;22:3-10.

156. Michenfelder JD et al. Evaluation of an ultrasonic device (precordial Doppler) for the diagnosis of venous air embolus. *Anesthesiology.* 1972;36:164-167.

157. Voorhies RM et al. Prevention of air embolism with positive-end expiratory pressure. *Neurosurgery.* 1983;12:503-506.

158. Adornato DC et al. Pathophysiology of intravenous air embolism in dogs. *Anesthesiology.* 1978;49:120-127.

159. Standiferd M et al. The sitting position in neurosurgery: a retrospective analysis of 488 cases. *Neurosurgery.* 1984;14:649-659.

160. Matjasko J et al. Anesthesia and surgery in the seated position: analysis of 554 cases. *Neurosurgery.* 1985;17:695-702.

161. Young ML et al. Comparison of surgical and anesthetic complications in neurosurgical patients experiencing venous air embolism in the sitting position. *Neurosurgery.* 1986;18:157-161.

162. Perkins-Pearson NAK et al. Atrial pressures in the seated position: implications for paradoxical air embolism. *Anesthesiology.* 1982;57:493-498.

163. Butler BD, Hills BA. The lungs as a filter for microbubbles. *J Appl Physiol.* 1979;47:537-543.

164. Todd MM. Monitoring in neuroanesthesia. In: Saidman L, Smith T, eds. *Monitoring in Anesthesia.* 4th ed. Boston: Butterworth-Heinemann; 1993:180.

165. Culley DJ, Crosby G. Anesthesia for posterior fossa surgery. In: Newfield P, Cottrell JE, eds. *Handbook of Neuroanesthesia.* 3rd ed. Philadelphia: Lippincott Williams & Wilkins; 2007:133-142.

166. Tinker JH. Detection of air embolism: a test for positioning of right atrial catheter and Doppler probe. *Anesthesiology.* 1975;43:104-106.
167. Cucchiara RF et al. Air embolism in upright neurosurgical patients: detection and localization by two-dimensional transesophageal echocardiography. *Anesthesiology.* 1984;60:353-355.
168. Munson ES, Merrick HC. Effect of nitrous oxide on venous air embolism. *Anesthesiology.* 1966;27:783-787.
169. Smith DS, Osborn I. Posterior fossa: anesthetic considerations. In: Cottrell JE, Smith DS, eds. *Anesthesia and Neurosurgery.* 4th ed. St Louis: Mosby; 2001:335-352.
170. Colohan AR et al. Intravenous fluid loading as prophylaxis for paradoxical air embolism. *J Neurosurg.* 1985;62:839-842.
171. Durant TM et al. Pulmonary (venous) air embolism. *Am Heart J.* 1947;33:269.
172. Liutkus D et al. The sitting position in neurosurgical anaesthesia: a survey of French practice. *Ann Fr Anesth Reanim.* 2003;22:296-300.
173. Schveibman DL, Matijasko MJ. Tumors: pathophysiology. In: *Handbook of Neuroanesthesia.* 4th ed. Philadelphia: Lippincott Williams & Wilkins; 2007:187-196.
174. Neal JG et al. Comparison of techniques of transsphenoidal pituitary surgery. *Am J Rhinol.* 2007;21(2):203-206.
175. Cucchiara RF et al. Evaluation of esmolol in controlling increases in heart rate and blood pressure during endotracheal intubation in patients undergoing carotid endarterectomy. *Anesthesiology.* 1986;65:528-531.
176. Matjasko MJ. Anesthetic considerations in patients with neuroendocrine disease. In: Cottrell JE, Smith DS. *Anesthesia and Neurosurgery.* 4th ed. St Louis: Mosby; 2002:591-610.
177. Frost E. Management of neurosurgical anesthesia: aneurysms. *Curr Rev Clin Anesth.* 1991;11:125-132.
178. Herrick LA, Gelb AW. Anesthesia for intracranial aneurysm surgery. *J Clin Anesth.* 1992;4:73-85.
179. Guy J, Gelb AW. Perioperative management of intracranial aneurysms. *Curr Rev Clin Anesth.* 1993;14:1-8.
180. Taneda M. Effect of early operation for ruptured aneurysms on prevention of delayed ischemic symptoms. *J Neurosurg.* 1982;57:622-628.
181. Newfield P. Perioperative management of intracranial aneurysms. *ASA Annu Refresher Course Lect.* 1993;22:13-26.
182. Macdonald RL et al. Etiology of cerebral vasospasm in primates. *J Neurosurg.* 1991;75:415-424.
183. Chyatte D. Antiinflammatory agents and cerebral vasospasm. *Neurosurg Clin North Am.* 1990;1:433-450.
184. Petruk KC et al. Nimodipine treatment in poor-grade aneurysm patients: results in a multicenter double-blind placebo-controlled trial. *J Neurosurg.* 1988;68:505-517.
185. Pickard JD et al. Effect of oral nimodipine on cerebral infarction and outcome after subarachnoid haemorrhage: British aneurysm nimodipine trial. *BMJ.* 1989;298:636-642.
186. Meyer FB. Calcium antagonists and vasospasm: cerebral vasospasm. *Neurosurg Clin North Am.* 1990;1:367-376.
187. Veyna RS et al. Magnesium sulfate therapy after aneurismal subarachnoid hemorrhage. *J Neurosurg.* 2002;96(3):510-514.
188. Schmid-Eliaesser R et al. Intravenous magnesium versus nimodipine in treatment of patients with aneurismal subarachnoid hemorrhage: a randomized study. *Neurosurgery.* 2006;58(6):1054-1065.
189. Solomon RA et al. Early aneurysm surgery and prophylactic hypervolemic hypertensive therapy for the treatment of aneurysmal subarachnoid hemorrhage. *Neurosurgery.* 1988;23:699-704.
190. Frazer D et al. Coiling versus clipping for the treatment of aneurismal subarachnoid hemorrhage: a longitudinal investigation into cognitive outcome. *Neurosurgery.* 2007;60(3):434-441.
191. Van Gijn J et al. Subarachnoid hemorrhage. *Lancet.* 2007;369(9558):306-318.
192. Gerlach R et al. Treatment-related morbidity of unruptured intracranial aneurysms: results of a prospective single centre series with an interdisciplinary approach during a six year period (1999-2005). *J Neurol Neurosurg Psychiatry.* 2007;78:864-871.
193. Molyneux AJ et al. International Subarachnoid Aneurysm Trial (ISAT) Collaborative Group. International subarachnoid aneurysm trial (ISAT) of neurosurgical clipping versus endovascular coiling in 2143 patients with ruptured intracranial aneurysms: a randomized comparison of effects on survival, dependency, seizures, rebleeding, subgroups an aneurysm occlusion. *Lancet.* 2005;366(9488):809-817.
194. Davies KR et al. Cardiac function in aneurysmal subarachnoid hemorrhage: a study of electrocardiographic and echocardiographic abnormalities. *Br J Anaesth.* 1991;67:58-63.

195. Keane JF et al. Monitoring of brainstem auditory evoked potentials during induced hypotension for cerebral aneurysm surgery. *Can Anaesth Soc J.* 1984;31:584-585.
196. Brown MM et al. The effect of suxamethonium on intracranial pressure and cerebral perfusion pressure in patients with severe head injuries following blunt trauma. *Eur J Anaesthesiol.* 1996;13:474-477.
197. Minton MD et al. Intracranial pressure after atracurium in neurosurgical patients. *Anesth Analg.* 1985;64:113-116.
198. Clancy M et al. In patients with head injuries who undergo rapid sequence intubation using succinylcholine, does pretreatment with a competitive neuromuscular blocking agent improve outcome? A literature review. *Emerg Med J.* 2001;18:373-375.
199. Yasargil MF, Fox JL. The microsurgical approach to intracranial aneurysms. *Surg Neurol.* 1975;3:7-14.
200. Lagerkranser M. Controlled hypotension in neurosurgery. *J Neurosurg Anesthesiol.* 1991;3:150-152.
201. Charbel FT et al. Temporary clipping in aneurysm surgery: technique and results. *Surg Neurol.* 1991;36:83-90.
202. Karibe H et al. Use of mild intraischemic hypothermia versus mannitol to reduce infarct size after temporary middle cerebral artery occlusion in rats. *J Neurosurg.* 1995;83(1):93-98.
203. Todd MM et al. Mild intraoperative hypothermia during surgery for intracranial aneurysm. *N Engl J Med.* 2005;352(2):135-145.
204. Dodson BA. Interventional neuroradiology and the anesthetic management of patients with arteriovenous malformations. In: Cottrell JE, Smith DS, eds. *Anesthesia and Neurosurgery.* 4th ed. St Louis: Mosby; 2001:399-424.
205. Brain Trauma Foundation; American Association of Neurological Surgeons; Congress of Neurological Surgeons; Joint Section of Neurotrauma and Critical Care, AANS, CNS. Guidelines for the management of severe traumatic brain injury. VIII. Intracranial pressure thresholds. *J Neurotrauma.* 2007;24(Suppl 1):S55-S58.
206. Grande CM et al. Appropriate techniques for airway management of emergency patients with suspected spinal cord injuries [letter]. *Anesth Analg.* 1988;67:714-715.
207. Becker P et al. Complement activation following head and brain trauma. *Anaesthetist.* 1987;36:301-305.
208. Konig SA et al. Coagulopathy and outcome in patients with chronic subdural haematoma. *Acta Neurol Scand.* 2003;107:110-116.
209. Caird J et al. The impact of antithrombotic therapy on neurosurgical emergency referral load. *Ir Med J.* 2006;99(7):206-208.
210. Konig SA et al. Coagulopathy and outcome in patients with chronic subdural hematoma. *Acta Neurol Scand.* 2003;107(2):110-116.
211. Dara SI et al. Fresh frozen plasma transfusion in critically ill medical patients with coagulopathy. *Crit Care Med.* 2005;33(11):2667-2671.
212. Aguilar MI et al. Treatment of warfarin-associated intracerebral hemorrhage: literature review and expert opinion. *Mayo Clin Proc.* 2007;82(1):82-92.
213. Yusim Y et al. The use of recombinant factor VIIa (NovoSeven) for treatment of active or impending bleeding in brain injury: broadening the indications. *J Clinc Anesth.* 2006;18(7):545-551.
214. Altman R et al. Recombinant factor VIIa reverses the inhibitory effect of aspirin or aspirin plus clopidogrel on in vitro thrombin generation. *J Thromb Haemost.* 2006;4(9):2022-2027.
215. Jantzen JP. Prevention and treatment of intracranial hypertension. *Best Pract Res Clin Anaesthesiol.* 2007;21(4):517-538.
216. White H et al. The use of hypertonic saline for treating intracranial hypertension after traumatic brain injury. *Anesth Analg.* 2006;102(6):1836-1846.
217. Ware ML et al. Effects of 23.4% sodium chloride solution in reducing intracranial pressure in patients with traumatic brain injury: a preliminary study. *Crit Care Med.* 1998;26(6):1118-1122.
218. Suarez JI et al. Treatment of refractory intracranial hypertension with 23.4% saline. *Crit Care Med.* 1998;26(6):1118-1122.
219. Wakai A et al. Mannitol for acute traumatic brain injury. *Cochrane Database Syst Rev.* 2007;24(1):CD001049.
220. Kobayashi S et al. Clinical value of serial computed tomography with severe head injury. *Surg Neurol.* 1983;20:25-29.
221. Sakabe T, Bendo AA. Anesthetic management of head trauma. In: Newfield P, Cottrell JE, eds. *Handbook of Neuroanesthesia.* 4th ed. Philadelphia: Lippincott Williams & Wilkins; 2007:91-110.
222. Frankville DD, Drummond JC. Hyperkalemia after succinylcholine administration in a patient with closed head injury without paresis. *Anesthesiology.* 1987;67:264-266.

CHAPTER 30

RENAL ANATOMY, PHYSIOLOGY, PATHOPHYSIOLOGY, AND ANESTHESIA MANAGEMENT

Sandra Maree Ouellette

The kidneys are paired organs that lie retroperitoneally on both sides of the vertebral column. They function to excrete the end products of bodily metabolism and thereby control the concentration of constituents of body fluids. A rich blood supply to these vital organs, coupled with the physiologic processes of filtration, reabsorption, secretion, and excretion, maintains homeostasis of the fluid that bathes each cell. For management of anesthetized patients to be optimal, the anesthetist must be familiar with physiologic mechanisms that allow the kidneys to control the body's intracellular and extracellular environments.

This chapter addresses the effect of anesthesia and surgery on the normal and the diseased kidney. After a discussion of the anatomic structure and physiologic mechanisms of the kidney, the effects of anesthesia on normal renal function are addressed. Pathophysiologic mechanisms associated with acute and chronic renal failure are discussed. Preoperative renal assessment and anesthetic considerations for patients with impaired renal function are emphasized, and pertinent anesthetic considerations for common urologic procedures are identified.

STRUCTURE OF THE KIDNEY

The kidneys are bean-shaped, reddish-brown organs located in the posterior part of the abdomen on both sides of the vertebral column (Figure 30-1). These organs extend from the 12th thoracic vertebra to the 3rd lumbar vertebra; each weighs approximately 125 to 170 g in men and 115 to 155 g in women. Each kidney is about 11.25 cm long, 5 to 7.5 cm wide, and 2.5 cm thick. The right kidney's position is slightly lower than the left because of hepatic displacement. The kidneys and their vessels are embedded in fatty tissue (perirenal fat) and enclosed in renal fascia. Renal fascia and large vessels hold the kidneys in position.

The anterior and posterior surfaces, upper and lower poles, and lateral margin of the kidney have convex contours. The medial margin is concave because of the presence of the hilus. Structures that enter or leave the kidney through the hilus include the renal artery and vein, nerves, lymphatics, and ureters.

A longitudinal section of the kidney reveals two distinct regions—the outer cortex and the inner medulla (Figure 30-2). The medulla is divided into 8 to 18 triangular wedges called *pyramids*. The base of each pyramid is directed toward the renal cortex, and the apexes converge toward the renal pelvis.

Pyramids have a striated appearance because they contain the loop of Henle and collecting ducts of the nephron. The apex of each pyramid, called the *papilla*, is composed of many collecting ducts. Papillary ducts empty into a cup-shaped structure known as the *minor calyx*. Several minor calyces join to form major calyces, which come together as the renal pelvis. The renal pelvis is the major reservoir for urine. Ureters connect the renal pelvis to the bladder.

Nephron

The functional unit of the kidney is the *nephron*. Approximately 1,250,000 of these units are present in each kidney. The shape of the nephron is unique, unmistakable, and admirably suited for its function. Each area of the nephron is selective with regard to its performance. Nephrons hold the filtrate that has been filtered from the blood. End products of metabolism are excreted, and metabolically important substances such as water are reabsorbed as needed.

The nephron (Figure 30-3) begins in the cortex at the glomerulus and ends where the tubule joins the collecting duct at the papilla. The glomerulus is a tuft of capillaries derived from the afferent arteriole. Blood is brought to the glomerulus by the afferent arteriole; blood that is not filtered returns to the circulation by way of the efferent arteriole. The filtrate from the glomeruli enters the Bowman capsule, or capsula glomeruli, flows through a tortuous tube, or proximal convoluted tubule, and then goes to the loop of Henle, distal convoluted tubule, and collecting duct.

The nephron, which changes in shape and direction as it follows its course, is contained partly in the renal cortex and partly in the medulla (Figure 30-4). The cortex contains the Bowman capsule, glomerulus, and proximal and distal tubules. The thin, descending loop of Henle comes from the proximal tubule and dips toward the pyramid. At some point it bends on itself and forms an enlarged, ascending loop of Henle. The ascending limb joins the distal convoluted tubule.[1]

The kidneys have two kinds of nephrons: cortical nephrons, which extend only partially into the medulla, and juxtamedullary nephrons, which lie deep in the cortex and extend deep into the medulla. One fifth to one third of the nephrons are juxtamedullary and play an important role in concentration of urine.

Renal Blood Supply

To understand how the kidneys function, it is essential to know how blood is brought to them. The kidneys are highly vascular. Although they represent only 0.5% of body weight, they receive 1100 to 1200 mL of blood per minute, or 20% to 25% of the cardiac output. Blood reaches these organs through the renal arteries. At the hilus of the kidney, the renal artery divides into several lobar arteries and then subdivides again into interlobar arteries, which run between the pyramids. When these vessels reach the corticomedullary zone, they make well-defined arches over the bases of the pyramids. These vessels, known as *arcuate arteries*, give off a series of vessels known as *interlobular arteries*. An interlobular artery may terminate as an afferent arteriole or as a nutrient artery to the tubule.

The afferent arterioles form the high-pressure capillary bed within the Bowman capsule called the *glomerulus*. Because little or no oxygen is removed in the glomerulus, the blood that is not filtered begins its passage to the venous system via the efferent arteriole. The efferent arteriole is smaller than the afferent arteriole, thereby affording some resistance to blood flow. The efferent vessel soon becomes a plexus of capillaries again, and this low-pressure bed is known as the *peritubular capillary*. The peritubular capillary bed winds and twists around the proximal and distal tubule. At one point, a few hairpin loops called *vasa recta* dip down among the loops of Henle. Anatomic arrangements of these capillary beds and the renal tubules set the stage for filtration, reabsorption, and concentration of urine.

After leaving the peritubular capillary, blood returns to the central circulation via the veins. Renal veins are named in reverse order of the arteries, and therefore are the interlobular, arcuate, interlobar, lobar, and renal veins. The renal vein leaves the kidney at the hilus and empties into the inferior vena cava.

The portion of the cardiac output that passes through the kidney is called the *renal fraction*. Because cardiac output in a 70-kg man is approximately 5600 mL/min, and blood flow through both kidneys is 1200 mL/min, the normal renal fraction is 21%. This flow may vary from 12% to 30%. Distribution of renal blood flow is to the renal cortex and the medulla, with the cortex receiving the larger amount. Values obtained from dogs indicate that 3 to 5 mL/g/min are distributed to the cortex, 1 to 2 mL/g/min to the outer medulla, and 0.3 to 0.6 mL/g/min to the inner medulla. Only a small portion of blood (1% to 2%) flows through the vasa recta in the medulla.

Regulation of Renal Blood Flow

Blood flow to any organ is determined by the arteriovenous pressure difference across the vascular bed and is given by the following relationship:

Equation 30-1

$$\text{Renal blood flow} = (\text{MAP} - \text{VP}) \times \text{VR}$$

where MAP is the mean arterial pressure, VP is the venous pressure, and VR is the vascular resistance. Renal blood flow is regulated by intrinsic autoregulation and neural regulation.

Autoregulation of renal blood flow implies that blood flow remains normal despite a considerable change in pressure. With a MAP between 75 and 160 mm Hg, renal blood flow to both kidneys remains 1200 mL/min. If mean systemic blood pressure falls below 60 mm Hg, filtration ceases. Afferent arteriole vasodilation and myogenic mechanisms are responsible for autoregulation.

When renal blood flow decreases, glomerular filtration is reduced. A reduction in glomerular filtration leads to dilation

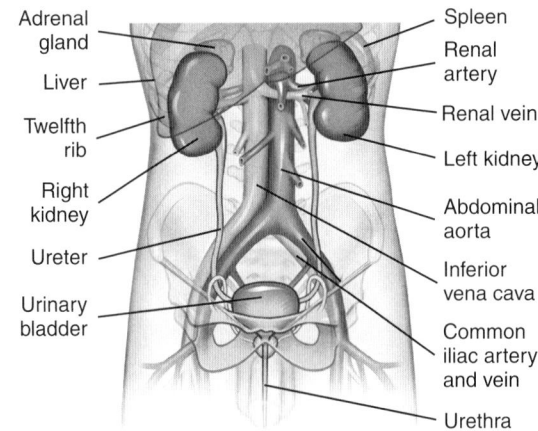

FIGURE **30-1** Kidney position. (*From Thibodeau GA, Patton KT. Anatomy & Physiology. 6th ed. St Louis: Mosby; 2007:1034*).

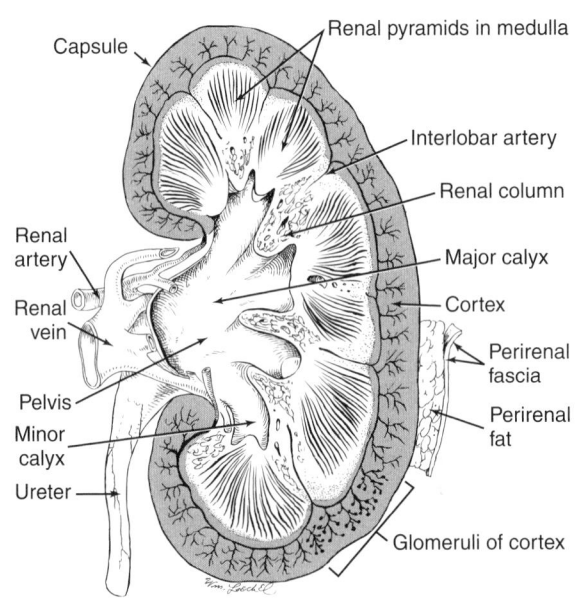

FIGURE **30-2** Longitudinal section of the kidney.

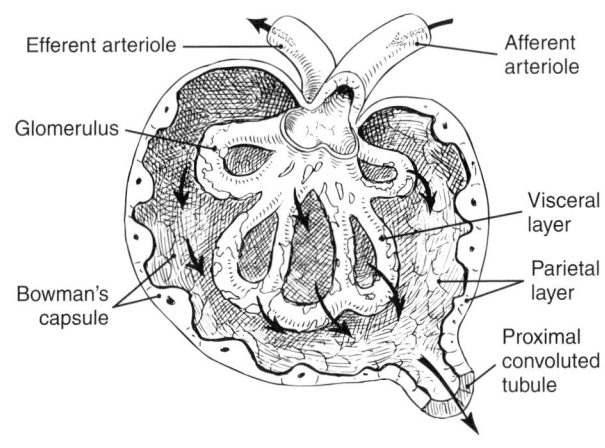

FIGURE **30-3** The nephron.

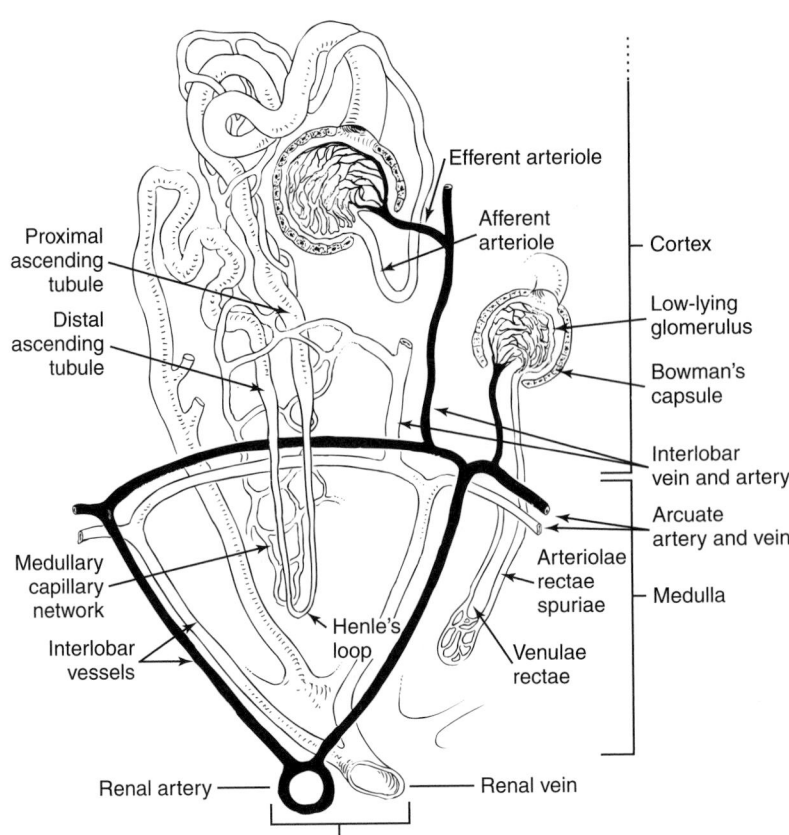

Proximal ascending tubule

Distal ascending tubule

Efferent arteriole

Afferent arteriole

Cortex

Low-lying glomerulus

Bowman's capsule

Interlobar vein and artery

Arcuate artery and vein

Medullary capillary network

Interlobar vessels

Henle's loop

Arteriolae rectae spuriae

Medulla

Venulae rectae

Renal artery

Renal vein

Hilus

FIGURE **30-4**   Renal filtration.

of the afferent arteriole. An increase in blood flow to the glomerulus returns glomerular filtration to normal.

Myogenic mechanisms also play a role in renal autoregulation. When arterial pressure rises, the arterial wall is stretched, the vessel constricts, and blood flow remains normal. When arterial pressure decreases, the opposite effect occurs. Therefore renal blood flow remains constant over a wide range of pressure changes.

Neural regulation also has a role in renal blood flow. The sympathetic nervous system innervates both the afferent and efferent arterioles. Although autoregulation overrides the adrenergic system with mild stimulation, acute sympathetic stimulation with its associated vasoconstriction can decrease renal blood flow substantially. The parasympathetic nervous system is not physiologically significant.

RENAL PHYSIOLOGY

The kidneys maintain a steady state essential to life. This is accomplished by three major mechanisms: filtration, reabsorption, and tubular secretion. What is filtered or secreted but not reabsorbed is excreted as urine.

Filtration

Filtration, which results from pressures that force fluids and solutes through the glomerulus, is the first step in the formation of urine. The quantity of glomerular filtrate formed each minute in all nephrons is called the *glomerular filtration rate* (GFR). The *filtration fraction* is the quantity of renal plasma flow that becomes filtrate and is defined as GFR divided by the flow to one kidney. Because the GFR is approximately 125 mL/min, and the flow to one kidney is 650 mL/min, the filtration fraction is 125/650, or 19% (approximately one fifth) of plasma flow. Of the 125 mL/min (or 180 L/day) of this protein-free filtrate made, 99% is reabsorbed from the renal tubules, and the remaining small portion is excreted as urine.

Regulation of Glomerular Filtration Rate

Glomerular filtration is also dependent on several physiologic factors:

- The pressure inside the glomerular capillaries
- The pressure in the Bowman capsule
- The colloid osmotic pressure of the plasma proteins

The pressure inside the high-pressure glomerulus (60 mm Hg) is an outward force, whereas the colloid osmotic pressure created by proteins in the glomerulus (28 mm Hg) is an inward force that tends to hold fluid within the glomerulus. Pressure in the Bowman capsule (18 mm Hg) opposes filtration. As illustrated in Figure 30-4, filtration pressure is the pressure that forces fluid through the glomerular membrane. It is equal to the glomerular pressure minus the sum of the glomerular colloid osmotic pressure and the capsular pressure. With the values given, the normal filtration pressure is 10 mm Hg. Several factors can alter GFR. Increased renal blood flow, dilation of the afferent arteriole, and increased resistance in the efferent arteriole increase GFR. Afferent arteriole constriction and efferent arteriole dilation tend to decrease GFR.

A special structure called the *juxtaglomerular complex* regulates GFR. At the juxtaglomerular complex, the distal convoluted tubule lies between the afferent and efferent arterioles. Cells of the distal tubule coming into contact with the arterioles are dense and therefore are referred to as the *macula densa*. Smooth muscle cells of both the afferent and efferent arterioles consist of juxtaglomerular cells, which contain renin. Anatomically this structure is arranged to allow fluid in the distal tubule to alter afferent or efferent arteriolar tone and thus regulate GFR.

Decreased glomerular filtration causes overabsorption of sodium ions (Na^+) and chloride ions (Cl^-) in the ascending limb of the loop of Henle and therefore a reduction in the delivery of these ions to the macula densa. Decreases in the concentrations of sodium and chloride cause afferent arterioles to dilate and thus increase renal blood flow and GFR. Sympathetic stimulation and decreased delivery of sodium and chloride to the macula densa also cause the juxtaglomerular cells to release renin. Renin clears angiotensinogen from the liver to form angiotensin I. In the lung, angiotensin I is changed into angiotensin II under the influence of a converting enzyme. In addition to having a generalized vasoconstricting effect, angiotensin II causes constriction of the efferent arteriole. This causes the pressure in the glomerulus to increase and the GFR to return to normal.

Filtrate Composition

Although permeability at the glomerulus is 100- to 500-fold greater than that of most capillaries, filtration at the glomerulus is a selective process. The process by which some substances are filtered and others are not is incompletely understood. It is thought that the glomerular capillary contains pores that are negatively charged. These pores, which are 70 to 100 nm in size, are freely permeable to water, some ions, and small molecules. Molecules with diameters up to 80 nm that do not have a negative charge are easily filtered. The glomerulus is almost impermeable to all plasma proteins but highly permeable to most other dissolved substances. Glomerular filtrate is therefore similar to plasma, except that it lacks significant amounts of proteins.

Tubular Reabsorption and Secretion

Conversion of glomerular filtrate to urine is the result of filtration at the glomerulus, tubular reabsorption or transport from the tubular lumen to the renal cell, and secretion or transport from the renal cell to the filtrate. Of all that is filtered or secreted, 99% is reabsorbed as the filtrate moves along the nephron.

Tubular reabsorption permits conservation of essential substances such as water, glucose, amino acids, and electrolytes. Some substances, such as water and sodium, are reabsorbed throughout the nephron, whereas others, such as glucose, are completely reabsorbed when plasma concentrations are low. Certain substances have a reabsorption maximum value. After it is reached, excess filtered material is excreted, regardless of plasma concentration. This maximum value is termed *maximum transport*. Maximum transport occurs because of saturation of a carrier for a particular substance.

By the time the blood has reached the peritubular capillary, one fifth of the plasma has been filtered into the Bowman capsule. The hydrostatic pressure in this low-pressure capillary bed has dropped to 13 mm Hg, whereas the osmotic pressure has increased to 30 to 32 mm Hg. The peritubular capillaries are extremely porous compared with those in other body tissues, and their proximity to the proximal and distal tubule sets the stage for movement of water and solutes from the tubule to the peritubular capillary bed. Anatomic location and the colloid osmotic pressure of plasma proteins account for the rapid absorption required in this area.

Transport Mechanisms

Basic mechanisms of transport through the tubular membrane can be divided into active transport and passive transport. Active transport is the net movement of particles across a membrane against an electrochemical gradient, generally at the cost of metabolic energy. Passive transport involves the movement of substances across membranes and relies on either concentration gradients or chemical gradients. Active transport can be further divided into primary active transport, which requires energy, and secondary active transport, which does not require energy. Most primary active transport is for sodium. Secondary active transport is a result of the movement of sodium from the tubular lumen to the interior of the cell. For example, the active transport of sodium pulls glucose and amino acids with it. Because a carrier protein in the membrane combines with sodium and glucose, the process is termed *cotransport*. In addition to glucose and amino acids, chloride, phosphate, calcium, magnesium, and hydrogen ions are cotransported.

Some substances are secondarily actively secreted into the renal tubule. Hydrogen, potassium, and urate ions are secreted in this manner. Hydrogen and potassium are generally secreted in exchange for sodium in a process termed *countertransport*.

When substances are actively transported from the tubule to the peritubular capillary bed, a concentration gradient that causes passive absorption of water by osmosis is established. When positive ions are actively transported, negative ions follow to maintain electrical neutrality. Chloride ions and urea are examples of substances that are passively absorbed.

Proximal Tubule

Each portion of the renal nephron is selective with regard to what is reabsorbed or secreted. Active transport of sodium is the primary function of the proximal tubule. Water, most electrolytes, and organic substances are cotransported with sodium. The osmotic force generated by active sodium transport promotes passive diffusion of water out of the tubules into the peritubular capillaries. Passive transport of water is further enhanced by the elevated osmotic pressure of the blood in the peritubular capillaries. Reabsorption of water leaves an increased concentration of urea within the tubular lumen, thereby creating a gradient for its passive diffusion into the peritubular plasma. As positively charged sodium ions leave the tubular lumen, negatively charged chloride ions passively follow to maintain electroneutrality. Hydrogen ions are actively secreted in exchange for sodium. Secretory transport of sodium also occurs in the proximal tubule.

As the filtrate passes along the proximal tubule, 60% to 70% of filtered sodium and water, 50% of urea, and potassium, calcium, phosphate, uric acid, and the bicarbonate (HCO_3) form of carbon dioxide (CO_2) have been reabsorbed. Glucose, proteins, amino acids, acetoacetate ions, and vitamins are completely or almost completely reabsorbed by active processes. Because protein molecules are too large to be reabsorbed by normal mechanisms, a special mechanism called *pinocytosis* is used to save proteins. In this process, the tubular membrane engulfs the protein and internalizes it. Once inside the cell, the protein is digested into amino acids that can then be absorbed into the interstitial fluid.

Loop of Henle

The primary function of the loop of Henle is establishing a hyperosmotic state within the medullary area of the kidney, a mechanism vital to conservation of salt and water.

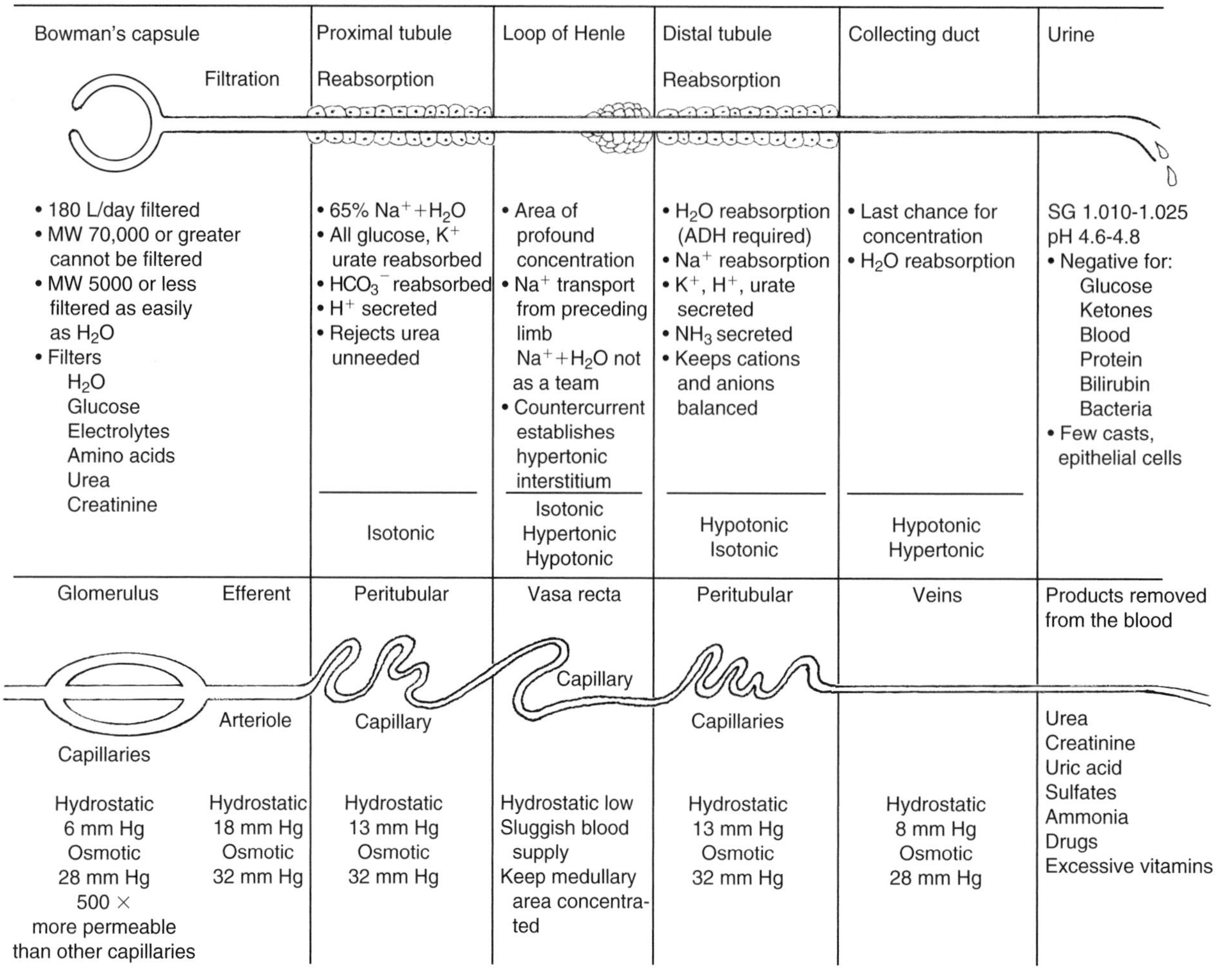

Bowman's capsule — Filtration	Proximal tubule — Reabsorption	Loop of Henle	Distal tubule — Reabsorption	Collecting duct	Urine
• 180 L/day filtered • MW 70,000 or greater cannot be filtered • MW 5000 or less filtered as easily as H_2O • Filters H_2O, Glucose, Electrolytes, Amino acids, Urea, Creatinine	• 65% $Na^+ + H_2O$ • All glucose, K^+ urate reabsorbed • HCO_3^- reabsorbed • H^+ secreted • Rejects urea unneeded	• Area of profound concentration • Na^+ transport from preceding limb $Na^+ + H_2O$ not as a team • Countercurrent establishes hypertonic interstitium	• H_2O reabsorption (ADH required) • Na^+ reabsorption • K^+, H^+, urate secreted • NH_3 secreted • Keeps cations and anions balanced	• Last chance for concentration • H_2O reabsorption	SG 1.010-1.025 pH 4.6-4.8 • Negative for: Glucose, Ketones, Blood, Protein, Bilirubin, Bacteria • Few casts, epithelial cells
	Isotonic	Isotonic Hypertonic Hypotonic	Hypotonic Isotonic	Hypotonic Hypertonic	
Glomerulus — Efferent	Peritubular	Vasa recta	Peritubular	Veins	Products removed from the blood
Capillaries — Arteriole	Capillary	Capillary	Capillaries		
Hydrostatic 6 mm Hg / Osmotic 28 mm Hg / 500 × more permeable than other capillaries	Hydrostatic 18 mm Hg / Osmotic 32 mm Hg (Efferent)	Hydrostatic 13 mm Hg / Osmotic 32 mm Hg	Hydrostatic low / Sluggish blood supply / Keep medullary area concentrated	Hydrostatic 13 mm Hg / Osmotic 32 mm Hg	Hydrostatic 8 mm Hg / Osmotic 28 mm Hg	Urea, Creatinine, Uric acid, Sulfates, Ammonia, Drugs, Excessive vitamins

FIGURE 30-5 Renal blood flow, filtration, reabsorption, and secretion. *ADH*, Antidiuretic hormone; *SG*, specific gravity.

Water conservation and the production of a concentrated urine involve a countercurrent exchange system in which a concentration gradient causes fluid to be exchanged across parallel pathways. The fluid moves up and down the parallel sides of the hairpin loop of Henle in the medulla. The longer the loop, the greater the concentration gradient, because the gradient increases from the cortex to the medulla. Sluggish blood flow in the vasa recta helps maintain the gradient.

Countercurrent exchange begins in the thick, ascending limb of the loop of Henle with the active transport of sodium and chloride out of the tubular lumen and into the medullary interstitium. Because the lumen in this area is impermeable to water, water cannot follow. The tubular fluid becomes hypoosmotic, and the medullary interstitium hyperosmotic. The descending limb of the loop is highly permeable to water but does not actively transport sodium and chloride. Sodium and chloride diffuse into the interstitium, the hypertonic interstitium causes water to move out, and the remaining fluid in the descending loop becomes concentrated at the tip of the medulla. As the tubular fluid rounds the loop and enters the ascending limb, water is retained, and sodium and chloride are removed. The filtrate therefore is very dilute as it reaches the distal tubule. The thick segment of the loop of Henle has a powerful role in renal mechanisms for diluting or concentrating the urine.

Late Distal Tubule

In the late distal tubule, sodium, under the influence of aldosterone, is reabsorbed. In this area, potassium is secreted into the lumen in exchange for sodium. It is mainly by this means that the potassium concentration is controlled in the extracellular fluids of the body.

The late distal tubule also secretes hydrogen against a concentration gradient. This function has a role in acid-base balance and the final degree of urine acidification. The late distal tubule reabsorbs 10% of filtered water. This area is permeable to water only in the presence of antidiuretic hormone (ADH).

Collecting Duct

The permeability of the collecting duct to water also is controlled by ADH. When this neurohypophyseal hormone is present, water is reabsorbed into the medullary interstitium, and the urine volume is reduced and concentrated. The collecting duct can also secrete hydrogen and therefore has a role in acid-base balance. Figure 30-5 illustrates renal blood flow, filtration, reabsorption, and secretion.

Renal Secretion

In addition to renin, hydrogen, and potassium, the kidneys release erythropoietin, a glycoprotein that stimulates red-blood-cell production in the bone marrow. Any condition that causes the quantity of oxygen transported to the tissues to decrease stimulates the release of erythropoietin, production of red blood cells, and correction of hypoxia. When both kidneys are destroyed by renal disease, the person invariably becomes very anemic.

Renal Hormones
Aldosterone
A number of hormones affect renal function. Aldosterone, the chief mineralocorticoid produced by the adrenal cortex, affects the distal segment of the nephron, causing the reabsorption of sodium and water. Several physiologic control systems regulate aldosterone release: potassium concentration in extracellular fluid; the renin-angiotensin system; and sodium concentration in extracellular fluid. Of these, potassium is the stronger trigger, followed by renin and then sodium.

Antidiuretic Hormone
ADH, a hormone synthesized in the hypothalamus but released from the neurohypophysis, also has the distal nephron as its target tissue. Because the distal tubule and collecting ducts are almost totally impermeable to water in the absence of ADH, water is not reabsorbed and is lost in the urine. In the presence of ADH, tubular permeability is increased, and water is reabsorbed. The release of ADH is controlled by the osmotic concentration of the extracellular fluids. Osmoreceptors located near the hypothalamus sense extracellular fluid concentration and release ADH accordingly. ADH is inhibited by stretch of atrial baroreceptors.

Angiotensin
Angiotensin is a hormone that has a direct renal effect, as well as a general systemic effect. As previously discussed, renin is a small protein enzyme released by the kidneys. Stimuli for the release of renin include β-adrenergic stimulation, decreased perfusion to the afferent arterioles, and reduction in sodium delivery to the distal convoluted tubule. Once released, renin acts on hepatic angiotensinogen to form angiotensin I. Angiotensin I is converted by an enzyme in the lung to form angiotensin II. In addition to causing powerful vasoconstriction, angiotensin II stimulates the release of aldosterone from the adrenal cortex. Aldosterone increases salt and water retention by the kidneys. Both of these actions increase arterial pressure.[2]

Atrial Natriuretic Factor
Atrial natriuretic factor (ANF) is a peptide hormone synthesized, stored, and secreted by the cardiac atria.[3] It acts on the kidney to increase urine flow and sodium excretion, and it may enhance renal blood flow and GFR. In addition, ANF antagonizes both the release and end-organ effects of renin, aldosterone, and ADH. The stimulus for ANF release is atrial distention, stretch, or pressure.[4] It is one of the most potent diuretics known. Inhibition of plasma renin, angiotensin, and aldosterone can produce a dose-dependent decrease in blood pressure.

Vitamin D
Vitamin D, along with parathyroid hormone and calcitonin, has a vital role in calcium metabolism. Vitamin D or cholecalciferol is obtained in the diet or synthesized by the action of ultraviolet radiation on cholesterol in the skin. To become active, cholecalciferol is first hydroxylated in the kidney to 25-hydroxycholecalciferol, then in the liver to 1,25-dihydroxycholecalciferol. Patients with advanced renal disease often have abnormal serum calcium levels.

Prostaglandins
Prostaglandins (PGs) such as PGE_2 and thromboxane A_2 modulate the renal effects of other hormones. PGE_2 is a vasodilator, and thromboxane A_2 produces contraction of vascular smooth muscle. Renal PGs influence renal excretion.

Renal Regulation of Acid-Base Balance
The kidneys, along with the body's fluid buffers and respiratory system, play a major role in regulating acid-base balance. Epithelial cells of the proximal tubules, the thick portion of the loop of Henle, distal tubules, and collecting ducts secrete hydrogen into the tubular fluid. This secretory process actually begins with CO_2 in the epithelial cells, where under the influence of carbonic anhydrase, CO_2 combines with water to form carbonic acid (H_2CO_3). H_2CO_3 dissociates into HCO_3 and hydrogen ions, and hydrogen ions are actively secreted into tubular fluid in exchange for sodium ions. This exchange maintains appropriate electrical balance between anions and cations in the tubular fluid.

An increase in HCO_3 in alkalosis means that the amount of HCO_3 filtered exceeds the amount of hydrogen secreted. Because excess HCO_3 must react with hydrogen ($HCO_3^- + H^+ \rightarrow H_2CO_3 \rightarrow CO_2^- + H_2O$) and be absorbed as CO_2, excess HCO_3 ions are lost in the urine along with sodium. In this way, sodium and excess HCO_3 are removed from the extracellular fluid.

In acidosis the concentration of hydrogen ions increases to a level far greater than that of HCO_3 in the tubules. Excess hydrogen ions are lost in the urine through the phosphate or ammonia (NH_3) buffer system.

The phosphate buffer is composed of hydrogen phosphate (HPO_2^-) and dihydrogen phosphate (H_2PO_4). Both of these ions become concentrated in the tubular fluid because of poor reabsorption. The quantity of HPO_2^- is normally fourfold greater than that of H_2PO_4. Excess hydrogen ions entering the tubules combine with monohydrogen phosphate to form H_2PO_4, which is lost in the urine. A sodium ion is absorbed into the extracellular fluid in exchange for hydrogen. It combines with HCO_3, which was formed in the process of secretion of the hydrogen, and sodium bicarbonate is added to the extracellular fluid.

NH_3, which is synthesized by all epithelial cells except those in the thin segment of the loop of Henle, is also secreted into the tubules. NH_3 reacts with hydrogen to form the ammonium ion (NH_4). Ammonium ions are lost in the urine with chloride and other tubular anions.

The kidneys control extracellular fluid hydrogen concentration by excreting an acidic or basic urine. Excretion of acidic urine removes excess acid from the extracellular fluid, whereas loss of basic urine removes base from the extracellular fluid.

Concentration and Dilution of Urine
The kidneys have the ability to respond to the changing tonicity of body fluids by excreting dilute or concentrated urine. This function involves a countercurrent exchange system in which a concentration gradient causes fluid to be exchanged across parallel pathways (Figure 30-6). In a countercurrent exchanger, reversal of flow in one stream results in the formation of a gradient that allows water and solutes to be exchanged along the length of the tube. The countercurrent exchanger in the kidney is the descending and ascending loop of Henle. The concentration gradient increases from the cortex to the tip of the medulla. The anatomic arrangement of this part of the nephron and sluggish blood flow in the vasa recta help maintain the gradient.

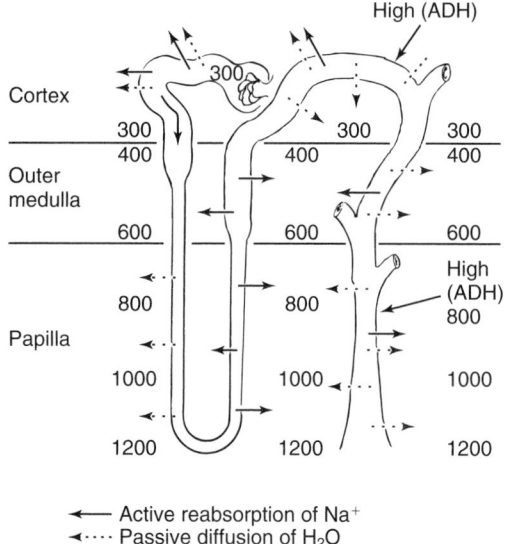

High (ADH)

Cortex

Outer medulla

Papilla

← Active reabsorption of Na⁺
◄···· Passive diffusion of H₂O

FIGURE **30-6** The countercurrent mechanism. *ADH*, Antidiuretic hormone.

Plasma water filtered at the glomerulus is isotonic with plasma. The daily urinary output is approximately 1.5 L/day, and its osmolarity may vary from 40 to 1400 mOsm/L, depending on water intake or loss. This is possible because of the countercurrent mechanism.

Approximately two thirds of the tubular fluid is reabsorbed between the glomerulus and the end of the proximal tubule. The tonicity of the filtrate in this area is the same as that of the surrounding tissue, or 300 mOsm. As the filtrate leaves the proximal tubule, it passes through an increasingly more concentrated medulla. Changes in the thick ascending limb of the loop of Henle are responsible for the hypertonicity.

The thick ascending limb of the loop of Henle is responsible for the active transport of sodium and chloride into the medullary interstitium. In contrast to the descending limb of the loop of Henle, the tonicity of which is in equilibrium with that of the interstitium, the ascending loop has a low permeability to water. The active transport of sodium and chloride produces a gradient between the ascending loop of Henle on one side and the descending loop and interstitium of the renal medulla on the other. The descending limb is highly permeable to water but does not actively transport sodium and chloride. The hyperosmotic interstitium causes water to move out of the descending limb, and the filtrate in the descending tubule is concentrated to 1200 mOsm at the tip of the medulla. As the tubular fluid rounds the loop and enters the ascending limb, active transport of sodium and chloride and retention of water create a hypoosmotic fluid of 100 mOsm at the distal tubule.

The hypoosmotic fluid of the distal tubule is delivered to the collecting duct, where the final adjustments of urine volume and concentration take place. In the absence of ADH water permeability is low, and water is not reabsorbed. Because sodium and chloride can be reabsorbed, the osmolality decreases to below that of the distal tubule, and the urine is dilute. When the need for water conservation develops, ADH is secreted, permeability of the collecting duct increases, and water diffuses out of the duct into the hyperosmolar environment of the medullary extracellular fluid. In this way urine is concentrated and its volume is reduced.

The sluggish blood supply of the vasa recta in the medulla allows blood to flow through the medullary tissue without disturbing the osmotic gradient. If blood flow were rapid, the medullary concentration gradient and the ability to concentrate the urine would be lost.

EFFECTS OF ANESTHESIA ON NORMAL RENAL FUNCTION

Before considering anesthetic implications for patients with renal disease, it is important to review the effects of anesthesia and surgery on normal renal function. Numerous studies have attempted to identify the effects of anesthesia on renal function, and although some have contributed to a better understanding of this area, differences among the studies in premedication, depth of anesthesia, fluid regimens, and other aspects of the experimental protocol allow only the broadest comparisons.

Anesthetic Effects

General anesthesia is associated with a temporary depression of renal blood flow, GFR, urinary flow, and electrolyte excretion. Although similar changes occur after spinal and epidural anesthesia, the magnitude of change tends to parallel the degree of sympathetic block and blood pressure depression. This consistent and generalized depression of renal function has been attributed to a number of factors, including type and duration of surgical procedure, physical status of the patient, volume and electrolyte status, depth of anesthesia, and choice of agent.[5]

Anesthesia may alter renal function by direct or indirect effects. Indirect effects are mediated through changes in the circulatory, endocrine, or sympathetic nervous system. Anesthetic drugs alter the circulatory system by decreasing renal perfusion, increasing renal vascular resistance, or a combination of both. Drugs associated with catecholamine release lead to vasoconstriction, an increase in renal vascular resistance, a decrease in renal blood flow, and a decrease in renal function. Volatile agents such as halothane and isoflurane cause a mild to moderate increase in renal vascular resistance as a compensatory response to decreased perfusion pressure secondary to alterations in cardiac output or systemic vascular resistance.[6-10] Desflurane has been shown to produce hemodynamic effects comparable to those produced by isoflurane.[11] It increases heart rate and decreases both mean arterial pressure and systemic vascular resistance while maintaining cardiac output. In some studies, but not all, desflurane maintains arterial pressure and systemic vascular resistance to a greater degree than equianesthetic concentrations of isoflurane. Otherwise, desflurane and isoflurane have similar effects on most vascular beds, including the renal circulation. Although earlier studies suggested that renal blood flow was reduced with sevoflurane, no renal functional or morphologic defects were noted after administration of this agent. Issues regarding the renal effects of the release of free fluoride ion associated with sevoflurane metabolism have been debated. Historically, high fluoride ion concentrations in the range of 60 to 90 μmol/L after methoxyflurane metabolism have led to nephrotoxicity characterized by polyuria. Sevoflurane has not acted in the same way as methoxyflurane. Intrarenal production of inorganic fluoride may be a more important factor than hepatic metabolism for the nephrotoxicity that causes increased serum fluoride concentration. Sevoflurane is not associated with nephrotoxicity.[12,13]

Changes in renal function during barbiturate, opiate, and nitrous oxide anesthesia are similar to those observed during the administration of low-dose volatile anesthesia.[14] Preoperative hydration, lower concentrations of volatile anesthetics, and maintenance of normal blood pressure attenuate reductions in renal blood flow and GFR.[15]

High levels of spinal or epidural anesthesia can impair venous return, diminish cardiac output, and reduce renal perfusion.[16] Epidural blocks at thoracic levels with epinephrine-containing local anesthetics cause moderate reductions in renal blood flow and GFR that parallel the decrease in mean blood pressure.[17] Epidural blocks performed with epinephrine-free solutions generate little change in systemic hemodynamics and only a small decrease in renal blood flow and GFR in animal models.[18]

In summary, virtually all anesthetics have the potential to alter the cardiovascular system and affect renal blood flow, GFR, and urinary output. Although arterial blood pressure may not fall below 80 to 90 mm Hg, renal blood flow may be decreased by 30% to 40% after the administration of various anesthetics. This suggests impairment of autoregulation. In most cases, changes in renal function are transient and reversible. If they persist into the postoperative period, the cause is often a combination of factors such as preexisting renal or cardiovascular disease, severe fluid imbalance, or mismatched blood, and the importance of the anesthetic effects is decreased.

Physiologic Responses

The renal vasculature is richly innervated by the sympathetic nervous system. Drugs or perioperative events that stimulate this system cause an increase in renal vascular resistance and a decrease in renal blood flow and glomerular filtration. Surgical stress may also alter autonomic and neuroendocrine responses. Norepinephrine from sympathetic postganglionic nerve fibers and epinephrine and norepinephrine from the adrenal medulla shift blood away from the cortical nephrons; this results in decreases in renal blood flow, GFR, electrolyte excretion, and urinary output. Catecholamines also stimulate the release of renin, which ultimately leads to the production of angiotensin II, a potent vasoconstrictor.

Endocrine changes associated with anesthesia and surgical stress involve ADH, aldosterone, and the renin-angiotensin-aldosterone system. Although the perioperative period is associated with high circulating levels of ADH and aldosterone, it is not clear whether anesthetics stimulate the release or the release is secondary to the surgical stress response. General anesthetics and narcotics are thought to be minor stimuli of the release of ADH, but the results of studies in this area are inconsistent.[19] Clinical studies have shown that induction of anesthesia with thiopental, nitrous oxide, and halothane does not elicit a significant release of ADH, but that blood loss and traction on abdominal viscera result in large elevations in blood levels.[20] Other investigations have shown that ADH levels do not change after the induction of anesthesia but do change in lightly anesthetized patients.[21]

It is clear that ADH release is modulated by blood volume changes that are sensed by stretch receptors in the atrial wall. Hemorrhage, positive pressure ventilation, and the upright position increase ADH release.[22] A decrease in arterial pressure stimulates ADH release. Distention of a balloon in the atrium, negative pressure ventilation, and immersion in water up to the neck decrease ADH release.

Renin-angiotensin levels may be elevated during the perioperative period, but the role of anesthetics and stress is not clear. Some studies have reported large increases in plasma renin levels associated with the use of anesthetics, whereas others reported only small increases.[23-26] The influence of renin-angiotensin on the renal effects of anesthetic agents needs further clarification.

Renin levels have been shown to increase during halothane anesthesia when sodium depletion is present. Preoperative hydration is thought to be important in the intraoperative release of renin.

Aldosterone, a hormone released from the adrenal gland, is responsible for the precise control of sodium excretion. It is not known whether anesthetic agents act directly on the adrenal gland to cause aldosterone release. They probably act indirectly through the neuroendocrine system and the renin-angiotensin-aldosterone system. Stimulation of the sympathetic nervous system causes renal vasoconstriction, which is a trigger for the renin-angiotensin-aldosterone system. Aldosterone leads to sodium and water reabsorption and can be associated with decreased urinary output.

Nephrotoxicity of Anesthetic Agents

The kidneys are extremely vulnerable to toxicity because of their rich blood supply and the increase in the concentration of excreted compounds that occurs in the renal tubules during the process of reabsorption. Medullary hyperosmolality encourages concentration of all substances, including toxins. The amount of renal damage associated with nephrotoxic agents depends on the concentration of the toxins, the degree of toxin binding to plasma proteins and nonrenal versus renal tissue, and the length of exposure of the kidneys to the toxin. The nephrotoxicity of anesthetic agents became fully appreciated in 1966, when vasopressin resistant–polyuria renal insufficiency was reported in patients receiving prolonged methoxyflurane anesthesia for abdominal surgery.[27] Evidence gathered indicated that the release of the inorganic fluoride ions (F^-) in the metabolism of this fluorinated anesthetic was the causative agent in nephrotoxicity.

Fluoride Ion Toxicity

Fluoride alters renal concentration mechanisms by interfering with active transport of sodium and chloride in the medullary portions of the loop of Henle. It also acts as a potent vasodilator, resulting in increased blood flow in the vasa recta and washout of medullary solute. Fluoride is a potent inhibitor of many enzyme systems, including those involving ADH, and it is necessary for distal nephron reabsorption of water. Proximal tubular swelling and necrosis associated with fluoride ions also contribute to nephrotoxicity. Signs and symptoms of fluoride nephrotoxicity include polyuria, hypernatremia, serum hyperosmolality, elevations in blood urea nitrogen (BUN) and serum creatinine levels, and decreased creatinine clearance. The extent of nephrotoxicity in general surgical patients has been correlated with dosage or maximum allowable concentration hours (MAC-hours), duration, and peak fluoride concentrations.[28]

Methoxyflurane

Methoxyflurane, an anesthetic no longer used, was the first anesthetic associated with serious nephrotoxicity. The serum fluoride concentration after methoxyflurane anesthesia showed positive correlation with the degree of renal dysfunction.[29] Vasopressin-resistant polyuria similar to that seen after methoxyflurane anesthesia was later produced in Fischer 344 rats injected with sodium fluoride.[30] After 2.5 to 3 MAC-hours of methoxyflurane anesthesia, fluoride concentration was 50 to 80 μmol, and subclinical toxicity evidenced by a delayed return to maximum preoperative urine osmolarity and decreased urate clearance were noted. At 5 MAC-hours, fluoride concentration was 90 to 120 μmol, and mild nephrotoxicity with serum hyperosmolality, hypernatremia, polyuria, and urinary hypoosmolality was noted. At 7 to 9 MAC-hours, fluoride concentration was 175 μmol, and marked nephrotoxicity was noted. Patients vary in nephrotoxic susceptibility, with genetic heterogeneity, preexisting renal disease, and drug interactions all contributing to toxicity. For example, the combination of methoxyflurane and aminoglycoside antibiotics encourages toxicity.[31]

Isoflurane

Isoflurane is metabolized only slightly and defluorinated much less than other halogenated agents. In one report of nine surgical patients, mean peak serum fluoride concentration measured 6 hours after anesthesia was only 4.4 μmol.[32] Clinical experience has indicated that renal toxicity is unlikely after the administration of isoflurane.[33]

Desflurane

The metabolism of desflurane has been assessed in both animals and humans with the appearance of fluoride metabolites (fluoride ion, nonvolatile organic fluoride, trifluoroacetic acid) in blood and urine. Administration of desflurane to rats that were either pretreated or not pretreated with phenobarbital or ethanol for 3.2 MAC-hours, as well as to swine for 5.5 MAC-hours, produced fluoride levels in blood that were almost indistinguishable from values measured in control animals.[34] In human studies, desflurane administered to patients for 3.1 MAC-hours and volunteers for 7.3 MAC-hours resulted in postanesthesia serum fluoride concentrations that did not differ from background fluoride concentrations. Similarly, postanesthesia urinary excretion rates of fluoride and organic fluoride in volunteers were comparable with preanesthetic excretion rates.[35-37] Small but statistically significant increases in the levels of trifluoroacetic acid were found in both the serum and urine of volunteers after exposure to desflurane. Although these increases in trifluoroacetic acid were statistically significant, they were approximately one tenth the levels seen after exposure to isoflurane. Desflurane strongly resists biodegradation, and only a small amount is metabolized in animals and humans.[38]

Sevoflurane

Sevoflurane undergoes approximately 5% metabolism, and the primary metabolites are fluoride and hexofluro-2-propranolol (HFIP). The oxidative defluorination of sevoflurane in the liver with the liberation of free fluoride ions raised concerns that sevoflurane, like methoxyflurane, might impair the ability of the kidneys to concentrate urine. Earlier research indicated that with methoxyflurane, renal dysfunction was likely to occur when plasma fluoride levels exceeded 50 μmol. The same does not appear to be true with sevoflurane.

Preliminary investigations with sevoflurane found that some adult patients receiving the drug had plasma fluoride levels that exceeded 50 μmol. However, renal function, assessed by BUN, creatinine, and decrease in urine osmolality, was not different from that in patients receiving similar amounts of other fluorinated anesthetics. In one study, serum fluoride levels averaged 29 μmol after 1 to 7 MAC-hours of anesthesia. The fluoride levels peaked 2 hours after the end of anesthesia and decreased by 50% within 8 hours.[39] The fast decline in plasma fluoride levels was attributed to insolubility of the agent and rapid pulmonary elimination of sevoflurane.

Numerous published reports indicate the absence of renal toxicity after sevoflurane anesthesia.[40-43] An explanation for the absence of fluoride-induced nephrotoxicity may be that intrarenal production of fluoride ion is important in the pathogenesis of this complication. The intrarenal metabolism of methoxyflurane is four times greater than that of sevoflurane.[13]

Studies of surgical patients receiving intermediate-duration sevoflurane with high and low fresh gas flow and long-duration sevoflurane with high fresh gas flow included sensitive measures of renal function or injury. These studies also indicate the absence of renal toxicity after sevoflurane anesthesia.[44-49]

In addition to release of inorganic fluoride ion resulting from biotransformation, CO_2 absorbents degrade sevoflurane, resulting in production of a vinyl ether called compound A. Factors associated with the generation of higher levels of compound A during administration of sevoflurane to patients include (1) a high concentration of agent, (2) increased temperature in the CO_2 absorbent, (3) low fresh gas flow rates, and (4) increased states of CO_2 production. The potential for compound A nephrotoxicity exists, particularly in the animal model.

Because the potential for renal injury exists with sevoflurane, studies in volunteers have raised the question of whether it is important to apply more sensitive measures of renal function in evaluation of this drug. Such tests have included urine concentrations or excretion of enzymes, albumin, protein, and glucose and creatinine clearance.[50] Two studies of volunteers receiving prolonged sevoflurane anesthesia with fresh gas flow no greater than 2 L/min concluded that the potential for adverse renal effects of sevoflurane may exist.[51-52] However, other studies of volunteers did not find the same results.[53-56]

A number of reports describe instances in which sevoflurane has been given to patients with renal dysfunction and other conditions that might enhance renal injury. Such conditions include patients who are hypotensive, hypertensive, elderly, or obese or who have renal insufficiency.[57-64] The only proved direct toxic effect of any anesthetic agent is the fluoride-related toxicity of methoxyflurane.[65]

Because the amount of compound A produced increases with lower gas flows, the package insert at one time recommended flows of 2 L/min or more. Several studies indicate no effect of low-flow sevoflurane on renal function, even those with moderate renal insufficiency.[66,67] Today the U.S. Food and Drug Administration recommends the use of sevoflurane for a minimum of 1 L/min of fresh gas flow and advises that 2 MAC-hours at this flow rate should not be exceeded.[68] Other countries have not recommended such limitations on the use of sevoflurane, and problems have not been noted.

ACUTE RENAL FAILURE

Acute renal failure (acute tubular necrosis, vasomotor neuropathy, lower nephron necrosis) is defined as the sudden inability of the kidneys to vary urine volume and content appropriately in response to homeostatic needs. Perioperative acute renal failure accounts for half of all patients who require dialysis and is associated with a 50% mortality rate.[69-72] A recent report confirmed earlier findings. A literature review spanning 47 years, or from 1956-2003, revealed no evidence of improved outcome from acute renal failure during this period. Mortality rates remained about 50% despite new approaches to general management, such as monitoring and management of the complication.[71]

Classification

Acute renal failure is classified according to its predominant cause or on the basis of urine flow rates. The cause of acute renal failure has prenal, renal, or postrenal origins. Prenal failure results from hemodynamic or endocrine factors that

---

Etiology of Acute Renal Failure

Hypovolemia
Impaired renal perfusion
Sepsis
Drugs
   1. Radiocontrast media
   2. Antimicrobials
Hepatic dysfunction
Vascular occlusion
Obstruction of collecting system
Primary renal disease

Classification of Acute Renal Failure

I. Prerenal Failure
  A. Hypoperfusion or hypovolemia
    1. Skin losses
    2. Fluid losses
    3. Hemorrhage
    4. Sequestration
  B. Cardiovascular failure
    1. Myocardial failure
    2. Vascular pooling
    3. Vascular occlusion
      a. Thromboembolic phenomena
      b. Aortic renal artery clamping
II. Renal or Acute Tubular Necrosis
  A. Prolonged renal ischemia
  B. Nephrotoxic injury
    1. Heme pigments
    2. Some anesthetics
    3. Antibiotics
    4. Radiocontrast dyes
    5. Chemotherapeutic agents
  C. Miscellaneous
    1. Cellular debris
    2. Acute interstitial nephritis
    3. Hypersensitivity reactions
    4. Acute glomerulonephritis
III. Postrenal Failure
  A. Obstruction
    1. Calculi
    2. Blood clots
    3. Neoplasm
  B. Surgical ligation
  C. Edema

---

impair renal perfusion, renal failure results from tissue damage, and postrenal failure results from urinary tract obstruction. Prerenal or postrenal failure is reversed with attention to hemodynamics or relief of obstruction. Acute renal failure caused by parenchymal disease or damage is more serious and often requires hemodialysis. Common causes are listed in Box 30-1.

Failure classified according to urine flow rates is known as *oliguric, nonoliguric,* or *polyuric failure. Oliguria* is defined as a urinary flow rate less than 0.5 mL/kg/hr in a patient subjected to acute stress. This rate is higher than that seen in unstressed patients because acutely stressed patients cannot maximally concentrate urine. Polyuric failure is associated with elevations of BUN and serum creatinine levels and is characterized by urine flow rates that exceed 2.5 L/day.

Conditions that lead to prerenal oliguria include acute reductions in GFR, excessive reabsorption of salt or water, or both. Increases in circulating levels of catecholamines, ADH, or aldosterone are physiologic factors that can decrease urinary output. Hypotension may or may not be present in the initiation of acute renal failure. If not reversed, prerenal oliguria may progress to parenchymal damage and tubular necrosis.

Acute tubular necrosis may be produced by a variety of factors that interfere with glomerular filtration or tubular reabsorption. The pathogenesis of acute tubular necrosis may be divided into an initiation period, a maintenance period, and a recovery period. Renal hypoperfusion or a nephrotoxic insult may initiate renal failure. Surgical patients with external and internal fluid losses or sepsis may have renal hypoperfusion. The renal medulla, with its sluggish blood supply and active transport mechanisms, is especially susceptible to even moderate renal ischemia.

The initiating insult culminates in the development of one or more maintenance factors, such as decreased tubular function, tubular obstruction, and sustained reductions in renal blood flow and glomerular filtration. Urine flow and solute excretion are reduced. Once the maintenance period has begun, pharmacologic interventions to improve renal blood flow do not reverse the failure.

Prerenal oliguria is associated with physiologic mechanisms that conserve salt and water. In this case urine has low sodium levels and high osmolality. Patients with parenchymal disease have trouble concentrating the urine. Urine sodium levels are high, and osmolality is low. Renal damage is also associated with a progressive rise in serum urea, creatinine, uric acid, and

polypeptide levels. Serum potassium levels may increase by 0.3 to 3 mEq/L/day, and a decrease occurs in the serum levels of sodium, calcium, and proteins such as albumin. Assessment of renal dysfunction perioperatively is difficult. Arterial blood gas analysis, which allows the anesthetist to detect pulmonary dysfunction quickly, has no renal equivalent. Exogenous factors may alter BUN level, and subtle changes in serum creatinine concentration are easily ignored. The creatinine clearance remains the single most helpful test in defining renal status and predicting the prognosis in cases of severe renal dysfunction. It has been suggested that incorporation of a creatinine clearance test with a threshold less than 60 mL/min in the preoperative assessment would facilitate identification of high-risk patients for renal-protective interventions during high risk surgery.[72]

Risk Factors

A number of conditions may place patients at high risk for acute renal failure (Box 30-2). Renal reserve decreases progressively with age. For each year after 50 years of age, creatinine clearance decreases by 1.5 mL and renal plasma flow by 8 mL. Older patients are less able to cope with fluid and electrolyte imbalance and are more prone to renal damage. Overall mortality rates associated with acute renal failure increase from 50% for those younger than age 40 years to 80% for those older than age 60 years.

Patients with preexisting renal dysfunction are also at high risk. Cardiac and hepatic failure is associated with abnormal renal hemodynamics. Cortical redistribution of blood flow, salt and water retention, and reduced GFR are all increased by anesthetics, stress, and hypovolemia, and therefore the incidence of postoperative renal failure increases. Bilirubin is nephrotoxic, and levels greater than 8.5 mg/dL are associated with elevated levels of endotoxin that may cause renal dysfunction.

Certain surgical procedures are associated with a higher risk of acute renal failure. Although cardiac surgery has only a 2% to 4% incidence of this complication, the risk increases in patients with preoperative ventricular dysfunction or bacterial endocarditis, in those undergoing emergency procedures, and in those who have procedures in which cardiopulmonary bypass lasts longer than 2 hours. Postoperative bleeding with reexploration and low cardiac output requiring use of the intraaortic balloon pump also carry a higher incidence of failure.

A ruptured abdominal aortic aneurysm implies hypovolemia, shock, and the need for high aortic cross-clamping. Of these patients, 40% have renal damage, and 11% develop acute renal failure with an associated mortality rate of 80%. Renal dysfunction after elective surgery is less profound if attention is given to adequate hydration and if a brisk diuresis is established before and maintained during aortic cross-clamping. The proximity of the aortic clamp to the renal arteries is critical. Aortic arteriography performed just before surgery also increases risk. Predisposing factors are preexisting renal disease with serum creatinine levels greater than 3 mg/dL, proteinuria, diabetes, and hypovolemia. Risk is reduced by minimizing the amount of dye given, maintaining hydration, and using diuretics such as mannitol to promote diuresis. Acute postoperative renal failure is a common complication of thoracic aorta, thoracoabdominal aorta, and aortic arch surgeries. It is observed in 6% to 18% of such surgical procedures. Predisposing factors for this complication include age older than 50, preoperative renal dysfunction, duration of renal ischemia, and amount of blood transfused.[73]

Mechanical obstruction by calculi or prostatic disease is the most common cause of obstructive uropathy. Risk is increased by the frequent presence of hypovolemia and electrolyte imbalance and by preoperative diagnostic studies that involve the use of dye.

Hypovolemia, hemolysis, disseminated intravascular coagulopathy, and acidosis are key factors in the development of acute renal failure in septic patients. The use of vasoconstrictive adrenergic agonists and antibiotics with nephrotoxic potential compounds the problem. Complications of pregnancy such as hemorrhage, amniotic fluid embolus, and toxemia carry a high risk of renal failure, but because patients are usually young and healthy, mortality in this group is reduced.

Prevention and Management

The old saying that an ounce of prevention is worth a pound of cure is especially true with regard to acute renal failure, because prevention is far more successful than management. Prevention can be based on the following generalizations:

1. The most common cause of failure is prolonged renal hypoperfusion.
2. Prophylaxis reduces mortality more effectively than dialytic therapy.
3. The duration and magnitude of the initiating renal insult are critical in determining the severity of failure.

A key strategy in reducing the incidence of renal failure is limiting the magnitude and duration of renal ischemia. Although a number of preventive strategies have been described, none apart from maintenance of normovolemia appears to be effective.[74] Prevention begins in the preoperative period.

Preoperative Strategies

In the preoperative preparation of surgical patients, high-risk patients and procedures should be identified. Reversible renal dysfunction should be sought, and fluid losses and hypovolemia should be corrected by intravenous fluids. Perioperative ADH and renin-angiotensin-aldosterone secretion can be minimized with adequate hydration before anesthetic induction. Administration of saline rather than solutions low in sodium is helpful in prevention of aldosterone secretion, hyponatremia, and oliguria.

Oliguria often signals inadequate systemic perfusion, and prevention of acute renal failure requires its rapid recognition through adequate monitoring. In addition to standard monitors and a urinary catheter, monitors for patients with questionable cardiac and pulmonary function should include a direct arterial line for blood pressure monitoring and a central venous pressure (CVP) or pulmonary artery catheter, when appropriate, for assessment of cardiac function and volume status. The hemodynamic endpoint should be adequate cardiac output and renal perfusion, not pulmonary dysfunction (e.g., pulmonary edema). Pulmonary edema can be supported with mechanical ventilation and is associated with a lower mortality rate than is acute renal failure.

Perioperative Strategies

Use of a urinary catheter is the only means of monitoring renal function in the operating room. A fluid challenge is necessary if hourly urinary output decreases to below acceptable levels.

The use of diuretics in the face of inadequate urinary output must be carefully evaluated. Although the administration of furosemide (Lasix) and mannitol decreases experimental renal failure in animals subjected to fixed insults, it worsens hypoperfusion and renal ischemia in hypovolemic patients.[75-77] Although diuretics may not be effective during the initiation of failure, large doses of furosemide may convert oliguric renal failure into nonoliguric failure, which is easier to manage.[78] In the maintenance phase, doses of furosemide in excess of 1 g may be required to convert oliguric failure to nonoliguric failure.[79] Little evidence suggests that doses smaller than 100 mg alter the course of renal failure. Diuretic therapy must be associated with aggressive monitoring and intravascular volume expansion. Prophylactic administration of mannitol and/or furosemide might prevent renal damage in hydrated patients.

Although the mechanism is unknown, prophylactic administration of mannitol in well-hydrated patients protects renal function. Loop diuretics may also prevent acute renal failure. Mechanisms for protection include the inhibition of sodium reabsorption and the prevention of tubular obstruction through the maintenance of high flow and pressure within the tubules and the reversal of intrinsic renal vasoconstriction. Prophylactic use of diuretics may be of benefit in the case of jaundice in surgical patients, excessive exposure to contrast media, hyperuricemia, or the presence of pigment in the urine. Fenoldopam, a dopamine receptor agonist also may be helpful.

Fenoldpam mesylate (Corlopam) is a selective DA_1 receptor agonist. It causes both systemic and renal arteriolar vasodilation and has no effect on DA_2, α-adrenergic, or β-adrenergic receptors. Unlike dopamine, which causes renal vasoconstriction at higher doses, fenoldopam at high dose produces even greater renal vasodilation.[80] Fenoldopam is more than 6 times as potent as dopamine in increasing renal blood flow.[81] Some investigators believe it is safer and more consistently effective as a renal protective agent than low-dose dopamine,[82] but this belief is controversial. Others found no difference between dopamine and fenoldopam in renal protection in high-risk procedures. A recent study found that fenoldopam had no greater renal protection in patients undergoing infrarenal aortic cross-clamping for abdominal reconstruction than sodium nitroprusside and dopamine. Selection of equivalent therapies may have relevance in an increasingly more cost-conscious health-care environment.[83]

Management of Acute Renal Failure

If acute renal failure develops, it progresses through four distinct phases: onset, the oliguric phase, the diuretic phase, and the recovery phase. Onset, or the initiation phase, precedes actual necrotic injury and correlates with a major alteration in renal hemodynamics. The oliguric phase reflects four pathophysiologic processes:

1. Obstruction of tubules by cellular debris, tubular casts, or tissue swelling
2. Total reabsorption or back leak of urine filtrate through damaged tubular epithelium and into the circulation
3. Tubular cell damage with leakage of adenosine triphosphate (ATP) and potassium and edema
4. Continuation of renal vasoconstriction

The diuretic phase signifies that tubular function is returning. It is marked by large daily urinary output (more than 3 L) secondary to the osmotic diuretic effect produced by an elevated BUN and impaired ability of tubules to conserve sodium and water. The recovery phase is characterized by gradual improvement of renal function over 3 months to 1 year.

After renal failure is established, the primary consideration in management is the maintenance of fluid and electrolyte balance. The early use of hemodialysis for the prevention of severe fluid and electrolyte imbalance is necessary during the oliguric and diuretic phases. The most common complication that results in death is infection.[84] Once identified, infection must be aggressively treated with antibiotics. A clinical algorithm for perioperative management of oliguria is found in Box 30-3.

CHRONIC RENAL FAILURE

Chronic renal failure is a slow, progressive, irreversible condition characterized by diminished functioning of nephrons and a decrease in renal blood flow, GFR, tubular function, and reabsorptive capacity. Although many conditions may lead to renal failure, primary causes include glomerulonephritis, pyelonephritis, diabetes mellitus, vascular or hypertensive insults, and congenital defects. Table 30-1 outlines the systemic effects of chronic renal failure.

The general course of progressive renal failure may be divided into three stages: decreased renal reserve, renal insufficiency, and end-stage renal failure or uremia. As the number of functioning nephrons declines, the signs, symptoms, and biochemical abnormalities become more severe.

Clinical signs or laboratory evidence of renal disease are absent until less than 40% of normal-functioning nephrons remain. Loss of nephron function without symptoms is known as the *decrease in renal reserve*. Renal insufficiency occurs when only 10% to 40% of nephrons are functioning adequately. Nocturia occurs secondary to a decrease in concentrating ability. Although affected patients seem well compensated when

BOX 30-3

Algorithm for Clinical Management of Perioperative Oliguria

- Oliguria is less than 0.5 mL/kg but may be 1-2 mL/kg in a patient who has received mannitol.
- Assume oliguria is prerenal until proven otherwise.
- Do not give a diuretic to "make urine" in face of intravascular hypovolemia or hypotension.
- Do give diuretics if there are signs of fluid overload or if oliguria persists despite fluid challenges and stabilized hemodynamics or if there is pigment nephropathy.
- If improvement is not noted with fluid challenge or diuretics, institute invasive hemodynamic monitoring.
- Maximize renal blood flow by enhancing cardiac function: normalize preload, heart rate, rhythm, afterload reduction with vasodilators or inodilator agents.
- Prophylactic pharmacologic agents may be used when renal risk is high but there is little evidence to suggest they are better at maintaining glomerular filtration rate than volume.
- Diuretic resistance may be related to:
  1. Acute tolerance induced by hypovolemia
  2. Chronic tolerance
  3. Refractory states

TABLE 30-1   Systemic Effects of Renal Disease

System	Effects
Cardiovascular	Hypertension Congestive heart failure Peripheral and pulmonary edema Pericarditis Coronary artery disease
Hematologic	Normochromic, normocytic anemia Platelet dysfunction Leukocyte, immunologic dysfunction
Neurologic	Encephalopathy Peripheral and autonomic neuropathy
Endocrine	Hyperparathyroidism Adrenal insufficiency
Respiratory	Pneumonitis Pulmonary edema
Gastrointestinal	Bleeding Nausea, vomiting Delayed gastric emptying
Metabolic	Acidosis Electrolyte imbalance

excretory capacity is unstressed, little renal reserve is present. Elimination of a large protein load or excretion of certain drugs is impaired, and preservation of remaining nephron function is a major goal. Toxic substances such as aminoglycosides potentiate existing damage, and aminoglycoside toxicity is enhanced in the presence of either volume depletion or arterial hypotension.[85] Radiocontrast exposure in patients with chronic renal insufficiency often causes further reversible decreases in renal function in those with either myocardial failure or diabetes mellitus.[86]

As renal function deteriorates further, end-stage renal disease develops. In this stage, concentrating and diluting properties of the kidney are severely compromised, and electrolyte, hematologic, and acid-base disturbances are common. The loss of 95% of functioning nephrons culminates in uremia, which is associated with volume overload and congestive heart failure. Uremia, which can be viewed as urine in the blood, adversely affects almost every organ system. Death occurs unless dialysis is performed.

Dialytic Therapy

Approximately 350,000 people in the United States today require chronic dialysis, and the end stage renal disease population is projected to grow about 7% per year. Thirty patients in 1 million receive dialysis for acute renal failure per year, and half of these patients require treatment early in the postoperative period.[87]

Dialysis Techniques

Dialysis is a general term used to describe therapy in which solute moves from blood through a semipermeable membrane into a chemically prescribed solution. The movement of solute, which is called *diffusive transport*, depends on differences in molecular concentration between the blood compartment and the dialysate. *Ultrafiltration* is a technique in which a hydraulic pressure difference across a semipermeable membrane causes the bulk removal of fluid and solute by convective transport.

Major types of dialysis include hemodialysis and peritoneal dialysis. In hemodialysis, blood moves through a device that exposes it to an individually prescribed dialysate solution across a semipermeable membrane. The hollow fiber type of dialyzer provides a membrane area of 0.8 to 2 m^2. Blood flow occurs through multiple channels and runs in a direction opposite to the flow of the dialysate. Both convective and diffusive movement of solute occurs. Hemodialysis requires systemic or regional anticoagulation.

In peritoneal dialysis, the blood compartment is the peritoneal microvasculature, and the semipermeable membrane is the peritoneal lining. The dialysate is infused into and withdrawn from the abdominal cavity. Movement of water occurs down an osmotic gradient from blood to dialysate and may be increased with an increase in the glucose concentration of the dialysate. Diffusive transport is influenced by the solute concentration within the dialysate.

Physiologic Effects

Dialysis and ultrafiltration are associated with a number of physiologic effects and complications. Major systems involved include the nervous system, cardiovascular system, and respiratory system. The disequilibrium syndrome is the most severe central nervous system (CNS) effect of dialysis. This syndrome is associated with a rapid increase in brain intracellular volume as serum sodium and BUN levels are reduced. Predisposing factors include a BUN concentration greater than 150 mg/dL, hypernatremia, severe acidemia, and preexisting brain disease. The syndrome may be mild or may progress to seizures, stupor, and coma. The incidence is reduced by the avoidance of high rates of hemodialysis therapy in high-risk patients.

Hemodialysis is associated with a 30% incidence of hypotension. Contributing factors include reduced plasma volume and blunted sympathetic nervous system response associated with

uremia. Acetate from the dialysate moves into the blood and contributes to the hypotension by causing vasodilation and cardiac depression.

The incidence of hypotension with dialysis is less in patients who have fasted than in those who have not. Fasting prevents the contribution to hypovolemia of increased gastrointestinal blood flow and the secretion of isotonic intestinal juices. Anemia should be corrected if the hematocrit is less than 20%. Leg elevation, a decrease in dialyzer transmembrane pressure, or the use of volume expanders or vasoconstrictors usually corrects hypotension. Substitution of HCO_3 for acetate in the dialysate decreases the incidence.

Hypoxemia is a common side effect of hemodialysis and may be seen during peritoneal dialysis.[88,89] During hemodialysis, arterial oxygen tension often decreases by 5 to 20 mm Hg. Pulmonary leukostasis and extracorporeal loss of CO_2 with a reduction in minute ventilation have been implicated. Hypoxemia is managed by increasing the inspired oxygen concentration during dialysis. The use of HCO_3 in place of acetate limits extracorporeal losses of CO_2 and reduces the incidence of hypoxemia.

Muscle cramping is the most common neuromuscular complication of dialysis. It is seen almost exclusively with hemodialysis and results from the rapid reduction of intravascular volume and serum sodium level. Intravenous administration of hypertonic saline relieves muscle cramping.

The nutritional depletion common in dialysis-dependent patients may be caused by the primary disease, dietary restrictions, or the loss of protein associated with peritoneal dialysis. Protein depletion may produce hypoalbuminemia and immunocompromise. The large quantities of hypertonic glucose solutions absorbed with peritoneal dialysis contribute to obesity, hyperglycemia, and hyperlipidemia. Insulin controls hyperglycemia, and exercise limits hyperlipidemia.

PREOPERATIVE RENAL ASSESSMENT

Preoperative assessment of the patient with suspected or known renal dysfunction must include a thorough history and physical examination, as well as appropriate laboratory evaluation (Box 30-4). The medical history is the single most important source of information in establishing the presence or absence of renal disease. Poorly controlled hypertension, trauma to the urinary system, prior renal surgery, or systemic disease (e.g., diabetes) may be associated with renal impairment. A history that arouses suspicion should lead to a more thorough evaluation of renal function.

Although abnormalities are commonly found on urinalysis, the quality of urinalysis results obtained by dipstick technique varies.[90-92] Because abnormal results on urinalysis usually fail to lead to a change in management, the test is generally omitted. If the test is available, attention should be directed to the following:

1. *Specific gravity.* Specific gravity, a measurement of solutes in the urine, indicates the ability of the kidney to excrete concentrated or dilute urine. It is a reflection of tubular function and normally varies from 1.003 to 1.030, depending on fluid intake and the presence or absence of high-molecular-weight substances such as glucose or mannitol. In the absence of such substances, a specific gravity of 1.018 or greater after overnight dehydration indicates reasonable function. A low specific gravity is meaningless if the condition under which the sample was collected is not known.

2. *Urine osmolality.* Osmolality, or the number of moles of solute (measured in osmoles) per kilogram of solvent, is

BOX **30-4**

Preoperative Assessment and Preparation of the Patient with End-Stage Renal Disease

I. Clinical History
  A. Document central nervous system deficits.
  B. Review cardiovascular history; look for significant hypertension, accelerated atherosclerosis, pericarditis, tamponade; assess extent, stability, and management of coronary artery disease.
  C. Look for history of excessive bleeding; if present consider use of desmopressin.
  D. Assess intravascular volume; correlate body weight changes with changes in blood pressure and heart rate before and after dialysis.
  E. Review pulmonary history.
  F. Dialyze 24 hr or less before surgery; ideal weight preoperatively is 1-2 kg above "dry" weight.
II. Physical Examination
  A. Locate and check patency of arteriovenous fistula or shunt.
  B. Evaluate vessels for venous or arterial access.
  C. Look for signs of congestive heart failure, pericarditis, or cardiac tamponade.
  D. Look for evidence of noncardiogenic pulmonary edema or aspiration.
III. Laboratory Tests
  A. Electrocardiography, chest radiography
  B. Blood urea nitrogen, creatinine
  C. Complete blood count with platelet count
  D. Bleeding time; prothrombin time; partial thromboplastin time
  E. Hematocrit; red-blood-cell index
  F. Electrolytes (especially potassium)
  G. Acid-base status
  H. Hepatitis antigen status

more specific than specific gravity. Excretion of concentrated urine (specific gravity 1.030; 1400 mOsm/kg) indicates excellent tubular function, whereas urinary osmolality fixed to that of plasma (serum gravity 1.010; 290 mOsm/kg) suggests tubular concentrating defects. Urinary diluting mechanisms are present after concentrating ability is lost.

3. *Proteinuria.* Proteinuria exists when more than 150 mg of protein is excreted per day. Massive proteinuria or the renal loss of more than 750 mg/day is always abnormal and usually indicative of severe glomerular damage. In addition to its association with glomerular damage, proteinuria may also be present with abnormal plasma proteins or increased concentrations of normal proteins or when the renal tubules fail to reabsorb the small amount of protein that may be filtered. Patients can have proteinuria without renal disease under conditions of stress, fever, dehydration, exercise, or congestive heart failure. Patients who have significant proteinuria are more likely to develop acute renal failure postoperatively than those who do not. The incidence of hypoalbuminemia and its consequences is increased in patients with severe proteinuria. In a concentrated urine sample, trace or 1+ proteinuria is a nonspecific finding, whereas 3+ or 4+ proteinuria suggests glomerular disease.

The kidneys share regulation of acid-base balance with the lungs. Because they provide the sole pathway for the excretion of the 60 mEq of hydrogen ions produced per day, urinary pH is a reflection of the ability of the kidneys to acidify urine. The inability to excrete an acid urine in the presence of systemic acidosis is indicative of renal insufficiency.

Laboratory Tests for Renal Function

Patients with suspected or known renal disease should be tested preoperatively to evaluate GFR and renal tubular function. Although urine specific gravity (1.003 to 1.030), urine osmolality (65 to 1400 mOsm/L), and urine sodium concentration (130 to 260 mEq/day) reflect renal tubular function, BUN concentration (10 to 20 mg/dL), plasma creatinine level (0.7 to 1.5 mg/dL), and creatinine clearance (110 to 150 mL/min) are necessary for the evaluation of GFR.

Blood Urea Nitrogen

Urea, the chief end product of protein metabolism, is formed in the liver. It is excreted by glomerular filtration, but significant amounts of urea are reabsorbed along the renal tubule. Although the normal range for BUN level is 10 to 20 mg/dL, it is altered by a variety of factors, including ingestion of protein, anabolic and catabolic states, GFR, state of hydration, and reabsorption of urea by the nephrons. Because of the numerous extrarenal factors that can influence BUN, it is a better indicator of uremic symptoms than of GFR. Levels below 8 mg/dL suggest overhydration or underproduction of urea, whereas those between 20 and 40 mg/dL suggest dehydration, high nitrogen levels, or decreased GFR. Levels higher than 50 mg/dL almost always indicate decreased glomerular filtration. Elevations of BUN level in the presence of normal serum creatinine concentration suggest a nonrenal cause of the elevation. In general, BUN level is a late indicator of renal disease because it does not increase in most patients until the GFR is reduced by more than 50%.

Serum Creatinine

Creatinine is a metabolite of creatine, a major muscle constituent. The daily rate of production of creatinine is constant and determined by skeletal muscle mass. Because body creatinine is eliminated almost entirely by glomerular filtration, its steady-state concentration in the serum has been used as a marker of glomerular function. Normal values range from 0.7 to 1.5 mg/dL, but the serum concentration can be lower in the elderly or in women who have reduced muscle mass. Patients with muscle wasting have lower levels, whereas those who are heavily muscled or those in acute catabolic states have higher values because of more rapid muscle breakdown. Because the production and release of creatinine are relatively stable throughout the day and from day to day, serum levels are inversely related to GFR if a steady state exists. In other words, for every 50% reduction in GFR, creatinine level doubles. Excretion of drugs dependent on glomerular filtration may be significantly decreased despite only a slight elevation in serum creatinine level.

An elevation of both BUN and serum creatinine levels provides more information than an elevation of either level alone. The usual ratio of urea nitrogen to creatinine in the serum is 10:1. Increased ratios are seen with increased urea input, decreased circulatory blood volume, and obstructive uropathy. Decreased ratios are seen with decreased urea input, increased creatinine production, and volume expansion.

Creatinine Clearance

Creatinine clearance is a specific test of GFR and the most reliable assessment tool for renal function. This test measures the ability of the glomeruli to excrete creatinine into the urine for a given plasma creatinine concentration. Although it does not depend on corrections for age or the presence of a steady state, a disadvantage of this test is the need for accurate 24-hour urine specimens. Creatinine clearance is calculated according to the following formula:

Equation 30-2

$$GFR = (Urine\ creatinine \times Urine\ volume) \times Serum\ creatinine$$

A 2-hour urine sample collected through a urinary catheter permits acceptable accuracy. In the absence of urine volume, creatinine clearance can be approximated with use of the following formula:

Equation 30-3

$$GFR = \frac{([140 - Age] \times Lean\ body\ weight)}{(72 \times Serum\ creatinine)}$$

where weight is expressed in kilograms. To compensate for their smaller muscle mass, when values for women are calculated, the weight should be multiplied by 0.8.[93]

The normal range for creatinine clearance is 95 to 150 mL/min. Mild renal dysfunction is present when creatinine clearance is 50 to 80 mL/min, and moderate dysfunction is present at values below 25 mL/min. In patients with dysfunction, the administration of drugs that depend on renal excretion should be reduced, and fluid and electrolyte balance should be carefully monitored. Patients with creatinine clearance less than 10 mL/min are anephric and require dialysis for fluid and water hemostasis.

Other Tests

Advanced renal disease affects most organ systems. Additional tests that may be useful in patients with advanced renal disease include chest radiography, electrocardiography, complete blood count, serum electrolytes, and acid-base studies.

Systemic Abnormalities and Advanced Renal Disease

Renal failure is characterized by a wide variety of biochemical disturbances. Although most organ systems are involved (see Table 30-1), only those most relevant to anesthetic management are discussed in this section.

Cardiovascular Alterations

Cardiovascular disease accounts for approximately 50% of all deaths in patients on hemodialysis.[94] Hypertension and congestive heart failure often accompany end-stage renal disease. Ninety percent of the hypertension is volume dependent and related to sodium and water retention. The remainder can be attributed to high circulatory levels of renin. The combination of hypertension, anemia, hypoalbuminemia, and circulatory overload secondary to salt and water retention contributes to peripheral and pulmonary edema and to an increased risk of congestive heart failure.

In nonsurgical settings, ischemic heart disease is the most common cause of death in patients with chronic renal failure. Multiple risk factors such as hypertension, hyperlipidemia, and abnormal carbohydrate metabolism contribute to this high incidence of ischemic heart disease.[95] The anesthetist should assume that clinically significant coronary artery disease exists and should evaluate the extent and stability of the disease. Several uncontrolled studies suggest that correction of coronary lesions with coronary artery bypass grafting is associated with better outcomes than coronary angioplasty in patients on hemodialysis.[96] Improvement of symptoms is common after coronary artery bypass grafting. A rate of restenosis of 80% within 6 months is seen with coronary angioplasty.[97]

A fibrous pericarditis is clinically evident in approximately 50% of patients with severe uremia. Signs and symptoms may include pain on deep inspiration or when lying down and a friction rub over the pericardium. An enlarged cardiac silhouette on chest radiography indicates pericardial effusion. Patients with uremic pericarditis occasionally develop a massive hemorrhagic effusion and cardiac tamponade, especially when anticoagulants are used for hemodialysis.

Uremic patients exhibit a wide range of hemodynamic abnormalities when studied during hemodialysis.[98,99] The striking feature of these studies is that the peripheral vasculature responds abnormally to hypovolemia induced by dialysis. Hypovolemia decreases arterial pressure without increasing heart rate. Peripheral VR is unchanged or decreased, and cardiac output is increased.

Because the potential for significant cardiovascular complications exists, patients with advanced renal disease should undergo chest radiography and electrocardiography preoperatively. Administration of antihypertensive drugs should be continued, blood pressure should be monitored, and signs and symptoms of cerebrovascular disease should be recorded. The blood pressure should be normal or slightly elevated before induction. Because adequate intravascular volume is necessary for hemodynamic stability, the patient's weight should ideally be 1 to 2 kg more than dry weight at the end of the last dialysis before anesthetic induction.

Hematologic Changes

Normochromic, normocytic anemia is an inevitable finding in advanced renal disease. Hematocrit levels often decrease to the 20% to 30% range and generally parallel the degree of azotemia. The primary reason for anemia is a decrease in erythrocyte formation secondary to a decrease in production by the failing kidney.[100] Also, some evidence suggests that uremic toxins may inactivate erythropoietin or suppress the response of the bone marrow to its action. A second factor that contributes to the anemia in uremic patients is reduction of the life span of the erythrocyte because of an increase in hemolysis secondary to the presence of an abnormal chemical environment. Additionally, blood loss from frequent sampling for laboratory tests, loss in hemodialysis tubing, and a tendency for gastrointestinal bleeding further aggravate anemia.

Hematocrit and red-blood-cell indexes should be measured preoperatively, and their values should be checked against dialysis records to ensure that no acute changes have occurred. Preoperative hematocrit levels that are similar to those of a patient maintained on dialysis suggest that the patient can withstand the chronic anemia, and routine transfusion of blood preoperatively is not recommended for these patients. If transfusion is necessary because of acutely decreased or poorly tolerated hematocrit values, no need exists to withhold red-blood-cell transfusions for fear of sensitization to histocompatibility antigens.[101]

Exogenous administration of human recombinant erythropoietin corrects the anemia associated with chronic renal failure.[102-106] Adequate iron stores and good dialysis are essential if the response to recombinant erythropoietin or epoetin is to be maximized.[105] Endogenous erythropoietin levels and hematocrit values increase to normal after successful renal transplantation.[106]

Patients with chronic uremia have a tendency to bleed excessively. Although platelet counts are only mildly reduced, a defect in platelet function appears to be responsible for a prolonged bleeding time and a tendency for excessive bleeding.[107] Dialysis partially corrects platelet dysfunction, and dialysis 24 hours or less before surgical intervention is recommended.[108,109]

Desmopressin is known to shorten bleeding time and increase circulating levels of factor VIII, the von Willebrand antigen, in uremic patients. Desmopressin is the agent of choice because of its rapid onset and minimal side effects.[110,111] Repeated doses over time may increase bleeding time between treatments. Cryoprecipitate and conjugated estrogens also shorten bleeding time and may reduce blood loss.[112,113]

Gastrointestinal Effects

Patients on dialysis have a high incidence of gastrointestinal mucosal inflammatory changes and are at high risk of gastrointestinal bleeding perioperatively. The use of histamine-2 (H_2) blocking drugs or antacids is recommended throughout the perioperative period for decreasing the incidence of stress ulcers.[114,115]

Infections

Infectious complications are common in patients with renal failure and represent a leading cause of death in dialysis-dependent patients. Protein malnutrition and abnormalities in neutrophil, monocyte, and macrophage function contribute to this problem.[116-118] Mechanisms that lead to leukocyte dysfunction and increased susceptibility to infection are not known but may be related to uremia, immunosuppressive therapy, and increased exposure to invasive therapy. Frequent exposure to blood and blood products increases the risk of infection with hepatitis B and C and the human immunodeficiency viruses. Universal precautions are mandatory for the protection of both patients and health-care providers.[119]

Neurologic Effects

Neurologic symptoms associated with end-stage renal disease roughly parallel the degree of azotemia. Early symptoms include apathy, decreased mental acuity, and lethargy. Fatigue and weakness are early complaints, and untreated patients eventually become confused and comatose. Seizures may be associated with hypertensive encephalopathy. Peripheral and autonomic nervous system neuropathy is common. Autonomic neuropathy is associated with delayed gastric emptying and places the patient at risk for aspiration pneumonitis.

Endocrine Abnormalities

Endocrine abnormalities in patients with end-stage renal disease include hyperparathyroidism and adrenal insufficiency. Hypocalcemia is common in patients with advanced renal disease, and hyperparathyroidism represents an appropriate compensatory increase in parahormone in response to a reduction in serum calcium levels. Adrenal insufficiency often is secondary to exogenous steroid administration.

Respiratory Effects

Respiratory complications associated with renal failure include pneumonitis and the "uremic lung." Chest radiographs of the uremic lung reveal bilateral butterfly-shaped infiltrates indicative of pulmonary edema. Pulmonary congestion and edema usually are related to volume overload.

Electrolyte Abnormalities

Abnormalities of water, electrolyte, and acid-base balance become more common as the degree of renal failure increases. With a normal diet, the kidneys typically excrete 40 to 60 mEq of hydrogen ions per day to prevent acidosis. Impaired ability of the kidney to excrete hydrogen ions with renal failure results in metabolic acidosis characterized by decreases in plasma pH and HCO_3 concentration. Acidosis is usually moderate, but symptoms of anorexia, nausea, vomiting, and lethargy, which are common in uremic patients, may be partly related to acidosis.

Sodium ion excretion by the kidney normally varies according to intake. Patients with chronic renal failure lose this flexibility and have sodium wasting or retention. In early renal insufficiency with polyuria, an increased solute load for each intact nephron results in sodium wasting. In renal failure, the patient is more likely to retain sodium. Salt and water retention leads to circulatory overload, hypertension, edema, and congestive heart failure.

Although the ability to excrete magnesium is reduced in uremic patients, hypermagnesemia is generally not a serious problem. Magnesium intake is usually reduced because of anorexia, reduced protein intake, and decreased absorption from the gastrointestinal tract.

Calcium balance is controlled by parathyroid hormone, calcitonin, and vitamin D. Vitamin D, or cholecalciferol, is inactive until it has been hydroxylated in the liver and kidney. Inability of the diseased kidney to hydroxylate 25-hydroxycholecalciferol to 1,25-dihydroxycholecalciferol (active vitamin D) results in hypocalcemia. Patients with chronic renal failure have skeletal disorders or osteodystrophy, and defective mineralization of bone predisposes patients to fractures. Special precautions should be taken when these patients are moved and positioned.

Potassium imbalance is one of the most serious disturbances that occurs in patients with renal failure. Although hypokalemia may be associated with the polyuria of renal insufficiency, end-stage renal disease invariably leads to hyperkalemia. Although the major mechanism for hyperkalemia is the inability of distal nephrons to secrete potassium in exchange for calcium, systemic acidosis also contributes to potassium imbalance. Acidosis causes potassium ions to shift from intracellular to extracellular fluid.

Fatal dysrhythmias or cardiac standstill can occur when serum potassium levels reach 7 to 8 mEq/L. Dialysis is the most effective means of managing perioperative hyperkalemia, and hemodialysis is indicated when serum potassium exceeds 6 mEq/L. Other techniques for treating hyperkalemia include insulin in glucose infusions (25 to 50 g of glucose with 10 to 20 units of regular insulin) and administration of bicarbonate. These measures promote rapid translocation of extracellular potassium to the intracellular space during hyperkalemic emergencies. Hyperventilation of the lungs with respiratory alkalosis lowers serum potassium concentration by approximately 0.5 mEq/L for every 10-mm Hg change in arterial CO_2 tension. Life-threatening cardiac dysrhythmias are treated with intravenous administration of calcium chloride. A typical dose may be 1 g in adults. Although calcium does not change the serum concentration of potassium, it antagonizes the cardiotoxic effects of hyperkalemia.

Unexpected hyperkalemia can develop rapidly, so it is important to measure potassium even when dialysis has been performed within 6 to 8 hours of surgery. Hyperkalemia occurs early postoperatively and is the primary reason patients with renal failure require dialysis within the first 24 hours after surgery.[120]

Surgical procedures are becoming increasingly more common in anephric patients. The perioperative course of these patients may be complicated by a high incidence of untoward events that increase morbidity and mortality. These complications are related to the abnormal physiology of the anephric state. They are predictable and can be minimized by preoperative evaluation and preparation. Pertinent points in the preoperative assessment and preparation of patients with end-stage renal disease are listed in Box 30-4.

ANESTHETIC MANAGEMENT OF PATIENTS WITH ADVANCED RENAL DISEASE

Preoperative preparation of patients with advanced renal disease should include an evaluation of recent laboratory measurements, coexisting diseases, and current medications. Patients with end-stage renal disease should undergo determination of BUN and serum creatinine levels, complete blood count, bleeding-time measurement, and electrolyte studies preoperatively. Special attention should be given to serum potassium, the type of and schedule for dialysis, and volume status.

Discussions regarding premedication should take into consideration unexpected sensitivity to CNS depressants and delayed gastric emptying. Benzodiazepines are useful as premedicants because of their oral route of administration and hepatic metabolism. Diazepam has active and long-lasting metabolites, and its action is prolonged in renal failure. Midazolam has virtually no active metabolites, and its half-life is only slightly prolonged in renal failure. Although this drug is useful when it is carefully titrated, patients with renal disease may be more susceptible to the sedative-hypnotic effects of benzodiazepines than those without renal dysfunction.[121]

Reduced protein binding may be responsible for increased sensitivity to these drugs in patients with advanced renal disease. Protein binding of morphine (Table 30-2) decreases by 10% in the presence of chronic renal failure.[122] This alters the free fraction only slightly because morphine generally is protein bound to such a small extent. Because morphine is almost completely metabolized in the liver to the inactive glucuronide, premedicant doses in patients with renal failure should not cause prolonged depression. However, one report has described severe respiratory and cardiovascular depression in a patient with renal failure who received 8 mg of morphine.[123] Excessive depression in these patients is thought to result from high brain levels of metabolites. These metabolites are pH dependent, and their concentration does not increase with respiratory alkalosis. Morphine is not removed by dialysis.

Meperidine is more lipophilic than morphine. It is 60% protein bound and is metabolized to renally eliminated compounds that are less potent respiratory depressants than morphine. Meperidine can cause convulsions when used in high concentrations, and it cannot be removed by dialysis.[124] Meperidine should be avoided in patients with renal failure.

Approximately 20% to 50% of a dose of atropine or glycopyrrolate is recovered unchanged in the urine, so the dose should be reduced.[125] Although only one tenth as much scopolamine is recovered from the urine, CNS effects prohibit its use when large or repeated doses of an anticholinergic are required.

Gastric hyperacidity and gastrointestinal bleeding are common in patients with renal failure. H2 blockers and magnesium-free antacids should be considered. Cimetidine has been used, but renal elimination accounts for 80% of total elimination, and elimination is impaired with reduced renal function. Although newer H2 antagonist are now available, all H2-receptor

TABLE 30-2	Protein Plasma Binding of Some Important Anesthetic Drugs
Drug	**Percent Bound**
Alfentanil	92
Atropine	39
Bupivacaine	95
Etidocaine	95
Etomidate	71-75
Fentanyl	84
Ketamine	26
Lidocaine	60-80
Remifentanil	66-93
Meperidine	42-60
Methohexital	73
Midazolam	94
Morphine	35
Pancuronium	11-29
Propofol	98
Ropivacaine	95
Sufentanil	93
Thiopental	80-84
Vecuronium	30

From Bovill JG, Howie MB. Clinical Pharmacology for Anaesthetists. London: Saunders; 1999.

blockers are very dependent on renal excretion. Metoclopramide is partly excreted unchanged in the urine and will accumulate in patients with renal failure.

Intraoperative Monitoring

The selection of monitors for a patient with diminished or absent renal function is based on the physiologic status of the patient and the proposed surgical procedure. Frequent measurements of blood pressure and continuous recording of temperature and heart rate and rhythm are essential. Electrocardiography may allow early detection of hyperkalemia.

Because these patients are often chronically anemic, a further reduction in oxygen delivery secondary to hypoxia can be extremely hazardous. Pulse oximetry is helpful for the early detection of arterial desaturations. Pulse oximetry and capnography are useful and required in all patients. Minor surgical procedures in stable patients can be monitored noninvasively.

The decision to use invasive monitors depends on the patient's functional cardiac reserve and the severity and control of hypertension. Continuous monitoring of intraarterial blood pressure is helpful when major surgical procedures are performed. A femoral or dorsalis pedis artery is sometimes used for cannulation, because vessels in the upper extremities may be needed later for vascular shunts. Vascular volume and fluid replacement can be guided by CVP or pulmonary artery catheter monitoring. A pulmonary artery catheter is useful if interpretation of the CVP is questionable or cardiac disease is present.

Vascular shunts and fistulas must be protected. Patency is easily monitored with Doppler imaging. Because of the immunocompromised state of these patients, strict aseptic technique is required during the placement of vascular catheters.

Regional Anesthesia

Regional anesthesia is tolerated by patients with advanced renal disease, provided no significant coagulation disorder is present and mean arterial pressure is maintained. Regional techniques avoid most of the pharmacokinetic and pharmacodynamic problems associated with general anesthetics and sedative drugs. Major concerns regarding this type of anesthesia include psychologic intolerance, coagulation abnormalities, the presence of peripheral neuropathies, difficulty in making intravascular volume adjustments, and risk of infection.

Arteriovenous shunts or fistulas may be surgically created with the use of local infiltration or brachial plexus block. In addition to providing analgesia, brachial blocks improve surgical conditions by providing maximum vascular vasodilation and abolishing vasospasm. Studies have shown that brachial plexus block is associated with greater brachial artery blood flow than local anesthesia, but this effect is not significant enough for the technique to be recommended over another.[126] Both brachial plexus block and local infiltration are good alternatives to general anesthesia for creation of arteriovenous fistula. Age, American Society of Anesthesiologists (ASA) class, and cardiac status were the determining factors for choice of anesthetic technique.[127]

The duration of brachial plexus block has been reported to be shortened by 40% in patients with chronic renal failure.[128] The reason for this reduction was thought to be an elevation in tissue blood flow secondary to an increase in cardiac output and a more rapid clearance of local anesthetics from active sites. A shortened duration of action would support the use of a longer-acting local anesthetic, such as bupivacaine, especially if prolonged surgery is anticipated. However, data suggest a similar duration of anesthesia with brachial plexus blocks in patients with renal failure and normal renal function.[129] High-dose mepivacaine has been used for brachial plexus block in patients with end-stage chronic renal failure. Brachial plexus anesthesia with 650 mg of plain mepivacaine did not result in serious systematic toxicity in these patients despite high mepivacaine plasma concentrations.[130] Levobupivacaine 0.5%, 50 to 60 mL, has also been used for axillary brachial plexus block in patients with renal disease and was well tolerated.[131] The use of clonidine (150 mcg) as an adjuvant for lidocaine in axillary blocks for arteriovenous fistula construction prolongs blockade, decreases heart rate and blood pressure, and provides sedative effects.[132]

With regard to spinal or epidural anesthesia, patients with long-standing renal disease often have undergone multiple procedures and prefer general anesthetic techniques. In addition to the history, the uremic patient's bleeding time, platelet count, prothrombin time, partial thromboplastin time, and fibrinogen level should be evaluated before subarachnoid or epidural catheters are placed. Paraplegia secondary to hematoma formation with spinal anesthesia has been reported in patients with chronic renal failure and clotting abnormalities.[133] A case of epidural hematoma in a surgical patient with chronic renal failure and epidural postoperative analgesia has been reported. The only risk factor for development of epidural hematoma was a history of chronic renal failure. High-risk patients should be monitored closely for early signs of cord compression such as severe back pain and motor or sensory deficits. An opioid or opioid and local epidural solution rather than local solution alone allows continuous monitoring of neurologic function. If spinal hematoma is suspected, the patient should undergo immediate MRI or CT scan, and decompressive laminectomy should be performed without delay.[134]

Peripheral neuropathies should be discussed with the patient and documented before regional anesthesia is undertaken. The incidence of hypotension with subarachnoid or epidural blockade may be increased because of effects of chronic hypertension or hypovolemia related to recent dialysis. Correction of hypovolemia postoperatively is hazardous. Recession of the sympathetic block in patients who cannot undergo diuresis may lead to pulmonary edema. One must weigh the advantages of fluid infusion against the effects of pressor drugs with these factors in mind.

Patients with end-stage renal disease are often acidotic, and local anesthetic toxicity may be increased with acidosis. The onset and duration of blocks have also been shown to vary in these patients. Subarachnoid blockade induced with 3 mL of 0.75% bupivacaine developed more rapidly, attained a greater level, and was of shorter duration in patients with renal failure than in control patients.[135] The slower onset of epidural anesthesia is of advantage in these patients.

General Anesthesia
Intravenous Drugs

Intravenous anesthetics can be used in patients with advanced renal disease, but the response of these patients may be more variable than normal. Variability arises from a complex interplay among changes in volume of distribution (which is often increased), protein binding (which may be low), low pH, and dependence on renal excretion for the parent drug or metabolites.

The action of many drugs is potentiated by metabolic abnormalities associated with renal failure. Highly protein-bound drugs (see Table 30-2) have more target-organ effect in the presence of hypoalbuminemia. The acidemic state associated with renal failure increases the proportion of the agent that is un-ionized and unbound and therefore more available to target tissue. Anemia associated with renal failure increases cardiac output and enhances delivery to the brain. Uremia alters the blood-brain barrier; this also increases the sensitivity to intravenous drugs.

From 75% to 85% of sodium thiopental is normally bound to albumin. It may have an exaggerated effect in renal failure, owing to decreased protein binding and an altered blood-brain barrier.[136] Ketamine and benzodiazepines are less heavily protein bound. The sympathomimetic effects of ketamine are frequently associated with an increase in blood pressure and cardiac output, which may be deleterious in hypertensive patients who are at risk for coronary artery disease or decreased left ventricular function. In addition, metabolites of ketamine depend on renal excretion and can accumulate in patients with renal failure.

The pharmacokinetic profile of narcotics can be altered in the presence of renal disease. Fentanyl is metabolized in the liver, and 85% of it appears in the urine and feces as inactive metabolites. Its slow elimination half-life is the result of a large volume of distribution. The effect is exaggerated in renal failure. Chronic renal failure is associated with a decrease in alfentanil plasma protein binding, but it does not change plasma clearance of the drug. The volume of distribution at steady state is greater in patients with renal failure. Altered protein binding of alfentanil must be considered in patients with renal failure.[137] Although the pharmacokinetics of sufentanil do not appear to be altered in patients with advanced renal disease, clearance and half-life are more variable in this group. Sufentanil should be carefully administered to these patients.[138] Remifentanil, which is metabolized by nonspecific plasma esterases and is not dependent on renal function for elimination, is a logical choice for renally compromised patients.

Propofol has gained wide acceptance for both induction and maintenance of anesthesia and appears to be safe. Induction doses of 2.5 mg/kg in patients with normal renal function or renal failure resulted in no significant difference between the groups in quality of induction or hemodynamics.[139] Studies suggest, however, that patients with end-stage renal disease require a higher dose to achieve hypnosis. A hyperdynamic circulation in these anemic patients may be responsible.[140] The half-life did not differ significantly between the groups, although the values were longer with propofol in patients with renal failure. Propofol has been used for induction and maintenance for 3- to 8-hour kidney transplant procedures. No accumulation of the drug occurred, and no unusual hemodynamic effects were observed. Emergence was rapid, and resumption of diuresis was satisfactory. The pharmacokinetics of propofol do not appear to be significantly altered in patients undergoing kidney transplantation.[141]

Uremic patients are generally anemic and may require high inspired oxygen concentrations. Because intravenous anesthesia is often supplemented with nitrous oxide, the inspired concentration of oxygen is reduced. Volatile agents are more reliable in controlling hypertension, and their action is more easily reversed. For these reasons, inhalation agents may be preferable for general anesthesia.

Volatile Anesthetic Agents

Inhalation agents offer some advantage in patients with renal failure. Although biotransformation of some agents may produce metabolites excreted by the kidneys, elimination of volatile agents does not rely on renal function. Volatile agents potentiate neuromuscular blocking drugs, allowing administration of reduced doses. Although the potency of these agents allows them to be administered without nitrous oxide, excessive depth of anesthesia may lead to a depression of cardiac output. Reductions in cardiac output and tissue blood flow must be avoided in these anemic patients if tissue oxygen delivery is to be maintained.

A disadvantage of inhalation agents relates to their biotransformation and nephrotoxic potential. The nephrotoxic threshold for fluoride of 50 μmol is rarely reached with current agents. Fluoride levels after isoflurane anesthesia increased by only 1 to 2 μmol, and desflurane is metabolized approximately one tenth as much as isoflurane. It is the least metabolized of the currently available volatile agents. In studies of patients and volunteers administered desflurane for prolonged periods, no evidence of renal, hepatic, or hematologic toxicity was observed.[142]

Some practitioners may avoid use of sevoflurane in patients with renal dysfunction because of the potential for nephrotoxicity. Studies do not support this concern. One study compared renal function after long-duration, low-flow (<1 L/min) sevoflurane and isoflurane anesthesia in surgical patients with normal renal function. Postoperative renal function was no different as assessed by serum creatinine and BUN levels and urinary excretion of protein and glucose, suggesting that low-flow sevoflurane is as safe as low-flow isoflurane.[143] Another study concluded that prolonged low-flow sevoflurane anesthesia had the same effect on renal and hepatic function as high-flow sevoflurane and low-flow isoflurane anesthesia. During low-flow sevoflurane, intake of compound A reached 277 ppm/hr, but the effect on the kidney and liver was the same in high-flow sevoflurane and low-flow isoflurane anesthesia.[144]

In summary, both regional and general anesthesia have been used successfully in patients with advanced renal disease. Advantages and disadvantages of both techniques are listed in Table 30-3.

Neuromuscular Blocking Drugs

The appropriate use of neuromuscular blocking drugs in patients with advanced renal disease has received much attention over the years. At one time, caution was advised in all cases of the use of a muscle relaxant in patients with renal disease. Because these drugs are ionized, water-soluble compounds freely filtered at the glomerulus, it was believed that their action would be prolonged. It was further theorized that as the anticholinesterase or relaxant

TABLE **30-3**	Regional versus General Anesthesia	
Technique	**Advantages**	**Disadvantages**
Regional	Patient responsiveness Minimal changes in renal hemodynamics	Presence of peripheral neuropathy Tendency for bleeding Patient anxiety Prolonged procedures Hypotension with sympathetic block; may cause reluctance to expand volume
Volatile anesthetics	Good airway control Blood pressure control Duration not dependent on urinary excretion Less neuromuscular blocking with drugs required F_{IO_2} can be increased because N_2O not necessary	Alterations in renal hemodynamics Decreased cardiac output Hypotension Biodegradation and potential nephrotoxicity; halothane 15%-20%; sevoflurane 5%; isoflurane 0.2%; desflurane 0.02%
Intravenous anesthetics	Hemodynamic stability	Unpredictable response Hypertension Greater need for N_2O and neuromuscular blockers

F_{IO_2}, *Fraction of inspired oxygen;* N_2O, *nitrous oxide.*

antagonist level decreased, the patient would be at risk of "recurarization," or reappearance of neuromuscular blockade. It is now known that renal excretion is of major importance for cholinesterase inhibitors as well. Approximately 50% of neostigmine and 70% of edrophonium and pyridostigmine are excreted in the urine.[145-147] Excretion of all cholinesterase inhibitors is delayed to the same or to a greater extent than muscle relaxants in patients with renal impairment.

Succinylcholine. Several problems have been associated with the use of succinylcholine in patients with renal failure. Succinylcholine is metabolized by hepatic-derived pseudocholinesterase to succinic acid and choline. A metabolic precursor of these two compounds is succinylmonocholine, which has nondepolarizing blocking activity and is eliminated by the kidneys. Large doses administered over prolonged periods of time, as may be seen with succinylcholine infusions, may lead to accumulation of the metabolite. Introduction of newer drugs eliminates the risk of prolonged blockade from succinylcholine infusions.

When succinylcholine is given after anticholinesterase administration, the action of succinylcholine is prolonged. An explanation for this prolongation is the alteration in pharmacokinetics of both drugs in patients with renal failure and their prolonged duration of action. Patients with renal failure who require muscle relaxants are at greater risk for prolonged succinylcholine blockade than normal individuals if they have recently undergone anticholinesterase-induced reversal of neuromuscular blockade.[148] Prolongation of succinylcholine has also been associated with depressed levels of pseudocholinesterase in uremic patients who require hemodialysis. Newer methods of hemodialysis have no effect on cholinesterase levels.[149,150]

Serum potassium increases by approximately 0.5 mEq/L in both normal patients and those with renal failure. This elevation in extracellular potassium is not prevented by pretreatment with a nondepolarizing muscle relaxant. The rise in serum potassium level is particularly dangerous in uremic patients who are hyperkalemic. The use of succinylcholine is inadvisable unless a patient has undergone dialysis within 24 hours before surgery and the potassium concentration is less than 5.5 mEq/L. Succinylcholine is safe in normokalemic patients who have recently undergone dialysis.[151-153]

Pancuronium. Approximately 40% to 50% of pancuronium is excreted in the urine. Biliary excretion accounts for much of the nonrenal elimination.[154,155]

A significant portion of the renal excretion of pancuronium occurs after its biotransformation to a less active metabolite.[156,157] Pancuronium has a prolonged terminal elimination half-life in patients with reduced renal function and should be administered cautiously.

Atracurium and Cisatracurium. Atracurium and vecuronium were introduced into clinical practice in the late 1980s. Initial reports indicated that the action of neither atracurium nor vecuronium was prolonged in patients with decreased renal function; however, it now appears that this is true only for atracurium.[158-160] Atracurium and cisatracurium are broken down by enzymatic ester hydrolysis and by nonenzymatic alkaline hydrolysis, or Hoffman elimination, to inactive products. This process is not dependent on renal excretion for termination of action. Onset, duration, and recovery are the same in patients with and without renal disease, and it is the drug of choice in patients with renal failure. Metabolism of atracurium and to a lesser extent cisatracurium produces the CNS excitant laudanosine, which is renally excreted and accumulates in patients with

renal failure.[161] The clinical significance of this finding is yet to be determined.

Vecuronium. Vecuronium is excreted renally, and the duration of neuromuscular blockade is longer in patients with renal failure than in those without renal failure.[162] This accumulation is presumed to be the result of the gradual saturation of peripheral storage sites.[163] Prolonged neuromuscular block may result from the use of an infusion or from large doses of vecuronium in patients with severely impaired renal function.[164] An 81-year-old patient with renal failure and subclinical, chronic hepatic cirrhosis remained paralyzed for 13 days after vecuronium infusion.[165] Prolonged blockade with vecuronium has also been reported in an 11-day-old infant with renal failure. In this case, an initial dose of 97 mg/kg was followed by complete neuromuscular blockade for 210 minutes.[166] If vecuronium is used, a low dose is recommended, and repeated administration should be avoided. Neuromuscular blockade is rapidly reversible with dialytic treatment.[167,168]

Rocuronium. Rocuronium bromide is a nondepolarizing neuromuscular blocking drug released for clinical use. It has a rapid onset of action, and in humans it produces good to excellent conditions for tracheal intubation in 60 to 90 seconds.[169] It has one fifth to one sixth the potency of vecuronium, few to no cardiovascular effects, and an intermediate duration of action.[170,171] Studies indicate that the pharmacokinetics and onset of action of twice the effective dose to produce a 95% response (ED_{95}) dose of rocuronium are not altered in patients with renal failure who are undergoing renal transplantation. Whether these results can be applied to patients with renal failure who undergo surgery other than renal transplantation is unknown. Rocuronium is suitable for patients with renal failure who undergo renal transplantation and may be particularly desirable in those patients in whom rapid onset of neuromuscular blockade is desired.[172] A rapid onset is particularly attractive in these patients because they are subject to autonomic neuropathy and delayed gastric emptying.

INTRAVENOUS FLUID MANAGEMENT

Perioperative management of fluids and electrolytes in patients with renal disease is critical. The state of hydration affects renin, aldosterone, and antidiuretic levels. Dehydration and hypovolemia lead to elevations in these hormones and to a decline in urinary output.

Perioperative Renal Function

Surgical patients at high risk for acute renal failure or those with advanced disease who do not require hemodialysis present unique challenges. Preservation of renal function intraoperatively is a major goal. Preservation of renal function is dependent on the maintenance of intravascular volume and cardiovascular stability and on the avoidance of events that cause renal vasoconstriction. Preoperative hydration with 10 to 20 mL of balanced salt solution per kilogram may be helpful. Intraoperatively, urinary output is the only time monitor for renal function. A urinary output of 0.5 to 1 mL/kg/hr intraoperatively and postoperatively is recommended in these patients.

Although urinary output seems to be a reasonable reflector of renal function intraoperatively, its value as a sole indicator of adequate volume resuscitation in patients undergoing aortic surgery has been questioned. In one study, intraoperative urinary output was not predictive of postoperative changes in renal function.[173] In this study, pulmonary artery occlusion pressure and blood pressure were maintained in the normal range with the infusion of fluids and blood. If urinary flow decreased to below 0.125 mg/kg/hr, the patient was treated with crystalloid solution, mannitol, furosemide, or nothing. Postoperative BUN and serum creatinine levels were similar among treatment groups and did not correlate with intraoperative urinary flow rates. Serum creatinine rose by 0.5 mg/dL in 21 patients, 17 of whom had preoperative renal dysfunction. This study highlighted the increased risk of renal dysfunction in patients with preexisting disease and emphasized that maintenance of intravascular volume guided by adequate hemodynamic monitoring is as important as maintaining an arbitrary urinary flow rate.

Renal Pathology
Patients with renal disease progress through several stages: decreased renal reserve, renal insufficiency, renal failure, and uremia.

Decreased Renal Reserve
The goal of fluid management in patients with decreased renal reserve is maximizing renal perfusion. Basal fluids should be replaced; 5% dextrose in water (D_5W) with 50 to 70 mEq of Na^+ per liter is appropriate. Potassium should be administered as needed to sustain a normal plasma level. Deficit and intraoperative losses should be replaced as for a normal patient. Third-space losses can be replaced with balanced salt solution. Although it is better to err on the side of excess with respect to volume replacement in these patients, if the ratio of replacement crystalloid solution to lost blood exceeds 3:1, consideration should be given to the judicious use of a colloid solution. The administration of huge volumes of crystalloid solution may be associated with pulmonary edema as fluids are mobilized. This generally occurs on the second to the fourth postoperative day.

Renal Insufficiency
In patients with renal insufficiency, volume deficits should be replaced preoperatively, as in normal patients. Basal fluids must be carefully regulated because these patients cannot tolerate much deviation. Overall basal fluid requirements must be related to metabolic rate and designed to provide an overall fluid balance that allows an isotonic urine to carry excreted electrolytes and waste products. Intraoperative losses greater than 10% to 15% of the blood volume should be replaced with colloid solution on a 1:1 basis after red-blood-cell losses are corrected. Smaller losses can be replaced with the usual 3:1 ratio of crystalloid infusion to blood loss. Third-space losses are ideally replaced initially with crystalloid solution without potassium or excess chloride. Initial third-space losses should be replaced with crystalloid solution at a rate of 2 to 3 mL/kg/hr. The critical goal in patients with renal insufficiency is sustaining blood volume. Monitoring of colloid osmotic pressure and hemoglobin can guide the choice between crystalloid and colloid infusions. If hemoglobin and colloid osmotic pressure are increasing, crystalloid solution is clearly indicated. If they are decreasing, crystalloid solution should be withheld in favor of colloid solution. Close monitoring of blood pressure, heart rate, CVP, pulmonary artery occlusion pressure, and cardiac output also guides fluid titration. This is especially true in patients with cardiac or respiratory compromise.

End-Stage Renal Disease
With regard to perioperative fluid management, patients with end-stage renal disease who are hemodialysis dependent require special attention. Although these patients are similar to normal patients in terms of fluid deficit, basal, and third-space requirements, they have a narrow margin of safety. The patient's ability to compensate for either fluid excess or fluid deficiency progressively declines as renal function is lost.

Fluid deficits must be replaced preoperatively in patients with end-stage renal disease. If deficits exceed 10% to 15% of the blood volume, invasive monitoring is justified. Dialysis is recommended on the day before anesthesia to allow time for equilibration of fluid and electrolyte shifts that are common with dialysis. Electrolyte levels must be checked before anesthesia.

Basal fluids in patients with end-stage renal disease should be replaced in a manner similar to that for patients with renal insufficiency. Volume restriction is recommended for intraoperative losses. Third-space losses should be replaced with a balanced salt solution that contains no potassium and small amounts of chloride. Close monitoring of hemoglobin and cardiac filling pressures is indicated for all major procedures. Patients with end-stage renal disease generally require dialysis within 24 to 36 hours after major surgery.

Uremia
Deficit replacement in patients with uremia must be guided by hemodynamic monitoring. Basal fluids should be replaced with red blood cells, fresh frozen plasma, or colloid solutions. Third-space losses are best replaced with crystalloid solutions in association with frequent monitoring of hemoglobin and cardiac filling pressures. A moderate degree of volume overload is not a grave problem. Many uremic patients require dialysis within 24 to 36 hours for the removal of mobilized fluid and the control of hypertension.

Although volume overload is most often emphasized in patients with end-stage renal disease, complications of hypovolemia are also serious. Hypotension associated with hypovolemia increases the risk of thrombosis of the arteriovenous fistula and predisposes to cardiac and cerebral ischemia. Hemodynamic goals include the avoidance of hypotension and gross fluid overload. This can be accomplished only through careful titration with the patient well monitored.

ANESTHESIA FOR RENAL TRANSPLANTATION
Transplantation Procedure
Renal transplantation has been performed for nearly a century and is an accepted means of replacing kidney function in patients with end-stage renal disease who are on maintenance dialysis. In this procedure, the donor kidney is placed extraperitoneally in the recipient's iliac fossa. The renal artery is anastomosed to the internal iliac artery, the renal vein to either the external or the common iliac vein, and the ureter to the bladder. The anesthesia provider plays a vital role in management of the viability of the transplanted kidney. Three interrelated variables affect surgical outcomes: management of the donor, preservation of the harvested organ, and perioperative care of the transplant recipient.[174] Additionally, improved surgical and immunosuppressive techniques have contributed to better outcomes in terms of graft survival.[175]

Harvested Organ Preservation
Ischemic time, beginning with the clamping of the donor's renal vessels and ending with the vascular anastomosis in the recipient, is a crucial factor in graft preservation. When renal ischemic time is less than 30 minutes, diuresis begins quickly, but if it is 2 hours

or longer, a variable period of oliguria or anuria may occur according to the following ischemic times:

Warm

Begins: Clamping of donor vessels; initial placement in recipient

Ends: Vascular anastomosis in recipient; interrupted with perfusion of cold preservation solution

Cold

Perfusion of harvested organ with cold preservation solution; storage at 4° C

Perfusion by recipient

Donor Preparation

Choice of anesthesia for the living, related donor is not critical. Adequate amounts of balanced salt solution should be administered to ensure a brisk diuresis from the donor kidney and to offset reduced venous return resulting from use of the flank position.[174] The greatest risk to the donor is hemorrhage. Adequate intravenous access and blood must be available in the event that transfusion becomes necessary.

If the donor kidney is obtained from a brain-dead patient, preservation of graft function is the highest priority. The loss of sympathetic tone after brain death may produce mild hypotension, despite adequate volume replacement. Many patients with irreversible cerebral dysfunction are hypovolemic and require vigorous fluid resuscitation. If pharmacologic support of the cardiovascular system is necessary, a dopamine infusion at a rate of 1 to 3 mcg/kg/min is recommended. Renal vasoconstrictive properties of high-dose vasopressors reduce immediate allograft function and increase the risk of kidney damage. Maintenance of urinary output is paramount and may warrant the use of diuretics and a low-dose dopamine infusion.[174-176]

Recipient Preparation

Because cadaveric kidneys can be preserved for 36 to 48 hours with cold perfusion, time is sufficient for optimal preparation of the transplant recipient (Box 30-5). The recipient should be free of acute illness and infections because of the likelihood of their spread during immunosuppressive therapy. Acute alterations in fluid and electrolyte balance should be corrected with dialysis carried out 24 hours before transplantation.

BOX 30-5

Anesthesia for Renal Transplantation

I. Preoperative Assessment and Preparation
   A. Clinical evaluation
      1. Evaluate status of coexisting diseases.
         a. Diabetes mellitus
         b. Hypertension
         c. Cardiac disease
         d. Hyperparathyroidism
         e. Pericardial tamponade
      2. Perform dialysis within 24 hr of transplantation; check weight.
      3. Evaluate tolerance to chronic anemia.
   B. Laboratory evaluation
      1. Complete blood count with platelet count
      2. Prothrombin time, partial thromboplastin time, bleeding time
      3. Blood urea nitrogen, creatinine, calcium, fluid balance
      4. Electrocardiography; chest radiography
   C. Type and cross-match 2 units of washed, packed red blood cells.
   D. Determine current drug regimen
   E. Premedication
      1. Benzodiazepines, narcotics
      2. Antacids, histamine-2 antagonist, metoclopramide
II. Monitors
   A. Electrocardiography
   B. Indirect or direct blood pressure measurement
   C. Precordial, esophageal stethoscope
   D. Neuromuscular blockade evaluation
   E. Foley catheter
   F. Central venous, pulmonary capillary wedge pressure measurement, if required

III. Anesthetic Management
   A. Regional techniques
      1. Continuous spinal or epidural
      2. Advantages
         a. No need for muscle relaxants
         b. Potential respiratory tract infection from intubation is avoided
         c. Amount of local anesthetic required is small
         d. Patients awake and comfortable postoperatively
      3. Disadvantages
         a. Patient anxiety
         b. Uncomfortable surgical positions, especially for donor
         c. Coagulation abnormalities present
         d. Fluid management with sympathetic blockade a challenge
         e. Unprotected airway in patients with delayed gastric emptying
   B. General anesthesia
      1. Induction with thiopental, propofol or etomidate
      2. Maintenance with volatile anesthetic (isoflurane, or desflurane) or narcotic-based technique
      3. Neuromuscular blockers
         a. Succinylcholine
         b. Atracurium and cisatracurium
         c. Vecuronium
IV. Miscellaneous Drugs
   A. Mannitol or furosemide
   B. Prednisone or methylprednisolone
   C. Azathioprine
   D. OKT3
   E. Cyclosporine

Postdialysis laboratory values should be checked, and serum potassium (K^+) level should be below 5.5 mEq/L. Coagulation studies and acid-base status should be normal. Serum creatinine concentration should be below 10 mg/dL, and BUN level below 60 mg/dL after dialysis.

Chronic anemia is common, and transfusion is not required if oxygen delivery is adequate. Because of the danger of volume overload, anemia should be corrected during dialysis with transfusion of packed red blood cells. It was formerly thought that multiple blood transfusions increased the risk of kidney rejection secondary to sensitization of the human leukocyte antigen system, but this belief has been disproved. Studies have shown a lower survival rate for transplanted kidneys in nontransfused patients and in those receiving leukocyte-poor blood.[177]

Abnormal platelet function, as well as ineffective production of factor VIII and von Willebrand factor, accounts for the syndrome of uremic coagulopathy seen in patients with renal failure. Correction of coagulation abnormalities has been accomplished through dialysis and administration of conjugated estrogen and desmopressin as seen in the following chart[178]:

Treatment	Effect
Dialysis	Improves platelet formation
Conjugated estrogen	Decreases transfusion need
Desmopressin	Increases factor VIII and von Willebrand factor

Acceptance of kidney transplantation in patients with type 1 diabetes mellitus is widespread. This is not the case, however, in patients with type 2 diabetes, because this condition carries increased risk for poor postoperative outcomes, largely because of the propensity for associated coexisting disease in such patients. One researcher found that patients with type 2 diabetes who had a history of stroke or myocardial infarction had a poorer prognosis than those patients without coexisting vascular disease.[179]

Patients should fast for 6 to 8 hours if possible. Premedication may include narcotics or benzodiazepines in usual to reduced doses, depending on the status of the patient. The use of antacids, H_2 antagonists, and metoclopramide should be considered if gastric emptying is delayed; however, reduced doses should be considered because these drugs depend on the kidney for excretion, and metoclopramide is partially excreted unchanged in the urine.[174]

In addition to routine monitors, a Foley catheter is inserted for the assessment of graft function. Although CVP lines are not routinely inserted, their use may indirectly improve graft function by improving the assessment of hydration status. A pulmonary artery catheter is useful if cardiac compromise is suspected or if the kidney is expected to have delayed graft function. Protection of vascular access and fistula patency is of prime importance with the use of blood pressure cuffs or if arterial cannulation is necessary. Sterile precautions during insertion of invasive lines are extremely important because transplant patients are immunocompromised. Strict adherence to aseptic technique is mandatory in the management of these lines, catheters, and endotracheal tubes. Commitment to aseptic technique on the part of the entire team may make the difference between safe transplantation and death for the patient.

Fluid management may be generous or conservative. Fluid replacement should be with normal saline or with dextrose in saline, generally at a maintenance infusion rate. Immediate function of the transplanted kidney cannot be guaranteed, and excessive intraoperative fluid replacement can lead to pulmonary edema and swelling of the grafted kidney.

Anesthesia
Regional Anesthesia
Both regional and general anesthesia have been used successfully for renal transplantation. Spinal and epidural anesthesia are both satisfactory, and because the procedure is extraperitoneal and in the lower half of the abdomen, the block can be kept low.[180,181] Advantages of regional anesthesia include a more aseptic technique, avoidance of the use of muscle relaxants and other drugs excreted by the kidney, and the fact that endotracheal intubation is not required. Intubation may increase the risk of nosocomial pneumonia. Pulmonary infection occurs in 10% to 15% of transplant recipients and is associated with a high mortality rate.[182] An additional advantage of regional anesthesia is postoperative analgesia.

Disadvantages of regional anesthesia techniques in these patients include hypotension associated with sympathetic blockade, the length of the procedure, and heparinization of the kidney. Sympathetic blockade can make control of blood pressure difficult in patients who may be hypovolemic. Given that transplantation procedures may last several hours, large amounts of sedation may be needed to supplement regional techniques. Because local heparinization of the kidney is often used, the use of continuous regional techniques may be contraindicated. For these reasons, general anesthesia is now the preferred approach in patients who undergo transplantation.

General Anesthesia
Volatile Agents. When general anesthesia is used, nitrous oxide combined with volatile agents (particularly isoflurane) or short-acting opiates is well tolerated. The skeletal muscle relaxant properties and minimal metabolism make isoflurane an attractive choice. Reductions in cardiac output secondary to the negative inotropic effects of volatile drugs must be minimized if suboptimal tissue oxygenation is to be avoided in these anemic patients.

Although no studies describe use of sevoflurane during kidney transplantation, researchers have reported on its effects on the kidney with impaired function. Evidence of increased plasma fluoride concentrations has been the predominant finding.[183,184] Also, compared with isoflurane, no significant difference in other renal function markers was found.[184] Although limited by a small sample size of chronic renal failure patients, Nishiyama and colleagues[185] found that these patients had significantly lower levels of urine fluoride than control subjects. The data suggest that fluoride kinetics in patients with chronic renal failure might be different from fluoride kinetics in patients with normal renal function.[185] These findings may facilitate further research in this area.

Muscle Relaxants. The choice of muscle relaxant must take into consideration the unpredictable nature of renal function after transplantation. Relaxants that are independent of renal function for plasma clearance, such as atracurium and cisatracurium, are excellent for this patient population.[157,158] Cisatracurium, one of 10 isomers of atracurium, represents approximately 15% of the total atracurium mixture.[186] It is three times more potent than atracurium. The processes of Hoffman elimination and ester hydrolysis are the elimination pathway for both drugs. No significant differences have been found in the duration of action of cisatracurium among patients with and without renal failure. However, variability in recovery times has been seen in patients with renal failure.[186-188] The pharmacokinetics of anticholinesterase drugs used for antagonizing nondepolarizing muscle relaxants is unchanged within 1 hour after renal transplantation.[146] Succinylcholine can be used to facilitate intubation if serum K+ level is normal.

Other Drugs. Mannitol is included in many transplant protocols. It does not depend on renal tubular concentrating mechanisms to promote urinary formation, and it facilitates urinary output and a reduction in tissue and intravascular volume. The effect of low-dose dopamine administration on cadaver graft function has also been evaluated. An infusion rate of 1 to 3 mcg/kg/min preoperatively does not affect early or late graft function. These findings are true in normovolemic, hemodynamically stable patients without severe vascular disease. In these circumstances, early graft function is dependent on ischemic changes, and late graft function is dependent on the management of rejection.[189]

Cardiac arrest has been reported after completion of the renal artery anastomosis to the transplanted kidney.[190] Arrest occurred at the time the occlusion clamp was released and was attributed to hyperkalemia from washout of the K+-containing solutions used to preserve the kidney. If clamping of the external iliac artery is necessary during the procedure, K+ can be released from the ischemic limb.[191] Unclamping may also result in hypotension from the release of vasodilating substances from ischemic limbs and the subsequent increase in vascular capacity.

Immunosuppressants

Tacrolimus (Prograf). Tacrolimus is indicated for the prophylaxis of organ rejection in patients receiving allogenic liver or kidney transplants. It is recommended that tacrolimus be used concomitantly with adrenal corticosteroids. Because of the risk of anaphylaxis, tacrolimus injection should be reserved for patients unable to take tacrolimus capsules orally. To avoid excess nephrotoxicity, tacrolimus should not be used simultaneously with cyclosporine. The recommended starting oral dose of tacrolimus is 0.2 mg/kg/day administered every 12 hours in 2 divided doses. The initial dose of tacrolimus may be administered within 24 hours of transplantation but should be delayed until renal function has recovered (as indicated for example by a serum creatinine <4 mg/dL). In patients unable to take oral tacrolimus capsules, therapy may be initiated with tacrolimus injection. The initial dose of tacrolimus should be administered no sooner than 6 hours after transplantation. The recommended starting dose of tacrolimus injection is 0.03 to 0.05 mg/kg/day as a continuous IV infusion.

Sirolimus (Rapamune). Sirolimus is indicated for the prophylaxis of organ rejection in patients receiving renal transplants. It is recommended that this agent be used initially in a regimen with cyclosporine and corticosteroids. In patients at low to moderate immunologic risk, cyclosporine should be withdrawn 2 to 4 months after transplantation, and the sirolimus dose should be increased to reach recommended blood concentrations. Sirolimus inhibits T-lymphocyte activation and proliferation that occurs in response to antigenic and cytokine (Interleukin [IL]-2, IL-4, and IL-15) stimulation by a mechanism that is distinct from that of other immunosuppressants. The drug also inhibits antibody production. Sirolimus is to be administered orally once daily at 2 mg following initial loading.

Mycophenolate Mofetil (CellCept). Mycophenolate mofetil inhibits immunologically mediated inflammatory responses and tumor development. It is a selective, noncompetitive, and reversible inhibitor of inosine monophosphate dehydrogenase

(IMPDH). Mycophenolic acid (MPA), the active metabolite, inhibits the de novo synthesis pathway of guanosine nucleotides without being incorporated into DNA. Because T and B lymphocytes are critically dependent for their proliferation on de novo synthesis of purines, whereas other cell types can use salvage pathways, MPA has potent cytostatic effects on lymphocytes. MPA inhibits proliferative responses of T and B lymphocytes to both mitogenic and allospecific stimulation.

Mycophenolate mofetil is indicated for the prophylaxis of organ rejection in patients receiving allogenic renal, cardiac or hepatic transplants. It should be used concomitantly with cyclosporine and corticosteroids.

Mycophenolate mofetil IV is an alternative dosage form to mycophenolate mofetil capsules, tablets, and oral suspension. The IV preparation should be administered within 24 hours following transplantation. Mycophenolate mofetil IV can be administered for up to 14 days, but patients should be switched to oral mycophenolate mofetil as soon as they can tolerate oral medication.

Azathioprine. Immunosuppression is critical for graft survival, and most patients receive several immunosuppressive drugs. Azathioprine (Imuran) is a bone marrow—toxic derivative of 6-mercaptopurine. Although its mechanism of action is unknown, a single dose of 5 mg/kg is administered intravenously at the time of transplantation. The drug is added to an intravenous drip chamber and administered over 10 to 30 minutes. Maintenance doses of 2 mg/kg/day are used thereafter if the leukocyte count is greater than 4000. Imuran is associated with dose-dependent neutropenia and occasionally with thrombocytopenia.

Orthoclone (OKT3). OKT3 is a mouse monoclonal antibody to the T3 antigen or human lymphocyte. It is administered daily by slow intravenous injection. A standard dose in patients who weigh more than 25 kg is 5 mg given by slow intravenous push. This drug is given only intravenously and is administered for 14 days. Patients receiving OKT3 are given antibiotics to minimize the risk of opportunistic infection. Risks associated with the use of this drug include anaphylaxis, pulmonary capillary leak, and fluid overload.

Cyclosporine. Cyclosporine is a fungal metabolite that suppresses interleukin II production and amplification of cell-mediated immunity. Side effects include nephrotoxicity, hypertension, hirsutism, tremor, and anaphylaxis. Use of the drug early after transplantation delays recovery of allograft function. It is not administered until renal allograft function has reduced serum creatinine level to half of the admission value. The induction dose is 12 mg/kg in two divided doses, and plasma levels are maintained by periodic intravenous or oral doses. The anesthetic action of drugs may be altered in individuals who receive even a single dose of cyclosporine. Several animal studies have shown that a single dose of this immunosuppressant increases the hypnotic effects of phenobarbital and the analgesic effect of fentanyl.[192] The drug also enhances the neuromuscular blockade produced by vecuronium and atracurium.[193]

Steroids. Steroid administration is common in patients who undergo renal transplantation. Both prednisone and methylprednisolone sodium succinate (Solu-Medrol) have potent antiinflammatory and immunosuppressive effects. They are also associated with impaired fibroblast proliferation and function and with impaired wound healing. Prednisone administration is initiated with a dose of 2 mg/kg given daily and slowly tapered to maintenance doses. Adjustments in the dosage of prednisone must be made according to the clinical situation.

Methylprednisolone is used prophylactically in a dose of 2 mg/kg intravenously. It is also used for treatment of acute allograft rejection at a dose of 0.5 to 1 g/day for 3 days. The maximum dose is 6 g.

EXTRACORPOREAL SHOCK-WAVE LITHOTRIPSY

Extracorporeal shock-wave lithotripsy (ESWL) is a technique that uses high-energy shock waves to fragment renal calculi into small particles. A biplanar fluoroscopy unit is used to focus the shock wave on the target stone. The shock wave is repeated several thousand times and causes the stone to disintegrate.

Water Immersion Effects

The original ESWL procedure required patients to be strapped in a chair in a semireclining position, followed by submersion in water up to the clavicle. This technique is rarely used today, but the principles underlying the surgical procedure are similar. The focused, reflected shock wave passes through the water and enters the body through the flank. Immersion in water has significant physiologic effects on cardiovascular and respiratory function and on temperature regulation (Box 30-6). Studies of healthy volunteers after immersion in water up to the neck demonstrated an increase in central blood volume of up to 700 mL and an increase in preload, stroke volume, and cardiac output. Although significant increases in CVP and pulmonary artery pressures occur, no changes in heart rate or arterial pressure occur.[194-196] Increased cardiac filling pressures may precipitate cardiac failure in patients with cardiac compromise.

Hydrostatic pressure on the chest estimated at 20 cm H_2O decreases functional residual capacity by 30% to 35%. Similar changes are noted in expiratory reserve volume and expiratory lung volumes. These changes encourage ventilation/perfusion mismatch. If spontaneously ventilating, awake patients are sedated while immersed, the likelihood of a reduction in oxygen saturation is increased. Supplemental oxygen is recommended.

Because the lungs are filled with air, they present a different acoustic impedance to the shock wave. If not protected, the lungs may be injured. A thick sheet of Styrofoam should be placed between the shock wave and lung tissue. Observation of fluoroscopy during ventilation ensures that the lungs are not in the path of the shock wave.

Diuresis, natriuresis, and kaliuresis have been observed after patients have been immersed in the water bath. These changes are thought to be related to ADH suppression or an increase in renal PG levels. If the patient is well hydrated before immersion, the diuresis that follows vasopressin suppression is reduced.

Immersion lithotripsy units require that the entire body except the head and neck be submerged. Changes in the temperature of the water bath affect the patient's temperature. Both general and epidural anesthesia are associated with vasodilation and loss of shivering. This loss encourages heat transfer between the patient and the water. Both hypothermia and hyperthermia have been reported.[197-200] The temperature of the water bath should be maintained at 35° to 37° C and should be continuously monitored.

Newer second- and third-generation lithotriptors do not require the patient to be submerged in water. Although they do use water for the production of shock waves, a membrane over the shock-wave generator encapsulates the fluid. Transmission of shock waves to the patient is ensured by the use of coupling gel between the patient and the generator membrane.[199]

Patient Monitoring

Electrocardiography, automated cuff measurement of blood pressure, and pulse oximetry are indispensable during lithotripsy. The electrocardiograph must be of good quality because the R wave is used to trigger the shocks. Synchronization of the shock wave to the electrocardiograph has reduced the incidence of cardiac dysrhythmias but has not totally eliminated them. These dysrhythmias are attributed to mechanical stimulation of the heart. Supraventricular premature complexes and premature ventricular complexes are the most common dysrhythmias noted. Atropine or glycopyrrolate may be given to increase the heart rate and thus the shock-wave rate.[200]

Patient Movement

For lithotripsy to be most effective, the stone must remain at the focal point. Because patient movement and patterns of respiration can change kidney and stone position, movement must be minimized and ventilation carefully controlled. The number and intensity of shock waves can be reduced when stone movement is minimized.[201]

Although high-frequency jet ventilation (HFJV) has been used to decrease stone movement during this procedure, its effectiveness is controversial.[202] Benefits of HFJV include less stone movement, less tissue trauma, and less stone disintegration, but its use is not without risk. Complications associated with HFJV include air trapping, bronchoconstriction, failure to adequately ventilate patients, and inaccurate delivery of anesthetic gases.[203,204] Heart-synchronized ventilation, by which the electrocardiograph signal from the patient has been used to trigger both the inspiratory cycle of the ventilator and the firing of shock waves, has improved the HFJV technique.[205] Conventional mechanical ventilation with respiratory rates of 20 to 80 breaths per minute and smaller tidal volumes has also been used for reducing stone movement.

Anesthetic Techniques

Various anesthetic techniques have been used for ESWL. General anesthesia is advantageous because of its rapid onset and control of patient movement. It also allows the use of HFJV. Other techniques include spinal or epidural anesthesia, patient-controlled analgesia (PCA), monitored anesthesia care, and topical anesthesia with eutectic local anesthetics. Continuous infusions of propofol, methohexital, ketamine, and alfentanil have been used alone or with midazolam for ESWL anesthesia.[206-208]

BOX 30-6

Side Effects Associated with Extracorporeal Shock Wave Lithotripsy

- Hypothermia, hyperthermia
- Cardiac dysrhythmias
- Hemorrhagic blisters of skin
- Renal edema
- Renal hematoma
- Lung injury
- Flank pain
- Hypertension, hypotension
- Autonomic hyperreflexia
- Nausea, vomiting

Spinal anesthesia has the advantage of rapid onset, and a pure opiate spinal using sufentanil is a common technique. Disadvantages include hypotension, spinal headache, and the inability to reinforce the block. Use of intrathecal opioids has also been evaluated. Lau and co-workers[208] compared 5% lidocaine with sufentanil 20 mcg and found no differences in pain perception between groups of patients who received the two agents. However, they also noted earlier discharge times in the sufentanil group.[209] Data from a study by Eaton and Kristensen[210] yielded similar results. Patients in the sufentanil group were discharged 52 minutes earlier than those who received lidocaine. The magnitude of hypotension was less in the sufentanil group, yet pruritus, at times intractable, was a common side effect.[209-211]

Although epidural anesthesia is associated with a slower onset, hypotension is less, and the block can be reinforced as needed. A dermatomal level of T6 or T4 must be achieved to ensure patient comfort. Air bubbles in Micropore foam tape used to secure epidural catheters, as well as within the catheter itself, have been associated with attenuation of shock-wave energy at the stone and with a reduction in success rate.[212] Changes in compliance in the epidural vicinity of air bubbles or epidural catheters have been blamed for failure of epidural anesthesia on subsequent ESWL treatments.[212,213] Studies comparing general and regional anesthesia indicate that no differences exist with regard to morbidity with ESWL. Both methods have been found to be effective techniques, with general anesthesia producing more rapid recovery.[214] Zeitlin and Roth[215] found no differences in the long-term effectiveness of ESWL, comparing epidural and general anesthesia with conventional low-volume ventilation or HFJV. Epidural opiates have also been used successfully as an alternative to general anesthesia or in combination with traditional epidural anesthesia.[215,216]

Eutectic mixture of local anesthetics (EMLA) is a local anesthesia cream that contains a mixture of lidocaine and prilocaine. Monk and colleagues[217] investigated the efficacy of EMLA in minimizing the pain associated with shock waves and found that EMLA significantly decreased the pain produced by test shocks greater than 15,000 V. Hemodynamic responses were comparable in EMLA cream and placebo groups. EMLA cream was significantly more effective in men than in women, possibly because of differences in pain perception, skin thickness, or dermal penetration.[217] Other investigators have concluded that although cutaneous anesthesia with lidocaine-prilocaine cream has significant effects on pain during ESWL, it does not eliminate the need for analgesic sedation. It can be used, however, for reducing the dose of analgesic and sedative drugs during ESWL performed with regional or general anesthesia and an unmodified Dornier HM3 lithotriptor.[218]

The effectiveness of PCA with and without the use of EMLA cream has been studied. Alfentanil has been used alone or in combination with midazolam or propofol. Although patient satisfaction scores were high, increased incidences of desaturation, bradypnea, and increased end-tidal CO_2 levels were found.[219] Ganapathy and co-workers[220] reported no difference in pain perception among groups treated with alfentanil PCA combined with EMLA cream and those treated with placebo. They also reported that the inclusion of EMLA cream did not facilitate early discharge from the postanesthesia care unit. Schelling and colleagues[221] found a gender-based relationship in patients treated with alfentanil PCA alone: men were found to have a higher pain tolerance than women.

PERCUTANEOUS NEPHROLITHOTOMY

Removal of kidney stones 25 mm or smaller can also be accomplished through percutaneous nephrolithotomy. This procedure requires general anesthesia and postoperative hospitalization. Stones are removed via a rigid operating scope inserted in the lower calyx of the kidney under fluoroscopy. Once located, calculi are pulverized by using laser, electrohydraulic, or ultrasound probes placed directly on the stones. The procedure is performed with the patient in the prone position; therefore associated anesthetic considerations apply (see following chart of complications of percutaneous nephrolithotomy).

Minor	Major
Pain	Septicemia
Fever	Bleeding
Urinary tract infection	Pelvic or ureteral tears
Renal colic	Pneumothorax
	Hemothorax
	Anaphylaxis secondary to contrast dye

TRANSURETHRAL RESECTION OF THE PROSTATE

Surgical Technique

Transurethral resection of the prostate (TURP) is one of the most commonly performed surgical procedures in men older than 60 years of age. These patients are often at greater anesthetic risk because they are more likely to have cardiovascular or pulmonary problems. The procedure consists of opening the outlet channel from the bladder with the use of a resectoscope in the urethra for electrically cutting away the obstructing median and lateral lobes of prostate tissue. Bleeding is controlled with a coagulation current. For visualization of the area, the bladder is distended, and continuous irrigation is used to wash away blood and dissected prostatic tissue.

Various types of irrigating fluid have been used. Although distilled water is associated with the least optical impairment, hemolysis of red blood cells is an unacceptable side effect. Normal saline or lactated Ringer's solution is highly ionized and promotes dispersion of high current from the resectoscope. For these reasons, irrigating solutions typically consist of sorbitol (2.70 g) and mannitol (0.54 g) in 100 mL of water (Cytal) or glycine 1.5%.[222,223] Glycine is slightly hypoosmolar to the blood but is used widely because of its low cost. Average features of a transurethral resection of the prostate are given in Table 30-4.

Complications

Fluid Absorption

A number of complications are associated with resection of the prostate (Box 30-7). Large amounts of irrigating solution can be absorbed through venous sinuses. The amount absorbed and the rate of absorption depend on the size of the gland to be resected, the congestion of the gland, the duration of resection, the pressure of the irrigating solution, the number of sinuses open at any one time, and the experience of the resectionist.[224] An average of 10 to 30 mL of fluid can be absorbed per minute of resection time, and 6 to 8 L can be absorbed in cases that last up to 2 hours.[225,226] In general, limiting resection time to 1 hour is desirable.

Complications specifically related to absorption of irrigating fluid include volume overload with pulmonary edema and dilutional hyponatremia. As fluid enters the vascular compartment, intravascular pressure and myocardial work increase. The fluid dilutes plasma proteins and electrolytes, and the change in intravascular pressure favors movement of fluid from the vascular to the interstitial compartment. This is poorly tolerated by patients with a high incidence of cardiovascular disease.

Absorption of irrigating fluid also leads to dilutional hyponatremia. Sodium is a major cation of extracellular fluid, and it is responsible for the depolarization of excitable cells and the production of action potentials. CNS symptoms associated with hyponatremia range from restlessness, headache, irritability, and confusion to blindness, coma, and seizures. Cardiac dysrhythmias may also develop.

Serum sodium (Na^+) concentrations of 120 mEq/L appear to be borderline for the development of severe reactions. Electrocardiographic changes characterized by widening of the QRS complex and ST-segment elevation are seen when the serum level decreases to 115 mEq/L. At levels less than 100 mEq/L, ventricular tachycardia and fibrillation can occur.[227] CNS symptoms associated with hypovolemia include restlessness, confusion, nausea, vomiting, coma, and convulsions. These symptoms can be detected more easily in patients receiving regional anesthesia. CNS symptoms are hidden under general anesthesia. Progressive increases in blood pressure, CVP, or pulmonary artery wedge pressure (when monitored) suggest hypervolemia.

Hyponatremia in such cases results from water excess rather than from Na^+ loss. Hypertonic saline (3% to 5% sodium chloride) and diuretics (furosemide, 0.15 to 0.5 mg/kg) are useful.

Bladder Perforation

Perforation of the bladder is another complication of prostatic surgery.[228] Symptoms vary, depending on whether the rupture is intraperitoneal or extraperitoneal (Box 30-8). These symptoms are better recognized when the patient has regional anesthesia if the regional technique does not produce a high block. With general anesthesia, only the surgeon can appreciate the inability to recover bladder fluid as a sign of perforation. Intraperitoneal fluid will be excreted by the kidney. However, if hemodynamic embarrassment occurs, suprapubic drainage is effective for removal of excess intraperitoneal fluid.

Glycine Absorption

Absorption of glycine has been associated with toxicity. Glycine, an amino acid normally found in the body, is a major inhibitory transmitter. Toxic effects have been produced in animals and humans. Signs and symptoms include nausea, vomiting, fixation and dilation of the pupils, weakness, and muscle incoordination. Transient blindness after TURP has been attributed to edema of the cortex, atropine, and hyponatremia.[229-231] Ovassapian and co-workers[232] reported five cases of transient blindness that they thought were attributable to glycine toxicity. Glycine may also result in CNS toxicity as a consequence of its biotransformation to NH_3.[233,234] NH_3 toxicity results in encephalopathy and delayed awakening in the postoperative period. NH_3 yields glutamine, which is metabolized to the inhibitory neurotransmitter serotonin. Hyperammonemia also decreases the production of dopamine and norepinephrine, which are central excitatory neurotransmitters.[235] Animal studies suggest that both glycine and NH_3 reduce the amplitude of the visual evoked potential and therefore have CNS effects.[236]

Skin Burns

The use of high voltage for cutting and coagulation during TURP may result in skin burns. Electrocardiography pads may be placed

TABLE 30-4	Average Parameters with a Transurethral Resection of the Prostate
Parameter	**Average**
Resection time	<77 min
Resect mass	20-48 g
Absorbed volume	1 L
Blood loss	176-534 mL
Speed of TURP syndrome onset	15 min
Serum sodium nadir	132-135 mmol/L

Adapted from Gravenstein D, Hahn RG. TURP syndrome. In: Lobato EB et al, eds. Complications of Anesthesiology. Philadelphia: Lippincott Williams & Wilkins; 2008:474-491.

BOX 30-7

Complications of Transurethral Resection of the Prostate

- Hypervolemia
- Hyponatremia
- Bladder perforation
- Hemorrhage
- Glycine toxicity
- Ammonia toxicity
- Electrical hazards
- Hypothermia
- Bacteremia

BOX 30-8

Symptoms of Bladder Perforation

Extraperitoneal
Periumbilical, inguinal, or suprapubic pain
Lower abdominal distention
Pain

Intraperitoneal
Abdominal rigidity, distention, pain
Referred shoulder pain
Hiccup, shortness of breath
Tachycardia
Hypotension or hypertension
Diaphoresis
Vomiting

at other sites so that potential burns are avoided. Many patients who undergo TURP have pacemakers. These devices must be converted to a fixed rate unless they are designed to operate in the presence of applied currents.[237]

Blood Loss

Blood loss during TURP generally is related to the weight of the resected tissue, operating time, and skill of the surgeon.[238-240] Assessment of blood loss is difficult because of the dilution of blood in irrigating fluid. Hematocrit may be increased, decreased, or unchanged, depending on the amount of fluid in the intravascular space at the time. Blood transfusion should be based on preoperative hematocrit, the duration and difficulty of resection, and a general assessment of the patient.

Anesthesia

Spinal anesthesia and general anesthesia have both been used for TURP procedures. Some clinicians believe that spinal anesthesia is ideal because with it, the signs and symptoms of hypervolemia and bladder perforation are more easily detected. As a result, a T10 sensory level is necessary for adequate anesthesia. Pain impulses from the bladder neck and prostate are propagated by afferent parasympathetic fibers originating primarily from the second and third sacral roots in concert with the pelvic splanchnic nerves. The sympathetic nerves via the hypogastric plexus, which is derived from T11 to L2 nerve roots, transmit sensation from the bladder.[241] Although general anesthesia may mask early complications, it may be desirable in the patient who requires pulmonary support or who cannot tolerate a fluid load for compensation of a loss of sympathetic tone. All inhalation agents have been used successfully. Some key points for anesthesia management of TURP are given in Box 30-9.

BOX 30-9

Key Points for Anesthesia Management of Transurethral Resection of Prostate

- TURP syndrome is caused by disturbance of intravascular volume and/or serum osmolality.
- Four questions to ask prior to a TURP:
  What is the irrigation fluid?
  What is the bag height over the prostate?
  What type of resectoscope is being used?
  In what mode is the resectoscope being used?
- Techniques for detection of pending TURP syndrome include measurement of serum sodium, measurement of breath alcohol levels by inserting 1% ethanol in the irrigating solution, and volumetric fluid balance.
- Treat symptomatic (mental status changes, seizures, hypotension) patients aggressively; treat asymptomatic aberrant lab values (hyponatremia, hyperglycemia) very slowly, if at all.
- Sodium loss is an important source of hyponatremia a few hours after a TURP during which absorption of an electrolyte-free irrigating fluid has occurred.

Adapted from Gravenstein D, Hahn RG. TURP syndrome. In: Lobato EB et al, eds. Complications of Anesthesiology. Philadelphia: Lippincott Williams & Wilkins; 2008:474-491.

LAPAROSCOPIC UROLOGIC SURGERY

Laparoscopy is the process of inspecting the abdominal cavity through an endoscope. Laparoscopy started in the mid-1950s when gynecologists began to use this technique to diagnose pelvic pain while reducing postoperative pain and length of hospital stay. Over the years, laparoscopy for general surgery has become a common procedure. Advantages of laparoscopic surgery are found in Box 30-10. Some examples of surgical procedures that can be done laparoscopically include varicocelectomy, percutaneous stone retrieval, nephrectomy, transplants, and radical prostatectomy.[242-244]

Carbon dioxide is the most universally used agent for insufflating the abdominal cavity to facilitate view during this procedure. Several pathophysiologic changes can occur after carbon dioxide pneumoperitoneum and the extremes of patient positioning required for the procedure. Most of the considerations for laparoscopic surgery are beyond the scope of this chapter, but two unique problems specific to urologic surgery are worth discussing.

The urogenital system is a retroperitoneal system. As such, carbon dioxide insufflated in this space communicates freely with the thorax and subcutaneous tissue. Subcutaneous emphysema can occur and may extend to the head and neck. In severe cases, it may lead to submucous swelling and airway compromise in the unprotected airway.[245]

In long cases, carbon dioxide may not be reabsorbed, and acidosis may develop. Because the carbon dioxide insufflation together with steep Trendelenburg position and long procedures may increase intraabdominal and intrathoracic pressure, controlled ventilation is mandatory. Increased pressure exerted by the insufflation may also affect renal and hepatic function. The pneumoperitoneum can cause renal cortical vasoconstriction due to activation of the sympathetic nervous system. Decreased renal perfusion activates the renin-angiotensin-aldosterone system, which causes vasoconstriction. These effects are additive to those seen with surgical stress. Renal and hepatic perfusion may be altered. Some suggestions to minimize the effect of positive pressure pneumoperitoneum are (1) lower insufflation pressures, (2) operate in a gasless environment, (3) substitute inert gas for carbon dioxide, (4) use drugs to antagonize the neuroendocrine response, (5) expand volume, and (6) use mechanical devices. It has been reported that the use of intermittent sequential pneumatic compression (ISPC), activated over the lower limbs 15 minutes after the pneumoperitoneum, improves splanchnic and renal perfusion. This technique augments cardiac output and lowers systemic vascular resistance.[246]

BOX 30-10

Advantages of Laparoscopic Surgery

1. Reduced postoperative pain
2. Better cosmetic results
3. Quicker return to normal activities
4. Reduction in hospital length of stay
5. Reduction on cost of care
6. Less intraoperative bleeding
7. Less postoperative pulmonary infections
8. Less postoperative wound infections
9. Reduced metabolic derangements
10. Better postoperative respiratory function

ROBOTIC UROLOGIC SURGERY

Robotic-assisted surgery is an emerging technique for managing various urologic procedures such as prostatectomy. One of the commercially available systems is the da Vinci surgical system (Intuitive Surgical Mountain View, CA, USA). It consists of a surgeon's console for surgical work, a surgical cart that houses the video and lighting equipment, and a robotic tower that supports three or four robotic arms.

The surgeon's console provides the surgeon with a three-dimensional, 10-times magnified view through a binocular viewpoint. Interaction is through "masters" into which the surgeon's hands are inserted. Free movement is possible from the masters to robotic instruments. Endoscopic instruments include graspers, hooks, scissors, knives, and surgical energy devices.[247]

Robotic surgery necessitates a coordinated approach by anesthetist and surgeon because the surgery is performed using a modified laparoscopic technique and can be very long in duration. A Trendelenburg position is used. Major complications of surgery in the Trendelenburg position include (1) neuropathies, (2) CVP elevation, (3) intraocular/intracranial pressure elevation, (4) increased pulmonary venous pressure, (5) decreased pulmonary compliance, (6) reduced functional residual capacity (FRC), and (7) swelling of the face, eyelids, conjunctivae, and tongue. Facial swelling may preclude immediate extubation at the end of the procedure. Major anesthetic considerations for robotic procedures are summarized in Box 30-11.

SUMMARY

Anesthetic management of the patient during the perioperative period for renal procedures depends upon an understanding of both normal renal function and pathophysiologic changes in

---

BOX 30-11

Anesthesia for Robotic Surgery

1. There is risk of thromboembolism due to lengthy procedures in Trendelenburg position. Use thrombo-embolic stockings to reduce risk.
2. Maximize protection over pressure areas to avoid nerve injury.
3. General anesthesia or general and regional combined may be used.
4. Difficulties inherent in patients having prolonged surgery in Trendelenburg position with lower limbs in lithotomy are present.
5. Difficulties with peritoneal insufflation are present.
6. Blood pressure augmentation with vasoconstrictors may be necessary, probably due to prolonged pneumoperitoneum.
7. A high volume requirement is required.
8. Urine output may be sluggish and generally responds to a fluid challenge.

---

the organ system. In addition to normal anatomy and physiology, this chapter highlighted ways to assess renal function and changes in renal function secondary to anesthetics. Various stages of renal pathology were identified and management of patients with acute and chronic renal failure emphasized. Rare and common urologic procedures were identified and pertinent anesthetic considerations discussed for each procedure.[248,249]

REFERENCES

1. Guyton AC. *Textbook of Medical Physiology.* 11th ed. *Philadelphia: Saunders.* 2006:291-305.
2. Mirenda JV, Grisson TE. Anesthetic implications of the renin-angiotensin system and angiotensin converting enzyme inhibitors. *Anesth Analg.* 1991;72:667-683.
3. Ballermann BJ, Brenner BM. Role of arterial peptides in body fluid homeostasis. *Circ Res.* 1986;58:619-630.
4. Mcloughlin TM, Watkins DW. Atrial natriuretic peptide: the state of the art. *Semin Anesth.* 1988;7:243-250.
5. Sladen RN. Renal physiology. In: Miller R, ed. *Anesthesia.* 6th ed. New York: Churchill Livingstone; 2005:777-812.
6. Price HL et al. Sympathoadrenal responses to general anesthesia in man and their relation to hemodynamics. *Anesthesiology.* 1959;20:563-575.
7. Cousins MJ et al. Metabolism and renal effects of enflurane in man. *Anesthesiology.* 1976;44:44-53.
8. Mazze RI et al. Renal function during anesthesia and surgery. I. The effects of halothane anesthesia. *Anesthesiology.* 1963;24:279-284.
9. Deutsch S et al. Effects of halothane anesthesia on renal function in normal man. *Anesthesiology.* 1966;27:793-804.
10. Mazze RI et al. Renal effects and metabolism of isoflurane in man. *Anesthesiology.* 1974;40:536-542.
11. Warltier DC, Pagel PS. Cardiovascular and respiratory actions of desflurane: is desflurane different from isoflurane? *Anesth Analg.* 1992;75:S17-S31.
12. Hines RL, Marschall KE. *Anesthesia Disease and Coexisting Diseases.* 5th ed. Philadelphia: Saunders; 2008:323-348.
13. Kharasch ED et al. Human kidney methoxyflurane and sevoflurane metabolism: intrarenal fluoride production as a possible mechanism of methoxyflurane nephrotoxicity. *Anesthesiology.* 1995;90:505-508.
14. Deutsch S et al. The effects of anaesthesia with thiopentone, nitrous oxide, narcotics, and neuromuscular blocking drugs on renal function in normal man. *Br J Anaesth.* 1969;41:807-815.
15. Barry KG et al. Prevention of surgical oliguria and renal hemodynamic suppression by sustained hydration. *N Engl J Med.* 1964;270:1371-1377.
16. O'Hara JF et al. The renal system and anesthesia for urologic surgery. In: Barash et al, eds. *Clinical Anesthesia.* 5th ed. Philadelphia: Lippincott Williams & Wilkins; 2006:1013-1034.
17. Kennedy WF Jr et al. Systemic cardiovascular and renal hemodynamic alterations during peridural anesthesia in normal man. *Anesthesiology.* 1969; 31:414-421.
18. Sivarajan M et al. Systemic and regional blood flow during epidural anesthesia without epinephrine in the rhesus monkey. *Anesthesiology.* 1976;45:300-310.
19. Bachman L. The antidiuretic effect of anesthetic agents. *Anesthesiology.* 1955;16:939-949.
20. Moran WH Jr et al. The relationship of antidiuretic hormone secretion to surgical stress. *Surgery.* 1964;56:99-108.
21. Philbin D, Coggins CH. Plasma antidiuretic hormone levels in cardiac surgical patients during morphine and halothane anesthesia. *Anesthesiology.* 1978;49:95-98.
22. Kharasch ED et al. Atrial natriuretic factor may mediate the renal effects of PEEP ventilation. *Anesthesiology.* 1988;69:862-869.
23. Pettinger WA. Anesthetics and the renin-angiotensin-aldosterone axis. *Anesthesiology.* 1978;48:393-396.
24. Miller ED Jr et al. The effect of ketamine on the renin-angiotensin system. *Anesthesiology.* 1975;42:503-505.
25. Miller ED et al. The regulatory function of the renin-angiotensin system during general anesthesia. *Anesthesiology.* 1978;48:399-403.
26. Udelsman R et al. Responses of the hypothalamic-pituitary-adrenal and renin-angiotensin axes and the sympathetic system during controlled surgical and anesthetic stress. *J Clin Endocrinol Metab.* 1987;64:986-994.
27. Crandell WB et al. Nephrotoxicity associated with methoxyflurane anesthesia. *Anesthesiology.* 1966;27:591-607.
28. Cousins MJ, Mazze RI. Methoxyflurane nephrotoxicity: a study of dose response to man. *JAMA.* 1973;225:1611-1616.
29. Mazze RI et al. Renal dysfunction associated with methoxyflurane anesthesia: a randomized prospective clinical evaluation. *JAMA.* 1971;216:278-283.
30. Mazze RI et al. Dose-related methoxyflurane nephrotoxicity in rats: a biochemical and pathologic correlation. *Anesthesiology.* 1972;36:571-587.

31. Mazze RI, Cousins MJ. Combined nephrotoxicity of gentamicin and methoxyflurane anesthesia in man: a case report. *Br J Anaesth.* 1973;45:394-397.
32. Hitt BA et al. Metabolism of isoflurane in Fischer 344 rats and man. *Anesthesiology.* 1974;40:62-67.
33. Davidkova T et al. Biotransformation of isoflurane: urinary and serum fluoride ion and organic fluorine. *Anesthesiology.* 1988;69:218-222.
34. Koblin DD et al. I-653 resists degradation in rats. *Anesth Analg.* 1988;67:534-538.
35. Jones RM et al. Biotransformation and hepatorenal function in volunteers after exposure to desflurane (I-653). *Br J Anaesth.* 1990;64:482-487.
36. Sutton TS et al. Fluoride metabolites after prolonged exposure of volunteers and patients to desflurane. *Anesth Analg.* 1991;73:180-185.
37. Smiley RM et al. Metabolism of desflurane and isoflurane to fluoride ion in surgical patients. *Can J Anaesth.* 1991;38:965-968.
38. Koblin DD. Characteristics and implications of desflurane metabolism and toxicity. *Anesth Analg.* 1992;75:510-516.
39. Frink EJ Jr et al. Plasma inorganic fluoride with sevoflurane anesthesia: correlation with indices of hepatic and renal function. *Anesth Analg.* 1992;74:231-235.
40. Blanco E et al. Comparison of maintenance and recovery characteristics of sevoflurane–nitrous oxide and enflurane–nitrous oxide anaesthesia. *Eur J Anaesthesiol.* 1995;12:517-523.
41. Goldberg ME et al. Sevoflurane versus isoflurane for maintenance of anesthesia: are serum inorganic fluoride ion concentrations of concern? *Anesth Analg.* 1996;82:1268-1272.
42. Newman PJ et al. Circulating fluoride changes and hepatorenal function following sevoflurane anaesthesia. *Anaesthesia.* 1994;49:936-939.
43. Wiesner G et al. Serum fluoride concentrations and exocrine kidney function with sevoflurane and enflurane. An open, randomized, comparative phase III study of patients with healthy kidneys. *Anaesthetist.* 1996;45:31-36.
44. Matsumura C et al. Serum and urine inorganic fluoride levels following prolonged low-dose sevoflurane anesthesia combined with epidural block. *J Clin Anesth.* 1994;6:419-424.
45. Highiyama T, Hirasakai A. Effects of sevoflurane anaesthesia on renal function—duration of administration and area under the curve and rate of decrease of serum inorganic fluoride. *Eur J Anaesthesiol.* 1995;12:477-482.
46. Bito H et al. Effects of low-flow sevoflurane anesthesia on renal function: comparison with high-flow sevoflurane anesthesia and low-flow isoflurane anesthesia. *Anesthesiology.* 1997;86:1231-1237.
47. Kobayashi Y et al. Serum and urinary inorganic fluoride concentrations after prolonged inhalation of sevoflurane in humans. *Anesth Analg.* 1992;74:753-757.
48. Higuchi H et al. Urine concentrating ability after prolonged sevoflurane anaesthesia. *Br J Anaesth.* 1994;73:239-240.
49. Higuchi H et al. Renal function in patients with high serum fluoride concentrations after prolonged sevoflurane anesthesia. *Anesthesiology.* 1995;83:449-458.
50. Frink EJ Jr et al. Sevoflurane degradation product concentrations with soda lime during prolonged anesthesia. *J Clin Anesth.* 1994;6:239-242.
51. Eger EI II et al. Dose-related biochemical markers of renal injury after sevoflurane versus desflurane anesthesia in volunteers. *Anesth Analg.* 1997;85:1154-1163.
52. Eger EI II et al. Nephrotoxicity of sevoflurane versus desflurane anesthesia in volunteers. *Anesth Analg.* 1997;84:160-168.
53. Frink EJ Jr et al. Renal concentrating function with prolonged sevoflurane or enflurane anesthesia in volunteers. *Anesthesiology.* 1994;80:1019-1025.
54. Munday IT et al. Serum fluoride concentration and urine osmolality after enflurane and sevoflurane anesthesia in male volunteers. *Anesth Analg.* 1995;81:353-359.
55. Ebert TJ et al. Absence of renal and hepatic toxicity after four hours of 1.25 minimum alveolar anesthetic concentration sevoflurane anesthesia in volunteers. *Anesth Analg.* 1998;86:662-667.
56. Ebert TJ et al. Absence of biochemical evidence for renal and hepatic dysfunction after 8 hours of 1.25 minimum alveolar concentration sevoflurane anesthesia in volunteers. *Anesthesiology.* 1998;88:601-610.
57. Frink EJ Jr et al. Plasma inorganic fluoride levels with sevoflurane anesthesia in morbidly obese and nonobese patients. *Anesth Analg.* 1993;76:1333-1337.
58. Bedford RF, Ives HE. The renal safety of sevoflurane. *Anesth Analg.* 2000;90:505-508.
59. Rooke GA et al. The hemodynamic and renal effects of sevoflurane and isoflurane in patients with coronary artery disease and chronic hypertension. Sevoflurane ischemic study group. *Anesth Analg.* 1996;82:1159-1165.
60. Conzen PF et al. Renal function and serum fluoride concentrations in patients with stable renal insufficiency after anesthesia with sevoflurane or enflurane. *Anesth Analg.* 1995;81:569-575.
61. Nishiyama T et al. Inorganic fluoride kinetics and renal tubular function after sevoflurane hemodialysis. *Anesth Analg.* 1996;83:574-577.
62. Tsukamoto N et al. The effects of sevoflurane and isoflurane anesthesia on renal tubular function in patients with moderately impaired renal function. *Anesth Analg.* 1996;82:909-913.
63. Artu AA. Renal effects of sevoflurane during conditions of possible increased risk. *J Clin Anesth.* 1998;10:531-538.
64. Hara T et al. Renal function in patients during and after hypotensive anesthesia with sevoflurane. *J Clin Anesth.* 1998;10:539-545.
65. Burchardi H, Kaczmarczyk G. The effects of anaesthesia on renal function. *Eur J Anaesthesiol.* 1994;11:163-168.
66. Higuchi H et al. The effects of low-flow sevoflurane and isoflurane anesthesia on renal function in patients with stable moderate renal insufficiency. *Anesth Analg.* 2001;92:650-655.
67. Conzen PF et al. Low-flow sevoflurane compared with low-flow isoflurane anesthesia in patients with stable renal insufficiency. *Anesthesiology.* 2002;97:578-584.
68. Gentz BA, Malan TP. Renal toxicity with sevoflurane: storm in a teacup? *Drugs.* 2001;61:2155-2162.
69. Kasiske BL, Kjellstrand CM. Perioperative management of patients with chronic renal failure and postoperative acute renal failure. *Urol Clin North Am.* 1983;10:35-50.
70. Ympa YP et al. Has mortality from acute renal failure decreased? A systematic review of the literature. *Am J Med.* 2005;118:827-832.
71. Wijeydundera DN et al. Improving the identification of patients at risk of postoperative renal failure after cardiac surgery. *Anesthesiology.* 2006;104:65-72.
72. Hou SH et al. Hospital-acquired renal insufficiency: a prospective study. *Am J Med.* 1983;74:243-248.
73. Godet G et al. Risk factors for acute postoperative renal failure in thoracic or thoracoabdominal aortic surgery: a prospective study. *Anesth Analg.* 1997;85:1227-1232.
74. Sear JW. Kidney dysfunction in the postoperative period. *Br J Anaesth.* 2005;95:20-32.
75. Hanley MJ, Davidson K. Prior mannitol and furosemide infusion in a model of ischemic acute renal failure. *Am J Physiol.* 1981;241:556-574.
76. De Torrente A et al. Effects of furosemide and acetylcholine in norepinephrine-induced acute renal failure. *Am J Physiol.* 1978;235:F131-F136.
77. Burke TJ et al. Ischemia and tubule obstruction during acute renal failure in dogs: mannitol in protection. *Am J Physiol.* 1980;238:F305-F314.
78. Kleinknecht D et al. Furosemide in acute oliguric renal failure: a controlled trial. *Nephron.* 1976;17:51-58.
79. Brown CV et al. High dose furosemide in acute renal failure: a controlled trial. *Clin Nephrol.* 1981;15:90-96.
80. Abay MC et al. Current literature questions the routine use of low-dose dopamine. *AANA J.* 2007;75:57-63.
81. Singer I, Epstein M. Potential of dopamine A-1 agonists in the management of acute renal failure. *Am J Kidney Dis.* 1998;31(5):743-755.
82. Mathur VS et al. The effects of fenoldopam, a selective dopamine receptor agonist, on systemic and renal hemodynamics in normotensive subjects. *Crit Care Med.* 1999;27:1832-1837.
83. Oliver WC et al. A comparison of fenoldopam with dopamine and sodium nitroprusside in patients undergoing cross clamping of abdominal aorta. *Anesth Analg.* 2006;103(4):833-840.
84. Wilson LM. Acute renal failure. *Pathophysiology: Clinical Concepts of Disease Processes.* 4th ed. St Louis: Mosby; 1992:704-710.
85. Moore RD et al. Risk factors for nephrotoxicity in patients treated with aminoglycosides. *Ann Intern Med.* 1984;100:352-357.
86. Shafi T et al. Infusion intravenous pyelography and renal function: effect in patients with chronic renal insufficiency. *Arch Intern Med.* 1978;138:1218-1221.
87. Tolkoff-Rubin N, Treatment of irreversible heart failure. In: Goldman L et al., eds. *Cecil Textbook of Medicine.* 23rd ed. Philadelphia: Saunders; 2008:936.
88. Sherlock J et al. Determinants of oxygenation during hemodialysis and related procedures: a report of data acquired under varying conditions and a review of the literature. *Am J Nephrol.* 1984;4:158-168.
89. Ganella S, Chang BS. Hemodialysis associated hypoxemia. *Am J Nephrol.* 1984;4:273-279.
90. Turnbull JM, Buck C. The value of preoperative screening investigations in otherwise healthy individuals. *Arch Intern Med.* 1987;147:101-105.
91. Lawrence VA, Kroenke K. The unproven utility of preoperative urinalysis: clinical use. *Arch Intern Med.* 1988;148:1370-1373.
92. Gold BD, Wolfersberger WH. Findings from routine urinalysis and hematocrit on ambulatory oral and maxillofacial surgery patients. *J Oral Surg.* 1980;38:677-678.
93. Morgan GE Jr et al. Anesthesia for patients with renal disease. *Clinical Anesthesiology.* New York: Lange Medical; 2006:742.

94. Ifudu O. Care of patients undergoing hemodialysis. *N Engl J Med.* 1998;339:1054-1062.
95. Rostand SG et al. Ischemic heart disease in patients with uremia undergoing maintenance hemodialysis. *Kidney Int.* 1979;16:600-611.
96. Owen CH et al. Coronary artery bypass grafting in patients with dialysis-dependent renal failure. *Ann Thorac Surg.* 1994;58:1729-1733.
97. Kahn JK et al. Short- and long-term outcome of percutaneous transluminal coronary angioplasty in chronic dialysis patients. *Am Heart J.* 1990; 119:484-489.
98. Endou K. Hemodynamic changes during hemodialysis. *Cardiology.* 1978;63:175-187.
99. Kinet J. Hemodynamic study of hypotension during hemodialysis. *Kidney Int.* 1982;21:868-876.
100. Eschbach JW. Correction of the anemia of the end-stage renal disease with recombinant erythropoietin: results of a combined phase I and II clinical trial. *N Engl J Med.* 1987;316:73-78.
101. Opelz G. Blood transfusion: current relevance of the transfusion effect in renal transplantation. *Transplant Proc.* 1985;27:1015-1022.
102. Erslev A. Erythropoietin coming of age. *N Engl J Med.* 1987;316:101.
103. Eschbach JW. Treatment of the anemia of progressive renal failure with recombinant human erythropoietin. *N Engl J Med.* 1989;321:158.
104. Eschbach JW. Recombinant human erythropoietin in anemic patients with end-stage renal disease: results of a phase III multicenter clinical trial. *Ann Intern Med.* 1989;111:992-999.
105. Ifudu O et al. The intensity of hemodialysis and the response to erythropoietin in patients with end-stage renal disease. *N Engl J Med.* 1996; 334:420-425.
106. Sun CH. Serum erythropoietin levels after renal transplantation. *N Engl J Med.* 1989;321:151-157.
107. Gafter U. Platelet count and thrombopoietic activity in patients with chronic renal failure. *Nephron.* 1987;45:207-209.
108. DiMinno G. Platelet dysfunction in uremia: multifaceted defect partially corrected by dialysis. *Am J Med.* 1985;79:552-559.
109. Remuzzi G. Bleeding in renal failure: altered platelet function in chronic uremia only partially corrected by haemodialysis. *Nephron.* 1978;22:347-353.
110. Kentro TB et al. Clinical efficacy of desmopressin acetate for hemostatic control in patients with primary platelet disorders undergoing surgery. *Am J Hematol.* 1987;24:214-218.
111. Mannucci PM. 1-Desamino-8-D-arginine vasopressin shortens the bleeding time in uremia. *N Engl J Med.* 1983;308:8-11.
112. Janson PA. Treatment of the bleeding tendency in uremia with cryoprecipitate. *N Engl J Med.* 1980;303:1318-1321.
113. Livio M. Conjugated estrogens for the management of bleeding associated with renal failure. *N Engl J Med.* 1986;315:731-735.
114. Margolis DM. Upper gastrointestinal disease in chronic renal failure: a prospective evaluation. *Arch Intern Med.* 1978;138:1214-1217.
115. Shuman RB et al. Prophylactic therapy for stress ulcer bleeding: a reappraisal. *Ann Intern Med.* 1987;106:562-566.
116. Young GA. Anthropometry and plasma valine, amino acids, and proteins in the nutritional assessment of hemodialysis patients. *Kidney Int.* 1992; 21:492-497.
117. Lewis SL, Van Epps DE. Neutrophil and monocyte alterations in chronic dialysis patients. *Am J Kidney Dis.* 1987;9:381-395.
118. Ruiz P et al. Impaired function of macrophage Fc receptors in end-stage renal disease. *N Engl J Med.* 1990;322:717-720.
119. Zeldis JB. The prevalence of hepatitis C virus antibodies among hemodialysis patients. *Ann Intern Med.* 1990;112:958-960.
120. Pinson CW et al. Surgery in long-term dialysis patients: experience with more than 300 cases. *Am J Surg.* 1986;151:567-571.
121. Vinik RH et al. The pharmacokinetics of midazolam in chronic renal failure patients. *Anesthesiology.* 1983;59:390-392.
122. Olsen GD et al. Morphine and phenytoin binding to plasma proteins in renal and hepatic failure. *Clin Pharmacol Ther.* 1975;17:677-681.
123. Don HF et al. Narcotic analgesics in anuric patients. *Anesthesiology.* 1975;42:745-747.
124. Kay J. Renal disorders. In: Cheng EY, Kay J, eds. *Manual of Anesthesia and the Medically Compromised Patient.* Philadelphia: Lippincott; 1990:244-264.
125. Gosselin RE et al. The fate of atropine in man. *Clin Pharmacol Ther.* 1960;1:597-603.
126. Mouquet C et al. Anesthesia for creation of a forearm fistula in patients with endstage renal failure. *Anesthesiology.* 1989;70:909-914.
127. Alsalti RA et al. Arteriovenous fistula in chronic renal failure patients: comparison between three different anesthetic techniques. *Middle East J Anesthesiol.* 1999;15:305-314.
128. Bromage PR, Gertel M. Brachial plexus anesthesia in chronic renal failure. *Anesthesiology.* 1972;36:488-493.
129. Martin R et al. Brachial plexus blockade and chronic renal failure. *Anesthesiology.* 1988;69:405-406.
130. Rodriquez J et al. High doses of mepivacaine for brachial plexus block in patients with end-stage chronic renal failure: a pilot study. *Eur J Anaesthesiol.* 2001;18:171-176.
131. Crews JC et al. Levobupivacaine for axillary brachial plexus block: a pharmacokinetic and clinical comparison in patients with normal renal function or renal disease. *Anesth Analg.* 2002;95:219-223.
132. Adnan T et al. Clonidine as an adjuvant for lidocaine in axillary brachial plexus block in patients with chronic renal failure. *Acta Anaesthesiol Scand.* 2005;49:563-568.
133. Grejda S et al. Paraplegia following spinal anesthesia in a patient with chronic renal failure. *Reg Anesth.* 1989;14:155-157.
134. Basta M, Sloan P. Epidural hematoma following epidural catheter placement in a patient with chronic renal failure. *Can J Anaesth.* 1999;46:271-274.
135. Orko R et al. Subarachnoid anesthesia with 0.75% bupivacaine in patients with chronic renal failure. *Br J Anaesth.* 1986;58:605-609.
136. Ghoreim MM, Pandya H. Plasma protein binding of thiopental in patients with impaired renal or hepatic function. *Anesthesiology.* 1975;42:545-548.
137. Chauvin M et al. Pharmacokinetics of alfentanil in chronic renal failure. *Anesth Analg.* 1987;66:53-56.
138. Davis PJ et al. Pharmacokinetics of sufentanil in adolescent patients with chronic renal failure. *Anesth Analg.* 1988;67:268-271.
139. Morcos WE, Payne JP. The induction of anaesthesia with propofol compared in normal and renal failure patients. *Postgrad Med J Suppl.* 1985;61:62-63.
140. Goyal P et al. Evaluation of induction dose of propofol: comparison between endstage renal disease and normal renal function patients. *Anaesth Intensive Care.* 2002;30:584-587.
141. Reiter V et al. Continuous flow propofol during kidney transplantation in the adult. *Can J Anesthesiol.* 1989;37:23-31.
142. Litz RJ et al. Renal responses to desflurane and isoflurane in patients with renal insufficiency. *Anesthesiology.* 2002;97:1133-1136.
143. Kharasch ED et al. Long-duration low-flow sevoflurane and isoflurane effects on postoperative renal and hepatic function. *Anesth Analg.* 2001; 93:1511-1520.
144. Obata R et al. The effects of prolonged low-flow sevoflurane anesthesia on renal and hepatic function. *Anesth Analg.* 2000;91:1262-1268.
145. Cronnelly R et al. Renal function and the pharmacokinetics of neostigmine in anesthetized man. *Anesthesiology.* 1979;51:222-226.
146. Cronnelly R et al. Pyridostigmine kinetics with and without renal function. *Clin Pharmacol Ther.* 1980;28:78-81.
147. Morris RB et al. Pharmacokinetics of edrophonium in anephric and renal transplant patients. *Br J Anaesth.* 1983;53:131-134.
148. Bishop MJ, Hornbein TF. Prolonged effect of succinylcholine after neostigmine and pyridostigmine administration in patients with renal failure. *Anesthesiology.* 1983;58:384-386.
149. Thomas JL, Holmes JH. Effects of hemodialysis on plasma cholinesterase. *Anesth Analg.* 1970;49:323-325.
150. Ryan DW. Preoperative serum cholinesterase concentration in chronic renal failure. *Br J Anaesth.* 1977;49:945-949.
151. Desmond JW, Gordon RA. The effect of haemodialysis on blood volume and plasma cholinesterase levels. *Can Anaesth Soc J.* 1969;16:292-301.
152. Miller RD et al. Succinylcholine-induced hyperkalemia in patients with renal failure? *Anesthesiology.* 1972;36:138-141.
153. Koide M, Waud BE. Serum potassium concentrations after succinylcholine in patients with renal failure. *Anesthesiology.* 1972;36:142-145.
154. Meijer DKF et al. Comparative pharmacokinetics of d-tubocurarine and metocurine in man. *Anesthesiology.* 1979;51:402-407.
155. Matteo RS et al. Pharmacodynamics and pharmacokinetics of metocurine in humans: comparison to d-tubocurarine. *Anesthesiology.* 1982;57:183-190.
156. Miller RD et al. The comparative potency and pharmacokinetics of pancuronium and its metabolites in anesthetized man. *J Pharmacol Exp Ther.* 1978;207:539-543.
157. Agoston S et al. The fate of pancuronium bromide in man. *Acta Anaesthesiol Scand.* 1973;17:267-275.
158. Hughes R, Chapple DJ. The pharmacology of atracurium: a new competitive neuromuscular blocking agent. *Br J Anaesth.* 1981;53:31-44.
159. Fahey MR et al. The pharmacokinetics and pharmacodynamics of atracurium in patients with and without renal failure. *Anesthesiology.* 1984;61:699-702.
160. Fahey MR et al. Pharmacokinetics of ORG NC 45 (Norcuron) in patients with and without renal failure. *Br J Anaesth.* 1981;53:1049-1053.
161. Fahey MR et al. Effects of renal failure on laudanosine excretion in man. *Br J Anaesth.* 1985;57:1049-1051.
162. Lynam DP et al. The pharmacodynamics and pharmacokinetics of vecuronium in patients anesthetized with isoflurane with normal renal function or with renal failure. *Anesthesiology.* 1988;69:231-277.

163. Bevan DR et al. Vecuronium in renal failure. *Can Anaesth Soc J.* 1984;31:491-496.

164. Slater RM et al. Prolonged neuromuscular blockade with vecuronium in renal failure. *Anaesthesia.* 1988;43:250-251.

165. Lagasse RS et al. Prolonged neuromuscular blockade following vecuronium infusion. *J Clin Anesth.* 1990;2:269-271.

166. Haynes SR, Morton NS. Prolonged neuromuscular blockade with vecuronium in a neonate with renal failure. *Anaesthesia.* 1990;45:743-745.

167. Rollino C et al. Is vecuronium toxicity abolished by hemodialysis? A case report. *Artif Organs.* 2000;24:386-387.

168. Sakamoto H et al. Increased sensitivity to vecuronium and prolonged duration of its action in patients with end-stage renal failure. *J Clin Anesth.* 2001;13:193-197.

169. Bartkowski RR et al. Rocuronium onset of action: a comparison with atracurium and vecuronium. *Anesth Analg.* 1993;77:574-578.

170. Foldes FF et al. The neuromuscular effects of ORG 9426 in patients receiving balanced anesthesia. *Anesthesiology.* 1991;75:191-196.

171. Agoston S et al. Clinical pharmacokinetics of neuromuscular blocking drugs. *Clin Pharmacokinet.* 1992;22:94-115.

172. Szenohradszky J et al. Pharmacokinetics of rocuronium bromide (ORG 9426) in patients with normal renal function or patients undergoing cadaver renal transplantation. *Anesthesiology.* 1992;77:899-904.

173. Alpert RA et al. Intraoperative urinary output does not predict postoperative renal function in patients undergoing abdominal aortic revascularization. *Surgery.* 1984;95:707-711.

174. Sprung J et al. Anesthesia for kidney transplant surgery. *Anesthesiol Clin North America.* 2000;18:919-951.

175. Tilney NL et al. Experience with cyclosporine and steroids in clinical renal transplantation. *Ann Surg.* 1984;200:605-613.

176. Opelz G, Terasaki PI. Poor kidney survival in recipients with frozen blood transfusions or no transfusions. *Lancet.* 1974;2:696-698.

177. Borland LM, Cook DR. Anesthesia for organ transplantation. *Advances in Anesthesia.* Chicago: Year Book; 1986:1-36.

178. Linke CL, Merin RG. A regional anesthetic approach for renal transplantation. *Anesth Analg.* 1976;55:69-73.

179. Hirsche MM. Renal transplantation in patients with type II diabetes mellitus. *Nephrol Dial Transplant.* 1995;10:58-60.

180. Strunin L. Some aspects of anaesthesia for renal homotransplantation. *Br J Anaesth.* 1966;38:812-822.

181. Katz J et al. Anesthetic considerations for renal transplant. *Anesth Analg.* 1967;55:69-73.

182. Munda R et al. Pulmonary infections in renal transplant recipients. *Ann Surg.* 1978;187:126-133.

183. Conzen PF et al. Renal function and serum fluoride concentrations in patients with stable renal insufficiency after anesthesia with sevoflurane or enflurane. *Anesth Analg.* 1995;81:569-575.

184. Tsukamoto N et al. The effects of sevoflurane anesthesia on renal tubular function in patients with moderately impaired renal function. *Anesth Analg.* 1996;82:909-913.

185. Nishiyama T et al. Inorganic fluoride kinetics and renal tubular function after sevoflurane anesthesia in chronic renal failure patients receiving hemodialysis. *Anesth Analg.* 1996;83:574-577.

186. Bluestein LS et al. Evaluation of cisatracurium, a new neuromuscular blocking agent, for tracheal intubation. *Can J Anaesth.* 1996;43:925-931.

187. Pollard BJ. Rocuronium and cisatracurium. *Br J Hosp Med.* 1997;57:346-348.

188. Schmith VD et al. Dose proportionality of cisatracurium. *J Clin Pharmacol.* 1997;37:625-629.

189. Kadieva VS et al. The effect of dopamine on graft function in patients undergoing renal transplantation. *Anesth Analg.* 1993;76:362-365.

190. Hirschman CA, Edelstein G. Intraoperative hyperkalemia and cardiac arrests during renal transplantation in an insulin-dependent diabetic patient. *Anesthesiology.* 1979;51:161-162.

191. Hirschman CA et al. Risk of hyperkalemia in recipients of kidneys preserved with an intracellular electrolyte solution. *Anesth Analg.* 1980;59:283-286.

192. Cirella VN et al. Effects of cyclosporine on anesthetic action. *Anesth Analg.* 1987;66:703-706.

193. Gramstad L et al. Interaction of cyclosporine and its solvent, Cremophor, with atracurium and vecuronium: studies in the cat. *Br J Anaesth.* 1986;58:1149-1155.

194. Behnia R et al. Hemodynamic and catecholamine responses associated with extracorporeal shock wave lithotripsy. *J Clin Anesth.* 1990;2:158-162.

195. Gissen D. Anesthesia for extracorporeal shock wave lithotripsy. *Semin Anesth.* 1987;6:57-60.

196. Behnia R et al. Hemodynamic responses associated with lithotripsy. *Anesth Analg.* 1987;66:354-356.

197. Malhotra V. Hyperthermia and hypothermia as complications of extracorporeal shock wave lithotripsy. *Anesthesiology.* 1987;67:448.

198. Higgins TL et al. Accidental hyperthermia as a complication of ESWL under general anesthesia. *Anesthesiology.* 1987;66:389-391.

199. Vandeursen H et al. Anesthesia-free extracorporeal shock wave lithotripsy in patients with renal calculi. *Br J Urol.* 1991;68:18-24.

200. Warner MA et al. Clinical efficacy of high frequency jet ventilation during extracorporeal shock wave lithotripsy of renal and ureteral calculi: a comparison with conventional mechanical ventilation. *J Urol.* 1988;139:486-487.

201. Schulte AM et al. Use of high-frequency jet ventilation in extracorporeal shockwave lithotripsy. *Anaesthesist.* 1985;34:294-298.

202. Perel A et al. High-frequency positive pressure ventilation during general anesthesia for extracorporeal shock wave lithotripsy. *Anesth Analg.* 1968;65:1231-1234.

203. Berger JJ et al. Failure of high-frequency jet ventilation to ventilate patients adequately during extracorporeal shock-wave lithotripsy. *Anesth Analg.* 1987;66:262-263.

204. Jansson L et al. Heart synchronized ventilation during general anesthesia for extracorporeal shock wave lithotripsy. *Anesth Analg.* 1988;67:706-709.

205. Harries A et al. Anesthesia for extracorporeal shock wave lithotripsy: a comparison of propofol and methohexitone infusions during high frequency jet ventilation. *Anaesthesia.* 1988;43:100-105.

206. Burmeister MA et al. A comparison of anaesthetic techniques for shock wave lithotripsy: the use of a remifentanil infusion alone compared to intermittent fentanyl boluses combined with a low-dose propofol infusion. *Anaesthesia.* 2002;57:877-881.

207. Monk TG et al. Comparison of alfentanil and ketamine infusion in combination with midazolam for outpatient lithotripsy. *Anesthesiology.* 1991;74:1023-1028.

208. Lau WC et al. Intrathecal sufentanil for extracorporeal shock wave lithotripsy provides earlier discharge of the outpatient than intrathecal lidocaine. *Anesth Analg.* 1997;84:1227-1231.

209. Eaton MP et al. Subarachnoid sufentanil versus lidocaine spinal anesthesia for extracorporeal shock wave lithotripsy. *Reg Anesth.* 1997;22:515-520.

210. Eaton MP, Kristensen EA. Subarachnoid sufentanil for extracorporeal shock lithotripsy. *Reg Anesth.* 1997;22:86-88.

211. Pandit SK et al. Epidural fentanyl is not effective for analgesia for extracorporeal lithotripsy (ESWL). *Anesthesiology.* 1988;68:176-177.

212. Korbon GA et al. Repeated epidural anesthesia for extracorporeal shock-wave lithotripsy is unreliable. *Anesth Analg.* 1987;66:669-672.

213. Kelly RE et al. Pulmonary function after extracorporeal shock wave lithotripsy: a comparison of general and regional anesthesia. *Can J Anaesth.* 1989;36:137-140.

214. Richardson MG, Dooley JW. The effects of general versus epidural anesthesia for outpatient extracorporeal shock wave lithotripsy. *Anesth Analg.* 1998;86:1214-1218.

215. Zeitlin GL, Roth RA. Effect of three anesthetic techniques on the success of extracorporeal shock wave lithotripsy in nephrolithiasis. *Anesthesiology.* 1988;68:272-276.

216. Kwa AM et al. Low-dose epidural lidocaine/sufentanil is effective for outpatient lithotripsy. *Middle East J Anesthesiol.* 1995;13:71-78.

217. Monk TG et al. Analgesic efficacy of EMLA during outpatient shock wave lithotripsy. *Anesth Analg.* 1992;74:213.

218. Tiselius HG. Cutaneous anesthesia with lidocaine-prilocaine cream: a useful adjunct during shock wave lithotripsy with analgesic sedation. *J Urol.* 1993;149:8-11.

219. Uyar M et al. Patient-controlled sedation and analgesia during SWL. *J Endourol.* 1996;10:407-410.

220. Ganapathy S et al. Eutectic mixture of local anaesthetics is not effective for extracorporeal shock wave lithotripsy. *Can J Anaesth.* 1996;43:1030-1034.

221. Schelling G et al. Patient-controlled analgesia for shock wave lithotripsy: the effect of self-administered alfentanil on pain intensity and drug requirement. *J Urol.* 1996;155:43-47.

222. Desmond J. Serum osmolality and plasma electrolytes in patients who develop dilutional hyponatremia during transurethral resection. *Can J Surg.* 1970;13:116-121.

223. Hesbit TE. The use of glycine in transurethral prostatic surgery. *J Urol.* 1948;59:1212-1216.

224. Desmond J. Complications of transurethral prostatic surgery. *Can Anaesth Soc J.* 1970;17:25-36.

225. Hagstrom RS. Studies on fluid absorption during transurethral prostatic resection. *J Urol.* 1955;73:852-859.

226. Henderson DJ, Middleton RG. Coma from hyponatremia following transurethral resection of the prostate. *Urology.* 1980;15:267-271.

227. Aasheim GM. Hyponatremia during transurethral surgery. *Can Anaesth Soc J.* 1973;20:274-280.

228. Kenyon HR. Perforation in transurethral operations: technique for immediate diagnosis and management of extravasations. *JAMA.* 1950;142:798-801.

229. Harrison RH et al. Dilutional hyponatremic shock: another concept of the transurethral prostatic resection reaction. *J Urol.* 1956;75:95-110.
230. Defalque KJ, Miller DW. Visual disturbances during transurethral resection of the prostate. *Can Anaesth Soc J.* 1975;22:620-621.
231. Gooding JM, Holcomb MC. Transient blindness following intravenous administration of atropine. *Anesth Analg.* 1977;56:872-873.
232. Ovassapian A et al. Visual disturbance: an unusual symptom of transurethral prostatic resection reaction. *Anesthesiology.* 1982;57:332-334.
233. Hoekstra PT et al. Transurethral prostatic resection syndrome: a new perspective: encephalopathy with associated hyperammonemia. *J Urol.* 1983;130:704-707.
234. Roesch RP et al. Ammonia toxicity resulting from glycine absorption during a transurethral resection of the prostate. *Anesthesiology.* 1983;58:577-579.
235. James JH et al. Hyperammonaemia, plasma amino acid imbalance, and blood-brain amino acid transport: a unified theory of portal-systemic encephalopathy. *Lancet.* 1979;2:772-775.
236. Wang JM et al. Effects of glycine on hemodynamic responses and visual evoked potentials in the dog. *Anesth Analg.* 1985;64:1071-1077.
237. Kellow NH. Pacemaker failure during transurethral resection of the prostate. *Anaesthesia.* 1993;48:136-138.
238. Madsen RE, Madsen PO. Influence of anesthesia form on blood loss in transurethral prostatectomy. *Anesth Analg.* 1967;46:330-332.
239. Perkins JB, Miller HC. Blood loss during transurethral prostatectomy. *J Urol.* 1969;101:93-97.
240. Levin K et al. Blood loss, tissue weight, and operating time in transurethral prostatectomy. *Scand J Urol Nephrol.* 1981;15:197-200.
241. Malhotra V. Transurethral resection of the prostate. *Anesthesiol Clin North America.* 2000;18:883-898.
242. Gettman MT, Blute ML. Critical comparison of laparoscopic, robotic and open radical prostatectomy: techniques, outcomes, and cost. *Curr Urol Rep.* 2006;7(3):193-199.
243. Mun SP et al. Minimally invasive video-assisted kidney transplantation (MIVAKT). *J Surg Res.* 2007;141(2):204-210.
244. Burgess NA et al. Randomized trial of laparoscopic v open nephrectomy. *J Endourol.* 2007;21(6):610-613.
245. Weingram J et al. Subcutaneous emphysema during laparoscopic pelvic lymph node dissection. *Anesth Analg.* 1993;76:S460.
246. Bickel A et al. Overcoming reduced hepatic and renal perfusion caused by positive-pressure pneumoperitoneum. *Arch Surg.* 2007;142:119-124.
247. Costello TG, Webb P. Anaesthesia for robot-assisted anatomic prostectomy: experience at a single institution. *Anaesth Intensive Care.* 2006;34:787-792.
248. Moitra V et al. Monitoring hepatic and renal function. *Anesthesiol Clin.* 2006;24(4):857-880, viii-ix.
249. Wagener G, Brentjens TE. Renal disease: the anesthesiologist's perspective. *Anesthesiol Clin.* 2006;24(3):523-547.

CHAPTER 31

HEPATOBILIARY AND GASTROINTESTINAL DISTURBANCES AND ANESTHESIA

Timothy J. Palmer

Several symptomatic manifestations are characteristic of gastrointestinal disease. A common finding is pain, which may be localized or referred and variable in intensity. Common symptoms include nausea and vomiting, abdominal distention, bloating, constipation, diarrhea, fever, and malaise. Clinical signs of gastrointestinal disease may range from occult, painless rectal bleeding to frank hemorrhage via the rectum or esophagus. Other signs of gastrointestinal disease include increased abdominal girth, petechiae, dehydration, jaundice, and evidence of malnutrition. Secondary organ system dysfunction due to gastrointestinal disease is evidenced by decreases in urinary output, alterations in cardiac rhythm, peripheral edema, pulmonary edema, perturbations in electrolyte balance, alterations in hemostatic function, and sepsis.

Planning and delivering anesthesia for patients with gastrointestinal disease must take into consideration whether the illness is acute or chronic. Initial assessment should include appraisal of the patient's compensatory status, particularly if secondary organ system involvement is apparent. The presence of preexisting, acquired, or age-related disease processes must also be determined in the patient's preanesthetic assessment. An anesthetic technique that preserves the patient's preexisting compensatory capabilities can therefore be undertaken.

Certain specific surgical procedures have benefited from advances in technology and technique. Laparoscopic-assisted, minimally invasive surgical methods continue to emerge. Extensive open procedures, formerly associated with potentially significant postoperative morbidity, can now be performed on an outpatient basis or with an abbreviated postoperative hospital stay. With less invasive surgical intrusion, outcome findings substantiate associated reductions in perioperative morbidity. Ongoing research continues to expand the complement of anesthesia delivery methods and mark the progress of standards and guidelines to accommodate emerging directions in surgery.

The purpose of this chapter is to give an overview of pathophysiologic processes specific to the hepatobiliary and gastrointestinal system commonly encountered by the anesthetist. Fundamental relevant anesthetic considerations are elucidated. For a more expansive understanding of the content presented, the reader is encouraged to consult chapters within the book that specifically address pertinent management issues related to associated comorbidities and emerging innovations in surgical strategies and technologies (e.g., laparoscopic surgery, endocrine disease, bariatric surgery, trauma, oncology, transplantation,

and fluid and electrolyte balance). Other resources that further elaborate on the topics discussed in this chapter may be found in the reference section.

PANCREATIC DISEASE

Physiologic Overview

The pancreas functions in both an endocrine and exocrine hormonal capacity. The exocrine function of the pancreas is primarily the continuous transductal secretion of 1500 to 3000 mL of pancreatic juice, normally clear and colorless with a pH of 8.3. The ionic composition consists largely of sodium, potassium, bicarbonate, and chloride, with smaller concentrations of phosphate, sulfate, zinc, and calcium. The principal function of pancreatic juice is to adjust the pH of the duodenal contents to promote optimal activity of pancreatic enzymes. Endocrine pancreatic function is represented by the direct (nonductal) elaboration of insulin and glucagon to conform to physiologic need. The physiology and diseases associated with pancreatic endocrine function receive specific discussion in Chapter 34.

Arrival of acidic chyme (partially digested gastric contents) into the duodenum and jejunum stimulates the release of the hormones cholecystokinin-pancreozymin (CCK-PZ) and secretin. Both hormones are produced in the duodenum, jejunum, and ileum. Secretin is responsible for stimulating the pancreas to release bicarbonate and water, and CCK-PZ, released in response to the presence of fats and partially digested proteins in the duodenum, stimulates elaboration of the pancreatic enzymes necessary for further intestinal digestive processes. Trypsinogen, produced by pancreatic cells, is converted to the active enzyme trypsin in response to the release of enterokinase by the gastric mucosa. Trypsin is responsible for the conversion of large ingested proteins into smaller peptides and amino acids in preparation for intestinal absorption. The major pancreatic enzyme groups are listed in Table 31-1.

Although control of pancreatic secretion is primarily hormonal, evidence suggests that a parasympathetic influence also exists. Administration of vagolytic agents (e.g., atropine, glycopyrrolate) or ganglionic blocking agents, along with physical interruption of the vagus nerve, may induce a decreased response to secretin. Vagotomy has also been shown to result in a decrease in the release of pancreatic bicarbonate in response to duodenal acidity.

Other factors influence pancreatic secretion. Fasting results in decreased secretion of pancreatic lipase and amylase. In protein

TABLE **31-1**	Major Pancreatic Enzyme Groups*
Enzyme Group	**Enzyme, Proenzyme, or Precursor**
Proteolytic	Trypsinogen (trypsin), chymotrypsinogen (chymotrypsin), procarboxypeptidase A (carboxypeptidase A), procarboxypeptidase B (carboxypeptidase B), proaminopeptidase (aminopeptidase), proelastase (elastase)
Amylolytic	α-Amylase
Lipolytic	Lipase, prophospholipase A$_2$ (phospholipase A$_2$), carboxylesterase lipase, procolipase (colipase)
Nucleolytic	Deoxyribonuclease, ribonuclease
Other	Trypsin inhibitor

Precursor molecules are listed, with products in parentheses.

malnutrition, as occurs in starvation and hypoalbuminemic states, a decrease in the secretion of pancreatic peptidases is typically seen. Severe protein-calorie malnutrition causes structural and functional changes within the pancreas. In general, acinar cell atrophy occurs, zymogen granules decrease, and the overall enzymatic activities of pancreatic juice decrease.[1] Therefore digestion of fat and protein is impaired.

The endocrine function of the pancreas consists primarily of regulation of the plasma glucose level. To do this, the pancreas releases hormones from the islets of Langerhans. Three types of these cells exist:

1. Beta cells are responsible for the secretion of insulin, facilitate use of carbohydrates, and suppress fat metabolism. Insulin enhances anabolism, inhibits catabolic processes (e.g., glycogenolysis, ketogenesis, and gluconeogenesis), and promotes glycogenesis and triglyceride storage.
2. Alpha cells are responsible for the secretion of glucagon, which basically acts in opposition to the effects of insulin.
3. Delta cells secrete the inhibitory hormone somatostatin (growth hormone–releasing inhibitory factor), which is responsible for controlling the plasma levels of both insulin and glucagon.

α-Adrenergic stimulation has been shown to be inhibitory to insulin secretion. β-Adrenergic and cholinergic blockade are inhibitory to insulin secretion as well. Arterial hypoxemia, hypothermia, traumatic stress, and surgical stress all suppress insulin secretion through α-adrenergic stimulation. Insulin secretion is enhanced by vagal stimulation, β$_2$-adrenergic activation, and cholinergic drug administration.

Anesthetic considerations in patients with derangements in pancreatic endocrine function, such as diabetes mellitus, are outside the scope of this chapter. The present discussion is directed toward anesthetic considerations germane to patients with inflammatory or neoplastic disease of the pancreas.

Acute Pancreatitis

The cause of pancreatitis is multifactorial. Common causes include alcohol abuse, direct or indirect trauma to the pancreas,

ulcerative penetration from adjacent structures (e.g., the duodenum), infectious processes, biliary tract disease, metabolic disorders (e.g., hyperlipidemia and hypercalcemia), and certain drugs (e.g., corticosteroids, furosemide, estrogens, and thiazide diuretics). Patients who have undergone extensive surgery involving mobilization of the abdominal viscera are at risk for development of postoperative pancreatitis, as are patients who have undergone procedures involving cardiopulmonary bypass. Patients who have received large doses of calcium intraoperatively, particularly after cardiopulmonary bypass, have also been shown to be at risk for development of postoperative pancreatitis.[1] A reasonable hypothetic pathophysiologic mechanism involves the imposition of a syndrome of induced autodigestion. Indeed, acute pancreatitis is characterized as a severe chemical burn of the peritoneal cavity.[2] Aberrant activation or release of pancreatic enzymes or injury to the acinar cells caused by one or more of the aforementioned etiologic factors produces a syndrome that results in hemorrhage, edema, and necrosis of the pancreas.

Enzymes implicated as major culprits in the syndrome of pancreatitis are those activated by trypsin, enterokinase, and bile acids. These enzymes are necessary for proteolysis, elastolysis, and lipolysis. The inappropriate elaboration of these enzymes results in pancreatic inflammation, which is caused by vascular breakdown, coagulation necrosis, fat necrosis, and parenchymal necrosis. Cardiovascular complications of acute pancreatitis can lead to pericardial effusions, alterations in cardiac rhythmicity, signs and symptoms mimicking acute myocardial infarction, thrombophlebitis, and cardiac depression. Acute pancreatitis also predisposes patients to the development of acute respiratory distress syndrome and disseminated intravascular coagulopathy.[3]

Pain is the foremost symptom of acute pancreatitis and may be variable in quality—localized or radiating, dull and tolerable, or severe and unremitting. Pancreatic pain may radiate from the midepigastric to the periumbilical region and may be more intense when the patient is in the supine position. Causes of pancreatitis include (1) obstruction and distention of the pancreatic ducts; (2) edema, with stretching of the pancreatic capsule; (3) edematous duodenal obstruction; (4) biliary tract obstruction; (5) inflammatory exudates, blood, and enzymes in the retroperitoneum; and (6) chemical peritonitis. Abdominal distention is often seen and is largely attributable to the accumulation of intraperitoneal fluid and paralytic ileus. Nausea, vomiting, and fever are common symptoms. Hypotension is seen in 40% to 50% of patients and is attributable to hypovolemia secondary to the loss of plasma proteins into the retroperitoneal space. Acute renal failure secondary to dehydration and hypotension may occur.

Hypocalcemia frequently develops in patients with acute pancreatitis, and this condition necessitates monitoring the electrocardiogram (ECG) for cardiac rhythm disorders (e.g., lengthened QT interval with possible reentry dysrhythmias). The clinician must also be observant for signs of tetany. Clinical shock may develop that is largely secondary to the effects of vasoactive kinin peptides (e.g., bradykinin) released during the inflammatory process; these peptides enhance vasodilation, vascular permeability, and leukocyte migration. Furthermore, the inappropriate release of pancreatic kinin peptides stimulates smooth muscle contraction and causes impairment in myocardial contractility.[4]

Elevated serum amylase levels are often present but do not necessarily indicate primary pancreatic disease. Such elevations may result from other intraabdominal disease processes such as biliary tract disease, tubo-ovarian disease, peptic ulcer disease, and acute bowel disease, including obstruction, inflammation, and ischemia.[5] Elevated serum lipase levels may also be observed. Disruption in the parenchymal integrity of the pancreas allows passage of enzymes into the venous blood and lymphatic stream. Passage of enzymes into the peritoneal cavity may occur, resulting in subsequent absorption into the general circulation. Compressive obstruction of the common bile duct by an edematous head of the pancreas contributes to elevations in serum bilirubin and alkaline phosphatase levels.

Radiographic and ultrasonographic findings aid in the differential diagnosis of pancreatic disease. Radiographic evidence of free intraperitoneal air suggests the presence of a perforated viscus. Pancreatic calcification also may be observed. Ultrasonography is useful in detecting the presence of concurrent (and perhaps causative) cholelithiasis, cholecystitis, and biliary obstruction due to stone or tumor. Computed tomography (CT) is highly effective in the diagnosis of an enlarged, edematous pancreatic head, typically seen in patients with pancreatitis.[5]

Initial therapy for acute pancreatitis is supportive. The regimen usually includes admission to an intensive care unit and may involve invasive monitoring, fluid and hemodynamic resuscitation, and interventions necessary for preserving perfusion and function of the abdominal viscera.[4] Severely ill, malnourished patients are often given parenteral nutritional support. Pain is controlled with synthetic opioids, such as fentanyl, which are preferable to morphine. Morphine-induced spasms of the Oddi sphincter may exacerbate bile obstruction and stasis. Normeperidine, the metabolite of meperidine, causes analeptic activity and makes meperidine unattractive for pain management in these patients. Epidural analgesia may be selectively appropriate.

If the cause of pancreatitis is obstructive biliary disease due to the presence of a stone in the common bile duct or inflammation of the gallbladder, cholecystectomy and possibly common bile duct exploration are indicated. The choice of anesthetic technique and the extent to which monitoring modalities are used are based on an assessment of the patient's history, the severity of disease, and the degree of preexisting physical compensation. Special attention should be paid to correcting significant intravascular volume deficits. The presence of labile hemodynamics and altered hepatic function must also be discerned and appropriate modifications made to the anesthetic plan—for example, ensuring stable arterial pressure, using anesthetic agents and adjuvants that require minimal hepatic biotransformation, ensuring adequate oxygenation, and replacing electrolytes and blood volume.

Chronic Pancreatitis

Chronic alcoholism is a common etiologic factor in chronic pancreatitis. This condition is strongly suggested by the classic diagnostic triad of steatorrhea, pancreatic calcification (evidenced radiographically), and diabetes mellitus. Individuals with chronic pancreatitis are often malnourished and emaciated. They are more often male than female. Besides chronic alcohol abuse, other conditions associated with the development of chronic pancreatitis include significant (and usually chronic) biliary tract disease and the effects of pancreatic injury sustained at an earlier age.[3]

Formation of a pseudocyst occurs in up to 8% of alcoholic patients after resolution of a bout of acute pancreatitis. Pancreatic abscess occurs in 3% to 5% of patients with acute pancreatitis but is present in 90% of patients dying as a result of acute pancreatitis.[5] Pancreatic pseudocyst is best evidenced through CT and may be continuous with the pancreatic ductal system. This collection of pancreatic fluid is not totally surrounded by an epithelial lining and therefore is not a true cyst. The mass consists of a collection of proteolytic enzymes that pose a potentially lethal danger to the patient should erosion or rupture occur, with consequent spillage into the abdominal cavity or other proximal intraperitoneal structures.

The clinical picture may also include hepatic disease, as evidenced by jaundice, ascites, esophageal varices, derangements in coagulation factors, serum albumin, and transferase enzymes. Perturbation in pancreatic exocrine function, with consequent enzymatic insufficiency, results in malabsorption of fats and proteins in the intestine. Patients with chronic pancreatitis also have a predisposition for pericardial and pleural effusions.[4]

Pancreatic abscesses develop from infected peripancreatic collections of fluid. Abscesses are usually secondary manifestations of chronic pancreatitis and warrant surgical drainage to prevent spread of the infectious contents to the subphrenic and pericolic spaces. Fistula formation is possible, particularly into the transverse colon. Severe intraabdominal hemorrhage is also possible as a result of erosion into major proximal arteries.

Surgical Therapy for Pancreatitis

Surgical drainage of a pancreatic pseudocyst is usually undertaken after a period of maturation of the cyst (usually 6 weeks). The procedure consists of formation of a cystogastrostomy, cystojejunostomy, cystoduodenostomy, or possibly distal pancreatectomy. The location of the pseudocyst dictates the extent and type of procedure used for providing drainage of cystic contents into the gastrointestinal tract. Percutaneous external drainage, guided by CT, is reserved for cases in which the pseudocyst is particularly friable. Spontaneous resolution of pseudocysts may be expected in 20% or more of patients who have undergone surgical drainage.[6]

Pancreatic Tumors

Adenocarcinoma of the pancreas arises most often from the ductal system (90%) and less frequently from the acini.[6] Patients with pancreatic carcinoma are typically 50 to 80 years of age, and the incidence is equal in men and women. Causation is multifactorial, but adenocarcinoma of the pancreas is associated with familial or genetic predisposition. Other etiologic factors include chronic diabetes, alcoholism, chronic pancreatitis, and heavy tobacco and caffeine use.

Because the head of the pancreas is most often the locus of the tumor, biliary obstruction is likely, resulting in progressive jaundice. The patient may have symptoms that are vague and nonspecific and include dull, aching, midepigastric or back pain. Anorexia and fatigue are often present and are associated with weight loss. Laboratory studies usually show elevated bilirubin and alkaline phosphatase levels. Radiographic evidence is generally nonspecific; needle biopsy during CT is most helpful in achieving diagnosis. Percutaneous transhepatic cholangiography and endoscopic retrograde cholangiopancreatography are useful diagnostic modalities. Endoscopic retrograde cholangiopancreatography is the most useful modality for defining lesions of the body and tail of the pancreas or of the duodenum and ampulla.[6]

Neoplastic involvement of beta cells is referred to as *insulinoma*. Hypersecretion of insulin is a major manifestation of this disease and results in profound hypoglycemia, which may lead to mental depression, seizures, and coma. Treatment of this disease is surgical excision, except in patients with advanced metastatic disease, and involves distal pancreatectomy, subtotal pancreatectomy, or removal of all but a small portion of pancreatic tissue around the rim of the duodenum (Child procedure).[6]

If neoplastic disease is determined to be resectable, that is, without involvement of mesenteric vessels or infiltration into the mesenteric arterial root or hepatobiliary structures, a pancreaticoduodenectomy (or a modification of this procedure) may be performed. This procedure involves excision of the antrum of the stomach with the duodenum, distal bile duct, and pancreatic head, along with reconstruction via choledochostomy and pancreaticogastrojejunostomy (Whipple procedure).[7]

Gastrinoma (Zollinger-Ellison syndrome) is associated with hypersecretion of gastrin, resulting in excessive stimulation of gastric acid secretion. Severe peptic ulcer disease is therefore a possibility, with marked potential for perforation and erosion into adjacent structures, a condition that results in severe hemorrhage. Diarrhea or steatorrhea is typical in this disease process. The culpable lesion is typically a non–beta-cell pancreatic tumor. These lesions are usually occult, slow growing, late metastasizing, and resistant to medical and surgical therapy. Surgical excision of the lesion is the treatment of choice in patients without metastatic disease. Total gastrectomy is infrequently performed because of the proven efficacy of histamine-2 (H_2) antagonists in the medical management of peptic ulcer disease.[5]

Anesthetic Considerations in Pancreatic Disease

The patient undergoing surgical treatment of pancreatic disease exhibits a variable clinical picture, from jaundiced and stable with a painless pancreatic mass to severely ill with multiorgan system involvement. Patients may have severe, acute abdominal pain with possible intestinal obstruction or ileus. Aspiration precautions should be in effect during induction of anesthesia and emergence from anesthesia. Because these patients are likely to be diabetic (secondary to beta-cell dysfunction) or hypoglycemic (as in the case of insulinoma), perioperative assessment of serum glucose and institution of appropriate control measures are warranted. Derangements in fluid and electrolyte balance must also be anticipated. Rigorous blood product and crystalloid resuscitation may be necessary throughout the perioperative period and likely will necessitate placing invasive hemodynamic lines to guide therapy and monitor central pressures.

Potential electrolyte disorders include hypocalcemia, hypomagnesemia, hypokalemia, and possibly hypochloremic metabolic alkalosis. The serum hematocrit value may be falsely increased secondary to hemoconcentration, or it may be decreased secondary to the presence of a bleeding diathesis. Coagulation parameters, including platelet count, prothrombin time (PT), activated partial thromboplastin time (aPTT), and fibrinogen level, should be assessed at regular intervals perioperatively. Preserving renal function mandates the preoperative assessment of blood urea nitrogen, serum creatinine, and 24-hour creatinine clearance (if possible); urinalysis should also be performed. Intraoperatively, a urine output of at least 0.5 to 1 mL/kg/hr should be maintained.

Thorough assessment of preexisting pulmonary status is vital. A significant incidence of postoperative respiratory morbidity is associated with upper abdominal surgery, especially in association with a preoperative debilitated state. Pulmonary assessment includes arterial blood gas analysis, chest radiography, and pulmonary function tests when appropriate. Considering the high incidence of pleural effusion that occurs secondary to pancreatic disease and a potential history of heavy tobacco use, the pulmonary assessment assumes added importance.

Cardiovascular assessment should assimilate related findings from the assessment of other organ systems so that the degree to which functional hemodynamic impairment may need to be corrected is fully appreciated. Correction of preexisting hemodynamic disturbances entails restitution of plasma volume and the oxygen-carrying capacity of the blood. Ischemic changes noted on the ECG must be treated promptly. ECG changes mimicking myocardial ischemia are often seen in pancreatitis.

General endotracheal anesthesia is the technique of choice. Preoperative placement of an epidural catheter allows greater flexibility in managing intraoperative pain and providing postoperative pain control. Patients undergoing extensive pancreatic surgery often require postoperative ventilatory support and intensive care unit monitoring because of the magnitude and length of the procedure, as well as the patient's preexisting cardiopulmonary status. Pancreatic transplants are discussed later in this chapter.

LIVER DISEASE

Physiologic and Pathophysiologic Considerations

The basic functional unit of the liver is the hepatic lobule. This structure is composed of cylindrically arranged hepatocytes that envelop a central vein that empties into hepatic veins and ultimately into the vena cava. Hepatic lobules number between 50,000 and 100,000 in the normal liver. Primary blood supply to the liver is furnished by the hepatic artery and the portal vein. The combined blood from both sources joins in the hepatic sinusoidal channels lying between the layer of cells in the lobule. These channels serve as capillaries. Endothelial cells and Kupffer cells line the sinusoids. Bile canaliculi are located between hepatocytes; these canaliculi empty into terminal bile ducts. A coalescence of central veins from hepatic lobules forms the hepatic veins, which empty into the inferior vena cava. An extensive arcade of lymphatic vessels is also present within the layer of cells.[7]

The liver is responsible for an enormous number of complex and interrelated functions. Because the liver possesses a large functional reserve, significant disease must be present before clinically apparent manifestations are seen. Hepatic dysfunction after anesthesia and surgery is therefore uncommon and, when discovered, is often related to preexisting hepatic disease processes.

The liver receives approximately 1500 mL of blood per minute, 25% to 30% from the hepatic artery and 70% to 75% from the portal vein. This represents 25% to 30% of the cardiac output.[3] The fact that most of the hepatic blood supply is derived from the gut permits speculation on the adequacy of hepatic oxygenation. Adequacy in hepatic oxygen delivery is not seen to be a prominent issue in the normal liver, given the large percentage of cardiac output that perfuses the liver, the great permeability of the hepatic sinuses, and the close proximity of the hepatic sinuses to hepatic cells, facilitating the processes of oxygenation, nutrient supply, and carbon dioxide and metabolic waste removal.

The filtering function of the liver has a prominent physiologic role. Blood from the gut contains large quantities of colonic bacilli; it is cleansed of more than 99% of the bacterial load by Kupffer cells (macrophages) that line the hepatic sinuses.[7] Endothelial cells that line the hepatic sinuses permit diffusion of large plasma proteins and other substances into the extravascular spaces in the liver. This phenomenon results in a large quantity of lymph that is nearly equal in protein concentration to plasma.

The low resistance of the hepatic sinusoids (7 to 10 mm Hg) to portal blood flow allows the liver to function as a circulatory reservoir. Up to 350 mL of blood may be delivered into the circulation in time of need, such as during hemorrhage. Splanchnic blood flow vessels, which provide the blood supply to the liver, gallbladder, omentum, spleen, and pancreas, are innervated by the splanchnic nerves derived from spinal nerves T3 through T11. Both α- and β-receptors are present in the hepatic arterial circulation, but only α-receptors are noted in the portal circulation. Hepatic arterial flow is autoregulated in accordance with metabolic demand, that is, oxygen consumption. Portal blood flow is dependent on the combined venous outflow from the spleen and gastrointestinal tract. A decrease in either portal or arterial blood flow affects a compensatory increase in blood flow delivered by the other system.[3]

Increased sympathetic nervous system outflow caused by factors such as hypotension, hypovolemia, hypoxia, hypercarbia, and light anesthesia produces hepatic arterial vasoconstriction. Abdominal surgery is recognized as the most profound etiologic factor that results in decreased hepatic blood flow, particularly if the liver is directly involved.

All volatile anesthetics are implicated in reduction of hepatic blood flow. Hepatic blood flow may be reduced as much as 25% with the use of halothane.[8] Although this impairment in hepatic blood flow is largely attributable to decreased systemic blood pressure, halothane is known to directly impair hepatic blood flow even further through abolition of the vasoconstrictor response to hypercarbia.[9] These changes reflect drug- or technique-induced alterations in splanchnic circulatory tone, perfusion pressure, or both. Indeed, hepatic blood flow may be reduced up to 30% in the absence of surgical stimulation when sympathectomy that results from regional lower extremity anesthesia (i.e., subarachnoid or epidural) is present.

Essential physiologic functions of the liver include bile production, protein synthesis, glycogen storage, protein metabolism, insulin clearance, lactate conversion into glucose, and drug metabolism and transformation. Glycogen, a storage form of glucose, is formed by the process of gluconeogenesis from lactate. Other substrates from which the liver manufactures glycogen include amino acids (particularly alanine) and glycerol. During periods of fasting, the liver maintains glucose levels at relatively normal levels through glycogenolysis. Hypoglycemia may therefore be encountered in patients with severe liver disease caused by derangements in insulin clearance, a decrease in glycogen capacities, and impairment in gluconeogenesis.

Bile is the primary secretion of the liver and is normally formed at a rate of approximately 1 L/day. Hepatocytes in each lobule continuously secrete fluid that contains phospholipids, cholesterol, conjugated bilirubin (the end product of hemoglobin metabolism), bile salts, and other substances. Bile is stored and concentrated in the gallbladder. In response to the intestinal hormone CCK, bile is released by the gallbladder. The presence of fat and protein in the duodenum initiates contraction of the gallbladder, which causes bile to flow via the common bile duct through the relaxed sphincter of Oddi and into the duodenum to assist in the absorption of fat and fat-soluble vitamins (vitamins A, D, E, K). The metabolic end products of many drugs are also removed via the bile. Liver disease may result in impaired bile production or flow, leading to steatorrhea, vitamin K deficiency, and delayed removal of active drug metabolites.

A deficiency in vitamin K results in coagulopathy due to impaired production of clotting factors II (prothrombin), VII, IX, and X. Indeed, except for factor VIII, which is produced in endothelial cells, all clotting factors are produced by the liver. Although only 50% of factor activity is typically necessary for normal clotting, liver disease often leads to derangements in coagulation. Hepatocellular disease therefore results in decreased clotting factor levels and abnormal bile production. A perturbation in bile production ultimately manifests as impaired production of vitamin K—dependent clotting factors.

Intrahepatic obstruction of blood flow ultimately causes portal hypertension. A consequence of the resultant transmission of backward pressure is congestive splenomegaly, leading to platelet sequestration and thrombocytopenia. Therefore, severe liver disease with portal hypertension induces coagulopathy not only as a result of impairment in hepatic coagulation factor production but also as a result of diminution in circulating functional platelets. In the presence of biliary deficiency, parenteral vitamin K administration helps correct coagulopathy. However, significant hepatocellular disease may dictate the need for fresh frozen plasma (FFP) for immediate correction of coagulation-factor deficits.

The use of subarachnoid and epidural blockade should be avoided in the presence of frank coagulopathy. Derangements in parameters such as PT, activated PTT, and platelet count are a relative contraindication to these techniques. Nasopharyngeal instrumentation and invasive procedures must be performed cautiously and carefully in the presence of increases in PT and activated PTT, a low platelet count, or other laboratory signs that arouse suspicion of coagulopathy.

With the exception of the immunoglobulins, the liver is responsible for the production of proteins. Therefore, decreased plasma oncotic pressure and impairment in drug binding are consequences of severe liver disease. In addition, overexpansion of the interstitial space and third-spacing secondary to derangements in plasma oncotic pressure result in a large increase in the volume of distribution of clinically used medications. Clinical concerns should therefore focus on the potential for an exaggerated effect with a given dose of drug, particularly a drug that is highly protein bound. Exaggeration of effect is particularly true with barbiturates. The amount of nondepolarizing muscle relaxant may also need to be increased to achieve a given level of blockade. This is secondary to an increased volume of distribution of the drug. Plasma cholinesterase, which is produced in the liver, may also be deficient. This condition may prolong the effects of succinylcholine as well as enhance the potential toxicity of ester local anesthetics.

Other roles in protein metabolism performed by the liver include synthesis of lipoproteins (important for lipid transport in the blood), deamination of amino acids into carbohydrates and fats for production of adenosine triphosphate (ATP) through citric acid cycle oxidation, and production of urea for the removal of ammonia, which is formed by hepatic deamination processes and bacteria in the gut.

The liver plays a prominent role in the biotransformation of many exogenous substances—in particular, most drugs. The end products of these processes are the result of deactivation and transformation of substances into benign by-products capable of being excreted in the bile or urine. Two types of biotransformative processes are predominant:

- Phase I reactions, which use oxidation, reduction, deamination, dealkylation, methylation, sulfoxidation, and hydrolysis to alter reactive chemical constituents. This phase is particularly important in the metabolism of most anesthesia-related drugs.
- Phase II reactions, which involve conjugation of the substance with glycine, sulfate, taurine, or glucuronide. Once conjugated the substance is ready for elimination in bile or urine.

Increased tolerance to certain drugs results from overproduction of enzymes within hepatic enzyme systems, including the cytochrome P-450 system. Drugs capable of inducing this process include ethanol, benzodiazepines, ketamine, barbiturates, and phenytoin. The result is an increased clinical requirement for certain drugs like sedatives, opioids, and muscle relaxants, such as vecuronium and rocuronium.

Hyperactivity of hepatic enzyme systems results in a state of increased pharmacokinetic tolerance or cross-tolerance to other drugs metabolized by the same enzyme system. Certain drugs, such as cimetidine and chloramphenicol, are noted to decrease the activity of these enzymes, thereby increasing the effects of other drugs. This effect assumes greater importance with the use of certain drugs known to yield metabolites that exert greater activity than the parent substrate drug or are potentially cytotoxic after phase-I hepatic metabolism. Such properties are associated with the drugs isoniazid, acetaminophen, and halothane.[10]

Certain drugs, such as lidocaine, morphine, meperidine, and propranolol, are highly dependent on hepatic extraction from the circulation for sufficient metabolism. Decreased blood flow to the splanchnic circulation, which occurs during hypotensive states and even during uneventful laparotomy, may decrease metabolic clearance of these drugs.

In addition to degrading insulin, the liver is also responsible for metabolizing other hormones, as well as vitamins and minerals. Triiodothyronine, the more active of the thyroid hormones, is produced from thyroxine in the liver. Degradation of thyroid hormone, steroid hormones (including aldosterone, cortisol, and estrogen), antidiuretic hormone, and glucagon is also primarily a function of the liver. The hepatocytes also function in the storage of vitamins A, B_{12}, E, and D. Metabolism of iron is affected through the hepatic synthesis of transferrin and haptoglobin. Ceruloplasmin produced in the liver is a necessary component in the process of copper metabolism.

Laboratory Evaluation of Liver Function

No single laboratory test reliably assesses liver function. As stated previously, the huge capacity and functional reserve of the liver allow for the presence of significant disease processes before evidence of liver failure is reflected in abnormal laboratory findings; abnormalities do, however, aid in differentiating parenchymal from obstructive disorders. Parenchymal disorders reflect dysfunction at the hepatocellular level, whereas obstructive disorders reflect disease processes caused by dysfunctional bile excretion. Table 31-2 notes the clinical significance of the liver function test.

Effects of Anesthesia on Liver Function

General as well as regional anesthetic techniques have been identified as inducing a reduction in hepatic blood flow. Both the direct effects of the anesthetics and the indirect sequelae of related adjunctive anesthetic activities (such as ventilatory techniques) have been implicated as contributing factors in a reduction of hepatic blood flow. Some locations of surgery, particularly the upper abdomen, have also been implicated as a cause of decreased hepatic blood flow.[8]

All of the volatile anesthetics have also been shown to reduce hepatic blood flow. Halothane causes the greatest reduction and isoflurane the smallest. The use of desflurane has been shown to have hepatic effects similar to those of isoflurane.[8] Sevoflurane appears to undergo hepatic biotransformation, rendering organic and inorganic fluoride ion. In human subjects, levels of serum inorganic fluoride ion secondary to sevoflurane metabolism are generally below nephrotoxic levels. Prolonged use of higher concentrations, however, may lead to problematic levels.

Studies continue with sevoflurane to determine the influence of biotransformation on renal and hepatic function, but no significant clinical toxicity has yet been reported.[11,12]

The reduction in mean arterial pressure and cardiac output frequently seen with the use of volatile anesthetics proportionately reduces hepatic blood flow. Another factor that impairs hepatic blood flow is the vasoconstrictive response of the splanchnic circulation; this response occurs as a sympathetic reflex to reduced mean arterial pressure. Isoflurane increases hepatic blood flow through direct vasodilatory properties. This effect is likely offset, however, by a reduction in portal blood flow. Hypotension secondary to regional anesthetic–induced sympathectomy (e.g., epidural or subarachnoid blockade) principally accounts for the reduced splanchnic blood flow associated with the use of these techniques.

Increased airway pressures associated with controlled mechanical ventilation may adversely affect venous delivery to the right atrium. Increased airway pressures also result in reduced cardiac output, with a consequent reduction in hepatic blood flow. Positive end-expiratory pressure further exacerbates this condition. Impairment in hepatic blood flow under these conditions may result from increased hepatic venous pressure from increased intrathoracic pressure and from increased reflex sympathetic tone caused by reduced cardiac output. Hypercapnia and acidosis have vasodilatory effects on the hepatic circulation that result in increased blood flow, whereas hypocapnia and alkalosis exert vasoconstricting effects that result in decreased flow. The interplay of various intraoperative variables (e.g., surgical site, ventilatory mode, direct and indirect effects of anesthetics used, physiologic responses to intraoperative events) influences the degree to which hepatic blood flow is compromised.

Other effects of anesthetics on hepatic function include a limited attenuation of the stress response usually associated with surgical trauma. With both general and regional techniques, the effects of increased levels of circulatory catecholamines, glucagon, and cortisol are partially blunted (all of which may compromise hepatic blood flow and metabolic activity).

New opioids have been implicated in causing spasm of the Oddi sphincter, with a resultant increase in biliary pressure. Judicious titration of opioids minimizes this occurrence. Opioids can be ranked in terms of their spasm-causing ability as follows, from greatest to least effect: fentanyl, alfentanil, sufentanil, remifentanil (morphine > meperidine > butorphanol > nalbuphine).[13] Spasm of the Oddi sphincter may cause biliary colic, or it may cause a false-positive result on intraoperative cholangiography.

Although the use of opioids is not discouraged, morphine is the opioid most associated with spasm and is best avoided with the preferential use of synthetic opioids. Spasm is low (3%) even when a fentanyl-based anesthetic is used. The cause of the spasm is unclear, and the spasm may have causes other than the anesthetic, such as surgical manipulation, cold irrigating solutions, and the irritant effect of contrast dye. The treatment of suspected spasm of the Oddi sphincter involves increases in the concentration of the volatile agent in use and administration of atropine or glycopyrrolate, glucagon, nitroglycerin, and naloxone or nalbuphine (if the spasm is related to prior opioid administration). Although direct inhibition in the metabolism of certain drugs (e.g., warfarin, ketamine, and phenytoin) occurs with the use of halothane, it is most likely the reduction of hepatic blood flow that indirectly causes altered drug metabolism through reduced drug delivery to appropriate hepatic enzyme systems.

Hepatic injury in the postoperative period, as evidenced only through nonspecific increased plasma lactic dehydrogenase and transaminase enzymes, is not uncommon. This is generally a subclinical and largely ambiguous finding. Its development is most likely the result of such factors as sympathetic stimulation, decreased splanchnic blood flow, location of the surgical site, and the procedure performed. Theories suggest that proximity of the surgical site to the liver may induce localized vasoconstriction, resulting in a variable degree of hepatocyte hypoxia. The consequence is a cellular injury pattern that is normally transient. Exacerbation of underlying hepatocellular disease is possible, however.

Significant, persistent postoperative hepatic dysfunction may be caused by preexisting liver disease, sepsis, drug reaction, surgical complications, and viral hepatitis (resulting from blood-product transfusion). Postoperative jaundice follows red-cell hemolysis related to transfusion reaction or hematoma reabsorption. Postoperative jaundice may also result from biliary obstruction. Causality must be determined through review of intraoperative events, to include adverse sequelae attributable to administration of blood products.

Though the clinical use of halothane as a volatile anesthetic agent has been superseded by the newer nonsoluble agents desflurane and sevoflurane, it is reasonable to presume that

TABLE 31-2   Clinical Significance of Liver Biochemical Tests

Test (Normal Range*)	Basis of Abnormality	Associated Liver Diseases	Extrahepatic Origin
Aminotransferases			
ALT (10-55 units/L) AST (10-40 units/L)	Leakage from damaged tissue	*Mild to moderate elevations:* many types of liver disease *Marked elevations:* hepatitis (viral, toxic, autoimmune, and ischemic) AST/ALT >2 suggests alcoholic liver disease or cirrhosis of any etiology	ALT more specific than AST for hepatic injury AST nonspecific: can originate from skeletal muscle, red blood cell, kidney, pancreas, brain, and myocardium
AP (45-115 units/L)	Overproduction and leakage into serum	*Moderate elevations:* many types of liver disease *Marked elevations:* extrahepatic and intrahepatic cholestasis, diffuse infiltrating disease (e.g. tumor, MAC), rarely alcoholic hepatitis	Bone growth or disease (e.g., tumor, fracture, Paget disease) placenta, intestine, and tumors
GGTP (0-30 units/L)	Overproduction and leakage into serum	Same as for AP; induced by ethanol and drugs GGTP/AP >2.5 suggests alcoholic liver disease	Kidney, spleen, pancreas, heart, lung, and brain
5' Nucleotidase (0-11 units/L)	Overproduction and leakage into serum	Same as for AP	Found in many tissues, but serum elevation is relatively specific for liver disease
Bilirubin (0.0-1.0 mg/dL)	Decreased hepatic clearance	*Moderate elevations:* many types of liver disease *Marked elevations:* extrahepatic and intrahepatic bile duct obstruction, viral alcoholic or drug-induced hepatitis, inherited hyperbilirubinemia	Increased breakdown of hemoglobin (resulting from hemolysis, disordered erythropoiesis, resorption of hematoma) or myoglobin (resulting from muscle injury)
Prothrombin time (PT) (10.9-12.5 seconds) (international normalized ratio [INR]: 0.9-1.2)	Decreased synthetic capacity	Acute or chronic liver failure (prolonged PT unresponsive to vitamin K) Biliary obstruction (prolonged PT usually responsive to vitamin K administration)	Vitamin K deficiency (secondary to malabsorption, malnutrition, antibiotics, consumptive coagulopathy
Albumin (3.5-5.0 g/dL)	Decreased synthesis; increased catabolism	Chronic liver failure	Decreased in nephritic syndrome, protein-losing enteropathy, vascular leak, malnutrition, malignancy, infections, and inflammatory states.

ALT, *Alanine aminotransferase;* AP, *alkaline phosphatase;* AST, *aspartate aminotransferase;* GGTP, *gamma glutamyl transpeptidase;* MAC, *mycobacterium avium complex.*
The normal values tabulated are for adult men and will vary with the methodology used in testing.

halothane is still in use in some countries. Continued awareness of the potentially deleterious effect of halothane on hepatic function is therefore justified. Though the clinical use of halothane is now more exceptional than routine, the cause and incidence of halothane hepatitis still continue to generate investigation. Liver damage after intraoperative exposure to halothane most frequently occurs in middle-aged, obese women of childbearing age. It is most common with repeat exposure within 28 days.[3,8] The incidence of hepatitis after halothane exposure is relatively low in octogenarians and children. Laboratory differentiation between halothane hepatitis and other forms of hepatitis has, however, been inconclusive. An estimated 1 in 10,000 patients develops postoperative jaundice after halothane exposure. In this population, a viral source of infection is more likely to be the cause—for instance, as a complication of intraoperative blood transfusion. According to epidemiologic studies, a mild form of halothane hepatitis may occur secondary to 20% of all halothane administrations. The incidence of fatal hepatic necrosis is only 1:35,000.[8]

Reduced hepatic perfusion related to halothane exposure causes hepatocyte hypoxia. The normal oxidative hepatic pathway for halothane metabolism is consequently converted to reductive pathways, and potentially hepatotoxic metabolites are produced.

Hypersensitive immune response to halothane exposure, producing an overabundance of antibodies that attack the hepatocytes, has also been implicated as an etiologic factor in the development of halothane-related hepatitis. Genetic susceptibility has also been studied.

Prevention of halothane hepatitis may be facilitated by:
- Limiting the use of halothane to prepubescent children
- Avoiding the use of halothane in patients with evidence or a history of liver dysfunction
- Avoiding the use of halothane in patients who have received it within the past month

The spectrum of severity of halothane hepatitis may extend from a mild increase in hepatic transaminase enzyme levels to fulminant hepatic failure. In the differential diagnosis, pathogenic sources such as viral hepatitis (types A, B, and C), Epstein-Barr virus, herpetic viruses, and cytomegalovirus must first be excluded. The introduction of sevoflurane has essentially made the modern use of halothane obsolete in the United States and most parts of the world. In recent years, it was generally avoided in adults but used for inhalation inductions in children; however, sevoflurane is a safe and effective alternative.

Hepatitis
Acute Hepatitis
Acute hepatitis presents a variable clinical picture. Manifestations may extend from mild inflammatory increases in serum transaminase levels to fulminant hepatic failure. The cause of this syndrome is usually exposure to an infectious virus. Other causes include exposure to hepatotoxic substances and adverse drug reactions.

Viral hepatitis may be attributable to exposure to one of a number of viruses, including hepatitis viruses (A, B, C [formerly referred to as non-A, non-B], D [delta virus], E [enteric non-A, non-B]), Epstein-Barr virus, herpes simplex virus, cytomegalovirus, and coxsackievirus. The most common culprits are hepatitis A, hepatitis B, and hepatitis C. Hepatitis A and E are transmitted by the oral-fecal route, and hepatitis B and C are transmitted by contact with body fluids and physical contact with disrupted cutaneous barriers.

The common clinical course of viral hepatitis begins with a 1- to 2-week prodromal period, the signs and symptoms of which include fever, malaise, and nausea and vomiting. Progression to jaundice typically occurs, with resolution within 2 to 12 weeks. However, serum transaminase levels often remain increased for up to 4 months. If hepatitis B or C is the cause, the clinical course is often more prolonged and complicated. Cholestasis may manifest in certain cases. Fulminant hepatic necrosis in certain individuals is also possible. Table 31-3 lists the major characteristics of hepatitis types A, B, C, D, and E.

Acute viral hepatitis may evolve into a chronic active syndrome, which develops in 3% to 10% of cases involving hepatitis B and in 10% to 50% of cases involving hepatitis C.[14] Many patients become asymptomatic infectious carriers of hepatitis B and C. These patients include many who are immunosuppressed or require chronic hemodialysis.

The B surface antigen (HBsAg) has been seen to persist in the blood of 0.3% to 30% of all patients previously infected with hepatitis B and C. Approximately 1% of patients infected with hepatitis C remain asymptomatic infectious carriers.[10] In view of the large number of asymptomatic and unrecognized carriers, avoiding exposure to blood and body fluids from high-risk patients (e.g., intravenous drug abusers, homosexual men, hemodialysis patients, patients residing in group homes,

TABLE 31-3	Five Causes of Acute Viral Hepatitis						
Hepatitis Virus	Size (nm)	Genome	Route of Transmission	Incubation Period (Days)	Fatality Rate	Chronic Rate	Antibody
A	27	RNA	Fecal-oral	15-45 (mean = 25)	1%	None	Anti-HAV
B	45	DNA	Parenteral Sexual	30-180 (mean = 75)	1%	2%-7%	Anti-HBs Anti-HBc Anti-HBe
C	60	RNA	Parenteral	15-150 (mean = 50)	<0.1%	70%-85%	Anti-HCV
D (delta)	40	RNA	Parenteral Sexual	30-150	2%-10%	2%-7% 50%	Anti-HDV
E	32	RNA	Fecal-oral	30-60	1%	None	Anti-HEV

From Hoofnagle JH. Acute viral hepatitis. In: Goldman L, Ausiello D, eds. Cecil Textbook of Medicine. 23rd ed. Philadelphia: Saunders; 2008:1101. Anti-HDV, Hepatitis D virus antibody; Anti-HEV, hepatitis E virus antibody; HAV, hepatitis A virus; HBc, hepatitis B core; HBe, hepatitis B e-antigen; HBs, hepatitis B surface; HCV, hepatitis C virus.

immunosuppressed patients) is an unreliable means of preventing exposure to hepatitis viruses. It therefore behooves all health-care personnel to adhere to universal precautions in performing patient care. Hepatitis vaccination is strongly recommended. Successful vaccination against hepatitis B (transmitted by parenteral and percutaneous routes) confers a limited measure of protection from hepatitis D, which requires hepatitis B for its expression.

Drug-Induced Hepatitis

Drug-induced hepatitis results from an idiosyncratic drug reaction, from direct hepatic toxicity, or from a combination of the two (Box 31-1). Clinically its manifestations resemble those of viral hepatitis, thereby complicating diagnosis. Alcoholic hepatitis is probably the most common form of drug-induced hepatitis and results in fatty infiltration of the liver (causing hepatomegaly), with impairment in hepatic oxidation of fatty acids, lipoprotein synthesis and secretion, and fatty acid esterification.[3]

BOX 31-1

Drugs and Substances Associated with Hepatitis

Toxic
Alcohol
Acetaminophen
Salicylates
Tetracycline
Trichloroethylene
Vinyl chloride
Carbon tetrachloride
Yellow phosphorus
Poisonous mushrooms
Amanita
Galerina

Idiosyncratic
Volatile anesthetics
Halothane
Phenytoin
Sulfonamides
Rifampin
Indomethacin

Toxic and Idiosyncratic
Methyldopa
Isoniazid
Sodium valproate
Amiodarone

Primarily Cholestatic
Chlorpromazine
Chlorpropamide
Oral contraceptives
Anabolic steroids
Erythromycin estolate
Methimazole

From Morgan GE, Mikhail MS. Anesthesia for patients with liver disease. In: Morgan GE, Mikhail MS. Clinical Anesthesiology. 4th ed. Norwalk, CT: Appleton & Lange; 2006:791.

Chronic Hepatitis

Chronic hepatitis does not occur in hepatitis A infections but does occur in 1% to 10% of acute hepatitis B infections and in 10% to 40% of hepatitis C infections.[3] Patients are classified as having one of three distinct syndromes, based on liver biopsy:
- Chronic persistent hepatitis
- Chronic lobular hepatitis
- Chronic active hepatitis

Chronic persistent hepatitis is relatively benign and confined to portal areas. Hepatic cellular integrity is preserved, and progression to cirrhosis is rare. Chronic lobular hepatitis involves recurrent exacerbations of acute inflammation; as in persistent hepatitis, progression to cirrhosis is rare.

The most serious form of chronic hepatitis is chronic active hepatitis, which is progressive and results in hepatocyte destruction, cirrhosis, and ultimately hepatic failure. Death often results from related manifestations of hepatic failure such as hemorrhage from esophageal varices, multiorgan system failure (e.g., hepatorenal syndrome), and encephalopathy. The typical etiologic agent is hepatitis B or hepatitis C virus. Autoimmune disorders (e.g., systemic lupus erythematosus) and exposure to certain drugs (e.g., methyldopa, isoniazid, and nitrofurantoin) have been implicated as etiologic factors as well.

Marked fatigue and jaundice are common in chronic hepatitis. Arthritis, neuropathy, myocarditis, thrombocytopenia, and glomerulonephritis may also be present. Plasma albumin levels are usually decreased, and PT is often prolonged.

Anesthetic Considerations in Hepatitis

Increased perioperative mortality (10%) and morbidity (12%) rates have been reported with surgery, particularly laparotomy, in patients with acute viral hepatitis. Operative procedures performed in patients with alcohol intoxication are also likely to be associated with increased perioperative complications. Surgery performed in those undergoing alcohol withdrawal is associated with a mortality rate as high as 50%.[10] With the acutely intoxicated alcoholic patient, certain anesthetic issues must be kept in mind: (1) less anesthetic is needed, (2) aspiration precautions must be implemented, (3) surgical bleeding may be increased as a result of interference with platelet aggregation, (4) the brain is less tolerant of hypoxia, and (5) the level of circulating catecholamines is increased, as evidenced by lability in vital signs and exaggerated responses to drugs and stimuli (probably indicating decreased neurotransmitter uptake).[3]

It is therefore prudent to postpone elective surgical procedures until liver function has been normalized. Surgery and anesthesia greatly increase the risk for further hepatic decompensation in patients with hepatitis; this risk may be compounded by the development of renal failure (hepatorenal syndrome), encephalopathy, and the decompensation of other organ systems.

If urgent or emergency surgery is necessary, as thorough a preoperative history as possible must be obtained. If serious time constraints are imposed, the preoperative evaluation should focus on signs and symptoms (e.g., encephalopathy, bleeding diatheses, jaundice, ascites, and hemodynamic findings) and on the results of laboratory studies (e.g., levels of electrolytes, blood urea nitrogen, creatinine, serum glucose, hemoglobin, hematocrit, liver enzymes, and bilirubin, as well as arterial blood gas determinations and coagulation studies). Other pertinent studies include chest radiography and ECG. If not previously ordered, blood typing and cross-matching are warranted, depending on the magnitude of the planned procedure. Any history of hospitalizations and anesthetic use

TABLE 31-4	Child-Turcotte-Pugh Score of Severity of Liver Disease		
Points	**1**	**2**	**3**
Encephalopathy	None	1-2	3-4
Ascites	Absent	Slight	Moderate
Bilirubin (mg/dL)	<2	2-3	>3
For PBC/PSC	<4	4-10	>10
Albumin (g/dL)	<3.5	2.8-3.5	>2.8
PT (INR)	<1.7	1.7-2.3	>2.3

INR, *International normalized ratio;* PBC, *primary biliary cirrhosis;* PSC, *primary sclerosing cholangitis.*

should also be obtained. In general, as much pertinent information as possible should be procured and recorded.

Dehydration and electrolyte derangements should be anticipated and corrected before surgery. Metabolic alkalosis and hypokalemia are often present as a result of vomiting. The presence of hypomagnesemia predisposes to the development of perioperative dysrhythmias. Elevated enzyme (e.g., alkaline phosphatase, alanine aminotransferase [ALT], aspartate aminotransferase [AST]) and serum bilirubin levels are nonspecific with regard to the degree of hepatic necrosis. Alcoholic hepatitis and obstructive hepatitis are commonly associated with an elevation in AST. Viral hepatitis and drug-induced hepatitis often reflect elevated ALT levels. The highest measured levels of AST are seen in viral hepatitis or in fulminant hepatic failure.

PT is a good indicator of the liver's ability to synthesize coagulation factors. Severe hepatic dysfunction results in a persistent prolongation of PT, even after the administration of vitamin K. Evaluation of serum albumin level is warranted, although deficiencies in serum albumin, as well as in all proteins synthesized by the liver (i.e., coagulation factors), are manifestations of severe hepatic dysfunction and malnutrition.

To prevent respiratory embarrassment or exacerbation of pre-existing encephalopathy, preoperative medication (e.g., sedation) is best avoided. Administration of FFP, vitamin K, and packed red blood cells may be necessary for the correction of coagulopathy and red-cell deficiency before surgery. Premedication with benzodiazepines and thiamine may be necessary for alcoholic patients in impending withdrawal. The Child classification system (Table 31-4) is useful in conjunction with other available assessment parameters for determining the degree to which liver disease influences surgical and anesthetic risk.

Cirrhosis

Cirrhosis is a progressive and ultimately fatal syndrome of hepatic failure. Chronic alcoholism is the most common cause of cirrhosis (Laënnec cirrhosis) in the United States. Cirrhosis is also caused by biliary obstruction, chronic hepatitis, right-sided heart failure, α_1-antitrypsin deficiency, Wilson disease, and hemochromatosis. Anatomic alterations secondary to hepatocyte necrosis are the primary cause of deterioration that occurs in liver function. Over time, the liver parenchyma is replaced by fibrous and nodular tissue, which distorts, compresses, and obstructs normal portal venous blood flow. Portal hypertension develops and impairs the ability of the liver to perform various metabolic and synthetic processes.

Obstructive engorgement of vessels within the portal system ultimately results in transmission of increasing back pressure within the splanchnic circulation. Therefore, splenomegaly, esophageal varices, and right-sided heart failure ensue in addition to deterioration in liver function.

The development of esophageal varices places the patient at risk for spontaneous, severe, upper-gastrointestinal hemorrhage. Fluid sequestration resulting from ascites causes consequent alterations in intravascular fluid dynamics and the renin-angiotensin system. Subsequent reduction in renal perfusion progresses to eventual renal failure concomitant with hepatic failure (hepatorenal syndrome). Failure of the liver to clear nitrogenous compounds (ammonia) from the blood contributes to the development of progressive mental-status changes (caused by encephalopathy), ultimately leading to coma.

It is interesting to note that the clinical manifestations of cirrhosis may not be strongly correlated with the severity of the disease process. Patients may have severe liver disease without overt jaundice and ascites. However, the eventual development of jaundice and ascites is observed in most patients as the disease process progresses. Other signs of severe liver disease include gynecomastia, spider angiomata, palmar erythema, and asterixis.[10]

Hepatic fibrosis results from the presence of other diseases; portal hypertension ensues, along with its sequelae. These diseases include Budd-Chiari syndrome (vena cava or hepatovenous obstruction), idiopathic portal fibrosis (Banti syndrome), schistosomiasis, and certain rare congenital fibrotic disorders. Veno-occlusive disease secondary to metastases, primary hepatic neoplasia, or thromboembolism is also associated with portal hypertension.[10]

Anesthetic preparation and management in cirrhosis is given in Box 31-2.

Perioperative Considerations in Liver Disease
Preoperative Assessment

The preoperative assessment of a patient with hepatic disease or insufficiency begins with a thorough history and proceeds in a systematic manner to include physical examination and laboratory studies. Assimilation of information pertaining to the presence of comorbidities assumes a prominent role in formulating the anesthetic plan. The range in health-care status of the patient can be impressive—from the cachectic patient with metastatic carcinoma or the patient exhibiting multisystem functional derangements associated with hepatic failure to the stable, ambulatory outpatient without overt signs and symptoms of hepatic disease. Considerations pertaining to potential impaired hepatic function should also be applied to the patient with a current history of alcohol or mood-altering substance abuse. Incidences of jaundice, ascites, hepatitis, blood transfusion, or substance abuse are important assessment findings, as is the patient's history of an alternative lifestyle (if the patient offers such information). Patients living in group or communal settings (e.g., special homes or halfway houses) are also at greater risk for hepatitis. Patients receiving outpatient renal dialysis should be considered potentially infectious for hepatitis. The history and outcome of prior anesthetics are also pertinent to the preoperative assessment.

Physical signs, such as petechiae, jaundice, ascites, dependent edema, altered mental status, and asterixis, suggest the presence of significant liver disease. Laboratory assessment includes:
- Albumin (normal, 3.5 to 5 g/dL)
- Complete blood count
- Coagulation studies

BOX **31-2**

Anesthetic Preparation and Management in Cirrhosis

Consider the same issues as in acute hepatitis.

Preserve hepatic blood flow.

Avoid halothane (isoflurane is best studied alternative; better preserves flow).

Consider regional anesthesia if procedure and coagulation allow.

Maintain normocapnia.

Avoid PEEP if possible.

Provide generous volume maintenance.

Avoid medications with situational potential hepatotoxicity when possible. Examples:

Acetaminophen, particularly in the alcoholic patient

Sulfonamides, tetracycline, and penicillins

Amiodarone

AND

Anticipate presence, development, or abnormalities of:

Coagulation

Attempt to correct prothrombin time to within 2 seconds of normal.

Consider cryoprecipitate if fresh frozen plasma is ineffective or fibrinogen abnormality exists.

Correct thrombocytopenia approximately for procedure.

Anticipate higher than normal blood loss for procedure.

Hemodynamics

Anticipate relative hypovolemia, worsened by treatment of ascites.

Assess for presence of high cardiac output, low peripheral resistance.

Suspect portal hypertension and/or variceal bleeding, even without history.

Anticipate depressed response to inotropes and vasopressors.

Consider invasive monitoring.

Pharmacokinetics and pharmacodynamics

Altered volume of distribution may occur.

Decreased serum albumin, increased gamma globulins

Intravascular volume unpredictable, especially with ascites treatment

Portosystemic shunted blood bypasses liver.

Drugs highly extracted by liver especially affected

Increased sensitivity to sedative medications may be present.

From Littlewood K, Nemergut EC. Liver disease. In: Fleisher LA. Anesthesia and Uncommon Diseases. 5th ed. Philadelphia: Saunders; 2005.

- Serum electrolyte and glucose levels
- Serum liver enzyme levels: ALT and AST (pathologic above 40 international units per liter [units/L]), alkaline phosphatase (pathologic above 115 units/L), lactic dehydrogenase (pathologic above 300 units/L), γ-glutamyl transpeptidase (pathologic above 85 units/L; often seen in chronic ethanol abuse)
- Blood type and screen

Serum ammonia level is a useful indicator of hepatic dysfunction; along with other parameters, it aids in detecting the presence of encephalopathy. A preoperative ECG is warranted, as are arterial blood gas determinations and pulmonary function tests in patients with suspected respiratory impairment. In the presence of suspected substance abuse, a toxicology screen is also useful in identifying intoxication and assessing the potential for acute withdrawal.

In patients without overt signs of hepatic disease but with a history of chronic alcohol or intravenous or ingested drug abuse, the issue of enzyme induction must be considered relative to clinical dosages of drugs necessary to achieve and maintain anesthesia. This is particularly true for sedatives, barbiturates, and opioids. These patients often require increased amounts of sedatives and anesthetic agents, which must be judiciously titrated to attain a therapeutic effect.

Patient history and preexisting physical status dictate the degree to which preoperative assessment should proceed, as well as the intensity with which perioperative monitoring modalities are instituted. Generally the preoperative degree of liver dysfunction is a major determinant of the patient's postoperative outcome. The greater the severity of liver disease, the greater the risk of exceeding the limited preexisting functional reserve. A greater potential for postoperative hepatic failure exists in patients with compromised hepatic function who undergo major surgery.

Liver Disease and Other Organ Systems
Perioperative Considerations

Cardiovascular System. Increased levels of endogenous vasodilators such as vasoactive intestinal peptide, ferritin glucagon, and others result in a hyperdynamic circulatory state, especially in the presence of cirrhotic liver disease. A high cardiac output and decreased systemic vascular resistance are present. Decreased blood viscosity and anemia contribute to the hyperdynamic circulatory state. The development of arteriovenous shunting occurs as a result of the development of extensive systemic collateral vessels. These vessels develop secondary to increased back pressure, reflected backward as a result of impaired hepatic circulation (portal hypertension). These collateral and frequently engorged vessels are well represented in the splanchnic circulation. Proliferation of collateral vessels also occurs in the lungs, skin, and musculature. Esophageal varices are a good example of this phenomenon. Chronic alcohol abuse predisposes a patient not only to hepatic cirrhosis but also to cardiomyopathy. Both conditions place the patient at risk for developing perioperative congestive heart failure.[10]

Hematologic Considerations. Anemia is a common finding, typically the upshot of hemorrhage, hemolysis, nutritional deficiencies, or bone-marrow suppression. Congestive splenomegaly contributes to the development of thrombocytopenia and leukopenia. Failure of hepatic synthetic processes results in clotting-factor deficiencies, decreased blood viscosity, and enhanced fibrinolysis due to decreased clearance of fibrinolytic factors.

In general, a growing body of evidence supports a prudent blood-product transfusion practice in accordance with a restrictive set of "transfusion triggers." The decision is based on awareness of potential negative sequelae that may follow even a moderate, controlled transfusion of blood products. In the setting of hepatic dysfunction, excessive blood transfusion may exacerbate encephalopathy, owing to the breakdown of red blood cells and the subsequent increase of protein-rich by-products in the plasma—by-products ordinarily metabolized by hepatocytes. When indicated, FFP, platelet, and cryoprecipitate transfusion should be undertaken to correct coagulation deficiencies before surgery. An acceptable preoperative hematocrit value in patients with liver disease is 30%. Particularly in the patient with concurrent uremia, both platelet quality and quantity must be considered. A platelet count of less than 100,000/mm^3 should be corrected before surgery, particularly when major blood loss is anticipated.[14,15]

Respiratory Considerations. Derangements in ventilatory mechanics and pulmonary gas exchange are commonly encountered in patients with liver disease. Right-to-left shunting secondary to arteriovenous shunting (attributable to increased circulating vasoactive substances normally metabolized by the liver) affects a hypoxemia that may involve up to 40% of the cardiac output. Ascitic impairment of diaphragmatic descent results in eventual development of a restrictive ventilatory defect. This defect causes decreased functional residual capacity and atelectasis, with subsequent alveolar hypoventilation.

Arterial blood gas determinations and chest radiographs are valuable additions to the preoperative assessment when the potential for perioperative respiratory embarrassment exists. Patients with a history of chronic alcoholism may also have a history of heavy tobacco use, suggesting the possible presence of obstructive pulmonary disease.

Fluid Balance and Renal Considerations. Ascites and edema offer distinct evidence of the presence of derangements in fluid balance in patients with liver disease. Hypoalbuminemia, sodium retention, and distortion in splanchnic intravascular hydrostatic pressure secondary to portal hypertension all contribute to alterations in renal perfusion, usually secondary to a state of hypoperfusion. The result is a progressive decline in renal function, as evidenced by decreased free water clearance, with resultant dilutional hyponatremia and hypokalemia.

Perioperative concerns focus on judicious correction of preexisting intravascular volume and electrolyte imbalances. Diuresis should be performed in a methodic and well-thought-out manner, and ample time should be taken to prevent hypotension and further electrolyte derangements. Perioperative preservation of adequate renal perfusion is of the utmost importance. Water restriction, controlled isotonic intravenous fluid administration, and potassium replacement may be necessary components of the preoperative plan of fluid therapy.

Intraabdominal ascites exerts a profound influence on many organ systems, including the renal system. Cirrhotic liver disease leads to development of excessive hydrostatic pressure within the hepatic venous and lymphatic systems. This phenomenon, coupled with impaired albumin synthesis, produces decreased plasma oncotic pressure within the liver parenchyma. An exudative process occurs across interstitial barriers and serosal liver surfaces, resulting in systemic edema, accumulation of protein-rich fluid within the peritoneum, and eventual electrolyte derangements. Ongoing exudation establishes an osmotic gradient for ongoing intraperitoneal filling, a relative intravascular hypovolemia, and sodium retention. Intraoperatively a sudden release of the tamponade effect of the ascitic abdomen during laparotomy can induce profound hypotension.

Sodium retention is explained by two theories. The underfilling theory describes sodium retention in terms of a discrepancy between total extracellular and plasma volumes and "effective" plasma volume. In this condition, an increased splanchnic vascular volume with resultant ascites causes a relative hypovolemia and consequent hyperaldosteronism. The reason is an imbalance in Starling forces brought about by a leakage of protein-rich fluid into the peritoneal cavity. The overflow theory establishes the cause of sodium retention as a primary event in the kidney in the presence of abnormal Starling forces, with ascites resulting from expansion of fluid volume. Leakage into the peritoneum then occurs via previously described exudative processes.[5]

Hepatorenal syndrome may occur as a consequence of gastrointestinal hemorrhage, sepsis, or surgery or as a result of aggressive diuretic therapy, all of which place patients at risk for derangements in renal perfusion. Characteristic signs include progressive ascites, azotemia, oliguria, and eventually multisystem organ failure. Institution of supportive therapy is undertaken until hepatic transplantation can be performed. Hepatic transplantation remains the only definitive treatment for this ultimately fatal syndrome.

Correction of volume status should be undertaken with attention to central filling pressures, electrolyte and coagulation status, and maintenance of adequate urinary output. Diuresis, after adequate cardiac preload is established, may be undertaken with the administration of mannitol (1 to 2 g/kg) or furosemide (0.3 to 4 mg/kg). Low-dose, or "renal," dopamine infusion (1 to 4 mcg/kg/min) was previously used for this purpose but has now largely fallen out of favor owing to reports indicating the imposition of renal tubular toxicity. This is theorized to be secondary to establishment of a hypotonic diuresis with concurrent intrarenal vasoconstriction. This has been shown to result in altered tubular ion exchange and solute retention.[16] Fenoldopam, a dopamine-1 agonist, administered by infusion (0.1 mcg/kg/min bolus with infusion 0.05 to 0.1 mcg/kg/min) is effective for inducing natriuresis, as well as diuresis. Alternative intravenous diuretic agents also include the loop diuretics ethacrynic acid and bumetanide and the potassium-sparing diuretics spironolactone, triamterene, and amiloride. Potentially nephrotoxic drugs should be avoided. These include nonsteroidal antiinflammatory drugs (NSAIDs), which inhibit renal prostaglandin synthesis. Interference with the production of prostaglandins results in renal artery and glomerular constriction, as well as interference with tubular sodium-potassium exchange.[16]

Central Nervous System Considerations. Encephalopathy is the most dramatic manifestation of CNS involvement during hepatic failure. Alterations in the function of the CNS are progressive and consist of neuromotor abnormalities, such as asterixis and hyperreflexia, and mental status changes. Ultimately the development of coma portends irreversible central nervous system failure and death. The degree of neurologic severity, however, correlates with the amount of portal blood deprived of the cleansing processes of the liver entering the systemic circulation.

Toxins delivered from the gastrointestinal tract implicated in the development of encephalopathy are substances normally metabolized by the hepatocytes. These nitrogenous substances include ammonia, aromatic amino acids, phenols, and short-chain amino acids (mercaptans). Buildup of these substances within the cerebral circulation contributes to the erosion of the blood-brain barrier. A markedly increased level of γ-aminobutyric acid is also noted, as are decreased levels of branched-chain amino acids.

The preoperative attenuation of encephalopathy is often undertaken through the administration of enteral lactulose or neomycin. These agents reduce the absorption of ammonia from the gastrointestinal tract. By altering the pH of the colon, lactulose enhances fecal elimination of ammonium, which is a poorly absorbable conversion product of ammonia. Neomycin interferes with the buildup of ammonia (converted from urea by bacterial ureases) by decreasing the amount of colonic bacteria. Potential precipitating factors associated with the development of encephalopathy should be corrected. These factors include gastrointestinal bleeding, metabolic alkalosis (e.g., from nausea and vomiting), infectious processes, progressive hepatic dysfunction, and a high level of dietary protein.

Cerebral uptake of benzodiazepines is greatly enhanced by a theoretically increased number of receptors or breakdown of the blood-brain barrier. Preoperative medication may be omitted altogether in the presence of encephalopathy.[5,8]

Intraoperative Anesthetic Considerations

Preoperative sedatives should be judiciously administered. Depending on the extent of mental impairment or obtundation, preoperative sedation may possibly be omitted altogether. Aspiration precautions should be used in patients with liver disease, even in those who have had nothing by mouth for an extended time. Patients with liver disease and concomitant ascites should be expected to have impaired gastric motility. An apparent lack of abdominal distention should not obviate this consideration. Variable incompetence of the lower esophageal sphincter (LES) should also be suspected. Hiatal hernia is also not uncommon in these patients. The presence of esophagitis with reflux should also be surmised in the course of the preoperative assessment, with provisions made to accommodate this information in planning anesthesia delivery. Intravenous metoclopramide, ranitidine, and famotidine are attractive considerations for aspiration prophylaxis before surgery and should be conscientiously administered. Oral ingestion of preinduction antacids for the purpose of increasing gastric pH are recognized to be equivocal in benefit for this purpose and may serve only to undesirably increase gastric volume. In the induction of general endotracheal anesthesia, best practice would support aspiration precautions that use either a rapid-sequence technique or its prudent modification, with both incorporating effectively applied cricoid pressure.

Standard monitoring procedures may be supplemented with more invasive modalities based on the perceived intraoperative risk of further decompensation—information the patient's preoperative assessment has disclosed. Pulmonary artery catheterization and central venous pressure monitoring add greater sensitivity to guide goal-directed volume and cardiopulmonary support. Arterial cannulation allows not only beat-to-beat arterial pressure assessment but also access through which laboratory studies may be readily obtained. Emerging minimally invasive hemodynamic monitoring technology, often using an arterial catheter with or without a central venous pressure line, is allowing acquisition of data of equal utility to that derived from more invasive modalities. Complications associated with central invasive lines such as infection, thromboembolism, vessel trauma, and hematoma may thus be significantly decreased. The option to use these modalities, if available, warrants consideration for not only their clinical utility but also for reducing the potential added risk of complications associated with invasive catheters in this susceptible subset of patients.[17,18]

Hypoxic injury to the liver occurs during surgery and anesthesia as a result of disturbances in oxygen supply-and-demand relationships. These disturbances are caused by inadequate ventilation, excessive bleeding, hypovolemia, hypotension, inadequate cardiac output, and iatrogenic disturbances in hepatic metabolic processes. Furthermore, a vasoconstrictive reduction in splanchnic perfusion occurs during intraabdominal surgery secondary to stimulation and manipulation of abdominal viscera. Efforts to attenuate these phenomena are directed toward optimizing central and systemic arterial perfusion pressures. This is accomplished with preferably minimal use of vasoconstricting agents (e.g., phenylephrine), as well as attenuation of the surgically induced stress response with an adequate anesthetized state.[18]

Arterial hypotension induces increased oxygen extraction by the tissues. This condition can have particularly deleterious consequences on the diseased liver, which is functioning with limited functional metabolic reserve. This places the liver in a particularly vulnerable state subject to further decompensation under hypoxic conditions. Reductions in cardiac output and arterial hypotension, therefore, warrant prompt correction.

Anesthetic Technique and Medication Choices

Regional anesthesia is used effectively for peripheral procedures if platelet and coagulation status is within acceptable parameters. Local anesthetic infiltration with judicious sedation may also be used for selected procedures. Certain medications, such as benzodiazepines, barbiturates, and some opioids, are highly protein bound; reduced concentrations of blood proteins call for a reduction in the usual dose. Patients with severe disease are theorized to have increased numbers of central benzodiazepine receptors, a phenomenon that also magnifies the effect of an administered dose. Therefore all sedatives, induction agents, and drugs known to depress organ and system function should be titrated carefully to achieve a therapeutic effect.

The use of succinylcholine during induction is acceptable; however, a prolonged effect is possible secondary to decreased levels of plasma cholinesterase, which is synthesized in the liver. In the hyperkalemic, immobile, or debilitated patient, the ramifications of exacerbated hyperkalemia must also be considered when administering an intubating dose of succinylcholine. A rapid-onset, nondepolarizing muscle relaxant such as rocuronium is capable of exhibiting prolongation of effect in patients with hepatic dysfunction. This must be expected with any muscle relaxant that requires hepatic clearance (e.g., vecuronium), making cisatracurium, which is relatively devoid of hepatic metabolic clearance mechanisms, an attractive choice.[19] Although reports have been published of hepatic dysfunction with the use of isoflurane, this agent may be used effectively. The nearly nonexistent hepatic metabolism and lipid solubility of desflurane makes this agent an unlikely direct cause of postoperative hepatic dysfunction and a particularly attractive choice as a volatile anesthetic in compromised patients. Use of sevoflurane has not been accompanied by reports of overt hepatic dysfunction directly attributable to the agent, but its metabolic by-products, particularly free fluoride ion and its association with renal toxicity, were thought to be a detraction to its use. Simple, recommended modifications in sevoflurane's delivery technique, however, have largely obliterated free–fluoride ion concerns. The low lipid solubility of sevoflurane also makes this agent suitable and attractive for patients with hepatic disease.

Nitrous oxide is not directly associated with an increased risk of postoperative hepatic dysfunction. Recognition of a mild to moderate sympathomimetic effect associated with the agent, potentially causing a variable degree of hepatic vasoconstriction, may invoke consideration of its inclusion for use in patients with hepatic impairment.

Opioids may be used effectively as adjunctive anesthetic agents in patients with liver disease. Fentanyl is relatively devoid of direct deleterious effects on hepatic blood flow, oxygen supply, and oxygen consumption. The commonly used volatile anesthetics and opioids exhibit equal effects on hepatic oxygen supply and demand. For this reason, isoflurane, desflurane, or sevoflurane used with judicious doses of fentanyl provide an appropriate and effective anesthetic technique. Sufentanil, alfentanil, and remifentanil are other suitable opioid alternatives. Morphine may be less appropriate, owing to its association with spasm of the sphincter of Oddi. Morphine also has the potential for inducing histamine release. Opioids (with the exception of remifentanil and to a lesser extent alfentanil) generally undergo hepatic metabolism, however. In this patient population, prolongation of effect—particularly with fentanyl and sufentanil—and side effects such as respiratory depression and hypotension are added concerns, even with small to moderate doses. Remifentanil, an ultrashort-acting opioid, possesses the advantage of nonspecific plasma esterase metabolism. It is therefore an attractive agent for use by infusion in patients with hepatic disease.

Selection of anesthetic agents in the presence of hepatic disease warrants attention to both pharmacokinetic and pharmacodynamic factors. In patients with hepatic disease, the typical existence of an increased volume of distribution directly affects distribution of an injected drug. This must be considered in addition to the intrinsic pharmacokinetics and pharmacodynamics of the injected drug and may entail the need for a larger initial dose to achieve desired clinical effect and smaller subsequent maintenance doses when indicated. Even with astute dosing discretion, aberrant prolongation of clinical effect should always be a consideration when administering a drug reliant upon hepatic metabolism and elimination.

Anesthetic management of patients undergoing hepatic surgery is often complicated by coagulopathy. This condition is caused by variable degrees of splenomegaly-induced thrombocytopenia and by decreased synthesis of clotting factors secondary to hepatic parenchymal destruction. This situation can also occur in patients with liver disease who are undergoing nonhepatic surgery. Yet another issue in the coagulopathic process in these patients involves the interaction of instilled blood in the peritoneal cavity with the collagen procoagulants found in peritoneal fluid. The result is a consumptive process involving platelets and fibrinogen. The clots formed are lysed by tissue plasminogen activator. A similar process results from exposure of ascitic fluid to blood in the general circulation. A clinical picture resembling disseminated intravascular coagulopathy results, with elevated international normalized ratio (INR), PT, and aPTT, decreased platelet count, decreased fibrinogen level, and increased levels of fibrin degradation products.[20]

Treatment of perioperative coagulopathy, as well as volume management, should always be goal directed. Correction of a coagulation deficiency is accomplished by blood product replacement that includes FFP, platelets, cryoprecipitate, and packed red blood cells, and only as indicated through laboratory findings. Other therapeutic options include the use of antifibrinolytic agents such as aminocaproic acid. Activities performed by the anesthetist in anticipation of major blood loss include (1) establishing large-bore intravenous lines suitable for rapid transfusion and (2) blood typing and cross-matching for an appropriate number of homologous units of packed red blood cells. Blood salvage techniques effectively minimize homologous blood product use.

Maintenance of normocarbia must be ensured for optimizing hepatic function, organ perfusion, and oxygen extraction. Hypothermia is particularly deleterious to coagulation processes. Convective warming measures, such as forced-air warming blankets and increased ambient room temperature, are most effective. Warming intravenous fluids, particularly blood products, contributes to promoting intraoperative normothermia.

Therapeutic Modalities for Portal Hypertension

Pharmacologic management of the patient with portal hypertension and acute variceal bleeding is considered secondary to

endoscopic treatment and traditionally consists of intravenous infusion of vasopressin or somatostatin. Vasopressin is a splanchnic vasoconstrictor but may also induce undesirable systemic vasoconstriction. Infusion of vasopressin is initiated at 0.1 to 0.4 unit/min. Concurrent infusion of nitroglycerin, titrated at around 40 mcg/min, may be used to attenuate coronary arterial vasoconstriction and control systolic blood pressure at 100 to 110 mm Hg.[20] In the presence of profound esophageal variceal exsanguination and hemodynamic instability, vasopressin may be used together with mechanical compression applied by inserting a triple-lumen Sengstaken-Blakemore tube. Use of this device also requires endotracheal intubation for airway support and prevention of pulmonary aspiration.

Octreotide, a somatostatin analog, has been shown to be equally as effective as vasopressin in pharmacologic control of variceal bleeding. Infused at 50 mcg/hr, octreotide acts as a potent and reversible inhibitor of gastrointestinal peptide hormone activity, thereby decreasing gut motility and venous return to the portal circulation. Octreotide has been shown to be as efficacious as sclerotherapy in acute treatment of variceal hemorrhage.[21]

Endoscopic sclerotherapy, usually performed with the patient under intravenous titrated sedation, has been recognized as the treatment of choice in definitive correction of variceal bleeding. Sclerotherapy is accomplished endoscopically by injecting a thrombosing agent either directly into the variceal bleeder or creating a fibrotic "overlayer" over the varix, accomplished by injection of the sclerosing agent proximal to the paravariceal mucosa. A course of treatments is usually necessary to reduce the incidence of rebleeding. Rebleeding, however, continues to be problematic in this subset of patients, with an incidence of up to 60%.[21,22]

SURGICAL DECOMPRESSION PROCEDURES

Transjugular intrahepatic portosystemic shunt (TIPS) is an interventional radiologic procedure that accomplishes portal decompression without undertaking major intraabdominal surgery. It was previously undertaken when endoscopic therapies such as sclerotherapy and drug therapies were unsuccessful in decompressing varices engorged secondary to portal hypertension. It now, however, has emerged as primary therapy for this purpose, usually as an elective procedure. The TIPS procedure is typically performed off-site under local anesthesia with sedation in the interventional radiology suite. During the TIPS procedure, a catheter/guidewire is placed from a right internal jugular vein insertion site and advanced under fluoroscopy via the inferior vena cava into a right hepatic vein. An intrahepatic channel is created within the liver parenchyma between the hepatic vein and a branch of the portal vein and kept patent through insertion of a reinforcing stent. The low-resistance conduit created promotes intrahepatic decompression by diverting blood flow directly into the systemic circulation. In doing so, portal back pressure is alleviated and both variceal blood flow and ascites formation are reduced. Shunted blood, however, is devoid of any benefit of hepatic metabolic processes, with the potential consequences. The onset of encephalopathy, nevertheless, is significantly less common compared with conventional anastomotic vascular shunts. Restenosis or occlusion within the first 6 months postinsertion has been problematic. The TIPS is strictly a palliative procedure and is largely considered a temporizing bridge until liver transplantation is performed. In patients undergoing the TIPS procedure, all anesthetic considerations appropriate to patients with end-stage hepatic disease must be attended to, particularly to the preference for agents with minimal hepatic pharmacokinetic dependence. Specific intraprocedural complications with the TIPS procedure include liver laceration, gallbladder perforation, oliguric renal failure (secondary to reaction to contrast dye), and stent embolization.[23-25]

Open portosystemic shunt procedures are considered either selective or nonselective, based on the degree to which portal venous blood is diverted from the diseased liver. The efficacy established in the TIPS procedure, however, has made this the intervention of choice for elective hepatic decompression. The unacceptably high morbidity and mortality associated with open, transabdominal procedures for the elective ablation of portal hypertension have largely resulted in their abandonment in most centers as an elective decompressive procedure. This has virtually relegated consideration of these procedures to drastic resuscitative measures in the moribund patient.

When used, a nonselective shunt diverts all portal blood from the liver. Examples of this kind of shunt are the portacaval shunt (end-to-side and side-to-side), mesocaval shunt (anastomosis of the mesenteric vein to the vena cava), and splenorenal shunt (anastomosis of the proximal splenic vein to the renal vein). An example of a selective portosystemic shunt is the Warren shunt, or distal splenorenal shunt. The significant feature of this shunt is that portal venous blood supply is preserved. It is therefore the preferred open surgical shunt procedure.[26] All such shunt procedures are palliative. The progression of morbidities such as encephalopathy, as well as other systemic sequelae of hepatic failure, are therefore only forestalled rather than corrected.

Anesthetic considerations in portosystemic shunt procedures include all perioperative accommodations made for patients with end-stage liver disease. Additionally, patients undergoing emergent open shunting procedures should be expected to be moribund or in an acute state of extremis. Preservation of systemic multiorgan function will thus be a monumental challenge. Particular concern focuses on the certainty of a precipitating hemorrhagic state and a coagulopathic diathesis necessitating massive transfusion of blood and blood products. These procedures are usually lengthy and as previously mentioned, primarily resuscitative in nature. Provisions for rapid infusion and adherence to a massive transfusion protocol will be required. Management of systemic organ function will typically include accommodations for preserving cardiovascular stability, hematologic parameters (hemoglobin, hematocrit, platelet count), coagulation status (INR, PT, aPTT), plasma osmolality, fibrinogen level, electrolyte levels, serum glucose level, and acid-base status. Urine output also must be meticulously monitored. Hemodynamic lability must be anticipated. Corrective therapy is accomplished by a goal-directed strategy. Hemodynamic assessment is best performed by means of information derived from an intraarterial line, as well as measures to determine central filling pressures, systemic perfusion, and cardiac contractility using invasive (and/or newer minimally invasive) monitoring modalities. The presence of bleeding esophageal varices, often the culpable etiologic factor for the surgical emergency, may preclude the use of transesophageal echocardiography to assess cardiac chamber filling and wall-motion abnormalities. The partial pressure of arterial carbon dioxide ($PaCO_2$) should be kept at 40 mm Hg or slightly above to optimize portal blood flow. Nitrous oxide is avoided to prevent bowel distention and maximize partial pressure of oxygen (PaO_2). This also serves to attenuate the effect of intrapulmonary shunting and ventilation-perfusion mismatch commonly found in patients with severe liver disease. Normothermia must be preserved through use of convective warming measures, warming of all infused volume, and increased ambient room temperature.[27]

Controversy exists regarding the choice of crystalloid intravenous solutions. Patients with hepatic failure may have preexisting metabolic alkalosis that may theoretically be exacerbated by the use of lactated Ringer's solution, which is metabolized into bicarbonate in the liver. Sodium retention is common in patients with hepatic disease and ascites. Research suggests that transfusing large quantities of normal saline may induce intraoperative hyperchloremic metabolic acidosis, which has been associated with inducing a variable degree of renal vasoconstriction in laboratory models.[28] Exacerbation of a preexistent hepatorenal syndrome is possible. When used as a primary intraoperative solution, normal saline (when compared with lactated Ringer's solution) has also been associated with a greater requirement for transfused blood products and sodium bicarbonate.[28] As a maintenance crystalloid, intravenous saline solutions should be used cautiously, with close scrutiny of electrolyte balance, particularly serum sodium and base excess. As in accepted, evidence-based, critical care management, perioperative glycemic management protocols should be placed into effect and strictly adhered to.

Current opinion supports the use of both lactated Ringer's and normal saline in a balanced ratio in surgical procedures involving extensive blood loss requiring aggressive volume management.[18] Other isotonic, isoosmolar intravenous solutions such as Plasma-Lyte merit consideration and may be used. Urinary output less than 50 mL/hr may warrant the use of agents to induce an osmotic diuresis. The potential for precipitation or exacerbation of acid-base and electrolyte derangements, as well as hepatorenal syndrome, justifies avoidance of overzealous efforts to accomplish this. Furosemide and loop diuretics should be used with trepidation and only when intravascular volume repletion is ensured.

DISEASES OF THE BILIARY TRACT

Biliary tract disease is a symptomatic expression of the presence of gallstones and/or an inflammatory process attributable to infection or ischemia. Gallstone formation is most likely caused by physicochemical derangements in the formation of bile. Approximately 90% of gallstones appear as radiolucent structures composed of hydrophobic cholesterol crystals. Calcium bilirubinate generally accounts for the composition of the remaining percentage. Stones composed of calcium bilirubinate are usually seen in patients with cirrhosis and hemolytic anemia. An estimated 15 to 20 million adults in the United States have biliary tract disease, as evidenced by the presence of gallstones.[29]

Anatomic and Physiologic Overview

The biliary tract is the excretory conduit for the liver. It is composed of (1) the intrahepatic ducts, which collect bile from the liver segments; (2) the coalescence of the intrahepatic ducts and the right and left hepatic ducts; (3) the common hepatic duct, which is formed by the junction of the right and left hepatic ducts in the liver hilum; (4) the gallbladder, which serves as a reservoir of bile; (5) the cystic duct, which joins the gallbladder to the common bile duct; and (6) the common bile duct, which begins at the junction of the cystic duct and the common hepatic duct and terminates in the lumen of the duodenum.[29]

The gallbladder is attached to the liver in a shallow fossa that lies at the junction of the right and left hepatic lobes. On gross examination, the gallbladder is a pear-shaped organ capable of holding 30 to 50 mL of fluid. The cystic duct is usually 2 to 3 cm

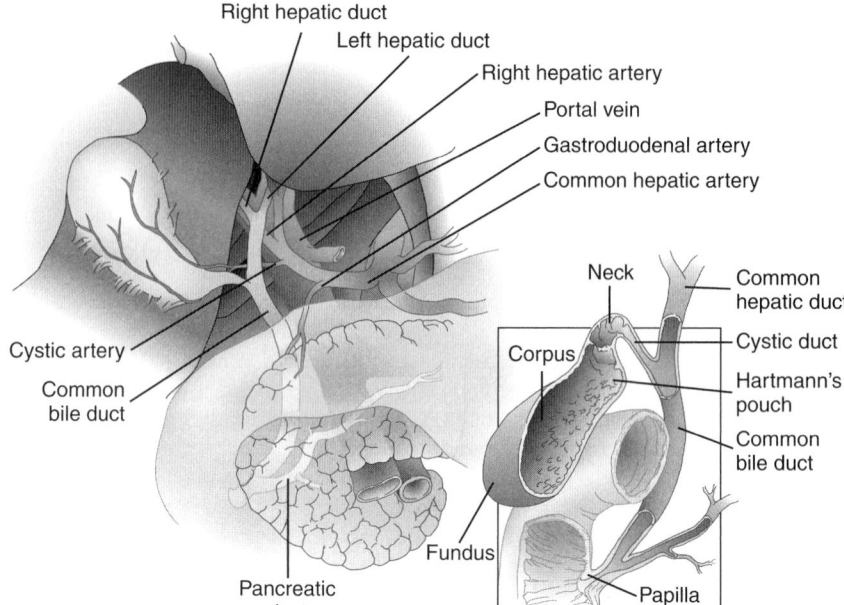

FIGURE **31-1**   Anatomy of the biliary tract. (*From Townsend CM et al, eds. Sabiston Textbook of Surgery: The Biological Basis of Modern Surgical Practice. 18th ed. Philadelphia: Saunders; 2008:1548.*)

long and arises from the narrow end, or infundibulum, of the gallbladder. The common bile duct is approximately 6 mm in diameter. It passes behind the duodenum to the right of the gastroduodenal artery, traversing the head of the pancreas before entering the second part of the duodenum. The common bile duct shares a channel with the main pancreatic duct. At the termination, these ducts are enveloped in smooth muscle, the sphincter of Oddi, which provides a barrier to intestinal bacteria for the sterile environment of the biliary tract. At this point, biliary tract obstruction can occur from a pancreatic tumor. Both the biliary and pancreatic tracts empty into the duodenum via the ampulla of Vater (Figure 31-1).

Arterial blood supply is furnished by the cystic artery, which is a branch of the right hepatic artery. The biliary ducts receive their blood supply from collateral branches of the hepatic artery and from small retroperitoneal vessels. Venous drainage flows into the portal vein. Lymphatic drainage flows into a cystic duct node located between the cystic duct and the common hepatic duct.

The gallbladder and the sphincter of Oddi are innervated by neurons of the enteric nervous system. This system, a hybrid of the sympathetic and parasympathetic nervous systems, is composed of neurons with cell bodies that lie in gut ganglia that are a component of the hypothalamic-pituitary axis.[29] A mediating component of this system is thus incorporated within the central nervous system. Neurons in the system are activated by neuropeptides, which are released under the influence of preganglionic fibers of both the sympathetic and the parasympathetic nervous systems. Reflex control of the gallbladder and the sphincter of Oddi is mediated by afferent fibers derived from the enteric nervous system.

Another structure, the porta hepatis, consists of an area bounded by the common bile duct, the cystic duct, and the undersurface of the liver. This area is known as the *cystohepatic triangle (Calot triangle)* and is a critical region that contains the cystic artery, the right hepatic artery, the cystic node, and sometimes an aberrant right segmental bile duct. This area must be

carefully dissected during cholecystectomy, so damage to these vital and friable structures is avoided.

The gallbladder mucosa secretes a protective mucus that prevents caustic damage by bile salts. After food is ingested, the gallbladder contracts, emptying its contents (bile) into the duodenum to assist in the digestive processes. Regulation of gallbladder contraction is primarily hormonal through the action of cholecystokinin. The release of cholecystokinin from duodenal cells is mediated by the presence of intraluminal amino acids and fat. Vagal stimulation also serves a role (secondary to the role of cholecystokinin). Indeed, vagotomy is associated with impaired gallbladder contraction and increased prevalence of gallstones.

Bile, the combined secretory product of the hepatocyte and biliary tract epithelial cell, has three main functions: (1) to emulsify and enhance absorption of ingested fats and fat-soluble vitamins; (2) to provide an excretory pathway for bilirubin, drugs and toxins, and immunoglobulin A (IgA); and (3) to maintain duodenal alkalization. The combined output of the ductal cells and hepatocytes is 500 to 1500 mL/day. The hepatocytes secrete bilirubin (the metabolic waste product of heme metabolism), cholesterol, bile salts, lecithin, water, and electrolytes. The epithelial cells contribute water and electrolytes. Vagal stimulation, secretin, cholecystokinin, and gastrin stimulate ductular cell secretion and increase bile flow. In addition, bile acids furnish a positive-feedback mechanism in the elaboration of hepatocyte and ductular secretion. Gallbladder filling during fasting occurs with relaxation and contraction of the sphincter of Oddi. Vasoactive intestinal peptide produces relaxation, whereas somatostatin, an inhibitory peptide, produces contraction. In states of prolonged fasting, the risk of gallstone formation increases because of the lack of cholecystokinin stimulation and consequent biliary stasis.[29]

Cholecystitis

Obstruction of the cystic duct by gallstones results in acute, severe, midepigastric pain, typically radiating to the right abdomen. Inspiratory effort usually accentuates the pain (Murphy sign). Increases in plasma bilirubin, alkaline phosphatase, and amylase levels frequently occur. Ileus and localized tenderness may indicate perforation with peritonitis. Leukocytosis and fever are often present. Jaundice indicates complete obstruction of the cystic duct. Symptoms are frequently confused with those of myocardial infarction. Differential diagnosis is accomplished through serial ECG evaluations and laboratory analysis of serum enzymes specific to cardiac muscle. Cholescintigraphy (a contrast study that evaluates gallbladder excretion of a radiographically labeled substance) and ultrasonography are often used for clinical confirmation of the diagnosis.

Patients with symptoms indicative of acute cholecystitis are often volume depleted because of intolerance of oral intake, vomiting, and possible preoperative nasogastric evacuation of gastric contents. Dehydration calls for preoperative intravenous fluid replacement. Gastric suction may be warranted in the presence of ileus. The presence of free abdominal air, as determined by abdominal radiography or symptoms of an acute abdomen (fever, ileus, rigid and painful abdomen, vomiting, dehydration), suggests a ruptured viscus, possibly including perforation of the gallbladder. Under these circumstances, emergency exploratory laparotomy is undertaken.

Cholelithiasis and Choledocholithiasis

Acute obstruction of the common bile duct often produces symptoms similar to those seen in patients with cholecystitis. Recurrent bouts of acute cholecystitis induce the development of fibrotic changes in gallbladder structure, thereby impeding the ability of the gallbladder to adequately expel bile. Presence of the Charcot triad (fever and chills, jaundice, upper quadrant pain) aids in establishing the diagnosis of acute ductal obstruction. Weight loss, anorexia, and fatigue complete the symptomatology. Diagnostic modalities include radiography, transhepatic cholangiography, ultrasonography, cholescintigraphy, and CT scan. A dilated common bile duct and biliary tree are typically observed in these studies.

Anesthetic Considerations in Gallbladder and Biliary Tract Disease

Removal of gallstones is undertaken not only for relief of symptoms but also for prevention of further sequelae, including cholecystitis, cholangitis, jaundice, pancreatitis, and peritonitis, all of which may result from stasis or impediment to bile flow. Diversity among patients who undergo biliary surgery is common; patients may range from otherwise healthy individuals with a history of recurrent bouts of cholecystitis to those who are desperately ill.

Cholecystectomy is now most commonly performed as an elective procedure through laparoscopy. Laparoscopic cholecystectomy is now often performed in the relatively healthy patient on an outpatient basis with either discharge later in the day of surgery or after an overnight stay in the hospital. Postoperative pain management is typically less challenging with laparoscopic surgery. Measures should be undertaken, however, to prevent postoperative nausea and vomiting. Patients undergoing laparoscopic cholecystectomy are at added risk of peritoneal irritation from insufflation of the abdomen with carbon dioxide. Other factors that need consideration are the (equivocal) role of nitrous oxide if used, the use of opioids, and the extent of intravascular volume repletion. Other factors may be demographic in nature (e.g., young, female, obese). Numerous preemptive, polymodal guidelines exist and should be considered.[30]

Open cholecystectomy may be indicated for patients who are emergently ill or in whom laparoscopy poses a particularly formidable technical challenge (e.g., in cases of morbid obesity or intraabdominal adhesions secondary to previous abdominal surgery or peritonitis). The use of abdominal carbon dioxide insufflation to effect adequate exposure of anatomic structures mandates general endotracheal intubation anesthesia to effectively seal the airway and prevent passive aspiration of gastric contents. Abdominal insufflation displaces the abdominal viscera and diaphragm in a cephalad direction, placing extra pressure on the lower esophageal sphincter (LES) and thereby increasing the risk of gastric reflux.

Insufflation of the abdomen with carbon dioxide also impedes diaphragmatic excursion, causing a decrease in functional residual capacity, closing capacity, and increased peak inspiratory pressure. A relative hypercarbia, as evidenced by increased end-tidal and arterial carbon dioxide levels, reflects variable uptake of insufflated carbon dioxide. Controlled ventilation is therefore necessary to minimize the development of atelectasis and prevent progressive hypercarbia. In the setting of intraabdominal insufflation, applying an alternative ventilatory strategy using pressure control ventilation (PCV) rather than a volume control mode may best serve to prevent alveolar derecruitment by providing a physiologic minute ventilation while minimizing the risk of barotrauma. The use of a reverse Trendelenburg position during laparoscopic cholecystectomy may also induce a variable degree of hemodynamic compromise by impeding venous return. Occult hemorrhage is also possible and may go undetected.

Patients who undergo open cholecystectomy often experience more complications, owing to preexisting pathologic medical conditions. There is also the greater likelihood of severe postoperative pain and respiratory splinting (caused by the use of a right subcostal or upper-abdominal midline incision), with the risk of postoperative respiratory embarrassment in the susceptible patient. The intraabdominal viscera is exquisitely sensitive to the effects of hemodynamic lability—in particular, derangements resulting in reduced perfusion pressure to this region. Patients who have experienced severe traumatic injury or who require aggressive intensive care for multiorgan disease are at particular risk for developing acute cholecystitis secondary to the stress of severe illness. Patients with significant comorbidities, including advanced age, who undergo prolonged or complex surgical procedures (e.g., trauma, cardiac surgery with cardiopulmonary bypass, abdominal aneurysm repair) that are complicated by perioperative hemodynamic lability have also been identified to be at added risk for ischemia of the abdominal viscera. The result may be the development of an acute, postoperative abdominal crisis. Under this circumstance, exploratory laparotomy for an acute abdomen may reveal necrosis and perforation of the gallbladder. This places the patient at extreme risk for developing peritonitis. The acute critical nature of the presenting illness, superimposed upon preexisting patient comorbidities, is another factor potentially complicating perianesthetic management of the patient.

Full-stomach precautions should be used during the induction of and emergence from anesthesia, particularly in the presence of abdominal distention or ileus. Patients with jaundice require a more thorough preparation, owing to the likelihood of a variable degree of hepatic dysfunction. This may make for greater susceptibility to hemorrhage, exaggerated drug effects, and fluctuation in hemodynamics. Institution of invasive hemodynamic monitoring and preparation for blood product transfusion are influenced by the patient's clinical status.

No strong clinically based evidence has contraindicated the use of nitrous oxide during laparoscopic surgery. However, reports of increased postoperative nausea and intraoperative expansion of bowel gas associated with its use are considerations. In the presence of hepatic dysfunction, isoflurane, desflurane, and sevoflurane are safe. The choice of muscle relaxant depends on the patient's ability to tolerate possible side effects of the drug (e.g., pancuronium-induced tachycardia), the drug's dependence on hepatic clearance, and the length of the procedure to be performed.[31]

Common bile duct exploration may be carried out in conjunction with cholecystectomy if necessary. Patients who require this intervention are often more ill and older; therefore a 1.5-times greater incidence of morbidity and mortality exists in patients who require this procedure in addition to cholecystectomy.[31] Severe postoperative pain may be reduced by patient-controlled analgesia, intercostal nerve blocks, or neuraxial opioid administration. Creation of a drainage conduit for the common bile duct may be performed through percutaneous choledochocystostomy. This is an option for the relief of common bile duct obstruction in the patient assessed to be unlikely to tolerate a more complex surgical procedure and may be performed with local anesthetic infiltration and intravenous sedation.

DISEASES OF THE ESOPHAGUS

Anatomic and Physiologic Overview

The esophagus originates at the pharynx at approximately the level of the sixth cervical vertebra and extends to the stomach. It can be divided into three functional zones: the upper esophageal sphincter (UES), the esophageal body, and the LES. The esophageal wall consists of an inner circular muscular layer, which consists of smooth and striated muscle, and an outer longitudinal layer, which is devoid of serosal covering. The mucosal lining consists of squamous epithelium, except for the distal 1 to 2 cm, which is composed of columnar epithelium. To reach the abdomen, the esophagus traverses a hiatus created by the right crus of the diaphragm. Intraabdominal length is variable.

The inferior thyroid arteries supply blood to the cervical region of the esophagus, and the aorta and esophageal branches from the bronchial arteries supply the thoracic region. The esophagus is well endowed with lymphatics, which run longitudinally along the esophageal wall before perforating the muscular layers to reach the regional lymphatics.

The esophagus has both intrinsic and extrinsic innervation. The intrinsic enteric innervating system consists of two interconnected plexuses, the myenteric (Auerbach plexus) and the submucosal (Meissner plexus). This system is a continuum that extends from the esophagus to the anus. Extrinsic innervation of the esophagus is derived from the sympathetic, parasympathetic, and somatic nervous systems. Parasympathetic stimulation by means of cranial nerves IX, X, and XI causes esophageal muscular contraction, but it also causes relaxation of the LES. Sympathetic fibers act on the myenteric plexus to modulate rather than control motor activity.

At rest the UES is closed, as is the LES. Excitatory stimulation of UES tone occurs with inspiration, esophageal distention, gagging, Valsalva maneuver, and acidity of gastroesophageal contents. Distention, belching, and vomiting reduce UES tone. Swallowing initiates peristaltic activity, which consists of a maximum pressure of 150 mm Hg, with an average velocity of 3 to 4 cm/sec. The exact mechanisms responsible for peristaltic activity, which include production, propagation, and regulation, remain controversial. It is clear, however, that peristaltic activity

is highly integrated and involves central and local mechanisms that are mediated largely through excitatory cholinergic neuronal activity.

The UES and upper portions of the esophageal body are composed of striated muscle, whereas the bulk of the LES and the esophageal body consist of smooth muscle. The tone of the LES is maintained at 20 mm Hg through a combination of intrinsic myogenic and excitatory neural mechanisms. Vagal mediation of the neuronal component is predominant. β-Blockade is seen to increase LES tone, an effect that suggests adrenergic inhibitory tone. Ingestion of a meal or increased intraabdominal pressure increases LES tone via vagal afferent pathways. Swallowing decreases LES tone within 1.5 to 2.5 seconds and is maintained for the duration of the peristaltic wave (approximately 6 to 8 seconds).[31]

Esophageal Disorders

A common symptom found in esophageal disease is dysphagia. The presentation of this disorder initiates pursuit of the underlying cause, often through barium contrast studies (e.g., barium swallow) and through endoscopic examination of the esophagus and stomach, with procurement of cytology and biopsy specimens when indicated.[31]

Chronic alcoholism is associated with impaired esophageal peristalsis and LES hypotonia. Degeneration of the Auerbach plexus is closely associated with this condition. Achalasia (failure of the LES to relax during swallowing, along with a lack of peristalsis) often develops secondary to systemic disease states, including diabetes, stroke, amyotrophic lateral sclerosis, and certain connective tissue diseases, such as amyloidosis and scleroderma. Regurgitation of food and liquid is common and places these patients at high risk for aspiration.

The formation of Barrett esophagus occurs when normal squamous epithelium changes to metaplastic columnar epithelium. Chronic exposure to acidic gastric contents due to reflux is a major etiologic mechanism. Other etiologies include chronic alcohol abuse and the use of tobacco. Esophagitis and hiatal hernia are also precipitating factors. Development of Barrett esophagus is closely correlated with eventual development of carcinoma of the esophagus. A Mallory-Weiss tear most commonly occurs at the gastroesophageal junction; it is secondary to persistent retching, most often due to chronic alcohol abuse. Pain and bloody vomitus may be noted with its presence. Surgical repair is usually not indicated.[32]

Esophageal dilation is moderately successful in the correction of achalasia. Dilatation may be performed on an outpatient basis, as an endoscopic procedure under sedation, or in conjunction with a definitive, corrective surgical procedure. Operative correction, consisting of esophagomyotomy with funduplasty, is associated with a reasonable success rate and is the definitive treatment for this syndrome.[33,34]

Surgery for gastroesophageal reflux disease (GERD) is now usually reserved as therapy when medical management fails. The need for increasing doses of antacid medications, such as proton pump inhibitors (PPIs), without relief of symptoms; progressive disease leading to esophageal erosion, ulceration, and stricture; and recurrence of symptoms despite aggressive full-spectrum medical therapy will often be decisive indicators for surgical intervention. Numerous procedures have been developed and used with positive outcome reports. Procedures such as the Nissen fundoplication, the Belsey procedure, and posterior gastropexy (Hill repair) have been used, studied, and modified over the years since their introduction. Different approaches have been incorporated into surgical procedures for GERD, including thoracotomy, thoracoscopy, and laparotomy (e.g., endoscopic or laparoscopic-assisted procedures). Emerging techniques are beginning to benefit from the incorporation of robotic-assisted technologies. Endoscopic techniques now being introduced not only serve to minimize the extent of surgical procedures but also enhance economy of time and resources, as well as raise patient satisfaction. Safer palliative procedures have also emerged and may be performed in medically compromised patients with severe esophageal disease (e.g., endoscopic mucosal resection [EMR]). Other endoscopic transluminal procedures that incorporate various banding and suturing devices and use local anesthesia with sedation have been used with success and are often undertaken in off-site anesthesia settings. Many of the new endotherapeutic techniques make use of devices that strengthen or support the LES. Newer procedures, minimally invasive procedures, and modifications of established surgical techniques have developed thanks to surgical research that has expanded understanding of the mechanisms responsible for reflux.[32]

Anesthetic Considerations in Esophageal Disease

Symptomatic patients who have peptic esophagitis associated with hiatal hernia or LES incompetence often take any number of oral antacids, proton-pump inhibitors (e.g., esomeprazole magnesium), or H_2 antagonists (e.g., cimetidine, ranitidine, nizatidine, famotidine). A history of symptoms that indicate the presence of gastric reflux warrants aspiration prophylaxis during induction of and emergence from general anesthesia. The safe maintenance of general anesthesia mandates the use of an endotracheal tube to effect a sealed airway so that the risk from passive regurgitation and aspiration is minimized. When general anesthesia is administered, a rapid-sequence induction technique should be used, with the application of cricoid pressure. The patient must be fully awake and have demonstrated conscious control of airway reflexes before extubation. Awake intubation also is an option before the induction of general anesthesia. In selected procedures, regional anesthesia may be used effectively. A sealed, secured airway in which a cuffed endotracheal tube is placed provides the safest method for providing ventilatory support during general anesthesia.

For elective procedures, administration of an H_2 antagonist the evening before surgery and again in the morning at least a half hour before surgery helps increase gastric pH. In urgent and emergency situations, preoperative oral administration of a clear, nonparticulate antacid such as sodium citrate is an option. This, however, may increase gastric pH only to a small or moderate extent and may serve to undesirably increase gastric volume. Administration of a gastrokinetic agent, such as metoclopramide, in conjunction with an H_2 antagonist stimulates gastrointestinal motility, which aids in the emptying of gastric contents. For best effect, metoclopramide should be administered at least 15 minutes before anesthetic induction.

Hiatal Hernia

A hiatal hernia consists of a weakness in the diaphragm that allows a portion of the stomach to migrate upward into the thoracic cavity. Two types of esophageal hiatal hernias are the sliding type (type I), formed by the movement of the upper stomach through an enlarged hiatus, and the paraesophageal type (type II), in which the esophagogastric junction remains in normal position but all or part of the stomach moves into the thorax and assumes a paraesophageal position.

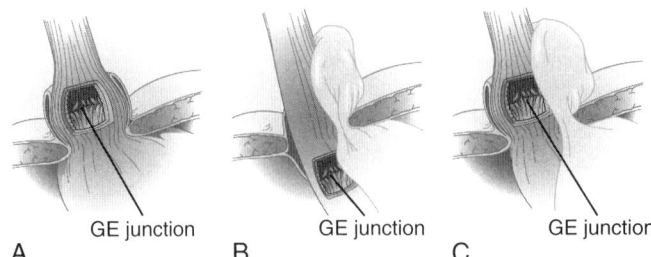

FIGURE 31-2   Three types of hiatal hernia. **A,** Type I, or *sliding hernia.* **B,** Type 2, or *rolling hernia.* **C,** Type 3, or *mixed hernia.* GE, Gastroesophageal. (*From Oelschlager BK et al. Hiatal hernia and gastroesophageal reflux disease. In: Townsend CM et al, eds. Sabiston Textbook of Surgery: The Biological Basis of Modern Surgical Practice. 18th ed. Philadelphia: Saunders; 2008:1109.*)

A third type of hiatal hernia (type III) has been identified that combines the features of sliding and paraesophageal hernias (Figure 31-2). A fourth type of hiatal hernia (type IV) occurs when other organs, such as the colon or small bowel, are contained in the hernial sac formed by a large paraesophageal hernia.[34] Hiatal hernia and peptic esophagitis often exist concurrently, although one does not cause the other. The major symptom is retrosternal pain of a burning quality that commonly occurs after meals. It is assumed that patients with a hiatal hernia are predisposed to developing peptic esophagitis, thereby providing a rationale for surgical correction of this condition. Most patients with hiatal hernia do not have symptoms of reflux esophagitis, however, and do not require H_2-agonist and oral antacid therapy. Nevertheless, implementation of aspiration precautions on induction of general anesthesia and emergence is strongly recommended.[32]

The primary goal in surgical correction of hiatal hernia is reestablishing gastroesophageal competence. This usually entails repair of the sliding hernia, reduction by 2 cm or more of the tubular distal esophagus below the diaphragm, and valvuloplasty. Abdominal, thoracic, or thoracoabdominal surgical approach may be selected. Common procedures for correction of hiatal hernia include the Nissen, Belsey, and Hill operations. Laparoscopically assisted fundoplication techniques are also more commonly being used. A gastroplasty may be performed (the Collis procedure) in association with repair of the hiatal hernia when indicated, usually in patients with a shortened esophagus. If a thoracic approach is selected, the patient must be assessed for ability to tolerate one-lung anesthesia.[34]

Esophageal Diverticula

Esophageal diverticula place the patient at risk for pulmonary aspiration of regurgitated food; another risk is posed from food and fluids ingested but sequestered within the diverticular pouch. Surgical correction may be performed in two stages, with the first stage involving mobilization of the pouch and the second stage entailing excision of the diverticulum, with esophageal repair. Esophageal diverticula are classified according to location. These classifications are epiphrenic (located near the LES), traction (in the midesophagus), and Zenker (upper esophagus). A Zenker diverticulum places the patient at greater risk of pulmonary aspiration.[33]

Esophageal Carcinoma

Patients undergoing surgical procedures for esophageal malignancy are often of advanced age, cachectic, malnourished, and suffering from disease processes that are both age related and relevant to other organ systems. To ensure safe and effective anesthesia in patients who undergo a curative or palliative procedure for this malady, consideration is given to adequate preoperative multisystem assessment and preparation.

Patients with esophageal carcinoma may have a significant associated history of alcohol and tobacco use. The presence of a variable degree of obstructive pulmonary disease or alcohol-related hepatic disease should be sought in the preoperative history, and findings should be incorporated into the anesthetic plan. Advanced age may also be a finding and considered a comorbidity. Furthermore, by the time the diagnosis of esophageal carcinoma is made, metastasis to adjacent lymph nodes and structures may have occurred. The absence of a serosal esophageal layer and the presence of abundant lymphatic networks facilitates rapid metastatic spread to the lungs and liver from a primary esophageal site. Preoperative radiation and chemotherapy also introduce potential complexity into the anesthetic plan, in particular the untoward side effects of those treatments. An added measure of comorbidities, to include bone marrow depression, intrathoracic and pulmonary fibrosis, and increased friability of the tissues, is thus brought to bear. These situations predispose the patient to potential intraoperative ventilatory difficulty, cardiac impairment, hematologic dyscrasias, and increased bleeding. Other side effects, particularly those related to chemotherapy, include induced cardiomyopathy (associated with daunorubicin and doxorubicin [Adriamycin] therapy) and pulmonary fibrosis (associated with bleomycin therapy). Chemotherapy-induced lung pathology results in a restrictive lung defect and an increased potential for oxygen toxicity. Patients with esophageal carcinoma may undergo any of a number of palliative or diagnostic endoscopic procedures performed either in the operating room or in an off-site setting. The frequently encountered debilitated state of these patients, often with additional imposition of coexisting disease, places them at particular risk for untoward complications that may require emergent surgical intervention. An example is the elderly patient who undergoes dilatation for strictures or complicated achalasia and sustains an esophageal perforation requiring emergent thoracotomy. The preoperative metabolic state may predispose to impaired wound healing, placing the patient at risk for dehiscence and anastomotic breakdown. The degree of comorbidity associated with the patient's history may merit performing a procedure in the operating room setting, rather than an off-site location where the particular procedure is typically undertaken.

A curative procedure may be attempted in a patient whose preoperative physical condition and tumor characteristics indicate the potential for long-term survival. This procedure involves en bloc resection of the esophagus for tumors in the lower third of the thoracic esophagus, along with reestablishment of gastrointestinal continuity through left colon interposition. This procedure involves a staged laparotomy and anterior thoracotomy.[35]

DISEASES OF THE STOMACH

Anatomic and Physiologic Overview

The stomach is essentially composed of two sections. The thin-walled and distensible fundus is located in the upper abdomen and has primarily a storage function. The thick-walled distal portion of the stomach is responsible for the mixing of food

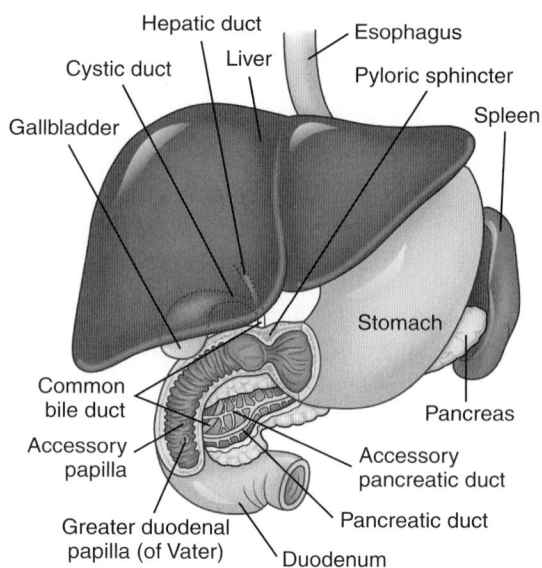

FIGURE **31-3** Position of the stomach relative to the other principal organs of the upper abdomen. (*From Huether SA, McCance KL. Understanding Pathophysiology. 4th ed. St Louis: Mosby; 2008: 925.*)

and its slow release through the pyloric sphincter into the duodenum. The liver is positioned right and ventral to the stomach and the spleen left and lateral. The biliary tract courses posterior to the stomach (Figure 31-3).

The blood supply of the stomach flows primarily from four major arteries: the right and left gastric arteries and the right and left gastroepiploic arteries (Figure 31-4). An extensive submucosal arterial arcade is also present. Major autonomic innervation is furnished by two branches of the vagus nerve, the right posterior (celiac) branch and the left anterior (hepatic) branch.

The gastric wall consists of an external serosal layer that covers an inner oblique, a middle circular, and an outer longitudinal layer of smooth muscle. The submucosa and mucosa provide a continuous inner integument that is separated by a thin sheet of muscularis mucosae (smooth muscle).

Within the gastric mucosa reside the glands responsible for the significant physiologic role played by the stomach during the digestive processes. Within the fundic mucosa lie mucus-secreting glands that provide a protective barrier to the acid outflow of the parietal cells, which are located in the same region of the stomach. The endocrine function of the stomach is apparent through the secretions (pepsinogen) of the chief cells and the secretions (serotonin) of other cells. Within the antrum are cells that secrete mucus (surface epithelial cells and mucous cells) and gastrin (G cells). The two important sphincters are the LES at the gastroesophageal junction and the pyloric sphincter at the gastroduodenal junction.

The stomach normally stores food for up to 4 hours. The sight and smell of food stimulate acid and pepsinogen production. Gastrin is released by the G cells in response to gastric distention, which stimulates parietal-cell acid (hydrochloric acid) secretion. The duodenum and upper jejunum also secrete a small amount of gastrin. Luminal acid suppresses gastrin feedback (negative feedback).

Pepsinogen and gastrin release are vagally mediated. Acid in duodenal contents induces the release of secretin, an effect that

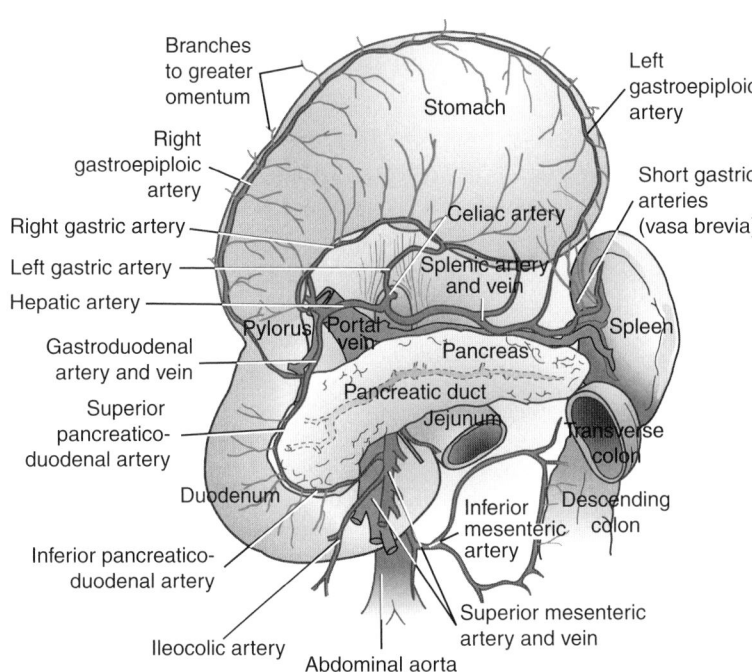

FIGURE **31-4** Blood supply to the stomach and duodenum with anatomic relationships to the spleen and pancreas. (*From Zuidema G. Shackelford's Surgery of the Alimentary Tract. 4th ed. Philadelphia: Saunders; 1995.*)

inhibits gastrin release even more and inhibits further acid production. Pancreatic bicarbonate release is also stimulated by duodenal acidity.

The acidic secretion of the parietal cells occurs through a hydrogen/potassium (H^+/K^+) exchange pump, which requires ATP. Release is mediated by vagal stimulation (from acetylcholine), gastrin, and histamine. Administration of H_2 antagonists such as cimetidine and ranitidine, H^+/K^+–ATP inhibitors such as omeprazole, and prostaglandins inhibits acid secretion. Vagotomy greatly diminishes parietal-cell response to gastrin and histamine. Anticholinergic agents, however, have only a minor influence on parietal-cell secretion.

Other gastric functions include providing a barrier against ingested pathogens. This goal is accomplished through the maintenance of a highly acidic environment and through a functional role in immunosurveillance. The stomach heats or cools ingested substances as needed for the maintenance of normothermia. Parietal cells also secrete intrinsic factor (in addition to hydrochloric acid), which facilitates ileal vitamin B_{12} absorption.

Peptic Ulcer Disease

Vagal stimulation causes elaboration of gastrin from antral cells. Gastrin, after entering the circulation, induces parietal-cell hydrochloric acid secretion. Secretion of hydrochloric acid also occurs in response to H_2-receptor activation. A chronic overabundance of hydrochloric acid and pepsin (from various causes) results in erosion of the protective mucous layer of the stomach and duodenum. Subsequent ulceration occurs in time, with lesions extending beyond the mucosal barrier into the submucosa and muscularis epithelial layers and sometimes into the serosal layer. In the case of LES incompetence, ulcerative involvement of the esophagus may develop.

A chronic ulcerative lesion in the duodenum constitutes duodenal ulcer disease. Because of similarity of symptoms and responses to therapy, this classification is also placed on lesions that occur before the pylorus in the lower antrum of the stomach. Men 45 to 65 years of age and women older than 55 years of age

have the highest incidence of duodenal ulcer disease. Chronic use of NSAIDs is the second most common cause of ulcer disease after *Helicobacter pylori* infection. Alcohol and corticosteroids are relatively minor etiologic factors.[3] Affected patients possess twice the number of acid-secreting parietal cells.[36]

H. pylori has been identified as a major etiologic factor of gastritis-associated disease, as well as gastric and duodenal ulcers and gastric carcinoma. Epidemiologic findings indicate a higher prevalence of this organism in older adults, individuals of lower socioeconomic status, and those born outside the United States. Infected patients undergoing stress are at greatest risk for exacerbation of the infection, with potential development of gastric and duodenal ulceration. At present, despite the numerous exposures of anesthesia providers to potential oral and ambient routes of transmission, *H. pylori* has not been recognized as a serious occupational hazard.[37]

Gastric mucosal acidosis has been commonly reported in critically ill patients, patients undergoing prolonged, complex surgical procedures, and patients undergoing cardiopulmonary bypass. Gastritis associated with gastric mucosal acidosis is associated with increased perioperative morbidity and mortality. The splanchnic viscera is particularly vulnerable to decreased circulatory blood flow, with the potential for breakdown of intestinal barrier function. This occurrence results in translocation of bacteria and endotoxin into the bloodstream, with consequent systemic sepsis. Ischemia and acidosis of the gut is the primary causative factor for erosion of gut barrier function.

Studies using gastric tonometry have correlated measurement of gastric mucosal pH (pHi) with indices of systemic acid-base balance. Measurement of gut pHi has been recognized as an earlier indicator of perturbations in acid-base balance than conventional blood gas analysis. The attractiveness in pHi measurement of the gut is threefold. First, the splanchnic circulation is reduced during stress in an effort to preserve more vital myocardial and cerebral circulation. Second, the gut villus is particularly susceptible to reduced blood flow. Third, the gut is readily accessible for regional monitoring via transesophageal or rectal probe.

Numerous studies have also demonstrated improvement in outcome in acutely ill patients who received pHi-directed therapy. However, controversy persists regarding how therapy should be guided and what pHi values are acceptable. Therefore, until the various clinical controversies are resolved and suitable technology developed that is adaptable to the needs of perioperative monitoring, efforts should be directed toward optimizing systemic perfusion. This is accomplished through optimization of hemodynamics and assurance of adequate oxygen-carrying capacity.

Patients in intensive care units who experience acute major illness or sustain major traumatic injury are at high risk for the development of acute, typically painless, erosive gastritis (Curling ulcer). This lesion is associated with a significant mortality rate because of the consequent severe hemorrhagic diathesis that often accompanies it. Other disease entities previously implicated as etiologic factors in gastritis and peptic ulcerative disease include hepatic cirrhosis, hyperparathyroidism, obstructive airway disease, and rheumatoid arthritis. Lifestyle-related factors such as emotional stress and alcohol consumption have been shown to be weak correlates with the development of peptic ulcer disease.[38] Therefore, the role of gastric hyperacidity in and of itself in predisposing a patient to duodenal ulcer disease is controversial.

A condition of reduced duodenal buffering, as is seen in biliary diversion away from the duodenum, has a greater likelihood of predisposing a patient to duodenal ulceration. Another example of reduced duodenal buffering with the potential for inducing ulcer formation in the duodenum occurs in a reduction in the flow of alkaline pancreatic juice, as would occur in a patient with chronic pancreatitis or pancreatic resection.[31]

Therapeutic Options in Peptic Ulcer Disease

Oral antacids, H_2-receptor antagonists, proton pump inhibitors, sucralfate, and antibiotics are the major medical therapies and treatments of choice used for the control of peptic ulcer disease. The proton pump inhibitor omeprazole is now being used in duodenal ulcer management. Surgical treatment is no longer considered primary treatment; it is reserved for patients who continue to experience intractable symptoms despite aggressive medical therapy and for treatment of complications. These complications are often of an urgent nature and consist of gastrointestinal hemorrhage, ulcerative perforation into adjacent structures such as the pancreas or jejunum, and obstruction.[38]

The use of antacids in the medical treatment of peptic ulcer disease has potential complications of interest to the anesthetist. Antacids may produce an acid rebound in which gastric acid secretion may increase after acid is neutralized by calcium-containing antacids. Another condition that may result from antacid therapy is the milk-alkali syndrome. In this condition, hypercalcemia, alkalosis, and an elevated blood urea nitrogen level may develop from the daily ingestion of large quantities of calcium-containing antacids and milk. Manifestations of this syndrome include skeletal muscle weakness and polyuria. Ingestion of large quantities of aluminum-containing antacids may result in acute hypophosphatemia due to increased binding of intestinal phosphorus. Skeletal muscle weakness and fatigue follow chronic overuse, resulting in pathologic fractures and osteoporosis.

The secretion of hydrochloric acid is blocked by H_2 antagonists, thereby promoting the healing of duodenal ulcers. A noteworthy side effect is seen in the alteration of cytochrome P-450 enzyme activity in the liver; this alteration may result in prolongation of the effects of concurrently administered drugs that rely on hepatic metabolism and elimination by means of this mechanism. Famotidine is the H_2 antagonist least likely to cause this effect. Other side effects include decreased hepatic blood flow, leukopenia and thrombocytopenia, mental confusion, interstitial nephritis, hepatitis, bradycardia, and hypotension.

The proton pump inhibitors are the most effective antisecretory agents and are listed in Table 31-5. Sucralfate, the aluminum salt of sulfated sucrose, not only binds to ulcers but also increases the gastric mucous layer, thereby promoting healing processes. It has been shown to be equally efficacious when used with H_2 antagonists and antacids and is relatively devoid of side effects.

Misoprostol is a synthetic prostaglandin and may be used as a secondary therapy to prevent ulcers in patients taking NSAIDs. *H. pylori* is a species of gram-negative spiral bacteria sensitive to combination therapy with a variety of antibiotics. Laparoscopic repair is indicated when medical therapy is unsuccessful.

Gastric Ulcer Disease

Gastric ulcers develop as a result of degeneration of the stomach's mucosal barrier to gastric acid. In patients with this condition, normal acid secretion and hypochlorhydria are present, phenomena that differentiate this condition from duodenal ulcer disease. Pain and anorexia predispose the patient to metabolic derangements and weight loss. Surgery, consisting of antrectomy with pyloroplasty and vagotomy, is undertaken if the patient's condition does not respond to medical therapy.

Parietal-cell vagotomy is another surgical option. In this procedure, selective sectioning of vagal fibers of the gastric fundus and parietal cells is performed, but the fibers innervating the antrum are preserved. However, mixed results regarding the efficacy of the procedure have been reported.

Gastric Neoplastic Disease

Most gastric neoplasms are malignant. The incidence of these neoplasms according to type is adenocarcinoma, 95%; lymphoma, 4%; and leiomyosarcoma, 1%. Signs and symptoms, such as anorexia and weight loss, may occur late. They serve as poor prognostic indicators of curative surgical treatment because of probable metastases to adjacent peritoneal organs and structures.

Gastric carcinoma is treated primarily through either total or subtotal gastrectomy. In addition, omentectomy, lymph node dissection, and splenectomy are considered to depend on the extent of spread, the patient's condition, and the preference of the surgeon.[39]

Gastrinoma, a neoplasm arising from the pancreas or duodenum, releases overabundant quantities of gastrin, resulting in the secretion of massive quantities of hydrochloric acid from the parietal cells (Zollinger-Ellison syndrome). This condition is associated with severe, intractable ulcer pain. If other endocrine neoplasias are present (i.e., thyroid or parathyroid adenoma, pituitary adenoma, insulinoma), the condition is referred to as *multiple endocrine neoplasia type I.*

Definitive therapy for gastrinoma is surgical excision. During anesthetic induction for excision of gastrinoma, a rapid-sequence technique is recommended because of the likelihood of a large volume of stagnant, acidic intragastric fluid. Electrolyte and intravascular volume derangements (e.g., from severe diarrhea) should be anticipated and corrected before surgery. Attention should also be given to intraoperative monitoring of electrolyte and fluid balance. Hypokalemia and metabolic alkalosis are likely to be present if the patient has been vomiting and is dehydrated. Furthermore, preparations for the treatment of patients with

TABLE **31-5**	Proton Pump Inhibitors				
Generic Name	**Trade Name**	**Adult Dosage Range**	**Available Dosage Forms***	**Dose Adjustment in Renal Dysfunction**	**Drug Interactions and Comments**
Esomeprazole	Nexium	20 mg daily	Capsule: 20, 40 mg	No	Cefuroxime, cefpodoxime, digoxin, dihydropyridine calcium channel blockers, iron salts, itraconazole, ketoconazole, sucralfate
Lansoprazole	Prevacid	15-30 mg daily or bid	Capsule: 15, 30 mg	No	Same as esomeprazole plus theophylline
Omeprazole	Prilosec	20-40 mg daily or bid	Capsule: 10, 20, 40 mg	No	Same as esomeprazole plus benzodiazepines, cilostazol, citalopram, clarithromycin, cyclosporine, disulfiram, methotrexate, phenytoin, sulfonylureas, theophylline, warfarin
Pantoprazole	Protonix, Protonix IV	40-80 mg daily	Tablet: 40 mg Injection: 40 mg/vial	No	Same as esomeprazole
Rabeprazole	Aciphex	20 mg daily	Tablet: 20 mg	No	Same as esomeprazole plus cyclosporine

Data from Mosby's Drug Consult. St Louis: Mosby; 2007.
*All oral forms are delayed release.

known or suspected derangements in endocrine function must be included in the anesthetic plan, to include blood glucose monitoring, vigilance for and timely correction of swings in vital signs and physiologic parameters, maintenance of normothermia and normocarbia, maintenance of an appropriately anesthetized state, and maintenance of renal function.

Anesthetic Considerations in Gastric Disease
Patients undergoing surgery for gastric disease are generally either acutely ill and require emergency surgery, as in the case of a bleeding gastric ulcer, or stable and require elective surgical treatment of gastric carcinoma or intractable ulcer disease. Many procedures are performed laparoscopically. Acutely ill patients are more likely to be hemodynamically unstable and dehydrated. Elective surgical patients may have a variable degree of debilitation and anemia. Aspiration precautions in both groups are warranted during anesthesia.

Hypovolemia should be corrected with the administration of appropriate colloid, crystalloid, or blood products before the induction of anesthesia. Clinical anemia and coagulopathy should be corrected with packed red blood cells and appropriate blood products (FFP, cryoprecipitate, platelets). The degree to which invasive monitoring (i.e., that using a pulmonary artery catheter, central venous pressure line, or arterial line) is used is determined by the presence of preexisting, age-related, or acquired compromise in the function of other organ systems. Preparations for the perioperative transfusion of blood products must be undertaken before anesthesia and surgery. Potential postoperative complications include hemorrhage, hypovolemia, hypothermia, atelectasis, and ileus. A postoperative stay in the intensive care unit may be necessary.

The anesthetic technique used in gastrectomy may include preoperative epidural catheter placement for intraoperative use—for instance, as an adjunct to general endotracheal anesthesia. Postoperative analgesia is also administered through an epidural catheter.

Procedures other than total and partial gastrectomy performed for gastric disease include:
- Billroth I: resection of the distal stomach with reconstruction via end-to-end gastroduodenostomy
- Billroth II: resection of the distal stomach with reconstruction via end-to-side gastrojejunostomy
- Laparotomy with oversewing of the ulcer and application of an omental patch

Vagotomy is usually performed during gastric ulcer surgery to decrease gastric acid secretion.

Postgastrectomy Syndromes
Surgical procedures are undertaken for the treatment of peptic ulcer disease to reduce the acid-secreting capabilities while preserving antral function and the gastric reservoir of the stomach. Untoward side effects of these procedures may result from loss of pyloric sphincter function, loss of the stomach's reservoir function, and as a secondary result of parasympathetic denervation. These sequelae may occur in combination or alone and are termed *postgastrectomy syndromes*.

Recurrent ulcer disease after operation for duodenal ulcer is occasionally seen in patients in whom vagotomy has been performed without partial gastrectomy (e.g., antrectomy). Symptoms include onset of typical ulcer pain, and diagnostic confirmation is made through endoscopic examination. Other causes of recurrent ulcer disease may be an unrecognized gastrinoma, the presence of an excessively long afferent limb after gastroenterostomy, or the retention of acid-secreting antral tissue at the duodenal stump (causing hypergastrinemia). Initial treatment is with H_2-receptor blocking agents, followed by repeat vagotomy with antrectomy if medical interventions fail.[39]

In the most commonly occurring postgastrectomy syndrome, early postprandial dumping occurs. The syndrome consists of gastrointestinal signs and symptoms that include nausea, cramping abdominal pain, weakness, and explosive diarrhea occurring within the first half hour after ingestion of a meal. Diaphoresis, dizziness, flushing, and palpitations indicate vasomotor instability. The syndrome results from rapid gastric emptying of hyperosmolar chyme from the residual stomach into the small intestine. Osmotic movement of fluid from the extracellular spaces into the intestine to achieve isotonicity is theorized to be responsible for the vasomotor aberrations that occur in patients with the syndrome. Increased proximal small-intestine hormone release brought about by distention probably accounts for the other clinical signs; this hormone release induces facial flushing, increased small-intestine motility, and explosive diarrhea. Many patients with this syndrome may be treated effectively without surgery. In other patients, surgery may be necessary, including revision of the gastroenterostomy, typically to a Roux-en-Y reconstruction. A Roux-en-Y gastroenterostomy provides a peristaltic conduit for drainage of pancreatic and biliary secretions into the jejunum and significantly attenuates the incidence of reflux.[39]

Late postprandial dumping syndrome occurs less commonly than early postprandial syndrome. Diaphoresis, tremulousness, and dizziness usually occur 1 to 3 hours after ingestion of a high-carbohydrate meal. The symptoms occur secondary to rapid gastric emptying and absorption of a high-carbohydrate load in the intestine, with resultant hyperglycemia. Overshoot of insulin release occurs in response to the development of hypoglycemia. Symptoms similar to insulin shock may become clinically manifest. Treatment is primarily medical.

Intermittent or complete obstruction of the afferent limb of a gastroenteric anastomosis (as seen in gastrectomy with a Billroth II reconstruction) may result in distention of the loop and a subsequent increase in hepatobiliary and pancreatic secretion. This condition, termed *afferent loop syndrome*, occurs after ingestion of a meal and is relieved by projectile, bilious vomiting. The vomitus typically lacks ingested food content because the food passes into the intestine and is absorbed. Definitive treatment of this condition is surgical reconstruction of the afferent limb, that is, creation of a long-limb Roux-en-Y.

Excessive reflux may occur from the intestinal tract into the stomach after gastrectomy and gastroenterostomy. A high incidence of excessive reflux is seen after gastrojejunostomy. Signs and symptoms include epigastric pain, bilious vomiting, anemia, and weight loss. Under these circumstances, conversion of the previous reconstruction to a Roux-en-Y has a high success rate.

Anesthetic considerations for postgastrectomy syndrome must include a thorough appreciation of the patient's nutritional and metabolic status. Involvement of the stomach remnant in the disease process may result in pernicious anemia due to insufficient secretion of intrinsic factor, the glycoprotein required for vitamin B_{12} absorption. Measures for the prevention of aspiration (i.e., full-stomach precautions) should be in effect perioperatively. Aggressive preoperative and intraoperative fluid and electrolyte replacement may be necessary and should be anticipated.

Signs and symptoms similar to those seen in postgastrectomy syndrome are consistent with complications associated with bariatric surgical procedures. For example, patients who have a history of previous laparoscopic bariatric surgery may present for open laparotomy Roux-en-Y revision, for bowel resection, or for relief of biliary duct obstruction. Surgery of a more urgent or emergent nature may be required for signs and symptoms of acute abdominal disease attributed to perforation or ischemia. The anesthetic management of the patient who has a history of uncomplicated bariatric surgery, as well as for the patient presenting for surgery secondary to complications of bariatric surgery, should always be guided by aspiration precautions and those considerations consistent with anesthetic management of the morbidly obese.

Gastrostomy

Gastrostomy consists of the surgical placement of a tube through the abdominal wall for the purpose of gastric decompression and nutritional support. Patients who require placement of a gastrostomy tube (permanent or temporary) are often neurologically incapacitated or otherwise markedly debilitated and are likely to have compromised command of their airway reflexes. This situation places them at greater risk for aspiration.

Gastrostomy placement is performed percutaneously at the bedside, in the endoscopy suite, or in the operating room. Endoscopic guidance is used with percutaneous placement of the gastrostomy tube. This may also be accomplished through a small laparotomy incision. A gastrostomy tube may be placed as an additional procedure in the course of laparotomy for resection for either temporary or permanent postoperative nutritional support. As a primary procedure, gastrostomy placement is commonly undertaken with sedation and local anesthetic site infiltration. General endotracheal anesthesia is indicated in patients who require laparotomy in conjunction with endoscopic placement and in those for whom percutaneous placement under local anesthesia with sedation may be contraindicated (e.g., the comatose patient).

PERITONEUM

The peritoneum consists of two double-layered sheets of cells with separately derived neural innervation. The visceral peritoneum is adherent to the intraabdominal organs, with the parietal peritoneum covering the inner surface of the abdominal wall. Innervation of the visceral peritoneum consists of autonomic sympathetic and parasympathetic fibers. Pain perceived is nonspecific, dull, and cramping and is mediated by C fibers. Parietal visceral innervation derives from somatic spinal fibers originating at levels T7 through L2. Pain transmitted is sharp and exquisite, mediated by A delta fibers.

Most intraabdominal organs are insensitive to many forms of stimulation (e.g., cutting, electrical), except for distention, stretch, torsion, and compression. Ischemic and inflammatory pain may be diffuse and indistinct. Only when visceral stimulation becomes transmural or affects the parietal peritoneum does pain become localized. Because a common nerve plexus is shared, pain from visceral structures may be referred to another intraperitoneal region. An example is seen in pain originating from the kidneys, ureters, or bladder. These structures have not only visceral autonomic innervation but also fibers from the celiac plexus, the thoracic and lumbar splanchnic nerves, and the intermesenteric and superior hypogastric plexus.[40]

Peritonitis

The peritoneal circulation cleans contaminants from the peritoneal cavity but may also facilitate transmission of pathologic substances to other regions of the abdomen. The peritoneum is secretory, hence the role it serves in the development of ascites and its utility in peritoneal dialysis. Only the surface of the diaphragm is absorptive. Ventilatory mechanics power fluid absorption via lacunae (channels of small openings) into subphrenic lymphatic channels. In this manner, pathologic processes, including dissemination of infectious and metastatic substances, may occur.

Under normal conditions the peritoneum is considered a sterile environment. Peritonitis (inflammation of the peritoneal cavity) signals a disruption in normal peritoneal barrier function and may be either primary or secondary. Primary peritonitis is the rarer of the two types, with immunocompromised individuals and those with cirrhotic liver disease at highest risk. Primary peritonitis follows direct bacterial contamination of the peritoneum; usually due to exudation across a compromised gut wall. Secondary peritonitis is usually a result of soiling due to perforation of the gut, with translocation of bacterial flora and toxins. Pathology responsible for secondary peritonitis includes inflammation and neoplasia, resulting in ischemia and necrosis, as well as traumatic gut and peritoneal perforation.[41]

DISEASES OF THE INTESTINAL TRACT

Anatomic and Physiologic Overview of the Small Intestine

The small intestine has three functional anatomic and physiologic subdivisions. In adults the first division, the duodenum, has a length of approximately 20 cm. The duodenum is followed by the second division, the jejunum, which has a length of approximately 100 to 110 cm. The third and longest division of the small intestine is the ileum, which has a length of approximately 150 to 160 cm. The jejunoileum extends from the ligament of Treitz (at the duodenojejunal junction) to the ileocecal valve. The jejunum is larger and thicker than the ileum and possesses a less extensive blood supply (one or two vascular networks versus four or five in the ileum).[42]

The mesentery, which is rich in lymphatics and blood vessels, tethers the small intestine. The superior mesenteric artery provides the primary arterial supply to the jejunum and ileum and to the proximal transverse colon. The mesentery supplies a vast network of collateral arterial supply as well. Venous drainage is primarily furnished by the superior mesenteric vein. This vessel joins the splenic vein posterior to the pancreas, which is joined into the portal vein. Lymphatic drainage from the bowel wall originates from the central bowel wall lacteal and continues through the superior mesenteric nodes into the cisterna chyli and ultimately the thoracic duct.

Histologic composition of the small bowel consists of a serosal outermost layer that is composed of visceral peritoneum. This layer is formed in the jejunum, ileum, and anterior duodenum. The muscular layer is made up of an outer longitudinal layer and a thin circular layer, both composed of smooth muscle. The Auerbach (myenteric) plexus, which primarily controls gastrointestinal motility, lies between the two muscular layers. The strongest component of the bowel wall is the submucosa, which consists of fibroelastic connective tissue. Within it lies the Meissner plexus, which controls local blood flow and gastrointestinal secretions. The innermost layer, the mucosa, is composed of transverse folds with millions of villi. These intraluminal projections greatly increase the absorptive surface of the small intestine.

The mucosa is further subdivided into three distinct layers:
1. Muscularis mucosae. The deepest layer, composed of a thin muscular sheet.
2. Lamina propria: A continuous connective tissue layer between the muscularis mucosae and the epithelium. This layer serves as a support epithelium and immunogenic barrier. Constituents of this layer include plasma cells, macrophages, fibroblasts, lymphocytes, eosinophils, and smooth muscle.
3. Epithelial layer. Covers the villi and lines the Lieberkühn crypts (which contain mucus-producing goblet cells, enterochromaffin [endocrine] cells, zymogen granules [Paneth cells], and basal undifferentiated cells). Cell turnover takes 3 to 7 days. The villi contain goblet, absorptive, and endocrine cells. Absorptive cells contain digestive enzymes and specific absorption receptors.[42]

Innervation of the small intestine is essentially parasympathetic through the vagus nerve and celiac ganglia. Parasympathetic stimulation is responsible for motility and secretion. Splanchnic nerves from the celiac plexus provide sympathetic innervation, which controls secretion, vascular integrity, and bowel motility. Sympathetic nerve tracts are also responsible for carrying afferent pain impulses. Physiologic functions of the small intestine are summarized in Box 31-3.

The intestinal mucosa provides a barrier to the entry of pathogens. The lamina propria provides a rich reservoir of IgA (the secretory immunoglobulin) and plasma cells (responsible for synthesis of IgA). IgA antigen binding initiates mucus secretion, which prevents intestinal bacterial and viral uptake. Furthermore, IgA binds with, incapacitates, and facilitates enzymatic destruction of bacteria. Binding with and preventing entry of toxins is another role of IgA. Lymphocytes, which are instrumental in the elaboration of a specific antibody to a given antigen, are found in Peyer patches, which are located in the intestinal wall.[42]

The mucosa of the small intestine provides a rich supply of hormones that regulate gastrointestinal function (Table 31-6).

A basic electrical rhythm in the longitudinal smooth muscle layer initiates action potentials in the circular muscular layers of the small intestine after feeding. This activity sets forth the muscular contractions that constitute small-bowel motility. Both segmental contractions, which mix chyme with digestive enzymes and expose it to absorptive surfaces, and peristaltic (propulsive) contractions are noted.

Autonomic functions have a major influence on intestinal motility. Sympathetic influence generally inhibits motility, whereas parasympathetic activity increases it. The intestinal inhibitory reflex responds to abnormal distention by decreasing motility proximal to the locus of distention. This reflex may have significant indirect clinical implications (e.g., aspiration risk).[42]

Malabsorption Syndromes

Numerous disorders of the small intestine manifest as derangements in absorption. Primary clinical signs include unexplained weight loss, steatorrhea, and diarrhea. These disorders affect the absorption of the major constituents of ingested nutrients, including amino acids, carbohydrates, and fats. Gluten-sensitive enteropathy is a disorder of malabsorption formerly referred to as *celiac sprue* and *tropical sprue*. It is characterized by the eventual development of megaloblastic anemia, fatigue, and weight loss and is managed through regulation of the diet (i.e., removal of dietary gluten) and administration of steroids (i.e., prednisone).

BOX 31-3

Synopsis of Physiologic Functions (Digestion and Absorption) of the Small Intestine

Protein
Initiated in the stomach
Completed in the duodenum and jejunum; further hydrolysis (via intracellular peptidases) of peptides to free amino acids occurs before entry into the portal vein (approximately 90% of intact peptides)

Carbohydrates
Initiated by salivary amylase
Digested by pancreatic amylase in the duodenum; absorption completed by brush border of the intestinal microvilli (through conversion of monosaccharides into absorbable hexoses)

Fats
Digestion and absorption of lipid (primarily triglycerides) occurs almost entirely in the small intestine by two processes:
• Lipolysis
• Formation of micelles
Facilitated by pancreatic bicarbonate and bile salts

Water and Electrolytes
10 L of water enters small bowel daily; most of this volume is absorbed
Net absorption of water facilitated primarily via osmosis; another mechanism involves passive diffusion through luminal pores under the influence of hydrostatic pressure
Sodium absorption occurs essentially in conjunction with bulk flow of water (primarily in the jejunum); this process occurs with concomitant hydrogen ion extrusion
Bicarbonate secretion and chloride ion absorption occur in conjunction with sodium absorption
Electrical neutrality is maintained
Calcium ion absorption (facilitated by an acidic environment) occurs primarily in the duodenum and jejunum via active transport; enhanced by vitamin D and parathyroid hormone
Passive potassium absorption occurs primarily in the jejunum
Absorption of iron occurs primarily in the duodenum

Other Vitamins and Minerals
Ascorbic acid—absorbed in the ileum and coupled to sodium
Cobalamin (vitamin B_{12})—absorbed in the distal ileum and linked to glycoprotein carrier molecules (especially intrinsic factor)
Folate—absorbed in the proximal jejunum in conjunction with sodium
Biotin—absorbed in the proximal small bowel as a result of sodium-linked active transport
Thiamine (vitamin B_1)—absorbed predominantly in the duodenum
Vitamin B_6—absorbed in the proximal small bowel
Niacin, pantothenate, and riboflavin—absorbed passively (mechanism incompletely understood)

Modified from Evers BM et al. Small intestine. In: Schwartz SI, et al, eds. Principles of Surgery. 7th ed. New York: McGraw-Hill; 1999:1217-1229.

Complications of gluten-sensitive enteropathy include small-bowel ulceration and a predisposition to malignancy, as well as megaloblastic anemia, fatigue, and weight loss. Treatment of this disorder is with administration of folic acid and antibiotics.[3]

Fat malabsorption results in deficiency of fat-soluble vitamins (vitamins A, D, E, and K). Deficiency in vitamin K manifests through hypoprothrombinemia. This condition is often evidenced through bleeding dyscrasias. Vitamin B_{12} deficiency results in anemia (which may also be encountered in patients with impaired iron absorption), neuropathy, and glossitis. Protein malabsorption may result in the development of peripheral edema and ascites. Tetany, osteomalacia, and pathologic fractures result from calcium deficiency caused by vitamin D malabsorption.[39]

The cause of malabsorption syndromes is multifactorial. The basic underlying defect is either disruption of intestinal mucosal integrity, such as from disease processes, or loss of absorptive surface area caused by extensive surgical resection of the small intestine (i.e., short gut syndrome). With regard to alterations in small-intestine absorption secondary to surgical resection, the particular part of the small bowel resected and the amount removed have a significant bearing on the degree to which deficiencies in minerals, vitamins, and electrolytes are clinically manifested.

Maldigestion Syndromes
Maldigestion syndromes are generally caused by derangements or deficiencies in pancreatic secretion. Diseases more likely to result in malabsorption syndromes may be differentiated from those responsible for maldigestion. The hallmark of maldigestion is steatorrhea. Significant pancreatic disease is usually present when a maldigestion syndrome exists, because the pancreas has a large functional reserve in both normal and disease states. Chronic pancreatitis is the major and most common cause of pancreatic insufficiency. Cystic fibrosis, fistulas, gallstones, ischemic enteritis, and neoplastic disease processes, however, are also etiologic factors.[42]

Anatomic and Physiologic Considerations of the Large Colon
The large colon is approximately 3 to 5 feet long and may be recognized not only by its size and position but also by the presence of three strips of longitudinal muscle and the numerous outpouchings (haustrations) throughout its length. The arterial supply comprises the superior mesenteric artery (which perfuses the right to the midtransverse colon), the inferior mesenteric artery (which perfuses the midtransverse colon to the superior rectum), and the internal iliac artery (which perfuses the middle and lower rectum). Venous drainage parallels arterial drainage, with the middle and superior veins contributing to the portal venous system. Sympathetic innervation is derived from T10 to T12 (right colon), L1 to L3 (left colon), and the presacral nerves arising within the preaortic plexuses (rectum). Parasympathetic innervation is primarily from the vagus nerve (right and transverse colon) and from nerve fibers arising from S2 to S4 (descending colon, sigmoid colon, and rectum). A rich endowment of lymphatics is present throughout the length of the colon and rectum.

The primary function of the large colon is to store and expel waste products. Another function performed largely in the right colon is the absorption of sodium and water. Most of the 1 to 2 L of ileal effluent presented to the large colon per day is absorbed, with the exception of 100 to 200 mL.

TABLE 31-6 Gastrointestinal Hormones

Hormone	Location	Major Stimulants of Peptide Secretion	Primary Effects	Diagnostic and Therapeutic Uses
Gastrin	Antrum, duodenum (G cells)	Peptides, amino acids, antral distention, vagal and adrenergic stimulation, gastrin-releasing peptide (bombesin)	Stimulates gastric acid and pepsinogen secretion; stimulates gastric mucosal growth	Gastrin analog (pentagastrin) used to measure maximal gastric acid secretion
CCK	Duodenum, jejunum (I cells)	Fats, peptides, amino acids	Stimulates pancreatic enzyme secretion; stimulates gallbladder contraction; relaxes sphincter of Oddi; inhibits gastric emptying	Biliary imaging of gallbladder concentration
Secretin	Duodenum, jejunum (S cells)	Fatty acids, luminal acidity, bile salts	Stimulates release of water and bicarbonate from pancreatic ductal cells; stimulates flow and alkalinity of bile; inhibits gastric acid secretion and motility and inhibits gastrin release	Provocative test for gastrinoma; measurement of maximal pancreatic secretion
Somatostatin	Pancreatic islet (D cells), antrum, duodenum	Gut: Fat, protein, acid, other hormones (e.g., gastrin, CCK) Pancreas: Glucose, amino acids, CCK	Universal "off" switch; stimulates release of all GI secretion and motility; stimulates gastric acid secretion and release of antral gastrin; stimulates growth of intestinal mucosa and pancreas	Treatment of carcinoid; diarrhea and flushing; decreases secretion from intestinal fistulas (particularly pancreatic fistulas); ameliorates symptoms associated with hormone overproducing endocrine tumors; treatment of esophageal variceal bleeding
Gastrin-releasing peptide (mammalian equivalent of bombesin)	Small bowel	Vagal stimulation	Universal "on" switch; stimulates release of all GI hormones (except secretin); stimulates GI secretin; stimulates growth of intestinal mucosa and pancreas	
Gastric inhibitory polypeptide	Duodenum, jejunum (K cells)	Glucose, fat, protein adrenergic stimulation	Inhibits gastric acid and pepsin secretion; stimulates pancreatic insulin release in response to hyperglycemia	
Motilin	Duodenum, jejunum	Gastric distention, fat	Stimulates upper GI tract motility; may initiate the migrating motor complex	
Vasoactive intestinal peptide	Neurons throughout GI tract	Vagal stimulation	Primarily functions as a neuropeptide; potent vasodilator	
Neurotensin	Small bowel (N cells)	Fat	Stimulates pancreatic and intestinal secretion; inhibits gastric acid secretion; stimulates growth of small and large bowel mucosa	
Enteroglucagon	Small bowel (L cells)	Glucose, fat	Glucagon-like peptide-1: stimulates insulin release; inhibits pancreatic glucagon release; Glucagon-like peptide-2: potent enterotropic factor	
Peptide YY	Distal small bowel, colon	Fatty acids, CCK	Inhibits gastric and pancreatic secretions; inhibits gallbladder contraction	

From Evers BM. Small intestine. In: Townsend CM et al, eds. Sabiston Textbook of Surgery: The Biological Basis of Modern Surgical Practice. 18th ed. Philadelphia: Saunders; 2008:1287.
CCK, Cholecystokinin; GI, gastrointestinal.

TABLE 31-7	Diagnosis of Crohn's Colitis versus Ulcerative Colitis	
Observation	**Crohn's Colitis**	**Ulcerative Colitis**
Symptoms and Signs		
Diarrhea	Common	Common
Rectal bleeding	Less common	Almost always
Abdominal pain (cramps)	Moderate to severe	Mild to moderate
Palpable mass	At times	No (unless large cancer)
Anal complaints	Frequent (>50%)	Infrequent (<20%)
Radiologic Findings		
Ileal disease	Common	Rare (backwash ileitis)
Nodularity, fuzziness	No	Yes
Distribution	Skip areas	Rectum extending upward and continuously
Ulcers	Linear, cobblestone, fissures	Collar-button
Toxic dilation	Rare	Uncommon
Proctoscopic Findings		
Anal fissure, fistula, abscess	Common	Rare
Rectal sparing	Common (50%)	Rare (5%)
Granular mucosa	No	Yes
Ulceration	Linear, deep, scattered	Superficial, universal

From Evers MB. Small intestine. In: Townsend CM et al, eds. Sabiston Textbook of Surgery: The Biological Basis of Modern Surgical Practice. 18th ed. Philadelphia: Saunders; 2008:1302.

Sodium absorption occurs through active transport against a gradient and is enhanced by minerals, corticoids, glucocorticoids, and fatty acids that are produced by indigenous bacteria. Potassium is passively absorbed and secreted, whereas chloride is absorbed in exchange for bicarbonate. Potassium is lost through passive diffusion in the colonic mucoid secretions. Significant potassium loss is likely to occur, therefore, in the presence of colitis and villous adenoma, two disease processes notable for mucoid stools. The colon is also involved in the enterohepatic circulation of bile acids (the greater degree of which occurs in the ileum). The colonic role in this process assumes greater importance in the presence of ileal disease or decreased ileal absorptive area. Conversion of primary bile acids to secondary bile acids also occurs in the colon.[43]

Conservation of sodium is so efficient in the large colon that a normal individual may require only 5 mEq/day in order to remain in sodium balance. Therefore, the presence of an ileostomy necessitates a greater intake of sodium (80 to 100 mEq/day) to approximate the high sodium content present as ileal effluent. The loss of the normal colonic reabsorption of sodium chloride and water (e.g., after colectomy) may eventually exceed the small intestine's capacity to increase absorption; clinical derangements in electrolyte balance follow.[41]

Inflammatory Bowel Disease

In the United States, between 200,000 and 300,000 individuals have inflammatory bowel disease, and approximately 30,000 new cases are diagnosed each year.[44] The two major types of inflammatory bowel disease are Crohn's disease and ulcerative colitis, which have different clinical features and manifestations (Table 31-7).

Crohn's disease involves primarily the distal ileum and large colon in approximately 50% of patients. The remainder of patients experience disease localized to either the colon or portions of the small intestine (regional enteritis). The deeper layers of the intestinal mucosa are typically involved, a situation that leads to derangements in colonic absorption. Owing to the loss of functional absorptive surfaces in the large colon, patients with Crohn's disease are often deficient in magnesium, phosphorus, zinc, and potassium. They also have deficiencies secondary to the loss of absorptive capability in portions of the small intestine. Protein-losing enteropathy is often encountered, as is anemia resulting from occult blood loss and deficiencies in vitamin B_{12} and folic acid. Iron deficiency secondary to insufficient intestinal absorption also contributes to development of an anemic state. Involvement of the distal ileum in the disease process results in deficiencies in vitamin B_{12} and nutrients dependent on bile acids for absorption. Disturbance in the enterohepatic circulation of bile in the terminal ileum is reflected in complex nutrient deficiencies, including proteins, zinc, magnesium, phosphorus, fat-soluble vitamins, and vitamin B_{12}. This state is typical of patients with chronic Crohn's disease. Folate deficiency may also be present in patients who receive sulfasalazine preparations.

Fistulas often develop between inflamed portions of the intestine and adjacent abdominal structures. Abdominal and pelvic abscesses, rectocutaneous fistulas, and perirectal abscesses have a high incidence in these patients. Increased calcium oxalate absorption in the terminal ileum frequently occurs, resulting in a high rate of renal calculi and cholelithiasis.[45,46]

Medical therapy for Crohn's disease includes a variety of drugs and is given in Box 31-4.

Surgery is warranted when medical treatment fails or when complications supervene. Although effective in the relief of complications, surgical resection of the diseased colon and ileum does not alter the progression of the disease. The primary principle of surgical management is to limit the operation to the

BOX 31-4

Agents Used to Treat Crohn's Disease

Agent

5-Aminosalicylates (5-ASAs)
Sulfasalazine
Sulfa-free (mesalamine, olsalazine, balsalazide)

Antibiotics
Metronidazole
Ciprofloxacin

Glucocorticoids
Classic
Novel (controlled ileal-release budesonide)

Immune Modulators
6-Mercaptopurine, azathioprine
Methotrexate
Cyclosporine

Biologic Response Modifiers
Infliximab

Sands BE. Crohn's disease. In: Feldman M et al, eds. Sleisenger & Fordtran's Gastrointestinal and Liver Disease. 8th ed. Philadelphia: Saunders; 2006:2480.

correction of the presenting complication, which could include bowel obstruction, fistulas, abscesses, and symptoms that indicate widespread symptomatic disease (for which total colectomy and ileal resection may be warranted).

Most patients with Crohn's disease undergo surgery, and a large number require repeat or continued procedures. The recurrence rate at 10 years after surgery is 50%. A high likelihood of repeat surgery involves areas of the remaining bowel proximal to the area of a previous anastomosis. Patients with a history of Crohn's disease are also shown to have a higher prevalence of bowel carcinoma.[47]

Ulcerative colitis is an inflammatory disease, primarily of the mucosa of the rectum and distal colon. It is a chronic disease that is fraught with remissions and exacerbations. It affects female patients more frequently than male patients and has a bimodal age distribution that shows a first peak incidence between ages 15 and 20 years and a second smaller peak between ages 55 and 60 years. The disorder is speculated to have a strong familial genetic predisposition, but psychologic factors have also been implicated in its cause.

Symptoms usually include abdominal pain, fever, and bloody diarrhea. Ulcerative colitis is typically chronic, with relatively low-grade symptoms, such as bloody stools, malaise, diarrhea, and pain. In approximately 15% of patients, however, ulcerative colitis that has acute, fulminating characteristics may occur. Under this circumstance, severe abdominal pain, profuse rectal hemorrhage, and high fever are seen. Associated symptoms include nausea and vomiting, anorexia, and profound weakness. Physical signs usually include pallor and weight loss.

Associated with an acute onset of fulminating ulcerative colitis is toxic megacolon, which is characterized by severe colonic distention that causes shock. In patients with this condition, the distended bowel lumen provides an environment conducive to bacterial overgrowth. This condition, coupled with erosive intestinal inflammation and perforation, allows for the systemic release of bacteria-produced toxins. Clinical signs and symptoms of toxic megacolon include fever, tachycardia, abdominal distention, pain, ileus, and dehydration. Electrolyte derangements, anemia, and hypoalbuminemia are also commonly present.[47]

Patients with ulcerative colitis are at increased risk for the development of carcinoma of the colon. An increased incidence of large-joint arthritis is seen in patients when the disease is clinically active. Concomitant liver disease, as evidenced by fatty infiltrates and pericholangitis, may also complicate the clinical picture. Other extracolonic manifestations of ulcerative colitis include iritis, erythema nodosum, and ankylosing spondylitis.[47]

Therapy for ulcerative colitis is initially medical. As with Crohn's disease, sulfasalazine preparations, antidiarrheal agents, and corticosteroids are the cornerstones of medical therapy. Both Crohn's disease and ulcerative colitis result in systemic disorders such as anemia and nutritional deficiencies, which are handled in the same supportive manner. In both diseases, surgical resection is reserved for patients with intractable complications. Whereas surgery for Crohn's disease is nondefinitive and complication oriented, proctocolectomy with ileostomy is generally curative for ulcerative colitis.[47]

Anesthetic Considerations in Inflammatory Bowel Disease

Anesthetic management of patients with inflammatory bowel disease begins with a thorough, systematic patient history, and particular attention is paid to the patient's fluid and electrolyte status. Possible extracolonic complications (e.g., sepsis, liver disease, anemia, arthritis, hypoalbuminemia, and other metabolic derangements) must also be considered during planning and perioperative management. Efforts to optimize the medical condition of such patients before elective surgery are strongly recommended.

Prophylactic steroid coverage is likely to be indicated, particularly in patients receiving long-term steroid therapy. Inclusion of nitrous oxide in anesthesia delivery should be reconsidered, with the possibility of bowel distention associated with its prolonged intraoperative use. Awareness of complications from parenteral nutritional therapy (e.g., hyperglycemia or hypoglycemia, increased carbon dioxide production, renal or hepatic dysfunction, nonketotic hyperosmolar hyperglycemic coma, and hyperchloremic metabolic acidosis) is also necessary for patients receiving total or partial parenteral nutritional support. Administration of a preexistent parenteral nutritional support infusion should be maintained throughout the perioperative period at the ordered infusion rate. Periodic laboratory assessment of metabolic status (i.e., serum glucose and electrolytes) should be performed and guide corrective interventions for detected derangements. The severity of extracolonic influence on the function of other organ systems dictates appropriate technique and drug selection, as well as the extent to which invasive monitoring is used. Correction of fluid, electrolyte, and hematologic derangements may be necessary before surgery. Increased intraluminal pressure caused by the administration of anticholinesterases for reversal of neuromuscular blockade has been shown to have no effect on colonic suture lines. No particular anesthetic technique is mandated; however, the use of a combined technique (epidural and general anesthesia) is attractive for both intraoperative use and postoperative analgesia needs.[47,48]

Diverticulitis and Diverticulosis

Diverticulosis of the colon is characterized by the presence of numerous mucosal outpouchings in the large colon, with the highest prevalence noted in the sigmoid colon (65%). Structural weakness of the colonic wall and increased intracolonic pressures are two mechanisms theorized to be responsible for the development of diverticulosis. Diverticulitis is inflammation of diverticula; this syndrome manifests as abdominal pain with ileus and other symptoms that indicate an acute abdomen, such as nausea, vomiting, rigid abdominal distention, and dehydration. Inflamed diverticula may be localized or more widespread and may involve the mesentery and other abdominal organs. Abscess formation and visceral perforation indicate the need for urgent surgical intervention.

Surgical treatment of diverticulosis is reserved for symptoms that are refractory to aggressive medical therapy. Intravenous corticosteroids, antibiotics, and fluid replacement are attempted initially. Exploratory laparotomy with colectomy may be necessary under emergent conditions of acute bleeding, recurrent bleeding that fails to cease spontaneously, or sepsis. The goals of surgical exploration include fecal diversion and abscess drainage, as well as resection of the diseased colon.

Complications of diverticulitis, which occur in up to 25% of patients, frequently necessitate surgical intervention. Such complications include bowel obstruction, fistulas, and abscesses. Abscess formation after colonic obstruction and perforation may involve such structures as the abdominal wall and the subdiaphragmatic spaces. Abscess formation may be extensive; it may include the deep pelvic organs and the hip and thigh.

Diverticulitis occurs in only 1% of patients with diverticulosis. Clinical symptoms of diverticulitis include abdominal pain, diarrhea, and fever. Progression of symptoms may lead to hypovolemia, hypokalemia, and shock. The presence of free intraperitoneal air, as evidenced on radiographic abdominal films, suggests perforation. Air in the retroperitoneum may be indicative of paracolic abscess. Both conditions require urgent surgical exploration.

Bleeding is uncommon in patients with diverticular disease, but when present, it often defies localization through endoscopy and even laparotomy. A bleeding diathesis in diverticular disease may be either occult or massive and is caused by erosion of the vessels adjacent to the diverticulum. Elective colon resection is usually considered in patients with recurrent episodes of acute diverticulitis. After a second attack of acute diverticulitis, the prevalence of complications associated with the disease approaches 50%, and the associated mortality rate is twice that of an initial attack. Diverticulitis, when present in the right colon or cecum, often mimics acute appendicitis. Surgery for appendectomy, therefore, may uncover the presence of an inflamed diverticulum or diverticulitis, necessitating extension of the procedure so that colonic resection can be performed.

In middle-aged and elderly patients, the clinical symptoms of diverticulitis may also be confused with those of Crohn's colitis. Some indications for surgery (e.g., obstruction and abscess) are similar in both diseases. Examination of the resected specimen differentiates the diagnoses. The patient may therefore be spared ineffective medical therapy for inflammatory bowel disease when a segmental colonic resection is potentially curative.[48]

Abdominal Compartment Syndrome

Increased abdominal pressure imposes profound effects on the circulation and systemic perfusion. Normal intraabdominal pressure is less than 10 mm Hg. At 10 mm Hg, hepatic arterial blood flow significantly decreases. Cardiovascular perturbations occur at 15 mm Hg. Oliguria occurs at 15 to 20 mm Hg and anuria at 40 mm Hg. The etiology of abdominal compartment syndrome (ACS) is multifactorial. Resuscitative efforts and exposure of the open abdomen induces mesenteric edema formation and bowel dilatation. Under these conditions, attenuation and prevention of worsening ischemic injury to the abdominal viscera are avoided through delayed closure until gross abdominal distention is resolved. Examples of conditions contributing to the development of acute ACS include intestinal obstruction, mesenteric arterial thrombosis, ruptured abdominal aortic aneurysm, and blunt or perforating abdominal trauma. Causes of chronic ACS include ascites, pregnancy, and intraabdominal tumors.

Cardiac output is decreased secondary to decreased cardiac preload (venous return), elevated systemic vascular resistance, and elevated intrathoracic pressure. Reflex tachycardia is a baroceptor-mediated response to decreased preload, with resultant diminished diastolic filling and coronary perfusion. Decreased thoracic compliance and decreased lung volumes result from impaired diaphragmatic descent. The outcome is increased pulmonary shunt fraction and atelectasis. Impairment in renal function results from compression of the kidney and diminished glomerular perfusion.

Treatment of ACS is undertaken urgently with decompressive laparotomy. Affected patients often have myriad medical problems that may significantly influence outcome. The possibility of ACS subsequent to resuscitative "damage-control" laparotomy used in the traumatically injured patient is always a consideration. Under this circumstance, immediate life-threatening injuries are primarily addressed, then the patient is returned to the operating room from the intensive care unit at a later date. This occurs after a period in which hemodynamic stabilization is accomplished. Definitive repairs of associated, less life-threatening injuries are then undertaken, often in stages. During this time, the abdomen may be left open but packed and sealed with sterile dressings, along with a drainage appliance to resolve post-resuscitation intraabdominal edema. The patient may undergo repeated returns to the operating room for dressing changes until conditions are conducive for abdominal wound closure. Providing anesthesia care for these patients can be extremely challenging. Intraoperative monitoring is directed toward maintenance of hemodynamic stability and includes knowledge of the patient's preoperative hemodynamic profile. If the patient is still receiving mechanical ventilatory support, it is of utmost importance to provide intraoperative ventilation as closely as possible to the mode being administered in the intensive care unit. This is particularly vital in the patient with adult respiratory distress syndrome (ARDS). This may require a modification of the anesthesia delivery ventilator to approximate as closely as possible the minute ventilation, FIO_2, I:E ratio, ventilatory rate, and level of positive end-expiratory pressure the patient has been receiving. In this way, the potential for perioperative deterioration of previously accomplished improvement in the patient's ventilatory status is minimized. Invasive monitors brought with the patient, such as an arterial line, central venous catheter, and pulmonary artery catheter, should be used for perioperative management. Opioids and inhalation agents are used with discretion in accordance with patient tolerance. Adequate muscle relaxation and amnesia with a benzodiazepine or scopolamine assume priority in the pharmacologic anesthetic management of the physiologically labile patient. Other vasoactive agents are included as indicated for hemodynamic support. Best practice caveats for the anesthetic management of these patients are provision of intraoperative stability and preservation of preoperative homeostatic compensation.[49]

Opening of the acute, hypertensive abdomen releases intraabdominal pressure and may have profound consequences on systemic perfusion. This results from release of the tamponade on a vast visceral vascular bed with a resultant reperfusion syndrome. Reperfusion washout of by-products of anaerobic metabolism releases an array of cardiac depressant and vasodilatory mediators into the general circulation. Proper preparation is mandated and includes optimization of intravascular volume, acid-base status, and arterial oxygenation.[49]

Mortality rate in ACS approaches 42%, with most patients succumbing to secondary systemic inflammatory response syndrome, sepsis, and multiple organ dysfunction syndrome. Other causes of death include respiratory failure (i.e., ARDS) and the consequences of added stress imposed on cardiac function in susceptible patients.[49]

Colonic Polyps

Colonic polyps are divided into two major groups: neoplastic (which includes the adenomas and carcinomas) and nonneoplastic. The adenomas and carcinomas share a common characteristic of cellular dysplasia. They may be subdivided according to the relative contribution of certain microscopic features. Non-neoplastic polyps may be grouped into several distinct categories, including hyperplastic polyps, mucosal polyps, juvenile polyps, inflammatory polyps, and others.[50]

Inflammatory polyps are typically small and have low potential for malignancy. The lesions are usually caused by chronic colitis. Hamartomatous polyps are usually small, juvenile polyps that have minor to nonexistent neoplastic potential (Peutz-Jeghers syndrome). Unclassified polypoid disorders include familial adenomatous polyposis coli. This disease is a genetic autosomal dominant disorder characterized by the presence of multiple adenomatous polyps. It has a very high neoplastic potential. Total colectomy with ileostomy is the treatment of choice in patients with this condition. Other familial polypoid disorders include Turcot syndrome (colonic polyps with central nervous system tumors) and Gardner syndrome (colonic polyposis with cutaneous tumors and osteosarcoma).

A common presenting sign in the diagnosis of polypoid colonic disease is painless frank or occult rectal bleeding. Such bleeding has the potential for causing anemia. Cramping abdominal pain may be present, particularly in children.

Anesthetic Considerations in Elective Surgery of the Colon

To prevent wound infection and facilitate healing of colorectal anastomoses, preoperative elimination of fecal mass and reduction of bacterial flora are undertaken, usually while the patient is in the hospital the evening before surgery or at home (by the patient) the night before admission. Lavage with isotonic and isosmotic solutions may be performed by the patient orally or instilled via nasogastric tube. Cleansing enemas may also be ordered. These techniques often are used for elective procedures in conjunction with dietary changes that emphasize the intake of fluids and low-residue foodstuffs and that culminate in the intake of only clear liquids for 24 to 48 hours before surgery. Intravenous and oral antibiotics used for bowel cleansing commonly include drugs of the aminoglycoside family (e.g., neomycin, erythromycin) and/or a combination of the cephalosporins and metronidazole.

The anesthetist must be aware of this preoperative preparation in patients who undergo elective surgery. Aggressive preoperative bowel preparation predisposes a patient to water and electrolyte imbalance that may have a deleterious influence on perioperative cardiovascular function, hemodynamics, and systemic organ perfusion, particularly if the patient is elderly or debilitated. Depending on the chronicity of the disease process, anemia resulting from frank or occult bleeding may be present. Malnutrition with hypoalbuminemia may also be present before surgery.

The presence of an adynamic colon or obstruction commonly necessitates evacuation of stagnant stomach and upper intestinal contents via nasogastric drainage. This preoperative intervention may be superimposed on a dehydrated patient or one who is electrolyte depleted. Fluid and electrolyte derangements therefore may be of sufficient magnitude to require postponement of the procedure until volume and electrolyte resuscitation has been accomplished.

Carcinoma of the Colon

Cancer of the colon is a highly treatable and often curable disease when localized to the bowel. It is the second most frequently diagnosed malignancy in the United States, as well as the second most common cause of cancer death. Surgery is the primary treatment and results in cure in approximately 50% of patients. Recurrence after surgery is a major problem and often is the ultimate cause of death. The prognosis of patients with colon cancer is clearly related to the degree of penetration of the tumor through the bowel wall and the presence or absence of nodal involvement.[44,51] Carcinoma of the colon accounts for approximately 60,000 deaths annually, and more than 140,000 new cases are diagnosed annually. The etiology is multifactorial and includes a strong correlation with diet (high red meat intake, low dietary fiber intake) and genetic predisposition. Inflammatory bowel disease is usually associated with a greater predisposition to colonic carcinoma. Occult stool testing for blood is a standard screening method. Rectal examination and colonoscopic examination with biopsy are important diagnostic modalities.

Right-sided colonic lesions often cause symptoms that may indicate the presence of an obstructive lesion because of their concentric characteristics. Right-sided lesions are also associated with a higher incidence of anemia and fatigue. Bleeding is usually less profuse than in patients with diverticular disease.[3]

Volvulus of the Colon

Obstruction of blood supply with subsequent necrosis may affect a given length of redundant bowel, which rotates and twists around the mesentery. This condition usually affects a freely mobile colonic segment and a fixed point or set of points about which the colon twists. Approximately 75% of colonic volvulus affects the sigmoid colon.[44,51]

Symptoms usually suggest the presence of acute bowel obstruction (e.g., acute, severe, colicky abdominal pain and distention). Acute strangulation of the bowel is suggested by generalized severe abdominal pain, hypovolemia, and fever. Initial therapy is attempted through endoscopic reduction via proctoscopy with rectal tube placement. This treatment has a high success rate (70% to 80%) and permits elective resection of the involved dysfunctional segment of the sigmoid colon with primary anastomosis at a later date. Failure of nonoperative detorsion necessitates surgical intervention. If gangrene is discovered on laparotomy, resection is carried out with the formation of an end colostomy and a mucous fistula (Hartmann procedure).[44,51]

Many patients with this condition are elderly or debilitated individuals and are referred from long-term care facilities. Associated disease processes include Alzheimer disease, Parkinson disease, multiple sclerosis, paralysis, pseudobulbar palsy, chronic schizophrenia, and dementia. Medications taken on a long-term basis by these patients may include neuropsychotropic drugs, which are known to alter bowel motility.

Pseudomembranous Colitis

Pseudomembranous colitis is associated with inflammatory bowel disease, uremia, intestinal ischemia, Hirschsprung disease, and shigellosis. It is characterized by mucosal exudate and plaque formation within the colon. It is also associated with antibiotic therapy, particularly with clindamycin and lincomycin.

Antibiotic-associated pseudomembranous colitis is usually caused by infection of the colonic mucosa caused by *Clostridium difficile* enterotoxin. Clinical manifestations include fever, diarrhea, abdominal pain, distention, and shock caused by dehydration and systemic bacterial dissemination.

Therapy begins with termination of the offending antibiotic. Supportive therapy and institution of antibiotic therapy (e.g., oral vancomycin, oral or parenteral metronidazole) directed against *C. difficile* often result in prompt clinical resolution. A 10% to 30% mortality rate is seen, however, in seriously ill patients.[50]

Ischemic Bowel Disease

Ischemic injury to the bowel occurs under numerous circumstances, including advanced atherosclerosis, shock, vasculitis, hypercoagulopathy, and amyloidosis. Surgical iatrogenic causes, such as interruption of the inferior mesenteric artery as a result of aortic cross-clamping during abdominal aortic surgery, are also culpable. Prolonged hemodynamic lability in patients with significant comorbidities such as advanced age, chronic diabetes, hypertension, and atherosclerotic disease places them at even greater risk for the consequences of ischemic bowel disease. The extent, severity, and prognosis of the syndrome of ischemic bowel disease are variable. Localized or segmental ischemia is often present. Differentiation of ischemic colitis from infectious processes, diverticulitis, or inflammatory bowel disease may be difficult. Definitive diagnosis depends on endoscopic examination with biopsy. Exclusion of bowel perforation in the differential diagnosis is made through radiographic or ultrasonographic examination of the abdomen for the presence of free air.

Patients with ischemic bowel disease are usually of advanced age. Symptoms typically include fever, vomiting, rectal bleeding, and abdominal cramping pain and may be present for weeks or months. The development of sudden rectal bleeding associated with left-sided abdominal pain and peritoneal signs strongly suggests the presence of this disease process. Concomitant ischemic heart disease and peripheral vascular disease are often present in these patients.[52] Supportive measures are initially undertaken if bowel necrosis is not suspected. This includes antibiotic therapy and fluid resuscitation. In patients in whom perforation or necrosis is suspected, emergency laparotomy is indicated, with possible bowel resection and temporary or permanent colostomy. Stable patients may be candidates for vascular reconstructive procedures.[3]

Diseases of the Rectum and Anus

Diseases of the anorectal region may include neoplastic lesions. If biopsy findings are consistent with localized adenocarcinoma, abdominal-perineal resection of the rectum and sigmoid colon with permanent colostomy may be curative. Squamous cell carcinomas of the rectum are effectively treated with chemotherapy and radiation, as well as local excision. Surgical proctectomy is another treatment option.

Other rectal diseases include rectal prolapse (repaired with rectosigmoidectomy or proctopexy), which is seen most often in the elderly. Perirectal disease may be manifested by abscess formation that requires drainage, which may be performed on either an inpatient or an outpatient basis.

Perirectal fistulas typically develop secondary to infectious disease processes that cause abscess formation. Four types are generally recognized: extrasphincteric, suprasphincteric, transsphincteric, and intersphincteric. Initial therapy is incision and drainage with delayed fistulectomy to facilitate healing of the abscess.

Hemorrhoidal disease is characterized by dilation of the perianal submucosal venous plexus. Internal hemorrhoids are often bleeding, prolapsed veins and generally painless. Treatment is usually by rubber band ligation or surgical excision. External hemorrhoids are associated with a greater tendency to thrombose and are typically painful. Surgical excision is the treatment of choice.[53]

Anesthesia for most perirectal and perianal procedures may be effectively provided by regional techniques such as spinal subarachnoid block or epidural blockade, as well as by local anesthesia infiltration with sedation. In some cases, general endotracheal anesthesia may be necessary. Anesthetic considerations must include the influence of patient position (e.g., prone or lithotomy position) on intraoperative cardiovascular and respiratory dynamics.

Radiation Enteritis

The colon is highly susceptible to radiation injury because of the normal rapid renewal of the intestinal epithelial lining. Radiation injury results from radiation therapy, usually for malignant disease of the bladder, uterus, ovaries, and cervix. Mucosal inflammation and atrophy cause symptoms similar to those seen in patients with idiopathic ulcerative colitis, and corticosteroid therapy may have only limited success. Strictures, obstruction, and secondary ulceration may develop in the colon; these conditions may require diverting colostomy or bowel resection for relief of symptoms, sometimes under emergent conditions. The presence of adhesions and the induced increased friability of the intestinal tissues predispose affected patients to increased intraoperative bleeding and tissue third spacing.

Appendicitis

The appendix arises from the cecum and is normally 5 to 10 cm long. It possesses a separate mesoappendix and derives its blood supply from an appendicular artery and vein, which are branches of the ileocolic vessels. The appendix may assume any of a number of positions that influence the quality of symptoms and the site of pain when inflammation occurs.

Appendicitis occurs most often in individuals in their late teens and early 20s. A slight prevalence for male patients over female patients exists. Obstruction of the appendiceal lumen is the usual cause. Obstruction is often the result of hyperplasia of lymphoid follicles, of which the lumen of the appendix is richly endowed. A fecalith is often the cause of obstruction as well, occurring in 35% of cases. The presence of foreign bodies, inflammatory strictures, and other rare factors (e.g., appendiceal carcinoma and Meckel diverticulum) can mimic the symptoms of appendicitis.[54]

Obstruction of the appendiceal lumen results in stasis of mucus secreted within the lumen. Bacterial overgrowth occurs secondarily and results in proliferation of secreted exotoxins and endotoxins that damage the epithelium. This condition leads to inflammation, ulceration, and eventual perforation. Depending on the time interval during which these events take place, either a walled-off abscess is formed or infective exudate is released into the peritoneum, resulting in generalized peritonitis. The latter condition, in which numerous intraperitoneal abscesses are formed, predisposes the patient to the development of systemic sepsis. The development of adhesions with bowel obstruction is also associated with peritonitis after rupture of an inflamed appendix.[55]

Symptoms of appendicitis include fever, nausea, vomiting, and localized, rebound, lower-right-quadrant pain. Leukocytosis is a common but nonspecific finding.

Other common clinical conditions with symptomatology similar to that of appendicitis include such gynecologic conditions as salpingitis, ovarian torsion, ruptured ovarian cyst, and ectopic pregnancy. In males, epididymitis and testicular torsion may mimic appendicitis. Other confounding clinical conditions include ureteral stones, cystitis, ruptured peptic ulcer, and mesenteric adenitis.[56]

Given the potentially life-threatening nature of the sequelae of untreated acute appendicitis, the diagnosis is made liberally, so 10% to 15% of patients exhibiting accepted clinical symptoms indicative of appendicitis are revealed to have a normal appendix at operation. If negative findings exist, other causes for the clinical symptoms are sought. This may necessitate further exploration and possibly extension of the laparotomy.

Definitive treatment of appendicitis is appendectomy, which may be performed with general or regional anesthesia. Laparoscopic techniques performed with the patient under general anesthesia also are now commonly used.[57] Patients are frequently dehydrated and may be febrile, thereby requiring preoperative volume replacement. Antibiotic therapy is usually initiated before surgery. If general anesthesia is selected, aspiration precautions that include a rapid-sequence induction should be considered.

SPLENIC DISEASE

Anatomic and Physiologic Overview

The spleen is located in the left upper quadrant of the abdomen and is surrounded by the fundus of the stomach (medially), the splenic flexure of the colon (inferiorly), the left kidney and adrenal gland (posteriorly), and the diaphragm (superiorly). Attachment to these organs via suspensory ligaments, which are vascular except for the gastrosplenic ligament, provides protection and support of this organ.

The splenic artery arises from the celiac plexus. The splenic vein joins the superior mesenteric vein to contribute to portal venous blood flow. The parenchyma of the spleen is divided into three zones, which are surrounded by a 1- to 2-mm capsule. These zones are (1) the red pulp, which consists of large, thin-walled, branching vessels, also known as the *splenic sinusoids*; (2) the white pulp, which consists of end-arterial branches of the central arteries and contains lymphocytes, plasma cells, and macrophages; and (3) the marginal zone, an ill-defined vascular space that connects the white pulp with the red pulp.

Total splenic blood flow is approximately 300 mL/min. The splenic artery divides into several branches within the

splenorenal ligament before entering the splenic hilum, where they branch again into these trabeculae as they enter the splenic pulp. Small arteriolar branches leave the trabeculae, and their adventitial coat becomes replaced by a sheath of lymphatic tissue that accompanies the vessels and their branches until they divide into capillaries. It is these lymphatic sheaths that make up the white pulp of the spleen and are interspersed along the arteriolar vessels as lymphatic follicles. The central arteries branch into vessels that enter the marginal zone and red pulp, ultimately collecting in the splenic sinusoid. From this juncture, blood flows via pulp veins, traverses the trabecular veins, and enters into the main splenic vein.

The spleen functions in several physiologic capacities, including blood filtering and immune processing of blood-borne foreign antigens. The spleen is also involved in hematopoiesis in the fetus. In filtering blood, the splenic sinusoids remove nuclear remnants and excess cell membrane found in immature erythrocytes. Abnormal blood cells, such as those found in sickle cell disease and spherocytosis, are filtered and removed by macrophages and other cells of the reticuloendothelial system. Aged red blood cells (older than 120 days) are removed by the same processes.

The spleen has an important role in specific and nonspecific immune responses. Macrophages and specialized histiocytes engulf and remove foreign cells, particularly those with a layer of affixed antibody. The production of specific antibody (immunoglobulin M [IgM]) is facilitated in the white pulp through the processing of foreign antigens.

The spleen has a minor role as a reservoir of platelets. This function, however, is important in only a few pathologic conditions. No significant reservoir function of red blood cells is performed by the spleen.[58]

Correction or amelioration of certain hematologic and immunologic disorders may be attempted through splenectomy. Despite its important and myriad functions, the spleen is not essential for life. Commonly accepted medical disease processes for which splenectomy is considered include idiopathic thrombocytopenic purpura, thrombotic thrombocytic purpura, Hodgkin disease, lymphoma, certain leukemias, hereditary spherocytosis, hereditary hemolytic anemia, idiopathic autoimmune hemolytic anemia, and hypersplenism. Splenectomy may also be performed in treatment of thalassemia and sickle cell disease when these diseases are refractory to medical management and when hypersplenism supervenes. The development of primary (having no identifiable underlying cause) or secondary (having a known cause) hypersplenism may warrant splenectomy. Symptoms of hypersplenism include fatigue, malaise, recurrent infection, and easy or prolonged bleeding. These symptoms occur from a hyperfunctional spleen that removes and destroys normal blood cells. In portal hypertension, transmitted back pressure results in hypersplenism, which leads to congestive failure of splenic function. Treatment of the primary disease process usually provides relief of symptoms. Splenectomy, however, is often a necessary part of therapy; particularly with long-standing disorders.[59]

Splenic Trauma

Blunt or penetrating abdominal trauma may involve the richly vascular spleen, thereby necessitating splenectomy as part of resuscitative measures, such as control of hemorrhage. Any patient who has sustained blunt abdominal trauma and who has left upper quadrant pain should be suspected of having sustained splenic injury. Conservative, nonoperative treatment (with avoidance of splenectomy) may be elected in minor splenic injury. Splenectomy is generally avoided in children because of the greater importance of splenic function (i.e., immunologic function) in growth and development in patients of this age group.[60]

In the presence of impending shock, emergency exploratory laparotomy is carried out to diagnose and treat all injuries to the abdominal viscera, including the spleen. Anesthetic management in these cases is directed by considerations given all unstable patients undergoing emergency laparotomy; particularly hemodynamic stability and renal function. A paramount consideration is maintaining physiologic hemoglobin and hematocrit levels and arterial blood pressure. Hemoglobin and hematocrit are decreased in the emergent setting, not only by hemorrhagic diathesis but also from dilution secondary to aggressive volume resuscitation with crystalloid solutions. These considerations assume an integral part in the decision to implement perioperative blood product transfusion.

Anesthetic Considerations in Elective Splenectomy

Elective splenectomy necessitates a thorough hematologic assessment in the patient's preoperative history. For example, precautions to prevent sickling crisis are an important part of the anesthetic plan in patients with sickle cell disease. Likewise, patients receiving bone marrow–suppressant drugs, as in cases of malignancy, may also exhibit derangements in physiologic levels of blood constituents.

Often these patients are in generally good health apart from the primary disease. The ability to transfuse blood products when indicated should be accommodated with the insertion of at least one large-bore intravenous line for this purpose. The extent of monitoring modalities is dictated by the patient's preexisting condition and anticipated perioperative course.

Patients who have been receiving chemotherapy for diseases such as Hodgkin and non-Hodgkin lymphoma, leukemia, or myeloid metaplasia may exhibit peripheral neuropathies (e.g., those associated with vincristine and cisplatin), hepatotoxicity (associated with methotrexate), and nephrotoxicity (associated with methotrexate and cisplatin). All derangements present preoperatively must be noted and documented. Appropriate measures must also be implemented intraoperatively to prevent any further deterioration in preexisting function. These measures include careful patient positioning, administering appropriate intravenous fluids, maintaining adequate urine output, monitoring hemoglobin and hematocrit levels, and avoiding anesthetics and adjuvants that place an extra metabolic burden on the renal or hepatic system.

CARCINOID TUMORS AND CARCINOID SYNDROME

Carcinoid tumors consist of slow-growing malignancies composed of enterochromaffin cells usually found in the gastrointestinal tract. They may also occur in the lung, pancreas, thymus, and liver. Carcinoid tumors have a low incidence rate of 1.9 per 100,000. The overall incidence appears to have increased since the early 1970s, which may at least partly reflect better diagnosis and awareness.[61] Speculation is that the advent and increasing use of proton-pump inhibitors is a major contributory factor to that increased incidence.[62] A delay of several years frequently occurs before a diagnosis of carcinoid tumor is made. The gastrointestinal tract accounts for about two thirds of carcinoids. Within the gastrointestinal tract, most tumors occur in the small intestine (41.8%), rectum (27.4%), and stomach (8.7%). Distant metastases may be evident at the time of diagnosis in 12.9% of patients, but better diagnostic techniques have contributed to improved survival rates. A 5-decade analysis of 13,715 carcinoid tumors showed an overall 5-year survival rate of 67.2%, with the best survival rates being recorded for patients with rectal (88.3%), bronchopulmonary (73.5%), and appendiceal (71.0%) carcinoids. Two markers are primarily used to diagnose and follow carcinoid tumors: 5-hydroxyindoleacetic acid (5-HIAA) and chromogranin A (CgA). The use of the radionuclide In-pentetreotide is one of the most important imaging investigations for identifying and staging carcinoid tumors of the gastrointestinal tract. An OctreoScan (Mallinckrodt, St. Louis, MO, U.S.A.) can show early evidence of lesions not revealed by other procedures. The results are particularly helpful if surgery is being considered.[61] The tumors can secrete several biologically active substances, including serotonin (5-hydroxytryptamine), kallikrein, histamine, prostaglandins, adrenocorticotropic hormone, gastrin, calcitonin, and growth hormone, among others (Box 31-5). These substances are capable of producing profound deleterious effects on cardiovascular homeostasis, although under normal circumstances the effects of the release of these substances are usually insignificant because of their hepatic metabolism. In the event that hepatic metastatic disease or processes cause impairment in liver function, the ability of the liver to clear these substances may be compromised and overwhelmed. This results in manifestations of the carcinoid syndrome (Box 31-6). Approximately 5% to 10% of patients with carcinoid tumors develop carcinoid syndrome.[63]

BOX 31-5

Secretory Products of Carcinoid Tumors

Amines	**Tachykinins**	**Peptides**	**Other**
Serotonin	Kallikrein	Pancreatic polypeptide (40%)	Prostaglandins
5-HIAA (88%)	Substance P (32%)	Chromogranins (100%)	
5-HTP	Neuropeptide K (67%)	Neurotensin (19%)	
Histamine		hCG$_\alpha$ (28%)	
Dopamine		hCG$_\beta$	
		Motilin (14%)	

From Eyers MB. Small intestine. In: Townsend CM et al., eds. Sabiston Textbook of Surgery: The Biological Basis of Modern Surgical Practice. 18th ed. Philadelphia: Saunders; 2008:1314.
hCG$_\alpha$, *Human chorionic gonadotropin alpha subunit;* hCG$_\beta$, *human chorionic gonadotropin beta subunit.*

Vasoactive peptides released from carcinoid tumors located in the bronchi and ovaries exert a faster effect because of their direct drainage into the portal vein. Carcinoid tumors are also functionally autonomous. Two factors that enhance release of carcinoid hormones are direct physical manipulation of the tumor and β-adrenergic stimulation.[63,64]

Bronchospasm occurs in response to carcinoid hormonal activity on histamine receptors. Patients with carcinoid tumors are also known to be at greater risk for the development of supraventricular tachydysrhythmias and atrial ectopy. Distortion of the cusps of the tricuspid valve or pulmonic valve results in failure in valvular function, with development of deleterious sequelae, such as valvular regurgitation. Flushing, diarrhea, and edema may be in evidence, as well as hypotension and decreased cardiac output. These signs and symptoms are caused by the exaggerated level of bradykinin activity. Abdominal pain and diarrhea are indicative of increased serotonin levels. Serotonin mimics epinephrine in its role in stimulating glycogenolysis and gluconeogenesis, thereby resulting in hyperglycemia. Clinical hypoalbuminemia may be present as a result of the diversion of tryptophan from protein synthesis to serotonin production.[3]

Patients with carcinoid syndrome may undergo primary resection of the carcinoid tumor. Examples of other procedures that these patients often undergo include cardiac valve replacement and hepatic resection (e.g., lobectomy) for excision of metastases.[64]

Particular discretion should be exercised in the use of drugs requiring significant hepatic biotransformation and elimination, particularly for patients with hepatic neoplasia or metastases who exhibit signs of carcinoid syndrome. Consideration is also given to patients with tumors in areas that drain into the portal circulation (e.g., the mesentery and spleen).

Many anesthetic techniques have been used successfully in the treatment of patients with carcinoid syndrome (Box 31-7). Preoperative preparation of the patient requires correction of deficiencies in circulating volume and electrolyte levels. Use of histamine-releasing agents such as morphine, thiopental, and atracurium should be avoided. Fasciculations may induce release

of carcinoid hormones and are therefore prevented by avoidance of succinylcholine, although it has been used successfully many times, especially for rapid-sequence induction.

Etomidate may be used for induction, but thiopental should be avoided because of associated histamine release. Propofol in both bolus and infusion doses has also been frequently used. Because it may produce hypotension, judicious use is advised. Vecuronium and cisatracurium may be safely used for neuromuscular blockade. Rocuronium is an attractive alternative when rapid onset is desired.

Vecuronium, cisatracurium, and rocuronium are virtually devoid of activity that invokes histamine release or hemodynamic changes. The piperidine-derivative opioids fentanyl, sufentanil, alfentanil, and remifentanil are suitable for use because of their lack of histamine-releasing properties and their innocuous effect on hemodynamics. Isoflurane, desflurane, and sevoflurane may all be safely used. No one anticholinesterase neuromuscular relaxant reversal agent is thought to have advantage over any other. However, glycopyrrolate, used as an adjunct to attenuate vagolysis, may be more desirable than atropine if a significantly increased heart rate is to be avoided. Ketamine activates the sympathetic nervous system, and catecholamine release may activate the kallikreins and other vasoactive substances and therefore should be avoided. The desire to avoid the use of

---

BOX 31-6

Signs and Symptoms of Carcinoid Syndrome

Episodic cutaneous flushing (kinins, histamine)
Diarrhea (serotonin, prostaglandins E and F)
Heart disease
Tricuspid regurgitation, pulmonic stenosis
Supraventricular tachydysrhythmias (serotonin)
Bronchoconstriction (serotonin, bradykinin, substance P)
Hypotension (kinins, histamine)
Hypertension (serotonin)
Abdominal pain (small bowel obstruction)
Hepatomegaly (metastases)
Hyperglycemia
Hypoalbuminemia (pellagra-like skin lesions resulting from niacin deficiency)

Modified from Stoelting RK, Dierdorf SF. Diseases of the gastrointestinal system. In: Anesthesia and Co-Existing Disease. 4th ed. New York: Churchill Livingstone; 2002:333.

BOX 31-7

Anesthetic Considerations in Carcinoid Syndrome

- The most common clinical signs are flushing, wheezing, blood pressure and heart rate changes, and diarrhea.
- Preoperative assessment should include complete blood count, measurement of electrolytes, liver function tests, measurement of blood glucose, electrocardiogram (echocardiogram if indicated), and determination of urine 5-HIAA levels.
- Optimize fluid and electrolyte status and pretreat with octreotide as noted. Continue octreotide throughout the postoperative period. Interferon-α has shown success in controlling some symptoms.
- Both histamine-1 and histamine-2 receptor blockers must be used to fully counteract histamine effects.
- Avoid histamine-releasing agents such as morphine, thiopental, and atracurium. Avoid sympathomimetic agents such as ketamine and ephedrine.
- Treat hypotension with an α-receptor agonist such as phenylephrine.
- General anesthesia is preferred over regional anesthesia. Patients with high serotonin levels may exhibit prolonged recovery; therefore, desflurane and sevoflurane, which have rapid recovery profiles, may be beneficial.
- Aggressively maintain normothermia to avoid catecholamine-induced vasoactive mediator release.
- Monitor intraoperative plasma glucose, as these patients are prone to hyperglycemia. Treat with insulin as is customary.

Modified from Vaughan DJ, Brunner MD. Anesthesia for patients with carcinoid syndrome. Int Anesthesiol Clin. 1997;35:129-142.
HIAA, 5-Hydroxyindoleacetic acid.

sympathomimetics such as ephedrine to treat hypotension makes the use of regional anesthesia controversial. Epidural anesthesia, cautiously administered, may be a reasonable technique for lower extremity and abdominal procedures. Severe and possibly refractory hypotension resulting from sympathectomy makes spinal anesthesia relatively contraindicated for use in carcinoid patients.

Octreotide, a somatostatin analog, is used to blunt the vasoactive and bronchoconstrictive effects of carcinoid tumor products. Octreotide mimics the inhibitory action of somatostatin on the release of several gastrointestinal hormones, as well as those derived from carcinoid tumors. Treatment for 2 weeks preoperatively with a dose of 100 mcg subcutaneously three times a day is standard. If prior therapy was not used, a dose of 50 to 150 mcg subcutaneously is given preoperatively. Intraoperative infusion may be continued at 100 mcg/hr. Bolus doses of 100 to 200 mcg given intravenously may be used for intraoperative carcinoid crises. Lantreotide, which is administered every 2 weeks, and octreotide LAR, which can be given monthly, are long-acting formulations that are superior in terms of patient acceptance and cost effectiveness.[61]

To avoid hormone release by β-adrenergic stimulation, hypotension should be treated with an α-adrenergic agonist (e.g., phenylephrine infusion). Bronchospasm resulting from histamine or bradykinin release has been shown to be resistant to ketamine and inhalation anesthetics. Low-dose β$_2$-agonists are effective in bronchodilation and have relatively little influence on carcinoid hormone release. In the presence of high levels of serotonin in carcinoid syndrome, adjustments in anesthetic selection and dosage must be considered if further compromise of cardiovascular function is to be prevented.[63-65]

TRANSPLANTATION

Liver Transplantation

Orthotropic liver transplantation (OLT) has emerged as a definitive treatment option for patients with end-stage hepatic disease. This is largely attributable to advances in surgical technique, immunosuppressive therapy, and donor organ procurement. Other contributing factors that have greatly attenuated the previously formidable morbidity and mortality associated with this procedure include advances made in technologic and perioperative management.

Patients with end-stage hepatic disease who experience progressive life-threatening complications that become increasingly refractory to medical intervention are the usual candidates for OLT.[66] Transplantation may also be considered a therapeutic option in patients with certain viral infections who respond poorly to medical management but are nevertheless deemed physiologically salvageable. In the adult population, postnecrotic (nonalcoholic) cirrhosis constitutes the most common indication for OLT, followed by (in decreasing occurrence) primary biliary cirrhosis, sclerosing cholangitis, and primary hepatic neoplasia. In the pediatric population, the most common indicator for OLT is biliary atresia, followed by various inborn errors of metabolism (Wilson disease, Crigler-Najjar syndrome, 1-antitrypsin deficiency) and postnecrotic cirrhosis.[67] Transplantation in patients with a history of alcoholic cirrhosis is performed but is a matter of considerable ethical debate. Current recommendation is to have the patient refrain from alcohol consumption for at least 6 months before surgery. Recidivism to active alcoholism after transplantation is the major stimulating factor in the ongoing controversy, although studies have shown that only 7% of those who refrain from alcohol for 6 months return to active alcoholism.[68,69]

The refinement of immunosuppressant therapy has been instrumental in the increasingly impressive survival rates in patients undergoing OLT. Key to this has been the use of cyclosporine, which interferes with helper T-cell activity and inhibits interleukin (IL)-2 and other proinflammatory cytokines. Cyclosporine is often used concurrently with azathioprine and corticosteroids. Anti-OKT3, a monoclonal antibody directed toward lymphocytes, has also shown efficacy in preventing acute rejection, particularly if it is steroid refractory. Tacrolimus (FK-506) is an effective alternative to cyclosporine.[70] Technical refinements in the procedure and development of more precise support modalities (e.g., venovenous bypass and rapid infusion technology) have also contributed to an overall improved outcome in patients undergoing OLT. Major categories of immunosuppressant drugs are given in Table 31-8.

Anesthesia-related concerns for patients undergoing OLT are consistent with those for patients undergoing major surgery with severe cirrhosis. The multisystem effects of cirrhosis are underscored. Profound hemodynamic derangements may preexist and are likely to be exacerbated by the numerous stressors imposed during particular phases of the procedure. These include the hemodynamic consequences of clamping and unclamping the portal vein and vena cava, as well as alterations in metabolism. Hyperkalemia and venous air embolism may be encountered with perfusion of the emplaced graft.

Frequently, optimal preoperative preparation of the patient is not possible. Priorities are therefore established and adhered to.

TABLE **31-8**	Major Categories of Immunosuppressant Drugs
Class of Immunosuppressant	**Immunosuppressant Agent**
General immunosuppressants	Corticosteroids
Calcineurin inhibitors	Cyclosporine (Sandimmune, Neoral)
	Tacrolimus (Prograf, FK506)
Antimetabolites	Azathioprine (Imuran)
	Mycophenolate mofetil (MMF)
Inhibitors of TOR (target of rapamycin)	Rapamycin (Sirolimus)
	Everolimus (RAD)
Antilymphocyte antibodies	
Polyclonal antibodies	Antilymphocyte serum (ALS)
	Antilymphocyte globulin (ALG)
Monoclonal antibodies	Antithymocyte globulin (ATG)
	OKT3
	Basiliximab (Simulect)
	Daclizumab (Zenapax)
	Alemtuzumab (Campath-1H)
Novel agents	Leflunomide
	FK778
	FK779
	FKY720

Krok KL, Thuluvath PJ. Perioperative and postoperative use of immunosuppressant agents in liver transplants. Int Anesthesiol Clin. 2006;44(3):53.

Patients with severe cirrhosis are typically coagulopathic to a variable extent (deficient in coagulation factors and thrombocytopenic). Massive blood loss should be anticipated. Red blood cells, FFP, platelets, and cryoprecipitate should be readily available. Blood-salvaging technology should also be used. Infusion of antifibrinolytics such as ϵ-aminocaproic acid may also be useful perioperatively in efforts to control hemorrhagic diatheses.

Invasive monitoring modalities are mandatory for OLT. These include intraarterial pressure monitoring and central venous or pulmonary artery catheterization. Owing to the profound fluid shifts and blood loss encountered in these procedures, direct measurement of central filling pressures assumes paramount importance for guiding volume and blood-product replacement. Large-bore (14- to 16-gauge) intravenous catheters and possibly an antecubital 8.5F catheter also may be used for administration of volume, which may be performed via a rapid infusion device. All administered fluids should be warmed to prevent hypothermia and its attendant effects on coagulation and metabolic processes. Other measures to maintain normothermia include forced-air surface warming and possibly increased ambient room temperature. All airway gases should be humidified. Urinary output, as measured via indwelling urinary catheter, should be maintained at a minimum of 0.5 mL/kg/hr.

Serial laboratory measurements are performed throughout surgery. These include measurements of arterial blood gases, electrolytes, and hemoglobin and hematocrit levels and metabolic studies assessing ionized calcium and serum glucose. Coagulation parameters are also closely assessed via activated PTT, PT, fibrinogen, and platelet count. Another useful monitoring modality for assessment of overall clotting capability, fibrinolysis, and platelet quality is thromboelastography (TEG).[71,72] Changes in commonly monitored parameters are shown in Table 31-9. Some coagulopathy associated with liver transplantations are noted int Table 31-10.

No single anesthetic technique is indicated for OLT. Patients undergoing OLT are considered at marked risk for aspiration of stomach contents because of the likelihood of abdominal distention or history of upper gastrointestinal bleeding. General anesthesia is therefore induced via rapid-sequence technique with cricoid pressure. Premedication may be administered but may be curtailed in the presence of marked encephalopathy. Sodium thiopental, ketamine, propofol, and etomidate are all

TABLE 31-10	Coagulopathy During Orthotropic Liver Transplantation
Stage	**Coagulopathy**
Dissection	Preexisting coagulopathy Dilution Fibrinolysis (mild) Ionized hypocalcemia Dilution
Anhepatic	Heparin effect (with venovenous bypass) Fibrinolysis (moderate) Hypothermia Ionized hypocalcemia Fibrinolysis (severe)
Early neohepatic	Heparin effect Intravascular coagulation Dilution Hypothermia Ionized hypocalcemia
Late neohepatic	Gradual recovery

Kang Y, Audu P. Coagulation and liver transplantation. Int Anesthesiol Clin. *2006;44(4):19.*

TABLE 31-9	Relative Changes in Various Parameters During Liver Transplantation*		
Variable	**Preanhepatic**	**Anhepatic**	**Neohepatic**
Glucose	+	−/+	+ +
Hemoglobin	−/− −	−	−/− −
Platelets	−	−	−
Urine output	+ +	− −	+/+ +
Cardiac index	+ +	+	+ + +
Systemic vascular resistance	− −	+ +	− − −
Peripheral vascular resistance	+	− −	+
Mean arterial blood pressure	−	− −	− − −/− followed by +
Lactate	+	+	+/+ +
K	+	+	+ + + followed by +
Ca	−	− −	−
Mg	−	− −	−
Na	+	+	+
Temperature	−	− − −	+

From Amand MS et al. Liver transplant. In: Sharpe MD, Gelb AW, eds. Anesthesia and Transplantation. *Boston: Butterworth-Heinemann; 1999:190.*

*Increases: + = mild, ++ = moderate, +++ = marked; decreases: − = mild, − − = moderate, − − − − = marked.

suitable hypnotic agents, but the requisite doses may be modified based on the patient's preexisting mental and hemodynamic status. Succinylcholine is used for rapid onset of neuromuscular blockade; however, rocuronium may also be used if no difficulty with intubation is anticipated. Maintenance of anesthesia is accomplished through the use of a volatile agent (e.g., isoflurane) and an intravenous opioid (usually sufentanil or fentanyl) by bolus administration or infusion. Patients with severe encephalopathy may have increased intracranial pressure requiring hyperventilation. The minimum alveolar concentration of volatile agent should also be reduced in these patients. The use of nitrous oxide is limited or avoided because of concerns pertaining to its capability to expand air bubbles that may reside in the nonperfused donor liver. Bowel distention is also a consideration with prolonged usage. Choice of neuromuscular relaxant is a relatively minor issue and is subject to individual preference. Patients undergoing OLT typically remain intubated and mechanically ventilated in the intensive care unit postoperatively.

Intraoperative anesthetic management is strongly influenced by the various hemodynamic manifestations presented during the three major phases of the procedure. During the preanhepatic (dissection) phase, a wide subcostal incision is used to provide optimal surgical exposure. Prior abdominal surgeries may have resulted in adhesion formation, thereby potentially increasing blood loss. The liver is still attached to the portal vein, inferior vena cava, biliary tract, and hepatic artery. During the anhepatic phase, the vena cava is clamped above and below the liver. The portal vein, common bile duct, and hepatic artery are also ligated. Total excision is then undertaken. Venovenous bypass is generally reserved for patients with pulmonary hypertension or significant cardiovascular disease. Removal of the liver may result in hypocalcemia because of loss of the liver's role in the metabolic removal of citrate from blood products that may have been administered. Hypocalcemia may also result in cardiac depression. Ionized calcium levels should be regularly assessed and should guide exogenous replacement (200 to 500 mg). Loss of hepatic clearance of acid metabolites from the gastrointestinal tract results in progressive acidosis. Sodium bicarbonate is administered judiciously to prevent hypernatremia, hyperosmolality, and metabolic alkalosis. Should large amounts of sodium bicarbonate be needed, tromethamine should be considered as an alternative. Hyperglycemia may be encountered more commonly than hypoglycemia because of the increased glucose load presented from large amounts of transfused blood products. In general, dextrose-containing intravenous fluids are avoided. Air emboli may result from air entrapped in venous sinusoids and released when the donor liver is reperfused. The incidence of air embolism is reduced by infusing cold crystalloid solution (e.g., Normosol, Plasma-Lyte) through the venous structures as the raft is being anastomosed. After the portal and suprahepatic caval anastomoses but before infrahepatic caval anastomosis is completed, the liver is flushed by portal blood through the incomplete infrahepatic anastomosis.

Caval clamping is associated with profound hemodynamic changes, particularly decreased cardiac output and hypotension. Renal perfusion may be adversely affected as well. Increased venous back pressure may also increase bleeding and impair splanchnic perfusion. The technique of venovenous bypass consists of cannulation of the inferior vena cava and portal vein and an axillary vein with the intention of diverting blood away from the liver and delivering it directly to the heart. Venovenous bypass is used to minimize hypotension, maintain

renal and splanchnic perfusion, and prevent gut edema and ischemia. Heparinization is not necessary because of circuit design technology. Venovenous bypass is associated with an element of risk, however. Venovenous bypass may lengthen operative time and subject the patient to increased risk of air embolic and thromboembolic events. Brachial plexus injury and hypothermia are also recognized side effects. Cannulation of the internal jugular vein rather than the axillary vein as a return circuit also has been used and has been shown to attenuate a number of the side effects of venovenous bypass. Percutaneous methods for establishing venous bypass also have been described. Prophylactic measures for preservation of renal perfusion include the use of mannitol and low-dose dopamine infusion (2 to 3 mcg/kg/min). Other agents that show promise in promoting renal protection include the dopaminergic receptor agonist (DA1 and DA2 with β_2-receptor agonist) dopexamine.[73] Another agent commercially available is the DA1 receptor agonist fenoldopam.[73,74] The lack of DA1, α-adrenergic, and β-adrenergic activity seen with the use of this agent makes it particularly attractive. Ultimately renal perfusion, as well as overall systemic organ perfusion, is best accomplished by optimizing cardiac output and systemic blood pressure. For this, any of a number of vasoactive and inotropic agents should be available and used as needed.

The consequent hypocalcemia and myocardial depression associated with removal of the liver is managed with the periodic administration of calcium chloride (200 to 500 mg), which is guided by assessment of serum ionized calcium concentration. Hyperkalemia may be a consequence of the progressive acidosis frequently encountered during the anhepatic stage. Symptomatic hyperkalemia may lead to cardiac dysrhythmias and refractory asystole. Treatment consists of the administration of calcium chloride, sodium bicarbonate, and glucose and insulin and the application of hyperventilation. Maintaining adequate diuresis throughout surgery is crucial to controlling hyperkalemia.

Fluid management presents a formidable perioperative challenge because of its unpredictability and variability. This is influenced in large part by the extent and magnitude of portal hypertension, the challenges in dissection, and the coagulation status. Ongoing goals are to maintain normovolemia, sustain organ system perfusion, and optimize oxygen-carrying capacity. Selection of crystalloid is based on these goals and preservation of electrolyte and acid-base balance. Lactated Ringer's solution may increase serum lactate levels and contribute to hyperkalemia. Normal saline may impose a hyperchloremic metabolic acidosis. Isotonic solutions with greater compatibility to normal osmolality are therefore preferred. Rapid-transfusion devices that allow the infusion of large volumes of warmed fluids and blood products should be used. Correction of acidosis may be accomplished by optimizing systemic perfusion, hyperventilation, and sodium bicarbonate. Excessive sodium bicarbonate may result in hyperosmolality, hypernatremia, central pontine myelinolysis, and metabolic acidosis. Before reperfusion of the grafted donor liver, correction of electrolyte and acid-base abnormalities should be undertaken. Central filling pressures should also be allowed to increase, and hyperventilation should be instituted. Preparation for rapid infusion of warmed blood products (e.g., salvaged blood and packed red blood cells), as well as for administration of indicated inotropic and vasoactive agents, allows prompt retrieval of hemodynamic parameters secondary to reperfusion hypotension. During the postanhepatic (revascularization-biliary reconstruction) phase, the venous anastomoses are completed, and circulation to the new liver is accomplished via the anastomosed hepatic artery. A Roux-en-Y choledocho-jejunostomy connects the bile duct to the recipient gastrointestinal tract. The reperfusion phenomenon can result in acidosis, hypotension, and electrolyte abnormalities; particularly hyperkalemia.[71]

Electrocardiographic aberrations may be noted: typically bradycardia. Management is largely supportive and consists of volume restoration by colloid or crystalloid (as directed by laboratory findings, central filling pressures and urinary output), calcium chloride, and sodium bicarbonate. Inotropic and vasoactive support may be indicated. This may entail a polypharmacologic approach because of the recipient's possible attenuated response to vasoactive agents. To optimize activity of these agents, existing acidosis must be corrected. A postperfusion coagulopathy is commonly encountered after reperfusion. This may be attributable to the release of sequestered heparin (administered during retrieval) in the donor liver or to activity of an endogenous heparinoid. Hyperfibrinolysis is frequently encountered subsequent to increased release of tissue plasminogen activator inhibitor during the anhepatic phase. The use of TEG furnishes a method for accurate detection of fibrinolysis and abnormalities in platelet activity and is valuable, in addition to laboratory findings, in directing blood and blood-component resuscitation. Platelets and FFP should be available. Cryoprecipitate may also be used for restoration of an adequate fibrinogen level in the presence of fibrinolysis. Desmopressin (DDAVP) may be administered to help improve platelet function. Overtransfusion with blood components and crystalloid should be avoided to prevent pulmonary edema, decreased oxygenation, peripheral edema, and prolonged intubation and ventilation and their attendant risks (e.g., pneumonia). Some common intraoperative complications and their management are noted in Table 31-11.

Postoperative problems may include persistent hemorrhage, volume overload, metabolic and electrolyte abnormalities (e.g., hyperglycemia, hyperkalemia, metabolic alkalosis), and infection. Neurologic complications include encephalopathy, seizures, cyclosporine neurotoxicity, and cerebrovascular hemorrhage. Surgical complications that may require return to the operating room for correction include anastomotic leak or stricture of the biliary reconstruction or dehiscence or thrombosis of the hepatic or portal vessels. Prophylactic antibacterial and antifungal agents are administered in addition to the immunosuppressive agents. The incidence of infection is high. The locus of infection may be an intraabdominal source, an indwelling catheter, the surgical wound, the urinary tract, or an intrapulmonary source. Numerous infective entities may be causative. Commonly encountered are fungi (e.g., *Candida* and *Aspergillus* species), gram-negative bacteria, viruses (e.g., cytomegalovirus), and parasites (e.g., *Pneumocystis*). Postoperative hepatitis may be caused by herpesvirus, Epstein-Barr virus, cytomegalovirus, adenovirus, or hepatitis B or C virus. Reactivation of a preexisting viral infection is also a causative possibility. Potential organ rejection is closely monitored and differentially determined by live biopsy. The most common period in which rejection occurs is during weeks 1 to 6 after transplant. Laboratory findings usually reflect a prodromal period before this occurs.

Considerations in addition to those for patients with hepatic failure apply to patients who undergo retransplantation. These patients are immunosuppressed and sensitized to antibodies, which makes type-matching and cross-matching more complex. A variable degree of renal insufficiency and hypertension secondary to cyclosporine toxicity may also be present. Patients on

TABLE **31-11**	Intraoperative Complications and Management
Complication	**Management**
Hypothermia	Use heat exchanger, fluid warmer, warming blanket, forced-air units, postoperative ventilation, warm blood flush
Hyperkalemia	Administer binding resins; perform diuresis, dialysis, hyperventilation; administer sodium bicarbonate, calcium chloride, insulin, or glucose
Hypocalcemia	Administer calcium chloride or gluconate by central line
Oliguria	Maintain adequate volume; increase renal perfusion pressure; administer mannitol, furosemide, and ethacrynic acid; avoid vasopressor use
Hypotension	Maintain adequate volume; check calcium and magnesium; rule out cardiac dysfunction; administer vasopressors; transfuse blood products if anemia or coagulopathy is present
Hypertension	Maintain adequate anesthetic depth; reduce filling pressures; avoid long-acting agents that are used to treat hypertension
Postreperfusion syndrome	Anticipate; ensure that volume loading is not excessive; administer calcium, vasopressors

From Amand MS et al. Liver transplant. In: Sharpe MD, Gelb AW, eds. Anesthesia and Transplantation. Boston: Butterworth-Heinemann; 1999:191.

immunomodulatory steroids who undergo retransplantation are considered steroid dependent and require steroid supplementation before surgery (e.g., methylprednisolone, 500 mg). Aseptic technique is mandatory and must be strictly adhered to.

Living donor hepatic transplantation is currently being undertaken in select centers and accounts for approximately 10% of all hepatic transplants internationally.[71] This modality has been made possible through research and experience-based advances in surgical, medical, and perianesthetic techniques and strategies. In living donor hepatic transplantation, the recipient typically receives the healthy right hepatic lobe from the donor. Besides the advantage of a closer graft match and decreased waiting time between donor and recipient, intraoperative ischemic time of the graft is significantly minimized. Recipient and donor hepatectomy are performed nearly simultaneously to reduce the time from donation to transplant. This assumes added importance with hepatic transplantation, owing to the limited ischemic reserve of the highly vascular liver. Anesthetic concerns for the donor will focus on the magnitude of perioperative management for hepatectomy but with the assurance of the presence of a minimal degree of potentially complicating comorbidities. Posttransplant regeneration of liver tissue within the donor is noted to occur within a year. Return of hepatic function to preoperative levels correlates with the amount of donor liver mass resected. The relative risk for complications in the donor are consistent with the degree of resection (e.g., right lobe donor, 31%; left lateral segmentectomy, 9%; left lateral lobe donation, 7.5%). Biliary complications (e.g., stricture and leakage), infection, and blood-product transfusion factors are major postoperative donor complications. Reoperation for complications (4.5%) may be necessary.[71]

In cadaveric liver transplantation, the time from retrieval to transplantation is limited to less than 6 hours, even under the most rigorous cooling and preservative protocols. Anesthetic considerations for the recipient of a cadaveric graft are consistent with those of the patient with end-stage liver disease. A summary of anesthetic management for orthotopic liver transplantation is noted in Table 31-12.

Pancreatic Transplantation

Pancreatic transplantation is increasingly becoming a treatment option in patients with insulin-dependent diabetes mellitus refractory to medical management. One-year graft and patient survival rates are currently 70% and 91%, respectively. The most common procedures include simultaneous pancreas and kidney transplant for uremic patients, pancreas after kidney transplant for immunocompromised patients (e.g., secondary to

TABLE 31-12 Anesthetic Management for Orthotopic Liver Transplantation

Management Issue and Common Practices	Comments
Hemodynamic Monitoring	
Direct intraarterial pressures: radial and/or femoral arteries	Two sites often used, heparin-free infusion in one for laboratory samples.
Pulmonary artery catheter	Continuous cardiac output and mixed venous saturation catheters allow rapid assessment of oxygen delivery and unitization.
Transesophageal echocardiography	Particularly useful for postpulmonary syndrome, reperfusion crisis, and suspected tamponade, as well as general cardiac function and fluid status. Risk of variceal bleeding in coagulopathic patients with esophageal varices.
Central Nervous System Monitoring	
Intracranial pressure monitoring	Indicated in fulminant liver failure with advanced encephalopathy if coagulopathy can be adequately corrected.
Laboratory Monitoring	
Standard coagulation profiles	Prothrombin and partial thromboplastin times, fibrinogen levels, degradation products, and platelet count.
Factor activity	Readily available in some centers, allows factor-specific determinations of abnormalities and therapeutic responses.
Thromboelastography (TEG)	TEG was commonly used in early transplantation series. Allows "bedside" evaluation of coagulation with patterns typical of factor and platelet deficiency and fibrinolysis. Allows in-vitro assessment of factor and antifibrinolytic therapy. Still used in many centers.
Potential for Massive Transfusion and Venovenous Bypass	
Extensive venous access	Peripheral large bore (8.5F or larger) catheters allow rapid volume infusion.
Blood bank protocol	10-20 units packed red blood cells, fresh frozen plasma, and platelets should be available. Many cases require that several units of cells and plasma be verified and at the bedside.
Rapid infusion devices	Many centers use rapid-infusion pump devices capable of infusing 1 L or more of fluid in a minute. Careful attention to overpressure alarms and catheter sites is important to avoid pressurized extravasation.
Cell salvage	Cell salvage is commonly used when cancer or infection is not suspected. Large volumes of processed cells will dilute platelets and coagulation factors. Effect on fibrinolysis is controversial.
Venovenous bypass	Utilization ranges from routine to selected or rare in different centers. Flow from femoral and portal vein to axillary or internal jugular vein maintains venous return during caval interruption. (Piggyback transplantation requires partial or short caval occlusion, typically venovenous bypass is not used.)

Littlewood K, Nemergut EC. Liver disease. In: Fleisher LA et al, eds. Fleisher Anesthesia and Uncommon Diseases. *5th ed. Philadelphia: Saunders; 2006:193.*

antirejection therapy), and pancreas transplantation alone for nonuremic patients.[75]

Preoperative screening is meticulous and thorough. One of the numerous laboratory-screening procedures is measurement of basal and stimulated C peptide. C peptide is the portion of the precursor insulin molecule used in production of circulating insulin. Functional pancreatic beta cells secrete C peptide in conjunction with insulin. The absence of C peptide serves as a strong marker for loss of endogenous insulin production and confirms absolute insulin deficiency (i.e., type 1 diabetes). Other assessments include evaluating the degree of secondary diabetic complications and (most prominently) detecting the presence of ischemic cardiac disease and renal insufficiency. Ischemic cardiac disease is common in diabetic patients who are considered candidates for pancreatic transplantation. The presence of silent coronary disease should be considered, particularly in candidates with preexisting peripheral neuropathy and uremia. Cardiac disease, the chief cause of morbidity and mortality in patients with end-stage renal disease, may often not be detected by means of ECG or the standard preoperative history and physical examination. Other complications of type 1 diabetes often detected during the preoperative assessment are peripheral vascular disease, ketoacidosis, chronic hypertension, chronic hyperglycemia, gastroparesis, and retinopathy. Such conditions may necessitate modifying the anesthetic plan. The reader is referred to Chapter 34 for specific anesthetic and perioperative considerations for patients with secondary complications of type 1 diabetes mellitus.

Airway evaluation is given special priority. Diabetic patients may pose a particular challenge with regard to intubation. The exact cause of increased difficulty in intubation of diabetic patients is not known. Contributing factors, however, may be contractures and general joint stiffness known to occur in diabetic patients. Joint stiffness involves the joints of the patient's head and neck, particularly those joints of the atlantooccipital axis. Neuropathy, both autonomic and systemic, is common in pancreatic transplant recipients and places affected patients at risk for wide swings in hemodynamic lability perioperatively. Denervation hypersensitivity of cardiac acetylcholine receptors may develop in diabetic patients and place them at risk for severe refractory bradycardia—a strong consideration when anticholinesterase reversal agents are used. Autonomic neuropathy may also affect patients' response to hypoxia, placing them at risk for pulmonary embarrassment. This could be of particular concern in the postoperative setting. Vagal neuropathy promotes gastroparesis, which places the patient at risk for aspiration of gastric contents. Motor and sensory neuropathy resulting from diabetes or uremia increases the risk of hyperkalemia subsequent to succinylcholine administration. Risk of postoperative neuropraxia must also be considered when preexisting deficits have been documented preoperatively. For the magnitude of autonomic dysfunction to be determined, the preoperative history should include history of nausea, diarrhea and bloating (indicative of intestinal involvement), hypotension on initiation of dialysis, esophageal dysfunction, and dizziness with position change. Orthostatic blood pressures and heart rate change also must be noted.[76]

Laboratory assay of metabolic status is also necessary preoperatively. Laboratory studies include baseline blood glucose, hemoglobinA1C, electrolytes, blood urea nitrogen, and creatinine and may include a liver function panel (i.e., bilirubin and transaminases). Hematologic and coagulation studies, as well as a type and screen should also be included. If severe hyperglycemia (blood glucose >500 mg/dL) is present, blood and urine should be analyzed for the presence of ketones, and an arterial blood gas evaluation should be performed to determine whether ketoacidosis is present. Surgery may be delayed until the patient's metabolic status is stabilized. With the high incidence of renal insufficiency in pancreatic transplant patients, many of these patients will be receiving hemodialysis preoperatively. It is important to determine when dialysis was last performed. The presence of hyperkalemia (serum potassium >5.5 mmol/L) should be assessed and appropriate corrective measures undertaken, such as administration of insulin (in the presence of hyperglycemia) with ion exchange resins (e.g., Kayexalate) or with dialysis.

Pancreatic transplantation, particularly when associated with renal transplantation, is a lengthy procedure. General anesthesia is administered in a standard manner with modifications in agent selection and administration consistent with planned preservation of the patient's hemodynamic status. Agents with a minimal direct depressant effect on cardiac function (e.g., etomidate, opioids) and minimal organ dependence on renal metabolism and elimination (e.g., cisatracurium, vecuronium) should be selected. Maintenance of general anesthesia is accomplished with volatile agents (e.g., isoflurane, sevoflurane, desflurane), low-dose opioids, and muscle relaxants. Aspiration precautions during induction and intubation should be in effect. Adjunctive airway devices should be readily available in the event of an anticipated or unanticipated difficult airway. Standard monitoring intraoperatively may be supplemented by the use of an arterial catheter for rapid detection of blood pressure changes and for laboratory sampling. A central venous catheter is also useful for administering immunosuppressive drugs, for inotropic support, and for assessment of central filling pressures.[77]

Intraoperative metabolic monitoring must include regular measurements of serum glucose. Hyperglycemia is often encountered secondary to the metabolic stress response and the hyperglycemic effect of administered corticosteroids or cyclosporine. Glucose determinations should be performed every half hour after allograft anastomosis is completed and reperfusion established. This is mandatory not only for optimization of the glucose level but also for determination of the level of function of the islet cells. Along with periodic monitoring of serum electrolytes and hemoglobin, periodic blood gas analysis is also recommended because of the common occurrence of metabolic acidosis in pancreatic transplant patients. This not only occurs as a result of systemic hypoperfusion but also may also be attributed to ketosis or renal insufficiency. Many patients with renal failure live with a compensated metabolic acidosis such that a mild acidosis may be tolerable and treatable with increased ventilation. Significant acidosis may require intravenous administration of sodium bicarbonate.[76,77]

It is imperative that hemodynamic status be optimized both before anastomosis of the allograft and after reperfusion has been established. A significant incidence of graft thrombosis and subsequent failure is attributed to hypotension. Vascular expansion must be directed judiciously, particularly in patients known to have cardiac insufficiency. In these patients, the use of a pulmonary artery catheter may be necessary to guide volume administration. Overzealous vascular expansion, particularly with crystalloid, may result in allograft edema, which may also result in vascular insufficiency, thrombosis, and failure. Prevention of graft edema and thrombosis may be accomplished by emphasizing colloid (including packed red blood cells for a hemoglobin less than 10 g/dL) rather than crystalloid transfusion and by administering sodium mannitol (25 g) before reperfusion. All patients receive antibiotics, usually broad spectrum. Low-dose heparin is usually administered at the discretion of the surgeon before the clamping of major vessels. Cyclosporine is most commonly started after surgery. Immunosuppression is often initiated intraoperatively with the use of agents such as tacrolimus, azathioprine, prostaglandin E_1 (PGE_1) and methylprednisolone. Hypotension and pulmonary edema are potential complications with the use of the immunosuppressant OKT3 (muromonab).

Postoperative extubation is accomplished only after reversal of neuromuscular blockade when the patient is hemodynamically stable and demonstrates control of airway reflexes. Monitoring of laboratory parameters (serum glucose, electrolytes, arterial blood gases, and hemoglobin) continues throughout the postanesthesia period. Infusions initiated intraoperatively, such as insulin for serum glucose management, supplemental dextrose, and vasoactive medications, should be adjusted as needed in accordance with metabolic and hemodynamic findings. Supplemental bicarbonate may be necessary for correction of acidosis secondary to losses of bicarbonate from pancreatic secretions into the urine and bladder. Pancreatic rejection is assessed via determinations of serum glucose and urinary amylase levels. Abdominal pain and distention serve as indicators of possible acute rejection syndrome, as well as other indicators such as hemodynamic compromise and signs and symptoms consistent with sepsis (e.g., fever and refractory hyperglycemia and ketosis). Under these circumstances, graft pancreatectomy is indicated, as is graft nephrectomy if necessary.[78-80]

Small Bowel Transplantation

Currently, small bowel transplantation (SBT) is performed at a limited number of centers. This largely controversial procedure may be considered an alternative therapy for select individuals with no prognosis for independence from total parenteral nutrition (TPN). The high morbidity and mortality associated with long-term TPN (e.g., secondary to infections, vascular occlusions, hepatobiliary dysfunction) may serve to make SBT an attractive option.[81,82]

Conditions that warrant chronic TPN are frequently those associated with short gut syndrome (SGS). The causes of SGS differ to an extent between adults and children. In children, SGS may result from necrotizing enterolysis, intestinal atresia, midgut volvulus, gastroschisis, and Hirschsprung disease. Crohn's disease eventually also may cause SGS in older children. Other syndromes associated with promotion of SGS in children include Gardner syndrome, with associated desmoid retroperitoneal tumors (causing abdominal vascular compression) and familial microvillus inclusion disease.

In adults, Crohn's disease and conditions that result in vascular occlusive disease in the gut, particularly of the superior mesenteric artery, are common causative factors in the development of SGS. In children and adults, a primary cause of SGS is surgical resection of the small bowel. Complications of SGS are basically the result of malabsorption and maldigestive syndrome resulting from loss of absorptive surface area. These syndromes may eventually result not only in malnutrition but also metabolic bone disease, electrolyte derangements, bile-salt deficiency, anemia, biliary lithiasis, and nephrolithiasis.

Preoperative assessment must take numerous issues into consideration, including the degree of debilitation of the patient, which factors prominently in evaluating the function and compensation of other organ systems (e.g., cardiopulmonary, renal, hematologic). Hepatobiliary function also requires careful assessment, particularly if the patient has been receiving long-term TPN. A combined liver transplant and SBT may be undertaken in patients with significant hepatic dysfunction. Adequate vascular access must be established. This may require central venous access because of obliteration of peripheral veins secondary to previous access attempts. Routine monitors are used, with consideration given to more aggressive hemodynamic monitoring (e.g., arterial, central venous, pulmonary arterial) if deemed appropriate. General anesthesia is used, and agent selection (e.g., muscle relaxants) must take into consideration any deficiencies in organ systems necessary for a particular drug's metabolism and elimination. A rapid-sequence induction is indicated.

Intraoperatively, central filling pressures are carefully monitored to facilitate maintenance of renal perfusion and hemodynamic stability. A balanced anesthetic technique is used, involving a volatile agent of low solubility and an opioid. Nitrous oxide may be avoided because of the long duration of the procedure and associated potential for bowel distention. Episodes of hemodynamic liability may be seen intraoperatively because of caval clamping during anastomosis and at the time of reperfusion of the graft after anastomosis. These periods may closely mimic those seen during resection of an abdominal aortic aneurysm and should be anticipated. Good communication among members of the anesthesia and surgical teams is requisite. Careful monitoring of electrolyte, hematologic, and metabolic (i.e., glucose) status should be performed. Blood loss may not be as great as that seen during liver transplantation but could be significant if there have been previous laparotomies with resultant significant peritoneal adhesion formation. Consideration should also be given to the patient's serum albumin status, which can have consequences that affect not only intravascular volume status but also the amount of available unbound circulating administered drugs. Optimization of intravascular volume status and central filling pressures is accomplished with the use of crystalloid (e.g., lactated Ringer's solution), albumin (especially in the presence of low serum albumin), and pentastarch (e.g., Hespan, Hextend).[83,84]

Immunosuppression is usually initiated with a tacrolimus-based regimen. Measures to prevent hypothermia are also of paramount importance. The major consequences of graft reperfusion on cardiac function are dysrhythmias and asystole, which result from acute hyperkalemia and hypothermia. Ionized serum calcium should be monitored and corrected if necessary. Metabolic acidosis is corrected by maintaining adequate perfusion pressures, optimizing ventilatory status, and judiciously using sodium bicarbonate. Hemodynamic stability ensures adequate graft perfusion.[79,80]

Postoperatively, patients are closely monitored in the intensive care unit. Derangements in metabolic, electrolyte, and volume status are corrected. A variable period of assisted positive-pressure ventilation is usually necessary because of the length of the procedure and secondary to edema from a large graft placed in a restrictive cavity (i.e., the abdomen). Analgesia is achieved via intravenous narcotics and eventually patient-controlled methods. Epidural catheter analgesia may be avoided because of possible coagulopathy in patients with hepatic insufficiency. Extubation of the trachea is performed only when the patient has attained adequate respiratory parameters and demonstrates control of airway reflexes.

SUMMARY

Surgical procedures for gastrointestinal disorders remain one of the most common interventions in clinical practice. Anesthetic management can be especially challenging because these patients may suffer from multiple medical problems. Along with the standard surgical and anesthetic considerations, anesthesia care often requires addressing long-standing and critical fluid, electrolyte, and nutritional imbalances. This chapter has addressed current approaches to successful treatment of these patients.

REFERENCES

1. Lobo DN et al. Evolution of nutritional support in acute pancreatitis. *Br J Surg.* 2000;87:695-707.
2. Michel M, Murr NJ. Acute pancreatitis. In: Greenfield LJ et al, eds. *Surgery: Scientific Principles and Practice.* 3rd ed. Philadelphia: Lippincott Williams & Wilkins; 2001:863-872.
3. Tantawy H. Diseases of the gastrointestinal system. 5th ed. New York: Churchill Livingstone; 2008:279-296.
4. Steer ML. Exocrine pancreas. In: Townsend CM et al, eds. *Sabiston Textbook of Surgery: The Biological Basis of Modern Surgical Practice.* 18th ed. Philadelphia: Saunders; 2008:1589-1623.
5. Sharp KW, Pofahl WE. Pancreas. In: Lawrence PF et al, eds. *Essentials of General Surgery.* 3rd ed. Philadelphia: Lippincott Williams & Wilkins; 2000:333-334.
6. Bergman S, Melvin WS. Operative and nonoperative management of pancreatic pseudocysts. *Surg Clin North Am.* 2007;87(6):1447-1460.
7. D'Angelica M, Fong Y. The liver. In: Townsend CM et al, eds. *Sabiston Textbook of Surgery: The Biological Basis of Modern Surgical Practice.* 18th ed. Philadelphia: Saunders; 2008:1463-1523.
8. Mushlin PS, Gelman S. Liver dysfunction after anesthesia. In: Benumof JL, Saiman LJ, eds. *Anesthesia and Perioperative Complications.* 2nd ed. St Louis: Mosby; 1999:441-470.
9. Mushlin PS et al. Acute liver dysfunction and anesthesia-induced hepatitis. In: Lobato EB et al. *Complications in Anesthesiology.* Philadelphia: Wolters Kluwer; 2008:590-601.
10. Morgan GE et al. Anesthesia for patients with liver disease. *Clinical Anesthesiology.* 4th ed. Norwalk, CT: McGraw-Hill; 2006:789-801.
11. Croinin DF, Shorten GD. Anesthesia and renal disease. *Curr Opin Anaesthesiol.* 2002;15(3):359-363.
12. Martin JL. Volatile anesthetics and liver injury: a clinical update, or what every anesthesiologist should know. *Can J Anaesth.* 2005;52(2):125-129.
13. Stoelting RK. Opioid agonists and antagonists. In: Stoelting RK, Hillier SC, eds. *Pharmacology and Physiology in Anesthetic Practice.* 4th ed. Philadelphia: Lippincott Williams & Wilkins; 2006:87-126.
14. Shaw BW et al. Diagnostic considerations in liver disease. In: Baker RJ, Fischer JE, eds. *Mastery of Surgery.* 4th ed. Philadelphia: Lippincott Williams & Wilkins; 2001:1060-1071.
15. Potts JR, Chapman WC. Liver. In: Lawrence PF et al, eds. *Essentials of General Surgery.* 3rd ed. Philadelphia: Lippincott Williams & Wilkins; 2000:343-347.
16. Janberg P. Renal protection strategies in the perioperative period. *Best Pract Res Clin Anaesthesiol.* 2004;18(4):645-660.
17. Shoemaker WC et al. Outcome prediction by a mathematical model based on noninvasive hemodynamic monitoring. *J Trauma.* 2006;60:82-90.
18. Littlewood K, Nemergut EC. Liver disease. In: Fleisher LA. *Anesthesia and Uncommon Diseases.* 5th ed. Philadelphia: Saunders; 2006:151-202.
19. Gao L et al. Rocuronium infusion requirements and plasma concentrations at constant levels of neuromuscular paralysis during three phases of liver transplantation. *J Clin Anesth.* 2003;15(4):257-266.
20. Keegan MT, Plevak DJ. Preoperative assessment of the patient with liver disease. *Am J Gastroenterology.* 2005;100(9):2116-2127.
21. Jenkins SA et al. A prospective randomized controlled trial comparing somatostatin and vasopressin in controlling acute variceal hemorrhage. *BMJ.* 1985;290:270-278.
22. Sarin SK. Long-term follow-up of gastric variceal sclerotherapy: an eleven year experience. *Gastrointest Endosc.* 1997;46(1):8-14.
23. Pivalizza EG et al. Anesthesia for transjugular intrahepatic portosystemic shunt placement. *Anesthesiology.* 1996;85:946-947.
24. Ochs A. Transjugular intrahepatic portosystemic shunt. *Dig Dis.* 2005;23(1):56-64.
25. LaBerge JM. Transjugular intrahepatic portosystemic shunt—role in treating intractable variceal bleeding, ascites, and hepatic hydrothorax. *Clin Liver Dis.* 2006;10(3):583-598.
26. Burroughs A et al. Randomized, double blind, placebo-controlled trial of somatostatin for variceal bleeding. Emergency control and prevention of early variceal rebleeding. *Gastroenterology.* 1990;99(5):1388-1395.
27. Rosado B, Kamath PS. Transjugular intrahepatic portosystemic shunts: an update. *Liver Transpl.* 2003;9(3):207-217.
28. Boldt J. Volume replacement in the surgical patient: does the type of solution make a difference? *Br J Anaesth.* 2000;84;783-793.
29. Chari RS, Shah SA. Biliary system. In: Townsend CM et al, eds. *Sabiston Textbook of Surgery: The Biological Basis of Modern Surgical Practice.* Philadelphia: Saunders; 2008:1547-1588.
30. Gan TJ et al. Society for Ambulatory Anesthesia guidelines for the management of postoperative nausea and vomiting. *Anesth Analg.* 2007;105(6):1615-28.
31. Leonard IE, Cunningham AJ. Anaesthetic considerations for laparoscopic cholecystectomy. *Best Pract Res Clin Anaesthesiol.* 2002;16:1-20.
32. Long JD, Orlando RC. Anatomy histology embryology and development anomalies of the esophagus. In: Feldman M et al, eds. *Sleisenger & Fordtran's Gastrointestinal and Liver Disease.* 8th ed. Philadelphia: Saunders; 2006:841-927.
33. Maish M. Esophagus. *Sabiston Textbook of Surgery: The Biological Basis of Modern Surgical Practice.* 18th ed. Philadelphia: Saunders; 2008:1049-1107.
34. Peters JH, DeMeester TR. Esophagus and diaphragmatic hernia. In: Brunicardi FC et al, eds. *Schwartz's Principles of Surgery.* 8th ed. New York: McGraw-Hill; 2005:835-932.
35. Ginsberg GC, Fleischer DE. Tumors of the esophagus. In: Feldman M et al, eds. *Sleisenger & Fordtran's Gastrointestinal and Liver Disease.* 8th ed. Philadelphia: Saunders; 2006:949-970.
36. Chey WD, Wong BC. Practice parameters of the Committee of the American College of Gastroenterology. *Am J Gastroenterol.* 2007;102(8):1808-1825.
37. Rokkas T et al. *Helicobacter pylori* and non-malignant diseases. *Helicobacter.* 2007;12(Suppl 1):20-22.
38. Cryer B, Spechler SJ. Peptic ulcer disease. In: Feldman M et al, eds. *Sleisenger & Fordtran's Gastrointestinal and Liver Disease.* 8th ed. Philadelphia: Saunders; 2006:1089-1110.
39. Mercer DW. Stomach. In: Townsend CM et al, eds. *Sabiston Textbook of Surgery: The Biological Basis of Modern Surgical Practice.* 18th ed. Philadelphia: Saunders; 2008:1223-1277.
40. Turnage RH et al. Abdominal wall, umbilicus, peritoneum, mesenteries, omentum, and retroperitoneum. *Sabiston Textbook of Surgery: The Biological Basis of Modern Surgical Practice.* 18th ed. Philadelphia: Saunders; 2008:1129-1154.
41. Rimola A et al. Diagnosis, treatment and prophylaxis of spontaneous bacterial peritonitis: a consensus document by the International Ascites Club. *J Hepatol.* 2000;32(1):142-53.
42. Evers BM. Small intestine. *Sabiston Textbook of Surgery: The Biological Basis of Modern Surgical Practice.* 18th ed. Philadelphia: Saunders; 2008:1278-1332.
43. Brown T, Windsor A. Surgical considerations in lower gastrointestinal surgery. In: Kumar CM, Bellamy M. *Gastrointestinal and Colorectal Anesthesia.* New York: Informa; 2007:25-32.
44. Fry R et al. The colon and rectum. *Sabiston Textbook of Surgery: The Biological Basis of Modern Surgical Practice.* 18th ed. Philadelphia: Saunders; 2008:1348-1432.
45. Hanaseur SB, Sandborn WJ. European evidence-based consensus on the diagnosis and management of Crohn's disease. *Gut.* 2007;56(2):161-163.
46. Baert F et al. Medical therapy for Crohn's disease: top-down or step-up? *Dig Dis.* 2007;25(3):260-266.
47. McLeod RS. Surgery for inflammatory bowel diseases. *Dig Dis.* 2003;21(2):168-179.
48. Murdoch SD. Anesthesia for colorectal surgery. In: Kumar CM, Bellamy M. *Gastrointestinal and Colorectal Anesthesia.* New York: Informa; 2007:285-298.
49. Cereda M et al. The critically ill injured patient. *Anesthesiol Clin.* 2007;25(1):13-21.
50. Itzkowitz SH, Rochester J. Colonic polyps and polyposis syndromes. In: Feldman M et al, eds. *Sleisenger & Fordtran's Gastrointestinal and Liver Disease.* 8th ed. Philadelphia: Saunders; 2006:2713-2758.
51. Stein U, Schlag PM. Clinical, biological, and molecular aspects of metastasis in colorectal cancer. *Recent Results Cancer Res.* 2007;176:61-80.
52. Storey EC, Lumb AB. Anesthesia for emergency exploratory laparotomy. In: Kumar CM, Bellamy M. *Gastrointestinal and Colorectal Anesthesia.* New York: Informa; 2007:347-362.
53. Bullard KM, Rothenberger DA. Colon, rectum and anus. In: Brunicardi FC et al, eds. *Schwartz's Principles of Surgery.* New York: McGraw-Hill; 2005:1055-1118.

54. Shelton T et al. Acute appendicitis: current diagnosis and treatment. *Curr Surg.* 2003;60:502-505.

55. Hsieh CH et al. Retroperitoneal abscess resulting from perforated acute appendicitis: analysis of its management and outcome. *Surg Today.* 2007; 37(9):762-767.

56. Pokala N et al. Complicated appendicitis—is the laparoscopic approach appropriate? A comparative study with the open approach: outcome in a community hospital setting. *Am Surg.* 2007;73(8):737-741.

57. Yau KK et al. Laparoscopic versus open appendectomy for complicated appendicitis. *J Am Coll Surg.* 2007;205(1):60-65.

58. McCance KL. Structure and function of the hematologic system. In: McCance KL, Heuther SE. *Pathophysiology: The Biological Basis of Disease in Adults & Children.* 5th ed. St Louis: Mosby; 2006:893-1028.

59. Tripathi D et al. Review article: recent advances in the management of bleeding gastric varices. *Aliment Pharmacol Ther.* 2006;24(1):1-17.

60. Wahl WL et al. Blunt splenic injury: operation versus angiographic embolization. *Surgery.* 2004;136(4):891-899.

61. Maroun J et al. Guidelines for the diagnosis and management of carcinoid tumors. Part 1: the gastrointestinal tract. A statement from a Canadian National Carcinoid Expert Group. *Curr Oncol.* 2006;13(2):67-76.

62. Modlin IM et al. A 50-year analysis of 562 gastric carcinoids: small tumor or larger problems? *Am J Gastroenterol.* 2004;99(1):23-32.

63. Vaughan DJ, Brunner MD. Anesthesia for patients with carcinoid syndrome. *Int Anesthesiol Clin.* 1997;35:129-142.

64. Kinney MA et al. Perianaesthetic risks and outcomes of abdominal surgery for metastatic carcinoid tumors. *Br J Anaesth.* 2001;87:447-452.

65. Jenset RT, Norton JA. Carcinoid tumors and the carcinoid syndrome. In: DeVita VT et al, eds. *Cancer Principles and Practice of Oncology.* 5th ed. Philadelphia: Lippincott-Raven; 1997.

66. Ahmed A, Keeffe EB. Current indications and contraindications for liver transplantation. *Clin Liver Dis.* 2007;11(2):227-247.

67. Otte JB. History of pediatric liver transplantation. Where are we coming from? Where do we stand? *Pediatr Transplant.* 2002;6:378-387.

68. Zetterman RK. Liver transplantation for alcoholic liver disease. *Clin Liver Dis.* 2005;9(1):171-181.

69. Webb K et al. Transplantation for alcoholic liver disease: report of a consensus meeting. *Liver Transpl.* 2006;12(2):301-305.

70. Herbert MF et al. Pharmacokinetics of cyclosporine pre- and post-liver transplantation. *J Clin Pharmacol.* 2003;43:38-42.

71. Merritt WT. Living donor surgery: overview of surgical and anesthesia issues. *Anesthesiol Clin North America.* 2004;22(4):633-650.

72. Murakawa M. Coagulation monitoring and management during liver transplantation. *J Anesth.* 2003;17:77-78.

73. Kaisers U et al. Dopamine, dopexamine and dobutamine in liver transplant recipients: a comparison of their effects on hemodynamics, oxygen transport and hepatic venous oxygen saturation. *Transpl Int.* 1996;9:214-220.

74. Mathur VS. The role of DA1 receptor agonist fenoldopam in the management of critically ill, transplant, and hypertensive patients. *Rev Cardiovasc Med.* 2003;4(Suppl 1):S35-S40.

75. Pavlakis M, Khwaja K. Pancreas and islet cell transplantation in diabetes. *Curr Opin Endocrinol Diabetes Obes.* 2007;14(2):146-50.

76. Halpern H et al. Anesthesia for pancreas transplantation alone or simultaneous with kidney. *Transplant Proc.* 2004;36(10):3105-3106.

77. Florina P, Secchi A. Pancreatic islet cell transplant for treatment of diabetes. *Endocrinol Metab Clin North Am.* 2007;36(4):999-1013.

78. Ryan EA et al. Current indications for pancreas islet transplant. *Diabetes Obes Metab.* 2006;8(1):1-7.

79. Pavlakis M, Khwaja K. Transplantation for type 1 diabetes: whole organ pancreas and islet cells. *Curr Diab Rep.* 2006;6(6):473-478.

80. Dieterie CD et al. Impaired glucose tolerance in pancreas-grafted diabetic patients is due to insulin secretory defects. *Exp Clin Endocrinol Diabetes.* 2007;115(10):647-653.

81. Fishbein TM. The current state of intestinal transplantation. *Transplantation.* 2004;78(2):175-178.

82. O'Keefe SJ. Candidacy for intestinal transplantation. *Am J Gastroenterol.* 2006;101(7):1633-1643.

83. Sudan DL. Treatment of intestinal failure: intestinal transplantation. *Nat Clin Pract Gastroenterol Hepatol.* 2007;4(9):503-510.

84. Fryer JP. Intestinal transplantation: current status. *Gastroenterol Clin North Am.* 2007;36(1):145-59.

ANESTHESIA FOR LAPAROSCOPIC SURGERY

Edward Waters

The word *laparoscopy* is derived from two Greek words: *laparo*, meaning "flank," and *skopein*, meaning "to examine."[1] Indeed, laparoscopy can be defined as the process of examining the contents of the abdominal cavity using a specially designed endoscope.[2] An important trend in surgery in recent decades has been the expanded use of laparoscopy by surgeons of many subspecialties as a tool in the diagnosis and treatment of many conditions.

Laparoscopic surgical techniques are central to the current emphasis on minimally invasive surgery. Surgeons in gynecologic, urologic, and general surgical disciplines currently use laparoscopic approaches to surgery. Common surgical applications of laparoscopy are noted in Box 32-1.

The advantages of laparoscopic surgery as compared with open techniques are numerous and include better aesthetic results (because the incisions are small), earlier postoperative mobility, and shorter hospital stays.[3-6] Many of the benefits of laparoscopic surgery are attributed to the reduced tissue trauma seen in it as compared with open surgery.[7] Studies of patients undergoing laparoscopic cholecystectomy have demonstrated significant improvement in postoperative pain control as compared with patients undergoing open cholecystectomy, as well as superior postoperative pulmonary function.[5,8]

The 1980s marked the beginning of a revolution in laparoscopic surgery. Before the 1980s, surgeons relied on a monocular laparoscope that provided a direct view of the abdomen.[11] The union of a small video camera with a laparoscope during the 1980s smoothed the progress of many improvements in laparoscopic surgery. Use of a video camera allowed much better ergonomics for the operator; perhaps more significantly, it allowed the entire surgical team to view and assist in the surgery. More complicated surgeries involving multiple assistant surgeons became possible and were facilitated by an ever-expanding variety of surgical instruments.[2,9]

An early result of the improved technology for laparoscopic surgery was the increased use of laparoscopy by general surgeons. The first four-trocar laparoscopic surgery, a laparoscopic cholecystectomy, was performed in France in 1987.[10] As general surgeons developed skills in laparoscopic cholecystectomies and other abdominal surgeries, a significant change in the patient population for laparoscopic surgery occurred.[1] No longer were laparoscopic cases limited to those of brief duration and reserved for women of childbearing age. More lengthy procedures of greater complexity began to be performed on patients such as the elderly and debilitated—sometimes in unusual positions like reverse Trendelenburg.[11,12]

CREATION OF THE PNEUMOPERITONEUM

One constant in laparoscopic surgery has remained over the years: the need to establish and maintain a pneumoperitoneum. The term *pneumoperitoneum* refers to air within the peritoneal cavity. Pneumoperitoneum is essential to the surgeon performing laparoscopic surgery. It provides the exposure necessary to clearly view the operative site and allows room for the surgeon to move instruments.[12] Pneumoperitoneum is the distinguishing feature of laparoscopic surgery as far as the anesthetist is concerned. But establishing a pneumoperitoneum brings with it the risk of severe, acute injury to the patient. The presence of a pneumoperitoneum is accompanied by physical stress to the body, and residual effects can persist into the immediate postoperative period, leading to patient morbidity.

Clinical experience shows that the patient who undergoes laparoscopic surgery is at the highest risk for serious complications during the initial establishment of the pneumoperitoneum.[13] At present, initial access to and insufflation of the abdominal cavity are accomplished in one of two manners: an "open" or a "closed" technique.

The older of the two techniques, the closed technique, involves the use of a spring-loaded needle to pierce the abdominal wall at its thinnest point—the infraumbilical region. The position of the Veress needle is confirmed by the injection of 10 mL of saline through the needle. The needle is assumed to be correctly placed if the surgeon is unable to aspirate the saline. An appropriate gas, usually carbon dioxide (CO_2), is then passed through the needle to create a space between the abdominal wall and organs. After insufflation of the abdomen, a trocar is blindly inserted to allow the surgeon to pass instruments into the abdominal cavity.[14]

The open or Hasson technique involves a small (1.5 to 3 cm) incision made immediately inferior to the umbilicus, through the skin and fascia. The surgeon then directly incises the peritoneum, and a trocar, the Hasson cannula, is placed. Once the Hasson cannula is placed, the abdomen is insufflated and the catheter sutured in place.[13]

The relative merits of the open technique over the closed technique for establishing pneumoperitoneum have been a source of debate among surgeons for some time. Proponents of the open technique argue that the Hasson technique, although not totally eliminating risk, minimizes the risk of major vascular injury (a grave complication) on induction of pneumoperitoneum.[15]

BOX 32-1

Applications of Laparoscopy

General Surgery
Diagnosis
Evaluation of abdominal trauma
Lysis of adhesions
Cholecystectomy
Appendectomy
Inguinal hernia repair
Bowel resection
Esophageal reflux surgery
Splenectomy
Adrenalectomy

Gynecologic Surgery
Diagnosis
Lysis of adhesions
Fallopian-tube surgery (sterilization, ectopic pregnancy surgery)
Fulguration of endometriosis
Ovarian cyst surgery
Laparoscopic-assisted hysterectomy

Urologic Surgery
Nephrectomy

Data from Soper NJ et al. Medical progress: laparoscopic general surgery. N Engl J Med. 1994;330:409-419; Smith I. Anesthesia for laparoscopy with emphasis on outpatient laparoscopy. Anesthesiol Clin North America. 2001;19:21-42; Ruurda JP et al. Robot-assisted surgical systems: a new era in laparoscopic surgery. Ann R Coll Surg Engl. 2002;84:223-226; Zupi E et al. Is local anesthesia an affordable alternative to general anesthesia for mini laparoscopy? J Am Assoc Gynecol Laparosc. 2000;7:111-114.

Investigators comparing open and closed techniques suggest that the open technique does have distinct practical advantages such as faster insufflation, which leads to a shorter operative time, as well as a lower rate of complications.[13,16] A review of the literature examining the incidence of complications on establishment of pneumoperitoneum concluded that visceral injuries were less frequent when an open technique was used but not at a level of statistical significance. The same review found a statistically significant reduction in major vascular injuries when the Hasson technique rather than a Veress needle was used to establish pneumoperitoneum.[17]

COMPLICATIONS OF LAPAROSCOPIC SURGERY

The potential for injury to the patient early in the course of a laparoscopic surgery is apparent when one considers the anatomic structures located in proximity to the infraumbilical puncture and incision site. The inferior vena cava, aorta, and iliac arteries and veins, as well as the bladder, bowel, and uterus are near the infraumbilical site. A subset of patients is at increased risk of injury during the establishment of pneumoperitoneum because of anatomic variations such as obesity, a very thin body habitus, adhesions, or distortion of the viscera as a result of masses such as neoplasms.[14] Iatrogenic injury can result from trauma to vascular structures, gas embolism, injury to abdominal and pelvic organs, and the migration of gas to extraperitoneal spaces.[18]

Vascular injury early in the intraoperative period resulting from trauma to the epigastric vessels is often minor,[6] but major vascular injuries occur in 0.02% to 0.9% of cases.[13] *Major vascular injury* refers to injury to the aorta, inferior vena cava, right renal artery, iliac arteries and veins, or mesenteric vessels. Estimates of mortality related to injury to these major vessels are as high as 15%.[13] Remarkably, trauma to major vessels may be occult because several of these vessels lie in the retroperitoneal space, which can contain significant hemorrhage. A case report[19] documented an incident in which a patient showed signs of cardiovascular decompensation, but observation of the abdominal cavity via the laparoscope failed to detect signs of bleeding. It was only on laparotomy that a large retroperitoneal hematoma resulting from laceration of the common iliac artery and vein was observed. In addition to concealed bleeding in the retroperitoneum, some authors state that venous bleeding may not be observed intraoperatively because of a tamponading effect resulting from the pneumoperitoneum-induced increase in intraabdominal pressure.[20]

A potentially catastrophic complication of laparoscopic surgery is gas embolism. This problem is quite rare, having a reported incidence of 1 occurrence in 77,604 cases[3] or 15 occurrences in more than 100,000 laparoscopies.[12] Gas embolism is most likely to occur during the initial insufflation of the abdomen.[20,21] It can result from the erroneous placement of a Veress needle or trocar into the lumen of an intraabdominal vessel or vascular organ (e.g., uterus or liver) and insufflation through that needle or trocar.[20] In the case of laparoscopic cholecystectomy, the patient is also at risk for gas embolism because the gallbladder is dissected away from the liver bed.[21]

Small gas bubbles can enter the pulmonary circulation, leading to pulmonary hypertension, right ventricular failure, and pulmonary edema. If the gas bubble is large enough, it can result in a "gas-lock" phenomenon, which obstructs right ventricular outflow.[20] Fortunately, catastrophic gas embolism that leads to cardiac arrest is exceedingly rare.[19]

Signs of a significant gas embolism include hypotension, dysrhythmia, and a distinctive "mill wheel" murmur, as well as cyanosis and pulmonary edema.[19] Management of gas embolism includes halting the insufflation of gas, eliminating nitrous oxide (N_2O) from the anesthetic gases, releasing the pneumoperitoneum, placing the patient in left lateral decubitus position (Durant maneuver), and aspirating the gas through a central venous catheter.[20] It should be noted that low central venous pressure (CVP) increases the risk of venous gas embolism.[21] Adequate hydration should therefore be provided for the patient undergoing laparoscopy. Box 32-2 lists the signs, symptoms, and treatment of gas embolism.

Visceral injuries can lead to significant morbidity and mortality in patients who undergo laparoscopy. The incidence of visceral injuries in patients in whom a pneumoperitoneum is created via the closed technique is in the range of 0.1% to 0.4%.[6,13] Trocar insertion has been associated with gastrointestinal tract perforation and hepatic and splenic tears.[11] Urinary bladder catheterization and nasogastric suction are often used in patients who undergo laparoscopy to reduce the risk of trauma to the bladder and stomach, respectively.[11,22]

Visceral lesions sustained during laparoscopic surgery are of particular concern because they are not always recognized at the time of surgery and tend to become symptomatic only after a period of time has elapsed postoperatively. Intraabdominal injuries can result in sepsis, fistulas, peritonitis, and abscesses.[3,13] Supporters of the open technique for creating pneumoperitoneum

BOX **32-2**

Gas Embolism

Signs and Symptoms
Hypotension
Dysrhythmia
Cyanosis
Hypoxia
Pulmonary edema
"Mill wheel" murmur

Treatment
Discontinue gas insufflation
Discontinue nitrous oxide
Administer 100% oxygen
Release pneumoperitoneum
Position patient in left lateral decubitus position
Attempt to aspirate gas via central venous catheter

Data from Noga J et al. Role of the anesthesiologist in the early diagnosis of life-threatening complications during laparoscopic surgery. Surg Laparosc Endosc. 1997;7:63-65; Beck DH, McQuillan PJ. Fatal carbon dioxide embolism and severe haemorrhage during laparoscopic salpingectomy. Br J Anaesth. 1994;72:243-245; Brimacomb JR, Orland H. Endobronchial intubation during upper abdominal laparoscopic surgery in the reverse Trendelenburg position. Anesth Analg. 1994;78:607.

contend that the use of this technique reduces the incidence of visceral trauma and has the advantage of causing lesions that are more easily recognized at the time of surgery.[13]

Another serious complication of pneumoperitoneum is pneumothorax. A retrospective review of 968 cases revealed an incidence of pneumothorax or pneumomediastinum in 1.9% of patients.[23] A subset of patients at increased risk for pneumothorax includes patients undergoing laparoscopic surgery for esophageal reflux disease.[21] Gas can enter the thoracic cavity by two mechanisms. In some cases, gas from a properly induced pneumoperitoneum can pass from the peritoneal cavity to the thoracic cavity via weak points in the esophageal or aortic hiatus.[24] Alternatively a pneumothorax can result from barotrauma secondary to the increased airway pressures and decreased pulmonary compliance typical of pneumoperitoneum.[25] Pneumothorax caused by CO_2 insufflation (perhaps more properly called *capnothorax*) may rapidly resolve both clinically and radiographically without intervention.[24,26] Pneumothorax resulting from barotrauma, such as a ruptured bleb, typically requires thoracentesis.[24]

A relatively minor complication of laparoscopic surgery is subcutaneous emphysema that occurs independently from a pneumothorax. Subcutaneous emphysema can be the result of trocar or Veress needle misplacement in subcutaneous tissue[21,27] and is characteristically manifested as crepitus.

The ideal gas for the creation and maintenance of pneumoperitoneum would demonstrate several properties, including colorlessness, lack of flammability in the presence of electrocautery, physiologic inertness, and excretion via a pulmonary route.[11] Several gases have been investigated in the search for the ideal gas for use in surgical peritoneum. The earliest laparoscopists used air to create a pneumoperitoneum; unfortunately air supports combustion and is poorly absorbed from the circulation, which leads to an unacceptably high risk of embolism.[22] N_2O is three

times more soluble than nitrogen; however, it supports combustion.[11] Helium was evaluated as a gas for abdominal insufflation. The potential suitability of helium lay in its inert physiochemical properties, but helium is not absorbable and could prove very dangerous if present in a gas embolism.[28]

The gas most commonly used in laparoscopic surgery today is CO_2. Although not an ideal gas for pneumoperitoneum, CO_2 is readily available and inexpensive, does not support combustion, and is rapidly absorbed from the vascular space,[7] as well as easily excreted by the respiratory system. When used in a pneumoperitoneum, CO_2 does have disadvantages that include an increased risk of hypercapnia (and subsequent respiratory acidosis) and the fact that CO_2 causes peritoneal and diaphragmatic irritation, which has been implicated in postoperative shoulder pain.[3,7,22]

PHYSIOLOGIC EFFECTS OF PNEUMOPERITONEUM

As laparoscopic surgery has progressed from simple gynecologic surgeries in a young, healthy population to more complicated surgical procedures in a population with increased incidence of systemic disease,[2] the need for an improved understanding of the physiologic effect of laparoscopic surgery has grown.

Patient response to laparoscopic surgery varies, depending on the interplay of numerous factors. The effect of pneumoperitoneum on the patient depends on the degree of intraabdominal pressure generated by the gas, the presence or absence of preexisting cardiopulmonary disease, intravascular volume status, and the duration of the surgery.[11] It is believed that pneumoperitoneum affects the body by means of three mechanisms: a direct mechanical effect, the presence of neurohumoral responses to the pneumoperitoneum, and the effects of absorbed CO_2.[5,21] In addition to experiencing pneumoperitoneum-induced physiologic changes, the patient undergoing laparoscopic surgery is affected by the anesthetic and ventilatory techniques used by the anesthetist, intraoperative positioning, and the surgical conditions (e.g., the presence of retractors and packing).[11,29]

A consistent finding in studies of the hemodynamic effects of pneumoperitoneum is increased systemic vascular resistance (SVR).[29] Increases in SVR in healthy human subjects have been documented at intraabdominal pressures of 14 torr.[22] Increases in SVR of as high as 65% have been documented in healthy human laparoscopy patients.[30]

Mechanical factors such as compression of the abdominal arteries, as well as humoral factors (e.g., vasopressin, renin), are implicated in the increased afterload observed in patients undergoing laparoscopic surgery.[5,22] The persistence of increased SVR observed in patients immediately after the release of pneumoperitoneum has been attributed to the action of humoral mediators. In healthy patients, the persistent influence of humoral mediators resolves within 30 minutes of the release of the pneumoperitoneum.[22]

The opinions of investigators regarding the influence of pneumoperitoneum on cardiac filling pressures are mixed. A study of swine in which a pneumoperitoneum of 15-torr pressure was created resulted in reports of increased pulmonary artery pressures.[10] Healthy human subjects undergoing laparoscopic surgery have demonstrated increased venous return when intraabdominal pressure was in the 14- to 20-torr range.[22,24,31] Although venous return improved in healthy gynecologic surgery patients with modestly elevated intraabdominal pressures, increasing the intraabdominal pressure to greater than 20 torr was found to decrease CVP. Motew reported a similar effect: an increased CVP in patients with an intraabdominal pressure of 20 torr and a decrease in CVP when intraabdominal pressure was 30 torr.[32]

Confounding factors such as the vasodilating actions of anes-thesia[5] and the effects of intraoperative positioning can alter cardiac preload. The reverse Trendelenburg position, so often used in laparoscopic cholecystectomy, tends to decrease venous return,[5] whereas the Trendelenburg position customarily used in gynecologic laparoscopy increases venous return.[22]

Two mechanisms have been proposed as reasons for the elevated filling pressures sometimes observed during laparoscopy. One theory proposes that increased intraabdominal pressure leads to compression of the abdominal venous beds, leading to a redistribution of blood to the central circulation. Another expla-nation suggests that the increased cardiac filling pressures are the result of increased intrathoracic pressure caused by elevated intraabdominal pressure. The increase in intrathoracic and cardiac filling pressures occurs in the absence of increased circu-lating volume.[5,33] The decreased filling pressures observed with grossly elevated intraabdominal pressures (e.g., >30 torr) have been explained as the result of compression of the vena cava.[12]

Reports of the effects of pneumoperitoneum on stroke volume uniformly record a reduction in stroke volumes.[12,22,33,34] In both human and animal studies, stroke volume was observed to decrease when intraabdominal pressure was in the range of 14 to 15 torr.[10,22] Decreases in stroke volume have been attenu-ated by interventions that increase the patient's circulating volume. Interventions to minimize the decrease in stroke volume include institution of the Trendelenburg position,[22] hydration with parenteral fluids, and compression of lower-extremity veins.[34] Despite preoperative expansion of intravascu-lar volume and wrapping legs with elastic bandages, the stroke volume in laparoscopic cholecystectomy patients (under general anesthetic and in reverse Trendelenburg) has been observed to decrease approximately 30%. Observations of laparoscopic cholecystectomy patients immediately after the release of pneu-moperitoneum and return to the supine position (from reverse Trendelenburg) typically find an increase in the stroke volume. This postpneumoperitoneum increase in stroke volume has been attributed to a return of blood to the systemic circulation from the lower extremities.[33]

The relationship of pneumoperitoneum to cardiac output (CO) and cardiac index (CI) is complex because of the multi-plicity of variables that influence CO. With a few exceptions, investigators report reduction of CO in the presence of pneumo-peritoneum.[29,31] In a canine model, decreased CO was noted at intraabdominal pressures of 8 to 12 torr, although significant reduction in CO was not observed until intraabdominal pressure reached 16 torr.[30] Patients undergoing laparoscopic gynecologic surgery have demonstrated decreases in CO associated with intraabdominal pressures in excess of 20 torr.[32,35,36] In patients undergoing laparoscopic cholecystectomy, decreases in CO of 50% have been observed.[34] The technique of optimizing intra-vascular volume and wrapping the patient's legs in elastic bandages has been shown to reduce the degree of decrease in CO in patients undergoing laparoscopic cholecystectomy. Healthy laparoscopic cholecystectomy patients with corrected hypovolemia and wrapped legs experienced a 20% drop in CO, as compared with a 50% drop in control patients.[22,33,24]

In clinical studies of human subjects, an initial decrease in CO is typically observed early in the course of surgery. This initial decrease is attributed to the mechanical effects of the pneumo-peritoneum plus any superimposed positional changes, such as the reverse Trendelenburg position, that may reduce venous return.[30] Five to ten minutes after this initial decrease, the CO tends to increase, partially reversing the initial reduction in CO.[5,29]

BOX 32-3

Hemodynamic Changes Associated with Pneumoperitoneum

- Central venous pressure ↑ or ↓,
- Mean arterial pressure ↑
- Stroke volume ↓
- Cardiac output ↑, ↓, or without change
- Systemic vascular resistance ↑
- Heart rate ↑

Data from Wahba RWM et al. Cardiopulmonary function and laparo-scopic cholecystectomy. Can J Anaesth. 1995;42:51-63; Coskun F, Salman M. Anesthesia for operative endoscopy. Curr Opin Obstet Gynecol. 2001;13:371-376; Nuzzo G et al. Routine use of open tech-nique in laparoscopic operations. J Am Coll Surg. 1997;184:58-62; Sharma KC et al. Cardiopulmonary physiology and pathophysiology as a consequence of laparoscopic surgery. Chest. 1996;110:810-815; O'Leary E et al. Laparoscopic cholecystectomy: haemodynamic and neuroendocrine responses after pneumoperitoneum and changes in position. Br J Anaesth. 1997;76:640-644; Hirvonen EA et al. Hemodynamic changes due to Trendelenburg positioning and pneumoperi-toneum during laparoscopy. Surg Endosc. 2000;14:272-277; Motew M et al. Cardiovascular effects and acid-base and blood gas changes during laparoscopy. Am J Obstet Gynecol. 1973;115:1002-1012.

↑, Increased; ↓, decreased.

This biphasic response is believed by some to be mediated by a neurohumoral response.[5] Aside from neurohumoral factors, an increased heart rate, usually observed in laparoscopy patients, helps reduce the decrease in CO that results from the diminished stroke volume seen in patients with pneumoperitoneum.[22]

Arterial blood pressure has been observed to rise in patients with intraabdominal pressures as low as 14 torr.[22] Some investi-gators have reported a 35% increase in mean arterial pressure associated with peritoneal insufflation.[31] The rise in arterial pressure seen in laparoscopy patients has been attributed to the increased afterload observed in patients with pneumoperitone-um.[5,31] Box 32-3 lists expected hemodynamic changes associated with pneumoperitoneum.

Humoral factors have been implicated in the increased after-load observed in patients with CO_2 pneumoperitoneum. Elevated levels of dopamine, vasopressin, epinephrine, norepinephrine, renin, and cortisol have been noted in laparoscopic cholecys-tectomy patients.[5,34] Vasopressin has been identified as a particularly significant mediator of hemodynamics in patients undergoing laparoscopy. Catecholamine levels in laparoscopy patients have been noted to be mildly elevated and may be related to a generalized stress response.[21] In animal models, catecholamine levels (epinephrine and norepinephrine) are unchanged at intraabdominal pressures of 10 torr but increase significantly at a pressure of 20 torr. Because equivalent results are noted whether N_2O, air, or CO_2 is used, the increases in catecholamines observed in swine undergoing intraperitoneal insufflation appear to be directly related to increased intra-abdominal pressure.[37]

An important cardiovascular effect of pneumoperitoneum is related to distention of the vagus nerve during insufflation. As the vagus is distended, bradycardia is sometimes observed in patients undergoing laparoscopic cholecystectomy.[21]

At an intraabdominal pressure of 14 torr, a reduction of lower-extremity blood-flow velocity has been observed similar to that seen in parturients and patients with ascites. The effect of decreased venous blood flow on the risk for thromboembolic events is not clear. One opinion holds that the laparoscopic technique in cholecystectomy has the net effect of reducing emboli by facilitating early ambulation.[8] Another researcher reports a lower incidence of deep vein thrombosis in gynecologic surgery and a higher incidence in laparoscopic surgery and attributes this difference to the lithotomy and Trendelenburg positions used in gynecologic surgery, as contrasted with the reverse Trendelenburg position used in laparoscopic cholecystectomy surgery.[38]

When compared with healthy patients, patients with significant comorbidity may exhibit exaggerated hemodynamic responses to pneumoperitoneum.[5] Specifically, the cumulative effects of CO_2 pneumoperitoneum and the reverse Trendelenburg position seen in laparoscopic cholecystectomy can result in moderate decreases in CO, as well as significant increases in filling pressures and afterload in sick patients.[39] A study by Safran and Orlando[12] found that in American Society of Anesthesiologists (ASA) class III and IV patients, an IAP of 15 torr resulted in significantly decreased CO and significantly increased MAP and SVR. The increased sensitivity of sick patients to the hemodynamic effects of pneumoperitoneum warrants careful intraoperative monitoring and preoperative attention to the patient's intravascular volume status.[5]

The relationship among intraabdominal, intrathoracic, and filling pressures in the presence of pneumoperitoneum was discussed previously. Serious reservations have been expressed regarding the use of direct measures of filling pressures to estimate intravascular volume. Several authors warn that measurements of CVP and pulmonary artery occlusion pressure are distorted in the presence of increased intraabdominal pressure.[33,34] One solution to this pressure-induced distortion is to calculate a transmural right atrial pressure (right atrial pressure [RAP] − extracardiac pressure) rather than relying on a directly measured RAP as an indication of preload.[33] Another approach involves echocardiographic observation of ventricular wall motion for signs of cardiac decompensation.[34] A pulmonary artery catheter may be of increased utility and its use more valid if serial measurements of CO and mixed venous oxygen saturation are carefully evaluated for signs of decreased cardiac performance.[5,22]

Compared with open surgery, laparoscopic surgery, and in particular laparoscopic cholecystectomy, has the advantage of a decreased incidence of postoperative pulmonary complications. However, relative to patients who undergo open surgery, those who undergo laparoscopic surgery are subjected to increased levels of intraoperative pulmonary dysfunction because of the mechanical effects of pneumoperitoneum and the introduction of exogenous CO_2 into the peritoneal space.[22]

CO_2 pneumoperitoneum is characteristically associated with increases in the partial pressure of arterial CO_2 ($PaCO_2$) and end-tidal CO_2 ($ETCO_2$), with or without acidosis.[12] The increase in $PaCO_2$ seen in CO_2 pneumoperitoneum is attributed primarily to absorption of the gas from the peritoneal surface.[12,40] Attribution of increased $PaCO_2$ levels to the presence of intraabdominal CO_2, not increased metabolism, is supported by studies that failed to find increased levels of oxygen consumption in animals undergoing abdominal insufflation.[12] Increased intraabdominal pressure in and of itself as a cause of hypercapnia was excluded by the findings of a study in which a helium pneumoperitoneum failed to increase $PaCO_2$.[5]

BOX 32-4

Pulmonary Function Changes Associated with Pneumoperitoneum

- Positive inspiratory pressure (PIP) ↑
- Pulmonary compliance dV/dP ↓
- Vital capacity ↓
- Functional residual capacity ↓
- Intrathoracic pressure ↑

Safran DB, Orlando R. Physiologic effects of pneumoperitoneum. Am J Surg. 1994;167:281-286.

↑, Increased; ↓, decreased; dV/dP, change in volume/change in pressure.

Maximum absorption of CO_2 is noted with an intraabdominal pressure of 10 torr. $PaCO_2$ levels are noted to reach a plateau approximately 40 minutes after the induction of the peritoneum.[21]

Compared with intraperitoneal insufflation of CO_2, extraperitoneal insufflation has been associated with an unusually rapid increase in $PaCO_2$ and exceptionally high levels of CO_2.[41,42] In addition to increased levels of CO_2, a study of retroperitoneal insufflation noted that compared to intraperitoneal insuflation, insufflation of the rertroperitoneal space resulted in a prolonged period of elevated CO_2[43]. A misplaced trocar can lead to CO_2 being inadvertently insufflated extraperitoneally, or the insufflation can be deliberate, as in herniorrhaphy and selected urologic procedures.[22,44] Researchers comparing laparoscopic hernia surgery and laparoscopic cholecystectomy have proposed that the increased $PaCO_2$ observed in patients undergoing extraperitoneal insufflation can be explained by the fact that the lack of containment of CO_2 by the peritoneum leads to an increased area for gas exchange.[45]

Mild hypercapnia (45 to 50 torr) is not believed to be clinically significant.[12] Hypercapnia in the range of 50 to 70 torr is associated with physiologic effects such as increased cerebral blood flow, peripheral vasodilation, pulmonary vasoconstriction, and increased risk of cardiac dysrhythmia.[5,8,22]

The mechanical effects of peritoneal insufflation inhibit ventilation. Insufflation of the peritoneum displaces the diaphragm in a cephalad direction.[5] The resulting compression of the basilar lobes of the lungs results in atelectasis,[21] decreased functional residual capacity (FRC), decreased vital capacity, and increased dead space ventilation.[12] Increased intraabdominal pressure also affects pulmonary compliance; in supine patients, pulmonary compliance has been observed to be reduced by 43%.[5] Pulmonary changes associated with pneumoperitoneum are listed in Box 32-4.

An additive effect is observed when general anesthesia, which in and of itself reduces FRC and pulmonary compliance, is combined with pneumoperitoneum.[5] Intraoperative positioning can either aggravate or attenuate pneumoperitoneum-induced pulmonary changes. The Trendelenburg position increases the effects of pneumoperitoneum on pulmonary mechanics. In laparoscopic hysterectomy, pulmonary compliance decreased 20% when the head of the bed was depressed and an additional 30% with peritoneal insufflation.[41] In contrast, the reverse Trendelenburg position partially counteracts the effects of pneumoperitoneum on the diaphragm and improves diaphragmatic function.[11]

One of the most common complications of pneumoperitoneum, endobronchial intubation, has been attributed to the cephalad displacement of the diaphragm caused by pneumoperitoneum. A study of 50 patients with an intraabdominal pressure of 15 torr and in the reverse Trendelenburg position found a 6% rate of right mainstem bronchial intubation.[46] Verification of bilateral breath sounds after insufflation is considered prudent practice by some authors.[38]

Controlled mechanical ventilation provides anesthetists a method for maintaining CO_2 homeostasis in patients undergoing laparoscopic surgery with CO_2 peritoneum. Studies of patients with pneumoperitoneum in the Trendelenburg position reveal that a 20% to 30% increase in minute volume is necessary if Pa_{CO_2} is to be maintained at prepneumoperitoneum levels.[40,47] Preinsufflation Pa_{CO_2} levels in patients who underwent surgery in the reverse Trendelenburg position were maintained by increasing minute volume by a factor of 12% to 16%.[47] Clinical studies of patients undergoing laparoscopic surgeries indicate that increasing the minute volume by preferentially increasing tidal volume rather than respiratory rate is the most effective way to speed CO_2 elimination.[40,47] Compared to normal weight patients, morbidly obese patients commonly experience lower Pa_{O_2} levels during laparoscopic surgery. Attempts to improve oxygenation by increasing tidal volume or respiratory rate have been unsuccessful.[48]

Laparoscopic surgical patients who have marginal cardiopulmonary function preoperatively are at risk of decompensation when faced with the stress introduced by increased intraabdominal pressure and exogenous CO_2. Patients particularly vulnerable to the effects of CO_2 peritoneum are those with increased metabolic rates (as in sepsis), large ventilatory dead space, and decreased CO.[12] Patients with pulmonary emphysema warrant special consideration. Studies in animals, as well as clinical studies in humans, indicate that whereas healthy patients experience minor changes in Pa_{CO_2} and Et_{CO_2} when confronted with CO_2 peritoneum, patients with obstructive lung disease have significantly increased levels of CO_2 retention that may lead to decreases in arterial pH.[11,28]

The high incidence of CO_2 retention observed in patients with chronic obstructive pulmonary disease demands careful intraoperative monitoring of CO_2 levels during laparoscopic surgery. Healthy, mechanically ventilated patients demonstrate a proportional relationship between Et_{CO_2} and Pa_{CO_2}; consequently, continuous Et_{CO_2} monitoring is widely accepted as a method for clinical monitoring.[5,11] In individuals with elevated Et_{CO_2}, the relationship between Et_{CO_2} and Pa_{CO_2} becomes inaccurate, with Et_{CO_2} underestimating Pa_{CO_2}.[22,47] This phenomenon is seen in patients with obstructive lung disease.[28] Direct measurement of Pa_{CO_2} with serial arterial blood gases may be warranted in patients with cardiopulmonary disease.[11]

Pulmonary dysfunction has been observed to persist into the immediate postoperative period in patients recovering from laparoscopic surgery. A slight restrictive breathing pattern in the postoperative period has been observed. Explanations for this aberrant breathing pattern include the residual effects of anesthesia, pain, and diaphragmatic dysfunction induced by stretching or reflex inhibition.[8] Furthermore, the postoperative patient may be subjected to an elevated CO_2 load. In the circumstance of prolonged CO_2 insufflation, CO_2 not excreted is stored in skeletal muscle and bone. It may take hours for this excess CO_2 to be excreted from the patient.[10,22]

The effect of abdominal insufflation on the kidneys often manifests as oliguria, probably because of three mechanisms:

compression of the kidneys (including the renal vasculature), compression of the inferior vena cava (with concomitant reduction in preload), and increased levels of antidiuretic hormone.[21] Significant reduction of renal blood flow was noted in pigs when intraabdominal pressure reached 24 torr.[49] In addition to the direct mechanical effects on the kidneys observed during pneumoperitoneum, humoral factors have an important effect on renal function. In laparoscopic cholecystectomy patients, plasma vasopressin levels were noted to be three times higher than preoperative levels at 30 minutes after insufflation and 20 times higher at 1 hour after insufflation.[50] Renin and aldosterone levels are also typically elevated in laparoscopic surgery patients, with a four-fold increase noted in laparoscopic cholecystectomy patients.[29]

The effects of increased intraabdominal pressure on hepatic and splanchnic blood flow have been the subject of both human and animal studies. In swine, an intraabdominal pressure of 16 torr and elevated head-of-bed position were associated with a 68% decrease in hepatic blood flow.[7] Use of low insufflation pressure has been demonstrated to attenuate the effect of CO_2 pneumoperitoneum on hepatic circulation. In a study of five healthy human subjects, splanchnic blood flow was not disrupted when intraabdominal pressure was maintained at 11 to 13 torr for 30 to 60 minutes.[50] An examination of hepatic blood flow in healthy subjects experiencing intraabdominal pressures of 12 torr noted increased hepatic perfusion.[51]

ANESTHETIC MANAGEMENT

Laparoscopic surgeries have been performed using local, regional, and general anesthetic techniques. The choice of technique is in large part dependent on the specifics of the surgery.

Local anesthesia with sedation has been used in patients undergoing minor gynecologic laparoscopic surgical procedures such as diagnostic laparoscopy or sterilization.[2,11] The use of local anesthesia is facilitated by surgical techniques such as the use of only one port (as in diagnostic laparoscopy) and small-diameter laparoscopes.[22,52] A randomized, controlled trial studied 164 women undergoing diagnostic laparoscopy for evaluation of infertility. Compared with patients who received general anesthetics, patients who received local anesthesia had shorter hospital stays and a reduction in anesthetic costs. The investigators did report limitations on the use of local anesthesia with sedation for laparoscopic surgery. In patients initially treated with local anesthesia, 5.5% required conversion to general anesthesia for completion of the surgery; furthermore, surgical exposure in patients who received local anesthesia with sedation was inferior to the surgical exposure in patients who received general anesthesia.[52]

Like the use of local anesthesia, the use of regional anesthesia for laparoscopic surgery tends to be limited to minor gynecologic surgical procedures. Shoulder and chest discomfort resulting from the pneumoperitoneum is not well managed by means of regional techniques.[25]

General anesthesia is the most practical technique for many if not most laparoscopic procedures.[2] General anesthesia facilitates managing the patient discomfort associated with pneumoperitoneum[11] and intraoperative positions such as steep Trendelenburg. General anesthesia also has the advantage of facilitating controlled ventilation[11] and the use of muscle relaxants,[5] which may help minimize, respectively, hypercapnia and abdominal insufflation pressure.

Use of the laryngeal mask airway (LMA) in patients receiving general anesthesia for laparoscopic surgery has been the subject of some controversy. Several authors have expressed concerns that the increased intraabdominal and intrathoracic pressures characteristic of pneumoperitoneum place the patient at increased risk of gastroesophageal reflux and pulmonary aspiration.[11,12]

Resistance to gastroesophageal reflux is quantified by the barrier pressure, which is the difference between the lower esophageal sphincter pressure and the gastric pressure.[53,54] A study examining the effect of laparoscopy on barrier pressure has shown that in endotracheally intubated patients undergoing gynecologic laparoscopy, an increase in intraabdominal pressure was accompanied by an adaptational increase in lower esophageal pressure, resulting in a net increase in barrier pressure.[54] However, concerns have been raised that use of LMAs impairs lower esophageal sphincter pressure, thereby reducing barrier pressure. Rabey and others, in a study of general and orthopedic surgery patients, did in fact observe reductions in lower esophageal sphincter pressures when an LMA was used as an airway in general anesthesia.[53]

Researchers have conducted studies to evaluate the safety and efficacy of LMAs in gynecologic laparoscopy. Authors of a retrospective study of 1469 gynecologic laparoscopies concluded that use of the LMA "appears safe."[55] A prospective study using direct fiberoptic examination of the laryngopharynx in 91 patients undergoing gynecologic laparoscopy with an LMA in place failed to identify a single incidence of regurgitation.[36] The efficacy of the LMA was evaluated in a randomized controlled trial that compared the performance of the LMA to endotracheal intubation (ETT) in 209 women undergoing gynecologic laparoscopy. The LMA compared favorably with ETT, with no statistical difference found in SpO_2, $ETCO_2$, or stomach size changes.[56] Researchers investigating the use of the ProSeal LMA in gynecologic laparoscopy found the device as efficacious as the classic LMA, with the added advantage that the ProSeal LMA resulted in a seal of the airway that was 10 cm H_2O pressure higher than the classic LMA.[57]

Authoritative sources suggest that under certain circumstances, LMA use may be appropriate during laparoscopy. Guidelines for use of the LMA in laparoscopy are given in Box 32-5. Brimacomb and Brain recommend that clinicians who use the LMA during laparoscopy should, among other considerations, be experienced and adhere to the "15" rule, which requires that the surgery not exceed 15 minutes' duration, the tilt of the bed be less than 15 degrees, and the intraabdominal pressure be less than 15 cm H_2O.[58] Although evidence can be presented to support the use of the LMA in pelvic surgery, research to support use of the LMA in upper-abdominal surgery is lacking. A consensus of clinicians fails to recommend the use of the LMA in upper-abdominal surgeries such as laparoscopic cholecystectomy.[2,55,58]

Use of N_2O in laparoscopic surgery has been a source of controversy because of beliefs that N_2O contributes to bowel distention and increases the incidence of nausea and vomiting. The effect of N_2O on bowel distention has been examined in two studies. A randomized controlled trial involving 50 patients undergoing laparoscopic surgery was conducted. Based on their observation of the bowel, surgeons were asked to determine whether or not the anesthetist was using N_2O. The surgeons, blinded to anesthetic technique, were unable to reliably detect the use of N_2O based on observation of the gut.[59] A similar study was conducted in 150 patients undergoing open colon surgery; again, surgeons blinded to anesthetic technique were unable to identify patients receiving N_2O based on clinical observation.[60]

BOX 32-5

Some Guidelines for Use of the Laryngeal Mask Airway During Laparoscopy

- Ensure that clinician is an experienced LMA user.
- Select patients carefully (e.g., fasted, not obese).
- Use correct size of LMA.
- Make surgeon aware of the use of LMA.
- Use total IV anesthetic technique or volatile agent.
- Adhere to "15" rule: <15 degree tilt; <15 cm H_2O intraabdominal pressure; <15 min duration.
- Avoid inadequate anesthesia during surgery.
- Avoid disturbance of the patient during emergence.

Maltby JR et al. LMA-Classic and LMA-ProSeal are effective alternatives to endotracheal intubation for gynecological laparoscopy. Can J Anaesth. 2003;50:71-77.

IV, *Intravenous;* LMA, *laryngeal mask airway.*

POSTOPERATIVE CONSIDERATIONS

Nausea and vomiting are common postoperative complaints from patients who have undergone laparoscopic surgery; some investigators report incidences of nausea and vomiting in postoperative laparoscopy patients to be as high as 50% to 62%.[21,61] The question of N_2O's role in postoperative nausea and vomiting remains controversial and is beyond the scope of this discussion. However, a brief review of studies examining the use of N_2O and postoperative nausea and vomiting in laparoscopy patients is in order. Three separate randomized controlled trials involving gynecologic laparoscopies enrolling a total of 640 patients failed to demonstrate a statistically significant increase in the rate of nausea and vomiting in patients receiving N_2O, as compared with patients not receiving N_2O.[62,63]

Postoperative pain after laparoscopic surgery is typically of a visceral quality on the day of surgery, with shoulder pain predominating on the first postoperative day.[64] Postoperative pain in laparoscopy patients is believed to be primarily the result of the pneumoperitoneum, rather than the incisions used to introduce trocars into the peritoneal space.[65] The pneumoperitoneum is believed to induce pain through both mechanical and chemical means. Insufflation of the abdomen is associated with distention of the peritoneum and abdominal wall, leading to traction of the nerves and trauma to blood vessels.[64] CO_2, commonly used as an insufflation gas, contributes to postoperative pain by decreasing intraperitoneal pH to as low as 6 in the immediate postoperative period.[65] This CO_2-induced intraperitoneal acidosis is believed to contribute to irritation of the phrenic nerve, which is manifested as shoulder pain often seen in postoperative laparoscopy patients.[46,64,65]

Management of postoperative pain in laparoscopy patients typically involves a multimodal approach including opioids, nonsteroidal antiinflammatory drugs (NSAIDs), and local anesthetics.[2] In a randomized controlled trial of laparoscopic cholecystectomy patients, the use of a multimodal technique was demonstrated to decrease levels of postoperative pain and nausea, as well as speed discharge.[61] A novel approach to control of pain in laparoscopy involved the preemptive administration of ketamine; this approach resulted in improved patient comfort in the immediate postoperative period.[66]

The use of NSAIDs in managing postoperative laparoscopic pain has been demonstrated to be of value. The efficacy of NSAIDs for postoperative laparoscopic pain has been repeatedly studied, and in all cases, NSAID performance was superior to placebo, although not always at a level of statistical significance.[64] Although NSAIDs are insufficiently potent to control laparoscopic pain as a single agent, they are often used in combination with opioids, with the resulting synergism leading to decreased opioid consumption.[64,65]

The efficacy of peripherally administered local anesthetics in the management of postoperative laparoscopy pain is a complicated question. A systematic review by Moiniche and colleagues evaluated 41 randomized controlled trials that studied pain control using local anesthesia in intraperitoneal and port-site infiltration, as well as mesosalpinx and fallopian-tube block. Moiniche concluded, after reviewing 11 studies of port-site infiltration, that the technique was without major effect. Evaluation of 12 trials of mesosalpinx and fallopian-tube blockade concluded that the treatment was of significant yet short-lasting value. Evaluation of studies of intraperitoneal local anesthesia injection characterized the intervention as statistically significant but questioned the clinical significance of the treatment effect.[67]

THE FUTURE OF LAPAROSCOPIC SURGERY

The dramatic growth in laparoscopy seen in the 1980s and early 1990s has reached a plateau, and the procedure has entered a period of incremental development. Recent innovations in technology that have advanced laparoscopy include systems such as EndoAssist and AESOP, which are computer-controlled laparoscopic camera holders.[9] Efforts to eliminate the need for pneumoperitoneum have led to the development of "gasless" laparoscopy. The gasless laparoscopy technique creates a working space for the surgeon by inserting a fan-shaped device into the abdomen to lift the abdominal wall away from the viscera. Gasless laparoscopic techniques have significant limitations, including the need to make multiple skin incisions to insert the lifting device, an increased risk of injury to the abdominal wall, and a quality of surgical exposure that is inferior to that associated with pneumoperitoneum.[18]

Standard laparoscopic techniques are limited in several ways. For example, two-dimensional television limits depth perception, and movement of standard laparoscopic instruments is counterintuitive (i.e., to move an instrument within a patient to the left, the operator moves his or her hand to the right).[4] Emerging technologies have the potential to allow surgeons to operate far more intuitively and with greater dexterity than traditional laparoscopic techniques.

Robotic surgery, perhaps more properly termed *telemanipulation* or *robotic-assisted surgery*, may permit surgeons to overcome some of the limitations imposed by standard laparoscopic technology. A surgeon using robotic-assisted technology (e.g., the daVinci surgical system) controls surgical instruments from a control console that may be immediately adjacent to the patient or at a site hundreds of miles away from the operating room. An important feature of telerobotic technology is three-dimensional imaging, which permits superior depth perception. The robot arms manipulated by the surgeon facilitate delicate surgery by simulating the motion of the human wrist and fingers and also allow scaling of the surgeon's movement (i.e., translation of the movement of a surgeon's hand into a finer movement of the instrument). The surgeon's dexterity is further improved by the robotic system's ability to factor out tremor. Robotic-assisted surgery offers the surgeon improved ergonomics, superior dexterity, and the ability to use traditional open surgical skills for laparoscopic operations. Surgeries using telerobotic technology have been performed in cardiac, general, gynecologic, and urologic surgical disciplines.[4]

Anesthetic management of robotic-assisted laparoscopic surgery is similar to standard laparoscopic surgery, but case reports have been published that note special considerations for this variation of laparoscopic surgery. Robotic-assisted radical prostatectomy requires a steep Trendelenburg tilt (30 to 45 degrees); this places patients at risk for laryngeal edema and brachial plexus injury.[68] A report describing a pediatric surgical experience noted that the setup of the robotic equipment (occurring after anesthetic induction) can take considerable time and impedes access to the patient. Because of the potential for limited access to patients undergoing robotic-assisted surgery, especially pediatric patients, careful contingency plans should be made by the surgical team should an intraoperative crisis call for immediate access to the patient.[69]

SUMMARY

As technology advances, one can anticipate even broader application of laparoscopy and other minimally invasive surgical techniques in the future. Providing safe and effective anesthetic care demands that the anesthetist understand the unique concerns of laparoscopic surgery, in particular the effect of abdominal insufflation on patient physiology.

REFERENCES

1. Soper NJ et al. Medical progress: laparoscopic general surgery. *N Engl J Med.* 1994;330:409-419.
2. Smith I. Anesthesia for laparoscopy with emphasis on outpatient laparoscopy. *Anesthesiol Clin North America* 2001;19:21-42.
3. Deziel DJ et al. Complications of laparoscopic cholecystectomy: a national survey of 4,292 hospitals and an analysis of 77,604 cases. *Am J Surg.* 1993;165:9-14.
4. Ruurda JP et al. Robot-assisted surgical systems: a new era in laparoscopic surgery. *Ann R Coll Surg Engl.* 2002;84:223-226.
5. Wahba RWM et al. Cardiopulmonary function and laparoscopic cholecystectomy. *Can J Anaesth.* 1995;42:51-63.
6. Lee VS et al. Complications of laparoscopic cholecystectomy. *Am J Surg.* 1993;165:527-532.
7. Chiu PT et al. Anesthesia for laparoscopic general surgery. *Anaesth Intensive Care.* 1993;21:163-174.
8. Goodale RL et al. Hemodynamic, respiratory and metabolic effects of laparoscopic cholecystectomy. *Am J Surg.* 1993;166:533-537.
9. Sackier JM, Wang Y. Robotically assisted laparoscopic surgery. *Surg Endosc.* 1994;8:63-66.
10. Ho H et al. Intraperitoneal carbon dioxide insufflation and cardiopulmonary function. *Arch Surg.* 1992;127:928-933.
11. Cunningham AJ, Brull SJ. Laparoscopic cholecystectomy: anesthetic implications. *Anesth Analg.* 1993;76:1120-1133.
12. Safran DB, Orlando R. Physiologic effects of pneumoperitoneum. *Am J Surg.* 1994;167:281-286.
13. Nuzzo G et al. Routine use of open technique in laparoscopic operations. *J Am Coll Surg.* 1997;184:58-62.
14. Rosen DM et al. Methods of creating pneumoperitoneum: a review of techniques and complications. *Obstet Gynecol Surv.* 1998;53:167-174.
15. Hanney RM et al. Use of the Hasson cannula producing major vascular injury at laparoscopy. *Surg Endosc.* 1999;13:1238-1240.
16. Sigman HH et al. Risks of blind verses open approach to celiotomy for laparoscopic surgery. *Surg Laparosc Endosc.* 1993;3:296-299.
17. Bonjer HJ et al. Open versus closed establishment of pneumoperitoneum in laparoscopic surgery. *Br J Surg.* 1997;84:599-602.

18. Canestrelli M et al. New techniques of gynaecologic laparoscopy, gasless, open Hasson, optic trocar. *Panminerva Med.* 1999;41:371-377.
19. Noga J et al. Role of the anesthesiologist in the early diagnosis of life-threatening complications during laparoscopic surgery. *Surg Laparosc Endosc.* 1997;7:63-65.
20. Beck DH, McQuillan PJ. Fatal carbon dioxide embolism and severe haemorrhage during laparoscopic salpingectomy. *Br J Anaesth.* 1994;72:243-245.
21. Koivusalo A, Lindgren L. Effects of carbon dioxide pneumoperitoneum for laparoscopic cholecystectomy. *Acta Anaesthesiol Scand.* 2000;44:834-841.
22. Sharma KC et al. Cardiopulmonary physiology and pathophysiology as a consequence of laparoscopic surgery. *Chest.* 1996;110:810-815.
23. Murdock CM et al. Risk factors for hypercarbia, subcutaneous emphysema, pneumothorax and pneumomediastinum during laparoscopic surgery. *Obstet Gynecol.* 2000;95:704-709.
24. Batra MS et al. Evanescent nitrous oxide pneumothorax after laparoscopy. *Anesth Analg.* 1983;62:1121-1123.
25. Collins L, Vaghadia H. Regional anesthesia for laparoscopy. *Anesthesiol Clin North America.* 2001;19:43-55.
26. Hasel R et al. Intraoperative complications of laparoscopic cholecystectomy. *Can J Anaesth.* 1993;40:459-464.
27. Lew JKL et al. Anaesthetic problems during laparoscopic cholecystectomy. *Anaesth Intensive Care.* 1992;20:91-92.
28. Fitzgerald SD et al. Hypercarbia during carbon dioxide pneumoperitoneum. *Am J Surg.* 1992;163:186-190.
29. O'Leary E et al. Laparoscopic cholecystectomy; haemodynamic and neuroendocrine responses after pneumoperitoneum and changes in position. *Br J Anaesth.* 1997;76:640-644.
30. Ishizaki Y et al. Safe intraabdominal pressure of carbon dioxide pneumoperitoneum during laparoscopic surgery. *Surgery.* 1993;114:549-554.
31. Joris JL et al. Hemodynamic changes during laparoscopic cholecystectomy. *Anesth Analg.* 1993;76:1067-1071.
32. Motew M et al. Cardiovascular effects and acid-base and blood gas changes during laparoscopy. *Am J Obstet Gynecol.* 1973;115:1002-1012.
33. Hirvonen EA et al. Hemodynamic changes due to Trendelenburg positioning and pneumoperitoneum during laparoscopy. *Surg Endosc.* 2000;14:272-277.
34. McLaughlin JG et al. The adverse hemodynamic effects of laparoscopic cholecystectomy. *Surg Endosc.* 1995;9:121-124.
35. Berridge JC. Anesthesia for laparoscopic surgery. In Kumar CM, Bellamy M, eds: *Gastrointestinal Colorectal Anesthesia,* New York: Informa; 2007:245-252.
36. Bapat PP, Verghese C. Laryngeal mask airway and the incidence of regurgitation during gynecological laparoscopies. *Anesth Analg.* 1997;85:139-143.
37. Mikami O et al. High intra-abdominal pressure increases plasma catecholamine levels during pneumoperitoneum for laparoscopic procedures. *Arch Surg.* 1998;133:39-43.
38. Rosen DM. Femoral venous flow during laparoscopic gynecologic surgery. *Surg Laparosc Endosc Percutan Tech.* 2000;10:158-162.
39. Fox LG et al. Physiological changes during laparoscopic cholecystectomy in ASA III and IV patients. *Anesthesiology.* 1993;79:A55.
40. Hirvonen EA et al. Ventilatory effects, blood gas changes and oxygen consumption during laparoscopic hysterectomy. *Anesth Analg.* 1995;80:961-966.
41. Wolf JS et al. Carbon dioxide absorption during laparoscopic pelvic operation. *J Am Coll Surg.* 1995;180:555-560.
42. Burton A, Steinbrook RA. Precipitous decrease in oxygen saturation during laparoscopic surgery. *Anesth Analg.* 1993;76:1177-1178.
43. Streich B et al. Increased carbon dioxide absorption during retroperitoneal laparoscopy. *Br J Anaesth.* 2003;91:793-796.
44. Mellinger JD, Ponsky JL. Recent publications in laparoscopic surgery: an overview. *Endoscopy.* 1996;28:441-451.
45. Liem MS et al. Does hypercarbia develop faster during laparoscopic herniorrhaphy than during conventional laparoscopic cholecystectomy? *Anesth Analg.* 1995;81:1243-1249.
46. Brimacomb JR, Orland H. Endobronchial intubation during upper abdominal laparoscopic surgery in the reverse Trendelenburg position. *Anesth Analg.* 1994;78:607.
47. Wahba RWM, Mamazza J. Ventilatory requirements during laparoscopic cholecystectomy. *Can J Anaesth.* 1993;40:206-210.
48. Sprung J et al. The effects of tidal volume and respiratory rate on oxygenation and respiratory mechanics during laparoscopy in morbidly obese patients. *Anesth Analg.* 2003;97:268-274.
49. Hashikura Y et al. Effects of peritoneal insufflation on hepatic and renal blood flow. *Surg Endosc.* 1994;8:759-761.
50. Odeberg S et al. Pneumoperitoneum for laparoscopic cholecystectomy is not associated with compromised splanchnic circulation. *Eur J Surg.* 1998;164:843-848.
51. Meierhenrich R et al. The effects of intraabdominally insufflated carbon dioxide on hepatic blood flow during laparoscopic surgery assessed by transesophageal echocardiography. *Anesth Analg.* 2005;100:340-347.
52. Zupi E et al. Is local anesthesia an affordable alternative to general anesthesia for mini laparoscopy? *J Am Assoc Gynecol Laparosc.* 2000;7:111-114.
53. Rabey PG et al. Effects of the laryngeal mask airway on lower oesophageal sphincter pressure in patients during general anesthesia. *Br J Anaesth.* 1992;69:346-348.
54. Jones MJ et al. Effects of increased intra-abdominal pressure during laparoscopy on the lower esophageal sphincter. *Anesth Analg.* 1989;68:63-65.
55. Verghese C, Brimacombe JR. Survey of laryngeal mask airway usage in 11,910 patients: safety and efficacy for conventional and non-conventional usage. *Anesth Analg.* 1996;82:129-133.
56. Maltby JR et al. LMA-Classic and LMA-ProSeal are effective alternatives to endotracheal intubation for gynecological laparoscopy. *Can J Anaesth.* 2003;50:71-77.
57. Lim Y et al. The ProSeal laryngeal mask airway is an effective alternative to laryngoscope-guided tracheal intubation for gynaecological laparoscopy. *Anaesth Intensive Care.* 2007;35:52-56.
58. Brimacomb JR, Brain AIJ. *The Laryngeal Mask Airway. A Review and Practical Guide.* London: Saunders; 1996.
59. Taylor E et al. Anesthesia for laparoscopic cholecystectomy: is nitrous oxide contraindicated? *Anesthesiology.* 1992;76:541-543.
60. Krogh B et al. Nitrous oxide does not influence operating conditions or postoperative course in colonic surgery. *Br J Anaesth.* 1996;72:55-57.
61. Michaloliakou C et al. Preoperative multimodal analgesia facilitates recovery after ambulatory laparoscopic cholecystectomy. *Anesth Analg.* 1996;82:44-51.
62. Arellano RJ et al. Omission of nitrous oxide from a propofol-based anesthetic does not affect the recovery of women undergoing outpatient gynecologic surgery. *Anesthesiology.* 2000;93:332-339.
63. Sukhani R et al. Propofol for ambulatory gynecological laparoscopy: does omission of nitrous oxide alter postoperative sequelae and recovery? *Anesth Analg.* 1994;78:831-835.
64. Alexander JI. Pain after laparoscopy. *Br J Anesth.* 1997;79:369-378.
65. Mouton W, Bessell JR, Otten KT, Madden GJ. Pain after laparoscopy. *Surg Endosc.* 1999;13:445-448.
66. Launo C et al. Preemptive ketamine during general anesthesia for postoperative analgesia in patients undergoing laparoscopic cholecystectomy. *Minerva Anestesiol.* 2004;70:727-734.
67. Moiniche S et al. Local anesthetic infiltration for postoperative pain relief after laparoscopy. *Anesth Analg.* 2000;90:899-912.
68. Phong SV, Koh LK. Anaesthesia for robotic-assisted radical prostatectomy: considerations for laparoscopy in the Trendelenburg position. *Anaesth Intensive Care.* 2007;35:281-285.
69. Mariano ER et al. Anesthetic concerns for robot-assisted laparoscopy in an infant. *Anesth Analg.* 2004;99:1665-1667.

CHAPTER 33

MUSCULOSKELETAL SYSTEM ANATOMY, PHYSIOLOGY, PATHOPHYSIOLOGY, AND ANESTHESIA MANAGEMENT

Mary C. Karlet

Somatic musculature is broadly classified into three compartments—skeletal, cardiac, or smooth—based on the muscles' anatomic and functional roles. Force generated by all these muscle types depends on the transient elevation of intracellular calcium (Ca^{2+}) and activation of actin and myosin filaments. Skeletal muscle is under voluntary control and is striated in appearance. Smooth muscle is found in most internal organs (except the heart), is under involuntary autonomic control, and is nonstriated. Cardiac muscle is striated in appearance and under control of an intrinsic pacemaker modulated by the autonomic nervous system.[1] The focus of this chapter is skeletal muscle, its function, and its neurologic control.

Skeletal muscle tissue includes muscles of the tongue and the soft palate, the extrinsic eye muscles, the muscles that move the scalp, all muscles attached to the skeleton, and the muscles in the pharynx and the upper third of the esophagus. Some skeletal muscles, such as those of the lips and the anus, serve as sphincters. Skeletal muscle is innervated by myelinated efferent motor nerve fibers called *alpha (α) motor neurons*. These fast-conducting somatic fibers arise from cell bodies located in the ventral horn of the spinal cord gray matter (Figure 33-1).

The motor nerve axon exits through the spinal cord ventral root and travels uninterrupted to the muscle through a mixed peripheral nerve. Inputs to the ventral horn motor nerve cell body are both excitatory and inhibitory. The inputs include neurons from the brain, neurons from other spinal cord segments, and afferent neurons from various sensory receptors (Figure 33-2). A motor neuron fires an action potential when the sum of the excitatory and inhibitory inputs depolarizes the nerve cell body to its critical threshold potential. Threshold depolarization of the cell body produces local electrical currents that spread to adjoining regions of the nerve membrane, leading to depolarization and action potential propagation down the axon.

At the muscle, each motor nerve divides into branches that enter the muscle and end on individual muscle cells called *muscle fibers*. A single motor neuron and all the muscle fibers it innervates are collectively called a *motor unit* (Figure 33-3). When a motor nerve fires, all the fibers within a single motor unit contract simultaneously.

Motor units exhibit considerable variability, and each unit usually contains between 100 and 200 muscle fibers. However, the motor unit may contain as few as two muscle fibers for fine, delicate movements or as many as a thousand for coarse movements.[1,2]

The strength of a muscle contraction is determined in large part by the number of motor units stimulated and the frequency of the stimulation. A minimal stimulus applied to a muscle may cause only a few muscle units to contract, with a weak overall response. As the stimulus is increased, more units are recruited, and a greater contraction of the muscle occurs.

Activation of nerve cell bodies in the ventral horn produces depolarization of the smallest motor units first. As the excitatory input into the motor neuron pool increases, larger motor units fire. The smaller motor units that are recruited first are resistant to fatigue. The larger motor units are less excitable, but they allow for more forceful contractions.[1,2]

OVERVIEW OF NEUROMUSCULAR TRANSMISSION

Skeletal muscles are normally relaxed and do not contract without nervous stimulation. At rest, the electrical potential difference across the muscle membrane is approximately -90 mV (inside negative). There is a high potassium ion (K^+) concentration inside the muscle cell and a high sodium ion (Na^+) concentration outside the cell.

The process of muscle contraction begins when the electrical activity of a *presynaptic* motor neuron communicates across a *junctional cleft*, or *synaptic gap*, to *postsynaptic* skeletal muscle fibers. The specialized conduction area, or *synapse*, where the axon of a motor neuron ends on a skeletal muscle fiber is called the *neuromuscular junction*, or *myoneural junction* (Figure 33-4). Each skeletal muscle fiber usually has only one neuromuscular junction, a notable exception being extraocular muscles that have multiple innervations per cell. The mediator substance that chemically transduces the axon's electrical message across the synaptic gap to the muscle is the neurotransmitter *acetylcholine* (ACh).[1-3]

Muscle contraction develops when the propagated action potential of the presynaptic motor neuron induces expulsion of the chemical mediator ACh into the junctional cleft. ACh binds to specialized receptors on the postsynaptic muscle membrane. If released from the axon nerve ending in sufficient quantity, ACh-receptor (AChR) occupation induces a transient change in the electrical property of the skeletal muscle membrane, and an action potential and muscle contraction follow.[2]

In the overall process of neuromuscular transmission, an action potential in the motor neuron induces the release of ACh into the junctional cleft, which evokes an action potential in the muscle. As described in greater detail in the following

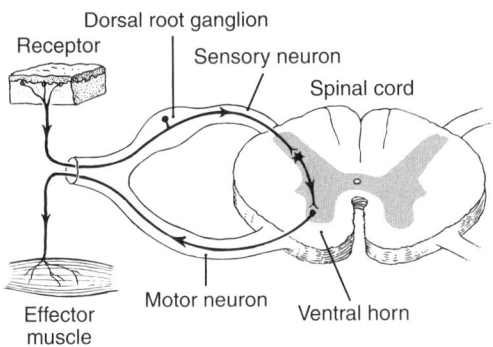

FIGURE **33-1** Spinal reflex arc. Sensory information from the skin is relayed to the motor neuron in the ventral horn of the spinal cord gray matter.

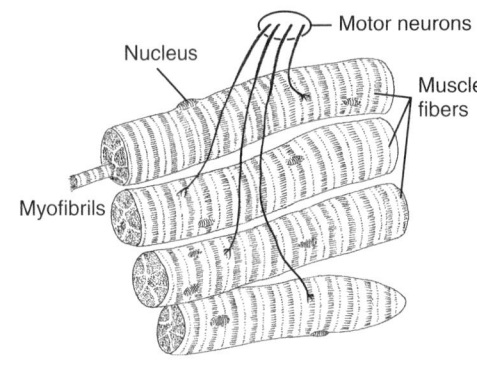

FIGURE **33-3** A motor unit. One motor neuron can synapse with several muscle fibers, which contract as a unit.

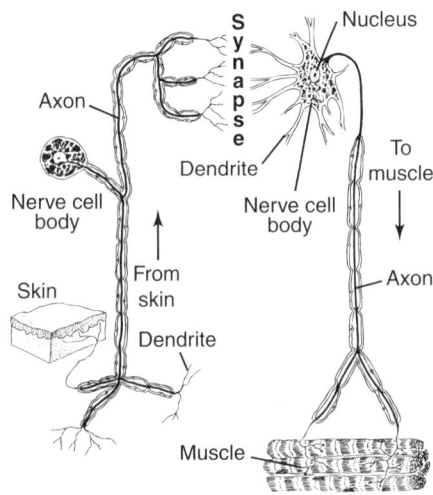

FIGURE **33-2** A sensory neuron synapsing with a motor neuron.

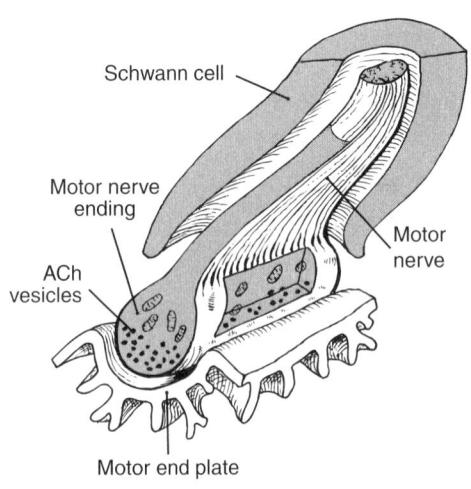

FIGURE **33-4** A cross-section of the neuromuscular junction. Acetylcholine (ACh) vesicles aggregate close to the nerve membrane.

sections, the end result of muscle membrane depolarization is muscle contraction.

Neuromuscular Junction

Motor nerve endings develop in intimate and precise proximity to skeletal muscle fibers. The motor axon terminal is separated from the muscle cell it innervates by a synaptic gap of only 20 to 50 nm.[2] A carbohydrate-rich, filamentous material in the synapse holds the nerve ending and its associated muscle cell in close alignment. This anatomic alliance increases the likelihood for prompt receptor activation after transmitter release.[2,4]

The synaptic gap is contiguous with the extracellular fluid, which provides a route for drugs or toxins to gain access to the neuromuscular junction. Botulinum toxin, for example, gains access to the junction through the extracellular fluid and produces its depressive neuromuscular effects by inhibiting ACh release from the nerve ending.[2]

Both sides of the neuromuscular junction, the presynaptic motor axon and the postsynaptic muscle cell, serve specialized functions (Figure 33-5). As it nears the neuromuscular junction, the motor nerve axon loses its myelin sheath and divides into many smaller nerve fibers, which terminate as *end-feet*.

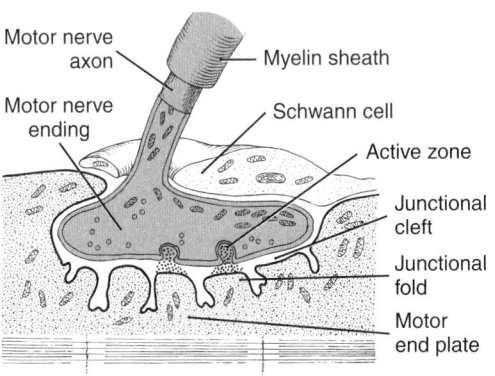

FIGURE **33-5** A longitudinal view of the neuromuscular junction. Nerve ending "active zones" are located opposite the junctional folds of the motor end plate. The motor end plate is distinct from the muscle contractile machinery. At the active zones, the ACh vesicles are shown discharging their ACh into the junctional cleft.

The motor nerve end-foot is distinct from the rest of the nerve. It is rich in mitochondria and the materials and support structures necessary for the synthesis, storage, mobilization, and release of the neurotransmitter ACh. Small, clear vesicles or granules are particularly numerous in the part of the nerve ending closest to the junctional gap. Each of these vesicles contains a small packet, or *quantum*, of ACh molecules. The ACh vesicles concentrate along the junctional surface of the nerve end-feet in areas called "active zones."[4]

At the neuromuscular junction, each motor nerve ending closely approximates with a thickened and highly convoluted portion of the postsynaptic membrane called the *motor end plate*. The motor end plate is physically and functionally demarcated from the surrounding muscle membrane. The many membrane convolutions at the end plate are known as *junctional folds*. ACh receptors are concentrated near the shoulders of the junctional folds, lying near the ACh release sites. The close approximation of ACh release site and target receptor site ensures little transmitter waste and direct coupling of nerve signal and muscle response.[5]

Acetylcholine Release

Physiologic transmission of the nerve message to the muscle begins with a Ca^{2+}-dependent mechanism for ACh release from the nerve terminal. When a nerve impulse arrives at a motor nerve ending, the action potential causes a transient increase in Ca^{2+} conductance across the nerve membrane by activating voltage-dependent Ca^{2+} channels. Both "fast" and "slow" Ca^{2+} channels appear to open, but it is primarily the fast ("N-type" and "P/Q-type") Ca^{2+} channels that are involved in depolarization-induced transmitter release.[6-8] Calcium enters the nerve terminal, flowing down its electrochemical gradient. The influx of Ca^{2+} causes ACh vesicles to fuse with the nerve plasma membrane and then expel their content into the synaptic cleft.[9] The amount of ACh released is influenced by the amount of Ca^{2+} that enters the nerve terminal during nerve stimulation. The more Ca^{2+} that enters the nerve terminal, the greater the amount of ACh released.

About 125 ACh vesicles, or quanta, are released with each nerve impulse. Each quantum in turn contains about 10,000 molecules of the neurotransmitter.[2] This amount of ACh and the normal abundance of postjunctional receptors at each neuromuscular junction readily ensure muscle activation. A considerable safety margin exists in the synaptic transmission. With each nerve impulse, excess ACh is released, and excess ACh receptors are available for occupation.[5,10,11]

Small concentrations of other divalent cations can compete with and limit Ca^{2+} influx into the nerve ending, decreasing ACh release and impairing neuromuscular transmission. When administered intravenously, magnesium sulfate, for example, can interfere with Ca^{2+} influx and produce muscle weakness by inhibiting ACh release.

Certain antibiotics, particularly the aminoglycosides, inhibit ACh release from the nerve terminal and can enhance neuromuscular blockade when administered concomitant with clinical dosages of neuromuscular blocking agents.

Calcium channel–blocking drugs used for the treatment of dysrhythmias and hypertension block Ca^{2+} conductance through so-called "slow" ("L-type") channels. Their primary action is on the slow Ca^{2+} channels of the heart and blood vessels, but they can inhibit prejunctional Ca^{2+} influx. The large safety margin inherent in normal neuromuscular transmission obscures any clinically detectable effect these drugs may have on neuromuscular transmission. However, with disorders associated with impaired neuromuscular transmission, such as myasthenic syndrome, the Ca^{2+} channel blocker's prejunctional attenuation of ACh release may be unmasked, and neuromuscular transmission may be further weakened.[12]

Acetylcholine Synthesis

Neurons that release the neurotransmitter ACh are called *cholinergic neurons*. Active cholinergic motor neurons replenish their ACh stores by continually resynthesizing the neurotransmitter. Many enzymes and other proteins needed by the nerve ending to synthesize, store, and release ACh are made in the motor nerve cell body and are transported distally to the nerve ending by a process called *axonal transport*.

In the axoplasm of the motor nerve ending, the enzyme *choline acetyltransferase* (CAT) catalyzes the reaction of two substrates, *acetyl coenzyme A* (acetyl CoA) and *choline*, to form ACh, as seen in Equation 33-1.

Equation 33-1

$$Choline + Acetyl\ CoA \rightarrow ACh + CoA$$

Choline is obtained locally by a Na^+-linked uptake into the cholinergic nerve ending. Acetyl CoA is synthesized from pyruvate in neuronal mitochondria. Mitochondria and other metabolic machinery used to synthesize ACh are abundant in the nerve ending (Figure 33-6).

About 80% of the newly synthesized ACh is stored within synaptic vesicles in the nerve terminal, positioned for release. Each nerve ending contains more than 300,000 of these vesicles. The remainder of the ACh is stored in a nonvesicular axoplasmic reserve.[2]

The ACh vesicles are released through exocytosis in response to action potential stimulation, but only a small fraction of the available vesicles is used to send each signal.[2]

Postjunctional End Plate

There is a distinction between the postjunctional cation channels of the muscle end plate and other cation channels of nerve and

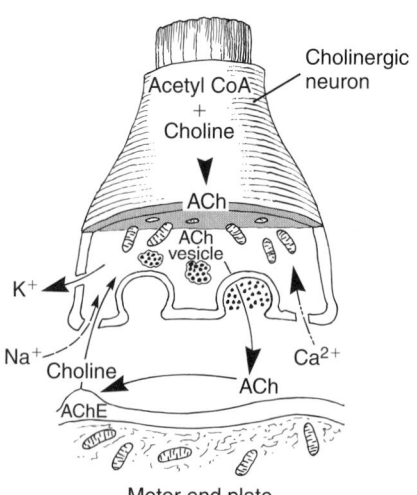

FIGURE **33-6** ACh synthesis from choline and acetylcoenzyme A (acetyl CoA) in the motor nerve ending. Calcium ion entry into the nerve ending causes the ACh vesicles to release their contents. Acetylcholinesterase (AChE) on the postjunctional membrane destroys ACh. Choline is recycled into the nerve ending by a sodium ion–linked transport mechanism.

muscle membranes. Motor end-plate cation channels are *ligand-gated*, that is, they are opened or closed by the action of a chemical. Cation channels of nerve axons, on the other hand, are *voltage-gated* by electrical changes in the membrane.[4]

The binding of ACh molecules to postsynaptic receptor proteins causes a transient increase in conductance in ligand (ACh)-gated cation channels at the postjunctional motor end plate. The cation flow at the end plate produces a net inward Na^+ current and a net outward K^+ current. The previously polarized end-plate membrane (resting membrane potential of approximately −90 mV) becomes transiently "depolarized." The resulting postjunctional membrane voltage change is called the *end-plate potential* (EPP).[4] The EPP does not begin until 0.5 millisecond after the arrival of the action potential at the presynaptic nerve ending. This *synaptic delay* arises from the relatively slow liberation and diffusion of ACh across the junctional cleft.[2,4]

EPPs vary in strength according to the quantity of ACh released. The more ACh released, the greater the postsynaptic end-plate voltage change. In other words, EPPs do not adhere to the "all-or-none" principle. EPPs can be summed, and their magnitude depends on the strength of the summed stimuli of ACh molecules.

Perijunctional Area

The postjunctional end-plate membrane does not fire action potentials. After it is depolarized by ACh-receptor occupation, the current sink created by the local EPP depolarizes the *adjacent* muscle membrane. If the depolarizing input is great enough and reaches threshold potential, action potentials are fired from either side of the end plate in both directions along the muscle fiber (Figure 33-7).[4]

The transition zone where the potential developed at the end plate is converted to an action potential is called the *perijunctional area*. A demarcation exists between the chemically sensitive AChR channels of the end plate and the chemically insensitive but electrically sensitive Na^+ channels in the perijunctional area of the muscle membrane. The membrane in the perijunctional area is rich in Na^+ channels, and this feature enhances its capacity to respond to an EPP and transform it to an action potential.

With a typical motor neuron's action potential, the EPP produced at the muscle end plate is usually sufficient to create an action potential at the muscle membrane, and muscle contraction is regularly produced.

Acetylcholine Receptor

Postjunctional neuromuscular ACh receptors have been extensively purified and studied in detail.[13] An estimated 50 million tightly packed nicotinic AChR sites are at each neuromuscular junction.

In fetal muscle, the ACh nicotinic receptor is a protein composed of five polypeptide subunits: two identical alpha (α) subunits, a beta (β) subunit, a gamma (γ) subunit, and a delta (δ) subunit. Figure 33-8 shows the receptor subunits organized in a pentagonal array around a central ion channel. Without ACh occupation, the central channel is closed; when open, small cations (Na^+ and K^+) are allowed to pass through the channel down their electrochemical gradients.[4]

In adults, the AChR protein structure is similar, except that the fetal γ subunit is replaced by an epsilon (ϵ) subunit.[14] The subunit's change produces an adult cholinergic junctional receptor that has an increased cation conductance and a shortened open time.

As noted earlier, the ACh receptors are located at the crests of the motor end-plate junctional folds, which directly approximate with nerve terminal release sites. In active adults, only the end-plate region of the muscle contains ACh receptors. As little as 200 μm away from the end plate, the muscle membrane becomes practically devoid of receptors.

The ACh receptors are synthesized in the muscle cells and then incorporated into the end-plate membrane as integral membrane proteins. The extracellular or junctional face of the receptor protrudes from the surface of the end-plate membrane, whereas the cytoplasmic surface of the receptor is more flush to the plasma membrane surface (Figure 33-9).

Activation of the postjunctional AChR and opening of the cation channel requires simultaneous ACh occupation at each of the two α-receptor subunits. The binding of two ACh molecules causes a conformational change in the α polypeptides, and the protein conformational change causes the central ion channel to open.[2] If only one α subunit site is occupied by the agonist, the channel remains closed. As described earlier, the open channel increases the conductance to positively charged ions, particularly Na^+, an effect that produces the net depolarizing potential, the EPP. When even one ACh molecule leaves the α subunit, the channel snaps shut and the current stops.

The α subunits are the sites of competition between the cholinergic agonist ACh and receptor antagonists, such as nondepolarizing neuromuscular blocking agents. The outcome of the competition, neuromuscular transmission or neuromuscular

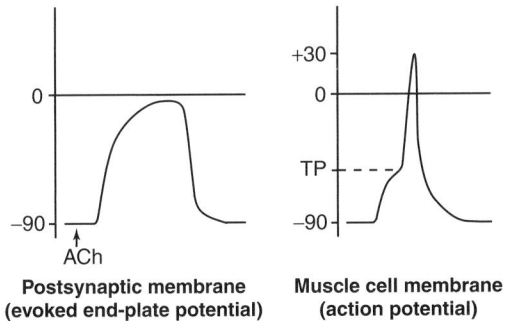

Postsynaptic membrane (evoked end-plate potential)   **Muscle cell membrane (action potential)**

FIGURE **33-7** Depiction of the depolarization characteristics (the end-plate potential) at the postsynaptic membrane in response to ACh and the depolarization and action-potential response at the adjacent, electrically excitable muscle membrane. *TP*, Threshold potential.

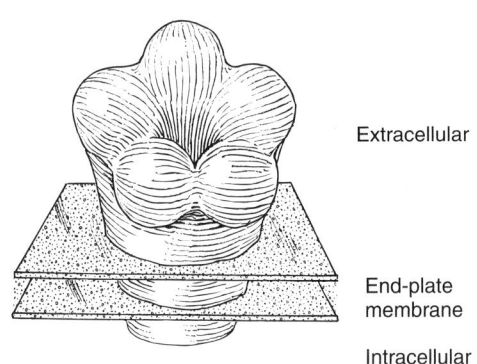

Extracellular

End-plate membrane

Intracellular

FIGURE **33-8** The ACh receptor. Five polypeptide subunits surround a central ion channel.

blockade, depends on the concentration of ACh and the relative concentration and binding properties of the antagonist involved.[3] Nondepolarizing muscle relaxants produce neuromuscular blockade, in part because they bind to one or both α subunit sites and, in so doing, prevent ACh from binding to both sites and opening the channel.

Prejunctional Receptors

Cholinergic receptors are also present at the prejunctional motor nerve ending. It is postulated that in addition to mediating nerve transmission at postjunctional receptor sites, ACh also acts on prejunctional receptors to enhance transmitter mobilization and release. Prejunctional cholinergic receptor occupation may transform the ACh pool from a reserve store to a readily releasable store so that transmitter output can keep pace with transmitter demand.[15]

All the nondepolarizing muscle relaxants used in anesthesia practice compete with ACh for postjunctional cholinergic receptor sites to produce neuromuscular blockade. Receptor antagonist effects at prejunctional receptors may augment nondepolarizing blockade by diminishing ACh output as well. Herein also lies an explanation for the *fade* that is observed with neuromuscular blockade monitoring of nondepolarizing muscle relaxers. Fade of tetanic and train-of-four stimulation may reflect the blockade of prejunctional ACh receptors by the muscle relaxant and failure of ACh release to keep pace with rapid stimulation.[16,17]

Acetylcholinesterase

As noted earlier, the combination of ACh with its muscle end-plate receptor causes a transitory depolarization of the end plate. The EPP is short-lived because soon after binding, ACh is rapidly destroyed by hydrolysis, and its depolarizing action halts.[4] Paradoxically, the rapid destruction and removal of ACh from the junctional cleft is critical for continued muscle contractile response. The ACh molecule must be off the muscle end-plate receptor for the perijunctional muscle membrane to repolarize, or "reset," in anticipation of further activation.

The hydrolysis of ACh to choline and acetate is rapid and efficient (Equation 33-2). Most ACh is destroyed within a few milliseconds after it is released into the junctional cleft.[2] The enzyme *acetylcholinesterase* (AChE), also known as *true* or *tissue cholinesterase*, catalyzes the hydrolysis.

Equation 33-2

$$\text{Acetylcholine} \xrightarrow{\text{Acetylcholinesterase}} \text{Choline} + \text{Acetate}$$

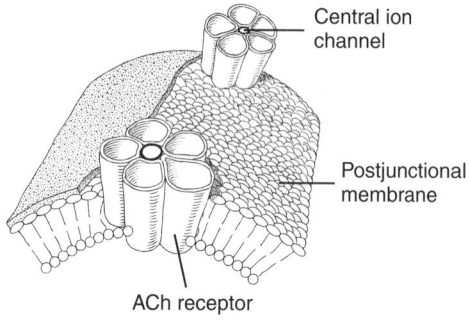

Central ion channel

Postjunctional membrane

ACh receptor

FIGURE **33-9** Two ACh receptors embedded in the postjunctional membrane.

Much of the choline by-product released by hydrolysis is efficiently drawn back within the prejunctional nerve terminal for use in the synthesis of new ACh. Acetylcholinesterase is present in high concentrations on the external surface of the postjunctional muscle membranes. The enzyme resembles a balloon-like structure and is loosely connected to the muscle end-plate membrane by thin stalks of collagen.

Without AChE, the concentration of ACh would become extremely high in the junctional cleft. Under these circumstances, ACh would maintain the muscle end plate in a state of persistent depolarization as ligand-gated cation channels remained open, yet the muscle itself would be paralyzed.[3] The reason for this seemingly illogical behavior (ACh-receptor occupation, end-plate depolarization, yet no muscle contraction) is that in the face of persistent end-plate depolarization, the Na^+ channels of the perijunctional muscle membrane do not reactivate or reset; these voltage-gated ion channels remain closed, impeding further muscle membrane depolarization. Thus, even with persistent end-plate depolarization, muscle contraction is prevented, and clinical weakness follows. A cyclic muscle membrane depolarization/repolarization sequence is necessary for normal muscle contraction to occur.

The mechanism of depolarizing muscle relaxants can, at least in part, be explained by a similar mechanism. Depolarizing muscle relaxants, such as succinylcholine, activate the muscle end plate in a manner similar to that of ACh, but they have a more protracted end-plate depolarizing response because they are less rapidly metabolized. AChR occupation by a depolarizing muscle relaxant causes a prolonged depolarization of the end plate, prohibits activation of perijunctional channels, and produces a depolarizing block.

Reversal of a nondepolarizing neuromuscular block may be accomplished by the use of cholinesterase inhibitors. Anticholinesterase agents inhibit the breakdown of ACh and, in so doing, increase the amount of ACh at the neuromuscular junction. The abundance of ACh in the synaptic gap changes the agonist-antagonist ratio and enables the agonist (ACh) to bind to the ACh receptor with greater frequency than the antagonist (nondepolarizing muscle relaxant). Hence, a higher ACh concentration can overcome the receptor occupation by the muscle relaxant, and neuromuscular transmission can be restored (see Chapter 13).

Various other esterases, in addition to AChE, are present throughout the body. One that is found in the plasma is *pseudocholinesterase*, or *nonspecific cholinesterase*. Like AChE, pseudocholinesterase is capable of hydrolyzing ACh, but it also has properties separate from those of AChE. One distinction particularly relevant to anesthesia practice is the ability of pseudocholinesterase to metabolize ester local anesthetics and the depolarizing muscle relaxant succinylcholine.

Extrajunctional Receptors

In utero, before muscle innervation occurs, the muscle cells of a fetus synthesize *extrajunctional receptors*. These fetal receptors are inserted over the entire length of the muscle cell. As the fetal neuromuscular junction develops, increasing motor nerve activity appears to have a trophic effect in restricting the ACh receptors specifically to the neuromuscular junction.[11] By the age of 2 years, the nerve-muscle contact is fully mature and active, and the extrajunctional receptors disappear from the peripheral part of the muscle. If neural activity is reduced or abolished and the neural trophic influence is lost, the muscle resorts to fetal-like synthesis of extrajunctional cholinergic receptors.[2]

Several situations, including stroke, spinal cord transection, thermal trauma, direct muscle damage, and prolonged immobility, have been associated with the accelerated spread of cholinergic receptors from the end-plate region to large areas of the skeletal muscle membrane. These so-called *denervation injuries* result in an abnormal excitability of the muscle and an increase in muscle sensitivity to ACh, a condition that is called *denervation hypersensitivity*.[14,18] The extrajunctional receptors may develop within 48 hours after diminution of nerve activity. Eventually, the number of aberrant receptors per muscle fiber may increase 5- to 32-fold.[18] These receptors disappear and muscle sensitivity returns to normal if neural input is reestablished. Extrajunctional and end-plate cholinergic receptors are similar in many ways, but an important distinction pertinent to anesthesia practice is their differing response to receptor agonists and antagonists.

Clinically, extrajunctional receptors demonstrate a resistance to nondepolarizing muscle relaxants. Hence, larger doses of nondepolarizing relaxants may be necessary to induce neuromuscular blockade—e.g., in an immobilized limb or in parts of the body affected by a stroke.[19,20] Monitoring a nondepolarizing neuromuscular block with a peripheral nerve stimulator in a paretic limb may result in an underestimation of the magnitude of neuromuscular blockade in nonparetic muscles.[19]

Conversely, extrajunctional receptors are more easily activated by agonists (e.g., ACh, succinylcholine) than junctional receptors. Moreover, each extrajunctional channel stays open about four times longer than junctional receptors, allowing more ions to flow (primarily Na^+ into the muscle cell and K^+ out) in response to agonist-induced depolarization.[21]

The clinical significance of denervation injuries and the proliferation of extrajunctional receptors becomes evident with the administration of succinylcholine, which can produce alarmingly high levels of plasma K^+ in these patients.[22] Succinylcholine-induced hyperkalemia reflects the extensive proliferation of extrajunctional receptors along the entire muscle membrane and their prolonged and exaggerated depolarization response to agonists. Succinylcholine stimulates the aberrant cholinergic receptors and triggers a protracted opening of the cation channels, allowing excess Na^+ movement into the cell and excess K^+ movement out, down their respective gradients.

Dangerous levels of succinylcholine-induced hyperkalemia have been observed within 4 days of denervation injury with doses of succinylcholine as low as 20 mg.[22] The pronounced release of K^+ in response to succinylcholine cannot be circumvented by the prior administration of nonparalyzing doses of nondepolarizing muscle relaxants.

MUSCLE PHYSIOLOGY

Skeletal muscle constitutes the greatest mass of somatic musculature. Skeletal muscle is composed of bundles of multinucleated, long, cylindrical cells. Because their length is much greater than their width, these cells are called *muscle fibers*. Each muscle fiber is a single cell surrounded by an electrically polarized cell membrane called the *sarcolemma*. The sarcolemma separates the extracellular space from the *myoplasm*, the muscle-fiber intracellular space.

Individual skeletal muscle cells are parallel to the muscle body and have no anatomic or functional bridges between them. The parallel arrangement helps maximize shortening capacity and velocity. The cells function independently so that the force of contraction of the total muscle is equal to the sum of individual fibers. This contrasts with smooth and cardiac muscle, in which

the muscle cells are interdependent and are mechanically coupled to adjacent cells.[1,2]

Bundles of cylindrical filaments called *myofibrils* run along the axis of the muscle fiber. Each skeletal muscle fiber contains several hundred myofibrils composed of contractile proteins that impart a striking, repetitive, light-and-dark banding pattern along the entire fiber length. The repeating unit, called a *sarcomere*, is the basic contractile unit of skeletal muscle. The alternating light-and-dark banding pattern is responsible for the classification called *striated muscle*. Cardiac muscle is also classified as striated muscle because it too has the repetitive pattern of light and dark bands.[1] The arrangement of the muscle fibers, myofibrils, and sarcomeres is shown in Figure 33-10.

Most skeletal muscles bridge two skeletal attachment points and are recruited to generate force and movement in actions ranging from chewing to walking. A muscle contraction that involves shortening of the muscle length to perform work is an *isotonic contraction*. A muscle contraction that produces increased tension but no appreciable decrease in length is an *isometric contraction*.

Structure of the Contractile Apparatus

The repeating, striated arrangement of the myofibril arises from the contractile filaments that compose the sarcomere: the *thick filaments* and the *thin filaments*.

The thick filaments, which are composed of the protein myosin, are in the central region of the sarcomere in a dark-colored area termed the *A band*. A densely staining *M line* in the middle of the A band contains proteins that link the thick filaments. The thin filaments are about half the diameter of the thick filaments and are composed of the proteins actin, troponin, and tropomyosin. Thin filaments, connected to *Z lines* or *Z disks*, normally interdigitate with the thick filaments in the relaxed muscle and to an even greater degree in the contracted muscle. The less dense areas of the sarcomere, which contain only thin filaments, are referred to as *I bands*. Two adjacent Z lines delimit each repeating sarcomere unit. The diagram of the sarcomere units in Figure 33-11 may merit careful study.

Cross-sections of the myofibril reveal that each thick filament is surrounded by a hexagonal arrangement of six thin filaments. The myosin and actin filaments are arranged to slide over one another, overlap, and create shortening of the sarcomere and the muscle[2] (Figure 33-12).

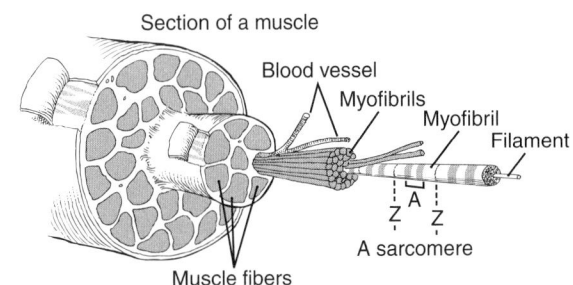

FIGURE **33-10**   The structural arrangement and organization at each level of the muscle assembly. The skeletal muscle is composed of muscle fibers that contain long, cylindrical myofibrils. Each myofibril is made up of precisely arranged thick and thin filaments that form repeating dark and light bands called *sarcomeres*.

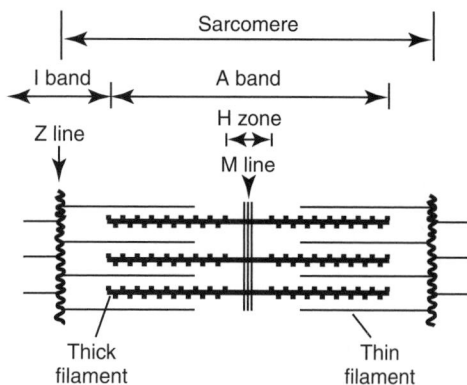

FIGURE **33-11** Longitudinal diagram of a sarcomere showing the arrangement of the thick filaments (myosin) and the thin filaments (primarily actin).

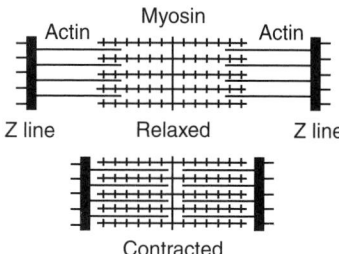

FIGURE **33-12** Actin filament sliding over myosin filament during muscle contraction.

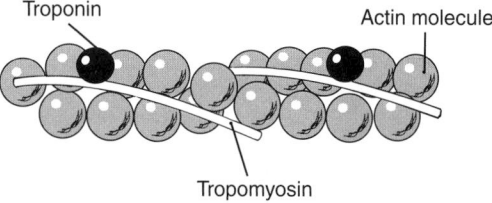

FIGURE **33-13** A thin filament. Globular actin molecules polymerize into a two-stranded, twisted filament. Rod-shaped tropomyosin molecules occupy the grooves between the two actin chains. The regulatory protein troponin binds to the tropomyosin component.

Thin Filament

The three major proteins that compose the thin filament—actin, tropomyosin, and troponin—each play a different role in the contractile process. Each thin filament includes two beadlike chains of polymerized *actin* twisted into a double helix. About 40 to 60 *tropomyosin* molecules are located along the groove between the two actin chains. Each rod-shaped tropomyosin molecule covers about six or seven individual actin proteins. The most important protein in the regulation of the contractile process is *troponin*.[1] As depicted in Figure 33-13, one molecule of troponin is bound to each tropomyosin molecule.

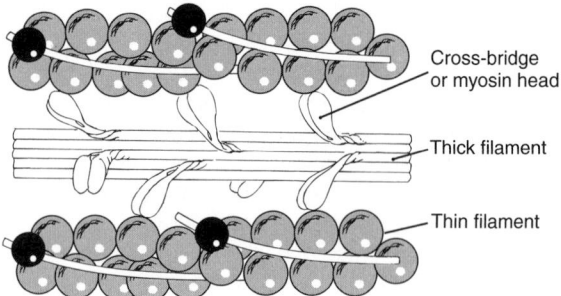

FIGURE **33-14** The tail regions of many myosin molecules intertwine to form a thick filament. The myosin heads, or cross-bridges, project out laterally toward the actin in the surrounding thin filaments.

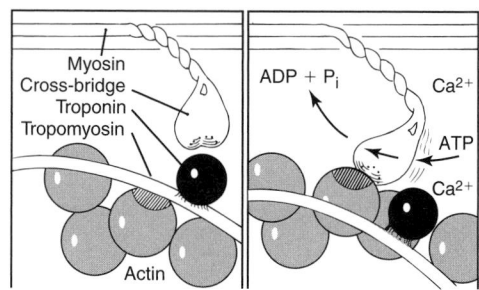

FIGURE **33-15** Formation of the actomyosin complex. Hydrolysis of adenosine triphosphate (ATP) leads to tipping of the myosin heads. *ADP*, Adenosine diphosphate; P_i, high energy phosphate.

Thick Filament

Myosin, the primary protein component of the thick filament, is a very large protein containing three pairs of polypeptides: one pair of heavy chains and two pairs of light chains. The six different polypeptides assemble to form the myosin protein, and each protein contains a long tail with two globular heads.

The tail regions of several hundred myosin molecules aggregate to form one thick filament. The globular heads project out laterally from the thick filament at regular intervals toward the six thin filaments surrounding it. In the relaxed muscle, the myosin heads are oriented toward but not attached to the thin filaments. The thick filament's globular projections are termed *cross-bridges* because they can link the thick and thin filaments. The cross-bridges in each half of the sarcomere are oriented in opposite directions away from the midpoint of the filament, which is important for their functional role in sarcomere shortening and muscle contraction.[1] The cross-bridge components are arranged as shown in Figure 33-14.

The myosin head and tail have a jointlike attachment, permitting a certain degree of movement. When muscle contraction is activated and myosin and actin link, the ability of the myosin head to swivel enables the attached actin filaments to slide over the thick myosin filaments (Figure 33-15).

Cross-Bridge Interaction and Cycling
Sliding Filament Mechanism

Physiologic contraction of striated muscle occurs when muscle fibers are depolarized to a threshold for action-potential formation. The excited muscle then transforms the chemical energy stored in adenosine triphosphate (ATP) directly into mechanical energy. The depolarizing wave initiated by AChR occupation at the motor end plate is carried along the muscle membrane surface from one Na^+ channel to the next. Action potential depolarization of the sarcolemma spreads rapidly to the muscle cell's interior through a reticular network of intracellular tubules that are contiguous with the cell membrane.

This network, composed of *transverse tubules*, or *T tubules*, forms a grid around the intracellular myofibrils and closely associates with the intracellular sarcoplasmic reticular membranes. The T tubules rapidly transmit the action potential from the sarcolemma to the myoplasm.

The *sarcoplasmic reticulum* is an irregular, closed membrane structure that weaves throughout the myoplasm of the muscle cell and contains large amounts of Ca^{2+}. The sarcoplasmic reticular membrane is active in sequestering Ca^{2+} by way of numerous high-affinity Ca^{2+} active-transport carriers in its membrane. These pumps maintain a high sarcoplasmic reticular store of Ca^{2+} and a very low resting myoplasmic Ca^{2+} concentration.[1,2]

The transit of an action potential along the sarcolemma and into the T-tubule system is detected by intracellular voltage sensors that trigger Ca^{2+} efflux from the sarcoplasmic reticular stores. The major Ca^{2+} release channels located on the sarcoplasmic reticumlum are called *ryanodine receptors*.[1] In response to action potential stimulation, the myoplasmic Ca^{2+} concentration rises several-fold from a resting value of less than 0.1 mmol. The overall effect is the discharge of Ca^{2+} from the sarcoplasmic reticulum into the myoplasm by the transit of an action potential into the muscle cell.

The Ca^{2+} released into the myoplasm binds to troponin, which acts as a switch that changes the conformation of the tropomyosin to which it is bound. The conformational change in the rod-shaped tropomyosin exposes myosin binding sites on the underlying actin. The myosin heads react by binding to the exposed thin filament sites, forming a reversible complex with actin—the *actomyosin complex*. The process of myosin-actin binding in response to elevated myoplasmic Ca^{2+} is termed *cross-bridge formation*.

The myosin filaments' heads contain not only an actin binding site but also a catalytic adenosine triphosphatase (ATPase) site that hydrolyzes the breakdown of ATP to adenosine diphosphate (ADP) and phosphate. Binding of a myosin head with an actin molecule is associated with ATP hydrolysis and energy release. ATP is essential for the sliding of the filaments and for muscle contraction. The energy yielded by the ATP breakdown is harnessed to tilt the myosin heads, drawing the thin actin filaments with them. The pull of the actin filaments accentuates the overlap of the thick and thin filaments, causing shortening of the sarcomere and culminating in muscle contraction (Figure 33-16).

The actomyosin complex is stable and can be broken only by a renewed binding of ATP to each myosin head. With the binding of ATP, the actomyosin cross-bridge dissociates, and the myosin heads are repositioned for another round of cross-bridge formation. If the intracellular Ca^{2+} concentration is still sufficiently high, which mainly depends on the frequency of incoming action potentials, the cycle begins again: myosin links to actin, swivels, detaches, and reconnects at the next actin site.

A single sliding cycle or myosin "rowing stroke" shortens the sarcomere's length by about 1%, causing the entire muscle fiber, which consists of a serial arrangement of sarcomeres, to also shorten by 1%. The sliding cycle has to be repeated about 50 times for full shortening of the muscle. The cycle continues until

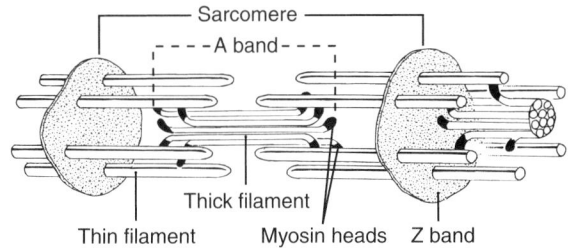

FIGURE **33-16** The basic contractile unit. The myosin heads at each end of the thick filaments are oriented in opposite directions. With cross-bridge formation, tilting of the myosin heads pulls the thin filaments along with them and causes sarcomere shortening.

BOX **33-1**

Outline of Neurohumoral Transmission and Excitation-Contraction Coupling

An action potential reaches the motor nerve ending.
Ca^{2+} enters the nerve ending; ACh is released into the synaptic cleft.
ACh binds to a postsynaptic cholinergic receptor at the motor end plate.
The motor end-plate membrane depolarizes (the EPP).
An action potential is generated at the perijunctional muscle membrane.
The action potential spreads along the muscle membrane and inward to the transverse tubules.
Depolarization of the T tubules causes Ca^{2+} release from the sarcoplasmic reticulum.
Ca^{2+} triggers actomyosin complex cross-bridge formation; the sarcomere shortens; the muscle contracts.

ACh, *Acetylcholine*; EPP, *end-plate potential*; T, *transverse*.

---

it is interrupted by the active removal of Ca^{2+} from the myoplasm or until the ATP is exhausted. Active Ca^{2+} removal from the cytoplasm back into the sarcoplasmic reticulum causes troponin, tropomyosin, and actin to return to a configuration that prohibits myosin binding, and the muscle relaxes.

The overall process by which depolarization of the muscle fiber causes Ca^{2+} release from the sarcoplasmic reticulum into the myoplasm to cause cross-bridge cycling and muscle contraction is called *excitation-contraction coupling*.

Box 33-1 summarizes the excitation-contraction coupling events. Box 33-2 summarizes the events leading to skeletal muscle relaxation.

Grading Contractile Force

Two major mechanisms grade skeletal muscle contractile force. One determining factor of muscle force is the number of motor units activated or recruited. With increasing voluntary effort, more and more motor units are recruited, and an increasing muscle force develops.

Outline of Skeletal Muscle Relaxation

ACh is hydrolyzed by AChE in the synaptic cleft.
The end plate and muscle membrane repolarize to their resting potentials.
Ca^{2+} is actively pumped back into the sarcoplasmic reticulum.
Myoplasmic Ca^{2+} concentration returns to a normal low level.
The muscle relaxes.

ACh, *Acetylcholine*; AChE, *acetylcholinesterase*; Ca^{2+}, *calcium ion.*

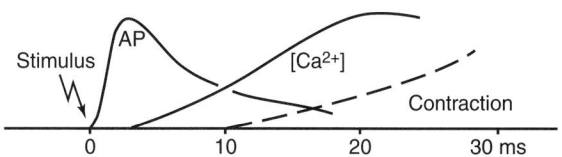

FIGURE **33-17** The electrical, ionic, and mechanical responses of a skeletal muscle to a single maximal stimulus. *AP,* Action potential.

The other mechanism by which skeletal muscle tension is graded is by varying the frequency of the action potential discharge to the muscle. A single action potential invariably liberates sufficient Ca^{2+} ions to activate skeletal muscle contraction. However, the Ca^{2+} ions are rapidly transported back into the sarcoplasmic reticulum before the muscle has time to develop maximal tension. The brief contraction that results from a single action potential is called a *twitch*.[2]

Unlike cardiac muscle, skeletal muscle does not have a refractory period. Because of this property, rapidly repeated electrical impulses can cause summation of contractions and greatly increase the muscle tension. Repetitive action potentials maintain a high Ca^{2+} concentration in the myoplasm. The greater the myoplasmic Ca^{2+} concentration, the more cross-bridge sites are exposed, and the stronger the force of the contraction. Maximal and sustained muscle tension without relaxation—produced by the fusion and summation of successive twitch responses—is called *tetanus*.[2]

Figure 33-17 shows the time course and relationship between a single action potential, the myoplasmic Ca^{2+} rise, and the resulting twitch response. The action potential lasts about 2 to 4 milliseconds. The twitch begins about 2 milliseconds after the start of the muscle membrane depolarization. The duration of the twitch varies with the type of muscle stimulated.

Slow Versus Fast Muscle

Skeletal muscle fibers are classified as type I ("slow fibers") or type II ("fast fibers"), based on different myosin isoenzymes that distinguish the two types. The two fiber types differ in their metabolic demands, their myosin ATPase activity, and their cross-bridge cycling rates. Muscles usually contain a mixture of both types of fibers, but one type often predominates.[23]

Slow (type I) muscle fibers are adapted for sustained movements, such as maintaining posture, and are resistant to fatigue. They have slow twitch durations, depend on oxidative phosphorylation for energy, have extensive blood supplies, and have rich concentrations of mitochondria.[1,2,23] Type I muscle is called "red" muscle because its high myoglobin content imparts a dark, rubrous color.

Fast (type II) muscle fibers usually predominate in "white" muscle and are primarily concerned with rapid or powerful movement. They have short twitch durations, depend on glycolytic pathways for energy, and are easily fatigued.[1] Muscles specialized for fine, skilled movement, such as extraocular muscles, and some muscles of the hand are in this category.

Infants have a greater tendency toward respiratory failure in part because only 25% of their diaphragm is composed of type I fatigue-resistant fibers, compared with 50% in the adult. Before 37 weeks' gestational age, type I slow fibers make up less than 10% of the total diaphragm muscle content. Intercostal muscles are more prone to fatigue than the diaphragm because they contain a higher proportion of type II fast fibers.[23]

Energy Sources for Skeletal Muscle

Muscle contraction requires a continual supply of energy at a rate proportionate to its energy consumption.[2] The energy consumed by skeletal muscle is used for (1) cross-bridge cycling during muscle contraction, (2) sarcoplasmic reticular resequestration of Ca^{2+} during muscle relaxation, (3) rephosphorylation of creatine to replenish creatine phosphate energy stores, (4) activation of the Na^+/K^+ pump to restore proper membrane polarization, and (5) resynthesis of muscle glycogen.

Muscle cells derive energy from three basic energy sources: creatine phosphate, carbohydrates, and free fatty acids and triglycerides.[1]

Creatine Phosphate (phosphocreatine)

The energy-rich phosphate bonds in muscle phosphocreatine supply a limited amount of energy to produce ATP in skeletal muscle. The hydrolysis of creatine phosphate to creatine and phosphate is an extremely rapid reaction that provides high-energy phosphates for the conversion of ADP to ATP. Creatine phosphate provides a stored source of energy that is used at the very beginning of muscle contraction while other, more sustainable, energy-regenerating systems are being turned on.[1]

Carbohydrates

Skeletal muscle stores glucose as energy-rich glycogen. With brief, intense muscle exertion, muscles meet their energy demands from the breakdown of glycogen (*glycogenolysis*) and the metabolism of glucose to pyruvate and lactate (*anaerobic glycolysis*). Anaerobic glycolysis is a rapid process, but it has a relatively small ATP yield and is limited by the cellular stores of glycogen, which can be depleted within a few hours of muscle contraction.[2] Additionally, the accumulation of lactate in the muscle produces an enzyme-inhibiting acidosis and causes the anaerobic pathway to be self-limiting.[1]

The presence of oxygen increases the ATP yield substantially. With adequate oxygen, pyruvate enters the mitochondrial citric acid cycle, liberating CO_2, water, and energy-rich ATP.

Fatty Acids and Triglycerides

When glucose is scarce but oxygen is plentiful, the skeletal muscle takes up free fatty acids and other substrates, such as amino acids or ketone bodies, and efficiently oxidizes them to CO_2, water, and ATP in the muscle fiber mitochondria, an energy-yielding process called *oxidative phosphorylation*. The oxidation of free fatty acids is a slow process, but it is usually sufficient to meet the more modest energy demands of the most frequently used skeletal muscle. Free fatty acids are the primary energy substrates for muscle cells during prolonged exercise and for steady-state requirements.[2]

MUSCULOSKELETAL PATHOPHYSIOLOGY AND ANESTHESIA

Musculoskeletal diseases have a wide variety of causes, ranging from autoimmune destruction of tissue, to genetically determined defects in muscle membrane proteins, to pharmacologically induced alterations in Ca^{2+} metabolism. Musculoskeletal defects may reside in the neuromuscular junction, the muscle infrastructure, or the skeletal support structures.

Myasthenia Gravis

Myasthenia gravis, a chronic disease of the neuromuscular junction, is manifested by increasing skeletal muscle weakness, fatigability on effort, and at least partial restoration of function after rest.

Incidence

In the United States, at least 1 in 7500 people have myasthenia gravis. In individuals younger than 50 years, the ratio of women to men with the disease is 3 to 2; however, in those older than 50 years, the disease is equally distributed between the sexes. Myasthenia gravis can begin spontaneously at any age, but it occurs most frequently between the ages of 30 and 40 years. The onset may be abrupt or insidious, and the course is fluctuating, marked by periods of exacerbation and remission.[24] Spontaneous remissions that do occur sometimes persist for years.

Pathophysiology

Electron microscopic examination of the neuromuscular junction of the patient with myasthenia gravis shows a decrease in the number of functional postsynaptic ACh receptors. The AChR lesion appears to be caused by immune-mediated destruction, blockage, or inactivation. The prejunctional ACh pool is normal.[24]

Myasthenia gravis is a prototype autoimmune disease. Circulating antibodies react with myoneural AChR proteins, leading to varying degrees of dysfunction. Anti-AChR antibodies (IgG) are found in the sera of 85% to 90% of patients with myasthenia gravis, but the antibody level does not necessarily correlate with the severity of the disease.[25-27] Most patients in clinical remission continue to show elevated serum levels of AChR antibodies.

The initiating stimulus for the production of anti-AChR IgG antibodies is unclear. A genetic cause or induction by microbial antigens has been postulated. The thymus gland seems to play a central role in the pathogenesis.[26,27]

Pregnancy exacerbates the symptoms of myasthenia gravis in 40% of pregnant women with the disease; however, other patients with the disease experience remission or no change in symptoms during pregnancy.[28] Anti-AChR antibodies that pass across the placenta may produce transitory symptoms of weakness in approximately 10% to 15% of infants born to mothers with myasthenia gravis. Signs of weakness (difficulty with breathing, ptosis, facial weakness) in the affected infant are usually present within the first few hours after birth. The condition lasts as long as 21 days, mirroring the half-life of the IgG antibodies.[27]

Clinical Manifestations

The clinical hallmarks of myasthenia gravis include generalized muscle weakness, which improves with rest, and an inability to sustain or repeat muscular contractions. Enhanced effort produces enhanced weakness. The severity of myasthenia gravis can range from mild (slight ptosis only) to severe (respiratory failure). Environmental, physical, and emotional factors seem to affect the disease process, although unpredictably.[28]

Mouth, eyes, pharynx, proximal limb, and shoulder girdle musculature are most often affected. Visual symptoms (ptosis and diplopia) from extraocular muscle weakness occur in more than 50% of patients with myasthenia gravis.[26] The disease is restricted to the extraocular muscles in 20% of patients. Sensation and cognition are not affected by the disease process.[27]

Thymus gland abnormalities are detectable in about 75% of patients with myasthenia gravis.[24,27] Other autoimmune disorders, such as thyroid disease, collagen vascular diseases, polymyositis, and rheumatoid arthritis, occur more frequently in patients with myasthenia gravis.[27]

Myocarditis may complicate myasthenia gravis, especially in patients with thymomas. Microscopic lesions of myasthenic cardiac muscles are similar to skeletal muscle lesions, indicating a common pathogenesis. The myocardial inflammation produces dysrhythmias, particularly atrial fibrillation and atrioventricular block.[29]

Treatment

Therapy for patients with myasthenia gravis is directed toward improving neuromuscular transmission and includes cholinesterase inhibitors, corticosteroids and other immunosuppressants, plasmapheresis, intravenous immunoglobulin, and thymectomy.[24,28]

Treatment with cholinesterase inhibitors can dramatically reduce the symptoms of myasthenia gravis by inhibiting the hydrolysis of ACh and therefore increasing the neurotransmitter's concentration at the neuromuscular junction. Increasing the synaptic concentration of ACh enhances the possibility of postsynaptic AChR occupation, which is critical for the production of a threshold-reaching EPP for muscle contraction. Anticholinesterase treatment is particularly successful in patients with milder disease.[24] The most commonly used anticholinesterase agent in the United States is oral pyridostigmine. An oral dose of 60 mg pyridostigmine lasts 3 to 4 hours and is equivalent to an intramuscular or intravenous dose of 2 mg pyridostigmine or 1 mg neostigmine.[30]

Titration of the anticholinesterase dose is challenging. Underdosing does not sufficiently retard the muscle weakness and can result in *myasthenic crisis*, a severe exacerbation of myasthenic symptoms. Overmedicating with a cholinesterase inhibitor can produce a surplus of ACh at the myoneural junction, causing a depolarizing-like block and augmenting skeletal muscle weakness. This situation is called *cholinergic crisis*. Muscarinic side effects (e.g., abdominal cramping, diarrhea, salivation, bradycardia, and miosis) predominate in a cholinergic crisis.

Corticosteroid therapy produces an 80% remission rate in patients with myasthenia gravis, in part by reducing AChR antibody levels. Glucocorticoid therapy is often used in combination with other agents. Use is limited by the side effects (e.g., osteoporosis, gastrointestinal bleeding, suppression of endogenous cortisol release, cataracts, increased susceptibility to acute infections, hypertension, and glucose intolerance) observed with long-term administration.

In patients with more debilitating, widespread disease, immunosuppresive drugs such as azathioprine (Imuran) and cyclosporine may induce remission by interfering with the production of AChR antibodies. Side effects of azathioprine include severe hemopoietic depression and liver dysfunction. Cyclosporine side effects include hypertension and nephrotoxicity.[24]

Excision of the thymus gland is recommended for adults with generalized disease and for patients with thymomas, thymus gland hyperplasia, or drug-resistant myasthenia gravis.[26,27] Thymectomy effectively arrests or reverses the myasthenic process by removing a major source of antibody production. Clinical improvement of myasthenic symptoms is seen in 75% to 96% of patients within weeks to months after surgery.[30]

Plasmapheresis (plasma exchange) arrests severe refractory myasthenia gravis by reducing the concentration of circulating antibodies. It is used primarily as a short-term treatment because the improvement that it produces in symptoms is generally short lived. Intravenous immunoglobulin may also be used for short-term control of symptoms prior to surgery.[24]

Anesthetic Implications

Several days before the operation and again immediately prior to surgery, the surgical candidate with myasthenia gravis should be evaluated for disease control and, if applicable, for stabilization of anticholinesterase dose.

The use of anticholinesterase medication in the immediate preoperative period is controversial.[31-34] Some experts feel that an awareness of drug mechanisms can enable anticholinesterase therapy to be safely continued into the preoperative period, especially in patients who depend on this therapy for their well-being. Others recommend discontinuing or tapering anticholinesterase medication before surgery to avoid complicating the anesthetic management. Patients with mild myasthenia gravis can usually tolerate the temporary disruption in treatment.[32]

The presence of cholinesterase inhibitors may potentiate vagal responses and beclouds both the intraoperative administration of muscle relaxants and the differential diagnosis and treatment of postoperative muscle weakness.

Emotional stress and surgery may precipitate or worsen skeletal muscle weakness. Pharyngeal and laryngeal muscle weakness, difficulty in eliminating oral secretions, and the risk of pulmonary aspiration should be considered in the anesthesia plan of care. Swallowing and respiratory muscle dysfunction account for much of the morbidity and potential mortality in patients with myasthenia gravis.[28]

Regional and local anesthesia with careful monitoring are the preferred anesthetic techniques when appropriate. If general anesthesia is indicated, the respiratory depressant effects of barbiturates, sedatives, narcotics, and volatile anesthetic agents, compounded by the presence of an already weakened respiratory system, must be carefully considered.[34,35]

In many patients, the relaxant effects of a volatile anesthetic in combination with the patient's preexisting skeletal muscle weakness are sufficient to facilitate intubation of the trachea.[32,34] Enhanced muscle relaxation may be seen with the administration of all the potent volatile anesthetics.[35]

Small doses of succinylcholine may be used to facilitate tracheal intubation, but the response may be unpredictable.[28] Untreated patients with myasthenia gravis appear to be two to three times more resistant to succinylcholine. Normal dosages of succinylcholine may not effectively depolarize the end plate because of the deficiency of viable AChRs. On the other hand, patients treated with cholinesterase inhibitors exhibit a normal or prolonged response to succinylcholine. Cholinesterase inhibitors block the effects of plasma cholinesterase, as well as those of true cholinesterase; hence, succinylcholine and other medications metabolized by plasma cholinesterase (e.g., ester local anesthetics)

may have a delayed hydrolysis and a prolonged duration of action.[32,36] The ester hydrolysis of atracurium is independent of plasma cholinesterase activity.

The deficient number of functioning AChRs in patients with myasthenia gravis produces an extraordinary sensitivity to nondepolarizing muscle relaxants. Small doses of nondepolarizing agents can produce a profound block with a prolonged effect, even in patients being treated with cholinergic drugs.[34] In one study of 11 myasthenic patients, the average ED_{95} value for vecuronium was 72% less in the myasthenic patient group than in the control group.[37] Some patients require no medication at all for surgical muscle relaxation.[38,39]

Generally, muscle relaxant requirements are widely variable in patients with myasthenia gravis, a characteristic that makes neuromuscular blockade monitoring an essential and integral part of the anesthetic management. The orbicularis oculi muscle may overestimate the degree of muscle relaxation in patients with myasthenia gravis.[40] This site may be the most ideal site to monitor neuromuscular blockade to avoid the possibility of undetected residual muscle weakness. When needed, the use of smaller doses (half to two thirds the normal dose) of shorter-acting nondepolarizing relaxants is the prudent choice.[25,41]

Reversal of neuromuscular blockade with an AChE inhibitor should be performed cautiously in patients with myasthenia gravis. Overtreatment with an anticholinesterase agent can precipitate a cholinergic crisis and aggravate rather than reverse the muscle weakness. In many circumstances, the neuromuscular block can be titrated to allow complete spontaneous recovery, avoiding the use of reversal.

Complete, sustained return of muscle strength must be demonstrated before extubation and resumption of spontaneous ventilation. The patient should be informed that postoperative tracheal intubation and ventilatory support may be required. Skeletal muscle strength may appear to be adequate shortly after surgery but may deteriorate a few hours later. A higher likelihood for postoperative ventilation can be predicted for patients undergoing transsternal thymectomy, duration of the disease longer than 6 years, a daily pyridostigmine dose greater than 750 mg, the presence of chronic obstructive pulmonary disease, and a preoperative vital capacity less than 2.9 L.[32,41]

Duchenne Muscular Dystrophy

Muscular dystrophy is a heterogeneous set of diseases that includes fascioscapulohumeral dystrophy, limb-girdle dystrophy, Becker muscular dystrophy, Duchenne muscular dystrophy, and others. *Duchenne muscular dystrophy* is the most common and most severe form.

Incidence

Duchenne muscular dystrophy (DMD) is an inherited, sex-linked, recessive disease that presents in early childhood between 3 and 6 years of age. It is clinically evident in males and has an incidence of 1 in 3500 live male births.[32] Females are generally unaffected but are carriers of the disorder. Mental retardation of varying degrees occurs in about 30% of patients with DMD.[42] There is no cure for the disease, but corticosteroid therapy improves muscle strength and slows disease progression in many patients.[42,43] Death often occurs in late adolescence or early adulthood and is usually caused by respiratory failure.

Pathophysiology

Patients with DMD experience an infiltration of fibrous and fatty tissue into the muscle, followed by a progressive and painless degeneration and necrosis of muscle fibers. Muscle weakness ends with muscle destruction.

In 1987, the abnormal gene responsible for DMD was identified. This gene is located on the X chromosome and is errant in coding for a vital protein called *dystrophin*. Dystrophin is normally bound to a complex of glycoproteins as a transmembrane structural component of the muscle-fiber sarcolemma.[44] Patients with DMD have an absence or a severe deficiency of the dystrophin protein, which alters sarcolemma integrity or stability.[43,45] The protein is present in low amounts or is structurally altered in Becker muscular dystrophy, a similar disorder that follows a milder, less progressive course than the Duchenne type.[44,45] Muscle biopsy remains the standard for diagnosis.

In the early stages of DMD, increased permeability of the sarcolemma and skeletal muscle necrosis are mirrored by elevated serum levels of the enzyme creatine kinase (CK) (formerly termed *creatine phosphokinase*). Serum CK levels are often 20 to 100 times normal levels (normal level, 40 to 150 units/L), but as muscle is lost to the destructive process, CK levels decrease.[42]

Clinical Manifestations

Duchenne muscular dystrophy is characterized by an unremitting weakness and a steady deterioration of the proximal muscle groups of the pelvis and shoulders. The child exhibits a clumsy, waddling gait and falls frequently. Weakness of the pelvic girdle leads to the classic finding of Gowers sign, in which patients use their hands to climb up their legs to arise from the floor. A steady deterioration of muscle strength forces most of these boys to be wheelchair bound by the age of 8 to 12 years.[42,46]

Skeletal muscle atrophy is usually preceded by fat and fibrous tissue infiltration, resulting in pseudohypertrophy. The infiltrative process is most apparent in the calf muscles, which become particularly enlarged.

Degeneration of respiratory muscles occurs and leads to a restrictive type of ventilatory impairment. Unopposed action by healthy, nondystrophic axial muscles predisposes these patients to kyphoscoliosis, which further decreases the pulmonary reserve.[42] Decreasing muscle strength also results in ineffective cough, impaired swallowing, and inability to mobilize secretions.[46]

More progressive forms of the disease affect not only skeletal muscle but also smooth muscle of the alimentary tract and cardiac muscle. Alimentary tract involvement can lead to intestinal hypomotility, delayed gastric emptying, and gastric dilation.[47,48]

Myocardial involvement occurs in almost all patients with progressive disease.[49] Studies by Nigro and coworkers established the presence of preclinical cardiac disease in 25% of patients with DMD who were younger than 6 years and in 59% of those between the ages of 6 and 10 years.[50] Myocardial pathology includes fibrotic changes localized primarily to the left ventricle (LV). Echocardiography can effectively evaluate LV function in patients with DMD and is recommended for operative patients.[32,51] Clinical symptoms of heart failure do not usually appear unless the patient is severely stressed or until advanced stages of the disease.

Electrocardiographic (ECG) changes characteristic of preclinical cardiomyopathy include a large or polyphasic R wave in lead V_1, deep Q waves in the lateral precordial leads (V_4 through V_6), premature beats (atrial and ventricular), and labile sinus or atrial tachycardia.[52]

Although often severe, compromised cardiac and respiratory conditions may be masked by the limited activity imposed by the patient's skeletal myopathy. Added stress, such as that produced by surgery and anesthesia, may suddenly increase cardiorespiratory demand and uncover the weakened cardiac and respiratory states.

Anesthetic Implications

Patients with DMD are susceptible to untoward anesthesia-related complications. When possible, local or regional anesthesia should be considered.[53]

Generalized muscle weakness, especially in the advanced stages of DMD, makes these patients exquisitely sensitive to the respiratory depressant properties of opioids, sedatives, and general anesthetic agents. Preoperative sedation should be omitted or minimal, and the smallest possible amounts of anesthetic agents should be used.

Preoperative and postoperative respiratory therapy can help maximize the patient's pulmonary condition.[32] In patients with more advanced disease, arterial blood gas determinations and preoperative pulmonary function studies may elucidate the extent of respiratory involvement and the amount of respiratory reserve. A preoperative forced vital capacity (FVC) of less than 35% of predicted has traditionally indicated a higher risk for postoperative pulmonary complications in patients with DMD. In one series, aggressive preoperative chest physiotherapy and incorporation of postoperative noninvasive ventilation enabled patients with preoperative FVC levels of 30% and below to successfully undergo corrective spinal surgery.[54] Assiduous attention to respiratory function must be continued into the postoperative period. Delayed pulmonary insufficiency as late as 36 hours after surgery has been reported.[32,47]

The effects of nondepolarizing muscle relaxants must be scrupulously monitored. There is enhanced muscle relaxant sensitivity, and recovery may be prolonged three to six times the normal duration in patients with DMD.[32,55] Short-acting nondepolarizing muscle relaxants that are carefully titrated with the use of a nerve stimulator are recommended.

A decreased cardiac reserve makes these patients sensitive to the myocardial depressant effects of general anesthetic agents, sedatives, and narcotics. Cardiac arrests associated with inhalation anesthetics have been reported.[56,57] A carefully titrated intravenous "balanced" technique may help provide a smoother cardiovascular course. Ketamine has been used successfully for anesthesia during diagnostic muscle biopsy in patients with DMD.[58] Judicious administration of intravenous fluids is warranted. The sudden occurrence of tachycardia during anesthesia may herald heart failure.

The potential for delayed gastric emptying, plus the presence of weak laryngeal reflexes, dictates that the anesthesia plan of care include measures for guarding against aspiration of stomach contents. Gastrokinetic agents and the prophylactic use of a nasogastric tube are recommended to avoid gastric dilation.[48]

Succinylcholine and the potent inhalational agents are not recommended for use in patients with muscular dystrophy; the altered sarcolemma can lead to rhabdomyolysis and myoglobin efflux with administration.[57,59] The resultant massive breakdown of the diseased muscle fibers produces a profound hyperkalemia that requires extensive and tenacious treatment with hyperventilation, calcium chloride, sodium bicarbonate, and glucose and insulin. Ventricular fibrillation or cardiac arrest occurring during general anesthesia has been associated with succinylcholine or potent inhalation agent administration to patients with diagnosed and undiagnosed muscular dystrophy.[56,60,61]

DMD is included among the myopathies that may be associated with malignant hyperthermia (MH).[60] Given the availabilities of safe anesthesia alternatives, the anesthetist should avoid MH-triggering agents and vigilantly observe for signs and symptoms of MH when these children undergo surgery. Dantrolene and other treatment modalities for MH should be readily available.[61]

Malignant Hyperthermia
Epidemiology/Incidence
Malignant hyperthermia is an uncommon, life-threatening, hypermetabolic disorder of skeletal muscle, triggered in susceptible individuals by potent inhalation agents, including sevoflurane, desflurane, isoflurane, and halothane, and the depolarizing muscle relaxant succinylcholine.[62-64] A review of published cases of MH by Strazis and Fox reported that about 52% of cases occur in patients younger than 15 years, with a mean age of 18.3 years.[65] The exact incidence of MH is unknown, but the rate of occurrence has been estimated to be 1 in 50,000 in adults and 1 in 15,000 in children.[62,63]

Susceptibility to MH is inherited in some families as an autosomal dominant pattern with variable penetrance.[62,64] A single defective gene is the basis for the underlying problem for many families, but in other families the genetic pattern has not been established.

The first formal case report of MH was of an Australian family, described by Denborough and colleagues over 40 years ago in the journal *Lancet*.[66] Since that time a great deal has been learned about the biochemical and physiologic components of the disease. Nonetheless, many questions remain regarding the pathophysiology, diagnosis, and significance of some clinical manifestations.

Pathophysiology
Although the cause of MH is not yet known with certainty, it is generally agreed that MH is an inherited disorder of skeletal muscle in which a defect in calcium regulation is expressed by exposure to triggering anesthetic agents; intracellular hypercalcemia results. The ryanodine receptor is the major calcium release channel of the sarcoplasmic reticulum, and much attention has been focused on this receptor as the site of the MH defect.[1,67] The defect involves skeletal muscle, and there is no evidence for a primary defect in cardiac or smooth muscle cells.

Malignant hyperthermia is initiated when specific triggering agents induce increased concentrations of calcium in the muscle cells of MH-susceptible (MHS) patients. Actomyosin cross-bridging, sustained muscle contraction, and rigidity result.[68] Energy-dependent reuptake mechanisms attempt to remove excess calcium from the myoplasm, increasing muscle metabolism two- to three-fold. The accelerated cellular processes increase oxygen consumption, augment carbon dioxide and heat production, deplete ATP stores, and generate lactic acid. Acidosis, hyperthermia, and ATP depletion cause sarcolemma destruction, producing a marked egress of potassium, myoglobin, and creatine kinase to the extracellular fluid.[64,68] Skeletal muscle constitutes 40% to 50% of our body mass, so relatively small changes in muscle metabolism may produce the dramatic systemic biochemical changes observed with MH.

Clinical Manifestations
Not all cases of MH are fulminant, but rather there is a spectrum or continuum of severity, ranging from an insidious onset with mild complications to an explosive response with pronounced rigidity, temperature rise, arrhythmias, and death.[62,69]

> ### BOX 33-3
>
> #### Clinical Events and Laboratory Findings During Malignant Hyperthermia
>
> **Clinical Events During MH**
> Unexplained, sudden rise in end-tidal CO_2 (>55 mm Hg)
> Unexplained tachycardia, tachypnea, labile blood pressure, or arrhythmias
> Masseter muscle or generalized muscle rigidity
> Unanticipated respiratory or metabolic acidosis
> Rising patient temperature
> Cola-colored urine (myoglobinuria)
> Mottled, cyanotic skin
> Decreased Sao_2
>
> **Laboratory Findings Consistent with MH**
> Arterial blood gases: $Paco_2$ >60 mm Hg, base excess more negative than −8 mEq/L, pH <7.25
> Serum potassium >6 mEq/L
> Creatine kinase >20,000 units/L
> Serum myoglobin >170 mcg/L
> Urine myoglobin >60 mcg/L

Although MH may present in several ways, a typical MH episode begins while the patient is under general anesthesia (GA) with a volatile anesthetic. Succinylcholine may or may not precede the MH episode.[62,68] The onset of MH symptoms may occur immediately after induction of anesthesia or several hours into the surgery.[69] Desflurane is a weaker MH trigger and has been associated with delayed onset of MH, as long as 6 hours after induction of anesthesia.[70-72] Succinylcholine appears to accelerate the onset and increase the severity of the MH episode.[62,68] The presentation of MH may follow a dose-dependent response, with lower concentrations of volatile anesthetics resulting in a more protracted onset of hypermetabolic symptoms.[69,70] Rarely, MH occurs in the recovery room, usually within 1 hour after general anesthesia.[68]

The clinical features of MH reflect increased intracellular muscle Ca^{2+} concentration and greatly increased body metabolism (Box 33-3). Common signs of MH include tachycardia, tachypnea, skin mottling, cyanosis, and total body or jaw muscle rigidity. Muscle rigidity is clinically apparent in 75% of cases.[68] The most sensitive indicator of MH is an unanticipated increase in end-tidal carbon dioxide ($ETco_2$) levels out of proportion to minute ventilation. The increased $ETco_2$ may be abrupt or it may rise gradually over the course of the anesthetic. Hyperthermia, which may climb at a rate of 1° to 2° C every 5 minutes and exceed 43.3° C (110° F), is often a late but confirming sign of MH.[62]

The combination of acidosis, hyperkalemia, and hyperthermia leads to cardiac irritability, a labile blood pressure, and arrhythmias that can rapidly progress to cardiac arrest. Laboratory findings mirror the muscle breakdown and include myoglobinuria and increased serum potassium and CK. Serum CK levels peak 12 to 24 hours after the onset of MH.[68] Myoglobin appears in the plasma within minutes of the hypermetabolic muscle response. Arterial and venous blood gas analysis reveals decreased oxygen

BOX 33-4

Manifestations That Mimic Malignant Hyperthermia—Signs and Symptoms

Tachycardia
Hypoxia
Hypercarbia
Hypovolemia
Insufficient anesthetic depth
Anticholinergics, sympathomimetics, cocaine
Pheochromocytoma

Hyperpyrexia
Heatstroke
Blood transfusion reaction
Infection
Drug reaction
Neuroleptic malignant syndrome
Serotonin syndrome
Hypermetabolic states (sepsis, thyroid storm, pheochromocytoma)

Tachypnea, Hypercapnia
Congestive heart failure, pulmonary edema
Hypermetabolic states
Intraperitoneal carbon dioxide insufflation
Airway obstruction, pneumothorax
Excess dead space, low minute volume

Masseter Muscle Rigidity
Insufficient neuromuscular blockade
Temporomandibular joint syndrome
Neuroleptic malignant syndrome
Myotonia

From Greenberg C: Diagnosis and treatment of hyperthermia in the post anesthesia care unit. Anesthesiol Clin North America. 1990;8:377-397.

tension and mixed metabolic and respiratory acidosis. Late complications may include cerebral edema, myoglobinuric renal failure, consumptive coagulopathy, hepatic dysfunction, and pulmonary edema.[62]

The variable time course and nonspecific clinical features and laboratory findings can make the diagnosis of MH difficult. Insufficient anesthetic depth, hypoxia, neuroleptic malignant syndrome, propofol infusion syndrome, thyrotoxicosis, pheochromocytoma, and sepsis can share several characteristics with MH, making the clinical picture ambiguous and the differential diagnosis challenging to even the most experienced practitioner[73,74] (Box 33-4). Surgical procedures performed of necessity in a darkened operating room can further compromise the practitioner's diagnostic acumen.

In addition to being a trigger of MH, succinylcholine may also induce hyperkalemic-mediated cardiac arrest in children with occult myopathies.[59,75] Because of this concern, most anesthetists use nondepolarizing muscle relaxants for elective intubation in children and reserve the use of succinylcholine for treatment of laryngospasm or emergency airway management. In 1994, the package insert for succinylcholine was modified to warn against the routine use of succinylcholine in children.

Preoperative Assessment and Prevention

Patients who are MH susceptible may be otherwise healthy and completely unaware of their risk until exposed to a triggering anesthetic.[65,76] Furthermore, not everyone who has the MH gene develops an MH episode upon each exposure to triggering anesthetics. It is estimated that about 21% of MHS patients have at least one uneventful anesthetic prior to having an MH episode.[65,68] Although MH susceptibility cannot be ruled out by history alone, every surgical patient should be questioned about:
- Family or personal history of muscle disorders
- Family history of unexpected intraoperative complications or deaths
- Family or personal history of muscle rigidity/stiffness or high fever under anesthesia
- Personal history of dark or cola-colored urine following surgery

Because MH is considered an inherited disorder, all members of a family in which MH has occurred must be considered MHS unless proven otherwise. Moreover, the absence of a positive family history does not preclude MH susceptibility.

There are certain disorders that should alert the anesthetist to an increased possibility of MH susceptibility. A clear genetic association between MH and the inherited myopathy *central core disease* has been demonstrated. Case reports have also linked MH or a MH-like disorder to Duchenne and Becker muscular dystrophy and forms of periodic paralysis and myotonia.[68] MH triggering agents should not be administered to patients with these disorders.[77] This caveat is especially consequential in patients undergoing outpatient procedures, who may have more limited postoperative observation.

All patients given general anesthesia for more than 30 minutes should have core temperature monitoring. The four true core temperature sites are nasopharyngeal, distal esophageal, tympanic, and pulmonary artery.[78] Intermediate temperature monitoring sites (oral, axillary, rectal, bladder, forehead) can be used to estimate core temperature with reasonable accuracy, except during extreme temperature changes.

Weglinski and others report that 50% of patients with unexplained CK elevation test positive for MH on biopsy.[65,79] However, as a diagnostic test for MH, CK levels are imprecise and nonspecific.

Stress, fever, prior exercise, and cocaine and alcohol ingestion have been implicated as causal factors of MH, but it is debated whether these factors cause, exacerbate, or have no effect on MH triggering in humans.[68]

Treatment

Enhanced patient monitoring, earlier diagnosis and treatment, and the introduction of dantrolene are responsible for the dramatic decrease in mortality from nearly 80% 20 years ago to less than 10% today.[62,68] Clearly, the nurse anesthetist plays a critical role in the early recognition and treatment of MH.

In 1979, dantrolene sodium was introduced as a treatment for MH. Since that time, dantrolene has contributed greatly to the dramatic decline in death and disability associated with MH. Dantrolene is a unique muscle relaxant that works by reducing the release of calcium from skeletal muscle sarcoplasmic reticulum, counteracting the abnormal intracellular calcium levels accompanying MH.[80,81] It does not work at the neuromuscular junction as do standard neuromuscular blocking drugs, but rather produces a direct or indirect inhibition of the ryanodine receptor, the major sarcoplasmic reticulum calcium-release channel.[81] At clinical concentrations, dantrolene does not render the muscle totally flaccid and without tone, but it may cause significant muscle weakness and respiratory insufficiency, especially in patients with preexisting muscle disease.

Dantrolene used with calcium channel blockers may induce life-threatening myocardial depression.[77,81]

The Malignant Hyperthermia Association of the United States (MHAUS) provides an "Emergency Therapy for MH" poster that should be posted in every surgical site. The following treatment sequence is recommended for an acute MH episode:

- Call for help and alert the surgeon to conclude the procedure promptly.
- Discontinue the volatile anesthetic and succinylcholine.
- Hyperventilate with 100% oxygen at high flows (at least 10 L/min) to improve tissue oxygenation and eliminate CO_2.
- Administer 2.5 mg/kg dantrolene IV bolus and repeat as necessary until symptoms abate.[77] Occasionally, a total dose greater than 10 mg/kg may be needed, but if greater than 20 mg/kg is given without reversal of symptoms, the diagnosis should be reassessed. The alkaline solution is highly irritating to vessels and should be administered into fast-running, large, peripheral veins or via central venous catheters.[81]
- Dysrhythmias will usually respond to treatment of acidosis or hyperkalemia. Treat persistent or life-threatening arrhythmias with standard antiarrhythmic agents (avoid calcium channel blockers).
- If fever is present, initiate cooling by lavage (orogastric, bladder, open cavities), administration of chilled intravenous normal saline, and surface cooling (hypothermia blanket; ice packs to the groin, axilla, and neck).
- Determine arterial blood gases, serum electrolytes, and blood glucose every 15 minutes until the syndrome stabilizes. Correct severe metabolic acidosis with sodium bicarbonate. Baseline values for coagulation studies, CK, myoglobin, and liver enzymes should be established.
- Treat hyperkalemia with hyperventilation, bicarbonate, and intravenous insulin and glucose.
- Maintain urine output greater than 2 mL/kg/hr with hydration and furosemide (0.5 to 1.0 mg/kg). Large losses of intravascular volume should be anticipated. Consider central venous or pulmonary artery hemodynamic monitoring.

Each vial of dantrolene must be reconstituted with 60 mL of sterile water, and its poor water solubility makes it very time consuming to mix and administer the requisite doses. During an MH emergency, the full-time efforts of additional medical personnel should be enlisted. Warming the diluent fluid to 41° C using an intravenous fluid warming device expedites dantrolene preparation.[82]

Documentation of an MH episode should include patient responses, personnel involved, medications, interventions, and patient outcomes.

Anesthesia for the Malignant Hyperthermia–Susceptible Patient

Standard intraoperative monitoring for the MHS surgical patient includes blood pressure, ECG, pulse oximetry, capnography, and continuous measurement of core body temperature. A cooling water mattress should be placed under the MHS patient at the start of the procedure. Dantrolene pretreatment for the MHS surgical patient is no longer routine. Inconsistent reports of emotional stress or anxiety predisposing a patient to MH have led to recommendations that anxiolytic agents be included in the premedication.[32]

BOX 33-5

Malignant Hyperthermia: Triggering and Nontriggering Agents

Triggering Agents
All volatile inhalation anesthetics (halothane, desflurane, isoflurane, sevoflurane)
Succinylcholine

Nontriggering Agents
Local anesthetics
Opioids
Nitrous oxide
Barbiturates, propofol, ketamine, etomidate
Benzodiazepines
Nondepolarizing skeletal muscle relaxants (vecuronium, atracurium, cisatracurium, pancuronium, rocuronium)
Digoxin, tricyclic antidepressants, magnesium
Anticholinesterase agents
Anticholinergic agents

If the surgical site permits, a regional or local anesthetic technique is preferable for the MHS patient. Local anesthetics (both amide and ester) are nontriggering drugs. Nontriggering general anesthetics can also be administered safely in concert with close monitoring of appropriate vital functions. The list of "nontriggering" anesthetic agents is comprehensive enough to meet most anesthetic requirements (Box 33-5). All volatile inhalation anesthetics and succinylcholine are MH triggers and should not be administered to the MHS patient.

Not all drugs have been thoroughly screened as potential MH triggers, but it is clear that the vast majority of prescription and nonprescription drugs are safe, including antibiotics, antihypertensive agents, and drugs used in the treatment of gastrointestinal disorders. Keys to successful perioperative outcome for the MHS patient include the following[77]:

- Avoidance of MH-triggering medications
- Preparation of an anesthesia machine by changing the soda lime and breathing circuits, removing or inactivating vaporizers, and flushing with oxygen or air at 10 L/min for at least 20 minutes, or 10 minutes if the fresh gas hose is also replaced
- Assiduous perioperative observation for signs of MH, including continuous intraoperative monitoring of the patient's $ETCO_2$, arterial oxygen saturation, and core temperature
- A full appreciation of a preestablished treatment protocol by all perioperative medical personnel

A machine to manufacture ice or the ready availability of ice, the ability to crush it, and a refrigerator containing at least 3000 mL of cold intravenous solution should be available.

Ambulatory surgery can be safely performed in most MHS patients, provided that appropriate monitoring is used and an adequate supply of dantrolene is available.[77,83] Yentis and others reviewed the medical records of 303 children labeled as MHS who underwent surgery with nontriggering anesthetics between 1981 and 1990. None of the children developed MH, and on the basis of their retrospective analysis, the authors concluded that admission to the hospital solely on the basis of the MHS label is not warranted.[84]

Patients known or suspected of having MH should be assessed well before their date of outpatient surgery so that anesthesia records and MH testing center reports (if available) can be collected to corroborate the history. As with any ambulatory procedure, patient selection for ouapatient surgery should be individualized.

Outpatient surgical cases for the MHS patient are best scheduled early in the day, allowing for at least 2.5 hours of post-anesthesia observation time, including a minimum initial recovery period of 1 hour of monitoring vital signs every 15 minutes.[77] Most MHS patients who experience uneventful outpatient surgery may be discharged on the day of surgery. Some experts recommend conservative management with over-night postoperative hospital admission for patients who have survived a previous fulminant or severe MH episode or when dantrolene prophylaxis is used.[68]

All locations where general anesthesia is administered should contain a fully stocked MH cart with drugs and supplies, including 36 vials of dantrolene. Each minute is critical in an MH emergency, so a dantrolene supply should not be shared with a nearby facility. Dantrolene should be kept in or very close to the operating room so it is available immediately if MH occurs.

Diagnostic Testing

The most accurate and commonly accepted test available for determining MH susceptibility is the caffeine halothane contracture test (CHCT). This test involves taking a biopsy of skeletal muscle from the patient's thigh and measuring its contractile response to caffeine, halothane, or both. Normal muscle contracts in response to caffeine or halothane, but this is augmented in the patient with MH. The test is available at eight medical centers in North America. Because it must be completed within hours after muscle biopsy, the patient must travel to the testing site. Patients who have survived an unequivocal episode of MH are considered MHS. The CHCT is indicated for family members of a MHS patient or for patients who have had a previous suspicious but undiagnosed reaction to anesthesia.

Intensive investigations have focused on identifying the gene or genes responsible for MH. Mutations in the gene(s) that encode the ryanodine receptor protein predispose patients to MH and central core disease.[85] For other MHS patients, the molecular genetic basis for the disease may be more heterogeneous, involving mutations at various sites on different chromosomes.[67,86,87] Molecular genetic testing and DNA-based mutation analysis reliably confirm MH susceptibility in approximately 50% of patients from families with known MH mutations.[88]

Postoperative Care

The patient who has experienced an acute MH episode should be observed in an ICU for at least 24 hours. Intravenous dantrolene should be continued, at approximately 1 mg/kg every 6 hours, for a minimum of 24 hours after control of the episode.[77] Recrudescence of an intraoperative episode may occur in 20% to 25% of cases.[89,90] Patients who experience recrudescence are more likely to have a muscular body type and to have had greater than 150 minutes transpire from induction to MH reaction.[90]

For the MHS patient who has undergone an uneventful surgical course, close observation and monitoring should continue into the postanesthesia care unit (PACU). Malignant hyperthermia can first manifest in the recovery room after uneventful surgery and anesthesia.

Masseter Muscle Rigidity

Masseter muscle rigidity (MMR) or trismus is a sustained and forceful contracture of the masseter muscle. The contracture may be severe enough to make opening the jaw impossible ("jaws of steel"). A mild increase in masseter muscle tone or incomplete jaw relaxation following succinylcholine is fairly common and may be a normal response, but severe jaw tightness that interferes with intubation may portend an episode of MH. If trismus is further accompanied by generalized body rigidity, MH is highly likely.[62,77]

Management of trismus in the surgical patient is a contentious issue, and authorities are divided on how to proceed after MMR.[77,91,92] Some experts recommend cautiously continuing the anesthetic with nontriggering agents after an episode of MMR, while monitoring for rhabdomyolysis and signs and symptoms of MH.[92] Others maintain that the safer course is to assume that trismus is a harbinger of MH, discontinue the anesthetic, and cancel elective surgery until results of a muscle biopsy are available.[77]

Because of the likelihood of MH and/or rhabdomyolysis, the surgical patient should be admitted to the hospital and observed for at least 24 hours following marked jaw rigidity and at least 12 hours after mild increase in jaw tension.[77] Myoglobinuria may be apparent in the recovery room, and inducing a brisk urine output may lessen the risk of myoglobinuric renal damage. Studies indicate that following MMR, if the CK is greater than 20,000 units/L and a concomitant myopathy is not present, the diagnosis of MH is likely.[62] Patients who have experienced MMR should be counseled concerning the possibility that they are MHS and should be referred to a well-informed primary or specialty care physician or genetic counselor for further investigation.

Information Resources

The Malignant Hyperthermia Association of the United States (MHAUS) provides educational and technical information to patients and health-care providers. Information is available via fax-on-demand (1-800-440-9990) or on the World Wide Web at http://www.mhaus.org. An MH hotline may be accessed for MH emergencies 24 hours a day at 1-800-MH-HYPER (1-800-644-9737). Health-care providers are encouraged to report MH episodes to the North American MH Registry.

Myotonic Dystrophy

The myotonias are a group of hereditary degenerative muscle diseases that include myotonic dystrophy, myotonia congenita (Thomsen disease), and paramyotonia congenita. A symptom common to all myotonias is the inability of skeletal muscles to relax after chemical or physical stimulation.

Myotonic dystrophy, also known as *Steinert disease*, *myotonia atrophica*, or *myotonia dystrophica*, is the most common and most severe form of the myotonias. It is characterized by skeletal muscles that are hypoplastic, dystrophic, and weak yet prone to persistent contraction. Although muscles are primarily affected, myotonic dystrophy is distinguished from nondystrophic myotonias by being a multisystem disease.[42,93]

Incidence

Myotonic dystrophy is inherited as an autosomal dominant trait. In most cases, an affected person has one affected parent. The onset of symptoms can occur at any age, but usually occurs in the second to third decade of life. A slow, progressive deterioration of skeletal, cardiac, and smooth muscle occurs, resulting in death by the sixth decade. An estimated 1 in 20,000 people worldwide have the disorder, with an equal occurrence in males and females. The severity of clinical symptoms usually increases with transmission to subsequent generations (*genetic anticipation*).[42,94,95] Myotonic dystrophy is the most common and severe inherited muscular dystrophy of adulthood.

Pathophysiology and Treatment

Myotonic dystrophy is a disorder of muscle membrane excitability that results in self-sustaining runs of depolarization. Electrophysiologic studies show a lowered resting membrane potential in muscle cells from patients with myotonic dystrophy. Therapeutic agents used to treat the myotonic contractures include quinine, procainamide, and phenytoin. These agents delay the return of membrane excitation by blocking rapid Na^+ influx into muscle cells.[42] Regional anesthesia and muscle relaxants do not prevent or relieve the recalcitrant contraction.[32] Dantrolene has also been ineffective in reversing myotonia. Warming the ambient temperature or injecting local anesthetics into the involved muscles may induce relaxation. Steroids and inhalation anesthetic agents may also attenuate the contraction in some patients. No treatment is available for the muscle weakness that develops with myotonic dystrophy.

Clinical Manifestations

A wide variety of symptoms are characteristic of myotonic dystrophy. Facial weakness ("expressionless facies"), ptosis, and sternocleidomastoid muscle and distal limb weakness are prominent features of the disease.[42,95] Frontal balding, cataracts, and testicular atrophy in males form a frequently recognized triad of characteristics. Endocrine abnormalities, such as diabetes mellitus and thyroid disease, occur with a greater frequency in this patient group than in the general population.[42]

Myotonia, the inability to relax a muscle, occurs in most symptomatic patients and may be worsened by pressure, touch, cold, or shivering.[95] Insidious muscle atrophy, particularly of the face, neck, pharynx, and distal limbs, causes severe muscle debility in the later stages of the disease.[42] Myotonic symptoms usually precede the atrophy and weakness.

Cardiac disturbances occur in most patients with myotonic dystrophy, often manifesting as conduction defects and arrhythmias.[42,95] Conduction defects were present in about 50% of the patients in one series.[96] First-degree atrioventricular block is the most common finding, but greater degrees of heart block are also seen.[42] Arrhythmias include sinus bradycardia, atrial flutter or fibrillation, and ventricular extrasystole.[96,97]

Weakening of the thoracic muscles, including the diaphragm, reduces the respiratory reserve and the vital capacity, and a restrictive type of ventilatory impairment develops with progression of the disease. Central sleep apnea and hypersomnolence cause hypoventilation and decreased ventilatory response to carbon dioxide.

Anesthetic Implications

Any drug that has the potential to depolarize skeletal muscle may produce an exaggerated contraction in patients with myotonic dystrophy. Administration of succinylcholine to these patients should be avoided because it can produce an intense generalized myotonic contracture that makes ventilation and intubation difficult or impossible. Agents associated with myoclonus (methohexital, etomidate) have the potential to produce similar effects.[32]

Nondepolarizing muscle relaxants may be used in these patients, as long as the degree of muscle wasting and weakness is appreciated. The dose of the nondepolarizer should be reduced according to the degree of muscle impairment, and the neuromuscular block should be monitored closely with a peripheral nerve stimulator.

An abnormal swallowing mechanism resulting from palatal, pharyngeal, and esophageal muscle involvement and gastrointestinal hypomotility renders myotonic dystrophy patients vulnerable to pulmonary aspiration of gastric contents.[32]

Reversal of neuromuscular blockade with anticholinesterase agents may theoretically precipitate skeletal muscle contraction by producing an ACh-induced depolarizing block.[32,98] Shorter-acting nondepolarizing muscle relaxants have the obvious advantage of being less likely to require reversal.

Hypothermia and shivering should be avoided by raising the room temperature, warming inhaled gases and intravenous fluids, and providing a forced-air thermal blanket.

Underestimating the severity of respiratory compromise is not uncommon in these patients. Preoperative arterial blood gas determinations and pulmonary function results may serve as useful baselines in the patient with advanced disease. The respiratory depressant effects of barbiturates, opioids, and volatile anesthetics may compromise already weakened respiratory musculature and lead to unexpected decompensation.[32,99] Even small doses of short-acting anesthetic agents may be associated with an exaggerated and prolonged anesthetic effect. Speedy reported on a typical case in which a 31-year-old man with myotonic dystrophy remained unconscious and unable to maintain a patent airway for 4 hours after receiving an anesthetic that consisted of 50 mg of propofol, 0.5% isoflurane, and 50% nitrous oxide in oxygen.[100] Completely uneventful responses to anesthesia in myotonic patients have also been reported.

Diligent monitoring of cardiovascular parameters should be maintained intraoperatively and postoperatively. Cardiac function that was clinically normal preoperatively may become unacceptably depressed when general anesthetic agents are administered. The patient should be questioned preoperatively about syncope, and the ECG should be examined closely for advanced conduction blocks to help ascertain the need for cardiac pacing. It may be wise to assume that even asymptomatic patients have some degree of cardiac involvement.

Pregnancy may exacerbate the symptoms of myotonia. Uterine atony, postpartum hemorrhage, and retained placenta have accompanied delivery in patients with myotonic dystrophy. Increased progesterone levels are linked to the deleterious effects.[101]

MH-triggering agents should be avoided in these patients, because associations between some forms of myotonia and MH have been described.[77,102]

Lambert-Eaton Myasthenic Syndrome
Incidence

Lambert-Eaton myasthenic syndrome (LEMS), is a rare autoimmune disease that classically occurs in patients with malignant disease, particularly small-cell carcinoma of the bronchi. One third to one half of patients, however, have no evidence of carcinoma.[103,104] Most patients with myasthenic syndrome are men between the ages of 50 and 70 years.

Pathophysiology

The basic defect associated with LEMS appears to be an autoantibody-mediated derangement in presynaptic Ca^{2+} channels leading to a reduction in Ca^{2+}-mediated exocytosis of ACh at neuromuscular and autonomic nerve terminals.[105]

The decreased release of ACh quanta from the cholinergic nerve endings produces a reduced postjunctional response. Unlike in myasthenia gravis, the number and quality of postjunctional AChRs remain unaltered, and the end-plate sensitivity is normal. The neuromuscular junction abnormality of LEMS is similar in location to that of Mg^{2+} intoxication or botulism poisoning, in which the release of presynaptic ACh is attenuated.

Clinical Manifestations and Treatment

Muscle weakness, fatigue, hyporeflexia, and proximal limb muscle aches are the dominant features of LEMS. The diaphragm and other respiratory muscles are also involved. Autonomic nervous system dysfunction is often present and is manifested as impaired gastric motility, orthostatic hypotension, and urinary retention.

Patients with LEMS experience a brief increase in muscle strength with voluntary contraction, distinguishing it from myasthenia gravis. Tetanic stimulation results in a progressive augmentation in muscle strength as the frequency of the stimulation is increased. Posttetanic potentiation is also enhanced.

There is no cure for LEMS. Treatment is aimed at improving muscle strength and reversing autonomic deficits.[106-108] 3,4-Diaminopyridine improves muscle strength in some patients by promoting presynaptic Ca^{2+} influx and increasing the number of ACh quanta that are liberated by a single nerve action potential. Anticholinesterase agents, plasmapheresis, corticosteroids, intravenous immunoglobulin, and immunosuppressive drugs provide improvement for some patients with LEMS.

Anesthetic Implications

An index of suspicion for LEMS should be maintained in surgical patients with a history of muscle weakness and suspected or diagnosed carcinoma of the lung. Patients with LEMS are extremely sensitive to the relaxant effects of both depolarizing and nondepolarizing muscle relaxants. Inhalational anesthetics alone may provide adequate relaxation, but if muscle relaxants are required, their dosages should be reduced and the neuromuscular blockade closely monitored.[109] Neuromuscular reversal with an anticholinesterase agent may be used. Prolonged ventilatory assistance may be required postoperatively.

Rheumatoid Arthritis

Rheumatoid arthritis (RA) is a chronic inflammatory polyarthropathy with myriad degrees of systemic involvement. The disease is multifactorial, and the clinical picture varies widely in severity, extent of involvement, and symptoms. The capricious course of the disease may be persistent and debilitating or relapsing and remitting.[110] With each successive exacerbation, new joints may become involved.

Incidence

Rheumatoid arthritis is the most common form of inflammatory arthritis, affecting approximately 0.8% of the U.S. population. The onset of RA can occur at any age, but most cases are diagnosed in patients between the ages of 35 and 50 years. RA is two to three times more likely to develop in women than in men. The life expectancy of patients with RA may be reduced by 3 to 7 years.[111]

Etiology

The exact cause of RA remains elusive, but heredity plays some role in increasing a person's susceptibility.[111,112] Impaired immunity, stress, and other environmental factors may precipitate or aggravate the disease.[111,113]

A viral or a bacterial infection that alters the immune system in a genetically susceptible host may play a role in the etiology.[111,113] The invading microbe may produce a protein similar to those in the body's own tissue, particularly joint tissue (*molecular mimicry*). To destroy the antigen, the immune system may mount an autoimmune response and mistakenly direct its attack against its own tissue. Circulating autoantibodies called *rheumatoid factors* are detectable in 70% to 80% of patients with RA.[111]

Clinical Manifestations

Joint Involvement. Inflammation and destruction of synovial tissues are responsible for most of the symptoms and chronic disability associated with RA. Joint involvement progresses in three main stages: (1) inflammation of the joint synovial membrane and infiltration by polymorphonuclear leukocytes; (2) rapid division and growth of cells in the joint (synovial proliferation and pannus formation); and (3) liberation of osteolytic enzymes, proteases, and collagenases, which damage small blood vessels, cartilage, ligaments, tendons, and bones. Collapse of normal cortical and medullary architecture leads to erosion and dislocation of bone that is contiguous with the inflammatory cell mass.

The onset of symptoms is most often insidious, evolving over a period of weeks to months.[111] The most common sites of onset are the hands, wrists, and feet. There is often symmetric joint involvement. Swelling, warmth, and pain in the affected joints are caused by the inflammatory process. Morning stiffness, weight loss, and fatigue are noted early in the disease course.

Dissolution of bone and disuse atrophy of bone (osteoporosis) are found in all seriously affected areas. Pain, inflammation, and erosion of bone and tissue may permanently limit the joint's full range of motion. Later stages of the disease are characterized by severe pain, joint instability, and crippling deformities.[111]

Nerve entrapment may occur at any site where peripheral nerves pass near the inflamed joint. Carpal tunnel syndrome is a common peripheral neuropathy.

Synovitis in the temporomandibular joint may limit jaw motion. An estimated 30% to 70% of patients with RA have involvement of the temporomandibular joint. As the disease progresses, flexion contractures and soft-tissue swelling may lead to a marked limitation in the patient's ability to open the jaw.

Although the thoracic and lumbar spine are usually spared, involvement of the cervical spine may be extensive and can lead to limited movement or deformity of the neck and to severe laryngeal deviation.[111,114] The most common site of cervical spine synovitis is C1-C2 (Figure 33-18).[114] Atlantoaxial (C1-C2) instability results from erosion and collapse of bone and from destruction of supporting cervical ligaments. Symptoms occur when excessive motion between C1 and C2 exerts pressure on the spinal cord (Figure 33-19). Additionally, separation of the atlanto-odontoid articulation may allow the odontoid process of the axis to impinge on the spinal cord, leading to neurologic damage. The atlantoaxial subluxation may also exert pressure and impair blood flow through the vertebral arteries (Figure 33-20).

Arthritis extends to the cricoarytenoid joint of the larynx in 40% of patients with severe RA.[115] The joint may become swollen, inflamed, and fixed in a position that obstructs airflow. Vocal cord nodules and polyps may also be present. Symptoms of cricoarytenoid arthritis include tenderness over the larynx, hoarseness, pain on swallowing, with radiation to the ear, and dyspnea or stridor. Patients with no overt clinical symptoms may also have significant laryngeal disease.

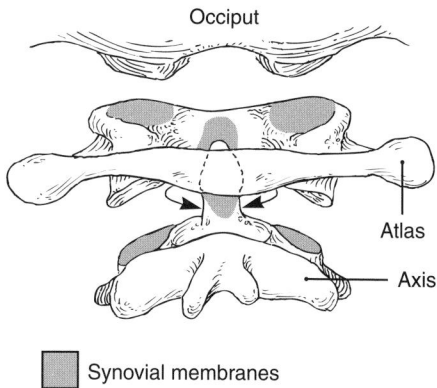

Occiput

Atlas

Axis

■ Synovial membranes

FIGURE 33-18   The relationship between the occiput, the atlas (C1), and the axis (C2). The atlas supports the head and rotates about the odontoid process of the axis. The occipitoatlantoaxial articulations are lined by synovial membranes and are firmly supported by surrounding ligaments (not shown).

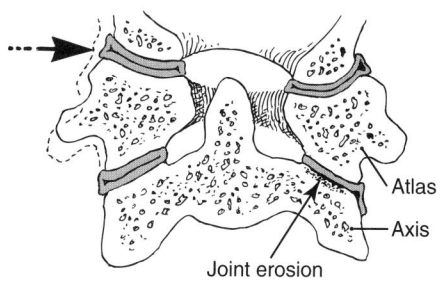

Atlas

Axis

Joint erosion

FIGURE 33-19   Erosion and collapse of C1 and C2 articular surfaces can lead to a shifting of the atlas over the axis. If the subluxation is pronounced, spinal cord compression may occur.

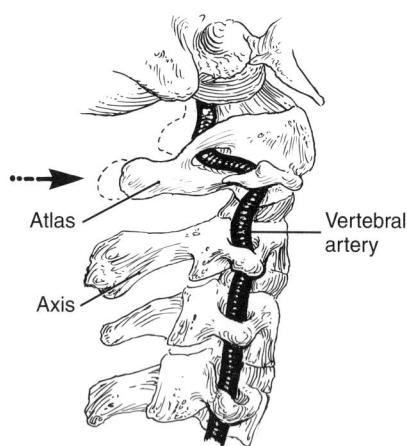

Atlas

Vertebral artery

Axis

FIGURE 33-20   Vertebral artery compression may result from atlantoaxial subluxation.

Systemic Involvement. Although the effects of RA are most clearly seen in joints, the disease is systemic. The immune-mediated destructive process affects a wide variety of organs, including the heart, lungs, muscle, vasculature, and eyes. The occurrence of extraarticular manifestations is usually associated with more active, erosive articular disease.

Firm, painless subcutaneous nodules occur in approximately 20% to 30% of patients with RA.[111] The nodules usually occur over pressure points, such as the occiput, the sacrum, the ulna, or the Achilles tendon, and may be associated with pressure ulcerations. Rheumatoid nodules can also occur in most visceral organs, including the lungs and the heart. Dural nodules can cause spinal cord compression and neurologic complications.

Pericarditis and pericardial effusion may accompany severe progressive RA and impair cardiac performance. Although rare, rheumatoid nodules have been isolated from the cardiac conduction system and may be associated with conduction defects.[111]

Pulmonary involvement manifests as pleural effusion, pneumonitis, pulmonary nodules, or interstitial fibrosis.[111,116] Decreased lung volume, diffusion capacity, and vital capacity may result from the lung alterations.

Rheumatoid myositis, which is characterized by muscle weakness and eventual muscle necrosis and atrophy, may accompany RA. Inflamed, painful, and underused joints contribute to the skeletal muscle atrophy.

Lacrimal duct and salivary gland destruction may result in dryness of the eyes and the mouth (Sjögren syndrome) in about 15% of patients with rheumatoid arthritis.[111]

Treatment

There is no cure for rheumatoid arthritis, and all treatment interventions are palliative. Medical therapy is directed toward relief of pain, nonspecific suppression of the inflammatory process, immunosuppression, prevention and correction of deformity, and control of systemic involvement.

Most patients, including those with mild to moderate disease, obtain some relief of symptoms with rest, joint immobilization, and use of nonsteroidal antiinflammatory drugs (NSAIDs). NSAIDs relieve joint pain, stiffness, heat, and swelling, in part by blocking cyclooxygenase and inhibiting prostaglandin, thromboxane, and prostacyclin synthesis. Despite their potent antiinflammatory properties, they do not alter the underlying disease process.[111]

Corticosteroids are potent antiinflammatory drugs that suppress many symptoms of RA. Long-term side effects (osteoporosis, predisposition to infection, suppression of endogenous cortisol release, cataracts, gastrointestinal bleeding, hypertension, and hyperglycemia), however, limit their use to isolated flares of the disease or to adjunctive rather than primary treatment.

Disease-modifying antirheumatic drugs (DMARDs) can slow the progressive damage and arrest the underlying disease process.[117,118] Agents such as the anticytokines etanercept (Enbrel), adalimumab (Humira), and infliximab (Remicade) work by interfering with the proinflammatory cytokine, tumor necrosis factor.[119-121] Notably, these drugs increase the risk of developing serious infection.

Biologic agents such as interleukin-1 receptor antagonists offer the potential for more effective treatment of RA.[122] Leflunomide (Arava) is a DMARD that inhibits the proliferation of T lymphocytes and slows disease progression. The major side effect of leflunomide is liver-enzyme elevation and liver disease.

The antimetabolite methotrexate (Rheumatrex) is widely used as an effective DMARD for patients with aggressive RA. Bone marrow suppression, oral ulcerations, pneumonitis, and hepatic damage are potential side effects of methotrexate.[123] Gold salts, sulfasalazine, antimalarial drugs, and penicillamine are effective DMARDs used when more conservative measures fail to retard symptoms.[111,117] Immunosuppressive drugs such as cyclophosphamide (Cytoxan) and cyclosporine (Sandimmune) and antimetabolites such as azathioprine (Imuran) are agents generally reserved for more refractory cases.[111]

Surgical interventions for relief of pain or correction or prevention of deformities include total joint replacement, synovectomy, and tenolysis.

Anesthetic Management

Overall, no individual anesthetic agent or mode of anesthesia is substantially safer than another for the patient with RA. Preoperative examination of an individual patient's disease course and medication history are likely to reveal specific features that affect the anesthesia or surgical course.

NSAID ingestion may result in platelet dysfunction. Mild anemia, a common finding in patients with RA, may be secondary either to the disease process or to drug therapy. Long-term NSAID therapy may exert harmful effects on the liver or kidney and exacerbate allergic rhinitis or asthma; these effects may influence the choice of anesthesia.

Patients receiving long-term corticosteroid therapy may develop hypophyseal-pituitary axis suppression, which may require perioperative steroid supplementation. Long-term administration of corticosteroids may increase the patient's susceptibility to infection by inhibiting normal host defense mechanisms. The newer tumor necrosis factor inhibitors are also associated with serious infections, mandating close attention to sterile techniques.

A thorough preoperative assessment of the airway is essential. Particular attention should be directed to the temporomandibular joints, cervical spine, and cricoarytenoid joints.

Range of motion of the temporomandibular joint must be assessed before anesthesia is induced. Patients with severe temporomandibular joint involvement may be unable to open their mouths more than 1 to 2 cm. In such cases, the use of a flexible fiberoptic bronchoscope or other optically guided instruments for tracheal intubation are of proven value.[114]

A thorough neurologic assessment and a radiographic evaluation of the cervical spine should be performed, especially for patients with advanced disease.[124] Some patients with significant radiographic evidence of atlantoaxial or subaxial instability may be entirely asymptomatic.[114,124]

Neck pain is an early symptom of cervical spine instability. Paresthesias into the shoulders and arms, muscle weakness,

paresis, and bowel or bladder dysfunction are some of the clinical manifestations of spinal cord compression secondary to atlantoaxial or subaxial subluxation. Compression on the vertebral arteries, with interruption of vertebral artery blood flow, may lead to symptoms such as nausea, vomiting, dysarthria, dysphagia, blurred vision, or transient loss of consciousness.

Altered cervical spine anatomy or laryngeal deviation can make intubation of the trachea an extreme challenge. Deviation of the larynx can frequently be detected preoperatively by palpating the location of the larynx in relation to the sternal notch. Flexion, extension, and rotation of the neck must be avoided in the presence of cervical instability. Such circumstances dictate fiberoptic-guided intubation of the trachea in the awake patient.

Hoarseness in a patient with RA should alert the anesthetist to possible cricoarytenoid joint involvement. Narrowing of the glottic opening may call for a smaller endotracheal tube. Laryngoscopy can assess normal cord motion and glottic patency. The patient should be observed closely for signs of airway obstruction after extubation.

Generalized demineralization of bone may increase the risk of fractures in patients with RA. Glucocorticoid therapy may aggravate the osteopenia. Proper patient positioning and padding of pressure points prevent nerve palsies, skin ulcerations, and further structural damage to the joints.

SUMMARY

Understanding the pathophysiologic characteristics, clinical presentation, and supporting laboratory studies of patients with musculoskeletal abnormalities is essential for safe and effective anesthetic management. A thorough preoperative assessment of this patient helps determine the extent of muscle, respiratory, and cardiac reserve and aids in anesthetic selection and planning for postoperative care.

Management of cases involving musculoskeletal pathology must take into account preoperative drug therapy for the disease and the potential effect this drug therapy may have on anesthetic agents and muscle relaxants. An anesthetic agent's margin of safety is often reduced in such patients; therefore, fixed dosage regimens should be avoided.

REFERENCES

1. Watras JM. Skeletal muscle physiology. In: Berne RM et al, eds. *Physiology.* 5th ed. St Louis: Mosby; 2004:223.
2. Guyton A, Hall J. Contraction of skeletal muscle. In: *Textbook of Medical Physiology.* 11th ed. Philadelphia: Saunders; 2006:72.
3. Donati F, Bevan DR. Neuromuscular blocking agents. In: Barash PG et al, eds. *Clinical Anesthesia.* 5th ed. Philadelphia: Lippincott Williams & Wilkins; 2005:421-452.
4. Kutchai HC. Synaptic transmission. In: Berne RM et al, eds. *Physiology.* 5th ed. St Louis: Mosby; 2004:44.
5. Guyton A, Hall J. Excitation of skeletal muscle. *Textbook of Medical Physiology.* 11th ed. Philadelphia: Saunders; 2006:85.
6. Katz E et al. Effects of Ca^{2+} channel blocker neurotoxins on transmitter release and presynaptic currents at the mouse neuromuscular junction. *Br J Pharmacol.* 1997;121:1531-1540.
7. Losavio A, Muchnik S. Spontaneous acetylcholine release in mammalian neuromuscular junctions. *Am J Physiol.* 1997;273:C1835-C1841.
8. Lin MJ, Lin-Shiau SY. Multiple types of Ca^{2+} channels in mouse motor nerve terminal. *Eur J Neurosci.* 1997;9:817-823.
9. Sheng ZH et al. Physical link and functional coupling of presynaptic calcium channels and the synaptic vesicle docking/fusion machinery. *J Bioenerg Biomembr.* 1998;30:335-345.
10. Paton WM, Waud DR. The margin of safety of neuromuscular transmission. *J Physiol.* 1967;191:59-90.
11. Ruff RL. Electrophysiology of postsynaptic activation. *Ann N Y Acad Sci.* 1998;841:57-70.
12. Tseng A et al. Respiratory failure in Lambert Eaton myasthenic syndrome precipitated by calcium-channel blockers: report of a case and literature review. *J Clin Neuromuscul Dis.* 2002;4:60-63.
13. Lindstrom J. Nicotinic acetylcholine receptors in health and disease. *Mol Neurobiol.* 1997;15:193-222.
14. Kopta C, Steinbach JH. Comparison of mammalian adult and fetal nicotinic acetylcholine receptors. *J Neurosc.* 1994;14:3922-3933.
15. Singh S, Prior C. Prejunctional effects of the nicotinic ACh receptor agonist dimethylphenylpiperazinium at the rat neuromuscular junction. *J Physiol (Lond).* 1998;511:451-460.
16. Prior C et al. Prejunctional actions of muscle relaxants: synaptic vesicles and transmitter mobilization as sites of action. *Gen Pharmacol.* 1995;26:659-666.
17. Storella RJ et al. Tetanic fade and acetylcholine release. *Anesthesiology.* 1993;79:A923.
18. Almon RR, Appel SH. Cholinergic sites in skeletal muscles: denervation effects. *Biochemistry.* 1976;15:3662-3667.
19. Moorthy SS, Hilgenberg JC. Resistance to non-depolarizing muscle relaxants in paretic upper extremities of patients with residual hemiplegia. *Anesth Analg.* 1980;59:624-627.
20. Gronert GA. Disuse atrophy with resistance to pancuronium. *Anesthesiology.* 1981;55:547-549.
21. Sastry BVR. Nicotinic receptor. *Anaesth Pharmacol Rev.* 1993;1:6-13.

22. Gronert GA. Use of suxamethonium in cord patients—whether and when. *Anaesthesia.* 1998;53:1035-1036.

23. Polla B et al. Respiratory muscle fibers: specialization and plasticity. *Thorax.* 2004;59:808-817.

24. Drachman DB. Myasthenia gravis and other diseases of the neuromuscular junction. In: Fauci AS et al, eds. *Harrison's Principles of Internal Medicine.* 17th ed. New York: McGraw-Hill; 2008:2672-2677.

25. Itoh H et al. Sensitivity to vecuronium in seropositive and seronegative patients with myasthenia gravis. *Anesth Analg.* 2002;95:109-113.

26. Zweiman B, Levinson AI. Immunologic aspects of neurological and neuromuscular diseases. *JAMA.* 1992;268:2918-2922.

27. Thanvi BR, Lo TCN. Update on myasthenia gravis. *Postgrad Med J.* 2004;80:690-700.

28. Dierdorf SF, Walton JS. Anesthesia for patients with rare and co-existing diseases. In: Barash PG et al, eds. *Clinical Anesthesia.* 5th ed. Philadelphia: Lippincott; 2005:502-528.

29. Hofstad H et al. Heart disease in myasthenia gravis. *Acta Neurol Scand.* 1984;70:176-184.

30. Lindberg C et al. Remission rate after thymectomy in myasthenia gravis when the bias of immunosuppressive therapy is eliminated. *Acta Neurol Scand.* 1992;86:323-328.

31. Ceremuga TE et al. Etiology, mechanisms, and anesthesia implications of autoimmune myasthenia gravis. *AANA J.* 2002;70:301-310.

32. Urban K, Lahlou S. Muscle disorders. In: Fleisher LA, ed. *Anesthesia and Uncommon Diseases.* Philadelphia: Saunders; 2006:303.

33. Froelich J. Anaesthetic management of a patient with myasthenia gravis and tracheal stenosis. *Can J Anaesth.* 1996;43:84-89.

34. Rusa R, Ulatowski JA. The patient with a neurologic disorder. *Problems in Anesthesia.* Philadelphia: Lippincott-Raven; 1997:221.

35. Nilsson E, Muller K. Neuromuscular effects of isoflurane in patients with myasthenia gravis. *Acta Anaesthesiol Scand.* 1990;34:126-131.

36. Baraka A. Suxamethonium block in the myasthenic patient: correlation with plasma cholinesterase. *Anaesthesia.* 1992;47:217-219.

37. Nilsson E, Meretoya OA. Vecuronium dose-response and maintenance requirements in patients with myasthenia gravis. *Anesthesiology.* 1990; 73:28-32.

38. Tortosa JA, Hernandeq-Palazon J. Anaesthesia for laparoscopic cholecystectomy in myasthenia gravis: a non-muscle relaxant technique. *Anaesthesia.* 1997;52:807-808.

39. Basaranoglu G et al. Anesthesia of a patient with cured myasthenia gravis [letter]. *Anesth Analg.* 2003;96:1842-1843.

40. Itoh H et al. Neuromuscular monitoring at the orbicularis oculi may overestimate the blockade in myasthenic patients. *Anesthesiology.* 2000;93:1194-1197.

41. Leventhal SR et al. Prediction of the need for postoperative mechanical ventilation in myasthenia gravis. *Anesthesiology.* 1980;53:26-30.

42. Brown RH et al. Muscular dystrophies and other muscle diseases. In: Fauci AS et al, eds. *Harrison's Principles of Internal Medicine.* 17th ed. New York: McGraw-Hill; 2008:2678-2695.

43. Palmieri B, Sblendorio V. Duchenne muscular dystrophy: an update. *J Clin Neuromuscul Dis.* 8:122-151, 2007.

44. Carlson CG. The dystrophinopathies: an alternative to the structural hypothesis. *Neurobiol Dis.* 1998;5:3-15.

45. Michalak M, Opas M. Functions of dystrophin and dystrophin associated proteins. *Curr Opin Neurol.* 1997;10:436-442.

46. Curran MJ. Muscular dystrophies and myotonic syndromes: anesthesia and musculoskeletal disorders. In: Lui ACP, Crosby ET, eds. *Problems in Anesthesia.* Philadelphia: Lippincott; 1991:124.

47. Staiano A et al. Upper gastrointestinal tract motility in children with progressive muscular dystrophy. *J Pediatr.* 1992;121:720-724.

48. Chung BC et al. Acute gastroparesis in Duchenne's muscular dystrophy. *Yonsei Med J.* 1998;39:175-179.

49. Sasaki K et al. Sequential changes in cardiac structure and function in patients with Duchenne type muscular dystrophy: a two-dimensional echocardiographic study. *Am Heart J.* 1998;135:937-944.

50. Nigro G et al. The incidence and evolution of cardiomyopathy in Duchenne's muscular dystrophy. *Int J Cardiol.* 1990;26:271-277.

51. Corrado G et al. Prognostic value of electrocardiograms, ventricular late potentials, ventricular arrhythmias, and left ventricular systolic dysfunction in patients with Duchenne muscular dystrophy. *Am J Cardiol.* 2002;89:838-841.

52. Perloff JK et al. The distinctive electrocardiogram of Duchenne's progressive muscular dystrophy. *Am J Med.* 1967;42:179-188.

53. Maccani RM et al. Femoral and lateral femoral cutaneous nerve block for muscle biopsies in children. *Paediatr Anaesth.* 1995;5:223-227.

54. Harper CM et al. The prognostic value of preoperative predicted forced vital capacity in corrective spinal surgery for Duchenne's muscular dystrophy. *Anaesthesia.* 2004;59:1160-1162.

55. Ririe DG et al. The response of patients with Duchenne's muscular dystrophy to neuromuscular blockade with vecuronium. *Anesthesiology.* 1998;88:351-354.

56. Nathan A et al. Hyperkalemic cardiac arrest after cardiopulmonary bypass in a child with unsuspected Duchenne muscular dystrophy. *Pediatr Anesth.* 2005;100:672-674.

57. Yemen TA, McCalin C. Muscular dystrophy, anesthesia and the safety of inhalational agents revisited; again. *Pediatr Anesth.* 2006;16:105-108.

58. Ramchandra DS et al. Ketamine monoanaesthesia for diagnostic muscle biopsy in neuromuscular disorders in infancy and childhood: floppy infant syndrome. *Can J Anaesth.* 1990;37:474-476.

59. Obata R et al. Rhabdomyolysis in association with Duchenne's muscular dystrophy. *Can J Anaesth.* 1999;46:564-565.

60. Larach MG et al. Hyperkalemic cardiac arrest during anesthesia in infants and children with occult myopathies. *Clin Pediatr (Phila).* 1997;36:9-16.

61. Smith W. Cardiac arrest during desflurane anaesthesia in a patient with Duchenne's muscular dystrophy [letter]. *Acta Anaesthesiol Scand.* 2005;49:268-269.

62. Rosenberg H et al. Malignant hyperthermia and other pharmacogenetic disorders. In: Barash PG, eds. *Clinical Anesthesia.* 5th ed. Philadelphia: Lippincott Williams & Wilkins; 2005:529-556.

63. Patel R et al. Evaluation of the difficult pediatric patient: ambulatory anesthesia. *Anesthesiol Clin North America.* 1996;14:753-767.

64. Malignant Hyperthermia Association of the United States. *Managing MH: Clinical Update Online Brochure.* Available at: http://www.info@mhaus.org. Accessed July 17, 2008.

65. Strazis KP, Fox AW. Malignant hyperthermia: a review of published cases. *Anesth Analg.* 1993;77:297-304.

66. Denborough MA et al. Anaesthetic deaths in a family. *Br J Anaesth.* 1962;34:395.

67. Manning BM et al. Identification of novel mutations in the ryanodine receptor gene (RYR1) in malignant hyperthermia: genotype-phenotype correlation. *Am J Hum Genet.* 1998;62:599-609.

68. Allen GC. Malignant hyperthermia susceptibility. *Anesthesiol Clin North America.* 1994;12:513-535.

69. Smith CA et al. Suspected malignant hyperthermia in a 13-month-old: today's "typical" episode—a case report. *AANA J.* 1997;65:247-249.

70. Michalek-Sauberer A et al. A case of suspected malignant hyperthermia during desflurane administration. *Anesth Analg.* 1997;85:461-462.

71. Uskova AA et al. Desflurane, malignant hyperthermia, and release of compartment syndrome. *Anesth Analg.* 2005;100:1357-1360.

72. Papadimos TJ et al. A suspected case of delayed onset malignant hyperthermia with desflurane anesthesia. *Anesth Analg.* 2004;98:548-549.

73. Stuebing VL. Differential diagnosis of malignant hyperthermia: a case report. *AANA J.* 1995;63:455-460.

74. Girard T, Urwyler A. Not every hypermetabolic state is due to malignant hyperthermia. *Anesth Analg.* 2007;104:1611-1612.

75. Sullivan M et al. Succinylcholine-induced cardiac arrest in children with undiagnosed myopathy. *Can J Anaesth.* 1994;41:497-501.

76. Bendixen D et al. Analysis of anesthesia in patients suspected to be susceptible to malignant hyperthermia before diagnostic in vitro contracture test. *Acta Anesthesiol Scand.* 1997;41:480-484.

77. Malignant Hyperthermia Association of the United States. *Managing MH: Clinical Update Online Brochure.* Available at: www.mhaus.org. Updated July 1, 2005.

78. Malignant Hyperthermia Association of the United States. *Temperature Monitoring.* Available at: www.mhaus.org. Updated February 18, 2004.

79. Weglinski MR et al. Malignant hyperthermia testing in patients with persistently increased serum creatine kinase levels. *Anesth Analg.* 1997; 84:1038-1041.

80. Nelson TE et al. Dantrolene sodium can increase or attenuate activity of skeletal muscle ryanodine receptor calcium release channel. *Anesthesiology.* 1996;84:1368-1379.

81. Krause T et al. Dantrolene: A review of its pharmacology, therapeutic use and new developments. *Anaesthesia.* 2004;59:364-373.

82. Baker KR et al. The Icarus effect: the influence of diluent warming on dantrolene sodium mixing time. *AANA J.* 2007;75:101-106.

83. McGoldrick K. Is malignant hyperthermia a contraindication for outpatient surgery? *Soc Ambul Anesth News.* 1992;7:11.

84. Yentis SM et al. Should all children with suspected or confirmed malignant hyperthermia susceptibility be admitted after surgery? A ten-year review. *Anesth Analg.* 1992;75:345-350.

85. Sei Y et al. Malignant hyperthermia in North America: genetic screening of the three hot spots in the type I ryanodine receptor gene. *Anesthesiology.* 2004;101:824-830.

86. Nelson TE et al. Genetic testing in malignant hyperthermia in North America [editorial]. *Anesthesiology.* 2004;100:212-214.

87. Reuter DA et al. The ryanodine contracture test may help diagnose susceptibility to malignant hyperthermia. *Can J Anaesth*. 2003;50:643-648.

88. Girard T et al. Molecular genetic testing for malignant hyperthermia susceptibility. *Anesthesiology*. 2004;100:1076-1080.

89. Greenberg C. Diagnosis and treatment of hyperthermia in the post anesthesia care unit. *Anesthesiol Clin North America*. 1990;8:377-397.

90. Burkman JM et al. Analysis of the clinical variables associated with recrudescence after malignant hyperthermia reactions. *Anesthesiology*. 2007; 106:901-906.

91. Orr RJ, Ramamoorthy C. Controversies in pediatric ambulatory anesthesia. *Anesthesiol Clin North America*. 1996;14:767-779.

92. O'Flynn RP et al. Masseter muscle rigidity and malignant hyperthermia susceptibility in pediatric patients: an update on management and diagnosis. *Anesthesiology*. 1994;80:1228-1233.

93. Ptacek LJ et al. Genetics and physiology of the myotonic muscle disorders. *N Engl J Med*. 1993;328:482-489.

94. Bruner HG et al. Brief report: reverse mutation in myotonic dystrophy. *N Engl J Med*. 1993;328:476-480.

95. Barohn RJ. Muscle diseases. In: Goldman L, Ausiello D, eds. *Cecil Textbook of Medicine*. 23rd ed. Philadelphia: Saunders; 2008:2817-2833.

96. Tokgozoglu LS et al. Cardiac involvement in a large kindred with myotonic dystrophy. Quantitative assessment and relation to size of CTG repeat expansion. *JAMA*. 1995;13:813-819.

97. Hawley RJ et al. Myotonic heart disease: a clinical follow-up. *Neurology*. 1991;41:259-262.

98. Schwartz JJ. Skin and musculoskeletal diseases. In: Hines RA, Marschall KE, eds. *Anesthesia and Co-existing Disease*. 5th ed. Philadelphia: Churchill Livingstone; 2008:437-468.

99. White RJ, Bass S. Anaesthetic management of a patient with myotonic dystrophy. *Paediatric Anaesth*. 2001;11:494-497.

100. Speedy HL. Exaggerated physiological responses to propofol in myotonic dystrophy. *Br J Anaesth*. 1990;64:110-112.

101. Blumgart CH et al. Obstetric anaesthesia in dystrophia myotonica. *Anaesthesia*. 1990;45:26-29.

102. Lehmann-Horn F, Iaizzo PA. Are myotonias and periodic paralyses associated with susceptibility to malignant hyperthermia? *Br J Anaesth*. 1990; 65:692-697.

103. Leonovicz B et al. Paraneoplastic syndromes associated with lung cancer: a unique case of concomitant subacute cerebellar degeneration and Lambert-Eaton myasthenic syndrome. *Anesth Analg*. 2001;93:1557-1559.

104. Gutman L, Phillips HG II. Trends in the association of Lambert-Eaton myasthenic syndrome with carcinoma. *Neurology*. 1992;42:848-850.

105. Leys K et al. Calcium channel autoantibodies in the Lambert-Eaton myasthenic syndrome. *Ann Neurol*. 1991;29:307-314.

106. Telford RJ, Hollway TE. The myasthenic syndrome: anaesthesia in a patient treated with 3,4 diaminopyridine. *Br J Anaesth*. 1990;64:363-366.

107. Oh SJ et al. Low-dose guanidine and pyridostigmine: relatively safe and effective long-term symptomatic therapy in Lambert-Eaton myasthenic syndrome. *Muscle Nerve*. 1997;20:1146-1152.

108. Muchnik S et al. Long-term follow-up of Lambert-Eaton syndrome with intravenous immunoglobulin. *Muscle Nerve*. 1997;20:674-678.

109. Itoh H et al. Neuromuscular monitoring in myasthenic syndrome. *Anaesthesia*. 2001;56:562-567.

110. Eberhardt K, Fex E. Clinical course and remission rate in patients with early rheumatoid arthritis: relationship to outcome after 5 years. *Br J Rheumatol*. 1998;37:1324-1329.

111. Lipsky PE. Rheumatoid arthritis. In: Fauci AS et al, eds. *Harrison's Principles of Internal Medicine*. 17th ed. New York: McGraw-Hill; 2008:2672-2677.

112. Shiozawa S et al. Identification of the gene loci that predispose to rheumatoid arthritis. *Int Immunol*. 1998;10:1891-1895.

113. Jeffries WM. The etiology of rheumatoid arthritis. *Med Hypotheses*. 1998;51:111-114.

114. Keenan MA et al. Acquired laryngeal deviation associated with cervical spine disease in erosive polyarticular arthritis. *Anesthesiology*. 1983; 58:441-449.

115. Khanan T. Anaesthetic risks in rheumatoid arthritis. *Br J Hosp Med*. 1994;52:320-325.

116. Tanoue LT. Pulmonary manifestations of rheumatoid arthritis. *Clin Chest Med*. 1998;19:667-685.

117. Mest CG. Osteoarthritis and rheumatoid arthritis. In: Arcangelo V, Peterson AM, eds. *Pharmacotherapeutics for Advanced Practice*. Philadelphia: Lippincott; 2001:515.

118. Rich E et al. Paucity of radiographic progression in rheumatoid arthritis treated with methotrexate as the first disease-modifying antirheumatic drug. *J Rheumatol*. 1999;26:259-261.

119. Lipsky PE et al. Infliximab and methotrexate in the treatment of rheumatoid arthritis. *N Engl J Med*. 2000;343:1594-1602.

120. Bathon JM et al. A comparison of etanercept and methotrexate in patients with early rheumatoid arthritis. *N Engl J Med*. 2000;343:1586-1593.

121. Adalimumab (Humira) for rheumatoid arthritis. *Medical Lett Drugs Ther*. 2003;45:25-28.

122. Bresnihan B et al. Treatment of rheumatoid arthritis with recombinant human interleukin-1 receptor antagonist. *Arthritis Rheum*. 1998;41: 2196-2204.

123. Hakim NS et al. Methotrexate-induced hepatic necrosis requiring liver transplantation in a patient with rheumatoid arthritis. *Int Surg*. 1998;83:224-225.

124. Kwek TK et al. The role of preoperative cervical spine X-rays in rheumatoid arthritis. *Anaesth Intensive Care*. 1998;26:636-641.

CHAPTER 34

THE ENDOCRINE SYSTEM AND ANESTHESIA

Mary C. Karlet

GENERAL PRINCIPLES OF ENDOCRINE PHYSIOLOGY

Body homeostasis is controlled by two major regulating systems: (1) the nervous system and (2) the endocrine or hormonal system. Both of these systems communicate, integrate, and organize the body's response to a changing internal or external environment.[1]

Organs that secrete hormones are called *endocrine glands*; collectively, these glands make up the *endocrine system*. The purpose of the endocrine system is regulation of behavior, growth, metabolism, fluid status, development, and reproduction. To accomplish these complex processes, multiple hormones interact to produce precise biochemical and physiologic responses.

Endocrine glands secrete their hormone products directly into the surrounding extracellular fluid. This distinguishes them from *exocrine glands*, such as salivary or sweat glands, whose products are discharged through ducts. Important endocrine glands include the pituitary gland, thyroid gland, parathyroid glands, adrenal glands, pancreas, ovaries and testes, and placenta.

Hormones

Endocrine function is mediated by hormones. Hormones are the signaling molecules or chemical messengers that transport information from one set of cells (endocrine cells) to another (target cells). Hormones are released from endocrine glands into body fluids in minute quantities but exert powerful control over most metabolic functions.[2,3]

Transmission of a hormonal signal through the bloodstream to a distant target cell (e.g., pituitary gland to the adrenal gland) is called an *endocrine function*. If a hormone signal acts on a neighboring cell of a different type (e.g., pancreas α cells to pancreas β cells), the interaction is termed a *paracrine function*. If the secreted hormone acts on the producer cell itself or on neighboring identical cells, the interaction is called an *autocrine function*.[1,2]

Types of Hormones

Hormones can be classified into three major categories: (1) proteins or peptides, (2) amines or amino acid derivatives, and (3) steroids.

Peptide or Protein Hormones. Most hormones have a peptide or protein structure. This group of hormones includes insulin, growth hormone, vasopressin (antidiuretic hormone), angiotensin, prolactin, erythropoietin, calcitonin, somatostatin, adrenocorticotropic hormone, oxytocin, glucagon, and parathyroid hormone. Peptide hormones are synthesized in endocrine cells as prehormones and prohormones. They are processed by the cell and stored in secretory granules within the endocrine gland.[1,2] The proper stimulus to secretion causes exocytosis of the peptide or protein hormone into the extracellular fluid.

Protein hormones, such as insulin, erythropoietin, and growth hormone, can now be synthesized for therapeutic purposes by recombinant deoxyribonucleic acid (DNA) techniques.

Amine- or Amino Acid–Derivative Hormones. Several hormones are amino acid or amine compound derivatives. Serotonin, important for its central nervous system effects, is synthesized from the naturally occurring amino acid tryptophan.[2] Thyroid hormones and catecholamine hormones (dopamine, epinephrine, and norepinephrine) are derived from the amino acid tyrosine. Thyroid hormones and catecholamine hormones are stored in the thyroid gland and adrenal medulla, respectively, and are released by the appropriate stimulation.[1]

Steroid Hormones. All steroid hormones are derived from cholesterol or have a chemical structure similar to that of cholesterol. Common steroid hormones include hormones of the adrenal cortex (e.g., cortisol, aldosterone) and reproductive hormones (e.g., estrogen, progesterone, testosterone). Active metabolites of vitamin D are also steroid hormones.[1] In contrast to most other hormones, steroid hormones are not stored in discrete secretory granules but are compartmentalized within the endocrine cell and released into the extracellular fluid by simple diffusion through the cell membrane.[1,2]

Circulating steroid and thyroid hormones are bound to *transport proteins*, whereas circulating catecholamine hormones and most protein hormones are not bound to carriers. Plasma protein binding protects hormones from metabolism and renal clearance.[2] The circulating half-life of steroid and thyroid hormones is therefore typically longer than that of peptide and catecholamine hormones. For example, the thyroid hormone thyroxine, which is 99.95% protein bound, has a plasma half-life of 6 days, whereas insulin, which has essentially no plasma protein binding, has a half-life of about 7 minutes.[1]

The major sites of hormone degradation and elimination are the liver and the kidneys. Some hormone degradation also occurs at target-cell sites.[1-3]

Hormone Receptors

Binding to a specific target-cell receptor is the primary event that initiates a hormone response.[2] The hormone receptor displays high specificity and affinity for the proper hormone ligand, and the location of the receptor directs the hormone to the specific target organ or target-cell site.[4] Some hormones, such as insulin and growth hormone, act on widespread target sites; others, such as thyroid stimulating hormone, act on one target tissue.[5] After binding, the hormone-receptor complex induces a cascade of intracellular events that produce specific physiologic responses in the target cell.[2]

Hormone Receptor Activation. Hormone receptors are located either on the surface of cells or inside cells.[3] Receptors for protein, peptide, and catecholamine hormones are located in or on the surface of the target-cell membrane. Hormone binding to a cell membrane receptor triggers a response by activating enzyme systems in or near the plasma membrane bilayer. The activated enzymes generate intracellular signals, called *second messengers*, which carry the hormone's message within the intracellular space.

Several different second-messenger systems operate in response to cell membrane receptor-hormone binding. Probably the most widely described second-messenger system is the *cyclic adenosine monophosphate (cAMP) system*. This hormone transduction mechanism is initiated when receptor occupation activates the plasma membrane enzyme *adenyl cyclase*. The membrane-bound adenyl cyclase then catalyzes the intracellular conversion of adenosine triphosphate (ATP) to cAMP; cAMP in turn becomes the hormone's intracellular messenger, activating intracellular enzymes, modifying cell-membrane permeability or transport, and altering cellular gene expression.[1] The enzyme phosphodiesterase catalyzes the hydrolysis of cAMP and terminates its intracellular actions. Hormones that use cAMP as their second messenger include thyroid stimulating hormone, vasopressin, parathyroid hormone, glucagon, some catecholamines, corticotropin, follicle-stimulating hormone, and luteinizing hormone.

Other intracellular second messengers include calcium, diacylglycerol, inositol triphosphate, and cyclic guanosine monophosphate. The primary intracellular messenger has not been identified for many hormones.

In contrast to peptide and catecholamine hormones, thyroid and steroid hormones produce the desired target-cell response chiefly by interacting with specific intracellular hormone receptors.[1] Thyroid and steroid hormones are small lipophilic molecules that enter target cells by simple diffusion or by special transport mechanisms. Once within the cell, these hormones occupy specific intracellular receptors.[2] In combination with their receptors, the hormones interact with DNA in the cell nucleus to enhance or suppress gene transcription or translation.[1,2]

Thyroid and steroid hormones enable the cell to alter gene expression, protein formation, and cell activity in response to environmental and developmental stimuli.[2]

Every hormone has a specific onset and duration of action.[3] Hormones that act by binding to cell membrane receptors (peptide, protein, and catecholamine hormones) usually generate a hormonal effect in seconds to minutes. Hormones that bind to intracellular receptors and activate the transcription processes of specific genes (thyroid and steroid hormones) may require several hours or even days to generate a hormonal response.[1,3]

Hormone Receptor Regulation. Receptors are dynamic molecules that are constantly being destroyed and replaced. The receptor for insulin, for example, has a normal half-life of only about 7 hours.[2] Hormone receptor destruction may be part of a normal endocrine response or part of an acquired or genetic disease state.

In many instances, the hormone receptor number is inversely related to the concentration of the circulating hormone. A sustained elevation of the plasma level of a given hormone may cause the target site to decrease the number of receptors per cell. This *downregulation* of receptor number serves to decrease the responsiveness of a target cell to hormone excess.[1] The insulin resistance observed in obesity and type 2 diabetes mellitus may be partly explained by downregulation of the insulin receptors in response to chronically high levels of circulating insulin.[2]

Conversely, a low circulating hormone concentration may cause the target gland to increase the number of hormone receptors per cell.[2] This *upregulation* of hormone receptor number amplifies the cell's sensitivity to hormone stimulation.[1,2]

The number of receptors in a target cell usually changes from day to day.[3] Regulation of receptor turnover, and thus hormone receptor number, is a mechanism by which hormone activity can be precisely modulated.[1]

Regulation of Hormone Secretion. The synthesis and secretion of hormones by endocrine glands are regulated by three general control mechanisms: neural controls, biorhythms, and feedback mechanisms.

Neural control can evoke or suppress hormone secretion. Pain, emotion, smell, touch, injury, stress, sight, and taste can alter hormone release through neural mechanisms.[1] Glucagon, cortisol, antidiuretic hormone, and catecholamines, for example, are all stimulated by the stress response to anesthesia, surgery, and trauma.

The secretion of many hormones is governed by genetically encoded or acquired *biorhythms*. These intrinsic hormonal oscillations may be circadian (e.g., the daily variability in glucocorticoid secretion), weekly (e.g., the menstrual cycle), or seasonal (e.g., thyroxine production).[1,4] The biorhythms may also vary at different stages of life (e.g., growth hormone secretion).[6]

Feedback control is another sophisticated mechanism through which a hormonal response is controlled. Many endocrine disorders arise from the breakdown of feedback loops.[2] *Negative feedback* acts to limit or terminate the production and secretion of a given hormone once the appropriate response has occurred. Negative feedback of a target-cell product to the hormone producer (the endocrine gland) limits or prevents hormone excess. When concentrations of the product are low, feedback inhibition to the endocrine gland is lessened and hormone secretion enhanced.

Virtually all hormones are controlled by some type of *negative feedback* mechanism.[3,4] For example, parathyroid hormone is controlled by calcium, insulin and glucagon are controlled by glucose, and vasopressin is controlled by serum osmolarity.[5] The negative feedback mechanism is a very important factor in the regulation of hormones of the hypothalamus and pituitary gland. Hypothalamic hormones stimulate the release of pituitary hormones from the pituitary gland. The pituitary hormones in turn may stimulate an output of product from peripheral target cells. Product from peripheral target tissues may then initiate feedback to the pituitary gland or the hypothalamus to inhibit pituitary or hypothalamic hormone synthesis and discharge.[1,2]

Positive feedback is a less common hormone-regulating mechanism in which a given hormone response initiates signals amplifying hormone release. The surge in luteinizing hormone (LH) that precedes ovulation is stimulated by LH; this is an example of positive feedback.[2]

PITUITARY GLAND

Relationship Between Pituitary Gland and Hypothalamus

The *pituitary gland*, or *hypophysis*, is known as the "master endocrine gland." It secretes hormones that have far-reaching effects

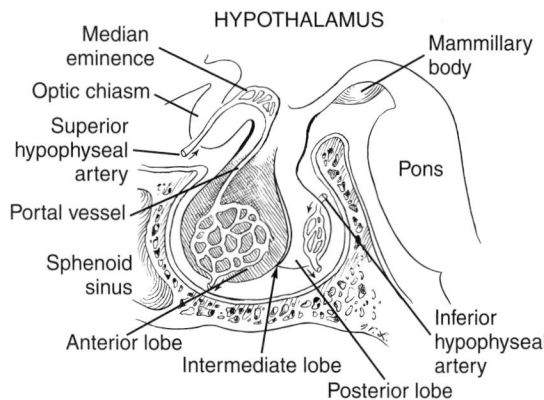

FIGURE **34-1** The pituitary gland is located at the base of the brain, enclosed within a cavity of the sphenoid bone called the *sella turcica*. It is connected to the overlying hypothalamus by the pituitary stalk.

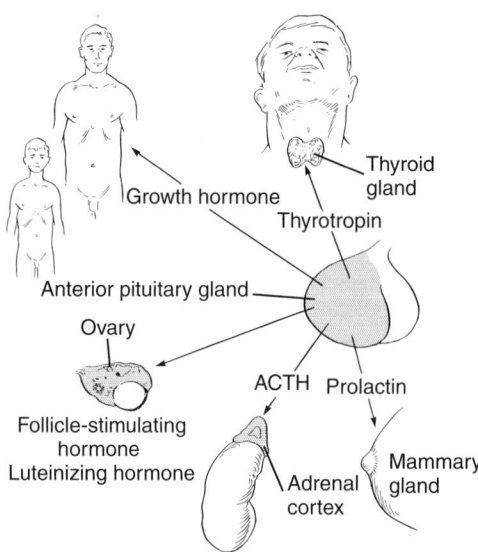

FIGURE **34-2** Major target sites for anterior pituitary hormones. *ACTH,* Adrenocorticotropic hormone.

on various homeostatic, developmental, metabolic, and reproductive functions of the body. The pituitary is a small endocrine gland (only 500 mg in weight and about the size of a pea) centrally located at the base of the brain. It is enclosed within a bony cavity of the sphenoid bone called the *sella turcica*.[5,6] The pituitary gland is connected to the overlying hypothalamus by the *hypophyseal stalk (pituitary stalk)*. The hypothalamus is located below the thalamus, behind the optic chiasm and between the optic tracts. The pituitary, hypothalamus, and some of the surrounding structures are shown in Figure 34-1.

The brain, via the hypothalamus, is an important regulator of pituitary gland secretion.[6] The hypothalamus collects and integrates information (pain, emotions, energy needs, water balance, olfactory sensations, electrolyte concentrations) from almost all parts of the body and uses this information to control the secretion of vital pituitary hormones.[5,6] Pituitary hormone secretion also is regulated by feedback control from peripheral target-organ hormones or other target-organ products.[5] The pituitary gland and hypothalamus have virtually no blood-brain barrier, allowing feedback products to exert potent effects.

Functionally and histologically, the pituitary gland is divided into two distinct portions: the *anterior lobe (adenohypophysis)* and the *posterior lobe (neurohypophysis)*.[6] The anterior pituitary lobe is embryologically derived from an upward invagination of pharyngeal epithelial cells. The posterior pituitary lobe develops from a downward outpouching of ectoderm from the brain. Blood supply to the anterior pituitary lobe is principally from the superior hypophyseal artery, which is a branch of the internal carotid artery. Blood supply to the posterior pituitary lobe is via the inferior hypophyseal artery.[5]

Anterior Pituitary Lobe

The anterior pituitary lobe, which constitutes about 80% of the pituitary gland by weight, secretes six primary hormones.[6] Target sites for the anterior pituitary hormones are shown in Figure 34-2.

1. *Growth hormone (GH)* promotes skeletal development and body growth and regulates protein and carbohydrate metabolism.
2. *Adrenocorticotropic hormone (ACTH)* regulates the growth of the adrenal cortex and the release of cortisol and androgenic hormones from the adrenal gland. ACTH possesses mild melanocyte-stimulating properties, resulting in skin pigmentation at high levels.
3. *Thyroid-stimulating hormone (thyrotropin or TSH)* controls the growth and metabolism of the thyroid gland and the secretion of thyroid hormones, which regulate the rates of most chemical reactions in the body.[5,6]
4. *Follicle-stimulating hormone (FSH)* stimulates ovarian follicle development in females and spermatogenesis in males.
5. *Luteinizing hormone (LH)* induces ovulation and corpus luteum development in females and stimulates the testes to produce testosterone in males.
6. *Prolactin* promotes mammary gland development and milk production (lactogenesis) by the breasts. Prolactin also exerts an effect on reproductive function by inhibiting the synthesis and secretion of LH and FSH. Prolactin synthesis is markedly increased during pregnancy.[5]

Several other less important or less well-defined hormones also are secreted from the anterior pituitary lobe.[6]

Anterior pituitary hormones are synthesized and secreted by at least five distinct cell types within the gland: *somatotrophs (acidophils)* synthesize GH; *gonadotrophs* synthesize the two gonadotropic hormones, LH and FSH; *thyrotrophs* synthesize TSH; *corticotrophs* synthesize ACTH; and *lactotrophs (mammotrophs)* synthesize prolactin. About 40% to 50% of the anterior pituitary cells are somatotrophs and about 20% are corticotrophs.[5]

Control of Anterior Pituitary Hormone Secretion

Synthesis of anterior pituitary hormones is controlled by signals from the hypothalamus. Neurosecretory cells in various hypothalamic nuclei respond to input from the body by synthesizing specific neurohormones that have corresponding anterior pituitary target-cell types.[6]

Hypothalamic neurohormones are released into a capillary bed of the hypothalamus in an area called the *median eminence*. The hypothalamic hormones travel from the capillary plexus of the median eminence, down the pituitary stalk, in a specialized vascular system called the *hypothalamic-hypophyseal portal vessels*.[6] At the anterior pituitary lobe, the hypothalamic hormones are released in high concentrations into capillary sinuses located among the glandular cells.[6] The hypothalamic hormones then locate and bind to their specific target-cell type.

| TABLE **34-1** | Hypothalamic Hormones and Corresponding Anterior Pituitary Hormones |

Hypothalamic Releasing/ Inhibiting Hormones	Anterior Pituitary Target-Cell Type	Anterior Pituitary Hormone Produced	Hormone Target Site
Thyrotropin-releasing hormone	Thyrotroph	Thyroid-stimulating hormone (TSH, thyrotropin)	Thyroid gland
Corticotropin-releasing hormone	Corticotroph	Adrenocorticotropic hormone (ACTH, corticotropin)	Adrenal gland
Gonadotropin-releasing hormone	Gonadotroph	Follicle-stimulating hormone Luteinizing hormone	Gonads (testes, ovaries)
Prolactin-releasing factor	Lactotroph (mammotroph)	Prolactin	Breasts
Prolactin-inhibitory factor (dopamine, PIF)	Lactotroph		
Growth hormone–releasing hormone	Somatotroph	Growth hormone	All tissues
Growth hormone–inhibitory factor (somatostatin)	Somatotroph	Growth hormone	All tissues

Specific hypothalamic hormones have either an inhibitory or a stimulatory effect on their corresponding anterior pituitary target cells. Synthesis and release of most anterior pituitary hormones depend on a positive stimulatory signal from a given hypothalamic hormone. Some anterior pituitary cells are subject to both inhibitory and stimulatory control by more than one hypothalamic neurohormone.[5]

Synthesis of prolactin from anterior pituitary lactotroph cells is unique in that it is tonically restrained by an inhibitory hormonal signal (dopamine) from the hypothalamus. In essence, dopamine serves as a "physiologic brake" for lactotroph growth and prolactin synthesis. The inhibitory effect of dopamine agonists, such as bromocriptine (Parlodel), is exploited therapeutically for suppressing pathologic production of prolactin from pituitary tumors.[5] Table 34-1 outlines the major hypothalamic releasing or inhibiting hormones and their corresponding anterior pituitary target sites.

Anterior Pituitary Disorders

Hyposecretion. Anterior pituitary hyposecretion may occur when large pituitary tumors (usually chromophobe adenomas) compress and destroy normal anterior pituitary cells. Postpartum shock (Sheehan syndrome), irradiation, trauma, and hypophysectomy are other causes of pituitary hormone deficiency states.[7] Generalized pituitary hypofunction (*panhypopituitarism*) is more common than reduced output of a single anterior pituitary hormone.[8]

Important effects of panhypopituitarism include a decrease in thyroid function due to reduction in levels of TSH, depression of glucocorticoid production by the adrenal cortex due to the lowering of ACTH levels, and suppression of sexual development and reproductive function due to deficient gonadotropic hormone secretion.[6] In addition, large pituitary tumors (macroadenomas >1 cm) may extend into or compress the surrounding brain tissue, producing diplopia, visual loss, facial numbness, facial pain, or (rarely) seizures.

Surgical intervention may be implemented to control bleeding or for decompression or removal of the pituitary tumor. Surgical patients with hypopituitary disorders may require thyroid

hormone replacement and corticosteroid coverage in the perioperative period.[9,10] Because of the possibility of diabetes insipidus after removal of the tumor, vasopressin should also be available.

Most pituitary adenomas are operated on via a transsphenoidal (transnasal) approach, and this route is generally well tolerated by most patients.[9-11] A sublabial transseptal hypophysectomy may be used for very large tumors with suprasellar extension.[9] Serious complications from transsphenoidal pituitary surgery (cerebral spinal fluid [CSF] leak, meningitis, ischemic stroke, visual loss) occur in less than 1.5% of cases.

For transsphenoidal pituitary surgery, the surgeon may request that the patient be placed in a half-sitting position, requiring appropriate monitoring (precordial Doppler, end-tidal CO_2, end-tidal N_2) to detect venous air entrainment. Infrequently, the approach and exposure of the tumor are associated with significant blood loss. The surgeon may use submucosal injection of epinephrine-containing solutions or topical vasoconstrictors to assist in hemostasis. Some surgeons place a lumbar intrathecal catheter to adjust CSF pressure by injecting saline or removing CSF, which assists with visualization of the tumor.[9] An anesthetic technique that incorporates muscle relaxation and allows for smooth extubation and rapid neurologic assessment is desirable. Nitrous oxide should be omitted from the anesthetic plan if air is injected surgically to aid with tumor visualization. Preparing the patient preoperatively for awakening with nasal packing is important.

Hypersecretion. Most pituitary tumors are hypersecreting pituitary adenomas. The three most common hypersecreting pituitary tumors are those that produce prolactin, ACTH, or GH. Tumors that secrete gonadotropin and thyrotropin hormones are rare.

Preparation of the patient awaiting pituitary surgery is guided in part by the results of preoperative endocrine tests. Hypersecreting pituitary tumors may become so large that they compress and destroy normal anterior pituitary cells, producing a deficiency in some anterior pituitary hormones.

Prolactin-secreting tumors commonly produce symptoms of galactorrhea, amenorrhea, and infertility in women and decreased libido and impotence in men. The dopamine agonist bromocriptine is used to control prolactin levels, decrease tumor size, and restore normal gonadal function. Patients who have a suboptimal response to medical therapy benefit from microsurgical removal of the pituitary tumor.[10]

Specific anesthetic management implications for patients with excess ACTH (Cushing disease) and excess GH (acromegaly) are described in this chapter.

Growth Hormone

Growth hormone (somatotropin) is synthesized and secreted by somatotroph cells of the anterior pituitary lobe and is under dual control by the hypothalamus.[6] Growth hormone–releasing hormone stimulates GH release, and growth hormone–inhibiting hormone *(somatostatin)* is a powerful inhibitor of GH release. Pulsatile fluctuations of the hypothalamic releasing and inhibiting hormones regulate somatotroph activity throughout the day.[5]

The GH secretion rate is generally increased in childhood, followed by a further increase in adolescence, a plateau in adulthood, and declining values in old age. In addition, GH secretion is stimulated by stress (including anesthesia and surgery), hypoglycemia, exercise, and deep sleep. GH release is inhibited by hyperglycemia and increased plasma free fatty acids.

Unlike the other anterior pituitary hormones, GH does not exert its principal effects through a specific target gland but functions through all or almost all tissues of the body; it promotes the growth and development of most tissues capable of growing.[6] Skeletal muscle, the heart, skin, and visceral organs undergo hypertrophy and hyperplasia in response to GH.

The most obvious effect of GH is on the skeletal frame. It produces linear bone growth by stimulating the epiphyseal cartilage or growth plate at the ends of long bones.[5,6] Throughout childhood, under the influence of GH, bones elongate at the epiphyseal plate, and the skeletal frame enlarges. After puberty, the growth plates unite with the shaft of the bone, bone lengthening stops, and GH has no further capacity to increase bone length.[6]

GH supports growth by increasing amino acid transport into cells and enhancing protein synthesis in the cell. It also decreases the catabolism of existing proteins by stimulating lipolysis and mobilizing free fatty acids for energy use, a protein-sparing effect.[6]

In addition to its growth-promoting activities, GH is said to be a "diabetogenic hormone." It increases blood glucose levels by decreasing the sensitivity of cells to insulin and inhibiting glucose uptake into cells.[6]

As is true of other anterior pituitary hormones, GH secretion is subject to negative feedback control. Somatomedins (growth factors) and GH itself exert negative feedback control on the hypothalamus and pituitary to inhibit GH secretion.

Hyposecretion. Deficient GH production in childhood can result in insufficient bone maturation and short stature, a condition known as *dwarfism*. Mild obesity, decreased lean body mass, and hypoglycemia are common in GH-deficient dwarfs. Puberty usually is delayed. Symptoms of GH deficiency may be the result of hypothalamic dysfunction, pituitary disease, failure to generate normal somatomedins, or GH-receptor defects.[6]

The biosynthesis of human GH by recombinant DNA techniques has enhanced the outlook for patients with GH deficiency. Treatment of these patients with GH leads to a positive nitrogen balance, accretion of lean body mass, and an improvement in metabolic homeostasis.[2]

Hypersecretion. Hypersecretion of GH, usually caused by a growth hormone–secreting pituitary adenoma (99% of cases), can produce a highly distinctive syndrome in adults

---

BOX **34-1**

Common Features of Acromegaly

Skeletal overgrowth (enlarged hands and feet, prominent prognathic mandible)
Soft-tissue overgrowth (enlarged lips, tongue, and epiglottis; distortion of facial features)
Visceromegaly
Osteoarthritis
Glucose intolerance
Peripheral neuropathy
Skeletal muscle weakness
Extrasellar tumor extension (headache, visual field defects)

---

called *acromegaly*. Acromegaly is produced by sustained hypersecretion of GH after adolescence. The condition occurs with equal frequency in both sexes.[12] If hypersecretion of GH occurs before puberty—that is, before closure of the growth plates—the individual grows very tall (8 to 9 feet), a rare condition known as *gigantism*.

Because growth plates close with adolescence, the excessive production of GH associated with acromegaly does not induce bone lengthening but rather enhances the growth of periosteal bone. Periosteal growth causes new bone to be deposited on the surface of existing bone.[6] The unrestrained bone growth in patients with acromegaly produces bones that are massive in size and thickness. Bones of the hands and feet *(acral)* become particularly large. Overgrowth of vertebrae may cause kyphoscoliosis and arthritis.

Soft-tissue changes are also prominent with GH hypersecretion. The patient develops coarsened facial features *(acromegalic facies)* that include a large, bulbous nose, supraorbital ridge overgrowth, dental malocclusion, and a prominent prognathic mandible.[12,13] The changes in appearance are insidious, and many patients do not seek treatment until the diagnosis is obvious and the disease course advanced.[12,13]

Overgrowth of internal organs is less apparent clinically but no less serious. The liver, heart, spleen, and kidneys become enlarged. Lung volumes increase, which may lead to ventilation-perfusion mismatch. Exercise tolerance may be limited due to increased body mass and skeletal muscle weakness.[12]

Cardiomyopathy, hypertension, and accelerated atherosclerosis in patients with acromegaly can lead to symptomatic cardiac disease (congestive heart failure, arrhythmias).[9,12,14] Echocardiography often shows left ventricular hypertrophy.[8] Resting electrocardiograms are abnormal in 50% of acromegalic patients. ST-segment and T-wave depression, conduction defects, and evidence of prior myocardial infarction may be present.[12]

The insulin-antagonistic effect of GH produces glucose intolerance in up to 50% of patients with acromegaly and frank diabetes mellitus in 10% to 25% of patients.[12]

Clinical manifestations resulting from the local effects of the expanding tumor may include headaches (55%), papilledema, and visual field defects (19%), which are caused by compression of the optic nerves and chiasm. Significant increases in intracranial pressure are uncommon. Compression or destruction of normal pituitary tissue by the tumor may eventually lead to panhypopituitarism.[12,13] Common features of acromegaly are summarized in Box 34-1.

Treatment for acromegaly is aimed at restoring normal GH levels. The preferred initial therapy for active acromegaly is microsurgical removal of the pituitary tumor, with preservation of the gland.[10,14,15] Surgical approach to the pituitary tumor most often is via the transsphenoidal route, with the patient in a semi sitting position.[9] Precautions associated with monitoring for venous air embolism should be part of the anesthesia management plan. Surgical ablation is usually successful in rapidly reducing tumor size, inhibiting GH secretion, and alleviating some symptoms.[16-18] Administration of octreotide (a long-acting somatostatin analog), pegvisomant (a GH-receptor antagonist), and gland irradiation are treatment options for patients who are not surgical candidates.[10,13]

Anesthetic Implications of Acromegaly. Preanesthetic assessment of patients with acromegaly should include a careful examination of the airway. Facial deformities and the large nose may hamper adequate fitting of an anesthesia mask.[15] Endotracheal intubation may be a challenge because of the patient's large and thick tongue (macroglossia), enlargement of the thyroid, obstructive teeth, hypertrophy of the epiglottis, and general soft-tissue overgrowth in the upper airway.[9,11,15] Subglottic narrowing and vocal-cord enlargement may dictate the use of a smaller-diameter endotracheal tube. Nasotracheal intubation should be approached cautiously because of possible turbinate enlargement.[8] Schmitt and colleagues reported intubation difficulties in 20% of the acromegalic patients classified preoperatively as Mallampati class 1 and 2.[16] As many as 70% of patients with acromegaly have a history of sleep apnea due to upper airway obstruction.[9] Preoperative dyspnea, stridor, or hoarseness should alert the anesthetist to airway involvement.[8] Indirect laryngoscopy, CT scan of the neck, and neck radiography may be performed for thorough assessment. If difficulties in maintaining an adequate airway are anticipated, optically guided intubation or fiberoptic-guided intubation in an awake patient is of proven value.[9] The endotracheal tube should remain in place until the patient is fully awake and has total return of reflexes. The predisposition to airway obstruction in these patients makes assiduous perioperative monitoring of the patient's respiratory status an absolute precaution.

The frequent occurrence of cardiac arrhythmias, coronary artery disease, and hypertension in acromegalic patients warrants a thorough preanesthetic cardiac evaluation. The increased risk of diabetes mellitus in these patients mandates careful perioperative monitoring of blood glucose and electrolyte levels.

If preoperative assessment reveals impairment of the adrenal or thyroid axis, stress-level glucocorticoid therapy and thyroid replacement should be implemented in the perioperative period.

Entrapment neuropathies, such as carpal tunnel syndrome, are common in patients with acromegaly. If arterial access is required, an Allen test should be performed before placement of a radial artery catheter; hypertrophy of the carpal ligament may cause inadequate ulnar artery flow. Alternatively, catheterization of other arterial sites should be considered.[8]

Posterior Pituitary Lobe

The posterior pituitary lobe secretes two important peptide hormones: *antidiuretic hormone (vasopressin* or *ADH)* and *oxytocin.* Oxytocin and ADH are structurally very similar, but they have quite different actions. ADH controls water excretion and reabsorption in the kidney and is a major regulator of serum osmolarity. Oxytocin stimulates contraction of myoepithelial cells of the breast for milk ejection during lactation. It also powerfully stimulates uterine smooth muscle contraction.[5]

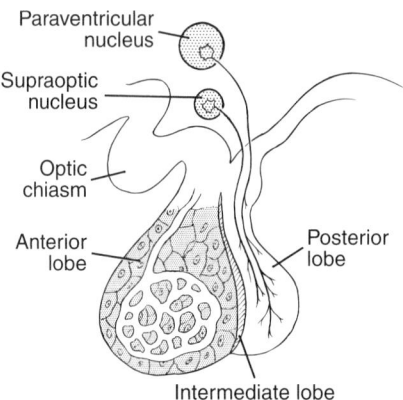

FIGURE **34-3** Nerve fibers arising from the supraoptic nucleus and the paraventricular nucleus transport antidiuretic hormone and oxytocin to the posterior pituitary.

Oxytocin and its derivatives are used clinically for inducing labor and decreasing postpartum bleeding.

In contrast to the anterior pituitary lobe, which communicates with the hypothalamus via a vascular system, the posterior pituitary lobe communicates with the hypothalamus through a neural pathway. Unlike anterior pituitary hormones, posterior pituitary hormones are not synthesized within the pituitary gland itself but rather within two large nuclei of the hypothalamus, the *supraoptic nucleus* and the *paraventricular nucleus.* ADH is chiefly synthesized in the supraoptic nucleus and oxytocin in the paraventricular nucleus.[5] As shown in Figure 34-3, nerve fibers arising from these hypothalamic nuclei transport ADH and oxytocin down the pituitary stalk by axoplasmic flow to the posterior pituitary lobe. There, the hormones are stored in secretory granules at the nerve terminals. With proper excitation, nerve impulses originating in the cell bodies of the supraoptic or paraventricular nucleus are transmitted down the pituitary stalk and stimulate the release of ADH or oxytocin from the posterior pituitary lobe. The hormones then diffuse into nearby blood vessels and are transported to their distant target sites.

Antidiuretic Hormone

ADH is the body's principal preserver of water balance. It acts on renal collecting ducts to increase the absorption of solute-free water from kidney tubules, thereby conserving water in the body and supporting normal body-fluid osmolarity. Without ADH, the collecting ducts are impermeable to water reabsorption; in this setting, water loss in the urine is excessive, and serious dehydration is provoked.[6]

ADH acts primarily to increase urine osmolarity, decrease serum osmolarity, and increase blood volume.[6] Additionally, high levels of ADH cause potent systemic vasoconstriction, especially in coronary, splanchnic, and renal vascular beds. ADH-induced vasoconstriction of splanchnic beds has been exploited therapeutically for the control of hemorrhage caused by esophageal varices. Current advanced cardiac life support protocols recommend vasopressin as an adrenergic alternative to epinephrine for promoting the return of spontaneous circulation after cardiac arrest. ADH also promotes hemostasis by increasing circulating levels of von Willebrand factor and factor VIII. Desmopressin (DDAVP), an arginine analog of ADH, is used to reverse coagulopathy associated with platelet adhesion defects.

Consonant with its role of maintaining normal fluid home-ostasis, ADH is secreted in response to an increase in plasma osmolarity or plasma sodium ion concentration, a decrease in blood volume, or a decrease in blood pressure.

The osmolarity of body fluids is the main variable controlling ADH secretion. Serum osmolarity changes as small as 1% to 2% are sensed by hypothalamic *osmoreceptors*, which in turn alter ADH synthesis and secretion.[5] The plasma *osmotic threshold* for ADH release is about 284 mOsm/L.[5] When the plasma tonicity reaches this level, healthy individuals release ADH into the blood.

The interplay between ADH and water is controlled by a delicate negative feedback loop. Water deprivation (increased plasma osmolarity) initiates signals in the hypothalamic osmo-receptors that cause ADH release from the pituitary gland to increase three- to five-fold. ADH, in turn, enhances renal tubular water reabsorption, dilutes the extracellular fluid, and restores normal osmotic composition.[6] Conversely, water inges-tion (decreased plasma osmolarity) suppresses the osmoreceptor signal for ADH release.

A 5% to 10% decrease in blood volume or blood pressure also provokes ADH release.[5] Changes in blood volume are sensed in peripheral baroreceptors (especially the great veins and pulmonary vessels) and atrial stretch receptors. When these baroreceptors sense underfilling (volume depletion), they transmit afferent signals through vagal and glossopharyngeal nerves to the hypothalamus.[5,17] The hypothalamus responds by increasing ADH synthesis and stimulating ADH release.

The perioperative period is characterized by enhanced ADH secretion. Pain, emotional stress, nausea, hemorrhage, and vari-ous drugs can be potent stimuli to ADH release. Positive-pressure ventilation enhances ADH release by reducing central blood volume.[7] The mild hyponatremia sometimes observed post-operatively may be at least partly explained on the basis of ADH action. Box 34-2 lists drugs that stimulate ADH release or enhance the action of ADH at the renal tubules.[11]

Thirst provides a second line of defense of water balance. It is stimulated when plasma osmolarity reaches the *thirst threshold* (about 285 mOsm/L).[5]

Deficient Antidiuretic Hormone and Anesthetic Impli-cations. Inadequate ADH secretion from the posterior pituitary lobe or the inability of renal collecting duct receptors to respond to ADH (impaired receptor sensitivity) results in a disorder called

---

BOX 34-2

Stimulators of Antidiuretic Hormone Enhancement or Release

Increased plasma sodium ion concentration
Increased serum osmolarity
Decreased blood volume
Decreased blood pressure
Pain
Stress
Nausea
Various medications (chlorpropamide, clofibrate, thiazide diuretics, carbamazepine, nicotine, cyclophosphamide, vincristine)
Angiotensin II
Positive-pressure ventilation

---

diabetes insipidus (DI). The former disorder is termed *neurogenic DI*, and the latter is called *nephrogenic DI.*

Common causes of neurogenic DI include severe head trauma, neurosurgical procedures (trauma to the median eminence, pitu-itary surgery), infiltrating pituitary lesions, and brain tumors.[5,7,17] Neurogenic DI that develops after pituitary surgery is usually transient and often resolves in 5 to 7 days.[9,11]

Nephrogenic DI may occur in association with an X-linked genetic mutation, hypercalcemia, hypokalemia, and medication-induced nephrotoxicity.[17] Ethanol, demeclocycline, phenytoin, chlorpromazine, and lithium all inhibit the action of ADH or its release.

The hallmark of DI is polyuria. The inability to produce a concentrated urine results in dehydration and hypernatremia. The syndrome is characterized by a urine osmolarity less than 300 mOsm/L, urine specific gravity less than 1.010, and urine volumes greater than 30 mL/kg each day. The tremendous urinary water loss produces serum osmolarities greater than 290 mOsm/L and serum sodium concentrations greater than 145 mEq/L. Neurologic symptoms of hypernatremia and neuronal dehydra-tion may be present and include hyperreflexia, weakness, lethargy, seizures, and coma.[17]

The thirst mechanism assumes a primary role in maintaining water balance in awake patients with DI. Ingestion of large volumes of water prevents serious hyperosmolarity and life-threatening dehydration.[11]

Treatment protocols for DI depend on the degree of ADH deficiency. Most patients have incomplete DI and retain some capacity to concentrate their urine and conserve water. Mild cases (incomplete DI) may be treated with medications that either augment the release of ADH or increase the receptor response to ADH. These drugs may include chlorpropamide (sulfonylurea hypoglycemic agent), carbamazepine (anticonvul-sant), and clofibrate (hypolipidemic agent).[14]

Significant deficiency (plasma osmolarity levels >290 mOsm/L) may be treated with various ADH preparations. Aqueous vasopressin is commonly used for short-term therapy and desmo-pressin is useful for long-term control.[11] Caution is advised when administering these drugs to patients with coronary artery dis-ease or hypertension because of the arterial constrictive action of ADH.[7,17] Desmopressin (5 to 10 mcg/day intranasally or 0.5 to 1 mcg twice daily subcutaneously) is often a preferred agent because it has less pressor activity, a prolonged duration of action (6 to 24 hours), and enhanced antidiuretic properties.[19]

Perioperative administration of vasopressin is usually not nec-essary in the patient with partial DI, because the stress of surgery causes enhanced ADH release.[11] The surgical patient with a total lack of ADH (complete DI) may be managed with desmopressin (1 mcg subcutaneously) or aqueous vasopressin (an intravenous bolus of 0.1 unit, followed by a continuous intravenous infusion of vasopressin at 0.1 to 0.2 unit/hr).[7,11] Plasma osmolarity, urine output, and serum sodium concentration should be measured hourly during surgery and in the immediate postoperative period. The surgical patient with DI receiving ADH replacement therapy should be monitored for ECG changes indicative of myo-cardial ischemia.

Isotonic fluids can generally be administered safely during the intraoperative period. If, however, the plasma osmolarity rises above 290 mOsm/L, hypotonic fluids should be considered and the vasopressin infusion increased above 0.2 unit/hr.[11]

Preoperative assessment of the patient with DI includes care-ful appraisal of plasma electrolytes (especially serum sodium), renal function, and plasma osmolarity. Dehydration will make these patients especially sensitive to the hypotensive effects of anesthesia agents. Intravascular volume should slowly be restored preoperatively over a period of at least 24 to 48 hours.

Hypersecretion of Antidiuretic Hormone and Anesthetic Implications. The *syndrome of inappropriate antidiuretic hormone (SIADH)* secretion is a disorder characterized by a high circulating vasopressin level relative to plasma osmolarity and serum sodium concentration. With SIADH, the kidneys, under ADH stimulation, continue to reabsorb water from the renal tubules despite the presence of hyponatremia and plasma hypotonicity.[11] Hormone-induced water reabsorption causes expansion of intracellular and extracellular fluid volumes, hemodilution, and weight gain. The urine is hypertonic relative to the plasma, and urine output is typically low.[7] An assay of high ADH levels in the blood confirms the diagnosis of SIADH. Table 34-2 compares SIADH and DI.

Clinical features of SIADH reflect water intoxication, dilutional hyponatremia, and resulting brain edema. The swelling of brain cells may cause lethargy, headache, nausea, and mental confusion, especially if the plasma osmolarity declines below 250 mOsm/L or the serum sodium concentration falls below 125 mEq/L.[18] Symptoms may progress to seizures and coma, particularly if the hyponatremia is severe and of rapid onset. Hypertension and peripheral edema are not common. Surgical patients may exhibit delayed awakening from anesthesia.[11]

Inappropriate hypersecretion of ADH can result from various pathologic processes, including hypothyroidism, pulmonary neoplasia, head trauma or infection, intracranial tumors, and following pituitary surgery.[7,8] Secretion of ADH by neoplasms, especially small-cell carcinomas of the lung, is a common cause of SIADH.[11] The ectopic ADH produced by these tumors is identical to the ADH of hypothalamic origin. Certain drugs are associated with enhanced ADH secretion or response; these include carbamazepine, tricyclic antidepressants, chlorpropamide, cyclophosphamide, nicotine, and clofibrate.[17].

The patient with mild SIADH not associated with symptoms of hyponatremia is often managed effectively with fluid restriction.[9] Rarely, surgical patients with profound hyponatremia (plasma Na⁺ <120 mEq/L) and acute neurologic symptoms may require more aggressive treatment with a slow intravenous infusion (rate ≤0.05 mL/kg/min) of hypertonic (3%) saline.[7,17,18] To prevent acute loss of brain water and possible permanent neurologic damage (*Central pontine demyelination syndrome*), the plasma sodium concentration must be corrected slowly —not greater than 0.5 to 1.0 mEq/L/hour or 6 to 8 mEq/L per day.[8,19,20] The infusion should be stopped as soon as the serum sodium increases to 130 mEq/L.

Demeclocycline, a tetracycline antibiotic, has been used to treat chronic SIADH by antagonizing the effects of vasopressin on the renal tubules.[11,18] Definitive treatment for SIADH is directed at the underlying disorder.

Stress and surgery may initiate or potentiate an inappropriate release of ADH. Clinical assessment of the patient's volume status is an essential part of the preoperative evaluation. Perioperative fluid management of the surgical patient with SIADH can usually be accomplished with fluid restriction that involves the use of isotonic solutions.[11] Estimating central volume status on the basis of central venous pressure or pulmonary artery catheter measurements can help guide fluid replacement. Frequent determinations of urine output, urine osmolarity, plasma osmolarity, and serum sodium concentrations can also help direct fluid management. Nausea should be prevented; it is a potent stimulus of ADH release.

PARATHYROID GLAND

The parathyroid glands are small (approximately 3 × 6 × 2 mm) oval bodies located on the posterior surface of the thyroid gland (Figure 34-4). Most individuals have four parathyroid glands, one on each pole of the thyroid, but approximately 6% of individuals have five glands and 13% have only three. Blood supply to the parathyroid glands is via the inferior thyroid arteries.

Calcium Regulation

The adult human body contains about 1 to 2 kg of the divalent cation calcium. Approximately 99% of the calcium exists in the bony skeleton, and about 1% is in the extracellular space and soft tissues.[7,21] Intracellular calcium is 10,000 times lower than ionized calcium concentration in the extracellular fluid.[7,22,23]

The concentration of the total serum calcium is tightly regulated within a range of 8.6 to 10.6 mg/dL (4.3 to 5.3 mEq/L).[22] Serum calcium exists in three different forms (Figure 34-5):
1. Approximately 10% exists in a nonionized, chelated form. This calcium is bound to diffusible anions such as citrate, bicarbonate, and phosphate.
2. Approximately 40% is combined with plasma proteins (primarily albumin) in a nonionized, nondiffusible complex.
3. Approximately 50% exists in an ionized and diffusible form (normal level 4.7 to 5.2 mg/dL).

TABLE **34-2**	Syndrome of Inappropriate Antidiuretic Hormone and Diabetes Insipidus	
	SIADH	**DI**
Serum osmolarity	<270 mOsm/L	>290 mOsm/L
Serum sodium	<130 mEq/L	>145 mEq/L
Urine volume	Low	High (4 to 8 L/day)
Urine osmolarity	High relative to plasma	Low relative to plasma
Treatment	Fluid restriction If serum Na⁺ <120 mEq/L, consider hypertonic saline	DDAVP or vasopressin

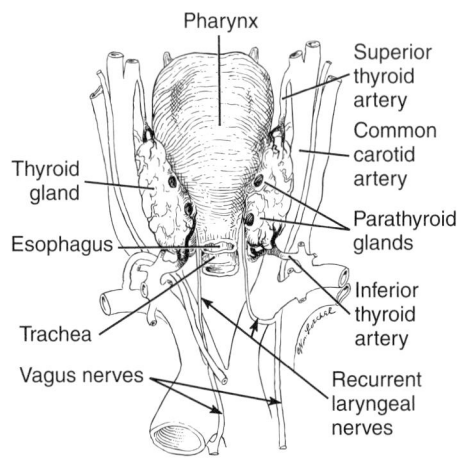

FIGURE **34-4** The four parathyroid glands are located on the posterior poles of the thyroid gland.

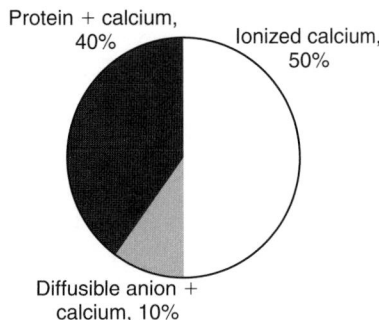

FIGURE **34-5** Serum calcium exists in three different forms: ionized, bound to serum proteins, and bound to diffusible anions. Only the ionized form of calcium exerts physiologic effects.

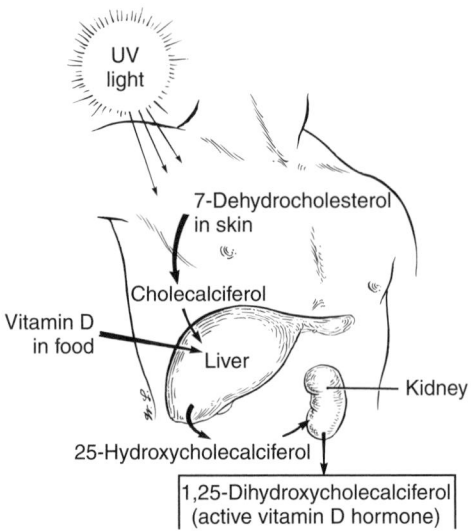

FIGURE **34-6** Conversion of cholecalciferol or vitamin D to an active form (1,25-dihydroxycholecalciferol) involves hydroxylation in the liver and kidneys. Active vitamin D is important in transporting calcium across the gastrointestinal tract. UV, Ultraviolet.

Only the free, ionized form of calcium exerts physiologic effects, hence measurement of serum ionized calcium levels provides the most clinically relevant determination.[7,21,22] Ionized calcium performs a wide range of vital physiologic functions, including hemostasis (platelet aggregation, blood coagulation), muscle contraction, neurotransmission, bone formation, cell division, and many other aspects of cell function.[21]

Total blood calcium levels may not always reflect the ionized calcium status. Changes in serum protein levels can alter total blood calcium levels without altering ionized calcium values. Changes in total calcium levels parallel the serum albumin.[22] A decrease in serum albumin of 1 g/dL, for instance, causes an associated decrease in total serum calcium of about 0.8 mg/dL.[7]

Alterations in the pH of blood affect ionized calcium levels. Plasma proteins are more ionized in an alkaline pH, providing an increase in the number of anion binding sites for the positively charged calcium. Alkalosis decreases ionized serum calcium by increasing protein-calcium binding. Acidosis, on the other hand, increases ionized serum calcium by decreasing calcium-protein binding.[22,23]

Two principal hormones, vitamin D and parathyroid hormone (PTH), operate in concert to regulate the plasma concentration of calcium. Both vitamin D and PTH raise serum calcium levels, but of the two, PTH has by far the strongest effect.

Vitamin D

Vitamin D compounds ingested from food or formed by the action of ultraviolet light on the skin are inactive prohormones.[22] Inactive vitamin D, called *cholecalciferol*, is converted by a series of reactions in the liver and kidneys to an active metabolite. The final step in the conversion of vitamin D to an active form is controlled in the kidneys by PTH. The in vivo conversion of inactive vitamin D to the final active product, *1,25-dihydroxycholecalciferol*, is shown in Figure 34-6.

Active vitamin D increases plasma calcium, magnesium, and phosphate ion concentrations by promoting their absorption across the intestinal epithelium to the extracellular fluid.

Inadequate vitamin D intake or absorption, or insufficient exposure to sunlight, can lead to poor intestinal absorption of calcium. In children, the resulting calcium deficiency leads to a defective mineralization of bone, a condition known as *rickets*.[21,22] In adults, vitamin D deficiency results in impaired bone mineralization, a condition known as *osteomalacia*.[23]

Parathyroid Hormone

PTH is secreted from *chief cells* of the parathyroid gland in response to low serum ionized calcium concentrations. Hyperphosphatemia (indirect effect) and acute hypomagnesemia also stimulate PTH secretion.[7,23]

PTH is the body's major hormonal regulator of calcium and phosphate metabolism. In PTH, the body possesses an extremely potent negative feedback agent for controlling serum calcium levels. In general, PTH increases the extracellular calcium concentration and decreases the extracellular phosphate concentration. A small decline in the level of circulating ionized calcium produces a rapid increase in PTH secretion from the parathyroid glands. A sustained deficit in serum calcium levels (lactation, pregnancy) produces hypertrophy of the parathyroid glands, sometimes five-fold or greater, in order to maintain adequate PTH output.[21,23]

An elevation in serum calcium ion concentration produces an abrupt decline in PTH synthesis and output. Conditions associated with chronic elevations of serum calcium (immobility, malignancy, Paget disease) provoke a blunted PTH output and a diminution in gland size. In contrast to *acute* magnesium deficiency, parathyroid gland function and PTH secretion are inhibited by severe and *chronic* hypomagnesemia.[23]

The increase in serum calcium level and the decline in serum phosphate level in response to PTH secretion are the result of the hormone's effect on bone, the kidney, and the intestinal tract.

Effect on Bone. Bone is a living tissue that is constantly being remodeled.[22] In the healthy adult, bone-forming cells called *osteoblasts* are balanced by bone-destroying cells called *osteoclasts*.[21] Exchangeable calcium in bone serves as a large, rapid buffer that plays a vital role in extracellular fluid calcium homeostasis. In addition to calcium, bone also provides an important reservoir for other ions such as magnesium and phosphorus.[23]

When ionized serum calcium levels decline, PTH is released and acts directly on bone to mobilize skeletal calcium stores.[22] PTH promotes the activation and proliferation of osteoclasts, stimulating rapid absorption of calcium (and phosphate) from bone tissue to the extracellular fluid. Over time, abnormally high levels of circulating PTH can produce extensive absorption of calcium from the bone matrix.[21]

The reservoir of calcium in bone is about 1000 times greater than the amount of calcium in the extracellular fluid. Only after sustained PTH activation, therefore, does bone erosion and destruction become apparent. With protracted PTH stimulation, however, the bones eventually become severely depleted of calcium.[21]

An increase in extracellular fluid calcium causes PTH levels to decline. Decreased PTH levels stimulate rapid deposition of calcium and phosphate bone salts, an effect that lowers serum calcium levels back to normal.

Effect on the Intestinal Tract. Parathyroid hormone indirectly enhances both calcium and phosphate absorption from the intestines by promoting formation of 1,25-dihydroxycholecalciferol, the active form of vitamin D. When the plasma calcium level is low, PTH stimulates 1α-hydroxylase, an enzyme in the kidney necessary for the formation of 1,25-dihydroxycholecalciferol. Active vitamin D in turn increases intestinal absorption of calcium and phosphate.[22]

In the absence of PTH, or in the presence of severe kidney disease, 1,25-dihydroxycholecalciferol is not formed, and vitamin D's effect on calcium and phosphate regulation is lost. Patients with chronic renal failure often suffer from hypocalcemia, in part because the diseased kidneys lose their ability to form active vitamin D. Consequently, these patients are unable to absorb a sufficient amount of calcium from the gastrointestinal tract.

Effect on the Kidney. PTH has two major effects on the kidney: it increases calcium reabsorption, and it increases phosphate excretion. PTH elevates serum calcium by augmenting the reabsorption of calcium from nephron tubules to the extracellular fluid. The major site of PTH-mediated calcium reabsorption is the distal convoluted tubule.[21]

Accompanying calcium reabsorption is enhanced phosphate excretion. PTH promotes phosphaturia by reducing phosphate ion reabsorption from the proximal convoluted tubule. The PTH-mediated phosphate loss from the kidney is generally strong enough to overcome the PTH-induced phosphate absorption from bone and intestines.[21]

Calcitonin
Calcitonin is a hormone secreted from the thyroid *parafollicular cells*, or *C cells*, in response to elevated serum ionized calcium.[22] It has an effect opposite that of the PTH system, lowering the serum ionized calcium concentration. Calcium levels are reduced by a calcitonin-mediated inhibition of bone osteoclasts, which shifts the balance toward osteoblasts and bone deposition.[22]

The serum calcium–lowering effect of calcitonin is weak. Its effect in lowering serum calcium is rapidly outweighed by the more powerful activity of PTH.[21] The rather weak effect of calcitonin is demonstrated by the observation that removal of the thyroid gland causes no significant alterations in bone density or long-term serum calcium levels.[21,22]

Parathyroid Gland Dysfunction
Hypoparathyroidism
Hypoparathyroidism is a disorder characterized by inadequate secretion of PTH or a peripheral resistance to its effect.[8] Patients with hypoparathyroidism typically have low serum calcium levels. The blood phosphate concentration may be elevated because of the decreased renal excretion of phosphate.

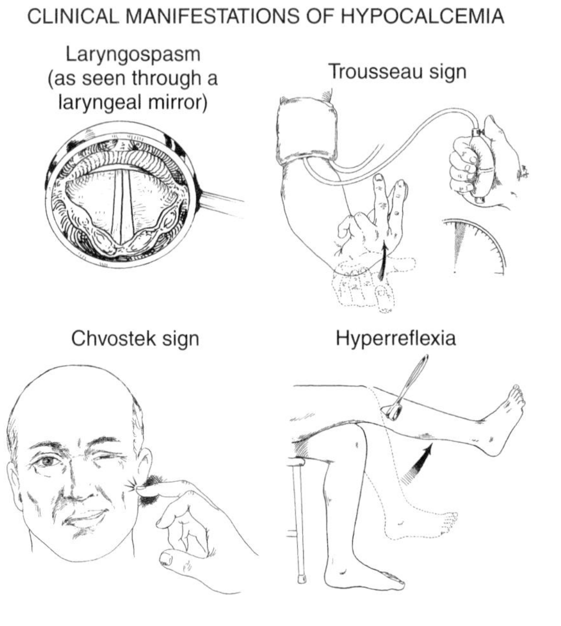

CLINICAL MANIFESTATIONS OF HYPOCALCEMIA

FIGURE **34-7** Hypocalcemia produces hyperexcitability of nerve and muscle cells. Chvostek sign and Trousseau sign are two classic manifestations of hypocalcemic tetany. Deep tendon reflexes may be hyperactive. Laryngeal muscles are sensitive to tetanic spasm.

Inadvertent removal of parathyroid tissue, parathyroid gland injury from irradiation or autoimmune destruction, and chronic severe magnesium deficiency (alcohol abuse, poor nutrition, malabsorption) are possible causes of hypoparathyroidism. Clinical signs of hypoparathyroidism reflect the degree of hypocalcemia and the rapidity of calcium decline. A sudden drop in ionized calcium usually produces more severe symptoms than a slow decline.[23] Treatment of chronic hypoparathyroidism includes vitamin D and calcium supplementation.

The decreased serum calcium ion concentration accompanying hypoparathyroidism produces hyperexcitability of nerve and muscle cells by lowering the threshold potential of excitable membranes. Cardinal features of neuromuscular excitability are muscle spasms and hypocalcemic tetany. Symptoms vary in severity and may take the form of muscle cramps, perioral paresthesias, numbness in the feet and toes, or hyperactive deep tendon reflexes. The patient may feel restless or hyperirritable. Life-threatening laryngeal muscle spasm may occur, producing stridor, labored respirations, and asphyxia.[23-26]

Two classic manifestations of latent hypocalcemic tetany are *Chvostek sign* and *Trousseau sign*. Chvostek sign is a contracture or twitching of ipsilateral facial muscles produced when the facial nerve is tapped at the angle of the jaw. Trousseau sign is elicited by the inflation of a blood pressure cuff slightly above the systolic level for a few minutes. The resultant ischemia enhances muscle irritability in hypocalcemic states and causes flexion of the wrist and thumb with extension of the fingers (*carpopedal spasm*).[23] Figure 34-7 illustrates some of the clinical manifestations of hypoparathyroidism and hypocalcemia.

Anesthesia Implications for Hypoparathyroidism. Temporary hypocalcemia often is observed after successful parathyroid surgery for hyperparathyroidism. This may occur within a few hours to a few days after surgery. The transient postoperative hypocalcemia is the result of parathyroid gland suppression (by preoperative hypercalcemia) and rapid bone uptake of calcium ("hungry bone syndrome").[23] Inadvertent removal of all parathyroid gland tissue induces a substantial decline in serum calcium concentration from normal levels (8.6 to 10.6 mg/dL) to 6 to 7 mg/dL. Even a small amount of remaining parathyroid tissue usually is capable of sufficient hypertrophy to preserve normal calcium-phosphate balance.[21]

Following parathyroid surgery, meticulous observation for signs of musculoskeletal irritability, as well as serial measurement of serum calcium, inorganic phosphate, magnesium, and PTH levels should be performed. The threshold for the development of signs of hypocalcemia is variable; however, manifestations of neuromuscular compromise often are observed at serum calcium levels of 6 to 7 mg/dL.[21]

Laryngeal muscles are especially sensitive to tetanic spasm, and laryngospasm may cause life-threatening airway compromise in the hypocalcemic patient.[21] Respiratory distress following parathyroid surgery may be secondary to laryngeal muscle spasm, edema or bleeding in the neck, or bilateral recurrent laryngeal nerve injury. Unilateral recurrent laryngeal nerve injury produces hoarseness and usually requires only close observation. Bilateral recurrent laryngeal nerve injury causes aphonia and requires immediate airway support and intubation.[11]

Hypocalcemia may be apparent on electrocardiographic tracings as a prolonged QT interval, reflecting delayed ventricular repolarization.[8] The cardiac rhythm usually remains normal. Decreased cardiac contractility and hypotension may occur, and congestive heart failure (although rare) is a danger.[23,26]

In addition to parathyroid surgery, circulating levels of ionized calcium can decline from other causes in the perioperative period. Precipitous increases in circulating levels of anions such as bicarbonate, phosphate, and citrate lower ionized calcium levels.[23] Hyperventilation, the rapid transfusion of citrated blood, or the rapid administration of bicarbonate may induce overt tetany in a previously asymptomatic hypocalcemic patient. Vigorous diuresis can also augment calcium loss.

Patients with confirmed symptomatic hypocalcemia require prompt therapy.[23,25] Acute hypocalcemia may be treated with an initial intravenous bolus of 10 to 20 mL of 10% calcium gluconate administered over 10 minutes, followed by 10 mL of 10% calcium gluconate in 500 mL solution over 6 hours.[11,23] Calcium, magnesium, phosphate, potassium, and creatinine levels should be monitored diligently during calcium replacement.[7] Chronic magnesium deficiency impairs the secretion of PTH and should be corrected.[22]

Hyperparathyroidism

Primary hyperparathyroidism is characterized and diagnosed by the presence of elevated serum PTH levels despite high serum calcium levels. It may result from a parathyroid adenoma, gland hyperplasia, or parathyroid cancer.[27] In approximately 80% of cases, primary hyperparathyroidism is caused by hypersecretion of a single parathyroid adenoma.[23,26,28] Hyperplasia of one or more parathyroid glands accounts for about 15% of cases. Carcinoma of the parathyroid gland is found in less than 1% of patients and is associated with particularly high serum calcium levels.[8,27,28] Hereditary hyperparathyroidism may exist as part of a multiple endocrine neoplastic syndrome (MEN-1, MEN-2A).[23]

The incidence of primary hyperparathyroidism in the United States is approximately 0.1% to 0.5%, with a higher occurrence in females and the elderly.[2] Stimulation of the parathyroid gland during pregnancy or lactation, prior neck irradiation, and a family history of parathyroid disease are predisposing etiologic factors.[27]

Sustained overactivity of the parathyroid glands is characterized by high serum calcium levels. Most patients remain asymptomatic until the total serum calcium level rises above 11.5 to 12 mg/dL.[7,29] Severe hypercalcemia (>14 to 16 mg/dL) may be life threatening and demands immediate attention.[7,26]

With the development of sensitive laboratory assays for calcium, today more than half of patients with hyperparathyroidism are asymptomatic at diagnosis. Over time, sustained high levels of PTH lead to exaggerated osteoclast activity in bone, resulting in diffuse osteopenia, subperiosteal erosions, and elevated extracellular calcium levels. As osteoblasts attempt to reconstruct the ravaged bone, they secrete large amounts of the enzyme *alkaline phosphatase*.[22] A heightened serum alkaline phosphatase level, therefore, is a significant diagnostic feature of hyperparathyroidism.[28] Despite an increased mobilization of phosphorus from bone, serum phosphate concentration usually remains normal or low as a result of increased urinary excretion.

The effect of hyperparathyroidism on bone becomes clinically apparent when osteoclastic absorption of bone overwhelms osteoblastic deposition. With severe and protracted disease, the weakened bones become filled with decalcified cavities, making them painful and susceptible to fracture. Owing to early diagnosis, the destructive bone disease associated with hyperparathyroidism, *osteitis fibrosa cystica*, is rare today.

Many of the nonskeletal manifestations of primary hyperparathyroidism are related to the accompanying hypercalcemia.[28] Sustained hypercalcemia may produce calcifications and other deleterious effects in the pancreas (pancreatitis), kidney (nephrolithiasis, nephrocalcinosis, polyuria), blood vessels (hypertension), heart (shortened ventricular refractory period, bradyarrhythmias, bundle branch block, heart block), and acid-producing areas of the stomach (peptic ulcer).[26,28] The mnemonic "stones, bones, and groans" summarizes renal, skeletal, and gastrointestinal features of advanced hyperparathyroidism. Profound muscle weakness, confusion, nausea, vomiting, and lethargy are additional features of the disorder. Figure 34-8 illustrates some of the clinical manifestations of hyperparathyroidism.

Secondary hyperparathyroidism develops in patients with chronically low levels of serum calcium, such as those with chronic renal failure and gastrointestinal malabsorption. A compensatory parathyroid response develops in response to the hypocalcemia. Their clinical course is marked by the same PTH-mediated skeletal assault seen in the primary form of the disorder, but because it is an adaptive response, secondary hyperparathyroidism is seldom associated with hypercalcemia.[26] Table 34-3 compares common clinical manifestations of hyperparathyroidism and hypoparathyroidism.

Anesthesia Implications for Hyperparathyroidism. The usual treatment for symptomatic primary hyperparathyroidism is surgical removal of abnormal parathyroid tissue. Surgical treatment for asymptomatic hyperparathyroidism is more controversial.[7] Parathyroidectomy may be performed with the patient under general anesthesia, but minimally invasive neck surgery using cervical plexus block anesthesia is increasingly used, especially for excision of a single adenoma.[29]

Parathyroid tissue resembles brown fat, and this can occasionally make it difficult for the surgeon to locate. Further, parathyroid tissue is sometimes footloose and can be found in such ectopic places as the deep recesses of the mediastinum, the carotid sheath, or the thymus gland.[22,23,30] Some surgeons use periodic intraoperative determinations of serum PTH and ionized calcium levels to help guide surgical resection.

Blood loss from parathyroid surgery is usually minimal, and advanced monitoring is not required based on the surgical procedure. Serum calcium, magnesium, and phosphorus levels should be monitored in the postoperative period until stable. In most cases, serum calcium levels start to decline within 24 hours and return to normal within 3 to 4 days after successful surgery.[7,8]

With current methods of detection, most patients with hyperparathyroidism are asymptomatic; however, erosive effects of elevated PTH on bone and the systemic effects of chronic hypercalcemia should be considered in the anesthetic plan for patients with severe untreated disease.

Severe or symptomatic hypercalcemia (>14 to 16 mg/dL) is treated aggressively. Isotonic saline hydration and loop diuretics (Lasix, 40 to 80 mg) can rapidly decrease serum calcium levels by hemodilution, increased glomerular filtration, and enhanced excretion.[8,11,26] Less frequently, corticosteroids or drugs that inhibit osteoclastic bone resorption (bisphosphonates, pamidronate, plicamycin, calcitonin) are used.[11,26,31]

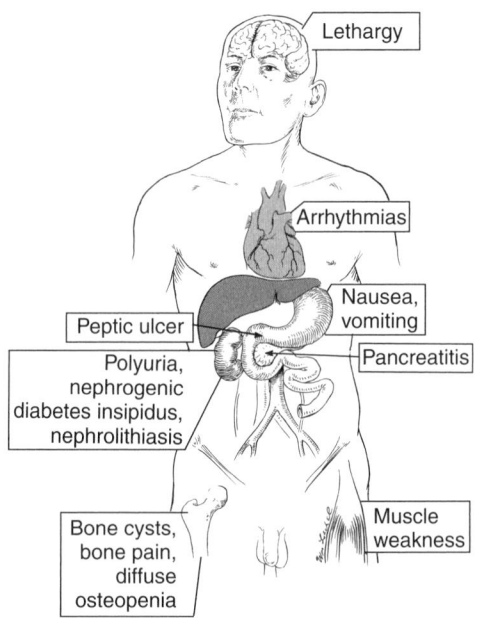

FIGURE **34-8** The patient with hyperparathyroidism exhibits manifestations of hypercalcemia. With severe, protracted disease, skeletal destruction becomes evident.

The hypercalcemic patient may be dehydrated because of anorexia, vomiting, and the impaired ability of the kidneys to concentrate urine.[31] In these patients, hydration with non–calcium-containing solutions should be maintained throughout the perioperative period to dilute serum calcium, maintain adequate glomerular filtration and calcium clearance, and ensure adequate intravascular volume. Vigorous hydration dictates the use of bladder catheterization, central venous pressure monitoring, and frequent determinations of serum electrolytes.[7]

Elevated calcium levels may depress the central and peripheral nervous systems.[21,24] The use of preoperative sedatives in the hypercalcemic patient who appears lethargic or confused should be avoided. General anesthetic requirements may be decreased as well.[8]

Careful review of the patient's renal status is especially crucial in patients with secondary hyperparathyroidism. Associated complications of renal impairment (volume overload, anemia, electrolyte derangements) may affect anesthetic medication dosages and selection.[24,32]

Cardiac conduction disturbances such as a shortened QT interval and a prolonged PR interval are observed with hypercalcemia.[8] Dysrhythmias and hypertension may respond to calcium channel antagonists (e.g., verapamil, 5 to 10 mg IV).

Awareness of the effects of pH on the ionized portion of plasma calcium is important. Alkalosis shifts ionized calcium to the protein-bound form and decreases serum levels.

The response to neuromuscular blockade may be unpredictable.[8,24] Muscle weakness, hypotonia, and muscle atrophy may increase the patient's sensitivity to nondepolarizing skeletal muscle relaxants. Careful titration of muscle relaxants with use of a peripheral nerve stimulator is prudent.[8]

Patients with clinically significant bone disease are susceptible to fractures, and care must be exercised in positioning and padding.[7]

Hyperparathyroid patients are prone to postoperative nausea and vomiting.[33] Prophylactic antiemetic medications are advisable.

PANCREAS

The *pancreas* is a flattened, elongated, retroperitoneal organ that has both exocrine and endocrine functions. *Acinar cells*, which make up the exocrine portion of the pancreas, account for about 98% of the gland's weight. Digestive enzymes and bicarbonate are synthesized in acinar cells and secreted into the pancreatic ducts to aid the digestive process.

TABLE **34-3**	Clinical Features of Hyperparathyroidism and Hypoparathyroidism	
System	**Hyperparathyroidism**	**Hypoparathyroidism**
Cardiovascular	Hypertension, cardiac conduction disturbances, shortened QT interval	Prolonged QT interval, hypotension, decreased cardiac contractility
Musculoskeletal	Bone pain, pathologic fractures, muscle weakness, muscle atrophy	Neuromuscular excitability
Neurologic	Somnolence, cognitive impairment, depression, hypotonia	Tetany, paresthesias, numbness in fingers and toes, seizures
Gastrointestinal	Anorexia, nausea, vomiting, constipation, abdominal pain, pancreatitis, peptic ulcer	None significant
Renal	Tubular absorption defects, diminished renal function, kidney stones, polyuria	None significant

Islets of Langerhans

The *islets of Langerhans,* which make up 1% to 2% of the pancreas's weight, constitute the endocrine pancreas. The islets are microscopic collections of cells scattered throughout the gland. They produce hormones that do not enter ducts but rather are secreted directly into capillary blood vessels. Each islet cell has an abundant blood supply. Venous blood from the islets drains into the hepatic portal vein and then into the general circulation.[34]

At least four distinct cell types are found in the islets of Langerhans, identified as α (alpha), β (beta), δ (delta), and PP (pancreatic polypeptide) cells. Each cell type secretes a different peptide hormone. The *β cells* account for 60% to 70% of the islet mass and secrete the hormone *insulin.* The *α cells* constitute about 25% of the islet cells and secrete the hormone *glucagon.* The *δ cells* represent about 10% of total cells and secrete the hormone *somatostatin.*[35]

Insulin and glucagon are crucial in regulating carbohydrate, fat, and protein metabolism. Their secretion is part of a hormonal regulatory system that accommodates repeated periods of feast and fasting throughout the day. Somatostatin may play a role in regulating gastrointestinal function by restraining the rate at which nutrients are digested and absorbed.[35] Somatostatin also is distributed throughout the central nervous system and, as noted earlier in this chapter, is a hypothalamic inhibitor of anterior pituitary GH release. Pancreatic peptide inhibits exocrine pancreatic secretion.

Energy Balance

Glucose is the body's most abundant circulating fuel. The breakdown of glucose into simpler compounds releases energy the body uses for cellular metabolism. The energy-yielding breakdown of glucose to pyruvate or lactate is called *glycolysis* or the *Embden-Meyerhof pathway.*

Despite daily fluctuations between feeding and fasting states, plasma glucose concentration is maintained within an amazingly narrow range. This is accomplished by the counterbalancing effect of multiple hormones that control the storage of glucose and other nutrient fuels after meals and regulate fuel mobilization between meals. In most healthy individuals, the liver stores enough glycogen to maintain a normal plasma glucose during 8 to 12 hours of fasting.[36] An overnight fast usually lowers the blood glucose to 80 to 90 mg/dL. The blood glucose concentration increases briefly to 120 to 140 mg/dL after a meal before returning to control levels.[35] In a person with impaired glucose tolerance, the fasting plasma glucose (FPG) level is above 100 mg/dL, and in the diabetic patient, the FPG is equal to or greater than 126 mg/dL.[35,37]

Certain metabolic processes ensure the efficient storage of nutrients so they can be available for later use. *Glycogenesis,* or the storage of glucose as glycogen, occurs primarily in the liver and muscle. *Lipogenesis,* which represents the formation and storage of fat as triglycerides, occurs primarily in adipose tissue.

Other metabolic processes work in the opposite direction, providing adequate energy sources during times of fasting. *Gluconeogenesis* is the formation of glucose from lactate, pyruvate, amino acids, and glycerol; it is an important hepatic glucose production mechanism during fasting and starvation. *Glycogenolysis,* the breakdown of glycogen into glucose, occurs primarily in the liver. *Lipolysis,* the breakdown of stored triglycerides to free fatty acids and glycerol, is stimulated by the enzyme *hormone-sensitive lipase.*

The rates of glycogenesis, lipogenesis, gluconeogenesis, glycogenolysis, and lipolysis are determined largely by the actions of insulin and the opposing actions of so-called "counterregulatory hormones" (GH, cortisol, epinephrine, and glucagon). Insulin plays an important role as an *anabolic hormone.* It promotes growth and the constructive phase of metabolism. The potent anabolic effects of insulin are balanced by the opposing *catabolic actions* of the counterregulatory hormones. These hormones mobilize fuel substrates from protein, carbohydrate, and fat stores to meet the energy demands of various tissues.[34]

The "push and pull" effect of these two hormone systems helps maintain normal glucose concentrations in the healthy individual. In diabetes, when insulin concentrations are low or absent, the unopposed counterregulatory hormones begin to exert more prominent metabolic effects.

Obligate Versus Facultative Tissue

Different tissues have different glucose requirements, and some tissues are able to adapt to alternative sources of fuel when glucose is scarce. Muscle and most other tissues in the body are said to be *facultative* glucose organs. They use glucose for energy when it is available, but they can also shift to alternative sources of fuel (amino acids or fat) in the absence of glucose.

The brain is unique in that it is one of the few organs that uses only glucose for energy. It is said to be an *obligate* glucose organ.[35] Erythrocytes and the adrenal medulla also depend on glucose as their sole source of energy. Unlike most other tissues, such as muscle, obligate glucose organs cannot immediately switch to alternative fuels when glucose levels fall. The brain's absolute, uninterrupted requirement for glucose dictates that the blood glucose concentration be maintained above a critical level. The central nervous system accounts for about 70% of total body glucose utilization, and normal cerebral function requires the delivery of about 125 to 150 g of glucose per day. During prolonged starvation, ketone bodies can substitute for glucose as cerebral fuel.

Insulin

Of the hormones secreted from the islet cells, insulin is of greatest physiologic importance. In 1922, Banting and Best first isolated this critical hormone from the pancreas in its pure form. The clinical importance of this event is demonstrated by insulin's history of lifesaving effects in diabetes mellitus (DM), a previously uniformly fatal disease.

Insulin was the first mammalian peptide hormone produced with the use of recombinant DNA techniques. Genetically engineered insulin does not differ in biologic or chemical characteristics from pancreatic human insulin.

Storage and Release

Insulin is synthesized within the β cells of the pancreas, and it is packaged and stored in membrane-lined vesicles within the β-cell cytoplasm. About 200 units of insulin are stored in the pancreas in this form. With stimulation, insulin is released via exocytosis from the β cell to the surrounding capillaries, where it enters the portal circulation. In the first pass through the hepatic circulation, the liver removes 50% of the insulin delivered to it. Total daily insulin secretion is estimated to be about 60 units, but the total daily peripheral delivery is about 30 units.[34]

Insulin circulates unbound to any carrier protein. The circulating half-life of insulin is only 5 to 8 minutes, and the biologic half-life is about 20 minutes.[34] Almost all tissues in the body can metabolize insulin, but the major sites of hormone degradation

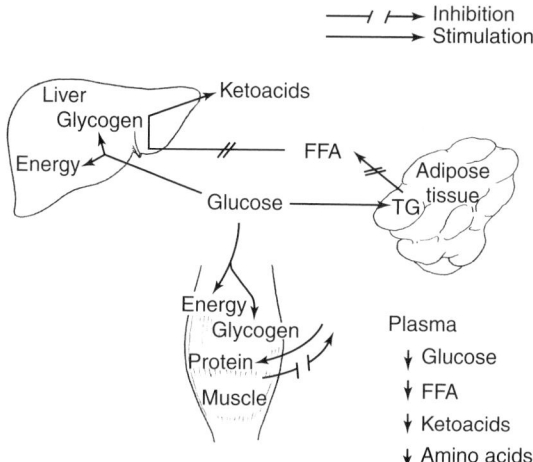

—⊣ ⟼ Inhibition
——⟶ Stimulation

FIGURE 34-9 The effect of insulin on the overall flow of metabolic substrates. Insulin promotes the uptake of glucose into insulin-responsive tissue to meet energy needs. In the liver and skeletal muscle, insulin promotes the storage of excess glucose as glycogen. In adipose tissue, excess glucose is stored as triglyceride (TG). Insulin inhibits the breakdown of triglyceride into glycerol and free fatty acids (FFA). Amino acid uptake into muscle is increased for protein synthesis, and protein breakdown is inhibited.

are the liver and the kidney.[35] Very little insulin is excreted unchanged in the urine.

Effects of Insulin

Insulin is a hormone of energy or fuel storage. It is important to many cellular mechanisms related to growth, and it is intimately involved in the regulation of carbohydrate, fat, and protein metabolism.

Following ingestion of a meal, insulin levels increase sharply in response to stimulation by abundant circulating nutrient substrates. Insulin promotes the storage of carbohydrate, fat, and protein for future use when substrate supply is low.[35] Figure 34-9 outlines the effects of insulin on nutrient substrates.

The peripheral effects of insulin are initiated by a reversible binding to specific cell-membrane insulin receptors. Most cells in the body have insulin receptors, but the major targets of insulin action are the liver, muscle, and adipose tissue.[34]

Effects on Carbohydrate Metabolism. Insulin is the body's key hormone controlling glucose removal from the plasma. It facilitates the disposition of glucose by stimulating its uptake into liver, muscle, and adipose tissue. The brain is one of the few tissues in the body that does not require insulin for glucose transport into its cells.[35]

In the liver, and to a lesser extent in muscle cells, insulin promotes the efficient storage of excess glucose in the form of glycogen (glycogenesis).[34] Under normal circumstances, about 60% of the glucose ingested with a meal is stored in the liver as glycogen. In addition to promoting hepatic glucose storage, insulin limits hepatic glucose output by inhibiting enzymes responsible for gluconeogenesis.[34,35]

Between meals, when the blood glucose and blood insulin levels decrease, the stored glucose can be released back into the blood (through gluconeogenesis and glycogenolysis) and be made available for local energy use or delivery to the central nervous system.

Effects on Protein Metabolism. Insulin's actions on protein metabolism are also directed toward nutrient storage and growth (anabolism). Insulin stimulates the uptake of amino acids from the extracellular fluid to the cell. Once inside the cell, it promotes the synthesis of specific proteins. Insulin also conserves amino acids in existing proteins by inhibiting the breakdown of protein stores. Because insulin is required for protein synthesis, it is firmly established as an essential hormone for normal development and maintenance of healthy tissues.[35]

Effects on Fat Metabolism. The acute effects of insulin on fat metabolism are not as readily apparent as the effects on carbohydrate metabolism, but in the long run they are no less important.

Insulin favors fat storage. After a meal, carbohydrates not utilized for energy or stored as glycogen are converted, under the direction of insulin, to fatty acids and glycerol. These two substances combine in adipose tissue to form triglyceride, the storage form of fat. Insulin not only stimulates triglyceride storage in adipose tissue but also strongly inhibits the breakdown of stored triglyceride to free fatty acids and glycerol. Insulin blocks triglyceride hydrolysis and the liberation of free fatty acids into the circulating blood by suppressing the enzyme *hormone-sensitive lipase*. Under ordinary conditions, insulin continually exerts a "braking" effect on free fatty acid release. A major consequence of lower concentrations of circulating free fatty acids is the decreased use of fatty acids for fuel.[34] Insulin suppresses fatty acid mobilization in the fed state when glucose is readily available to meet energy needs.

In the fasted state, when insulin levels are low, free fatty acid release is accelerated to provide metabolic fuel. The oxidation of fatty acids for energy during fasting spares glucose use.[34,35] Organic acids called *ketoacids* or *ketone bodies* are generated in the liver from fatty acid oxidation. Ketoacid production is increased in the fasted state when insulin levels are low, and it is markedly reduced when insulin levels are high. Insulin is the body's major antiketogenic hormone.[35]

Effects on Ion Transport. Insulin stimulates the translocation of vital electrolytes from the extracellular compartment into cells. Potassium, phosphate, and magnesium uptake into cells is mediated by an insulin mechanism.[34] Exogenous insulin administration may appreciably lower serum potassium, phosphate, and magnesium levels. The precipitation of hypokalemia secondary to vigorous insulin treatment can be of great clinical significance.

Insulin's actions are complex and wide ranging. Overall, insulin promotes the formation of complex molecules for nutrient storage and growth and fosters glucose utilization, instead of fat or protein, for energy.

Control of Insulin Secretion

Insulin synthesis and secretion are stimulated by "feast" or energy abundance. Ingestion of a meal (fuel excess) increases the rate of insulin secretion four- to five-fold.[37] Plasma insulin levels rise, reaching peak values 30 to 60 minutes after eating is initiated.[34] High insulin levels in turn direct nutrients to appropriate storage sites.

Between meals, insulin levels drift downward, the storage process is reversed, and metabolic substrates are mobilized in the form of glucose, free fatty acids, and amino acids. Plasma glucose is by far the most important stimulator of insulin release. Elevated plasma glucose levels directly activate β cells of the pancreas, stimulating insulin synthesis and secretion. Low plasma glucose concentrations inhibit this response. A maximal insulin response occurs at blood glucose levels of about 300 mg/dL.[34] Very little insulin is secreted at plasma glucose levels of 50 mg/dL and below.[34]

Amino acids also are potent stimulators of insulin release, although the β-cell response to amino acids is not as pronounced as the response to glucose. Fat has little if any stimulating effect on insulin release.[34]

Both adrenergic and cholinergic fibers of the autonomic nervous system innervate the islets. Parasympathetic vagal activity and β-adrenergic receptor stimulation increase insulin release. A general sympathetic discharge has a suppressive effect on insulin release through α-adrenergic receptor stimulation.[11] Pancreatic insulin secretion, however, does not *require* intact autonomic innervation; appropriate secretion responses occur in the transplanted pancreas as well.

Gastrointestinal hormones that accompany the digestive process potentiate insulin secretion. Food ingestion seems to send an "anticipatory" signal to the pancreas to discharge insulin in preparation for the absorption of glucose and amino acids.[35] Box 34-3 lists some of the factors that influence insulin secretion.

Glucagon

Glucagon is a linear polypeptide hormone produced by the α cells of the pancreatic islets as a biologic antagonist to insulin.[34,35] The most important role of glucagon is to enhance hepatic glucose output and increase plasma glucose. A decrease in blood glucose concentration below 90 mg/dL increases the plasma glucagon level by several-fold. Hyperglycemia, on the other hand, decreases glucagon release from the α cells.

Insulin and glucagon have opposing biologic actions. Whereas insulin is considered a hormone of energy storage, glucagon is considered a hormone of energy release.[35] Between meals, when blood glucose levels are low, the concentration of glucagon increases to maintain fuel production at a level that meets the energy needs of the individual. Special priority for glucose delivery is given to the brain.

Glucagon works in concert with the counterregulatory hormones epinephrine, GH, and cortisol. These hormones are strong defenders against hypoglycemia and are critical in restoring normal glucose levels during periods of hypoglycemic stress. They also are secreted in response to various other stresses such as infection, toxemia, severe injury, and surgery.[34] Nondiabetic surgical patients experience an increased plasma blood glucose, as much as 60 mg/dL above their preoperative levels, in response to surgical stress.[38]

DIABETES MELLITUS

Diabetes mellitus is a complex metabolic derangement caused by relative or absolute insulin deficiency. Diabetes has been called "starvation in a sea of food." Glucose is present in abundance, but because of insulin lack or insulin resistance, it is unable to reach cells for energy provision. Guidelines for diagnosing diabetes include an FPG level of 126 mg/dL or greater or a random glucose level above 200 mg/dL. The FPG diagnostic level was reduced from a previous value of 140 mg/dL based on findings that patients with an FPG of 126 mg/dL are at risk for diabetes-related complications.[39]

The incidence of diabetes has increased dramatically over the last 40 years. Today it affects nearly 21 million people in the United States; almost 7% of our population.[40] The rise can be attributed to a combination of three factors: (1) an overweight population, (2) more sedentary lifestyles, and (3) a rise in the effect of elderly.[41] As more of our population advances in age into the decades in which most cases of diabetes occur, the effect of the disease will become even more alarming. As outlined in Figure 34-10, many pathophysiologic features of DM are directly attributable to a lack of the normal effects of insulin on carbohydrate, fat, and protein metabolism.

Type 1 Diabetes Mellitus

About 5% to 10% of diabetic patients have *type 1 DM*. This type of diabetes was formerly known as *insulin-dependent diabetes* or *juvenile-onset diabetes*. Individuals with type 1 DM have an absolute deficiency of insulin and are therefore entirely dependent on exogenous insulin therapy. In the absence of sufficient exogenous insulin, the disease course may be complicated by periods of ketosis and acidosis.

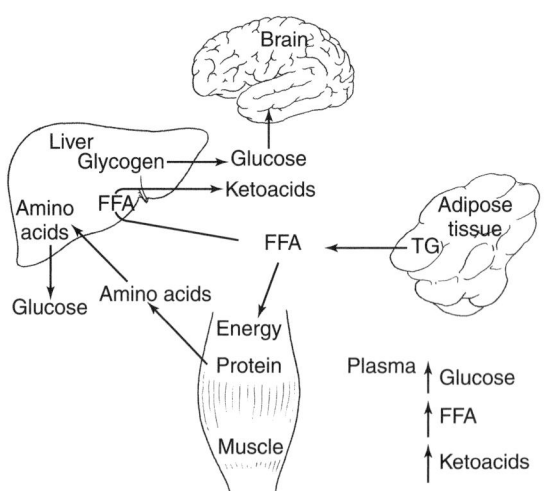

FIGURE **34-10** The pattern of substrate flow in the diabetic state. Lack of insulin enhances hepatic glucose production because of increased gluconeogenesis and glycogenolysis. The diabetic state promotes protein breakdown, and the released amino acids are converted to glucose in the liver (gluconeogenesis). Lipolysis is augmented, and this increases free fatty acid supply to the liver, resulting in enhanced ketogenesis. Free fatty acids provide an energy source to muscle and other facultative tissue. Glucose uptake by the brain is sustained. *FFA*, Free fatty acids; *TG*, triglyceride.

BOX **34-3**

Factors That Influence Insulin Release

Stimulators
Glucose, mannose, fructose
Amino acids
Gastrointestinal hormones
Acetylcholine (parasympathetic stimulation)
β-Adrenergic stimulation

Inhibitors
Hypoglycemia
Somatostatin
Glucagon, cortisol, growth hormone
α-Adrenergic stimulation

In most cases, type 1 DM is caused by an unusually vigorous autoimmune destruction of the β cells of the pancreatic islets. Environmental factors such as infection or exposure to specific antigenic proteins are cited as possible initiators of the immune assault.[42] Type 1 DM patients are also more likely to have other autoimmune diseases such as thyroid disease or Addison disease.[43] A genetic predisposition for development of the disease also is involved.[37]

Type 1 DM usually develops before the age of 30 years, but it can develop at any age. The classic symptoms of type 1 DM appear only when at least 80% of the β cells are destroyed.[37] The remaining β cells usually are eliminated inexorably over 2 or 3 years. In patients with type 1 DM, daily exogenous insulin therapy is essential for life. Some type 1 DM patients may be candidates for pancreatic transplant. The transplantation of isolated pancreatic islets has been plagued by graft survival and islet isolation setbacks, but it holds out promise for a future cure.

Type 2 Diabetes Mellitus
About 90% to 95% of the patients with diabetes have *type 2 DM*. Type 2 DM is characterized by impaired insulin secretion, peripheral insulin resistance (a decreased number of insulin receptors or an insulin receptor or postreceptor defect), and excessive hepatic glucose production.[37] This form of diabetes was formerly known as *non–insulin-dependent diabetes or maturity-onset diabetes*.

Type 2 DM occurs in patients who have some degree of endogenous insulin production but produce quantities insufficient for sustaining normal carbohydrate homeostasis. Insulin levels may be low, normal, or even elevated, but a *relative* insulin deficiency exists. The ultimate expression is a hyperglycemic state.

Typically, type 2 DM occurs in patients who are older than 30 years, obese (80%), and with a family history of the disease.[37] Type 2 DM has an insidious onset; indeed, it is estimated that half of those who have type 2 DM are not even aware of it. The disease course is rarely associated with ketosis or acidosis, but it may be complicated by a nonketotic, hyperosmolar, hyperglycemic state.

Treatment for this class of diabetes consists primarily of oral hypoglycemic agents, exercise, and diet therapy. Weight reduction in the obese diabetic patient improves tissue responsiveness to endogenous insulin and often restores normoglycemia.

The distinction between *insulin-treated* diabetics and *insulin-dependent* diabetics is important. Some type 2 diabetics may benefit from exogenously administered insulin, especially during times of illness or stress. Type 1 diabetics, on the other hand, are insulin-dependent and require exogenous insulin daily to live.

Diabetes Associated with Other Conditions
Diabetes may result from other conditions such as pancreatectomy, cystic fibrosis, or severe pancreatitis. Certain endocrine conditions, including Cushing syndrome, glucagonoma, pheochromocytoma, and acromegaly may also be associated with a diabetic condition. Steroid-induced diabetes may occur in the patient taking supraphysiologic doses of glucocorticoids. Gestational diabetes occurs in approximately 4% of pregnancies in the United States.[37] Women who have had gestational DM have a 20% to 50% chance of developing type 2 DM 5 to 10 years postpartum.[40,41]

Insulin Deficiency
Effect of Insulin Deficiency on Carbohydrates
Insulin deficiency results in a decreased uptake and use of glucose by insulin-sensitive cells. Glycogen storage is decreased, and gluconeogenesis is uninhibited with insulin lack, causing the liver to increase its glucose output. This produces an intracellular deficit and an extracellular surplus of glucose.[34]

The hyperglycemia produced by insulin lack has immediate adverse consequences. When the blood glucose concentration increases to a threshold level (about 180 to 200 mg/dL), the amount of glucose filtered at the kidney glomerulus cannot be totally reabsorbed. The excess filtered glucose spills into the urine (*glucosuria*) and acts as an osmotic diuretic, pulling water with it. The increased urine output (*polyuria*) contributes to extracellular dehydration and electrolyte depletion. Intracellular dehydration also occurs because of the osmotic transfer of water out of cells and into the hypertonic extracellular fluid. In an attempt to compensate for the hypovolemia, the diabetic patient may drink large quantities of water (*polydipsia*).[34,35]

Effect of Insulin Deficiency on Fat
As the diabetic state evolves, glucose-deprived cells meet their energy requirements by drawing on fat and protein reserves. Fat breakdown occurs normally between meals, when insulin levels are low, but it is enhanced greatly in diabetes. The lack of insulin activates hormone-sensitive lipase, which causes uninhibited lipolysis of stored triglycerides to free fatty acids and glycerol. This fat mobilization increases circulating lipids and may contribute to the atherosclerotic and angiopathic changes that complicate the disease course.[35]

Insulin deficiency produces a shift from carbohydrate to fat metabolism. Free fatty acids become the main energy substrate for essentially all tissues (the brain excluded). With uncontrolled diabetes, the excess free fatty acids are converted in the liver to ketone bodies (*acetoacetic acid, β-hydroxybutyric acid*, and *acetone*). This ultimately leads to greater circulating levels of ketoacids and an elevated hydrogen ion concentration in body fluids. The ketone body acetone is a volatile acid and is excreted via the lungs. Consequently, one can frequently identify ketonemia in uncontrolled diabetes by detecting a fruity "acetone breath."

Effect of Insulin Deficiency on Protein
The insulin deficiency of diabetes causes protein storage to halt and catabolism to ensue. When insulin levels are low or absent, the plasma amino acid concentration increases, and the excess circulating amino acids are converted in the liver to glucose (gluconeogenesis). The protein-wasting effects accompanying diabetes lead to weight loss, weakness, and widespread organ dysfunction. The diabetic may attempt to compensate for the protein loss and caloric drain by increasing food intake (*polyphagia*).

Many proteins, including hemoglobin and structural tissue proteins, become glycosylated in the presence of high circulating blood glucose levels. Glucose adducts can alter protein function and may contribute to the organ damage and functional derangements observed in individuals with longstanding diabetes.[34]

Long-Term Diabetic Complications
Diabetic patients are subject to long-term complications that confer substantial morbidity and premature mortality. These complications include extensive arterial disease, cataracts, sensory and motor neuropathy, infection, and autonomic nervous system dysfunction.

Arterial thrombotic lesions in the diabetic population are widely distributed in the extremities, kidneys, eyes, skeletal muscle, myocardium, and nervous system. Owing to these diffuse lesions, diabetes carries a serious risk for the development of microvascular (nephropathy, retinopathy, neuropathy) and macrovascular (atherosclerosis, stroke, coronary artery disease) complications.[44,45]

Cardiovascular disease is markedly increased in patients with DM. According to data from the Centers for Disease Control, the incidence of circulatory insufficiency to the legs and feet is four-fold to seven-fold greater in diabetic men and women compared with their nondiabetic counterparts. Gangrene is 17-fold more common in the diabetic than in the nondiabetic individual.[40,46] Not surprisingly, lower-extremity bypass grafting and amputations are common surgical procedures in the diabetic population. Heart disease is the leading cause of diabetes-related deaths. Adults with diabetes have heart disease death rates about two to four times higher than adults without diabetes.[40] Systolic dysfunction, decreased ejection fraction, and congestive heart failure may occur with severe and longstanding disease.

Further, more than 70% of diabetic individuals have a medical history of hypertension, a rate of occurrence two- to three-fold that for nondiabetic people. In many of these patients, the hypertension is uncontrolled. The risk of stroke is two to four times higher in people with diabetes, and their recovery rate after a stroke is poor.[46]

The eyes are vulnerable to vascular disease because of the dense network of capillary vessels in the retina. Individuals with DM are 25 times more likely to be legally blind than individuals without DM.[37] Diabetic retinopathy is characterized by microaneurysm formation, swelling and narrowing of retinal blood vessels, and neovascularization. These vascular lesions may result in vitreous hemorrhage and retinal scarring or detachment. Loss of vision from diabetic retinopathy is the leading cause of new cases of blindness in people aged 20 to 74 years in the United States.[40]

Diabetic renal disease is the leading cause of end-stage renal disease in the United States.[37,46] The nephropathy may be caused by hemodynamic alterations, inflammation and thickening of the glomerular capillary basement membrane and other structural changes in the glomerulus.[37] Renal insufficiency or chronic renal failure is often the end result. Diabetics commonly are candidates for kidney transplantation.

The diabetic process also interferes with normal nerve function. Diabetic neuropathy occurs in over 50% of individuals with longstanding disease.[37,40,41] Both the peripheral and autonomic nervous systems may be involved. Vagal denervation may occur early in the course of the disease. Dysfunction of the cardiac vagus nerve may be manifested as resting tachycardia, cardiac dysrhythmias, and the absence of heart-rate variability with deep breathing. Postural hypotension may occur in the diabetic with autonomic neuropathy as a result of dysfunctional sympathetic nervous system vasoconstrictive processes. Manifestations of orthostatic hypotension may include postural syncope, dizziness, and lightheadedness.

Diabetic patients with autonomic neuropathy are at increased risk for developing painless myocardial ischemia. The possibility of a myocardial infarction should be considered in the presence of unexplained hypotension in these patients.[47]

Other signs of autonomic neuropathy in the diabetic patient include early satiety, lack of sweating, impotence, and nocturnal diarrhea.[11] The patient with diabetic autonomic neuropathy has impaired gastric emptying and is at risk for aspiration of stomach contents in the perioperative period. Box 34-4 summarizes major chronic complications of DM.

BOX 34-4

Chronic Complications of Diabetes Mellitus

Microvascular
Retinopathy
Neuropathy (sensory, autonomic, motor)
Nephropathy

Macrovascular
Coronary artery disease
Peripheral vascular disease
Cerebrovascular disease

Other
Infection
Cataracts
Stiff joint syndrome
Glaucoma
Poor wound healing

There is a strong relationship between the hyperglycemia of diabetes and end-organ diseases. Sustained hyperglycemia seems to be prerequisite for significant nephropathy, retinopathy, and neuropathy to occur in type 1 and type 2 diabetes.[44,48,49] Other factors—genetic, environmental, or both—may have roles in determining end-organ complications. The hemoglobin A_{1c} test, or glycosylated hemoglobin level, provides an estimate of the patient's overall plasma glucose control during the past 2 to 3 months. A value less than 7.0% suggests adequate blood glucose control.[37]

Anesthetic Management of the Diabetic Patient

Diabetes is the most common endocrine disorder encountered in surgical patients. Long-standing diabetes predisposes the patient to many diseases that require surgical intervention. Cataract extraction, kidney transplantation, ulcer debridement, and vascular repair are some of the operations frequently performed on diabetic patients.

Diabetic patients have higher morbidity and mortality in the perioperative period compared with nondiabetics of similar age. Increased complications are not because of the disease itself but primarily because of organ damage associated with long-term disease.[11] Ischemic heart disease is the most common cause of perioperative mortality in the diabetic patient.[8]

Preoperative Considerations

The diabetic patient may come to the operating room with a spectrum of metabolic aberrations and end-organ complications that warrant careful preanesthetic assessment.

Cardiovascular complications account for most of the surgical deaths in diabetic patients.[11] The presence of hypertension, coronary artery disease, or autonomic nervous system dysfunctions can result in a labile cardiovascular course during anesthesia. It is essential that the cardiovascular and volume status of the patient be thoroughly evaluated before surgery. Preoperative electrocardiography is advised for all adult diabetic patients because of the high incidence of cardiac disease.

Autonomic nervous system dysfunction may result in delayed gastric emptying, making these patients prone to aspiration, nausea and vomiting, and abdominal distention. Preoperative aspiration prophylaxis with H_2-receptor blockers, gastroprokinetic agents, and/or preinduction antacids are recommended for patients with a prolonged history of poor glycemic control.[11,49] Intubation during general anesthesia is a logical choice for the patient with gastroparesis.

Patients with significant autonomic neuropathy may have an impaired respiratory response to hypoxia. These patients are especially sensitive to the respiratory-depressant effects of sedatives and anesthetics and require particular vigilance in the perioperative period.[8,11]

Peripheral neuropathies (paresthesias, numbness in the hands and feet) should be adequately documented in the preanesthetic evaluation. Their presence may affect the decision to use regional anesthesia. Neuraxial blockade may exacerbate neural deficits in patients with diabetic polyneuropathy.[50]

Glycosylation of tissue proteins may produce a stiff-joint syndrome in diabetics. An estimated 30% to 40% of type 1 diabetics demonstrate restricted joint mobility.[8] Limited motion of the atlantooccipital joint can make endotracheal intubation difficult.[51,52] Demonstration of the "prayer sign," an inability to approximate the palms of the hands and fingers, may help identify patients with tissue protein glycosylation and potentially difficult airways.

Evidence of kidney disease should be sought, and basic tests of renal function (urinalysis, serum creatinine, blood urea nitrogen) evaluated preoperatively. The presence of renal impairment may influence the choice and dosage of anesthetic agents, and potentially nephrotoxic drugs should be avoided. Patients should be well hydrated after radiocontrast dye exposure.

The anesthetist should examine the patient's history of glycemic control, including a fasting blood sugar on the morning of surgery, to ensure preoperative optimization of the patient's metabolic state. It is not clear what level of glycemic control is associated with the best risk/benefit ratio in the perioperative period, but a recommended target blood glucose range is 80 to 180 mg/dL.[53,54]

Sustained hyperglycemia with attendant osmotic diuresis should alert the anesthetist to possible fluid deficits and electrolyte depletion. Preoperative electrolyte levels should be evaluated. Lactate-containing intravenous solutions are generally avoided because lactate conversion to glucose may contribute to hyperglycemia.

An important part of the preoperative evaluation is a review of oral hypoglycemic and insulin regimens.

Oral Glucose-Lowering Agents. Oral glucose-lowering agents and insulin are used as adjuncts to diet therapy and exercise for treating type 2 DM. Currently available oral hypoglycemic agents fall into the following classifications: (1) sulfonylureas, (2) α-glucosidase inhibitors, (3) thiazolidinediones, (4) biguanides, (5) nonsulfonylurea secretagogues, and (6) others. Often patients are on a combination of therapeutic agents. Table 34-4 lists medications commonly used to treat type 2 diabetes.[55]

Sulfonylurea agents increase the secretion of insulin from the pancreas and thus require the presence of functioning β cells. These agents are not effective in patients with type 1 DM. Persistent and severe hypoglycemia is a possible adverse effect of sulfonylureas.[55] The syndrome of inappropriate ADH secretion and hyponatremia has been associated with chlorpropamide, a first-generation sulfonylurea.

Newer non-sulfonylurea secretagogues such as the *meglitinides* (repaglinide) and *D-phenylalanine* (nateglinide) increase insulin

TABLE **34-4**	Oral Drugs for Type 2 Diabetes
Drug	**Usual Daily Dosage**
DPP-4 Inhibitor	
Sitagliptin (Januvia)	100 mg once
Sulfonylurea: First Generation	
Chlorpropamide (Diabinese)	250 to 375 mg once
Tolazamide (Tolinase)	250 to 500 mg once or divided
Tolbutamide	1000 to 2000 mg divided
Sulfonylurea: Second Generation	
Glimepiride (Amaryl)	1 to 4 mg once
Glipizide (Glucotrol)	10 to 20 mg once or divided
(Glucotrol XL sustained-release tablets)	5 to 20 mg once
Glyburide (DiaBeta, Micronase)	5 to 20 mg once or divided
(Glynase micronized tablets)	3 to 12 mg once or divided
Alpha-glucosidase Inhibitors	
Acarbose (Precose)	50 to 100 mg tid with meals
Miglitol (Glyset)	50 to 100 mg tid with meals
Thiazolidinediones	
Rosiglitazone (Avandia)	4 to 8 mg once or divided
Pioglitazone (Actos)	15 to 45 mg once
Biguanides	
Metformin (Glucophage)	1500 to 2550 mg divided
(Glucophage XR)	1500 to 2000 mg once
Metformin/glyburide (Glucovance)	500 mg/5 mg bid
Metformin/rosiglitazone (Avandamet)	500 mg/2 mg bid
Metformin/Glipizide (Metaglip)	500 mg/2.5 mg bid
Nonsulfonylurea Secretagogues	
Repaglinide (Prandin)	1 to 4 mg tid before meals
Nateglinide (Starlix)	60 to 120 mg tid before meals
Other	
Exenatide (Byetta)	10 mcg subQ bid before breakfast and dinner
Pramlintide (Symlin)	60-120 mcg subQ tid before main meals
Colesevelam (Welchor)	3.8 g once or divided bid

Modified from Drugs for type 2 diabetes. Treat Guidel Med Lett. *2008;6(71):47-54.*
DPP-4 inhibitor, *Dipeptidyl-peptidase.*

production by pancreatic β cells in a manner similar to the sulfonylureas.[37,55]

Acarbose (Precose) and miglital (Glyset) are α-*glucosidase inhibitors*. These medications block the intestinal enzymes that digest starches into absorbable monosaccharides, resulting in a slower and lower rise in postprandial plasma glucose.

TABLE **34-5**	Pharmacokinetics of Insulin Preparations				
Insulin Type	**Onset**	**Peak**	**Duration**	**Route**	
Long-Acting					
Insuling detemir—*Levemir* (Novo Nordisk)	1 hr	Relatively flat	12-20 hr	subQ	
Insulin glargine—Lantus (Sanofiaventis)	1-2 hr	No peak	22-24 hr	subQ	
Rapid-Acting					
Insulin aspart—Novolog (Novo Nordisk)	10-30 min	30-60 min	3-5 hr	subQ	
Insulin lispro—Humalog (Lilly)	10-30 min	30-60 min	3-5 hr	subQ	
Insulin glulisine—Apidra (Sanofiaventis)	10-30 min	30-60 min	3-5 hr	subQ	
Regular Insulin					
Humulin R (Lilly)	30-60 min	1½-2 hr	5-8 hr	IV, subQ, IM	
Novolin R (Novo Nordisk)	30-60 min	1½-2 hr	5-8 hr	IV, subQ, IM	
Intermedlate-Acting NPH					
Humulin N	1-2 hr	4-8 hr	10-20 hr	subQ	
Novolin N	1-2 hr	4-8 hr	10-20 hr	subQ	

Adapted from Drugs for type 2 diabetes. Treat Guidel Med Lett. 2008;6(71):47-54.
IM, *Intramuscular;* IV, *intravenous;* subQ, *subcutaneous;* NPH, *neutral protamine Hagedorn. Time course is based on subcutaneous administration.*

Rosiglitazone (Avandia) and pioglitazone (Actos) are *thiazol-idinedione derivatives*. Thiazolidinediones decrease hepatic glucose output and reduce insulin resistance in the type 2 DM patient by sensitizing the insulin receptor for glucose uptake.[55] Liver enzymes must be monitored closely with these agents. The thiazolidinedione *troglitazone* (Rezulin) was withdrawn from the U.S. market for serious liver complications associated with the drug. In August 2007, the U.S. Food and Drug Administration (FDA) issued a "black box" warning on the drugs Avandia, Actos, and combination drugs that include these agents because of a significant increase in the risk of heart failure in patients taking these medications.

Metformin, a *biguanide*, decreases hepatic glucose production and increases peripheral insulin utilization. Lactic acidosis, a rare but potentially fatal problem, has been reported with biguanides. Lactic acidosis is precipitated by drug accumulation; therefore, even mild renal impairment or nephrotoxicity is a contraindication to metformin therapy. Metformin is also not prescribed to patients with conditions that predispose to acidosis (e.g., liver disease, congestive heart failure).[56,57]

Newer drugs for patients with type 2 DM include pramlintide, exenatide, and sitagliptin phosphate. Pramlintide (Symlin) is an injected antihyperglycemic medication for use in patients with type 2 or type 1 diabetes treated with mealtime insulin. Pramlintide is a synthetic analog of human amylin, a naturally occurring hormone synthesized from pancreatic β cells that contributes to glucose control during the postprandial period. Amylin, similar to insulin, is absent or deficient in patients with diabetes.

Exenatide (Byetta) is the first in a new class of drugs called *incretin mimetics*. The drug is approved as an alternative to starting insulin in type 2 DM and is only available as a subcutaneous injection. Exenatide is derived from the saliva of the gila monster, with an amino acid sequence similar to that of human glucagon-like peptide. In the presence of glucose, the drug stimulates insulin release and lowers serum glucagon levels.[55]

In October 2006, the FDA approved sitagliptin phosphate (Januvia), the first in a new class of oral glucose-lowering drugs known as *DPP-4 (dipeptidyl peptidase-4) inhibitors* that enhance insulin release from the pancreas in response to hyperglycemia.

Insulin Preparations. Insulin preparations are generated today by DNA recombinant technology, mimicking the amino acid sequence of human insulin. All insulin formulations in the United States are prepared as U-100 (100 units/mL).

Insulin preparations differ in onset and duration after subcutaneous administration. In addition to subcutaneous injections, insulin delivery devices (implantable pumps, mechanical syringes) are used to facilitate exogenous administration. The greatest risk with all forms of insulin is hypoglycemia. Table 34-5 identifies major classes of exogenous insulin: regular, rapid-acting, inhaled, intermediate-acting, and long-acting.

It is imperative to know the surgical patient's normal insulin dosage regimen and treatment compliance. Some diabetic patients are on a fixed regimen that consists of a mixture of rapid- and intermediate-acting insulins taken before breakfast and again at the evening meal.[8] Other patients are on multiple injection regimens designed to provide more physiologic glycemic control.[37]

Insulin glargine (Lantus) and insulin detemir (Levemir) are biosynthetic human insulin analogs taken once a day. These insulins have delayed absorption from subcutaneous tissue, which prolongs their effects. Unlike NPH and Lente, they have no peak effects, but rather provide steady plasma concentrations.[58]

Exubera was the first FDA-approved inhaled insulin in the United States, but it was discontinued by the manufacturer in September 2008.

Continuous subcutaneous insulin infusion is increasingly used by motivated patients desiring an optimal physiologic regimen.[59] Sophisticated infusion devices deliver small doses (microliters/min) of rapid-acting insulin lispro or insulin aspart at various programmable delivery rates. The pumps may be discontinued and a continuous insulin infusion implemented for the perioperative period. Alternatively, if continued into the perioperative period, the pump can be programmed to deliver a basal insulin dose supplemented with dextrose and potassium as needed, with rate adjustment based on serial blood-glucose measurements.[37,60]

Intraoperative Management

The diabetic surgical patient's operation should be scheduled early in the day if possible to minimize disruptions in treatment and nutrition regimens. Surgery produces a catabolic stress response and elevates stress-induced counterregulatory hormones.[8] In the diabetic patient, the hyperglycemic, ketogenic, and lipolytic effects of the counterregulatory hormones compound the state of insulin deficiency. For this reason, perioperative hyperglycemia and other metabolic aberrations are common in the surgical diabetic patient.

No specific anesthetic technique is superior overall for diabetic patients. Both general anesthesia and regional anesthesia have been used safely. General anesthesia, however, has been shown to induce hormonal changes that accentuate glycogenolysis and gluconeogenesis, compounding the diabetic patient's hyperglycemic state. Regional anesthesia may produce fewer deleterious changes in glucose homeostasis.[54,61,62]

The Certified Registered Nurse Anesthetist (CRNA) must be especially careful in positioning and padding the diabetic patient on the operating table. Decreased tissue perfusion and peripheral sympathetic neuropathy may contribute to the development of skin breakdown and ulceration.

Diabetic patients represent a heterogeneous group requiring individualized perioperative care. The specific approach to metabolic management depends on the type of diabetes (type 1 or type 2), the history of glycemic control, and the type of surgery being performed. Frequent blood glucose determinations are an integral part of any diabetic management technique. A glucose meter or other accurate and rapid means of monitoring blood glucose levels should be available. During a long surgical procedure or for major surgery, at least hourly intraoperative blood glucose measurement is the prudent course for the brittle diabetic patient.

Strict control of even short-term elevations in blood glucose improves perioperative morbidity.[63,64] Persistent hyperglycemia has been shown to impair wound healing and wound strength.[65] In addition, reports suggest that postoperative infection is more prevalent in diabetic patients with uncontrolled blood sugar levels.[66,67] Studies also provide evidence that hyperglycemia worsens the neurologic outcome after ischemic brain injury.[68-70] Avoiding perioperative hyperglycemia is advisable, especially in patients at risk for acute neurologic insult (carotid endarterectomy, intracranial surgery, cardiopulmonary bypass).

Various regimens have been tendered on how to best manage the metabolic changes that occur in the surgical diabetic patient.[11,71-75] Experts differ on optimal protocols for case management and precisely defined target glucose levels. Current debate centers on the risk/benefit ratio of intensive or "tight" blood glucose control versus "nontight" control during surgery. The universal goal with all techniques is to avoid hypoglycemia and minimize metabolic derangements. Patients under anesthesia are generally maintained with a mild transient hyperglycemia to avoid the potentially catastrophic effects of hypoglycemia.[11,53] Frequent blood glucose determinations during surgery and in the immediate postoperative period are central to safe practice.[11]

Following are three different approaches to the metabolic management of the adult surgical diabetic patient, but the reader should note that there are numerous variations.

Intermediate-Acting Insulin Use. This is a traditional nontight method of managing the surgical diabetic patient and involves less intensive control of plasma glucose but aims to avoid marked hyperglycemia and dangerous hypoglycemia. Variations of this technique are used for stable diabetics undergoing elective operative procedures.[8,11]

1. On the morning of surgery, fasting blood sugar level is measured.

2. An intravenous (IV) infusion containing 5% dextrose is started at 100 to150 mL/hr.

3. After the IV infusion is started, half of the patient's normal morning intermediate- or long-acting insulin dose is administered subcutaneously.

4. The glucose-containing IV infusion is continued throughout surgery. Additional fluid requirements are met with the administration of a second glucose-free infusate.

5. Blood glucose levels are checked every 1 to 2 hours during surgery.

6. If the blood glucose level exceeds an established maximum level, commonly 180 mg/dL, regular insulin is administered according to an established "sliding scale." Insulin sensitivity varies markedly from one patient to the next, but on the average, 1 unit of regular insulin can be expected to decrease the blood glucose level 40 to 50 mg/dL.[76]

This time-tested regimen is easy to implement, and it is usually successful in preventing significant hypo- or hyperglycemia.[11,77,78] The disadvantages of this technique are:

1. Absorption of preoperatively administered subcutaneous insulin is unpredictable and erratic in the surgical patient because of blood pressure, blood flow, and temperature variations that occur with anesthesia.

2. The onset and peak effect of the preoperative intermediate-acting insulin may not correspond to the time of surgical stress, especially if the operation is delayed or prolonged.

3. The half-life of regular insulin is short, and a "rollercoaster" glucose profile may occur. Plasma glucose levels will vary considerably.

Insulin Infusion. An insulin infusion management technique may be used to maintain the blood glucose concentration within relatively narrow boundaries. Intensive perioperative regulation of blood glucose prevents hyperglycemia, but it carries the risk of hypoglycemia, and therefore necessitates more frequent blood glucose assays.[11,54,63] Regular insulin infusion may range from 0.5 to 5 units/hr, depending on the clinical situation and insulin resistance.[37]

Intraoperative insulin infusion may be considered for the type 1 diabetic having major or prolonged surgery, the poorly controlled diabetic, the pregnant diabetic, the diabetic undergoing coronary artery bypass grafting, and the diabetic with serious concurrent illness.[11] An example of this regimen would be[11]:

1. On the morning of surgery, a fasting blood glucose level is measured.

2. An infusion of 5% dextrose is started at a rate of 100 to 150 mL/hr.

3. A regular insulin infusion is begun, piggy-backed to the glucose infusion. The insulin infusion rate is set at: insulin (units/hr) = last plasma glucose (mg/dL) ÷ 150. (If the patient is obese, has infection, or is on corticosteroids, the divisor is changed to 100.)

4. Blood glucose levels are measured every hour during insulin infusion and potassium levels checked after the first hour of the infusion.

5. Additional fluid requirements are met with the administration of a second glucose-free infusate.

Blood glucose levels less than 80 mg/dL may be treated with $D_{50}W$ and remeasured in 30 minutes. In a 70-kg patient, 15 mL of $D_{50}W$ can be expected to raise the blood glucose concentration by about 30 mg/dL. Surgical patients undergoing renal transplantation or coronary artery bypass graft procedures, obese and septic patients, and patients on steroid therapy usually have higher insulin-infusion requirements.[11,74]

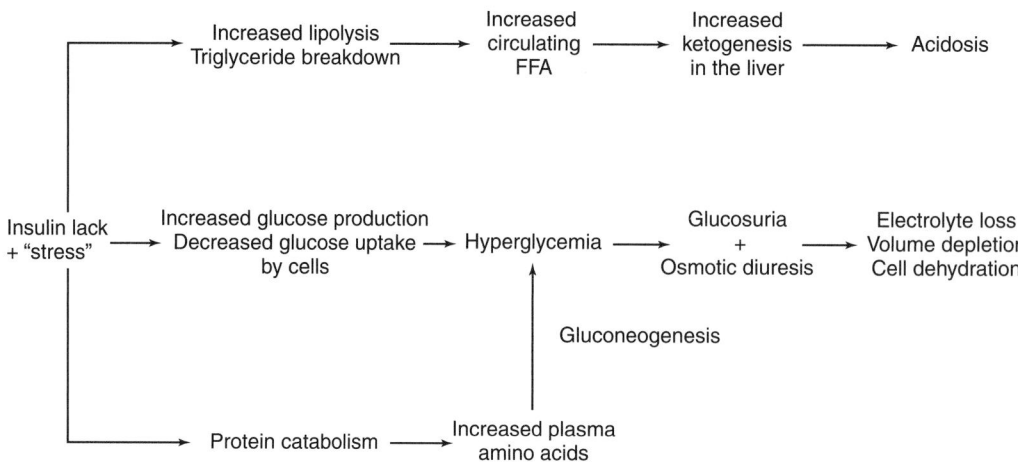

FIGURE **34-11**   Diabetic ketoacidosis. *FFA,* Free fatty acid.

The advantages of tight glucose management in the perioperative period are that:

1. The insulin infusion can be finely regulated to correspond to hourly variations in blood glucose levels.
2. Periods of hyperglycemia are less likely. Deleterious effects of hyperglycemia (hyperosmolarity, osmotic diuresis, impaired wound healing, infection) may be prevented.
3. The insulin-glucose infusion can be continued into the postoperative period until the patient is ready to eat, at which time subcutaneous insulin or an oral hypoglycemic agent can be reinstated.

Type 2 Diabetes and Oral Hypoglycemic Agents. Patients treated with oral hypoglycemic agents demand the same individualized perioperative management as those with type 1 diabetes. The duration of action of the patient's oral agent must be noted. Discontinuing long-acting agents 2 to 3 days before surgery and converting to shorter-acting agents or insulin affords better perioperative glucose control.[7,73] Metformin should be discontinued 2 days or more before surgery because the surgical risks of hypotension and renal hypoperfusion place patients on this drug at increased risk for lactic acidosis.[56,57]

For the well-controlled surgical patient with type 2 diabetes who is scheduled for minor to moderate surgery, the patient's oral hypoglycemic agent may be continued until the evening before surgery. Glucose-containing fluids may be administered intraoperatively to protect against possible residual effects of oral hypoglycemic agents. Other experts adhere to a "no glucose, no insulin" technique for well-controlled type 2 diabetic patients. Regardless of the technique chosen, plasma glucose should be measured regularly throughout the procedure and hyperglycemia treated with insulin on a "sliding" scale.[77,78]

Acute Derangements in Glucose Homeostasis
Hypoglycemia
Hypoglycemia is encountered more frequently in the diabetic patient than in the healthy adult, and it can develop insidiously during the perioperative period.

Medications (insulin, sulfonylureas, β-adrenergic receptor blocking agents) and toxins (ethanol) are common causes of hypoglycemia. Severe liver disease (impaired hepatic glucose output), the altered physiology associated with gastric bypass surgery, sepsis, or an insulin-secreting tumor of the islets of Langerhans (an insulinoma) are conditions that are often complicated by hypoglycemia.

The blood glucose concentration at which signs and symptoms of hypoglycemia appear varies widely from one person to the next, but blood glucose levels in the range of 45 to 50 mg/dL commonly produce mild symptoms in the otherwise healthy patient. Because the brain is the predominant organ of glucose consumption, it is most sensitive to glucose deprivation.[35,36] Manifestations of impaired cerebral function (confusion, dizziness, headache, weakness) are associated with glucose lack. As the blood sugar level declines below 50 mg/dL, aberrant behavior, seizures, and loss of consciousness may occur. Other signs of hypoglycemia (tachycardia, diaphoresis, anxiety, tremors, piloerection, pupillary dilation, and vasoconstriction) reflect sympathetic-adrenal hyperactivity.[35] Acute treatment for the hypoglycemic surgical patient is the intravenous administration of 25 to 50 mL of 50% dextrose, followed by a continuous infusion of 5% dextrose.[8,37] Unless prompt glucose therapy is provided, irreversible brain damage may result.

Hypoglycemia is potentially catastrophic during surgery because most of the neural indications of glucose lack are masked by general anesthesia. Signs of sympathetic adrenal discharge may also be blunted by general anesthesia or severe diabetic autonomic neuropathy, making the diagnosis of hypoglycemia extremely difficult. β-Adrenergic receptor blocking agents can reduce the hyperglycemic effects of epinephrine, in addition to diminishing the symptomatic warning signs of hypoglycemia.[36,37] Frequent blood glucose determinations, maintenance of mild hyperglycemia, and diligent monitoring help to avoid this serious complication during anesthesia.

Diabetic Ketoacidosis
Diabetic ketoacidosis (DKA) is a medical emergency triggered by a hyperglycemic event, usually in a patient with type 1 DM. Treatment errors, critical illnesses (myocardial infarction, trauma, cerebral vascular accident, burns), and infections are common precipitants of DKA.[79-81]

Stressful events stimulate the release of hyperglycemic counterregulatory hormones (glucagon, GH, epinephrine, cortisol).[35,37] The insulin-dependent diabetic is unable to secrete insulin to counterbalance the serum elevations of glucose, free fatty acids, and ketone bodies produced by these stress-induced hormones. Unless exogenous insulin is provided, the glycemic event may progress to severe ketoacidosis, dehydration, and acute metabolic decompensation.

TABLE **34-6**	Features of Diabetic Ketoacidosis (DKA) and Hyperglycemic Hyperosmolar Syndrome (HHS)	
	DKA	**HHS**
Plasma glucose	>250 mg/dL	>600 mg/dL
pH	<7.3	>7.3
Serum bicarbonate	<18 mmol/L	>15 mmol/L
Serum osmolarity	+	++
Ketonemia	++	Normal or slight +
Mental obtundation	Variable	Present
Hypovolemia	Present	Present

+, *Increase;* ++, *large increase.*

DKA usually develops over 24 hours. Major signs and symptoms include hyperglycemia, volume depletion (average fluid deficit 5 L), tachycardia, metabolic acidosis, a calculated anion gap greater than 10, electrolyte depletion, hyperosmolarity (>300 mOsm/L), nausea and vomiting, abdominal pain, and lethargy.[37,82] Blood levels of ketone bodies are elevated, and the patient's breath may have a fruity odor from excess acetone production. The respiratory center is typically stimulated by the low plasma pH, resulting in rapid, deep breathing (*Kussmaul respiration*). Acidosis, hyperosmolarity, and dehydration may depress consciousness to the point of coma.[37,79-82] Figure 34-11 outlines the pathophysiologic events leading to diabetic ketoacidosis.

Gangrene and infection of an ischemic lower extremity are common surgical conditions associated with DKA. Preoperative management of the surgical patient with DKA requires an aggressive approach to restore intravascular volume, correct electrolyte abnormalities, improve acid-base balance, and reduce blood glucose levels with intravenous insulin.[79,82] The airway must be protected in the obtunded patient. Once the surgical problem that initiated DKA has resolved, medical management often is more effective.[11,79]

Hyperglycemic Hyperosmolar State

Hyperglycemic hyperosmolar state (HHS) is a life-threatening hyperosmolar condition triggered by a hyperglycemic event. This syndrome commonly occurs in elderly patients with type 2 DM, but it also develops in patients with no history of diabetes. Patients generally have some endogenous insulin secretion, but the hyperglycemic episode overwhelms the pancreas and produces severe hyperglycemia and glucosuria. The amount of insulin secreted is usually sufficient to prevent lipolysis and ketone production. Therefore unlike DKA, this syndrome usually is not associated with acidosis or significant ketogenesis. Table 34-6 compares common features of diabetic ketoacidosis and HHS.

Common precipitating factors of HHS include infection, sepsis, pneumonia, stroke, and myocardial infarction.

A spectrum of symptoms is associated with HHS, culminating in mental confusion, lethargy, and coma.[37,82] Profound dehydration is present, resulting in hypotension and tachycardia. Laboratory evaluation may reveal a biochemical profile of marked hyperglycemia, normal arterial pH, absent or minimal ketonemia, and hyperosmolarity (>330 mOsm/L).[14,52] Despite depleted total body potassium stores, the serum potassium levels at presentation may be normal or elevated due to acidosis and insulin-lack.[37]

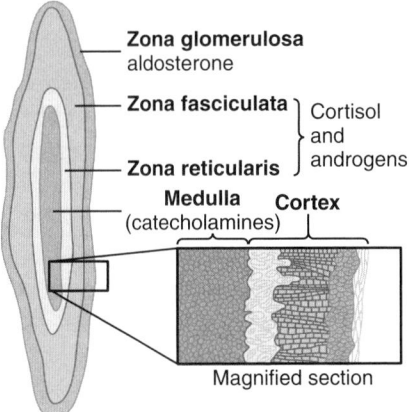

FIGURE 34-12 Secretion of adrenocortical hormones by the different zones of the adrenal cortex and secretion of catecholamines by the adrenal medulla. (*From Guyton AC, Hall JE. In:* Textbook of Medical Physiology. *11th ed. Philadelphia: Saunders; 2006:945.*)

Even with appropriate treatment, the mortality figures for HHS are substantially higher (15%) than those for DKA (<5%), in part because HHS commonly affects an older patient population, often with accompanying comorbidities.[8,37,82]

Treatment goals are similar to those for DKA and include identification and management of the precipitating problem, vigorous isotonic rehydration (average total body water deficit 9 L), correction of hyperglycemia, and electrolyte replacement.[80,82] The hazards inherent in aggressive fluid administration in the elderly patient dictate central hemodynamic monitoring during treatment.

ADRENAL GLANDS

The adrenal glands are located at the superior poles of each kidney and consist of two distinct anatomic and physiologic entities, the adrenal cortex and the adrenal medulla. The *adrenal medulla* comprises the central 20% of the adrenal gland and secretes the hormones epinephrine and norepinephrine. The *adrenal cortex* constitutes the outer part of the adrenal gland and secretes three main types of hormones: mineralocorticoids (aldosterone), glucocorticoids (cortisol), and androgenic hormones (dehydroepiandrosterone).[83]

Adrenal Cortex

The adrenal cortex is composed of three layers, each having distinct properties. The *zona glomerulosa* is the outermost tissue of the cortex; it secretes mineralocorticoid hormones. The *zona fasciculata* is the middle layer; it secretes primarily cortisol and other glucocorticoid hormones. The *zona reticularis* is the innermost layer of the adrenal cortex; it secretes primarily adrenal androgenic hormones[83] (Figure 34-12).

Hormones Secreted from the Adrenal Cortex

All hormones secreted from the adrenal cortex have a steroidal structure and share a common cholesterol backbone. As a group, these hormones are termed *corticosteroids*. Corticosteroids have similar chemical structures but widely diverse functions.

Glucocorticoid and androgenic hormone production and release is controlled in large part by ACTH from the anterior pituitary gland. ACTH stimulates glucocorticoid hormone synthesis by activating the enzyme desmolase. Desmolase causes the conversion of cholesterol to pregnenolone, the first step in corticosteroid hormone synthesis (Figure 34-13). ACTH has little or

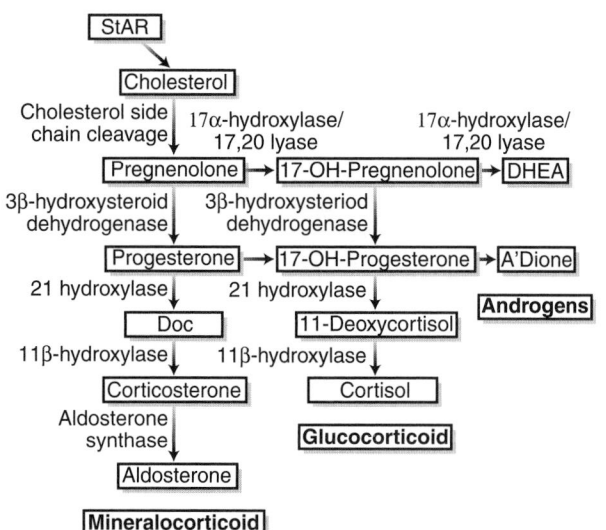

FIGURE **34-13** Adrenal steroidogenesis. Aldosterone, cortisol, and adrenal androgens are synthesized by a series of steroidogenic enzymes in a zone-specific fashion. *A'Dione*, Androstenedione; *DHEA*, dehydroepiandrosterone; *Doc*, deoxycorticosterone. (*From Stewart PM. The adrenal cortex. In: Kronenberg HM et al. Williams Textbook of Endocrinology. 11th ed. Philadelphia: Saunders; 2008:449.*)

BOX 34-5

Control of ACTH Hormone Secretion

Stimulation
Corticotropin-releasing hormone
Sleep-to-waking period
Stress
Hypoglycemia
Sepsis
Trauma
Decreased plasma cortisol
α-Adrenergic receptor stimulation

Inhibition
Elevated plasma cortisol
Opioids

---

no effect on mineralocorticoid secretion.[84] In the *zona glomerulosa*, angiotensin II stimulates the initial conversion of cholesterol to pregnenolone.[84]

The adrenal androgens, of which dehydroepiandrosterone is the most important, have effects similar to the male sex hormone testosterone and account for secondary sexual characteristics in females.[83] The glucocorticoids and mineralocorticoids are discussed in more detail in the following sections.

Glucocorticoids. The adrenal cortex synthesizes more than 30 types of steroid hormones. Cortisol (hydrocortisone) is the prototypical glucocorticoid, and it accounts for 95% of the glucocorticoids released from the adrenal cortex.

Cortisol secretion is largely controlled by ACTH, and in turn, cortisol is the most potent regulator of ACTH. Cortisol has a direct negative feedback effect on the hypothalamus, inhibiting the release of CRH, and on the anterior lobe of the pituitary gland, decreasing ACTH synthesis and release. When cortisol concentration is high, the feedback system reduces ACTH production. Secretion rates of CRH, ACTH, and cortisol follow a circadian rhythm: levels are elevated in the early morning and decrease in the evening.[84]

The daily cortisol production is 15 to 30 mg, and most of this is produced and released between 5 AM and 9 AM.[85] Physical and mental stress increase the secretion of CRH, ACTH, and cortisol (Box 34-5). Stress can raise cortisol production levels to more than 250 mg/day.[83,84]

After release from the adrenal cortex, cortisol circulates in the blood as free cortisol (the physiologically active form) or bound to cortisol-binding globulin (transcortin) or albumin. Ninety-four percent of cortisol is transported in the bound form, and 6% is free. Cortisol is cleared from the blood in 1 to 2 hours but has a prolonged end-organ effect. It is inactivated mainly in the liver and excreted in the urine as 17-hydroxycorticosteroids. The normal cortisol blood concentration averages 12 mcg/dL.[84]

Cortisol Actions. Glucocorticoids are essential to maintain life. They are needed for the proper use of proteins, carbohydrates, and fats by the body. They mediate catecholamine-induced effects on the heart and vasculature and are central to the body's response to physical and mental stress.[83,84] Almost any stress, psychologic or physical, causes an immediate and marked increase in ACTH and cortisol secretion. Important perioperative stressors may include pain, anxiety, trauma, infection, heat or cold, and surgery. Inadequate cortisol during critical illness and surgery can lead to hypotension, shock, and death.[83,85]

Glucocorticoids have some mineralocorticoid and androgenic effects that may become apparent with hormone excess or supraphysiologic replacement dosages.

Effect on Carbohydrate Metabolism. Overall, glucocorticoids enhance the production of high-energy fuel for metabolic needs.[83] A key function is their ability to stimulate gluconeogenesis in the liver. The rate of gluconeogenesis increases 6- to 10-fold in the presence of cortisol. Further, cortisol mobilizes amino acids from extrahepatic tissues (mainly muscle), making them available for gluconeogenesis and glycogenesis in the liver. In extrahepatic tissues, cortisol moderately decreases the rate of glucose uptake and use. Cortisol is called "diabetogenic" because it increases blood glucose concentrations. Typically, a single dose of glucocorticoid raises blood glucose for 12 to 24 hours.[11]

Effect on Protein Metabolism. Cortisol decreases protein synthesis and increases protein catabolism in essentially all body cells except those of the liver. In the presence of sustained cortisol excess, the catabolic effects are marked. This is especially apparent in skeletal muscles, which become weak and atrophic.

Effect on Fat Metabolism. Plasma free fatty acids are mobilized from adipose tissue under cortisol's effect. Cortisol also enhances oxidation of fatty acids in the cells. In times of starvation or other stress, these two effects help shift metabolic systems to the use of fatty acids instead of glucose for energy. Excess cortisol results in a distinctive obesity, with chest, abdominal, interscapular, and facial fat expansion, leading to a "buffalo-like" torso and "moon facies."[83-85]

Effect on Inflammation and Immunity. Cortisol can diminish the body's inflammatory responses by suppressing proinflammatory cytokines. Migration of white blood cells into the inflamed area is also decreased. At pharmacologic doses, cortisol stabilizes lysosomal membranes and decreases antibody production.[83] These effects are the basis for therapeutic use of corticosteroids to reduce inflammatory responses associated with asthma, allergic reactions, and other inflammatory disorders.

Cortisol decreases the number of eosinophils and lymphocytes in the blood. T lymphocyte and antibody output are decreased

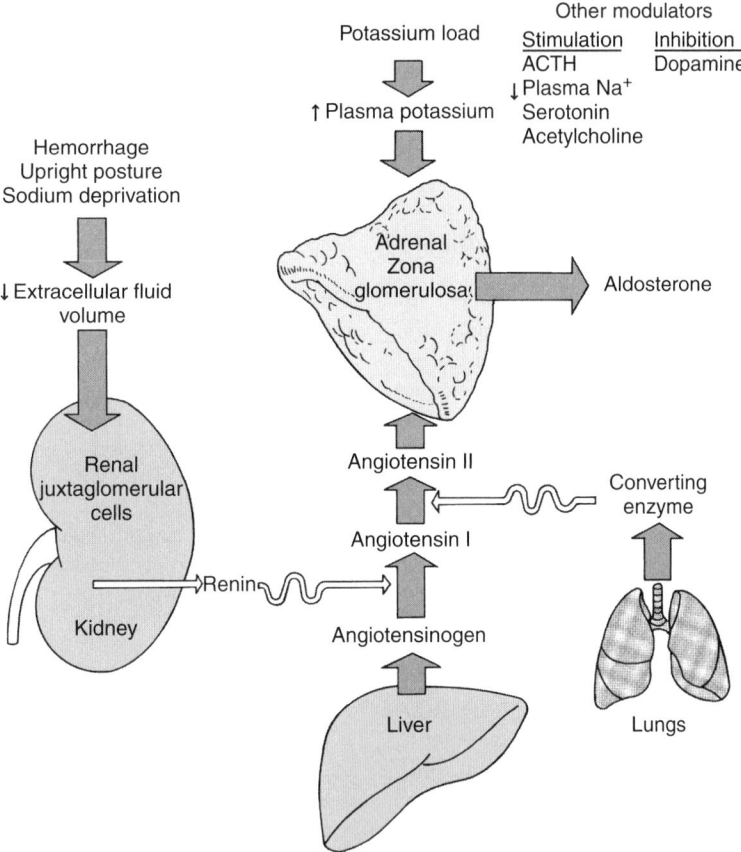

FIGURE **34-14** Regulation of aldosterone secretion. Hyperkalemia and activation of the renin-angiotensin system in response to hypovolemia are the predominant stimuli to aldosterone production. Adrenocorticotropin hormone (ACTH) has a minor tonic stimulatory effect. (*From Berne RM et al, eds. Physiology. 5th ed. St Louis: Mosby; 2004:905.*)

from the atrophy of lymphoid tissue. As a result, with pharmacologic doses of cortisol, the level of immunity to foreign invaders of the body is reduced, and infection may ensue from infection that would otherwise not be pathologic. The ability of cortisol and other glucocorticoids to suppress immunity makes exogenous administration of these hormones useful in preventing the immunologic rejection of transplanted organs and in treating several autoimmune disorders.

Mineralocorticoids. *Mineralocorticoids* are required for life. They play a major role in the regulation of extracellular sodium and potassium ion concentrations and total body fluid balance. *Aldosterone* is the body's principal mineralocorticoid. It is secreted from the zona glomerulosa, the thin zone of cells on the surface of the adrenal cortex. In large part, this zone functions autonomously of the other two adrenal cortex zones. Most distinctly, control of aldosterone secretion from the zona glomerulosa is relatively independent of ACTH control (Figure 34-14). Following secretion from the adrenal cortex, aldosterone circulates 60% bound to serum proteins; it reaches its target sites within 30 minutes.

The four main physiologic stimulants of aldosterone release are, in order of importance[86]:

1. Hyperkalemia
2. Angiotensin II (activation of the renin-angiotensin system)
3. Hyponatremia
4. ACTH

With a total loss of mineralocorticoid secretion, death would ensue within days without treatment.[84,85]

Aldosterone Functions. One of our body's most significant protectors of volume status is the renin-angiotensin-aldosterone system. Renin is a proteolytic enzyme released from the *juxtaglomerular cells* of the kidney afferent arteriole in response to hypovolemia, sympathetic nervous system stimulation, hypotension, or hyponatremia[87,88]. Renin acts on the plasma protein angiotensinogen to form angiotensin I (a 10–amino acid peptide), which is acted on by *angiotensin-converting enzyme* (primarily in the lung) to form angiotensin II (an 8–amino acid peptide). Angiotensin II is an extremely powerful vasoconstrictor and a potent stimulus of aldosterone synthesis and release.

Aldosterone's primary target cells are *principal cells*, located in the kidney distal convoluted tubules and cortical collecting ducts. Here, aldosterone causes the reabsorption of Na^+ from the tubular fluid and in exchange, secretion of K^+ (or H^+) into the tubular fluid for excretion. Aldosterone's effect on the extracellular sodium ion *concentration* is limited because simultaneous with the Na^+ absorption is absorption of nearly equivalent amounts of water. Sodium and water reabsorption expands the extracellular fluid volume and elevates arterial blood pressure.

Aldosterone's action on sweat and salivary glands is similar to that on renal tubules. The effect on sweat glands is important in hot environments, where body salt conservation is needed.

Disorders Associated with the Adrenal Cortex

An excess or deficiency of corticosteroids is associated with distinctive clinical syndromes.

Primary Aldosteronism. J.W. Conn described the first case of primary mineralocorticoid excess in 1954, a year after the biochemical composition of aldosterone was identified.[86] *Conn syndrome*, the most common form of *primary aldosteronism*, results from hypersecretion of aldosterone from an adrenal adenoma independent of stimulus. Primary aldosteronism may also be caused by adrenocortical hyperplasia or rarely carcinoma.[83] An increase in the plasma concentration of aldosterone and an increase in the urinary excretion of potassium with coexisting hypokalemia are pathognomonic of hyperaldosteronism.[83]

Manifestations of the syndrome reflect the exaggerated effects of aldosterone. Diastolic hypertension and hypernatremia are usually present. Aldosterone's action of promoting renal excretion of K^+ (or H^+) in exchange for Na^+ results in hypokalemic metabolic alkalosis. Hypertension associated with Conn syndrome results from aldosterone-induced sodium retention and subsequent increase in extracellular fluid volume.[87,88] Primary aldosteronism accounts for approximately 1% of all cases of hypertension.[83]

Primary aldosteronism is associated with low renin levels, a result of the elevated blood pressure's negative feedback to the juxtaglomerular cells. With *secondary hyperaldosteronism* the stimulus of excess aldosterone resides outside of the adrenal gland and is often associated with an increase in circulating renin levels.[83]

Treatment. Treatment of primary aldosteronism involves surgical removal of the adenoma or medical management. Surgical intervention is more successful for primary aldosteronism caused by adrenocortical adenoma than for gland hyperplasia because adenomas are almost always unilateral. When the affected adrenal gland is removed, the patient is cured in most cases. For patients with adrenal hyperplasia, medical management has been used successfully to treat primary aldosteronism.[83,89,90]

Management of Anesthesia. Preoperative management of the patient with Conn syndrome includes correcting electrolyte and blood glucose levels and managing hypertension.[8,11] Potassium should be replaced slowly to allow for equilibration of intracellular and extracellular potassium stores. Hypokalemia may alter nondepolarizing muscle relaxant responses, making peripheral nerve stimulation monitoring especially valuable. Electrocardiographic signs of potassium depletion include prominent U waves and arrhythmias. Plasma electrolyte concentrations and acid-base status should be checked often during the perioperative period. Inadvertent hyperventilation may further decrease plasma potassium concentration.

Hypertension may be controlled preoperatively with sodium restriction and aldosterone antagonists such as spironolactone.[7,91,92] Spironolactone, 25 to 100 mg every 8 hours, slowly increases potassium levels by inhibiting the action of aldosterone on the distal convoluted tubule. Patients with primary aldosteronism have a higher incidence of left ventricular hypertrophy, albuminuria, and stroke than patients with essential hypertension.[83,91,92] Measurement of cardiac filling pressures may be needed to assess fluid volume status in the perioperative period.[8]

Laparoscopic adrenalectomy is currently advocated as the operation of choice for surgically remediable mineralocorticoid excess. Compared with open laparotomy, patients who undergo laparoscopic adrenalectomy have similar improvement in blood pressure control and correction of hypokalemia.[93-95]

Glucocorticoid Excess (Cushing Syndrome). *Cushing syndrome* is a diverse complex of symptoms, signs, and biochemical abnormalities caused by excess glucocorticoid hormone. Clinical features reflect cortisol excess, either from overproduction of the adrenal cortex or exogenously administered glucocorticoid. The clinical picture includes central obesity with thin extremities, hypertension, glucose intolerance, plethoric facies, purple striae, muscle weakness, bruising, and osteoporosis.[84] Mineralocorticoid effects include fluid retention and hypokalemic alkalosis. Women manifest a degree of masculinization (hirsutism, hair thinning, acne, amenorrhea), and men manifest a degree of feminization (gynecomastia, impotence) due to androgenic effects of glucocorticoid excess. The catabolic effects of cortisol result in skin that is thin, atrophic, and unable to withstand the stresses of normal activity. Patients with Cushing syndrome typically gain weight and develop a characteristic redistribution of fat.[96,97]

The most common cause of Cushing syndrome today is the administration of supraphysiologic doses of glucocorticoids for conditions such as arthritis, asthma, various autoimmune disorders, allergies, and myriad other diseases.[9,98,99]

Endogenous Cushing syndrome is most often the result of one of three distinct pathogenic disorders: pituitary tumor (Cushing disease), adrenal tumor, or ectopic hormone production.

Cushing disease specifically denotes an anterior pituitary tumor cause of the syndrome. The pituitary tumor produces excessive amounts of ACTH and is associated with bilateral adrenal hyperplasia.[83] Patients often develop skin pigmentation as a result of excess ACTH. Cushing disease is the most common cause of endogenous Cushing syndrome.[88]

Adrenal Cushing syndrome is caused by autonomous corticosteroid production (ACTH-independent) by an adrenal tumor, usually unilateral. This form of hyperadrenalism accounts for 20% to 25% of patients with Cushing syndrome and is usually associated with suppressed plasma ACTH levels.[83,84] Adrenal tumors that are malignant are usually large by the time Cushing syndrome becomes manifest.[96,97]

Ectopic Cushing syndrome results from autonomous ACTH and/or CRH production by extrapituitary malignancies, producing markedly elevated plasma levels of ACTH. Bronchogenic carcinoma accounts for most of these cases. Carcinoid tumors and malignant tumors of the kidney, ovary, and pancreas also can cause ectopic production of ACTH.[83]

Diagnosis. A widely used test for the diagnosis of hyperadrenocorticism is measurement of the plasma cortisol concentration in the morning after a dose of dexamethasone. Dexamethasone suppresses plasma cortisol secretion in normal patients but not in those with endogenous hyperadrenocorticism. Diagnosis of Cushing syndrome is also based on elevated levels of plasma and urinary cortisol, plasma ACTH, and urinary 17-hydroxycorticosteroids.[8,89]

Treatment. Treatment for Cushing syndrome depends on the cause.[98,99] Transsphenoidal hypophysectomy is a primary treatment option for Cushing disease. Complications occur in less than 5% of patients and include diabetes insipidus (usually transient), cerebrospinal fluid rhinorrhea, and hemorrhage.[99]

Adrenal Cushing syndrome may be treated by surgical removal of the adrenal adenoma. Because the contralateral adrenal gland is preoperatively suppressed, glucocorticoid replacement may be necessary for several months after surgery until adrenal function returns. Bilateral adrenalectomy in the patient with Cushing syndrome is associated with a high incidence of complications and permanent corticosteroid deficiency.[98,100]

The treatment of choice for an ectopic ACTH-secreting tumor is surgical removal, but this may not always be feasible because of the nature of the underlying process (e.g., metastatic carcinoma). Metyrapone, an 11-β-hydroxylase inhibitor, and mitotane, an agent that blocks steroidogenesis at several levels, may be used to help normalize cortisol levels.[83]

Management of Anesthesia. Important perioperative considerations for the patient with Cushing syndrome include normalizing blood pressure, blood glucose levels, intravascular fluid volume, and electrolyte concentrations.[7,9,11,14] The aldosterone antagonist spironolactone effectively decreases extracellular fluid volume and corrects hypokalemia under these conditions.

Osteopenia is an important consideration in positioning the patient for the operative procedure. Special attention must be given to the patient's skin, which can easily be abraded by tape or minor trauma. Glucocorticoids are lympholytic and immunosuppressive, placing the patient at increased risk for infection and mandating particular enforcement of aseptic techniques as indicated.[83]

The choice of drugs for induction and maintenance of anesthesia is not specifically influenced by the presence of hyperadrenocorticism.[8] Muscle relaxants may have a more exaggerated effect in patients with preexisting myopathy, and a conservative approach to dosing is warranted when significant skeletal muscle weakness is present.

If adrenal resection is planned, glucocorticoids may be indicated postresection, administered at doses equivalent to adrenal output for maximum stress (hydrocortisone, 100 mg IV, followed by 100 to 200 mg IV over 24 hours, and then reduced over 3 to 6 days postoperatively until a maintenance dose is reached).

Thromboembolic phenomena occur more frequently in patients with Cushing syndrome, with an 11% incidence of deep venous thrombosis and a 2% to 3% incidence of pulmonary embolus postoperatively. The thromboembolic events are believed to be secondary to the prevalence of obesity, hypertension, elevated hematocrit, and increased factor VIII levels.[101,102]

Primary Adrenocortical Insufficiency (Addison Disease). In 1855, an English physician, Dr. Thomas Addison, first described a relatively rare clinical syndrome characterized by wasting and skin hyperpigmentation and identified its cause as destruction of the adrenal glands. *Primary adrenocortical insufficiency (Addison disease)* becomes apparent when 90% of the gland is destroyed. Tuberculosis is a common cause of primary adrenocortical insufficiency worldwide, but in the United States, most cases are the result of autoimmune dysfunction.[83] Primary adrenocortical insufficiency may also be associated with other autoimmune disorders, such as type 1 diabetes and Hashimoto thyroiditis. Less commonly, primary adrenal insufficiency is congenital or caused by sarcoidosis, human immunodeficiency virus infection, adrenal hemorrhage, malignancy, or trauma.[103,104]

Clinical symptoms of Addison disease reflect destruction of all cortical zones, resulting in adrenal androgen, glucocorticoid, and mineralocorticoid hormone deficiency (Box 34-6).

Weakness and fatigue are cardinal features. Reduced appetite with weight loss, vomiting, abdominal pain, and diarrhea are frequently reported. Hypoglycemia is often present.[103,104]

Volume depletion is a common feature of the disease and may be manifested by orthostatic hypotension. Hyponatremia and hyperkalemia are commonly revealed by laboratory screening.[103,104]

The adrenal-pituitary axis is intact in primary adrenal insufficiency, and ACTH concentrations are elevated as a result of the reduced production of cortisol. Increased melanin formation in the skin and hyperpigmentation of the knuckles of the fingers, toes, knees, elbows, lips, and buccal mucosa may be evident.

Treatment. Treatment for adrenal insufficiency aims to replace both glucocorticoid and mineralocorticoid deficiency.[83] Normal adults secrete 15 to 30 mg of cortisol (hydrocortisone) and 50 to 250 mcg of aldosterone per day (Table 34-7). Corticosteroids used for therapy have varying degrees of mineralocorticoid and glucocorticoid effects (Table 34-8).[83,85]

A typical oral replacement dose for Addison disease may consist of prednisone, 5 mg in the morning and 2.5 mg in the evening, or hydrocortisone, 20 mg in the morning and 10 mg in the evening. If indicated, mineralocorticoid replacement may

---

BOX 34-6

Clinical Features of Primary Adrenocortical Insufficiency

Asthenia
Weakness
Anorexia
Hypoglycemia
Hypotension
Hyponatremia
Nausea
Vomiting
Abdominal pain
Mucosal and skin pigmentation
Weight loss
Hyperkalemia

TABLE **34-7**	Physiologic Effects of Endogenous Corticosteroids			
Corticosteroid	**Daily Secretion (mg)**	**Mineralocorticoid Effect***	**Glucocorticoid Effect***	**Antiinflammatory Effect***
Aldosterone	0.125	3000	0	Insignificant
Desoxycorticosterone		100	0	0
Cortisol	20	1	1	1
Corticosterone	Minimal	15	0.35	0.3
Cortisone	Minimal	0.8	0.8	0.8

Adapted from Stoelting RK, Hillier SC. Pharmacology and Physiology in Anesthetic Practice. 4th ed. Philadelphia: Lippincott Williams & Wilkins; 2006:809.
*Relative to cortisol.

TABLE **34-8**	Comparative Pharmacology of Endogenous and Synthetic Corticosteroids				
	Common Name	**Glucocorticoid Effect***	**Mineralocorticoid Effect***	**Equivalent Dose (mg)**	**Duration of Action (hr)**
Cortisol	Hydrocortisone	1	1	20	8-12
Cortisone	Cortone	0.8	0.8	25	8-36
Prednisolone	Prelone	4	0.8	5	12-36
Prednisone	Deltasone	4	0.8	5	18-36
Methylprednisolone	Medrol, SoluMedrol	5	0.5	4	12-36
Betamethasone	Diprosone, Celestone	25	0	0.75	36-54
Dexamethasone	Decadron	25	0	0.75	36-54
Triamcinolone	Aristocort, Kenalog	5	0	4	12-36
Fludrocortisone	Florinef	10	250	2	24

Modified from Stoelting RK, Hillier SC. Pharmacology and Physiology in Anesthetic Practice. 4th ed. Philadelphia: Lippincott Williams & Wilkins; 2006:462.
*Relative to cortisol.

consist of 0.05 to 0.2 mg/day of fludrocortisone.[7,8] Standard glucocorticoid doses should be supplemented during periods of surgical stress (see Perioperative Steroid Replacement).

Secondary Adrenocortical Insufficiency. Secondary adrenocortical insufficiency is caused by ACTH deficiency from two primary etiologies: (1) hypothalamic-pituitary-adrenal (HPA) axis suppression after exogenous glucocorticoid therapy, and (2) ACTH deficiency secondary to hypothalamic or pituitary gland dysfunction (tumor, infection, surgical or radiologic ablation). Long-term treatment with glucocorticoids for any cause results in negative feedback to the hypothalamus and pituitary, decreased ACTH output, and eventual adrenal cortex atrophy.[104] The longer the duration of glucocorticoid administration, the greater the likelihood of suppression, but the precise dose or duration of therapy that produces adrenal suppression is unknown. Sustained and clinically important adrenal suppression usually does not occur with treatment periods less than 14 days. Treatment periods long enough to provoke signs of Cushing syndrome are usually associated with adrenal suppression of clinical importance.[7,104,105]

Clinical manifestations of secondary adrenal insufficiency resemble the primary disease, except secondary insufficiency is less likely to be associated with severe hypovolemia, hyperkalemia, or hyponatremia because mineralocorticoid secretion is usually preserved.[8,105] Hyperpigmentation is absent because ACTH levels are low.

Acute Adrenal Crisis. Acute adrenal crisis is a sudden exacerbation or onset of severe adrenal insufficiency. It is a rare event associated with high morbidity and mortality if allowed to progress unrecognized.[106,107] A patient with chronic adrenal insufficiency may deteriorate rapidly into an acute insufficiency state as a result of some superimposed stress, such as infection, acute illness, or sepsis. The stress of surgery or trauma in the patient with inadequate adrenal reserves can precipitate acute adrenal crisis in the perioperative period.[11,106,107]

Symptoms of adrenal crisis reflect acute deficiency of corticosteroids and include severe weakness, nausea, hypotension, fever, and decreasing mental status. In the surgical setting, hemodynamic instability or cardiovascular collapse may herald adrenal crisis. The index of suspicion for adrenal crisis should be particularly high if the patient has hyperpigmentation,

hyponatremia, and/or hyperkalemia; a history of autoimmune disease (hypothyroidism, diabetes); or recent prior use of exogenous steroids.[103,104,106,107] The anesthetist should be mindful of the adrenal suppressive effects of etomidate. Even a single dose of etomidate for induction of anesthesia can cause acute adrenocortical insufficiency and should be avoided in patients susceptible to adrenal insufficiency.[108]

Acute adrenal crisis is a medical emergency requiring aggressive treatment of the steroid insufficiency and associated hypoglycemia, electrolyte imbalance, and volume depletion. Early recognition and intervention are crucial steps in altering the course of acute adrenal insufficiency. Initial therapy begins with rapid intravenous administration of a glucose-containing isotonic crystalloid solution.[106,107] If the patient is hemodynamically unstable, advanced hemodynamic monitoring and inotropic support may be necessary. Steroid replacement therapy begins with hydrocortisone, 100 mg IV, followed by hydrocortisone, 100 to 200 mg IV over 24 hours. Mineralocorticoid administration is unnecessary with large doses of steroids (hydrocortisone 100 to 200 mg) because mineralocorticoid effects are present at these doses.[83]

Perioperative Steroid Replacement. Case reports of perioperative cardiovascular collapse in surgical patients on supraphysiologic doses of glucocorticoids were first reported in 1952.[109] These reports and subsequent knowledge regarding the stress response associated with surgery and the suppression of the HPA-axis with supraphysiologic doses of corticosteroids has led to the practice of administering perioperative glucocorticoids to patients who have taken steroids in the preoperative period.

Several reports have suggested that clinically important suppression of the HPA axis is uncommon and that levels of glucocorticoids required for surgical stress are much lower than previously believed.[8,109-111] Debate exists regarding who should receive perioperative steroid coverage, what the appropriate steroid dose should be, and the time period for recovery of normal HPA-axis responsiveness.

Patients who have received pharmacologic doses of glucocorticoids (greater than 5 mg prednisone-equivalent per day) for more than 2 weeks during the 12 months before surgery may have HPA-axis suppression.[11,101] Under these circumstances, inadequate perioperative replacement of corticosteroids can

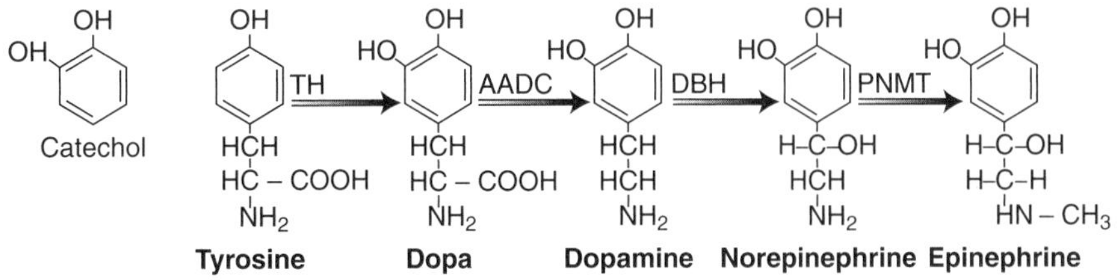

FIGURE **34-15** Biosynthetic pathway for catecholamines. The term *catecholamines* comes from the catechol (ortho-dihydroxybenzene) structure and a side chain with an amino group—the "catechol nucleus" (*left*). Tyrosine is converted to 3,4-dihydroxphenylanine (dopa) (rate-limiting step) by tyrosine hydroxylase (TH); TH inhibitor, α-methyl-para-tyrosine (metyrosine). Aromatic L-amino acid decarboxylase (AADC) converts dopa to dopamine. Dopamine is hydroxylated to norepinephrine by dopamine β-hydroxylase (DBH). Norepinephrine is converted to epinephrine by phenylethanolamine N-methyltransferase (PNMT); cortisol serves as a cofactor for PNMT, which is why epinephrine-secreting pheochromocytomas are almost exclusively localized to the adrenal medulla. (*From Kronenberg HM et al, eds.* Williams Textbook of Endocrinology. *11th ed. Philadelphia: Saunders; 2008:506.*)

lead to adrenal crisis and death.[106,107] The benefits of perioperative steroid supplementation are tempered by the potentially negative effects of decreased glucose tolerance, induction of stress ulcers, infection, and impaired wound healing. Because acute adrenal crisis is life threatening, most clinicians believe that the potential risks associated with short-term glucocorticoid administration are outweighed by the benefits.[7,8,11]

The adrenal glands secrete 116 to 185 mg of cortisol per day in the perioperative period in response to stress.[11] In general, major surgery of long duration produces a greater adrenal output response than minor surgery of short duration. For the adult patient who has received supraphysiologic doses of glucocorticoids (oral, topical, or inhaled) during the year preceding surgery, supplemental intravenous administration of hydrocortisone is advocated to compensate for the amount the body manufactures in response to maximal stress.[7,109-111] A common perioperative protocol for major surgical stress is the administration of hydrocortisone, 100 mg IV at induction, followed by 100 to 200 mg IV over 24 hours. A more recently proposed "low-dose" regimen calls for hydrocortisone, 25 mg IV at induction, followed by hydrocortisone, 100 mg IV infusion over the next 24 hours.[8] If the surgical patient is undergoing treatment with glucocorticoids at the time of surgery, supplemental doses are administered in addition to the patient's daily maintenance dose.[11] Therapeutic aims are to tailor the steroid dose considering the length and severity of surgical stress, while administering the minimal dose that will fully protect the patient.[105,111]

Adrenal Medulla

The adrenal medulla is a catecholamine-producing endocrine gland that is derived embryologically from neuroectodermal cells. The gland is enervated by preganglionic cholinergic fibers of the sympathetic nervous system and can be thought of as analogous to a postganglionic neuron. Preganglionic fibers bypass the paravertebral ganglia and run directly from the spinal cord to the adrenal medulla. Epinephrine accounts for approximately 80% of the hormone secreted by the adrenal medulla, and norepinephrine accounts for 20%. The majority of norepinephrine synthesized in the adrenal medulla is converted to epinephrine by the enzyme *phenylethanolamine-N-methyltransferase*. The ability of the adrenal medulla to synthesize epinephrine is probably influenced by the flow of glucocorticoid-rich blood from the cortex through the medulla because high concentrations of glucocorticoids stimulate the enzyme (Figure 34-15). Catecholamines in the adrenal medulla are stored in chromaffin granules.[112]

Stimulation of the sympathetic nerves to the adrenal medulla causes large quantities of epinephrine and norepinephrine to be released into the circulation. The effects of circulating epinephrine and norepinephrine are similar to the effects of direct sympathetic stimulation but last 5 to 10 times longer because of the slow removal of these hormones from the blood. Norepinephrine and epinephrine are metabolized in the liver and kidney by the enzyme *catechol-O-methyltransferase*. The by-products of metabolism, vanillylmandelic acid (VMA) and metanephrines, and free unchanged catecholamines are excreted in the urine (Figure 34-16).[7,112]

Norepinephrine stimulates α- and β-adrenergic receptors. It causes constriction of most blood vessels of the body, increasing total peripheral resistance. High circulating norepinephrine levels increase the heart's activity, inhibit gastrointestinal function, and dilate the pupils. Epinephrine has a greater affinity for β-adrenergic receptors. Its actions are seen primarily in the heart, producing chronotropic and inotropic effects. Epinephrine causes less constriction of blood vessels than norepinephrine. Norepinephrine and epinephrine release from the adrenal medulla can increase the metabolic rate of the body by as much as 100% above normal.

Pheochromocytoma

In 1905, the term *pheochromocytoma* was first used to describe the appearance of a tumor noted during autopsy resection to be a dusky (*pheo*) color (*chromo*). Cesar Roux of Lausanne, Switzerland, and Charles Mayo of the United States were the first surgeons to successfully remove a pheochromocytoma (Figure 34-17).

Pheochromocytomas are catecholamine-secreting tumors derived most commonly from adrenomedullary chromaffin cells. The tumors synthesize, store, and secrete catecholamines, mostly norepinephrine and epinephrine. Unlike a normal adrenal medulla, most of these tumors predominantly secrete norepinephrine. In the majority of cases, however, it is impossible to predict the precise catecholamine secretion from the clinical features. The tumors are not innervated, and neural stimulation does not stimulate hormone release.[113]

Pheochromocytomas are sometimes broadly defined as following the "rule of 10s." They involve both adrenal glands in 10% of adult patients with the tumor, approximately 10% of the tumors arise from extraadrenal chromaffin cells, approximately 10% of the tumors are in children (Tables 34-9 and 34-10), and malignant spread of pheochromocytomas occurs in less than 10%

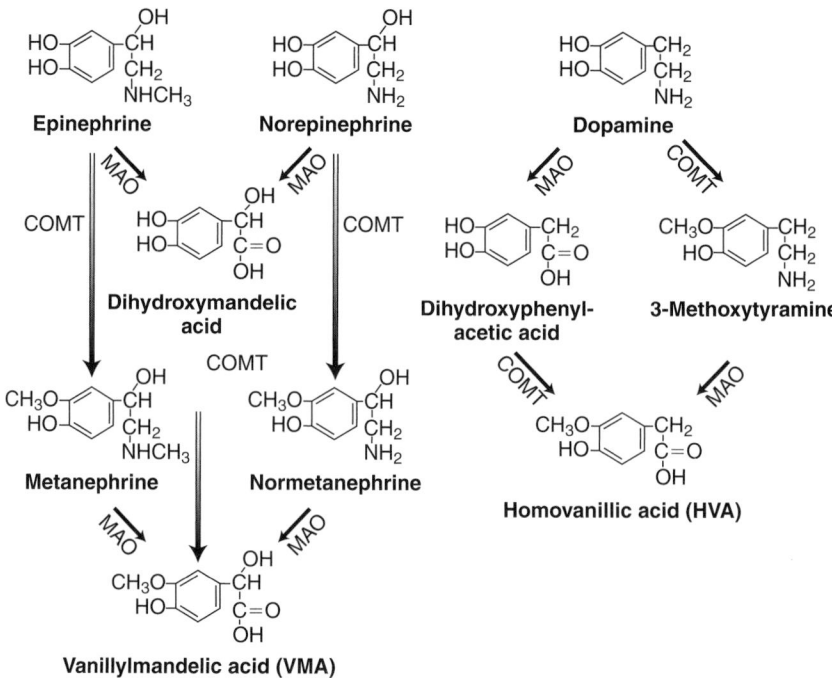

FIGURE **34-16** Catecholamine metabolism. Metabolism of catecholamines occurs through two enzymatic pathways. Catechol-O-methyltransferase (COMT) converts epinephrine to metanephrine and converts norepinephrine to normetanephrine by meta-O-methylation. Metanephrine and normetanephrine are oxidized by monoamine oxidase (MAO) to vanillylmandelic acid (VMA) by oxidative deamination. MAO also may oxidize epinephrine and norepinephrine to dihydroxymandelic acid, which is then converted by COMT to VMA. Dopamine is also metabolized by MAO and COMT to the final metabolite homovanillic acid (HVA). (*Modified and redrawn from Dluhy RG, Lawrence JE, Williams GH. Endocrine hypertension. In: Larsen PR, et al. Williams Textbook of Endocrinology, 10th ed. Philadelphia: Saunders; 2003:555*).

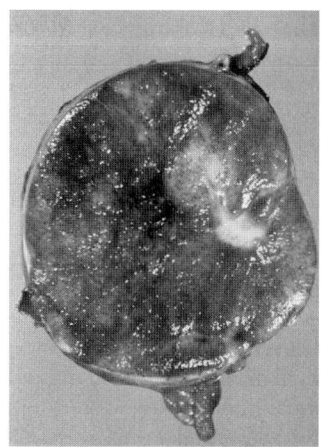

FIGURE **34-17** Pheochromocytoma of the adrenal gland. (*Courtesy of Dr. Terri L. Johnson, Department of Pathology, Henry Ford Hospital, Detroit, Michigan.*)

TABLE **34-10**	Locations of Extraadrenal Pheochromocytomas	
Location		**%**
Cervical		2
Thoracic		10-20
Intraabdominal		70-80
Upper abdomen		40
Organ of Zuckerkandl		30
Bladder		15

From Landsberg L, Young JB. Catecholamines and the adrenal medulla. In: Wilson JD, Foster DW, eds. Williams Textbook of Endocrinology. 9th ed. Philadelphia: Saunders; 1998:707.

TABLE **34-9**	Locations of Pheochromocytomas		
	Percentage		
Location	**Total**	**Familial**	**Children**
Solitary adrenal	80	<50	50
Extraadrenal	10	<10	25
Bilateral adrenal	10	>50	25

From Landsberg L, Young JB. Catecholamines and the adrenal medulla. In: Wilson JD, Foster DW, eds. Williams Textbook of Endocrinology. 9th ed. Philadelphia: Saunders; 1998:707.

of cases.[113] Malignant pheochromocytomas are more often extraadrenal and secrete norepinephrine exclusively[114]; metastasis usually proceeds via venous and lymphatic channels to the liver.[113]

Diagnostic tests for detecting a catecholamine tumor include measurements of urinary or plasma catecholamines and their metabolites, vanillylmandelic acid and metanephrine. Free norepinephrine measurement in a 24-hour urine sample is a sensitive index of pheochromocytoma (Table 34-11).

Incidence and Associated Diseases. Pheochromocytomas are rare, occurring in approximately 0.1% of hypertensive patients.[113,115] These tumors may be associated with neurocutaneous syndromes such as von Hippel-Lindau disease, tuberous sclerosis, and Sturge-Weber syndrome. The tumors may also be a component of multiple endocrine neoplasia (MEN) type 2A or 2B[116,117] (Table 34-12). Patients with a family history of MEN

TABLE **34-11**	Values for Catecholamines and Catecholamine Metabolites
Hormone/Metabolite	**Normal Value**
Vanillylmandelic acid, urine	2-7 mg/24 hr
Metanephrines, urine	<1.3 mg/24 hr
Norepinephrine, urine	<100 mcg/24 hr
Norepinephrine, plasma	150-450 pg/mL
Epinephrine, plasma	<35 pg/mL
Catecholamines, free urinary	<110 mcg/24 hr

TABLE **34-12**	Manifestations of Multiple Endocrine Neoplasia*
Syndrome	**Manifestations**
MEN type 1 (Wermer syndrome)	Hyperparathyroidism, pituitary adenomas, pancreatic islet-cell tumors
MEN type 2A (Sipple syndrome)	Medullary thyroid cancer, hyperparathyroidism, pheochromocytoma
MEN type 2B (mucosal neuroma syndrome)	Medullary thyroid tumor, pheochromocytoma, neuromas of the oral mucosa, marfanoid habitus

Multiple endocrine neoplasia (MEN) is a group of rare diseases caused by genetic defects that lead to hyperplasia and hyperfunction of two or more components of the endocrine system.

TABLE **34-13**	Frequency of Symptoms in 100 Patients with Pheochromocytoma		
Symptom	**%**	**Symptom**	**%**
Headache	80	Chest pain	19
Excessive perspiration	71	Dyspnea	19
Palpitation (with or without tachycardia)	64	Flushing or warmth	18
Pallor	42	Numbness or paresthesia	11
Nausea (with or without vomiting)	42	Blurring of vision	11
Tremor or trembling	31	Tightness of throat	8
Weakness or exhaustion	28	Dizziness or faintness	8
Nervousness or anxiety	22	Convulsions	5
Epigastric pain	22	Neck-shoulder pain	5
		Extremity pain	4
		Flank pain	4

From Landsberg L, Young JB. Catecholamines and the adrenal medulla. In: Wilson JD, Foster DW, eds. Williams Textbook of Endocrinology. 8th ed. Philadelphia: Saunders; 1998:706.

syndrome should be regularly screened for pheochromocytoma. Twenty-five percent of pheochromocytomas occur as part of an inherited autosomal dominant trait.[113]

Pheochromocytomas can occur at any age, but usually occur within the third to the fifth decade of life, with equal frequency in both sexes in adults.[7,9]

Clinical Manifestations. Manifestations of a pheochromocytoma reflect massive catecholamine release and include hypertension, diaphoresis, headache, tremors, and palpitations.[118] Hypertension may be paroxysmal or sustained.[113] The combination of paroxysmal diaphoresis, tachycardia, and headache in the hypertensive patient is a recognized triad of symptoms for pheochromocytoma.[7,8,11,115]

A catecholamine-mediated paroxysm typically consists of a sudden and alarming increase in blood pressure, a severe throbbing headache, profuse sweating, palpitations, tachycardia, a sense of doom, anxiety, pallor (rarely flushing), and nausea.[113] Orthostatic hypotension may result from plasma volume deficit or a lack of tone in the postural reflexes that defend upright blood pressure, due to the sustained excesses of catecholamines. Paroxysmal symptoms may last several minutes to days and are often followed by physical exhaustion. The frequencies of clinical symptoms associated with pheochromocytoma are outlined in Table 34-13.

A paroxysm may be triggered by abdominal palpation, defecation, or any event that provokes pressure on the tumor.[113] Micturition may trigger symptoms if the pheochromocytoma is present in the urinary bladder wall. In some patients, no clearly defined precipitating factor can be found. Mental or psychologic stress does not usually initiate a crisis.[113]

Owing to the predominance of norepinephrine secretion, the symptoms associated with a pheochromocytoma reflect α-adrenergic activity over β-adrenergic effects.[8] As a result of α-adrenergic inhibition of insulin and enhanced hepatic glucose output, hyperglycemia may be present. The cardiac output and heart rate may be significantly increased. An overall increase in metabolism accelerates oxygen consumption and can cause hyperthermia. Vasoconstriction in the extremities may produce pain, paresthesias, intermittent claudication, or ischemia.

Hypertension is the most common symptom, occurring in more than 90% of patients.[7,8] Severe paroxysmal hypertension is present in approximately 40% of patients and is a distinctive manifestation of the disease.[7,113] Sustained hypertension is often resistant to conventional treatment. When pheochromocytomas are predominantly epinephrine secreting, hypertension can alternate with periods of hypotension associated with syncope. Hypotension reflects surges of epinephrine, causing disproportionate β-adrenergic stimulation with vasodilation in the presence of a contracted vascular space.

A catecholamine-induced increase in myocardial oxygen consumption, hypertension, and coronary artery spasm can precipitate myocardial infarction or congestive heart failure even in the absence of coronary artery disease.[8,113] ECG changes are common. Nonspecific ST-segment and T-wave changes and prominent U waves may be seen.[8] Sinus tachycardia, supraventricular tachycardias, and premature ventricular contractions are commonly noted. Right and left bundle branch blocks and

| TABLE 34-14 | Drugs Used in the Management of Pheochromocytoma | | | |

Drug	Action	Pressor Crisis	Preoperative Blood Pressure Control	Comment
Phentolamine	α-Blocker	IV 2-5 mg	—	Rapid onset, short-acting; bolus every 5 min or infuse initially 1 mg/min^{-1}
Phenoxybenzamine	α-Blocker	—	Oral 30 mg·day^{-1}, increasing daily dosage by 30 mg	Long half-life; may accumulate; administer two or three times daily
Doxazosin	Selective α$_1$ antagonist	1 mg/day PO up to 8 mg/day PO	—	First-dose phenomenon; may cause syncope
Propanolol	β-Blocker	IV 1-mg bolus to total of 10 mg	Oral 40 mg bid; increase to 480 mg·day^{-1}	Should not be administered without first creating α blockade
Atenolol	β-Blocker	—	Oral 50 mg·day^{-1} initially; may increase to 100 mg·day^{-1}	Long-acting, selective β$_1$ antagonist eliminated unchanged by kidney
Esmolol	β-Blocker	IV 500 mcg/kg^{-1}/min^{-1} loading followed by maintenance infusion	—	Ultrashort-acting selective β$_1$ antagonist; may be used during anesthesia
Labetalol	α-and β-Blocker	IV 10-mg bolus to 150 mg	Oral 200 mg tid	A much weaker α-blocker than β-blocker; may cause pressor response in pheochromocytoma
Nitroprusside	Vasodilator	IV infusion initially 0.5-1.5 mcg/kg^{-1}/min^{-1}	—	Powerful vasodilator; short-acting; may be used during anesthesia
Magnesium sulfate	Vasodilator	IV 40-60 mg/kg^{-1} bolus followed by 2 g/hr^{-1} and additional 20 mg/kg^{-1} boluses as needed	—	May potentiate neuromuscular blockade
Nicardipine	Calcium channel blocker	IV 2-6 mcg/kg^{-1}/min^{-1}	—	Better vasodilator than diltiazem
α-Methyl-tyrosine	Inhibitor of biosynthesis of catecholamines	—	Oral 1-4 g·day^{-1}	Suitable for patients not amenable to surgery; may be nephrotoxic

Modified from Schwartz JJ, Rosenbaum S. Anesthesia and the endocrine system. In: Barash PG et al, eds. Clinical Anesthesia. 5th ed. Philadelphia: Lippincott; 2006:1143.
adm., *Administer*; IV, *intravenous*.

ventricular strain sometimes occur. Ventricular tachycardia also has been reported.[119-121]

Preoperative Management. The pharmacologic effects of released catecholamines present major anesthetic challenges. Medical management prior to tumor excision aims to reverse the effects of excessive adrenergic stimulation. Preoperative antihypertensive therapy and volume replacement have helped to decrease the surgical mortality rate from about 50% to the current 1% to 3%.[11] The preoperative use of α-adrenergic antagonists in concert with reexpansion of the intravascular fluid compartment greatly improves cardiovascular stability intraoperatively.[122,123] Myocardial infarction, congestive heart failure, cardiac dysrhythmias, and cerebral hemorrhage decrease in frequency when the patient has been treated preoperatively

with α-adrenergic receptor antagonists. Table 34-14 outlines drugs used in the management of pheochromocytoma.

α-Adrenergic Receptor Blockade. Phenoxybenzamine (Dibenzyline) is the drug of choice for preoperative α-adrenergic blockade and blood pressure stabilization. It is a noncompetitive presynaptic (α$_2$) and postsynaptic (α$_1$) adrenergic receptor antagonist of long duration (24 to 48 hours).[7] Most patients with pheochromocytoma require an oral dose between 60 and 250 mg/day.[11,113] Postural hypotension is a common side effect of treatment.

Typically, patients require 10 to 14 days of α-adrenergic antagonist therapy to stabilize blood pressure, restore fluid volume, and decrease symptoms. Establishing normotension facilitates reexpansion of the intravascular fluid compartment.

Satisfactory α-adrenergic blockade is implied if the hematocrit decreases by 5% during treatment.[8] Half to two thirds of the normal oral phenoxybenzamine dose may be given the morning of surgery.[11]

Prazocin (Minipress), a specific postsynaptic α₁-adrenergic receptor antagonist, has also been used successfully to treat the hypertension of pheochromocytoma preoperatively. Labetalol (Trandate, Normodyne), a mixed α- and β-receptor antagonist, has not been as effective as a first-line drug in controlling the blood pressure response, but it may be used as an adjunctive agent.[7,8,124]

β-Adrenergic Receptor Blockade. A β-adrenergic receptor antagonist is usually introduced in the preoperative period for control of tachycardia, hypertension, and catecholamine-induced supraventricular dysrhythmias. An important caveat is that β-adrenergic receptor antagonists should not be administered until after α-adrenergic blockade is established. Blocking β-receptor–mediated vasodilation in skeletal muscle without prior α-adrenergic blockade can increase the blood pressure even further in the patient with pheochromocytoma.[118]

Other Treatment Regimens. Calcium channel blockers and magnesium sulfate infusion have been used with variable success as monotherapy for the perioperative management of pheochromocytoma.[125] Some regimens use these agents in conjunction with adrenergic blocking drugs.

Metyrosine (Demser) is used for patients requiring long-term therapy—for instance, the patient for whom surgery is contraindicated.[123,126] The drug competitively inhibits catecholamine formation by blocking tyrosine hydroxylase, the rate-limiting enzyme in catecholamine synthesis.[113]

The following criteria are proposed as end-points for the patient awaiting surgery for pheochromocytoma resection[11]:

1. No in-hospital blood pressure reading higher than 160/90 mm Hg 24 hours prior to surgery.
2. No blood pressure on standing lower than 80/45 mm Hg.
3. No ST-segment or T-wave abnormality on the ECG that cannot be attributed to a permanent defect.
4. No marked symptoms of catecholamine excess; no more than one premature ventricular contraction every 5 minutes.

Anesthetic Management. Effective anesthetic management is based on (1) selecting drugs that do not stimulate catecholamine release and (2) implementing monitoring techniques that facilitate early and appropriate intervention when catecholamine-induced changes in cardiovascular function occur.[7]

Pheochromocytomas are excised by open laparotomy or laparoscopy.[127-131] Postoperative morbidity is similar with both approaches.[130,131] During pneumoperitoneum for laparoscopy, significant catecholamine release has been reported.[128]

A number of drugs and conditions can precipitate hypertension in the surgical patient with pheochromocytoma. Dopamine antagonists (metoclopramide, droperidol), radiographic contrast media, indirect-acting amines (ephedrine, methyldopa), drugs that block neuronal catecholamine reuptake (tricyclic antidepressants, cocaine), histamine, and glucagon may enhance the physiologic effect of tumor product.[8,113,132,133]

Pheochromocytomas are vascular tumors. Large-bore intravenous lines and a peripheral arterial catheter should be established preoperatively. A central venous pressure or pulmonary artery catheter should be placed to help guide fluid management and intervention with inotropes or vasoactive drugs.[7,8] Arterial blood gases, electrolyte concentrations, and blood glucose levels should be assessed regularly during the anesthetic.

Critical intraoperative junctures are (1) during induction and intubation of the trachea, (2) during surgical manipulation of the tumor, and (3) after ligation of the tumor's venous drainage.

Anesthesia induction may be accomplished with barbiturates, etomidate, or propofol. Anesthetic depth can be enhanced by mask ventilation of the lungs with a volatile anesthetic prior to laryngoscopy and intubation. Lidocaine (1 to 2 mg/kg IV) administered 1 minute prior to intubation may help attenuate the hemodynamic response to laryngoscopy. Rapid-acting vasodilating drugs such as nitroprusside should be readily available to treat hypertension.[8] Short-acting opioids, such as fentanyl or remifentanil, administered prior to intubation may also help blunt the blood pressure responses to intubation.[8] Morphine sulfate should be avoided because of its propensity for histamine release.

Sevoflurane and short-acting opioids (such as remifentanil) provide cardiovascular stability and possess the ability to rapidly change anesthetic depth—attractive features in the anesthetic management of the patient with pheochromocytoma.[7,8,11,134] The tachycardia associated with desflurane makes it a less desirable choice for these cases.

The use of succinylcholine has been questioned because compression of an abdominal tumor by drug-induced skeletal muscle fasciculations may provoke catecholamine release. However, a predictable adverse effect of succinylcholine has not been supported clinically when administered to patients with pheochromocytoma. Skeletal muscle paralysis with a nondepolarizing muscle relaxant devoid of vagolytic or histamine-releasing effects is desirable. Pancuronium should be avoided for its known chronotropic effect.[7,8,11]

The anesthetist should anticipate a labile cardiovascular course during surgery. Hypertension can be treated with intravenous nitroprusside and high concentrations of inhaled anesthetic.[7,8,11] Propranolol, lidocaine, labetalol, or esmolol may be given intravenously to decrease tachydysrhythmias. β-Adrenergic antagonists must be used cautiously in patients with catecholamine-induced cardiomyopathy because even minimal β-adrenergic blockade can accentuate left ventricular dysfunction.[7,8] The short half-life of esmolol makes it an advantageous choice for β-adrenergic blockade. Dysrhythmias associated with hypertension may be resolved by simply lowering an abnormally high blood pressure. Indirect-acting sympathomimetics have an unpredictable pressor effect in these patients and should be avoided.

After surgical ligation of the veins that drain a pheochromocytoma, the rapid decrease in circulating catecholamines and the associated downregulation of adrenergic receptors may precipitate a decrease in blood pressure.[135] During this juncture, close communication with the surgical team is important. Decreasing the inhaled anesthetic agent concentration and increasing the administration of intravenous crystalloid or colloid solution should adequately increase blood pressure. Intravenous administration of phenylephrine hydrochloride (Neo-Synephrine) or dopamine may be needed until the peripheral vasculature can adapt to the decreased level of endogenous α-stimulation.[8]

Hyperglycemia is common before excision of the pheochromocytoma. With tumor removal, the sudden withdrawal of catecholamine stimulation can result in hypoglycemia. Further, β-adrenergic blockade impairs hepatic glucose production. β-Adrenergic blockers may also mask hypoglycemic signs by preventing tachycardia and tremor. Blood glucose levels should be monitored at frequent intervals intraoperatively and postoperatively.

Some pheochromocytomas may first present as a hypermetabolic state during anesthesia for unrelated surgery.

The hypertension, tachycardia, hyperthermia, and respiratory acidosis of a pheochromocytoma may mimic light anesthesia, thyroid crisis, malignant hyperthermia, or sepsis.[118,136]

Postoperative Management. Fluid shifts, pain, hypoxia, hypercapnia, autonomic instability, urinary retention, or residual tumor are all causes of postoperative hypertension. Invasive monitoring is indicated during the initial postoperative period to assess blood pressure changes and cardiac status.[7,8] Fifty percent of patients remain hypertensive during the immediate postanesthesia recovery period, despite removal of the pheochromocytoma.[8] Transient hypertension postoperatively usually reflects fluid shifts and autonomic instability. Postoperative catecholamine levels decrease to normal over several days. In 75% of patients, normal blood pressure returns within 14 days postsurgery.[113]

Relief of postoperative pain can be accomplished with neuraxial opioids and may contribute to early tracheal extubation in otherwise healthy patients.

THYROID GLAND

The thyroid gland is an endocrine gland located anterior to the trachea between the cricoid cartilage and suprasternal notch. It produces and secretes two important thyroid hormones: 3,5,3-triiodothyronine (T_3) and thyroxine (T_4). The vascular supply to the gland is derived from the superior and inferior thyroid arteries. Blood flow is equivalent to about five times the weight of the gland, which is a blood supply as rich as almost any tissue in the body. The gland consists of two lobes and an isthmus. The recurrent laryngeal nerves run along the lateral borders of each thyroid lobe.

Microscopically, the thyroid is divided into lobules, each of which is composed of 20 to 40 follicles. The follicles are lined by epithelial cells that surround central deposits of a secretory substance called *colloid*. The major constituent of the colloid is a large glycoprotein called *thyroglobulin*, which serves as the backbone for the synthesis and storage of thyroid hormones.[137,138]

Synthesis of Thyroid Hormones
Iodide Trapping
Approximately 1 mg of ingested iodine is required each week to form normal quantities of thyroid hormones. Dietary iodine is then reduced in the gastrointestinal tract to *iodide*. Common table salt is iodized with sodium iodide for the prevention of iodine deficiency.

The first stage of thyroid hormone formation is the transport of iodides from the extracellular fluid into the thyroid cells and follicles. About one fifth of the circulating iodide is removed from the blood by the thyroid cells and used for the synthesis of thyroid hormones, a process called *iodide trapping*. The iodide pump normally concentrates the iodide to about 30 times its concentration in the blood. Iodide trapping is the rate-limiting step in thyroid hormone synthesis and is under the control of TSH from the anterior pituitary. Once inside the thyroid gland, iodide ions are oxidized back to iodine.

Thyroid Hormone Formation
Thyroid hormones are formed in the follicles of the thyroid gland under the control of TSH. Thyroglobulin contains the amino acid tyrosine, which combines with iodine to form various iodotyrosines, including the two major thyroid hormones. Thyroxine and triiodothyronine remain part of the thyroglobulin molecule, stored as colloid within the thyroid follicle until release. Enough hormone is synthesized and stored under basal conditions to

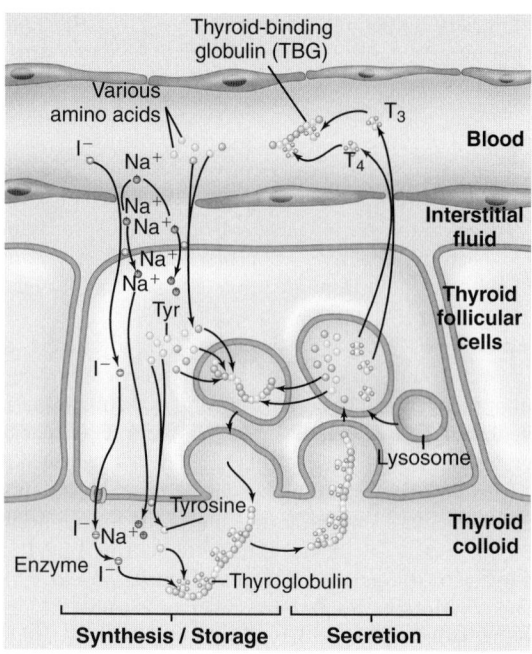

FIGURE **34-18** Thyroid hormone biosynthesis consists of four stages: (1) iodide trapping, (2) oxidation, (3) coupling, and (4) release and recycling. (*From Thibodeau GA, Patton KT. Anatomy & Physiology. 6th ed. St Louis: Mosby; 2007:615.*)

supply the body with its normal hormone requirements for 2 to 3 months.[137,138]

Although iodine is required for hormone synthesis, paradoxically, excess iodine can inhibit gland production of thyroid hormone.

Release of Thyroxine and Triiodothyronine
TSH controls the release of hormones from the thyroid gland. On release, T_4 and T_3 are cleaved from the thyroglobulin molecule and secreted into the circulating blood. Thyroglobulin remains within the colloid.

Under normal conditions, about 90% of the hormone released from the thyroid gland is T_4 and 10% T_3. The secretion of T_4 from the thyroid gland is 80 to 100 mcg/day. When thyroid hormones reach their target tissues, most of the T_4 is deiodinated to T_3, T_4 serving mostly as a hormone precursor. Triiodothyronine is more potent and less protein bound than T_4 and is the primary metabolically active hormone that stimulates target tissues. Figure 34-18 summarizes the biosynthesis and chemical structure of thyroid hormones.

Transport of Thyroxine and Triiodothyronine to Tissues
Thyroid hormone exists in circulation in both free and bound forms. The amount of free hormone, which is the metabolically active fraction, is extremely small, less than 0.03% of total circulating T_4 and 0.3% of total circulating T_3. The majority of circulating hormone (99.9%) is bound to thyroid-binding proteins. Eighty percent of thyroid hormones bind to the circulating protein *thyroxine-binding globulin* and the remainder to *transthyretin* and *albumin*.[139]

Because of the very high affinity of the plasma-binding proteins for thyroid hormones, the hormones are released to the tissue cells very slowly. The half-life of T_4 in the circulation is 6 to 7 days, and the half-life of T_3 is 24 to 30 hours.[9,137,138]

Functions of Thyroid Hormones
Increased Cellular Metabolic Activity
Thyroid hormones initiate protein formation in virtually all cells of the body. Consequently, the level of enzymes, structural proteins, transport proteins, and other substances increases considerably under the direction of T_4 and especially T_3. The net result is a generalized increase in metabolic activity, heat production, and oxygen consumption of all or almost all tissues in the body.[139,140] The basal metabolic rate can increase by as much as 60% to 100% above normal when large quantities of thyroid hormones are secreted. The rate and depth of respiration increase due to the enhanced metabolic rate and increased oxygen use and carbon dioxide formation by cells. The use of energy substrates is greatly accelerated. Protein synthesis is increased; however, protein catabolism also is increased. When the quantity of thyroid hormone is slightly increased, the muscles react with vigor; however, when the quantity is excessive, muscles become weakened from excess protein catabolism.

Effect of Thyroid Hormone on Growth
Thyroid hormones are necessary for normal growth in infants and children. In a hypothyroid state, the rate of tissue growth is greatly reduced. Thyroid hormone is required for normal growth and development of the brain during fetal life and for the first few years of postnatal life.[137,138]

Effect of Thyroid Hormone on Specific Systems
Thyroid hormones have a direct effect on the excitability of the heart by increasing the number of β-adrenergic receptors. The heart rate and the force of contraction are augmented with increasing thyroid hormone production.[141]

Thyroid hormones increase the rate of hormone secretion from most endocrine glands, especially the pancreas. The heightened cellular requirement for glucose mandates higher insulin secretion. Thyroid hormones also enhance the secretion of digestive juices and the motility of the gastrointestinal tract, in addition to increasing an individual's appetite and food intake. In adults, thyroid hormones enhance the rapidity of cerebration.

Regulation of Thyroid Hormone Secretion
Specific feedback mechanisms operate through the hypothalamus and anterior pituitary gland to precisely control the rate of thyroid secretion. Thyrotropin-releasing hormone (TRH) from the hypothalamus causes cells of the anterior pituitary lobe to produce and secrete TSH. TSH increases all known activities of thyroid gland cells, resulting in increased hormone synthesis and release. Circulating thyroid hormones inhibit the secretion of TSH and TRH through a negative feedback effect on the anterior pituitary lobe and hypothalamus.

Thyroid Gland Disorders
Thyrotoxicosis and Graves Disease
Hyperthyroidism is defined as thyroid gland hyperactivity. *Thyrotoxicosis* is more specifically defined as a state of thyroid hormone excess.[139] The most common cause of thyrotoxicosis in the United States is *Graves disease*. Graves disease is an autoimmune disease in which TSH-receptor antibodies bind to and stimulate the thyroid gland, causing excessive production and secretion of T_4 and T_3.[142] Immunoglobulin G (IgG) autoantibodies mimic the action of TSH, but their effects are longer, lasting up to 12 hours compared with 1 hour for normal TSH.[142]

The aberrant immunologic response associated with Graves disease targets primarily the thyroid gland but also other tissues, including extraocular muscles and skin. There is a familial tendency and a higher incidence of other autoimmune disorders in patients with Graves disease.[143] The disease occurs most often in women (prevalence 1% to 3% in women; 0.1% in men) and between 20 and 50 years of age.[139] Graves disease has an unpredictable course, marked by relapses and exacerbations.

Thyrotoxicosis can also be caused by benign follicular adenomas, which are not believed to have an autoimmune etiology. Exogenous iodine excess (radiocontrast agents or angiography dye) or the administration of thyroid hormones may induce iatrogenic thyrotoxicosis. The antiarrhythmic agent amiodarone is iodine rich and may cause either hypothyroidism or hyperthyroidism.[11,24,144] Toxic multinodular goiter, subacute viral thyroiditis, postpartum thyroiditis, TSH-secreting pituitary tumors, and thyroid cancer are less common causes of thyrotoxicosis.

Signs and Symptoms. Clinical manifestations associated with thyrotoxicosis reflect the widespread hypermetabolic effects of excess thyroid hormones. Physical signs include tachycardia, tremor, goiter, and muscle weakness. Sleep is often difficult. Weight loss (despite increased food consumption), anxiety, fatigue, and heat intolerance are symptoms of thyrotoxicosis.

Signs of ophthalmopathy and dermopathy are associated with Graves disease.[139] Thyroid-associated ophthalmopathy may cause proptosis, eye redness, and a gritty sensation in early stages, with diplopia, ocular pain, and (rarely) loss of visual acuity in more advanced stages. Graves ophthalmopathy results from cytokine-mediated inflammation and swelling of the periorbital connective tissue and extraocular muscles.[139]

The blood volume increases slightly under the influence of excess thyroid hormone, a result of vasodilation. Mean arterial pressure usually remains unchanged, but the pulse pressure increases. The systolic blood pressure is typically elevated 10 to 15 mm Hg, and the diastolic pressure is reduced. Blood flow to the skin increases in response to the increased need for heat elimination.

The effects of thyrotoxicosis on the heart are pronounced. Palpitations, tachycardia, and cardiac dysrhythmias affect most patients. The cardiac output increases, sometimes to 60% or more above normal. About 10% of thyrotoxic patients have atrial fibrillation. Mitral valve prolapse is more common in patients with Graves disease than in the general population. With protracted high thyroid hormone levels, heart muscle strength may become depressed due to protein catabolism. Diagnosis of thyrotoxicosis is more difficult in the elderly because many of the hyperkinetic manifestations of hyperthyroidism are absent.[145] Elderly patients may initially present with myocardial failure.[8]

The hyperthyroid individual may feel constant fatigue from the exhausting effect of thyroid hormone on the musculature and the central nervous system.

Diagnosis. The diagnosis of primary disease is biochemically established in most cases by the combined findings of an abnormally high total and unbound serum T_4 assay and depressed TSH levels. With Graves disease, the diagnosis may be supported by the presence of stimulatory TSH-receptor autoantibodies. An elevated uptake of radioactive iodine (^{131}I, ^{123}I) by the thyroid gland may be used to confirm gland hyperactivity. Serum alkaline phosphatase and calcium concentrations are mildly elevated in approximately 20% of patients with Graves disease.

Other autoimmune diseases such as myasthenia gravis, rheumatoid arthritis, systemic lupus erythematosus, and DM are more common in patients with Graves disease.

Treatment. A variety of treatment options are available for patients with Graves disease. The three primary treatment options for thyrotoxicosis are radioactive gland ablation, surgery, and antithyroid drug therapy.[139,143,146-149]

Radioactive Iodine. A common therapy for Graves disease is ablation of the thyroid gland with radioactive iodine (Na[131]I). Two to four months is needed to reverse the hyperthyroidism. Hypothyroidism is common following treatment. Use of Na[131]I is contraindicated in pregnancy.[143,149]

Subtotal Thyroidectomy. Surgery for treatment of Graves disease is an option when antithyroid drugs are ineffective, if radioiodine treatment is refused, in children or pregnant women, or if the thyroid goiter is exceptionally large. Patients should be treated preoperatively with antithyroid medication and rendered euthyroid prior to surgery. Complications associated with thyroid surgery occur in less than 1% of cases and include damage to the recurrent laryngeal nerve, hypoparathyroidism, and neck hematoma.

Antithyroid Drugs and β-Adrenergic Receptor Blockade. The main class of antithyroid medications is the *thionamides*, which include propylthiouracil (PTU), methimazole, and carbimazole. All thionamides inhibit thyroid hormone synthesis by interfering with the incorporation of iodine into tyrosine residues of thyroglobulin. PTU also inhibits conversion of T_4 to T_3. A euthyroid state is usually obtained in 6 to 7 weeks. Hepatitis and agranulocytosis are the most serious side effects of these drugs.

About 10 days before surgery, oral potassium iodide (SSKI, Lugol solution) is added to the course of therapy to decrease gland vascularity and block hormone synthesis and release. Propranolol is added to the antithyroid regimen to reduce cardiovascular symptoms and inhibit the peripheral conversion of T_4 to T_3.[7,8,147,148]

Preoperative Assessment—Hyperthyroidism. The key to successful preoperative preparation of the hyperthyroid surgical patient is a careful assessment of the extent of thyrotoxicosis and the severity of end-organ manifestations.[24] Thyrotoxicosis is associated with increased operative risk, so elective surgery should not proceed until the patient has been rendered euthyroid by medical management.[139] Antithyroid medications should be continued through the morning of surgery.[7]

Hyperthyroid patients have increased blood volume, decreased peripheral resistance, and a wide pulse pressure. The cardiac output, heart rate, and systolic blood pressure may be increased. Appropriate corrections of the patient's fluid volume and electrolyte status should be accomplished before surgery.

A careful preoperative evaluation of the airway is mandatory in all hyperthyroid patients undergoing surgery. Thyroid gland enlargement can cause tracheal deviation and tracheoesophageal compression. Hoarseness, sore throat, a feeling of pressure in the neck, coughing, or dyspnea suggests tracheal compression that can be caused by thyromegaly. Chest and airway radiographs and computed tomography (CT) scans are useful to detect tracheal deviation and compression.[150]

A patient with a large goiter and an obstructed airway poses the same challenge as any other patient in whom airway management is problematic.[11] An awake fiberoptic intubation with topical anesthesia is of proven value under these conditions. Tracheomalacia weakens thyroid cartilage from chronic pressure, and its presence may necessitate a more prolonged intubation and vigilant observation after surgery.

Only life-threatening emergency surgery should be performed in an untreated symptomatic hyperthyroid patient.[7,8,11] In an emergency situation, the otherwise healthy patient can be expeditiously prepared for surgery with the oral administration of potassium iodide (3 to 5 drops every 6 hours) and carefully titrated intravenous propranolol (1 to 10 mg) or esmolol (50 to 300 mcg/kg).[11] Elderly patients who require emergency surgery and have rapid ventricular rates require central pressure monitoring to guide therapy.

Intraoperative Management. A major goal of the perioperative management of the hyperthyroid patient is prevention of sympathetic nervous system stimulation. This is accomplished by providing sufficient anesthetic depth and avoiding medications that stimulate the sympathetic nervous system.[7,8,11]

A preoperative anxiolytic medication is generally warranted. Atropine should be avoided as an antisialagogue because of its vagolytic effects and its ability to impair sweating.

Induction of anesthesia may be achieved with a number of intravenous medications. Thiopental is an attractive choice for induction because of its antithyroid activity, although significant antithyroid effect with a single induction dose is probably unlikely.[8] Ketamine should be avoided because it can stimulate the sympathetic nervous system.[151]

If the airway is not compromised by an enlarged goiter, administration of a muscle relaxant can facilitate intubation of the trachea. Pancuronium should be avoided because it has the potential to increase the heart rate. Because of the increased incidence of myasthenia gravis and skeletal muscle weakness in the hyperthyroid patient, precaution dictates careful titration of muscle relaxant doses with use of a peripheral nerve stimulator.[7,8]

Isoflurane or sevoflurane are attractive choices for inhalation anesthetics because of their ability to offset sympathetic nervous system responses to surgical stimulation and because they do not sensitize the myocardium to catecholamines. Hyperthyroid patients do not generally require a higher MAC for inhalational anesthesia.[140] The increased cardiac output accompanying hyperthyroidism may accelerate the uptake of an inhaled anesthetic, resulting in the need to increase the delivered concentration, and this may be perceived clinically as an increased anesthetic requirement.[8,11]

Monitoring of the hyperthyroid patient should focus on early recognition of increased thyroid gland activity suggesting the onset of thyroid storm. Core body temperature should be monitored closely. The ECG should be assessed for tachycardia or dysrhythmias. Hypotension occurring during surgery is better treated with direct-acting vasopressors than with indirect-acting vasoactive drugs that stimulate the release of catecholamines.[7] Hypercarbia and hypoxia should be stringently avoided because they stimulate the sympathoadrenal axis.

Meticulous care of the eyes is required. The patient with proptosis is at risk for corneal exposure and damage, so special care should be taken to lubricate and protect the eyes perioperatively. Box 34-7 summarizes key anesthesia implications for patients with hyperthyroidism.

Thyroid Storm. A feared complication in the hyperthyroid patient is *thyroid storm* or *thyrotoxic crisis*. Thyroid storm is a rare event that is caused by acute stress in the previously undiagnosed or incompletely treated hyperthyroid patient. Precipitating events may include trauma, surgery (especially thyroid surgery), the peripartum period, radioiodine treatment, acute illness, and infection.[11,152,153]

Thyroid storm is a life-threatening medical emergency that represents a severe exacerbation of hyperthyroid signs and symptoms. The clinical manifestations may include marked tachycardia, hyperthermia, hypertension, atrial fibrillation, sweating, tremor, vomiting, weakness, agitation, shock, and congestive heart failure (Box 34-8). Metabolic acidosis may be

Anesthesia Implications for the Hyperthyroid Patient

Determine the extent of thyrotoxicosis and end-organ complications.
Ensure a euthyroid state prior to surgery.
Evaluate the airway closely.
Avoid sympathetic nervous system activation and sympathomimetic drugs.
Titrate muscle relaxants carefully, considering possible myopathy and myasthenia gravis.
Position carefully (decreased bone density and predisposition to osteoporosis)
Monitor closely for early signs of thyroid storm.
Pad and protect the eyes.

Clinical Manifestation of Thyroid Storm

Fever >38.5° C
Tachycardia
Confusion and agitation
Dysrhythmias
Nausea and vomiting
Hypertension
Congestive heart failure
Abnormal liver function tests

present secondary to increased lactate production from overactive metabolism. Similarities exist between the clinical features of thyroid storm and those of pheochromocytoma, neuroleptic malignant syndrome, light anesthesia, and malignant hyperthermia, making clinical diagnosis challenging in some cases.[11]

Thyroid storm associated with surgery may occur anytime in the perioperative period but is more likely to occur 6 to 18 hours after surgery.[8] To prevent substantial morbidity and mortality, treatment must be initiated as soon as the diagnosis is made. Mortality rates are as high as 30%, even with early diagnosis and management.[139] The high mortality associated with thyroid storm underscores the importance of achieving a euthyroid state before surgery.

Management of perioperative thyroid storm includes identifying and treating the precipitating cause, administering antithyroid medications, and providing hemodynamic support. Carefully titrated β-adrenergic receptor blockers, potassium iodide, and antithyroid drugs (PTU or methimazole) block thyroid hormone synthesis and adrenergic manifestations.[82,154] Supplemental glucocorticoids should be administered because the turnover of endogenous steroids is accelerated by the hypermetabolism of thyrotoxicosis.

Supportive measures include intravenous hydration with glucose-containing crystalloid solutions, correction of electrolyte and acid-base imbalances, and management of hyperthermia. Salicylates may displace T_4 from its carrier protein; therefore, acetaminophen is the recommended antipyretic for lowering body temperature. Adequate oxygenation is of paramount importance during thyroid storm. Vasoactive medications and advanced hemodynamic monitoring may be necessary to help manage the labile cardiovascular course.

Hypothyroidism

Hypothyroidism is a state of thyroid gland hypofunction resulting in decreased circulating concentrations of thyroid hormones. Laboratory findings show decreased plasma T_4 concentrations and increased TSH levels in patients with primary hypothyroid disease.[139] The clinical spectrum of thyroid hormone deficiency can range from the asymptomatic patient with no overt physical findings to the classic myxedematous patient with profound symptoms.[155] Hypothyroidism is the most common disorder of thyroid function, occurring in 5% to 10% of women and 0.5% to 2% of men.[139]

Primary hypothyroidism accounts for 95% of all cases of hypothyroidism. An autoimmune-mediated destruction of the thyroid gland, known as *Hashimoto thyroiditis*, is the most common form of hypothyroidism in the United States.[156] The disorder most often occurs in females of middle age and is associated with other autoimmune disorders such as myasthenia gravis and adrenal insufficiency.

Primary hypothyroidism may also be the result of severe iodine deficiency, previous thyroid surgery, neck irradiation, or treatment for hyperthyroidism (radioiodine therapy).[24,155] The antiarrhythmic agent amiodarone is associated with hyper- and hypothyroidism. Lithium inhibits the release of thyroid hormone and causes hypothyroidism in some patients.

Rarely, secondary hypothyroidism is the result of pituitary or hypothalamic disorders. Secondary hypothyroidism is associated with decreased concentrations of both thyroid hormones and TSH. Regardless of the etiology, the clinical manifestations of hypothyroidism are similar.

Signs and Symptoms. Most cases of hypothyroidism are subclinical, with laboratory findings of increased plasma TSH but no overt signs. Patients with more significant disease develop signs and symptoms that reflect a slowed metabolism and impaired cellular functions. The thyroid gland usually is enlarged, nontender, and firm. Patients may have dry skin, cold intolerance, paresthesias, slow mental functioning, ataxia, puffy face, and constipation. Lack of thyroid hormones causes the muscles to become sluggish. Patients with severe hypothyroidism may be hypersomnolent with a decreased ventilatory response to hypoxia and hypercarbia. The hair and nails frequently are brittle.[11,155-157]

The accumulation of proteinaceous fluid in serous body cavities is a well-recognized feature of hypothyroidism. The most common sites of effusions associated with hypothyroidism are the pleural, pericardial, and peritoneal cavities.[158] Inappropriate ADH secretion and impaired free water clearance can lead to hyponatremia. Accumulation of mucopolysaccharides and fluid imparts the characteristic edematous appearance called *myxedema*.[24]

Cardiovascular complications include sinus bradycardia, dysrhythmias, cardiomegaly, impaired contractility, congestive heart failure, and labile blood pressure.[11,155] Symptoms of low exercise tolerance and shortness of breath with exertion may be partially the result of decreased cardiac function. Chronic vasoconstriction produces diastolic hypertension and decreases the intravascular fluid volume.[24,159] The autonomic nervous system response is blunted, and there is a decrease in the sensitivity and number of β-receptors.[159,160]

Overt hypothyroidism is associated with a number of abnormalities in lipid metabolism that may predispose patients to accelerated coronary artery disease. Hypothyroidism is associated with anemia and decreased erythrocyte production of 2,3-diphosphoglycerate, leading to a leftward shift of the oxyhemoglobin dissociation curve.

These "classic" clinical features of hypothyroidism are often lacking in the elderly hypothyroid patient. In the older patient, thyroid status cannot always be predicted from clinical signs and symptoms; diagnosing hypothyroidism is more difficult.[161,162]

Treatment. Treatment of hypothyroidism requires replacement with thyroid hormone. The agent of choice is synthetic *levothyroxine sodium* (T4) because of its long half-life (7 days) and its ability to attain physiologic levels of T3. Replacement dosages range from 75 to 150 mcg/day, depending on the underlying autonomous thyroid function.

An area of particular concern during thyroid hormone replacement is the effect on the cardiovascular system. Initiation of thyroid hormone replacement in a patient with coexisting angina pectoris or underlying risk factors for coronary artery disease is potentially hazardous and requires careful monitoring of both cardiovascular and thyroid status. Myocardial oxygen consumption is augmented by thyroid hormone, and a hypothyroid patient with deficient coronary artery circulation may not tolerate full replacement doses.[163]

Anesthetic Management—Hypothyroidism. Patients with subclinical disease have an overall low risk of complications when undergoing anesthesia and surgery.[24] These patients should receive a careful preoperative evaluation and preoperative continuation of levothyroxine therapy.[8] Patients with severe hypothyroidism are predisposed to multiple complications with anesthesia. Depression of myocardial function, abnormal baroreceptor function, and reduction in plasma volume may be present.[7,8,11,155] Slowed hepatic metabolism and renal clearance of injected drugs may prolong their effects, but MAC is not decreased significantly.[140] Elective surgical procedures should be postponed in the presence of severe or symptomatic hypothyroidism until normal thyroid status can be restored.[11]

All patients with hypothyroidism should undergo careful preoperative evaluation of the airway. A large goiter may cause airway compromise in the form of tracheal deviation or compression. In some patients with severe hypothyroidism, adequate air exchange may be compromised by an enlarged tongue and myxedematous infiltration of the vocal cords.[164] Depression of the ventilatory responses to hypoxia and hypercarbia must be considered. Preoperative sedation should be avoided in the patient with macroglossia or preexisting hypoventilation. The risk of pulmonary aspiration is increased because of associated somatic obesity and delayed gastric emptying.[11]

Hypothyroid patients may respond to opioids with increased central nervous system and respiratory depression and to volatile agents with increased hypotension and myocardial depression. Although ketamine has been proposed as the ideal induction agent, even ketamine can produce cardiovascular depression in the absence of a robust sympathetic nervous system.[7,8]

BOX 34-9

Anesthesia Implications for the Hypothyroid Patient

Delay elective surgery for the patient with severe symptomatic disease.

Evaluate the airway closely.

Monitor for exaggerated central nervous system depression with anesthetic agents.

Titrate muscle relaxants carefully, considering possible coexisting muscle weakness.

Consider decreased hepatic metabolism and renal elimination when dosing medications.

Maintain normothermia.

Monitor ventilation closely, considering blunted ventilatory response to hypercarbia and hypoxia.

Intubation of the trachea may be facilitated by the administration of succinylcholine or a nondepolarizing muscle relaxant; however, hypothyroid patients may be more sensitive to standard doses of nondepolarizing muscle relaxants because of coexisting muscle weakness and decreased hepatic metabolism and renal elimination of these drugs.[11] Maintaining muscle paralysis with minimal doses of muscle relaxants is an appropriate goal.

Supplemental perioperative cortisol should be considered in the patient with symptomatic disease, because there exists a potential for adrenal insufficiency with stress.[7,11,157]

In hypothyroidism, the number of β-receptors is diminished, and responses to inotropic drugs and sympathetic stimulation may be influenced by the altered β-receptor pool.

Body temperature should be monitored closely in hypothyroid patients, and mechanisms for warming the patient should be used during surgery. Box 34-9 summarizes the anesthesia implications of hypothyroidism.

Myxedema Coma. Myxedema coma is a rare syndrome that reflects the end stage of untreated hypothyroidism. The presence of coma is a marker of the patient's clinical deterioration rather than a primary effect of hypothyroidism. A critical insult (infection, surgery, cerebrovascular accident, pneumonia, gastrointestinal bleeding, cold exposure) can precipitate myxedema coma in a patient with hypothyroidism.[24,139]

Generally the patient is elderly, has severe clinical features of hypothyroidism, and is hypothermic, hypoventilating, and hyponatremic. The response to hypoxia and hypercapnia is measurably decreased, and mechanical ventilation may be required. The patient is typically lethargic or stuporous. The skin often is pale as a result of cutaneous vasoconstriction.[139]

Myxedema coma is a medical emergency. Vigorous therapeutic attention should be paid to body temperature, shock, and ventilatory failure. Treatment consists of hemodynamic and ventilatory support and the intravenous administration of levothyroxine (300 to 500 mcg), with continuous ECG monitoring for myocardial ischemia.[11] Supplemental cortisol is appropriate because the myxedematous patient may have adrenal atrophy and decreased adrenal reserve. Because these patients may be vulnerable to water intoxication and hyponatremia, meticulous fluid replacement is important.[7] Only lifesaving surgery should proceed in a patient with myxedema coma.[8,11,139]

SUMMARY

The number and variety of patients with endocrine disorders presenting to surgery remains a consistent challenge for the practicing anesthesia provider. Our ability to diagnose and treat these disorders continues to evolve. Several advances in imaging and genetic profiling have yielded improved preoperative diagnostics. The increase in knowledge of the pathophysiology associated with each patient's individual condition will result in better anesthesia management.

REFERENCES

1. Genuth SM. General principles of endocrine physiology. In: Berne RM et al, eds. *Physiology*. St Louis: Mosby; 2004:719.
2. Jameson JL. Principles of endocrinology. In: Fauci AS et al, eds. *Harrison's Principles of Internal Medicine*. 17th ed. New York: McGraw-Hill; 2008:2187-2194.
3. Guyton AC, Hall JE. Introduction to endocrinology. In: Guyton AC, Hall JE, eds. *Textbook of Medical Physiology*. 11th ed. Philadelphia: Saunders; 2006:905.
4. Kronenberg HM et al. Principles of endocrinology. In: Kronenberg HM et al, eds. *Williams Textbook of Endocrinology*. 11th ed. Philadelphia: Saunders; 2008:3-11.
5. Genuth SM. The hypothalamus and pituitary gland. In: Berne RM et al, eds. *Physiology*. St Louis: Mosby; 2004:819.
6. Guyton AC, Hall JE. The pituitary hormones and their control by the hypothalamus. In: Guyton AC, Hall JE, eds. *Textbook of Medical Physiology*. 11th ed. Philadelphia: Saunders; 2006:918.
7. Schwartz JJ, Rosenbaum S. Anesthesia and the endocrine system. In: Barash PG et al, eds. *Clinical Anesthesia*. 5th ed. Philadelphia: Lippincott Williams & Wilkins; 2006:1129-1151.
8. Wall RT. Endocrine disease. In: Hines RL, Marschall KE, eds. *Anesthesia and Co-existing Disease*. 5th ed. Philadelphia: Churchill Livingstone; 2008:365-406.
9. Nemergut EC et al. Perioperative management of patients undergoing transsphenoidal pituitary surgery. *Anesth Analg*. 2005;101(4):1170-1181.
10. Klibanski A, Zervas NT. Diagnosis and management of hormone-secreting pituitary adenomas. *N Engl J Med*. 1991;324:822-831.
11. Roizen MF, Enany NM. Diseases of the endocrine system. In: Fleisher LA, ed. *Anesthesia and Uncommon Diseases*. 5th ed. Philadelphia: Saunders; 2006:413.
12. Molitch ME. Clinical manifestations of acromegaly. *Endocrinol Metab Clin North Am*. 1992;21:597-614.
13. Melmed S. Acromegaly. *N Engl J Med*. 2006;355:2558-2572.
14. Fahlbusch R et al. Surgical management of acromegaly. *Endocrinol Metab Clin North Am*. 1992;21:669-691.
15. Baxter MA. Acromegaly and transsphenoidal hypophysectomy: a case report. *AANA J*. 1994;62:182-185.
16. Schmitt H et al. Difficult intubation in acromegalic patients: incidence and predictability. *Anesthesiology*. 2000;93:110-114.
17. Robertson GL. Disorders of the neurohypophysis. In: Fauci AS et al, eds. *Harrison's Principles of Internal Medicine*. 17th ed. New York: McGraw-Hill; 2008:2217-2223.
18. Ayus JC, Arieff AI. Pathogenesis and prevention of hyponatremic encephalopathy. *Endocrinol Metab Clin North Am*. 1993;22:425-446.
19. Sterns RH. Severe hyponatremia: the case for conservative management. *Crit Care Med*. 1992;20:534-539.
20. Berl T. Treating hyponatremia: what is all the controversy about? *Ann Intern Med*. 1990;113:417-419.
21. Guyton AC, Hall JE. Parathyroid hormone, calcitonin, calcium and phosphate metabolism, vitamin D, bone, and teeth. In: Guyton AC, Hall JE, eds. *Textbook of Medical Physiology*. 11th ed. Philadelphia: Saunders; 2006:978.
22. Genuth SM. Endocrine regulation of calcium and phosphate metabolism. In: Berne RM et al, eds. *Physiology*. St Louis: Mosby; 2004:794.
23. Bringhurst FR et al. Bone and mineral metabolism in health and disease. In: Fauci AS et al, eds. *Harrison's Principles of Internal Medicine*. 17th ed. New York: McGraw-Hill; 2008:2365-2376.
24. Edwards R. Thyroid and parathyroid disease. In: Desborough J, ed. *International Anesthesiology Clinics*. Philadelphia: Lippincott-Raven; 1997:63.
25. DeRubertis FR. Recognition and reversal of hypocalcemia. *Hosp Med*. 1990;26:125-148.
26. Al-Zahrani, Levine MA. Primary hyperparathyroidism. *Lancet*. 1997;349:1233.
27. Lufkin KG. Primary hyperparathyroidism. *Hosp Med*. 1991;27:98-116.
28. Irvin GL III et al. Progress in the operative management of sporadic primary hyperparathyroidism over 34 years. *Ann Surg*. 2004;239:704-711.
29. Ditkoff BA et al. Parathyroid surgery using monitored anesthesia care as an alternative to general anesthesia. *Am J Surg*. 1996;172:698-700.
30. Jossart GH, Clark OH. Thyroid and parathyroid procedures—surgical techniques. *Sci Am*. 1997;7:1-8.
31. Nussbaum SR. Pathophysiology and management of severe hypercalcemia. *Endocrinol Metab Clin North Am*. 1993;22:343-361.
32. Tominaga Y et al. Surgical treatment of renal hyperparathyroidism. *Semin Surg Oncol*. 1997;13:87-96.
33. Sonner JM et al. Nausea and vomiting following thyroid and parathyroid surgery. *J Clin Anesth*. 1997;9(5):398-402.
34. Genuth SM. Hormones of the pancreatic islets. In: Berne RM, Levy NM, eds. *Physiology*. St Louis: Mosby; 2004:766.
35. Guyton AC, Hall JE. Insulin, glucagon, and diabetes mellitus. In: Guyton AC, Hall JE, eds. *Textbook of Medical Physiology*. 11th ed. Philadelphia: Saunders; 2006:961.
36. Cryer PE. Hypoglycemia. In: Fauci AS et al, eds. *Harrison's Principles of Internal Medicine*. 17th ed. New York: McGraw-Hill; 2008:2305-2309.
37. Powers AC. Diabetes mellitus. In: Fauci AS et al, eds. *Harrison's Principles of Internal Medicine*. 17th ed. New York: McGraw-Hill; 2008:2275-2304.
38. Clarke RSJ. The hyperglycemic response to different types of surgery and anaesthesia. *Br J Anaesth*. 1970;42:45.
39. American Diabetes Association. Report of the expert committee on the diagnosis and classification of diabetes mellitus. *Diabetes Care*. 1997;20(7):1183-1197.
40. Centers for Disease Control and Prevention. *National Diabetes Fact Sheet: General Information and Estimates on Diabetes in the United States, 2005*. Atlanta, GA: U.S. Department of Health and Human Services, CDC; 2005.
41. Centers for Disease Control and Prevention: *The Public Health of Diabetes in the United States: Surveillance Report 2006*. Atlanta, GA: U.S. Department of Health and Human Services, CDC; 2006.
42. MacLaren N, Atkinson M. Is insulin-dependent diabetes mellitus environmentally induced? *N Engl J Med*. 1992;327:348-349.
43. Barker JM. Type 1 diabetes-associated autoimmunity: natural history, genetic associations, and screening. *J Clin Endocrinol Metab*. 2006;91(4):1210-1217.
44. The Writing Team for the Diabetes Control and Complications Trial, Epidemiology of the Diabetes Interventions and Complications Research Group. Effect of intensive therapy on the microvascular complications of type 1 diabetes mellitus. *JAMA*. 2002;287:2563.
45. UK Prospective Diabetes Study Group. Intensive blood-glucose control with sulphonylureas or insulin compared with conventional treatment and risk of complications in patients with type 2 diabetes. *Lancet*. 1998;352:1998.
46. National Diabetes Data Group, eds. *Diabetes in America* [NIH Publication No. 95-1468:339-48]. 2nd ed. Washington, DC: U.S Department of Health and Human Services, National Institutes of Health, National Institute of Diabetes and Digestive and Kidney Diseases; 1995.
47. Mangano DT. Diabetic silent hearts and anesthesia: the duty to assess. *J Clin Anesth*. 1998;10:610-612.
48. Tamborlane WV, Ahern J. Implications and results of the diabetes control and complications trial. *Pediatr Clin North Am*. 1997;44:285-299.
49. Scott JW et al. Effect of metoclopramide on gastric fluid volumes in diabetic patients who have fasted before elective surgery. *Anesthesiology*. 2005;102(5):904-909.
50. Hebl JR et al. Neurologic complications after neuraxial anesthesia or analgesia in patients with preexisting peripheral sensorimotor neuropathy or diabetic polyneuropathy. *Anesth Analg*. 2006;103(5):1294-1299.
51. Salzarulo HH, Taylor LA. Diabetic "stiff joint syndrome" as a cause of difficult endotracheal intubation. *Anesthesiology*. 1986;64:366-368.
52. Reissell E et al. Predictability of difficult laryngoscopy in patients with long-term diabetes mellitus. *Anaesthesia*. 1990;45:1024.
53. Zulfiqar A et al. Advances in diabetic management: implications for anesthesia. *Anesth Analg*. 2005;100:666-669.
54. Robertshaw HJ et al. Strategies for managing the diabetic patient. *Best Pract Res Clin Anaesthesiol*. 2004;18(4):631-643.
55. Abramowicz M. Drugs for diabetes. *Treat Guidel Med Lett*. 2005;3(36):57-62.
56. DeFronzo RA, et al. Efficacy of metformin in patients with non-insulin-dependent diabetes mellitus. *N Engl J Med*. 1995;333:541-549.

57. Vreven R, DeKock M. Metformin lactic acidosis and anesthesia: myth or reality? *Acta Anaesthesiol Belg.* 2005;56:297-302.

58. Abramowicz M. Insulin glargine (Lantus), a new long-acting insulin. *Med Lett.* 2001;43:1110.

59. White WA et al. Continuous subcutaneous insulin infusion during general anesthesia: a case report. *AANA J.* 2004;72(5):353-357.

60. Connery LE, Coursin DB. Assessment and therapy of selected endocrine disorders. *Anesthesiol Clin North America.* 2004;22(1):93-123.

61. Weissamn C. The metabolic response to stress: an overview and update. *Anesthesiology.* 1990;73:308.

62. Engquist A et al. The blocking effect of epidural analgesia on the adrenocortical and hyperglycemic responses to surgery. *Acta Anaesthesiol Scand.* 1977;21:330-335.

63. Turina M et al. Diabetes and hyperglycemia: strict glycemic control. *Crit Care Med.* 2006;34(9):S291-S300.

64. Ouattara A et al. Poor intraoperative blood glucose control is associated with a worsened hospital outcome after cardiac surgery in diabetic patients. *Anesthesiology.* 2005;103:687-694.

65. McMurry JF Jr. Wound healing with diabetes mellitus: better glucose control for better wound healing in diabetes. *Surg Clin North Am.* 1984;64:769-778.

66. Lazar HL et al. Tight glycemic control in diabetic coronary artery bypass graft patients improves perioperative outcomes and decreases recurrent ischemic events. *Circulation.* 2004;109:1497-1502.

67. Knight JW et al. Epidural abscess following epidural steroid and local anaesthetic injection. *Anaesthesia.* 1997;52:576-578.

68. Longstretch WT, Invi TS. High blood glucose level on hospital admission and poor neurological recovery after cardiac arrest. *Ann Neurol.* 1984;15:59-63.

69. Pulsinelli WA et al. Increased damage after ischemic stroke in patients with hyperglycemia with or without established diabetes mellitus. *Am J Med.* 1983;74:540-544.

70. Rovlias A, Kotson S. The influence of hyperglycemia on neurological outcome in patients with severe injury. *Neurosurgery.* 2000;46(2):335-342.

71. Maser RE et al. Glucose monitoring of patients with diabetes mellitus receiving general anesthesia: a study of the practices of anesthesia providers in a large community hospital. *AANA J.* 1996;64:357-361.

72. Eldridge AJ, Sear JW. Perioperative management of diabetic patients: any changes for the better since 1985? *Anaesthesia.* 1996;51:45-51.

73. Kerner PA. Perioperative management of the diabetic patient. *Exp Clin Endocrinol Diabetes.* 1995;103:213-218.

74. Hirsch IB, Paauw DS. Diabetes management in special situations. *Endocrinol Metab Clin North Am.* 1997;26:631-645.

75. Raucoules-Aime M et al. Comparison of two methods of IV insulin administration in the diabetic patient during the perioperative period. *Br J Anaesth.* 1994;72:5-10.

76. Nolte MS. Insulin therapy in insulin-dependent (type I) diabetes mellitus. *Endocrinol Metab Clin North Am.* 1992;21:281-303.

77. Raucoules-Aime M et al. Use of IV insulin in well-controlled non-insulin-dependent diabetics undergoing major surgery. *Br J Anaesth.* 1996;76:198-202.

78. Hemmerling TM et al. Comparison of a continuous glucose-insulin-potassium infusion versus intermittent bolus application of insulin on perioperative glucose control and hormone status in insulin-treated type 2 diabetics. *J Clin Anesth.* 2001;13:293-300.

79. Fleckman AM. Diabetic ketoacidosis. *Endocrinol Metab Clin North Am.* 1993;22:181-207.

80. Siperstein MD. Diabetic ketoacidosis and hyperosmolar coma. *Endocrinol Metab Clin North Am.* 1992;21:415-432.

81. Kitabchi AE, Wall BM. Diabetic ketoacidosis. *Med Clin North Am.* 1995;79:9-37.

82. Kearney T, Dang C. Diabetic and endocrine emergencies. *Postgrad Med J.* 2007;83(976):79-86.

83. Williams GH, Dluhy RG. Disorders of the adrenal cortex. In: Fauci AS et al, eds. *Harrison's Principles of Internal Medicine.* 17th ed. New York: McGraw-Hill; 2008:2247-2268.

84. Guyton AC, Hall JE. The adrenocortical hormones. In Guyton AC, Hall JE, eds. *Textbook of Medical Physiology.* 11th ed. Philadelphia: Saunders; 2006:944.

85. Genuth SM. The adrenal glands. In: Berne RM et al, eds. *Physiology.* 5th ed. St Louis: Mosby; 2004:883.

86. Conn JW. Part I. Painting background. Part II. Primary aldosteronism, a new clinical syndrome, 1954 [historical article]. *J Lab Clin Med.* 1990;116:253-267.

87. Stewart PM. Mineralocorticoid hypertension. *Lancet.* 1999;353(9161):1341-1347.

88. Schamess A et al. Refractory hypertension due to Conn's syndrome. *Postgrad Med.* 1994;95(4):199-200, 203-206.

89. Bravo EL. Primary aldosteronism: issues in diagnosis and management. *Endocrinol Metab Clin North Am.* 1994;23(2):271-283.

90. Favia G et al. Adrenalectomy in primary aldosteronism: a long-term follow-up study in 52 patients. *World J Surg.* 1992;16:680-684.

91. Nishimura M et al. Cardiovascular complications in patients with primary aldosteronism. *Am J Kidney Dis.* 1999;33(2):261-266.

92. Rossi GP et al. Changes in left ventricular anatomy and function in hypertension and primary aldosteronism. *Hypertension.* 1996;27(5):1039-1045.

93. McLeod MK. Complications following adrenal surgery. *J Natl Med Assoc.* 1991;83:161-164.

94. Shen WT et al. Laparoscopic vs open adrenalectomy for the treatment of primary hyperaldosteronism. *Arch Surg.* 1999;134(6):628-631.

95. Puccini M et al. Conn syndrome: 14 years' experience from two European centers. *Eur J Surg.* 1998;164(11):811-817.

96. Hutter AM, Kayhoe DE. Adrenal cortical carcinoma: clinical features of 138 patients. *Am J Med.* 1966;41:572.

97. Goldfard DA. Contemporary evaluation and management of Cushing's syndrome. *World J Urol.* 1999;17(1):22-25.

98. Ernest I, Ekman H. Adrenalectomy in Cushing's disease: a long-term follow-up. *Acta Endocrinol Suppl.* 1972;160:3.

99. Tyrrell JB et al. Cushing's disease: selected trans-sphenoidal resection of pituitary microadenomas. *N Engl J Med.* 1978;298:753.

100. Kemink L et al. Residual adrenocortical function after bilateral adrenalectomy for pituitary-dependent Cushing's syndrome. *J Clin Endocrinol Metab.* 1992;75:1211-1214.

101. Small M et al. Thromboembolic complications in Cushing's syndrome. *Clin Endocrinol (Oxf).* 1983;19:503-511.

102. Dal Bo Zanon R et al. Increased factor VIII associated activities in Cushing's syndrome: a probable hypercoagulable state. *Thromb Haemost.* 1982;47:116-117.

103. Oelkers W. Adrenal insufficiency. *N Engl J Med.* 1996;335:1206.

104. Arit W, Allolia B. Adrenal insufficiency. *Lancet.* 2003;361:1881.

105. Glowniak JV, Loriaux DL. A double-blind study of perioperative steroid requirements in secondary adrenal insufficiency. *Surgery.* 1997;121:123.

106. Werbel SS, Ober KP. Acute adrenal insufficiency. *Endocrinol Metab Clin North Am.* 1993;22:303-328.

107. Chin R. Adrenal crisis. *Crit Care Clin.* 1991;7:23.

108. Lundy JB et al. Acute adrenal insufficiency after a single dose of etomidate. *J Intensive Care Med.* 2007;22(2):111-117.

109. Salem M et al. Perioperative glucocorticoid coverage. A reassessment 42 years after emergence of a problem. *Ann Surg.* 1994;219(4):416-425.

110. Udelsman R et al. Adaptation during surgical stress: a re-evaluation of the role of glucocorticoids. *J Clin Invest.* 1986;77:1377-1381.

111. Henriques HF III, Lebovic D. Defining and focusing perioperative steroid supplementation. *Am Surg.* 1994;61(9):809-813.

112. Guyton AC, Hall JE. The autonomic nervous system and the adrenal medulla. In: Guyton AC, Hall JE, eds: *Textbook of Medical Physiology.* 11th ed. Philadelphia: Saunders; 2006:748.

113. Neumann HP. Pheochromocytoma. In: Fauci AS et al, eds. *Harrison's Principles of Internal Medicine.* 17th ed. New York: McGraw-Hill; 2008:2269-2274.

114. Young WF. Endocrine hypertension. In: Kronenberg HM et al, eds. *Williams Textbook of Endocrinology.* 11th ed. Philadelphia: Saunders; 2008:505-537.

115. Geoghegan JG et al. Changing trends in the management of phaeochromocytoma. *Br J Surg.* 1998;85:117.

116. Dougherty TB, Cronau LH Jr. Anesthetic implications for surgical patients with endocrine tumors. *Int Anesthesiol Clin.* 1998;36(3):31-44.

117. Neumann HP et al. Pheochromocytoma, multiple endocrine neoplasia type 2, and von Hippel-Lindau disease. *N Engl J Med.* 1993;329:1531-1538.

118. Reisch NA et al. Pheochromocytoma: presentation, diagnosis and treatment. *J Hypertension.* 2006;24(12):2331-2339.

119. Cheng TO, Bashour TT. Striking cardiographic changes associated with pheochromocytoma masquerading as ischaemic heart disease. *Chest.* 1976;70:397.

120. Kaul U et al. Pheochromocytoma presenting as recurrent syncope resulting from ventricular tachycardia: an annual presentation. *Indian Heart J.* 1984;36:118-120.

121. Shub C et al. Echocardiographic findings in pheochromocytoma. *Am J Cardiol.* 1986;57:971-975.

122. Ulchaker JC et al. Successful outcomes in pheochromocytoma surgery in the modern era. *J Urol.* 1999;161(3):764-767.

123. Sand J et al. Preoperative treatment and survival of patients with pheochromocytomas. *Ann Chir Gynaecol.* 1997;86(3):230-232.

124. Briggs RSJ et al. Hypertensive response to labetalol in pheochromocytoma. *Lancet.* 1978;1:1045-1046.

125. Colson P et al. Haemodynamic heterogeneity and treatment with the calcium channel blocker nicardipine during phaeochromocytoma surgery. *Acta Anaesthesiol Scand.* 1998;42(9):1114-1119.

126. Perry RR et al. Surgical management of pheochromocytoma with the use of metyrosine. *Ann Surg.* 1990;212(5):621-628.

127. Pujol J et al. Laparoscopic adrenalectomy: a review of 30 initial cases. *Surg Endosc.* 1999;13(5):488-492.

128. Joris JL et al. Hemodynamic changes and catecholamine release during laparoscopic adrenalectomy for pheochromocytoma. *Anesth Analg.* 1999;88(1):16-21.

129. Col V et al. Laparoscopic adrenalectomy for pheochromocytoma: endocrinological and surgical aspects of a new therapeutic approach. *Clin Endocrinol (Oxf).* 1999;50(1):121-125.

130. Jaroszewski DE et al. Laparoscopic adrenalectomy for pheochromocytoma. *Mayo Clin Proc.* 2003;78:1501-1504.

131. Kalady MF et al. Laparoscopic adrenalectomy for pheochromocytoma. A Comparision to aldosteronoma and incidentaloma. *Surg Endosc.* 2004; 19(4):621-625.

132. Fraley DS et al. Severe hypertension associated with pancuronium bromide. *Anesth Analg.* 1978;7:265-267.

133. Plouin PF et al. Hypertensive crisis in patient with pheochromocytoma given metoclopramide. *Lancet.* 1976;2:1357.

134. Bakan M et al. Anesthesia management with short acting agents for bilateral pheochromocytoma removal in a 12-year-old boy. *Ped Anesth.* 2006;16: 1184-1189.

135. Roth JV. Use of vasopressin bolus and infusion to treat catecholamine-resistant hypotension during pheochromocytoma resection. *Anesthesiology.* 2007;106(4):883-884.

136. Allen GC, Rosenberg H. Pheochromocytoma presenting as acute malignant hyperthermia: a diagnostic challenge. *Can J Anaesth.* 1990;37: 593-595.

137. Guyton AC, Hall JE. The thyroid metabolic hormones. In: Guyton AC, Hall JE, eds. *Textbook of Medical Physiology.* 11th ed. Philadelphia: Saunders; 2006:931.

138. Genuth SM. The thyroid glands. In Berne RM, Levy MN et al, eds. *Physiology.* 5th ed. St Louis: Mosby; 2004:860.

139. Jameson JL, Weetman AP. Disorders of the thyroid gland. In: Fauci AS et al, eds. *Harrison's Principles of Internal Medicine.* 17th ed. New York: McGraw-Hill; 2008:2224-2246.

140. Babad AA, Eger EI. The effects of hyperthyroidism and hypothyroidism on halothane and oxygen requirements in dogs. *Anesthesiology.* 1969;29: 1087-1093.

141. Bilezikian J, Loeb JN. The influence of hyperthyroidism and hypothyroidism on alpha and beta adrenergic receptor systems and adrenergic responsiveness. *Endocr Rev.* 1983;4:378.

142. Smith BR et al. Autoantibodies to the thyrotropin receptor. *Endocr Rev.* 1988;9:106-120.

143. Caruso DR, Mazzaferri EL. Intervention in Graves' disease: choosing among imperfect but effective treatment options. *Postgrad Med.* 1992;92:117-134.

144. Surks MI, Sievert R. Drugs and thyroid function. *N Engl J Med.* 1995;333:1688.

145. Rehman S et al. Thyroid disorders in elderly patients. *South Med J.* 2005;98(5):543-549.

146. Gittoes NJL, Franklyn JA. Hyperthyroidism: current treatment guidelines. *Drugs.* 1998;55:543.

147. Farling PA. Thyroid disease. *Br J Anaesth.* 2000;85:15-28.

148. Geffner DL, Hershman JM. Beta-adrenergic blockade for the treatment of hyperthyroidism. *Am J Med.* 1992;93:61.

149. Tsuruta M et al. Long-term follow-up studies on iodine-131 treatment of hyperthyroid Graves' disease based on the measurement of thyroid volume by ultrasonography. *Ann Nucl Med.* 1993;7:193-197.

150. Shaha AR. Surgery for benign thyroid disease causing tracheoesophageal compression. *Otolaryngol Clin North Am.* 1990;23:391-401.

151. Kaplan JA, Cooperman LH. Alarming reactions to ketamine in patients taking thyroid medication: treatment with propranolol. *Anesthesiology.* 1971;35:229-230.

152. Rufener S et al. Thyroid storm precipitated by infection: an atypical case involving multisystem organ dysfunction. *Endocrinologist.* 2005;15(2):111-114.

153. Hirvonen EA et al. Thyroid storm prior to induction of anaesthesia. *Anaesthesia.* 2004;59:1020-1022.

154. Thorne AC, Bedford RF. Esmolol for perioperative management of thyrotoxic goiter. *Anesthesiology.* 1989;71:291-294.

155. Lindsay RS, Toft AD. Hypothyroidism. *Lancet.* 1997;349:413.

156. Toft AD. Subclinical hypothyroidism. *N Engl J Med.* 2001;345:512-516.

157. Mokshagundam S, Barzel SE. Thyroid disease in the elderly. *J Am Geriatr Soc.* 1993;41:1361-1369.

158. Kabadi VM, Kumar SP. Pericardial effusion in primary hypothyroidism. *Am Heart J.* 1990;120:1393-1395.

159. Whitten CW et al. Anesthetic management of a hypothyroid cardiac surgical patient [review]. *J Cardiothorac Vasc Anesth.* 1991;5:156-159.

160. Kunos G et al. Effects of thyroid state on adrenoreceptor properties. *Nature.* 1974;250:779-781.

161. Bemben DA et al. Thyroid disease in the elderly: prevalence of undiagnosed hypothyroidism. *J Fam Pract.* 1994;38(6):577-582.

162. Bemben DA et al. Thyroid disease in the elderly: predictability of subclinical hypothyroidism. *J Fam Pract.* 1994;38(6):583-588.

163. Toft AD. Thyroxine therapy. *N Engl J Med.* 1994;331:174.

164. Meares N et al. Massive macroglossia as a presenting feature of hypothyroid-associated pericardial effusion. *Chest.* 1993;104:1632-1633.

CHAPTER 35

HEMATOLOGY AND ANESTHESIA

Judith A. Franco

When disruptions within the endothelial lining of blood vessels occur, the breach in vessel-wall integrity can be due to spontaneous plaque disruption, trauma, or iatrogenic reasons such as venous access or surgical intervention. Vessel-wall injury initiates an extraordinary chain of events that causes the cessation of bleeding with the formation of a clot, allowing the site of injury to heal. This event is followed by clot dissolution. *Hemostasis* is the process by which the body maintains the delicate balance between bleeding and clotting. Were it not for this balance, hemorrhage or thrombosis would ensue and be disastrous.

The focus of this chapter is to review the normal and abnormal processes of hemostasis, emphasizing the (1) vessel wall, (2) platelet, (3) coagulation cascade, (4) emerging cell-based theory of coagulation, and (5) fibrinolytic system. An in-depth discussion surrounding the importance of hemostatic assessment and management during the perioperative period, with particular attention to transfusion practices and guidelines, will follow. A discussion concerning the patient with special hematologic circumstances concludes the chapter.

THE NORMAL VESSEL WALL

The normal blood vessel acts as a conduit to maintain a state of fluidity within the vascular system. Blood vessels are cylindrical and consist of three distinct layers—the intima, the media, and the adventitia (Figure 35-1).

The intima (the inner layer) is the lining separating the flowing blood from the vessel; it is made up primarily of endothelial cells. These endothelial cells play an important role in the modulation of hemostasis by synthesizing and secreting many procoagulants (initiators of coagulation), anticoagulants (inhibitors of coagulation), and fibrinolytics (to dissolve the clot) (Table 35-1). One of the important mediators, von Willebrand factor (vWF), is a necessary cofactor for the adherence of platelets to the subendothelial layer. Tissue factor (a cofactor from the coagulation cascade) activates the clotting cascade pathway when injury to the vessel occurs. Some of these mediators (thromboxane A_2, adenosine diphosphate [ADP]) control blood flow by influencing vasoconstriction. Other mediators (nitric oxide, prostacyclin) control blood flow by vasodilation of blood vessels. Endothelial cells can also suppress activation of the coagulation system by their expression of many coagulation inhibitors such as tissue factor pathway inhibitor.[1]

One of the most important yet simple functions of the endothelial lining is that of forming a barrier separating the fluid contents within the blood vessel (red blood cells, white blood cells, albumin, globulins, fibrinogen, platelets, etc.) from the highly thrombogenic material (collagen and procoagulants) that lies beneath, within the subendothelial space. The smooth endothelial lining physically repels the blood components away from the vessel wall, preventing activation of the clotting mechanism. When the endothelial wall is damaged, the above properties no longer apply.

The second layer of the vessel wall, the subendothelial layer, is extremely thrombogenic and very active. The subendothelial layer contains collagen, a potent and important stimulus for platelet attachment to the injured vessel wall. The subendothelial layer also contains fibronectin, which facilitates the anchoring of fibrin during the formation of a hemostatic plug.

The third layer, the adventitia, participates in the control of blood flow by influencing the vessel's degree of contraction. The endothelial cells produce nitric oxide and prostacyclin, which influence the adventitia. Nitric oxide affects platelet function by inhibiting platelet adhesion, aggregation, and the binding of fibrinogen between glycoprotein IIb/IIIa complex (GpIIb-IIIa) pseudopods. Nitric oxide's ability to influence and promote smooth-muscle relaxation results in vascular vasodilation. Once the vessel vasodilates, the increase in blood flow limits the activity of procoagulant mediators by simply washing the procoagulant mediators away. This metabolic reaction occurs within the endothelial lining (Figure 35-2). Under the influence of nitric oxide synthetase (NOS), L-arginine is converted to nitric oxide (NO). Nitric oxide then diffuses into the muscle cells and activates soluble guanylate cyclase, subsequently producing a second messenger, cyclic guanosine monophosphate, that causes muscle relaxation.[1]

Prostacyclin is a lipid molecule produced in the endothelial cells from prostaglandin. A powerful vasodilator, prostacyclin also interferes with platelet formation and aggregation.

Platelets are an essential component of the thrombogenic response to bleeding. Platelets are round and disklike and circulate freely within the blood. They are formed in the bone marrow from megakaryocytes, maintain a concentration count of approximately 150,000 to 300,000/mm^3, and survive approximately 8 to 12 days.[2] Platelets are constantly working to "patch" thousands of minute vascular injuries that occur in perpetuity. Approximately 7.1×10^3 are used each day.[3]

The platelets flow along the vessel surface. Because they are smaller than some other constitutes in fluid blood (e.g., RBCs, WBCs), they tend to be pushed aside, strategically positioned near the vessel-wall surface where they can then "react" in the event of injury (Figure 35-3).

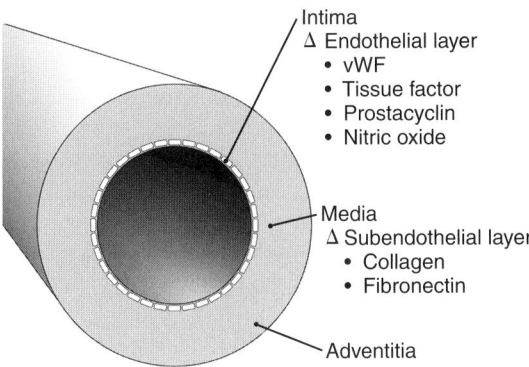

FIGURE 35-1 Schematic of vessel layers and some important mediators. *vWF*, Von Willebrand factor.

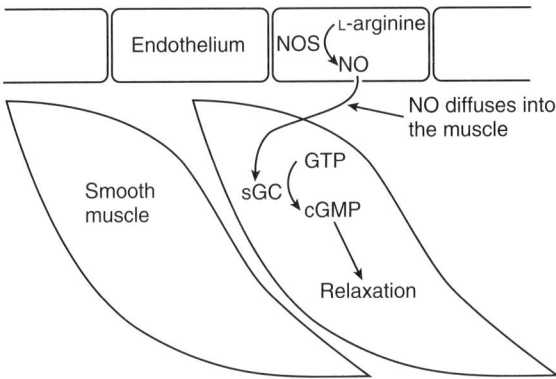

FIGURE 35-2 Nitric oxide influences vessel-wall vasodilatation by causing muscle relaxation. *cGMP*, Cyclic guanosine monophosphate; *GTP*, guanosine triphosphate; *NO*, nitric oxide; *NOS*, nitric oxide synthetase; *sGC*, soluble guanylate cyclase.

TABLE 35-1	Mediators Responsible for Procoagulant, Anticoagulant, and Fibrinolytic Activities	
Property	**Mediator**	**Function**
Procoagulant	Coagulation factors	Coagulation
	Collagen	Tensile strength
	vWF	Adhesion
	Protein C	Degrades factors V and VII
	Protein S	Cofactor for protein C
	Fibronectin	Mediates cell adhesion
	Thrombomodulin	Regulates anticoagulant pathway
Anticoagulant	Antithrombin III	Degrades factors XII, XI, X, IX, II
	Tissue pathway factor inhibitor	Inhibits tissue factor
Vasodilation	Nitric oxide	Vasodilates
	Prostacyclin	Vasodilates, inhibits aggregation
		Both promote smooth-muscle relaxation
Vasoconstriction	Thromboxane A$_2$	Vasoconstriction
	ADP	Vasoconstriction
	Serotonin	Vasoconstriction
Fibrinolytic	Plasminogen	Converts to plasmin
	tPA	Activates plasmin
	Urokinase	Activates plasmin
Antifibrinolytic	Plasminogen activator inhibitor	Inactivates tPA, urokinase
	α-Antiplasmin	Inhibits plasmin

ADP, Adenosine diphosphate; tPA, tissue plasminogen activator.

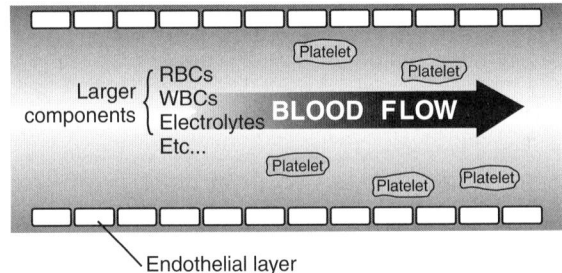

FIGURE 35-3 Position of platelets flowing in the blood vessel.

contractile proteins, store large amounts of calcium and various enzymes, and require the use of their phospholipids' surface to promote cellular activity. Platelets contain alpha (α) granules that store proteins (vWF, fibrinogen, fibronectin, platelet factor 4, and platelet growth factor) and dense granules that store nonproteins (serotonin, ADP, adenosine triphosphate [ATP], histamine, and epinephrine).[2] Many of these granules synthesize prostaglandins that enable the platelets to promote vascular and local tissue reactions.[2,4] Platelets also produce thrombin. In the platelet, thrombin's role is to activate some of the coagulation factors and to influence recruitment of platelets to the site of injury. All the contents in the cytoplasm of the platelet participate in regulating hemostasis. Platelets do not contain a nucleus, RNA, or DNA, so they do not reproduce.[2]

Platelets are largely inactive unless they become activated as a result of vascular trauma. Adequate hemostasis is not possible in the absence of an adequate quality or quantity of activated platelets. It is important to note that platelets do not work independently to achieve hemostasis. They work in conjunction with plasma proteins of the coagulation cascade (discussed under Vessel Injury) to build a stable clot when injury to the vascular integrity occurs.

VESSEL INJURY

Clot formation in response to injury has traditionally been described to include the adherence of the platelet to the injured vessel wall and the response of the clotting cascade to form a stable clot and stop the progress of bleeding. When the

The membrane surface of the platelet serves as a physical barrier between platelet cytoplasm and the surrounding plasma. Platelets contain mitochondria in their cytoplasm, enabling them to participate in aerobic metabolism, and have glycogen stores that allow for anaerobic metabolism.[4] Platelets also contain

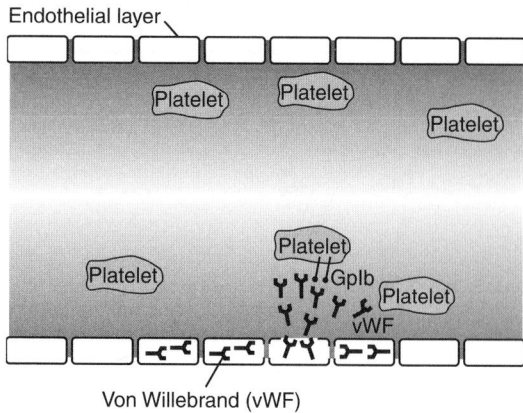

FIGURE **35-4** Von Willebrand factor is responsible for adhesion of platelets.

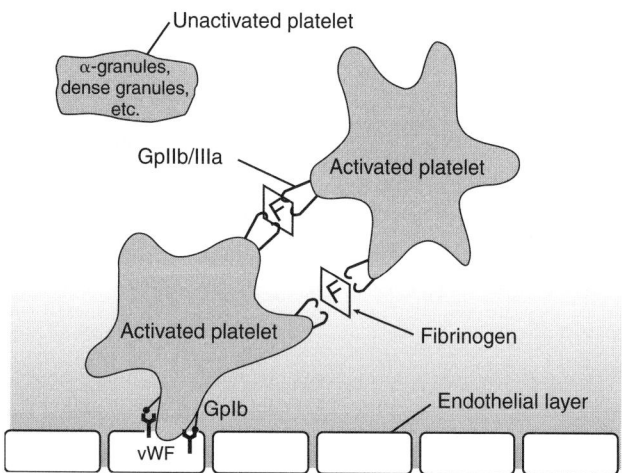

FIGURE **35-5** Glycoprotein IIb/IIIa complex (GpIIb-IIIa). Pseudopods link activated platelets together with fibrinogen to form a mound to "patch" injury to vessel walls. *GpIIb-IIIa*, Glycoprotein IIb/IIIa complex; *VIII*, factor VIII; *vWF*, von Willebrand factor.

endothelial lining is disrupted, as it might be by plaque dislodgement, surgical instrumentation, or trauma, an intricate process to maintain hemostasis and promote clot formation is initiated.

The vessel wall immediately contracts to cause a tamponade, decreasing blood flow. This contraction is a result of autonomic nervous system reflexes and the expression of thromboxane A_2, and ADP.[2,5] The area adjacent to the injury vasodilates and distributes blood to the surrounding organs and tissues. Contraction is followed by three separate stages in the formation of a primary plug: adhesion, activation, and aggregation.

In the adhesion stage, vWF mobilizes from within the endothelial cells and emerges from the endothelial lining. Glycoprotein Ib (GpIb) receptors emerge from the surface of the platelet (Figure 35-4). The purpose of GpIb is to attach to vWF and attract platelets to the endothelial lining; vWF makes platelets "sticky" and allows them to adhere to the site of injury.

Under the influence of tissue factor (a cofactor of the extrinsic clotting pathway), the platelet then undergoes a conformational transformation as it becomes activated (Figure 35-5). The once disklike structure swells and becomes oval and irregular. From the platelet surface, two other major glycoproteins, IIb and IIIa, project themselves outward. The purpose of the GpIIb-IIIa receptor complex is to link other activated platelets together in an effort to form a primary platelet plug. When this action is complete, the platelets form a mound whose only goal is to seal and heal the site of injury within the blood vessel.

As platelets undergo this metamorphosis, they release the alpha and dense granules, the contractile granules, thrombin, and many important mediators into the blood in an effort to promote procoagulant activity. All these mediators are responsible for platelet aggregation to form a primary unstable clot. When injury is minute and less threatening, this primary plug is enough to maintain hemostasis. When the injury is large, activation of the coagulation clotting cascade is required for permanent repair to create and stabilize a secondary clot to cease bleeding.[2]

The coagulation cascade illustrates the activation of cofactors (also referred to as *zymogens*) and their role in this process of hemostasis. Most cofactors are enzymes, with some exceptions (e.g., factors V and VIII). The coagulation factors circulate as inactive cofactors until they are activated to assist in the process of coagulation (Table 35-2). Activation of cofactors results from either tissue or organ damage and sets in motion a process that terminates in stabilization of hemorrhagic conditions in the absence of pathology. The factors are identified with Roman numerals for ease of interpretation.

The clotting pathways are thought to be two separate and distinct pathways (extrinsic and intrinsic) that worked independently of each other but in conjunction with platelet activity and the common coagulation pathway (Figure 35-6). The extrinsic pathway (tissue factor pathway) became activated by the release of tissue factor when injury occurred outside the vessel wall (with organ trauma or crushing injuries). This section of the coagulation cascade consisted of factor III (tissue factor or thromboplastin) and factor VII (proconvertin).

When damage occurs outside of blood vessels, tissue factor (factor III) activates proconvertin (factor VII), changing it to activated (a) factor VII (VIIa). (When factor III activates factor VII, it is immediately inhibited by tissue factor pathway inhibitor, so only a predetermined amount of factor VII is activated.) Once factor VII is activated, it in turn activates factor X (Stuart-Prower) of the common pathway. Factor X forms a complex with factor V (proaccelerin, a prothrombinase complex), activating factor II (prothrombin), which when activated becomes factor IIa (thrombin). Thrombin in turn activates factor I (fibrinogen) to form activated factor I (Ia, fibrin).

The intrinsic pathway (contact activation pathway) is initiated when damage occurs to the blood vessels themselves. The intrinsic pathway is initiated by prekallikrein, high-molecular-weight kininogen (HMWK), and by the activation of factor XII (Hageman). With the help of calcium (factor IV), the coagulation pathway initiates a domino effect. Each factor, once activated, affects its subsequent factor. Factor XII (Hageman) activates factor XI (plasma thromboplastin antecedent), which activates factor IX (Christmas), which then activates factor VIII (antihemophiliac factor) and ultimately (similar to the extrinsic pathway) merges at the common pathway and activates factor X. The result is the generation of fibrin from the activation of prothrombin to thrombin.

Conversion of prothrombin to thrombin is an important reaction for both coagulation pathways. Thrombin activates factors V, VIII, I, and XIII and influences the recruitment of platelets to

TABLE **35-2**	Coagulation Table			
Factor	**Factor Name**	**Synthesized**	**Vitamin K Dependent**	**Action**
I	Fibrinogen	Liver	No	Forms a clot
II	Prothrombin	Liver	Yes	When in active form, activates I, V, VII, XIII, platelets, and protein C
III	Tissue factor or thromboplastin	Vascular wall and extravascular cell membranes; released from traumatized cells	–	Cofactor of VII
IV	Calcium	Diet	–	Promotes clotting reactions
V	Proaccelerin	Liver	No	Cofactor of X; forms a prothrombinase complex
VI	(Unassigned)	–	–	–
VII	Proconvertin	Liver	Yes	Activates IX and X
VIII	Antihemophiliac	Liver	No	Cofactor to IX
vWF	Von Willebrand	Endothelial cells	–	Mediates adhesion
IX	Christmas	Liver	Yes	Activates X
X	Stuart-Prower	Liver	Yes	Activates II, forms a prothrombinase complex with V
XI	Plasma thromboplastin antecedent	Liver	No	Activates IX
XII	Hageman	Liver	No	Activates XI
XIII	Fibrin stabilizing	Liver	No	Crosslinks fibrin
Prekallikrein	Fletcher		–	Activates XII, cleaves HMWK
High-molecular-weight kininogen (HMWK)	Contact activation factor		–	Supports activation of prekallikrein, XII, XI

the injured area. Enough thrombin must be present to activate adequate fibrin to form a stable clot.

When thrombin behaves as an anticoagulant it (1) prevents runaway clot formation by releasing tissue plasminogen activator (tPA) from endothelial cells, (2) stimulates protein C and protein S to inhibit clot formation, and (3) forms a relationship with antithrombin III to interfere with coagulation.[1] The common pathway is the terminal pathway of the coagulation cascade. In the common pathway, factor X has been activated by the intrinsic and extrinsic pathways. Factor X requires the help of factor V (proaccelerin) and calcium to convert factor II (prothrombin) to its active-state thrombin (IIa). Thrombin then activates factor I (fibrinogen) to its active form, Ia (fibrin). Factor XIII (fibrin stabilizing factor) is required to ensure the platelet plug will hold. Factor XIII helps form a cross-linked mesh within the platelet plug, increasing its strength. Fibrin (factor Ia) in conjunction with factor XIII finally secures a stable secondary plug, and bleeding stops. Once a clot is made, it retracts, eliminating its serum. As it retracts, it weaves the edges of the vessel together, healing the site of injury.[2]

Most of the coagulation proteins are synthesized in the liver. Calcium, which is not a true factor, comes from diet; it is needed

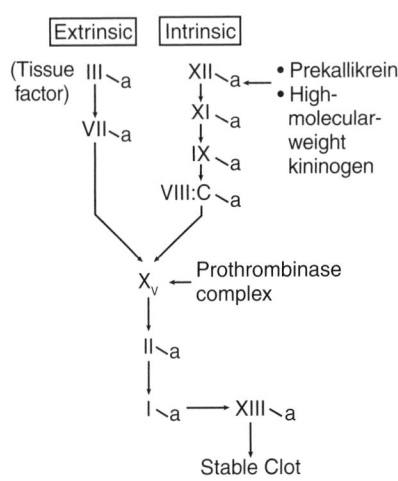

FIGURE 35-6 Schematic of the coagulation cascade (extrinsic intrinsic and common pathways). *a*, Active form.

to "position" the coagulation factors on the surface of the platelet so clotting will ensue. von Willebrand is synthesized in the endothelial cells, and factors II, VII, IX and X are dependent on vitamin K for utilization.

CELL-BASED THEORY OF COAGULATION

The cell-based theory is a newer concept for explaining the platelet and clotting cascades' involvement in hemostasis. It hypothesizes *why* platelets and the extrinsic and intrinsic pathways of coagulation cascade do not work independently of one another but form a very interdependent relationship.[6] The theory posits that coagulation takes place on different "cell surfaces" that bear tissue factor (TF). These surfaces play a pivotal role in factor expression leading to hemostasis. The cell-based theory describes hemostasis as taking place in three phases: initiation, amplification, and propagation.

The initiation phase is triggered by injury to the endothelial surface (Figure 35-7). When injury occurs, TF is exposed at the site of injury. In its presence, the endothelial surface of the blood vessel changes, becoming acidic and making its phospholipid surface less repellent to platelets. TF downregulates anticoagulants that reside in the subendothelial layer (e.g., antithrombin III, thrombomodulin) in an effort to promote coagulation.[7] This new medium enhances the many enzymatic processes that work to maintain hemostasis by encouraging aggregation and the activation of clotting factors to the site of injury. TF recruits platelets and activates factor VII.

In the cell-based theory, TF/VII reaction results in the activation of factors X (common pathway) *and* IX (intrinsic pathway). Factor X forms a complex with factor V, and together these two activated factors are able to generate a *small* amount of thrombin for clot formation.[8] Only a small amount of thrombin is created because this reaction terminates almost immediately when tissue factor pathway inhibitor (TFPI) limits the amount of TF expressed. The activation of factor IX from the TF/VII complex does not participate in this initiation stage because IX does not act on TF-bearing cell surfaces.[7]

It is on the platelet cell surface that factor IX (generated from TF/VII) exerts its coagulation contribution to hemostasis. Factor IX attaches to the activated platelet cell surface and binds with a receptor, resulting in the activation of factor VIII, which in turn activates factor X. Additional thrombin is then produced.

As injury perpetuates and TF is expressed, platelets mobilize to the site of injury.[7] It is during the amplification phase that thrombin generation gains momentum, and acceleration and activation of clotting factors persists. Thrombin activates factors V, VIII, and IX.[6] Activated factor XI assists in generating even more IX on the platelet surface.[9] Von Willebrand factor promotes platelet aggregation through its adhesive properties with GpIb, and the expression of the GpIIb-IIIa pseudopods from the surface of platelets facilitates aggregation of additional platelets.

During the propagation phase, all coagulation factors are actively influencing one another, promoting coagulation and finally activating prothrombin, resulting in a large "*burst*" of thrombin. Remember, enough thrombin must be present to convert fibrinogen to fibrin to form a stable secondary hemostatic plug. This burst of thrombin does just that.

The cell-based theory is a means of providing a more thorough understanding and an innovative interpretation of coagulation. It explains how cell surfaces do not just express coagulation factors; these surfaces participate in conjunction with platelets and the coagulation cascade pathways to maintain hemostasis. This theory also explains why certain deficiencies fail to cause

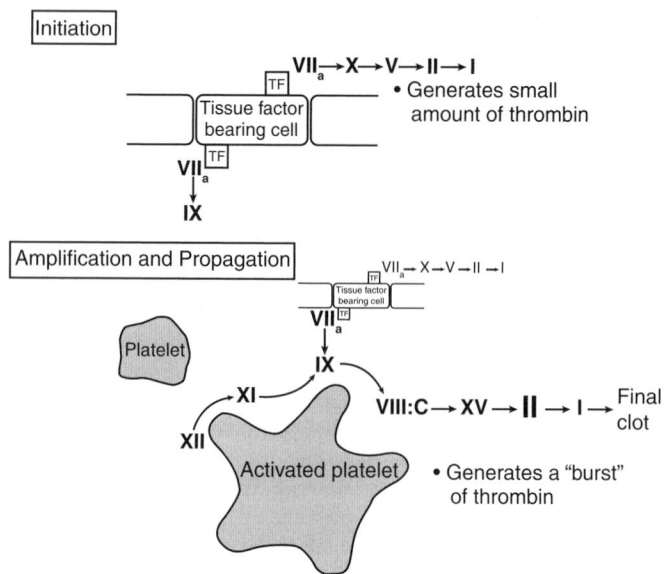

FIGURE **35-7** Cell-based theory of coagulation. (*Adapted from Hoffman M, Monroe D. Coagulation 2006: a modern view of hemostasis.* Hematol Oncol Clin North Am. 2007;21(1):1-11.)

bleeding, despite changes in laboratory values such as the PT prothrombin time (PT) or activated partial thromboplastin time (aPTT), indicative of coagulation problems.[6]

FIBRINLOYTIC SYSTEM

Once a disrupted vessel is sealed, there is no longer a need for a hemostatic plug. A counterbalance mechanism, the fibrinolytic system, exists to degrade fibrin. Initially there is an increase in blood flow at the site of injury. This increase in blood flow washes away ADP and thromboxane A_2 and other procoagulant mediators, which were initially present to encourage hemostasis and limit the size of the clot. Thrombin, which initially behaved as a procoagulant, now acts as an anticoagulant and activates additional anticoagulant mediators. TFPI stops the action of TF. Protein C and protein S inhibit coagulation factors III, V, and VIII. Antithrombin III inhibits thrombin activity by sequestering factors XII, XI, IX, and X. Antithrombin III is a mediator that corrals some of the factors present in the clotting cascade and takes them out of the clotting equation (Figure 35-8). The clot manufactured is disrupted.

The process of fibrinolysis is highly regulated by plasma proteins (Figure 35-9). A clot is composed primarily of plasminogen, plasmin, fibrin, and fibrin degradation products. Plasminogen is an enzyme synthesized in the liver. It is stored like the clotting factors in an inactive form. While the clot is forming, plasminogen incorporates itself into the clot. With the assistance of the body's own tPA and urokinase, plasminogen is activated to plasmin. Plasmin then acts on the fibrin, causing fibrin to degrade into fibrin degradation products. The circulatory system removes the waste products of the clot. α-Antiplasmin and tissue plasminogen activator inhibitor are important fibrinolytic mediators that stop the process of fibrinolysis when the clot has been digested.

Platelets, coagulation cofactors, and the fibrinolytic systems are dependent on each other to ensure a person does not bleed to death or clot to death at any given moment. This system of checks and balances maintains hemostasis when a breach in vascular integrity occurs.

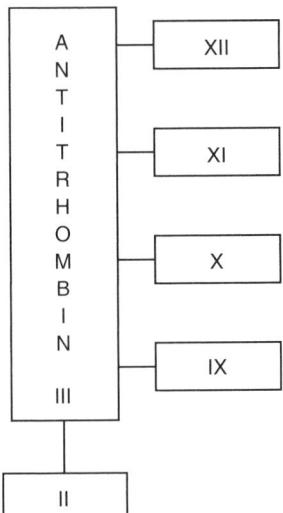

FIGURE **35-8** Antithrombin III corrals clotting factors XII, XI, IX, X. This influences factor II.

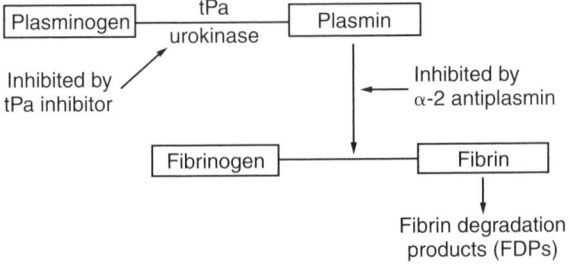

FIGURE **35-9** Schematic of the fibrinolytic system. *tPA*, Tissue plasminogen activator.

ANESTHETIC IMPLICATIONS

Preoperative Considerations

The preoperative interview is the ideal time for the anesthesia provider to gather detailed information regarding the patient's health status. A thorough history and physical is the best way to identify patients at risk for surgical bleeding or those patients with thrombopoietic tendencies.[10] It is also during the interview that additional laboratory tests can be ordered if necessary to identify potential defects in hemostasis and to guide the decision whether to order and/or administer blood products.

During the preoperative interview, it is important to ask questions directly related to bleeding: (1) Does the patient experience unusual bleeding or bruising (e.g., bleeding gums, epistaxis, mucous membrane bleeding, or melena)? (2) Is there a history of previous bleeding with dental procedures? (3) Are there repeated spontaneous bleeding episodes or a history of excess bleeding that may have occurred after a minor procedure or childhood trauma? (4) Do familial bleeding tendencies exist? (5) Has there been a time when expected bleeding from a surgical procedure was more than anticipated?[4,11] These questions can reveal an undiagnosed inherited disorder of coagulation. Patients who have undiagnosed inherited coagulopathies may complain of hematomas, runaway bruising, and oozing, even after the most minor injuries. An undetected preoperative bleeding tendency can lead to life-threatening blood loss during surgery.[4]

Laboratory evaluation of platelets, coagulation, and fibrinolytic components can be screened with the commonly available coagulation tests.

When approaching the patient scheduled for surgery, a physical examination with a complete systems approach is necessary. The anesthesia provider must be alert to potential disruptions in hemostasis. Any overt physical sign of bleeding such as the appearance of bruising or petechial hemorrhages on the chest, abdomen, or upper extremities warrants further investigation. Small hemorrhages on the skin may indicate the presence of small hemorrhages on other organs as well. Remember, the questionable coagulopathy can be related to any number of disruptions in the hemostasis process: a platelet problem, a factor deficiency, an inherited disorder of coagulation, the presence of circulating anticoagulants, or a disturbance in the fibrinolytic system.

During the physical assessment, disorders of malnutrition or liver insufficiency suggesting a vitamin K deficiency may be revealed. These disorders can influence coagulation and explain increased bleeding, even for the simplest surgery. Vitamin K is created from bacteria in the gut and is necessary for the formation of factors II, VII, IX, and X. When illness such as liver insufficiency, cirrhosis, absorption problems, and failure to secrete bile are present, the patient will be unable to form and use these factors for effective coagulation.

Patients with preexisting inherited disorders of coagulation must undergo an adequate preoperative workup prior to surgery. Consultation with a hematologist or transfusion specialist is strongly recommended. Patients with preexisting coagulation disorders require considerable attention in the operating room. If general surgery is anticipated, special attention must be made to ensure no damage to soft tissues occurs. Damage to tissues may transpire during direct laryngoscopy, endotracheal intubation, peripheral or central line placement, and positioning or moving to and from the operating-room table.

The preoperative use of many medications—prescribed, over the counter, and herbal remedies—can interfere with normal platelet function and coagulation (Box 35-1). The anesthesia provider must ascertain whether the patient regularly ingests medications that might interfere with normal coagulation and when the last time the medications or herbals were taken. For example, many patients take aspirin for a number of reasons. Historically it has been recommended that aspirin be held for 7 to 10 days prior to surgery. Current recommendations are discussed in detail later in this chapter. Aspirin directly affects the life of the platelet by *irreversibly* inhibiting cyclooxygenase, resulting in decreased platelet function.[12] Nonsteroidal antiinflammatory drugs (NSAIDs) also inhibit cyclooxygenase, albeit *reversibly*, and the recommendation is to withhold NSAIDs for approximately 24 to 48 hours to avoid any bleeding effects in surgery[13,14] (Figure 35-10).

A preoperative discussion between the patient, surgeon, and anesthesia provider must occur regarding transfusion requirements during surgery. Informing patients about the safety, screening measures, and risks of blood administration cannot be ignored. A small percentage of patients will have to contend with the negative sequelae of transfusion therapy (hepatitis, human immunodeficiency virus, and bacterial transmission), despite careful screening and handling. In situations with emergent or trauma patients, many times a preoperative interview is unattainable, and the provider must rely purely on information supplied by family members (if present), physical assessment, and lab analysis.

BOX 35-1

Frequently Encountered Medications That Influence Coagulation

Anticoagulants
- Heparins
- Low-molecular-weight heparins
- Coumarin derivatives
- Direct thrombin inhibitors

Procoagulants
- Vitamin K

Antiplatelets
- Nonsteroidal antiinflammatory drugs
- Persantine
- Thienopyridine (Plavix and Ticlid)

Antifibrinolytics
- Amicar
- Tranexamic acid

Nonherbal Dietary
- Vitamin K
- Vitamin E
- Coenzyme Q10
- Zinc
- Omega-3 fatty acids

Herbal
- Garlic
- Ginger
- Ginkgo
- Feverfew
- Fish oil
- Flaxseed oil
- Black cohosh
- Cranberry

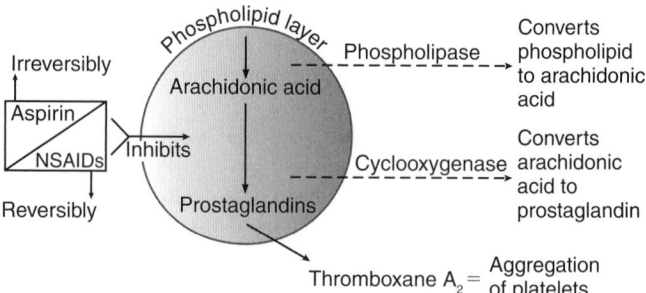

FIGURE 35-10 Schematic illustration depicting the mechanism and site of action of aspirin and nonsteroidal antiinflammatory drugs (NSAIDs).

Laboratory Tests

Routine laboratory tests must be evaluated preoperatively. They serve to guide the clinician in determining whether a coagulation disorder exists (Table 35-3). Laboratory tests should be ordered on an individual basis, considering the patient's history and planned surgical procedure.

The most frequently assessed tests are the bleeding time, platelet count, PT, aPTT, and thrombin time (Table 35-4). Together, these tests evaluate vascular contraction, platelet function, coagulation, and the fibrinolytic system. Results of these routine tests must fall within the normal range. If they are outside normal range, there must be a reasonable explanation, and adequate measures must taken to correct or control hemostasis before bringing the patient into the operating room. For example, if the patient requires surgery but not emergently, vitamin K can be administered 4 to 6 hours prior to surgery. If the risk of bleeding is moderate, a type and crossmatch may be preferred to a type and screen. If the patient requires surgery emergently, ordering blood components such as packed red blood cells, FFP, platelets, and cryoprecipitate may be advisable.

The bleeding time evaluates the capability of microvascular contraction and the function of platelets. When vascular injury occurs, the initial response from the blood vessels is to contract, and the response of the platelets is to adhere to the site of injury. If either of these two processes is compromised, prolonged bleeding will occur, resulting in inadequate hemostasis.

The bleeding time was once thought to be the best indicator of bleeding risk. The use of a bleeding time test, however, is open to much scrutiny, and there are many reasons to question its use and interpretation.[17] In the absence of drug ingestion, a prolonged bleeding time suggests primary hemostasis abnormality, and further investigation is recommended. Although the bleeding time is a means of evaluating vascular integrity and platelet function, it is important to appreciate that a prolonged bleeding time is not a good predictor of bleeding or a sign that an abnormality is present.[18] In addition, an isolated prolonged value is not a reason to cancel or delay a surgical procedure.

The platelet count is the actual number of platelets present in blood per cubic millimeter. A normal platelet count does not imply normal platelet function exists, only how many platelets are present in plasma. It is used to evaluate patients who present with petechiae or unexplained spontaneous bleeding and to monitor thrombocytopenia (low platelet count). The platelet's

Careful consideration must be given to the patient who refuses blood component therapy for personal or religious reasons. This patient can be an ethical challenge to health-care providers, especially when refusal may mean a greater chance for mortality because a high-risk procedure may incur greater blood loss. In these special situations, an inclusive discussion of potential or available options must be addressed. If the patient is a candidate, there are alternatives available such as erythropoietin administration, acute normovolemic hemodilution, cell salvage, recombinant factor VII or VIII, and topical coagulants. Pharmacologic alternatives (Amicar, tranexamic acid) can also be means of stabilizing coagulation when significant blood loss is anticipated.

Most anesthesia providers are familiar with the Jehovah Witness population and their refusal of blood transfusion or derived components. However, it is important to consider that some Jehovah Witness will accept certain fractions of primary blood components (albumin, leukocyte-depleted red cells, platelets, solvent-treated fresh frozen plasma [FFP], and recombinant products) or alternatives to allogenic transfusions, as long as blood remains continuous with the body.[15] Advice regarding available management options should be discussed, especially with high-risk blood-loss procedures.[16]

TABLE 35-3 Possible Causes and Treatment of Hemostatic Disorders

Clinical Coagulation Tests							
BL	aPTT	PT	BT	PC	Fib	Possible Cause	Treatment
	Abn					Factor VIII, heparin, "lupus anticoagulant," poor sample	No treatment
+	Abn					Factors XI, IX, VIII, heparin therapy	FFP, protamine
+	Abn	Abn				Factors V, X, II, dysfibrinogenemia, heparin, coumarins	FFP, cryoprecipitate, protamine
+		Abn				Factor VII	FFP
+	Abn		Abn			Von Willebrand disease	Desmopressin acetate, cryoprecipitate
+	Abn	Abn	Abn		Low	Hypofibrinogenemia	FFP, cryoprecipitate
+			Abn	Abn		Thrombocytopenia	Platelet concentrate (8-10 units)
+			Abn			Thrombocytopathy, aspirin, NSAIDs	Platelet concentrate
+	Abn	Abn	Abn	Abn	Abn	DIC, severe liver disease, dilutional coagulopathy	FFP, cryoprecipitate, platelet concentrate, whole blood

+, *Increased clinical bleeding;* Abn, *abnormal result;* aPTT, *activated partial thromboplastin time;* BL, *bleeding;* BT, *bleeding time,* DIC, *disseminated intravascular coagulation;* FFP, *fresh frozen plasma;* Fib, *fibrinogen;* NSAIDs, *nonsteroidal antiinflammatory drugs;* PC, *platelet count;* PT, *prothrombin time.*

TABLE 35-4 Coagulation Tests

Laboratory Test	Value*	Description
Bleeding time	3-7 minutes	Measures platelet function: adhesion, aggregation Not considered a routine test Modest prolongations do not predict surgical bleeding * Altered by aspirin and NSAIDs
Platelet count	150,000-350,000 mm³	Thrombocytopenic: <100,000 mm³ Surgical risk: <50,000 mm³ Spontaneous bleeding: <20,000 mm³
Prothrombin time (PT)	Normal: control Average normal: 12-14 seconds	Value is reagent dependent Prolonged with: • extrinsic pathway disorder • common pathway disorder * Altered by coumarin derivatives
Activated partial thromboplastin time (aPTT) (intrinsic and common pathway)	Average normal: 25-32 seconds	Prolonged with: • intrinsic pathway disorder • common pathway disorder * Altered by heparin and Lovenox
Thrombin time (common pathway)	8-12 seconds	Measures fibrinogen-to-fibrin reaction
Activated clotting time (ACT)	80-150 seconds	Guides anticoagulation dosing
Fibrinogen	>150 mg/dL; 200-350 mg/mL	Measures fibrinogen level
Fibrinogen (degradation products)	<10 mcg/mL	Measures by-products from clot dissolution
D-Dimer	<500 mg/mL	Measures degradation products secondary to fibrinolysis
Thromboelastogram		Measures global hemostasis
Antithrombin III	80%-120%	Measures antithrombin III levels; decreased level may explain subtherapeutic heparin Severely depressed in DIC

DIC, *Disseminated intravascular coagulation;* NSAIDs, *nonsteroidal antiinflammatory drugs;* TEG, *thromboelastogram.*

primary role is to maintain vascular integrity, aggregate when a plug is necessary to stop bleeding, and help initiate the clotting pathways. A normal platelet count is 150,000 to 300,000/mm^3.[2] Patients are considered thrombocytopenic at counts less than 100,000 mm^3. There are varying degrees of thrombocytopenia that must be considered preoperatively. Platelet counts greater than 100,000 are sufficient for hemostasis. When the platelet count declines to 50,000/mm^3, spontaneous bleeding rarely occurs, but one should suspect prolonged bleeding under surgical conditions.[19] A platelet count less than 20,000 is considered a critical level, and spontaneous bleeding is likely to occur.[20,21]

The PT is used to evaluate the efficiency of the extrinsic factors (III and VII) and common coagulation pathway (factors X, V, II, I) in generating enough thrombin to form fibrin to create a stable clot. The PT is specific to the extrinsic pathway of the clotting cascade. It is the most commonly used test to monitor oral anticoagulant therapy (e.g., the coumarin derivatives). The PT will be prolonged when patients have abnormalities or are deficient in factors specific to the extrinsic and common clotting pathways (III, VII, X, IX, II, I).[5]

Despite the frequent assessment of the PT value preoperatively, this lab value has drawbacks. The PT is not a very sensitive test. The PT also fails to identify the specific factor defect in the hemostatic system. It only identifies an existing problem that may or may not cause bleeding.

The international normalized ratio (INR) evaluates the extrinsic and common pathway independently of various reagents used in different laboratory settings and in different areas of the world. The normal INR is 1.5 to 2.5. Many institutions report both PT and INR values.

The aPTT is a test used to evaluate the efficiency of the intrinsic coagulation pathway (factors XII, XI, IX, and VIII) and the common coagulation pathway (factors X, V, II, I, and ultimately XIII) to form fibrin and eventually a stable clot. The aPTT can identify abnormalities in all factors except III and VII. It is also used to monitor anticoagulation status when heparin therapy is used. The aPTT can be prolonged by abnormalities, deficiencies, or inhibitors of any intrinsic or common pathway defect. Factor concentration must be decreased 30% before evidence of a prolonged PT or an aPTT can be appreciated.[1,19]

Any factor deficiency in either limb of the clotting cascade can alter the PT and/or aPTT, but this does not imply that any prediction of an individual patient risk of bleeding can be anticipated.[7] For example, a decrease in factor XII will demonstrate an increase in aPTT but will not cause bleeding.[6] A decrease in factor XI may or may not cause abnormal bleeding. However, a decrease in either factor VIII or IX will definitely cause bleeding with injury. This is seen in hemophilia.

The activated clotting time (ACT) is a simple, quick test that can be used in surgery to monitor the blood's ability to clot. The ACT is also used to regulate heparin therapy. The normal ACT is 90 to 150 seconds. The ACT is not, however, a sensitive test.

The thrombin time is a screening tool for assessing the ending phase of coagulation. Because fibrinogen can be assessed directly, analysis of the thrombin time is less emphasized.

The thromboelastogram (TEG) measures the process of clot formation over time. The benefit of this test is its ability to evaluate (1) platelet reactions, (2) coagulation and, (3) fibrinolysis. A blood specimen is collected and placed in a machine that measures the speed at which a clot forms. The results of the TEG provide an indication of (1) clot strength, (2) platelet number and function, (3) intrinsic pathway defects, (4) thrombin formation, and (5) the rate of fibrinolysis. The results of this test can be used to guide blood component therapy and possibly decrease the amount of transfusion products administered.[2]

Lab tests are only as good as the individual interpreting them and many times will not adequately reflect the potential to bleed or thrombose. The use of coagulation tests is best interpreted when patients are without pathology, are not on any medications that could disrupt the lab value measured, and are assessed in conjunction with physical assessment and clinical judgment. It is prudent to consult with a hematologist when there is any suspicion of the potential for abnormal bleeding in surgery or if a coagulation disorder exists. Coagulation tests can be performed in the operating room; however, lengthy delay in reporting their values during a time of critical volume loss and coagulopathic alterations can render the value ineffective. Coagulation tests initiated in the operating room may nevertheless serve as a guide.

Intraoperative Period

One main focus of the surgeon and the anesthesia practitioner in the operating room is to recognize and efficiently control blood loss. Frequent evaluation of the patient's clinical status, surgical site, sponges, canisters, and the operating room floor cannot be overemphasized.[19] The surgeon and anesthesia provider are equally responsible in communicating that persistent oozing or frank bleeding is occurring. It is this open communication that helps the surgical team recognize problems and rapidly intervene by having blood components in the room, rechecking ABO compatibility, and anticipating the need for coagulation-factor replacement if transfusion therapy is necessary.

There are many potential adverse effects associated with the administration of blood component therapy. Despite the presence of screening tests, hepatitis and human immunodeficiency virus (HIV) transmission continue to influence patients' decisions about whether they wish to receive blood components. But the incidence of hepatitis and HIV is low when compared with the frequency of other adverse reactions to blood component therapy. Transfusion therapy is also associated with acute hemolytic transfusion reactions, nonhemolytic reactions, viral transmission, transfusion-related acute lung injury, parasite transmission, and bacterial transmission.

The most commonly transfused blood components are red blood cells, platelets, fresh frozen plasma, and cryoprecipitate (Table 35-5). The major reasons for transfusion therapy in the operating room are to replace volume and coagulation factors and improve oxygen-carrying capacity.[22] Each component carries its own concerns.

Packed red blood cells (PRBCs) are transfused to improve tissue oxygenation. Although the oxygen-carrying capacity of red cells decreases with the length of storage, it improves when 2,3 diphosphoglycerate (2,3 DPG) is regenerated once transfused. Platelets are provided to patients when a deficit is appreciated or when massive transfusion is required. Platelets can be given as a single-donor plateletpheresis pack or collected and pooled from multiple donors (random-donor platelets).

The recommended dose for platelet replacement is one plateletpheresis pack per each 10 kg patient weight. This dose should increase the platelet count by approximately 5000 to 10,000 mm^3.[5,19] Whereas the normal life span of a platelet is 7 to 10 days, the life span of a donated platelet is only 4 to 5 days.[9]

The Anesthesia Task Force recommends (1) the use of platelets in the operating room for microvascular bleeding, regardless of platelet count, and (2) the use of clinical judgment based on the risk of bleeding and the length of the surgery when the platelet count falls between 50,000 and 100,000/mm^3.

TABLE **35-5**	Blood Components		
Blood Component	**Definition**	**Surgical Indications**	**Dose**
PRBC	1. Red blood cells anticoagulated in plasma	1. Bleeding 2. Increase O_2 carrying capacity	1 unit increases Hb by 1 g/dL and Hct by 3%
FFP (all factors)	1. Plasma separated from RBC and platelets 2. Contains ALL clotting factors 3. Contains naturally occurring inhibitors 4. Source of antithrombin III 5. One bag = 200-250 mL 6. Expires 12 months post-donation	1. Microvascular bleeding 2. Coagulopathy due to factor deficiency 3. PT/aPTT >1.5 normal 4. Massive blood transfusions 5. Reversal of warfarin 6. Acquired coagulopathy 7. Von Willebrand disorder unresponsive to DDAVP 8. Antithrombin deficiency	10-15 mL/kg
Platelets	1. Obtain from whole blood or plateletpheresis donations 2. Contain platelets only 3. One bag = random volume 4. One bag pheresis = 250-300 mL	1. Massive blood transfusion 2. Active bleeding 3. <5000 = spontaneous hemorrhage 4. 10-50,000 = variable bleeding risk 5. >50,000 = spontaneous bleeding unlikely due to platelets	1 unit/10 kg body weight One unit increases platelet level 5000-10,000/mm^3
Cryoprecipitate	1. Protein fraction taken off the top of FFP when being thawed 2. Then refrozen up to 1 year 3. Contains factors I, vWF, VIII, fibrinogen, XIII 4. One bag = 10-20 mL	1. Microvascular bleeding 2. Von Willebrand disease unresponsive to DDAVP	1 bag/5 mg body weight 1 unit raises fibrinogen by 50 mg/dL

DDAVP, *Desmopressin acetate*; FFP, *fresh frozen plasma*; Hct, *hematocrit*; Hb, *hemoglobin*; PRBC, *packed red blood cells*; vWF, *von Willebrand factor*.

Prophylactic administration of platelets may not be necessary, especially when the cause of thrombocytopenia is destruction of platelets (e.g., heparin-induced thrombocytopenia, idiopathic thrombocytopenia purpura, thrombotic thrombocytopenia purpura) or when the count is greater than 100,000.[19,22] Although there are varying degrees of thrombocytopenia, if persistent bleeding or oozing occurs in the operating room, a transfusion might be considered despite a platelet count greater than 50,000. Compatible plateletpheresis is recommended, but when matched platelets are unavailable, unmatched platelets can be given; however, this incompatibility shortens the life span of the platelet.[3,23] When pooled platelets are administered to women of childbearing age, Rh sensitization can occur, and administration of Rh$_O$(D) immune globulin may be necessary prior to discharge.

Platelets carry the greatest risk of bacterial transmission.[23,24] Platelets are stored for 4 to 5 days at room temperature, providing an excellent medium for the growth and reproduction of bacteria. Standard protocols for blood banks and transfusion services require that a method be in place to detect bacterial contamination of platelets.[23,25]

Fresh frozen plasma is the fluid portion of whole blood, separated then frozen to preserve coagulation factors and subsequently thawed on use. FFP contains all the clotting factors and naturally occurring inhibitors.[26] It does not provide platelet replacement. The average volume in a unit of FFP is 200 to 250 mL. FFP must be ABO plasma compatible whenever possible.

FFP is transfused (1) for microvascular bleeding, (2) when the concentration of coagulation factors is deficient, (3) to patients with an inherited coagulopathy, (4) for the reversal of warfarin administration, and (5) for a deficiency resulting from a dilutional coagulopathy[19,21,26] (assuming the patient's preoperative lab values were normal). Dilutional coagulopathies increase when blood is diluted to at least 30% or when a patient loses more than one volume of blood, indicating only a third of the coagulation factors are present.[27] This deficit is reflected in lab values. Lab analysis will reveal the need for FFP by a PT and aPTT prolonged more than 1.5 times normal. The use of FFP for volume replacement is contraindicated. Safety screening for FFP is the same as for RBCs.

Cryoprecipitate is the precipitate collected off the top of FFP as it is thawed. Cryoprecipitate is then refrozen and thawed on use. It is rich in fibrinogen and contains factors VIII, XIII, and fibronectin. The current guidelines recommend cryoprecipitate for (1) microvascular bleeding in conjunction with FFP, (2) patients with von Willebrand disease or hemophilia when concentrates are unavailable, (3) suspected factor deficiencies, and (4) prophylaxis when a fibrinogen defect is present.[21] Despite cryoprecipitate's ability to decrease factor deficiencies, more studies are required to ascertain the effectiveness of cryoprecipitate in clinical outcome.

It is preferable to transfuse platelets, FFP, and cryoprecipitate with adherence to ABO compatibility to avoid hemolytic reactions, but there are times when this practice is impractical. When massive transfusion occurs, one should be alert to the risk of hemolytic reaction. In addition to viral screening for donor units, the institution of solvent detergents, psoralen derivatives, and methylene blue are being evaluated as means to decreasing emerging viral contaminations, especially when blood products are pooled. The effect of these additives on platelets, FFP, and cryoprecipitate is still under investigation.[23,25]

Despite policies, procedures, and screening modalities, there may never be a time when blood component therapy will be without risk.[23,28] New illnesses and viruses emerge as quickly as the old ones are controlled. Additionally, human error influences the incidence of transfusion reactions. Nevertheless, blood component therapy is still often necessary in the operating room.

Transfusion Guidelines

There is no magic number or an absolute transfusion "trigger" for blood-component administration. There are few if any fixed guidelines or practice standards for transfusion therapy. There are, however, many suggested guidelines and protocols that vary among individual institutions. Past literature recommends a hemoglobin of 10 g/dL as an indicator for red-blood-cell transfusion, but transfusion delivery based on one isolated lab value without regard to the patient's overall health status is irresponsible.[29] A hemoglobin value of 8 g/dL and even 6 g/dL may be acceptable when ischemia or risk factors for cardiovascular disease are not evident.[19,22]

Blood components should be initiated when blood loss is real, when there is a need to increase oxygen-carrying capacity, and when patient hemodynamics reflect instability from blood loss (decreased blood pressure, increased heart rate, decreased saturation, low central venous pressure, and low urine output).[19] Transfusion of blood products may also be given for anticipated blood loss. Prophylactic blood transfusion may be indicated under certain circumstances to improve platelet count, correct a coagulopathy, or increase oxygen-carrying capacity prior to the procedure.

It is prudent to consider the patient's vital signs, age, and medical history as reflections of blood-loss tolerance. A tachyarrhythmia may imply that a state of hypovolemia exists in the absence of pain or light anesthesia. The same may be true for a patient experiencing hypotension. Although evaluation of vital signs and urinary output provide the chief indicators of volume status or bleeding, administration of medications can manipulate or mask reflections of hypovolemia. Many medications blunt reflexes or block heart rates that would otherwise alert the anesthesia provider to intolerant hypovolemia, especially when blood loss is sequestered under and between the sterile drapes.[22] Communication with the surgeon, evaluation of lab analysis, and assessment of the clinical profile are crucial when the decision is being made to transfuse.

Some simple interventions may reduce the need for blood transfusions and the risks that accompany them. Serial hemoglobin and hematocrit, PT, and aPTT can be used more frequently to guide replacement therapy. Using an approved blood filter or warming the blood can deter coagulopathies that persist in the operating room.[22]

There are also alternatives available to reduce or allay allogenic component replacement: preoperative autologous donation (PAD), acute normovolemic hemodilution (ANH), blood-cell salvage (BCS), and recombinant factor VII. If the patient is a candidate and time permits, PAD collection for transfusion in surgery is an option. Candidates must be healthy, have an elective procedure scheduled ahead of time, be undergoing a procedure in which the necessity for transfusion is likely, have a hemoglobin greater than 10 g/dL, and be without medical conditions (coronary artery disease or infection) that would contraindicate donating autologous blood.[29]

PAD can be used alone or in combination with other alternative means for transfusion. Patients who donate benefit from the reduction in some adverse affects that accompany transfusion therapy but are not spared the possibility of bacterial contamination. Importantly, the availability of autologous blood does not guarantee allogenic blood transfusion will not be necessary. Autologous donation is not necessary when the expected blood loss for a particular surgery is low. Additionally, collection and processing can be a financial disadvantage, especially when the blood units are discarded and not returned to the blood pool.

Acute normovolemic hemodilution (ANH) is a form of autologous blood transfusion that may substitute for allogenic blood replacement. In ANH, a predetermined number of blood units are withdrawn from the patient shortly after induction but before incision. The blood is removed to a target hematocrit 25% to 35% of the preoperative value.[30] The units are placed in standard collection bags containing an anticoagulant (citrate), labeled with the patient's name and medical record number, dated, and timed. The collected blood units remain in the operating room and can be stored for up to 8 hours at room temperature and up to 24 hours when refrigerated.[30-32] Patients who are candidates for ANH are generally healthy, without cardiovascular risk factors, and must be able to tolerate a decreased blood volume. Blood retrieved by ANH has normal levels of coagulation factors and functioning platelets, assuming the patient was without factor deficiency prior to entering the operating room. ANH is used when blood loss in surgery is likely to be greater than 20% of the patient's blood volume.[25,30,31] It is also a useful alternative when compatible blood is unavailable or when there is a delay or a problem in crossmatching blood components. Because viral transmission and antibody issues are nonexistent, patients are spared some of the risks of infection and immunologic side effects. The need for ANH is based on surgical risk and not on its availability. Good communication between the anesthesia provider and the surgeon is recommended.[31]

The physiologic theory supporting ANH is that decreasing the number of red cells by dilution with crystalloid or colloid translates into a decreased RBC loss (fewer RBCs in circulation). By decreasing the blood's viscosity, a reciprocal increase in oxygen delivery occurs. Although ANH offers an alternative to the administration of allogenic blood transfusion, in times of emergency when massive blood loss is present, allogenic blood replacement may be the only option.

Intraoperative blood-cell salvage (BCS) devices are more common as a strategy for autologous transfusion. The patient's blood is collected from the surgical field, citrated, filtered, and washed with saline. Salvaged blood is then concentrated and returned to the patient. BCS is considered when the expected blood loss is greater than 20% of blood volume.[16] BCS can lower allogenic requirements and is ideal when massive blood loss occurs and blood is not readily available. It provides an alternative for the patient who refuses blood products. Salvaged blood is deficient in clotting factors and platelets; patients may become hypofibrinogenemic, as well as thrombocytopenic.[32] BCS does not require viral screening, adding to its attractiveness as a substitute for allogenic products. Hemolyzed red blood cells may exacerbate renal failure when insufficiency preexists.

The use of cell salvage is contraindicated when bacteria have contaminated the wound, malignancy exists, blood contains fat or amniotic fluid, or synthetic clotting agents have been placed on tissues.[25,30] Despite the recovery of intraoperative blood, allogenic replacement is still necessary in many cases of trauma and massive blood loss.

The administration of recombinant factor VII is another alternative therapy to boost coagulation. Recombinant factor VII was approved by the U.S. Food and Drug Administration (FDA) in 1999 for hemophilia A (factor VIII) and B (factor IX), inhibitor disorders of factor VIII and IX, factor VII deficiency, and as a universal hemostatic agent.[8,33-35] Its off-label use has successfully treated coagulation insufficiencies associated with platelet dysfunction, intracranial hemorrhage, prostate surgery, and trauma.[36]

The exact mode of action of factor VII is undetermined. Both the classic coagulation cascade and the cell-based theory agree that factor VII enhances thrombin generation by augmenting TF/VII at the site of vessel injury and on the surface of the platelet.[6,33,34] Administration ultimately boosts thrombin to form fibrin for clot stabilization. The recommended dose of factor VII for hemophilia is 90 to 120 mcg/kg. There is no definitive dose for use in the operating room for patient without prior coagulation disorders, but 20 to 45 mcg/kg has been suggested.[8]

Factor VII will reverse prolonged INR, but it fails to replace all the clotting factors.[33] The anesthesia provider must remain vigilant intraoperatively, providing interventions that would prevent acidosis and hypothermia, both of which can interrupt the efficacy of the drug.[33,34,37] Patients have experienced cerebrovascular accidents, myocardial infarctions, pulmonary emboli, and arterial and venous thromboemboli. Factor VII should be used cautiously in any patient predisposed to thrombosis.[19,26,35,36,38]

The indications for the use of factor VII remain limited, and the expense of the drug (more than $9000 for a 4.8-mL vial) can affect its use.[37] The utilization of factor VII should not be initiated in a desperate effort to improve outcome but rather as a means of adjunctive therapy when other conventional interventions have not sufficiently induced hemostasis. Consultation with a hematologist or transfusion specialist should be considered.[35] Factor VII should be initiated following specific guidelines of the institution. Additional studies on patients without coagulopathies will better assess factor VII's safety and efficacy and lead to development of more specific guidelines for its use.[35,38]

Postoperative Management

Patients should be reassessed in the postanesthesia care unit and again within 24 hours of surgery. Unrecognized bleeding can thus be identified and corrected before the patient deteriorates. Evaluations of (1) the patient's color and mentation, (2) trends in vital signs (with specific attention to tachycardia or hypotension), (3) urine output, (4) hypothermia, (5) hemodynamic values such as CVP, (6) lab values, and (7) dressings and/or drain volume must be judiciously monitored.

SPECIFIC DISORDERS

Bleeding diathesis can result from any number of deficiencies in coagulation. A few disorders encountered in practice are described here, as well as points to consider when dealing with a patient requiring anticoagulant therapy.

Von Willebrand Disease

Von Willebrand disease (vWD) has traditionally remained the most common inherited coagulation diathesis. Von Willebrand factor (vWF) is a heterogeneous multinumeric glycoprotein that serves two main functions: to facilitate platelet adhesion and to behave as a plasma carrier for factor VIII of the coagulation cascade.[39] Synthesis of vWF takes place in the endothelial cells and megakaryocytes.[40] An acquired form of vWD is seen with lymphomyeloproliferative or immunologic disease states secondary to antibodies against vWF.[41]

Similar to many coagulopathies, vWD has varying degrees of severity—mild, moderate, and severe. In the milder or moderate forms, regular or spontaneous bleeding is not evident but is likely after surgery or when trauma occurs.[10] In the more severe form of vWD, spontaneous epistaxis and oral, gastrointestinal, and genitourinary bleeding can be relentless.

Most patients with vWD exhibit a prolonged bleeding time, a deficiency in vWF and factor VIII, decreased vWF activity measured by a ristocetin (an antibiotic) cofactor (RCoF) assay, and decreased factor VIII coagulant activity (VIII:C). The recommended treatment for vWD is supplementation with recombinant factor VIII-vWF concentrate preoperatively and during surgery to raise the levels of circulating factor VIII and vWF. Cryoprecipitate is another means of acquiring factor VIII; however, there is attendant risk of viral transmission. Desmopressin acetate (DDAVP), a synthetic vasopressin, is an excellent option for the milder forms of vWD and should not be overlooked. DDAVP helps increase plasma levels of vWF and augment aggregation.[42]

Hemophilia

Hemophilia is an X-linked hematologic recessive disorder characterized by unpredictable bleeding patterns. Patients are either deficient in factor IX (hemophilia A) or factor VIII (hemophilia B). Hemophilia affects males almost exclusively, although females carry the gene for the disease. Patients with hemophilia A are grouped as mild (excessive bleeding after trauma or surgery), moderate (rarely have extensive, unprovoked bleeding), and severe (absence of factor VIII in the plasma). Hemophiliacs exhibit spontaneous bleeding, muscle hematomas, and pain at joint sites. Continued joint bleeding often results in decreased range of motion and progressive joint arthropathy and often requires orthopedic surgical intervention throughout life.[43]

In the past, the life expectancy for the hemophiliac was short. Because hemophiliacs were deficient in factors VIII and IX, they required blood-component transfusion to replace the deficient or missing factors. The only factor components available were FFP and cryoprecipitate. Screening tests for donated blood units were unavailable, and patient mortality was high. Many hemophiliacs contracted transmissible diseases such as hepatitis and HIV and ultimately died from sequelae of blood transfusion therapy.[43] Furthermore, hemophiliacs were termed "high risk" for most surgical procedures and often turned down for many elective procedures. Today, blood components undergo extensive screening, and newer and safer treatment modalities exist. Most surgeries are available to hemophiliacs, with little risk of uncontrolled bleeding.[44]

For patients with hemophilia or a family history of hemophilia, a preoperative assessment of hemostasis is imperative. Preoperative lab tests should include a platelet count and function, a coagulation panel (PT, aPTT, factor VIII, factor IX, and fibrinogen), as well as an inhibitor test.[44] If the hemophiliac was given a test dose of factor VII preoperatively, the response to the test dose should be evaluated. The patient should be typed and crossmatched, because even a low-risk procedure can be catastrophic for the hemophiliac.

A clearly defined anesthesia plan is essential for the hemophiliac; uncontrolled bleeding is certainly a possibility. Factor VIII concentrate can be given prior to surgery. Factor VII is administered intraoperatively to augment thrombin generation and deter bleeding. The dose should be precalculated and vial availability confirmed prior to going into the operating room. Desmopressin (0.3 mcg/kg) can also be administered to increase plasma levels of factor VIII and vWF for mild to moderate hemophiliacs.[39,45] There is no risk for viral transmission when either of these drugs is initiated.

OTHER CONSIDERATIONS

Perioperative Management of Patients Taking Anticoagulant Drugs

The preoperative discontinuation of anticoagulation therapy is currently a controversial topic with no absolute universal guidelines. Excessive bleeding may occur if the anticoagulation medications are not discontinued before surgery. This may lead to potentially serious intraoperative and postoperative complications or the need for transfusion of blood and blood products. Withholding anticoagulant medications places the patient at increased risk for myocardial infarctions, cerebrovascular accidents, arterial or venous thromboembolism, pulmonary embolism, or death.[46-48] Situation-specific considerations are leading to new recommendations on surgical management of anticoagulated patients.

A study by Dunn and Turpie demonstrates safety with uninterrupted administration of anticoagulant therapy specifically for *low*-risk procedures such as dental events, arthrodesis, cataracts, and diagnostic endoscopies. A thorough assessment of the patient history, diagnosis, and procedure must be made to weigh the risks of potential stroke, myocardial infarction, and thromboembolism for both cardiac and noncardiac surgeries. Complications of any kind translate into increased cost and prolonged hospitalizations.[11] Common anticoagulants, doses, and indications are given in Table 35-6.

Antiplatelet Drugs and Noncardiac Surgery: Patients with Coronary Stents

Anesthesia providers routinely manage patients with coronary artery disease who have had coronary stents placed and are receiving dual antiplatelet therapy with aspirin and thienopyridines. Coronary stents are placed to improve coronary artery flow in patients with stable but symptomatic coronary artery disease or acute coronary syndromes, including unstable angina, non–Q wave myocardial infarction, and ST-elevation acute myocardial infarctions. Once the coronary stent is placed in the lumen of the coronary artery, endothelialization of the stent begins.

There are two distinct complications associated with stent placement: acute stent thrombosis and in-stent restenosis. Acute stent *thrombosis* may lead to abrupt closure of the coronary artery and an acute coronary syndrome such as myocardial infarction. Thrombosis can occur anytime after stent implantation and anytime antiplatelet medications are discontinued. Most of these events occur in the first 30 days after stent placement, usually in the first week. *Restenosis* of a stent is a slowly developing occlusion directly related to excessive endothelial growth over time. In most cases, it peaks between 6 and 9 months after stent implantation. Symptoms of restenosis can be insidious and lead to symptoms of coronary insufficiency or be silent and (less frequently) lead to acute myocardial infarction.[46-48]

There are two types of stents available: bare-metal stents (BMS) and drug-eluting stents (DES). Bare-metal stents are made of a steel or cobalt alloy. The endothelialization process takes approximately 2 to 4 weeks. For drug-eluting stents, the process is significantly slower and in some cases may be incomplete. A polymer attached to the stent releases a drug designed to stop cell division and therefore excessive endothelial growth.[49] Patients receive concomitant aspirin and a thienopyridine such as clopidogrel as antiplatelet therapy. The risk of acute stent thrombosis is relatively low but may occur more commonly with DES. The most common cause is premature cessation of antiplatelet therapy. In the case of DES, the delayed or incomplete endothelialization process is felt to be a risk factor for acute stent thrombosis, especially when clopidogrel is stopped. Stents require dual antiplatelet therapy to prevent stent thrombosis. Clopidogrel is recommended for 4 to 6 weeks for bare-metal stents and for at least 1 year for drug-eluting stents. Aspirin is used indefinitely. Additional risk factors for acute stent thrombosis include inadequate stent expansion, the use of multiple stents, stenting across coronary side branches, small-diameter stents, and long stented segments (>33 mm). For these reasons, it is prudent to consult a cardiologist for guidance regarding preoperative and postoperative management of antiplatelet therapy. Box 35-2 outlines the duration of antiplatelet therapy for different situations after percutaneous coronary interventions.

This patient population requires special attention preoperatively. Important information should include the date of stent implantation, the type of stent deployed, and antiplatelet therapy if applicable. Additional points to consider are the type of operation planned and the risk of bleeding. The current medication regimen must be assessed; many patients have discontinued their antiplatelet medications preoperatively, but others continue them at the request of their cardiologist. Surgery in which the risk of bleeding is low may not require discontinuation of antiplatelet therapy. Patients who require emergent surgery should be evaluated on a case-by-case basis, weighing the risks of bleeding against the risks of thrombosis. The American Heart Association/American College of Cardiology (AHA/ACC) Science Advisory and the Society of Cardiovascular Angiography DES Task Force have recently updated their guidelines for management of patients with drug-eluting stents (Box 35-3). Their additional recommendations include:

- Aspirin as a lifelong therapy; it should not be stopped before surgery when it is prescribed as a secondary prevention after stroke, angina, myocardial infarction, or revascularization. When used as a primary prevention, it can be withdrawn 1 week before surgery.
- If clopidogrel is prescribed for unstable angina or during the reendothelialization period of a stent, it should not be stopped before a noncardiac procedure. This period lasts 2 to 4 weeks after simple dilatation, 6 weeks after a bare-metal stent is placed, and up to 12 months after a drug-eluting stent is placed, and may be prolonged in unstable situations.
- In tonsillectomy or surgery in closed spaces, the least postoperative hemorrhage might have disastrous consequences, particularly in neurosurgery. Continue aspirin but withdraw clopidogrel for 1 week before intracranial open-skull surgery; meanwhile, it would be safer to give low-molecular-weight heparin (LMWH), although the degree of protection is inferior. In the case of stereotaxic intracranial procedures, aspirin should also be interrupted, but if possible, postpone the operation until the patient can safely stop all antiplatelet medication.
- If it is essential to continue antiplatelet therapy for as long as possible, intravenous infusion of GpIIb-IIIa inhibitors may be used (See Table 35-6.).

TABLE **35-6**	Anticoagulants: Dosages and Indications				
Anticoagulant	**Prophylactic Dosage**	**Therapeutic Dosage**	**FDA-Approved Prophylactic Conditions**	**FDA-Approved Therapeutic Conditions**	
Warfarin (Coumadin)	Usual maintenance: 2-10 mg daily	Usual maintenance: 2 to 10 mg daily	—	—	
Unfractionated heparin	5000 units every 8 to 12 hours	For DVT, start with 80 units per kg bolus, then 18 units/kg/hr infusion	Prophylaxis for patients at risk of developing DVT and PE Prophylaxis of peripheral artery embolization	Treatment of DVT and PE Atrial fibrillation with embolism Prevention of clotting during arterial and cardiac surgery Treatment of peripheral artery embolization Treatment of consumptive coagulopathies	
Low-molecular-weight heparin (dalteparin [Fragmin])	5000 international units daily	100 international units/kg every 12 hours or 200 international units/kg every 24 hours	Unstable angina and non–Q wave MI with aspirin Conditions that predispose to DVT: joint replacement surgery, abdominal surgery, immobilized medical patients	None	
Enoxaparin (Lovenox)	40 mg daily	1 mg/kg every 12 hours or 1.5 mg/kg every 24 hours	Unstable angina and non–Q wave MI with aspirin Conditions that predispose to DVT: joint replacement surgery, abdominal surgery, immobilized medical patients	Inpatient treatment of DVT with and without PE with warfarin Outpatient DVT without PE with warfarin	
Tinzaparin (Innohep)	3500 international units daily	175 international units/kg per 24 hours	None	Treatment of DVT and PE with warfarin	
Bivalirudin (Angiomax)	—	1 mg/kg IV bolus 2.5 mg/kg/hr for 4 hours; with ASA 325 mg May continue with 0.2 mg/kg for up to 20 hours	None	During PTCA for unstable angina	

Adapted from du Breuil AL, Umland EM. Outpatient management of anticoagulation therapy. Am Fam Physician. 2007;75(7):1031-1042; Drugs for percutaneous coronary interventions. Med Lett. 2004;46(1197/1198):100-103.
ASA, Aspirin; DVT, deep vein thrombosis; HIT, heparin-induced thrombocytopenia; MI, myocardial infarction; PCI, percutaneous coronary intervention; PE, pulmonary embolism; PTCA, percutaneous transluminal coronary angioplasty.
Continued

TABLE 35-6   Anticoagulants: Dosages and Indications—cont'd

Anticoagulant	Prophylactic Dosage	Therapeutic Dosage	FDA-Approved Prophylactic Conditions	FDA-Approved Therapeutic Conditions
Desirudin (Iprivasc)	15 mg every 12 hours	—	DVT prophylaxis after hip replacement	None
Lepirudin (Refludan)	—	0.4 mg/kg bolus (maximum: 45 mg) *or* 0.15 mg/kg/hr (maximum: 16.5 mg) for 2 to 10 days	Prophylaxis of venous thromboembolism in patients with HIT	Treatment of thrombosis in patients with HIT
Argatroban (Acova)	—	2 mcg/kg/min	Prophylaxis of venous thromboembolism in patients with HIT	Treatment of thrombosis in patients with HIT
Fondaparinux (Arixtra)	2.5 mg daily	5 mg for a patient less than 50 kg 7.5 mg for 50 to 100 kg 10 mg for more than 100 kg	DVT prophylaxis after hip or knee replacement or abdominal surgery	
Glycoprotein IIb-IIIa Inhibitors				
Abciximab (ReoPro)	—	0.25 mg/kg IV bolus, then 0.125 mcg/kg/min IV (max 10 mcg/min)	Percutaneous coronary intervention (PCI)	Prevent platelet aggregation Administered 10-60 minutes prior to PCI
Eptifibatide (Integrilin)	—	180 mcg/kg IV bolus × 2, 10 min apart, then 2 mcg/kg/min IV	Acute coronary syndromes; PCI	Prevent platelet aggregation Administered immediately prior to PCI
Tirofiban (Aggrastat)	—	0.4 mcg/kg/min for 30 min, then 0.1 mcg/kg/min	Acute coronary syndromes	Prevent platelet aggregation Administered prior to PCI

BOX 35-2

Duration of Antiplatelet Therapy After Percutaneous Coronary Intervention

- Dilatation without stenting: 2-4 weeks
- Bare-metal stent: 4-6 weeks
- Drug-eluting stent (sirolimus: Cypher): 3 months
- Drug-eluting stent (paclitaxel; Taxus, Achieve, V-flex): 6 months
- Brachytherapy: 12 months
- Safety precaution after drug-eluting stent: clopidogrel up to 12 months
- Aspirin: lifelong therapy

From Chassot PG et al. Perioperative use of anti-platelet drugs. Best Pract Clin Anaesthesiol. 2007;21(2):241-256; Antiplatelet therapy for patients with stents. Med Lett. 2008;50(1292):61-63.

BOX 35-3

Recommendations for Management of Patients with Drug-Eluting Stents

12 months of dual antiplatelet therapy after DES and postponement of all elective operations for 1 year

Antiplatelet regimen should not be modified perioperatively

Low-dose aspirin (≤300 mg/day) in secondary prevention should never be stopped

Clopidogrel must be maintained in unstable coronary syndromes and during the reendothelialization phase of stents (6 to 24 weeks)

If hemorrhage in a closed space is feared, the combined treatment of aspirin–clopidogrel may be reduced to aspirin alone and heparin

During the first 6 to 12 weeks after PCI and stent, only lifesaving operations should be performed

During PCI, the type of stent (if any) should be adapted to the presumed subsequent noncardiac surgery

Modified from Grines CL et al. Prevention of premature discontinuation of dual antiplatelet therapy in patients with coronary artery stents. A science advisory from the American Heart Association, American College of Cardiology, Society of Cardiovascular Angiography and Interventions, American College of Surgeons, and American Dental Association, with representation from the American College of Physicians. J Am Coll Cardiol. 2007;49:734-739; Hodgson JMcB et al. Late stent thrombosis: considerations and practical advice for use of drug-eluting stents. A report from the Society for Cardiovascular Angiography and Interventions Drug-Eluting Stent Task Force [clinical alert]. Catheter Cardiovasc Interv. 2007;69:327-333.

DES, Drug-eluting stent; mg/day, milligrams per day; PCI, percutaneous coronary intervention.

Outpatients Requiring Noncardiac Surgery

The Eighth American College of Chest Physicians (ACCP) Conference on Antithrombotic and Thrombolytic Therapy provides guidelines for outpatient management of anticoagulation therapy and thromboembolism (Table 35-7).[50] No prospective, double-blind, randomized controlled studies have been performed

to evaluate these bridge therapies. Recent trials suggest that the bleeding risk using perioperative unfractionated heparin or LMWH may lead to more bleeding complications than previously thought. For these reasons, bridging anticoagulation should be approached cautiously, using patient input once risks and benefits have been discussed. There is room for interpretation by the physician managing anticoagulation and the surgeon and anesthesia providers.

Disseminated Intravascular Coagulation

Disseminated intravascular coagulation (DIC) is a coagulation disorder characterized by ongoing activation of the coagulation cascade in response to a clinical or systemic event. Organ damage and death are the result of widespread microvascular bleeding and thrombosis. Historically, the concept of DIC was established from reports of gynecologic diseases, leukemias, and cancers.[51] As the pathogenesis was explored, different concepts emerged, such as intravascular fibrin formation, systemic inflammatory response syndrome (SIRS) related to sepsis, and sepsis-related organ failure.

The diagnosis of DIC is usually secondary to a systemic illness or insult (Box 35-4). Coagulation activation ranges from mild thrombocytopenia and prolongation of clotting times to acute DIC characterized by extensive bleeding and thrombosis.[52] During overactive coagulation, available platelets and coagulation factors are consumed. This consumption along with fibrinolysis exhausts the hemostatic balance. Rarely is the primary culprit a coagulation deficiency or dysfunction.

Intravascular Coagulation

Several factors play an important role in the pathogenesis of DIC, including the propagation of thrombin, alteration in anticoagulant activity, impaired functioning of the fibrinolytic system, and the release of cytokines.[5,53] TF release is considered to play the most important role in the development of a hyperthrombinemia in DIC. Mediators such as antithrombin and TFPI that normally inhibit coagulation are altered. Reasons for this alteration include septicemia, liver impairment, capillary leakage, and the release of endotoxins and proinflammatory cytokines. Experimental models of septicemia have shown increased fibrinolytic activity due to the acute release of tPA from the endothelium. The initial increased fibrinolytic activity is followed by the release of plasminogen activator inhibitor type 1 (PAI-1), which in turn impairs fibrinolysis and leads to accelerated thrombus formation in DIC. And lastly, activated protein C mediates the release of inflammatory cytokines such as tumor necrosis factor and interleukins from endothelial cells. Complement activation and kinin generation increase the coagulation response, leading to subsequent vascular occlusion.

A diagnosis of DIC is made by considering the patient's clinical picture in conjunction with laboratory tests (platelet count, aPTT, PT, fibrin-related markers such as fibrin degradation products (FDP), D-dimer, fibrinogen, and antithrombin). Additionally, a scoring system developed by the International Society of Thrombosis and Haemostasis (ISTH) assists with the diagnosis.[54] Overt (acute) DIC is characterized by ecchymosis, petechiae, mucosal bleeding, depletion of platelets and clotting factors, and bleeding at puncture sites. A score of 5 or greater indicates overt DIC. Non-overt (chronic) DIC is characterized by thromboembolism accompanied by evidence of activation of the coagulation system. A score less than 5 suggests nonovert DIC.

The management and treatment of DIC always depend on the underlying cause. In obstetric catastrophes, DIC may resolve as a

TABLE 35-7	Bleeding Risk Associated with Invasive Procedures and Recommendations for Perioperative Management	

Bleeding Risk (Category)	Invasive Procedures	Recommendations
High	Cardiac surgery, abdominal aortic aneurysm repair, neurosurgery, most cancer surgery, bilateral knee replacement, TURP, kidney biopsy	*Low-risk thromboembolism:* Stop warfarin 5 days before surgery and allow INR to return to near normal Restart warfarin 12-24 hours after surgery Use prophylactic dosages of LMWH or unfractionated heparin if procedure predisposes to thrombosis *Intermediate-risk thromboembolism:* Stop warfarin therapy 5 days before surgery Consider no bridging versus starting prophylactic LMWH or unfractionated heparin 2 to 3 days before surgery After surgery, restart warfarin and prophylactic LMWH or unfractionated heparin Alternatively follow bridge protocol *High-risk thromboembolism:* Follow bridge therapy protocol Await hemostasis before restarting LMWH; consider using therapeutic dosages of LMWH or unfractionated heparin
Intermediate (surgical)	Abdominal surgery, hemorrhoidal surgery, axillary node dissection dilatation and curettage, hydrocele repair, orthopedic surgery, pacemaker insertion, internal cardiac defibrillator insertion, endarterectomy or carotid bypass surgery, noncataract eye surgery (complex lid, lacrimal, orbital), extensive dental surgery (multiple tooth extractions)	*Low-risk thromboembolism:* Stop warfarin 4 to 5 days before surgery and allow INR to return to near normal Restart warfarin after surgery Use prophylactic LMWH or unfractionated heparin if procedure predisposes to thrombosis *Intermediate-risk thromboembolism:* Stop warfarin 4 to 5 days before surgery Consider no bridging versus starting prophylactic LMWH or unfractionated heparin 2 to 3 days before surgery After surgery, restart warfarin and prophylactic LMWH or unfractionated heparin Alternatively follow bridge therapy protocol *High-risk thromboembolism:* Follow bridge therapy protocol Await hemostasis before restarting LMWH; consider using therapeutic dosages of LMWH or unfractionated heparin
Intermediate to low (nonsurgical)	Coronary angiography with or without percutaneous coronary intervention, noncoronary angiography, upper endoscopy with endosphincterotomy, colonoscopy with polypectomy, bronchoscopy with or without biopsy, biopsy (prostate, bladder, thyroid, breast, lymph node, pancreas)	*Low-risk thromboembolism:* Stop warfarin 5 days before surgery and allow INR to return to near normal Restart warfarin after surgery Use prophylactic dosages of LMWH or unfractionated heparin if procedure predisposes to thrombosis *Intermediate-risk thromboembolism:* Stop warfarin therapy 5 days before surgery Consider no bridging versus starting prophylactic LMWH or unfractionated heparin 2 to 3 days before surgery After surgery, restart warfarin within 12 to 24 hours, and/or prophylactic LMWH or unfractionated heparin Alternatively follow bridge protocol

From du Breuil AL, Umland EM. Outpatient management of anticoagulation therapy. Am Fam Physician. 2007;75(7):1031-1042. Geerts WH et al. Prevention of venous thromboembolism: American College of Chest Physicians Evidence-Based Clinical Practice Guidelines. (8th ed.). Chest. 2008 Jun;133(6 Suppl):381S-453S
INR, International normalized ratio; LMWH, low-molecular-weight heparin; TURP, transurethral resection of the prostate.

Continued

TABLE 35-7	Bleeding Risk Associated with Invasive Procedures and Recommendations for Perioperative Management—cont'd	
Bleeding Risk (Category)	**Invasive Procedures**	**Recommendations**
		High-risk thromboembolism: Follow bridge therapy protocol Await hemostasis before restarting LMWH; consider using therapeutic dosages of LMWH or unfractionated heparin
Low to minimal	Arthrocentesis, general dental treatment (hygiene, restorations, endodontics, prosthetics, minor periodontal therapy, and uncomplicated extractions), ophthalmic procedures (cataract, trabeculectomy, vitreoretinal), TURP with laser surgery, upper and lower gastrointestinal endoscopy with or without mucosal biopsy	*All risks of thromboembolism:* Continue warfarin therapy Continue aspirin therapy Check INR the day of or the day before surgery to be sure not supratherapeutic

---

BOX 35-4

Clinical Conditions Associated with Disseminated Intravascular Coagulation

Sepsis
  Gram negative
  Gram positive
Cancers
Trauma
  Burns
  Cerebral injury
Obstetric complications
  HELLP syndrome
  Amniotic fluid embolism
  Placenta abruptio
  Fetal death in utero
  Preeclampsia
Inflammatory diseases
Liver failure
Cerebral injury
Viremias
  HIV
  Hepatitis
  Varicella
  Cytomegalovirus
Prosthetic devices
Snake venom
Toxic or immunologic reactions

HELLP, *Hemolysis, elevated liver enzymes, low platelet count.*

result of prompt delivery. Treatment of sepsis with antibiotic therapy may halt the progression of DIC. Restoration of physiologic anticoagulant pathways with activated protein C in the treatment of sepsis with overt DIC holds promise.[52] Activated protein C inactivates factors Va and VIIIa, resulting in decreased thrombin formation. Its use in treating DIC patients with severe sepsis has been approved by the FDA. For individuals requiring surgery who are bleeding or at risk for active bleeding, correction of coagulopathy with platelets, FFP, and/or cryoprecipitate must be used. Continued replacement of blood products should be based on the clinical picture and reassessment of laboratory results.[5]

The use of anticoagulants for DIC remains controversial, especially for a patient who is prone to bleeding. Antithrombin III concentrates may prove effective in inhibiting coagulation; however, their use is still under investigation.[53]

Sickle Cell Disease. Sickle cell disease is one of the more commonly inherited hemoglobinopathies. It is a disorder transmitted as an autosomal recessive trait that causes an abnormality of the globin genes in hemoglobin. A person who is homozygous for hemoglobin S manifests the disorder. Individuals may have the sickle cell trait or sickle cell disease. The sickle cell trait is a heterozygous disorder seen in 10% of African Americans.[39] Their hemoglobin S levels are normally 30% to 50%, and sickling is seen with a P_{O_2} of 20 to 30 mm Hg. Sickle cell disease is a homozygous disorder seen in 0.5% to 1.0% of African Americans. The majority of the hemoglobin molecule is hemoglobin S, and sickling is seen with a P_{O_2} of 30 to 40 mm Hg. A crisis may be caused by a decrease of oxygen saturation and temperature, infections, dehydration, stasis, and acidosis. These complicated scenarios translate into perioperative mortality rates of 10% and postoperative complications of 50%.[55,56] Suggestions for intraoperative management of patients with sickle cell disease are given in Box 35-5.

There is no universal method for caring for patients with a sickle cell disorder. It is suggested that patients with a preoperative hemoglobin A level of at least 50% and a hematocrit of at least 35% may have less risk of an intraoperative crisis as an effort is made to correct anemia.[55,57] Providing preoperative transfusion supplementation always carries a risk of increasing the blood's viscosity and causing end-organ damage. The National Preoperative Study in Sickle Cell Disease concluded that a conservative transfusion regimen was as effective as an aggressive regimen in preventing perioperative complications.[55]

From Lewis MA, Goodwin SR. Sickle cell disease and acute porphyria. In: Lobato EB et al, eds. Complications in Anesthesiology. Philadelphia: Lippincott Williams & Wilkins; 2008:550.
ASA, American Society of Anesthesiologists.

Anesthesia management that includes adequate hydration, saturation, normothermia, normal acid base balance, proper positioning, and analgesia may interrupt intraoperative and postoperative crisis.[58]

Heparin-Induced Thrombocytopenia. Heparin-induced thrombocytopenia (HIT) is a disorder of coagulation that is a direct consequence of heparin therapy. The anticoagulant properties of heparin were first noted in 1916 and introduced into clinical practice in 1937.[59] Heparin continues to be used because of its rapid onset, easy reversibility, and moderate therapeutic window with relatively few side effects. One of the few relative (versus absolute) contraindications for heparin is a history of HIT.

HIT results in thrombocytopenia, tachyphylaxis, and arterial and venous thrombosis. Of all patients who receive heparin therapy for 5 days, 5% to 28% are at risk of developing thrombocytopenia.[5,12,45,60,61] HIT typically manifests 7 to 10 days after heparin exposure and is caused by the formation of IgG

antibodies directed against platelet-factor-4 heparin complexes. These complexes bind and activate platelets, fix complement, and generate platelet aggregation.[60] The proliferation of platelet aggregation is associated with major morbidity and mortality when arterial thrombus formation occurs in critical organ beds and/or distal extremities. In the United States, a yearly estimate of 600,000 new cases of HIT occur, with as many as 300,000 patients developing thrombotic complications and 90,000 patients dying.[62] Patients are often suspected to have HIT when the platelet count suddenly and unexplainably decreases 50% from the admission platelet count. Diagnosis of HIT can be difficult in the patient without a diagnosis of thrombocytopenia.[5] However, the anesthesia provider needs to be aware of the potential of HIT in any patient who is receiving heparin therapy.

Clinical understanding of HIT continues to grow in clinical medicine. Hemostasis plays a pivotal role in surgery, critical care, trauma, perioperative medicine, and hematology. Understanding the clinical event and therapeutic approaches to diagnosing and treating HIT is important. During the preoperative interview, the anesthesia provider needs to review current labs and medications. HIT should be considered in all patients with complications or thrombosis (with or without thrombocytopenia) in the presence of heparin therapy. If HIT is suspected, a hematologist should be consulted. HIT is a rare occurrence within the operating room, but the complications of HIT may warrant emergency surgery (e.g., thrombectomy of a postoperative-day-5 femoro-popliteal graft). Treatment entails withdrawal of heparin (including heparin flush bags) and consideration of an alternate anticoagulant. Standard management for HIT includes direct thrombin inhibitors and heparinoids (hirudin, argatroban, lepirudin, bivalirudin, danaparoid), with the exception of LMWH.[5] There is no point-of-care test available to diagnose HIT, but the reaction should be suspected when the platelet count decreases 50% from the admission count after heparin exposure.

SUMMARY

Each time patients agree to a surgical intervention, the hemostatic system is challenged. An understanding of the normal hemostatic system, ways to deter bleeding and decrease transfusion requirements, and alternatives to blood transfusions can only enhance patient care and safety when providing anesthesia care.

REFERENCES

1. Cobas M. Assessment of coagulation disorders. In: Hurford W, Gilbertson L, eds. International Anesthesia Clinics. Philadelphia: Lippincott; 2001:1-15.
2. Guyton AC, Hall JE. Hemostasis and blood coagulation. In: Guyton AC, Hall JE, eds. Textbook of Medical Physiology. 11th ed. Philadelphia: Saunders; 2006:457-468.
3. Brecher ME. The platelet prophylactic transfusion trigger: when expectations meet reality. Transfusion. 2007;47:188-191.
4. Hillman RS, Ault KA. Hematology in Clinical Practice: A Guide to Diagnosis and Management. New York: McGraw-Hill; 1998:409-429, 472-489.
5. Drummond JC, Petrovich CT. Hemotherapy and hemostasis. In: Barash PG, ed. Clinical Anesthesia. 5th ed. Lippincott Williams & Wilkins; 2006:208-244.
6. Hoffman M. A cell-based model of coagulation and the role of factor VIIa. Blood Rev. 2003;17:S1-S5.
7. Adams GL et al. The balance of thrombosis and hemorrhage in surgery. Hematol Oncol Clin North Am. 2007;21:13-23.
8. Welsby IJ et al. Recombinant activated factor VII and the anaesthetist. Anaesthesia. 2005;60:1203-1212.
9. Becker RC. Cell-based models of coagulation: a paradigm in evolution. J Thromb Thrombolysis. 2005;20(1):65-68.
10. Koh MBC, Hunt BJ. The management of perioperative bleeding. Blood Rev. 2003;17:179-185.
11. Dunn AS, Turpie AG. Perioperative management of patients receiving oral anticoagulants: a systematic review. Arch Intern Med. 2003;163:901-908.
12. Opie LH. Drugs for the Heart. 5th ed. Philadelphia: Saunders; 2001:273-313.
13. Goldenberg NA et al. Brief communication: duration of platelet dysfunction after a 7-day course of ibuprofen. Ann Intern Med. 2005;142(7):506-509.
14. Braganza A et al. The effect of nonsteroidal antiinflammatory drugs on bleeding during periodontal surgery. J Periodontol. 2005;76(7):1154-1160.
15. Sniecinski R, Levy JH. What is blood and what is not? Caring for the Jehovah Witness patient undergoing cardiac surgery. Anesth Analg. 2007;104:753-754.
16. Marsh JCW, Bevan DH. Haematological care of the Jehovah Witness patient. Br J Haematol. 2002;119:25-37.
17. Rohrer MJ et al. A prospective evaluation of the efficacy of preoperative coagulation testing. Ann Surg. 1988;208:554-557.
18. Harrison P. Platelet function analysis. Blood Rev. 2005;19:111-123.
19. American Society of Anesthesiologists Task Force on Perioperative Blood Transfusion and Adjunctive Therapy. Practice guidelines for perioperative blood transfusion and adjuvant therapy. (An updated report.) Anesthesiology. 2006;105:198-208.
20. Stehling L et al. Guidelines for blood utilization review. Transfusion. 1994;34:438-448.

21. American Society of Anesthesiologists Task Force on Blood Component Therapy. Practice guidelines for blood component therapy: a report. *Anesthesiology.* 1996;84(3):732-747.

22. Nuttall GA et al. American Society of Anesthesiologists Committee on Transfusion Medicine. Current transfusion practices of members of the American Society of Anesthesiologists. *Anesthesiology.* 2003;99(6):1433-1443.

23. McLennan S, Williamson LM. Risk of fresh frozen plasma and platelets. *J Trauma.* 2006;60(6):S46-S50.

24. Easley RA et al. Blood components: development of proficiency testing for detection of bacterial contamination of platelet products. *Transfusion.* 2007;47:251-255.

25. Goodnough LT et al. Transfusion medicine—blood conservation—second of two parts. *N Engl J Med.* 1999;340:525-533.

26. Lundberg GD. Practice parameters for the use of fresh frozen plasma, cryoprecipitate and platelets. *JAMA.* 1994;271(10):777-781.

27. Sphan DR. Physiologic transfusion triggers. Do we have to use (our) brain? *Anesthesiology.* 2006;104:905-906.

28. Weiskopf RB. More on the changing indications for transfusion of blood and blood components during anesthesia. *Anesthesiology.* 1996;84:498-501.

29. Hasley PB et al. The necessary and unnecessary transfusion: a critical review of appropriateness rates and criteria for red cell transfusions. *Transfusion.* 1994;34:110-115.

30. Napier JAF et al. British Committee for Standards in Haematology, Blood Transfusion Task force. Guidelines for autologous transfusion. II. Perioperative haemodilution and cell salvage. *Br J Anaesth.* 1977;78:768-771.

31. Levack ID, Gillon J. Intraoperative conservation of red cell mass, controlled hypotension or haemodilution—not necessarily mutually exclusive. *Br J Anaesth.* 1999;82:161-163.

32. National Heart, Lung, and Blood Institute Expert Panel on the Use of Autologous Blood. Transfusion alert: use of autologous blood. *Transfusion.* 1995;35:703-711.

33. Alexander E. Emerging role of recombinant factor VIIa in neuroscience. *AACN Adv Crit Care.* 2006;17:363-367.

34. Grounds M. Recombinant factor VIIa (rFVIIa) and its use in severe bleeding in surgery and trauma: a review. *Blood Rev.* 2003;17:S11-S21.

35. Criddle LM. Recombinant factor VIIa and the trauma patient. *J Emerg Nurs.* 2006;32:404-408.

36. Mayer SA et al. Recombinant activated factor VII for acute intracerebral hemorrhage. *N Engl J Med.* 2005;352:777-785.

37. Dutton RP et al. Recombinant factor VIIa for control of hemorrhage: early experience in critically ill trauma patients. *J Clin Anesth.* 2003;15:184-188.

38. Yusim Y et al. The use of recombinant factor VII (NovoSeven) for treatment of active or impending bleeding in brain surgery: broadening the indications. *J Clin Anesth.* 2006;18:545-551.

39. Fleisher LA. Hematologic diseases In: *Anesthesia and Uncommon Diseases.* 5th ed. 2006:362-368, 372.

40. Holmberg L, Nilsson IM. Von Willebrand disease. *Eur J Haematol.* 1992;48:127-141.

41. Maddox JM et al. Management of acquired von Willebrand's syndrome in a patient requiring major surgery. *Haemophilia.* 2005;11:633-637.

42. Michiels JJ et al. Intravenous DDAVP and factor VIII-von Willebrand factor concentrate for the treatment and prophylaxis of bleedings in patients with von Willebrand disease type 1, 2 and 3. *Clin Appl Thromb Hemost.* 2007;13(1):14-34.

43. Hoyer LW. Hemophilia A. *N Engl J Med.* 1994;330:38-47.

44. Ingerslev J, Hvid I. Surgery in hemophilia. The general view: patient selection, timing, perioperative assessment. *Semin Hematol.* 2005;S23-S26.

45. Hamidovic A. Coagulation disorders. In: Chisholm-Burns MA et al, eds. *Pharmacotherapy Principles and Practice.* New York: McGraw-Hill; 2008:987-1002.

46. Chassot PG et al. Perioperative use of antiplatelet drugs. *Best Pract Res Clin Anaesthesiol.* 2007;21(2):241-256.

47. Chassot PG et al. Perioperative antiplatelet therapy: the case for continuing therapy in patients at risk of myocardial infarction. *Br J Anaesth.* 2007;99(3):316-328.

48. du Breuil AL, Umland EM. Outpatient management of anticoagulation therapy. *Am Fam Physician.* 2007;75(7):1031-1042.

49. Dalal AR et al. Brief review: coronary drug-eluting stents and anesthesia. *Can J Anaesth.* 2006;53:1230-1243.

50. Dunn A. Perioperative Management of oral anticoagulation: when and how to bridge. *J Thromb Thrombolysis.* 2006;21:85-89.

51. Wada H. Disseminating intravascular coagulation: a review. *Clinica Chim Acta.* 2004;344:13-21.

52. Levi M. Disseminating intravascular coagulation, what's new? *Crit Care Clin.* 2005;21:449-467.

53. Saba H, Morelli GA. The pathogenesis and management of disseminating intravascular coagulation. *Clin Adv Hematol Oncol.* 2006;4(12):919-926.

54. Bakkhtiari K et al. Prospective validation of the International Society of Thrombosis and Haemostasis scoring system for disseminated intravascular coagulation. *Crit Care Med.* 2004;32(12):2416-2421.

55. Vichinsky EP et al. A comparison of conservative and aggressive transfusion regimes in the perioperative management of sickle cell disease. *N Engl J Med.* 1995;333:206-213.

56. Lewis MA, Goodwin SR. Sickle cell abnormalities and acute porphyria. In: Lobato EB et al, eds. *Complications in Anesthesiology.* Philadelphia: Lippincott Williams & Wilkins; 2008:546-553.

57. Schmalzer EA et al. Viscosity mixtures of sickle and normal red cells at varying hematocrit levels: implications for transfusion. *Transfusion.* 1987;27:228-233.

58. Firth PG, Head CA. Sickle cell disease and anesthesiology. *Anesthesiology.* 2004;101:766-785.

59. McLean J. The discovery of heparin. *Circulation.* 1959;19:75.

60. Youngberg JA. *Cardiac, Vascular and Thoracic Anesthesia.* New York: Churchill Livingstone; 2000.

61. Taylor FB et al. Scientific and Standardization Committee. Communications towards a definition, clinical and laboratory criteria, and a scoring system for DIC, on behalf of the International Society on Thrombosis and Haemostasis. *Thromb Haemost.* 2001;86:1327-1330.

62. Levy JH. Hemostatic agents. *Transfusion.* 2004;44:58S-61S.

CHAPTER 36

THERMAL INJURY AND ANESTHESIA

Julie Ann Lowery

In the 1950s, there were fewer than 10 recognized burn centers in the United States. This number now exceeds 120, with established burn centers now located across the country in virtually every major metropolitan area. For an institution to receive verification as a burn center, it must submit to a vigorous review by both the American Burn Association (ABA) and the American College of Surgeons (ACS). Burn center verification establishes that this facility provides high-quality, specialized care of burned individuals and maintains the necessary resources and medical services rendered mandatory by ABA guidelines.[1]

Recent statistics reveal a decline in the national incidence of burn injury and burn care use during the past 2 decades. This progress coincides with an increased national focus on burn prevention. Smoke detectors have come into widespread use, fire and burn prevention education has expanded, and regulation of consumer products and occupational safety has increased significantly. Nevertheless, in the United States, more than 1.25 million people sustain burn injuries annually.[2] The ABA 2007 fact sheet estimates that 500,000 receive medical treatment, with 40,000 requiring acute hospital admission and 25,000 of these individuals being admitted to specialized burn centers. Approximately 4000 die from the burn injury—3500 from residential fires and 500 from motor vehicle or aircraft crashes.[3] Roughly 35% of all burn victims are younger than 17 years of age, with more than 15,000 children requiring hospitalization as a result of their burn injuries. Scald injuries predominate among small children, with a progressive increase in the frequency of thermal-related burns in the elderly.[4] The major causes of death in burn patients are multiple organ failure and infection. Death following a burn injury is not related to the toxic biologic effects of thermally injured skin but to the shock associated with metabolic and infectious consequences of a large open wound, depletion of the patient's resistance to infection, inhalation injury, and extensive malnutrition, which cumulatively set the stage for life-threatening bacterial sepsis originating from the burn wound.[5]

CLASSIFICATION OF BURN INJURY

Burn injuries, regardless of their etiology, are classified according to the depth and extent of skin and tissue destruction, as well as the total body surface area (TBSA) involved. First-degree (superficial) burns are limited to the epidermis, which is the outermost layer of skin. The epidermis is primarily thin and avascular. First-degree burns heal spontaneously and usually do not require any medical intervention. Second-degree burns are also known as deep and superficial *partial-thickness burns*. They extend into the dermis, which lies below the epidermis. In contrast with the epidermis, the dermis is very vascular and contains numerous blood vessels and nerves. The severity of the type of burn varies, depending on the amount and depth of the dermal tissues involved. If the epithelial basement membrane of the dermis is intact, the skin will regenerate, and grafting may not be required. Third-degree or *full-thickness burns* extend into the subcutaneous tissue lying below the dermis. The entire skin thickness is destroyed with third-degree burns.[6] Skin grafting is required for these types of burns because the epithelium and the dermal appendages are destroyed. A fourth-degree burn classification is used by some institutions to describe structures burned below the dermis, such as muscle, fascia, and bone. Table 36-1 classifies burns according to depth of skin layers affected, and Figure 36-1 illustrates the layers of burn injury.

The burn team assesses the extent of a burn and plans initial resuscitation efforts. Burn wounds can be readily quantified, but estimation of the burn size remains subjective and assessor related. The most widely used estimation is the "rule of nines," which was first described by Lund and Browder (Figure 36-2). The body is divided into regions that represent 9% or a multiple of 9% of the TBSA. Specific modifications apply to children, because the surface areas of their heads and trunks are proportionally larger than their extremities.[7] The rule of nines is a quick method to visually estimate a burn size; however, it is not definitive. The extensiveness of a burn injury can be more specifically quantified using the Lund and Browder chart. Figure 36-3 demonstrates the Lund and Browder method. Although more time-consuming to use, determining a burn victim's injury extent via this method is much more accurate, especially in the pediatric patient.

According to the ABA's injury severity grading system, a *major burn* is (1) a second-degree burn involving more than 10% of the TBSA in adults or 20% at extremes of age, (2) a third-degree burn involving more than 10% of the TBSA in adults, (3) any electrical burn, or (4) a burn complicated by smoke inhalation. Associated mortality estimates follow a burn formula derived from the National Burn Registry: if the age of the patient plus percentage TBSA of burn exceeds 115, the mortality is greater than 80%. Additionally, clinical observations estimate that the mortality of a burn victim is approximately doubled if inhalation injury is sustained in conjunction with a thermal burn.

ETIOLOGIES OF BURN INJURIES

On a patient's admission to the burn unit, it is vital for the burn team to ascertain the etiology of the thermal injury. Specific

TABLE **36-1**	Degrees of Burn Injury	
Classification	**Tissue Level Involvement**	**Appearance**
Superficial, first-degree burn	Epidermis destroyed	Skin, red tone (sunburn); painful with erythema and blisters; heals spontaneously with no scarring
Partial-thickness, second-degree burn		
Superficial dermal	Epidermis and some (upper) dermis destroyed	Red or pale ivory with a moist, shiny surface; painful, immediate blisters with minimal scarring
Deep dermal	Epidermis and deep dermis	Mottled with white, waxy, dry surface; blisters may or may not appear; significant scarring
Full-thickness, third-degree burn	All epidermis and dermis	White, cherry red, or black; dry, tissue-paper skin; grafting necessary; decreased scarring with early excision
Fourth-degree burn	Muscle, fascia, bone	Complete excision required; limited function

Modified from Faldmo L, Kravitz M. Management of acute burns and burn shock resuscitation. AACN Clin Issues Crit Care Nurs. 1993;4:351-366.

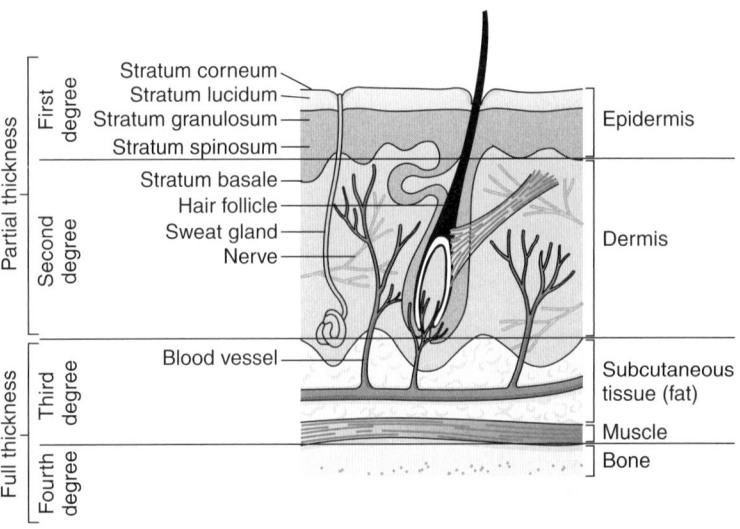

FIGURE **36-1** Depth of a thermal injury determines whether a burn will heal without grafting. Superficial and partial-thickness burns do not destroy the dermal appendages and thus are able to heal readily. Full-thickness burns, particularly when they reach the muscle and bone, require skin grafting to prevent infection and promote healing. (*From Beare PG, Myers JL. Adult Health Nursing. 3rd ed. St Louis: Mosby; 1998.*)

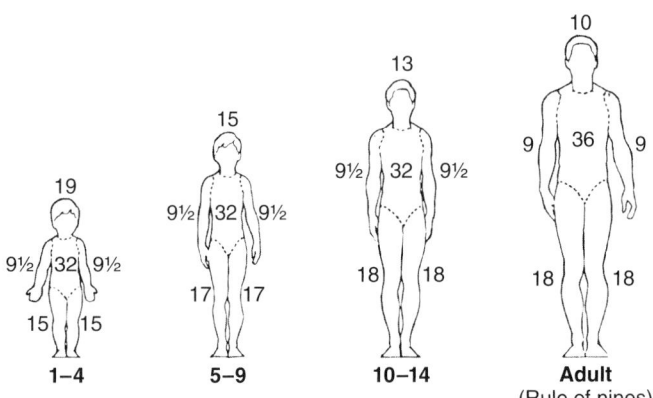

FIGURE **36-2** Burn assessment chart with body proportions. Numbers under figures indicate age; other numbers indicate percent body surface. (*Modified from Palmisano BW, Rusy LM. Anesthesia for plastic surgery. In: Gregory GA, ed. Pediatric Anesthesia. 4th ed. Philadelphia: Churchill Livingstone; 2002:733, with permission.*)

pathophysiologic sequelae can be expected after an electrical burn, others after a thermal burn. The overall circumstances behind the burn injury must be examined. An individual burned in a contained space such as a house fire, for example, should be suspected of having an inhalation injury as well.

There are four types of burn injuries: chemical, electrical, thermal/heat (also referred to as *flame* or *scald*), and inhalation. Chemical burns commonly occur in a laboratory setting or industrial environment. These types of burns occur when a noxious chemical substance comes into contact with the skin. Tissue damage and destruction result from the reaction of the chemical with the tissue proteins and cellular components. Skin disruption will continue until the chemical irritant is removed or neutralized. Initial treatment is with copious amounts of water or normal saline irrigation. Chemical burns are uncommon in children, although they can occur.

Electrical burns can be the most damaging to skin and surrounding tissues. The extent of the burn depends on the amount of thermal energy conducted through the skin, based on the voltage and duration of contact with the electrical source. Significant tissue disruption can occur where the electric current is the most concentrated—at the points of entry and exit, although two wounds are not always evident. Initially, the

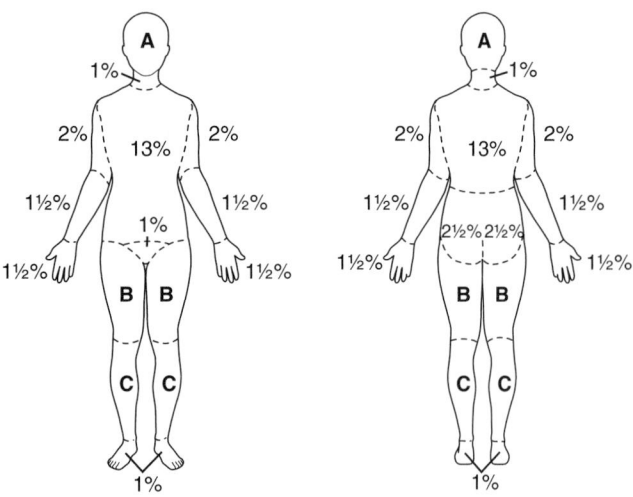

Area	Age 0	1	5	10	15	Adult
A - ½ of head	9½%	8½%	6½%	5½%	4½%	3½%
B - ½ of one thigh	2¾%	3¼%	4%	4¼%	4½%	4¼%
C - ½ of one leg	2½%	2½%	2¾%	3%	3¼%	3½%

FIGURE **36-3** Lund-Browder chart. (*From National Association of EMTs. PHTLS: Prehospital Trauma Life Support. 6th ed. St Louis: Mosby/JEMS;2007:338.*)

extensiveness of skin and underlying tissue involvement may be hard to diagnose, because surface damage may not reflect all tissue damage, and the entrance wounds may appear superficial. Electrical burns can cause severe damage to bones, blood vessels, muscle, and nerves. If the amount of muscle damaged from the conducted electric current is significant, myoglobin can be released into the circulation. Myoglobinemia places the electrical burn patient at great risk for developing renal failure secondary to myoglobinuria, which affects nephron and renal tubular function.

Thermal-related burns, or burns sustained from any heat source, commonly occur in and around the home. In children between 1 and 4 years of age, fires and burns are the second leading cause of accidental death. Scald burns in children remain one of the most common injuries resulting from abuse.[8]

Inhalation burn injuries often accompany thermal burns and should be suspected until aggressively ruled out.[9-11] Damage to the airway can vary, depending on whether the upper airway or lower airway is affected. Upper airway injuries result from inhalation of superheated air or steam and toxic compounds found in smoke.[12] Brief exposure of the epiglottis or larynx to either dry air at 300° C or steam at 100° C can lead to massive edema and rapid airway obstruction.[13] As mentioned, the addition of an inhalation injury to a cutaneous burn of any size doubles the mortality rate[14] and is a stronger determinant of death than the size of the burn wound.[5] Inhalation of heated air can result in direct injury to the face, oropharynx, and upper trachea, with sparing of the lower airway. It is speculated that the heat entrained is readily dissipated in the upper airway, and there is reflex closure of the vocal cords. These features are thought to protect the lower airways from heat-related injury. However, true thermal injury from exposure to live steam can occur in the lower respiratory tract because the heat-exchange mechanisms of the airway are unable to cool the gas sufficiently as it is inhaled. Obstruction of the

upper airway is mainly due to excessive edema, macroglossia, and swelling of the pharyngeal soft tissue. Lower airway injuries more commonly arise from the inhalation of soot particles and/or chemicals produced by a fire. In the lower airways, the inhaled toxins react with the airway mucosa, forming acidic and alkali substances. Capillary permeability is increased. Extensive alveolar and epithelial damage can occur, with the trachea and bronchi becoming necrotic. Warning signs of respiratory injury include hoarseness, sore throat, dysphagia, hemoptysis, tachypnea, the use of accessory muscles, wheezing, carbonaceous sputum production, and elevated carbon monoxide levels.[15]

Treatment of the burn patient involves three distinct phases: the resuscitative phase, débridement and grafting, and the reconstructive phase. Each phase has its own unique problems the anesthesia provider must identify when developing an anesthetic plan.

TREATMENT OF THE BURN PATIENT

Resuscitative Phase

As for any trauma patient, the initial treatment of the burn patient should involve attention to the airway, breathing, circulation, and coexisting trauma. All burn patients must be considered at risk for pulmonary compromise, especially if the percentage of TBSA involved is significant, and signs of inhalation injury are present.

Airway Injury

It is necessary to aggressively rule out upper airway injury in patients at risk (e.g., involving a fire that occurred in a closed space or the development of unconsciousness or stupor that prevented the patient from protecting his or her airway). Diagnosis is made by the history, the circumstances surrounding the burn injury, and physical examination. This is best achieved by direct visualization of the airway with a laryngoscope or fiberoptic bronchoscopy.[16] The chest radiograph is usually normal in the early phase of inhalation injury (unless aspiration of gastric or pharyngeal contents occurred during the accident), becoming abnormal once pulmonary edema or infiltration develops. Treatment of upper airway injury involves *early* endotracheal intubation, even if the burn patient is not yet demonstrating any signs of airway decompensation. Even in the absence of an inhalation injury, the lungs are at risk for compromise if the burn is large.

Thermal damage to the soft tissues of the respiratory tract and trachea can make intubation an almost impossible task because of the malalignment of structures, swelling, and bleeding of the tissues involved. Intubation of the trachea is much easier to perform earlier rather than later, when there may be glottic or facial edema, which worsens after fluid resuscitation.[17] In the pediatric population, intubation should be performed with an uncuffed endotracheal tube, usually one size smaller than expected according to age and weight. Nasotracheal intubation in children is generally preferred; it is better tolerated by the child, and tube displacement with movement is less likely.[18,19]

In the absence of an airway abnormality, early tracheal intubation can usually be achieved using a rapid-sequence technique with an intravenous (IV) induction agent and a rapidly acting muscle relaxant. There is general agreement that succinylcholine administration to patients more than 24 hours after burn injury is unsafe,[20,21] although some authors extend this safe period to several days.[22] It is speculated that a denervation-like phenomenon occurs following a burn, with a proliferation of acetylcholine receptors throughout the muscle membrane. Succinylcholine is structurally similar to acetylcholine and can cause potassium (K⁺) release from the entire muscle membrane rather than from discrete end-plate junctions, leading to hyperkalemia and possibly cardiac arrest.[23] The magnitude of K⁺ elevation appears to be related to the size of the burn. This process of receptor proliferation takes several days to develop, allowing an initial 24-hour window of safety. It is wise to avoid the use of succinylcholine in a burn patient more than 24 hours after injury[24] until complete wound closure has occurred and the patient is gaining weight.[25] Administering high doses of nondepolarizing muscle relaxants (e.g., rocuronium, vecuronium, or cisatracurium) is an alternative to succinylcholine.

Variations in acetylcholine receptors—specifically, an increased number of nicotinic acetylcholine receptors[26]—along with a change in volume and distribution associated with alterations in plasma protein binding may account for decreased sensitivity to nondepolarizing drugs. Both the dose administered and the serum concentrations required in the burn patient may be increased two- to three-fold to achieve the desired paralysis with a nondepolarizer.[25]

With an abnormal airway or upper airway obstruction, the safest way to secure the airway is with the patient awake. Key actions include effective topical anesthesia, patient positioning, and supplemental oxygenation. Administration of sedatives may worsen airway obstruction and should be given cautiously. However, IV opioid administration may be appropriate for the alert patient in pain. Methods to secure the airway include flexible fiberoptic bronchoscopy, direct laryngoscopy, laryngeal mask airway, blind nasal intubation, and other adjunct airway devices. When the upper airway is badly damaged and endotracheal intubation is not possible, a direct surgical approach is indicated: needle cricothyroidotomy, surgical cricothyroidotomy, or tracheotomy. This should *only* be considered as a last resort.

For the most part, after airway management, the burn patient is taken to the intensive care unit and placed on ventilatory support.[27] Inspired gases should be humidified to aid clearing of tracheobronchial debris and prevent drying of secretions. The endotracheal tube must be kept in place until the surrounding laryngeal edema has subsided. A progressive air leak around the endotracheal tube, especially in uncuffed pediatric sizes, is an indication that edematous tissue is returning to normal.

Carbon Monoxide Poisoning
Any burn victim rescued from an enclosed-space fire should be considered at high risk for carbon monoxide poisoning. It is estimated that 50% to 60% of all fire victims die from carbon monoxide poisoning.[28] Symptoms depend on the carboxyhemoglobin level, although it is actually the tissue carbon monoxide level that determines the toxicity of carbon monoxide (Table 36-2).

Carbon monoxide binds to the hemoglobin molecule with 200 times greater affinity than oxygen,[29] leading to a fall in oxyhemoglobin saturation as tissues become unable to extract oxygen. The end result is a disruption in oxidative phosphorylation and metabolic acidosis at the cellular level. Analysis of blood gases reveals a normal arterial oxygen tension but a decreased total oxygen content, indicating that the hemoglobin oxygen saturation is markedly reduced.[25] Carbon monoxide increases the stability of the oxyhemoglobin molecule, decreasing the release of oxygen to the tissues—a leftward shift in the oxyhemoglobin curve (Figure 36-4). Pulse oximeters do not detect carboxyhemoglobin and give falsely elevated readings for oxygen saturation in its presence. A co-oximeter, which measures the percentages of

TABLE 36-2	Clinical Manifestations of Carbon Monoxide Exposure
Carboxyhemoglobin Level (%)	**Clinical Manifestations**
0-5	None
5-10	Mild headache, confusion
11-20	Throbbing headache, blurred vision
21-40	Disorientation, nausea, vomiting, irritability, syncope
41-60	Tachycardia, tachypnea, agitation, combativeness, hallucination
>60	Death

Modified from Sharar SR et al. Management of inhalation injury in patients with and without burns. In: Haponik EF, Munster AM, eds. Respiratory Injury: Smoke Inhalation and Burns. New York: McGraw-Hill; 1990.

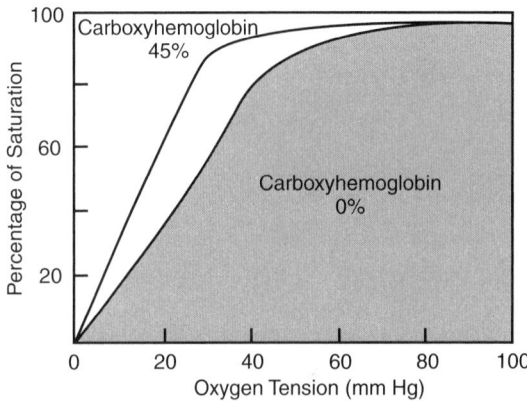

FIGURE **36-4** Shift of the oxyhemoglobin dissociation curve to the left by 45% carboxyhemoglobin. (*From Jackson DL, Menges H. Accidental carbon monoxide poisoning. JAMA. 1980;243:772. Copyright 1980, American Medical Association.*)

hemoglobin, oxyhemoglobin, carboxyhemoglobin, and methemoglobin, is needed to obtain an accurate oximetry saturation.[30]

Treatment is to displace the carbon monoxide molecule from the hemoglobin. Typical interventions include administering 100% oxygen via face mask or an endotracheal tube. The half-life of carboxyhemoglobin is 250 minutes in room air. Oxygen displaces the carbon monoxide and shortens its half-life to 40 to 60 minutes.[17,29] Hyperbaric oxygen treatments are an alternative therapy and may be required if the carboxyhemoglobin level exceeds 25% or if clincial signs of toxicity are evident. The debate continues over the effectiveness of hyperbaric oxygen (HBO) to treat carbon monoxide poisoning. The major question is whether HBO reduces the incidence of delayed neurologic sequelae. Studies have been inconclusive.[16,31-33]

Hypovolemic Shock Associated with Thermal Injury
After the airway has been secured and other life-threatening injuries have been managed, the burn patient must be resuscitated with large volumes of fluid. Aggressive fluid administration

and restoration of the blood volume are critical interventions for improving the patient's survival chances and preventing renal failure. Fluid losses are greatest in the first 12 hours after the burn and then begin to stabilize after 24 hours. Fluid losses occur secondary to direct transudation of plasma and plasma proteins from the wound and from diffuse capillary leakage that shifts fluid from the intravascular space into the interstitium of unburned tissue. Capillary leak results from the loss of endothelial integrity and from reduction of intravascular oncotic pressure as plasma proteins are lost through the burn wound and incompetent capillary beds.[34] The end result of the changes in microvasculature caused by thermal injury is disruption of normal capillary barriers separating intravascular and interstitial compartments and rapid equilibration of these compartments. This causes severe depletion of plasma volume and a marked increase in extracellular fluid, clinically manifested as hypovolemia and burn-induced edema.

Inflammatory mediators are released from burned tissues following the injury, causing localized inflammation and burn-wound edema. Localized mediators include oxygen radicals, arachidonic acid metabolites, histamine, prostaglandins, leukotrienes, products of platelet activation, and the complement cascade.[17,28,34] In minor burns, the inflammatory process remains sequestered in the wound itself. However, in major burn insults, this local injury signals the release of systemic circulatory mediators. This results in a systemic response to the burn.

Fluid Resuscitation

Within seconds after an acute burn injury, massive fluid shifts begin to occur. Therefore, fluid resuscitation and airway management are the hallmarks of initial therapy and should be instituted by the first-response emergency medical providers. There are many formulas for calculating a burn patient's initial fluid resuscitation requirements. The current ABA consensus formula for fluid resuscitation and urine output in burn patients is given in Box 36-1. Table 36-3 lists other commonly used fluid protocols. Common to all of these formulas is the need to know the patient's weight in kilograms and the percentage of TBSA involved. The American College of Surgeons Committee on Trauma has advocated that only crystalloid formulas be used for all burn resuscitation. Colloid solutions are not advocated in the first 24 hours because capillary permeability remains enhanced, and any colloids administered will not remain in the intravascular space. It is important to remember that the formulas for fluid guidelines are only that—guidelines. Individual factors must also be taken into account. It is crucial to resuscitate the patient with fluids according to patient response, hemodynamic variables, sensorium, and urinary output (0.5 to 1 mL/kg/hr in adults and 1 mL/kg/hr in children weighing less than 60 pounds),[34] instead of by a fixed formula.[17,25] Fluid resuscitation in children requires extreme precision, owing not only to their

---

BOX 36-1

Consensus Formula for Fluid Resuscitation and Urine Output in Burn Patients (American Burn Association)

Adults: Ringer's lactate 2-4 mL × kg body weight × percent TBSA burned*

Children: Ringer's lactate 3-4 mL × kg body weight × percent TBSA burned*†

*One half of the estimated volume of fluid should be administered in the first 8 hours after the burn. The remaining half should be administered over the subsequent 16 hours of the first postburn day.

†Infants and young children should receive fluid with 5% dextrose at a maintenance rate in addition to the resuscitation fluid noted above.

Minimum Urinary Output in Burn Patients

Adults: 0.5 mL/kg/hr
Children weighing less than 30 kg: 1 mL/kg/hr
Patients with high-voltage electrical injuries: 1-1.5 mL/kg/hr

Modified from American Burn Association. Advanced Burn Life Support Course Provider's Manual. *Chicago: American Burn Association; 2005.*

TBSA, *Total body surface area.*

TABLE 36-3	Fluid Resuscitation Formulas for Burn Patients	
Formula	**First 24 Hours**	**Second 24 Hours**
Brooke Crystalloid	2 mL LR/% burn per kg ½ in first 8 hr ½ in next 16 hr	D₅W maintenance
Colloid	None	0.5 mL/% burn per kg
Parkland Crystalloid	4 mL LR/% burn per kg ½ in first 8 hr ½ in next 16 hr	D₅W maintenance
Colloid	None	0.5 mL/% burn per kg
MGH Crystalloid	1.5 mL LR/% burn per kg ½ in first 8 hr ½ in next 16 hr	Not specified
Colloid	0.5 mL LR/% burn per kg None in first 4 hr ½ in second 4 hr ½ in next 16 hr	Not specified
Evans Crystalloid	1 mL LR/% burn per kg ½ in first 8 hr ½ in next 16 hr	D₅W maintenance
Colloid	1 mL LR/% burn per kg ½ in first 8 hr ½ in next 16 hr	Not specified

D_5W, *5% dextrose in water;* LR, *lactated Ringer's solution;* MGH, *Massachusetts General Hospital.*

size but also their limited physiologic reserve. Because infants and small children have high volume-to-surface-area ratios, formulas that base fluid requirements on surface area burned and weight may underestimate need. The ABA recommends that to counteract the rapid use of glycogen stores and prevent the development of hypoglycemia, a dextrose-containing IV solution be administered for maintenance purposes in burned children in the immediate postburn period.[35]

Invasive hemodynamic monitoring (central venous pressure, pulmonary artery catheterization) is indicated in patients who do not respond to fluid resuscitation or who have preexisting cardiopulmonary disease. Catheters should be removed as quickly as possible to minimize the risk of local and systemic infection.

Hypermetabolic/Hyperhemodynamic Phase
Once a burn victim survives the initial 48 hours after the burn insult, a systemic inflammatory syndrome is noted: the hypermetabolic/hyperhemodynamic phase. The hypermetabolic phase is associated with increased blood flow to organs and tissues. The exact cause remains unclear, but it may be related to heat loss from burned tissue and increased intrinsic sympathetic nervous system activity.[36] The state is manifested by hyperthermia, tachypnea, tachycardia, increased serum catecholamine levels, increased oxygen consumption, increased catabolism, and increased basal metabolic rate. The state persists for several weeks, gradually receding to normal when the wound healing is well underway.[25]

Pathophysiologic Changes
As with any disease entity, certain pathophysiologic alterations occur after an acute burn injury (Table 36-4). It is important for the anesthetist to understand the basis for these changes because many of these changes must be managed intraoperatively and reflected in the anesthetic plan.

TABLE 36-4	Pathophysiologic Effects of Major Burns	
System	**Considerations**
Respiratory	
Upper airway	Thermal damage to soft tissue and respiratory tract requires early endotracheal intubation
Carbon monoxide poisoning	Considered in all victims of enclosed fires; treatment with 100% oxygen by mask or endotracheal tube
Cardiac	
Burn shock phase (0 to 48 hr)	Hypovolemia is a major concern; fluid resuscitation mandatory; expect impaired cardiac contractility
Hypermetabolic phase (after 48 hr)	Increased blood flow to organs and tissues; manifested by hyperthermia, tachypnea, tachycardia, increased oxygen consumption, and increased catabolism
Renal	
Early	
Reduced renal blood flow	Secondary to hypovolemia and decreased cardiac output; adequate fluid resuscitation and diuresis prevents renal failure
Electrical burns and muscle necrosis damage renal tubules	Intravenous administration of sodium bicarbonate to alkalize the urine
Late	
Increased renal blood flow	Variable drug clearance
Nutrition	
Increased caloric requirements	Limited to no nothing-by-mouth (NPO) status required
Ileus and duodendal ulcers	Treatment with H_2 blockers and antacids
Pharmacokinetics	
Decreased albumin	Benzodiazepines, phenytoin, and salicylic acid have an increase in the free fraction and thus a larger volume of distribution
Increased α_1-acid glycoprotein	Lidocaine, meperidine, and propranolol have the opposite effect
Denervation phenomenon with spreading of acetylcholine receptors	Succinylcholine avoided 24 hours after injury.
Increased nicotinic acetylcholine receptors	Requires a two-fold to three-fold increased concentration of nondepolarizer for paralysis
Skin Integrity	
Vulnerable to nosocomial infections	Strict adherence to aseptic individual patient rooms; wound care, including topical antimicrobial agents and early excision/grafting of the burn wound

Cardiovascular System. The cardiovascular system is greatly affected in the burn patient. Almost immediately after an acute burn injury, intravascular fluid losses begin. Etiologies for this include the loss of vascular and endothelial integrity and the release of circulating mediators described earlier. The loss of plasma proteins from within the intravascular compartment (due to disruption of the endothelium) persists for up to 36 hours after the initial burn injury. Hypovolemia results, with subsequent hypotension and circulatory compromise. The size and extent of the burn determine the magnitude of this development. Hence, burn victims can develop "burn shock" within the first 24 to 36 hours following an acute burn injury. A reduction in cardiac output is a hallmark of burn shock and appears to occur within minutes after the injury. It is initially preserved via catecholamine responses—tachycardia and vasoconstriction. However, with the progressive loss of intravascular fluids and proteins, left ventricular filling declines, leading to a reduction in cardiac output. Additionally, cardiac output is thought to be depressed from the release of a myocardial depressant factor or proteins from burned tissues. The cardiovascular response to catecholamines is attenuated after a burn injury as the result of reduced adrenergic-receptor affinity and decreased secondary-messenger production. Coronary blood flow can be reduced, further decreasing cardiac function. Systemic vascular resistance increases.

Aggressive fluid resuscitation administered over the first 24 to 36 hours aims to restore intravascular volume and cardiac function. What is seen is a systemic inflammatory response syndrome, characterized by increased cardiac output, tachycardia, and a reduction in systemic vascular resistance. The patient becomes hypermetabolic, with an increase in oxygen consumption and carbon dioxide production.

Children with extensive burn injuries can become quite hypertensive weeks after their injury. A definite etiology is not clear but is speculated to be a result of increased catecholamine production, hypervolemia, and/or activation of the renin-angiotensin system during the postburn period. This occurs primarily within the first 2 weeks and can last for several weeks.[8]

Pulmonary System. The pulmonary system is greatly affected in burn patients, with resulting pathophysiologic changes. Pulmonary function may decrease markedly, even in the absence of inhalation injury. Functional residual capacity is reduced, and both lung and chest-wall compliance decrease. The latter can be severely compromised if the chest is circumferentially burned. With progressive fluid shifts and interstitial edema formation in cases with eschar formation, the inability to adequately expand the lungs impairs ventilation. In some cases, escharotomies are necessary to alleviate pressure in the tissues to improve oxygenation and ventilation. The oxygen gradient between alveoli and arterial blood increases as well. Ventilation can increase to as much as 40 L/min from a normal rate of 6 L/min.[25]

As stated, the lungs are at risk for compromise even without an inhalation injury. There are many mechanisms involved. A primary factor is the effect released mediators have on the lung. Plasma oncotic pressure greatly decreases after a burn, owing to the loss of plasma proteins in both burned and nonburned tissues. Impaired vascular and capillary permeability, combined with the large amount of fluid resuscitation needed, sets the stage for pulmonary edema.[29]

Patients with varying degrees of hypoxemia and respiratory insufficiency require mechanical support and ventilation. High-frequency percussive ventilation may be superior to conventional, volume-controlled mechanical ventilation, presumably because barotrauma is minimized.[37,38] In severely burned patients, especially if there is an inhalation injury, prolonged endotracheal intubation and mechanical ventilation are likely. Despite this, early or routine tracheostomy placement in burned patients has not been shown to improve the overall outcome in this patient population.[39]

Immune System. Burn victims, regardless of age, are particularly susceptible to infection. The protective barrier of the skin has been destroyed, and the doorway to microbial invasion is wide open. Altered immune responses are also present and begin within hours after the burn injury. Leukocyte activity is depressed, as well as humoral and cellular responses. Burn eschar is a prime medium for bacterial growth. Colonization of gram-negative bacteria increases mortality. These patients often become septic and are vulnerable to pneumonia, especially if prolonged endotracheal intubation is required. Strict asepsis is required. Of those patients who die after sustaining a burn, infection is the leading cause of death over the long term in nearly 100% of children and 75% of adults.

Renal System. The development of acute renal failure (ARF) after acute burn injury is a serious complication that increases mortality rates.[18] Decreases in renal blood flow can occur immediately after a burn injury, leading to alterations in glomerular filtration. Causes include the large intravascular depletion, hypovolemia, decreased cardiac output, and increased circulating plasma catecholamine levels. The renin-angiotensin-aldosterone system and the release of ADH are stimulated and act to conserve sodium and water.[40] Subsequently, alterations in electrolyte balance can take place. Electrical burns with massive muscle necrosis can result in myoglobinemia, which may damage renal tubules and impair renal function. Intravenous administration of sodium bicarbonate to alkalize the urine protects the kidneys by preventing the formation of myoglobin casts. With adequate fluid resuscitation, renal blood flow and glomerular filtration are preserved. Hourly urine output measurements remain the gold standard for assessing adequate fluid replacement and resuscitation (see Box 36-1).

Acute renal failure can also occur 2 to 3 weeks after the burn injury. Associated causes include sepsis and delayed wound excision. Delayed renal failure in children is rare and usually not a problem.

Gastrointestinal System/Nutrition. Caloric requirements for a patient with a 40% thermal injury are estimated to be 132% higher than basal energy expenditure, compared with a 79% increase for sepsis and a 25% increase for major elective surgery.[41] The increased energy expenditure enhances a period of negative nitrogen balance and causes an erosion of lean body mass, requiring intensive nutritional support. This nutritional support is essential for immune-system function, wound healing, and the prevention of catabolism. In patients with large burns and a pronounced hypermetabolic response, carbohydrate is more effective than fat in maintaining body protein.[42] The burn patient has an injury-induced resistance to the action of insulin in the liver and skeletal muscle. Ongoing assessment of blood glucose, with administration of exogenous insulin may be necessary.

The necessity for continued adequate caloric intake cannot be ignored during the preanesthetic evaluation. Because of the importance of nutrition, it is unwise to arbitrarily stop enteral feedings the night before surgery. This can result in an excessive loss of calories, especially if the patient must undergo multiple burn débridements in a short period. Preoperative nothing-by-mouth (NPO) status must be kept at a safe minimum to prevent the patient from reverting to a catabolic state. Tracheally intubated patients do not need the enteral feedings discontinued before surgery, and unintubated patients can remain on nutritional support as late as 4 hours before the scheduled surgical procedure.[43] This practice improves preoperative nutrition without increasing the risk for aspiration. On admission to the operating room, the nonintubated patient's nasogastric tube should be suctioned and induction tailored to ensure rapid protection of the airway.[36] If the patient is not receiving enteral feedings, but rather parenteral feedings via a central venous catheter, the parenteral nutrition line should not be used for administering fluids or drugs during anesthesia. Parenteral hyperalimentation and lipid infusions need not be discontinued intraoperatively.

Burn patients demonstrate a decrease in gastrointestinal function. If the percentage of TBSA involved is greater than 20%, the development of ileus is common.[44] Other gastrointestinal sequelae are acute ulcerations of the gastric and/or duodenal mucosa. These are known as *Curling ulcers*. Treatment primarily entails the administration of H_2 blockers and antacids.[17] However, there has been an associated increased incidence of pulmonary infection with *Pseudomonas* in intensive-care-unit patients treated with such medication. The clearance of cimetidine (but not ranitidine) is increased, so appropriate dosage adjustments are required.[26]

Pharmacokinetics. Burn injury causes considerable changes in plasma protein levels, with significant consequences for the protein binding of drugs. In general, patients with burns exhibit decreased albumin and increased α_1-acid glycoprotein (AAG) levels.[26,45,46] Because the pharmacologic effect is often related to the unbound fraction of a drug, alterations in protein binding can also affect the efficacy and tolerability of drug treatment in patients with burns. This alteration causes the plasma binding of predominantly albumin-bound drugs (e.g., benzodiazepines, phenytoin, salicylic acid) to be decreased, resulting in an increase in the free fraction and thus a larger volume of distribution for the drug. Drugs primarily bound to AAG (e.g., lidocaine, meperidine, propranolol) have the opposite effect.

Volume of distribution (V_d) may be increased or decreased in patients with burns. In general, two factors may cause alteration in V_d: changes in extracellular fluid volume and changes in protein binding.[26] Fluid loss to the burn wound and edema can decrease plasma concentrations of many drugs. After the initial resuscitation state, cardiac output increases as the hypermetabolic phase develops. This increases blood flow to the kidneys and liver, with increased drug clearance. Dosage requirements may change if the drug has a small V_d and a narrow therapeutic range. Overall, there is significant patient variability based on fluid status and phase of recovery.

Burn Management: Surgical Débridement and Grafting

Of all of the surgical procedures performed, the débridement and grafting of burn wounds is one an anesthetist must understand well. The course and dynamics of the surgical procedure can affect the anesthetic in many ways. Additionally, good communication with the surgeon regarding the patient's hemodynamic tolerance must be maintained.

A goal of burn therapy is to rapidly restore skin integrity after the burn. After thorough cleansing, the burn wound should be treated with antimicrobial agents as early as possible to limit bacterial proliferation on the wound surface and to avoid bacterial wound invasion. Wounds have been shown to reepithelialize more rapidly with less pain and inflammation when they are occluded and a thin layer of wound fluid is maintained in contact with the surface. Subsequent treatment involves surgical procedures such as amputation, grafting, and multiple skin débridements.[47]

There is varying opinion on the timing of burn wound excision, débridement, and grafting. Some surgeons favor early excision and grafting of the wound within the first 24 to 48 hours after injury. This point of view reflects the philosophy that the earlier the dead eschar is removed, the less time elapses for bacterial colonization to take place. Some authors suggest that this time frame appears to decrease the mortality rate,[5,48,49] shorten the hospital stay,[47-49] improve cellular immunity, and provide a better cosmetic outcome.[5] Conversely, there is the opinion that deferring surgical treatment of the burn wounds until at least 1 week to (up to 3 weeks) after the initial burn injury is the best approach. With this option, it is possible that some marginal burned sites may heal and/or tissue granulation will occur, reducing the amount of skin harvesting and grafting and promoting better skin-graft adherence.[50,8]

Independent of the timing, a common shared approach entails an initial waiting period to stabilize and fluid-resuscitate the patient, followed by excision and grafting of the wound. The primary goals are to control infection and remove sloughing burn eschar. Limiting an operation to approximately 20% of body surface is suggested[17]; however, larger areas may be excised depending on the patient's preoperative and perioperative hemodynamic stability and coagulation status. Additional surgery end-points include a time of 2 to 3 hours if the patient's core temperature decreases to 35° C or less or if there has been a blood loss requiring 10 units or more of packed red blood cells.[51] Usually the patient will be taken to the operating room every 2 to 3 days, with staging of the burn wound excisions until full grafting has been completed.

In patients with extensive burns and limited donor sites, biologic dressings provide temporary coverage for the excised wound. One effective biologic dressing is homograft (or cadaveric) skin, which derives a temporary blood supply from the underlying wound bed. New alternatives for the management of burns are being developed. Results with the use of recombinant human growth hormone have been encouraging, especially in children.[52] Artificial skin substitutes such as Integra provide an outer silicone layer for wound closure, and an inner layer establishes a vascular supply.[42,53] The outer layer is removed after 2 weeks and replaced with thin autologous skin grafts.

Anesthetic Implications

There are many anesthetic implications that accompany caring for the burn patient—not only in the operating room but beforehand as well. To facilitate the delivery of a safe and effective anesthetic, the astute anesthetist will view the global picture of this patient, including the preoperative status.

Preoperative Evaluation. The burn patient requires a thorough and complete preoperative assessment. A complete medical history, including laboratory studies, and a brief physical examination with lung auscultation, assessment of chest compliance, and inspection of the neck and oral cavity to evaluate for difficulties with intubation or reintubation should be implemented. There are specific data unique to the burn patient that the anesthesia provider should know, such as the underlying trauma, mechanism of burn (electrical, inhalation), percentage of TBSA burned, location of the burn sites, the area and amount the surgeon intends to débride, and whether the patient will be grafted during the perioperative course. Assimilation of this information affects the anesthetic plan in terms of anesthetic

---

agents selected, appropriate monitoring, positioning, vascular access, and blood-product requirements. A review of prior anesthetic records can be helpful in determining the anesthetic plan. Quite often this is possible to do because more often than not, these patients make several trips to the operating room.

The Set-Up and Preparation. A successful anesthetic for the excision and grafting of a burn wound requires planning and preparation of necessary equipment (Box 36-2). There are specific anesthetic interventions that should be done for this patient before arrival in the operating room.

Intraoperative Management

Equipment and Monitoring. Burn patients require all of the standard monitors intraoperatively. It can be challenging at times to adapt standard monitors to the burned patient. Electrocardiogram (ECG) leads are often difficult to place because of a lack of intact skin. It may be necessary to staple the lead electrodes to the skin or use needle electrodes on the patient to obtain an acceptable ECG tracing. Ideally, blood pressure cuffs should be placed on an unaffected limb or at a nonsurgical site. If the planned amount of surgical débridement is extensive or if manipulation of the patient's limbs intraoperatively limits the accuracy of noninvasive cuff readings, the placement of an arterial line for blood pressure monitoring may be warranted, even in the healthy patient. In large burns that are greater than 20% to 30% TBSA, invasive blood pressure monitoring should be instituted after induction if not in place preoperatively. Rapid blood losses, the potential for hemodynamic swings, and the need to check intraoperative laboratory values all validate this requirement. The standard sites for pulse oximetry placement may not be available. Alternative sites include the nose, ear, and cheek. Any preexisting invasive monitors such as an arterial line or central venous or pulmonary artery catheters should be continued in the operating room. Accurate temperature monitoring is essential because burn patients can become very hypothermic intraoperatively. Temperature measurements should be obtained via an esophageal stethoscope. Skin temperature devices are highly inaccurate and there may not be a suitable place to apply one.

Critically ill burn patients are usually transported by the anesthesia provider directly to the operating room from the burn intensive care unit (and vice versa postoperatively). These patients are usually intubated or have a tracheostomy, are on continuous infusions of pharmacologic agents, and have invasive lines in place. Astute monitoring of the patient's vital signs during transport is mandatory. Care must be taken while transporting to not disrupt or dislodge any invasive lines or IVs. A portable oxygen delivery system is another component of required transport equipment. Careful handling and vigilant guarding of the airway are vital. The anesthetist must also consider the patient's comfort and privacy during transport. Amnestic and analgesic drugs should be administered as needed.

Airway Management. Acute airway problems are usually handled on the patient's admission to the burn unit. In the patient with a major burn or inhalation injury, preoperative intubation is likely. In the nonintubated patient without an inhalation injury and whose airway is normal, induction and intubation of the airway can proceed as with any other anesthetic (except no succinylcholine). Preoperative airway evaluation is necessary as with any other patient. The anesthetist should exert good judgment in determining the degree of intubation difficulty. If the airway appears difficult, fiberoptic intubation should be considered or at least be readily available.

In the severely burned patient who is intubated preoperatively, vigilance is required to protect the airway from accidental extubation. Because of edema of the airway structures, loss of the airway in this patient may be impossible to regain. Securing such an airway can be challenging; tape does not readily stick to burned skin. The use of soft beard straps to secure an endotracheal tube is a good option, especially if the plan is to extubate the patient at the end of the procedure. Cloth ties encircling the head are frequently used in the burn unit to secure endotracheal tubes and should not be disrupted.

Temperature Regulation. Depending on the percentage TBSA affected by the burn, temperature regulation can be problematic in the burn patient. These patients are at high risk for hypothermia development due to the loss of the skin's insulating mechanisms, radiation and evaporative heat losses, and the large amount of body surface area exposure intraoperatively. The temperature in the operating room should be above 28° C.[25,28,41] Intravenous solutions and skin preparations should be warmed. All methods of heat conservation should be used while the patient is in the operating room. The use of inline humidivents or low gas flows reduces evaporative respiratory tract heat loss. Forced-air warming blankets are very effective, but their use can be limited. Over-body heating lamps can be used but need to be at a safe distance above the patient to prevent further skin burns. Plastic bags can also be helpful to insulate any exposed body parts not requiring surgical access (the "plastic approach").

It is suggested that keeping a patient warm is more beneficial than rewarming. With hypothermia, vasoconstriction occurs, which may curtail any warming efforts later on. It has been shown that slow rewarming postoperatively in critically ill burn patients leads to an increase in mortality.[54] If the patient becomes hypothermic despite the best efforts at prevention, the surgeon needs to be advised to stop the procedure.

Fluid and Blood Replacement. Surgical burn débridements may be extraordinarily bloody operations. Wound management involves removal of the burn eschar layer until brisk bleeding of the dermis is reached.[25] The surgical team may remove the eschar so rapidly that it becomes difficult to keep up with the massive blood loss, resulting in a suddenly hypovolemic patient.

Some institutions stop the surgical procedure after 2 hours if more than two blood volumes have been lost or if the body temperature falls to 35° C or by greater than 1.5° C from baseline.

There are many formulas to approximate the amount of potential blood loss for a burn débridement. These vary from 200 to 400 mL of blood loss for each 1% of BSA excised and grafted[28] to as high as 4% to 15% of the patient's blood volume for every percentage of skin débrided.[18] During and especially after the excision and débridement, gauzes soaked in a vasoconstrictor[17] (e.g., epinephrine, phenylephrine) are placed on the newly excised wound to control the bleeding. However, this may result in systemic absorption of vasoconstrictors, causing elevation of the patient's blood pressure, even in the face of hypovolemia. Thrombin-soaked sponges may be preferred for patients in whom systemic absorption of epinephrine may cause myocardial ischemia or arrhythmias.[28]

Preoperative anemia is another indicator for the frequent need for transfusion and is commonly seen in thermally burned patients with greater than 10% TBSA involvment.[55-57] There are several reasons for its development. There is acute destruction of red blood cells immediately following the burn and inflammatory process. Later, red blood cells accumulate in the thrombosed microcirculation of burned tissues, leading to an erythroctye loss of up to 18% in full-thickness burns greater than 15% TBSA.[58] Bone-marrow response to above-normal production of erythropoietin is suppressed following a burn injury. In addition, patients with extensive burns undergo numerous operative procedures, all of which result in blood loss and further anemia.

Adequate venous access is critical prior to the initiation of surgical débridement. The size and extent of the burn will mandate how much access is needed. One intravenous catheter is adequate for the induction of anesthesia in most burned patients, but at least two large-bore intravenous catheters are necessary before beginning a major excision. Obtaining sufficient IV access can be challenging and time consuming, depending on the extent and location of the burn. Critically ill patients or those with limited peripheral sites for IV access will often have a central venous catheter in place (i.e., triple-lumen catheter), and although this catheter is adequate in the intensive care unit setting, it is not ideal in the operating room when fluid and blood replacement are needed quickly.

The readiness of blood products should be ascertained before the patient is taken to the operating room. Ideally, blood supplies should be in the operating room, checked, and ready to go at the beginning of the surgical procedure. This is particularly vital in pediatric patients. If there are no blood products prepared for the pediatric patient who is about to undergo a significant burn excision, the anesthetist should consider canceling the case or delaying the surgical start until adequate blood products are on hand. Some practitioners initiate blood transfusions before the beginning of surgical débridement and apply compression dressings after excision and grafting.

Careful planning is necessary to manage the hemorrhage and potential complications associated with massive transfusion (citrate toxicity, loss of clotting factors) during débridement. Visual estimation of blood loss is subjective at best and prone to be miscalculated. Suction is not used during débridements. Sponges may be accidentally thrown away or covered up. Blood may drip onto the floor, may be covered up in the surgical drapes, or leak under the patient. It is possible to be lulled into a false sense of security immediately after the eschar incision. Proper monitoring of the patient's urinary output, hematocrit, and hemodynamic status is crucial to keeping the patient within normal limits.

The Anesthetic Agents

Induction. There is no single best anesthetic agent to administer to the burn patient. The anesthetic is individualized and should be based on the patient's preoperative status and medical history. The acute burn patient seldom comes to the operating room immediately after the injury. Patients are usually admitted and stabilized in the burn unit. If the patient requires immediate surgery, the anesthetist must realize that the burn patient is both fragile and labile within the first 24 hours of injury. Anesthetic agents can exert extreme depressant effects, especially if fluid resuscitation is not adequate or has not been fully completed. The loss of intravascular volume coupled with the potential for a depressed myocardium can result in a hemodynamically unstable patient under general anesthesia. Careful and slow titration of all anesthetic agents is vital. Premedicating stable patients with a benzodiazepine or a narcotic decreases anxiety and makes transfer to the OR tolerable. Anxiety, depression, and pain are interrelated in patients with burns.[59,60] Induction can be performed while the patient is in the ICU bed. The subsequent move onto the OR table will provoke minimal discomfort.

Regional anesthesia is sometimes considered for burn trauma limited to a small area or an extremity or for surgery during the reconstructive phase. One advantage of the technique is prolonged postoperative analgesia, but variables in this patient population restrict its application. The anesthesia provider must avoid performing any regional technique through burned tissue because of the potential for the spread of infection. There is an almost universal presence of hypotension (hypovolemia) and vasodilation (with or without sepsis), which is a relative contraindication to the use of spinal or epidural routes for pain control until the burn wound is closed. Coagulopathy and cardiorespiratory instability are also reasons to avoid a regional anesthetic technique. The greatest limitation to the use of regional anesthesia is the extent of the surgical field. The anesthetized region must include both the area to be excised and the area to be harvested for donor skin.

In children, regional anesthesia blocks are sometimes a viable option for postoperative analgesia. A tried-and-true regional block to institute in children undergoing débridements in the lower extremities or skin harvesting from the buttocks or thighs is a single-shot caudal injection. This can be placed either after the induction of general anesthesia or at end of the case before emergence. Injection of 0.25% bupivacaine with added epinephrine 1:200,000 has proved safe and effective. The volume of local anesthetic injected into the caudal space is determined by the child's weight in kilograms and the analgesia level to be covered by the block. If the child is to be admitted postoperatively, the addition of morphine, 30 to 50 mcg/kg, or clonidine, 1 to 2 mcg/kg, can be considered.

The standard induction drugs are all acceptable to use. Sodium thiopental is well tolerated, but it may require higher than normal dosages.[23] The use of this agent may produce hypotension on induction if the patient has not received adequate intravascular replacement.[57] Etomidate maintains hemodynamic stability during induction and produces less respiratory depression than barbiturates.[23] However, repeated doses may inhibit adrenocortical function. Propofol has greater negative inotropic effects than either thiopental or etomidate, which may lead to hypotension after induction. The high lipid content of propofol may limit its use during initial resuscitation and in septic patients.[61]

Another intravenous anesthetic is ketamine, a phencyclidine derivative, that produces a dissociative anesthetic state of relatively short duration. Ketamine offers the advantage of stable hemodynamics and analgesia. Low doses produce adequate amnesia and analgesia for the débridement of superficial burns; higher doses may be administered for more extensive procedures such as eschar excisions.[17,25,55] Hallucinogenic episodes can be minimized with the administration of benzodiazepines in small doses, and an anticholinergic prevents excessive pharyngeal and tracheobronchial secretions. In the pediatric burn patient, an inhalation induction with sevoflurane is certainly acceptable if the child does not have intravenous access prior to induction and if the airway appears normal.

Anesthesia should be maintained with opioid or inhalation agents as the hemodynamic status of the patient permits. Inhaled volatile agents have proved to be safe and effective, allowing rapid adjustment of anesthetic depth and administration of high oxygen concentrations. The burn patient may be sensitive to the cardiovascular depressant effects of inhaled anesthetics, especially if acute fluid resuscitation is incomplete.[28] Inhaled agents do not provide analgesia during the postsurgical period. Intubated burn patients may require the continuance of specialized critical-care ventilators (e.g., percussive ventilators) intraoperatively to maintain adequate oxygenation and ventilation. In this instance, a total intravenous anesthetic is indicated.

The main group of anesthetic agents that can exert altered effects in the burn patient are the muscle relaxants. Within the first 24 hours following burn injury, the burn is considered stable. Succinylcholine is probably safe to use within this time frame. As stated previously, the postjunctional acetylcholine receptors begin to proliferate soon after a burn injury occurs. This phenomenon is thought to be fully complete by 7 days after the acute injury. Succinylcholine given after the initial 24-hour window has produced significant hyperkalemia as a result of this upregulation of receptors.

Nondepolarizing muscle relaxants are safe to use with the burn patient, but the anesthetist should realize that the patient may demonstrate a resistance to their effects. Higher dosing or more frequent redosing may be necessary. Again, the phenomenon is thought to result from the increase in postjunctional acetylcholine receptors. Because responses to the nondepolarizers can vary significantly, neuromuscular blockade monitoring should always be used.

Pain Management. The increased requirement for narcotics by the burn patient[17,59,61] may be accounted for by the activation of endogenous opioid pathways during stress-induced analgesia.[25,60] Pain sensations associated with a serious burn injury may start within a few minutes of trauma or may be delayed for several hours.[59,61] The intravenous route (patient-controlled analgesia) is preferred early in the course of burn care, because the absorption from intramuscular sites may be erratic or too slow for rapid control of pain.[59]

Narcotics are a very important component in the anesthetic care of the burn patient. These are painful procedures. Pain from skin harvest sites frequently exceeds that from burned, débrided, and grafted areas. Morphine, fentanyl, and sufentanil all provide intraoperative and postoperative analgesia and are acceptable choices. Remifentanil, a short-acting opioid, may be used for dressing changes. Many times, burn patients will be on narcotic infusions preoperatively for pain control and/or sedation. One option is to continue these infusions during the operative procedure, with narcotic bolus supplementation. Narcotic-based anesthetics provide the advantage of minimal cardiac depression. In addition, postoperative analgesia must be a vital constituent incorporated into the anesthetic plan.

Nonsteroidal antiinflammatory agents can work peripherally to reduce pain through control of inflammation. However, these agents also inhibit the synthesis of thromboxane A, resulting in the failure of platelet aggregation, with potentially disastrous effects on hemostasis. This may cause problems during the surgical procedure, precluding their routine use to control peripheral pain.

Concern about possible addiction or the inability of burn patients to eliminate opioids has led to undermedication[41,59,60,62]; yet surveys have not indicated a high prevalence of iatrogenic addiction. Painful procedures include multiple dressing changes, débridements, nursing care, hydrotherapy, physiotherapy, and surgical procedures. The profound level of pain associated with these treatments, together with the fact that they are inflicted repeatedly (sometimes twice a day or more) over long periods of time, explains why patients require medication. However, inadequate pain management is a problem in many burn units.[60]

Emergence from Anesthesia. The postoperative anesthetic course should be planned in advance and is frequently intuitive. Critically ill and intubated burn patients are kept intubated postoperatively and directly transported to the burn unit. The anesthetist should safeguard the airway and be respectful of the patient's need for sedation and analgesia during this terminal phase of the anesthetic.

If the patient is to be extubated, emergence from anesthesia should be planned in advance as with any other patient undergoing an anesthetic procedure. Neuromuscular blockade should be adequately reversed and (if possible) the patient allowed to begin spontaneously breathing at an appropriate time. Narcotics for postoperative analgesia should be titrated according to the patient's respiratory status. Keep in mind that these are painful procedures, and the patient's narcotic requirements can be tremendous.

Reconstructive Phase

It is important to address the ongoing effect a burn injury can have on an individual. After all of the skin grafting and surgery have been completed and some healing has taken place, scarring may remain. To optimize function and prevent contractures and deformity, physical and occupational therapy are very important assists for these individuals. For months to years after hospital discharge, victims of major burns return for reconstructive procedures to remove or reduce scar tissue. Such procedures improve cosmetic and functional outcomes. Patients may experience anxiety, stress, and depression from undergoing repeated procedures over a long period of time. The most important anesthetic concern is management of the airway, particularly if contractures of the face and neck are present. An awake fiberoptic technique may be the safest method of intubating the patient.

Invisible scars may remain as well. Psychologic issues must be explored as needed while the patient is in the hospital. This effort is especially important when dealing with children. Recreational therapists can help them reveal their feelings and fears. Once the child is at home and healed, group settings such as burn camps can offer opportunities to be around other children who have suffered burn injuries. In such a place, a child can experience freedom from judgment and need not feel ashamed of the burn scars.

SUMMARY

Anesthetic implications for the burn patient are numerous and can be challenging. As burn centers continue to improve in their ability to extend life after a severe burn injury, the likelihood of an anesthesia provider being involved in the care of a patient with thermal injury increases. We must always remember that these patients are being challenged not only physically but also emotionally. For many, the road to recovery is long and painful. As both anesthesia providers and patient advocates, it is important that we take into account the unique aspects of the burn patient's needs. And although we may play a small, temporary part in helping such a patient on the difficult journey to recovery and healing, it is nonetheless a role with many rewards.

REFERENCES

1. American Burn Association website. http://www.ameriburn.org/. Updated continually. Accessed August 12, 2008.
2. Brigham P, McLoughlin E. Burn incidence and medical care use in the United States: estimates, trends, and data sources. *J Burn Care Rehabil.* 1996;17:95-107.
3. American Burn Association. Burn Incidence and Treatment in the US: 2007 Fact Sheet. Available at: http://www.ameriburn.org/resources_factsheet/. Accessed August 12, 2008.
4. Saffle J et al. Recent outcomes in the treatment of burn injury in the US: a report from the American Burn Association patient registry. *J Burn Care Rehabil.* 1995;16:219-231.
5. Donati P. Survival and therapy of burn patients at the threshold of the twenty first century: a review. *J Chemother.* 1995;7:475-502.
6. Kane A, Kumar V. Environmental and nutritional pathology. In: Cotran R et al, eds. *Robbins Pathologic Basis of Disease.* 6th ed. Philadelphia: Saunders; 1999:433-444.
7. Palmisano B, Rusy L. Anesthesia for plastic surgery. In: Gregory GA, ed. *Pediatric Anesthesia.* 4th ed. Philadelphia: Churchill Livingstone; 2002: 707-745.
8. Clarke H, Chalain T. Burns and post-burn care: surgical considerations. In: Bissonnette B, Dalens B, eds. *Pediatric Anesthesia Principles and Practice.* New York: McGraw-Hill; 2002:1414-1427.
9. Weiss Sm, Lakshminarayan S. Acute inhalation injury. *Clin Chest Med.* 1994;15(1):103-116.
10. Paus S, Bueno R. The burned trachea. *Chest Surg Clin North Am.* 2003;13(2):343-348.
11. Lee-Chiong TL Jr. Some inhalation injury. *Postgrad Med.* 1999;105(2):55-62.
12. Haponik EF, Summer W. Respiratory complications in burned patients, pathogenesis and spectrum of inhalation injury. *J Crit Care.* 1987;2:49-74.
13. Moritz AR et al. The effects of inhaled heat on the air passages and lungs: an experimental investigation. *Am J Pathol.* 1945;21:311.
14. Tredget EE et al. The role of inhalation injury in burn trauma. *Ann Surg.* 1990;212:720-727.
15. Haponik EF, Lykens MG. Acute upper airway obstruction in patients with burns. *Crit Care Rep.* 1990;2:28-49.
16. Sharar S, Hudson DH. Toxic gas, fume, and smoke inhalation. In: Parrillo JE, Bone RC, eds. *Critical Care Medicine: Principles of Diagnosis and Management.* St Louis: Mosby; 1995:849-866.
17. MacLennan N, et al. Anesthesia for major thermal injury. *Anesthesiology.* 1998;89:749-770.
18. Berger M, Bernath M. Burns and post-burn care: anesthetic considerations and postoperative management. In: Bissonnette B, Dalens B, eds. *Pediatric Anesthesia Principles and Practice.* New York: McGraw-Hill; 2002:1428-1446.
19. Eckhauser FE et al. Tracheostomy complicating massive burn injury: a plea for conservation. *Am J Surg.* 1974;127:418-423.
20. Huggins RM et al. Cardiac arrest from succinylcholine-induced hyperkalemia. *Am J Health Syst Pharm.* 2003;60(7):694-697.
21. Maclennan N et al. Anesthesia for major thermal injury. *Anesthesiology.* 1998;89(3):749-770.
22. Gronert GA. Succinylcholine hyperkalemia after burns. *Anesthesiology.* 1999;91(1):320-322.
23. Martyn JA et al. Neuromuscular effects of mivacurium in 2- to 12-year-old children with burn injury. *Anesthesiology.* 2000;92(1):31-37.
24. Diefenbach C, Busello W. Muscle relaxation in patients with neuromuscular disease. *Dir Anaesthetist.* 1994;43:283-288.
25. Sartain-Spivak E. Anesthesia for the burn patient. In: Nagelhout J, Zaglanicny K, eds. *Nurse Anesthesia.* Philadelphia: Saunders; 1997:988-995.
26. Jaehde U, Sorgel F. Clinical pharmacokinetics in patients with burns. *Clin Pharmacokinet.* 1995;29:15-28.
27. Clark WR. Smoke inhalation: diagnosis and treatment. *World J Surg.* 1992;16:24-29.

28. Creasman M, Bradshaw MJ. AANA journal course: update for nurse anesthetists—anesthetic considerations for the burn patient. *AANA J.* 1995;63:257-265.
29. Morgan GE et al. Smoke inhalation. *Clinical Anesthesiology.* 4th ed. New York: McGraw-Hill; 2006:1043-1045.
30. Vegfors M, Lennmarken C. Carboxyhemoglobinaemia and pulse oximetry. *Br J Anaesth.* 1991;66:625.
31. Weaver LK et al. Neuropsychologic and functional recovery from severe carbon monoxide poisoning without hyperbaric oxygen therapy. *Ann Emerg Med.* 1996;27:736-740.
32. Thom SR et al. Delayed neuropsychologic sequelae after carbon monoxide poisoning: prevention by treatment with hyperbaric oxygen. *Ann Emerg Med.* 1995;25:474-480.
33. Norkool DM. Treatment of acute carbon monoxide poisoning with hyperbaric oxygen: a review of 115 cases. *Ann Emerg Med.* 1985;14: 1168-1171.
34. Carleton S et al. The cardiovascular effects of environmental traumas. *Cardiol Clin.* 1995;13:257-262.
35. American Burn Association. *Advanced Burn Life Support Course Provider's Manual.* Chicago: ABA; 2001:33-39.
36. Funke D. The burn patient. *Nurse Anesthetist Forum.* 1997;1:4-12.
37. Monafo WW. Initial management of burns. *N Engl J Med.* 1996;335: 1581-1586.
38. Rue LW et al. Improved survival of burned patients with inhalational injury. *Arch Surg.* 1993;128:772-780.
39. Saffle J et al. Early tracheostomy does not improve outcome in burn patients. *J Burn Care Rehabil.* 2002;23:431-438.
40. Aikawa N et al. Regulation of renal function in thermal injury. *J Trauma.* 1990;30:174-178.
41. Davis S, Kingsley C. Update on perioperative care of the burned patient. In: Lake C, ed. *Advances in Anesthesia.* St Louis: Mosby; 1996:149-191.
42. Shirani K et al. Update on current therapeutic approaches in burns. *Adv Burn Ther.* 1996;5:1-16.
43. Pearson KS et al. Continuous enteral feeding and short fasting periods enhance perioperative nutrition in patients with burns. *J Burn Care Rehabil.* 1992;14:477-481.
44. Lee C et al. Pediatric diseases. In: Hines RL, Marschall KE, eds. *Stoelting's Anesthesia and Co-existing Disease.* 5th ed. Philadelphia: Churchill Livingstone; 2008:581-638.
45. Zini R et al. Disease-induced variations in plasma protein levels. Implications for drug dosage regimens. *Clin Pharmacokinet.* 1990;19:147-159.
46. Martyn JA et al. Plasma protein binding of drugs after severe burn injury. *Clin Pharmacol Ther.* 1984;35:539.
47. Heimbach DM. Early burn excision and grafting. *Surg Clin North Am.* 1987;67:93-107.
48. Deitch EA. A policy of early excision and grafting in elderly burn patients shortens hospital stay and improves survival. *Burns Incl Therm Inj.* 1985;12:109-114.
49. Still J Jr et al. Decreasing length of hospital stay by early excision and grafting of burns. *South Med J.* 1996;89:578-582.
50. Caldwell FT Jr et al. Sequential excision and grafting of the burn injuries of 1507 patients treated between 1967 and 1986: end results and the determinants of death. *J Burn Care Rehabil.* 1996;17:137-145.
51. Yim KK, Berhow MT. Burn surgery. In: Jaffe RA, Samuels SI, eds. *Anesthesiologist's Manual of Surgical Procedures.* 3rd ed. Philadelphia: Lippincott Williams & Wilkins; 2004:927-932.
52. Lal SO et al. Growth hormone, burns and tissue healing. *Growth Horm IGF Res.* 2000;10(Suppl B):S39-43.
53. Heimbach D et al. Artificial dermis for major burns. A multi-center randomized clinical trial. *Ann Surg.* 1988;208:313-320.
54. Shiozaki T et al. Recovery from postoperative hypothermia predicts survival in extensively burned patients. *Am J Surg.* 1993;165:326, 1993.

55. Shankar R et al. Hematologic, hematopoietic, and acute phase response. In: Herndon DN, ed. *Total Burn Care.* 2nd ed. London: Saunders; 2002:331-332.

56. Topley E et al. Assessment of red cell loss in the first two days after severe burns. *Ann Surg.* 1962;155:581-590.

57. Loebl EC et al. Erythrocyte survival following thermal injury. *J Surg Res.* 1974;16:96-101.

58. Kwan P et al. Safe and successful restriction of transfusion in burn patients. *J Burn Care Res.* 2006;27(6):826-834.

59. Ashburn M. Burn pain: the management of procedure-related pain. *J Burn Care Rehabil.* 1995;46:365-371.

60. Latarjet J, Choiner M. Pain in burn patients. *Burns.* 1995;71:344-348.

61. Beushausen T, Mucke K. Anesthesia and pain management in pediatric burn patients. *Pediatr Surg Int.* 1997;12:327-333.

62. Kealey GP. Pharmacologic management of background pain in burn victims. *J Burn Care Rehabil.* 1995;16:358-362.

TRAUMA ANESTHESIA

Charles R. Barton, Brian P. Radesic

The term *trauma system* denotes an integrated approach to the care of the critically injured patient. The ideal system should include (1) triage and in-field treatment, (2) a communications network, (3) air and ground transportation, (4) patient treatment within the hospital, (5) education of paramedical personnel and the public on trauma care and accident prevention, and (6) evaluation of care.

Trauma is responsible for more than 150,000 deaths and more than 3 million nonfatal injuries per year in the United States. Each year, approximately 340,000 individuals are disabled as a result of trauma.[1,2] In 2005, there were 43,443 deaths and 2.7 million injuries from motor vehicle crashes in the United States. Firearm injuries included 29,797 fatal and 64,000 nonfatal injuries. Trauma patients are hospitalized for 19 million days annually—more than the total days required for all heart patients and four times the days required for cancer patients. Because the increase in the incidence of trauma is projected to continue and emergency medical care is improving dramatically, the number of severely injured trauma patients admitted to trauma facilities will continue to rise. Accidents cost the nation approximately $480.5 billion a year in medical fees, hospital expenses, and lost productivity.[2]

Trauma is the leading cause of death in individuals younger than 45 years in the United States. When patients of all ages are included in the overall mortality rate, it is the fifth leading cause of death, following heart disease, cancer, cerebrovascular disease, and chronic lower respiratory disease.[3] Unlike the diseases of advancing age, trauma strikes mainly between the ages of 1 and 37 years. Recognition of the tremendous loss of life in this age group prompted a group of concerned anesthesia professionals to form the International Trauma Anesthesia and Critical Care Society in 1988. The society has worked with several other groups of anesthesia and critical care providers who dedicate most or all of their professional attention to the care of trauma patients. This international society works to compile and share the collective knowledge and experience gained in trauma anesthesia and critical care management.

PATHOPHYSIOLOGIC CHANGES ARISING FROM TRAUMATIC INJURY

Cell injury can be defined as an alteration of normal homeostasis that leads to unfavorable consequences for the organism.[4] Depending on the severity of cell injury, various morphologic and biochemical changes occur. After traumatic injury, these changes may lead to eventual restoration of the cell or to ultimate death of the cell. When shock and hypoxia are involved, injured tissues that require high oxygen consumption are more vulnerable to injury and subsequent death. Metabolic rates, not tissue mass, are related to oxygen consumption. Consequently, tissues with the highest metabolic demand are likely to suffer damage and death. Providing early intervention, adequate ventilation, oxygenation, and perfusion to the trauma patient is vital.

The body's response to trauma and shock has been described as a complex series of neural and hormonal reflexes that are induced by injury. They result in an integrated attempt by the organism to preserve oxygen delivery, mobilize energy substrates, and reduce pain.[5] These reflexes intensify correspondingly with greater levels of traumatic injury. A point is eventually reached at which the reflexes can no longer compensate for disturbances caused by the traumatic insult. This irreversible condition eventually leads to death.

Trauma causes the body to call on many physiologic defense mechanisms, including fever, immune system activation, leukocytic and reticuloendothelial cell changes, metabolic effects, responses by the brain and autonomic nervous system, release of various hormones, and sometimes the activation of the coagulation, complement, and kinin systems.[6] These responses include a general acceleration of body metabolism, a catabolic degradation of skeletal muscle protein, the production of needed extra energy substrates from endogenous sources, and the production of new body cells and molecular products as needed for host defense and the healing process. Other responses include certain transient derangements in electrolyte and water metabolism, a redistribution of certain minerals and trace elements, a need for the elimination of toxic waste products and metabolites, and the direct participation of body cells in defensive mechanisms such as inflammatory processes, immune responses, and tissue repair.

When trauma results in hemorrhagic blood loss or sequestration of extracellular fluid in the injured tissues, the loss of circulating volume triggers a response by low-pressure baroreceptors in the right atrium and high-pressure baroreceptors in the carotid arteries and aorta.[7,8] When the blood volume is reduced, the venous return and cardiac output are similarly diminished. This effect in turn results in a neuroendocrine response that increases secretion of adrenocorticotropic hormone (ACTH), vasopressin, and growth hormone through central pathways and the secretion of epinephrine, norepinephrine, renin, and glucagon through peripheral sympathetic pathways. In turn, some of these hormones stimulate a further hormonal response that inhibits pancreatic secretion of insulin secondary to the release of epinephrine or stimulation of adrenocortical secretion of aldosterone by ACTH and renin-angiotensin.[9] Pain, which is an

---

BOX 37-1

Conditions Presented by Trauma Patients That Contraindicate the Use of Specific Anesthetic Agents

Shock

Most anesthetic agents cause dose-related cardiovascular depression. Intravenous induction agents are used cautiously in small incremental doses. Inhalation agents are added slowly as cardiovascular stability improves. Use of histamine-releasing muscle relaxants (e.g., atracurium) and narcotics (e.g., morphine, codeine) that aggravate shock are avoided.

Head Injury

Ketamine causes increases in ICP. N_2O causes increases in pneumocephalic tension. All inhalation agents tend to increase ICP as a result of increases in cerebral blood volume. However, inhalation agents decrease $CMRO_2$. The effects are temporarily attenuated by moderate hyperventilation of patients to Pa_{CO_2} levels of 30 to 35 mm Hg. Succinylcholine causes rises in ICP that may be detrimental in certain situations of significant ICP elevation. Hyperventilation with a Pa_{CO_2} of 25 mm Hg or less is not recommended.[12]

Burns, Spinal Cord Injury, and Crush Injuries

In these categories, succinylcholine can produce dangerous rises in potassium levels if it is administered approximately 24 hours after the injury. This problem can occur indefinitely in patients with permanent spinal cord injuries (e.g., paraplegics, quadriplegics).

Pneumothorax, Pneumocephalus, and Pneumoperitoneum

N_2O causes a wide variety of problems in the trauma patient to the extent that it is not used in the acute anesthetic management of trauma patients. N_2O tends to accumulate in closed spaces, aggravating conditions such as pneumothorax, pneumocephalus, and distention of the bowel. N_2O exaggerates the effects of air embolism.

Malignant Hyperthermia

All potent inhalation agents are absolutely contraindicated. Succinylcholine is known to trigger malignant hyperthermia and is absolutely contraindicated.

$CMRO_2$, *Cerebral metabolic rate of oxygen saturation;* ICP, *intracranial pressure;* N_2O, *nitrous oxide;* Pa_{CO_2}, *partial pressure of arterial carbon dioxide.*

---

almost universal finding after injury, stimulates a neuroendocrine response. Pain causes activation of nociceptive fibers, resulting in the release of endogenous opiates, vasopressin, ACTH, catecholamines, and other hormones.[10,11]

CHARACTERISTICS OF TRAUMA PATIENTS

Trauma patients often present to surgery and anesthesia with many unique characteristics. These differences are not always immediately apparent in a cursory evaluation. Frequently, trauma patients arrive in an obtunded state and are unable to supply information about past medical history, possible allergies, or previous response to anesthesia. The trauma patient frequently has a full stomach and is at high risk for developing aspiration pneumonitis if aspiration occurs during induction and emergence of anesthesia. In dealing with trauma, medical personnel are frequently confronted with an acute disease process that is occurring in a previously healthy patient. Compensatory mechanisms cannot offset impairment as they often do in chronic disease processes. If the popliteal artery is traumatically disrupted, for example, collateral circulation cannot develop as it might in a chronic vascular disease state such as coronary artery disease. Unlike elective surgery, anesthesia and surgery in the trauma patient generally cannot be postponed if an optimal outcome is to be achieved. The compensatory mechanisms that evolve during the shock state may eventually cause death. Injured tissues release factors or toxins that affect the metabolic and physiologic functioning of other organ systems. These factors include tissue thromboplastin, prostaglandin, myocardial toxic factor, and endotoxins released from dead gram-negative bacteria in the gut. In the past, clinicians tended to look only at the injured organ when treating traumatic injuries. It is currently known that trauma often leads to depression of multiple organs

and physiologic systems. Trauma has both direct and indirect effects on organs not directly involved with the trauma (e.g., severe brain injury may lead to diabetes insipidus due to pituitary gland damage). Disseminated intravascular coagulation may occur as a result of tissue thromboplastin release. Neurogenic pulmonary edema may occur after head injury. In addition, the trauma patient often has many conditions that may contraindicate the use of specific anesthetic agents (Box 37-1)[12].

IDEAL TRAUMA CARE

In the ideal trauma center, anesthesia-care providers are anesthesiologists and nurse anesthetists working together as a team to offer the best possible anesthesia care to the trauma patient.[13] As key members of the trauma team, these individuals bring a wealth of experience and expertise to this patient population. In few other anesthesia situations do the two specialties better complement each other. The role of the anesthetist in the care of trauma patients begins at the earliest possible moment when the patient is transported to the trauma facility. As a member of the admissions team, the anesthetist meets the patient immediately at the heliport or ambulance entrance. Radio transmissions from the field may give advance notice of the nature of the injuries so that the anesthetist and other trauma team members can be prepared to deal with the specific needs of the patient.

In a well-managed trauma center approach, assessment and treatment often have to be carried out in rapid succession. The anesthetist is primarily concerned with managing the airway and ventilation during the initial resuscitation efforts. After these tasks are accomplished, highly skilled anesthesia practice is required for providing intraoperative critical care so that prompt surgical intervention can occur. Effects of anesthesia care delivery are manifested not only during the surgery but also long beyond the operative period. Therefore, proper anesthesia management in trauma patients must be conducted from the time of initial resuscitation and treatment to the completion of initial and follow-up surgical procedures and possible reconstructive procedures.

TRAUMA SYSTEMS AND LEVELS OF CARE

Trauma centers are classified into three levels—level I, level II, and level III—representing the best possible use of community resources. The organization of trauma services within the community or region must address the development of a good *prehospital* system. The practice of taking the severely injured patient to the nearest hospital is no longer acceptable.

Death resulting from trauma has a trimodal distribution.[14] The initial peak in deaths is within seconds or minutes of injury. Invariably, these deaths are due to lacerations of the brain, brainstem, upper spinal cord, heart, or aorta or other large vessels. Few of these patients can be saved.

The second peak in deaths occurs within the first 2 hours after injury. Death is usually caused by subdural and epidural hematomas, hemopneumothorax, ruptured spleen, liver lacerations, fractured femur, or multiple injuries associated with significant blood loss. These patients, whose numbers are significant and who can usually be saved, benefit most from regionalized trauma care.

The third peak in deaths occurs days or weeks after the injury; these deaths usually result from sepsis and multiple organ failure. These patients can benefit also from a trauma center in which the concentration of the expertise of surgeons, anesthesia professionals, and other specialists allows for a rational therapeutic approach that positively affects patient outcomes.[15]

Level I and Level II Trauma Care

The goals of the Committee on Trauma of the American College of Surgeons are (1) improved care of the injured patient, (2) education for all personnel involved in trauma care, and (3) research in trauma. In keeping with these goals, the committee believes that the commitment to quality of patient care should be identical in level I and level II hospitals. Training and research programs are essential parts of level I and level II facilities. Invariably, in the planning for regional trauma needs, physicians, administrators, and health planners must decide how many hospitals should be so designated. Factors they must consider include the maintenance of skills and experience, cost, population density, and geography.

Injuries can be divided into three general categories: severe, urgent, and nonurgent. *Severe injuries* are those that are immediately life threatening (Box 37-2). Although they represent only 5% of all injuries, they account for 50% of all trauma deaths. *Urgent injuries* are those that are not immediately life threatening but may become so or result in significant disability. Urgent injuries account for approximately 10% to 15% of all injuries, whereas *nonurgent injuries* account for 80% of all injuries. These injuries are not immediately life threatening, nor do they present a risk of permanent disability.

Level III Trauma Care

The level III hospital generally serves communities that do not have resources for a level I or level II institution. Planning care for the injured in small community or suburban settings usually calls for transfer agreements and protocols for the most severely injured.

In the ideal system, the capability of the hospital and its personnel precisely matches the severity of the injury. Improved care for the seriously injured, with maximum efficiency and minimal costs in terms of life, disability, and dollars, depends on the appropriate use of trained personnel, specific trauma facilities, and equipment.

STAGES IN TRAUMA CARE

Initial Resuscitation and Stabilization

At the scene of an accident, emergency medical technicians attempt to stabilize the patient. The major concern is ensuring a patent airway so the patient can breathe adequately. At times, endotracheal intubation may be initiated before the patient is transported to the treatment facility. However, if the patient has adequate respiratory exchange, intubation should be performed at the trauma center, ideally after stabilization. Other advanced life support procedures that can be applied before the patient is transported include control of bleeding points and initiation of intravenous fluid resuscitation.

Resuscitation efforts should occur within minutes of the team members' arrival at the scene. Speed is essential. Prompt, appropriate treatment provided during the first 60 minutes after a severe traumatic injury often determines whether a patient will survive. Not all trauma patients are in shock, but for patients who are in hemorrhagic shock, the time to adequate resuscitation is critical. If the effects of shock are not sufficiently corrected within the first 60 to 90 minutes, the mortality rate rises substantially. The term *golden hour* denotes the principles developed by R. Adams Cowley, MD, founder of the University of Maryland Shock Trauma Center. This principle demonstrates that as more time elapses between the moment a trauma patient develops hemorrhagic shock and the beginning of resuscitation, the rate of survival decreases.[16] The highest rate of mortality occurs at approximately 60 minutes. Awareness of the golden hour principle encourages trauma-care providers to begin aggressive resuscitation efforts at the earliest possible moment.

Because trauma patients are susceptible to infection, vascular lines placed in the field under less than ideal conditions are replaced at the trauma center when possible. At the trauma center, arterial, central venous, and pulmonary artery catheters are inserted using aseptic technique. Numerous factors are considered in preparing the trauma patient for surgery and anesthesia (Box 37-3). Fluid status is monitored, and appropriate fluid replacement is continued. Monitoring oxygenation enables early diagnosis of acute respiratory distress syndrome and a previously undiagnosed pneumothorax or other forms of pulmonary dysfunction.

BOX 37-3

Preoperative Anesthetic Considerations and Preparations for Trauma Patients

Obtain initial radio or telephone report of patient's condition from field providers.

Prepare anesthesia machine and ventilator and anticipated drugs, equipment, and supplies.

Prepare for standard endotracheal intubation and alternative airway interventions.

Have proper monitoring equipment and supplies, as well as equipment for rapid infusion of blood and fluids.

Use gloves, gowns, proper eyewear protection, and universal precautions for contact with patient during placement of invasive lines, endotracheal intubation, and surgical procedures.

Evaluate at the earliest feasible point after arrival of the patient to the trauma facility (e.g., at heliport or ambulance entrance).

Elicit appropriate information from patient at the earliest possible time to ascertain current and past history of trauma, surgeries, medical conditions, current medications, allergic reactions, previous anesthesia experiences, and current mechanism of injury.

Evaluate airway and ventilation for adequacy of presenting status and need for immediate or delayed interventions.

Evaluate airway to determine anticipated relative difficulty and plan for primary and possible secondary maneuvers for securing the airway.

Determine the Glasgow Coma Scale score and Trauma Severity score at the time of arrival.

Secure intravenous access with two or more large-bore catheters, and initiate the use of fluid warmer as soon as possible.

Obtain venous and arterial blood samples for typing and crossmatch, CBC, electrolyte levels, blood glucose levels, coagulation profile, toxicology screen, and blood gas analysis.

Have appropriate crystalloids, colloids, and blood components available for use.

Formulate the plan for use of anesthetic agents and techniques appropriate for the patient.

Provide airway and anesthesia support as necessary for diagnostic procedures (e.g., CT, MRI, angiography, ultrasonography, diagnostic peritoneal lavage, laparoscopy, examination during general anesthesia).

Exercise care during transport of the trauma patient within the trauma facility to protect the spine, ensure adequate ventilation, maintain hemostasis, maintain fluid infusion, and maintain drug therapies.

CBC, *complete blood count;* CT, *computed tomography;* MRI, *magnetic resonance imaging.*

Airway Management

It is beyond the scope of this chapter to provide a detailed description of specific techniques of airway management for all situations encountered in trauma patients (Boxes 37-4 and 37-5). General guidelines are given in this chapter; the clinician's sound judgment for each trauma situation takes precedence. Anesthesia care of the trauma patient demands an individualized approach with the goal of properly assessing and securing the airway as quickly as possible.

Rapid control of the airway and ventilation with oxygen is critical for traumatic shock resuscitation (Box 37-6). Although in certain critical situations tracheal intubation must be accomplished immediately, intubation conditions generally improve after initial fluid resuscitation and general stabilization. If the patient can maintain adequate spontaneous respiration, the patient's cervical spine is radiographed before intubation to detect possible cervical-spine injuries. Arterial blood gas values are obtained immediately after the patient arrives, and the results are used to guide subsequent airway interventions. Placing the patient on a known fraction of inspired oxygen (FiO_2) before the arterial blood gases are measured is advantageous so the adequacy of oxygen exchange can be evaluated.[17]

With a cervical collar in place and the patient lying on a long spinal board, well-maintained axial stabilization of the head (in-line stabilization with the head in the neutral position) should be performed in all trauma patients with suspected or confirmed cervical-spine injuries. In most situations, direct laryngoscopy and intubation is accomplished, even when there is a limited view of the larynx.[18] However, when this is not the case,

BOX 37-4

Factors Considered in Securing the Airway of the Trauma Patient

Severity of deterioration of ventilation and oxygenation
Need for rapid assessment and intervention in a limited time
Full stomach
Hemorrhagic shock and/or cardiovascular instability
Influence of alcohol and/or "street drugs"
Burns and/or inhalation injuries
Head injury and/or obtunded or combative patient
Maxillofacial and laryngeal injuries
Neck injuries and/or cervical-spine injuries
Chest injuries to lungs, major airways, heart, great vessels
Penetrating eye injuries
Near-drowning
Anatomic distortion
Existing medical problems
Prior medication administration

other airway adjuncts such as the GlideScope have the advantage of providing a better view of the glottis.[19] Although awake nasal intubation is often considered ideal in patients with possible cervical-spine injuries, it is often difficult to carry out in the inebriated, obtunded, frightened, or confused trauma patient.

BOX 37-5

Airway Evaluation and Interventions in the Trauma Patient

Administer oxygen immediately while the evaluation is being conducted.

Evaluate the patency of the natural airway and the adequacy of ventilation.

Evaluate the quality of gas exchange visually and with pulse oximetry and arterial blood gas analysis.

When the patient's oxygenation and general condition appear adequate, one or more of the following imaging techniques are employed prior to securing the airway: three-view cervical spine series, thin-cut axial computed tomography (CT) images with sagittal reconstruction.

Evaluate the neurologic status (e.g., level of consciousness, ability to follow commands, presence of head and spinal cord injury).

Evaluate blunt or penetrating facial and throat injuries that may complicate airway function or interventions.

Evaluate for evolving edema that may compromise the airway.

Evaluate complicated airway injuries with a surgeon who is prepared to establish an invasive primary or alternative "backup" airway (e.g., cricothyroidotomy, tracheostomy, or laryngeal mask airway) in the event that standard noninvasive attempts are ineffective.

Perform oral endotracheal intubation after induction of anesthesia and use an appropriate neuromuscular blocking agent with application of cricoid pressure and in-line axial immobilization of the cervical spine in most situations.

Awake oral or nasal intubation can be attempted in cooperative patients who are adequately oxygenated and hemodynamically stable; nasal intubation is contraindicated in head-injured patients who may have cribriform plate injuries because of the potential for the endotracheal tube to enter the brain vault.

Intubation over a flexible fiberoptic bronchoscope (if no active bleeding exists that can obscure visualization) using a flex-tip (Parker-Tube) is useful to increase initial success.

Placement of chest tubes in the presence of a pneumothorax is completed before, or simultaneously with intubation in order to avoid acceleration of the size of the pneumothorax, with the potential development of mediastinal shift and hemodynamic compromise.

Modified from Nelson LA. Airway trauma. Int Anesthesiol Clin. 2007;45(3):99-118; Kristensen MS. The Parker Flex-Tip tube versus a standard tube for fiberoptic orotracheal intubation: a randomized double-blind study. Anesthesiology. 2003;(2):354-358.

BOX 37-6

Recommended Equipment and Drugs for Emergency Airway Management

Face masks for adults and children

Oropharyngeal and nasopharyngeal airways

Long- and short-handled laryngoscopes

Blades of several sizes and shapes

Endotracheal tubes with stylets sized appropriately for adults and children

Elastic bougie (Eschmann) intubating style—when only the epiglottis is viewed, usually allows entry into trachea with bumping of tracheal rings to help confirm placement; then acts as guide for endotracheal tube placement over the introducer into the glottic opening

Laryngeal mask airways appropriately sized for temporary airway rescue

Suction with large-bore openings connected to a vacuum source

Self-inflating positive-pressure bag

Local and topical anesthetics for infiltration and spraying

Water-soluble lubricant for endotracheal tubes

Pro-Seal LMA (for use only when standard endotracheal intubation fails)

Drugs appropriate for sedation, analgesia, induction, and production of neuromuscular blockade; drying agents

---

When it is difficult to obtain a secure airway with an endotracheal tube, a Pro-Seal laryngeal mask airway (LMA) is useful as a temporary measure to oxygenate or assist intubation in patients who are in life-threatening situations. The concept that all trauma patients are considered to have a "full stomach" precludes long-term use of the LMA. Once the Pro-Seal LMA is placed, a fiberoptically-assisted intubation with a microlaryngeal tube is accomplished.

Awake nasal intubation may be ideal for patients who are about to undergo elective procedures; however, it is often not feasible in an emergency. Topical anesthesia and nerve blocks obtund the patient's cough reflex and potentially increase the chance of aspiration. Fiberoptic-guided nasal intubation should be attempted only in cooperative patients. A lighted wand may be helpful for guiding intubation of the trachea. This technique is based on transillumination of the soft tissues of the neck.

Nasal intubation has several disadvantages. It is time consuming, it depends on the patient's respiratory effort, and it commonly causes nosebleeds. Furthermore, foreign material may enter the brain through a basilar skull fracture. Muzzi and associates[20] published a case report involving a trauma patient with a basilar skull fracture in whom a nasopharyngeal airway was inserted into the cranial vault via a cribriform plate fracture. Additionally, the presence of an endotracheal tube in the nose can cause a sinus infection (and eventually late sepsis) because of prolonged obstruction of sinus drainage. These complications can be avoided with the oral intubation route.

Oral tubes also have disadvantages. They get in the way if surgery of the mouth is necessary, they make oral hygiene difficult, and they are not ideal for long-term use postoperatively.

This unprepared emergency patient, who frequently has a full stomach, is often uncooperative and thrashes about during attempts at awake intubation. Local and topical anesthesia can obtund protective laryngeal reflexes and contribute to the possibility of pulmonary aspiration. Additionally, head-injured patients with suspected basilar skull fractures (e.g., those with raccoon eyes, Battle sign, cerebrospinal fluid from the nose or ears) benefit from oral intubations to avoid penetration of the cribriform plate and subsequent entry of foreign material into the brain through the fracture site.

However, in overall consideration, these disadvantages are minor, and oral intubation is usually preferable to nasal intubation in the trauma patient.

Many trauma patients have inadequate respiratory function and are hypoxic on arrival at the trauma center. Until the trachea can be intubated, these patients undergo continuous ventilation with a mask. Cricoid pressure is applied to occlude the esophagus when anesthesia is induced; this averts regurgitation of gastric or esophageal contents and prevents gastric distention. Maintaining continuous ventilation with cricoid pressure prevents further hypoxic insults that can otherwise occur during the apneic period between administration of a neuromuscular-blocking agent and completed intubation. If an intubation attempt fails, cricoid pressure is continued, and mask ventilation is resumed before the next attempt. It is often helpful to gently lift the mandible forward and bring the patient's face upward to meet the mask; otherwise, the pressure of the tongue against the posterior pharyngeal wall may obstruct the airway. Typically, until trauma patients can be intubated, they undergo continuous ventilation with a mask.

The efficacy of cricoid pressure in preventing aspiration has been questioned, but it still remains a common practice. It is important to apply sufficient pressure to the cricoid ring to press the esophagus firmly against the anterior vertebral bodies to seal it against possible regurgitation.[21] Delivering oxygen with mask-and-bag ventilation while applying cricoid pressure to protect the airway improves oxygenation before endotracheal intubation is performed. The feasibility of performing ventilation on a given patient is assessed ("testing the airway"); if the airway allows ventilation, muscle relaxants are used. Muscle relaxants are not administered before the airway is opened and ventilation ensured by visible rising of the chest. This gives the anesthetist the knowledge that the patient can undergo adequate ventilation if attempts at intubation fail.[22]

Testing the airway allows the anesthetist to assess his or her ability to support ventilation when intubation proves difficult or infeasible. It also ensures the ability to continue ventilation after failed intubation while the patient is prepared for emergency tracheostomy or cricothyroidotomy. Again, all trauma patients are considered to have full stomachs. Early intubation often prevents potential long-term problems such as those caused by aspiration or hypoxic insult.

If endotracheal intubation is made impossible by severe facial injuries or other causes, and if ventilatory effort is poor or absent because of partial or complete obstruction, an emergency cricothyroidotomy, tracheotomy, or percutaneous tracheal catheter is placed to allow adequate oxygenation. Emergency supplies and equipment are readily available for this possibility. After intubation, general anesthesia may be initiated to facilitate further diagnostic workup with or without subsequent surgery.

Verification by end-tidal CO_2 concentration with normal waveform morphology is now considered the gold standard for ensuring proper placement of an endotracheal tube in the trachea. In conjunction with pulse oximetry and arterial blood gas determinations, end-tidal CO_2 values also serve as a guide for adequate ventilation. During cardiac arrest, the endotracheal tube can be correctly placed, yet end-tidal CO_2 is not observed by capnography. With minimal or no perfusion (as with cardiac arrest), CO_2 is not delivered to the lungs. As perfusion improves, CO_2 levels again begin to rise. Conversely, the endotracheal tube can be placed in the esophagus, and CO_2 may be initially detected. This phenomenon can occur if the patient previously swallowed air or ingested a carbonated beverage. Generally, the

waveform observed in this situation is flattened and is generally nonexistent after a few attempts at ventilation.

In cases of penetrating chest injury, a chest tube is ideally placed in patients with a pneumothorax before the endotracheal tube is placed. When intubation is done first, a chest tube is placed immediately after intubation is completed. This measure helps prevent rapid progression of a tension pneumothorax accelerated by positive-pressure ventilation. The progression can lead to mediastinal shift, reduced venous return, reduced cardiac output, and cardiac arrest.

Monitoring the Trauma Patient

Initial noninvasive monitoring procedures include continuous core temperature measurements, pulse oximetry, continuous end-tidal CO_2 monitoring, end-tidal agent measurements, and automatic blood pressure cuff monitoring. An indwelling urinary catheter is usually part of trauma fluid-management monitoring.

Arterial, central venous, and pulmonary artery catheters are inserted. Fluid status is continuously assessed as appropriate fluid resuscitation is accomplished. Initially volume replacement is guided by monitoring mean arterial pressure (MAP), pulse rate, central venous pressure (CVP), urinary output, and peripheral arterial oxygen saturation values. Measurements of cardiac index and derived hemodynamic variables help guide fluid and vasoactive drug management. Restoration of these values to normal ranges is a major goal of resuscitation. Sudden changes in any of the parameters being monitored are evaluated carefully because they may indicate the presence of significant clinical problems requiring prompt treatment (Box 37-7). A reasonable approximation of intravascular volume can be determined by observation of central venous and arterial pressure, pulse rate, external bleeding, chest-tube drainage, and the rate and total volume of fluid infused. During resuscitative efforts, venous and arterial lines should be evaluated for continued proper placement and function. The electrocardiogram is monitored for heart rate, arrhythmias, and ST-T–segment abnormalities. The urinary output is monitored for volume, concentration, and color.

Initial laboratory screening should include complete blood count, coagulation profile, electrolyte levels, blood glucose level, toxicology screen, blood alcohol level, serum osmolality, and arterial blood gas analysis. An upright chest radiograph is obtained to screen for acute pathology, including pneumothorax, hemothorax, pulmonary contusion, and widening of the mediastinum that may suggest cardiac or major vascular injury.

TRAUMA-INDUCED SHOCK

Shock is considered a generalized state of severe circulatory inadequacy due to reduced perfusion and inadequate delivery of oxygen and nutrients to tissues. Shock results in a profound and sustained loss of effective circulating blood volume. It leads to hypoperfusion of peripheral tissues and to a deficit in transcapillary exchange function.[23] Traumatic shock that follows severe hemorrhage inevitably leads to depression of physiologic systems in multiple organs. The faster emergency intervention begins, the greater the patient's chances for survival. Rapid control of the airway, ventilation with oxygen, and appropriate fluid replacement are critical for traumatic shock resuscitation. Venous access is rapidly established by use of several large-bore plastic cannulas. This measure facilitates volume restoration with appropriately selected fluids and provides a route for the administration of drugs. The rapid infusion of large volumes of fluid and blood can be optimized by pressurization of the fluid containers with an automated device (e.g., level I infuser).

BOX **37-7**

Assessment and Interventions for Common Problems in Trauma

Hypotension

The most common cause of hypotension is generally hypovolemia. Fluid resuscitation is initiated and continued as the underlying causes of the hypovolemia are investigated. Disruptions of major vessels in the chest, abdomen, and pelvis are the most common causes of hypovolemia. Cardiac tamponade is considered as a cause of persistent hypotension. Inotropes and vasopressors are seldom indicated in managing hypotension in the trauma patient. Exceptions may include the patient in spinal shock or the patient who has sustained myocardial contusion.

Desaturation

Desaturation is usually noted first by pulse oximetry measurements and/or arterial blood gas determination. Check for adequate FIO_2, ventilation, and perfusion. Check breath sounds. Check for endobronchial intubation. Look for signs of pneumothorax (i.e., distended neck veins and increased resonance on affected side, tracheal deviation). Desaturation may be due to pulmonary contusion, often treated with increasing levels of PEEP to open atelectatic areas. Copious secretions and mucous plugs are considered potential causes. A chest radiograph is helpful for ruling out many potential causes of desaturation. Aspiration of blood, stomach contents, or foreign bodies and postobstructive pulmonary edema are considered. Fiberoptic bronchoscopy can be diagnostic and therapeutic. Consider the possibility of air embolism, especially in cases of penetrating injuries.

Hypertension

Trauma patients frequently become hyperdynamic after resuscitation; this problem is usually treated with adequate levels of anesthesia, including moderately large doses of potent narcotics such as fentanyl or sufentanil. Use of antihypertensive agents may need to be considered.

Tachyarrhythmias and Bradyarrhythmias

Hypoxemia and hypercarbia must be considered first. Myocardial injury is also considered. 12-lead ECG is obtained. Consider performing echocardiography to assess cardiac motion and possible tamponade.

Sudden Cardiac Arrest

Check for obvious causes using ABCs (**A**irway patency, **B**reathing adequacy, and **C**irculatory adequacy). Sudden cardiac arrest is often a strong indication for open thoracotomy to inspect the heart for pericardial tamponade or other injuries or to perform open-chest cardiac massage; abdominal incision may also be indicated to look for other sources of bleeding; rapid blood and fluid resuscitation are continued as indicated.

ECG, *Electrocardiogram;* FIO_2, *inspired concentration of oxygen;* PEEP, *positive end-expiratory pressure.*

During cardiopulmonary resuscitation (CPR), placement of a 16-gauge or larger catheter in the largest accessible peripheral vein is preferred. Ideally the antecubital veins are used for drug administration during CPR.[24] Insertion of a central line may hamper CPR. After restoration of spontaneous circulation, a central venous catheter is placed. Efforts at cannulating subclavian or internal jugular veins for central-line placement are contraindicated during CPR because of the danger of inducing pneumothorax when these measures are attempted in the patient who is being bounced by cardiac compressions.[25] Attempts at inserting central lines during CPR often interfere with ventilation, oxygenation, and cardiac compressions. It is advantageous to have at least one large-bore intravenous catheter above and below the diaphragm in patients with injuries to the abdomen or pelvis. If injuries to the superior or inferior vena cava are present, venous return is ineffective from catheters placed distal to vena caval disruptions. Use of lower-extremity veins is generally not suitable because these veins are often smaller and may be occluded from chronic venous stasis.

Three Phases of Shock

Stage I

Stage I of the three stages of shock is often called *nonprogressive shock* or *compensated shock.*[26] A negative-feedback control mechanism of the circulation tries to return the cardiac output and arterial pressure to normal levels. This phenomenon is mediated through the baroreceptor reflexes, central nervous system (CNS) ischemic responses, contraction of blood vessels, release of vasopressin (antidiuretic hormone), formation of angiotensin, and compensation mechanisms that tend to return the blood volume back toward normal by mobilizing fluids from other spaces of the body.

Stage II

Stage II of shock is also known as *progressive shock.* A positive-feedback mechanism comes into play with this phase of shock. When shock becomes severe enough, components of the cardiovascular system start to deteriorate. This deterioration is associated with cardiac depression caused by ischemia, vasomotor failure, thrombosis of small vessels, increased capillary permeability, release of endotoxins by ischemic tissues, and generalized cellular degeneration.

Stage III

Stage III of shock is also called *irreversible shock.* This stage occurs when adenosine triphosphate reserves are depleted. Death follows as the natural consequence of unsuccessfully halting progressive shock.

Fluid Management and Resuscitation

The mortality rate for shock is approximately 50% if treatment is initiated 30 minutes from onset; the rate increases to 90% if 1 hour elapses.[14,15] This high mortality rate associated with the delayed treatment of shock is the basis for initiating fluid resuscitation in the field. At the trauma center, red blood cells (RBCs) are replaced to provide adequate oxygen-carrying capacity. Blood loss is replaced with a 1:1 volume of packed RBCs and a 3:1 volume of crystalloids. Evaluation of the patient's fluid

Advanced Trauma Life Support Classification of Hemorrhagic Shock

	CLASS I	CLASS II	CLASS III	CLASS IV
Blood loss (mL)	≤750	750-1500	1500-2000	≥2000
Blood loss (% blood volume)	≤15	15-30	30-40	≥40
Pulse rate (per min)	<100	>100	>120	≥140
Blood pressure	Normal	Normal	Decreased	Decreased
Pulse pressure	Normal or increased	Decreased	Decreased	Decreased
Respiratory rate (breaths/min)	14-20	20-30	30-40	>35
Urine output (mL/hr)	≥30	20-30	5-15	Negligible
Mental status	Slightly anxious	Mildly anxious	Anxious, confused	Confused, lethargic
Fluid replacement	Crystalloid	Crystalloid	Crystalloid + blood	Crystalloid + blood

Modified from American College of Surgeons Committee on Trauma. Shock. In: American College of Surgeons, eds. Advanced Trauma Life Support Course for Physicians. *7th ed. Chicago: American College of Surgeons; 2004:74.*

status is accomplished in part with CVP monitoring, pulmonary artery catheter monitoring (or both), and observing clinical signs for return of the heart rate and blood pressure to normal levels.

Serial electrolyte levels, hemoglobin and hematocrit levels, and arterial blood gas analysis are obtained approximately every hour in severely injured, unstable patients in surgery until the patient is stable. Coagulation parameters are closely observed in patients with signs of active bleeding. Colloids usually allow rapid restoration of intravascular volume but can contribute to a later episode of pulmonary edema in some patients. Balanced electrolyte solutions are given to help maintain the CVP between 1 and 15 mm Hg (8 to 10 mm Hg in anesthetized patients). Up to 1500 mL of 5% plasma protein fraction (Plasmanate) or hetastarch (Hespan) is infused initially to rapidly restore intravascular volume in unstable patients. Fresh frozen plasma is indicated in single or multiple coagulation deficiencies. It should not be used for volume replacement or any other nonspecific use.

Dextrose-containing solutions are generally undesirable for use in initial resuscitation fluid administration. Rapid determination of blood glucose levels is critical in patients with diabetes and in children. Traumatized infants and children in shock may rapidly consume their gluconeogenic substrate, allowing significant hypoglycemia to occur.[26] Although patients are more likely to become hyperglycemic than hypoglycemic after traumatic injury, hypoglycemia can occur. Significant hyperglycemia is associated with further neurologic injury.[27] Traumatically induced hyperglycemia is so common it is often called *diabetes of injury*.[28] Withholding glucose or giving it in moderate amounts to maintain blood glucose levels at less than 150 mg/dL is advisable if brain ischemia occurs. Data have shown that preexisting hyperglycemia increases the damage of ischemic or hypoxic events.[29]

Dilutional thrombocytopenia is the most common cause of coagulopathy in the trauma patient, followed by hypofibrinogenemia. These conditions are treated with pooled platelets, fresh frozen plasma, or cryoprecipitate, as indicated. Cryoprecipitate is the most concentrated source of fibrinogen, and it is also given when von Willebrand factor is needed. Administration of supplemental platelets is considered when the platelet count drops to less than 50,000/μL. If signs of unaccountable bleeding are present during surgical procedures, platelets are replaced at levels below 70,000/μL. An autotransfusion device is an excellent alternative to homologous transfusions, considering the risks associated with banked blood (e.g., type-and-cross mismatches or transmission of infectious diseases). Autotransfused blood has several advantages, including a higher oxygen-carrying capacity and elimination of incompatibilities and disease transmission. An aseptic approach should be used for starting all invasive lines. Trauma patients are at greater risk for to infection. Meticulous preparing and draping while gloves are worn are imperative for the initiation of any vascular line.

Hemorrhagic shock is evaluated clinically using physiologic parameters commonly observed. Box 37-8 gives the Advanced Trauma Life Support classification of hemorrhagic shock. Changes in heart rate, blood pressure, pulse pressure, respiratory rate, urine output, and mental status are used to determine the severity of hemorrhagic shock.[30]

Continued use of military antishock trousers (MAST) is controversial. In theory, inflated MAST will compress arterial inflow to the legs and effectively raise both the arterial resistance and the blood pressure as measured in the arms. However, complications observed with the use of MAST include ischemia of the skin and superficial tissues, acidosis, hyperkalemia, ventilatory embarrassment from pressure on the abdomen, muscle damage, increased capillary permeability, coagulopathy, and elevated levels of thrombolytic products. Initially, the MAST device was viewed as a panacea for hypovolemic trauma patients.[31] However, it has proven deleterious to trauma patients with moderate hypotension (systolic BP 50 to 90 mm Hg) who have a relatively short transport time to a hospital. Its role in patients with severe hypotension or long prehospital transport times remains unclear.

MECHANISM OF INJURY

An understanding of the mechanism of injury is crucial because it predicts the pattern of injuries that can be anticipated from a given type of traumatic insult. To effectively resuscitate and provide anesthesia care for the trauma patient, the anesthetist needs a basic knowledge of the various mechanisms of injury. Research and experience have demonstrated that certain types of injuries generally produce predictable pathophysiologic changes. At the earliest feasible time in the assessment and treatment of the trauma patient, a careful history of the sequence of physical events leading to the traumatic injury is conducted.[32]

This information may be obtained from many sources, including the patient (if he or she is conscious and coherent), paramedics, other rescue workers, police, and eyewitnesses.

Blunt trauma is caused by high-velocity or low-velocity impact, generally from dull objects. Penetrating trauma usually results from the piercing of tissue by sharp objects such as knives or bullets. Mixed blunt and penetrating injuries are often seen in impalement injuries. Falls from substantial heights can cause vertical high-velocity injuries. Burns are caused by thermal, electrical, or chemical exposure. Airway burns and smoke inhalation injuries are often associated with carbon monoxide poisoning. Chemical, biologic, and nuclear injuries are other forms of trauma that have a known basis. Environmental injuries can be caused by such events as poisonous insect bites, animal bites, or snake bites with venom.

Penetrating Injuries

With *neck penetration injuries*, large arteries and veins, nerves, and the vertebral column can be damaged from either direct impact or from the effects of cavitation. The airway can be damaged by either effect as well. With *penetrating head injuries*, cavitation within the brain from a high-velocity missile can cause massive damage, if not instant death. Transmitted energy from a tangential missile injury can cause skull fractures, brain contusions, or lacerations. Penetration of the chest cavity can cause severe injuries. A high-velocity missile can shatter the heart, causing instantaneous death. Low-velocity missiles may cause small holes in the heart that are usually repairable if tamponade or hemorrhage is not excessive. Major vessel penetration frequently causes death unless tamponade is sufficient to contain the hemorrhagic state. Isolated lung injuries can often be treated by placement of a chest tube. Significant major airway or blood-vessel damage may require lobectomy. A high-velocity missile may rupture the diaphragm and cause damage to the upper abdominal organs from cavitation effect. Penetrating injuries to the abdomen by high-velocity bullets cause temporary cavity formation as they pulp the liver, spleen, and kidney. Low-velocity bullets usually produce less severe drill-hole injuries unless blood vessels are directly hit.

Injury from a high-velocity missile can produce trauma to the entire extremity. Low-velocity missiles cause drill-hole injuries through muscle, bone, and subcutaneous tissues. The presence or absence of a pulse distal to an injury is not necessarily a reliable indicator of vascular integrity.

Classification of Penetrating Trauma

Penetrating injuries can range from a simple pinprick to high-velocity projectile injury. Damage depends on three interactive factors[33]:

- The type of wounding instrument (e.g., knife, missile, fragment)
- The velocity of the missile at time of impact
- The characteristics of tissue through which it passes (e.g., bone, muscle, fat, blood vessels, nervous tissues, and organs)

The crush component of penetrating injuries causes destruction by fraying of the tissues as they are stretched to accommodate the wounding instrument (e.g., as occurs when a car falls onto the leg of an individual working under it). The blunter the penetrating instrument, the greater the crushing.

The science of ballistics classifies the types of penetrating wound missile injuries. The characteristics of ballistic injuries are studied in either animal models or artificial models, such as the "ordnance gelatin" model, while being photographed by high-speed cinematography. These types of injuries can be *penetrating*, in which only an entrance wound is present, because the missile remains in the body. Conversely, they can be *perforating*, in which both entrance and exit wounds are present. High-velocity projectiles generally produce massive exit wounds, based on the following formula:

Equation 37-1

$$\text{Kinetic energy} = MV^2/2$$

As a result, doubling the mass (M) of a projectile doubles its energy, but doubling its velocity (V) quadruples its energy.

In perforating trauma, the energy deposited in the tissues equals the difference between the amount of energy a missile had before it entered the body and the energy it retains after it leaves the body. In penetrating trauma, all the energy the missile possesses at the time of impact is transferred to the body. Low-velocity and high-velocity bullets differ in the amount and pattern of damage they create. Low-velocity bullets usually cut and crush tissues to form a drill hole, known as a *permanent cavity*, that approximates the same diameter as the missile. A high-velocity bullet creates a temporary cavity in addition to the permanent cavity. The temporary cavity forms in the wake of the high-velocity bullet, which creates a shock wave with a series of rapid tissue expansions, followed by collapse. This *cavitation effect* causes stretching and tearing of tissues as far as 10 cm from the permanent cavity.

High-velocity bullets pulp less elastic organs, such as the liver, spleen, kidney, brain, or heart, as a result of the temporary cavity effect. More elastic tissues, such as the lung, bowel, skin, and muscle, tend to sustain less damage from high-velocity missiles.

Blunt Trauma

Direct impact, deceleration, continuous pressure, shearing, and rotary forces may all contribute to the resulting *blunt trauma*. These factors are related to the high levels of energy associated with high-speed collisions and falls from substantial heights. Newton's first law can explain how most traumatic injuries occur: an object tends to remain in motion until it is affected by an outside force. Abrupt deceleration creates negative gravitational forces. As the human body decelerates, the internal organs continue forward at the original velocity. The organs that continue to move forward are torn from their attachments through rotary and shearing forces. These forces often cause disruption of connective tissue, blood vessels, and nerves.

Motor Vehicle Accident Trauma

The five types of *motor vehicle accidents* are classified as head-on, rear impact, side impact, rotational impact, and rollover. Because passengers are traveling in the same direction as the vehicle they are in, they often have injury locations similar to that of the vehicle. In addition, contralateral injuries can result. Depending on the passenger's position and the presence or absence of seat belts, various injuries can occur. "Down-and-under" injuries begin with the passenger slumping into the seat or dashboard with the knees moving forward. Forces can cause injuries to the knees, femurs, and acetabula. The upper portion of the body may collide with the dashboard, steering wheel, or windshield, resulting in injuries of the head, neck, chest, abdomen, and upper extremities. Physical evidence of this down-and-under pattern includes imprints of the knees in the dashboard, starburst patterns in the windshield, and steering-wheel imprints on the chest. "Up-and-over injuries" result when the body arcs forward; the head suffers the first point of contact, usually with the windshield, and the thorax follows. The cervical spine absorbs a large energy impact. Resultant vertebral injuries are common as a result of hyperflexion, hyperextension, or direct compression. Direct impact to the trachea frequently produces laryngeal fractures (*padded dash syndrome*).

The greater the anesthetist's knowledge of the many factors involved in a specific injury, the more appropriate the anesthesia care plan will be. A complete understanding of the details of a particular traumatic injury can permit every health-care provider involved after the event to see the complete picture and not just the aftermath.

Thoracic Trauma

Blunt thoracic trauma often results when drivers who are not wearing safety belts collide with the steering wheel during a motor vehicle accident. Penetrating and blunt trauma to the chest may injure vital structures and thus compromise optimal resuscitation. These structures include the chest wall, lungs and airways, heart and pericardium, and great vessels of the thorax. Injuries to thoracic structures compromise anesthesia care by affecting gas exchange and cardiac output.

If the trauma patient is still in shock despite vigorous resuscitative measures, the differential diagnosis of traumatic shock must be reviewed again, other causes must be sought aggressively, and specific injuries may need to be treated immediately. Both blunt and penetrating chest injuries may be responsible for continued hemodynamic and ventilatory compromise. These problems can be caused by direct effects on the lungs and airways or by indirect effects (e.g., pulmonary dysfunction due to cardiovascular pathology).[34]

Several life-threatening conditions require immediate interventions in patients with chest injuries. A *tension pneumothorax* develops when the pleural cavity is punctured, creating a one-way valve that controls the flow of air into this cavity. With each breath, more air becomes trapped in this space, increasing intrapleural pressure to the point that it eventually exceeds all other intrathoracic pressures. The enlarging pleural cavity then collapses the ipsilateral lung and shifts structures of the mediastinum (e.g., trachea, great vessels, heart) into the opposite hemithorax, thereby compressing the contralateral lung. The size of a pneumothorax rapidly increases during positive-pressure ventilation, especially if nitrous oxide is used for analgesia in the field or during anesthesia in the trauma facility. Patients with a pneumothorax often present with hypotension, subcutaneous emphysema of the neck or chest, unilateral decrease in breath sounds, diminished chest-wall motion, hyperresonance to percussion of one hemithorax, distended neck veins, or tracheal shift. An upright expirational chest radiograph provides definite information if the problem is significant. However, if the trauma patient is unstable, a large-bore intravenous catheter is inserted into the second superior portion of the intercostal space along the midclavicular line. A hissing sound may be created by air escaping under pressure. The catheter is attached to an underwater seal system. Initially the catheter can be temporarily attached to a length of intravenous-line extension tubing and an underwater seal created by placing the tubing in a bottle of sterile water positioned beneath the level of the patient.

Certain thoracic injuries are life threatening. *Massive hemothorax*, which can be caused by bleeding from the heart and great vessels, is treated immediately. Adequate fluid resuscitation is accomplished before placement of chest tubes. Chest tubes allow drainage of blood from the pleural cavity but can lead to

more extensive bleeding and hypotension. *Pericardial tamponade* that restricts filling of the cardiac chambers during diastole and produces a fixed low cardiac output is also a life-threatening emergency that requires immediate correction with pericardiocentesis. Patients with *cardiac rupture* without pericardial tamponade seldom survive; exsanguination is extremely rapid in this situation. If complete, *traumatic aortic rupture* is usually fatal, but with an intimal tear in a dissecting aneurysm, the patient can be saved if the diagnosis and repair are performed promptly during well-managed fluid resuscitation and anesthesia care. Management of these cases requires rapid and accurate assessment and appropriate surgical and anesthesia intervention. *Partial disruption of the trachea or major bronchi* often is managed by securing the airway (by intubation or tracheostomy) and surgical correction. *Total disruption of the trachea* is often fatal unless rapid surgical retrieval of the distal disrupted airway segment is accomplished to allow lifesaving mechanical ventilation.

Diagnosis of stable chest injuries is frequently enhanced by computed tomography (CT), magnetic resonance imaging (MRI), angiography, and other radiologic studies. Upright chest radiographs (in contrast to flat plate views) frequently reveal widening of the mediastinum in the patient who has mediastinal bleeding from any cause. Radiographs taken with the patient in an upright position generally display a narrow profile of the mediastinum because of the effects of gravity on the mediastinal contents. Widening of the mediastinum in an upright radiograph warrants a high index of suspicion for a life-threatening condition such as disruption of a major vessel like the aorta. Chest radiographs are also helpful in the diagnosis of hemothorax and pneumothorax. Arterial blood gas analysis facilitates assessment of ventilation and treatment of acid-base disturbances. Serial evaluation of the hematocrit and coagulation profile helps guide fluid and blood-component replacement.

Abdominal Trauma

In stable trauma patients with abdominal injuries, abdominal sonography, CT scan, MRI, or angiography may offer help in diagnosing specific injuries. Extremely unstable patients with abdominal trauma need immediate surgery. Placement of a diagnostic peritoneal catheter for lavage and subsequent analysis of the obtained fluid can guide the decision about whether to perform exploratory laparotomy in patients with *abdominal trauma* (Box 37-9). The incidence of false-positive results from lavage is less than 2%.[35,36] This procedure can be performed with local anesthesia and intravenous analgesia as appropriate. Peritoneal washings are analyzed for the presence of RBCs, white blood cells, amylase, bacteria, feces, or bile. Peritoneal lavage is unreliable in patients with gunshot wounds of the lower chest and abdomen; in these patients, false-negative rates may reach 25%.[36-38]

Both blunt and penetrating injuries of the abdomen can cause substantial bleeding or other damage that requires exploratory surgery. Retroperitoneal injuries can damage the abdominal aorta, inferior vena cava, kidneys, pancreas, and duodenum. Intraperitoneal injuries can occur to the spleen, liver, stomach, small bowel, colon, or rectum. In addition to abdominal sonography, peritoneal lavage and CT with contrast enhancement are considered for evaluation of abdominal trauma. Knowing the mechanism of injury and performing a meticulous physical examination can yield valuable information regarding abdominal injuries.

Anesthetic problems in patients with abdominal trauma include hemorrhage, hypothermia, sepsis, and interference

---

BOX **37-9**

Sonography, CT, Diagnostic Peritoneal Lavage, and Laparoscopy

In hemodynamically stable patients, abdominal sonography is faster and less expensive than conventional invasive and noninvasive approaches, but it cannot reliably detect intestinal trauma unless there is associated bleeding.

CT scan is indicated in hemodynamically stable patients with blunt abdominal trauma.

When patients with suspected blunt abdominal injuries present with cardiovascular instability, diagnostic peritoneal lavage (DPL) is indicated in some trauma center protocols, though it is being used less frequently.

Laparoscopy provides direct assessment of patients who have sustained abdominal trauma. It can miss retroperitoneal injuries but avoids laparotomy in more than 60% of patients.

Other diagnostic approaches to abdominal trauma include serial hematocrit determinations, serial abdominal examinations, and MRI of the abdomen.

BOX **37-10**

Preventing and Treating Hypothermia in the Trauma Patient

Remove all wet clothing and bedding and dry skin as soon as possible at the time of admission.

Warm the admission, surgery, and recovery areas.

Warm all fluids and blood products with an effective system (e.g., level I fluid warmer).

Warm irrigating fluids and topical cleansers.

Use in-line heat-moisture exchangers in the breathing circuit.

Use convection warm-air devices

During rewarming, use neuromuscular blocking agents to prevent shivering—shivering may increase oxygen consumption by 200% to 400% without improving oxygen delivery.

---

with ventilation. Major hemorrhage is associated with injuries to solid organs, liver, spleen, and kidney and with vascular injuries. In the patient with significant abdominal trauma, an indwelling arterial line is placed to allow close monitoring of blood pressure and to provide a route for sampling blood for blood gas, hematologic, and chemistry analysis. Placement of a central line facilitates CVP measurements for volume assessment and provides a route for obtaining venous blood samples.

Hypothermia is a common complication of abdominal trauma surgery because of increased heat loss through the open mesentery and reduced heat production associated with shock and anesthesia. All intravenous fluids are warmed with an efficient system, and factors that tend to encourage heat loss must be guarded against in patients who have sustained major trauma (Box 37-10). Use of heat-moisture exchangers in the airway circuit is beneficial for preventing direct delivery of dry, cool gas to the lungs.

Orthopedic Trauma

Although most *orthopedic injuries* are not usually immediately life threatening and are considered in the secondary evaluation of the trauma patient, they can be associated with significant hemorrhage and other extensive systemic physiologic derangements such as shock, fat emboli, and thromboembolic hypoxic respiratory failure. Major hemorrhage associated with fractures requires massive intraoperative fluid resuscitation, although rapid exsanguination from major fractures is unlikely. Modern intramedullary rodding devices often allow patients to ambulate within 24 hours of surgery, drastically reducing the incidence of thrombophlebitis and its subsequent morbidity.[39]

Because the ideal time to repair open fractures operatively is within the first few hours after injury, all patients taken to the operating room for emergency surgical repairs are considered to have full stomachs and are anesthetized with techniques aimed at reducing the risk of aspiration. Certain secondary vascular injuries commonly occur with specific fracture sites because the sharp edges of fractured bones are forced into blood vessels and nerves in proximity to the fracture site.[40] Massive hemorrhage can be associated with pelvic fractures. The displaced pelvic fragments can sever arteries, veins, and nerves that exit the pelvis to the perineum and the lower extremities. This can result in major blood loss into the retroperitoneal space, with continued hemorrhage from movement of unstable fragments that shear away hemostatic elements that have formed in these ruptured blood vessels. Although blood loss from pelvic fractures involving the iliac artery is notorious, significant blood loss can also occur from fractures associated with disruption of the axillary, brachial, femoral, and popliteal arteries. Severe shock can result from major bleeding into fracture sites, particularly in pelvic and long-bone fractures. Close monitoring and replacement of initial and ongoing blood loss are needed during the anesthetic management of these cases.

Hypoxic respiratory failure is a common sequela of long-bone fractures. The hypoxia results from continuous seeding of marrow fat into the venous circulation. All patients with major fractures, especially fractures of the pelvis and femur, receive frequent assessment of arterial blood gases. Endotracheal intubation and mechanical ventilation are recommended for the treatment of fracture-induced hypoxia and prevention of further lung damage. If patients are extubated immediately after fracture fixation, despite evidence of poor oxygenation and a large pulmonary venous admixture, they may develop acute respiratory distress syndrome and fat emboli syndrome. These patients benefit from continued mechanical ventilation and positive end-expiratory pressure (PEEP) that is titrated for the reduction of intrapulmonary shunting.[41]

Head Injury

Patients with *head injury* may sustain initial damage from trauma that is beyond response to treatment. The goal of care is the prevention of secondary brain damage resulting from intracranial complications aggravated by intracranial bleeding, edema, and resultant increased intracranial pressure (ICP). Common extracranial causes of death in head-injured patients are hypoxia and shock. Anesthesia management of the head-injured patient includes early control of the airway to maintain SpO_2 greater than 90% and establishing cardiovascular stability. Blood pressure is monitored, intracranial hypertension (≥ 20 mm Hg) and systolic hypotension (<90 mm Hg) should be avoided. Baseline evaluation of the patient's Glasgow Coma Scale score, pupillary reactivity, and motor function should be carefully documented before therapeutic maneuvers are initiated. Early oral endotracheal intubation with normoventilation helps in the reduction of hypercarbia and hypoxemia and contributes to the reduction of intracranial pressure. Judicious use of induction agents and neuromuscular blocking agents can facilitate a straightforward intubation. Attempts to perform an awake intubation in an obtunded, semicomatose, head-injured patient may promote coughing, bucking, and thrashing about, along with concomitant increases in ICP that carry the risk of tentorial herniation. In the head-injured patient with a possible basilar skull fracture, nasal intubation may be problematic because it can facilitate contamination and ultimate sepsis from nasal microorganisms introduced into the cranial vault. Late sepsis can also occur from a sinus infection caused by prolonged nasal tracheal intubation. Gastric tubes are placed orally in head-injured patients for the same reasons.[42]

Patients with a suspected open- or closed-head injury are placed in a head-up position to help promote venous drainage and reduce ICP. Placement of an ICP measurement device is indicated for the monitoring of ICP changes in patients with a severe traumatic brain injury. Treatment is initiated when ICP exceeds 20 mm Hg. The goal in treating intracranial hypertension is to promote adequate oxygenation and nutrient supply by maintaining cerebral perfusion pressure (CPP), oxygenation, and glucose supply without hyperglycemia. Therapeutic maneuvers involve one or more of six treatment options: (1) decrease cerebral blood volume, (2) decrease cerebral spinal fluid volume, (3) diuretics, (4) decompressive craniectomy, (5) resection of injured tissue, and (6) resection of hematomas. Moderate short-term hyperventilation to a $PaCO_2$ of 30 to 35 mm Hg helps reduce increased ICP. However, excessive or prolonged hyperventilation ($PaCO_2$ of 25 mm Hg) or less is not recommended. Hyperventilation is recommended as a temporizing measure for the reduction of elevated ICP and is avoided during the first 24 hours after injury, when cerebral blood flow (CBF) is often critically reduced. If hyperventilation is used, jugular venous oxygen saturation (SjO_2) measurement or brain-tissue oxygen monitoring is recommended.[11,12] Prompt endotracheal intubation, administration of hyperosmotic diuretics, consideration of moderate short-term hyperventilation, and possible cerebrospinal fluid drainage are considered to reduce cerebral swelling and prevent further brain injury.

A judicious induction dose of thiopental, propofol, or etomidate is usually suitable in the preparation of the head-injured patient for intubation. Succinylcholine has traditionally been used for facilitating intubation in these patients, with the reminder, however, that succinylcholine may increase ICP, especially if already elevated. Preceding succinylcholine administration with an induction agent and a pretreatment dose of a nondepolarizing muscle relaxant may minimize possible ICP increases. When contraindications to the use of succinylcholine exist, nondepolarizing neuromuscular blocking agents, which do not increase ICP, may be safely used.[43-45] Rocuronium exhibits the fastest onset among the nondepolarizing neuromuscular blocking agents. At a dose of 0.6 to 0.9 mg/kg, rocuronium facilitates good to excellent intubation conditions in 60 seconds with a duration of approximately 60 minutes. Reasonably rapid recovery from neuromuscular blockade allows early neurologic evaluation of the head-injured patient.

Patients with significant head injury benefit from the placement of an arterial line in addition to standard monitoring, which should include capnography and pulse oximetry. Placing an ICP monitoring device facilitates the observation of changes in ICP

dynamics that are influenced by drug administration and other manipulations. Intracranial hypertension exists when the ICP is at a sustained elevation of greater than 15 mm Hg. Therapeutic maneuvers are aimed at maintaining cerebral perfusion pressure (CPP) within a range of 50 to 70 mm Hg and oxygen delivery SpO_2 of 90% or greater.[11] The safety of isoflurane, desflurane, and sevoflurane has been demonstrated. Avoidance of nitrous oxide is recommended, at least until the full extent of injuries is known, because it may aggravate potential pneumocephalus and pneumothorax in the traumatized patient. In the head-injured patient, ketamine is generally avoided, because it tends to increase the ICP. Temporary reduction of ICP is often achieved using small, incremental doses of thiopental or propofol, moderate levels of hyperventilation (short-term), mannitol and/or furosemide for diuresis, and elevation of the patient's head in relation to the heart for a beneficial gravitational influence. Owing to its minimal hemodynamic effects, etomidate has been advocated for use in trauma patients. Blood pressure is monitored carefully to avoid hypotension (systolic blood pressure less than 90 mm Hg). Etomidate may inhibit the adrenocortical response to stress.[46] Although no significant clinical effects have been reported from single doses of etomidate, long-term use may be associated with increased mortality in multiple-trauma patients.[47] Hyperosmolar therapy with mannitol 0.25 to 1 g/kg is effective for control of elevated ICP. Steroids have not been shown to improve outcome or reduce ICP.[48]

Spinal Cord Injury

Approximately 10,000 *spinal cord injuries* (SCIs) occur each year in the United States, and the median age at injury is 25 years. There are more than 250,000 spinal injury patients living in the United States. The leading cause of death in patients with SCI at the scene is aspiration pneumonia. Most injuries occur in young males in the second and third decades of life, and SCIs are usually sustained from motor vehicle accidents, falls, assaults, diving injuries, and other sport injuries. Few severe injuries have as devastating physical and psychologic effects as those caused by spinal cord trauma. Eventual outcome after an acute SCI depends on three factors: (1) the severity of the acute injury, (2) the prevention of exacerbation of the injury during rescue, transport, and hospitalization, and (3) the avoidance of hypoxia and systemic hypotension, which can further compromise neural function.[49] Table 37-1 lists the common classification of SCI.

Spinal cord injury should be ruled out in any traumatized individual. The nature of the accident and the mechanism of injury should help guide the diagnosis. If an individual has been thrown from an automobile, a 1 in 13 chance exists that a cervical fracture has been sustained. If the victim remains in the car, the chance of such an injury rises to 1 in 436.[50] Cervical SCI should be assumed to be present in any patient who has sustained trauma to the head or face, in any unconscious trauma patient, and in any patient who complains of pain before or after careful palpation of the cervical spine. The anesthetist should be aware of the six conditions that are highly correlated with SCIs: paralysis, pain, position, paresthesias, ptosis, and priapism (Box 37-11).

If SCI is suspected, care should be taken to prevent further extension of the injury. A properly fitted cervical collar should be carefully placed before the patient is moved or extricated.

Precautions should be taken to prevent further extension of actual or potential neurologic deficits. Spinal immobilization should be completed before the patient is moved. The head should be stabilized in neutral alignment with no extension, flexion, or rotation. Stabilization can be accomplished by placing a

TABLE **37-1**	Classification of Spinal Injuries

Mechanisms of Spinal Injury	Stability
Flexion	
Wedge fraction	Stable
Flexion teardrop fracture	Extremely unstable
Clay shoveler's fracture	Stable
Subluxation	Potentially unstable
Bilateral facet dislocation	Always unstable
Atlantooccipital dislocation	Unstable
Anterior atlantoaxial dislocation with or without fracture	Unstable
Odontoid fracture with lateral displacement fracture	Unstable
Fracture of transverse process	Stable
Flexion-rotation	
Unilateral facet dislocation	Stable
Rotary atlantoaxial dislocation	Unstable
Extension	
Posterior neural arch fracture (C1)	Unstable
Hangman's fracture (C2)	Unstable
Extension teardrop fracture	Usually stable in flexion; unstable in extension
Posterior atlantoaxial dislocation with or without fracture	Unstable
Vertical compression	
Bursting fracture of vertebral body	Stable
Jefferson fracture (C1)	Extremely unstable
Isolated fractures of articular pillar and vertebral body	Stable

From Hockberger RS et al. Spinal injuries. In: Marx JA et al, eds. Rosen's Emergency Medicine. 6th ed. St Louis: Mosby; 2006:399.

BOX **37-11**

Six Signs and Symptoms Correlated with Spinal Cord Injuries

Paralysis
Inability to move the arms or legs should always raise suspicion of spinal cord injury.

Pain
Conscious patient may complain of pain localized at the site of the spinal injury.

Position
Patient holding the head upright or the neck with both hands may be indicating a Jefferson-type C1 fracture; the "hold-up" position (arms and hands held over the head as in a robbery) can indicate a C4, C5 fracture; the "prayer position" (arms folded across chest) indicates a possible C5, C6 fracture.

Paresthesias
Complaints of numbness, a "pins-and-needles" sensation, a burning sensation (dysesthesia), or a feeling of electric shock passing down the vertebral column or of water flowing down the back may indicate the presence of a spinal cord injury.

Ptosis
Drooping eyelid and myotic pupil, which are signs of Horner syndrome, may indicate a cervical spinal cord injury.

Priapism
Penile erection occurs in about 3% to 5% of spinal cord injuries. Its presence indicates that the sympathetic nervous system is involved.

cervical collar on the patient, splinting, and/or sandbagging the head in neutral alignment. The patient should be secured on a long spinal backboard before being moved.[50]

All patients with suspected SCI must be assessed for adequacy of a patent airway. Care should be used to avoid extension, flexion, or rotation of the neck in the attempts to open the airway. A gentle "chin lift" maneuver may be adequate for securing a patent airway without disturbing the neutral neck position. Oxygen should be administered by mask immediately in the patient whose airway is secured at the scene. Hypoxia and hypercarbia can further accentuate the damage sustained with SCIs. Injuries at the C1 or C2 level result in complete respiratory paralysis. Death follows within a few minutes if artificial ventilation is not commenced rapidly. In such patients, an LMA or a Combitube may be placed at the scene by paramedics. Although these devices initially may be adequate for allowing transport to a medical facility, they are replaced with an endotracheal tube as quickly as possible after the patient is admitted to a treatment facility. The head is maintained in a neutral position with in-line axial immobilization during the intubation. The anterior portion of the cervical collar is removed before intubation so that

movement of the mandible is facilitated. If the patient with an SCI is breathing spontaneously on arrival at the treatment facility, the anesthetist must evaluate the adequacy of ventilation. If the patient is not able to protect the airway (i.e., is unconscious or semiconscious, has an absent or diminished gag reflex or cough, or has intraoral or facial injuries with significant edema, bleeding, or both), rapid intubation is needed. If ventilation appears to be reasonable, chest and cervical spine radiographic evaluation and neurologic examinations can be started while an arterial blood gas determination is completed. A lateral view of the cervical spine can be obtained quickly, and it reveals most unstable fractures. For a complete evaluation of the cervical spine, multiple films or CT scanning or MRI may be required. Adequate evaluation must include all seven cervical vertebrae; C7 is the most common site of injury. In the stable, cooperative patient with an SCI, awake nasal intubation is the method of choice.[51] The nasal intubation can be accomplished blindly with the use of an Endotrol tube that has a trigger device that allows the tip of the endotracheal tube to be positioned with relative ease. The tube can also be guided by use of a direct fiberoptic laryngoscope. Sedation may be accomplished with small doses of midazolam and fentanyl. Topical anesthesia can be useful, but transtracheal injection should be avoided in patients with a possible full stomach because the possibility of pulmonary aspiration is increased in this situation. In children and uncooperative adults or in patients in whom awake intubation fails, a carefully selected dose of thiopental or propofol and a neuromuscular blocking agent is used for inducing general anesthesia for the intubation. Special care is given in the situation that requires oral intubation. SCI patients have the best chance of recovery if hypoxia, hypercarbia, and hypotension are avoided or rapidly corrected if encountered. Arterial blood gas values indicating that ventilation is suboptimal are corrected by intubation and mechanical ventilation. If there is a delay in establishing the airway, the patient is given ventilation by mask while cricoid pressure is maintained until the airway is secured. Severely traumatized patients who are hypoxic on arrival undergo ventilation by mask with application of cricoid pressure until the intubation is completed. This method prevents further hypoxic insults that can occur during the apneic period between the administration of a muscle relaxant and the completed intubation. Often, time does not allow the luxury of adequate preoxygenation in an already compromised hypoxic patient with respiratory inadequacy. To prevent further hypoxic insult and the resultant potential life-threatening dysrhythmias, these patients are continuously ventilated while cricoid pressure is applied. This measure helps maintain or improve oxygenation until laryngoscopy and intubation are completed.

Use of Muscle Relaxants in Patients with Spinal Cord Injury

Succinylcholine may precipitate cardiac arrest in patients with massive muscle injury or denervation, such as that seen in patients with SCIs, crush injuries of muscles, or burns.[45] The basis for this problem involves supersensitivity of the neuromuscular junction to the depolarizing effect of both acetylcholine and succinylcholine. This phenomenon results in the release of large quantities of potassium during muscle contraction. Normal depolarization results in a small potassium flux across the muscle-cell membrane. If a muscle is crushed, burned, or denervated, acetylcholine receptors proliferate around the injured cell, so that when the muscle is depolarized, the flux of potassium is increased significantly. The problem is thought to develop in response to succinylcholine several days after the injury. Succinylcholine is not recommended for intubation of the patient with acute SCI because muscle fasciculation may exacerbate the SCI.[52] A conservative approach to caring for patients with SCI would be to avoid the use of succinylcholine by using nondepolarizing muscle relaxants or nonrelaxant-assisted airway control techniques.

Spinal Shock

A triad of *hypotension*, *bradycardia*, and *hypothermia* frequently results from a relative sympathectomy in SCI patients. The *spinal shock* is progressively intensified the more cephalad the SCI. Patients with SCIs at the T6 level or higher have severely impaired CNS function. Sympathetically mediated cardioaccelerator responses no longer oppose vagal innervation, allowing the heart rate to slow dramatically. Loss of sympathetic tone allows vasodilation, pooling of the peripheral circulation, and decreased venous return to the heart. This situation results in decreased cardiac output and hypotension. The SCI also interrupts sympathetic pathways from the hypothalamus (temperature-control center) to peripheral blood vessels. The patient in spinal shock is unable to constrict vessels or shiver to produce heat or to dilate vessels to dissipate heat. The patient's body temperature has a tendency to migrate toward the environmental temperature.

Treatment

Patients in spinal shock are hypotensive and bradycardic with warm, pink extremities. In contrast, patients in hemorrhagic shock tend to be hypotensive and tachycardic with cold, clammy skin. Use of invasive monitoring is critical for fluid resuscitation and appropriate intervention with vasoactive drugs. An indwelling arterial catheter is mandatory in the acute phase of spinal shock. Moment-to-moment control of arterial blood pressure is essential for the replacement of fluids and the use of vasoactive drug therapy. In addition, arterial blood gas assessments are facilitated by an indwelling arterial catheter.

A pulmonary artery catheter may be helpful for managing fluid and drug therapy. It allows for measurement of the cardiac output and derived hemodynamic variables needed for proper therapy. SCI patients can readily develop pulmonary edema if their fluids and vasoactive drug therapy are not guided by the variables derived from use of a pulmonary artery catheter. A general principle in any therapeutic protocol is to prevent secondary deterioration that may worsen neurologic status after an acute SCI. In severe SCIs, electrical conduction through the injured cord segment ceases as a result of direct tissue disruption from the trauma and the secondary concussion effect. Vasomotor reactivity of the injured cord is lost, leading to changes in the spinal cord flow. These local injury changes in the microcirculation may be compounded by cardiovascular instability secondary to the trauma itself. The resultant ischemia from these factors causes the accumulation of metabolic toxins and sets in motion a biochemical sequence of events that leads to further ischemia and irreversible damage. Because some of these secondary events are avoidable or reversible, recovery from SCI is limited but possible. Oxygen is supplemented by mask or endotracheal tube, with arterial blood gas values used for determining the approximate FIO_2.

The SCI patient is frequently unable to maintain adequate cardiac filling pressures. However, overaggressive fluid therapy can precipitate pulmonary edema. For the maintenance of adequate arterial blood pressure and cord perfusion, pressor therapy may be initiated.

Patients with a high cervical SCI who manifest cardiovascular instability are not placed on a Stryker frame because of the rapid change in cardiovascular status turning may cause. These patients are placed on a Roto-Rest bed or a regular bed after their spinal column has been stabilized.

Other Considerations

Patients with SCI are extubated as quickly as possible after spinal stabilization surgery. If the patient requires intubation because of associated pulmonary injuries or dysfunction, then a weaning program is started when it is tolerated by the patient. With frequent assessment of respiratory status, this weaning is usually begun within the first few days. Useful guidelines for assessing the adequacy of ventilation include measurement of the tidal volume (>5 mL/kg), negative inspiratory force (−20 to 25 cm H_2O pressure—needed for adequate cough), and vital capacity (>15 mg/kg).

Patients with a high SCI often lose innervation of the intercostal and abdominal musculature. Continued assessment of adequate diaphragmatic innervation, a function essential to generating adequate ventilation, is mandatory. Some patients require tracheostomies. Chest physiotherapy is initiated for all patients as soon as possible to reduce the risk of pulmonary congestion and infection. Oral or nasogastric tubes are placed for decompressing the stomach. This measure eases diaphragmatic excursion for improved ventilation and reduces the risk of aspiration. Peptic ulceration with loss of sympathetic innervation in the patient with a high SCI is a well-described complication, especially in patients receiving steroids.

Surgical Intervention and Anesthesia Approach

Although external immobilization devices (e.g., halo vest) are sometimes used, many neurosurgeons believe that prolonged use of external fixation devices is contraindicated in patients with unsatisfactorily reduced spines. Frequently, spinal stabilization and/or decompression procedures are performed after initial resuscitation and diagnostic workup.

The neurosurgeon and anesthesia team document the current neurologic status and note any deficits before the start of anesthesia and intubation. In an awake intubation, the patient is assessed before and after endotracheal tube placement and after the patient is positioned for surgery.

Whether an anterior or a posterior surgical approach is used in cervical SCI depends on the nature of the injury. For stabilization of lower SCIs, internal fixation devices are commonly placed in the acute phase. At times, these procedures can be associated with significant surgical blood loss. Careful monitoring and replacement of blood loss are essential. Use of an autotransfusion device often saves considerable bank blood use in these procedures.

In patients deferred for elective spinal stabilization procedures, awake nasal intubations are performed. In controlled conditions, this measure allows the use of local, topical, and transtracheal anesthesia without the risk of pulmonary aspiration that is present in emergency procedures. Glycopyrrolate is given before localizing the airway. Once moderate sedation is accomplished, superior laryngeal nerve block and topical oropharyngeal and transtracheal sprays are administered. Oxymetazoline (Afrin) nasal spray is helpful in reducing nasal congestion. Topical 4% cocaine to both nares provides good topical anesthesia and helps constrict the nasal mucosa. Serial dilation of the nares with increasing sizes of soft nasopharyngeal airways helps facilitate passage of the endotracheal tube. Endotracheal tubes that have a trigger mechanism to help control the tube tip position are helpful. Nasal intubation is accomplished efficiently with fiberoptic guidance. Anesthetic techniques that avoid hypotension and provide good cardiovascular stability are recommended. Baseline analgesia is provided with opioids (generally fentanyl or sufentanil). Muscle relaxation is provided with a nondepolarizing neuromuscular blocking agent to promote cardiovascular stability. Following a spinal cord injury with permanent neuromuscular deficits, succinylcholine must be avoided for the patient's remaining lifetime. Because many SCI patients may have a head injury or possible pneumothorax, nitrous oxide may also be avoided. Following head injury, nitrous oxide can cause a pneumocephalus to develop, with a subsequent rise in the intracranial pressure. Following injury to the chest wall, use of nitrous oxide with positive pressure can cause rapid expansion of a subclinical pneumothorax into a rapidly increasing and life-threatening pneumothorax with mediastinal shift. Ketamine can be useful as an induction agent in unstable chest trauma patients, but because it increases ICP, it is contraindicated if an associated head injury may be present.

Autonomic Hyperreflexia (Mass Reflex)

Trauma centers frequently deal with acute trauma patients not only during the initial hospitalization but for future related surgery. In this setting, the anesthesia plan addresses the implications of *autonomic hyperreflexia*. Autonomic hyperreflexia is a sudden massive sympathetic discharge resulting from stimulation below the level of spinal-cord transection.[53] Hyperreflexia is seen in 85% of SCI patients with lesions above T5. Signs of this condition include paroxysmal hypertension, bradycardia, and cardiac dysrhythmias in response to stimuli below the level of transection, such as bladder catheterization, distention of the bladder or rectum, defecation, childbirth, and even cutaneous stimulation. Hyperreflexia is not observed until the spinal shock phase has passed. It is therefore usually seen when patients return to surgery for such procedures as cystoscopies, performed later in their recovery phase. It can occur intraoperatively with local, spinal, and nitrous oxide–opioid general anesthesia. If autonomic hyperreflexia occurs, is treated by removing the stimulus, deepening anesthesia, and administering direct-acting vasodilators. Untreated, the hypertension crisis may progress to seizures, intracranial hemorrhage, or myocardial infarction. No episodes have been reported with the use of potent inhalation anesthetics. Bradycardia is treated with atropine or glycopyrrolate.

Radiologic Studies

Diagnostic workup of suspected SCI patients consists of various radiographic imaging techniques and multidetector CAT scan (MDCT). Chest, pelvic, and skull imaging techniques are performed in that sequence. Upright chest radiographs are not taken until cervical imaging evaluation has been determined to be normal. Lumbar and thoracic spine radiographs are obtained if the workup suggests the presence of a lesion in these areas. If a question exists about pathologic findings in the cervical spine radiograph, the patient is accompanied by anesthesia personnel to CT for management of the airway, anesthesia, and vasoactive drug therapy.

SELECTION OF ANESTHETIC AGENTS FOR THE TRAUMA PATIENT

Trauma patients arriving in the admitting area are frequently unable to provide reliable information about their past medical history. The anesthetist may have no knowledge of the patient's possible allergies or previous response to anesthesia. Moreover, 30% to 50% of trauma patients are intoxicated, usually with ethyl alcohol and sometimes with illicit "street drugs." These substances may alter a patient's response to drugs administered during anesthesia; postoperative hallucinations or delayed recovery from anesthesia may occur. In shock trauma patients, maintaining cardiovascular stability is the major criterion in formulating a safe plan for anesthesia management.

Because of the many problems that can occur if nitrous oxide is used, other techniques are preferable in acutely injured patients. Its affinity for diffusing into closed spaces makes it contraindicated when pneumothorax, closed-head injury with possible pneumocephalus, or bowel injury has occurred. Because ruling out such conditions in acute trauma cases is often difficult, nitrous oxide should generally be avoided in trauma management.

Isoflurane, desflurane, and sevoflurane may all be used successfully, and anesthesia can be maintained with a mixture of oxygen and air to achieve an appropriate FiO_2 concentration. Vecuronium, rocuronium, and cisatracurium are very useful during induction and maintenance of anesthesia in the trauma patient. They are not associated with histamine release that may cause bronchospasm and hypotension. Rocuronium has the fastest onset in intubating doses.

During the preoperative phase, midazolam in small doses helps provide consistent amnesia during the insertion of invasive monitoring lines. A narcotic such as fentanyl, sufentanil, or remifentanil can be used for supplementing the induction and maintenance of anesthesia.

Propofol or thiopental may be used as induction agents in standard doses in stable trauma patients and in reduced doses in unstable patients. They can be helpful in patients with brain injuries, because they tend to reduce cerebral metabolic rate, ICP, and cerebral blood flow. To avoid the risk of increased ICP, ketamine is not used in any patient with suspected head injury. Etomidate may be valuable in the very unstable patient. Propofol is a very effective agent for use in postacute trauma patients who may undergo numerous follow-up corrective procedures following primary surgical procedures performed on admission to the trauma facility. Use of propofol in these patients allows for a rapid recovery with minimal residual drowsiness. This is in sharp contrast to the somnolence usually seen following use of thiopental.

Postoperative Analgesia

Trauma patients frequently experience severe postoperative pain. Intravenous narcotics, such as fentanyl and sufentanil, often help alleviate that pain. Patient-controlled analgesia systems can also maintain a stable level of pain relief. Alternatively, morphine can be continuously administered via epidural catheters.

Continuous intercostal catheter techniques can be used for injecting local anesthetic agents in patients with chest injuries

SUMMARY

Trauma care is an important specialty of modern anesthesia practice. The organization of trauma care in the United States has substantially improved survival and quality of outcomes for traumatically injured patients. The anesthetist's involvement begins as soon as the patient reaches the trauma facility. The major concern is evaluating the patient's airway and maintaining ventilation until endotracheal intubation can be performed. The principles of successful management of the trauma patient are based on organization and preparation, assessment of the patient's injuries, proper priority for therapeutic interventions, achievement and maintenance of a patent airway, fluid resuscitation, application of appropriate continuous invasive and noninvasive monitoring, correction of acid-base and electrolyte disturbances, and careful titration of anesthetic and adjunctive agents. The degree of functional outcome of trauma patients is largely dependent on the early involvement of sound principles of anesthesia care in the resuscitation and overall anesthetic management during the perioperative period. In a well-managed team approach, assessment and treatment are carried out in rapid succession or even simultaneously.

REFERENCES

1. Barker SJ. Anesthesia for trauma: a fresh look. *ASA Annual Refresher Course Lectures.* Park Ridge, IL: ASA; 1999:244.
2. American Association for the Surgery of Trauma. *Trauma Facts.* Available at: www.aast.org. Accessed November 7, 2007.
3. Gin-Shaw SL, Jorden RC. Multiple trauma. In: Marx JA et al, eds. *Rosen's Emergency Medicine.* 6th ed. St Louis: Mosby; 2006:300-328.
4. Lee CC et al. A current concept of trauma-induced multiorgan failure. *Am Emerg Med.* 2001;38(2):170-176.
5. Johnson D, Mayers I. Multiple organ dysfunction syndrome: a narrative review. *Can J Anaesth.* 2001;48(5):502-509.
6. Baranov D, Neligan P. Trauma and aggressive homeostasis management. *Anesthesiol Clin North America.* 2007;25(1):49-63.
7. Guyton AC, Hall JE. Nervous regulation of the circulation and rapid control of arterial pressure. *Textbook of Medical Physiology.* 11th ed. Philadelphia: Saunders; 2006:204-215.
8. Marieb EN, Hoehn K. Heart physiology. In: Marieb EN, Hoehn K, eds. *Human Anatomy and Physiology.* 7th ed. San Francisco: Pearson, Benjamin Cummings; 2007:692-704.
9. Keel M, Tentz O. Pathophysiology of polytrauma. *Injury.* 2005;36(6):691-709.
10. Grundy PL et al. The hypothalamo-pituitary-adrenal axis response to experimental traumatic brain injury. *J Neurotrauma.* 2001;18(12):1373-1381.
11. Kofke WA, Stiefel M. Monitoring and intraoperative management of elevated intracranial pressure and decompressive craniectomy. *Anesthesiol Clin.* 2007;25(3):579-603.
12. Bullock R et al. Guidelines for the management of severe traumatic brain injury. *J Neurotrauma.* 2007;24:S87-S90.
13. Howie WO. Anesthesia "Go Team" for trauma patients: field-based anesthesia. *AANA J.* 2007;75(2):107-110.
14. Trunkey DD. Trauma centers and trauma systems. *JAMA.* 2003;289(12):1566-1567.
15. Trunkey DD. History and development of trauma care in the United States. *Clin Orthop.* 2000;374:36-46.
16. Olson CJ. Time to death of hospitalized injured patients as a measure of quality of care. *J Trauma.* 2003;55(1):45-52.
17. Nelson LA. Airway trauma. *Int Anesthesiol Clin.* 2007;45(3):99-118.
18. Kristensen MS. The Parker Flex-Tip tube versus a standard tube for fiberoptic orotracheal intubation: a randomized double-blind study. *Anesthesiology.* 2003;(2):354-358.
19. Smith CE et al. Evaluation of tracheal intubation difficulty in patients with cervical spine immobilization. Fiberoptic (WuScope) versus conventional laryngoscopy. *Anesthesiology.* 1999;91:1253.
20. Muzzi DA et al. Complication from a nasopharyngeal airway in a patient with a basilar skull fracture. *Anesthesiology.* 1991;74:366-368.
21. Ewart L. The efficacy of cricoid pressure in preventing gastro-oesophageal reflux in rapid sequence induction of anaesthesia. *J Perioper Pract.* 2007;17(9):432-436.
22. Dutton RP, McCunn M. Anesthesia for trauma. In: Miller RD, ed. *Anesthesia.* 6th ed. New York: Churchill Livingstone; 2005:2451.
23. Pinsky MR. Targets for resuscitation from shock. *Minerva Anaestesiol.* 2003;69(4):237-244.
24. American Heart Association. *Guidelines for cardiopulmonary resuscitation and emergency cardiac care: adult advanced cardiac life support.* ACLS Provider Manual 2006. St Louis: Mosby; 2006.
25. Babbs CF. Interposed abdominal compression CPR: a comprehensive evidence based review. *Resuscitation.* 2003;59(1):71-82.
26. Circulatory shok and physiology of its treatment. In: Guyton AC, ed. *Textbook of Medical Physiology.* Philadelphia: Saunders; 2006:278-287.
27. Sperry JL et al. Early hyperglycemia predicts multiple organ failure and mortality but not infection. *J Trauma.* 2007;63(3):487-493.
28. Bochicchio GV et al. Early hyperglycemic control is important in critically injured trauma patients. *J Trauma.* 2007;63(6):1353-1358.
29. Oddo M et al. Glucose control after severe brain injury. *Curr Opin Clin Nutr Metab Care.* 2008;11(2):134-139.
30. American College of Surgeons Committee on Trauma. Shock. In: American College of Surgeons, eds. *Advanced Trauma Life Support Course for Physicians.* Chicago: American College of Surgeons; 2004:108.
31. Frank LR: Is MAST in the past? The pros and cons of MAST usage in the field. *J Emerg Med.* 2000;25(2):38-41, 44-45.
32. Colwell C et al. Detecting mechanism of injury. *Emerg Med Serv.* 2003;32(5):52-58.
33. Moloney JT et al. Anesthetic management of thoracic trauma. *Curr Opin Anaesthesiol.* 2008;21(1):41-46.
34. Liman ST et al. Chest injury due to blunt trauma. *Eur J Cardiothorac Surg.* 2003;23(3):374-378.
35. Demetriades D, Velmahos G. Technology-driven triage of abdominal trauma: the emerging era of nonoperative management. *Annu Rev Med.* 2003;54:1-15.
36. Stengel D et al. Emergency ultrasound-based algorithms for diagnosing blunt abdominal trauma. *Ann Emerg Med.* 2007;49(3):364-366.
37. Steve JK, Grande CM. Anesthesia for trauma patients. In: Longnecker DE et al, eds. *Anesthesiology.* New York: McGraw-Hill; 2008:1660-1673.
38. Villavicencio RT, Aucar JA. Analysis of laparoscopy in trauma. *J Am Coll Surg.* 1999;189:11.
39. Litchtblau S. Hip fracture: surgical decisions that affect medical management. *Geriatrics.* 2000;55(5):50-5255-56.
40. Stone WM et al. Upper extremity trauma: current trends in management. *J Cardiovasc Surg (Torino),* 2007;48(5):551-555.

41. Dutton RP, McCunn M. Anesthesia for trauma. In: Miller RD, ed. *Anesthesia.* 6th ed. New York: Churchill Livingstone; 2005:2451-2496.

42. Parikh S et al. Traumatic brain injury. *Int Anesthesiol Clin.* 2007;45(3): 119-135.

43. Marvez E et al. Predicting adverse outcomes in a diagnosis-based protocol system for rapid sequence intubation. *Am J Emerg Med.* 2003;21(1):23-29.

44. Kofke WA, Stiefel M. Monitoring and intraoperative management of elevated intracranial pressure and decompressive craniectomy. *Anesthesiol Clin.* 2007;25(3):579-603.

45. Perry J et al. Rocuronium versus succinylcholine for rapid-sequence induction intubation. *Cochrane Database Syst Rev.* 2003;(1):CD002788.

46. Absalom A et al. Adrenocortical function in critically ill patients 24 h after a single dose of etomidate. *Anaesthesia.* 1999;54(9):861-867.

47. Schenarts CL et al. Adrenocortical dysfunction following etomidate induction in emergency department patients. *Acad Emerg Med.* 2001;8(1):1-7.

48. Bullock R et al. Guidelines for the management of severe traumatic brain injury. *J Neurotrauma.* 2007;24:S14-S20, S91-S95.

49. McKinley WO et al. Long-term medical complications after traumatic spinal cord injury: a regional model systems analysis. *Arch Phys Med Rehabil.* 1999;80:1402-1410.

50. Stier GR et al. Spinal cord: injury and procedures. In: Newfield P, Cottrell JE, eds. *Handbook of Neuroanesthesia.* 4th ed. Philadelphia: Lippincott Williams & Wilkins; 2007:216-255.

51. Fuchs G et al. Fiberoptic intubation in 327 neurosurgical patients with lesions of the cervical spine. *J Neurosurg Anesthesiol.* 1999;11(1):11-16.

52. Vuksanj D, Fisher DM. Pharmacokinetics of rocuronium in children aged 4-11 years. *Anesthesiology.* 1995;82:1104-1110.

53. George E. Evaluation of the trauma patient. In: Longnecker DE et al, eds. *Anesthesiology.* New York: McGraw-Hill; 2008:1784-1796.

CHAPTER 38

OUTPATIENT ANESTHESIA

Rex A. Marley

The concept of outpatient anesthesia is not unique to the past 3 decades. It was introduced in dentists' offices with the administration of nitrous oxide. Physicians' offices were next to offer this type of service for superficial procedures that required at most the administration of local anesthesia. In 1909, Nicoll[1] first reported on 8988 outpatient surgical procedures performed at the Glasgow Royal Hospital for Sick Children. In 1916 in Sioux City, Iowa, Waters[2] opened the first freestanding unit designed for outpatient surgery.

The evolution of and demand for outpatient care have not slowed since first described by these pioneers. Ambulatory surgery has become well established as the needs of the patient and medical community have been realized. Approximately 82% of all procedures were performed as outpatient surgery by the year 2005.[3,4] The patient is expected to enter the outpatient surgical care facility, undergo the procedure, and then be released without needing an overnight stay. Outpatient surgery includes the "23-hour observation" patient, who may be admitted to the inpatient or overnight facility yet is discharged before staying in the hospital 24 hours. Surgical procedures requiring the expertise of an anesthesia provider in the office setting are becoming increasing popular. Office-based surgery can be performed more efficiently and at lower cost than in the hospital.[5] Presently, 10 million operations are performed annually in the office-based setting.[6]

FEATURES OF OUTPATIENT SURGERY

Advantages

Financial

An advantage of ambulatory surgical settings has been the economic benefit for consumers, third-party payers, and medical facilities. Patients may benefit not only from reduced medical cost but also from minimized costs of outside child care and from resumption of normal living activities at an earlier time. Third-party payers concerned about cost containment are increasingly identifying procedures that may be performed only in the outpatient setting. Cost savings exceeding 50% have been reported for selected surgeries (e.g., laparoscopic cholecystectomy) performed on an outpatient basis.[7]

Medical

One medical advantage of ambulatory surgery is the increased availability of hospital beds for patients requiring hospital admission. For patients who are susceptible to infection (e.g., children, immunosuppressed patients, cancer patients, and transplant recipients), minimizing time and contact in the inpatient hospital setting may decrease the risk of nosocomial infections.[8]

Social

Children benefit from outpatient surgery because it minimizes separation from parents and causes less disruption in a child's feeding schedule. The continued presence and care offered by the parents are beneficial for children with mental or physical impairments. Geriatric patients show better cognitive and physical capacity when separation from familiar surroundings and family is minimized.[9] The elderly are better able to maintain their normal living routines (e.g., diet, medication, and sleep pattern). Postoperative confusion is decreased in geriatric patients undergoing outpatient procedures because they receive less medication and are returned to a familiar environment sooner than their inpatient counterparts.

Staffing

The ambulatory surgery setting is more convenient than the inpatient surgery setting for the staff because it offers better use of time, uniform work schedules, and more predictable surgical outcomes.

Disadvantages

The outpatient setting may have several disadvantages:

1. The degree of patient privacy is less than that in the inpatient setting.
2. The patient must make multiple trips to the physician's office or the ambulatory setting for evaluation and screening.
3. Adequate home care must be ensured once the patient is discharged from the facility after surgery.
4. Compliance and efficacy related to preoperative and postoperative instructions may not be as good as when the patient is admitted to the hospital before surgery.
5. Because of the emphasis on efficiency, children have less time to adapt to the surgical setting than they would as inpatients.
6. Observation time and monitoring for the occurrence of adverse events are decreased in the outpatient setting.

Demographic Considerations

Patient Age

Patients receiving outpatient anesthesia can be any age. Approximately 30% of outpatients are younger than 12 years,[10] and more than 10% are at least 60.[11]

Surgical Length

Earlier guidelines recommended limiting the length of outpatient surgery to less than 1.5 to 2 hours.[12] Reasoning was that the longer surgery lasts, the more likely patients will experience severe pain.[13] Surgical time exceeding 2 hours was also thought to be a strong predictor for unplanned hospital admission postoperatively.[14] However, other factors such as the skill of the surgeon, the type of surgery performed, the patient's condition, and the anesthetic technique used must be considered. Arbitrarily limiting the length of surgery to less than 2 hours is no longer considered necessary; procedures exceeding 4 hours are routinely performed without complications in ambulatory centers.

Suitable Procedures

The list of procedures suitable for the ambulatory setting is constantly evolving. Ophthalmologic procedures are the most common type of outpatient procedure, and gynecologic surgery is the second.[15] The outpatient surgical procedure should not involve extensive blood loss or physiologic shifts of considerable fluid volumes because these processes necessitate protracted patient observation and hydration. In the past, the potential for blood transfusion implied the need for the procedure to be conducted at an inpatient facility. The increasing popularity of autologous blood donation for future transfusion has led to the application of transfusion during or after the outpatient surgery.[16]

Acceptable surgical procedures are expanding and routinely include such surgeries as laparoscopic cholecystectomy,[17] lumbar laminectomy,[18] cervical laminectomy and fusion,[19] thyroidectomy,[20] vaginal hysterectomy,[21] craniotomy for tumor,[22,23] and tonsillectomy.[17,24] The 23-hour observation area, which is designed for extended patient inspection, is popular for outpatient tonsillectomy.

Procedures requiring prolonged immobilization are best conducted on an inpatient basis. For procedures associated with postoperative discomfort, arrangements for parenteral opioid therapy in the home may be made, provided that adequate pain relief can be achieved with safe doses of opioids.

PATIENT SELECTION

Proper patient selection minimizes the number of hospital admissions that follow outpatient surgery. Evaluation of which patients are appropriate for outpatient surgery and anesthesia requires consensus and cooperation between the surgical and anesthesia staff. Factors to consider in determining the suitability of a patient for outpatient surgery include:

1. *The anticipated surgical procedure for the patient.* The proposed surgery should have an insignificant incidence of intraoperative and postoperative problems and should not require intense postoperative patient management.
2. *The physical and psychosocial health of the patient.* The patient is ideally in his or her usual good health, or if ill, the condition should be under proper control. The patient and family should be receptive to the outpatient philosophy and the perioperative adaptations that will be required of them.
3. *The surgeon's skills and cooperation.* Early referral to the anesthesia department for patients of questionable appropriateness helps streamline the outpatient process and minimize delays on the day of surgery.

Selection Criteria
Acute Substance Abuse

The patient with a history of substance abuse should be evaluated before the day of surgery. Counseling for such patients includes the warning that preoperative substance abuse will lead to cancellation of the surgery. A distinction between long-term and acute substance abuse must be made. A urinary drug screen should be performed in patients suspected of substance abuse. The patient with signs of acute substance intoxication is an inappropriate ambulatory surgery candidate because of the increased likelihood of impaired autonomic and cardiovascular responses. The surgery should be rescheduled after the patient is detoxified and treated. Patient management strategies should emphasize methods of minimizing postoperative pain, because substance abusers are typically intolerant to pain. Regional or local anesthetic techniques, if their use is suitable to the surgeon and appropriate for the type of operation being performed, may be used if the patient wishes to abstain from sedatives and opioids. Postoperatively, pain may be minimized by the use of local wound infiltration and the prophylactic use of nonsteroidal analgesics. Placing a catheter in the wound and instilling local anesthesia, either continuously or intermittently, has been shown to prolong pain relief and improve patient satisfaction and should be considered in this population.[25]

Age

Patient age by itself should not be the deciding factor for outpatient suitability. Meridy[26] retrospectively examined the charts of patients ranging in age from 9 months to 92 years and noted that most perioperative complications occurred in the 20- to 49-year age group.

Premature Infant. The premature infant (gestational age of 37 weeks or less at birth) is an inappropriate candidate for outpatient surgery because of potential physiologic aberrations. The premature infant may:

1. Exhibit anemia
2. Not have fully developed gag reflexes (and thus be more prone to aspiration of liquid or solid food)
3. Have immature temperature control and be susceptible to the effects of hypothermia, which could contribute to postoperative apnea
4. Demonstrate immature brainstem functioning, which predisposes the infant to pathologic respiratory conditions

The infant with a hemoglobin value less than the predicted normal value for that age will require additional evaluation before surgery. Hemoglobin values in the premature infant may drop to between 7 and 8 g/100 mL 1 to 3 months after birth.[27] The presence of anemia (hematocrit less than 30%) may increase the incidence of apnea in the newborn.[28] Some investigators have recommended delaying elective surgery until the hematocrit is increased to greater than 30% through supplementation of iron intake.[29]

In the perioperative period, the preterm infant is at greater risk for developing respiratory complications, including apnea, than is the full-term infant.[30] The preterm infant is susceptible to short apnea (6 to 15 seconds), prolonged apnea (>15 seconds), or periodic breathing (three or more periods of apnea of 3 to 15 seconds separated by less than 20 seconds of normal respiration). Short or prolonged apnea and periodic breathing predispose the infant to hypoxemia and bradycardia. An obstructive component that leads to quicker oxyhemoglobin desaturation appears to be part of postoperative apnea in these infants.[31] These infants have developed prolonged apnea as late as 12 hours after surgery.[30]

The older the infant, the less likely that respiratory complications such as apnea will occur. In evaluating the suitability of a former preterm infant for outpatient surgery, conservative measures are best; inpatient status should be assigned if significant concerns exist. These patients benefit from the intensive monitoring available in the inpatient setting. Much discussion has been held as to the postgestational age (gestational age plus postnatal age) at which the former preterm infant may safely undergo outpatient anesthesia. Healthy former premature infants whose postgestational age is less than 50 to 60 weeks[32,33] should be admitted to the hospital for extended monitoring. Postoperative apnea has even been described in the full-term infant.[34] Our ability to exactly predict the susceptibility of an infant to postoperative apnea is lacking.[35] Patients should be evaluated individually for appropriateness for outpatient surgery, and consideration should be given to growth and development, feeding problems, upper respiratory tract infections (URTIs), apneic history, and disorders of metabolic, endocrine, neurologic, or cardiac systems. All infants with a history of prematurity should be closely observed for signs of apnea and bradycardia. If any of these signs are evidenced in the postanesthesia care unit, patients should be admitted and observed. An infant with a history of apnea or bradycardia must be apnea free and without monitoring for at least 6 months to be considered for outpatient surgery.[36] Efforts should be made to schedule surgery for these patients as early in the day as possible to allow for extended observation time.

Beyond simply delaying surgery, attempts to minimize the likelihood of postoperative apnea in susceptible infants have been examined. Spinal anesthesia without sedation resulted in less prolonged apnea, oxyhemoglobin desaturation, and bradycardia than did general anesthesia[37] or spinal anesthesia with ketamine sedation.[38] However, apnea and delayed respiratory failure have been reported in children who have had spinal or caudal anesthesia.[39-42] Infants treated with endotracheal intubation or mechanical ventilation (or both) for respiratory distress syndrome at birth have been shown to have abnormal arterial blood gas values and abnormal pulmonary function results as late as 1 year after treatment.[43] Infants exhibiting signs of bronchopulmonary dysplasia should not be considered for outpatient surgery.[44] Patients with a history of bronchopulmonary dysplasia are at risk for sudden infant death.[45]

Infants with a history of apneic events or with siblings who developed sudden infant death syndrome (SIDS) are at risk for SIDS. The greatest at-risk age for the development of SIDS is between 1 month and 1 year of age.[46] In infants who have lost a sibling to SIDS, the risk of dying from the same syndrome is four to five times that of the general population.[47] Patients at risk for the development of SIDS should not be considered for outpatient surgical procedures until they are at least 6 months[48] to 1 year old.[49]

Full-Term Infant. Healthy, full-term infants (greater than 37 weeks' gestational age at birth) at least 2 weeks[50] to 4 weeks[16] of age can be considered for minor outpatient surgery. Full-term infants with histories of apneic episodes, failure to thrive, and feeding difficulties are not suitable candidates for outpatient surgery. Infants with a history of respiratory difficulties at birth are not suitable outpatient candidates unless they are free of respiratory symptoms at the time of surgery and at the time of hospital discharge.[48]

Geriatric Patient. The decision whether ambulatory surgery should be performed in a geriatric patient (age 65 years or older) should be individualized and based on physiologic age rather than on chronologic age. Existing medical problems are a concern when considering the geriatric patient for outpatient surgery. There are more concomitant age-related diseases that should be optimally treated preoperatively in this group of patients. Patient age exceeding 85 years is a predictor of hospital admissions following outpatient surgery.[51] Appropriate home care and

transportation to and from the outpatient center with a responsible caregiver must be ensured.

Special Considerations

Convulsive Disorders. Surgery for patients with seizure disorders should be scheduled early in the day so patients can be observed for 4 to 8 hours after the operation before they are discharged.[52] It is important to establish the patients' ability to maintain their schedule for anticonvulsant medications. Patients with uncontrolled seizure activity are not deemed appropriate for outpatient surgery by most institutions.

Cystic Fibrosis. The extent of pulmonary involvement is the primary determinant of appropriateness for ambulatory surgery in patients with cystic fibrosis. Such patients should be evaluated several days before the proposed surgery; patients with symptomatic respiratory distress are better treated in an inpatient setting, where appropriate respiratory-care management and hydration can be administered.[53]

Malignant Hyperthermia Susceptibility. A malignant hyperthermia (MH)—susceptible patient is defined as having one or more of the following[54]:
1. A previous episode of MH
2. Masseter muscle rigidity with previous anesthesia
3. A first-degree relative with history of an MH episode or positive muscle biopsy

The MH-susceptible patient who has received a trigger-free anesthetic does not require overnight hospitalization based exclusively on being MH susceptible. The ambulatory facility should have the requisite monitoring and resuscitation capabilities, including a minimum of 36 vials of dantrolene, for managing the MH patient.[55] The patient should be scheduled as early in the day as possible to allow for extended patient observation for at least 2.5 hours after surgery, and the lack of symptoms of MH should be ensured before discharge is considered. A patient who exhibits marked rigidity of the jaw muscles should not be discharged. Overnight observation is required for temperature rise, myoglobinuria, elevated CK levels, or progression to an MH episode. Patients who experience milder increases in jaw tension should be observed for signs and symptoms of MH for at least 12 hours. If there is evidence of myoglobinuria (dark, cola-colored urine), elevated temperature and pulse rate, or abnormality of acid-base balance, the patient should be admitted and observed overnight.[56] Written discharge instructions should include (1) how to monitor the patient's temperature at home, (2) how to recognize the signs and symptoms of MH, and (3) contact information if emergency medical advise is required.[57]

Morbid Obesity. The uncomplicated morbidly obese patient is an appropriate candidate for select outpatient surgery.[58,59] However, morbidly obese patients with significant preexisting cardiac, hepatic, pulmonary, or renal disease should be managed as inpatients. Late problems are more likely to occur when the body mass index reaches 35 to 40 kg/m^2; this is considered by some to be the cutoff point for ambulatory surgery.[17,60] The laparoscopic adjustable gastric banding procedure has opened the door for bariatric surgery to be performed on an outpatient basis, because this procedure does not open the digestive tract.[58,61-64] The ability to sufficiently manage postoperative pain and address postoperative ambulation should be discussed preoperatively by the surgeon and anesthesia provider. The morbidly obese patient is at risk for persistent hypoxemia in the postanesthesia care unit (PACU), which may necessitate overnight supplemental oxygen therapy.

BOX 38-1

Ambulatory Surgery Considerations for the Patient with Obstructive Sleep Apnea

Ambulatory Surgery Center

The facility should have (a) a transfer agreement with an inpatient facility in place, (b) emergency difficult-airway equipment, (c) consensus on availability of respiratory care equipment (i.e., nebulizers, CPAP equipment, ventilators), (d) radiology facilities (for portable chest radiograph), and (e) clinical laboratory facilities (for blood gases, electrolytes).

Patient

Acceptability dependent on (a) sleep apnea status, (b) anatomic and physiologic abnormalities, (c) status of coexisting diseases, (d) anticipated need for postoperative opioids, and (e) patient age.

Procedure (Type of Surgery/Anesthesia)

Acceptable:

Superficial surgery/local or regional anesthesia
Minor orthopedic surgery/local or regional anesthesia
Lithotripsy
No consensus (equivocal):
Superficial surgery/general anesthesia
Tonsillectomy in children >3 years old
Minor orthopedic surgery/general anesthesia
Gynecologic laparoscopy

Unacceptable:

Airway surgery (adult, e.g., UPPP)
Tonsillectomy in children <3 years old
Laparoscopic surgery, upper abdomen

Postoperative

Supplemental oxygen should be administered as needed to maintain acceptable oxyhemoglobin saturation. It may be discontinued when baseline saturations are maintained on room air.
CPAP or NIPPV should be administered as soon as feasible postoperatively to patients with OSA who were receiving it preoperatively.

Discharge Considerations:

Baseline room air oxyhemoglobin saturation should return to baseline
When left undisturbed, patients should not exhibit hypoxemia or clinical airway obstruction
Anticipate longer phase II recovery stays, median of 7 hours after last episode of airway obstruction or hypoxemia while breathing room air in an unstimulating environment.
Ensure adequate postdischarge observation.

Modified from American Society of Anesthesiologists Task Force on Perioperative Management. Practice guidelines for the perioperative management of patients with obstructive sleep apnea: a report by the American Society of Anesthesiologists Task Force on Perioperative Management of Patients with Obstructive Sleep Apnea. Anesthesiology. 2006;104:1081-1093.
CPAP, *Continuous positive airway pressure;* NIPPV, *noninvasive positive pressure ventilation;* OSA, *obstructive sleep apnea;* UPPP, *uvulopalatopharyngoplasty.*

Morbid obesity is associated with an increased risk of obstructive sleep apnea.[59] Preoperative airway evaluation (e.g., Mallampati classification, nuchal girth, redundant pharyngeal tissue) is important. An assessment of intubating conditions in the patient with obstructive sleep apnea found a 22% incidence of difficult endotracheal intubation.[65] The likelihood of a difficult airway has to be assessed preoperatively and the ability to manage the difficult airway ensured. If continuous positive airway pressure (CPAP) is part of the patient's management of obstructive sleep apnea, it should be available for use in the immediate postoperative recovery phase. Opioids should be avoided in these patients and pain controlled with alternative techniques (e.g., nonopioid analgesics, local wound infiltration with local anesthesia).[66] One retrospective study of patients with confirmed obstructive sleep apnea found no increase in hospital admissions following ambulatory surgery.[67] The decision whether to provide for the patient with obstructive sleep apnea in the ambulatory setting should be contingent on certain criteria being met (Box 38-1).[68] Consideration should be given to scheduling these patients early in the day to allow for prolonged observation.

Reactive Airway Disease. Before surgery is performed, the severity of reactive airway disease must be assessed, and optimal disease management should be achieved. A chest radiograph is indicated only if the patient is suspected of having an acute infiltrative process or if deterioration in the patient's physical condition has occurred. Likewise, arterial blood gases are indicated when signs and symptoms of chronic respiratory insufficiency are suspected. The patient may be best managed as an inpatient if indications for a chest radiograph or arterial blood gases are met. Consultation with the patient's internist may help in formulating therapeutic modalities and establishing baseline conditions for this patient. Patients receiving long-term medication therapy should continue to take their medications until the time of surgery. All parties involved must anticipate the possibility of admitting the patient to the hospital should the symptoms of the disease become exacerbated.

Sickle Cell Disease. The possibility of sickle cell hemoglobinopathy should be considered in every African American when obtaining the preoperative medical history. If individual or family history is suggestive of the disease, a Sickledex may be obtained in children 6 months of age and older to determine the presence of sickle-shaped red blood cells.[69] The patient with sickle cell disease is at risk for crisis development should acidosis, dehydration, or hypoxia occur. The select patient diagnosed with sickle cell disease is an acceptable outpatient candidate, but this patient is not without risk.[70] Sickling of the red blood cells may occur when the patient with sickle cell trait is subjected to hypoxia.[71] If the patient with sickle cell anemia is to be cared for in the ambulatory setting, certain criteria must be satisfied[72]:

1. The patient should have no major organ disease as a result of the sickle cell disease.
2. The patient should have not had a sickle cell crisis for at least 1 year.

3. The patient should be compliant with the prescribed medical care.
4. On discharge, the patient should be within 15 minutes' travel time to a facility prepared to care for the patient.
5. The patient should receive close follow-up postoperative care.

The procedure should not be a prolonged surgery that is associated with blood loss. The patient should arrive earlier than normal so adequate intravenous hydration can be established. The patient's surgery should be scheduled early in the day to allow for extended postoperative monitoring before the patient is discharged from the ambulatory center.

Social Considerations

Factors other than physical condition must be weighed in considering a patient for outpatient surgery (Box 38-2). The lack of appropriate home conditions and care makes the outpatient option less desirable.

Unacceptable Patient Conditions for Ambulatory Surgery

Certain situations make ambulatory surgery impractical. Each patient must be considered individually for acceptability as an outpatient surgical candidate. Adult patients believed to be unacceptable candidates[73] are those with any of the following:

- Unstable American Society of Anesthesiologists (ASA) physical status classification III or IV (e.g., cardiac, renal, endocrine, pulmonary, hepatic, or cancer diagnoses)
- Active substance/alcohol abuse
- Psychosocial difficulties (see Box 38-2)
- Poorly controlled seizures
- Previously unevaluated and managed obstructive sleep apnea
- Uncontrolled diabetes
- Current sepsis or infectious disease necessitating separate isolation facilities
- Anticipated postoperative pain not expected to be controlled with oral analgesics or local anesthesia techniques

PATIENT EVALUATION AND PREPARATION

To recognize anesthetic risks and determine the patient's suitability for the planned procedure, preoperative evaluation is mandatory for all patients preparing to undergo outpatient anesthesia and surgery. Challenges for the outpatient team will be organizing and accomplishing all the necessary tests and evaluations while causing the least inconvenience to the patient and maintaining an expedient surgical process. The preoperative interview gathers pertinent patient information and clarifies risk factors that may affect surgery and outcome. Additionally, by obtaining a thorough current and past medical history— including a personal and family anesthetic history—the staff may determine what further patient workup is required before surgery. A formalized preanesthesia assessment clinic is the

most comprehensive and cost-effective process for preoperative evaluation and preparation.[74] Preoperative screening also allows the staff to communicate what will be expected of the patient in the perioperative phases. Consultations, laboratory tests, and diagnostic procedures should be performed based on clinical findings rather than on a preestablished regimen of "standard" tests. Without any discoveries from the medical history and physical examination, the probability of observing a significant abnormality is negligible in diagnostic procedures, including electrocardiogram, chest radiograph, and laboratory tests. Abnormal tests results obtained from routine testing potentially alter patient care only 0.22% to 0.56% of the time.[75,76] Routine preoperative laboratory screening is neither cost-effective nor predictive of postoperative complications.[77,78]

Patient Interview

Patient screening should take place sufficiently in advance of the scheduled surgery to allow time for necessary risk assessment, preoperative testing, specialty consultations, and adjustments in patient care. Proper timing of the patient assessment, particularly for the patient with complex medical conditions, minimizes surgical delays and cancellations. The high-risk patient should be evaluated at least 1 week before the scheduled procedure. With respect to client convenience, the otherwise healthy individual who does not have the opportunity to visit the clinic can be evaluated on the day of surgery. In this circumstance, there is a higher potential for surgical postponement or cancellation with last-minute discovery (e.g., inappropriate fasting, suspected difficult airway).

Patient Orientation

The preoperative interview allows the staff to convey what is expected of the patient and what the patient can expect perioperatively. Providing instructions to the patient, verbally and in writing, results in improved patient compliance. An information packet given to the patient at the interview is beneficial. It should detail specific instructions and concerns related to the procedure (Box 38-3).

At the time of the patient interview, or at a mutually agreeable time, patients and family members should have the opportunity to become acquainted with the ambulatory surgery facilities and the anticipated sequence of events. This includes orientation to the laboratory and procedure areas, changing areas, waiting room, play areas, and the short-stay area, where the patient remains after surgery until discharge. This orientation is designed to reduce patient and family fear by providing relevant perioperative information (e.g., directions, anticipated schedule, instructions for physiologic preparation of the child, expected postoperative course, and discharge instructions), offering reassurance, and enhancing coping skills through familiarity. A variety of techniques may be incorporated to prepare the child for the operative procedure. Children can be oriented to equipment that is commonly used in the perioperative setting (e.g., anesthetic mask, intravenous therapy equipment, the anesthesia machine and circuit, blood pressure cuff, thermometer, and postoperative oxygen therapy devices). Children can be told when and where they will be reunited with their parents after surgery.

History and Physical

A thorough medical history and physical examination performed by a member of the medical staff should be available in the patient's chart before the surgery is performed. A separate anesthesia history should be incorporated into a questionnaire

---

BOX 38-3

Preoperative Patient Instructions

Preoperative Instructions
Tell the patient when and where laboratory tests, consultations, and diagnostic procedures will be completed.
Clarify the appropriate time for the patient to be without food and drink.

Registration on the Day of Surgery
Tell the patient the time to report for surgery, and mention that a wait can normally be expected.
Describe the location of the parking areas.
Tell the patient where to report for surgery.

Ambulatory Center Policies
Inform the patient and family about expected conduct.
Explain the ambulatory facility policies to the patient and family.
Describe the family waiting area and services (e.g., dining areas).
Review advance-directive information as required by law in some states.
Review the patient's right-to-privacy policies.
Outline the facility's cancellation policies: late arrival, nonadherence to fasting guidelines, inappropriate transportation home, lack of responsible person to help patient postoperatively, interim changes in patient's health status (e.g., upper respiratory tract infection [URTI]).

Personal Considerations
Tell patient to wear comfortable, loose-fitting clothing that may be easily stored.
Instruct patient to wear no jewelry or makeup (remove nail polish from at least one nail).

Instruct patient to bring personal toilet items (e.g., comb, brush, toothbrush) as required.
Caution patient to leave valuables at home.
Tell caregiver to bring child's favorite toy, comforter, or pacifier, or light reading material for the older patient.

Postoperative Considerations
Inform patient and family of the discharge time, including the time spent in the postanesthesia care unit and the customary length of stay until discharge.
Instruct patient in the manner of discharge, the appropriate transportation arrangements, and the necessity for the presence of a responsible caregiver.
Give the patient postoperative instructions: no driving, alcohol, or major decisions postoperatively for at least 24 to 48 hours after anesthesia. (See Box 38-11 for additional information.)
Inform the patient where, how, and to whom complications should be reported. Supply telephone numbers.
Indicate the possibility of hospital admission.

Considerations if the Patient's Physical Condition Changes
Tell the patient to contact the surgeon.
Tell the patient to contact the anesthetist.
Tell the patient to call regarding cancellations or physical condition changes (e.g., URTI).

---

specifically designed for preanesthetic evaluation; the anesthesia provider should review this history with the patient. Such a review may be accomplished in a written format and would include a general review of the major systems, history of allergies, current medicines, past and present medical problems, laboratory and diagnostic test results, and patient and family response to previous anesthetics. Prior anesthesia records should be examined for complications, response to anesthesia, and postoperative course. Patient evaluation should be conducted within 30 days of the scheduled surgery for medically stable patients and within 72 hours of the scheduled surgery for high-risk patients. The clinician should determine whether any changes might have occurred since the original history and physical examination were performed, and an update note should be made on the day of the procedure. A review of current vital signs, laboratory test results, diagnostic reports, and fasting status should be made.

Laboratory Evaluation
Each ambulatory center should have a consensus regarding the minimum testing requirement for surgery. These testing criteria depend on the proposed surgical procedure, the patient's medication history, and the patient's physical condition. Certain states and regions have established minimum testing requirements. However, conducting a battery of preoperative laboratory

tests without specific indications has not been shown to reduce patient morbidity,[76] is not cost-effective, and may even place the patient at increased risk.[79] Discriminating laboratory testing, based on findings from the history and physical examination and primarily designed to evaluate a patient's comorbidities and surgical risk, seems to be indicated. Normal laboratory test and diagnostic procedure results are deemed current if the tests are performed within 6 months of surgery if the patient's physical condition remains stable.[80] Exceptions include serum potassium level determinations, which should be obtained within 7 days of surgery for patients receiving diuretics or digitalis, and blood glucose level determinations, which should be obtained on the same day of surgery for patients with diabetes controlled by medication. Physical conditions and systemic illnesses in which preoperative laboratory testing is appropriate are listed in Box 38-4.

Pregnancy Testing
The medical facility should have established guidelines delineating when testing for pregnancy is appropriate. If the medical history and physical examination indicate that the patient may be pregnant, or if pregnancy might complicate the surgery, then pregnancy testing should be performed. It is important that the patient be educated as to the potential risks of exposing a fetus

BOX 38-4

Indications for Laboratory Testing

Complete Blood Count
Hematologic disorder
Vascular procedure
Chemotherapy
Unknown sickle cell syndrome status

Hemoglobin/Hematocrit
Age <6 months (<1 yr if born premature)
Hematologic malignancy
Recent radiation or chemotherapy
Renal disease
Anticoagulant therapy
Procedure with moderate to high blood loss potential
Coexisting systemic disorders (e.g., cystic fibrosis, prematurity, severe malnutrition, renal failure, liver disease, congenital heart disease)

White Blood Cell Count
Leukemia and lymphomas
Recent radiation or chemotherapy
Suspected infection that would lead to cancellation of surgery
Aplastic anemia
Hypersplenism
Autoimmune collagen vascular disease

Blood Glucose Level
Diabetes mellitus
Current corticosteroid use
History of hypoglycemia
Adrenal disease
Cystic fibrosis

Serum Chemistry
Renal disease
Adrenal or thyroid disease
Chemotherapy
Pituitary or hypothalamic disease
Body fluid loss or shifts (e.g., dehydration, bowel prep)
Central nervous system disease

Potassium
Digoxin therapy
Diuretic therapy

Creatinine and Blood Urea Nitrogen
Cardiovascular disease (e.g., hypertension)
Renal disease
Adrenal disease
Diabetes mellitus
Diuretic therapy
Digoxin therapy
Body fluid loss or shifts (e.g., dehydration, bowel prep)
Procedure requiring radiocontrast

Liver Function Tests
Hepatic disease
Exposure to hepatitis
Therapy with hepatotoxic agents

Coagulation Studies

Prothrombin Time and Activated Partial Thromboplastin Time
Leukemia
Hepatic disease
Bleeding disorder
Anticoagulant therapy
Severe malnutrition or malabsorption

Platelet Count and Bleeding Time
Bleeding disorder
Abnormal hemorrhage, purpura, easy bruisability

Urinalysis
Not indicated as a routine screening test

Pregnancy
Possibility of pregnancy

Serum Medication Levels
Monitor for medications (e.g., theophylline, phenytoin, digoxin, carbamazepine) if patient exhibits signs of ineffective therapy, potential drug side effects, poor drug compliance, or has recently changed medication therapy without documentation of drug level

Modified from Marley RA. Preoperative preparation. In: Zaglaniczny K, Aker J, eds. Clinical Guide to Pediatric Anesthesia. Philadelphia: Saunders; 1999:34-35.

to an anesthetic. Whenever possible, especially in the adolescent population, a female staff member should question the patient in the absence of family members.

Diagnostic Procedures

Chest Radiography. Performing routine preoperative chest radiography is not recommended without specific indications from the history and physical examination. Its value as a screening tool has been questioned, and some contend that the history and physical examination are as efficient as chest radiography for screening for chronic lung pathology.[79] In asymptomatic individuals younger than 75 years of age, the risk involved in obtaining

a routine preoperative chest radiograph is greater than the benefit.[81] Box 38-5 cites indications for obtaining a preoperative chest radiograph or electrocardiogram.

Electrocardiography. Few data support the routine performance of 12-lead electrocardiographic screening before surgery, because it has not been shown to be cost-effective,[82-84] is a poor predictor of perioperative complications,[85,86] and is of limited value in detecting ischemia[87] in asymptomatic individuals. The use of age as a criterion for obtaining baseline electrocardiograms has recently been questioned[85,88]; however, if a minimum age criterion is deemed appropriate, it has been argued that it should be raised to 60 years of age.[88-90] It has been proposed

---

BOX 38-5

Indications for Diagnostic Procedures

Chest Radiograph

Previous abnormal results on chest radiography

History of malignancy in which pulmonary metastasis might alter surgical therapy

History of tuberculosis or positive skin test result for tuberculosis for which no treatment was given

History suggestive of pulmonary infection (e.g., new or chronic productive cough or blood-tinged or purulent-appearing sputum)

Suspected intrathoracic pathologic condition (e.g., tumors, vascular ring)

History of congenital heart disease

History of prematurity associated with residual bronchopulmonary dysplasia

Severe obstructive sleep apnea (may have cardiomegaly)

Down syndrome (may have asymptomatic subluxation of the atlantoaxial junction)

Symptomatic or debilitating asthma, chronic obstructive pulmonary disease, or cardiovascular disease

Electrocardiogram

Patients at risk for cardiovascular disease (e.g., cocaine abuse, hypertension, renal disease, circulatory disease, thyroid disease, diabetes mellitus [age 40 years or older], significant pulmonary disease)

History of previously unevaluated pathologic-sounding murmur or palpitation

Family history reveals possibility of inherited prolonged QT syndrome

History of moderate to severe sleep apnea or chronic anatomic airway obstruction (e.g., Pierre Robin syndrome) may present risk for right-sided heart strain

From Marley RA. Preoperative preparation. In: Zaglaniczny K, Aker J, eds. Clinical Guide to Pediatric Anesthesia. Philadelphia: Saunders; 1999:29-45; Cassidy J, Marley RA. Preoperative assessment of the ambulatory patient. J Perianesth Nurs. 1996;11:334-343.

BOX 38-6

Risk Factors for Pulmonary Aspiration

Age extremes (<1 yr or >70 yr)

Anxiety

Ascites

Collagen vascular disease (e.g., scleroderma)

Depression

Esophageal surgery

Exogenous medications (opioids or premedications [e.g., barbiturates] and anticholinergics)

Failed intubation or difficult airway history

Gastroesophageal junction dysfunction (e.g., hiatal hernia)

Mechanical obstruction (e.g., pyloric stenosis, duodenal ulcer)

Metabolic disorders (e.g., hypothyroidism, chronic diabetes, hepatic failure, hyperglycemia, obesity, renal failure, and uremia)

Neurologic sequelae (e.g., developmental delays, head injury, hypotonia, seizures)

Pain

Pregnancy

Prematurity with respiratory problems

Smoking

Type and composition of gastric contents (e.g., solid foods, milk products)

---

that routinely acquiring a preoperative electrocardiogram is not indicated in the elderly patient for ambulatory surgery.[91] Box 38-5 cites indications for obtaining a preoperative electrocardiogram.

Fasting Status and Aspiration Risk

Part of the preoperative evaluation process identifies patients at risk for aspirating gastric contents into the lungs and developing aspiration pneumonitis. Factors associated with an increased risk of pulmonary aspiration of gastric contents[92-103] are listed in Box 38-6.

Recent ingestion of food and liquid before surgery contributes to an increased risk of aspiration. Solid foods must be digested to a bolus diameter of less than 2 mm before the food can pass through the pylorus.[104] This process normally takes several hours for solids, whereas liquids pass through the pylorus in 1 to 2 hours. Historically, patients have been required to fast for extended periods in an attempt to ensure an empty stomach. However, sustained fasting does not ensure that the stomach will be empty at the time of surgery.[105] The traditional policy

of fasting after midnight fails to address several variables that influence gastric emptying for surgery:

- The time of the scheduled surgery
- The time at which the patient retired for the night
- The variability of gastric emptying for solids and fluids across individuals

Several problems have been associated with prolonged fasting:

- Dehydration
- Hypoglycemia[106]
- Hypovolemia
- Increased irritability
- Enhanced preoperative anxiety[107]
- Reduced compliance with preoperative fasting orders
- Thirst and related discomfort (e.g., hunger, headache, unhappiness)

Data suggest that liquids (e.g., clear apple juice, clear broth, coffee, gelatin, Popsicles, pulp-free orange juice, water, and weak tea) may be given to healthy, unpremedicated patients up to 2 hours[108-110] to 3 hours[111,112] before surgery without placing them at increased risk for aspiration. There is no increase in gastric volume, nor is there a decrease in gastric pH, at the time of elective surgery. The studies that allowed patients to consume clear liquids until 2 to 3 hours before surgery demonstrated that although the patients appeared to be at no greater risk of aspirating gastric contents, the pH of the stomach contents remained less than 2.5. In light of these findings, recommended fasting guidelines for the otherwise healthy individual have been liberalized (Table 38-1).[113]

Special Considerations

Daily Medications

Patients should continue to take their prescribed cardiopulmonary medications on the morning of the surgery. The medications

TABLE 38-1	Fasting Guidelines for Healthy Patients Undergoing Elective Procedures	
Ingested Material	**Minimum Fasting Period (hr) All Ages**	
Clear liquids*	2	
Breast milk	4	
Infant formula	6	
Nonhuman milk†	6	
Light meal‡	6	

From Warner MA, et al. Practice guidelines for preoperative fasting and the use of pharmacologic agents to reduce the risk of pulmonary aspiration: application to healthy patients undergoing elective procedures. Anesthesiology. 1999;90:896-905.
*Examples of clear liquids include water, fruit juices without pulp, carbonated beverages, clear tea, and black coffee.
†Because nonhuman milk is similar to solids in gastric emptying time, the amount ingested must be considered when determining an appropriate fasting period.
‡A light meal typically consists of toast and clear liquids. Meals that include fried or fatty foods or meat may prolong gastric emptying time. Both the amount and type of foods ingested must be considered when determining an appropriate fasting period.

may be taken with a minimum of water (up to 150 mL in adults and up to 75 mL in children) up to 1 hour before anesthesia.[114]

Warfarin Sodium. An early decision of whether the administration of warfarin sodium should be continued must be made in consultation with the surgeon and the patient's internist. The question of whether the disadvantages of stopping the administration of this medication before surgery outweigh any advantage must be addressed. If the decision to withhold warfarin is made, the drug should be discontinued for 4 to 5 days before the scheduled surgery,[115] and a prothrombin time or international normalized ratio (INR) should be determined on the day of surgery.[116] A bridging program involving low molecular-weight heparin may be indicated, and a medical consult should be considered. Tinker and Tarhan[117] withheld oral anticoagulants preoperatively for 1 to 3 days, then reinstated the anticoagulant between 1 and 7 days after surgery; the investigators did not observe an increase in thromboembolic problems.

Diabetes

Recommended care for the diabetic patient who is undergoing ambulatory surgery is a subject of debate and lacks clear guidelines. The patient with diabetes should receive an early and thorough preoperative evaluation, including electrocardiography, history and physical examination, and laboratory analysis. The patient with insulin-dependent diabetes whose diabetes is not well controlled and whose serum glucose levels are prone to wide fluctuations may be best treated in the inpatient setting. Considerations for care of the patient with diabetes who is undergoing ambulatory surgery include:

1. Scheduling the patient early in the day
2. Instructing the patient to have nothing to eat or drink after midnight the night before surgery if the procedure is scheduled early in the day
3. Monitoring the patient's blood or serum glucose levels on arrival to the ambulatory center by use of a capillary test strip or laboratory analysis

4. Preventing hypoglycemia while maintaining blood glucose levels at less than 180 mg/dL[118]
5. Returning the patient to preoperative activities of daily living (e.g., baseline activity status, nutrition habits) as soon as possible
6. Making the patient aware that admission to the hospital is likely if persistent nausea and vomiting prevent resumption of normal dietary intake

Heart Murmur

The surgical patient with a heart murmur requires further workup if the condition was previously undetected. Heart murmurs are categorized as innocent or pathologic. Pathologic murmurs may be due to complex congenital malformations or heart disease and have accompanying physical dysfunction, whereas with innocent murmurs, the patient may be completely asymptomatic.[119] Whether the murmur is benign, functional, or caused by organic heart disease, cardiologic assessment should be obtained before the induction of anesthesia.

Rhinorrhea

From 20% to 30% of all children display symptoms of rhinorrhea a good portion of the year. Children younger than 2 years of age are prone to 5 to 10 viral respiratory infections annually.[120] For the child undergoing ambulatory surgery, individual patient evaluation is required for a runny nose. The history and physical examination are beneficial in determining the cause. The differential diagnosis of rhinorrhea should include[50]:

- Allergic (seasonal) rhinitis
- Bacterial infection (early stages)
- Flu syndrome
- URTI
- Vasomotor rhinitis
- Nothing found

The clinician obtaining the patient history should try to ascertain the allergic or acute nature of the runny nose and determine whether it is normal for the child or an illness has recently developed and worsened. Recently acquired (within 12 to 24 hours of surgery) rhinorrhea[50] or chronic rhinorrhea[121] in the otherwise fit child is not a contraindication to surgery. The differentiation between a noninfectious and an infectious runny nose might influence the decision of whether the procedure should be delayed (Box 38-7). Surgery might be delayed for only 2 weeks in the child with localized infectious rhinorrhea.[122]

Considerations for Postponing Surgery

Lack of Drug Compliance

The patient with uncontrolled hypertension or diabetes who has wide swings in blood pressure or blood glucose levels may not be suitable for outpatient surgery; such conditions should be optimally managed before outpatient surgery and anesthesia are performed.

Fasting Status

For safety reasons, the patient not adhering to the fasting guidelines should not undergo surgery, and the rationale of not eating before surgery should be reinforced.

Suspicion of Pregnancy

If the patient responds that she may be pregnant or if clinical signs are indicative of pregnancy, surgery should be delayed until determination of whether the patient is pregnant can be made. Decisions about whether surgery should be performed and what

Differential Diagnosis of Rhinorrhea

Noninfectious Runny Nose
Allergic rhinitis
    Seasonal
    Perennial
Vasomotor rhinitis
    Emotional (crying)
    Temperature

Infectious Runny Nose
Viral infections
    Nasopharyngitis (common cold)
    Contagious disease (e.g., chickenpox, measles)
Acute bacterial infections
    Streptococcal tonsillitis
    Meningitis

From Berry FA. Pre-existing medical conditions of pediatric patients. Semin Anesth. 1984;3:24-31.

type of anesthesia should be used can be based on pregnancy test results.

Upper Respiratory Tract Infection

URTI is the most common reason for delaying surgery in children.[123] In patients with an acute infection, differentiating between a bacterial infection as causative of the URTI and other causes—such as uncomplicated viral infection (afebrile, clear secretions) or allergic conditions—is important. Differentiating between a noninfectious process and an infectious process is paramount in the decision whether the procedure should be performed. This differentiation may be difficult to make early in the course of the disease. Symptoms of URTI include the following:

1. Elevated white blood cell count (greater than 12,000 with a left shift)
2. Mucopurulent nasal secretions
3. Inflamed and reddened mucosa (nasopharyngeal and oropharyngeal) (with allergic rhinitis, the nasal mucosa is ashen and boggy)
4. Positive chest findings (e.g., congestion, rales)
5. Temperature of 37.5° C to 38° C (greater than 38° C usually associated with lower respiratory tract involvement)
6. Tonsillitis
7. Viral ulcers in the oropharynx

Other accompanying symptoms may include conjunctivitis, coughing (nonproductive), fatigue, itching, laryngitis, malaise, myalgias, sneezing, and sore throat. Laboratory and diagnostic testing in children with suspected URTI includes nasal or throat cultures if signs of an infectious process are observed. A chest radiograph is not warranted, especially if chest sounds are clear.[124] Similarly, the value of obtaining a white blood cell count has been challenged because the results may be normal and typically do not influence whether to proceed with the surgery.[124]

Anesthetizing the patient who has a URTI has been shown to increase the incidence of respiratory-associated complications two- to seven-fold.[125] The anesthetized patient with a URTI is more prone to experience breath holding, bronchospasm,

coughing, hypoxemia, increased secretions, laryngospasm, pneumonia, atelectasis, croup, and stridor.[126,127] Risk factors for the development of perioperative adverse respiratory events in children with URTI include endotracheal intubation (<5 years of age), history of prematurity, history of reactive airway disease, paternal smoking, surgery involving the airway, the presence of copious secretions, and nasal congestion.[128] A minimum of 4 hours of postoperative observation is appropriate before the patient is considered for discharge from the ambulatory setting. Each case should be reviewed individually. The decision to operate frequently depends on the urgency of the surgery, the duration and complexity of the surgery, and the need for instrumentation of the airway.[129]

Children with uncomplicated URTIs may undergo elective procedures without significantly increasing anesthesia complications.[130] Guidelines for deciding whether surgery should be performed in children with URTI apply to both the symptomatic and the asymptomatic child. In the case of the symptomatic child (fever >38° C, mucopurulent sputum or secretions, wheezing, generally seems sick), the surgery should be canceled and rescheduled to at least 4 weeks later.[131] For the asymptomatic child (nonpurulent nasal secretions, unremarkable chest examination), anesthesia and surgery can be performed if the following conditions are met:

1. The child is older than 1 year.
2. The surgery is not of the thorax or abdomen.
3. The child is otherwise healthy; no other illness that might complicate perioperative patient management exists.
4. Endotracheal intubation is not planned. The laryngeal mask airway has been found to contribute to fewer adverse respiratory events than the endotracheal tube.[132] Endotracheal intubation in a child increases the risk of adverse respiratory complications 11-fold.[125]

Each case has to be reviewed individually and consideration given to the urgency of the surgery, the duration and complexity of the surgery, the number of times the procedure has been canceled, and the wishes of the family and patient.

PREMEDICATION

Premedicating the ambulatory surgery patient with sedative agents remains controversial. The concern about giving anxiolytic and sedative medications is related to their potential to prolong the patient's stay. Nonsteroidal antiinflammatory drugs (NSAIDs) given orally, when indicated, should be considered preoperatively.[17] Preemptive analgesia may reduce postoperative pain by preventing surgically induced peripheral and central sensitization.[133] Lower postoperative pain scores and less opioid use have been seen when NSAIDs were given prior to surgery.[134] The use of premedication should not become routine; rather, the decision to administer these agents should be based on individual need and desired benefit. Common indications for preoperative medication are:

- To decrease patient anxiety and fear
- To facilitate smooth induction and emergence from anesthesia
- To supplement anesthesia and reduce the need for general anesthetic agents
- To reduce the volume and acidity of gastric contents
- To provide a more pleasant stay in the PACU

Pulmonary Aspiration Prophylaxis

Patients at higher risk for aspirating gastric contents should be given medications before surgery to raise gastric pH and lower gastric volume, with the hope of minimizing their risk for pulmonary aspiration. Pulmonary aspiration prophylaxis in the patient not at risk is not recommended.[102]

Antacids

The value of oral antacids lies in their ability to rapidly reduce gastric acidity; they are effective in raising pH in 15 to 20 minutes.[135] This characteristic is useful in emergency situations, but it is of limited application in the ambulatory setting. Although oral antacids raise gastric pH, they have the disadvantage of increasing gastric volume. Clear, nonparticulate oral antacids (e.g., two tablets of Alka-Seltzer Gold in 30 mL of water; 30 mL [0.4 mL/kg pediatric dose] of 0.3 M sodium citrate [Bicitra]) are preferred over particulate antacids, such as Maalox or Mylanta, because particulate antacids may produce pulmonary injury if aspirated.[136]

Gastrokinetics

Reducing the volume of gastric fluid with the gastrokinetic agent metoclopramide (Reglan) should help minimize the risk of aspiration. Metoclopramide has been demonstrated to decrease gastric fluid volume by reducing gastric emptying time without increasing pH in adults[137] and in children.[138] Metoclopramide may also reduce the risk of pulmonary aspiration by increasing lower esophageal sphincter tone.[139] It has been suggested to exert a central antiemetic effect (which is a dopaminergic receptor–blocking property of chemoreceptor trigger zone).[140] The antiemetic effect of metoclopramide has not been confirmed by other authors.[141] The combination of metoclopramide with a histamine$_2$ (H$_2$)-receptor antagonist has been shown to be effective in raising gastric volume pH and decreasing gastric volume content.[142]

The intramuscular dose is 10 mg for adults (0.1 mg/kg for children[98]), given at least 45 minutes before surgery.[143] The intravenous dose is 10 to 20 mg (0.15 to 0.2 mg/kg) given over the course of 3 to 5 minutes[144] at least 30 minutes[145] to 45 minutes[143] before surgery. These regimens allow sufficient time for the desired results to be achieved. The oral dose, 10 mg for adults (0.1 mg/kg for children[98]), achieves peak plasma concentrations 40 to 120 minutes after administration.[146]

H$_2$ Receptor Antagonists

Selective and competitive H$_2$-receptor antagonists, such as cimetidine (Tagamet), famotidine (Pepcid), and ranitidine (Zantac), block hydrogen ion release by gastric parietal cells.[147] These drugs do not alter the pH of gastric fluid already present in the stomach. These medications may be administered the night before surgery, on the day of surgery, or both, to reduce gastric acidity. Famotidine and ranitidine have longer durations of action,[148] are more potent,[149] and exhibit a lower potential for side effects than cimetidine.[150]

Cimetidine. In one study, an intravenous adult cimetidine dose of 300 mg helped reduce the risk of pulmonary aspiration.[151] The oral dose is 300 mg (3 to 4 mg/kg) for adults[152] and 7.5 mg/kg for children,[153] given from 1.5 to 3 hours before surgery. This is effective in reducing the risk of chemical pneumonitis should pulmonary aspiration occur.

Famotidine. The intravenous dose of famotidine is 20 mg for adults, given 15 to 30 minutes before surgery; this is effective in increasing gastric pH.[154] When given electively, oral famotidine (40 mg) is given the night before surgery and on arising the morning of surgery. This results in a mean gastric pH of 6.2 and a gastric fluid volume of 7.8 mL at the time of the outpatient surgery.[150] When compared with ranitidine, famotidine was slower in raising the gastric pH to safe levels.[155]

Ranitidine. The intravenous dose of ranitidine is 50 to 100 mg[151] or 1 to 2.5 mg/kg.[156] This drug decreases the risk associated with pulmonary aspiration. The oral dose of 150 to 300 mg for adults (2.5 mg/kg for children[98]), given 1 to 3 hours before surgery, increases gastric pH, whereas gastric fluid volume may not be less than 25 mL.[157,158] Comparable results were noted when ranitidine (150 mg) was given at bedtime and again on arising the morning of surgery[150] or when it was given orally 1 to 2 hours before surgery.[157]

Gastric Proton-Pump Inhibitors

Omeprazole. Omeprazole (Prilosec) causes dose-dependent intracellular inhibition of gastric acid secretion in humans without affecting gastric volume.[159] Omeprazole has a longer duration of action than the H$_2$-receptor antagonist agents in suppressing gastric acid secretion[160] and appears to cause no significant side effects.[161]

The intravenous dose of omeprazole is 40 mg, administered after the induction of anesthesia. This is as effective as ranitidine in raising gastric pH above 2.5.[162]

The oral dose is 80 mg, given the evening before surgery. This has increased mean gastric pH to 4.56, compared with the pH of 2.05 that was achieved with the administration of a placebo.[159] Orally administered omeprazole, 40 mg, was not found to be as effective as either famotidine, 40 mg, or ranitidine, 300 mg, in protecting against pulmonary aspiration in parturients.[163]

Lansoprazole and Rabeprazole. Orally administered lansoprazole (Prevacid), 30 mg, and rabeprazole (Aciphex), 20 mg, given the day prior to surgery and on the morning of surgery were not as effective in raising pH and lowering gastric volume as a single morning-of-surgery dose of ranitidine, 150 mg.[164]

Pantoprazole. Pantoprazole (Protonix) is marketed as an intravenous solution, as well as tablets, which may prove useful for perioperative use. Intravenously administered pantoprazole, 40 mg, was comparable with ranitidine, 50 mg, in increasing pH and reducing gastric fluid volume.[165]

ANESTHETIC CONSIDERATIONS

Anesthetic techniques suitable for outpatient surgery include general anesthesia, regional anesthesia, and monitored anesthesia care. The goals for outpatient anesthesia, regardless of the type administered, are listed in Box 38-8, and factors influencing the choice of anesthesia are shown in Box 38-9. The ideal anesthetic agent for ambulatory anesthesia—whether it is administered inhalationally, intravenously, locally, or regionally—is one with the appropriate pharmacokinetic traits (i.e., rapid onset and offset, short beta-elimination half-lives, inert metabolites, and insignificant side effects).

BOX **38-8**

Goals of Outpatient Anesthesia

Minimize the physiologic changes associated with anesthesia.
Provide a fast, smooth onset of anesthetic action.
Promote intraoperative amnesia and analgesia.
Afford suitable operating circumstances.
Minimize perioperative anesthetic side effects.
Allow rapid offset of anesthetic influence while maintaining patient comfort.

General Anesthesia

General anesthesia is the most widely used anesthetic technique for ambulatory surgery. General anesthesia should be achieved with the less soluble inhalation agents or with short-acting intravenous agents that have the capability of reversal if required. A combination of potent rapid-onset and rapid-offset inhalation agents (e.g., desflurane, sevoflurane), along with intravenous agents (e.g., propofol, intravenous opioids, short-acting muscle relaxants, NSAIDs), comprise general anesthesia in contemporary practice. The popularity of general anesthesia in the ambulatory setting is related to its acceptance by the patient, the anesthesia provider, and the surgeon, and to the consistent pace that can be maintained with regard to achieving a satisfactory state of anesthesia.

Depth-of-Anesthesia Monitoring

Recent advances in depth-of-anesthesia monitoring technology have made their presence felt in ambulatory anesthesia. With appropriate application of depth-of-anesthesia monitoring principles, rapid emergence and recovery from ambulatory anesthesia may be optimized, thus promoting beneficial turnover and discharge times.[166] Bispectral Index (BIS) monitoring has been found to correlate well with levels of sedation and amnesia.[167] Some of the purported advantages of BIS monitoring in the outpatient setting include reducing the amount of anesthetic agent required,[168] faster emergence from anesthesia,[169-173] and a reduction in phase II vomiting.[174] Not all studies in ambulatory populations have shown an enhanced recovery or quicker discharge home with the use of the BIS monitor.[175-177]

Airway Management

Issues regarding the use of general anesthesia with a face mask, a laryngeal mask airway (LMA), or an endotracheal tube in patients undergoing outpatient surgery are the same as those in patients undergoing inpatient surgery. The indications for intubating the trachea depend on the constraints of the surgery and the individual patient concerns (e.g., risk of regurgitation and aspiration, hypoventilation, access to the airway, use of muscle relaxants, and airway obstruction).

Drawbacks to endotracheal intubation specific to the outpatient setting must be considered. Resumption of dietary intake is prolonged in patients in whom the trachea was intubated for surgery.[178] More medications are administered to patients who require endotracheal intubation than to those who receive anesthesia through a mask.[179] The delayed oral intake and the increased total amount of medications required by endotracheal intubation may delay patient discharge. Irritation and trauma to the upper airway and trachea are a concern, especially in children. The development of postextubation croup is rare (0.1%),[180] but the potential for its occurrence must be considered in the plan for discharging the patient. Careful attention paid to minimizing intubating trauma, ensuring that an air leak is present at less than 40 cm H_2O,[179] and avoiding large-diameter endotracheal tubes helps reduce the incidence of postextubation croup in children.

The LMA has proven to be a popular and cost-effective airway management tool in the ambulatory setting.[25] Additional reported advantages of the LMA include less coughing, analgesic requirement, and sore throats following ambulatory surgery.[181,182]

Intravenous Fluid Therapy

Debate exists over whether all patients undergoing brief (less than 15 minutes) anesthesia require intravenous cannulation for uncomplicated surgery in which rapid recovery is expected. If an intravenous catheter is not inserted in children undergoing general anesthesia, the equipment and personnel trained in intravenous line placement should be immediately available in case they are needed. Generous intravenous fluid hydration, administered either preoperatively or intraoperatively, has several benefits. Keane and Murray[183] found quicker postoperative recovery (i.e., earlier discharge from the facility, earlier return to work) in fasting adult patients who received 2 L of intravenous fluid than in patients in whom fluids were withheld. Healthy adult outpatients were found to have fewer problems after surgery if they received 20 mL/kg of lactated Ringer's solution (with or without dextrose) prior to surgery[184] or throughout the perioperative phase.[185] These patients were less thirsty; reported a lower incidence of sore throat; and were not as prone to dizziness, drowsiness, and faintness on standing compared with patients for whom fluids were withheld perioperatively. Less thirst, dizziness, and drowsiness were observed in ambulatory patients undergoing short surgical procedures who were given 20 mL/kg of intravenous fluids, compared with patients who only received 2 mL/kg.[186] Less nausea and vomiting was reported in patients receiving liberal (15 to 30 mL/kg) intravenous solution, compared with patients who received 10 mL/kg.[187-190]

Intravenous cannulation should be used, and perioperative fluid should be administered in the following situations:

1. Procedures lasting longer than 30 minutes. Longer surgical times increase the risk of hypothermia, increase the amount of anesthetics delivered to the patient, and result in a delay of resumption of normal diet.
2. Procedures with an increased incidence of postoperative nausea and vomiting. Intravenous access permits the administration of antiemetic medications and allows hydration.
3. Procedures associated with postoperative discomfort. If anticipated postoperative pain is unlikely to be controlled by nonintravenous means, an avenue should be established for the administration of intravenous analgesics.
4. Prolonged fasting before surgery. If the child has been fasting for more than 15 hours, intravenous hydration is desirable for the maintenance of fluid and glucose homeostasis.
5. Procedures associated with intraoperative and postoperative bleeding.
6. Procedures associated with the use of perioperative antibiotics or patients who require the perioperative administration of antibiotics.

BOX 38-9

Considerations for Choice of Anesthetic

Surgical requirements
Skill of anesthesia provider
Patient choice
Patient age
American Society of Anesthesiologists physical status classification
Level of care available once patient is discharged from outpatient facility

Regional Anesthesia

The use of regional anesthesia in the ambulatory setting is well established. Local wound infiltration, peripheral nerve block, intravenous regional anesthesia, ophthalmic blocks (e.g., retrobulbar or periorbital), brachial plexus anesthesia, spinal anesthesia, and epidural anesthesia are all successfully used for outpatient surgery. The proper application of outpatient regional anesthesia requires knowledge of the anticipated surgical procedure (e.g., anesthesia requirements, length of procedure), proper patient selection, and skillful anesthesia providers who are capable of providing the required block. The shortest-acting agent capable of providing satisfactory central neuraxial blockade should be used in the ambulatory setting if unreasonable delays in discharge are to be avoided. Peripheral nerve blockade with longer-acting local anesthetics can provide up to 24 hours of analgesia postoperatively. The advantages and disadvantages of the use of outpatient regional anesthesia are listed in Box 38-10.

Patients must understand and be willing to accept this type of anesthesia before it is used. Special consideration must be given to senile and mentally disabled patients. Preanesthesia patient education and appropriately administered sedation with continual reassurance and support promote patient acceptance, cooperation, and understanding regarding regional anesthesia. Patients' orientation to regional anesthesia can appropriately begin with support and an introductory dialogue with their surgeon.

BOX 38-10

Advantages and Disadvantages of Outpatient Regional Anesthesia

Advantages

Recovery times are shorter than those of general anesthesia.[191]

Unanticipated admission to the hospital is reduced.

Phase I recovery bypass (fast-track) eligibility is high.[191]

Provides excellent immediate postoperative pain relief[192]

Results in better postoperative pain scores than general anesthesia[191]

Common side effects associated with general anesthesia (e.g., airway trauma, dizziness, "hangover," myalgia, nausea and vomiting, pharyngitis) are minimized.

The patient who fears general anesthesia or "loss of control" has a satisfactory alternative.

Disadvantages

Cooperation of the patient and the surgeon is required.

Regional anesthesia may require more time to provide than general anesthesia. In an ambulatory setting, where surgeries and patient stays tend to be of short duration, regional anesthesia may not be as well received. If a team approach is used, patient stays may be minimized by early placement of the proposed regional anesthetic if appropriate.

Inherent problems associated with regional anesthesia, regardless of inpatient or outpatient status, include the sympathetic block associated with spinal and epidural anesthesia, which may complicate the discharge course if residual block results in orthostatic hypotension.

The various types of regional anesthesia suitable for ambulatory surgery are reviewed in this chapter for their relevance to outpatient management.

Brachial Plexus Anesthesia

Brachial plexus anesthesia—involving the axillary, interscalene, and supraclavicular or infraclavicular approaches—is ideal for ambulatory surgery on the arm or shoulder.[193] The interscalene block is the most popular nerve block for shoulder surgery.[194] A potential drawback for brachial plexus anesthesia is the length of time (longer than 15 minutes) required before complete anesthesia is achieved. This lengthy interval makes advance placement of the block in the preoperative area attractive. It does not appear that the addition of sodium bicarbonate to lidocaine[195] or bupivacaine[196] is beneficial in shortening the onset of the brachial plexus block, yet it appears to be of some benefit when mepivacaine is used as the anesthetic.[197,198] The shortest-acting agent for the surgical length should be used unless prolonged analgesia is desired. Indwelling brachial plexus catheters to permit the continued use of local anesthetic have been shown effective in minimizing postdischarge pain.[199,200] If discharge is considered before sensory and motor functions return, meticulous verbal and written instructions should be provided to the patient and the guardian, and the arm should be supported in a sling. Approximately 85% of clinicians performing axillary or interscalene block with long-acting local anesthesia routinely discharge patients home with a persistent block.[201]

For surgeries involving the forearm or hand, the axillary approach is the preferred method for use in outpatients and the least likely to create complications. Ideal for surgeries involving the arm, the supraclavicular approach is associated with a small likelihood of pneumothorax, which may become apparent after the patient is discharged from the surgical facility.[202] The risk of development of a pneumothorax is enhanced if the patient becomes quite active after these blocks are performed.[203] The interscalene approach, which is ideal for surgeries involving the shoulder, has a lower incidence of pneumothorax than the supraclavicular approach[204] and has been shown to promote earlier discharge and have fewer side effects (e.g., less pain and nausea) than general anesthesia.[205,206] However, the interscalene approach is associated with intradural injection of local anesthetic, vertebral artery puncture, and stellate ganglion, phrenic nerve, or recurrent laryngeal nerve block.[207]

Caudal Anesthesia

Although caudal anesthesia does not provide the same quality of block as that provided by spinal anesthesia, it is occasionally used in outpatients undergoing pelvic and perineal surgery[208] and in children requiring intraoperative and postoperative analgesia.[209,210] An advantage of caudal anesthesia in the geriatric patient is the absence of hypotension after the administration of this block.[10] Additionally, caudal analgesia has been shown to offer superior recovery features.[211] Caudal anesthesia appears to offer no advantage in preventing postoperative pain, compared with treating the patient with intravenous ketorolac[212] or local anesthesia nerve block with wound infiltration.[213]

Epidural Anesthesia

Epidural anesthesia is successfully used in the ambulatory setting. The advantages of epidural anesthesia in this setting include a reduced incidence of nausea and vomiting and other problems that could delay discharge. With the epidural approach, the incidence of postdural puncture headache (PDPH) is lower, the control over level of block is greater, and the changes in blood pressure are fewer. Titration of a short- to intermediate-acting local anesthetic agent (e.g., 2-chloroprocaine, lidocaine, mepivacaine) through a continuous catheter technique is appropriate for outpatient surgery. Predictable surgical procedures, proper agent selection, and consideration for the addition of epinephrine may negate the necessity of catheter placement in favor of one-time injection. Disadvantages of outpatient epidural anesthesia include slower onset of anesthesia and a less reliable block than with spinal anesthesia.

Intravenous Regional Anesthesia

Intravenous regional anesthesia (Bier block) is suitable for some outpatient surgical procedures because it is simple to perform, it has a rapid onset with reliable results, and it has a rapid offset once the tourniquet is deflated. In the outpatient setting, it has been shown to cost less (approximately one half), be associated with fewer postoperative complications, and yield shorter discharge times when compared with general anesthesia.[214] The use of intravenous regional anesthesia need not be limited to adults. This type of block is successful in children undergoing outpatient surgery on an upper extremity.[215]

Ankle Nerve Block

An ankle block is a simple, safe, and effective means of providing anesthesia and postoperative analgesia (12 to 24 hours with long-acting agents) for operations involving the foot. Popliteal fossa and sciatic nerve blocks also provide complete anesthesia distal to the knee and are appropriate for procedures on the foot and ankle.[216] Continuous infusion of local anesthesia via a catheter in the popliteal fossa is effective in managing postoperative pain following foot and ankle surgery.[217] Limiting factors for an ankle block are the time it takes to block the nerves individually and the delayed onset of anesthetic action. This makes early placement of the block desirable in the busy ambulatory setting. If the ankle and foot continue to be numb at the time of discharge, instructions on patient protection should be provided and emphasized.

Sciatic, Femoral, Lateral Femoral Cutaneous, and Obturator Nerve Blocks

Blocking these nerves singularly or (more commonly) in combination provides appropriate anesthesia and postoperative analgesia for procedures involving a lower extremity.[218] The anesthesia given by this type of block may be extensive and is appropriate for longer procedures. When performed for complex knee surgeries, femoral or sciatic nerve blocks were associated with less postoperative pain in phase II recovery and fewer unplanned hospital admissions.[193] Discharge from the unit can be prolonged as a result of loss of coordination and loss of strength in the leg.[219] When proper preparation for home discharge with an insensate extremity is ensured, the likelihood of patient injury is minimal.[220]

Spinal Anesthesia

For the busy ambulatory surgery setting, a subarachnoid block may be preferable to epidural anesthesia because delays in the onset of block that result from epidural anesthesia may increase the time each patient spends in the preoperative holding room. The side effects of spinal anesthesia—such as orthostatic hypotension, PDPH, urinary retention, and transient neurologic sequelae following concentrated hyperbaric local anesthetic agents—are of particular concern for the patient who expects same-day discharge. The geriatric patient exhibits prolonged sympathetic block and thus is more prone to orthostatic hypotension and urinary retention than the younger patient.[221]

The choice of appropriate local anesthetic agents helps minimize the side effects associated with spinal anesthesia.[222] Lidocaine and procaine are the preferred shorter-acting agents, whereas tetracaine and bupivacaine, because of their prolonged duration of effect, are best avoided.[204] If spinal anesthesia is deemed necessary for a procedure lasting longer than 1.5 to 2 hours, the use of bupivacaine or tetracaine may be required. In this instance, the surgery should be scheduled early in the day so sufficient time is allowed for recovery. The use of lidocaine alone is appropriate for surgeries anticipated to last less than 1 hour. The addition of epinephrine (0.2 to 0.3 mg) or phenylephrine (1 to 5 mg) to lidocaine should prolong the anesthesia for procedures lasting between 1 and 2 hours. The addition of vasoconstrictive agents is not recommended for the longer-acting agents.[208] Should the surgical procedure last longer than anticipated, the surgeon may perform local wound infiltration with a longer-lasting local anesthetic agent to provide the anesthesia necessary for the completion of the surgery.

Efforts to optimize spinal anesthesia (i.e., minimize recovery time) in ambulatory surgery have placed increasing emphasis on maintaining patient comfort while reducing the total amount of the local anesthetic agent (lidocaine,[223-225] bupivacaine,[226-233] or ropivacaine[234]) administered plus the addition of intrathecal opioids to augment the sensory block.[223,224,230,231,235,236] Lidocaine remains the most useful local anesthetic for spinal anesthesia in the outpatient setting.[237]

Orthostatic Hypotension. Residual autonomic blockade, as manifested by such signs as dizziness or fainting, may be problematic when attempts are made to have the patient ambulate prior to discharge. These patients should be scheduled early in the day to allow recovery from the effects of sympathetic block. The use of short-acting local anesthetics is preferred to minimize the duration of sympathetic block. The longer-lasting local anesthetic agents, which have a prolonged duration of action and recovery time, are not desirable for outpatient spinal anesthesia.

Postdural Puncture Headache. The likelihood of PDPH occurrence remains the major concern regarding the use of spinal anesthesia in the outpatient setting. With the use of smaller-gauge, noncutting spinal needles, the incidence of PDPH is very low. The overall incidence of PDPH in the ambulatory population is 0% to 2%,[237,238] with less than 1% requiring management with an epidural blood patch.[239] Patient selection is important if spinal anesthesia is considered for ambulatory surgery. If the patient requires early resumption of normal activities without interference from the anesthesia, spinal anesthesia may not be the appropriate choice, because incapacitating headache may occur. The patient should be informed preoperatively that PDPH may occur and that treatment may be required. For this reason, patients receiving spinal anesthesia should remain within a convenient distance from the ambulatory surgery center for at least 72 hours in case treatment is required.[48]

Prior to discharge, the patient should be educated as to the typical presenting symptoms of a PDPH. Part of the patient's discharge instructions will include information on how to access assistance should a headache occur. If the patient complains of headache, conservative measures for mild symptoms (e.g., analgesics, bed rest, oral hydration, or oral caffeine) may be sufficient treatment. If an epidural blood patch is required, this may be easily performed on an outpatient basis.

Specific patient instructions should be reviewed before the patient is discharged from the ambulatory surgery center. Patients should be informed that lying flat is not required, because this measure does not affect the occurrence of PDPH.[240]

Transient Neurologic Symptoms. The term *transient neurologic symptoms* refers to a set of temporary pain or dysesthesia symptoms involving the back and legs after complete resolution of a spinal anesthetic.[241] The mechanism of this transient neural insult is believed to be a result of direct action on sensory neurons from a lidocaine-induced increase in intracellular calcium.[242] The symptoms appear between 1 and 24 hours following the spinal block resolution and usually resolve within 1 week. Risk factors for the development of transient neurologic symptoms include (1) certain types of surgeries (e.g., knee arthroscopy with the use of a tourniquet and urologic or gynecologic procedures performed in the lithotomy position), and (2) outpatient status (associated with early ambulation), especially in the obese patient. Transient neurologic symptoms have been observed with local anesthetics other than lidocaine,[243-246] but lidocaine has the highest reported incidence (up to 33%) following ambulatory knee arthroscopy.[247] Clinical management typically involves the use of NSAIDs and the more potent analgesics the patient might possess as a result of the surgery. See Chapter 11 for further discussion of transient neurologic symptoms.

Urinary Retention. Transient urinary retention secondary to sympathetic and parasympathetic block at the S2-S4 level of the nerves innervating the bladder, detrusor, and sphincter muscles results in loss of bladder tone and thus in loss of the reflex to void. This problem may require bladder catheterization and may prolong discharge or lead to hospital admission.[227] The incidence of urinary retention after regional anesthesia is affected by the type and the site of the surgery,[248] is higher in male patients, and is influenced by the duration of the sympathetic block.[249] Strategies to reduce the incidence of urinary retention following spinal anesthesia include:

- Reduce the total amount of local anesthesia used for the spinal anesthetic.[250]
- Use the shorter-acting local anesthetic agent (e.g., lidocaine, chloroprocaine) as opposed to the longer-acting agents (e.g., tetracaine).[251,252]
- Add fentanyl to the local anesthesia agent.[253,254] Reducing the total amount of lidocaine (from 50 mg to 20 mg) by adding fentanyl (10 mcg to 25 mcg) had a beneficial effect of reducing the time to patient voiding by approximately 30 minutes.[235]
- Omit the addition of epinephrine to the lidocaine, because it prolongs the block and thus the time to micturition.[228,255]
- Careful attention to intravenous fluid administration and the avoidance of bladder distention.[256]

If these strategies are incorporated into the spinal anesthetic plan and the surgical procedure is not associated with a high incidence of urinary retention (high-risk surgeries include rectal and inguinal hernia operations), the patient can be discharged without voiding.[257]

Concomitant Sedation

Comfort and safety are premier concerns in the care of patients undergoing regional or local anesthesia with monitored anesthesia care. Patients frequently verbalize their anticipated anxiety relating to discomfort and awareness during the time of the block and the procedure. The anesthesia provider's role during these procedures is to maximize patient comfort while ensuring patient protection. The anesthetist's continued presence, along with verbal reassurance and patient education, helps foster acceptance in the patient. Even so, the use of agents that promote amnesia, analgesia, anxiolysis, and sedation is often required to create the ideal conditions for the patient and the surgical team. Several suitable techniques incorporating benzodiazepines, analgesics (opioid and nonopioid), and subhypnotic doses of intravenous anesthetic agents have been described that provide patient sedation during monitored anesthesia care for outpatient procedures. Alternate routes of drug administration (e.g., transmucosal) may have a place, but at present, the intravenous route remains the most popular means of administering these agents.

Some investigators have described the use of benzodiazepines (e.g., diazepam and midazolam) alone[258] or in combination with opioid analgesics (e.g., fentanyl),[259] nonopioid analgesics (e.g., ketorolac and dezocine),[260] and hypnotics (e.g., propofol).[261] Because of its superior recovery profile, midazolam may be the preferred benzodiazepine in the ambulatory setting. It is now available in an easily administered oral formulation, as well as the traditional intravenous preparation. The use of other agents such as opioid analgesics (e.g., remifentanil) and hypnotic agents (e.g., etomidate, methohexital,[258] and propofol[262]), administered by bolus or continuous infusion, have been described for outpatient surgery. Propofol is associated with a more rapid recovery than that afforded by midazolam,[261] but the pain on injection and the short amnesia time it causes may contribute to diminished patient acceptance.[263] Opioid agents, when used in combination with benzodiazepines, have the advantage of promoting patient comfort. The shorter-acting opioid analgesics may be titrated until their therapeutic effect is demonstrated for procedures such as brachial plexus block, in which paresthesias are likely to be elicited. The patient should be comfortable, yet able to readily respond to a paresthesia. Patient-controlled analgesia may be desirable for some patients because it allows them additional control over their surgical experience.

POSTOPERATIVE CONSIDERATIONS

After the surgical procedure, care is provided in either the PACU (phase I) or the short-stay unit (phase II) until the patient is ready for discharge from the ambulatory setting. The location and the level of nursing care required vary according to the patient undergoing the procedure, the type of anesthesia used, and the surgical procedure. Properly addressing potential or realized complications in the most efficient manner possible expedites patient management and promotes a timely discharge process. Complications that might delay the patient's departure from the ambulatory facility include nausea, vomiting, and pain. Each outpatient facility has specific criteria for discharge that should be met before the patient is released from the facility.

Postanesthesia Care Unit

The care afforded to the recovering outpatient should be of the same quality as that afforded to comparable inpatients; patient monitoring capability and resuscitative equipment should be similar in both environments. These capabilities include methods of monitoring the patient's circulation, oxygenation, temperature, and ventilation. Respiratory care includes means of delivering supplemental oxygen therapy to the intubated and the nonintubated patient, as well as a method for evaluating the adequacy of such care. Mechanical ventilatory support should be available for the patient requiring postoperative ventilatory assistance.

An increasingly popular concept in ambulatory care relates to the bypassing of phase I recovery by taking select patients directly to the phase II recovery area.[264] This concept has seen increased popularity as a result of faster awakening times secondary to the rapid-offset anesthetic agents[265] and the ability to more accurately titrate the amount of anesthesia required by the patient as a result of intraoperative electroencephalogram monitoring.[266,267] "Fast-tracking" is designed to improve efficiency and reduce health-care expenses. A $50,000 to $160,000 per year savings was reported at institutions participating in the early evaluation of the fast-track concept.[268] A study in a community hospital–based ambulatory setting found 83% of their healthy outpatients could safely bypass phase I recovery.[269] Although this technique can significantly reduce the time patients spend in the PACU (variable cost savings), it is likely to have little effect on PACU productivity or labor costs (fixed costs).[270] An evaluation of lower-extremity surgeries in a freestanding facility found successful bypass rates of 87% but noted that more nursing interventions were required for these patients in phase II than for patients who came to phase II after initially recovering in the phase I area.[271] Phase I bypass eligibility criteria should be established to gauge the appropriateness of patients going directly to the phase II area, where less intensive monitoring typically occurs (Table 38-2).[272]

Postoperative Complications and Management

With today's standard of anesthesia care, major morbidity and mortality following ambulatory surgery are extremely rare. A review of ambulatory surgical care encompassing 45,090 patients during a 3-year period at a rural-based referral center found most major postoperative morbidities (myocardial infarction, stroke, pulmonary embolism, respiratory failure) to occur within the first 48 hours.[273] Shnaider and Chung reported on a variety of adverse postoperative events (Box 38-11),[274] of which pain and vomiting occurred most frequently.[57] Awad and colleagues described a 2.2% hospital admission rate from the short-stay unit for their pediatric population (Table 38-3).[275] Recent publications have cited overall unanticipated hospital admissions following ambulatory surgery to range between 0.2% and 2.9%.[275-280] Postoperative nausea and vomiting and pain are the most common reasons requiring hospitalization following ambulatory surgery. Certain procedures (laparoscopic sterilization; laparoscopic inguinal herniorrhaphy; head and neck; ear, nose, and throat; urologic; orthopedic) are associated with a higher incidence of hospital admissions; otherwise, the hospital admission rate following ambulatory surgery approaches 0.5% to 1.5%.[14,281]

Nausea and Vomiting

Persistent nausea and vomiting are responsible for delays in discharge and for increases in patient cost[282] and are a prominent factor in unanticipated hospital admission after outpatient surgery.[283] The reported incidence of postoperative nausea and vomiting ranges from 18% to 28% in adult patients[284,285] and 25% to 39% in children.[286,287] Nearly 50% of patients who

TABLE 38-2	White's Fast-Tracking Scoring System	
Criterion		**Score***
Level of Consciousness		
Awake and oriented		2
Arousable with minimal stimulation		1
Responsive only to tactile stimulation		0
Physical Activity		
Able to move all extremities on command		2
Some weakness in movement of extremities		1
Unable to voluntarily move extremities		0
Hemodynamic Stability		
Blood pressure ± 15% of baseline		2
Blood pressure ± 30% of baseline		1
Blood pressure ± 50% of baseline		0
Respiratory Stability		
Able to breathe deeply		2
Tachypnea with good cough		1
Dyspnea with weak cough		0
Oxygen Saturation		
Maintains value >92% on room air		2
Requires supplemental oxygen		1
Saturation <92% with supplemental oxygen		0
Pain Assessment		
None or mild discomfort		2
Moderate to severe pain controlled with analgesics		1
Persistent severe pain		0
Emetic Symptoms		
None or mild nausea with no active vomiting		2
Transient vomiting or retching		1
Persistent moderate severe nausea and vomiting		0

From Watkins AC, White PF. Fast-tracking after ambulatory surgery. J Perianesth Nurs. 2001;16:379-387.
*Total possible score is 14. A minimum score of 12 (with no score less than 1 in any category) would be required at the time the patient is transferred from the OR after general anesthesia.

BOX 38-11	
Risk Factors for Unanticipated Hospital Admission	

Surgical
Pain
Bleeding
Extensive surgery
Surgical complications
Abdominal surgery
ENT and urology surgery

Anesthesia
Nausea and vomiting
Somnolence
Aspiration

Social
Discharge without escort

Medical
Medical complications related to DM, IHD, and sleep apnea
Medication error

From Shnaider I, Chung F. Outcomes in day surgery. Curr Opin Anaesthesiol. 2006;19:622-629.
DM, Diabetes mellitus; ENT, otorhinolaryngology; IHD, ischemic heart disease.

TABLE **38-3**	Reasons for Admission of Children to the Hospital Following Ambulatory Surgery	
Reason	**Number of Patients (%) (*n* = 10,772)**
Unanticipated admission	242 (2.2)
Surgical Pain Complications Need for observation More extensive surgery Oozing	146 (54)
Anesthesia Nausea and vomiting Complications Somnolence	44 (16)
Social Surgery after 1500	38 (14)
Medical	31 (11)
Unclassified	10 (4)

From Awad IT, et al. Unplanned hospital admission in children undergoing day-case surgery. Eur J Anaesthesiol. 2004;21:379-383.

experience vomiting in phase I or II recovery will continue to vomit once discharged.[288] A third of patients who vomited in phase III did not experience any nausea or vomiting prior to discharge.[289] Many anesthetic-related and nonanesthetic-related factors affect the susceptibility of patients to postoperative nausea and emesis.[290-292] Nonanesthetic-related factors contributing to increased episodes of emesis include:

1. *Age.* There is a higher incidence of postoperative vomiting in children,[293-295] particularly between 3 and 12 years of age.[286,296,297] A gradual decrease in the incidence of postoperative nausea and vomiting has been shown after 50 years of age.[298,299]
2. *Apprehension.* Preoperative anxiety may increase the likelihood of vomiting.[300] Proposed mechanisms by which apprehension contributes to vomiting include swallowed air,[301] with resultant abdominal distention,[302] increased gastric volume,[303,304] and increased catecholamine levels.[305]
3. *Gastroparesis*[306] is associated with several pathologic conditions, such as ileus, bowel obstruction, diabetes mellitus, muscular dystrophies, collagen vascular disorders, uremia, raised intracranial pressure, and pregnancy.[290] The accompanying delayed gastric emptying means a greater gastric content and thus a greater chance of vomiting.[306,307]
4. *Gender.* Emesis occurs in adult females more than in males.[308,309] After 70 years of age, gender is no longer a distinction for developing postoperative nausea and vomiting.[294]
5. *Individual predisposition.* Patients relating a previous history of nausea and vomiting after anesthesia or motion sickness are at increased risk for nausea and vomiting after subsequent anesthetics.[308,309]
6. *Food ingestion.* Recent ingestion of food before undergoing anesthesia increases the probability of vomiting,[310,311] as does vomiting during the induction of anesthesia.

7. *Nonsmoking status.* Cigarette smokers seem to experience less postoperative nausea and vomiting than nonsmokers.[299,308,309]
8. *Type of surgery.* Prolonged surgical times correspond to an increased risk of vomiting.[299,308,309] Certain surgical procedures—for example, arthroscopy, laparoscopy, lithotripsy, intestinal operations, ovum retrieval, orchiopexy, otoplasty, retinal detachment, tonsillectomy with or without adenoidectomy, and strabismus—are associated with an increased incidence of postoperative vomiting.[308]

Anesthetic-related factors contributing to emesis include:

1. *Premedications.* Preoperatively administered opioid analgesics, primarily the longer-lasting agents,[312] can increase postoperative vomiting.[313,314] The proposed mechanisms for this to occur include opioid receptor site stimulation,[294] impaired gastric motility,[315] release of serotonin from the small intestine,[316] and vestibular system sensitization.[317]
2. *Induction of anesthesia.* Inhalation induction may result in gastric distention from positive pressure ventilation via the anesthesia face mask and is known to increase postoperative vomiting.[305] This coincides with increased vomiting in cases in which the anesthesia provider is relatively inexperienced and not familiar with proper mask ventilation technique.[318] For intravenous induction of anesthesia, propofol has been found to result in less postoperative vomiting than the other common hypnotic agents (e.g., etomidate, thiopental, ketamine, methohexital).[319-321]
3. *Maintenance of anesthesia.* Several variables are known to increase the incidence of postoperative vomiting:
   - Longer anesthesia times[299,308,309]
   - General anesthesia when compared with regional or local anesthetic techniques[322]
   - Older inhalation anesthetic agents (isoflurane) when compared with the newer volatile agents (e.g., desflurane,[323] sevoflurane[324])
   - Volatile inhalation anesthetics when compared with intravenous hypnotic agents[308,312]
   - Intraoperative opioid administration[299,308,309]
   - Nitrous oxide[25,299,308]; the proposed mechanisms leading to increased postoperative vomiting with nitrous oxide include increased middle-ear pressure,[325,326] distention of the gut by nitrous oxide diffusing into the gastrointestinal tract, interaction with opioid receptors,[327] and sympathetic nerve activation.[328]

Postanesthetic-related factors contributing to emesis include the following:

1. *Ambulation.* More commonly seen in phase II recovery when the patient is mobilized in preparation for discharge, especially in patients receiving opioid analgesics.
2. *Postural hypotension.* Dizziness, syncope, and nausea may be a problem if there is a significant reduction in blood pressure on standing.[305]
3. *Uncontrolled pain.*[329] Etiologic factors may include increased catecholamine concentrations, increased level of consciousness, or peripheral sensitization after direct tissue injury with the resultant release of endogenous nociceptor activators (i.e., serotonin).
4. *Postoperatively administered opioid analgesics.*[299,330]
5. *Oral intake* before discharge from phase II recovery results in approximately a 50% greater incidence of vomiting or prolonged phase II stay than in counterparts who only drank if they desired.[331-333] When oral fluids were held postoperatively for 4 to 6 hours, the incidence of postoperative nausea and

vomiting was reduced in children from 56% to 38%.[334] In children receiving opioids, withholding of oral fluids saw a further reduction in vomiting from 73% to 36%.

6. *Lower inspired oxygen concentrations.* Higher concentrations (50% to 80%) of intraoperative and postoperative supplemental oxygen therapy have been suggested to reduce the incidence of vomiting following laparoscopic and open abdominal surgical procedures where subtle intestinal ischemia is likely.[335] Systematic reviews of all studies have failed to demonstrate any benefit in reducing overall nausea and vomiting by supplementing oxygen.[336,337] If supplemental oxygen is beneficial, it appears to be of short-term benefit: once oxygen therapy is discontinued, the incidence approaches that of those breathing reduced concentrations of oxygen.[338] One study conducted in ambulatory patients found no benefit of supplemental oxygen in reducing the incidence of postoperative vomiting.[339]

7. *Reversal agents.* Opioid and benzodiazepine receptor antagonists and neuromuscular reversal agents may increase nausea and vomiting.[290] In regard to neuromuscular reversal, it appears that only higher doses of neostigmine (>2.5 mg) may demonstrate emetic tendencies.[308,340]

Suggested management of nausea and vomiting involves perioperatively administered pharmacologic interventions. However, evaluating the efficacy of these agents is difficult because the cause of nausea and vomiting is multifactorial. Oral fluids should be withheld, and intravenous fluid hydration can be maintained with normal saline or lactated Ringer's solution until the emesis is controlled. Patients at high risk for postoperative nausea and vomiting will benefit from prophylactic antiemetic therapy. Prophylactic antiemetic therapy has been shown to be cost-effective in ambulatory surgery and is recommended to prevent postoperative nausea and vomiting.[340] Antiemetic drugs should be administered singularly or in combination, based on the number of identified risk factors. Patients at high risk will benefit from combination drug therapy as limitations of single treatment interventions are realized.[25,341] Combination therapy permits targeting multiple receptors, as well as administering agents with prolonged effects to complement medications with rapid-onset properties.[341] When postoperative nausea and vomiting does occur in the postoperative phase, pharmacologic treatment should consist of medications from a different pharmacologic class than from the prophylaxis antiemetic administered.[342] Circumstances that benefit from the perioperative administration of medications for the control of nausea and vomiting include:

- A history of protracted postoperative emesis
- Operations associated with a high incidence of nausea and vomiting
- Mandibular surgery when the jaws are wired shut
- Increased intracranial pressure
- Circumstances in which retching could jeopardize the surgical result (gastric, esophageal, plastic, or eye procedures)

Acupressure/Acupuncture. P6 acupoint stimulation can be effective in preventing or minimizing postoperative nausea and vomiting.[340,343-346] The mechanism of action is uncertain, but endorphin release or serotonin changes have been suggested.[340]

Aprepitant. Aprepitant is a recently introduced antiemetic that works as a neurokinin-1 receptor antagonist.[347] Oral administration of 40 mg within 3 hours of induction of anesthesia is recommended for high-risk, nonpregnant patients. Aprepitant has been shown to be more effective than ondansetron for preventing postoperative nausea and vomiting,[348] especially in the first 48 hours.[349,350]

Dexamethasone. Studies have found dexamethasone to be effective in reducing the incidence of postoperative nausea and vomiting.[351-355] For adults, dexamethasone, 5 to 10 mg, given alone or in combination with antiemetic agents,[356,357] was effective in reducing postoperative vomiting. In children, 0.0625 mg/kg was as effective as 1 mg/kg intravenously in preventing vomiting following tonsillectomy.[358] The earlier dexamethasone is given, the more effective it appears to be.[359] Administering dexamethasone immediately after induction of anesthesia avoids the perineal pruritus seen when the drug is administered to an awake patient.[360] Dexamethasone may be beneficial in the treatment of postoperative nausea and vomiting when used in combination therapy with other agents.[361,362] The time until discharge from the phase II recovery area has been shortened following ambulatory surgery in patients receiving dexamethasone.[363,364] The incidence of vomiting in phase III is reduced if dexamethasone is administered during surgery. This beneficial effect could be secondary to its long duration of action. Adverse effects from a single dose of dexamethasone have not been reported.[365]

Dolasetron. Dolasetron (a selective serotonin type 3 receptor antagonist), 12.5 mg given intravenously, is effective in preventing[366] and treating[367] postoperative vomiting. Dolasetron should be administered within 15 minutes before the end of anesthesia.[368] A single oral dose of 100 mg of dolasetron given 1 to 2 hours before surgery is effective for the prevention of postoperative vomiting.[369] One comparative study found 50 mg of dolasetron given intravenously to be as effective as 4 mg of ondansetron for the prevention of postoperative nausea and vomiting.[370]

Droperidol. Droperidol (Inapsine, a butyrophenone/dopamine receptor antagonist), 10 to 20 mcg/kg given intravenously, has been effective in reducing vomiting.[371] Prophylactically administered droperidol, 20 mcg/kg given intravenously immediately after induction, was superior to metoclopramide, 5 or 10 mg orally, in reducing postoperative vomiting.[141] This dose appears to offer a compromise between reducing vomiting and extending the patient's stay owing to prolonged sedation.[372] Caution should be exercised with the use of larger doses of droperidol (50 to 75 mcg/kg), because the occurrence of side effects (anxiety, dizziness, drowsiness, extrapyramidal symptoms, hypotension) and the potential to delay discharge may be increased. In 2001, the Food and Drug Administration (FDA) placed a "black box" advisory on the packaging label regarding the use of droperidol and risk of fatal dysrhythmias. The FDA recommends 12-lead electrocardiographic monitoring of patients for 2 to 3 hours following drug administration, which creates concerns over time efficiency in the ambulatory setting.[373] The FDA has recently agreed to reassess this issue, given that the overwhelming consensus among anesthesiologists and nurse anesthetists is that droperidol is safe when used in small doses as an antiemetic. Since the FDA-mandated advisory, the use of droperidol in anesthesia has decreased significantly[374]. A further discussion of the clinical use of droperidol can be found in Chapter 10.

Ephedrine. Ephedrine (an indirect-acting sympathomimetic agent), 0.5 mg/kg given intramuscularly at the end of surgery, was found to be as effective as droperidol, 40 mcg/kg given intramuscularly, in minimizing nausea and vomiting while producing less sedation.[375] Similarly, ephedrine, 0.5 mg/kg given at the end of abdominal surgery, reduced the incidence of nausea and vomiting during the first 3 hours postoperatively.[376] Ephedrine, 10 to 25 mg given intravenously, has been recommended for the treatment of nausea and vomiting associated with the postural hypotension of ambulation before the patient is discharged from the facility.[377]

Gastric Suctioning. Intraoperative insertion of a gastric tube into the stomach to suction out the contents is commonly advocated as being beneficial in reducing postoperative nausea and vomiting. Prospective clinical trials that support any reduction in postoperative vomiting with intraoperative gastric aspiration are lacking. Existing clinical evaluations have failed to show beneficial results with this maneuver,[378-381] and it may actually increase the incidence of emesis.[382]

Metoclopramide. Metoclopramide (a benzamide) exerts beneficial gastric effects by increasing lower esophageal sphincter tone, promoting gastric emptying by increasing gastric and small-bowel motility, presumably through antidopaminergic and antiserotonin (at higher doses) receptor effect.[290,383] Conflicting reports have been published about the efficacy of metoclopramide as an antiemetic. A review of placebo-controlled studies involving metoclopramide failed to find any clinically significant antinausea effect at low dosages.[384] Metoclopramide is ineffective as an antiemetic at lower dosages (e.g., 10 mg) in the adult population[385] unless used in combination with other antiemetics (e.g., dexamethasone).[386] Larger doses of metoclopramide (0.4 to 0.5 mg/kg or generic 50 mg IV) in the adult patient may offer some antinausea benefit individually and when used in conjunction with ondansetron or dexamethasone.[387,388] By itself, even at moderate doses of 0.5 mg/kg, metoclopramide is not as effective as ondansetron.[389] An advantage of metoclopramide is its lack of sedative traits; this quality reduces the potential for delaying patient discharge. The intravenous administration of 0.15 mg/kg of metoclopramide has been recommended for the treatment of nausea and vomiting in patients in the PACU who appear sedated.[390] Metoclopramide is not without side effects; extrapyramidal symptoms have been associated with its use.[391]

Midazolam. Benzodiazepines have been shown to reduce nausea and vomiting resulting from chemotherapy and anesthesia.[392-396] Midazolam (pediatric dose: 50 to 75 mcg/kg IV; adults: 2 mg IV) is effective in reducing the incidence of postoperative nausea and vomiting when given as a premedication,[397] intraoperatively,[398,399] or as rescue therapy postoperatively.[400] Possible methods of this antinausea and vomiting effect relate to GABA receptor antagonism, inhibition of dopamine release, and anxiolytic effects.[397] Combination antiemetic therapy of midazolam with dexamethasone reduced the incidence of postoperative nausea and vomiting to zero following strabismus surgery in children.[401]

Ondansetron. Ondansetron (a selective serotonin type 3 receptor antagonist), 0.15 mg/kg given intravenously over the course of 2 to 5 minutes, has been popular for the management of chemotherapy-induced nausea and vomiting, and recent studies have demonstrated its effectiveness in the treatment of anesthesia-related emesis. When administered preoperatively (intravenously[402] or orally[403]), ondansetron appears to be effective in preventing vomiting intraoperatively and postoperatively.[404] It also appears to be effective in treating postoperative vomiting.[405] This drug is most effective at preventing postoperative nausea and vomiting when administered at the end of the surgical procedure.[406] In the adult patient, 4 mg of ondansetron appears to be as effective as 8 mg when it is administered intravenously in the PACU as a treatment for nausea and vomiting.[407,408] A repeat dose, given either intravenously or orally 8 hours later, has been used as part of an antiemetic management regimen. Under select conditions, ondansetron was more effective in reducing the early (within the first 4 hours postoperatively) incidence of postoperative vomiting when compared with droperidol[402,408-411] and metoclopramide.[402,410,412]

Promethazine. Blanc and colleagues found that promethazine (a phenothiazine/dopamine receptor antagonist), in doses of 0.5 mg/kg given intravenously and 0.5 mg/kg given intramuscularly for strabismus repair before extraocular muscle manipulation, reduced the overall incidence of vomiting to 10%, compared with a 56% incidence for droperidol, 75 mcg/kg, given intravenously.[413] The only difference in side effects between these agents was increased restlessness in the promethazine group. The likelihood of significant sedation—especially when used in patients receiving opioids—is significant, thus limiting the utility of this drug in routine ambulatory surgery.[340] The potential for delays in recovery secondary to sedative and extrapyramidal effects must be taken into account. Recently, low-dose promethazine (5 to 10 mg IV) has been recommended both for prophylaxis and for rescue, secondary to the antihistamine effects.[340] Promethazine 6.25 mg was more effective than ondansetron for treating postoperative vomiting after failed ondansetron prophylaxis.[414]

Scopolamine. Transdermal scopolamine has a 2- to 4-hour onset of action and should be applied before surgery (preferably the night prior).[308,342] Timing of the patch placement may be challenging in the ambulatory setting. Side effects, including dry mouth, drowsiness, contact dermatitis, and visual disturbances, are generally mild. Toxic psychosis has been reported in pediatric and elderly populations.[415]

Postoperative Pain

Appropriate postoperative pain management helps minimize the stress of surgery, thereby fostering a quicker convalescence. Uncontrolled postoperative pain causes triggering of the stress response (i.e., elevated catecholamine release, increased oxygen consumption, increased cardiac work, tachycardia),[416] patient uneasiness, neurohumoral response (i.e., increased production of adrenocortical hormone, aldosterone, antidiuretic hormone, cortisol, follicle-stimulating hormone, growth hormone, luteinizing hormone, plasma renin activity, prolactin),[417] increased nausea and vomiting, psychologic distress,[418] discharge delays,[419] and unanticipated hospital admission.[26] Forty-five percent of discharged ambulatory surgical patients reported moderate to severe pain up to 48 hours postoperatively.[289] Pain management should begin with the use of wound infiltration with local anesthesia, the use of peripheral or regional nerve block, perineural, incisional, or intra-articular local anesthesia catheters, and the administration of opioid and nonopioid (i.e., NSAIDs) analgesics preoperatively or intraoperatively, particularly in procedures associated with discomfort after emergence from anesthesia. These practices decrease analgesic requirements in the immediate recovery period, resulting in reduced pain scores and decreased postoperative nausea and vomiting (Box 38-12).[420]

The severity and onset of postoperative discomfort are influenced by previously administered analgesics. Immediate control of pain in the PACU can be achieved by incremental titration of small intravenous doses of a short-acting opioid analgesic such as fentanyl (12.5 to 75 mcg) or alfentanil (50 to 300 mcg) every 2 to 3 minutes until nociceptive pain relief has been achieved.[421] Nonopioid analgesics should be considered to treat inflammatory pain or neuropathic pain. They have the advantage of improving overall analgesia, promoting early mobilization, and minimizing opioid-related side effects. Once patient discomfort has been controlled and the patient is tolerating oral fluids, early management of pain with oral analgesics (similar to those the patient will be taking after discharge) should be considered. This allows for evaluation of the analgesic's effect on pain alleviation, the

BOX **38-12**

Advantages of Local/Regional Anesthesia

Patient Advantages
Avoidance of general anesthetic with its related complications
Minimal incidence of nausea and vomiting
Improved postoperative pain relief
Shortened recovery room time (can bypass phase I recovery)
Patient communication with staff during surgery
Patient observation of the procedure (arthroscopy)
Earlier mobilization, including immediate physiotherapy

Surgeon Advantages
Accurate assessment of function before end of surgery
Discussion of operative findings and treatment options at surgery

Facility Advantages
Options of direct transfer to phase II recovery
Shortened patient recovery room time
Reduced postoperative nursing requirements
Fewer hospital admissions (shoulder surgery, breast augmentation surgery)
Overall reduction in facility costs

From Rawal N. Postoperative pain treatment for ambulatory surgery. Best Pract Res Clin Anaesthesiol. 2007;21:129-148.

TABLE **38-4**	Postanesthesia Discharge Scoring System (PADS) for Determining Home Readiness	
Criterion		**Score***
Vital Signs		
Vital signs must be stable and consistent with age and preoperative baseline.		
Blood pressure and pulse within 20% of preoperative baseline		2
Blood pressure and pulse 20%-40% of preoperative baseline		1
Blood pressure and pulse >40% of preoperative baseline		0
Activity Level		
Patient must be able to ambulate at preoperative level.		
Steady gait, no dizziness, or meets preoperative level		2
Requires assistance		1
Unable to ambulate		0
Nausea and Vomiting		
The patient should have minimal nausea and vomiting before discharge.		
Minimal: successfully treated with oral medication		2
Moderate: successfully treated with intramuscular medication		1
Severe: continues after repeated treatment		0
Pain		
The patient should have minimal or no pain before discharge.		
The level of pain the patient has should be acceptable to the patient.		
Pain should be controllable by oral analgesics.		
Location, type, and intensity of pain should be consistent with anticipated postoperative discomfort.		
Acceptability		
Yes		2
No		1
Surgical Bleeding		
Postoperative bleeding should be consistent with expected blood loss for the procedure.		
Minimal: does not require dressing change		2
Moderate: up to two dressing changes required		1
Severe: more than three dressing changes required		0

From Marshall S, Chung F. Assessment of "home readiness": discharge criteria and postdischarge complications. Curr Opin Anaesthesiol. 1997;10:445-450.
*Total possible score is 10. Patients who score 9 or 10 are considered fit for discharge.

patient's mental condition, and the patient's respiratory drive. The outpatient's analgesic medication should be safe and easily managed by the patient or caregiver once the patient is discharged from the facility.

Discharge Criteria

Before the patient is discharged from the ambulatory facility, he or she must meet certain criteria of recovery from the effects of surgery and anesthesia. An organized approach to patient evaluation postoperatively allows for the most comprehensive and efficient means of judging the patient's readiness to be "weaned" from the immediate care of the anesthetist without compromising the patient's safety. A consistent method of evaluating the patient for discharge readiness offers the advantages of reproducibility, standardization, and objectivity; however, no universally accepted standard exists for determining discharge readiness. Several methods of patient evaluation have been proposed. Aldrete and Kroulik[422] were the first to describe a means of postoperative patient evaluation that was appropriate for all types of anesthesia; this method is based on physical signs that are frequently monitored. A minimum total Aldrete postanesthetic recovery (PAR) score of 8 is required before the patient is considered for discharge from phase I recovery.[423] More recently, Aldrete[424] has updated his original phase I PAR score to reflect the contemporary ability to monitor oxygenation in a more exact fashion with the use of pulse oximetry. The Aldrete phase I PAR scoring system is not meaningful for the phase II ambulatory population in regard to comprehensive "home readiness." Newer, more discriminating models such as the postanesthesia discharge scoring system (PADS) for determining home readiness[425] (Table 38-4) and Aldrete's phase II postanesthetic recovery score[424] (Table 38-5) address items

TABLE **38-5**	Aldrete's Phase II Postanesthetic Recovery Score	
Patient Sign	**Criterion**	**Score***
Activity	Able to move 4 extremities (voluntarily or on command)	2
	Able to move 2 extremities (voluntarily or on command)	1
	Able to move 0 extremities (voluntarily or on command)	0
Respiration	Able to breathe deeply and cough	2
	Dyspnea, limited breathing, or tachypnea	1
	Apneic or on mechanical ventilator	0
Circulation	Blood pressure ± 20% of preanesthesia level	2
	Blood pressure ± 20%-49% of preanesthesia level	1
	Blood pressure ± 50% of preanesthesia level	0
Consciousness	Fully awake	2
	Arousable on calling	1
	Not responding	0
Oxygen saturation	SpO_2 >92% on room air	2
	Requires supplemental O_2 to maintain SpO_2 >90%	1
	SpO_2 <90% even with O_2 supplement	0
Dressing	Dry and clean	2
	Wet but stationary or marked	1
	Growing area of wetness	0
Pain	Pain free	2
	Mild pain handled by oral medications	1
	Severe pain requiring IV or IM medications	0
Ambulation	Can stand up and walk straight†	2
	Vertigo when erect	1
	Dizziness when supine	0
Fasting-feeding	Able to drink fluids	2
	Nauseated	1
	Nauseated and vomiting	0
Urine output	Has voided	2
	Unable to void but comfortable	1
	Unable to void and uncomfortable	0

From Aldrete JA. Discharge criteria. In: Thomson D, Frost E, eds. Baillieres Clinical Anaesthesiology—Postanaesthesia Care. *London:* Bailliere Tindall; 1994:763-773.
*Total possible score is 20. A score of 18 or greater is required before patient discharge.
†May be replaced by Romberg's test, or picking up 12 clips in one hand.

specific to suitability for home discharge (i.e., ambulation, bleeding, comfort level, and nausea and vomiting). Although significant progress has been made in attempts to develop a meaningful discharge scoring system for the ambulatory surgical population, a definitive tool that is sensitive to the patient, surgical procedure, and anesthetic technique, as well as compatible with today's economic concerns, has yet to be finalized.

For discharge to occur, the patient must be clinically stable and able to continue the recovery process at a remote recovery location. The decision to discharge is best made on objective criteria outlined in the policies of each ambulatory surgical facility. Distinct objective discharge criteria must be addressed when assessing home readiness of the patient. (*Note:* Before discharge from phase I, the patient's vital signs will be stable, there will be no respiratory impairment, protective reflexes of swallow and cough will be present, and the patient will be oriented to his or her preoperative level. It is assumed that the status of these parameters will not deteriorate during the patient's stay in phase I.) Individually, the following clinical markers should be evaluated in an organized, concise manner:

1. Vital signs should be stable and age appropriate.
2. The patient should be oriented to person, place, and time or at a level appropriate for the patient's developmental and preoperative status.
3. Ambulation can be affected by the surgical procedure and the patient's developmental level. If assistance to ambulate is required, the home caregiver must be capable of meeting this need.
4. There should be no respiratory distress.
5. Swallowing and coughing protective airway reflexes must be present.
6. Bleeding should be minimal or appropriate for the surgical procedure.
7. Pain should be minimal or controlled with an appropriate analgesic regimen.
8. Nausea and vomiting should be minimal.
9. Oral intake prior to discharge is not necessary unless crucial to the patient's continued convalescence at home (e.g., diabetic patient, patient requiring oral analgesics).[57]
10. Voiding is not mandatory before discharge, except for patients at high risk for postoperative urinary retention (e.g., history of postoperative urinary retention, pelvic or urologic surgery, perioperative catheterization).[57]
11. A responsible caregiver should be available.

Discharge Considerations

During the preparatory phase, the availability of a responsible person who will oversee the patient's care once the patient is discharged should be ascertained before surgery. In some cases, inpatient admission may be necessary if a responsible individual cannot be located. Postoperative care may be required for up to 48 hours in such cases, especially in elderly patients.[426] The patient and responsible person should be provided with written instructions that are verbally reinforced before the patient is discharged. This information should include the physician's telephone numbers and steps to be taken if questions or complications arise. Once the patient has satisfied the criteria for discharge from the outpatient facility, certain discharge instructions should be reviewed to expedite and streamline the discharge process (Box 38-13).

The period of patient recovery after discharge from the ambulatory facility until resumption of normal activities is termed

---

BOX **38-13**

Key Education Points for Discharge Instructions

Medications

Detail the name, purpose, and dosage schedule for each medication. Emphasize the importance of following the directions on the label.

The patient should resume medications taken before surgery per the physician's order.

If pain medication is not prescribed, nonprescription, nonaspirin analgesics (e.g., acetaminophen, ibuprofen) may be effective on mild aches and pains.

Additional pain medication may be ordered by the physician after surgery. The patient should take these medications as directed, preferably with food to prevent gastrointestinal upset.

Activity Restriction

Caution the patient to take it easy for the remainder of the day following surgery. Postoperative dizziness or drowsiness is not unusual after surgery and anesthesia and may last several days.

For the next 24 hours, the patient should not drive a vehicle, operate machinery or power tools, consume alcohol (including beer), make important personal or business decisions, or sign important documents.

Describe the permissible activity level in specific behavioral terms (e.g., do not lift objects greater than 20 lb); describe any limitation of activities.

Diet

Explain any dietary restrictions or instructions.

If no dietary restriction, instruct the patient to progress as tolerated to a regular diet.

Surgical and Anesthesia Side Effects

Anticipated sequelae of surgery, such as bleeding and pain, should be delineated.

Common side effects associated with anesthesia include dizziness, drowsiness, myalgia, nausea and vomiting, and sore throat.

Possible Complications and Symptoms

Instruct the patient and responsible caregiver in pertinent signs and symptoms that could be indicative of postoperative complications.

The patient should call his or her physician if any of the following develop:

Fever >38.3° C (>101° F) orally

Persistent, atypical pain

Pain not relieved by pain medication

Bleeding that does not stop or prolonged, unexpected drainage from the wound

Extreme redness/swelling around the incision, drainage of pus

Urinary retention after 8 hours or as otherwise instructed

Unremitting nausea or vomiting

Treatment and Tests

Procedures the patient or responsible caregiver are expected to perform, such as dressing changes or the application of warm, moist compresses, should be described in detail.

A complete list of necessary supplies should be included.

If any postoperative tests are to be conducted, instructions as to the date, time, test location, and any pre-visit preparation should be listed.

Access to Postdischarge Care

The telephone number of the responsible and available physician

The telephone number of the ambulatory center and the hours of operation

The name, address, and telephone number of the appropriate emergency care facility

Follow-up Care

Identify the date, time, and location of the patient's scheduled return visit to the clinic or surgeon.

From Marley RA, Moline BM. Patient discharge issues. In: Burden N, ed. Ambulatory Surgical Nursing. 2nd ed. Philadelphia: Saunders; 2000.

---

phase III. This is an important and often forgotten aspect of postoperative ambulatory care. Patient-care issues requiring attention continue to be important. Up to 86% of all outpatients report minor complications following anesthesia and surgery.[427] Common postdischarge reports after outpatient surgery include pain (45%), nausea (17%), vomiting (8%), nonspecific headaches (17%), PDPH (9%), postdural puncture backache (27%), drowsiness (42%), dizziness (18%), and fatigue (21%).[289] Thirty percent of discharged ambulatory surgical patients report moderate to severe pain 24 hours postsurgery. Greater than 60% of outpatients required 3 days of recuperation before they were able to resume their usual daily activities.[427] It is important to convey to patients that it will take several days before they begin to feel as they did before surgery.

SUMMARY

The numbers and types of surgeries performed on an ambulatory basis will continue to increase, as will the ability of facilities to appropriately treat these patients. As anesthetic techniques and agents are refined, thereby increasing the safety and efficiency of patient care and discharge, new groups of patients will be evaluated for their appropriateness for outpatient surgery. These new groups will continue to challenge our resources for providing ambulatory anesthesia.

REFERENCES

1. Nicoll JH. The surgery of infancy. *BMJ.* 1909;2:753-754.
2. Waters RM. The down-town anesthesia clinic. *Am J Surg.* 1919;33(Anesth suppl):71-73.
3. Friedman Z et al. Ambulatory surgery adult patient selection criteria—a survey of Canadian anesthesiologists. *Can J Anesth.* 2004;51:437-443.
4. Bian J, Morrisey MA. Freestanding ambulatory surgery centers and hospital surgery volume. *Inquiry.* 2007;44(2):200-210.
5. Hancox JG et al. The safety of office-based surgery: review of recent literature from several disciplines. *Arch Dermatol.* 2004;140:1379-1382.
6. American Society of Anesthesiologists: *Office-based Anesthesia and Surgery.* Available at: http://www.asahq.org/patientEducation/officebased.htm. Accessed July 8, 2008.
7. Fleisher LA et al. Is outpatient laparoscopic cholecystectomy safe and cost-effective? A model to study transition of care. *Anesthesiology.* 1999; 90:1746-1755.
8. Gilmartin J, Wright K. The nurse's role in day surgery: a literature review. *Int Nurs Rev.* 2007;54:183-190.
9. Canet J et al. Cognitive dysfunction after minor surgery in the elderly. *Acta Anaesthesiol Scand.* 2003;47:1204-1210.
10. Polaner DM. Anesthesia for pediatric same-day surgical procedures. In: Motoyama EK, Davis PJ, eds. *Smith's Anesthesia for Infants and Children.* 7th ed. St. Louis: Mosby; 2006:874-894.
11. Federal Ambulatory Surgery Association. *FASA Special Study I.* Alexandria, VA: FASA; 1986.
12. Epstein BS. Outpatient anesthesia. In: Hershey SG, ed. *ASA Refresher Courses in Anesthesiology.* Philadelphia: Lippincott; 1984:85-95.
13. McGrath B, Chung F. Postoperative recovery and discharge. *Anesthesiol Clin North America.* 2003;21:367-386.
14. Fleisher LA et al. A novel index of elevated risk of inpatient hospital admission immediately following outpatient surgery. *Arch Surg.* 2007;142:263-268.
15. Henderson JA. Ambulatory surgery: past, present, and future. In: Wetchler BV, ed. *Anesthesia for Ambulatory Surgery.* 2nd ed. Philadelphia: Lippincott; 1991:1-27.
16. Bogetz MS. Outpatient surgery. In: Stoelting RK, Miller RD, eds. *Basics of Anesthesia.* 5th ed. Philadelphia: Churchill Livingstone; 2007:538-549.
17. Smith I. Dissecting the myths of day surgery: the anaesthetist. *J Perioper Pract.* 2006;16:244-248.
18. Scanlon J, Richards B. Development of a same-day laminectomy program. *J Perianesth Nurs.* 2004;19:84-88.
19. Erickson M et al. Outpatient anterior cervical discectomy and fusion. *Am J Orthop.* 2007;36:429-432.
20. Inabnet WB et al. Safety of same-day discharge in patients undergoing suture-less thyroidectomy: a comparison of local and general anesthesia. *Thyroid.* 2008;18:57-61.
21. Campo V, Campo S. Hysteroscopy requirements and complications. *Minerva Ginecol.* 2007;59:451-457.
22. Bernstein M. Outpatient craniotomy for brain tumor: a pilot feasibility study in 46 patients. *Can J Neurol Sci.* 2001;28:120-124.
23. Blanshard JH et al. Awake craniotomy for removal of intracranial tumor: considerations for early discharge. *Anesth Analg.* 2001;92:89-94.
24. Brigger MT, Brietzke SE. Outpatient tonsillectomy in children: a systematic review. *Otolaryngol Head Neck Surg.* 2006;135:1-7.
25. Gupta A. Evidence-based medicine in day surgery. *Curr Opin Anaesthesiol.* 2007;20:520-525.
26. Meridy HW. Criteria for selection of ambulatory surgical patients and guidelines for anesthetic management: a retrospective study of 1553 cases. *Anesth Analg.* 1982;61:921-926.
27. Stockman JA III. Anemia of prematurity: current concepts in the issue of when to transfuse. *Pediatr Clin North Am.* 1986;33:111-128.
28. Welborn LG et al. Anemia and postoperative apnea in former preterm infants. *Anesthesiology.* 1991;74:1003-1006.
29. Welborn LG, Greenspun JC. Anesthesia and apnea: perioperative considerations in the former preterm infant. *Pediatr Clin North Am.* 1994;41:181-198.
30. Kurth CD et al. Postoperative apnea in preterm infants. *Anesthesiology.* 1987;66:483-488.
31. Kurth CD, LeBard SE. Association of postoperative apnea, airway obstruction, and hypoxemia in former premature infants. *Anesthesiology.* 1991;75:22-26.
32. Stierer T, Fleisher LA. Challenging patients in an ambulatory setting. *Anesthesiol Clin North America.* 2003;21:243-261.
33. Fishkin S, Litman RS. Current issues in pediatric ambulatory anesthesia. *Anesthesiol Clin North America.* 2003;21:305-311.
34. Karayan J et al. Postoperative apnea in a full-term infant. *Anesthesiology.* 1991;75:375.
35. Fisher DM. When is the ex-premature infant no longer at risk for apnea? *Anesthesiology.* 1995;82:807.
36. Stierer T, Fleisher LA. Challenging patients in an ambulatory setting. *Anesthesiol Clin North America.* 2003;21:243-261.
37. Krane EJ et al. Postoperative apnea, bradycardia, and oxygen desaturation in formerly premature infants: prospective comparison of spinal and general anesthesia. *Anesth Analg.* 1995;80:7-13.
38. Welborn LG et al. Postoperative apnea in former preterm infants: prospective comparison of spinal and general anesthesia. *Anesthesiology.* 1990;72:838-842.
39. Watcha MF et al. Postoperative apnea after caudal anesthesia in an ex-premature infant. *Anesthesiology.* 1989;71:613-615.
40. Cox RG, Goresky GV. Life-threatening apnea following spinal anesthesia in former premature infants. *Anesthesiology.* 1990;73:345-347.
41. Tobias JD et al. Apnea following spinal anaesthesia in two former pre-term infants. *Can J Anaesth.* 1998;45:985-989.
42. Kunst G et al. The proportion of high-risk preterm infants with postoperative apnea and bradycardia is the same after general and spinal anesthesia. *Can J Anesth.* 1999;46:94-95.
43. Bryan MH et al. Pulmonary function studies during the first year of life in infants recovering from the respiratory distress syndrome. *Pediatrics.* 1973;52:169-178.
44. Berry FA. Pre-existing medical conditions of pediatric patients. *Semin Anesth.* 1984;3:24-31.
45. Garg M et al. Hypoxic arousal responses in infants with bronchopulmonary dysplasia. *Pediatrics.* 1988;82:59-63.
46. Valdes-Dapena MA. Sudden infant death syndrome: a review of the medical literature 1974-1979. *Pediatrics.* 1980;66:597-614.
47. Guntheroth WG et al. Risk of sudden infant death syndrome in subsequent siblings. *J Pediatr.* 1990;116:520-524.
48. Litchtor JL. Anesthesia for ambulatory surgery. In: Barash PG et al, eds. *Clinical Anesthesia.* 5th ed. Philadelphia: Lippincott Williams & Wilkins; 2006:1229-1245.
49. Rockoff MA, McCann ME. Case report no 12. From Wong HC, Nkana CA. In the real world. In: Wetchler BV, ed. *Anesthesia for Ambulatory Surgery.* 2nd ed. Philadelphia: Lippincott; 1991:509-511.
50. Berry FA. Preoperative assessment of pediatric outpatients. In: White PF, ed. *Outpatient Anesthesia.* New York: Churchill Livingstone; 1990:147-162.
51. Fleisher LA et al. A novel index of elevated risk of inpatient hospital admission immediately following outpatient surgery. *Arch Surg.* 2007; 142:263-268.
52. Pasternak LR. Case report no 18. From Wong HC, Nkana CA. In the real world. In: Wetchler BV, ed. *Anesthesia for Ambulatory Surgery.* 2nd ed. Philadelphia: Lippincott; 1991:525-528.
53. Karlet MC. An update on cystic fibrosis and implications for anesthesia. *AANA J.* 2000;68:141-148.
54. McGoldrick K. Is malignant hyperthermia a contraindication for outpatient surgery? *Soc Ambulatory Anesth Newslett.* 1992;7:11.
55. Pollock N et al. Malignant hyperthermia and day stay surgery. *Anaesth Intensive Care.* 2006;34:40-45.
56. Malilgnant Hyperthermia Association of the United States. *Medical Professional's FAQs.* Available at: http://medical.mhaus.org/index.cfm/fuseaction/Content.Display/PagePK/MedicalFAQs.cfm. Accessed June 29, 2008.
57. Awad IT, Chung F. Factors affecting recovery and discharge following ambulatory surgery. *Can J Anesth.* 2006;53:858-872.
58. Servin F. Ambulatory anesthesia for the obese patient. *Curr Opin Anaesthesiol.* 2006;19:597-599.
59. Marley RA et al. Perianesthesia respiratory care of the bariatric patient. *J Perianesth Nurs.* 2005;20:404-431.
60. Gupta A. Strategies for outpatient anaesthesia. *Best Pract Res Clin Anaesthesiol.* 2004;18:675-692.
61. McCarty TM et al. Optimizing outcomes in bariatric surgery. *Ann Surg.* 2005;242:494-501.
62. McCarty T. Can bariatric surgery be done as an outpatient procedure? *Adv Surg.* 2006;40:99-106.
63. Montgomery KF et al. Outpatient laparoscopic adjustable gastric banding in super-obese patients. *Obes Surg.* 2007;17:711-716.
64. Wasowicz-Kemps DK et al. Laparoscopic gastric banding for morbid obesity: outpatient procedure versus overnight stay. *Surg Endosc.* 2006; 20:1233-1237.

65. Siyam MA, Benhamou D. Difficult endotracheal intubation in patients with sleep apnea syndrome. *Anesth Analg.* 2002;95:1098-1102.

66. Bryson GL et al. Patient selection in ambulatory anesthesia—an evidence-based review: part I. *Can J Anesth.* 2004;51:768-781.

67. Sabers C. The diagnosis of obstructive sleep apnea as a risk factor for unanticipated admissions in outpatient surgery. *Anesth Analg.* 2003;96:1328-1335.

68. American Society of Anesthesiologists Task Force on Perioperative Management. Practice guidelines for the perioperative management of patients with obstructive sleep apnea: a report by the American Society of Anesthesiologists Task Force on Perioperative Management of Patients with Obstructive Sleep Apnea. *Anesthesiology.* 2006;104:1081-1093.

69. Aker J. Sickle cell disease: implications for perioperative care. *J Perianesth Nurs.* 1999;14(4):221-227.

70. Firth PG, Head CA. Sickle cell disease and anesthesia. *Anesthesiology.* 2004;101:766-785.

71. McCormick F. Abnormal hemoglobins. II. The pathology of sickle cell trait. *Am J Med Sci.* 1961;92:329.

72. Pasternak LR. Sickle cell disease. In: Schmitter CR Jr, ed. *Ambulatory surgery: is it for everyone? Soc Ambulatory Anesth Newslett.* 1992;7:2.

73. Twersky RS. Ambulatory surgery update. *Can J Anaesth.* 1998;45(Suppl):R76-R83.

74. Lew E et al. Outpatient preanaesthesia evaluation clinics. *Singapore Med J.* 2004;45:509-516.

75. Perez A et al. Value of routine preoperative tests: a multicentre study in four general hospitals. *Br J Anaesth.* 1995;74:250-256.

76. Kaplan EB et al. The usefulness of preoperative laboratory screening. *JAMA.* 1985;253:3576-3581.

77. Velanovich V. Preoperative laboratory screening based on age, gender, and concomitant medical diseases. *Surgery.* 1994;115:56-61.

78. Ransom SB et al. Cost-effectiveness of routine blood type and screen testing before elective laparoscopy. *Obstet Gynecol.* 1995;86:346-348.

79. Roizen MF, Rupani G. Preoperative assessment of adult outpatients. In: White PF, ed. *Outpatient Anesthesia.* New York: Churchill Livingstone; 1990:181-200.

80. Pasternak LR et al. Practice advisory for preanesthesia evaluation: a report by the American Society of Anesthesiologists Task Force on Preanesthesia Evaluation. *Anesthesiology.* 2002;96:485-496.

81. Roizen MF, Cohn S. Preoperative evaluation for elective surgery: what laboratory tests are needed? In: Stoelting RK, ed. *Advances in Anesthesia.* St Louis: Mosby; 1993:25-47.

82. Rabkin SW, Horne JM. Preoperative electrocardiography: its cost-effectiveness in detecting abnormalities when a previous tracing exists. *Can Med Assoc J.* 1979;121:301-306.

83. Gold BS et al. The utility of preoperative electrocardiograms in the ambulatory surgical patient. *Arch Intern Med.* 1992;152:301-305.

84. Turnbull JM, Buck C. The value of preoperative screening investigations in otherwise healthy individuals. *Arch Intern Med.* 1987;147:1101-1105.

85. Tait AR et al. Evaluation of the efficacy of routine preoperative electrocardiograms. *J Cardiothorac Vasc Anesth.* 1997;11:752-755.

86. Munro J et al. Routine preoperative testing: a systematic review of the evidence. *Health Technol Assess.* 1997;1:i-iv;1-62.

87. Orkin FK, Gold B. Selection. In: Wetchler BV, ed. *Anesthesia for Ambulatory Surgery.* 2nd ed. Philadelphia: Lippincott; 1991:81-129.

88. Callaghan LC et al. Utilisation of the pre-operative ECG. *Anaesthesia.* 1995;50:488-490.

89. Wagner JD, Moore DL. Preoperative laboratory testing for the oral and maxillofacial surgery patient. *J Oral Maxillofac Surg.* 1991;49:177-182.

90. Haug RH, Reifeis RL. A prospective evaluation of the value of preoperative laboratory testing for office anesthesia and sedation. *J Oral Maxillofac Surg.* 1999;57:16-20.

91. Luirink MR, Pfaff A. Routine electrocardiography in elderly patients for ambulatory surgery. *Br J Anaesth.* 1999;82:6.

92. Cote CJ. Aspiration: an overrated risk in elective patients. In: Stoelting RK, ed. *Advances in Anesthesia.* St Louis: Mosby; 1992:1-26.

93. Yogendran S, Chung FF. How long should we fast our patients? *Soc Ambulatory Anesth Newslett.* 1992;7:10.

94. Simpson KH, Stakes AF. Effect of anxiety on gastric emptying in preoperative patients. *Br J Anaesth.* 1987;59:540-544.

95. Borland LM et al. Pulmonary aspiration in pediatric patients during general anesthesia: incidence and outcome. *J Clin Anesth.* 1998;10(2):95-102.

96. Nimmo WS. Drugs, diseases and altered gastric emptying. *Clin Pharmacokinet.* 1976;1:189-203.

97. Morgan M. Anaesthetic contribution to maternal mortality. *Br J Anaesth.* 1987;59:842-855.

98. Morrison JE Jr, Lockhart CH. Preoperative fasting and medication in children. *Anesthesiol Clin North America.* 1991;9:731-743.

99. Cote CJ. Changing concepts in preoperative medication and "NPO" status of the pediatric patient. *ASA 1992 Annual Refresher Course Lectures.* Philadelphia: Lippincott; 1992:132.

100. Hinder RA, Kelly KA. Canine gastric emptying of solids and liquids. *Am J Physiol.* 1977;233:E335-E340.

101. Warner ME. Risks and outcomes of perioperative pulmonary aspiration. *J Perianesth Nurs.* 1997;12:352-357.

102. Nagelhout JJ. Aspiration prophylaxis: is it time for changes in our practice? *AANA J.* 2003;71:299-303.

103. Soreide E et al. Pre-operative fasting guidelines: an update. *Acta Anaesthesiol Scand.* 2005;49:1041-1047.

104. Minami H, McCallum RW. The physiology and pathophysiology of gastric emptying in humans. *Gastroenterology.* 1984;86:1592-1610.

105. Farrow-Gillespie A et al. Effect of the fasting interval on gastric fluid pH and volume in children. *Anesth Analg.* 1988;67:S59.

106. Dose VA, White PF. Effects of fluid therapy on serum glucose levels in fasted outpatients. *Anesthesiology.* 1987;66:223-226.

107. Sutherland AD et al. Effects of preoperative fasting on morbidity and gastric contents in patients undergoing day-stay surgery. *Br J Anaesth.* 1986;58:876-878.

108. Read MS, Vaughan RS. Allowing pre-operative patients to drink: effects on patients' safety and comfort of unlimited oral water until 2 hours before anaesthesia. *Acta Anaesthesiol Scand.* 1991;35:591-595.

109. Shevde K, Trivedi N. Effects of clear liquids on gastric volume and pH in healthy volunteers. *Anesth Analg.* 1991;72:528-531.

110. Splinter WM, Schaefer JD. Unlimited clear fluid ingestion two hours before surgery in children does not affect volume or pH of stomach contents. *Anaesth Intensive Care.* 1990;18:522-526.

111. Maltby JR et al. Gastric fluid volume and pH in elective patients following unrestricted oral fluid until three hours before surgery. *Can J Anaesth.* 1991;38:425-429.

112. Splinter WM, Schaefer JD. Ingestion of clear fluids is safe for adolescents up to 3 h before anaesthesia. *Br J Anaesth.* 1991;66:48-52.

113. American Society of Anesthesiologists. Practice guidelines for preoperative fasting and the use of pharmacologic agents to reduce the risk of pulmonary aspiration: application to healthy patients undergoing elective procedures. *Anesthesiology.* 1999;90:896-905.

114. Fasting S et al. Changing preoperative fasting policies. *Acta Anaesthesiol Scand.* 1998;42:1188-1191.

115. Majerus PW, Tollesfen DM. Blood coagulation and anticoagulant, thrombolytic, and antiplatelet drugs. In: Brunton LL et al, eds. *Goodman and Gilman's The Pharmacological Basis of Therapeutics.* 11th ed. New York: McGraw-Hill; 2006:1467-1488.

116. Park S, Warren L. Ambulatory anesthesia. In: Dunn PF, ed. *Clinical Anesthesia Procedures of the Massachusetts General Hospital.* 7th ed. Philadelphia: Lippincott Williams & Wilkins; 2007:563-569.

117. Tinker JH, Tarhan S. Discontinuing anticoagulant therapy in surgical patients with cardiac valve prostheses: observations in 180 operations. *JAMA.* 1978;239:738-739.

118. Graham GW et al. Perioperative management of selected endocrine disorders. *Int Anesthesiol Clin.* 2000;38:31-67.

119. Saunders NR. Innocent heart murmurs in children: taking a diagnostic approach. *Can Fam Physician.* 1995;41:1507-1512.

120. Monto AS, Ullman BM. Acute respiratory illness in an American community: the Tecumseh study. *JAMA.* 1974;227:164-169.

121. Bailey AG, Valley RD. Myths in pediatric anesthesia. In: Spielman FJ, ed. *Problems in Anesthesia: Myths in Anesthesiology.* Philadelphia: Lippincott; 1991:483-496.

122. Elwood T, Bailey K. The pediatric patient and upper respiratory infections. *Best Pract Res Clin Anaesthesiol.* 2005;19:35-46.

123. Abu_Shahwan I. Ambulatory anesthesia and the lack of consensus among Canadian pediatric anesthesiologists: a survey. *Ped Anesth.* 2007;17:223-229.

124. Tait AR, Malviya S. Anesthesia for the child with an upper respiratory tract infection. *Curr Rev Nurse Anesth.* 1999;21:170-175.

125. Cohen MM, Cameron CB. Should you cancel the operation when a child has an upper respiratory tract infection? *Anesth Analg.* 1991;72:282-288.

126. Rolf N, Cote CJ. Incidence of hypoxemic events during anesthesia in children with upper respiratory infection. *Anesthesiology.* 1990;73:A1124.

127. Malviya S et al. Risk factors for adverse postoperative outcomes in children presenting for cardiac surgery with upper respiratory tract infections. *Anesthesiology.* 2003;98:628-632.

128. Tait AR et al. Risk factors for perioperative adverse respiratory events in children with upper respiratory tract infections. *Anesthesiology.* 2001;95:299-306.

129. Tait AR, Malviya S. Anesthesia for the child with an upper respiratory tract infections: still a dilemma? *Anesth Analg.* 2005;100:59-65.

130. Serafini G et al. Upper respiratory tract infections and pediatric anesthesia. *Minerva Anestesiol.* 2003;69:457-459.

131. Tait AR et al. Perioperative considerations for the child with an upper respiratory tract infection. *J PeriAnesth Nurs.* 2000;15:392-396.

132. Tait AR et al. Use of the laryngeal mask airway in children with upper respiratory tract infections: a comparison with endotracheal intubation. *Anesth Analg.* 1998;86:706-711.

133. Kamming D et al. Pain management in ambulatory surgery. *J Perianesth Nurs.* 2004;19:174-182.

134. Reuben SS et al. The preemptive analgesic effect of rofecoxib after ambulatory arthroscopic knee surgery. *Anesth Analg.* 2002;94:55-59.

135. Solanki DR et al. Comparative effects of oral sodium citrate and oral cimetidine on gastric pH in pediatric patients. *Anesth Analg.* 1986;65:S147.

136. Murrell GC, Rosen M. In vitro buffering capacity of Alka-Seltzer Effervescent: a comparison with magnesium trisilicate mixture BP and sodium citrate 0.3 M. *Anaesthesia.* 1986;41:138-142.

137. Manchikanti L et al. Effect of preanesthetic ranitidine and metoclopramide on gastric contents in morbidly obese patients. *Anesth Analg.* 1986;65:195-199.

138. Christensen S et al. Effects of ranitidine and metoclopramide on gastric fluid pH and volume in children. *Br J Anaesth.* 1990;65:456-460.

139. Brock-Utne JG et al. The effect of metoclopramide on the lower oesophageal sphincter in late pregnancy. *Anaesth Intensive Care.* 1978;6:26-29.

140. Diamond MJ, Keeri-Szanto M. Reduction of postoperative vomiting by preoperative administration of oral metoclopramide. *Can J Anaesth.* 1980;27:36-39.

141. Pandit SK et al. Dose-response study of droperidol and metoclopramide as antiemetics for outpatient anesthesia. *Anesth Analg.* 1989;68:798-802.

142. Dimich I et al. The effects of intravenous cimetidine and metoclopramide on gastric pH and volume in outpatients. *J Clin Anesth.* 1991;3:40-44.

143. Meyer PD. Preoperative interview and medication. In: McGough EK, Monroe MC, eds. *Problems in Anesthesia: Preoperative Evaluation.* Philadelphia: Lippincott; 1991:541-549.

144. Stoelting RK, Hillier SC. Antacids and gastrointestinal prokinetics. In: Stoelting RK, Hillier SC, eds. *Pharmacology and Physiology in Anesthetic Practice.* 4th ed. Philadelphia: Lippincott Williams & Wilkins; 2006:504-526.

145. Wyner J, Cohen SE. Gastric volume in early pregnancy: effect of metoclopramide. *Anesthesiology.* 1982;57:209-212.

146. Schulze-Delrieu K. Drug therapy: metoclopramide. *N Engl J Med.* 1981;305:28-33.

147. Stoelting RK, Hillier SC. Histamine and histamine receptor antagonists. In: Stoelting RK, Hilllier SC, eds. *Pharmacology and Physiology in Anesthetic Practice.* 4th ed. Philadelphia: Lippincott Williams & Wilkins; 2006:429-443.

148. McCullough AJ. A multicenter, randomized, double-blinded study comparing famotidine and ranitidine in the treatment of active duodenal ulcer disease. *Am J Med.* 1986;81(suppl 4B):17-24.

149. Ostro MJ. Pharmacodynamics and pharmacokinetics of parenteral histamine (H$_2$)-receptor antagonists. *Am J Med.* 1987;83(Suppl 6A):15-22.

150. Dubin SA et al. Comparison of the effects of oral famotidine and ranitidine on gastric volume and pH. *Anesth Analg.* 1989;69:680-683.

151. Lam AM et al. The effects of cimetidine and ranitidine with and without metoclopramide on gastric volume and pH in morbidly obese patients. *Can J Anaesth.* 1986;33:773-779.

152. Stoelting RK. Gastric fluid pH in patients receiving cimetidine. *Anesth Analg.* 1978;57:675-677.

153. Goudsouzian N et al. The dose-response effects of oral cimetidine on gastric pH and volume in children. *Anesthesiology.* 1981;55:533-536.

154. Tatekawa S et al. Comparison of effects of intravenous versus intramuscular famotidine on pH and volume of gastric juice. *Masui.* 1990;39:1619-1625.

155. Gardner JD et al. Determination of the time of onset of action of ranitidine and famotidine on intra-gastric acidity. *Aliment Pharmacol Ther.* 2002;16:1317-1326.

156. Manchikanti L et al. Dose-response effects of intravenous ranitidine on gastric pH and volume in outpatients. *Anesthesiology.* 1986;65:180-185.

157. Manchikanti L et al. Ranitidine and metoclopramide for prophylaxis of aspiration pneumonitis in elective surgery. *Anesth Analg.* 1984;63:903-910.

158. Escolano F et al. The efficacy and optimum time of administration of ranitidine in the prevention of the acid aspiration syndrom. *Anaesthesia.* 1996;51:182-184.

159. Haskins DA et al. Single-dose oral omeprazole for reduction of gastric residual acidity in adults for outpatient surgery. *Acta Anaesthesiol Scand.* 1992;36:513-515.

160. Gin T et al. Effect of oral omeprazole on intragastric pH and volume in women undergoing elective caesarean section. *Br J Anaesth.* 1990;65:616-619.

161. Ewart MC et al. A comparison of the effects of omeprazole and ranitidine on gastric secretion in women undergoing elective caesarean section. *Anaesthesia.* 1990;45:527-530.

162. Atanassoff PG et al. Effects of single-dose intravenous omeprazole and ranitidine on gastric pH during general anesthesia. *Anesth Analg.* 1992;75:95-98.

163. Escolano F et al. Effects of omeprazole, ranitidine, famotidine and placebo on gastric secretion in patients undergoing elective surgery. *Br J Anaesth.* 1992;69:404-406.

164. Nishina K et al. A comparison of rabeprazole, lansoprazole, and ranitidine for improving preoperative gastric fluid property in adults undergoing elective surgery. *Anesth Analg.* 2000;90:717-721.

165. Memis D et al. The effect of intravenous pantoprazole and ranitidine for improving preoperative gastric fluid properties in adults undergoing elective surgery. *Anesth Analg.* 2003;97:1360-1363.

166. Chikungwa M, Smith I. Controversial issues in ambulatory anesthesia. *Anesthesiol Clin North America.* 2003;21:313-327.

167. Liu J et al. Electroencephalographic bispectral index correlates with intraoperative recall and depth of propofol-induced sedation. *Anesth Analg.* 1997;84:185-189.

168. Anez C et al. The effect of encephalogram bispectral index monitoring during total intravenous anesthesia with propofol in outpatient surgery. *Rev Esp Anestesiol Reanim.* 2001;48:264-269.

169. Song D et al. Titration of volatile anesthetics using bispectral index facilitates recovery after ambulatory anesthesia. *Anesthesiology.* 1997;87:842-848.

170. Pavlin DJ et al. The effect of bispectral index monitoring on end-tidal gas concentration and recovery duration after outpatient anesthesia. *Anesth Analg.* 2001;93:613-619.

171. Messieha ZS et al. Bispectral Index System (BIS) monitoring reduces time to extubation and discharge in children requiring oral presedation and general anesthesia for outpatient dental rehabilitation. *Pediatr Dent.* 2005;27:500-504.

172. Messieha ZS et al. Bispectral Index System (BIS) monitoring reduces time to discharge in children requiring intramuscular sedation and general anesthesia for outpatient dental rehabilitation. *Pediatr Dent.* 2004;26:256-260.

173. White PF et al. Does the use of electroencephalographic bispectral index or auditory evoked potential index monitoring facilitate recovery after desflurane anesthesia in the ambulatory setting? *Anesthesiology.* 2004;100:811-817.

174. Nelskyla KA et al. Sevoflurane titration using bispectral index decreases postoperative vomiting in phase II recovery after ambulatory surgery. *Anesth Analg.* 2001;93:1165-1169.

175. Zohar E et al. Bispectral index monitoring does not improve early recovery of geriatric outpatients undergoing brief surgical procedures. *Can J Anaesth.* 2006;53:20-25.

176. Avidan MS et al. Anesthesia awareness and bispectral index. *N Engl J Med.* 2008;358(11):1097-1108.

177. Orser BA. Depth of anesthesia monitoring and the frequency of intraoperative awareness. *N Engl J Med.* 2008;358(11):1189-1191.

178. Tomlin PJ et al. Postoperative atelectasis and laryngeal incompetence. *Lancet.* 1968;1:1402-1405.

179. Kurer FL, Welsh DB. Gynaecological laparoscopy: clinical experiences of two anaesthetic techniques. *Br J Anaesth.* 1984;56:1207-1212.

180. Litman RS, Keon TP. Postintubation croup in children. *Anesthesiology.* 1991;75:1122-1123.

181. Cork RC et al. Prospective comparison of use of the laryngeal mask and endotracheal tube for ambulatory surgery. *Anesth Analg.* 1994;79:719-727.

182. Joshi GP et al. Use of the laryngeal mask airway as an alternative to the tracheal tube during ambulatory anesthesia. *Anesth Analg.* 1997;85:573-577.

183. Keane PW, Murray PF. Intravenous fluids in minor surgery: their effect on recovery from anaesthesia. *Anaesthesia.* 1986;41:635-637.

184. Chohedri AH et al. The impact of operative fluids on the prevention of postoperative anesthetic complications in ambulatory surgery—high dose vs low dose. *Middle East J Anesthesiol.* 2006;18:1147-1156.

185. Cook R et al. Intravenous fluid load and recovery: a double-blind comparison in gynaecological patients who had day-case laparoscopy. *Anaesthesia.* 1990;45:826-830.

186. Yogendran S et al. A prospective randomized double-blinded study of the effect of intravenous fluid therapy on adverse outcomes on outpatient surgery. *Anesth Analg.* 1995;80:682-686.

187. Magner JJ et al. Effect of intraoperative intravenous crystalloid infusion on postoperative nausea and vomiting after gynaecological laparoscopy: comparison of 30 and 10 ml kg(-1). *Br J Anaesth.* 2004;93:381-385.

188. Ali SZ et al. Effect of supplemental pre-operative fluid on postoperative nausea and vomiting. *Anaesthesia.* 2003;58:780-784.

189. Holte K et al. Liberal versus restrictive fluid management in knee arthroplasty: a randomized, double-blind study. *Anesth Analg.* 2007;105:465-474.

190. Holte K et al. Liberal versus restrictive fluid administration to improve recovery after laparoscopic cholecystectomy: a randomized, double-blind study. *Ann Surg.* 2004;240:892-899.

191. Mulroy MF, Salinas FV. Neuraxial techniques for ambulatory anesthesia. *Int Anesthesiol Clin.* 2005;43:129-141.
192. Gebhard RE. Outpatient regional anesthesia for upper extremity surgery. *Int Anesthesiol Clin.* 2005;43:177-183.
193. Klein SM et al. Peripheral nerve block techniques for ambulatory surgery. *Anesth Analg.* 2005;101:1663-1676.
194. Julien RE, Williams BA. Regional anesthesia procedures for outpatient shoulder surgery. *Int Anesthesiol Clin.* 2005;43:167-175.
195. Chow MY et al. Alkalinization of lidocaine does not hasten the onset of axillary brachial plexus block. *Anesth Analg.* 1998;86:566-8.
196. Candido KD et al. Addition of bicarbonate to plain bupivacaine does not significantly alter the onset or duration of plexus anesthesia. *Reg Anesth.* 1995;20:133-138.
197. Tetzlaff JE et al. Alkalinization of mepivacaine accelerates onset of interscalene block for shoulder surgery. *Reg Anesth.* 1990;15:242-244.
198. Quinlan JJ et al. Alkalinization of mepivacaine for axillary block. *Anesth Analg.* 1992;74:371-374.
199. Bryan NA et al. Indwelling interscalene catheter use in an outpatient setting for shoulder surgery: technique, efficacy, and complications. *J Shoulder Elbow Surg.* 2007;16:388-395.
200. Russon K et al. Postoperative shoulder surgery initiative (POSSI): an interim report of major shoulder surgery as a day case procedure. *Br J Anaesth.* 2006;97:869-873.
201. Klein S et al. Peripheral nerve blockade with long-acting local anesthetics: a survey of the Society for Ambulatory Anesthesia. *Anesth Analg.* 2002;94:71-76.
202. Philip BK. Regional anaesthesia for ambulatory surgery. *Can J Anaesth.* 1992;39:R3-R6.
203. Litchtor JL, Kalghatgi SV. Outpatient anesthesia. In: Longnecker DE et al, eds. *Anesthesiology.* New York: McGraw-Hill; 2008:1608-1624.
204. Mulroy MF. Regional anesthesia for adult outpatients. In: White PF, ed. *Outpatient Anesthesia.* New York: Churchill Livingstone; 1990:293-311.
205. D'Alessio JG et al. A retrospective comparison of interscalene block and general anesthesia for ambulatory surgery shoulder arthroscopy. *Reg Anesth.* 1995;20:62-68.
206. Brown AR et al. Interscalene block for shoulder arthroscopy: comparison with general anesthesia. *Arthroscopy.* 1993;9:295-300.
207. Davis WJ et al. Brachial plexus anesthesia for outpatient surgical procedures on an upper extremity. *Mayo Clin Proc.* 1991;66:470-473.
208. Philip BK, Covino BG. Local and regional anesthesia. In: Wetchler BV, ed. *Anesthesia for Ambulatory Surgery.* 2nd ed. Philadelphia: Lippincott; 1991:309-374.
209. Wolf AR et al. Bupivacaine for caudal analgesia in infants and children: the optimal effective concentration. *Anesthesiology.* 1988;69:102-106.
210. Jamali S et al. Clonidine in pediatric caudal anesthesia. *Anesth Analg.* 1994;78:663-666.
211. May AE et al. Analgesia for circumcision in children: a comparison of caudal bupivacaine and intramuscular buprenorphine. *Acta Anaesthesiol Scand.* 1982;26:331-333.
212. Splinter WM et al. Reducing pain after inguinal hernia repair in children. *Anesthesiology.* 1997;87:542-546.
213. Splinter WM et al. Regional anaesthesia for hernia repair in children: local vs. caudal anaesthesia. *Can J Anaesth.* 1995;42:197-200.
214. Chilvers CR et al. Pharmacoeconomics of intravenous regional anaesthesia vs. general anaesthesia for outpatient hand surgery. *Can J Anaesth.* 1997;44:1152-1156.
215. Olney BW et al. Outpatient treatment of upper extremity injuries in childhood using intravenous regional anaesthesia. *J Pediatr Orthop.* 1988;8:576-579.
216. Shah S et al. Outpatient regional anesthesia for foot and ankle surgery. *Int Anesthesiol Clin.* 2005;43:143-151.
217. Ilfeld BM et al. Popliteal sciatic perineural local anesthetic infusion: a comparison of three dosing regimens for postoperative analgesia. *Anesthesiology.* 2004;101:970-977.
218. Williams BA et al. Femoral-sciatic nerve blocks for complex outpatient knee surgery are associated with less postoperative pain before same-day discharge: a review of 1,200 consecutive cases from the period 1996-1999. *Anesthesiology.* 2003;98:1206-1213.
219. Nakamura SJ et al. The efficacy of regional anesthesia for outpatient anterior cruciate ligament reconstruction. *Arthroscopy.* 1997;13:699-703.
220. Klein SM et al. Ambulatory discharge after long-acting peripheral nerve blockade: 2382 blocks with ropivacaine. *Anesth Analg.* 2002;94:65-70.
221. Felts JA. Outpatient anesthesia in the geriatric patient. *Clin Anesthesiol.* 1986;4:1025-1034.
222. Korhonen A-M. Use of spinal anaesthesia in day surgery. *Curr Opin Anaesthesiol.* 2006;19:612-616.
223. Vaghadia H et al. Small-dose hypobaric lidocaine-fentanyl spinal anesthesia for short duration outpatient laparoscopy. I. A randomized comparison with conventional dose hyperbaric lidocaine. *Anesth Analg.* 1997;84:59-64.
224. Chilvers CR et al. Small-dose hypobaric lidocaine-fentanyl spinal anesthesia for short duration outpatient laparoscopy. II. Optimal fentanyl dose. *Anesth Analg.* 1997;84:65-70.
225. Pollock JE et al. A comparison of two regional anesthetic techniques for outpatient knee arthroscopy. *Anesth Analg.* 2003;97:397-401.
226. Kokki H et al. Spinal anaesthesia for paediatric day-case surgery: a double-blind, randomized, parallel group, prospective comparison of isobaric and hyperbaric bupivacaine. *Br J Anaesth.* 1998;81:502-506.
227. Tarkkila P et al. Home-readiness after spinal anaesthesia with small doses of hyperbaric 0.5% bupivacaine. *Anaesthesia.* 1997;52:1157-1160.
228. Moore JM et al. The effect of epinephrine on small-dose hyperbaric bupivacaine spinal anesthesia: clinical implications for ambulatory surgery. *Anesth Analg.* 1998;86:973-977.
229. Ben-David B et al. Spinal bupivacaine in ambulatory surgery: the effect of saline dilution. *Anesth Analg.* 1996;83:716-720.
230. Ben-David B et al. Intrathecal fentanyl with small-dose dilute bupivacaine: better anesthesia without prolonging recovery. *Anesth Analg.* 1997;85(3): 560-565.
231. Liu SS. Optimizing spinal anesthesia for ambulatory surgery. *Reg Anesth.* 1997;22:500-510.
232. Korhonen AM et al. Intrathecal hyperbaric bupivacaine 3 mg + fentanyl 10 microg for outpatient knee arthroscopy with tourniquet. *Acta Anaesthesiol Scand.* 2003;47:342-346.
233. Gupta A et al. Low-dose bupivacaine plus fentanyl for spinal anesthesia during ambulatory inguinal herniorrhaphy: a comparison between 6 mg and 7.5 mg of bupivacaine. *Acta Anaesthesiol Scand.* 2003;47:13-19.
234. Buckenmaier CC III et al. Small-dose intrathecal lidocaine versus ropivacaine for anorectal surgery in an ambulatory setting. *Anesth Analg.* 2002;95:1253-1257.
235. Ben-David B et al. A comparison of minidose lidocaine-fentanyl and conventional-dose lidocaine spinal anesthesia. *Anesth Analg.* 2000;91: 865-870.
236. Ben-David B et al. A comparison of minidose lidocaine-fentanyl spinal anesthesia and local anesthesia/propofol infusion for outpatient knee arthroscopy. *Anesth Analg.* 2001;93:319-325.
237. Urmey WF. Spinal anaesthesia for outpatient surgery. *Best Pract Res Clin Anaesthesiol.* 2003;17:335-346.
238. Santanen U et al. Comparison of 27-gauge (0.41-mm) Whitacre and Quincke spinal needles with respect to post-dural puncture headache and non-dural puncture headache. *Acta Anaesthesiol Scand.* 2004;48:474-479.
239. Mulroy MF. Extending indications for spinal anesthesia. *Reg Anesth Pain Med.* 1998;23:380-383.
240. Carbaat PA, van Crevel H. Lumbar puncture headache: controlled study on the preventive effect of 24 hours' bed rest. *Lancet.* 1981;2:1133-1135.
241. Sime AC. Transient neurologic symptoms and spinal anesthesia. *AANA J.* 2000;68:163-168.
242. Gold MS et al. Lidocaine toxicity in primary afferent neurons from the rat. *J Pharmacol Exp Ther.* 1998;285:413-421.
243. Hampl KF et al. Transient neurologic symptoms after spinal anesthesia: a lower incidence with prilocaine and bupivacaine than with lidocaine. *Anesthesiology.* 1998;88:629-633.
244. Freedman JM et al. Transient neurologic symptoms after spinal anesthesia: an epidemiologic study of 1,863 patients. *Anesthesiology.* 1998;89:633-641.
245. Liguori GA et al. Transient neurologic symptoms after spinal anesthesia with mepivacaine and lidocaine. *Anesthesiology.* 1998;88:619-623.
246. Hodgson PS et al. Procaine compared with lidocaine for incidence of transient neurologic symptoms. *Reg Anesth Pain Med.* 2000;25:218-222.
247. Casati A et al. Spinal anesthesia with lidocaine or preservative-free 2-chlorprocaine for outpatient knee arthroscopy: a prospective, randomized, double-blind comparison. *Anesth Analg.* 2007;104:959-964.
248. Harris AP. Spinal anesthesia: it works. *Anesthesiol Rep.* 1990;3:56.
249. Bridenbaugh LD. Catheterization after long- and short-acting local anesthetics for continuous caudal block for vaginal delivery. *Anesthesiology.* 1977;46:357-359.
250. Ben-David B et al. Spinal bupivacaine in ambulatory surgery: the effect of saline dilution. *Anesth Analg.* 1996;83:716-720.
251. Kamphuis ET et al. Recovery of storage and emptying functions of the urinary bladder after spinal anesthesia with lidocaine and with bupivacaine in men. *Anesthesiology.* 1998;88:310-316.
252. Frey K et al. The recovery profile of hyperbaric spinal anesthesia with lidocaine, tetracaine, and bupivacaine. *Reg Anesth Pain Med.* 1998;23: 159-163.

253. Turker G et al. Effects of adding epinephrine plus fentanyl to low-dose lidocaine for spinal anesthesia in outpatient knee arthroscopy. *Acta Anaesthesiol Scand.* 2003;47:986-992.

254. Vath JS, Kopacz DJ. Spinal 2-chloroprocaine: the effect of added fentanyl. *Anesth Analg.* 2004;98:89-94.

255. Kito Km et al. The effect of varied doses of epinephrine on duration of lidocaine spinal anesthesia in the thoracic and lumbosacral dermatomes. *Anesth Analg.* 1998;86:1018-1022.

256. Breebaart MB et al. Urinary bladder scanning after day-case arthroscopy under spinal anaesthesia: comparison between lidocaine, ropivacaine, and levobupivacaine. *Br J Anaesth.* 2003;90:309-313.

257. Mulroy MF et al. Ambulatory surgery patients may be discharged before voiding after short-acting spinal and epidural anesthesia. *Anesthesiology.* 2002;97:315-319.

258. Urquhart ML, White PF. Comparison of sedative infusions during regional anesthesia: methohexital, etomidate, and midazolam. *Anesth Analg.* 1989;68:249-254.

259. Tucker MR et al. Arterial blood gas levels after midazolam or diazepam administered with or without fentanyl as an intravenous sedative for outpatient surgical procedures. *J Oral Maxillofac Surg.* 1986;44:688-692.

260. Ramirez-Ruiz M et al. Monitored anesthesia care: use of ketorolac, dezocine, and fentanyl. *Anesthesiology.* 1992;77:A27.

261. White PF, Negus JB. Sedative infusions during local and regional anesthesia: a comparison of midazolam and propofol. *J Clin Anesth.* 1991;3:32-39.

262. Church JA et al. Propofol for sedation during endoscopy: assessment of a computer-controlled infusion system. *Gastrointest Endosc.* 1991;37:175-179.

263. Patterson KW et al. Propofol sedation for outpatient upper gastrointestinal endoscopy: comparison with midazolam. *Br J Anaesth.* 1991;67:108-111.

264. White PF. Ambulatory anesthesia—fast tracking concepts. IARS 1998 Review Course Lectures. *Anesth Analg.* 1998;March(Suppl):153-156.

265. Song D et al. Fast-track eligibility after ambulatory anesthesia: a comparison of desflurane, sevoflurane, and propofol. *Anesth Analg.* 1998;86:267-273.

266. Gan TJ et al. and the BIS Utility Study Group. Bispectral index monitoring allows faster emergence and improved recovery from propofol, alfentanil, and nitrous oxide anesthesia. *Anesthesiology.* 1997;87:808-815.

267. Song D et al. Is the bispectral index useful in predicting fast-track eligibility after ambulatory anesthesia with propofol and desflurane? *Anesth Analg.* 1998;87:1245-1248.

268. Apfelbaum JL. Bypassing PACU: a cost effective measure. *Can J Anaesth.* 1998;45:R91-R92.

269. Duncan PG et al. A pilot study of recovery room bypass ("fast-track protocol") in a community hospital. *Can J Anaesth.* 2001;48:630-636.

270. Macario A et al. What can the PACU manager do to decrease cost in the PACU? *J Perianesth Nurs.* 1999;14(5):284-293.

271. Williams BA et al. PACU bypass after outpatient knee surgery is associated with fewer unplanned hospital admissions but more phase II nursing interventions. *Anesthesiology.* 2002;97:981-988.

272. Watkins AC, White PF. Fast-tracking after ambulatory surgery. *J PeriAnesth Nurs.* 2001;16:379-387.

273. Warner MA et al. Major morbidity and mortality within 1 month of ambulatory surgery and anesthesia. *JAMA.* 1993;270:1437-1441.

274. Shnaider I, Chung F. Outcomes in day surgery. *Curr Opin Anaesthesiol.* 2006;19:622-629.

275. Awad IT et al. Unplanned hospital admission in children undergoing day-case surgery. *Eur J Anaesthesiol.* 2004;21:379-383.

276. Junger A et al. Factors determining length of stay of surgical day-case patients. *Eur J Anaesthesiol.* 2001;18:314-321.

277. Fleisher LA et al. Inpatient hospital admission and death after outpatient surgery in elderly patients. *Arch Surg.* 2004;139:67-72.

278. Twersky R et al. What happens after discharge? Return hospital visits after ambulatory surgery. *Anesth Analg.* 1997;84:319-324.

279. Mezei G, Chung F. Return hospital visits and hospital readmissions after ambulatory surgery. *Ann Surg.* 1999;230:721-727.

280. Scarlett M et al. Paediatric day surgery: revisiting the University Hospital of the West Indies experience. *West Indian Med J.* 2007;56:320-325.

281. Woods DM et al. Ambulatory care adverse events and preventable adverse events leading to a hospital admission. *Qual Saf Health Care.* 2007;16:127-131.

282. Green G, Jonsson L. Nausea: the most important factor determining length of stay after ambulatory anaesthesia: a comparative study of isoflurane and/or propofol techniques. *Acta Anaesthesiol Scand.* 1993;37:742-746.

283. Westman HR. Postoperative complications and unanticipated hospital admissions. *Semin Pediatr Surg.* 1999;8:23-29.

284. Forrest JB et al. Multicenter study of general anesthesia. II. Results. *Anesthesiology.* 1990;72:262-268.

285. Larsson S, Lundberg D. A prospective survey of postoperative nausea and vomiting with special regard to incidence and relations to patient characteristics, anesthetic routines and surgical procedures. *Acta Anaesthesiol Scand.* 1995;39:539-545.

286. Karlsson E et al. Postanesthetic nausea in children. *Acta Anaesthesiol Scand.* 1990;34:515-518.

287. Cohen MM et al. Pediatric anesthesia morbidity and mortality in the perioperative period. *Anesth Analg.* 1990;70:160-167.

288. Kotiniemi LH et al. Postoperative symptoms at home following day-case surgery in children: a multicentre survey of 551 children. *Anaesthesia.* 1997;52:963-969.

289. Wu CL et al. Systematic review and analysis of postdischarge symptoms after outpatient surgery. *Anesthesiology.* 2002;96:994-1003.

290. Marley RA. Postoperative nausea and vomiting: the outpatient enigma. *J Perianesth Nurs.* 1996;11:147-161.

291. Norred CL. Antiemetic prophylaxis: pharmacology and therapeutics. *AANA J.* 2003;71:133-140.

292. Cameron D, Gan FJ. Management of postoperative nausea and vomiting in ambulatory surgery. *Anesthesiol Clin North America.* 2003;21:347-365.

293. Muir JJ et al. Role of nitrous oxide and other factors in postoperative nausea and vomiting: a randomized and blinded prospective study. *Anesthesiology.* 1987;66:513-518.

294. Purkis IE. Factors that influence postoperative vomiting. *Can Anaesth Soc J.* 1964;11:335-353.

295. Bellville JW et al. Postoperative nausea and vomiting IV: factors related to postoperative nausea and vomiting. *Anesthesiology.* 1960;21:186-193.

296. Lerman J. Surgical and patient factors involved in postoperative nausea and vomiting. *Br J Anaesth.* 1992;69(suppl):24S-32S.

297. Rowley MP, Brown TC. Postoperative vomiting in children. *Anaesth Intensive Care.* 1982;10:309-313.

298. Sinclair DR et al. Can postoperative nausea and vomiting be predicted? *Anesthesiology.* 1999;91:109-118.

299. Murphy MJ et al. Identification of risk factors for postoperative nausea and vomiting in the perianesthesia adult patient. *J PeriAnesth Nurs.* 2006;21:377-384.

300. Quinn AC et al. Studies in postoperative sequelae: nausea and vomiting—still a problem. *Anaesthesia.* 1994;49:62-65.

301. Eger EI II. Nitrous oxide transfer to closed gas spaces. *Anesthetic Uptake and Action.* Baltimore: Williams & Wilkins; 1974:171-183.

302. Foldes FF et al. Severe gastrointestinal distention during nitrous oxide and oxygen anesthesia. *JAMA.* 1965;194:1146-1148.

303. Ong BY et al. Gastric volume and pH in out-patients. *Can Anaesth Soc J.* 1978;25:36-39.

304. White PF, Shafer A. Nausea and vomiting: causes and prophylaxis. *Semin Anesth.* 1987;6:300-308.

305. Watcha MF, White PF. Postoperative nausea and vomiting: its etiology, treatment, and prevention. *Anesthesiology.* 1992;77:162-184.

306. Read NW, Houghton LA. Physiology of gastric emptying and pathophysiology of gastroparesis. *Gastroenterol Clin North Am.* 1989;18:359-373.

307. Varis K. Diabetic gastroparesis. *Scand J Gastroenterol.* 1989;24:897-903.

308. Gan TJ et al. Society for Ambulatory Anesthesia guidelines for the management of postoperative nausea and vomiting. *Anesth Analg.* 2007;105:1615-1628.

309. Gan TJ. Risk factors for postoperative nausea and vomiting. *Anesth Analg.* 2007;102:1884-1898.

310. Bodman RI et al. Vomiting by outpatients after nitrous oxide anaesthesia. *BMJ.* 1960;30:1327-1330.

311. Riding JE. The prevention of postoperative vomiting. *Br J Anaesth.* 1963;35:180-188.

312. Pandit SK, Kothary SP. Intravenous narcotics for premedication in outpatient anaesthesia. *Acta Anaesthesiol Scand.* 1989;33:353-358.

313. Gerwels JW et al. Oral transmucosal fentanyl citrate premedication in patients undergoing outpatient dermatologic procedures. *J Dermatol Surg Oncol.* 1994;20:823-826.

314. Shafer A et al. Outpatient premedication: use of midazolam and opioid analgesics. *Anesthesiology.* 1989;71:495-501.

315. Andrews PLR. Physiology of nausea and vomiting. *Br J Anaesth.* 1992;69(suppl):2S-19S.

316. Racke K, Schworer H. Regulation of serotonin release from the intestinal mucosa. *Pharmacol Res.* 1991;23:13-25.

317. Rubin A, Winston J. The role of the vestibular apparatus in the production of nausea and vomiting following the administration of morphine to man. *J Clin Invest.* 1950;29:1261-1266.

318. Hovorka J et al. The experience of the person ventilating the lungs does influence postoperative nausea and vomiting. *Acta Anaesthesiol Scand.* 1990;34:203-205.

319. de Grood PM et al. Anaesthesia for laparoscopy: a comparison of five techniques including propofol, etomidate, thiopentone and isoflurane. *Anaesthesia.* 1987;42:815-823.

320. Chittleborough MC et al. Double-blind comparison of patient recovery after induction with propofol or thiopentone for day-case relaxant general anaesthesia. *Anaesth Intensive Care.* 1992;20:169-173.

321. Jobalia N, Mathieu A. A meta-analysis of published studies confirms decreased postoperative nausea/vomiting with propofol [abstract]. *Anesthesiology.* 1994;81:A33.

322. Cheng KP. A prospective, randomized, controlled comparison of retrobulbar and general anesthesia for strabismus surgery. *Ophthalmic Surg.* 1992;23:585-590.

323. Ghouri AF et al. Recovery profile after desflurane-nitrous oxide versus isoflurane-nitrous oxide in outpatients. *Anesthesiology.* 1991;74:419-424.

324. Johannesson GP et al. Sevoflurane for ENT-surgery in children: a comparison with halothane. *Acta Anaesthesiol Scand.* 1995;39:546-550.

325. Davis I et al. Nitrous oxide and the middle ear. *Anaesthesia.* 1979;34:147-151.

326. Perreault L et al. Middle ear pressure variations during nitrous oxide and oxygen anaesthesia. *Can Anaesth Soc J.* 1982;29:428-434.

327. Gillman MA. Possible mechanisms of action of nitrous oxide at the opioid receptor. *Med Hypotheses.* 1984;15:109-114.

328. Jenkins LC, Hahay D. Central mechanisms of vomiting related to catecholamine response: anaesthetic implications. *Can Anaesth Soc J.* 1971;18:434-441.

329. Andersen R, Krohg K. Pain as a major cause of postoperative nausea and vomiting. *Can J Anaesth.* 1976;23:366-369.

330. Rose DK et al. Reducing postoperative nausea and vomiting: what works and what doesn't [abstract]. *Anesth Analg.* 1995;80:S403.

331. Byers GF et al. Postoperative nausea and vomiting in paediatric surgical inpatients. *Paediatr Anaesth.* 1995;5:253-256.

332. Schreiner MS et al. Should children drink before discharge from day surgery? *Anesthesiology.* 1992;76:528-533.

333. Jin F et al. Should adult patients drink fluids before discharge from ambulatory surgery? *Anesth Analg.* 1998;87:306-311.

334. Kearney R et al. Withholding oral fluids from children undergoing day surgery reduces vomiting. *Paediatr Anaesth.* 1998;8:331-336.

335. Kabon B, Kurz A. Optimal perioperative oxygen administration. *Curr Opin Anaesthesiol.* 2006;19:11-18.

336. Orhan-Sungur M et al. Supplemental oxygen does not reduce postoperative nausea and vomiting: a systematic review of randomized controlled trials. *Anesthesiology.* 2005;103:A626.

337. Kranke P et al. A qualitative systematic review on supplemental perioperative oxygen to reduce the incidence of postoperative nausea and vomiting. *Eur J Anaesthesiol.* 2005;22(suppl 34):4.

338. Purhonen S et al. Supplemental oxygen for prevention of nausea and vomiting after breast surgery. *Br J Anaesth.* 2003;91:284-287.

339. Purhonen S et al. Supplemental oxygen does not reduce the incidence of postoperative nausea and vomiting after ambulatory gynecologic laparoscopy. *Anesth Analg.* 2003;96:91-96.

340. Skledar SJ et al. Eliminating postoperative nausea and vomiting in outpatient surgery with multimodal strategies including low doses of nonsedating, off-patent antiemetics: is "zero tolerance" achievable? *Sci World J.* 2007;7:959-977.

341. Kranke P et al. Recent advances, trends and economic considerations in the risk assessment, prevention and treatment of postoperative nausea and vomiting. *Expert Opin Pharmacother.* 2007;8:3217-3235.

342. Golembiewski J, Tokumaru S. Pharmacological prophylaxis and management of adult postoperative/postdischarge nausea and vomiting. *J PeriAnesth Nurs.* 2006;21:385-397.

343. Turgut S et al. Acupressure for postoperative nausea and vomiting in gynaecological patients receiving patient-controlled analgesia. *Eur J Anaesthesiol.* 2007;24:87-91.

344. Streitberger K et al. Acupuncture for nausea and vomiting: an update of clinical and experimental studies. *Auton Neurosci.* 2006;129:107-117.

345. Hickman AG et al. Acupressure and postoperative nausea and vomiting. *AANA J.* 2005;73:379-385.

346. Rowbotham DJ. Recent advances in the non-pharmacological management of postoperative nausea and vomiting. *Br J Anaesth.* 2005;95:77-81.

347. Alvaro G, Di Fabio R. Neurokinin 1 receptor antagonists—current prospects. *Curr Opin Drug Discov Devel.* 2007;10:613-621.

348. Diemunsch P et al. Preventing postoperative nausea and vomiting: post hoc analysis of pooled data from two randomized active-controlled trials of aprepitant. *Curr Med Res Opin.* 2007;23:2559-2565.

349. Diemunsch P et al. Single-dose aprepitant vs. ondansetron for the prevention of postoperative nausea and vomiting: a randomized, double-blind phase III trial in patients undergoing open abdominal surgery. *Br J Anaesth.* 2007;99:202-211.

350. Gan TJ et al. A randomized, double-blind comparison of the NK1 antagonist, aprepitant, versus ondansetron for the prevention of postoperative nausea and vomiting. *Anesth Analg.* 2007;104:1082-1089.

351. Warren A, King L. A review of the efficacy of dexamethasone in the prevention of postoperative nausea and vomiting. *J Clin Nurs.* 2008;17:58-68.

352. Bianchin A et al. Postoperative vomiting reduction after laparoscopic cholecystectomy with single dose of dexamethasone. *Minerva Anestesiol.* 2007;73:343-346.

353. Fazel MR et al. The effect of dexamethasone on postoperative vomiting and oral intake after adenotonsillectomy. *Int J Pediatr Otorhinolaryngol.* 2007;71:1235-1238.

354. Fujii Y, Nakayama M. Dexamethasone for reduction of nausea, vomiting and analgesic use after gynecological laparoscopic surgery. *Int J Gynaecol Obstet.* 2008;100:27-30.

355. Fujii Y, Nakayama M. Reduction of postoperative nausea and vomiting and analgesic requirement with dexamethasone in women undergoing general anesthesia for mastectomy. *Breast J.* 2007;13:564-567.

356. Liechti M et al. Prevention of postoperative nausea and vomiting in children following adenotonsillectomy, using tropisetron with or without low-dose dexamethasone. *J Anesth.* 2007;21:311-316.

357. Kim EJ et al. Combination of antiemetics for the prevention of postoperative nausea and vomiting in high-risk patients. *J Korean Med Sci.* 2007;22:878-882.

358. Kim MS et al. There is no dose-escalation response to dexamethasone (0.0625-1.0 mg/kg) in pediatric tonsillectomy or adenotonsillectomy patients for preventing vomiting, reducing pain, shortening time to first liquid intake, or the incidence of voice change. *Anesth Analg.* 2007;104:1052-1058.

359. Wang JJ et al. The effect of timing of dexamethasone administration on its efficacy as a prophylactic antiemetic for postoperative nausea and vomiting. *Anesth Analg.* 2000;91:136-139.

360. Neff SP et al. Excruciating perineal pain after intravenous dexamethasone. *Anaesth Intensive Care.* 2002;30:370-371.

361. Rusch D et al. The addition of dexamethasone to dolasetron or haloperidol for treatment of established postoperative nausea and vomiting. *Anaesthesia.* 2007;62:810-817.

362. Koc S et al. The preoperative use of gabapentin, dexamethasone, and their combination in varicocele surgery: a randomized controlled trial. *Anesth Analg.* 2007;105:1137-1142.

363. Coloma M et al. Dexamethasone facilitates discharge after outpatient anorectal surgery. *Anesth Analg.* 2001;92:85-88.

364. Coloma M et al. Dexamethasone in combination with dolasetron for prophylaxis in the ambulatory setting: effect on outcome after laparoscopic cholecystectomy. *Anesthesiology.* 2002;96:1346-1350.

365. Steward DL et al. Steroids for improving recovery following tonsillectomy in children. *Cochrane Database Syst Rev.* 2003;1:CD003997.

366. Kranke P et al. Dolasetron in the prevention of postoperative nausea and vomiting: a meta-analysis of randomized controlled trials. *Anasthesiologie Intensivmedizin.* 2002;43:413-427.

367. Korttila K et al. Intravenous dolasetron and ondansetron in prevention of postoperative nausea and vomiting: a multicenter, double-blind, placebo-controlled study. *Acta Anaesthesiol Scand.* 1997;41:914-922.

368. Philip BK et al. Dolasetron for the prevention of postoperative nausea and vomiting following outpatient surgery with general anaesthesia: a randomized, placebo-controlled study. The Dolasetron PONV Prevention Study Group. *Eur J Anaesthesiol.* 2000;17(1):23-32.

369. Philip BK et al. Pooled analysis of three large clinical trials to determine the optimal dose of dolasetron mesylate needed to prevent postoperative nausea and vomiting. The Dolasetron Prophylaxis Study Group. *J Clin Anesth.* 2000;12(1):1-8.

370. Walker JB. Efficacy of single-dose intravenous dolasetron versus ondansetron in the prevention of postoperative nausea and vomiting. *Clin Ther.* 2001;23:932-938.

371. Valanne J, Korttila K. Effect of a small dose of droperidol on nausea, vomiting and recovery after outpatient enflurane anaesthesia. *Acta Anaesthesiol Scand.* 1985;29:359-362.

372. Lee Y et al. A dose ranging study of dexamethasone for preventing patient-controlled analgesia-related nausea and vomiting: a comparison of droperidol with saline. *Anesth Analg.* 2004;98:1066-1071.

373. Young D. FDA advisory panel discusses droperidol concerns. *Am J Health Syst Pharm.* 2004;61:219-220.

374. Wax D et al. Changing patterns of postoperative nausea and vomiting prophylaxis drug use in an academic anesthesia practice. *J Clin Anesth.* 2007;19:356-359.

375. Rothenberg DM et al. Efficacy of ephedrine in the prevention of postoperative nausea and vomiting. *Anesth Analg.* 1991;72:58-61.

376. Hagemann E et al. Intramuscular ephedrine reduces emesis during the first three hours after abdominal hysterectomy. *Acta Anaesthesiol Scand.* 2000;44:107-111.

377. Wetchler BV. Management of nausea and vomiting in the ambulatory surgical patient. *Soc Ambulatory Anesth Newslett.* 1988;3:2-3.

378. Heyman HJ et al. Does gastric suction enhance the efficacy of droperidol prophylaxis of post-operative nausea and vomiting? *Anesthesiology.* 1990;73:A19.

379. Hovorka J et al. Gastric aspiration at the end of anaesthesia does not decrease postoperative nausea and vomiting. *Anaesth Intensive Care.* 1990;18:58-61.

380. Kakinohana M et al. The effect of intraoperative gastric juice retention on the incidence of postoperative nausea and vomiting. *Masui.* 1995;44:119-123.

381. Jones JE et al. Efficacy of gastric aspiration in reducing posttonsillectomy vomiting. *Arch Otolaryngol Head Neck Surg.* 2001;127:980-984.

382. Trepanier CA, Isabel L. Perioperative gastric aspiration increases postoperative nausea and vomiting in outpatients. *Can J Anaesth.* 1993;40:325-328.

383. Albibi R, McCallum RW. Metoclopramide: pharmacology and clinical application. *Ann Intern Med.* 1983;98:86-95.

384. Henzi I et al. Metoclopramide in the prevention of postoperative nausea and vomiting: a qualitative systematic review of randomized placebo-controlled studies. *Br J Anaesth.* 1999;83:761-771.

385. Oksuz H et al. Comparison of the effectiveness of metoclopramide, ondansetron, and granisetron on the prevention of nausea and vomiting after laparoscopic cholecystectomy. *J Laparoendosc Adv Surg Tech A.* 2007;17:803-808.

386. Nesek-Adam V et al. Comparison of dexamethasone, metoclopramide, and their combination in the prevention of postoperative nausea and vomiting after laparoscopic. *Surg Endosc.* 2007;21:607-612.

387. Wallenborn J et al. Prevention of postoperative nausea and vomiting by metoclopramide combined with dexamethasone: randomized double blind multicentre trial. *BMJ.* 2006;333:324.

388. Gunter JB et al. A factorial study of ondansetron, metoclopramide, and dexamethasone for emesis prophylaxis after adenotonsillectomy in children. *Paediatr Anaesth.* 2006;16:1153-1165.

389. Bolton CM et al. Randomized, double-blind study comparing the efficacy of moderate-dose metoclopramide and ondansetron for the prophylactic control of postoperative vomiting in children after tonsillectomy. *Br J Anaesth.* 2007;99:699-703.

390. Wetchler BV. Recovery room: the anesthesiologist's role as a problem solver in ambulatory surgery. In: Barash PG, ed. *ASA Refresher Courses in Anesthesiology.* Philadelphia: Lippincott; 1991:207-216.

391. Caldwell C et al. An unusual reaction to preoperative metoclopramide. *Anesthesiology.* 1987;67:854-855.

392. Rodola F. Midazolam as an anti-emetic. *Eur Rev Med Pharmacol Sci.* 2006;10:121-126.

393. Dikmen Mentes S et al. Effect of sedation with midazolam or propofol on patient's comfort during cancer chemotherapy infusion: a prospective, randomized, double-blind study in breast cancer patients. *J Chemother.* 2005;17:327-333.

394. Mandala M et al. Midazolam for acute emesis refractory to dexamethasone and granisetron after highly emetogenic chemotherapy: a phase II study. *Support Care Cancer.* 2005;13:375-380.

395. Ozcan AA et al. Using diazepam and atropine before strabismus surgery to prevent postoperative nausea and vomiting: a randomized, controlled study. *J AAPOS.* 2003;7:210-212.

396. Khalil SN et al. The antiemetic effect of lorazepam after outpatient strabismus surgery in children. *Anesthesiology.* 1992;77:915-919.

397. Heidari SM et al. Effect of intravenous midazolam premedication on postoperative nausea and vomiting after cholecystectomy. *Acta Anaesthesiol Taiwan.* 2004;42:77-80.

398. Jung JS et al. Prophylactic antiemetic effect of midazolam after middle ear surgery. *Otolaryngol Head Neck Surg.* 2007;137:753-756.

399. Lee Y et al. Midazolam vs ondansetron for preventing postoperative nausea and vomiting: a randomized controlled trial. *Anaesthesia.* 2007;62:18-22.

400. Unlugenc H et al. Comparative study of the antiemetic efficacy of ondansetron, propofol and midazolam in the early postoperative period. *Eur J Anaesthesiol.* 2004;21:60-65.

401. Riad W et al. Effect of midazolam, dexamethasone and their combination on the prevention of nausea and vomiting following strabismus repair in children. *Eur J Anaesthesiol.* 2007;24:697-701.

402. Alon E, Himmelseher S. Ondansetron in the treatment of postoperative vomiting: a randomized, double-blind comparison with droperidol and metoclopramide. *Anesth Analg.* 1992;75:561-565.

403. Leeser J, Lip H. Prevention of postoperative nausea and vomiting using ondansetron, a new, selective, 5-HT$_3$ receptor antagonist. *Anesth Analg.* 1991;72:751-755.

404. Monk TG et al. Ondansetron reduces nausea following outpatient lithotripsy. *Anesthesiology.* 1992;77:A19.

405. Larijani GE et al. Treatment of postoperative nausea and vomiting with ondansetron: a randomized, double-blind comparison with placebo. *Anesth Analg.* 1991;73:246-249.

406. Tang J et al. The effect of timing of ondansetron administration on its efficacy, cost-effectiveness, and cost-benefit as a prophylactic antiemetic in the ambulatory setting. *Anesth Analg.* 1998;86:274-282.

407. Scuderi P et al. Treatment of postoperative nausea and vomiting after outpatient surgery with the 5-HT$_3$ antagonist ondansetron. *Anesthesiology.* 1993;78:15-20.

408. Kovac A et al. Prophylactic intravenous ondansetron in female outpatients undergoing gynaecological surgery: a multicentre dose-comparison study. *Eur J Anaesthesiol.* 1992;9(suppl 6):37-47.

409. Davis PJ et al. Effect of antiemetic therapy on recovery and hospital discharge time: a double-blind assessment of ondansetron, droperidol, and placebo in pediatric patients undergoing ambulatory surgery. *Anesthesiology.* 1995;83:956-960.

410. Paxton LD et al. Prevention of nausea and vomiting after day case gynaecological laparoscopy: a comparison of ondansetron, droperidol, metoclopramide and placebo. *Anaesthesia.* 1995;50:403-406.

411. Splinter WM et al. Ondansetron is a better prophylactic antiemetic than droperidol for tonsilectomy in children. *Can J Anaesth.* 1995;42:848-851.

412. Malins AF et al. Nausea and vomiting after gynaecological laparoscopy: comparison of premedication with oral ondansetron, metoclopramide and placebo. *Br J Anaesth.* 1994;72:231-233.

413. Blanc VF et al. Antiemetic prophylaxis with promethazine or droperidol in paediatric outpatient strabismus surgery. *Can J Anaesth.* 1991;38:54-60.

414. Habin AS et al. A comparison of ondansetron with promethazine for treating postoperative nausea and vomiting in patients who received prophylaxis with ondansetron: a retrospective database analysis. *Anesth Analg.* 2007;104:548-551.

415. Nachum Z et al. Transdermal scopolamine for prevention of motion sickness: clinical pharmacokinetics and therapeutic applications. *Clin Pharmacokinet.* 2006;45:543-566.

416. Tyler DC, Krane EJ. Postoperative pain management in children. *Anesthesiol Clin North America.* 1989;7:155-170.

417. Boss MJ et al. Pain management in the PACU. In: Drain CB, Odom-Forren J, eds. *Perianesthesia Nursing: A Critical Care Approach.* St Louis: Saunders; 2009:437-457.

418. Egan KJ. Psychological issues in postoperative pain. *Anesthesiol Clin North America.* 1989;7:183-192.

419. Pavlin DJ et al. A survey of pain and other symptoms that affect recovery process after discharge from an ambulatory surgery unit. *J Clin Anesth.* 2004;16:200-206.

420. Rawal N. Postoperative pain treatment for ambulatory surgery. *Best Pract Res Clin Anaesthesiol.* 2007;21:129-148.

421. Wetchler BV. What are the problems in the recovery room? *Can J Anaesth.* 1991;38:890-894.

422. Aldrete JA, Kroulik D. A postanesthetic recovery score. *Anesth Analg.* 1970;49:924-934.

423. Klepper ID. Paediatric patients. In: Klepper ID et al, eds. *Ambulatory Anaesthesia and Sedation: Impairment and Recovery.* Boston: Blackwell Scientific; 1991:191-204.

424. Aldrete JA. Discharge criteria. In: Thomson D, Frost E, eds. *Baillieres Clinical Anaesthesiology—Postanaesthesia Care.* London: Bailliere Tindall; 1994:763-773.

425. Marshall S, Chung F. Assessment of "home readiness." *Curr Opin Anaesthesiol.* 1997;10:445-450.

426. Philip BK. Patient's assessment of ambulatory anesthesia and surgery. *J Clin Anesth.* 1992;4:355-358.

427. McGrath B et al. Thirty percent of patients have moderate to severe pain 24 hr after ambulatory surgery: a survey of 5,703 patients. *Can J Anesth.* 2004;51:886-891.

CHAPTER 39

ANESTHESIA FOR EAR, NOSE, THROAT, AND MAXILLOFACIAL SURGERY

Gary D. Clark, Julie A. Stone

The practice of anesthesia for the ear, nose, throat (ENT) patient is challenging and rewarding. Decisions regarding difficult airway management are often necessary, as are the knowledge and skills to navigate abnormal and difficult anatomy. As a specialty, ENT presents specific concerns to the anesthetist for the preparation and management of surgical procedures (Box 39-1). There are several essential goals when providing anesthesia for ENT and maxillofacial (i.e., plastics and dental) surgical procedures:

1. Possessing a thorough knowledge of the airway anatomy and function
2. Selecting appropriate technique(s) and approach for airway management
3. Preventing and managing potential airway complications
4. Producing profound selective muscle relaxation during periods of extreme stimulation (e.g., suspension laryngoscopy)
5. Maintaining cardiovascular stability during periods of potent surgical stimulation
6. Omitting neuromuscular relaxation for surgical procedures that require isolation of nerves
7. Preventing and containing an endotracheal tube fire
8. Minimizing intraoperative and postoperative blood loss
9. Preventing adverse respiratory and cardiac responses resulting from manipulation of the carotid sinus and body
10. Taking the appropriate postoperative measures to prevent and treat postsurgical airway obstruction
11. Avoiding or limiting the use of nitrous oxide during tympanoplasty or other closed-space grafting

Surgical intervention for ENT procedures uses a variety of specialty equipment, including lasers, endoscopes, and specialized endotracheal tubes (e.g., laser and microlaryngeal tube). The basis of many ENT and maxillofacial surgical procedures include endoscopic examination of the sinuses; tissue tumors of the head, neck, and oral cavity; abscesses; surgery to the middle ear; papillomas of the airway; hypertrophic tonsils and adenoids; acute epiglottitis; and traumatic or congenital facial deformities. The majority of these procedures involve the nose, facial and frontal sinuses, larynx, oropharynx, nasopharynx, tongue, trachea, mandible, and maxilla, as well as other supporting structures of the head and neck. These procedures necessitate sharing the airway with the surgeon and may lead to a tenuous airway and significant challenges for the anesthetist. Airway compromise in ENT patients may be subtle and can take several forms.

This chapter describes the pertinent anatomy and physiology of the head and neck for the anesthetist, reviews specialized anesthetic considerations, reviews surgical and anesthesia equipment used during ENT procedures, analyzes some of the common pharmacologic agents used for ENT procedures, and discusses principles of anesthesia for ENT.

FUNCTIONAL ANATOMY OF THE HEAD AND NECK

A fundamental knowledge of the anatomic and physiologic function of the structures of the head and neck is essential for dealing with the myriad decisions arising perioperatively during these procedures. Commonly, the ENT surgical procedure is being performed because the anatomic structures are abnormal, distorted, or deviated. Having a working knowledge of the structures and their relationships before subjecting the patient to respiratory changes produced by anesthesia is imperative.

The anatomic structures of the head and neck and their relationships are complex (Figure 39-1). The sensory and motor supply of the upper airway originates from cranial nerves and includes the trigeminal, glossopharyngeal, facial, and vagus nerves (Figure 39-2). Understanding the sensory supply allows the anesthetist to provide sufficient local and regional anesthesia. Likewise, motor function can be evaluated following surgical procedures that may yield trauma or damage to muscles and the nerves controlling their function.

The relationships of the oropharynx, nasopharynx, nasal chambers, sinuses, esophagus, and lower airway structures such as the larynx, cricoid, thyroid, and vocal cords provide a basis for directing and providing care for the patient receiving ENT surgery. The nose is a major anatomic structure that is responsible for warming, filtering, and providing humidity to the air taken in during inspiration. The structures of the nose include the external nose, the nasal cavity, and frontal, maxillary, and ethmoid sinuses. The nares or nostrils are separated by the septum. The lateral margins of the nares are cartilaginous structures and extend posteriorly over the hard palate, leading to a confluence at the soft palate, oropharynx, and base of the tongue. The oropharynx rests superior to the epiglottis, vocal cords, larynx, and trachea.

The external nose is composed largely of cartilage supported primarily by soft connective tissue and delicate mucous membranes, as is the nasal septum. The nasal cavities are hollow structures formed by a floor, roof, lateral wall, and the septum. The lateral aspects of the nasal cavities contain concha or turbinates. The turbinates are highly vascular and are divided into three separate compartments: the superior, middle, and inferior.

The turbinates greatly increase the surface area of the nasal cavities, aiding in filtration and humidification of inspired gases. The extensive vascular supply of the turbinates may lead to severe bleeding if the endotracheal tube is not inserted along the superior margin of the hard palate. Congestion of the mucosal veins in the turbinates of the nose causes swelling of these tissues, reducing the size of the nasal cavity (most notably, the paranasal sinuses) and thus creating the feeling of "congestion" during respiration. These paired sinuses include the sphenoid, ethmoid, frontal, and maxillary sinuses. They not only serve as resonators for the voice but also filter, humidify, and warm the air during inspiration. These hollow structures are formed of low-density bone and lined with a thin layer of mucous membranes, reducing the weight of the skull but making these bones more susceptible to fractures secondary to facial trauma.

The pharynx is composed of the terminal end of the nasopharynx, the oropharynx, and laryngopharynx or hypopharynx

---

BOX **39-1**

Special Considerations for ENT Procedures

Use of specialized ventilation techniques
  Insufflation
  Intermittent apnea
  Apneic oxygenation
Prevention of endotracheal tube fire
Shared airway
Surgical field avoidance
Restricted use of nitrous oxide
Restricted use of muscle relaxants
Use of specialized equipment
  Laser
  High-frequency jet ventilation (HFJV)
High percentage of pediatric patients
Minimizing blood loss

---

extending to the sixth cervical vertebra. The medulla inhibits respiration with swallowing; the pharynx then serves as a muscular tube that constricts, allowing the passage of food. The pharynx allows the smooth passage of air and functions as a modulator for the voice. The nasopharynx is continuous with the internal nasal cavities and extends to the soft palate. The nasopharynx communicates with the oropharynx and forms the posterior aspect of the throat. Major structures of the oropharynx include the base of the tongue, soft palate, uvula, and lymphatic structures (tonsils). The tonsils are the most sensitive areas of the oropharynx. Beginning with the anterior margin and progressing bilaterally and posteriorly, the oropharynx is defined by the soft palate, base of the tongue, uvula, palatine tonsils, and adenoids, forming Waldeyer's ring.[1,2]

Hypertrophy of the palatine and adenoid tonsils (exaggerated many times by chronic infection) and of the soft palate and uvula can pose serious airway compromise, particularly in young children. The generous blood supply to the tonsils from branches of the external carotid, maxillary, and facial arteries and their close proximity to the facial and internal arteries are matters of concern regarding potential bleeding during "routine and simple" tonsillectomy. The laryngopharynx includes the epiglottis, which provides protection for the vocal cords, and is the region shared by the esophageal orifice and larynx.

The complexity of the neuromuscular system, which controls the epiglottis, allows the isolation of the trachea from the esophagus during swallowing.[1] Any interruption of this coordinated neuromuscular function of the epiglottis or of any other protective reflexes can provide a dangerous opportunity for the entrance of food or liquid into the larynx and lower airway. As food is squeezed posteriorly, an automatic swallowing reflex is initiated. The larynx is pulled superiorly, allowing the epiglottis to cover and protect the opening of the larynx.[1] The epiglottis does not operate as a movable lidlike structure that falls to close the larynx during swallowing, as is often claimed. Passage of food into the trachea can occur if the muscles and protective elevation of the larynx become rigid or are changed due to nerve

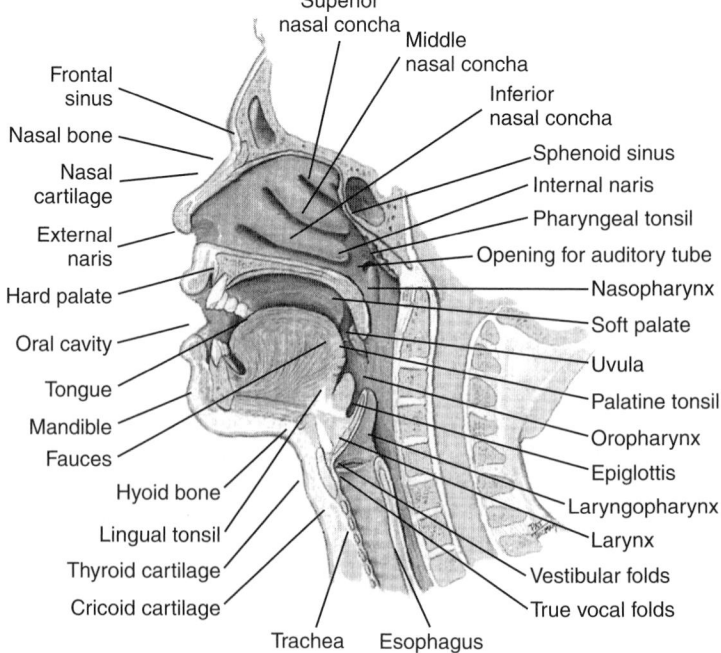

FIGURE **39-1** Anatomic features of human head and neck. (*From Applegate EJ. The Anatomy and Physiology Learning System. Philadelphia: Saunders; 1995:307.*)

interruption. A series of reflex and involuntary processes mediated by the superior laryngeal, recurrent laryngeal, and glossopharyngeal nerves coordinates and regulates glottic closure during swallowing. Structures that provide both sensory and motor nerve innervation and functionality to the larynx are listed in Table 39-1.

The larynx is a rigid organ composed of three paired and three unpaired cartilages (arytenoid, corniculate, and cuneiform and thyroid, cricoid, and epiglottis, respectively) and is supported by the hyoid bone. This hollow structure forms a reservoir distal to Waldeyer's ring and provides the connection of the oropharynx to the trachea (Figure 39-3). The primary functions of the larynx are vocalization and articulation; secondarily, it provides protection of the airway and allows respiration.[1] In the adult, the area of the vocal cords, or rima glottis, is the narrowest portion of the larynx. In children, the cricoid ring is the narrowest portion of the airway until approximately 10 years of age. Cuffed tubes are then generally recommended for those older than 8 to 10 years of age to allow for a better seal of the airway, prevent subglottic edema, and reduce the incidence of postoperative airway compromise.[3]

Specific nervous structures of the head and neck are worthy of note because of their superficial location or proximity to operative sites. Surgeons may use audible or visual nerve-locating devices to find these nerves and their appropriate branches. To accurately locate these nerves, neuromuscular blocking agents should be avoided during the maintenance of general anesthesia. The facial nerve (VII) has six major branches: four anterior (temporal, zygomatic, buccal, and mandibular), one inferior (cervical), and one posterior (posterior auricular) branch. The facial nerve located at the tragus of the ear is the motor and sensory supply to the muscles for facial expressions. The zygomatic branch leaves the skull via the stylomastoid foramen and advances anteriorly over the maxilla. The corda tympani branch of the facial nerve conveys taste from the anterior two thirds of the tongue, and the more superficial tri-branched facial nerve controls facial expression. The trigeminal nerve begins at the gasserian ganglion and divides into three branches; they are the ophthalmic (the first division, V_1), maxillary (the second division, V_2), and mandibular (the third division, V_3). All

three divisions provide sensory and motor innervation to the nose, sinuses, palate, and tongue. They aid in the motor control of the face and in mastication. The glossopharyngeal nerve provides motor and sensory innervation for the base of the tongue and nasopharynx and oropharynx. The glossopharyngeal nerve is responsible for eliciting the gag reflex during instrumentation of the posterior pharynx and vallecula. The superior laryngeal and recurrent laryngeal nerves are both branches of the vagus (X). The superior laryngeal nerve descends to the hyoid bone and then branches into the internal laryngeal nerve, which passes through the thyrohyoid membrane, and the exterior laryngeal nerve, which descends over the lateral thyroid cartilage to the distal trachea. The recurrent laryngeal nerve ascends from the vagus up the distal trachea, passing through the cricothyroid ligament into the proximal trachea and vocal cords. The recurrent laryngeal nerve lies between the trachea and esophagus and supplies sensory innervation to the trachea and vocal cords. This branch of the vagus nerve also affects vocal cord closure and sensory function up to the inferior aspect of the epiglottis. Stimulation of the epiglottis with the tip of a straight laryngoscope, blades, suction catheters, and placement of an endotracheal tube in the trachea can produce a vagal response.[3]

PREPARATION AND CONSIDERATIONS FOR EAR, NOSE, AND THROAT PROCEDURES

The Shared Airway and Considerations for Positioning

Operative procedures involving the airway, mouth, or bony structures of the face involve a true sharing of the airway between the surgeon and the anesthetist. Therefore, proper preparation requires planning and communication between the surgeon, surgical personnel, and the anesthetist prior to the surgical procedure. Sharing the airway with the surgeon also requires preparing and planning the use of the appropriate equipment. For example, during laryngoscopy the endotracheal tube may have to be smaller in diameter and moved to one side of the oropharynx to allow the surgeon to work around the tube and to facilitate the surgery. Many times the head of the table is rotated 90 to 180 degrees away from the anesthetist, resulting in a vulnerable airway to which the anesthetist may have little or no access. Of particular concern are the maintenance of adequate ventilation and

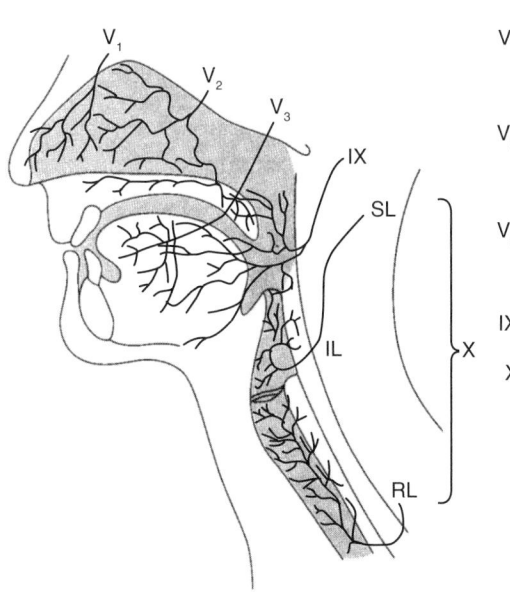

V_1 Ophthalmic division of
       trigeminal nerve
       (anterior ethmoidal nerve)

V_2 Maxillary division of
       trigeminal nerve
       (sphenopalatine nerves)

V_3 Mandibular division of
       trigeminal nerve
       (lingual nerve)

IX   Glossopharyngeal nerve

X   Vagus nerve
    SL Superior laryngeal
        branch of the vagus
        nerve
    IL Internal laryngeal
        nerve
    RL Recurrent laryngeal
        nerve

FIGURE **39-2** Sensory nerve supply of the airway. (*From Morgan GE et al. Clinical Anesthesiology. 3rd ed. New York: McGraw-Hill; 2002:62.*)

TABLE **39-1**	Structures and Innervation of the Larynx

Cartilages

Paired	Unpaired
Arytenoid	Thyroid
Corniculate	Cricoid
Cuneiform	Epiglottis

Nerves

Nerve	Motor	Sensory	Innervation
Internal laryngeal (vagus)		X	Laryngeal mucosa above vocal cords (inferior epiglottis)
Recurrent laryngeal		X	Laryngeal mucosa below vocal cords
Glossopharyngeal		X	Superior aspect of epiglottis and base of tongue
Recurrent laryngeal	X		All intrinsic muscles except cricothyroid
External laryngeal	X		Cricothyroid muscles

Muscles Controlling The Laryngeal Inlet

Muscle	Action
Oblique arytenoids	Approximates aryepiglottic folds, narrows inlet
Aryepiglottic	Narrows inlet
Thyroepiglottic	Widens inlet by pulling aryepiglottic folds apart

Muscles Controlling Movements of Vocal Folds

Muscle	Action
Cricothyroid	Tenses vocal cords; tilts cricoid and arytenoids posteriorly
Thyroarytenoid	Relaxes vocal cords; pulls arytenoids forward
Vocalis	Relaxes vocal cords; pulls arytenoids forward
Lateral cricoarytenoid	Adducts vocal ligaments
Posterior cricoarytenoid	Abducts vocal ligaments
Transverse arytenoids	Closes posterior part of rima glottis

Modified from Snell RS, Katz J. Clinical Anatomy for Anesthesiologists. Norwalk, CT: Appleton & Lange; 1988:17,25-26.

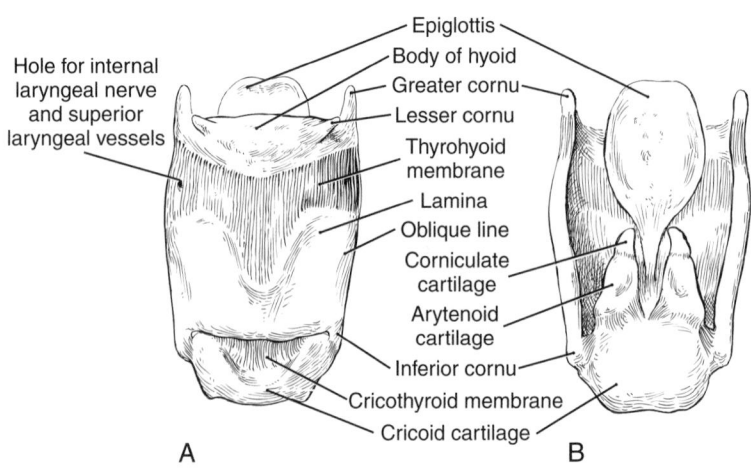

FIGURE **39-3** The larynx and its ligaments. **A,** Anterior view. **B,** Posterior view. (*From Snell RS, Katz J. Clinical Anatomy for Anesthesiologists. Norwalk, CT: Appleton & Lange; 1988.*)

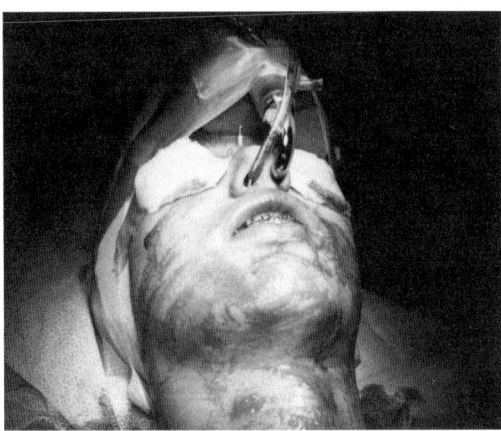

FIGURE **39-4**   Illustration of secured airway for a patient undergoing face, neck, or maxillofacial surgical procedures. Note that the tube is positioned to prevent pressure on the lip, nose, or forehead and secured with tape to prevent movement during surgery. The connection is covered by sterile surgical drapes and allows only limited access during the surgical procedure.

patency of the anesthesia circuit and endotracheal tube. Extubation, disconnects, and leaks must be prevented. Adequacy of ventilation is constantly assessed by observing chest movement, auscultation, pulse oximetry, end-tidal CO_2, and blood gas analysis.[4] A sudden loss of breath sounds, rising inspiratory pressures, or a reduction in end-tidal CO_2, particularly in the presence of a sharp reduction in inspiratory effort, may be due to a deflation of the endotracheal tube cuff, obstruction of the endotracheal tube, dislodgment of the endotracheal tube, a disconnection of the anesthesia circuit, or severing of the endotracheal tube during surgical dissection.[5] When coupled with vigilance, the precordial or esophageal stethoscopes are simple devices that should not be overlooked in favor of more sophisticated mechanical devices.

Assessment of the airway prior to induction is critical in most ENT patients. Although the induction of anesthesia and securing of the airway are performed in the usual manner (with the anesthetist at the head of the table), the management of the airway can become questionable and difficult while at a distance. Obtaining a thorough history and performing an extensive evaluation of the airway for the ENT patient is crucial. A good examination of the airway will (1) allow for a careful and deliberate approach to airway management, (2) aid in evaluating the need for additional equipment and assistance, and (3) include alternative approaches for the difficult airway should the initial plan not be successful. Once the induction is complete and the airway established, the anesthetist must be prepared to provide adequate ventilation, deliver necessary anesthetic and adjunct agents, place invasive lines, and safely monitor the patient while remaining at a distance and isolated from the airway.

Orchestrating turning of the patient so that the patient's head is away from the anesthetist demands clear planning. The endotracheal tube should be secured with tape or suture to prevent removal. The invasive line tubing, intravenous access lines, monitoring devices, and breathing circuit require added length to extend to the patient without creating tension at the site before induction. The patient's entire head is frequently draped and prepped into the surgical field, limiting access to the endotracheal tube and breathing circuit connections (Figure 39-4).

When repositioning of the head is necessary, communication between the surgeon and anesthetist is important to reduce the possibility of extubation or position change or occlusion of the endotracheal tube. Signs of air leaks around the endotracheal tube (bubbling, the sound of air escaping, or the smell of anesthetic agent from the patient's mouth) may well be more sensitive indicators than mechanical airway monitors. Occlusion of the endotracheal tube is best prevented but can be determined by good auscultation, watching chest wall motion, and monitoring inspiratory pressures and morphology of CO_2 waveforms. The surgeon must communicate, and the anesthetist must be aware of any changes in the surgical field, such as changing the position of a suspended or fixed laryngoscope, dark blood, manipulation of carotid bodies, or the need for a change in the patient's head position.[6] Increased inspiratory pressures or a rapid loss of inspiratory pressure, decreased oxygen saturation, changes in end-tidal CO_2 measurements, or diminished breath sounds should in turn be communicated to the surgeon by the anesthetist so that inspection of the airway and anesthesia circuit may be undertaken. If unable to arrive at a cause, undraping the patient may become necessary for a thorough examination of tube placement and connections or to find a leak in the anesthesia circuit that could compromise patient ventilation.

Procedures of the head and neck typically require access to all planes of the head by several members of the surgical team.[7] Because of the number of problems that can be encountered with the patient intubated during the surgical procedure, the surgeon may elect to perform a tracheostomy, then place and suture a flexible endotracheal tube in a fixed position during the procedure. The anesthetist should remain in a heightened state of vigilance for occlusions from mucous plugs or blood, disconnects, and other problems that may arise during the anesthetic. During some ENT procedures, the surgical team may also need access to the chest and abdomen for securing grafts for the esophagus or oral cavity. Often this requires the anesthetist to take residence at either the side of the patient or at the foot of the operating table (Figure 39-5). Providing a smooth transition with protection of the established airway and prevention of hypoxia are the primary concerns during movement of an operating table with an anesthetized patient.

The anesthesia circuit and other monitors should be temporarily and briefly disconnected before the bed is turned. This will prevent undue tension on the circuit and other lines that could lead to traumatic extubation or loss of access. Ventilation of the patient with 100% oxygen and adequate tidal volumes for 3 to 5 minutes before disconnection will denitrogenate the functional residual volume and provide an extra reservoir of oxygen during the turn, preventing even a short period of hypoxia. However, if a volatile agent is the primary source of anesthesia, the addition of intravenous anesthesia during this preoxygenation is necessary to maintain an adequate level of anesthesia and/or amnesia during this period. A saturation of 100% is a reasonable goal before the disconnection and table movement.

The degree of table movement should be discussed with the surgeon before any interruption in the anesthesia or the breathing circuit. Turning of the operating table should be a well-organized procedure, understood by all members of the surgical team, that takes the minimum amount of time. Following relocking the bed, reconnection of the anesthesia circuit must be immediate. Reevaluation and assessment of the tube placement, breath sounds, chest expansion, oxygen saturation, anesthetic level, line and intravenous access, and end-tidal CO_2 should be performed *before* prepping and draping is begun. Once adequate

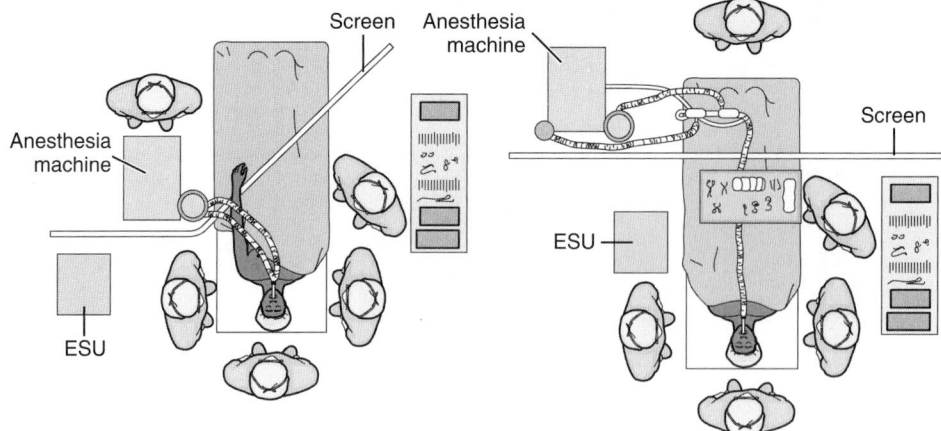

FIGURE **39-5**   Position of the anesthetist for surgery of the head and neck. *Left,* The anesthetist is positioned at the side of the table and using a standard circle circuit. *Right,* The anesthetist is positioned at the foot of the bed and using a coaxial (Bain) circuit. *ESU,* Electrosurgical unit (*From Phillips N. Berry & Kohn's Operating Room Technique. 11th ed. St Louis: Mosby; 2007:877.*)

ventilation is established, the use of an "artificial nose" or airway humidifier will help in preserving heat and moisture during long periods of anesthesia.

Attention to simple practical points may prevent airway mishaps. At least one large-bore intravenous line, as well as arterial and central venous pressure lines, should be started on the non-operative side, if possible the side of the patient that will be nearest to the anesthetist during the procedure. This will prevent obstruction of flow due to the surgical procedure, afford easier access for drug administration and blood sampling, facilitate the manipulation or maintenance of lines during surgery, and allow the surgeon easy access to the operative field. If such lines must be placed on extremities opposite the anesthetist or if the anesthetist is located a distance from the site, to reduce the chance of lines being removed, infiltrating, or becoming disconnected during movement, adequate Luer-Lok extensions should be placed before a change in position of the table. The calf of the leg may be used for noninvasive blood pressure measurements to prevent dampening of intravenous fluid flows in the upper extremities. Monitoring of neuromuscular relaxation may be performed at locations other than the adductor pollicis. Stimulation of the tibial nerve produces flexion of the big toe and is similar to that of the adductor pollicis.[8] Recent investigations have indicated small differences in the response to train-of-four (TOF) nerve stimulation in the arm (adductor pollicis muscle) and the leg (flexor hallucis brevis muscle); these differences are probably of little clinical significance.[10] Because ENT procedures may take more than 2 hours and can require significant fluid administration, monitoring urinary output with a Foley catheter may be included in the plan.

SPECIALIZED EQUIPMENT FOR EAR, NOSE, AND THROAT PROCEDURES

Endotracheal Tubes Designed for ENT Surgery

There are a number of endotracheal tubes to select from to secure an airway. Standard endotracheal tubes equipped with flexible or straight connectors are acceptable for many ENT procedures. The diameter and length of the endotracheal tube (ETT) will affect ventilation and seal of the airway. Using a small-diameter ETT in a large adult airway will not only lead to less ventilation through increased resistance but also will allow only a small portion of the cuff to contact the trachea. Using specialized tubes with small diameters (e.g., the microlaryngeal tube [Mallinckrodt MLT]) allows more even distribution of the cuff over the trachea

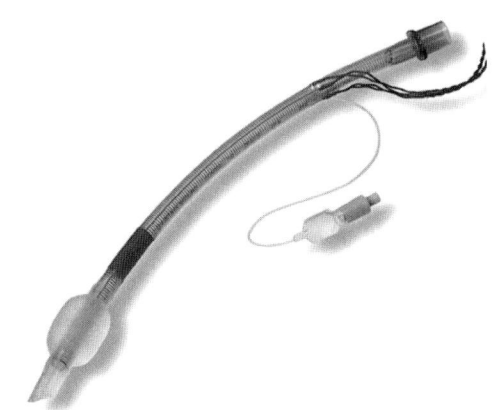

FIGURE **39-6**   NIM-EMG Reinforced endotracheal tube. Two wire electrodes allow for monitoring vocal cords and recurrent laryngeal activity.

during inflation. Several of these specially designed ETTs have found wide acceptance in ENT anesthesia. A variety of designs are used by the nurse anesthetist to limit encroachment of the ETT into the surgical field, prevent kinking of the ETT when severe angles are necessary, prevent fires in the airway during laser therapy, and provide maximal patient ventilation and safety.[10]

A number of ETTs have been introduced for use in ENT anesthesia. Since the red rubber ETT was introduced in the 1960s, there have been several types of ETT cuffs that have evolved. These ETT cuffs are the low-volume, high-pressure cuff; the high-volume, low-pressure cuff; the self-inflating foam (Bivona) cuff; and automatic regulating cuff.[11] The purpose for the evolution of these various types of ETT cuffs was to reduce cuff pressure on the tracheal wall and allow for improved tracheal perfusion and reduced tracheal injury. However, unless the pressure of these cuffs was checked frequently, nitrous oxide, improper inflation techniques, failure of the autoregulating system, and movement of the ETT changed the pressures in these cuffs or allowed the cuff to leak.

A recent arrival is the NIM-EMG ETT (Figure 39-6), used to assess recurrent laryngeal and vocal cord function during surgery.[11,12] Injury during certain types of ENT surgical procedures can lead to hoarseness, aphonia, and (although rare) difficulty with ventilation as a result of permanent adduction of the cords.

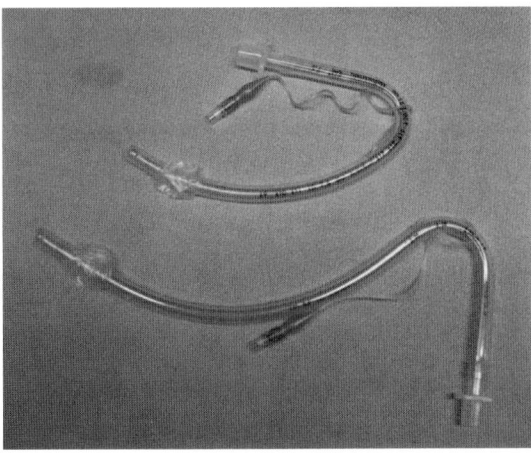

FIGURE **39-7** Preformed RAE endotracheal tubes for procedures of the head, neck, and airway. *Top,* Oral RAE. *Bottom,* Nasal RAE.

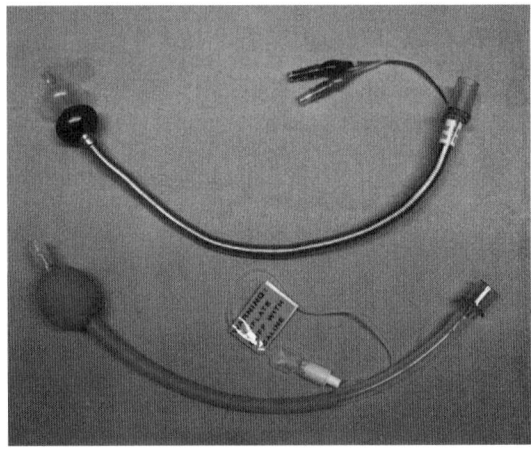

FIGURE **39-8** Endotracheal tubes for laser surgery of the airway.

The major advantage of using the NIM-EMG ETT is that it allows the surgeon the capability of identifying the recurrent laryngeal nerve prior to traction or severing the nerve.

Preformed right-angled ETTs, in cuffed and noncuffed types, are available for either oral or nasal intubation of adults or children (Figure 39-7). Oral Ring, Adair, and Elwyn (RAE) tubes are an excellent choice for cleft palate repair, tonsillectomy, uvulopalatopharyngoplasty, and procedures of the eye or upper face. Nasal RAE tubes are particularly well suited to maxillofacial surgery that does not allow for oral intubation. The nasal RAE can be used for cosmetic procedures of the face, surgical procedures of the oral cavity and mandible, or to correct malocclusion. However, although the preformed bend in the RAE tube prevents the ETT from kinking in many instances, the preformed bend may be too distal or proximal for an individual patient's airways. This then allows the tip of the ETT to rest well below or above the carina. A careful check of the breath sounds and inspiratory pressures is imperative following intubation with the RAE to ensure proper positioning. Nasal intubation and placement of a nasogastric tube in the unconscious patient with facial trauma is best avoided to prevent possible penetration of the brain.[13]

Anode, armored, reinforced, and Kant Kink tubes all have an embedded coiled wire or plastic coil strand to produce a tube with greater flexibility and memory. Armored tubes for oral or nasal intubation resist kinking and retain their original integrity. They are useful when acute neck flexion or severe angles of the ETT are required, as in procedures involving the base of the skull or posterior aspect of the neck. However, there are several reports in the literature that suggest even the edentulous patient can on occasion occlude a reinforced ETT.[14] Several varieties of metal-impregnated tubes are available for use with laser surgery and are designed to reduce the occurrence of an airway fire (Figures 39-8, 39-9, 39-10, and 39-11). The cuff of the laser tube is usually filled with saline to dampen or prevent the ignition. Wrapping a standard ETT with reflective tape is not an adequate alternative to these commercially prepared tubes because the wrapped standard ETT will dry and lead to greater flammablility.[14,15]

The Carden tube, or the Xomed-Treace Mon-Jet Tube (Figure 39-12), is a small-diameter, cuffed tube specifically

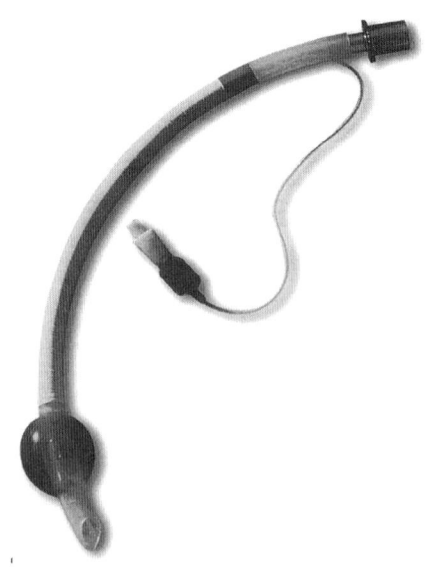

FIGURE **39-9** Laser-Shield II is a silicone tube with an aluminum inner shield. (*Courtesy of Xomed-Treace Inc, Jacksonville, FL.*)

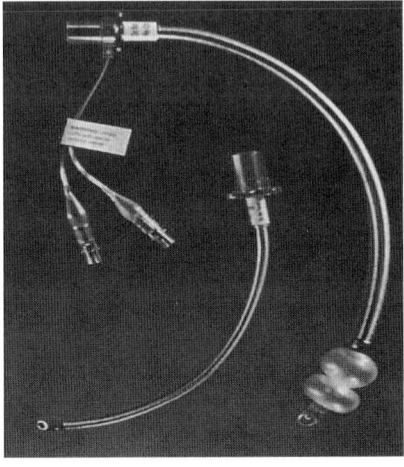

FIGURE **39-10** The Laser Flex endotracheal tube comes with a double cuff or no cuff. The double cuff is typically filled with normal saline. (*Courtesy of Mallinckrodt Inc.*)

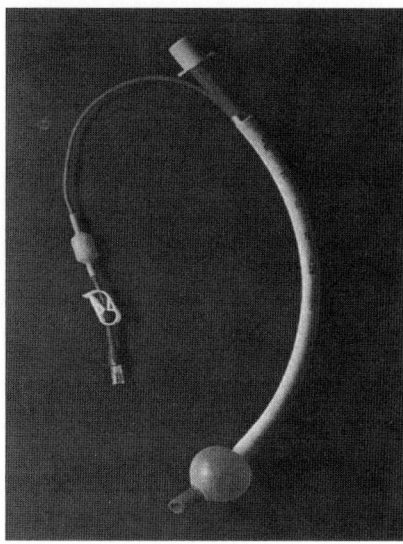

FIGURE **39-11**   Sheridan's Laser Trach tube has a copper foil and outer fabric wrapping. (*Courtesy Kendall Healthcare, Mansfield, MA.*)

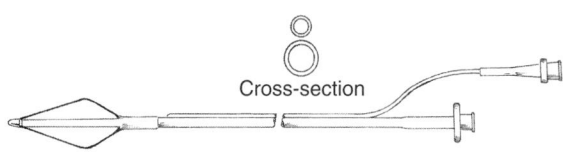

Cross-section

FIGURE **39-12**   Schematic drawing of the Xomed-Treace Mon-Jet Tube for jet ventilation.

designed to be used with high-flow jet ventilation for procedures of the larynx or subglottic area. A second method uses hand-controlled Venturi jet ventilation through needle tip. The needle fits into a side port of the laryngoscope or bronchoscope and entrains air for delivery as it exits at a high pressure. The jet ventilation system allows the intermittent delivery of oxygen and anesthetic gases during the procedure.

Although not classified as an endotracheal tube, the laryngeal mask airway (LMA) and intubating laryngeal mask airway (ILMA) may be used to facilitate intubations, as well as diagnostic fiberoptic laryngoscopy and bronchoscopy[16] (Figure 39-13). The LMA is designed to be used for anesthesia when the patient is spontaneously breathing; it is particularly well suited for visualization of the vocal cords or their function. The ILMAs or FastTrac LMAs have gained further popularity and acceptance in anesthesia as a means of establishing ventilation and intubation in patients with a difficult airway. With the use of a Portex connector that has a diaphragm port, a fiberoptic scope may be inserted into the lumen of the LMA without interrupting ventilation. The anesthetist must remember that the patient will be susceptible to laryngospasm if anesthesia is light or inadequate. The ILMA has a small flap that moves and is more conducive to placement of a laryngoscope or ETT. The LMA does not provide protection of the airway and thus is not comparable to the ETT. The incidence of complications (e.g., aspiration of gastric contents, injury to the airway, dislodgment, failure of the device, and damage to the device) is reported to be related to the experience and expertise of the clinician.[17-21]

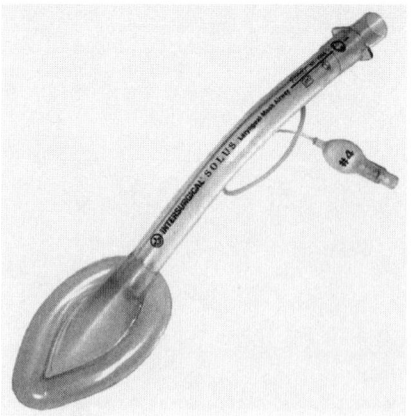

FIGURE **39-13**   Laryngeal mask airway (LMA).

SPECIAL CONSIDERATIONS FOR EAR, NOSE, AND THROAT PROCEDURES

Pharmacologic Considerations

The use of local anesthetics is particularly prevalent during nasal and sinus surgery. The most commonly used local anesthetics for ENT surgery include the amide-based drugs. Many procedures are performed using topical and local anesthesia as the sole agent, in combination or supplemented with monitored anesthesia care, intravenous sedation, or general anesthesia. Local anesthetics are drugs that produce reversible conduction blockade of impulses along central and peripheral nerve pathways. The anesthetist using these agents or caring for patients receiving these drugs should be well versed in their pharmacology, duration of action, metabolism, toxicity, and effects on other anesthetics and dosages (Table 39-2). The anesthetist should also be familiar with physiologic changes such as acidosis, infection, and hyperthermia that will change or alter the effects of local anesthetic drugs. A practical point to remember is that the total dose based on patient weight must be determined prior to injection and must take into account all local anesthesia used during the case by the surgeon and anesthetist. Additionally, multiple or large injection sites, hypercarbia, hypovolemia, and liver disease lower the toxic threshold of local anesthetics and are important considerations in calculating total dose. It has been suggested that mixing an ester and an amide may prevent the toxic effects of each and allow the better effects to prevail. For example, mixing 2-chloroprocaine with bupivacaine allows a quick onset of action and an extended block. Mixing of agents may reduce the effectiveness of the block.[22]

Vasoactive Drugs

The duration of action of a local anesthetic is proportional to the time the drug is in contact with nerve fibers. For this reason, epinephrine in varying concentrations (1:200,000 or 5 mcg/mL; 1:100,000 or 10 mcg/mL; and 1:50,000 or 20 mcg/mL) may be added to local anesthetic solutions to produce vasoconstriction. Vasoconstriction limits systemic absorption and maintains a higher drug concentration in the vicinity of the nerve fibers to be anesthetized, thus extending the effects of the local anesthetic.[23,24] Addition of epinephrine to a lidocaine solution prolongs the duration of conduction blockade by approximately 50% and decreases systemic absorption and plasma concentrations of local anesthetics by approximately one third.[25,26]

TABLE 39-2	Topical Anesthetic Drugs		
Drug	**Concentration**	**Dose**	**Notable Features**
Cocaine	4%	3 mg/kg	Only local anesthetic with vasoconstrictive ability Blocks reuptake of norepinephrine and epinephrine at adrenergic nerve endings
Lidocaine	2% and 4% solution 2% viscous solution 10% aerosol 2.5% and 5% ointment 10%, 15%, 20%	4 mg/kg plain 7 mg/kg epinephrine 250-300 mg	Rapid onset Suitable for all areas of the tracheobronchial tree
Benzocaine	*Cetacaine contains:* 14% benzocaine, 2% butamben, and 2% tetracaine		Short duration of action (10 min) Can produce methemoglobinemia
Bupivacaine	0.25%, 0.5%, 0.75%	2.5 mg/kg plain	Slow hepatic clearance Long duration of action
Mepivacaine	1%, 2%	4 mg/kg	Intermediate potency with rapid onset
Dyclonine	0.5%, 1%	300 mg maximum	Topical spray or gargle Frequent use for laryngoscopy Absorbed through skin and mucous membranes

A generally accepted "safe" total dose of epinephrine is 200 mcg, or 1.5 mcg/kg. The presence of volatile anesthetics may accentuate toxic reactions to epinephrine.[27-29] Caution must be exercised when using epinephrine in combination with volatile anesthesia agents. It has been reported that the dosages of epinephrine injected submucosally and necessary to produce ventricular dysrhythmias in 50% of patients anesthetized with 1.25 times the minimum alveolar concentration of halothane or isoflurane is 2.1 or 6.7 mcg/kg, respectively.[29]

It is estimated that in the United States, topical cocaine (4% to 10% solution) anesthesia is used in more than 50% of ENT procedures performed annually—specifically rhinolaryngology procedures.[30] Cocaine is a naturally occurring ester of benzoic acid that is hydrolyzed by plasma cholinesterase. Applied topically, it is an excellent local anesthetic and vasoconstrictor. The duration of action is approximately 45 minutes.[31] Cocaine produces vasoconstriction by blocking catecholamine reuptake into the adrenergic nerve ending, resulting in vasoconstriction and shrinking of the mucosa. Epinephrine is also injected for ENT procedures and is usually injected shortly after the application of cocaine. This combination of cocaine and epinephrine sets the stage for a significant interaction. Because cocaine that is absorbed into the plasma can block the uptake of epinephrine systemically, a toxic effect of epinephrine can result from the injection. This interaction can result in severe headaches, hypertension, tachycardia, and dysrhythmias.[32,33]

Anticholinergics

Anticholinergics were used liberally in the early days of anesthesia, predominantly because of the excessive mucus production caused by older volatile inhalation agents. With the advent of newer anesthetic agents, mucus production is lower, and the need for anticholinergics has been diminished. Premedication with anticholinergics helps reduce or diminish vagal tone, reduces

secretions, and increases bronchodilation. The antisialagogue effects may be desired for intraoral procedures that require a drier operative field. The addition of anticholinergics and the use of dry gases during anesthesia can increase the viscosity of secretions during long cases, limiting the evacuation of mucus or even creating a mucous plug in the bronchus or ETT. Anticholinergics can also precipitate closed angle glaucoma and should be avoided in patients with a known history. When choosing an anticholinergic, glycopyrrolate may be a better choice than atropine. In comparison to atropine and scopolamine, glycopyrrolate does not readily cross the blood-brain barrier and thus lacks sedative effects. It is also less likely to raise intraocular pressure than atropine.

Corticosteroids

Glucocorticoids may be administered preoperatively and intraoperatively to decrease laryngeal edema formation, reduce nausea and vomiting, and prolong the analgesic effects of local anesthetics. They should be administered as early as possible in the perioperative period so as to reach their peak effect prior to initiating surgery. The use of steroids may reduce the nausea and vomiting experienced following surgery. In a recent study, dexamethasone was also reported to prolong the analgesic effects of local anesthetics.[34] It has been asserted that prostaglandins, histamine, and other mediators increase the permeability of local vessels, changing the nociception at the site of trauma and leading to the sensation of pain. Steroids inhibit the production of prostaglandins and therefore reduce pain. Although the use of steroids may be beneficial, they can also create sufficient immunosuppression to mask inflammation or infection.

Postoperative Nausea and Vomiting

All patients are at risk for postoperative nausea and vomiting (PONV). ENT procedures, particularly of the middle ear, are associated with a high incidence of PONV. Patients experiencing PONV are uncomfortable after surgery, their discharge may be delayed from the postanesthesia care unit (PACU), or they may have an unscheduled hospital admission. The accumulation of blood in the posterior oropharynx, which may drain into the stomach or be swallowed during the postoperative period, can lead to PONV. This frequently occurs during throat procedures such as tonsillectomy. Packing the back of the throat with surgical packs during the procedure can prevent some drainage into the stomach. Care must be taken that the patient is awake, all surgical packs are removed, and suctioning of the airway precedes the extubation process, producing a clear airway and ensuring the control of protective airway reflexes. A multimodal approach is advocated to attenuate PONV in ENT patients.[35]

Special Anesthetic Techniques Associated with Ear, Nose, and Throat Procedures
Deliberate Controlled Hypotension
Extensive dissection is required for head and neck tumors, with operative times extending to 12 or more hours. Considerable fluid replacement, blood loss, electrolyte imbalances, and cardiovascular and respiratory changes may occur during surgery. The surgeon may request deliberate controlled hypotension to reduce blood loss. Patients must be individually evaluated prior to controlled hypotension to determine a safe mean pressure. The effects of common intravenous controlled hypotensive techniques are compared in Table 39-3.[36-39] The practice of controlled hypotension focuses on reducing the mean arterial pressure to some predetermined level related to the limits of cerebral and

systemic autoregulation. The mean pressure is not usually allowed to fall below 60 mm Hg, maintaining cerebral and renal autoregulation, as well as adequate coronary artery blood flow. Patients with chronic hypertension may require a higher mean pressure to maintain adequate perfusion.[39] Regardless of the technique or medication chosen, it is imperative that urine output, mean arterial blood pressure, cerebral and cardiac perfusion pressure, and arterial blood gases be closely monitored and maintained. Owing to the high acuity of this technique and the need for accurate blood pressure monitoring and frequent sampling for blood gases and electrolytes, an arterial line will provide the minute-to-minute access required during controlled hypotension.

SELECT TECHNIQUES COMMONLY USED IN EAR, NOSE, AND THROAT PROCEDURES
Laser Surgery
Anesthesia and laser surgery is also discussed in Chapter 43. However, there are some specific issues the nurse anesthetist faces during ENT surgery. Laser technology has been used in medicine for more than 25 years. The two most common lasers used in ENT surgery are the CO_2 and Nd:YAG (neodymium-doped yttrium aluminum garnet); recently the argon laser has gained popularity.[40] Laser light is different from standard light. Whereas standard light has a variety of wavelengths, lasers have only one wavelength (monochromatic). Laser light oscillates in the same phase, or all the photons are moving in the same direction (coherent), and its beam is parallel (collimated). The wavelength of the Nd:YAG laser beam is shorter as it passes through the garnet than that of the CO_2 laser. The shorter

TABLE **39-3**	Common Intravenous Agents for Hypotensive Techniques	
Drug and Dosage	**Advantages**	**Disadvantages**
Sodium Nitroprusside Variable age- and anesthetic-dependent effects; *Young adults:* 1-5 mcg/kg/min *Children:* 6-8 mcg/kg/min	Potent; reliable; rapid onset and recovery; cardiac output well preserved	Reflex tachycardia; rebound hypertension; pulmonary shunting; cyanide toxicity possible
Esmolol 200 mcg/kg/min to achieve 15% reduction of mean arterial pressure	Particularly useful to control tachycardia	Potential for significant cardiac depression
Nitroglycerin *Adults:* 125-500 mcg/kg/min *Children:* 10 mcg/kg/min	Preserves myocardial blood flow; reduces preload; preserves tissue oxygenation	Increases intracranial pressure; highly variable dosage requirements
Fenoldopam 0.5-22 mcg/kg/min	Preserves renal blood flow	Reflex tachycardia; rebound hypertension; increased pulmonary shunting
Nicardipine 5 mcg/kg/min	Ca++ channel blocker Preserves cerebral blood flow	
Remifentanil with Propofol Remi: 1 mcg/kg IV then continuous infusion 0.25-0.5 mcg/kg/min Prop: 2.5 mg/kg IV then infusion of 50-100 mcg/kg/min	Remifentanil reduces middle ear blood flow, creating a dry surgical field for tympanoplasty Propofol may help reduce PONV	No analgesic effect once remifentanil infusion discontinued

Modified from DeGoute CS. Controlled hypotension: a guide to drug choice. Drugs. 2007;67(7):1053-1076.
PONV, *Postoperative nausea and vomiting.*

wavelength allows less absorption by water and therefore less tissue penetration. For example, the shorter wavelength of the Nd:YAG allows the laser light to pass through the cornea, whereas the longer wavelength of the CO_2 laser would burn the cornea. Laser light emits a small amount of radiation and can be infrared, visible, and ultraviolet in the spectrum. Lasers enable very precise excision, produce minimal edema and bleeding, and are favored by surgeons for resection of tumors and other obstructions of the airway. For operations in and around the larynx, the CO_2 laser is most often used because of its shallow depth of burn and extreme precision.[41] The CO_2 laser produces a beam with a relatively long wavelength that is absorbed almost entirely by the surface of these tissues, vaporizing cellular water. Intermittent bursts of the CO_2 laser produce intense, precisely directed energy that results in a clean cut through the target tissue with minimal amount of penetration of surrounding tissue. A low-energy helium-neon laser is commonly used to aim or direct CO_2 laser beams.

Laser light beams are primarily used for their thermal effect and can be used to cut, coagulate, or vaporize tissues. The exact tissue interaction of a laser is dependent on several variables, including the types of tissues being irradiated, the wavelength of the emitted beam, and the power of the beam.

The use of laser technology mandates taking measures to ensure the safety of the patient and operating room personnel (Box 39-2). Specific concerns include eye protection with appropriate colored glasses, avoidance of the dispersion of noxious fumes, and fire prevention. Stray or reflected beams of the Nd:YAG laser are capable of traversing the eye to the retina; therefore, green-lensed eye protection for all personnel is mandatory during its use. All persons in the operating room must wear goggles specifically designed to absorb Nd:YAG laser beams. The required protective eyewear for CO_2 can be any clear glass or plastic that surrounds the face. Orange-red eye protection is required for the potassium-titanyl phosphate (KTP) laser and orange glasses for the argon laser.

When tissues are cut by a laser, the smoke and vapors that are formed are called laser "plume." This plume is an environmental concern and potentially toxic to operating room personnel. When the tissues vaporized by the laser are malignancies or viral papilloma, the concern arises as to whether these vapors are even more dangerous to operating room personnel if not removed from the environment. Because this issue remains under investigation, it is judicious to suction the laser plume and not allow it to circulate into the room.

The prevention of combustion within the airway is of primary concern to the anesthetist. Fire in the airway is relatively uncommon (0.4%), and it is usually due to penetration of the laser through the ETT, which exposes the beam to a rich oxygen supply. Nitrous oxide, although not flammable, also supports combustion and can propagate the flame.[42] Positive pressure ventilation in the presence of intraluminal combustion produces a blowtorch effect with serious damage to the respiratory tract of the unfortunate patient.[43] Steps to reduce the possibility of fire include using the lowest concentration of oxygen appropriate for a particular patient, avoiding paper surgical drapes, spraying the flame with a 60-mL syringe filled with normal saline, and using water-based rather than oil-based lubricants. Once a flame has been ignited, the ETT should be immediately removed and replaced with a new ETT large enough to allow the surgeon to assess the lungs with a bronchoscope.

The "perfect" ETT for use with lasers remains a major discussion (Table 39-4). However, several manufacturers have attempted to produce a laser-compatible ETT that allows for adequate ventilation during the laser procedure but reduces the risk of airway fire injury. However, there is no guaranteed method of preventing an airway fire.[11] The necessity of an inflatable cuff is a point of debate, although its ability to better ventilate the patient and keep the field free of combustible gases is an advantage. Cuff material must be made of thinner substance than the tube body, making it more susceptible to laser penetration. When filled with air, the cuff becomes a generous reservoir of combustion-supporting gas. If a cuffed tube is used, inflation with methylene blue–tinged normal saline is encouraged. If a laser beam contacts the cuff, the colored liquid will absorb and disperse heat, alerting the surgeon and anesthetist to the penetration; the liquid will reduce combustion.[44] High-frequency jet ventilation can also be used but poses several problems. Many systems use oxygen only, which dries the tissues quickly and provides gases for ignition in the open airway.[45-47]

The American Society for Testing and Materials (ASTM) Subcommittee F29.02.10 of the Anesthesia Patient Safety Foundation developed guidelines for the provision of safe anesthesia during laser surgery for the upper airway. These guidelines compare and comment on the advantages and disadvantages of several anesthetic techniques and laser-resistant ETTs.[46]

Endoscopy

Endoscopic surgery includes panendoscopy, laryngoscopy, microlaryngoscopy (laryngoscopy aided by an operating microscope), esophagoscopy, and bronchoscopy. All of these procedures can be performed using a rigid or flexible endoscope. If the rigid laryngoscope is used, the laryngoscope may be suspended from an arching support anchored to the patient's abdomen/chest or from a Mayo stand over the patient. One of the most common endoscopic procedures performed is the endoscopic sinus surgery. Endoscopic sinus surgery is often associated with multiple and seasonal allergies leading to polyps. Patients undergoing surgery are often also being evaluated for pathology responsible for hoarseness, stridor, or hemoptysis. Other possible reasons for endoscopic examination include foreign-body aspiration, papillomas,

---

BOX 39-2

General Safety Protocol for Surgical Lasers

- Post warning signs outside any operating area: "WARNING: LASER IN USE."
- Patient's eyes should be protected with appropriate colored glasses and/or wet gauze.
- Matte-finish (black) surgical instruments reduce beam reflection and dispersion.
- Use the lowest concentration of oxygen possible.
- Avoid using N_2O, because it supports combustion.
- Lasers should be placed in STANDBY mode when not in use.
- Use an endotracheal tube specifically prepared for use with lasers.
- Inflate cuff of laser tube with normal saline.
- All adjacent tissues should be shielded by wet gauze to prevent damage by reflected beams.
- Plume should be suctioned and evacuated from the surgical field.

TABLE 39-4	Advantages and Disadvantages of Commonly Available Laser-Resistant Tracheal Tubes	
Tube Type	**Advantages**	**Disadvantages**
Metal	Atraumatic external surface Double cuff maintains seal even if punctured by laser Kink resistant	Thick-walled nonflammable cuff reflects laser and transfers heat Cuff difficult to deflate if punctured Metal may reflect beam onto non-targeted tissue
Polyvinyl chloride (PVC)	Inexpensive Nonreflective Maintains shape well Double cuff maintains seal after proximal cuff puncture	Burns vigorously and yields pulmonary toxin (hydrogen chloride) Cuffed version contains flammable material
Red rubber	Wrapping protects flammable material but dries tube Maintains structure Nonreflective	Red rubber itself is highly flammable Tubes are thick walled
Silicone rubber	Wrapping protects flammable material Methylene blue aids in detection of cuff perforation Nonreflective	Contains flammable material Turns to toxic ash Single cuff is vulnerable to laser damage

Data from Pashayan A. Laser safety in the operating room. Curr Rev Nurs Anesth. 1995;18:11-19; Sois MB. Which is the safest endotracheal tube for use with CO$_2$ laser?: a comparative study. Clin Anesth. 1992;4:217; Sois M, Heller S. A comparison of five metallic tapes for endotracheal tube protection during CO$_2$ laser surgery. Can J Anaesth. 1988;35:S63.

trauma, tracheal stenosis, obstructing tumors, or vocal cord dysfunction. Several complications can arise with endoscopic surgery: eye trauma, epistaxis, laryngospasm, bronchospasm, and excessive plasma levels of local anesthesia and epinephrine have been reported.[48,49] Preoperatively, the patient should be examined for any signs of airway obstruction and proper measures taken to ensure safe and controlled airway management. Knowledge of the location and size of a mass is important, and discussion with the surgeon about chest roentgenogram, magnetic resonance imaging (MRI), and computed tomography (CT) scan results can be invaluable.[48]

Light sedation is suggested for premedication, because older children and adults may experience respiratory depression and worsening of airway obstruction. The airway must be protected from aspiration of gastric contents, especially during prolonged airway manipulation and deeper sedation. Premedication with an antisialagogue to dry secretions and a full regimen of acid aspiration prophylaxis in aspiration-prone patients may be indicated. An awake oral or nasal intubation with minimal sedation and topical anesthesia of the oral cavity, pharynx, larynx, and nasopharynx may be indicated. For shorter ENT procedures, anesthesia should be maintained with short-acting inhalation and intravenous agents to (1) avoid patient movement and vocal cord movement and (2) control sympathetic nervous system response to brief periods of extreme stimulation, as in laryngoscopy.

Good muscle relaxation of the vocal cords is an essential part of anesthesia management for microsurgery of the larynx. A short-acting relaxant or infusion may be considered for brief cases. If the procedure is expected to last 30 minutes or more, use of an intermediate-duration neuromuscular-blocking drug such as vecuronium, atracurium, cisatracurium, or rocuronium for the initial tracheal intubation allows the return of muscle strength and spontaneous respiration to meet extubation criteria

at the end of the surgical procedure. Emergence should include adequate oropharyngeal suctioning, humidified oxygenation, and observation in the PACU for laryngeal spasm or postextubation croup.

One of the greatest management challenges during endoscopic procedures is to share the airway continuously with the surgeon. Several methods have been used to provide oxygenation and ventilation during the procedures. One method is to control the airway by using a small, cuffed ETT (5.0 to 6.0 mm for an adult). Because the 5.0- and 6.0-mm ETTs are designed for smaller patients, a better ETT selection might include the microlaryngeal endotracheal tube (MLT). The MLT in similar sizes (5.0 to 6.0 mm) has a cuff that is larger than the small standard ETTs (5.0 to 6.0 mm), allowing for a larger cuff distribution across the surface of the trachea and creating a wider field of pressure on the tracheal surface. There are some distinct advantages of an ETT, including a secure airway with easily controlled ventilation, a cuff to protect the lower airway from debris, monitoring of end-tidal CO$_2$, and the ability to administer inhalational anesthetics. Several drawbacks include the potential for extubation and loss of airway, complications during laser surgery, and interference with the operative field by the ETT.

Intermittent apnea is also used as a technique to ventilate patients in this shared space. The anesthetist or the surgeon repeatedly removes the ETT, operates during a brief period of apnea, and then allows the anesthesia provider to reintubate and ventilate the patient. One advantage of the technique is that no special equipment is needed to ventilate the patient. Many patients undergoing these procedures have a long history of heavy smoking and alcohol use, which predisposes them to cardiovascular disease and labile vital signs. Some of the disadvantages of this approach include difficulty in reintubation and the time allotment between ventilations while preventing desaturations. The procedure must be interrupted frequently to ventilate the patient, and the airway is unprotected while the ETT is removed. During this technique, the blood pressure and heart rate tend to fluctuate widely. The procedure resembles a series of stress-filled laryngoscopies and intubations, separated by varying periods of minimal surgical stimulation. Intravenous administration or topical application of agents such as lidocaine; small doses of alfentanil, remifentanil, sufentanil, or fentanyl; and/or β-adrenergic receptor blocking drugs such as esmolol may help moderate the sympathetic response.

Jet Ventilation

Jet ventilation has been used extensively for laryngeal surgery. When the trachea is not intubated, a metal needle mounted in the operating laryngoscope or passed through the cords can be used for jet ventilation. Jet ventilation may be performed manually, using a simple hand valve attached to an appropriate oxygen source, or together with various mechanical devices that allow for adjustment of rate and oxygen concentration. Because oxygen can support combustion, the anesthetist should consider as low a concentration of oxygen as is possible. Many patients will tolerate an FIO_2 of 30% or less; however, oxygen requirements for each patient should be considered for their individual needs. Using lower levels of oxygen will be less likely to create a fire.

High-frequency jet ventilation (HFJV) was originally used as a technique to provide adequate oxygenation and alveolar ventilation for rigid bronchoscopy and laryngeal surgery. HFJV is typically ventilation at low tidal volumes with high respiratory rates. A needle connected to a high-pressure hose with a regulator to adjust rate and volume is used to deliver the ventilation. With the tip of the needle either above or below the glottis, the anesthetist directs a high-velocity jet stream of oxygen into the airway lumen. The lungs are ventilated as the mixture of oxygen forces air into the lumen. Introduction of high-pressure (up to 60 psi) jet-injected oxygen entrains room air into the lung, allowing the jet stream of gases into the airway for ventilation.[47,48] Whereas inspiration is accomplished by HFJV pressurizing gas into the airway, the expiration is passive. Therefore, some pauses in ventilation may be necessary to provide adequate time for expiration, particularly in patients with severe respiratory disease.

If an airway mass lies above the level of delivery of the gas jet, it may be easy to force the gas down the trachea during inspiration, but the gases will be trapped during expiration. This air trapping can lead to increased airway pressure, subcutaneous emphysema, and pneumothorax, particularly in patients with bullae. The anesthetist or surgeon may also find it difficult to aim the jet into the airway lumen, leading to hypoxia. If the jet is not accurately aimed, gastric distention, subcutaneous emphysema, or barotrauma may result. Patients with decreased pulmonary compliance or increased airway resistance from bronchospasm, obesity, or chronic obstructive pulmonary disease (COPD) are at high risk for hypoventilation with jet techniques. Jet ventilation is contraindicated in any situation in which an unprotected airway is a concern (e.g., full stomach, hiatal hernia, or trauma).[48,49]

Adequacy of ventilation is assessed by observing chest movement, auscultation with the precordial stethoscope, and a pulse oximeter. Total intravenous anesthesia (TIVA) is the primary anesthesia technique used with HFJV, because volatile agents cannot be delivered, and environmental contamination is a concern. TIVA with short-acting agents such as propofol, alfentanil,

fentanyl, and remifentanil provide an excellent anesthetic for these procedures.

Foreign-Body Aspiration

Aspiration of foreign bodies is a common problem that carries high morbidity and mortality, particularly in children. Some common aspirants include peanuts, popcorn, jelly beans, coins, and bites of meat and hot dogs. The majority of aspirated items are food particles; however, beads, pins, and small toys are not unusual. A common site of foreign body aspiration is the right bronchus. If the patient is supine when the aspiration occurs, the object will most likely be found in the right upper lobe. If the patient is standing, the right lower lobe is most likely to be affected. Signs of aspiration include wheezing, choking, coughing, tachycardia, aphonia, and cyanosis. These signs indicate an obstructive severe irritation and swelling in the airway. As a result of the swelling, air may be trapped in the lungs, not allowing adequate expiration.

Anesthetic management depends on the location of the airway obstruction, the size and location of the object, and the severity of the obstruction. If the foreign body is located at the level of the larynx, a simple laryngoscopy with Magill forceps should allow for easy removal of the object. Care must be taken not to dislodge the object and allow it to fall deeper into the airway. If the foreign body is located in the distal larynx or trachea, the patient should have an inhalation induction performed in the operating room, maintaining spontaneous respiration. With the patient spontaneously breathing, the surgeon will most likely use a rigid bronchoscope for extraction of the foreign body. Usually, a gentle mask induction without cricoid pressure or positive pressure ventilation is the preferred induction technique.[50] The anesthetist should not assist with respirations, because this may cause the object to move farther into the airway and compromise ventilation with occlusion. Patients should be placed in the sitting position because it is known to produce the least adverse effect on airway symptoms. An antisialagogue, H_2 antagonist, and metoclopramide are often administered intravenously to decrease secretions and promote gastric emptying; the secretions may obscure the view through the bronchoscope. Patients with full stomachs who are induced with a rapid sequence must be prepared for complete occlusion of the airway.

Direct and sometimes rigid laryngoscopy is typically performed. A rigid bronchoscope is also used and passed through the vocal cords into the trachea. Ventilation is accomplished through a side port of the laryngoscope or bronchoscope that can be attached to the anesthesia circuit. If a foreign body is present, the telescope eyepiece within the bronchoscope is removed and optical forceps are inserted through the bronchoscope for retrieval of the item. When the telescopic eyepiece is being changed, a leak is present in the ventilation system, and protracted periods can lead to hypoxia. When an anesthesia gas machine circuit is used, high fresh gas flow rates, large tidal volumes, and high concentrations of inspired volatile anesthetic agents are often necessary to compensate for leaks around the ventilating bronchoscope. Coughing, bucking, or straining during instrumentation with the rigid bronchoscope may cause difficulty for the surgeon and result in damage to the patient's airway; these must be avoided. The best anesthesia technique for rigid laryngoscopy and bronchoscopy is total intravenous anesthesia, allowing greater control of cardiovascular stability and relaxation for short periods, as well as ventilation with 100% oxygen, allowing longer periods of hypoventilation without hypoxia.

A rigid bronchoscopy can lead to several complications, including damage to dentition, gums, and upper lips and chipped or damaged teeth, all of which can be prevented to some degree with the use of a mouth guard and vigilance. Vagal stimulation may be noted from the extreme head extension, and tracheal tears can occur with the introduction of the bronchoscope. Inadequate ventilation manifests as hypoxemia, hypercarbia, barotrauma, and dysrhythmias. The surgeon must be prepared to perform an emergency tracheotomy or cricothyrotomy if partial obstruction suddenly becomes complete.

At the conclusion of the procedure, patients can be intubated to provide ventilation until returning to consciousness. Allow the patient to return to consciousness as quickly as possible, with airway reflexes intact prior to extubation. Laryngeal and subglottic edema may occur for 24 hours after removal of a foreign body. To check for airway edema, the cuff of the ETT can be deflated if not contraindicated, and the lumen of the ETT should be occluded for one or two breaths during inspiration and expiration while listening for air movement around the tube. If there is no air escaping around the ETT, postoperative sedation and ventilation might be considered. Close observation and use of humidified oxygen are suggested during the recovery period. Some additional supportive measures that can alleviate some of the postoperative complications that occur include racemic epinephrine, bronchodilators, and steroids.

PROCEDURES OF THE EAR AND FACE

Some of the common surgical procedures for the ear and face include myringotomy with insertion of tubes, mastoidectomy, acoustic neuroma, stapedectomy, and tympanoplasty. During ear surgery, the anesthetist must be concerned with four major issues: (1) nerve preservation (particularly cranial nerves VII, IX, X, XI, and XII), (2) the effect of nitrous oxide on the middle ear, (3) control of bleeding, and (4) PONV.

Anesthesia Considerations
Nerve Preservation
Surgical procedures of the ear and face involve meticulous identification and preservation of the facial and other cranial nerves, especially during resection of a glomus tumor or an acoustic neuroma. The identification of these nerves requires the surgeon to isolate and verify function by means of an electrical stimulation. One method used for nerve isolation is the brainstem auditory evoked potential and electrocochleogram monitoring. It has been documented that the facial nerve is more sensitive to the train-of-four than is the ulnar nerve. Studies have also concluded that reliable intraoperative facial nerve monitoring may be performed despite significant neuromuscular blockade detected by conventional ulnar train-of-four monitoring.[51,52] However, profound skeletal muscle relaxation should be avoided, and a volatile anesthetic drug (because of the muscle-relaxant properties) should be used judiciously as a primary anesthetic. If an opioid-relaxant technique is chosen, a minimum of 30% muscle response using the peripheral nerve stimulator should be preserved.[53] Selecting and using a combined or balanced technique may provide adequate anesthesia with minimal muscle relaxation, producing better outcomes. Opioids used with low-dose volatile agents may provide nerve integrity, allowing better assessment of function, and provide anesthesia adequate enough for the procedure.

Effect of Nitrous Oxide on the Middle Ear
Nitrous oxide is more soluble than nitrogen in blood. Therefore, nitrous oxide diffuses into air-containing cavities more rapidly than the bloodstream can absorb nitrogen. Normally, pressure increase in the middle ear is vented by the eustachian tube into the nasopharynx. Yawning and swallowing actively open the eustachian tubes, but these equalizing maneuvers cannot occur in anesthetized patients. Additionally, pressure may also be increased in the middle ear with positive pressure ventilation by forcing air into the compartment through the eustachian tubes.

During tympanoplasty, the middle ear is opened to the atmosphere, and there is no pressure buildup. Once the surgeon has replaced a tympanic membrane graft, the middle ear becomes a closed space. If nitrous oxide is allowed to diffuse into this space, middle ear pressure will rise,[54] and the graft may be displaced. Conversely, administering nitrous oxide then discontinuing the gas after the graft has been placed will create a negative pressure in the middle ear that may last up to 6 weeks postoperatively. Either scenario may contribute to the development of serous otitis, disarticulation of the stapes, displacement of grafts, and impaired hearing.[55] There is no evidence that using N_2O 50% or less for general anesthesia for type 1 tympanoplasty interferes with the graft placement or changes the outcome of the surgical procedure.[55,56] To avoid complications if N_2O is used, the anesthesia provider should discontinue the administration of N_2O at least 15 minutes before closure of the middle ear.

Control of Bleeding
During microscopic ear surgery, even a small drop of blood can make the procedure difficult. Injecting the ear with an epinephrine-containing solution (often in concentrations of 1:1000; 1:50,000; 1:100,000; and 1:200,000) is performed in the area of the tympanic vessels to produce vasoconstriction. Mild head elevation to decrease venous pressure, lowering of arterial pressure with volatile agents, and (although somewhat controversial) deliberate hypotensive techniques are other methods used to decrease blood loss during these procedures. At the completion of the surgical procedure, the patient's head is lifted and usually wrapped with a bandage. The anesthetist will want to avoid excessive coughing and bucking of the patient during this period. Provided there are no contraindications, a deep extubation might be considered.

Myringotomy and Tube Placement
Most often, patients scheduled for myringotomy are young and healthy patients. A myringotomy allows the pressure to equalize between the middle ear and the atmosphere, reducing the pressure in the middle ear compartment. Simple tubes with a lumen are placed through the patient's tympanic membrane to alleviate the pressure created in the middle ear usually seen with chronic serous otitis media or recurrent otitis media. Chronic otitis media is manifested as fluid in the middle ear. Recurrent otitis media, a common pediatric disorder, is defined as six or more episodes of otitis media over the prior year. Untreated otitis media may lead to permanent middle ear damage and hearing loss; therefore, prompt treatment is necessary. Children with chronic otitis frequently have accompanying recurrent upper respiratory infections (URIs). Intervals between URIs may be brief, and the patient is usually on a regimen of antibiotics. Scheduling surgery during these interludes is often impractical. Frequently, the eradication of middle ear fluid and inflammation resolves the URI; therefore, surgery should not be delayed.

Bilateral myringotomies with tube insertions are typically very short operations. Sedative premedications may outlast the procedure and are usually not necessary. Mask or IV induction and maintenance using oxygen, nitrous oxide, and a volatile inhalation agent such as sevoflurane is routine. If IV access is established, it is usually after mask induction in children and may include fluid therapy or an injection cap for temporary access and administration of drugs. IVs are not usually necessary unless another procedure is performed in addition to positron emission tomography. N_2O is often avoided in surgeries that involve the middle ear, because it is 34 times more soluble in blood than nitrogen and can create pressure in the closed space.[55,56] But given that the myringotomy surgical procedure is relatively short, and a tube will be placed through the tympanic membrane into the middle ear to relieve pressure, the effects of N_2O are often not relevant. For bilateral procedures, the inhalation anesthetic is discontinued during the second myringotomy to facilitate prompt emergence. N_2O is continued until the completion of the surgery. Intubation is performed only if airway difficulties are anticipated or encountered, but airway equipment is always prepared and available. The procedure is typically without much risk of bleeding, but the patient's head must be held still, particularly when the myringotomy knife is being used.

The patient is supine with the head turned to expose the ear to the microscope. An ear speculum is inserted into the ear canal, cerumen is removed, and an incision is made in the tympanic membrane. Fluid is sometimes suctioned from the middle ear, and then a tympanostomy tube is inserted through the incision into the middle ear, straddling the tympanic membrane. Antibiotic and steroid eardrops frequently are inserted into the external auditory canal. The surgeon moves to the other side of the table, the microscope is repositioned, the head is turned, and the procedure is repeated in the other ear.

Tonsillectomy and Adenoidectomy

The lateral tonsils, tonsillar tissue at the base of the tongue, and adenoids form a tonsillar "ring" around the oropharynx that can lead to significant airway challenges following surgical intervention. An adenotonsillectomy, although often considered a simple procedure, requires a great degree of finesse by the anesthetist. Considerations of airway obstruction, shared airway, mechanical suspension of the airway, management of intubation and extubation, pain management, and the desire for a rapid awakening are all subtleties of anesthesia that challenge the anesthetist. In adult patients, a tonsillectomy may also accompany a uvulopalatopharyngoplasty (UPPP) for pickwickian syndrome or obstructive sleep apnea (OSA). OSA is typically seen with obesity and redundant pharyngeal tissue. OSA patients can also present with a history of right heart failure and congestive heart failure (CHF), which is not uncommon.[57-59]

The patient undergoing a tonsillectomy and/or adenoidectomy will probably have a higher incidence of airway obstruction because of the hypertrophied tissues. Chronic obstruction and infections of the tonsils can lead to systemic involvement, producing additional cardiac and respiratory anomalies. In the case of suspected airway obstruction, the clinician must choose wisely among routine intravenous induction, inhalation induction, awake intubation, or fiberoptic-assisted intubation before induction. Adult patients with severe obstructive sleep apnea may require a tracheostomy under local anesthesia in advance to secure the airway before the induction of general anesthesia. Such determination is based on the degree of obstruction, physical examination of the airway, and the clinical judgment of the anesthetist. Regardless of the induction technique chosen, the use of an antisialagogue is strongly encouraged.

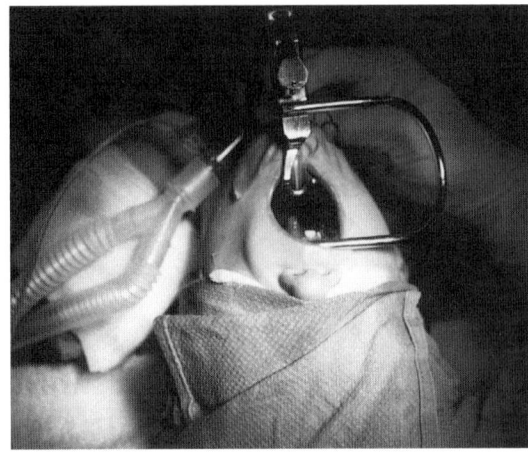

FIGURE 39-14 Superior view of the suspension technique for tonsillectomy using the Crowe-Davis mouth gag. Note use of preformed RAE orotracheal tube.

In children, anesthesia is usually induced with a volatile drug, oxygen, and N_2O by mask. Some institutions allow parental presence in the operating room during induction to prevent separation anxiety in the child. Tracheal intubation in children is best accomplished under deep inhalation anesthesia or aided by a short-acting nondepolarizing muscle relaxant. The airway generally is secured with an oral RAE or reinforced tube. A cuffed tube is recommended in those older than 8 to 10 years of age,[4] with continued attention to inflation pressures of the cuff. A properly sized pediatric ETT should allow a leak at 20 cm H_2O airway pressure, which reduces the likelihood of postoperative croup and edema. The tube must be secured midline. A simple yet effective method of securing the oral RAE tube is to apply a strip of tape directly to the chin, incorporating the ETT and another strip of tape over the tube. The first strip provides a secure base for the second strip, which actually holds the tube.

After the airway is secured, the mouth gag is inserted by the surgeon. An adequate depth of anesthesia is needed to facilitate gag insertion. The gag, designed to maintain an open mouth and tongue retraction, is equipped with a groove for the ETT to rest in (Figure 39-14). The airway should be reevaluated at the time the gag is placed to ensure that the tube has not been moved from its original position and that occlusion of the ETT has not occurred as a result of compression from the gag. The table is frequently turned 45 to 90 degrees away from the anesthetist just prior to incision.

The choice of techniques varies for the maintenance of anesthesia. There are four major goals to consider when choosing an anesthetic: (1) provide a depth of anesthesia adequate to blunt strong reflex activity elicited by the procedure, (2) a rapid return of protective reflexes, (3) good postoperative analgesia, and (4) reduced postoperative bleeding. The use of intermediate-acting muscle relaxants is acceptable, but their action must be completely reversed at the end of the case. Judicious narcotic supplementation will reduce the total amount of inhalation agent required and provide analgesia with minimal postoperative respiratory depression. Although postoperative bleeding has been a concern in the past regarding the use of ketorolac, it has been successfully used as an alternative to opioids, has not been found to accentuate bleeding, and has lead to shortened hospital stays following tonsillectomy.[60,61]

Blood loss during tonsillectomy is difficult to assess but has been estimated to average 4 mL/kg or 5% of blood volume.[7] Average blood loss during UPPP is slightly higher because the procedure frequently is performed in conjunction with adenotonsillectomy. Replacement for blood loss of less than 10% of the calculated volume may be accomplished with the administration of 3 mL of crystalloid per mL of blood loss. Although younger, healthier patients can tolerate greater volumes of blood loss, transfusion should be considered if blood loss exceeds 10% of calculated preoperative blood volume.

At the end of the surgical procedure, the surgeon may release tension on the mouth gag to ensure that all bleeding has been controlled. The insertion of an orogastric tube and some irrigation may be used to remove blood and secretions from the stomach and oropharynx. This is thought to reduce the incidence of postoperative nausea and vomiting. Suctioning of the oropharynx and nares should be done very gently and briefly, avoiding the surgical beds to prevent disruption and mucosal bleeding. Vigorous suctioning may induce laryngospasm and bronchospasm.

During emergence from anesthesia after tonsillectomy or UPPP, the anesthetist should ensure that all protective reflexes have returned, the airway is free of blood and debris, and an adequate breathing pattern is present before the removal of the ETT. A topical spray of 2% lidocaine (maximum 3 mg/kg) on the glottic and supraglottic areas before intubation prevents postextubation stridor and laryngospasm following adenotonsillectomy. This approach has proved as effective as administering lidocaine (1 mg/kg IV) before extubation but without higher sedation scores.[62]

The postoperative tonsillectomy patient should be transported to the recovery in the "tonsil position"—that is, on one side with the head slightly down. This allows blood or secretions to drain out of the mouth rather than flow back onto the vocal cords. Adults, however, frequently prefer a middle- or high-Fowler position following UPPP. This position aids in ventilation and lessens the feeling of asphyxiation in the immediate postoperative period. The anesthetist must, however, make sure the patient is awake enough to manage his or her own airway. To hydrate the airway, 100% oxygen with a high-humidity mist is given by face mask or face tent. The pharynx should be rechecked directly for bleeding and edema before discharge from the recovery room.

Increasingly, tonsillectomy is being performed as an outpatient procedure. Although postoperative bleeding is the most serious complication, persistent vomiting and poor oral intake are the most common reasons for unscheduled overnight admission after ambulatory surgery. The incidence of postoperative nausea and vomiting can be as high as 70% during the first 24 hours after tonsillectomy.[63] As discussed previously, it is important to develop anesthetic techniques that incorporate the use of antiemetics to minimize episodes of nausea and vomiting.

Bleeding Tonsil

The incidence of post-tonsillectomy bleeding that requires surgery is 0.3% to 0.6%. Approximately 75% of the postoperative tonsillar hemorrhages that occur are within 6 hours of the surgical procedure. The remaining 25% of the postoperative bleeds occur within the first 24 hours of surgery, although bleeding may be noted up until the sixth postoperative day.[64] Because cautery is used for control of bleeding instead of ligatures, a slow oozing

of the tonsillar bed is far more common than profuse bleeding. One concern is that these patients may swallow large volumes of blood before bleeding is actually discovered. The patient may present with signs of hypovolemia evidenced by tachycardia, hypotension, and agitation. If the blood is swallowed, the patient may have nausea and vomiting. Appropriate laboratory tests (e.g., hemoglobin and hematocrit) should be performed to determine replacement. If reoperation is deemed necessary, restoration of intravascular volume and/or blood based on the volume lost should precede induction. It is important to evaluate the adequacy of intravenous access (two lines may be appropriate), assess the coagulation variables, and be prepared to transfuse blood. All such patients should be assumed to have a significant amount of blood in the stomach, and an awake intubation of the trachea should be an initial consideration to maintain reflexes. At induction of anesthesia, an additional person should be available to provide suctioning of blood from the oropharynx. If an awake technique is not practical, a rapid-sequence induction with cricoid pressure should be implemented. The patient should be placed in a slight head-down position to protect the trachea and glottis from aspiration of blood. A nasogastric tube may be placed to remove stomach contents prior to induction and then removed after induction. The induction agent selected is based on the hemodynamics and condition of the patient.

Cleft Palate and Lip

Cleft Palate (Hard Palate and Soft Palate)

Cleft palate repair is usually performed in stages, depending on the extent of the defect. For more severe deformities, the initial operation repairs the lip and anterior portion of the hard palate. The soft palate and other deformities are usually corrected later, after 6 months of age. Infants with cleft lip deformities can have difficulty feeding and may be prone to malnutrition and congenital (heart) anomalies and disease.[65]

Intubation may sometimes be difficult if the laryngoscope blade slips into the cleft. However, packing the cleft with gauze may prevent this from occurring. An oral RAE tube or flexible connector is used and secured at the midline of the lower lip. A specialized mouth gag is used to hold the mouth open and the ETT in place during cleft-palate surgery. All air bubbles should be carefully removed from IV lines to prevent air embolus, owing to the incidence of associated cardiac anomalies (e.g., atrioventricular defect [AVD]) that may lead to air crossing from the venous to the arterial circulation. Congenital heart disease may influence drugs that are selected for maintenance of anesthesia and infiltration of the operative site, particularly if epinephrine is selected. Care must be implemented to protect the child's eyes because accidental damage may occur during the surgical procedure. Before emergence, a suture is often placed through the tip of the tongue and taped to the cheek. This suture eliminates the need for an oral airway and prevents damage to the palatal repair. If soft-tissue obstruction occurs during emergence or recovery, traction on the suture can alleviate the problem. If edema occurs, a more aggressive and immediate airway management technique should be used. Copious secretions and blood may cause laryngospasm after extubation, and therefore a clear airway is imperative.

Cleft Lip

Patients who have a documented URI prior to surgery may have perioperative respiratory complications, so surgery should be postponed until the symptoms of the cold subside.[66] Management of unilateral cleft lip repair consists of routine induction followed by oral intubation using an RAE tube or a flexible connector. Secure the tube to the lower lip and midline via tape. To decrease tension on the surgical sutures at the end of the procedure, the surgeon may place a Logan bow across the upper lip of the patient.[67] When the Logan bow is placed, mask ventilation during emergence will become impaired or impossible. Extubation must be performed only with the patient fully awake and reflexes intact. The child's surgical site must also be protected from finger and hand manipulation. Some hospitals recommend the use of hand mittens or taping the extremities onto armboards during the postoperative period. Close monitoring of respiration should proceed into the postoperative period.

Dental Restoration Procedures

Dental restoration procedures are performed under general anesthesia for a multitude of reasons. These include rampant cavities, history of cerebral palsy or Down syndrome, and an uncooperative patient who would not be an appropriate candidate for local anesthetic and an office procedure.

Mentally disabled patients typically develop a close relationship with either a family member or their long-term health-care worker. It is often suggested that this individual accompany the patient to decrease anxiety and communicate a health history to the anesthesia provider. A thorough airway assessment should be performed before considering induction. Oral midazolam (0.5 mg/kg) or ketamine (3 to 4 mg/kg IM) is most effective in sedating children in the preoperative arena. Because many patients requiring dental restoration have congenital anomalies, it is not uncommon to find a small oropharynx, enlarged tonsils, a large tongue, and increased secretions. Atlantoaxial instability and congenital heart disease should also be considered in the preoperative preparation and anesthetic management.[65,68,69] Preparation and appropriate airway management must be planned and implemented for these patients. Patients who receive phenytoin to control seizures may have gingival hyperplasia. Because the gingiva is highly vascular, any surgical manipulation during restoration may lead to significant blood loss.

In patients with normal airways, a standard induction is appropriate, and a nasal intubation usually facilitates the dental procedure. The application of a topical vasoconstrictive nasal spray during the preoperative period reduces or prevents bleeding during the insertion of the nasotracheal tube. Following loss of consciousness, lubricated intranasal trumpets may be inserted into the most patent nasal airway. Starting with a smaller nasal trumpet, several are placed in increasing sizes to dilate the airway. When full dilation of the nares has occurred, a well-lubricated ETT is passed through the nose into the trachea, either blindly or assisted by Magill forceps under direct laryngoscopy. The nasal ETT is preferably placed on the side opposite where the surgeon will be working. The ETT is often sewn to the nasal septum by the surgeon. Throat packs may be placed to prevent blood from entering the stomach and causing nausea and vomiting; monitoring their removal is essential to preventing respiratory obstruction following extubation.

Sinus and Nasal Procedures

Nasal and sinus procedures for drainage of chronic sinusitis, polyp removal, repair of a deviated septum, or closed reduction of fractures generally involves the young and healthy patient population. Many patients who undergo sinus and nasal surgery have chronic environmental and drug allergies; therefore, there is an increased incidence of reactive airway disease in these patients. Nasal polyp removal, for example, may be necessitated by Samter syndrome. A patient with Samter syndrome or triad presents with nasal polyps, asthma, and an aspirin allergy. The nasal polyps, if symptomatic, are removed surgically. The use of fiberoptics or functional endoscopic sinus surgery for nasal and sinus surgery has become a popular treatment for chronic sinusitis.

Nasal surgery may be successfully accomplished with local anesthesia, local combined with intravenous sedation, or general anesthesia. All three methods of anesthesia require profound vasoconstriction. The mucous membranes of the sinuses and nose are highly vascular, and blood loss may be significant if vasoconstriction is not used. The surgeon may select to control vasoconstriction with epinephrine or cocaine. Recently, Bizikas and colleagues found when comparing cocaine and tetracaine, using tetracaine 2% with epinephrine produces superior anesthesia and vascular control for rhinoplasty.[70] The anesthetist may be asked to use a hypotensive technique or slight head elevation (10 to 20 degrees) during the procedure. Using general anesthesia has been associated with increased blood loss, even with the use of an epinephrine injection. This exaggerated blood loss may be related to the vasodilatory properties of inhalation agents. Delivering general anesthesia for sinus surgery with propofol, as well as other intravenous anesthetic techniques for the maintenance of anesthesia, has been associated with less blood loss than occurs with the use of volatile agents for maintenance.[68] The placement of an oropharyngeal pack and light suctioning of the stomach at emergence may attenuate postoperative retching and vomiting. After all of the packing is removed, extubation should be performed on the awake patient who has regained control of protective reflexes.[69] The use of intravenous or topical lidocaine may reduce some of the coughing prior to extubation, leading to less bleeding in the postoperative period.

Trauma
Initial Assessment

Traumatic disruption of the bony, cartilaginous, and soft-tissue components of the face and upper airway challenge the anesthesia provider to recognize the nature and extent of the injury and consequent anatomic alteration. It is imperative to create an anesthetic plan for securing the airway without promoting further damage or compromising ventilation. Possible mechanisms by which the upper or lower airway may become obstructed include edema, bleeding from the oral mucosa and palate, intraoral fracture sites, distortion of the nasal passages, injury of the pharynx and sinuses, open lacerations, and the presence of foreign bodies such as avulsed teeth, blood clots, or bony fragments.[71]

Initial management of the airway depends on the situation at hand. In the case of severe facial or neck trauma, alternative methods of tracheal intubation (e.g., fiberoptic laryngoscopy, retrograde wire placement, jet ventilation via cricothyrotomy or emergent tracheostomy) may be necessary to secure the airway.

Injuries of the head and neck should alert the anesthetist to possible cervical spine injury. Although a complete evaluation of all cervical vertebrae is ideal, inspection of a lateral radiograph of the cervical spine is judicious to determine the presence or absence of dislocations and fractures. All seven cervical vertebrae must be visible in such studies. The seventh cervical vertebra is the most common site of traumatic fracture of the spine.[72] Vertebral artery injury must be suspected with a cervical injury, because these fractures can lead to vertebral artery tear or occlusion. If deteriorating respiratory function requires immediate airway management and intubation, the head should be maintained in a fixed position before any manipulation of the airway is performed. The use of manual in-line axial stabilization (MAIS) (by a qualified assistant) and/or a rigid cervical collar in place is recommended. The removal of the anterior segment of the collar can facilitate intubation and manipulation of the soft tissues of the neck.[72,73]

Blunt trauma to the face or anterior neck may produce rapid airway occlusion secondary to soft-tissue edema or hematoma formation secondary to trauma of the vascular structures of the neck. The patient exhibiting smoke or blistering in the area of the mouth and nares or with a history of inhalation of toxic by-products of combustion should be intubated immediately. Edema of the face and glottis, which may lack symptoms in the early stages, has the potential to produce serious airway compromise several hours after injury. Securing the airway by either oral or nasal intubation is preferable to tracheostomy, which is associated with a higher incidence of complications.[74]

Maxillofacial Trauma and Orthognathic Surgery

Le Fort[75] determined the common fracture lines of the maxilla and face by experimentation on cadavers in 1901. The fractures are divided into Le Fort I, II, and III[75,76] (Figure 39-15). The Le Fort I fracture is a horizontal fracture of the maxilla extending from the floor of the nose and hard palate, through the nasal septum, and through the pterygoid plates posteriorly. The palate, maxillary alveolar bone, lower pterygoid plate, and part of the palatine bone are all mobilized. The Le Fort II fracture is a triangular fracture running from the bridge of the nose, through the medial and inferior wall of the orbit, beneath the zygoma, and through the lateral wall of the maxilla and the pterygoid plates. The Le Fort III fracture totally separates the midfacial skeleton from the cranial base, traversing the root of the nose, the ethmoid bone, the eye orbits, and the sphenopalatine fossa.[76]

A Le Fort I fracture generally causes little difficulty for the anesthesia provider. Patients may be intubated orally or nasally and the airway secured without a problem. The Le Fort II and Le Fort III fractures are of particular concern to the anesthetist contemplating nasal intubation. In both of these fractures, disruption of the cribriform plate may occur, opening the underside of the cranial cavity. The presence of cerebral fluid in the nose, blood behind a tympanic membrane, periorbital edema, or "raccoon-eyes" hematoma are indications that attempts to pass an endotracheal tube or nasogastric tube through the nares could lead to inadvertent intracranial placement.[76] Although the insertion of a nasal tube may aid the surgeon, an attempted

nasotracheal intubation of a patient with a basal skull fracture involves the very serious risk of introducing the tube into the skull, bringing contaminated material into the subarachnoid space and causing meningitis. The tube may also inflict damage to the brain itself.[77]

The forces required to produce facial fractures are considerable and may be associated with other trauma. It is important that cervical spine injury, subdural hematoma, pneumothorax, and intraabdominal bleeding be investigated. Soft-tissue injury to the airway and blood or debris in the oropharynx may make visualization impossible. If in doubt while in the emergency department, a tracheostomy under local anesthesia or an awake oral intubation with topical anesthesia should be considered. These patients should be treated with full stomach precautions.

As with any trauma victim, attention is first directed toward maintaining the ABCs: airway, breathing, and circulation. The repair of the facial fracture may be carried out at a later time. Once the patient arrives in the operating room for surgery (sometimes 24 to 48 hours after insult), it may be challenging to open the patient's mouth for intubation because of edema, pain, or trismus. It is necessary to differentiate the cause of the small mouth opening because it may be pain related or mechanical in nature. The administration of a short-acting narcotic or midazolam will sometimes assist the anesthesia provider in determining the cause of the restriction, which greatly influences the induction chosen. In mandibular or maxillary fractures, nasal intubation is usually best, because the patient's teeth are brought together via wires or rubber bands at the conclusion of surgery (intermaxillary fixation). Anesthesia is induced with an IV agent and maintained with narcotics, muscle relaxants, and inhalation agents. Blood loss from facial fractures can be extensive. The patient's blood should be typed and crossmatched so that blood is immediately available. The fixation process closes the teeth in proper occlusion and prevents access to the oropharynx. Masking the patient at emergence requires that the patient be awake with intact reflexes at extubation. It also requires that wire cutters or scissors be available to cut the wire or rubber bands fixing the mandible to the maxilla in case an airway emergency occurs in the recovery area.[78]

Orthopedic orthognathic procedures often require sagittal splitting of the mandible to move the lower jaw either forward or back. A Le Fort I or Le Fort II osteotomy may be purposefully performed to move the maxilla in any direction to correct anomalies. Many of these patients have anomalies of the mandible and maxilla, small mouth openings, and appliances that make intubation difficult and airway management challenging. Because many of the malocclusions are treated orally, a nasal endotracheal tube is usually preferred over an oral intubation. Securing the nasotracheal tube away from the surgical field without causing necrotic injury of the nares is vital. Because blood loss during these procedures can be extensive, the patient is typed and crossmatched, and deliberate hypotensive anesthetic techniques are often used. Rigid external or internal fixation devices are used to maintain stability in both the mandible and maxilla postoperatively; therefore, the proper cutting tools should be at the patient's bedside for emergency airway issues. The anesthetist must also consider that edema will often be extensive and progress over the first 24 hours following orthognathic surgery. To prevent postoperative respiratory problems, the patient may remain intubated for several days. If extubation is necessary, it should only be done when the patient is awake and in full command of protective reflexes.

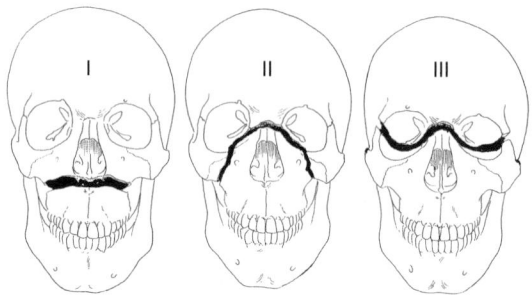

FIGURE **39-15**   Examples of Le Fort I, II, and III facial fractures (*left to right*).

Radical Neck Dissection

Radical neck dissection is required when cancerous tumors have invaded the musculature and other structures of the head and neck. Neoplastic growths can occur anywhere within the upper airway and may achieve significant size with little evidence of airway penetration or obstruction. Such tumors are often friable and bleed readily. These patients are frequently heavy drinkers and smokers who have bronchitis, pulmonary emphysema, or cardiovascular disease. If the tumor interferes with eating, associated weight loss, malnutrition, anemia, dehydration, and electrolyte imbalance can be significant. Patients who have had radiation treatments of the neck and jaw prior to surgical intervention will have soft tissues that are less mobile, making intubation more difficult. Many of these patients are older. The number of complications in patients age 65 and older are nearly double those of younger patients.[79,80] Attempted tracheal intubation can induce significant hemorrhage and edema, causing severe compromise of the airway.

Determining the appropriate techniques for airway management entails consultation with the surgeon as to the nature, extent, and location of the tumor; therapy administered (radiation or chemotherapy); CT results; history and physical examination; and relevant preoperative lab values.

Head and neck reconstruction is an integral part of surgical removal of head and neck tumors. Traditional methods of reconstruction include regional pedicle flaps with microvascular reconstruction. Flaps include the pectoralis major myocutaneous flap, trapezius flap, and local rotational flaps (e.g., forehead flap). Additionally, small bowel may be harvested to reconstruct the oropharynx and esophagus. The anesthesia team plays an important role in maximizing the overall success rate of a free flap and microvascular flow of the flap.[78] The anesthetist must communicate with the surgeon regarding the planned donor site, which will limit the available sites to place lines necessary for monitoring and venous access. Although the choice of monitoring is largely dependent on the general condition of the patient, the placement of a central venous pressure (CVP) line, a Foley catheter, and an arterial line (beat-to-beat and arterial blood gas trends) is suggested, particularly if deliberate hypotension during anesthesia is used. A pulmonary artery catheter may be useful if a history of cardiac problems is present. The internal jugular approach should be avoided because of proximity to the surgical site. Sites commonly used for the CVP and pulmonary catheter placement when the internal jugular is not accessible are the subclavian and femoral veins, respectively.

Maintenance of anesthesia is often performed with an inhalation agent and supplemental narcotics. The use of a nondepolarizing muscle relaxant must be discussed with the surgical team preoperatively because a nerve stimulator is frequently used (by the surgeon) to locate nerves distorted by the tumor during the procedure. Significant blood loss can be a problem; sometimes a controlled hypotension technique may be requested.[79,80] At least one and preferably two large-bore peripheral IV lines (16 to 14 gauge) should be in place. The patient's blood should be typed and crossmatched, with blood readily available. It is important to replace blood loss, but not to the point of overloading the patient. Monitoring estimated blood loss and measuring the hematocrit may provide some guidelines for replacement of blood. A positive fluid balance in the postoperative phase can result in edema and congestion of the flap, predisposing it to vascular compromise. Colloids may be used to help limit the amount of crystalloid required during the procedure. Patients undergoing a radical neck dissection are frequently hypovolemic and have electrolyte imbalances. This requires some fluid replacement and electrolyte balance intraoperatively to maintain cardiovascular stability.

In preparation for a tracheostomy or total laryngectomy to be performed during the surgical procedure, the patient should receive 100% oxygen. The trachea will be transected by the surgeon, which requires that the anesthesia provider suction the airway and remove the ETT only to a level above the tracheal incision. Once the tracheostomy tube has been placed by the surgeon and ventilation validated, the ETT can then be completely removed. A reinforced tube is usually placed in the distal airway by the surgeon and connected to the anesthesia machine. A reassessment of the ventilation should be performed, including the entire procedure of listening to bilateral breath sounds, observing chest excursion, and checking end-tidal CO_2 and positive inspiratory pressure (PIP) or negative inspiratory pressure (NIP). After the anesthesia provider has validated tube placement, the ETT is sutured to the chest wall for the entire surgical duration. At the end of surgery, the reinforced tube may be switched for a tracheostomy cannula.

During radical lymph node dissection of the neck for carcinoma, manipulation of the carotid sinus may elicit a vagal reflex, causing bradycardia, hypotension, or cardiac arrest. Small doses of local anesthetic injected near the carotid sinus or administration of an anticholinergic may block vagal reflexes. Owing to the long duration of the surgery and interruption of venous flow, venous thrombus is commonly seen in patients who are undergoing radical neck dissection. The head-up position and open neck veins during surgery may lead to venous air embolism. Careful monitoring with precordial Doppler sonography or transesophageal echocardiography (TEE) provides the best detection of air embolism. Immediate removal of the air through the CVP is essential. Laryngeal edema, vascular occlusion, and obstruction can also occur as a result of the venous stasis that follows major disruptions in venous flow during surgery or with trauma. Continual review of complications and follow-up treatments are necessary.[78-80]

Postoperative considerations consist of tracheostomy care, controlled ventilation, chest roentgenogram (to rule out pneumothorax, hemothorax, pulmonary edema), and monitoring for laryngeal edema induced by thrombosis. Postoperative characteristics of various surgical laryngectomy procedures are given in Table 39-5. It is suggested that these patients be admitted overnight in the intensive care unit because they have undergone major fluid and electrolyte shifts and altered ventilation-perfusion status and have spent an extensive time under the influence of anesthesia.

SUMMARY

Administering anesthesia for ENT and maxillofacial procedures requires knowledge in both basic and advanced anesthesia techniques. Using these techniques demands the best skills of even a seasoned and experienced nurse anesthetist. The usual tenets of safe practice must often be adhered to while remaining at a distance from the airway. Delivering anesthesia for ENT and maxillofacial surgery can be very rewarding but also complex and difficult. Good preparation remains imperative. These patients require high levels of clinical proficiency and vigilance. Cooperation and communication between the surgeon and anesthetist maintain a vital link for all concerned, especially those patients in their charge.

TABLE 39-5	Laryngectomy	
Structures Removed	**Structures Remaining**	**Postoperative Conditions**
Total Laryngectomy		
Hyoid bone Entire larynx (epiglottis, false cords, true cords) Cricoid cartilage Two or three rings of trachea	Tongue Pharyngeal wall Lower trachea	Loses voice; breathes through tracheostomy; no problem swallowing
Supraglottic or Horizontal Laryngectomy		
Hyoid bone Epiglottis False vocal cords	True vocal cords Cricoid cartilage Trachea	Normal voice; may aspirate occasionally, especially liquids; normal airway
Vertical (or HEMI-) Laryngectomy		
One true vocal cord False cord Arytenoid One half thyroid cartilage	Epiglottis One false cord One true vocal cord Cricoid	Hoarse but serviceable voice; normal airway; no problem swallowing
Laryngofissure and Partial Laryngectomy		
One vocal cord	All other structures	Hoarse but serviceable voice; occasionally almost normal voice; no airway problem; no swallowing problem
Endoscopic Removal of Early Carcinoma		
Part of one vocal cord	All other structures	May have a normal voice; no other problems

From Drain CB. Perianesthesia Nursing. 5th ed. St Louis: Saunders; 2009:470.

REFERENCES

1. Guyton A, Hall J. Respiration. *Textbook of Medical Physiology.* 11th ed. Philadelphia: Saunders; 2006:471-522.
2. Marieb E, Hoehn K. Functional anatomy of the respiratory system. *Human Anatomy and Physiology.* 7th ed. Menlo Park, CA: Benjamin/Cummings Science; 2007:831-845.
3. Murphy TM. Somatic blockade of the head and neck. In: Cousins MJ, Bridenbaugh PO, eds. *Neural Blockade in Clinical Anesthesia and Management of Pain.* 3rd ed. Philadelphia: Lippincott-Raven; 1998:493-505.
4. Motoyama EK et al. Induction of anesthesia and maintenance of the airway in infants and children. In: Motoyama E, Davis P, eds. *Smith's Anesthesia for Infants and Children.* 7th ed. St Louis: Mosby; 2006:319-358.
5. Kagan B. Anesthesia for otorhinolaryngolic (ear, nose and throat) surgery. In: Longnecker D et al, eds. *Anesthesiology.* New York: McGraw-Hill; 2008:1582-1607.
6. Philip J et al. Monitoring anesthetic and respiratory gases. In: Blitt C, Hines R, eds. *Monitoring in Anesthesia and Critical Care Medicine.* 3rd ed. New York: Churchill Livingstone; 1995:375.
7. Everett LL. Anesthesia for children. In: Longnecker D et al, eds. *Anesthesiology.* New York: McGraw-Hill; 2008:1520-1540.
8. Sopher MJ et al. Neuromuscular monitoring comparing the flexor hallucis brevis and adductor pollicis muscles. *Anesthesiology.* 1988;69:129.
9. Brown ACD. Anesthesia. In: Cummings CW et al, eds. *Otolaryngology: Head and Neck Surgery.* Vol 1. 2nd ed. Philadelphia: Mosby; 1993.
10. Jaeger JM, Durbin CG. Special purpose endotracheal tubes. *Respir Care.* 1999;44(6):661-683.
11. Medtronic Xomed: *NIM EMG [product insert].* Minneapolis, MN: Medtronic ENT; 2000.
12. Maloney RW et al. A new method for intraoperative recurrent laryngeal nerve monitoring. *Ear Nose Throat J.* 1994;73(1):30-33.
13. Gregory JA et al. A complication of nasogastric intubation: intracranial penetration. *J Trauma.* 1978;18:822.
14. Kervin MW. Occlusion of a wire-reinforced endotracheal tube in an almost completely edentulous patient. *Mil Med.* 2003;168(5):422.
15. Muzzi DA et al. Complications from nasopharyngeal airway in a patient with a basilar skull fracture. *Anesthesiology.* 1991;74:366.
16. Patel KF, Hicks JN. Prevention of fire hazards associated with the use of carbon dioxide lasers. *Anesth Analg.* 1981;60:885.
17. Wat LI. The laryngeal mask airway for oral and maxillofacial surgery. *Int Anesthesiol Clin.* 2003;41(3):29-56.
18. Lopez-Gil M et al. Laryngeal mask airway in pediatric practice: a prospective study of skill acquisition by anesthesia residents. *Anesthesiology.* 1996;84:807-811.
19. Wender R, Goldman AJ. Awake insertion of the fibreoptic intubating LMA CTrach in three morbidly obese patients with potentially difficult airways. *Anaesthesia.* 2007;62(9):948-951.
20. Dhonneur G et al. Tracheal intubation of morbidly obese patients: LMA CTrach vs direct laryngoscopy. *Br J Anaesth.* 2006;97(5):742-745.
21. Hagberg CA et al. Instruction of airway management skills during anesthesiology residency. *J Clin Anesth.* 2003;2:15.
22. de Jong RH, Bonin JD. Mixtures of local anesthetics are no more toxic than the parent drugs. *Anesthesiology.* 1981;54:177.
23. Heavner JE. Local anesthetics. *Curr Opin Anaesthesiol.* 2007;20(4):336-342.
24. Anderhuber W et al. Plasma adrenaline concentrations during functional endoscopic sinus surgery. *Laryngoscope.* 1999;109:204-207.
25. Stoelting R. Local anesthetics. *Pharmacology and Physiology in Anesthetic Practice.* 3rd ed. Philadelphia: Lippincott Williams & Wilkins; 2006:179-207.
26. Catterall W, Mackie K. Local anesthetics. In: Brunton LL et al, eds. *Goodman and Gilman's Pharmacological Basis of Therapeutics.* 11th ed. New York: McGraw-Hill; 2006:369-386.
27. Rosenberg PH et al. Maximum recommended doses of local anesthetics: a multifactorial concept. *Reg Anesth Pain Med.* 2004;29(6):564-575.
28. Bridenbaugh PO et al. Anesthesia for otolaryngologic procedures. In: Paperella MM et al, eds. *Otolaryngology.* Vol 1. 3rd ed. Philadelphia: Saunders; 1991.
29. Imamura S, Ikeda K. Comparison of the epinephrine-induced arrhythmogenic effect of sevoflurane with isoflurane and halothane. *J Anesth.* 1987;1(1):62-68.
30. Harper SJ, Jones NS. Cocaine: what role does it have in current ENT practice? A review of the current literature. *J Laryngol Otol.* 2006;120(10):808-811.
31. Gallo JA Jr. Catecholamine anesthetic interaction in ENT surgery. *Contemp Anesth Pract.* 1997;9:7-30.
32. Myburgh JA et al. The cerebrovascular effects of adrenaline, noradrenaline and dopamine infusions under propofol and isoflurane anaesthesia in sheep. *Anaesth Intensive Care.* 2002;30 (6):725-733.

33. Lange RA, Hillis LD. Cardiovascular complications of cocaine use. *N Engl J Med.* 2001;345:351-358.
34. Kim MS et al. There is no dose-escalation response to dexamethasone (0.0625-1.0 mg/kg) in pediatric tonsillectomy or adenotonsillectomy patients for preventing vomiting, reducing pain, shortening time to first liquid intake, or the incidence of voice change. *Anesth Analg.* 2007;104(5):1052-1058.
35. Kranke P et al. Algorithms for the prevention of postoperative nausea and vomiting: an efficacy and efficiency simulation. *Eur J Anaesthesiol.* 2007; 24(10):856-867.
36. Degoute CS. Controlled hypotension: a guide to drug choice. *Drugs.* 2007;67(7):1053-1076.
37. Goldberg ME et al. A comparison of labetalol and nitroprusside for inducing hypotension during major surgery. *Anesth Analg.* 1990;70:537-542.
38. Degoute CS et al. Remifentanil and controlled hypotension; comparison with nitroprusside or esmolol during tympanoplasty. *Can J Anaesth.* 2001; 48(1):20-27.
39. Kim KH et al. Nicardipine hydrochloride injectable phase IV open label clinical trial: study on the antihypertensive effects and safety of nicardipine for acute aortic dissection. *J Int Med Res.* 2002;3(30):337-345.
40. Poe DS et al. Laser eustachian tuboplasty: a preliminary report. *Laryngoscope.* 2003;113(4):583-591.
41. Baxter DA. Laser safety in the operating room. *Insight.* 2006;31(4):13-14.
42. Neuman GG et al. Laparoscopy explosive hazards with nitrous oxide. *Anesthesiology.* 1993;78:875-879.
43. Dullenkopf A et al. Nitrous oxide diffusion into tracheal tube cuffs. Comparison of five different tracheal tube cuffs. *Acta Anaesthesiol Scand.* 2004;48(9):1180-1184.
44. Sesterhenn AM et al. Value of endotracheal tube safety in laryngeal laser surgery. *Lasers Surg Med.* 2003;32(5):384-390.
45. Houck PM. Comparison of operating room lasers: uses, hazards, guidelines. *Nurse Clin North Am.* 2006;41(2):193-218.
46. Pashayan AG et al. Anesthetic management guidelines for laser airway surgery: ASTM subcommittee. *Anesth Patient Saf Found Newsl.* 1993;8:13.
47. Bourgain JL et al. Transtracheal high frequency jet ventilation for endoscopic airway surgery: a multicentre study. *Br J Anaesth.* 2001;87:870-875.
48. Treggiari MM, Deen S. Anesthesia and critical care medicine. In: Barash P et al, eds. *Clinical Anesthesia.* 5th ed. Philadelphia: Lippincott Williams & Wilkins; 2006:1473-1498.
49. Chang JL et al. Severe abdominal distention following jet ventilation during general anesthesia. *Anesthesiology.* 1978;49:216.
50. Soysal O et al. Tracheobronchial foreign body aspiration: a continuing challenge. *Otolaryngol Head Neck Surg.* 2006;135(2):223-226.
51. Le Corre F et al. Visual estimation of onset time at the orbicularis oculi after five muscle relaxants: application to clinical monitoring of tracheal intubation. *Anesth Analg.* 1999;89(5):1305-1310.
52. Pathak D et al. A comparison of the response of hand and facial muscles to non-depolarizing relaxants. *Anaesthesia.* 1988;43:747-748.
53. Levine RA et al. Auditory evoked potential and other neurophysiologic monitoring techniques during tumor surgery in the cerebellopontine angle. In: Loftus CM, Traynelis VC, eds. *Intraoperative Monitoring Techniques in Neurosurgery.* New York: McGraw-Hill; 1994:175.
54. Chinn K et al. Middle ear pressure variation: effects of nitrous oxide. *Laryngoscope.* 1997;107:357.
55. Stein SN et al. Complications rare and unusual. *Semin Anesth.* 1996;15:238.
56. Doyle WJ, Banks JM. Middle ear pressure change during controlled breathing with gas mixtures containing nitrous oxide. *J Appl Physiol.* 2003;94(1):199-204.

57. Strollo PJ, Rogers RM. Obstructive sleep apnea. *N Engl J Med.* 1996;334:99.
58. Sabers C et al. The diagnosis of obstructive sleep apnea as a risk factor for unanticipated admissions in outpatient surgery. *Anesth Analg.* 2003; 96(5):1328-1335.
59. Benumof JL. Obstructive sleep apnea in the adult obese patient: implications for airway management. *Anesthesiol Clin North America.* 2002;20(4):789-811.
60. Agrawal A et al. Postoperative hemorrhage after tonsillectomy: use of ketorolac tromethamine. *Otolaryngol Head Neck Surg.* 1999;120(3):335-339.
61. Kokki H. Nonsteroidal anti-inflammatory drugs for postoperative pain: a focus on children. *Paediatr Drugs.* 2003;5(2):103-123.
62. Koc C et al. The use of preoperative lidocaine to prevent stridor and laryngospasm after tonsillectomy and adenoidectomy. *Otolaryngol Head Neck Surg.* 1998;118:880.
63. Bolton CM et al. Randomized, double-blind study comparing the efficacy of moderate-dose metoclopramide and ondansetron for the prophylactic control of postoperative vomiting in children after tonsillectomy. *Br J Anaesth.* 2007;99(5):699-703.
64. Crysdale WD, Russel D. Complications of tonsillectomy and adenoidectomy in 9409 children observed overnight. *Can Med Assoc J.* 1986;135:1139.
65. Lee C et al. Pediatric diseases. In: Hines RL, Marschall KE, eds. *Stoelting's Anesthesia and Co-existing Disease.* 5th ed. Philadelphia: Churchill Livingstone; 2008:612.
66. Takemura H et al. Correlation of cleft type with incidence of perioperative respiratory complications in infants with cleft lip and palate. *Paediatr Anaesth.* 2002;12(7):585-588.
67. Gotta A et al. Otolaryngologic and maxillofacial surgery. In: Kirby R, Gravenstein N, eds. *Clinical Anesthesia Practice.* 2nd ed. Philadelphia: Saunders; 2002:1420-1441.
68. Blackwell K et al. Propofol for endoscopic sinus surgery. *Am J Otolaryngol.* 1993;14:262-266.
69. Fedok FG et al. Operative times, postanesthesia recovery times, and complications during sinonasal surgery using general anesthesia and local anesthesia with sedation. *Otolaryngol Head Neck Surg.* 2000;4(122):560-566.
70. Bizakis JG et al. Cocaine flakes versus tetracaine/adrenalin solution for local anesthesia in septoplasty. *Rhinology.* 2004;42(4):236-238.
71. Phero JC et al. Anesthesia for maxillofacial/mandibular trauma. *Otolaryngol Head Neck Surg.* 1993;11:509-523.
72. Veras LM et al. Vertebral artery occlusion after acute cervical spine trauma. *Spine.* 2000;25(9):1171-1177.
73. Parks RE, Livoni JP. Detection of cervical spine injury in the multi-trauma patient. In: Baisdell FW, Trunkey KK, eds. *Trauma Management III: Cervical Thoracic Trauma.* New York: Thieme Medical; 1986:56.
74. Eckhauser FE et al. Tracheostomy complicating massive burn injury: a plea for conservation. *Am J Surg.* 1974;127:418.
75. Le Fort R. The classic reprint. Experimental study of fractures of the upper jaw. I and II. *Plast Reconstr Surg.* 1972;50(5):497-506.
76. Gotta AW. *Management of the traumatized airway.* ASA Refresher Course. Park Ridge, IL: American Society of Anesthesiologists; 1996:121.
77. Tintinali JE, Claffey J. Complications of nasotracheal intubation. *Ann Emerg Med.* 1981;10:142.
78. van Aalst JA et al. Reconstructive considerations in the surgical management of melanoma. *Surg Clin North Am.* 2003;83:187-230.
79. Supkis DE Jr et al. Anesthetic management of the patient undergoing head and neck cancer surgery. *Int Anesthesiol Clin.* 1998;36(3):21-29.
80. Arosarena OA. Perioperative management of the head and neck cancer patient. *J Oral Maxillofac Surg.* 2007;65(2):305-313.

CHAPTER 40

ANESTHESIA FOR OPHTHALMIC PROCEDURES

Randolf R. Harvey

Ophthalmic anesthesia continues to be an exciting and challenging segment of nurse anesthesia practice. Ophthalmologists recognize the value anesthesia practitioners provide to their patients and practice. Newer surgical techniques for eye surgery have reduced the need for traditional injection eye blocks (i.e., peribulbar and retrobulbar blocks) and increased the popularity of topical anesthesia. Topical anesthesia, used frequently for cataract surgery, challenges the anesthetist to provide care in a high-volume ambulatory surgery center (ASC) environment. Practice varies widely according to surgeon preference, but some surgeons continue to request ocular regional blocks for cataract, glaucoma, adult muscle, corneal transplants, and retinal procedures. Today, more than a million ocular blocks are performed annually for surgical procedures. Thanks to ophthalmic anesthesia educational programs, we are administering safer ocular blocks today, along with providing efficient patient care. There are a growing number of nurse anesthetists throughout the United States who have chosen to perform ophthalmic blocks. This expertise in eye anesthesia has spurred a high demand for their services, especially with the proliferation of ASCs to meet the public's demand for ophthalmic surgery.

OPHTHALMIC ANATOMY

Extraocular Muscles

Six extraocular muscles exist (Figures 40-1 through 40-3). The *superior rectus muscle* is located at the 12-o'clock position on the globe. This muscle moves the eye upward, or *supraducts* the eye. The *inferior rectus muscle* is located at the 6-o'clock position on the globe. This muscle moves the eye downward, or *infraducts* the eye. The *medial rectus muscle* is located 90 degrees medially to the 12-o'clock position on the globe and moves the eyeball nasally, or *adducts* the eye. The *lateral rectus muscle* is located 90 degrees laterally to the 12-o'clock position on the globe and moves the eyeball *laterally*, or *abducts* the eye. The *superior oblique muscle* is located on the superior aspect of the eye. This muscle rotates the eyeball on its horizontal axis toward the nose, or *intorts* the eye, and depresses the eyeball. The *inferior oblique muscle* is located on the inferior aspect of the globe. This muscle rotates the eyeball on its horizontal axis temporally, or *extorts* the eye, and elevates the eyeball (Table 40-1).

All the ocular muscles except the inferior oblique originate in the orbital apex around the annulus of Zinn (Figure 40-4), which is a fibrinous ring that encircles the optic foramen. The four rectus muscles move forward in a conal pattern that forms the muscle cone around the globe. These muscles, which are about 40 mm long, insert into the globe just anterior to its equator.[1] The superior oblique muscle arises just superior to the annulus of Zinn and moves forward, becoming a tendon. This tendon passes

through a cartilaginous ring called the *trochlea*, which is located on the medial supranasal orbital wall. After passing through the trochlea, the tendon is redirected in a posterolateral direction and inserts on the superolateral aspect of the globe under the superior rectus muscle. The inferior oblique muscle originates from the anterior nasal orbit and moves in a posterolateral direction to the globe, inserting along the lateral aspect of the globe. The arching of both the inferior and the superior oblique muscles around the globe allows for the torsional movements of the eye.

Eyelid Muscles

The levator muscle of the upper eyelid is the primary muscle used for raising the upper eyelids. This muscle originates near the annulus of Zinn (see Figure 40-1). It moves forward just superior and slightly medial to the superior rectus muscle, inserting into the upper eyelid. Because the levator muscle only retracts and does not contract the eyelid, akinesia of this muscle is not necessary.

The *orbicular muscle* of the eye (Figure 40-5) causes the eyelids to contract. This muscle has three divisions—*orbital*, *palpebral*, and *tarsal*—which are concentrically arranged around the eyelid. Akinesia of these muscles is generally desired for ocular procedures, because if the muscles were allowed to contract around the globe, intraocular pressure would increase. However, the recent success of cataract and glaucoma procedures performed with the use of topical and subconjunctival anesthesia has demonstrated that akinesia of the orbicular muscle of the eye is not always mandatory.

Cranial Nerves

The orbital portion of the *optic nerve* (cranial nerve II) (Figure 40-6) is from 25 to 30 mm long and travels posteriorly within the muscle cone from the globe into the cranial cavity. This distance is actually longer than that from the posterior portion of the globe to the orbital apex, giving the optic nerve an S-shaped configuration. This shape allows free movement of the nerve so that the many positions of the eye are accommodated. The optic nerve is myelinated and is about 4 mm in diameter.[2] The optic nerve extends through the *optic canal* and continues until it meets the *optic chiasm* intracranially. The optic chiasm is the junction of both optic nerve tracts. Here, suspended in and surrounded by cerebrospinal fluid, the optic nerve fibers partially decussate, sending visual fibers to the contralateral eye.

According to Wolff, the optic nerve is not a true cranial nerve but is actually an outgrowth of the brain.[1] As a result, the optic nerve is also covered by the *meninges*, the fibrous wrappings of the arachnoid, dura, and pia mater, which envelop the central nervous system (CNS). Therefore, any anesthetic agent injected into the optic nerve sheath can find its way back to the midbrain

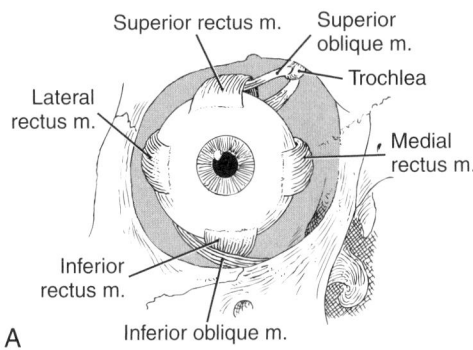

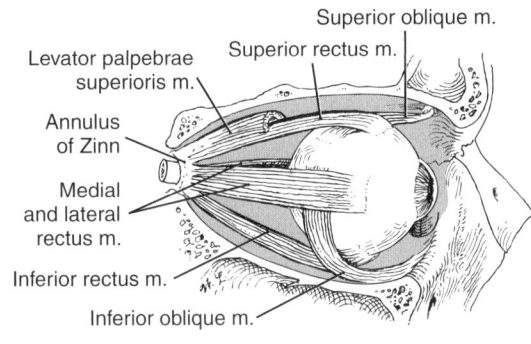

FIGURE **40-1** **A,** Frontal view of the orbit. **B,** Lateral view of the orbit. *m.,* Muscle.

TABLE **40-1**	Orbital Muscles and Innervation	
Muscle	**Function**	**Cranial Nerve**
Superior rectus	Supraduction	III
Inferior rectus	Infraduction	III
Medial rectus	Adduction	III
Lateral rectus	Abduction	VI
Superior oblique	Intorsion Depression	IV
Inferior oblique	Extorsion Elevation	III

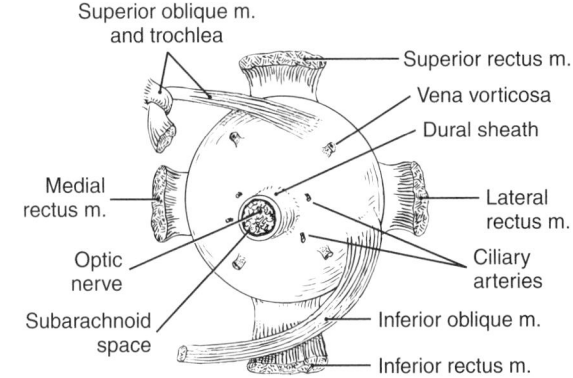

FIGURE **40-3** Posterior view of the globe. *m.,* Muscle.

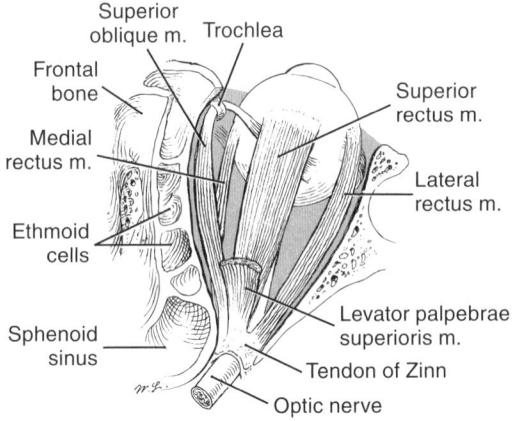

FIGURE **40-2** Superior view of the orbit. *m.,* Muscle.

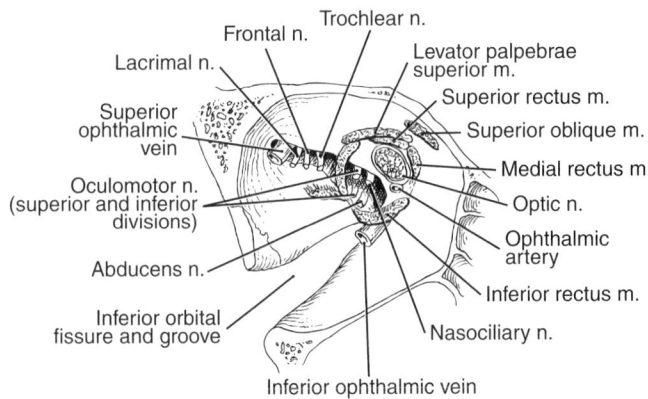

FIGURE **40-4** View of the orbital apex. *m.,* Muscle; *n.,* nerve.

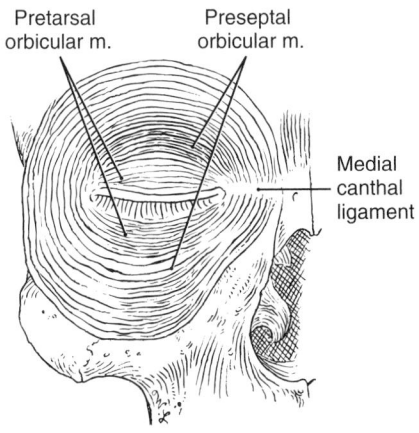

FIGURE **40-5** Orbicularis oculi muscles. *m.,* Muscle.

through the cerebrospinal fluid and result in CNS depression and even lead to respiratory arrest. The optic nerve also carries the central retinal artery and vein into the globe. The central retinal artery and vein exit the optic nerve about 8 to 15 mm posterior to the globe.[3]

The *oculomotor nerve* (cranial nerve III) innervates the following muscles of the orbit: the superior rectus muscle, the inferior rectus muscle, the inferior oblique muscle, the medial rectus muscle, and the levator muscle of the upper eyelid. The oculomotor nerve is the primary motor nerve to the extraocular muscles of the orbit; this nerve branches superiorly and inferiorly

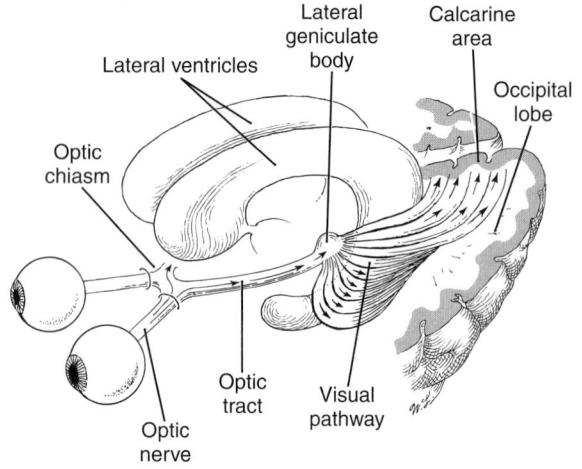

FIGURE **40-6**   Intraorbital and intracranial view of the optic nerve.

(Figure 40-7). The superior branch innervates the superior rectus muscle and the levator muscle of the upper eyelid. The inferior branch of the oculomotor nerve innervates the medial rectus muscle, the inferior rectus muscle, and the inferior oblique muscle. This nerve also sends parasympathetic fibers to the ciliary ganglion (Figure 40-8), which is located adjacent to the optic nerve in the posterior portion of the orbit. The ciliary ganglion receives parasympathetic fibers from the oculomotor nerve and also sympathetic fibers from the carotid artery plexus and a sensory branch from the nasociliary nerve, a branch of the ophthalmic nerve. The parasympathetic fibers move from the ciliary ganglion forward to innervate the iris sphincter muscles, which cause constriction of the pupil. The sympathetic motor fibers move forward to control the radial muscle of the iris for pupillary dilation.

The *trochlear nerve* (cranial nerve IV) (see Figure 40-7) provides the motor fibers for the superior oblique muscle. This nerve enters the orbit through the superior orbital fissure outside the muscle cone. It is the only orbital cranial motor nerve that enters the orbit outside the muscle cone. Once inside the orbit, the

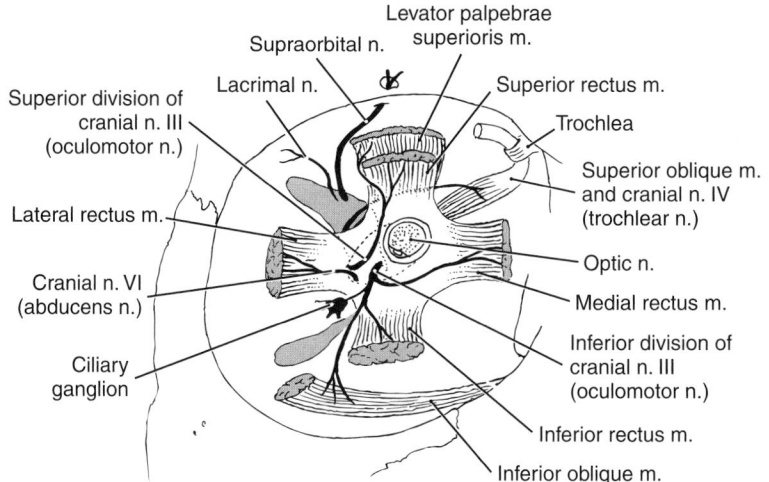

FIGURE **40-7**   Frontal view of the posterior orbit with its motor nerves and the extraocular muscles. *m.*, Muscle; *n.*, nerve.

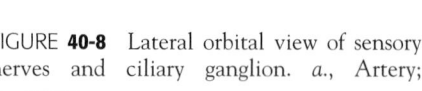

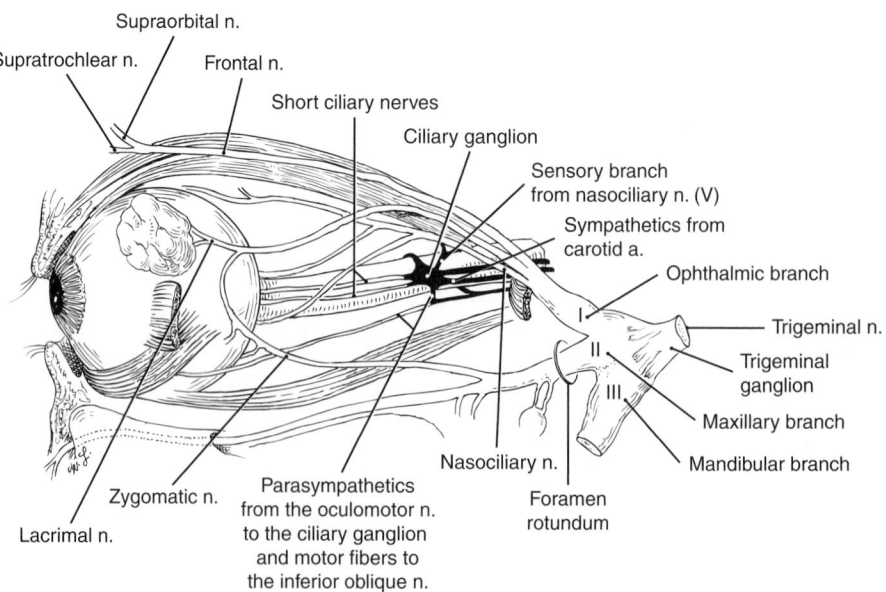

FIGURE **40-8**   Lateral orbital view of sensory nerves and ciliary ganglion. *a.*, Artery; *n.*, nerve.

nerve root moves in a medial direction to innervate the superior oblique muscle.

The *trigeminal nerve* (cranial nerve V) (see Figure 40-8) has sensory and motor components. In ocular anesthesia, the sensory component is of primary importance. The intracranial portion of the nerve forms the trigeminal ganglion, which has three main divisions: the ophthalmic, the maxillary, and the mandibular nerves. The ophthalmic branch provides for the sensation of pain, touch, and temperature to the cornea, ciliary body, iris, lacrimal gland, conjunctiva, nasal mucosa, eyelid, eyebrow, forehead, and nose. The maxillary branch provides for the sensation of pain, touch, and temperature to the upper lip, nasal mucosa, and scalp muscles.[4]

The *ophthalmic nerve* has three main branches: lacrimal, frontal, and nasociliary. The *lacrimal nerve branch* innervates the lacrimal gland in the superior lateral aspect of the orbit. The frontal branch is the largest branch of the ophthalmic nerve. This branch enters the orbit outside the muscle cone through the superior orbital fissure and travels anteriorly outside the muscle cone superior to the levator muscle. The frontal nerve itself splits into two branches. The larger, supraorbital branch continues forward into the orbit and exits the orbit through the supraorbital notch; this branch innervates the forehead. The smaller branch is the supratrochlear nerve, which moves in a medial direction, supplying nerve roots to the forehead and the medial portion of the upper eyelid. The *nasociliary nerve branch* enters the orbit inside the muscle cone and crosses over the optic nerve, sending nerve fibers medially and to the ciliary ganglion. The fibers to the ciliary ganglion form the short ciliary nerves, which continue anteriorly, penetrating the posterior portion of the globe near the optic nerve. The nasociliary nerve also gives rise to the long ciliary nerves, which continue anteriorly and enter the posterior portion of the globe supplying the ciliary muscle, iris, and cornea. The long ciliary nerves also carry sympathetic fibers to the dilator muscle of the iris from the superior cervical ganglion. The nasociliary nerve continues along the medial aspect of the orbit just superior to the medial rectus muscle until it passes through the orbital septum to become the *infratrochlear nerve*. The infratrochlear nerve provides sensory input to the side of the nose, the medial aspect of the eyelids, the medial conjunctiva, the caruncle, and the lacrimal sac.

The *abducens nerve* (cranial nerve VI) (see Figure 40-7) provides motor function to the lateral rectus muscle. The nerve enters through the superior orbital fissure within the muscle cone and continues along the conal surface of the lateral rectus muscle, eventually inserting in the posterior one third of that muscle.

The *facial nerve* (cranial nerve VII) (Figure 40-9) is predominantly a motor nerve for the muscles of the face. This nerve exits from the stylomastoid foramen. The facial nerve travels underneath the external auditory canal to the parotid gland, where it divides into an upper and a lower branch. Ocular anesthesia is more concerned with the upper branch of the facial nerve than with the lower. The upper branch further divides into the temporal and zygomatic branches, which innervate the orbicular muscle of the eye, the superficial facial muscles, and the scalp muscles.

The *vagus nerve* (cranial nerve X) provides motor function to the intrinsic muscles of the larynx and the heart; it provides major parasympathetic visceral innervation elsewhere. It is also the efferent pathway for the oculocardiac reflex, which can result in bradycardia and dysrhythmias.

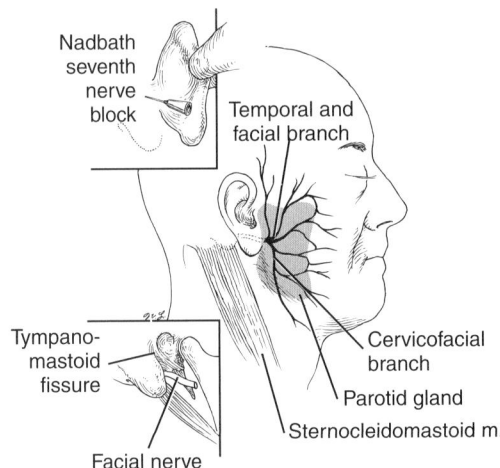

FIGURE **40-9** The origin and branches of the facial nerve. *Upper inset*: Needle placement for the Nadbath seventh nerve block. *m.*, Muscle.

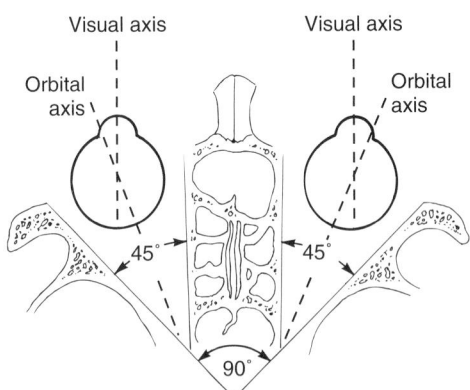

FIGURE **40-10** Superior view of the bony orbit, demonstrating the orbital and visual axes.

Orbital Fossa

The *orbital fossa* has been described as pear shaped. The medial walls of the orbit extend almost straight back, whereas the lateral walls diverge medially at about a 90-degree angle to each other (Figure 40-10). The *superior* and *inferior orbital fissures* are in the orbital apex, which is located in the posterior orbit. These fissures are the entry portals for the orbital nerves and vessels (Figure 40-11). The *optic foramen* lies just medial to the superior orbital fissure and is the entry portal for the optic nerve and the ophthalmic artery from the intracranial to the intraorbital area. In the medial nasal aspect of the fossa, just behind the orbital rim, is the *lacrimal bone*, which is used as a landmark for the medial peribulbar block (Figure 40-12). The *ethmoid bone* is just posterior to the lacrimal bone.

The *supraorbital nerve* exits the orbit in the supraorbital notch, which is in the superior nasal aspect of the orbital rim. The *infraorbital foramen*, where the infraorbital nerve and artery exit, is just below the infraorbital rim at about the 6-o'clock position. The *infraorbital nerve* is the sensory branch of the maxillary nerve. The *lacrimal*, *frontal*, and *trochlear nerves* all enter through the superior orbital fissure outside the muscle cone. The *oculomotor*, *abducens*, and *nasociliary nerves* all enter the orbit inside the muscle cone.

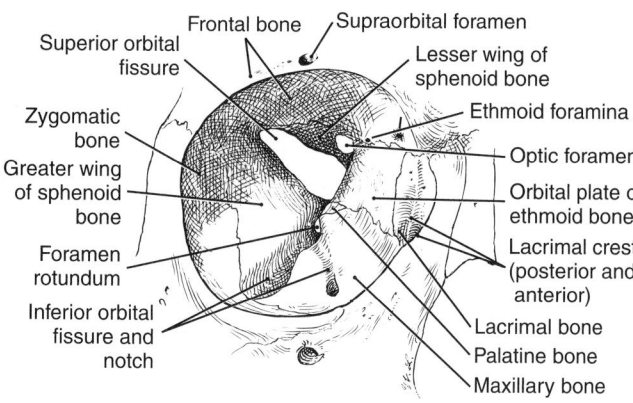

FIGURE **40-11**　Frontal view of the orbital bones.

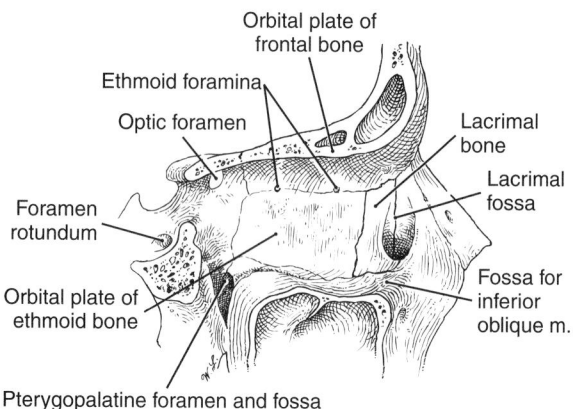

FIGURE **40-12**　Lateral view of the orbital bones. *m.*, Muscle.

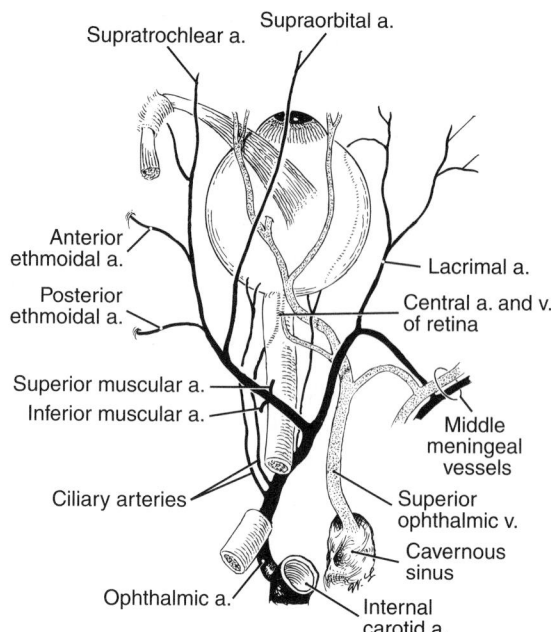

FIGURE **40-13**　Superior view of the orbital arteries and veins. *a.*, Artery; *v.*, vein.

The *ophthalmic artery* (Figure 40-13), which is the first branch of the internal carotid artery, passes into the orbit through the optic canal. The ophthalmic artery usually lies just inferolateral to the optic nerve. The artery extends along the optic nerve for a short distance, crossing over it in most cases and continuing medially.[5] The first branch of the ophthalmic artery is usually the *central retinal artery*. The central retinal artery moves in an anterior direction underneath the optic nerve, usually entering the optic nerve on its inferomedial side 8 to 15 mm posterior to the globe.[3] The artery continues forward into the optic nerve head and branches into the retinal arteries. The ophthalmic artery gives rise to the long and short posterior ciliary arteries. The short posterior arteries move anteriorly and divide into many small branches that penetrate the globe close to the optic nerve and supply the choroid and the optic nerve head. The ophthalmic artery also provides branches to the optic nerve. The orbital branches of the ophthalmic artery include branches to the supraorbital arteries, the rectus muscles, and the lacrimal gland.

The *lacrimal artery* moves anteriorly along the superior aspect of the lateral rectus muscle to the lacrimal gland. The *supraorbital artery* branches from the ophthalmic artery as it crosses over the optic nerve and extends just medial to the superior rectus and levator muscles. It continues forward on a superior nasal route and exits through the *supraorbital notch* or *foramen*.

The *dorsal nasal artery* is one of the terminal branches of the ophthalmic artery. It exits the orbital septum above the medial canthal tendon and joins with the *angular artery*, thus establishing

communication between the internal and external carotid arteries.[1] The *external carotid artery* gives branches to the facial artery (the external maxillary artery). The *facial artery* originates near the angle of the mandible, extends toward the stylohyoid muscles, and then proceeds forward to the lower border of the mandible. The artery then turns upward and moves toward the nose, where it joins with the dorsal nasal artery in the medial canthal area. The inferior orbital fissure is the entrance site for the *infraorbital artery*. This artery moves anteriorly through the infraorbital canal and exits to the face through the infraorbital foramen.

The venous drainage system (see Figure 40-13) for the orbit includes the superior and inferior ophthalmic veins, which drain into the cavernous sinus that is located intracranially. Radiographic studies have demonstrated a unique characteristic of the orbital vascular system: the orbital veins are independent of the orbital arteries.[5] The venous system of the orbit is valveless, and blood flow in this area is determined by pressure gradients. The primary vein of the orbit is the *superior ophthalmic vein*. This vein travels posteriorly to the medial side of the superior rectus muscle, then beneath the superior rectus muscle inside a support hammock. The vein then emerges on the muscle's lateral aspect. The vein continues its posterior direction along the lateral aspect of the superior rectus, exiting the orbit through the superior orbital fissure, and terminating in the cavernous sinus.[5]

Several veins enter into the superior ophthalmic vein: the *ciliary veins*, the *lacrimal veins*, and the *superior vortex veins*, which are located on the posterior quadrants of the globe and drain the choroid, or second layer, of the globe. The *inferior ophthalmic vein* originates from a diffuse plexus on the floor of the orbit. This vein receives several branches, including the extraocular muscles and the inferior vortex veins located on the inferoposterior quadrants of the globe. The primary branch of the inferior ophthalmic vein also drains into the *superior ophthalmic vein* before the entrance of the superior ophthalmic vein into the cavernous sinus. The *central retinal vein* exits the globe inside the optic nerve. The central retinal vein then exits the optic nerve

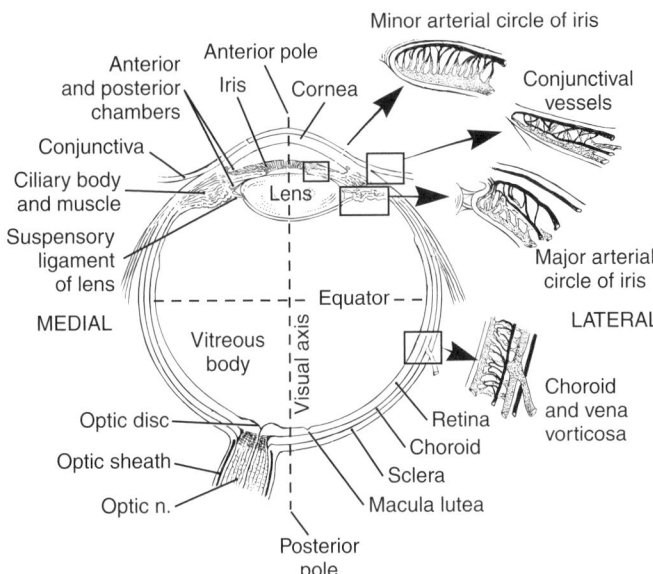

FIGURE **40-14** Cross-sectional view of the globe.

and enters the orbit between 8 and 15 mm posterior to the globe[3] and usually passes directly to the cavernous sinus.[1]

Orbit

An evaluation of the patient's orbit and globe size is important before ocular anesthesia is conducted. The usual volume of the orbit is 30 mL (Box 40-1). The volume of a typical globe (which has a diameter of about 25 mm) is 6.5 to 7 mL.[5] The balance of the orbital volume is approximately 23 mL and is composed of muscles, vessels, nerves, and fat. Katsev and associates[6] measured 120 orbits from 60 adult skulls and found an average orbital depth of 48 mm. The distance from the middle third and lateral third of the infraorbital rim to the superior aspect of the optic foramen was also measured and ranged from 42 to 52 mm. This distance should not be confused with the depth of the orbital floor. Because of the pear shape of the orbit, the orbital floor does not extend directly to the orbital apex. The orbital floor extends only to the posterior wall of the maxillary sinus, about two thirds of the depth of the orbital apex.

Orbital fat is contained in both the extraconal and the intraconal areas. The orbital fat encircles and encapsulates all these areas of the orbit.

The *orbital septum* is a fibrinous tissue that defines the anatomic anterior boundary of the orbit and keeps the adipose tissue from protruding forward. The *visual axis* (also known as the *optic axis* or the *geometric axis*) is an imaginary line from the midpoint of the cornea (anterior pole) to the midpoint of the retina or macula (posterior pole) (Figure 40-14). The horizontal (anteroposterior) diameter of the globe is an important consideration for ocular blocks. This measurement of the visual axis is referred to as the *axial length*. The axial length is measured preoperatively to determine the appropriate intraocular lens that should be placed in the eye after cataract removal. The axial length of the globe can be used *only* when measurements for intraocular lens implants are performed by the ophthalmologist. Normal axial lengths range from 23 to 23.5 mm. In the hyperopic (farsighted) eye, the globe is less than 22 mm long. This shorter eye length may allow a little more working area behind the eye during an ophthalmic block; however, this advantage may be offset by a smaller overall orbit.

The main concern regarding ophthalmic blocks involves the longer, myopic (nearsighted) eye, whose axial length is greater than 24 mm. As the globe stretches, it is believed that the fibrinous scleral layer thins, making the globe easier to penetrate by the needle. This increased posterior length of the globe also increases the chance of globe puncture. Therefore, because of a greater chance of contact in the posterior aspect of the orbit, the axial length of the eye (if this measurement is available) should be considered in the planning for ocular block. If the axial length is unknown, which may be the case in glaucoma surgery, corneal

transplants, retinal procedures, or muscle surgery, the practitioner's preoperative questions should include history of nearsightedness, previous retinal procedures, and general appearance of the eye.

The separate *coats*, or *tunics*, of the eyeball (see Figure 40-14) start with the *sclera*, which is the outer, fibrinous protective layer. The sclera is white and opaque and lies just posterior to the cornea. The *cornea* is the outer, fibrinous protective layer located anteriorly, and it is transparent and colorless. The middle, or vascular, layer is called the *choroid*. The *retina* is the inner layer of the posterior half of the eye. The *limbal area* is defined as the area at the junction between the cornea and the sclera.[1] The *conjunctiva* is a thin, transparent mucous membrane that covers the posterior surface of the eyelids and the anterior surface of the sclera.

A *staphyloma* is a bulging of the uvea, which comprises the iris, the ciliary body, and the choroid, into a thin and stretched sclera. Staphylomas may occur in the anterior, equatorial, and posterior areas.[2]

Tissue Systems of the Orbit

Three connective tissue systems within the orbit have been defined by Koornneef.[7] They are the Tenon capsule, the orbital connective tissue, and the fascial sheaths of the extraocular muscles (Figure 40-15).

Tenon Capsule. The *Tenon capsule* (bulbar fascia) consists of fibrous connective tissue that covers the eyeball from near the corneal limbus, where it is fused to the conjunctiva, and extends behind the eye, with openings for the extraocular muscles and the optic nerve. The Tenon capsule serves primarily as a cavity in which the eye moves.

Orbital Connective Tissue. Koornneef demonstrated the presence of *connective tissue* attachments between both the globe and the periorbital area. The connective tissue begins at the orbital apex and continues anteriorly, becoming more complex and more clearly defined at the level of the globe. Koornneef[7] also noted that the tissue septa are in a 360-degree encapsulation of the globe (Figure 40-16). These connective tissue septa encircle and support the globe within the bony

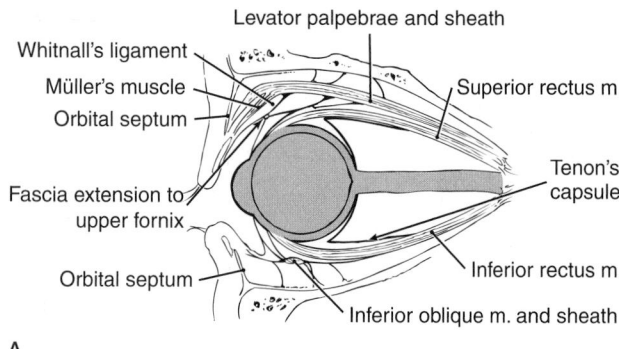

A

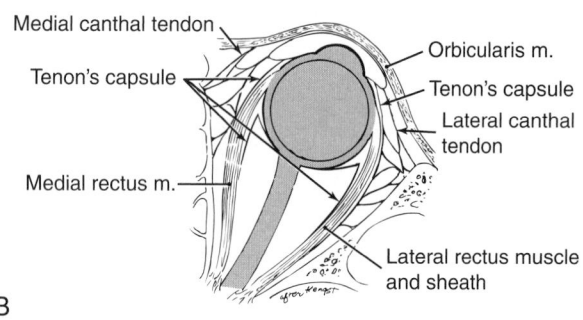

B

FIGURE **40-15** **A,** Lateral view of the orbital connective tissue. **B,** Superior view of the orbital connective tissue. *m.,* Muscle.

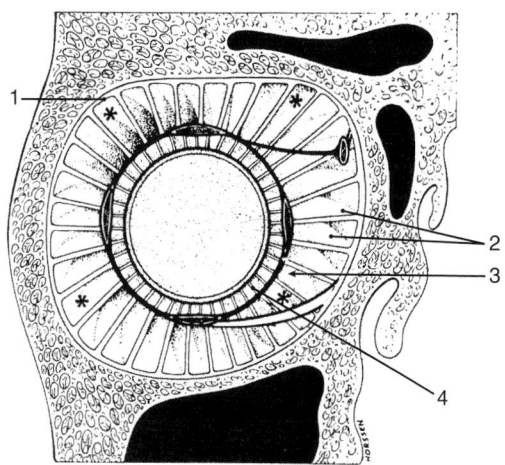

FIGURE **40-16** Schematic representation of the anterior orbital connective tissue septa. *1,* Periorbital; *2,* common muscle sheath around the eye; *3,* fibrous septa; *4,* orbit. *(From Koornneef L. New insights in the human orbital connective tissue: results of a new anatomic approach. Arch Ophthalmol. 1977;95:1269. Copyright 1977, American Medical Association.)*

orbit. Connective tissue septa were also noted between the superior and inferior oblique muscles, the Tenon capsule, the rectus muscles, and the ligaments stabilizing the globe within the orbit. This connective tissue septa meshwork limits displacement of the globe.

Fascial Sheaths. The *intermuscular membrane* is a fibrous membrane that connects the four rectus muscle sheaths.

Numerous extensions from these muscle sheaths form an intricate system of fibrinous attachments that interconnect the muscles into the orbit, support the globe, and check the ocular movements.

In the posterior orbit, the fascial sheaths of the extraocular muscles are not as well defined as they are immediately behind the globe.[8] Koornneef was not able to identify a common muscle cone throughout the orbit (Figure 40-17). The muscle sheaths themselves contribute fibrinous septa to the periorbit; these septa serve as ligaments for the extraocular muscles. These fascial extensions promote the efficiency of the extraocular muscle functions.[7-10]

PHARMACOLOGY: OCULAR MEDICATIONS AND ANESTHETIC AGENTS

Ocular medications are listed in Table 40-2.

Mydriatic Agents

Mydriatic agents cause pupillary dilation by direct or indirect effect on the dilator muscle of the iris.

Phenylephrine

Phenylephrine (Neo-Synephrine) is a commonly used and effective mydriatic and vasoconstrictor that has no cycloplegic effects. The 2.5% concentration is generally safe for use in children and the elderly. The 10% solution may contain up to 5 mg per drop of phenylephrine. However, few adverse effects have been reported with 10% phenylephrine drops. The most common and generally transient responses are headache, tremors, hypertension, and tachycardia that may be accompanied by reflex bradycardia. More severe reactions include ventricular dysrhythmias and myocardial infarctions, including some that have been fatal. One case of acute hypertension secondary to concomitant use of 10% phenylephrine drops and systemic β-blockers resulted in the rupture of a congenital cerebral aneurysm. The vasopressor response may also be potentiated by reserpine, methyldopa, tricyclic antidepressants, monoamine oxidase inhibitors, and atropine-like drugs. If treatment becomes necessary, small doses of α-adrenergic blocking agents, such as phentolamine (Regitine), chlorpromazine (Thorazine), or droperidol, have been suggested.[11]

Tropicamide

Tropicamide (Mydriacyl), available in strengths of 0.5% to 1%, is a synthetic antimuscarinic compound that provides good mydriatic activity but has weak cycloplegic effects.

Epinephrine

For ocular procedures requiring continued mydriasis, such as cataract extraction, epinephrine is commonly placed in the intraocular irrigating solution. Fiore and Cinotti[12] studied the effects of epinephrine in intraocular irrigating solutions. They concluded that solutions containing low-dose epinephrine, specifically 0.5 mL of 1:1000 epinephrine in 500 mL of solution, were probably safe for maintaining surgical mydriasis and did not appear to cause systemic side effects. However, a sudden onset of epinephrine-induced side effects may warrant discontinuation of the solution.

Cycloplegic Agents

The *cycloplegic agents*, also referred to as *parasympatholytic compounds*, cause a temporary paralysis of the ciliary muscle and the muscles of accommodation.

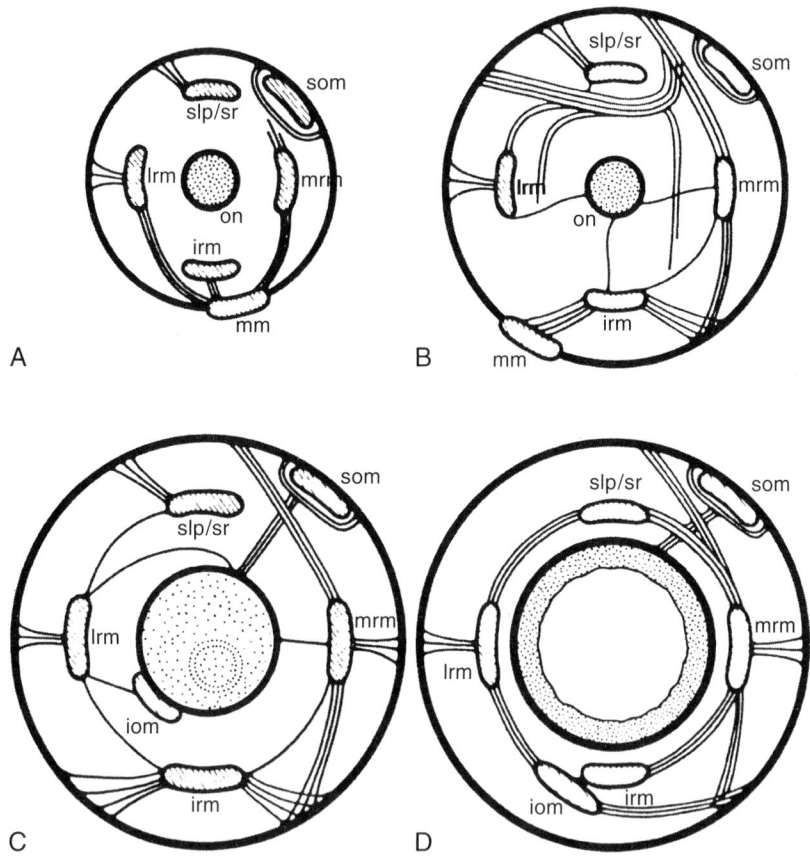

FIGURE **40-17** Extraocular muscle connective tissue system. Highly schematic representation of the connective tissue system of the extraocular muscles. **A,** Coronal section near the orbital apex. **B,** Coronal section near the posterior portion of the globe. **C,** Coronal section lying just anterior to the posterior portion of the globe. **D,** Coronal section near the equator of the globe. *iom,* Inferior oblique muscle; *irm,* inferior rectus muscle; *lrm,* lateral rectus muscle; *m,* Müller's muscle; *mrm,* medial rectus muscle; *on,* optic nerve; *slp/sr,* levator palpebrae superioris–superior rectus complex; *som,* superior oblique muscle. (*From Koornneef L. Orbital septa: anatomy and function. Ophthalmology. 1979;86:876. Courtesy of Ophthalmology.*)

Atropine

Topical atropine (1%) causes both mydriasis and cycloplegia, resulting in pupillary dilation. Intravenous atropine in doses of 0.4 to 0.6 mg has minimal ocular effects[13,14]; however, caution is advised in patients with narrow-angle glaucoma. Side effects of atropine include thirst, flushing, dry skin, tachycardia, irritability, and delirium.

Homatropine

Homatropine, available in strengths of 2% to 5%, is a topical cycloplegic with a rapid onset. Accommodation of the eye usually returns within 24 hours when the 2.5% concentration is used.

Cyclopentolate

Cyclopentolate (Cyclogyl), available in strengths of 0.5% to 2%, is a commonly used synthetic antimuscarinic agent that possesses potent mydriatic and cycloplegic properties. Reported toxic effects of cyclopentolate include speech impairment, disorientation, convulsions, and psychotic reactions.

Topical Nonsteroidal Agents

Flurbiprofen sodium 0.03% (Ocufen) is a topical nonsteroidal antiinflammatory agent for ophthalmic use. Flurbiprofen is given preoperatively to reduce the production of prostaglandins, which are potent mediators of miosis, during surgical manipulation.

Osmotic Diuretic Agents
Mannitol

Mannitol (20% solution in water) is an effective agent for reducing intraocular pressure before surgery or in an acute glaucoma attack. The usual dosage is 1.5 to 2 g/kg, administered over a period of 30 to 60 minutes.[15] Maximum ocular hypotensive effects should be seen about 1 hour after the administration of the drug. This large dose must be carefully infused because rapid infusion can lead to electrolyte imbalance, hypertension or hypotension, pulmonary edema, congestive heart failure, and renal failure resulting from osmotic overload.

Glycerin

Glycerin (Osmoglyn), an osmotic diuretic, may be taken orally before ophthalmic procedures in dosages of 1 to 1.5 g/kg. This agent can increase the risk of aspiration with general anesthesia. The metabolism of glycerin may result in hyperglycemia and glycosuria. Common side effects of all osmotic diuretics include headache, nausea, and vomiting.

Glaucoma Medications
α_2-Agonists

α_2-Agonists (Alphagan) lower intraocular pressure by reducing the formation and increasing the uveoscleral outflow of aqueous humor by their selective action on the α_2-receptors.

β-Adrenergic Blockers

β-Blockers are thought to work by reducing aqueous humor production; however, the exact mechanism is not known.

Timolol Maleate and Levobunolol

Timolol maleate (Timoptic) and levobunolol (Betagan) are topical medications, available in strengths of 0.25% or 0.5%. They are potent, nonselective β-blocking agents used to treat glaucoma.

TABLE 40-2	Ocular Medications	
Class	**Generic Name (Trade Name)**	**Comments**
α₂-Agonist	brimonidine tartrate (Alphagan P)	Glaucoma: reduces aqueous humor production Contraindicated with MAO inhibitors
Cholinesterase inhibitors	echothiophate iodide (Phospholine Iodide)	Glaucoma: produces miosis by allowing acetylcholine to continually stimulate iris and ciliary muscles, improving uveoscleral outflow of aqueous humor May prolong effects of succinylcholine; however, rarely used
β-Blockers	timolol (Timoptic) levobunolol (Betagan Liquifilm) betaxolol (Betoptic) metipranolol (OptiPranolol)	Glaucoma: reduces aqueous humor production Caution in patients with asthma, COPD, heart block, heart failure, and hypotension
Carbonic anhydrase inhibitors	acetazolamide (Diamox) dorzolamide (Trusopt) brinzolamide (Azopt)	Glaucoma: reduces aqueous humor production
Cholinergic agonists	pilocarpine, topical carbachol (Miostat), intraocular acetylcholine chloride (Miochol-E), intraocular	Miotics; used to constrict pupil for surgical procedures
Cycloplegics	atropine homatropine cyclopentolate	Pupillary dilators; cause temporary paralysis of ciliary muscle and muscles of accommodation
Intraocular gases	sulfur hexafluoride perfluoropropane	Retinal detachment: intravitreal insufflation to tamponade retina in place **Avoid nitrous oxide**
Mydriatics	phenylephrine tropicamide epinephrine	Pupillary dilators; cause either a direct or indirect effect on dilator muscle of iris
Nonsteroidal antiinflammatory agents	flurbiprofen sodium (Ocufen)	Preserves pupillary dilation during surgical procedure by inhibiting prostaglandins which cause miosis
Osmotic diuretics	glycerin (oral agent) mannitol	Reduce intraocular pressure
Prostaglandins	latanoprost (Xalatan) bimatoprost (Lumigan) travoprost (Travatan)	Glaucoma; promotes uveoscleral outflow of aqueous humor
Viscoelastics	hyaluronate sodium (Healon, Amvisc)	Protect endothelial cells of cornea during surgical procedures

MAO, *Monoamine oxidase.*

Betaxolol Hydrochloride

Betaxolol hydrochloride 0.5% (Betoptic) is a cardioselective β₁-adrenergic receptor blocking agent with an efficacy comparable to that of timolol for the treatment of glaucoma.

Usually, β-blockers do not cause systemic problems, although the anesthetist must consider the patient's age, drug sensitivity, and underlying pulmonary and cardiovascular pathology before administering these drugs because in some patients generalized systemic effects may occur. Contraindications for β-blockers are asthma, severe sinus bradycardia, heart block, burns more severe than first degree, hypotension, and severe heart failure.[16]

Cholinesterase Inhibitors
Echothiophate Iodide

Echothiophate iodide (Phospholine Iodide), 0.03% to 0.25% is a topical eye medication absorbed into the system through the lacrimal apparatus. After covalently bonding with

pseudocholinesterase, the drug begins to deactivate the enzyme within several days to a few weeks. The activity of the enzyme has been reported to take 3 to 6 weeks to return to normal after administration of the medication is discontinued. Therefore, the anesthesia practitioner may anticipate prolonged apnea with the use of succinylcholine and delayed metabolism with the use of the local ester anesthetics.[13] These agents are largely historic and rarely used in modern ophthalmic practice.

Carbonic Anhydrase Inhibitors

Carbonic anhydrase inhibitors temporarily inhibit the enzyme carbonic anhydrase. This inhibition decreases the production of aqueous humor by the ciliary body.

Acetazolamide

Acetazolamide (Diamox), a sulfonamide derivative, is a potent carbonic anhydrase inhibitor. It is effective in treating acute increased intraocular pressure by decreasing the production of aqueous humor. It is also a mild diuretic. It may be administered orally or intravenously. An injection of up to 500 mg should provide a rapid onset of action with a peak effect within 20 minutes of administration.

Dorzolamide (Trusopt) and brinzolamide (Azopt) are topical carbonic anhydrase inhibitors for the treatment of glaucoma. Side effects are rare; however, fatigue and loss of appetite have been reported.[17]

Prostaglandins

Prostaglandins reduce intraocular pressure by normalizing the uveoscleral outflow tract and thereby reduce the buildup of aqueous humor in the eye.

Latanoprost, Bimatoprost, and Travoprost

At present, the prostaglandin analogs latanoprost (Xalatan), bimatoprost (Lumigan), and travoprost (Travatan) are taking precedence over β-blockers for the treatment of glaucoma and ocular hypertension. They are very effective at reducing intraocular pressure but are contraindicated in narrow-angle glaucoma.[18] Significant systemic effects have not been reported.[17]

Cholinergic Agonists

The miosis that results from cholinergic agonists may be used to constrict the pupil for operative procedures such as secondary intraocular lens implants, trabeculectomies, and corneal transplants without an intraocular implant.

Pilocarpine

Pilocarpine (Isopto Carpine) 0.5% to 4% is a topical muscarinic alkaloid that causes pupillary constriction or miosis. Pilocarpine may cause irritation and redness of the eye. If redness is present before the ocular block is administered, one must determine whether the redness of the eye is from the medication or from an infection.

Carbachol

Carbachol (Isopto Carbachol) 0.75% to 3% topical or (Miostat) 0.01% intraocular is a synthetic carbamyl ester of choline. Its actions result from the endogenous release of acetylcholine at the terminal ending of the cholinergic fibers.

Acetylcholine

Acetylcholine (Miochol-E) is an intraocular agent used to cause pupillary constriction, usually after cataract lens extraction. Adverse effects of this cholinergic agent are uncommon, although bradycardia and bronchospasm have been reported. These symptoms respond well to intravenous atropine.

Viscoelastics

Hyaluronate sodium (Healon, Amvisc) is a physiologic viscoelastic substance that is distributed throughout the connective tissues in animals and humans. It is used for maintaining a deep anterior chamber and for protecting the endothelial cells of the cornea from surgical instrumentation and the intraocular lens in ocular surgery.

Intraocular Gases

Sulfur hexafluoride and perfluoropropane are gases that are used for the insufflation of the vitreous cavity and for the tamponade of a retinal detachment. For maintenance of the appropriate-sized bubble, nitrous oxide should be turned off 15 minutes before the gas is injected. The rest of the procedure should be performed with 100% oxygen and a volatile agent. Nitrous oxide should not be used for at least a minimum of 10 days after the injection of sulfur hexafluoride or perfluoropropane.[14]

Topical Local Anesthetic Agents
Cocaine

Cocaine has limited use in ophthalmology today because of its many serious side effects. However, it still may be used in a nasal pack for dacryocystorhinostomy procedures. The maximum recommended dose for clinical use is 1.5 to 3 mg/kg. When used in conjunction with inhalation anesthetics, the dose should be cut in half. Intravenous labetalol has been recommended for the treatment of cocaine's cardiovascular side effects.[19-21]

Tetracaine

Tetracaine (Pontocaine), which is available in strengths of 0.5% to 1%, is an ester-linked local anesthetic. Each milliliter of the 0.5% solution contains 5 mg of tetracaine hydrochloride. As a topical agent, its onset is seen within 1 minute of administration, and its effects last about 30 minutes. Tetracaine tends to cause more stinging on instillation than proparacaine. Although very rare, topical dosages have been associated with systemic toxicity, usually seen as CNS stimulation followed by CNS and cardiovascular depression.

Proparacaine Hydrochloride

Proparacaine hydrochloride (Alcaine, Paracaine) is a benzoate ester; however, it is chemically different from tetracaine and is much less irritating to the eye. The onset of action ranges from 13 to 20 seconds, and the duration of action is about 15 minutes.

Amide Anesthetic Agents

Bupivacaine, lidocaine, and ropivacaine are amide local anesthetics used in ophthalmic surgery. Bupivacaine (0.75%) may be used by itself or combined with lidocaine as a means of decreasing its time of onset. In ophthalmic blocks, complete ocular analgesia usually precedes the onset of extraocular muscle akinesia. Therefore, the presence of akinesia determines the adequacy of the block, and analgesia must be assumed, yet not guaranteed. The use of long-acting bupivacaine in ocular anesthesia generally provides the patient with adequate postoperative pain relief.[21-23] Patients may also experience postoperative diplopia of 24 to 48 hours' duration with this agent. Diplopia after eye muscle surgery may affect the postoperative evaluation by the surgeon; for this reason, a preoperative discussion with the ophthalmologist regarding the duration of action of the planned local anesthetic is in the patient's best interest.[23]

Although allergies to local anesthetics are rare, patients whose skin test results were positive for the preservative-free amides have been encountered and a few others seen whose results were positive for the preservative agents. For ocular anesthesia, local anesthesia may be used separately or in any combination to achieve the desired effect, as long as the total drug dosage does not exceed the recommended doses for the anesthetic administered.

Sodium Bicarbonate

Alkalization of local anesthesia with sodium bicarbonate may decrease the onset time and improve the quality of neural blockade. The primary ocular anesthetic bupivacaine readily precipitates when alkalization dosages less than those recommended are used. The pH threshold for bupivacaine precipitation has been measured at between 6.7 and 6.9.[24] In clinical experience with

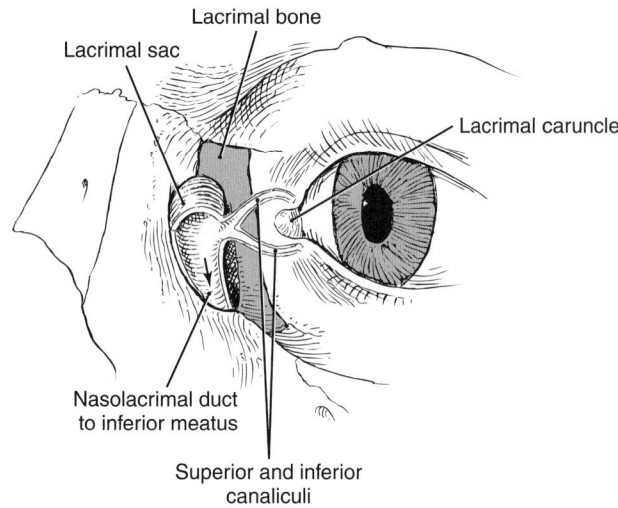

Lacrimal bone

Lacrimal sac

Lacrimal caruncle

Nasolacrimal duct
to inferior meatus

Superior and inferior
canaliculi

FIGURE **40-18** Frontal view of the lacrimal drainage system.

properly placed modified retrobulbar anesthesia, lidocaine-bupivacaine results in an ocular block onset time of within 2 minutes, with minimal to no patient discomfort from the anesthetic solution. However, a study performed by Zahl and co-workers[25] on the effects of bicarbonate on peribulbar anesthetic mixtures demonstrated a measurable decrease in onset time of 2.9 to 4.5 minutes. Therefore, alkalization of ocular anesthetics may be of benefit, depending on the type of block used and its time of onset.

Hyaluronidase

Hyaluronidase (Amphadase, Vitrase) is a protein enzyme that hydrolyzes hyaluronic acid, the cellular cement between connective tissue. This enzyme promotes the spread of local anesthesia. Clinical experience has demonstrated that hyaluronidase speeds up the onset of action of ocular anesthesia. It may also improve the quality of the block, especially the peribulbar type, by promoting a more uniform spread of anesthesia throughout the orbital fossa.[26] Recommended dosage is less than 2 units/mL for the modified retrobulbar block and less than 15 units/mL for the peribulbar block. Hyaluronidase may be omitted from a subcutaneous eyelid block.

Systemic Absorption of Eye Drops

The *lacrimal apparatus* includes the lacrimal gland, the puncta, the inferior and superior canaliculus, the common canaliculus, the lacrimal sac, and the nasolacrimal duct (Figure 40-18). The lacrimal gland is located in a depression of the frontal bone in the superior temporal orbit.[20] The gland has several ducts that lead to the conjunctival surface of the upper eyelid. Tears pass from the lacrimal gland through the ducts, over the cornea and conjunctiva, keeping the eye moist. Near the medial canthus, tears enter the puncta, travel through the canaliculus to the lacrimal sac, and drain into the nasolacrimal duct before entering the nasal mucosa.

Topical eye medications enter the bloodstream through the outer eye membrane and the lacrimal apparatus. The following measures reduce the amount of topical medications that enter the bloodstream:

1. Have the patient close the eyes for 60 seconds after drops are instilled to encourage absorption by the eye and minimize drainage to the nasal mucosa.
2. Have the patient avoid blinking, which rapidly moves the medication into the tear outflow canal and the systemic circulation.

3. Block the tear outflow canal by placing the index finger over the medial canthus after the eye is closed.[2]

Patients may complain of a metallic taste after the administration of ocular anesthetics. This precursor to a toxic anesthetic level needs further evaluation. However, it is usually the result of the local anesthesia passing into the nasal mucosa.

SELECT OCULAR ANESTHESIA TECHNIQUES

Ophthalmic Block Techniques
Topical/Intraocular Anesthesia

Cataract and vitreoretinal surgeries are the most frequently performed intraocular surgical procedures.[27,28] Topical anesthesia for cataract surgery (e.g., 2% lidocaine) has proved to be effective in providing adequate analgesia for the surgical procedure and is commonly used with phacoemulsification. Topical anesthesia is applied as drops or gels and may be supplemented by intracameral injection by the surgeon for better intraoperative pain control. Vitreoretinal surgery usually requires at least a sub-Tenon block and more frequently injection anesthetic techniques.[28] Today's smaller-incision surgical techniques with foldable intraocular lenses provide a safer surgical experience for the patient and a more rapid recovery. Intraocular anesthesia can further enhance the analgesia for the surgical procedure; 1% lidocaine (preservative free) has been studied and recognized as safe for intraocular administration.[29] However, topical anesthesia may not be appropriate in all cases for the surgeon or the patient, because it provides a lesser degree of analgesia and no akinesia of the ocular muscles or eyelids. There is wide variability in operative conditions, sensations, and pain relief, depending on the type of local anesthesia administered for intraocular surgery. Using published data that present the strength of evidence as "strong evidence," "weak evidence," or "no evidence," the differences between local/regional anesthetic techniques for variables such as pain (during placement of the block and during the surgery), eye akinesia, eyelid sensation, and visual sensations were quantified on a + or − scale, and the conflicts of evidence are presented as a range in Table 40-3.[28]

Sub-Tenon Block

The sub-Tenon block will produce a more profound analgesia; however, motor movement of the globe may still be present. The Tenon tissue, as described earlier, encapsulates the globe posteriorly and fuses with the conjunctiva anteriorly. Anteriorly it is inferior to the conjunctiva. The sub-Tenon block is a procedure performed between the rectus muscles of the globe. The conjunctiva is incised, the Tenon tissue is elevated and incised, and a short cannula is inserted into the sub-Tenon space. Local anesthetic is injected with the objective of a posterior spread of the agent. The dose is usually 3 to 4 mL to achieve analgesia; however, larger doses of up to 10 mL have been reported to achieve some degree of akinesia.[30]

OCULAR REGIONAL ANESTHESIA

The ocular regional needle block still remains the most common and effective way to consistently produce a profound analgesia and akinesia of the eye and eyelids.

The term *ocular local anesthesia* has been used to refer to retrobulbar or peribulbar blocks. More correctly, local anesthesia should be defined as *superficial*, *topical*, or *cutaneous anesthesia*, used, for example, when skin-laceration suturing is performed that poses minimal risks both to the body as a whole and to proximate vital organs.

Retrobulbar and peribulbar injections are categorized under regional anesthesia methods. These blocks are designed to

TABLE **40-3**	Comparisons of Local/Regional Anesthesia Techniques			
	Topical	**Sub-Tenon Block**	**Peribulbar Block**	**Retrobulbar Block**
Pain on administration	0 or −	+ or ++	++ or +++	+++
Surgical pain prevented	− −	+++	++	++
Eye akinesia	− − −	0 or +	++	++
Eyelid sensation blocked	− − −	+	+	+
Visual sensations experienced	+++	++ or +	+	+

From Vann MA et al. Sedation and anesthesia care for ophthalmologic surgery during local/regional anesthesia. Anesthesiology. 2007;107(3):502-508.
+ Represents strength of affirmative evidence; 0 represents insufficient evidence; − represents strength of contrary evidence.

anesthetize multiple cranial nerves (III, IV, V, VI, and VII). As described earlier, the optic nerve is a continuation of the brain. The dura mater divides at the entrance of the optic nerve into the orbit. The visceral layer of the dura covers the intraorbital part of the optic nerve, and the parietal layer blends into the periosteum of the orbit.[1] Therefore, by anatomic definition, this procedure is performed in the orbital epidural space. As has been demonstrated in the anatomic reviews by Koornneef, no true muscle cone exists, especially in the posterior portion of the orbit.[7-10] Therefore, old anatomic concepts such as the image of an intact muscle cone must be set aside in favor of concepts that illustrate a communication throughout the orbit.

Techniques and Modifications

The term *retrobulbar block* refers to an ophthalmic block technique originally described by Atkinson in 1936. The patient is instructed to look up and nasally (supranasal position). A 23-gauge retrobulbar (dull) needle is inserted through the skin in the inframtemporal area, just above the inferior orbital rim and advanced toward the orbital apex 35 mm (1.38 inches) deep into the muscle cone (retrobulbar space). After negative aspiration, 2 to 4 mL of anesthetic solution is injected into the muscle cone. After the injection is completed, the eyelids are closed, and digital pressure is applied over the globe to the orbit. A few minutes later, the eyelids are opened, and the globe is inspected for akinesia.[31,32] The popularity of the retrobulbar block for ophthalmic procedures grew, with more than 1 million blocks performed annually in the 1940s. Unfortunately, so also did the complication rates.

The reported complications from retrobulbar anesthesia include trauma to the optic nerve, the blood vessels, and the globe, all of which can lead to loss of vision. Respiratory arrest may result when anesthetic agents enter the cerebrospinal fluid of the optic nerve. Seizures may occur when even small amounts of local anesthetic are injected intravascularly.

As a result of the increasing number of complications being reported, practitioners began to alter the Atkinson retrobulbar technique in an effort to increase the margin of safety for ocular anesthesia.[33] Three major problem areas in the Atkinson technique are identified in this chapter, and technique modifications are discussed (Figure 40-19).

Eye Position

The position of the eye during retrobulbar block anesthesia is an important consideration. When the patient looks upward and nasally, the optic nerve and blood vessels are placed in the path of the needle. Tension is created on the optic nerve and the surrounding vasculature, making the orbital structures more susceptible to trauma. In this position, the posterior pole of the globe also moves into the needle path. As a means of avoiding this

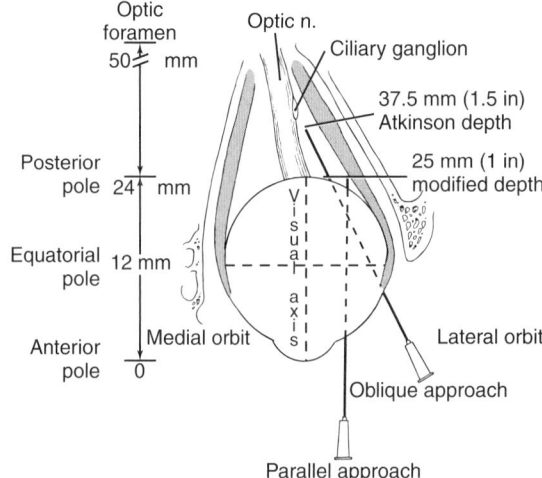

FIGURE **40-19** Superior view of the parallel and oblique approach to retrobulbar anesthetic blocks.

problem, the following modification in technique has been recommended.

The primary gaze position, in which the patient is looking directly forward, allows the optic nerve to maintain its S–shaped curvature and also releases the tension on the blood vessels. The down-and-out gaze position allows the optic nerve and vessels to rotate toward the optic foramen and farther away from the needle path. Both of these eye positions have the potential disadvantage of needle visualization by the patient. The upward-gaze position should only be used as described by Gills and Lloyd.[33] Their technique allows the use of the upward-gaze position because the needle is placed lateral and parallel to both the optic nerve and the vessels.

Needle Depth

A second problem is the depth of the needle insertion. The vital structures in the ocular anatomy are more crowded in the posterior orbit. Deep needle penetration in the orbit increases the likelihood of trauma to the optic nerve and vessels. If the depth of the needle insertion is decreased to approximately 25 mm (1 inch), the needle would lie just posterior to the globe, thereby reducing the risk of puncture of the vital structures. Studies have demonstrated that because of the wide variation in orbital and globe sizes, a needle depth of 19 to 31 mm (0.75 to 1.25 inches) is the safest.[6]

Needle Tip Shape

A pertinent issue debated in the literature is the use of sharp versus dull needles for ocular blocks. Dull or flat-grind needles made specifically for retrobulbar anesthesia are touted by some clinicians as the only safe needles for use in ocular blocks. Grizzard and colleagues[34] noted that it is not so much the type of needle but where the needle is placed that increases the risk. Dull retrobulbar needles may not be tolerated as well by awake patients because of the sensation of pressure they create on insertion. Other needles proposed for ocular blocks include a curved retrobulbar needle[35] and a dull pinhead needle, in which the injection port is proximal to the head of the needle.[36]

Needle Angle

The angle of the needle is a third very important area that should be considered for modification. The original Atkinson technique uses an oblique approach; that is, the needle is inserted in the infratemporal area just above the inferior orbital rim and is directed toward the orbital apex. This pathway tracts the needle tip toward the posterior pole of the globe, arteries, and the optic nerve.

However, Gills and Lloyd[33] developed a technique that takes into consideration not only the aforementioned changes but also the length and spherical shape of the globe. This technique changes the oblique approach to a parallel approach. The lateral limbic margin (corneoscleral junction) is identified, and the needle is inserted in the inferotemporal area transconjunctivally, just lateral and parallel to the lateral limbic margin. The needle is inserted to a depth of approximately 25 mm (1 inch), entering the muscle cone just behind the globe. The advantages of this technique result from the needle position, which lies lateral and parallel to the optic nerve, the vasculature, and the posterior pole of the globe.

The original retrobulbar block technique described by Atkinson can be made safer by modification of the technique. Modifications that decrease the risk of adverse effects are:

1. Position the globe to decrease tension on the vital orbital structures and position them farther away from the needle—for example, the primary gaze position.
2. Use a depth of needle insertion of about 25 mm (1 inch), which places the needle just behind the globe itself and avoids the structures deep in the orbit.
3. Consider using a more lateral to parallel approach to the orbit than was originally demonstrated by Atkinson.

Some practitioners, in an effort to further improve the safety of ocular blocks, have advocated the use of extraconal peribulbar blocks.[37-41] The literature describes these techniques as directing the needle outside the muscle cone, or *extraconal*. The anesthetic is injected, creating a positive extraconal pressure that spreads the agent inside the muscle cone to anesthetize the cranial nerves. To accomplish this, the needle is inserted parallel to, or is angled away from, the visual axis of the globe in an effort to remain outside the muscle cone. Peribulbar injections may be performed in the superior temporal, medial, and inferior temporal orbital areas. Peribulbar anesthesia requires larger volumes of anesthetic agents (8 to 12 mL). Owing to the many septal divisions of the orbit, the anesthetic flow may not adequately diffuse into the intramuscle cone. Therefore, extraconal peribulbar anesthetic injections, as described in the literature, may not consistently produce adequate akinesia and may necessitate multiple repeat injections.[38]

Patients who may benefit from the extraconal peribulbar approach are those at increased risk for globe puncture, such as those with high myopia resulting in long axial lengths, significant enophthalmos, previous scleral buckling procedures, and staphylomas. However, peribulbar blocks have also been used in patients with globe punctures.[42]

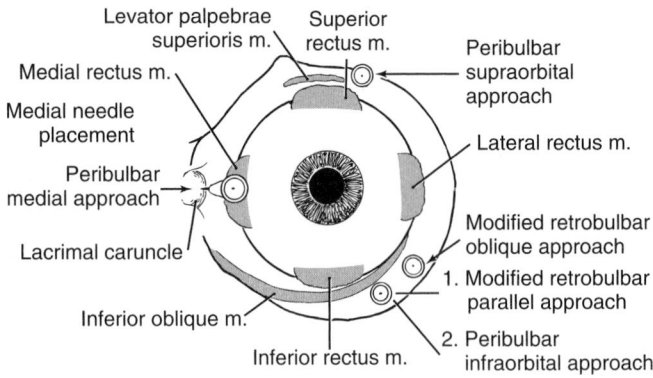

FIGURE **40-20** Frontal view of needle placement for retrobulbar and peribulbar anesthetic blocks. *m.*, Muscle.

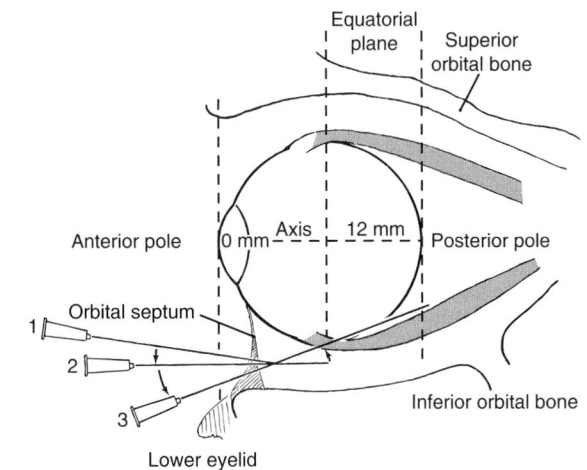

FIGURE **40-21** Lateral view of needle angles for a modified retrobulbar block.

The primary goal of extraconal peribulbar blocks is the avoidance of the muscle cone and its vital structures. With modified retrobulbar blocks, the goal is not only to avoid the vital structures but also to enter the muscle cone just posterior to the globe.

The least vascular areas in which ocular blocks can be performed were described by Koornneef and Kramer[9] (Figure 40-20). The inferotemporal area can be used for both the intraconal modified retrobulbar and the extraconal peribulbar technique. The superior orbital area just lateral to the 12-o'clock position through the skin and the medial orbital area through the caruncle conjunctiva may be accessed for the extraconal peribulbar technique.

The most important considerations for ocular blocks are the position of the eye and the depth and angle of the needle. Needle placement should avoid the optic nerve, the arteries and veins, the globe, and the extraocular muscles.

Anesthesia Techniques
Gills-Lloyd Modified Retrobulbar Technique[33]
Equipment List
One 3-mL syringe
One 6-mL syringe
One 25- or 27-gauge needle
1-inch paper tape
One 4 × 4 gauze pad
Description. Figures 40-21 and 40-22 and Box 40-2 present valuable reference aids for the Gills-Lloyd modified retrobulbar technique.

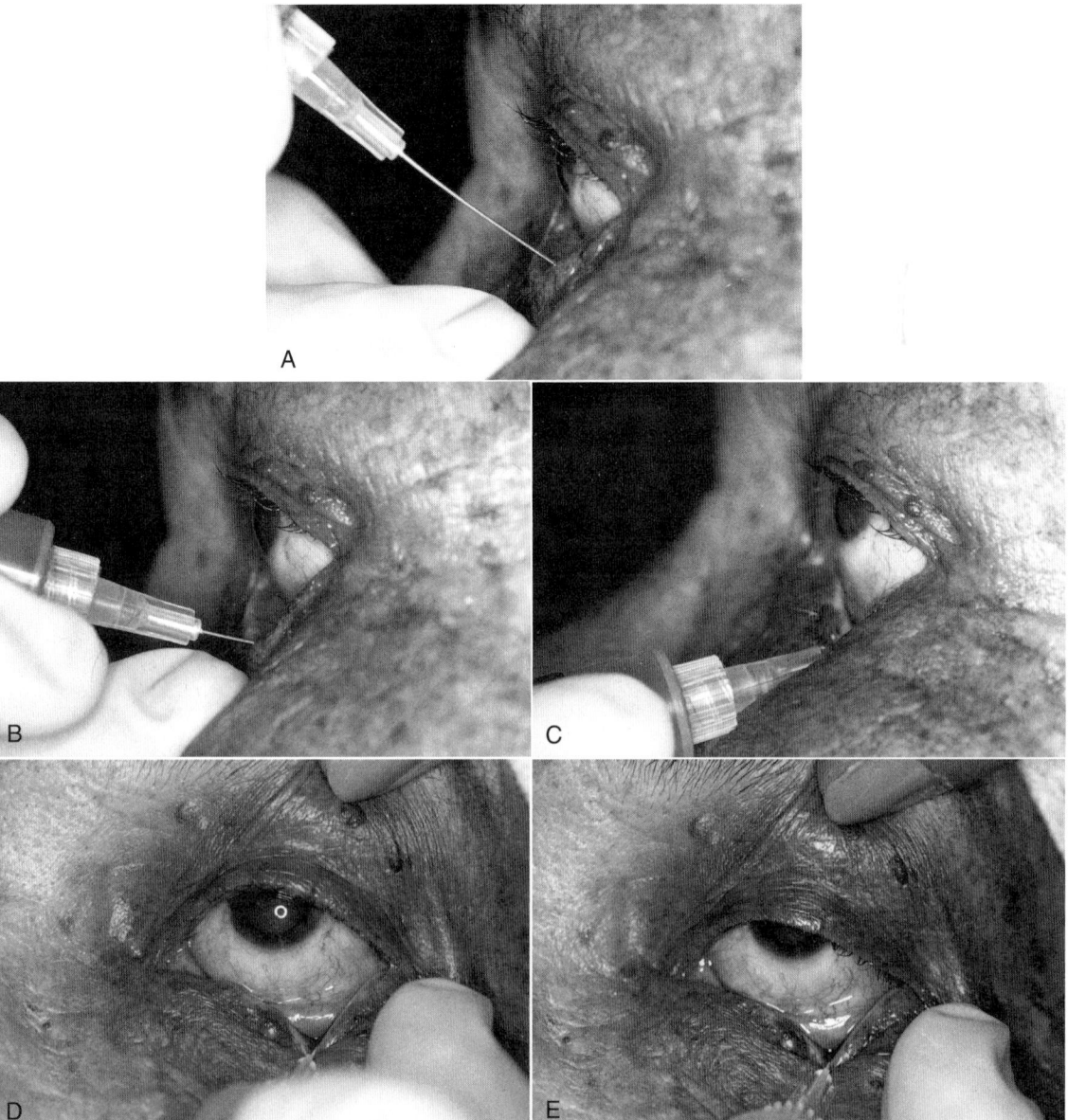

FIGURE **40-22** **A,** In the Gills-Lloyd modified retrobulbar technique, the needle should be inserted transconjunctivally or transcutaneously, angled away from the visual axis of the globe toward the orbital floor until the orbital septum is penetrated. **B,** After penetrating the orbital septum, the needle should be redirected parallel to the visual axis to a depth of about 12 mm (0.5 inch) to the equatorial plane of the globe. **C,** At the equatorial plane of the globe, the needle should be redirected toward the visual axis to a depth of about 25 mm (1 inch). At this point, the needle enters the muscle cone, and the medication is injected. **D,** Needle placement, which is lateral and parallel to the lateral limbic margin. **E,** Completion of the modified retrobulbar block. Some degree of globe proptosis and drooping of the upper eyelid should be expected.

The patient should be in a comfortable, reclining position. Anesthetic drops are placed in the conjunctiva, the eyelids are closed, and the outer eyelids are cleansed. The patient is asked to look directly overhead and to stare at a finger or other object. The eye should not look inward but may look somewhat outward. Needle insertion through the skin is preferably avoided in this technique so that patient discomfort is minimized. The lateral limbic margin (corneoscleral junction) is identified. The lower eyelid is everted and controlled with a finger. The needle is placed in the bevel-up position just above the inferior orbital rim, just lateral and parallel to the lateral limbic margin. The

needle is then inserted through the conjunctiva and directed toward the orbital floor until the orbital septum is penetrated. The needle is then redirected parallel to the visual axis of the globe to a depth of 25 mm (1 inch). At this time, 1 to 1.5 mL of lidocaine, 1% to 2%, is injected after negative aspiration is performed. This initial extraconal peribulbar technique is effective in reducing the potential discomfort from the needle and the anesthetic injection of the modified retrobulbar block in the awake patient.

The eye is closed briefly in preparation for the modified retrobulbar injection. The lower eyelid is again everted and

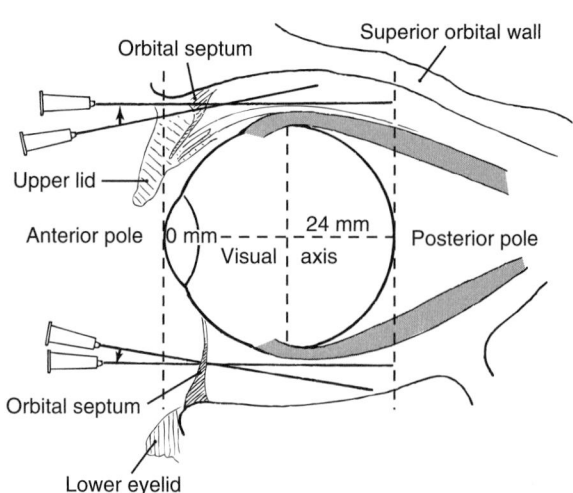

FIGURE **40-23** Lateral view of needle angles for peribulbar block.

BOX **40-2**

The Gills-Lloyd Modified Retrobulbar Technique: Parallel Approach

Insert the needle transconjunctivally or transcutaneously, lateral to the lateral limbic margin and angled away from the visual axis of the globe toward the orbital floor, until the orbital septum is penetrated (see Figure 40-22, A).

After penetrating the orbital septum, redirect the needle parallel to the visual axis to a depth of about 12 mm (0.5 in) past the equatorial plane of the globe (see Figure 40-22, B).

Past the equatorial plane of the globe, redirect the needle toward the visual axis to a depth of about 25 mm (1 in), entering the muscle cone while remaining lateral to the lateral limbic margin, and inject the medications (see Figure 40-22, C).

---

controlled with a finger. The needle is placed bevel up, just above the inferior orbital rim, just lateral and parallel to the lateral limbic margin. The needle is then inserted through the conjunctiva and directed toward the orbital floor until the orbital septum is penetrated. The needle is then redirected parallel to the visual axis of the globe past its equatorial plane, about 12 mm deep. At this point, the needle is rotated cephalad between the lateral and inferior rectus muscles. Resistance may or may not be felt as the needle enters the muscle cone. The needle should be inserted about 25 mm (1 inch), depending on the size of the orbit and the globe (range, 19 to 31 mm). After negative aspiration, the anesthetic agent is injected slowly, 1 mL/10 sec, until the orbit is filled. Orbital size governs the total amount of anesthetic injected; however, 4 to 6 mL usually suffices. Once the orbit is full of anesthesia, as indicated by orbital tension, the needle is withdrawn. The eyelids are closed, a 4 × 4 gauze is placed over the eye, and positive digital pressure is applied. The pressure helps spread the anesthetic and detect any increasing orbital pressure, which might indicate a retrobulbar hemorrhage.

The initial needle insertion is directed away from the globe so that the risk of globe puncture is decreased. Resistance may or may not be felt as the needle enters the muscle cone, depending on the presence or absence of the fibrinous connective tissue in the area behind the globe, as described by Koornneef and Kramer.[9] The sharper the needle, the less resistance felt by the practitioner and the less discomfort felt by the patient. By comparison, use of dull needles results in more resistance, potentially resulting in greater patient discomfort. Patients have described this resistance to the needle as *pressure pain*. Because a pop may or may not be felt as the needle enters the muscle cone, attention to needle depth is extremely important for the avoidance of deep penetration into the orbit.

During injection, the patient is told to inform the practitioner if any discomfort, such as stinging or a mild headache, is experienced. If this occurs, the injection should be stopped to allow the agent to take effect. The pressure sensation appears to result from the local agent's spreading throughout the orbital area. The stinging is noticed more when the agent moves into the peripheral area along the upper and lower eyelids. This slow injection process is continued until the orbit is filled with the anesthetic agent. When the anesthetic is placed into the muscle cone, the effects are seen rapidly, and the block can be evaluated for akinesia after about 2 minutes. Generous traction must be applied

to the lower eyelid, because this technique is performed before the orbicular muscles of the eyelids are anesthetized (seventh nerve block). Seventh nerve blocks can be very painful and are not well tolerated by patients. These blocks generally precede retrobulbar or peribulbar blocks but may not be necessary, because the anesthetic agent from the modified retrobulbar or peribulbar block spreads randomly throughout the orbit and eyelids, providing adequate akinesia of the eyelids.[42,43]

Peribulbar Extraconal Techniques

Description. Figures 40-23 and 40-24 and Box 40-3 serve as valuable reference aids for the peribulbar technique.

Extraconal peribulbar blocks may be performed using different techniques. One is a supraorbital-only technique of injecting a large volume (10 to 12 mL) of anesthetic agent, which should distribute throughout the orbit for completion of the block. An inferotemporal-only technique also involves injection of a large volume (10 to 12 mL) of anesthesia, which should distribute throughout the orbit and anesthetize the eye. A more reproducible approach to extraconal peribulbar anesthesia is the use of both the inferior and superior approaches. Each of these injections may be performed with a 6-mL syringe for a total volume of 10 to 12 mL. The combination technique generally provides a more consistent result. It is usually easier to handle a 6-mL syringe than a 10-mL syringe around the eye.

Infraorbital and Supraorbital Extraconal Peribulbar Anesthesia
Equipment List
One 10-mL syringe or two 6-mL syringes
One or two 25- or 27-gauge needles
One 4 × 4 gauze pad
1-inch paper tape
One alcohol or povidone-iodine (Betadine) wipe

Description. For the *infraorbital peribulbar technique*, the lateral limbic margin is identified, and the patient is asked to look directly overhead. The lower eyelid is everted and controlled with a finger. The needle is placed bevel up just above the inferior orbital rim, lateral and parallel to the lateral limbic margin. The needle is then inserted, bevel up, through the anesthetized conjunctiva and directed toward the orbital floor until the orbital septum is penetrated. The needle is then redirected parallel to, or angled away from, the visual axis of the globe to a depth of about 25 mm (1 inch). After the syringe is secured and negative

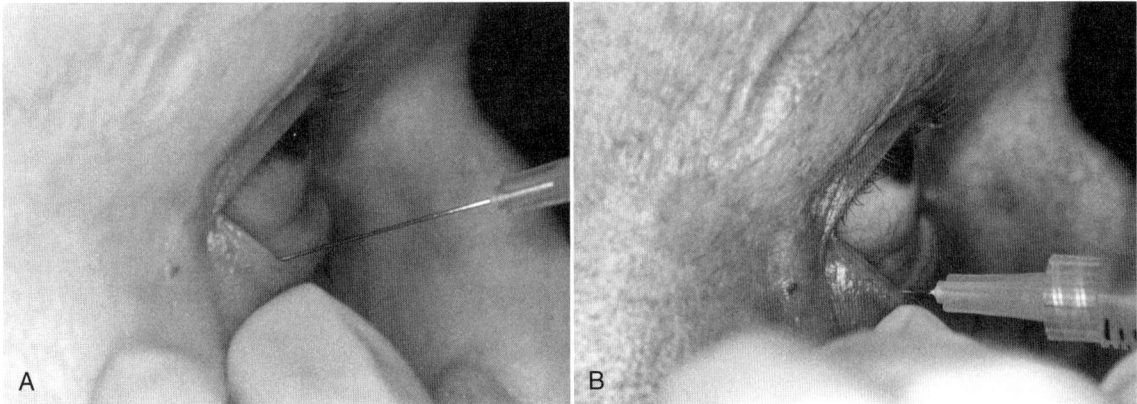

FIGURE **40-24** **A,** In the infraorbital approach, the needle is inserted transconjunctivally or transcutaneously and angled away from the visual axis of the globe toward the orbital floor to a depth of about 25 mm (1 inch), and the medications are injected. **B,** After penetration of the orbital septum, as shown in **A,** the needle is redirected parallel to the visual axis to a depth of about 25 mm (1 inch), and the medications are injected.

BOX **40-3**

Peribulbar Techniques

Infraorbital Approach
Insert the needle transconjunctivally or transcutaneously, lateral to the lateral limbic margin and angled away from the visual axis of the globe toward the orbital floor, to a depth of about 25 mm (1 inch), and inject the medications (see Figure 40-24, *A*).
OR
After penetrating the orbital septum, as described in item 1, redirect the needle parallel to the visual axis to a depth of about 25 mm (1 inch), and inject the medications (see Figure 40-24, *B*).

Supraorbital Approach
Insert the needle only transcutaneously, just inferior to the supraorbital rim, just lateral to the 12-o'clock position and superior to the globe. Angle away from the visual axis of the globe toward the orbital ceiling, to a depth of about 25 mm (1 inch), and inject the medications.
OR
After penetrating the orbital septum, as described in item 3, redirect the needle parallel to the visual axis to a depth of about 25 mm (1 inch), and inject the medications.

---

aspiration is performed, 6 mL of the anesthetic agent is slowly (1 mL/10 sec) injected. The rate of injection is determined by patient comfort. After the injection, the eyelids are closed, and positive pressure is applied for dispersal of the medication.

The *supraorbital peribulbar injection* is performed just inferior to the supraorbital rim, just lateral to the 12-o'clock position and superior to the globe. The needle is inserted bevel down through the skin. This area is generally anesthetized from the original inferotemporal injection. The needle is inserted parallel to, or angled away from, the visual axis of the globe to a depth of about 25 mm (1 inch). After negative aspiration is performed, the anesthetist may begin a slow injection of 4 to 6 mL of anesthetic solution until a tense orbital area is observed. A more tense orbit

should be expected to result from the peribulbar technique because of the increased extraconal pressure necessary to move the anesthetic intraconally.

Once this technique is completed, the eyelids are closed and taped shut. A 4 × 4 gauze pad is placed over the closed eye. A positive-pressure device is now placed over the eye to help distribute the agent throughout the orbit and achieve the desired analgesia and akinesia. The positive-pressure device also decreases intraocular pressure to an acceptable surgical level. To avoid corneal abrasion, the eyelids must completely cover the eye. It may take up to 20 minutes for satisfactory surgical anesthesia to be established from an extraconal peribulbar block. Should the peribulbar block fail to attain adequate akinesia within 10 to 20 minutes, the appropriate muscles must be reblocked by use of the inferior technique for the inferior rectus, inferior oblique, and lateral rectus muscles. The superior technique is used for the superior rectus, superior oblique, and medial rectus muscles. The supraorbital approach should not be attempted through the conjunctiva because of the potential for damage to the levator muscle of the upper eyelid; such damage may result in upper eyelid ptosis.

Medial Extraconal Peribulbar Block
Equipment List
One 3-mL syringe
One 30-gauge, ½-inch needle
Description. Figures 40-25 and 40-26 and Box 40-4 serve as valuable reference aids for medial peribulbar anesthesia.

The *medial peribulbar area* is a rather avascular fatty compartment that lies just medial to the medial rectus muscle. This area narrows significantly as it approaches the posterior surface of the globe, with the medial rectus muscle lying next to the bony orbit. Superior to the medial peribulbar area is the supranasal area. This area contains a portion of the superior ophthalmic vein and branches of the ophthalmic artery and should be avoided when ophthalmic blocks are performed.

The medial area also has herniated orifices within the connective tissue that communicate anteriorly to the posterior surface of the orbicular muscle of the eye. Therefore, the anterior spread of the anesthetic agent also provides satisfactory akinesia of the eyelids for surgery. The medial peribulbar technique can also be used with minimal discomfort to provide eyelid akinesia before a modified retrobulbar block is performed; in this case,

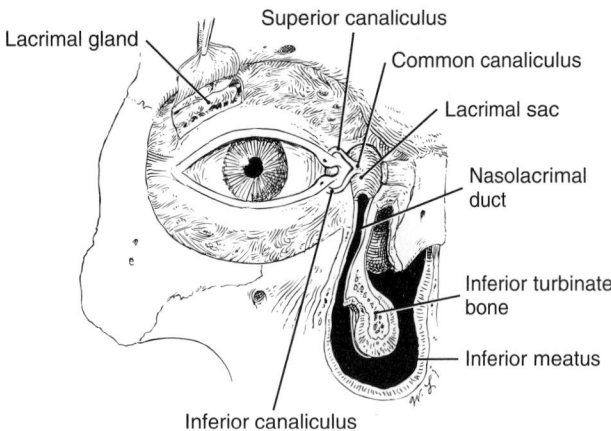

FIGURE **40-25**   Frontal view of the lacrimal drainage system.

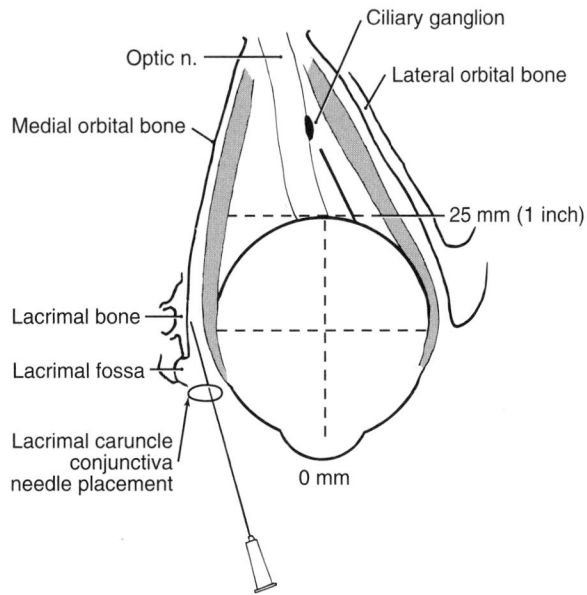

FIGURE **40-26**   Superior view of the needle angle for a medial peribulbar block. *n.*, Nerve.

BOX **40-4**

Medial Peribulbar Block

Penetrate the caruncle conjunctiva with the bevel of the needle toward the globe and the needle angled toward the lacrimal bone, to a depth of approximately 12 mm (0.5 inch), and inject the medications.

---

proparacaine drops are applied to the caruncle before the block is administered. The anesthetic agent is injected into the periorbital space that exists between the medial wall of the bony orbit and the medial rectus muscle. The technique is very effective as a secondary block both for incomplete akinesia of the medial rectus muscle and the superior oblique muscle and as a primary block for the orbicular muscles of the eyelid.

To avoid needle injuries to the medial rectus muscle, a modified insertion site, needle length, and angle may enhance the

ease of needle placement and safety. The landmark for the modified technique is the *caruncle*, a small mound at the inner canthus of the eye formed by a conjunctival fold at its junction with the skin. The needle is inserted through the caruncle conjunctiva, tangential to the globe, and is directed medially and posteriorly toward the lacrimal bone, which is just posterior to the lacrimal sulcus. Care must be taken to avoid trauma to the puncta, the lacrimal cuniculi, and the lacrimal sac. To avoid contact with the medial rectus muscle, it is important to keep the needle angled toward the lacrimal bone and away from the visual axis. Insert the needle to a depth of about 12 mm (0.5 inch). After negative aspiration is performed, 3 mL or more of anesthetic agent may be injected for facilitation of the desired effect. After the block is completed, the eyelid should be closed and light pressure applied to reduce the incidence of bleeding.

Ocular Block Evaluation

After an ophthalmic block is performed, partial movement of one or more of the ocular muscles may occur. Residual movement should be assessed to determine which muscles are involved and whether additional anesthesia is required. Analgesia of the globe generally precedes akinesia of the eye muscles. Therefore, analgesia of the globe may be assumed, but not guaranteed, in the presence of an akinetic muscle. The effectiveness of a modified retrobulbar block may be evaluated 2 minutes after it is administered (and a peribulbar block 10 to 20 minutes after it is administered) by observing for eye movement in all four quadrants.

Eyelid Block

Once satisfactory akinesia of the globe is established, evaluation for movement of the eyelids is necessary. Partial to complete akinesia of the orbicular muscle is generally found after the ocular block, especially when the medial peribulbar block is used. If incomplete akinesia occurs after an ocular block, an additional seventh nerve block may be necessary. Several seventh nerve blocks are described in the literature, including those by Van Lint, O'Brien, Nadbath, and Hustead.[40,44,45]

The O'Brien and Nadbath techniques block the seventh cranial nerve proximally, resulting in unilateral facial paralysis. The O'Brien and Nadbath techniques are still used; however, their popularity is decreasing because of their systemic side effects and patient discomfort. The Van Lint technique more appropriately addresses the need for eyelid akinesia, with less potential for adverse effects, by blocking the temporal and zygomatic branches of the facial nerve to the orbicular muscles. However, it is very painful. A variation of these techniques may be used for *orbicularis oculi block*. This technique has the advantage of being safer, less painful, and better accepted by the awake patient than the Van Lint block, but it requires injections through the skin and has the potential for causing patient discomfort and eyelid ecchymosis. The preferred technique for eyelid akinesia remains the medial peribulbar block.

Orbicularis Oculi Block
Equipment List
One 6-mL syringe
One 30-gauge, ½-inch needle
One alcohol wipe
Description. Figure 40-27 and Box 40-5 serve as valuable reference aids for the orbicularis oculi block.

This technique is performed after a modified retrobulbar or peribulbar block in which residual eyelid movement remains. The first injection is made inferotemporally in the lower eyelid.

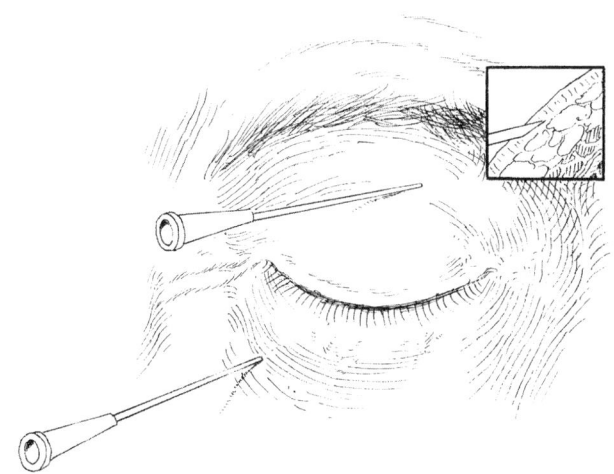

FIGURE **40-27** Frontal view of the needle placement for an orbicularis oculi block.

BOX **40-5**

Orbicularis Oculi Block

Lower Lid: Insert the needle subcutaneously, bevel down and tangential to the lid in the infratemporal area, and inject the medications.

Upper Lid: While slightly depressing the globe, insert the needle subcutaneously, bevel down and tangential to the lid in the supranasal area, and inject the medications.

The needle is inserted bevel down, subcutaneously and tangentially to the lower eyelid, and 1 to 2 mL of the anesthetic agent is injected just under the skin of the eyelid. After the needle is removed, the local anesthesia should be digitally spread to the medial and the lateral canthi; this measure avoids running the needle across the lower eyelid. The second injection is made supranasally in the upper eyelid. A finger should be placed over the closed eyelid, slightly depressing the globe. The needle is again inserted, bevel down, subcutaneously and tangentially to the eyelid, and 1 to 2 mL of the agent is injected just under the skin of the eyelid. After the needle is removed, the local anesthetic is digitally spread to the medial and lateral canthi. Once the anesthetic is spread throughout the eyelids, light to moderate pressure is applied over the eyelids for prevention or reduction of superficial bleeding.

Van Lint Technique

Equipment List

One 6-mL syringe

One 25- or 27-gauge, 1.5-inch needle

One alcohol or povidone-iodine wipe

One 4 × 4 gauze pad

Description. A 37.5-mm (1.5-inch) needle is inserted inferotemporally into the subcutaneous tissue of the lateral canthus. The first injection of 1 to 2 mL of anesthetic agent is directed nasally along the lower margin of the orbit and then withdrawn to its origination point. The second injection of 1 to 2 mL of anesthetic agent is directed upward along the supratemporal margin of the orbit. After the block is completed, light pressure is applied over the closed eyelids to disperse the medication and decrease ecchymosis.

POSITIVE ORBITAL PRESSURE

The increased volume of local anesthetic required for both modified retrobulbar and peribulbar anesthetics causes an increase in orbital and intraocular pressures. The anesthetic agent not only tracks along and penetrates the fascial sheaths behind the globe, it also moves anteriorly underneath the conjunctiva, producing chemosis (subconjunctival edema) of the eye. These events may make the surgical procedure more difficult to perform. However, the random diffusion of the orbital anesthetic cannot be controlled. The agent merely tracks along the path of least resistance. Clinically, chemosis can begin with the injection of as little as 1 to 2 mL of anesthetic. In other instances, chemosis has not been seen even after the injection of as much as 12 mL of anesthetic agent.

Positive-pressure devices are used to reduce increased intraocular/intraorbital pressures and chemosis. Such devices are placed directly over the globe and orbit to enhance the orbital spread of anesthetic agent and return the orbital anatomy to a softer, more normal state for surgery. Positive-pressure devices deepen the anterior chamber by further reducing the intraocular pressure, thus allowing greater room for surgical intervention.

Positive-Pressure Device

Honan Intraocular Pressure Reducer

The Honan Intraocular Pressure Reducer, or Honan balloon, is an inflatable pneumatic device used to apply ocular compression after retrobulbar or peribulbar anesthetic injection. A rubber head strap is placed behind the head. The eye is taped closed, and a folded 4 × 4 gauze pad is placed over the eye. The Honan cuff is placed over the gauze pad and secured with the Velcro head strap. The pressure gauge is inflated to 30 mm Hg, a value marked in yellow on the gauge.

ANESTHESIA MANAGEMENT

Preoperative Preparation

Ophthalmic procedures are most commonly performed on young children and elderly persons. Each age group has a unique set of physical problems. For the young child, the questions regarding the patient's history should include any congenital, metabolic, and musculoskeletal abnormalities, such as malignant hyperthermia, that may affect anesthesia care. In the elderly patient, multisystem medical problems may be present, and drug interactions from multiple medication regimens may exist. A thorough patient history is therefore paramount.

Admissions on the Day of Surgery

Anesthesia practitioners must not forget how stressful a surgical procedure on the eye can be for patients. A kind and professional attitude on the part of all those providing care will help patients deal more effectively with personal stress. The proper use of progressive relaxation and hypnotic techniques further helps alleviate their anxiety. Establishing a good patient-provider relationship works synergistically with pharmacologic agents in promoting the best possible surgical environment. On admission, the patient's mental and physical status, vital signs, and ECG should be reviewed for any changes that may require postponement.

Regional versus General Anesthesia

Patients undergoing regional block, in which they are awake for the procedure, must be evaluated for claustrophobia, severe arthritis, tremors, and any other physical derangements that

---

BOX **40-6**

Indications for General Anesthesia

Pediatric patient
Patient's lack of cooperation
Severe claustrophobia
Inability to communicate
Inability to lie flat
Open-eye injuries
Procedures with durations greater than 2 hours

BOX **40-7**

Disadvantages of General Anesthesia

Nausea/vomiting
Retching/bucking
Increased intraocular pressure
Aspiration
Complications secondary to other medical problems
  (e.g., cardiovascular disease)
Time and expense

---

may make it difficult for them to lie supine. Patients' mental status must also be evaluated so that their degree of cooperation and ability to follow commands can be determined.

Elderly patients often take multiple medications and may not remember all of them. Patients should be instructed to bring their medications to the surgery center the day of surgery. A preoperative visit to the primary care physician is advised to confirm that the patient's overall medical condition is optimized for the planned surgical procedure.

The attending surgeon, in collaboration with the anesthesia practitioner, will make the final evaluation as to the patient's fitness on the day of surgery. An electrocardiogram (ECG) performed within the past year should augment medical evaluation. The preoperative ECG assessment furnishes a baseline of what is optimal for the individual patient. Comparing the baseline ECG against the patient's ECG on the day of surgery helps determine whether any further preoperative testing is warranted.[46] For patients receiving regional anesthesia, routine laboratory tests are not ordered unless they are medically necessary.[47] *Appropriate laboratory data are necessary when general anesthesia is planned.*[48]

After the patient history and physical examination are completed, the anesthetist can formulate the appropriate anesthesia plan. General anesthesia should be used for infants and young children. General anesthesia is also indicated for patients with severe claustrophobia, a history of uncontrolled acute anxiety attacks, or inability to cooperate, communicate, or lie flat (Box 40-6). It is also a consideration for procedures of greater than 2 hours' duration.[49] Most adults tolerate ophthalmic procedures well when regional anesthesia is used. Given the potential risks associated with general anesthesia (Box 40-7), regional anesthesia should be considered the anesthetic of choice in ophthalmic procedures.

Regional Anesthesia
Regional Block with Minimal Sedation

Nothing-per-Mouth (NPO) Status. The views of anesthesia practitioners vary on the advisability of NPO status prior to ocular procedures, especially cataracts. Some practices allow patients undergoing surgery in the morning to eat a light breakfast the day of surgery. Those undergoing surgery in the afternoon may be told to eat a light lunch. Patients may also be encouraged to consume clear fluids until they are admitted to the facility.[50-52] However, practitioners may also mandate a strict NPO protocol.

Patients are requested to take their medications as usual on the day of surgery. An exception may be patients who complain of a frequent need to urinate after taking diuretic medications. Antiglycemic agents may be reduced or held when patients are NPO. Antiplatelet drugs (e.g., aspirin, Clopidogrel) and anticoagulants (e.g., warfarin, [Coumadin]) are not mandatory to discontinue. Retrospective studies have shown no increase in hemorrhagic complications either operatively or postoperatively when these drugs were taken.[53-55] In addition, the risk of systemic complications, such as cardiovascular accidents and myocardial infarctions, is potentially greater if administration of these products is discontinued. Continuing anticoagulant administration, however, requires consultation and agreement between the anesthesia practitioner and the surgeon. If bleeding occurs, it may be more severe; therefore, patients also need to be made aware of the risk and benefits of continuing their anticoagulants. Patients who are receiving or have previously been treated with chemotherapy may also have prolonged bleeding times.

Regional Block Environment
Ocular blocks are commonly performed outside the operating room. This method facilitates a more efficient case flow and a more comfortable environment for the patient. The potentially life-threatening effects of orbital epidural blocks require that appropriate resuscitative equipment and trained personnel are available to monitor the patient. The area used for performing ocular blocks should have the following:

Oxygen
Bag-valve mask
Suction
Airways
ECG equipment
Blood pressure cuff
Oxygen saturation monitor
Intravenous access tubing
Canthotomy set
Ammonia capsules
Nitroglycerin tablets
Atropine
Glycopyrrolate

Additional resuscitative equipment and medications as recommended by advanced cardiac life support guidelines should be available.

Sedation for Regional Blocks and Ophthalmic Procedures
The goal of conscious sedation is to help patients gain and maintain control by reducing their heightened state of anxiety. This enhances their cooperation and ability to tolerate the awake surgical procedure.

Many techniques have been advocated to relax the patient prior to the ocular block and during the surgical procedure.[56,57] Conscious sedation techniques have included the use of benzodiazepines, narcotics, barbiturates, and nonbarbiturates. When

---
BOX **40-8**

Sedation Techniques

Good rapport between patient and clinician—minimizes
 medications necessary
Intravenous benzodiazepine administration
Intravenous narcotic administration
Intravenous barbiturate or nonbarbiturate (propofol or
 narcotic) administration

BOX **40-9**

Causes of Discomfort Resulting from Regional Blocks

Needle injection through the skin
Needle penetration of the conjunctiva
Needle penetration of the intermuscular membrane
Rapid injection of anesthetic
Stinging from peripheral spread of anesthetic

BOX **40-10**

Procedure for Patient Who Is Asleep During
Regional Block

Tilt head to maintain patent airway
Open patient's eye in primary gaze position
Administer regional block
Administer incremental sedation as required

---

these medications are properly tailored by the anesthesia practitioner, they are tolerated well by the elderly patient. Sedation techniques should be designed to decrease anxiety (Box 40-8) and reduce the discomfort of the block (Box 40-9). When the block is less painful, patients require less sedation for comfort. The surgeon's preference for an awake, relaxed, or sleeping patient during the procedure should also be considered. Sleeping patients often snore and may have sudden head movements on awakening.

If the patient is to be asleep during the block, fasting before the procedure consistent with the facility's criteria for general anesthesia should be followed (Box 40-10). Propofol is an excellent choice for this technique because of its short duration of action.[58]

Sedation is typically effective and safe for ocular blocks and intraoperative use but necessitates provider vigilance and monitoring to recognize and treat any of the adverse medical events that may occur.[59]

Monitoring for Regional Anesthesia

Communication is the cornerstone of dealing with the patient who is awake. Informing the patient what to expect and what to do if he or she experiences any problems is mandatory. Questions and instructions must be clear and specific, especially if the patient is hearing impaired or if a language barrier exists.

The positioning of the patient is very important. Pillows may be used under the knees to decrease back strain. The patient with severe arthritis must be carefully padded and positioned. The patient's head and neck should be placed in a satisfactory surgical position. The practitioner should ensure that the patient is warm and as comfortable as possible. Nasally administered oxygen is recommended. Monitoring equipment should consist of electrocardiograph, blood pressure, and oxygen saturation monitor. Observing the surgical procedure on a television monitor is preferable to not seeing the surgery. This allows the anesthetist to follow the surgical progress and visualize critical points in the procedure at which patient movement would be most detrimental.

The surgical draping placed over the patient's face should be tented, and high-flow air may be used to decrease expired carbon dioxide. Claustrophobia can be a problem for awake patients, and some patients experience it for the first time during this procedure. Techniques for dealing with claustrophobia include taping the nonsurgical eye or adjusting the drape so that the patient can see the room with the nonsurgical eye. If a patient experiences a claustrophobic attack, the surgical drapes should be tented away from the face immediately, while the sterile field is maintained, and verbal control of the patient is gained. At this point, the anesthetist must determine whether the patient can proceed with surgery under regional block. Rarely, the patient may experience incomplete ocular analgesia, even in the presence of muscle akinesia. This problem responds well to tetracaine or proparacaine drops or subconjunctival anesthetic injection.

Acute increased intraocular pressure during the surgical procedure can be catastrophic and cause loss of ocular contents. This problem can be created by coughing or a choroidal hemorrhage. The increased intrathoracic pressure created during coughing is reflected through the valveless orbital veins, resulting in an acutely increased intraocular pressure of 40 mm Hg or greater.[12] A choroidal hemorrhage occurs when a vessel in the vascular choroidal layer of the eye ruptures, bleeding into the closed cavity and creating an acute rise in intraocular pressure with potential expulsion of eye contents unless the eye is closed quickly. In the acute phase, medications that lower intraocular pressure may be of minimum benefit.

If the patient has a history of postnasal drip, vasoconstrictive nose drops may be given preoperatively. If the patient complains of a dry throat, small amounts of water may be given. These two remedies are helpful in reducing the incidence of coughing intraoperatively. The patient must also be instructed to give notice before he or she coughs. Instructing the patient to clear his or her throat effectively reduces the forcefulness of the cough. Quick, shallow breaths have been reported to help suppress the cough reflex.[60] Sedating the patient or using intravenous lidocaine to prevent further coughing can help but has minimal effect during an active coughing episode.[61]

After the surgery is completed, the patient is transported from the operating room to postanesthesia recovery (PAR). Postoperative recovery time should be in accordance with the individual patient's physical and mental status and the amount of medication administered.

Postoperative nausea noted immediately after surgery may result from the sedative medications, increased intraocular pressure, or ocular pain.[62,63] On the afternoon or evening after their surgery, patients are generally called at home for evaluation of their status. A sudden onset of nausea at home after the procedure is more likely associated with increased intraocular pressure than anesthetic medications. Patients are usually examined the following day by the surgeon and are requested to fill out questionnaires regarding their experience on the day of surgery.

General Anesthesia

For general anesthesia, preoperative patient preparation should include the appropriate fasting guidelines for the patient's age and physical condition (e.g., diabetes). The patient should be reminded that the surgical eye will be patched when he or she awakens. Sedation should be administered as needed to help the patient relax. Benzodiazepines such as midazolam are effective in low doses. For reduction in the incidence of postoperative nausea, the use of 5-HT3-receptor antagonists, histamine-2 antagonists, metoclopramide, and other antiemetics should be considered. Induction of general anesthesia with propofol or any of the intravenous barbiturates or nonbarbiturates is recommended because they all decrease intraocular pressure. In infants and children, inhalation induction also decreases intraocular pressure. Because of their emetic effect, narcotics should be used in low doses. Other than during examinations under anesthesia, endotracheal intubation is indicated for maintenance of the airway.

Succinylcholine causes a transient increase in intraocular pressure; however, it can be used safely for ocular procedures. Some caveats include:

1. The sustained contracture of the extraocular muscles after succinylcholine could cause an expulsion of the intraocular contents. This assumption is theoretical and it is now felt that succinylcholine may be safely used in eye surgery. See full discussion below.
2. In eye muscle surgery, the sustained contraction may interfere with the forced duction test used by the surgeon for the treatment plan.
3. Patients taking long-acting glaucoma medications, such as echothiophate, may have prolonged apnea.

Nondepolarizing muscle relaxants are also satisfactory for induction and have the advantage of decreasing intraocular pressure.[64] Laryngoscopy, especially with light anesthesia, increases intraocular pressure, but intravenous lidocaine (1.5 to 2 mg/kg), given 1 to 1.5 minutes before laryngoscopy, helps attenuate this response. Inhalation anesthetics, which also decrease intraocular pressure, are commonly used for the maintenance of general anesthesia.

For intraocular procedures, the continued use of nondepolarizing muscle relaxants is recommended for the maintenance of an akinetic eye and a satisfactory intraocular pressure. The anesthetist must be aware of the adverse ECG changes that may result from the oculocardiac reflex, which may be elicited when traction is exerted on the extraocular muscles and orbital structures. Patients undergoing eye-muscle surgery have an increased incidence of malignant hyperthermia and postoperative nausea. In retinal procedures in which sulfur hexafluoride or perfluoropropane is used as an intraocular gas, the use of nitrous oxide should be discontinued 15 minutes before injection.

When spontaneous ventilation returns after neuromuscular blockade is reversed, the patient may be extubated while receiving deep anesthesia with 100% oxygen and placed in the lateral position until he or she awakens. In the patient with a difficult airway, full stomach, or incompetent esophageal sphincter, gastric suction and intravenous lidocaine (1.5 to 2 mg/kg) may be given before the patient is extubated awake. This method helps reduce the incidence of coughing and vomiting, along with their deleterious effects.

Postoperative care, with attention paid to the alleviation of pain and control of nausea, will help maintain a satisfactory intraocular pressure. The ophthalmologist should be made aware of continued postoperative nausea, because it may be the result of acute increased intraocular pressure.[62,63]

Open-Eye Injury and the Use of Succinylcholine

Traumatic eye injuries can be categorized as either open- or closed-globe injuries. Open-eye injury in a patient with a full stomach is at best a difficult situation for the anesthesia provider. These injuries are commonly considered emergencies requiring general anesthesia. The clinician must protect the patient from aspiration and yet avoid increased intraocular pressure that could result in expulsion of intraocular contents. Authors have traditionally debated the risks and advantages of using succinylcholine for this procedure.[65,66] Normal intraocular pressure (IOP) is 10 to 22 mm Hg, with slight diurnal and positional changes of 1 to 6 mm Hg. It is physiologically determined by aqueous humor dynamics, changes in choroidal blood volume, central venous pressure, and extraocular muscle tone. The most important determinant of IOP is the balance between production and elimination of aqueous humor, maintaining an average volume of 250 mL. Aqueous humor is formed in the ciliary process from capillaries by diffusion, filtration, and active secretion. It flows through the posterior chamber, around the iris, and into the anterior chamber. It is eliminated through the spaces of Fontana and canal of Schlemm at the iridocorneal angle, where it flows into the episcleral venous system. Any increase in venous pressure (e.g., cough, strain, head-down position) will increase IOP. Additionally, any decrease in cross-sectional area of the spaces of Fontana (e.g., mydriatic drugs) will increase IOP.[67-71] Administration of succinylcholine increases IOP within 1 minute and peaks at an increase of 9 mm Hg within 6 minutes after succinylcholine administration. The exact mechanism of this increase is unknown. Some feel that tonic contractions of the extraocular muscles may explain this IOP increase. It is now thought, however, that succinylcholine-induced IOP increase is a vascular event, with choroidal vascular dilatation or a decrease in drainage secondary to elevated central venous pressure, temporarily inhibiting the flow of aqueous humor through the canal of Schlemm.[68]

It is clear that succinylcholine raises IOP. However, at induction of general anesthesia, there are many activities that raise IOP to a much greater degree than succinylcholine, including crying, Valsalva, forceful blinking, rubbing of the eyes, and coughing or bucking during poor intubating technique. Therefore, the increase in IOP due to succinylcholine may be inconsequential if optimal intubating conditions are not provided.

Moreno wrote: "This observation, coupled with the lack of any documented cases of extrusion of intraocular contents in open globes of humans when succinylcholine is used, causes us to question the traditional teaching that succinylcholine should be avoided in all cases when open globe is suspected or known."[67]

Chidiac and Raiskin have stated that two questions need to be asked before the decision about the use or avoidance of succinylcholine in open-globe surgeries is made: Is this an easy airway; and Is the eye viable?[68] If the airway assessment shows that intubation should be easy, then regardless of the patient's aspiration risk, and regardless of the viability of the eye, succinylcholine can be avoided and replaced with rocuronium. If the airway assessment shows that this could be a difficult intubation, regardless of the patient's aspiration risk, then the second question becomes important: Is the eye viable? If the ophthalmologist feels that the eye is viable, use of succinylcholine is recommended. Pretreatment with drugs that attenuate the intraocular pressure effect of succinylcholine, such as a small dose of nondepolarizing agent and lidocaine, should be used.

Choosing or avoiding succinylcholine is a matter of balance of risk. To control IOP at induction, there must be adequate dosing of drugs timed appropriately to coincide with the three potent stimuli: the administration of succinylcholine, the laryngoscopy, and the endotracheal intubation. It is clear that succinylcholine increases IOP, but this increase can be attenuated with various pretreatments, is less than increases seen with inadequate paralysis at the time of laryngoscopy and intubation, and is unimportant when weighed against the risk of loss of the airway. Therefore, in the situation of "difficult airway, eye viable," one should use succinylcholine.

Closed-globe injuries require significant planning and preparation to prevent further damage to the eye by an increase in IOP. They also require smooth induction and emergence because patient coughing or bucking will cause a detrimental increase in IOP.[69]

OPHTHALMIC ANESTHESIA COMPLICATIONS

Anxiety coupled with underlying cardiovascular disease may promote marked hypertension, cardiac dysrhythmias, or angina in the patient before surgery. Vasovagal responses (e.g., fainting) secondary to anxiety are not unusual. Ammonia capsules are effective in preventing and treating fainting episodes.

Chronic coughing secondary to chronic obstructive pulmonary disease, asthma, or postnasal drip must be evaluated. Vasoconstrictive nose drops effectively decrease postnasal drip. Coughing and deep breathing before surgery help clear the lungs of excess mucus in patients with chronic pulmonary disease. Proper evaluation and treatment help reduce undesired perioperative systemic and ocular sequelae.

Most complications of regional ocular anesthetics can be attributed to direct traumatization of the orbital vessels, the globe, and the optic nerve. Trauma to these structures can result whenever a needle is placed near the eye. Frequently, the cause of complications during general anesthesia is patient movement.

Retrobulbar Hemorrhage

Retrobulbar hemorrhage results from trauma to an orbital vessel. The retrobulbar bleeding moves the eyeball forward (proptosis), and a subconjunctival hemorrhage is usually present. Venous hemorrhages are typically slow in onset, but arterial hemorrhage has a rapid onset and more pronounced proptosis and subconjunctival hemorrhage. Ecchymosis of the eyelids and orbit is usually present. The pressure caused by the bleeding in the bony orbital cavity produces increased orbital pressure on the optic nerve, vessels, and globe. This pressure usually resolves without problems but may result in an occlusion or spasm of the central retinal artery or vein, resulting in partial to complete loss of vision.[72] One may detect a progressively increasing orbital pressure when digital pressure is applied over the eye after an ocular block. Continuous digital pressure may be all that is required for stopping a venous hemorrhage.[33] If the orbital pressure continues to increase in the presence of digital pressure, a lateral canthotomy should be performed immediately, and the ophthalmologist should be notified. *Canthotomy* is a procedure performed to increase the orbital space by cutting the lateral canthus. This procedure reduces the orbital pressure that results from a retrobulbar hemorrhage.

Anesthesia practitioners who perform ocular blocks should consider being instructed in the performance of a canthotomy, and a canthotomy set should be readily available (Box 40-11). The ophthalmologist should examine the central retinal artery and vein for patency. Occlusion of these vessels may warrant

---

BOX 40-11

Canthotomy Procedure

Equipment
1 straight hemostat
1 plastic scissors

Procedure
If possible, inject lidocaine along the lateral canthus.
Place the hemostat in a temporal direction along the lateral canthus 4-6 mm, and clamp the hemostat.
Remove the hemostat.
Use the plastic scissors to incise only in the crush marks left by the hemostat.
Control local bleeding with the hemostat or with digital pressure.

BOX 40-12

Measures for Preventing Retrobulbar Hemorrhage

Choose least vascular areas for needle placement
Avoid deep orbital injections
Avoid supranasal position of gaze
Use primary gaze position
Use upward-gaze position (Gills-Lloyd technique only)
Insert needle slowly

---

further surgical intervention for reduction of elevated orbital pressure.

A localized episcleral hemorrhage also causes subconjunctival bleeding. In this situation, however, no proptosis of the globe or increase in orbital pressure is noted. These episcleral vessels are the same ones the ophthalmologist cauterizes after a conjunctival incision. The vessels break as a result of the spread of local anesthesia through the subconjunctival area and are of no consequence. However, the ophthalmologist should be notified of their presence before the procedure begins.

Retrobulbar hemorrhage remains the most common sequela for ocular blocks (Box 40-12). Peribulbar injections can also cause orbital hemorrhages.[42] Retrobulbar hemorrhages have been reported to occur in 1% to 3% of cases.[73]

Intravascular Injection

Grand mal seizures have been reported to occur after retrobulbar injections with lidocaine and lidocaine-bupivacaine combinations.[74,75] Seizures may result from a less-than-toxic dose of local anesthesia by direct intraarterial injection, resulting in retrograde flow to the cerebral circulation (Box 40-13). Mathers[76] surveyed 200 ophthalmologists. Sixty-six responded and reported three seizures occurring after retrobulbar injections. From these data, it appears that seizures after retrobulbar anesthesia may occur more frequently than reported in the literature. A reaction after an orbital vein injection has also been reported: the patient experienced uncontrolled shivering and rigor approximately 15 seconds after the retrobulbar injection. These symptoms resolved within 2 minutes of onset.[77]

BOX 40-13

Measures for Preventing Seizures Resulting from Intravascular Injection

Choose least vascular areas for needle placement
Avoid deep orbital injections
Avoid supranasal position of gaze
Insert needle slowly
Aspirate gently before injection; negative aspiration is no guarantee that you are not in a blood vessel.
Avoid injection against resistance
Avoid forceful rapid injections

BOX 40-14

Measures for Preventing Globe Puncture

Use caution in patients with increased axial length
Avoid supranasal position of gaze
Direct needle away from axis of globe during insertion through the orbital septum
Observe globe movement with needle insertion
Insert needle slowly
Never forcefully inject anesthetic
Use modified retrobulbar and peribulbar techniques (although globe punctures have also been reported with these)

BOX 40-15

Signs and Symptoms of Globe Puncture*

Increased resistance to injection
Immediate dilation and paralysis of the pupil
Rapid increase in intraocular pressure with edematous cornea
Subconjunctival hemorrhage
Pain and agitation
Hypotony of the globe
Intraocular hemorrhage

Patient may or may not exhibit signs and symptoms of a puncture immediately.

---

confirmed a lack of safety with the use of blunt needles. The investigators quoted multiple authors who reported optic nerve penetration, ocular perforation, and CNS complications resulting from the use of blunt needles. The surgeon should be notified if a globe puncture is suspected (Box 40-15).

Optic Nerve Sheath Trauma

To review, the *optic nerve sheaths* surround the optic nerve and are composed of the meninges of the brain. The outer sheath contains the *dura mater* and the inner sheath consists of the *arachnoid mater* and *pia mater*. The subarachnoid space contains cerebrospinal fluid and is continuous with the optic chiasm. The dura splits into two layers at the optic foramen. The outer dural layer becomes continuous with the orbital periosteum. The inner layer forms the dural covering of the optic nerve, creating the orbital epidural space.[1] Anesthetic agents injected into the subdural or subarachnoid space may track back to the optic chiasm. Here, the anesthetic can affect the contralateral eye by blocking cranial nerves II and III as they proceed through the subdural or subarachnoid space; this block can result in contralateral amaurosis.[84-86] The condition can be a precursor to the continued migration of the anesthetic to the respiratory centers of the midbrain, resulting in respiratory arrest.[72,87,88]

The anesthetist should observe the contralateral pupil before an ocular block is performed. The pupil may be dilated from accidental administration of preoperative eye drops, a preoperative examination, or existing pathology. If the contralateral pupil is constricted before the ocular block and dilates after the ocular block (contralateral amaurosis), one must assume that subarachnoid or subdural injection has occurred and be prepared to treat a respiratory arrest.

The onset of *respiratory arrest* is usually within 2 to 5 minutes after injection; however, it may occur as late as 10 to 17 minutes after injection. Spontaneous ventilation usually returns in 15 to 20 minutes but may take up to 55 minutes for complete recovery. Treatment includes appropriate ventilatory and cardiovascular support, supplemental oxygen with oxygen saturation monitoring, ECG monitoring for cardiac dysrhythmias, and blood pressure monitoring. The surgeon should be notified immediately so the eye can be examined for any optic-nerve trauma that may require surgical intervention.

A retrobulbar hemorrhage resulting in increased extravascular pressure may result in occlusion of the central retinal artery or vein, or both. Also, direct trauma to the ophthalmic artery or the optic nerve by the retrobulbar needle may cause artery or vein occlusion without causing retrobulbar hemorrhage[89] (Box 40-16).

Globe Puncture

Multiple reports have been published regarding globe perforations. Both sharp and dull needles have either penetrated or perforated the eye during retrobulbar and peribulbar injections. Although rare, globe punctures have occurred in the hands of experienced practitioners who have performed many thousands of ophthalmic blocks. The literature also notes that patients may or may not exhibit signs and symptoms of a puncture immediately, and the diagnosis has been made anywhere from 1 to 14 days after the event.[34,78-81] The most devastating globe injury reported, fortunately rare, is an ocular explosion. The globe can literally burst apart from the intraocular pressure exerted by the local anesthesia injection.[82-83]

The myopic eye has an increased axial length of greater than 24 mm. Scleral thinning may result from this increased anteroposterior diameter. A previous scleral buckling procedure also increases the anteroposterior diameter of the eye. *Staphyloma*, a bulging of the sclera, may also predispose the patient to globe puncture. The risk of puncture increases when this abnormality is located inferoposteriorly on the globe. *Enophthalmos* is a recession of the eyeball into the orbit. This condition decreases the distance between the posterior pole of the globe and the posterior orbital wall. The supranasal gaze position rotates the posterior pole of the globe in line and closer to the retrobulbar needle path. Multiple orbital injections have also been cited as a factor in globe punctures, along with unexpected patient movement (Box 40-14).

The choice of sharp versus dull retrobulbar needles is highly debated. The literature reviewed appears to draw conclusions based more on opinion than on fact. In 1991 Grizzard and colleagues[34] published a detailed review of the literature; this review

Ocular Ischemia

Retinal vascular occlusion or thrombosis has been reported after ocular blocks.[90,91] Studies have also discovered a decrease in the pulsatile ocular blood flow after ocular blocks, secondary to the pressure exerted by the volume of local anesthesia injected into the orbit. However, the same orbital injection volume did not cause a significant rise in the intraocular pressure. Even though not contraindicated, caution should be exercised in patients with preexisting compromised ocular circulation.[92-95] Some authors have advocated not using epinephrine in the local anesthetic solution.[96,97]

Optic nerve atrophy has been reported after intraocular surgery with either *regional block or general anesthesia.*[72] Direct trauma to the optic nerve may result in transient symptoms, such as contralateral amaurosis or respiratory arrest, or it may result in vascular occlusion or thrombosis, or both, with partial to complete loss of vision.

Extraocular Muscle Palsy and Ptosis

Inferior muscle palsy has been reported after retrobulbar anesthesia. Segmental inferior rectus muscle enlargement was noted posterior to the globe deep in the orbit.[98] The complication has not been reported to occur after general anesthesia.[99] The initial signs and symptoms of this problem manifest after surgery as persistent vertical diplopia. Surgical intervention is indicated for correction of this condition. Trauma to the superior oblique tendon–trochlea complex has also been reported to occur with peribulbar anesthesia[100] (Box 40-17).

Carlson and colleagues performed experiments on the rectus muscle of monkeys and humans and demonstrated minimal myotoxic damage to ocular muscles after retrobulbar administration of local anesthetics. Typically after the injection of local anesthesia, the surface muscle fibers degenerate, then regenerate. However, direct injections of local anesthesia into the rectus muscle resulted in massive internal muscle lesions that were large enough to produce noticeable functional deficit. The myotoxicity of local anesthetics may also play a role in postoperative ptosis, especially in the elderly, because regeneration of their muscle fibers may not be as complete as that in younger patients.[101] However, ptosis is also associated with the superior rectus stay suture and the eyelid speculum. Postoperative ptosis may take as long as 6 months to resolve.

Facial Nerve Blocks

Patients commonly experience discomfort as a result of seventh nerve blocks. Prolonged Bell's palsy has been seen after Nadbath and O'Brien blocks, probably secondary to direct nerve trauma.[102] Several authors have reported cases of dysphagia,

blocks (Box 40-18). They noted that these symptoms were consistent with paresis of the vagus, glossopharyngeal, and spinal accessory nerves. These nerves exit the skull about 10 mm medial to cranial nerve VII. Therefore, anesthesia injected for the seventh nerve block could also reach these nerves and result in unilateral vocal cord paralysis.[103,104]

Patients have also complained of jaw ache with movement for several weeks after the seventh nerve block. Grand mal seizure has rarely occurred (1 report) when 3 mL of 2% lidocaine with epinephrine (1:200,000) was injected using the Nadbath technique.

Zaturansky and Hyams reported an ocular perforation that occurred when a modified Van Lint procedure was performed after a retrobulbar block. The needle penetrated the proposed eye just under the insertion of the lateral rectus muscle.[105]

Oculocardiac Reflex

The *oculocardiac reflex* is a trigeminal-vagal reflex that was first described in 1908 by Aschner. The stimulus for this reflex is generated by pressure on the globe, the orbital structures (e.g., the optic nerve), or the conjunctiva, or by traction on the extraocular muscles (particularly the medial rectus muscle). The afferent pathway for the stimulus is via the long and short ciliary nerves to the ciliary ganglion and then through the gasserian ganglion along the ophthalmic division of the trigeminal nerve terminating in the main trigeminal sensory nucleus in the floor of the fourth ventricle. The efferent pathway consists of the vagus nerve to the cardioinhibitory center.

The reflex may be elicited during local infiltration anesthesia, retrobulbar or peribulbar blockade, and general anesthesia. The occurrence of the reflex in ocular procedures is variable, but it is commonly seen in muscle procedures performed in children. The oculocardiac reflex reveals itself most often as an acute sinus bradycardia. However, it may also cause a wide variety of other cardiac dysrhythmias, such as nodal rhythms, atrioventricular block, ventricular ectopy, idioventricular rhythm, and asystole. Continuous ECG monitoring is essential for the diagnosis of dysrhythmias that result from the oculocardiac reflex. If cardiac dysrhythmias are observed, the surgeon must be instructed to immediately cease all pressure or traction on the orbit. Simultaneously, the patient should be assessed for adequate oxygenation and ventilation and for adequate anesthetic depth because one or more of these may be an underlying cause for the dysrhythmia. The aberrant rhythm usually resolves without intervention within a few seconds. However, if the aforementioned measures are taken and the dysrhythmia continues, thus threatening to cause hemodynamic instability, intravenous atropine should be administered. Atropine, 2 to 3 mg, may be required for complete vagal blockade. Caution should be exercised with the administration of atropine, because atropine itself may induce cardiac dysrhythmias. The surgeon may proceed only after the dysrhythmia is resolved. If the reflex recurs, the aforementioned process should be repeated. The oculocardiac reflex, however, appears to fatigue with continued manipulations. The use of intravenous atropine or intravenous glycopyrrolate just before surgery may help reduce the incidence of the reflex, especially in children.[106,107]

Other Complications

Corneal abrasion is the most common injury occurring after general anesthesia. It is believed to result from the drying of the exposed cornea or from direct trauma, such as an anesthesia-mask injury. Ensuring that the eyelids are closed and secured with tape should provide satisfactory protection of the cornea. *Movement during ocular surgery was identified as the single most common mechanism of injury.* Movement was described as coughing and bucking, which resulted in poor visual outcome. In these reported cases, muscle relaxants were used less than 50% of the time, and nerve stimulators were omitted. Chemical injury can result from spillage of cleaning materials or preparatory solutions into the eye. In these cases, the eye should be flushed immediately with saline.[108]

Central retinal artery occlusion may result from prolonged pressure on the eye.[109] This type of injury may result with the patient in the prone position. Careful attention to padding and periodic checks of the eyes are necessary, especially for long procedures. Eye protectors, along with foam headrests or gel donuts for the face, may help prevent eye trauma. It is prudent to request an ophthalmic examination immediately after surgery if the patient complains of any eye problems or if the anesthesia provider suspects a problem.

SUMMARY

Anesthesia management for ophthalmic procedures has changed rapidly in the last few years. Surgical procedures have improved, and many ophthalmologists are using simple local anesthesia. Some are predicting that treatments such as cataract repair will become totally office-based procedures not requiring the participation of an anesthesia provider. Anesthesia for more complex surgery or as a result of ocular trauma will continue to occupy an important place in clinical practice.

REFERENCES

1. Marieb EN, Hoehn K. The eye and vision. In: *Human Anatomy and Physiology.* 7th ed. San Francisco: Pearson, Benjamin Cummings; 2007.
2. Vaughn D, Asbury T: *General Ophthalmology.* 11th ed. Norwalk, CT: Appleton-Century-Crofts; 1986.
3. Scheie H, Albert D. Anatomy of the human eye. In: *Textbook of Ophthalmology.* 9th ed. Philadelphia: Saunders; 1977:45-78.
4. Netter F: *Nervous System.* Vol 1. 11th ed. Summit, NJ: Ciba Pharmaceutical; 1972.
5. Doxanas MT, Anderson RL: *Clinical Orbital Anatomy.* Baltimore: Williams & Wilkins; 1984.
6. Katsev D et al. An anatomic study of retrobulbar needle path length. *Ophthalmology.* 1989;96:1221-1224.
7. Koornneef L. New insights in the human orbital connective tissue: results of a new anatomic approach. *Arch Ophthalmol.* 1977;95:1269.
8. Koornneef L. Orbital septa: anatomy and function. *Ophthalmolgy.* 1979;86:876.
9. Koornneef L, Kramer N: *Anatomy and Anesthesia [videotape].* The Netherlands: University of Amsterdam, Orbita Centrum; 1988.
10. Ettl A et al. High resolution magnetic resonance imaging of the orbital connective tissue system. *Ophthal Plast Reconstr Surg.* 1998;14(5):323-327.
11. McGoldrick K. Principles of ophthalmic anesthesia. *J Clin Anesth.* 1989;1: 297-312.
12. Fiore P, Cinotti A. Systemic effects of intraocular epinephrine during cataract surgery. *Ann Ophthalmol.* 1988;20:23-25.
13. Henderer JD, Rapuano CJ. Ocular pharmacology. In: Brunton LL et al, eds. *Goodman and Gilman's Pharmacological Basis of Therapeutics.* 11th ed. New York: McGraw-Hill; 2006:1707-1737.
14. McGoldrick KE, Gayer S. Anesthesia and the eye. In: Barash P et al, eds. *Clinical Anesthesia.* 5th ed. Philadelphia: Lippincott Williams & Wilkins; 2006:974-996.
15. Mauger TF et al. Intraocular pressure, anterior chamber depth and axial length following intravenous mannitol. *J Ocul Pharmacol Ther.* 2000;16(6):591-594.
16. Frishman WH et al. Cardiovascular considerations in using topical, oral, and intravenous drugs for the treatment of glaucoma and ocular hypertension: focus on beta-adrenergic blockade. *Heart Dis.* 2001;3:386-397.
17. Lichter P et al. Intraocular pressure effects of carbonic anhydrase inhibitors in primary open-angle glaucoma. *Am J Ophthalmol.* 1989;107:11-17.
18. Nordstrom Bl et al. Persistence and adherence with topical glaucoma therapy. *Am J Ophthalmol.* 2005;140(4):598-606.
19. McGoldrick K. Ocular drugs and anesthesia. *Int Anesthesiol Clin.* 1990; 28:72-77.
20. Paulsen F. The human nasolacrimal ducts. *Adv Anat Embryol Cell Biol.* 2003;170:iii-xi, 1-106.
21. Naor J, Slomovic AR. Anesthesia modalities for cataract surgery. *Curr Ophthalmol.* 2000;11(1):7-11.
22. Huha T et al. Clinical efficacy and pharmacokinetics of 1% ropivacaine and 0.75% bupivacaine in peribulbar anaesthesia for cataract surgery. *Anaesthesia.* 1999;54(2):137-141.
23. Nicholson G et al. Comparison of 1% ropivacaine with 0.75% bupivacaine and 2% lidocaine for peribulbar anaesthesia. *Br J Anaesth.* 2000;84(1):89-91.
24. Peterfreund R et al. pH adjustment of local anesthetic solutions with sodium bicarbonate: laboratory evaluation of alkalinization and precipitation. *Reg Anesth.* 1989;14:74.
25. Zahl K et al. Peribulbar anesthesia effect of bicarbonate on mixtures of lidocaine, bupivacaine, and hyaluronidase with or without epinephrine. *Ophthalmology.* 1991;98:239-242.
26. Kallio H et al. Hyaluronidase as an adjuvant in bupivacaine-lidocaine mixture for retrobulbar/peribulbar block. *Anesth Analg.* 2000;91(4):934-937.
27. Jacobi PC et al. Cataract surgery under topical anesthesia in patients with co-existing glaucoma. *J Cataract Refract Surg.* 2001;27(8):1207-1213.
28. Vann MA et al. Sedation and anesthesia care for ophthalmologic surgery during local/regional anesthesia. *Anesthesiology.* 2007;107(3):502-508.
29. Iradier MT et al. Intraocular lidocaine in phacoemulsification. *Ophthalmology.* 2000;107(5):896-901.
30. Kumar CM et al. A review of sub-Tenon block: current practice and recent development. *Eur J Anaesth.* 2005;22:567-577.
31. Atkinson WS. Anaesthesia LA in ophthalmology. *Trans Am Ophthalmol Soc.* 1934;32:399-451.
32. Atkinson WS. *Anaesthesia in Ophthalmology.* Springfield, MO: Charles C. Thomas; 1955.
33. Gills J, Lloyd T. A technique of retrobulbar block with paralysis of orbicularis oculi. *J Am Intraocul Implant Soc.* 1983;9:339-340.
34. Grizzard WS et al. Perforating ocular injuries caused by anesthesia personnel. *Ophthalmology.* 1991;98:1011-1016.
35. Straus J. A new retrobulbar needle and injection technique. *Ophthalmic Surg.* 1988;19:134-138.

36. Simonson D. Retrobulbar block: a review for the clinician. *AANA J.* 1990;58:456-461.

37. Davis D, Mandel M. Posterior peribulbar anesthesia: an alternative to retrobulbar anesthesia. *J Cataract Refract Surg.* 1986;12:182-184.

38. Wang H. Peribulbar anesthesia for ophthalmic procedures. *J Cataract Refract Surg.* 1988;14:441-443.

39. Bloomberg L. Anterior periocular anesthesia: five years' experience. *J Cataract Refract Surg.* 1991;17:508-511.

40. Hustead RF et al. Periocular local anesthesia: medial orbital as an alternative to superior nasal injection. *J Cataract Refract Surg.* 1994;20:197-201.

41. Leonardo R et al. Peribulbar anesthesia: a percutaneous single injection technique with a small volume of anesthetic. *Anesth Analg.* 2005;100:94-96.

42. Shriver P et al. Prospective study of the effectiveness of retrobulbar and peribulbar anesthesia for anterior segment surgery. *J Cataract Refract Surg.* 1992;18:162-165.

43. Martin S et al. Retrobulbar anesthesia and orbicularis akinesia. *Ophthalmic Surg.* 1986;17:232-233.

44. Hustead R, Johnson R. The history of ophthalmic anaesthesia: clinical perspectives. In: Kumar C et al, eds. *Ophthalmic Anesthesia.* Lisse, Netherlands: Swets & Zeitlinger BV; 2002:1-12.

45. Nadbath RP, Rehman I. Facial nerve block. *Am J Ophthalmol.* 1963;55:143-146.

46. Glantz L et al. Perioperative myocardial ischemia in cataract surgery patients: general versus local anesthesia. *Anesth Analg.* 2000;91(6):1415-1459.

47. MacPherson R. Structured assessment tool to evaluate patient suitability for cataract surgery under local anaesthesia. *Br J Anaesth.* 2004;93:521-524.

48. Schein OD et al. The value of routine preoperative medical testing before cataract surgery: Study of Medical Testing for Cataract Surgery. *N Engl J Med.* 2002;342(3):168-175.

49. McGoldrick KE, Foldes PJ. General anesthesia for ophthalmic surgery. *Ophthalmol Clin North Am.* 2006;19(2):179-191.

50. Maltby J. Preoperative fasting guidelines undergo revision: report on the annual meeting of the Society for Ambulatory Anesthesia. *Excerpta Medica.* 1991;21:3-14.

51. Daughtery J. Clear liquids before surgery offer ASCs more flexibility. *Same Day Surg.* 1991;15:105-107.

52. Practice guidelines for preoperative fasting and the use of pharmacologic agents to reduce the risk of pulmonary aspiration: application to healthy patients undergoing elective procedures: a report by the American Society of Anesthesiologists Task Force on Preoperative Fasting. *Anesthesiology.* 1999;90(3):896-905.

53. Narendran N, Williamson TH. The effects of aspirin and warfarin therapy on haemorrhage in vitreoretinal surgery. *Acta Ophthalmol Scand.* 2003;81(1):38-40.

54. Katz J, Feldman MD. Risks and benefits of anticoagulant and antiplatelet medication use before cataract surgery. *Ophthalmology.* 2003;110:1784-1788.

55. Hirschman DR, Morby LJ. A study of the safety of continued anticoagulation for cataract surgery patients. *Nurse Forum.* 2006;41(1):30-37.

56. Balken BK et al. Comparison of sedation requirements for cataract surgery under topical anesthesia or retrobulbar block. *Eur J Ophthalmol.* 2004;14(6):473-477.

57. Vann MA et al. Sedation and anesthesia care for ophthalmologic surgery during local and regional anesthesia. *Anesthesiology.* 2007;107(3):502-508.

58. Habib NE et al. Efficacy and safety of sedation with propofol in peribulbar anaesthesia. *Eye.* 2003;16(1):60-62.

59. Katz J et al. Adverse intraoperative medical events and their association with anesthesia management strategies in cataract surgery. *Ophthalmology.* 2001;108(10):1721-1726.

60. Romano P. Coughing and the open eye [letter]. *Ophthalmic Surg.* 1983;14:1041-1042.

61. Stewart RH et al. Lidocaine: an antitussive for ophthalmic surgery. *Ophthalmic Surg.* 1988;19:130-131.

62. Gross JG et al. Increased intraocular pressure in the immediate postoperative period after extracapsular cataract extraction. *Am J Ophthalmol.* 1988;150:466-469.

63. Knopf H. Periocular anesthesia for relief of pain. *Ann Ophthalmol.* 1987;19:181.

64. Vinik HR. Intraocular pressure changes during rapid sequence induction and intubation: a comparison of rocuronium, atracurium, and succinylcholine. *J Clin Anesth.* 1999;11(2):95-100.

65. Poterack KA. How controversial are anesthetic controversies? *J Clin Anesth.* 1997;9(4):266-269.

66. Vachon CA et al. Succinylcholine and the open globe. Tracing the teaching. *Anesthesiology.* 2003;99:220-223.

67. Moreno R et al. Effect of succinylcholine on the intraocular contents of open globes. *Ophthalmology.* 1991;98:636-638.

68. Chidiac EJ, Raiskin AO. Succinylcholine and the open eye. *Ophthalmol Clin North Am.* 2006;19(2):279-285.

69. Kohli R et al. The anesthetic management of ocular trauma. *Int Anesthesiol Clin.* 2007;45(3):83-98.

70. Libonati MM et al. The use of succinylcholine in open eye surgery. *Anesthesiology.* 1985;62:637-640.

71. Morsman C. Succinylcholine in open eyes [letter]. *Ophthalmology.* 1991;98:1607-1608.

72. Ben-David B. Complications of regional anesthesia: an overview. *Anesthesiol Clin North America.* 2002;20(3):427-429.

73. Mullins RM. Retrobulbar block. In: Atlee JL, ed. *Complications in Anesthesia.* Philadelphia: Saunders; 1999:782-784.

74. Gomez RS et al. Brainstem anaesthesia after peribulbar anaesthesia. *Can J Anaesth.* 1997;44(7):732-734.

75. Rozentsveig V et al. Respiratory arrest and convulsions after peribulbar anesthesia. *J Cataract Refract Surg.* 2001;27(6):960-962.

76. Mathers W. Occasional seizures that can follow retrobulbar anesthesia with bupivacaine 0.75%. *Ann Ophthalmol.* 1987;19(3):91.

77. Pearson PA et al. Contralateral cavernous sinus syndrome after retrobulbar anesthetic injection. *Am J Ophthalmol.* 1991;111:773-774.

78. Duker J. Inadvertent globe perforation during retrobulbar and peribulbar anesthesia. *Ophthalmology.* 1991;98:519-526.

79. Hay A et al. Needle penetration of the globe during retrobulbar and peribulbar injections. *Ophthalmology.* 1991;98:1017-1024.

80. Rinkoff J et al. Management of ocular penetration from injection of local anesthesia preceding cataract surgery. *Arch Ophthalmol.* 1991;190:1421-1425.

81. Joseph JP et al. Perforation of the globe—a complication of peribulbar anaesthesia. *Br J Ophthalmol.* 1991;75(8):504-505.

82. Magnante DO et al. Ocular explosions after peribulbar anesthesia: case report and experimental study. *Ophthalmology.* 1997;104:608-615.

83. Bullock JD et al. Ocular explosions from periocular anesthetic injections. A clinical, histopathologic, experimental, and biophysical study. *Ophthalmology.* 1999;106:2341-2353.

84. Friedberg H, Kline O. Contralateral amaurosis after retrobulbar injection. *Am J Ophthalmol.* 1986;101:688-690.

85. Follette J, LoCascio J. Bilateral amaurosis following unilateral retrobulbar block [letter]. *Anesthesiology.* 1985;63:237-238.

86. Antoszyk A, Buckley E. Contralateral decreased visual acuity and extraocular muscle palsies following retrobulbar anesthesia. *Ophthalmology.* 1986;93:462-465.

87. Loken RG et al. Respiratory arrest following peribulbar anesthesia for cataract surgery: case report and review of the literature. *Can J Ophthalmol.* 1998;33(4):225-226.

88. Korbet K. Cerebral spinal fluid recovery of lidocaine and bupivacaine following respiratory arrest subsequent to retrobulbar block. *Ophthalmic Surg.* 1987;18:11-13.

89. Paulter SE et al. Blindness from retrobulbar injection into the optic nerve. *Ophthalmic Surg.* 1986;17:334-337.

90. Cowley M et al. Retinal vascular occlusion without retrobulbar or optic nerve sheath hemorrhage after retrobulbar injection of lidocaine. *Ophthalmic Surg.* 1988;19:859-861.

91. Hersch M et al. Optic nerve enlargement and central retinal artery occlusion secondary to retrobulbar anesthesia. *Ann Ophthalmol.* 1989;21:195-197.

92. Jindra L. Blindness following retrobulbar anesthesia for astigmatic keratotomy. *Ophthalmic Surg.* 1989;20:433-435.

93. Brod R. Transient central retinal artery occlusion and contralateral amaurosis after retrobulbar anesthetic injection. *Ophthalmic Surg.* 1989;20:643-646.

94. Watkins R et al. Intraocular pressure and pulsatile ocular blood flow after retrobulbar and peribulbar anaesthesia. *Br J Ophthalmol.* 2001;85:796-798.

95. Coupland SG et al. Intraocular pressure and pulsatile ocular blood flow during regional orbital anesthesia. *Can J Ophthalmol.* 2001;36:140-144.

96. Mori F et al. Factors affecting pulsatile ocular blood flow in normal subjects. *Br J Ophthalmol.* 2001;85:529-530.

97. Huber KK, Remky A. Colour Doppler imaging before and after retrobulbar anaesthesia in patients undergoing cataract surgery. *Graefes Arch Clin Exp Ophthalmol.* 2005;243(11):1141-1146.

98. Jan-Tjeerd H et al. Inferior rectus muscle palsy after retrobulbar anesthesia for cataract surgery [letter]. *Am J Ophthalmol.* 1991;112:209-211.

99. Hamed L, Mancuso A. Inferior rectus muscle contracture syndrome after retrobulbar anesthesia. *Ophthalmology.* 1991;98:1506-1512.

100. Erie JC. Acquired Brown's syndrome after peribulbar anesthesia [letter]. *Am J Ophthalmol.* 1990;109:349-350.

101. Carlson BM et al. Extraocular muscle regeneration in primates. *Ophthalmology.* 1992;99:582-589.

102. Spaeth G. Total facial nerve palsy following modified O'Brien facial nerve block. *Ophthalmic Surg.* 1987;18:518-519.

103. Koenig SB et al. Respiratory distress after a Nadbath block. *Ophthalmology.* 1988;95:1285-1287.
104. Birt CM et al. Vocal cord paralysis with Nadbath facial block. *Can J Ophthalmol.* 1994;29(5):231-233.
105. Zaturansky B, Hyams S. Perforation of the globe during the injection of local anesthesia. *Ophthalmic Surg.* 1987;18:585-588.
106. Barnard NA, Bainton R. Bradycardia and the trigeminal nerve. *J Craniomaxillofac Surg.* 1990;18:259-360.
107. Fayon M et al. Intraoperative cardiac arrest due to the oculocardiac reflex and subsequent death in a child with occult Epstein Barr virus myocarditis. *Anesthesiology.* 1995;83:622-624.
108. Gild WM et al. Eye injuries associated with anesthesia: a closed claims analysis. *Anesthesiology.* 1992;76:204-208.
109. Locastro A et al. Central retinal artery occlusion in a child after general anesthesia [letter]. *Am J Ophthalmol.* 1991;110:91-92.

CHAPTER 41

ANESTHESIA FOR ORTHOPEDICS AND PODIATRY

Joseph Anthony Joyce

Historically, anesthesia has been closely associated with the field of orthopedic surgery from the first attempted anesthetic for rapid amputations using ethyl alcohol or laudanum. Most often this "anesthetic technique" was a futile effort that frequently resulted in a delirious patient and the surgeon or assistants being injured over the course of the surgical procedure.

Orthopedics is the branch of medicine that deals with maladies of the bones and joints, including congenital deformities, diseases, and injuries. The term *orthopedics* derives from the Greek words *orthos*, "straight," and *paideia*, "rearing of children"; thus a literal translation would be "straight rearing of children."[1] In fact, in its infancy, orthopedics dealt predominantly with children by attempting to correct maladies or deformities now known to have resulted from nutritional and congenital abnormalities—rickets, for example. Over the past 20 to 30 years, this medical specialty has grown enormously. The development of metal prostheses for joint replacement and the refinement of the arthroscope have been the leading advances responsible for the tremendous growth in the field of orthopedics. Complete replacement of joints has allowed improvement in the quality of life for patients suffering from many forms of degenerative joint disease. The increasing refinement of arthroscopic procedures has reduced the invasive nature of many orthopedic procedures. The arthroscope allows the practitioner direct visualization of the affected area, such as the shoulder or knee, via comparatively small incisions. Patients undergoing arthroscopic procedures also benefit from greater mobility immediately postoperatively, reduced discomfort in the surgical area, and reduced length of hospitalization. Patients having arthroscopic procedures often receive treatment on an outpatient basis and may be discharged on the day of surgery or on the first postoperative day. Since the intense interest in arthroscopy was renewed in the 1970s, this subspecialty has continually expanded to include the foot, ankle, wrist, elbow, and shoulder in addition to the knee.

The choice of anesthetic technique to facilitate performance of the proposed orthopedic procedure mirrors that of other surgical specialties. General anesthesia, regional anesthesia, a combination of regional and general anesthesia, and monitored anesthesia care are possible.

The appropriate technique should take into consideration the following: the proposed procedure itself, the anticipated length of the procedure, the patient's position required to accomplish the procedure, the patient's state of health (including body habitus), and the patient's acceptance of the proposed anesthesia technique. There remain patients for whom no anesthetic other than general anesthesia is acceptable, despite the tremendous advances in regional anesthesia and reassurances given by the nurse anesthetist.

PNEUMATIC TOURNIQUET

As with any surgical procedure, one of the concerns when caring for the orthopedic surgical patient is estimation of blood loss. A relatively bloodless surgical field is the desire of virtually any surgeon. The orthopedic surgeon can accomplish this by using a pneumatic tourniquet during many surgical procedures performed on the extremities. The pneumatic tourniquet consists of an inflatable cuff similar to the sphygmomanometer, a pressurization source, connecting tubing, a pressure display, and a pressure regulator. The inflatable cuff differs from that of a sphygmomanometer in that it should provide at least 3 but no more than 6 inches of overlap. The width of the cuff should cover approximately 50% of the target extremity, as opposed to two thirds for the sphygmomanometer. The area covered by the inflatable cuff must be padded using either stockinette or cotton wadding. The nurse anesthetist should take care to avoid wrinkling of the padding material, because wrinkles may result in formation of bullous lesions while the cuff is pressurized.[2] The cuff should then be applied in such a manner that the cuff overlap is opposite the neurovascular bundle of the target extremity.[2] For example, for the upper extremity, when the cuff is applied to the humerus, the overlap should be situated on the lateral aspect of the humerus, which is 180 degrees away from the brachial plexus. After the cuff is properly and satisfactorily positioned, it is connected to the pressure source via the connecting tubing, and the appropriate inflation pressure is determined. A guide to determining appropriate inflation pressure is the initial systolic blood pressure measured before induction of anesthesia or administration of regional anesthesia. Adding 90 to 100 mm Hg of pressure to this initial systolic blood pressure has been demonstrated to effectively control hemostasis in lower extremities.[3] Inflation pressures for upper and lower extremities should not exceed 300 mm Hg and 500 mm Hg, respectively.[2] Before inflation of the pneumatic tourniquet, the operative extremity should be exsanguinated. Exsanguination is accomplished by very tightly wrapping the extremity with an Esmarch bandage, beginning with the digits and continuing proximally up to and including the distal edge of the inflatable cuff. While holding the Esmarch bandage in place, the cuff should be inflated to the predetermined pressure. The cuff should be palpated to ensure that inflation has occurred before the Esmarch bandage is removed. Additional checks of circulatory isolation can be accomplished by palpation of the arterial supply, such as the radial artery for the upper extremity or the popliteal artery for the lower extremity, or using the pulse oximeter to note its inability to obtain a reading. The use of the pneumatic tourniquet provides the advantages of dramatically reduced surgical blood loss and a virtually bloodless operative field, which helps reduce operative time. However, the

BOX 41-1

Physiologic Changes Caused by Limb Tourniquets

Neurologic Effects

Abolition of somatosensory evoked potentials and nerve conduction occurs within 30 minutes.

Application for more than 60 minutes causes tourniquet pain and hypertension.

Application for more than 2 hours may result in postoperative neuropraxia.

Evidence of nerve injury may occur at the skin level underlying the edge of the tourniquet.

Muscle Changes

Cellular hypoxia develops within 2 minutes.

Cellular creatinine value declines.

Progressive cellular acidosis occurs.

Endothelial capillary leak develops after 2 hours.

Systemic Effects of Tourniquet Inflation

Elevation in arterial and pulmonary artery pressures develops. This is usually slight to moderate if only one limb is occluded. The response is more severe in patients undergoing balanced anesthesia that does not include a potent anesthetic vapor.

Systemic Effects of Tourniquet Release

Transient fall in core temperature occurs.

Transient metabolic acidosis occurs.

Transient fall in central venous oxygen tension occurs, but systemic hypoxemia is unusual.

Acid metabolites (e.g., thromboxane) are released into the central circulation.

Transient fall in pulmonary and systemic arterial pressures occurs.

Transient increase in end-tidal carbon dioxide occurs.

---

technique is not without potential problems and complications. Box 41-1 lists the physiologic changes that occur with pneumatic tourniquets.

Tourniquet Pain

Probably the best-known problem encountered with the pneumatic tourniquet is the experience of tourniquet pain. When tourniquets were first used in surgery and potential complications unknown, inflation pressures commonly exceeded 500 mm Hg. In 1944, Denny-Brown and Brenner[4] reported the first investigation into the cause of tourniquet discomfort. They listed characteristic anatomic changes associated with tourniquet ischemia that were due to acute compression of the nerves under the inflated cuff. Compression of the intraneural blood vessels caused a secondary ischemia of the nerve fibers. The subjective discomfort occurred under the cuff and distal to the tourniquet. Similar reports of "tourniquet discomfort" or "aching" despite adequate spinal anesthesia prompted considerable attention toward discovering appropriate pressures required for both hemostasis and minimizing subjective discomfort. Interestingly, from the first reports of tourniquet discomfort, the time to onset of subjective symptoms has been from 45 to 60 minutes. The first use of the term *tourniquet pain* was in 1952.[5]

Subsequent research into the cause of tourniquet pain, conducted between 1953 and 1979, resulted in reduction of effective pressures and accompanying reduction in the incidence of tourniquet pain. Not until 1979 and 1980, however, did reduction in tourniquet pressure become common practice. Patterson and Klenerman[6] reported histologic destruction of the ultrastructure of skeletal muscle under the tourniquet cuff in 1979. Based on this discovery and subsequent measurements of "occlusive pressure" in 1979, Klenerman and Hulands[7] suggested using tourniquet pressures of two times the patient's systolic blood pressure to minimize the subjective discomfort and destruction of tissues. Klenerman[8] modified this recommendation in 1980 to between 50 and 75 mm Hg more than the patient's systolic pressure.

The ischemic pain associated with tourniquet application is similar to that of thrombotic vascular occlusion and peripheral vascular disease.[9] At about 45 to 60 minutes after tourniquet pressurization, patients report various symptoms associated with dull aching that progress to burning and excruciating pain that may require general anesthesia. Once the pain begins, it is often resistant to analgesics and anesthetic agents, despite the anesthetic technique. Even with a well-controlled general anesthetic at the time of tourniquet inflation, ischemic pain may begin during this same time interval and may cause increasing heart rate and blood pressure that require pharmacologic intervention.[10]

Although specific neural and metabolic factors responsible for tourniquet pain are still unknown, several researchers have identified the nerve fibers responsible for transmission of the impulses. The burning and aching pain corresponds to the activation of the small, slow-conducting, unmyelinated C fibers. The pinprick, tingling, and buzzing sensations that frequently accompany tourniquet application, often even after deflation, correspond to activation of the larger and faster myelinated A-delta fibers.

Activation of C fibers in which theorized metabolic effects of tourniquet ischemia were reproduced has been performed in the laboratory setting. In a study by MacIver and Tanelian[9] in 1992, hypoglycemia increased the activation of C fibers by more than 650% in as little as 15 minutes. Hypoxia increased the activation of C fibers by more than 200%, but when combined with hypoglycemia, it increased the activation of C fibers by more than 670%. Acidosis from pH 6.9 to 7.4 did not increase the activation of C fibers. Hypoxia and hypoglycemia, either alone or together, did not increase the activation of A-delta fibers.

Myelinated A-delta and unmyelinated C fibers differ in their sensitivity to local anesthetics. As the concentration of local anesthetic decreases, the activation of C fibers increases, but the A-delta fiber activation is still suppressed. This means that C fibers may be more difficult to anesthetize than A-delta fibers, and tourniquet pain therefore seems more consistent with pain sensation carried by C fibers.[9] Other research has shown that certain local anesthetics enhance the effect of the blockade in the presence of increased stimulation of the isolated nerve fiber. For example, the potency of bupivacaine is enhanced by an increase in the rate of nerve stimulation and may offer an advantage by lowering the incidence of tourniquet pain.[11]

Some of these impulses travel with the sympathetic trunk and enter the spinal cord above the level of the sensory block with spinal or epidural anesthesia, but the incidence of tourniquet pain does not seem to be related to this level. It is apparent that a high-quality blockade of the sacral roots is more important than the thoracic sensory level in reducing the incidence of tourniquet pain, because the intensity of pain may be due to ischemia of the entire leg, as well as under the cuff.[12] The addition of opioids to local anesthesia solutions used for spinal and epidural anesthesia improves the quality of the block and may reduce the incidence of tourniquet pain.[13] If time permits, the superficial application of a eutectic mixture of local anesthetic (lidocaine-prilocaine [EMLA]) cream before tourniquet application may increase the time before onset of tourniquet pain.[14]

Postoperative Tourniquet Paresthesias

Properly placed tourniquets inflated to appropriate pressures rarely cause injury. The use of excessive tourniquet pressure for a prolonged time may cause postoperative paresthesias that are frustrating to treat and very painful for the patient. Excessive tourniquet pressure causes deformation of the underlying nerves—the myelin may be stretched on one side of the node and invaginated on the other. Nerve damage due to rupture of the Schwann cell membrane may be present. Use of proper padding, appropriate choice of tourniquet size, and adherence to recommendations of appropriate pressure and time minimize the incidence of this complication.

Tourniquet Inflation and Deflation

During the time of inflation, physiologic changes consistent with anaerobic metabolism occur in the exsanguinated limb. The nurse anesthetist must be aware of these changes (see Box 41-1) to anticipate the release of cold, acidotic metabolites into the patient's circulation when the tourniquet is released. Common effects of tourniquet release and reperfusion include serum potassium, bicarbonate, and carbon dioxide level increases and decreased pH, arterial oxygen partial pressure, and core temperature (0.6° C) for each hour of tourniquet time.[13]

The patient may experience lability in the blood pressure and heart rate as 300 to 500 mL of blood is acutely returned to systemic circulation on exsanguination and cuff inflation. Under general anesthesia, inflation may cause increased vascular resistance and blood pressure, especially if the patient has preexisting cardiovascular disease. At the end of the procedure, sudden deflation of the tourniquet allows an acute reperfusion of the exsanguinated limb; this situation results in a decrease in the circulating blood volume by as much as 500 mL and washing out of the anaerobic metabolites. This change may cause transient hypotension and bradycardia, rapidly increased end-tidal carbon dioxide levels,[15] and dysrhythmias that may or may not require treatment.

Although exsanguination of the extremity is an important part of tourniquet application, several cases of fatal pulmonary embolism have been reported at tourniquet inflation.[16] The pathologic mechanism in these cases involved dislodgement of preexisting thrombi, either by use of the Esmarch bandage or inflation of the tourniquet.[17] Fat embolism syndrome is evident in 0.5% to 2% of patients with long-bone fractures, as evidenced by preoperative blood gas analysis.[18] Caution must be exercised in the use of tourniquets for patients with fractures, patients who are elderly, and patients with a history of risk factors for emboli formation, such as prolonged bed rest or immobilization.

Tourniquet Time

The research into complications associated with excessive tourniquet pressure also elucidated problems associated with excessive inflation time. Histologic and serum testing documented reversible changes that varied with changes in inflation duration. In 1977, Tountas and Bergman[19] reported that no significant changes relative to ischemia occurred in patients subjected to 2 hours of tourniquet time, but that permanent nerve damage sometimes occurred if tourniquet time was 4 hours. In 1980, Klenerman[8] measured biochemical changes in patients' blood

---

---

that were associated with tourniquet ischemia during and serially after tourniquet deflation. He reported that serum parameters completely returned to normal in 20 minutes if the tourniquet was deflated at the end of 1 hour, but that parameters took 40 minutes to return to normal if the tourniquet was deflated at the end of 3 hours. Histologic changes, however, took 24 hours to return to normal if the tourniquet remained inflated for 3 hours. If the tourniquet was inflated for longer than 3 hours, muscle power in the extremity did not return to normal for 1 week. Klenerman recommended that the "safe" tourniquet time be no longer than 3 hours. Subsequent research has verified Klenerman's recommendations, and current "safe" tourniquet time should not exceed 2 hours routinely.[20] Safety measures for preventing or minimizing complications associated with the pneumatic tourniquet are listed in Box 41-2.

PATIENT POSITIONING

The discipline of orthopedic surgery is probably unique for the variety of patient positioning that may be used to facilitate a proposed surgical procedure. Patient positioning is a crucial component in the successful completion of an orthopedic procedure. Appropriate patient positioning must allow optimal exposure of the surgical site. Additionally, such positioning must afford adequate, appropriate monitoring throughout the procedure, provide good access to the patient's airway, provide comfort and warmth, minimize or prevent physiologic functioning compromise, protect all body systems, and maintain patient dignity.[21] Often surgery on one site (e.g., the elbow) may be accomplished using any one of the three main patient positions—that is, supine, lateral decubitus, or prone. The choice of patient position is dictated to a great extent by the nature of the surgery itself and to a somewhat lesser extent by the personal preference of the individual surgeon. For these reasons, good communication among the nurse anesthetist, operating room staff, and the surgeon is imperative.

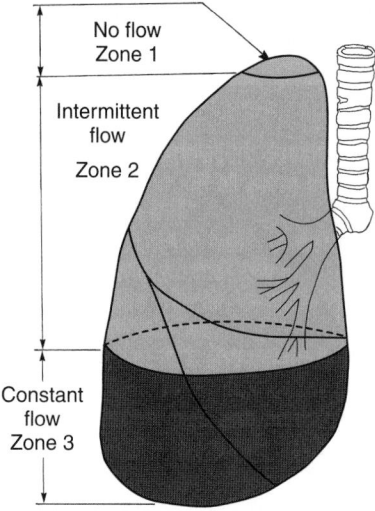

FIGURE **41-1** Lung zones: the effect of gravity on ventilation-perfusion.

The anesthetist is ultimately responsible for proper positioning of the patient on the operating room table. Changes from the usual upright or erect position bring with them a multitude of potential injuries to the patient, as well as physiologic changes the nurse anesthetist must be prepared to prevent or treat. Physical injury is deemed preventable, and the anesthetist must be meticulous in ensuring that relatively normal anatomic positioning of the patient is maintained. Chapter 22 provides an excellent overview of the myriad potential injuries attributable to patient positioning. Physiologic changes are the areas about which the nurse anesthetist must demonstrate knowledge and understanding to adequately prepare for their occurrence and respond with appropriate measures to maintain homeostasis.

Over the millennia, human physiology has adapted to being in an upright or erect position for the majority of the wakeful hours. For example, in the upright position there are three zones of ventilation-perfusion within the lungs: (1) areas where alveolar pressure is greater than arterial pressure, (2) areas of complex, variable pressure gradients between alveolar and arterial components, and (3) areas where arterial pressure is greater than alveolar pressure.[22] Figure 41-1 illustrates lung zones 1, 2, and 3. Another example of physiologic adaptation are the valves found in dependent areas of the venous system, such as the extremities, and the absence of valves in nondependent areas, such as the cranium. Changes from the upright position produce corresponding physiologic changes.[21,23]

Supine Position

In the upright position, the majority of ventilation-perfusion distribution occurs in the variable, complex alveolar-arterial gradients known as *zone 2* (Figure 41-2).[21] The supine position redistributes the lung fields into predominately zone-3 ventilation-perfusion distribution.[24] The ventilation-perfusion distribution dynamics are further disturbed by an average 800-mL reduction in functional residual capacity (FRC) that accompanies being in the supine position[25]; if general anesthesia is used, the patient's FRC is further reduced by an average of 400 mL.[26-28] The initial FRC reduction is presumably the result of pressure being exerted on the diaphragm by the abdominal contents. The FRC reduction is further compounded by diaphragmatic relaxation brought about

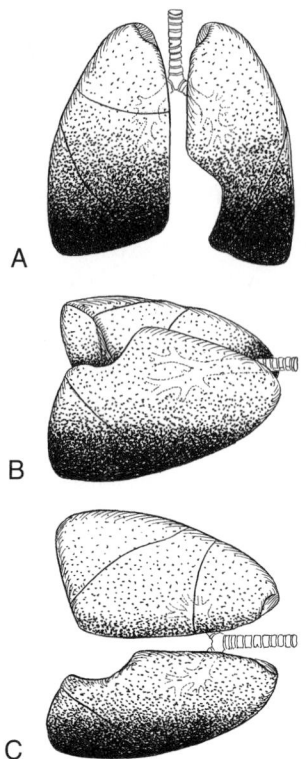

FIGURE **41-2** Gravity dependence of ventilation and perfusion as noted by lungs depicted in the standing (**A**), supine (**B**), and lateral (**C**), positions.

by general anesthesia. Furthermore, induction of general anesthesia results in almost immediate formation of areas of atelectasis, predominantly in the dependent lung fields.[29] The areas of atelectasis are absolute or true shunting areas within the lung capillary bed—blood passes the capillary/alveolar interface without gas exchange occurring. However, with the change from upright posture to the supine position, the diaphragm demonstrates posterior displacement in a cephalad direction, which increases with unparalyzed general anesthesia and is further displaced with paralysis.[23] This diaphragmatic displacement produces greater muscle fiber stretch, which in turn improves efficiency of muscle shortening. As a result of the greater efficiency of muscle fiber shortening, a greater portion of ventilation is directed to the dependent areas of the lung where gravity has already redistributed a larger portion of pulmonary blood flow; therefore, ventilation-perfusion is more closely matched than in the upright position.[23]

The central nervous system undergoes some dynamic changes when the patient is placed in the supine position. Both blood and cerebrospinal fluid drainage from the enclosed cranial vault are via valveless systems, which are gravity dependent. The directional forces of gravity within the cranial vault shift from parallel to the patient's position to perpendicular to that position when the supine position is assumed. These forces can be effectively reversed if the Trendelenburg variation of the supine position is used. Directional changes in the forces of gravity can increase the patient's intracranial pressure, which may in turn reduce the cerebral perfusion pressure (cerebral perfusion pressure equals mean arterial pressure minus intracranial pressure). Such changes in dynamics are of particular concern if the patient has or is suspected of having any form of closed head injury or pathology.

Lateral Decubitus Position

Placing the patient in a lateral decubitus position produces physiologic changes similar to those found in the supine patient. Although the majority of organ systems are unaffected, the physiologic alterations of most concern to the nurse anesthetist revolve around pulmonary and cardiovascular functioning.[30] Remember, in the upright position there are three zones of ventilation-perfusion distribution. Placing the patient in the lateral decubitus position results in a significantly greater proportion of the uppermost lung being classified as *zone 1*, where ventilation is more abundant than pulmonary blood flow, as well as a large portion of the dependent lung being classified as *zone 3*, where pulmonary blood flow exceeds alveolar ventilation[22] (see Figure 41-2). In addition, the percentage of the zone 2 areas of the lung fields is reduced and split between the lungs, with the larger amount being in the dependent lung.

The alteration in ventilation-perfusion distribution is accompanied by reductions in vital capacity and tidal volume. On assuming the lateral decubitus position, healthy, conscious individuals experience about a 10% reduction in vital capacity[31] as a result of reduced anterior, as well as lateral, movement of the dependent rib cage along with restriction of the dependent hemidiaphragm.[32] Ventilation-perfusion distribution may be further altered by the shift in the mediastinum toward the dependent side, which rotates the heart on its axis.[30] This cardiac rotation can impede venous return, reducing cardiac output. The reduced cardiac output can produce hypotension, which must be judiciously treated with either fluid challenges or small doses of vasoactive medication.[30]

Prone Position

Physiologically and mechanically, the ventral surface of the thorax is not adapted to being a weight-bearing surface. Its structures are significantly more mobile than those of the dorsal surfaces.[33] However, placing a patient in the prone position puts just such requirements on the ventral structures. Maintaining normal cardiovascular function while in the prone position assumes the pressure of skeletal flexibility, normal muscle tone, cardiovascular reflexes that are intact, and sufficient energy reserves to increase ventilatory effort by lifting the torso.[33] Induction of general anesthesia or high levels of regional anesthesia nullifies most and sometimes all of those assumptions.

Cardiovascular functioning remains relatively normal when the patient is placed in the prone position so long as occlusive pressure to the inferior vena cava and femoral veins is avoided.[33] If these routes of venous return become occluded—partially or completely—collateral routes must accomplish the task. However, the available collateral venous system has a greatly reduced capacity to accommodate the induced increase in flow rate,[34,35] and a reduction in venous return ensues, resulting in reduced cardiac output. In addition, placing a patient in the prone position produces significant increases in both systemic and pulmonary vascular resistance. These increases lead to significant decreases in stroke volume and cardiac index.[36] It must be ensured that minimal pressure is exerted on the aforementioned vascular structures to maintain cardiac output as close to normal as possible.

Respiratory dynamics are greatly affected by placing the patient in the prone position. The three-zone model discussed earlier is rearranged. The proportion of zone 2 reduces, whereas that of zone 3 increases.[22] The spontaneously breathing patient must expend greater amounts of his or her energy reserves to elevate the weight of the thorax, as well as push the abdominal viscera back caudally, to inflate the lungs. This extra energy expenditure is of greatest concern to the nurse anesthetist when caring for patients with any type of limitation to energy reserves, such as the elderly, the very young, and patients with moderate to severe chronic obstructive pulmonary disease or cardiac disease. The effort required to push the abdominal viscera back in a caudal direction during inspiration can be lessened by allowing the abdomen to rest free from pressure as much as possible; less pressure on the abdomen produces less intrusion of the viscera on the diaphragm. With general anesthesia, the patient's ventilatory effort is often abdicated to the nurse anesthetist, who assumes that role via positive-pressure ventilation. The prone position necessitates higher airway pressures to achieve adequate ventilation. With the increased airway pressure in the prone position, the nurse anesthetist must be cognizant of the increased potential for barotrauma, particularly if the patient is not properly positioned.[33]

Finally, the prone position can alter CNS dynamics more than the supine position, which is of particular concern if head injury or closed head pathology is present or suspected. The anterior neck is particularly supple without considerable bony structural and protective support. In the spontaneously ventilating patient not under general anesthesia or unconscious, sensorium and protective reflexes remain largely intact. Such patients can assist the nurse anesthetist with positioning their head in a manner that is comfortable but does not alter blood flow via the carotid or vertebral arteries. With the unconscious patient or one under general anesthesia, head rotation during positioning must be done with great care. Should the patient's head be rotated 60 degrees, compression of the contralateral vertebral artery begins to constrain blood flow; if rotated 80 degrees, the contralateral vertebral artery becomes completely occluded.[37] The carotid artery and jugular vein on the upper side of the neck can become compressed by extreme degrees of head rotation, and those on the down side of the neck may become compressed by inappropriate head support.[33] Compression of the arterial supply to the brain can produce alterations in consciousness in the awake patient. Under general anesthesia or with a patient whose level of consciousness is already altered, the alteration in arterial blood supply to the brain may not be easily recognized. Therefore, patients in whom any aberration in carotid blood flow is suspected or who have head injury should probably have the head maintained in a neutral anatomic alignment while in the prone position. In addition, even if no arterial or venous compression occurs, if the patient's head rests below the level of the heart, both blood and cerebrospinal fluid may accumulate within the closed cranial vault solely as a result of gravitational direction changes.[33] Such an accumulation can result in increased intracranial pressure and may reduce the cerebral perfusion pressure. Several recent cases of postoperative blindness following prone position surgery have been reported. This complication is discussed in Chapter 22.

As stated, orthopedics has experienced virtually exponential growth in surgical procedures over the past 20 to 30 years. Three surgical areas are at the forefront of the growth in this field: arthroscopy, arthroplasty, and spinal/back surgery.

ARTHROSCOPY

Dorland's Pocket Medical Dictionary defines arthroscopy as "examination of the interior of a joint with an endoscope."[38] The concept of arthroscopy was first described and demonstrated by Takagi in 1918.[39,40] The concept was introduced into the United States in 1926.[41] However, without the availability of

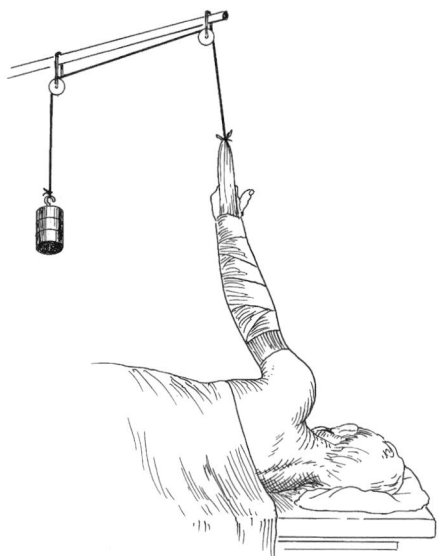

FIGURE **41-3**   Shoulder arthroscopy positioning.

Anesthetic Selection in Orthopedics

What is the proposed surgical procedure?
How long is the procedure estimated to take?
What patient position will be necessary to accomplish the procedure?
Is this patient's overall health status sufficient to remain in the required position for an extended period of time without general anesthesia?
Is this patient receptive to an anesthesia technique (or techniques) other than general anesthesia?

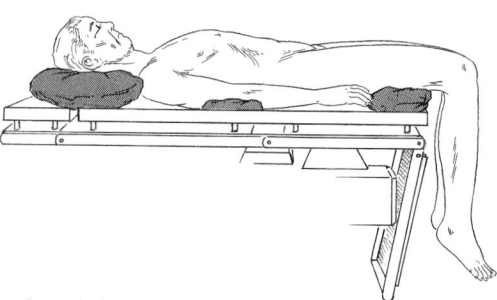

FIGURE **41-4**   Positioning for knee procedures.

practical sources of illumination, arthroscopy languished. The development of fiberoptic light sources in the 1970s brought a resurgence of interest in the utilization of arthroscopy. Takagi's descriptions and demonstrations were predicated on using the techniques on the knee joint. Indeed, on the resurgence of interest in arthroscopy, the knee was the primary site for the procedure and currently remains the most common site for arthroscopy. Initially, arthroscopy was used to obtain definitive diagnosis of a patient's orthopedic malady so a definitive, corrective surgical procedure could be performed. As interest in the procedure and technique increased, coupled with development of the necessary smaller surgical instrumentation, previously open surgical procedures on the knee, such as partial or complete meniscectomy, loose-body removal, or cruciate ligament repair or reconstruction, were attempted and refined solely via the arthroscope.

Successful performance of arthroscopic procedures on the knee produced several benefits for the patient, including reduced blood loss, less postoperative discomfort, reduced length of hospitalization, and reduced length of rehabilitation. The success achieved with arthroscopic procedures on the knee led to application of the principles and techniques to other joints (e.g., the shoulder, elbow, wrist, hip, ankle, and phalangeal joints of the foot). Through the middle portion of the 1990s, application of arthroscopic procedures focused on the shoulder. Accordingly, shoulder arthroscopy use ranges from tendon débridement to rotator cuff repair.[40,41] The development and refinement of shoulder arthroscopic procedures mirrors that of knee arthroscopic procedures; that is, as more skill and comfort are obtained with initial procedures, more traditionally open surgical treatments are attempted solely via the arthroscope. Arthroscopic techniques are being developed, refined, and expanded for the elbow, wrist, hip, and ankle.[40]

Anesthetic Management

Arthroscopic procedures may be anesthetically managed by almost any of the available anesthesia techniques (general anesthesia, regional anesthesia, combined regional and general anesthesia, local blockade, and sometimes monitored anesthesia care). Patient selection for a given anesthetic technique is crucial with arthroscopic procedures, as with all operative procedures.

As previously mentioned, for some patients there is absolutely no substitute for receiving general anesthesia. Critical factors in the selection and presentation of the available anesthesia techniques appropriate for arthroscopic procedures are the patient positioning necessary to facilitate the proposed arthroscopic procedure and the overall state of health of the patient. For example, shoulder arthroscopy uses one of two positions to accomplish the surgery, either lateral decubitus or modified Fowler's ("beach chair") position.[41] The choice of position is determined in part by the nature and extent of the malady being surgically addressed. For some shoulder arthroscopy procedures, supplemental traction with weights and abduction may be necessary to provide optimum operative visualization (Figure 41-3); for others, the modified Fowler's position may be used with the force of gravity or manual traction providing sufficient operative visibility. Reviewing the patient's chart and (most important) personally interviewing the patient, along with understanding the physiologic changes associated with various positions, will assist the nurse anesthetist in offering the best suggestion for anesthesia care for each patient. Box 41-3 lists important factors in this decision.

Patient positioning for arthroscopic procedures can encompass virtually the entire gamut of possible operative positions. Most often, arthroscopic procedures for lower extremity joints use the supine position, as do most arthroscopic procedures on the upper extremities. Arthroscopy on the knee requires the supine position with the foot of the operating room bed lowered (Figure 41-4). The nonoperative leg should either be wrapped with an elastic bandage or have some form of antiembolic stocking in place to reduce pooling of blood and the potential for thrombus formation. At times, patients undergoing elbow arthroscopy may be placed in the supine, lateral decubitus, or prone position; the position is dictated by operative necessity and surgeon preference (Figures 41-5 and 41-6). The prone

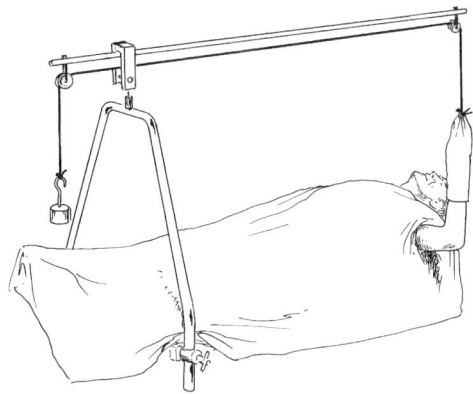

FIGURE **41-5** Supine position for elbow surgery.

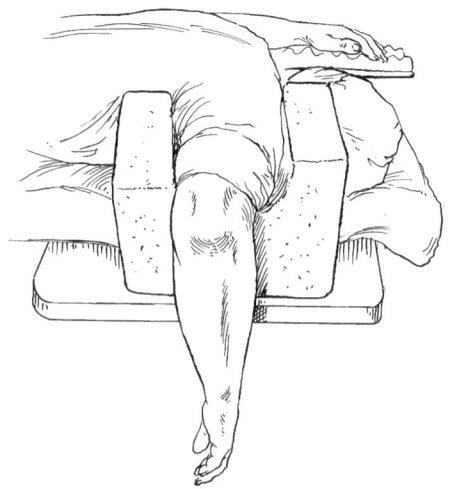

FIGURE **41-6** Prone position for elbow surgery.

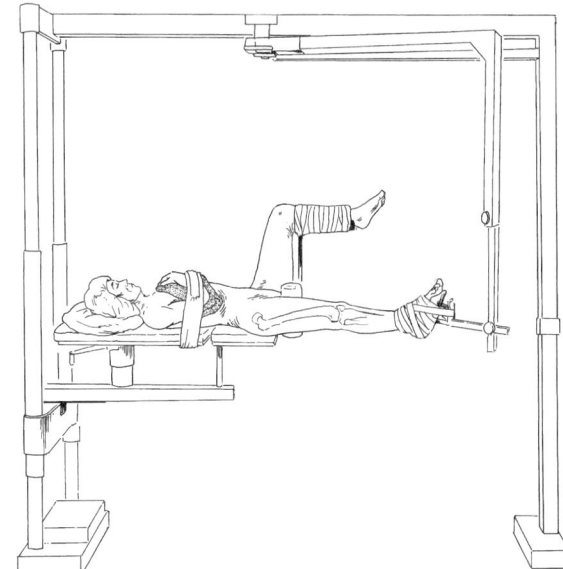

FIGURE **41-7** Fracture table. Allows easy access for x-ray equipment.

position is more advantageous primarily because of the better limb stability during the procedure.[42] Shoulder arthroscopy is usually accomplished via either the modified Fowler's position or the lateral decubitus position, based on optimal access to the injury and surgeon preference (see Figure 41-3).[41] Hip arthroscopy is also typically accomplished via the lateral decubitus or the supine position, with the patient on a fracture table[43] (Figure 41-7). The fracture table is used to provide greater stability while traction is applied, using either weights and counterweights (lateral decubitus position) or mechanical traction attached to the leg-holding device of the fracture table (supine position).[43] Wrist arthroscopy is seldom performed, but when used, the patient need only be in the supine position.

Complications from arthroscopic procedures represent a small percentage of the total number of procedures performed.[44-47] Accordingly, complications resulting from arthroscopic procedures that particularly concern the nurse anesthetist are relatively few. The full range of potential anesthetic complications associated with patient positioning apply (e.g., inadvertent extubation, eye or corneal injury, and nerve injury from improper patient positioning). Because of the less invasive nature of arthroscopic procedures, concerns over blood loss are typically minimal. However, sudden, sustained hypotension is a cause for immediate investigation. With many arthroscopic procedures, the pneumatic tourniquet may be used to provide a clear, bloodless

surgical field. Perforation of a major blood vessel may occur during trocar insertion and may not be detected until the tourniquet is deflated. Such vascular injury may result from pressure exerted by excess extravasated irrigation fluid during the procedure.[39] In the case of shoulder or hip arthroscopy, procedures in which pneumatic tourniquet use is not possible, any major vascular injury will be recognized significantly earlier than completion of the procedure.

To provide optimal visualization of joint structures during arthroscopic procedures, the irrigating fluid used to distend the operative joint is instilled under pressure. Pressurization of the irrigating solution is accomplished either by hanging the solution 3 to 4 feet higher than the operative joint or by using a mechanical pump device. Hanging the irrigation fluid 3 to 4 feet above the operative joint produces almost 90 mm Hg of fluid pressure entering the joint space.[39] Alternatively, mechanical pumps specifically designed for arthroscopic procedures are set to deliver fluid pressurized to between 60 and 80 mm Hg. As a result of the pressurization of the irrigating fluid, extravasation is not uncommon during arthroscopic procedures. The typical irrigation setup uses large bags of irrigating solution, 3 to 5 L in volume. The nurse anesthetist should take note of any deficits of inflow versus outflow of irrigating solution throughout the procedure. Depending on the severity or complexity of the arthroscopic procedure, a large number of irrigation fluid bags may be required. Therefore, even small individual inflow/outflow deficits may result in significant fluid absorption by the patient over the course of an extended procedure. Fluid absorption is of particular concern to the nurse anesthetist for shoulder or hip arthroscopic procedures in which fluid absorption is not relatively limited by the use of the pneumatic tourniquet. Absorption of excessive extravasated fluid may lead to the development of signs and symptoms of congestive heart failure, pulmonary edema, volume overload, or hyponatremia (if a "salt-poor" fluid is used). Should the patient experience these symptoms, treatment with fluid restriction, supplemental oxygen, and diuresis should be instituted.

Although the mechanism of occurrence has not been delineated, subcutaneous emphysema, tension pneumothorax, and pneumomediastinum have been reported during shoulder

Signs and Symptoms of Tension Pneumothorax

Sudden, inexplicable hypoxemia
Elevated central venous pressure
Tachycardia
Absent breath sounds on the affected side
Tracheal shift
Agitation (may be observed in patients receiving regional anesthesia)
Hypotension
Jugular vein distention
Increased airway pressure
Asymmetric chest wall movement
Percussive hyperresonance over the affected side
Extreme anxiety (may be observed in patients receiving regional anesthesia)

arthroscopy, specifically subacromial decompression.[47] These complications appear to be associated at least in part with the use of mechanical irrigation pumps and power-saver suction. The nurse anesthetist must be alert to the signs and symptoms of these complications to alert the surgeon to the need for immediate termination of the use of these arthroscopic adjunct devices and initiation of appropriate treatment measures. Box 41-4 lists the signs and symptoms of tension pneumothorax. Because tension pneumothorax is a potentially life-threatening event, early recognition and treatment are paramount. Ideally, placement of a chest tube is most desirable to relieve the pent-up intrathoracic pressure. However, an immediate and very effective treatment is needle decompression with a 14- to 18-gauge intravenous stylet placed into either the second or third intercostal space anteriorly or the fourth or fifth intercostal space laterally.[48,49] Successful decompression is accompanied by a sudden rush of air, as well as readjustment of physical symptoms and vital signs back toward the patient's normal parameters. After successful decompression, the intravenous catheter stylet should remain in place and be covered or capped to prevent air from being sucked back into the chest cavity until a chest tube can be properly inserted.

ARTHROPLASTY

Arthroplasty is the surgical replacement of all (total arthroplasty) or part (hemiarthroplasty) of a joint to achieve a return of natural motion and function of the joint, as well as restoration of the controlling function of the surrounding soft tissues (i.e., muscles, ligaments, and tendons). The goals of arthroplasty are pain relief, stability of joint motion, and deformity correction.[50] In the 1940s and 1950s, hemiarthroplasty was heavily investigated using molded metal alloy prosthetics as an alternative to interpositional grafting arthroplasty. Still, long-term results continued to be unsatisfactory. Finally, in the 1960s, Sir John Charnley developed a system for hip joint replacement that consisted of a metal alloy femoral component that articulated with a "plastic" or high-density polyethylene acetabular prosthesis. The "metal-to-plastic" system produced both the short- and long-term goals desired since the mid-1800s. Charnley's system was subsequently adapted for other joint replacements, including the knee, shoulder, elbow, ankle, and finger.[18,50]

The original hip prosthesis was fabricated from stainless steel. Prostheses currently in use are stronger metal alloys, most of which are based on cobalt or titanium. These alloys demonstrate greater tensile strength and are more resistant to fatigue than the original stainless steel. Indeed, the search for metal alloys with even greater tensile strength and more resistance to fatigue is an area of continued intense research.[50]

Lower Extremity Arthroplasty

Hip Arthroplasty

The hip joint is one of the most frequently replaced joints. It is classified as a major surgical undertaking. Typically, the patient is placed in the lateral decubitus position, which offers greater range of motion and visibility throughout the surgical procedure. This procedure requires a large incision, extending from near the iliac crest across the joint to the midthigh level. Several large muscle groups must be incised and dissected through to gain access to the joint, after which the joint is disarticulated. The femoral head and neck are excised, leaving the femoral canal open. The femur is filled with rich marrow, being one of the erythrocyte-production areas for the body; therefore, it is also richly vascular. The acetabulum is a part of the pelvic girdle, also one of the erythrocyte-production areas, and is richly vascular as well. After the femoral head and neck are removed, the femoral canal is reamed to the appropriate diameter to accommodate the prosthetic head and neck. The acetabulum is then reamed in a similar manner to accommodate its own prosthesis. During the reaming for both prosthetic components, bone is shaved from the canal and acetabulum to produce a smoother bony surface to achieve better adherence of the prosthetic device and cement. Also during the reaming process, venous sinuses within these bony structures are opened and often destroyed, which can result in significant blood loss. After the femoral canal has been satisfactorily prepared, the canal is cleaned out using pulse irrigation, which forces irrigation solution deep within the femoral canal under pressure in a high-frequency, pulsatile stream. The canal is further cleaned with a sponge, after which methylmethacrylate (MMA) cement may be instilled into the femoral canal. For some procedures, usually in younger or very physically active patients, MMA is not used to secure the femoral prosthesis, and the prosthesis is referred to as being *press-fit*. After instillation of the MMA cement, the femoral prosthesis is inserted into the canal and forcibly "seated" with a mallet. The acetabular component is secured in place with screws and bone grafting. The dislocated joint is reduced, and the soft tissues are returned to normal anatomic position during wound closure.

Knee Arthroplasty

Total knee arthroplasty is the other frequently performed joint replacement procedure. A pneumatic tourniquet is typically used to provide a relatively bloodless surgical field. Nevertheless, blood loss as a result of total knee arthroplasty can be up to 2 units.[18] During the procedure, the articulating surfaces of the femur and tibia are excised via precise angular cuts, and the patellar articulating surface is shaved, all to conform the bones to the inner surfaces of the prostheses. Both the femoral and tibial surfaces are covered with MMA cement, and the individual prosthesis components are forcibly seated with a mallet. The high-density polyethylene patellar component is cemented and seated with a viselike clamp. The medial and lateral menisci are replaced with a conforming wedge of high-density polyethylene.

Ankle Arthroplasty

Because of the success rate of total knee arthroplasty, ankle arthroplasty proponents were originally filled with high hopes and expectations. Over the ensuing years, ankle arthroplasty has succumbed to an exceedingly high failure rate, which is attributable to various causes, from prosthetic loosening to infection.[51] As a result, ankle arthroplasty is sparingly to rarely performed.

Anesthetic Management

Anesthetic management of the patient undergoing arthroplasty of the lower extremity is nearly the same as that of the patient scheduled for lower extremity arthroscopy. In the case of arthroplasty surgery, general, spinal, continuous epidural, or combined regional and general anesthesia may be used with equal expectations from the standpoint of anesthesia and analgesia. As mentioned, for some patients no anesthesia technique other than general anesthesia is acceptable. Such patients usually voice strong concerns, both about having a needle placed in their back and being awake enough to hear the sawing and drilling that are integral parts of joint replacement surgery. Almost invariably, the patient's concern about having a needle placed in the back has its genesis in a family member, close friend, or associate who has intimated a particularly unpleasant experience with a spinal or epidural anesthetic in the distant past. Such reluctance to receive a regional anesthetic may also be the result of a personally unpleasant experience in the distant past. Nevertheless, general anesthesia is the only technique to which such a patient is amenable. As with any general anesthetic, the patient is unable to inform the nurse anesthetist of anything that is painful during the procedure; specifically, the anesthetist must be fastidious and vigilant regarding patient positioning throughout the procedure. The nurse anesthetist is charged with maintaining, as nearly as possible, normal anatomic alignment to minimize the potential for injury. These considerations are particularly relevant for the total hip arthroplasty patient who must be placed in the lateral decubitus position. Airway patency must be maintained during the positioning of the patient under general anesthesia, being sure to carefully and gently control the patient's head and neck during transfer to the operating room bed to prevent inadvertent extubation, endobronchial intubation, or neck injury.

Other patients may initially be hesitant with regard to receiving either spinal or epidural anesthesia for lower extremity arthroplasty. Often, this patient's hesitance stems from the same concerns related previously; however, this patient will ask for more information about regional anesthesia for arthroplasty procedures. The patient's questions and concerns must be addressed in a frank, forthright, and reassuring manner by explaining the advantages and disadvantages of regional anesthesia. Patients will be encouraged to learn that regional anesthesia will still be in effect immediately postoperatively, and there will be little to no pain on admission to the postanesthesia care unit. The patient needs to understand that the nurse anesthetist will be in attendance throughout the procedure to ensure comfort and safety at all times and that the surgical procedure will not commence until the regional anesthetic is fully in effect.

One patient concern is blood loss and the need for transfusion. Total hip arthroplasty can result in significant blood loss—up to about 6 units.[18] The supply of donated blood has never been safer than at the present time. In addition to being typed and crossmatched according to individual antibodies, donated blood is tested for numerous transfusion-related diseases, including human immunodeficiency virus (HIV) and hepatitis. The patient is encouraged to make an autologous blood donation, whereby 1 or 2 units of the patient's own blood is placed in the hospital's blood bank before the anticipated date of surgery, provided there is no conflict with the patient's religious beliefs. There are several ways to reduce both blood loss and the need for transfusion. The nurse anesthetist can help reduce the blood loss during the procedure by using deliberate hypotension during the surgery. Other avenues to reduce the need for blood transfusion include (1) use of the cell saver, which may be particularly desirable for patients whose religious beliefs forbid transfusions, (2) reducing the "transfusion point" to a hematocrit of less than 30%, and (3) maintaining normothermia. Less blood loss occurs in patients receiving regional anesthesia than in those receiving general anesthesia.[52-56]

It is important to be particularly cognizant of the possible occurrence of hypotension, hypoxia, and (potentially) cardiovascular collapse. These complications are observed most often during insertion of the femoral prosthesis during total hip arthroplasty but may be observed soon after tourniquet deflation during total knee arthroplasty. Possible etiologies of these complications include the MMA cement, fat embolism, air embolism, thromboembolism, and bone marrow embolism.[57-62] MMA has been demonstrated to produce significant increases in both pulmonary vascular resistance (PVR) and pulmonary wedge pressure, while decreasing systemic vascular resistance (SVR), cardiac output, and arterial pressure.[57] Deep vein thrombosis (DVT) is a precursor to pulmonary embolism (PE) development. DVT has been demonstrated in 40% to 60% of patients undergoing total hip arthroplasty and approximately 80% of patients having total knee arthroplasty. From within the two patient populations, PE is believed to develop 1% to 5% of the time.[51]

Upper Extremity Arthroplasty

Arthroplasty in the upper extremity makes up a low percentage of the number of joint arthroplasties performed each year. Of the two more commonly replaced upper extremity joints, the shoulder and the elbow, shoulder arthroplasty accounts for approximately 5% of the number of total joint replacements performed annually.[63] The primary goal of shoulder arthroplasty is relief of pain, with the secondary goal being improvement in overall joint functioning. Indications for shoulder arthroplasty include glenohumeral joint destruction due to osteoarthritis, complex proximal humerus fractures, rheumatoid arthritis, avascular necrosis of the humeral head, and malunion or nonunion of the proximal humerus.[64-66] Shoulder arthroplasty is performed with the patient in either the lateral decubitus or modified Fowler ("beach chair") position (see Figure 41-3). Because a pneumatic tourniquet cannot be used, shoulder arthroplasty tends to result in significant intraoperative blood loss.

Elbow arthroplasty is performed with less frequency than shoulder arthroplasty. The goals for elbow arthroplasty are much the same as for shoulder arthroplasty: pain relief and improvement in joint function. The indications for elbow arthroplasty include rheumatoid arthritis, traumatic arthritis, and ankylosis of the joint.

Anesthetic Management

Patients undergoing total shoulder arthroplasty can be managed by general anesthesia, interscalene blockade, or supraclavicular blockade. Box 41-3 lists questions and factors to aid the nurse anesthetist in presentation of the most appropriate anesthetic technique for each patient. If general anesthesia is chosen, it is important to be mindful of the ongoing potential for inadvertent extubation as a result of the surgical manipulations necessary while in close proximity to the patient's head and neck. The patient's neck may be subjected to excessive stretch during the surgical manipulations, and if the patient's head becomes dislodged from the supportive device used, there is the potential for cervical spine injury.

For the patient undergoing shoulder arthroscopy, pulmonary function will more closely resemble "normal" function as a result of being in the modified Fowler's position. However, the nurse anesthetist must be aware that as a result of that position, the potential for venous air embolism is somewhat increased over other positions. The risk of fat or bone marrow embolism and thromboembolism incumbent with the required reaming of the shaft of one of the body's long bones. The potential cardiovascular effects of MMA cement must also be considered if the humeral component is cemented in place.

Blood loss during shoulder arthroplasty can be significant, just as it can with hip arthroplasty. The anesthetist should use the same measures for minimizing blood loss and transfusion that apply during hip arthroplasty (e.g., deliberate hypotension and autologous donation).

Elbow arthroplasty can be performed in any of three positions: supine, lateral decubitus, or prone. The deciding factors on which position will be used for this procedure are surgeon preference and the health of the patient. Elbow arthroplasty can be managed by general anesthesia or supraclavicular, intraclavicular, interscalene, or axillary blockade. During elbow arthroplasty, the pneumatic tourniquet will probably be used to minimize blood loss and provide a clear surgical field. It is necessary to be prepared to treat the patient's tourniquet pain whenever regional anesthesia is used. There is also an increased risk of thromboembolism development when the pneumatic tourniquet is used,[67] particularly in patients with a history of DVT.

SPINAL SURGERY

Spinal surgery is the third area within this specialty in which the greatest developments are occurring. Back injuries account for a large percentage of work-related injuries and are a leading cause of work absences. Estimates are that 80% of the population will experience some type of back problem. The resultant medical costs are estimated at greater than $25 billion per year, and the related costs of lost employee productivity are estimated at $60 billion.[68,69] Virtually every industry now provides employees with education on body mechanics to attempt to reduce the number of back injuries.

In the past, laminectomies required large incisions to afford the surgeon optimal visualization of the affected area of the spinal column. The large incision resulted in greater amounts of blood loss, prolonged wound healing, and lengthy hospitalization. Over the past decade, orthopedic surgeons have incorporated operative microscopes on an ever-increasing basis. Use of the operative microscope affords the surgeon better visualization while eliminating the need for the large incisions that were commonplace in the recent past, even for straightforward, "simple" lumbar laminectomies. In addition, the smaller incision results in reduced blood loss, faster wound healing, less trauma to surrounding soft tissues, shorter recovery, shorter length of hospitalization, and quicker return to a preinjury level of activity. Owing to refined surgical techniques, straightforward, "simple," single-level lumbar laminectomy patients are discharged from the hospital on the first postoperative day and on occasion may be discharged the same day of surgery.

The most common reasons for spinal surgery are intervertebral disk herniation and spinal stenosis. These maladies can occur anywhere along the spinal column from C2-C3 through the L5-S1 vertebrae. Surgical intervention via the posterior approach consists of a midline incision and tissue dissection to expose the disk herniation or stenotic areas. The disk herniation is excised, or the neuroforaminal space is enlarged, to relieve compression of the nerve root. For the posterior approach, the patient is positioned prone. At times, other conditions exist that necessitate fusion of two vertebrae. Vertebral fusion is accomplished by a number of methods: bone grafting, either autologous or cadaveric; plate and screws; or the newest method, interbody cage devices. The goal is to prevent further degeneration and loss of the surgical correction achieved. Interbody cage devices facilitate fusion of the specific vertebral joint. They are designed to enhance the symptomatic relief that precipitated the fusion by restoring normal disk height, maintaining anatomically normal tension in the annular fibers, restoring lordosis in the affected segment, reducing subluxed facet joints, providing neuroforaminal space enlargement, and returning normal weight-bearing proportion through the anterior spinal column.[70] Interbody cage procedures, done by experienced surgeons, are more quickly accomplished than the previously standard bone-grafting procedure, are less costly, provide greater stability, and afford faster recovery and rehabilitation times.[69,70] In contrast to interbody cage devices and procedures, total disk replacement procedures are accomplished most commonly via an anterior approach. This approach may require the orthopedic surgeon enlist the assistance of a general or vascular surgeon—someone more proficient or comfortable with manipulating the abdominal viscera or major abdominal vascular structures—to secure an adequate surgical field around the targeted vertebral body or bodies.[71-76] Eight prosthesis designs are being investigated[74] (Box 41-5). These prosthetic devices are reported to afford even greater stability within the spinal column, in a fashion similar to the benefits derived from the interbody cage devices. Fusion within the cervical spine is most frequently accomplished by initial diskectomy followed by a wedge of bone graft, often cadaveric, or by fusion of the joint with a plate and screws.

Scoliosis is lateral curvature of the spinal column. It is classified as either idiopathic, for which the cause is not known, or from a known cause.[77] The majority (75% to 80%) of scoliosis cases are idiopathic. The remaining 20% to 25% can be identified as resulting from such conditions as congenital skeletal abnormalities (vertebral or extravertebral), neuromuscular disease, neurofibromatosis, arthrogryposis, trauma, and irritative phenomena resulting from nerve root compression or spinal cord tumor.[77] Untreated, scoliosis can lead to complex deformity in two planes (sagittal and coronal), chronic pain, neurologic and cardiopulmonary compromise, and cosmetic concerns.[78] Treatment pathways

---

BOX 41-5

Types of Total Disk Replacement Prosthetics

Prosthetic Disc Nucleus
Aquarelle
NeuDisc
Newcleus
Regain
IPD
Dascor Disk Arthroplasty Device
BioDisc

are determined by the severity and cause of the deformity and may be nonsurgical or surgical. Surgical intervention consists primarily of fusion of multiple joint spaces, with or without anterior release, and may include extensive instrumentation (e.g., Harrington rods and Dewer or Luque instrumentation). These surgical interventions may involve anterior or posterior approaches. Either approach is a major surgical intervention, but the anterior approach is more technically involved. The anterior approach to the thoracic spine requires performing a thoracotomy.

In conjunction with the development of "cage" technology, the principles of laparoscopy/endoscopy are being adapted and applied to spinal surgery. The first use of laparoscopy for lumbar discectomy was reported by Obenchain[79] in 1991. Laparoscopic techniques were first used by Mack and coworkers[80] for thoracic spinal surgery in 1993. Application of laparoscopic principles and techniques offers numerous advantages to anterior vertebral joint fusion (Box 41-6), not the least of which are dramatically reduced blood loss, improved ventilation (both intraoperatively and postoperatively), and reduced overall medical costs. The major disadvantage of utilizing laparoscopic techniques in spinal surgery is the necessity for the surgeon's acquisition of the technical skills and level of comfort with the procedural requirements, which in large part are dependent on the frequency with which the newly acquired skills are used.

At present, not all patients should be considered for laparoscopic spinal surgery. For lumbar spinal surgery candidates, laparoscopy is currently contraindicated for patients with severe abdominal adhesions resulting from inflammatory processes, previous laparotomy, or severe abdominal trauma and patients with marked cardiac or pulmonary disease processes who may not be able to tolerate the hypercarbia that can result from abdominal insufflation of carbon dioxide, particularly during longer procedures.[81] For thoracic spinal surgery candidates, laparoscopy is currently contraindicated for patients unable to tolerate one-lung ventilation and those with severe or acute respiratory insufficiency, high positive airway pressures, and pleural symphysis. Patients who have required previous thoracotomy or chest-tube placement must be more extensively evaluated preoperatively to determine if thorascopic spinal surgery will be used. Also, at present, patients in need of internal fixation with extensive instrumentation of the anterior spine are not considered candidates for thorascopic spinal surgery.[81]

Anesthetic Management

Almost all spinal surgery procedures are managed using general anesthesia, because this technique affords a more secure airway and the greatest degree of control over the patient's reflexive actions. Spinal anesthesia may be combined with general anesthesia when a lighter plane of anesthesia with a more secure airway would be better tolerated by the patient and produce a better postoperative course, as in a patient with severe chronic obstructive pulmonary disease.

A major anesthesia concern during spinal surgery centers on patient positioning. For spinal surgery involving the posterior approach, the patient will of necessity be placed in the prone position. While placing the patient in the prone position, the clinician must be vigilant in maintaining the security and integrity of the patient's airway so that inadvertent extubation, endobronchial intubation, or endotracheal tube kinking does not occur. The potential for eye or corneal injury is high in the prone position. It is important to avoid extremes in flexion or extension of the patient's neck and ensure proper alignment and padding of the patient's upper extremities. When positioned prone, the patient's abdomen should not be compressed, because compression of the abdominal cavity will displace the organs and therefore the diaphragm cephalad, producing reduced functional residual capacity, reduced tidal volume, and increased airway pressures. Abdominal compression also contributes to engorgement of the epidural venous network and can be a contributing factor to greater blood loss during the surgical procedure. To avoid abdominal compression, the abdomen must be elevated from the surface of the operating room bed.

Numerous methods and devices can be used to greatly reduce or eliminate abdominal compression. The simplest method is the use of bilateral "prone rolls," which are firm but compressible pads that extend from the shoulder to the iliac crest (Figure 41-8). Other devices include the Wilson frame (Figure 41-9), the Relton adjustable pedestal frame (Figure 41-10), and the Andrews frame, or spinal-surgery table (Figure 41-11). Each of these positioning devices is designed to allow the abdomen to

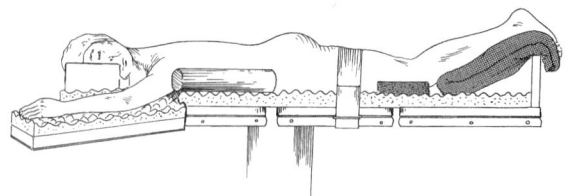

FIGURE **41-8** Prone position using chest rolls.

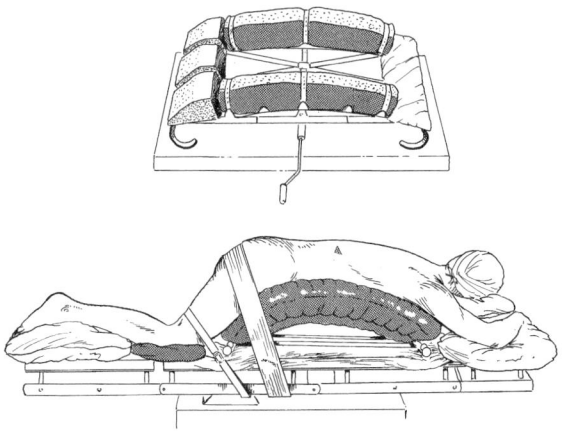

FIGURE **41-9** Spinal operations using a convex saddle frame (Wilson frame).

BOX **41-6**

Advantages of Laparoscopy for Anterior Spinal Surgery

Enhanced visualization
Decreased potential for infection
Reduced trauma to surrounding soft tissues
Shorter hospitalization
Shorter rehabilitation period
Decreased blood loss
Improved intraoperative and postoperative ventilation
Reduced intensive care unit time
Better cosmetic appearance
Reduced overall costs

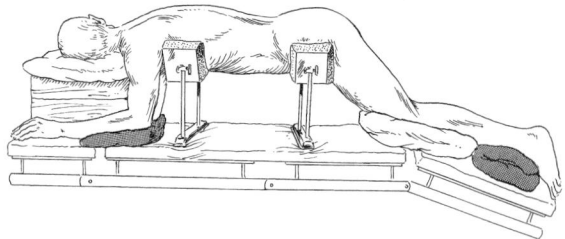

FIGURE **41-10**   The Relton adjustable pedestal frame.

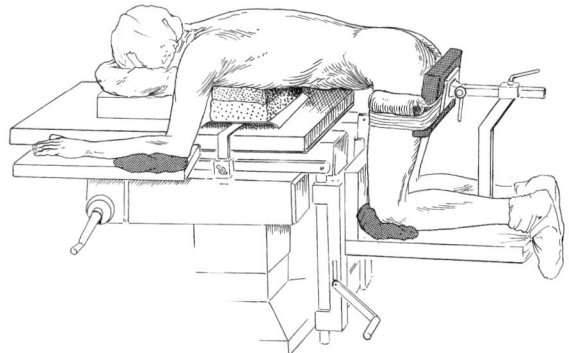

FIGURE **41-11**   The Andrews frame.

"hang" freely and reduce the possibility of compressing major vascular structures.

The Andrews spinal surgery table is the most complex of the positioning devices. With the Andrews table, as with the other positioning devices, the patient is induced and intubated on the transportation stretcher, after which he or she is lifted onto the table. On initial positioning on the Andrews table, the patient lies flat with the legs resting perpendicular to the plane of the table. A buttock support is securely attached to the framework of the table, and the bony prominences of the hips and, particularly, the knees are adequately padded. The leg portion of the table is then lowered until the weight of the lower body rests on the knees, resulting in the patient's hips and knees being flexed at 90 degrees. This table produces a modified knee-chest position, allows the abdomen to "hang" freely, and greatly reduces the potential for compression of the major vascular structures of the lower abdomen and pelvic region (femoral arteries and veins). This position also maximizes the surgeon's visualization of the surgical site. Blood loss is decreased by using the Andrews spinal surgery table.[82] However, hypotension occurs frequently when using this table as a result of blood pooling in the dependent lower extremities. Antiembolic stockings may help counteract the tendency for blood to pool in the lower extremities, and any hypotensive event may be treated by judicious use of fluid challenges or small doses of vasoactive medications, such as ephedrine.

Scoliosis correction with large-scale instrumentation (e.g., Harrington instrumentation) is a major surgical intervention. The surgeon may choose a posterior, anterior, or thoracoabdominal approach to accomplish the procedure, depending on the location and severity of the defect. The posterior approach requires the patient to be in the prone position. Scoliosis of the lower thoracic to upper lumbar spine may necessitate a thoracoabdominal incision and require the patient to be placed in a semilateral position. Scoliosis exclusively of the thoracic spine requires the patient to be placed in the lateral decubitus position.

Entry into the thoracic cavity necessitates placement of a double-lumen endobronchial tube so the ipsilateral lung can be deflated to facilitate visualization of the thoracic spine. Intubation may be difficult at best if the patient has a severe deformity. If the deformity has already produced significant cardiopulmonary compromise, the nurse anesthetist should carefully evaluate the anesthetic plan, specifically because the patient's cardiopulmonary reserves may already be extremely poor to nonexistent, and a more prudent course of action may be an awake, fiberoptic intubation. Endobronchial intubation can result in a host of untoward sequelae, including tracheal dissection and pneumomediastinum, right mainstem bronchus occlusion, and bronchial tree rupture or tear. For surgical correction of scoliosis by spinal fusion with anterior release, the patient is placed in the lateral decubitus position for the thoracotomy incision and requires endobronchial intubation. Depending on the direction of curvature of the thoracic spine, the heart may necessarily be manipulated, which may produce cardiac dysrhythmias.

With the large incision and complex dissection required for the multilevel spinal fusions and instrumentation needed to surgically correct the scoliosis, the nurse anesthetist should be prepared for a significant volume of blood loss. Blood transfusion is virtually ensured during the course of the procedure. Patient concerns about receiving a blood transfusion may be reduced by being encouraged to make an autologous blood donation of 1 to 2 units to the blood bank before the anticipated surgery date, assuming there are no conflicts with the patient's religious convictions. The nurse anesthetist can be instrumental in reducing the blood loss by maintaining the patient as nearly as possible at normothermia, using deliberate hypotension, and using the cell saver to minimize net blood loss incurred during the procedure.

As described, laparoscopic principles and techniques are beginning to be applied more frequently to spinal-fusion surgery. Spinal fusion via laparoscopy provides the surgeon with enhanced visualization of the surgical site, reduces operative time once the surgeon and staff have acquired and are comfortable with the necessary skills, results in greatly reduced trauma to the surrounding soft tissues, produces dramatically less blood loss, reduces recovery and rehabilitation time, greatly reduces medical costs, contributes to an earlier return to preinjury level of activity, and is aesthetically more pleasing to the patient. It is important to compensate for any hypercarbia that may accompany insufflation of carbon dioxide, particularly during long procedures.

Sudden, dramatic, unanticipated, sustained hypotension requires rapid intervention and assessment of cause. The surgeon should be informed, and together a plan to rapidly determine the cause and initiate appropriate effective treatment measures may be instituted. Because of the close proximity to the spinal column, injury to the aorta can occur during surgery on the thoracic or lumbar spine. In addition to aortic injury, the inferior vena cava, iliac vessels, and common femoral vessels may be damaged as a result of traction during laparoscopic spinal procedures.[81] Injury to these vascular structures can be a truly emergent situation. If the patient is in the prone position, rapid closure of the surgical wound is imperative so the patient can be repositioned to facilitate repair to the damaged vessel. Large volumes of crystalloids, colloids, or blood transfusions may be required to maintain the patient's circulating blood volume and perfusion pressures while access to and repair of the injured vessel is achieved. If the patient has not been crossmatched, the worst-case scenario may involve transfusion of O-negative blood until crossmatched, banked blood becomes available.

FOOT AND ANKLE SURGERY

The feet and ankles are the supports on which the remainder of the body rests. Surgical correction of maladies and deformities of the feet and ankles falls under the scope of practice of two specialists: the orthopedic surgeon and the doctor of podiatric medicine (DPM), or podiatrist. Both of these specialists are highly skilled in the surgical correction of the multitude of problems that occur with the feet and ankles.

The most commonly performed procedures on the ankle involve surgical repair of ankle fractures and fusion of the ankle joint. The Achilles tendon is also a frequent focus of surgery, particularly on more physically active individuals. The most widely known surgical procedures on the feet are bunionectomy (with or without fusion), correction of hammertoe deformities (with or without fusion), and plantar fasciotomy (either open or endoscopic).

Open repair of ankle fractures is usually accomplished using plates and screws to hold the bone fragment in proper alignment until the fragments grow back together. Ankle fusion (arthrodesis) is performed for a multitude of medical reasons and may involve two or three bones being fused together to provide pain relief and greater joint stability. Incisions are usually made on both the medial and lateral aspects of the ankle joint to allow for optimal surgical access to the involved bones. The fracture is reduced, after which a plate is placed across the fracture site or sites. Holes are drilled with the plate acting as the template, and screws are placed into these holes. For ankle fusions, incisions are typically made across the medial and lateral aspects of the joint, and Kirschner wires or screws are used to fuse the appropriate bones in place. The incisions are closed, and some type of inflexible stabilizing device is applied (e.g., cast or plaster splints or ambulatory boot) while under anesthesia. Pneumatic tourniquets are almost always used to keep blood loss at a minimum and provide a clear surgical field.

Bunion deformity usually involves the first, or great, toe. Incision is made along the anterior surface from about midtoe across the metatarsophalangeal joint. The bony deformity is excised. Depending on the variation of the bunionectomy procedure chosen, excision of the bony deformity may be the totality of the procedure, or the angular deformity may be corrected with a screw or Kirschner-wire fusion.

Hammertoe deformity correction involves incision of the anterior surface of the malformed toe or toes. The incision crosses the joint containing the bony deformity. The surgeon dissects down to the joint and excises the bony deformity. Depending on the severity of the deformity, the interphalangeal joint may be fused by inserting a Kirschner wire.

Plantar fasciotomy is indicated for severe foot pain during or after ambulating or on arising after sleep. Pain results from chronic plantar fasciitis that has not responded to conservative therapy. Open fasciotomy is accomplished via a small incision along the posterior surface of the calcaneus. The plantar fascia is incised to relieve the tension across the plantar arch. Endoscopic plantar fasciotomy is accomplished via two "miniature" incisions, one medial and one lateral, at the beginning of the plantar arch. A small trocar is inserted through these incisions. The sheath of the trocar is slotted to allow visualization of the plantar fascia with the endoscope. The full thickness of the plantar fascia is incised, and the skin incisions are closed.

Anesthetic Management

Patients scheduled for foot or ankle surgery are excellent candidates for regional anesthesia. Most surgical procedures on the foot or ankle can be accomplished within a 2-hour time frame, often on an outpatient basis. Spinal anesthesia provides sufficient surgical anesthesia to allow completion of most procedures. However, the postanesthesia recovery phase may be unacceptably long and require an overnight stay in the hospital or outpatient facility, which may be unacceptable to the patient.

Nerve blocks are especially effective for surgical procedures on the foot or ankle. Posterior tibial nerve block, Mayo blockade, and Bier block are examples of blocks that are effective for foot and ankle procedures. Intravenous sedation by either continuous infusion or intermittent bolus can provide amnesia and minimize or eliminate any anxiety the patient may have. The surgeon can inject the surgical site with long-acting local anesthetic (e.g., bupivacaine) to maintain the patient's comfort immediately and for several hours postoperatively.

FOREARM AND HAND SURGERY

Surgical procedures on the hand or forearm may be precipitated by violent trauma resulting in complex or dislocated fractures to the bones of the forearm, hand, or fingers, or may be performed to alleviate numbness of the hand resulting from compression of the nerves of the forearm or wrist, as in carpal tunnel syndrome. Procedures on the fingers and hand are often relatively quick, requiring 1 hour or less to complete, whereas surgical correction of complex or dislocated fractures of the forearm may require considerable instrumentation and time to complete. For virtually all surgical procedures of the hand and forearm, the pneumatic tourniquet is used.

Anesthetic Management

Patients scheduled for surgical procedures on the forearm or hand are well-suited candidates for regional anesthesia. Axillary blockade and Bier block provide excellent surgical anesthesia for most surgical procedures of the forearm and hand anticipated to require 1 hour or less to accomplish.

For procedures that may require considerable amounts of time to accomplish—those precipitated by traumatic injury, such as complex, comminuted fractures or reconstruction of the vascular and nerve structures of the hand or forearm, for example—the better anesthetic choice may be general anesthesia. Tourniquet pain becomes an issue with longer procedures if regional anesthesia is chosen. Also, for the patient requiring surgery as the result of traumatic injury, the issue of the patient's nothing-by-mouth (NPO) status becomes important. Frequently, trauma patients have eaten or ingested liquids close to the time of the injury. Alcohol ingestion may be involved as well. For these reasons, rapid-sequence induction of general anesthesia may be a more appropriate anesthetic course.

ARTHRITIC SYNDROMES

Of the many arthritic syndromes, two are especially disconcerting: rheumatoid arthritis (RA) and ankylosing spondylitis (AS). Both of these arthritic conditions extend beyond the primary affliction to the skeletal system and orthopedic medicine.

Rheumatoid arthritis is a chronic inflammatory process that primarily affects the synovial tissues. Even though RA has been investigated for decades, the etiology of the disease has yet to be delineated. Diagnosis of this malady is not made on the basis of a single biochemical, histologic, or immunologic entity; rather, it is confirmed by a series of symptomatologic entities listed in Box 41-7.[83] Four criteria must be present (symptoms A through D) for a minimum of 6 weeks. One of the characteristics of RA is its spontaneous exacerbations and remissions. The chronic

American College of Rheumatology Criteria for Diagnosis of Rheumatoid Arthritis

A. One hour or more of morning stiffness around joints
B. Simultaneous swelling or presence of fluid at three or more joint areas, including the right and left proximal interphalangeal (PIP), metacarpophalangeal (MCP), wrist, elbow, knee, ankle, and metatarsophalangeal joints
C. Swelling or fluid in at least one wrist, MCP, or PIP joint area
D. Symmetric swelling or presence of fluid simultaneously at right and left target joint areas listed in criterion B
E. Subcutaneous rheumatoid nodules
F. The presence of serum rheumatoid factor determined by a laboratory test in which less than 5% of the normal control population is positive
G. Posteroanterior hand and wrist radiographs demonstrating erosions or unequivocal bony decalcifications

Classifications of Pulmonary Disease in Rheumatoid Arthritis Patients

Pleural effusion
Intrapulmonary nodules
Rheumatoid pneumoconiosis (Caplan syndrome)
Interstitial lung disease
Vasculitis
Obliterative bronchiolitis
Upper lobe fibrosis
Pulmonary infections
Bronchogenic carcinoma

inflammatory processes at work destroy and remodel the articular surfaces, weaken surrounding soft tissues, and contribute to joint subluxation and muscle contractures.

Of particular concern are the effects of RA on the cervical spine, temporomandibular joint, larynx, and pulmonary system. Deposition of rheumatoid nodules causes inflammation of the intervertebral disks and dura, which is expressed as atlantoaxial joint subluxation. The synovium of the temporomandibular joint is also affected by RA and can result in severe limitation of joint range of motion. The cricoarytenoid joints are common sites for rheumatoid nodule deposition. The resultant chronic synovitis may cause fixation of the vocal cords in adduction and airway obstruction. Finally, RA is associated with nine forms of pulmonary disease, including pleural effusion, interstitial lung disease, obliterative bronchiolitis, and vasculitis (Box 41-8).

Ankylosing spondylitis is also a chronic inflammatory process. The primary target is the spinal column and surrounding soft tissues. The progressive nature of AS means the spine can be injured by seemingly inconsequential trauma. Patients with AS also experience cardiac valvular dysfunction, conduction delays, bundle branch blocks, and restrictive lung disease.

Anesthetic Management

The primary concern when caring for a patient with either RA or AS is the patient's airway. The mobility of the patient's cervical spine must be meticulously evaluated during the preoperative interview. Any neurologic symptoms that occur during movement of the cervical spine must be thoroughly documented at that time. As a result of RA or AS, cervical mobility may be

severely restricted; therefore, the patient may prove to be extremely difficult to intubate. Because of the high risk to these patients from cervical-spine manipulation during direct laryngoscopy for tracheal intubation, awake fiberoptic intubation may be the safer course of action. The prudent anesthetic course may also include positioning the patient such that neurologic symptoms remain absent before induction of general anesthesia. The cervical spine must be neutrally positioned throughout any surgical procedure, during emergence, and during transfer to the postanesthesia care unit. Regional anesthesia is a safe approach to extremity surgery in these patients.[84,85]

SUMMARY

Orthopedic surgical procedures allow and require the nurse anesthetist to be proficient in more general and regional anesthetic techniques than in any other specialty. The patient's health history and acceptability of various anesthetic techniques, the proposed surgery and its duration, the patient's intraoperative position, and the need for postoperative pain management are important considerations in the planning and preparation for a safe and comfortable outcome. The anesthetic plan must adapt to the needs of the patient and the proposed surgery rather than expect the patient to adapt to one anesthetic technique. The nurse anesthetist would do better to anticipate problems and avoid them than have to treat them when they occur.

The innovations of orthopedic surgical procedures over the past 20 to 30 years have provided opportunities and challenges. Many procedures are now performed with the aid of the arthroscope in same-day surgery, and anesthesia practice has adapted by introducing short-acting anesthetic agents with fewer residual side effects and by providing various regional anesthesia techniques. Trauma and high-profile surgeries corresponding to the increasing geriatric population have challenged nurse anesthetists to adapt techniques that reduce complications and provide postoperative pain management.

REFERENCES

1. Barnhart CL, Barnhart RK, eds. The World Book Dictionary. Vol 2. Chicago: World Book; 1990:1468.
2. Aker J. Pneumatic tourniquet application in the perioperative period. Curr Rev Nurse Anesth. 1997;20:1-8.
3. Estersohn HS, Sourifman HA. The minimum effective mid-thigh tourniquet pressure. J Foot Surg. 1982;21:281-284.
4. Denny-Brown D, Brenner C. Paralysis of nerve induced by direct pressure and by tourniquet. Arch Neurol Psychiatry. 1944;51:1-26.
5. Cole F. Tourniquet pain. Anesth Analg. 1952;31:63-64.
6. Patterson S, Klenerman L. The effect of pneumatic tourniquets on the ultrastructure of skeletal muscle. J Bone Joint Surg Br. 1979;61:178-183.
7. Klenerman L, Hulands GH. Tourniquet pressures for the lower limbs. J Bone Joint Surg Br. 1979;61:124-127.
8. Klenerman L. Tourniquet time. how long? Hand. 1980;12:231-234.
9. MacIver MB, Tanelian DL. Activation of C fibers by metabolic perturbations associated with tourniquet ischemia. Anesthesiology. 1992;76:617-623.

10. Wakai A et al. Pneumatic tourniquets in extremity surgery. *J Am Acad Orthop Surg.* 2001;9(:5):345-351.
11. Strichartz GR, Zimmerman M. An explanation for pain originating from tourniquets during regional anesthesia. *Reg Anesth.* 1984;94:44-48.
12. Bridenbaugh PO et al. Addition of glucose to bupivacaine in spinal anesthesia increases incidences of tourniquet pain. *Anesth Analg.* 1986; 65:1181-1185.
13. Bailey PD, Tobin JR. Evaluation of the patient with neuromuscular and skeletal disease. In: Longnecker DE et al, eds. *Anesthesiology.* New York: McGraw-Hill; 2008:156-172.
14. Lowire A et al. Effect of a eutectic mixture of local anesthetic agents (EMLA) on tourniquet pain in volunteers. *Br J Anaesth.* 1989;63:751-753.
15. Bourke SL et al. Respiratory responses associated with release of intraoperative tourniquet. *Anesth Analg.* 1989;69:541-544.
16. Hofmann AA, Wyatt RWB. Fatal pulmonary embolism following tourniquet inflation: a case report. *J Bone Joint Surg Am.* 1985;67:633-634.
17. Pollard BJ et al. Fatal pulmonary embolism secondary to limb exsanguination. *Anesthesiology.* 1983;58:373-374.
18. Martin G et al. Anesthesia for orthopedic surgery. In: Longnecker DE et al, eds. *Anesthesiology.* New York: McGraw-Hill; 2008:1541-1557.
19. Tountas CP, Bergman RA. Tourniquet ischemia: ultrastructural and histochemical observations of ischemic human muscle and of monkey muscle and nerve. *J Hand Surg.* 1977;2:31-37.
20. Kam PC et al. The arterial tourniquet: pathophysiological consequences and anaesthetic implications. *Anaesthesia.* 2001;56(:6):534-545.
21. Hoshowsky VM. Surgical positioning. *Orthop Nurs.* 1998;17:55-65.
22. Shapiro BA et al: *Clinical Application of Blood Gases.* 3rd ed. Chicago: Year Book Medical; 1982:55-66.
23. O'Brien TJ, Ebert TJ. Physiologic changes associated with the supine position. In: Martin JT, Warner MA, eds. *Positioning in Anesthesia and Surgery.* 3rd ed. Philadelphia: Saunders; 1997:27-36.
24. West JB et al. Distribution of blood flow in isolated lung: relation to vascular and alveolar pressures. *J Appl Physiol.* 1964;19:713.
25. Froese AB, Bryan CA. Effects of anesthesia and paralysis on diaphragmatic mechanics in man. *Anesthesiology.* 1974;41:242-255.
26. Fratacci MD et al. Diaphragmatic shortening after thoracic surgery in humans. Effects of mechanical ventilation and thoracic epidural anesthesia. *Anesthesiology.* 1993;79:654-655.
27. Rehder K et al. General anesthesia and the lung. *Am Rev Respir Dis.* 1975;112:541-563.
28. Vellody VP et al. Effects of body position change on thoracoabdominal motion. *J Appl Physiol.* 1978;45:581-589.
29. Klingstedt C et al. The influence of body position and differential ventilation on lung dimensions and atelectasis formation in anesthetized man. *Acta Anaesthesiol Scand.* 1990;34:315-322.
30. Lawson NW, Meyer DJ Jr. Lateral positions. In: Martin JT, Warner MA, eds. *Positioning in Anesthesia and Surgery.* 3rd ed. Philadelphia: Saunders; 1997: 127-152.
31. Courington FW, Little DM Jr. The role of posture in anesthesia. *Clin Anesth.* 1968;3:23-54.
32. Campos JH. Lung isolation techniques. *Anesthesiol Clin North America.* 2001;19:455-474.
33. Martin JT. The ventral decubitus (prone) positions. In: Martin JT, Warner MA, eds. *Positioning in Anesthesia and Surgery.* 3rd ed. Philadelphia: Saunders; 1997:155-195.
34. Batson OV. Function of the vertebral veins and their role in the spread of metastases. *Ann Surg.* 1940;112:138.
35. Toyota S, Amaki Y. Hemodynamic evaluation of the prone position by transesophageal echocardiography. *J Clin Anesth.* 1998;10(:1):32-35.
36. Backofen JE, Schauble JF. Hemodynamic changes with prone positioning during general anesthesia. *Anesth Analg.* 1985;64:194.
37. Toole JF. Effects of change of head, limb, and body position on cephalic circulation. *N Engl J Med.* 1968;279:307-311.
38. *Dorland's Pocket Medical Dictionary.* 27th ed. Philadelphia: Saunders; 2004:88.
39. Phillips BB. General principles of arthroscopy. In: Canala ST, ed. *Campbell's Operative Orthopaedics.* Vol 3. 10th ed. St Louis: Mosby; 2003:2497-2514.
40. Miller GK. Operative arthroscopy into the next century. *Compr Ther.* 1998;24:383-387.
41. Long JS. Shoulder arthroscopy. *Orthop Nurs.* 1996;15:21-31.
42. Baker CL, Brooks AA. Arthroscopy of the elbow. *Clin Sports Med.* 1996;15: 261-281.
43. Phillips BB. Arthroscopy of lower extremity. In: Canala ST, ed. *Campbell's Operative Orthopaedics.* Vol 3. 10th ed. St Louis: Mosby; 2003:2515-2612.
44. Small NC. Complications in arthroscopy: the knee and other joints. Committee on Complications of the Arthroscopy Association of North America. *Arthroscopy.* 1986;2:253-258.
45. Small NC. Complications in arthroscopic surgery performed by experienced arthroscopists. *Arthroscopy.* 1988;4:215-221.
46. Blumenthal S et al. Severe airway obstruction during arthroscopic shoulder surgery. *Anesthesiology.* 2003;99:1455-1456.
47. Lee HC et al. Subcutaneous emphysema, pneumomediastinum, and potentially life threatening tension pneumothorax. *Chest.* 1992;101:1265-1267.
48. Nagelhout JJ. Respiratory anatomy, physiology, and pathophysiology. In: Nagelhout JJ, Zaglanicnzy KL, eds. *Nurse Anesthesia.* 3rd ed. St. Louis: Saunders; 2005:511-573.
49. Higgins TL, Yared J-P. Postoperative respiratory care. In: Kaplan JA, ed. *Kaplan's Cardiac Anesthesia.* 5th ed. Philadelphia: Saunders; 2006:1087-1102.
50. Harkess JW, Daniels AU. Introduction and overview (arthroplasty). In: Canala ST, ed. *Campbell's Operative Orthopaedics.* Vol 1. 10th ed. St Louis: Mosby; 2003:223-242.
51. Sharrock NE et al. Anesthesia for orthopedic surgery. In: Miller RD, ed. *Anesthesia.* 6th ed. Philadelphia: Churchill Livingstone; 2005:2409-2434.
52. Scilco TP, Ranawat C. The use of spinal anesthesia for total hip replacement. *J Bone Joint Surg.* 1975;57:173-177.
53. Thornburn R et al. Spinal and general anesthesia in total hip replacement: frequency of deep vein thrombosis. *Br J Anaesth.* 1980;52:1117-1121.
54. Keith I. Anaesthesia and blood loss in total hip replacement. *Anaesthesia.* 1977;32:444-450.
55. Modig J et al. Thromboembolism after total hip replacement: role of epidural and general anesthesia. *Anesth Analg.* 1983;62:174-180.
56. Modig J et al. Comparative influences of epidural and general anesthesia on deep vein thrombosis and pulmonary embolism after total hip replacement. *Acta Chir Scand.* 1981;147:125-130.
57. Fallon KM et al. Fat embolization and fatal cardiac arrest during hip arthroplasty with methylmethacrylate. *Can J Anaesth.* 2001;48:626-629.
58. Dandy DJ. Fat embolism following prosthetic replacement of the femoral head. *Injury.* 1971;3:85-88.
59. Sevitt S. Fat embolism in patients with fractured hips. *BMJ.* 1972;2:257-262.
60. Anderson KH. Air aspirated from the venous system during total hip replacement. *Anaesthesia.* 1983;38:1175-1178.
61. Evans RD et al. Air embolism during total hip replacement: comparison of two surgical techniques. *Br J Anaesth.* 1989;62:243-247.
62. Ngai SH et al. Air embolism during total hip arthroplasties. *Anesthesiology.* 1974;40:405-407.
63. Deuschle JA, Romeo AA. Understanding shoulder arthroplasty. *Orthop Nurs.* 1998;17:7-15.
64. Neer CS et al. Recent experience in total shoulder replacement. *J Bone Joint Surg.* 1982;64:319-337.
65. Gartsman GM et al. Modular shoulder arthroplasty. *J Shoulder Elbow Surg.* 1997;6:333-339.
66. Wilde AH. Shoulder arthroplasty: what is it good for and how good is it? In: Matsen FA et al. *The Shoulder: A Balance of Mobility and Stability.* Rosemont, IL: American Academy of Orthopedic Surgeons; 1992:459-481.
67. Muntz JE. The risk of venous thromboembolism in non-large-joint surgeries. *Orthopedics.* 2003;26:s237-242.
68. Rucker S et al. Perioperative care of patients undergoing spinal stabilization with internal fixation. *Today's OR Nurse.* 1994;16:8-13.
69. Lestini WF. "Cage" technology revolutionizes approach to spinal fusion surgery. *N C Med J.* 1988;59:101-104.
70. Wener BK, Fraser RD. Spine update: lumbar interbody cages. *Spine.* 1998;23:634-640.
71. Zdeblick T, Phillips FM. Interbody cage devices. *Spine.* 2003;28(:15S):S2-S7.
72. Kulkami AG, Diwan AD. Prosthetic lumbar disc replacement for degenerative disc disease. *Neurology India.* 2005;53(:4):499-505.
73. Bajnoczy S. Artifical disc replacement—evolutionary treatment for degenerative disc disease. *AORN J.* 2005;82(2):191-206.
74. DiMartino A et al. Nucleus pulposus replacement: basic science and indications for clinical use. *Spine.* 2005;30(16S):S16-S22.
75. Guyer RD, Ohnmeiss DD. Intervertebral disc prostheses. *Spine.* 2003;28(15S):S15-S23.
76. Christie SD et al. Dynamic interspinous process technology. *Spine.* 2005;30(16S):S73-S78.
77. Freeman BL. Scoliosis and kyphosis. In: Canala ST, ed. *Campbell's Operative Orthopaedics.* Vol 2. 10th ed. St Louis: Mosby; 2003:1751-1954.
78. Hellman EW et al. Clinical outcome after fusion of the thoracic or lumbar spine in the adult patient. *Orthop Clin North Am.* 1998;29:859-869.
79. Obenchain TG. Laparoscopic lumbar discectomy. *J Laparoendosc Surg.* 1991;1:145-149.
80. Mack MJ et al. Application of thoracoscopy for diseases of the spine. *Ann Thorac Surg.* 1993;56:736-738.
81. Regan JJ, Guyer RD. Endoscopic techniques in spinal surgery. *Clin Orthop Relat Res.* 1997;335:122-139.

82. Bostman O et al. Blood loss, operating time, and positioning of the patient in lumbar disc surgery. *Spine*. 1990;15:360-363.

83. Arnett FC et al. The American Rheumatism Association 1987 revised criteria for the classification of rheumatoid arthritis. *Arthritis Rheum*. 1988;31: 315-324.

84. Brill S et al. Bier's block; 100 years old and still going strong! *Acta Anaesthesiol Scand*. 2004;48:117-122.

85. Holmes C. Intravenous regional blockade. In: Cousins MJ, Bridenbaugh PO, eds. *Neural Blockade in Clinical Anesthesia and Management of Pain*. 3rd ed. Philadelphia: Lippincott 1998:395-409.

CHAPTER 42

THE IMMUNE SYSTEM AND ANESTHESIA

Michael P. O'Donnell

The field of immunology addresses the body's defense mechanisms against pathogens, such as bacteria and viruses, that have the potential to trigger tissue injury and disease. Protection from infection and disease depends on the functions of particular leukocytes, the phagocytes and lymphocytes, with the assistance of auxiliary cells such as mast cells, basophils, and platelets.[1-3] Immune responses involve not only these various cell types, but also soluble mediator molecules secreted by the cells (Table 42-1). Lymphocytes secrete antibodies or cytokines, whereas auxiliary cells secrete proinflammatory mediators, one purpose of which is to attract leukocytes to a site of infection or tissue injury.

Two components of immunity provide defense against invading pathogens: the innate immune system and the adaptive (acquired) immune system. This chapter highlights immune system physiology and pathology, including the effects of human immunodeficiency virus (HIV) on the immune system, with particular consideration of the effects of anesthesia on immune function.

THE IMMUNE SYSTEM

Innate Immune System

Innate immunity is nonspecific, that is, it provides defense against a very large number of pathogens, rather than being directed at one specific microorganism or type of microorganism. Components of innate immunity include physical barriers such as the skin and lung alveoli, the pathogen-hostile environment of the gastrointestinal tract, leukocytes whose primary function is phagocytosis and destruction of invading pathogens, and soluble molecules such as interferons and the complement system.[1-3]

Phagocytes

Polymorphonuclear neutrophils (PMNs) and macrophages are the primary phagocytes of the immune system. Polymorphonuclear neutrophils and monocytes, the cellular precursors of tissue macrophages, are generated from pluripotent hematopoietic stem cells in the bone marrow (Figure 42-1). Both cell types are continually released to the blood, and many are stored in the marrow until mobilized for defense. Chemical substances known as *colony-stimulating factors* that enter the circulation from an area of infection are transported to the marrow to stimulate production and release of PMNs and monocytes. Colony-stimulating factors are members of the cytokine superfamily, a very large collection of peptides that regulate the activity of immune system cells (Box 42-1).

After release from bone marrow, PMNs and monocytes circulate for a short time (<24 hours) in the blood before moving either directly across, or through pores between, venule endothelial cells to enter tissues. This process is known as *diapedesis*. Transendothelial movement of PMNs and monocytes and their subsequent movement within tissue to a site of inflammation are not random events, but rather are orchestrated by numerous chemotactic substances that include chemokines produced by endothelial cells, bacterial and viral components, and products C3a and C5a of the blood complement system (Figure 42-2). Production of endothelial-cell chemokines and adhesion molecules, which permit leukocytes to "stick" to the endothelium prior to diapedesis, is stimulated by proinflammatory cytokines, in particular tumor necrosis factor alpha (TNF-α) produced by activated macrophages (Figure 42-3).

The primary function of PMNs and macrophages is phagocytosis of pathogens such as bacteria and viruses. In this process, the phagocyte engulfs and destroys the foreign agent. Of critical importance is the ability of the phagocyte to distinguish between what is foreign and what is self. To this end, phagocytes have receptors that recognize carbohydrate and lipid moieties, known as *pathogen-associated molecular patterns* (PAMPs), present on cell surfaces of many pathogens but typically not on cells of the host. An example of a microbial PAMP is lipopolysaccharide in the cell walls of gram-negative bacteria. Phagocyte recognition of PAMPs permits the phagocyte to bind directly to the pathogen.

Phagocyte selectivity can also be provided by the process of opsonization, in which serum components bind to the pathogen and permit indirect recognition by phagocytes. Antibodies directed against a pathogen (and produced as part of acquired immunity) act as opsonins by binding to the pathogen and subsequently to antibody receptors on the phagocyte cell membrane (Figure 42-4). Alternatively, the complement product C3b may act as an opsonin, with subsequent binding of C3b to its receptors on phagocyte cell membranes. Phagocyte binding to a pathogen is followed by endocytosis of the pathogen and its intracellular destruction by lysosomal enzymes and products of the phagocyte respiratory burst, which include superoxide ion, hydrogen peroxide, and nitric oxide (Figure 42-5).

Although some macrophages are mobile and migrate through tissues in response to chemotactic signals, many are fixed within tissues for long periods of time (resident macrophages) as part of the mononuclear phagocyte system (also called the *reticuloendothelial system*; Figure 42-6). This system includes the network of monocytes, mobile macrophages, and fixed macrophages that provides phagocytic function in body tissues. The resident macrophages are particularly important in those tissues potentially exposed to large amounts of pathogens, that is, skin, lymph nodes, lung alveoli, liver sinusoids, and the spleen. When these macrophages encounter a pathogen, a number of responses are

TABLE **42-1**	Cellular Components of Immunity
Components	**Functions**
Phagocytes	
Polymorphonuclear neutrophils (PMNs)	Phagocytosis and destruction of microorganisms; contain bactericidal substances and produce bactericidal reactive oxygen molecules
Monocytes	Circulating cells of the mononuclear phagocyte system; after entering tissues, monocytes mature into macrophages
Macrophages	Mobile and fixed tissue cells of the mononuclear phagocyte system; perform phagocytosis and destruction of microorganisms, present antigen to helper T (T_H) cells and secrete cytokines
Eosinophils	Provide defense against parasitic infections and perform phagocytosis of allergen-antibody complexes formed in an allergic response
Lymphocytes	
Natural killer (NK) cells (also called *large granular lymphocytes* [LGLs])	Destruction of virus-infected "self" cells and tumor cells; secrete cytokines
B lymphocytes	Differentiate into plasma cells that secrete antibodies; present antigen to T_H cells
Helper T lymphocytes (T_H cells)	Secrete cytokines that stimulate T_H cell proliferation and activation of B lymphocytes, cytotoxic T lymphocytes, and macrophages
Cytotoxic T lymphocytes (CTLs)	Engage antigen and secrete pore-forming proteins known as *perforins* into foreign cell membrane; secrete granzymes that destroy the targeted cell
Auxiliary Cells	
Mast cells and basophils	Release histamine and other proinflammatory mediators responsible for hyperemia, increased vascular permeability, and pain
Dendritic cells	Present antigen to T_H cells
Platelets	Participate in coagulation and "walling off" areas of inflammation; secrete proinflammatory mediators

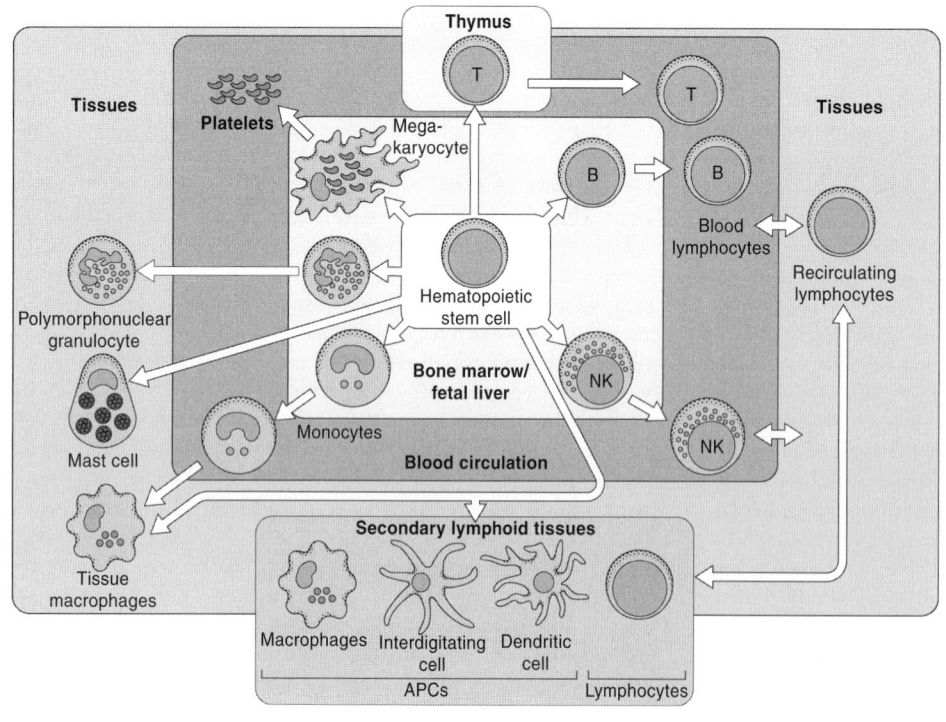

FIGURE **42-1** All immune cells originate from hematopoietic stem cells. Polymorphonuclear cells and monocytes are released from bone marrow to the circulation and then pass into tissues. B cells mature in the fetal liver and postnatal bone marrow, and T cells mature in the thymus gland. These lymphocytes are released into the circulation and pass into tissues. Other cells that originate from hematopoietic stem cells include mast cells, platelets, antigen-presenting cells (APCs), and natural killer (NK) cells. (*From Male D et al. Immunology. 7th ed. Philadelphia: Mosby; 2006:20.*)

Cytokines

- Cytokines are peptide molecules that regulate the action of immune system cells.
- The cytokine superfamily includes tumor necrosis factor-alpha (TNF-α), interleukins, colony-stimulating factors (CSFs), interferons (IFNs), and chemokines (chemotactic cytokines).
- Cytokines act in complex interconnecting networks involving leukocytes, vascular endothelial cells, mast cells, and hematopoietic stem cells to control immune cell proliferation, differentiation, and activation.
- TNF-α, interleukin-1 (IL-1), interleukin-6 (IL-6), and interleukin-12 (IL-12) are important proinflammatory cytokines.
- Interleukin-2 (IL-2) promotes T-lymphocyte proliferation, and interleukin-4 (IL-4) activates B lymphocytes.
- Granulocyte, monocyte, and granulocyte-monocyte CSFs are released from activated macrophages and vascular endothelial cells and stimulate bone marrow to release PMNs and monocytes into the circulation.
- IFNs have antiviral activity and act to suppress spread of viral infection; IFN-α and IFN-β are produced by cells already infected by virus, and IFN-γ is produced by activated NK cells and helper T (T$_H$) cells.
- Chemokines are produced by venule endothelial cells and activated macrophages and act to attract leukocytes to an area of infection.

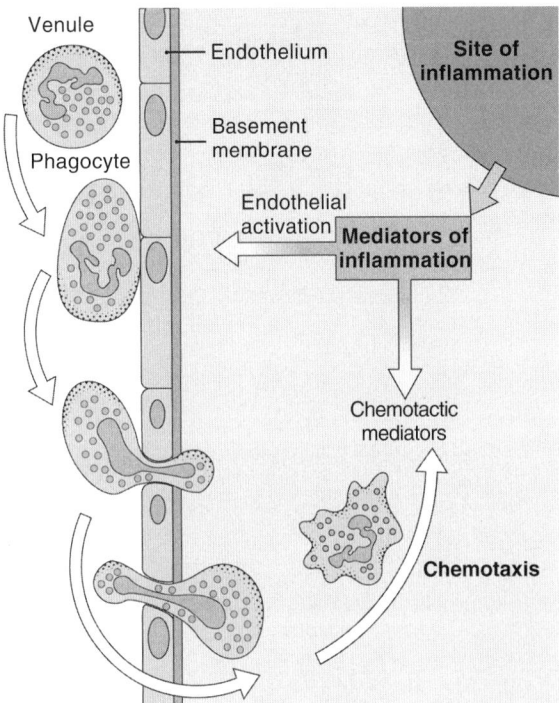

FIGURE **42-2** Infection or tissue injury causes inflammation and release of inflammatory mediators, some of which stimulate chemotaxis of phagocytes to the site of inflammation. Chemokines stimulate phagocytes to stick to the venular endothelium and undergo migration across the vessel wall (diapedesis). Phagocytes then move to the site of inflammation in response to a concentration gradient of chemotactic molecules such as complement product C5a. (*From Male D et al.* Immunology. *7th ed. Philadelphia: Mosby; 2006:16.*)

rapidly set into play: (1) phagocytosis of the pathogen, which provides a first line of defense against infection, (2) secretion of chemotactic mediators that promote infiltration of leukocytes to the site of infection, (3) secretion of colony-stimulating factors that mobilize PMNs and monocytes from the bone marrow, and (4) secretion of proinflammatory cytokines such as TNF-α and interleukin-1 (IL-1). Neutrophil infiltration provides a rapid second line of defense against the pathogen, while a delayed but potent third line of defense occurs as infiltrating monocytes mature into macrophages, and lymphocytes migrate to the area of infection.

Phagocytosis and breakdown of pathogens also permits macrophages to present chemical components (e.g., peptide fragments) of pathogens to cells of the acquired immune system. In this way, macrophages behave as "antigen-presenting cells" to recruit the acquired immune system and greatly augment the body's defense responses to pathogens.

Natural Killer Cells

Another cellular component of the innate immune system is the natural killer (NK) cell. These cells have some morphologic resemblance to lymphocytes, and hence are also referred to as *large granular lymphocytes* (see Table 42-1). NK cells develop in the bone marrow (see Figure 42-1), though the exact mechanism of their differentiation from precursor cells is not well understood. NK cells are potent killers of virus-infected "self" cells. Although leukocytes known as *cytotoxic T lymphocytes* (CTLs; discussed later) destroy many virus-infected cells, some viruses (e.g., herpes simplex virus [HSV]) evade detection by these lymphocytes. Fortunately, NK cells can recognize and kill HSV-infected cells. The mechanism by which NK cells kill virus-infected cells is the same as that by which CTLs destroy

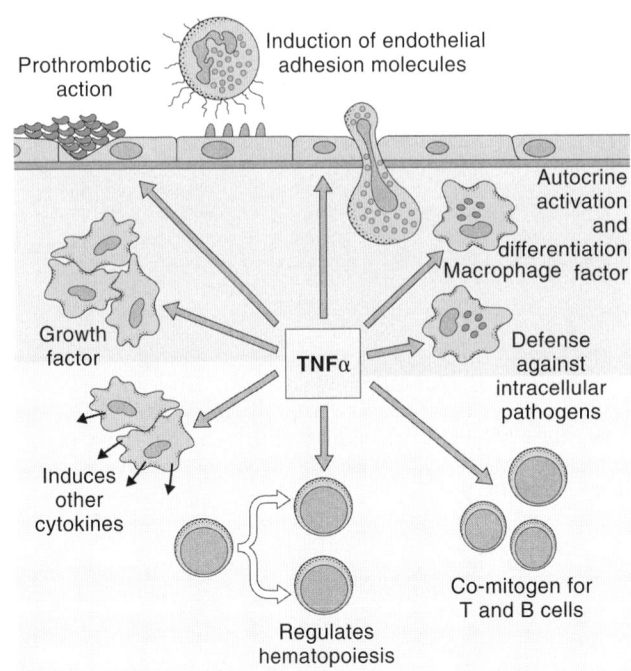

FIGURE **42-3** The cytokine TNF-α plays a central role in inflammation. Among its proinflammatory actions, it promotes clotting, leukocyte adhesion and diapedesis, macrophage activation, and cytokine production by other cells. (*From Male D et al.* Immunology. *7th ed. Philadelphia: Mosby; 2006:130.*)

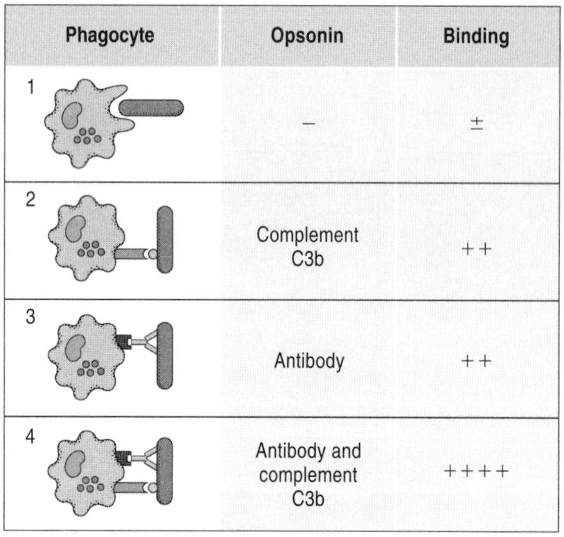

Phagocyte	Opsonin	Binding
1 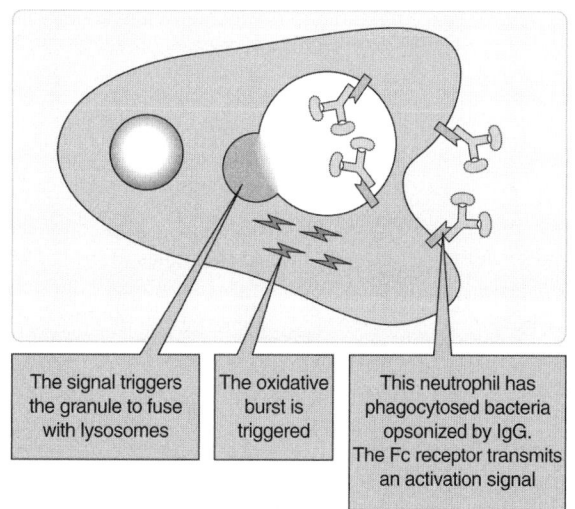	–	±
2	Complement C3b	+ +
3	Antibody	+ +
4	Antibody and complement C3b	+ + + +

FIGURE **42-4** Phagocytes have some intrinsic ability to bind and phagocytize pathogens *(1)*. Phagocytosis is enhanced if the pathogen has been opsonized by complement product C3b *(2)* or antibody *(3)*. Phagocytes have C3b and Fc receptors that bind opsonized pathogens. Phagocytosis is greatly enhanced if both C3b and antibody opsonize the pathogen *(4)*. *(From Male D et al. Immunology. 7th ed. Philadelphia: Mosby; 2006:11.)*

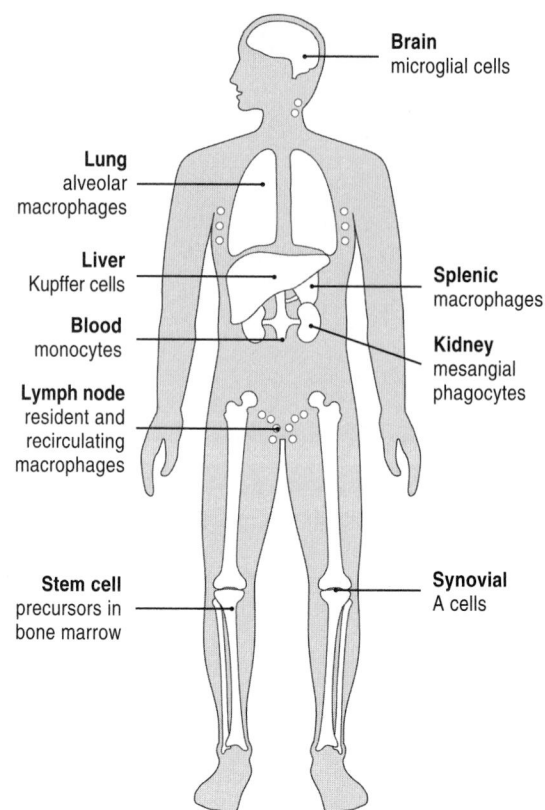

The signal triggers the granule to fuse with lysosomes

The oxidative burst is triggered

This neutrophil has phagocytosed bacteria opsonized by IgG. The Fc receptor transmits an activation signal

FIGURE **42-5** Mechanism of phagocyte killing of pathogen. Opsonized pathogen undergoes phagocytosis, triggering the respiratory (oxidative) burst and fusion of the phagocytic granule with intracellular lysosomes, which digest the pathogen. *(From Nairn R, Helbert M. Immunology for Medical Students. 2nd ed. Philadelphia: Mosby; 2007:155.)*

FIGURE **42-6** Cells of the mononuclear phagocyte system are located in many tissues and organs. These cells all derive from blood monocytes that originate from hematopoietic stem cells in the bone marrow. *(From Male D et al. Immunology. 7th ed. Philadelphia: Mosby; 2006:5.)*

infected self-cells and foreign cells. The NK cell binds to the infected cell, secretes a pore-producing protein known as *perforin* into the infected cell membrane, and then releases cytotoxic proteolytic enzymes into the infected cell.

Natural killer cells have other key functions. They are the main immune cells of the pregnant uterus, where they act to protect the uterus and the fetus from viral infections during pregnancy. NK cells are very important in the surveillance of tumor cells (i.e., transformed self-cells) and can destroy some tumor cells. They also release cytokines that influence the immune response to pathogens. One key cytokine released by NK cells is interferon-gamma (IFN-γ).

Interferons

As noted in Box 42-1, the interferons (IFNs) are cytokines with antiviral activity. Indeed, the name *interferon* derives from the ability of these substances to "interfere" with viral replication. There are two main IFN families: type I and type II. Type I IFNs include IFN-α and IFN-β, which are released from many cell types within hours after initiation of viral infection. These cytokines act on neighboring noninfected cells in a paracrine fashion to prevent spread of the viral infection. In addition, type I IFNs promote proliferation and activation of NK cells, which can bind to and destroy virus-infected cells. Synthetic IFN-α produced by recombinant technology is used to treat hepatitis B infection and some neoplasms. Recombinant IFN-β has been used successfully to reduce nervous system inflammation in some patients with multiple sclerosis.

Type II IFN is IFN-γ released from activated NK and T lymphocytes. Like the type I IFNs, IFN-γ can exert protective antiviral activity in noninfected cells, but more importantly it serves to activate macrophages, promote further NK-cell activity, and stimulate differentiation of T lymphocytes. Synthetic IFN-γ is used for treatment of chronic granulomatous disease (discussed later).

Complement

The complement system is a collection of plasma proteins produced mainly by the liver; it plays a key role in both innate and acquired immunity. When the complement system is activated, a

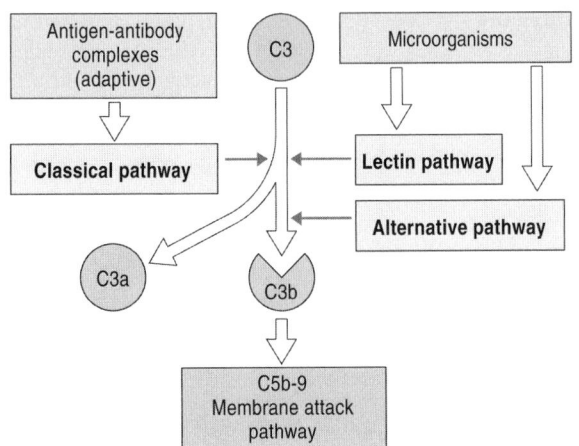

FIGURE **42-7** Three pathways can serve to activate the complement cascade. Antigen-antibody reaction typically activates the classical pathway. The alternative and lectin pathways do not require antibody and are directly activated by chemical groups on the pathogen surface. Thus the alternative and lectin pathways serve innate immunity, whereas the classical pathway is linked to the adaptive immune system. All three pathways convert C3 to C3b as the central event of the complement cascade. C3b can then promote the formation of the membrane attack complex. (*From Male D et al. Immunology. 7th ed. Philadelphia: Mosby; 2006:88.*)

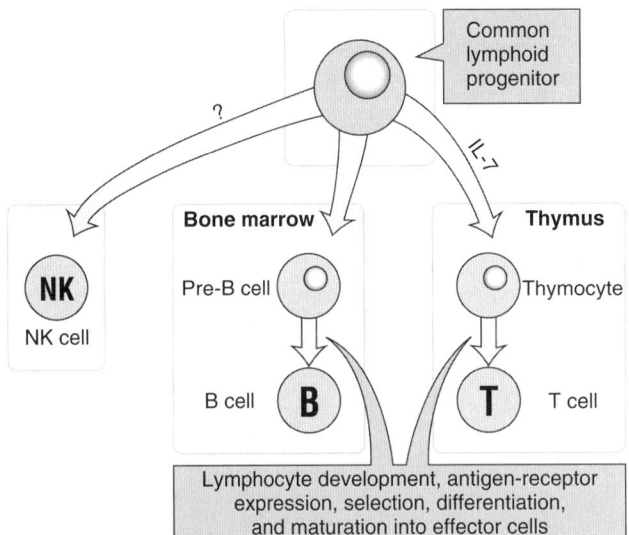

FIGURE **42-8** Development of B cells, T cells, and natural killer (NK) cells from a common lymphoid progenitor. B cells begin maturation in the bone marrow, and T cells mature in the thymus gland. NK cells develop in the bone marrow, though the mechanism of their differentiation is unclear. (*From Naim R, Helbert M. Immunology for Medical Students. 2nd ed. Philadelphia: Mosby; 2007:79.*)

cascade of reactions occurs in which a particular complement component catalyzes the production of the next component in the cascade and so on until the final product is produced. The main proteins of the complement system are labeled C1 through C9. The complement cascade can be triggered by an antigen-antibody reaction that activates C1 (the classical pathway) or by direct microorganism interaction with C3 (the alternative and lectin pathways). In either case, activation of the complement cascade generates products that cause opsonization, chemotaxis, and activation of mast cells and basophils. The final product of the cascade is a complex of five complement factors—C5b6789—that acts as a membrane attack complex by inserting cytolytic pores into pathogen cell membranes (Figure 42-7).

Acquired Immune System

Acquired, or adaptive, immunity is specific, that is, the immune responses are directed against a particular antigen, which is usually a component of a microorganism or foreign tissue.[1-3] In some cases, though, a "self" antigen may generate an autoimmune response that results in tissue injury. By one definition, an antigen is a chemical substance with a molecular weight greater than or equal to 8000 Da, and thus antigens are typically polypeptides or large polysaccharides.[3] Acquired immunity directed against a particular antigen is usually directed at one or more small regions, known as *epitopes*, within the antigen structure.[1-3]

Acquired immunity depends fundamentally on lymphocytes, which comprise approximately 30% of circulating leukocytes. There are two main families of lymphocytes: B lymphocytes (B cells) and T lymphocytes (T cells). B lymphocytes are responsible for humoral immunity, which is provided by soluble antibodies directed against a particular antigen. T lymphocytes are responsible for cell-mediated immunity directed against a particular antigen.

Maturation of lymphocytes occurs in primary lymphoid tissues: the thymus gland, fetal liver, and bone marrow. Initially, some pluripotent hematopoietic stem cells differentiate to become lymphoid progenitor cells, which in turn differentiate to become

either pre-T cells (thymocytes) or pre-B cells (Figures 42-1 and 42-8). Pre-T cells migrate from the marrow to the thymus gland, where they are processed to become mature T cells directed against specific antigens. T-cell maturation is characterized in part by the appearance of T-cell receptors (TCRs) on the cell membranes. Specificity of a particular T cell for an antigen reflects the specificity of its TCRs to recognize and bind that antigen. As a critical part of thymic processing, T cells that recognize and bind self-antigens undergo programmed cell death, known as *apoptosis*, while T cells that recognize foreign antigens expand and migrate to secondary lymphoid tissues—lymph nodes, adenoids and tonsils, submucosal lymph tissue, and the spleen. Literally thousands of different T-cell clones develop in the thymus gland, each clone having TCRs directed against a particular antigen.

Distinct populations of T cells are produced during thymic maturation. The two main populations are CD4+ T cells, also known as *helper T* (T_H) *cells*, and CD8+ T cells, also known as *cytotoxic T lymphocytes* (CTLs). (The abbreviation CD refers to "cluster of differentiation" and indicates a particular cell-membrane marker molecule that can be used to identify the hematopoietic cell type.) Helper T cells can further differentiate into T_H1 and T_H2 cells, based on the nature of an ongoing immune response and cytokines present in the local environment (Figure 42-9). T_H1 cells assist the function of the mononuclear phagocytes, and T_H2 cells assist the function of B lymphocytes.

Development of B cells begins in the fetal and postnatal bone marrow and is completed in secondary lymphoid tissues such as the spleen and lymph nodes (Figure 42-10). As maturation proceeds, B cells that recognize self-antigens undergo apoptosis and are not released into the blood. Those B cells that do leave the bone marrow and migrate to secondary lymphoid tissue acquire two types of immunoglobulin (Ig) molecules on the cell surface, IgM and IgD. These surface-bound Ig molecules are functionally analogous to the TCRs on surfaces of mature T cells, that is, they recognize and bind specific antigens. Other Ig molecules that may be expressed on B-cell surfaces include IgA, IgG, and IgE.

Similar to the situation for T cells, thousands of different B-cell clones are produced, each clone having surface Ig molecules directed against a particular antigen.

Humoral Response to Antigen

When a mature B cell encounters and binds antigen, it proliferates and differentiates into plasma cells that secrete soluble antibodies directed against the antigen. In addition, memory B cells are produced that expand the clone of B cells directed against that antigen. The secreted antibodies are Ig molecules and are members of the gamma globulin fraction of serum proteins. Five main classes of Ig molecules exist, which differ substantially in molecular size and charge: IgA, IgD, IgE, IgG, and IgM. Immunoglobulin G comprises approximately 70% of serum immunoglobulins, whereas IgA and IgM comprise approximately 20% and 10%, respectively. Normally, serum levels of IgD and IgE are very low. Rather, IgD is located primarily on B-cell surfaces, where it serves to bind antigen, while IgE is found primarily on the surfaces of tissue mast cells and circulating basophils and plays a role in hypersensitivity reactions.

An Ig molecule consists of two or more pairs of light chain–heavy chain polypeptide combinations. The variable, or Fab, regions of an Ig molecule are regions in which the amino acid sequence permits specific, high-affinity binding to antigen (hence, the variable regions "vary" in amino acid sequence among antibody molecules). The constant, or Fc, portion of Ig molecules has a relatively "constant" amino acid sequence that can bind to Fc receptors on phagocyte cell membranes (Figure 42-11).

Antibodies promote antigen removal by different mechanisms, including activation of the classical complement pathway, opsonization of a pathogen for phagocytosis, and binding to a pathogen to permit recognition by NK cells. Recently, monoclonal antibodies (mAbs) (i.e., antibodies with very high specificity for antigen)

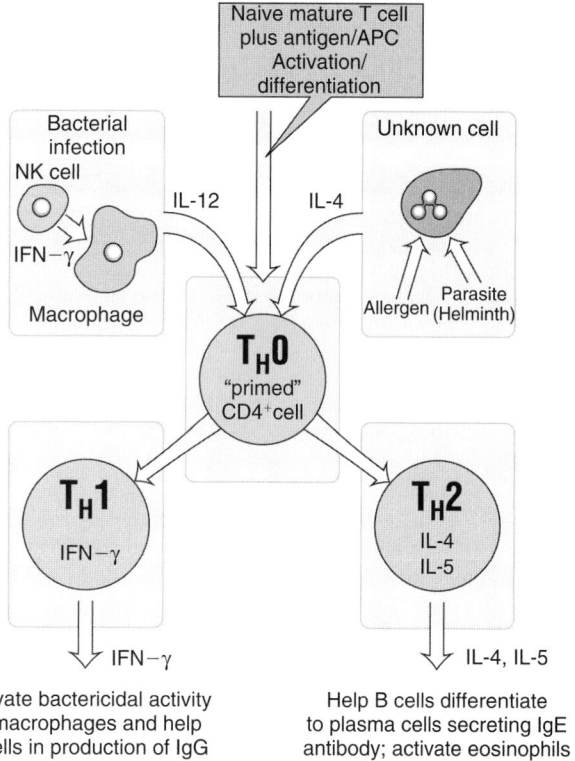

FIGURE **42-9**   Differentiation of T helper subsets. When a naïve, mature T_H cell is presented antigen by an antigen-presenting cell (APC), it becomes "primed" to differentiate into either a T_H1 or T_H2 cell. Preference of differentiation is driven by the nature of the infection and the local cytokine environment. After differentiation, T_H1 cells secrete interferon-gamma (IFN-γ) and promote cellular immunity, and T_H2 cells secrete interleukin (IL)-4 and -5 and promote humoral immunity. (*From Nairn R, Helbert M. Immunology for Medical Students. 2nd ed. Philadelphia: Mosby; 2007:114.*)

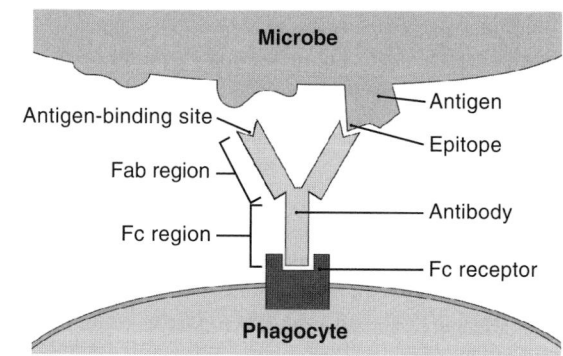

FIGURE **42-11**   The Fab region of an antibody binds to a small portion (epitope) of an antigen on the pathogen surface. The "stem" of the antibody is its Fc region, which binds to phagocyte Fc receptors to promote phagocytosis. (*From Male D et al. Immunology. 7th ed. Philadelphia: Mosby; 2006:11.*)

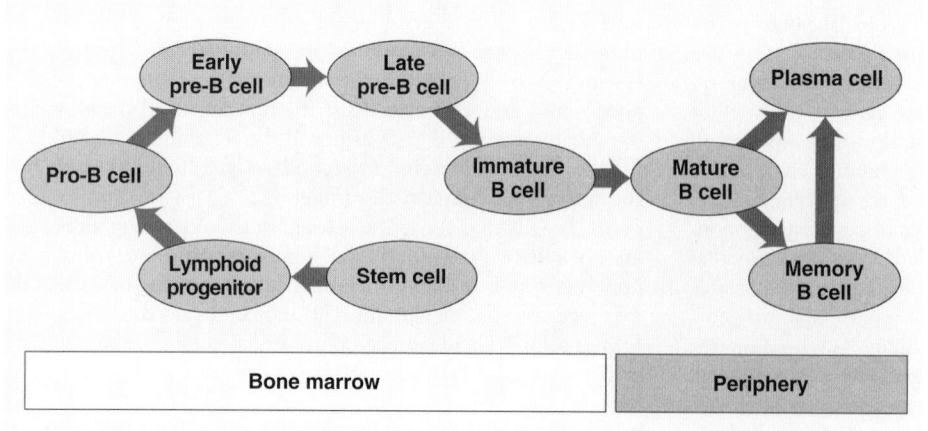

FIGURE **42-10**   Stages of B-cell development. After B-cell release from the bone marrow, maturation is completed in the periphery. When activated by exposure to antigen, mature B cells differentiate into antibody-secreting plasma cells and proliferate to form memory B cells that provide for clonal expansion. (*From Nairn R, Helbert M. Immunology for Medical Students. 2nd ed. Philadelphia: Mosby; 2007:96.*)

have been developed by recombinant technology for treatment of diseases such as rheumatoid arthritis, Crohn's disease, and breast cancer, as well as for other applications (Box 42-2). Adalimumab and infliximab are mAbs directed against the proinflammatory mediator TNF-α.

Antibodies can provide effective defense against toxins or pathogens in the extracellular compartment. However, many pathogens exist within cells of the host, and defense against these pathogens requires a second component of the adaptive immune response—cell-mediated immunity provided by T lymphocytes.

T-Lymphocyte Response to Antigen

Cell-mediated immunity requires "presentation" of antigen to T lymphocytes by infected cells or antigen-presenting cells (APCs)

BOX 42-2

Monoclonal Antibodies

The monoclonal antibodies (mAbs) are genetically engineered immunoglobulins (IgGs) that react with specific molecular targets. They may be part mouse/part human (termed *chimeric* or *humanized*, depending on the degree of mouse Ig sequences) or fully human. In chimeric and humanized mAbs, antigen-recognizing portions of mouse antibodies are joined to the framework of a human IgG molecule.

- **Abciximab:** chimeric mAb against the clotting receptor GpIIb-IIIa on platelets; used to prevent clotting in patients undergoing coronary angioplasty.
- **Adalimumab:** humanized mAb against the cytokine TNF-α used for rheumatoid arthritis.
- **Alemtuzumab:** humanized mAb against an antigen on T and B lymphocytes; used to treat B-cell leukemia.
- **Basiliximab:** chimeric mAb against the receptor for the cytokine interleukin-2 on activated T cells; used in acute rejection of kidney transplants.
- **Daclizumab:** humanized mAb against the receptor for the cytokine interleukin-2 on activated T cells; used in acute rejection of kidney transplants.
- **Gemtuzumab:** humanized mAb against an antigen on leukemia cells; used to treat relapsed acute myeloid leukemia.
- **Infliximab:** chimeric mAb against the cytokine TNF-α; used for rheumatoid arthritis and Crohn's disease.
- **Muromonab (Orthoclone OKT3):** murine mAb to the CD3 antigen of human T cells; that functions as an immunosuppressant in heart, kidney and liver transplants.
- **Omalizumab:** humanized mAb against the binding of IgE to the high-affinity IgE receptor on the surface of mast cells and basophils; used for the treatment of asthma.
- **Palivizumab:** humanized mAb against a protein of respiratory syncytial virus (RSV); used to treat RSV infection in children.
- **Rituximab:** humanized mAb against the cytokine CD20 receptor on B cells; used in non-Hodgkin lymphoma.
- **Satumomab:** conjugate produced from a murine mAb; used for imaging and diagnostics.
- **Trastuzumab:** mAb against HER2; used for breast cancer treatment.

Modified from Mosby's Drug Consult. St Louis: Mosby; 2007; Rang HP et al. Pharmacology. 6th ed. Edinburgh, Scotland: Churchill Livingstone; 2007:773.

---

such as dendritic cells, macrophages, and B lymphocytes. What is actually presented to the T cell is a small portion of the parent antigen that has been processed, or degraded, by the presenting cell. The antigen fragment is presented bound to a major histocompatibility (MHC) molecule on the presenting cell surface. T-cell receptors on T cells directed against the antigen then recognize and bind the antigen-MHC complex (Figure 42-12).

The MHC is a collection of genes that serve immune recognition in all mammals. There are two types of MHC molecules that function in immune recognition. Class I molecules are present on the surfaces of all nucleated cells, and class II molecules are present on the surfaces of APCs. In humans, the MHC is known as the *human leukocyte antigen* (HLA). Three regions, or loci, on the HLA encode for MHC class I molecules found on nucleated cell surfaces. Collectively, these three regions comprise more than 100 genes and are known as *HLA-A, HLA-B,* and *HLA-C.* A separate region on the HLA, known as *HLA-D*, encodes for MHC class II molecules found on APCs. Within this region are three loci, known as *HLA-DP, HLA-DQ,* and *HLA-DR.* A key characteristic of the HLA is the high degree of polymorphism of the MHC molecules for which it encodes. An individual's HLA type (haplotype) is determined by the MHC molecules expressed on that person's cell membranes. Genetic variability in HLA type influences susceptibility to infection and autoimmune disease and rejection of transplanted tissue. Tissue typing prior to organ transplantation involves characterization of the HLA types of donor and recipient to determine if an acceptable "match" is present.

MHC class I molecules present antigen derived from an intracellular pathogen, such as a virus, that has infected the cell. The antigen-MHC class I complex is presented to CTLs, which bind the complex and destroy the infected cell. MHC class II molecules present antigen derived from pathogens that have undergone phagocytosis and subsequent processing. The antigen-class II complex is presented to T_H cells, which function to augment the overall immune response to the antigen. Two subsets of T_H cells, T_H1

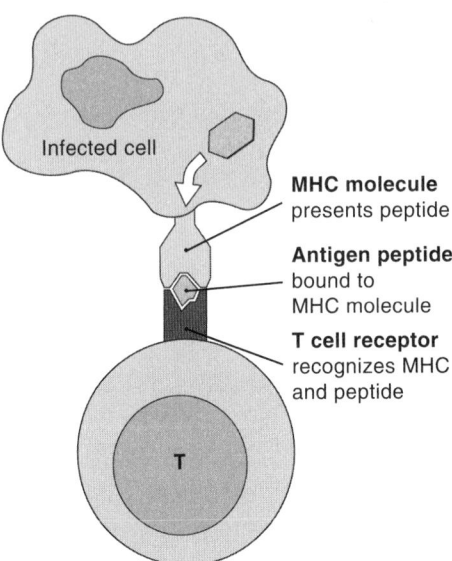

FIGURE 42-12 General mechanism of antigen presentation to T cells. A surface major histocompatibility complex (MHC) molecule presents a peptide portion of pathogen in an infected cell. The T-cell receptor recognizes and binds the MHC molecule/peptide combination. (*From Male D et al. Immunology. 7th ed. Philadelphia: Mosby; 2006:12.*)

and T$_H$2 cells, can be generated in response to antigen presentation (see Figure 42-9). The T$_H$1/T$_H$2 ratio is determined by the nature of the immune response and the local cytokine environment. T$_H$1 cells secrete IFN-γ, which activates mononuclear phagocytes. T$_H$2 cells secrete IL-4 and IL-5, which promote conversion of B lymphocytes to antibody-secreting plasma cells and stimulate mast cells to release inflammatory mediators. Activation of T cells in response to antigen also promotes T-cell production of IL-2, which acts locally to promote T-cell proliferation and augment the immune response to the antigen.

Vaccination

A key characteristic of the immune response to antigen is clonal expansion of specific B and T lymphocytes directed at the antigen. Clonal expansion allows a more rapid and vigorous immune response on subsequent exposure to the antigen. Vaccination is a process that produces acquired immunity against specific diseases by deliberate exposure of an individual to particular antigens. Vaccination against diseases such as typhoid, cholera, pertussis, and influenza is accomplished by administration of dead organisms that have retained their chemical antigens (epitopes), yet cannot cause an actual disease state. Toxoid vaccines are chemical modifications of toxins produced by pathogens such as tetanus and diphtheria. Attenuated microorganisms are mutated pathogens that themselves do not readily produce disease, but may be used to produce immunity against diseases such as poliomyelitis, measles, rubella, and smallpox.

Passive immunity is produced by administering preformed antibody to provide protection against an invasive pathogen or toxin, often as a lifesaving maneuver. For example, passive immunity may be a maneuver used to treat botulism, diphtheria, or snakebite. Preformed antibodies are obtained from human or animal blood following immunization against a particular antigen.

Inflammation

Inflammation is the collective response to tissue injury, which can be caused by invasion of infectious microorganisms, toxins, or trauma. The inflammatory response consists of several components: localized vasodilatation and increased blood flow; increased capillary permeability and extravasation of plasma proteins, including complement and coagulation factors; and chemotactic movement of leukocytes to the site of injury. The clinical manifestations of inflammation include erythema, localized edema, and pain.[1,2]

Both the innate and acquired immune systems participate in the production of inflammation. Communication between the two immune systems is provided by a network of chemical substances known as *cytokines* (see Box 42-1). Normally these substances act locally to regulate the immune response and may exert synergistic or inhibitory interactions in the regulation of immune cell activity. If produced in high amounts during an exuberant inflammatory response, though, some cytokines may demonstrate measurable blood levels and exert adverse systemic effects.

When resident macrophages encounter a pathogen, they become activated to phagocytize the pathogen and secrete proinflammatory cytokines such as TNF-α, IL-1, IL-6, and IL-12. Among its various actions, TNF-α stimulates the production of endothelial-cell adhesion molecules and chemokines, which are necessary for leukocyte infiltration to the site of infection (see Figure 42-3). Overproduction of TNF-α can have deleterious local and systemic effects. Indeed, high circulating levels of TNF-α are characteristic of chronic major illness and systemic inflammatory response syndrome.

Like TNF-α, IL-1 stimulates endothelial-cell adhesion molecule production. It also has other actions, one of which is to alter the hypothalamic core temperature set-point and produce fever. One important consequence of increased body temperature is more rapid lymphocyte proliferation to combat infectious microorganisms. IL-1 also activates T lymphocytes, thereby recruiting those cell types against the infection. IL-12 promotes preferential differentiation of T$_H$ cells to the T$_H$1 subtype and activates NK cells. Both T$_H$1 cells and NK cells release IFN-γ, which enhances NK-cell activity and inhibits T$_H$2 cell function. IL-6 stimulates B lymphocytes and may play a role in wound healing. In addition, a recent study in mice has provided evidence that IL-6 can directly stimulate adrenocortical secretion of glucocorticoids, providing a unique mechanism by which the inflammatory response can provoke stress hormone secretion.[4]

TNF-α, IL-1, and IL-6 stimulate production of acute-phase proteins.[1,2] These serum proteins are produced by hepatocytes, and their serum levels increase rapidly with the onset of infection. One acute-phase protein of particular importance is C-reactive protein (CRP), which derives its name from its affinity for the C protein of pneumococci. Indeed, CRP serves to opsonize pneumococci and promote their phagocytosis by macrophages. The serum CRP level is often used as a clinical measure of inflammation and may have particular prognostic significance. A number of large, prospective studies have demonstrated the serum CRP level to be an independent predictor of cardiovascular risk.[5,6] It has also been suggested that elevated serum CRP levels might be predictive of perioperative morbidity. One recent study found an association between elevated CRP level and increased length of hospital stay in patients with medium cardiovascular risk undergoing orthopedic procedures.[7]

If the immune response is successful in clearing the pathogen and allowing recovery of tissue function, the inflammatory response is termed *acute inflammation*.[1,2] In some situations, though, the initial immune response does not completely remove the pathogen, and infection persists, causing chronic inflammation to develop. Chronic inflammation is characterized by greater numbers of macrophages and CTLs, compared with the leukocyte population seen with acute inflammation. One concern with chronic inflammation is that it can cause significant injury to host tissues. Chronic bacterial infection, such as occurs with tuberculosis, can lead to the formation of granulomas. These structures are composed of a central core of macrophages and epithelioid cells (produced from activated macrophages) surrounded by infiltrating T lymphocytes. TNF-α is a key cytokine responsible for granuloma formation. Chronic viral infections can also cause tissue injury, such as occurs with chronic hepatitis B virus infection.

Auxiliary cells, such as tissue mast cells, circulating basophils, and platelets, play a key role in inflammation and mobilization of immune responses (see Table 42-1). Mast cells and basophils can be activated by allergens that cross-link antibody molecules bound to the cell surface (to be discussed), by complement products C3a and C5a, by particular drugs such as codeine, morphine, and vancomycin, and by radiocontrast media. Once activated, mast cells and basophils undergo rapid release of proinflammatory substances such as histamine and serotonin and slower de novo production and release of leukotriene D$_4$ (a powerful bronchoconstrictor) and cytokines TNF-α and IL-4 (Figure 42-13).

Blood platelets can be activated in several ways, including contact with damaged endothelial cells, by IgG immune complexes, and by platelet activating factor released from activated macrophages. Activated platelets can aggregate and help to "wall off' an area of inflammation. In addition, activated platelets release serotonin, which acts to increase capillary permeability.

IMMUNE SYSTEM PATHOLOGY

Hypersensitivity and Allergic Reactions

In some cases, the immune response to antigen is greatly exaggerated, a situation referred to as *hypersensitivity*.[1,2] In 1963, Coombs and Gell classified hypersensitivity reactions into types

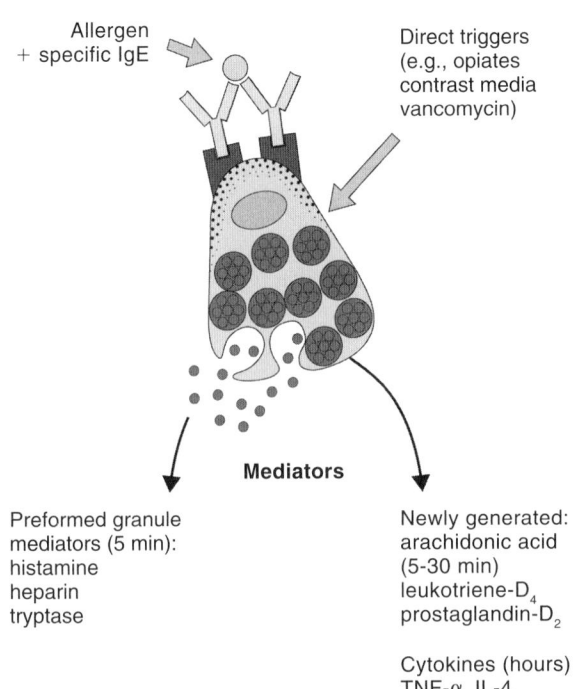

Triggering mechanisms

Allergen + specific IgE

Direct triggers (e.g., opiates contrast media vancomycin)

Mediators

Preformed granule mediators (5 min): histamine heparin tryptase

Newly generated: arachidonic acid (5-30 min) leukotriene-D$_4$ prostaglandin-D$_2$

Cytokines (hours) TNF-α, IL-4

FIGURE 42-13   Release of proinflammatory mediators after binding of antigen to IgE molecules on mast cell membranes. Preformed mediators such as histamine are rapidly released, whereas de novo synthesis delays release of other mediators such as leukotrienes and cytokines. Mast cells can also be directly activated by agents such as opioids, vancomycin, radiocontrast media, and complement products C3a and C5a. Similar events occur in response to activation of circulating basophils. (*From Male D et al. Immunology. 7th ed. Philadelphia: Mosby; 2006:435.*)

I, II, III, and IV (Figure 42-14). Recently, however, it has been recognized that this classification system is somewhat artificial, as there are overlapping mechanisms of action in types I, II, and III.

Sensitivity Types

Type I Hypersensitivity.   Type I hypersensitivity is a rapidly developing reaction that results from antigen-antibody interaction in an individual who has been previously exposed and sensitized to the antigen. The responsible antigen, referred to as an *allergen*, reacts with specific IgE antibodies on tissue mast cells and circulating basophils to trigger mediator release (see Figure 42-13) and an allergic response. A key mediator of allergic symptoms is histamine (Box 42-3). Chemically, allergens are usually proteins, and a multitude of environmental factors, including grass, pollen, dust, mites, molds, and animal dander, can generate type I hypersensitivity reactions.

Allergic reactions present with symptoms such as rhinitis, conjunctivitis, urticaria, pruritus, and possibly anaphylaxis. The term *anaphylaxis* refers to a severe, generalized, immediate hypersensitivity reaction that includes pruritus, urticaria, angioedema (especially laryngeal edema), hypotension, wheezing and bronchospasm, and direct cardiac effects, including arrhythmias. A shocklike state can develop from hypotension secondary to systemic vasodilatation and extravasation of protein and fluid. Clinical manifestations of an allergic reaction can present in various combinations and usually occur within minutes of exposure to the precipitating antigen(s). In some cases, though, the onset of signs and symptoms may be delayed for an hour or longer. Signs and symptoms can be protracted and variably responsive to treatment. Biphasic anaphylaxis can also occur, in which early signs and symptoms clear, either spontaneously or after acute therapy, and symptoms recur several or many hours later. Generally, the severity of an anaphylactic event relates to the suddenness of its onset and to the magnitude of the challenge, that is, the bigger the provocative stimulus, the more severe the reaction. However, anaphylaxis can occur after exposure to minute amounts of allergen in highly sensitive individuals.

Anaphylactoid reactions are caused by mediator release from basophils, but not from mast cells, in response to a non–IgE-mediated triggering event. Such reactions present with similar clinical manifestations as those with anaphylaxis, though it has been reported that cutaneous symptoms are more frequent, and cardiovascular collapse is less frequent, in patients experiencing

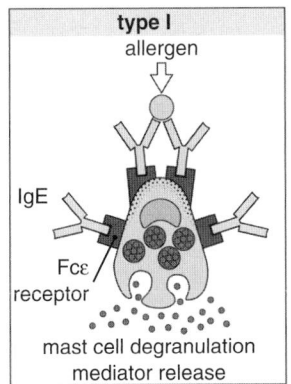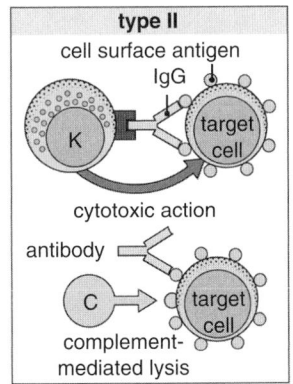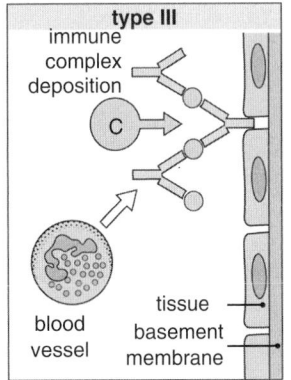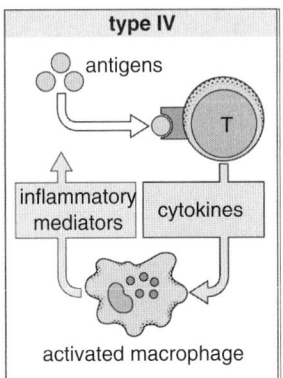

type I
allergen
IgE
Fcε receptor
mast cell degranulation
mediator release

type II
cell surface antigen
IgG
K
target cell
cytotoxic action
antibody
C
target cell
complement-mediated lysis

type III
immune complex deposition
C
blood vessel
tissue basement membrane

type IV
antigens
T
inflammatory mediators
cytokines
activated macrophage

FIGURE 42-14   The Coombs and Gell classifications of the four types of hypersensitivity reactions. Type I reactions are immediate hypersensitivity reactions, and type IV reactions are delayed-type hypersensitivity reactions. See discussion in text for characteristics of each type of reaction. (*From Male D et al. Immunology. 7th ed. Philadelphia: Mosby; 2006:424.*)

Adapted from Rang HP et al. Pharmacology. 6th ed. Edinburgh, Scotland: Churchill Livingstone; 2007:214.

anaphylactoid reactions versus those experiencing anaphylactic reactions.[8]

Tryptase is a marker for mechanistic delineation of an allergic response. It is an enzyme released from mast cells, along with histamine and other inflammatory mediators, during an allergic response. Tryptase has a half-life of several hours and is stable at room temperature. It demonstrates a positive predictive value of 92.6% and a negative predictive value of 54.6% as an indicator of an immunologically mediated event. Thus a significantly elevated tryptase level (>25 mcg/L) strongly suggests an allergic mechanism. The presence of a normal tryptase level, however, does not exclude an immunologic reaction because elevated tryptase levels are not found in almost one third of anaphylactic cases. Although diagnosis of anaphylaxis should not rely on a single test, the high positive predictive value of tryptase makes it useful medicolegally and for subsequent patient management.[8,9]

Type II Hypersensitivity. Type II hypersensitivity reactions result from IgG and IgM antibodies binding to antigens on cell surfaces or extracellular tissue components such as basement membrane (see Figure 42-14).[1,2] The antigen-antibody reaction activates the complement cascade, causing production of C3a and C5a, which attract PMNs and macrophages, and production of the C5b5789 membrane attack complex that inserts into target cell membranes. Examples of type II hypersensitivity reactions include transfusion reactions, autoimmune hemolytic anemia, myasthenia gravis, and Goodpasture syndrome.

Type III Hypersensitivity. Type III hypersensitivity represents immune complex disease, in which antigen-antibody complexes deposit in tissues and cause injury (see Figure 42-14). Normally, immune complexes are cleared by the mononuclear

phagocyte system shortly after their formation. In some situations, however, immune complexes persist and deposit in tissues. Protracted infections or autoimmune processes can lead to type III reactions. The mechanism of tissue injury is similar to that in type II reactions, involving activation of complement and recruitment of phagocytes. Systemic lupus erythematosus, rheumatoid arthritis, and glomerulonephritis are examples of immune complex diseases.

Type IV Hypersensitivity. Type IV hypersensitivity is also referred to as *delayed-type hypersensitivity* (see Figure 42-14). By the strict Coombs and Gell definition, type IV reactions require at least 12 hours after contact with antigen. Migration of antigen-specific CD4+ lymphocytes to the reaction site is followed by cytokine release and a local inflammatory response. Contact hypersensitivity is one form of type IV reaction and occurs where skin has come into contact with antigen. Contact dermatitis and the response to poison ivy are examples of contact hypersensitivity. Another form of type IV hypersensitivity is granulomatous hypersensitivity, in which chronic infection leads to the formation of granulomas in tissues. Granulomatous diseases include tuberculosis, sarcoidosis, and Crohn's disease.

Drug Reactions

Predicting who will react adversely to a drug or combination of drugs is difficult. Fortunately, life-threatening adverse reactions to drugs and products used during anesthesia and surgery are very uncommon, with the overall incidence estimated to be 1 in every 5000 to 10,000 anesthetics.[9] Much of the information regarding the epidemiology of adverse reactions to anesthetic agents derives from a series of French studies initiated in 1989. Mertes and colleagues have shown that two thirds of adverse reactions to anesthetic agents were found to be immune-mediated (anaphylactic reactions), whereas the other one third were classified as anaphylactoid reactions.[8] Of anesthetic drugs that triggered anaphylactic reactions, neuromuscular blocking agents (NMBAs) did so most frequently, with rocuronium implicated in more than 40% of cases (Table 42-2). Anaphylactic and anaphylactoid reactions occurred more frequently in female patients, which is thought to be due to chemical epitopes that NMBAs and many cosmetics have in common. This observation may also explain why many patients generate an allergic response to NMBAs on their first exposure to the drug. In the same study, antibiotics were involved in 15% of anaphylactic reactions, with penicillins and cephalosporins most often responsible. Anaphylactic reactions to local anesthetics were rare, and the authors suggested that adverse reactions to local anesthetics most often result from accidental intravascular injection of the local anesthetic or absorption of epinephrine co-administered with the anesthetic.

Persons who have an increased allergic tendency are termed *atopic* and exhibit a genetic predisposition to such events. Atopic patients frequently present with some history of hay fever, rhinitis, asthma, or food or drug allergy. There has been long-standing concern as to whether such patients are at increased risk for an anaphylactic or anaphylactoid reaction during anesthesia. Such a relationship does appear to exist for latex allergy, in which a history of generalized atopy or specific allergy to certain fruits, such as kiwi, avocado, or figs, is recognized as a significant risk factor for latex reactions.[8,9] By contrast, a generalized history of allergy does not necessarily predispose a patient to anaphylactic or anaphylactoid reactions to anesthetic drugs. However, if a patient has a history of sensitivity to a particular anesthetic drug, such as a muscle relaxant, that individual may well be at increased risk for allergic responses to other agents in that class.

TABLE **42-2**	Agents Involved in Anaphylactic Reactions During Anesthesia	
Causal Agent		**Percentage**
Neuromuscular Blocking Agents		58.2 (total)
Rocuronium		43.1
Succinylcholine		22.6
Atracurium		19.0
Vecuronium		8.5
Pancuronium		3.3
Cisatracurium		0.6
Latex		16.7
Antibiotics		15.1 (total)
Penicillin		41.8
Cephalosporin		39.2
Vancomycin		11.4
Quinolone		5.1
Rifamycin		1.3
Aminoglycosides		1.3
Hypnotics		3.4 (total)
Propofol		66.7
Thiopental		16.7
Midazolam		16.6
Opioids		1.3
Nalbuphine		
Fentanyl		
Sufentanil		
Remifentanil		
Colloids		4.0 (total)
Gelatin		95.0
Hetastarch		5.0
Other Agents		1.3
Protamine		
Ketoprofen		
Methylene blue		
Ethylene oxide		

From Mertes PM et al. Anaphylactic and anaphylactoid reactions occurring during anesthesia in France in 1999-2000. Anesthesiology. 2003;99:536-545.

Indeed, the Mertes study reported cross-reactivity among NMBAs to be 75%.[8]

While anaphylactic reactions to local anesthetics are uncommon, ester local anesthetics are more likely than amide agents to elicit an allergic response.[10] Ester local anesthetic metabolites, such as para-aminobenzoic acid, have been identified to be responsible for this higher incidence of allergic response. Local anesthetic solutions containing methylparaben and propylparaben as preservatives may induce allergic responses in susceptible individuals. Thus administration of preservative-free local anesthetic solutions may reduce the likelihood of an allergic response. Recent theories suggest that allergies to various antioxidants and certain sulfite components may be responsible for some degree of allergic reactions to local anesthetic preparations.

Avoiding known causal agents (particularly those that induce histamine release), combined with careful selection and application of additional drugs, can reduce risk of adverse reactions. A thorough history and discussion with the patient or the patient's guardian can usually reveal the potential for untoward drug effects and alert the anesthesia provider to avoid suspicious agents. Patients frequently mistake drug sensitivity or an unpleasant response for an allergy. This is especially true with local anesthetic solutions containing epinephrine or administered with opioids. Careful investigation and cautious interviewing techniques are usually beneficial in clarifying these questionable areas. Reviewing past procedural notes and anesthesia records, and possible consultation with an allergist when appropriate, can further help in determining situational specifics and facilitate appropriate planning. The administration of H_1 and H_2 receptor antagonists preemptively may prevent allergic reactions in many cases when a known or suspected sensitivity is present.

Treatment of Allergic Reactions

Patients who do not appear to have life-threatening symptoms on initial presentation may nonetheless progress to life-threatening anaphylaxis. Early administration of medications may be beneficial in halting this progression. Standard therapy for non–life-threatening situations includes the following:

1. Epinephrine: The initial adult dose may range from 100 to 500 mcg subcutaneously or intramuscularly. This dose may be repeated every 10 to 15 minutes as needed up to a maximum of 1 mg per total dose. The dose in children is 10 mcg/kg up to a maximum of 500 mcg per total dose. The total dose can be repeated every 15 minutes for two doses and then every 4 hours as needed. There is evidence that more rapid systemic absorption and higher peak plasma levels occur after intramuscular administration than after subcutaneous administration.
2. Diphenhydramine: 1 to 2 mg/kg or 25 to 50 mg/dose (parenterally).
3. Glucocorticoids (Table 42-3) may also be administered. However, the efficacy of glucocorticoids in treating acute anaphylaxis or in reducing a late anaphylactic reaction has not been clearly established.

Life-threatening anaphylaxis requires immediate administration of epinephrine and may require other immediate measures for support of cardiorespiratory status. Cardiopulmonary resuscitation (CPR) should be instituted if there is loss of circulation or respiration. Oxygen (100%) should be administered and the airway secured. Hypotension should be addressed by administration of vasopressors and infusions of large volumes of intravenous fluids and/or colloids to compensate for peripheral vasodilation and intravascular fluid loss. Bronchospasm should be treated with inhaled bronchodilators, theophylline, or both.

Patients experiencing anaphylaxis may not always respond adequately to one injection of epinephrine. Epinephrine has a rapid onset but a short duration of action. At the same time, mediator release from mast cells and basophils may be prolonged, producing biphasic or protracted anaphylaxis. Moreover, patients who are taking β–adrenergic blocking agents may not respond to epinephrine and may require substantial fluid replacement. For patients with life-threatening anaphylaxis who are poorly responsive to initial doses of epinephrine, more frequent or higher doses may be required. If the patient does not respond to subcutaneous epinephrine, intravenous administration of epinephrine must be initiated. Bolus doses of 50 to 100 mcg should be titrated

	TABLE 42-3	Comparison of Select Glucocorticoid Agents			

Compound	Equivalent Dose (mg) Oral and IV	Relative Antiinflammatory Potency	Duration of Action after Oral Dose*	Comments
Hydrocortisone (cortisol)	20	1	S	Drug of choice for replacement therapy
Cortisone	25	0.8	S	Inexpensive; inactive until converted to hydrocortisone; not used as antiinflammatory because of mineralocorticoid effects
Prednisolone	5	4	I	Drug of choice for systemic antiinflammatory and immunosuppressive effects
Prednisone	5	4	I	Inactive until converted to prednisolone
Methylprednisolone	4	5	I	Antiinflammatory and immunosuppressive
Triamcinolone	4	5	I	Relatively more toxic than others
Dexamethasone	0.75	25	L	Antiinflammatory and immunosuppressive; used especially when water retention is undesirable, e.g., cerebral edema; drug of choice for suppression of ACTH production
Betamethasone	0.75	30	L	Antiinflammatory and immunosuppressive; used especially when water retention is undesirable

Modified from Chrousos GP. Adrenocorticosteroids and adrenocortical antagonists. In: Katzung BG, ed. Basic and Clinical Pharmacology. 10th ed. New York: McGraw-Hill; 2007:651; Schimmer BP, Parker KL. Adrenocorticotropic hormone, adrenocortical steroids, and their synthetic analogues: inhibitors of the synthesis and actions of adrenocortical hormones. In: Brunton LL et al. Goodman and Gilman's The Pharmacological Basis of Therapeutics. 11th ed. New York: McGraw-Hill; 2006:1602.
Hydrocortisone is the standard for comparison.
*Duration of action (hours): S, short, 8-12; I, intermediate, 12-36; L, long, 36-72.

to effect. Epinephrine infusion should initially be administered at 1 mcg/min, which can be increased to 2 to 10 mcg/min. For refractory cardiorespiratory arrest in children, the initial intravenous epinephrine dose is 10 mcg/kg. Subsequent doses of 100 mcg/kg can be administered every 3 to 5 minutes, and, if the patient is still refractory, the dose may be increased to 200 mcg/kg.

A good clinical response represents resolution of the allergic reaction. If there is partial resolution or concern about biphasic anaphylaxis, continuous monitoring is suggested. Additional history might reveal previous episodes of anaphylaxis or asthma. Antihistamines may be useful in the treatment of anaphylaxis, particularly for symptoms of urticaria and angioedema. An H_1-receptor antagonist, alone or in combination with an H_2-receptor antagonist, may be useful in reversing hypotension refractory to epinephrine and intravascular fluid replacement. Glucocorticoids, such as 200 mg of intravenous hydrocortisone, may reduce the risk of recurring or protracted anaphylaxis, although direct clinical evidence for this has not been clearly established.

Transfusion Reactions
Because of advances in technologic capabilities and quality-control practices, blood transfusion reactions are fortunately not a common occurrence. The relative risk of an allergic transfusion reaction of mild severity (urticaria and pruritus) is approximately 1:500, whereas a fatal hemolytic reaction occurs in approximately 1 in 250,000 to 600,000 transfusions administered nationally. The mechanism responsible for most transfusion reactions involves ABO incompatibility. Transfusion of incompatible blood type causes recipient antibodies to react with donor red blood cells, causing their destruction and the potential for

significant consequences. Disseminated intravascular coagulation, renal failure, and death are not uncommon following this type of reaction. Because the most common cause for a major hemolytic transfusion reaction is human error, it should never be assumed that another person is solely responsible for checking blood that one is preparing to administer to a patient.

Transfusion reactions are frequently masked, or at least delayed appreciably, during anesthesia. Hallmark symptoms of cardiovascular instability such as hypotension, as well as fever, hemoglobinuria, and bleeding diathesis, are indicative of a transfusion incompatibility and should be immediately treated.[11]

Latex Allergy
Allergies to latex-containing products continue to be a source of significant problems for specific populations. Health-care workers and certain patients, particularly those with congenital neural tube deficits and those who have undergone multiple surgical procedures, have shown particular sensitivity to latex-containing products.

It has been estimated that approximately 0.8% of the general population has some form of sensitivity to latex. Atopic persons who react with skin dermatitis and who are allergic to certain fruits (particularly kiwi and bananas) should be further evaluated for latex allergy. Health-care workers and patients who experience frequent exposure to devices and products that contain latex also exhibit such allergic reactions.[12] The incidence of health-care worker allergy to latex-containing products ranges between 8% and 25%. The most frequent clinical manifestations of latex reactions include some form of contact dermatitis, type I hypersensitivity reaction with the potential for anaphylaxis, or type IV

BOX **42-4**

Latex Reactions

Awake Patient	Anesthetized Patient
Itchy eyes	Tachycardia
Generalized pruritus	Hypertension
Shortness of breath	Wheezing
Feeling of faintness	Bronchospasm
Feeling of impending doom	Cardiorespiratory arrest
Nausea	Flushing
Vomiting	Facial edema
Abdominal cramping	Laryngeal edema
Diarrhea	Urticaria
Wheezing	

BOX **42-5**

Immunosuppressant Drugs

Most immunosuppressant drugs act in the induction phase of the immunologic response to reduce lymphocyte proliferation; some also inhibit aspects of the effector phase. The drugs used for immunosuppression can be roughly divided into agents that:
- Inhibit cytokine gene expression, e.g., glucocorticoids
- Inhibit purine or pyrimidine synthesis, e.g., azathioprine, mycophenolate mofetil
- Block intracellular signal transduction, e.g., cyclosporine, tacrolimus, rapamycin
- Block T-cell surface molecules involved in signaling, e.g., monoclonal antibodies

Immunosuppressant drugs are used:
- To suppress rejection of transplanted organs and tissues (kidneys, bone marrow, heart, liver, etc.)
- To suppress graft-versus-host disease in bone marrow transplants
- To treat conditions with an autoimmune component in their pathogenesis, including idiopathic thrombocytopenic purpura, some forms of hemolytic anemia, some forms of glomerulonephritis, myasthenia gravis, systemic lupus erythematosus, rheumatoid arthritis, psoriasis, and ulcerative colitis.

Therapy of autoimmune disease often involves a combination of glucocorticoid and cytotoxic agents.

For transplantation of organs or bone marrow, cyclosporine is usually combined with a glucocorticoid, a cytotoxic drug, or an antilymphocyte immunoglobulin.

Modified from Rang HP et al. Pharmacology. 6th ed. Edinburgh, Scotland: Churchill Livingstone; 2007:243.

hypersensitivity reaction. Mertes and associates found latex reactions to be the second most common cause of anaphylactic reactions during anesthesia and surgery.[8] Box 42-4 lists clinical manifestations of latex reactions in both awake and anesthetized patients.

Preventive procedures and recommended protocols have been established for the management of latex allergies that can have significant anaphylactic consequences. The incidence of latex allergies increased proportionately with the 10-fold increase in medical glove usage to accommodate universal precautions and barrier protection during anesthesia, surgery, and obstetric care. Using gloves that do not contain latex (e.g., gloves processed from polyvinyl or neoprene) can prevent this source of latex exposure. Although skin prick, patch testing, and radioallergosorbent tests for latex allergy are available, all present various challenges in qualifying a conclusive diagnosis. The American Association of Nurse Anesthetists (AANA) Latex Protocol provides a detailed plan to avoid and treat latex allergic responses.[13]

DISEASES OF THE IMMUNE SYSTEM

Autoimmune Disease

In the process of lymphocyte maturation, there normally occurs negative selection (apoptosis) of most cells that react against self-antigens.[1,2] Despite the efficiency of this self-tolerance mechanism, however, individuals normally display detectable levels of autoreactive B cells and T cells, which are usually not activated, owing to inadequate presentation of self-antigen or other factors that prevent autoreactivity. Impairment in the mechanisms that act to prevent autoreactivity can lead to production of excess amounts of autoreactive antibodies and T cells and autoimmune disease. Examples of such diseases are Hashimoto thyroiditis, insulin-dependent diabetes mellitus (IDDM), myasthenia gravis, rheumatoid arthritis, and systemic lupus erythematosus (SLE).

There is much evidence that certain HLA haplotypes predispose to autoimmune disease. Rheumatoid arthritis, for example, associates with certain HLA-DR haplotypes, and the risk of IDDM is greatly increased in persons with certain HLA-DQ haplotypes. The majority of autoimmune diseases affect women more often than men; in particular, they affect women of childbearing and working age. Moreover, it is not uncommon for an individual to have more than one autoimmune disease.

In some cases, autoimmune disease may result secondarily from an infection in which microbial antigens contain epitopes that are shared with self-antigens. Presentation of microbial antigen to T_H cells as part of the normal response to infection then triggers activation and proliferation of lymphocytes directed against not only the microbe but also self-antigens in tissues. This process of microbial cross-reactivity is the basis of rheumatic heart disease that develops in some individuals after a streptococcal infection. In this case, antibodies produced against streptococcal antigens cross-react with certain heart valve antigens. Microbial cross-reactivity may also play a role in the development of rheumatoid arthritis and ankylosing spondylitis.

Treatment of autoimmune disease depends in part on whether the disease is organ-specific (e.g., hypothyroidism, myasthenia gravis, IDDM) or systemic (e.g., rheumatoid arthritis, SLE). Organ-specific disease may be treated with discrete strategies, for example, cholinesterase inhibitors used to treat myasthenia gravis and exogenous insulin used to treat IDDM. Systemic disease may be treated with antiinflammatory and/or immunosuppressive regimens. Antiinflammatory agents that may be used include cyclooxygenase inhibitors, corticosteroids (see Table 42-3), and more recently monoclonal antibodies directed against the inflammatory mediator TNF-α (see Box 42-2). Treatment with immunosuppressant drugs (Box 42-5) may reduce the immune response but carries significant risk of opportunistic infections.

Immunodeficiency

Primary immunodeficiency is caused by deficient function of lymphocytes, the complement system, or phagocytes.[1,2] Deficient B-cell and antibody function can predispose to pyogenic infections, in which bacterial infection causes pus accumulation. IgA deficiency is a primary disorder and is the most common immunodeficiency syndrome. It occurs almost exclusively in Caucasians, with a prevalence of 1 in 700, and affected individuals are prone to develop type III hypersensitivity reactions. Approximately one fifth of patients with IgA deficiency also have deficient production of two IgG subclasses, IgG2 and IgG4, which makes them susceptible to pyogenic infections. Individuals with deficient antibody responses are prone to recurring respiratory infections with encapsulated bacteria such as *Streptococcus pneumoniae* and *Haemophilus influenzae*. Such recurrent infections can result in bronchiectasis and chronic obstructive pulmonary disease.

Individuals who lack T cells or who have deficient T-cell function are prone to opportunistic infections by environmental pathogens such as yeast and chickenpox, microorganisms to which normal individuals develop prompt immunity. Because T cells support (in part) B-cell function, T-cell defects may also be accompanied by deficient humoral immunity. Individuals born with severe combined immunodeficiency (SCID) have low levels of circulating lymphocytes, lymphoid tissue that is virtually devoid of lymphocytes, and an immature thymus gland. A number of genetic mutations, including X-linked and autosomal recessive genes, can cause SCID. Affected infants are prone to develop diarrhea and pneumonia and usually do not survive more than 2 years unless treated with a bone-marrow transplant. T-cell deficiency also accompanies the DiGeorge syndrome, which results from abnormal development of the thymus and parathyroid glands, structures that originate from the same embryonic tissue. The syndrome is characterized by an "elfin-like appearance," with eyes set widely apart and a shortened infranasal depression. Structural micrognathia is frequently associated with this syndrome and can hinder laryngoscopy and airway management efforts. Congenital cardiac abnormalities and tetany secondary to deficient parathyroid gland function are also characteristic of DiGeorge syndrome.

Genetic abnormalities in complement proteins may cause primary immunodeficiency syndromes. Hereditary angioneurotic edema (HAE) is caused by absent or defective C1 inhibitor, a protein that normally acts to control complement activation and coagulation mechanisms. Deficient C1 inhibitor activity can lead to kinin accumulation, angioedema, and upper airway obstruction. Exogenous C1 inhibitor can be administered to treat acute angioedema.

Deficiencies in PMNs or the mononuclear phagocyte system can result in severe, life-threatening infections. Neutropenia represents a variable reduction in PMNs, which can predispose the affected individual to severe bacterial infections. Chronic granulomatous disease (CGD) results when defective PMNs are unable to generate a bactericidal respiratory burst after bacterial phagocytosis. Ingested pathogens that survive within the phagocytes trigger a cell-mediated immune response against the phagocytes and formation of granulomas. Symptoms of CGD in pediatric patients include pneumonia and abscesses in various tissues.

Secondary immunodeficiency can result as an adverse effect of immunosuppressive drugs administered to prevent graft rejection or to treat autoimmune disease (see Box 42-5). Glucocorticoids have potent immunosuppressive effects (see Table 42-3).

These steroid agents markedly reduce circulating levels of lymphocytes and monocytes, inhibit immune cell cytokine production, and inhibit T-cell activation. Lymphocytopenia and monocytopenia result within hours after a single dose of glucocorticoid and resolve within 24 hours. Azathioprine is a cytostatic immunosuppressive agent that is effective only on dividing lymphocytes, reducing levels of both B and T lymphocytes. Mycophenolate mofetil inhibits lymphocyte proliferation by blocking the last step of purine synthesis necessary for DNA replication. Cyclosporine, tacrolimus (formerly known as *FK-506*), and rapamycin bind to cytoplasmic proteins known as *immunophilins*, causing blockade of signal transduction pathways from the cell membrane and inhibition of T-cell proliferation.

Human Immunodeficiency Virus

Secondary immunosuppression can also result from infection that causes depletion of immune cells. In this regard, infection with HIV is the most significant etiology. The virus exists as two main types, HIV-1 and HIV-2. Of the two, HIV-1 is more prevalent and more pathogenic. The primary targets of HIV infection are CD4$^+$ lymphocytes. A glycoprotein on the viral envelope binds to the CD4 antigen to allow the virus to enter the T cell. HIV is a retrovirus, that is, its genome contains two strands of single-stranded RNA. After the virus enters the host cell, its RNA undergoes reverse transcription to produce complementary DNA that is incorporated into the host-cell DNA. Synthesis of new viral RNA then occurs in the host cell, followed by formation of new virus particles and their release to infect other CD4$^+$ cells. Infection with HIV alters T-cell function and causes cytotoxicity, leading to the characteristic decline in CD4$^+$ cells. Exactly how HIV infection kills T cells, though, is not known and may involve several mechanisms. Ultimately, with a sufficient fall in CD4$^+$ cells, individuals become susceptible to life-threatening opportunistic infections.

Epidemiology

The epidemiologic basis for HIV infection begins with transmission of the virus through certain body fluids. Box 42-6 lists the potential sources of transmission of HIV, which can enter the body through blood contact, sexual transmission, and perinatal exposure. In 2004, it was estimated that 40 million individuals worldwide were infected with HIV, with an annual incidence of 5 million cases. Infection with HIV can progress to acquired immune deficiency syndrome (AIDS) and fatal disease.[14] While more than 25 million individuals have died as a result of AIDS complications since the first description of the disease, early detection, evaluation, and pharmacologic intervention have become very successful in controlling HIV infection in many individuals while preserving immune system integrity.

Acute infection with HIV is characterized by a mononucleosis-like illness, in which release of inflammatory mediators, including IL-1 and TNF-α, causes symptoms such as malaise, fever, myalgias, and rash. At the same time, a transient decline in circulating CD4$^+$ cells occurs. Over several weeks following the primary infection, antibodies directed against virus envelope proteins are produced, and CTLs begin to kill infected T cells that display HIV peptides. These immune responses permit resolution of the symptoms of acute infection, however, anti-HIV antibodies and CTLs become overwhelmed by viral replication and mutation, and progression of HIV infection occurs.

BOX **42-6**

Routes of HIV Transmission

Absolute
Blood
Body fluids containing blood

Possible
Cerebrospinal fluid
Pericardial fluids
Amniotic fluids
Semen, vaginal secretions
Synovial fluid
Pleural fluid

Remote
Feces
Saliva
Sputum
Sweat
Tears
Urine
Wound drainage
Nasal secretions

Not Implicated in Health-Care Settings
Human breast milk

BOX **42-7**

Treatment of HIV/AIDS

Antiretroviral Therapy of HIV Infection Is Based on the Following Principles:
- Start treatment before immunodeficiency becomes evident
- Aim to reduce plasma viral concentration as much as possible for as long as possible
- Use a combination of three or four antiretroviral drugs, i.e., highly active antiretroviral therapy (HAART)
- Monitor plasma viral load and CD4$^+$ cell count
- Change to a different regimen if plasma viral concentration increases

Drugs Used for Treatment of HIV Infection:
- Nucleoside reverse transcriptase inhibitors (NRTIs): zidovudine, lamivudine, didanosine, emtricitabine, stavudine, and abacavir
- Nonnucleoside RTIs (NNRTIs): delavirdine, efavirenz, and nevirapine
- Protease inhibitors: amprenavir, indinavir, ritonavir, saquinavir, and tipranavir
- Fusion inhibitors: enfuvirtide

Spontaneous resolution of the acute symptoms of HIV infection is followed by a variable period of asymptomatic infection. If the infection is not treated, a gradual, progressive fall in CD4$^+$ cells occurs in conjunction with a gradual increase in the plasma viral load. Progression to AIDS in untreated individuals occurs in an average time of 10 years, though in some individuals progression may occur much more rapidly or perhaps not at all. With respect to the latter possibility, there are reports of individuals who have not developed AIDS despite multiple exposures to HIV, suggesting that the adaptive immune system in some individuals may provide chronic protection by an as yet undefined mechanism. Clinically, AIDS is defined as a CD4$^+$ cell count less than 200 cells/μL or by the presence of an AIDS-indicator condition (discussed later).

Treatment Modalities

Many years of research have produced numerous agents for combating HIV infection. Most current therapies involve a "cocktail" of antiretroviral agents that can include nucleoside reverse transcriptase inhibitors (NRTIs), nonnucleoside reverse transcriptase inhibitors (NNRTIs), protease inhibitors (PIs), and a fusion inhibitor (Box 42-7). A combination of three or four agents, known as *highly active antiretroviral therapy* (HAART), is now the usual therapeutic approach.[1,2]

Nucleoside Reverse Transcriptase Inhibitors. The NRTIs bind to and inhibit the viral reverse transcriptase enzyme responsible for production of HIV RNA. The prototype agent in this class is zidovudine, also known as *AZT*, which was the first antiretroviral drug to be approved by the U.S. Food and Drug Administration for treatment of HIV infection. Resistance to zidovudine may occur with certain HIV strains, and the most significant side effect of AZT therapy is bone-marrow suppression, which causes anemia and neutropenia.

Nonnucleoside Reverse Transcriptase Inhibitors. Like the NRTIs, the NNRTIs bind to and inhibit the viral reverse transcriptase enzyme but at a different molecular site. Resistance to NNRTI monotherapy can readily occur, and adverse effects include skin rash and (uncommonly) Stevens-Johnson syndrome. NNRTIs are metabolized by hepatic CYP3A4, and agents can either induce or inhibit this cytochrome P-450 isoform. Thus the practitioner should be prepared for possible interactions with other drugs, including some anesthetic agents that are metabolized by CYP3A4.

Protease Inhibitors. The viral enzyme protease catalyzes production of viral core structural proteins from immature polypeptide precursors. By inhibiting this enzyme, the PIs cause production of altered, noninfectious virions. Adverse effects of the PIs include Cushing-like signs and symptoms (e.g., central obesity, buffalo hump, glucose intolerance). Like the NNRTIs, the PIs can either induce or inhibit CYP3A4, and drug interactions should be anticipated.

Fusion Inhibitors. The newest class of antiretroviral agents is the fusion inhibitors, which prevent viral adherence to and entry into the host cell. Enfuvirtide is the prototype fusion inhibitor. It is injected subcutaneously, and clearance does not involve cytochrome P-450 enzymes.

Therapeutic modalities may fail owing to patient nonadherence, inadequate potency of antiretroviral agents, or viral resistance. Ongoing research continues to address resistance and investigate multiple strains of the virus that may not respond to current therapeutic modalities. Ultimately, of course, the goal is to develop a cure for HIV. In this regard, global clinical trials of HIV vaccine have been initiated in numerous locations around the world.[15] Unfortunately, a significant setback in this direction occurred recently when it was announced that the STEP study, an international HIV vaccine clinical trial conducted by the National Institute of Allergy and Infectious Diseases and the pharmaceutical company Merck & Co., Inc. was to be discontinued.[16] In a review of interim data, an independent monitoring board determined that the vaccine did not

TABLE 42-4	Common Abdominal Pathogens That May Necessitate Surgical Intervention in AIDS Patients
Pathogen	**Effects**
Virus	
Cytomegalovirus	Most common reason for surgery; potentially serious colitis, peritonitis, diarrhea, fever, hematochezia, gastrointestinal perforation, ulceration, ischemia resulting in small-bowel resection with diversion; acute cholecystitis
Tumors	
Kaposi sarcoma	Gastrointestinal and biliary tree involvement results in hemorrhage, perforation; represents end stage of disease, so laparotomy for obstruction results in limited resection with reanastomosis
Lymphoma	Extranodal masses, usually distal to esophagus; presents with abdominal pain, mass, bowel obstruction, hemorrhage, and peritonitis from perforation; most common presenting symptom is small-bowel obstruction resulting in emergency laparotomy
Bacteria	
Mycobacterium	Disseminated disease of liver, spleen, lymph nodes, and small intestine; very poor prognosis, with limited surgical intervention
Coexisting Gastrointestinal Pathogens	
Viruses	
Adenovirus	Colon involvement, chronic watery, nonbloody, nonmucoid diarrhea with weight loss
Herpes simplex	Chronic cutaneous ulcers; perianal lesions, proctitis; esophagitis
Protozoa	
Cryptosporidium	Debilitating, chronic, voluminous, watery diarrhea; severe dehydration; electrolyte imbalance and wasting; occasional biliary tract obstruction; malabsorption syndrome
Microsporidium	Nonbloody, nonmucoid diarrhea, often requiring fluid and electrolyte replacement; patient retains good appetite
Bacteria	
Mycobacterium avium-intracellulare	Most common systemic bacterial infection
Salmonella *Shigella* *Campylobacter*	All bacterium-caused diarrhea requires rehydration and electrolyte supplementation, as well as drugs to inhibit intestinal motility and secretion; occasional need for total parenteral nutrition
Fungal	
Candida albicans	Invasive disease in oral cavity and esophagus

Modified from Smith PD et al. NIH conference. Gastrointestinal infections in AIDS. Ann Intern Med. 1992;116:63-77; Lowy AM, Barie PS. Laparotomy in patients infected with human immunodeficiency virus: indications and outcome. Br J Surg. 1994;81(7):942-945.

prevent HIV infection or affect the course of the disease in those who became infected with HIV. The STEP study had included 3000 participants in nine countries including the United States. A separate clinical trial in South Africa, known as the *Phambili study* and using the same candidate HIV vaccine, was also suspended.

Anesthesia Management

The HIV-infected patient may require a variety of surgical interventions (Table 42-4). Although several studies have evaluated the effects of surgery and anesthesia in HIV-infected patients, to date there is no conclusive evidence to support any particular set of recommendations. Most alterations caused by various anesthetic agents and techniques are transient and have not been shown to contribute to any adverse outcome.

It is important to understand the patient's status both in response to and application of antiretroviral therapy and other treatments when an operative procedure is planned. Appreciation of both recent and past therapeutic efforts and the patient's response is important in preparing the HIV-infected patient for anesthesia and related care. Consultation with and participation of the patient's primary care provider in the planning process can be beneficial.

When anesthesia care is planned, attention should focus on possible end-organ and systemic dysfunction. Clinically significant alterations occur in many organ systems, particularly in the advanced disease stages of HIV infection, when vigilant monitoring and at times intensive intervention may be necessary. The patient (or his or her legal representative or caregiver) should be included in the planning and evaluation of potential care options. Informed consent may be the responsibility of a legal guardian or durable power of attorney designee for the patient who may be mentally incompetent.

The immunocompromised patient may have combined deficiencies that predispose to significant or fatal outcomes. It is important to remember that microorganisms that are not routinely pathogenic can cause the demise of these patients. Meticulous implementation of infection control measures throughout the perioperative period should be a primary focus in the care of these vulnerable patients. Respiratory isolation should be used when it is either known or suspected that airborne pathogens may be transmitted. Examples of such pathogens include the causative agents of tuberculosis and varicella. The immune-system compromise resulting from HIV infection markedly increases the susceptibility to tuberculosis, and recurrent or newly acquired tuberculosis is frequently the cause of death for persons infected with HIV. A striking clinical feature of tuberculosis in HIV-infected patients is a high incidence of extrapulmonary involvement, usually with concomitant pulmonary presentation.[17-19]

Although equipment preparedness is important for every patient to whom anesthesia is administered, it is of particular significance with the immunocompromised patient. Meticulous attention to behaviors and adherence to strict aseptic technique in providing care to these most vulnerable patients is paramount to safe practice and quality patient care. The anesthesia machine and its multitude of components should be adequately maintained, cleaned, and disinfected, and appropriate sterile components should be changed between each use, in accordance with both approved infection control practices and manufacturers' recommendations.

A multitude of clinical presentations have the potential to affect anesthesia management in the patient infected with HIV. Oxygenation and metabolic functions are frequently impaired during progressive HIV infection. Pulmonary infections can alter both gas exchange and lung perfusion and create ventilation-perfusion mismatch. Dehydration and hypovolemia secondary to gastrointestinal disturbances can further complicate the patient's clinical course. A thorough preoperative assessment, including current physical examination, laboratory results, and radiographic examination, combined with other studies as indicated by patient presentation and current disease state, is critical prior to anesthesia.

Complications from HIV

Wasting syndrome may be seen in HIV-infected patients and results from disturbances in food absorption and metabolism. This syndrome is defined as profound, involuntary weight loss greater than 10% of baseline body weight. Chronic diarrhea frequently contributes to this scenario. Parenteral nutrition and appetite stimulation are usually required when this syndrome is persistent. Preoperative assessment should include evaluation of volume status and related physiologic studies to plan appropriate management.

Neurologic evaluation is essential for HIV-infected patients. Both the central and peripheral nervous systems can be impaired due to direct disease effects, concomitant opportunistic infections, or adverse effects of therapeutic agents used to combat viral insult. Peripheral neuropathies may result in considerable discomfort or physical limitations, and autonomic neuropathy may result in some degree of cardiovascular instability requiring immediate or continuous intervention. AIDS-related dementia can influence both motor and cognitive states, particularly in advanced disease states.

Non-Hodgkin lymphoma, manifesting as a space-occupying lesion within the central nervous system, may require surgical or chemotherapeutic intervention. Kaposi sarcoma, a cancer that invades endothelial tissues, can attack both skin and internal organs. Women infected with HIV may develop cervical dysplasia and cancers.

As HIV infection progresses to AIDS, advanced disease combinations emerge that would otherwise be resisted in the immunocompetent host. These opportunistic disease processes increase in both manifestation and severity as the immune system fails.

Both acute and chronic bacterial infections tend to plague HIV-infected individuals. *Mycobacterium avium-intracellulare* (MAI) infection is characterized by intractable diarrhea and resultant wasting states. Splenic and pulmonary infections with MAI lead to severe thrombocytopenia and tuberculosis. MAI attacks the immunosuppressed host easily and is transmissible.

Several viral infections can occur or recur from previously dormant states as HIV disease progresses. Herpes simplex and varicella infections can invade oral and esophageal tissues and the central nervous system. Cytomegalovirus can affect the gastrointestinal and pulmonary systems, resulting in colitis and pneumonia. Retinal invasion may lead to marked visual disturbances and blindness. Ganciclovir is used to treat cytomegalovirus infection.

Opportunistic protozoal infections can develop in persons with advanced HIV infection. *Pneumocystis jiroveci* pneumonia is responsible for the majority of deaths secondary to opportunistic infection in HIV-infected persons. Fever and impaired gas exchange frequently result in hypoxemia, and pneumothorax is not uncommon. Toxoplasmosis encephalitis can affect both central nervous system function and the sensorium. Cryptosporidiosis can trigger considerable diarrhea, resulting in significant dehydration and related electrolyte imbalance. Volume status must be judiciously evaluated and monitored.

Fungal infection is responsible for histoplasmosis and aspergillosis pneumonia in the HIV-infected patient. Such insults can result in significant febrile and hypoxic states, with impairment of gas exchange and overall sensorium. Disseminated candidiasis infections are responsible for oropharyngeal and esophageal pathology that includes stomatitis, dysphagia, and esophagitis. Patients with cryptococcal meningitis can experience increased intracranial pressure.

Childbearing women constitute a significant portion of reported cases of HIV and AIDS. This is of considerable significance in that perinatal transmission accounts for greater than 80% of all pediatric AIDS cases that have been reported in the United States. The pregnant patient with HIV presents unique challenges for health maintenance. Anemia can be particularly significant in advanced states of HIV infection, frequently necessitating transfusion therapy. Elective cesarean section in the HIV-positive parturient appears to reduce the risk of HIV transmission from mother to neonate.[20] However, complications of cesarean section, including blood loss and wound infection, may be exaggerated in HIV-infected parturients as a result of immunosuppression.[21] Avidan and colleagues recently reported no increase in intra- or postoperative complications associated with spinal anesthesia and cesarean section in HIV-infected parturients who were receiving effective antiretroviral therapy and who received preoperative broad-spectrum antibiotics.[22] Such an approach may be effective in reducing risk of perinatal HIV transmission in parturients in whom antiretroviral therapy is effective and spinal anesthesia is not contraindicated.

Because many physical manifestations of HIV-related illness involve neuromuscular disorders, pain management can be a difficult challenge in patients with advanced HIV infection. Both routine analgesic modalities and analgesic agents combined with the use of various chemotherapies, nerve blocks, and complementary therapies have been beneficial in treating acute postoperative and obstetric pain in HIV-infected patients.[23]

Managing HIV Infection

Occupational Safety. The primary emphasis in managing HIV infection during anesthesia and other aspects of patient care is an effective prevention program. Because the routes of

HIV transmission are well known, an appropriate infection control program, with consistent application of proven blood and body substance precautions, can prevent disease transmission. Universal precautions were developed after known modes of transmission of both HIV and hepatitis B virus (both blood-borne pathogens) were clarified. More recent efforts to apply this practice throughout all patient care areas have resulted in the consistent application of standard precautions during patient care. The basic premise on which these guidelines is based is the prevention of parenteral, mucous membrane, and nonintact skin exposure to blood and certain body fluids from all patients. Guidelines include the following:

1. Gloves must be worn when contact with body substances is suspected or possible.
2. A plastic gown or apron must be worn when soiling with body substances is likely.
3. Protective masks and eyewear must be worn in the presence of airborne disease or for preventing splash or aerosolization of body substances to eyes or mucous membranes.
4. Hands must be thoroughly washed before and after body substances or articles possibly covered with body substances have been handled and after gloves have been removed at the completion of each task or procedure.
5. Uncapped needles and syringes must be discarded in puncture-resistant receptacles placed as close to their point of use as is practical.
6. Trash and linens must be discarded in impervious, sealed plastic bags that are labeled as infectious and transported according to standard precautions.

Self-protection against HIV and all other infectious blood-borne pathogens such as hepatitis B and C viruses is an essential element of safe practice. The Occupational Safety and Health Administration (OSHA) Act, which became effective in 1992, mandates that employers minimize occupational exposure to all blood-borne pathogens in workplaces where a potential for such exposures exists. Known or suspected exposure to blood-borne pathogens should be responded to immediately with appropriate action, as recommended by OSHA and institutional infection control standards. The AANA infection control guide details recommended practices for managing blood-borne pathogens during anesthesia care.[24] Current HIV/AIDS treatment guidelines and protocols may be obtained from the National HIV/AIDS Clinicians' Consultation website at http://www.ucsf.edu/hivcntr.

HIV Postexposure Prophylaxis. As of December 2001, the Centers for Disease Control and Prevention (CDC) had received voluntary reports of 57 documented cases of HIV seroconversion temporally associated with occupational exposure to HIV among U.S. health-care personnel.[25,26] An additional 138 infections among health-care personnel were considered possible cases of occupational HIV transmission. Because there is no cure or effective vaccine for HIV, optimal postexposure care, including the administration of antiretroviral drugs, remains a high priority for protecting health-care personnel.[27]

Percutaneous injury with a hollow-bore needle is the most common mechanism of occupational HIV transmission. The CDC estimates that more than 380,000 needle-stick injuries occur in U.S. hospitals each year; approximately 61% of these injuries are caused by hollow-bore devices.[28] The proportion of injuries involving exposure to blood from HIV-infected sources is not known, but each exposure is an urgent health issue for the exposed person.

Pooled data from several prospective studies of health-care personnel suggest that the average risk of HIV transmission is approximately 0.3% after a percutaneous exposure to HIV-infected blood and approximately 0.09% after a mucous membrane exposure.[25] The average risk associated with exposure of nonintact skin and exposure to HIV-infected fluids and tissues other than blood or bloody fluids is too low to be estimated in prospective studies. In a retrospective study, the CDC found that the risk of HIV transmission to health-care workers was increased when the device causing the injury was visibly contaminated with blood or was used for insertion into a vein or artery, when a deep injury occurred, or when the source patient died within 2 months after the exposure.[29] A low plasma HIV RNA titer does not exclude the possibility of transmission, especially because this measurement does not account for cell-associated HIV. Transmission from source patients with undetectable HIV RNA has been documented.[25]

Suture needles have not been implicated as a source of infection in prospective studies, but occupational HIV infection has been reported among surgical personnel, and suture needles are one potential source of such infection. Exposure of intact skin to contaminated blood has not been identified as a risk for HIV transmission.

Evidence suggests that postexposure prophylaxis (PEP) with antiretroviral drugs soon after occupational exposure to HIV decreases risk of infection. The pathogenesis of the initial infection provides suggestive evidence that there is a window of opportunity in which antiretroviral treatment can prevent infection or abort it before irreversible systemic infection and HIV seroconversion occur. In a retrospective case-control study of health-care personnel, PEP with zidovudine was associated with an 81% reduction in the risk of HIV infection.[30] However, there are no data from randomized, controlled trials. Data from clinical trials of prophylaxis against perinatal HIV transmission consistently demonstrate that antiretroviral treatment can prevent HIV infection after exposure, even among neonates who are not treated until after birth.[31-33] The relevance of this clinical situation to occupational exposure, however, is not known.

Although data are encouraging, it is clear that protection afforded by PEP is not absolute. Twenty-one cases of HIV infection have been reported in health-care personnel in the United States and elsewhere, despite postexposure antiretroviral treatment that included two or more antiretroviral drugs in some cases.[25,34-36] A variety of factors may have contributed to the treatment failure, including an intrinsic lack of efficacy of prophylactic antiretroviral treatment and resistance to antiretroviral drugs.

It is unclear why 99.7% of occupational injuries involving percutaneous exposure to HIV do not transmit infection, and an assessment of the risk of transmission remains imprecise. The most effective and safest antiretroviral regimen for exposed persons also remains uncertain. Current PEP guidelines and treatment protocols can be found at the National HIV/AIDS Clinicians' Consultation website. A combination of antiretroviral agents is usually advised for the treatment of HIV infection, but such combinations are not universally effective in preventing infection after occupational exposure. Indeed, of five health-care workers known to have acquired HIV infection despite PEP with more than one antiretroviral drug, three individuals received three or more drugs.[37]

ANESTHESIA AND THE IMMUNE SYSTEM

The effects of anesthesia on the immune system have been investigated for more than 30 years. For two reasons, however, no clear picture regarding how anesthetic agents alter immune function has emerged. First, anesthesia is administered in the context of surgery, which itself strongly activates the body's stress response to cause reversible immunosuppression. Second, many in vitro studies have been performed to examine the effects of anesthetic agents on immune components in controlled, experimental situations. Results of these in vitro studies, although possibly yielding mechanistic insights, do not always agree with in vivo observations. The focus of this final section of the chapter is to describe the relationship between stress and the immune system and to summarize the results of in vitro and in vivo studies of the effects of individual anesthetic agents on the principal components of the immune system, that is, phagocytes, lymphocytes, and soluble mediators.

Surgical Stress and the Immune System

The immune response to surgery is variable and can involve several components. Surgical trauma may provoke or inhibit production of particular cytokines and cause perioperative immunosuppression characterized by depressed cell-mediated immunity.[38] Tissue trauma strongly stimulates the body's stress response, which can produce immunosuppression by several mechanisms. First, activation of the hypothalamic-pituitary-adrenal axis causes release of the glucocorticoid cortisol from the adrenal cortex. As discussed, glucocorticoids have potent immunosuppressive activity (see Table 42-3). In addition, sympathetic nervous system activation increases catecholamine secretion from the adrenal medulla. Some immune cells display adrenergic receptors by which circulating catecholamines can alter cell function. Activation of β-adrenergic receptors has been found to suppress in vitro monocyte production of the proinflammatory cytokines TNF-α and IL-1 and PMN production of reactive oxygen molecules.[39,40] Moreover, lymphoid tissue receives sympathetic innervation, and stress-induced release of norepinephrine there can alter immune cell activity.[41]

The stress response to surgery may be associated with alterations in lymphocyte subtypes. In particular, stress may reduce the T_H1/T_H2 cell ratio through actions of both catecholamines and glucocorticoids. Elenkov and colleagues treated whole blood with bacterial lipopolysaccharide (endotoxin) to stimulate monocyte cytokine production.[42] Dexamethasone, used to mimic the in vivo effects of cortisol, inhibited monocyte IL-12 production but had no effect on IL-10 production. The catecholamines epinephrine and norepinephrine also inhibited IL-12 production and increased IL-10 production. The effects of the catecholamines were blocked by the β-adrenergic antagonist propranolol. IL-12 induces T_H cell differentiation to T_H1 cells and promotes cellular immunity. By contrast, IL-10 inhibits T_H1 cell function and promotes T_H2 cell responses and humoral immunity. The authors suggested that stress hormones might shift the T_H1/T_H2 cytokine balance to a pattern that predisposes to infections by pathogens that would normally be intercepted by cellular immunity.

Evidence from animal and human studies indicates that the magnitude of the surgical stress can influence postoperative immune responses. Anesthetized animals that underwent experimental laparoscopy had preserved postoperative cellular immunity compared with animals that underwent more invasive laparotomy.[43,44] Similarly, in humans, open cholecystectomy was associated with greater postoperative suppression of T-cell proliferation than was laparoscopic cholecystectomy.[45]

Anesthesia may attenuate the stress response to surgically induced tissue injury, and this may be of greater significance with regional anesthesia, which is generally associated with less stress response to surgery than is general anesthesia. However, anesthetic agents themselves may have immunomodulatory activity, which must be considered in formulating an overall picture of how anesthesia affects the immune system.

Effects of Anesthesia and Anesthetic Agents on Immune Function

Lymphocyte Number and Function

Several studies have found that anesthesia and surgery together can alter the levels of circulating lymphocytes. In patients undergoing elective abdominal surgery with isoflurane general anesthesia, arterial blood lymphocytes were increased at 5 minutes after induction of anesthesia, 5 minutes after skin incision, and 5 minutes after peritoneal incision.[46] Unfortunately the authors did not measure lymphocyte levels later in the surgical procedure or in the postoperative period. An early rise in circulating lymphocytes might be transient; several studies indicate that perioperative lymphopenia can occur in patients undergoing general anesthesia and surgery.[47] Rem and colleagues reported decreased blood lymphocytes at 6 and 9 hours after skin incision in women undergoing hysterectomy with general anesthesia.[48] Similarly, Corsi and co-workers found reduced number and function of T_H cells at 10 minutes after the initiation of hysterectomy surgery in patients anesthetized with isoflurane.[49] In these studies, the lymphopenia resolved by 48 hours after surgery. These findings of perioperative lymphopenia in patients undergoing surgery with general anesthesia are consistent with data showing reduced plasma levels of IL-2, a key cytokine responsible for T-cell proliferation, in patients undergoing isoflurane anesthesia.[50] Plasma IL-2 was reduced at the end of surgery and had returned to the preinduction level at 24 hours postoperatively.

In patients undergoing craniotomy, the postoperative T_H1/T_H2 cell ratio was reduced in patients anesthetized with isoflurane but not in patients anesthetized with propofol.[51] Because IL-2 also promotes T-cell differentiation to T_H1 cells, these results are consistent with isoflurane anesthesia suppression of IL-2 production and observation that total intravenous anesthesia (TIVA) with propofol can increase perioperative IL-2 production.[50,52] It was suggested that propofol anesthesia might be more appropriate in patients with particular diseases, such as HIV-infected patients, in whom a decrease in the T_H1/T_H2 cell ratio could accelerate the rate of disease progression. A trend toward reductions in both the T_H1 cell count and the postoperative T_H1/T_H2 cell ratio was observed in patients undergoing isoflurane general anesthesia for transurethral resection of the prostate (TURP), though the reductions did not achieve statistical significance.[53]

Anesthesia and surgery together may also affect T-cell function. Previous studies suggest that impaired perioperative lymphocyte proliferation may occur in surgical patients. Hole and Unsgaard isolated lymphocytes from patients undergoing total hip replacement under either general or epidural anesthesia.[54] Lymphocytes were then treated with phytohemagglutinin (PHA), which is an agent commonly used to provoke in vitro T-cell proliferation. PHA-induced T-cell proliferation was depressed during and after surgery in patients receiving general anesthesia but not in patients receiving epidural anesthesia. In a separate study, serum obtained from patients undergoing general anesthesia, but not that from patients undergoing epidural anesthesia, showed suppressed proliferation of T cells when compared to cells obtained from healthy, nonsurgical volunteers.[55] These results suggested that one or more circulating factors associated with general anesthesia may suppress lymphocyte function.

Such factors might include intravenous and inhalation anesthetic agents and hormones such as cortisol and catecholamines released as components of the stress response.

Some studies have suggested that induction agents may have immunosuppressive activity. Devlin and colleagues treated blood obtained from healthy volunteers with PHA to provoke in vitro T-cell proliferation.[56] Several intravenous induction agents—thiopental, methohexital, etomidate, and propofol—inhibited T-cell proliferation at concentrations representative of those achieved in the blood during anesthesia. In a follow-up study by the same group, blood was collected from healthy volunteers who received intravenous injections of either thiopental or etomidate but did not undergo surgery.[57] Although the authors found no alteration of PHA-stimulated in vitro T-cell proliferation, they did find depression of delayed-type hypersensitivity (DTH) reactions to allergens, suggesting that in vivo T-cell function was impaired by administration of the induction agents. These latter results are of potential clinical significance because there has been reported an association between depressed DTH reactions and increased postoperative mortality.[58]

Although intravenous anesthetic agents may exert some immunosuppressive effect on T-cell function, inhalation anesthetics alone may be insufficient to cause postoperative impairment of T-cell proliferation. Indeed, PHA-induced proliferation of lymphocytes obtained from volunteers administered inhalation anesthesia with enflurane or halothane, but who did not undergo surgery, was not impaired.[59]

Studies of B-cell function, though limited, suggest that postoperative reduction of B-cell numbers[47] and suppression of B-cell function[60] can occur in surgical patients. Such responses, though, appear to result primarily from the stress of the surgical procedure. In anesthetized patients, B-cell function was not altered until after the surgical procedure was initiated. Moreover, neither thiopental nor halothane had a significant effect on the in vitro response of B cells to mitogen.[61,62] Procopio and co-workers reported no change in antibody responses to antigen in healthy volunteers who received either general anesthesia (thiopental/isoflurane) or lumbar epidural anesthesia (lidocaine) but did not undergo surgery.[63]

Anesthesia and surgery may alter NK-cell number and function. Both NK-cell number and in vitro cytotoxic activity were reduced after upper abdominal surgery in patients receiving general anesthesia.[64,65] Opioids in particular may exert an immunosuppressive effect on NK-cell function. Patients who received either low- or high-dose fentanyl during surgery demonstrated postoperative suppression of NK-cell cytotoxic activity, the duration of which was greater in those patients who received high-dose fentanyl.[66] Healthy volunteers administered intravenous morphine, but who did not undergo surgery, demonstrated reduced NK-cell cytotoxicity that persisted for as long as 48 hours.[67] Procopio and colleagues reported increased NK-cell cytotoxicity in healthy volunteers who received either general anesthesia (thiopental/isoflurane with no opioid) or lumbar epidural anesthesia (lidocaine) but did not undergo surgery.[63]

Phagocyte Function

Numerous studies indicate that anesthesia and surgery can impair phagocyte function and that this effect may result in part from a direct effect of anesthetic agents on PMNs and monocytes/macrophages. Inhalational agents may have suppressive effects on PMN function. Halothane, isoflurane, and sevoflurane inhibit in vitro adhesion of PMNs to endothelial cells,[68] and halothane and isoflurane inhibit in vitro PMN superoxide ion production,

that is, the "respiratory burst" important for killing pathogens.[69] Heine and colleagues studied PMNs isolated from surgical patients and found in vitro phagocytosis and respiratory burst to be suppressed after 4 hours of isoflurane anesthesia.[70] Inhalational agents also impair in vitro monocyte chemotaxis,[47] and Kotani and colleagues found decreased phagocytic activity of alveolar macrophages isolated from patients undergoing orthopedic surgery with isoflurane anesthesia.[71]

Intravenous agents used in anesthesia may alter phagocyte function. Propofol, etomidate, ketamine, and thiopental were found to suppress in vitro PMN phagocytosis and superoxide production.[72-75] Neutrophils isolated from surgical patients displayed reduced in vitro phagocytosis and respiratory burst after 4 hours of propofol anesthesia.[70] The effects of propofol on PMN function might depend on its lipid carrier. Propofol dissolved in long-chain triglycerides (LCTs) suppressed in vitro PMN superoxide formation and phagocytosis. By contrast, propofol dissolved in a mixture of LCTs and medium-chain triglycerides (MCTs) enhanced PMN production of reactive oxygen molecules.[73] Similarly, etomidate dissolved in a LCT/MCT mixture enhanced PMN function, whereas etomidate dissolved in conventional propylene glycol solvent modestly suppressed PMN function. Interestingly, and of potential clinical significance, the α_2-agonist sedative agents clonidine and dexmedetomidine do not suppress in vitro PMN phagocytosis or superoxide ion formation, despite the fact that PMNs do display α_2 adrenoceptors.[76]

Intravenous anesthetic agents may also impair monocyte/macrophage function. Ketamine and midazolam reduced in vitro monocyte chemotaxis and proliferation, and thiopental, etomidate, and propofol inhibited proliferation of cultured monocytes.[77,78] Kotani and colleagues found decreased phagocytic activity of alveolar macrophages isolated from patients undergoing orthopedic surgery with propofol anesthesia.[71]

Although evidence suggests that fentanyl may suppress NK-cell function,[66] it appears that among the opioids commonly used in anesthesia and surgery, morphine may be the only agent that suppresses PMN function. Welters and co-workers demonstrated dose-dependent reduction of PMN phagocytosis and respiratory burst in vitro by morphine action on μ-3 opioid receptors on PMN cell membranes. The inhibitory effects of morphine were linked to nitric oxide production and were blocked by the μ-receptor antagonist naloxone.[79] By contrast, fentanyl had no effect on in vitro PMN function. These results are consistent with reports that fentanyl does not bind to the μ-3 receptor[80] and that fentanyl and alfentanil do not affect PMN phagocytosis and killing of bacteria in vitro.[81]

Cytokines

Production and release of proinflammatory cytokines such as TNF-α, IL-1, IL-6, and IL-12 is a key component of host defense against infectious pathogens and the tissue response to physical trauma. Suppression of proinflammatory cytokine release in the perioperative period might predispose to particular infections.

Several studies have found no changes in plasma levels of IL-1 or TNF-α in patients undergoing anesthesia and surgery.[38,50,82-84] Low perioperative plasma levels of TNF-α is not necessarily surprising because TNF-α typically acts as a local proinflammatory mediator, and high circulating levels of TNF-α are more characteristic of major illness and systemic inflammatory response syndrome. Low perioperative plasma levels of IL-1 and TNF-α might reflect suppressed production due to a combination of catecholamine[39] and anesthetic agent effects on mononuclear cells. In a small sample of patients undergoing major vascular surgery, Kruimel and colleagues measured ex vivo production of both IL-1 and TNF-α in whole blood samples obtained from the study patients and stimulated with bacterial endotoxin.[82] Production of both TNF-α and IL-1 was reduced immediately after intubation and fell to less than 10% of baseline production at the end of surgery. Cytokine production was still depressed on postoperative day 1 and recovered to baseline levels by postoperative day 6. It is possible that one or more anesthetic agents present in the blood were partially responsible for the attenuated cytokine response to endotoxin, at least during the intraoperative period; unfortunately, the anesthetic regimen was not described. However, other studies have demonstrated effects of volatile anesthetic agents, particularly sevoflurane, to suppress in vitro TNF-α and IL-1 production by human peripheral blood mononuclear cells.[85] In mechanically ventilated rats, halothane reduced TNF-α secretion into bronchoalveolar lavage fluid in response to an endotoxin challenge.[86] By contrast, intravenous anesthetic agents may have a stimulatory effect on production of proinflammatory cytokines. Rossano and colleagues found propofol, thiopental, and ketamine to increase in vitro monocyte production of TNF-α, IL-1, and IL-6.[87]

In contrast to the above studies, Koksal and colleagues found increased plasma levels of TNF-α and IL-1 at the end of surgery in patients undergoing tympanoplasty with either desflurane or sevoflurane anesthesia.[88] Moreover, the increases in plasma TNF-α and IL-1 levels were greater in the patients who received desflurane anesthesia. It is unclear why patients in this study demonstrated elevated plasma levels of TNF-α and IL-1, though considering the relatively minor surgical procedure, it might be argued that the stress response was minimal and did not suppress production of the two cytokines.

There appears to occur consistently in surgical patients a perioperative increase in plasma levels of the proinflammatory cytokine IL-6.[38,83,84,88] Moreover, the degree to which the plasma IL-6 level increases during surgery appears to correlate with the magnitude of the surgical stress. The plasma IL-6 concentration may be the most sensitive and reliable cytokine indicator of a perioperative inflammatory response.[83] IL-6 is a potent stimulator of hepatic production of acute phase proteins such as CRP and may serve to stimulate adrenal glucocorticoid secretion.[4]

Gilliland and colleagues found postoperative plasma levels of IL-10 to be increased in patients who had undergone elective hysterectomy.[38] As discussed earlier, IL-10 produced by activated macrophages acts to inhibit T_H1 function and promote T_H2 cell function and is considered to be an "antiinflammatory" cytokine. Although the postoperative increase in plasma IL-6 was similar between patients who received either isoflurane anesthesia or total intravenous anesthesia (TIVA) with propofol, the postoperative increase in plasma IL-10 was greater in the patients who received TIVA. The authors suggested that compared with inhalational anesthesia with isoflurane, TIVA might provide an advantage of greater postoperative antiinflammatory cytokine response.

Regional Anesthesia and Analgesia

In a comprehensive review article, Hollmann and Durieux have described numerous antiinflammatory actions of local anesthetics.[89] Both in vivo and in vitro studies indicate that local anesthetics can suppress release of proinflammatory mediators and inhibit phagocyte migration and function. Therapeutic administration of local anesthetics has been found to attenuate inflammatory disease in both humans and experimental animal models. Despite potential benefits, though, the authors caution

that administration of local anesthetics to achieve systemic levels capable of antiinflammatory activity might at the same time increase risk of infection.

Neuraxial administration of local anesthetics may have little or no effect on immune function. Procopio and co-workers found no change in PMN phagocytosis and increased NK-cell cytotoxicity in healthy volunteers who received epidural lidocaine anesthesia but did not undergo surgery.[63] The authors concluded that epidural anesthesia in itself has minor, reversible effects on immune system function. Nonetheless, it is generally agreed that the stress response to surgery is less with neuraxial anesthesia than with general anesthesia. Neuraxial anesthesia can be very effective in attenuating postoperative pain, which is a potent activator of the stress response and probable contributor to postoperative immunosuppression. Not unexpectedly, a number of studies have shown that that neuraxial anesthesia can prevent, or reduce the degree of, perioperative immune dysfunction.

In a study of women undergoing elective hysterectomy, Rem and colleagues demonstrated that epidural anesthesia prevented postoperative lymphopenia that occurred in patients who underwent general anesthesia.[48] Moreover, epidural anesthesia reduced by approximately 60% the peak postoperative increase in granulocytes (i.e., PMNs) that occurred in patients who received general anesthesia. In another study of patients undergoing hysterectomy, epidural anesthesia prevented changes in lymphocyte subpopulations and NK-cell activity.[64] Le Cras and colleagues found the postoperative T_H1/T_H2 cell ratio to be increased in TURP patients who received spinal anesthesia, compared with a trend for reduced T_H1/T_H2 cell ratio in patients who received isoflurane general anesthesia.[53] The authors suggested that one advantage of spinal anesthesia over general anesthesia may be less postoperative immunosuppression.

Postoperative immune function may be influenced by the type of postoperative pain management, and independently of the degree of postoperative pain. In a recent study, patients who underwent general anesthesia (propofol/fentanyl) for major spine surgery were randomly assigned to receive either patient-controlled intravenous analgesia (PCIA; morphine) or patient-controlled epidural analgesia (PCEA; ropivacaine/sufentanil).[90] Patients who received PCEA had significantly less postoperative pain through postoperative day 3. However, in both groups, postoperative levels of neutrophils increased comparably and remained elevated through postoperative day 7. Postoperative levels of T_H cells decreased in patients receiving PCIA, but not in those receiving PCEA. By contrast, postoperative NK-cell counts decreased in the patients receiving PCEA but remained near baseline levels in patients receiving PCIA. The authors speculated that the reduction in postoperative NK-cell number with PCEA might result from administering local anesthetic in the epidural space. Postoperative plasma levels of IL-6 and IL-10 increased comparably in both groups, and thus epidural analgesia did not appear to modify postoperative inflammatory (IL-6) and antiinflammatory (IL-10) responses. The finding that PCEA preserved postoperative T_H-cell number, along with another report that PCEA preserves in vitro mitogen-stimulated lymphocyte proliferation more so than PCIA,[91] suggests that one benefit of epidural analgesia might be better resistance against postoperative infection.

Evidence suggests that the nature of the surgical procedure can affect the extent to which regional anesthesia attenuates postoperative immune dysfunction. Yokoyama and colleagues randomly assigned patients undergoing radical esophagectomy with isoflurane general anesthesia to receive either continuous epidural infusion initiated during surgery and continued into the postoperative period or postoperative continuous intravenous morphine.[92] Two epidural catheters were placed in the patients receiving epidural infusion to achieve an extensive analgesic area extending from C3 to L2. This maneuver was performed to address a report that block of phrenic nerve sensory fibers is necessary to block the stress response to upper abdominal surgery.[93] The epidural infusion consisted of lidocaine/fentanyl during surgery and ropivacaine/fentanyl in the postoperative period. Postoperative pain immediately after surgery was greater in patients receiving intravenous morphine but was not different between the two groups on postoperative days 1 to 3. Epidural analgesia prevented a perioperative rise in plasma catecholamines but not an intraoperative rise in plasma cortisol. A decline in circulating total lymphocytes and the percentage of lymphocytes composed of NK cells was similar in both groups through postoperative day 3. Plasma levels of IL-1, IL-6, and IL-10 were comparably elevated in both groups through postoperative day 3. These results suggest that epidural analgesia, even though effective in suppressing postoperative pain, may not completely block the endocrine stress response and prevent immune system alterations in patients undergoing upper abdominal surgical procedures.

SUMMARY

Two components of immunity provide defense against invading pathogens: the innate immune system and the adaptive immune system. Innate immunity is nonspecific, and adaptive, or acquired, immunity is specifically directed against a particular antigen.

Both the innate and acquired immune systems participate in the production of inflammation, which is the collective response to tissue injury caused by infectious microorganisms, toxins, or trauma. In some cases, the immune response can be greatly exaggerated, a situation referred to as *hypersensitivity*. Anaphylaxis is a severe and potentially life-threatening type I hypersensitivity reaction.

Immune system dysfunction can manifest as autoimmune disease or immunosuppression. Impairment in mechanisms that normally act to prevent autoreactivity of the immune system can lead to autoimmune disease. Primary immunodeficiency is caused by deficient function of lymphocytes, the complement system, or phagocytes.

Secondary immunodeficiency can result as an adverse effect of immunosuppressive drugs administered to prevent graft rejection or treat autoimmune disease or from infection that causes depletion of immune cells, such as occurs with human immunodeficiency virus-1 (HIV-1) infection. Numerous clinical presentations have the potential to affect anesthesia management in the patient infected with HIV. Percutaneous injury with a hollow-bore needle is the most common mechanism of occupational HIV transmission.

Surgery strongly stimulates the body's stress response, which can produce immunosuppression by release of cortisol from the adrenal cortex and catecholamine secretion from the adrenal medulla. Perioperative lymphopenia commonly occurs in patients undergoing general anesthesia and surgery, and surgical stress may reduce the T_H1/T_H2 cell ratio and predispose to certain infections. Impaired lymphocyte proliferation has been reported in surgical patients and may be caused by circulating factors such as intravenous and inhalation anesthetic agents and stress hormones. Opioids in particular appear to suppress NK cell activity.

Neuraxial anesthesia may prevent, or reduce the degree of, perioperative immune dysfunction. Spinal and epidural anesthesia have been found to prevent postoperative lymphopenia and adverse changes in lymphocyte subpopulations and NK-cell activity that occur in patients who undergo general anesthesia. Thus one potential advantage of neuraxial anesthesia over general anesthesia may be less postoperative immunosuppression. The nature of the surgical procedure, however, may affect the extent to which regional anesthesia and analgesia attenuates postoperative immune dysfunction.

REFERENCES

1. Male D et al. *Immunology*. 7th ed. Philadelphia: Mosby; 2006:3-491.
2. Nairn R, Helbert M. *Immunology for Medical Students*. 2nd ed. Philadelphia: Mosby; 2007:2-293.
3. Guyton AC, Hall JE. *Resistance of the body to infection, parts I and II. Textbook of Medical Physiology*. 11th ed. Philadelphia: Saunders; 2006: 429-450.
4. Silverman MN et al. Characterization of an interleukin-6- and adrenocorticotropin-dependent, immune-to-adrenal pathway during viral infection. *Endocrinology*. 2004;145:3580-3589.
5. Pai JK et al. Inflammatory markers and the risk of coronary heart disease in men and women. *N Engl J Med*. 2004;351:2599-2610.
6. Ridker PM et al. Plasma concentration of C-reactive protein and risk of developing peripheral vascular disease. *Circulation*. 1998;97:425-428.
7. Ackland GL et al. Pre-operative high sensitivity C-reactive protein and postoperative outcome in patients undergoing elective orthopaedic surgery. *Anesthesia*. 2007;62:888-894.
8. Mertes PM et al. Anaphylactic and anaphylactoid reactions occurring during anesthesia in France in 1999-2000. *Anesthesiology*. 2003;99:536-545.
9. Moss J. Allergic to anesthetics. *Anesthesiology*. 2003;99:521-523.
10. Cox B et al. Toxicity of local anesthetics. *Best Pract Res Clin Anaesthesiol*. 2003;17:111-136.
11. Miller RD. Transfusion therapy. In: Miller RD, ed. *Miller's Anesthesia*. 6th ed. Philadelphia: Churchill Livingstone; 2005:1799-1830.
12. Parisian S. Latex allergies causing more anesthesia problems. *Anesth Patient Safety Found Newsl*. 1992;7:1-12.
13. American Association of Nurse Anesthetists. *Latex Protocol*. Park Ridge, IL: AANA; 1998.
14. Statistics from the World Health Organization and the Centers for Disease Control. *AIDS*. 1989;2:145-149.
15. Tramont EC, Johnston MI. Progress in the development of an HIV vaccine. *Expert Opin Emerg Drugs*. 2003;8:37-45.
16. News Release. Vaccination and enrollment are discontinued in phase II of Merck's investigational HIV vaccine candidate. *HIV Vaccine Trials Network*. Sept 21, 2007.
17. Barnes PF et al. Tuberculosis in patients with human immunodeficiency virus infection. *N Engl J Med*. 1991;324:1644-1650.
18. Nicoll A, Godfrey-Faussett P. HIV and tuberculosis in the commonwealth. *BMJ*. 1999;319:1086.
19. Telenti A, Iseman M. Drug-resistant tuberculosis: what do we do now? *Drugs*. 2000;59:171-179.
20. The International Perinatal HIV Group. The mode of delivery and the risk of vertical transmission of human immunodeficiency virus type 1: a meta-analysis of 15 prospective cohort studies. *N Engl J Med*. 1999;1:977-987.
21. Grubett TA et al. Complications after caesarean section in HIV-1-infected women not taking antiretroviral treatment. *Lancet*. 1999;6:354:1612-1613.
22. Avidan M et al. Low complication rate associated with cesarean section under spinal anesthesia for HIV-1-infected women on antiretroviral therapy. *Anesthesiology*. 2002;97:320-324.
23. Newshan G. Pain management in HIV and AIDS. *GMHC Treat Issues*. 1995;9:5:10-12.
24. American Association of Nurse Anesthetists. *Infection Control Guide*. Park Ridge, IL: AANA; 1997.
25. Centers for Disease Control and Prevention. Updated U.S. Public Health Service guidelines for the management of occupational exposures to HBV, HCV, and HIV and recommendations for postexposure prophylaxis. *MMWR Morb Mortal Wkly Rep*. 2001;50(RR-11):1-52.
26. Centers for Disease Control and Prevention. HIV/AIDS Surveillance Report 2000. Vol 12. Issue 2. Atlanta, GA: U.S. Department of Health and Human Services, Public Health Service; 2000:24.

27. Gerberding JL. Occupational exposure to HIV in health care settings. *N Engl J Med.* 2003;348:826-833.

28. Occupational Safety and Health Administration. *Selected Cost and Benefit Implications of Needlestick Prevention Devices for Hospitals (Publication No. GAO-01-60R).* Washington, DC: General Accounting Office; 2000.

29. Cardo DM et al. A case-control study of HIV seroconversion in health care workers after percutaneous exposure. *N Engl J Med.* 1997;337:1485-1490.

30. Busch M et al. Time course of detection of viral and serologic markers preceding human immunodeficiency virus type 1 seroconversion: implications for screening of blood and tissue donors. *Transfusion.* 1995;35:91-97.

31. Public Health Service Task Force. Recommendations for use of antiretroviral drugs in pregnant HIV-1-infected women for maternal health and interventions to reduce perinatal HIV-1 transmission in the United States (revised November 3, 2000). *HIV Clin Trials.* 2001;2:56-91.

32. Wade NA et al. Abbreviated regimens of zidovudine prophylaxis and perinatal transmission of the human immunodeficiency virus. *N Engl J Med.* 1998;339:1409-1414.

33. Jackson JB et al. Intrapartum and neonatal single-dose nevirapine compared with zidovudine for prevention of mother-to-child transmission of HIV-1 in Kampala, Uganda: 18-month follow up of the HIVNET 012 randomized trial. *Obstet Gynecol Surv.* 2004;59:183-185.

34. Jochimsen EM. Failures of zidovudine postexposure prophylaxis. *Am J Med.* 1997;102(suppl 5B):52-55.

35. Perdue B et al. HIV-1 transmission by a needlestick injury despite rapid initiation of four-drug postexposure prophylaxis. *Program and Abstracts of the 6th Conference on Retroviruses and Opportunistic Infections.* Chicago, IL: Foundation for Retrovirology and Human Health; 1999. Abstract 107.

36. Beltrami EM et al. HIV transmission after an occupational exposure despite postexposure prophylaxis with a combination drug regimen. *Infect Control Hosp Epidemiol.* 2002;23(6):345-348.

37. Beltrami EM et al. Antiretroviral drug resistance in HIV-infected source patients for occupational exposures to healthcare workers. *Infect Control Hosp Epidemiol.* 2003;24(10):724-730.

38. Gilliland HE et al. The choice of anesthetic maintenance technique influences the antiinflammatory cytokine response to abdominal surgery. *Anesth Analg.* 1997;85:1394-1398.

39. Yoshimura T et al. Inhibition of tumor necrosis factor-alpha and interleukin-1-beta production by beta-adrenoceptor agonists from lipopolysaccharide-stimulated human peripheral blood mononuclear cells. *Pharmacology.* 1997;54:144-152.

40. Weiss M et al. Is inhibition of oxygen radical production by neutrophils by sympathomimetics mediated via beta-2 adrenoceptors? *J Pharmacol Exp Ther.* 1996;278:1105-1113.

41. Kelbel I, Weiss M. Anesthetics and immune function. *Curr Opin Anaesthesiol.* 2001;14:685-691.

42. Elenkov IJ et al. Modulatory effects of glucocorticoids and catecholamines on human interleukin-12 and interleukin-10 production: clinical implications. *Proc Assoc Am Physicians.* 1996;108(5):374-381.

43. Trokel MJ et al. Preservation of immune response after laparoscopy. *Surg Endosc.* 1994;8:1385-1387.

44. Gitzelman CA et al. Cell-mediated immune response is better preserved by laparoscopy than laparotomy. *Surgery.* 2000;127:65-71.

45. Griffith JP et al. Influence of laparoscopic and conventional cholecystectomy upon cell-mediated immunity. *Br J Surg.* 1995;82:677-680.

46. Kim C, Sakamoto A. Differences in the leukocyte response to incision during upper abdominal surgery with epidural versus general anesthesia. *J Nippon Med Sch.* 2006;73:4-9.

47. Hunter JD. Effects of anaesthesia on the human immune system. *Hosp Med.* 1999;60(9):658-663.

48. Rem J et al. Prevention of postoperative lymphopenia and granulocytosis by epidural analgesia. *Lancet.* 1980;1(8163):283-284.

49. Corsi M et al. Influence of inhalational, neuroleptic and local anesthesia on lymphocyte subset distribution. *Int J Tiss Reac.* 1995;17:211-217.

50. Helmy SA, Al-Attiyah RJ. The effect of halothane and isoflurane on plasma cytokine levels. *Anaesthesia.* 2000;55:899-910.

51. Inada T et al. Effect of propofol and isoflurane anaesthesia on the human immune response to surgery. *Anaesthesia.* 2004;59:954-959.

52. Helmy SAK et al. The effect of anaesthesia and surgery on plasma cytokine production. *Anaesthesia.* 1999;54:733-738.

53. LeCras AE et al. Spinal but not general anesthesia increases the ratio of T helper 1 to T helper 2 cell subsets in patients undergoing transurethral resection of the prostate. *Anesth Analg.* 1998;87:1421-1425.

54. Hole A, Unsgaard G. The effect of epidural and general anaesthesia on lymphocyte functions during and after major orthopedic surgery. *Acta Anesthesiol Scand.* 1983;27:135-141.

55. Hole A. Pre- and postoperative monocyte and lymphocyte functions: effects of sera from patients operated under general or epidural anesthesia. *Acta Anesthesiol Scand.* 1984;28(3):287-291.

56. Devlin EG et al. Effect of four i.v. induction agents on T-lymphocyte proliferations to PHA in vitro. *Br J Anaesth.* 1994;73:315-317.

57. Devlin EG et al. The effects of thiopentone and propofol on delayed hypersensitivity reactions. *Anaesthesia.* 1995;50:496-498.

58. Christou NV et al. The delayed hypersensitivity response and host resistance in surgical patients. 20 years later. *Ann Surg.* 1995;222:534-546.

59. Duncan PG et al. Failure of enflurane and halothane anesthesia to inhibit lymphocyte transformation in volunteers. *Anesthesiology.* 1976;45:661-665.

60. Eskola J et al. Impaired B lymphocyte function during open-heart surgery. Effects of anesthesia and surgery. *Br J Anaesth.* 1984;56:333-338.

61. Salo M. Effects of thiopentone on immunoglobulin production in vitro. *Br J Anaesth.* 1989;63:716-720.

62. Stevenson GW et al. The effect of anesthetic agents on the human immune response. *Anesthesiology.* 1990;72:542-552.

63. Procopio MA et al. The in vivo effects of general and epidural anesthesia on human immune function. *Anesth Analg.* 2001;93:460-465.

64. Tonnesen E, Wahlgreen C. Influence of extradural and general anesthesia on natural killer cell activity and lymphocyte subpopulations in patients undergoing hysterectomy. *Br J Anaesth.* 1988;60:500-507.

65. Tonnesen E et al. Natural killer cell activity in patients undergoing upper abdominal surgery: relationship to the endocrine stress response. *Acta Anaesth Scand.* 1984;28:654-660.

66. Beilin B et al. Effects of anesthesia based on large versus small doses of fentanyl on natural killer cell cytotoxicity in the perioperative period. *Anesth Analg.* 1996;82:492-497.

67. Yeager MP et al. Morphine inhibits spontaneous and cytokine-enhanced natural killer cell cytotoxicity in volunteers. *Anesthesiology.* 1995;83:500-508.

68. Mobert J et al. Inhibition of neutrophil activation by volatile anesthetics decreases adhesion to cultured human endothelial cells. *Anesthesiology.* 1999;90:1372-1381.

69. Nakagawara M et al. Inhibition of superoxide production and Ca^{+2} mobilization in human neutrophils by halothane, enflurane, and isoflurane. *Anesthesiology.* 1986;64:4-12.

70. Heine J et al. Anaesthesia with propofol decreases FMLP-induced neutrophil respiratory burst but not phagocytosis compared with isoflurane. *Br J Anaesth.* 2000;85:424-430.

71. Kotani N et al. Intraoperative modulation of alveolar macrophage function during isoflurane and propofol anesthesia. *Anesthesiology.* 1998;89:1125-1132.

72. Krumholz W et al. Inhibition of phagocytosis and killing of bacteria by anesthetic agents in vitro. *Br J Anaesth.* 1995;75:66-70.

73. Heine J et al. Flow cytometry evaluation of the in vitro influence of four i.v. anaesthetics on respiratory burst of neutrophils. *Br J Anaesth.* 1996;77:387-392.

74. Mikawa K et al. Propofol inhibits human neutrophil functions. *Anesth Analg.* 1998;87:695-700.

75. Weigand MA et al. Ketamine modulates the stimulated adhesion molecule expression on human neutrophils in vitro. *Anesth Analg.* 2000;90:206-212.

76. Nishina K et al. The effects of clonidine and dexmedetomidine on human neutrophil functions. *Anesth Analg.* 1999;88:452-458.

77. Krumholz W et al. The influence of several intravenous anaesthetics on the chemotaxis of human monocytes in vitro. *Eur J Anaesthesiol.* 1999;16:547-549.

78. Chanimov M et al. Substances used for local and general anaesthesia in major surgery suppress proliferative responsiveness of normal rat peripheral blood mononuclear cells in culture. *Eur J Anaesthesiol.* 2000;17:248-255.

79. Welters ID et al. Morphine suppresses complement receptor expression, phagocytosis, and respiratory burst in neutrophils by a nitric oxide and μ_3 opiate receptor-dependent mechanism. *J Neuroimmunol.* 2000;111:139-145.

80. Krumholz W et al. The effects of midazolam, droperidol, fentanyl, and alfentanil on phagocytosis and killing of bacteria by polymorphonuclear leukocytes in vitro. *Acta Anaesthesiol Scand.* 1995;39:624-627.

81. Bilfinger TV et al. Morphine's immunoregulatory actions are not shared by fentanyl. *Int J Cardiol.* 1998;64:561-566.

82. Kruimel JW et al. Depression of plasma levels of cytokines and ex-vivo cytokine production in relation to the activity of the pituitary-adrenal axis, in patients undergoing major vascular surgery. *Cytokine.* 1999;11:382-388.

83. Goto Y et al. General versus regional anaesthesia for cataract surgery: effects on neutrophil apoptosis and the postoperative pro-inflammatory state. *Eur J Anaesthesiol.* 2000;17:474-480.

84. Hogevold HE et al. Changes in plasma IL-1β, TNF-α and IL-6 after total hip replacement surgery in general or regional anaesthesia. *Cytokine.* 2000;12:1156-1159.

85. Mitsuhata H et al. Suppressive effects of volatile anesthetics on cytokine release in human peripheral blood mononuclear cells. *Int J Immunopharmacol.* 1995;17:529-534.

86. Giraud O et al. Halogenated anesthetics reduce interleukin-1β-induced cytokine secretion by rat alveolar type II cells in primary culture. *Anesthesiology.* 2003;98:74-81.
87. Rossano F et al. Anesthetic agents induce human mononuclear leucocytes to release cytokines. *Immunopharmacol Immunotoxicol.* 1992;14:439-450.
88. Koksal GM et al. Effects of sevoflurane and desflurane on cytokine response during tympanoplasty surgery. *Acta Anaesthesiol Scand.* 2005;49: 835-839.
89. Hollmann MW, Durieux ME. Local anesthetics and the inflammatory response. A new therapeutic indication? *Anesthesiology.* 2000;93:858-875.
90. Volk T et al. Postoperative epidural anesthesia preserves lymphocyte, but not monocyte, immune function after major spine surgery. *Anesth Analg.* 2004;98:1086-1092.
91. Beilin B et al. The effects of postoperative pain management on immune response to surgery. *Anesth Analg.* 2003;97:822-827.
92. Yokoyama M et al. The effects of continuous epidural anesthesia and analgesia on stress response and immune function in patients undergoing radical esophagectomy. *Anesth Analg.* 2005;101:1521-1527.
93. Segawa H et al. The role of phrenic nerves in stress response in upper abdominal surgery. *Anesth Analg.* 1996;82:215-1224.

CHAPTER 43

ANESTHESIA AND LASER SURGERY

Bernadette T. Higgins Roche

Although Albert Einstein first described theoretic stimulated emission of radiation in 1917, it was nearly 40 years before Arthur Schawlow and Charles Townes developed the first laser. In 1964, Townes won the Nobel Prize in physics for his work on masers and lasers. The term *laser* is an acronym for *light amplification by the stimulated emission of radiation.*[1] The first laser, a 694-nanometer (nm) ruby laser, was built by Theodore Maiman in 1960.[2] Shortly after, a near-infrared laser (1060 nm) was developed with glass rods doped with neodymium (Nd:Glass laser). Initially, lasers appeared to primarily have industrial applications, but they quickly found widespread use in a variety of unrelated fields, including construction, communications, the military, energy production, and the entertainment industry. In addition, lasers have major medical applications and make it possible to treat conditions that previously were untreatable. The surgical laser is a standard surgical instrument in any operating room and offers distinct advantages over traditional surgical techniques, including improved access to operative sites and precision in tissue destruction and removal. Surgical lasers have revolutionized the field of dermatology and esthetic surgery.[3,4]

Medical lasers were introduced in the mid-1960s when the ruby and the argon-ion lasers were first used in retinal surgery. The neodymium:yttrium-aluminum-garnet (Nd:YAG) and the carbon dioxide (CO_2) lasers found early applications in otolaryngology and gynecology. In the early 1980s, smaller and more powerful lasers were developed for the new field of laparoscopic surgery. The original surgical lasers were continuous wave (CW) and had limited use because of nonselective heat injury. Pulsed dye lasers were introduced in the late 1980s after it was discovered that "pulsing" of the laser beam allowed selective destruction of abnormal tissue. They quickly became invaluable for the treatment of pigmented skin lesions such as port-wine stains. Q-switched lasers were introduced soon after and were used to remove permanent tattoos. Scanning devices, introduced in the early 1990s, allowed computerized control of the laser beam and had a significant impact on the use of surgical lasers, especially in cosmetic surgery. Because of the unique hazards associated with surgical lasers, it is imperative that the anesthetist have an understanding of the basic physics of lasers, injuries associated with the laser beam, and the anesthetic implications of laser surgery.

BASIC PRINCIPLES OF LASERS

Light

Electromagnetic radiation is a broad spectrum of heat energy composed of radio waves, microwaves, infrared waves, visible light waves, ultraviolet waves, x-rays, and gamma rays (Figure 43-1). A wavelength is defined as the distance between two successive points on a periodic wave that has the same phase. There is a progressive decrease in wavelength and an increase in frequency as the electromagnetic spectrum moves from radio waves to gamma waves. The optical portion of the electromagnetic spectrum is composed of ultraviolet, visible, and infrared waves with a wavelength range of 200 to 1000 nm. The visible light spectrum that can be seen or sensed by the human eye constitutes a very small portion of the electromagnetic spectrum. Visible light includes a rainbow of colors—red, orange, yellow, green, blue, indigo, and violet—with a very narrow range of wavelengths of 400 nm (violet) to 700 nm (red). Both infrared and ultraviolet waves are invisible to the human eye, but certain fish, reptiles, and insects can sense ultraviolet waves. Although the infrared portion of the optical spectrum is perceived as heat, ultraviolet waves cause a chemical reaction in human skin with little heat production. Incandescent light is white and actually composed of several different wavelengths.

Light can be described as both a wavelength and a particle, or quantum, of energy called a *photon*. The energy of an electromagnetic wave is proportional to its frequency and inversely proportional to its wavelength. Because of its short wavelength and high frequency, ultraviolet radiation contains a lot of energy that can damage the skin. The energy of a photon is defined as the energy emitted when an electron falls from an excited orbit to one of lower energy; the energy between the two orbits defines the wavelength of the emitted photon.[5] The relationship between the energy and the wavelength of light is expressed by the following equation:

Equation 43-1

$$E = hc/\lambda$$

where E = energy in joules, h = Planck's constant (6.63×10^{-34} J-s), c = the speed of light (2.998×10^{-8} m/s), and λ = wavelength in meters.

Spontaneous Absorption and Emission of Energy

Electrons of an atom occupy shells, or orbits, and each orbit has a different energy. The higher the orbit, the greater the energy. The ground state is an atom's lowest energy state. Electrons can move from one orbit or energy level to another by the *spontaneous absorption or emission of energy.* When an electron absorbs energy, it can jump to a higher energy (metastable) state; conversely, it emits energy if it falls to a lower orbit. Electrons have a tendency to return to the ground state spontaneously, releasing a photon of light energy in the process. This is called *spontaneous emission of radiation.* The energy of the photon and therefore its wavelength is dependent on the energy levels between the two orbits. When several atoms undergo spontaneous decay at the same time, the emitted photons will not be in phase with each other. Light produced by fluorescent lights or incandescent bulbs is a result of electrons changing orbits and returning to ground state; in the process they release photons that radiate randomly in all directions. The energy of the photon and the wavelength of the light are proportional to the energy difference between the excited state and the ground state of the atom. The light produced by spontaneous emission is composed of different wavelengths and frequencies; the photons oscillate randomly (noncoherence), and the light disperses as it travels.

Laser Radiation

An atom can be "pumped" up to a higher energy level by a stimulating photon if the energy of the stimulating photon is the same as the energy level between the two orbits. Likewise, a stimulating photon can cause an electron in an excited state to undergo decay. Laser light requires stimulated emission of energy. When a stimulating photon strikes an atom in the excited state,

the atom decays back to its ground state, emitting a second photon. If the energy of the stimulating photon is equal to the energy difference between the excited and ground states of the atom, the atom emits a photon of the same wavelength, energy, frequency, and direction and in phase with the stimulating photon. This process is known as *stimulated emission of radiation* (Figure 43-2). The two photons can strike other excited atoms, stimulating further emission of photons. This process produces a sudden burst of coherent radiation as all the atoms return to ground state in a rapid chain reaction.

Properties of laser light that differentiate it from fluorescent or incandescent light include coherence, directionality, and monochromaticity. Unlike natural light, laser beam photons have the same wavelength and oscillate synchronously in identical phase with one another (coherence). Laser light displays minimal dispersion and moves in a parallel, narrow beam (spatial coherence) over long distances. This spatial coherence, known as *collimation*, allows the laser to be focused on a very small area (Figure 43-3). Reflectors placed on the moon allow calculation of the distance from the moon to the earth by measuring the amount of time it takes for a laser light to return to earth. Reflection of a laser beam can reduce the collimation and increase the dispersion, especially if the reflecting surface has a matte or dull finish; however, the reduction in collimation and increased dispersion of a reflected laser beam is insignificant if the reflecting surface is smooth and shiny. Laser light is composed of specific and discrete wavelengths; consequently the light emitted is monochromatic and

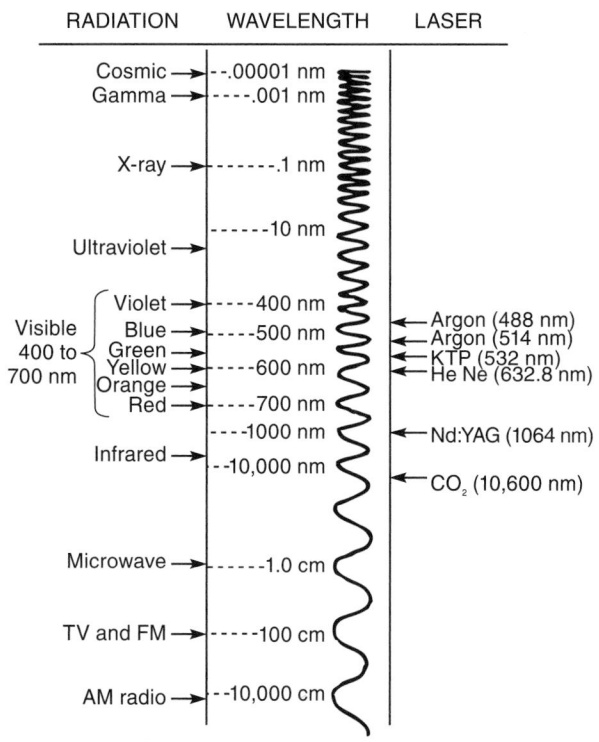

FIGURE **43-1** Electromagnetic spectrum. (*Modified from Arndt KA et al, eds.* Lasers in Cutaneous and Aesthetic Surgery. *Philadelphia: Lippincott-Raven; 1997:4.*)

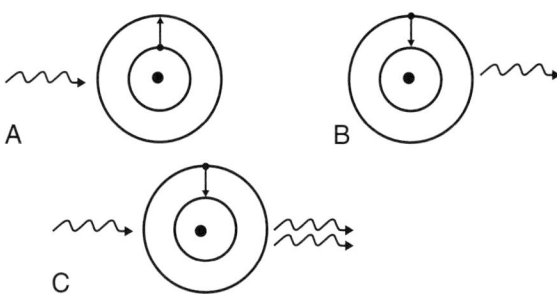

FIGURE **43-2** **A,** Spontaneous absorption of energy. Absorption of energy from a striking photon will allow electrons to move a higher energy (metastable) state. **B,** Spontaneous release of energy. As an atom decays back to its ground state, an electron falls to a lower orbit and releases a photon of energy. **C,** Stimulated emission of energy. When an excited atom is stimulated by a striking photon, it releases a photon of the same wavelength and frequency that travels in phase and in the same direction as the stimulating photon.

FIGURE **43-3** Characteristics of light. Incandescent (white) light **(A)** is composed of different wavelengths and frequencies. It is noncoherent and disperses as it travels (noncollimation). In contrast, laser light **(B)** is monochromatic. It is composed of photons with the same wavelength and frequency (coherence) and displays minimal dispersion as it travels (collimation).

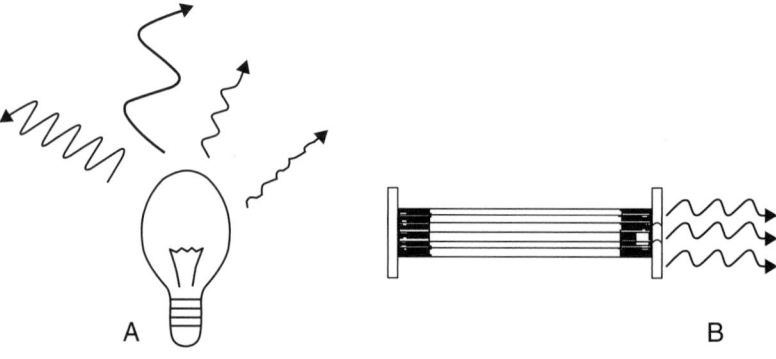

specific for each laser. Just as white light is composed of multiple colors, some lasers are tunable and can emit light at several different wavelengths. However, tunable lasers can only emit one color or wavelength at a time. A typical light bulb is more powerful than a laser, but its light is not collimated, and the dispersion of the light reduces its intensity. In contrast, the intensity of a 1-milliwatt (mW) laser can be six times that of a 100-watt (W) incandescent bulb. Although a typical laser emits only a few milliwatts of power, from a distance of 100 feet lasers can produce a highly intense beam of 1 to 2 mm that can be 1 million times more concentrated than light from an incandescent source.

Components of a Laser

A laser is a device that creates and amplifies a narrow, intense beam of coherent light. It consists of an energy source, an optical resonating cavity, and a laser medium to create the laser light (Figure 43-4).[6]

Energy Source

Lasers require an external energy source for excitation of the lasing medium. Flash lamps, continuous light, high-voltage discharge, diodes, and, in some cases, another laser can be used as the energy source. The external energy is used to transfer or pump up the energy of the laser medium. The electrons in the lasing medium absorb the energy and move to a higher energy state. Electric current is used to excite gas lasers, such as carbon dioxide (CO_2) and argon (Ar) lasers. Liquid and solid state lasers, such as the KTP laser, require activation by a flash lamp or another laser.

Optical Resonating Cavity

The optical resonating cavity is a tubelike structure that provides optimal amplification of the laser beam. It contains the lasing medium and a mirror at each end of the tube. When the lasing medium is excited by the outside energy source (e.g., flash lamp, electric current), the atoms are "pumped" to a higher energy level, increasing the number of atoms in the excited state. Population inversion is necessary for stimulated emission of radiation, and it occurs when more atoms are in an unstable excited state than the resting state. When one of the atoms spontaneously decays back to its ground state, it releases a photon that "stimulates" another excited molecule to decay back to its ground state, releasing another photon. The wavelength, frequency, phase, and direction of the second photon are identical to those of the first photon. The mirrors reflect the excited photons back into the resonating cavity at approximately 186,000 miles per second, where they travel back and forth in a parallel fashion, stimulating the release of more photons from other excited atoms. A cascade effect occurs, and the resultant light is amplified. One of the mirrors is partially transparent and allows a portion of the coherent, collimated, and monochromatic laser light to escape in a very thin beam that can be easily focused on a very small area.

Laser Medium

The laser medium can be a solid, gas, liquid, or semiconductor that is stimulated to a metastable state when pumped with an external energy source. Lasers are commonly named after the laser medium, and the medium determines the wavelength output of the laser. Solid-state lasers such as the Nd:YAG laser use a solid matrix that is doped with a small amount of impurity (dopant). It is the impurity, neodymium (Nd), that provides the energy source for the laser. Solid-state lasers are more powerful than gas lasers and require optical pumping. Gas lasers use a variety of gases as lasing media, including argon, CO_2, helium, helium-neon, and krypton. An electrical source of energy is required for pumping. Complex dyes, dissolved in a liquid such as alcohol, constitute the lasing media in liquid lasers. Optically pumped, liquid lasers are tunable over a broad range of wavelengths, mostly in the visible spectrum. Excimer lasers use electrical stimulation to produce a dimer of a halogen such as chlorine and fluorine and an inert gas such as argon, krypton, or xenon. The dimer is unstable and quickly breaks down into its constituent atoms, releasing energy in the form of light. Semiconductor lasers, also called *diode lasers*, are composed of semiconductor crystals that are pumped by a high-intensity current. They are commonly used in compact disk players, laser printers, and laser pointers. The gallium-arsenide laser is an example of a semiconductor laser.

Modes of Operation

Most medical lasers deliver only one wavelength, so laser selection is dependent on the desired effect on the targeted tissue. The wavelength or color of the laser light is dependent on the laser medium, and the effect on tissue is dependent on the wavelength. In addition to selecting the appropriate wavelength, the surgeon must use the appropriate exposure time and energy density (power setting) to achieve the intended photomechanical, photothermolytic, or photochemical effect.

A laser beam can be delivered in a continuous wave (CW), pulsed-wave, or Q-switched mode. In the CW mode, the laser emits a steady beam for as long as the laser medium is excited. The power output of a CW laser is measured in watts and can vary significantly among lasers. The power of the helium-neon laser is measured in milliwatts, whereas the output of the more powerful CO_2 laser is measured in kilowatts. Power density of the beam (irradiance or flux) varies from a few watts per square centimeter to hundreds of watts per square centimeter. Collateral tissue damage can be expected if the laser beam is held on

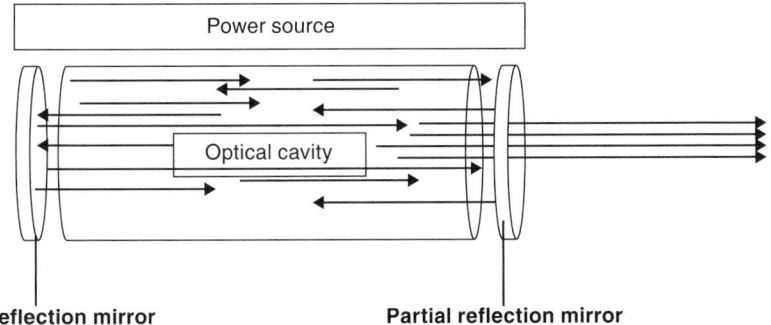

100% Reflection mirror   **Partial reflection mirror**

FIGURE **43-4** Basic components of a laser. The optical cavity contains the lasing medium (solid, liquid, gas). The power source (flashlamp, electric current, other laser) pumps up the electrons in the lasing medium to a higher energy state. Two mirrors reflect the photons back into the cavity, where they stimulate other excited atoms to emit identical photons. One mirror is partially transparent and allows a portion of the laser beam to exit the cavity in a narrow beam.

tissue longer than the thermal relaxation time (time it takes for 50% of the laser energy to be thermally conducted to surrounding tissue). Pulsing the laser beam or scanning a continuous beam allows time for concentration of the energy, limits the exposure time, and minimizes thermal damage. In the pulsed mode, the laser emits peak energy levels in individual pulses from femtoseconds (quadrillionths of a second) to seconds. The power of a pulsed laser is measured in joules, and energy intensity is expressed as joules per square centimeter. The duration of the laser beam is limited by computerized scanning of the laser beam in a preset pattern before delivery of the beam to the tissue. In the Q-switched mode, the laser emits high-energy, ultrashort pulses (approximately 10 to 250 nanoseconds [nsec]). A shutter is placed in the optical path to allow the buildup of a large population inversion. After release of the shutter, the electrons fall rapidly to ground state, releasing a large amount of energy that is measured in megawatts. The effects of the laser on the tissue can be controlled by the mode of delivery. The Nd:YAG laser can be used in CW mode for coagulation of tumors, in the pulsed mode for hair removal, and in the Q-switched mode for tattoo removal. In the CW mode, the CO_2 laser can be focused very tightly and used for incision, much like a scalpel. In contrast, the defocused CO_2 laser can be used to vaporize a larger area. When delivered through a scanning device, the laser beam can remove a predetermined thickness of skin.

Fiberoptic cables are used for delivery of laser beams with visible and near-infrared wavelengths. Articulated arms with reflecting mirrors mounted in tubes are used to direct the beam of a far infrared laser (CO_2). Additional devices may be attached to the fiberoptic cables or articulated arms, including slit lamps (for use on the eye), operating microscopes, and insulated fibers (for use with endoscopes). Contact laser probes (sapphire) attached to the distal end of a fiberoptic bundle transform the light energy into heat for precise cutting and reduced penetration. Because of drastic increases in temperature ($> 800°$ C), the probes require a compressed gas or liquid jet cooling system.

MEDICAL LASERS

Because of their ability to cause rapid and precise vaporization or coagulation of tissues, lasers are commonly used in a variety of unrelated diagnostic and therapeutic procedures. Laser light is monochromatic and has very selective effects on biologic tissues. The degree of laser light transmission, scattering, reflection, or absorption is dependent on the tissue and the wavelength. Light absorption is necessary for the laser to be effective; if the tissue transmits, reflects, or scatters the light, the laser will have little or no effect on the tissue. A specific wavelength may be absorbed by one type of tissue and transmitted by another. Biologic tissues can be thought of as an aqueous solution of light-absorbing molecules. Chromophores, such as hemoglobin and melanin, and water are the main absorbing components, and they determine the reaction of the tissue to the light. To be effective, the laser light must match the absorptive property of the tissue. When absorption occurs, the laser light is converted to heat. If the temperature reaches 100° C, vaporization or ablation of the tissue occurs. As the tissue is vaporized, the thermal energy of the laser beam cauterizes capillaries and provides immediate hemostasis. A lower temperature will produce tissue coagulation or denaturation rather than ablation.

A tissue's reaction to light absorption depends on the wavelength, intensity, and exposure time of the light. Powerful, short pulses of laser light cause an explosive tissue expansion (photomechanical reaction), whereas low-power, long pulses cause a rapid increase in temperature (photothermal reaction) that results in tissue vaporization and coagulation. When applied for longer durations, low-power lasers can cause a chemical reaction or change in specific molecules (photochemical reaction). Laser light can also be used to activate a photosensitizing medication that is selectively absorbed by a specific tissue (photodynamic reaction). The effectiveness of nonthermal laser-assisted techniques is dependent on the ability of special drugs (photosynthesizers) to produce cytotoxicity in the presence of oxygen (O_2) after stimulation with light of an appropriate wavelength.

Tissue absorption is greatest with longer wavelengths such as the far-infrared wavelength of the CO_2 laser (10,600 nm). The CO_2 laser beam is completely absorbed by water in the first few cellular layers, resulting in explosive vaporization of the top layer but little or no damage to the underlying tissues. Excimer lasers (ultraviolet) are associated with an even more superficial effect because of their strong absorption by water. The light from lasers with visible wavelengths, such as the ruby, argon, and krypton lasers, is transmitted by water and absorbed by cells that contain dark pigment. It can penetrate the skin and the cornea to coagulate pigmented or vascular lesions. The light from near-infrared lasers, such as the Nd:YAG, is transmitted rather than absorbed by water. Because they have a greater tissue penetration, near-infrared lasers are better suited for deeper procedures such as tumor debulking. Advantages of lasers include precision, access to remote sites in the body, reduced blood loss, reduced damage to adjacent tissue, and improved patient satisfaction. A disadvantage of laser therapy may be delayed wound healing.[7,8]

Ophthalmology was the first medical specialty to adopt laser therapy. Lasers continue to play a major role in ophthalmology, with the excimer laser used for vision correction. Urology was another area of medicine in which lasers found early application, and such therapy continues to be a treatment option for a variety of urologic problems, including strictures, genital condylomas, prostatic hypertrophy, urethral calculi, and interstitial cystitis. Laser surgery of the upper and lower airways offers definite advantages over traditional surgery, including access, precision, anatomic preservation, and controlled hemostasis. Both fiberoptic and rigid bronchoscopes allow laser resection of endobronchial lesions. Interstitial laser thermotherapy is used for destruction of both superficial and deep solid tumors.[8] In orthopedics, lasers are used in endoscopic laser-assisted disk surgery and arthroscopic procedures.[9,10] They also have several applications in cardiovascular surgery, including transmyocardial laser revascularization and percutaneous transluminal angioplasty.[11-13] Lasers have revolutionized dermatology and plastic surgery and are indispensable in oral surgery and otolaryngology.[4,14] Dentists and periodontists incorporate lasers in their practice for gum reshaping, drilling, and whitening of teeth. Low-power laser therapy appears to be useful in the management of chronic low back pain.[15]

Types of Medical Lasers

The major types of lasers used in medicine are far-infrared (CO_2), mid-infrared (erbium [Er]:YAG, holmium [Ho]:YAG, Nd:YAG), near-infrared (diode), visible (ruby, krypton, argon, copper, and gold vapor), and ultraviolet (excimer). Commonly used surgical lasers are listed in Table 43-1.

Carbon Dioxide Laser

The most commonly used surgical laser is the CO_2 laser. The infrared light produced by the CO_2 laser (10,600 nm) is invisible

TABLE **43-1**	Common Surgical Lasers	
Laser	**Wavelength**	**Applications**
Far Infrared		
CO_2	10,600 nm	Multiple uses: general surgery, orthopedics, gynecology, urology, otolaryngology, plastic surgery
Mid-Infrared		
Nd:YAG	1064 nm	Multiple uses: gastroenterology, pulmonology, urology, ophthalmology, dermatology
Ho:YAG	2070 nm	Orthopedics, urology
Er:YAG	2940 nm	Dermatology
Near Infrared		
Diode	800-900 nm	Multiples uses: ophthalmology, otolaryngology, periodontics, cosmetic surgery, pain management. Multiple nonmedical applications
Visible		
Argon	488 and 514 nm	Multiple uses: ophthalmology, plastic surgery, dermatology, gynecology, otolaryngology
Krypton	476, 521, 568 nm	Dermatology
Copper bromide	511 and 577 nm	Dermatology, photosynthesizer
KTP	532 nm	Dermatology
Pulsed dye	577-585 nm	Dermatology
Gold	578-628 nm	Oncology
Ruby	694 nm	Dermatology
Alexandrite	755 nm	Dermatology
Ultraviolet (Excimer)		
Argon-fluoride	193 nm	Multiple uses: ophthalmology, dermatology
Krypton-fluoride	249 nm	Dermatology
Xenon-chloride	308 nm	Multiple uses: dermatology, ophthalmology, dermatology
Xenon-fluoride	351 nm	Multiple uses: angioplasty, ophthalmology, dermatology

to the human eye, and a low-power helium-neon (He-Ne) laser (633 nm) is incorporated to provide a visible red beam for surgical aim. Because it emits light in the infrared region of the electromagnetic spectrum, the CO_2 laser is a powerful but dangerous laser. Infrared radiation is heat, and this laser basically melts through whatever its beam is focused on, including steel. It is a very precise laser; with the lateral zone of damage less than 0.5 nm from the area of incision.[1] The CO_2 laser beam is not transmitted by quartz, glass, or other transparent material and must be delivered as a free beam or through a rigid endoscope with a mirrored, articulated arm.

Light from the CO_2 laser is strongly absorbed by water, and vaporization of cells occurs within the first 100 to 200 µm of the irradiated surface. It can be used in both the CW and pulsed-wave mode. Blood loss is minimal during CO_2 laser procedures. Focused into a tight beam, the CO_2 laser can be used for cutting. Defocusing the beam decreases the power density, and the tissue will be vaporized, or *ablated*. The CO_2 laser is used extensively in general surgery, orthopedics, gynecology, urology, and otolaryngology. When used with a scanning device, thin layers of the skin are ablated for skin resurfacing, such as in plastic surgery. Because of its high power, the CO_2 laser is widely used in industry for cutting, drilling, and welding.

Yttrium-Aluminum-Garnet Lasers

The lasing medium of a yttrium-aluminum-garnet laser is a YAG crystal rod doped with atoms of rare earth minerals, which accounts for the different properties of the YAG lasers. YAG lasers can be used in the CW, pulsed-wave, or Q-switched mode.

Neodymium:Yttrium-Aluminum-Garnet Laser. The Nd:YAG laser emits a near-infrared invisible light at 1064 nm and requires the addition of a visible aiming beam. It has a penetration of 5 to 7 mm and can be used to cut or coagulate tissue. In the Q-switched mode, the laser removes black tattoo ink and hair. The Nd:YAG laser has important applications in internal debulking or destruction of lesions and is used to treat gastrointestinal and tracheobronchial tumors and genitourinary lesions. The pulsed and Q-switched Nd:YAG laser is used in ophthalmology. The energy of the Nd:YAG beam is more widely dispersed, and damage to adjacent tissues may not be evident for hours after the laser treatment.

Holmium:Yttrium-Aluminum-Garnet Laser. When doped with holmium (Ho) the YAG laser emits a mid-infrared beam at 2070 nm that is strongly absorbed by water. Output in the mid-infrared spectrum requires a coincident aiming beam. The Ho:YAG is used to vaporize, cut, coagulate, and sculpt avascular tissue with a minimal amount of thermal necrosis. The primary applications of the Ho:YAG laser are in endoscopic orthopedic procedures (bone and cartilage ablation) and urology (stone removal and transurethral resection of the prostate [TURP]).

Erbium:Yttrium-Aluminum-Garnet Laser. When the YAG laser is doped with erbium (Er), it emits a mid-infrared beam at 2940 nm (peak absorption of water). Because the infrared beam is not transmitted by quartz or glass, the Er:YAG can be used only as a free beam or through a rigid endoscope. It has limited penetration and excellent precision. It is used extensively in laser resurfacing of the skin and vaporization of fibrous tissue, cartilage, and bone. Because of its ability to penetrate dental tissue, the Er:YAG is also used in microdentistry for cavity fillings, root canals, and treatment of gum disease.

Diode Lasers

Diode lasers are semiconductors. They emit a near-infrared light (800 to 900 nm) when pumped with a high-intensity electric current. Medical uses include ophthalmology, dermatology (hair removal), and periodontal surgery. Diode lasers are also used to "pump" other laser media such as YAG rods. They have multiple nonmedical applications and are used in laser printers, music recordings, and fiberoptic communication systems.

Visible Lasers

Argon Laser. In an argon laser, the argon gas has lost one or more of its electrons, and the positive ions are excited by a large electrical discharge. The argon ion laser emits visible blue-green light with wavelengths of 488 nm and 514 nm simultaneously. The laser light is transmitted by water and absorbed by hemoglobin and melanin, where the main effect is photocoagulation. Penetration is approximately 1 to 2 millimeters (mm), but this can vary depending on the degree of pigmentation. The beam passes through quartz optical fibers, allowing the laser to be used with a microscope or endoscope. The argon laser is used in ophthalmology, plastic surgery, dermatology, gynecology, and otolaryngology. A forced-air or water-cooling system is required for this laser.

Krypton Laser. The active medium, krypton, is also a rare gas with one or more electrons removed, and the krypton ions are excited by an electrical discharge. The laser produces visible green and blue light at 476, 521, and 568 nm. It is absorbed by hemoglobin and used for photocoagulation of vascular or pigmented lesions.

Ruby Laser. The ruby laser uses a synthetic ruby crystal of aluminum oxide doped with chromium. It emits a red light with a wavelength of 694 nm and has a penetration greater than 1 mm. The ruby laser light is absorbed by melanin and blue, green, and black pigment. It is very effective for tattoo removal, hair removal, and treatment of pigmented lesions such as freckles, liver spots, and nevi (Q-switched mode). Because the ruby laser has a low efficiency and requires a cooling system, its use has declined in favor of newer and more powerful lasers.

Alexandrite Laser. Named after Czar Alexander II, the solid-state laser contains a rod of synthetic chrysoberyl doped with chromium. It emits a deep red light at 755 nm, and frequency doubling of the alexandrite laser produces a tunable laser output of 360 to 400 nm. Blue and black pigments absorb the beam, with a lesser degree of absorption by melanin. Properties and uses are similar to those of the ruby laser.

Metal Vapor Lasers

The active medium of metal vapor lasers is a neutral metal heated beyond its vapor point. A pulsed electrical discharge is used for excitation of the vapor. Vaporized copper bromide emits green light at 511 nm and yellow light at 577 nm. It is used to treat vascular lesions. It also has applications for facial resurfacing. The gold vapor laser (578 to 628 nm) is used in photodynamic therapy for cancer.

Potassium-Titanyl-Phosphate Laser (KTP)

The wavelength of the Nd:YAG laser is halved when it is passed through a potassium-titanyl-phosphate (KTP) crystal. A solid-state laser, the KTP laser is similar to the argon gas laser. The beam is transmitted by water and absorbed within 1 to 2 mm of vascular or pigmented tissue. A bright green light (532 nm) delivered through fiberoptics, scanners, or microscopes is used to cut tissue (CW mode) and remove vascular lesions (pulsed mode) and red-orange and black tattoo ink (Q-switched mode). Although the power density of the KTP laser is sufficient to cut vascular tissue, it is insufficient to achieve effective hemostasis.

Dye Lasers

Dye lasers use organic fluorescent materials dissolved in a solvent such as methanol and are typically pumped with a flashlamp or another laser. The energy levels of the dyes are very close to one another and allow the lasers to release a wide range of wavelengths. In the CW and pulsed mode, dye lasers have wavelengths of 400 to 1000 nm. They can produce extremely short pulses (measured in trillionths of a second [picoseconds]). The major advantage of the dye laser is the ability to tune the wavelength to maximize the laser-tissue interaction. Dye lasers are used in dermatology for excision of vascular and pigmented lesions, in urology for treatment of urinary calculi, and in oncology for photodynamic therapy. The pulsed dye laser (PDL) uses a rhodamine dye to emit a yellow laser beam at 577 to 585 nm (peak absorption of hemoglobin). It is the laser of choice for treatment of port-wine stains in children and thick, red scars.

Excimer Lasers

Derived from the terms *excited* and *dimer*, excimer lasers use a medium composed of a reactive noble gas (chlorine or fluorine) and an inert halogen gas (argon, krypton, or xenon). When the medium is electrically stimulated, an unstable pseudomolecule (dimer) is produced. As the dimer breaks down to its constituent atoms, it releases light in the ultraviolet range that is strongly absorbed by water. Excimer lasers have a photochemical effect on targeted tissues (pulsed mode), with minimal thermal effect on the underlying tissue. The very short wavelength (ultraviolet) is capable of high resolution and has applications in microscopic surgery. Excimer lasers are currently used in ophthalmology for photorefractive keratectomy (PRK) and laser in situ keratomileusis (LASIK). Other uses include removal of arterial plaques and treatment of psoriasis. Examples of excimer lasers are the argon-fluoride (193 nm), krypton-fluoride (249 nm), xenon-chloride (308 nm) and xenon-fluoride (351 nm) lasers.

Cold Lasers

Cold lasers, also known as *low-level laser therapy (LLLT)* and *soft lasers*, use diodes to produce visible to infrared light. The laser beam can penetrate up to 2 inches without damaging tissues or producing a significant amount of heat. Through biostimulation of cellular metabolism, cold lasers speed up the healing process. They are used for treatment of carpal tunnel syndrome and other soft-tissues injuries.

Photodynamic Therapy (PDT)

Photosensitizers such as porfimer sodium (Photofrin) are attracted to cancer cells. Approximately 72 hours after intravenous administration, when the photosensitizer has left normal cells but remains in cancer cells, the tumor is exposed to laser light with a red wavelength. The photosensitizer absorbs the light and produces an active form of oxygen that destroys cancer cells. Currently PDT is used to treat esophageal and pulmonary tumors and has potential for application in dermatology and ophthalmology.

LASER SAFETY

The Bureau of Radiological Health (BRH) assigns lasers and laser systems to four categories (Table 43-2), Class I to IV, according to their potential for causing biologic damage. Class I lasers are incapable of producing damaging radiation and are exempt from radiation hazard controls. This classification includes CD players and laser printers; supermarket laser scanners are classified as IA. Class II lasers emit radiation in the visible portion of the electromagnetic spectrum but at a radiant power less than 1 mW. The human aversion reaction to bright light will protect the eyes, but injury can occur if the beam is viewed directly for an extended period of time. Class II lasers include laser pointers and scanners. Class III lasers can cause eye injury when viewed directly and include spectroscopy and light shows. The direct beam and reflected beam of Class IV lasers are hazardous to the eye and are potential fire and skin hazards. Reflected beams are specular and maintain the beam coherence; diffuse beams are scattered when they are reflected from a rough or matte surface. Most medical lasers are Class IV; these lasers also create hazardous airborne contaminants and require a high-voltage power supply. The U.S. Food and Drug Administration (FDA) regulates the manufacturing and marketing of lasers used in medicine; however, it does not regulate laser safety. The American National Standards Institute's (ANSI) Z136.3–2005 is the most commonly used laser standard addressing medical laser safety.[16] Compliance with the ANSI guidelines is voluntary. The Occupational Safety and Health Administration (OHSA) has

identified the hazards associated with the use of medical lasers and has developed safety standards to protect patients and operating room personnel.[17] ANSI requires a Laser Safety Officer (LSO) at institutions that utilize Class IIIB or Class IV lasers. The LSO is responsible for overseeing operation, maintenance, safety, and servicing of medical lasers. A number of professional organizations have also developed recommendations for laser safety. Physicians who use lasers should have appropriate training and institutional privileges for laser use.

Only qualified personnel should operate laser equipment. An aiming beam should be used if the laser does not produce a visible light. When not in use, the laser should be disabled and stored in a secure location. When the laser is in use, appropriate laser warning signs should be posted inside and outside the laser area (Figure 43-5). Doors should remain closed during laser operation, and windows should be covered to prevent the transmission of a misdirected laser beam. Safety controls should limit access to the laser area through the use of a safety interlock system that will prevent unexpected entry or trigger a shut-off device for the laser if the door is unexpectedly opened. Lasers require high power and carry the potential for electrical injury. In addition, liquid gases

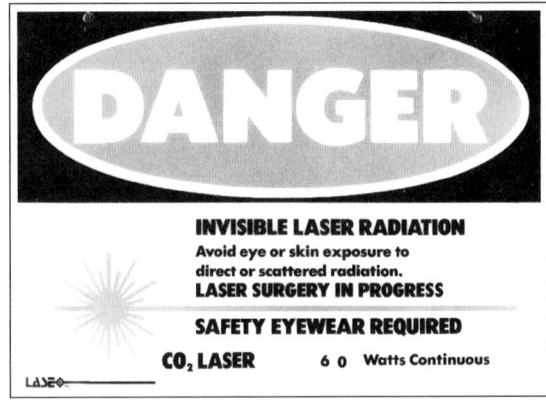

FIGURE **43-5** Danger sign indicating laser procedure in progress.

TABLE **43-2**	Laser Classification
Class I	Do not emit hazardous radiation and are exempt from radiation hazard controls. Typically continuous wave of 0.4 µW at visible wavelengths. Examples: CD players and laser printers, CD-ROM devices, geologic survey equipment, and laboratory analytical equipment.
Class IA	Includes lasers that are not intended for viewing. Maximum power is 4.0 mW. Example: supermarket laser scanners.
Class II	Do not cause ocular injury unless viewed directly for an extended period. The normal aversion response to bright light protects the eye from a brief exposure. Class II lasers only operate in the visible range (400-700 nm). Maximum power is ≤1 mW. Examples: helium-neon lasers and some laser pointers.
Class IIA	Special-purpose lasers not intended for viewing. Power output is less than 1 mW. Ocular injury can occur if viewed directly for more than 1000 seconds over an 8-hour day, not continuous exposure. Examples: scanners and bar-code readers.
Class IIIA	Do not pose a serious eye hazard unless viewed through optical instruments (e.g., microscopes). Power outputs for CW lasers operating in the visible range are between 1 and 5 mW. Examples: solid-state laser pointers.
Class IIIB	Direct beam viewing or specular reflections will result in ocular injury. Power output between 5 and 500 mW for CW lasers and <0.125 J within 0.25 second for a pulsed laser. Do not produce a hazardous diffuse reflection and are not considered fire hazards. Examples: spectroscopy, stereolithography, and entertainment light shows.
Class IV	Significant ocular injury can result from direct beam viewing, specular reflections, and diffuse reflections. These lasers require significant controls. Power output >500 mW for a CW laser and >0.125 J within 0.25 second for a pulsed laser. Skin and fire hazards are also present with Class IV lasers. Examples: medical lasers and industrial lasers (drilling, cutting, and welding).

used for cooling of the laser medium, especially liquid nitrogen, are hazardous to the skin if accidentally spilled. Vaporization of liquid nitrogen also decreases the ambient O_2 concentration, and its use should be limited to well-ventilated spaces. Some of the chemicals used in dye lasers can be toxic and hazardous to handle.

Although lasers pose a variety of risks to humans and equipment, the most common hazards of medical lasers are thermal trauma, eye injury, perforation of organs or vessels, gas embolization, pollution, and fire. The majority of laser-related accidents and injuries can be attributed to inappropriate use or intentional use of malfunctioning equipment.[18] In addition to the risk of laser trauma incurred by patients, significant risks exist for operating room personnel secondary to misdirected beams during laser procedures. The laser beam is transmitted through air and reflected by smooth metal surfaces such as metal cabinets and large surgical instruments such as retractors.

LASER HAZARDS AND PRECAUTIONS

Thermal Trauma

The most common cause of laser-induced tissue damage is thermal in nature. Tissue proteins are denatured after absorption of the laser energy, and tissue damage can range from mild reddening of the skin to blistering and charring.[19] Skin trauma is dependent on the energy and wavelength of the laser. Longer wavelengths have a deeper skin penetration than shorter wavelengths; shorter wavelengths (400 to 700 nm) are nearly completely absorbed in the first 4 mm of the skin. Burns occur with exposure times greater than 10 μsec and wavelengths ranging from the near ultraviolet to the far infrared (315 to 10,300 nm). Ultraviolet-A (315 to 400 nm) exposure causes hyperpigmentation and erythema, but the greatest skin damage is caused by ultraviolet-B (UV-B) radiation (280 to 315 nm). In addition to thermal trauma, carcinogenesis is a potential risk of UV-B exposure. Exposure to ultraviolet-C (UV-C) waves (200 to 280 nm) is less harmful to the skin because they are predominantly absorbed in the outer dead layers of the epidermis. Exposure to visible and near-infrared lasers can cause photosensitive reactions and burns. The major skin damage associated with mid- and far-infrared lasers is burns. Lasers may also precipitate the development of or exaggerate existing skin lesions, including reactivation of viral infections.[20]

Patients should have saline-soaked towels applied to the skin surrounding the path of the laser beam. Jackets and gloves will provide skin protection for operating room personnel. Topical sunblock cream will protect against ultraviolet radiation for patients undergoing repeat laser treatments.[17]

Eye Trauma

The human eye is extremely vulnerable to laser beams. Laser radiation is coherent, and all of its energy can be focused on a very small portion of the cornea or retina. The eye is not harmed by incandescent and fluorescent light because those lights are incoherent, and only a small portion of the energy is spread out over the retina. Eye trauma from laser light is dependent on the intensity and wavelength of the laser and the exposed tissue. Pulsed-mode lasers present an additional hazard to the eye. Laser pulses less than 10 microseconds induce shock waves that rupture tissue, resulting in a larger area of permanent retinal damage.

Mid- and far-infrared wavelengths are absorbed by water. Damage to the cornea, and to a lesser extent the lens, can occur if the unprotected eye is exposed to an aberrant laser beam from a mid- or far-infrared laser with wavelengths less than 400 nm or greater than 1400 nm. Ultraviolet (200 to 315 nm) and mid-infrared (1400 to 3000 nm) radiation are absorbed by the cornea and can cause corneal photokeratitis (Figure 43-6). Both wavelengths increase the opacity of the lens, resulting in traumatic cataracts.[21] Far-infrared radiation (3000 to 10,000 nm) is absorbed by the cornea and can result in corneal burn and potential loss of vision. Inadvertent exposure to the invisible CO_2 laser beam (10,600 nm) causes burning pain of the cornea or sclera. There are no immediate signs of exposure to ultraviolet radiation, but severe eye pain and a sensation of sand in the eye may be present later. After minor injury, regeneration of the epithelium occurs without any permanent abnormality, but corneal scarring and cataract formation may result with more extensive injury.

The retina is composed of two types of photoreceptors, rods and cones. Rods make up over 95% of the retina. They are sensitive to light but not color. Cones make up less than 5% of the total retinal area and are responsible for color and fine detail. They are heavily concentrated in the fovea centralis, an area associated with the sharpest and most brilliantly colored vision. Retinal damage is associated with visible and near-infrared (400 to 1400 nm) lasers. Their light is transmitted by the cornea and focused by the lens to produce an intense concentration of light energy on a small portion of the pigmented retina. Focusing of the laser by the lens amplifies the irradiance on the retina 100,000 times (see Figure 43-6). The conversion of the light energy to heat can cause retinal burns, visual loss, or total blindness. One milliwatt of visible laser radiation entering the eye deposits 100 W/cm^2 at the retina. Wavelengths less than 400 nm and greater than 1400 nm are not associated with retinal damage.

A visible laser beam produces a bright color flash of the emitted wavelength followed by an afterimage of its complementary color (e.g., a green, 532-nm laser light would produce a green flash followed immediately by a red afterimage). If the individual's cones are damaged by a green laser light, he or she may have difficulty discriminating blue and green colors. The Q-switched Nd:YAG laser beam (1064 nm) is especially hazardous to the eye because the beam is invisible, and the retina lacks sensory innervation. Visual disorientation resulting from retinal damage may not be apparent until considerable thermal damage has occurred. Unlike corneal injuries, laser damage to the retina is permanent.

FIGURE **43-6** Laser-associated eye injury. **A,** Mid- and far-infrared wavelengths (<400 nm and >1400 nm) are absorbed by the cornea and associated with corneal injury. **B,** Retinal injury is associated with visible and near-infrared (400-1400 nm) wavelengths.

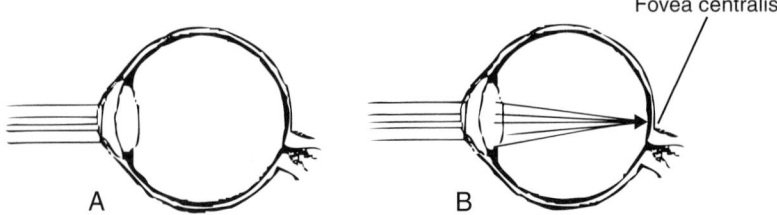

Perforation

Operator error, such as a misdirected laser beam or failure to check for proper laser function before use, accounts for the majority of laser perforations of a viscus or vessel. A pneumothorax can be a life-threatening complication of a misdirected laser beam, especially during the administration of nitrous oxide (N_2O). Lasers cannot photocoagulate blood vessels larger than 5 mm, and unexpected or excessive bleeding may accompany an accidental perforation with a misdirected beam. Because of greater tissue penetration and dissemination, perforation with the laser beam of the Nd:YAG laser is associated with delayed tissue damage. Perforation, bleeding, or edema may not be apparent for hours to days. Patients undergoing Nd:YAG laser surgery of the airway should be monitored for 24 to 48 hours after the procedure.[22]

Embolism

Although it is a rare event, venous gas embolism is a potential fatal hazard of laser procedures. Coronary and cerebral embolisms have occurred during endobronchial Nd:YAG therapy, and transmyocardial laser revascularization is also associated with cerebral microembolization. Venous air embolisms have even been reported with diode lasers. Hysteroscopy also carries the risk of a venous air embolism. A liquid coolant will reduce the risk of air embolism. CO_2 emboli appear to be less damaging than air or nitrogen emboli.

Pollution

Thermal destruction of tissue with a laser creates a smoke plume that may contain toxic gases and vapors, including benzene, hydrogen cyanide, formaldehyde, bioaerosols, dead and live cellular material, and viruses.[23] The CO_2 laser produces the greatest amount of smoke. During the use of the CO_2 laser, the amount of smoke produced from one gram of tissue is equivalent to the smoke from three to six cigarettes. The smoke plume may contain fine particulates (0.3 µm) that can be deposited in the lower airways. In addition to ocular and respiratory irritation, the smoke plume has the potential for causing cellular mutations. Because lasers are commonly used to vaporize tumors and viral lesions, concern exists that the laser plume may contain infectious material and viral DNA.[24]

The National Institute for Occupational Safety and Health (NIOSH) recommends the use of a local exhaust ventilation system—for example, a portable smoke evacuator—as the most efficient method to control laser-generated smoke.[23] An in-line smoke filter attached to wall suction can be used for laser procedures that produce a small smoke plume. A triple filtration smoke evacuator is indicated for evacuation of a large smoke plume. The Filtresse Smoke Filtration System (Utah Medical Products, Midvale, Utah) and the SmartVac Smoke Evacuation System (Niche Medical, Warwick, RI) are three-stage disposable filter systems composed of a high-efficiency particulate air (HEPA) filter that can filter 0.3-µm particulate matter, a layer of activated charcoal for odor absorption, and an ultra–low-penetration air filter (ULPA) that can filter particulate matter as small as 0.01 µm. For maximum effectiveness, the smoke evacuator inlet must be kept within 2 inches of the site of laser application and should be activated any time airborne particles are produced during the laser procedure. The Laparoshield (Pall Medical, East Hills, NY) is a three-stage filter designed for use during laparoscopic procedures. High-filtration masks (0.3 µm) should be worn by operating room personnel to filter out particulate matter and noxious odors. A close-fitting, surgical mask can filter particulate matter as small as 5 µm but is ineffective when moist. Box 43-1 includes recommendations for laser safety.

Fire

Historically, surgical fires were associated with the use of explosive or flammable anesthetics. When the use of these anesthetics was discontinued in the 1970s, sensitivity of the operating room staff to the possibility of a fire decreased. However, the risk of a surgical fire is still a very real but preventable hazard of modern surgery. The number of surgical fires has increased and is primarily associated with the use of electrocautery units and surgical lasers. Surgical fires occur most frequently during upper airway surgery, tracheostomies, and bronchoscopies; 21% to 34% percent of these fires occur in the airway, and 28% occur on the head or neck area. Only 14% of all fires are internal in nature.[25,26] Immediate recognition and management of a surgical fire can limit patient injury, whereas delayed recognition and response can be fatal for the patient. More than 50 million combined inpatient and outpatient surgeries are performed annually in the United States. Every year there are approximately 100 surgical fires[26]; 20% involve a serious injury, and 1% to 2% result in patient death. Injuries are not limited to burns. Inhalation of toxic products of combustion, carbon monoxide, ammonia, hydrogen chloride, and cyanide can cause significant airway and pulmonary damage. According to the American Society of Anesthesiologists (ASA) Closed Claims Project database, 2.2% of the total claims were attributed to thermal injury. Of 145 thermal injuries, 27 were due to electrocautery fires, and three involved laser surgery of the airway. One death resulted from an airway fire that occurred during laser surgery. The other two airway fires resulted in significant morbidity and lifelong disability. The highest payments, with a median $167,000, were for airway fires.[27]

BOX **43-1**

Laser Safety Precautions

- Restrict access to laser area.
- Close all doors and cover windows.
- Post Laser Warning signs outside laser area.
- Use appropriate LSE.
- Provide eye protection for patients.
- Cover all exposed skin.
- Minimize the potential for specular reflections by removal of unnecessary shiny surfaces.
- Avoid wearing bright, reflective jewelry or watches.
- Maintain room lights as bright as possible to constrict the pupils.
- Adjust brightness of patient monitors to ensure appropriate degree of visibility with LSE.
- Require surgeon to warn of activation of laser and to keep the beam path above or below normal eye level (<4.5 feet or >6.5 feet).
- Ensure operational warning devices are installed for lasers with invisible beams.
- Do not position self near anticipated path of the beam.
- Avoid looking into the primary beam at all times.
- Do not leave an active laser unattended.

LSE, *Laser safety eyewear.*

For a fire to occur, three components of the fire triangle must be present: a fuel source, an ignition source, and an oxidizer. All three components are frequently present in the operating room, and a fire can occur any time the three components are allowed to interact. The oxidizers, air, O_2, and N_2O, are under control of the anesthetist. Oxygen is heavier than air and tends to accumulate in low-lying areas such as surgical drapes. In an oxygen-rich environment, materials ignite faster, burn quickly with greater intensity, release more heat, and are more difficult to extinguish. The surgeon controls the source of ignition, an ESU, fiberoptic light sources or cables, defibrillators, high-speed drills, and lasers. However, sevoflurane and desiccated soda lime or baralyme can also be a source of ignition in the breathing circuit. Baralyme use has subsequently been discontinued. Fuel sources are abundant in the operating room and are predominantly under the control of the nursing staff. They include surgical prep solutions, petroleum-based ointments, facial hair, surgical drapes, gloves, ointments, sponges, dressings, endotracheal tubes, laryngeal mask airways, breathing circuits, nasogastric tubes, suction catheters, pneumatic tourniquet cuffs, Silastic stents, suction catheters, and tracheostomy tubes. Bowel gas, which contains methane and hydrogen, also provides a fuel source during intraabdominal laser procedures. Volatile organic chemicals such as alcohol, acetone, and ether are common components of skin preps, tinctures, degreasers, suture pack solutions, and liquid wound dressings. Alcohol and alcohol-based solutions are very volatile and pose a significant fire hazard in the operating room. If adequate drying time is not provided, the laser can ignite the vapors. This is more likely to occur in a confined space (e.g., tented drapes) and an oxygen-enriched environment. Care must be taken to ensure that the surgical prep solution does not pool under the patient or saturate the drapes. Alcohol-based hand sanitizers may also release alcohol vapor, are flammable, and pose a new fire hazard in operating rooms.[28-30] Although they will resist ignition and slow the spread of a flame in room air, fire-retardant drapes and materials are not fireproof. Materials considered nonflammable may ignite easily and burn more quickly and at a higher temperature when exposed to an oxidizer-enriched environment.

Everyone in the operating room must understand the fire hazards presented by all three sides of the fire triangle, including those not under their direct control. Vigilance is key, and communication among all members of the surgical team is mandatory. The risk of fire is greatest during head and neck surgery, in which oxygen can build up under the surgical drapes, creating an oxidizer-enriched environment. An oxidizer-enriched environment is associated with 75% of surgical fires, whereas in 10% of the fires, lasers provided the ignition source.[26] It is imperative that all surgical personnel are aware of the hazards of fire during laser procedures and know how to prevent and manage operating room fires.

Laser-related fires are not confined to the airway, but airway fires can cause extensive damage and can contribute to significant patient morbidity and mortality.[18,31] The incidence of airway fires in the United States is probably underreported, primarily because of liability issues. During airway surgery, fire can occur if the laser beam or the reflected laser light comes into direct contact with the endotracheal tube. Localized thermal trauma occurs if the fire is contained to the outside of the endotracheal tube. Rupture of the endotracheal-tube cuff allows leakage of anesthetics gases into the path of the laser beam, increasing the risk of an ignition. If the fire burns through to the inner side of the tube, an intraluminal fire occurs, fed by both the anesthetic gases and the volatile products of combustion of the endotracheal-tube wall. The intraluminal flame will travel toward the source of the oxidizer. A secondary flame can shoot out of the distal end of the endotracheal tube like a blowtorch and cause extensive lower airway damage.

Prevention of a Surgical Fire

Operating room personnel must be educated on the prevention of surgical fires. They need to understand the fire triangle, be able to identify the procedures that present a risk of fire, understand their role in preventing a surgical fire, and know how to respond to a surgical fire. Every operating room should have a fire safety plan in place that includes periodic fire drills.[32,33] Surgical personnel must be familiar with the location and function of fire alarms, fire extinguishers, and emergency exits and should know how to shut off electrical and medical gas supplies. They should be aware of the fire hazards present in the laser area, such as anesthetic gases, skin prep solutions, adhesive plastic tape, and surgical drapes. Oil-based lubricants should be avoided, and alcohol-based preparation solutions should be allowed adequate drying time before the patient is covered by drapes. Patients' eyes must be protected with laser safety eyewear (LSE) or saline-moistened pads and laser eye shields. Fire-resistant drapes are mandatory, and saline-soaked towels should be placed on the skin surrounding the path of the laser beam. Additional precautions are required for the possibility of an airway fire, including laser-resistant endotracheal tubes and limited O_2 concentration. The use of 5 to 10 cm H_2O positive end-expiratory pressure (PEEP) has been advocated during laser surgery of the airway to prevent the hot, toxic gases from reaching the lower airways. Application of a water-soluble surgical lubricant to a facial beard will reduce the possibility of ignition.

Having a preplanned method of responding to a surgical fire is vital. A basin of water or normal saline should be available during laser procedures to extinguish a burning endotracheal tube or other material. Two syringes filled with normal saline should be readily available to extinguish an endotracheal tube fire.[34] Use of excessive tape to secure the endotracheal tube should be avoided to allow easier removal of the tube in the event of an airway fire. Emergency supplies, including a rigid bronchoscope and forceps, should also be readily available. A carbon dioxide fire extinguisher (Class BC) is appropriate for extinguishing surgical fires. The BC fire extinguisher leaves no residue and will not damage human tissue. Dry powder extinguishers (Class ABC) are inappropriate as the first response because the powder (ammonium phosphate) contaminates all surfaces, is a respiratory irritant, and may interfere with visibility.[26] The Joint Commission requires health-care organizations to have an educational and prevention program in place for surgical staff. Recommendations for prevention of surgical fires are listed in Box 43-2.

Management of a Surgical Fire

During any laser procedure, everyone in the operating room must be alert to the possibility of a fire and be prepared to respond quickly. Communication among all members of the surgical team is vital for the prevention of a surgical fire.[35] In most cases, a towel, gloved hand, water, or saline can be used to extinguish small surgical fires. Focus should be on eliminating oxidizers, extinguishing the burning materials, and assessing the patient for thermal trauma. In the event of an airway fire, the anesthetist has approximately 6 seconds for recognition and removal of an endotracheal tube that has ignited. Signs of an airway fire include darkening of the endotracheal tube or breathing circuit with soot,

---

BOX 43-2

Prevention of Surgical Fires

- Educate surgical personnel.
- Schedule annual fire drills, and include evacuation of anesthetized patients in the event of an uncontrolled surgical fire.
- Identify location of fire alarms and extinguishers and O_2 and N_2O shut-off valves.
- Use pulse oximetry to identify patients who can tolerate brief periods of ventilation with air, as well as patients who may benefit from supplemental O_2.
- Question need for 100% oxygen during airway/facial/head surgery.
- Limit supplemental O_2 to 30%.
- Alert surgical team members to potential sources of fire: oxidizers, fuels, and source of ignition.
- Avoid pooling of prep solutions and allow adequate drying time before draping patient.
- Coat facial hair with a water-soluble surgical lubricant during head and neck surgery.
- Use flame-retardant drapes or moistened sponges in the area of the laser.
- Use laser-resistant endotracheal tubes during laser surgery of the upper airway. Inflate the cuff with saline and dye to allow early recognition of tube rupture.

- Use moistened sponges to prevent air leaks, especially when using uncuffed tubes during airway surgery. Sponges and pledgets should also be moistened to resist ignition.
- Use a properly applied incise drape to help isolate head, neck, and upper-chest incisions from oxygen-enriched atmospheres and flammable vapors.
- Minimize the buildup of O_2 and N_2O beneath the drapes.
- Have immediately available a container of water to extinguish burning materials. Two syringes of sterile saline should be prepared prior to laser surgery of the airway.
- Have fire extinguishers available in the room or immediately accessible.
- Use deep oropharyngeal suction to scavenge gases from the oropharynx of an intubated patient during laser surgery of the airway.
- If possible, discontinue supplemental oxygen at least 1 minute before and during laser use for head and neck surgery, and especially surgery of the airway.
- Place laser in standby mode when it is not in active use.

---

an orange or red glow to the endotracheal tube, and the presence of flames in or around the endotracheal tube. The endotracheal tube acts like a blowtorch, with high concentrations of O_2 adding to the intensity of the fire. Within seconds the flames can reach a height of 5 to 10 inches. Intraluminal fires will spread toward the proximal end of the tube—the source of the O_2. Severe thermal or chemical trauma is unlikely to occur if the flame is vented through the tube or oropharynx. Downstream gases contain the products of oxidation and little O_2, but a free-end fire can occur if the products of oxidation ignite in the O_2-rich alveoli.

In rapid succession, ventilation should be discontinued, the breathing circuit disconnected from the patient, all gases and volatile anesthetics discontinued, and the endotracheal tube removed and extinguished in a basin of water. A continuing airway fire should be extinguished with normal saline, and any residual smoldering material removed from the airway. The patient should be mask ventilated with air until all burning has stopped, at which time ventilation with 100% O_2 should be instituted. Removal of the endotracheal tube is controversial, especially if it is not burning and complete loss of the airway is a real concern.[36] A tube exchanger or tracheostomy can be used to replace the damaged tube without the risk of losing the airway completely. Recommendations for management of an airway fire are listed in Box 43-3. In the event the fire spreads, the acronym *RACE* is applicable: **R**escue the patient, **A**lert other staff and **a**ctivate the fire alarm systems, **C**onfine the fire by shutting doors, closing off gas supplies and electrical power, and using fire extinguishers, and **E**vacuate the room. Should a surgical fire occur, all equipment and materials involved in the fire should be retained for further inspection.

Anesthesia should be continued to allow evaluation of the airway for direct thermal trauma, chemical inhalation injury, and smoke inhalation. Direct visualization of the tracheobronchial tree with a rigid bronchoscope is recommended for assessment of thermal injury and removal of foreign material. A flexible bronchoscope may be necessary for evaluation of distal airways, and tracheobronchial lavage with saline solution should be considered. After reintubation with a smaller tube, a chest x-ray (CXR) examination and evaluation of arterial blood gases (ABGs) are indicated to guide postoperative management. Carboxyhemoglobin (COHb) levels are needed for assessment of smoke inhalation.

After an airway fire, 24-hour observation of the patient is indicated. For minor burns, the patient should be monitored for development of laryngeal-tracheal edema following extubation. A patient with severe burns should remain intubated and receive 30% to 60% humidified O_2. A tracheostomy and mechanical ventilation with positive end-expiratory pressure (PEEP) should be a definite consideration. Corticosteroids have been recommended for the treatment of both smoke inhalation and the bronchospasm that may be precipitated in patients with irritable airways. Additional treatment is dependent on the extent of the injury and the response of the patient. Complications may be delayed, and tracheal stenosis has been documented 14 weeks after an airway fire.[37] A monthly laryngoscopy or bronchoscopy may be indicated for up to 6 months.[38] All surgical fires should be reported to The Joint Commission as sentinel events.

Eye Protection

All medical lasers are Class IV lasers. Their use poses an eye, skin, and fire hazard, so the use of protective eyewear is required to

---

BOX **43-3**

Management of Airway Fires

- Discontinue use of laser.
- In rapid succession, stop ventilation, disconnect breathing circuit from the patient, turn off all gases and volatile anesthetics, and remove ETT.*
- Extinguish burning ETT/LMA in basin of water
- Extinguish airway fire with normal saline.
- Assume mask ventilation with air. Ventilate with 100% O_2 once the fire is extinguished.
- Reintubate with a smaller ETT, and continue anesthetic.
- Examine airway and remove residual debris with rigid bronchoscope. Consider lavage with normal saline.
- Examine small and distal airways with flexible fiberoptic bronchoscope.
- Assess extent of thermal trauma with ABG, carboxyhemoglobin levels, and CXR.

- Extubate patient, and administer humidified O_2 by mask if airway damage is minimal and risk of laryngeal edema is low.
- Keep patient intubated and administer 40% to 60% humidified O_2 if airway burn is present or suspected.
- Consider tracheostomy and mechanical ventilation for postoperative management.
- Consider administration of steroids.
- Admit patient to ICU for a minimum 24-hour observation.
- Retain all equipment and materials involved in the fire for further inspection.
- Reassemble surgical team to identify the sequence of events that led to the surgical fire.
- Report fire as a sentinel event to The Joint Commission, ECRI, and the FDA.

ABG, *Arterial blood gas;* CXR, *chest x-ray;* ECRI, *Emergency Care Research Institute;* ETT, *endotracheal tube;* FDA, *Food and Drug Administration;* ICU, *intensive care unit;* LMA, *laryngeal mask airway;* O_2, *oxygen.*
*Extubation may not be indicated if a risk of total loss of the airway is present.

---

protect against reflected and diffuse laser light. Laser beams can be reflected off any reflective surface, including surgical instruments, watches, and jewelry. Anodized, dull, nonreflective, or matte-finished equipment should be used whenever possible to decrease reflectivity of the beam. Laser safety eyewear (LSE) protects against accidental exposure to a laser beam but will not protect against intra-beam or direct viewing of a laser beam. The aversion or blink response of 0.25 second is triggered by bright, visible light only. It will not prevent the trauma of visible laser beams and provides no protection against lasers with a wavelength of 700 to 1400 nm. The aversion response is absent or sluggish under general anesthesia. In an operating room that is darkened for video and microscope use, the pupils of the eyes will be dilated, increasing the risk for laser exposure for surgical personnel and awake patients. The awake patient's eyes must be protected with LSE. An anesthetized patient's eyes should be covered with saline-moistened eye pads and laser shields. Petroleum-based eye ointments should not be used during laser procedures because they may cause severe burns if ignited by a misdirected laser beam.

During laser procedures, access to the laser area should be restricted to authorized personnel. Individuals entering a laser area must wear LSEs specific for the type of laser in use. The LSE must have the appropriate optical density (OD) and reflective properties for the wavelengths of the beams encountered, the beam intensity, and the expected exposure conditions. *Optical density* refers to the attenuation or absorption of the laser light and transmission of sufficient ambient light for safe visibility. Medical LSEs are typically 4 to 7 OD An increase of 1 OD will result in a 10-fold increase in ability to block light. The higher the OD, the greater the protection, but the lower the visibility. Historically, operating room personnel have relied on the color of the lenses to indicate their use for specific lasers. However, there is no current standard for protective lenses, and there is an apparent lack of consensus among LSE manufacturers. For example,

Nd:YAG laser protection can be provided with green lenses or specially coated clear lenses. Surgical personnel should not rely on the color of the lens to indicate use for specific lasers. They should check the O.D. and wavelength on the lenses relative to the laser in use. For example, protective eyewear for the Nd:YAG should be marked "OD5 or greater for 1,064 nm." Vision correction glasses may attenuate the effect of the CO_2 laser beam but do not completely protect the eye from direct or reflected laser beams because they lack protective side shields. The side shields on laser glasses provide additional protection against accidental laser exposure. Tunable lasers, such as the titanium-doped sapphire laser, have tunable wavelengths of 700 to 1000 nm. More than one type of LSE may be required during use of a tunable laser because the output wavelength can vary. Currently there are no laser glasses available that protect against all types of laser beams. LSE that cover several wavelengths would require very dark filters, which would interfere with visual acuity. CO_2 lenses are usually clear and do not affect color perception, but tinted or colored lenses can affect color perception. Some Nd:YAG LSE can significantly dim the green color on monochrome monitors, tempting the anesthesia provider to remove the glasses while the laser is in use. Prior to anesthetizing a patient for a laser procedure, the anesthetist should observe the monitors through the LSE to ascertain the effect of the colored lenses on the visibility of the displayed parameters. Display lights and alarms of patient monitors should be set to maximum brightness or otherwise adjusted to compensate for the color restriction. Audible alarms should be adjusted to the loudest setting. Warning signs posted on the inside and outside of all entrances should include the type and wavelength of the laser in use, as well as the wavelength and specific LSE required for everyone entering the laser area (see Figure 43-5). Entryway controls must be in place, such as a nondefeatable control on the door that cuts off the beam when the door is opened. All other optical paths (windows) should be covered to reduce the transmitted intensity of the laser radiation.

A variety of laser-absorbing glass, plastics, laser safety curtains and screens are available. These interact with laser energy in a manner similar to LSE. If only CO_2 lasers are used, window coverings are not necessary, because glass absorbs laser energy at 10,600 nm. If a Nd:YAG or a laser with a similar wavelength is used, a laser-blocking shield is necessary to stop accidental exit of the laser beam. A windowless room provides the maximum protection.

SPECIAL ANESTHETIC CONSIDERATIONS

Anesthetic Gases

Oxygen concentration should be the lowest possible to support acceptable patient oxygenation and should not exceed 30%. The practice of administering supplemental O_2 via nasal cannula to every patient under local anesthesia needs to be reevaluated, especially if the surgical drapes promote the accumulation of O_2 during laser procedures.[39] Preanesthetic patient evaluation should include an assessment of the patient's need for supplemental oxygen, because many patients can easily tolerate short periods of ventilation with air.[40] Pulse oximetry should be used to identify the patient who may benefit from supplemental O_2, as well as the patient who can tolerate short periods of ventilation with room air. Rarely is supplemental O_2 indicated. If supplemental O_2 is necessary, it should be discontinued at least 1 minute before and during laser use.

Nitrous oxide readily supports combustion and should be avoided during laser procedures. Suitable gases include O_2 and air, O_2 and nitrogen, and O_2 and helium. Helium has a high thermal conductivity and is more resistant to ignition. In addition, its lower viscosity can help overcome the increased resistance resulting from smaller internal diameter (ID) tubes or airway obstruction. Volatile anesthetics are nonflammable, but their use is not recommended during airway laser procedures because they may deteriorate to potentially toxic compounds in the presence of a fire.

Endotracheal Tubes

Polyvinyl chloride (PVC) tubes ignite easily. In addition to thermal trauma, PVC tubes produce toxic materials that can increase the amount of damage to the airway.[41] PVC tubes appear to be more susceptible to damage by the CO_2 laser; however, the presence of blood on the tube makes a PVC tube also susceptible to damage by the Nd:YAG laser. The radiopaque barium sulfate strip found on most PVC tubes has a faster ignition rate than the PVC. Red rubber tubes appear to be more resistant to initial ignition, have a slower rate of burn, and produce less toxic smoke. However, they tend to melt and can produce carbon monoxide. Although silicone tubes are also less combustible, inhalation of silica ash may produce pulmonary damage.[34] Laser procedures of the airway require use of an endotracheal tube with a small ID, which increases resistance, as well as a tendency to kink.

Laser-resistant endotracheal tubes should be used during laser surgery. The Laser-Flex Tracheal Tube (Nellcor) is a flexible stainless steel tube with a matte finish that is resistant to the CO_2 and KTP lasers. In the event of a proximal-cuff rupture with a laser beam, the distal cuff will maintain a tracheal seal and prevent anesthetic gases from leaking into the path of the laser beam. The Lasertubus (Rüsch) is a soft, white rubber tube that is resistant to the argon, Nd:YAG, and CO_2 lasers. The lower 17 cm of the tube is covered with a Merocel wrap that dissipates the laser light and prevents backscatter. Soaking the tube in water will reduce ignition potential. The Lasertubus has two high-volume cuffs, one inside the other. The Bivona Fome-Cuff (Portex), a silicone and aluminum spiral tube, is designed for use with the CO_2 laser. It has a polyurethane self-inflating foam cuff covered with silicone that is designed to maintain a tracheal seal in the event of a cuff rupture. Inability to deflate the foam following cuff rupture is a recognized problem with this tube. The Laser Shield II (Medtronic), a reflective aluminum-wrapped silicone tube with a smooth fluoroplastic covering, is specific for use with CO_2 and KTP lasers. The cuff is designed to be inflated with saline, and methylene blue is present in the inflation valve for immediate detection of cuff rupture. The Laser-Trach (Kendall/Sheridan) is a red rubber tube with an embossed copper foil for use with CO_2 and KTP lasers.

Application of a metallic foil wrap (aluminum or copper) or a thin metal-coated plastic tape has been used to protect PVC and red rubber endotracheal tubes during laser surgery of the airway, but this practice should be discouraged. Recognized problems with foil wrappings include laser reflection damage, potential areas of exposed tube, unprotected cuff, the need to use a smaller ID tube, and airway damage from the sharp edges of the foil wrap. Only the Merocel Laser-Guard Endotracheal Tube Wrap (Medtronic) has FDA approval for endotracheal-tube protection.

Laser-resistant endotracheal tubes are not laser-proof and carry the inherent risk of ignition. When exposed to the CO_2 laser (CW) in room air, silicone tubes ignite in 0.3 seconds, unwrapped PVC tubes ignite in 0.8 seconds, and the Laser Shield II ignites in 5 seconds. The Laser-Flex does not ignite after 30 seconds.[41] The Nd:YAG laser (CW) will ignite clear PVC, red rubber, silicone, and laser-resistant tubes, including the Bivona Fome-Cuff and Laser-Flex tubes. The clear PVC tube can withstand the pulsed Nd:YAG, but it is prone to ignition if blood is present on the tube or if the tube has radiopaque markings. The Nd:YAG laser does not appear to ignite aluminum- and copper-wrapped red rubber tubes.[42]

Endotracheal-tube cuffs, including those on the laser-resistant tubes, are not laser resistant, and cuff rupture is often the prelude to an airway fire. The cuffs should be inflated with normal saline. The addition of methylene blue may alert the surgeon to cuff rupture. The endotracheal-tube cuff should be fully inflated and a stethoscope used to confirm the absence of a leak before the laser is used. Saline-moistened cotton gauze should be placed proximal to the endotracheal-tube cuff. The gauze and the attached cotton strings should be constantly remoistened. At least 1 minute should elapse before a laser is used after reinflation of an endotracheal-tube cuff or repositioning of the endotracheal tube for correction of a leak.

Laryngeal mask airways (LMAs) have been tested with the KTP and Nd:YAG lasers. The tube of the standard silicone mask is more resistant to the laser beams than the disposable PVC tube, but the PVC cuff is more resistant than the silicone cuff. The intubating LMA (silicone and steel) is more sensitive to the KTP laser. The presence of blood increases the vulnerability of all the LMAs, especially with the KTP laser.[43] Additional precautions for use of an LMA during laser procedures include inflation of the cuff with saline and methylene blue and protection of the cuff with moistened gauze.

ANESTHESIA FOR LASER PROCEDURES

Anesthesia is frequently required for laser procedures, and most anesthetic techniques are suitable for laser procedures. Although they may appear to be less invasive, laser procedures have complications similar to those of traditional surgery. Major anesthetic concerns exist when the airway is shared between the anesthetist and the surgeon during a laser procedure. The proximity of the endotracheal tube and anesthetic gases to the laser beam creates a very real hazard of airway fire. Communication between the surgeon and the anesthetist is paramount to ensure patient safety, maximize surgical access, and avoid complications.

Ventilation techniques during laser procedures of the airway depend on surgeon preference and the site of the laser application. For the patient receiving supplemental O_2 during monitored anesthesia care (MAC), good communication between the surgeon and anesthetist is mandatory. To reduce the risk of fire, supplemental O_2 should be discontinued 1 minute before and during laser use. Pulse oximetry will allow monitoring of the patient's response to the decrease in O_2 concentration. To maximize surgical view and access, small-sized endotracheal tubes are necessary, and the anesthetist must be prepared to deal with the associated increase in resistance to ventilation. Some surgeons may prefer an apneic technique, in which case the airway is alternately shared between the surgeon and the anesthetist. After induction of general anesthesia and the administration of a muscle relaxant, the patient is hyperventilated by mask after brief periods of laser application. The pulse oximeter must be monitored closely and ventilation immediately resumed if oxygenation decreases 2% to 3% below the patient's initial saturation or when 1.5 to 2 minutes have elapsed. A disadvantage of

this technique is the potential aspiration of blood and resected tissue. An alternative approach is the use of a jet ventilator to deliver O_2 through the operating laryngoscope.[44] Because the entrainment of room air (Venturi effect) dilutes the final oxygenation concentration delivered to the patient, 100% O_2 should be used during jet ventilation.

SUMMARY

Because of their ability to cut, coagulate, vaporize, and selectively destroy abnormal tissue, medical lasers have numerous applications in all surgical specialties. They are an integral part of a surgeon's armamentarium, and newer and more powerful lasers are in development. Anesthetists are involved on a daily basis with patients undergoing laser procedures, both in the operating room and in off-site locations. Safe provision of anesthetic care requires knowledge of laser physics, as well as the potential hazards associated with the use of medical lasers. In addition to the threat of thermal and eye trauma, the anesthetist must be acutely aware of the risk of fire during laser procedures, especially laser surgery of the airway. The anesthetist must be prepared to identify preventive safety measures, as well as institute definitive treatment should a fire occur.

REFERENCES

1. Absten GT. *Laser Medicine and Surgery. Fundamentals for the Operating Room and Clinics.* 2004. Available at: www.lasertraining.org.
2. Anderson RR. Dermatologic history of the ruby laser: the long story of short pulses. *Arch Dermatol.* 2003;139:70-74.
3. Cantatore JL, Kriegel DA. Laser surgery: an approach to the pediatric patient. *J Am Acad Dermatol.* 2004;50:165-184.
4. Tanzi EL et al. Lasers in dermatology: four decades of progress. *J Am Acad Dermatol.* 2003;49:1-34.
5. Davidovits P. *Physics in Biology and Medicine.* San Diego: Harcourt Academic; 2001.
6. Waynant RW, Merberg GN. Basics of Lasers. In: Waynant RW, ed. *Lasers in Medicine.* Boca Raton, FL: CRC; 2002.
7. Spector N et al. Reduction in lateral thermal damage using heat-conducting templates: a comparison of continuous wave and pulse CO_2 lasers. *Lasers in Surgery and Medicine.* 2003;32:94-100.
8. Lippert BN et al. Wound healing after laser treatment of oral and oropharyngeal cancer. *Lasers Med Sci.* 2003;18:36-42.
9. Joseph TA et al. Laser capsulorrhaphy for multidirectional instability of the shoulder. An outcomes study and proposed classification system. *Am J Sports Med.* 2003;31:26-35.
10. Sherk HH et al. Electromagnetic surgical devices in orthopaedics: lasers and radiofrequency. *J Bone Joint Surg.* 2002;84-A:675-681.
11. Aaberge L et al. Continued symptomatic improvement three to five years after transmyocardial revascularization with CO_2 laser: a late clinical follow-up of the Norwegian randomized trial with transmyocardial revascularization. *J Am Coll Cardiol.* 2002;39:1588-1593.
12. Huikeshoven M et al. Transmyocardial laser revascularization and other treatment modalities for angina pectoris. *Lasers Med Sci.* 2003;18:2-11.
13. Nahrendorf M et al. Effects of transmyocardial laser revascularization on myocardial perfusion and left ventricular remodeling after myocardial infarction in rats. *Radiology.* 2002;225:487-493.
14. Newman J, Anand V. Applications of the diode laser in otolaryngology. *Ear Nose Throat J.* 2002;81:850-851.
15. Gur A et al. Efficacy of low power laser therapy and exercise on pain and function in chronic low back pain. *Lasers Surg Med.* 2003;32:233-238.
16. American National Standards Institute. *Safe Use of Lasers in Health Care Facilities* (Publication No. Z136.3-2005). Washington, DC: Laser Institute of America; 2005. Available at: http://www.laserinstitute.org/store/ANSI/113.
17. U.S. Department of Labor Occupational Safety and Health Administration. Laser hazards. In: *OSHA Technical Manual* [Section II, Chapter 6]. Washington, DC: OSHA; 1999. Available at: http://www.osha.gov/pls/osha-web/owadisp.show_document?p_table DIRECTIVES&P_ID = 1705. Accessed July 23, 2008.

18. Barat K. Laser accidents: occurrence and response. *Health Phys.* 2003;84: 593-595.
19. Grossman PH, Grossman AR. Treatment of thermal injuries from CO_2 laser resurfacing. *Plast Reconstr Surg.* 2002;109:1435-1445.
20. Stratigos AJ et al. Rapid development of nonmelanoma skin cancer after CO_2 laser resurfacing. *Arch Dermatol.* 2002;138:696-698.
21. Foroozan R et al. Traumatic cataract after inadvertent laser discharge. *Arch Ophthalmol.* 2003;121:286-287.
22. Albelmalak B et al. Respiratory arrest after successful neodymium:yttrium-aluminum-garnet laser treatment of subglottic tracheal stenosis. *Anesth Analg.* 2002;95:485-486.
23. National Institute for Occupational Safety and Health. *Control of Smoke from Laser/Electric Surgical Procedures.* Washington, DC: NIOSH; 1998. Available at: http://www.cdc.gov/niosh/hc11.html. Accessed May-June 28, 2008.
24. Garden JM et al. Viral disease transmitted by laser-generated plume (aerosol). *Arch Dermatol.* 2002;138:1303-1307.
25. Singla AK et al. Surgical field fire during a repair of bronchoesophageal fistula. *Anesth Analg.* 2005;100:1062-1064.
26. ECRI. Surgical Fires. *Healthcare Risk Control.* 2006;2:1-17.
27. Kressin KA. Burn injury in the operating room: a closed claims analysis. *ASA Newsl.* 2004;68. Available at: www.asahq.org/Newsletters/2004/06_04/kressin06_04.html. Accessed June 28, 2008.
28. Spigelman AD, Swan JR. Skin antiseptics and the risk in operating theatre fires. *ANZ J Surg.* 2005;75:556-558.
29. Prasad R et al. Fires in the operating room and intensive care unit: awareness is the key to prevention. *Anesth Analg.* 2006;102:172-174.
30. PA-PSRS Patient Safety Advisory. *Risk of fire from alcohol-based solutions.* 2005;2:1-2.
31. Niskanen M et al. Fatal injury caused by airway fire during tracheostomy. *Acta Anaesthesiol Scand.* 2007;51:509-513.
32. Flowers J. Code red in the OR—implementing an OR fire drill. *AORN J.* 2004;79:797-805.
33. ECRI. Surgical fire safety. *Health Devices.* 2006;35:45-66.
34. Lierz P et al. Management of intratracheal fires during laser surgery. *Anesth Analg.* 2002;95:502.
35. Bruley ME. Surgical fires: perioperative communication is essential to prevent this rare but devastating complication. *Qual Saf Health Care.* 2004;13:467-471.
36. Ng J, Hartigan PM. Airway fire during tracheostomy: should we extubate? *Anesthesiology.* 2003;98:1303.
37. Ilgner J et al. Long-term follow up after laser-induced endotracheal fire. *J Laryngol Otol.* 2002;116:213-215.
38. Pollack GS. Eliminating surgical fires: a team approach. *AANA J.* 2004;72:294-298.

39. Lampotang S et al. Reducing the risk of surgical fires: supplying nasal cannulae with sub-100% O_2 gas mixtures from anesthesia machines. *Anesth Analg.* 2005;101:1407-1412.

40. Lupson ML et al. Preventing surgical fires: who needs to be educated? *Jt Comm J Qual Patient Saf.* 2005;31:522-527.

41. Lai HC et al. Fires of endotracheal tubes of three different materials during carbon dioxide laser surgery. *Acta Anaesthesiol Sin.* 2002;40:47-51.

42. Edwards BE et al. Medical laser safety hazard evaluation. *Health Phys.* 2002;83:S36-S44.

43. Keller C et al. Liability of laryngeal mask airway to thermal damages from KTP and Nd:YAG lasers. *Br J Anaesth.* 1999;82:29.

44. Unzueta MC et al. Endobronchial high-frequency jet ventilation for endobronchial laser surgery: an alternative approach. *Anesth Analg.* 2003;96:298-300.

CHAPTER 44

OBESITY AND ANESTHESIA PRACTICE

Maura S. McAuliffe, Paul Gregg Gambrell, Melydia J. Edge

OVERVIEW

Obesity is a complex, multifactorial, chronic disease that develops from an interaction between the genotype and the environment.[1-6] It is the second leading cause of preventable death in the United States.[1] The prevalence of overweight and obesity has increased significantly during the last 3 decades. Obesity is associated with an increased incidence of a wide spectrum of medical and surgical conditions and morbidity. As a result, anesthetists can expect to encounter overweight and obese patients frequently in their practices. These patients may provide the anesthetist with a considerable challenge. A thorough understanding of the pathophysiology, pharmacology, and specific anesthetic considerations associated with obesity will promote optimal anesthesia care.

Statistics

The prevalence of obesity around the world continues to rise, and in the United States, millions of Americans are considered to be severely obese. Current estimates are that 65% of U.S. adults are classified as overweight or obese, and more than 30% of adults are classified as obese, which means the prevalence of obesity has doubled over the past 20 years.[7] In nationwide data from 2004, 7% of women and 3% of men were extremely obese. There are an estimated 23 million people in the United States with a body mass index (BMI) of no less than 35 kg/m[2], and 8 million with a BMI of 40 kg/m[2] or higher.[8]

For persons ages 20 years and older, there has been an increase in the proportion of obese adults from a previous level of 23% in 1994 to a new level of approximately 32% (Table 44-1).

Obesity is not confined to the United States; it is a health problem that is increasing at an alarming rate throughout the world. Globally there are approximately 2 billion individuals documented as overweight (BMI of 25 kg/m[2] to 29.9 kg/m[2]), which approximates the number of individuals who are starving worldwide.[9] It is estimated that there are more than 300 million obese people worldwide,[10] and three countries report that more than 50% of their population is obese. In most countries, obesity appears to be more common in women than in men (Figure 44-1). The World Health Organization (WHO) has predicted that the number of severely overweight adults is expected to double by 2025.[11] Concerns about the global obesity crisis are growing, and WHO reports that obesity accounts for more than 400,000 deaths annually, second only to tobacco-related disease as a cause of preventable and premature death.[11]

In the United States, individuals who are obese have a 10% to 50% percent greater risk of death from all causes, compared with healthy-weight individuals (BMI 18.5 to 24.9). Obesity is associated with about 112,000 excess deaths per year.[12] Most of the increased risk is due to cardiovascular causes.[13]

Cost of Obesity

Public awareness of the problems that arise from obesity is corroborated by the $100 billion spent annually on medical treatment, weight-reduction programs, exercise equipment, low-fat diet products, pharmacologic agents, advertising, and marketing.[14] Obesity is a major health concern, and obese patients admitted for surgery may exhibit one or more medical conditions in addition to the primary underlying problem.[15] Clearly, identification of obesity-related conditions is vital to the safe administration of an anesthetic.

Definitions

BMI is the accepted measure of body habitus that normalizes adiposity for height.[1] BMI can be calculated according to the following formulas:
- BMI = Weight (in kilograms)/Height (in meters)[2]
- BMI = (Body weight [in pounds]/Height [in inches][2]) × 703

Overweight is defined as a BMI of 25 to 29 kg/m[2], and *obesity* as a BMI of 30 kg/m[2].[1-3] The rationale for these definitions is based on epidemiologic data that reveal increasing mortality with BMIs over 25 kg/m[2].[6] For individuals with a BMI greater than 30 kg/m[2], mortality rates for a number of conditions, especially those associated with cardiovascular disease, are increased 50% to 100% above rates in individuals of normal weight. A person's degree of obesity is commonly defined using the body mass index, as classified in Table 44-2. A BMI greater than or equal to 25 is considered "overweight," a BMI of greater than or equal to 30 is considered "obese," and a BMI greater than or equal to 40 is classified as "extremely obese." We are now seeing references to "super-obese" (BMI >50) and "super-super-obese" (BMI >60).[16]

Ideal body weight (IBW) is a term used interchangeably with the terms *normal weight*, *lean body weight*, and *desirable weight*.[1-3] IBW is a measurement of height and body mass that exhibits the lowest morbidity and mortality for a given population.[2] Determination of IBW is especially useful in calculating drug and intravenous infusion doses in morbidly obese patients. Certain drugs, if administered according to actual body weight, can produce toxicity, renal damage, or hemodynamic instability. Conversely, some drugs must be given according to actual body weight if therapeutic effects are to be achieved. The formula for IBW (in kilograms) is as follows:
- For men: IBW = Height (in centimeters) − 100
- For women: IBW = Height (in centimeters) − 105

Risk Factors

Obesity is associated with an increase in the incidence of more than 30 medical conditions (Box 44-1). The risk for cardiovascular disease, certain cancers, diabetes, and overall mortality is

TABLE **44-1**	Age-Adjusted* Prevalence of Overweight and Obesity Among U.S. Adults, Age 20 Years and Over			
	NHANES III (1988-94) (n = 16,679)	**NHANES** (1999-2000) (n = 4117)	**NHANES** (2001-02) (n = 4413)	**NHANES†** (2003-04) (n = 4431)
Overweight or obese (BMI ≥ 25)	56.0	64.5	65.7	66.3
Obese (BMI ≥ 30)	22.9	30.5	30.6	32.2

From *http://www.cdc.gov/nchs/products/pubs/hestats/overweight/overwght_adult_03.htm. Accessed August 31, 2007.*
NHANES, *National Health and Nutrition Examination Survey.*
Age-adjusted by the direct method to the year 2000 U.S. Bureau of the Census estimates using the age groups 20-39, 40-59, and 60 years and over.
†*Crude estimates (not age-adjusted) for 2003-2004 are 66.5% with a BMI ≥25 and 32.3% with a BMI ≥30.*

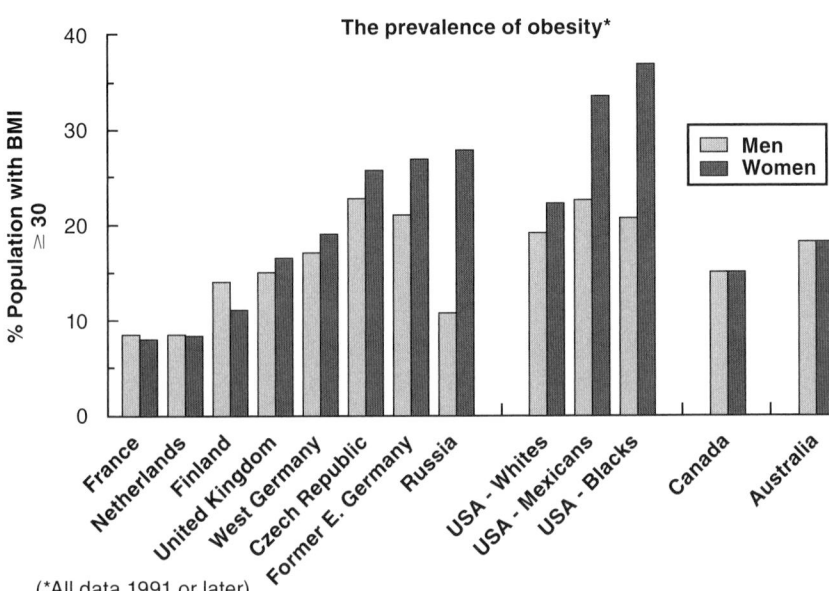

FIGURE **44-1** The increasing prevalence of obesity in adults worldwide. (*Data from http://www.iuns. org/features/obesity/obesity.htm; http://www.iuns.org/ features/obesity.tabfig.htm; and International Obesity Task Force www.iotf.org. Accessed August 31, 2007.*)

TABLE **44-2**	Classification of Overweight and Obesity by Body Mass Index		
	Obesity Class	**Body Mass Index (kg/m²)**	**Risk of Disease**
Underweight	—	<18.5	Increased
Normal	—	18.5-24.9	Normal
Overweight	—	25-29.9	Increased
Obesity	I	30-34.9	High
	II	35-39.9	Very high
Extremely obese	III	> 40	Extremely high
Superobese		> 50	Extremely high
Super-super obese		> 60	Extremely high

Data from *National Institutes of Health. Clinical Guidelines on the Identification, Evaluation, and Treatment of Overweight and Obesity in Adults: the Evidence Report (Publication No. 98-4083). Washington, DC: National Institutes of Health; 1998; Klein S, Romijn J. Obesity. In: Kronenberg HM et al. Williams Textbook of Endocrinology. 11th ed. Philadelphia: Saunders; 2008:1563-1589; Flier JS, Maratos-Flier. Biology of obesity. In: Fauci AS et al, eds. Harrison's Principles of Internal Medicine. 17th ed. New York: McGraw-Hill; 2008:462-468. Brodsky JB, Lemmens HJM. Is the superobese patient different? Obes Surg. 2004;1428.*

linearly related to weight gain.[1-3] Type 2 diabetes, coronary heart disease, hypertension, and hypercholesterolemia are prominent conditions in overweight and obese patients.[1-3] With increasing weight gain and increased adiposity, glucose tolerance deteriorates, blood pressure rises, and the lipid profile becomes more atherogenic.[2] Using BMI, age, and gender as independent variables, a multiple logistic regression model established that males (P = 0.021), those with higher BMI (P <0.0001), and those of older age (P <0.0001) tended to have more comorbid illness. These data suggest that age, male gender, and extent of obesity are risk factors because they are markers for sicker patients.[17] Hormonal and nonhormonal mechanisms contribute to the greater risk of breast, gastrointestinal, endometrial, and renal cell cancers.[6] Psychologic health risks often stem from social ostracism, discrimination, and impaired ability to participate fully in activities of daily living. Coexistent feelings of worthlessness and low self-esteem can lead to depression that not only magnifies anesthetic morbidity, but also contributes to an increased incidence of suicide among morbidly obese persons.

ADIPOSE TISSUE

Adipose tissue has major integrative physiologic functions, secretes numerous proteins, and is considered an endocrine organ.[2] Its major functions as an organ are to provide a reservoir of readily convertible and usable energy and to maintain heat insulation.[2,3,18] Functions associated with liver fat metabolism include degradation of fatty acids into usable units of energy,

---

BOX 44-1

Conditions Associated with Obesity

Type 2 diabetes
Coronary heart disease
Hypertension
Dyslipidemia
Cerebrovascular disease
Thromboembolic disease
Restrictive lung disease
Obesity hypoventilation syndrome
Obstructive sleep apnea
Gout
Infertility
Impaired immune response
Wound infections
Depression

Osteoarthritis
Cancer: esophageal, gallbladder, colon, breast, uterine,
  cervical, prostate, renal
Chronic venous insufficiency
Deep vein thrombosis
Gallbladder disease
Urinary incontinence
Gastroesophageal reflux disease
Pancreatitis
Nonalcoholic fatty liver disease: steatosis, cirrhosis,
  hepatomegaly
Low back pain
Obstetric complications
Surgical infections

Data from *National Institutes of Health*. Clinical Guidelines on the Identification, Evaluation, and Treatment of Overweight and Obesity in Adults: the Evidence Report *(Publication No. 98-4083)*. *Washington, DC: National Institutes of Health; 1998; Klein S, Romijn J. Obesity. In: Kronenberg HM et al. Williams Textbook of Endocrinology. 11th ed. Philadelphia: Saunders; 2008:1563-1589; Flier JS, Maratos-Flier E. Obesity. In: Fauci AS et al, eds. In: Harrison's Principles of Internal Medicine. 17th ed. New York: McGraw-Hill; 2008:462-468.*

---

synthesis of triglycerides from carbohydrates and proteins, and synthesis of other lipids from fatty acids, particularly cholesterol and phospholipids.[18] The ability of the liver to desaturate fatty acids is tremendously important because all cells contain some unsaturated fats synthesized by the liver.

Body fat is also important in heat regulation and insulation. Fat cells, which arise from modified fibroblasts, enlarge and fill with liquid triglycerides to nearly 95% of their storage capacity.[18,19] During exposure of the skin to cold (several weeks), the fatty acid chains of the triglycerides shorten, or become more unsaturated.[3] This phenomenon lowers their melting point, which allows the fat in the fat cells to maintain a liquid state. Metabolically, this is significant. Only liquid fat can be hydrolyzed and transported from the cells to be used for energy.[3]

Body Fat Distribution

In early childhood, fat-cell formation occurs rapidly.[2] Overfeeding during this time accelerates fat storage and triggers hyperproliferation of fat cells. During adolescence, the number of fat cells stabilizes and remains constant throughout adult life. Children become obese through an increase in fat-cell numbers, whereas adults become obese through hypertrophy of existing fat cells.[2,3] The distribution of body fat, however, is a clearer indicator of increased health risk.[19]

Central, android, or abdominal visceral obesity ("apple" shape), with a waist/hip ratio greater than 0.85 in men and 0.92 in women, is perceived as a malignant form of fat accumulation[2,20] (Figure 44-2, A). Waist/hip ratio is calculated by dividing the narrowest waist measurement by the broadest hip measurement while the patient is standing.[2] Waist circumference is the newly established standard used as a marker for abdominal obesity. In men a waist circumference greater than 102 cm (40 inches) and in women a waist circumference of 88 cm (35 inches) denote increased risk for certain diseases and conditions.[2,18] These include ischemic heart disease, diabetes mellitus, hypertension, dyslipidemia, and death.[1-3]

Peripheral gynecoid, or gluteal femoral obesity ("pear" shape), with a waist/hip ratio below 0.76 is associated with varicose vein development, joint disease, and reduced incidence of

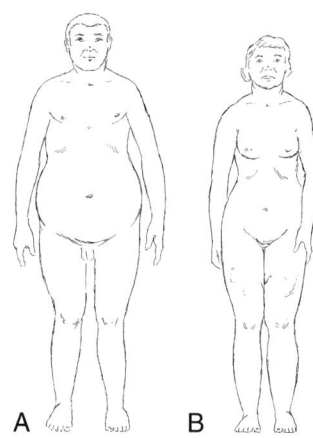

FIGURE **44-2** Obesity. **A,** Central android, or abdominal visceral. **B,** Peripheral gynecoid, or gluteal.

non–insulin-dependent diabetes mellitus (Figure 44-2, B). Medical risks accompanying gynecoid fat deposition are less perilous than those associated with the android pattern.[1,4]

Differences in morbidity between android and gynecoid fat distribution are caused by metabolic attributes of the adipose and tissues adjacent to it. Gynecoid repositories of fat, found primarily in women, are metabolically static and are proposed to function as energy depots for pregnancy and lactation.[3,4] Android fat distribution, typically seen in males, is metabolically active with regard to free fatty acid (FFA) release.[2] When elevated levels of FFAs are mobilized from adipose tissue, portal venous drainage delivers high concentrations of FFAs to the liver. Continual delivery of excessive FFAs stimulates hepatic synthesis of very-low-density lipoproteins (VLDLs) and circulation of low-density lipoproteins (LDLs). Hepatic exposure to high concentrations of FFAs also increases gluconeogenesis and inhibition of insulin uptake, which induces non–insulin-dependent diabetes mellitus. Although VLDLs, LDLs, and hyperglycemia are catalysts for the formation of associated cardiovascular and cerebrovascular disease, some studies support the possibility that hyperinsulinemia alone may cause hypertension.[2,3]

CAUSES OF OBESITY

Body size is dependent on genetic and environmental factors. Genetic predisposition, believed to be a primary factor in the development of obesity, explains only 40% of the variance in body mass.[6] The significant increase in the prevalence of obesity has resulted from environmental factors that result in increased calorie intake and reduced physical activity.[6,18] Other factors such as socialization, age, sex, race, and economic status affect its progression. In the United States, food consumption has risen as a result of the "super-sizing" of portions and the availability of high-fat fast food and snacks. Physical activity has been reduced as a result of modernization (television and computers) and sedentary lifestyle and work activities. Cultural and lifestyle variations play an important role in the development of obesity.[6] For example, some ethnic foods contain high levels of fats and carbohydrates, whereas others (e.g., Asian) focus on low-fat foods such as fish and vegetables.

Since the discovery of the adipose tissue protein leptin, advances have been made in understanding the molecular basis of body fat regulation. In 1994, the *ob* gene was identified in mice and was shown to control the production of the protein leptin.[21] Genetically obese *ob/ob* mice produce insufficient leptin and tend to overeat, which leads to obesity. Exogenous leptin reverses hyperphagia and induces weight loss. However, serum leptin levels increase exponentially with fat mass, suggesting that most obese patients are resistant or insensitive to weight regulation by exogenous leptin. Leptin is a regulator between fat storage and the brain. Brain resistance to leptin may contribute to excessive caloric intake and morbid obesity.

There is increased interest in the role of inflammation in obesity. Several inflammatory mediators such as angiotensinogen (AGT), transforming growth factor beta (TGF-β), tumor necrosis factor alpha (TNF-α), and interleukin 6 (IL-6) are elevated in morbidly obese patients. Weight loss results in a reduction in both the inflammatory mediators and comorbidities associated with obesity.[22] Continued investigation into genetic-environmental interactions may provide further understanding and treatment of obesity.[4,20,21]

PATHOPHYSIOLOGY OF OBESITY

A number of pathophysiologic changes occur as a result of overweight and obesity.[23] These changes involve all of the major body organ systems, leading to an increase in morbidity and premature death. The risk of many of the medical conditions associated with obesity increases linearly with BMI.[2-4]

Cardiovascular Considerations

Cardiovascular considerations are predominantly a reflection of the progressive compensatory processes that evolve to meet the increased metabolic demands of the fat organ.[2-4,24] Cardiovascular disease dominates the morbidity and mortality in obesity and manifests in the form of ischemic heart disease, hypertension, and cardiac failure.[15] Development and sustenance of the fat mass necessitates formation of extra blood vessels and increased circulatory, pulmonary, central, and peripheral blood volume.[2-4] For every 13.5 kg of fat gained, an estimated 25 miles of neovascularization occurs to provide blood flow at a rate of 2 to 3 mL/100 g of tissue per minute. This represents an increased cardiac output of 0.1 L/min for each kilogram of fat acquired.[3] Expansion of blood volume, stimulated by hypoxia-induced chronic

respiratory insufficiency, is seen in severe obesity. Accelerated renin-angiotensin activity and the perfusion requirements of the fat organ further increase the vascular fluid compartment.[2-4,24]

Movement of the expanded blood volume through extensive vascular tissue, under compression by adipose tissue, places greater demand on the myocardium. Increased workload caused by elevation of the basal metabolic rate is reflected in increased cardiac output, increased oxygen (O_2) consumption, increased carbon dioxide production, and normal or slightly abnormal arteriovenous O_2 difference.[2,25] Chronically elevated cardiac output precedes increased left-sided heart pressures and left ventricular hypertrophy. Because heart rate usually remains the same, cardiac output must be augmented by an increase in stroke volume. Therefore, cardiomegaly, atrial and biventricular dilation, and biventricular hypertrophy ensue. These contribute to the development of hypertension and eventual congestive heart failure[2-4,24] (Figure 44-3).

Hypertension is defined as a systolic pressure greater than 140 mm Hg, a diastolic pressure greater than 90 mm Hg, or both.[3] The prevalence rates of hypertension in obese patients are more than twice as high as those in lean men and women.[24,26] Blood pressure has been shown to increase 6.5 mm Hg for every 10% increase in body weight.[27] In the nonhypertensive remainder of the severely obese, decreased systemic vascular resistance may serve to facilitate forward blood flow through the doubled body habitus.[2,4] Hypertension is precipitated by increased blood viscosity, catecholamine kinetics, and possibly increased estrogen concentrations. Hyperinsulinemia, elevated mineralocorticoids, and abnormal sodium reabsorption are also implicated as causes of hypertension. Hypercholesterolemia (defined as a cholesterol level greater than 250 mg/dL) often coexists with hypertension, thereby predisposing obese patients to atherosclerosis and cerebrovascular accident.[25,26] Arrhythmias may occur as a result of hypoxemia, hypercapnia, electrolyte disorders, sleep apnea, ventricular hypertrophy, hypertension, and coronary artery disease.[28]

Coronary artery disease in the obese is a frequently associated but independent risk factor. It appears with or without hypertension, hypercholesterolemia, diabetes mellitus, hyperlipidemia, or sedentary lifestyle.[2-4,29] Obesity coincident with coronary artery disease results in frequent angina, congestive heart failure, acute myocardial infarction, and sudden death.[15,24,25] Ischemic heart disease is more common in those obese individuals with a central distribution of fat.[24]

Respiratory Considerations

Compromise of respiratory function results from the compression of fat on abdominal, diaphragmatic, and thoracic structures. Over time, thoracic kyphosis and lumbar lordosis develop, resulting in impaired rib movement and fixation of the thorax in an inspiratory position.[1,3] As a result, chest wall, lung, parenchyma, and pulmonary compliance is reduced to 35% of predicted values.[29,30] Metabolic needs of the fat organ and the greater mechanical work of breathing stimulate increased myocardial O_2 consumption. Increases in carbon dioxide production and retention, coupled with decreased ventilation, coincide with reduced respiratory muscle efficiency.[2] Lung inflation is inhibited, which causes declinations in functional residual capacity (FRC) to less than closing capacity. Premature airway closure increases dead space and causes carbon dioxide retention, ventilation-perfusion mismatch, shunting, and hypoxemia[1,20] (Figure 44-4). Morbid obesity is associated with reductions in FRC, expiratory reserve volume (ERV), and total lung capacity.[29-31] FRC declines exponentially with increasing BMI.[2] A recent study of pulmonary function in morbidly obese patients indicates that forced vital

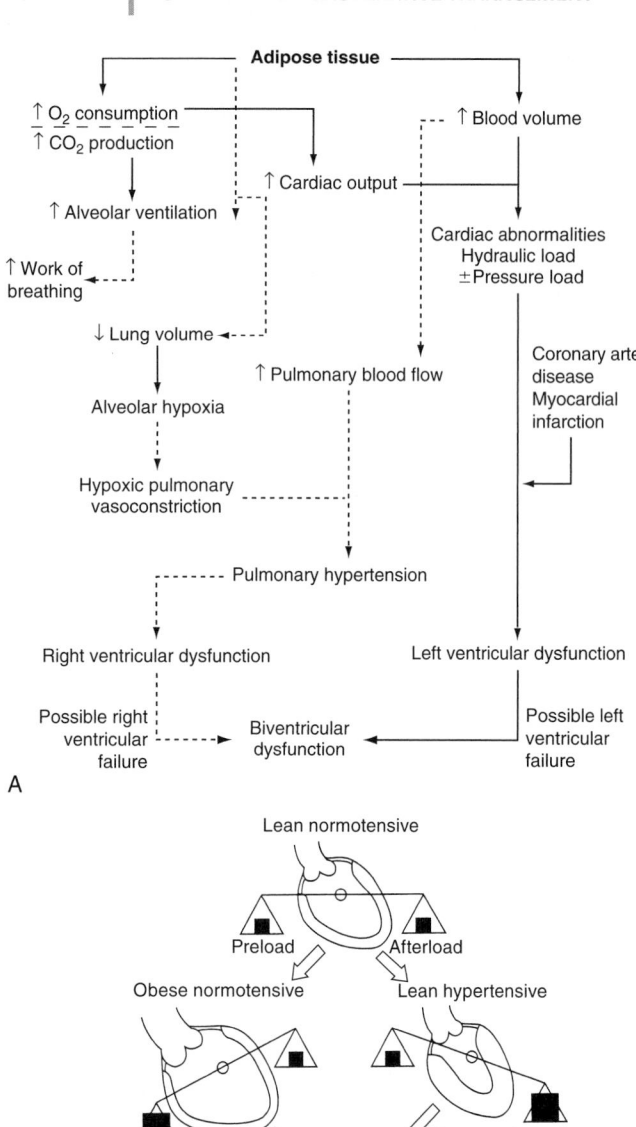

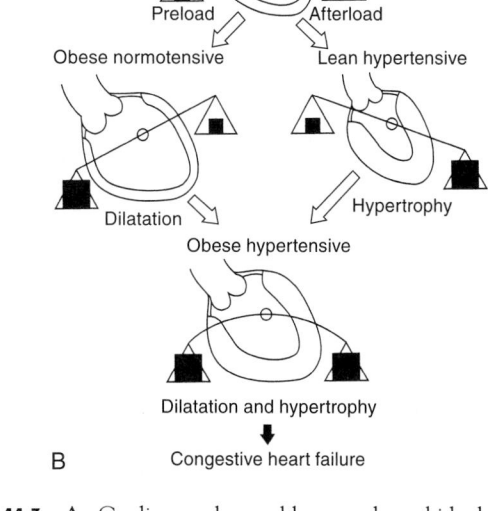

FIGURE **44-3** **A,** Cardiovascular problems and morbid obesity. **B,** Adaptation of the heart to obesity, hypertension, and a combination of the two. Although hypertension produces concentric hypertrophy only, obesity plus hypertension produces hypertrophy and dilation (eccentric hypertrophy), associated with a high incidence of congestive heart failure. (**A,** *Modified from Vaughan RW. Anesthetic management of the morbidly obese patient. In: International Anesthesia Research Society 1987 Review Course Lectures. New York: International Anesthesia Research Society; 1987:11-18.* **B,** *From Messerli FH. Cardiovascular effects of obesity and hypertension. Lancet. 1982;1:1165.*)

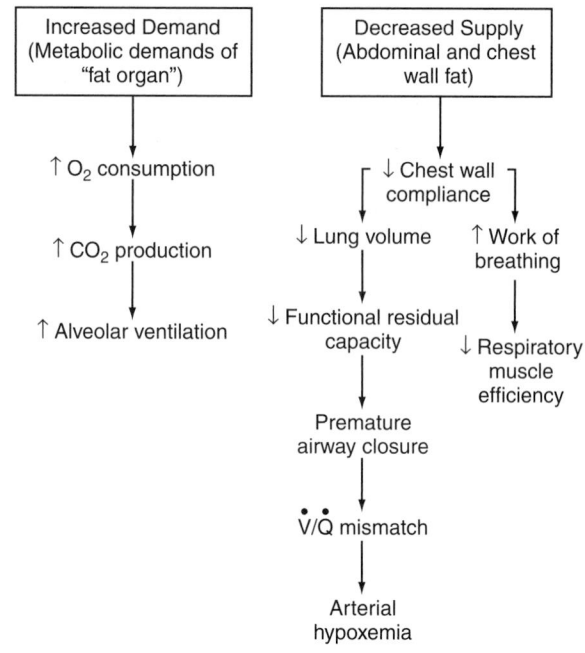

FIGURE **44-4** Pulmonary problems and morbid obesity. (*Modified from Vaughan RW. Pulmonary and cardiovascular derangements in the obese patient. In: Brown BR Jr, ed. Anesthesia and the Obese Patient: Contemporary Anesthesia Practice. Philadelphia: FA Davis; 1982:19-41.*)

capacity varies inversely with BMI, and patients with a very high BMI, even when asymptomatic, will have major reductions in lung function.[32]

Concomitant diminution of vital capacity, total lung capacity, ERV, and inspiratory capacity are demonstrated by rapid, shallow breathing. These ventilation patterns are characteristic of restrictive lung disease.[2,30,31] Eventual hypoventilation, hypercarbia, and acidosis result from depression of central nervous system responsiveness to chronic hypoxia.[3] Recurrent hypoxemia leads to secondary polycythemia and is associated with an increased risk of coronary artery disease and cerebrovascular disease.[19] Respiratory muscle dysfunction also has been reported with obesity[33] and may result from an inefficiency secondary to changes in chest-wall compliance or the lower lung volumes found in obesity. These abnormalities predispose obese patients to respiratory failure in the setting of even mild pulmonary or systematic insults.[34]

Obstructive Sleep Apnea

Obesity is a well-established risk factor for sleep apnea, with the incidence of obstructive sleep apnea (OSA) increasing in direct proportion with the level of obesity. Patients characterized with OSA have a BMI greater than 30 kg/m^2, abdominal fat distribution, and a large neck girth (>17 inches in men and >16 inches in women).[2] For patients with clinically severe obesity (BMI $\geq 35 \text{ kg/m}^2$) who present for bariatric surgery, the incidence of sleep apnea ranges from 71% to 77%.[35-57]

Approximately 5% of morbidly obese patients have OSA. OSA is characterized by excessive episodes of apnea (10 seconds) and hypopnea during sleep that are caused by complete or partial upper airway obstruction.[38] Findings from one recent study indicated that approximately 25% of all surgical patients are at high risk of OSA.[39] Obstructive sleep apnea is characterized by intermittent closure or narrowing of the upper airway during sleep, which leads to episodes of apnea-hypopnea, arousal, and oxygen desaturation.[40] This disorder is pervasive and affects nearly

18 million Americans.[41] As many as 80% to 95% of persons with OSA are undiagnosed.[42]

Apnea is the cessation of airflow at the nose and mouth for more than 10 seconds.[43] Apnea is considered obstructive if there is continued respiratory effort despite airflow cessation. Hypopnea is defined as a 50% reduction in airflow for 10 seconds for 15 or more times per hour of sleep associated with snoring and a 4% decrease in oxygen saturation. It connotes a transient reduction in airflow caused by increased upper airway resistance.[42] OSA syndrome is diagnosed by polysomnography using an apnea-hypopnea index (AHI).[44] OSA is diagnosed by the presence of at least five obstructive apneas, hypopneas, or both per hour while the patient is sleeping. OSA is graded into three levels of severity: mild (AHI of $\geq$5 but <15 events per hour); moderate (AHI of 15 to 30 events per hour); and severe (AHI of >30 events per hour). Research findings reveal that significant clinical sequelae occur even with mild OSA.[45]

The pathogenesis of OSA is likely multifactorial.[46] Contributing factors include airway anatomy, the state-dependent control of the upper airway dilator muscles, and ventilatory stability. The site of upper airway obstruction typically lies in the pharynx. The pharyngeal luminal area during inspiration reflects a balance between collapsing intrapharyngeal negative suction pressure and dilating forces provided by the pharyngeal muscles.[45] In awake human subjects, the patency is maintained by the central nervous system's continually mediated contraction of the tensor muscles. These dilator muscles oppose the negative collapsing force developed during inspiration.[42] This activation of muscle tone is typically reduced during sleep and in many individuals leads to compromised patency of the upper airway with turbulent airflow and snoring. In obese patients, more adipose tissues in the pharyngeal structures increase the likelihood that relaxation of the upper airway muscles will cause collapse of the soft-walled oropharynx between the uvula and the epiglottis. Extraluminal pressure is increased by superficially located masses, and the upper airway is compressed externally.[40,42,47,48]

While sleeping, any and all of these mechanical, neural, and structural factors may contribute to upper airway collapse that either interferes with or eliminates ventilation, which results in a surge of pharyngeal dilator muscle activity that subsequently opens the airway. A period of hyperventilation then follows, which reverses hypercarbia, and then correspondingly the central respiratory drive is reduced. The process can repeat itself continually throughout the night, causing intermittent hypoxia and hypercarbia, fragmenting sleep, and triggering adrenergic surges with each cycle.[42,43,45] Clinically significant episodes of 5 or more per hour or more than 30 per night result in hypoxia, hypercapnia, systemic and pulmonary hypertension, and cardiac arrhythmias.[19,30,31,38]

One study series of patients undergoing ECG Holter monitoring showed that nocturnal paroxysmal asystole, episodic bradycardia, and sinus node dysfunction were more prevalent in patients with OSA.[49] Study of OSA patients with permanent atrial pacemakers demonstrated that subjects had fewer episodes of OSA if their pacemakers were set to increase their heart rate during the night. It is hypothesized that the increased vagal tone accompanying bradycardia also affects airway patency.[50]

Patients with OSA also have a higher incidence of comorbidities. Approximately 50% to 60% of patients with OSA are hypertensive, and an estimated 50% of hypertensive patients have sleep apnea.[51]

Because 80% to 95% of all patients with OSA are undiagnosed and untreated, many patients who present for surgery will not be diagnosed. During preanesthetic evaluation, patients should be asked about their sleeping patterns, and anesthesia providers should have a high index of suspicion for OSA in all obese patients.[52] Some advocate that all obese patients, or those who observe them while they sleep, be routinely asked about nocturnal snoring or apnea, arousals, and diurnal sleepiness.[53]

Obese Hypoventilation (Pickwickian) Syndrome

Obesity hypoventilation syndrome (OHS), or pickwickian syndrome, is a complication of extreme obesity characterized by OSA, hypercapnia, daytime hypersomnolence, arterial hypoxemia, cyanosis-induced polycythemia, respiratory acidosis, pulmonary hypertension, and right-sided heart failure. At its extreme there is evidence of nocturnal episodes of central apnea, apnea without respiratory efforts, reflecting progressive desensitization of the respiratory centers to nocturnal hypercarbia.[30,31,38,47]

OHS, which occurs in 8% of the obese population, is clinically distinct from simple obesity.[31] With simple obesity, the partial pressure of arterial carbon dioxide, pH, and pulmonary compliance are within normal ranges.[29] Hypoxia may be present, but no evidence of cardiac failure or arterioalveolar O_2 difference exists. In contrast, OHS is diagnosed when the morbidly obese patient exhibits inappropriate and sudden somnolence, sleep apnea, hypoxia, and hypercapnia.[3] Alveolar ventilation is reduced because of shallow and inefficient ventilation related to decreased tidal volume, inadequate inspiratory strength, and inadequate elevation of the diaphragm. Cardiac enlargement, cyanosis, polycythemia, and twitching also are evident on physical examination.[4] Activities of daily living are altered by the somnolent episodes. Operating machinery or driving a vehicle may cause injury or death.

Gastrointestinal Disease

The incidence of gastroesophageal reflux disease, gallstones, and pancreatitis increases with obesity. Obesity is associated with a number of liver abnormalities referred to as *nonalcoholic fatty liver disease* (NAFLD).[54] NAFLD includes steatosis, steatohepatitis, fibrosis, cirrhosis, hepatomegaly, and abnormal liver biochemistry. Liver impairment in severely obese patients is caused by infiltration of hepatocytes with triglycerides. Continued deposition of lipid ruptures the cellular wall of the hepatocyte, causing extrusion of serum lactic dehydrogenase and aspartate aminotransferase.[3] Triglycerides block bile canaliculi and cause elevated serum alkaline phosphatase. Lipid-induced inflammation of the hepatic lobules degenerates to necrosis and intralobular collagen deposition. Portal inflammation or fibrosis ensues in 29% of these patients, and 3% develop cirrhosis.[4] In obese patients the mortality rate from liver cirrhosis is 1.5 to 2.5 times higher than in nonobese persons.[19]

Gallstones

Gallstones are 30% more prevalent in obese than nonobese women, and this prevalence increases linearly with BMI.[4] Higher concentrations of cholesterol in the bile and an increased ratio of bile salts to lecithin are responsible for the development of gallstones.[55] Jaundice may also accompany bile duct obstruction. Laparoscopic and open cholecystectomies are commonly performed in this group of patients because of the increased incidence of gallbladder disease in the obese. Although technically more difficult for both surgical and anesthesia teams, the benefits of laparoscopic gallbladder removal (reduced postoperative pain, shorter hospitalization, earlier return to activities of daily living) may outweigh the risks.

Endocrine and Metabolic Disease

Obesity is seldom the result of primary endocrine dysfunction. Thyroid, adrenocortical, and pituitary function should be investigated with obesity that manifests atypical symptoms.[3] Menstrual problems such as oligomenorrhea, amenorrhea, menorrhagia, and the presence of hirsutism may herald hypothalamic-pituitary abnormalities.[4] Obese men may experience decreased libido or impotence indicative of hypogonadism. Low serum follicle-stimulating hormone and testosterone levels are evident.[4]

Within groups of individuals demonstrating non–insulin-dependent diabetes mellitus, 80% are obese. The risk of type 2 diabetes increases linearly with BMI.[4] Hyperinsulinemia and impaired insulin-receptor sensitivity lead to hyperglycemia and glycosuria. A metabolic or insulin-resistant syndrome, or "syndrome X," has been described in patients with abdominal obesity. It is characterized by insulin resistance, impaired glucose tolerance, type 2 diabetes, dyslipidemia, and hypertension.[2]

Orthopedic and Joint Disease

Obese persons often develop osteoarthritis from continued mechanical stress on weight-bearing joints. A linear relationship between degree of arthritis and weight exists.[2-4] Ankles, hips, knees, and lumbar spine are frequently burdened. Bone resorption secondary to limited physical activity may also reduce bone density and contribute to stress fractures. Reduction of weight can curb orthopedic injury and lessen the discomfort in the back and lower extremities.

PEDIATRIC OBESITY

Obesity is a growing problem among U.S. children. In 1994, one in five children between the ages of 6 and 17 was overweight, doubling the rate of 30 years ago.[56] The 2004 National Center of Health Statistics (NCHS) report shows 17.1% of children and adolescents 2 to 19 years of age are overweight, and that 4% of adolescents have BMIs greater than 40. Adolescents are more overweight then preschool children.[57] The percentage of overweight adolescent girls increased from 13.8% to 16.2%, and overweight adolescent boys increased from 14% to 18.2%.[58] These adverse trends in obesity have potentially profound effects on children's health now and for their long-term health outlook.

Obesity is clinically diagnosed as a weight-for-height greater than the 90th percentile or a BMI greater than or equal to the 95th percentile, age and sex specific. Pediatric obesity is recognized by BMI greater than the 95th percentile on the Centers for Disease Control and Prevention (CDC) growth chart. Evidence-based guidelines and expert committee recommendations have repeatedly stressed that the BMI for age should be the basis of our definitions of pediatric overweight and obesity.

Studies document links between early childhood and adolescent obesity and adult obesity:

- Obese adolescents have a 70% to 80% chance of being obese adults.[59]
- Childhood obesity is associated with a higher chance of premature death and disability in adulthood, particularly in urban areas.[60]
- Childhood and adolescent overweight and obesity are linked with adult cardiovascular and endocrine problems.[61]
- Obese children are three to five times more likely to suffer a heart attack or stroke before they reach the adult age of 65.[61]
- Being overweight as young as age 18 could be the strongest predictor of future hip replacement because of osteoarthritis.[62]

Determinants of obesity are multifactored and include genetics, biology, and social and environmental behaviors that may begin in early childhood. The escalating national and global epidemics of obesity and sedentary lifestyle warrant increased attention by physicians and other health-care professionals. The health goals for obese children and adolescents should be to develop healthy eating habits, maintain weight or reduce the rate of gain, and to be active rather than sedentary.[63]

Some specific problems obese children face related to the health care community are the following:

- Pediatric obesity is more common than diabetes, human immunodeficiency virus (HIV), cystic fibrosis, and all childhood cancers combined.
- Primary hypertension in children has become increasingly common in association with obesity and risk factors such as a family history of hypertension and an ethnic predisposition to hypertensive disease. Obese children are at approximately a three-fold higher risk for hypertension than nonobese children.[64]
- Most children with type 2 diabetes are overweight or obese at diagnosis and usually have a family history of type 2 diabetes. Americans of African, Hispanic, Asian, and American Indian descent are disproportionately represented.[65]
- OSA sleep disorder was very common in a clinical sample of overweight children. OSA is not associated with abdominal obesity. On the contrary, higher levels of abdominal obesity and fat mass are associated with central sleep apnea.
- Bariatric surgery may be useful but only with carefully selected obese children with serious comorbidities and unresponsiveness to interventions. The biggest barrier seems to be the psychosocial aspect, although complications from child bariatric surgery may include leaks, deep vein thrombi, micronutrient deficiency, bleeding, and infection.[66]
- Psychosocial disorders may result when obese children are treated differently. This may be the most devastating effect of obesity on children. They may feel isolated and lonely and have self-esteem and identity problems. It is important for the health-care professional to be sensitive to this issue and understand that an individual's confidence, especially a child's, is affected by self-image and perceptions of peers.[67]

Unfortunately, children with long-standing obesity (especially morbidly obese) develop medical problems previously seen in adulthood. Medical effects of obesity such as hypertension, insulin resistance, coronary artery disease, and metabolic syndrome previously reserved for adults are on the rise in children and adolescents.[68,69]

The prevalence of the metabolic syndrome is high among obese children and adolescents and increases with worsening obesity. Diagnosis of metabolic syndrome in children and adolescents is only now receiving greater attention, and there does not seem to be consensus on precise standards of treatment. The dominant underlying risk factors for this syndrome appear to be abdominal obesity, insulin resistance, hypertriglyceridemia, hypertension, and proinflammatory and prothrombotic states. Insulin resistance, in which the body cannot use insulin efficiently, is why metabolic syndrome is also called *insulin-resistance syndrome*.[69]

Studies show that obesity increases the burden of disease for children and adolescents, and special attention has been given to clinical complications for that population. These include cardiovascular disease (dyslipidemia and hypertension), respiratory disease (sleep apnea, snoring, asthma), orthopedic conditions (Blount's disease, slipped capital femoral epiphysis), gastrointestinal disease (gallbladder, steatohepatitis), and endocrine disease (insulin resistance, hyperinsulinism, impaired glucose tolerance, and type 2 diabetes that is normally reserved for adults). Other conditions in adolescent females include polycystic ovarian syndrome and menstrual irregularity. Studies also include psychosocial conditions such as depression, eating disorders, and social isolation.[70]

MATERNAL OBESITY

Obstetric complications of maternal obesity correlate more to pregravid obesity rather than excessive weight gain during gestation. Maternal obesity, not diabetes, seems to be the most important link to the nation's increase in mean birth weight. Mean increase in birth weight in the past 30 years was 116 at 37 to 41 weeks gestation.[71]

Prepregnancy obesity significantly increases the parturient risk for cesarian delivery.

Both first and second stages of labor are longer in obese women. Obesity is a risk factor for developing gestational hypertension, insulin-treated gestational diabetes, and hydramnios. However, neonatal outcome of obese women is comparable to women with normal prepregnancy body mass index.[72]

The National Institutes of Health (NIH) recognizes many risk factors associated with maternal obesity. Outcomes in pregnancy complicated by obesity include gestational diabetes, preeclampsia, preterm labor, cesarean delivery, postpartum hemorrhage, infection, pregnancy-induced hypertension (PIH), and macrosomic infants. The American College of Obstetricians and Gynecologists (ACOG) reports increased risk for spontaneous abortion and miscarriage rates of almost double that of nonobese women in the first 6 weeks of pregnancy.[71] Metabolic syndrome in pregnancy manifests as preeclampsia, gestational hypertension, insulin resistance, and diabetes. Preeclampsia increases further in obese women with gestational diabetes mellitus (GDM) that is poorly controlled, a previous history of GDM, family history of type 2 diabetes, and history of a macrosomic fetus.[68]

Newborns considered large for gestational age (LGA), or macrosomic, are at long-term risk for adolescent and adult obesity. Weiss and associates defined *fetal macrosomia* as birth weight greater than 4000 g. The study found the rate of macrosomia to be 8.3% in nonobese parturients, 13.3% in those who were obese, and 14.6% in the morbidly obese.[73] These increased birth weights have been linked to increased adolescent metabolic syndrome and type 2 diabetes. By age 4, 25% of these children have impaired glucose tolerance. Children born to mothers with BMIs greater than 30 in the first trimester are more likely to show fetal overgrowth and adiposity beginning in utero and continuing into the first years of life. The results of one study demonstrated that at ages 2, 3, and 4, growth was increased by 15.1%, 20.6%, and 24.1%, respectively.[74]

Peripartum risks associated with maternal obesity include:

- Cesarean delivery and associated morbidity (approaches 40% in severely obese)
- Difficult placement of epidural and spinals, requiring multiple attempts
- Difficult intubation risk, usually in an emergent setting (twice the risk as nonobese)
- Decreased ability of ultrasound to detect cardiac and craniospinal abnormalities
- Increased postoperative complications, longer surgery times, wound infection and breakdown, endometritis, antepartum venous thrombi/emboli (VTE), and excessive blood loss during surgery but no increased risk of postpartum hemorrhage

Bariatric Surgery for Obese Women: Gestational Considerations

Owing to limited success with lifestyle changes, more obese women of reproductive age are seeking bariatric surgery as an alternative. Previous reports showed complications during pregnancy after these malabsorptive procedures included increase in premature rupture of membranes, small bowel ischemia, nutrient deficiencies and fetal abnormalities.[71] Cesarean deliveries increased in women who had previous bariatric surgery. Gestational diabetes and PIH disorders were significantly reduced in women having laparoscopic adjustable gastric banding procedures. There were no significant differences in placental abruption and previa, labor dystocia, or perinatal complications with bariatric surgery prior to conception.

Recommendations by ACOG[75] include weight screening annually, especially for women of childbearing age with a family history of cardiovascular disease and diabetes mellitus. They recommend physical activity, proper diet, behavioral therapy, and bariatric surgery for women with BMIs greater than 40 with comorbidities prior to pregnancy. After delivery, continued exercise and diet, as well as breastfeeding the infant, are beneficial. During pregnancy, weight gain should be limited following the IOM suggestions: 25- to 35-lb increase in nonobese women, 15 to 25 lb in overweight women, and 15 lb in obese women.

Genetic predisposition, physiology, and mechanisms related to maternal and fetal-placental interaction are important to the growth and development of children. Maternal obesity is shown to be a significant risk factor in adverse outcomes in pregnancy. Higher birth weights have a definite connection to overgrowth in children and obesity in adolescents.

TREATMENT OF OBESITY

A multimodal approach in the treatment of obesity includes dietary intervention, increased exercise, behavior modification, drug therapy, and surgery. Weight-loss programs are individualized to each patient based on the degree of obesity and coexisting conditions. Drug therapy is initiated in patients with a BMI greater than 30 kg/m² or a BMI between 27 and 29.9 kg/m² with a coexisting medical condition.[2-4] Pharmacologic management includes the administration of anorexiant drugs that affect the monoamine oxidase system. Through interactions with norepinephrine, dopamine, and serotonin, anorexiant agents affect satiation (level of fullness), satiety (level of hunger after eating), or both.[2] A commonly used anorexiant drug is sibutramine hydrochloride (Meridia). Recently, gastrointestinal lipase inhibitors such as orlistat (Xenical) have been used to block the absorption of dietary fat. Overweight and obese patients may self-prescribe "natural" herbs and plant concoctions such as ma huang or diet teas that contain ephedra and unknown quantities of other stimulants.

Surgical Treatment

Besides common surgeries performed within the general population, obese persons undergo additional procedures to ameliorate obesity-related diseases (Box 44-2). Surgical approaches designed to treat obesity can be classified as malabsorptive or restrictive.[18-21] Malabsorptive procedures, which include jejunoileal bypass and biliopancreatic bypass, are rarely used at the present time. Restrictive procedures include the vertical banded gastroplasty (VBG) and gastric banding, including adjustable gastric banding (AGB). Roux-en-Y gastric bypass (RYGB) combines gastric restriction with a minimal degree of malabsorption. VBG, AGB, and RYGB can all be performed laparoscopically. RYGB, the most commonly performed bariatric procedure in the United States, involves anastomosis of the proximal gastric pouch to a segment of the proximal jejunum, bypassing most of the stomach and the entire duodenum.[76-79] It is the most effective bariatric

BOX 44-2

Obesity-Related Diseases Treated Surgically

Metabolic
Cholelithiasis
Thromboembolism
Peripheral vascular disease
Urolithiasis

Mechanical
Osteoarthritis
Varicose veins
Esophagitis
Hiatal hernia
Abdominal wall hernia

Neoplastic
Cancer (endometrial, breast, prostate, colorectal, renal)
Fibroadenoma of the breast

Gynecologic
Uterine fibroma
Ovarian cysts
Cesarean section
Stress urinary incontinence

From Kral JG. Obesity. In: Lubin MF et al. Medical Management of the Surgical Patient. 4th ed. New York: Cambridge University Press; 2006:467-478.

procedure for production of short-term and long-term weight loss in severely obese patients.[77]

Advances in laparoscopic surgery have significantly improved surgical procedure times, morbidity, and mortality related to bariatric surgery. If the operation is performed using the "closed" method, the negative impact of pneumoperitoneum on respiratory system mechanics and oxygenation during laparoscopy can be seen. Ezri and colleagues demonstrated that the endotracheal tube moves more often in obese patients undergoing laparoscopy compared with those having open abdominal surgery.[80] Patients appreciate laparoscopic bariatric surgery because it reduces postoperative pain and the duration of convalescence.[81] Many studies show reductions in overall morbidity when a laparoscopic technique is used.[82] Postoperative lung volumes and pulmonary function are reduced by about 50% after open bariatric surgery and by about 40% after minimally invasive bariatric procedures.[83] The peak decline in postoperative lung function occurs in the first 24 hours after surgery. Identifying patients with reduced lung volumes preoperatively will facilitate postextubation treatments such as the use of continuous positive airway pressure (CPAP). Laparoscopy is usually well tolerated as long as the pneumoperitoneum pressure is maintained at less than 15 mm Hg.[82]

Patients selected for weight-loss surgery are generally younger than 65 years of age and weigh 100 lb or more above IBW.[77] Previous attempts to lose weight must be documented.[76-79] A thorough examination must be performed to rule out underlying physiologic diseases or psychologic disorders.[78] Failure to assess appropriate candidates for surgical intervention and long-term follow-up care may lead to recidivism. Poor compliance with postoperative dietary and exercise regimens can negate any benefit derived from surgical intervention.

Postoperatively, patients must stay in close contact with multidisciplinary team members. Rehabilitation of previous lifestyle patterns is achieved through counseling and support provided by psychologists, dietitians, physical therapists, and internists.[77-79] Most patients who are monitored for as long as 5 years postoperatively, achieve losses from their original weight of as much as 40% to 45% with gastric partitioning and 55% to 65% with gastric bypass.[3,77-79]

PHARMACOLOGIC CONSIDERATIONS

Obesity is associated with significant alterations in body composition and function that can alter the pharmacodynamics and pharmacokinetics of drugs. Alterations in the volume of distribution are related to size of the fat organ, increased blood volume, increased cardiac output, decreased total body water, alterations in protein binding, and lipophilicity of the drug.[84]

Highly lipophilic drugs have an increased volume of distribution in obese persons compared with normal-weight individuals.[76] The increased volume of distribution requires higher doses of lipophilic drugs to produce the required pharmacologic effect and prolongs the elimination of certain drugs such as pentothal and benzodiazepines. Factors such as protein binding and end-organ clearance affect volume of distribution.

No systemic relationship exists between the solubility and the distribution of some highly lipophilic drugs (digoxin, remifentanil, and procainamide) in obese patients.[85] Determination of dosage according to IBW is appropriate with these drugs. Dosages of drugs with weak or moderate lipophilicity are usually determined on the basis of IBW or lean body mass. Recommendations for determining the dosages of commonly used anesthetics are listed in Table 44-3.[76,84-88] Clinical judgment guides the determination of dosages for individual patients and the administration of pharmacologic agents in overweight and obese patients. In obese patients, larger fat stores provide an increased volume of distribution for lipid-soluble drugs (e.g., narcotics and benzodiazepines). Thus maintenance doses should be administered less frequently because clearance would be expected to be slower. The amount of intraoperative opioids administered has been correlated with complications during the immediate postoperative period.[43]

Fentanyl is a highly lipophilic synthetic opiate, and its clearance is not linearly correlated with TBW greater than 70 kg. The use of a formula for calculating the dosage of fentanyl based on weight has recently been validated. This "dosing weight" is the body mass into which the drug distributes and has been coined *pharmacokinetic mass*.[89] Rough approximations of pharmacokinetic mass of fentanyl for patients weighing 70, 100, 120, 140, 160, 180 and 200 kg are 65, 83, 93, 99, 104, 107 and 109 kg, respectively.[90] The actual dose in micrograms per hour equals 1.22 multiplied by the pharmacokinetic mass.

Sufentanil is also highly lipid soluble, and pharmacokinetic dosing parameters for this drug were also derived from nonobese subjects. These do accurately predict plasma sufentanil concentrations in morbidly obese subjects, but with increasing BMI they overestimate plasma sufentanil concentration rises.[86] Dexmedetomidine, an α_2-agonist with sedative and analgesic properties, provides hemodynamic stability without myocardial depression. It does not contribute to clinically significant respiratory depression, which makes it an attractive agent for use as an anesthetic adjunct in obese patients.[91] Further, it reduces postoperative opioid requirements and their attendant respiratory-depressant effects.[92,93] Another fat-soluble drug is propofol.

TABLE **44-3**	Guidelines for Dosages of Intravenous Anesthetics in Obese Patients	
Anesthetic Agent	**Basis for Calculation of Dosage**	**Guidelines**
Midazolam	TBW	Increase central V_D; increase initial dose to achieve therapeutic effect; prolonged sedation
Thiopental	TBW	Increase V_D; increase initial dose; prolonged time to awakening
Propofol	TBW (initial and infusion)	Increase V_D; increase initial dose; high affinity for fat; high hepatic extraction
Fentanyl	TBW	Increase V_D; increase elimination half-time
Sufentanil	TBW	Increase V_D; increase elimination half-time
Remifentanil	IBW	Consider age and lean body mass
Cisatracurium	TBW	No difference from patients with normal weight
Vecuronium	IBW	Increase V_D; impaired hepatic clearance; prolonged duration of action
Rocuronium	IBW	Faster onset and similar duration of action than normal weight patient
Succinylcholine	TBW	Increase plasma pseudocholinesterase activity; increase dose

Data from Ogunnaike BO et al. Anesthetic considerations for bariatric surgery. Anesth Analg. 2002;95:1793-1805; Hunter JD et al. Anesthetic management of the morbidly obese patient. Hosp Med. 1998;59:481-483; Song D et al. Remifentanil infusion facilitates early recovery for obese outpatients undergoing laparoscopic cholecystectomy. Anesth Analg. 2000;90:111-113; Slepchenko G et al. Performance of target-controlled sufentanil infusion in obese patients. Anesthesiology. 2003;98:65-73; Puhringer FK et al. Pharmacokinetics of rocuronium bromide in obese female patients. Eur J Anaesthesiol. 1999;16:507-510; Salihoglu Z et al. Total intravenous anesthesia versus single breath technique and anesthesia maintenance with sevoflurane for bariatric operations. Obes Surg. 2001;11:496-501.
IBW, *Ideal body weight;* TBW, *total body weight;* V_D, *volume of distribution.*

The dosage for propofol is based on corrected body weight: CBW = ideal body weight (IBW) + (0.4 × excess weight).[94]

In contrast, water-soluble drugs, such as neuromuscular blocking agents, have a much more limited volume of distribution, and maintenance doses should be based on IBW to avoid overdosing. One study compared the effects of rocuronium dosage based on TBW with effects based on IBW and concluded that rocuronium dosage in obese patients should be guided by IBW to avoid significant prolongation of the duration of action (55 minutes versus 22 minutes, until 25% twitch tension return).[95] These researchers also demonstrated that the duration of cisatracurium may be prolonged in obese females, and thus dosages should be guided by IBW.[96]

Although a systematic review demonstrated that intubating conditions of rocuronium and succinylcholine are similar,[97] many believe succinylcholine is the gold standard for rapid-sequence induction. However, obese patients may react differently than lean patients when given succinylcholine. In one study of 14 morbidly obese patients who received succinylcholine without pretreatment with a nondepolarizing blocking agent, only 3 patients had gross fasciculations, and only 2 of the 14 developed myalgia, suggesting that the morbidly obese do not develop fasciculations to the same degree as the nonobese. Because succinylcholine also concomitantly increases the lower esophageal sphincter pressure, the decrease in barrier pressure might be less than anticipated (see Table 44-3).

Inhalation agents have all been used successfully in obese and morbidly obese patients. Studies comparing the effects of isoflurane and sevoflurane in morbidly obese patients showed faster emergence after surgery with sevoflurane.[98,99] When comparing sevoflurane and desflurane in obese patients, a recent study showed faster emergence and marginally higher oxygen saturation in patients treated with desflurane.[100] The pharmacokinetic characteristics of the newer volatile anesthetics offer the possibility of a more rapid emergence and faster immediate recovery. All modern anesthetic vapors are safe to use in obese patients.[101]

Elimination of drugs in obese individuals is normal or increased in phase I reactions (oxidation, reduction, hydrolysis) and increased in phase II reactions (metabolism). Renal clearance is increased because of augmented renal blood flow and glomerular filtration rate.[2]

Parenteral Drug Administration

The intravenous route allows dependable and precise drug administration in morbidly obese patients. Patient-controlled analgesia, commonly used in postoperative pain management, is an example of intravenous administration technology. Caution must be observed, however, when drugs are injected via the subcutaneous or intramuscular route. If the drug is deposited into adipose tissue, absorption and efficacy of the drug is unpredictable because of reduced vascularization. As a result, the patient may not receive adequate analgesia or maximum therapeutic drug response. Use of a longer needle inserted into the muscle with the least fat (deltoid) may be more reliable.

Biotransformation of Inhaled Anesthetics

Intraoperative hepatic concerns stem from alterations in biotransformation and metabolism of drugs. Isoflurane, desflurane and sevoflurane have been used with minimal complications in overweight and obese patients.[98,102,103]

Sevoflurane is pleasant smelling and nonirritating to the airway. Sevoflurane causes increased levels of serum inorganic fluorides to be metabolized at a rate 100% faster in obese patients than in nonobese patients.[98,102,103] Its potential ability to enhance fluoride ion concentrations in obese patients with marginal renal function (creatinine greater than 1.5 mg/dL) and production of compound A (with low fresh gas flows less than 2 L/min) may necessitate the use of another inhalation agent.[102]

Sevoflurane and desflurane are the least soluble of all the potent inhalation anesthetics. Of the two, desflurane is the more resistant to hepatic degradation (less than 0.02% with desflurane versus 0.2% with sevoflurane). With its low solubility profile, rapid washout, absence of hepatic and renal toxicity, and support of blood pressure, desflurane may be the preferred inhalation agent in morbidly obese patients.[98,102,103]

ANESTHETIC MANAGEMENT: PREANESTHETIC EVALUATION

The goals of the preanesthetic evaluation are to obtain pertinent data regarding the patient's medical or surgical history, to optimize current physiologic functioning, and to determine an appropriate anesthetic plan (see Chapter 20). Of paramount importance is the need to establish a nonjudgmental and trusting relationship with the patient. Explanations of anticipated events during preoperative preparation (multiple venipunctures, central and arterial line insertions, awake intubation, pain management) and protection of the patient's privacy will allay anxiety.

Medications

Obese persons must be queried for concurrent use of weight-reducing substances, herbal supplements, and anorexiant drugs. Chronic use of noradrenergic and serotonergic therapy can produce hypertension, tachycardia, anxiety, psychosis, and catecholamine depletion. Patients who take over-the-counter drugs, including herbal medications, often forget or are afraid to reveal that they are taking these preparations, which can have deleterious consequences on induction. Catecholamine depletion can summate in profound hypotension during induction and maintenance of anesthesia, which is refractory to indirect-acting vasopressors such as ephedrine. Phenylephrine hydrochloride (Neo-Synephrine) is usually effective in reversing low blood pressure. At least 2 weeks of abstinence from the drugs is recommended for adequate catecholamine levels to be recovered.[84] Patients' usual medications should be continued until the time of surgery, with the possible exception of insulin and oral hypoglycemics. Antibiotic prophylaxis is important because of an increased incidence of wound infections in the obese.[104]

Laboratory Tests

Given the current climate of cost-consciousness and cost-efficiency, only the laboratory tests appropriate in light of the patient's history, physical examination, and planned surgery should be ordered.[15] In morbidly obese patients, baseline studies that may be directly affected by associated medical conditions are performed. Routine testing includes assessment of a complete blood count and electrolyte panel. Complete blood cell counts may reveal hematocrits as high as 65%, which can result from contracted blood volume or polycythemia associated with cardiopulmonary disease.[15,29] Leukocytosis (greater than 11,000 μL) is a strong predictor of risk for acute myocardial infarction independent of tobacco smoking.[18]

Arterial blood gas analysis that compares samples taken with the patient lying supine and sitting while breathing room air provides baseline values and can distinguish simple obesity from OHS. The renal panel may reflect abnormal glucose and potassium levels, which are indicators of insulin resistance and potentiation of myocardial irritability. Concomitant use of diuretics and certain cardiac medications can exacerbate electrolyte disturbances.[15] Blood urea nitrogen (BUN) and creatinine levels may be elevated in response to dehydration or renal dysfunction. Liver function tests are typically elevated in obese patients. This is generally not the result of hepatic disease but of infiltration of the hepatocytes with triglycerides (fatty liver, liver steatosis). The severity of fatty infiltration may alter pharmacologic effects of many anesthetic drugs, thereby requiring dose reductions.[84]

Coagulation studies are necessary if regional anesthesia is planned or if coagulopathy exists. Patients taking anticoagulants for treatment of deep vein thrombosis or atrial fibrillation may exhibit elevated prothrombin and partial thromboplastin times. Use of nonsteroidal antiinflammatory drugs (NSAIDs) may prolong bleeding times and affect surgical hemostasis.

In obese patients undergoing abdominal or thoracic surgery, pulmonary function tests are invaluable and essential for anesthetic planning; for selected procedures, the tests may be waived.[19] Chest radiography is necessary to determine the presence of cardiomegaly, pulmonary infiltrates, and evidence of chronic obstructive pulmonary disease.

Cardiac Assessment

Evaluation of cardiac function is essential in overweight and obese patients undergoing surgery. Investigation of prior myocardial infarction and the presence of hypertension, angina, or peripheral vascular disease is crucial. Limitations in exercise tolerance, history of orthopnea, and paroxysmal nocturnal dyspnea may indicate left ventricular dysfunction.[2-4] A careful elicitation of drug history is invaluable in garnering clues about the patient's coexistent diseases. When possible, cardiac medications should be continued up to and including the morning of surgery.

An electrocardiogram (ECG) is essential for determination of resting rate, rhythm, and ventricular hypertrophy or strain. Because of the increased incidence of coronary artery disease and myocardial infarction in this population, the preoperative ECG is also helpful in providing a reference for comparison in the event that myocardial ischemia is suspected in the perioperative period. Beyond this, there is no reason to believe that extensive preoperative testing to detect coronary artery disease (CAD) is indicated based solely on a patient being obese.[105] Ischemic changes or evidence of coronary artery disease must be investigated.[15,29] The ECG may be of low voltage because of the excess overlying tissue and therefore might result in underestimation of the severity of ventricular hypertrophy. Axis deviation and atrial tachyarrhythmias are relatively common.[4]

QT-interval prolongation, discovered retrospectively in severely obese patients who died from refractory dysrhythmias, is a marker for sudden cardiac arrest.[3] In cases of fatal and nonfatal dieting, prolonged QT intervals were also exhibited on patient ECGs.[4] In addition, sudden cardiac death is more prevalent in morbidly obese patients with left ventricular hypertrophy and ventricular ectopy.[5] If right ventricular hypertrophy is suspected, echocardiography is useful. Tricuspid regurgitation on echocardiography is the most confirmatory test of pulmonary hypertension when combined with clinical evaluation.[106]

Exercise testing may elicit valuable information about myocardial function in morbidly obese patients. Most are physically unable, however, to achieve adequate levels of exercise stress to make the studies worthwhile.[15] Alternative tests using dipyridamole-thallium are satisfactory for determining myocardial adequacy. In addition, echocardiography is useful for determining whether akinesis or wall-motion abnormalities are present in the obese myocardium.

Cardiomegaly, pulmonary congestion, elevated diaphragm, and a tortuous aorta can be identified by use of chest radiography. Results of radiographic studies serve to guide preoperative pharmacologic and medical management (diuretics, β₁-agonists, antibiotics). Repeated radiographs may be required to obtain adequate penetration and visualization of all lung fields.[84] Unfortunately, standard stationary and portable x-ray machines cannot accommodate massively obese persons. As a result, diagnostic x-ray examinations or evaluation of central line placement may be impossible. Under these circumstances, clinical expertise and management of subtle symptoms are invaluable. If it is indicated, the patient should be referred to a cardiologist for further investigation and optimization of his or her condition (e.g., control of blood pressure, treatment of heart failure, or coronary angioplasty).[107]

Respiratory Evaluation

Careful preoperative evaluation of the patient's respiratory function identifies potential problems. A patient who becomes dyspneic and desaturates when recumbent experiences the same symptoms during induction in the supine position.[108] Questions must elicit information regarding the presence or absence of orthopnea, wheezing, sputum production, or smoking history. Recent upper respiratory infection, snoring, or sleep disturbances may indicate obstructive processes. The potential for difficult mask ventilation should also be considered during the preoperative visit. Obesity has been identified as an independent risk factor for difficult face mask ventilation. Increasing this risk would be findings such as presence of a beard, lack of teeth, and history of snoring.[109] Room air pulse oximetry saturations and blood gases obtained in supine and upright positions may reflect disturbances in cardiac compensation.[31]

Airway Evaluation

A thorough airway evaluation is warranted for determination of the optimal airway management technique in overweight and obese patients.[108] A variety of assessment criteria have been evaluated for prediction of difficult intubation in obese patients.[110-112] Most practitioners use evaluation of multiple patient physical characteristics to identify potential airway problems indicative of the unanticipated difficult airway. These include measurement of interincisor distance, thyromental distance, head and neck extension, Mallampati classification, body weight, and most importantly a history of difficult airway.[110-112] Inspection of the oropharynx is necessary to determine Mallampati classification for intubation difficulty (Figure 44-5).[110] The value of oropharyngeal Mallampati classification alone is low. Evaluation of the length of upper incisors, visibility of the uvula, shape of the palate, compliance of the mandibular space, and length and thickness of the neck provide further criteria for assessment.

Opinions differ about the use of a patient's weight (BMI) as an independent predictor of difficulty in intubation. Some have demonstrated that difficult intubation is more common in obese patients.[113] Others have demonstrated that increased BMI per se is not a predictor of difficult intubation.[114] Variables determined likely to predict difficulty in intubation of the obese patient include increased neck circumference, Mallampati classification greater than 3, increased age, male sex, temporomandibular joint (TMJ) pathology, a history of OSA, and abnormal upper teeth.[114,115] Of these, a high Mallampati score (≥3) with a large neck circumference and a history of sleep apnea were in the aggregate found to be good predictors of difficulty in intubation.[110]

Fat rolls around the neck (restricting neck motion) and fat in the airway (decreasing glottic opening) together increase the difficulty of successfully intubating the trachea. The larger the neck circumference, the more difficult the laryngoscopy and intubation. Neck circumference of 40 cm was associated with a 5% probability of difficult intubation, and neck circumference of 60 cm was associated with a 35% probability of difficult intubation.

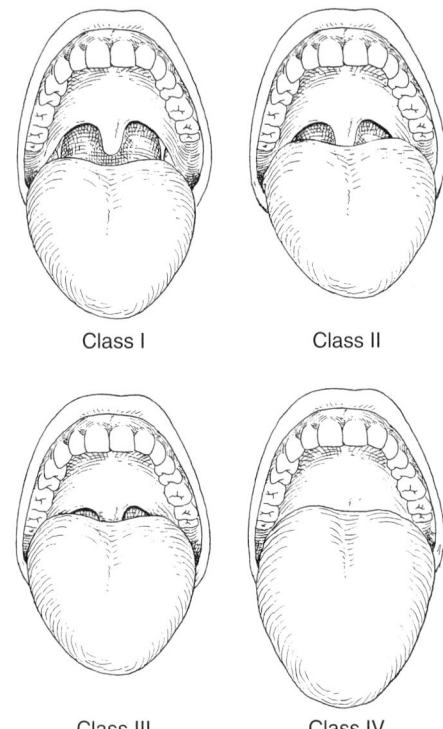

Class I Class II

Class III Class IV

FIGURE **44-5** Mallampati classification for intubation difficulty. *(From Mallampati SR et al. A clinical sign to predict difficult tracheal intubation: a prospective study. Can Anaesth Soc J. 1985;32:429-434.)*

A normal neck circumference in a 70 kg man is about 35 cm. Other researchers, using ultrasound to quantify the amount of anterior neck soft tissue, produced data that support these findings.[116]

Anatomic aberrations of the upper airway induced by severe obesity include reduced temporomandibular and atlantooccipital joint movement. Unsatisfactory mouth opening, presence of neck or arm pain, or inability to place the head and neck into "sniffing position" may indicate the need for awake fiberoptic intubation. Extreme airway narrowing in conjunction with shortened mandibular-hyoid distance (less than three fingerbreadths) can complicate mask ventilation and intubation. Presence of a short, thick neck, pendulous breasts, hypertrophied tonsils and adenoids, or a beard can contribute to a difficult airway. Marginal room air pulse oximeter saturations, abnormal arterial blood gases, and history of complicated airway management also indicate a potentially difficult intubation.[110-112] (Refer to Chapter 23 for a full description of the assessment and management of a difficult airway.) Airway management techniques should be explained to the patient, with emphasis on awake intubation and the need for postoperative ventilation.[117,118]

Vascular Access

Venipuncture can be challenging in overweight and obese patients with excessive fat that obscures blood vessels from visualization and palpation.[15] Central cannulation of vessels is impeded by distortions of the underlying anatomy by adipose tissue.[119] Hemorrhage, hypothermia, and trauma further reduce the likelihood of accessing vessels with ease. Use of a portable ultrasound machine may improve central venous catheter placement. As in all patients, iatrogenic pneumothorax must be avoided. Morbidly obese patients are less able than nonobese patients to tolerate the ensuing respiratory impairment.

ANESTHETIC MANAGEMENT: PREPARATION

Operating Room Equipment

In preparation for either emergent operating room procedures or nonemergent hospital admission, appropriate equipment must be readied. Newer-model operating room tables can accommodate up to 600 lb of weight. Older-model standard operating room tables could hydraulically elevate 300 to 350 lb of weight. In cases of extreme morbid obesity, "big boy" hydraulic beds are obtained and used in the operating room. Heavy-duty stirrups, extra-large retractors, elongated instruments, arm sleds, doubled armboards, and extremity tourniquets must be obtained. Sometimes a sanitized engine crane or other hoisting device must be used to suspend the panniculus adiposus for optimal surgical exposure.

Extra-large thigh cuffs can be used on the upper arm or the lower leg (over the posterior tibial artery). A regular-size or large blood pressure cuff can be used on the forearm over the radial artery until arterial cannulation for blood pressure monitoring can be performed. Bed-warming devices, fluid warmers, and warm airflow blankets should be used to prevent hypothermia, which can occur rapidly when large areas of body surface are exposed.

Airway Equipment

An equally important part of airway assessment is the preparation of equipment and personnel necessary to ventilate and intubate the morbidly obese patient. An assortment of blades, laryngoscopy handles, endotracheal tubes, masks, oral and nasopharyngeal airways, and stylets should be assembled. Laryngeal mask airways (LMAs), intubating laryngeal mask airways (ILMA), fiberoptic and bronchoscopic devices, Eschmann introducers, a jet ventilator (or Venturi apparatus), and emergency tracheotomy and cricothyrotomy kits must be available in the event that ventilation by mask or endotracheal tube is unsuccessful. Most departments have a difficult-airway cart that has all of the available equipment that should be placed in the operating room. Recently the ILMA and LMA CTrach (a modified version of the intubating LMA that allows continuous videoendoscopy of the tracheal intubation procedure) have been advocated as particularly useful tools for ventilating and intubating morbidly obese patients.[120,121]

Monitoring

Intraoperative monitoring, both basic and advanced, should address the specific needs of the patient.[84] Selection of electrocardiographic leads, when possible, should enhance detection of myocardial ischemia and pathology (leads II and V_5). Needle electrodes may be useful for obtaining a better tracing. Cuffs with bladders that encircle a minimum of 75% of the upper arm circumference but preferably the entire arm should be used. Forearm measurements with a standard cuff overestimate both systolic and diastolic blood pressures in obese patients.[122] Placement of an arterial catheter is appropriate for monitoring hemodynamic status and is advocated for all but the most minor procedures in the morbidly obese.[19] Use of central venous and pulmonary artery catheters should be considered in patients undergoing extensive surgery or those with serious cardiorespiratory disease.[84,119]

Aspiration Prophylaxis

Anesthesia providers have traditionally considered obese patients to be "full stomach" patients and at risk for regurgitation and subsequent pulmonary aspiration.[123-125] It is known that gastroesophageal reflux and hiatal hernia are more prevalent in the obese, and this may predispose them to esophagitis and pulmonary aspiration.[2] More recent data, however, have demonstrated that obese patients (BMI >30 kg/m^2) may have a lower incidence of "at-risk" stomach contents compared to lean patients.[126] In one study, researchers evaluated gastric contents of 232 surgical patients. Only 20 of 75 obese patients (27%) had high-volume, low-pH stomach contents, compared with 66 of 157 (42%) of lean patients. More recent studies have also demonstrated that obese patients who are fasting may not have gastric pH and volumes that would put them at risk for pulmonary aspiration.[127,128]

There is no consensus on whether obese patients have delayed, normal, or accelerated gastric emptying.[129] Current recommendations are that obese patients should follow the same fasting guidelines as nonobese patients. All patients should be allowed to drink as much as 300 mL of clear liquids until up to 2 hours before elective surgery; that volume has been demonstrated to not adversely affect the pH and volume of gastric contents at induction of anesthesia.[130]

Obesity is significantly related to gastroesophageal reflux disease (GERD).[131] Although increased body mass has been shown by some researchers to correlate directly with an increased incidence of reflux symptoms,[132] others have demonstrated the opposite and question the routine use of rapid-sequence induction on all patients who present with a diagnosis of GERD.[133]

Owing to the more recent and favorable data, some advocate the avoidance of rapid-sequence induction technique on obese patients as standard protocol, citing that is a common misperception that all obese patients should be viewed as "full stomach" patients, and in the event of failed intubation, obese patients may have poorer outcomes.[120,134] Although obese patients and patients with sleep apnea syndrome are prone to GERD, and both groups may also have an increased risk of difficult intubation, in the case of elective surgery in a fasted patient with no risk factors other than obesity or sleep apnea syndrome, the requirement for rapid-sequence induction is debatable.[135]

However, if symptoms are present in obese patients with GERD disease, the potential increased risk of aspiration should be discussed with the patient, and prophylactic measures (cricoid pressure, H_2 blockers, and proton-pump inhibitors) should be considered.[136] Although it is unclear which if any of these measures are effective,[137] they are within the current standard of care. Timely preinduction administration of histamine-2 and dopamine receptor antagonists coupled with oral administration of nonparticulate antacids has been demonstrated to decrease morbidity resulting from pulmonary aspiration and Mendelson syndrome.

Although rapid-sequence induction may be safe for some obese patients, its safety in superobese patients has been questioned. For patients with a BMI greater than 50 kg/m^2, or lower but with risk factors such as sleep apnea syndrome (SAS) or large neck circumference, either an awake intubation (with local anesthesia) on spontaneous respiration of the patient or intubation without relaxants (after only propofol administration) is suggested.[138]

Patient Positioning for Induction

It is essential that optimal patient positioning for laryngoscopy is ensured prior to induction of anesthesia. This includes the placement of towels under the patient's shoulders and head and putting the operating room table in reverse Trendelenburg to

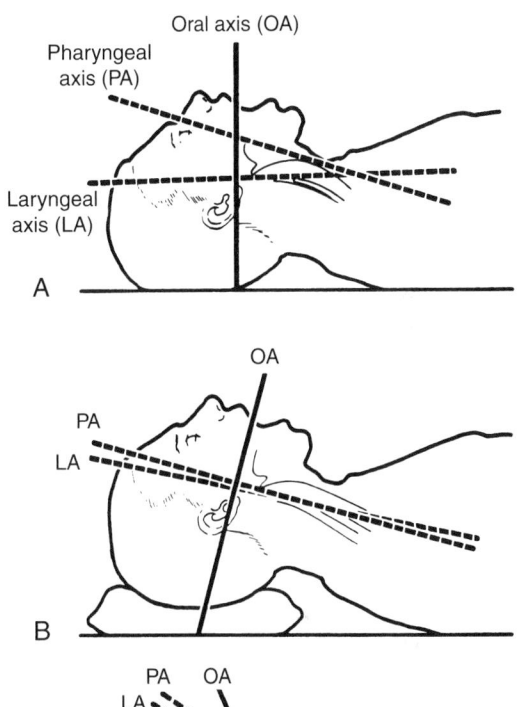

FIGURE **44-6** **A,** Supine position. **B,** Sniffing position.

increase the patient's FRC. The term *HELP* (Head Elevated Laryngoscopy Position) reminds clinicians of the importance of patient positioning for successful laryngoscopy.[139] This position generally improves the view during laryngoscopy and contributes to increasing the safety period until patients demonstrate signs of oxygen desaturation. This position is also a better patient position for using rescue ventilation techniques, such as bag-valve mask ventilation or insertion of an LMA, should they be required.

One study described positioning morbidly obese patients with the head, upper body, and shoulders significantly elevated above the chest, such that an imaginary horizontal line could connect the patient's sternal notch with the external auditory meatus. Positioning patients in this manner resulted in successful intubation in 99 of 100 morbidly obese patients, with all having a Cormack Grade I view.[140]

Others have also concluded that the "ramped" position (with blankets used to elevate both the upper body and head of the patient) improves laryngeal view in obese patients when compared with a conventional 7-cm cushion under the patient's head (sniffing position), which should result in fewer failed intubations[141] (Figure 44-6). Without proper support and alignment of the oropharynx and trachea (Figure 44-7), ventilation may be obstructed, and visualization of the laryngeal structures may be obscured.

The importance of proper positioning and the difficulty of repositioning morbidly obese patients during failed intubation can be underestimated by practitioners who are not experienced in airway management in obese patients. If direct laryngoscopy is unsuccessful, LMAs can be effective for establishing ventilation and should be immediately available.[117,130] In one study, the use of an intubating laryngeal mask resulted in better patient oxygenation compared with intubation through direct laryngoscopy in morbidly obese patients.[121]

During a rapid-sequence induction, cricoid pressure is applied while the patient's trachea is intubated. Landsman examined the topic of cricoid pressure and provided comprehensive review, describing the advantages and risks associated with the technique.[142]

In theory, when pressure is applied to the cricoid cartilage, it causes an occlusion in the esophagus between the cricoid cartilage and the vertebral body. However, it has been demonstrated that the application of cricoid pressure results in a reduction in lower esophageal sphincter pressure in anesthetized patients, but gastric pressure is reportedly less than the esophageal pressure, and the barrier to reflux remains intact.[143]

Researchers have determined that during rapid-sequence induction, gastric pressure is about 14 mm Hg or less and that gastric barrier pressure is less than 15 mm Hg. These researchers

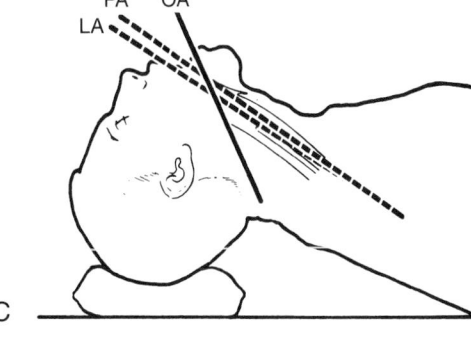

FIGURE **44-7** Schematic diagram demonstrating head position for endotracheal intubation. **A,** Successful direct laryngoscopy for exposure of the glottic opening requires alignment of the oral, pharyngeal, and laryngeal axes. **B,** Elevation of the head approximately 10 cm, with pads under the occiput and shoulders remaining on the table, aligns the laryngeal and pharyngeal axes. **C,** Subsequent head extension at the atlantooccipital joint serves to create the shortest distance and most nearly straight line from the incisor teeth to the glottic opening. *(From Gal TJ. Airway management. In: Miller RD, ed. Anesthesia. 6th ed. New York: Churchill Livingstone; 2005:1622.)*

concluded that the amount of cricoid pressure that is adequate to protect most anesthetized patients from regurgitation is 20 Newtons (N), increasing the force to 30 N as loss of consciousness occurs.[144]

The theory, however, has been challenged. In a recent study of awake patients using magnetic resonance imaging (MRI), it was demonstrated that when applying cricoid pressure, the esophagus may actually be displaced laterally. The lateral laryngeal displacement was noted in 67% of the subjects with cricoid pressure, and airway compression of at least 1 mm was demonstrated in 81% of the subjects as a result of cricoid pressure.[145]

ANESTHETIC MANAGEMENT: MAINTENANCE

Intubation

For airway management to be facilitated, the obese patient should be positioned with the head elevated (reverse Trendelenburg position) on the operating room table. This position promotes patient comfort, reduces gastric reflux, provides easier mask ventilation, improves respiratory mechanics, and helps maintain FRC. The reduced FRC in obese patients contributes to the rapid desaturation that occurs with induction of general anesthesia.[146] To attenuate the desaturation and maximize O_2 content in the lungs, patients are preoxygenated with 100% mask O_2 for at least 3 to 5 minutes.[147] Adequate preoxygenation is vital in obese patients because of rapid desaturation after loss of consciousness secondary to increased oxygen consumption and decreased FRC. Application of positive-pressure ventilation during preoxygenation decreases atelectasis and improves oxygenation in morbidly obese patients. A recent study[148] in morbidly obese individuals (limited to 160 kg by the weight limit of the computed tomography scanner) has demonstrated that the administration of continuous positive airway pressure (CPAP) during the preoxygenation period and gentle ventilation with positive end-expiratory pressure (PEEP) during anesthetic induction significantly reduce atelectasis, as documented by chest CT scans. An associated benefit to the reduced atelectasis was a significantly increased average PaO_2 (457 ± 130 pascals [Pa] versus 315 ± 100 Pa, P = 0.035) in those subjects who received CPAP-PEEP versus the control subjects. Theoretically, the increase in PaO_2 would increase the apneic time to oxygen desaturation if an airway event were to occur.[149]

Some practitioners advocate the use of an "awake look" to visualize the difficulty of the airway.[110-112,117,118] Careful administration of sedative drugs and application of topical anesthesia to the oropharyngeal structures, possibly including transtracheal and superior laryngeal nerve blocks, are performed. Nasal O_2 is used as a supplement during awake laryngoscopy. If the epiglottic and laryngeal architecture is easily visualized, successful asleep intubation can be done. If the airway structures cannot be visualized, an intubating LMA or awake fiberoptic intubation should be used.[117,150,151] The endotracheal tube must be safely secured to prevent movement during positioning and surgery.[80]

The surgeon and another skilled anesthesia provider must also be in attendance during the induction. Muscle hypotonus in the floor of the mouth, followed by rapid occurrence of soft-tissue obstruction and hypoxia, requires one person to support the mask and airway while another person bag-ventilates the patient.[84] In the case of inability to ventilate or intubate, the American Society of Anesthesiologists' difficult airway algorithm should be followed (see Chapter 23). Intubation of the obese patient can be safely accomplished with careful assessment

and planning and use of airway techniques familiar to the anesthetist.

Effects of General Anesthesia on Respiration

General anesthesia depresses respiration in normal subjects, so any preexisting pulmonary dysfunction is exaggerated by anesthesia.[19] The type of surgery, positioning, and underlying disease pathology further compound the undesirable respiratory responses caused by obesity and anesthesia.[152-157] General anesthesia causes a 50% reduction in FRC in the obese anesthetized patient, as compared with a 20% reduction in anesthetized nonobese patients.[80] Airway collapsibility is likely due to the decreased lung volume associated with deeper anesthesia as the end-expiratory esophageal pressure is reduced with lighter planes of anesthesia.[158] FRC can be increased by ventilating with large tidal volumes (15 to 20 mL/kg), although this has been shown to improve arterial O_2 tension only minimally.[76,152] In contrast, the addition of PEEP achieves an improvement in both FRC and arterial O_2 tension but only at the expense of cardiac output and O_2 delivery.[154,155] Current ventilation recommendations include using tidal volumes of 10 to 12 mL/kg to avoid barotrauma.[76] During laparoscopic surgeries, the respiratory rate should be 12 to 14 breaths per minute.[75]

Prolonged (longer than 2 to 3 hours) and extensive procedures (those involving the abdomen, thorax, and spine) negatively influence respiratory function. Subdiaphragmatic packing, cephalad displacement of organs, and surgical retraction cause decreased alveolar ventilation, atelectasis, and pulmonary congestion.[152,153] Recumbent or Trendelenburg positioning further reduces diaphragmatic excursion, which is already impaired by the weight of the panniculus (which can be very large) (Figure 44-8). Trendelenburg positioning also causes elevated filling pressures, which then increase right ventricular preload. Subsequently, myocardial O_2 consumption, cardiac output, pulmonary artery occluding pressures, peak inspiratory pressures, and venous admixtures are increased above upright-sitting values.[154]

In a normal-weight person, cardiac output increases in response to supine posturing to maintain hemodynamic stability. By increasing left ventricular output, the centrally located circulating volume is propelled forward, thereby minimizing pulmonary congestion and hypoxia. In a severely obese patient, positive-pressure ventilation (which impedes venous return)

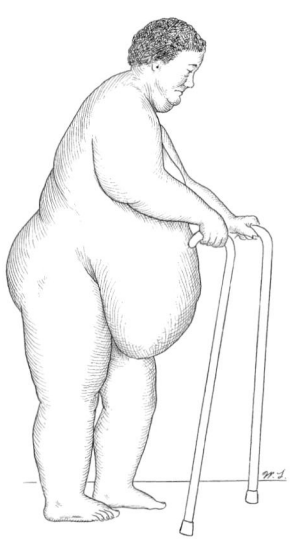

FIGURE **44-8** Panniculus in a standing patient.

and inability to increase cardiac output may result in cardiopulmonary decompensation.[155,156] This is exhibited intraoperatively by hypoxia, rales, ventricular ectopy, congestive heart failure, and hypotension.[157] Bag ventilation by hand may be useful to attenuate hypotension resulting from positive pressure.

Use of ventilators powerful enough to inflate the morbidly obese thorax is critical to minimizing hypoxia. Pressure- or volume-controlled ventilators can be used to maintain adequate oxygenation and normocapnia. Avoidance of prolonged prone, Trendelenburg, or supine positioning also decreases ventilation-perfusion mismatch. Optimization of oxygenation by using no less than 50% flow of inspired O_2 is emphatically recommended.[19,31,76] Intermittent manual "sighs" of large volume can also augment the FRC.

Application of PEEP can reduce venous admixture and support adequate arterial oxygenation. PEEP, however, can impair arterial oxygenation in some patients when it is superimposed on large tidal volumes.[156] For these reasons, PEEP that exceeds 15 cm H_2O is not recommended.

Other intraoperative events, such as hemorrhage or hypotension, further impair ventilatory homeostasis and result in hypoxemia that extends into the postoperative period.[30] A vertical abdominal incision, compared with a horizontal (transverse) incision, also prolongs postoperative hypoxia.[108] Pain causes further reductions in diaphragmatic excursion and vital capacity, leading to atelectasis and ventilation-perfusion mismatch.[19,76] For these reasons, 24-hour postoperative admission to a monitored bed is prudent for severely obese patients, who already exhibit higher morbidity and mortality apart from anesthesia and surgery.

Choice of Anesthetic Technique

Selection of the anesthetic technique is dependent on the patient, coexisting history, planned surgical procedure, anesthetist skill and preference, and patient preference. Diverse anesthetic techniques have been described for use with obese patients undergoing surgical and diagnostic procedures.[159-165] Anesthetic management of obese patients can include local or monitored anesthesia, general (narcotic, inhalation) anesthesia, regional blocks, or a combination of techniques.

No demonstrable difference in emergence from inhalation versus narcotic technique has been discerned in the obese patient.[19,85,98,103] The use of short-acting, water-soluble anesthetics facilitates smooth anesthetic induction, maintenance, and emergence from anesthesia.[85,98,103] Objectives for maintenance of anesthesia in the obese patient include strict maintenance of airway, adequate skeletal muscle relaxation, optimum oxygenation, avoidance of the residual effects of muscle relaxants, provision of appropriate intraoperative and postoperative tidal volume, and effective postoperative analgesia.[19,76] Depending on the patient's condition, these can be achieved by either general or regional anesthesia. An epidural anesthetic with concomitant "light" general anesthesia is frequently chosen. A light general anesthetic can facilitate management of the airway, ventilation, and the patient's level of consciousness, whereas the epidural provides surgical analgesia and anesthesia. The epidural catheter can be used for postoperative analgesic administration and will enhance earlier resumption of deep breathing and coughing maneuvers.

Volume Replacement

Despite the augmentation of circulatory fluid that accompanies morbid obesity, the estimated blood volume is actually diminished.[23] Fat, which contains only 8% to 10% water, contributes less fluid to total body water than equivalent amounts of muscle. The normal adult percentage of total body water is 60% to 65%.[19] In the severely obese, it is reduced to 40%. Therefore, calculation of estimated blood volume should be 45 to 55 mL/kg of actual body weight rather than the 70 mL/kg apportioned in nonobese adults.[18] Use of reduced parameters for volume replacement and avoidance of rapid rehydration lessen cardiopulmonary compromise. Fluid management is guided by blood pressure, heart rate, and urine output measurements. Volume expanders, such as hetastarch (Hespan), should not be administered at greater than recommended volumes per kilogram of IBW (20 mL/kg). Dilutional coagulopathy, factor VIII inhibition, and decreased platelet aggregation can result from excessive administration. Albumin 5% and 25% should be used as indicated to support circulatory volume and oncotic pressure. When blood loss is replaced with crystalloid, the 3:1 ratio (3 mL of crystalloid to 1 mL of blood loss) is applicable in severely obese patients. Blood products, after careful identification, should be replaced according to the patient's laboratory values and hemodynamic or surgical need. No difference in the criteria between the administration of blood products in normal-weight patients versus severely obese patients has been identified.

Intraoperative Positioning

Surgical positioning of morbidly obese patients necessitates extra precautions for the prevention of nerve, integumentary, and cardiorespiratory compromise. The type of surgery, combined with inordinate stretching or compression of nerve plexuses and prolonged immobility, cause local tissue ischemia and damage, which begins at the cellular level. Hypothermia, hypotension, table positioning, and the hydraulic pressure effect the adipose tissue places on orthopedic or cardiopulmonary structures potentiate impairment.[164]

Although many peripheral nerves are subjected to possible ischemia or necrosis, the ulnar, brachial plexus, radial, peroneal, and sphenoid nerves are the most vulnerable to injury in any anesthetized patient. In morbidly obese patients, the incidence may be increased because of excessive weight on the anatomic structures.[164] Care is necessary when one is positioning obese extremities in slings, draping them on Mayo stands, or securing them in lithotomy stirrups. Excess weight and loose skin may "strangle" or macerate tissues on the dangling ankle or wrist. Cavalier draping of heavy upper extremities atop poorly secured Mayo stands can cause cuts, bruises, or abrasions of the arm, breast, or abdomen, as well as obscure early signs of skin breakdown or circulatory compromise.

Prolonged hyperextension, external rotation, or abduction greater than 90 degrees overstretches the brachial plexus and can cause postoperative muscle pain, nerve palsies, or paralysis. Often obese patients do not have the range of motion that nonobese individuals possess. Therefore, less flexion or abduction and rotation of hips, legs, and arms may be necessary. Frequent palpation of pulses, generous padding, correct alignment, and repeated inspection of extremities for color and temperature can help diminish the incidence of positioning-related injuries.[165]

Lower back pain can be aggravated by both spinal and general anesthesia because of ligamentous relaxation that results in loss of lumbar curvature. Surgical towels placed under the lumbar spine before induction will enhance lordosis and reduce postoperative discomfort.[164]

Treatment of the panniculus is often a major concern for both anesthetist and surgeon. Extra-long straps and wide adhesive tape can secure the panniculus and reduce shifting when the operating table is changed. If Trendelenburg positioning is anticipated, some means to prevent its sliding cephalad must be devised. The head-down position, coupled with the crushing weight of the thorax and panniculus, compresses the brachial neurovascular bundle between the clavicle and first rib. If the patient requires a fracture table, ensure that sufficient padding encircles the pole adjacent to the patient's vulva or penis.[165] Genital and pudendal nerve injury can be profound if adipose tissue surrounding the thigh is not carefully distracted to reveal proper placement of the padding.

Integumentary Concerns

Decubitus ulcers, skin infection, and wound dehiscence are exceedingly common in the severely obese. Decubitus ulcers arise from prolonged immobility and compression of the fat on bony prominences and vessels. Traction, external fixation devices, and straps may cause certain types of injury. Creases of the skin are subject to erosion and ulceration from sweat and constant friction of opposing skin surfaces. Inability to perform hygiene under the breasts, between neck folds, or beneath the abdominal pannus accommodates organism proliferation. Concomitant diabetes, which interferes with leukocyte function, further accelerates the growth of bacterial or fungal infections.[2,3] As a result, wound dehiscence, particularly in the abdomen, can occur after suboptimal surgical closure in compromised skin. A poorly vascularized panniculus and torsion on the wound by the weight of the fat apron also contribute to malunion of the tissue.[165] Although atelectasis and hypoxia are less frequent with a horizontal laparotomy, a vertical laparotomy approach is often preferred by the surgical team. Compression of abdominal contents on superficial wound layers is lessened during ambulation and therefore may reduce the occurrence of dehiscence.[78]

Extubation

The risk of airway obstruction after extubation is increased in obese patients.[166] A decision to extubate depends on evaluation of the ease of mask ventilation and tracheal intubation, the length and type of surgery, and the presence of preexisting medical conditions, including OSA. Criteria for extubation include an awake state, tidal volume and respiratory rate at preoperative levels, ability to sustain head lift or leg lift for at least 5 seconds, strong and constant hand grip, effective cough, adequate vital capacity of at least 15 mL/kg, and inspiratory force of at least −25 to −30 cm H_2O. Patients must be placed with the head up or in a sitting position. If doubt exists regarding the ability of the patient to breathe adequately, the endotracheal tube is left in place and extubation over an airway exchange catheter or via a fiberoptic bronchoscope may be performed.[166,167]

Regional Anesthesia

Regional anesthesia can be used as the primary anesthetic in selected cases or as an accompaniment to postoperative pain and mobility management.[19,25,165] Difficulties are frequently encountered, though, in severely obese patients. Anatomic landmarks used to guide conduction blockade are not easily visualized or palpable. Brachial plexus anesthesia can be hampered by adipose tissue in the axillary region, inability to position the arm, and an undetectable pulse. Full-term pregnancy, obesity, and the coincident discomfort of active labor further inhibit the discernment of spinous processes and posterior iliac crests. Redundant rolls of fat, unsatisfactory ventilation, and inability of the patient to sustain optimal positioning make neuraxial anesthesia even more challenging.

For subarachnoid or epidural anesthesia, it is recommended that the patient sit upright so that landmarks such as C7 or L3 to L4 can be more easily identified.[79] In addition, skin-fat folds will fall toward the operating table, and respiratory ventilation will be enhanced. A selection of longer needles (7 inches) should also be available before anesthetic administration is begun. Generous infiltration with local anesthetic will provide greater patient comfort during insertion of the "finder," Tuohy, or spinal needle. The importance of generous administration of local anesthetic cannot be overemphasized because repeated insertions and repositioning of the needle or introducer may be required before access to the epidural (or subarachnoid) space is achieved.

Another consideration regarding subarachnoid or epidural anesthesia in severely obese pregnant or surgical patients is the lack of predictability of spread of local anesthetic.[166] Obese patients will also experience greater respiratory embarrassment from a high regional block than normal-weight patients will.[168] Successful laparotomy procedures have been described after epidural anesthesia.[169]

In obese parturients, a cesarean section can be performed under spinal or epidural anesthesia. Performing epidural analgesia in morbidly obese patients requires an experienced anesthetist and proper equipment (extra-large needle: 16G, 11 cm long). A significant correlation exists with increased body mass and rostral spread of epidural subarachnoid anesthetics when a patient is positioned supine.[166] Undesirable cephalad spread of local anesthetics can be obviated by reducing the volume and increasing the patient's upright sitting time.

ANESTHETIC MANAGEMENT: POSTOPERATIVE CARE

Pain Management

Optimal postoperative pain management is facilitated by the use of oral analgesics, NSAIDs, narcotics, patient-controlled analgesia, local infiltration of the surgical site, and epidural anesthesia. Obese patients are more sensitive to the respiratory-depressant effects of opioid analgesics; therefore, caution and close monitoring are warranted. Supplemental O_2 and pulse oximetry monitoring are mandated.[29] If the patient was on CPAP (nasal or face mask) preoperatively, CPAP should be applied at all rest times in the early post–general anesthetic period. The CPAP protects the patient with OSA against airway obstruction during sleep by pneumatically splinting the oropharynx.[43] Postoperative opioids must be used judiciously.

Postoperative Complications

Morbidity and mortality rates are higher in obese patients than in normal-weight patients. Various studies have reported that the mortality rate during the perioperative period has decreased among morbidly obese patients.[170] Older age, a high BMI, and male gender have been confirmed as proven surgical risk factors for obese patients undergoing gastric bypass surgery.[171,172] Other factors that have been shown to increase mortality risk include hypertension, postoperative leak, and thromboembolism.[173] Those with major comorbid diseases had a higher BMI, a higher mortality, a greater leak rate, and a higher rate of surgical site infections.[174] Ventilation abnormalities are exacerbated in obese patients with OSA and OHS and may last for several days. The maximum decrease in partial pressure of arterial oxygen occurs 2 to 3 days postoperatively.[29] In one study, morbidly obese subjects had a mean maximal oxygen uptake that was similar to patients with severe heart failure (mean ejection fraction 21.5 ± 8%).[175] The same investigators studied cardiorespiratory fitness in 109 patients prior to laparoscopic gastric bypass.

They found that severe complications and mortality were more common in patients whose maximum oxygen uptake was less than 15.8 mL/kg/min than in those whose maximum oxygen uptake was more than 15.8 mL/kg/min (P = 0.02).[176] This may be a promising way to identify high-risk patients and perhaps monitor their preoperative progress. Blouw and co-workers tried to identify factors influencing the frequency of respiratory failure in patients with morbid obesity. They found that a higher rate of respiratory failure is associated with BMI greater than 43 kg/m^2.[177]

Rhabdomyolysis is a complication in about 1.4% of bariatric surgeries, owing to high pressures exerted on deep tissues. Serum CPK measured pre- and postoperatively aids in early diagnosis and treatment, which helps reduce further complications such as myoglobinuric acute renal failure that can be as high as 30% with serum CPK greater than 5000 units/L.[178] A recent report[179] describes rhabdomyolysis of the gluteal muscles leading to renal failure in several morbidly obese patients who were supine for 5-hour gastric bypass operations. Another case report[180] describes rhabdomyolysis leading to renal failure and death after bariatric surgery.

The risk of thromboembolism, wound infections, and atelectasis is amplified in patients with increased BMI.[29,167] Thromboembolism is facilitated by immobility (venous stasis), increased blood viscosity (polycythemia, hypovolemia), increased abdominal pressure, and abnormalities in serum procoagulants and anticoagulants.[6] Obesity is an independent risk factor for development of venous thromboembolism (VTE).[181] Thromboembolism is reported to be the most common cause of postoperative mortality after bariatric surgery, accounting for as many as 50% of all deaths.[182]

Four important risk factors, namely venous stasis disease, BMI $\geq$60, truncal obesity, and obesity hypoventilation syndrome (OHS)/SAS are significant in the development of postoperative venous thromboembolism, and if present, preoperative prophylactic placement of an inferior vena cava (IVC) filter should be considered. Venous stasis disease, BMI greater than 60, truncal obesity, OHS, OSA, a previous incidence of pulmonary embolism, and hypercoagulable states have been suggested as factors that increase the baseline risk of perioperative pulmonary embolism in obese patients after bariatric surgery.[183] Administration of minidose heparin (5000 units administered subcutaneously twice per day), low-molecular-weight heparin, antiembolic stockings, and correctly fitting pneumatic compression boots can lessen the occurrence of deep vein thrombosis in the early postoperative period. Early ambulation and maintenance of vascular volume further attenuate the likelihood that clots will develop. Wound infections and pulmonary embolism are 50% higher in obese patients than in normal-weight patients.

In one multicenter retrospective examination of bariatric surgical patients in whom enoxaparin was given for VTE prophylaxis, it was reported that enoxaparin administered at a dose of 30 mg and begun preoperatively or given 40 mg every 12 or 24 hours postoperatively resulted in no reported deep venous thrombosis and a low occurrence of pulmonary embolisms (0% to 2%). Severe bleeding, largely gastrointestinal in origin, occurred in only 0.9% of the entire study population.[184] In another study, enoxaparin dosed 1.5 mg/kg once or 1 mg/kg twice daily in obese patients did not result in supratherapeutic anti-Xa activity, thus supporting the safety of the higher dosing regimens.[185]

Post–Gastric Bypass Anastomotic Leaks

In a recent series of more than 3000 gastric bypass patients from four centers, the anastomotic leak rate was 2.1%.[186] The most common signs and symptoms of a leak were tachycardia (72%), fever (63%), and abdominal pain (54%). An upper gastrointestinal series was positive in 17 of 56 patients. Tachycardia is the most sensitive sign of an anastomotic leak, and a heart rate greater than 120 beats per minute should prompt an investigation, even if the patient looks and feels well. Tachypnea or decreasing oxygen saturations can also signal early sepsis from a leak and may be clinically indistinguishable from pulmonary embolism.

In general, morbidly obese patients have higher rates of postoperative and intensive care unit (ICU) complications and may require more intensive care and increased staffing requirements.[187] Investigations in surgical/trauma ICU patients universally report an adverse effect of obesity on outcomes. In a surgical ICU, investigators reported that morbid obesity conferred elevated odds of death after 4 days of ICU stay,[188] and among blunt-trauma patients, obese patients suffered more frequent complications (multiple-system organ failure, acute respiratory distress syndrome, myocardial infarction, and renal failure), including the need for more vasopressors, additional days of ventilator support, and more often failed extubation. Among survivors, obese patients had a higher ICU and hospital length of stay.[189]

SUMMARY

Obesity is a complex and multifactorial disease, and its incidence is continuing to increase in the U.S. patient population. Through an understanding of the implications of associated conditions in obesity, the anesthetist can promote more favorable anesthetic outcomes. Consideration of the physiologic and pharmacologic changes and their implications for optimal anesthetic management guides clinical practice.[190]

REFERENCES

1. National Institutes of Health. *Clinical Guidelines on the Identification, Evaluation, and Treatment of Overweight and Obesity in Adults: the Evidence Report* (Publication No. 98-4083). Washington, DC: National Institutes of Health; 1998.
2. Klein S, Romijn J. Obesity. In: Kronenberg HM et al, eds *Williams Textbook of Endocrinology.* 11th ed. Philadelphia: Saunders; 2008:1563-1588.
3. Flier JS, Maratos-Flier E. Biology of obesity. In: Fauci AS et al, eds. *Harrison's Principles of Internal Medicine.* 17th ed. New York: McGraw-Hill; 2008:462-468.
4. *American Obesity Association Fact Sheet.* Available at: http://www.obesity.org/subs/fastfacts/obesity_US.shtml. Accessed August 29, 2008.
5. Flegal KM et al. Prevalence and trends in obesity among US adults, 1999-2000. JAMA. 2002;288:1723-1727.
6. Colditz GA. Epidemiology of obesity. In: Gumbiner B. *Obesity.* Philadelphia: American College of Physicians–American Society of Internal Medicine; 2001:1-22.
7. Ogden CL et al. Prevalence of overweight and obesity in the United States. 1999-2004. JAMA. 2006;295:1549-1555.
8. CDC/NHANES. *Overweight and Obesity: Obesity Trends: U.S. Obesity Trends 1985-2005.* Available at: http://www.cdc.gov/nccdphp/dnpa/obesity/trend/maps/index.htm. Accessed April 7, 2008.
9. International Union of Nutritional Sciences, The Global Challenge of Obesity and International Obesity Task Force. *Projected Prevalence of Obesity in Adults by 2025.* Available at: http://www.iuns.org/features/obesity/obesity.htm. Accessed April 7, 2008.
10. Wyatt HR. The prevalence of obesity. *Prim Care Clin Office Pract.* 2003;(30): 267-279.
11. World Health Organization. Obesity: preventing and managing the global epidemic: report of a WHO consultation. *World Health Organ Tech Rep Ser.* 2000;894:1-253.
12. Flegal KM et al. Excess deaths associated with underweight, overweight, and obesity. JAMA. 2005;293(15):1861-1867.

13. National Institutes of Health; National Heart, Lung, and Blood Institute. *Clinical Guidelines on the Identification, Evaluation, and Treatment of Overweight and Obesity in Adults—The Evidence Report.* September 1998. Available at: www.nhlbi.nih.gov/guidelines/obesity/ob_gdlns.htm. Accessed August 29, 2008.

14. Devlin MJ et al. Obesity: what mental health professionals need to know. *Am J Psychiatry.* 2000;157:854-866.

15. Roizen MF. Anesthetic implications of concurrent diseases. In: Miller RD, ed. *Anesthesia.* 6th ed. New York: Churchill Livingstone; 2005:1017-1149.

16. Brodsky JB, Lemmens HJM. Is the superobese patient different? *Obes Surg.* 2004;14:1428.

17. Benotti PN et al. Obesity disease burden and surgical risk. *Surg Obese Relat Dis.* 2006;2:600-606.

18. Jensen M. Obesity. In: Goldman L, Ausiello D, eds. *Cecil Textbook of Medicine.* 23rd ed. Philadelphia: Saunders; 2008:1643-1654.

19. Adams JP, Murphy PG. Obesity in anaesthesia and intensive care. *Br J Anaesth.* 2000;85:91-108.

20. Woods SC et al. Signals that regulate food intake and energy homeostasis. *Science.* 1998;280:1378-1386.

21. Comuzzie AG, Allison DB. The search for human obesity genes. *Science.* 1998;280:1374-1377.

22. Cottam DR et al. The chronic inflammatory hypothesis for the morbidity associated with morbid obesity: implications and effects of weight loss. *Obes Surg.* 2004;14:589-600.

23. Kuchta KF. Pathophysiologic changes of obesity. *Anesthesiol Clin North America.* 2005;23:421-429.

24. Lean JM. Obesity and cardiovascular disease: the wasted years. *Br J Cardiol.* 1999;6:269-273.

25. Rosenbaum M et al. Obesity. *N Engl J Med.* 1997;337:396-407.

26. Brown CD et al. Body mass index and the prevalence of hypertension and dyslipidemia. *Obes Res.* 2000;8:605-619.

27. Pi-Sunyer X. Body mass index as a risk factor for incident hypertension. *Nat Clin Pract Endocrinol Metab.* 2007;3(11):742-743.

28. Kannel W et al. The relationship of adiposity to blood pressure and development of hypertension. The Framingham Study. *Ann Intern Med.* 1967;67:48-59.

29. Stoelting RK, Dierdorf SF. *Anesthesia and Co-existing Diseases.* 4th ed. New York: Churchill Livingstone; 2002:441-451.

30. Wilson WC, Benumof JL. Respiratory physiology and respiratory function during anesthesia. In: Miller RD, ed. *Anesthesia.* 6th ed. New York: Churchill Livingstone; 2005:679-722.

31. Biring MS et al. Pulmonary physiologic changes of morbid obesity. *Am J Med Sci.* 1999;318:293-297.

32. Santana AN et al. The effect of massive weight loss on pulmonary function of morbid obese patients. *Respir Med.* 2006;100:1100-1104.

33. Jubber AS. Respiratory complications of obesity. *Int J Clin Pract.* 2004;58(6):573-580.

34. Parameswaran K et al. Altered respiratory physiology in obesity. *Can Respir J.* 2006;13:203-210.

35. Frey WC, Pilcher J. Obstructive sleep-related breathing disorders in patients evaluated for Bariatric surgery. *Obes Surg.* 2003;13:676-683.

36. O'Keefe T, Patterson EJ. Evidence supporting routine polysomnography before bariatric surgery. *Obes Surg.* 2004;14:23-26.

37. Hallowell PT et al. Potentially life-threatening sleep apnea is unrecognized without aggressive evaluation. *Am J Surg.* 2007;193:364-367.

38. Benumof JL. Obstructive sleep apnea in the adult obese patient: implications for airway management. *J Clin Anesth.* 2001;13:144.

39. Murphy G, Vender J. *Abstracts on Patient Safety Presented at the 2004 American Society of Anesthesiologists Annual Meeting.* Available at: http://www.apsf.org/resource_center/newsletter/2004/winter/04abstracts.htm. Accessed August 29, 2008.

40. Krimsky WR, Leiter JC. Physiology of breathing and respiratory control during sleep. *Semin Resp Crit Care Med.* 2005;26(1):5-12.

41. Willard RM, Dreher MH. Wake-up call for sleep apnea. *Nursing.* 2005;35(3):49.

42. Benumof JL. Obesity, sleep apnea, the airway, and anesthesia. *Curr Opin Anesthesiol.* 2004;17(1):21-30.

43. Moos, DD et al. Are patients with obstructive sleep apnea syndrome appropriate candidates for the ambulatory surgical center? *AANA J.* 2005;73(3):197-204.

44. Nguyen A et al. Laryngeal and velopharyngeal sensory impairment in obstructive sleep apnea. *Sleep.* 2005;28(5):585-593.

45. Den Herder C et al. Hyoidthyroidpexia: a surgical treatment for sleep apnea syndrome. *Laryngoscope.* 2005;115(4):740-745.

46. Pashayn AG et al. Pathophysiology of obstructive sleep apnea. *Anesthesiol Clin North America.* 2005;23:431-443.

47. Macey, PM et al. Aberrant neural responses to cold pressor challenges in congenital central hypoventilation syndrome. *Pediatr Res.* 2005;57(4):500-509.

48. Marcus, CL et al. Upper airway dynamic responses in children with obstructive sleep apnea syndrome. *Pediatr Res.* 2005;57(1):99-107.

49. Roche F et al. Relationship among the severity of sleep apnea syndrome, cardiac arrhythmias, and autonomic imbalance. *Pacing Clin Electrophysiol.* 2003;26:669-677.

50. Garrigue S et al. Benefit of atrial pacing in sleep apnea syndrome. *N Engl J Med.* 2002;346:404-412.

51. Phillips C et al. Diurnal and obstructive sleep apnea influences on arterial stiffness and central blood pressure in men. *Sleep.* 2005;28(5):604-609.

52. Meoli AL et al. Upper airway management of the adult patient with obstructive sleep apnea in the perioperative period—avoiding complications. *Sleep.* 2003;26(8):1060-1065.

53. Paje DT, Kremer MJ. The perioperative implications of obstructive sleep apnea. *Orthop Nurs.* 2006;25(5):291-297.

54. Matteoni C et al. Nonalcoholic fatty liver disease: a spectrum of clinical pathological severity. *Gastroenterology.* 1999;116:1413-1419.

55. Aria HE. Pitfalls in the diagnosis of gall bladder disease in clinically severe obesity. *Obes Surg.* 1998;8:444-451.

56. Nelson et al. Diet, activity and overweight among preschool age children enrolled in the special supplement nutrition program for women, infants and children (WIC). *Prev Chronic Dis.* 2006;3(2):1-12.

57. Fowler-Brown A. Prevention and treatment of overweight in children and adolescents. *Am Fam Physician.* 2004;69(11):2591-2598.

58. National Center for Health Statistics. *2004 Fact Sheet: Obesity Still a Major Problem. Prevalence of Overweight Among Children and Adolescents: United States, 2003-2004.* Available at: http://www.cdc.gov/nchs/pressroom/o4facts/obesity.htm. Accessed August 29, 2008.

59. Satcher D. *The Surgeon General's Call to Action to Prevent and Decrease Overweight and Obesity* Available at: http://www.surgeongeneral.gov/topics/obesity/calltoaction/facts_adolescents. Accessed August 29, 2008.

60. Demarco, Gail. (2003 June 10). *Childhood obesity. Statement of New York State Nurses Association.* Available at: http://www.nysna.org/advocacy/testimonies/child_obesity.htm. Accessed August 29th, 2008.

61. Budd G, Freedman D. The relation of cardiovascular risk factors among children and adolescents. *J Cardiovasc Nurs.* 2006;21(6):437-441.

62. Harms S et al. Obesity increases the likelihood of total joint replacement surgery among younger adults. *Int Orthop.* 2007; 31(1):23-26. Epub 2006 May 11.

63. Galvez et al. Obesity in the 21st century. *Environ Health Perspect.* 2003;111(13):A684-A685.

64. Sorof et al. Overweight ethnicity and the prevalence of HTN in school aged children. *Pediatrics.* 2004;113:475-482.

65. Goran M et al. Obesity and risk of type 2 diabetes and cardiovascular disease in children and adolescents. *Clin Endocrinol Metab.* 2003;88(4):1417-1427.

66. Inge TH et al. Bariatric surgery for severely overweight adolescents: concerns and recommendations. *Pediatrics.* 2004;114(1):217-223.

67. Hesketh et al. Body mass index and parent report self esteem in elementary school children: evidence for causal relationship. *Int J Obes.* 2004;28(10):1233-1237.

68. Brenn MD, Randall B. Anesthesia for pediatric obesity. *Anesthesiol Clin North America.* 2005;23(4):745-764.

69. Grundy SM et al. Definition of metabolic syndrome. *Arterioscler Thromb Vasc Biol.* 2004;24:e13-18.

70. Narayan KM et al. Lifetime risk for diabetes mellitus in the United States. *JAMA.* 2003;290(14):1884-1890.

71. Catalano PM. Management of obesity in pregnancy. *Obstet Gynecol.* 2007;109(1):419-433.

72. Burstein E et al. Pregnancy outcome among obese women: a prospective study. *Am J Perinatol.* 2008;25(9):561-566. Epub 2008 Sept 3.

73. Weiss JL et al. Obesity, obstetric complications and cesarean delivery rate: a population-based screening study. *Am J Obstet Gynecol.* 2004;190:1091-1097.

74. Mokdad AH et al. Diabetes trends in the U.S. 1990-1998. *Diabetes Care.* 2000;23:1278-1283.

75. ACOG Committee. The overweight adolescent: prevention, treatment, and obstetric-gynecologic implications [editorial]. *Obstet Anesth Digest.* 2007;27(1):7.

76. Ogunnaike BO et al. Anesthetic considerations for bariatric surgery. *Anesth Analg.* 2002;95:1793-1805.

77. Provost DA, Jones DB. Minimally invasive surgery for the treatment of severe obesity. *Dallas Med J.* 1999;87:110-113.

78. Balsiger BM et al. Bariatric surgery: surgery for weight control in patients with morbid obesity. *Med Clin North Am.* 2000;84:477-489.

79. Scott DJ et al. Laparoscopic Roux-en-Y gastric bypass for morbid obesity. *Surg Rounds.* 2000;23:177-189.

80. Ezri T et al. The endotracheal tube moves more often in obese patients undergoing laparoscopy compared with open abdominal surgery. *Anesth Analg.* 2003;96:278-282.

81. Nguyen NT. Open vs. laparoscopic procedures in bariatric surgery. *J Gastrointest Surg.* 2004;8:393.

82. Lamvu G et al. Obesity: physiologic changes and challenges during laparoscopy. *Am J Obstet Gynecol.* 2004;191(2):669-674.

83. Nguyen NT et al. Comparison of pulmonary function and postoperative pain after laparoscopic versus open gastric bypass: a randomized trial. *Am J Surg.* 2001;192:469-477.

84. Hunter JD et al. Anesthetic management of the morbidly obese patient. *Hosp Med.* 1998;59:481-483.

85. Song D et al. Remifentanil infusion facilitates early recovery for obese outpatients undergoing laparoscopic cholecystectomy. *Anesth Analg.* 2000; 90:111-113.

86. Slepchenko G et al. Performance of target-controlled sufentanil infusion in obese patients. *Anesthesiology.* 2003;98:65-73.

87. Puhringer FK et al. Pharmacokinetics of rocuronium bromide in obese female patients. *Eur J Anaesthesiol.* 1999;16:507-510.

88. Salihoglu Z et al. Total intravenous anesthesia versus single breath technique and anesthesia maintenance with sevoflurane for bariatric operations. *Obes Surg.* 2001;11:496-501.

89. Shibutani K et al. Accuracy of pharmacokinetic models for predicting plasma fentanyl concentrations in lean and obese surgical patients: derivation of dosing weight ('pharmacokinetic mass'). *Anesthesiology.* 2004;101: 603-613.

90. Shibutani K, et al. Pharmacokinetic mass of fentanyl for postoperative analgesia in lean and obese patients. *Br J Anaesth.* 2005;95::377-383.

91. Ramsay MS et al. Hemodynamic and respiratory changes related to the use of dexmedetomidine in bariatric surgical patients. *Anesthesiology.* 2002;96:A165.

92. Hofer RE et al. Anesthesia for a patient with morbid obesity using dexmedetomidine without narcotics. *Can J Anesth.* 2005;52:176.

93. Ramsey MA et al. Tracheal resection in morbidly obese patient: the role of dexmedetomidine. *J Clin Anesth.* 2006;18(6):452-454.

94. Servin F et al. Propofol infusion for maintenance of anesthesia in morbidly obese patients receiving nitrous oxide. *Anesthesiology.* 1993;78:657-665.

95. Leykin Y et al. The pharmacodynamic effects of rocuronium when dosed according to real body weight or ideal body weight in morbidly obese patients. *Anesth Analg.* 2004;99(4):1086-1089.

96. Leykin Y et al. The effects of cisatracurium on morbidly obese women. *Anesth Analg.* 2004;99:1090.

97. Perry J et al. Rocuronium versus succinylcholine for rapid sequence induction intubation. *Cochrane Database Syst Rev.* 2003;1:CD002788.

98. Torri G et al. Randomized comparison of isoflurane and sevoflurane for laparoscopic gastric banding in morbidly obese patients. *J Clin Anesth.* 2001;13(8):565-570.

99. Sollazzi L et al. Volatile anesthesia in bariatric surgery. *Obes Surg.* 2001;11(5):623-626.

100. Strum EM et al. Emergence and recovery characteristics of desflurane versus sevoflurane in morbidly obese adult surgical patients: a prospective, randomized study. *Anesth Analg.* 2004;99(6):1848-1853.

101. Passannante AN, Rock P. Anesthetic management of patients with obesity and sleep apnea. *Anesthesiol Clin North America.* 2005;23:479-491.

102. Bedford RF, Ives HE. The renal safety of sevoflurane. *Anesth Analg.* 2000;90:505-508.

103. Juvin P et al. Postoperative recovery after desflurane, propofol, or isoflurane anesthesia among morbidly obese patients: a prospective, randomized study. *Anesth Analg.* 1999;91:714-719.

104. Kabon B et al. Obesity decreases perioperative tissue oxygenation. *Anesthesiology.* 2004;100:274.

105. Ramaswamy A et al. Extensive preoperative testing is not necessary in morbidly obese patients undergoing gastric bypass. *J Gastrointest Surg.* 2004;8(2):159-164.

106. Elliot C, Kiely DG: Pulmonary hypertension: diagnosis and treatment. *Clin Med.* 2004;4:211.

107. Chung F et al. Pre-existing medical conditions as predictors of adverse events in day-case surgery. *Br J Anesth.* 1999;83:262-270.

108. Dominguez-Cherit G et al. Anesthesia for morbidly obese patients. *World J Surg.* 1998;22:1182.

109. Cartagena R. Preoperative evaluation of patients with obesity and obstructive sleep apnea. *Anesthesiol Clin North America.* 2005;23:464-478.

110. Brodsky JB et al. Morbid obesity and tracheal intubation. *Anesth Analg.* 2002;94:732-736.

111. Siyam MA, Benhamou D. Intubation in morbidly obese patients. *Anesth Analg.* 2002;94:732-736.

112. Ezri T et al. Prediction of difficult laryngoscopy in obese patients by ultrasound quantification of anterior neck soft tissue. *Anaesthesia.* 2003;58:1101-1118.

113. Juvin P et al. Difficult tracheal intubation is more common in obese than in lean patients. *Anesth Analg.* 2003;97:595-600.

114. Ezri T et al. Increased body mass index per se is not a predictor of difficult laryngoscopy. *Can J Anaesth.* 2003;50:179-183.

115. Siyam M, Benhamou D. Intubation in morbidly obese patients. *Anesth Analg.* 2003;96:913.

116. Ezri T et al. Prediction of difficult laryngoscopy in obese patients by ultrasound quantification of anterior neck soft tissue. *Anaesthesia.* 2003;58(11):1111-1114.

117. Frappier J et al. Airway management using the intubating laryngeal mask airway for the morbidly obese patient. *Anesth Analg.* 2003;96:1510-1515.

118. Brodsky JB et al. Anesthetic considerations for bariatric surgery: proper positioning is important for laryngoscopy. *Anesth Analg.* 2002;95:1793-1805.

119. Jefferson P, Ball DR. Central venous access in morbidly obese patients. *Anesth Analg.* 2001;93:1363.

120. Erert TJ et al. Perioperative considerations for patients with morbid obesity. *Anesthesiol Clin North America.* 2006;24(3):621-636.

121. Dhonneur G et al. Tracheal intubation of morbidle obese patients: LMA CTrach vs direct laryngoscopy. *Br J Anaesth.* 2006;97(5):742-745.

122. Pierin AM et al. Blood pressure measurement in obese patients: comparison between upper arm and forearm measurements. *Blood Press Monit.* 2004;9:101.

123. Mendelson CL. Aspiration of stomach contents into lungs during obstetric anesthesia. *Am J Obstet Gynecol.* 1946;53:196-205.

124. Sellick BA. Cricoid pressure to control regurgitation of stomach contents during induction of anesthesia. *Lancet.* 1961;2:404-406.

125. Juvin P et al. Gastric residue is not more copious in obese patients. *Anesth Analg.* 2001;93:1621-1622.

126. Harter RL et al. A comparison of the volume and pH of gastric contents of obese and lean surgical patients. *Anesth Analg.* 1998;86:147-152.

127. Abeidi AM et al. Gastric volumes in obese patients presenting for day case surgery: no need for rapid sequence induction. *Anesthesiology.* 2005; 103:A632.

128. van den Berg et al. Gastric volume in diabetic patients presenting for day case surgery: no need for rapid sequence induction? *Anesthesiology.* 2005;103:A629.

129. Jackson SJ et al. Delayed gastric emptying in the obese: an assessment using the non-invasive (13)C-octanoic acid breath test. *Diabetes Obes Metab.* 2004;6(4):264-270.

130. Maltby JR et al. Drinking 300 ml of clear fluid two hours before surgery has no effect on gastric fluid volume and pH in fasting and non-fasting obese patients. *Can J Anesth.* 2004;51:111.

131. Murray L et al. Relationship between body mass and gastro-oesophageal reflux symptoms. The Bristol Helicobacter Project. *Int J Epidemiol.* 2003;32(4):645-650.

132. Nilsson M et al. Obesity and estrogen as risk factors for gastroesophageal reflux symptoms. *JAMA.* 2003;290(1):66-72.

133. van den Berg A et al. Gastric volumes in patients with gastro-esophageal reflux disease: Is rapid sequence indicated? *Anesthesiology.* 2005;103:A628.

134. Ezert TJ et al. Perioperative anesthesia considerations for the morbidly obese. *Bariatric Times.* May 2006;14-17.

135. Fried EB. The rapid sequence induction revisited: obesity and sleep apnea syndrome. *Anesthesiol Clin North America.* 2005;23:551-564.

136. Suter M et al. Gastro-esophageal reflux and esophageal motility disorders in morbidly obese patients. *Obes Surg.* 2004;14(7):959-966.

137. Kalinowski CP, Kirsch JR. Strategies for prophylaxis and treatment for aspiration. *Best Pract Res Clin Anaesthesiol.* 2004;18(4):719-737.

138. Gaszynski T et al. General anesthesia with remifentanil and cisatracurium for superobese patient. *Eur J Anaesthesiol.* 2003;20:77-78.

139. Levitan RM et al. Head elevated laryngoscopy position: improving laryngeal exposure during laryngoscopy by increasing head elevation. *Ann Emerg Med.* 2003;41:322-330.

140. Brodsky JB. Anesthetic considerations for bariatric surgery: proper positioning is important for laryngoscopy. *Anesth Analg.* 2003;96(6):1841-1842.

141. Collins JS et al. Laryngoscopy and morbid obesity: a comparison of the "sniff" and "ramped" positions. *Obes Surg.* 2004;14(9):1171-1175.

142. Landsman I. Cricoid pressure: indications and complications. *Paediatr Anaesth.* 2004;14:43-47.

143. Garrard A et al. The effect of mechanically induced cricoid force on lower oesophageal sphincter pressure in anesthetized patients. *Anaesthesia.* 2004;59:435-439.

144. Haslam N et al. Intragastric pressure and its relevance to protective cricoid force. *Anaesthesia.* 2003;58(10):1012-1015.

145. Smith KJ et al. Cricoid pressure displaces the esophagus: an observational study using magnetic resonance imaging. *Anesthesiology.* 2003;99:60-64.

146. Boyce JR et al. A preliminary study of the optimal anesthesia positioning for the morbidly obese patient. *Obes Surg.* 2003;13:4-9.

147. Cressey DM et al. Effectiveness of continuous positive airway pressure to enhance pre-oxygenation in morbidly obese women. *Anesthesia.* 2001;56:680-684.

148. Coussa M et al. Prevention of atelectasis formation during the induction of general anesthesia in morbidly obese patients. *Anesth Analg.* 2004;98:1491-1495.

149. Coussa M et al. Prevention of atelectasis formation during the induction of general anesthesia in morbidly obese patients. *Anesth Analg.* 2004;98:101.

150. Keller C et al. The laryngeal mask airway ProSeal as a temporary ventilatory device in grossly and morbidly obese patients before laryngoscope-guided tracheal intubation. *Anesth Analg.* 2002;94:737-740.

151. Natalini G et al. A comparison of the standard laryngeal mask airway and the ProSeal laryngeal mask airway in obese patients. *Br J Anesth.* 2003;90:323-326.

152. Sprung J et al. The impact of morbid obesity, pneumoperitoneum, and posture on respiratory system mechanics and oxygenation during laparoscopy. *Anesth Analg.* 2002;94:1345-1350.

153. Sprung J et al. The effects of tidal volume and respiratory rate on oxygenation and respiratory mechanics during laparoscopy in morbidly obese patients. *Anesth Analg.* 2003;97:268-274.

154. Perilli V et al. The effects of the reverse Trendelenburg position on respiratory mechanics and blood gases in morbidly obese patients during bariatric surgery. *Anesth Analg.* 2000;91:1520-1525.

155. Auler JO Jr et al. The effects of abdominal opening on respiratory mechanics during general anesthesia in normal and morbidly obese patients: a comparative study. *Anesth Analg.* 2002;94:741-748.

156. Pelosi P et al. Positive end-expiratory pressure improves respiratory function in obese but not in normal subjects during anesthesia and paralysis. *Anesthesiology.* 1999;91:1221-1231.

157. Tsueda K. Obesity supine death syndrome: report of two morbidly obese patients. *Anesth Analg.* 1979;58:345-347.

158. Jordan, AS et al. Recent advances in understanding the pathogenesis of obstructive sleep apnea. *Curr Opin Pulm Med.* 2003;9(6):459-464.

159. Coker LL. Continuous spinal anesthesia for cesarean section for a morbidly obese parturient patient: a case report. *AANA J.* 2002;70:189-192.

160. Kadar AG et al. Anesthesia for electroconvulsive therapy in obese patients. *Anesth Analg.* 2002;94:360-361.

161. Ranucci M et al. Obesity and coronary artery surgery. *J Cardiothorac Vasc Anesth.* 1999;13:280-284.

162. Michaloudis D et al. Continuous spinal anesthesia/analgesia for perioperative management of morbidly obese patients undergoing laparotomy for gastroplastic surgery. *Obes Surg.* 2000;10:220-229.

163. Lippmann M et al. An alternative anesthetic technique for the morbidly obese patient undergoing endovascular repair of an abdominal aortic aneurysm. *Anesth Analg.* 2003;97:981-983.

164. Warner MA. Patient positioning. In: Barash PG et al, eds. *Clinical Anesthesia.* 5th ed. Philadelphia: Lippincott; 2006:643-667.

165. Brodsky JB. Positioning the morbidly obese patient for anesthesia. *Obes Surg.* 2002;12:751-758.

166. Benumof JL. Airway exchange catheters: simple concept potentially great danger. *Anesthesiology.* 1999;91:342-344.

167. Eichenberger A et al. Morbid obesity and postoperative pulmonary atelectasis: an underestimated problem. *Anesth Analg.* 2002;95:1788-1792.

168. von Ungern-Sternberg BS et al. Impact of spinal anaesthesia and obesity on maternal respiratory function during elective Caesarean section. *Anaesthesia.* 2004;59(8):743-749.

169. Loo K et al. Epidural analgesia for a laparotomy in a morbidly obese patient with a history of difficult intubation. *Can J Anaesth.* 2003;50:312-313.

170. Dindo D et al. Obesity in general elective surgery. *Lancet.* 2003;361:2032-2035.

171. Livingston EH et al. Male gender is a predictor of morbidity and age a predictor of mortality in patients undergoing bypass surgery. *Ann Surg.* 2002;236:576-582.

172. Benotti PN. Perioperative outcomes and risk factors in gastric surgery for morbid obesity; a 9-year experience. *Surgery.* 2006;139:340-346.

173. Fernandez AZ et al. Multivariate analysis of risk factors for death following gastric bypass for treatment of morbid obesity. *Ann Surg.* 2004;239:698-703.

174. Jamal MK et al. Impact of major comorbidities on mortality after gastric bypass. *Surg Obes Relat Dis.* 2005;1:511-516.

175. Gallagher MJ et al. Comparative impact of morbid obesity vs. heart failure on cardiorespiratory fitness. *Chest.* 2005;127:2197-2203.

176. McCullough PA et al. Cardiorespiratory fitness and short-term complications after bariatric surgery. *Chest.* 2006;130:517-525.

177. Blouw EL et al. The frequency of respiratory failure in patients with morbid obesity undergoing gastric bypass. *AANA J.* 2003;71:45-50.

178. Mognol P et al. Rhabdomyolysis after laparoscopic bariatric surgery. *Obes Surg.* 2004;14:19.

179. Bostanjian D et al. Rhabdomyolysis of gluteal muscles leading to renal failure: a potentially fatal complication of surgery in the morbidly obese. *Obes Surg.* 2003;13(2):302-305.

180. Collier B et al. Postoperative rhabdomyolysis with bariatric surgery. *Obes Surg.* 2003;13(6):941-943.

181. Goldhaber SZ et al. A prospective study of risk factors for pulmonary embolism in women. *JAMA.* 1997;277:642-645.

182. Pieracci FM et al. Critical care of the bariatric patient. *Crit Care Med.* 2006;34:1796-1804.

183. Sapala JA et al. Fatal pulmonary embolism after bariatric operations for morbid obesity: a 24-year retrospective analysis. *Obes Surg.* 2003;13(6):819-825.

184. Hamad GG, Choban PS. Enoxaparin for thromboprophylaxis in morbidly obese patients undergoing bariatric surgery: findings of the prophylaxis against VTE outcomes in bariatric surgery patients receiving enoxaparin (PROBE) study. *Obes Surg.* 2005;15:1368-1374.

185. Bazinet A et al. Dosage of enoxaparin among obese and renal impairment patients. *Thromb Res.* 2005;116:41-50.

186. Gonzalez R et al. Diagnosis and contemporary management of anastomotic leaks after gastric bypass for obesity. *J Am Coll Surg.* 2007;204:47-55.

187. Rose MA et al. Nurse staffing requirements for care of morbidly obese patients in the acute care setting. *Bariatr Nurs Surg Patient Care.* 2006;1(2):115-121.

188. Nasraway SAJ et al. Morbid obesity is an independent determinant of death among surgical critically ill patients. *Crit Care Med.* 2006;34:964-970.

189. Brown CV et al. The impact of obesity on severely injured children and adolescents. *J Pediatr Surg.* 2006;41:88-91.

190. McAuliffe MS, Edge MJ. Perioperative and anesthesia considerations on obese patients. *Bariatr Nurs Surg Patient Care.* 2007;2(2):123-130.

CHAPTER 45

REGIONAL ANESTHESIA: Spinal and Epidural Anesthesia

R. Lee Olson, Joseph E. Pellegrini, Beth Ann Movinsky

Spinal and epidural blocks are known collectively as *central neuraxial blockade* (CNB) because they involve the placement of local anesthetic solution onto or adjacent to the spinal cord. Both spinal and epidural blocks share much of the same anatomy and physiology but are distinct from one another due to their unique anatomic, physiologic, and clinical features.

The person most credited with introducing spinal anesthesia is Augustus Bier, who in 1898 described the injection of cocaine into the spinal column and its potential for use as a surgical anesthetic technique. When cocaine was introduced into the subarachnoid space, anesthesia lasted approximately an hour. With the development of newer and safer anesthetic drugs, needles, and techniques, regional anesthesia expanded to include many neural blocks for the enhancement of surgery and obstetrics and the management of pain.[1,2] Modern procedures have simplified, refined, and increased the safety and success of regional anesthesia techniques.[2]

APPLIED ANATOMY AND PHYSIOLOGY OF THE CENTRAL NEURAXIS

Knowledge of anatomic landmarks and underlying structures aids the anesthetist in forming a three-dimensional "mind's-eye" picture. This picture, coordinated with the "feel" of the structures and tissues against the needle and a steady, sensitive hand, facilitates accurate placement of the needle tip and administration of appropriate techniques and medications. Although anatomy is the oldest of medical sciences (with detailed descriptions of the spinal column dating from the 19th century), modern imaging methods like computed tomography, magnetic resonance imagining, and endoscopic examination have permitted in vivo investigations that further our understanding of spinal anatomy. The following is therefore a current review of applied anatomy of the central neuraxis.

The sequential interconnectivity of the 33 bones called *vertebrae* form the spinal, or vertebral, column, which anesthetists use as a bony reference during the placement of various anesthetics or analgesics. This column is located in the posterior midline of the trunk and allows for truncal flexibility because movable joint surfaces and cartilaginous vertebral bodies exist between 24 of the 33 vertebrae (Figure 45-1). The vertebral column extends from the base of the skull and the foramen magnum to the tip of the coccyx. The vertebral bodies are stacked on top of one another, separated by fibrocartilaginous intervertebral disks that provide support for the cranium and trunk. In general, each vertebra can be visualized as having two parts. The anterior, cylindric portion of the vertebra is solid and called the *body*. This heavier portion of the vertebra forms the anterior portion of the vertebral arch. The body of each vertebra is contiguous with two pedicles that stretch in a posterior and slightly lateral direction, joining to two laminae that stretch posteriorly and

medially to complete an arch, creating an oval-triangular foramen. This foramen, known as the *vertebral foramen*, allows for the passage and protection of the spinal cord. Transverse processes on both sides of the pedicles allow for muscular attachments and the control of movement. A spinous process projects along the median plane from the union of the laminae in a posteroinferior direction. The spinous process is the long, slender, bony prominence that can often be seen and felt along the midline of the back. The spinous process also provides a place for muscular attachment and movement control. In addition, the inferior angle of the bone creates an overlap that further protects the spinal cord (Figure 45-2).[3]

The pedicles and processes of each vertebra have superior and inferior articular surfaces and lateral notches. The superior notch is shallow when compared with the deeper inferior notch. When the vertebrae are stacked, the notches and the articulating surfaces, known as *zygapophyseal* or *facet joints*, form the intervertebral foramina. The intervertebral foramina provide safe passage for spinal nerves passing from the spinal cord to the rest of the body. The articular surfaces of the facet joints are covered with hyaline cartilage, which permits a gliding motion between the vertebrae. Because the facet joints are innervated by branches from closely associated spinal nerves, these joints often become clinically important. When the joint is injured, the associated spinal nerves may also be affected, leading to pain along associated dermatomes or muscle spasm along associated myotomes.[3]

The size and shape of vertebral lamina and spinous processes differ among the thoracic, lumbar, and sacral regions, and variation exists within each region. Knowledge of these variations is important in the practice of regional anesthesia in selection and administration of spinal and epidural anesthesia. For instance, cervical and thoracic vertebrae have spinous processes that angle acutely in a caudad direction such that the process of the superior vertebra overlaps the inferior vertebra and its process. This construction adds protection to the spinal cord when an individual stands erect. When attempts are made to insert a needle into the cervical or thoracic regions, the tight construction and angles of the vertebral column must be considered.

In the lumbar region the vertebrae are larger, and the spinous processes become shorter and broader and have a posterior orientation with less overlap than in other vertebrae. Relatively large gaps, bridged by ligaments, exist between the spinous processes in the lumbar area. This provides the anesthesia practitioner easier access for needle placement, catheter passage, and the instillation of anesthetic into the epidural or subarachnoid space for surgical or obstetric procedures.

The sacrum is a triangle-shaped section of fused bodies of vertebrae. The broader portion is the base, which tapers as it approaches the coccyx. The sacrum is shaped so the weight of the body forces the base of the sacrum downward and forward. It is wedged tightly between the two iliac crests by the downward forces exerted on the spinal column. The lamina of the last sacral vertebra is incomplete and bridged only by ligaments. This area is known as the *sacral hiatus* (Figure 45-3). The coccyx is composed of four small segments of bone that become fused into two bones as an individual ages; between the ages of 25 and 30 years, fusion is complete. The bodies of the vertebrae can

be identified with the transverse processes and articular processes. No pedicles or spinous processes are present. The last, or fourth, bone is small and is similar to a nodule. The changing size of the bone from the first to the fourth vertebra gives the coccyx the appearance of a triangle. The projections of the rudimentary articular processes are known as the *cornua*, and the superior pair is the most pronounced. These sacral cornua are the "horns" or bony protuberances that guard the area of the sacral hiatus.[3] Because they can be easily palpated in children and in most adults, they are important surface anatomic landmarks for the performance of a caudal anesthetic procedure.

Of the more than 35 pairs of muscles and ligaments in the back, the supraspinous ligaments, the interspinous ligaments, and the ligamenta flava (yellow ligaments) are of special significance to the anesthesia practitioner. These three structures act as landmarks that help in identification of and access to the epidural and subarachnoid spaces. The supraspinous ligament is a strong

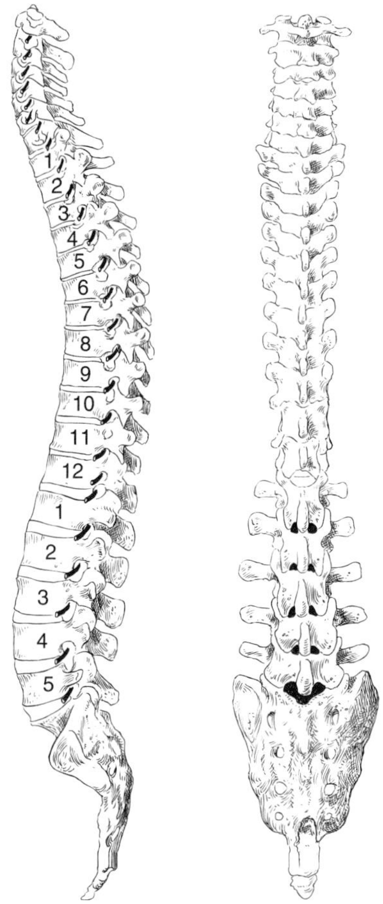

FIGURE **45-1**   The spinal, or vertebral, column with its 33 vertebrae.

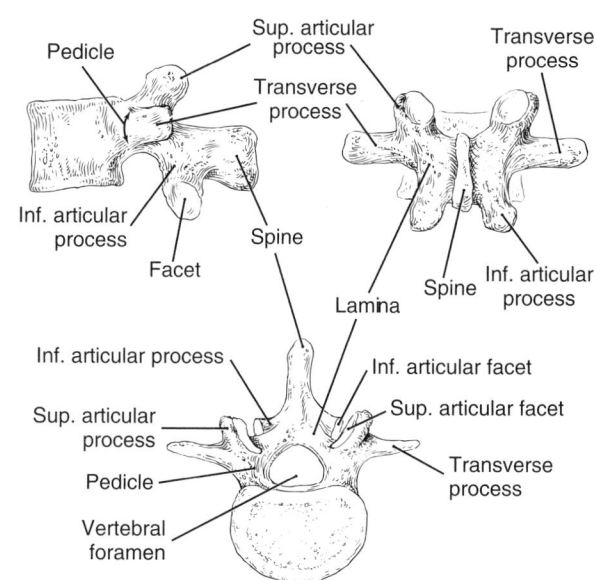

FIGURE **45-2**   Articular surfaces, transverse processes, and spinous process. *Inf*, Inferior; *Sup*, superior.

FIGURE **45-3**   Sacrum and coccyx.

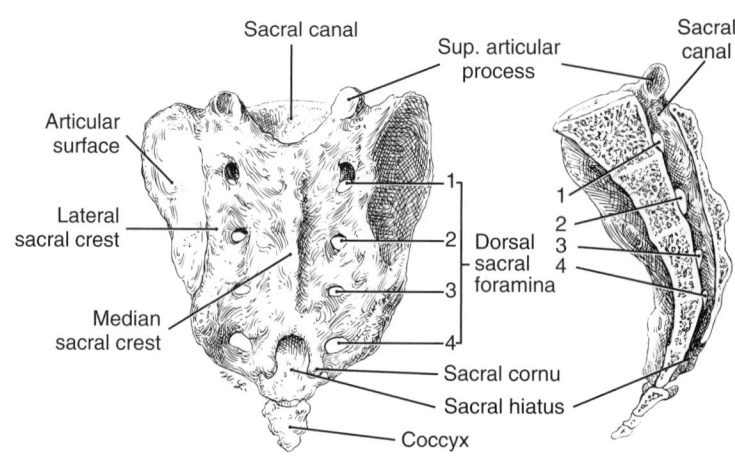

cordlike ligament that connects the apices of the spinous processes; it is thick and serves as the major ligament in the cervical and upper thoracic regions. The supraspinous ligament consists of three layers: the superficial layer extends over several vertebral spinous processes, the middle layer connects two or three spinous processes, and the inner layer connects only the neighboring spinous processes. The ligament blends at all levels with the thin interspinous ligaments that run between adjacent spinous processes. The interspinous ligaments are usually absent or of poor quality in the cervical region and can be exceptionally thin in the lumbar area, even in young people. The ligamenta flava are the strongest of the posterior ligaments. These broad elastic bands join the vertebral arches through vertical extensions from adjacent lamina. The ligamenta flava are paired flat ligaments that run caudad from the inferior border of one lamina to the upper border of the lower lamina on both sides of the midline. The two ligaments almost fill the space, leaving only a separation in the midline and thereby creating a V or wedge that points posteriorly to align with the interspinous and supraspinous ligaments. The V is thin on the lateral edge and thickest midline—in an adult approximately 3 to 5 mm at the L2-L3 interspace. The ligaments extend from each lamina with an overlapping of fibers that creates the appearance of a contiguous ligament from one vertebral body to the next. The ligament is thicker in the lumbar area than in the cervical area and is responsible for maintenance of upright posture. The ligaments' color comes from their high content of yellow elastic tissue.[4]

The spinal cord itself is a cylindrical structure extending from the medulla oblongata through the spinal foramen to the level of the L2 vertebra in most adults and ranges from 42 to 45 cm in length (Figure 45-4). Because the vertebral column grows more rapidly than the spinal cord, the spinal cord in children extends initially to the level of the third lumbar vertebra.

In approximately 1% of adults, the spinal cord may extend below L2 and rarely to the level of L3. The spinal cord tapers to the conus medullaris, and nerve pathways continue in a collection of rootlets called the *cauda equina* or *horse's tail*, which extends from L1 to S5. The spinal cord is enlarged in two regions. The first, called the *cervical enlargement*, extends from the spinal segments C4 to T1. The ventral rami of the spinal nerves in this enlargement form the brachial plexus of nerves that innervates the upper limbs. The second enlargement stretches from segments L2 to S3. This lumbosacral enlargement contributes corresponding nerves to create the lumbar and sacral plexuses. It is important to note that the spinal cord levels do not directly correspond with vertebral levels. For example, in adults the lumbosacral enlargement (L2 to S3) usually extends from the body of the T11 vertebra to the body of the L1 vertebra.[3]

The spinal cord is enveloped by the same three membranes that line the cranium, and they are collectively called the *meninges*. The meninges are nonnervous support tissues that provide a protective covering for the cord and nerve roots from the foramen magnum to the base of the cauda equina. The linings are identified as the *dura mater*, the *arachnoid mater*, and the *pia mater*. The dura mater is the outermost layer. It is a thick, tough membrane that provides most of the protection for the central cord structures. The nerve roots are covered with dura mater while inside the spinal canal. As the roots exit the canal via the intervertebral foramen, the dura blends into the root at a junction referred to as a *dural cuff* or *root sleeve*. The arachnoid mater is a thin, spiderweb-like covering that forms the middle layer. Beneath the arachnoid mater is a space that is continuous with the central canal of the cord and the ventricles. This space, which is filled with cerebrospinal fluid (CSF) is known as the *subarachnoid space*. This mater and the fluid protect the spinal cord from shock injuries and are the medium for the interaction with local anesthetics and opioids that occurs during the administration of regional anesthesia. The innermost layer, the pia mater, is thin and is in direct contact with the outer surface of the spinal cord (Figure 45-5).[3]

The epidural space is a potential space outside the dural sac but inside the vertebral canal and is continuous from the base of the cranium to the base of the sacrum at the sacrococcygeal membrane. The epidural space contains epidural veins, fat, lymphatics, segmental arteries, and nerve roots. Fat in the epidural

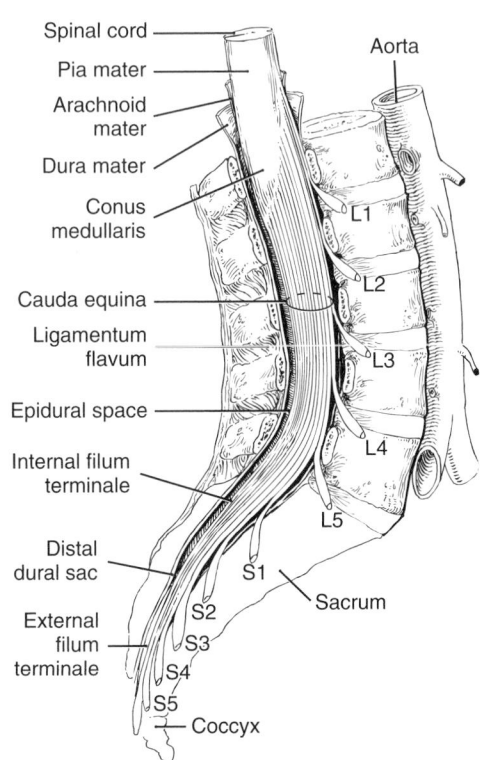

FIGURE **45-4** Extension of the spinal cord to the second lumbar vertebra.

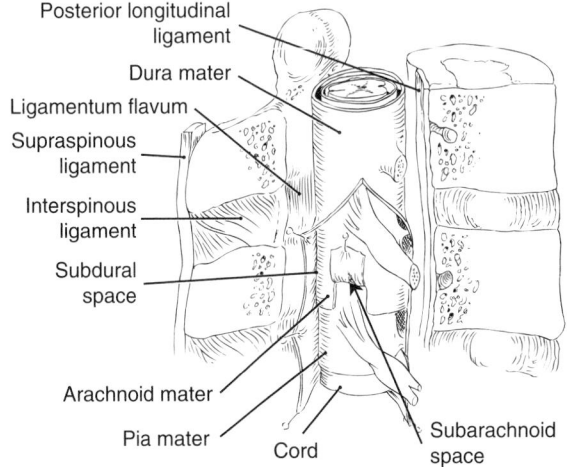

FIGURE **45-5** The linings of the spinal cord and the posterior ligaments of the spinal column.

spaces is physiologically fluid, acting as a pad and lubricant for the movement of neural structures within the canal. The posterior epidural space, as it is approached by the anesthetist's advancing needle, is protected by the ligamenta flava, the lamina, and the spinous processes. It is easy but inaccurate to depict the epidural space as a uniform column surrounding an equally uniform and tapering spinal cord. A better mental picture is provided by a "look" along the longitudinal axes. The epidural space can be envisioned as a series of lateral, posterior, and anterior compartments existing among the vertebral body, lamina, and pedicles. The compartments, occupied mostly by fat but also by nerves and fibrous tissue, repeat at each segment in a metameric fashion. Of greatest interest to the anesthetist, the posterior epidural space is a series of fat-filled tripodial pads, shaped like a three-sided sand dune. The pad stretches and narrows in a caudad direction as it approaches the next inferior lamina. In areas of the vertebral canal surrounded by bone, the dura actually contacts bone, leaving only a potential epidural space that physically separates the epidural fat-containing compartments. The posterior epidural space, therefore, is a discontinuous group of tapering fat pads that repeat throughout the length of the spinal canal and are separated by a potential space that allows the passage of fluids or small catheters.[4-7]

The distance from the skin to the epidural space and the depth of the epidural space, or the distance to the dura, is of interest to one wishing to avoid needle injury of neural and vascular tissues. The distance to the epidural space varies with vertebral level and is loosely correlated with patient weight. The distance from skin to the lumbar epidural space using a midline approach varies from 2.5 cm to 8 cm, with an average of 5 cm. Because the space itself is not uniform in shape, the depth of the epidural space from the ligamenta flava to the dura varies considerably. Given the tripodial, dunelike shape of the epidural space, expect the space to narrow considerably when approaching laterally to the midline and in more caudad areas in the space. The depth of the epidural space is also relative to the vertebral level of approach and angle of needle entry, but some clinical generalizations can be made. The epidural space is largest (posterior to anterior) in the midline of the midlumbar region, at 5 to 6 mm. The midline thoracic region epidural space may be 3 to 5 mm deep and is narrower there (lateral width). Caution must be exercised when one approaches the lower cervical region because the epidural space is very small (only 1.5 to 2 mm), leaving little room for error.[5]

In addition to a larger epidural space, another anatomic reason to stay midline with an approaching anesthetic needle is the presence of the epidural veins. The epidural veins are valveless veins that form a plexus draining the blood from the spinal cord and the linings of the cord. The plexus is most prominent in the lateral portion of the epidural space. In pregnant or obese patients, the epidural veins become engorged and swollen as increased intraabdominal pressure results in venous congestion of the lumbar and sacral vessels. The potential for injury or accidental cannulation of these vessels is increased because of this physiologic compensation.[3,4,6]

A final anatomic consideration for neuraxial anesthesia is the existence of normal and abnormal curvatures of the spinal column. A median-plane longitudinal view of the vertebral column reveals four curvatures in the normal adult. The thoracic and sacral curvatures have posterior curvatures (concave anteriorly), whereas the cervical and lumbar regions have anterior curvatures (concave posteriorly). In a supine patient, the apex of the lumbar curve is usually at L3 to L4, and the trough of the

thoracic curve is at T4.[8] *Scoliosis*, the most common abnormal curvature, is a lateral curvature of the spine, and *kyphosis* is an excessive posterior curvature or hump, usually of the thoracic region. Excessive *lordosis*, or hollowing of the back, may occur as a result of obesity as the body attempts to restore the center of gravity. A temporary lordosis may also occur during pregnancy. Changes in these anatomic curves will challenge the anesthesia practitioner during the performance of epidural or spinal anesthetic techniques. Clear knowledge of the curves is also important when anticipating the spread of local anesthetics in the subarachnoid space relative to the site of injection and the patient's position.[3]

Neuroanatomic Mapping and Evaluation of Neuraxial Anesthesia

The goal of neuraxial anesthesia is to block pain transmission from areas of injury, disease, or surgical intervention. Therefore, it is clinically useful to have knowledge of the innervations of body structures being operated on in relation to spinal nerve location within the vertebral column. Anatomic maps have been generated based on cutaneous sensation alone. These sensation maps are referred to as *dermatomal maps, charts,* or *levels.* A *dermatome* is defined as the area of cutaneous sensation supplied by a spinal nerve that is anatomically identified as it passes through an intervertebral foramen. For example, the umbilical area is directly anterior to the L3 vertebra but receives cutaneous innervations from T7 to T11, depending on the dermatomal map consulted (Figure 45-6).

For the practical clinician, use of accepted anatomic landmarks and test methods is perhaps the best method for documenting the functional level of blockade—the level of the loss of sensation achieved. The level of anesthetic can be evaluated in many ways, and tests can be used to evaluate several components of the neuraxial anesthetic. For motor function, a straight leg

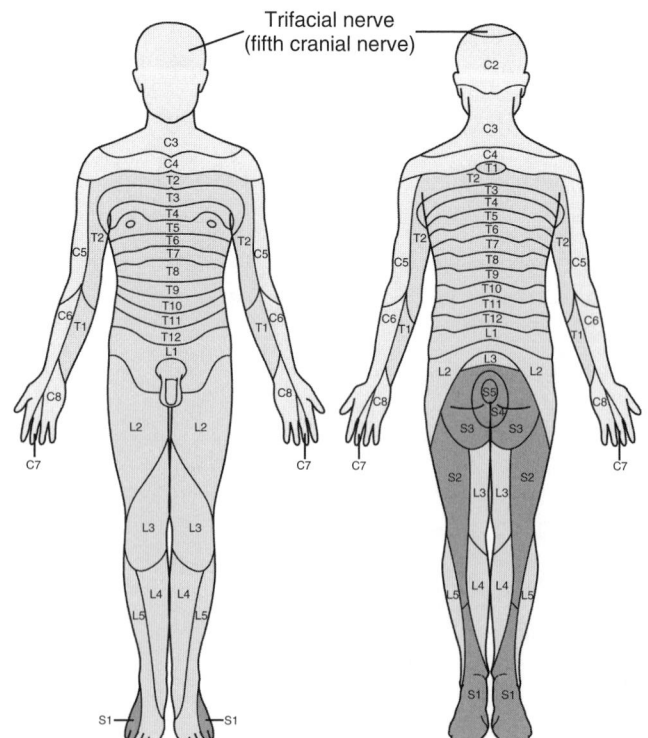

FIGURE **45-6**   Dermatomes.

raise or a request to "step on the gas" works well as a clinical measure. Cutaneous sensation can be evaluated through use of a Wartenberg pinwheel, a Semmes-Weinstein Monofilament Aesthesiometer or (more practically and simply) with the stylet from the spinal or epidural needle, a portion of a broken wooden tongue blade, or even a peripheral nerve stimulator. Such "pressure" or "scratch" tests are done using two surface-anatomy points for comparison. Inform the patient that the sensation on a normal area, such as the skin surface of the shoulder, is scratchy or sharp. Next, scratch or press an area expected to be numb, such as the lateral thigh. Gradually work cephalad in 2- or 3-inch bands until the patient notices a change in sensation. Note the level of the change in sensation relative to a dermatomal map. This approximates the upper level of sensory loss. Skin refrigerant, ice cubes, and alcohol pads can be used in a similar manner to identify changes in temperature sensation.

Physiology and Purported Mechanisms of Action

Despite more than 90 years of research and experience with spinal and epidural anesthesia, much speculation remains regarding the exact cellular locations and molecular mechanisms involved when local anesthetics, opioids, and other pharmacologically active agents bind to produce spinal analgesia and anesthesia.[9,10] For a thorough review of local anesthetics and details on mechanism of action please see Chapter 11. What is known and clinically important about spinal and epidural anesthesia is that the primary site of action for local anesthetics is on the nerve roots within the spinal cord. When a drug is injected directly into the CSF, the drug distributes through the subarachnoid space based on the physical and chemical properties of that injectant and the characteristics of the space in which it must spread. When the drug concentration reaches a minimal effective concentration, neuronal transmission is altered in a manner that clinically provides anesthesia. Neurons—some myelinated, others not; some relatively large, others smaller—differ in susceptibility to drugs such as local anesthetics, and these pharmacodynamic relationships are not easily explained (Table 45-1). The processes involved at the cellular level are very complex, and *blockade* is perhaps a confusing term. It is more accurate to say that anesthetic drugs alter nerve transmission, predominantly by affecting sodium ion channels and inhibiting the units of information that are transferred along the spinal cord. Complete blockade or a "chemical transection" of the cord is an oversimplification. For example, somatosensory evoked potentials have been recorded in individuals made functionally insensate from lidocaine epidural anesthesia. This suggests that neural transmissions are reaching the brain without causing sensory perceptions.[4,11]

When a local anesthetic interrupts nerve transmission of autonomic nerves but not sensory nerves or motor nerves (because of a variation in susceptibility), a "differential block" is said to have occurred. A differential block is seen in the more rostral spinal segments of a spinal anesthetic. As the spinal anesthetic spreads from the epicenter of injection, the distal reaches of drug distribution are presumably of lesser concentrations. A differential block is clinically important when sensory anesthesia is desired at a specific level; however, sympathetic blockade could be deleterious in a patient with coexisting disease. The level of sympathetic blockade could be as high as six or more dermatomal levels above the level of sensory blockade and therefore contribute to hypotension and bradycardia.[10]

Drug injected into the epidural space is distributed to the same sites of action as a spinal anesthetic but in a slightly different manner. The drug must first distribute along the epidural space then diffuse through the meninges and dural cuffs to reach the nerve roots or reach the spinal cord through absorption into the radicular arteries.[12] Data exist to support the clinical impression that spinal anesthesia is generally more effective or complete from the patient's perspective than epidural anesthesia and therefore referred to as a more "dense" anesthetic. Epidural local anesthetics first act at sites such as the dural cuffs, at which spinal nerves pass through the peridural spaces. This is consistent with the segmental onset often associated with epidural anesthesia. If the concentration and volume of the anesthetic agent are increased, or if time is allowed for the drug to diffuse into the CSF or pass via radicular arteries into the spinal cord, the epidural anesthetic can become more dense.[4,8]

Central Neuraxial Blockade: Indications and Preoperative Considerations

Spinal and epidural anesthesia (central neuraxial blocks) can be used successfully for a variety of inpatient or ambulatory surgical procedures involving the lower extremities, perineum, and abdomen. In addition, spinal and epidural anesthesia or analgesia is used for the treatment of acute and chronic pain syndromes, for obstetric procedures and labor analgesia, and can be applied in patients at the extremes of age.[13] Spinal anesthesia techniques may also be used in combination with other techniques, such as epidural catheter techniques, general or intravenous anesthetic techniques, and with the use of a laryngeal mask airway, to provide anesthesia during surgery. Such combinations, or balanced techniques, minimize the side effects of any one anesthetic technique, maximize the benefits, and offer options in the selection of anesthesia or analgesia for surgical or obstetric procedures.[14]

TABLE **45-1**	Classification of Nerve Fibers			
		Conduction		
Nerve Fiber	**Myelination**	**Diameter (μm)**	**Velocity (m/sec)**	**Function**
A-α	Heavy	15-20	70-120	Motor
A-β	Moderate	5-12	30-70	Touch and pressure
A-γ	Moderate	5-10	30-70	Proprioception
A-δ	Light	2-5	12-30	Pain and temperature
B	Light	1-4	3-15	Preganglionic, autonomic
C	None	0.5-1	0.5-2	Pain and temperature

As with any anesthetic plan, proper preparation, patient selection, education, and collaboration with surgeons and nurses are the keys to success. Often the best time to obtain a truly informed consent is during the preoperative visit. It is important to establish rapport with patients to gain their trust and cooperation. Patients eager to be involved in their own care often have the emotional maturity to understand the benefits of their anesthetic options and make rational choices. Anticipate patients' fears and anxieties; they are often easily dealt with through education and the reassurance provided by the calm voice of a confident and competent anesthetist.

Before presenting the option of a regional anesthetic to the patient, the anesthesia practitioner should answer the following three important questions about the procedure:

1. Will the patient be comfortable having this surgical procedure performed with the proposed regional anesthetic technique?
2. Will the patient be able to remain in the required position without difficulty for the length of the procedure?
3. Does this regional anesthetic technique outweigh the risks of performing this procedure using an alternate anesthetic technique?

The answers to these questions directly affect the choice of anesthetic techniques offered to the patient. When recommending any anesthetic technique to the patient, the practitioner has a responsibility to educate the patient, the patient's family, and other interested parties about the anesthesia procedure and the potential outcomes. One can then obtain an informed consent and garner the trust of the patient before performing any technique. Without this trust, even the best anesthetic technique may be a failure.

Potential advantages of neuraxial anesthesia include less nausea, vomiting, and urinary retention; a reduced total opioid requirement; and greater mental alertness compared with patients who have received general anesthesia alone. After regional anesthesia, patients are quick to eat, void, and ambulate. Ambulatory surgical patients may or may not be discharged any sooner after spinal anesthesia when compared with those who have undergone general anesthesia, but they can avoid unnecessary overnight admissions resulting from complications of general anesthesia. A growing body of evidence also supports improved outcomes for selected patients and situations. Spinal and epidural anesthesia blunt the body's stress response to surgery and may offer preemptive analgesia. In addition, studies have shown neuraxial anesthetics to decrease intraoperative blood loss, lower the incidence of postoperative thromboembolic events and postoperative ileus, increase patency of vascular grafts, improve respiratory function and cardiac stability, and improve outcome in high-risk surgical patients.[15] Although headache remains a small concern, this risk is greatly reduced.[16]

Another group of patients well known to benefit from the use of CNB techniques are patients who require anesthesia for obstetric procedures. One primary example is the administration of an epidural anesthetic to the patient in labor. No other modality can provide the parturient with relative relief from the most severe discomfort and still permit the baby and mother to interact immediately after delivery, all with minimal possibility of respiratory distress or depression. Also, epidural techniques in labor allow a safe conversion of the analgesia to a surgical anesthetic should a cesarean section become necessary.[17,18]

Patient safety may also be increased with spinal or epidural anesthesia. Urologic procedures such as cystoscopic examinations and transurethral resections of the prostate (TURP) are most often performed with the use of spinal anesthesia. When awake

and anesthetized to the level of the dome of the bladder (T10), the patient may verbally respond to bladder overdistention, thereby helping the urologist minimize the potential for bladder rupture. In addition, the mental status and sensorium of a responsive patient can easily be monitored and the development of conditions associated with TURP syndrome such as hypervolemia, hyponatremia, and ammonium toxicity are more readily detected.[19]

Safety is also an issue when the patient is placed in the prone or jackknifed position as for perianal procedures. A patient in such a position under general anesthesia is at risk for inadvertent extubation and positioning injury. A hypobaric spinal anesthesia technique offers several advantages. The anesthetic procedure can be performed after the patient is positioned and has verbalized that he or she is comfortably padded. With hypobaric spinal anesthesia, the spread of the local anesthetic is controlled, and spontaneous ventilation is maintained.

Additionally, patients often fear postoperative discomfort.[20] Therefore, another advantage of spinal anesthesia is the ability to administer long-acting opioid analgesics or clonidine. Epidural catheter placement allows for opioids, low concentrations of local anesthetics, or mixtures containing both solutions to be continuously infused or administered by patient-controlled devices, thereby keeping patients comfortable well into the postoperative period. Because the total doses of opioids and local anesthetics are small, the patient remains alert and possibly ambulatory while receiving analgesia with minimal side effects.[4,8] The patient's right to be fully informed also necessitates a discussion of the disadvantages of CNB. Consider the patient's perspective, and keep in mind that the disadvantages and risks inherent in any anesthetic plan are relative only to those of another anesthetic option. For example, patients with a history of headaches or backaches are at increased risk for experiencing these problems after spinal and epidural analgesia but may also have exacerbations of these problems after a general anesthetic. Such patients should be evaluated and counseled regarding this potential problem before the administration of any anesthetic. A thorough history of the patient's previous pattern of headaches or backaches is essential when faced with the challenge of evaluating similar symptoms in the postoperative period.

To many patients, the risk of paralysis is the most important concern, despite the extreme rarity of any neurologic sequela. The incidence rate of persistent paresthesia and sensory or motor dysfunction is less than 0.1%.[4,21-23] Common patient questions may also include the following:

- "Will the injections hurt?"
- "How long will I be numb?"
- "I am afraid of hearing (or smelling or feeling) the surgery. Can I be asleep?"

Patient perceptions can be corrected with thoughtful explanation and discussion of the clinician's expectations regarding the patient's case. Additional discussion should include the topic of intraoperative risks, such as the inability to obtain adequate anesthesia, paresthesia, hypotension, dyspnea, high or total spinal anesthesia, nausea and vomiting, use of additional sedation, and allergic reactions. Postoperative complications may include backache, postdural puncture headache (PDPH), hearing loss, transient neurologic symptoms, infection, and peridural abscess or hematoma formation.[5,16,21,24,25]

Before administration of any anesthetic, a thorough preoperative history and physical examination must be conducted. During this part of the preoperative patient visit, any concerns regarding administration of spinal anesthesia can be identified.

Often the terms *absolute* and *relative contraindications* are used; the definition of these categories varies, and their use is therefore controversial. It is more important to think of the anesthetic risks and associated complications relative to the possible benefits of the proposed anesthetic technique. An obvious example is patient refusal or lack of cooperation. Other preoperative concerns include increased intracranial pressure, significant preexisting or therapeutic coagulopathy, skin infection at the site of injection, hypovolemia, spinal cord disease, patients with a fixed-volume cardiac state such as idiopathic hypertrophic subaortic stenosis (IHSS) or severe atrial stenosis, and an anticipated lengthy surgical time. Finally, if a difficult airway is anticipated, the plan of care must be discussed with both patient and surgeon.

Neurologic diseases are often listed as potential, absolute, or relative contraindications for neuraxial anesthesia, but data are often mixed. A dural puncture by a spinal needle or a larger epidural needle creates a rent in dural tissue that may or may not leak CSF. In patients with a preexisting increase in intracranial pressure, the risk of brain herniation is increased. In the case of epidural catheter placement or epidural blood patch, the addition of large volumes of fluid into the epidural or subarachnoid spaces could increase already elevated intracranial pressures.[4,8]

Musculoskeletal deformities such as severe kyphoscoliosis, arthritis, osteoporosis, and fusion and scarring of the vertebrae are considered relative contraindications to neuraxial anesthesia. The location of the epidural or subarachnoid spaces by needle tip may be technically difficult, and spread of anesthetic agents may be limited by anatomic alterations.[21] However, a large retrospective study surmises that osteoporosis may be an important risk factor for CNB complications.[26]

Peripheral neuropathies can be the result of metabolic, autoimmune, infectious, or hereditary etiologies. A presumption is that patients with preexisting neural compromise are more susceptible to and less able to recover from injury when exposed to a secondary insult, compared with patients with healthy tissues. Also, abnormal tissues may not respond to pharmacologic agents in predictable ways. Secondary insults might stem from needle or catheter trauma, ischemic injury from the use of vasoconstrictors, or direct local anesthetic neurotoxicity. For example, diabetes mellitus (DM) is the most prevalent cause of peripheral polyneuropathy, with most patients having some abnormalities in nerve conduction. A study by Hebl and colleagues supports the increased risk of the "double-crush" phenomenon, finding that 0.4% of patients with diabetic polyneuropathy experience new or progressive changes in their neurologic deficits. This suggests that spinal or epidural anesthesia may worsen or exacerbate conditions such as a gradually progressive diabetic neuropathy. However, the same group of investigators also took a retrospective look at central nervous system (CNS) diagnoses such as post-poliomyelitis, multiple sclerosis, traumatic spinal cord injury, and amyotrophic lateral sclerosis. The nature of their study did not permit definitive recommendations, yet they found no patients with exacerbations or deterioration of symptoms. Additionally, they note that their results suggest the safety of CNB in these patients and that their findings were supported by other studies. Until further prospective study can support definitive conclusions, the decision to perform a CNB technique must be made by weighing the relative risks to the individual patient's neurologic disease against the potential benefits of minimizing the anesthetic effects on their coexisting diseases.[27] Because few objective data are available, use of CNB in such patients becomes a medicolegal risk, especially if blame is incorrectly placed on the anesthetic. If a neuraxial block is the appropriate anesthetic choice, then precise documentation of the patient's preexisting disease state and existing neurologic compromise is a mandatory precaution, as is attentive follow-up care.[4,8,21,24]

The existence of a significant preexisting or therapeutic coagulopathy increases the risk of spinal or epidural hematoma formation in a patient receiving a CNB. Spinal or epidural hematoma is a rare but devastating complication, possibly resulting in permanent neurologic injury. Therefore, central neuraxial anesthesia should be avoided in any patient with a known coagulopathy. Insufficient data are available to quiet the controversy surrounding absolute laboratory values below which the practitioner should avoid CNB. In determining whether a CNB technique should be avoided, Winnie suggested using arbitrary values for platelet counts of less than 100,000 and prothrombin time (PT), activated partial thromboplastin time (aPTT), and bleeding times that are greater than two times normal values. For a spinal anesthetic, this is perhaps an overly conservative guide.[28] However, severe bleeding with or without symptomatic hypovolemia or the potential for severe bleeding is a possible contraindication to the administration of a regional anesthetic because the sympathectomy caused by CNB further aggravates severely contracted volume states.

Much discussion has arisen regarding the use of spinal and epidural anesthesia when coagulopathy for thromboprophylaxis or for therapeutic treatment of coexisting disease has been initiated, planned, or is ongoing because the therapies, timing, and the effects on coagulation are highly varied. For example, the use of platelet inhibitors, like aspirin or nonsteroidal antiinflammatory drugs (NSAIDs), do not appear to be a contraindication to spinal and epidural anesthesia. Even planned intraoperative anticoagulation with heparin is reasonably safe following atraumatic dural puncture if the patient presents with a normal coagulation profile. Traditionally, a patient's bleeding time was obtained prior to administration of neuraxial anesthesia, but the predictive value of bleeding time has not been established in patients taking aspirin and NSAIDs.[29,30] Also, with the increased use of natural and herbal medicines, anesthetists must be alert to the possibility of drug interactions. Alone, herbal supplements appear not to increase the risk of spinal hematoma; however, data on combinations of herbal and other anticoagulants are not available. Still, if basic precautions are followed, many thromboprophylaxis strategies have had an extensive safety record when co-administered with neuraxial anesthetics. With heparin, the usual recommendation is to place a needle or catheter at least 1 hour before administration. Anticoagulation should be monitored, aPTT should be measured, and any catheters used should be pulled when heparin activity is at a minimal level, an hour before any subsequent dose. A similar approach is used with the oral anticoagulant warfarin. Coagulation should be closely monitored (via assessment of PT and international normalized ratio [INR]) because of considerable variability in patient response to this drug. Generally, the need for acute pain management exists within the first few days after surgery. If warfarin is started in the postoperative period, the epidural catheter is removed before warfarin has reached a therapeutic level. It is also important to remember that the tissue trauma and bleeding associated with needle placement and catheter insertion are as likely with catheter removal. Therefore, documentation of normal coagulation for catheter removal is a reasonable goal. This goal, however, may need to be weighed against the risks of ongoing trauma from an indwelling catheter and the need for ongoing coagulation.[23]

In 1993, the first low-molecular-weight heparin (LMWH) was approved by the U.S. Food and Drug Administration (FDA) for

TABLE **45-2**	Low-Molecular-Weight Heparin Guidelines in Regional Anesthesia	
Postoperative LMWH Regimen	**Timing of Initial Dose(s) of LMWH**	**Use of Catheters**
Twice-daily dosing	Administer first dose no earlier than 24 hours postoperatively, regardless of anesthetic technique and only in the presence of adequate hemostasis	Remove indwelling catheters before initiation of LMWH therapy. When a continuous epidural catheter technique is used, catheters may be left indwelling overnight and removed the following day. The first dose of low-molecular weight heparin (LMWH) should be administered 2 hours after catheter removal.
Once-daily dosing	Administer first dose 6-8 hours postoperatively, and administer second dose no sooner than 24 hours after first dose.	Indwelling catheters may be safely maintained but should be removed at a minimum of 10-12 hours after last LMWH medication is given. Initiate any subsequent LMWH dosing a minimum of 2 hours after the catheter has been removed.

thromboembolism prophylaxis, and use became extensive. However, within the first several years, the FDA compiled a total of 60 cases of spinal hematoma that occurred in patients who had received LMWH and CNB. This reflected an increase in the incidence of spinal hematomas in the United States from an estimated rate of approximately 1:200,000 to a rate between 1:1000 and 1:10,000.[23] This prompted the manufacturers of LMWH medications to revise their warnings to include a precaution against regional anesthesia in patients receiving LMWH medications.[31] In 1998, a set of guidelines was made available to clinicians to use in their clinical practice. It was noted that following publication of these guidelines, the cases of spinal hematoma decreased significantly but did not totally disappear from the clinical landscape. In response to these findings and a second consensus conference, an updated guideline on neuraxial anesthesia and anticoagulation was published by the American Society of Regional Anesthesia (ASRA) in 2003.[32] The 2003 guideline supports safe administration of regional anesthesia in patients in receipt of LMWH prophylaxis with caveats on the calibration of the total daily dose, the timing of the doses of LMWH, and the placement and maintenance of neuraxial anesthesia. The guidelines are readily available for review on the Internet and cover the range of regional anesthesia in the anticoagulated patient. Because this can be a very complex issue, patient management goals must keep in focus the individual patient's condition, the risks of CNB versus the benefits, alternative anesthetic techniques, and a plan for vigilance during postoperative care to ensure the early detection and treatment of neurologic compromise. Table 45-2 summarizes LMWH guidelines, and the following practice guide is a condensed list of the recommendations of the ASRA conference:

1. The surgeon and anesthesia practitioner should consider the potential benefit versus risk before neuraxial intervention for patients who have been or will be anticoagulated for thromboprophylaxis.
2. Patients not receiving anticoagulant therapy and with no history or clinical signs of coagulopathy (easy bruising, bleeding gums, small cuts that bleed profusely) may be offered regional anesthetic options as appropriate.
3. Patients receiving NSAIDs, including aspirin, may receive CNB anesthesia regardless of when they received the last dose. Herbal therapy alone does not seem to be a specific concern.

4. Subcutaneous or minidose heparin thromboprophylaxis does not preclude the use of neuraxial techniques.
5. Patients receiving intravenous heparin therapy before surgery should not receive CNB anesthesia until a normal aPTT can be documented. When a CNB is used and intraoperative anticoagulation is initiated, it is recommended that heparin dosing be held for at least 1 hour after the placement of a neuraxial anesthetic. Indwelling catheters should be removed 2 to 4 hours after the last heparin dose and the patient's coagulation status is known. Heparinization can again occur 1 hour after catheter removal.
6. Warfarin therapy and CNB remains controversial. Patients receiving chronic warfarin therapy should have this medication stopped at least 4 days before surgery. If a patient receives a dose of warfarin within 24 hours of surgery, an INR should be checked immediately before the scheduled procedure. CNB anesthesia may be administered if the preoperative INR is less than 1.5. The PT and INR values in patients with epidural catheters for continuous postoperative epidural analgesia should be evaluated daily. The catheter should not be pulled until the INR is less than 1.5.
7. Patients receiving fibrinolytic or thrombolytic drug therapy should not receive neuraxial anesthesia for 10 days. If the uses of such medications are anticipated in the postoperative period, these neuraxial techniques should be avoided.
8. Data on the risk of spinal hematoma associated with thienopyridine therapy (ticlopidine and clopidogrel) and GP IIb-IIIa antagonists (abciximab, eptifibatide, and tirofiban) are lacking. Consensus management suggests discontinuation of ticlopidine 14 days, and clopidogrel 7 days, prior to CNB. Normal platelet aggregation occurs 24 to 48 hours after abciximab and 4 to 8 hours after eptifibatide and tirofiban. Use of GP IIb-IIIa antagonists is contraindicated for 4 weeks after surgery.
9. Limited information is available on newer anticoagulants such as desirudin, lepirudin, bivalirudin, and argatroban, and risk assessment statements have yet to be made.
10. Fondaparinux, a factor Xa inhibitor, has a black box warning similar to that of LMWH and has been used safely in clinical trials with spinal techniques of single-pass, atraumatic needle placement.

11. Combinations of the previously listed medications place the patient at greater risk for the development of complications such as spinal or epidural hematoma formation and permanent neurologic injury. Therefore, risks and benefits must be carefully weighed on an individual basis.

12. Patients who have received a CNB anesthetic and who are anticoagulated should be closely monitored for signs and symptoms of neurologic impairment. Neurologic assessments are recommended at 2-hour or more frequent intervals. Any noted neurologic compromise is to be immediately reported, and emergent treatment is required.

By following evidence and consensus-based precautions, the low incidence of permanent neurologic complications can be decreased. A meta-analysis by Brull and colleagues identified the risk of permanent neurologic injury after spinal anesthesia at 1 to 4.2:10,000 and after epidural anesthesia at 0 to 7.6:10,000.[33] Because complications are very infrequent, risk factor identification is difficult, and vigilant care must be maintained for all patients. Analysis of known case reports found the median time to onset of neurologic dysfunction after initiation of LMWH therapy to be 3 days. Scrupulous postoperative nursing surveillance is also required to support patient safety. The initial complaint may be of new-onset weakness to the lower limbs and sensory deficit, although bowel and bladder dysfunction and new-onset back pain may occur. If emergent neurosurgical care is required, recovery is unlikely if surgical decompression of the hematoma is delayed more than 8 hours.[23,26,33]

The etiology of neuraxial infection is based on the theory that needle placement disrupts the body's physiologic protective mechanisms and deposits infectious or noxious agents beyond the skin into underlying tissues and the peridural space and past the blood-brain barrier into subarachnoid spaces. Indeed, skin infection at the site of injection increases the risk of meningitis or epidural abscess formation. Although infectious complications of CNB are rare, the practitioner must maintain aseptic technique during the preparation and administration of any regional anesthetic to minimize the potential for infection. Septic meningitis or epidural abscess due to bacterial contamination, and the consequences of persistent neurologic deficits such as loss of bowel and bladder control, chronic pain, and lower extremity weakness or paraplegia, can be devastating. Other factors that increase the risk of infection include dermatologic conditions such as psoriasis that prevent aseptic skin preparation, underlying sepsis, diabetes, immunologic compromise, steroid therapy, and the preexistence of chronic infections such as human immunodeficiency virus (HIV) or herpes simplex virus (HSV). Because meningitis after spinal or epidural anesthesia is so rare, it has been difficult to directly attribute causality to the anesthetic or to identify significant risk factors. In fact, based on the limited data available it would appear that regional anesthesia is safe in cases of secondary HSV infection and reasonable for patients in the early stages of HIV infection. Again, vigilance must be emphasized. Known predisposing factors include advanced age, diabetes, alcoholism, cancer, and AIDS. Patients are monitored for signs of meningeal irritation, fever, increasing back pain, neurologic changes, and local tenderness to injection sites. Although classic symptoms such as high fever, nuchal rigidity, and severe headache may be present, less alarming symptoms can occur, resulting in misdiagnosis. Although α-hemolytic streptococci is commonly seen in spinal block meningitis, *Staphylococcus aureus* is the most common causative organism in epidural abscesses, and iatrogenic methicillin-resistant. *S. aureus* is a growing concern. Epidural abscess, like epidural

hematomas with evidence of neurologic deficit, can best be diagnosed by MRI. Early, aggressive surgical intervention and antibiotic administration are vital.[4,21,26,34-36]

Arachnoiditis and aseptic meningitis are rare but can occur when foreign substances irritate the meninges. As the needle is inserted, precautions must be taken to avoid introduction of glass or metal particles, highly concentrated local anesthetics or dextrose solutions, detergents or antiseptics, and a core of epidermis. Indwelling catheters, previous myelography, and hemorrhages into the subarachnoid or epidural space have also been associated with meningeal irritation and scarring. Modern technology and techniques incorporate the use of disposable equipment, needles with matched stylets, filter needles, and improved pharmacologic agents that make this complication rare.[37]

Shock and severe uncorrected hypovolemia are contraindications to spinal or epidural anesthesia, because both techniques cause sympathetic blockade. The resulting vasodilation prevents physiologic compensation and may worsen hypotension. In addition, management of shock and hypovolemia often requires aggressive fluid therapy and multisystem treatments that are often physiologically and psychologically uncomfortable for the aware patient.[4,8,21]

Patients with a fixed-volume cardiac state such as IHSS or severe atrial stenosis do not tolerate bradycardia, decreases in systemic vascular resistance, or decreases in venous return and left ventricular filling—all physiologic changes that can be anticipated with neuraxial block by local anesthetics. In these patients, even transient episodes of hypotension can cause serious coronary hypoperfusion and cardiac arrest. Therefore spinal, and usually epidural, anesthesia, are avoided; however, few things in anesthesia are truly absolute. For example, epidural administration of opioids has been used to provide obstetric analgesia and may provide cardiac benefit for these patients. Precautions in such a scenario might include close hemodynamic monitoring with an arterial line and pulmonary artery catheter, careful titration of the anesthetic, intravascular volume expansion, and use of ephedrine or phenylephrine to treat hypotension.[23]

Spinal anesthesia is typically a singular deposit of local anesthetic and therefore provides anesthesia for a fixed duration. If uncertainty exists about the anticipated length of surgery, epidural catheter placement is more appropriate to allow for the additional administration, or continuous infusions, of anesthetic agents. If the extent of the surgery is unknown, a neuraxial anesthetic may be initiated only to be converted at a later time to a general anesthetic when the surgeon exceeds the limits of the anesthetic block. This is rarely an ideal situation; the patient may experience discomfort, albeit brief, and the anesthesia practitioner must contend with less-than-ideal intubating conditions. Despite the advantages of neuraxial anesthesia, many patients such as the elderly and those with arthritis or musculoskeletal limitations of the neck and upper extremities poorly tolerate prolonged immobility. The judicious use of conscious sedation can quickly devolve into a "room air general," placing the patient at risk for hypoventilation, hypoxia, and hypercarbia. To avoid such circumstances, combined neuraxial and general anesthetic techniques are advocated and offer advantages by minimizing the total dose of general anesthetic used. Such techniques lower the risk of secondary effects of general anesthesia (e.g., nausea and vomiting) while gaining the advantages associated with neuraxial anesthesia, such as attenuation of the stress hormone response and improved postoperative pain relief.[8]

The administration of spinal or any regional anesthesia to patients with a difficult airway or full stomach requires careful consideration. The use of spinal anesthesia permits the patient to retain upper airway and pharyngeal reflexes that block the sympathetic nervous system. This theoretically results in increased gastric and intestinal motility, causing the stomach to empty. However, such benefits may be negated by the perception of pain and anxiety that accompanies illness or injury. If sedation is used to counter such perceptions, the airway may again become compromised. Furthermore, if hypotension develops from the resulting sympathectomy, the patient may experience nausea and vomiting. When an injury has occurred after the ingestion of alcohol or if the patient received opioid analgesics, the pain caused by the injury may be the only stimulus for consciousness.

When spinal or other regional anesthesia is instituted, the reticular activating centers in the brain receive less input. This often results in somnolence in a normal patient but can result in unconsciousness in the overly sedated or inebriated patient. In addition, spinal or epidural anesthesia may reach an undesirably high level that is physically and psychologically intolerable for the patient and can even become a "total spinal." A total spinal is characterized by unresponsiveness accompanied by cardiac and respiratory compromise. In such situations airway support is required, and the emergent management of any airway can severely compromise patient safety. Therefore, regional anesthesia is not an alternative to a secure airway. For patients identified as potentially difficult to intubate, equipment should be immediately available to secure the airway in a safe manner. Advances in airway management such as the laryngeal mask airway, improved fiberoptics, laryngoscopes, and light wands may tip the risk-benefit scale in favor of regional anesthesia.[8,10,37]

SPINAL ANESTHESIA

Spinal anesthesia became popular after the discovery of the local anesthetic properties of cocaine, the invention of the hollow needle and syringe, and the written descriptions of the first lumbar puncture. The first clinical application of the technique was reportedly performed in the late 1890s. However, spinal anesthesia's prominence was short lived. The introduction of specific, reversible, neuromuscular blocking drugs and concurrent improvements in inhalation agents for general anesthesia soon displaced its popularity. Only recently has it regained popularity, in large part because of the introduction of newer agents, equipment, and techniques.

Equipment and Techniques

Preparation for spinal anesthetic procedures, like that for any other regional technique, requires the immediate availability of emergency equipment and supplies should emergent resuscitation be required. Usually spinal anesthetics are administered in the operating room where the minimal requirements—functional laryngoscopes, endotracheal tubes, induction agents, cardiovascular drugs including atropine and ephedrine or phenylephrine, suction, oxygen and ventilation equipment, a noninvasive blood pressure monitor, and pulse oximetry and electrocardiographic monitoring equipment—are readily available.

The original spinal technique, performed by August Bier in 1898, has been continually examined and modified in hope of reducing the incidence of complications—primarily that of PDPH. The goal of needle design has been to create a needle that minimally rends, tears, or cuts dural tissues. As technology has improved, the use of sterile, disposable procedure trays containing needles, syringes, catheters, and drugs has virtually eliminated problems previously associated with dull needles or contaminated equipment and has allowed for the development

of innovative needles. Currently, two main types of needles are available for use in spinal anesthesia. Needles such as the Quincke-Babcock or Pitkin have a *cutting bevel tip*. These needles have matching stylets, which minimizes tissue coring, and the tip's cutting angle is blunter than that of a standard needle. The newer *noncutting-tip needles* are either pencil-point shaped with lateral openings (e.g., Sprotte, Whitacre, or Pencan needles) or have the rounded bevel tip of the Greene-type needle and an opening at the needle's end. Several of the more popular types of spinal needles are shown in Figure 45-7. Spinal needles also have matched stylets and are marketed for spinal anesthesia use in sizes ranging from 22 to 29 gauge and in lengths of approximately 3.5 inches (88 mm) and 5 inches (120 mm). Most blocks are performed using 25- to 27-gauge, 3.5-inch (88 mm) needles.[21,37]

Recent data support the use of noncutting-tip needles over cutting needles for several reasons. Cadaver lumbar punctures performed with sharp cutting needles show piercing of the cauda equina roots without resistance appreciated by the practitioner. This does not occur with pencil-point needles. The bevel of cutting-tip needles encourages tip deviation on insertion, whereas symmetric noncutting needles stay midline. The use of a beveled needle requires holding the bevel direction parallel to longitudinal dural tissue fibers to minimize the risk of PDPH. Noncutting needles may drag fewer skin contaminants into subdermal tissue than cutting needles. Pencil-point needles pierce the dura with a clearly perceptible "click" or "pop" not as easily noticed with cutting needles. Newer, thin-walled noncutting needles have improved CSF flow rates without compromise to strength. This allows for their use for CSF diagnostic procedures and helps simplify the identification of the intrathecal space by permitting quick return of CSF after stylet removal. Finally, unless prohibitively small cutting needles are used, the incidence of PDPH is clearly reduced with the use of noncutting needles. Pencil-point needles are associated with less than a 1% risk of PDPH and a failure rate of approximately 5%.[8,21,38,39]

After the patient arrives in the surgical or obstetric preoperative area, the consents for surgery and anesthesia should be checked, and any further patient questions or concerns should be addressed. Review of the anesthetic preoperative history and physical examination should include the addition of any last-minute changes in patient status and notation of recently obtained diagnostic results. Intravenous access is achieved, and a continuous crystalloid infusion is begun. Preoperatively, most patients benefit from low-dose anxiolysis. With the increased emphasis on same-day admission, surgery, and discharge, long-acting agents are avoided. A rapid-acting benzodiazepine with a relatively short duration, such as midazolam, is highly titratable in 0.5- to 1-mg increments given intravenously and minimally alters the patient's hemodynamic status when used in low doses. The drug's effects can be reversed with flumazenil.

Monitors appropriate to the patient's physical status should be applied and at minimum include blood pressure monitoring, a continuous electrocardiogram, and pulse oximetry. For the purpose of baseline comparisons, vital signs must be assessed with the patient in both the supine position and the position in which the block will be administered.

The surgical or obstetric procedure to be performed helps determine the patient's position for the administration of the block. For example, if vaginal or urologic surgery is planned, a "saddle" block with the patient in a sitting position may be indicated. The prone position is useful for rectal surgery, because the patient can be placed in position before the block

Cutting-point tips   Pencil-point tips

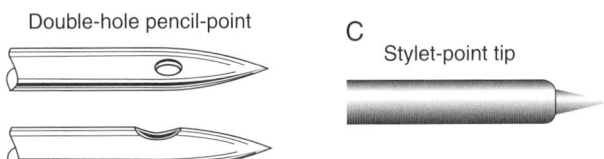

25-gauge Quincke   25-gauge Whitacre   24-gauge Sprotte

Double-hole pencil-point   C
                                        Stylet-point tip

FIGURE **45-7**   Graphic representations of spinal needle design features. **A,** Cutting-point tips. **B,** Pencil-point tips. **C,** Stylet-point tip. (**A** *from Chestnut DH. Obstetric Anesthesia: Principles and Practice. 3rd ed. Philadelphia: Mosby; 2004;* **B** *from Chestnut DH. Obstetric Anesthesia: Principles and Practice. 3rd ed. Philadelphia: Mosby; 2004. And from CSEN International. Eldor Spinal Needle. Available at: http://www.csen.com.*)

is implemented. This reduces the time required for positioning by permitting the patient to move with minimal assistance and to personally verify comfort and adequacy of padding. A lateral position favors spinal drug spread for right- or left-sided extremity or abdominal procedures. When the patient is in the lateral position, a pillow placed under the head and perhaps shoulders helps maintain neutral alignment of the spinal column. Surgical table height or patient position may need to be adjusted to compensate for variations in anatomic structure or physiologic limitations and to maximize anesthetist ergonomics. To maximize the space between spinous processes, the patient should arch the back (with assistance from the clinician) into a C shape or "like a Halloween cat." Once the patient is positioned, anatomic surface landmarks are used to identify the lumbar region of the back to be used for dural puncture, a point below the end of the spinal cord (L2). The line formed between the tops of the iliac crests, called the *intercristal line* or *Tuffier's line*, crosses the vertebral column as high as the L3 to L4 disk or as low as the L5 to S1 disk (Figure 45-8). The accuracy of predicting the precise level of needle insertion is at best 50%. This fact may account for variability in the spinal anesthesia level ultimately achieved, yet this landmark has been clinically useful since the advent of spinal anesthesia.[7] The skin overlying a prominent spinous process at this level is marked for easy identification after the skin is prepared and draped. A surgical skin-marking pen is useful for this purpose, with caution exercised to avoid scratching the skin surface and predisposing the patient to infection.

Next, the spinal anesthesia tray is opened, and sterile gloves are donned. The patient is prepared with an antiseptic solution such as Betadine, a povidone-iodine solution that releases a concentration of 1% free iodine as it dries on a surface. The solution must remain in contact with the skin for at least 1 minute to be effective, and then the dry residue can be wiped away with sterile gauze to help prevent a chemical arachnoiditis. Do not use alcohol to remove residue because alcohol neutralizes the iodine solution and minimizes its antiseptic effect. Maintain aseptic technique, and apply the sterile drape to the back. Many spinal

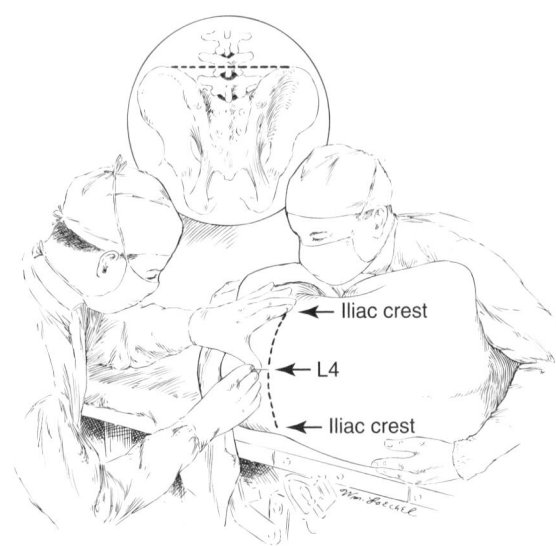

FIGURE **45-8**   Patient positioning and identification of landmarks in the lumbar region of the back.

and epidural drapes have a circular window that is placed over the area of anticipated injection and adhesive strips to simplify application to the patient's back. Avoid touching the adhesive, because this has been shown to create small holes in gloves, which increases the risk of infection in both the patient and anesthesia practitioner.[40]

A rapid-acting local anesthetic such as 1% lidocaine is used for local infiltration of the area just caudad to the identified spinous process. Approach the skin of the back with the bevel of the needle facing away from the skin and at a 15- to 30-degree angle from the skin. Start injecting before the bevel of the needle is completely through the skin, and raise a skin wheal to place local anesthetic into subdermal tissues most likely to

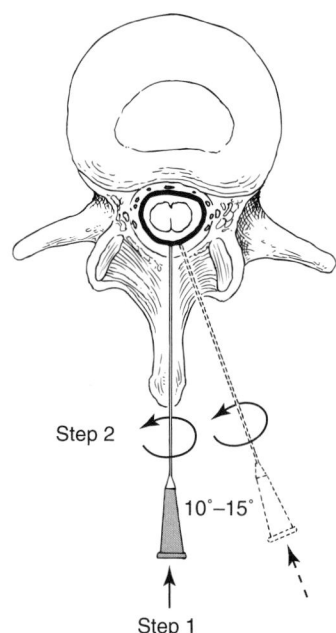

FIGURE **45-9**   Insertion of the needle between the spinous processes and toward the umbilicus.

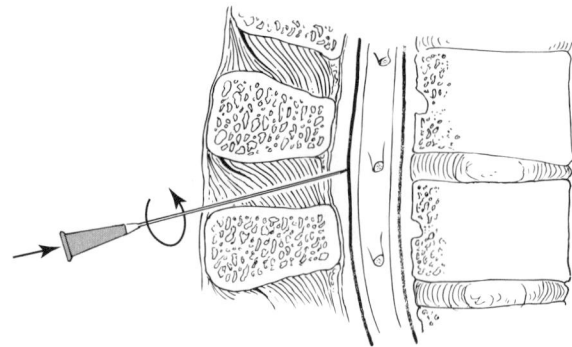

FIGURE **45-10**   Spinal needle rotated 360 degrees to aid evaluation of tip location within the subarachnoid space.

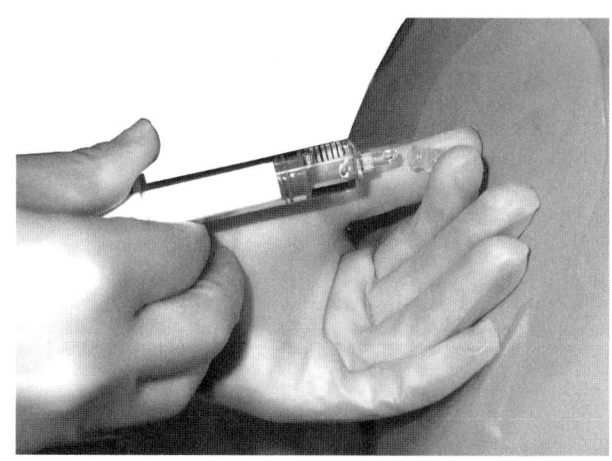

FIGURE **45-11**   The Bromage grip, showing needle control and syringe connection.

contain nociceptors. Deep tissues, including the supraspinous ligament, can be anesthetized by spreading 3 to 5 mL of local anesthetic through the tissues in a fan pattern.[8,21]

Larger 22- to 25-gauge spinal needles and epidural needles (used for continuous spinal anesthetic techniques) have tensile strength sufficient to permit introduction of the needle without additional support. However, spinal needles smaller than 25 gauge often require an "introducer" needle to help stabilize the needle during insertion and minimize infection in the surrounding dermis. The introducer is typically an 18- or 20-gauge needle with a "B" or blunt bevel. Introducer needles are approximately 3.8 cm long and matched to the spinal needles. The introducer is inserted through the skin and supraspinous ligament and into the interspinous ligament. Care must be taken, especially in thin individuals, not to enter the subarachnoid space with the introducer needle; the dura may be only 2.5 cm beneath the skin. Depth to the epidural space and the nearby dura correlates with weight but typically averages approximately 4 to 5 cm and rarely exceeds 9 cm. An introducer needle placed into the subarachnoid space would be likely to cause a PDPH.[4,8,14,21]

Several common spinal anesthesia techniques can be used, including a straight midline approach. With this easy-to-learn technique, the anesthesia practitioner inserts the needle directly midline between the spinous processes and toward the umbilicus perpendicularly to all planes or at the lumbar level with a slight cephalad angle (Figures 45-9 and 45-10). If bone is encountered early, the needle is withdrawn into the introducer and subcutaneous tissue. The introducer is then redirected in small angular increments in a cephalad direction. If bone is encountered when the needle is deeply inserted, the needle should be withdrawn and redirected caudad. As the tip of the spinal needle passes through the ligamenta flava, the sensation is similar to that felt when a needle is passed through a pencil eraser. As the needle tip passes through the dura, the anesthesia practitioner may sense a "pop" or "click." The stylet is removed, and several seconds are given for CSF to return through the small-gauge needle. Once CSF return is confirmed, some authors recommend rotating the needle 360 degrees in 90-degree increments to ensure that the needle tip is seated well within the subarachnoid space (see Figure 45-10). Other authors suggest that such needle manipulation risks a larger dural rent or needle dislodgement. Whichever method is used, secure needle handling is important. As shown in Figure 45-11, firmly place the dorsum of one's nondominant hand against the patient's back and below the spinal needle. Grasp the needle hub between the thumb and index finger. With this *Bromage* type of grip, the patient's body then acts as a firm support for the needle-stabilizing hand and helps prevent advancement or withdrawal of the needle tip from the subarachnoid space when the syringe is applied to inject the anesthetic agent.

A second technique is called the *paramedian approach*. With this technique, the needle is inserted 1 cm or approximately one fingerbreadth lateral to the caudad aspect of the interspace. The needle is directed toward the spinal canal and angled slightly cephalad and then medially approximately 10 to 15 degrees (see Figure 45-10). Elderly and arthritic patients may have decreased back flexibility and degenerating, calcified ligaments. For such patients, this approach may be the only possible means of entering the subarachnoid space because it aims for the largest area between processes and avoids calcified interspinous ligaments. A third approach to the subarachnoid space, known as the *Taylor approach*, takes advantage of the L5 interspace, which is the largest interlaminar space. A point 1 cm medial and 1 cm caudad to the posterior superior iliac spine is located, and the needle is angled medially and cephalad at a 55-degree angle toward the fifth lumbar interspace. The Taylor approach is best used for pelvic and perineal surgical procedures.[4,7,8,14,21]

Intrathecal Drugs, Spread, and Block Levels

Once the anesthetic solution is delivered into the CSF, the distribution of its active molecules through the subarachnoid space is dependent on the chemical and physical characteristics of the solution in relation to the chemical and physical characteristics of the patient's CSF and the subarachnoid space. In adults, approximately 500 mL of CSF is produced each day, predominantly by the choroid plexuses of the cerebral ventricles. Much of the CSF is reabsorbed by arachnoid granulations along the sagittal sinus to regulate CSF pressure to 10 to 20 cm H_2O. At any given time, a total of approximately 140 mL of CSF flows by bulk flow through the subarachnoid spaces, the central canal of the cord, and the ventricles of the brain. It is estimated that only 30 to 80 mL of the total CSF is present in the spinal canal. However, this quantity is difficult to measure, variable among individuals, and uncontrollable by the clinical anesthetist.[3,4,41]

The density of a substance compared with the density of water is a ratio known as *specific gravity*. The specific gravity of CSF is 1.004 to 1.009 and can vary depending on variations in temperature and location of the fluid within the subarachnoid space. For example, the specific gravity of CSF sampled from the lumbar area is slightly greater than that of CSF from the ventricles. This difference is directly dependent on the protein in the CSF, as well as on the effects of gravity and the position of the patient. The specific gravity of CSF also tends to increase as patient age increases, correlating to increases in glucose and protein. Hyperglycemia and uremia increase specific gravity of CSF, whereas jaundice and related liver problems may decrease specific gravity. The change in specific gravity is related to the presence of bilirubin within the CSF. An increase in a solution's temperature decreases its specific gravity. This decrease averages 0.001 point for each degree rise in Celsius temperature. Although all of these factors have been thought to influence the distribution of an anesthetic solution injected into the CSF, they are usually beyond the control of the anesthetist.[4,8,14,21,41]

A closely related concept, *baricity*, refers to the resting position of two fluids with differing specific gravities when the fluids are mixed in a single container, such as CSF and an anesthetic agent in the subarachnoid space. The baricity of the injected solution is compared with that of the CSF. Knowledge about the baricity of an injected solution provides the practitioner with information that helps determine the potential spread of the anesthetic mixture in the subarachnoid space. Therefore, when several medications are combined, the specific gravity of the combined solution at body temperature should be considered when the spread of the medication is anticipated. Unfortunately these bedside mixtures are rarely controlled or measured, and use becomes reliant on practical experience. When baricity (the ratio of specific gravity of local anesthetic to patient CSF) equals 1, the solution is referred to as being *isobaric*. Because the specific gravity of CSF is variable, it is not possible to prepare a solution that is precisely isobaric. Near-isobaric solutions remain and act in approximately the same location in which they are injected. A *hyperbaric* solution has a specific gravity that is greater than that of CSF. The solution would fall, or sink to the lowest anatomic

point at which CSF is contained within the subarachnoid space in relation to gravity and the patient's position (presuming that, as previously mentioned, drug preparations are corrected for body temperature). *Hypobaric* solutions that are less dense than CSF rise or float to the highest anatomic position possible when injected into the subarachnoid space. Because the normal range for the specific gravity of CSF is variable, local anesthetics, opioids, or other solutions injected into the CSF must be predictably hypobaric or hyperbaric. By tradition, hypobaric solutions are defined as having a baricity of less than 0.999, and hyperbaric solutions have a baricity of greater than 1.0015. Clinically this is accomplished by dissolving the drug in either sterile water to create a hypobaric solution or 5% to 8% dextrose solutions to create a hyperbaric solution. If CSF or normal saline is added to the medications, the specific gravity of the solution is similar to that of CSF, and the drugs remain approximately where injected.[4,8,14,21,41]

More than 23 factors, including CSF density and local anesthetic baricity, have been thought to affect the spread of local anesthetics in CSF and therefore affect the level and quality of the anesthesia achieved. Less than half of these factors have been found to have clinical significance, and an even smaller number are controllable by the anesthetist performing the anesthetic procedure.[21] Clinically the most important factors are those that can be manipulated by the anesthesia practitioner. These are the total dose of the local anesthetic, the site of injection, the baricity of the drug (drug choice), and (when nonisobaric solutions are used) the position or posture of the patient during and after injection.[41]

The duration of a spinal anesthetic is based primarily on local anesthetic choice and total dose. Highly protein-bound drugs, such as tetracaine, bupivacaine, and ropivacaine, have long durations of action compared with less protein-bound drugs such as lidocaine and mepivacaine. Vasoconstrictors such as 0.1 to 0.2 mL of 1:1000 (1 mg/mL) epinephrine solution are sometimes added to the local anesthetic solution to prolong the duration of action. Epinephrine is thought to prolong the duration of spinal anesthesia by causing vasoconstriction, thereby delaying normal uptake of local anesthetics, by direct antinociceptor action, or by a combination of these effects. The effect of added epinephrine on the prolongation of anesthesia is greatest with tetracaine, less with lidocaine, and minimal with bupivacaine. In addition, local anesthetic solutions may include opioids (10 to 25 mcg fentanyl, 10 mcg sufentanil, or 250 mcg preservative-free morphine) or the α-agonist clonidine, 150 mcg, to prolong duration. These agents act at opioid and α_2-adrenergic receptors, respectively. The exact nature of the synergistic effect among opioids, α_2-agonists, and the local anesthetics is not clear, but the result is again prolonged spinal anesthesia. Volume in the tested range of 1 to 14 mL, and therefore concentration, minimally affects the duration of anesthesia or the final sensory level achieved. Increasing the total dose of a spinal local anesthetic will increase its duration of action and affect the sensory level achieved. Duration of sensory and motor blockade for local anesthetics has been shown to be predictable. For example, increasing the dose of hyperbaric bupivacaine from 10 mg to 15 mg prolongs the duration of sensory block by 50% and increases the maximum sensory level achieved. Based on these principles Table 45-3 offers administration suggestions to achieve an approximate sensory level and duration of spinal anesthesia in a typical clinical setting.[41,42]

Selecting the precise site of injection, as mentioned, is technically inaccurate at the clinical level.[7] The higher the site of heartsuitinjection, obviously, the higher the level of sensory

TABLE **45-3**	Choice of Medication for Spinal Anesthesia Used for Surgical Procedures				
Procedure	Medication*	Dosage	Duration Without Epinephrine	Duration With Epinephrine
Vaginal delivery	Tetracaine	5 mg	1-1.5 hr	2.5-3 hr
	Bupivacaine	5-7 mg	1 hr	1.5 hr
	Lidocaine	25 mg	15-25 min	45 min-1 hr
Cesarean section	Tetracaine	8 mg	1-1.5 hr	2.5-3 hr
	Bupivacaine	10 mg	1-1.25 hr	1.5-2 hr
	Lidocaine	50-75 mg	30-45 min	1-1.25 hr
Anorectal surgery	Tetracaine (hyperbaric)	6 mg	1-1.5 hr	3 hr
	Tetracaine (hypobaric)	6 mg	1 hr	3 hr
	Bupivacaine	8 mg	1 hr	1.5-2 hr
	Lidocaine	25-50 mg	15-30 min	45 min
Genital or lower-extremity procedure	Tetracaine	6-10 mg	1.5 hr	2-3 hr
	Bupivacaine	8-12 mg	1.5 hr	2 hr
	Lidocaine	75-100 mg	45-60 min	1.25-1.5 hr
Hernia, pelvic procedure	Tetracaine	10-12 mg	1.5 hr	2-3 hr
	Bupivacaine	12-15 mg	1.5 hr	2 hr
	Lidocaine	100 mg	45-60 min	1.25-1.5 hr
Intraabdominal surgery	Tetracaine (by patient height)	5 ft to 5 ft 5 in = 12 mg 5 t 6 in to 6 ft = 15 mg >6 ft = 18 mg	1.5 hr	2-3 hr
	Bupivacaine (by patient height)	5 ft to 5 ft 5 in = 15 mg 5 ft 6 in to 6 ft = 18 mg >6 ft = 20 mg	1.5 hr	2 hr
Back and spine surgery	Tetracaine	10-15 mg	1-1.5 hr	2-2.5 hr
	Bupivacaine	15-20 mg	1-1.5 hr	1.5-2 hr

Local anesthetic solutions administered to intrathecal or epidural spaces must be sterile and preservative free.

block, but this is limited by the anatomy of the spinal cord and the anesthetist's desire to approach the subarachnoid space below the termination of the spinal cord. Theoretically, if a patient is administered a hyperbaric solution at the L3 level and placed supine, the local anesthetic would flow both cephalad and caudad from the relative peak of the lumbar lordosis to the troughs of the thoracic kyphosis and sacral regions. If a hyperbaric drug is placed below L3 with the patient in a sitting position, and the patient is left sitting for 5 minutes, a lumbar and sacral-root anesthetic known as a *saddle block* will occur. However, even under experimental conditions using the second to fifth lumbar interspace, the data on the ability to control the maximum sensory block level achieved are inconsistent. Therefore, the site of injection can be a poor predictor of the final level of sensory anesthesia achieved.[41]

Several authors suggest that the level of the anesthetic can be adjusted or modified by use of position changes within the first few minutes after injection or until the medication becomes fixed on the nerve roots and the spinal cord. Some have even found that changes in position as late as 60 minutes after injection can alter the level of block achieved. For example, one of the suggested methods used to modify the level of the anesthetic is to raise a supine patient's legs 45 degrees. This position is thought to increase blood flow through the epidural venous plexus,

indirectly altering CSF pressures. Such a position also flattens the lumbar lordosis, altering flow of hyperbaric local anesthetic within the subarachnoid space. The combined effects result in further cephalad spread of local anesthetic solutions. If one uses a similar line of thought, morbid obesity and third trimester pregnancy also are associated with epidural venous engorgement when the patient is supine, and a slightly higher level of spinal anesthesia is found when compared with controls. With traditional hyperbaric solutions, the block achieved may range from T3 to T6. Therefore, the anesthetist's ability to precisely control the level of sensory anesthesia through baricity and changes in posture is associated with great variability and low predictability from patient to patient.[21,41] Once achieved, the final level of sensory blockade should be determined as discussed previously, then documented.

Continuous spinal anesthetics are administered with the same techniques used to establish a spinal or epidural anesthetic. A small epidural needle is used for the procedure, with the bevel turned parallel to dural fibers to help minimize the risk of PDPH. After the needle is inserted into the subarachnoid space, the bevel of the needle is turned either caudad or cephalad to facilitate passage of an epidural catheter into the subarachnoid space. The catheter is inserted only 2 to 3 cm into the subarachnoid space. Further insertion could result in advancement of the catheter along a nerve root or in curling of the catheter. The incidence of headache is minimal in elderly patients or when the catheter can remain in the subarachnoid space for at least 40 hours. Because of reports of cauda equina syndrome, in 1992 the FDA removed from the U.S. market small needles and microcatheters designed to further reduce the risk of PDPH. *Cauda equina syndrome*, or persistent paralysis of the nerves of the cauda equina with resultant lower extremity weakness and bowel and bladder dysfunction, has subsequently been attributed to the deposition of neurotoxic concentrations of hyperbaric local anesthetics, particularly 5% lidocaine.[4,8,16,25,37,42]

This same solution of lidocaine in varying concentrations has been associated with *transient neurologic symptoms* (TNS). Symptoms are usually described as pain originating in the gluteal region that radiates to both lower extremities. Symptoms appear within a few hours up to 24 hours after recovery and spontaneously disappear in virtually all cases in 10 days. The symptoms range from mild to severe radicular back pain in up to 30% of patients, and although NSAIDs are the usual treatment, opioids may be required. Changing concentrations of lidocaine does not seem to affect the incidence of transient symptoms. Although not unique to lidocaine use, the risk of developing TNS is approximately seven times greater after lidocaine administration than after bupivacaine, prilocaine, and procaine administration. The incidence of TNS may be similar with the use of mepivacaine. Other factors have been implicated as contributing to TNS and include knee and hip flexion (presumably stretching nerve roots), obesity, and ambulatory surgery. This complication has prompted many practitioners to modify their use of lidocaine by limiting the dose to a single, rapid, cephalad injection of less than 100 mg when the benefit of a short-acting anesthetic is desired or to avoid its use altogether.*

Physiologic Alterations and Their Management

Spinal anesthesia causes several physiologic changes that are predictable and can usually be readily managed through anticipation and prevention or with minimal intervention. Physiologic changes include effects on the central nervous system, cardiovascular system, respiratory system, and gastrointestinal (GI) system. In addition, physiologic alterations caused by central neural blockade affecting neuroendocrine, renal, and hepatic function are mentioned.

The obvious central nervous system effect of spinal anesthesia is the inhibition of nerve impulse conduction, resulting in spinal anesthesia. This occurs when the local anesthetic concentration exceeds the minimal blocking concentration of the particular nerve exposed to the drug. Neurons have different levels of susceptibility to local anesthetics, and this partially explains the differential block seen with spinal and epidural anesthesia. As a local anesthetic spreads from the epicenter of its injection site, the concentration of molecules decreases. As the local anesthetic spreads rostral and the concentration gradient lessens, only the most susceptible neurons will be blocked, and a differential block occurs. With spinal anesthesia, typically kinesthetic sense is inhibited at a dermatomal level higher than light touch or cold sensation, which in turn is inhibited at a more rostral dermatomal level than pinprick anesthesia. Therefore, a differential blockade among the levels of sympathetic, somatic sensory, and somatic motor fibers can be identified. Attempts to demonstrate the numbers of segments between areas of differential blockade have

found that sympathetic fibers are blocked a mean of six or seven segments higher than somatic sensory fibers.[9,10]

The reticular excitatory area in the brainstem is responsible for the brain's overall state of alertness or arousal. The primary determinant of the activity of the reticular excitatory area is the amount of sensory input from the body. Because spinal anesthesia greatly decreases the number of sensory impulses to the reticular excitatory area, normal patients often experience somnolence. Caution must be taken during administration of spinal anesthesia to a patient in pain and already under the influence of central depressants such as alcohol or opioids. The pain caused by the injury may be the only stimulus for consciousness, and when spinal or other regional anesthesia is instituted, unconsciousness may ensue.[10]

Spinal or epidural techniques using local anesthetics block sympathetic nerve transmission in addition to blocking sensory and motor fibers. Therefore, the sum effect of neuraxial anesthesia on the cardiovascular system depends primarily on the overall degree of sympathetic blockade in terms of the rostral spread of the anesthetic and partially on the degree of patient sedation and central sympathetic inhibition. Blockade of the sympathetic nervous system causes arterial vasodilation, decreased systemic vascular resistance, venous pooling, and a reduction in venous return. These changes cause a redistribution of blood that often results in hypotension. If the block is high enough, the sympathetic nerve fibers that innervate the heart, known as the *cardiac accelerators* (T1 to T4), become anesthetized. An imbalance occurs between vagal fibers, and the heart rate often slows, further contributing to hypotension. Baroreceptor reflexes, volume receptor reflexes, and decreased central sympathetic outflow all contribute to the complexity of the cardiovascular response to neuraxial anesthesia. The overall result is loss of normal cardiovascular homeostatic reflexes and the ability to compensate for minor cardiovascular stresses.[45,46] Rapid changes in position, changes in skeletal muscle tone caused by relaxation, decreased venous return, low preoperative volume status, reflex surgical stimulation, preoperative medications (especially opioid and sedative-hypnotics), and concurrent conditions such as pulmonary embolism, pregnancy, and systemic reactions to medications have all been implicated in increased severity of perioperative hypotension.[10,45]

Hypotension is immediately relevant to the perfusion of critical organs like the heart and brain and is important to all organs in maintaining near homeostasis. Although normotensive patients have been shown to maintain cerebral blood flow despite a moderate decrease in blood pressure, hypertensive subjects may have altered cerebral blood flow autoregulation and are less tolerant of changes in mean arterial pressures.[10] A similar situation exists with elderly patients and patients with known coronary disease. With these caveats in mind, most clinicians allow a decrease in blood pressure of 20% from a patient's baseline before initiating treatment. Clinicians continue to debate the optimal treatment of spinal anesthesia–induced hypotension and bradycardia. The treatment is often dependent on coexisting disease, but some general recommendations can be made. Preventive management of hypotension includes the administration of glucose-free crystalloid or colloid solutions in volumes of approximately 15 mL/kg 15 minutes before the start of the anesthetic procedure to maintain preload to the heart. This initial infusion should include replacement of any fluid deficit caused by restricted oral intake and has been shown to help prevent immediate cardiovascular side effects. Continuous infusions of α-adrenergic vasoconstrictors and sympathomimetic agents have been used to maintain volume preload by increasing central volume and have been shown to help reduce the incidence of

---

*References 4, 8, 14, 21, 23, 25, 38, 43, 44.

cardiovascular side effects requiring treatment. Should the treatment of hypotension become necessary, the ongoing administration of intravenous solution is often the first response; however, excessive fluid therapy can lead to fluid overload and urinary retention, especially in the elderly.[45] Continued treatment is guided by the patient's presenting symptoms and coexisting disease. The heart rate can be used to help guide pharmacologic intervention. Ephedrine (a mixed α- and β-agonist) in 5 to 10 mg intravenous boluses is the agent of choice in patients with symptomatic bradycardia. Ephedrine's indirect effects cause an increase in peripheral vascular resistance and heart rate. If the heart rate is normal or elevated, an α-agonist, such as 50 to 100 mcg of intravenous phenylephrine, causes increased systemic vascular resistance without further increasing the heart rate. The use of phenylephrine may therefore be more efficacious in the elderly. Bradycardia is treated with intravenous atropine 0.4 to 0.8 mg. Severe hypotensive events should be treated vigorously with medication and fluids, because mortality from rare cardiac arrests increases when treatment is delayed.[4,10,14,45]

Most studies demonstrate that midthoracic levels of either spinal or epidural anesthesia have minimal effects on tidal volume, respiratory rate, minute ventilation, and arterial blood gas tensions in otherwise healthy individuals. The phrenic nerve is rarely paralyzed, even when sensory levels reach the cervical dermatomes. However, the accessory abdominal and intercostal muscles for ventilation are impaired, and the ability to cough and clear secretions is inhibited. With the loss of perception of intercostal and abdominal wall muscle movement and the inability to cough, the patient may begin to feel dyspneic. Caution must be exercised if the accompanying anxiety is treated with large doses of sedatives or opioids. They may worsen ventilation and result in hypoxia. Although regional techniques have been shown to have minimal effects, adequate ventilatory ability during surgery is dependent on multiple factors, and improved pulmonary outcomes have not been clearly demonstrated. Some of the factors that affect ventilatory ability under spinal or epidural anesthesia include the presence of coexisting disease, depressant medications, patient position, type and location of the surgery and incision, and presence of hypotension and hemorrhage. The anesthetic plan must be adapted to the patient and the operation.[9,10]

The GI tract is regulated by the parasympathetic and sympathetic nervous systems. The parasympathetic innervation of the GI tract is primarily via the vagus nerves and is composed of both afferent and efferent fibers. Parasympathetic afferent nerves transmit sensations of satiety, distention, and nausea, whereas efferent outflow generally increases GI activities such as tonic contractions, sphincter relaxation, peristalsis, and secretion. Sympathetic innervation of the GI tract stems from the T5 to L2 spinal cord segments and via prevertebral ganglia. Sympathetic afferent nerves are responsible for transmitting pain information; efferent nerves inhibit peristalsis and gastric secretion and cause sphincter contraction and vasoconstriction. When spinal and epidural anesthesia cause a sympathetic blockade, the result is unopposed or dominant parasympathetic activity. The neuraxial sympatholysis results in a generalized constriction of the bowel, normal to increased peristalsis, increased intraluminal pressure, and increased GI blood flow.[9,10,14] The combination of abdominal muscle relaxation and a contracted bowel offers improved operating conditions for intraabdominal procedures, but because gastric motility can be increased, some clinicians have questioned the risk of wound disruption. Several studies have reported that the intraoperative and postoperative use of neuraxial anesthesia does not increase the risk of wound

breakdown. Steinbrook and other researchers suggest that continued postoperative analgesia, especially with a thoracic epidural and local anesthetic infusion, has beneficial effects on the recovery of bowel function after major abdominal surgery.[9,10,47]

Nausea and vomiting are associated with neuraxial block in up to 20% of patients. Nausea and vomiting are primarily related to the GI hyperperistalsis of parasympathetic dominance, although other contributing factors may include hypoxemia, hypotension, systemic medications (opioids or rapidly infused antibiotics), and psychologic stimuli. A cardiac mechanism associated with spinal anesthesia, as proposed by some authors, may also lead to nausea and vomiting. Theoretically, cardiac vagal afferent nerves can be activated in response to a decrease in venous return via ventricular mechanoreceptors, especially with high block levels. Therefore, the vagolytic properties of atropine provide indirect acting antiemetic effects in the treatment of the nausea and vomiting associated with high spinal anesthesia.[10,14]

The neuroendocrine stress response is a combination of responses of the body to tissue trauma (like surgery) or critical illness. The response includes components of neural, immune, endocrine, metabolic, and inflammatory systems that are closely integrated through a complex mechanism of hormones, neurotransmitters, and receptors that affect cells throughout the body. These systems are activated in proportion to the level of critical illness or tissue injury experienced by the body.[10] The stress response is usually associated with increases in blood concentrations of adrenocorticotropins, cortisol, insulin, growth hormone, aldosterone, and glucose. Initially a protective response—the stress response—can lead to tachycardia, hypertension, catabolism, immunosuppression, and hypercoagulability.[9] Regional blocks such as spinal and epidural techniques moderate the stress response to surgery. Although spinal anesthesia blocks this response only for the duration of the anesthetic administration, the use of continuous epidural analgesia well into the postoperative period has the potential to improve perioperative outcome.

Renal blood flow and function are well preserved during spinal anesthesia when blood pressure is maintained. Hepatic blood flow is directly proportional to the mean arterial pressure and therefore depends on the treatment of any hypotension associated with the spinal or epidural anesthetic.[9] Spinal and epidural anesthetics block sympathetic fibers, thereby increasing the tone of the internal urethral sphincter; in addition, neuraxial opioids cause a decrease in detrusor contraction and an increase in bladder capacity. These changes in the genitourinary system can result in the rare complication of urinary retention.

Complications of Spinal Anesthesia
Postdural Puncture Headache
PDPH is perhaps the most commonly discussed and managed complication of neuraxial anesthesia, with a documented incidence that has varied over the years from 0.2% to 24%. Theoretically PDPH is caused by a decrease in the CSF available in the subarachnoid space through a leak created by the dural puncture with an intruding needle. The medulla and brainstem, having lost their hydraulic support, drop into the foramen magnum, stretch the meninges and pull on the tentorium. This pulling, further irritated by movement and the upright position, causes a characteristic headache.[4,16,21,48] A contributing theory suggests that cerebrovasodilation may result from low CSF pressure. This theory is supported by the beneficial effects of vasoconstrictor drugs such as caffeine and theophylline.[48]

Several factors are known to increase the incidence of PDPH. The use of large, non–pencil-point needles or a cutting-needle bevel direction that is perpendicular to the long axis of the body will make larger holes in the dural fibers and create larger CSF leaks. Multiple punctures also increase CSF leak and the risk of headache. In addition, female patients are more likely than male patients to get a PDPH, and the young are more likely than the elderly to experience this complication. Most studies also demonstrate a higher incidence of PDPH in the pregnant population. Patients with a history of PDPHs are predisposed to another headache after a subsequent spinal anesthetic procedure. However, one should keep in mind that not all headaches that follow spinal anesthetic procedures are PDPHs. It is common for patients to experience headaches after surgery and even after general anesthetics. Factors that contribute to headaches may include anxiety, interrupted sleep, dehydration, hypoglycemia, and even simply the lack of normal morning caffeine intake. A differential-diagnosis approach should be taken to identify serious complications such as subdural hematoma, subarachnoid hemorrhage, meningitis, sinusitis, or subarachnoid hemorrhage.[14,16,21,39,48]

Fortunately, PDPHs have several characteristic features that aid in diagnosis. Usually PDPHs occur within several hours to the first or second postoperative day. Historically, bed rest was thought to help prevent PDPH, but subsequent studies found that avoiding early ambulation simply postponed the onset of PDPH. The headache is typically described as a mild to incapacitating bilateral frontal headache that radiates from behind the eyes and across the head toward the occiput and often into the neck and shoulders. The headache is considered positional, because it completely subsides when the patient is lying down. The only other form of headache that has this positional component is caused by pneumocephalus. Other symptoms that may be associated with PDPH include nausea and vomiting, appetite loss, blurred vision or photophobia, a sensation of a plugging of the ears and loss of hearing acuity, tinnitus, vertigo, and depression.[8,16,21,48]

Although PDPHs are self-limiting and often resolve in less than 10 days, early identification and prompt treatment are essential if complications of immobility, depression, and patient dissatisfaction (a potential reason for litigation) are to be avoided. Conservative management includes a horizontal position, adequate hydration, oral analgesics, and the administration of 500 mg intravenous caffeine benzoate, 300 mg of oral caffeine, or theophylline. The horizontal position is impractical for most patients, especially mothers of newborns, and encourages further complications of immobility.[48] Abdominal binders, thought to increase epidural venous plexus blood flow and therefore CSF pressure, are also uncomfortable and often impractical. Increasing fluids during the evaluation and early management period was thought to increase the central volume and increase the secretion of CSF from the choroid plexus, but this is not well supported in the literature. However, adequate hydration should be maintained in all patients.[21] Caffeine and theophylline are both methylxanthine derivatives that cause cerebral vasoconstriction and central nervous system stimulation. Caffeine therapy, both oral and parenteral, is the most commonly used pharmacologic treatment modality; however, theophylline and sumatriptan are promising agents for the treatment of PDPH.[30,39] Caffeine has been shown to eliminate headache in up to 70% of patients, but this effect may be transient. Still, Panzer and co-authors suggested that prophylactic intravenous caffeine administration may safely minimize PDPHs.[49]

An epidural blood patch is considered the definitive treatment for PDPH. Thought to work via clot formation that seals the dural rent and increases CSF pressure, the epidural blood patch is associated with a greater than 90% cure rate. Clinically an epidural blood patch is performed in a manner similar to that of placing an epidural catheter. First, the availability of intravenous access is identified, usually in the antecubital fossa, and informed consent is obtained. Both the patient's back and intravenous access site are prepared and draped in an aseptic manner. An insertion site at or below the level of the lowest initial needle insertion is chosen, because blood has been shown to spread in a predominantly cephalad direction within the epidural space. The epidural space is identified by use of either loss-of-resistance or hanging-drop technique (discussed in the section on epidural anesthesia). Autologous venous blood (approximately 20 mL) is withdrawn from the vein and then slowly injected through the epidural needle into the epidural space. The injection proceeds until the patient senses pressure in the back, buttocks, or legs. Typically, this occurs at a volume of 12 to 15 mL, which is sufficient blood to patch most patients. A supine position should be maintained for $1/2$ to 1 hour before the patient ambulates. Relief of the headache is often instantaneous. In the rare case in which an epidural blood patch fails, a repeat blood patch may be attempted in 24 hours, with a similar success rate.[16,21,48]

The success rate and excellent safety record of the epidural blood patch encourages the use of this therapeutic option early in the treatment of PDPH. However, some risks, although minor or rare, are associated with this more invasive procedure. Backache, often associated with the administration of general, spinal, or epidural anesthetic techniques, occurs in up to 35% of patients after an epidural blood patch. Although rarely as debilitating as a PDPH, backache risk should be explained to the patient. The most common cause of backache is relaxation of the muscles of the back and flattening of the normal lordotic curve. As the muscles stretch, injury to tendons and ligaments can occur. The position of the patient might increase the severity of the problem. An exaggerated lithotomy position or a completely supine position can further increase tension on tendons, resulting in increased trauma to both the muscles and the tendons. Trauma from multiple punctures, hemorrhage, infections, use of large needles, retractors, and forceps; extremes of positions; preexisting diseases such as arthritis and osteoporosis; and prolonged labor can contribute to backaches that may persist well into the postoperative period.[21,48]

Management of backache includes the use of antispasmodics and NSAIDs to reduce discomfort, permit ambulation, and promote a more rapid recovery. In addition, authors have reported a 5% incidence of transient (24- to 48-hour) temperature elevation, a 1% incidence of neck ache, radicular pain, nerve root irritation, cranial nerve palsy, and meningitis, although the cause of meningitis was unproven.[21,48]

Several caveats regarding the treatment of PDPH are worth mentioning. Systemic infection, perhaps indicated by fever, presents a relative contraindication to epidural blood patch and warrants a trial of pharmacologic intervention. The risk of neurologic sequelae after epidural blood patch in the presence of HIV infection or sepsis is controversial, because few data are available, leading some authors to suggest alternative therapies such as epidural 0.9% sodium chloride or dextran.[14,35,48] Prophylactic epidural blood patch placement has not been shown to be consistently successful.[16] In light of the relatively low incidence of PDPH and the effectiveness of the epidural blood patch, treatment should not begin until the problem exists. Finally, an alternative diagnosis should be sought if two epidural blood patches fail to resolve the patient's symptoms.[21,48]

Nausea

As with general anesthesia, intraoperative and postoperative nausea and vomiting (PONV) associated with CNB is a complex issue. Although it is believed that PONV is less common with regional anesthesia techniques than general anesthesia techniques, agents such as propofol have considerably narrowed the incidence gap. Although not life-threatening, PONV remains a significant concern for patients and clinicians. General strategies can be implemented to help reduce the incidence of this unpleasantness.

Nausea immediately after the initiation of CNB is often considered a sign of significant hypotension and a climbing block level. Resulting cerebral ischemia affects the vomiting centers of the medulla, possibly triggering nausea. Others posit that gut ischemia leads to the release of emetogenic substances like serotonin. Fluid and sympathomimetic administration treats the hypotension, and the nausea resolves. Another contributing element may result from the sympathectomy caused by the onset of CNB. The resulting unopposed parasympathetic activity in the gastrointestinal tract results in hyperactivity, possibly contributing to nausea. Evidence that this may be the case is that vagolytic agents such as atropine are efficacious in treating this nausea.[50]

Avoiding hypotension, providing adequate hydration, and supporting perfusion with supplemental oxygen are the basis of an antiemetic plan for CNB. Premedication and intraoperative sedation can significantly affect the incidence of intraoperative and PONV. Clonidine does not influence the incidence of PONV, and evidence supports that propofol and midazolam have antiemetic effects. The addition of epinephrine to local anesthetics administered intrathecally for spinal anesthesia increases the incidence of nausea. Also, a dose-dependent increase in PONV occurs when intrathecal morphine is used. However, the addition of 20 mcg fentanyl or 2.5 to 5 mcg of sufentanil to spinal bupivacaine results in less intraoperative nausea compared with placebo. Similar strategies apply to epidural anesthesia, although opioid use must be matched to patient and case type to maximize analgesia while minimizing secondary effects.[50]

Urinary Retention

Urinary retention can occur after anesthesia and surgery because spinal or epidural anesthetics block sympathetic fibers and increase the tone of the internal urethral sphincter. However, other factors often contribute to the risk of urinary retention after surgery and anesthesia. These include the type of surgical procedure, bladder distention from the administration of large volumes of intravenous fluids, bladder trauma, prolonged hypotension, incision pain, urethral edema caused by prolonged labor, benign prostatic hypertrophy, and the use of neuraxial or intraoperative opioids. Some authors suggest that spinal anesthesia may even carry a lower risk of urinary retention when compared with general anesthesia. In any case, urinary retention and subsequent catheterization can lead to complications such as urinary tract infections and urethral strictures. Attempts should first be made to allow the patient every opportunity to void in a natural position. Save urethral catheterization as a last resort.[15]

Neurologic Risk

Patients greatly fear the perceived risk of paraplegia resulting from neuraxial anesthetics, and the seriousness of such complications warrants concern. However, several very large series have shown that the incidence of persistent motor paralysis is exceedingly rare (<1 per 10,000). Because neurologic sequelae are rare, the knowledge base of complications comes from case studies, and often the cause is not proved but rather inferred by association. Direct needle or catheter nerve injury, drug-related neurotoxicity, anterior spinal artery syndrome, undiagnosed neurologic disease, intraneural or intramedullary injections, the presence of blood in the CSF, patient positioning, hematomas, and abscesses are associated with permanent neurologic deficits. Therefore, good clinical practice depends on (1) the use of appropriate anesthetic techniques that minimize risk and (2) the conduct of postoperative assessments in a manner that promotes early detection, diagnosis, and treatment—especially because reversibility of complications is often time dependent.[14,21,23,51] Transient neurologic symptoms are discussed in Chapter 11.

Unexpected Cardiac Arrest

Cardiac arrest associated with neuraxial anesthesia is often sudden and unexpected and can result in severe neurologic injury and death. Additionally, this undesired complication occurs in a significant number of young, previously healthy patients. Estimates of occurrence have ranged from 0.04:10,000 to 6.25:10,000 for spinal anesthesia and slightly less for epidural anesthesia. This suggests that cardiac arrest is not such a rare event in neuraxial anesthesia. How then might it be differentiated from arrests under general anesthesia (5.5:10,000)?[52] Because unexpected cardiac arrest with spinal anesthesia has been reported in previously healthy patients, some authors consider this a physiologic response to neuraxial blocks. Other authors suggest a pattern of presentation with a gradual downward trend in heart rate followed by an abrupt onset of severe bradycardia or asystole.[10] Spinal anesthesia cardiac arrest can occur well after the onset of spinal blockade. Large and recent retrospective studies note that arrests can occur 20 to 60 minutes after the onset of spinal blockade and are frequently associated with intraoperative events such as significant blood loss and orthopedic cement placement.[53] Liguori and Sharrock's review of 12 epidural anesthetic cases with arrest found that severe bradycardia or asystole could develop in seconds or minutes from a stable heart rate, a downward trend, or even increasing heart rate trends.[54] Asystole or bradycardia may occur as late as 3 hours after epidural injection. Although it has been hypothesized that the Bezold-Jarisch reflex (BJR) is the predominant reflex involved, evidence to support this idea is minimal. Current speculations suggest at least two or more mechanisms are involved in addition to a paradoxical BJR. These include activation of low-pressure right atrial baroreceptors, activation of receptors within myocardial pacemaker cells, a high sympathetic level, sedation, hypoxemia, and hypercarbia—which all contribute to decreased ventricular filling pressures, bradycardia, and asystole.[52,53] Vigilance, awareness, and aggressive treatment are essential because prophylaxis with volume loads, chronotropic support, or vagolysis remains unproven in the complete prevention of this untoward complication. In addition to pacing and cardiopulmonary resuscitation, pharmacologic intervention should be aggressive and include intravascular fluids, atropine, and cardiac resuscitation doses of epinephrine.[10,54]

Auditory, Ocular, and Facial Complications

Unexpected complications or complications that a patient may not ascribe to anesthesia may be unreported or underreported, especially if they are transient in nature and not life threatening.

The complications of transient hypoacusis or hearing loss and retinal hemorrhage are thought to be caused by changes in CSF pressure, either from postdural puncture leaks or increases in pressure from the epidural administration of a large volume of solution. Epidural injection of 8 to 16 mL of fluid can increase CSF pressure by 85 cm H_2O for several minutes before compensation occurs. Horner syndrome (ptosis, miosis, anhidrosis, and enophthalmos) and trigeminal nerve palsy probably result from a high spread of local anesthetic to the sympathetic fibers of the head and neck and to cranial nerve V, respectively. These problems are usually self-limiting; however, knowledge of their previous occurrence enables the compassionate anesthetist to provide counsel and reassurance to anxious patients.[25,55]

EPIDURAL ANESTHESIA

Epidural anesthesia is a central neuraxial block that can be used for a wide variety of procedures. Unlike spinal anesthesia that results in an all-or-none block, epidural anesthesia can be titrated to deliver either analgesia or anesthesia for a wide variety of surgical and analgesic procedures. Epidural anesthesia allows the anesthesia practitioner better control of the extent of sensory and motor blockade than is offered by spinal anesthesia. The luxury of placing an epidural catheter that can be used before, during, and for an extended period following any surgical procedure is another advantage. The general indications for epidural anesthesia are the same as those outlined for spinal anesthesia, with the distinct difference that epidural anesthesia allows for continuous anesthesia secondary to placement of an epidural catheter. This makes epidural anesthesia more suitable for procedures of long duration and for extended use in the postoperative period to deliver long-term, titratable analgesia.

Local anesthetics or other analgesic solutions injected into the epidural space spread anatomically. Horizontally, medication spreads to the regions of the dural cuffs, where it is able to diffuse into the CSF and leak into the intravertebral foramen and paravertebral spaces to achieve analgesia/anesthesia. Longitudinally, medication spreads in a cephalad direction, with possible sites of anesthetic action along the paravertebral nerve trunks, intradural spinal roots, dorsal and ventral spinal roots, the dorsal root ganglia, the spinal cord, and the brain. Initial blockade is probably a result of anesthetic blockade at the spinal roots within the dural sleeves.[4] The dural cuffs or sleeves have a proliferation of arachnoid villi and granulations that effectively reduce the thickness of the dura mater, permitting rapid diffusion of anesthetics from the epidural space through the dura and into the CSF. Differences in physicochemical properties of anesthetics (e.g., lipid solubility) may account for the differences in diffusion rates across the dura, which contributes to the variances seen in sensory, motor, and sympathetic blockade.[5] Because epidural anesthesia is diffusion dependent, relatively large volumes (20 mL) of local anesthetics must be used to achieve anesthesia as compared with spinal anesthesia, which routinely only requires 1 to 2 mL. In addition, because epidural anesthesia requires that the medication be delivered to the subarachnoid space by the process of diffusion and spread, anesthesia takes significantly longer to achieve than spinal anesthesia. Given these caveats, any procedure that can be done with the patient under spinal anesthesia can also be done under epidural anesthesia.[4] However, epidural techniques allow for the placement of a continuous catheter, which is especially useful in cases of unpredictable duration, for prolonged postoperative analgesia, and for chronic pain control. In addition, labor epidural analgesia is the only method currently available that can relieve most of the discomfort of labor while minimally affecting maternal or fetal physiology. Labor epidural analgesia is highly satisfactory in these patients because it permits their participation in a comfortable delivery and allows maternal-infant bonding after delivery. Labor analgesia also satisfies obstetricians and anesthesia practitioners in that its flexibility allows quick conversion from an analgesic technique to a surgical anesthetic technique for cesarean section.

Equipment and Techniques

Patient preparation and positioning and the availability of emergency equipment and monitors are similar to the preparation for a spinal anesthetic. With a spinal anesthetic, the practitioner seeks CSF by piercing the dura, while the tip of the epidural needle seeks the fat-filled space deep to the ligamenta flava and shallow to the dura. The standard epidural needle is typically 16 to 18 gauge and 3 inches long, with a blunted bevel and gentle curve of 15 to 30 degrees at the tip. This blunt bevel and curve allow the needle to pass through the skin and ligamenta flava and abut against the dura, or push away from the dura, rather than penetrate through the dura. The two most common epidural needles used in clinical practice with a curvature at the blunt bevel are the Tuohy and Hustead needle designs. The Tuohy needle has the most pronounced curvature (30 degrees) at the tip and is often cited as the easiest for beginning practitioners to place because it allows directional placement of the epidural catheter into the space and the curved, blunt tip is less likely to penetrate into the subarachnoid space. However, it has also been noted that placement of the Tuohy needle can be more difficult because the tip's exaggerated curvature is too blunt, inhibiting penetration through the skin and ligamenta flava as compared with other needle tips. The Hustead needle is an intermediate needle with a less pronounced 15-degree curvature that can more easily pass though skin and ligamenta flava.

A third epidural needle is the Crawford needle. It is a thin-walled epidural needle that does not have the curvature of the Tuohy or Hustead needle. The straight tip may allow easier access through the skin into the epidural space. The Crawford needle is preferred by practitioners when catheter advancement into the epidural space is difficult or the angle of approach is steep, as encountered with thoracic epidural catheter placement. Because the Crawford needle lacks the curvature at the bevel end, it also has been implicated in a higher ratio of accidental dural punctures and is typically not used by beginning practitioners. These three common epidural needles are shown in Figure 45-12. Smaller-gauge (20 to 22 gauge) epidural needles are available in each needle design for pediatric catheter techniques, regional blocks, and specialty use. Many needle designs incorporate wings near the base or hub. The wings provide a grip for the practitioner that permits distribution of pressure equally over the needle during insertion. The wings and notches in the hub also align with the stylet and needle tip to indicate the direction of the needle tip's bevel and lumen. Needles may also have clear hubs to allow early detection of blood or CSF, plastic stylets to prevent coring, and 0.5- or 1-cm depth markings along the needle shaft.

Epidural catheters also come in a variety of materials and designs. Typically, catheter diameter is 2 gauges smaller than the needle. For example, a 20-gauge catheter would be used with an 18-gauge Tuohy needle. Catheters are constructed of physiologically inert materials designed to resist kinking, compression, and stretching and should be radiopaque. The two most common epidural catheters used in clinical practice are the single-holed, open-ended (uniport) and lateral-holed, closed tip

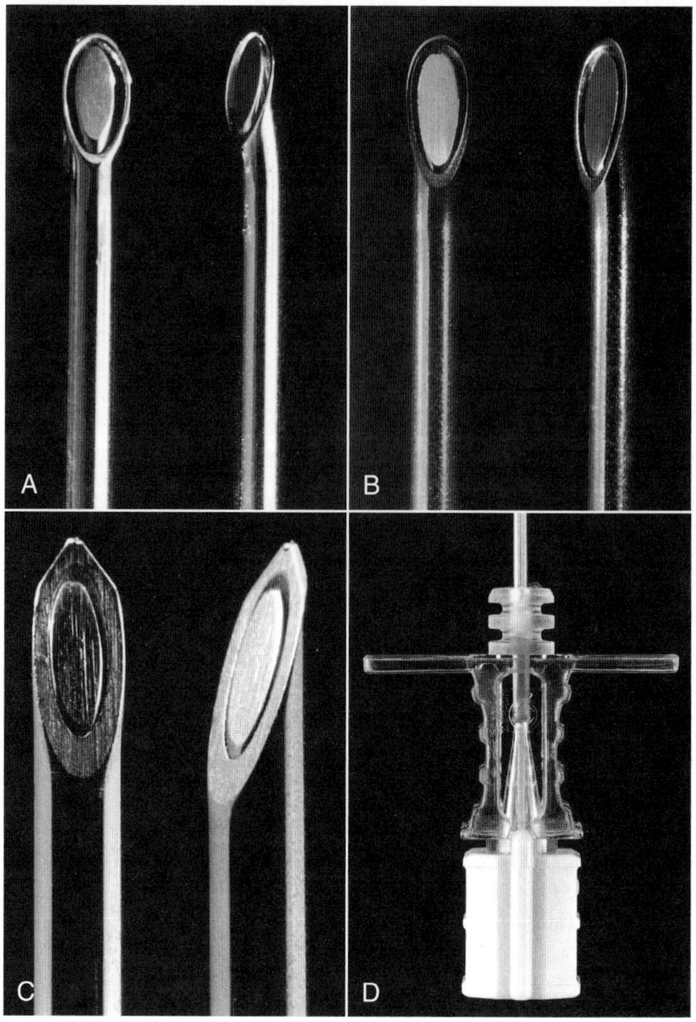

FIGURE **45-12** Epidural needle design features. **A,** Hustead. **B,** Tuohy. **C,** Crawford. **D,** Weiss-style "winged" epidural needle hub with tab and notch stylet. (From Miller RD. Miller's Anesthesia. 6th ed. Philadelphia: Churchill Livingstone; 2005:1666,1671).

(multiport) epidural catheters. Each catheter design is reported to offer several advantages and disadvantages. Studies that have compared the differences in catheter designs show a significantly lower incidence of inadequate analgesia with multiport catheters but a higher incidence of inadvertent intravenous cannulation.[56] Catheters have markings that identify the tip of the catheter to help verify removal of the catheter and identify when the catheter is at the tip of the needle, with 1-cm markings to measure depth of catheter placement. The depth that a catheter should be threaded beyond the needle tip and into the epidural space is often a controversial topic. Manufacturers of epidural catheters recommend that a catheter should be threaded 1 to 3 cm into the epidural space to avoid possible migration into an epidural vein or through an intravertebral foramen.[14,57] However, in clinical practice practitioners noted that when an epidural catheter was only threaded 1 to 3 cm, a higher incidence of epidural catheter failure could result. Many practitioners reported anecdotally that when the catheter was threaded 3 to 5 cm into the epidural space, a higher success rate without a resultant increase in migration into an epidural vein or intravertebral foramen occurred. This routine clinical practice was validated by Beilin and colleagues. They reported that a catheter insertion of less than 3 cm resulted in a higher incidence of inadequate analgesia, and an insertion depth of more than 5 cm resulted in an increase in inadvertent

intravenous cannulation. They recommended that optimal catheter insertion should be 3 to 5 cm into the epidural space.[57]

Proper patient positioning is important to ensure successful catheter placement. Epidural anesthesia is most often instituted with the patient in the sitting or lateral decubitus position and the landmarks, aseptic preparation, draping, and localization are similar to those for a spinal anesthetic. The spine should be in proper alignment, using pillows or pads if necessary, and intervertebral spaces need to be identified and marked prior to preparation of the patient's back (see Figure 45-8). In contrast to thin, flexible spinal needles, epidural needles are larger and more rigid. Therefore, placement of the epidural needle does not require an introducer needle and offers better directional control; however, all needle-handling techniques must anticipate patient movement. Whether inserting a spinal or epidural needle into a patient, a similar controlled grip is used to accommodate for potential patient movement. This grip, described earlier as the *Bromage grip* (see Figure 45-11), allows the patient's body to act as a firm support for the needle-stabilizing hand and helps prevent advancement or withdrawal of the needle tip from its position (1) if the patient should move, (2) when the syringe is applied, and (3) as a catheter is passed into the epidural space. The needle is placed bevel tip cephalad through the supraspinous ligament and seated in the interspinous ligament before the stylet is removed. After the stylet is removed, the needle is slowly advanced by use of either the hanging-drop technique or the loss-of-resistance technique into the epidural space.[5]

After the needle is seated in the interspinous ligament, the hanging-drop technique is accomplished by filling the hub of the needle with saline. The surface tension of the saline creates a droplet hanging on the needle hub. The needle is then advanced slowly in a slight cephalad orientation toward the epidural space. As the needle is advanced through the ligamentous structures, the drop should not move; however, as the tip of the needle enters into the epidural space, the negative pressure within the space will cause the drop of fluid to be drawn into the needle. This aspiration of the hanging drop into the needle signifies that the needle has successfully entered the epidural space. It should be noted that if the needle becomes plugged or the negative pressure in the epidural space is very low, the drop will not be drawn into the hub of the needle and passage into the epidural space will not be recognized. A dural puncture could result. Therefore, the hanging-drop technique is not recommended for the novice practitioner.[5]

The loss-of-resistance technique is the most common method used to enter the epidural space. The epidural needle is placed through the dermis into the interspinous ligament or ligamenta flava, at which time the stylet of the epidural needle is removed. Once the needle has been firmly seated into ligament, a loss-of-resistance syringe (plastic or glass) containing 2 to 3 mL of normal saline or air and a freely movable plunger is attached. If the needle is properly seated in the ligament, it should be difficult to inject the normal saline or air, and slight pressure on the syringe plunger should result in the plunger springing back to its original position. Some practitioners use a combination of saline and air in the syringe during the loss-of-resistance technique, using approximately 3 mL of normal saline and a small air bubble (0.1 to 0.3 mL). They report that this provides them with a more compressible feel for entry into the ligamenta flava. If the air bubble cannot be compressed without injecting the normal saline, the needle is most likely not seated into the ligamenta flava and may still be in the interspinous ligament or off midline into the paraspinous muscles. The needle is advanced toward the epidural space by application of pressure to the needle, not the syringe or syringe plunger. If normal saline is used, constant pressure may be applied to the syringe plunger. Contact with the needle or needle wings is maintained to control needle advancement. As the needle passes through the ligamenta flava, resistance increases, and it is very difficult to inject either saline or air. Once the bevel of the needle completes the passage through the ligamenta flava and enters the epidural space, an immediate loss of resistance occurs. The contents of the syringe can then be injected gently and without resistance. After the syringe is removed from the needle, an outward rush of a small amount of air or fluid may occur. Penetration of the dura with a large epidural needle usually results in profuse return of CSF; the needle should be removed immediately to minimize CSF loss.

The loss of resistance experienced by a beginning practitioner, or by the experienced practitioner with a patient with difficult anatomy, may not be easily discerned. Sometimes it may be necessary to further evaluate the needle tip's location. For example, several mL of air can be injected through the needle while the soft tissue lateral to the spinous process is palpated. If crepitus is felt, the needle is most likely located in the tissues adjacent and shallow to the spinous process. If fluid returns from either the needle or catheter, CSF can be distinguished from normal saline

(NS) or local anesthetic. CSF is warm to the forearm, compared with recently administered room-temperature fluids. Glucose test paper will detect the glucose in CSF. Local anesthetics mixed with a similar volume of thiopental will immediately form a precipitate. Multiple tests should be used to achieve the most accurate confirmation of fluid type.

Once the practitioner is reassured of the needle tip's position, an epidural catheter is threaded through the needle and into the epidural space to a depth of 3 to 5 cm. As the catheter is passed into the epidural space, it is important to warn the patient that a "funny bone" sensation may be experienced down one or both legs. This is a paresthesia that may indicate that the catheter has brushed by a nerve root as it was passing into the epidural space or perhaps even lodged into the nerve root. If the paresthesia is persistent prior to or following needle removal, the catheter must be withdrawn and replaced. Injection of medication into a patient complaining of persistent paresthesias can result in nerve-root damage or even nerve-root death and cause long-term morbidities. If the catheter is being replaced secondary to a persistent paresthesia, it is best to move to a new interspace to avoid oversensitized nerve roots. It is important that the needle remain stabilized during catheter advancement. Often if a patient does experience a paresthesia during threading of the catheter, the patient will move reflexively. Unanticipated movement and an uncontrolled needle could result in inadvertent subarachnoid puncture. Once the catheter is threaded approximately 3 to 5 cm, the needle is withdrawn slowly over the catheter. It is common practice to note the depth of the catheter at the level of the skin (by noting the cm-depth mark on the catheter) both prior to and following removal of the epidural needle. Once the epidural needle is removed, the catheter depth should be noted and documented. If the catheter was inadvertently threaded deeper than desired into the epidural space, it should be slightly withdrawn to the desired depth as noted at the level of the skin. If the catheter migrated out of the epidural space, again the depth should be observed and recorded. Finally, if the depth into the epidural space is less than 1 cm, replacement of the catheter should be considered before any attempts are made to inject through the catheter. Never attempt to withdraw the catheter through the needle! This can shear the catheter and embed foreign material in the patient's back. Surgical intervention may be required for catheter remnant removal.

Once a catheter is placed and the needle removed safely, a catheter-to-syringe adapter is placed on the free catheter end. Observe the clear catheter as it enters the back. Look for backflow of CSF or blood. Owing to the greater resistance of a long and narrow catheter compared with a needle, gravity flow alone may not reveal the presence of blood or CSF. Therefore, gentle syringe aspiration is applied to the catheter via the adapter. Because tissue at the catheter tip may create a ball-valve effect, CSF or blood may not flow out; therefore, a negative aspiration test does not guarantee that the catheter tip is in the epidural space. Only if fluids do return does this test confirm that the catheter tip is placed either into an epidural vein or the subarachnoid space. The return of CSF or blood indicates that the catheter should be removed and replaced at a different interspace. To avoid this ball-valve effect or to dislodge any skin or tissue that may have lodged at the catheter tip, some practitioners advocate injection of 1 to 2 mL of normal saline solution through the catheter to confirm catheter patency before injection of medications. After needle removal, the catheter should be taped away from the midline of the back to avoid spinous processes and minimize the risks of catheter displacement from the epidural space or pressure injuries over bony prominences.

Prior to injection of a large amount of medication into an epidural space, a test dose of a small amount of medication is administered to determine if the catheter or needle has inadvertently entered the subarachnoid space or possibly threaded into an epidural vein. A test dose of 3 mL of a rapid-acting, low-toxicity local anesthetic agent with or without a small concentration of epinephrine is most typically used. A lidocaine 1.5% with 1:200,000 epinephrine solution provides 45 mg of lidocaine with 15 mcg of epinephrine per 3 mL dose. If the needle or catheter tip is in the subarachnoid space, this dose will result in spinal anesthesia within 3 minutes. If the same test dose is injected into a blood vessel, the 15 mcg of epinephrine will result in a 20% rise in heart rate and systolic blood pressure within 30 seconds. The patient may also experience sensations from the intravascular lidocaine, describing symptoms such as tinnitus, a metallic taste, circumoral numbness, or a rushing sound in the ears. The duration of these test-dose effects is less than 5 minutes. After the test dose is injected, vital signs are reassessed. Additionally, 100 mcg of undiluted fentanyl can be injected as a test dose to avoid potential complications caused by even low doses of epinephrine. If the needle or catheter is intravascular, the patient will experience immediate dizziness and sleepiness from the opioid. Despite all efforts to avoid them, systemic toxic reactions can still occur. Be vigilant, be cautious, and be prepared to handle emergencies.[58,59]

Epidural anesthesia can also be administered by direct injection through the needle once it has been placed into the epidural space. This is called a "single shot" epidural anesthesia technique, and the same contraindications and safety precautions apply as those already reported for catheter insertion. Once the needle is placed into the epidural space, the end of the open needle is observed for the presence of blood or CSF. Allow a few seconds for gravity flow of fluids to detect blood or CSF when the single-shot technique is used, then attach a syringe for medication administration using needle control techniques previously discussed.

Epidural anesthesia can be performed at any of the four segments of the spine but is most typically performed at the lumbar level. As with spinal anesthesia, there are two approaches, the midline and paramedian approach, that are used to facilitate placement of the epidural needle into the epidural space. The most common approach is the midline approach because it is the easiest to perform and helps place the catheter in the medial region of the epidural space. The paramedian approach is usually selected when surgery or degenerative joint disease contraindicate the midline approach. Using the paramedian approach is more difficult for the beginner because advancement into the interspinous ligament does not occur. The needle advances primarily through paraspinous muscle mass, and resistance is only felt when entering the ligamenta flava. The technique for paramedian placement involves identification of the desired interspace and the spinous process. The skin surface area approximately 3 cm lateral to the lowest aspect of the spinous process is prepped and anesthetized. The epidural needle is then placed through the anesthetized region and directed toward the midline using a slight cephalad orientation. Once the dermal levels are penetrated and the paraspinous muscle mass encountered, the needle stylet is removed and attached to a syringe containing either air or normal saline (or both) and advanced. The midline of the spine should be encountered approximately 3 to 5 cm from the entry point. The needle is advanced slowly using the incremental approach described earlier through ligamenta flava and then into the epidural space. When a paramedian approach is required by difficult surface anatomy or a steep approach to the thoracic levels is anticipated, the Crawford needle may be preferred. The Crawford needle's straight, blunt bevel allows the catheter to pass directly through the end of the needle, thus facilitating threading of the catheter.

Epidural Drugs, Spread, and Block Levels

As with any anesthetic technique, the clinical success of epidural anesthesia is often dependent on experience because multiple factors must be managed and balanced to provide safe patient care. Two of these factors, dose and the site of injection, are the most important factors in determining the extent of dermatomal blockade. It should be remembered that the size of the segmental epidural spaces increases down the spinal cord as the spinal cord occupies less and less space. For example, when a very small volume of local anesthetic is injected into the cervical region, it will spread across a larger number of segments as compared with when the same volume is injected into the thoracic region. This is also true when comparing the dermatomal spread between the thoracic and lumbar or caudal regions. The suggested dose of local anesthetic is dependent on the location of the catheter tip as it lies in the epidural space. Common clinical practice is to insert the epidural needle at a vertebral interspace such that the catheter tip falls near the middle of the spinal dermatomes of the proposed surgical incision. For example, an epidural catheter placed for labor or lower abdominal anesthesia would be placed at the L2 or L3 interspace. Placement would be at T8 to T10 for upper abdominal surgery; T4 to T5 for thoracic surgery; and C7 to T1 for chronic pain treatments or surgeries of the arms, shoulders, or upper chest. This has several advantages. The catheter tip, being at the relative center of the spread of the local anesthetic, creates an area of high concentration at the spinal nerves specific to the site of the operation with the least amount of local anesthetic. This high concentration at a specific location results in rapid block onset and greater block density, which often creates a differential blockade that can be controlled by dose. Dose is described as volume multiplied by concentration. The concentration of the local anesthetic generally affects the density of the block, whereas the volume, within limits, affects the spread from the needle or catheter tip throughout the epidural space. Successful analgesia can be achieved with relatively small volumes and high concentrations of local anesthetics. Clinically useful doses are based on volumes that permit an even filling of the anterior and posterior epidural spaces at the level of insertion. For example, the suggested volumes per segment at the cervical and thoracic levels are 0.7 to 1 mL per segment, remembering that the spread will occur in both a cephalad and caudad fashion. Therefore, an initial total dose, usually less than 10 mL, will achieve a 10- to 14-dermatomal spread of local anesthetic. In contrast, when the local anesthetic is injected at the lumbar level, the volume of local anesthetic required is 1.25 to 1.5 mL per segment. A typical initial volume of 15 to 20 mL is required to ensure adequate anesthesia by blocking a total of 12 to 16 segments (6 to 8 segments above and below the catheter tip). Also, it should be remembered that spread of blockade tends to occur faster in the cephalad direction from the catheter tip, possibly because thoracic nerve roots are smaller in diameter than large lumbar and sacral nerve roots.[4,5,8]

Other factors thought to affect the level of blockade achieved with epidural anesthesia include height, weight, age, patient position during injection, pregnancy, and the speed or mode of injection. However, the clinical significance of these factors has been challenged. Correlations between patient height and weight and the spread of the epidural block are clinically insignificant, except, perhaps, in the extremely tall, short, or morbidly obese. Studies have examined patients in the sitting and lateral positions during administration of epidural anesthetics and found small differences in spread and onset that favor the dependent portion of the patient's body. Therefore, provision of anesthesia to the sacral roots might be facilitated by having the patient sit up during the injection. In addition, leaving the patient on the operative side after the solution is injected may speed onset. However, these are clinically small differences and may not always be effective. Drugs should be injected slowly into the epidural space to avoid rapid increases in CSF pressure, headache, and increased intracranial pressure. A rapid speed of injection has not been shown to increase the spread of anesthetic. Also, incremental or bolus injection modes appear to have no influence on spread. The spread of epidural anesthetics may be three or four dermatomes greater in elderly patients, because age-related tissue changes create a less compliant and less leaky epidural space. Although conflicting data exist, some studies suggest that the epidural spread of anesthetics is greater in pregnant patients.[4,5,8] Therefore, it is recommended that the volume of anesthetic solution administered to pregnant patients and elderly patients should initially be limited to 0.5 to 1 mL per segment when injected at lumbar levels. The density of block is also more dependent on the concentration of local anesthetic used. The lower the concentration, the lower the effect the local anesthetic will have on the degree of sensory and motor blockade. Routinely a lower concentration of local anesthetic is used to facilitate analgesia (as in laboring analgesia) or to provide a sympathectomy. If the primary purpose of the epidural is to provide complete surgical anesthesia, higher concentrations must be used. Table 45-4 lists recommended volumes of local anesthetic based on the position of the catheter and the location of the intended surgical intervention.

All solutions should be injected in increments of 3 to 5 mL every 3 minutes and titrated to the desired anesthetic level. With loading doses and intermittent injections, aspiration of the catheter should occur before any injection. This gradual administration of the medication slows the rate of onset of the anesthetic level and controls the development of the sympathetic blockade. After a loading dose is given, the anesthetic is maintained with either intermittent dosing or a continuous infusion technique. Intermittent injections are most often used when high concentrations of local anesthetic (2% lidocaine or 0.5% ropivacaine) are administered. A continuous infusion is more appropriate when the goal of the epidural is to provide a consistent level of analgesia. Continuous infusions typically use a lower concentration of local anesthetic solution (0.0625% to 0.125% bupivacaine or 0.1% to 0.2% ropivacaine), and the level of block is monitored on a regular interval basis. A continuous opioid infusion may also be used either as a sole agent or as an admixture with low concentrations of local anesthetic. Typical infusion rates range from as low as 2 mL/hr for concentrated hydrophilic opioid solutions, such as preservative-free morphine, up to 20 mL/hr for dilute solutions of local anesthesia (0.125% bupivacaine or 0.1% ropivacaine) used for postoperative or labor analgesia. Often, continuous infusions will contain a dilute concentration of local anesthetic solution with an admixture of a low-dose lipophilic opioid such as fentanyl, 1 to 5 mcg/mL, or sufentanil, 1 to 1.5 mcg/mL. Epidural infusions of these mixtures augment the quality

TABLE **45-4**	Recommended Doses for Epidural Analgesia		
Procedure	**Position of Catheter**	**Dose (mL)**
Chest	T12-L2	8-12
Upper Abdomen		
Cholecystectomy	L2	12-16
Gastric resection	L2	12-16
Incisional pain	L2	7-10
Lower Abdomen		
Colon resection	L2	12-16
Repair of aortic aneurysm	L2	12-16
Retropubic prostatectomy	L3	12-16
Herniorrhaphy	L3	8-12
Incisional pain	L3	8-12
Pancreatic pain	L3	5-7
Hysterectomy	L3	10-14
Lower Extremities		
Anesthesia	L4	10-14
Sympathetic block	L2	5-7
Perineum		
Transurethral resection of prostate	L4	8-12
Vaginal hysterectomy	L4	8-12
Back and Flank		
Nephrectomy	L2	10-14
Vaginal Delivery		
First-stage labor	L3	5-7
Second-, third-stage labor	L3	10-12

and duration of analgesia while limiting the side effects of any one drug.

Epidural Opioids

Opioids placed into the epidural space may undergo uptake into the epidural fat, systemic absorption, or diffusion across the dura into the CSF.[60] When administered via the epidural route, opioids produce considerable CSF concentrations of drug. Penetration of the dura from the epidural space into the subarachnoid space is influenced by lipid solubility and molecular weight. The administration of an epidural opioid by either an intermittent or continuous infusion has become common in many anesthesia practices. When an opioid is administered epidurally, it needs to cross from the epidural space through the dura to reach the opioid receptors located in the substantia gelatinosa in the spinal cord. Besides the physical barrier of the dura, epidural opioids may also be deposited in the fat and connective tissues in the epidural space, which may significantly increase the opioid dose required to achieve analgesia. In fact, in order to achieve adequate analgesia from epidurally administered opioids, the dose is increased by approximately 10 times the opioid dose administered intrathecally. Also, the epidural space is highly vascularized, and there is significant absorption of the opioids into the systemic circulation; however, the rate of absorption is dependent on individual pharmacokinetics and lipid solubility of the opioid. For example, epidural administration of fentanyl and sufentanil (highly lipid-soluble opioids) results in a serologic level of opioid similar to that produced when the drugs are administered intravenously.[60] When an opioid is administered by the epidural route, the onset of action and duration are dependent on the type of drug used. A faster onset and analgesic peak effect is achieved when a more lipophilic opioid is used versus an opioid that is more lipophobic. Epidural opioids can be administered by either a single bolus dose or a continuous infusion. A continuous infusion provides easier analgesic titration to patient requirements, which is especially important when a shorter-acting opioid such as fentanyl is used. Epidural opioids can also be administered using patient-controlled (assisted) epidural analgesia (PCEA), which is a hybrid of continuous infusion and patient-assisted boluses to titrate analgesic requirements based on individual patient needs. The goal is to establish a continuous or "basal rate" infusion to optimize the analgesic effect. The PCEA bolus component can then be preset by the anesthesia practitioner to meet individual patient requirements and use in the event of breakthrough pain.[60] Table 45-5 lists the opioids and dosages most commonly used to achieve epidural-based analgesia.

Extended-Release Epidural Morphine (DepoDur). A sustained-release formulation of morphine sulfate (DepoDur; SkyPharma, San Diego, CA) is newly available for use in the treatment of acute postoperative pain. DepoDur consists of microscopic spherical particles with integral aqueous chambers separated by lipid membranes containing an encapsulated dose of morphine. DepoDur is unique in that it delivers standard morphine sulfate using DepoFoam technology. DepoFoam (also from SkyPharma) is a drug-delivery system composed of multivesicular lipid particles containing nonconcentric aqueous chambers that encapsulate the morphine sulfate, allowing the morphine to be released over an extended period of time (up to 48 hours) without a requirement for subsequent dosing.[60,61] The half-life of DepoDur is dose dependent, but the DepoFoam technology allows for larger doses to be administered than could be given when conventional epidural injection is used. For example, a study done by Carvalho and co-workers compared analgesia and side effects in groups of cesarean section patients receiving either a single epidural injection of 5 mg of preservative-free morphine or 5, 10, or 15 mg of DepoDur. After cord clamp, the authors noted that patients who received the 10- and 15-mg doses of DepoDur had significantly lower pain scores and analgesic requirements for the first 48 hours following cesarean delivery.[61]

DepoDur is intended to be used as a sole agent and cannot be administered concomitantly with a local anesthetic solution. Because DepoDur is encapsulated by DepoFoam technology, studies have shown that administration of any local anesthetic solution may elicit a physicochemical interaction and cause a reduction in the sustainability of the DepoFoam to release the morphine over an extended period of time. This can result in an increase in the quantity of the encapsulated morphine released to the systemic circulation and place the patient at increased risk for respiratory depression and hypotension. The full extent of this interaction is being investigated by the manufacturer. This recommendation for not mixing with local anesthetics does not preclude the anesthetist from testing the epidural catheter for possible subarachnoid or intravascular migration preceding injection, and it is recommended that a routine test dose be performed prior to injection of the DepoDur, with some added precautions. The manufacturer recommends that the test dose be administered

using prescribed techniques, then the catheter should be flushed with at least 1 mL of 0.9% NaCl solution a minimum of 15 minutes prior to injection of the DepoDur.[61] It has also been recognized that sustained levels of analgesia from DepoDur require a minimum dose of 10 mg. Current research shows that when a dose of 5 mg of DepoDur is administered, the terminal half-life of the morphine is comparable to a similar 5-mg dose of standard morphine.[61]

Management of Epidural Anesthesia

After epidural administration of local anesthetic, the spread of the dermatomal block will continue and peak in an amount of time dependent on the factors previously mentioned and the local anesthetic solution used. Typically the time to maximal spread is between 10 and 25 minutes, and the level of the block will regress over time; therefore, consistent monitoring of sensory dermatomal level should be performed. When the sensory level of the block has diminished by one or two dermatomes, as detected by the "scratch" or "ice" test used to denote dermatomal level, then another dose, 30% to 50% of the initial dose, is given to reestablish the initial level of anesthesia. It is important to perform consistent monitoring of the anesthetic level because tachyphylaxis, or the need for an increase in the dosage required to maintain an adequate level of blockade, may occur if the regression is allowed beyond two dermatomal segments. The phenomenon of tachyphylaxis is poorly understood but is more likely to occur with short-acting amides such as lidocaine or mepivacaine. It can be avoided by using longer-acting agents (bupivacaine, ropivacaine, and tetracaine) or using a continuous infusion device.

One of the most frustrating problems that can occur with epidural anesthesia is the phenomenon of an inadequate block, a one-sided block or single-sensory dermatome segment that fails to achieve adequate anesthesia. A variety of techniques are used to deal with this phenomenon. Some anesthetists will attempt to increase the spread of the local anesthetic to the area of missed dermatomes by repositioning the patient with the unblocked side down (dependent) or by administering more local anesthetic solution. An inadequate block could be secondary to coiling of the epidural catheter or an anatomic abnormality. However, inadequate anesthesia during epidural anesthesia placement may be secondary to the technique used during identification of the epidural space. Studies have shown that using air during the loss-of-resistance technique may be a contributing factor in missed dermatomal spread of the local anesthetic. Studies by Beilin and colleagues[62] Valentine and colleagues[63] and Shenouda and Cunningham[64] report that when air was used during a loss-of-resistance technique, a significant number of patients experienced "missed" dermatomal spread of the local anesthetic solution. They recommend using normal saline during catheter placement to minimize this complication.[62-64]

Rarely an epidural catheter passes through dura but without penetrating the arachnoid membrane. This is sometimes thought of as intradural placement. Spread of the injected anesthetic in this situation can be very unpredictable. Anesthesia can range from a patchy, inadequate block to a rapid and high level of anesthesia requiring ventilatory support, similar to the total-spinal anesthetic complication. Fortunately, intradural catheter placement is rare, and complications can be avoided by the careful use of test doses, maintained vigilance, and a high index of suspicion. If an intradural catheter placement is suspected, the catheter needs to be removed and replaced after resolution of any side effects (hypotension, bradycardia). Additionally, it is

TABLE 45-5 Recommended Doses of Epidural Opioids

Agent	Analgesia				Continuous Infusion Rate			
	Bolus Dose	Onset (min)	Peak (min)	Duration (hours)	Range (mL/hr)	Basal Rate (mL/hr)	PCEA Bolus (mL)	Interval (min)
Morphine	2-5 mg	20-30	30-60	12-24				
Morphine 0.05%-0.1% solution					1-6			
Morphine 0.05%-0.1% + bupivacaine 0.0625%-0.125%					3-6	3-4	1	20
Meperidine	25-100 mg	5-10	10-30	4-6				
Meperidine 0.1%-0.25% bupivacaine 0.0625%-0.125%					2-10	5	1	12
Hydromorphone	1 mg	10-15	20-30	8-15				
Hydromorphone 0.05%					0.8			
Fentanyl	50-100 mcg	5-10	20	2-6				
Fentanyl 0.001%-0.002%					4-12			
Fentanyl 0.001% + bupivacaine 0.0625%-0.1%					4-10	5	1	12
Sufentanil	10-60 mcg	5-10	20-30	4-6				
Sufentanil 0.0001%					10			

Modified from Cousins MJ, Mather LE. Intrathecal and epidural administration of opioids. Anesthesiology. 1984;61;276.

recommended that the catheter be replaced at a dermatomal level more cephalad to the interspace previously attempted.[5,13]

Complications of Epidural Anesthesia

As with spinal anesthesia, the hemodynamic changes seen with epidural anesthesia are attributed to sympathetic blockade and subsequent arterial and venous dilation. Use of plain local anesthetic solutions in the epidural space to create a high level of blockade will decrease the mean arterial pressure, cardiac output, stroke volume, heart rate, and peripheral vascular resistance. The addition of epinephrine (usually a 1:200,000 to 1:400,000 solution) to the epidural local anesthetic solution diminishes and slows systemic uptake, resulting in lower plasma levels of the local anesthetic and prolongation of its duration of action. However, the epinephrine is thought to be absorbed systemically in low levels, thereby causing β_2-adrenergic vasodilatation. The result is lower arterial pressure and peripheral resistance when compared with spinal anesthesia. Treatments of these hemodynamic alterations are very similar to those used for effects of spinal anesthesia. They include ephedrine 5 to 10 mg, phenylephrine 50 to 100 mcg, or a low- to moderate-rate infusion of dopamine, keeping in mind the caveats for use of these potent vasopressors. Atropine or glycopyrrolate is also useful for the treatment of bradycardia.[4,8]

One complication that is more prevalent with epidural anesthesia than spinal anesthesia is backache. The incidence of back pain following epidural anesthesia is between 30% and 45%, especially in the obstetric patient.[14] There have been several studies that have identified various techniques to use to decrease the incidence and severity of back pain following epidural anesthesia. For example, Todd and colleagues[65] analyzed what effect the addition of ketorolac to the dermal anesthesia solution would have on the overall incidence and severity of back pain following laboring epidural placement and delivery. These authors reported that the addition of 2 mg/kg of ketorolac to the 1% lidocaine dermal anesthetic solution resulted in a decrease in the incidence and severity of back pain in the postpartum period as compared with a similar group receiving 1% lidocaine solution alone for dermal anesthesia prior to entry of the epidural needle through the skin.[65]

Other complications associated with epidural catheters are similar to those associated with spinal anesthesia and have already been discussed. Like spinals, the overall risk of PDPH is low. For epidural catheters the PDPH rate is 1% to 2% with the placement of an epidural catheter. However, epidural needles are large in diameter compared with spinal needles. Although the goal of an epidural catheter technique is to avoid puncture of the dura, an inadvertent rent created by a 17-gauge Tuohy is a rather large dural perforation and is referred to as a "wet tap" for the quite brisk free flow of CSF that can escape through the needle. With such a rent in the dura, the incidence of PDPH can be as high as 75% in young patients. Epidural catheters are also more likely to place a patient at risk for neuraxial anesthesia complications than the single passage of a smaller-gauge spinal needle because the catheter acts as a foreign body that remains within the patient. The catheter causes mechanical tissue disruption, acts as a physical irritant, may provide a path for infection, and will cause tissue trauma on removal—perhaps as much trauma as that associated with catheter placement. Therefore, although complications are rare overall, patients must be followed closely in the postoperative period for signs and symptoms of neurologic compromise such as spine ache, root pain, weakness, and bowel or bladder dysfunction.

COMBINED SPINAL AND EPIDURAL ANESTHESIA

First described in 1937, the combined spinal epidural anesthesia (CSE) technique has risen in popularity and is used successfully for orthopedic, urologic, and gynecologic surgeries, and for providing postoperative pain relief. It has also gained favor in the obstetric suite for providing anesthesia and analgesia for labor and delivery and for cesarean section.[66-70]

CSE anesthesia and analgesia offers the advantages of each technique while reducing or eliminating disadvantages.[5,42] The CSE technique is appropriately used in any setting in which the practitioner plans a spinal or epidural anesthetic and desires to exploit the advantages of each technique—usually the quicker onset of the spinal anesthetic combined with the flexibility of an epidural catheter.

History and Development

In 1937, Soresi described the sequential injection of local anesthetic, first into the epidural space, then into the subarachnoid space, using the same small-gauge spinal needle. Soresi described placing an epidural needle (without a stylet) into the epidural space using a hanging-drop technique and injecting 7 to 8 mL of procaine, then advancing the needle into the subarachnoid space, where he injected 2 additional mL of procaine. He reported the anesthesia lasted between 24 to 48 hours. His experience using this technique in more than 200 patients led him to state that "by combining the two methods many of the disadvantages of both methods are eliminated and their advantages are enhanced to an almost incredible degree."[71]

In 1979, Curelaru reported application of the CSE technique in 150 patients. He used a two-puncture technique; he placed an epidural catheter first, using a standardized epidural needle, followed by a subarachnoid puncture, using a spinal needle one or two interspaces below the level of the epidural puncture. Advantages of the technique included "the possibility of obtaining a high quality conduction anesthesia, virtually unlimited in time, the ability to extend over several anatomic regions the surgical field, minimal toxicity, the absence of postoperative pulmonary complications and the economy." Disadvantages included "the need for two vertebral punctures, the longer induction time of anesthesia and some difficulty in finding the subarachnoid space after catheterization of the epidural space."[72]

Finally, in 1982 Coates and Mumtaz and colleagues used a single-space technique in which a long spinal needle was inserted through the epidural needle to provide the spinal component of the CSE technique.[67,68] Coates stated that the technique was "simple, reliable and quick to perform." He was, however, concerned that "the theoretical hazards of this technique include the possible passage of the epidural catheter through the hole in the dura mater and the possibility of subarachnoid effects from epidurally injected drugs by passage through the hole in the dura." Eldor described finding metallic particles while using the needle-through-needle technique, supposedly formed by abrasion of the inner surface of the epidural needle by the passage of the spinal needle.[69] They were concerned that these particles might be introduced into the epidural space. In addition, they were concerned that uneven distribution of the spinal local anesthetic was possible. The delay, they theorized, inherent in introducing the epidural catheter after intrathecal administration of local anesthetic could affect the spread of the anesthetic. These concerns led to the development of a combined spinal-epidural needle with two separate conduits to allow the epidural catheter to be placed first, followed by the spinal puncture. Because the needle had two conduits, it allowed both techniques to be performed with one puncture at one interspace. This innovation led to the development of several needle types, each of which sought to improve on the others.

Equipment and Techniques
Two-Level Technique

The two-level technique is unique in that each component is performed separately at two different interspaces. An epidural catheter is inserted first, followed by a spinal anesthesia needle placed one or two interspaces lower. The primary advantage of this technique is the ability to insert and test the epidural catheter first, then place the spinal anesthetic needle. Once the spinal needle is placed, no delay occurs in positioning the patient, which may be an important factor when using a hyperbaric spinal anesthetic solution. Prior placement of the epidural catheter is not entirely benign. Potential problems include the inability to distinguish the epidural test dose from the spinal block, inability to differentiate the epidural test dose from CSF, epidural catheter laceration by the spinal needle, misdirection of the spinal needle by the catheter, inability to obtain CSF because of compression of the dural sac by the test dose, and an increased risk of dural puncture by the epidural catheter.[66] Other disadvantages include increased discomfort, tissue trauma, and morbidity associated with multilevel interspinous space penetration (e.g., backache, epidural venous laceration, hematoma, infection, and technical difficulties).[70]

Single-Level Technique: Needle Through Needle

First described in 1982, the needle-through-needle technique involves insertion of an epidural needle at the appropriate interspace and then using the epidural needle as a guide for the spinal needle.[67,68] A small (25-, 27-, or 29-gauge) pencil-point spinal needle is inserted through the epidural needle into the subarachnoid space, and local anesthetic is injected. The spinal needle is removed, and an epidural catheter is threaded into the epidural space. The epidural needle is removed, and the catheter is secured. The main advantages are related to performance of a single interspace insertion (e.g., less tissue trauma, backache, and associated morbidity). Disadvantages include the possibility of inadequate spinal block if catheter placement is delayed, potential for increased nerve-root trauma if paresthesias occur during catheter insertion, and the inability to reliably test the catheter with a preexisting spinal block. Inability to obtain CSF because of inadequate spinal needle length is a risk avoided by the use of the appropriate specialized needles.

Specialized Needles

Eldor was the first to develop and patent a combined spinal-epidural needle with two channels—one for the epidural catheter, the other for the spinal needle.[69] The needle is placed at the selected interspace, the epidural catheter is inserted through its designated conduit, and then the spinal needle is placed through its conduit. Once CSF is obtained, the chosen local anesthetic is injected, and the needle is removed. The catheter is taped in place, and the patient is positioned. Purported advantages and disadvantages are similar to those described for the single-level technique. Although the risk of metallic particle formation may be reduced, the risk of trauma to the interspinous ligaments is increased because of a larger needle diameter.

Several other needles have been developed, all seeking to minimize or eliminate potential problems.[69] To reduce external size, decrease needle abrasion, and allow for a direct angle of approach to the dura, a Tuohy needle was modified with a

separate back-eye at the bend of the needle, thereby permitting straight passage of the spinal needle. These needles are subject to their own limitations and failure rates as well. The spinal needle can miss the back-eye hole and exit the epidural needle through the main orifice, as occurs in the needle-through-needle technique.

Sequential Technique

Rawal and colleagues described a single-level "sequential" technique that was developed to minimize the hypotensive effects of the spinal component of CSE anesthesia for cesarean section. An epidural needle is placed at the selected interspace and a low-dose (7.5 mg of hyperbaric bupivacaine) spinal anesthetic is placed using the needle-through-needle technique. The spinal needle is removed, the catheter is inserted and taped in place, and the patient is placed in the supine position with a left lateral tilt. After 15 minutes, the block is extended by titrating epidural local anesthetic until the desired level is achieved (1.5 to 2 mL for each unblocked segment). Although this technique takes longer to perform, it has been shown to decrease the frequency and severity of the hypotension seen with spinal anesthesia. This technique has also been applied in other types of surgery.[66]

Agents

As discussed, local anesthetic agents and their concentration are chosen depending on the effects desired. Appropriate anesthetics for the spinal component include isobaric or hyperbaric 5% lidocaine with or without epinephrine, hyperbaric 0.75% (spinal) bupivacaine, and isobaric or hyperbaric 1% tetracaine. Appropriate anesthetics for the epidural component include 2% lidocaine with or without epinephrine, 0.5% or 0.75% bupivacaine, 2% or 3% 2-chloroprocaine, and 1% ropivacaine. The concentration of these agents may be adjusted to provide postoperative analgesia in combination with opioids such as morphine and fentanyl. All agents should be preservative free to reduce or eliminate any neurotoxic effects.

Management of CSE Anesthesia

Although the CSE technique may be used in any type of surgical procedure in which a spinal or epidural would be acceptable, this technique may be particularly well suited to providing analgesia and anesthesia in obstetric patients. The CSE technique offers several potential advantages over conventional epidural anesthesia and analgesia.[66]

- Rapid onset of the intrathecal component for women who are in the later stages of labor and in significant pain and distress.
- The use of intrathecal opioids (fentanyl, sufentanil, morphine, and meperidine) in early labor; the minimal to absent motor block associated with intrathecal opioids allows the patient to ambulate while in labor.

The CSE technique for the laboring patient usually involves the placement of an epidural needle at the selected (usually lumbar) interspace, followed by the placement of the spinal needle using the needle-through-needle technique. Intrathecal opioids (5 to 15 mcg of sufentanil or 25 to 50 mcg of fentanyl) may be given alone or in combination with a small dose (2.5 mg of bupivacaine) of local anesthetic, saline, or both. The spinal needle is withdrawn, and the epidural catheter is inserted. The epidural needle is removed, and the catheter is taped in place. The catheter can be activated at any time should supplemental analgesia or anesthesia be required. Standard testing of the epidural catheter before use is always recommended.

The CSE technique can also be used to provide anesthesia for cesarean section if required. If the patient already has an epidural catheter in place, a test dose (3 mL 1.5% lidocaine with 1:200,000 epinephrine) is given to rule out intrathecal and intravascular placement. After a negative test dose, incremental administration of 2% lidocaine, 0.5% bupivacaine, or 3% 2-chloroprocaine can be used to establish a level of surgical anesthesia.

If a catheter has yet to be placed, and if time allows, proceed as with any new patient. After the spinal needle is placed, an intrathecal dose of local anesthetic (12 to 15 mg of 0.75% bupivacaine) with or without opioid (10 to 15 mcg of fentanyl, 0.2 to 0.3 mg of preservative-free morphine, or both) is given. The catheter is inserted and taped in place. The spinal anesthetic will set up quickly and allow for urgent (but maybe not emergent) delivery.

Despite the utility and flexibility of the CSE technique, several concerns related to its use exist. The first of these concerns is related to the use of intrathecal sufentanil and its associated hypotension.[73] Controversy exists with regard to whether intrathecal sufentanil causes clinically significant changes in blood pressure and fetal heart rate (fetal bradycardia). Purported mechanisms include pain relief, mild sympatholysis, and uterine hypertonus.[74-76] Studies show no differences in outcome between CSE using intrathecal sufentanil and epidural anesthesia.[77,78]

A second concern with CSE analgesia is the ability to ambulate after receiving intrathecal narcotics. The concern is related to possible motor weakness if low-dose local anesthetic is added and regarding the effects on blood pressure.[79] Hypotension appears within the first 30 minutes after intrathecal fentanyl but remains stable through ambulation and follow-up doses of epidural local anesthetic. Studies demonstrate the safety of allowing ambulation with no apparent deleterious effects.[80]

A third concern with CSE technique in laboring patients is related to complications. Overall, the complications of itching and hypotension, although bothersome, do not appear to significantly affect outcome or patient satisfaction.[62] CSE anesthesia is associated with faster onset, denser motor block, lower anxiety, lower preoperative and intraoperative pain scores, and greater patient satisfaction preoperatively. There were no significant differences in the incidence or severity of hypotension or nausea, the need for supplemental analgesics, or the postoperative assessments of intraoperative pain, anxiety, and satisfaction.[81,82]

Complications of CSE Anesthesia

Spinal and epidural anesthesia both have their own associated complications as discussed. The CSE technique has the same complications and some additional unique complications. Therefore, as always, vigilance is prudent.

Failure to Obtain a Subarachnoid Block

The failure rate for subarachnoid block alone ranges from 3.1% to 17%.[83-85] With the single-level CSE technique for anesthesia, the range is 0% to 24.5%, and for the two-level technique, the range is 1.6% to 4%.[84-86] Failure with the single-level CSE technique may occur because the epidural needle is not in the epidural space, because the epidural needle is off midline, because the spinal needle is too short (or dull) and does not penetrate the dura, or because the angle of approach of the spinal needle is too oblique to puncture the dura.

One of the most important considerations is the length of the spinal needle—specifically, the length of needle that extends beyond the tip of the epidural needle.[70] Studies have shown an increased success rate when the tip of the spinal needle extends 7 to 15 mm beyond the tip of the epidural needle.[85,87] The angle at which the spinal needle approaches the dura may also be important. As the spinal needle exits a standard epidural needle tip, the angle caused by the epidural needle's curve may be 4 to 5 degrees or more.[88] This factor, combined with inadequate needle length, may result in failure to obtain CSF. This situation has led to the development of a modified Tuohy needle that has a separate back-eye at the bend of the needle to allow for a straight-on approach to the dura. Pan determined that the success rate for the needles exiting the correct hole ranged from 50% to 67%.[89] The success rate can be improved to 81% to 94% by bending the spinal needle slightly in the direction of the epidural needle bevel and to 91% to 96% by orientating the epidural needle bevel upward.

Failure rates may also be directly related to level of experience with the technique and are not easily correctable. The problem of spinal needle displacement during connection of the syringe, aspiration, or injection of the local anesthetic has led to the development of "locking" devices that fix the spinal needle in the epidural needle once the dura has been punctured. Their efficacy has not yet been confirmed.

Catheter Migration

Another problem with the needle-through-needle technique is the possibility of catheter migration through the dural puncture caused by the introduction of the spinal needle.[90] Studies that assessed the risk of catheter migration through a dural puncture site demonstrated little to no risk if the dural puncture was made with a 25-gauge or smaller spinal needle, but an increased risk if the dural puncture was made by a larger (18-gauge) Tuohy needle.[90-92] Many factors may result in catheter placement in, or migration into, the subarachnoid space, including patient movement, undetected dural puncture with the epidural needle with subsequent catheter placement, and (least likely) diffusion of local anesthetic from the epidural space into the subarachnoid space through the dural puncture. The prudent practitioner is advised to adopt a conservative approach that includes a high index of suspicion and frequent aspiration and testing of the catheter.

However, even the question of when to test the epidural catheter can be problematic. The purpose of the epidural catheter test dose is to rule out inadvertent placement or migration of the catheter into the subarachnoid space or into an epidural vein. A preestablished subarachnoid block may preclude the ability to reliably test for subarachnoid catheter placement and mask intravascular placement. To date, no published studies have demonstrated reliable detection of inadvertent subarachnoid catheter placement in someone with a preexisting spinal block.

Increased Spinal Level After Epidural Administration

The CSE technique is known to cause an increased spread of spinal anesthesia after injection of solutions through the epidural catheter. Although controversial, several theories may help explain this phenomenon. The first, the "volume effect" theory, states that the volume of fluid injected into the epidural space compresses the subarachnoid space and the CSF within it, thereby increasing the spread of the intrathecal local anesthetic. This effect has been documented clinically and by the use of contrast media and radiography.[93,94] The second theory presupposes a "leak" or flow of local anesthetic from the epidural into the subarachnoid space through the dural puncture.

This effect has also been demonstrated clinically and by radiography.[95,96] Other radiographic studies have been unable to confirm these results.[92,97]

Metallic Particles
Eldor and Levine noted the production of metallic particles when passing a spinal needle through a Tuohy epidural needle.[83] Subsequently, Eldor has implied that scratches in the spinal needle and metallic particles may be associated with an increase in aseptic meningitis and cancer in patients who have received CSE anesthesia via the needle-through-needle technique.[98,99] No studies have been published to support these assertions, but several studies have examined the issue of metallic particle formation.[100] These studies used electron microscopy, atomic absorption spectrography, photomicrography, and microscopy; none were able to detect metallic particle formation.[92,101]

Postdural Puncture Headache
Conflicting evidence exists regarding whether a greater risk of PDPH is associated with the CSE technique compared with conventional epidural anesthesia and analgesia. Both techniques involve the placement of an epidural needle, with its attendant risk of dural puncture. In addition, the CSE technique involves a dural puncture, usually with a small-gauge, pencil-point spinal needle. Because this type of spinal needle is associated with an extremely low incidence of PDPH, one would expect an equally low incidence with the CSE technique. A review of the literature on the CSE technique shows a PDPH rate between 0% and 2.3% in laboring patients.[102] Theoretic reasons for a low incidence with the CSE technique include:

- The epidural needle serves as an introducer for the smaller-gauge spinal needles and allows for a straight approach at the dura.
- CSF leakage through the dural puncture is abated because of the presence of the epidural catheter and fluids, which increases pressure in the epidural space.
- The spinal needle penetrates the dura at a slight angle, which may help dural fibers seal the hole on withdrawal.

Studies suggest that the use of intrathecal opioids as part of the CSE technique may offer a protective effect from PDPH.[103,104] In addition, the success rate in obtaining CSF may be higher when the patient is in the sitting, rather than the lateral position.[59] The sitting position allows for correct midline placement of the epidural needle and makes it more likely that CSF will be obtained with the spinal needle (higher hydrostatic pressure). Both of these factors contribute to minimization of the number of dural punctures and may decrease the risk of PDPH.

Infection
The incidence of infectious complications associated with epidural and spinal anesthesia has always been considered to be very low—in the range of 0% to 0.04%.[23,105,106] However, perhaps because of close monitoring of this newer technique, an increase has occurred in the number of case reports of patients who have developed complications that may be associated with the use of the CSE technique. Bouhemad and co-workers cite several cases (three between 1994 and 1998) of bacterial meningitis associated with the use of CSE. The authors believed that potentially infectious skin matter was first introduced into the epidural space during the insertion of the epidural needle and was then introduced into the CSF by the passage of the spinal needle into the subarachnoid space.[107] Because the CSE technique requires invasion of both the epidural and subarachnoid spaces, strict aseptic

technique should be practiced. As with other complications associated with the use of CSE, further study of this area is warranted.

Neurologic Injury
Neurologic injury associated with spinal and epidural anesthesia is also very low, ranging from 0.02% to 0.1%, and is usually transient in nature.[5] Although there does not appear to be any increased risk inherent in the CSE technique as compared with either spinal or epidural anesthesia alone, there have been several case reports of cauda equina syndrome in patients who underwent CSE anesthesia.[108,109] In none of these cases was the cause ever identified. Possible causes include preexisting spinal deformity (present in one case), use of lidocaine (present in one case), and an intrathecal catheter (never proved or disproved).

A final concern with the use of the CSE technique is paresthesia on epidural catheter insertion. A preexisting spinal block may mask a significant paresthesia on catheter insertion and result in neurologic injury. Paresthesias during epidural catheter placement range in frequency from 20% to 44%.[110] However, studies show no significant difference in the frequency of paresthesias reported for either technique.[85,110]

CAUDAL ANESTHESIA
Caudal anesthesia can be thought of as a distal approach to the epidural space. Therefore, anesthetics administered or catheters placed via the caudal route will act as epidural administered anesthetics, but first on the sacral dermatomes. A caudal technique is useful for perirectal surgery, urologic surgery, and orthopedic surgery of the lower extremity. Caudal techniques are especially useful in pediatrics but can also be used for labor and delivery and for chronic pain states. With the success of lumbar epidural catheters for labor and delivery, caudal anesthesia is rarely used in this population currently and is less likely to be used in the adult population in general. After the age of 12, sacral anatomy changes and bone growth makes identification of the epidural space by this approach difficult and the spread of anesthesia less reliable.[8] Therefore, caudal anesthesia is most often used in combination with a light general anesthetic to augment postoperative analgesia in preadolescent pediatric patients.

Equipment and Techniques
The patient can be placed either prone or in a lateral position. The posterior iliac spines and the sacral hiatus are identified. Positioning the patient prone with the legs slightly apart, the heels rotated outward, and a pillow under the buttocks facilitates the palpation of the cornua of the sacral hiatus. In the lateral, Sims, or knee-chest position, identification of the cornua can be enhanced by adjusting the amount of hip flexion. Excess flexion can stretch the skin, making landmark identification difficult. An assistant is often useful when one is positioning patients who are anesthetized.

In pediatric patients, general anesthesia is usually induced, the airway and intravenous access secured, and the patient turned prone or placed in a lateral decubitus position. After aseptic preparation is performed, the index and second fingers of one hand are placed on the cornua of the sacrum, with the hand cephalad and against the patient's back. A 22- to 25-gauge short needle attached to a 10-mL syringe filled with local anesthetic is inserted midline between the cornua at a steep angle to the skin into the sacral hiatus. Alternatively, a 20-gauge over-the-needle intravenous catheter is sufficiently long enough for the block, and the catheter can be passed into the epidural space while the needle is removed. This allows the anesthetist better control when administering the local anesthetic. The needle is inserted, with the bevel of the needle directed toward the sacrum. As the membranes are penetrated and the ventral canal of the sacrum is entered, a popping sensation can be felt. At this point the needle angle is lowered parallel to the sacrum and the spinal canal. The needle is advanced into the epidural space for a distance of 1 to 3 cm but no farther than the second sacral interspace. The second sacral interspace lies 1 to 2 cm below a line drawn between the posterior iliac spines. The needle position is evaluated for entrance into the subarachnoid space or epidural veins via gentle aspiration and examination for CSF or blood return through the needle. Once the appropriate location of the needle is verified, the anesthetic is incrementally injected as with an epidural. During injection the skin area above the end of the needle is palpated. Bulging over the needle tip indicates subcutaneous or superficial injection rather than injection into the epidural space. If the needle is in the subperiosteal area, resistance to injection is felt, and the needle must be repositioned.

Agents

In children, 0.5 to 1 mL of solution per kilogram of body weight is injected to reliably achieve a level of analgesia to the umbilicus. Bupivacaine or ropivacaine, in concentrations of 0.125% to 0.5%, are usually administered with epinephrine 1:200,000, to a maximum dose of 2.5 mg/kg body weight. Additionally, levobupivacaine 0.2% has been compared with equal concentrations of ropivacaine and bupivacaine and been found effective. These dosing regimens have been shown effective for children undergoing subumbilical surgical procedures providing analgesia or anesthesia for the lower extremities and the abdomen, urogenital surgery, inguinal hernia repair, or orthopedic procedures with analgesia that lasts 3 to 5 hours postoperatively.[8,111,112] Clonidine 1 mcg/kg of body weight added to the local anesthetic has been shown to be comparable with opioids that are added to enhance analgesia. Clonidine has fewer side effects than caudal opioids (e.g., delayed recovery, respiratory depression, and nausea).[113] Some patients may be unable to tolerate the loss of lower-extremity motor control. These patients should be identified before the anesthetic is administered and be offered another technique. For example, infants too young to walk greatly benefit from caudal analgesia, but toddlers may be frightened by their inability to move their legs. Ropivacaine and levobupivacaine may have benefit over bupivacaine, because analgesia in the postoperative period is equivalent, but ropivacaine and levobupivacaine offer shorter duration of motor blockade and less risk of CNS and cardiotoxicity.[8,111,112,114,115]

In adults, the principles of epidural drug administration should be followed, with use of a 3-mL test dose and incremental injections and aspiration. Only 12 to 15 mL is necessary for sacral anesthesia, and up to 20 to 30 mL offers sufficient spread for lower-extremity procedures to approximately the 10th thoracic dermatome. The spread of drug, duration of anesthesia, and desired level of anesthesia are less predictable than with epidural anesthesia because of the variability in the volume, content, and leakage of the caudal canal. The maximum recommended dose of lidocaine or mepivacaine is 10 mg/kg of body weight and 2.5 mg/kg of body weight for bupivacaine.[8] All agents injected into the epidural or subarachnoid spaces should be preservative free.

Management of Caudal Anesthesia

Caudal anesthesia, like epidural anesthesia, is adaptable to a continuous catheter technique. However, if a Tuohy needle is used, the angle of the tip must be kept in mind when one attempts to pass the catheter into the epidural space. Management is similar to that with an epidural catheter.

Complications of Caudal Anesthesia

Caudal anesthesia has complications that are very similar to those of epidural anesthesia. The caudal canal has a sacral epidural venous plexus with vessels that can be unintentional recipients of a needle or catheter tip, with subsequent intravenous injection of local anesthetic. Dural puncture is also possible, although the dural sac usually ends in adults at the lower border of L2, and in infants the sac can extend to S4. High spinal punctures are less likely but have been reported. In addition, the anatomy of caudal anesthesia is variable enough, especially in adults, to cause a high (10% to 15%) failure rate as the needle is unintentionally inserted into false passages. The proximity of the caudal canal to the rectum theoretically makes infection a potential risk, although clinically significant infection is rarely reported.[8,116] The risk of infections, perhaps, will best be shown to be minimized with the use of chlorhexidine solutions instead of povidone-iodine solutions.[117]

In 1899, Alice Magaw described the job of an anesthetist and best summarized the reality of the practice of regional anesthesia. She stated, "While one should be competent in the theoretical part of this important work, there is nothing so helpful to the anesthetist as the hard school of practical experience."[118]

SUMMARY

Regional anesthesia techniques are a vital part of modern anesthesia practice. Our ability to understand and apply neuraxial anesthesia continues to evolve. These techniques are increasingly being used for all types of anesthetics, including many outpatient procedures. Their utility in providing for perioperative pain management has greatly enhanced our ability to provide comfort to our patients.

REFERENCES

1. Thomas SJ, Orkin FK. Scope of modern anesthetic practice. In: Miller RD, ed. Anesthesia. 6th ed. New York: Churchill Livingstone; 2005:55-66.
2. Brown DL, Fink BR. History of neural blockade and pain management. In: Cousins MJ, Bridenbaugh P, eds. Neural Blockade in Clinical Anesthesia and Management of Pain. 3rd ed. Philadelphia: Lippincott; 1998:3-34.
3. Moore KL. The spinal cord. In: Moore KL, ed. Clinically Oriented Anatomy. Baltimore: Williams & Wilkins; 1992.
4. Bernards CM. Epidural and spinal anesthesia. In: Barash PG et al, eds. Clinical Anesthesia. 5th ed. Philadelphia: Lippincott Williams & Wilkins; 2006:691-717.
5. Cousins MJ, Veering BT. Epidural neural blockade. In: Cousins MJ, Bridenbaugh P, eds. Neural Blockade in Clinical Anesthesia and Management of Pain. Philadelphia: Lippincott-Raven; 1998:243-321.
6. Portnoy D, Vadhera RB. Mechanisms and management of an incomplete epidural block for cesarean section. Anesthesiol Clin North America. 2003;21:39-57.
7. Hogan Q. Anatomy of spinal anesthesia: some old and new findings. Reg Anesth Pain Med. 1998;23:340-343.
8. Stevens RA. Neuraxial blocks. In: Brown DL, ed. Regional Anesthesia and Analgesia. Philadelphia: Saunders; 1996:319-355.
9. Butterworth J. Physiology of spinal anesthesia: what are the implications for management? Reg Anesth Pain Med. 1998;23:370-373.
10. Mackey DC. Physiologic effects of regional blocks. In: Brown DL, ed. Regional Anesthesia and Analgesia. Philadelphia: Saunders; 1996:397-422.
11. Strichartz GR, Berde CB. Local anesthetics. In: Miller RD, ed. Anesthesia. 6th ed. New York: Churchill Livingstone; 2005:573-604.
12. Harrington BE. Postdural puncture headache and the development of the epidural blood patch. Reg Anesth Pain Med. 2004;29:136-163.

13. Mulroy M. Extending indications for spinal anesthesia. *Reg Anesth Pain Med.* 1998;23:380-383.

14. Brown DL. Spinal, epidural and caudal anesthesia. In: Livingstone C, ed. *Anesthesia.* New York: Churchill Livingstone; 2000:1491-1519.

15. Greenberg CP. Practical, cost-effective regional anesthesia for ambulatory surgery. *J Clin Anesth.* 1995;7:614-621.

16. Turnbull DK, Shepherd DB. Post-dural puncture headache: pathogenesis, prevention and treatment. *Br J Anaesth.* 2003;91:718-729.

17. Ng K et al. Spinal versus epidural anaesthesia for caesarean section. *Cochrane Database Syst Rev.* 2004;2:CD003765.

18. Reynolds F. Epidural analgesia in obstetrics. *BMJ.* 1989;297:751-752.

19. O'Hara JF et al. The renal system and anesthesia for urologic surgery. In: Barash PG et al, eds. *Clinical Anesthesia.* 5th ed. Philadelphia: Lippincott, Williams & Wilkins; 2006:1013-1039.

20. Shevde K, Panagopoulos G. A survey of 800 patients' knowledge, attitudes, and concerns regarding anesthesia. *Anesth Analg.* 1991;73(2):190-198.

21. Bridenbaugh PO et al. Spinal (subarachnoid) neural blockade. In: Cousins MJ, Bridenbaugh PO, eds. *Neural Blockade in Clinical Anesthesia and Management of Pain.* 3rd ed. Philadelphia: Lippincott-Raven; 1998:203-241.

22. Liu SS et al. The efficacy of epinephrine test doses during spinal anesthesia in volunteers: implications for combined spinal-epidural anesthesia. *Anesth Analg.* 1997;84:780-783.

23. Horlocker T, Wedel DL. Spinal and epidural blockade and perioperative low molecular weight heparin: smooth sailing on the Titanic. *Anesth Analg.* 1998;86:1153-1156.

24. Veering BT et al. Pharmacokinetics of bupivacaine during postoperative epidural infusion: enantioselectivity and role of protein binding. *Anesthesiology.* 2002;96:1062-1069.

25. Gielen M. Spinal anesthesia: hearing loss, failure, and transient radicular irritation (TRI). *Anaesthesia.* 1998;53:23-25.

26. Moen V et al. Severe neurological complications after central neuraxial block-ades in Sweden 1990-1999. *Anesthesiology.* 2004;101(4):950-959.

27. Hebl JR et al. Neurologic complications after neuraxial anesthesia or analgesia in patients with preexisting peripheral sensorimotor neuropathy or diabetic polyneuropathy. *Anesth Analg.* 2006;103(5):1294-1299.

28. Gogarten W. Spinal anaesthesia for obstetrics. *Best Pract Res Clin Anaesthesiol.* 2003;17:377-392.

29. Horlocker TT et al. Risk assessment of hemorrhagic complications associated with nonsteroidal anti-inflammatory medications in ambulatory pain clinic patients undergoing epidural steroid injection. *Anesth Analg.* 2002;95:1691-1697.

30. Horlocker TT et al. Does preoperative antiplatelet therapy increase the risk of hemorrhagic complications associated with regional anesthesia? *Anesth Analg.* 1990;70:631-634.

31. Lumpkin MM. FDA public health advisory. *Anesthesiology.* 1998;88(2):27A-28A.

32. Horlocker TT et al. Regional anesthesia in the anticoagulated patient: defining the risks (the second ASRA Consensus Conference on Neuraxial Anesthesia and Anticoagulation). *Reg Anesth Pain Med.* 2003;28:172-197.

33. Brull R et al. Neurological complications after regional anesthesia: contemporary estimates of risk. *Anesth Analg.* 2007;104(4):965-974.

34. Wulf H. Epidural anaesthesia and spinal haematoma. *Can J Anaesth.* 1996;43:1260-1271.

35. Royakkers AA et al. Catheter-related epidural abscesses: don't wait for neurological deficits. *Acta Anaesthesiol Scand.* 2002;46:611-615.

36. Kindler CH et al. Epidural abscess complicating anesthesia and analgesia. *Acta Anaesthesiol Scand.* 1998;42:614-620.

37. Mulroy MF. Peripheral nerve blockade. In: Barash PG et al, eds. *Clinical Anesthesia.* 5th ed. Philadelphia: Lippincott Williams & Wilkins; 2006:718-745.

38. Rosenberg PH. Novel technology: needles, microcatheters, and combined techniques. *Reg Anesth Pain Med.* 1998;23:363-369.

39. Spencer HC. Postdural puncture headache: what matters most in technique. *Reg Anesth Pain Med.* 1998;23:374-379.

40. Cork RC et al. Leak rate of latex gloves after tearing adhesive tape. *Am J Anesthesiol.* 1995;22:133-137.

41. Stienstra R, Veering BT. Intrathecal drug spread: is it controllable? *Reg Anesth Pain Med.* 1998;23:347-351.

42. Veering BT, Stienstra R. Duration of block: drug, dose, and additives. *Reg Anesth Pain Med.* 1998;23:352-356.

43. Liu SS. Drugs for spinal anesthesia: past, present, and future. *Reg Anesth Pain Med.* 1998;23:344-346.

44. Zaric D et al. Transient neurologic symptoms after spinal anesthesia with lidocaine versus other local anesthetics: a systematic review of randomized, controlled trials. *Anesth Analg.* 2005;100(6):1811-1816.

45. Critchley LA. Hypotension, subarachnoid block and the elderly patient. *Anaesthesia.* 1996;51:1139-1143.

46. Guyton AC, Hall JE. Nervous regulation of the circulation, and rapid control of arterial pressure. In: Guyton AC, Hall JE, eds. *Textbook of Medical Physiology.* 11th ed. Philadelphia: Saunders; 2006:204-215.

47. Steinbrook RA. Epidural anesthesia and gastrointestinal motility. *Anesth Analg.* 1998;86:837-844.

48. Weeks SK. Postpartum headache. In: Chestnut DH, ed. *Principles and Practice of Obstetric Anesthesia.* 3rd ed. Philadelphia: Mosby; 2004:562-578.

49. Panzer O et al. Shivering and shivering-like tremor during labor with and without epidural analgesia. *Anesthesiology.* 1999;90:1609-1616.

50. Borgeat A et al. Postoperative nausea and vomiting in regional anesthesia: a review. *Anesthesiology.* 2003;98(2):530-547.

51. Liu SS et al. Epidural anesthesia and analgesia. Their role in postoperative outcome. *Anesthesiology.* 1995;82:1474-1506.

52. Campagna JA, Carter C. Clinical relevance of the Bezold-Jarisch reflex. *Anesthesiology.* 2003 May;98(5):1250-1260.

53. Kopp SL et al. Cardiac arrest during neuraxial anesthesia: frequency and pre-disposing factors associated with survival. *Anesth Analg.* 2005;100(3):855-865.

54. Liguori GA, Sharrock NE. Asystole and severe bradycardia during epidural anesthesia in orthopedic patients. *Anesthesiology.* 1997;86:257-264.

55. Day CJ, Shutt LE. Auditory, ocular, and facial complications of central neural block. *Reg Analg.* 1996;21:197-201.

56. D'Angelo R et al. A comparison of multiport and uniport epidural catheters in laboring patients. *Anesth Analg.* 1997;84:1226-1229.

57. Beilin Y et al. The optimal distance that a multiorifice epidural catheter should be threaded into the epidural space. *Anesth Analg.* 1995;81:301-304.

58. Mulroy M et al. Safety steps for epidural injection of local anesthetics: review of literature and recommendations. *Anesth Analg.* 1997;85:1346-1347.

59. Norris MC et al. Complications of labor analgesia: epidural versus combined spinal epidural techniques. *Anesth Analg.* 1994;79:529-537.

60. Chaney MA. Side effects of intrathecal and epidural opioids. *Can J Anaesth.* 1995;42:891-903.

61. Carvalho B et al. for the DepoDur Study Group. Single-dose, sustained-release epidural morphine in the management of postoperative pain after elective cesarean delivery: results of a multicenter randomized controlled study. *Anesth Analg.* 2005;100:1150-1158.

62. Beilin Y et al. Quality of analgesia when air versus normal saline is used for identification of the epidural space in the parturient. *Reg Analg.* 2000;24:596-599.

63. Valentine SJ et al. Comparative study of the effects of air or saline to identify the extradural space. *Br J Anaesth.* 1991;6:224-227.

64. Shenouda PE, Cunningham BJ. Assessing the superiority of saline versus air for use in the epidural loss of resistance technique: a literature review. *Reg Anesth Pain Med.* 2003;28:48-53.

65. Todd G et al. Intradermal ketorolac for reduction of epidural back pain. *Int J Obstet Anesth.* 2002;11:100-104.

66. Rawal N et al. Combined spinal-epidural technique. *Reg Analg.* 1997;22:406-423.

67. Coates MB. Combined subarachnoid and epidural techniques: a single space technique for surgery of the hip and the lower limb. *Anesthesiology.* 1982;37:89-90.

68. Mumtaz MH et al. Combined subarachnoid and epidural techniques: another single space technique for orthopaedic surgery. *Anaesthesia.* 1982;37:90.

69. Eldor J. The evolution of combined spinal-epidural anesthesia needles. *Reg Analg.* 1997;22:294-296.

70. Joshi G, McCaroll S. Evaluation of combined spinal-epidural anesthesia using two different techniques. *Reg Analg.* 1994;19:169-174.

71. Soresi AL. Episubdural anesthesia. *Anesth Analg.* 1937;16:306-310.

72. Curelaru I. Long duration subarachnoid anesthesia with continuous epidural blocks. *Prakt Anaesth.* 1979;14:71-78.

73. D'Angelo R, Eisenach JC. Severe maternal hypotension and fetal bradycardia after a combined spinal epidural anesthetic. *Anesthesiology.* 1997;87:166-168.

74. Shnider S et al. Maternal catecholamines decrease during labor and after lumbar epidural anesthesia. *Am J Obstet Gynecol.* 1983;16:13-15.

75. Van de Velde M et al. Intrathecal sufentanil and fetal heart rate abnormalities: a double-blind, double placebo-controlled trial comparing two forms of combined spinal epidural analgesia with epidural analgesia in labor. *Anesth Analg.* 2004;98:1153-1159.

76. Clarke V et al. Uterine hyperactivity after intrathecal injection of fentanyl for analgesia during labor: a cause for fetal bradycardia? *Anesthesiology.* 1994;81:1083.

77. Albright GA, Forster RM. Does combined spinal-epidural analgesia with subarachnoid sufentanil increase the incidence of emergency cesarean delivery? *Reg Analg.* 1997;22:400-405.

78. Nielsen PE et al. Fetal heart rate changes after intrathecal sufentanil or bupivacaine for labor analgesia: incidence and clinical significance. *Anesth Analg.* 1996;83:742-746.

79. Nageotte MP et al. Epidural analgesia compared with combined spinal-epidural analgesia during labor in nulliparous women. *N Engl J Med.* 1997;337:1715-1719.

80. Nageotte MP et al. Epidural analgesia compared with combined spinal-epidural analgesia during labor in nulliparous women. *N Engl J Med.* 1997;337:1715-1719.

81. Davies SJ et al. Maternal experience during epidural or combined spinal-epidural anesthesia for cesarean section: a prospective, randomized trial. *Anesth Analg.* 1997;85:607-613.

82. Collis RE et al. Randomized comparison of combined spinal-epidural and standard epidural analgesia in labor. *Lancet.* 1995;345:1413-1416.

83. Eldor J, Levine S. Failed spinal anesthesia in combined spinal-epidural anesthesia. *Anaesth Intensive Care.* 1997;25:312-331.

84. Urmey WF et al. Combined spinal-epidural anesthesia for outpatient surgery: dose response characteristics of intrathecal isobaric lidocaine using a 27-gauge Whitacre spinal needle. *Anesthesiology.* 1995;83:528-534.

85. Casati A et al. A clinical comparison between needle-through-needle and double segment techniques for combined spinal and epidural anesthesia. *Reg Anesth Pain Med.* 1998;23:390-394.

86. Lyons G et al. Combined epidural/spinal anesthesia for caesarian section. Through needle or in separate spaces? *Anaesthesia.* 1992;47:199-201.

87. Hoffman V et al. A new combined spinal-epidural apparatus: measurement of the distance to the epidural and subarachnoid spaces. *Anesthesiology.* 1997;52:350-355.

88. Westbrook J et al. An evaluation of a combined spinal/epidural needle set utilising a 26-gauge, pencil point spinal needle for caesarean section. *Anaesthesia.* 1992;47:990-992.

89. Pan P. Laboratory evaluation of single lumen, dual orifice combined spinal-epidural needles: effects of bevel orientation and modified technique. *J Clin Anesth.* 1998;10:286-290.

90. Robbins PM et al. Accidental intrathecal insertion of an extradural catheter during combined spinal-extradural anaesthesia for cesarean section. *Br J Anaesth.* 1995;75:355-357.

91. Holmstrum B et al. Risk of catheter migration during combined spinal epidural block: Percutaneous epiduroscopy study. *Anesth Analg.* 1995;80:747-753.

92. Holst D et al. No risk of metal toxicity in combined spinal-epidural anesthesia. *Anesth Analg.* 1999;88:393-397.

93. Blumgart C et al. Mechanism of extension of spinal anesthesia by extradural injection of local anaesthetic. *Br J Anaesth.* 1992;69:457-460.

94. Takiguchi T et al. The effect of epidural saline injection on analgesia level during combined spinal and epidural anesthesia assessed clinically and myelographically. *Anesth Analg.* 1997;85:1097-1100.

95. Stienstra R et al. Mechanism of action of an epidural top-up in combined spinal epidural anesthesia. *Anesth Analg.* 1996;83:382-386.

96. Leach A, Smith G. Subarachnoid spread of epidural local anesthetic following dural puncture. *Anaesthesia.* 1988;43:671-674.

97. Vartis A et al. Potential intrathecal leakage of solutions injected into the epidural space following combined spinal epidural anesthesia. *Anaesth Intensive Care.* 1998;26:256-261.

98. Eldor J. Metallic particles in the spinal-epidural needle technique. *Reg Analg.* 1994;19:219-220.

99. Eldor J, Guedj P. Aseptic meningitis due to metallic particles in the needle-through-needle technique. *Reg Analg.* 1995;20:360.

100. Birnbach D, Danzer B. Comments on combined spinal-epidural anesthesia. *Reg Analg.* 1996;21:275.

101. Herman N et al. No additional metal particle formation using the needle-through-needle combined epidural/spinal technique. *Acta Anaesthesiol Scand.* 1996;40:227-231.

102. McLoughlin L. Combined spinal-extradural analgesia in labour and post-dural puncture headache. *Br J Anaesth.* 1998;80:123-124.

103. Boskovski N, Lewinski A. Epidural morphine for the prevention of headache following dural puncture. *Anaesthesia.* 1982;37:217-218.

104. Johnson M et al. Intrathecal fentanyl may reduce the incidence of spinal headache [abstract]. *Anesthesiology.* 1989;71:A911.

105. Scott D, Hibbard B. Serious non-fatal complications associated with extra-dural block in obstetric practice. *Br J Anaesth.* 1990;64:537-541.

106. Horlocker T et al. A retrospective review of 4767 consecutive spinal anesthetics: central nervous system complications. *Anesth Analg.* 1997;84:578-584.

107. Bouhemad B et al. Bacterial meningitis following combined spinal-epidural analgesia for labor. *Anaesthesia.* 1998;53:292-295.

108. Kubina P et al. Two cases of cauda equina syndrome following spinal-epidural anesthesia. *Reg Analg.* 1997;22:447-450.

109. Paech MJ. Unexplained neurologic deficit after uneventful combined spinal and epidural anesthesia for cesarean delivery. *Reg Analg.* 1997;22:479-482.

110. Levin A et al. Does combined spinal-epidural analgesia alter the incidence of paresthesia during epidural catheter placement? *Anesth Analg.* 1998;86:448-449.

111. Ivani G et al. Caudal anesthesia for minor pediatric surgery: a prospective randomized comparison of ropivacaine 0.2% vs levobupivacaine 0.2%. *Paediatr Anaesth.* 2005;15(6):491-494.

112. Breschan C et al. A prospective study comparing the analgesic efficacy of levobupivacaine, ropivacaine and bupivacaine in pediatric patients undergoing caudal blockade. *Paediatr Anaesth.* 2005;15(4):301-306.

113. Vetter TR et al. A comparison of single-dose caudal clonidine, morphine, or hydromorphone combined with ropivacaine in pediatric patients undergoing ureteral reimplantation. *Anesth Analg.* 2007;104(6):1356-1363.

114. Karmakar MK et al. Ropivacaine undergoes slower systemic absorption from the caudal epidural space in children than bupivacaine. *Anesth Analg.* 2002;94(2):259-265.

115. Knudsen K et al. Central nervous and cardiovascular effects of i.v. infusions of ropivacaine, bupivacaine and placebo in volunteers. *Br J Anaesth.* 1997;78:507-514.

116. Kost-Byerly S et al. Bacterial colonization and infection rate of continuous epidural catheters in children. *Anesth Analg.* 1998;86(4):712-716.

117. Kinirons B et al. Chlorhexidine versus povidone iodine in preventing colonization of continuous epidural catheters in children: a randomized, controlled trial. *Anesthesiology.* 2001;94(2):239-244.

118. Koch E. Alice Magaw and the great secret of open drop anesthesia. *AANA J.* 1999;67:33-38.

CHAPTER 46

REGIONAL ANESTHESIA: Upper and Lower Extremity Blocks

Joseph F. Burkard, Charles A. Vacchiano

Anesthesia practice has seen significant change in the last decade, challenging the anesthesia provider to be proficient in regional anesthesia. The advantages of regional techniques are fewer recovery room admissions, decreased nausea and vomiting, decreased urinary retention, and improved postoperative analgesia. The introduction of long-acting local anesthetics and placement of peripheral nerve catheters have improved the ability to provide postoperative pain relief for several hours to several days. Clinical research has spawned new and more effective techniques for upper and lower extremity blocks. The development and increased use of catheter techniques and ultrasonography for nerve location will undoubtedly revolutionize regional anesthesia.

HISTORY OF REGIONAL ANESTHESIA

The contributions of many practitioners have brought regional anesthesia techniques to the state of the art that exists today. Much of the early motivation for the investigation of regional anesthesia came about because of the risks and mortality associated with general anesthesia. The early inhalation agents were difficult to administer, and toxicity was common.[1]

Without the contributions of LaFargue in 1836, Rynd in 1844, and Pravaz in 1851, regional anesthesia would not have advanced so quickly. Until that time, opiates and other medications were applied to or rubbed into open wounds to provide analgesia. LaFargue devised a needle trocar for depositing morphine under the skin. Rynd invented the hollow needle, which was used for delivering hypodermic medications. Pravaz invented the hypodermic syringe, which was improved by Wood in 1854.[1,2]

SELECTION OF REGIONAL ANESTHESIA TECHNIQUES

When regional anesthesia is chosen for management of pain, the technique should be discussed with the patient before surgery. The patient is informed of all optional procedures available, their potential risks, and their potential complications before an anesthesia technique is selected. Once the patient is thus advised, the most appropriate anesthesia technique can be selected, and true informed consent can be obtained. Regional anesthesia is used extensively for surgical procedures involving the extremities or the lower abdomen, for the management of labor pain, for the management of obstetric procedures, and for the control of chronic pain syndromes. Frequently, regional anesthesia techniques are used in combination with other techniques to provide analgesia or anesthesia during surgical or obstetric procedures. Regional anesthesia may be the technique of choice when local anesthesia requires supplementation with heavy sedation. These techniques provide the patient with increased anesthesia options when selecting an anesthetic for surgical or obstetric procedures.[3,4] It is the preferred technique for obstetrics and many other types of procedures such as certain urologic surgeries.[5-8]

The administration of regional anesthesia to patients with a difficult airway or a full stomach presents both additional benefits and potential risks. The use of regional anesthesia, when appropriate, permits the patient to retain upper airway and pharyngeal reflexes while providing surgical anesthesia. Unless the sedation is reduced to a minimum, the airway may not be protected after the administration of the regional technique. Furthermore, block of the sympathetic nervous system theoretically results in increased gastric and intestinal motility, causing the stomach to empty sooner. However, this benefit may be negated by the perception of pain and anxiety that accompanies injury. If hypotension develops, the patient may have increased nausea and vomiting. When the block is instituted, the patient may lose consciousness as a result of the effects of the alcohol. At this point, airway support is required, and other problems may arise as well.[3,8]

Regional anesthesia should not be considered an alternative to securing the airway. If the patient's airway cannot be secured in a safe manner in an emergent situation, use of a regional anesthetic should be avoided. The airway concerns must be addressed before the anesthetic technique is initiated so that the patient's ability to survive is maximized.[3,8]

Absolute Contraindications

Contraindications to the selection of regional anesthesia techniques are few, and some remain controversial. Absolute contraindications include patient refusal, uncorrected coagulation deficiencies, and infection at the site of the block. The most significant absolute contraindication to regional anesthesia is patient refusal. Each patient must be informed of the acceptable techniques that will provide analgesia or anesthesia, as well as significant risks and potential benefits. The discussion must include the advantages and disadvantages of each proposed technique. The patient's questions should be answered completely. This level of communication helps the practitioner uncover misconceptions while educating the patient about regional anesthesia.[8]

Another absolute contraindication is systemic anticoagulation in the patient. Certain drugs and systemic diseases can cause alterations in the coagulation profile. The long-term or extended use of aspirin products or nonsteroidal antiinflammatory drugs (NSAIDs) can prolong bleeding time without significantly altering other laboratory data. The patient's medical and pharmacologic history may provide information about increased bleeding time. Asking the patient about frequent bruising without injury may reveal the first indication of a problem. For instance, physical evaluation of the skin may show evidence of bruising or subcutaneous bleeding of which the patient may not recall the cause. If injury to a large epidural vessel were to occur during the performance of either a spinal or an epidural technique, significant bleeding could develop in the epidural space. A similar injury to the axillary artery in the confined space of the axilla might result in a hematoma that would produce further complications. Injury to a large vessel in the neck during an interscalene technique could result in compromise of the airway.[8]

In determining whether a regional anesthetic technique should be avoided, Winnie suggested using arbitrary values for platelet counts of less than 100,000 and prothrombin time (PT), activated partial thromboplastin time (aPTT), and bleeding times that are greater than two times normal values.[4,8] Severe bleeding with or without symptomatic hypovolemia or the potential for severe bleeding is a contraindication to the administration of a regional anesthetic. The contraindication can be considered either absolute or relative, depending on the clinical presentation of the patient. Trauma, along with physiologic or pathophysiologic conditions that cause contracted volume states and abruptio placentae, can result in the development of significant hypotension and tachycardia after the initiation of regional anesthesia, especially spinal or epidural anesthesia. A blockade of the sympathetic nervous system quickly develops, resulting in significant relaxation of the smooth muscles of the vascular bed. The extent of this block is dependent on the regional anesthesia technique, the dose of medication, and the volume of solution used when the procedure is performed.

When the patient demonstrates symptoms of hypovolemic shock on evaluation, his or her ability to safely tolerate peripheral vasodilatation and the subsequent reduction in systemic vascular resistance is reduced. The anesthetist's inability to compensate for falling blood pressure by increasing systemic vascular resistance places the patient at risk for potential hypoperfusion to vital organs and subsequent hypoxic tissue injury.

When an obstetric patient experiences abruptio placentae with or without fetal distress, the anesthesia practitioner must consider other anesthetic procedures. These alternatives should be considered so that hypotension and the compromise to fetal oxygen supply that results from decreased uterine blood flow can be minimized. Regional techniques require time to administer in addition to the reduction in blood pressure that occurs with establishment of the block. Uterine blood flow is dependent on arterial pressure and has few autoregulatory capabilities. However, when an epidural anesthetic has been established for labor, the time required for surgical anesthesia to be instituted may be less with epidural than with general anesthesia. The choice of anesthesia technique must focus on the possible effects of the sympathectomy, even if its development can be slowed or controlled. With the onset of the sympathetic blockade, the fall in blood pressure may be more than the mother and baby can tolerate. The anesthesia practitioner caring for the patient, in consultation with the patient's obstetrician, must decide whether administration of the regional anesthetic should be continued or whether another anesthesia procedure should be selected.[3-6,8]

If an active infectious process is present near the location at which regional anesthesia is to be performed, another anesthetic should be chosen.

Relative Contraindications and Precautions

One relative contraindication to regional anesthesia is patient age. In neonates with impairment in ventilatory regulation,

regional anesthesia techniques are recommended when either surgery or pain management is required. The knowledge and the abilities of the practitioner are more important considerations, however.[4,7,8]

Small children tolerate the administration of a combination anesthetic for many surgical procedures, including hernia procedures, extremity procedures, and circumcision. A general anesthetic can be administered for the surgical procedure, and a regional technique can be used for postoperative pain management. Anatomic landmarks are easily identified in children, which permits implementation without extensive difficulty. Precautions must be taken when the patient is of short stature. This technique should be avoided in children who are unable to tolerate the loss of feeling and strength in the legs. As children begin to acquire independence through increased ambulation, the loss of feeling and movement in the legs may increase their fear. This phenomenon is especially common in children between the ages of 3 and 9 years.[7]

Interscalene and axillary blocks have been used to permit immobilization and analgesia of the upper extremity for extended periods of time. Intravenous regional anesthesia (Bier block) has been used in small children aged 8 to 12 years; in these cases a reduced amount of local anesthetic medication is used for the reduction of an arm fracture.[9]

Patients who have difficulty understanding the procedures to be performed or who are unable to cooperate with the practitioner should undergo another type of anesthesia. Such patients may respond negatively to the presence of anyone behind them who may create confusion or cause discomfort; they could perceive this presence as an imminent threat and could respond inappropriately.

Patients with a history of headaches or backaches are at increased risk for experiencing these problems after spinal and epidural analgesia or anesthesia. Such patients should be evaluated and counseled regarding this potential before the administration of subarachnoid or epidural anesthesia. Postanesthesia symptoms of backache or headache become difficult to evaluate without information about the patient's previous pattern of headaches or backaches. Information about the position of the patient during the surgical or obstetric procedure assists in the evaluation of the patient.[4-6,10]

Patients with chronic neurologic disorders must be well informed of the potential effects of the regional anesthetic technique. The regional anesthetic may not cause an increase in the patient's symptoms; however, if symptoms of the disorder increase or deterioration results, the regional anesthetic technique may be identified as the cause of the problem.

Patients with a history of a documented local anesthetic allergy should undergo further evaluation in a controlled situation by an allergist. A true allergy to local anesthetic agents is rare. The problem may be caused by a preservative in the anesthetic solution or by a metabolic product of local anesthetic hydrolysis (para-aminobenzoic acid [PABA]). Skin testing is helpful but not always accurate. Patients may have a negative skin test but have a reaction when a concentration of the local anesthetic sufficient for the provision of anesthesia is administered. Alleged allergic reactions may be related to an intravenous injection of a local anesthetic solution that contains epinephrine.[11-13]

If a regional technique is used in a patient with an allergy, a local anesthetic that is unrelated to the suspected agent should be selected. For example, if the patient is allergic to an ester anesthetic, an amide anesthetic agent should be chosen. Before the anesthetic is administered, the patient should be medicated with histamine-1 and histamine-2 receptor blockers.

When the patient has a history of Mobitz type I, Mobitz type II, or third-degree heart block without a pacemaker, it may be advisable to choose another technique. In patients with increased plasma levels of local anesthetic after large-volume local anesthetic administration, stabilization of the cardiac cellular membrane may result in an increase in the degree of heart block.[3,8]

Patients with fixed-volume cardiac states are at risk for cardiovascular compromise after the initiation of a regional anesthetic. If the patient is unable to respond to changes in systemic vascular resistance by increasing stroke volume as a means of maintaining cardiac output, selected regional anesthesia techniques, including spinal and epidural anesthesia, should be reconsidered. As the heart rate increases to compensate for the falling pressure, the heart may fail, or ischemia may develop.[14]

COMPLICATIONS OF REGIONAL ANESTHESIA

Complications of regional anesthesia can be immediate or delayed. Cardiovascular problems are the most critical immediate complications. However, effects on the respiratory and gastrointestinal (GI) systems can have equally serious consequences. Delayed complications include problems involving the cardiovascular, musculoskeletal, genitourinary, and neurologic systems.

Immediate Complications

The potential of an intravascular injection is increased when local anesthetics are injected into the tissues around nerves and blood vessels or in high volumes. If lidocaine is injected into the intravascular space, central nervous system toxicity can occur. The patient may first complain of tingling of the lips, a strange taste in the mouth, ringing in the ears, and then visual disturbances. Seizures may also occur. In patients receiving an intravenous injection of 0.5% to 0.75% bupivacaine (Marcaine), the first symptom of intravascular injection may be a cardiac dysrhythmia. The most common dysrhythmias are of ventricular origin. Local anesthestic toxicity may progress from the symptoms noted above to seizure activity to respiratory and cardiovascular collapse. However, if the local anesthetic concentration in the brain rises rapidly, the initial expression of toxicity can be complete cardiovascular collapse.[4,8,10-15]

Delayed Complications

The anesthesia practitioner must be prepared to manage complications that occur after the block has been established or during the postanesthesia recovery period. Some complications are less difficult to manage than are others.

Complications Associated with Continuous Peripheral Nerve Blocks

Continuous peripheral nerve blocks (CPNBs) have been shown to improve postoperative pain control and hemodynamic stability, reduce opioid requirements, and decrease nausea and vomiting. There are few studies at present in the literature evaluating the adverse effects and complications of this technique. Wiegel and colleagues[16]. analyzed 1398 CPNBs performed in 849 orthopedic patients. The CPNBs included interscalene, femoral, sciatic, and a combination of femoral and sciatic blocks performed preoperatively in addition to general or spinal anesthesia. The standard technique included use of a nerve stimulator, injection of a bolus of local anesthetic, placement of the catheter, application of a transparent dressing, a single dose of antibiotic prophylaxis, and infusion of 0.2% ropivacaine at 5 to 8 mL per hour

commencing in the postanesthesia care unit for a period of 24 hours. Following this period, bolus doses of 0.2% ropivacaine (10 to 20 mL) were administered every 6 hours on an orthopedic ward. Patients were questioned about complications during their 3-month postoperative visit. The primary study end-point was the rate of complications, including nerve injury, bleeding requiring surgical intervention, catheter-associated infection, dyspnea, pneumothorax, and local anesthetic toxicity. A unique feature of this study was the extended period of time catheters remained in situ—up to 12 days in some cases. Local inflammation at the catheter insertion site occurred in 9 patients (0.6%), and local infection occurred in 3 patients (0.2%; all femoral CPNBs). There were 12 patients with transient neurologic deficits (0.9%), and 1 with a permanent neurologic deficit (0.1%). Vascular puncture occurred at a rate of 5.2%, and a catheter was broken in one patient as a result of withdrawing the catheter back into the needle, a practice that should always be avoided. The authors found that while major complications of CPNBs are rare, minor adverse events are not uncommon.[16]

Technical Difficulties

Technical problems include difficulties with equipment and supplies. Broken needles, broken catheters, glass in the epidural and subarachnoid spaces, and injection of the wrong drugs are some of the problems that can be encountered.

Disposable needles are made in two parts: the hub and the barrel. The two parts are joined together and then fused to create a single unit. The weakest point on the needle is at the joint with the hub. Precautions should be taken so that the needle is not inserted so far that the hub abuts the skin surface. In addition, the needle should not be bent. If extreme force is used while the needle is being inserted, the needle is stressed at the hub; this stress could cause the needle to break at the hub. If the needle is not inserted with the hub abutting the skin surface, some portion of the needle can be secured and removed, thus preventing its loss.[8,15,17]

Broken or sheared catheters are a concern in continuous regional anesthesia techniques. A visual inspection of the catheter should occur before it is inserted. The portion of the catheter that is inserted should have a radiopaque marker on the tip. Markings are placed at 1-cm divisions along the catheter, thereby providing an approximate measure for estimations of the length of the catheter that is inserted into the epidural or intrathecal space. When removed, the catheter should be inspected and its intactness verified and recorded on the patient's record. An epidural catheter should not be pulled back through the needle once the tip has passed beyond the bevel opening. The point where the two sides of the bevel join is the sharpest point of the entire needle. As the catheter is pulled back, it is forced against the joint and may be sheared off. If the catheter is sheared off, radiography can be used to locate the catheter, verify its position, and document the shearing. Catheters in use today have a radiopaque tip and are made of a material of low tissue reactivity. Surgical procedures used in the search for a catheter can delay a patient's recovery. The patient should be told of the problem, where the catheter is located, the composition of the catheter, and any other information that might help reduce concerns about the catheter's location. Most catheters can remain in place without causing problems. However, when the remaining catheter is located in the subarachnoid space, it must be retrieved. The potential exists for the catheter to migrate cephalad, causing further problems once it reaches the level of the spinal cord or is directed through a foramen into a nerve root.[4,8,15,17]

BOX 46-1

Regional Anesthesia Discharge Information Sheet

What is regional anesthesia?
Regional anesthesia is the injection of a local anesthetic (like Novocaine) near the nerves that sense pain from the area of your body that had surgery. Regional anesthesia is the same as a dentist injecting local anesthesia into your mouth—it numbs an area of your body so that procedures won't hurt.

What should I expect after regional anesthesia?
After regional anesthesia, the area of your body that had surgery will be numb for several hours. In fact, the area may be numb for up to 24 hours. The block will wear off slowly, and your first sensations will be a tingling feeling in the area that was numb.

What should I do when the block starts to wear off?
As soon as you develop any feeling in the numb area, begin taking the pain medications your surgeon has prescribed. It is much easier to treat pain before it begins than try to catch up later.

What should I be careful about after regional anesthesia?
Because part of your body is numb, you won't know if you injure it. You should take care to protect that part of your body from being bumped, cut, and otherwise harmed, and you should look at it frequently to make sure it isn't injured. You should also avoid lying on the numb area while you sleep.

What complications should I watch for after regional anesthesia?
The site of your body where the injection was made will be sore for a few days. This pain should go away with any over-the-counter pain-relief medicine (Tylenol, Advil, Motrin, etc.). It is not uncommon for the area that was numb to have some strange sensations (mild numbness, tingling, etc.) for a few days after the block.

If you experience any of the following changes, you should immediately phone your health-care provider:
- Sensation doesn't begin to return to the numb area after 24 hours.
- The area that was numb regained sensation but is becoming numb again.
- The skin in the numb area turns blue or feels cool.
- There is persistent pain in the area that was numb, even several days after the surgery.

Glass from broken ampules can be injected into the subarachnoid or epidural space or in the area of the nerve if care is not exercised during preparation of the medication. Ampules should be broken away from the tray and enclosed within a sponge that is then discarded. A filter needle should be used during the withdrawal of all medications from ampules. The filter needle should then be discarded to prevent injection of the particles that have been filtered. The glass particles may act as a foreign body, causing a local reaction and the development of a sterile abscess.[4,8]

Discharge Information

A useful tool to provide patients who have received a regional anesthetic is a discharge information sheet (Box 46-1). This sheet provides the patient with information about the nature of the anesthetic and what to expect as the block resolves. Most importantly it should alert the patient to contact the anesthesia provider in the event certain symptoms, which may indicate a potential complication of the regional anesthetic, occur following discharge.

PHARMACOLOGY OF LOCAL ANESTHETICS

See Chapter 11 for a complete discussion of the pharmacology of local anesthetics. To briefly review, local anesthetic agents temporarily block the transmission of a stimulus along the path of a nerve fiber through interference with the local ionic gradient across the cell membrane. Each nerve is composed of a cell body and an extension of the cell body known as an *axon*. Many nerves are covered with a sheath that is made of a phospholipid known as *myelin*. The sheath is produced by Schwann

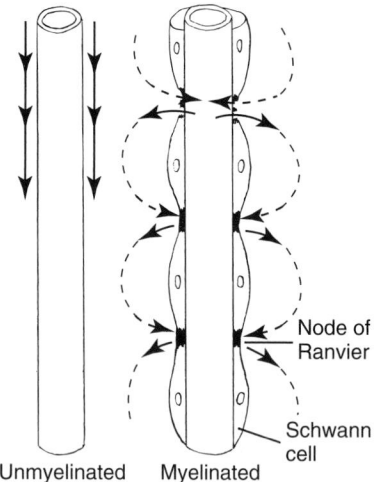

FIGURE **46-1** Unmyelinated and myelinated nerve fibers. In myelinated fibers the stimulus is transmitted from one node of Ranvier to the next in a hopping fashion, resulting in saltatory conduction.

cells in peripheral nerves and is interrupted in areas along the axon known as *nodes of Ranvier*. Electrical transmission along a myelinated fiber is different from that along an unmyelinated nerve fiber. In a myelinated fiber, the stimulus is transmitted from node of Ranvier to node of Ranvier in a hopping fashion (Figure 46-1). This phenomenon results in a more rapid transmission of the nerve impulse known as *saltatory conduction*.[17]

TABLE **46-1**	Local Anesthetic Drugs						
Local Anesthetic	pK$_a$	Nonionized Drug at pH 7.4 (%)	Mean Onset (min)	Mean Subarachnoid Block Onset (min)	Mean Epidural Onset (min)	Mean Brachial Plexus Duration (min)	Maximum Dose (mg) Without Epinephrine
Esters							
Procaine	8.9	3	45-60	2-5	NA	NA	1000
Tetracaine	8.6	14	7-10	7-10	NA	60-180	100; 1-1.5 mg/kg
Chloroprocaine	9.8	2	6-12	5-12	5-12	30-45	800-1000
Amides							
Lidocaine	7	24	3-7	5-10	5-15	60-120	300-500; 3 mg/kg without epi; 7 mg/kg with epi
Mepivacaine	7.6	39	5-7	10-20	5-15	90-180	300-500; same as lidocaine
Bupivacaine	8.1	17	8-15	2-5	10-20	240-480	175-225
Chirocaine	8.1	17	8-15	2-5	10-20	240-480	175-225
Ropivacaine	8.1	17	5-13	2-5	11-26	3-8	300
Prilocaine	7.9	24	5-20	5-15	5-15	60-120	400-600; 8 mg/kg with epi

Data from Mosby's Drug Consult. *St Louis: Mosby; 2007.*
epi, *Epinephrine;* NA, *not applicable.*

In an unmyelinated nerve fiber, the stimulus is transmitted continuously along the fiber.[11,18-21]

The cell membrane of the axon is important for the conduction of the stimulus. Several theories about the actual structure of the membrane have been proposed. A predominant theory postulates that the cell membrane has two layers that are made up of lipid molecules with protein molecules interspersed throughout the space. The protein molecules contain small openings known as *pores* or *channels* that are the size of small ions. Access to these channels is controlled by gates. These gates restrict the movement of ions between the intracellular and extracellular spaces. The gates are influenced by changes in the electrical field of the cell membrane.[19-21]

The primary function of most of the gates is to restrict the movement of sodium into the cell. Because the gates do not restrict the movement of potassium, it can freely move in and out of the cell. Potassium moves out of the cell when the cell is at rest, producing an internal environment that is negatively charged compared with the external milieu. Several selective cells and conducting tissues have gates that regulate the flow of other ions, such as calcium and magnesium. One of the methods of action of the local anesthetics is the stabilization of the gate by maintaining it in the closed position. This action may be accomplished by the fixing of the local anesthetic with intracellular calcium, which creates a large molecule and closes the gate. With the gate closed, sodium ion movement from the extracellular to the intracellular space is prevented. This stops the internal milieu of the cell from becoming relatively more positive, a process known as *depolarization*, and prevents the transmission of the impulse along the axon. The failure to alter the resting potential results in interference with the action potential cycle of the cell.[11,20-22]

Current thoughts on the action of local anesthetic agents suggest that the following events occur:

1. Calcium ions are displaced from a receptor site at the cell membrane as a result of the local anesthetic moiety.
2. Reduction in cell permeability to sodium ions results.
3. The rate of depolarization of the membrane action potential is decreased.

4. The degree of depolarization of the cell is insufficient for reaching the threshold potential of the cell.
5. A propagated action potential does not occur.
6. Conduction blockade is the end result.

The synthetic local anesthetics are weakly basic tertiary amines that are not readily soluble in water. Solubility is achieved by dissolving the local anesthetics in hydrochloric acid, producing a highly water-soluble and stable hydrochloride salt. When in an aqueous solution, the anesthetic compound dissociates into a positively charged quaternary amine (cation) and an uncharged tertiary amine base (free base).[12,13]

The direction of the reaction depends on the pH of the solution. Each anesthetic has a pK$_a$, which is the negative logarithm of the dissociation constant. Based on the Henderson-Hasselbalch equation, when the pK$_a$ of the drug equals the pH of the solution, 50% of the salt exists as a cation, and 50% exists as an uncharged free base. Because the pK$_a$ for a specific compound is constant, the amount of free base or charged cation is dependent on the pH of the solution.[12,13] As the pH of the solution decreases and the hydrogen ion concentration increases, the balance shifts, and more charged cation is present.

The positively charged cation is responsible for the ability of the local anesthetic to prevent the entrance of sodium ions into the cell. However, the positively charged cation is unable to penetrate the lipid soluble membrane and therefore cannot pass into the intracellular space. The uncharged free base is lipid soluble and is able to diffuse into the axon. Once the uncharged free base has crossed the cell membrane it dissociates, generating a proportion of cations. The cation acts to stabilize (close) the sodium channel gate, resulting in a block of movement of ions through the gate (Table 46-1). Therefore, the free base allows the local anesthetic access to the intracellular portion of the axon, where it dissociates into a percentage of cations that produce the conduction block. This dissociation is enhanced by the relatively lower pH that exists in the axon as compared with the extracellular fluid pH.

Both forms of the local anesthetic are necessary for the action of the medication to occur. One of the hindrances to the

TABLE 46-2	Local Anesthetics Classified by Duration and Potency	
Medication	**Duration**	**Potency**
Procaine	Short	Low
2-Chloroprocaine	Short	Moderate
Lidocaine	Moderate	Moderate
Prilocaine	Moderate	Moderate
Mepivacaine	Moderate	Moderate
Tetracaine	Long	High
Bupivacaine	Long	High
Ropivacaine	Long	High
Chirocaine	Long	High

administration of a local anesthetic drug is an acidic medium. When the tissues are acidotic, as is seen during an infection, the local anesthetic has difficulty diffusing across the cellular membrane and having sufficient positively charged cations to cause membrane stabilization.[11,23]

Each local anesthetic contains an aromatic derivative of benzoic acid or alanine that is lipophilic, as well as a hydrophilic teritary amine group. The hydrophilic portion is an amine derivative of ethyl alcohol or acetic acid. The two parts are linked by a hydrocarbon chain that contains an ester or an amide bond. Changing a portion of the chain alters the activity of the compound. Within limits, lengthening the chain increases the potency of the compound. Surpassing this limit results in a decrease in the potency of the anesthetic. Chemical alterations to the compounds that change the protein-binding characteristics change the duration of action of the local anesthetic (Table 46-2).[11,15,22]

Procaine, tetracaine, and 2-chloroprocaine are all ester-linked local anesthetics that are metabolized by hydrolysis by plasma cholinesterases. This rapid chemical reaction results in the metabolism of the local anesthetic once it is absorbed into the vascular space. There are no plasma cholinesterases in either the epidural space or the CSF. Lidocaine, bupivacaine, mepivacaine, etidocaine, levobupivacaine, and ropivacaine are amide-linked drugs. The amide-linked local anesthetics are metabolized by liver microsomes, and extended use of the medication in either repeated bolus doses or continuous infusions results in possible accumulation and toxicity. With the use of the short-acting, ester-linked, local anesthetic 2-chloroprocaine, accumulation and eventual toxicity are unlikely to occur because of its almost immediate hydrolysis in the plasma.[11,23,24]

Etidocaine was developed by modification of the lidocaine molecule. A propyl group is substituted for an ethyl group at the amine end. One ethyl group is added to an alpha carbon in the intermediate chain. This medication is more soluble and more highly protein bound, and it has a greater potency and a longer duration of action than the parent compound. The affinity of etidocaine is higher for motor neurons when compared with sensory neurons. When a butyl group was added to the aromatic end of the procaine molecule, tetracaine was synthesized. Tetracaine has a greater potency, a longer duration of action, and a higher toxicity than procaine.

Changing the chemical structure of the compound results in changes in its intrinsic toxicity and duration of action. Tetracaine is hydrolyzed more slowly than procaine and has a greater potential for toxicity. 2-Chloroprocaine is rapidly

hydrolyzed and is the least toxic of the ester-linked anesthetics. Prilocaine is an amide-linked local anesthetic that is rapidly metabolized; it has a smaller potential for toxicity than any other agent in this group.[11-13,23-25]

The potential for allergic reaction is greatest in the ester-linked group of local anesthetics. Drugs in this group are derivatives of PABA. The ester-linked local anesthetics are hydrolyzed by plasma cholinesterases, resulting in the formation of PABA. This compound can produce an allergic reaction in some individuals.

The metabolism of amide-linked local anesthetics does not produce PABA. The documented incidence of allergic reactions to amide local anesthetics continues to be rare. Local anesthetics that are prepared for multiple-dose regimens contain a stabilizing agent that can be an allergen. Individuals who have allergic reactions to amide local anesthetics may have received an injection with either PABA in the solution or another antigen. Patients may believe that an intravenous injection of an epinephrine-containing solution causes an allergic reaction because of the symptoms (increased heart rate) that may occur.[24]

The absorption and duration of action of local anesthetics are functionally dependent on the pharmacology of the agent, the dose administered, the anesthetic procedure performed, and the use of a vasopressor mixed with the solution. This may not be true of ropivacaine.[23]

In a study comparing solutions containing bupivacaine with those containing bupivacaine and epinephrine, no change in the duration of the anesthetic was observed when the epinephrine-containing solutions were used.[23] However, ropivacaine can produce a reduction in the blood flow to the area of the injection, resulting in a reduction of the absorption of the medication when a vasopressor agent was not used concomitantly.

Pharmacologically, each drug's duration of action is related to the protein-binding characteristics of the local anesthetic compound, the direct action of the agent, the pH of the solution (as well as of the area surrounding the injection), the rate of metabolism, the excretion of the agent or metabolites, the degree of vasodilatation in the area, and the specific tissue being injected.

Tetracaine, bupivacaine, levobupivacaine, and ropivacaine are highly protein bound; this quality results in a significantly greater duration of action than those of the medications that are less protein bound. Among the ester-linked anesthetics, tetracaine is 10 times more protein bound and has a duration of action three to four times greater than that of procaine. Among the amide-linked local anesthetics, bupivacaine, ropivacaine, and levobupivacaine are highly protein bound, whereas mepivacaine and lidocaine are relatively less protein bound. As a result, the duration of action of bupivacaine, levobupivacaine, and ropivacaine is two to three times longer than that of lidocaine and mepivacaine.[26]

Vasodilatory activity and metabolic rate also influence the duration of action of the local anesthetic. When lidocaine and procaine are compared in vitro, they are very similar; however, when they are compared in vivo, the duration of procaine is much shorter than that of lidocaine because of the vasodilator effects of procaine. When 2-chloroprocaine is compared with procaine, it has a shorter duration of action because of its rapid rate of metabolism.

Most local anesthetic agents produce vasodilatation as a result of direct smooth-muscle relaxation. However, cocaine and ropivacaine cause vasoconstriction. Cocaine inhibits the uptake of norepinephrine, resulting in vasoconstriction. The mechanism by which ropivacaine produces vasoconstriction in some tissues remains under investigation. Because of the potent vasodilatory effects of tetracaine, epinephrine or another vasoconstrictor is typcially used when this medication is administered outside the subarachnoid or epidural space. Lidocaine is a more potent vasodilator than prilocaine. No significant difference occurs in the vasodilatation seen with either bupivacaine or etidocaine.[20]

Adding a vasoconstrictor to a local anesthetic slows the uptake of the local anesthetic. Vasoconstriction decreases vascular absorption and removal of the local anesthetic from the local vicinity of the nerve, resulting in an increased intensity of the block and an increased duration of action. The duration of action of levobupivacaine and bupivacaine is minimally affected by the addition of epinephrine. However, the absorption of the anesthetic solution is delayed, an effect that reduces the plasma levels of the medication. When epinephrine is added to the local anesthetic, fresh epinephrine solutions rather than prepared solutions should be used. Commonly used concentrations of epinephrine include 1:200,000 or 1:400,000. The pH of a prepared local anesthetic stock solution containing epinephrine is lower than that of a freshly mixed local anesthetic and epinephrine solution, resulting in more of the cation moiety per milligram of drug and a potentially slower onset. Additionally, phenylephrine (100 mcg) can be used in place of epinephrine as a vasoconstrictor.[22]

Absorption of the local anesthetic determines its duration of action. The site of the injection directly affects the absorption of the agent. Local anesthetic injected into the intercostal nerve area results in the most rapid absorption. The slowest absorption results from cutaneous injections in areas of the body that have reduced blood supply. The rate of uptake changes the response to the medication. If the uptake is rapid, a less than toxic dose can cause toxic symptoms because of the rapid rise in the blood level of the medication.

As with other medications, local anesthetics are distributed throughout the body based on the rules of diffusion and redistribution. The highest concentrations of local anesthetics are found in vessel-rich tissues, and the lowest concentrations are found in vessel-poor tissues. Bupivacaine's affinity for cardiac muscle tissue is one of the many factors that contribute to the increased toxicity of this drug, especially in cardiac tissue.

Placental transfer of local anesthetics is dependent on the rate of diffusion and protein binding.[19] After epidural injection, bupivacaine and levobupivacaine appear to have the lowest concentrations in the umbilical vein, whereas lidocaine and mepivacaine have moderate concentrations. Agents that are highly protein bound in the mother, a quality that results in a low maternal plasma concentration, may have a higher concentration in the fetal circulation. Medication chosen for obstetric use should have reduced ability to cross the placenta.[10,27]

Excretion depends on metabolism of the drug. The metabolism of both groups of local anesthetics is dependent on liver function, either through direct degradation or through the production of pseudocholinesterases. The ester-linked local anesthetics are hydrolyzed by plasma pseudocholinesterase into PABA and diethylamino-ethanol. The amide-linked local anesthetics undergo degradation via hydrolysis in the liver. The rate of hydrolysis has a direct effect on toxicity. Prilocaine is the most rapidly metabolized and the least toxic of this group.

Although metabolites of the amide-linked local anesthetics have been found, the complete mechanism of degradation has not yet been identified. Lidocaine oxidizes to become monoglycinexylidide. In normal patients, little concern exists regarding the toxic or pharmacologic effects of the residual metabolite. However, in patients with renal failure, this metabolite may accumulate and play a role in increased toxicity. Prilocaine is metabolized to o-toluidine, which can cause the development of methemoglobin, thus resulting in methemoglobinemia. This condition may develop when the dose of the local anesthetic exceeds 400 mg. Treatment of methemoglobinemia consists of administration of methylene blue, 1 to 5 mg/kg.

In addition, excretion of the local anesthetics is dependent on renal function. Less than 2% of procaine is excreted unchanged, whereas 100% of cocaine is excreted unchanged. An inverse relationship exists between renal clearance of the amide-linked local anesthetics and the degree of protein binding. Prilocaine is less protein bound than lidocaine, which results in more rapid renal clearance of prilocaine.[11]

ELECTRICAL STIMULATORS IN REGIONAL ANESTHESIA

Peripheral nerve stimulators have become an indispensable tool in the practice of regional anesthesia. Knowledge and in-depth understanding of how they function is required if their full potential in a clinical setting is to be realized.[28]

Electrical translocation devices provide a controlled stimulating pulse of variable amplitude that is administered through a conducting device. Location of neural fibers is improved without the need for eliciting repeated paresthesias. Specialized shielded needles have been designed to localize the distribution of the stimulating charge to the tip of the needle. This characteristic reduces confusion from wide-field stimulation of the area around the nerve, thereby enhancing the isolation of the appropriate nerve fibers. If specialized sheathed needles are not available, the alternative is preparation of a shielded needle through the use of an intravenous catheter and a short-beveled needle. The needle must be advanced slowly, and the amplitude of the unit must be adjusted as the needle approaches the nerve.

The electrical device must be equipped with an accurately adjustable amplitude from 0 to 5 mÅ. When a device is being selected for use with electrotranslocation techniques, it is advantageous to choose a device with a digital readout of the amplitude of the stimulus being delivered. The negative lead is attached to the skin with an electrocardiogram electrode, and the positive lead is attached to the needle. When this technique is used, the stimulator should not be turned on until the needle has entered the skin. This measure reduces the discomfort experienced by the patient during the initial advancement of the needle. The patient must be instructed to identify discomfort verbally and to not move during the advancement of the needle.[18,28-30]

Limiting the sedation helps the patient tolerate the procedure, maintain sufficient alertness to respond to the stimulus, and be cooperative. Use of an electrotranslocation device can assist the practitioner during the administration of nerve block anesthesia to patients with sensory perception difficulties or neural degeneration, such as that experienced during end-stage renal disease.

The stimulator is adjusted to deliver 2 mÅ after the needle has been introduced into the subcutaneous tissues. As the needle approaches the sheath, the amplitude is continuously reduced so that the muscle response to the stimulus is maintained. When the needle enters the sheath, the amplitude should be reduced to 0.5 mÅ. The muscle response to the stimulus continues to be the same as that obtained when the needle is outside of the sheath. The lower amplitude decreases the discomfort experienced by the patient while enhancing the anesthetist's ability to accurately identify the neurovascular bundle.

The use of an electrotranslocation device should not be restricted to brachial plexus techniques. Such a device can be used for enhancing any technique in which identification of specific nerve roots improves the success of the block and reduces the amount of medication required for anesthesia of the nerve root.

Electrotranslocation devices or a peripheral nerve stimulator can be used with continuous spinal and epidural techniques for monitoring the level of the motor or sensory block. After the desired level of block is established, the nerve stimulator can be used for monitoring the block. The stimulator leads are connected to the patient at the lowest level of motor block desired. When the patient responds to the stimulus at this level, local anesthetic can be administered to increase the level of the block. With the electrodes in place, a stimulus is applied at an amplitude of 2.5 mA for 15 seconds at intervals of 10 to 15 minutes.

A peripheral nerve stimulator or an electrotranslocation device can be used for determining the level of the anesthetic with single-shot spinal and epidural techniques. If the patient is unable to interpret changes in temperature, single twitches or tetanus that results from lowered settings can provide information on the level of the block. This technique can minimize the patient's discomfort during the evaluation period. Patients may complain of aching or weakness along the path of the stimulated nerve after the regional anesthesia is terminated. This phenomenon is seen after the posterior tibial or the common peroneal nerves are stimulated. Severe or prolonged discomfort occurs when the stimulus is delivered over a long period or at a high current. The response to a stimulus with a lower amplitude is often adequate and results in less discomfort. Placement of the negative electrode has been important in the enhancement of electrotranslocation of the nerve. If the path of the nerve fiber is located under the negative electrode, a lesser stimulus produces a significant response.

ULTRASOUND-GUIDED REGIONAL ANESTHESIA

The technology and clinical understanding of anatomic sonography has evolved greatly over the past decade. In anesthesia departments throughout the United States, ultrasonography has become a routine technique for regional anesthetic nerve block. Recent studies have shown that direct visualization of the distribution of local anesthetics with high-frequency probes can improve the quality and avoid the complications of upper/lower extremity nerve blocks and neuroaxial techniques. Ultrasound guidance enables the anesthetist to secure an accurate needle position and monitor the distribution of the local anesthetic in real time. The advantages over conventional guidance techniques, such as nerve stimulation and loss-of-resistance procedures, are significant. Considering ultrasound's enormous potential, these techniques should have a role in the future training of anesthesia providers. The key requirement for successful regional anesthetic block is to ensure optimal distribution of local anesthetic around nerve structures. This goal is most effectively achieved under sonographic visualization. Over the past decade, the Vienna study group has demonstrated that ultrasound guidance can significantly improve the quality of nerve block in almost all types of regional anesthesia. In addition, complications such as intraneuronal and intravascular injection can be reduced. The use of ultrasound guidance in daily clinical practice requires high-level ultrasonographic equipment and a high degree of training. Anesthetists need to develop a thorough understanding of the anatomic structures involved, and they need to acquire both a solid grounding in ultrasound technology and the practical skills to visualize nerve structures. The successful performance of nerve block under direct ultrasonographic guidance varies with the operator's skill in a given regional anesthetic technique.

Experience suggests that it is best to begin learning ultrasonographic blocks on peripheral nerves under supervision before going on to more central blocks. Despite a lack of specific learning curves for ultrasonographically guided regional anesthetic nerve blocks, studies have shown a rapid increase in the number of successful blocks performed by anesthetists experienced in regional anesthesia, always depending on individual ability. Prior to using ultrasonographic regional anesthesia techniques, anesthetists should acquire the necessary skills by attending hands-on workshops. High success rates can be achieved compared with conventional guidance techniques using nerve stimulation. Significant improvements can be obtained in sensory and motor onset times. This superior quality of perioperative analgesia has greatly improved patient satisfaction among adults.[31]

UPPER-EXTREMITY BLOCK

Frequent injury of the hand, arm, and shoulder, combined with the accessibility of the nerves of the brachial plexus, has encouraged the development of regional anesthesia techniques for surgical procedures of the upper extremity, as well as the diagnosis and control of pain.[29,30,32-36] The widespread use of upper-extremity regional anesthesia is the result of numerous factors, including the availability of equipment to locate and deliver local anesthetics to the nerves of the plexus, the development of local anesthetics that can be applied alone and in combination to produce an appropriate duration of action for the procedure at hand, and the variety of techniques and approaches that can be used. The four primary approaches to block the brachial plexus are axillary, interscalene, supraclavicular, and infraclavicular. Because of the ease of performance, the relatively high success rate and low incidence of complications, and the ability to produce anesthesia of the forearm and hand, the most frequently used technique is the axillary approach. The requirement for anesthesia of the upper arm and shoulder is most often met through use of the interscalene approach. This is because of the potential complications associated with needle placement in close proximity to the apex of the lung necessary with supraclavicular and infraclavicular block. However, the decision to use one approach rather than another when both will produce satisfactory anesthesia of a specific region of the upper extremity is often driven by the training and experience of the anesthesia provider. The decision to use regional anesthesia rather than general anesthesia (which may be viewed by the surgeon as failure-free and more expedient) for elective and emergency surgical procedures of the upper extremity requires a strong commitment to and expertise in the use of these techniques. A practitioner who rarely uses these techniques during "normal" working hours does a disservice to both the patient and the surgical team by selecting brachial plexus block for the patient with upper extremity trauma who requires emergent surgery in the middle of the night. Moreover, the astute practitioner with experience and expertise in regional anesthesia does not lose sight of the fact that even in the most skilled hands, upper extremity block is associated with a degree of failure. In this regard, one can never rule out the potential requirement for conversion to general anesthesia and therefore must be cognizant of elements of the patient's history and physical examination that would affect the ability to manage the airway and deliver general anesthesia safely.[29,30,32-36]

Despite the fact that existing patient pathology may suggest a regional anesthetic, it is unwise to base the decision to use an upper extremity block (or any regional technique) solely on the

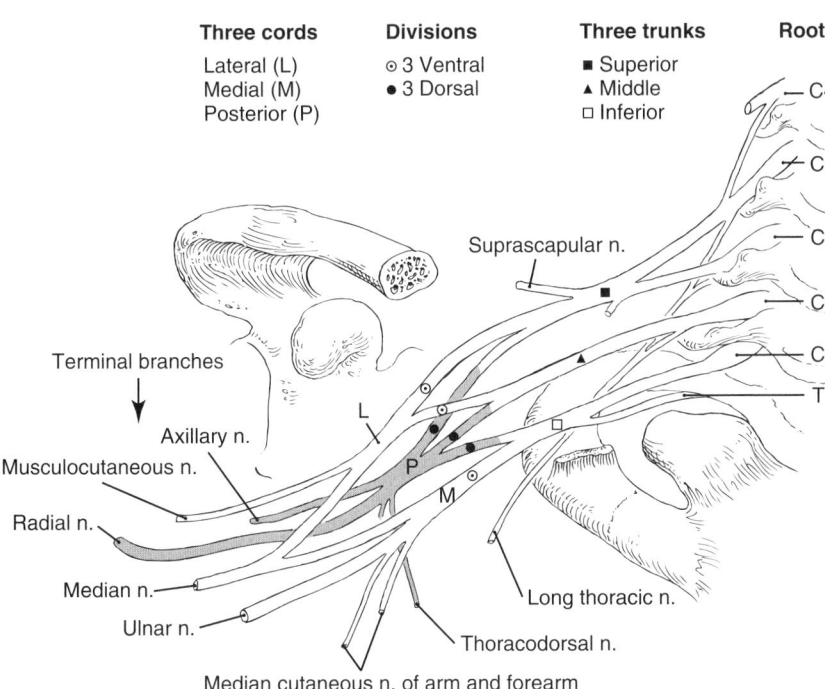

Three cords
Lateral (L)
Medial (M)
Posterior (P)

Divisions
⊙ 3 Ventral
● 3 Dorsal

Three trunks
■ Superior
▲ Middle
□ Inferior

Roots

C4
C5
C6
C7
C8
T1

Suprascapular n.

Terminal branches

Axillary n.

Musculocutaneous n.

Radial n.

Median n.

Ulnar n.

Thoracodorsal n.

Long thoracic n.

Median cutaneous n. of arm and forearm

FIGURE **46-2** Derivation of the brachial plexus from the cervical spine. *n*, Nerve.

premise that general anesthesia should be avoided, because ultimately it may be unavoidable. The circumstances should dictate the degree to which "plan B" is considered and executed before administration of the block.[29,30-36]

Brachial Plexus Anesthesia
Applied Anatomy of the Brachial Plexus
An understanding of brachial plexus anatomy is mandatory if effective clinical application of regional block techniques of the upper extremity is to be achieved. This includes familiarity with muscle, facial, and vascular anatomy in relation to the origin and distribution of the brachial plexus. However, intimate knowledge of many of the anatomic details with regard to the evolution of nerve roots distributed to the brachial plexus and ultimately to peripheral nerves is not clinically essential for successful blockade. The brachial plexus is a large network of nerves that extend from the neck through the axilla and innervate the upper extremity (Figure 46-2). It is composed of ventral rami, trunks, divisions, cords, and their branches. The supraclavicular portion of the plexus, including the five primary ventral rami and the three nerve trunks and their six divisions, lies in the posterior triangle of the neck. The infraclavicular portion of the plexus, including the three cords and their four terminal branches, lies in the axilla. These nerves combine, divide, recombine, and divide again as they pass between the anterior and middle scalene muscles, through the posterior triangle of the neck, and into the axilla, where they end in the four terminal branches that supply the upper extremity. The resulting nerve pathway, when pictured and contemplated in two dimensions and without the associated bone, muscle, and vascular structures, often leads to difficulty in understanding and applying this textbook anatomy in the clinical setting. When learning brachial plexus blockade, the value of augmenting written material with an apprenticeship at the hands of a master of the art cannot be overestimated.[29,30-36]

The archetypal brachial plexus is formed by the rami from the fifth (C5) to the eighth (C8) cervical nerves and the first thoracic (T1) nerve. In a small percentage of individuals, the fourth cervical (C4) or the second thoracic (T2) nerve or a combination

of the two contributes to the plexus. After the rami pass the lateral border of the scalene muscles, they reorganize into trunks. The rami from C5 and C6 combine to form the superior or upper trunk, and the ramus from C7 continues alone as the middle trunk. The rami from C8 and T1 combine to form the inferior or lower trunk, which lies on the first rib posterior to the subclavian artery. The nerve trunks are enveloped by a fascial "sheath," the origins of which are from the posterior fascia of the anterior scalene muscle and the anterior fascia of the middle scalene muscle. This forms a closed space at this level known as the *interscalene space*, or more generally as the *sheath of the brachial plexus*. Cadaver studies have demonstrated the existence of extensive velamentous septa that can form compartments around the contents of this sheath. These septa appear to be incomplete and therefore may not function as mechanical barriers to the spread of local anesthetics. Indeed, a single injection of local anesthesia into this sheath commonly produces complete block of the upper extremity. Nevertheless, anatomic variations do exist, and it is possible that in certain individuals, septa occur that isolate nerves, resulting in so-called "patchy blocks" by preventing exposure to the injected local anesthetic. It has also been shown that injection even outside the sheath can produce neural blockade, albeit with a considerably greater latency period. The lesson to be learned with regard to clinical application of this information is that failure to allot a sufficient amount of time to perform an upper extremity block, and in particular to allow it to "set up," generally produces an unsatisfactory result.[29,30,32-36]

At the lateral border of the first rib and posterior to the clavicle, each of the three trunks divides into ventral and dorsal divisions. These divisions are of significant clinical importance to application and evaluation of brachial plexus blockade, because the ventral divisions generally supply the ventral (flexor) portion of the upper extremity, and the dorsal divisions generally supply the dorsal (extensor) portions. As these divisions enter the axilla, the three posterior divisions combine to form the posterior cord, the anterior divisions of the superior and middle trunks combine to form the lateral cord, and the anterior division of the inferior trunk continues to become the medial cord. At that point, the cords are named according to their position in relation to the axillary artery. At the lateral border of the pectoralis minor muscle, each of these cords divides into two branches that reorganize to form the peripheral nerves of the upper extremity. The lateral cord divides and generates the musculocutaneous nerve and the lateral root of the median nerve. The medial cord divides and generates the ulnar nerve and the medial root of the median nerve. The posterior cord divides to generate the axillary and the radial nerves.

Understanding the anatomic relationships that result as the nerve cords give rise to the nerve branches and knowing the areas of the upper extremity these branches innervate are of paramount importance in the clinical application, evaluation, and supplementation of brachial plexus block. The branches of the lateral and medial cords (median, ulnar, and musculocutaneous nerves) predominantly supply the ventral portions of the upper extremity, and the branches of the posterior cord (radial and axillary nerve) predominantly supply the dorsal portions. However, in certain areas of the upper extremity, such as the posterior portion of the fingers and hand, there exists considerable cutaneous representation of the "predominantly ventral" median and ulnar nerves.

The radial nerve (C5 to C8 and Tl) is the major nerve supply to the dorsal extensor muscles, such as the triceps, of the upper limb below the shoulder. It supplies sensory innervation to the extensor region of the arm, forearm, and hand. The musculocutaneous nerve (C5 to C7) supplies the flexor muscles, such as the biceps, brachialis, and coracobrachialis, of the ventral portion of the arm. It supplies sensory innervation to the lateral aspect of the forearm between the wrist and elbow as the lateral antebrachial cutaneous nerve. The median and ulnar nerves pass through the arm and provide sensory and motor innervation to the forearm and hand. The median nerve (C6 to Tl) is better represented than the ulnar nerve in the forearm, where it supplies most of the flexor and pronator muscles. It also supplies sensory innervation to the ventral portion of the thumb, the first and second fingers, the lateral half of the third finger, and the palm of the hand. The ulnar nerve (C8 and Tl) is better represented than the median nerve in the hand, where it supplies motor innervation to most of the small flexor muscles. It has no sensory innervation of the forearm but supplies sensation to the medial part of the third finger, the entire fourth finger, and the remaining portion of the palm of the hand.

Approaches to Brachial Plexus Block

There are multiple approaches to local anesthetic block of the brachial plexus and various techniques applied with each approach. The choice of approach should be based on several factors, including patient considerations, the location of the planned surgical intervention, and especially the skill and experience of the anesthesia practitioner. Although surgical site and practitioner preference often drive the decision as to which approach and technique are used, the patient's body habitus, comfort, and coexisting disease and the nature and location of the injury are as important, if not more so, than these other concerns. Patient-related considerations should be weighed in the context of the risk of potential complications associated with a given approach, technique, and local anesthetic solution. The following discussion provides a practical approach to anesthesia of the brachial plexus, with a focus on axillary and interscalene approaches.[29,30,32-36]

Axillary Approach. The axillary approach to anesthesia of the brachial plexus is best suited to surgical procedures at or

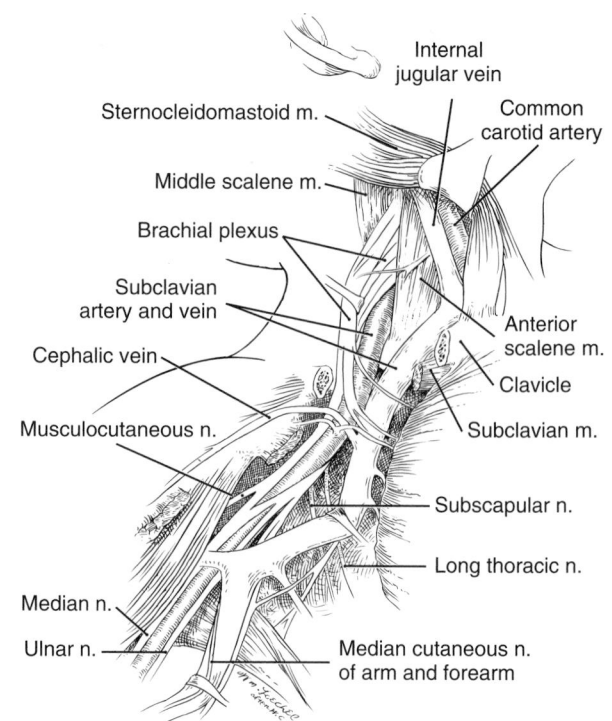

FIGURE **46-3**   The brachial plexus at the axilla. *m*, Muscle; *n*, nerve.

below the elbow (hand and forearm). However, an injury to the hand or forearm such as a fracture—which also limits the range of motion of the extremity because of patient discomfort—reduces the versatility of this approach. Under these conditions, patient comfort must be weighed against the need for profound anesthesia of the hand or forearm, often in the presence of a full stomach and the desire to avoid general anesthesia. In this instance, access to the axilla can generally be gained by the judicious use of intravenous opioids before slow, careful positioning and support of the extremity in preparation for placement of the block.[29,30,32-34,36]

The patient is placed in the supine position, with the arm to be blocked abducted 90 degrees from the body. The forearm is flexed to 90 degrees and rested parallel to the long axis of the body. The anesthetist uses the index and third fingers to identify the axillary artery, starting at the lateral margin of the pectoralis major muscle and tracing the artery into the mid- to lower axilla (Figure 46-3). Needle insertion need not occur high in the axilla, as some authors suggest, for successful block. Insertion in the mid- to lower axilla is just as effective; however, it reduces the chances that a local anesthetic will reach the point at which the musculocutaneous nerve leaves the sheath. A well-defined, localized pulsation of the axillary artery is more important to successful blockade than the point at which needle insertion occurs within the axilla. After appropriate preparation of the skin, a local anesthetic intradermal skin wheal is raised just proximal and superior to the palpating index finger. During needle insertion, moderate digital pressure should be applied to the artery to minimize the distance between the skin and subcutaneous tissue and the neurovascular bundle. An appropriate needle connected to a sterile extension tubing and syringe containing 50 mL of local anesthetic is inserted through the skin wheal. At this point the technique diverges, depending on the endpoint used to determine when the needle tip lies within the sheath. These end-points include loss of resistance to the advancing

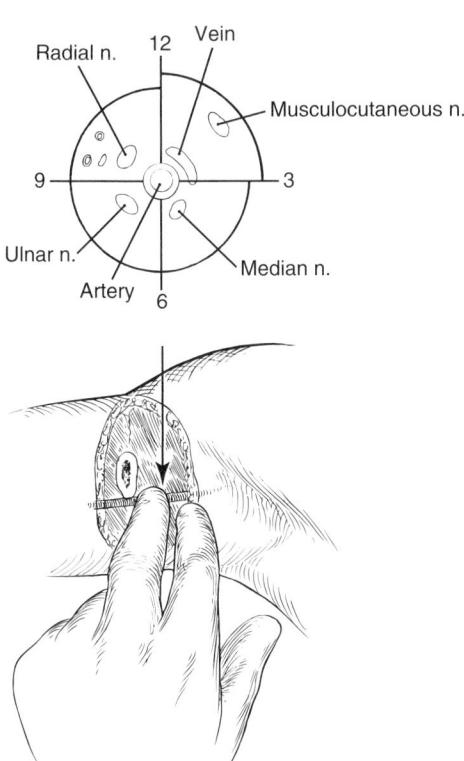

FIGURE **46-4** Identification of the intercostobrachial and brachial cutaneous nerves after completion of the axillary block. *n*, Nerve.

needle, penetration of the axillary artery, and elicitation of a paresthesia.[29,30,32-34,36-49]

Loss-of-Resistance Technique. The loss-of-resistance technique uses a distinct change in tissue resistance often described as a "pop" as the needle penetrates the fascia and enters the sheath. After the axillary artery is identified, a 22-gauge, 1½-inch, short-bevel ("B-bevel") needle is inserted medially at approximately a 20-degree angle to the skin and parallel to the longitudinal course of the artery (Figure 46-4). Use of a short-bevel needle enhances the loss-of-resistance sensation on penetration of the sheath; however, the drag associated with the attachment of an extension tubing decreases this sensation. Some practitioners disconnect the extension tubing and observe the free needle for a pulsatile movement associated with the needle tip's close proximity to the axillary artery. This is considered a further indication of correct needle placement within the sheath, but it does not guarantee proper placement. The needle is then advanced medially an additional ½ to 1 inch parallel to the axillary artery at an acute angle to the skin. Before local anesthesia is injected, the patient is instructed to immediately inform the anesthetist if symptoms indicative of rapid intravascular uptake or direct intravascular injection occur. These include dizziness, tinnitus, metallic taste in the mouth ("mouth full of nickels"), circumoral numbness or tingling, visual disturbances, and muscle twitching. If epinephrine has been added to the local anesthetic to reduce vascular absorption of the solution, the patient may also be instructed to report the sensation of having a "rapid" or "hard" heartbeat. The needle is held fixed in position, and an assistant gently aspirates the syringe while the operator observes for blood in the extension tubing, which would indicate that the needle has entered the axillary artery or vein. In the absence of frank blood in the aspirate, a 3- to 5-mL test

dose of the local anesthetic solution is injected and the patient observed and queried for the existence of any of the vascular warning symptoms for a minimum of 1 minute. Barring an untoward event, the remainder of the local anesthetic solution is injected in 5-mL increments, with each injection preceded by gentle aspiration and observation for blood in the extension tubing. During the injection, firm pressure should be applied with several fingers to the area immediately behind the needle insertion site to prevent retrograde flow of the anesthetic solution. Injection of each 5 mL of local anesthetic should be considered a "test dose," because unrecognized penetration of the artery or rapid uptake of the local anesthetic remains a possibility throughout the procedure. When 40 mL of the local anesthetic solution has been injected, the needle is withdrawn to the level of the skin in preparation for field block, if desired, of the musculocutaneous, medial brachial cutaneous, and intercostobrachial nerves (see Figure 46-4). These nerves may require individual blockade because they exit the sheath high in the axilla (musculocutaneous and medial brachial cutaneous) or lie outside the sheath altogether (intercostobrachial). If care is taken to apply continuous digital pressure immediately below the site of needle insertion during injection of a 40-mL bolus of local anesthetic solution, and the arm is adducted after injection, anesthesia of the musculocutaneous nerve and its terminal distribution, the lateral antebrachial nerve (sensory innervation to the lateral forearm from the elbow to the wrist), can be achieved. Before the needle is withdrawn from the skin, the musculocutaneous nerve can be independently blocked by injecting 3 to 5 mL of the remaining local anesthetic into the body of the coracobrachialis muscle. The coracobrachialis muscle is located immediately superior to the axillary artery and inferior to the biceps brachialis muscle. After block of the musculocutaneous nerve has been performed, the needle is again withdrawn to the level of the skin and redirected inferior and perpendicular to the artery into the subcutaneous tissue. The remaining 3 to 5 mL of local anesthetic is injected into the subcutaneous tissue as the needle is advanced to the hub. This subcutaneous "bracelet" of local anesthetic produces conduction block of the medial brachial cutaneous and intercostobrachial nerves necessary to prevent discomfort if a tourniquet is to be used. After completion of the block, the arm is immediately adducted and held close to the body to promote the cephalad spread of the local anesthetic solution, which can be obstructed by the abducted humeral head.[29,30,32-34,39]

Transarterial Technique. The transarterial technique uses intentional penetration of the axillary artery and aspiration of blood as the end-point for determining that the needle is within the sheath. After the axillary artery is identified, a local anesthetic skin wheal is raised directly above the artery at the planned point of needle insertion (see Figure 46-4). A 21-gauge, 1½-inch needle is inserted perpendicularly to the skin and advanced slowly until blood is aspirated into the extension tubing by an assistant, who provides gentle aspiration of the syringe. The needle is then advanced along the same plane until blood can no longer be aspirated because the bevel has exited the posterior wall of the artery. Care must be taken to avoid advancing the needle through the posterior wall of the sheath after the artery is exited, which would result in deposition of the local anesthetic outside the sheath. Failure rate of the transarterial technique has been shown to be significantly reduced when a 26-gauge, ½-inch needle is used as opposed to a 22-gauge, 1½-inch needle.[33] Presumably the shorter needle reduces the chance of exiting the posterior wall of the sheath and deposition of local anesthetic outside the sheath. Before local anesthetic is injected, the patient is instructed to immediately inform the anesthetist if symptoms indicative of rapid intravascular uptake or direct intravascular injection occur. The needle is held fixed in position, and an assistant gently aspirates the syringe while the operator observes for blood in the extension tubing, which would indicate that the needle has entered the axillary artery or vein. In the absence of frank blood in the aspirate, a 3- to 5-mL test dose of the local anesthetic solution is injected, and for a minimum of 1 minute, the patient is observed for and queried regarding the existence of any of the symptoms previously noted. Barring an untoward event, the remainder of the local anesthetic solution is injected in 5-mL increments, with each injection preceded by gentle aspiration and observation for blood in the extension tubing. Again, to prevent retrograde flow of the anesthetic solution, firm pressure with several fingers should be applied to the area immediately behind the needle insertion site during the injection. Injection of each 5 mL of local anesthetic should be considered a "test dose," because unrecognized penetration of the artery or rapid uptake of the local anesthetic remains a possibility throughout the procedure. When 40 mL of the local anesthetic solution has been injected, the needle is withdrawn to the level of the skin in preparation for field block, if desired, of the musculocutaneous, medial brachial cutaneous, and the intercostobrachial nerves, as noted previously.[29,30,32-34,36]

Interscalene Approach. The interscalene approach to the brachial plexus was first described in 1970 by Dr. Alon Winnie. The interscalene approach is the most proximal brachial plexus block and is typically used to provide anesthesia for surgical procedures involving the shoulder and proximal humerus. It is the only technique that can provide adequate anesthesia and analgesia to the shoulder and the rest of the upper extremity. The catheter is placed at the level of the trunks, where the brachial plexus is relatively compact in size.[37] With the patient in the supine position, the anesthetist asks the patient to lower the shoulder on the side of the proposed anesthetic and surgery site to pull the shoulder away from the brachial plexus, intentionally trying to stretch the neck muscles and improve visualization and access. The patient's head can then either be turned so that the patient looks away from the area of the anesthetic or moved laterally away from the site, maintaining forward vision.

The cricoid cartilage ring is then palpated just below the thyroid cartilage. This anatomic landmark correlates to the vertebral body of C6 and the corresponding area of the transverse process called *Chassaignac's tubercle*. A straight line is drawn posteriorly to cross over the sternocleidomastoid (SCM) muscle, and the lateral border of the SCM is palpated. If this border is difficult to assess, the patient can be asked to raise the head against gentle resistance and then relax. Posterior to this border, the anesthetist palpates for the groove between the anterior and middle scalene muscles with two fingers (Figure 46-5). This is the level of the trunks of the brachial plexus (Figure 46-6).

After cleansing the patient's skin, an intradermal skin wheal of local anesthetic is made at this point on the groove. A 22-gauge, insulated B-bevel needle, usually 1½ inches long, is inserted gently through the skin wheal perpendicularly to the skin and then angled slightly caudad. The needle is attached to an intravenous extension tube with an anesthetic-filled syringe. The patient is told what to expect, and the needle is slowly advanced until a motor twitch response is elicited. The nerve stimulator current is lowered from 1 to 0.5 mA to minimize excessive current to the patient and to ensure proper needle position. After gentle aspiration is negative for blood or CSF, a test dose of 1 mL of local anesthetic solution is injected. A fade will

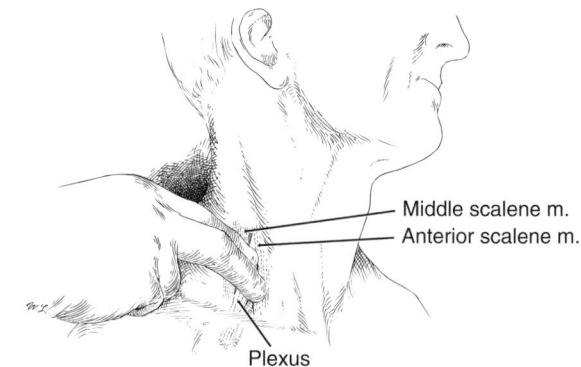

FIGURE **46-5**   Technique for identifying the anterior and middle scalene muscles and the major vessels so the interscalene perivascular technique can be accomplished. *m*, Muscle.

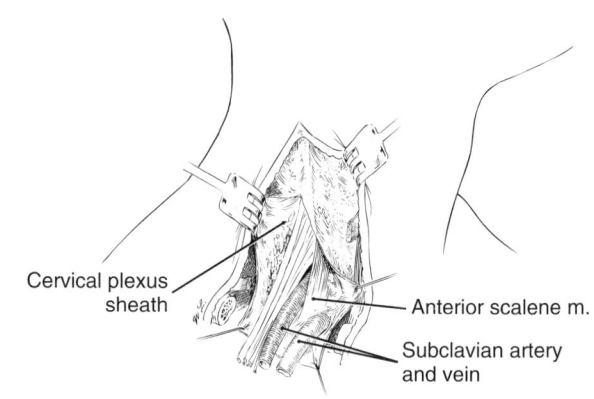

FIGURE **46-6**   Three trunks of the cervical plexus are revealed lying alongside the subclavian vessels. *m*, Muscle.

be observed in the quality of the motor twitch experienced by the patient. This indicates that the needle is probably within the brachial plexus sheath. If no subjective symptoms of toxicity reaction are present, incremental injections of 3 to 5 mL of local anesthetic, each followed by aspiration to detect blood, are administered until the intended volume is given. In adult patients, the volume is usually 30 to 35 mL.[29,30,32-34,36,39]

Subclavian Approach. The patient is positioned and prepared as for the interscalene approach (Figure 46-7). In addition, some practitioners may place the patient's bed in a 30- to 45-degree head-up position or place a pillow under the patient's shoulder to accentuate the anatomy. The area above and including the clavicle on the surgical side is cleansed and draped.

The pulsations of the subclavian artery in the plexus are behind and below the clavicle, just above the superior surface of the first rib and between the scalene muscles; the artery is palpated behind the midpoint of the clavicle. The anesthetist uses the nondominant hand to palpate for pulsations behind and 1 to 2 cm above the clavicle at this point and uses the dominant hand to place a skin wheal of local anesthetic immediately lateral to this site. Through the skin wheal, the 22-gauge, insulated B-bevel needle, attached to a nerve stimulator, is advanced perpendicularly to the skin, inward, and caudad until a motor twitch is noted in the lower portion of the upper extremity (Figure 46-8). The nerve stimulator current is lowered from 1 to 0.5 mA to minimize excessive current to the patient and to ensure proper needle position. After gentle aspiration is negative

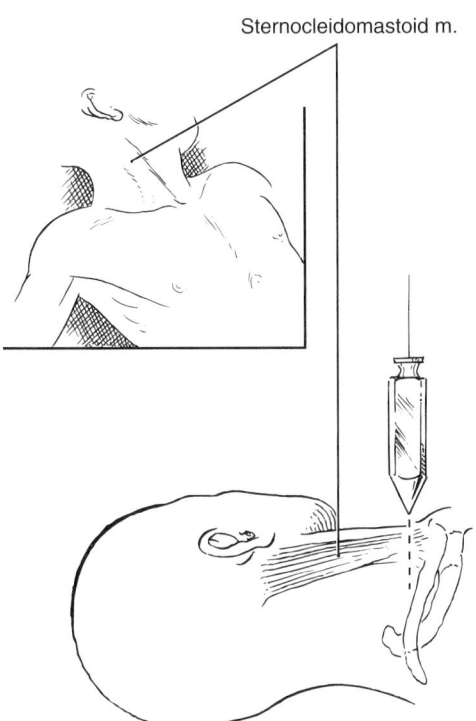

FIGURE **46-7** The patient is placed in the supine position with the head supported and turned toward the opposite shoulder. *m.*, Muscle.

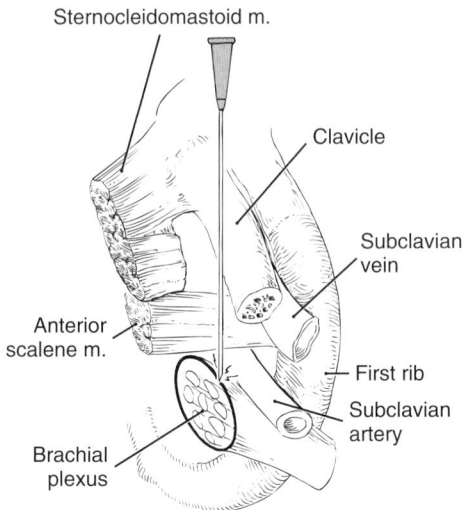

FIGURE **46-8** The needle enters the sheath of the brachial plexus at the farthest possible distance from the subclavian artery. *m*, Muscle.

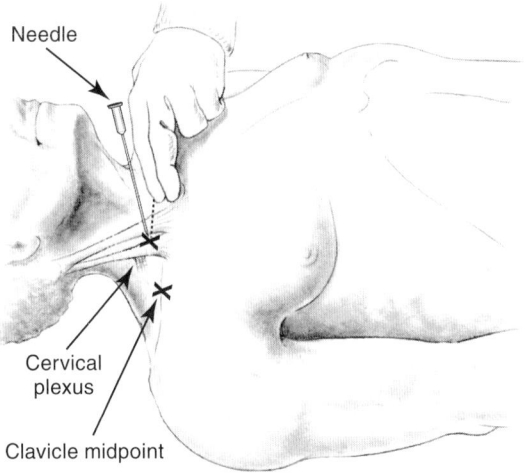

FIGURE **46-9** Technique for intersternocleidomastoid block of the brachial plexus.

for blood, a test dose of 1 mL of local anesthetic solution is injected. A fade will be observed in the quality of the motor twitch experienced by the patient. This indicates that the needle is probably within the brachial plexus sheath. If no subjective symptoms suggesting toxicity reactions are present, incremental injections of 3 to 5 mL of local anesthetic followed by aspiration to detect blood are administered until the intended volume is given. In adult patients, the volume is usually 30 to 35 mL.

The anesthetist must watch for the onset of Horner syndrome (triad of miosis, partial ptosis, and loss of hemifacial sweating) as a positive sign of a successful block. The most important

complication of the supraclavicular approach is pneumothorax. The pleura of the lung is immediately inferior to the first rib, and careful needle placement as described previously is imperative. If landmarks are difficult to define, if the patient is very thin, or if the pleura of the lung is unusually high, the incidence of pneumothorax may increase. The increased incidence of pneumothorax with the supraclavicular approach and the high incidence of Horner syndrome with the interscalene approach led to Charles Pham Dang's development in 1997 of a new approach to the brachial plexus called the *intersternocleidomastoid* (ISCM) *block*.

Intersternocleidomastoid Approach. In the newest supraclavicular approach to the brachial plexus, the ISCM, the puncture site is situated between the heads of the SCM muscle. The novelty of the technique arises from many features, including simple surface landmarks, minimized risk of pleural puncture, and no risk of epidural, subarachnoid, or intravertebral artery injection or catheterization of the perineural space.

Depending on the direction of the needle with the ISCM approach, the brachial plexus can be reached at the level of the trunks (i.e., superior, middle, and inferior). The needle passes successively between the heads of the SCM, behind the clavicular head, through the middle cervical fascia, next to the phrenic nerve, and through the anterior scalene muscle before arriving at the brachial plexus. The following nerves can be reached and stimulated, depending on the direction of the needle, at a depth varying from 3 to 8 cm: suprascapular nerve, superior trunk, middle trunk, and the divisions and cord.[29,30,32-34,36,39,40]

The patient lies supine with the head turned away, arm at the side, and hand positioned on the abdomen. The anesthetist stands next to the patient's head, opposite the side to be blocked. The sternal and clavicular heads of the SCM, as well as the midclavicle, are marked. The puncture site is situated two fingerbreadths above the sternal notch, between the heads of the SCM, medial to the clavicular head. After disinfection and skin-wheal infiltration, the stimulating needle of appropriate length is introduced behind the posterior border of the clavicular head of the SCM. The needle, practically leaning on the sternal head, is advanced laterally, posteriorly, and caudally in the direction indicated by a point situated 1 cm lateral to the midclavicle. The needle makes an angle of 45 degrees to the table and 15 degrees to the clavicle (Figure 46-9). This initial orientation of the needle leads to the suprascapular nerve, the stimulation of which evokes glenohumeral coaptation and contraction of the supraspinatus and infraspinatus muscles. Stimulation of the superior trunk evokes contraction of the biceps brachii and deltoid muscles, elbow flexion, and abduction of the arm. Stimulation of the middle trunk evokes contraction of the triceps brachii muscle and elbow extension. Stimulation of the divisions and cord evokes flexion pronation of the hand and digit flexion in conjunction with pectoral contraction. Movements of the abdomen can be seen from stimulation of the phrenic nerve. They imply withdrawal and redirection of the needle. These motor responses are obtained at a depth of 2 to 8 cm, depending on the collar size. The nerve stimulator current is lowered from 1.0 to 0.5 mA to minimize excessive current to the patient and ensure proper needle position. After gentle aspiration is negative for blood, a test dose of 1 mL of local anesthetic solution is injected. A fade will be observed in the quality of the motor twitch experienced by the patient. This indicates that the needle is probably within the brachial plexus sheath. If no subjective symptoms suggesting are present, incremental injections of 3 to 5 mL of local anesthetic followed by aspiration to detect blood are administered until the intended volume is given. In adult patients, the volume is usually 30 to 35 mL.

Continuous Catheter Technique. Postoperative pain control after upper extremity surgery requires adequate analgesia not only at rest but also for incident pain. Especially after joint surgery, mobilization is required, as is the need to assess neurologic function. The use of brachial plexus catheters for the surgical anesthetic can have significant benefits by reducing postoperative analgesic requirements, including superior control of incident pain, and can be extended to aid in postoperative rehabilitation of the patient.[33]

Continuous administration of local anesthetics via a brachial plexus catheter inserted at the cervical level can markedly improve analgesia and decrease opioid requirements. The advent of cheaper and reliable pump technology has given rise to a significant growth in the use of continuous peripheral nerve blocks in general, especially continuous brachial plexus blocks.[33]

Under strict sterile technique, a 22-gauge, insulated block needle should be advanced at the level of C6 or the cricoid cartilage into the anterior and middle scaline groove and directed 45 degrees in a caudal, dorsal, and medial angle to reduce the risk of a punctured vertebral artery or inadvertent subarachnoid or epidural placement. The practitioner may feel a slight "pop" as the needle enters the sheath. Before placement of the catheter, the patient should be instructed to report any paresthesia experienced. Use of an insulated needle and a nerve stimulator or ultrasound technology may allow more accurate placement, reduce the risk of intraneuronal injection and trauma, and reduce time for placement of the catheter. When the desired motor stimulation is identified—movement in the upper or lower arm—the current should be gradually reduced to 0.5 mA with continued stimulation to ensure close proximity to the neural target. Normal saline, 5 to 10 mL, should then be injected incrementally with intermittent aspiration to guard against accidental intravascular injection. The addition of normal saline will expand the sheet and allow for the passage of the continuous catheter. The catheter should be inserted 3 to 5 cm and secured at the skin. Local anesthetic solution in a volume of 30 to 35 mL should now be injected incrementally, with intermittent aspiration to guard against accidental intravascular injection and to ensure that the continuous catheter works. Continuous infusions

of 0.125 to 0.25 at a rate of 4 to 6 mL/hr have been shown to be very effective.[33,37,38]

Selective Blocks at the Elbow

Several other blocks of the upper extremity can be of benefit and may become techniques of choice, especially in outpatients. Selective blocks at the elbow and wrist permit the surgeon to complete the procedure while minimizing the amount of anesthesia administered. The blocks at the elbow and wrist are primarily sensory blocks. The patient retains the ability to move the hand during the procedure. Reduction of the area anesthetized, the amount of sedation administered, and the potential for complications minimizes the patient's stay in the outpatient center. The mastery and use of selective nerve blocks of the upper extremity avoids the use of a general anesthetic when the regional anesthetic technique fails to completely block all the nerves that innervate the surgical site.[4,15,41]

Each nerve that supplies sensory branches to the arm can be blocked at the elbow and the wrist. Use of a nerve locator at the level of the elbow (for the median and radial nerves) and at the level of the wrist (for the ulnar and median nerves) can improve the success rate of the block.

When a tourniquet is used during the surgical procedure, the intercostobrachial nerve and the brachial cutaneous nerve should be blocked in the axilla. These blocks provide sufficient anesthesia to permit the patient to tolerate a tourniquet. The coracobrachial muscle can also be blocked at the level of the shoulder to provide anesthesia so the patient may better tolerate the tourniquet.

Ulnar Nerve Block at the Elbow

As the ulnar nerve traverses the ulnar sulcus of the humerus, it is tightly fixed in the groove. Performing a regional anesthetic technique in this location can increase the for nerve entrapment. The volume of the solution should be limited to reduce the amount of pressure exerted on the nerve and the ischemia that could develop from injection of a large volume (>3 mL).[4,15,41]

The technique should be performed 1 to 2 cm proximal to the sulcus. The patient's elbow is flexed 90 degrees, and the medial condyle of the humerus is identified. A finger is placed in the ulnar sulcus, extending approximately 1 cm proximal to the condyle (Figure 46-10). The insertion point for the needle is between the medial condyle of the humerus and the olecranon process of the ulna. The needle is inserted at a 45-degree angle to the skin and perpendicularly to a line drawn between the medial condyle and the olecranon process. If a paresthesia is elicited on introduction of the needle, the needle is withdrawn approximately 1 mm, and 2 to 3 mL of the solution is injected. If a paresthesia is not elicited, the volume of the solution can be increased. The total volume of the local anesthetic solution is 3 to 5 mL. The onset of action is determined by the local anesthetic used for the procedure. Epinephrine can be used at this level; however, this agent delays the onset.

Median Nerve Block at the Elbow

Anesthesia of the forearm and hand can be achieved by a combination of median and ulnar nerve block as either a supplement to another technique or as a primary anesthetic technique. The combination of median and ulnar nerve block provides adequate anesthesia for procedures on the cutaneous portions of the lower forearm, the hand, and the second, third, and fourth fingers. The median nerve block can be used to supplement a partially

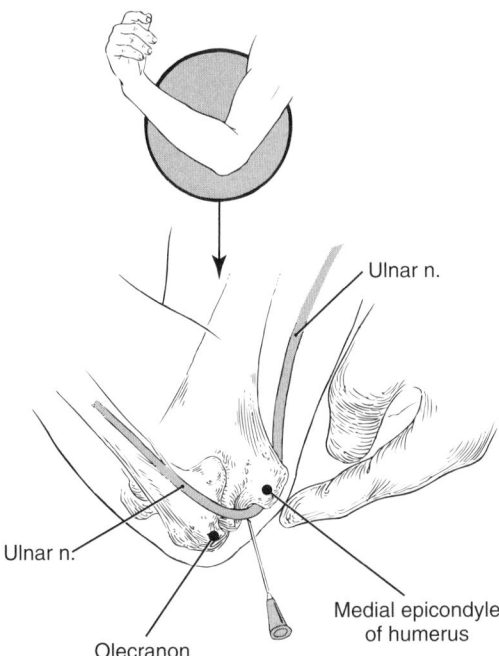

FIGURE **46-10** Technique of ulnar block at the elbow. The patient's elbow is flexed 90 degrees, and the medial condyle of the humerus is identified. *n*, Nerve.

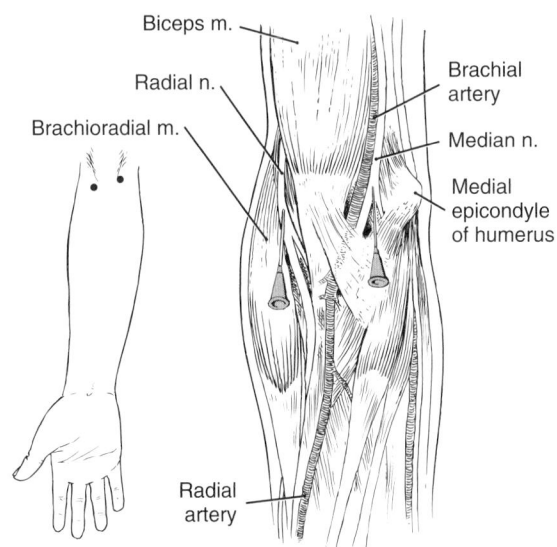

FIGURE **46-11** Performance of median nerve block, positioning the patient's arm on a stable surface with the elbow slightly flexed. After the brachial artery is identified, a short B-bevel needle is inserted slightly medial to the brachial artery. *m*, Muscle, *n.*, nerve

successful brachial plexus block. The median nerve block should be avoided in patients with carpal tunnel syndrome, if neuritis is present, or if the artery is perforated. If anesthesia is administered to two of the three nerves in the foramen, limited function of the hand remains.

The median nerve block is performed by positioning the patient's arm on a stable surface with the elbow slightly flexed. A line is drawn from the medial to the lateral condyles of the humerus on the anterior surface of the elbow. The brachial artery is then identified as it crosses this line (Figure 46-11). A short B-bevel needle is inserted slightly medial to the brachial artery to a depth of 0.5 to 0.75 cm. Median nerve blocks at the elbow can be facilitated with the use of a nerve locator. When the nerve locator is used, a stimulus of low amplitude elicits a response along the path of the median nerve. If a nerve locator is not used, a paresthesia can be elicited by fan-wise movement of the needle. Identification of the median nerve is necessary for a successful block. Local anesthetic solution (3 to 5 mL) is injected after the nerve is located. As the needle is withdrawn through the fascia, an additional 1 to 2 mL of solution is injected to block cutaneous branches of the nerve.

Radial Nerve Block at the Elbow
Block of the radial nerve can be used as an adjunct to axillary perivascular techniques. This block can also be used for surgery of the forearm and hand that is within the distribution of the radial nerve or in conjunction with other nerve blocks.

With the elbow extended and stabilized on a firm surface, the brachioradialis muscle and biceps tendon are identified. The radial nerve is located in the groove formed by the fascial border of the brachioradialis muscle (see Figure 46-11) on the lateral edge and the biceps tendon medially. A line is drawn between the medial and lateral condyles. A short B-bevel needle is inserted along the medial border of the brachioradialis muscle toward the lateral condyle at the point at which the line

between the condyles crosses the facial groove. The needle is directed toward the anterior aspect of the lateral condyle so that gentle contact occurs. After contact with the condyle, the needle is withdrawn 2 mm. Local anesthetic solution (3 to 5 mL) is injected. This procedure is repeated two or three times while the needle is moved slightly more proximally for each injection. As the needle is withdrawn into the subcutaneous tissue, 3 to 5 mL of local anesthetic is injected.

An alternate approach to the radial nerve requires identification of the lateral border of the brachioradialis muscle. Measuring 3 to 5 cm proximal from the lateral condyle along the border of the brachioradialis muscle enables palpation of the radial nerve as it parallels the humerus. The nerve is adherent to the bone at this level and can be easily injured during trauma or during the performance of the regional anesthesia. By slight movement of the nerve, a paresthesia can be elicited. A short B-bevel needle is inserted in a plane perpendicular to the humerus and advanced to the proximity of the identified radial nerve. Because of its fixation against the humerus, the needle must be advanced slowly and the position evaluated to avoid injury to the nerve.

Selective Blocks at the Wrist
Selective blocks of the ulnar, median, and radial nerves at the wrist can be used for supplying limited anesthesia for the outpatient or as a supplement to brachial plexus anesthesia. Procedures that require a motor block in addition to the sensory blockade should be accomplished by use of another anesthesia technique. Epinephrine is not included in solutions used in nerve blocks below the elbow because of the relatively small blood vessels of the wrist, hand, and fingers and the risk of compromising circulation to these areas.

Ulnar Block at the Wrist
With the wrist slightly flexed and stabilized on a firm surface, the ulnar flexor muscle of the wrist is identified (Figure 46-12). A line is then drawn across the forearm at the level of the styloid process of the ulna. A short B-bevel needle is inserted perpendicularly to the skin on the radial side of the ulnar flexor muscle of

the wrist, where it is crossed by the line. At this location, the needle is slightly lateral to the ulnar artery, and a small deviation medially can place the needle over the artery. The ulnar artery can be palpated when the wrist is in moderately exaggerated extension. However, severe extension causes the artery to collapse. After the needle is inserted, 2 to 4 mL of local anesthetic solution is injected. An additional 2 mL is injected as the needle is withdrawn from the deep fascia. The dorsal branch of the ulnar nerve is blocked by injection of 3 to 5 mL of local anesthesia in a half-ring around the ulnar aspect of the wrist. The needle is placed subcutaneously at the radial margin of the ulnar flexor muscle of the wrist and advanced to the midportion of the dorsal aspect of the wrist.

Median Block at the Wrist

The wrist is stabilized on a firm surface and slightly flexed against resistance. When the wrist is flexed, the long palmar muscle and the radial flexor muscle of the wrist are easily identified (see Figure 46-12). A line is drawn across the wrist that parallels the proximal crease. A short B-bevel needle is inserted perpendicularly to the skin between the two tendons to a distance of 0.5 to 1 cm. The carpal tunnel is a tightly confined space. The nerve is located in the superficial portion of the carpal tunnel. A paresthesia can be elicited during the performance of the procedure. If the sensation persists, the needle must be withdrawn and repositioned. Local anesthetic solution (2 to 5 mL) is injected within the carpal tunnel, and another 2 to 3 mL is injected after the needle is withdrawn from the fascia of the carpal tunnel.

Radial Block at the Wrist

The sensory fibers of the radial nerve to the hand are superficial branches at the wrist. Anesthesia of the radial fibers is achieved through the injection of a subcutaneous ring of local anesthetic solution, beginning at the radial flexor muscle of the wrist and extending to the dorsal surface of the ulnar styloid (Figure 46-13). The anesthetist should avoid the formation of a continuous ring of local anesthetic around the wrist when this procedure is accomplished in conjunction with an ulnar block because circulation to the hand could be compromised.

Another approach to anesthesia of the radial nerve is the identification of the brachioradialis muscle proximal to the wrist. Approximately 6 to 8 cm proximal to the wrist, 5 to 7 mL of local anesthetic solution is injected under the brachioradialis muscle. This technique is the least well tolerated of all of the supplemental blocks and has limited success.

INTRAVENOUS REGIONAL ANESTHESIA (BIER BLOCK)

Intravenous regional block is a technically simple, safe, and rapid means of producing surgical anesthesia of the extremity. The technique is best suited for upper extremity (hand and wrist)

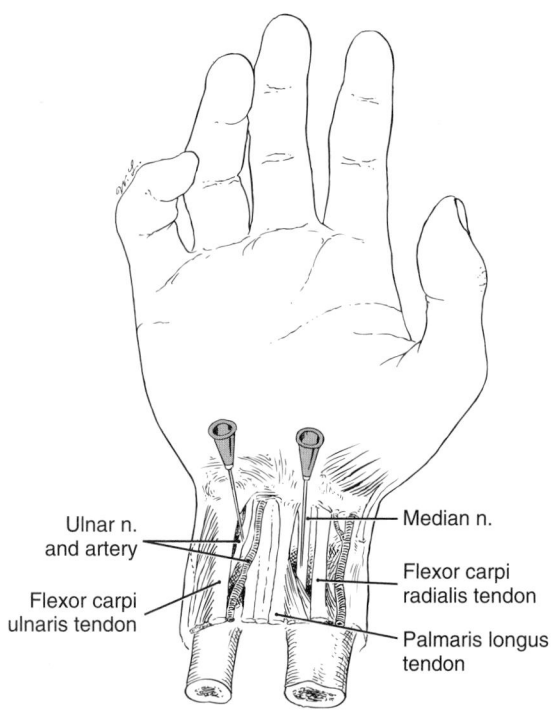

FIGURE 46-12   With the patient's wrist slightly flexed and stabilized on a firm surface, the ulnar flexor muscle of the wrist is identified. A short B-bevel needle is inserted perpendicular to the skin on the radial side of the ulnar flexor muscle of the wrist. *n*, Nerve.

FIGURE 46-13   Anesthesia of the radial fibers is achieved by injecting a subcutaneous ring of local anesthetic solution at the radial flexor muscle of the wrist, extending to the dorsal surface of the ulnar styloid. *n.*, Nerve.

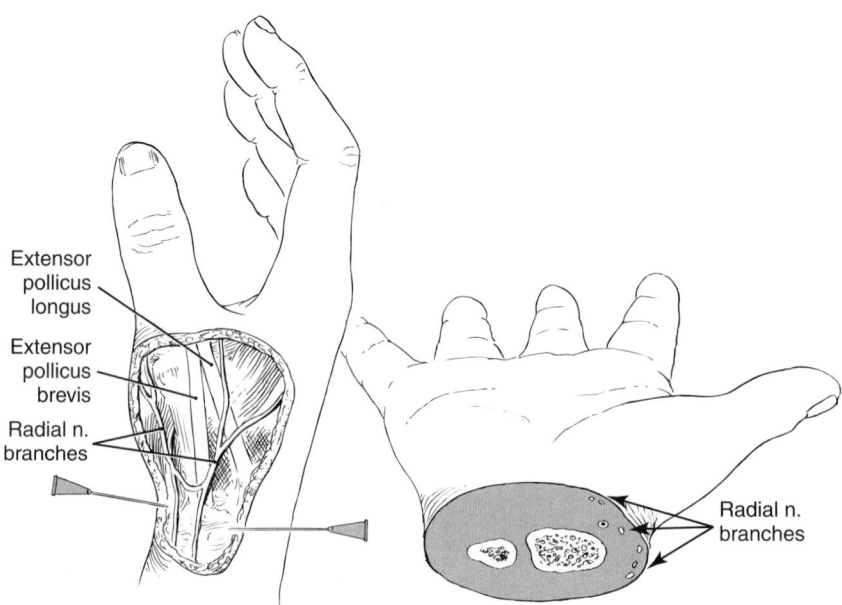

soft-tissue surgical procedures of 1 hour or less; however, it has also been used for lower extremity surgical procedures of the foot and ankle. The factor limiting the duration of anesthesia to approximately 1 hour is most commonly discomfort produced by the tourniquet required to initiate and maintain the block. Use of a dual tourniquet system and preoperative and or intraoperative administration of small doses of opioids may extend this time limit to 1½ hours or longer. The greatest risk associated with intravenous regional anesthesia (IVRA) is the potential for rapid transfer of a large volume of local anesthetic from the extremity to the central circulation in the event of an improperly fitted or inflated tourniquet or tourniquet failure. Therefore, it is important to have emergency equipment, medications, and monitors immediately available when this block is administered. Because of the rapid onset of the block and the limited duration, it is almost always performed in the operating area, where the emergency items needed are readily available. The necessity for intravenous access and manipulation of the affected extremity, the prerequisite for a tourniquet, and the density and duration of the block influence the clinical application of this technique.[29,30,32,42,43]

Intravenous Regional Anesthesia: Upper Extremity Block

A small-bore intravenous catheter is placed in a distal vein of the affected extremity and secured in place, and a heparin lock is attached and flushed with normal saline. The preferred location for access to the venous system of the upper extremity is the dorsum of the hand; however, forearm and antecubital fossa veins have been used. Evidence suggests that use of forearm or antecubital fossa veins increases the possibility of a partial or complete failure of the block when the hand or wrist is the surgical target. It is reasonable to assume that consideration should be given to the area on which surgery is to be performed with regard to access to the venous system because attainment of surgical anesthesia is predicated on the adequate spread of the injected local anesthetic. The patient is placed supine, and several layers of a suitable padding material are wrapped around the arm in preparation for application of the tourniquet. Although a single tourniquet can be used, a dual tourniquet is recommended because it provides a means to extend the length of the block after the initial onset of tourniquet pain. After application of the tourniquet, the extremity is elevated and exsanguinated. Exsanguination is accomplished by wrapping an Esmarch bandage at close overlapping intervals tightly around the arm, starting at the fingertips and continuing until the bandage overlies the tourniquet itself. In cases in which application of an Esmarch bandage would cause undue discomfort, exsanguination by simple elevation of the extremity for a minimum of 5 minutes may be attempted. This method may or may not result in adequate block. In addition, an air-inflated splint may be used as an alternative to the Esmarch bandage. After exsanguination, the proximal tourniquet is inflated to 250 mm Hg or 100 mm Hg above systolic blood pressure, and the Esmarch bandage is removed. A total of 50 mL of 0.5% lidocaine is then injected via the intravenous catheter. The local anesthetic should be free of preservatives (methylparaben, metabisulfite) and contain no vasoconstrictor. The patient should be carefully monitored during the injection for signs of local anesthetic toxicity. An alternative technique uses an additional "tourniquet" (Penrose drain) applied at midforearm in the manner used to start an intravenous line after primary distal tourniquet inflation. Half of the 50-mL volume of local anesthetic is injected with the forearm tourniquet in place; the tourniquet is removed, and the remaining local

anesthetic is injected. This technique results in a faster onset and a denser block. The addition of 15 to 30 mg of ketorolac to the local anesthetic solution can provide a degree of postoperative analgesia without increasing the risk of postoperative bleeding.

Intravenous Regional Anesthesia: Lower Extremity Block

Indications for IVRA of the lower extremity include orthopedic surgery of short duration on the foot, removal of fixation plates and screws from the bones below the knee, and foreign body removal from the foot.

Two significant differences exist between IVRA of the upper and lower extremities. First, the local anesthetic volume (and dose) for IVRA of the lower extremity is approximately double that used for the arm. This obviously increases the risk of local anesthetic intoxication resulting from leakage under the inflated cuff and from release of a large bolus dose of local anesthetic when the cuff is deflated. Second, in order to occlude the arterial inflow at the thigh level (femoral artery), the tourniquet pressure must be higher than in the arm (usually 350 to 400 mm Hg), which increases the occurrence and intensity of tourniquet pain.

Two separate 9-cm-wide tourniquet cuffs (adult patient) are applied, and care must be taken that the pneumatic parts of the tourniquets surround the thigh by more than 1.5 turns. Otherwise, the technique is similar to that described for IVRA of the arm.

During brief surgical procedures of the foot or the ankle, the distal tourniquet cuff may be applied on the calf, clearly below the head of the fibula (away from the peroneal nerve), and the proximal cuff left on the thigh. The local anesthetic solution is injected with the distal tourniquet cuff inflated; therefore, the volume and the dose can be the same as for the arm of an adult, that is, 35 to 45 mL of 0.5% lidocaine. The proximal tourniquet is usually not inflated but can be rapidly inflated in the event the distal tourniquet fails.

INTERCOSTAL NERVE BLOCKS

The use of the intercostal nerve block has increased in the past several years. The anatomic landmarks are easily identified, thereby facilitating the performance of the block. The procedure is not extremely painful, has a high rate of success, has a low incidence of complications, and provides the patient with significant analgesia. The most common complications are pneumothorax and toxicity from the local anesthetic. The patient who has pain with respiratory effort is able to cough and breathe deeply with reduced discomfort. In the outpatient or ambulatory care setting, surgical procedures can be accomplished with the aid of this regional anesthesia technique.[44-46]

The use of multiple-level intercostal nerve block can lead to the highest local anesthetic plasma levels of any regional techniques. The high vascularity of the area and large intercostal veins contribute to high plasma levels of local anesthetic. The high plasma concentration can produce toxicity with lower-than-toxic injected doses.

Intercostal nerve block is used for supplementing balanced anesthesia techniques to increase tolerance of the surgical procedure. Sufficient analgesia can be provided to permit the performance of surgical procedures involving the abdominal wall without the need for supplemental blocks. For more involved procedures, additional anesthesia may be required.

Intercostal nerve block can provide analgesia for postoperative pain control when epidural analgesia is not desired or possible.

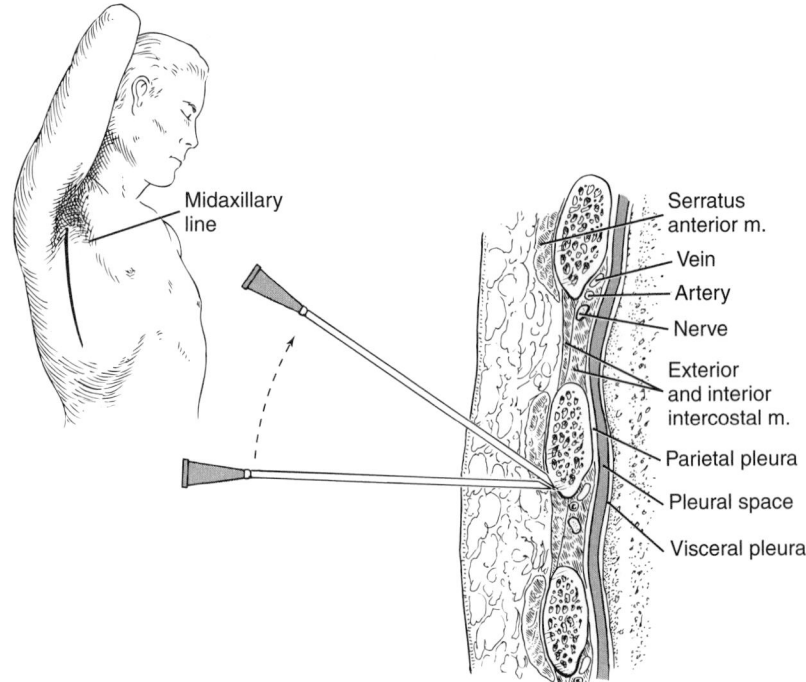

FIGURE **46-14** A 22-gauge, B-bevel needle is inserted perpendicular to the rib and advanced until contact is made with the rib. The needle is slowly walked caudad off the rib. *m.*, Muscle.

Labels on figure: Midaxillary line; Serratus anterior m.; Vein; Artery; Nerve; Exterior and interior intercostal m.; Parietal pleura; Pleural space; Visceral pleura

The procedure can provide analgesia during or after chest-tube insertion to limit the patient's discomfort. The landmarks are easily identified in most patients. The procedure can be accomplished with the patient prone, in the lateral position, or sitting comfortably with the upper body supported over a table or a stand. Having obese patients sit up enables easier identification of landmarks. One advantage of using multiple-level intercostal nerve blocks is the reduction in the amount of pain medication required to facilitate normal respiration in the postoperative period. These factors result in a reduction in the potential development of respiratory depression related to the use of intravenous or intramuscular opioids, especially in obese patients.

The intercostal nerve emerges from the intervertebral foramen and follows the rib in the costal groove. This groove is located on the anteroinferior aspect of the rib. The intercostal artery and vein accompany the nerve in the groove. Medial to the posterior angle of the rib, the neurovascular bundle lies between the pleura and the internal intercostal fascia. As the nerve passes the angle of the rib, it begins to run between the two layers of the internal intercostal muscle. At the midaxillary line, the nerve branches send sensory fibers anteriorly and posteriorly to supply skin and subcutaneous tissue. Fibers also provide motor and sensory innervation to the bundles of the superior rectus muscle in the upper abdomen.

Positioning the patient may require modification to facilitate breathing during the procedure. The area of pain may have to be splinted, or other measures may need to be taken to reduce pain-induced movement during the procedure. Ideally the patient should be positioned in the prone position with the arms hanging down. This position pulls both scapulas away from the midline and permits the practitioner to perform the block as the nerve root begins to travel in the intercostal groove.

The block can be performed with the patient lying on the unaffected side with the arm extended over the head. This technique is helpful in obese patients and in patients experiencing severe pain, especially when such a patient is prone. When the patient is in the lateral position, preservation of circulation in the downward arm must be preserved.

In postoperative patients, the supine position can be used with the anterior approach to the intercostal nerve. This position is less satisfactory and is associated with a higher incidence of complications.

The rib is palpated posterior to the midaxillary line in the prone patient so that the appropriate landmarks can be identified. In this position, the rib becomes superficial to the muscle bodies. The lateral border of the sacrospinal muscle must be identified before the block is attempted. The sacrospinal muscle lies approximately 7 to 10 cm from the midline.

With a small-gauge (27- to 30-gauge) needle, a skin wheal is raised over the point chosen for the injection. A 22-gauge, B-bevel needle is then inserted perpendicularly to the rib through the skin wheal and advanced until contact with the rib is made. The needle is slowly walked caudad off the rib. As the edge of the rib is cleared, the needle is advanced another 2 to 3 mm (Figure 46-14). The needle should be gently aspirated for verification of needle placement. Use of a "free needle," as described in brachial plexus anesthesia, can facilitate the maneuverability of the needle and increase control.

Once the needle is located in the appropriate location, 3 to 5 mL of the local anesthetic solution is injected. The procedure can be repeated for anesthesia at each dermatome level. If resistance is encountered during the injection, the injection should be terminated and the needle repositioned. If the patient begins to cough or move, the needle position should be reevaluated before injection. Advancing the needle several millimeters can place the needle within the nerve itself, resulting in severe pain or direct injury to the nerve.

Procaine, bupivacaine, tetracaine, and lidocaine have all been used for blocking the intercostal nerves, with varying effects. Because the goal is to provide the patient with extended pain relief, a longer-acting agent is most commonly used. An injection of 3 mL of bupivacaine (0.5%) into the tissues surrounding the intercostal nerve provides the patient with 3 to 9 hours of anesthesia and analgesia. Patient factors such as temperature, presence of infection, and the response to local anesthetics affect the duration of action. The addition of low-molecular-weight dextran to the solution in a ratio of 1 mL of dextran to 3 mL of bupivacaine further extends the duration of action. Dextran slows the absorption of the local anesthetic, thereby reducing the plasma level of the anesthetic and permitting more of the concentrated local anesthetic solution to remain in close proximity to the neural tissue.

Epinephrine 1:200,000 or 1:400,000 should be added to the local anesthetic solution. Bupivacaine's duration of action may be unchanged; however, the rise in the plasma concentration of the local anesthetic is slowed. The addition of epinephrine to tetracaine or lidocaine prevents the rapid absorption of the anesthetic and increases the duration of action. With the use of epinephrine, increased vasoconstriction occurs, an effect that reduces absorption of the local anesthetic. The increased contact time between the neural tissue and the local anesthetic increases the amount of local anesthetic present to be absorbed into the neural fibers.

In addition to the single-shot technique described previously, a continuous intercostal block can be used for providing additional pain relief. The technique was originally described in the mid-1960s. However, it did not gain popularity until 1983, when it was reintroduced as a "new" technique. The continuous technique permits the reinjection of the intercostal fibers without the need for additional invasive procedures. Opioids have been injected in the intercostal nerve sheath with limited enhancement of the analgesia.

The continuous intercostal technique is performed by use of an epidural needle and a catheter in place of a single-shot needle technique. The intercostal groove is located using the technique described for the single-shot technique. When an epidural needle is used for the procedure, resistance is met as the needle passes through the sheath. The nerve can also be identified with a nerve locator or nerve stimulator. After the intercostal neural sheath is identified, the needle is adjusted so that the bevel of the needle directs the catheter toward the midline posteriorly. The epidural catheter is inserted slowly along the intercostal groove 2 to 3 cm. If severe pain or discomfort occurs during advancement of the catheter, the procedure is terminated, and the catheter is removed. Advancement of the catheter may produce electric-like shocks as the catheter brushes the nerve fibers. Severe pain should alert the practitioner of the possibility of an intraneural injection.

As the medication is injected, a band of analgesia develops along the path of the catheter and spreads anteriorly and posteriorly. Other than the direct action of the local anesthetic on the neural fibers, the exact mechanisms of action are unknown. However, paravertebral or epidural distribution of the local anesthetic may facilitate and enhance the block. The medication is injected in 3-mL increments until the desired level and intensity of block are achieved.

Tachyphylaxis develops with repeated injections of local anesthetic. Permitting resolution of the block before reinjection or using another local anesthetic reduces this effect. If an ester is used for the initial blockade, an amide local anesthetic can be used when symptoms of tachyphylaxis develop.

Small doses of fentanyl and morphine have been injected through the catheter. However, the uptake of medication into the vascular compartment is rapid, essentially negating the advantages of this route of administration. The use of opioids in the intercostal space may increase the incidence of complications, including respiratory embrassement.

The likelihood of complications, such as pleural injection and pneumothorax, can be reduced by use of a short B-bevel needle. To avoid an intraneural injection, the needle is directed cephalad as it passes over the ridge of the rib. A symptomatic pneumothorax can occur; however, use of a single 22-gauge, short-beveled needle reduces the risk. A leak created by this needle can be minimal. When a larger or A-bevel needle is used, the risk of complications is increased.

In most patients a small leak of air does not cause a symptomatic pneumothorax. Most patients are able to compensate for any reduced ventilatory capacity, and the pneumothorax resolves without intervention. In a small percentage of patients, intervention is needed for relief of the discomfort and dyspnea. Radiologic studies should be performed after completion of the procedures so the status or occurrence of a pneumothorax can be established. The studies can be used during follow-up evaluations and therapy if required.

The use of intercostal nerve block has enhanced the practice of anesthesia and pain control. This technique provides the patient with increased flexibility in the control of pain and reduces the need for opioids. In the ambulatory surgery center, this technique offers increased options to the patient who desires a regional anesthetic technique.

LOWER-EXTREMITY BLOCK

Lower-extremity nerve blocks are well described and can provide high-quality anesthesia and analgesia for lower-extremity surgical procedures. Lower-extremity nerve blocks, although underused, have significant advantages compared with central neuraxial techniques, especially in the ambulatory setting.

Advantages of lower-extremity nerve block include reduced recovery room admissions, decreased nausea and vomiting and urinary retention, and improved postoperative analgesia. These benefits may translate into shortened hospital stays, decreased probability of hospital admission, and an overall reduction in hospital costs and patient charges.

Anatomy of the Lumbar Plexus

The lumbar plexus is formed from the first, second, third, and fourth lumbar nerve roots. Contributions to the plexus originate in the twelfth thoracic nerve. The plexus is formed in front of the quadratus lumborum muscle and behind the psoas major muscle (Figure 46-15). As the major branches from the plexus begin their descent into the leg, the muscle bodies and the connecting fascia tightly bind them. The lateral femoral cutaneous nerve is formed from the second and third lumbar nerves and is the first to leave the compartment. It emerges from the lateral border of the psoas major at its midpoint. The nerve then traverses the iliac muscle obliquely toward the anterior iliac spine. The lateral femoral cutaneous nerve passes under the lateral border of the inguinal ligament and provides the sensory innervation to the lateral aspect of the thigh (Figure 46-16).

The obturator nerve arises from the second, third, and fourth lumbar nerves as an extension of the lumbar plexus. It emerges from the medial border of the psoas major at the level of the sacroiliac joint and is covered by the external iliac artery and vein. The nerve passes into the pelvis minor and runs anteroinferiorly to the obturator canal, which it traverses near the obturator vessels. Because of the proximity of the nerve to the external iliac artery, it can be injured during surgical procedures. This nerve is frequently injured when patients undergo extensive pelvic surgery. The obturator nerve is primarily a motor nerve that has some mixed sensory fibers to the hip, the medial aspect

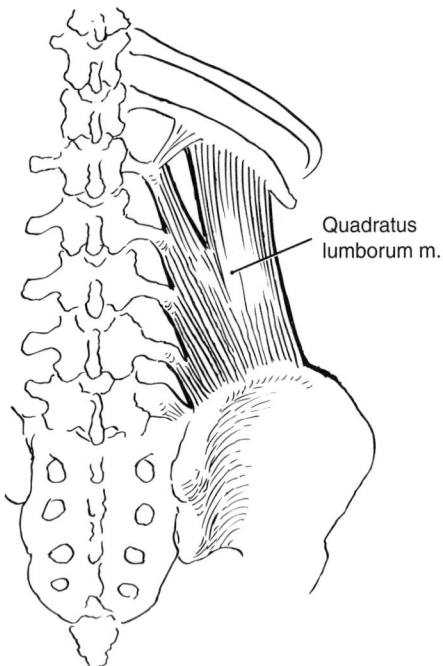

FIGURE **46-15** Location of the lumbar plexus. *m.*, Muscle.

of the femur, and the skin and soft tissue of the lower portion of the thigh. The third nerve in the lumbar plexus is the femoral nerve, which is formed from the contributions of the second, third, and fourth lumbar nerve roots. This nerve forms and appears at the junction of the middle and lower third of the psoas major muscle. It remains within the groove of the psoas major and the iliac muscles and runs deep under the inguinal ligament, where it comes to lie anterior to the iliopsoas muscle and lateral to the femoral artery. The femoral nerve forms two branches: the anterior and the posterior bundles. This formation usually occurs just after the nerve passes under the inguinal ligament but may occur before it passes under the ligament. The anterior branch provides innervation to the anterior surface of the thigh and the sartorius muscle. The posterior branch provides innervation to the quadriceps muscles, the knee joint, and its medial ligament and is the origin of the saphenous nerve. The femoral nerve is bound by several structures above and below the inguinal ligament. Above the inguinal ligament, the iliaca fascia encapsulates the femoral nerve laterally, the psoas fascia medially, and the transverse fascia anteriorly. The posterior border of this capsule or sheath is made up of the bony structure of the pelvis. As the femoral nerve joins the femoral artery to enter the leg, the iliopsoas fascia forms the posterolateral wall. The inguinal ligament and the fascia lata form the anterior wall, and the iliopectineal fascia forms the medial wall of the capsule. Winnie and associates suggested that the neural sheath originating with the femoral artery in conjunction with the fascial attachments form a structure similar to the neural sheath in the brachial plexus.[8] With this anatomic design, anesthesia can be provided

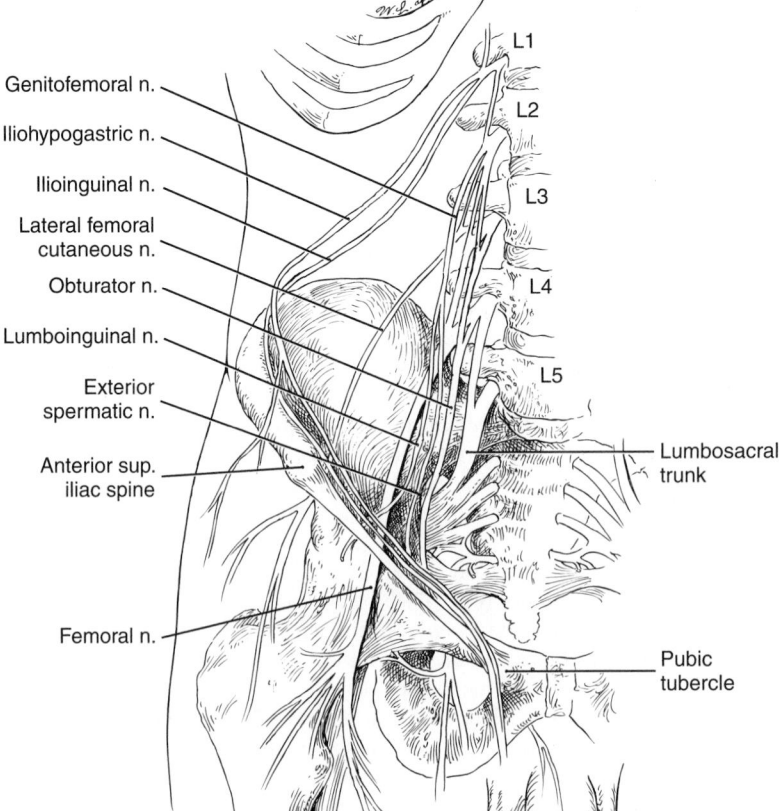

FIGURE **46-16** Origin and position of the nerves of the lower extremity. *n*, Nerve.

for the lower extremity through techniques used in upper extremity anesthesia.

Psoas Compartment Block

Immediately after emerging from the intervertebral foramina, the nerve roots form the lumbar plexus. Blockade of the lumbar plexus as a unit can be accomplished by injecting local anesthetic into the fascial sheath surrounding the plexus. This can be done at the level of the psoas compartment.[18,29-30]

This approach attempts to block the plexus as it lies in the fascial plane bordered medially by the vertebral column, dorsally by the quadratus lumborum muscle, and ventrally by the psoas major muscle.

The patient is placed in either the lateral or sitting position. If placed in the lateral position, the patient should be in a relaxed but curled position similar to that used for spinal or epidural anesthesia, with the operative side uppermost (Figure 46-17).

From the spinous process of L4, a 3-cm line is drawn caudally in the interspinal line. From the end of this line, a 5-cm line is drawn perpendicularly and laterally toward the side to be blocked, usually ending at the medial edge of the iliac crest. This spot identifies the point of needle insertion. A 120-cm insulated block needle is used. A skin wheal is raised, and the needle is inserted perpendicularly to all planes and advanced until contact with bone is made, which identifies the transverse process of L5 and usually occurs at a depth of 5 to 10 cm.

The needle is then withdrawn, redirected slightly cephalad, and advanced until it slides over the transverse process of L5. Using the loss-of-resistance technique, the psoas compartment is usually encountered at the depth of 8 to 12 cm. The tip of the needle now lies in the psoas compartment. Needle placement can be confirmed with the aid of a nerve stimulator, by checking for stimulation of the quadriceps muscles, by eliciting paresthesias into the thigh, or by advancing the needle slightly into the psoas muscle and reconfirming a loss of resistance while withdrawing the needle slightly into the psoas compartment.

After the needle is properly placed, and after careful aspiration, 30 to 40 mL of local anesthetic is injected in 5-mL divided doses. It is often helpful to have the patient remain in the lateral position for a few minutes after injection to limit spread of the drug.

Inguinal Perivascular Technique and Femoral Nerve Block

The inguinal perivascular technique, described by Winnie, is also known as the *three-in-one block* of the lower extremity.

The lumber plexus is "sandwiched" among the psoas major, quadratus lumborum, and iliacus muscles and is enclosed by the fascia of these three muscles.[47,48]

After the patient is positioned supine, the groin is prepared and draped by use of aseptic technique. One possible complication is contamination of the deeper tissues. An immobile needle can be used for improved control of the needle.

The site of injection is 1 cm lateral to the femoral artery and 1 cm inferior to the inguinal ligament. The identified area is prepped with a povidone-iodine (Betadine) solution and then infiltrated with 2 to 3 mL of 1% lidocaine solution subcutaneously. A 22-gauge, 4-cm insulated B-bevel needle is advanced perpendicularly to the skin just lateral to the artery until the femoral nerve is located with the aid of a peripheral nerve stimulator. With a stimulation frequency of 2 Hz, the intensity level is set at 1 mA until quadriceps extension is elicited, then decreased to less than 0.5 mA. Local anesthetic solution (20 to 30 mL) is injected in 3-to 5-mL increments, with intermittent syringe aspiration. Digital pressure is applied firmly but gently distal to the needle. This action assists in limiting the distal spread of the anesthetic solution by forcing it proximal into the channel formed by the neural sheath and other structures. Digital pressure is continued after the injection for approximately 5 to 10 minutes. Winnie and associates indicated that the total volume of anesthetic solution required to maximize the block must exceed 20 mL. Volumes of less than 20 mL provide a spotty and unpredictable block. Increasing the volume of the solution to 30 mL increases the ability of the solution to contact all three nerves. Bupivacaine (0.5%), ropivacaine (0.5%), levobupivacaine (0.5%), and lidocaine (1.5%) are commonly used for this procedure. Anesthesia to the sciatic distribution does not occur with this technique. If the surgical procedure requires anesthesia along the sciatic distribution, a separate procedure must be performed (Figure 46-18).[8,47,48]

Continuous Femoral Nerve Block

Extension of the anesthesia and analgesia provided by a femoral nerve block through the use of a continuous catheter technique following surgical procedures of the femur and knee has grown in popularity and application. The success rate is high as long as the surgical procedure does not extend beyond the innervations of the femoral nerve. The landmarks are readily identifiable and include the femoral artery and the femoral crease immediately inferior to the inguinal ligament.

The patient is placed in the supine position and the skin is thoroughly prepped with an antiseptic solution. The practitioner stands on the side to be blocked. Sterile gloves are donned, and the needle insertion site is located at the lateral border of the

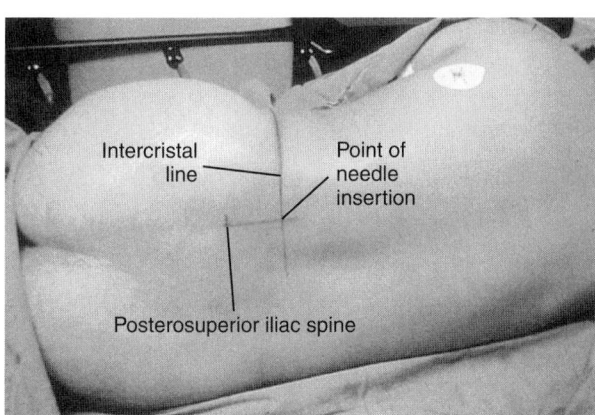

FIGURE **46-17** Lumbar plexus block.

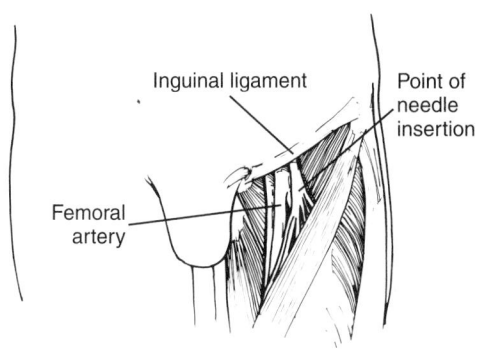

FIGURE **46-18** Femoral nerve block.

femoral artery (approximately 1 cm lateral to the arterial pulse) in the femoral crease. A 17-gauge, 3½-inch insulated needle connected to a nerve stimulator set at 1 mÅ, 2 Hz, 100-300 μsec is inserted and advanced in the sagittal plane at a 45- to 60-degree cephalad angle. The technique is similar to single-injection femoral nerve block except for the more acute cephalad angle of needle insertion to facilitate threading of the catheter. Following a quadriceps muscle twitch (patellar twitch) at 1 mÅ, the current is reduced to 0.5 mÅ, and the twitch response is reestablished. If a quadriceps twitch is not elicited following initial needle placement, the needle should be withdrawn and redirected slightly more lateral to the femoral artery until the desired twitch response is achieved. An initial bolus of local anesthetic (15 to 20 mL) is injected slowly after negative aspiration for blood, and the catheter is then threaded 5 to 10 cm beyond the tip of the needle. The nerve stimulator can be connected to the catheter to confirm that the tip lies in close proximity to the femoral nerve. The catheter is then secured by one of several mechanisms. Kits available for continuous nerve block often contain a securing device, but the catheter may be secured through use of a suture and/or a clear dressing applied over the catheter. The continuous infusion of local anesthetic is initiated immediately after the bolus injection at a rate of 8 to 10 mL per hour. Typical local anesthetics and concentrations used for this purpose are 0.2% ropivacaine and 0.25% bupivacaine or levobupivacaine.

Strict aseptic technique should be adhered to during placement and maintenance of the catheter, and it has been recommended that the catheter be removed after 48 hours. In addition, as with all peripheral nerve blocks, complaints of pain during needle insertion or injection suggest intraneural penetration. In this event, the needle should be withdrawn and redirected. Insertion of the needle medially is likely to produce femoral artery and or vein penetration. If this occurs, constant pressure should be applied to the site for a period of not less than 2 to 3 minutes prior to another attempt at locating the nerve. The patient should be counseled with regard to the extended loss of sensation and motor control of the extremity and what action to take in the event of a potential complication upon discharge (see Box 46-1).

Fascia Iliaca Compartment Block

The fascia iliaca compartment block is an anterior lumbar plexus approach with a puncture point distant from the neurovascular sheath. A nerve stimulator is not necessary for this procedure. Described for the first time in children in 1989, fascia iliaca compartment block is widely used for postoperative analgesia after lower limb surgery in children and adults and provides effective postoperative analgesia after hip, femoral shaft, or knee surgery. Compared with three-in-one block, it provides a faster and more consistent simultaneous blockade of the lateral femoral cutaneous and femoral nerves. The fascia iliaca compartment block is performed as described by Dalens and colleagues.[49-51] With the patient in a supine position, a projection of the inguinal ligament is drawn on the skin from the pubic tubercle to the anterior superior iliac spine and trisected. The puncture site is marked 1 cm caudal to the point at which the lateral meets the middle third of the inguinal ligament line. After disinfecting the skin using topical 10% povidone-iodine, a short-bevel needle (24 gauge, 50 mm) is inserted at a 90-degree angle to the skin. An initial loss of resistance is felt as the needle tip crosses the fascia lata. The needle is advanced at the same angle until a second loss of resistance is felt as the fascia iliaca is pierced (a paresthesia is not intentionally elicited), and 30 mL of local anesthetic is injected.

Sciatic Nerve Block

Sciatic nerve blocks, in combination with lumbar plexus, femoral, or saphenous nerve blocks, provide complete anesthesia and postoperative analgesia for lower-extremity surgery. Contrary to common belief, sciatic nerve block is relatively easy to accomplish and master.[52] In a recent review of outpatients undergoing complex knee surgery, it was noted that among the patients who received a combination sciatic nerve block with a femoral nerve block, a lower incidence of nursing interventions for pain occurred in the step-down unit.[48] In addition, patients had fewer hospital admissions and were more satisfied with their surgical procedures.[47,48]

Anatomy of the Sciatic Nerve

The sciatic nerve is the continuation of the upper division of the sacral plexus and is the largest nerve trunk in the body. It supplies the muscles of the back of the thigh, the skin of the leg, and the muscles of the lower leg and foot. It passes out of the pelvis through the great sacrosciatic foramen, below the piriform muscle. It descends between the major trochanter and the tuberosity of the ischium to the lower third of the thigh, where it divides into the internal and external popliteal nerves.[25,29,47,48]

Technique of Sciatic Nerve Block

Although posterior and lateral popliteal approaches to the sciatic nerve are performed most commonly for ankle and foot surgery, and higher approaches to the sciatic nerve are performed more commonly for surgery below, above, and at the knee, there is no clinical evidence to support one particular sciatic approach over another. The indications for a given approach are based on the specific surgical requirement (Figure 46-19).[47,48]

After standard monitors are placed, the patient is positioned in the Sims position with the operative leg positioned superiorly and flexed at the knee. A line is drawn from the posterior superior iliac spine to the greater trochanter of the femur. A second line is drawn from the sacral hiatus to the greater trochanter, and a third line is drawn perpendicular to and bisecting the first line. The intersection of the second and third lines is the point of needle entry. The identified area is prepared with a Betadine solution and then infiltrated with 2 to 3 mL of 1% lidocaine solution subcutaneously. A 22-gauge, 10-cm insulated B-bevel needle, inserted perpendicularly to the skin, is advanced until the posterior tibial nerve distribution is elicited with the aid of a peripheral nerve stimulator. A stimulation frequency of 2 Hz and an intensity level of 1 mÅ is used until a plantar flexion

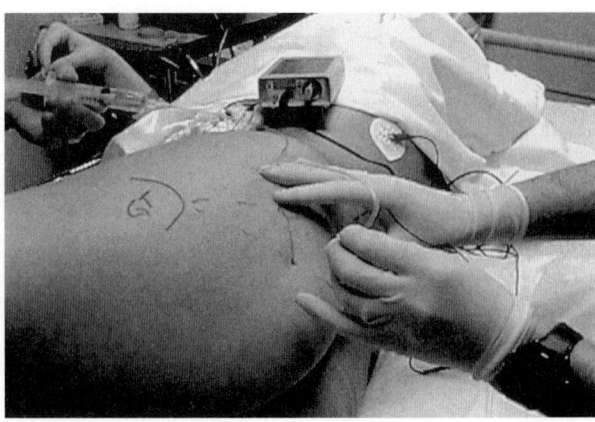

FIGURE **46-19** Sciatic nerve block.

motor response is elicited. The intensity level is decreased to less than 0.5 mÅ as long as motor response is still present. Local anesthetic solution (10 mL) is injected in 5-mL increments, with intermittent syringe aspiration. The needle is redirected laterally and advanced until peroneal nerve distribution is elicited with the aid of a peripheral nerve stimulator. A stimulation frequency of 2 Hz and an intensity level of 1 mÅ is used until a dorsal flexion motor response is elicited. The intensity level is decreased to less than 0.5 mÅ as long as motor response is still present. Local anesthetic solution (10 mL) is injected in 5-mL increments, with intermittent syringe aspiration. Bupivacaine (0.5%), ropivacaine (0.5%), Chirocaine (0.5%), and lidocaine (1.5%) are commonly used for this procedure.

Popliteal Fossa Block

This approach is based on the use of the three anatomic landmarks that define the posterior popliteal fossa: the popliteal crease, the medial border of the femoris biceps muscle laterally, and the tendon of the semitendinous muscle medially.

A line is drawn joining the medial border of the femoris biceps muscle laterally and the lateral border of the semitendinous muscle medially at the level of the popliteal crease. From the middle of this line, a perpendicular line is extended 15 cm cephalad. The site of insertion of the needle is 1 cm laterally. A 10-cm insulated needle connected to a nerve stimulator is introduced through a skin wheal of local anesthesia at a 45- to 60-degree anterosuperior angle. The sciatic nerve usually is located at a depth of 1 to 2 cm in an adult. After careful aspiration, 35 to 40 mL of a local anesthetic is injected (Figure 46-20).

Ankle Blocks

The ability to administer anesthesia to patients who require surgery of the foot offers additional regional block options to anesthesia practitioners. Either a complete or partial block of the foot can provide adequate anesthesia for many of the surgical procedures performed by podiatrists and orthopedic surgeons. The nerves are easy to locate, and the procedures can be rapidly accomplished. This tool can prove invaluable in the care of certain patients, such as those with gangrene of the foot or those with diabetes who have foot ulcers, in whom a local anesthetic procedure would be inadequate.[53-55]

Anatomy of the Ankle

The ankle block is performed by the blocking of five nerves at the level of the ankle: the tibial nerve, the sural nerve, the superficial peroneal nerve, the deep peroneal nerve, and the saphenous nerve.[53-55]

Tibial Nerve. The tibial nerve arises from the nerve roots of the fourth and fifth lumbar roots, along with the first, second, and third sacral roots. It is the larger of the two branches of the sciatic nerve. The path of this nerve lies on the medial side of the Achilles tendon. It passes into the ankle with the posterior tibial artery (Figure 46-21). At the level of the ankle this nerve lies behind the posterior tibial artery and between the tendons of the long flexor muscles of the toes and the long flexor muscles of the great toe. The nerve is covered by the flexor retinaculum. Several branches leave the neural bundle at the level of the medial malleolus. Two of the branches, the medial and the lateral plantar nerves, traverse the ankle, following under the cover of the abductor hallucis. They provide sensory innervation to the foot.

Sural Nerve. The sural nerve is formed from the union of a branch of the tibial nerve and the common peroneal nerve. This nerve travels superficially with the short saphenous nerve behind the lateral malleolus into the ankle, where it provides the sensory innervation to the posterior portion of the sole of the foot, as well as to the posterior portion of the heel and the portion of the Achilles tendon immediately above the ankle (Figure 46-22).

Superficial Peroneal Nerve. The superficial peroneal nerve arises from the roots of the fourth and fifth lumbar nerve roots, as well as the first and second sacral nerve roots. The nerve becomes superficial in the middle two thirds of the lower leg and remains subcutaneous as multiple branches proceed into the dorsum of the foot. Just above the ankle (Figure 46-23) the nerve begins to branch; for this reason a single injection site does not provide sufficient anesthesia.

Deep Peroneal Nerve. The deep peroneal nerve arises from the same nerve roots as the superficial peroneal nerve. However, it remains within the protection of the anterior tibial muscle and

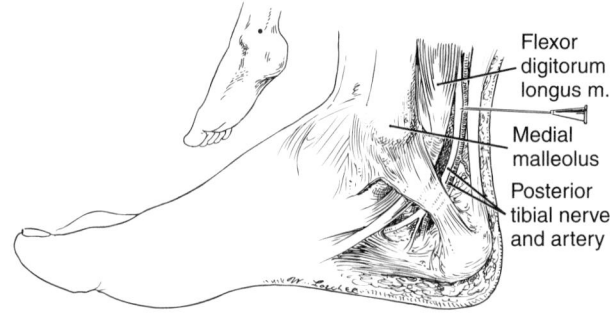

FIGURE **46-21** Path of the posterior tibial nerve, with the posterior tibial artery past the Achilles tendon. M, Muscle.

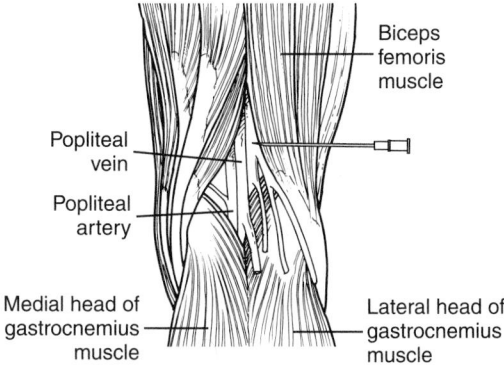

FIGURE **46-20** Popliteal nerve block.

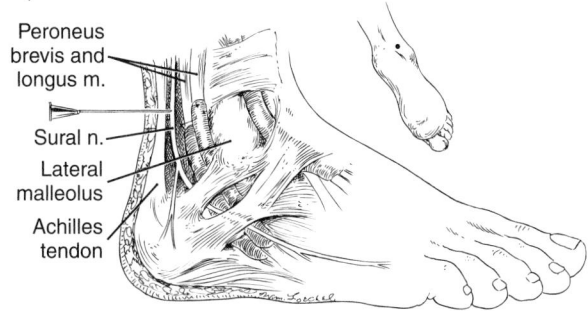

FIGURE **46-22** Path of the sural nerve behind the lateral malleolus into the ankle. M, Muscle; n, nerve.

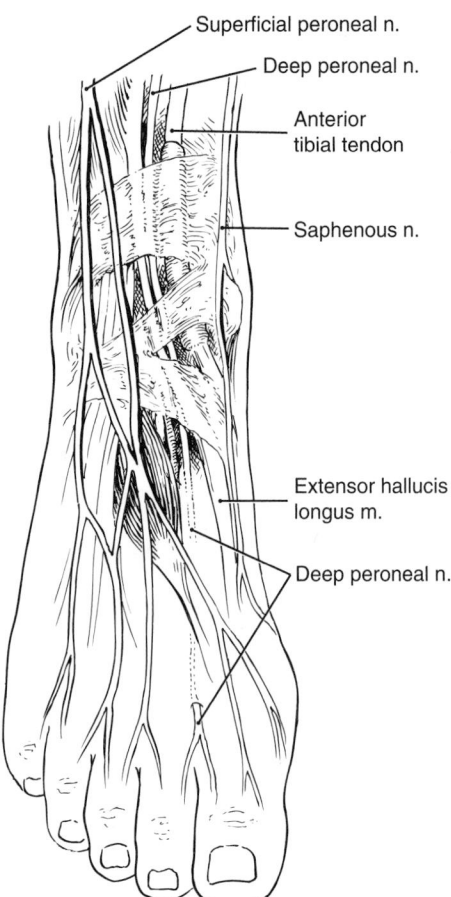

FIGURE **46-23**   The superficial peroneal nerve proceeds to the dorsum of the foot subcutaneously through multiple branches. *n*, nerve.

the long extensor muscle of the great toe (see Figure 46-23) as it traverses the leg and into the ankle. As it crosses the ankle, it is covered by the extensor retinaculum. The deep peroneal nerve provides innervation to the short extensors of the toes and provides sensory innervation to the skin on the lateral side of the hallux and on the medial side of the second digit. The nerve and the artery cross each other, so the nerve lies lateral to the anterior tibial artery and medial to the long extensor muscle of the great toe that is in the ankle. This nerve is frequently missed when regional anesthesia is administered to the ankle.

Saphenous Nerve. The saphenous nerve is the terminal branch of the femoral nerve and travels subcutaneously from the lateral side of the knee joint. It follows the greater saphenous vein to the medial malleolus and provides sensory innervation to the medial side of the malleolus and the skin of the medial aspect of the lower leg (see Figure 46-23). If the block of this nerve is inadequate, the patient is unable to tolerate a tourniquet above the ankle.

Ankle Block Technique

The approach to both the sural and the posterior tibial nerves can be enhanced by placing the patient in the prone position. However, this is not always the most comfortable position. Therefore, the patient should be placed in the most comfortable position that permits sufficient mobility of the foot. Rotation of the foot from side to side can be facilitated by turning the patient

onto either side or elevating the foot on towels or pillows. The posterior tibial artery is palpated at the level of the superior portion of the medial malleolus. After the artery is located, the needle is inserted lateral to the artery in a line drawn from the superior portion of the medial malleolus to the lateral malleolus across the Achilles tendon. If the artery is not palpated, the needle is inserted lateral to the Achilles tendon at the level of the superior portion of the medial malleolus. The needle is advanced toward the medial malleolus and lateral to the position of the posterior tibial artery. As the needle is advanced toward the outer aspect of the medial malleolus, a paresthesia may be elicited. If this occurs, 5 mL of the anesthetic solution is injected with the needle held in position, and an additional 3 mL is injected as the needle is withdrawn. If a paresthesia is not elicited, the medial malleolus is gently contacted with the needle tip and withdrawn 2 mm from the bone. The anesthetic solution is slowly injected at this position, and the location is gently massaged after the injection.

With the patient in the same position, the line from the medial malleolus across the Achilles tendon is identified on the lateral malleolus. The needle is inserted under the skin along the lateral border of the Achilles tendon in the plane with the line that is between the medial and lateral malleoli. The needle is advanced subcutaneously toward the superior edge of the lateral condyle, and 5 mL of solution is injected in the subcutaneous tissues as the needle is withdrawn. The solution must reach the superior edge of the lateral malleolus to anesthetize all the fibers of the sural nerve.

The patient is then placed in the supine position, and the anterior ankle is prepared for the block. For blocking of the deep peroneal nerve, a line is drawn from the superior edge of the medial malleolus to the superior border of the lateral malleolus across the anterior portion of the ankle. The tendons of the anterior tibial muscle and the long muscles of the great toe are identified by having the patient flex the foot against resistance. Where the line crosses the midpoint between the two tendons, the needle is inserted toward the tibia (Figure 46-24). As the needle advances through the fascia, a paresthesia may be elicited. If the paresthesia is not obtained, the needle is slowly advanced until the needle gently contacts the tibia. As the needle is withdrawn from contact with the tibia, 5 mL of anesthetic solution is injected. The needle is then withdrawn through the fascia, and an additional 3 mL of solution is injected.

With the needle remaining in the subcutaneous tissue, the needle direction is changed. The needle is advanced toward the inferior border of the lateral malleolus. The superficial peroneal nerve is located in subcutaneous tissue at this level. While the needle is withdrawn, 5 mL of anesthetic solution is injected. A subcutaneous ring develops that should reach the lateral malleolus.

The needle is withdrawn to the midpoint, and the needle direction is again changed. The needle is redirected to the inferior border of the medial malleolus. The saphenous nerve is in the subcutaneous tissue, superficial to the saphenous vein. If the needle is not superficial, the saphenous vein is entered. Five milliliters of solution is injected toward the medial malleolus. As the needle is withdrawn, 3 mL is injected.

The deep peroneal and the posterior tibial nerves are the only nerves of the ankle that are not in the subcutaneous tissue. The nerve locator can be used for facilitating the identification of the nerves and improving the chances of success with the block. The technique of electrotranslocation of the

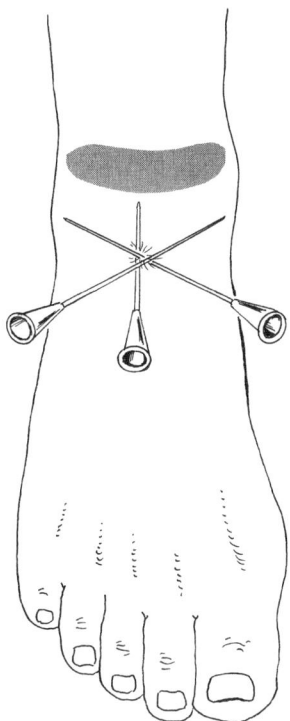

FIGURE **46-24** Direction and redirection of the needle in the ankle block technique.

nerves is similar to the technique used with brachial plexus block.[3,53-55]

REGIONAL ANESTHESIA AND TRAUMA

Regional anesthesia techniques have become preferred for surgical procedures when the injury involves either the lower extremities or a single upper extremity. Postoperative pain management can be provided for the patient with an epidural catheter. Regional anesthesia to an extremity can provide muscle relaxation and sensory block while the patient remains awake and able to maintain protective reflexes.[56]

When the patient is experiencing severe pain, technical difficulties may be encountered. Both the injury and the pain restrict movement of the extremities, making adjustments in position difficult or impossible. In patients who are experiencing pain, it is generally difficult to optimize their position to facilitate the implementation of regional anesthesia.

Patel and associates[56] suggest that an epidural technique may be more advantageous than a subarachnoid block during the perioperative period. Many surgical procedures change once the full extent of the trauma is evaluated. These changes may require additional surgical and anesthesia time. With the gradual onset of a sympathetic block, management of changes in sympathetic tone and systemic vascular resistance can be more easily controlled.

The patient may be confused because of the effects of alcohol or drugs in addition to the effects of the trauma itself. Use of epidural opioids in the postoperative period permits the surgeon and the anesthesia practitioner to evaluate the mental and physical status of the patient without having to be concerned about the cerebral effects of opioids.

In the presence of alcohol, drugs, or other sedation, the patient's ability to provide the anesthesia practitioner with an informed consent for the procedure must be evaluated. In this situation, patient refusal may not be an indication of the patient's actual desires. However, a regional technique is significantly more difficult to manage in a noncooperative patient than in a cooperative one.

Sympathetic stimulation occurs with trauma, and this response must be considered during the initial evaluation and care of the patient. The patient's pulse and blood pressure may be maintained through this stimulation. Symptoms of hypovolemia and shock are masked by artificially induced hypertension mediated through high circulating catecholamine levels. When regional anesthesia is administered to such a patient, elimination of the stimulation to the sympathetic nervous system may precipitate hypotension. Decompensation can occur rapidly after the reduction of circulating catecholamines. The extent and rapidity of the decompensation are dependent on the type of regional technique used, the type of local anesthetics chosen, and the sedation administered to the patient when the block is instituted. When symptoms of hypovolemic shock are present, the patient is unable to compensate for the reduction in systemic vascular resistance.[56]

Winnie and colleagues have found that initial alterations in blood pressure and heart rate occur during positioning. They suggest that the patient receive additional fluid boluses to compensate for this problem. Positioning the patient before administering the regional anesthetic minimizes this response. For example, hypobaric spinal anesthesia may be administered to a patient with a fractured femur. The patient is positioned for the surgical procedure, and the anesthetic is administered after the patient is stabilized.[8]

The administration of regional anesthesia to the patient with a full stomach must be a cause for concern to the practitioner. Regional techniques can provide anesthesia to the injured area while maintaining upper airway and pharyngeal reflexes. Theoretically a block of the sympathetic nervous system increases gastric and intestinal motility, causing the stomach to empty sooner. In practice this advantage is rarely seen. The development of hypotension after the administration of the anesthetic results in a higher incidence of nausea. If the patient's clinical situation is complicated by the ingestion of alcohol or the use psychopharmaceutical substances, pain from the injury may be the only stimulus that causes the patient to maintain consciousness. After the regional anesthesia is administered, the patient may lose consciousness and require airway support.[4]

When the patient has a difficult airway that prevents or limits the clinician's ability to secure it in an emergency, regional anesthesia should be avoided. The airway concerns must be addressed before anesthesia is administered.[4]

SUMMARY

Regional anesthesia techniques for upper- and lower-extremity blocks can be invaluable for specialized surgical procedures and immediate and long-term pain relief. There are a wide variety of techniques to achieve regional anesthesia: subarachnoid, epidural, caudal, brachial plexus, lumbar plexus, selective block of the upper- and lower-extremity nerves, intravenous infusion, intercostal nerve block, and specialized trauma techniques. Placement of these blocks can be facilitated by technology such as the peripheral nerve stimulator and ultrasonographic nerve location. Regional block may be used alone or in combination with general anesthesia and offers patients and surgeons excellent options for safe, effective anesthesia and analgesia.

REFERENCES

1. Thomas SJ, Orkin FK. Scope of modern anesthetic practice. In: Miller RD, ed. *Anesthesia*. 6th ed. New York: Elsevier, Churchill Livingstone; 2005:55-66.
2. Brown DL, Fink BR. History of neural blockade and pain management. In: Cousins MJ, Bridenbaugh P, eds. *Neural Blockade in Clinical Anesthesia and Management of Pain*. 3rd ed. Philadelphia: Lippincott; 1998:3-34.
3. Mulroy MF. Peripheral nerve blockade. In: Barash PG et al, eds. *Clinical Anesthesia*. 5th ed. Philadelphia: Lippincott Williams & Wilkins; 2006: 718-745.
4. Winnie AP. Brachial plexus anesthesia. In: Winnie AP, ed. *Brachial Plexus Anesthesia*. Philadelphia: Saunders; 1987.
5. Ng K et al. Spinal versus epidural anaesthesia for caesarean section. *Cochrane Database Syst Rev.* 2004;2:CD003765.
6. Reynolds F. Epidural analgesia in obstetrics. *BMJ.* 1989;297:751-752.
7. O'Hara JF et al. The renal system and anesthesia for urologic surgery. In: Barash PG et al, eds. *Clinical Anesthesia*. 5th ed. Philadelphia: Lippincott Williams & Wilkins; 2006:1013-1039.
8. Gogarten W. Spinal anaesthesia for obstetrics. *Best Pract Res Clin Anaesthesiol.* 2003;17:377-392.
9. Broadman LM, Rice LJ. Neural blockade for pediatric surgery. In: Cousins MJ, Bridgenbaugh P, eds. *Neural Blockade in Clinical Anesthesia and Management of Pain*. 3rd ed. Philadelphia: Lippincott; 1998:615-638.
10. Bromage P, Levinson G: Choice of local anesthetics in obstetrics. In: Wilkins W, ed. *Anesthesia for Obstetrics*. Baltimore: Williams & Wilkins; 1993:83-102.
11. Liu SS, Joseph RS. Local anesthetics. In: Barash PG et al, eds. *Clinical Anesthesia*. 5th ed. Philadelphia: Lippincott Williams & Wilkins; 2006: 453-474.
12. Catterall WA, Mackie K. Local anesthetics. In: Brunton LL et al, eds. *Goodman and Gilman's The Pharmacological Basis of Therapeutics*. 11th ed. New York: McGraw-Hill; 2006:369-386.
13. Strichartz GR, Berde CB. Local anesthetics. In: Miller RD, ed. *Anesthesia*. 6th ed. New York: Churchill Livingstone; 2005:573-604.
14. Guyton AC, Hall JE. Nervous regulation of the circulation. In: Guyton AC, Hall JE, eds. *Textbook of Medical Physiology*. 11th ed. Philadelphia: Saunders; 2006:204-214.
15. Veering BT et al. Pharmacokinetics of bupivacaine during postoperative epidural infusion: enantioselectivity and role of protein binding. *Anesthesiology.* 2002;96:1062-1069.
16. Wiegel M et al. Complications and adverse effects associated with continuous peripheral nerve blocks in orthopedic patients. *Reg Anesth.* 2007;104(6): 1578-1582.
17. Turnbull DK, Shepherd DB. Post-dural puncture headache: pathogenesis, prevention and treatment. *Br J Anaesth.* 2003;91:718-729.
18. Harrington BE. Postdural puncture headache and the development of the epidural blood patch. *Reg Anesth Pain Med.* 2004;29:136-163.
19. Hawkins JM, Moore PA. Local anesthesia: advances in agents and techniques. *Dent Clin North Am.* 2002;46:719-732, ix.
20. Wood M. Local anesthetic agents. In: Wood M, Wood AJ, eds. *Drugs and Anesthesia: Pharmacology for Anesthesiologists*. Baltimore: Williams & Wilkins; 1990:319-346.
21. Butterworth JF IV, Strichartz GR. Molecular mechanisms of local anesthesia: a review. *Anesthesiology.* 1990;72:711-734.
22. Nau C, Strichartz GR. Drug chirality in anesthesia. *Anesthesiology.* 2002; 97:497-502.
23. Heavener JE. Pharmacology of local anesthetics. In: Longnecker DE et al, eds. *Anesthesiology*. New York: McGraw-Hill; 2008:954-973.
24. Cox B et al. Toxicity of local anaesthetics. *Best Pract Res Clin Anaesthesiol.* 2003;17:111-136.
25. Hickey R et al. Plasma concentrations of ropivacaine given with or without epinephrine for brachial plexus block. *Can J Anaesth.* 1990;37:878-882.
26. Tetzlaff JE. *Clinical Pharmacology of Local Anesthetics*. Boston: Butterworth-Heinemann; 2000:47-54.
27. Arthur GR et al. Comparative pharmacokinetics of bupivacaine and ropivacaine, a new amide local anesthetic. *Anesth Analg.* 1998;67:1053-1058.
28. Visan A et al. Peripheral nerve stimulators technology. *Tech Reg Anesth Pain Manag.* 2002;6:155-157.
29. Hahn MB et al. *Regional Anesthesia: An Atlas of Anatomy and Techniques*. St Louis: Mosby; 1996.
30. Brown DL, ed. *Atlas of Regional Anesthesia*. 3rd ed. Philadelphia: Saunders; 2006.
31. Marhofer P et al. Ultrasound guidance in regional anaesthesia. *Br J Anaesth.* 2004;94:7-17.
32. Pollock JE. Regional anesthesia for hand surgery. *Tech Reg Anesth Pain Manag.* 1999;3:79-84.
33. Panchal SJ. Upper extremity techniques for postoperative analgesia. *Tech Reg Anesth Pain Manag.* 2002;6:56-59.
34. Pham-Dang C et al. A novel supraclavicular approach to brachial plexus block. *Anesth Analg.* 1997;85:111-116.
35. English LA et al. Effect of needle size on success of transarterial axillary block. *AANA J.* 2004;72(1):57-60.
36. Narchi P et al. A new approach to axillary brachial plexus block. *Tech Reg Anesth Pain Manage.* 1997;1:178-180.
37. Urmey WF. Interscalene block. *Tech Reg Anesth Pain Manage.* 1999;3:207-211.
38. Winnie AP. An "immobile needle" for nerve blocks. *Anesthesiology.* 1969;31:577-578.
39. Urmey WF. New considerations in brachial plexus anesthesia. *Tech Reg Anesth Pain Manag.* 1997;1:185-193.
40. Pham Dang C. A novel supraclavicular approach to the brachial plexus. *Anesth Analg.* 1997;85:111-116.
41. Lofstrom B. Nerve block at the elbow. In: Eriksson E, ed. *Illustrated Handbook in Local Anesthesia*. Copenhagen, Denmark: Munksgaard; 1969.
42. Saga-Rumley SA. Intravenous regional anesthesia. *Curr Rev Nurse Anesth.* 1997;19:217-228.
43. Marchant AE, McConachie I. Intravenous regional anesthesia. *Curr Anaesth Crit Care.* 2003;14:32-37.
44. Bernards CM. Epidural and spinal anesthesia. In: Barash PG et al, eds. *Clinical Anesthesia*. 5th ed. Philadelphia: Lippincott; 2006:691-717.
45. Lofstrom B. Intercostal nerve blocks. In: Eriksson E, ed. *Illustrated Handbook in Local Anesthesia*. Copenhagen, Denmark: Munksgaard; 1969:93-95.
46. Debreceni G et al. Continuous epidural or intercostal analgesia following thoracotomy: a prospective randomized double-blind clinical trial. *Acta Anaesthesiol Scand.* 2003;47:1091-1095.
47. Nielsen KC et al. Femoral nerve blocks. *Tech Reg Anesth Pain Manag.* 2003;7:8-17.
48. Williams BA et al. Femoral-sciatic nerve blocks for complex outpatient knee surgery are associated with less postoperative pain before same-day discharge. *Anesthesiology.* 2003;98:1206-1213.
49. Dalens B et al. Comparison of the fascia iliaca compartment block with the 3-in-1 block in children. *Anesth Analg.* 1989;69:705-713.
50. Capdevila X et al. Comparison of the three in one fascia iliaca compartment blocks in adults: clinical and radiographic analysis. *Anesth Analg.* 1998;86:1039-1044.
51. Lopez S et al. Fascia iliaca compartment block for femoral bone fractures in prehospital care. *Tech Reg Anesth Pain Manag.* 2003;28:203-207.
52. Chelly JE. Sciatic nerve block. *Tech Reg Anesth Pain Manag.* 2003;7:18-25.
53. Lofstrom B. Nerve block at the ankle. In: Eriksson E, ed. *Illustrated Handbook in Local Anesthesia*. Copenhagen, Denmark: Munksgaard; 1969:112-119.
54. Hadzic A, Vloka JD. Anesthesia for ankle and foot surgery. *Tech Reg Anesth Pain Manag.* 1999;3:113-119.
55. Kay J. Ankle block. *Tech Reg Anesth Pain Manag.* 1999;3:3-8.
56. Patel KP et al. Musculoskeletal injuries. In: Capan L et al, eds. *Trauma: Anesthesia and Intensive Care*. Philadelphia: Lippincott; 1991:511-546.

CHAPTER 47

OBSTETRIC ANESTHESIA

Lisa A. Osborne

As anesthetic techniques have advanced in the modern day, so have the attitudes toward anesthesia during childbirth. Consequently, the demand for obstetric anesthesia services has made this a large part of most anesthesia practices. An in-depth understanding of the physiologic changes of pregnancy and the associated anesthesia considerations are vital to providing safe anesthesia for this special high-risk population.

ANATOMIC AND PHYSIOLOGIC CHANGES DURING NORMAL PREGNANCY

Physiologic changes in pregnancy are related to increased metabolic demands, hormonal changes, and anatomic changes. These changes begin early in pregnancy and continue into the postpartum period. The marked changes have significant anesthesia implications.

Cardiovascular Changes

Cardiovascular changes begin as early as 4 weeks of pregnancy and continue into the postpartum period.[1] Heart rate increases 20% in the first trimester, but normal heart rate variability does not appear to be changed until late in pregnancy, when tachyarrhythmias may be seen.[2] Cardiac output increases by approximately 40% over nonpregnant values. This increase in cardiac output begins at the 5th week, and is mostly due to the increase in stroke volume (SV) and to a lesser extent an increase in heart rate (HR). The increase in cardiac output continues until about the 32nd week, where it is stable until labor and delivery.[3,4] Immediately after delivery, cardiac output may increase further to as much as 180% above baseline because of the increase in fluid load from the now empty uterus and relief of aortocaval compression. This postpartum increase in cardiac output is the reason pregnant cardiac patients are at greatest risk right after delivery. Cardiac output remains elevated for approximately 24 hours postpartum and returns to baseline 10 days later as HR and SV normalize.[5]

During pregnancy the heart enlarges, and ventricular walls thicken. End-diastolic volume increases. These changes cause the physical examination of the pregnant patient to appear abnormal. A loud, split first heart sound, an S_3, or a benign systolic murmur grade 1 or 2 may be heard on auscultation. The normal pregnant patient may report having signs of cardiac abnormality such as exercise intolerance, shortness of breath, and edema.[6] However, if the systolic murmur is greater than grade 3 or accompanied by chest pain or syncope, further evaluation is necessary. Diastolic murmurs are considered pathologic.

Blood volume increases throughout pregnancy up to 45% by term (85 to 100 mL/kg). A relative (dilutional) anemia results because the actual red-cell volume increases by just 30%. Average hemoglobin is 11.6 g/dL and hematocrit 35.5%.[7] Venous return (preload) increases as a result of the change in the rennin-angiotensin system. At delivery, preload increases to a greater extent because of an autotransfusion of blood from the contracting uterus. Pregnant women have greater baroreflex-mediated changes in HR at term than at 6 to 8 weeks postpartum.[8] This increase in baroreceptor responsiveness persists for even longer periods after delivery in some women.[9]

Systemic vascular resistance (SVR) decreases as much as 21% by term pregnancy, owing in large part to decreased resistance in the uteroplacental, pulmonary, renal, and cutaneous vascular beds.[10,11] Baseline central sympathetic outflow is twice as high in normal, term pregnant women as in nonpregnant women.[12] The venous capacitance system loses tone, allowing pooling of the larger blood volume. This decrease in SVR results in little overall systolic blood pressure changes during normal pregnancy, despite increases in blood volume.[13] A decrease in diastolic blood pressure of up to 15 mm Hg may occur, resulting in a decrease in mean pressure.

Renin

The pregnant woman is more dependent on the renin-angiotensin system for maintenance of blood pressure than her nonpregnant counterpart.[14] Plasma levels of renin and angiotensin II are increased during pregnancy,[8] despite the increase in blood volume. Baseline plasma renin activity in the third trimester is 12 times greater than that in nonpregnant control women. Vascular sensitivity to angiotensin II is both clinically and statistically significantly reduced in third-trimester pregnant women,[15-17] whereas sensitivity to norepinephrine is unchanged. The magnitude of the reduction in sensitivity to angiotensin varies throughout the day in a diurnal pattern.[18]

Clearly, some dramatic changes occur in both vascular sensitivity to angiotensin II and plasma levels of renin and angiotensin II during pregnancy. What is not known is if a cause-and-effect relationship exists between these changes. Causes become exceedingly important when the effects of epidural anesthesia on renin release are considered. Because the renin-angiotensin system provides support for mean arterial pressure (MAP) in the absence of sympathetic nervous system—controlled vasoconstriction, understanding the cause of reduced vascular sensitivity to and increased plasma levels of angiotensin becomes important in the context of epidural anesthesia and maternal hypotension.

Vasopressin

The clearance of vasopressin at 36 to 38 weeks' gestation is three to four times greater than that observed before pregnancy (P <0.01).[19] Vasopressinase levels increase by a factor of 50 between early and term pregnancy, likely accounting for the increased clearance rate observed. The vasopressin system is important because it is one of three systems with which the body defends against decreases in MAP.

Aortocaval Compression

In the early 1950s, a syndrome of supine hypotension was identified in term or near-term pregnant women.[20-21] This syndrome is caused by compression of the vena cava by the gravid uterus, which restricts venous return to the heart when the parturient lies in the supine position. Compression is more severe when the abdomen is tense or when the uterus is larger than normal, as in polyhydramnios or multiple gestation. Decreased venous return results in a significant reduction in SV and cardiac output. Figure 47-1 depicts typical changes in vital signs during supine hypotension. The resultant hypotension can be severe enough to cause loss of consciousness in some women. Maximal decreases in blood pressure may require up to 10 minutes to develop; however, some women experience the decrease almost immediately. The normal physiologic responses to caval compression are tachycardia and vasoconstriction of the lower extremities. Despite this attempted compensation, uterine blood flow and therefore fetal oxygenation are reduced.[22] Figure 47-2 depicts changes in aortocaval compression with changes in position.

In addition to compressing the vena cava, the gravid uterus may compress the abdominal aorta. For this reason, supine hypotensive syndrome is more correctly referred to as *aortocaval compression*. When the abdominal aorta is compressed, upper-body blood pressure remains relatively normal, whereas blood pressure distal to the L3 to L4 site of aortic compression (uterus and lower extremities) may be significantly reduced. It is by this mechanism that uterine blood flow and therefore fetal oxygenation may suffer, despite the presence of an apparently normal maternal systemic blood pressure.

Compression of the aorta and vena cava can usually be relieved by shifting the uterus to the left (left uterine displacement) or, even more effectively, by lying on the side.[23] Left uterine displacement can be accomplished by rotation of the operating room table 15 degrees to the left or by placing a 15-cm-high wedge under the parturient's right hip and back, as shown in Figure 47-2. Care should be taken to ensure adequate left uterine displacement because most anesthetists have been shown to underestimate the angle of tilt they have provided.[24] In women with an exceptionally large uterus, greater displacement may be necessary to be effective. In a small percentage of women, right uterine displacement may be more effective than left displacement, although in the majority of cases, right uterine displacement results in SVs that are no better than those measured with the patient in the supine position.[23]

Left uterine displacement or the side-lying position is an essential component of obstetric care, especially when labor epidural analgesia (LEA) is administered. LEA defeats compensatory lower-extremity vasoconstriction by blocking the sympathetic nerves responsible for vasoconstriction, resulting in even greater hypotension.

Respiratory Changes

Term pregnancy is accompanied by an increase in O_2 demand of up to 33% at baseline and 100% during the second stage of labor.

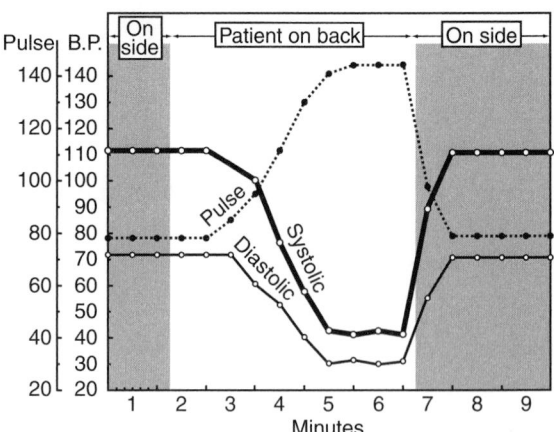

FIGURE **47-1** Typical vital sign pattern in supine hypotensive syndrome. (*From Howard BK et al. Supine hypotensive syndrome in late pregnancy.* Obstet Gynecol. 1953;1:371-377.)

At term, minute ventilation is increased by 50%, primarily due to an increase in tidal volume (increased by 40%), whereas the respiratory rate is increased by only 10%. The parturient's breathing pattern becomes more diaphragmatic because of the enlarging uterus. By 12 weeks, the normal arterial partial pressure of CO_2 ranges from 30 to 32 mm Hg, and this continues through term. The normal arterial partial pressure of O_2 is greater than 100 mm Hg.

The functional residual capacity (FRC), expiratory reserve, and residual volume are decreased primarily as a result of upward pressure on the diaphragm, with results functionally similar to restrictive lung disease. The decrease in functional residual capacity (20%), which is an important O_2 reserve, and the increase in O_2 consumption that occur in pregnancy commonly result in rapid arterial desaturation in the apneic pregnant patient. Closing capacity (CC) does not change, which results in a decreased FRC/CC ratio often leading to small-airway closure before the tidal volume has been exhaled. This mechanism may explain the observation of reduced O_2 saturations in parturients during natural sleep. Compared with nonpregnant controls, whose average oxygen saturation as measured by pulse oximetry (SpO_2) during sleep was 98.5%, healthy near-term pregnant women averaged only 95.2%, with temporary desaturations below 90% being not uncommon.[25] However, oxygen transport is maximized by an increased cardiac output and a shift to right in the oxyhemoglobin dissociation curve.

During labor, increases in minute ventilation of up to 300% may occur in response to pain and may occasionally cause maternal arterial partial pressure of CO_2 to drop below 15 mm Hg. Some evidence indicates that hyperventilation may cause a decrease in uterine blood flow. However, in animal studies this finding has usually been associated with stressful events such as intubation and invasive procedures. In pregnant, laboring human volunteers, hyperventilation to an arterial partial pressure of CO_2 of 20 mm Hg does not seem to harm the fetus. Specifically, the fetus does not develop hypoxia or acidosis as determined by analysis of a scalp blood sample. However, a situation in which both hyperventilation and extreme stress are present is potentially detrimental to the fetus. When an anesthetized parturient is hyperventilated during stress, the neonate may be at risk of acidosis and hypoxia.

In addition to the respiratory changes in pregnancy, there are changes to the airway itself. There is narrowing of the glottic

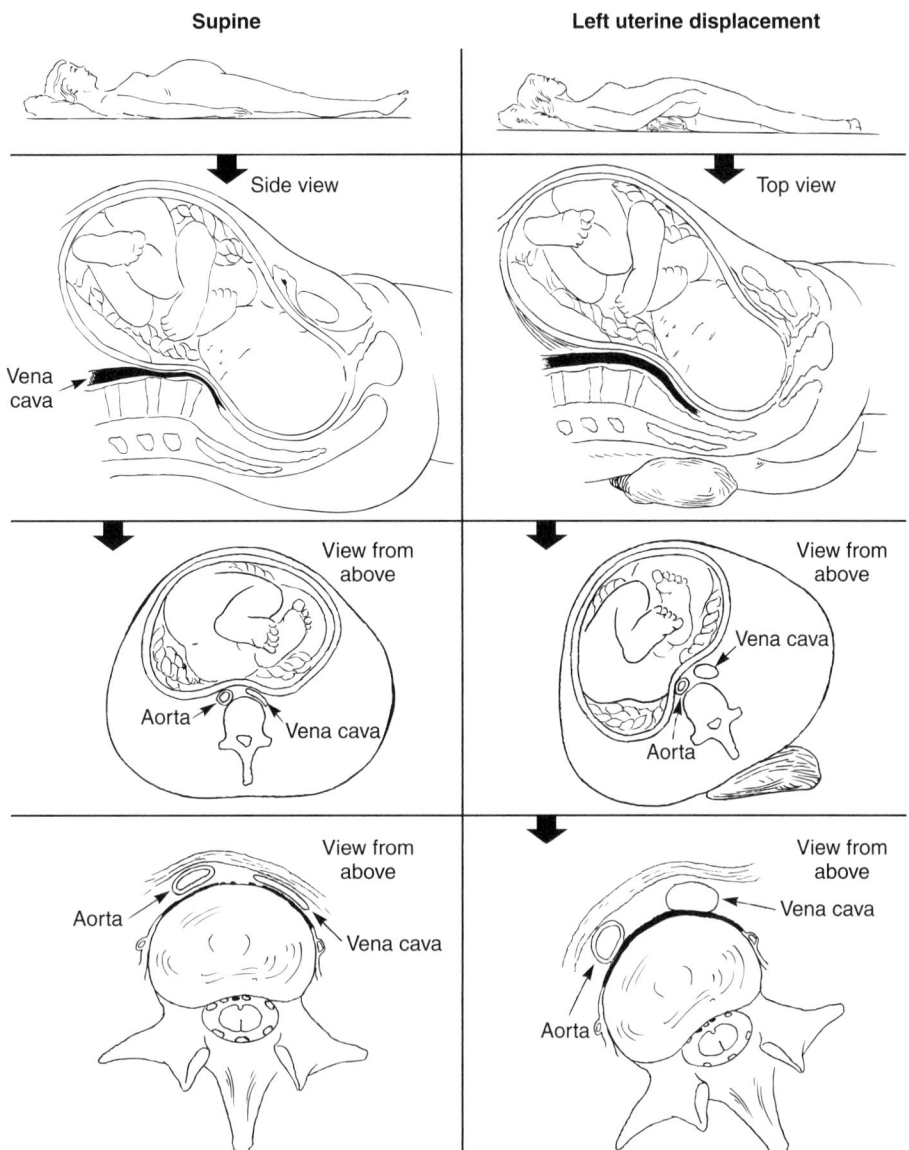

FIGURE **47-2**   Effects of left uterine displacement on the diameter of the abdominal aorta and vena cava.

opening and generalized edema that is a result of capillary engorgement. These changes make the airway friable and can result in a difficult intubation. Care must be taken during placement of airway adjuncts, or bleeding may result. Nasal intubation in the parturient should generally be avoided.

Coagulation Changes

In general, the parturient is said to be "hypercoagulable." Levels of several clotting factors, including platelets, factor VII, and fibrinogen are increased. The increased levels, when combined with venous pooling, place the parturient at risk for deep venous thrombosis. Thromboembolic events remain one of the leading causes of maternal mortality. In the nonpregnant state, fibrinogen levels average from 200 to 400 mg/dL. Late in pregnancy, fibrinogen levels are normally at least 400 mg/dL and may be as high as 650 mg/dL. Platelet counts are also elevated at term and may be as high as 400,000.

Several pathologic conditions during pregnancy are associated with decreased levels of fibrinogen, platelets, or both.

The incidence of low platelets in a normal pregnancy is about 8%.[26] Low platelets in relationship to preeclampsia is discussed later in the chapter. In the parturient, platelet and fibrinogen levels that are within normal ranges for the nonpregnant state may actually represent a decrease from the parturient's baseline values; this has important implications if regional anesthesia is being considered.

Nervous System Changes

Pregnant women have an increased sensitivity to local and general anesthetics from early in pregnancy.[27-30] The exact mechanism remains unclear, but animal studies have demonstrated a variable reduction in the minimum alveolar concentration (MAC) of inhalation agents in rabbits chronically exposed to progesterone.[27] In pregnant rats, the effects of endorphins on pain thresholds are also demonstrated, which may also be an important factor. Additionally, research and clinical experience have demonstrated an increase in the sensitivity of nerves to local anesthetic blockade during pregnancy.[27-31]

Gastrointestinal Changes

The parturient is at increased risk for regurgitation and aspiration of gastric contents because of anatomic and physiologic changes associated with pregnancy. A significant number of pregnant women, and women immediately postpartum, have gastric volumes in excess of 25 mL and gastric pH below 2.5.[32] Ultrasound has demonstrated solid food in the stomach of almost two thirds of women in whom LEA had been instituted and in the stomach of more than 40% of laboring women who had not eaten in 12 to 24 hours.[33] Increased levels of gastrin during pregnancy result in greater gastric volume and lower pH. Upward displacement of the stomach by the gravid uterus may result in mechanical obstruction to outflow through the pylorus, delayed gastric emptying, and increased intragastric pressure. Elevated levels of progesterone, a smooth-muscle relaxant, also decrease gastric motility and cause a reduction in lower-esophageal sphincter tone. This explains the heartburn frequently experienced by pregnant women. Gastrointestinal changes do not completely normalize until several weeks postpartum.

The onset of labor is accompanied by a further reduction in the rate of gastric emptying. If not contraindicated, administration of a histamine-2 (H_2) blocker and metoclopramide may benefit patients prior to anesthesia. The use of these drugs is advocated in the event that a general anesthetic or airway management becomes necessary. Ranitidine has been shown to reduce the acidity of gastric contents in the parturient within 30 minutes after an intravenous (IV) dose.[34] Unlike cimetidine, ranitidine does not inhibit the metabolism of amide local anesthetics. Metoclopramide and ranitidine are compatible with most IV solutions.

Hepatic Changes

During pregnancy, levels of aspartate aminotransferase, alanine aminotransferase, lactate dehydrogenase, and alkaline phosphatase increase to the upper limits of nonpregnant normal levels. Serum albumin concentration decreases somewhat, and this decrease may result in increased free fractions of highly protein-bound drugs. Serum cholinesterase activity decreases by 30% or more during the first or second trimester; it recovers slightly by term, although it is still reduced compared with normal cholinesterase activity. Within a few days after delivery, cholinesterase levels dip again before returning to normal nonpregnant values over a few weeks. Despite decreases in cholinesterase activity, clinically relevant prolongation of the duration of action of drugs that depend on cholinesterase for elimination, such as succinylcholine, is uncommon in women with genotypically normal cholinesterase enzymes

Renal Changes

During pregnancy, increased cardiac output leads to increased renal plasma flow and increased glomerular filtration rate. Creatinine clearance rises to 140 to 160 mL/min. As a result, the level of blood urea nitrogen decreases to approximately 8 mg/dL and that of creatinine to approximately 0.5 mg/dL. Low levels of glucosuria and proteinuria commonly are present in the absence of disease and are attributable to increased glomerular filtration rate (GFR) and reduced renal absorption. The gravid uterus may produce mechanical obstruction of a ureter.

Musculoskeletal Changes

To maintain the center of gravity with the weight of the enlarging fetus, lumbar lordosis becomes increasingly exaggerated. The shoulders are typically slumped and rotated back. The hormone relaxin results in increased mobility of joints, including the sacroiliac, sacrococcygeal and pubic joints. This results in a widening of the pelvis in preparation for the birth. These changes have implications for neuraxial anesthesia. The increased lordosis can result in a narrowing of the interspinous space, potentially resulting in a difficult spinal or epidural placement. The widening of the pelvis can result in a difficulty with patient positioning for neuraxial techniques in the side-lying position.

Uterine Changes

The uterus is altered tremendously during pregnancy. The uterus enlarges, and its blood flow increases to meet both uterine and fetal metabolic demands. Uterine blood flow is supplied by two uterine arteries that are thought to be maximally dilated throughout pregnancy. Placental blood flow on the uterine side is supplied via the maternal arcuate, radial, and spiral arteries. The spiral arteries expel blood into the intervillous space. The maternal venous sinuses receive blood from the intervillous space and return it to the general circulation. Uterine blood flow increases to a maximum of 800 mL/min (approximately 10% of maternal cardiac output). Of this, approximately 150 mL/min supplies nutritive flow to the myometrium, and 100 mL/min flows to the decidua (the lining of the uterus); the remainder flows to the intervillous space.

The fetus sends O_2-poor blood to the placenta via two umbilical arteries. These vessels perfuse capillary networks within placental villi that protrude into the pool of maternal blood. Placental villi are small, fingerlike projections, the purpose of which is to maximize the placental surface area in contact with maternal blood. Each villus contains a capillary network that exchanges respiratory gases, nutrients, and wastes with maternal blood (Figure 47-3). Both O_2 and CO_2 diffuse through placental tissue quickly. For clinical purposes, diffusion does not limit the transfer of these gases. Both O_2 and CO_2 are said to be "perfusion limited," because their transfer to the fetus is limited only by the perfusion of the placenta, not by the rate of diffusion of the gases. Therefore, decreases in maternal uterine artery blood flow or increases in placental vascular resistance will decrease fetal oxygenation.

Autoregulation of intervillous blood flow does not seem to occur. Spiral arteries, however, do constrict in response to α-agonists. Evidence of fetal embarrassment occurs if maternal systolic blood pressure drops below 100 mm Hg in awake, healthy patients during epidural anesthesia. Patients with preeclampsia (formerly called *pregnancy-induced hypertension*, or PIH) can develop placental insufficiency at systolic pressures greater than 100 mm Hg. Unlike patients who receive LEA, patients receiving inhalation anesthesia seem to maintain adequate placental blood flow, despite somewhat reduced blood pressure; this may be a function of altered uterine blood flow, altered fetal O_2 requirements, or both.

Placental Transfer and Fetal Effects of Drugs

Placental transfer of free (non–protein-bound) drug is dependent on the magnitude of the concentration gradient, molecular weight, lipid solubility, and drug ionization state. Drugs with molecular weights greater than 1000 daltons (Da) cross the placenta poorly, whereas drugs with weights less than 500 Da cross easily. Most drugs that are administered to the parturient are relatively small compounds and able to cross to the placenta. However, size is only one of the determinants of permeability.

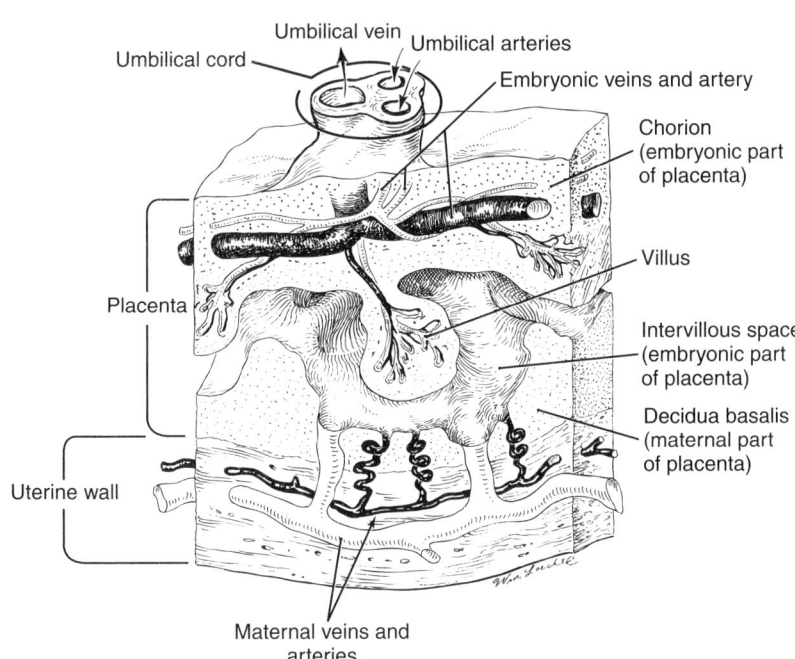

Umbilical vein
Umbilical cord
Umbilical arteries
Embryonic veins and artery
Chorion
(embryonic part
of placenta)
Placenta
Villus
Intervillous space
(embryonic part
of placenta)
Decidua basalis
(maternal part
of placenta)
Uterine wall
Maternal veins and
arteries

FIGURE **47-3**   Cross-section of the uteroplacental inter-face and the maternal and fetal blood supply.

Because cell membranes consist primarily of phospholipids, lipid solubility favors passage of drugs through cell membranes. Highly lipid-soluble drugs such as thiopental cross readily. Ionized molecules are polar and water soluble, which inhibits diffusion through lipophilic cell membranes. The degree of ionization of a drug will affect the amount of drug allowed to cross, because the nonionized portion crosses readily. Nondepolarized muscle relaxants are an example of a large ionized drug that is inhibited from crossing to the placenta.

After drugs have crossed the placenta, a variety of factors minimize their effects on the fetus. The chief factor responsible for minimizing these effects is dilution. Before reaching the fetus, a drug is diluted in intervillous blood, absorbed by the placenta, further diluted in placental blood, and circulated to the fetus. Once in the fetus, the drug is distributed within the fetal intravascular volume and redistributed to fetal tissues. Several other minor factors limit the effects of maternally administered drugs on a fetus. Some drugs, such as thiopental, are partially taken up by the fetal liver before gaining access to the general fetal circulation. Approximately one fifth of the fetal cardiac output returns directly to the placenta because of shunt flow through the foramen ovale and ductus arteriosus. This shunted blood does not circulate, and any drug it contains does not have a systemic fetal effect.

The acid-base status of the fetus may affect the accumulation of a drug. A fetus who has become acidotic will alter the degree of ionization of a drug, potentially resulting in "ion trapping" leading to accumulation. For a complete discussion of fetal ion trapping see Chapter 11. Some key points to remember regarding physiologic changes in pregnancy are given in Box 47-1.

STAGES OF LABOR AND DELIVERY

The experience of pain is a highly personal phenomenon. Pain tolerance varies widely from one individual to the next. There are also many factors that are related to the perception of pain during labor that range from social support factors to physical factors such as fetal presentation. A few women are able to tolerate labor and delivery without significant discomfort; others experience pain in excess of their ability to cope. The combination of lack of control over the process in which the body is engaged, exhaustion, frustration, and seemingly unending pain can result in hyperventilation, screaming, cursing, and physical aggression. Effective labor analgesia not only makes the birth process more enjoyable but also provides women with more opportunity for control over their bodies and the environment, allowing them to maintain personal dignity.

In the absence of effective analgesia, the onset of labor brings with it an intensification of many of the physiologic alterations of pregnancy. Serum catecholamine levels increase in response to pain, stress, and uterine activity. Whole-body O_2 demand increases an additional 60% during painful contractions. Each uterine contraction expels blood from the uterus into the general circulation, acutely increasing venous return to the heart and therefore SV. Cardiac output in the first stage of labor increases 40% to 80% during contractions and returns to pregnant baseline between contractions.

As stated, increases in minute ventilation of up to 300% may occur in response to pain and may occasionally cause maternal arterial partial pressure of CO_2 to drop below 15 mm Hg. Hyperventilation may cause a decrease in uterine blood flow, and in situations in which both hyperventilation and extreme stress are present, it may be detrimental to the fetus, who is at risk for acidosis and hypoxia.

Labor is generally divided into three stages. The first stage begins at the onset of contractions, which progressively results in complete dilation of the cervix. The first stage of labor is further divided into the latent and active phases. The beginning of this stage is considered the latent phase because initially there is little dilation of the cervix; however, it does become softer. The active phase is associated with regular cervical dilation in response to uterine contractions.

The second stage begins at full cervical dilation (10 cm) and ends with delivery of the infant. The third stage encompasses the delivery of the placenta. The length of time it takes to progress through these stages is dependent on parity, effective uterine contractions, the size and type of pelvis, and fetal presentation. The Friedman curve is used to track normal progress of labor. Cervical dilation is generally 1 to 1.2 cm/hr during the active phase of labor. When labor progress no longer follows the normal pattern, it is considered a "dysfunctional labor," and may require the use of oxytocin to augment contractions. Abnormal labors are classified as *slow latent phase*, *arrest of active phase*, and *arrest of descent*.

First Stage of Labor

During the late 1950s and early 1960s, it was demonstrated that the pain of labor and delivery is mediated by T10 to L1 sympathetic nerve fibers and S1 to S4 somatic nerve fibers (Box 47-2 and Figure 47-4). The nerves at the T10 to L1 level were shown to be responsible for carrying pain sensation from cervical dilation, whereas those at the S1 to S4 level mediated vaginal and perineal pain perception.

Cervical dilation and possibly uterine muscle ischemia during contraction cause nonspecific nociceptor stimulation that is mediated by small, unmyelinated "C fibers." Pain transmission to the spinal cord occurs via nerves at the T10 to L1 level. Two modes of pain are perceived by laboring women: a nonlocalized cramping referred to the appropriate surface dermatomes on the abdomen from the level of the umbilicus to the inguinal ligament; and so-called "back labor," a sharp localized back pain that results from referred pain to dermatomes (cutaneous innervation) and sclerotomes (innervation of the bone and muscle). Sclerotomes are located several inches below the actual vertebral level of involvement, causing the pain to be felt over the L5 to S1 region. This pathway can be interrupted by a lumbar sympathetic block, a pericervical block, or an epidural sympathetic block with a local anesthetic level up to the T10 sensory dermatome.

BOX 47-2

Pain Pathways During Labor

Area	Innervation	Comments
Uterus and cervix	T10 to L1-L2	Pain impulses carried in visceral afferent type C fibers
Perineum	S2, S3, and S4	Pain impulses carried by somatic nerve fibers; pudendal nerves

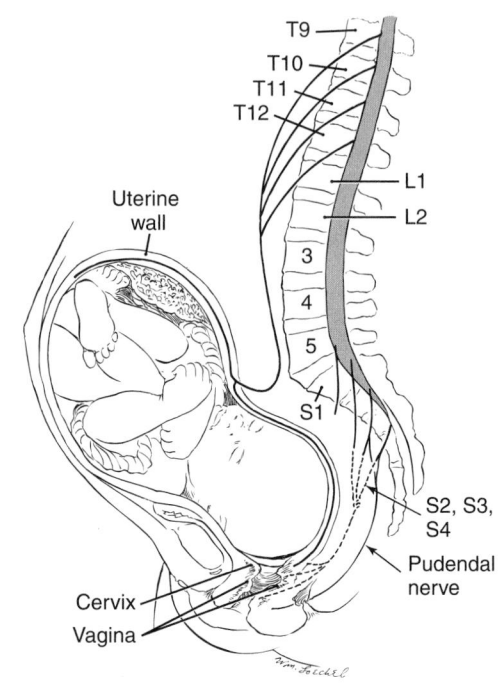

FIGURE **47-4** Lower thoracic, lumbar, and sacral regions of the spine showing spinal cord, nerve roots, and sensory innervation to the uterus, cervix, and vagina.

Second Stage of Labor

As cervical dilation progresses and the fetal head descends into the pelvis, a second pain pathway becomes important. Compression and stretching of pelvic musculature and ligaments produce pain that is mediated by the sacral plexus. This pain can be eliminated with blockade of the pudendal nerve. In a normal laboring patient, a lumbar epidural block effectively relieves the pain of uterine contraction and cervical dilation and under some circumstances also provides effective sacral analgesia. When sacral analgesia is not achieved with the epidural block, a pudendal block (usually placed by the obstetrician) provides nearly complete sacral relief.

Occasionally during labor, other sources of pain not mediated by these two pathways occur. They usually are mediated by lumbar somatic fibers and less frequently by sacral and thoracic somatic fibers. Such pain usually occurs in labors with abnormal presentations (e.g., occiput posterior presentation) or in cases of cephalopelvic disproportion.

PREPARATION FOR ANESTHETIC INTERVENTION

History and Physical

The anesthetist should begin, as with any other patient, with an appropriate history-taking and physical examination. It is easier for a mother to cooperate during history-taking if she is not experiencing the pain of labor. Therefore it is helpful if the history is taken early in the labor and delivery process, often long before regional anesthesia is indicated. An added benefit of an early history-taking is that if anesthesia is needed emergently for fetal distress or maternal bleeding, much more is known about the patient than if history-taking had been postponed. For this reason, obtaining a history early is helpful in parturients in whom obstetricians suspect the possibility of problems.

Taking the history should include general questions about systemic disease and an assessment of problems related to pregnancy and fetal well-being. If the history is taken early, a reassessment of fetal well-being is necessary just before an anesthetic intervention. In a healthy parturient who desires labor analgesia, a preanesthetic evaluation should include the following additional information: the extent of the patient's cervical dilation and percent effacement; the station of the fetal presenting part; the fetal heart rate (FHR) and an assessment of FHR variability; whether the amniotic membrane is ruptured or intact; the gestational age of the fetus; and the parturient's gravidity and parity. Some centers record the last of these using the designation $G_xP_xAb_x$, for gravidity (the number of conceptions), *parity* (the number of live births), and *abortus* (the number of preterm dead births), with the subscript after each abbreviation representing the number of each. Other centers use the FPAL system (*full-term, premature, abortus,* and *living* children), documenting only the numbers for each category. Any previous analgesic interventions should be noted.

The parturient should be questioned about problems with previous pregnancies, deliveries, or anesthetics during pregnancy. Because a regional anesthetic is the most widely used technique, she should be asked specifically about bleeding or back problems. An assessment of her state of hydration is especially important, because obstetric patients are prone to increased fluid losses resulting from mouth-breathing and panting and may have taken nothing by mouth for an extended period. Oxygenation of the fetus is dependent on maintenance of an adequate maternal blood pressure, and epidural analgesia may produce significant hypotension in the presence of dehydration. Review of baseline laboratory values before the institution of LEA in healthy patients is not mandatory. In circumstances of little to no prenatal care, however, baseline laboratory values may be indicated because of the increased possibility of an undiagnosed complication. In a 1995 survey of private-practice anesthesiologists, 68% said they checked a complete blood cell count before administration of LEA, and 31% checked a platelet count.[35] If preeclampsia or other pathology with anesthetic implications is present, the performance of the anesthetic procedure should generally be delayed until appropriate laboratory results (e.g., coagulation studies) are available.

At some point during the interview, a general discussion of LEA that includes an explanation of both risks and benefits should be conducted with the parturient. Methods of pain relief that are available should be addressed. The depth of this discussion may be guided by the stage of labor because the parturient may be experiencing a great deal of pain. However, even the most insistent parturient normally should be informed of the risks of the anesthetic procedure. Any problem for which the parturient is particularly at risk should be also be discussed. The risks of LEA should be discussed to the extent to which the parturient is comfortable and to her satisfaction.[36] It is not necessary to secure consent for the anesthesia accompanying a surgical procedure (e.g., cesarean section) at this time, but if the potential for a problem does exist, the anesthetist may request consent for anesthesia in the event of an emergency situation in which delay for a complete discussion would endanger the mother or her baby.

It is good to remember that communication between the anesthesia and obstetric personnel is a critical aspect of safe care. Although attempts should be made to prepare for the provision of pain relief as quickly as possible, rushing through the history-taking process or failing to adequately communicate with staff can result in injury to the patient. It is better to have a few women deliver without epidural analgesia than to cause injury to a mother or fetus because of inadequate preparation.

The choice of anesthetic depends on many factors related to the labor pattern, cervical dilation, and fetal well-being. Therefore the preanesthesia assessment must include a fetal assessment as well. FHR monitoring provides useful information about how the fetus is tolerating the current circumstances. A basic understanding of the information contained in the FHR tracing allows the anesthetist to better plan for and assess anesthetic intervention in the pregnant patient.

Fetal Assessment

Although the FHR is not a specific predictor of fetal well-being, it is the most readily available method for the assessment of fetal condition. From the FHR, information about the baseline status of a fetus can be obtained during a preanesthesia assessment. The FHR also reveals information about the fetal response to anesthetic intervention. This information is useful during LEA, anesthesia for assisted or operative delivery, and anesthesia for nondelivery surgery. Important information on which to build an anesthetic plan and evaluate its effects on both mother and fetus is available to the anesthetist knowledgeable in FHR monitoring.

The FHR is recorded on a graph running at 3 cm/min. Uterine tone, or pressure, is recorded concurrently on a second channel below the FHR tracing. In this way it is possible to relate FHR changes to uterine contractions. Two methods of detecting the FHR are used clinically. The first is noninvasive, using an abdominal ultrasound probe aimed at the fetal heart. Heart movement during each cardiac cycle is counted as a heartbeat, and the interval between beats is used to calculate the number of beats per minute. The FHR can also be measured invasively by inserting a spiral electrode approximately 2 mm into the fetal scalp. This method requires a ruptured amniotic sac and a partially dilated cervix through which the electrode is inserted.

Given a reasonable maternal O_2 saturation, fetal oxygenation is limited primarily by uteroplacental blood flow, not maternal oxygenation. Anything that decreases maternal blood pressure or uterine artery blood flow also decreases uteroplacental blood flow. This results in fetal hypoxia and eventually acidosis. Hypoxia results in FHR changes, and acidosis has been correlated with specific FHR responses.

The normal FHR in a term fetus is 120 to 160 beats per minute (bpm). An immature fetus has a higher HR. Fetal bradycardia down to 100 bpm is generally well tolerated if it lasts less than 2 minutes. Fetal bradycardia less than 100 bpm is cause for concern, and bradycardia less than 80 bpm is severe regardless of duration.

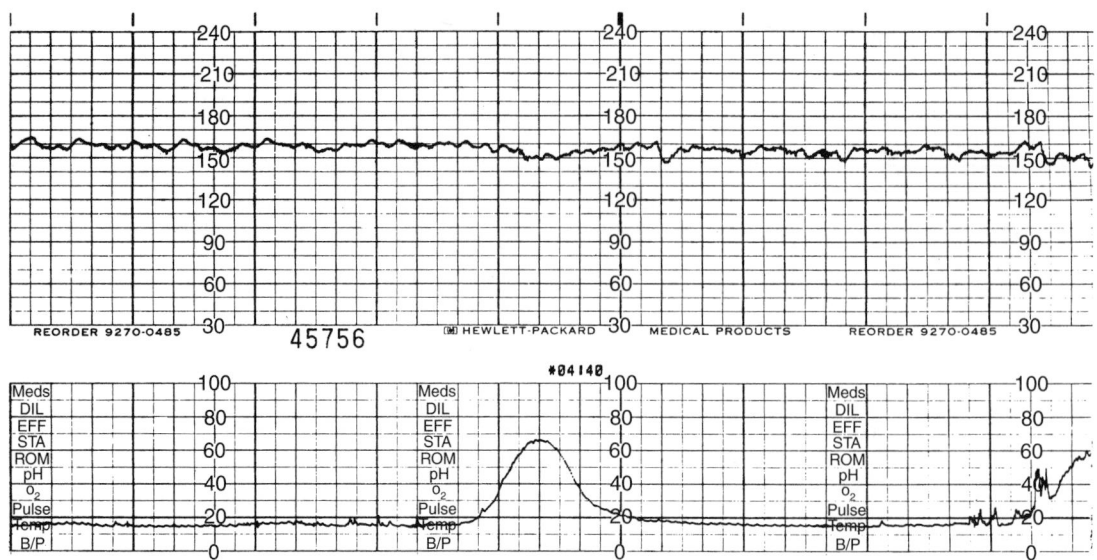

FIGURE **47-5**   Normal beat-to-beat and long-term variability with fetal heart rate (FHR) of 150 to 160 beats per minute (bpm). The distance between the heavy vertical lines represents 60 seconds. The lighter vertical lines are 10 seconds apart. The top graph is the FHR tracing; the bottom graph is intrauterine pressure. The rise in the bottom graph under the time stamp *04:40 represents a uterine contraction. Both FHR and uterine pressure are measured directly. *(From Fiedler MA. An introduction to fetal heart rate monitoring. AANA J. 1989;57:257-264.)*

Changes in Fetal Heart Rate

Fetal tachycardia is defined as an HR higher than 160 bpm in a term fetus. In a few circumstances, it may be the result of fetal hypoxia but never when normal variability is present. More common causes of fetal tachycardia include fever, fetal arrhythmias, immaturity, and drugs such as terbutaline and atropine. Ephedrine, for example, can increase both FHR and variability if given to the parturient in large enough doses.[37]

Fetal bradycardia is present when the FHR is less than 120 bpm. Transient decreases to as low as 100 bpm are generally not a cause for concern as long as FHR variability remains normal. Bradycardia can be caused by arrhythmias, drugs, and hypoxia or asphyxia. Prolonged bradycardia is the result of maternal hypoxemia or a sustained decrease in blood flow to the placenta.

Heart Rate Variability

Variability is a term used to describe small changes in the FHR. In general, baseline FHR variability increases with advancing gestational age. Short-term or beat-to-beat variability is the instantaneous change in rate that occurs between two consecutive heartbeats. The FHR monitor calculates HR based on the interval between two successive R waves on the fetal electrocardiogram. It records this rate on graph paper as a horizontal line. If each successive R wave–to–R wave interval is the same, then the HR is the same, and the line on the graph is flat. If successive R wave–to–R wave intervals are slightly different, then the resultant FHR calculation is different, and the line on the graph is irregular. This irregularity is the beat-to-beat variability. Indirect or external ultrasound monitoring of the FHR results in artifacts that can look very much like normal variability. For this reason, beat-to-beat variability can be accurately assessed only by direct FHR monitoring with a fetal scalp electrode.

Long-term variability, also called *reactivity*, is the acceleration of the FHR for short periods followed by a return to baseline HR. It often is associated with fetal movement. Long-term variability

is described as "normal" when the baseline HR varies by 15 bpm for 15 seconds on a frequent and regular basis. Variability is decreased or absent when the baseline rate changes are less than this. During fetal sleep, beat-to-beat variability should continue, but long-term variability normally decreases for periods of up to 40 minutes. Examples of both normal beat-to-beat and long-term variability are shown in Figure 47-5.

FHR variability is the single best noninvasive clinical indicator of fetal well-being. In general, beat-to-beat variability and long-term variability are seen to occur together. They probably represent the presence of an intact central nervous system (CNS) regulatory mechanism. Changes in beat-to-beat variability are vagally mediated. Hypoxia causes CNS depression, which results in decreased variability. Other causes of decreased variability include fetal sleep, acidosis, anencephaly, drugs (CNS depressants or autonomic agents), and defects of the fetal cardiac conduction system. Administration of opioids to the mother, for example, decreases FHR variability for up to 30 minutes.[38-41] Maternal magnesium sulfate administration also may attenuate HR variability.[42]

FHR variability is indicative of fetal reserve. The presence of normal variability is a good sign that the fetus is either healthy or well compensated. Although nonpathologic causes of decreased FHR variability exist, decreased variability may be a sign that the fetus is beginning to decompensate. This is especially true when variability decreases in conjunction with variable or late FHR decelerations. Evidence shows that both beat-to-beat variability and long-term variability decrease when the fetal scalp pH is 7.2 or less. A fetus that is in trouble almost always loses variability before death occurs. Figure 47-6 shows an example of poor beat-to-beat variability and almost no long-term variability.

Sinusoidal Fetal Heart Rate Pattern. An uncommon variant of FHR variability is the sinusoidal pattern (Figure 47-7). The cause of this variant is unknown in most circumstances but may be associated with fetal anemia. The sinusoidal FHR tracing is a

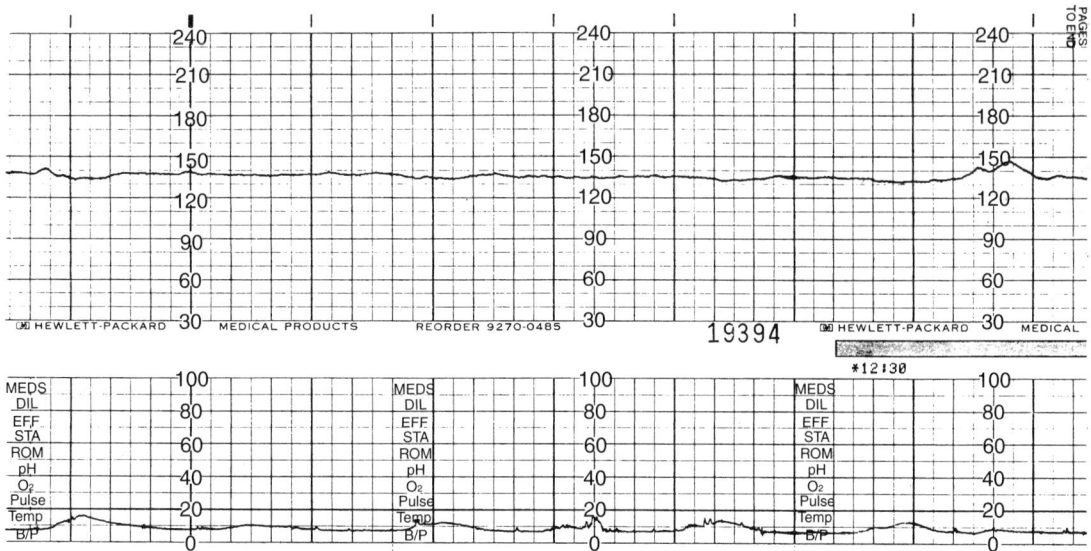

FIGURE **47-6** Poor beat-to-beat and long-term variability. The fetal heart rate was measured with a scalp electrode. (*From Fiedler MA. An introduction to fetal heart rate monitoring. AANA J. 1989;57:257-264.*)

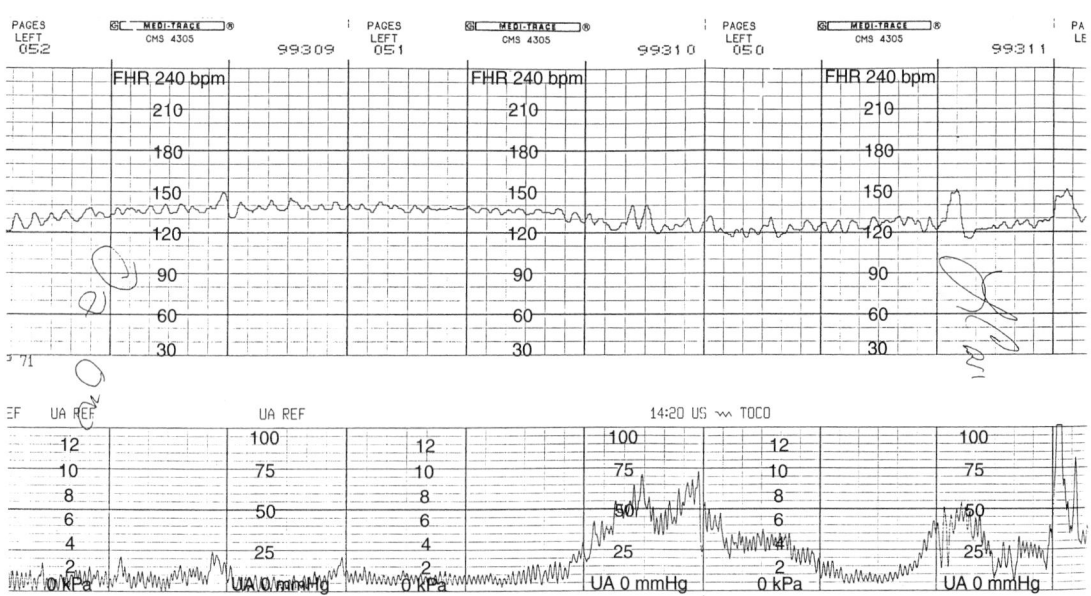

FIGURE **47-7** Sinusoidal fetal heart rate pattern in a healthy 15-year-old primigravida who later delivered a healthy infant. Monitoring is external. (*From Fiedler MA. An introduction to fetal heart rate monitoring. AANA J. 1989;57:257-264.*)

pattern of consistent, repeating variability superimposed on a background of a normal FHR. It resembles a sine wave with a frequency of two to five cycles per minute and a wave amplitude of 5 to 10 bpm. The administration of as little as 0.5 mg of butorphanol (Stadol), an opioid agonist/antagonist commonly used for relief of obstetric pain, has been strongly associated with a sinusoidal FHR pattern.[43] The reported onset and duration of the sinusoidal pattern after butorphanol administration are highly variable, with the former ranging from 2 to 36 minutes and the latter from 10 to 92 minutes.

Early Decelerations

Early decelerations occur in concert with uterine contractions. The deceleration begins when the contraction begins, and it returns to baseline when the contraction ends. Early decelerations are smooth in appearance, and the change in HR is mild, usually no more than 20 bpm. An early deceleration occurs with each uterine contraction and has the same appearance from one contraction to the next. Compression of the fetal head as it passes through the birth canal is thought to be the cause of early decelerations via vagal stimulation. Early decelerations may be a sign

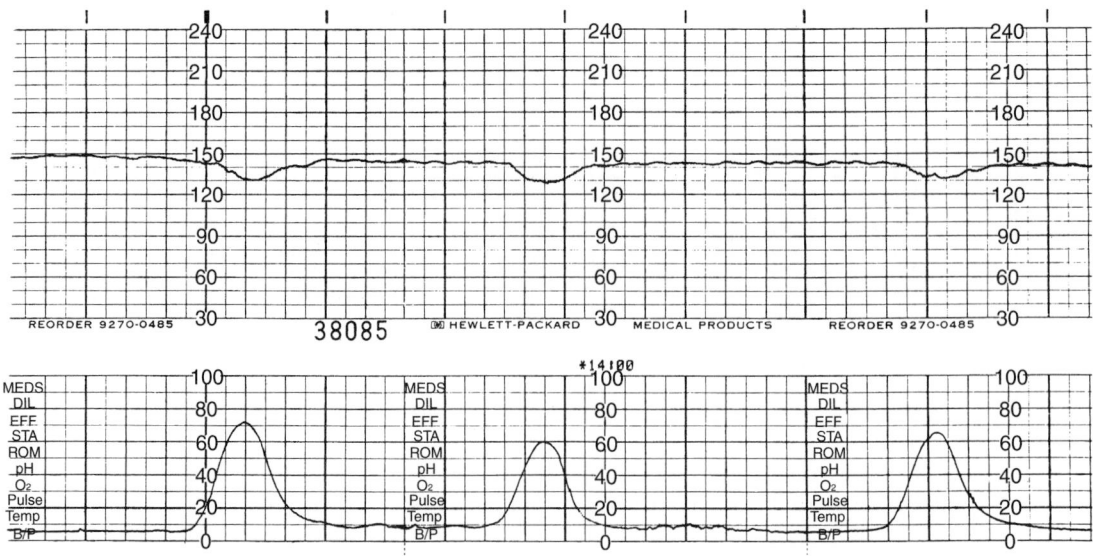

FIGURE **47-8** Early decelerations with each of three uterine contractions and poor fetal heart rate variability. (*From Fiedler MA. An introduction to fetal heart rate monitoring. AANA J. 1989;57:257-264.*)

that the parturient is pushing too early against a less than fully dilated cervix, or they may be a late sign of impending delivery. In either case, early decelerations are physiologic unless they are seen with fetal tachycardia or loss of variability. Figure 47-8 shows early decelerations with poor baseline variability.

In summary, early decelerations have the following characteristics:

- Occur with each uterine contraction
- Start and end with the contraction
- Gradually decrease in rate and then end in a return to baseline
- Are uniform in appearance
- Are associated with a mild decrease in FHR (20 bpm or less)
- Are accompanied by a loss in beat-to-beat variability during the deceleration

Variable Decelerations

Variable decelerations occur with uterine contractions but usually not with every uterine contraction. The deceleration may begin when the contraction begins, or it may begin late. Also, a variable deceleration may end after the contraction ends, sometimes with a transient tachycardia. Variable decelerations are abrupt in both onset and recovery; at times the FHR plunges 60 bpm in only 1 or 2 seconds. Variable decelerations are variable in occurrence, onset, depth, duration, and appearance. Normally, beat-to-beat variability is still present during the decelerations. Variable decelerations are thought to be caused by a baroreflex-mediated response to umbilical cord compression. Variable decelerations are termed *severe* if the FHR decreases by 60 bpm from the baseline, if the FHR drops below 60 bpm, or if the decelerations are sustained for 60 seconds or longer. Less severe variable decelerations are still of concern if beat-to-beat variability is absent. If the fetus is compromised, then the recovery phase of the deceleration may be delayed. Figure 47-9 shows a variable deceleration on a baseline of good variability.

In summary, variable decelerations have the following characteristics:

- Vary in appearance, duration, depth, and shape
- Demonstrate abrupt onset and recovery
- Maintain beat-to-beat variability with the deceleration

- Are classified as severe if the FHR decreases by 60 bpm, if the FHR decreases to less than 60 bpm, or if the decelerations last 60 seconds or longer

If variable decelerations continue to occur or are severe, the anesthetist should anticipate the possibility of obstetric intervention for which anesthesia will be required. Figure 47-10 shows two variable decelerations, the second of which is severe.

Late Decelerations

Late decelerations occur with a uterine contraction. In contrast to early decelerations, late decelerations begin between 10 and 30 seconds after the onset of the uterine contraction (Figure 47-11). Like early decelerations, they are smooth in both onset and recovery. Late decelerations are regular in occurrence. They occur with each uterine contraction, and they appear similar from one contraction to the next (however, as the fetus decompensates, recovery takes longer). Beat-to-beat variability may or may not be present during the deceleration, depending on the baseline level of fetal oxygenation. A fetus with late decelerations and absent variability is much more likely to have metabolic acidosis than one in which variability is still present. When late decelerations are noted, it is important to evaluate beat-to-beat and long-term variability as well. The absence of variability in combination with late decelerations may indicate the presence of hypoxic myocardial depression.

In summary, late decelerations have the following characteristics:

- Occur with each uterine contraction
- Start between 10 and 30 seconds after the uterine contraction
- Gradually decrease in rate and end in a return to baseline
- Are uniform in appearance
- Vary in depth according to the strength of the uterine contraction
- May or may not be accompanied by beat-to-beat variability
- Are classified as severe if the FHR decreases by more than 45 bpm

Late decelerations are probably caused by a problem in the uteroplacental interface that results in fetal hypoxia and acidosis. Any late deceleration is a reason for concern. Even small,

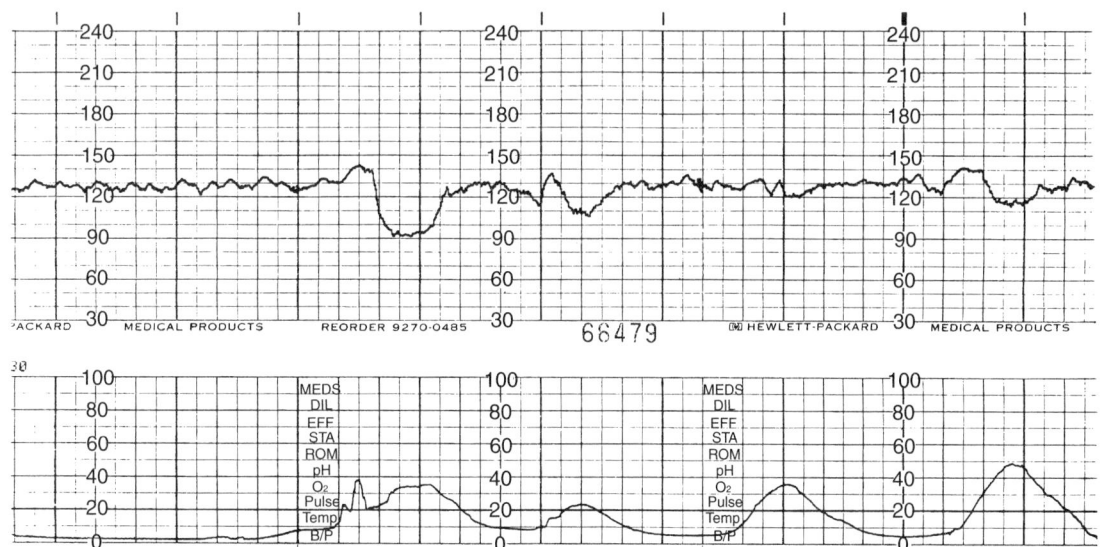

FIGURE **47-9** Variable deceleration superimposed on a baseline of good variability. Note the quick descent and recovery characteristic of variable decelerations, as well as the presence of beat-to-beat variability within the deceleration. The two peaks on the upslope of the uterine contraction are artifacts. (*From Fiedler MA. An introduction to fetal heart rate monitoring. AANA J. 1989;57:257-264.*)

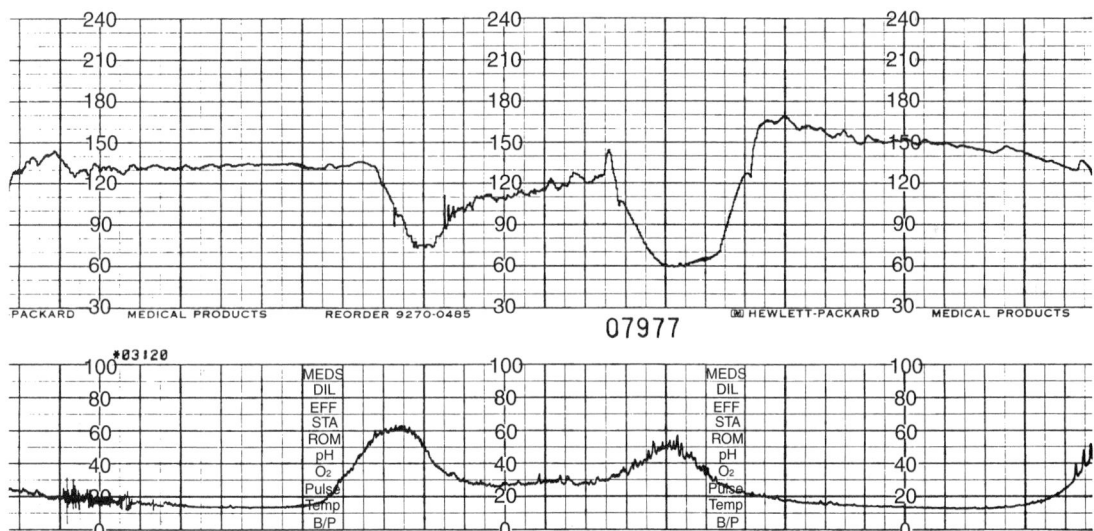

FIGURE **47-10** Two variable decelerations on a baseline of poor long-term variability. The first deceleration recovers slowly, probably indicating fetal decompensation. Before recovery is complete, a second uterine contraction occurs, prompting another variable deceleration. The second deceleration meets the criteria for severity. The FHR drops by more than 60 bpm or to 60 bpm, and the deceleration persists for longer than 60 seconds. Note that the first uterine contraction did not relax to baseline before the second one began. The irregularity of the uterine pressure graph is artifact. (*From Fiedler MA. An introduction to fetal heart rate monitoring. AANA J. 1989;57:257-264.*)

almost imperceptible late decelerations may represent severe fetal decompensation when they are combined with the absence of FHR variability. Intervention is needed to correct any cause of fetal hypoxia. If these efforts are not successful, the anesthetist should be prepared for emergency obstetric intervention for which anesthesia will be required.

Anesthetic Considerations

If the FHR tracing made during the preanesthesia assessment suggests hypoxia, caution should be used in making the decision to proceed with epidural analgesia. Careful consideration must be given to the severity of the fetal hypoxia and to the possibility that it may be worsened by anesthetic intervention.

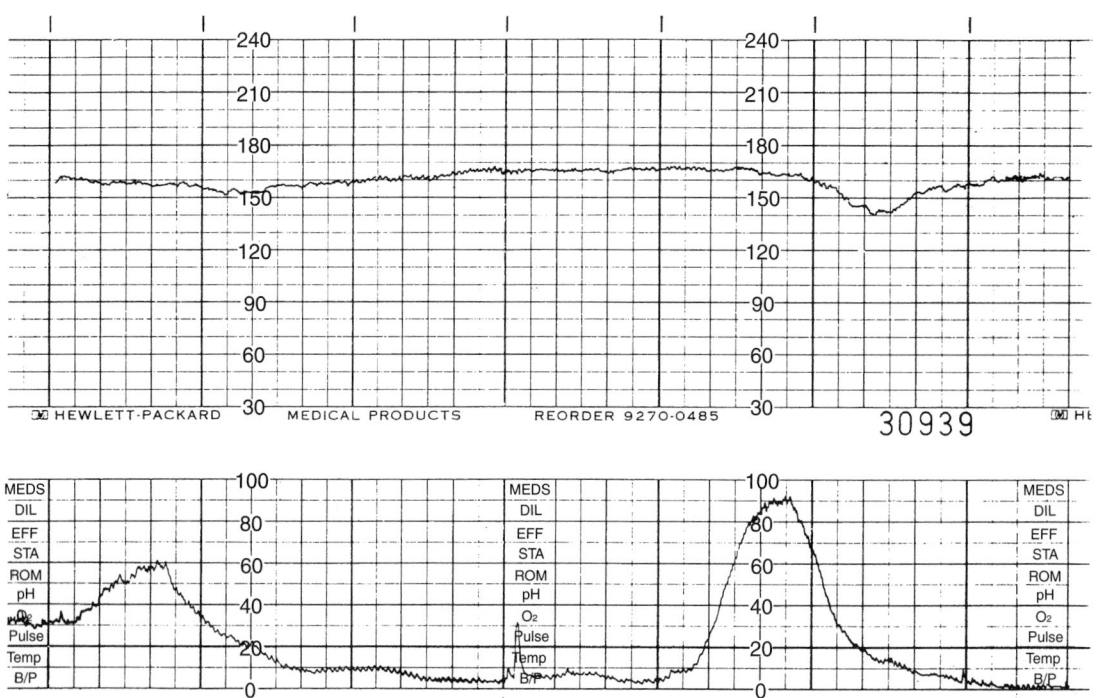

FIGURE **47-11**   Two late decelerations in a woman with a placental abruption. The first deceleration is significant, even though it is only 10 bpm in depth. Any late deceleration is a poor sign. Note the poor variability, which indicates that the fetus is already decompensated. (*From Fiedler MA. An introduction to fetal heart rate monitoring. AANA J. 1989;57:257-264.*)

Thoughtful consultation with the anesthesiologist or obstetrician involved is warranted.

Thoughtful consideration of the anesthetic technique to be used should include the following factors:

1. Cervical dilation and effacement
2. Parity
3. Adherence to normal labor pattern
4. Fetal tolerance to labor and well-being
5. Obstetrician assessment of potential for problematic delivery and/or cesarean delivery
6. Patient desire or willingness for a technique

Anesthetic Effects on the Progress of Labor

For years, controversy has surrounded whether LEA prolongs labor or increases the need for assisted or operative delivery. The number of variables involved and the diversity of both patients and study methods make this a difficult topic about which to draw valid conclusions. It is generally accepted that LEA probably prolongs latent stage labor, but if properly conducted has little effect on active labor. Even if LEA does prolong labor (and this "fact" is not universally accepted), most laboring women would agree that a slightly longer comfortable labor is preferable to a slightly shorter uncomfortable one.

An unnecessarily dense block may affect stage two labor in many women. Complete sensory anesthesia eliminates a woman's signal to push and at best results in uncoordinated and less effective pushing during the second stage of labor. At worst it removes the urge to bear down; therefore some women will not participate in the second stage of labor, leading to an increased risk of an instrumented delivery.[44] If the block is dense enough to include an effective motor block, even the most motivated, well-coached, and involved parturient may be unable to push. The goal of LEA is to provide analgesia for labor that does not remove maternal

awareness of uterine contractions and that does not cause motor block. A minimally effective concentration of local anesthetic, perhaps in combination with an opioid, decreases the likelihood that LEA will interfere with the birth process.

INTRAVENOUS ANALGESIA IN THE PARTURIENT

Although less effective, IV opioids are still used for labor pain relief when LEA is unavailable, refused, or contraindicated. From an anesthesia perspective, the use of IV opioids presents several disadvantages. The pain relief they afford is often inadequate, and fetal CNS depression, maternal respiratory depression, nausea, vomiting, and decreased lower esophageal sphincter tone may result. Nevertheless, IV analgesia can sometimes be a bridge to LEA or a necessary supplement to achieve complete anesthesia during cesarean section with the patient under regional anesthesia.

All opioids are lipid soluble and small (<500 Da), therefore, they cross rapidly to the placenta. Opioids may be administered by IV bolus or patient-controlled analgesia (PCA). The advantage of the PCA is it allows the parturient greater control over drug dosing and has resulted in greater patient satisfaction. However, in one study PCA was compared with nurse-administered boluses, and there was no difference in pain scores or maternal and fetal side effects.[45] Although many infants do not exhibit respiratory depression after delivery, naloxone must be available for the depressed infant if maternal IV opioid drugs are administered.

Opioids

Fentanyl

Fentanyl is a desirable drug for labor because of its potency and short duration. It can be detected in fetal circulation after 1 minute of IV administration, and depressant effects, including a reduction in beat-to-beat variability, may be seen.[46] Dosages for labor are either 50 to 100 mcg IV every hour[47] or 25 mcg with a lockout of 10 minutes for PCA.[48]

Butorphanol

Butorphanol is an opioid agonist-antagonist that is useful in labor. The typical dose for labor is 1 to 2 mg IV. Two milligrams of butorphanol is equal to approximately 10 mg of morphine in analgesic potency and respiratory depression, although higher doses of butorphanol do not result in equally greater respiratory depression. The half-life of butorphanol is 3 hours. Unlike morphine, butorphanol increases pulmonary artery pressure and myocardial work. Butorphanol is a better sedative than pure opioids; unlike opioids, it has a ceiling effect for respiratory depression. One study comparing butorphanol IV to fentanyl IV demonstrated improved analgesic scores with butorphanol.[47] Butorphanol has no active metabolites.

Meperidine

Meperidine crosses the placenta easily and has been recovered from the fetus within 2 minutes of IV administration. Like all opioids, it is capable of causing neonatal respiratory depression, although less so than morphine or methadone. Because of differences in pH and protein binding, the level of meperidine in the fetus is likely to be higher than the maternal blood level. Normeperidine is an active metabolite of meperidine with an elimination half-life of 30 hours. Normeperidine remains in the neonate for several days after delivery and may lead to depression of neonatal behavioral assessment scores.[49]

Historically, larger doses of meperidine were used during labor than are used now, often in combination with other depressant drugs. With contemporary doses (generally <100 mg in total), neonatal depression is less of a problem. The interval from administration of the drug to delivery of the infant is important, however. A drug-to-delivery interval of 2 to 3 hours results in the greatest neonatal depression. Both meperidine and normeperidine can be antagonized by naloxone.

Morphine

Morphine also crosses the placenta easily and has a maternal/fetal ratio of 0.96. It has been used in early labor at dosages of up to 10 mg IV to provide sedation or a period of rest for the parturient, but this practice has been associated with complications and is no longer widely used. It is notable, however, that the kinetics of morphine appear to be different in the parturient. Gerdin and co-workers showed that the elimination half-life is significantly shorter in the parturient, and the infants in this study were not depressed.[50]

Ketamine

In appropriate doses, ketamine can be used advantageously in obstetric anesthesia without emergence reactions. In fact, many women report pleasant thoughts after receiving low doses of ketamine for sedation and analgesia. The use of ketamine for labor, especially early labor, is limited by its short duration of action of 5 minutes. Certain special circumstances may warrant the use of ketamine.

Ketamine produces a centrally and peripherally mediated sympathomimetic effect. Ketamine is a good bronchodilator and therefore may be helpful when pregnancy complicates asthma or other airway diseases. Ketamine may also be used for the dose-dependent increase in blood pressure, but it is best avoided in preeclampsia patients. Although catecholamines may cause uterine vasoconstriction via an α-agonist effect, uterine arterial blood flow does not decrease after ketamine administration as it does with sympathomimetics; in fact, it may increase slightly.[51,52] Neonatal depression has not been demonstrated after maternal ketamine doses of up to 1 mg/kg. Blood pressure will increase unless the sympathomimetics are already fully activated; if so, no additional sympathomimetic effect will be caused by ketamine. The temptation to exceed 1 mg/kg should be avoided. Because it has a high lipid solubility, ketamine crosses the placenta easily; larger doses result in neonatal depression and chestwall rigidity and may cause maternal dysphoric reactions.

Low-dose ketamine often preserves airway reflexes while causing somatic analgesia or anesthesia, sedation, increased blood pressure, and a dreamlike state appropriate for the second stage of labor. All these effects are dose dependent. Low IV doses of ketamine are within the range of 10 to 25 mg, up to a total of 1 mg/kg. Onset of drug action is within 1 minute, and duration is dose dependent (usually 5 to 15 minutes at these doses).

REGIONAL ANALGESIA AND ANESTHESIA FOR LABOR AND VAGINAL DELIVERY

Regional anesthesia is a superior method of pain relief for labor and delivery. Contraindications to neuraxial anesthesia include patient refusal, severe hypovolemia, bleeding diathesis, elevated intracranial pressure, infection at the site of injection, and severe stenotic valvular heart disease. The anesthetic history and physical are performed as described previously. After consultation with the obstetrician and a full assessment of the parturient, LEA may be begun. The American College of Obstetricians and Gynecologists (ACOG) offers guidelines for assessing the obstetric patient (Box 47-3).[53]

Active labor is generally present when cervical dilation is 4 cm in the primiparous patient or 3 cm in the multiparous patient. The woman's pain perception should also be considered in the timing of LEA. Epidural analgesia can be initiated earlier if a particular woman perceives a significant amount of pain and the obstetrician agrees. It is difficult to determine the effect of the early administration of an epidural on the progress of labor. The results of such studies may easily be skewed by the fact that the more painful labor requiring an epidural is more likely to be dysfunctional to begin with.

Before epidural block is administered, the room should be inspected for the presence of resuscitation supplies, an O_2 source, and ready-to-use suction. A large-bore IV catheter should be in place.

Vascular Access

Generous venous access is recommended for any pregnant patient because of the potential for significant blood loss. Sites above the wrist are preferred because wrist movement often causes fluid flow to be position dependent. The back of the hand is an undesirable IV site; mechanical irritation of the vein by the end of the catheter can result in perforation of the vein and subcutaneous infiltration. An IV catheter should be placed in a proximal location that is least affected by the movement of the arms that occurs during vigorous pushing.

Drugs and Equipment

Emergency equipment and drugs for airway management, treatment of local anesthetic toxicity, maintenance of vital signs, and cardiopulmonary resuscitation (CPR) should always be immediately available wherever regional or general anesthesia is performed in the labor and delivery area. Carts containing

BOX 47-3

American College of Obstetricians and Gynecologists (ACOG) Guidelines for Assessment of the Obstetric Patient

Major Recommendations
The following recommendations are based on good and consistent scientific evidence (Level A):

- Regional anesthesia provides a superior level of pain relief during labor when compared with systemic drugs and therefore should be available to all women.
- Parenteral pain medications for labor pain decrease fetal heart rate variability and may limit the obstetrician-gynecologist's ability to interpret the fetal heart rate tracing.
- Consideration should be given to other drugs in the setting of diminished short or long-term heart rate variability.

The following recommendations are based on limited or inconsistent scientific evidence (Level B):

- Patients with platelet counts of 50,000 to 100,000/µL may be considered candidates for regional analgesia.
- Regional anesthesia is preferred in women with preeclampsia unless a contraindication to regional analgesia is present.
- Breastfeeding does not appear to be affected by the choice of anesthesia; therefore, the choice should be based on other considerations.

The following recommendations are based primarily on consensus and expert opinion (Level C):

- It is not necessary to routinely obtain a platelet count before administration of regional anesthesia in a pregnant patient without complications.
- Clear liquid intake may be allowed in patients in labor without complications.
- Sodium citrate should be administered promptly to neutralize gastric contents following the decision to perform a cesarean delivery.
- Identifying women with risk factors for failed intubation or other complications of anesthesia and referring them for antepartum consultation may reduce this risk.
- To avoid respiratory depression, close monitoring of the cumulative narcotic dosage given to a patient antepartum, intrapartum, and postpartum is essential.
- The decision of when to place epidural analgesia should be made individually with each patient, with other factors, such as parity, taken into consideration. Women in labor should not be required to reach 4 to 5 cm of cervical dilation before receiving analgesia.

American College of Obstetricians and Gynecologists (ACOG). Guidelines for Assessment of the Obstetric Patient. Obstetric Analgesia and Anesthesia ACOG Practice Bulletin No. 36. Washington, DC: ACOG; 2002:15

epidural anesthesia trays, local anesthetics, tape, and other supplies are wheeled from room to room for epidural insertions. These carts also contain an Ambu bag, O_2 tubing, an anesthesia mask, oral and nasal airways, endotracheal tubes, two laryngoscope handles, and Miller and Macintosh blades. Emergency drugs ready for use should include atropine, an induction drug (for terminating local anesthetic–induced seizure), succinylcholine, ephedrine, epinephrine, calcium chloride (for treating magnesium sulfate overdose), and sodium bicarbonate. A "crash cart" with a defibrillator must be available. Automatic blood pressure machines are required in each labor and delivery room, and pulse oximetry should be readily available. Operating rooms in the labor and delivery suite should be equipped exactly as main operating rooms and include up-to-date anesthesia machines, anesthesia gas analysis, pulse oximetry, and O_2 concentration monitoring. Although many institutions require that emergency drugs be discarded and replaced at 24-hour intervals because of infection control concerns, many emergency drugs (thiopental, succinylcholine, ephedrine, atropine, lidocaine, and oxytocin) have been shown to remain sterile for up to 8 days in the obstetric anesthesia setting.[54] However, other reasons exist for replacement of emergency drugs. The concentration of atropine in a plastic syringe has been shown to decrease by 44% over 24 hours because of drug adsorption to the inner surface of the syringe.[55]

Personnel

In addition to proper drugs and equipment, knowledgeable assistants are essential for the safe insertion of an epidural catheter. A competent obstetric nurse who is capable of assisting with fetal heart rate monitoring is mandatory. Additionally, it is impossible to place an epidural catheter with strict sterile technique and at the same time steady a sitting parturient. If the patient becomes faint or apneic or has a seizure, a minimum of two professionals are needed to manage the situation. An additional anesthetist (either a physician or a certified registered nurse anesthetist) who is available to respond quickly to help with an emergency is also desirable.

Local Anesthetics

For years, the mainstay of LEA has been bupivacaine. Bupivacaine is not, however, the ideal obstetric local anesthetic. It tends to produce motor block, which is bothersome to many parturients, and can at times interfere with or prolong the second stage of labor. When excessive systemic absorption or intravascular injection occurs, bupivacaine also produces potent cardiac toxicity, which is worsened in pregnant women because of the increased level of progesterone. Although the incidence of cardiac toxicity is relatively low, given the risk of morbidity and mortality when it does occur in the parturient, consideration should be given to using a less cardiotoxic local anesthetic for LEA.

Ropivacaine is a pure S-isomer, rather than a racemic mixture of both isomers as is bupivacaine. The elimination half-life of ropivacaine in pregnant women is 5.2 hours, compared with 10.9 hours for bupivacaine.[56] This reduced elimination half-life makes it less likely that ropivacaine will accumulate to toxic levels over the course of a long labor epidural infusion. Ropivacaine produces approximately one third less motor block[57] and has a reduced potential to produce CNS and cardiac toxicity than does bupivacaine. A ropivacaine motor block develops more slowly, goes away more quickly, and is approximately one third less dense than that produced by bupivacaine.[57-60]

Only slightly less potent than bupivacaine, ropivacaine is markedly less toxic,[61,62] and ropivacaine toxicity regresses more quickly once administration of the drug is terminated.[62] Whereas bupivacaine cardiac toxicity is enhanced in the parturient, that of ropivacaine is not.[63,64] Accidental intravascular injection of as little as 15 mL of 0.5% or 6.6 mL of 0.75% bupivacaine has resulted in maternal death,[65] whereas up to 20 mL of intravascular ropivacaine has resulted only in tinnitus.[66]

Epidural Insertion

Epidural insertion should be preceded by skin surface disinfection using a newly opened container of povidone-iodine (single-use container). Solution from single-use containers provides more effective skin disinfection than that from previously opened containers. Of cultures taken after two applications of povidone-iodine from previously opened containers, 40% grew bacterial colonies, fungal colonies, or both, and 70% of those grew multiple colonies. Only 5% of cultures taken after skin surface disinfection with solution from previously unopened containers grew any colonies at all, and when they did, they grew only one colony each. Although intuitively it would seem as though a container of povidone iodine should "self-sterilize," preventing growth of infectious organisms, this is not the case. Of cultures taken from the lid of previously opened povidone-iodine bottles, 40% had a positive result, but there was no growth from any unopened container.[67]

Baseline blood pressure should be measured, and blood pressure should be checked at regular intervals once the epidural anesthetic is begun. If the parturient is having difficulty cooperating because of her perception of pain, administration of 50 to 100 mcg of IV fentanyl (limit 1 mcg/kg) often provides significant relief while the epidural anesthetic is being administered. This dose has been shown to present little risk to the neonate,[68] especially when the fentanyl is given more than 2 hours before delivery. Although of shorter duration than meperidine, fentanyl results in fewer maternal side effects.[40,69]

Often the sitting position is easiest for the patient to maintain and usually offers the anesthetist the maximum interspace width. A knowledgeable obstetric nurse who helps to steady the parturient in the proper position while offering comfort is a great asset. If the patient is having a difficult time holding still during contractions, then placing her in the lateral position may help limit motion. A comforting attitude, patience, understanding, and complete explanation of what the anesthetist is doing often help minimize the parturient's fears.

When placing the epidural catheter, the anesthetist should take into consideration stage of the labor and delivery. If the parturient is in the early stages of labor, several hours of labor analgesia will be necessary. In this case, introducing the catheter as high as safely possible (usually at the L2-3 interspace) and inserting it in a cephalad direction will be most likely to result in an optimal final catheter tip position of L1-2. From this position, as little as 6 mL of local anesthetic volume may provide a truly segmental epidural block from T10 to L4, covering the nerves carrying pain from cervical dilation and uterine contractions (Figure 47-12). If the catheter is inserted at a point lower than L2-3, a greater volume of local anesthetic will be necessary to achieve a block up to the T10 dermatome. For optimal performance, multiple side-hole catheters (closed end) should be inserted 5 cm into the epidural space,[70] and single end-hole catheters should be inserted 2 to 4 cm. Once inserted part of the way, the epidural catheter should not be pulled back through the needle or it may shear off in the patient.

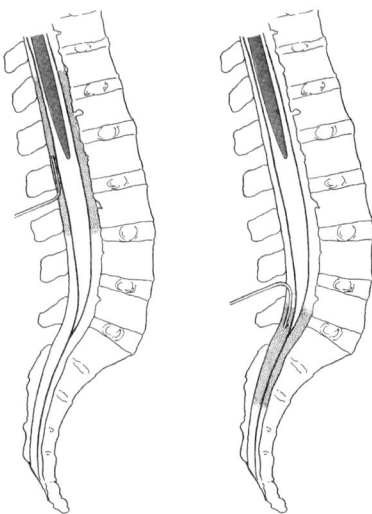

FIGURE **47-12** Effect of epidural catheter position and direction on the spread of local anesthetic.

Rather, the needle and catheter should be withdrawn together and another attempt made.

In the circumstance in which the epidural block is to be performed late in labor, and analgesia is desired mainly for perineal pain caused by stretching and episiotomy, placing the catheter as low as possible (generally at L4-5) and directing it caudad results in a greater chance that a sacral block will be achieved. A sacral block can sometimes be difficult to achieve with epidural anesthesia and may require large volumes of local anesthetic. If epidural anesthesia has been established early in labor and a local anesthetic has been infusing for several hours, a sacral block is usually achieved before stage two (delivery of the fetus), when sacral analgesia is needed.

It has long been observed that the failure rate of epidural anesthetics is greater in the obese patient. It has been shown that the distance from the skin to the epidural space varies with changes in body position and more so in the obese. The greatest increase in the distance from the skin to the epidural space is associated with a change from the sitting, flexed position to lying with the legs straight out. Because epidural catheters are usually secured to the back while the parturient is sitting up in a flexed position, when the parturient lies back down and the distance from the skin to the epidural space increases, the catheter can actually be pulled out of the epidural space. The average increase in skin-to-epidural-space distance in those with a body mass index (BMI; equal to weight in kilograms divided by height in meters squared) between 25 and 30 is 0.75 cm, with a range of up to 2.72 cm. The average increase in distance in those with a BMI greater than 30 is 1.04 cm, with a range of up to 4.28 cm.[71] Withdrawing the epidural catheter a centimeter or more could certainly result in one or more of its openings exiting the epidural space. This problem can be avoided by having the patient lie on her side and straighten her legs before the epidural catheter is secured to the back, thereby allowing the catheter to be pulled in a bit as the distance to the epidural space increases. In obese patients it is possible to visualize the epidural catheter being "sucked in" during this position change.

The type of epidural catheter used has an influence on the effectiveness of the block. The incidence of unilateral or spotty epidural blocks is highest when a single-end hole catheter is used.

Fewer unsatisfactory blocks occur when a closed-end catheter with several side holes is used.[72-74]

Test Doses

The test dose is designed to reveal subarachnoid or intravascular injection of local anesthetic without producing systemic toxicity or widespread subarachnoid block. The key is to think of the test dose as the amount of drug in milligrams required to produce a detectable effect either spinally or systemically. Unlike spread of local anesthetic within the epidural space, volume has little to do with the effectiveness of a test dose. It is generally agreed that 30 mg of lidocaine is an effective test dose for subarachnoid injection. Alternatively, 10 mg of bupivacaine has been shown to produce a noticeable increase in foot temperature and motor block at the ankle 4 minutes after subarachnoid but not epidural injection.[75] Disagreement exists regarding how best to test for intravascular injection. The most widely accepted test dose involves the administration of 15 mcg of epinephrine, which has been shown to reliably increase HR in nonpregnant patients when injected intravascularly. However, this test dose is not universally accepted for obstetric anesthesia. In the laboring parturient, increases in HR are a less specific indicator because of the changes in HR that occur during uterine contractions. Furthermore, concern exists that epinephrine may cause significant uterine artery constriction in a few patients,[76,77] resulting in a decrease in fetal O_2 delivery.

Given the limitations and occasional hazards of the epinephrine test dose, in laboring patients an alternative method of detecting intravascular or subarachnoid placement would be desirable. Two nonpharmacologic methods have been described. Both rely on the detection of blood or cerebrospinal fluid (CSF) in the epidural catheter to indicate a positive test result.[78,79] Observing for blood or CSF while aspirating the epidural catheter had a 0% false-positive rate and a 0.2% false-negative rate in over 1000 women in whom 60 intravascular or subarachnoid catheter placements were performed.[79] Ideally, the administration of every dose should be observed as a test dose, with the anesthetist checking for signs of intravascular and subarachnoid injection with each dose administered. One of the most important factors in the safe administration of epidural analgesics is the physical presence of an observant anesthetist during administration and for a period of time after its completion.

Minor CNS local-anesthetic side effects are easily observed when they occur. With the exception of those related to bupivacaine, they carry little risk as long as administration is stopped when they become evident. Given this, an alternative test for intravascular injection is the slow administration of lidocaine or 2-chloroprocaine while the patient is observed for CNS side effects. For this technique to be successful, one must pay close attention and constantly stay in verbal communication with the patient. For example, CNS changes after the IV administration of 60 mg of 2-chloroprocaine often include ringing in the ears, auditory changes, or changes in mental functioning. Because of the rapid intravascular metabolism of 2-chloroprocaine, these changes are very transient and may be missed if the anesthetist is not observant. The transient nature of the changes is an advantage, however, as any problem that develops resolves quickly.

Some clinicians differentiate between the small doses of local anesthetic used for a laboring epidural and the larger doses given for cesarean delivery. The incidence of inadvertent dural puncture in pregnant women is rare; the reported rate is 0.6%-1.6%. It is believed that by using multiorifice catheters and giving small doses of local anesthetic for sensory analgesia during labor, an epinephrine test dose is unjustified. The risk of compromise in uteroplacental blood flow by epinephrine injection outweighs the benefits. Observation for failure to produce sensory analgesia is sufficient. When administering larger doses such as those given for an epidural for cesarean delivery, however, an epinephrine test dose is reasonable.[78]

Administration of the Epidural Anesthetic

The spread of analgesia when an epidural catheter is placed is primarily determined by the volume of local anesthetic solution injected. It is important to note that this is different from a subarachnoid block, in which the dose in milligrams, the baricity of the local anesthetic, and the patient's position are the chief determinants of the extent of the anesthesia. In a normal, young, healthy, term parturient, an average of approximately 1 mL of local anesthetic is required for each dermatomal level of local anesthetic spread. This is an average volume per segment. Because the lumbar epidural space is larger than, for example, the thoracic epidural space, a larger volume of local anesthetic is required for the spread of analgesia across one level in the lumbar epidural space than in the thoracic epidural space. Therefore, if the catheter is placed at L2, an average of 16 mL is required for spread up to T6 and down to S4.

Adequate analgesia must be balanced against loss of the sensation of labor, which is not desirable during the second stage, and motor block, which is bothersome to the mother during labor and prevents expulsive efforts during delivery. There are many ways to approach epidural administration. The amount and concentration of the drug for a laboring epidural vary from one anesthesia provider to another, and from one institution to another, so the following is only a recommendation.

After the epidural catheter has been inserted and a test dose performed, 6 to 12 mL of either 0.1% to 0.2% ropivacaine or 0.125% to 0.25% bupivacaine may be injected incrementally through the catheter. Slow injection results in markedly lower peak plasma local anesthetic concentrations than rapid injection.[80] Alternatively, the bolus feature of an epidural pump can be used to inject the initial bolus slowly over several minutes, with monitoring performed by the anesthetist. The addition of small amounts of fentanyl to the initial local anesthetic dose speeds the onset, intensifies the analgesia provided, and allows the anesthetist to decrease the concentration of local anesthetic without reducing pain relief. Up to 100 mcg of fentanyl can be included in the epidural bolus dose without producing adverse fetal or neonatal effects,[81] but a smaller dose is frequently effective.

If a patient admitted for delivery is very early in labor and perceiving a great deal of pain, the anesthetist might consider placing an epidural catheter and initially using plain narcotic until the labor becomes more active. In this situation, the patient should receive 100 mcg of fentanyl. This dose commonly results in approximately 1 hour of good analgesia that is superior to IV opioids. Once active labor is present, the local anesthetic may be given in the usual fashion. If an additional dosage of opioid is necessary in the interim, 50 to 75 mcg of fentanyl can be used at hourly intervals without danger of depressing a healthy fetus.

Although the small amount of epinephrine present in an IV test dose should be safe for a healthy fetus, the larger amounts present in the volume of local anesthetic used to maintain LEA carry some risk of umbilical artery constriction in some parturients.[82] For this reason, routine use of epinephrine-containing solutions is not recommended, especially in the preeclamptic patient.

To avoid aortocaval syndrome, after epidural analgesia has been instituted, the patient should be not be allowed to lie on her back. A hip roll or wedge is necessary to maintain left (or right) uterine displacement. The anesthetist should remain aware of cervical dilation and the progress of labor after the epidural catheter has been placed. Communication with obstetric personnel is important to prevent use of a drug, dose, or concentration of local anesthetic that is inappropriate for the patient's circumstances. For example, readministration of 0.5% bupivacaine at the beginning of the second stage of labor is likely to result in a motor block that causes the patient to be unable to push or sense contractions.

Maintaining Epidural Analgesia for Labor and Delivery

Although it is possible to maintain LEA with intermittent bolus administration, less local anesthetic is administered and more effective analgesia achieved when analgesia is maintained with a continuous epidural infusion. Historically the most commonly chosen local anesthetic for epidural infusion has been bupivacaine, but ropivacaine produces less motor block and carries a lesser risk of life-threatening cardiotoxicity. During labor, the minimal effective concentration of local anesthetic should be used so that the risk of motor block is minimized. Ropivacaine or bupivacaine in concentrations of 0.0625% to 0.2% is commonly used. The lower concentration may be effective in mild to moderate labors as long as adequate spread is achieved. Maintaining an adequate sensory level usually necessitates an infusion rate of 10 to 15 mL/hr. In the majority of women, this dilute concentration is associated with minimal motor block, although block will become denser as the infusion is maintained. A higher concentration may be needed as labor intensifies or in women who experience greater pain.

The addition of fentanyl to the local anesthetic speeds the onset, increases the density, and prolongs the duration of analgesia. In an epidural infusion, this maximizes the pain relief while minimizing the concentration of local anesthetic needed. An epidural maintenance infusion of 0.1% or 0.15% ropivacaine or bupivacaine combined with 1 or 2 mcg/mL of fentanyl at a rate of 10 to 15 mL/hr produces better pain relief than higher concentrations of local anesthetic alone. However, even these low concentrations can result in motor block when they are infused for many hours. If the labor is prolonged, it may be necessary to decrease the concentration of local anesthetic over time.

If the onset of the second stage of labor occurs during a stable labor epidural block, and if the patient has good motor function, the block may be maintained while the patient pushes. The ideal block provides analgesia for labor pain, dense analgesia of the perineum for delivery, and little motor block. If motor block hinders pushing or if sensory block prevents the parturient from sensing contractions and therefore knowing when to push, the epidural infusion may be turned off or changed to a more dilute solution. If necessary, the block can be supplemented when the baby is beginning to crown or when perineal analgesia is needed. At that time perineal anesthesia, if lacking, can usually be achieved with the injection of 10 mL of 1.5% lidocaine with epinephrine, 2% 2-chloroprocaine, or 0.25% bupivacaine. If a more dense analgesia is needed, the addition of up to 100 mcg of fentanyl will produce very dense analgesia. If anesthesia is needed for a mid- or high-forceps delivery and the obstetrician does not need the parturient to push, the concentrations of

bupivacaine, lidocaine, and 2-chloroprocaine are increased to 0.5%, 2%, and 3%, respectively, with or without fentanyl added.

Patient-Controlled Epidural Analgesia

Continuous infusion of local anesthetic solution into the epidural space is probably the most common method of maintaining analgesia during the first stage of labor. Several investigations of the efficacy of patient-controlled epidural analgesia (PCEA) have been conducted. PCEA may afford some advantages during labor, because it has been associated with a reduced need for top-up doses,[83,84] a high degree of patient satisfaction,[83-86] and a reduction in total doses of bupivacaine required.[83,86]

Intrathecal Anesthesia and Analgesia

A single-shot spinal is not often an appropriate anesthetic choice for the laboring patient because of the disadvantage of the finite duration. For this reason, this technique is generally reserved for multiparous patients in stage two. An opioid (see regional opioid section) combined with a small amount of local anesthesia (hyperbaric bupivacaine 2.5mg) is administered for perineal anesthesia.

A continuous spinal is rarely used for labor and delivery; it is only used for a patient with a difficult anatomic variation or morbid obesity. Microcatheters for this purpose are no longer available because of the incidence of cauda equina syndrome.[87] However, continuous spinal catheters can be performed with epidural catheters. The morbidly obese parturient is at greater risk of cesarean delivery and at greater risk of failed regional technique.[88] The need for replacement of the epidural catheter is also greater in the morbidly obese parturient. Therefore, a continuous spinal catheter may be indicated in the morbidly obese parturient due to the difficulty of the regional technique and the increased morbidity and mortality of general anesthesia; 0.5 to 1.5 mL of 0.25% bupivacaine is used for intermittent boluses. The level of the block must be carefully monitored, and it is highly recommended that this catheter be labeled as a spinal catheter.

Combined Technique

A combined technique has become a popular technique that has the advantage of the speed of onset of an intrathecal administration and the flexibility of an epidural catheter. The epidural needle is placed first to identify the epidural space. The spinal needle is then introduced through the epidural needle and opioid, and a small amount of local anesthetic is introduced. The spinal is then withdrawn and an epidural catheter is placed.

The combined technique is most useful in very early labor or in stage two. In early labor the administration of an intrathecal opioid is often administered without local anesthetic. After the patient begins to complain of pain, the epidural is then dosed and an infusion is started.

In stage two of labor, the intrathecal is dosed with opioid and local anesthetic and provides excellent anesthesia for the perineal area. The epidural catheter is used if the stage is prolonged or if a cesarean delivery is necessary.

Regional Opioids

One of the chief advantages of combining local anesthetics and opioids in obstetric pain relief is that the use of opioids allows the concentration of local anesthetic to be decreased; this results in less motor blockade but equal relief. The onset of relief is also faster. Although opioids have centrally mediated effects, several areas in the spinal cord, including the substantia gelatinosa within the dorsal horn, are known to possess opioid receptors. These receptors can be stimulated by the application of opioids by the subarachnoid or epidural routes. Epidurally administered opioids are believed to be absorbed into the CSF, and ultimately the spinal cord, to exert their action on spinal opioid receptors.

Fentanyl

When used in combination with local anesthetics, fentanyl in epidural doses of 50 to 100 mcg and subarachnoid doses of 10 to 25 mcg produces good to excellent analgesia in 5 to 15 minutes. Administration of these doses, repeated as often as every 90 minutes in women in labor, has been shown not to affect Apgar scores, umbilical cord blood analysis, or neurobehavioral test results for up to 24 hours after delivery.[89-91] Fentanyl 100 mcg in the epidural space has been shown to be undetectable in breast milk.[92] Much higher doses of opioids are needed to provide labor analgesia if opioids are given alone, and even these higher doses are not entirely effective during the second stage of labor. When analgesia from fentanyl administration is at its peak, serum fentanyl levels are lower than those known to produce equivalent analgesia after IV administration. In fact, most women have undetectable plasma fentanyl levels after receiving 100 mcg of epidural fentanyl.[93]

The duration of action of fentanyl is 3 to 4 hours. Because fentanyl is so much more lipid soluble than morphine, it is absorbed into neural tissue faster, therefore it has a faster onset and shorter duration of action than morphine. As a result the cephalad migration of fentanyl is much less than that of morphine; therefore fentanyl is associated with a significantly lower incidence of CNS side effects. This is probably why respiratory depression has rarely been reported after subarachnoid or epidural administration of fentanyl. In fact, subarachnoid doses of fentanyl up to 0.75 mcg/kg (much higher than the absolute limit of 25 mcg observed by most clinicians) result in a decrease in respiratory rate without undue respiratory depression.[94] An exceptionally high block with fentanyl, however, can result in respiratory depression. A young parturient who received 100 mcg of fentanyl and 0.5% bupivacaine in the epidural space for a cesarean section experienced a C4 block; this patient became apneic 100 minutes after the injection of the fentanyl. Spontaneous respirations resumed after the IV administration of naloxone.[95]

For continuous LEA, fentanyl concentrations up to 2.5 mcg/mL of local anesthetic can be used without adversely affecting neonatal respiration or neurobehavioral scores.[96] Bupivacaine (up to 0.125%) or ropivacaine (up to 0.2%) with 1 to 2 mcg/mL of fentanyl is a widely used combination.[97-100]

Sufentanil

Sufentanil is highly lipid soluble, has a high receptor affinity, and is very potent. When injected into the epidural space, 98% of the dose is absorbed either by epidural fat or into epidural veins. Little sufentanil reaches the CSF. As a result, relatively higher plasma levels of sufentanil are achieved compared with those of fentanyl after the epidural injection of equipotent doses. When sufentanil is injected directly into the subarachnoid space, plasma levels of the drug are much lower than its CSF levels. One advantage of sufentanil is that it has a shorter plasma half-life than fentanyl; therefore, accumulation should be even less likely to occur when it is used instead of fentanyl.

Sufentanil, 50 mcg, administered in the epidural space in combination with bupivacaine has been shown to decrease the slope of the CO_2 response curve by an average of approximately 40% (by <30% in patients who received 30 mcg). In a similar population of post–cesarean section women who received conventional subcutaneous morphine analgesia, the average decrease in the slope of the CO_2 response curve was 50%.[101,102]

Morphine

Morphine can be used in epidural doses of up to 5 mg to provide analgesia for 24 hours or longer. Subarachnoid administration of morphine, in doses of 0.1 to 1 mg, also may be used. With both epidural and subarachnoid blocks, a trend toward the use of lower doses is occurring in an effort to limit side effects. Morphine is lipid insoluble; therefore its onset of action after an epidural dose (approximately 1 hour) is longer than that of other opioids. Fentanyl has been added to the subarachnoid morphine infusion in healthy parturients in an effort to speed the onset of analgesia. Probably because of its limited lipid solubility, morphine continues to move cephalad long after injection into the subarachnoid or epidural space. It is thought that this mechanism accounts for respiratory depression, which can begin 12 hours or longer after epidural or subarachnoid morphine administration. Because of the long duration of action and absence of motor effects, epidural morphine is an excellent postoperative analgesic. Only preservative-free preparations should be used.

Many patients do not require any additional pain relief within the first 24 hours; the average duration of pain relief is 14 hours. The most common side effects are pruritus (42%), followed by vomiting (18%) and nausea (13%).[103] All the patients should have monitoring for respiratory depression, especially the obese and those with a history of airway obstruction during sleep.

Side Effects of Regional Opioids

Side effects of epidural and subarachnoid opioid administration include respiratory depression, itching, urinary retention, nausea, and vomiting. These effects occur more commonly when the opioid is given by the subarachnoid than by the epidural route. IV doses of an opioid antagonist (naloxone) or agonist-antagonist (nalbuphine) are effective at reducing or eliminating the undesirable effects without antagonizing the analgesia and often are more effective against pruritus than an antihistamine.

The incidence and severity of pruritus after epidural morphine administration are greater in patients who have had epinephrine in their local anesthetic doses.[104] As little as 15 mcg of epinephrine in a test dose results in an increase in itching, even if the morphine is not given for up to 65 minutes after the epidural administration of epinephrine. Of interest, in some studies the incidence of shivering in parturients was decreased after administration of epidural fentanyl[105] or sufentanil,[106] but other investigations do not arrive at this conclusion.[107] As with other drugs, anaphylaxis is a rare risk of fentanyl administration. At least two cases of fentanyl-related anaphylaxis have been reported.

Hypotension

The accepted cause of hypotension during regional anesthesia in obstetric patients has long been the fact that the block results in a sympathectomy that causes peripheral venous pooling, a reduction in venous return to the heart, reduced preload, reduced SV, and therefore reduced cardiac output and a fall in blood pressure. From this it followed that simply infusing additional volume would restore venous return to the heart and preserve cardiac output, thereby preventing hypotension. The most common measure undertaken to prevent maternal hypotension after epidural block has therefore been the infusion of IV fluid in an attempt to replace volume thought to pool because of sympatholytic-induced vasodilation.

Numerous studies have reported the incidences and magnitude of hypotension after IV infusion of various solution types, volumes, and methods of administration. No study has identified a volume of intravascular fluid that comes close to eliminating hypotension in pregnant women undergoing regional anesthesia. Volume preload regimens have inconsistent efficacy and do not eliminate maternal hypotension.[108,109]

Crystalloid IV preloads with solutions such as lactated Ringer's of up to 30 mL/kg are commonly associated with an incidence of maternal hypotension of approximately 50%, often not statistically different from the incidence in controls who receive no preload at all.[110,111] One reason crystalloid preloads may be ineffective is that they remain in the circulation for a short period of time. Only 28% of 1.5 L of lactated Ringer's solution infused over 30 minutes remains in the maternal circulation at the end of the 30-minute infusion period.[112] Preloading with colloid solutions to prevent epidural anesthetic–induced hypotension nets a modest improvement in prevention of hypotension. Studies comparing preloads with hetastarch versus crystalloid solution often do show a significant difference between groups, but the incidence of hypotension remains high.[113] In addition, a study in which 1 L of 6% hetastarch was administered *in addition to* crystalloid solution as an IV preload still yielded 17% hypotension.[112] Clinically, colloid IV preloads are uncommonly used. They do not eliminate hypotension, and practitioners are often hesitant to use them because of their greater cost, and the small but important chance of anaphylaxis. In clinical practice, crystalloid solutions are used almost exclusively. The overall incidence of maternal hypotension is probably at least 38%, given the infrequent use of colloids.

A mechanism exists to suggest that aggressive crystalloid preloading may contribute to maternal hypotension during subarachnoid or epidural block. Administering volume in excess of that needed to replace the deficit acquired during an overnight fast may play a role in maternal hypotension in the presence of subarachnoid or epidural block. The level of block necessary for effective anesthesia for cesarean section attenuates the ability of the sympathetic nervous system and the renin-angiotensin system to maintain normotension. The vasopressin system remains to support blood pressure. Vasopressin and antidiuretic hormone (ADH) are the same hormones, called by different names according to the context of the discussion. On the whole, the body is more responsive to the antidiuretic role of ADH than it is to the vasoconstrictive role of vasopressin, with small reductions in plasma colloid osmotic pressure resulting in strong inhibition of ADH release. Vasopressin release in response to loss of intravascular volume, on the other hand, requires a fairly strong stimulus. Animal studies[114] have shown that infusion of 10 mL/kg of dextran 40 in lactated Ringer's solution results in a 30% decrease in circulating vasopressin during mock operation, as opposed to a 250% increase during mock operation without dextran infusion. Three healthy nonpregnant women had vasopressin levels assayed before and after ingestion of 20 mL of water per kilogram.[19] Two hours after water ingestion, vasopressin had decreased to immeasurable levels. Therefore, it is possible that the volumes of crystalloid IV preload commonly used in an effort to prevent maternal hypotension may actually inhibit the body's efforts to support blood pressure by delaying or reducing the magnitude of the vasopressin response.

Prevention and Treatment of Maternal Hypotension. Hypotension is probably the most frequent complication in obstetric anesthesia. It can cause discomfort for the mother and result in dangerous decreases in fetal oxygenation by decreasing

uteroplacental blood flow. Intervillous blood flow is dependent on maternal MAP.[115] Furthermore, in the presence of reasonable maternal arterial partial pressure of oxygen (PaO$_2$), fetal oxygenation is dependent on intervillous blood flow and maternal MAP. Maternal hypotension of sufficient magnitude and duration results in fetal hypoxia, which if allowed to progress results in fetal academia and death.[116-118] In a healthy pregnant woman, the critical duration of hypotension is probably greater than 2 minutes.[117] For many years, the accepted critical magnitude of hypotension is a systolic blood pressure less than 100 mm Hg.[119] Because of pregnancy-related changes in vascular tone and cardiovascular dynamics, the parturient is more dependent on vascular tone for maintenance of blood pressure than a nonpregnant woman. In pregnant women receiving either subarachnoid or epidural block for cesarean section, which involves wide areas of chemical sympathectomy, hypotension is more likely than in nonpregnant patients who have received the same block.[120]

Ephedrine. Ephedrine is a synthetic, nonselective, noncatecholamine sympathomimetic drug. Doses of 5 to 25 mg intravenously are used to treat acute decreases in blood pressure. The duration of ephedrine's cardiovascular effects varies with the dose given. The effect of a 5- or 10-mg IV dose usually persists for 5 minutes. Tachyphylaxis can occur with repeated administration of small doses, resulting in a noticeably reduced clinical effect after subsequent dosing. Ephedrine is metabolized in the liver, and up to 40% is excreted unchanged by the kidneys. It has an elimination half-life of 3 hours.

Ephedrine causes direct β stimulation and indirect α stimulation through the release of endogenous norepinephrine. It has been the favorite vasoactive agent in obstetric anesthesia because it was thought to affect uterine artery blood flow less than other vasoactive drugs in pregnant ewes.[121] However, more recent evidence has shown that this is not entirely true in humans, and in fact, there is a greater incidence of fetal acidosis in parturients treated with ephedrine than compared with phenylephrine.[122]

Phenylephrine. Based on animal studies, α-agonists were previously thought to cause fetal acidosis, but phenylephrine has been shown to be safe for the treatment of maternal hypotension during regional anesthesia.[122] Neonatal blood gas values and Apgar scores remain within normal limits in all healthy subjects after the administration of 80-mcg[123] or 100-mcg[102] bolus doses of phenylephrine. Other investigators have also found reassuring results with the use of phenylephrine in healthy parturients.[122-125] The vasopressor choice should now be based on the heart rate. Phenylephrine is now the drug of choice for maternal hypotension and often used with ephedrine for heart rate management.

Cesarean section is indicated for many reasons, such as labor classified as failure to progress, fetal bradycardia or nonreassuring fetal heart tones, and malpresentation of fetus. The degree of urgency of the cesarean section is not always the same, so the anesthetist must communicate with the obstetrician before deciding the anesthesia technique. When possible, regional techniques are desirable because of the increased morbidity and mortality of general anesthesia in this population. Regional techniques also offer the ability for the parturient to participate in the cesarean birth process.

SURGICAL CONSIDERATIONS AND COMPLICATIONS FOR OBSTETRIC PATIENTS

Aspiration Risk

From an anesthetic point of view, all obstetric patients have a full stomach. Routine measures to prevent aspiration pneumonitis in the obstetric patient are warranted. Unless contraindicated, a clear oral antacid, IV H$_2$ blocker, and IV metoclopramide are recommended for obstetric patients undergoing surgical procedures. Thirty milliliters of sodium citrate (Bicitra) effectively raises the pH of gastric contents for up to 1 hour and is best administered near the time of the induction of anesthesia. The very sour taste of Bicitra is unpleasant, and it is better tolerated when gulped or given over crushed ice. Bicitra is most effective when thoroughly mixed with gastric contents. The use of particulate antacids is best avoided, because animal studies have shown that they cause pulmonary damage when aspirated.

Ranitidine inhibits gastric acid secretion, thereby reducing future gastric volume. It can be given orally (150 or 300 mg) or intravenously (50 mg IV piggyback). A single oral or IV dose of ranitidine has been shown not to affect uterine contractions or neonatal neurobehavioral scores.[126] Unlike cimetidine, ranitidine does not inhibit the elimination of amide local anesthetics.[127] Metoclopramide (10 mg intravenously) increases gastric motility and increases sphincter tone between the esophagus and the stomach but should be administered slowly so that agitation and psychosis are avoided.[128] Metoclopramide inhibits the enzyme pseudocholinesterase (PCHE) and to a lesser degree acetylcholinesterase. By itself, this effect is unlikely to prolong the duration of succinylcholine to a clinically significant degree, but it does add to the depression of PCHE activity normally present at term pregnancy. Prolongation of neuromuscular block because of preeclampsia or magnesium administration could be intensified.

Positioning

During positioning of the parturient on the operative table, left uterine displacement should be provided as soon as possible. The table should be rolled to the left or a wedge placed under the right hip of the patient in order to shift the uterus off the inferior vena cava and abdominal aorta, thereby preserving fetal oxygenation. Fetuses delivered of mothers with left uterine displacement have a lower incidence of CNS depression and acidosis than those delivered of mothers in the supine position.[129]

Surgical Blood Loss

Blood loss during cesarean section is usually less when regional anesthesia is used than when general anesthesia is used. On average, approximately 500 mL of blood is lost during cesarean section with regional anesthesia and approximately 700 mL with general anesthesia. Despite this average, the range of blood loss is great—in one study, from 164 to 1438 mL.[130] Many factors affect the volume of blood lost during cesarean section, including surgical time, surgical technique, blood pressure, fetal lie, fetal size, placental implantation, maternal coagulation status, and the ability of the uterus to contract after the placenta has been delivered. Statistically determined risk factors for excessive bleeding during cesarean section (with odds ratios) include general anesthesia (2.94), amnionitis (2.69), preeclampsia (2.18), protracted active phase of labor (2.4), second-stage arrest (1.9), and Hispanic ethnicity (1.82).[131]

General Anesthesia

Regional anesthesia is generally preferred for cesarean section. Properly conducted regional anesthesia may yield less neonatal depression (at least in the short term), and the mother is usually able to enjoy experiencing her newborn sooner.[132-135] Also, surgical blood loss is less when regional anesthesia rather than general anesthesia is used. A general anesthetic is indicated for cesarean section when the anesthetist is not knowledgeable in regional anesthetic techniques, when regional anesthesia is contraindicated, when the patient refuses regional anesthesia, or when anesthesia must be induced emergently.

Airway Management

When general anesthesia is chosen, use of a cuffed endotracheal tube is indicated, and rapid-sequence induction should be performed unless it is contraindicated. An airway evaluation is an important part of the preparation for anesthesia in any patient and even more so in the parturient. Airway problems tend to occur more frequently in obstetric patients than in other healthy patients; failure to intubate has been reported to occur as frequently as 1 in 250 obstetric patients.[136] This is true at least in part because of the soft-tissue edema often present in the hypopharynx. Breast enlargement and cephalad displacement of the thorax often make maneuvering the laryngoscope into the mouth difficult. Placement of a rolled towel lengthwise along the thoracic spine or widthwise under the shoulders helps to elevate the chest off the operating table. This makes it possible to flex the neck at the shoulders and extend the neck at the head more optimally, facilitating insertion of the laryngoscope blade and improving visualization of the glottis. Some anesthetists find short-handled laryngoscopes easier to use in these patients. Positioning for the obese parturient for laryngoscopy is shown in Figure 47-13.

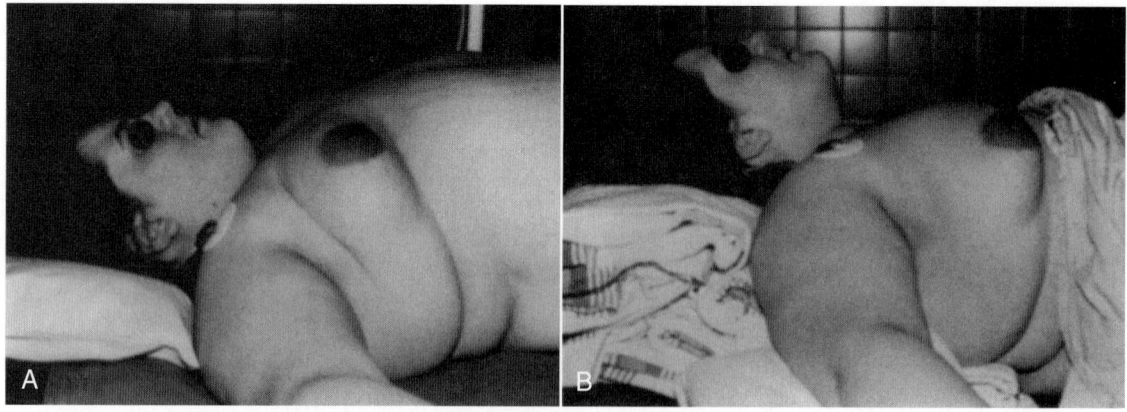

FIGURE **47-13** Positioning for the obese parturient for laryngoscopy. **A,** Standard positioning. **B,** Improved positioning with the elevation of the torso and head. (*From Hagberg CA. Benumof's Airway Management. 2nd ed. Philadelphia: Mosby; 2007:844.*)

Induction

Induction of general anesthesia proceeds in the usual rapid-sequence manner, with cricoid pressure after denitrogenation and generous preoxygenation. Appropriate induction agents in the healthy parturient include thiopental, ketamine, etomidate, and propofol. Propofol produces no greater neonatal depression than thiopental and is rapidly cleared from the neonate.[137-139] It is cleared from the parturient more quickly than thiopental, resulting in more rapid emergence.[138,139] Some studies have shown less variation in vital signs with the use of propofol than with thiopental.[140] Thiopental is usually used in doses of approximately 3 to 5 mg/kg. Ketamine, up to 1 mg/kg, is especially useful in patients who have airway disease or are hypotensive. It has also been associated with lower analgesic demands during the first 24 hours postoperatively compared with demands in women induced with thiopental.[141] The indirect sympathomimetic effect of ketamine helps support blood pressure until adequate volume can be replaced. The 1-mg/kg upper limit on ketamine should be observed to prevent depression of the neonate and maternal emergence reactions. Up to 0.3 mg/kg of etomidate can be used; the indications are the same in pregnant patients as they are in nonpregnant patients. All these lipid-soluble induction drugs cross the placenta rapidly, but neonatal depression is infrequently a problem when the cited doses are used.

Traditionally, induction of anesthesia has been delayed until preparation for surgery is completed. Surgery starts immediately after verification of proper endotracheal tube placement. The reasoning behind this practice has been that the dose of depressant drugs to which the fetus is exposed before delivery should be minimized. An interesting study has called this practice into question because of concerns over maternal awareness during surgical incision. King and co-workers[142] have reported that as many as 96% of women given 3 mg of thiopental per kilogram, 50% nitrous oxide, and 0.5% halothane (the vaporizer setting, not the end-tidal concentration) with a 5-L fresh gas flow obeyed commands during skin incision; as many as 20% still responded 2 minutes after incision. They suggested that other means of providing anesthesia at skin incisions should be considered, such as the use of local infiltration or opioids. Perhaps ketamine should be used more often to induce anesthesia; ketamine is a good amnestic and, unlike thiopental, provides somatic analgesia.

Neonatal depression during routine cesarean section has not been observed, despite anesthetic induction-to-delivery intervals of up to 10 minutes.[143] If this induction-to-delivery interval is safe, and if maternal awareness is a problem at the time of incision when traditional anesthetic techniques are used, then another alternative might simply be to delay incision until 3 minutes after anesthetic induction in healthy women.

Intubation

Succinylcholine remains the preferred muscle relaxant during induction of general anesthesia in the parturient. If the use of succinylcholine is contraindicated, a fast-acting nondepolarizer may be judiciously administered, or an awake intubation may be attempted. Although intubation can be accomplished quickly with a fast-onset nondepolarizing muscle relaxant, the duration of action will be longer than with succinylcholine.

Succinylcholine is metabolized by PCHE. PCHE activity is normally decreased approximately 30% in a healthy pregnant woman at term. If the parturient also has preeclampsia, PCHE levels may be decreased by 60%. Although a 30% decrease in PCHE has little clinical significance, a 60% decrease may prolong recovery time after succinylcholine neuromuscular blockade.

Although magnesium sulfate seems to have no effect on PCHE activity, succinylcholine's duration of action is prolonged in patients receiving magnesium sulfate. Metoclopramide may also prolong the action of agents eliminated through ester hydrolysis.[144]

After adequate relaxation has been achieved, the trachea should be intubated expeditiously. Because the parturient's functional residual capacity is decreased by 25% and her whole-body O_2 demand is up to 30% greater than normal, desaturation occurs rapidly. Once apnea occurs, maternal O_2 partial pressure drops three times as quickly as it would in a nonpregnant woman.

The Difficult Airway

Airway problems resulting in a failure to oxygenate and ventilate the obstetric patient are still a significant anesthesia-related cause of maternal mortality. Although rapid-sequence induction is the technique most commonly used to minimize the risk of gastric aspiration during induction of general anesthesia, it is *not* indicated if the laryngoscopist has doubts about his or her ability to intubate the patient. In such a case an alternative method, such as awake intubation, may be necessary. Blind nasal intubation should be performed cautiously, if at all, in the parturient, who commonly has swollen nasal mucosa that is prone to bleeding.

The anesthetist should be familiar with and able to perform the steps in an obstetric failed intubation algorithm (Figure 47-14). Those skilled with the laryngeal mask airway (LMA) would probably want to insert its use in the algorithm before cricothyrotomy. Pulse oximetry and capnography are essential monitors.

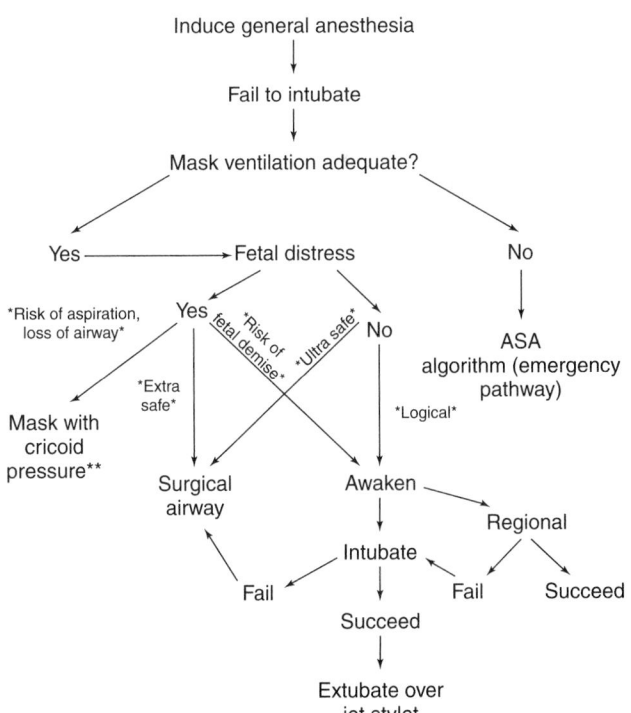

FIGURE **47-14** Supplement to the difficult airway management algorithm, with special reference to the presence or absence of fetal distress. This algorithm includes options in the management of a recognized difficult airway in an uncooperative patient or in a cooperative patient with dire fetal distress. (*From Chestnut DH. Obstetric Anesthesia: Principles and Practice. 3rd ed. Philadelphia: Mosby; 2004.*)
Denotes implications of this choice.
**Conventional face mask or laryngeal mask airway.*

ANESTHESIA FOR CESAREAN SECTION

Maintenance of Anesthesia Before Delivery

General anesthesia can be maintained by one of several methods. If propofol was used for induction, it can be used as an infusion for maintenance in the usual doses. Low doses of an inhalation agent also are appropriate. Up to two thirds MAC of an inhalation agent (0.75% isoflurane, 1.7% sevoflurane, 4.8% desflurane) has a long, safe history of use during cesarean section. However, all inhalation agents cause uterine relaxation, and the uterus must contract after delivery of the placenta to stop bleeding. Two thirds MAC inhalation agent depresses uterine contractility by approximately 25%,[145] and this amount of uterine relaxation usually can be overcome with clinically used doses of oxytocin.[145-147] If the woman has been laboring for an extended period, has received high doses of oxytocin before delivery, or has a uterus that has been stretched by multiple fetuses or hydramnios, her uterus will not contract well. In these circumstances, it is important to have as much of the inhalation agent as possible eliminated at the time of delivery. Under normal circumstances, low MAC levels of inhalation agent can be washed out quickly enough at delivery for undesirable uterine relaxation and bleeding to be avoided.

Disagreement exists regarding whether nitrous oxide should be used before delivery during cesarean section. If fetal distress is present or if maternal O_2 saturation is below 97%, high concentrations of O_2 should be used without nitrous oxide. Administering 100% O_2 does result in improved fetal oxygenation compared with 50% O_2,[148] but questions have been raised about the danger of free radical activity in neonates born to women administered greater than 50% O_2.[149] However, 50% nitrous oxide usually has been "allowable" during cesarean section in healthy women because it is believed that 50% O_2 is adequate if the fetus is healthy. Comparisons of Apgar scores, umbilical venous O_2 tension, time to breathing, and resuscitation efforts in neonates has revealed that infants born to women given 100% O_2 before delivery have a slightly better outcome.[150-152] Little benefit is associated with the discontinuation of nitrous oxide in order to deliver 100% O_2 only during the time from hysterotomy to delivery.[133]

After induction, if muscle relaxation is needed it can be accomplished with either a succinylcholine drip or a nondepolarizing agent. The duration of action of at least some nondepolarizers is slightly shorter than normal in a healthy term parturient.[153] A final consideration should be whether a muscle relaxant is needed at all. Because a woman's skin and abdominal muscles are so stretched during pregnancy, the surgeon may not need additional muscle relaxation to perform the procedure if adequate anesthesia is provided.

Tasks at Delivery and Postdelivery Maintenance

The length of time from uterine incision to delivery has been shown to correlate with the degree of neonatal acidosis.[154] The interval should be recorded. An interval of 3 minutes seems to be the critical value[155]; neonates delivered later than 3 minutes after uterine incision are more likely to be depressed.

After the umbilical cord has been clamped, the anesthetist's options for anesthetic maintenance increase because the administered drugs will no longer reach the baby. If adequate uterine contraction is achieved with oxytocin, there is no reason why the use of an inhalation anesthetic cannot be continued. A low-dose inhalation agent (up to 1 MAC), with or without nitrous oxide, and either fentanyl or sufentanil work well. The obstetrician also

may want an antibiotic to be given. If uterine tone does not allow the use of an inhalation agent, an opioid technique is useful. When opioids are used, nitrous oxide is usually needed. If nitrous oxide is not used, the anesthetist may consider giving a small dose of midazolam for amnesia. Opioid administration should be customized to the circumstances. One option is giving up to 5 mcg of fentanyl per kilogram or 0.5 mcg of sufentanil per kilogram, adjusting the dose according to the expected duration of the case and the patient's response. Another opioid choice is morphine 10 mg intravenously and 10 mg intramuscularly. One of these options should be selected and nitrous oxide added. If midazolam is used, the dose of opioid should be reduced. If an inhalation agent is not used, paralysis must be maintained in order to prevent patient movement.

After the placenta has been delivered, oxytocin should be given immediately unless the obstetrician's plan for uterine contraction calls for the use of another agent. Pitocin is the clinically available synthetic equivalent of oxytocin, a naturally occurring hormone synthesized in the supraoptic and paraventricular nuclei of the hypothalamus. In the mature uterus of a pregnant woman, oxytocin causes an increase in the frequency and strength of uterine contractions. Endogenous oxytocin release occurs with stimulation of the cervix, vagina, and breasts.

The half-life of oxytocin varies from 4 to 17 minutes. It is metabolized by liver, kidney, and plasma enzyme pathways in the parturient. Commercially available preparations of oxytocin contain a preservative that causes systolic and especially diastolic hypotension, flushing, and tachycardia when infused at high doses.[156] The amount of oxytocin added to the IV solution should be tailored to the volume of solution remaining in the bag, the flow rate of the IV, and the patient's condition. If the IV bag is nearly empty or if IV solution is being administered rapidly, less oxytocin should be added to the bag. In general, the obstetrician is likely to desire the administration of 30 to 40 units of oxytocin over the first hour postpartum. If an unusually large blood loss results in hypotension, and if fluid resuscitation is needed, it may be helpful to infuse the oxytocin at an appropriate rate and to start a second IV line for administering fluid volume at a rapid rate. If the solution with the added oxytocin is infused fast enough to replace volume, it is likely that the high dose of oxytocin may cause further hypotension.

If oxytocin does not adequately stimulate uterine contraction, the next drug used is usually an ergot alkaloid (Methergine, Ergotrate). Because of their potent vascular effects, ergot alkaloids are not administered intravenously. Ergot alkaloids normally cause an increase in blood pressure, central venous pressure, and pulmonary capillary wedge pressure. IV administration may result in arterial and venous constriction, coronary artery constriction, severe hypertension, cerebral bleeding, headache, nausea, and vomiting. An intramuscular dose of 0.2 mg is commonly administered for stimulating uterine contractions. In some cases the obstetrician may choose to administer oxytocin or ergotamine directly into the uterine muscle to maximize effect. Ergot alkaloids are metabolized and eliminated chiefly by the liver. The plasma half-life is approximately 2 hours, but uterine effects last much longer.

Ergot alkaloids potentiate sympathomimetics, especially α-agonists (including ephedrine). Severe hypertension, cerebrovascular accidents, and retinal detachment have occurred when the two drugs were used simultaneously. These effects may persist even when the vasopressor is given well after the last dose of methylergonovine maleate.

When the uterus does not contract well despite the use of oxytocin and ergot alkaloids, prostaglandin F_{2a} (Hemabate; 250 mcg) is administered either intramuscularly or directly into the uterine muscle. Prostaglandins are potent stimulators of uterine contractions. The contractions induced by prostaglandins are strong and painful. Nausea, vomiting, and diarrhea are frequent side effects. In addition to causing uterine contractions, prostaglandins may cause hypotension by relaxing vascular smooth muscle; however, cases of severe hypertension after prostaglandin administration have also been reported.[157-159] Prostaglandins may cause a recalcitrant uterus to contract and stop bleeding. If they do not, the surgeon is likely to extend the procedure and include hysterectomy, for which the anesthetist must be prepared.

Emergence from Anesthesia

Even with the administration of metoclopramide, the parturient often has a large volume of gastric contents. Suctioning of the stomach with an orogastric tube while the patient is anesthetized decreases the incidence of vomiting after awake extubation. Before extubation, the anesthetist should verify full recovery of neuromuscular function. Because cesarean section is usually a brief procedure involving fairly limited exposure to anesthetic, emergence is often quick. Advance preparation limits patient discomfort before extubation. A suggested method for providing general anesthesia for cesarean section is given in Box 47-4.

BOX 47-4

General Anesthesia for Cesarean Section

Histamine$_2$-receptor antagonist or proton pump inhibitor and/
  or metoclopramide intravenously
Clear antacid orally
Left uterine displacement
Application of monitors
Denitrogenation (administration of 100% oxygen)
• Traditional 3 to 5 minutes versus four vital-capacity breaths
Cricoid pressure
Intravenous induction
• Thiobarbiturate, propofol, ketamine, or etomidate
• Succinylcholine (rocuronium or vecuronium if
  succinylcholine is contraindicated)
Intubation with a 6.0- to 7.0-mm cuffed endotracheal tube
Administration of 30% to 50% nitrous oxide in oxygen and a
  low concentration (e.g., 2/3 minimum alveolar
  concentration MAC) of a volatile halogenated agent.
After delivery
• Increased concentration of nitrous oxide, with or without a
  low concentration of a volatile inhalation agent
• Opioid titrated as needed
• Intravenous hypnotic agent (e.g., benzodiazepine,
  barbiturate, propofol), if needed
• Muscle relaxant (e.g., succinylcholine boluses or infusion,
  rocuronium, cisatracurium, vecuronium)
Extubation awake with intact airway reflexes

Modified from Kuczkowski KM et al. Anesthesia for cesarean section. In: Chestnut DH, ed. Obstetric Anesthesia. 3rd ed. Philadelphia: Mosby; 2004:434.

Epidural Block

Several local anesthetics are safe and effective for use in a cesarean section. Bupivacaine 0.5% provides good motor block and dense anesthesia but may require up to 30 minutes to take effect. The long time to onset is often considered a disadvantage. However, the sympathetic block also occurs more slowly; this means that there is more time to react to hemodynamic changes than when agents with a more rapid onset are used. Lidocaine 2% provides good motor block and dense anesthesia and has an onset time of approximately 10 minutes. If 1 mEq of sodium bicarbonate is added to each 10 mL of lidocaine solution, the onset time shortens to 5 minutes or less. Adding sodium bicarbonate increases the pH of the solution and shifts the equilibrium toward a greater percentage of nonionized local anesthetic base, thereby facilitating local anesthetic spread. Adding 1 mEq of sodium bicarbonate to each 10 mL of lidocaine solution results in faster onset of the block[160,161] and denser sensory[162] and motor[161] block. The density of motor block varies with the concentration of local anesthetic used but should be expected to be greater in the bicarbonate solution for any given concentration. A solution of lidocaine and sodium bicarbonate has a shelf life of at least 7 days and noticeably reduces stinging when it is injected in cutaneous and subcutaneous tissues.[163] Because bicarbonated lidocaine speeds the onset of sympathetic block, hypotension may develop quickly (Figure 47-15). No advantage is gained from the addition of sodium bicarbonate to bupivacaine; also, it is difficult to combine the two without causing precipitation. 2-Chloroprocaine 3% provides good motor block and dense anesthesia and has a very short time to onset, but bicarbonated lidocaine acts nearly as quickly. The use of 2-chloroprocaine 3% probably offers no clinical advantage other than its ester hydrolysis elimination pathway; also, its low pH results in a high incidence of backache.

Women not in labor, such as most of those undergoing elective cesarean sections, have been shown to have a greater

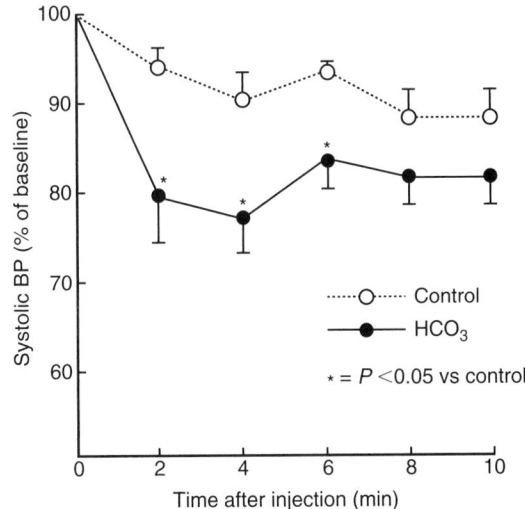

FIGURE **47-15** Time course of average systolic blood pressure *(BP)* readings *(mean SEM)* expressed as a percentage of the baseline value after epidural injections of lidocaine alone or lidocaine with added sodium bicarbonate. *(From Parnass SM et al. Incidence of hypotension associated with epidural anesthesia using alkalinized and nonalkalinized lidocaine for cesarean section. Anesth Analg. 1987;66:1148-1150. Reprinted with permission from the International Anesthesia Research Society.)*

BOX **47-5**

Epidural Anesthesia for Cesarean Section

Metoclopramide 10 mg intravenously
Clear antacid orally
Intravascular volume replacement with Ringer's lactate or
  normal saline (15-20 mL/kg)
Application of monitors
Supplemental oxygen by face mask or nasal prongs
Epidural catheter at L2-L3 or L3-L4
Left uterine displacement
Test dose
Therapeutic dose
• 5-mL boluses of 2% lidocaine + 1:400,000 epinephrine
  Alternatively, 5-mL boluses of:
  • 0.5% Bupivacaine *or*
  • 0.5% Ropivacaine *or*
  • 3% 2-chloroprocaine (boluses of lidocaine or
    2-chloroprocaine every 1-2 minutes, boluses of
    bupivacaine or ropivacaine every 2-5 minutes)
Aggressive treatment of hypotension:
• Exaggerated left uterine displacement
• Intravenous fluids
• Ephedrine and/or low-dose phenylephrine

Modified from Kuczkowski KM et al. Anesthesia for cesarean section. In: Chestnut DH, ed. Obstetric Anesthesia. 3rd ed. Philadelphia: Mosby; 2004:431.

BOX **47-6**

Spinal Anesthesia for Cesarean Section

Metoclopramide 10 mg intravenously
Clear antacid orally
Intravascular volume replacement with Ringer s lactate or
  normal saline (15-20 mL/kg)
Application of monitors
Supplemental oxygen by face mask or nasal prongs
Lumbar puncture at L3-L4
• Right lateral or sitting position
• 25- or 24-gauge Sprotte needle or 27- or 25-gauge
  Whitacre needle
• Bupivacaine 12 mg in 8.25% dextrose
  • Morphine 0.1 to 0.25 mg for postoperative analgesia
• Left uterine displacement
Aggressive treatment of hypotension
• Exaggerated left uterine displacement
• Intravenous fluids
• Ephedrine and/or phenylephrine titrated to effect

Modified from Kuczkowski KM et al. Anesthesia for cesarean section. In: Chestnut DH, ed. Obstetric Anesthesia. 3rd ed. Philadelphia: Mosby; 2004:429.

incidence of hypotension after the institution of epidural anesthesia than women in labor.[116] This may be because of the lack of autologous transfusion provided to the woman in labor each time the uterus contracts and squeezes blood into the general circulation.

Although it may be tempting to administer epidural anesthesia for cesarean section through the Tuohy needle rather than an epidural catheter in order to save time, this administration technique has distinct disadvantages. If a complication related to the site of injection (e.g., intravascular injection) is going to occur, it will occur more quickly and be more severe when this technique is used. The incidence of hypotension after administration through the Tuohy needle is greater than it is when the dose is administered incrementally through the epidural catheter.[164]

The duration of action of bupivacaine and lidocaine, as well as the density of the block that they provide, can be increased by the addition of 5 mcg/mL or less of epinephrine.[165] Adding epinephrine to local anesthetics during cesarean section has been shown to be safe in healthy women with a healthy fetus.[166] An epidural anesthetic with added epinephrine may be preferable to spinal anesthesia with respect to the incidence of hypotension, umbilical artery Doppler pulsatility, FHR, and umbilical artery blood pH.[107]

In years past, women have almost universally complained of a diffuse, difficult-to-describe painful or noxious feeling during cesarean section despite "good," dense local anesthetic blocks. This uncomfortable feeling most commonly occurred during exteriorization of the uterus. Experience and scientific studies have verified that the use of local anesthetic solutions containing an opioid, both for epidural and subarachnoid blocks, significantly reduces this discomfort and results in greater patient satisfaction without danger of neonatal depression.[93,94] The addition of 100 mcg of fentanyl to the epidural local anesthetic also

results in less nausea and vomiting between delivery and the end of surgery.[167] A suggested method for epidural anesthesia for cesarean section is given in Box 47-5.

Subarachnoid Block

Both bupivacaine and lidocaine are good choices for cesarean section with subarachnoid block. Tetracaine 10 to 15 mg provides a block that lasts approximately 90 minutes within 15 minutes after administration. Bupivacaine, 10 to 15 mg, provides a solid anesthetic block and less motor blockade than tetracaine, and its duration of action is approximately 90 minutes. Bupivacaine sets up noticeably faster than tetracaine. A factor to consider when using bupivacaine is that in a patient placed in the lateral position for performance of the block the dose should be reduced compared with that in a patient in the sitting position. Failure to reduce the administered dose results in a noticeably higher spread of anesthetic block. Lidocaine, 75 to 100 mg, provides a block in 5 minutes or less, and the block lasts from 50 minutes to 1 hour. Transient neurologic symptoms appear not to be a concern in women undergoing cesarean section with lidocaine subarachnoid block.[168,169] Addition of fentanyl to either a subarachnoid or epidural block prolongs the block duration and increases its density, but without prolonging motor block or urinary retention as epinephrine does. A suggested method for spinal anesthesia for cesarean section is given in Box 47-6.

ANESTHETIC COMPLICATIONS

From 1987 to 1990, anesthesia complications accounted for 2.5% of all maternal deaths in the United States,[170] down from 3.3% for the 7 years preceding 1986.[171] Most anesthesia-related deaths were associated with general anesthesia for cesarean section. Although the overall reduction in maternal deaths related to anesthesia is encouraging, complications of anesthesia resulted in maternal death six to seven times more frequently in African American women than in Caucasian women.[170] The anesthesia-related maternal mortality rate decreased from 4.3 per million live births in 1979 to 1981 to 1.7 per million in 1988 to 1990. This change is attributed to the increased use of regional anesthetic techniques in obstetrics. The number of regional anesthesia related deaths has continuously decreased since 1984.[172]

Nausea and Vomiting

Nausea and vomiting caused by anesthesia in the obstetric setting often are closely related to hypotension. The aggressive treatment of hypotension prevents much vomiting. Some clinicians believe that a sympathetic block results in unopposed gastrointestinal vagal stimulation, which predisposes the patient to nausea. The administration of an antimuscarinic agent (atropine, glycopyrrolate) before the institution of either an epidural or subarachnoid block may prevent nausea by this mechanism. Opioids administered in either the epidural or subarachnoid space may cause nausea. Scopolamine transdermal patches have been shown to significantly reduce the incidence of post–cesarean section nausea and vomiting resulting from regional opioids.[173] The transdermal scopolamine patch begins to be effective in 2 to 4 hours. Although this onset time is long, the duration of the scopolamine patch (48 hours or longer) makes it a desirable choice. The patch delivers a much smaller dose over time than parenteral administration of scopolamine, and some women may experience side effects such as dry mouth or dizziness, which for some patients will outweigh the benefits of scopolamine.

Postdural Puncture Headache

Postdural puncture headache (PDPH) results from a loss of CSF from within the dural and arachnoid membrane that surrounds the brain and spinal cord. The total volume of CSF present within this sac in an adult is approximately 150 mL. Approximately 500 mL of CSF is produced and reabsorbed each day.

PDPH occurs when CSF leaks out through a hole in the dura made during the performance of a subarachnoid block or accidentally during the attempted performance of an epidural block. Because the Tuohy needle used to place an epidural catheter has a large diameter, puncture of the dura with a Tuohy results in the loss of a significant volume of CSF. Loss of CSF is not the only cause of headache after regional anesthesia in the obstetric patient. Meningitis, although rare, can develop despite the adherence to aseptic technique, and this disease shares many of the signs and symptoms of PDPH (headache, nausea, and photophobia) in the initial stages.

Incidence

The incidence and severity of PDPH vary with factors thought to be related to the volume and rate of CSF leakage out of the subarachnoid space. PDPH is infrequent in the elderly and most frequent in young adults. Women seem to be slightly more susceptible than men. In general, the use of large needles is more likely to be associated with PDPH than use of small ones. Even so, an 11% incidence of "mild and transient" headache was reported among 50 women undergoing cesarean section after dural puncture with a 30-gauge needle.[174] The configuration of the tip of the needle is also important. Other factors being equal, the use of beveled needles, like the Quincke needle, result in headache more frequently than the use of pencil-point or bullet-tip needles, like the Whitacre or Sprotte needle (Figure 47-16). No PDPH occurred in 38 patients after dural

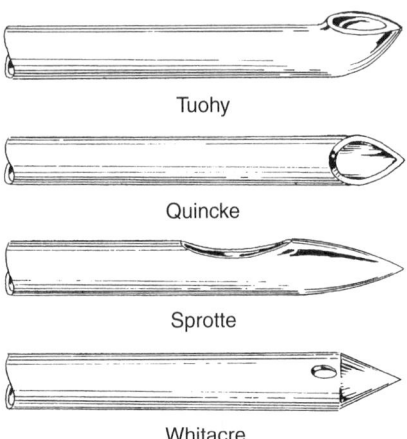

FIGURE **47-16** Physical characteristics of four different types of spinal and epidural needles. Needle diameters are not to scale.

puncture with a 26-gauge pencil-point Portex needle.[175] Only one case of PDPH was reported in 50 parturients after dural puncture with a 26-gauge Becton-Dickinson needle,[176] and only one "slight" headache was reported in 271 parturients after dural puncture with a 24-gauge Sprotte needle.[177] In a retrospective study of 366 obstetric patients, the incidence of PDPH after the use of a Sprotte needle was 1.5%, compared with 9% after the use of a beveled Quincke needle of similar gauge.[178] The orientation of the needle as it punctures the dural fibers also may be important. Spreading the fibers along their cephalad-to-caudad axis may result in less CSF leakage than cutting the fibers by inserting the bevel perpendicular to the axis of the dural fibers. In support of this theory, electron microscopy has confirmed that elastic fibers in the dura are arranged longitudinally.[179] Of course, this is true only with the use of beveled needles, not that of pencil-point or bullet-tip needles. The angle at which the needle approaches the dura may also modify the amount of CSF leakage and therefore the incidence of PDPH; however, the angle of approach most often is dictated by anatomy and therefore is difficult for the anesthetist to modify effectively.

Clinical Appearance

The hallmark of a PDPH is its postural nature. The headache is relieved by lying down and returns on sitting or standing up. It is commonly fronto-occipital and sometimes is associated with neck and shoulder stiffness. Photophobia may be present in patients with severe headaches, whereas double vision occurs less frequently. Temporary deafness has occurred rarely. The onset of the headache is usually not immediate, but may take 1 to 2 days to become bothersome. It may be mild or severe, and it often becomes worse if the patient feels sick and does not consume liquids.

Treatment

Patients should be given a choice of treatments ranging from the most conservative to the most aggressive. PDPH may be a mild irritation for a few days, or it may be debilitating. Patients with a mild PDPH may elect to rest in bed because the horizontal position often provides complete relief from the headache, or to take over-the-counter analgesics if they are up and about. Adequate hydration should be encouraged. In hospitalized patients who are not taking fluids by mouth, IV hydration is warranted. Liberal hydration does not increase the production of CSF; however, it is important that the patient not be allowed to become dehydrated, because dehydration does decrease CSF production.

Caffeine is a cerebral vasoconstrictor and is effective in preventing or treating PDPH in some patients. In one trial, 90% of patients with documented PDPH who were given 300 mg of caffeine showed significant improvement, compared with only 60% of patients who received a placebo.[180] For reference, Vivarin contains 200 mg of caffeine, NoDoz 200 mg, a cup of coffee approximately 100 mg, and slightly less in certain soft drinks. Like caffeine, serotonin also causes cerebral vasoconstriction. Case reports of serotonin type-1δ receptor agonists (sumatriptan) successfully relieving PDPH have also been published.[181]

The most effective treatment available for PDPH is an epidural blood patch. This treatment entails some risk because it is invasive; also, the headache is likely to become worse if another dural puncture is made in the course of placing the epidural (with a 17- or 18-gauge Tuohy needle). The usual contraindications to an epidural procedure also apply to this treatment.

A blood patch is performed by placing a Tuohy needle in the epidural space, preferably at the same interspace as the dural puncture or one interspace below. Once the Tuohy needle is in place, an assistant performs a peripheral venipuncture and draws 20 mL of the patient's own blood using strict aseptic technique. The blood is slowly injected into the epidural space. The ideal volume for injection appears to be between 15 and 20 mL; the use of smaller volumes is associated with a significantly lower success rate, especially in the placement of prophylactic blood patches.[182,183] If discomfort develops in the back or neck, the injection is temporarily stopped. After the discomfort has passed, injection of the target volume of 15 to 20 mL may continue (unless discomfort returns). After the desired volume is injected, the Tuohy needle is withdrawn, and the patient should lie quietly for at least 1 hour.[184] For the next several hours, the patient should rest and not be overly active. This may need to be specifically discussed with the patient, because she may feel quite well for the first time in days and therefore may want to be more active. Excessive activity before complete clot consolidation may result in the clot being dislodged from the dural puncture site, allowing CSF leakage to resume.

The epidural blood patch is thought to plug the dural rent with a fibrin clot; the injected volume of blood applies pressure to the dura, in effect "autotransfusing" the cerebrum with CSF from around the spinal cord. An epidural blood patch is effective in more than 90% of patients when it is performed 24 hours after the dural puncture. A second patch is effective in approximately half of those who do not obtain relief from the first; this brings the total success rate to approximately 95%. Placing further patches does not increase the success rate significantly. Some authorities recommend earlier or prophylactic blood patches; however, the results obtained with them have been mixed. It is clear, however, that the success rate with early or prophylactic blood patches is not as high as that of blood patches performed 24 hours or more after the dural puncture. Still, only 21% of parturients who received a prophylactic blood patch after accidental dural puncture with a Tuohy needle experienced headache, compared with 80% of those who did not.[185] Likewise, in a study of 10 obstetric patients who received a prophylactic epidural blood patch after dural puncture with an 18-gauge Hustead needle, only one patient reported a "mild" headache; this patient's headache did not require further treatment.[186]

Accidental Intravascular Injection

Intravascular injection of local anesthetic may have CNS or cardiovascular consequences. CNS signs generally occur at lower plasma concentrations than does cardiovascular depression, although the effects of bupivacaine may be an exception to this rule at times. The first signs include ringing in the ears or other changes in hearing, confusion, inability to speak, a metallic taste in the mouth, or circumoral numbness. Higher blood levels eventually cause seizure and cardiovascular collapse. Obviously, the first step to be taken when any of these complications occurs is discontinuation of the injection of local anesthetic. If a seizure occurs, both mother and fetus are at risk of hypoxia. Quick action involving the administration of a barbiturate or benzodiazepine is necessary to end the seizure and control the airway with an endotracheal tube. Thiopental, atropine, ephedrine, a self-inflating breathing bag, an anesthesia mask, laryngoscopes, oral and nasal airways, endotracheal tubes, and stylettes should all be on epidural insertion carts. Cardiovascular support is provided symptomatically, if needed. Positive-pressure ventilation through an endotracheal tube should be instituted as soon as possible. After this has been accomplished, maternal O_2 saturation, blood pressure, and pulse should be checked, and FHR and variability assessed.

Accidental Subarachnoid Injection

Subarachnoid injection results in a denser and more widespread block and one of more rapid onset than does epidural injection; therefore it may lead to the rapid onset of dyspnea, hypotension, or both. Treatment is directed at relief of symptoms. These complications may occur quickly after a bolus injection through a supposedly epidural catheter or insidiously after catheter migration in a patient receiving a continuous infusion of local anesthetic. The harmful effects of accidental subarachnoid injection can be greatly reduced if the anesthetic is administered through the catheter in increments no greater than 5 mL.

Accidental Subdural Injection

Occasionally the epidural catheter may be placed accidentally in the subdural space between the dura and the arachnoid membranes. After a negative intravascular and subarachnoid test dose, anesthetic is administered through the supposed epidural catheter in the normal fashion. After a delay of 10 to 25 minutes, a sudden excessive spread of the block is noted,[187] primarily in the cephalad direction.[188] The magnitude of the spread of the local anesthetic block is significantly greater than would be anticipated if the catheter were in the epidural space and very similar to what would be expected with a subarachnoid injection. Hypotension caused by extensive sympathetic block is usually the primary problem and is treated with ephedrine or other vasopressors as needed. If the block is sufficiently extensive to compromise respiration or airway maintenance, endotracheal intubation is necessary. This complication is uncommon and quite possibly unpreventable. The possibility of respiratory compromise emphasizes the necessity of being prepared to manage such a complication as well as the need for close monitoring after epidural administration.

Electrocardiographic Changes During Regional Anesthesia for Cesarean Section

In a series of 93 healthy parturients undergoing "routine" cesarean section, a 47% incidence of electrocardiographic (ECG) changes "characteristic" of myocardial ischemia was noted.[189] Although not all of the women with ECG changes had associated subjective complaints, 86% of the women with complaints of chest pain, pressure, nausea and vomiting, or dyspnea did have associated ECG changes. The investigators speculated that the superimposition of large fluid shifts involved with regional anesthesia on the already increased cardiac workload associated with term pregnancy may have resulted in myocardial ischemia. Further investigations of ECG changes during cesarean section have concluded that ST-segment changes are not caused by myocardial ischemia.[190] Observations of wall motion have shown no abnormality during ST changes, nor have myocardial-specific creatine kinase levels. Further studies indicate that few ST changes during regional anesthesia for cesarean section in healthy women are actually caused by myocardial ischemia.[191,192]

Cardiopulmonary Resuscitation of the Pregnant Patient

CPR has been accomplished successfully early in pregnancy, but use of the technique is problematic at best in the near-term parturient. The fetus does not tolerate decreases in maternal oxygenation and blood pressure well. The mother has a high O_2 demand and a small O_2 reservoir (residual volume). Perhaps most important, the term or near-term uterus obstructs central venous return in the supine parturient.[193-195] It follows that left uterine displacement is important to the success of CPR in pregnant women. However, lateral tilt has been shown to decrease the force of cardiac compressions and presumably their effectiveness. Chest compressions done on a patient in 27-degree lateral tilt have only 80% of the force of compressions performed on a patient in the supine position.[196] As a result, a wedge that displaces the uterus while allowing closed-chest compressions has been developed. Presumably, any handy wedge that is positioned under the right hip would displace the uterus to the left while leaving the thorax fairly supine for effective chest compressions. In any case, when the near-term parturient does not respond to resuscitative efforts within 5 minutes, emergent cesarean section is often indicated. This makes possible direct oxygenation of the neonate and has resulted in substantially improved venous return in the mother,[194,195] ultimately allowing for successful resuscitation of her as well.

OBSTETRIC COMPLICATIONS

From 1982 to 1996, the maternal mortality rate in the United States was 7.5 per 100,000 live births.[196] Yet the range of mortality rates varied greatly by state and ethnicity (1987 to 1996), with a low of 2.7 for Caucasian women in Massachusetts to a high of 28.7 for African American women in New York.[197] The most common causes of maternal death (from most to least) include hemorrhage, embolism, preeclampsia, infection, and cardiomyopathy.

Prematurity

Premature delivery is a leading cause of perinatal morbidity and mortality. Premature delivery is implicated in more than 50% of all perinatal deaths. The frequency of preterm birth in the United States increased from 10.7% in 1992 to 12.3% in 2003. Premature labor is an even more frequent occurrence.

Premature labor is defined as regular uterine contractions that occur between 20 and 37 weeks of gestation and that result in dilation or effacement of the cervix. When labor begins prematurely, the ability to halt it can allow the fetus additional time to mature. Stopping labor is termed *tocolysis* (from the Greek *tokos*, meaning "childbirth," and *lysis*, meaning "breaking up"). The cause of preterm labor is not well understood; however, four pathways are supported by a considerable body of clinical and experimental evidence: excessive myometrial and fetal membrane overdistention, decidual hemorrhage, precocious fetal endocrine activation, and intrauterine infection or inflammation. The processes leading to preterm parturition may originate from one or more of these pathways. Common risk factors include women with multifetal pregnancies, presumably owing to pathologic uterine overdistention. Women with preterm rupture of membranes or preterm labor at a very early gestational age (e.g., 24 to 28 weeks) are at increased risk for having underlying intrauterine infection, one of the four common pathways mentioned previously. Other noted risk factors may include race, weight, drug use, stress, parity, multiple gestation, extremes of maternal age, and the presence of additional obstetric complications.[198,199]

Methods of Tocolysis

Historically, ethyl alcohol was used to stop premature labor. Ethanol depresses myometrial contractility and suppresses the release of oxytocin from the posterior pituitary. It was, however, the cause of many dangerous side effects, including increased gastric volume, depression or obliteration of airway reflexes, vomiting, lactic acidosis, and fluid and electrolyte abnormalities.

Although more than 80% of women with preterm labor who are treated with tocolytics have their pregnancies maintained for 24 to 48 hours, few data suggest that tocolysis maintains pregnancy for a longer period. A critical goal of tocolysis is to delay delivery long enough to allow for the administration of corticosteroids, which reduces the risks of the neonatal respiratory distress syndrome, intraventricular hemorrhage, necrotizing enterocolitis, and overall perinatal death. The initial benefit of corticosteroid therapy occurs approximately 18 hours after administration of the first dose with maximal benefit at about 48 hours. Thus treatment of acute preterm labor may allow time for the onset of the therapeutic effect of corticosteroids.

A variety of agents are used as tocolytics. These include β-adrenergic receptor agonists, nitric oxide donors, magnesium sulfate, calcium channel blockers, prostaglandin synthesis inhibitors, and oxytocin antagonists. Labor-inhibiting drugs are only marginally effective. Tocolytics act by two primary mechanisms: through generation or alteration of intracellular messengers or by inhibiting the synthesis or blocking the action of a known myometrial stimulant.

Magnesium Sulfate. Magnesium sulfate has been used for decades as a tocolytic, but recently it has been noted that given its lack of benefit, possible harms, and expense, magnesium sulfate should not be used for tocolysis.[200] Others feel it is still of some benefit when used properly.[201] Magnesium causes relaxation of vascular, bronchial, and uterine smooth muscle by altering calcium transport and availability. Motor end-plate sensitivity and muscle membrane excitability also are depressed. Magnesium hyperpolarizes the plasma membrane and inhibits myosin light-chain kinase activity by competing with intracellular calcium, which in turn reduces myometrial contractility.

The normal serum magnesium level during pregnancy is 1.8 to 3 mg/dL. A serum magnesium level of 4 to 8 mg/dL is therapeutic as a tocolytic, but even toxic levels do not eliminate uterine contractility. At 10 to 12 mg/dL, the patellar reflex is eliminated. Levels above 12 mg/dL cause respiratory depression; at approximately 18 mg/dL, respiratory depression progresses to apnea. The presence of higher levels (25 mg/dL) can cause cardiac arrest.

Side Effects. The side effects of magnesium sulfate administration are dose dependent. As magnesium levels increase, skeletal muscle weakness increases and CNS depression and vascular dilation occur. Magnesium sulfate infusion commonly results in a slight decrease in blood pressure during epidural anesthesia.

Magnesium antagonizes the vasoconstrictive effect of α-agonists, so ephedrine and phenylephrine are likely to less effectively increase maternal blood pressure when administered concomitantly with magnesium. Cardiac muscle is not affected to a clinically evident degree when magnesium is administered at therapeutic levels, although magnesium can have profound myocardial effects during a gross overdose. Magnesium is eliminated unchanged by the kidneys. In a patient who is receiving a maintenance infusion of magnesium and who has decreasing urine output, blood levels of magnesium quickly increase, as do related side effects.

Side effects of magnesium sulfate include the following:
- Cutaneous vasodilation with flushing
- Headache and dizziness
- Nausea
- Skeletal-muscle weakness
- Depression of deep tendon reflexes
- Respiratory depression
- ECG changes

Patients on magnesium sulfate therapy have partial, if subclinical, neuromuscular blockade. Both depolarizing and nondepolarizing[202,203] neuromuscular blocking drugs are potentiated by magnesium. Administration of priming or defasciculating doses of neuromuscular blocking drugs may cause significant paralysis when combined with magnesium therapy. The neuromuscular blocking effects of magnesium can be at least partially antagonized by calcium.

Magnesium sulfate overdose is treatable. In an excellent case report, a 23-year-old gravida received a 20-g bolus of magnesium sulfate superimposed on a therapeutic magnesium (Mg^{2+}) level. She attained a magnesium level of 38.7 mg/dL.[204] She had a respiratory arrest, became hypotensive and bradycardic, and developed a prolonged QRS complex. Resuscitation was successfully accomplished with discontinuation of the magnesium administration, endotracheal intubation and ventilation, IV administration of calcium chloride, and diuresis to facilitate the elimination of magnesium. Vital signs improved dramatically with ventilation and calcium administration, and the woman was extubated 8 hours later after her magnesium level had declined to a therapeutic level.

Neonatal side effects after maternal magnesium administration are rare. A few cases of hypotonia and respiratory depression in neonates after prolonged high-dose maternal magnesium administration have been reported; however, in general, magnesium administration is safe for the neonate. Magnesium is also used in the treatment of preeclampsia, a vasospastic disease of pregnancy that can result in severe hypertension, coagulopathy, and seizure. Magnesium sulfate causes relaxation of vascular smooth muscle, a decrease in SVR, and a decrease in blood pressure. At serum levels of 7 to 9.5 mg/dL, it is an anticonvulsant. It also decreases fibrin deposition, improving circulation to visceral organs that are vulnerable to vasospasm and failure.

β-Agonists. Stimulation of the $β_2$-receptor system causes smooth muscle relaxation, including relaxation of the uterus. The myometrium has $β_2$-receptors in cell membranes. Stimulation of these receptors triggers a cascade of biochemical effects, resulting in inhibition of myometrial contractility at the cellular level. $β_2$ Stimulation also causes an increase in progesterone production. Progesterone in turn causes histologic changes in myometrial cells that limit the spread of contractile impulses. The β-adrenergic receptor agonists cause myometrial relaxation by binding to $β_2$-adrenergic receptors and subsequently increasing the levels of intracellular cyclic adenosine monophosphate

(AMP), which activates protein kinase, inactivating myosin light-chain kinase, thus diminishing myometrial contractility.

The administration of β-agonists results in downregulation of β-receptors over time. This results in a decreased tocolytic effect during long-term β-agonist therapy that has been demonstrated in animals after as few as 24 hours of ritodrine administration.

Maternal Side Effects. All currently available β-agonists have both $β_1$ and $β_2$ effects, although some agents are fairly selective for one receptor subset over the other. The side effects of β-agonist therapy can be predicted on the basis of a knowledge of systemic β effects. Cardiovascular effects are generally the most clinically important and troublesome. $β_1$ Stimulation causes an increase in HR, myocardial contractility, and myocardial O_2 demand. Palpitations and premature ventricular contractions are not uncommon. $β_2$ Stimulation causes vascular dilation, bronchial dilation, an increase in secretions, and various metabolic effects.

In one published case, a young, healthy parturient received an overdose of ritodrine (50 mg) in an IV bolus; the overdose resulted in flushing, tremor, tachycardia, and hypotension that lasted for 6 hours. She recovered with supportive treatment.

Maternal side effects of β-agonists include the following:
- Cerebral vasospasm
- Chest pain or tightness
- Glucose intolerance
- Hypokalemia
- Ileus
- Myocardial ischemia
- Nausea
- Palpitations
- Pulmonary edema
- Restlessness
- Tremor
- Ventricular arrhythmias

By the 24th week of gestation, maternal cardiac output is increased by up to 50% as a result of an increase in both HR and SV. β-Agonist therapy further increases the demand on the cardiovascular system. Complaints of palpitations and chest pain are not uncommon. ECG changes are sometimes seen, although myocardial ischemia is not always documented.

Both ritodrine and terbutaline can antagonize hypoxic pulmonary vasoconstriction through $β_2$-mediated vasodilation. Hypoxic pulmonary vasoconstriction causes pulmonary arteries that lead to areas of the lung with low O_2 tension to constrict and divert blood flow to well-oxygenated areas of lung. In patients with a significant degree of hypoxic pulmonary vasoconstriction, such as those with underlying pulmonary disease or pulmonary edema, dilation of constricted pulmonary arteries may result in a significant decrease in maternal O_2 tension.

Metabolic Effects. β Stimulation increases blood glucose and insulin levels. When a β-agonist infusion is started, the blood glucose level increases within a few hours and returns to baseline within 72 hours without treatment. Potassium is redistributed from the extracellular to intracellular compartments. This results in a decrease in serum potassium level, sometimes to less than 3 mEq/L. As with glucose levels, serum potassium levels return to normal within 72 hours after initiation of β-agonist therapy.

Pulmonary Edema. There is a small but notable incidence of pulmonary edema among healthy parturients receiving β-agonists. The mechanism for the development of pulmonary edema in these patients is unclear. Fluid overload resulting from a physiologic increase in intravascular volume, antidiuresis, and IV fluid administration may have a role. Myocardial fatigue caused by tachycardia also has been suggested as a possible cause. Pulmonary artery pressures are not uniformly elevated, however, and sometimes they are low; this finding can be used to argue against both of these hypotheses. However, it is clear that the danger of pulmonary edema increases when parturients receiving β-agonists are preloaded for regional anesthesia.

Risk factors associated with pulmonary edema during β-agonist tocolysis include the following:

- Anemia
- Fluid overload
- Magnesium
- Multiple gestation
- Prolonged maternal tachycardia

Fetal and Neonatal Side Effects. Clinically used β-agonists cross the placenta and have fetal and neonatal effects. Fetal tachycardia (FHR >160 bpm) is common. Neonatal hypoglycemia may result, especially if maternal serum glucose is elevated at delivery. When maternal and therefore fetal blood glucose levels are elevated, the fetus increases insulin release in response. After delivery the neonate continues to release insulin at an increased rate, even though it is no longer receiving a glucose load from the mother. After the excess circulating glucose has been used up, continued release of insulin causes a rebound hypoglycemia. Because delivery of the infant during tocolysis is not the goal, these side effects are seldom a concern.

Ritodrine (Yutopar) is a selective β$_2$-agonist. Ritodrine therapy increases maternal HR by an average of 40 bpm. Systolic blood pressure commonly increases, and diastolic pressure decreases. The manufacturer's literature recommends that patients on ritodrine therapy receive no more than 2 L of IV fluid over 24 hours. Before spinal or epidural anesthesia for cesarean section is initiated, it is not uncommon for a 2-L IV preload to be given in less than 30 minutes. However, even smaller IV preloads are not recommended in patients receiving ritodrine until use of the drug has been discontinued for at least 1 hour. Ritodrine is eliminated by the kidneys and has an elimination half-life of approximately 30 minutes.

Terbutaline (Brethine, Bricanyl) is a synthetic, relatively β$_2$ receptor–selective, noncatecholamine sympathomimetic amine. When administered parenterally, terbutaline is less β$_2$ receptor–selective than ritodrine. Arrhythmias are more likely to occur with terbutaline use than during ritodrine administration, and tachycardia can be a problem. Terbutaline is approximately 50% eliminated by the kidneys and has a half-life of up to 16 hours. Like ritodrine, terbutaline has been associated with pulmonary edema when it is used for tocolysis.

Nitric Oxide Donors. Nitric oxide is a vasodilator that is essential for the maintenance of normal smooth-muscle tone and is produced in a variety of cells. Nitric oxide increases cyclic guanosine monophosphate (cGMP) content in smooth-muscle cells that inactivates myosin light-chain kinases, leading to smooth-muscle relaxation. In a comparison of nitroglycerin, which is a nitric oxide donor, and magnesium sulfate, the latter was more likely to delay delivery for at least 12 hours. However, transdermal nitroglycerin was superior to placebo in prolonging pregnancy for 48 hours.[199]

Calcium Channel Blockers. Nifedipine is the most commonly used agent as it can be administered orally. The calcium channel blockers inhibit the influx of calcium ions through the cell membrane and the release of intracellular calcium from the sarcoplasmic reticulum. This decreases intracellular free calcium, leading to inhibition of calcium-dependent myosin light-chain kinase–mediated phosphorylation, resulting in myometrial relaxation.

Cyclooxygenase Inhibitors. Cyclooxygenase converts arachidonic acid to prostaglandin H$_2$. Prostaglandin H$_2$ serves as a substrate for tissue-specific enzymes, which is critical in parturition. Prostaglandins enhance the formation of myometrial gap junctions and increase available intracellular calcium by raising transmembrane influx and sarcolemmal release of calcium. Indomethacin is the most commonly used tocolytic agent in this class.

Oxytocin Receptor Antagonists. Atosiban is an oxytocin receptor antagonist that blocks the normal effects of oxytocin in the uterus. Normally, oxytocin stimulates contractions by inducing the conversion of phosphatidyl inositol triphosphate to inositol triphosphate, which binds to a protein in the sarcoplasmic reticulum, causing the release of calcium into the cytoplasm. Reports of excess fetal and infant deaths with the administration of atosiban before 28 weeks of gestation has limited the use of this agent.

Therapy Recommendations. Nifedipine appears to be a reasonable choice for initial tocolysis, given the oral route of administration, low frequency of side effects, and efficacy in reducing neonatal complications. Nifedipine can be used at any gestational age when labor-inhibition therapy is being considered. For pregnancies of less than 32 weeks' gestation, an alternative to nifedipine is indomethacin. These agents have been shown to be more effective than the β-adrenergic receptor agonists in comparative studies. Indomethacin should be avoided in women with a platelet dysfunction or bleeding disorder, hepatic or renal dysfunction, gastrointestinal ulcerative disease, or asthma (in women with hypersensitivity to aspirin). The use of β-adrenergic–receptor agonists is an alternative to therapy with nifedipine and indomethacin. The side-effect profile of this class of drugs is less favorable than that of nifedipine, but their effectiveness in stopping contractions appears to be similar.[195]

Anesthetic Considerations

When an anesthetic intervention is planned for a patient who is receiving a tocolytic agent, knowledge of maternal and fetal physiology and of the pharmacology of the tocolytic agent must be integrated.

Regional Anesthesia

When tocolysis fails, preterm deliveries are often accomplished by cesarean section. In this situation, 1- and 5-minute Apgar scores have been shown to be higher in neonates delivered with epidural anesthesia than in those delivered with general anesthesia.[205] Patients on magnesium therapy are often candidates for subarachnoid or epidural blocks as long as careful attention is devoted to volume status. Magnesium causes vasodilation, and maternal hemorrhage is tolerated poorly by parturients on magnesium and their fetuses.[206,207] Subarachnoid block has the advantage of involving very small amounts of local anesthetic, and this reduces the chance for fetal local anesthetic toxicity. Epidural anesthesia can be used throughout labor for analgesia and can be induced slowly; this minimizes the risk of sudden hypotension caused by sympathetic block.

Even when volume status is accurately assessed, IV preloads before subarachnoid or epidural anesthesia are associated with an increased risk of pulmonary edema in parturients receiving β-agonist drugs. Use of ritodrine (and perhaps terbutaline) should almost always be discontinued, and enough time for the drug to be largely eliminated should be allowed to pass before regional anesthesia is induced. If time constraints do not permit the needed delay, induction of general anesthesia for an urgent or emergent procedure is almost always preferable. If the patient is already in pulmonary edema or has marginal to poor uterine artery blood flow because of vascular constriction, slowly induced epidural anesthesia may provide a beneficial vasodilation. Anesthesia-induced hypotension must be carefully avoided, however, because almost all therapies directed at restoration of blood pressure would be detrimental. Ephedrine could increase an already rapid HR, and IV fluid administration could precipitate or worsen pulmonary edema. A low dose of an α-agonist (e.g., 50 to 100 mcg of phenylephrine given intravenously) may be the least detrimental choice.

General Anesthesia

Succinylcholine is the muscle relaxant of choice during the rapid-sequence induction of an obstetric patient. In patients on magnesium therapy, defasciculation with a small dose of a nondepolarizing neuromuscular blocking agent is not recommended because significant paralysis may result, increasing the risk of aspiration of gastric contents. Magnesium potentiates depolarizing and, especially, nondepolarizing relaxants.[202,203] The amount of potentiation is variable, and a peripheral nerve stimulator is invaluable. The duration of paralysis after administration of a standard dose of succinylcholine may give a clue as to how much longer than normal the effect of a nondepolarizer will last.

Induction of general anesthesia in a patient receiving a β-agonist tocolytic can present a challenge. As with regional anesthesia, there are advantages to delaying induction of general anesthesia whenever possible until ritodrine has been largely eliminated (at least an hour).[208] Thiopental has a long, safe history of use in obstetric anesthesia, and its cardiovascular depression may offset some of the cardiac stimulation caused by the β-agonist. Propofol may also be used. The use of a vagolytic, such as atropine, glycopyrrolate, or pancuronium bromide, is counterproductive.

Induction of general anesthesia should usually be delayed until the patient has been prepared and the operating surgeon and assistants are ready for incision. Preterm neonates have a significantly higher incidence of low Apgar scores at 1 minute. Reducing the interval from the induction of anesthesia to the delivery of the infant minimizes the depressant effects of the anesthetic that the neonate must overcome.

In nonpregnant patients, opioids such as the fentanyl analogs are often used to blunt the sympathetic response to laryngoscopy and intubation. In pregnant patients, effective doses of fentanyl (5 to 8 mcg/kg) cross the placenta and result in significant neonatal depression. Fentanyl, 1 mcg/kg, administered before the induction of general anesthesia for cesarean section has been shown not to affect the Apgar score or neurobehavioral test results of neonates significantly.[209] By itself, this dose is certainly not enough to blunt the sympathetic response to laryngoscopy and intubation but will contribute to the goal. Of course, as more depressants are added, the option to allow the parturient to awaken and breathe spontaneously if it is impossible to intubate or ventilate her is less conceivable.

Finally, because the tocolytic effect of a β-agonist is no longer needed, β-blockers may be used carefully before the induction of anesthesia and instrumentation of the airway. Labetalol, a selective α₁- and nonselective β-receptor antagonist, has been used successfully to decrease maternal blood pressure while uteroplacental blood flow is maintained.[210,211] Neonatal side effects (hypotension, bradycardia) are apparently minimal.[212] In women with preeclampsia, labetalol has been administered before the induction of general anesthesia in order to decrease mean blood pressure at induction and during the first 10 minutes of anesthesia.[213]

Magnesium reduces the MAC of inhalation agents in rats to a clinically significant degree; ritodrine does not. Anesthetic depth has important implications for fetal oxygenation. Light anesthesia results in maternal catecholamine outflow in response to surgical stimulation, which in turn results in uterine artery constriction and a decrease in uterine artery blood flow. Anything that decreases uterine artery blood flow decreases uteroplacental blood flow and therefore results in fetal hypoxia.

Embolism

Thromboembolism

Thrombotic pulmonary embolism occurs in pregnant individuals five times more often than it does in nonpregnant individuals and is more likely to occur postpartum than antepartum. It is associated with prolonged inactivity, cesarean delivery, obesity, and increasing age and parity. The patient with pulmonary embolism may have a few minor complaints or a massive cardiovascular collapse. Pleuritic chest pain, dyspnea, hyperventilation, hypocapnia, coughing, hemoptysis, and distention of neck veins are associated with the disorder. Thromboembolism is a major cause of maternal mortality, but while the parturient is in the delivery area, it is less likely to occur than either amniotic fluid or air embolism.

Venous Air Embolism

Venous air embolism can occur during labor, spontaneous vaginal delivery, and operative delivery and is frequently associated with placenta previa. The overall incidence of subclinical venous air embolism in the parturient has been reported to be as high as 29%[214,215]; during general anesthesia, the incidence in the parturient may be as high as 97%.[216,217] Most venous air emboli are detected between delivery and uterine repair.[215,216] Air is entrained into open maternal venous sinuses in the uterine wall when the placenta separates or at the site of a surgical incision. Air returning to the heart may pass through a patent foramen ovale and form an embolism in any organ in the body. More often it passes through the right atrium and ventricle and lodges in the pulmonary arteries, impeding blood flow through the lungs. The resultant increase in pulmonary vascular resistance causes an increase in central venous pressure. A heavy, nonradiating, retrosternal chest pain may persist for 10 minutes after even a small venous air embolism. End-tidal CO_2 drops, because CO_2 cannot return to the lungs. A mill-wheel murmur may be heard over the precordium as a frothy air-blood mixture moves through the heart. This murmur is most pronounced when a large volume of air becomes trapped in the right ventricle. Dyspnea is common. If a sufficient number of pulmonary arteries are affected, cardiovascular collapse will occur.

The signs and symptoms of venous air embolism are as follows:
- Mill-wheel murmur detected over the precordium
- Chest pain
- Dyspnea
- Decreased end-tidal CO_2
- Elevated central venous pressure

Amniotic Fluid Embolism

Although rare, amniotic fluid embolism is almost uniformly fatal. It may occur during labor, vaginal delivery, or operative delivery and is associated with placental abruption. The pathogenesis is almost identical to that of venous air embolism except that patients who develop amniotic fluid embolism are prone to develop disseminated intravascular coagulation (DIC) if they survive the initial embolism. Signs and symptoms of amniotic fluid embolism include a chill, shivering, anxiety, cough, dyspnea, cyanosis, tachypnea, pulmonary edema, and cardiovascular collapse. O₂ saturation has been reported to decrease quickly.[217] This cascade often leads to death within a few minutes.

Anesthetic Implications

The incidence of postpartum thromboembolism can be affected by anesthetic interventions. Cesarean sections performed with general anesthesia are associated with accelerated maternal coagulation compared with those performed with regional anesthesia,[218] so the use of regional anesthesia may help reduce the incidence of postoperative thromboemboli. The anesthetist can help prevent prolonged inactivity in those who have had a cesarean section by providing analgesia sufficient to allow comfortable ambulation. Use of epidural opioid analgesia is often an appropriate solution to this problem. It may be specifically indicated in those at risk for thromboembolism, even if it must be administered after a general anesthetic has been given.

Because air embolism occurs when open veins are above the level of the heart, raising the head of the bed in order to position the uterus below the heart would seem to be useful for preventing embolization. However, a head-up tilt of between 5 and 10 degrees does not appear to decrease the incidence of venous air embolism during cesarean section and has increased the incidence of hypotension.[216,219] If embolism is suspected during spontaneous or operative delivery, the obstetrician should be informed immediately. The obstetrician can take steps to stop the entrainment of air or amniotic fluid, which include flooding the surgical field with saline, returning the uterus to within the abdomen, and stimulating uterine contractions.

One hundred percent O₂ should be administered by positive-pressure ventilation through a cuffed endotracheal tube. Nitrous oxide administration should be discontinued; it rapidly expands the volume of an air embolus and prevents the delivery of 100% O₂. An arterial line may be needed for monitoring of oxygenation and blood pressure. IV fluids are administered as needed to bolster central venous pressure. A generous preload is necessary to enable the right side of the heart to pump volume forward against increased pulmonary vascular resistance. If the fetus has not been delivered, left uterine displacement improves uterine blood flow and facilitates venous return to the heart. Pharmacologic support of the cardiovascular system is likely to be needed.

Patient position has been suggested to hinder the movement of the foreign substance into the pulmonary arteries. A slight anti-Trendelenburg (head-up) position with left lateral tilt of at least 15 degrees is designed to trap air in the right atrium, from which it can be aspirated via a central venous catheter. Unfortunately, it often is difficult to place the patient in this position and insert a central line in time to prevent pulmonary artery embolization.

In the case of amniotic fluid embolism, prompt recognition and action is necessary to prevent maternal mortality. Immediate support of maternal circulation is necessary. Inotropic support should not be delayed (epinephrine, dopamine). Treatment for coagulopathy must also begin immediately and ideally with the consultation of a hematologist. Large volume infusion devices may also be helpful for the resuscitation effort.

Blood Loss

Blood loss is difficult to estimate in the obstetric patient. Often, lost blood is hidden inside the women's body, soaked in laparotomy sponges, absorbed by drapes, or spilled onto the floor. In general, approximately 500 mL is lost during a spontaneous vaginal delivery and approximately 700 mL during a cesarean section with general anesthesia; 1500 mL or more is lost if a hysterectomy is performed during cesarean section. Because the term parturient has a 50% increase in blood volume, a great amount of blood can often be lost before the vital signs begin to change in response to the loss; 15% of the total blood volume may be lost without the occurrence of any compensatory tachycardia or vasoconstriction.[220] Hypotension may not occur until 30% of the total blood volume has been lost. Approximately 4% of all parturients who deliver vaginally experience excessive postpartum bleeding.[221]

Placenta Previa

When the placenta has implanted on the lower uterine segment and either partially or completely covers the opening of the cervix, placenta previa is present. Placenta previa has an incidence of up to 1%, and the mortality rate for those with it approaches 1%. Placenta previa is more common in women who have had it during a prior pregnancy. It most often results in painless vaginal bleeding before the onset of labor that may stop without intervention or hemodynamically significant blood loss. The potential exists, however, for *sudden* loss of large amounts of blood. The risk of bleeding increases if the placenta is disturbed by manual examination or cervical dilation. Postpartum bleeding is often increased as well because the lower uterine segment, where the placenta previa was implanted, does not contract as well as the rest of the uterus. Three variations of placenta previa are shown in Figure 47-17.

Anesthetic Implications

The diagnosis of placenta previa normally indicates an operative delivery. The anesthetist should prepare for heavy blood loss. The anesthetist may choose either a general or regional anesthetic technique, taking into consideration the parturient's current volume status and the potential for blood loss. Regional techniques should be performed only by an anesthetist who is very experienced with regional anesthesia and only after careful assessment and preparation.

Abnormal Placental Implantation

The placenta normally implants into the endometrium. A placenta implanted on or in the myometrium, the underlying

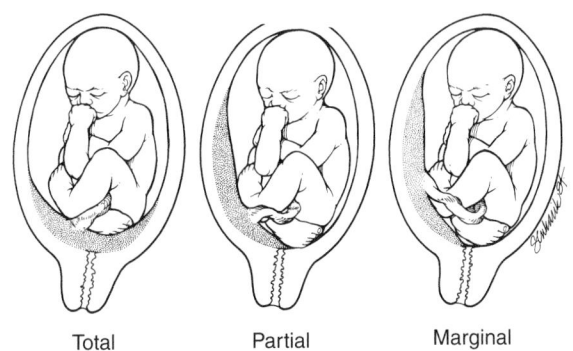

FIGURE **47-17** Three variations of placenta previa. (*From Chestnut DH. Obstetric Anesthesia: Principles and Practice. 3rd ed. Philadelphia: Mosby; 2004:663.*)

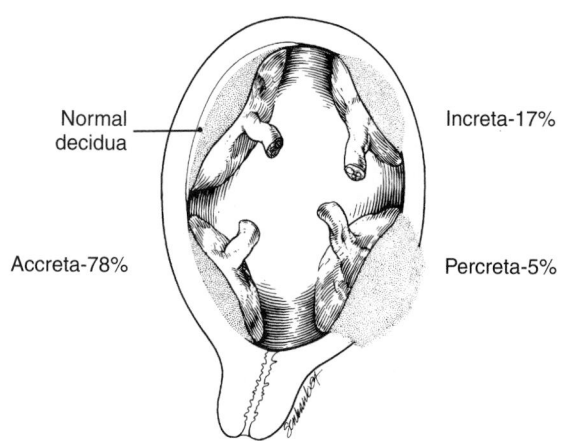

FIGURE **47-18**   An example of placenta increta, percreta and accreta. (*From Chestnut DH. Obstetric Anesthesia: Principles and Practice. 3rd ed. Philadelphia: Mosby; 2004:673.*)

muscular layer of the uterus, is termed *placenta accreta* (on the myometrium), *placenta increta* (into the myometrium), or *placenta percreta* (completely through the myometrium). Any of these abnormal placental implantations means that separation of the placenta from the uterine wall will be difficult and that separation may be accompanied by severe bleeding. Placenta accreta, placenta increta, and placenta percreta (Figure 47-18) are commonly associated with placenta previa and are more common in women who have had a previous cesarean section than in those who have not. The anesthetic implications are the same as those for other causes of increased blood loss.

Placental Abruption

Abruption occurs when the placenta begins to separate from the uterus before delivery; this allows bleeding behind the placenta and jeopardizes the fetal blood supply. Placental abruption results in bleeding (often hidden), uterine irritability (often hypertonic), abdominal pain, and fetal distress or death. Open venous sinuses in the uterine wall may allow products of hemostasis and amniotic fluid to enter the maternal circulation; this results in an incidence of DIC of up to 50%. The reported incidence of abruption in the general population varies widely but is much higher in women with hypertension (up to 23% among women with preeclampsia). When fetal death occurs, maternal mortality can exceed 10%.

Anesthetic Implications

In cases of placental abruption without fetal distress, vaginal delivery may still be possible. Because fetal distress can occur without warning, the anesthetist should be prepared to administer anesthesia for an emergency cesarean section. Taking an anesthetic history as soon as the diagnosis of placental abruption becomes known and checking for adequate IV access are recommended. If the mother is unstable or if fetal distress is present, operative delivery is necessary. Regional anesthesia usually is not indicated because of the potential for coagulopathy and because of the uncertainty of uteroplacental blood flow and therefore of fetal oxygenation. Generous venous access should be established as soon as possible. Although placental abruption does not usually result in sudden blood loss, a large volume of blood may be lost. When abruption results in fetal death, the volume of lost maternal blood can be as great as 5 L, all of which may be

concealed. Volume resuscitation should begin as soon as IV access has been secured. Large volumes of crystalloid and colloid solutions and of red blood cells may be needed.

General anesthesia can be induced with ketamine, up to 1 mg/kg. If the uterus is hypertonic, another drug should be chosen because the use of ketamine may further increase uterine tone, decreasing fetal O_2 supply. An alternate choice is etomidate, 0.3 mg/kg. If uterine tone is excessive, a volatile inhalation agent may be useful for maintenance of anesthesia and uterine relaxation. After the baby has been delivered, the uterus often becomes atonic; therefore, the use of inhalation agents should normally be discontinued. IV or intramyometrial oxytocin and intramyometrial ergotamine may be used with uterine massage to facilitate uterine contraction and to halt bleeding.

Postpartum Bleeding

Postpartum bleeding in moderate amounts is a normal event. Excessive bleeding may occur because of uterine atony (which accounts for 80% of all postpartum bleeding), placental retention, abnormalities of the uterus, lacerations of the delivery channel, uterine inversion, and abnormalities of coagulation. Uterine atony is associated with multiparity, prolonged infusions of oxytocin before delivery, polyhydramnios, and multiple gestation. A retained placenta or retained placental fragments must be removed manually to stop the bleeding. In the past, this has often required the administration of an inhalation agent for uterine relaxation. Nitroglycerin, a potent uterine relaxant with a relatively short duration of action, has been used successfully to provide uterine relaxation adequate for placental extraction. A dose of approximately 1 mcg/kg intravenously appears to be adequate.[222,223] Sublingual nitroglycerin spray has also been used effectively and offers the added benefits of long shelf life and a ready-to-use preparation.[224] Because nitroglycerin is a potent venodilator when given at low doses and is an arteriolar dilator when administered intravenously at a rate of 1 mcg/kg/min or higher, care should be taken to ensure that intravascular volume is adequate before this drug is administered. Analgesia for the procedure can be accomplished with a variety of methods, including the use of an already established epidural catheter or the administration of small IV doses of ketamine.

Anesthetic Implications

When postpartum bleeding is excessive, the anesthetist performs fluid resuscitation while simultaneously working with the obstetrician to eliminate the cause of the bleeding. Fundal massage, IV oxytocin, intramuscular methylergonovine maleate, or intramuscular prostaglandin often is all that is needed. In some cases anesthesia may be necessary for an additional procedure.

Uterine Rupture

Uterine rupture is most commonly associated with labor in the presence of a previous uterine incision (vaginal birth after cesarean, or VBAC) but may occur in an unscarred uterus.[225] The incidence of uterine rupture during attempted VBAC is approximately 0.6%.[226] Uterine rupture has also been associated with cocaine abuse during pregnancy.[227] The classic description of complete uterine rupture includes sudden, severe, tearing abdominal pain in a multiparous woman in hard labor. The pain may break through labor epidural anesthesia. Next, labor stops, and shock and fetal distress rapidly develop. Unfortunately, uterine rupture often does not present classically. For example, some ruptures occur during periods of mild labor.[228] The clinical finding most commonly associated with uterine rupture is an abnormal FHR tracing.[229,230] Whatever the presentation, bleeding is often severe. The uterus receives approximately 800 mL of blood per minute (approximately 10% of the cardiac output); therefore, a tear in this organ holds the potential for rapid exsanguination. Mortality from uterine rupture accounts for half of the maternal deaths attributed to blood loss each year. Fetal mortality after uterine rupture is nearly 80%.

Anesthetic Implications

Uterine rupture requires surgery for hemostasis and, often, for delivery. Anesthetists should be prepared for heavy bleeding commensurate with any severe abdominal trauma. In the operating room, as much as 3500 mL of blood has been found in the abdomen at incision.

Cesarean Hysterectomy

After delivery, when hemostasis is unobtainable despite the use of some combination of oxytocin, ergot alkaloids, and prostaglandin, the surgeon performs a hysterectomy to stop uterine bleeding. An atonic uterus, especially an incised uterus, can lose several liters of blood within a few minutes, outpacing the ability of even the most prepared anesthesia providers to replace intravascular volume. Anesthesia at this point becomes trauma anesthesia, the primary purpose of which is the maintenance of vital signs, vital organ perfusion, and oxygenation; maternal analgesia and amnesia are important but secondary concerns. Etomidate, ketamine, benzodiazepines, and opioids are useful because they cause minimal hemodynamic depression. If rapid blood loss begins during cesarean section with regional anesthesia, the anesthetist should consider the rapid induction of general anesthesia. It is difficult to manage volume resuscitation and to keep an awake patient both mentally and physically comfortable.

Disseminated Intravascular Coagulation

DIC is a generalized activation of the clotting system. It can occur when a large portion of the vascular system suffers damage or when thromboplastic material enters the general circulation. DIC is frequently associated with three obstetric problems: retention of a dead fetus, placental abruption, and amniotic fluid embolism. Circulatory shock, which often accompanies DIC, worsens the problem by decreasing peripheral and hepatic blood flow and causing further cell damage. Renal failure may result from the deposit of fibrin and cellular debris in the filtration system. Clinically the patient with DIC has uncontrolled bleeding because of the consumption of clotting factors. Laboratory studies show decreased levels of fibrinogen and platelets, increased prothrombin and partial thromboplastin times, and excessive amounts of fibrin degradation products.

Anesthetic Implications

The patient with DIC needs fluid resuscitation, and she almost always is hemorrhaging. Increasing intravascular volume dilutes activated clotting factors and slows the clotting process. Increased peripheral and hepatic perfusion limits cellular damage and improves clearance of activated clotting factors. Because the patient is bleeding and many clotting factors are depleted, it appears as if repletion of clotting factors is necessary; however, administration of clotting factors fuels an already out-of-control coagulation process. Definitive treatment of DIC first requires elimination of the cause. Replacement of clotting factors in the obstetric patient should probably be postponed until the DIC has subsided.

Breech Presentation

Many obstetricians now choose to deliver fetuses in breech presentations by cesarean section. In this case, cesarean section usually is elective, and either a regional or a general anesthetic can be used. If the baby is to be delivered vaginally, an epidural anesthetic may be requested and in fact is considered strongly indicated at some centers. The muscle relaxation that it provides is helpful, and some sort of analgesia is required, at least for the forceps delivery of the fetal head. Breech deliveries often result in laceration of the birth canal and therefore cause more bleeding than head-first deliveries.

Multiple Gestation

Multiple-gestation pregnancies carry higher risk for both mother and fetuses than singleton pregnancies. Many of the risk factors affect anesthetic management. Multiple-gestation pregnancies, especially rare monoamniotic pregnancies, are associated with complications requiring emergent surgical intervention more often than singleton pregnancies. The anesthetist should constantly be prepared to provide anesthesia for an emergency cesarean section. The multiple fetuses are often small and premature. The large uterus compounds the problems of aortocaval compression; therefore, left uterine displacement should be maintained at all times when the parturient is not lying on her side. If the fetuses are to be delivered vaginally, an epidural is valuable for maternal analgesia and neonatal safety. Because the neonate often is small and premature, a slow, controlled delivery through a well-relaxed birth canal makes birth trauma less likely. The epidural provides pelvic relaxation and reduces maternal discomfort, decreasing the likelihood that pain will induce a forceful reflexive expulsion of the fetus. Either regional or general anesthesia is appropriate for a cesarean section. After the babies have been delivered, the uterus may not contract well because it has been overstretched for many weeks. Larger than usual doses of oxytocin may be needed to induce the uterus to contract well and to stop bleeding. However, it is imperative that oxytocin administration not be started until after all the neonates have been delivered. Strong uterine contractions before the delivery of all neonates deprive any remaining fetuses of blood supply and oxygenation.

Prolapsed Umbilical Cord

A prolapsed umbilical cord is present when the cord protrudes through the cervix ahead of the fetus. Danger arises when compression of the cord against the wall of the cervix by the presenting part cuts off blood flow and oxygenation to the fetus. The obstetrician attempts either to restore blood flow in the umbilical cord by pushing the presenting part back into the uterus or to deliver the fetus abdominally before asphyxia causes permanent injury. In the first situation, anesthesia is likely to be needed for uterine relaxation; in the second it is necessary for emergent cesarean section.

Preeclampsia
Description

Preeclampsia is a vasospastic disease of pregnancy that affects 2.6% to 6% of parturients. The incidence of preeclampsia is highest in primigravidas younger than 20 years or older than 35 years of age and in women who have had preeclampsia during a previous pregnancy. The exact cause of preeclampsia is unknown but probably involves an abnormality in the ratio of thromboxanes to prostacyclins. Thromboxanes are potent vasoconstrictors and platelet aggregators, whereas prostacyclins have the opposite effect. Thromboxane A_2 and prostacyclin levels normally increase during pregnancy. An imbalance of prostacyclins and thromboxanes, both of which are produced by the placenta, has been demonstrated in preeclampsia.[231-233]

Preeclampsia results in hypertension, 1+ to 2+ proteinuria, and edema after the 20th week of gestation. Generally the diagnosis of preeclampsia is made when two of the three signs are present. Hypertension is defined as a blood pressure greater than 140/90 or more than 30 mm Hg above systolic baseline and more than 15 mm Hg above diastolic baseline.

Severe preeclampsia is said to exist when the following conditions are present: maternal blood pressure greater than 160/110, 3+ or 4+ proteinuria, urine output less than 20 mL/hr, CNS signs (blurred vision or changes in mentation), pulmonary edema, and epigastric pain. Blood pressure monitoring is a key indicator because it is technically easy to perform, and the severity of the hypertension frequently parallels the severity of the disease.

Preeclampsia results in maternal, fetal, and neonatal morbidity and mortality. The chief cause of maternal mortality is cerebral hemorrhage caused by hypertension. Pulmonary edema, renal failure, hepatic rupture, cerebral edema, and DIC also may cause maternal death. Brain edema results in CNS irritability, seizures (a significant percentage of which occur postpartum), and an increase in sensitivity to depressant drugs. Fetal death results primarily from placental abruption or infarct. Delivery of the fetus is curative.

Pathophysiology

No uniform agreement exists with regard to the pathophysiology of preeclampsia. One view is that preeclampsia is a hyperdynamic state involving an early increase in cardiac output and elevated SVR.[234,235] Another view is that preeclampsia is characterized by an increase in SVR and variable decrease in cardiac output.[236-239] In fact, SVRs of up to 4168 dyne • sec/cm^5 have been reported.[234] Thromboxane A_2 is found in increased levels during preeclampsia and has been correlated with disease severity.[240]

Increased vascular permeability results in extravasation of fluid and protein (proteinuria in the kidneys). Hypertension results in compensatory decreases in circulating blood volume and a loss of intravascular water and electrolytes via the kidney. Capillary injury stimulates platelet aggregation and fibrin deposition and may result in thrombocytopenia and, occasionally, DIC. It also results in multiple organ system dysfunction. Often, total body water is increased. Intravascular volume may decrease by as much as 40%. Marked peripheral and end-organ vasoconstriction is common, and it either causes or occurs in response to the decrease in vascular volume. An increased vascular sensitivity to vasopressin, angiotensin, and catecholamines has been demonstrated. Catecholamine levels often increase, and this results in decreased perfusion to the uterus, placenta, and fetus. Arteriolar constriction increases left ventricular work. When preeclampsia becomes severe, intravascular volume is either contracted or shifted centrally.

Central venous pressure may be low because of a contracted blood volume, or it may be relatively normal because of a redistribution of vascular volume into the central circulation. Pulmonary capillary occlusion pressure may be normal or high because of left-sided heart failure and often does not correlate well with the central venous pressure.

Uteroplacental insufficiency can result from a combination of decreased intravascular volume, vascular intimal deterioration, and increased vascular resistance. Placental perfusion in the preeclampsia patient may decrease by 70% compared with that in a healthy parturient. Decreased placental perfusion leads to intrauterine growth restriction and can cause fetal hypoxia and placental infarction.

Platelet aggregation and fibrin deposition increase in preeclampsia. Platelet counts may drop as the platelets are consumed; however, even in the presence of a normal platelet count, platelet function may be below normal.

Obstetric Management

Magnesium sulfate is almost always administered to women with preeclampsia in the United States. Although it is not curative, it has been shown to reduce the likelihood of eclampsia by 58% and the risk of maternal death by 45%.[241] Delivery presently is the only definitive way of ending the disease process of preeclampsia. When a fetus is at a gestational age of more than 37 weeks, obstetricians generally proceed with delivery. If the fetus is immature, delivery is delayed to allow the fetus time to mature. If preeclampsia is severe or fetal distress occurs, delivery is usually accomplished expeditiously. In any case, obstetric treatment is aimed at preventing eclampsia (seizures), avoiding decreases in uteroplacental blood flow, and maximizing organ perfusion. Magnesium sulfate, which is also used as a tocolytic, causes venodilation, mild CNS depression, a decrease in the rate of fibrin deposition, and a reduction in uterine activity, if present. Decreasing fibrin deposition prevents further decay in organ perfusion and often greatly decreases liver pain in parturients with hemolysis, elevated liver enzymes, and a low platelet count (HELLP syndrome). Magnesium therapy is continued after delivery for the suppression of seizures.

Regional Anesthesia and Preeclampsia

Epidural analgesia and anesthesia generally are preferred for both spontaneous vaginal delivery and cesarean section in the preeclampsia patient when they are not contraindicated. A carefully initiated epidural infusion helps control maternal hypertension and may improve organ blood flow. Characteristic changes in vital signs in women with preeclampsia before volume expansion, after volume expansion, and after institution of epidural analgesia are shown in Figure 47-19. Careful initiation of the block is necessary in women with preeclampsia, because their mean blood pressure tends to decrease more than that of healthy parturients (Figure 47-20). During a cesarean section, epidural anesthesia avoids stimulation of the airway, which can aggravate hypertension and possibly cause cerebral bleeding. During a vaginal delivery, epidural analgesia allows a slower, more controlled expulsion of the premature infant and decreases the likelihood of trauma to the fetal head. Even these advantages, however, must be weighed against the risks of regional anesthesia, primarily hypotension and bleeding.

Because thrombocytopenia and other coagulation problems are associated with preeclampsia, careful consideration should be given to the patient's coagulation status before regional anesthesia is begun. A careful history of bleeding should be taken and a platelet count evaluated before insertion of an epidural catheter in a patient with a diagnosis of preeclampsia. Coagulation problems are found almost exclusively in women with platelet counts below 100,000/mm^3.[242,243] Several studies indicate that significant decreases in platelet count occur almost exclusively in women with severe preeclampsia (diastolic blood pressure

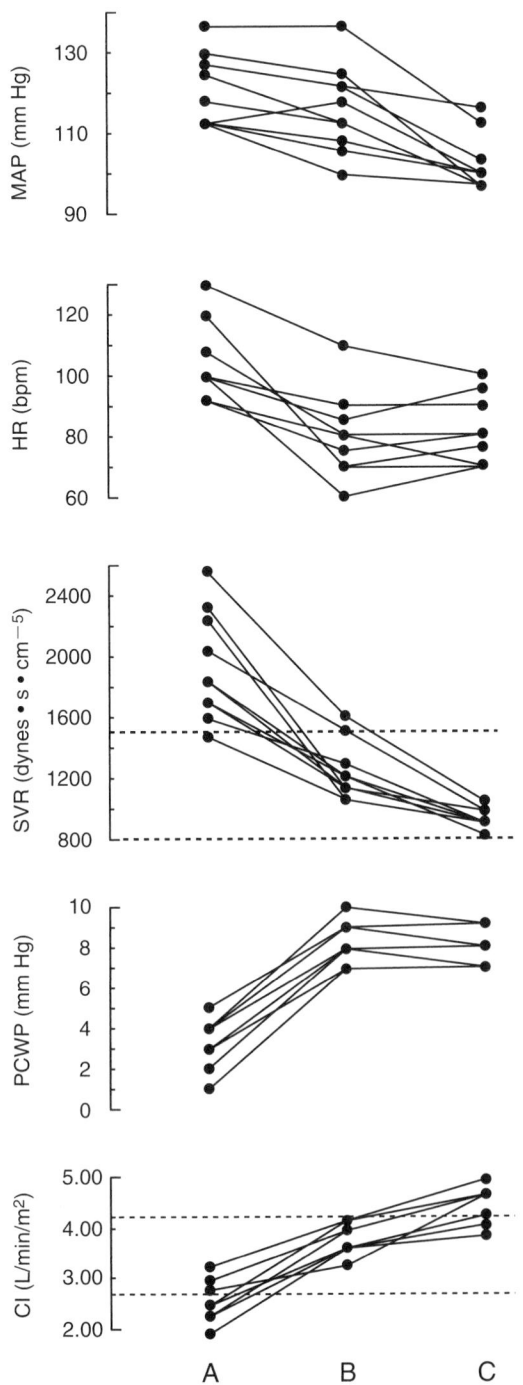

FIGURE **47-19**   Individual hemodynamic values before (**A**) and after (**B**) volume expansion and after vasodilation (**C**) in women with pregnancy-induced hypertension. The dotted lines represent the normal range for nonpregnant individuals. *CI,* Cardiac index; *HR,* heart rate; *MAP,* mean arterial pressure; *PCWP,* pulmonary capillary wedge pressure; *SVR,* systemic vascular resistance. (*From Groenendijk R et al. Hemodynamic measurements in preeclampsia: preliminary observations. Am J Obstet Gynecol. 1984;150:232-236.*)

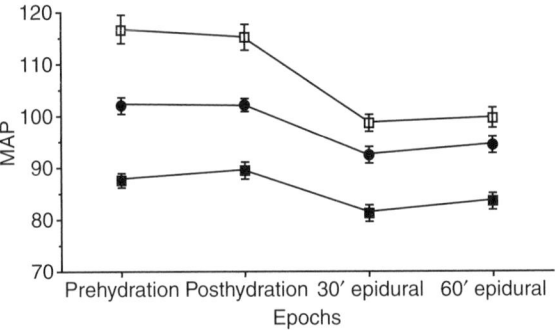

FIGURE **47-20**   Mean arterial pressure (MAP) of three study groups compared over four epochs. All values are expressed as group means; the bars represent standard errors. Maternal MAP decreased significantly in all groups after epidural blockade was established. *Closed circles,* Chronic hypertension; *closed squares,* normal; *open squares,* preeclampsia. (*From Ramos-Santos E et al. The effects of epidural anesthesia on the Doppler velocimetry of umbilical and uterine arteries in normal and hypertensive patients during active term labor. Obstet Gynecol. 1991;77:20-25. Reprinted with permission from The American College of Obstetricians and Gynecologists.*)

women with mild preeclampsia and 34% of women with severe preeclampsia had prolonged bleeding times.[245] The platelet count correlated with prolongation of the bleeding time only when it was less than 100,000/mm^3.[244] When the platelet count falls below 100,000/mm^3, it is not likely to recover until several days after delivery.[246]

Some evidence indicates that epidural analgesia can improve uteroplacental perfusion, and therefore fetal oxygenation, by decreasing plasma catecholamines.[247,248] Epidural analgesia causes vascular dilation; this decreases blood pressure while maintaining—and, in some cases, improving—perfusion of the uterus and other organs, as long as hypotension is not allowed.[247-255] Uterine artery systolic/diastolic ratios in women with preeclampsia decrease after the initiation of epidural analgesia, suggesting that resistance to blood flow is lowered.[248] Diastolic blood pressure should not be reduced to less than 90 mm Hg in women with severe preeclampsia, because such a reduction will probably result in inadequate uteroplacental blood flow. Hypotension is a significant concern in the parturient with severe preeclampsia because of the sometimes constricted intravascular volume and the likelihood that the patient has already received an antihypertensive agent such as hydralazine or labetalol. When hypotension does occur, ephedrine and other vasopressors should be used cautiously, because they may produce an exaggerated response in the preeclampsia patient.

Epidural anesthesia can be accomplished safely in these patients if careful attention is devoted to volume status. Most but not all preeclampsia patients have a contracted blood volume.[254] IV preloading may be necessary because of the constricted intravascular volume; however, some patients have a normal central venous pressure or left ventricular dysfunction. Preloading in these patients can result in pulmonary edema. Placement of a central venous pressure line or pulmonary catheter may be indicated in severe preeclampsia when the patient is oliguric or hypoxic. Central line insertion probably is not indicated for anesthesia alone unless the line is needed for a general anesthetic and operative delivery. If so, the anesthetist must balance the benefits of infusing platelets and inserting a central

>110 mm Hg and urinary protein of at least 2+). Others do not believe that any correlation exists between the severity of preeclampsia and platelet count.[244] The normal bleeding time in healthy pregnant women appears to be approximately 5 minutes. When the platelet count was greater than 100,000/mm^3, 13% of

line against the risks. The most useful platelet count is one of a continuous series and is as recent as possible, because the count may decrease precipitously as the disease progresses.

Bupivacaine is usually the local anesthetic of choice because of its long history of safe use in preeclampsia patients and because it has a slower onset than lidocaine and chloroprocaine. The slower onset allows time for the anesthetist to react to hemodynamic changes. Often, it is necessary to begin administering epidural anesthesia slowly with bupivacaine in these patients without any intravascular prehydration. Small incremental doses of bupivacaine can be administered and fluid given intravenously as needed when and if changes in blood pressure occur.

After epidural analgesia or anesthesia has been instituted, the sympathectomy should not be allowed to wear off abruptly, because the increased intravascular volume could precipitate a hypertensive crisis or pulmonary edema. Instead, the block should be allowed to recede slowly, when the body is able to eliminate the intravascular fluid load and adequate monitoring is available.

General Anesthesia and Preeclampsia

Coagulopathy or decay in maternal or fetal condition is the most common indication for general anesthesia in the patient with preeclampsia. The maternal brain is edematous and more sensitive to CNS-depressant drugs. Induction of general anesthesia is hazardous in persons with preeclampsia. Their exaggerated hypertensive response to laryngoscopy and endotracheal intubation is potentially lethal. Compounding the problem, upper airway swelling may make identification of landmarks and intubation more difficult. Swelling may preclude the insertion of an endotracheal tube of normal size. Difficulty in intubation increases the duration of airway stimulation and worsens hypertension. The challenge during induction of general anesthesia is prevention of a further increase in blood pressure, which may result in intracranial hemorrhage. Antihypertensives have long been used to control blood pressure during preeclampsia. Nevertheless, an average increase of 56 mm Hg in systolic blood pressure has been reported after induction of general anesthesia despite the use of β-blockers, trimethaphan, or both.[255] Comatose patients have even greater increases in systolic blood pressure (up to 70 mm Hg). Control of blood pressure during induction of general anesthesia in these patients demands careful planning and skill in implementation.

Opioids to Control Blood Pressure

Opioids have long been known to attenuate the sympathetic response to laryngoscopy and intubation. Fentanyl, 5 to 8 mcg/kg, has been shown to be effective in nonpregnant individuals, but this dose is infrequently used in obstetrics for fear of neonatal respiratory depression. For many years opioids were simply not used in obstetric anesthesia. However, studies have shown that small doses of fentanyl or alfentanil given before induction of general anesthesia help attenuate the sympathetic response to laryngoscopy without causing neonatal respiratory depression.[256-259] Figure 47-21 shows the changes in systolic and diastolic blood pressure with and without the administration of 10 mcg of alfentanil per kilogram 1 minute before the induction of general anesthesia for cesarean section. The data in these figures were collected from healthy women undergoing cesarean section. Blood pressure changes in women with preeclampsia are likely to be more pronounced. Table 47-1 provides neonatal data for both control (no alfentanil before induction) and

alfentanil induction groups. Using opioids to blunt blood pressure increases is not without risk. If the anesthetist is unable to manage the airway after a rapid-sequence induction, the chance that the woman will reawaken and breathe in a reasonable amount of time is decreased.

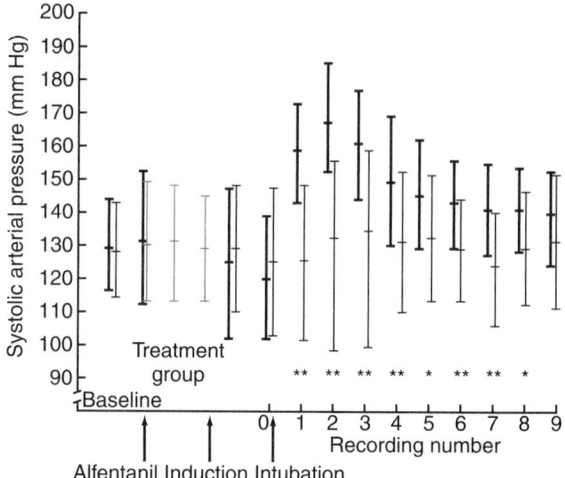

FIGURE **47-21** Changes (1 SD) in systolic blood pressure before and after the induction of anesthesia, in the control group (*bold bars*) and the treatment group (*narrow bars*). The shaded area represents the time from the administration of alfentanil to the administration of thiopental and therefore is of significance only for the treatment group. By *t*-test: *P.05; **P.01; others not significant. (*From Dann WL et al. Maternal and neonatal responses to alfentanil administered before induction of general anesthesia for cesarean section. Br J Anaesth. 1987;59:1392-1396.*)

TABLE **47-1**	Neonatal Results after Maternal Administration of Alfentanil, 10 mcg/kg, 1 Minute before Induction of General Anesthesia	
	Control (n = 16)	**Alfentanil (n = 21)**
Induction-to-delivery interval (min, mean [SD])	10.4 (2.6)	11.8 (2.5)
Weight (g, mean [SD])	3280 (690)	3240 (600)
Intubated	0	0
Received naloxone	0	0
Admitted to special baby unit	1	2
Apgar score at 1 min		
Median	9	9
Range	4-10	5-10
Apgar score at 10 min		
Median	10	10
Range	(All 10)	9-10

From Dann WL et al. Maternal and neonatal responses to alfentanil administered before induction of general anesthesia for cesarean section. Br J Anaesth. 1987;59:1392-1396.

Antihypertensives to Control Blood Pressure

Labetalol, a combined selective α_1- and nonselective β-antagonist, is widely used in obstetric anesthesia. Uteroplacental blood flow is maintained or increased when a total of up to 1 mg of labetalol per kilogram is used for treatment of preeclampsia.[210,211,213,260,261] Neonatal side effects (hypotension, bradycardia, hypoglycemia) are apparently minimal when this dose is used.[212,262-264] The fetal-to-maternal ratio of plasma levels for labetalol has been reported to be 0.5.[265] In women with preeclampsia, the administration of labetalol before induction of general anesthesia results in a lower mean blood pressure at induction and during the first 10 minutes of anesthesia.[213,266] Although the elimination half-life of labetalol is between 5 and 8 hours in nonpregnant adults, it is only 1.7 hours in pregnant adults.[265]

Hydralazine increases splanchnic, coronary, cerebral, uterine, and renal blood flow as long as hypotension is not allowed. Resistance vessels in these vascular beds are more affected than those of the skin and skeletal muscle. Hydralazine is favored in the preeclampsia patient because it may actually improve uteroplacental circulation. It is also a potent pulmonary arterial dilator. The long onset time (10 to 20 minutes) probably precludes use immediately before an emergent cesarean section.

IV nitroglycerin has a quick onset, but its antihypertensive effect is less predictable than that of other drugs. Nevertheless, it is widely used for this purpose. The fetal-to-maternal ratio of nitroglycerin blood levels in sheep is only 0.04.[267] If this is true in humans, it represents very low placental passage and could give nitroglycerin a significant advantage over other antihypertensives.

In one study, when a nitroglycerin infusion was begun before induction, the maximum MAP after intubation was 119 mm Hg in the nitroglycerin group and 155 mm Hg in the control group.[268] Nitroglycerin may, however, result in an increase in intracranial pressure in women with severe preeclampsia.

Nitroprusside has a fast onset and is easily titratable. Although at least theoretic concerns regarding neonatal cyanide toxicity exist, this should not be a problem if the drug is used briefly during the induction of anesthesia. Nitroprusside has been used for intracranial procedures during pregnancy without fetal toxicity. Probably to a greater degree than even nitroglycerin, nitroprusside may cause deleterious increases in maternal intracranial pressure.

Esmolol was initially thought to hold promise for attenuating the hypertension and tachycardia of laryngoscopy in preeclampsia patients because (1) early investigations reported the inability to measure any esmolol in fetal sheep 10 minutes after the discontinuation of an esmolol infusion, and (2) immature neonatal red blood cells hydrolyzed esmolol. A subsequent case report of a woman who was 22 weeks pregnant and underwent repair of a cerebellar arteriovenous malformation demonstrated only a mild effect on FHR both preoperatively and intraoperatively.[269] Unfortunately, more detailed studies have shown that except at very low doses, esmolol does cross the placenta and may result in clinically significant fetal β-blockade.[270]

Whichever antihypertensive drug is used, it is wise to perform a test run before the induction of general anesthesia. This test indicates whether the agent will yield the desired result and also allows estimation of the proper dose.

Muscle Relaxants

Nondepolarizing relaxants are markedly potentiated in women with preeclampsia and therapeutic levels of magnesium. In these patients, half of an effective dose in 95% of the population dose produced 100% block for 35 minutes.[203] In healthy parturients not receiving magnesium sulfate, the same dose on average produced 42% blockade for approximately 9 minutes. Reduced doses of nondepolarizers can be used, if desired, but these drugs yield a longer-than-usual block.

HELLP Syndrome

HELLP syndrome consists of *h*emolysis, *e*levated *l*iver enzymes, and a *l*ow *p*latelet count. From 5% to 10% of the sickest women with preeclampsia develop HELLP syndrome. Clinical signs of HELLP syndrome include epigastric pain, upper abdominal tenderness, proteinuria, hypertension, jaundice, nausea, and vomiting. Rarely, HELLP syndrome may result in liver rupture. Some experts believe that a degree of compensated DIC is present in all patients with HELLP syndrome.

ANESTHESIA FOR THE PREGNANT PATIENT UNDERGOING A NONOBSTETRIC PROCEDURE

Occasionally anesthetists must provide anesthesia care for a pregnant woman having nonobstetric emergency procedures. Some key points are noted in Box 47-7.

> **BOX 47-7**
>
> **Key Points for the Pregnant Patient Undergoing Nonobstetric Procedure**
>
> - A significant number of women undergo anesthesia and surgery during pregnancy for procedures unrelated to delivery.
> - Maternal risks are associated with the anatomic and physiologic changes of pregnancy (e.g., difficult intubation, aspiration) and with the underlying maternal disease.
> - The diagnosis of abdominal conditions often is delayed during pregnancy, which increases the risk of maternal and fetal morbidity.
> - Maternal catastrophes involving severe hypoxia, hypotension, and acidosis pose the greatest acute risk to the fetus.
> - Other fetal risks associated with surgery include increased fetal loss, increased incidence of preterm labor, growth restriction, and low birth weight. Clinical studies suggest that anesthesia and surgery during pregnancy do not increase the risk of congenital anomalies.
> - It is unclear whether adverse fetal outcomes result from the anesthetic, the operation, or the underlying maternal disease.
> - No anesthetic agent is a proven teratogen in humans, although some anesthetic agents, specifically nitrous oxide, are teratogenic in animals under certain conditions.
> - Many anesthetic agents have been used for anesthesia during pregnancy, with no demonstrable differences in maternal or fetal outcome.
> - The anesthesia management of the pregnant surgical patient should focus on the avoidance of hypoxemia, hypotension, acidosis, and hyperventilation.

From Naughton NN, Cohen SE. Nonobstetric surgery during pregnancy. In: Chestnut DH, ed. Obstetric Anesthesia. 3rd ed. Philadelphia: Mosby; 2004:269.

NEONATAL RESUSCITATION

All labor and delivery personnel should be trained in basic neonatal resuscitation, including anesthetists. The drugs and equipment must be readily available for all deliveries (Box 47-8). The anesthetist in clinical practice may participate in neonatal resuscitation, but a single anesthetist is responsible for attending to the care of the mother.

Approximately 15% of newborns require resuscitation, but this can generally be predicted from the known risk factors (Box 47-9). Tactile stimulation of the newborn will often result in spontaneous respiration. If spontaneous respiration is delayed after stimulation, initiation of assisted ventilation should begin.

The Apgar scoring system is widely used to assess newborns. The score is derived from five parameters including heart rate, respiratory rate, muscle tone, reflex irritability, and color. The assessment is performed at 1 minute and again at 5 minutes. The score is used to guide resuscitation. A score of 8 to 10 is considered normal, 4 to 7 indicates moderate distress or impairment, and 0 to 3 indicates the need for immediate resuscitation.

If the parturient has received prenatal care, there may be previous knowledge or suspicions of a congenital anomaly that may be used to guide resuscitation. In the event of little or no prenatal care, this information may be unavailable. Special circumstances of resuscitation are shown in Table 47-2 that can be used to identify clinical signs of various conditions and the resuscitative action required.

SUMMARY

Nurse anesthetists play a major role in the provision of obstetric anesthesia care. The practice of obstetric anesthesia has the additional challenge of the safety of the newborn. The satisfaction attained from successful maternal and fetal outcomes is like no other in medicine. Advances in monitoring and prenatal care have allowed for continuous refinements in regional and, when necessary, general anesthesia management of these patients.

BOX 47-8

Equipment and Drugs Needed for Neonatal Resuscitation

Suction Equipment
Bulb syringe
Mechanical suction and tubing
Suction catheters, 5F or 6F, 8F, and 10F or 12F
8F feeding tube and 20-mL syringe
Meconium aspiration device

Bag-and-Mask Equipment
Neonatal resuscitation bag with a pressure-release valve or pressure manometer (the bag must be capable of delivering 90% to 100% oxygen)
Face masks, newborn and preterm sizes (masks with cushioned rim preferred)
Oxygen with flowmeter (flow rate up to 10 L/min) and tubing (including portable oxygen cylinders)

Intubation Equipment
Laryngoscope with straight blades, No. 0 (preterm) and No. 1 (term)
Extra bulbs and batteries for laryngoscope
Tracheal tubes, 2.5, 3.0, 3.5, and 4.0 mm ID
Stylet (optional)
Scissors
Tape or securing device for tracheal tube
Alcohol sponges
CO_2 detector (optional)
Laryngeal mask airway (optional)

Medications
Epinephrine 1:10,000 (0.1 mg/mL): 3- or 10-mL ampules
Isotonic crystalloid (normal saline or Ringer's lactate) for volume expansion: 100 or 250 mL

Sodium bicarbonate 4.2% (5 mEq/10 mL): 10-mL ampules
Naloxone hydrochloride 0.4 mg/mL: 1-mL ampules (or 1 mg/mL: 2-mL ampules)
Normal saline, 30 mL
Dextrose 10%, 250 mL
Normal saline "fish" or "bullet" (optional)
Feeding tube, 5F (optional)
Umbilical vessel catheterization supplies
Sterile gloves
Scalpel or scissors
Povidone-iodine solution
Umbilical tape
Umbilical catheters, 3.5-F, 5-F
Three-way stopcock
Syringes, 1, 3, 5, 10, 20, and 50 mL
Needles, 25-, 21-, and 18-gauge, or puncture device for needleless system

Miscellaneous
Gloves and appropriate personal protection
Radiant warmer or other heat source
Firm, padded resuscitation surface
Clock (timer optional)
Warmed linens
Stethoscope
Tape, ½- or ¾-inch
Cardiac monitor and electrodes and/or pulse oximeter with probe (optional for delivery room)
Oropharyngeal airways

From Niermeyer S et al. International guidelines for neonatal resuscitation: an excerpt from the Guidelines 2000 for Cardiopulmonary Resuscitation and Emergency Cardiovascular Care: International Consensus on Science. Pediatrics. 2000;106:E29:1-16.

BOX **47-9**

Risk Factors Suggesting an Increased Need for Neonatal Resuscitation

Antepartum Risk Factors
Maternal diabetes
Pregnancy-induced hypertension
Chronic hypertension
Chronic maternal illness
Cardiovascular
Thyroid
Neurologic
Pulmonary
Renal
Anemia or isoimmunization
Previous fetal or neonatal death
Bleeding in second or third trimester
Maternal infection
Polyhydramnios
Oligohydramnios
Premature rupture of membranes
Postterm gestation
Multiple gestation
Size-dates discrepancy
Drug therapy, e.g.:
    Lithium carbonates
    Magnesium
    Adrenergic-blocking drugs
Maternal substance abuse

Fetal malformation
Diminished fetal activity
No prenatal care
Age <16 or >35 years

Intrapartum Risk Factors
Emergency cesarean section
Forceps or vacuum-assisted delivery
Breech or other abnormal presentation
Premature labor
Precipitous labor
Chorioamnionitis
Prolonged rupture of membranes (>18 hours before delivery)
Prolonged labor (>24 hours)
Prolonged second stage of labor (>2 hours)
Fetal bradycardia
Nonreassuring fetal heart rate patterns
Use of general anesthesia
Uterine tetany
Narcotics administered to mother within 4 hours of delivery
Meconium-stained amniotic fluid
Prolapsed cord
Abruptio placentae
Placenta previa

From Niermeyer S et al. International guidelines for neonatal resuscitation: an excerpt from the Guidelines 2000 for Cardiopulmonary Resuscitation and Emergency Cardiovascular Care: International Consensus on Science. Pediatrics. 2000;106:E29:1-16.

TABLE **47-2** Special Circumstances in Resuscitation of the Newly Born Infant

Condition	History/Clinical Signs	Actions
Mechanical Blockage of the Airway		
Meconium or mucus blockage	Meconium-stained amniotic fluid Poor chest-wall movement	Intubation for suctioning/ventilation
Choanal atresia	Pink when crying, cyanotic when quiet	Oral airway Endotracheal intubation
Pharyngeal airway malformation	Persistent retractions, poor air entry	Prone positioning, posterior nasopharyngeal tube
Impaired Lung Function		
Pneumothorax	Asymmetric breath sounds Persistent cyanosis/bradycardia	Needle thoracentesis
Pleural effusions/ascites	Diminished air movement Persistent cyanosis/bradycardia	Immediate intubation Needle thoracentesis, paracentesis Possible volume expansion
Congenital diaphragmatic hernia	Asymmetric breath sounds Persistent cyanosis/bradycardia Scaphoid abdomen	Endotracheal intubation Placement of orogastric catheter
Pneumonia/sepsis	Diminished air movement Persistent cyanosis/bradycardia	Endotracheal intubation Possible volume expansion
Impaired Cardiac Function		
Congenital heart disease	Persistent cyanosis/bradycardia	Diagnostic evaluation
Fetal/maternal hemorrhage	Pallor; poor response to resuscitation	Volume expansion, possibly including red blood cells

From Niermeyer S et al. International guidelines for neonatal resuscitation: an excerpt from the Guidelines 2000 for Cardiopulmonary Resuscitation and Emergency Cardiovascular Care: International Consensus on Science. Pediatrics. 2000;106:E29:1-16.

REFERENCES

1. Capeless EL, Clapp JR. Cardiovascular changes in the early stages of pregnancy. Am J Obstet Gynecol. 1989;161:1439.
2. Widerhorn J et al. WPW syndrome during pregnancy: increased incidence of supraventricular arrhythmias. Am Heart J. 1992;123:796.
3. Mabie WC et al: A longitudinal study of cardiac output in normal human pregnancy. Am J Obstet Gynecol. 1994;170:849.
4. Hennessy TG et al. Serial changes in cardiac output during normal pregnancy: a Doppler ultrasound study. Eur J Obstet Gynecol Reprod Biol. 1996;70:117-122.
5. Robson SC et al. Maternal hemodynamics after normal delivery and delivery complicated by postpartum hemorrhage. Obstet Gynecol. 1989;74:234-239.
6. Cole PL, St John Sutton M. Normal cardiopulmonary adjustments to pregnancy: cardiovascular evaluation. Cardiovasc Clin. 1989;19:37.
7. Conklin KA. Maternal physiological adaptations during gestation, labor and the puerperium. Semin Anesth. 1991;10:221-234.
8. Schrier RW, Briner VA. Peripheral arterial vasodilation hypothesis of sodium and water retention in pregnancy: implications for pathogenesis of preeclampsia-eclampsia. Obstet Gynecol. 1991;77:632-639.
9. Leduc L et al. Baroreflex function in normal pregnancy. Am J Obstet Gynecol. 1991;163:886-890.
10. van Oppen AC et al. A longitudinal study of maternal hemodynamics during normal pregnancy. Obstet Gynecol. 1996;88:40-46.
11. Clark SL et al. Central hemodynamic assessment of normal term pregnancy. Am J Obstet Gynecol. 1989;161:1439-1442.
12. Greenwood JP et al. Sympathetic neural mechanisms in normal and hypertensive pregnancy in humans. Circulation. 2001;104:2200-2204.
13. van Mook WN, Peeters L. Severe cardiac disease in pregnancy, part I: hemodynamic changes and complaints during pregnancy, and general management of cardiac disease in pregnancy. Curr Opin Crit Care. 2005;11:430-434.
14. August P et al. Role of renin-angiotensin system in blood pressure regulation in pregnancy. Lancet. 1995;345:896-897.
15. Magness RR et al. Angiotensin II metabolic clearance rate and pressor responses in nonpregnant and pregnant women. Am J Obstet Gynecol. 1994;171:668-679.
16. Lumbers ER. Peripheral vascular reactivity to angiotensin and noradrenaline in pregnant and non-pregnant women. Aust J Exp Biol Med Sci. 1970;48:493-500.
17. Chesley LC et al. Vascular reactivity to angiotensin II and norepinephrine in pregnant and nonpregnant women. Am J Obstet Gynecol. 1965;91:837-842.
18. Delemarre FM et al. Diurnal variation in angiotensin sensitivity in pregnancy. Am J Obstet Gynecol. 1996;174:259-261.
19. Davison JM et al. Changes in the metabolic clearance of vasopressin and in plasma vasopressinase throughout human pregnancy. J Clin Invest. 1989;83:1313-1318.
20. Howard BK et al. Supine hypotensive syndrome in late pregnancy. Obstet Gynecol. 1953;1:371-377.
21. McRoberst WA Jr. Postural shock in pregnancy. Am J Obstet Gynecol. 1951;62:627.
22. Pirhonen JP, Erkkola RU. Uterine and umbilical flow velocity waveforms in the supine hypotensive syndrome. Obstet Gynecol. 1990;76:176-179.
23. Bamber JH, Dresner M. Aortocaval compression in pregnancy: the effect of changing the degree and direction of lateral tilt on maternal cardiac output. Anesth Analg. 2003;97:256-258.
24. Jones SJ et al. Comparison of measured and estimated angles of table tilt at caesarean section. Br J Anaesth. 2003;90:86-87.
25. Bourne T et al. Nocturnal hypoxaemia in late pregnancy. Br J Anaesth. 1995;75:678-682.
26. Tygart SG et al: Longitudinal studies of platelet indices during normal pregnancy. Am J Obstet Gynecol. 1986;154:883-887.
27. Datta S et al. Chronically administered progesterone decreases halothane requirements in rabbits. Anesth Analg. 1989;68:46-50.
28. Palahniuk RJ et al. Pregnancy decreases the requirements for inhaled anesthetic agents. Anesthesiology. 1974;41:82-83.
29. Flanagan HL et al. Effect of pregnancy on bupivacaine-induced conduction blockade in the isolated rabbit vagus nerve. Anesth Analg. 1987;66:123-126.
30. Butterworth JF et al. Pregnancy increases median nerve susceptibility to lidocaine. Anesthesiology. 1990;72:962-965.
31. Gintzer AR. Endorphin-mediated increases in pain threshold during pregnancy. Eur J Pharmacol. 1989;159:205-209.
32. Wyner J, Cohen SI. Gastric volume in early pregnancy: effect of metoclopramide. Anesthesiology. 1982;57:209-212.
33. Carp H et al. Ultrasound examination of the stomach contents of parturients. Anesth Analg. 1992;74:683-687.
34. Rout CC et al. Intravenous ranitidine reduces the risk of acid aspiration of gastric contents at emergency cesarean section. Anesth Analg. 1993;76:156-161.
35. Beilin Y et al. Practice patterns of anesthesiologists regarding situations in obstetric anesthesia where clinical management is controversial. Anesth Analg. 1996;83:735-741.
36. Clarke S. Informed consent without bureaucracy. J Clin Neurosci. 2003;10:35-36.
37. Wright RG et al. The effect of maternal administration of ephedrine on fetal heart rate and variability. Am J Obstet Gynecol. 1981;57:734-738.
38. Petrie RH et al. The effect of drugs on fetal heart rate variability. Am J Obstet Gynecol. 1978;130:294-299.
39. Zimmer EZ et al. Influence of meperidine on fetal movements and heart rate beat-to-beat variability in the active phase of labor. Am J Perinatol. 1988;5:197-200.
40. Rayburn WF et al. Randomized comparison of meperidine and fentanyl during labor. Obstet Gynecol. 1989;74:604-606.
41. Alahuhta S et al. Epidural sufentanil and bupivacaine for labor analgesia and Doppler velocimetry of the umbilical and uterine arteries. Anesthesiology. 1993;78:231-236.
42. Petrikovsky BM, Vintzileos AM. Magnesium sulfate and intrapartum fetal behavior. Am J Perinatol. 1990;7:154-156.
43. Hatjis CG, Meis PJ. Sinusoidal fetal heart rate pattern associated with butorphanol administration. Obstet Gynecol. 1986;67:377-380.
44. Amin-Somuah M et al. Epidural versus non-epidural or no analgesia in labour. Cochrane Database Syst Rev. 2005;4:CD000331. DOI: 10.1002/14651858.CD000331.pub 2.
45. Rayburn WF et al. Comparison of patient-controlled and nurse administered analgesia using fentanyl during labor. Anesthesiol Rev. 1991;18:31-36.
46. Smith CV et al. Influence of intravenous fentanyl on fetal biophysical parameters during labor. J Maternal-Fetal Med. 1996;2:89-92.
47. Atkinson BD et al. Double-blind comparison of intravenous butorphanol (Stadol) and fentanyl (Sublimaze) for analgesia during labor. Am J Obstetr Gynecol. 1994;171:993-998.
48. Rosaeg OP et al. Maternal and fetal effects of intravenous patient-controlled fentanyl analgesia during labour in a thrombocytopenic parturient. Can J Anaesth. 1992;39:277-281.
49. Kuhnert BR et al. Effects of low doses of meperidine on neonatal behavior. Anesth Analg. 1985;64:335-342.
50. Gerdin E et al. Maternal kinetics of morphine during labor. J Perinatal Med. 1990;18:478-487.
51. Craft JB Jr et al. Ketamine, catecholamines, and uterine tone in pregnant ewes. Am J Obstet Gynecol. 1983;146:429-434.
52. Levinson G et al. Maternal and fetal cardiovascular and acid-base changes during ketamine anaesthesia in pregnant ewes. Br J Anaesth. 1973;45:1111-1115.
53. American College of Obstetricians and Gynecologists. Obstetric analgesia and anesthesia. Washington, DC: American College of Obstetricians and Gynecologists, Medical Specialty Society; 2002. NGC:003123.
54. Driver RP Jr et al. Sterility of anesthetic and resuscitative drug syringes used in the obstetric operating room. Anesth Analg. 1998;86:994-997.
55. Lewis B et al. Atropine and ephedrine adsorption to syringe plastic. AANA J. 1994;62:257-260.
56. Datta S et al. Clinical effects and maternal and fetal plasma concentrations of epidural ropivacaine versus bupivacaine for cesarean section. Anesthesiology. 1995;82:1346-1352.
57. Lacassie HJ et al. The relative motor blocking potencies of epidural bupivacaine and ropivacaine in labor. Anesth Analg. 2002;95:204-208.
58. Scott DA et al. Pharmacokinetics and efficacy of long-term epidural ropivacaine infusion for postoperative analgesia. Anesth Analg. 1997;85:1322-1330.
59. Etches RC et al. Continuous epidural ropivacaine 0.2% for analgesia after lower abdominal surgery. Anesth Analg. 1997;84:784-790.
60. Gautier P et al. A double-blind comparison of 0.125% ropivacaine with sufentanil and 0.125% bupivacaine with sufentanil for epidural labor analgesia. Anesthesiology. 1999;90:772-778.
61. Scott DB et al. Acute toxicity of ropivacaine compared with that of bupivacaine. Anesth Analg. 1989;69:563-569.
62. Knudsen K et al. Central nervous and cardiovascular effects of IV infusions of ropivacaine, bupivacaine and placebo in volunteers. Br J Anaesth. 1997;78:507-514.
63. Moller RA, Covino BG. Effect of progesterone on the cardiac electrophysiologic alterations produced by ropivacaine and bupivacaine. Anesthesiology. 1992;77:735-741.

64. Moller RA et al. Effects of progesterone on the cardiac electrophysiologic action of bupivacaine and lidocaine. *Br J Anaesth.* 1992;76:604-608.

65. Reiz S, Nath S. Cardiotoxicity of local anaesthetic agents. *Br J Anaesth.* 1986;58:736-746.

66. Morton CP et al. Ropivacaine 0.75% for extradural anaesthesia in elective caesarean section: an open clinical and pharmacokinetic study in mother and neonate. *Br J Anaesth.* 1997;79:3-8.

67. Birnbach DJ et al. Povidone iodine and skin disinfection before initiation of epidural anesthesia. *Anesthesiology.* 1998;88:668-672.

68. Kleiman SJ et al. Patient-controlled analgesia (PCA) using fentanyl in a parturient with a platelet function abnormality. *Can J Anaesth.* 1991;38:489-491.

69. Rayburn W et al. Fentanyl citrate analgesia during labor. *Am J Obstet Gynecol.* 1989;161:202-206.

70. Beilin Y et al. The optimal distance that a multiorifice epidural catheter should be threaded into the epidural space. *Anesth Analg.* 1995;81:301-304.

71. Hamilton CL et al. Changes in the position of epidural catheters associated with patient movement. *Anesthesiology.* 1997;86:778-784.

72. Michael S et al. A comparison between open-end (single hole) and closed-end (three lateral holes) epidural catheters. Complications and quality of sensory blockade. *Anaesthesia.* 1989;44:578-580.

73. D'Angelo R et al. A comparison of multiport and uniport epidural catheters in laboring patients. *Anesth Analg.* 1997;84:1276-1279.

74. Dickson MAS et al. Comparison of single, end-holed and multi-orifice extradural catheters when used for continuous infusion of local anaesthetic during labour. *Br J Anaesth.* 1997;79:297-300.

75. Dalal P et al. Assessing bupivacaine 10 mg/fentanyl 20 mcg as an intrathecal test dose. *Int J Obstet Anesth.* 2003;12:205-255.

76. Hood DD et al. Maternal and fetal effects of epinephrine in gravid ewes. *Anesthesiology.* 1986;64:610-613.

77. Chestnut DH et al. Effect of intravenous epinephrine upon uterine blood flow velocity in the pregnant guinea pig. *Anesthesiology.* 1986;65:633-636.

78. Guay J. The epidural test dose: a review. *Anesth Analg.* 2006;102(3):921-929.

79. Norris MC et al. Labor epidural analgesia without an intravascular "test dose". *Anesthesiology.* 1998;88:1495-1501.

80. Jiang X et al. The plasma concentrations of lidocaine after slow versus rapid administration of an initial dose of epidural anesthesia. *Anesth Analg.* 1997;84:570-573.

81. Viscomi CM et al. Fetal heart rate variability after epidural fentanyl during labor. *Anesth Analg.* 1990;71:679-683.

82. Marx GF et al. Effects of epidural block with lignocaine and lignocaine-adrenaline on umbilical artery velocity wave ratios. *Br J Obstet Gynaecol.* 1990;97:517-520.

83. Purdie J et al. Continuous extradural analgesia: comparison of midwife top-ups, continuous infusions and patient controlled administration. *Br J Anaesth.* 1992;68:580-584.

84. Viscomi C, Eisenach JC. Patient-controlled epidural analgesia during labor. *Obstet Gynecol.* 1991;77:348-351.

85. Gambling DR et al. Comparison of patient-controlled epidural analgesia and conventional intermittent "top-up" injections during labor. *Anesth Analg.* 1990;70:256-261.

86. Sia AT et al. A comparison of a basal infusion with automated mandatory boluses in parturient-controlled epidural analgesia during labor. *Anesth Analg.* 2007;3:673-677.

87. Rigler ML et al. Cauda equine syndrome after continuous spinal anesthesia. *Anesth Analg.* 1991;72:275-281.

88. Hood DD, Dewan DM. Anesthetic and obstetric outcome in morbidly obese parturients. *Anesthesiology.* 1993;79:1210.

89. Celleno D, Capogna G. Epidural fentanyl plus bupivacaine 0.125% for labour analgesic effects. *Can J Anaesth.* 1988;35:375-378.

90. D'Athis F et al. Epidural analgesia with bupivacaine-fentanyl mixture in obstetrics: comparison of repeated injections and continuous infusion. *Can J Anaesth.* 1988;35:116-122.

91. Jones G et al. Comparison of bupivacaine and bupivacaine with fentanyl in continuous extradural analgesia during labour. *Br J Anaesth.* 1989;63:254-259.

92. Madej TH, Strunin L. Comparison of epidural fentanyl with sufentanil. *Anaesthesia.* 1987;42:1156-1161.

93. Paech MJ et al. A double-blind comparison of epidural bupivacaine and bupivacaine-fentanyl for caesarean section. *Anaesth Intensive Care.* 1990;18:22-30.

94. Ackerman WE et al. Epidural fentanyl for the management of the pain caused by uterine manipulation during epidural anesthesia for elective cesarean section. *Anesthesiol Rev.* 1989;16:41-45.

95. Brockway MS et al. Profound respiratory depression after extradural fentanyl. *Br J Anaesth.* 1990;64:243-245.

96. Porter J et al. Effect of epidural fentanyl on neonatal respiration. *Anesthesiology.* 1998;89:79-85.

97. Yau G et al. Obstetric epidural analgesia with mixtures of bupivacaine, adrenaline, and fentanyl. *Anaesthesia.* 1990;45:1020-1023.

98. Yee I et al. A comparison of two doses of epidural fentanyl during caesarean section. *Can J Anaesth.* 1993;40:722-725.

99. Malinow AM et al. Does pH adjustment reverse Nesacaine antagonism of postcesarean epidural fentanyl analgesia? *Anesth Analg.* 1988;67(Suppl):1376.

100. Camann WR et al. Chloroprocaine antagonism of epidural opioid analgesia: a receptor-specific phenomenon? *Anesthesiology.* 1990;73:860-863.

101. Vertommen JD et al. The effects of intravenous and epidural sufentanil in the chronic maternal-fetal sheep preparation. *Anesth Analg.* 1995;80:71-75.

102. Abboud TK et al. Mini-dose intrathecal morphine for the relief of postcesarean section pain: safety, efficacy, and ventilatory responses to carbon dioxide. *Anesth Analg.* 1988;67:137-143.

103. Abouleish E et al. The addition of 0.2 mg subarachnoid morphine to hyperbaric bupivacaine for cesarean delivery: a prospective study of 856 cases. *Reg Anesth.* 1991;16:137-140.

104. Douglas MJ et al. The effect of epinephrine in local anaesthetic on epidural morphine-induced pruritus. *Can Anaesth Soc J.* 1986;33:737-740.

105. Shehabi Y et al. Effect of adrenaline, fentanyl and warming of injectate on shivering following extradural analgesia in labor. *Anaesth Intensive Care.* 1990;18:31-37.

106. Sevarino FB et al. The effect of epidural sufentanil on shivering and body temperature in the parturient. *Anesth Analg.* 1989;68:530-533.

107. Robson SC et al. Maternal and fetal hemodynamic effects of spinal and extradural anesthesia for elective cesarean section. *Br J Anaesth.* 1992;68:54-59.

108. Morgan PJ et al. The effects of an increase of central blood volume before spinal anesthesia for cesarean delivery: a qualitative systematic review. *Anesth Analg.* 2001;92:997-1005.

109. Kubli M et al. A randomised controlled trial of fluid pre-loading before low dose epidural analgesia for labour. *Int J Obstet Anesth.* 2003;12:256-260.

110. Park GE et al. The effects of varying volumes of crystalloid administration before cesarean delivery on maternal hemodynamics and colloid osmotic pressure. *Anesth Analg.* 1996;83:299-303.

111. Rout CC et al. A reevaluation of the role of crystalloid preload in the prevention of hypotension associated with spinal anesthesia for elective cesarean section. *Anesthesiology.* 1993;79:262-269.

112. Ueyama H et al. Effects of crystalloid and colloid preload on blood volume in the parturient undergoing spinal anesthesia for elective cesarean section. *Anesthesiology.* 1999;91:1571-1576.

113. Riley ET et al. Prevention of hypotension after spinal anesthesia for cesarean section: six percent hetastarch versus lactated Ringer's solution. *Anesth Analg.* 1995;81:838-842.

114. Shiraishi Y et al. Vasopressin and atrial natriuretic peptide release in cardiopulmonary denervated dogs. *Am J Physiol.* 1990;258:R704-R710.

115. Jouppila R et al. Placental blood flow during caesarean section under lumbar extradural analgesia. *Br J Anaesth.* 1978;50:275-279.

116. Brizgys RV et al. The incidence and neonatal effects of maternal hypotension during epidural anesthesia for cesarean section. *Anesthesiology.* 1987;67:782-786.

117. Corke BC et al. Spinal anaesthesia for caesarean section: the influence of hypotension on neonatal outcome. *Anaesthesia.* 1982;37:658-662.

118. Antoine C, Young BK. Fetal lactic acidosis with epidural anesthesia. *Am J Obstet Gynecol.* 1982;142:55-59.

119. Hon EH et al. The electronic evaluation of fetal heart rate. II. Changes with maternal hypotension. *Am J Obstet Gynecol.* 1960;79:209-215.

120. Goodlin RC. Venous reactivity and pregnancy abnormalities. *Acta Obstet Gynecol Scand.* 1986;65:345-348.

121. Ralston DH et al. Effect of equipotent ephedrine, metaraminol, mephentermine, and methoxamine on uterine blood flow in the pregnant ewe. *Anesthesiology.* 1974;40:354-370.

122. Cooper DW et al. Effect of intravenous vasopressor on spread of spinal anesthesia and fetal acid-base equilibrium. *Br J Anaesth.* 2007;98;5:649-656.

123. Lee A et al. A quantitative, systematic review of randomized controlled trials of ephedrine versus phenylephrine for the management of hypotension during spinal anesthesia for cesarean delivery. *Anesth Analg.* 2002;94:920-926.

124. Moran DH et al. Phenylephrine in the prevention of hypotension following spinal anesthesia for cesarean delivery. *J Clin Anesth.* 1991;3:301-305.

125. Ramanathan S, Grant GJ. Vasopressor therapy for hypotension due to epidural anesthesia for cesarean section. *Acta Anaesthesiol Scand.* 1988;32:559-565.

126. McAuley DM et al. Ranitidine as an antacid before elective caesarean section. *Anaesthesia.* 1983;38:108-114.

127. Brashear WT et al. Effect of ranitidine on bupivacaine disposition. *Anesth Analg.* 1991;72:369-376.

128. Caldwell C et al. An unusual reaction to preoperative metoclopramide. *Anesthesiology.* 1987;67:854.
129. Crawford JS. Anesthesia for section: further refinements of a technique. *Br J Anaesth.* 1973;45:726-731.
130. Duthie SJ et al. Intra-operative blood loss during elective lower segment cesarean section. *Br J Obstet Gynaecol.* 1992;99:364-367.
131. Combs CA et al. Factors associated with hemorrhage in cesarean deliveries. *Obstet Gynecol.* 1991;77:77-82.
132. Marx GF et al. Foetal-neonatal status following caesarean section for foetal distress. *Br J Anaesth.* 1984;56:1009-1013.
133. Ong BY et al. Anesthesia for cesarean section—effects on neonates. *Anesth Analg.* 1989;68:270-275.
134. Morgan BM et al. Anaesthesia for emergency caesarean section. *Br J Obstet Gynaecol.* 1990;97:420-424.
135. Evans CM et al. Epidural versus general anaesthesia for elective caesarean section. Effect on Apgar score and acid-base status of the newborn. *Anaesthesia.* 1989;44:778-782.
136. Hawthorne L et al. Failed intubation revisited: 17-year experience in a teaching maternity unit. *Br J Anaesth.* 1996;76:680-684.
137. Dailland P et al. Intravenous propofol during cesarean section: placental transfer, concentrations in breast milk, and neonatal effects. A preliminary study. *Anesthesiology.* 1989;71:827-834.
138. Gin T et al. Pharmacokinetics of propofol in women undergoing elective caesarean section. *Br J Anaesth.* 1990;64:148-153.
139. Valtonen M et al. Comparison of propofol and thiopentone for induction of anaesthesia for elective caesarean section. *Anaesthesia.* 1989;44:758-762.
140. Gin T et al. The haemodynamic effects of propofol and thiopentone for induction of caesarean section. *Anaesth Intensive Care.* 1990;18:175-179.
141. Ngan Kee WD et al. Postoperative analgesic requirement after cesarean section: a comparison of anesthetic induction with ketamine or thiopental. *Anesth Analg.* 1997;85:1294-1298.
142. King HK et al. Adequacy of general anesthesia for cesarean section. *Anesth Analg.* 1993;77:84-88.
143. Bernstein K et al. Influence of two different anaesthetic agents on the newborn and the correlation between foetal oxygenation and induction delivery time in elective caesarean section. *Acta Anaesthesiol Scand.* 1985;29:157-160.
144. Kao YJ et al. Dose-dependent effect of metoclopramide on cholinesterase and suxamethonium metabolism. *Br J Anaesth.* 1990;65:220-224.
145. Munson ES, Embro WJ. Enflurane, isoflurane, and halothane and isolated human uterine muscle. *Anesthesiology.* 1977;46:11-14.
146. Karaman S et al. The maternal and neonatal effects of the volatile agents desflurane and sevoflurane in caesarean section: a prospective randomized clinical study. *J Int Med Res.* 2006;34:183-192.
147. Dogru K et al. The direct depressant effects of desflurane and sevoflurane on spontaneous contractions of isolated gravid rat myometrium. *Int J Obstet Anesth.* 2003;12:74-78.
148. Ngan Kee WD et al. Randomized, double-blind comparison of different inspired oxygen fractions during general anaesthesia for caesarean section. *Br J Anaesth.* 2002;89:556-561.
149. Khaw KS et al. Effects of high inspired oxygen fraction during elective caesarean section under spinal anaesthesia on maternal and fetal oxygenation and lipid peroxidation. *Br J Anaesth.* 2002;88:18-23.
150. Piggott SE et al. Isoflurane with either 100% oxygen or 50% nitrous oxide in oxygen for caesarean section. *Br J Anaesth.* 1990;65:325-329.
151. Bogod DG et al. Maximum FiO2 during caesarean section. *Br J Anaesth.* 1988;61:255-262.
152. Perrault C et al. Maternal inspired oxygen concentration and fetal oxygenation during cesarean section. *Can J Anaesth.* 1992;39:155-157.
153. Dailey PA et al. Pharmacokinetics, placental transfer, and neonatal effects of vecuronium and pancuronium administered during cesarean section. *Anesthesiology.* 1984;60:569-574.
154. Bader AM et al. Maternal and fetal catecholamines and uterine incision-to-delivery interval during elective cesarean. *Obstet Gynecol.* 1990;75:600-603.
155. Datta S et al. Neonatal effect of prolonged anesthetic induction for cesarean section. *Obstet Gynecol.* 1981;58:331-335.
156. Rosaeg OP et al. The effect of oxytocin on the contractile force of human atrial trabeculae. *Anesth Analg.* 1998;86:40-44.
157. Veber B et al. Severe hypertension during postpartum haemorrhage after IV administration of prostaglandin E2. *Br J Anaesth.* 1992;68:623-624.
158. Silva D et al. Acute hypertensive response to prostaglandin F2 alpha during anaesthesia administration. *J Reprod Med.* 1987;32:700-702.
159. Partridge BL et al. Life-threatening effects of intravascular absorption of PGF2 alpha during therapeutic termination of pregnancy. *Anesth Analg.* 1988;67:1111-1113.
160. Parnass SM et al. Incidence of hypotension associated with epidural anesthesia using alkalinized and nonalkalinized lidocaine for cesarean section. *Anesth Analg.* 1987;66:1148-1150.
161. Benzon HT et al. Onset, intensity of blockade and somatosensory evoked potential changes of the lumbosacral dermatomes after epidural anesthesia with alkalinized lidocaine. *Anesth Analg.* 1993;76:328-332.
162. Curatolo M et al. Adding sodium bicarbonate to lidocaine enhances the depth of epidural blockade. *Anesth Analg.* 1998;86:341-347.
163. Bartfield JM et al. Buffered lidocaine as a local anesthetic: an investigation of shelf life. *Ann Emerg Med.* 1992;21:16-19.
164. Crochetière CT et al. Epidural anaesthesia for caesarean section: comparison of two injection techniques. *Can J Anaesth.* 1989;36:133-136.
165. Ohno H et al. Effect of epinephrine concentration on lidocaine disposition during epidural anesthesia. *Anesthesiology.* 1988;68:625-628.
166. Alahuhta S et al. Effects of extradural bupivacaine with adrenaline for cesarean section on uteroplacental and fetal circulation. *Br J Anaesth.* 1991;67:678-682.
167. Vincent RD Jr et al. Does epidural fentanyl decrease the efficacy of epidural morphine after cesarean delivery? *Anesth Analg.* 1992;74:658-663.
168. Aouad MT et al. Does pregnancy protect against intrathecal lidocaine-induced transient neurologic symptoms? *Anesth Analg.* 2001;92:401-404.
169. Philip J et al. Transient neurologic symptoms after spinal anesthesia with lidocaine in obstetric patients. *Anesth Analg.* 2001;92:405-409.
170. Koonin LM et al. Pregnancy-related mortality surveillance—United States, 1987-1990. *MMWR CDC Surveill Summ.* 1997;46:17-36.
171. Atrash HK et al. Maternal mortality in the United States, 1979-1986. *Obstet Gynecol.* 1990;76:1055-1060.
172. Gottumukkala V et al. Evaluation of anesthesia risk. In: Lobato EB et al, eds. *Complications in Anesthesiology.* Philadelphia: Lippincott Williams & Wilkins; 2008:15-41.
173. Kotelko DM et al. Transdermal scopolamine decreases nausea and vomiting following cesarean section in patients receiving epidural morphine. *Anesthesiology.* 1989;71:675-678.
174. Lesser P et al. An evaluation of a 30 gauge needle for spinal anaesthesia for cesarean section. *Anaesthesia.* 1990;45:767-768.
175. Carrie LES, Donald F. A 26-gauge pencil point needle for combined spinal-epidural anaesthesia for cesarean section. *Anaesthesia.* 1991;46:230-231.
176. Barker P. Are obstetric spinal headaches avoidable? *Anaesth Intensive Care.* 1990;18:553-554.
177. Cesarini M et al. Sprotte needle for intrathecal anaesthesia for caesarean section: incidence of postdural puncture headache. *Anaesthesia.* 1990;45:656-658.
178. Ross BK et al. Sprotte needle for obstetric anesthesia: decreased incidence of postdural puncture headache. *Reg Anesth.* 1992;17:29-33.
179. Fink BR, Walker S. Orientation of fibers in human dorsal lumbar dura mater in relation to lumbar puncture. *Anesth Analg.* 1989;69:768-772.
180. Camann WR et al. Effects of oral caffeine on postdural puncture headache: A double-blind, placebo-controlled trial. *Anesth Analg.* 1990;70:181-184.
181. Carp H et al. Effects of the serotonin-receptor agonist sumatriptan on postdural puncture headache: report of six cases. *Anesth Analg.* 1994;79:180-182.
182. Palahniuk RJ, Cumming M. Prophylactic blood patch does not prevent post lumbar puncture headache. *Can Anaesth Soc J.* 1979;26:132-133.
183. Loeser EA et al. Time vs success rate for epidural blood patch. *Anesthesiology.* 1978;49:147-148.
184. Martin R et al. Duration of decubitus position after epidural blood patch. *Can J Anaesth.* 1994;41:23-25.
185. Colonna-Romano P, Shapira BE. Unintentional dural puncture and prophylactic epidural blood patch in obstetrics. *Anesth Analg.* 1989;69:522-523.
186. Cheek TG et al. Prophylactic extradural blood patch is effective. *Br J Anaesth.* 1988;61:340-342.
187. Elliott DW et al. Sudden onset of subarachnoid block after subdural catheterization: a case of arachnoid rupture? *Br J Anaesth.* 1996;76:322-324.
188. Mehta M, Maher R. Injection into the extra-arachnoid subdural space. Experience in the treatment of intractable cervical pain and in the conduct of extradural (epidural) analgesia. *Anaesthesia.* 1977;32:760-766.
189. Palmer CM et al. Incidence of electrocardiographic changes during cesarean delivery under regional anesthesia. *Anesth Analg.* 1990;70:36-43.
190. Zakowski MI et al. Electrocardiographic changes during cesarean section: a cause for concern? *Anesth Analg.* 1993;76:162-167.
191. Eisenach JC et al. Is ST segment depression of the electrocardiogram during cesarean section merely due to cardiac sympathetic block? *Anesth Analg.* 1994;78:287-292.
192. Burton A, Camann W. Electrocardiographic changes during cesarean section: a review. *Int J Obstet Anesth.* 1996;5:47-53.
193. Rees GA, Willis BA. Resuscitation in late pregnancy. *Anaesthesia.* 1988;43:347-349.

194. Lee RV et al. Cardiopulmonary resuscitation of pregnant women. *Am J Med.* 1986;81:311-318.

195. Katz VL et al. Perimortem cesarean delivery. *Obstet Gynecol.* 1986;68:571-576.

196. Anonymous. Maternal mortality—United States, 1982-1996. *MMWR Morb Mortal Wkly Rep.* 1998;47:705-707.

197. State-specific maternal mortality among black and white women—United States, 1987-1996. *MMWR Morb Mortal Wkly Rep.* 1999;48:492-496.

198. Giles W, Bisits A. The present and future of tocolysis. *Best Pract Res Clin Obstetr Gynaecol.* 2007;20(20):1-12.

199. Simhan HN, Caritis SN. Prevention of preterm delivery. *N Engl J Med.* 2007;357;5:477-487.

200. Grimes DA, Nanda K. Magnesium sulfate tocolysis: time to quit. *Obstet Gynecol.* 2006;108(4):986-989.

201. Perkins RP. Magnesium sulfate tocolysis: time to quit. *Obstet Gynecol.* 2007;109(3):778-779.

202. Kussman B et al. Administration of magnesium sulphate before rocuronium: effects on speed of onset and duration of neuromuscular block. *Br J Anaesth.* 1997;79:122-124.

203. Baraka A, Yazigi A. Neuromuscular interaction of magnesium with succinyl-choline-vecuronium sequence in the eclamptic parturient. *Anesthesiology.* 1987;67:806-808.

204. Bohman VR, Cotton DB. Supralethal magnesemia with patient survival. *Obstet Gynecol.* 1990;76:984-986.

205. Rolbin SH et al. The premature infant: anesthesia for cesarean delivery. *Anesth Analg.* 1994;78:912-917.

206. Chestnut DH et al. Does the intravenous infusion of ritodrine or magnesium sulfate alter the hemodynamic response to hemorrhage in gravid ewes? *Am J Obstet Gynecol.* 1988;159:1467-1473.

207. Reynolds JD et al. Magnesium sulfate adversely affects fetal lamb survival and blocks fetal cerebral blood flow response during maternal hemorrhage. *Anesth Analg.* 1996;83:493-499.

208. Shin YK, Kim YD. Ventricular tachyarrhythmias during cesarean section after ritodrine therapy: interaction with anesthetics. *South Med J.* 1988;81:528-530.

209. Baraka A et al. Supplementation of general anaesthesia with tramadol or fentanyl in parturients undergoing elective caesarean section. *Can J Anaesth.* 1998;45:631-634.

210. Jouppila P et al. Labetalol does not alter the placental and fetal blood flow or maternal prostanoids in pre-eclampsia. *Br J Obstet Gynaecol.* 1986;93:543-547.

211. Lubbe WF. Hypertension in pregnancy. Pathophysiology and management. *Drugs.* 1984;28:170-188.

212. Macpherson M et al. The effect of maternal labetalol on the newborn infant. *Br J Obstet Gynaecol.* 1986;93:539-542.

213. Ramanathan J et al. The use of labetalol for attenuation of the hypertensive response to endotracheal intubation in preeclampsia. *Am J Obstet Gynecol.* 1988;159:650-654.

214. Malinow AM et al. Precordial ultrasonic monitoring during cesarean delivery. *Anesthesiology.* 1987;66:816-819.

215. Fong J et al. Are Doppler-detected venous emboli during cesarean section air emboli? *Anesth Analg.* 1990;71:254-257.

216. Lew TWK et al. Venous air embolism during cesarean section: more common than previously thought. *Anesth Analg.* 1993;77:448-452.

217. Quance D. Amniotic fluid embolism: detection by pulse oximetry. *Anesthesiology.* 1988;68:951-952.

218. Sharma SK, Philip J. The effect of anesthetic techniques on blood coagulability in parturients as measured by thromboelastography. *Anesth Analg.* 1997;85:82-86.

219. Karuparthy VR et al. Incidence of venous air embolism during cesarean section is unchanged by the use of a 5 to 10 degree head-up tilt. *Anesth Analg.* 1989;69:620-623.

220. Breheny F, McCarthy J. Maternal mortality. A review of maternal deaths over twenty years at the National Maternity Hospital, Dublin. *Anaesthesia.* 1982;37:561-564.

221. Combs CA et al. Factors associated with postpartum hemorrhage with vaginal birth. *Obstet Gynecol.* 1991;77:69-76.

222. Abouleish AE, Corn SB. Intravenous nitroglycerin for intrapartum external version of the second twin. *Anesth Analg.* 1994;78:808-809.

223. Dayan SS, Schwalbe SS. The use of small-dose intravenous nitroglycerin in a case of uterine inversion. *Anesth Analg.* 1996;82:1091-1093.

224. Redick LF, Livingston E. A new preparation of nitroglycerin for uterine relaxation. *Int J Obstet Anesth.* 1995;4:14-16.

225. Schrinsky DC, Benson RC. Rupture of the pregnant uterus: a review. *Obstet Gynecol Surv.* 1978;33:217-232.

226. Chauhan SP et al. Maternal and perinatal complications with uterine rupture in 142,075 patients who attempted vaginal birth after cesarean delivery: a review of the literature. *Am J Obstet Gynecol.* 2003;189:408-417.

227. Gonsoulin W et al. Rupture of unscarred uterus in primigravid woman in association with cocaine abuse. *Am J Obstet Gynecol.* 1990;163:526-527.

228. Chazotte C, Cohen WR. Catastrophic complications of previous cesarean section. *Am J Obstet Gynecol.* 1990;163:738-742.

229. Flamm BL et al. Vaginal birth after cesarean delivery: results of a 5-year multicenter collaborative study. *Obstet Gynecol.* 1990;76:750-754.

230. Johnson C, Oriol N. The role of epidural anesthesia in trial of labor. *Reg Anesth.* 1990;15:304-308.

231. Friedman SA. Preeclampsia: a review of the role of prostaglandins. *Obstet Gynecol.* 1988;71:122-137.

232. Walsh SW. Preeclampsia: an imbalance in placental prostacyclin and thromboxane production. *Am J Obstet Gynecol.* 1985;152:335-340.

233. Fitzgerald DJ et al. Decreased prostacyclin biosynthesis preceding the clinical manifestation of pregnancy-induced hypertension. *Circulation.* 1987;75:956-963.

234. Phelan JP, Yurth DA. Severe preeclampsia. I. Peripartum hemodynamic observations. *Am J Obstet Gynecol.* 1982;144:17-22.

235. Mabie WC et al. The central hemodynamics of severe preeclampsia. *Am J Obstet Gynecol.* 1989;161:1443-1448.

236. Zemel MB et al. Altered platelet calcium metabolism as an early predictor of increased peripheral vascular resistance and preeclampsia in urban black women. *N Engl J Med.* 1990;323:434-438.

237. Groenendijk R et al. Hemodynamic measurements in preeclampsia: preliminary observations. *Am J Obstet Gynecol.* 1984;150:232-236.

238. Belfort M et al. Haemodynamic changes in gestational proteinuric hypertension: the effects of rapid volume expansion and vasodilator therapy. *Br J Obstet Gynaecol.* 1989;96:634-641.

239. Gant NF et al. A study of angiotensin II pressor response throughout primigravid pregnancy. *J Clin Invest.* 1973;52:2682-2689.

240. Fitzgerald DJ et al. Thromboxane A2 synthesis in pregnancy-induced hypertension. *Lancet.* 1990;335:751-754.

241. Anonymous. Do women with pre-eclampsia, and their babies, benefit from magnesium sulphate? The Magpie Trial: a randomised placebo-controlled trial. *Lancet.* 2002;359:1877-1890.

242. Barker P, Callander CC. Coagulation screening before epidural analgesia in pre-eclampsia. *Anaesthesia.* 1991;46:64-67.

243. Leduc L et al. Coagulation profile in severe preeclampsia. *Obstet Gynecol.* 1992;79:14-18.

244. Schindler M et al. Thrombocytopenia and platelet functional defects in pre-eclampsia: implications for regional anaesthesia. *Anaesth Intensive Care.* 1990;18:169-174.

245. Ramanathan J et al. Correlation between bleeding times and platelet counts in women with preeclampsia undergoing cesarean section. *Anesthesiology.* 1989;71:188-191.

246. Neiger R et al. The resolution of preeclampsia-related thrombocytopenia. *Obstet Gynecol.* 1991;77:692-695.

247. Jouppila P et al. Lumbar epidural analgesia to improve intervillous blood flow during labor in severe preeclampsia. *Obstet Gynecol.* 1982;59:158-161.

248. Ramos-Santos E et al. The effects of epidural anesthesia on the Doppler velocimetry of umbilical and uterine arteries in normal and hypertensive patients during active term labor. *Obstet Gynecol.* 1991;77:20-26.

249. Moore TR et al. Evaluation of the use of continuous lumbar epidural anesthesia for hypertensive pregnant women in labor. *Am J Obstet Gynecol.* 1985;152:404-412.

250. Jouppila R et al. Epidural analgesia and placental blood flow during labour in pregnancies complicated by hypertension. *Br J Obstet Gynaecol.* 1979;86:969-972.

251. James FM III, Davies P. Maternal and fetal effects of lumbar epidural analgesia for labor and delivery in patients with gestational hypertension. *Am J Obstet Gynecol.* 1976;126:195-201.

252. Giles WB et al. The effect of epidural anaesthesia for caesarean section on maternal uterine and fetal umbilical artery blood flow velocity waveforms. *Br J Obstet Gynaecol.* 1987;94:55-59.

253. Hollmen AI et al. Effect of extradural analgesia using bupivacaine and 2-chloroprocaine on intervillous blood flow during normal labour. *Br J Anaesth.* 1982;54:837-842.

254. Clark SL et al. Severe preeclampsia with persistent oliguria: management of hemodynamic subsets. *Am J Obstet Gynecol.* 1986;154:490-494.

255. Connell H et al. General anaesthesia in mothers with severe pre-eclampsia/eclampsia. *Br J Anaesth.* 1987;59:1375-1380.

256. Cartwright DP et al. Placental transfer of alfentanil at caesarean section. *Eur J Anaesthesiol.* 1989;6:103-109.

257. Lawes EG et al. Fentanyl-droperidol supplementation of rapid sequence induction in the presence of severe pregnancy-induced and pregnancy-aggravated hypertension. *Br J Anaesth.* 1987;59:1381-1391.

258. Rout CC, Rocke DA. Effects of alfentanil and fentanyl on induction of anaesthesia in patients with severe pregnancy-induced hypertension. *Br J Anaesth.* 1990;65:468-474.

259. Dann WL et al. Maternal and neonatal responses to alfentanil administered before induction of general anaesthesia for caesarean section. *Br J Anaesth.* 1987;59:1392-1396.

260. Eisenach JC et al. Maternal and fetal effects of labetalol in pregnant ewes. *Anesthesiology.* 1991;74:292-297.

261. Michael CA. The evaluation of labetalol in the treatment of hypertension complicating pregnancy. *Br J Clin Pharmacol.* 1982;13:127S-131S.

262. Mabie WC et al. A comparative trial of labetalol and hydralazine in the acute management of severe hypertension complicating pregnancy. *Obstet Gynecol.* 1987;70:328-333.

263. Pickles CJ et al. The fetal outcome in a randomized double-blind controlled trial of labetalol versus placebo in pregnancy-induced hypertension. *Br J Obstet Gynaecol.* 1989;96:38-43.

264. Plouin PF et al. Comparison of antihypertensive efficacy and perinatal safety of labetalol and methyldopa in the treatment of hypertension in pregnancy: a randomized controlled trial. *Br J Obstet Gynaecol.* 1988;95:868-876.

265. Rogers RC et al. Labetalol pharmacokinetics in pregnancy-induced hypertension. *Am J Obstet Gynecol.* 1990;162:362-366.

266. Lavies NG et al. Hypertensive and catecholamine response to tracheal intubation in patients with pregnancy-induced hypertension. *Br J Anaesth.* 1989;63:429-434.

267. de Rosayro M et al. Plasma levels and cardiovascular effect of nitroglycerin in pregnant sheep. *Can Anaesth Soc J.* 1980;27:560-564.

268. Hood DD et al. The use of nitroglycerin in preventing the hypertensive response to tracheal intubation in severe preeclampsia. *Anesthesiology.* 1985;63:329-332.

269. Losasso TJ et al. Response of fetal heart rate to maternal administration of esmolol. *Anesthesiology.* 1991;74:782-784.

270. Eisenach JC, Castro MI. Maternally administered esmolol produces fetal beta-adrenergic blockade and hypoxemia in sheep. *Anesthesiology.* 1989;71:718-722.

CHAPTER 48

NEONATAL ANESTHESIA

Theresa L. Culpepper

The neonatal period is generally regarded as the first 28 days of extrauterine life. Anesthesia for the neonate is often required as the result of an urgent or life-threatening illness that requires surgical intervention. The normal human neonate is remarkably resilient and well equipped to survive in this hostile environment. The differences between the baby and the adult, however, are clearly greatest in the neonatal period, especially if birth occurs before term. The neonate that is born prematurely and ill is not as resilient as the full-term infant. Therefore, the neonatal anesthetist must have a thorough understanding of normal growth and development, the anatomic and physiologic differences during various stages of maturation, and how immature organ systems affect anesthetic pharmacokinetics and pharmacodynamics. Anesthetic management of the neonate requires integration of this specialized knowledge and refinement of acquired technical skills.

In the past, neonates and in particular preterm, sick neonates were anesthetized with the "Liverpool Technique," which consisted of oxygen, nitrous oxide, and curare. Volatile anesthetics and opioids were not used, and the "stable" state that resulted was due to a sympathetic system in overdrive. However, in the last 3 decades, our understanding of neonatal physiology, particularly neurobiology, has led to an active program of research in the field of neonatal anesthesia. Neonates, term and preterm, respond to painful stimuli.[1] Signs of distress are clearly evident when neonates are exposed to stimuli that are painful. The behavioral, physiologic, and humoral signs are similar to those seen in older children and adults.[2] Therefore, all neonates require anesthesia for surgery except under extraordinary circumstances. Physiologic development is in a transitional state, and congenital anomalies may be present. There is a 10-fold incidence of intraoperative morbidity and mortality in neonates when compared with other age groups of pediatric patients.[3]

DEVELOPMENTAL CONSIDERATIONS

Fetal Circulation

The fetal circulatory system relies on the placenta for delivery of oxygen and transport of carbon dioxide (CO_2). The chorionic villus is the functional unit of the placenta. Normally, fetal blood is separated from the maternal blood in the placenta by a thin layer of cells known as *syncytial trophocytes*. Oxygen, CO_2, and small nonionized particles readily pass through this layer, whereas substances with a larger molecular weight are prevented from diffusing across the syncytial trophocytes. Fetal circulation is characterized by high pulmonary vascular resistance (uninflated atelectatic lungs and hypoxic vasoconstriction) and low systemic circulatory resistance (high flow and low impedance of the placental vessels). Fetal deoxygenated blood travels down the aorta and through the internal iliac arteries, arriving in the placenta via paired umbilical arteries. The umbilical arteries divide, forming the arterioles, capillaries, and venules of the intervillous placental space. Oxygenated blood is delivered to the fetus from the placenta via a single umbilical vein. This oxygenated blood bypasses the lungs by flowing through extracardiac (ductus arteriosus, ductus venosus) and intracardiac (foramen ovale) shunts, forming a parallel circulation. The ductus venosus routes oxygenated blood away from the sinusoids of the liver. The oxygenated blood in the inferior vena cava is directed by the eustachian valve toward the atrial septum and passes through the foramen ovale to enter the left side of the circulation. Oxygenated blood passes into the left ventricle and exits the aorta, supplying the coronary arteries. Blood entering the pulmonary artery from the right ventricle flows to the aorta via the ductus arteriosus. Only 5% to 10% of the combined ventricular output flows through the pulmonary circulation.

Transitional Circulation

The transitional circulation is established at the time of birth. With the cessation of placental blood flow, aortic pressure increases. Clamping of the umbilical vein doubles systemic vascular resistance. Pulmonary vascular resistance falls with lung expansion, and increasing partial pressure of arterial oxygen (PaO_2) produces pulmonary vasodilation, resulting in further decreases in pulmonary resistance. These changes in systemic and pulmonary blood flow produce corresponding changes in intracardiac pressure. Decreases in right atrial pressure with accompanying increases in left atrial pressure change the direction of blood flow through the foramen ovale, resulting in the closure of the foramen ovale as left atrial pressure increases. The foramen ovale may reopen if right atrial pressure is greater than left atrial pressure (e.g., pulmonary hypertension), permitting venous blood to flow from right to left. Within a period of 2 to 3 months the foramen ovale will be permanently closed. Up to 25% of adult patients may demonstrate a probe patent foramen ovale at autopsy.[4] Closure of the ductus arteriosus is precipitated in part by the increase in systemic vascular resistance and decrease in pulmonary vascular resistance. In utero prostaglandins maintain the patency of the ductus arteriosus. Within a few hours after birth, the muscular wall of the ductus arteriosus constricts, preventing the retrograde flow of blood from the aorta into the pulmonary artery. This functional closure (thrombosis) occurs within 1 to 8 days. Anatomic closure (fibrosis of the ductus arteriosus) requires

1 to 4 months. Ductus closure may be influenced by elevations in the systemic PaO_2 that occur after birth. The majority of portal blood flow continues to enter the ductus venosus after interruption of umbilical vein blood flow. Although the cause of the initiating mechanisms of ductus venosus closure is unknown, the muscular wall of the ductus venosus begins to constrict 1 to 3 hours postnatally. Blood flow is directed into the liver, and portal venous pressure increases.

Persistent Pulmonary Hypertension of the Newborn

During fetal development, pulmonary vascular resistance (PVR) is high but rapidly decreases at birth to near normal levels, allowing the lungs to become a gas exchanging organ. Before anatomic closure of the extracardiac and intracardiac shunts, fetal circulation may be reestablished and persist. Persistent pulmonary hypertension of the newborn (PPHN) (formerly persistent fetal circulation) is manifest by increases in pulmonary vascular resistance and accompanying pulmonary hypertension, which produces a right-to-left shunt across the foramen ovale and the ductus arteriosus, with resultant cyanosis. The presence of congenital cardiovascular or pulmonary disease inhibits functional and anatomic closure of these aforementioned fetal shunts. Persistent fetal circulation is common in preterm infants and infants with metabolic derangements (asphyxia, sepsis, meconium aspiration, congenital diaphragmatic hernia). Hypoxemia, acidosis, pneumonia, and hypothermia are primary precipitating factors of PPHN. Oxygenation, the avoidance of acidosis, and maintenance of normothermia will attenuate the increase in pulmonary vascular resistance. Continual increases in pulmonary vascular pressure and resistance will precipitate the development of right ventricular hypertrophy (cor pulmonale). Although pulmonary vasodilators may have some utility in decreasing pulmonary vascular resistance, concurrent reductions in systemic vascular resistance can occur and may worsen the shunt. Nitric oxide (NO), a specific, short-acting pulmonary vasodilator, decreases pulmonary vascular resistance and produces antegrade flow through the ductus arteriosus while avoiding changes in systemic vascular resistance. Other pharmacologic treatment options are magnesium,[5] prostacyclin,[6] adenosine,[7] or atrial natriuretic peptide (ANP).[8] High-frequency oscillatory ventilation (HFOV) and extracorporeal membrane oxygenation are technologic treatment options that may be performed to maintain oxygenation in infants with PPHN and severe respiratory dysfunction.[9,10]

GROWTH AND DEVELOPMENT

Cardiovascular System

The myocardium of the newborn is immature. The neonatal heart contains the essential structural elements of the adult heart, however there is cellular disorganization and fewer myofibrils. Although the ventricles are of equal size and shape, the contractile components (sarcoplasmic reticulum and T-tubule system) are immature. Accordingly the neonatal heart is less capable of generating a response to an increase in resistive load (increase in stroke volume) and is dependent on free ionized calcium for contractility. Despite this immaturity, the neonatal heart is capable of limited increases in stroke volume up to left atrial pressures of 10 to 12 mm Hg when afterload remains low.[11] This information suggests that the neonatal heart is operating near the peak of the Frank-Starling curve because there is a limited reserve to increases in both preload and afterload.

During maturation, the left ventricle will hypertrophy through an increase in the number and size of myofibrils. This maturation

is a consequence of left ventricular contraction against a higher postnatal systemic pressure. Acute increases in afterload (acidosis, hypothermia, pain) will produce further reductions in cardiac output. In the immediate postnatal period, left ventricular compliance is low. The neonate may develop congestive heart failure because the stiff left ventricle will not stretch to accommodate large fluid loads. Left ventricular distention from volume overload compresses the adjacent right ventricle, producing additional embarrassment to cardiac output. Likewise, ventilation with high peak pressure will produce left ventricular dysfunction and overload of the right ventricle.

Owing to the immaturity of the contractile elements of the neonatal myocardium, it has been believed that pediatric cardiac output was solely dependent on heart rate. Atropine is frequently administered for the treatment of decreased cardiac output. However, marked increases in heart rate fail to a large extent to produce further increases in cardiac output. Although the neonatal myocardium will develop less stretch with volume loading than the older child or adult, volume expansion remains important, albeit to a smaller extent than in the adult in increasing cardiac output.[11] The combination of hypovolemia and bradycardia produce dramatic decreases in cardiac output that threaten organ perfusion. Epinephrine rather than atropine increases contractility and heart rate and is now advocated for the treatment of bradycardia and decreased cardiac output in pediatric patients. The baroreceptor reflex is not completely developed, limiting the neonate's ability to compensate for hypotension with the reflex tachycardia expected in the older child and adult.

Autonomic innervation of the neonatal heart is predominantly controlled by the parasympathetic nervous system; the sympathetic nervous system is immature at birth. Parasympathetic dominance produces bradycardia with minor clinical interventions such as pharyngeal suctioning and laryngoscopy. Marked variation in the newborn heart rate and rhythm occur secondary to changes in autonomic tone. The electrocardiogram (ECG) recording in the newborn reflects the immaturity of the conduction system. The ECG axis is shifted to the right but shifts to the left with maturation and accompanying hypertrophy of the left ventricle. The P wave is evident; the PR is less than 0.12 second and increases until adolescence. T waves are upright in the recorded chest leads, reflecting right ventricular domination. The newborn heart rate averages 120 beats per minute during the first day of life, increasing to 160 beats per minute at 1 month of age, then steadily decreases to an average of 75 beats by the adolescent period. Sleep may produce heart rates lower than 100 beats per minute, whereas pain increases the rate up 200 beats per minute.

Blood pressure increases immediately after birth, rising to a mean systolic of 70 to 75 mm Hg within the first 48 hours. Blood pressure is lower in the preterm infant. As the heart rate decreases with maturation, there is an accompanying increase in blood pressure. Hypotension in an anesthetized newborn is defined as a systolic blood pressure of less than 60 mm Hg. In a 1-year-old, hypotension is defined as systolic pressure less than 70 mm Hg. In the older child, hypotension is determined as a systolic pressure of 70 mm Hg plus twice the child's age in years. Table 48-1 shows values for heart rate and blood pressure at different ages.

Fetal hemoglobin is the predominant hemoglobin species in the newborn contributing between 70% and 90% of the total. This amounts to a hemoglobin of between 18 and 20 g/dL at birth. Fetal hemoglobin has a higher affinity for oxygen than

TABLE 48-1	Age-Related Changes in the Cardiovascular System		
Age	**Heart Rate**	**Systolic BP**	**Diastolic BP**
Neonate	140	70-75	40
12 mo	120	95	65
3 yr	100	100	70
12 yr	80	110	60

BP, *Blood pressure.*

TABLE 48-2	Estimated Blood Volumes by Age
Age Group	**Volume (mL/kg)**
Premature	90-100
Newborn (less than 1 mo of age)	80-90
Infants 3 mo–3 yr of age	75-80
Children older than 6 yr of age	65-70

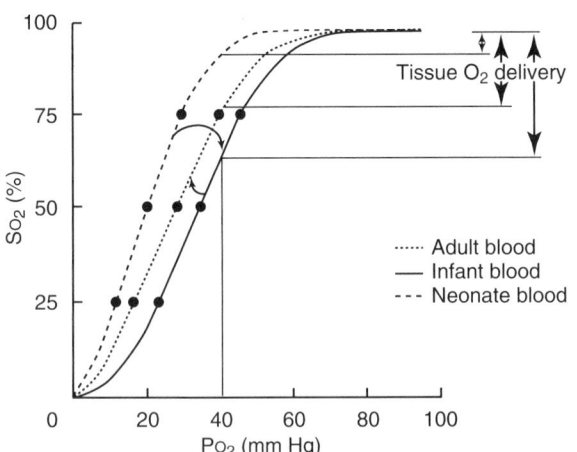

FIGURE 48-1 Schematic representation of oxyhemoglobin dissociation curves with different oxygen affinities. *Top arrows,* Direction of rightward shifting of the oxyhemoglobin dissociation curve (and P50) after birth. By 10 weeks of age, the adult position of the curve is reached. (*From Motoyama EK. Respiratory physiology in infants and children. In: Motoyama EK, David PJ, eds.* Smith's Anesthesia for Infants and Children. *5th ed. St Louis: Mosby; 1990:11-76. With permission.*)

adult hemoglobin. In utero, this increased oxygen affinity facilitates oxygen uptake as fetal blood circulates through the placenta, increasing the binding of oxygen to fetal hemoglobin and allowing the fetus to exist in a relatively low PaO_2 environment. There is a rapid change in the fetal hematopoietic physiology in the oxygen-rich extrauterine environment. The increased arterial oxygen content after birth results in a decrease in erythroid activity, and hematopoiesis ceases. A decrease in erythropoiesis and decreased life span of the newborn's red blood cells (RBCs) produces a progressive decrease in hemoglobin, reaching a nadir by age 3 months. This "physiologic anemia of infancy" does not compromise the delivery of oxygen, because the oxyhemoglobin dissociation curve shifts to the right and RBC concentrations of 2,3-diphosphoglycerate increase (Figure 48-1). Fetal hemoglobin is replaced by adult hemoglobin during the first 3 to 6 months, producing a rightward shift of the oxyhemoglobin dissociation curve.[12]

It is important to note that the premature infant may experience a dramatic fall in hemoglobin because of insufficient body stores of iron. Newborns should receive vitamin K prophylaxis, because the concentration of vitamin K–dependent clotting factors (II, VII, IX, and X) are 20% to 50% of adult levels. Premature infants generally have lower levels of vitamin K–dependent clotting factors. Maternally ingested drugs such as warfarin and isoniazid may precipitate the development of a coagulopathy.

The newborn's blood volume is dependent on the time of cord clamping (transfusion from the placenta). Blood volume is approximately 80 to 90 mL/kg but may be as high as 100 mL/kg in the premature neonate. The intravascular volume decreases 25% in the immediate postnatal period with the loss of intravascular fluid. Blood volume increases over the next 2 months, peaking at 2 months of age. Table 48-2 provides an estimate of circulating blood volume development.

Respiratory System
The fetal lungs are physically and metabolicaly active. Respiratory movements have been observed early in the first trimester of pregnancy During intrauterine development, the fetal lungs are filled with liquid secreted by the pulmonary epithelium. The volume and rate at which the liquid is secreted into the fetal lungs are calibrated to maintain lung volume at about functional residual capacity, and are the major determinants of normal lung growth.[13] At birth this fetal pulmonary fluid is replaced by air, much of it being pushed out of the mouth by the force of the uterine contractions acting on the chest wall and the remainder being absorbed by pulmonary lymphatic and blood vessels. Early in fetal development, the bronchial tree begins to develop the respiratory bronchioles, and they are formed by 24 to 26 weeks, gestation. Extrauterine survival of the fetus is possible at this time. Surfactant production begins during the 30th week of gestation via Lamellar bodies, reaching satisfactory levels at approximately 35 weeks. A postnatal increase occurs in the number of alveoli, as does vascularization. During maturation the pulmonary vasculature and airway smooth muscle proliferates with extension to the alveoli. Prenatal lung development may be affected by congenital defects, such as congenital diaphragmatic hernia that produces a hypoplastic lung. Congenital heart lesions may also inhibit the maturation of the pulmonary vasculature and result in either a decrease or increase in pulmonary blood flow.

Anatomy
At birth the neonatal larynx is small compared with the mouth and pharnyx. The epiglottis is short and small and the vallecula is shallow so that the tongue approximates the epiglottis. The larynx is pointed toward the nasopharynx, facilitating nasal breathing. The arytenoids are large in proportion to the lumen of the larynx. The subglottic region is smaller than the glottic opening with the cartilages telescoping into one another forming a conical shape.[14] The cricoid cartilage is the narrowest portion of the airway. In one study it was determined that the cricoid lumen is not a round but mostly an ellipsoid structure.[15] It is lined with pseudostratified epithelium that is easily injured, resulting in significant edema and stridor.

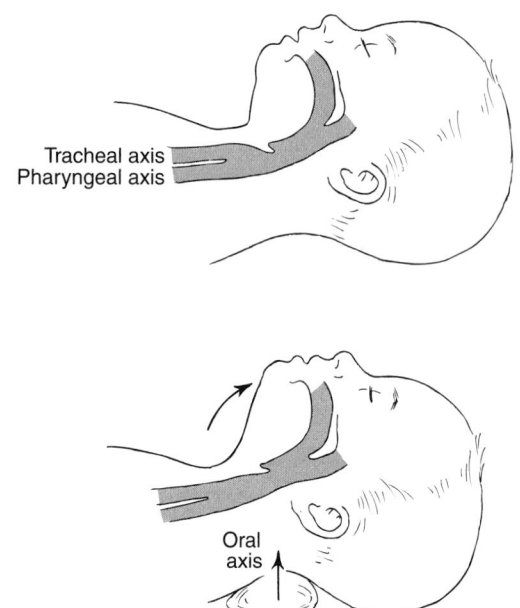

FIGURE **48-2** Alignments of visual, oral, and laryngeal axes during laryngoscopy.

TABLE **48-3**	Differences Between the Adult and the Pediatric Airway	
	Pediatric	**Adult**
Laryngeal location	C2-C4	C3-C6
Narrowest location of airway	Cricoid	Glottis
Shape of epiglottis	Longer, more narrow	V-shaped
Right mainstem bronchus	Less vertical	More vertical

The newborn tongue is large and difficult to manipulate because of the position of the hyoid. In addition, a smaller potential submental space is present in which to displace the tongue during laryngoscopy. The anterior position of the larynx and the large tongue increase the potential difficulty of mask ventilation.

The larynx is located more cephalad and anterior, extending from the second to the fourth cervical vertebrae (C2 to C4). The anesthetic implication of the more cephalad location is that placing a neonate in the "sniffing position" for laryngoscopy and intubation will only move the larynx in an anterior direction.

The occiput of the newborn's head is large and prominent. The placement of a rolled towel under the shoulders aids in the visual alignment of the oral, pharyngeal, and laryngeal axes during laryngoscopy (Figure 48-2 and Table 48-3).

Mechanics of Breathing

The neonate's chest wall is pliable for lack of developed musculature and a skeletal structure primarily composed of cartilage. The ribs are horizontal in orientation, providing minimal assistance in the expansion of the chest wall with inspiration. During inspiration the compliant chest wall is noted to collapse inward during respiration (paradoxical breathing). To maintain negative intrathoracic pressure in the face of a compliant chest wall, the neonate and infant actively recruit accessory muscles of respiration (i.e., intercostal muscles). Additionally, exhalation is limited by the adductor muscles of the larynx, which contract and serve as an expiratory valve or brake to maintain end-expiratory pressure. These structural differences are responsible for the decrease in functional residual capacity (FRC) with administration of general anesthesia in the neonate and infant. The previously cited muscular activity responsible for maintaining FRC is lost with the administration of sedatives, inhalation anesthetics, and neuromuscular relaxants. Rapid hypoxemia follows the loss of FRC. FRC may be restored with the application of continuous positive airway pressure or controlled ventilation. The premature infant has even a more pliable chest wall, and paradoxical chest movement may occur with breathing during rest.

The diaphragm contributes to the differences in respiratory function of the neonate and infant. Unlike the adult diaphragm, which is dome-shaped, the diaphragm of the neonate and infant is relatively flat. Accordingly, its anterior insertion on the chest wall fails to contribute any mechanical advantage with contraction. In addition, the infant diaphragm is composed of just 10% to 30% slow-twitch, high-oxidative, fatigue-resistant type I fibers as opposed to the adult diaphragm, whose composition is approximately 60%. This inherient structural composition predisposes the neonate and infant diaphragm to fatigue in the face of an increasing work of breathing.

Control of Breathing

The control of breathing is dependent on the PaO_2 sensed via the peripheral chemoreceptors (carotid and aortic bodies), the partial pressure of arterial CO_2 ($PaCO_2$) and pH, which influence the central chemoreceptors within the respiratory control center of the medulla. Increases in $PaCO_2$ produce corresponding increases in tidal volume and respiratory rate, although this response is not as vigorous as in the adult. Increases in PaO_2 will depress the ventilatory response in the newborn, whereas a decreased PaO_2 will increase the ventilatory response. The ventilatory response to hypoxemia produces two distinctly different responses. Initially hypoxemia stimulates an increase in ventilation for the first minute but produces ventilatory depression with a decreasing response for the next 3 to 5 minutes. This response is more robust in the premature infant than in the newborn. Ventilatory depression is more profound in the hypothermia, acidotic or hypercarbic neonate.

Respiratory depression and/or apnea may develop in the newborn following stimulation of the carina and/or the superior laryngeal nerve, following upper airway obstruction or following lung inflation (Hering-Breuer reflex). The newborn may exhibit periodic breathing with inspiratory pauses lasting 10 seconds, followed by abrupt increases in ventilation. Periodic breathing is more common in the premature infant and occurs more often during rapid eye movement sleep. Apneic episodes are not uncommon in the premature infant and produce arterial desaturation. Bradycardia and cardiac arrest may follow these apneic episodes. The suspected causes of apnea in premature infants include immature responses of the respiratory control center to hypercarbia or hypoxic stimuli and respiratory fatigue. Infants who have experienced apneic or bradycardic episodes are at risk for these episodes after general anesthesia.

Lung Volumes

The mean values for pulmonary function in the newborn and adult are shown in Table 48-4. The infant's metabolic rate and

TABLE **48-4**	Mean Values for Normal Pulmonary Function in the Newborn and the Adult		
		Newborn	**Adult**
Body weight (kg)		3	70
Tidal volume (mL/kg)		6	6
Respiratory rate (bpm)		35	15
Alveolar ventilation (mL/kg/min)		130	60
Oxygen consumption (mL/kg/min)		6.4	3.5
Total lung capacity (mL/kg)		63	86
Functional residual capacity (mL/kg)		30	34
Vital capacity (mL/kg)		35	70
Residual volume (mL/kg)		23	16
Closing capacity (mL/kg)		35	23
Arterial pH		7.38-7.41	7.35-7.45
$Paco_2$		30-35	35-45
Pao_2		60-90	90-100
Sao_2 (%)		95-100	95-100

$Paco_2$, *Partial pressure of arterial carbon dioxide;* Pao_2, *partial pressure of arterial oxygen;* Sao_2, *oxygen saturation.*

oxygen consumption are approximately twice those of the adult. The decreased reservoir for oxygen (decreased FRC), coupled with the increased demand for oxygen (increased metabolic rate), results in rapid desaturation when ventilation is interrupted. Airway closure produces a mismatching of ventilation and perfusion. The volume of these poorly ventilated alveoli that contribute to intrapulmonary shunting is greater in neonates than in adults. In addition, increased pulmonary vascular resistance can produce a right-to-left shunt through the foramen ovale or a patent ductus arteriosus, resulting in the rapid development of cyanosis.

Airway Dynamics

Airway resistance is greater in neonates and declines markedly with growth from 19 to 28 cm H_2O/L/sec to less than 2 cm H_2O/L/sec in adults[16,17] According to Poiseuille's law, airway resistance is inversely proportional to the fourth power of the radius of the airway during laminar flow. A neonate must overcome the resistance to airflow, as well as the elastic recoil of the lungs and chest wall. The rate of ventilation that uses the least amount of muscular energy and generates a satisfactory tidal volume has been found to be 37 breaths per minute in the healthy newborn.

The metabolic cost of breathing in the neonate is similar to an adult, approximately 0.5 mL per 0.5 L of ventilation. This is equivalent to 1% of their metabolic energy. The premature neonate's metabolic cost of breathing is 0.9 mL/0.5 L, almost double the metabolic price. If the neonate has pulmonary problems, the cost could go even higher.[18]

Airway resistance changes with age. Although the larger airway resistance remains constant, airway resistance in the smaller airways is increased. The increase in airway resistance increases the work of breathing in the neonate. Small airway disease (e.g., pneumonia) produces additional increases in the work of breathing.

Nervous System

The central nervous system in the newborn differs from the older child in the degree of myelination, muscle tone and reflexes, and development of the cerebral cortex. In the peripheral nervous system, myelination begins in the motor roots and progresses to the sensory roots. In contrast, the myelination in the cerebral sensory systems precedes that of the central motor systems. This incomplete myelination is associated with those reflexes that are used to measure neural development, the Moro and grasp reflexes. Myelination of the nervous system is not complete until age 3.

Development of Neuromuscular Junction

The neuromuscular junction (NMJ) undergoes developmental changes during the first 2 months of life. During the maturation process, the NMJ differs in several ways. There is a difference in the maturity, density, sensitivity and distribution of the post-synaptic acetylcholine receptors, in the rapidity of neuromuscular transmission, and in muscle fiber type.[19] What differentiates the immature receptors from the developed ones is a functional difference that is due to a prolonged opening of the ionic channels. This prolonged channel opening allows the immature muscles to be more easily depolarized. These receptors also have a greater affinity for depolarizing agents and a lower affinity for nondepolarizing muscle relaxants (NDMRs). The clinical implication of these maturational changes is that neonates can have a greater variability in their responses to nondepolarizing muscle relaxants and in the monitoring of the NMJ via a peripheral nerve stimulator. Neuromuscular immaturity may be demonstrated with the appearance of fade after tetanic stimulation in the absence of neuromuscular blocking drugs. It is also worth noting that the type I fibers are more sensitive to NDMRs when compared with type II fibers. The clinical relevance of this difference is that with the diaphragm of a neonate has fewer type I fibers as compared to a diaphragm of a toddler or an adult. This makes the diaphragm of a neonate more responsive to NDMRs than his own peripheral musculature.[20]

Pain Sensitivity

Pathways required for pain perception can be traced from sensory receptors in the skin to sensory areas in the cerebral cortex of newborn infants. These pain pathways have been demonstrated in the perioral area as early as 7 weeks gestation. With position emmission tomography scans, neonates demonstrate maximal metabolic activity in the regions associated with sensory perception, such as the cortex, thalamus and midbrain—brainstem regions. Neonatal anesthesia providers have seen newborns exhibit signs of increased sympathetic activity (tachycardia and hypertension) in response to surgical stimulation with inadequate anesthesia. The risks associated with inadequate or absent pain control expose the neonate to noxious stimulation that can have significant physiologic consequences. Those consequences in the presence of abnormal cerebral autoregulation could result in intraventricular hemorrhage and pulmonary hypertension.[21]

Lack of development of inhibitory tracts may actually increase the intensity and duration of the painful stimulus. It has been suggested that newborn infants may develop prolonged responses to painful procedures that far outlast the stimuli by hours or days. This is illustrated by several examples. Premature infants mount a metabolic stress response that can be blocked with opioids, increased crying, interrupted sleep patterns and behavioral changes have been shown to occur for days after circumcision,[22] and with repeated heel lancing there appeared to be a hyperalgesic response to injury.[23] Other physiologic alterations that have been demonstrated are increased right-to-left shunting, hypoxemia, acidosis, and intraventricular hemorrhage.[21]

Cranium

The skull of the neonate is less rigid and has a short-term ability to expand and accommodate increases in cerebral volume by expansion of the fontanelles. The anterior fontanelle closes at approximately 18 to 20 months of age. The "fullness" of the fontanelle can be used as an indicator of fluid volume status. In the full-term, healthy neonate, the brain accounts for approximately 10% of the total birth weight.

The spinal cord ends at approximately L3, reaching the adult level of L1 by age 8. This is an important consideration during lumbar puncture and spinal anesthesia in the neonate.

Cerebral Metabolic Requirement

Because of the rapid maturation of the central nervous system (CNS) during infancy and childhood, proper nutrition is essential to ensure normal development. With maturation there is an increase in the metabolic demands of the CNS. The primary fuel for the brain is glucose, and in the neonate there are decreased stores of glycogen, making hypoglycemia a major source of morbidity causing apnea, hypotension, bradycardia, convulsions and brain injury.

Cerebral Blood Flow

Cerebral blood flow (CBF) is closely coupled with cerebral metabolic rate of oxygen consumption ($CMRO_2$). CBF in the premature infant is 40 mL/100 g/minute, and in older children approaches the adult level of 100 mL/100 g/min. Autoregulation of CBF refers to the ability of the CNS to regulate CBF over a wide range of cerebral perfusion pressures. CBF autoregulation is thought to take place in the neonate, but the specific limits are unknown. Complete loss of cerebral autoregulation may occur with hypoxia, severe hypercapnia (>80 mm Hg), blood-brain barrier disruption following head trauma, subarachnoid or intracerebral hemorrhage, or cerebral ischemia, or following the administration of high concentrations of potent inhalation anesthetics and vasodilators (nitroprusside). Changes in CBF will parallel changes in cerebral blood volume, except when cerebral perfusion decreases and auroregulation produces vasodilation to maintain a constant flow. The cerebral vessels are very fragile in preterm and low-birth-weight infants. This fragility predisposes neonates to intracranial hemorrhage. Intracranial hemorrhage may be precipitated by hypoxia, hypercarbia, hyperglycemia, hypoglycemia, hypernatremia, and wide swings in arterial or venous pressure. The intravenous administration of hypertonic solutions may damage these fragile vessels. Therefore, adult-strength sodium bicarbonate should not be administered to neonates.

Renal System

The fetus does not worry about its fluid balance, because water and electrolytes equilibrate across the placenta in response to growth and metabolic demands. The fetal kidneys make urine that passes into the amniotic cavity to compose one half of the amniotic fluid, which is then swallowed and absorbed in the gut. Structurally the kidney is different in the neonate. Nephrons are still being formed up to 35 weeks' gestation. The resulting glomerular filtration rate is much lower in a preterm (0.55 mL/min/kg) than a full-term baby (up to 1.6 mL/min/kg) or a 2-year-old child (2 mL/min/kg). Decreased systemic arterial

TABLE 48-5	Daily Electrolyte Requirements of the Newborn	
Electrolyte	**Daily Requirement**
Sodium	2-3 mEq/kg
Potassium	1-2 mEq/kg
Calcium	149-200 mg/kg

pressure, increased renal vascular resistance, and decreased permeability of the glomerular capillaries contribute to the low glomerular filtration rate (GFR). In addition to the stiff, noncompliant myocardium, the neonate is unable to tolerate fluid overload because of the lower GFR. GFR reaches adult levels by 6 to 12 months. The renal medulla is not completely mature, and the potential effect of antidiuretic hormone is diminished. However, all of the hormones that affect the kidney are active even in a very immature infant, albeit with reduced potency. Neonates are *obligate sodium excreters* because of their inability to conserve sodium, even in cases of severe sodium depletion. The renin-angiotensin-aldosterone system (RAA) acts to reduce sodium loss from the distal tubule, but the immature renal tubules fail to respond. In addition, the renal tubules have a limited ability to reabsorb glucose. Increasing plasma glucose concentrations may elicit an osmotic diuresis, depleting intravascular volume. Table 48-5 lists the daily electrolyte requirements for the newborn. Renal tubular function is immature until the age of 2 to 3 years. The neonate has a limited ability to concentrate urine compared with an adult (700 vs 1200 mOsm/L). Overall, the neonate has a tendency to accumulate sodium because it is essential for growth. Atrial natriuretic peptide is present, but its effects are blunted. In effect, the neonatal kidney is able to excrete water and sodium but cannot conserve them like the kidney of an older child.[24]

By the end of the first month of life, renal function is approximately 70% of adult levels and by the end of the first year, renal function reaches adult levels.

Fluid Balance

Neonates have a high turnover of fluid. After the first week, a baby needs 150 mL/kg/day of fluid (equivalent to 20 pints a day for an adult). This is because milk has a low concentration of energy compared with solid food, and the neonate cannot physiologically reduce urine output below 1 mL/kg/hr. Neonates also have high insensible losses, particularly from evaporation, as a result of a high surface area/body-weight ratio (four times higher than an adult) and immature skin. These problems are accentuated for the preterm baby. Thirst mechanisms are poorly developed and are affected by sepsis or respiratory distress syndrome. Also, a surge of antidiuretic hormone at birth causes oliguria over the first few days. Table 48-6 summarizes indicators of fluid balance.

Hepatic System

The liver begins to develop at 10 weeks' gestation, and by 12 weeks' gestation it has already begun to function. Gluconeogenesis and protein synthesis are under way, and by 14 weeks glycogen is found in liver cells. The fetal liver has the ability to synthesize glycogen. Glycogen storage capacity is greatly increased just before birth. Approximately 98% of this stored glycogen is released from the liver within the first 48 hours of life, and glycogen levels are not restored to adult levels until the third week of life. Glycogen stores are not as large in preterm or small-for-gestational-age

TABLE 48-6	Indicators of Fluid Balance
Parameter	**Normal Range**
Sodium	133-144 mmol/L
Body weight	Should fall by up to 10% below birth, by 1 week, then increase
Hematocrit	Increases (without transfusion) suggest dehydration
Creatinine	Should fall from maternal levels to <50 μmol/L after 5 days

(SGA) infants. Therefore preterm and SGA infants should be monitored for the development of hypoglycemia.

The synthetic function of the liver is decreased, and the capability for biotransformation is decreased, with oxidative activities approximately one quarter to one half of adult values.[25] The capacity to enzymatically break down proteins is depressed at birth as a result of a decrement in quantity and quality of hepatic enzymes. Albumin, an essential protein that regulates colloidal osmotic pressure, is produced beginning at 3 to 4 months of gestation, reaching adult levels at the time of birth. Plasma levels of albumin and other necessary proteins for binding of drugs are lower in newborns and even lower in premature infants. The lower ability of the newborn to bind drug to plasma proteins results in greater levels of free drug. At approximately 2 years of age, its activity reaches adult levels.

There is little glucuronyl transferase activity in the fetal liver. This enzyme is responsible for the metabolic breakdown of bilirubin. Hyperbilirubinemia may develop in term infants within the first days of life. Bilirubin production as a result of the breakdown of RBCs and enterohepatic circulation are increased because of the aforementioned depressed activity of glucuronyl transferase that is required for hepatic conjugation. Bilirubin levels of 6 to 8 mg/100 mL are not uncommon in term infants. However, premature infants may have levels as high as 10 to 12 mg/mL on the third day of life. Phototherapy and, in rare cases, exchange transfusion are used to avoid the development of encephalopathy (kernicterus). In infants with hyperbilirubinemia, it is imperative that a determination of physiologic versus pathologic jaundice be determined.

Concentrations of clotting factors in the premature infant and the newborn are low; however, hepatic synthesis of essential clotting factors reaches adult levels during the first week after birth. In utero, the liver is the organ responsible for hematopoiesis, but by 4 to 6 weeks after birth, this function is assumed by the bone marrow.

Temperature Regulation

The neonate is decidedly disadvantaged in the regulation of body temperature. Large surface area, poor insulation, a small mass from which heat is generated, and the inability to shiver contribute to the problem of thermoregulation.

The neonate has a minimal ability to shiver, so sympathetic stimulation of brown fat metabolism (non-shivering thermogenesis [NST]) increases heat production. NST is the neonate's defense against hypothermia. It is metabolically driven heat production that does not involve muscular work. Brown fat stores located in the scapulae, axillae, the mediastinum, and in the retroperitoneal space surrounding the kidneys are

metabolically active and contain a high density of mitochondria. Hypothermia stimulates the release of norepinephrine, which acts on brown fat to uncouple oxidative phosphorylation.[26] Heat production follows an increase in the basal metabolic rate stimulated through the release of anterior pituitary hormones.

Perioperative hypothermia has many contributing causes, including a cold operating room environment, anesthetic-induced vasodilation, the infusion of room-temperature intravenous fluids, evaporative heat loss from opened body cavities, use of cool irrigating solutions, and the inspiration of cool/dry anesthetic gases.

It is well recognized that the thermoregulatory response is inhibited by anesthetic agents. Core body temperature may decrease as much as 1° C to 3° C. Heat loss occurs as a result of the internal redistribution of heat, reduced metabolism and heat production, increased heat loss to the environment, and the effects of anesthetic agents on thermoregulatory control. Heat loss occurs more rapidly in neonates because of limited heat production (NST) and the body surface/body weight ratio. The skin (particularly the premature neonate) is thinner and has less subcutaneous tissue, increasing the rate of evaporative heat loss.[27]

Radiant heat loss is responsible for the majority of heat loss.[28] Placing a neonate on a cold operating table results in heat transfer from the neonate to the table, with a resultant drop in core body temperature. In this example, radiant heat loss may be minimized by wrapping the neonate in a warm blanket and isolating from the cold operating table, effectively decreasing the transfer of heat. Radiant heat lamps may be used to maintain temperature during surgical positioning and preparation. Radiant heat lamps increase the temperature of the air between the neonate and the lamps, thereby minimizing radiant heat loss. However, radiant heat lamps are ineffective when operating room personnel or large objects are placed between the lamp and the patient. In addition, the placement of a radiant heat lamp in close proximity to the neonate may produce thermal injury.

Conductive heat loss occurs with the transfer of heat to the environment and is dependent on the temperature differences between the neonate and the environment. Conductive heat loss is minimized with the use of warmed irrigating solutions, the use of warm blankets or heated forced-air blankets to cover the nonoperative areas of the patient, and the prewarming of the operating room. Covering the head with a stockinette or reflective cap dramatically decreases conductive heat loss. The neonate's head may account for up to 60% of the total heat loss during the perioperative period.[29,30]

Convective heat loss is precipitated by moving air currents. The operating room air circulation is changed 6 to 12 times per hour and, in conjunction with cool ambient temperatures, increases heat loss. The air surrounding the body is warmed and subsequently rises, being replaced by the cooler ambient air. To minimize convective heat loss, the ambient air temperature must be increased. Prudent practice is to preheat the operating room to 26° C for premature and neonatal surgical patients. The premature infant or neonate arrives in the operating room in a heated isolette and is immediately covered with a warm blanket before being transferred to the operating table. Convective heat loss may be increased when wet cloth is in contact with the infant. Wet diapers and blankets soiled with preparation solutions must be replaced and not allowed to remain in contact with the skin.

Evaporative heat loss occurs through the vaporization of liquid from body cavities and the respiratory tract. Evaporative heat loss is either sensible loss (the evaporation of sweat) or insensible loss (the evaporation of water through the skin). The thin-skinned premature infant is particularly susceptible to insensible evaporative heat loss. Sensible evaporative heat loss may be prevented by removing wet clothing or blankets and thoroughly drying the neonate. Insensible evaporative heat loss may be mitigated by increasing the relative humidity of the operating room, covering the patient with a plastic barrier, and using warmed irrigating solutions. Insensible respiratory tract evaporative heat loss may be prevented with humidification of the inspired gases, which requires attentive temperature monitoring to avoid superheating of airway gases and subsequent airway burns. The addition of in-line humidifiers to the patient breathing circuit adds to the complexity and weight, perhaps increasing the likelihood of unintended tracheal extubation. These humidifiers may also contribute to unintended increases in core body temperature during lengthy surgical procedures. The use of a passive heat and moisture exchanger, added between the patient circuit and endotracheal tube, has been of questionable efficacy.[31,32]

Iatrogenic increases in core body temperature also may occur. Attentiveness in covering the neonate may result in progressive increases in core temperature during prolonged surgical procedures. These steady increases in core temperature may be aggravated by the previous administration of atropine. Surgical procedures may also affect thermoregulation.

ANESTHETIC PHARMACOLOGIC CONSIDERATIONS IN THE NEONATE

Physiologic characteristics that modify the pharmacokinetic (what the body does to the drug) and pharmacodynamic (what the drug does to the body) activity in the neonate include differences in total body water (TBW) composition; immaturity of metabolic degradation pathways; reduced protein binding; immaturity of the blood-brain barrier; greater proportion of blood flow to the brain, heart, liver and lungs; reduced glomerular filtration; smaller functional residual capacity; and increased minute ventilation.

Pharmacokinetics

Several age-related differences in absorption, distribution, and elimination effect pharmacologic responses in the neonate. Absorption and distribution are increased via an increased cardiac output per kilogram of body weight, protein binding limits, body composition, and the maturity of the blood-brain barrier. Elimination is many times decreased due to immature metabolic pathways and renal immaturity.

Cardiac Output

Resting cardiac output in the newborn is approximately 200 mL/kg/min. This means faster circulation times that are capable of delivering and removing drugs from their sites of action at a higher rate.

Body Composition

A large proportion of the neonate's body weight is water. As a result, water-soluble medications, such as neuromuscular blockers, will have a larger volume of distribution in this group of patients, possibly requiring a higher loading dose per kilogram of body weight to achieve the desired serum level and clinical response.[33] Table 48-7 illustrates the changes in TBW, intracelluar fluid (ICF) and extracellular fluid (EXF) during stages of maturation.

Protein Binding

Protein binding of parenterally administered drugs can be diminished in the neonate. The two plasma proteins to which drugs

TABLE **48-7**	Fluid Compartment Volumes			
	Premature	**Infant**	**Child**	**Adult**
Total body water (TBW)	80%-90%	75%	65%-70%	55%-60%
Extracellular fluid (ECF)	50%-60%	40%	30%	20%
Intracellular fluid (ICF)	60%	35%	40%	40%

From Aker J et al. Pediatric fluid and blood therapy. In: Zaglaniczny K, Aker J, eds. Clinical Guide to Pediatric Anesthesia. *Philadelphia: Saunders; 1999:85.*

bind, primarily albumin and α_1-acid glycoprotein, are decreased in quantity and quality. Drugs that are normally highly protein bound can have a greater free fraction of the drug and a greater pharmacologic effect.

Blood-Brain Barrier

The blood-brain barrier is not fully developed in the neonate. This barrier is relatively impermeable to most ionized substances and other large molecules when fully developed. In newborns and neonates, this immature blood-brain barrier results in greater uptake by the brain of certain drugs that are partially ionized, such as morphine.

Metabolism

Generally, owing to a large proportion of the cardiac output that traverses the liver in the neonate, there is a more rapid clearance of drugs. However, phase I (cytochrome-dependent) reactions (e.g., oxidation, reduction, hydrolysis) are not fully developed, making some anesthetic-related drugs last longer than anticipated. These processes are fully developed within the first week of life, with remaining cytochrome-dependent metabolic pathways continuing to increase during the first 3 months of life.[34] Phase II reactions (conjugation reactions) make many agents water soluble to promote renal excretion, and this process is underdeveloped in neonates. Consequently, normal pediatric doses should not be given until the infant has reached the age of 1 month. Certain cytochrome-dependent reactions can be induced prior to delivery when the mother is exposed to certain drugs and cigarette smoke.

The neonate lacks the capacity to efficiently conjugate bilirubin (decreased glucuronyl transferase activity) and metabolize acetaminophen, chloramphenicol, and sulfonamides. Although the necessary enzyme systems are present at birth, enzyme activity is reduced, increasing drug elimination half-lives. Drugs that produce a prolonged plasma half-life in the newborn/neonate include bupivacaine (25 hours),[35] mepivacaine (8.5 hours),[36] diazepam (up to 100 hours),[37] indomethacin (15 to 20 hours),[38] meperidine (22 hours), and phenytoin (21 hours).[39]

Excretion

Most anesthesia-related drugs are eliminated by the kidney. In the neonate, GFR and tubular function is reduced, particularly in those infants born at less than 34 weeks. However, renal function reaches adult levels by 8 to 12 months of age. Healthy preterm and full-term neonates have relatively normal renal drug clearance by 3 to 4 weeks of age.

Pharmacodynamics

Pharmacodynamics describes what the drugs do to the body. The actions of a drug and its receptor are influenced by number, type, and affinity of the receptor and availability of ligands.

Nicotinic Acetylcholine Receptor

In its fetal form, this receptor remains open longer after binding the acetylcholine, protecting or increasing the safety factor of neuromuscular transmission and could account for the neonate's resistance to muscle relaxants.[40] As it transitions into its adult form, the receptor open time is decreased after binding, resulting in less propensity for generation of an action potential, manifesting as less resistance to muscle relaxants. There is also a reduction in acetylcholine release in the neuromuscular junction in the neonate, which could account for the increased sensitivity to nondepolarizing muscle relaxants.[41] These opposing factors make a neonate's response to a neuromuscular blocking agents occasionally unpredictable.

Opioid Receptors

The mu and kappa receptors are responsible for the respiratory depression associated with opioids. In the neonate, changes in the number and affinity of these receptors may account for the respiratory depression that results when opioids are used.

γ-Aminobutyric Acid Receptor

Conventional thought is that the action of general anesthetics may be associated with activation of γ-aminobutyric acid (GABA) receptors.[42] There are only one third the number of the $GABA_A$ receptors in the neonate as compared with the adult, and half of these receptors have a high affinity for binding with benzodiazepines and other anesthetics.[43] The potency of anesthetics and benzodiazepines in these patients could be explained by the high affinity of these receptors.

DRUGS USED IN NEONATAL ANESTHESIA

Inhalation Agents

Inhaled anesthetic agents equilibrate more rapidly in neonates due to an increased level of ventilation in relation to FRC; increased cardiac output, which is directed mainly to the vessel-rich group of tissues; and reduced solubility of the inhaled anesthetics in blood. In addition, their decreased distribution of adipose tissue and decreased muscle mass affect the rate of equilibration among the alveoli, blood, and brain. Neonates have a somewhat lower minimum alveolar concentration (MAC), which peaks at around 30 days of age and decreases thereafter (Figure 48-3). The anesthetic implication is that induction in this patient population is more rapid and the development of cardiovascular side effects occurs sooner. The margin of safety between adequate anesthesia and significant cardiopulmonary depression is very narrow. Removal of inhalation agents, and therefore recovery, is also rapid, provided that cardiopulmonary function is not depressed.

In neonates there is both left-to-right and right-to-left intracardiac shunting. In the presence of a left-to-right shunt, there is no increase in anesthetic uptake due to no changes in anesthetic partial pressure when the recycled blood returns to the lungs. However, when there is a right-to-left shunt, there is a slowing of the rate of rise of the alveolar concentration of inhaled agent due to the decrease in the anesthetic concentration in the blood of the arterial system. The clinical implication of a right-to-left intracardiac shunt is that the neonate could have a prolonged induction time.

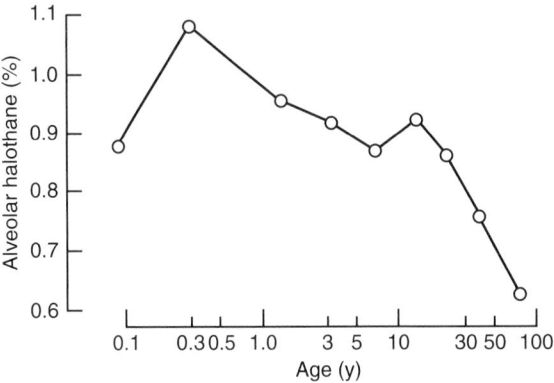

FIGURE **48-3** Effects of age on maximum alveolar concentration. (*Modified from Gregory GA et al. The relationship between age and halothane requirement in man. Anesthesiology. 1969;30:488-491; Lerman J et al. Anesthetic requirements for halothane in young children 0 to 1 month and 1 to 6 months of age. Anesthesiology. 1983;59: 421-424.*)

Potent inhalation agents all depress ventilation in a dose-dependent manner and increase the risk of apnea. Likewise, they readily depress the myocardium and blood pressure because of immature compensatory mechanisms.

Intravenous Agents

Neonates and infants have a higher proportion of cardiac output delivered to vessel-rich tissues (i.e., heart, brain, kidneys, and liver). Intravenously administered drugs are readily taken up by these tissues and are subsequently redistributed to tissues less well perfused (muscle and fat). Intravenously administered drugs may have a prolonged duration of action in neonates and infants because of decreased percentages of muscle and fat. The CNS effects of opioids and barbiturates may also be prolonged because of the immaturity of the blood-brain barrier.[44] Anesthetists have historically been hesitant to use opioids because of their toxicity profile in neonates, particularly morphine. It is less lipid soluble, and this allows it greater access through the immature blood-brain barrier and may result in proportionately greater levels in the brain. Fentanyl is well tolerated even in the sickest neonates. Yaster reported that fentanyl 10 mcg/kg produced cardiovascular stability in neonates undergoing repair of congenital anomalies.[45] Even doses as high as 30 to 50 mcg/kg have been reported in patent ductus arteriosus ligation.[46,47] Although this evidence suggests that intravenously administered anesthetic doses should be reduced, one must also recall the effect of increased body water. Increased doses of thiopental, propofol, and ketamine are required, presumably because of a greater volume of distribution.[48]

In most circumstances when a neonate requires some type of surgical intervention, intravenous access is established prior to arrival in the operating room. If the access is peripheral, it can be used for induction of anesthesia with intravenous agents. However, if the vascular access is central, it should not be used for induction unless thorough aseptic technique is observed. If the central line is being used for hyperalimentation, it should not be used.

Neuromuscular Blocking Drugs

Neuromuscular blocking drugs are highly ionized and have a low lipophilicity, which limits their ability to cross the blood-brain barrier. These pharmacologic properties restrict the distribution

TABLE 48-8	Effective Doses (ED95) of Clinical Neuromuscular Blocking Drugs (mcg/kg)			
	Neonate	**Infant**	**Child**	**Adult**
Succinylcholine*	620	729	423	290
Atracurium	120	156-175	170-350	110-280
Vecuronium	47	42-47	56-80	27-56
Rocuronium	600	600	600	300
Pancuronium	–	55	55-81	49-70

*Should be used for emergency airway stabilization in children younger than 12 years. Not for routine intubation.

of neuromuscular blockers to the ECF compartment, which is larger in the neonate and infant than in the child and adult (see Table 48-7). Increases in ECF volume and the ongoing maturation of neonatal skeletal muscle and acetylcholine receptors affect the pharmacokinetics and pharmacodynamics of neuromuscular blockers. The dose requirements are similar to those of adults because of the combined effects of a larger volume of distribution and increased sensitivity to the drug. The result is neuromuscular blockade at a lower plasma concentration. The variation in response to these relaxants could be due to each neonate's volume of distribution, as well as the presence of a higher proportion of extra junctional receptors. Table 48-8 references the effective doses of neuromuscular blocking drugs in various age groups.

The neuromuscular junction is incompletely developed at birth. The presynaptic release of acetylcholine is slowed at birth compared with that in the adult, which explains the decreased margin of safety for neuromuscular transmission in the neonate. The acetylcholine receptors of the newborn are anatomically different from the adult receptors, which may explain the sensitivity of the neonate to the nondepolarizing class of neuromuscular blockers.

- Neonates are more resistant to the effects of succinylcholine than children and adults. This sensitivity is illustrated by the intravenous ED_{95} for neonates (620 mcg/kg), infants (729 mcg/kg), children (423 mcg/kg), and adults (290 mcg/kg) (see Table 48-8). The increase in dose requirement is in part a result of the increased volume of distribution within the large extracellular compartment.[49] Plasma cholinesterase activity is reduced in neonates; however, the duration of action after a single dose is of expected duration (6 to 10 minutes). A longer duration of action after a single bolus dose suggests the presence of an inherited deficiency of plasma cholinesterase activity.
- Neonates are sensitive to the effects of nondepolarizing neuromuscular blocking drugs. This apparent sensitivity may be explained in part by the larger volume of drug distribution.

The selection of a nondepolarizing neuromuscular blocker should take into consideration the desired degree and duration of skeletal muscle paralysis, the immaturity of organ systems, and the associated side effects of the selected relaxant. Interpatient variability in response to these drugs is greater, particularly in premature infants and neonates. Monitoring of neuromuscular function must be used to guide repeated administration of these drugs in all neonatal patients (and should be used in all patients requiring neuromuscular blockade).

Reversal of Neuromuscular Blockade

The neonate is more vulnerable if respiration is impaired even to a mild degree; more alveoli will collapse, leading to hypoxia and progressive acidosis, potentiating and prolonging the blockade. Neuromuscular blockade should always be reversed unless mechanical ventilation in the postoperative period is planned. Rackow and colleagues found that 20% of neonates required assisted ventilation postoperatively when neuromuscular blockade was not reversed.[50] Antagonism can be negatively impacted if the patient is hypothermic (<35° C) or has been on aminoglycosides (neomycin, gentamicin, tobramycin). Hypocalcemia has a deleterious effect on muscular contraction and can potentiate neuromuscular blockade. It is usually the result of some type of metabolic problem. Calcium chloride 3 to 5 mg/kg can be administered slowly while observing return of muscle tone. The safest treatment of prolonged apnea is sedation and controlled ventilation until the neuromuscular blocker is eliminated.

It can be difficult to judge adequacy of reversal in neonates. The rule of thumb is to observe flexion of the elbows and hips, return of abdominal muscle tone, and presence of facial grimacing. Another measurement is the ability to generate a maximum inspiratory force (MIF) greater than 25 cm of water or a crying capacity of more than 15 mL/kg.[51] Neonates are capable of generating an MIF of −70 cm H_2O with the first few breaths after birth.[52] An MIF of at least −32 cm H_2O has been found to correspond with leg lift, which is indicative of the adequacy of ventilatory reserve required before tracheal extubation.[53] If a peripheral nerve stimulator is used, the train-of-four should demonstrate four equal contractions.

There are two commonly used anticholinesterase drugs for reversal of neuromuscular blockade; neostigmine (0.05 to 0.07 mg/kg) and edrophonium (0.5 to 1.0 mg/kg). An anticholinergic agent, atropine (0.02 mg/kg) or glycopyrrolate (0.01 mg/kg), should be given prior to the anticholinesterase to prevent vagotonic bradycardia. It has been reported that owing to similarities in time to onset and duration of action, glycopyrrolate can be given with neostigmine and atropine with edrophonium. However, the gold standard is to administer the anticholinergic agent, observe for any increase in heart rate, and then administer the anticholinesterase. This technique guarantees the arrival of the anticholinergic drug prior to the anticholinesterase, thereby avoiding the muscarinic effects.

Drug Preservatives

Premature neonates have a reduced ability to metabolize the preservatives benzyl alcohol and sodium benzoate. This accumulation of benzoic acid results in the "benzyl alcohol gasping syndrome," with deterioration of multiple organ systems, severe metabolic acidosis, and gasping respirations. These agents can produce severe CNS toxicity, seizures, and permanent brain damage. Use of preservative-free drugs and solutions is essential.

FLUID MANAGEMENT

Neonatal fluid management varies based on gestational age, birth weight, rate of caloric expenditure and growth, ratio of evaporative surface area to body weight, the degree of renal functional maturation and reserve, and the TBW.[54] Total body water accounts for approximately 75% of body weight in the neonate. This high percentage of TBW results from expansion of the extracellular fluid compartment, which may account for 50% of the TBW. In the first few days of life, a term neonate can lose 5% to 15% of its body weight. Urine output is low and if kept warm and covered, fluid requirements are relatively low, as little

---

BOX 48-1

Common Intravenous Fluid and Electrolyte Requirements in the Newborn

Glucose

Most newborns require 2-4 mg/kg/min.

SGA/LGA infants may require >15 mg/kg/min on days 1 to 3 of life.

Glucose tolerance may fluctuate significantly in very low- and extremely low-birth-weight (VLBW and ELBW) infants.

Sodium

Most neonates require no sodium for the first 24 hours of life.

On day 2 and beyond, most newborns receive 2 to 4 mEq/kg/day.

Sodium requirement may change dramatically in response to gastrointestinal, genitourinary, or transcutaneous losses or drug or metabolic effects.

The ELBW infant may have huge transcutaneous losses, requiring meticulous monitoring and replacement.

Potassium

Requirements for potassium are minimal for the first 24 to 48 hours of life.

Subsequently, maintenance delivery is about 1 to 3 mEq/kg/day, always in the presence of a normal urine output.

Serum levels in the newborn, especially VLBW and ELBW, are higher than in older infants.

Replace gastrointestinal, genitourinary, or iatrogenic losses cautiously.

Calcium

Requirements for calcium range between 200 and 400 mg/kg/day (calcium gluconate).

Requirements for calcium vary with gestational age, history of asphyxia, growth disturbances (SGA, LGA).

Serum levels can be obtained for total Ca^{2+} and/or ionized Ca^{2+}.

From Brett C et al. Anesthesia for neonates and premature infants. In: Motoyama EK, Davis PJ, eds. Smith's Anesthesia for Infants and Children. 7th edition. St Louis: Mosby; 2006:534.

LGA, Large for gestational age; SGA, small for gestational age.

---

as 40 to 60 mL/kg/day.[55,56] Box 48-1 shows the common electrolyte requirements in the newborn.

Assessing Fluid Requirements

In the neonatal period, several physiologic and physical factors can affect fluid requirements. Basically, the smaller the infant the larger the percentage of body water to total body weight. With the smaller amount of body fat, the major part of body weight is body water. The combination of uncontrollable renal loss and a large insensible water loss make the neonate prone to dehydration and hemodynamic instability. There are numerous physical observations that can assist in estimating the fluid status of the patient. Table 48-9 illustrates some of those clinical signs.[57]

Anesthesia and surgery have a significant effect on fluid homeostasis and renal function. The combination of vasodilatation, myocardial depression and blood pressure changes may alter fluid compartment dynamics, vascular capacitance, and/or organ flood flow. The RAA system is inhibited as a result of anesthesia, as is GFR. The neonate is at risk for an increase in intravascular volume and eventually body water overload.

Water Requirements

Holliday and Segar published the seminal work identifying caloric requirements of the "average" hospitalized infant based on body weight.[55] A secondary finding was that the water requirement in milliliters was equivalent to the total energy expended in calories. However, the immature renal system cannot excrete large amounts of free water and their water requirements are less. Table 48-10 gives the water requirements of newborns.

Several things should be considered in planning the fluid management in the neonatal surgical patient:

- Dehydration present before preoperative fasting
- Fluid deficit due to fasting

TABLE **48-9**	Estimation of Degree of Dehydration		
	Degree of Dehydration		
Sign	<5%	5%-10%	10%-15%
Skin turgor	Good	Tenting	Poor
Feel of skin	Moist	Dry	Clammy
Mucous membranes	Moist	Dry	Parched
Eyeballs	Normal	Deep set	Sunken
Fontanelle	Flat	Soft	Sunken
CNS	Consolable	Irritable	Lethargy coma
CV	Normal	Normal	Decreased BP and capillary filling

From Bissonnette B. Fluid therapy. In: Hughes D et al, eds. Neonatal Anesthesia. London: Saunders; 1996.

CNS, Central nervous system; CV, cerebrovascular.

- Maintenance requirements during anesthesia/surgery
- Estimated third-space loss
- Alterations in body temperature

Because of the nature of the surgical interventions required by neonates, most will have had their fluid status managed in a neonatal unit. If that is not the case, during the time of preoperative evaluation, deficits should be determined and dehydration or electrolyte imbalance should be reversed. Other issues, not limited to acidosis, low hemoglobin, poor urine output, and poor perfusion should be resolved.[21]

Fasting times for the elective procedure should be as short as is safe for the patient. The standard is that the neonate can be formula fed up to 4 hours prior to anesthesia and given clear

TABLE 48-10	Water Requirements of Newborns		
	Water Requirement (mL/kg/24 hr) by Age		
Birth weight (g)	1-2 days	3-7 days	7-30 days
<750	100-250	149-300	120-180
749-1000	80-150	100-150	120-180
1000-1500	60-100	80-150	120-180
>1500	60-80	100-150	120-180

From Alexander DC, Robin B. Neonatology. In: Siberry GK, Iannone R, eds. The Harriet Lane Handbook. 15th ed. St Louis: Mosby; 2000.

liquids until 2 hours before surgery. The fasting requirements of the breastfed neonate can be controversial. Some anesthesia providers assert that breast milk is equivalent to formula or solids and should be stopped at 4 hours preoperatively. Others feel that it is somewhere between solids and clear liquids and will allow it up to 2 to 3 hours prior to surgery.[58]

Knowledge of the caloric requirements of the neonate can be used to estimate the maintenance fluid requirements. The classic "4-2-1" rule takes the caloric expenditure into consideration because it is calculated by body weight. A neonate weighing less than 10 kg will require 100 mL/kg/day or 4 mL/kg/hr.

Fluid deficits are a result of preoperative fasting or excessive gastrointestinal (GI) losses. Neonates receiving adequate preoperative maintenance will have no deficit and will require no deficit replacement calculated into the fluid management plan. If there has not been adequate maintenance, the fluid deficit can be calculated by multiplying the hourly maintenance rate by the number of hours without feeding. Total deficit restoration may require several hours or even days in the smallest babies. The goal is to restore and preserve the cardiovascular stability and renal perfusion.

In the presence of total parenteral nutrition (TPN), the amount of glucose/kg/min, as well as other components such as sodium, potassium, and calcium currently being administered, should be noted. If at all possible, the TPN should be maintained without interruption. If it must be discontinued, glucose must be monitored vigilantly and dextrose added to the fluid management plan.

Third-space losses need to be replaced with a solution that does not contain glucose (e.g., normal saline, lactated Ringer's or Plasma-Lyte). In those patients with abdominal lesions such as gastroschisis or necrotizing enterocolitis (NEC), the third-space losses can be very large. These babies may need as much as 25 to 100 mL/kg/hr to replace fluid loss.

Urine osmolality and specific gravity and serum osmolality are important indices in managing intraoperative fluids in neonates. They provide information as to the need for fluid, solute, and electrolyte replacement. Normal urine osmolality in the neonate ranges from 49 to 800 mOsm/L, with an average of 270 mOsm/L. Osmolality should be maintained between 200 and 400 mOsm/L and specific gravity between 1.006 and 1.012. Serum osmolality ranges between 270 and 280 mOsm/kg.[59] Hyperosmolar states can result in intraventricular hemorrhage or kidney damage.

Fluid Management of the Premature Infant

Proper fluid management of the premature infant requires an understanding of severable variables: the extensive variability in body fluid composition, renal maturation, neuroendocrine control of intravascular fluid status,[60] and insensible fluid loss with age.[61] Renal tubular function develops after the 24th week of gestation, and nephrons mature by the 36th week.[62,63] The premature infant has a lower GFR and immature tubular function. The immature kidneys are unable to excrete sodium and excess fluid. The inability to concentrate urine secondary to the inability to reabsorb sodium leads to the excretion of large quantities of dilute urine. Therefore, underestimation of fluid needs leads to more serious consequences than overestimation of fluid needs.[64]

Glucose homeostasis is volatile in the premature neonate. Hypoglycemia can be attributed to inadequate glycogen stores and deficient gluconeogenesis. Symptoms of hypoglycemia are jitteriness, cyanosis, apnea, lethargy, hypotonia, and seizures. If not treated rapidly, hypoglycemia in the preterm neonate can lead to neurologic damage. Preterm and SGA neonates can have a glucose requirement of 8 to 10 mg/kg/min to prevent hypoglycemia. Glucose as a D_5 or D_{10} solution followed by a 10% to 15% dextrose solution can be titrated to maintain a serum glucose level greater than 40 mg/dL.[21] It is as important to avoid hyperglycemia, which can result in intraventricular hemorrhage, osmotic diuresis, dehydration, and release of insulin, leading to hypoglycemia.

Electrolyte abnormalities are often seen in preterm neonates. Hypernatremia may result if water loss is greater than sodium depletion combined with abnormal renal tubular function. Hypokalemia can result from respiratory alkalosis or aggressive diuresis. Hyperkalemia can be caused by infusion of large amounts of potassium-containing fluids.

Blood Replacement

Over the first 6 months of life, many physiologic changes are occurring that can complicate the decision to replace blood in the neonatal surgical patient. Fetal hemoglobin (HbF), which has a higher affinity for oxygen than adult hemoglobin, can range from 70% to 80% of the neonate's total hemoglobin at birth. It can be as high as 97% in the preterm infant.[65] The clinical implication of this is that the younger the baby, the higher the fraction of HbF and thus the lower the oxygen-carrying capacity and oxygen delivery to the tissues.

Replacement of blood loss is critical in the surgical neonate, especially the preterm infant. Their blood volume is very small (85 to 100 mL/kg), and a loss of 10 mL could be approximately 10% of total blood volume. The clinical indication for blood administration should not be some predetermined percentage of total blood volume. Maintaining oxygen-carrying capacity and oxygen delivery to peripheral tissues and improving coagulation are the primary concerns. The transfusion trigger in this age group will need to be at higher hemoglobin levels than the older infant or child. Rapid blood loss in neonates can result in cardiovascular complications quicker than in the adult; therefore, transfusion may be required sooner. In the sick, surgical neonate and particularly the preterm baby, the hematocrit should be approximately 30% to 40%. The decision to transfuse should be based on the underlying and current cardiorespiratory status, ongoing blood loss, anticipated further blood loss, and baseline hemoglobin. Another concern is the presence of congenital heart disease or lung disease, resulting in a decreased ability to oxygenate blood.

The accurate measurement of blood loss in neonates and infants is crucial to any replacement regimen. The margin of safety is reduced in the neonate, and because the oxygen consumption is twice that of the adult, a smaller percentage of blood loss will result in cardiovascular instability. It has been reported as recently as August of 2007 in an article published by Bhananker and colleagues that 41% of all cardiac arrests in pediatric surgical patients were due to hypovolemia from blood loss and hyperkalemia from transfusion of stored blood.[66] It is mandatory to monitor loss by the weighing of sponges, the use of small calibrated suction containers, and vigilant visual estimation of ongoing blood loss. Every 1 of sponge weight is equal to 1 mL of blood loss.

Estimating Allowable Blood Loss

The estimated blood volume (EBV) and allowable blood loss (ABL) must be calculated prior to induction of anesthesia for any procedure where blood loss is expected. Estimated blood volume is calculated based on age and body weight (see Table 48-2).

A predetermined acceptable low hematocrit is identified based on the clinical situation and the baby's health. Maximum allowable blood loss (MABL) can be calculated with the formula below where Hct_0 is the original hematocrit, H_l is the lowest acceptable hematocrit, and H_a is the average hematocrit, $(Hc_{+0} + Hc_1)/2$.

Equation 48-1

$$MABL = wt\ (kg) \times EBV \times (Hct_0 - Hct_1)/Hct_a$$

Example: A surgical neonate who weighs 4 kg is going to have an abdominal procedure. Beginning hematocrit is 42%. The lowest acceptable hematocrit is 30%. The MABL for this patient is 106 mL.

$$MABL = 4 \times 320 \times (42 - 30)/(42 + 30)/2 = 106$$

When the blood loss equals or exceeds the calculated allowable loss, transfusion should be considered. The volume of packed RBCs to be infused may be determined by the following formula:

Equation 48-2

$$Packed\ RBCs\ (mL) =$$
$$\frac{(Blood\ loss - ABL) \times Desired\ hematocrit\ (30\%)}{Hematocrit\ of\ PRBCs\ (75\%)}$$

Using the previous example of a 4-kg infant, with a total blood loss of 100 mL, the volume of PRBCs would be $175 - 106 \times 30/75 = 27.6$ mL.

The administration of packed red cells can lead to a significant increase in the plasma potassium and cardiac arrest. Hyperkalemia associated with massive transfusion has been reported to be the most common cause of arrest in noncardiac procedures.[67] Rapid administration via handheld syringes and small gauge catheters (23-gauge or smaller) of packed cells stored less than 2 weeks have also be reported to result in hyperkalemia.[68] Hypocalcemia and cardiovascular instability can result from the rapid administration of blood due to the amount of citrate contained in the stored blood. Whole blood should not be used, and irradiated blood should be given only in immunocompromised patients. Irradiation accelerates the leakage of potassium from red cells into serum. To reduce the risk of hyperkalemia, washed or fresh (i.e., less than 7 days old) PRBCs should be used.[65]

ANESTHETIC EQUIPMENT

Anatomic differences in the face and upper airway affect the design of the masks, laryngoscopes, and tracheal tubes. Physiologically, the need to minimize the resistance and dead space has design implications for breathing systems, connectors,

TABLE **48-11**	Recommended Endotracheal Tube Sizes
Neonatal Age	**Endotracheal Tube Size**
Preterm neonate	2.0-3.0
Full-term neonate	3.0-3.5
3 months to 1 year	4.0

and tubes. Disposable, humidified pediatric circle systems are more commonly used in neonates for some important reasons. These systems have low compliance, they are lightweight, and with the addition of plastic valves have eliminated the high resistance associated with older systems. They also offer a more reliable method of monitoring end-tidal carbon dioxide. Ventilation is usually controlled in these patients, reducing the deleterious effects of the work of breathing in the spontaneously ventilating baby.

The anesthesia machine should be equipped to deliver air when nitrous oxide is not desirable, for example, in the neonate undergoing some type of abdominal procedure or when it is necessary to reduce the inspired oxygen concentration to avoid retinopathy of prematurity (ROP). Most patients are mechanically ventilated. The newest anesthesia machines have ventilators designed to deliver very small tidal volumes at appropriately high rates and pressures. It is also possible to adapt and use the ventilators used in the neonatal intensive care units (NICUs), However, this is not the most desirable method of mechanical ventilation in the operating room. In some pediatric centers, with the most critically ill neonates, certain operative procedures are actually performed in the NICU to avoid disturbing the delicately balanced ventilation patterns and to preserve cardiorespiratory stability.

The anatomy of the upper airway makes a straight blade preferable. The blade is placed along the right side of the mouth, sweeping the tongue to the left. The epiglottis is picked up with the tip of the blade and the tracheal inlet exposed. The tube is inserted with the convex side to the left. When the tip approaches the glottic opening, rotate the tube 90 degrees counterclockwise. There are several types of straight-bladed laryngoscopes: Anderson-Magill, Seward, Flagg, Robertshaw, and Miller. The advantage of one over to another is the characteristic that allows the large tongue of the neonate to be manipulated out of the visual field. There are also modifications of straight blades that allow insufflation of oxygen into the pharynx during intubation.

Oral endotracheal tube (OET) size for neonates cannot be calculated by formula because of the rapid growth during the immediate postnatal period. It can be determined from a table based on kilogram weight (Table 48-11). It is common for the full-term neonate to accommodate a 3.0 mm OET and a premature infant (<2 kg) to need a 2.5-mm OET. A clinical shortcut is to look at the size of the tip of the 5th ("pinkie") finger. It is wise to select a tube that will result in an air leak at 20 to 30 cm H_2O pressure to avoid postextubation airway edema.

The length of the trachea (vocal cords to carina) in neonates and infants up to 1 year varies from 5 to 9 cm. Insertion distance of an oral endotracheal tube should be less than 10 cm, falling within the 8 to 10 cm range.

Traditionally it was taught that in pediatric patients up to 8 years of age, the use of an uncuffed endotracheal tube was the accepted method for endotracheal airway management. The standard of practice in neonatal anesthesia has been the use of uncuffed endotracheal tubes for reasons of airway resistance and tracheal damage from inflated cuffs. In light of new scientific evidence, the proper use of cuffed endotracheal tubes under certain clinical situations is acceptable. In 2004, in an article published in the British journal *Pediatric Anesthesia*, the authors stated that a cuffed OET is appropriate and should be the first choice when an OET of greater than 3.5 mm inner diameter is contemplated for use. It concluded that the advantages of decrease in air pollution, the use of lower fresh gas flow rates (more economical), and the possible avoidance of repeated laryngoscopy and intubation to seal the leak enable better control of ventilation. The negatives associated with using cuffed OETs less than 3.5 mm for prolonged periods include the risk of tube blockage and increasing the work of breathing (WOB). However, because most neonatal patients will have their ventilation controlled, the problems with WOB can be overcome with appropriate ventilator settings.[69]

Monitoring of the neonate during anesthesia is important in detecting those small changes that can be very significant because of their smaller physiologic margin of safety. The anesthetist should not devalue the use of clinical observation skills—hearing, seeing, touching, and the rest. Even the most sophisticated electronic monitor can never replace the anesthetist's touch on the baby.

The precordial or esophageal stethoscope, as the case allows, is a simple means of assessing heart rate, rhythm, sound, and secondarily extrapolate vascular volume. Continuous ECG monitoring is used for monitoring of not only heart rate but also for detection of arrhythmias, particularly in the baby that has electrolyte imbalances. Pulse oximetry is the standard of care for all patients in a critical care or surgical environment. The other standard monitoring parameters are blood pressure; inspired oxygen concentration; end-tidal carbon dioxide and inhalation agent concentration; and peak airway and end-expiratory pressure monitoring. Neuromuscular monitoring is technically difficult in the neonate, particularly preterm and very low-birth-weight babies, owing to their small muscle mass. The use of needle electrodes must be justified because of the risk of infection and bleeding.[21] The monitoring of urine output is next to impossible because of technical problems of size of the catheters and accessibility of the patient.

PREOPERATIVE ASSESSMENT

The perioperative management of any neonate is determined by the nature of the surgical procedure, the gestational age at birth, postgestational age at surgery, and associated medical conditions.

Gestational Age and Postgestational Age at Surgery

The gestational age and postgestational age are critical to the determination of the physiologic development of the neonate. The history of the delivery and the immediate postdelivery course can influence the choice of anesthetic technique and assist in anticipating possible postoperative complications.

Preterm neonates are classified as *borderline preterm* (36 to 37 weeks gestation); *moderately preterm* (31 to 36 weeks gestation); and *severely preterm* (24 to 30 weeks gestation).[70] Neonates can be classified according to their weight, as well as their gestational age. Full term is considered to be 37 to 42 weeks' gestation. However, even full-term neonates that are SGA often present with conditions requiring surgical intervention. SGA neonates have different pathophysiologic problems from preterm infants (<37 weeks' gestation) of the same weight.[71] Gestational age and neonatal problems are closely related. Maternal health problems also

TABLE 48-12	Maternal History with Commonly Associated Neonatal Problems
Maternal History	**Anticipated Neonatal Sequelae**
Rh-ABO incompatibility	Hemolytic anemia Hyperbilirubinemia Kernicterus
Toxemia	Small for gestational age and its associated problems Muscle relaxant interaction after magnesium therapy
Hypertension	Small for gestational age and its associated problems
Drug addiction	Withdrawal and small for gestational age
Infection	Sepsis, thrombocytopenia, viral infection
Hemorrhage	Anemia, shock
Diabetes	Hypoglycemia, birth trauma, large or small for gestational age and associated problems
Polyhydramnios	TE fistula, anencephaly, multiple anomalies
Oligohydramnios	Renal hypoplasia, pulmonary hypoplasia
Cephalopelvic disproportion	Birth trauma, hyperbilirubinemia, fractures
Alcoholism	Hypoglycemia, congenital malformation, fetal alcohol syndrome, small for gestational age and associated problems

Adapted from Cote CJ et al. Preoperative evaluation of pediatric patients. In: Cote CJ et al, eds: A Practice of Anesthesia for Infants and Children. 3rd. Philadelphia: Saunders; 2001:39.
TE, *Transesophageal.*

can have significant implications for all neonates. Table 48-12 lists several common maternal problems and the possible associated neonatal sequelae.

Prematurity

Because of advances in neonatal medicine, many preterm babies born at exceptionally early gestational age and extremely low birth weights are surviving to be challenged with a plethora of unique diseases and pose many anesthetic challenges. The premature infant is not an infrequent visitor to the operating room for either elective or emergent surgical intervention. Prematurity presents its own set of complications, which include anemia, intraventricular hemorrhage, periodic apnea accompanied by bradycardia, and chronic respiratory dysfunction. It is beyond the scope of this chapter to address all issues regarding preterm neonates and anesthetic implications.

Premature neonates are challenging to evaluate, and considerable controversy exists regarding the appropriateness of elective surgical intervention and proper postoperative care. Postgestational age (gestational age + postnatal age) should be determined at the time of the anesthetic evaluation. Premature infants of less than 60 weeks postgestational age have the greatest risk of experiencing postanesthetic complications. The manifestations

From Aker J. Preoperative preparation of the pediatric patient: capsules and comments. Nurse Anesth. 1996;1:1.

of prematurity are thought to occur as a result of inadequate development of respiratory drive and immature cardiovascular responses to hypoxia and hypercapnia. Therefore, premature infants have a significant risk of postoperative apnea and bradycardia during the first 24 hours after general anesthesia.[72-74] Box 48-2 lists contributing factors that may influence the occurrence of apnea in premature infants.

Apnea in the Premature Infant

Some generalities regarding the frequency of postoperative apnea can be made.[75-76] The incidence of apnea in the postoperative period is inversely related to postgestational age and is most frequent in infants of less than 50 weeks postgestational age. Apnea may still occur when regional anesthetic techniques have been substituted for general anesthesia. Premature infants without a history of apnea or bradycardia may still experience postoperative apnea. Premature infants with histories of respiratory distress, concurrent respiratory disease, and periods of apnea are twice as likely to develop postoperative apnea.[77] Concurrent anemia (hematocrit <30%) places additional risk for the occurrence of postoperative apnea.[74]

Kurth recommends in-house admission of all premature infants of less than 60 weeks postgestational age after general anesthesia, with continuous monitoring for apnea and bradycardia for at least the first 24 hours. Such children should have a minimum of 12 apnea-free hours before dismissal.[77] Welborn recommends deferral of elective surgical procedures until 44 weeks postgestational age. Infants younger than 44 weeks postgestational age should be admitted postoperatively and monitored for at least 12 hours for the occurrence of apnea and bradycardia.[76] The care of these infants is further clouded by a recent report suggesting the need for oxygen monitoring in the postoperative period. Prolonged periods of hypoxemia may be unaccompanied by bradycardia or apnea in healthy premature infants.

Outpatient surgical care is usually not an acceptable venue for premature infants. Although the literature supports an increased risk for premature infants up to 60 weeks postgestational age, debate continues as to when this risk decreases. Mestad and colleagues found that premature infants at 40 weeks postgestational age without a history of apnea or bradycardia can be safely discharged after outpatient anesthesia.[78]

Apnea Prevention and Treatment. Much is written about the use of caffeine in the prevention and treatment of apnea in the preterm neonate. Historically, theophylline had been used, and in 1981 it was reported that the same results could be seen with caffeine. It was determined that preterm neonates methylate theophylline into caffeine (owing to the immature demethylation and oxidation pathways in the liver) and that even at high concentrations (50 mg/L), there were no toxic effects. Conversely, theophylline demonstrated cardiovascular toxicity at much lower levels.[79-81] The standard doses of caffeine and theophylline are 10 mg/kg and 6 mg/kg, respectively. Both have been shown to reduce the incidence of idiopathic apnea of prematurity and reduce the occurrence of apnea after surgery in the premature baby.

Preanesthetic Assessment and Neonatal Anesthetic Implications

The anesthesia provider is responsible for coordinating preoperative evaluation and acting as a gatekeeper to ensure that undue risks are minimized. Valuable information is obtained from those caring for the baby in the NICU. It is often best to alter the infant's plan of therapy as little as possible (i.e., management of ventilation, acid base status, glucose, etc). Consultation with the neonatologist will be helpful.

A maternal drug history is very important. In presence of illicit drugs, such as heroin and cocaine, the baby could be withdrawing from the drug at the time of surgery. Particularly with cocaine, there is an increased incidence of pulmonary hypertension and bowel perforation. Some mothers take large doses of aspirin or acetaminophen during pregnancy. Their infants could also exhibit pulmonary hypertension and persistent fetal circulation during the first few days of life.[82]

All of the information gathered during the assessment will lead to the anesthetic plan based on the implications of all the transitioning body systems. Table 48-13 gives the characteristics of the body system and the anesthetic implications.

System Review and Examination

The two body systems that are of primary interest in a preanesthetic system review are the respiratory and cardiovascular systems. However, there are other important metabolic and structural problems that can have a significant impact on the anesthesia plan. When performing a physical assessment, one should look carefully for congenital anomalies. A rule of thumb is that if there is one anomaly present, there are probably more because many occur in clusters, labeled a syndrome. These problems can occur most often in small and large for gestational age neonates (Box 48-3) and should be analyzed and understood.

Head and Neck Abnormalities

Any abnormality of the head and/or neck should raise the concerns regarding airway management. The shape and size of the head, with or without the presence of pathology, can make airway management difficult. The small mouth and large tongue can obstruct the airway during mask ventilation. Neonates have very small nares, and when obstructed by an anesthesia face mask, they do not convert to mouth breathing, particularly if the mouth is being held closed. A nasogastric tube can obstruct half of the neonat's airway and should be placed orally. A small and/or receding chin, as seen in Pierre Robin and Treacher

Collins syndromes, may make direct laryngoscopy and visualization of the glottis impossible, requiring other types of airway management. Cleft lip, with or without cleft palate may complicate intubation. Anomalies such as cystic hygroma or hemangioma of the neck can produce upper airway obstruction. In the case of a preterm neonate, it should also be determined if the patient has retinopathy of prematurity (ROP), cataracts or glaucoma. Atropine administration could result in significant increases in intraocular pressure and further damage to the eye.

Respiratory System Abnormalities

The incidence of respiratory distress syndrome (RDS) and bronchopulmonary dysplasia (BPD) is inversely related to gestational age at birth. The onset of RDS can be as early as 6 hours after birth. The symptoms include tachypnea, retractions, grunting, and oxygen desaturation. BPD is a disease of the newborn that manifests as a need for supplemental oxygen, lower airway obstruction and air trapping, carbon dioxide retention, atelectasis, bronchiolitis, and bronchopneumonia. Oxygen toxicity,

TABLE 48-13	Preanesthetic Assessment and Neonatal Anesthetic Implication	
System	**Characteristics**	**Anesthetic Implications**
Central Nervous System		
	Incomplete myelination	Judicious use of muscle relaxants
	Lack of cerebral autoregulation	Cerebral perfusion pressure control
	Cortical activity	Pain relief/adequate level of anesthesia
	ROP	Oxygen saturation (94%-98%)
Respiratory		
Mechanical	↓ Lung compliance	Assist or control ventilation during G/A
	↓ Elastic recoil	
	↓ Rigidity of chest wall	
	↓ V̇/Q̇ due to lung fluid	
	↑ Fatigue of respiratory muscles	
	↓ Coordination, nose/mouth breathing	Do not obstruct nasal passages
Anatomic	Large tongue	
	Position of larynx, epiglottis, vocal folds, subglottic region	
Biochemical	Response to hypercapnia not potentiated by hypoxia	Avoid hypoxia Maintain normothermia
Reflex	Hering-Breuer reflex	Apnea/no desaturation/
	Periodic breathing	stimulation
	Apnea	Stimulation/airway support
Cardiovascular		
	↓ Myocardial contractility/↓ myocardial compliance	Maintain adequate volume Maintain heart rate
	CO rate dependent	Use vagolytic agents
	Vagotonic	
	Limited sympathetic innervation	
	Reactive pulmonary vasculature	Avoid hypoxemia resulting in ↓ PBF & possible
	PDA/FO shunting	shunting
Renal		
	↓ GFR	Maintain vascular volume/CO
	↓ Tubular function	Avoid overhydration
	Low glucose threshold	Avoid excess glucose (0.5-1.0 g/kg)
Hepatic		
	Depressed hepatic enzymes	Judicious use of drugs metabolized by liver
	↓ Metabolism & clearance of drugs	
	Altered (decreased) protein binding	
	Hypoglycemia due to ↓ glycogen stores	
	Low prothrombin levels	Vitamin K (1 mg) before surgery
Hematologic		
	Fetal hemoglobin (does not readily release O_2 to tissues)	Avoid hypoxia
	Oxyhemoglobin curve shifted left	

In Culpepper TL. Neonatal anesthesia. In: Zaglaniczny K, Aker J, eds. Clinical Guide to Pediatric Anesthesia. Philadelphia: Saunders; 1999:395-396. CO, Cardiac output; G/A, general anesthesia; GFR, glomerular filtration rate; PBF, pulmonary blood flow; PDA/FO, patent ductus arteriosus/foramen ovale; ROP, retinopathy of prematurity.

barotrauma of positive-pressure ventilation on immature lungs and endotracheal intubation have been reported as causative factors. Management of the patient's oxygenation can be challenging. Careful monitoring of the acid-base status, the use of increased peak inspiratory pressure, and positive end-expiratory pressure may be needed to maintain oxygenation during surgery.

Cardiovascular System Abnormalities

In evaluation of the neonate's cardiovascular system, several variables should be examined: heart rate, blood pressure patterns, skin color, intensity of peripheral pulses, and capillary filling time. Presence of a murmur or abnormal heart sound, low urine output, metabolic acidosis, dysrhythmias, or cardiomegaly, alone or in combination, raises the concern of some type of congenital heart lesion, and these patients should be evaluated with a chest x-ray, ECG, and echocardiogram. The results of these diagnostic tests will allow for effective planning of the anesthetic, decreasing the possibility of complications (Table 48-14).

It is beyond the scope of this chapter to discuss all anesthetic implications of congenital heart disease in the neonate; however, there are some important assessment points.

1. Direction and flow through any shunt
2. Baseline oxygenation
3. Dependence of the systemic or pulmonary circulation on flow through the ductus arteriosus
4. The presence and size of any obstruction to blood flow
5. Heart failure (high output, low output, or hypoxic)
6. Drug therapy
7. Antibiotic prophylaxis against bacterial endocarditis[83]

Central Nervous System Abnormalities

An assessment of the CNS should include the status of the infant's intracranial pressure and intracranial compliance. Intraventricular hemorrhage (IVH) is almost exclusively seen in preterm babies. There is spontaneous bleeding into and around the lateral ventricles of the brain. The more preterm the neonate is and the smaller the weight, the more likely it is that intraventricular hemorrhage will be found. The hemorrhage is usually the result of RDS, hypoxic-ischemic injury, and/or episodes of acute blood pressure fluctuation that rapidly increase or decrease cerebral blood flow. The classic example is laryngoscopy in the presence of inadequate anesthesia.[84] The symptoms of IVH include hypotonia, apnea, seizures, loss of sucking reflex, and a bulging anterior fontanelle. Particular evaluation of the neonate with myelomeningocele (spina bifida) will be discussed subsequently.

Preoperative Labs

Neonates who are premature (<60 weeks postgestational age), those with concurrent cardiopulmonary disease, and babies in whom major blood loss is anticipated during the surgical procedure should have serial hematocrit, electrolytes, blood gases, and serum osmolality measured. The test values will assist in the fluid, electrolyte, and blood replacement during the surgical procedure.

BOX 48-3

Common Metabolic and Structural Problems in Small- and Large-for-Gestational Age (SGA and LGA) Infants

SGA
Congenital anomalies
Chromosomal abnormalities
Chronic intrauterine infection
Heat loss
Asphyxia
Metabolic abnormalities (hypoglycemia, hypocalcemia)
Polycythemia/hyperbilirubinemia

LGA
Birth injury (brachial, phrenic nerve, fractured clavicle)
Asphyxia
Meconium aspiration
Metabolic abnormalities (hypoglycemia, hypocalcemia)
Polycythemia/hyperbilirubinemia

From Brett CM et al. Anesthesia for neonates and premature infants. In: Motoyama EK, Davis PJ, eds. Smith's Anesthesia for Infants and Children. *7th ed. Philadelphia: Mosby; 2006:524.*

TABLE 48-14	Syndromes Associated with Cardiac Defects	
Syndrome/Malformation	**Cardiac Defect**	**Other Associated Conditions**
Beckwith-Wiedemann	Miscellaneous	Macroglossia, exomphalos, hypoglycemic
CHARGE syndrome	Tetralogy of Fallot, PDA, double outlet RV with AV canal, ASD, VSD	Choanal atresia, micrognathia, coloboma, cleft palate
Treacher Collins'	Miscellaneous	Facial and pharyngeal hypoplasia, microsomia, cleft palate, choanal atresia
VATER	VSD	Vertebral anomalies, TEF, renal anomalies, imperforate anus, absent radius
Trisomy 21 (Downs syndrome)	AV canal, ASD, VSD, PDA, TOF	Bowel atresia, large tongue, atlantoaxial instability
Trisomy 18 (Edwards syndrome)	VSD, PDA	Micrognathia, renal malformations
Trisomy 13 (Patau syndrome)	VSD, dextrocardia, ASD	Microcephaly, micrognathia, cleft lip & palate

Reproduced with permission from Peutrell JM, Weir P. Basic principles of neonatal anesthesia. In: Hughes DH et al, eds. Handbook of Neonatal Anesthesia. *London: Saunders; 1996:166.*
ASD, Atrial septal defect; AV, artioventricular, PDA, patent ductus arteriosus; RV, right ventricle; TOF, tetralogy of Fallot, VSD, ventricular septal defect.

TABLE 48-15	Preoperative Treatment of Significance for Anesthesia
Drug	**Implication**
Diuretics for heart failure bronchopulmonary dysplasia (BPD)	Hypokalemia
Digoxin for heart failure	ECG abnormalities
Steroids for BPD	Hyperglycemia Immunocompromised
Anticonvulsants	Cardiac arrhythmia Potent inducer of hepatic enzymes
Indomethacin	Increase risk of bleeding Displaces bilirubin from protein-binding sites Transient hyponatremia Renal impairment
Theophylline or caffeine	Significant toxic side effects; convulsions, tachycardia, tremor
Prostaglandins E_1 or E_2	Ventilatory depression and apnea Hypotension Cerebral irritability Seizures Tachycardia Pyrexia
Tolazoline	Systemic hypotension Cardiac irritability Transient oliguria Increased gastric acid
Prostacyclin	Hypotension Inhibition of platelet aggregation Rebound PPHN with withdrawal

PPHN, *Persistent pulmonary hypertension of the newborn.*

Preoperative Treatment of Significance for Anesthesia

Many of the preexisting conditions in the neonate will require medical treatment. Table 48-15 illustrates some of the preoperative drugs and their anesthetic implications.

Parental preparation is important. In the case of institutions that do not have a NICU, the patient will have been transferred in from another institution, and the parents may still be in the institution where the baby was delivered. It is imperative that the parents be prepared and the informed consent for anesthesia be obtained. Often this must be done via telephone or from the father, who may have accompanied the neonate to the NICU. The anxiety of the parents of a newborn with a serious illness requiring surgical intervention is very high. The anesthetist will foster trust and confidence through a courteous and understandable explanation of the anesthetic experience.

Regional Anesthesia in the Neonate

Regional anesthesia in the neonate is an acceptable option when for anatomic or physiologic reasons, the risks of complications during or after general anesthesia and endotracheal intubation are very high. These techniques have allowed surgical procedures to be done on critically ill neonates under minimal general anesthesia, with considerable reduction in the need for CNS depressant drugs. The preterm baby with respiratory distress syndrome and the former preterm baby who is at higher risk for post anesthetic apnea are example candidates for regional anesthesia. An additional benefit to the use of regional anesthesia in this age group is postoperative pain control. The two most common techniques used in the neonate are the spinal and caudal epidural blocks.

Anatomic differences in the neonate must be considered, particularly the location of the terminal end of the spinal cord, the dural sac, and the volume of cerebrospinal fluid (CSF). The spinal cord extends as far as L3 in the newborn and does not reach the adult position of L1 until 1 year of age. The dural sac extends to S3-S4 in these babies and does not reach the adult position of S1 until approximately 1 year of age (Figure 48-4). The volume of CSF is twice that of the adult (4 mL/kg vs 2 mL/kg). This dilutes

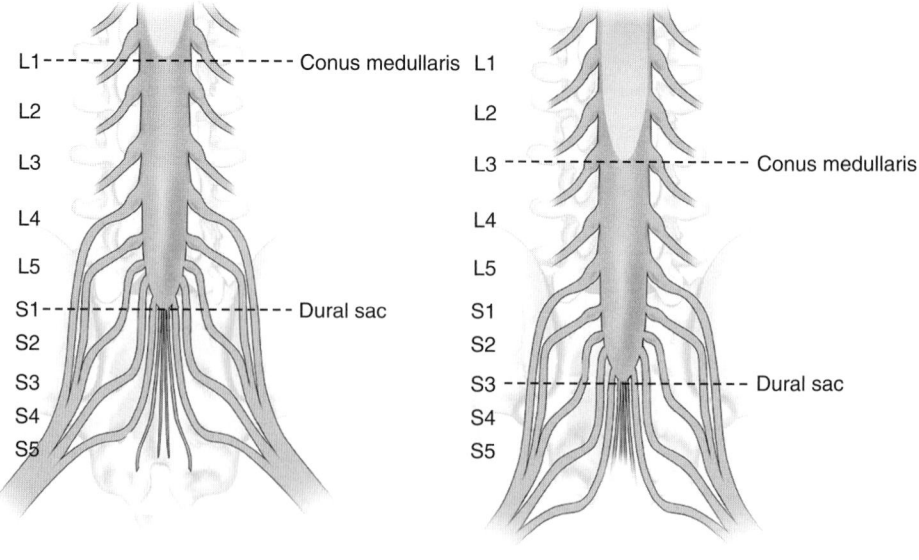

FIGURE 48-4 Comparison of levels of the conus medullaris and the dural sac in the infant and the older child or adult. (*From Motoyama EK, Davis PJ. In: Smith's Anesthesia in Infants and Children. 7th ed. St Louis: Mosby; 2006:466.*)

the local anesthetics injected and could explain the higher dose requirements and shorter duration of analgesia.

The physiologic considerations—cardiovascular, ventilatory and hormonal—are very important to the neonatal anesthetist. Patients in this age group have been reported to have remarkably stable cardiovascular responses to regional anesthesia. Bradycardia and hypotension are not often seen. It is thought that this could be due to the immature sympathetic nervous system or the proportionately small blood volume in the lower limbs, decreasing the amount of venous pooling.[85,86] The ventilatory response to the regional anesthetic is related to the level of the block. With a level as high as T2-T4, there could be intercostal muscle weakness that requires the dependence on diaphragmatic movement for tidal breathing, but tidal volume and respiratory rate are not usually affected.[87]

There are pharmacologic considerations when regional anesthesia is used in neonates. The extracellular space is larger. This means the initial dose of local anesthetic will be diluted into a larger volume of distribution, resulting in a lower initial plasma peak concentration. Neonates have diminished concentrations of albumin and alpha acid glycoprotein, resulting in reduced protein binding of local anesthetics and significant increases in the concentration of free drug, which could increase the risk of CNS and cardiac toxicity. Local anesthetics, particularly the amides, are broken down slower in neonates due to immature hepatic degradation. The major elimination pathway for ester local anesthetics is hydrolysis via plasma cholinesterases, and these levels are lower in the neonate as well. The demonstrations of the previous differences are shorter duration of blocks when compared with adults and larger initial doses of local anesthetic per kilogram to achieve the same extent of blockade.

Most neonates will have a regional technique performed after the induction of general anesthesia because of the age of the patient and the possibility of agitation and continuous movement affecting the placement and success of the block. The possible complications of regional anesthesia in newborns that have been reported by several sources are neurologic injury due to intraneural injection of local anesthetic and the inability to detect intravascular injection of local anesthetic.[88] The use of ultrasonography has decreased the risk of complications associated with the placement of spinal and epidural needles and catheters, as well as enabled monitoring the spread of local anesthetics.[89] It is difficult to assess a dermatome level, because these patients are nonverbal.

Spinal Anesthesia

The use of spinal anesthesia in neonates and infants was common in the early part of the 20th century, but its use declined with the advent of safer general anesthesia in this young age group. In the early 1980s, Gregory and Steward studied the incidence of life-threatening apnea in preterm babies less than 60 weeks postgestational age after general anesthesia,[90] and the result was the increased use of spinal anesthesia for preterm neonates and infants when presenting for surgical procedures of the lower abdomen.

Spinal anesthesia can be performed in the sitting or lateral position; however, the neck should be extended to prevent airway obstruction (Figure 48-5). The lumbar puncture is performed at the L3-L4 or L4-L5 interspace because the spinal cord ends at L3 in the neonate. A 1½-inch, 22-gauge needle is inserted, and even with this small needle, resistance can be felt when the needle enters the ligamentum flavum, and the characteristic "pop" occurs when the needle enters the

subarachnoid space. The distance is approximately 1 cm.[91] The most common local anesthetics are tetracaine 1% and bupivacaine 0.5% to 0.75% at doses of 0.4 to 1.0 mg/kg. When the local anesthetic is injected, the neonate should be immediately placed in the supine position, and the legs should be secured with tape to prevent them from being raised for any reason.

Caudal Anesthesia

Caudal anesthesia is the most commonly used regional block in pediatric anesthesia. It can be used for any procedure involving innervation from the sacral, lumbar, or lower-thoracic dermatomes.[86] In the youngest patients, the caudal block can be used as an adjunct to general anesthesia or solely for postoperative analgesia. In the neonate, it is most often placed after induction of general anesthesia prior to the beginning of the surgical procedure.

The patient is placed in the lateral position with the upper knee flexed. (Figure 48-6). The landmarks are identified: the tip of the coccyx to fix the midline and the sacral cornua on either side of the sacral hiatus. These landmarks form the points of an equilateral triangle with the tip resting over the sacral hiatus. A 22-gauge needle is placed bevel up at a 45-degree angle to the skin. When the sacrococcygeal membrane is punctured, a distinctive loss of resistance is felt, and the angle of the needle is reduced and advanced cephalad. With aspiration, if there is not CSF or blood, the local anesthetic can be administered. Any local anesthetic can be used. The volume of the local anesthetic determines the height of the block. Volumes of 1.2 to 1.5 mL/kg provide analgesia and anesthesia to the T-4 to T-6 dermatome. No matter which local anesthetic is used, the concentration is adjusted to deliver no more than 2.5 mg/kg. The addition of epinephrine (1:200,000) or clonidine (1 to 2 mcg/kg) will prolong the block significantly.

Any regional technique can theoretically be used in neonates, with careful attention to the potential for toxicity of local anesthetics and careful dosing parameters.

ANESTHETIC CONSIDERATIONS FOR SELECTED CASES

Gastrointestinal

Anesthesia and surgery in neonates and infants present unique challenges. The acuity of intraabdominal procedures can range

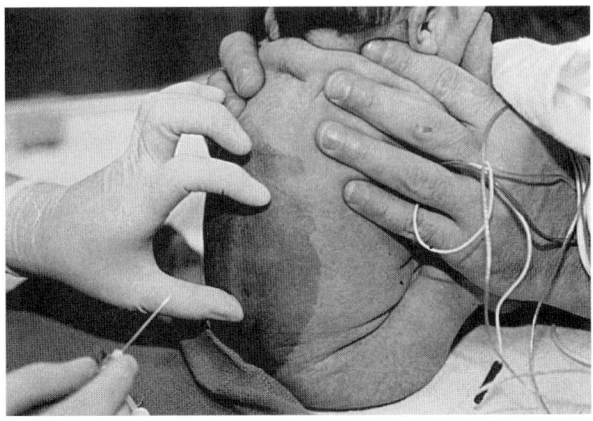

FIGURE **48-5** Spinal block performed in sitting position. Note that the head is in neutral position to prevent airway obstruction. (*From Cote CJ et al, eds. A Practice of Anesthesia for Infants and Children. 2nd ed. Philadelphia: Saunders; 1993.*)

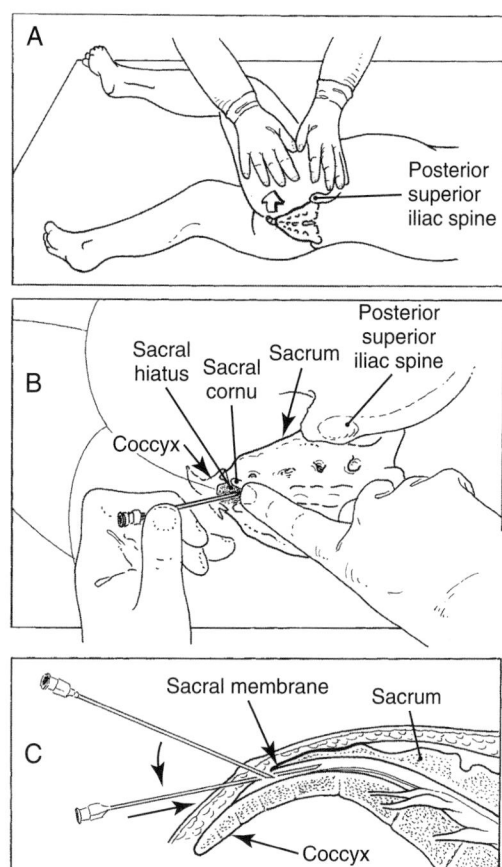

FIGURE **48-6** Performing a caudal block. (*From Cote CJ et al, eds. A Practice of Anesthesia for Infants and Children. 2nd ed. Philadelphia: Saunders; 1993.*)

from a simple hernia repair in a healthy neonate to a complex abdominal/thoracic procedure in a critically ill preterm infant.

Pyloric Stenosis

Pyloric stenosis is an obstructive lesion characterized by an "olive shaped" enlargement of the pylorus muscle. It is a common gastrointestinal anomaly, particularly in males. It is usually diagnosed between 2 to 12 weeks of life, and clinical symptoms include nonbilious postprandial emesis that becomes more projectile with time, a palpable pylorus, and visible peristaltic waves. The procedure to correct the problem is a pyloromyotomy.

Historically, pyloric stenosis was considered an emergency situation. However, as with medical progress on many fronts, the procedure is now considered semi-elective. It is not wise to anesthetize a neonate emergently for this procedure if the baby is dehydrated or has electrolyte abnormalities. Fluid, electrolyte, and acid-base balance should be corrected prior to anesthesia.

Prior to induction, the neonate's stomach must be emptied via orogastric tube. Some anesthetists will irrigate the stomach via the orogastric tube with warm normal saline until the aspirate is clear and minimal. Others will tilt the baby in various directions to evacuate the remaining contents.

After preoxygenation, the induction should be a modified rapid sequence with properly applied cricoid pressure and gentle positive pressure ventilation via mask. (Many practitioners still perform an awake oral or a true rapid-sequence.) Oral endotracheal intubation is mandated to protect the airway from any gastric contents that may be residual. Maintenance can be with inhalation anesthetics or in combination with intravenous drugs. These babies should be extubated awake.

Postoperatively, these patients, particularly a preterm or SGA neonate, could exhibit drowsiness, lethargy, or apnea. This could be attributed to electrolyte abnormalities and/or postgestational age.

Inguinal Hernia

Inguinal hernia is particularly prevalent in the preterm infant. The surgical problem presents the possibility of incarceration of the small bowel in the hernia defect, resulting in ischemia and tissue death. Also of concern is the potential injury to the ipsilateral testicle. These babies routinely have hernia repair prior to discharge from the NICU, and the anesthetist is faced with all the usual problems of prematurity, such as bronchopulmonary dysplasia (BPD). The surgical approach can be the standard abdominal incision or in some centers, laparoscopy is the preferred technology. In most situations, the contralateral side is explored to rule out the presence of another defect because of the high incidence of bilateral involvement. When this procedure is performed by a urologist, the contralateral side is most often not explored.

Because of the many possible patient issues, the anesthetic technique must be tailored for each patient. Inhalation or intravenous induction is acceptable, as well as airway management with a mask, laryngeal mask airway (LMA), or endotracheal tube. The use of the laparoscopic approach will necessitate the use of the endotracheal tube. Maintenance can be with inhalation anesthetics or in combination with intravenous drugs. Small neonates who are at risk for postoperative apnea may benefit from spinal anesthesia.

Congenital Diaphragmatic Hernia

A congenital diaphragmatic hernia (CDH) is a defect of the diaphragm that allows extrusion of the abdominal contents into the thoracic cavity. This disorder has an incidence of 1 in 2500 live births.[92,93] The herniated abdominal contents act as a space-occupying lesion and prevents normal lung growth and development. Most of theses defects are left-sided via the foramen of Bochdalek, and the lung affected to the greatest extent is on the ipsilateral side, but the other lung can be affected as well. The lungs have reduced-sized bronchi, less bronchial branching, decreased alveolar surface area, and abnormal pulmonary vasculature. There is a thickening of the arteriolar smooth muscle extending to the capillary level of the alveoli. This results in increased pulmonary artery pressure and causes right-to-left shunting.[94]

Neonates with CDH present immediately after birth with dyspnea, tachypnea, cyanosis, absence of breath sounds on the affected side, and severe retractions. Their physical appearance is a scaphoid abdomen and a barrel chest. Diagnosis is confirmed by chest radiograph documenting bowel in the thoracic cavity and a gasless abdominal cavity. Between 44% and 66% of neonates with CDH have other anomalies, particularly heart lesions.

The emergent nature of the repair has been reexamined in the past decade, and more emphasis is now placed on stabilizing pulmonary hypertension and other medical issues. Studies published by Azarow and colleagues and Jona in the late 1990s demonstrated that the ventilation parameters were a major factor in survival of these babies. Permissive hypercarbia with high frequency, oscillatory ventilation was most successful in improving outcomes.[95,96] Extracorporeal membrane oxygenation (ECMO) is one method of bridging the gap between birth and surgical repair, but it is not the mode of treatment for all patients. In 1999, the CDH study group published their findings in the pediatric surgery literature indicating that ECMO babies had an overall lower survival rate than non-ECMO babies, except in those neonates with a very high mortality risk.[97]

A thorough assessment of the baby, including laboratory, radiographic, and physical symptoms, is mandatory. Listening to breath sounds will assist in evaluating the degree of ventilation on each side of the chest after intubation. Because of the respiratory manifestations of the problem, most of the patients will be already intubated and have intravenous access and arterial lines in place when they arrive in the operating room. If they are not intubated, an endotracheal tube should be placed after a rapid-sequence induction. If a difficult airway is suspected, an awake intubation should be done.

It is important in these patients to administer an anticholinergic (atropine 0.02 mg/kg) intravenously just prior to induction to prevent the bradycardia during induction. If an awake intubation is planned, some type of analgesia should be used to decrease the stress response of airway instrumentation. Ventilation should be delivered gently to avoid inflating the stomach with air, further compromising the pressure in the chest.

The patient's hemodynamic stability should determine the anesthetic drugs used. A high-dose narcotic technique is commonly used (fentanyl, 15 to 25 mcg/kg) if tolerated. The use of inhalation agents must be judicious because they pose significant risk to the baby's cardiovascular stability. Nitrous oxide should be avoided because it will increase the volume of gastrointestinal tissue and further impair ventilation.

Monitoring must include blood pressure, ECG, pulse oximetry, capnography, temperature, and heart rate. To monitor for right-to-left shunting, oximeter probes should be placed preductal (right upper extremity) and postductal (lower extremity). The use of arterial blood pressure monitoring will not only allow beat-to-beat assessment of blood pressure but also provide an outlet for easier blood sampling. All conditions that can increase pulmonary vascular resistance—hypoxia, hypothermia, or acidosis—must be avoided. Carbon dioxide should be kept at normal or slightly elevated levels and oxygen saturation maintained above 80 mm Hg. Any derangement of electrolytes must be corrected quickly and any significant blood loss replaced.

In the event that cardiorespiratory instability prevents the neonate from being transported to the operating room, the anesthetist might be required to administer anesthesia in the NICU while the baby is still on ECMO. Under these circumstances, the recommended anesthetic choice is an opioid and nondepolarizing muscle-relaxant technique instead of an inhalation agent. Postoperative ventilation is required, with the goal of keeping the arterial oxygenation greater than 150 mm Hg and slowing weaning to lower oxygen concentrations over a 48- to 72-hour period.[94]

Omphalocele and Gastroschisis

These anomalies are both defects in the abdominal wall that occur during gestation when the visceral organs fail to move from the yolk sac back into the abdominal cavity. It is more common to encounter omphalocele in term newborns and gastroschisis in preterm newborns. The primary difference in the two defects is the presence of a membrane (the peritoneum) covering the extruded abdominal contents in the baby with omphalocele and the lack of membrane in the baby with gastroschisis (Figures 48-7 and 48-8). The defects occur at the insertion of the umbilicus. They are often associated with other anomalies. Some of

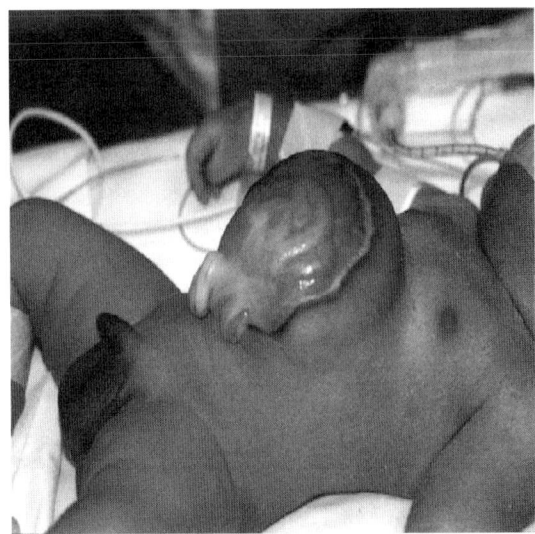

FIGURE **48-7** Omphalocele. (*Courtesy Dr. William Hardin, The Children's Hospital of Alabama.*)

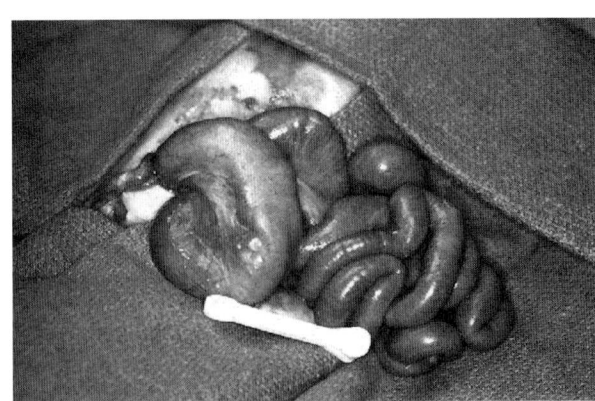

FIGURE **48-8** Gastroschisis. (*Courtesy Dr. William Hardin, The Children's Hospital of Alabama.*)

those anomalies might be cardiac, genitourinary (bladder exstrophy), metabolic (e.g., Beckwith-Wiedemann syndrome with macroglossia, hypoglycemia, organomegaly, gigantism), malrotation, Meckel's diverticulum, and intestinal atresia. When the omphalocele is in the epigastric region, cardiac and thoracic problems are more prevalent. If the omphalocele is located in the hypogastric area, cloacal anomalies and exstrophy of the bladder are seen more often.[92] Both gastrointestinal anomalies, although very different in presentation, are almost identical in anesthetic management.

A newborn with an omphalocele or gastroschisis is usually brought to the operating room very soon after birth to minimize the possibility of infection, the loss of fluid and heat, and the possible death of bowel tissue. A thorough preoperative evaluation must be done to identify the presence of any of the previously mentioned associated anomalies. Historically, the surgical approach was to immediately attempt primary closure of the defect. This entailed placing a large amount of abdominal contents into a cavity that was not usually large enough, and the result was a significant increase in intraabdominal pressure, which impeded ventilation and caused profound hypotension secondary to aortocaval compression. Over the past decade, surgeons

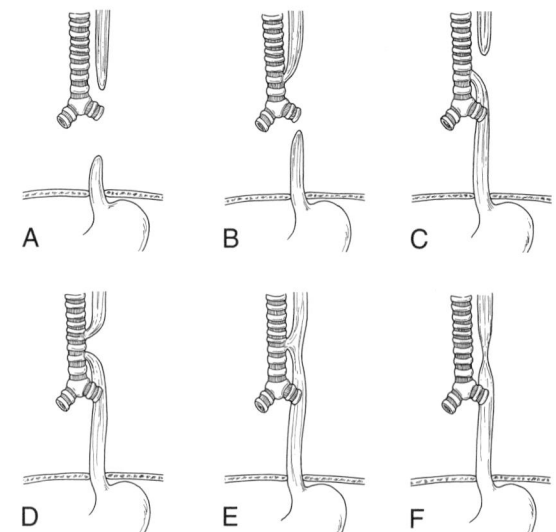

FIGURE 48-9   Five types of tracheoesophageal fistula. Illustration C is the most common form. (*From Tobias JD, Maxwell LG. Anesthesia for pediatric thoracic surgery. In: Litman RS, ed. Pediatric Anesthesia: The Requisites in Anesthesiology. Philadelphia: Mosby; 2004:298.*)

have opted for a staged closure, using a Silastic silo as a temporary housing for the bowel. This silo is sutured to the defect, and over the next 3 to 7 days, the silo is reduced to allow for accommodation of the gastric contents and abdominal-wall stretching. The neonate is usually then brought for complete closure. In the event primary closure is attempted, it should be noted that exceeding certain criteria can increase the possibility of unsuccessful completion of the closure (Box 48-4).[98-100]

The choice of anesthetic agent and technique is determined by several guiding principles: severe dehydration and massive fluid loss from exposed viscera and internal third-spacing of fluid due to bowel obstruction, hypothermia, the potential for sepsis, associated anomalies, and postoperative ventilation requirements. It is not uncommon for the anesthetist's choice to be an opioid and nondepolarizing muscle relaxant technique; however, even with the use of muscle relaxants, the abdominal wall may not allow primary closure. Ventilatory compromise and decreased organ perfusion are major problems as intraabdominal pressure increases. It is imperative to have adequate intravenous access to infuse large amounts of fluid quickly and invasive monitoring to guide the replacement. A pulse oximeter probe on a lower extremity will indicate if there is compromise in the perfusion to the lower extremities due to obstruction of venous return.

Postoperative ventilation is mandatory on all of these babies, requiring the continued use of paralytics and sedation with an opioid until their clinical status stabilizes.

Tracheoesophageal Fistula and Esophageal Atresia

Esophageal atresia (EA), with or without tracheoesophageal fistula (TEF), is normally diagnosed immediately after birth when an orogastric tube cannot pass into the stomach, when there is coughing and choking after the first feeding, or after recurrent pneumonia associated with feedings.[92] In the past this condition was often lethal. Today there is an expectation of almost 100% survival.[96]

There is a significant association of other serious congenital anomalies in these babies. Some sources report as high as 30% to 50% of newborns with AE and TEF have other anomalies, particularly VACTERL (vertebral anomalies, anal atresia, cardiac, tracheoesophageal fistula, renal and limb malformations) syndrome.

Esophageal atresia with a distal fistula is the most common presentation of TEF in approximately 80% to 90% of patients.[92] The esophagus ends in a blind pouch, and the distal esophagus forms a fistula with the trachea, usually above the carina. There are five other configurations of this anomaly, varied by the location of the fistula and the presence or absence of EA (Figure 48-9). The morbidity and mortality of TEF are directly related to the resulting pulmonary complications from aspiration of feedings.[101] The focus of the preoperative preparation should

be to minimize the pulmonary complications by discontinuing oral feedings, placement of a tube to suction nasopharyngeal secretions that accumulate in the blind esophageal pouch, maintain the infant in a semirecumbent position to minimize aspiration of secretions, and placement of a gastrostomy tube to prevent excess gastric distention from impairing ventilation. The surgical procedure is performed via a thoracotomy incision, usually on the right side. The sequence of the repair is the ligation of the fistula and then anastomosis of the two ends of the esophagus if possible.

Standard monitors should be used. The precordial stethoscope should be placed in the left axilla after induction to allow for monitoring of ventilation and heart sounds. The cardiorespiratory condition of the neonate should dictate the use of more invasive monitoring techniques such as an arterial line, umbilical or radial. In the youngest, critically ill patients, preductal and postductal oximeter probes may be used.[21]

The technique of induction should be based on the clinician's evaluation of the airway. When there is concern of a difficult airway an "awake intubation" should be performed. This technique minimizes the gastric distention from anesthetic gases passing through the fistula and allows proper placement of the endotracheal tube without positive-pressure ventilation. When airway management is determined to be routine, an inhalation induction with gentle positive-pressure ventilation and intubation can be used. To further minimize the distention of the stomach, spontaneous ventilation to an adequate depth of anesthesia followed by endotracheal intubation could be carried out. If this technique is used, care must be taken to avoid hypoxemia that will result from the respiratory depression produced by high concentrations of inhalation agents. Another accepted technique is the intravenous rapid-sequence induction with endotracheal intubation. With any of the described techniques, once the endotracheal tube is placed, proper position must be verified. A common method of verifying the correct position is to actually intubate the right mainstem bronchus and then withdraw the endotracheal tube until breath sounds are heard on the left side of the chest. The tip of the tube is likely between the fistula and

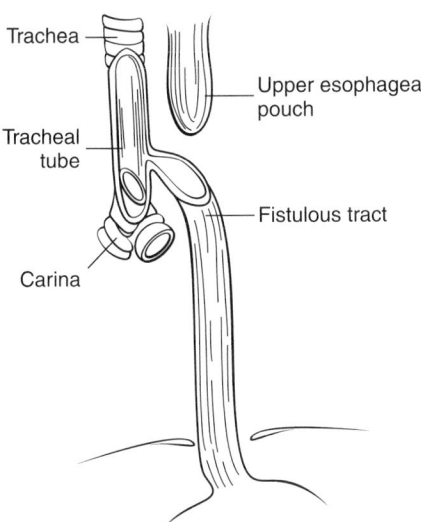

Trachea

Tracheal tube

Carina

Upper esophageal pouch

Fistulous tract

FIGURE **48-10** Correct placement of endotracheal tube—between fistula and carina.

the carina (Figure 48-10). Another method, if there is a gastrostomy in place, is to submerge the gastrostomy tube in water and if there are bubbles on ventilation, the fistula is being ventilated and the tube must be repositioned. The bevel of the endotracheal tube should be turned anteriorly to allow the posterior surface of the endotracheal tube to occlude the fistula. In one configuration of TEF, the fistula is located very close to the carina. In this case, the endotracheal tube may need to be placed in the bronchus of the nonoperative lung until the fistula can be ligated. After ligation, the tube can be withdrawn to above the carina.

During the procedure, it is essential to monitor ventilation very carefully. Airway obstruction can occur if the trachea is compressed or if secretions or blood block the openings of the endotracheal tube. This must be corrected immediately.

The neonate without significant pulmonary complications who is awake and moving vigorously is most often extubated in the operating room. Blood and secretions may be present in the endotracheal tube and should be suctioned gently prior to removal. If there is any concern about airway obstruction or impaired ventilation, mechanical ventilation should be continued. It is thought that should bag-and-mask ventilation or reintubation be required, undue stress could be placed on the suture lines of the repair with laryngoscopy and neck extension, resulting in damage to the esophagus, necessitating further surgical procedures. Another problem that can occur with early extubation in smaller neonates is an inability to maintain the work of breathing due to preoperative lung disease. If postoperative mechanical ventilation is needed, the endotracheal tube should be positioned 1 cm away from the fistula repair to allow for healing of the suture line. A suction catheter should be clearly marked with a distance for insertion that approximates the distance just above the anastomotic repair.[102] Postoperative pain can be managed with opioids and/or a caudal epidural, placed intraoperatively.

Complications may occur later that could influence anesthetic management. Neonates who have had EA/TEF repair early in life can develop a diverticulum at the site of the old tracheal fistula. This could present problems in the future if inadvertent intubation of the diverticulum occurs. Esophageal stricture could develop at the site of esophageal anastomosis requiring repeated dilation or possible resection.[103]

Malrotation and Midgut Volvulus
As the intestine is moving from its extraabdominal location during the first trimester of gestation, it can become twisted. The result can be a compromised superior mesenteric artery and intestinal ischemia. This ischemia can cause bowel strangulation, bloody stools, peritonitis, and hypovolemic shock. When this occurs, it is termed *volvulus*. According to some sources, this is a true emergency.[94]

Many of these neonates are diagnosed in the first week of life when the neonate presents with bilious vomiting, a tender and distended abdomen, and increasing hemodynamic instability. The surgical procedure relieves the obstruction by reducing the volvulus, dividing the fixation bands between the cecum and the duodenum or jejunum, and widening the base of the mesentery.

The major concerns in anesthetic management are airway management, fluid and electrolyte replacement, treatment of sepsis and postoperative pain management. Any baby with intestinal obstruction will likely have abdominal distention (which could impede diaphragmatic movement) and is at higher risk for aspiration of gastric or intestinal contents. This necessitates the use of a rapid-sequence induction with the proper application of cricoid pressure. If there is concern for difficult airway, awake intubation should be considered. There is likely volume depletion due to peritonitis, ileus, bowel manipulation, and sepsis. It is absolutely necessary to have adequate intravenous access, and it is desirable to have a central line and an arterial line.

The choice of anesthetic agents should be dependent on the neonate's condition. It is not advisable to use nitrous oxide, but other inhalation agents could be acceptable. As with other emergent abdominal procedures, postoperative mechanical ventilation could be required, making the intraoperative choice of an opioid and nondepolarizing muscle relaxant a good choice (Box 48-5). Although anesthetic agent choice is not critical, the maintenance of an adequate circulating volume and red blood cells is vital to ensure perfusion of vital organs.

Necrotizing Enterocolitis
NEC is an intestinal inflammation that can become a life-threatening emergency situation. It occurs primarily in preterm babies with a gestational age of less than 32 weeks and a weight of less than 1500 g. The etiology of the problem is reported to be secondary to bowel ischemia and immaturity, probable bacterial invasion, and premature oral feeding.[92,94] Box 48-6 lists the common symptoms of NEC. Diagnosis is confirmed by abdominal

radiography that shows fixed dilated intestinal loops, pneumatosis intestinalis, portal vein air, ascites, and pneumoperitoneum. Accompanying lab values might evidence hyperkalemia, hyponatremia, metabolic acidosis, hyperglycemia or hypoglycemia, and, in the most serious cases, signs of disseminated intravascular coagulation.

When an attempt at medical management is unsuccessful, surgical intervention consists of an exploratory laparotomy with resection of dead bowel, usually a colostomy, and peritoneal lavage.

These neonates are very sick and usually come to the operating room already intubated and on ventilator support. If they are not intubated, a rapid-sequence induction or awake intubation is indicated. The anesthetic drugs chosen should depend on the patient's condition, but a common choice is a narcotic and relaxant technique. These are thought to be the safest choice in the presence of cardiovascular instability because the inhalation agents may further depress the myocardium and lower the blood pressure to unacceptable levels. Nitrous oxide is avoided, and if there is concern over high oxygen concentrations, compressed air can be added to the gas mixture. If cardiac output is low and renal perfusion is below normal, dopamine may be indicated. The amount of third-space loss in these patients is very large and may require multiple blood volumes of crystalloid and colloid combinations to replace intravascular volume. Red blood cells, fresh frozen plasma, and platelets may also be required to increase oxygen-carrying capacity or to treat factor deficiency.[92,94]

The postoperative care should focus on continuation of the fluid resuscitation and cardiorespiratory support and mechanical ventilation until the baby stabilizes.

Imperforate Anus

During the first few days after birth, when there is no passage of meconium, the diagnosis of imperforate anus is considered. The degree of this anomaly can range from a mild stenosis to complete anal atresia that is associated with other anomalies. The VACTERL (vertebral anomalies, anal atresia, cardiac, tracheoesophageal fistula, renal, and limb malformations) syndrome contains all the above-mentioned anomalies.[104] In male newborns the operative procedure may be urgent to allow the passage of meconium via a colostomy. In female newborns, owing to the usual presence of a rectovaginal fistula, the procedure can be

delayed for a few weeks. The anesthetic considerations for this neonate are based on the existence of associated anomalies and fluid and electrolyte balance.

Other Intestinal Obstructive Lesions

Duodenal obstruction, jejunoileal atresia, and meconium ileus can all result in a complete intestinal obstruction. Although each of these pathologies are different in etiology and presentation, the anesthetic management is very much like that for the previously mentioned midgut volvulus.

Neurosurgical

Neonatal Hydrocephalus

Hydrocephalus is usually the result of some existing pathologic process. It is usually due to an obstruction in the CSF or an inability to absorb CSF. The standard treatment is the placement of a shunting catheter from the ventricle of the brain to another location to allow absorption of the fluid. Most often the shunt is placed from the ventricle to the peritoneal cavity. Occasionally the catheter is placed in the right atrium or pleural cavity. In the newborn and neonate, if the hydrocephalus develops slowly, the cranial vault will expand to accommodate the increase in brain bulk. When there is no more ability to expand, intracranial pressure (ICP) begins to increase, and the baby could be in serious trouble. The signs and symptoms of increasing intracranial pressure are a tense anterior fontanelle, irritability, somnolence, and/or vomiting.

Anesthetic management is directed at controlling the ICP and relieving the obstruction. The urgency of the procedure is determined by the preanesthetic assessment of the ICP. The major risk associated with delay is the possible herniation of the brain due to increasing pressure in the cranial vault. Comorbidities such as prematurity and all associated problems must be addressed.

Induction in the presence of increased ICP is usually a rapid-sequence induction and tracheal intubation. A variety of anesthetic agents are acceptable for maintenance, with the goal being to extubate the patient at the end of the procedure. If the neonate is preterm, it is advisable to adjust the oxygen concentration to maintain oxygen saturation at 95% to 97%. This decreases the risk of ROP. The neurologic status of the neonate could affect the decision to extubate immediately, and mechanical ventilation could be required.

Myelomeningocele

Myelomeningocele is the most common CNS defect that occurs during the first month of gestation. Another common name for this defect is *spina bifida*. It is failure of the neural tube to close, resulting in herniation of the spinal cord and meninges through a defect in the spinal column and back. If the herniation only contains meninges, it is a meningocele. If the herniation contains meninges and neural elements, it is a myelomeningocele. These lesions mostly occur in the lumbosacral region but can occur at any level of the neuroaxis. The repair of the defect is considered urgent and is usually undertaken with the first 24 hours of life to avoid the increasing risk of bacterial contamination of the spinal cord and further deterioration of neural and motor function (Figure 48-11). Most newborns with myelomeningoceles do not have other associated anomalies or congenital heart disease. These neonates, however, often have an Arnold-Chiari malformation. The Arnold-Chiari malformation is a result of the hindbrain being displaced downward into the foramen magnum, resulting in hydrocephalus. This will necessitate the placement of a ventriculoperitoneal shunt, usually during the

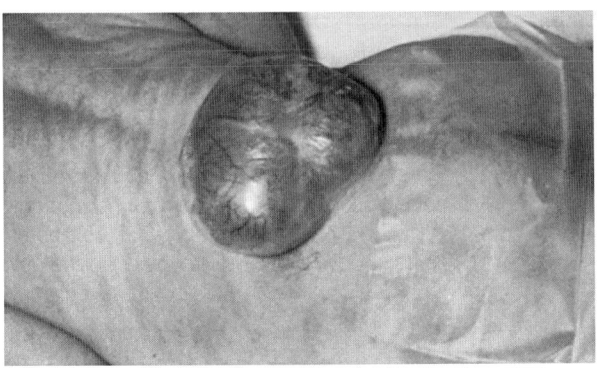

FIGURE **48-11** A lumbar myelomeningocele is covered by a thin layer of skin. *(From Kinsman et al. Nelson Textbook of Pediatrics. 18th ed. Philadelphia: Saunders; 2007:2446.)*

myelomeningocele repair. There are usually significant neurologic deficits below the level of the lesion, and evaluation of the degree of deficit is important to anesthetic decision making. Preoperative assessment should include a thorough review of all other organ system to rule out additional congenital anomalies. Minimal lab work should include a blood count and a type of screen for blood.

Routine neonatal monitoring is necessary, and the use of invasive monitoring techniques should be based on a risk/benefit analysis. Positioning and airway management is one of the biggest challenges for the anesthetist. Most of these babies can be induced and intubated in the supine position with the lumbosacral defect supported in a "donut" ring or with strategically placed towels to avoid direct pressure on the dural sac. If the defect is very large or if there is accompanying severe hydrocephalus, it may be necessary to place the neonate in the lateral position for induction and intubation. If there is a suspicion of a difficult airway, the endotracheal tube may be placed with the patient awake, after administration of atropine and preoxygenation. Adequate intravenous access is essential because of the possibility of significant blood loss during the procedure. If the defect is large, the surgeon may be required to undermine a large amount of tissue for closure, resulting in a large blood loss.

Anesthesia can be induced with an inhalation or intravenous technique. After the endotracheal tube is placed, the procedure is performed in the prone position with appropriate protection of all body parts. In some institutions, the use of muscle relaxants is discouraged to allow for stimulation and identification of neural tissue. Anesthesia can be maintained with a variety of drugs, keeping in mind the goal of extubation at the end of the procedure and the possibility of postoperative apnea.

These patients are prone to hypothermia, and conservation of body heat should include warming the operating room to at least 80° F before the procedure and until the baby is draped. Radiant heat lamps should be used during the preparation and positioning of the patient. A forced-air warmer should also be placed underneath the neonate to maintain body temperature. Anesthetic gases should be humidified to prevent heat loss and minimize pulmonary complications. There has been reported an increased sensitivity to latex in these babies. As a precaution, they should be treated as latex allergic, avoiding all products that contain latex.[105]

SUMMARY

Despite the advances in neonatal medicine, surgery, and particularly anesthesia, the anesthetic management of critically ill neonates continues to be a challenge. A thorough knowledge of developmental physiology and knowledge of neonatal disease states and their treatment is imperative to safe anesthesia. Many conditions that were once thought to be a death sentence for neonates are now surgically treated with increasingly good outcomes. Neonatal anesthesia requires the anesthetist to have astute clinical observation skills, to be intensely vigilant, and to be capable of sound judgments.

REFERENCES

1. Anand K, Hickey P. Pain and its effects in the human neonate and fetus. *N Engl J Med.* 1987;(317):1321-1329.
2. Davidson AJ. The aims of anesthesia in infants: the relevance of philosophy, psychology and a little evidence. *Pediatr Anesth.* 2007;17:102-108.
3. Cohen MC et al. Pediatric anesthesia morbidity and mortality in the perioperative period. *Anesth Analg.* 1990;70:160-167.
4. Konstadt S et al. Intraoperative detection of patent foramen ovale by transesophageal echocardiography. *Anesthesiology.* 1991;74:212-216.
5. Tolsa JJ et al. Magnesium sulphate as an alternative and safe treatment for severe persistent pulmonary hypertension of the newborn. *Arch Dis Child Fetal Neonatal Ed.* 1995;72:184-187.
6. Simonneau G et al. Continuous subcutaneous infusion of treprostinil, a prostacyclin analogue, in pateints with pulmonary arterial hypertension: a double-blind, randomized, placebo-controlled trial. *Am J Resp Crit Care Med.* 2002;165:800-804.
7. Konduri G et al. Adenosine infusion improves oxygenation in term infants with respiratory failure. *Pediatrics.* 1996;97:295-300.
8. Petros A, Pierce D. The management of pulmonary hypertension. *Pediatr Anesth.* 2006;16:816-821.
9. Kinsella J et al. Randomized multi-center trial of inhaled nitric oxide and high frequency ventilation in severe persistent pulmonary hypertension of the newborn. *J Pediatr.* 1997;131:55-62.
10. Group U.C.E.T. UK collaborative trial of neonatal extracorporeal membrane oxygenation. *Lancet.* 1996;348:75-82.
11. Van Hare et al. The effects of increasing mean arterial pressure on left ventricular output in newborn lambs. *Circ Res.* 1990;67(1):78-83.
12. Bell C, Kain Z, eds. *The Pediatric Anesthesia Handbook.* St Louis: Mosby; 1997.
13. Riggato H. Control of ventilation in the newborn. *Ann Rev Physiol.* 1984;46:661.
14. Vries PD, Bries CD. Embryology and development. In: Gans S, ed. *The Pediatric Airway.* Vol 4. Philadelphia: Saunders; 1991.
15. Litman R et al. Developmental changes of laryngeal diminesions in unparalyzed, sedated children. *Anesthesiology.* 2003;98:41-45.
16. Taussig LT et al. Lung function in infants and young children: functional residual capacity, tidal volume and respiratory rates. *Am Rev Respir Dis.* 1977;116:233-239.
17. Karlburg P, Koch G. Development of mechanics of breathing during the first week of life: a longitudinal study. *Acta Paediatr Scand.* 1962;51:121-129.
18. Steward D, Lerman J, eds. Anatomy and physiology in relation to pediatric anesthesia. In: Steward D, Lerman J, eds. *Manual of Pediatric Anesthesia.* New York: Churchill Livingstone; 2001:22.
19. Everett LL. Anesthesia for children. In: Longnecker D et al, eds. *Anesthesiology.* 2008, New York: McGraw-Hill; 2008:1520-1540.
20. Martin J et al. Up and down regulation of skeletal muscle acetylcholine receptors. *Anesthesiology.* 1992;76:822-843.
21. Brett C et al. Anesthesia for neonates and premature infants. In: Motoyama E, Davis P, eds. *Smith's Anesthesia for Infants and Children.* Philadelphia: Mosby; 2006:564.
22. Emde ER et al. Stress and neonatal sleep. *Psychosom Med.* 1971;33:491.
23. Field T, Goldson F. Pacifying effects of nonnutritive sucking on term and preterm neonates during heelstick procedures. *Pediatrics.* 1984;74:1012.
24. Round J. Neonatal physiology. *Surgery.* 2004;22(10):242-248.
25. Thaler M. Liver function and maturation in the perinatal period. In: Lebenthal E, ed. *Textbook of Gastroenterology and Nutrition in Infancy.* New York: Raven; 1981:177.
26. Plattner O et al. Lack of nonshivering thermogenesis in infants anesthetized with fentanyl and propofol. *Anesthesiology.* 1997;86:772-777.
27. Rutter N, Hull D. Water loss from the skin of term and preterm babies. *Arch Dis Child.* 1979;54:858.

28. Jessen K. An assessment of human regulatory non-shivering thermogenesis. *Acta Anaesthesiol Scand.* 1980;24:138-143.
29. Dick W et al. Prevention of heat loss during anesthesia and operation in the newborn baby and small infant. *Acta Anaesthesiol Scand.* 1970;37(Suppl):134.
30. Tempelman M, Bell E. Head insulation for premature infants in servocontrolled incubators, and radiant warmers. *Am J Dis Child.* 1986;140:940.
31. Arndt K. Inadvertent hypothermia in the OR. *AORN J.* 1999;70(2):204-206.
32. Bissonnette B et al. Inspired gas humidification prevents intraoperative hypothermia in infants and children. *Anesth Analg.* 1989;68:258.
33. Besumder J et al. Principles of drug biodisposition in the neonate: a critical evaluation of the pharmacokinetic-pharmacodynamic interface. Part I. *Clin Pharmacokinet.* 1988;14:189-216.
34. Kearns G et al. Developmental pharmacology: drug disposition, action, and therapy in infants and children. *N Engl J Med.* 2003;349:1157-1167.
35. Caldwell JJ et al. Pharmacokinetics of bupivacaine administered epidurally during childbirth. *Br J Pharmacol.* 1976;3:956-957.
36. Gunter J. Benefit and risks of local anesthetics in infants and children. *Paediatr Drugs.* 2002;4:649-672.
37. Morselli P et al. Clinical pharmcokinetics in newborns and infants. *Clin Pharmacokinet.* 1980;5:485-527.
38. Jacqz-Aigrain E et al. Clinical pharmacokinetics of sedatives in neonates. *Clin Pharmacokinet.* 1996;31:423-443.
39. Battino D et al. Clinical pharmacokinetics of antiepileptic drugs in paediatric patients. Part II: phenytoin, carbamazepine, sulthiame, lamotrigine, vigabatrin, oxcarbazepine and felbamate. *Clin Pharmacokinet.* 1995;29:341-369.
40. Meakin G et al. Age-dependent variation in response to tubocurarine in the isolated rat diaphragm. *Br J Anaesth.* 1992;68:161-163.
41. Wareham A et al. Low quantal content of the endplate potential reduces safety factory for neuromuscular transmission in the diaphragm of the newborn rat. *Br J Anaesth.* 1994;72:205-209.
42. Franks N, Lieb W. Molecular and cellular mechanisms of general anaesthesia. *Nature.* 1994;367:604-617.
43. Brooks-Kayal A et al. Developmental changes in human aminobutyric acid receptor subunit composition. *Ann Neurol.* 1993;34:687-693.
44. Raddle I, McKerchner H. Transport through membranes and the development of membrane transport. In: Macleod S, Raddle I, eds. *Textbook of Pediatric Clinical Pharmacology.* Littleton, MA: PSG; 1985:.
45. Yaster M. The dose response of fentanyl in neonatal anesthesia. *Anesthesiology.* 1987;66:433-435.
46. Robinson S, Gregory G. Fentanyl-air-oxygen anesthesia for ligatin of patent ductus arteriosus in preterm infants. *Anesth Analg.* 1981;60:331-334.
47. Shew S et al. Ligation of a patent ductus arteriosus under fentanyl anesthesia improves protein metabolism in premature neonates. *J Pediatr Surg.* 2000;35:1277-1281.
48. Cook D. Neonatal anesthetic pharmacology. *Anesth Analg.* 1974;(53):544-548.
49. Meakin G et al. Dose-response curves for suxamethonium in neonates, infants and children. *Br J Anaesth.* 1989;55:599-602.
50. Rackow H et al. Modern concepts in pediatric anesthesiology. *Anesthesiology.* 1969;30:208.
51. Shimada Y et al. Crying vital capacity and maximal inspiratory pressure as clinical indicators of readiness for weaning of infants less than a year of age. *Anesthesiology.* 1979;51:456-459.
52. Shoults D et al. Maximum inspiratory force in predicting successful neonate tracheal extubation. *Crit Care Med.* 1979;7:485-486.
53. Brandom B, Fine G. Neuromuscular blocking drugs in pediatric anesthesia. *Anesthesiol Clin North America.* 2002;20:45-58.
54. Ellis D. Regulation of fluids and electrolytes in infants and children. In: Motoyama E, Davis P, eds. *Smith's Anesthesia for Infants and Children.* Philadelphia: Mosby; 2006:.
55. Holliday M. Fluid and nutrition support. In: Holliday M, Barratt T, eds. *Pediatric Nephrology.* Baltimore: Williams & Wilkins; 1994:301.
56. Winters R. *Principles of Pediatric Fluid Therapy.* Boston: Little, Brown; 1982.
57. Bissonnette B. Fluid therapy. In: Hughes D et al, eds. *Neonatal Anesthesia.* London: Saunders; 1996:110-131.
58. Bliss A. Pre-operative starvation: have we changed our views since Emerson, Wrigley and Newton? *Pediatr Anesth.* 2002;12(9):829-830.
59. Rowe M et al. Clinical evaluation of methods to monitor colloid oncotic pressure in the surgical treatment of children. *Surg Gynecol Obstet.* 1974;139:889.
60. Siegel S et al. Serum aldosterone concentrations related to sodium balance in the newborn infant. *Pediatrics.* 1974;53:410-413.
61. Fanaroff A et al. Insensible water loss in low birth weight infants. *Pediatrics.* 1972;50:236-245.
62. Dabbagh D et al. Regulation of fluids and electrolytes in infants and children. In: Motoyama E, Davis P, eds. *Smith's Anesthesia for Infants and Children.* St Louis: Mosby; 1996:1062-1069.
63. McManus M. Pediatric fluid management. In: Cote C et al, eds. *A Practice of Anesthesia in Infants and Children.* Philadelphia, Saunders; 2001:216-234.
64. Edelmann CJ et al. Renal concentrating mechanisms in newborn infants: effect of dietary protein and water content, role of urea, and respnsiveness to antidiuretic hormone. *J Clin Invest.* 1960;39:1062-1069.
65. Bracelona S et al. Intraoperative pediatric blood transfusion therapy: a review of common issues. Part I: hemotologic and physiologic differences from adults; metabolic and infectious risks. *Pediatr Anesth.* 2005;15:716-726.
66. Bhananker S et al. Anesthesia-related cardiac arrest in children: update from the Pediatric Perioperative Cardiac Arrest Registry. *Anesth Analg.* 2007;105(2):301-303.
67. Brown K et al. Hyperkalemia during rapid blood transfusion and hypovolemic cardiac arrest in children. *Can J Anaesth.* 1990;37:747-754.
68. Miller M, Schlueter A. Transfusions via hand-held syringes and small-gauge needles as risk factors for hyperkalemia. *Transfusion.* 2004;44:373-381.
69. Fine G, Borland L. The future of the cuffed endotracheal tube. *Pediatr Anesth.* 2004;14:38-42.
70. Gregory G. Anesthesia for premature infants. In: Gregory G, ed. *Pediatric Anesthesia.* New York: Churchill Livingstone; 2002:345.
71. Lubchenco L et al. Intrauterine growth as estimated from live born birth-weight data at 24 to 42 weeks of gestation. *Pediatrics.* 1963;32:793.
72. Cote D et al. Postoperative apnea in former preterm infants after inguinal herniorrhaphy: a combined analysis. *Anesthesiology.* 1995;82:809-822.
73. Fisher D. When is the ex-premature infant no longer at risk for apnea? *Anesthesiology.* 1995;82:807-808.
74. Welborn L, Greenspun J. Anesthesia and apnea; perioperative considerations in the former preterm infant. *Pediatr Clin North Am.* 1994;41:181-198.
75. Cox R, Goresky G. Life-threatening apnea following spinal anesthesia in former premature infants. *Anesthesiology.* 1997;73:345-347.
76. Welborn L. Preoperative apnea in the preterm infant. *Anesthesiol Clin North America.* 1991;9:885-895.
77. Kurth C. Postoperative apnea in premature infants. *Anesthesiology.* 1987;66:483-487.
78. Mestad P et al. When is outpatient surgery safe in the preterm infant. *Anesthesiology.* 1988;69:744.
79. Aranda A et al. Pharmacologic considerations in the therapy of neonatal apnea. *Pediatr Clin North Am.* 1981;28:113.
80. Welborn L et al. The use of caffeine in the control of postanesthetic apnea in former premature infants. *Anesthesiology.* 1988;71:347.
81. Welborn L et al. High-dose caffeine suppresses postoperative apnea in former preterm infants. *Anesthesiology.* 1989;71:347.
82. Perkin R et al. Serum salicylate levels and right-to-left ductus shunts in newborn infants with persistent pulmonary hypertension. *J Pediatr.* 1980;96:721.
83. Peutrell J, Weir P. Basic principles of neonatal anesthesia. In: Hughes D et al, eds. *Handbook of Neonatal Anesthesia.* London: Saunders; 1996:166-167.
84. Litman R. The premature infant. In: Litman R, ed. *Pediatric Anesthesia: The Requisites in Anesthesiology.* Philadelphia: Mosby; 2004:76.
85. Somri M et al. The effectiveness and safety of spinal anesthesia in the pyloromyotomy procedure. *Pediatr Anesth.* 2003;13:32.
86. Ross A. Pediatric regional anesthesia. In: Motoyama E, Davis P, eds. *Smith's Anesthesia for Infants and Children.* Philadelphia: Mosby; 2006:473.
87. Pascucci R et al. Chest wall motion of infants during spinal anesthesia. *J Appl Physiol.* 1990;68:2087.
88. Tobias JD. Caudal epidural block: a review of test dosing and recognition of systemic injection in children. *Anesth Analg.* 2001;93:1156.
89. Willschke H et al. Epidural catheter placement in neonates: sonoanatomy and feasibility of ultrasonographic guidance in term and preterm neonates. *Surv Anesthesiol.* 2007;51(5):257-258.
90. Gregory G, Steward D. Life-threatening perioperative apnea in the "ex-premie." *Anesthesiology.* 1983;59:495-498.
91. Tobias J, Litman R. Pediatric regional anesthesia. In: Litman R, ed. *Pediatric Anesthesia: The Requisites in Anesthesiology.* Philadelphia: Mosby; 2004.
92. Liu L, Pang L. Neonatal surgical emergencies. *Anesthesiology Clinics of North America.* Philadelphia: Saunders; 2001:1-16.
93. Puri P, Wester T. Historical aspects of congenital diaphragmatic hernia. *Pediatr Surg Int.* 1997;12:95-100.
94. Wheeler M. Anesthesia for neonatal surgical emergencies. In: Schwartz A et al, eds. *ASA Refresher Courses in Anesthesiology.* Vol. 30(1). Philadelphia: Lippincott Williams & Wilkins; 2002:201-214.
95. Azarow K et al. Congenital diaphragmatic hernia—a tale of two cities: the Toronto experience. *J Pediatr Surg.* 1997;32:395-400.
96. Jona J. The incidence of positive contralateral inguinal exploration in preschool children: a combined retrospective and prospective study. *J Pediatr Surg.* 1996;31:656-660.

97. The Congenital Diaphragmatic Hernia Study Group. Does extracorporeal membrane oxygenation improve survival in neonates with congenital diaphragmatic hernia? *J Pediatr Surg*. 1999;34:720-724.

98. Lacey S et al. Bladder pressure monitoring significantly enhances care of infants with abdominal wall defects: a prospective clinical study. *J Pediatr Surg*. 1993;28:1370-1374.

99. Puffinbarger N et al. End-tidal carbon dioxide for monitoring primary closure of gastroschisis. *J Pediatr Surg*. 1996;31:280-281.

100. Yaster M et al. Prediction of successful primary closure of congenital abdominal wall defects using intraoperative measurements. *J Pediatr Surg*. 1989;24:1217-20.

101. Somppi E et al. Outcome of patients operated on for esophageal atresia: 30 years experience. *J Pediatr Surg*. 1998;33:1341-1346.

102. Tobias J, Maxwell L. Anesthesia for pediatric thoracic surgery. In: Hines R, ed. *Pediatric Anesthesia: The Requisites in Anesthesiology*. Philadelphia: Mosby; 2004:297-301.

103. Steward D, Lerman J. General and thoracoabdominal surgery. In: Steward D, Lerman J, eds. *Manual of Pediatric Anesthesia*. New York: Churchill Livingstone; 2001:291-292.

104. Litman R. Anesthesia for general and abdominal surgery. In: Hines R, ed. *Pediatric Anesthesia: The Requisites in Anesthesiology*. Philadelphia: Mosby; 2002:225-235.

105. Hepner D, Castells M. Latex allergy: an update. *Anesth Analg*. 2003;96:1219.

CHAPTER 49

PEDIATRIC ANESTHESIA

John G. Aker

Pediatric subspecialty practice requires the anesthetist to master the foundations of pediatric growth and development, the anatomic and physiologic differences during various stages of maturation, and the influence of immature organ systems on anesthetic pharmacokinetics and pharmacodynamics. Anesthetic management of the pediatric patient requires integration of this specialized knowledge, refinement of the acquired technical skills of adult anesthetic management, and the ability to apply this knowledge when caring for the pediatric patient.

The father of American pediatric care, Dr. Abraham Jacobi, declared that "pediatrics does not deal with miniature men and women, with reduced doses and the same class of disease in smaller bodies."[1] The frequently uttered adage that "children are simply small adults" represents a myopic view of the striking structural and physiologic differences between infants and adults. However, by the age of 5 years, these physiologic differences are almost insignificant.

It is impossible to provide a comprehensive discussion of the discipline of pediatric anesthesia within a single chapter; however, the content of this chapter provides an extensive discussion of the essentials for pediatric practice. The foundation of anesthetic management is developed through an understanding of pediatric anesthetic morbidity and mortality; the pharmacologic and physiologic differences among adults, infants and children; and a clinical strategy for anesthetic management.

PEDIATRIC ANESTHETIC MORBIDITY AND MORTALITY

Anesthetic morbidity and mortality differ between the pediatric and the adult patient. Accordingly, children require individualized and specialized anesthetic care. When compared with adults, children often present for surgery with unique symptoms. Their lack of ability to communicate effectively further complicates proper diagnosis and interventions. Fortunately, with a well-conducted history and physical and effective caregiver communication, a safe anesthetic may be planned and executed.

The anesthetic literature clearly suggests that pediatric patients have anesthetic experiences that are different from those of adults. Anesthetic morbidity and mortality are greater in pediatric patients.[2-4] Intraoperative bradycardia is more frequent in infants. Intraoperative bradycardia precipitated by the development of hypoxemia or following the delivery of high concentrations of inhalation agent is associated with significant morbidity. Keenan and co-workers found that morbidity accompanying intraoperative bradycardia (heart rate <100 beats/min during the first

year of life) included hypotension (32%), ventricular fibrillation or asystole (14%), and perioperative death (8%).[5]

A comparison of adult and pediatric closed claims reveals that respiratory complications occur with greater frequency in the pediatric population, and associated outcome is significantly worse.[2] In addition, these respiratory complications occur in healthy children of normal weight, as opposed to the adult populations with concurrent cardiopulmonary disease and obesity. Respiratory complications occur not only in the operating suite but also in the recovery room and more frequently in pediatric patients (13 in 10,000) than in adults (5.9 in 10,000).[3] A reported European estimate of serious injury or death among pediatric patients during anesthesia found a three-fold greater incidence in pediatric patients than in adults, from 1 in 20,000 to 1 in 100,000.[6]

In a 6-year prospective examination of more than 29,000 pediatric anesthetic procedures, Morray and colleagues found that children less than 4 weeks of age have the greatest risk of adverse events during the perioperative period and the greatest risk of perioperative death. These adverse events include hypotension, bronchospasm, laryngospasm, apnea, and cardiac arrest. Emergency surgical procedures increase risk in children. Patients between the ages of 1 month and 12 years experience the fewest perioperative anesthetic complications. Children between the ages of 1 and 5 and 6 and 10 have a greater incidence of intraoperative dysrhythmias than adults.[3]

Pediatric Cardiac Arrest

The Pediatric Perioperative Cardiac Arrest Registry (POCA), an ongoing database of pediatric cardiac arrest established in 1994, is a self-reporting, voluntary registry recording institutional cardiac arrests in children up to 18 years of age from as many as 80 participating institutions in Canada and the United States. The POCA data provide a retrospective assessment of contributing factors rather than determining causation of cardiac arrest. The initial registry results for the years 1994 to 1997 found 289 cardiac arrests in more than 1 million pediatric anesthetic experiences. One hundred and fifty (52%) were judged to be anesthesia related (1.4/10,000).[3] The resulting risk of anesthesia-related cardiac arrest was 1 in 7000, with a mortality rate of 26%.

Three important clinical caveats emerged from an analysis of these data. First, anesthesia-related cardiac arrest was more frequent in patients younger than 1 year of age. The infant and neonate accounted for 55% of all cardiac arrests. Second 32% of the cardiac arrests were from cardiovascular causes. This was markedly different from the 13% reported in the Pediatric Closed Claim study.[2] And third, previously healthy children (American Society of Anesthesiologists [ASA] 1 to 2) accounted for 33% of the cardiac arrests, whereas 67% occurred in children with an ASA classification of 3 to 5. Cardiac arrest occurred in 21% of those children during emergency surgical procedures, and interestingly, more frequently during urologic and general surgical procedures. In examining the time period of cardiac arrest, the majority occurred during anesthetic induction (37%), and during the maintenance phase of anesthesia (45%). Several clinical warning signs of impending cardiac arrest were identified and included bradycardia (54%), hypotension (49%), inability to obtain a blood pressure (52%), or an abnormality in the pulse oximeter.

Medication-related etiologies were the most common, accounting for 37% of all arrests. Cardiac arrest involved the administration of halothane alone, or halothane with an intravenous opioid and thiopental, or halothane with concomitant administration of bupivacaine for caudal anesthesia. The median age for these arrests was age 6 months; 66% of the arrests with halothane occurred during anesthetic induction, and 34% occurred during anesthetic maintenance. The common antecedent events were bradycardia and hypotension. Associated factors included assisted or controlled ventilation and difficult venous access requiring multiple attempts during mask ventilation. Sevoflurane was also implicated in anesthesia-related cardiac arrest in two ASA physical status 3 children. Both were successfully resuscitated.

Pediatric anesthesia practice has evolved in the past decade with the introduction of the inhalation agent sevoflurane. Many pediatric anesthetists have abandoned the use of halothane for sevoflurane. At the recent session of the Society of Pediatric Anesthesia, fewer than a dozen practitioners responded positively when asked if they use halothane for anesthetic induction (personal communication Dr. Leslie Friskel). There may be sound reasons for the abandonment of halothane, particularly in the neonate. The minimum alveolar concentration (MAC) of halothane in the neonate (<30 days of age) is 0.87%, and in infants age 1 to 6 months 1.08%,[7] whereas the MAC of sevoflurane is 3.3% up to age 1 month, decreasing to 3% for ages 1 to 6 months.[8] Studies suggest that an incremental sevoflurane induction produces less myocardial depression and less frequent instances of bradycardia than halothane.[9-11]

Bhananker and colleagues recently completed an analysis of cases submitted to the POCA registry for the years 1998 to 2004.[4] There were an additional 397 reported perioperative cardiac arrests, with 193 (49%) judged to be anesthesia related. Three quarters (75%) of the anesthesia-related arrests occurred in ASA physical status 3 to 5, compared with 67% incidence in the 1994 to 1997 data. Fifty-eight percent of all reported cardiac arrests developed during the maintenance of anesthesia. There were fewer medication-related cardiac arrests than the previous report of the years 1994 to 1997 (Figure 49-1, Table 49-1). The proportion of cardiac arrests following inhalation agent cardiac depression was 18%, compared with 37% for the years 1994 to 1997. Given the apparent change in practice since 1997 (the substitution of sevoflurane for halothane), the reduction in medication-related cardiac arrest may reflect the decreased use of halothane and increasing use of sevoflurane.

The cardiovascular etiologies of cardiac arrest accounted for 41% of the anesthesia-related arrests. Hypovolemia secondary to blood loss accounted for 12%. These arrests occurred during either spinal fusion (9 cases) or craniotomy (7 cases). Underestimation of blood loss and inadequate intravenous or

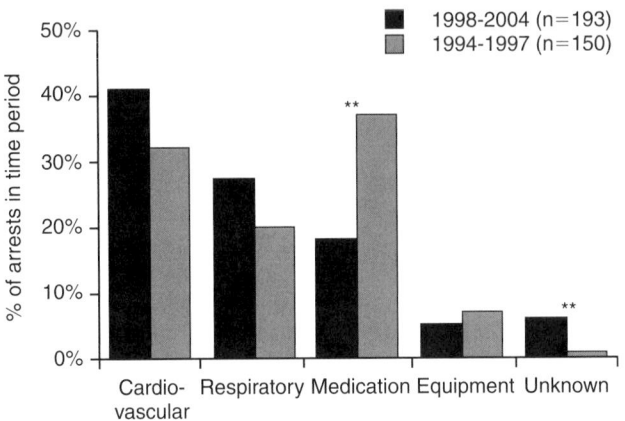

FIGURE **49-1** Etiology of cardiac arrest, 1994 to 1997 and 1998 to 2004. (*From Bhananker SM, Ramamoorthy C et al. Anesthesia-related cardiac arrest in children: update from the Pediatric Perioperative Cardiac Arrest Registry. Anesth Analg. 2007;105:344-350:346.*)

central venous access were contributory. It is important to point out that the etiology of cardiac arrest in 8 of every 10 children was the result of hyperkalemia following transfusion of banked blood.

Respiratory events were responsible for 27% (n = 53) of anesthesia-related arrests. Airway obstruction from laryngospasm was the most common etiology (11 cases). Laryngospasm occurred during anesthetic induction (4 cases) and during the immediate postoperative recovery (7 cases). All patients experiencing laryngospasm had oxygen desaturation below 85% and bradycardia prior to the arrest. All were resuscitated without sequelae.

Equipment failures accounted for 5% of the reported cardiac arrests. Complications related to the placement of central intravenous catheters (pneumothorax, hemothorax and hemopericardium), as well as bradycardia with catheter advancement, were reported. In addition, bradycardia and hypotension were reported with the abrupt cessation of inotropic support following inadvertent central venous catheter removal.

PEDIATRIC PHARMACOLOGIC CONSIDERATIONS

Immature organ systems are responsible for existing pharmacologic differences between the infant and child. Physiologic characteristics that modify the pharmacokinetic (what the body does to the drug) and pharmacodynamic (what the drug does to the body) activity include differences in total body water (TBW) composition, immaturity of metabolic degradation pathways, reduced protein binding, immaturity of the blood-brain barrier, greater proportion of blood flow to the vessel-rich organs (brain, heart, liver and lungs), reductions in glomerular filtration, a smaller functional residual capacity, and increased minute ventilation.

Water freely diffuses across cell membranes and is essential for the transport of cellular nutrients and substrates that support metabolic reactions. TBW, expressed in liters, is determined as a percentage of total body weight (1 L of water weighs 1 kg) and steadily decreases with increasing age and varies according to sex and body habitus. TBW is distributed into the intracellular fluid (ICF) compartment and the extracellular fluid (ECF) compartment. With maturation, there is an accompanying decrease in the relative fluid compartment volumes of TBW and ECF during the first year of life, followed by additional decreases in

TABLE 49-1	Causes of Cardiac Arrest, 1998-2004	
Cause		**n = 193 No. (% of 193)**
Cardiovascular		79 (41)
Hypovolemia associated with blood loss		23 (12)
Electrolyte imbalance		10 (5)
Hypovolemia (nonhemorrhage)		5 (3)
Air embolism		4 (2)
Other CV		11 (6)
Presumed CV unclear mechanism		26 (13)
Respiratory		53 (27)
Airway obstruction—laryngospasm		11 (6)
Airway obstruction—other		5 (3)
Inadequate ventilation or oxygenation		9 (5)
Inadvertent or premature extubation		7 (4)
Difficult intubation		4 (1)
Esophageal or endobronchial intubation		3 (2)
Bronchospasm		4 (2)
Pneumothorax		2 (1)
Aspiration		2 (1)
Other		1 (1)
Presumed respiratory, unclear mechanism		5 (3)
Medication		35 (18)
Halothane-induced CV depression		9 (5)
Sevoflurane-induced CV depression		6 (3)
Other single medication*		9 (5)
Medication combination		7 (3)
Allergic reaction		2 (1)
Intravascular injection of local		2 (1)
Equipment		9 (5)
Central catheter		5 (3)
Kinked or plugged ETT		2 (1)
Peripheral IV catheter		1 (1)
Breathing circuit		1 (1)
Multiple events		3 (2)
Miscellaneous		2 (1)
Unknown		12 (6)

From: Bhananker SM et al. Anesthesia-related cardiac arrest in children: update from the Pediatric Perioperative Cardiac Arrest Registry. Anesth Analg. 2007;105:344-350:346.
CV, Cardiovascular; ETT, endotracheal tube; IV, intravenous.
*Noninhalation agents.

TABLE 49-2	Fluid Compartment Volumes			
	Premature (%)	Infant (%)	Child (%)	Adult (%)
Total body water (TBW)	80-90	75	65-70	55-60
Extracellular fluid (ECF)	50-60	40	30	20
Intracellular fluid (ICF)	60	35	40	40

From Aker J et al. Pediatric fluid and blood therapy. In: Zaglaniczny K, Aker J, eds. Clinical Guide to Pediatric Anesthesia. Philadelphia: Saunders; 1999:85.

drug distribution. The infant has a larger extracellular fluid compartment and a greater total body water content. In addition, there is a greater adipose content and a higher ratio of water to lipid. Fat content is approximately 12% at birth, doubling by 6 months of age, and reaching 30% at 12 months of age.[12] These factors lower plasma drug concentrations when water-soluble drugs are administered according to weight. Accordingly, a larger drug loading dose is required to achieve the desired plasma concentration. An excellent example is the intramuscular dosage of the water-soluble depolarizing muscle relaxant succinylcholine (4 mg/kg). The effect of immaturity on the volume of distribution is not as evident for lipophilic drugs that are transported across cell membranes.

Protein Binding

Alterations in protein binding affect the availability of the free-drug fraction of protein-bound drugs. Reductions in plasma proteins (i.e., albumin) increase the free-drug fraction, increasing the availability of active drug. Total plasma protein is decreased in the infant, reaching equivalent adult concentrations by childhood. Albumin, the predominant plasma protein, is responsible for the binding of acidic pharmacologic compounds (benzodiazepines, barbiturates, acetylsalicylic acid), and α_1-acid glycoprotein (AAG) is responsible for the binding of basic pharmacologic compounds (local anesthetics, α-blockers, opioids, and neuromuscular relaxants). Both albumin and AAG concentrations are diminished at birth but reach the adult equivalency by infancy (age 4 weeks).[12] Recall that albumin concentrations may fluctuate, decreasing in chronic disease states with parallel increases in AAG concentration.

Metabolism

The administered drug must be metabolized to prepare for its elimination from the body. Drug metabolism takes place in the liver, gastrointestinal tract, gastric mucosa, and lungs. In most instances, metabolism reduces drug activity; however, the metabolite may have a greater increase in drug activity than the parent compound. The ultimate goal of drug metabolism is the production of a water-soluble compound that can be easily excreted.

Drug metabolism occurs in two phases. Phase I metabolism consists of three enzymatic reactions (oxidation, reduction, and hydrolysis) catalyzed by the P-450 enzyme system. Enzyme systems within the red blood cell, plasma, and other extrahepatic tissues are capable of hydrolyzing a variety of pharmacologic agents, including local anesthetics, the depolarizing relaxant succinylcholine, and the nondepolarizing relaxants atracurium and cisatracurium. Phase I reactions produce a water-soluble

ECF later in childhood. Table 49-2 illustrates the changes in TBW, ICF, and ECF during maturation.

Volume of Distribution

Drug distribution is best described by the apparent volume of distribution, which is determined by dividing the dose of the administered drug by the resulting plasma concentration. Accordingly, body water composition influences the volume of metabolic product with the introduction of polar hydroxyl, amino, sulfhydryl, or carboxyl groups for excretion within the bile or urine. Phase II reactions, which are immature at birth, consist of conjugation or synthesis. Conjugation couples the drug with an endogenous substrate (glucuronidation, methylation, acetylation, and sulfation) to facilitate excretion. The newborn lacks the capacity to efficiently conjugate bilirubin (decreased glucuronyl transferase activity), and metabolize acetaminophen, chloramphenicol, and sulfonamides.

Although the necessary enzyme systems are present at birth, enzyme activity is reduced, increasing drug elimination half-lives. Drugs that produce a prolonged plasma half-life in the include bupivacaine (25 hours),[13] mepivacaine (8.5 hours),[14] diazepam (up to 100 hours),[15] indomethacin (15 to 20 hours),[16] meperidine (22 hours), and phenytoin (21 hours).[17]

Drug Administration
Rectal and Oral Drug Administration
Rectal and oral drug administration are easy and convenient, compared with parenteral drug administration. Drugs are usually formulated as liquids for oral administration in children. Midazolam may be administered orally for premedication, and the rectal route may be selected for the administration of acetaminophen, opioids, barbiturates (thiopental and methohexital), and benzodiazepines. Both routes rely on passive diffusion for drug absorption. The resulting plasma drug concentration is dependent on the molecular weight, degree of drug ionization, and lipid solubility.

The degree of ionization of orally administered drugs is dependent on gastric pH levels. Acidic drugs are nonionized and are favorably absorbed in the low pH medium of the stomach. Basic drugs have more favorable absorption in the alkaline medium of the intestine. Orally administered drugs are generally reserved for older children because gastric pH is elevated in the neonate at birth (pH 6 to 8), and although decreased to a pH level of 1 to 3 within 24 hours, values that parallel adult gastric pH are not consistent until age 2.[18-20] Gastric absorption is reduced following oral administration of acidic drugs in infants. Gastric emptying time reaches adult values by 6 months of age. Although gastric emptying time does not affect drug absorption, it may alter peak drug concentration.

Rectal drug absorption is directly affected by drug formulation and rectal blood flow. The superior (upper third of the rectum), middle, and inferior rectal veins carry blood away from the rectal mucosa. The superior rectal vein empties into the portal system, whereas the middle and inferior rectal veins empty into the systemic circulation by way of the inferior vena cava. For example, the administration of acetaminophen into the upper third of the rectum results in a lower plasma concentration because of first-pass metabolism with drug transport to the liver.[13] Opioids, barbiturates, and midazolam undergo first-pass metabolism, and their administration into the upper third of the rectum should be avoided.

Acetaminophen, a metabolite of phenacetin, is a popular and safe analgesic and antipyretic commonly administered to children during the perioperative period. The inhibition of cyclooxygenase within the central nervous system is the proposed analgesic mechanism of action. Acetaminophen is capable of inducing dose-dependent hepatocyte injury. Acetaminophen toxicity following suicide attempts or exceeding the recommended daily dosage is the most common etiology of acute hepatic failure, accounting for 39% of cases in a survey of 17 tertiary care centers.[21] This drug deserves some discussion because of its popularity as an intraoperative analgesic in pediatric patients.

The analgesic and antipyretic effects of acetaminophen are equivalent to those of aspirin when the drugs are administered in equipotent dosages. Acetaminophen is metabolized by the hepatic microsomal enzyme system, and approximately 80% of the parent drug is conjugated with glucuronic acid and sulfate (phase II metabolism). Animal data suggest that a small amount of the parent drug is metabolized by the cytochrome P-450 enzyme system (phase I metabolism), producing an intermediate metabolite that undergoes conjugation with glutathione and is excreted in the urine. High doses of acetaminophen may deplete glutathione, increasing the accumulation of this intermediate metabolite, which is thought to be responsible for acetaminophen-induced liver necrosis. Glutathione depletion may develop with continued administration of high doses of acetaminophen.[22]

Suppositories should not be divided in an attempt to provide the exact calculated dose, because the suspended acetaminophen is distributed unevenly within the suppository. Recommended acetaminophen doses have been based on the age of the child, weight, body surface area calculations, and fractions of adult dosages. Doses calculated per patient weight are the most accurate for individual patients.[23] Currently recommended oral and rectal doses of acetaminophen range from 10 to 15 mg/kg every 4 hours.[24] Because of the variable absorption of acetaminophen suppositories, some practitioners have advocated the administration of larger initial rectal dosages. Birmingham and colleagues examined the 24-hour pharmacokinetics of rectal acetaminophen, and based on the observed kinetics, they recommend an initial dose of 40 mg/kg.[24,25] Analgesic efficacy was not studied, but rather the dosages were based on resultant serum acetaminophen concentrations of 10 to 20 mcg/mL, which have been determined to be essential for antipyretic activity. It should be emphasized that subsequent rectal doses should be decreased (20 mg/kg), and the dosing interval should be extended to every 6 to 8 hours.[24,25] Montgomery and colleagues administered 45 mg/kg of acetaminophen rectally to 10 pediatric patients who weighed between 13 and 15 kg.[26] Plasma sampling demonstrated a peak concentration that occurred 198 ± 70 minutes after administration. Resultant plasma concentrations were comparable to those after a 10 to 15 mg/kg oral dose, and attained plasma concentrations were not associated with acute toxicity.

Parents are likely to continue to administer acetaminophen following the surgical procedure. Following acetaminophen administered during the perioperative period, the parents should be informed as to the time of administration and be advised of appropriate acetaminophen dosages (60 to 65 mg/kg/day). The daily acetaminophen dosage administered either rectally or orally should be limited to 100 mg/kg/day for children and 75 mg/kg/day for infants. A recent case report by Morton and Arana highlights the dangers of exceeding this recommended dose.[27] A 2½-year-old female weighing 11.2 kg who had a viral febrile illness received 16 mg/kg every 4 hours for a period of 5 days (total dose of 5 g). She presented with hepatomegaly, encephalopathy, increased ammonia and transaminase levels, lactic acidosis and hypoglycemia. Recovery without sequelae followed 4 days of controlled ventilation and the administration of N-acetylcysteine, ranitidine, sucralfate, antibiotics, and vitamin K. The author has knowledge of one child requiring liver transplant following chronic administration of a cough syrup containing acetaminophen. There are additional examples of acetaminophen toxicity in the literature.[21]

Animal and human data are conflicting with regard to the effect of inhalation agents on the hepatic degradation of acetaminophen. Studies have suggested a decrease in acetaminophen conjugation,[28] an increase in acetaminophen metabolism via the oxidative metabolic pathway,[29] and an increase in hepatic metabolism on the first postoperative day.[30] Additional clinical studies are required to confirm the appropriate initial rectal dosages and the effect of inhalation anesthesia on serum acetaminophen concentrations and metabolism, as well as serum concentrations that provide optimum analgesia.

The vascular mucosa of the oral, nasal, and pulmonary passages is easily accessed. The advantage of transmucosal drug administration is the avoidance of first-pass metabolism. Sedation with nasally administered midazolam (0.2 mg/kg) may be achieved in as little as 10 to 20 minutes and is explained in part through drug absorption via the olfactory mucosa.[31,32] Nasal administration avoids first-pass metabolism but is unpleasant because the midazolam produces a burning of the nasal mucosa. Oral fentanyl, although effective in producing significant sedation, has been plagued by significant side effects, including facial pruritus (up to 80%) and postoperative nausea and vomiting, seven times greater than when a child receives an oral meperidine, midazolam, or atropine premedicant.[33] Recall that water-soluble drugs (atropine, fentanyl, lidocaine, morphine) may be administered via inhalation; however, only 5% to 10% of the administered dose will reach the systemic circulation.

Types of Agents
Inhalation Agents

The rapid increase in alveolar concentration of inspired anesthetic is quantified by the ratio of the alveolar to inspired concentration (F_A/F_I). Factors that affect the F_A/F_I ratio include the delivered inspired anesthetic concentration, the inhalation agent blood-gas partition coefficient, alveolar ventilation (V_A), cardiac output (Q), and the distribution of Q to the vessel-rich organs (i.e., heart, brain, kidneys, and liver). Although tidal volume is similar between children and adults (5 to 7 mL/kg), children have greater minute ventilation and a higher ratio of tidal volume to functional residual capacity (5:1) compared with the adult (1.5:1). The greater minute ventilation and higher Q in infants and children are responsible for rapid inhalation anesthetic uptake and rapidly increasing alveolar anesthetic concentration. In addition, their decreased distribution of adipose tissue and decreased muscle mass affect the rate of equilibration among the alveoli, blood, and brain. The percentage of blood flow to the vessel-rich organs is greater than in the adult, and the blood-gas partition coefficients are lower in infants and children.[34,35]

The MAC is an index of anesthetic potency and provides an appreciation of the concentration of a particular anesthetic, as well as an ability to compare the potency of different agents. Because it is widely accepted and universally applicable to all inhalation anesthetics, MAC can be used to evaluate the pharmacologic and physiologic factors that alter anesthetic requirement. Anesthetic requirements are known to change with age. Neonates have a somewhat lower MAC, which peaks at around 30 days of age (see Figure 49-2.) MAC is higher in infants from age 1 to 6 months of age; thereafter, MAC values are known to decrease with increasing age.[36,37]

Myocardial depression may be exaggerated when inhalation anesthetics are administered to pediatric patients.[38,39] A more rapid rise in F_A/F_I ratio, the greater percentage of blood flow to the vessel-rich organs, and higher administered anesthetic concentrations are central to the cause of myocardial depression. To summarize, inhalation induction is more rapid in pediatric patients and is accompanied by a higher incidence of myocardial depression than in adults.

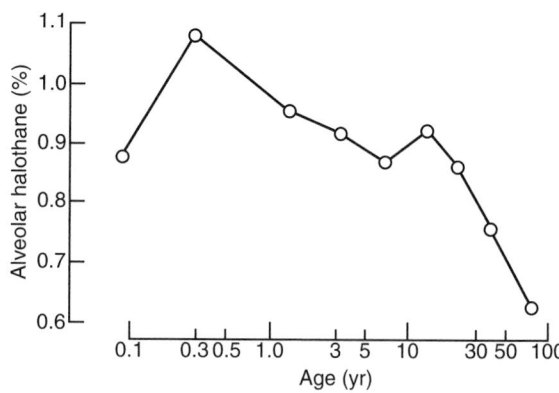

FIGURE **49-2** Effects of age on maximum alveolar concentration. (*Modified from Gregory GA et al. The relationship between age and halothane requirement in man. Anesthesiology. 1969;30:488-491; Lerman J et al. Anesthetic requirements for halothane in young children 0 to 1 month and 1 to 6 months of age. Anesthesiology. 1983;59:421-424.*)

Halothane. With the introduction of sevoflurane in the mid–1990s, the role of halothane in pediatric anesthesia has been reexamined. Contemporary anesthesia students no longer have the opportunity to administer halothane, and accordingly this discussion will likely be an academic exercise. The minimum alveolar concentration (MAC) of halothane in oxygen is 0.56% in the preterm, 0.87% in the full-term newborn, 1.2% in the 6-month-old infant, and 0.95% in the child. Halothane is less pungent than isoflurane and desflurane and is readily accepted for inhalation induction, yet it has a greater incidence of clinical significant cardiovascular depression, particularly when administered to the neonate. Children receiving halothane or sevoflurane have fewer airway-related incidents (bronchospasm, laryngospasm, breath-holding) compared with those induced with either isoflurane or desflurane.[40,41] Anesthetic induction is facilitated with increasing inspired concentrations of ½% every two or three breaths. Following the establishment of controlled ventilation and intravenous access, the inspired concentration must be reduced to prevent agent overdose, evidenced by accompanying bradycardia and hypotension.

Halothane sensitizes the myocardium to the effects of endogenous and exogenous catecholamines. Ventricular dysrhythmias may occur with inadequate depths of anesthesia and in the presence of hypercarbia, which stimulates the central release of catecholamines.[42] It has been suggested that epinephrine administration with local anesthetics should be limited to 10 mcg/kg body weight to minimize the potential of cardiac dysrhythmias.[43] As mentioned, halothane produces dose-dependent myocardial depression. The administration of high concentrations to infants and children will decrease cardiac output, blood pressure, mean arterial pressure, and heart rate. Systolic blood pressure may decrease by as much as 30% at 1 MAC end-tidal concentrations. Myocardial contractility and left ventricular stroke work are depressed, whereas peripheral vascular resistance is minimally altered. Atropine administration increases both heart rate and blood pressure.

Isoflurane. The MAC of isoflurane in oxygen is 1.6% in infants and children. Inhalation induction with isoflurane produces more adverse respiratory events (breath-holding, coughing, and laryngospasm with copious secretions) than either halothane or sevoflurane. Administration of isoflurane to adults produces dose-dependent decreases in peripheral vascular resistance, while increases in heart rate maintains blood pressure. This touted advantage (e.g., increase in heart rate to maintain blood pressure) does not occur in infants. Anesthetic induction in infants with isoflurane produces significant decreases in heart rate, blood pressure, and mean arterial pressure that are not corrected with prior atropine administration.[44]

Desflurane. The MAC of desflurane in oxygen is 9% for infants and 6% to 10% for children. Desflurane has the lowest blood-gas partition coefficient of all the inhalation anesthetics (0.42), which facilitates a rapid induction, rapid alterations in anesthetic depth, and emergence. Like isoflurane, desflurane is pungent and is associated with more adverse respiratory events during inhalation induction including breath-holding, laryngospasm, coughing, and increased secretions with accompanying hypoxia. Following inhalation induction with sevoflurane, desflurane is appropriate for the maintenance of general anesthesia with face mask, endotracheal tube, or laryngeal mask airway. As in the adult population, dramatic increases in desflurane concentrations may induce sympathetic stimulation evidenced by tachycardia and hypertension.[45,46]

Sevoflurane. The MAC of sevoflurane in oxygen is 3% for the infant up to 6 months of age, decreasing to 2.5% to 2.8% up to 1 year of age.[47] Sevoflurane produces a more rapid induction and emergence than halothane because of its low blood-gas partition coefficient.[48] Sevoflurane is readily accepted for mask induction, and its safe cardiovascular profile (when compared with halothane) is responsible for the increasing popularity of sevoflurane in pediatric anesthesia. During anesthetic induction, inspired concentrations in excess of 6% have been reported to produce seizure activity in an animal model. Seizure activity has been reported in two pediatric patients with epilepsy.[49,50]

Sevoflurane produces a greater depression of ventilation when compared with halothane. Both minute ventilation and respiratory rate are significantly lower after sevoflurane administration. With the introduction of high inspired concentrations, apnea is likely to occur.

Extreme reactions have developed with the exposure of sevoflurane to desiccated CO_2 absorbent (barium hydroxide), producing explosion and fire[51,52] and patient injury.[53] Sevoflurane is also unstable in CO_2 absorbent, producing fluoromethyl-2, 2-difluoro-1-(trifluoromethyl) vinyl ether, known as *compound A*. Animal data suggest that compound A concentrations between 50 and 100 ppm may produce renal toxicity.[54,55] Compound A may be formed during high-flow, low-flow, and closed-circuit anesthesia.[56-58] A limited study of 19 children who received a 4-hour sevoflurane anesthetic using a 2-L total flow via a circle system produced compound A concentrations of up to 15 ppm. A 24-hour follow-up concluded that there was no renal or hepatic dysfunction.[59] However, reports have suggested that subtle renal abnormalities, including albuminemia and altered renal thresholds for glucose, occur in adults who volunteered to receive a sevoflurane anesthetic without surgical intervention.[60,61]

Sevoflurane metabolism may produce concentration-dependent elevations in serum fluoride levels that decline when sevoflurane is discontinued. However, it is important to note that sevoflurane has been administered to thousands of patients without evidence of fluoride-induced renal dysfunction.

Some clinicians, when performing longer procedures, use sevoflurane for anesthetic induction and subsequently introduce either desflurane or isoflurane for anesthetic maintenance. This clinical decision reduces patient cost and limits sevoflurane exposure. Unlike halothane, sevoflurane does not sensitize the

TABLE **49-3**	The Pediatric Anesthesia Emergence Delirium (PAED) Scale
1. The child makes eye contact with caregiver.	
2. The child's actions are purposeful.	
3. The child is aware of his/her surroundings.	
4. The child is restless.	
5. The child is inconsolable.	

From Sikich N, Lerman J. Development and psychometric evaluation of the pediatric anesthesia emergence delirium scale. Anesthesiology. 2004;100:1138-1145.
Items 1, 2, and 3 are scored as follows: 4 = not at all, 3 = just a little, 2 = quite a bit, 1 = very much, 0 = extremely. For items 4 and 5, scoring is reversed: 0 = not at all, 1 = just a little, 2 = quite a bit, 3 = very much, 4 = extremely. The scores are summed to obtain a total. The degree of emergence delirium increases directly with total score.

myocardium to the effects of endogenous and exogenous catecholamines. However, not unlike halothane, concentration-dependent myocardial depression may occur. The MAC of sevoflurane in oxygen is 2% to 3%.

Emergence Delirium. Sevoflurane was introduced in Japan in 1992 and was subsequently licensed by the Food and Drug Administration for use in the United States in 1995. Following the U.S. and European introduction, case reports of postoperative agitation appeared in the literature, which were interestingly absent following the Asian introduction. It was noted that children quietly emerging from sevoflurane anesthesia would suddenly develop agitation, a state of excitement whereby the child failed to be consoled, requiring the attention of two postanesthesia care unit nurses. This phenomenon was well known from earlier epidemiologic studies that identified as many as 13% of children may experience postoperative agitation during emergence from anesthesia.[62,63]

A variety of terms are used interchangeably when referring to postoperative agitation. These include *emergence delirium*, *emergence agitation*, and *postanesthetic excitement*. These terms describe altered behavior in the immediate postoperative period manifested as nonpurposeful restlessness, crying, moaning, incoherence, and disorientation (known here as *emergence delirium* [ED]).[64,65] A report of three children and one adult who were able to describe their emergence experiences following a sevoflurane anesthetic suggests that ED may be the result of a short-lived misperception of environmental stimuli or paranoia.[66] The case reports also suggest that ED occurs more frequently in preschoolaged children (< age 6).[67] The reported incidence of ED is between 25% and 80%, although the incidence has been difficult to pinpoint because previous studies are confounded by the previously mentioned varying definitions.[68,69] This has prompted the development of a valid and reliable assessment tool (the Pediatric Anesthesia Emergence Delirium [PAED] scale) for the assessment of ED (Table 49-3).[70]

Emergence delirium is fortunately self-limiting but may manifest for as long as 45 minutes. It typically requires the attention of two postanesthesia care nurses, limiting the flow of patients into a busy postanesthesia care unit. ED may result in physical harm to the child (bleeding of the surgical site, loss of surgical drain or intravenous access, increased postoperative pain) and in rare instances result in injury to the postanesthesia recovery nurse[70,71] and delay discharge from the postanesthesia care unit.

In a search for the causation of ED, several emerging themes have been examined. Proposed etiologies include rapid emergence in a strange environment, pain on awakening, and preoperative behavior. The initial focus as to the cause of ED was rapid emergence following the administration of the insoluble agents sevoflurane and desflurane. However, both isoflurane and desflurane have been reported to have a similar incidence of ED in young children.[72-74] A comparison between propofol and sevoflurane in children ages 2 to 36 months found times to extubation and recovery were similar, yet ED was significantly higher in children who received sevoflurane (23%) versus propofol (3.7%).[75] This study seems to weaken the theme of rapid awakening as the etiology of ED in infants and children.

It has been argued that pain control is important in the avoidance of ED. Unpremedicated children clearly experience a higher incidence of emergence delirium.[66,69,76] Davis and colleagues found a decreased incidence of ED in patients receiving intravenous ketorolac for myringotomy and tube placement.[77] A similar study found that acetaminophen decreased ED following sevoflurane anesthesia.[78] Cravero and colleagues examined the incidence of ED in pediatric patients receiving either sevoflurane or halothane for magnetic resonance imaging (no surgical intervention). Painful stimuli were limited to intravenous access following inhalation induction. The incidence of ED was increased with the use of sevoflurane (as high as 33%).[69] In a follow-up study with the same patient population undergoing magnetic resonance imaging, Cravero and colleagues found that ED was significantly decreased and the time to discharge unchanged in children who received a sevoflurane anesthetic with the administration of 1 mcg/kg of fentanyl 10 minutes prior to the termination of anesthesia.[79] Aono demonstrated that children who received a regional anesthetic and were pain free experienced more agitation following sevoflurane compared with halothane.[67]

Lapin and colleagues found that children undergoing myringotomy and tube placement premedicated with midazolam before receiving sevoflurane experienced less postoperative agitation and cried less than their unpremedicated counterparts. These children had longer recovery times but experienced less ED, although it was still greater than that witnessed in the halothane group.[80] Of the unpremedicated children receiving sevoflurane, 67% experienced some degree of postoperative agitation.

In a prospective cohort examination of 521 children ages 3 to 7 years in the pediatric postanesthesia care unit, 18% exhibited ED (nonpurposeful restlessness, thrashing, crying, disorientation and incoherence) lasting up to 45 minutes. Pharmacologic intervention and supportive therapies were required in 52% of the children, prolonging the care in the postanesthesia recovery unit (117 ± 66 vs 101 ± 61 minutes for the nonagitated). Identified independent risk factors for the development of ED were otorhinolaryngologic (26%) and ophthalmologic surgical procedures (28%), rapid awakening, and the use of sevoflurane anesthesia (24%). In this study, ED was associated with four adverse outcomes (bleeding from the surgical site, removal of a surgical drain, increased pain, injury to the recovery room nurse, and prolonged recovery room stay).[71]

There appears to be no clearly delineated pathophysiologic explanation for ED. The evidence is fairly convincing that ED is the result of a specific effect of sevoflurane. Several strategies have been advocated for the prevention of ED, although a scientific, clinically tested strategy for prevention has yet to be advanced. Following inhalation induction with sevoflurane, propofol infusion for maintenance has been demonstrated to reduce ED.[81] Some anesthetists advocate the substitution of sevoflurane with isoflurane, yet there are no studies that detail the effectiveness of this strategy. All previous studies of ED have examined the use of a single anesthetic agent rather than combinations of inhalation agent.

The phenomenon of ED is clearly increased following the administration of sevoflurane (and likely desflurane). A pathophysiologic explanation is yet to be defined. Fortunately ED is a time-limited phenomenon.

Intravenous Anesthetics

As discussed previously, infants and children have a higher proportion of cardiac output delivered to vascular-rich tissues (i.e., heart, brain, kidneys, and liver). Intravenously administered drugs are readily taken up by these tissues and are subsequently redistributed to muscle and fat, tissues that are less well perfused. Intravenously administered drugs may have a prolonged duration of action in infants and children because of decreased percentages of muscle and fat. The central nervous system effects of opioids and barbiturates may also be prolonged because of the immaturity of the blood-brain barrier.[82] Although this evidence suggests that intravenously administered anesthetic doses should be reduced, one must also recall the effect of increased body water. Increased doses of thiopental, propofol, and ketamine are required, presumably because of a greater volume of distribution.[83,84]

Thiopental. Thiopental is supplied as a 2.5% solution. Intravenous induction dosages range from 4 to 6 mg/kg in children without significant cardiovascular disease.[85,86] Neonates have limited fat stores and may have an extended duration of action after thiopental administration. Thiopental, 25 to 30 mg/kg, may be administered rectally for anesthetic induction (see discussion of rectal induction).

Propofol. Propofol has a rapid onset and a short duration of action and has been established as a sole agent for induction and maintenance of general anesthesia, or may be combined with an opioid and nitrous oxide to provide total intravenous anesthesia. Propofol may be delivered as a continuous infusion for short diagnostic and radiologic procedures and is used as a primary sedative in chronically ventilated intensive care patients. Its antiemetic properties may reduce the incidence of postoperative nausea and vomiting in children undergoing strabismus correction.[87] Infants require larger induction doses (2.5 to 3 mg/kg) than children (2 to 2.5 mg/kg).[88,89] These induction doses produce moderate decreases in systolic blood pressure.[90] The pain that accompanies intravenous administration may be reduced with the addition of as little as 0.2 mg/kg of lidocaine. Additional strategies promulgated for decreasing the pain of injection include a slower injection of propofol into a rapid-running intravenous line or injection into larger intravenous catheters placed in the antecubital space.[91]

In 1992, Parke and colleagues reported the deaths of five children who received long-term, high-dose propofol infusions.[92] Additional case reports followed, further characterizing this serious reaction, subsequently referred to as *propofol infusion syndrome*.[93-96] Propofol infusion syndrome is characterized by severe lactic acidosis, followed by rhabdomyolysis and lipidemia, resulting in cardiovascular collapse and death. Propofol inhibits mitochondrial function, uncouples oxidative phosphorylation,[97-99] and inhibits the transport of long-chain acylcarnitine esters.[100] Children with mitochondrial defects may have an increased risk with propofol administration. In a prospective study of children undergoing short, elective surgical procedures, propofol administration did not produce acidosis or liver or myocardial injury.[101]

Neuromuscular Relaxants

Neuromuscular blocking drugs are highly ionized and have a low lipophilicity, restricting their distribution to the ECF compartment. Recall that the ECF compartment is larger in the neonate and infant than in the child and adult (see Table 49-4). Increases in ECF volume and the ongoing maturation of neonatal skeletal muscle and acetylcholine receptors affect the pharmacokinetics and pharmacodynamics of neuromuscular relaxants. Table 49-4 references the effective doses of neuromuscular blocking drugs in various age groups.

The neuromuscular junction is incompletely developed at birth, maturing after 2 months of age.[102] Skeletal muscle, acetylcholine receptors, and the accompanying biochemical processes essential in neuromuscular transmission mature during infancy into childhood.

The presynaptic release of acetylcholine is slowed compared with the adult, which explains the decreased margin of safety for neuromuscular transmission in the neonate. The acetylcholine receptors of the newborn are anatomically different from the adult receptors, which may explain the sensitivity of the neonate to the nondepolarizing class of neuromuscular relaxants.[103] This neuromuscular immaturity may be demonstrated with the appearance of fade after tetanic stimulation in the absence of neuromuscular blocking drugs.[102,104]

Succinylcholine. Succinylcholine is composed of two acetylcholine molecules united by an ester bond. Succinylcholine is metabolized into the inactive metabolites succinylmonocholine, choline, and succinic acid by plasma (butyryl) cholinesterase. Succinylcholine has a number of well-defined side effects, including increased intragastric pressure, increased intraocular and intracranial pressure, cardiac dysrhythmias, myalgia, and myoglobinemia.[105,106]

Because succinylcholine contains acetylcholine moieties, its intravenous administration will reproduce the effects of acetylcholine when it interacts with nicotinic and muscarinic receptors, provoking both sympathetic and parasympathetic cardiovascular responses. Stimulation of the parasympathetic ganglia or direct stimulation of cardiac muscarinic receptors will produce sinus bradycardia, junctional rhythms, unifocal premature ventricular contractions, and ventricular fibrillation.[107,108] The prior administration of 0.02 mg of atropine per kilogram will block cardiac muscarinic receptors and minimize the decreases in heart rate. Dysrhythmia is more common in children, particularly after repeated doses in the presence of hypoxia or concurrent electrolyte imbalance.

Myoglobinemia may occur in up to 20% of children who receive intravenous succinylcholine and in 40% of children who receive succinylcholine and halothane.[109] The prior administration of a small dose of a nondepolarizing neuromuscular blocking drug will modify the degree of myoglobinuria.[110]

Myalgia is common following succinylcholine administration. The etiology of succinylcholine-induced myalgia has recently been hypothesized to occur secondary to the production of prostaglandins.[111] This hypothesis was successfully tested with the intravenous administration of acetylsalicylic acid (aspirin), which effectively reduced the incidence and intensity of postoperative myalgia.

Succinylcholine is a known triggering agent for the development of malignant hyperthermia (MH).[112] The North American and European estimates of the frequency of MH in children are approximately 1 in every 15,000 anesthetic procedures. A resistance to mouth opening during endotracheal intubation has been described after succinylcholine administration. Increased masseter muscle tone, masseter muscle rigidity, or trismus occurs 0.2% of the time after the combination of halothane and succinylcholine.[113] Some clinical reports suggest that masseter spasm is a foreboding sign of MH and that as many as 50% of children with masseter muscle rigidity will develop MH.[114-117] This suggests that the incidence of MH is indeed higher than has been reported. It has been suggested that masseter muscle rigidity may occur as a result of inadequate succinylcholine intravenous doses in children.[116]

A variety of opinions exist regarding the clinical management of the child with masseter muscle rigidity. Clearly, signs of MH should be sought in the child experiencing masseter rigidity. If the jaw can be forcefully opened to allow endotracheal intubation, the anesthetic procedure may proceed, with vigilance for clinical signs of MH (increases in end-tidal CO_2, rigidity of other skeletal muscle groups, and an increase in core temperature). If the mouth cannot be forcefully opened, airway management may be difficult, necessitating the termination of the procedure. These children should undergo laboratory serial determinations of creatinine kinase, electrolytes, and myoglobin.

Neonates are more resistant to the effects of succinylcholine than children and adults. This sensitivity is illustrated by the ED_{95} for neonates (620 mcg/kg), infants (729 mcg/kg), children (423 mcg/kg), and adults (290 mcg/kg) (see Table 49-4).[117] The increase in dose requirement is in part a result of the increased volume of distribution within the large extracellular compartment.[118] Plasma cholinesterase activity is reduced in neonates; however, the duration of action after a single dose is of expected duration (6 to 10 minutes). A longer duration of action after a single bolus dose suggests the presence of an inherited deficiency of plasma cholinesterase activity.

Historically, succinylcholine has been the only available neuromuscular relaxant that can be administered intramuscularly to facilitate endotracheal intubation in the absence of intravenous access (see the discussion of rocuronium). Intramuscular succinylcholine may facilitate endotracheal intubation in children without suitable intravenous access. Because of the increased volume of distribution, a larger dose is required to achieve satisfactory relaxation. Although a dose of 3 mg/kg will produce satisfactory relaxation in 85% of patients, an intramuscular dose of 4 mg/kg in the deltoid muscle will provide skeletal muscle relaxation in all, with a duration of action of up to 21 minutes.[119,120] To attenuate the effects of succinylcholine at both the nicotinic and muscarinic receptors, atropine at a dose of 0.02 mg/kg may be combined in the same syringe with the calculated dose of succinylcholine or in an additional syringe, which is administered in a selected muscle group before succinylcholine administration.

TABLE **49-4**	Effective Doses (ED_{95}) of Clinical Neuromuscular Blocking Drugs (mcg/kg)			
	Neonate	**Infant**	**Child**	**Adult**
Succinylcholine*	620	729	423	290
Atracurium	120	156-175	170-350	110-280
Vecuronium	47	42-47	56-80	27-56
Rocuronium	600	600	600	300
Pancuronium	—	55	55-81	50-70

Should be used for emergency airway stabilization in children younger than 12 years. Not for routine intubation.

Unexpected cardiac arrest has been reported after the routine administration of succinylcholine, with less than 40% of patients successfully resuscitated. Boys younger than age 8 with undiagnosed Duchenne muscular dystrophy may experience hyperkalemia and subsequent cardiac arrest after succinylcholine administration. In November 1993, the U.S. Food and Drug Administration (FDA) relabeled succinylcholine, restricting its use to emergency endotracheal intubation in children and adults.[121,122] After lengthy discussions between the FDA and clinicians, this was changed to a strong "warning" that noted that succinylcholine should not be routinely used for airway management in children younger than 8 years of age.[122,123]

Nondepolarizing Neuromuscular Blocking Agents. Infants and children are more sensitive than adults to the effects of nondepolarizing neuromuscular blocking drugs (see Table 49-4). A lower plasma concentration of the selected neuromuscular relaxant is required to achieve the desired clinical level of neuromuscular blockade. This does not imply that the selected dosage should be decreased because infants have a greater volume of distribution. The larger volume of distribution and slower drug clearance result in longer half-life elimination, decreasing the need for repeated drug dosing (longer dosing intervals). Neuromuscular function monitoring must be used to guide repeated administration of these drugs in all pediatric patients. The selection of a nondepolarizing neuromuscular relaxant should take into consideration the desired degree and duration of skeletal muscle paralysis, the immaturity of organ systems, and the associated side effects of the selected relaxant.

Atracurium is an intermediate-acting neuromuscular relaxant that is metabolized by nonspecific esterases and spontaneous breakdown of the parent compound by Hofmann elimination. Cisatracurium also uses Hofmann elimination and nonspecific ester hydrolysis for the metabolism of the parent compound. The duration of action of atracurium is relatively the same as in the adult. The volume of distribution is greater in infants, yet the clearance is more rapid.[124] Accordingly, an intubating dose (0.5 mg/kg) may be administered in infants and children with the same expected duration of action. Atracurium (intubating dose 0.5 mg/kg, maintenance dose 0.2 to 0.3 mg/kg) and cisatracurium (intubating dose 0.1 mg/kg, maintenance dose 0.08 to 0.1 mg/kg) may be the drugs of choice for the infant because these drugs are independent of mature organ function for elimination.

Vecuronium produces minimal alterations in cardiovascular function and stimulates the release of histamine. Infants are more sensitive to the effects of vecuronium than children (ED95 0.047 vs 0.081 mg/kg).[125] Vecuronium may be administered as a continuous infusion at a rate of 0.8 to 1 mcg/kg/min. It is also important to note that prolonged infusions of vecuronium in the intensive care setting have been associated with prolonged paralysis.[126]

Rocuronium is an intermediate-acting neuromuscular blocker with a rapid to intermediate onset of 60 to 90 seconds after an intubating dose of 0.6 mg/kg. The potency of rocuronium is greater in infants than children; however, its onset is faster in children.[127] Unlike vecuronium, rocuronium in intubating doses may produce transient increases in heart rate.[128] Skeletal muscle relaxation can be maintained with repeat doses of 0.075 to 0.125 mg/kg. In clinical situations in which intravenous access is not available, rocuronium may be administered intramuscularly. Reynolds and colleagues found acceptable intubating conditions in lightly anesthetized infants 2.5 to 3 minutes after a deltoid intramuscular dose of 1000 mcg/kg and within 3 minutes

after 1800 mcg/kg in children. The onset of action approximates the onset of succinylcholine after intramuscular injection. Rocuronium injection into the deltoid muscle provided a faster onset of twitch and ventilatory depression than did injection into the quadriceps muscle group. A disadvantage of this route of administration is the accompanying prolonged duration of relaxation—in excess of 60 minutes.[129] Whether intramuscular rocuronium is appropriate for the treatment of laryngospasm in children with contraindications to succinylcholine has not been studied. Rocuronium may also be administered by continuous infusion at doses of 0.004 to 0.016 mg/kg/min.

Antagonism of Neuromuscular Blockade

Residual neuromuscular blockade places the infant and child at risk of hypoventilation and the inability to independently and continuously maintain a patent airway. Because of increased basal oxygen consumption, impaired respiratory function will lead to arterial oxygen desaturation and CO_2 retention. The resulting acidosis will potentiate residual neuromuscular blockade. Accordingly, the infant and child must have neuromuscular function restored at the conclusion of the surgical procedure. The detection of residual neuromuscular blockade requires the integration of clinical criteria and the assessment of neuromuscular blockade via a peripheral nerve stimulator. Conventional doses of the anticholinesterase inhibitors (50 to 60 mcg/kg of neostigmine; 500 to 1000 mcg/kg of edrophonium) combined with appropriate doses of atropine or glycopyrrolate are acceptable for antagonism of nondepolarizing neuromuscular blockade.

Voluntary clinical tests are obviously not applicable to the infant and young child. Useful clinical signs of successful antagonism of neuromuscular blockade include the ability to flex the arms, lift of the legs, and flexion of the thighs upon the abdomen, providing evidence of the return of abdominal muscle tone, in addition to the return of a normal train-of-four response as assessed by the peripheral nerve stimulator.[130] Neonates are capable of generating a negative inspiratory force (NIF) of −70 cm H_2O with the first few breaths after birth.[131] A negative inspiratory force of at least −32 cm H_2O has been found to correspond with leg lift, which is indicative of the adequacy of ventilatory reserve required before tracheal extubation.[132]

Clinical investigation is ongoing in examining a novel antagonist of neuromuscular blockade. Sugammadex, a water-soluble, modified γ-cyclodextrin, is being investigated as a reversal of steroidal neuromuscular blocking agents.[133] This water-soluble molecule encapsulates and forms a fixed complex with the steroidal neuromuscular relaxants (rocuronium>vecuronium>>pancuronium), preventing the availability of the neuromuscular relaxant to complex with acetylcholine receptor. The drug does not effect acetylcholinesterase, eliminating the need for the co-administration of an anticholinergic. As of this writing sugammadex is not available in the United States.

PERIOPERATIVE CARE

Pediatric Anesthesia Equipment

The child's age, weight, and proposed surgical procedure guide the selection of essential pediatric anesthesia equipment. The anesthesia workroom should be appropriately stocked with a variety of sizes of masks, airways, laryngeal mask airways (LMAs), laryngoscope blades, endotracheal tubes, endotracheal tube stylets, blood pressure cuffs, pulse oximeter probes, calibrated pediatric fluid sets, syringe pumps for the delivery of both fluids and drugs, an assortment of intravenous catheters, tape, and armboards.

Airway Equipment

The pediatric face mask is designed to fit the smaller facial features of the child and eliminate mechanical dead space. Contemporary masks are manufactured from transparent plastics and have a soft inflatable cuff that sits on the face (Figure 49-3). The transparent feature allows continuous observation of skin color and the appearance of gastric contents should vomiting occur.

Oral and Nasal Airways

Appropriately sized oral airways must be readily available (Figure 49-4, A). The relatively large infant tongue predisposes to airway obstruction after the induction of general anesthesia. Oral airways that are too large may produce airway obstruction, inhibit venous and lymphatic drainage, subsequently producing macroglossia and creating further airway compromise. The oral airway should be inserted with the aid of a tongue blade, displacing the tongue toward the floor of the mouth to allow smooth insertion of the airway. The insertion and rotation of an oral airway should be avoided in children because the rotation may dislodge loose deciduous teeth.

Nasal airways are infrequently used in children less than 1 to 2 years of age. The internal diameter of the nasal airway may unnecessarily increase the work of breathing. Adenoid hypertrophy may make nasal airway placement difficult and produce severe epistaxis. If a nasal airway is required, a suitably sized, well-lubricated uncuffed endotracheal tube ETT may be cut to desired length and inserted through the nares (Figure 49-4,B). Commercially available suitable nasal airways are also available.

Endotracheal Tubes. Traditional teaching since the 1960s has been that the use of a cuffed ETT in infants and children less than 8 to 10 years of age should be avoided. Although this adage is widely accepted, recent literature suggests that this belief is not universally applied, is empirical rather than scientifically based, and is a perpetuated "myth" of pediatric anesthesia. The age-old argument against the use of a cuffed ETT in infants and children is quite logical; the narrowest portion of the infant and child airway has traditionally been understood to be at the level of the cricoid cartilage. The lumen of the noncompressible

cricoid was thought to be round. This traditional teaching has recently been challenged (see discussion below). It is reasoned that the insertion of a properly sized uncuffed ETT will be "snug" at the cricoid, providing for assisted or controlled ventilation and protection of the trachea against foreign substances.

Historical Perspective. Endotracheal intubation was rarely performed in infants and children prior to the 1940s because the available tubes were not manufactured from proper material (reactive hard red rubber), and were poorly designed for application in the pediatric patient (length, diameter, position of low-pressure high-volume cuff). Cuffed ETTs were not favorable because the selection of a cuffed ETT required a smaller size (e.g., a smaller internal diameter), increasing resistance and the work of breathing in spontaneously ventilating children. The decreased internal diameter was also feared to increase the risk of obstruction from tracheal secretions. Consequently, long-term ventilatory management required tracheostomy, a procedure with significant complications. The development of softer and more pliable polyvinyl chloride tubes was a major technologic leap in pediatric airway management.

In 1965, two landmark papers reported the successful use of nasotracheal intubation for prolonged ventilatory management in the intensive care unit.[134,135] This management was unfortunately not without consequences. McDonald and Stocks reported the development of severe subglottic narrowing in a 2-year-old child. In their paper they opined:

> *"Choosing the proper tube requires care. It is important that the tube is not too large as to exert excessive pressure on the mucosa overlying the cricoid cartilage, the narrowest part of the larynx."*[134]

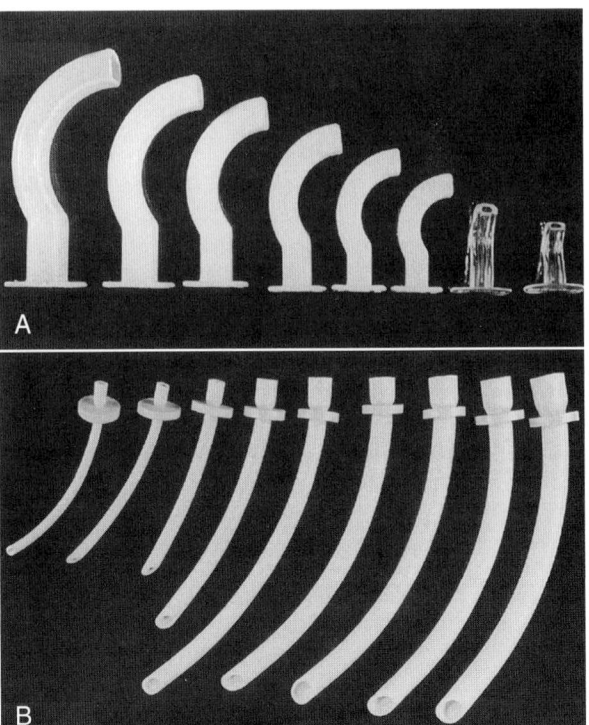

FIGURE 49-4 A, Oral airways. Sizes range from adolescent (*left*) to neonate (*right*). **B,** Nasal airways. Sizes range from infant to adolescent (*left to right*). (*From Boytim M. Pediatric equipment. In: Zaglaniczny K, Aker J, eds. Clinical Guide to Pediatric Anesthesia. Philadelphia: Saunders; 1999.*)

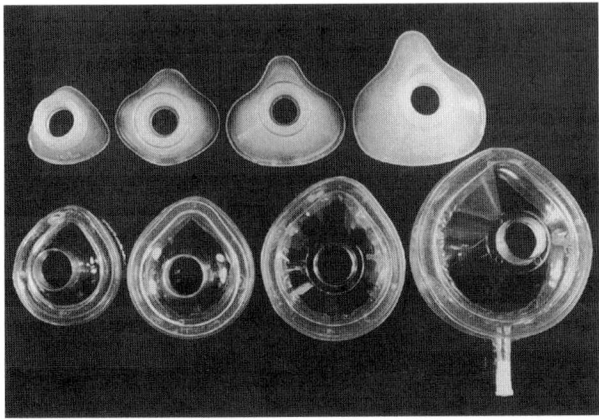

FIGURE 49-3 Types of pediatric face masks. *Top row,* Rendell-Baker-Soucek masks, which have a low profile and the least amount of dead space. *Bottom row,* Transparent masks with pneumatic cushions, which have more dead space but provide an effective seal for positive-pressure ventilation. (*From Boytim M. Pediatric equipment. In: Zaglaniczny K, Aker J, eds. Clinical Guide to Pediatric Anesthesia. Philadelphia: Saunders: 1999.*)

TABLE 49-5	Estimation of Endotracheal Tube Size by Age									
	28-34 Wk	Newborn	6 Mo	1 Yr	2 Yr	4 Yr	6 Yr	8 Yr	10 Yr	12 Yr
Endotracheal tube size	2.5-3	3	4	4	4.5-5	5-5.5	5.5-6	6-6.5	6.5 cuffed	6.5-7 cuffed
Suction catheter (F)	6-8	8	10	10	10	14	14	14	14	14
Laryngoscope blade	0	0-1	1	1½	1½	2	2	2	2-3	2-3

Allen and Stevens also reported "severe" cicatricial subglottic stenosis in a 4-year-old ventilated with an oversized ETT for a period of 6 days, and in an additional case, diffuse subglottic hemorrhagic necrosis in a deceased 6-year-old. They recognized that the etiology of these injuries were the result of the use of a "well-fitting tube to give some semblance of an airtight seal."[135] Significant laryngeal damage is known to develop with the use of uncuffed tubes, as evidenced by the development of subglottic stenosis in the preterm and neonate requiring prolonged ventilatory support. Holzki has reported that a large ETT was responsible for airway injury in 92% of 65 children under the age 8 years and in as many as 82% of 91 infants.[136] The characteristic laryngeal pathology develops following mucosal ulceration at the cricoid, and with continued compression, the ulceration may extend into the perichondrium. Collagen fibers are deposited to repair the mucosal defect, subsequently maturing into a fibrous scar. Contraction of this scar tissue creates subglottic stenosis. Clearly, the use of an oversized ETT for prolonged ventilation is associated with significant morbidity. Accordingly, the pediatric anesthetist has accommodated the shortcomings (air leak with environmental pollution of the operating room, required high inspired gas flow, inaccurate capnograph) of uncuffed ETTs. As James opined in a recent editorial, *"The little evidence we have is that cuffed tubes per se are not more dangerous than uncuffed tubes."*[137] To the author's knowledge, there are no case reports of the development of subglottic stenosis following intubation for short surgical procedures.

Sizing the Endotracheal Tube. Early detailed accounts of the laryngeal framework suggested that the larynx is shaped as a cone, with the apex at the level of the cricoid cartilage.[138,139] The compression of the tracheal mucosa at the level of the cartilaginous cricoid ring by an oversized ETT will produce mucosal edema. This traditional understanding has recently been challenged. Magnetic resonance imaging of sedated children ages newborn to 14 years has demonstrated that the lumen of the cricoid cartilage is not round but elliptical, with the narrowest dimension in the transverse plane at the level of the vocal cords.[140] Accordingly, the pressure exerted on the laryngeal and tracheal mucosa with the use of an uncuffed ETT is in the posterior-lateral position. This has been verified, as evidenced by the associated pathologic lesions found posteriorly in the subglottis. In addition, trauma that appears within the trachea occurs anteriorly from the impingement of the distal end of the ETT on the anterior tracheal wall.

The goal of ETT selection is the placement of an appropriately sized tube that allows controlled ventilation but minimizes laryngeal or tracheal injury. How is a properly sized ETT chosen? Because of patient variability many formulas exist for the determination of the correct ETT size and for the depth of insertion. Despite countless practitioner recommendations, there is no agreed standard formula.[141] In addition, may practitioners fail to appreciate the differences in the internal diameter of small ETTs.

ETTs for neonates are sized by the internal diameter, yet the external diameters may differ by as much as 0.9 mm among manufacturers in tubes with identical internal diameters.[142]

The approximate size of an ETT for children 2 years of age and older may be determined with the following formula: $16 + age \div 4$. To accommodate the variability in patient airway size, ETTs a half size larger and a half size smaller should be immediately available.

The depth of ETT insertion from the dental alveoli may be estimated using the "1, 2, 3, 4/7, 8, 9, 10" rule—for example, the ETT is inserted to a depth of 7 cm in a neonate weighing 1 kg and to a depth of 8 cm in a 2-kg neonate. Another approximate method is to insert the ETT to a depth in centimeters three times the internal diameter of the ETT in millimeters. For example, a 3-mm ETT should be inserted to a depth of 9 cm. Uncuffed ETTs are marked distally with a double black line that provides a visual indication of the depth of the ETT. During intubation, the ETT is passed until the double black line has reached the level of the vocal cords. In an evaluation of three methods for determining ETT depth (deliberate mainstem intubation with a subsequent 2-cm withdrawal, alignment of the double black line at the vocal cords, and placement with the use of the formula ETT internal diameter × 3), mainstem intubation with subsequent withdrawal was the most reliable in positioning the ETT above the carina.[143] Table 49-5 provides approximate sizes of ETTs, suction catheters, and laryngoscope blades for preterm infants through 12-year-old children.

Following intubation, what method can the clinician rely on in verifying the proper ETT size? Again, historic teaching is that the determination of a properly fitting ETT can be confidently demonstrated at the time of endotracheal intubation with a demonstrated air leak around the ETT, providing "clinical" evidence that the tracheal mucosa is not excessively compressed. This practice originated with the publication of a discussion of prolonged intubation and resulting subglottic stenosis by Stocks in 1966.[144] Stocks stated, *"... too small a tube will make intermittent positive pressure ventilation difficult because of the leakage of gases through the larynx. Too large a tube will make development of subglottic stenosis a possibility."*[144] Stocks modified his practice with the application of a "leak-test," allowing an audible leak with lung insufflation. This air leak traditionally sought is between 20 and 25 cm H_2O because it has been suggested that the laryngeal and tracheal mucosal capillary pressure is in this range (based on studies in rabbits), yet this value is not precisely known in the infant or child. An ETT with a demonstrable leak at a lower pressure (e.g., 10 cm H_2O) may be too small for the intended use (application of positive-pressure end-expiratory pressure, controlled ventilation during laparoscopy), whereas an ETT with an absence of leak may be argued to be too large, risking mucosal damage with prolonged use. Many anesthetists judge the size of the ETT using the "leak test"; however, Schwartz and colleagues found considerable variation between two experienced observers in deciding whether a the ETT passed the leak test.[145] As the leak-test pressure increased, there was greater disagreement between the observers.

At the author's institution, it is the practice to an select an uncuffed ETT for children younger than 8 years or until a 6- to 6.5-mm tube is required. The ETT is inserted below the level of the vocal cords. If resistance is encountered with laryngeal advancement of the ETT, it should be withdrawn, and an ETT a half size smaller in internal diameter should be selected. After proper placement is confirmed, the anesthetist should listen over the child's mouth (preferably with the aid of a stethoscope) while simultaneously squeezing the reservoir bag and noting the pressure at which an air leak is appreciated. Positive-pressure ventilation may be ineffective when an air leak is detected at 8 to 10 cm H_2O. A large or tight-fitting ETT that does not permit a detectable air leak until 25 to 30 cm H_2O may be too tight at the level of the cricoid cartilage, resulting in postintubation laryngeal edema ("croup"). The reader is referred to the comprehensive review of postextubation laryngeal edema by Marley.[146] If the intended operative procedure is a lengthy one, the anesthetist may elected to reintubate with either a smaller cuffed or an uncuffed ETT. The selected uncuffed or cuffed ETT should have a demonstratable air leak detected at 20 to 25 cm H_2O. Suominen and colleagues found that children who had an absent air leak at 25 cm H_2O had more adverse events (barking cough, obstructed or prolonged expiration, subcostal and sternal retractions, arterial desaturation and laryngospasm) following removal of the ETT.[147] It should be appreciated that a leak may not be detected immediately following endotracheal intubation. As anesthetic depth increases, laryngeal and tracheal relaxation may then produce a leak, necessitating an additional laryngoscopy and exchange of the ETT.

During confirmation of successful endotracheal intubation, inadvertent endotracheal extubation may occur. Small ETTs are easily kinked (particularly when warmed by the action of a forced-air blanket) or may be pulled from the mouth by the weight of the anesthesia breathing circuit. Following intubation, the ETT may be "pinned" against the palate at the desired depth of insertion with the index or middle finger of the left hand, freeing the right hand for stethoscope placement and manual compression of the breathing bag for confirmation of intubation. The ETT is secured with the application of an adhesive (tincture of benzoin) to both the face and the ETT prior to the application of cloth tape. The confirmation of breath sounds must be repeated after the application of tape, followed by documentation of the depth of insertion on the anesthesia record.

Specialized uncuffed and cuffed oral and nasal ETTs may be chosen for otolaryngologic, ophthalmologic, and dental procedures (Figure 49-5). The RAE (Mallinckrodt, Argyle, NY) ETT is premolded, with the acute angle of the tube designed to be positioned over the lower lip. The nasal RAE is premolded with a 180-degree bend that directs the tube toward the top of the head. These tubes facilitate the routing of the breathing circuit away from the surgical field. RAE tubes are longer than straight ETTs and place the distal end of the tube in closer proximity to the carina, thereby minimizing the chance of inadvertent extubation with neck extension. The RAE tube is designed with not one Murphy eye but two, located at the distal end of the tube to facilitate uninterrupted ventilation should the tube migrate in a caudad fashion. However, proper ETT placement must be determined with confirmation of bilateral breath sounds after intubation and repositioning of the head. The use of a precordial

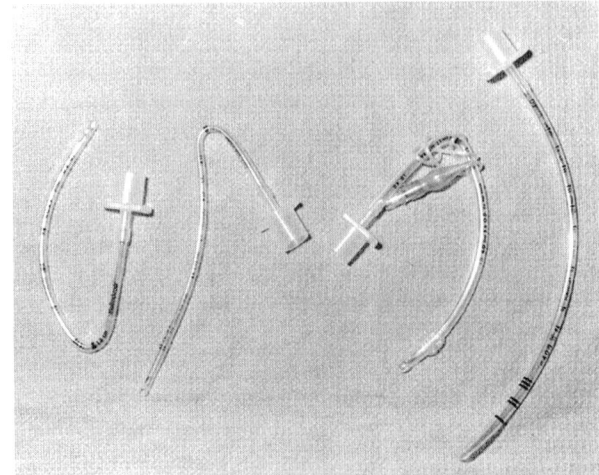

FIGURE **49-5** Common pediatric endotracheal tubes. From left, Uncuffed oral RAE, uncuffed nasal RAE, cuffed oral RAE, and uncuffed straight endotracheal tube. (*From Boytim M. Pediatric Equipment. In Zaglaniczny K, Aker J, eds.* Clinical Guide to Pediatric Anesthesia. *Philadelphia: Saunders; 1999.*)

stethoscope placed over the left anterior area of the chest will aid the detection of right bronchial migration of the RAE tube.

The clinical application of laser technology for the treatment of airway pathology necessitates the use of a specialized ETT. Endotracheal tube ignition may occur in as many as 1.5% of patients during CO_2 laser laryngeal procedures.[148] Modern polyvinyl chloride ETTs absorb infrared light and may be ignited with a direct hit from a CO_2 laser or as a result of burning material in close proximity to the tube. Laser-resistant or "laser-safe" ETTs are available from several manufacturers and marketed for specific laser applications (CO_2; neodymium-doped:yttrium-aluminum-garnet [Nd:YAG]; and potassium titanyl phosphate [KTP]). An alternative is wrapping the external surface of a polyvinyl chloride ETT with a metallic foil (Merocel Laser Guard, Merocel Corporation, Mystic, CT). An extensive discussion of anesthesia delivery for laser surgery may be found in Chapter 43.

Cuffed Endotracheal Tubes. The frequency of cuffed ETT use in pediatric patients within the United States is unknown. A recent survey of European pediatric anesthetists found that in France only 25% selected a cuffed ETT routinely in 80% of their patients.[149] The continuing argument regarding the use of cuffed ETTs is based on reports of laryngeal damage produced by overinflated cuffs.[150,151] Although there is a considerable body of evidence regarding the hazards of cuffed ETT use in infants and children, there is a growing body of literature suggesting that a cuffed ETT may be safely used in the operating room and intensive care unit.[152-154]

In 1997, Khine and colleagues published the results of a prospective randomized study of cuffed ETT versus uncuffed ETT use during general anesthesia in 488 children younger than 8 years of age. They found no difference in postoperative airway complications in children who were intubated with cuffed or uncuffed ETTs. Interestingly, children who were selected to receive an uncuffed ETT had multiple laryngoscopies for the selection of the proper-fitting ETT (23% vs 1.2%).[153] This may have been the result of a strict adherence to the formula for calculating ETT size. Clearly, one might argue that the initial use of a cuffed ETT is important because multiple laryngoscopies increase the risk of pharyngeal or laryngeal trauma. This paper stimulated the discussion reconsidering the argument against cuffed ETT use in children.

There are a number of design flaws evident when selecting a conventional adult manufactured cuffed ETT for the infant and child. As mentioned, there is variability in the outer diameter of uncuffed tubes among the same manufacturers with similar internal diameters (0 to 0.9 mm), as well as variation of the internal diameters between cuffed and uncuffed tubes (0 to 1.1 mm) of the same size. Cuff diameters and cross-sectional cuff area at an inflation pressure of 20 cm H_2O do not always cover the age-related tracheal diameters. Positioning of the ETT in the mid trachea with cuffed tubes with an internal diameter of 3, 4, or 5 may ultimately position the cuff within the larynx.[142] When the cuffed ETT is visually placed 1 cm below the level of the cricoid, the distal tip of the ETT is very close to the carina and may result in an inadvertent bronchial intubation. In addition, a manufacturer may or may not provide appropriately calibrated depth markings on the ETT. In an attempt to address these design flaws, new thin-walled tubes are being developed specifically for use in the pediatric patient (Microcuff, Weinheim, Germany; Microcuff, Kimberly-Clark, Roswell, GA). These tubes are constructed of polyurethane with short, thin-walled, high-pressure, low-volume cuffs with improved tracheal sealing characteristics.

There are a number of advantages for the use of a cuffed ETT for anesthetic management. A cuffed ETT has a smaller internal diameter and accordingly may not wedge within the delicate cricoid mucosa. The sealing of the ETT occurs with cuff inflation within the trachea and not at the level of the cricoid. Theoretically, this will place the distal tip of the ETT away from the anterior tracheal mucosa, minimizing tracheal damage. The cuffed ETT has an economic benefit in that it allows the use of lower inspired gas flows (minimal leak), decreasing the waste of expensive inhaled anesthetic agents. A proper seal provides a more accurate determination of end-tidal CO_2. The cuff volume may be adjusted during the operative period maintaining a leak at 15 to 25 cm H_2O. The use of a cuffed ETT decreases the risk of multiple laryngoscopies to replace ill-fitting tubes and the associated intubation trauma.[153] Finally, the presence of a cuff may reduce the risk of aspiration.[155]

Monitoring of cuff pressure is essential to minimize the risk of stenosis from pressure-induced mucosal ischemia.[156,157] It is certainly appreciated that an adult cuffed ETT may produce subglottic injury. The free inflation of the ETT cuff, assessed by some practitioners with palpation of the pilot balloon, may result in variable cuff pressures up to 120 cm H_2O.[158] This is particularly important when administering nitrous oxide, which diffuses into the cuff, further increasing cuff pressure.[153] The use of a manometer to monitor cuff pressure is particularly important with the new thin-walled cuffed ETT.[159]

At the author's institution the uncuffed ETT is the first choice in infants and children up to the age of 6 to 8 years, the age when a cuffed tube is chosen. When an unacceptable leak occurs, for instance in the child about to undergo laparoscopy, a cuffed tube may be selected (a half size smaller than the previously selected tube) to minimize repeat laryngoscopies. The cuff is inflated, allowing for a leak up to but no greater than 25 cm H_2O. For the majority of patients undergoing general anesthesia, an uncuffed ETT is easily and safely used, provided it is not too large.

Laryngeal Mask Airway. The original LMA device was intended as an alternative to the anesthesia face mask rather

TABLE 49-6	Laryngeal Airway Mask Sizes
Laryngeal Airway Mask Size	**Suggested Inflation Volume**
1	6 mL
1½	10 mL
2	15 mL
2½	21 mL
3	30 mL
4	45 mL
5	60 mL

From Brain AIJ et al. LMA-Classic and LMA-Flexible Instruction Manual. *San Diego: LMA North America; 1998.*

than endotracheal intubation. The LMA is used for short surgical procedures that do not require endotracheal intubation (herniorrhaphy, peripheral extremity surgical procedures) and resuscitation situations. The LMA is available in sizes specific for the neonate, infant, child, and adolescent (Table 49-6). Many alternative designs are being introduced because generic versions are now available. After inhalation or intravenous induction, the LMA is inserted (after lubrication of its posterior surface) by pressing the cuff against the posterior pharyngeal wall. The distal end of the cuff rests in the inferior aspect of the hypopharynx superior to the esophageal sphincter; however, isolation of the esophageal sphincter is not guaranteed. Regurgitation, vomiting, and aspiration have all been reported with the use of the LMA. With a syringe, the cuff is inflated with air, creating a pharyngeal seal. Spontaneous respirations are allowed to resume after insertion.

The inflation of the pharyngeal cuff can produce undue pressure on pharyngeal structures. Like the adult ETT cuff, the LMA cuff may be expanded during the course of the anesthetic procedure with the administration of nitrous oxide. The initial volume of air injected into the laryngeal cuff may be regulated by identifying the amount of air and airway pressure that produces an audible leak. This pressure is generally between 15 and 25 cm H_2O. Algren and colleagues recommend that the LMA cuff be inspected before each use, that the volume of air required for cuff inflation should not exceed the manufacturer's recommendation, and that the LMA cuff should be periodically checked during the administration of nitrous oxide to prevent overinflation.[160]

The LMA has traditionally been removed in the adult when airway reflexes return. Removal of the LMA in the pediatric patient is associated with biting, pulmonary edema, severe laryngospasm, and separation of the tube from the pharyngeal mask.[161,162] Several studies have examined the appropriate time of LMA removal in children. In one study, oxygen desaturation was more prevalent (31.3%) following awake removal, compared with removal in a deep anesthetic plane (4.5%), whereas airway obstruction occurred more frequently (20%) with deep removal.[163] Sinha and Sood found a 10% incidence of severe laryngospasm with awake removal, compared with 5% with deep removal.[164]

Pediatric Breathing Circuits. Oxygen, nitrous oxide, air, and potent inhalation agents are mixed by the anesthesia machine and delivered to the patient via the breathing circuit. The breathing circuit is essential for the removal of CO_2, the isolation of the anesthetic mixture from room air to prevent dilution of the desired anesthetic mixtures, and the maintenance of airway temperature and humidity. Spirometric and gas sampling connections to the breathing circuit allow the continuous monitoring of the end-tidal concentrations of oxygen, CO_2, nitrogen, and the potent inhalation agents. Additional accessories may be added to the breathing circuit, facilitating the pulmonary delivery of water-soluble and aerosol-derived pharmacologic agents.

The anesthesia machine should be equipped with an air flow-meter that allows the delivery of compressed air to the inspired mixture, drawn either from a central hospital supply or from an anesthesia machine–mounted cylinder. The blending of air with oxygen decreases the inspired concentration of oxygen, which is necessary for laser airway surgical procedures.

Adult anesthetists rarely contemplate the particulars of pediatric breathing circuits. The ideal pediatric breathing circuit should be lightweight, minimize dead space, have a low resistance and a low compressible volume, be adaptable for both spontaneous and controlled ventilation, be capable of providing humidification and warming of inspired gases, and permit the collection and scavenging of exhaled anesthetic gases.

An easy method to conceptualize pediatric breathing circuits is to characterize the circuit according to the presence of the number of valves within the circuit.[165] A circuit without valves is an open circuit. The Ayre's T-piece is an excellent example of an open circuit (Box 49-1). It is commonly used throughout hospitals to provide supplemental oxygen during patient transport. The T-piece was first used for the delivery of anesthesia to infants undergoing cleft palate and cleft lip repair. The T-piece, which is in a T configuration, is formed by an inspiratory limb for the delivery of oxygen and anesthetic gas, a limb directed to the patient for connection to a face mask or ETT, and an opposite expiratory limb that is open to the atmosphere for the removal of exhaled gas. This expiratory limb may also serve as a reservoir for oxygen that may be rebreathed. Because there are no valves inspired air is drawn from both the inspired limb and expiratory limb. The rebreathing of expired CO_2 can be prevented with the administration of fresh gas flows at least two times the patient minute ventilation. The T-piece can be configured to increase oxygen delivery or decrease PaCO₂.

The modification of the Ayre's T-piece with the addition of a single valve allows the delivery of positive-pressure ventilation. A variety of modifications of the Ayre's T-piece have been classified by Mapleson as A to F (Figure 49-6). The Mapelson A

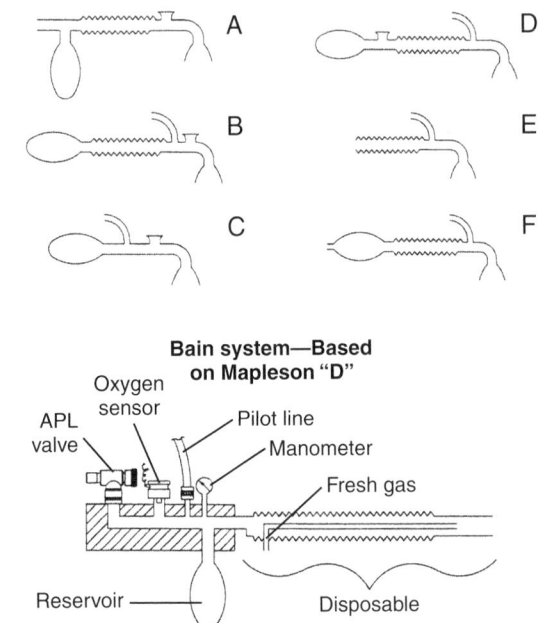

FIGURE 49-6 Mapleson's classification of breathing systems. Mapleson's systems **A-F** differ in the location and/or presence of fresh gas inlets, valves, and breathing bags. APL, Adjustable pressure limiting or "pop off" valve. *(From Zaglaniczny K, Aker J, eds.* Clinical Guide to Pediatric Anesthesia. *Philadelphia: Saunders; 1999.)*

circuit is best used for the spontaneously ventilating patient. The Mapleson D system contains an expiratory valve at the distal end of the expiratory limb and is used for controlled ventilation. The Mapelson B and C circuits are no longer in use. The Mapleson E system was modified by Jackson-Reese with the addition of a reservoir bag with an adjustable valve at the tail of the bag. Spontaneous ventilation is permitted with the opening of the adjustable valve, whereas closing the valve fills the reservoir bag, and repeated manual compression allows the delivery of continuous positive airway pressure (CPAP), or positive-pressure ventilation. With an expiratory pause of sufficient duration and sufficient fresh gas flows, exhaled CO_2 is washed from the reservoir tube, preventing the inhalation of exhaled CO_2 with subsequent inspiration. Fresh gas flows of two to three times the child's minute ventilation are required to prevent rebreathing of exhaled gases. Because of the required high fresh gas flow rates, this circuit is not economical for children who weigh more than 20 kg.

The Bain circuit is a coaxial modification of the Mapleson D circuit.[166,167] The inspiratory limb, which receives fresh gas from the anesthesia machine via a special adapter, is contained within the expiratory limb. The flow of expiratory gases over the inspiratory limb may aid in the warming of the inspired gas mixture and improve humidification. Recommended fresh gas flow rates producing normocarbia for spontaneous ventilation range from 200 to 300 mL $\cdot$ kg^{-1} and 70 to 100 mL $\cdot$ kg^{-1} for controlled ventilation. The circuit is lightweight and adaptable for the collection and scavenging of exhaled anesthetic gases. Disadvantages of the Bain circuit include practitioner unfamiliarity, misconnection to the adapter mounted to the anesthetic machine, and kinking of the inner inspiratory limb. The integrity of the inner inspiratory limb must be ensured, otherwise inspired fresh gas will enter the expiratory limb, creating a large dead space. Pethick's maneuver is used to test the integrity of the inspiratory limb.[168] The patient end of the inspiratory limb is occluded, and the reservoir bag is filled with the oxygen flush valve. The patient end is subsequently opened, and with continued high flow oxygen introduced from the oxygen flush, collapse of the reservoir bag (Venturi effect) should occur. If the inspiratory limb is fractured, the oxygen introduced via the oxygen flush will fill the reservoir bag.

We have briefly discussed the fresh gas flow requirements for spontaneous and controlled ventilation during the employment of the Mapleson F and Bain breathing circuits. The variables that must be considered to determine $PaCO_2$ during controlled ventilation when using these circuits include the ratio of dead space to tidal volume (V_D/V_T), the fresh gas flow rate, the child's CO_2 production, and the alveolar-to-arterial CO_2 difference. For children with decreased minute ventilation (recent opioid administration or high concentrations of potent inhalation agent), fresh gas flow rates may need to be increased or ventilation controlled.

The circle breathing system has become popular for anesthetic gas delivery in the past decade, because most pediatric centers have abandoned the use of the Bain or Mapelson F circuit for the circle system. The Mapelson F was described as the breathing circuit that met the ideal requirements for the pediatric patient.[169] Technologic advancements in anesthesia machine design have decreased the resistance imparted by the absorbent canisters and the one-way inspiratory and expiratory valves. The circle system compares in performance with the Mapleson F circuits that have comparable resistance and are acceptable for short periods of spontaneous ventilation in small infants.[170] Overall system compliance is greater than that of the Mapleson F circuit. The breathing tubing for the pediatric circle systems is a smaller diameter than the adult tubing and has a lower compression volume, allowing accurate delivery of desired tidal volumes. The circle breathing system is characterized by the presence of CO_2 absorbent canisters and a total of three valves (a one-way inspiratory valve, a one-way expiratory valve, and a pop-off or pressure-limiting [APL] valve) that directs exhaled gas to the scavenging system. Advantages of the circle system include the conservation of potent inhalation agents, the ability to retain heat and humidity, and the ease of collecting and scavenging waste gases.

The reservoir bag contains the anesthesia machine—delivered anesthetic mixture inspired by the patient and serves as a visual and tactile monitor of ventilation. Reservoir bags are shaped to allow compression with one hand and are constructed of rubber and latex, although latex-free bags are readily available. Reservoir bags range in size from 0.5 to 6 L. The selected reservoir bag must be appropriate for the patient's size, that is, capable of containing a volume in excess of the child's inspiratory capacity. The use of an inappropriately small reservoir bag may restrict respiratory efforts, and a large reservoir bag inhibits the ability to use the reservoir bag as a monitor of ventilation.

PREOPERATIVE PREPARATION

The process of preoperative preparation has undergone extensive change with the move to outpatient day-care surgery. The preoperative evaluation may take place during a scheduled clinic visit days or weeks before but typically is accomplished the morning of, and occasionally within minutes before, the scheduled operative procedure. The current time constraints of preoperative evaluation may disrupt the surgical schedule with cancellations for the medically unprepared or those who are acutely ill. Fortunately, the majority of pediatric surgical patients are in good health ASA classes 1 and 2). Accordingly, the preoperative evaluation is generally straightforward.[171]

Review of Systems

Appropriate anesthetic evaluation and management are dependent on a thorough understanding of the surgical and anesthetic requirements for the proposed procedure. All possible sources of medical information, including the patient chart, physical examination of the child, and the parental/guardian interview are essential. The review of the chart should focus on the medical history (beginning with the gestational history), previous hospitalizations, previous medical or surgical experiences, the presence of chronic illness or infectious disease, and any family history of anesthetic complications (e.g., family history of atypical pseudocholinesterase). The child should also be evaluated for proper growth and development as determined by a review of norms and percentages for age and gender. Developmental delay may suggest a prenatal pathologic condition, the presence of a chronic illness, or the presence of a concurrent neurologic or neuromuscular disease. The examination of any previous anesthetic records is invaluable in gleaning information regarding previous anesthetic encounters. The parent or guardian verifies information obtained during the chart review during the face-to-face interview and physical examination of the child.[172]

The physical examination allows the anesthetist to evaluate the child's general health. If not previously evaluated, the child's ears and nose should be examined. It is important to examine the throat for signs of redness when cough and rhinorrhea are present. This also provides the opportunity to evaluate the size of the pharyngeal tonsils, which may produce airway obstruction if hypertrophied. Airway obstruction secondary to adenotonsillar hypertrophy may be uncovered through a history of snoring with sleep. These children may also have obstructive sleep apnea and underlying pulmonary hypertension. Children between the ages of 5 and 9 should be examined for the presence of loose teeth, and these should be noted on the evaluation. A loose deciduous tooth that is in danger of being dislodged during airway management should be removed after anesthetic induction with the consent of a parent. Table 49-7 lists the anesthetic implications of the review of systems and history.

Preoperative Laboratory Testing

Preoperative laboratory tests should be ordered based on abnormal findings from the medical history and physical examination. Box 49-2 lists indications for preoperative laboratory testing. Preoperative hemoglobin determination has characteristically been obtained to provide an assessment of anesthetic fitness. An "adequate" hemoglobin concentration is essential for oxygen delivery and has been arbitrarily defined as a hemoglobin of 10 g/dL or a hematocrit of 30%. No scientific studies support or refute this "acceptable" quantity. The determination of an acceptable value requires an understanding of the child's current medical history, the proposed surgical procedure, and an understanding of global oxygen transport and use. The value of a routine hemoglobin determination has been questioned for some time and has been found rarely to affect the anesthetic management of children.[171,172] The frequency of asymptomatic anemia in a prospective study of 2649 pediatric outpatients was found to be less than 1%, with 7 of 14 anemic patients younger than 1 year of age. However, the frequency of anemia may be as high as 12% in immigrant and indigent children.[173]

Children who benefit from preoperative hemoglobin determinations include premature infants less than 60 weeks'. postconceptional age, children with concurrent cardiopulmonary disease, children with known hematologic dysfunction

TABLE 49-7   Medical History and Review of Symptoms: Anesthetic Implications

System	History	Possible Anesthetic Implications
Central nervous and neuromuscular	Seizures	Medications: drug interactions, possible inadequate serum levels, valproate-induced hepatitis
	Head trauma	Elevated intracranial pressure
	Hydrocephalus	Possible elevated intracranial pressure
	CNS tumor	Possible elevated intracranial pressure, chemotherapeutic drugs and interactions Possible risk of malignant hypothermia
Cardiovascular	Heart murmur	Septal defect, avoid air bubbles in IV line
	Cyanosis	Right-to-left cardiac shunt
	History of squatting	Possible tetralogy of Fallot
	Diaphoresis with feedings	Congestive heart failure
	Hypertension	Possible coarctation of the aorta; renal disease; pheochromocytoma
	Transplant recipient	Fixed heart rate; insensitivity to anticholinergic drugs
Respiratory	Prematurity	Increased risk of postoperative apnea; possible lower respiratory tract illness
	Bronchopulmonary dysplasia	Lower airway obstruction; reactive airways; possible subglottic stenosis; possible postoperative hypoxia and apnea; pulmonary hypertension
	Lower respiratory infection, cough	Reactive airways; bronchospasm; medication history; drug interactions
	Croup	Possible subglottic stenosis or anomaly
	Snoring, sleep apnea	Perioperative airway obstruction; hypoxia
	Asthma	β-Agonist or theophylline drugs; pulmonary hypertension or cor pulmonale; steroid use; adrenal insufficiency; postoperative hypoxia
	Cystic fibrosis	Drug interactions; pulmonary toilet; pulmonary dysfunction; reactive airways
	Recent cold	Possible lower respiratory tract infection; reactive airways
Gastrointestinal and hepatic	Vomiting, diarrhea	Electrolyte abnormality; dehydration; full stomach
	Growth failure	Possible anemia
	Gastroesophageal reflux	Risk of aspiration; reactive airways; hypoxia
	Jaundice	Altered drug metabolism; risk of hypoglycemia
	Liver transplant recipient	Altered drug metabolism; immunosuppression
	Frequency, nocturia	Unrecognized diabetes, urinary tract infection
	Renal failure or dialysis	Electrolyte abnormality; hypervolemia or hypovolemia; anemia; medication history
	Renal transplant recipient	Immunosuppression
Endocrine and metabolic	Hypoglycemia	Hypoglycemia
	Diabetes	Insulin requirement; intraoperative hypoglycemia
	Steroid therapy	Adrenal insufficiency
	Pregnancy	Teratogenic effects of N_2O and other drugs; risk of spontaneous abortion
Hematologic	Anemia	Transfusion requirement
	Bruising, excessive bleeding	Coagulopathy
	Sickle cell disease	Anemia; transfusion; hydration; oxygenation; orthopedic tourniquet use
	AIDS	Susceptibility to infection; infectious risk to medical personnel
Allergies	Medication history	Drug reactions; drug interactions
Dental	Loose teeth	Dental trauma; aspiration of tooth

Modified from Coté CJ et al, eds. A Practice of Anesthesia for Infants and Children. 3rd ed. Philadelphia: Saunders; 2001:40.
AIDS, Acquired immunodeficiency syndrome; CNS, central nervous system; IV, intravenous; N_2O, nitrous oxide.

BOX 49-2

Indications for Preoperative Laboratory Testing

Complete Blood Count
Hematologic disorder
Vascular procedure
Chemotherapy
Unknown sickle cell syndrome status

Hemoglobin and Hematocrit
<6 months of age (<1 year of age if born premature)
Hematologic malignancy
Recent radiation or chemotherapy
Renal disease
Anticoagulant therapy
Surgical procedures with potential for large blood loss
Coexisting systemic disorders (e.g., cystic fibrosis, prematurity, severe malnutrition, renal failure, hepatic disease, congenital heart disease)

White Blood Cell Count
Leukemia or lymphomas
Recent or concurrent radiation or chemotherapy
Suspected infectious process
Aplastic anemia
Hypersplenism
Autoimmune collagen vascular disease

Blood Glucose
Diabetes mellitus
Current corticosteroid use
History of hypoglycemia
Adrenal disease
Cystic fibrosis

Serum Chemistry
Renal disease
Adrenal or thyroid disease
Previous or concurrent hemotherapy
Pituitary or hypothalamic dysfunction
Body fluid loss or shifts (e.g., dehydration, bowel preparation)
Central nervous system disease

Potassium
Digoxin or diuretic therapy

Creatinine and Blood Urea Nitrogen
Hypertensive cardiovascular disease
Renal disease
Adrenal disease
Diabetes mellitus
Digoxin or diuretic therapy
Body fluid loss or shifts (e.g., dehydration, bowel preparation)
Administration of intravenous radiocontrast material

Liver Function Tests
Hepatic disease
Exposure to hepatotoxic agents

Coagulation Studies
Prothrombin time
Activated partial thromboplastin time (aPTT)
Leukemia
Hepatic disease
Known coagulation disorder (e.g., hemophilia, Christmas disease)
Concurrent anticoagulant therapy
Severe malnutrition or malabsorption

Platelet Count or Bleeding Time
Known coagulation disorder (e.g., hemophilia, Christmas disease)
Purpura (increase in bruising)

Pregnancy Test
Serum human chorionic gonadotropin (HCG) in menstruating, sexually active patient

Electrocardiogram
Family history of prolonged QT interval
Congenital heart disease
History of sleep apnea or chronic airway obstruction (adenotonsillar hypertrophy)
Possible previously undiagnosed heart murmur

Chest Radiograph
Suspected intrathoracic pathology (e.g., tumors, vascular ring)
Congenital heart disease
History of prematurity with residual bronchopulmonary dysplasia
Obstructive sleep apnea with cardiomegaly

Cervical Spine Radiograph
Down syndrome (rule out subluxation of atlantooccipital junction)

Modified from Cassidy J, Marley RA. Preoperative assessment of the ambulatory patient. J Perianesth Nurs. 1996;11:334-343.

(sickle cell disease), and children in whom major blood loss is anticipated during the surgical procedure.

The time constraints of preoperative evaluation hinder the child's psychological preparation, which has ostensibly become the responsibility of the parent or guardian and the surgeon. Children's exhibited behavior is age dependent and shaped by fears of parental separation, postoperative pain, the potential for disfigurement, and the loss of control. Children during the first 6 months of age readily accept strangers and can be separated from their parents, whereas children from 6 months to 5 years of age become distressed when separated from their parents.[174]

Parental preparation is important. One of the most important tasks is allaying the fear of the parent and family members. The anesthetist will foster trust and confidence through a courteous and understandable explanation of the anesthetic experience. Parental anxiety may be driven by personal past anesthetic experiences, such as painful intravenous catheter placement, coerced mask induction, and postoperative pain, nausea, and vomiting.

Parents offer invaluable information regarding their child's past anesthetic experiences. When the child appears for a repeat surgical procedure, the parents may have important information relative to what works and may be helpful in detailing a successful approach. Parental presence during anesthetic induction in preschool-aged and young children may allay the fears of separation for both the parent and the child. The reader is referred to the excellent article by Azarnoff and Woody for additional information on psychological preparation.[174]

Preoperative Fasting

Gastric regurgitation and pulmonary aspiration are known consequences of general anesthesia. Pathologic conditions that increase the risk of pulmonary aspiration include known difficult airway, impaired protective airway reflexes secondary to neurologic injury, gastroesophageal reflux, gastrointestinal obstruction, morbid obesity, chronic renal failure, and diabetes mellitus. Children undergoing emergency surgical intervention are also at risk. New guidelines for preoperative fasting have been published by the ASA (Table 49-8).

The risk of pulmonary aspiration in the pediatric patient is extremely low (1 in 10,000).[175] Accordingly, traditional fasting guidelines have become broader. Although the goal of preoperative fasting is to ensure an empty stomach at the time of anesthetic induction, consideration must be given to gastric volume and pH. The determination of risk is based on an experimentally derived case of gastric aspiration in Rhesus monkeys. These studies found that the development of Mendelson syndrome required a gastric volume of 0.4 mL/kg and a gastric pH of less than 2.5.[176] This benchmark is frequently quoted yet bears little resemblance to contemporary clinical practice. Gastric volume may be manipulated preoperatively with the administration of antacids (increases gastric pH) and metoclopramide 0.1 mg/kg (stimulates gastric emptying). Metoclopramide may be administered either intravascularly or intramuscularly. Antacids are generally refused by children preoperatively. Although the majority of children have a gastric pH of less than 2.5 and a gastric volume in excess of 0.4 mL/kg after an overnight fast, pulmonary aspiration remains an infrequent event.[177-179]

Prolonged fasting may produce irritability as a result of thirst and hunger. Prolonged fasting may also alter fluid balance, producing preinduction hypovolemia and hypoglycemia. Hypoglycemia is especially problematic in premature infants. Preoperative access to clear fluids (e.g., apple juice, water)

TABLE **49-8**	Preoperative Fasting Recommendations
Ingested Materials	**Minimum Fasting Period* (hr)**
Clear liquids†	2
Breast milk	4
Infant formula	6
Non-human milk‡	6
Light meal§	6

From *Summary of fasting recommendations to reduce the risk of pulmonary aspiration.* Anesthesiology. 1999;90(3):896-905.
These recommendations apply to healthy patients who are undergoing elective procedures. They are not intended for women in labor. Following the guidelines does not guarantee complete gastric emptying.
*The fasting periods noted above apply to all ages.
†Examples of clear liquids include water, fruit juices without pulp, carbonated beverages, clear tea, and black coffee.
‡Because non-human milk is similar to solids in gastric emptying time, the amount ingested must be considered when determining an appropriate fasting period.
§A light meal typically consists of toast and clear liquids. Meals that include fried or fatty foods or meat may prolong gastric emptying time. Both the amount and type of foods ingested must be considered when determining an appropriate fasting period.

2 hours before anesthetic induction has been shown to have a minimal effect on the resultant gastric volume and pH.[180]

Several factors, including glucose content, osmolarity, and concentrations of proteins and lipids, affect the gastric emptying of infant formula and milk. Litman and colleagues found that fasting intervals of 2 hours after breastfeeding result in high residual gastric volumes (>1 mL/kg).[181]

The new guidelines are known loosely as the *2, 4, 6, 8 guidelines* (see Table 49-8). Many institutions have liberalized fasting guidelines to reflect local practice with no increase in morbidity.[180] Heavy meals and fatty foods require an 8-hour fasting time.

Preoperative Controversies
Upper Respiratory Infection
Upper respiratory infections (URIs) are common in the pediatric age group, are seasonal in occurrence, and may be accompanied by cough, pharyngitis, tonsillitis, and croup. The child with an active or resolving URI has increased airway reactivity, a propensity for the development of atelectasis and mucous plugging of the airways, and the potential to experience postoperative arterial hypoxemia.[182] In addition, bronchial reactivity may persist for 6 to 8 weeks after a viral lower respiratory tract infection. The presence of chronic respiratory disease (asthma or bronchopulmonary dysplasia) requires a thorough assessment to ensure that the disease is well controlled and the child is not currently experiencing an exacerbation. The anesthetist must understand the child's routine pharmacologic management. A history of steroid use necessitates consideration of steroid supplementation throughout the perioperative period.

Healthy children who are scheduled for the placement of tympanostomy tubes frequently have rhinitis. In deciding whether to proceed with anesthesia, additional patient history must be obtained to differentiate between a chronic allergic or an acute infectious presentation and to determine whether there is lower-airway involvement. The assessment of the color and the duration of nasal drainage will assist in deciding whether

---

BOX 49-3

Recommendations for Patients With Upper Respiratory Tract Infections

These recommendations are neither clinical guidelines nor a consensus statement and should not replace clinical judgment, but they should serve as a guide to help make a rational decision with parents, surgeons, and patients. The absence of a visit for preoperative evaluation does not eliminate the need for an exchange of information between families and the center, which should occur before the day of surgery. Efforts should make parents aware of the problems with respiratory tract infections and anesthesia, and parents should be encouraged to call before the day of surgery to discuss the symptoms and possible need for delay of surgery. There may be a role for pediatricians and other primary care practitioners to play in the process of perioperative evaluation and education.

- First, an emergency case mandates judicious airway management and logically must proceed regardless of the presence or absence of respiratory symptoms. In patients presenting for elective (non-urgent) surgery, initial consideration should be with respect to the severity of respiratory tract symptoms.

- Acute symptoms, such as runny nose and cough, must be differentiated from chronic symptoms related to underlying diseases such as allergic rhinitis (clear runny nose) and asthma (cough).
- Often careful questioning of parents can differentiate acute from chronic symptoms.
- Patients with severe symptoms such as fever (>38.4° C), malaise, productive cough, wheezing, or rhonchi should be considered for delay of elective surgery. A reasonable period of delay would be 4 to 6 weeks.
- If mild symptoms are present, such as nonproductive cough, sneezing, or mild nasal congestion, surgery could proceed for those having regional or general anesthesia without endotracheal tube placement. However, those patients who require endotracheal tube placement for anesthesia, especially children less than 1 year of age, should be considered carefully for other risk factors such as passive smoke exposure and underlying conditions (i.e., asthma, chronic lung disease, etc.), because they may benefit from a slight delay of 2 to 4 weeks.

Modified From Easley RB, Maxwell LG. Should a child with a respiratory tract infection undergo elective surgery? In: Fleisher LA, ed. Evidence-Based Practice of Anesthesiology. Philadelphia: Saunders; 2004:424.

---

rhinorrhea is chronic or acute. Purulent nasal discharge associated with pharyngitis, cough, or fever may be indicative of a bacterial or viral URI. Additional information may be obtained by questioning the parents regarding their assessment of the child's current health. Helpful questions include the following: Does your child appear sick? Is your child eating, sleeping, and playing normally? Is there anyone in the family (including siblings) who is ill? Children with chronic allergic rhinorrhea who exhibit a clear nasal drainage without accompanying signs of illness (no cough, pharyngitis, wheezing, or associated fever) are probably in satisfactory condition for elective general anesthesia with no imposed increased risk.

Lower respiratory tract dysfunction typically accompanies viral or bacterial URI. This combination may be associated with a greater frequency of laryngospasm (5-fold greater incidence) and bronchospasm (10-fold greater incidence) during anesthetic management, particularly when endotracheal intubation is performed.[183] Although mild URI may be inconsequential during the intraoperative period, significant problems may develop in the immediate postoperative period. Studies have noted an increase in the incidence of postintubation croup, hypoxemia, and bronchospasm in patients with URIs compared with asymptomatic children.[183-185]

Multiple factors must be considered when one is deciding whether to cancel an elective procedure. Olsson noted persistent spirometric changes indicative of bronchial hyperactivity for up to 7 weeks after URI and recommend postponing surgery for this period of time.[186] Postponement for 7 weeks may not be practical, because children experience multiple URIs (as many as 6 to 8 per year). Children with signs and symptoms of acute airway dysfunction should have further medical evaluation by a pediatrician. A white blood cell count of 12,000 to 15,000/mm³ suggests the presence of infection, and the surgery should be canceled. Clearly, elective surgery should be postponed for children who have a cough and pharyngitis accompanied by fever and wheezing. Box 49-3 has recommendations based on a thorough review of the literature.

Heart Murmur

The parent may relay a previous history of a heart murmur, or a murmur may be discovered during the physical examination. A heart murmur may be detected in up to 50% of pediatric patients. It is important to properly classify the murmur as either innocent or pathologic prior to anesthetic intervention. The murmur may not impose a functional limitation; however, this may change with the physiologic trespass of an anesthetic. For example, the child with aortic stenosis may function appropriately as long as the heart rate is capable of sustaining a normal cardiac output. Children with functional murmurs are generally asymptomatic, without the presence of cyanosis, and are growing appropriately. An example of a functional murmur is the Still's vibratory systolic murmur, which is common in children between the ages of 2 and 6 years. It is important that a pediatrician or cardiologist evaluate previously undiagnosed murmurs prior to the induction of anesthesia. Although the murmur may not impose a perceptible functional limitation, this may change with the physiologic trespass of an anesthetic. For example, the child with aortic stenosis may function appropriately as long as the heart rate is normal and capable of sustaining a normal cardiac output. Decreases in heart rate or acute hypotension during the induction of anesthesia would be poorly tolerated in this child.

If the heart murmur has been previously detected and the child has undergone an evaluation, the parent may be able to provide the information as to the relevance of the murmur.

BOX **49-4**

Rationale for Obtaining Preoperative Cardiology Consultation

Patient History
Difficulty feeding, shortness of breath (infant)
Poor exercise tolerance, unable to match peers (child)
Family history of congenital heart disease (Down syndrome)
Cyanotic episodes

Physical Examination
Presence of a diastolic murmur
Loud murmur (Grade III or higher)
Abnormal or absent peripheral pulses

Adapted from Litman RS. Presence of cyanosis, pallor and poor capillary refill. In: Pediatric Anesthesia: The Requisites in Anesthesiology. Philadelphia: Mosby; 2004:92.

BOX **49-5**

Goals for Premedication

Anxiolysis
Amnesia (insertion of invasive monitoring)
Analgesia (children in pain)
Antisialagogue (airway manipulation)
Increase gastric pH
Reduction of gastric volume
Reduce anesthetic requirements
Blunting of central nervous system reflex responses
Prophylaxis
Subacute bacterial endocarditis
Allergic reactions (latex)
Postoperative nausea and vomiting
Infectious processes

Modified from Moline BM, Marley RA. Midazolam as a pediatric premedicant in the ambulatory setting. J Perianesth Nurs. 1997;12:42-47.

Previous records may also contain information as to the significance and whether additional testing was performed to assess the physiologic significance. Box 49-4 provides information suggesting when a preoperative cardiology consult is warranted.

The absence of a murmur during the physical examination does not preclude the presence of a serious cardiac defect. Pulmonary hypertension (increased pulmonary vascular resistance) that develops concurrently with chronic hypoxemia may reduce the left-to-right intracardiac shunt, reducing the quality of the murmur. The detection of a murmur in the individual with Down syndrome should trigger a consultation with a pediatric cardiologist to determine whether the murmur is innocent or pathologic in nature.

Smythe and colleagues have demonstrated that a clinical evaluation by a pediatric cardiologist provides an accurate assessment of heart murmurs in individuals up to 17 years of age.[187] In patients with heart murmur referred by the primary physician, the initial diagnosis was found to be incorrect 69% of the time as judged by the pediatric cardiologist. Auscultation by an experienced pediatric cardiologist had a sensitivity of 96%, a specificity of 95%, and negative predictive value of 98%. Although generally obtained with the clinical cardiology evaluation, the electrocardiogram was found to be helpful in shaping a lesion-specific diagnosis only when the murmur was judged to be pathologic in nature. This study concluded that echocardiography was not helpful in the diagnosis in individuals with clinically diagnosed innocent heart murmurs. Auscultation of the murmur and patient history may determine that the murmur is functional, and no additional studies will be required. However, the consultant may wish to obtain additional information by means of an echocardiogram prior to anesthetic. The reader is directed to an excellent review by Pelech of the evaluation of the pediatric patient with a cardiac murmur.[188]

Premedication

The selection and administration of premedication for the pediatric patient requires an understanding of the desired goals, the planned surgical procedure (inpatient or outpatient procedure), the familiarity and previous experiences with the particular drug, and the availability of nursing staff to monitor the child after the drug's administration (Box 49-5). The ideal premedicant should be dependable, with a rapid and reliable onset and offset, and

TABLE **49-9**	Commonly Prescribed Pediatric Premedicants—Premedicant Dose and Route of Administration
Anticholinergics	
Atropine	0.02 mg/kg PO, IV, IM
Glycopyrrolate	0.01 mg IV
Opioids	
Morphine sulfate	0.1-0.3 mg/kg IM
Meperidine	1.5-2 mg/kg PO 1-2 mg/kg IM
Benzodiazepines	
Diazepam	0.1-0.5 mg/kg PO
Midazolam	0.07-0.1 mg/kg IM 0.2 mg/kg nasally 0.025-0.05 mg/kg IV 0.25-0.5 mg/kg PO 0.5-1 mg/kg rectally
Barbiturates	
Methohexital (10%)	10 mg/kg IM 20-30 mg/kg rectally
Other	
Ketamine	3-6 mg/kg PO 3 mg/kg nasally 2-10 mg/kg IM

IM, *Intramuscular;* IV, *intravenous;* PO, *orally.*

should be devoid of undesirable effects. The use of "cookbook" doses of premedicant is hazardous and may produce general anesthesia in some children while producing ineffective sedation in others. Table 49-9 lists commonly prescribed pediatric premedicants.

Premedication must be individualized to account for differences in maturation and development and the child's previous surgical experiences. The reliance on pharmacologic premedication in preparing the child for the surgical experience should not be routine; rather, it should be reserved for children who are extremely apprehensive. Anxiolytics and sedatives may prolong the time to discharge, thereby increasing patient care costs.[189-191] Children older than 1 year of age may benefit from anxiolytic premedication to decrease preoperative anxiety and modify behavioral changes after discharge.[192]

Midazolam has great utility as a premedicant in the pediatric patient. This short-acting, highly lipophilic benzodiazepine produces amnesia and anxiolysis and in sufficient dosages may also produce sleep (hypnosis). Serious respiratory events (respiratory depression, airway obstruction, apnea, and oxygen desaturation) may develop after the administration of midazolam. Resuscitative equipment must be immediately available.

Midazolam may be administered by a variety of routes, including parenteral (intravenous, intramuscular), transmucosal (intranasal, rectal), and oral. The parents should be instructed to hold the child or place the child on a cart, preventing ambulation. Appropriate monitoring is imperative after midazolam administration. A health-care provider should remain within eye contact of the child, and continuous oxygen saturation monitoring should be initiated by pulse oximetry.

The dose for intramuscular midazolam ranges from 0.07 to 0.1 mg/kg, with an onset time between 30 and 60 minutes. The intramuscular route is the least desirable because of the anxiety and the pain associated with parenteral injection, but this route may be necessary in children who refuse to swallow a liquid. The crying that accompanies intramuscular injection has been reported to produce oxygen desaturation in children with congenital heart disease.[193]

The intravenous route is rapid and reliable and allows for the titration of additional drug. An intravenous dose of 0.025 to 0.05 mg/kg produces on onset of action within 1 to 2 minutes. However, intravenous access is generally not established before the induction of anesthesia and is rarely indicated for the administration of a premedicant.

Intranasal administration of midazolam avoids first-pass metabolism and provides a rapid onset. A dose of 0.2 mg/kg produces effective sedation in 2 to 10 minutes. The calculated dose may be administered via a syringe, alternating nares, but parental assistance is required (the parent holds the child's head). Children frequently object to this route of administration, and this practice is falling out of favor. Midazolam administered intranasally may produce nasal burning and an unpleasant taste (the intravenous formulation contains benzyl alcohol). The intranasal route of drug administration may be disagreeable to parents and anesthesia providers in that it is commonly associated with the self-administration of recreational drugs.

Oral premedicants are generally accepted by children, particularly after an unexpected nothing-by-mouth (NPO) period. Rapid absorption occurs after the oral administration of midazolam. Oral administration is the least threatening but can also be the most challenging in uncooperative children. It may be difficult to determine the ingested dose, as children may swallow only a portion of the desired dose and refuse the remainder or may expectorate the dose after tasting the mixture (formulation with benzyl alcohol). Before the recent release of an oral formulation, intravenous midazolam was mixed with a variety of oral fluids, including apple juice, acetaminophen elixir, cherry and chocolate syrups, and flavored gelatins, in an attempt to disguise the unpleasant taste. A cherry-flavored midazolam syrup is now available (Roche Laboratories) and appears to be more palatable than the intravenous preparation.

Monitoring

As previously discussed, anesthetic morbidity and mortality are greater in pediatric patients, and intraoperative vigilance is imperative if poor anesthetic outcomes are to be averted. Patient blood pressure and heart rate are monitored for the assessment of the cardiovascular system. Pulse oximetry and capnography are used for the assessment of the adequacy of oxygenation and ventilation, a temperature probe for intermittent or continuous assessment of core body temperature, and a neuromuscular function monitor for the evaluation of the child's response to the administration of neuromuscular blocking drugs. A precordial or esophageal stethoscope should be used for the continuous assessment of heart rate during anesthetic induction and throughout the perioperative period.

Pulse oximetry is essential for anesthetic induction. Artifactual alarms occur with excessive movement of the child, interference from environmental ultraviolet light and radiant lamps, and intermittent interference from electrocautery.[194] It may also be difficult to obtain an expired gas sample for accurate determination of end-tidal CO_2 when a nonrebreathing circuit is used. A more accurate determination may be obtained by sampling the expired gas as close as possible to the ETT or perhaps through aspiration from the ETT itself.[195,196] Thin sampling tubes are commercially available and may be inserted into the anesthesia circuit via the CO_2 sampling port and threaded into the ETT for the sampling of expired gases.

Some circumstances require the application of arterial and central venous pressure monitoring. Fluid overload from the continuous heparinized flush is a real danger in the pediatric patient and may produce an iatrogenic coagulopathy. Small multilumen catheters are available for the pediatric patient. These catheters are advantageous when large blood losses are expected (e.g., during burn débridement and skin grafting). However, these catheters have long, thin lumens that may severely limit the rate at which intravenous fluid or blood may be administered. When rapid flow is required, a peripheral intravenous line may be used for maintenance and deficit fluid replacement, and a single-lumen venous catheter placed within the femoral vein may be reserved for colloid and blood administration.

The precordial and esophageal stethoscopes are indispensable monitors for the pediatric anesthetist. The precordial stethoscope is ideally placed in the 3rd to 4th intercostal space to the left of the sternal border. The esophageal stethoscope is advanced to a depth where heart and breath sounds are maximal. In the infant, the esophageal stethoscope may be inadvertently advanced into the stomach. These instruments allow the continual assessment of breath sounds and the quality and character of heart tones during anesthetic induction, maintenance, and emergence, as well as during patient transport. A sudden change or absence in breath sounds may indicate a right mainstem intubation.

Anesthetic Induction
Mask Induction

Anesthetic induction may be accomplished in a variety of ways and is dependent on the child's current state of health, the age and level of anxiety, the proposed surgical procedure, and the parent's agreement with regard to the proposed anesthetic plan. Mask induction is the most popular and is easily accomplished in infants less than 8 months of age, as well as children. At the author's institution, mask induction is offered to children through the age of 16 years who have needle phobia. The essential monitoring modalities for inhalation induction include a precordial stethoscope and a pulse oximeter. The circulating nurse places the remaining monitors during the induction period, following the loss of consciousness. Anesthetic induction is begun with a 70:30 mixture of nitrous oxide and oxygen via mask or a cupped hand placed on the child's chin, with the anesthetic mixture directed toward the mouth and nose. A pacifier may quiet the infant during the induction, or the infant may suck on the end of the anesthetist's gloved finger. Sevoflurane is added to the nitrous oxide–oxygen mixture beginning with a 2% concentration, with a rapid increase to 8%. The mask may then be introduced as the inspired concentration is increased. The anesthetist should await the return of respiration and avoid the temptation to administer a breath because this may produce coughing and laryngospasm. Unconsciousness is produced with inspired sevoflurane concentrations 6% to 8%. Following the loss of consciousness, nitrous oxide is discontinued, and sevoflurane is administered in 100% oxygen. At this time the anesthetist should begin to assist respiration and promptly decrease the inspired anesthetic concentration of sevoflurane to 2% to 2.5%. Controlled ventilation with high-inspired concentrations of inhalation agent aggravates myocardial depression, precipitating the development of sudden cardiac arrest.[2,3,5,6]

During assisted ventilation, intravenous access should be established. The age of the child, proposed surgical procedure, and ease of airway management during induction are the determining factors for whether to proceed with intravenous access. Establishing intravenous access in all children before laryngoscopy and endotracheal intubation is advised. For elective surgical procedures, neonates may be managed with a 24-gauge catheter, infants with a 22-gauge catheter, and children with a 20-gauge catheter. Surgical procedures with expected large third-space fluid loss or blood loss require an additional intravenous catheter. Preferred sites for intravenous access include the nondominant upper extremity (dorsum of the hand, antecubital fossa) and the lower extremity (dorsum of the foot, the saphenous vein). The deep saphenous vein is most easily accessed with a 20- or 22-gauge catheter. This vein can be identified by placing the thumb over the medial malleolus and moving it toward the anterior portion of the tibia. By extending the foot and piercing the skin parallel to the tibia and passing subcutaneously, the saphenous vein may be entered. Tincture of benzoin is applied to the intravenous site and adjacent skin, and the catheter is secured with a sterile bioclusive dressing. The extremity is secured with a padded board, and the intravenous site is covered with a gauze dressing.

Following the establishment of intravenous access, preparations are made for endotracheal intubation. Intubation may be accomplished using the inhaled anesthetic agent without muscle relaxation or subsequent to the administration of a nondepolarizing neuromuscular relaxant. The administration of a neuromuscular relaxant decreases the potential for the cardiovascular depression that accompanies the administration of high concentrations of inhalation agents that may be required to facilitate laryngoscopy and intubation. The ED95 for acceptable intubating conditions with sevoflurane in children ages 1 to 8 years is 3.54 ± 0.25%.[197] The addition of 66% nitrous oxide decreases the ED95 by 40%.[197] A recent survey of members of the Society of Pediatric Anesthesia found that inhalation agent administration without neuromuscular blockade was used to facilitate endotracheal intubation 38% of the time in infants (0 to 12 months) and 43.6% of the time in children (1 to 7 years old).[198] Whatever method is selected, the inhalation agent should be discontinued immediately before laryngoscopy. This practice minimizes the contamination of the operating room with free-flowing inhalation agent from the patient's breathing circuit, and (more importantly) the delivery of high inspired

anesthetic concentrations is avoided immediately after intubation during the confirmation of ETT placement. Following confirmation the ETT is secured, and the position of the tube at the alveolar ridge or lip is noted on the anesthetic record.

Parental Presence During Anesthetic Induction

Children greater than 1 year of age may have difficulty with parental separation and may require premedication to ease their anxiety. In addition to preoperative medication, a new strategy some anesthetic departments have adopted is to have one parent present for anesthetic induction. Parents may stay with their children during diagnostic procedures such as bone-marrow biopsy, immunization, dental rehabilitation, and the induction of anesthesia.[199-201] Anesthesia departments may have age limitations, not allowing parental presence for children less than 12 to 18 months of age. Clearly the parent should not be invited to participate in the induction of a child with a full stomach or perhaps a child with a compromised airway.

Studies examining the effectiveness of parental presence are mixed. Parental presence has been demonstrated to reduce the child's anxiety, precluding the need for premedication.[202,203] However, in a randomized controlled trial, preoperative oral midazolam was found to be more effective for the control of the child's preoperative anxiety than parental presence. One should be aware that mothers who are motivated to be present in the operating room during the induction of anesthesia may be very anxious, and their children are likely to have high anxiety levels during anesthetic induction.[202]

Following a detailed account of anesthetic induction, one cooperative parent or guardian may be invited to "dress up" and accompany the child to the operating room. The child is placed in the lap of the parent, or the child may sit on the operating table while remaining in contact with the parent. Older children with previous anesthetic experience may find mask induction unpleasant but generally prefer this method over a frightening attempt at intravenous access. Preoperatively the anesthetist may allow the child to select a scented mask or to choose a favorite scented oil (banana, strawberry, orange, bubble gum), which is coated inside the mask (Loran Oils, Lansing MI). The child is persuaded to participate through conversation, and the parent or guardian is encouraged to participate (perhaps assist in holding the mask). The child is introduced to the pulse oximeter, because this is the minimum monitoring for the initial induction of children who resist the application of a precordial stethoscope, electrocardiogram (ECG) leads, and the noninvasive blood pressure cuff.

It should be emphasized that before entering the operating room with parent and child, a through explanation of the expected behavior of the child during anesthetic induction (excitement, spontaneous involuntary movements, snoring, floppy appearance with unconsciousness) should be provided to the parent or guardian. Despite these detailed conversations, the author has had parents who suddenly became uncomfortable and attempted to remove their child from the operating room during the excitement phase of anesthesia induction. It is important that a there be a clear line of communication between the anesthetist and the parent. In addition, the parent should agree to leave the operating room accompanied by an escort when the child has lost consciousness or when requested to do so by the anesthetist. Hospitals and anesthesia departments occasionally request the parent to sign a waiver of liability prior to accompanying the child to the operating room.

Induction begins with the introduction of a 70:30 mixture of nitrous oxide and oxygen via a cupped hand or the selected mask, with the subsequent introduction of sevoflurane as described previously. When the child becomes unconscious with a regular respiratory rate, he or she is carefully lifted from the lap of the parent or guardian and placed supine on the operating table (the parent is escorted out at this point). Subsequently the ECG and a noninvasive blood pressure cuff are applied, and intravenous access is established. Endotracheal intubation is accomplished as previously described.

Intravenous Induction

Intravenous induction is generally reserved for the child with an existing intravenous line. An intravenous induction may be clinically indicated when the child has a full stomach or a history of gastroesophageal reflux. Intravenous induction is quicker and more dependable, facilitating the rapid securing of the airway with endotracheal intubation. Venipuncture can be a frightening experience for the needle-phobic child. Oral premedication with midazolam before the child enters the operating room may be beneficial to decrease the child's anxiety and gain cooperation. The following describes a successful technique for venipuncture in nonemergent situations.

The child is taken to the operating room accompanied by two anesthesia providers and is encouraged to assume the supine position on the operating table. If the child is cooperative, the standard monitors are applied. One of the anesthetists is positioned on either side of the child and initiates a conversation. The pediatric breathing circuit is within easy reach of this anesthetist. The arm selected for venipuncture is positioned behind the hip of the anesthetist, minimizing the child's view of the preparations for venipuncture. During the casual conversation, the anesthetist grasps and squeezes the upper arm, providing a tourniquet effect. This eliminates the application of a tourniquet, which may increase the child's anxiety. The selected intravenous induction agent is drawn into a syringe and connected to the intravenous administration extension set through a stopcock. The venipuncture site is quickly prepared with alcohol, a subdermal injection of lidocaine is made with a 30-gauge needle, the selected intravenous catheter is inserted, the induction dose of propofol or thiopental is administered, and the intravenous catheter is secured with one strip of tape. Some anesthetists avoid the use of propofol in this situation because of the discomfort associated with its injection immediately after intravenous catheter insertion.

The pain associated with preoperative intravenous access may be eased with the subcutaneous injection of local anesthetic via a 30-gauge needle. Additional analgesia may be provided by an anesthetist via the administration of a 50:50 mixture of nitrous oxide and oxygen during venipuncture. Cautious administration of nitrous oxide is warranted in children with gastroesophageal reflux or impaired swallowing, because nitrous oxide may blunt the protective airway reflexes, increasing the risk of aspiration. The administration of concentrations in excess of 50% may produce significant disorientation and muscle rigidity, impeding the ability to obtain intravenous access. The timely application of a eutectic mixture of local anesthetic will also minimize the pain of venipuncture. Suitable intravenous sites are identified preoperatively and marked with an ink pen. The eutectic mixture of local anesthetic is applied well in advance (30 to 60 minutes) to ensure effectiveness and covered with a Tegaderm dressing.

Intramuscular Induction

On rare occasions, an intramuscularly administered drug may be required in uncooperative children or in children who refuse alternative routes (oral, nasal, or rectal) for premedication.

Ketamine, a derivative of phencyclidine, produces dose-dependent unconsciousness and analgesia via blockade of the excitatory neurotransmitter glutamic acid at the N-methyl-D-aspartate (NMDA) receptor. Following intramuscular administration, the child may appear to be in a catatonic state. Parents who witness the administration of ketamine should be warned that their child might exhibit spontaneous involuntary movements and nystagmus. Ketamine is a cardiac stimulant that produces an increase in systemic blood pressure and heart rate. Additional undesirable effects include bronchodilation, increases in intraocular and intracranial pressure, disorientation, unpleasant dreaming, and hallucinations. The psychogenic effects may be decreased with the concomitant administration of a benzodiazepine. Intramuscular ketamine in a dose of 2 to 3 mg/kg facilitates inhalation induction in children who are reluctant to be subjected to inhalation induction or venipuncture.[204] Ketamine doses between 5 and 10 mg/kg are associated with a lengthy recovery period and the inability to accept oral fluids.[205] Ketamine may be injected in a small volume; a variety of formulated concentrations exist. Ketamine is particularly advantageous in children with cardiovascular instability because the cardiovascular system is stimulated via the central nervous system (CNS).

Intramuscular midazolam may be used to induce sleep. Intramuscular midazolam (0.1 to 0.15 mg/kg) may also be used as a premedicant. Intramuscular induction is less reliable and more uncomfortable for the child.

PEDIATRIC AIRWAY MANAGEMENT

Respiratory complications are frequent in the pediatric patient during the perioperative period and may rapidly lead to the development of hypoxemia. Anatomic, physiologic, and technical challenges all interact to complicate airway management of the infant and child. Changes in the state of consciousness can rapidly lead to hypoxemia from upper airway obstruction. Bradycardia quickly follows decreasing cardiac output, producing acidosis and ultimately cardiac arrest.[4,184,206] Depending upon the child's underlying medical condition, the time from apnea to cardiovascular collapse occurs much quicker than in the adult. In a recent review of data from the Pediatric Perioperative Cardiac Arrest Registry (see discussion following), Bhananker and colleagues found that respiratory events were responsible for 27% (n = 53) of anesthesia-related cardiac arrests, with airway obstruction from laryngospasm the most common etiology.[4] Therefore, the maintenance of a patent pharyngeal airway with anesthetic induction and emergence is a formidable challenge when caring for the infant and child.[207]

The Normal Pediatric Airway

There are important anatomic and physiologic differences between the adult and pediatric airway (Table 49-10). These factors interact to maintain pharyngeal airway patency. The infant larynx is located in a more cephalad position (C3-C4 interspace), achieving the adult position (C5) by 6 years of age. This position allows the infant to swallow and breathe simultaneously. The epiglottis is described as omega or U-shaped, is short and stiff, and projects posteriorly at a 45-degree angle, increasing the difficulty of vocal cord visualization. Because of these anatomic differences, the use of a straight laryngoscope blade placed into the vallecula improves visualization of the glottic opening. The infant tongue is significantly larger in relation to the oral cavity, increasing the size of soft tissue within the oral cavity. Accordingly, there is a smaller submental space for displacement of the tongue during laryngoscopy. Unlike the

TABLE 49-10	Differences Between the Adult and the Pediatric Airways	
	Pediatric	**Adult**
Laryngeal location	C2-C4	C3-C6
Narrowest location of airway	Cricoid	Glottis
Shape of epiglottis	Omega-shaped	V-shaped
Right mainstem bronchus	Less vertical	More vertical

neonate or infant, the child has an increase in oropharyngeal tissue with the appearance and hypertrophy of the tonsils and adenoids between the ages of 2 and 7 years. The size of the tongue and the position of the epiglottis increase the difficulty of mask ventilation. Because of the more cephalad laryngeal position, the tongue lies closer to the palate and easily opposes it, producing upper airway obstruction and explaining why the neonate and small infant are obligate nose breathers. Attempted mask ventilation of the infant may be unsuccessful until the mouth is opened and the tongue swept away from the palate. These anatomic differences also make the airway appear more anterior during laryngoscopy. A complement of pediatric oral airways should be immediately available prior to the administration of sedatives or the induction of general anesthesia.

The infant head and occiput are large relative to the shoulders and upper body. With slight head extension, the infant will assume a proper intubating position (Figure 49-7). The maintenance of a neutral head position is more helpful than an exaggerated head tilt. Because of the higher position of the infant larynx and the larger occiput, the traditionally applied "sniffing position" may actually hinder glottic visualization.[169] The alignment of the pharyngeal and laryngeal axis is best achieved with support (perhaps a small towel) under the shoulders.

As previously discussed, the cricoid has been described as the narrowest portion of the pediatric airway. Cadaveric studies have described the larynx as conical in shape with the apex of the cone appearing at the nondistensible cricoid.[138,208] Litman and colleagues have found that the narrowest portion of the larynx is at the glottic opening and the immediate subglottic level, and this relationship does not change with maturation. The larynx can be viewed as a cone, with the apex at the level of the vocal cords rather than at the level of cricoid. This may explain glottic injury that occurs following chronic intubation in children.[140]

Maintenance of a Patent Airway

A variety of anatomic and neurologic interactions are essential for the maintenance of a patent pharyngeal airway. It is truly remarkable that airway patency is continuously maintained with changes in posture as well as extremes of head and neck position. The larynx is innervated by a variety of receptors that react to stretch, the flow of inspired and expired gas, and muscle movement. Airway patency is also dependent on lung stretch reflexes, central and carotid body chemoreceptor reflexes, and CNS arousal mechanisms. Pharyngeal patency is established and maintained through a delicate balance of CNS derived dilating and collapsing forces on the pharyngeal airway.[209,210] The pharynx may be conceptualized as a collapsible tube within a box, bordered by the tongue and soft palate, and enveloped by the bony elements of the mandible anteriorly and the cervical vertebrae posteriorly. Pharyngeal patency is a function of the

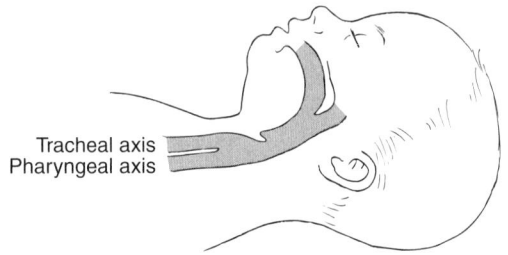
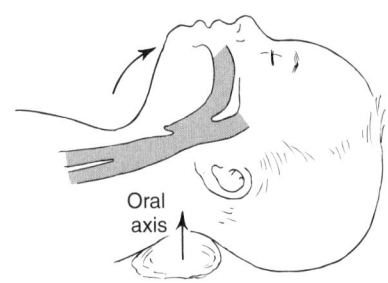

FIGURE **49-7** Alignments of tracheal, oral, and laryngeal axes during laryngoscopy.

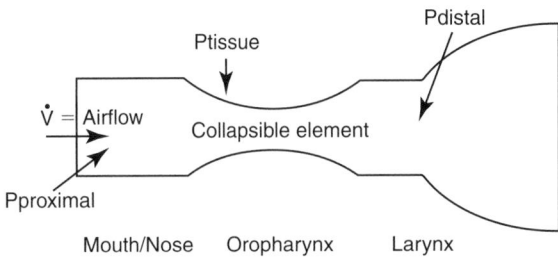

The oropharynx is open, partially open, or closed, depending on proximal pressure at Pproximal, distal pressure at Pdistal, and surrounding tissue pressure at Ptissue.

FIGURE **49-8** The Starling resistor. (*From: Stalford CB. The Starling resistor: a model for explaining and treating obstructive sleep apnea. AANA J; 2004;72:133-138.*)

overall size of this box, and the amount of soft tissue between the bony elements and the pharynx. An increase in the amount of soft tissue within the box (obesity, hypertrophy of adenoids and tonsils, large tongue), or a decrease in the size of the bony elements (small craniofacial structures or craniofacial deformity) will limit the content of the box, resulting in compression of the pharyngeal airway. In effect the pharyngeal airway functions as a Starling resistor.[211]

As detailed in Figure 49-8, the proximal pressure (Pproximal) must overcome the tissue pressure (Ptissue) of the soft-tissue contents of the box to prevent pharyngeal collapse. The central nervous system activity of the pharyngeal dilator muscles will overcome the collapsing pressure of the soft-tissue contents of the box. With the loss of consciousness following the onset of sleep or general anesthesia, the central nervous system activity of the pharyngeal dilator muscles decrease, yet there is continued activity driving the inspiratory pump muscles (diaphragm and external intercostal muscles), resulting in a narrowing or collapse of the pharyngeal airway.[207] The continued effort of the inspiratory pump muscles contributes to airway collapse as Ptissue is elevated and distal pressure (Pdistal) (the area below the vocal cords) is low.

Contraction of the inspiratory pump muscles produces a negative pharyngeal airway pressure, effectively collapsing the extra thoracic airway.[207] Pharyngeal collapse is opposed by the activity of pharyngeal airway dilator muscles.

As all anesthetists appreciate, general anesthesia affects pharyngeal patency. The CNS regulation of the inspiratory pump muscles and the pharyngeal dilator muscles are altered by the level of consciousness,[212] chemical stimuli (hypoxia, hypercarbia),[213,214] and airway reflexes.[215] In the examination of an animal model, Nishino and colleagues found that halothane, as well as thiopental and midazolam, produced a greater depression of hypoglossal rather than phrenic nerve activity.[216] These depressant effects are likely greater in neonates and the young infant who have an immature central nervous system.[217] During isoflurane anesthesia in adults with obstructive sleep apnea, pharyngeal collapse occurs at the level of the soft palate. However, as the depth of anesthesia is decreased, the pharynx is noted to be less collapsible, suggesting a strengthening regulation of pharyngeal dilator muscles with decreasing anesthetic depth.[218]

Intraoperative Airway Management
The Infant
In the awake infant and child, the tongue, the upper airway muscles (genioglossus, geniohyoid, sternohyoid, and sternothyroid) interact to tent the pharynx, preventing collapse. Anesthetic agents inhibit the neural activity of these airway muscles, resulting in pharyngeal narrowing or collapse.[216,217] The young infant depends on central nervous system compensatory mechanisms to maintain pharyngeal patency but is disadvantaged because of an anatomic imbalance (small maxilla and mandible, large cranium, large tongue).[207] As noted, a steadily increasing anesthetic depth during inhalation induction depresses these compensatory mechanisms, leading to pharyngeal narrowing and collapse. Incomplete airway obstruction may be clinically evident early in the inhalation induction as audible inspiratory or expiratory sounds evident through the precordial stethoscope. As the obstruction increases, the anesthetist may notice tracheal tug with attempted inspiration. The infant has a compliant chest wall, and because of forceful diaphragmatic contraction, the chest is noted to collapse with inspiratory efforts against partial pharynx collapse. With continued inspiratory attempts, a paradoxical movement of the chest and abdomen (the contraction of the chest with abdominal expansion) is also appreciated. This thoracoabdominal asynchrony is an important clinical sign of upper airway obstruction. With complete pharyngeal collapse, the audible signs of obstruction are no longer appreciated, and thoracoabdominal asynchrony continues. Perhaps as a result of immaturity, the CNS regulation of the pharyngeal dilator muscles is ineffective to open the pharyngeal airway in the infant.[219] The application of CPAP 5 to 10 cm H_2O is essential in the reestablishment of a patent pharyngeal airway until sufficiently anesthetized to allow the placement of an oral airway. The application of CPAP accompanied by airway opening maneuvers (more importantly a chin lift) will reverse the anatomic imbalance, increase tidal volume, and diminish thoracoabdominal asynchrony.[220] The chin lift is an important airway maneuver because it widens the anteroposterior (at the epiglottis) and transverse diameters (at the level of the soft palate) of the pharyngeal airway.[221]

Because of the general anesthetic depression of CNS compensatory mechanisms for the maintenance of a patent pharyngeal airway, tracheal extubation should be undertaken when the young infant is awake and has adequate respirations. Thoracoabdominal asynchrony appearing immediately following extubation is indicative of upper airway obstruction and is not accompanied by traditional sounds of upper airway obstruction (snoring) as in the adult. Following extubation, the lateral decubitus position may be advantageous in that it has been shown to decrease the compressive effects of soft tissue that surround the pharynx in individuals with obstructive sleep apnea.[222]

The Child
Pharyngeal patency improves during the first year of life as the anatomic imbalance is lessened with continued growth of the maxilla and mandible, and CNS regulation matures. This is evidenced by the fact that there is generally less airway obstruction with inhalation induction in older infants and children. However, when airway obstruction develops during inhalation induction, the obstruction is generally easily managed with the previously cited airway opening maneuvers. "Deep" extubation can be safely accomplished in children with the prior insertion of an oral airway, and following extubation, continued maintenance of pharyngeal patency may be facilitated with the application of airway-opening maneuvers previously discussed.

Laryngospasm
The larynx is the gatekeeper of the airway, protecting the lungs from the aspiration of foreign material. This function is most evident during swallowing, when the glottic closure reflex is initiated by stimulation of the superior laryngeal nerve facilitating sphincteric closure of the airway. Laryngospasm is a magnified glottic closure reflex in response to noxious stimuli of the superior laryngeal nerve and may persist despite the immediate removal of the stimuli. Laryngospasm precipitates a host of serious complications, including complete airway obstruction, gastric aspiration, postobstruction pulmonary edema, cardiac arrest, and death.[223]

Etiology
In a study of over 136,000 patients, Olsson and colleagues found that the frequency of laryngospasm in all patients was 0.87%. However, the frequency of laryngospasm in children ages 0 to 9 years was doubled (17.4/1000) and tripled in infants 0 to 3 months of age (28.2/1000).[223] Laryngospasm occurred following tracheal extubation (42/1000) and in children with a nasogastric tube (48/1000). The frequency of laryngospasm was the greatest in children with a concurrent upper respiratory tract infection (95.8/1000).[223] In examining the influence of tobacco-smoke exposure and airway irritability, Lakshmipathy and Bokesch discovered that children exposed to second-hand tobacco smoke have a 10-fold increase in the relative risk of laryngospasm (0.9% with no exposure, 9.4% with exposure).[224] Although laryngospasm may be self-limiting, the clinical importance of proper management is exemplified by the fact that five of every thousand children who experience laryngospasm have a subsequent cardiac arrest.[223]

The incidence of laryngospasm may be greater in the pediatric population because of specific practices in the anesthetic management of infants and children. Several factors are generally associated with the development of laryngospasm (Box 49-6).

The risk of laryngospasm is increased when airway instrumentation is attempted before an adequate depth of anesthesia has

---

BOX 49-6

Risk Factors for Laryngospasm

Preoperative Factors
Exposure to second-hand tobacco smoke
Concurrent or recent upper respiratory tract infection
Gastroesophageal reflux
Mechanical irritants (oropharyngeal secretions)

Intraoperative Factors
Excitement phase of inhalation induction
Tracheal intubation/extubation during "light" anesthesia
Upper airway surgical procedures (tonsillectomy,
   adenoidectomy, nasal/sinus procedures, palatal procedures,
   laryngoscopy/bronchoscopy)

BOX 49-7

Preventive Measures for Laryngospasm

Avoid noxious airway/surgical stimulation during "light"
   anesthesia
Assure sufficient anaesthesia prior to airway instrumentation
Topical application of lidocaine to suppress laryngeal sensory
   nerve activity
Intravenous lidocaine prior to extubation
Suction oral pharynx prior to extubation
Tracheal extubation when fully awake
Administer 100% oxygen for 3 to 5 minutes prior to
   extubation

---

been achieved, without the benefit of neuromuscular blocking drugs, and in infants and children with residual effects of previous upper respiratory tract infections.

Pathophysiology

The precise pathophysiologic mechanism responsible for laryngospasm remains illusive. To expand our understanding of laryngospasm and clinical management, it is best to revisit the original description provided by Fink in 1951.[225] The basic execution of laryngeal closure follows superior laryngeal nerve stimulation. The mechanism resembles a shutter, where the laryngeal inlet is closed by the action of the supraglottic folds, the false vocal cords, and the true vocal cords. Fink has suggested that glottic closure is a dual mechanism. The first response is the closure of the vocal cords (a shutter effect) followed by a ball-valve effect with closure of the false cords and the subsequent rounding of the supraglottic tissue following the shortening of the thyrohyoid muscle. This produces an envelopment of the laryngeal inlet by the supraglottic tissue with continued inspiratory effort, producing complete airway obstruction.

Prevention of Laryngospasm

The prevention of laryngospasm requires an understanding of the risk factors. Box 49-7 lists measures that may be undertaken for the prevention of laryngospasm.

Clinical Management

Algorithms for the management of incomplete and complete airway obstruction are provided in Figures 49-9 and 49-10. Prompt recognition and management are imperative to prevent hypoxemia and the subsequent development of bradycardia and cardiac arrest.

Incomplete airway obstruction may be evident as "grunting" or audible inspiratory and expiratory sounds as heard through a precordial stethoscope, accompanied by tracheal tug and thoracoabdominal asynchrony. Management consists of three essential processes. First, the responsible noxious stimuli should be discontinued (surgical stimulation, attempted airway instrumentation during "light" anesthesia, removal of pharyngeal secretions with gentle suctioning). Next, anesthetic depth should be increased by the delivery of increased concentration of inhalation agent or intravenous administration of a small dose of thiopental or propofol. And third, gentle positive-pressure ventilation using 100% oxygen should be attempted using a properly applied face mask with concurrent airway opening maneuvers (slight head extension, chin lift, and jaw thrust). On occasion, this may require two individuals, one to firmly apply the face mask and open the airway, and one individual to attempt positive-pressure ventilation.

The transition to complete airway obstruction becomes evident with the absence of inspiratory and expiratory sounds, as well as the inability to deliver positive-pressure ventilation. The application of positive airway pressure for the treatment of complete airway obstruction may not be successful. Further deterioration of arterial oxygen saturation with accompanying bradycardia may occur despite the continued application of positive-pressure ventilation, and the envelopment of the laryngeal inlet supraglottic tissue may be worsened. The administration of succinylcholine will then be required to break the laryngospasm.

Larson has advocated the direct application of pressure to the laryngospasm notch, bounded anteriorly by the mandibular rami, posteriorly by the mastoid process, and cephalad by the base of the skull (Figure 49-11). Bilateral firm and direct application of pressure toward the skull base produces an anterior displacement of the mandible. In addition to producing a jaw thrust, the intense stimulation with postcondylar pressure in the lightly anesthetized patient often produces a ventilatory sigh.[226] Larson and others have suggested that this maneuver is successful for the treatment of laryngospasm.[227,228]

Should complete airway obstruction continue unabated, intravenous administration of atropine and succinylcholine should be administered without delay. In the absence of intravenous access, intramuscular succinylcholine (4 mg/kg) is administered in the deltoid muscle. Following intramuscular administration the vocal cords will begin to relax within 60 seconds, permitting positive-pressure ventilation and relaxation to facilitate endotracheal intubation. With continued deterioration in arterial oxygen saturation, intubation may be required prior to the onset of skeletal muscle relaxation. In an extreme situation, the application of lidocaine to the vocal cords may produce sufficient relaxation allowing endotracheal intubation. As observed by Suzuki and Sasaki in an animal model, an alteration in superior laryngeal nerve conduction modifies the degree of laryngospasm. For example, severe hypoxia and hypercarbia are known to terminate laryngospasm.[229] Certainly these are not treatment options for laryngospasm.

The Difficult Pediatric Airway

Airway management of the infant and child requires a thorough understanding of the anatomic and physiologic differences

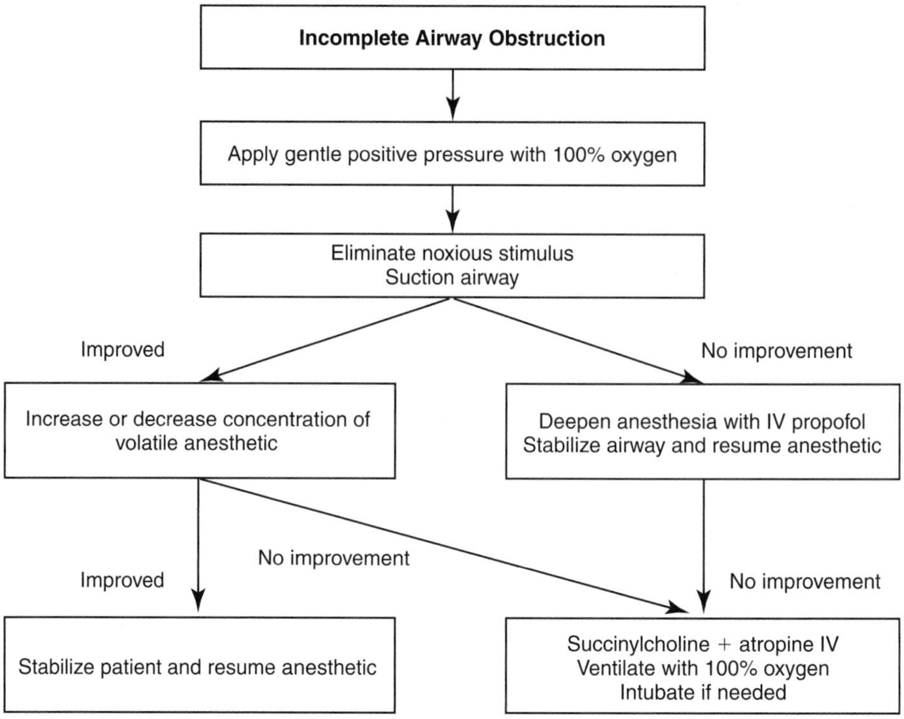

```
┌─────────────────────────────────────────┐
│       Incomplete Airway Obstruction       │
└─────────────────────────────────────────┘
                     │
                     ▼
┌─────────────────────────────────────────┐
│ Apply gentle positive pressure with 100% oxygen │
└─────────────────────────────────────────┘
                     │
                     ▼
┌─────────────────────────────────────────┐
│         Eliminate noxious stimulus         │
│              Suction airway                │
└─────────────────────────────────────────┘
```

Improved ← → No improvement

```
┌──────────────────────────────┐        ┌──────────────────────────────┐
│ Increase or decrease          │        │ Deepen anesthesia with IV      │
│ concentration of volatile     │        │ propofol                       │
│ anesthetic                    │        │ Stabilize airway and resume    │
│                               │        │ anesthetic                     │
└──────────────────────────────┘        └──────────────────────────────┘
```

Improved   No improvement   No improvement

```
┌──────────────────────────────┐        ┌──────────────────────────────┐
│ Stabilize patient and resume  │        │ Succinylcholine + atropine IV  │
│ anesthetic                    │        │ Ventilate with 100% oxygen     │
│                               │        │ Intubate if needed             │
└──────────────────────────────┘        └──────────────────────────────┘
```

FIGURE **49-9**   Incomplete airway obstruction algorithm. *(From Wittkugel E. Pediatric laryngospasm. In: Atlee JL, ed. Complications in Anesthesia. 2nd ed. Philadelphia: Saunders; 2007:601.)*

between the infant, child, and adult airway (see previous discussion). A *difficult airway* may be defined as difficulty in accomplishing mask ventilation and/or endotracheal intubation. The identification of the difficult pediatric airway begins with a thorough history followed by physical examination of the mouth, head and neck (Box 49-8).

A history of snoring, difficulty breathing with feeding, current or recent upper respiratory tract infection, and past history of croup should be obtained. Previous anesthetic records are an invaluable resource in determining the history of difficult airway management. However, a prior uneventful anesthetic does not preclude the possibility of difficulty of airway management with succeeding anesthetics. The physical examination should focus on the assessment of facial skeletal features, specifically the size and shape of mandible and maxilla, size of the tongue in relation to the oral cavity, absence of dentition, presence of loose dentition, and the range of motion of the neck. Box 49-9 lists pathologic conditions that affect pediatric airway management.

Classification

Following the completion of the history and physical examination the pediatric patient may be classified into one of four categories based on the noted airway pathology and degree of respiratory distress.[230]

Category I. These individuals have a normal-appearing airway, minimal or no sternal retractions, with an age-appropriate respiratory rate and normal arterial oxygen saturation.

Category II. These individuals present with moderate airway distress and/or significant airway disease (e.g., laryngeal papillomatosis). The anesthetic history demonstrates previous successful airway management.

Category III. The delineating characteristic of this group is an abnormal airway identified by physical examination (micrognathia, macroglossia, palate deformities, or prominent dentition).

Individuals with maxillary or mandibular pathology (e.g., Treacher Collins syndrome, Down syndrome) are grouped here. Included in this group are individuals with mediastinal mass.

Category IV. Individuals in this category have significant respiratory distress exemplified by marked sternal retractions, significantly decreased arterial oxygen saturations, and marked increases in respiratory rate that may ultimately lead to respiratory fatigue. An example is the pediatric patient presenting with an inhaled foreign body.

Anesthetic management is tailored according to the patient category. The majority of pediatric patients with respiratory embarrassment require definitive airway management. This is often best accomplished in a controlled environment (operating suite) with general anesthesia and the presence of surgical expertise to obtain a surgical airway should there be an inability to provide mask ventilation. For individuals who are categories I and II, an inhalation induction with sevoflurane, with the application of CPAP (5 to 10 cm H_2O) as previously described, minimizes soft tissue obstruction and pharyngeal collapse with increasing depths of anesthesia. Following confirmation of the ease of positive-pressure ventilation and acceptable arterial oxygen concentration, then and only then should a neuromuscular relaxant be administered to facilitate endotracheal intubation.

Individuals who are categories III and IV require advanced preparation for airway management and require the immediate availability of surgical expertise in airway management. Airway adjuncts including size-appropriate LMAs, oral airways, a light wand, and flexible fiberoptic bronchoscopes should be immediately available. A flexible fiberoptic bronchoscope with an external diameter of 2.2 to 4.0 mm will transverse a 2.5- to 4.5- mm internal diameter ETT. These individuals are best managed with spontaneous ventilation. A slow and deliberate inhalation induction is accomplished with sevoflurane. The administration of a neuromuscular relaxant must be avoided because total airway obstruction will follow the loss of pharyngeal and laryngeal tone.

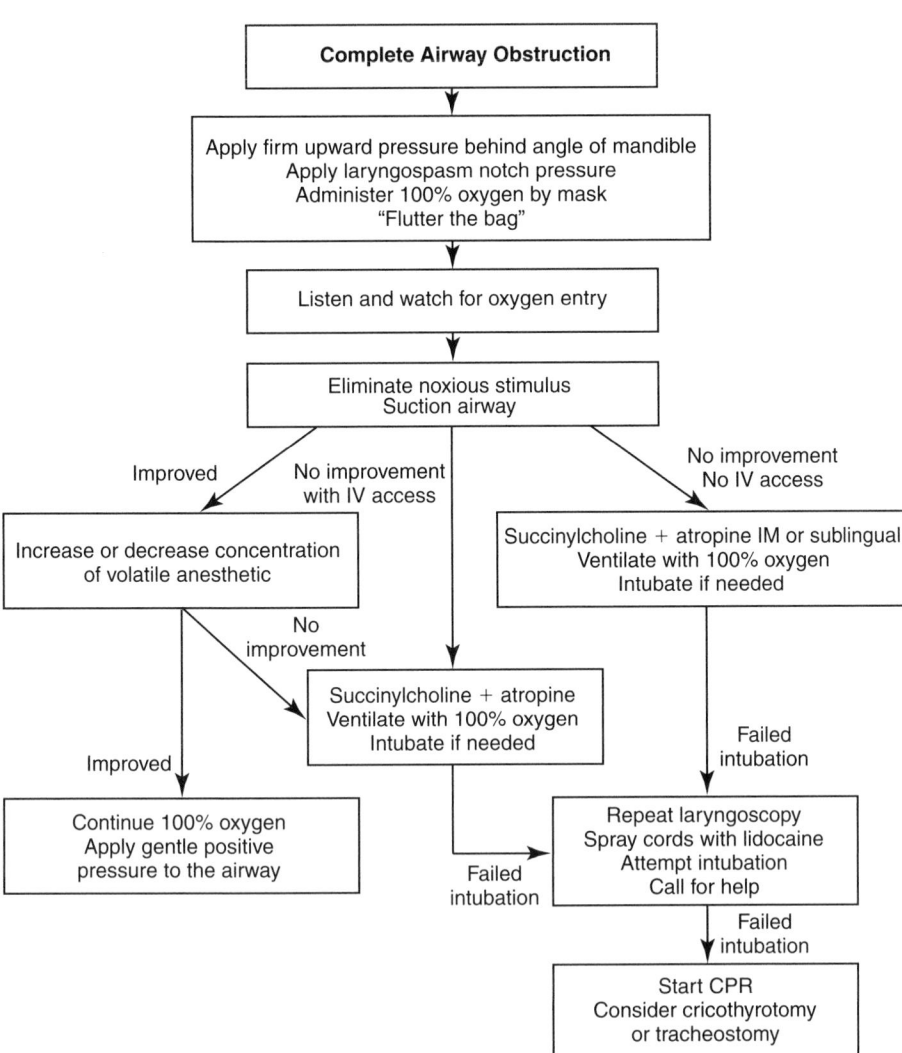

Complete Airway Obstruction

↓

Apply firm upward pressure behind angle of mandible
Apply laryngospasm notch pressure
Administer 100% oxygen by mask
"Flutter the bag"

↓

Listen and watch for oxygen entry

↓

Eliminate noxious stimulus
Suction airway

Improved → Increase or decrease concentration of volatile anesthetic

No improvement with IV access ↓

No improvement No IV access → Succinylcholine + atropine IM or sublingual
Ventilate with 100% oxygen
Intubate if needed

No improvement → Succinylcholine + atropine
Ventilate with 100% oxygen
Intubate if needed

Improved → Continue 100% oxygen
Apply gentle positive pressure to the airway

Failed intubation

Failed intubation → Repeat laryngoscopy
Spray cords with lidocaine
Attempt intubation
Call for help

Failed intubation ↓

Start CPR
Consider cricothyrotomy
or tracheostomy

FIGURE **49-10** Complete airway obstruction algorithm. (*From Wittkugel E. Pediatric laryngospasm. In: Atlee JL, ed.* Complications in Anesthesia. *2nd ed. Philadelphia: Saunders; 2007:600.*)

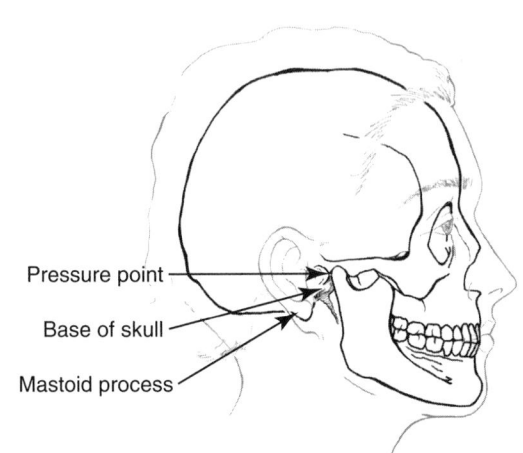

Pressure point
Base of skull
Mastoid process

FIGURE **49-11** The laryngospasm notch.

INTRAVENOUS FLUID AND BLOOD THERAPY

The maintenance of fluid homeostasis is essential in the comprehensive intraoperative care of the pediatric patient. The restoration and maintenance of pediatric intravascular volume is crucial if cardiac output is to be optimized and tissue oxygen delivery ensured.

BOX **49-8**

Physical Examination of the Pediatric Airway

Note the size and shape of the head
Facial features—size and shape of mandible and maxilla
Oral examination—size of tongue, loose or missing dentition, prominence of upper incisors
Range of motion of jaw and cervical spine

Intravascular fluid balance is influenced by a number of preoperative and perioperative circumstances. Preoperative intravenous fluid administration minimizes the degree of dehydration that accompanies the NPO period. Unless there exists a compelling reason to place an intravenous catheter preoperatively, intravenous therapy is generally avoided in the pediatric patient until general anesthesia has been induced via inhalation.

Perioperative fluid homeostasis is altered by a number of factors, including inhalation agent administration, the operating room environmental temperature, iatrogenic hyperventilation, and surgical stress. Potent inhalation agents produce peripheral vasodilation and varying degrees of myocardial depression, decreasing systemic blood pressure and end-organ perfusion.

Dehydration following prolonged preoperative oral fluid abstinence aggravates these decreases in systemic blood pressure. The delivery of cold, dry anesthetic gases via an ETT bypasses normal anatomic humidification, increasing the loss of fluid from the respiratory tract. These insensible respiratory fluid losses can be minimized with the use of active or passive humidification systems during the intraoperative period. The operating room temperature also influences fluid balance. Basal caloric and water requirements are increased in a cold environment. Increases in core body temperature of 1° C may increase caloric expenditure by 12% to 14%.

General anesthesia modifies the neuroendocrine control of fluid balance. Surgical stress increases plasma glucose levels. Hyperglycemia induces an osmotic-induced renal loss of free water. Anesthetic agents modify neuroendocrine regulation of fluids and electrolytes. Morphine and halothane have been demonstrated to increase the release of antidiuretic hormone (ADH) from the posterior pituitary.[231,232] ADH stimulates the release of aldosterone to conserve water through the renal reabsorption of sodium and water and the excretion of potassium. Decreased glomerular filtration, which parallels the decrease in renal perfusion, alters the kidneys' ability to handle administered fluid loads. Decreased renal perfusion stimulates the release of renin, which cleaves angiotensin I to form angiotensin II, a powerful vasoconstrictor that acts to increase systemic blood pressure. Renin stimulates the release of aldosterone.

Surgical trauma modifies fluid balance, the degree of which is dependent on the invasiveness of the surgical procedure. Intravenous fluids are used to replace intraoperative blood loss and fluid loss resulting from fluid shifts that develop from evaporative and third-space fluid losses. Physiologic parameters, such as heart rate, blood pressure, capillary refill time, urine output, and ongoing blood loss, are continually assessed. The rate of intraoperative fluid administration is continuously modified to maintain circulatory homeostasis. Peripheral surgical procedures (extremity procedures) have minimal evaporative or third-space fluid losses. However, intracavitary procedures (intraabdominal or intrathoracic procedures) are associated with greater blood loss, third-space fluid loss, and substantial evaporative fluid losses that approach 10 mL/kg of body weight per hour.

Pediatric Fluid Compartments

The growth of the newborn is accompanied by a decrease in the relative fluid compartment volumes of TBW and ECF volumes during the first year of life, followed by additional decreases in ECF later in childhood.[233] The TBW of the premature infant is as high as 80% of total body weight, whereas the TBW of the term infant is approximately 70% to 75% of total body weight. The adult value of TBW (55% to 60%) is reached between 6 months and 1 year of age. Knowledge of body fluid distribution is important when one is selecting specific fluids and volumes for administration. The differences in TBW, as well as in the ICF and ECF compartments in the premature, infant, child, and adult, can be found in Table 49-2.

Maintenance-Fluid Calculation

The most direct and widely accepted method for determining intravenous fluid requirements is based on body weight. Holiday and Segar proposed a formula for the calculation of hourly maintenance fluids based on caloric expenditure studies in children. The hourly maintenance fluid level is determined by the "4-2-1" formula and is calculated as follows (Table 49-11).[234] For the first 10 kg of body weight, 4 mL of crystalloid intravenous fluid (e.g., lactated Ringer's) is administered for each kilogram of body weight per hour. The hourly maintenance fluid requirement of a child who weighs 10 kg would be calculated as 10 kg × 4 mL/kg/hr = 40 mL/hr. Children weighing in excess of 10 kg but less than 20 kg would receive an additional 2 mL/kg/hr for body weight in excess of 10 kg. The child weighing 14 kg would receive 4 mL/kg/hr for the first 10 kg (40 mL) plus an additional 2 mL/kg/hr, for a total of 48 mL/hr. Children weighing in excess of 20 kg would receive an additional 1 mL/kg/hr in hourly fluid. This hourly maintenance fluid calculation serves as a basic guideline and does not take into account fluid deficits that develop during the NPO period and additional fluid losses (such as blood and third-space losses) that occur during the perioperative period.

Preoperative fluid deficits develop during the period of time in which the child has not received oral or intravenous maintenance fluids. The preoperative fluid deficit is calculated by determining the hourly maintenance fluid rate and multiplying this rate by the number of hours the child has been without intravenous or oral intake. The following calculations are used to

TABLE **49-11**	Hourly Fluid Requirements: The "4-2-1" Formula
Weight (kg)	**Fluid**
0-10	4 mL/kg/hr for each kg of body weight
10-20	40 mL + 2 mL/kg/hr for each kg >10 kg
>20	60 mL + 1 mL/kg/hr for each kg >20 kg
Sample Calculated Fluid Requirements	**Maintenance Fluid per Hour**
4 kg	16 mL
9 kg	36 mL
15 kg	50 mL
30 kg	70 mL

TABLE **49-12**	Fluid Replacement for Third-Space Fluid Losses	
Expected Surgical Trauma	**Administration Rate (mL/kg/hr)**	**Recommended Intravenous Fluid**
Minimal	3-4	Lactated Ringer's 0.9% NS, Plasma-Lyte
Moderate	5-6	Lactated Ringer's 0.9% NS, Plasma-Lyte
Severe	7-10	Lactated Ringer's 0.9% NS, Plasma-Lyte

NS, *Normal saline.*

determine the preoperative fluid deficit of an 8-kg child who has been NPO for 6 hours:

Equation 49-1

Maintenance fluid = 8 kg × 4 mL/kg/hr = 32 mL/hr
Deficit = NPO hours × maintenance fluid rate =
6hr × 32 mL/hr = 192 mL

The calculated fluid deficit is replaced following the guidelines of Furman[235]: half of the fluid deficit is replaced during the first hour, with the remainder divided in half and replaced in the subsequent 2 hours. Using the calculations just presented, the following plan for intravenous fluids is developed.

Weight = 8 kg	Hour 1	Hour 2	Hour 3
Maintenance fluid (mL/hr)	32	32	32
Deficit (mL/hr)	96	48	48
Hourly total (mL)	128	80	80

In addition to the calculated maintenance and deficit fluids necessary to replace insensible fluid losses, additional intravenous fluid is required to replace third-space fluid losses that occur with surgical trauma. Lactated Ringer's solution, 0.9% normal saline, and Plasma-Lyte are acceptable for the replacement of insensible and third-space fluid losses at the rate of 1 to 2 mL/kg/hr. Expected third-space fluid losses can be categorized as minimal surgical trauma (an additional 3 to 4 mL/kg/hr), moderate surgical trauma (5 to 6 mL/kg/hr), and major surgical trauma (7 to 10 mL/kg/hr; Table 49-12).

Glucose-Containing Solutions

Historically, glucose was administered during the perioperative period to prevent hypoglycemia, provide free water to replace the insensible water lost during the NPO period, conserve protein, and avert ketosis by preventing gluconeogenesis.[236] As previously discussed, surgical stress (e.g., surgical incision) elicits a neuroendocrine response, increasing plasma glucose levels. Despite extended periods of fasting, studies have noted that healthy pediatric patients infrequently become hypoglycemic.[237,238] However, very critically ill infants and those weighing less than 10 kg may develop hypoglycemia with prolonged periods of fasting. Most anesthetists administer a glucose-free intravenous solution

(lactated Ringer's) for maintenance fluid administration the replacement of third-space and intraoperative blood loss. If the child has had an extended NPO period, a plasma glucose level may be determined at the time of intravenous catheter insertion following inhalation induction.

Although the CNS is totally dependent on a continuous supply of exogenous glucose for the maintenance of cellular energy requirements, the continuous administration of glucose or elevated plasma glucose levels may worsen neurologic outcome in the event of an ischemic or hypoxic event. This association between hyperglycemia and worsened neurologic outcome has been noted in several reports.[239,240]

Hypoglycemia is likely to develop in a variety of clinical circumstances. Examples include infants who are premature, infants of diabetic mothers, children with diabetes who have received a portion of daily insulin preoperatively, and children who receive glucose-based parenteral nutrition. A glucose-containing intravenous solution is administered to these patients as a controlled piggyback infusion, with frequent plasma glucose determinations performed to avoid hyperglycemia. Infants born of mothers with diabetes and infants of mothers who receive glucose-containing solutions during labor may require a continuation of these solutions for the prevention of rebound hypoglycemia. Premature infants who have had less time to store glycogen in the liver than term infants are more susceptible to hypoglycemia. For this reason, premature infants receive an infusion of 10% dextrose in 0.2% normal saline.

Crystalloid Intravenous Fluids

Crystalloid intravenous fluids contain water, various concentrations of electrolytes, and varying amounts of glucose. These solutions move freely between the intravascular and interstitial fluid compartments. Crystalloid intravenous solutions are advantageous for perioperative administration because they are the least expensive of the available intravenous solutions and are acceptable for the replacement of preoperative, intraoperative, and postoperative isotonic fluid deficits. Unlike colloid solutions, crystalloid solutions do not produce allergic reactions.

Crystalloid intravenous solutions can be further subdivided by their tonicity in relation to plasma (hypotonic, isotonic, or hypertonic). Tonicity is a measurement of the comparative osmolarity of solutions, which is determined by the sodium chloride content. For example, a hypotonic solution (e.g., 0.45% normal saline) has a lower sodium concentration (<130 mEq/L) and an osmolarity

TABLE **49-13**	Physical Characteristics of Popular Intravenous Crystalloid Solutions						
	Na (mEq/L)	Cl (mEq/L)	K (mEq/L)	Ca (mg/mL)	Lactate (mg/mL)	Glucose (mg/dL)	mOsm/L
Hypotonic Solutions							
0.45% Normal saline	77	77					154
5% Dextrose in water						50	252
Isotonic Solutions							
0.9% Normal saline	154	154					308
Lactated Ringer's	130	109	4	3	28		273
Ringer's	130	109	4	3			309
Plasma-Lyte A	140	98	5				290
Hypertonic Solutions							
5% Sodium chloride	855	855					1700
7.5% Sodium chloride	1283	1283					2400

From Aker J. The selection and administration of intravenous fluids. Curr Rev Post Anesth Care Nurs. 1995;17:63.

less than 280 mOsm/L; an isotonic solution (e.g., lactated Ringer's) has a sodium concentration between 130 and 155 mEq/L and an osmolarity between 280 and 310 mOsm/L; a hypertonic solution (e.g., 3% normal saline) has a sodium concentration greater than 155 mEq/L and an osmolarity in excess of 310 mOsm/L. These sodium-containing solutions move freely about the extracellular space, whereas the sodium-free intravenous solutions such as 5% dextrose in water (D_5W), are distributed throughout all fluid compartments. Table 49-13 lists the physical constituents and the osmolarities of popular crystalloid solutions. An isotonic solution does not need to be equivalent to plasma in exact physical constituents (sodium, chloride, potassium) to be considered an isotonic solution because it is the number of particles dissolved in solution (principally sodium) that determines the osmolarity.

Estimation of Blood Volume

The goal of perioperative blood administration is the maintenance of acceptable oxygen-carrying capacity. Because pediatric patients have a relatively low intravascular volume compared with adults, vigilance and an accurate determination of intraoperative blood loss is fundamental to quality patient care.

The intravascular volume may be estimated by multiplying the child's weight by the estimated blood volume. The estimated blood volumes are as follows: premature infant, 90 to 100 mL/kg; full-term newborn, 80 to 90 mL/kg; infants 3 months to 3 years, 75 to 80 mL/kg; and child older than 6 years, 65 to 70 mL/kg (see Table 48-2). For example, the estimated blood volume of a 6-month-old infant who weighs 7 kg is 525 mL (7 kg × 75 mL/kg = 525 mL).

The determination of intraoperative blood loss is difficult. Subjective estimates of blood loss are grossly inaccurate. Blood collected from the surgical field in suction canisters can be easily measured, but up to one half of blood lost during surgery can be contained in items such as surgical drapes, sponges, and towels and is difficult to measure. Accurate accounting of surgical blood loss related to these items requires weighing them. The weight of the dry item is subtracted from the weight of a blood-soaked item. Every 1 g of weight is equal to 1 mL of blood loss. Ongoing surgical blood loss requires frequent reassessment of the child's physiologic responses. Moderate to severe decreases in intravascular volume produce tachycardia, hypotension, narrowed pulse pressure, low urine output, decreased central venous pressure, pallor, and slow capillary refill. A sudden decrease in blood pressure in neonates and infants with rate-dependent cardiac output is indicative of significant intravascular volume depletion.

Permissible Blood Loss

What amount of blood loss may be permitted while the patient still maintains adequate tissue oxygenation? No published studies are available to guide the anesthetist in determining the optimal and safe lower limits for hemoglobin concentration. Historically a hemoglobin of 10 g/L or a hematocrit of 30% triggered blood transfusion. This "transfusion trigger" has been redefined in light of the risks of blood-borne pathogen transmission. Permissible blood loss must be defined individually for each patient based on current medical condition, surgical procedure, and cardiovascular and respiratory function. Children with normal cardiovascular function may tolerate a lower hematocrit and may compensate with an increased cardiac output if a higher inspired oxygen concentration is provided to improve oxygen delivery. An exception is the premature infant. As discussed, the incidence of apnea is higher in neonates and the premature with hematocrit levels below 30%. The anesthetist, surgeon, and neonatologist should agree on a target hematocrit level, and this discussion should be documented in the medical record.

The permissible blood loss may be calculated by means of the following formula:

Equation 49-2

$$ABL = EBV \times (H_O - H_L)/(H_A)$$

where ABL = allowable blood loss, EBV = estimated blood volume, H_O = the original hematocrit, H_L = the lowest acceptable hematocrit, and H_A = the average hematocrit, or $(H_O + H_L)/2$. For a 6-month-old infant who weighs 7 kg, with a starting hematocrit of 35% and the selection of the lowest acceptable hematocrit of 25%, we calculate the following:

$$ABL = 525 \times (35 - 25)/(25 + 35)/2 = 174 \text{ mL}$$

Blood loss may be replaced with suitable crystalloid solutions (0.9% normal saline, lactated Ringer's) by administering 3 mL for each mL of blood loss. Recall that the intravascular volume is one third of the ECF volume. Accordingly, one must administer

3 mL of an intravenous crystalloid solution to replace each mL of blood loss. A blood loss of 100 mL therefore requires replacement with 300 mL of crystalloid solution. Blood loss that is less than the calculated permissible blood loss may be replaced with colloid (1 mL for every 1 mL of blood loss).

When the blood loss equals or exceeds the calculated allowable loss, transfusion should be considered. Before transfusion is performed, a current hemoglobin and hematocrit should be obtained. The surgeon should be included in the decision process. These discussions and the resultant hemoglobin and hematocrit are recorded in the anesthetic record. The volume of packed red blood cells (PRBC) to be infused may be determined by the following formula:

Equation 49-3

PRBCs (mL) =

$$\frac{(\text{Blood loss} - \text{ABL}) \times \text{Desired hematocrit (30\%)}}{\text{Hematocrit of PRBCs (75\%)}}$$

Using the previous example of a 7-kg infant, with a total blood loss of 300 mL the volume of PRBCs would be 300 − 174 × 30/75 = 50 mL.

Blood Transfusion

Before blood component therapy is initiated, the proper equipment (filters, infusion devices, blood warming devices) should be obtained and tested. Standard blood transfusion sets contain a 170- to 200-μm filter. Microaggregate filters (20 to 40 μm) may be placed between the blood-dispensing bag and the filtered infusion set, although no studies prove these filters to be of benefit over the standard 170- to 200-μm filter. Infusion pumps (syringe or piston driven) selected for the infusion of blood and blood products should be licensed for this function by the manufacturer. An excessive infusion rate can produce RBC lysis.

Blood is usually warmed before infusion. The American Association of Blood Banks has published standards for the use of blood-warming devices. Blood warmers must have a visible thermometer and an audible warning indicating excessive heating (>42° C). Warming devices for adult transfusions (in-line water baths, countercurrent heating with water through large-bore tubing) are cumbersome to use for the small volumes to be transfused in the pediatric patient. The selected blood-component containers may be placed under the forced-air warming blanket, or the measured aliquot of blood drawn into a syringe may be warmed with the hand. Syringes should not be placed into water baths because bacterial contamination may occur.

Blood administration need not be complicated. It is difficult to accurately determine the amount of blood administered when it is infused via adult-intended warming devices. Accurate accounting of transfused blood products is facilitated by drawing the measured quantity by syringe with subsequent delivery of the measured quantity. A suitable device is the Fenwal (Baxter Healthcare Corporation, Deerfield, IL) infusion set with an 80-μm blood component filter. This three-way infusion set is spiked into the blood component container, and the second limb of the set is placed into a stopcock, preferably located at the intravenous site. A syringe is attached to the remaining limb of the infusion set, allowing measured aliquots of blood to be drawn from the blood component container and then injected into the intravenous site.

The use of adult blood units is wasteful when a small infant requires transfusion. The blood bank can dispense small aliquots of blood into a calibrated syringe or provide 50- to 100-mL bags of the selected blood product transferred from an assigned donor unit. Blood used for neonatal transfusion is preferably less than

1 week old, to preserve 2,3-diphosphoglycerate levels, and irradiated to prevent graft-versus-host disease. When PRBCs are transfused, the blood should not be diluted prior to transfusion; this may contribute to hypervolemia.

PEDIATRIC REGIONAL ANESTHESIA

During the past 10 years, the use of pediatric regional anesthesia has become established. Regional anesthesia provides perioperative analgesia minimizing the risk of respiratory depression, modifies the metabolic responses to anesthesia and surgery, and improves patient outcome.[241,242] Although the popularity of combined regional anesthetic techniques for adults has increased, the use of pediatric regional anesthesia has been more limited. Valid considerations are that a limited number of anesthesia providers are properly trained in the administration of peripheral and central regional anesthesia in infants and children, regional anesthesia is generally performed during general anesthesia, the detection of intravascular injection and the signs of local anesthetic toxicity are masked during general anesthesia, there is a limited ability to properly assess the sensory level of block in the sedated preverbal child, the consequences of accidental dural puncture, and the ethical and medical legal implications of regional anesthetic administration in anesthetized children.

Unlike the adult patient, the pediatric patient will generally receive a peripheral or centrally administered regional anesthetic following the induction of general anesthesia. The inherent fear of needles and pain, the fear of neurologic injury in a combative child, and the difficulty in providing adequate sedation to ensure patient mobility during the introduction of the block often necessitate the safe execution of the regional anesthetic during general anesthesia. Perhaps the risk of neurologic injury is lower in the anesthetized child who is not resistant and combative during attempted epidural or caudal anesthesia. However, Bromage and Benumof report of a devastating neurologic injury in an adult after attempted epidural anesthesia.[243] These authors state that central neural axis techniques should not be attempted in patients who are under general anesthesia. A subsequent editorial in the same journal authored by a number of pediatric anesthesiologists experienced in pediatric regional anesthesia disagreed with this conclusion and proposed that the extrapolation of adult regional anesthetic experiences to children is inappropriate and may result in the denial of these beneficial procedures to children.[244] Regional anesthetic procedures in children should be performed only by anesthetists with previous training, demonstrated skill in adult regional anesthetic procedures, and knowledge of the appropriate applications of each technique.

The detection of intravascular injection in the child during the concurrent administration of inhalation agents has been the subject of several studies. Infants may have a greater risk of amide local anesthetic toxicity because of their decreased levels of AAG.[245] The routine administration of epinephrine-containing test doses of local anesthetics may be counterproductive during the concurrent administration of myocardial depressant drugs. Desparmet and colleagues found that the administration of halothane decreased the ability of epinephrine to produce tachycardia after intravascular injection.[246] Despite the intravascular injection of epinephrine, heart rate did not increase by greater than 10 beats per minute in 39% of the children studied. Desparmet and co-workers suggest that pretreatment with atropine increases the reliability of the detection of tachycardia after intravascular injection. In a study examining the reliability of an epidural test dose during sevoflurane administration, Tanaka and Nishikawa found that intravascular injection of epinephrine, when preceded by atropine administration, produced a heart rate increase exceeding 10 beats per minute and a systolic blood pressure increase of at least 15 mm Hg and concluded that an epinephrine test dose was a reliable indicator of intravascular injection.[247]

Fisher and colleagues have suggested that the ECG can be an effective marker of the intravascular injection of epinephrine.[248] They demonstrated that increased T-wave amplitude was a marker of intravascular injection, with the most prominent change in amplitude occurring within 15 to 45 seconds after intravascular injection.

SUMMARY

Anesthetic morbidity and mortality is greater in the pediatric patient and is multifactorial in origin. Pediatric subspecialty practice requires the anesthetist to master the foundations of pediatric growth and development, the anatomic and physiologic changes with maturation, and the influence of anesthetic agents on immature organ systems. Anesthetic management of the pediatric patient requires integration of this specialized knowledge, refinement of the acquired technical skills of adult anesthetic management, and the ability to apply this knowledge when caring for pediatric patients. This chapter has reviewed pediatric pharmacology, airway management, and fluid and blood product management for the pediatric patient.

REFERENCES

1. Halpern S: *American Pediatrics: The Social Dynamic of Professionalism, 1880-1980*. Berkeley: University of California Press; 1988.
2. Morray J et al. A comparison of adult and pediatric closed malpractice claims. *Anesthesiology*. 1993;78:461-467.
3. Morray J et al. Anesthesia-related cardiac arrest in children: initial findings of the Pediatric Perioperative Cardiac Arrest (POCA) Registry. *Anesthesiology*. 2000;93:6-14.
4. Bhananker S et al. Anesthesia-related cardiac arrest in children: update from the Pediatric Perioperative Cardiac Arrest registry. *Anesth Analg*. 2007;105:344-350.
5. Keenan R et al. Bradycardia during anesthesia in infants. *Anesthesiology*. 1994;80:976-982.
6. Morray J. Anesthesia-related cardiac arrest in children: an update. *Anesthesiol Clin North America*. 2002;20:1-28.
7. Learman J et al. Anesthetic requirements for halothane in young children 0-1 months and 1-6 months of age. *Anesthesiology*. 1983;59:421-424.
8. Learman J et al. The pharmacology of sevoflurane in infants and children. *Anesthesiology*. 1994;80:814-824.
9. Holzman R et al. Sevoflurane depresses myocardial contractility less than halothane during induction of anesthesia in children. *Anesthesiology*. 1996;85:1260-1267.
10. Wodey E et al. Comparative hemodynamic depression of sevoflurane versus halothane in infants: an echocardiographic study. *Anesthesiology*. 1997;87:795-800.
11. Green D et al. Nodal rhythm and bradycardia during inhalation induction with sevoflurane in infants: a comparison of incremental and high-concentration techniques. *Br J Anaesth*. 2000;85:368-370.
12. Mazoit J, Dalens BJ. Pharmacokinetics of local anesthetics in infants and children. *Clin Pharmacokinet*. 2004;43:17-32.
13. Caldwell J et al. Pharmacokinetics of bupivacaine administered epidurally during childbirth. *Br J Pharmacol*. 1976;3:956-957.
14. Gunter J. Benefit and risks of local anesthetics in infants and children. *Paediatr Drugs*. 2002;4:649-672.
15. Morselli P et al. Clinical pharmacokinetics in newborns and infants. *Clin Pharmacokinet*. 1980;5:485-527.
16. Jacqz-Aigrain E, Burtin P. Clinical pharmacokinetics of sedatives in neonates. *Clin Pharmacokinet*. 1996;31:423-443.
17. Battino D et al. Clinical pharmacokinetics of antiepileptic drugs in paediatric patients. Part II. Phenytoin, carbamazepine, sulthiame, lamotrigine, vigabatrin, oxycarbazepine, and felbamate. *Clin Phamacokinet*. 1995;29:341-369.
18. Kearns G, Reed MD. Clinical pharmacokinetics in infants and children: a reappraisal. *Clin Pharmacokinet*. 1989;17:29-67.
19. Milsap R, Jusko WJ. Pharmacokinetics in the infant. *Environ Health Perspect*. 1994;102(Suppl 11):107-110.
20. Certana P, Maurelli M. Rectal administration of anesthetic agents. *Minvera Anestesiol*. 1995;61:219-228.
21. Ostapowicz G et al. Results of a prospective study of acute liver failure a 17 tertiary care centers in the United States. *Ann Intern Med*. 2002;137:947-954.
22. Alcorn J, McNamara PJ. Pharmacokinetics in the newborn. *Adv Drug Deliv Rev*. 2003;55:667-686.
23. Temple A. Pediatric dosing of acetaminophen. *Pediatr Pharmacol*. 1983;3:321.
24. Birmingham P et al. Twenty-four hour pharmacokinetics of rectal acetaminophen in children: an old drug with new recommendations. *Anesthesiology*. 1997;87:244-252.
25. Anderson B et al. perioperative pharmacodynamics of acetaminophen analgesia in children. *Anesthesiology*. 1990;90:411-421.
26. Montgomery C et al. Plasma concentrations after high-dose (45 mg/kg) rectal acetaminophen in children. *Can J Anaesth*. 1995;42:982-986.
27. Morton N, Arana A. Paracetamol-induced fulminant hepatic failure in a child after 5 days of therapeutic doses. *Paediatr Anaesth*. 1999;9:463-465.
28. Bruun L et al. Hepatic failure in a child after acetaminophen and sevoflurane exposure. *Anesth Analg*. 2001;92:1446-1448.
29. Berde C, Sethna NF. Analgesics for the treatment of pain in children. *N Engl J Med*. 2002;347:1094-1103.
30. Ray K et al. Effect of halothane anesthesia on salivary elimination of paracetamol. *Eur J Clin Pharmacol*. 1986;30:371-373.
31. Geldner G et al. Comparison between three transmucosal routes of administration of midazolam in children. *Paediatric Anaesth*. 1997;7:103-109.
32. Weber F et al. Premedication with nasal S-ketamine and midazolam provides good conditions for induction of anesthesia in preschool children. *Can J Anaesth*. 2003;50:470-475.
33. Nelson P et al. Comparison of oral transmucosal fentanyl citrate and an oral solution of meperidine, diazepam, and atropine for premedication in children. *Anesthesiology*. 1989;70:616-621.
34. Eger E et al. The effects of age on the rate of increase of alveolar anesthetic concentration. *Anesthesiology*. 1971;35:365-372.
35. Goldman L. Anesthetic uptake of sevoflurane and nitrous oxide during an inhaled induction in children. *Anesth Analg*. 2003;96:400-406.
36. Lerman J et al. Effect of age on the solubility of volatile anesthetics in human tissues. *Anesthesiology*. 1986;65:307-311.
37. Lerman J et al. Anesthetic requirements for halothane in young children 0-1 months and 1-6 months of age. *Anesthesiology*. 1983;59:421-424.
38. Copnstant I et al. Changes in electroencephalogram and autonomic cardiovascular activity during induction of anesthesia with sevoflurane compared with halothane in children. *Anesthesiology*. 1999;91:1604-1614.
39. Friesen R, Lichtor JL. Cardiovascular depression during halothane anesthesia in infants: a study of three induction techniques. *Anesth Analg*. 1982;61:42-45.
40. Morimoto Y et al. Rapid induction of anesthesia with high concentrations of halothane or sevoflurane in children. *J Clin Anesth*. 2000;12:184-188.
41. Fisher D et al. Comparison of enflurane, halothane and isoflurane for diagnostic and therapeutic procedures in children with malignancies. *Anesthesiology*. 1985;63:647-650.
42. Rolf N, Cote CJ. Persistent cardiac arrhythmias in pediatric patients: effects of age, expired carbon dioxide values, depth of anesthesia, and airway management. *Anesth Analg*. 1991;73:720-724.
43. Karl H et al. Epinephrine-halothane interactions in children. *Anesthesiology*. 1983;58:142-145.
44. Friesen R, Lichtor JL. Cardiovascular effects of inhalation induction with isoflurane in infants. *Anesth Analg*. 1983;62:411-414.
45. Weiskopf R et al. Rapid increases in desflurane concentration is associated with greater transient cardiovascular stimulation than with rapid increases in isoflurane concentrations in humans. *Anesthesiology*. 1994;80:1035-1045.
46. Marret E et al. Accelerated idioventricular rhythm associated with desflurane administration. *Anesth Analg*. 2002;95:319-321.
47. Lerman J et al. The pharmacology of sevoflurane in infants and children. *Anesthesiology*. 1994;80:814-824.
48. Moore E et al. Anaesthetic agents in paediatric day case surgery: do they affect outcome? *Eur J Anaesthsiol*. 2002;19:9-17.
49. Osawa M et al. Effects of sevoflurane on central nervous system electrical activity in the cat. *Anesth Analg*. 1994;79:52-57.
50. Komatsu H et al. Electrical seizures during sevoflurane anesthesia in two pediatric patients with epilepsy. *Anesthesiology*. 1994;81:1535-1537.
51. Wu J et al. Spontaneous ignition, explosion, and fire with sevoflurane and barium hydroxide lime. *Anesthesiology*. 2004;101:534-537.

52. Castro B et al. Explosion within an Aestiva anesthesia machine: Baralyme, high fresh gas flows and sevoflurane concentration. *Anesthesiology.* 2004;101:537-539.

53. Fatheree R, Leighton BL. Acute respiratory distress syndrome after an exothermic Baralyme-sevoflurane reaction. *Anesthesiology.* 2004;101:531-533.

54. Baum J, Woehlck HJ. Interaction of inhalational anaesthetics with CO_2 absorbents. *Best Pract Res Clin Anaesthesiol.* 2003;17:63-76.

55. Stabernack C et al. Sevoflurane degradation by carbon dioxide absorbents may produce more than one nephrotoxic compound in rats. *Can J Anaesth.* 2003;50:249-252.

56. Gentz B, Malan TP Jr. Renal toxicity with sevoflurane: a storm in a tea cup? *Drugs.* 2001;61:2155-2162.

57. Conzen P et al. Low-flow sevoflurane anesthesia compared with low-flow isoflurane anesthesia in patients with stable renal insufficiency. *Anesthesiology.* 2002;97:578-584.

58. Versichelen L et al. Only carbon dioxide absorbents free of both NaOH and KOH do not generate compound A during in vitro closed-system sevoflurane anesthesia: evaluation of five absorbents. *Anesthesiology.* 2001;95:750-755.

59. Frick E et al. Compound A concentrations during sevoflurane anesthesia in children. *Anesthesiology.* 1996;84:566-571.

60. Eger E et al. Nephrotoxicity of sevoflurane versus desflurane anesthesia in volunteers. *Anesth Analg.* 1997;84:160-168.

61. Iwasaka H et al. Glucose intolerance during prolonged sevoflurane anesthesia. *Can J Anaesth.* 1996;43:1059-1061.

62. Smessaert A et al. Observations in the immediate postanaesthesia period II. Mode of recovery. *Br J Anaesth.* 1960;32:181-185.

63. Eckenhoff J et al. The incidence and etiology of postanesthesia excitement. *Anesthesiology.* 1961;22:667-673.

64. Armstrong T, Aitken HL. The developing role of play preparation in paediatric anaesthesia. *Paediatr Anaesth.* 2000;10:1-4.

65. Holm-Knudson R et al. Distress at induction of anaesthesia in children. A survey incidence, associated factors and recovery characteristics. *Paediatr Anaesth.* 1998;8:383-392.

66. Wells L, Rasch DK. Emergence "delirium" after sevoflurane anesthesia: a paranoid delusion? *Anesth Analg.* 1999;88:1308-1310.

67. Aono J et al. Greater incidence of delirium during recovery from sevoflurane anesthesia in preschool boys. *Anesthesiology.* 1997;87:1298-1300.

68. Galinkin J et al. Use of intranasal fentanyl in children undergoing myringotomy and tube placement during halothane and sevoflurane anesthesia. *Anesthesiology.* 2000;93:1378-1383.

69. Cravero J et al. Emergence agitation in pediatric patients after sevoflurane anesthesia and no surgery: a comparison with halothane. *Paediatr Anaesth.* 2000;10:419-424.

70. Sikich N, Lerman J. Development and psychometric evaluation of the pediatric anesthesia emergence delirium scale. *Anesthesiology.* 2004;100:1138-1145.

71. Voepel-Lewis T et al. A prospective cohort study of emergence agitation in the pediatric postanesthesia care unit. *Anesth Analg.* 2003;96:1625-1630.

72. Meyer R et al. Isoflurane is associated with a similar incidence of emergence agitation/delirium as sevoflurane in young children-a randomized controlled study. *Pediatr Anaesth.* 2007;17:56-60.

73. Welborn L et al. Comparison of emergence and recovery characteristics of sevoflurane, desflurane, and halothane in pediatric ambulatory patients. *Anesth Analg.* 1996;83:917-920.

74. Davis P et al. Recovery characteristics of desflurane versus halothane for maintenance of anesthesia in pediatric ambulatory patients. *Anesthesiology.* 1994;80:298-302.

75. Cohen I et al. Rapid emergence does not explain agitation following sevoflurane anaesthesia in infants and children: a comparison with propofol. *Paediatr Anaesth.* 2003;13:63-67.

76. Kain Z et al. Postoperative behavioral outcomes in children: effects of sedative premedication. *Anesthesiology.* 1999;90:758-765.

77. Davis P et al. Recovery characteristics of sevoflurane and halothane in preschool-aged children undergoing myringotomy and pressure equalization tube insertion. *Anesth Analg.* 1999;88:.

78. Johannesson G et al. Sevoflurane for ENT surgery in children: a comparison with halothane. *Acta Anaesthesiol Scand.* 1995;39:.

79. Cravero J et al. The effect of small dose fentanyl on the emergence characteristics of pediatric patients after sevoflurane anesthesia without surgery. *Anesth Analg.* 2003;97:364-367.

80. Lapin S et al. Effects of sevoflurane anesthesia on recovery in children: a comparison with halothane. *Paediatr Anaesth.* 1999;9:299-304.

81. Uezono S et al. Emergence agitation after sevoflurane versus propofol in pediatric patients. *Anesth Analg.* 2000;91:563-566.

82. Raddle I, McKerchner HG. *Transport through Membranes and the Development of Membrane Transport.* Littleton, MA: PSG; 1985.

83. Cook D. Neonatal anesthetic pharmacology: a review. *Anesth Analg.* 1974;53:622-623.

84. Lockhart C, Nelson WL. The relationship of ketamine requirements to age in pediatric patients. *Anesthesiology.* 1974;40:507-508.

85. Brett C, Fisher DM. Thiopental dose-response relations in unpremedicated infants, children and adults. *Anesth Analg.* 1987;66:1024.

86. Russon H, Bressolle F. Pharmacodynamics and pharmacokinetics of thiopental. *Clin Pharmacokinet.* 1998;35:95-134.

87. Olutoye O, Watcha MF. Management of postoperative vomiting in pediatric patients. *Anesthesiol Clin North America.* 2003;41:99-117.

88. Aun C et al. Induction dose-response of propofol in unpremedicated children. *Br J Anaesth.* 1992;68:64-67.

89. Hanallah R et al. Propofol: effective dose and induction characteristics in unpremedicated children. *Anesthesiology.* 1991;74:217-219.

90. Short S, Aun CS. Hemodynamic effects of propofol in children. *Anaesthesia.* 1991;46:783.

91. Picard P, Tramer MR. Prevention of pain on injection with propofol: a quantitative systematic review. *Anesth Analg.* 2000;90:963-969.

92. Parke T et al. Metabolic acidosis and fatal myocardial failure after propofol infusion in children: five case reports. *BMJ.* 1992;305:613-616.

93. Bray R. Fatal myocardial failure associated with a propofol infusion in a child. *Anaesthesia.* 1995;50:94.

94. Strickland R, Murray RJ. Fatal metabolic acidosis in a pediatric patient receiving an infusion of propofol in the intensive care unit: is there a relationship? *Crit Care Med.* 1995;23:405-409.

95. Plotz F et al. Fatal side effects of continuous propofol infusion in children may be related to malignant hyperthermia. *Anaesth Intensive Care.* 1996;24:724.

96. vanStraaten E et al. Rhabdomyolysis and pulmonary hypertension in a child, possibly due to long-term high-dose propofol infusions. *Intensive Care Med.* 1996;22:997.

97. Short T, Young Y. Toxicity of intravenous anaesthetics. *Best Pract Res Clin Anaesthesiol.* 2003;17:77-89.

98. Rigoulet M et al. Mechanisms of inhibition and uncoupling of respiration in isolated rat liver mitochondria by the general anesthetic 2,6-diisopropylphenol. *Eur J Biochem.* 1996;241:280-285.

99. Wolf A, Potter F. Propofol infusion in children: when does an anesthetic tool become an intensive care liability? *Paediatric Anaesth.* 2004;14:435-438.

100. Wolf A et al. Impaired fatty acid oxidation in propofol infusion syndrome. *Lancet.* 2001;357:606-607.

101. Ozlu O et al. Propofol anaesthesia and metabolic acidosis in children. *Paediatric Anaesth.* 2003;13:53-57.

102. Goudsouzian N. Maturation of neuromuscular transmission in the infant. *Br J Anaesth.* 1980;52:205-214.

103. Blount P, Merelis JP. Molecular basis of two nonequivalent ligand-binding sites of the muscle nicotinic acetylcholine receptor. *Neuron.* 1989;3:349.

104. Goudsouzian N, Standaert FG. The infant and the myoneural junction. *Anesth Analg.* 1986;65:1208-1217.

105. Sullivan M et al. Succinylcholine-induced cardiac arrest in children with undiagnosed myopathy. *Can J Anaesth.* 1994;41:497-501.

106. Gronert G. Cardiac arrest after succinylcholine: mortality greater with rhabdomyolysis than receptor upregulation. *Anesthesiology.* 2001;94:523-529.

107. Durant M, Katz RI. Suxamethonium. *Br J Anaesth.* 1982;54:195-208.

108. Nagiub M, Magboul MM. Adverse effects of neuromuscular blockers and their antagonists. *Drug Saf.* 1998;18:99-116.

109. Wong S, Chung F. Succinylcholine-associated postoperative myalgia. *Anaesthesia.* 2000;55:144-152.

110. Cozanitis D et al. Precurarisation in infants and children less than three years of age. *Can J Anaesth.* 1987;34:17-20.

111. Nagiub M et al. Effect of pretreatment with lysine acetyl salicylate on suxamethonium-induced myalgia. *Br J Anaesth.* 1995;59:606-610.

112. Blache J. *Anesthesia Related Malignant Hyperthermia—Clinical Forms.* Englewood, NJ: Normed Verlag; 1993.

113. Sambughin N et al. North American malignant hyperthermia population: screening of the ryanodine receptor gene and identification of novel mutations. *Anesthesiology.* 2001;95:594-599.

114. O'Flynn R et al. Masseter muscle rigidity and malignant hyperthermia susceptibility in pediatric patients: an update on management and diagnosis. *Anesthesiology.* 1994;80:1228-1233.

115. Ellis F, Halsall PJ. Suxamethonium spasm: a differential diagnosis conundrum. *Br J Anaesth.* 1984;56:381-384.

116. Hanallah R, Kaplan RF. Jaw relaxation after halothane/succinylcholine sequence in children. *Anesthesiology.* 1994;81:99.

117. Larach M et al. Prediction of malignant hyperthermia susceptibility by clinical signs. *Anesthesiology.* 1987;66:547-550.

118. Meakin G et al. Dose-response curves for suxamethonium in neonates, infants and children. *Br J Anaesth.* 1989;62:655-658.

119. Cook D, Fisher CG. Characteristics of succinylcholine in neonates. *Anesth Analg*. 1978;57:63-66.
120. Liu L et al. Dose response to intramuscular succinylcholine in children. *Anesthesiology*. 1981;55:599-602.
121. Rosenburg H, Fletcher JE. Masseter muscle rigidity and malignant hyperthermia susceptibility. *Anesth Analg*. 1986;65:161.
122. Morell R, Berman JM. Is succinylcholine safe for children? *Anesth Patient Saf Found Newsl*. 1994;9:1-3.
123. Morell R, Berman JM. Sux "contraindication" reduced to "warning." *Anesthesia Patient Saf Found Newsl*. 1995;10:1-3.
124. Fisher D et al. Pharmacokinetics and pharmacodynamics of atracurium in infants and children. *Anesthesiology*. 1990;73:33-37.
125. Meretoja O et al. Age-dependence of the dose-response curve of vecuronium in pediatric patients during balanced anesthesia. *Anesth Analg*. 1988;67:21.
126. Segredo V et al. Persistent paralysis in critically ill patients after long-term administration of vecuronium. *N Engl J Med*. 1992;327:524-528.
127. Tavainen T et al. Rocuronium in infants, children and adults during balanced anesthesia. *Paediatr Anaesth*. 1996;6:271-275.
128. Eikermann M et al. Optimal rocuronium dose for intubation during inhalation induction with sevoflurane in children. *Br J Anaesth*. 2002;89:277-281.
129. Reynolds L et al. Intramuscular rocuronium in infants and children. *Anesthesiology*. 1996;85:239-321.
130. Mason L, Betts EK. Leg lift and maximal inspiratory force: clinical signs of neuromuscular blockade reversal in neonates and infants. *Anesthesiology*. 1980;52:441-442.
131. Shoults D et al. Maximum inspiratory force in predicting successful neonate tracheal extubation. *Crit Care Med*. 1979;7:485-486.
132. Brandom B, Fine GF. Neuromuscular blocking drugs in pediatric anesthesia. *Anesthesiol Clin North America*. 2002;20:45-58.
133. Sparr H et al. Early reversal of profound rocuronium-induced neuromuscular blockade by Sugammadex in a randomized multicenter study. *Anesthesiology*. 2007;106:935-943.
134. McDonald I, Stocks JG. Prolonged nasotracheal intubation. A review of its development in a paediatric hospital. *Br J Anaesth*. 1965;37:161-172.
135. Allen T, Stevens IM. Prolonged endotracheal intubation in infants and children. *Br J Anaesth*. 1965;37:566-573.
136. Holzki J. Laryngeal damage from tracheal intubation. *Paediatric Anaesth*. 1997;7:435-437.
137. James I. Cuffed tubes in children. *Paediatric Anaesth*. 2001;11:259-263.
138. Wailoo M, Emery JL. Normal growth and development of the trachea. *Thorax*. 1982;37:584-587.
139. Eckenhoff J. Some anatomical considerations of the infant larynx influencing endotracheal anesthesia. *Anesthesiology*. 1951;12:401-410.
140. Litman R et al. Developmental changes of laryngeal dimensions in unparalyzed, sedated children. *Anesthesiology*. 2003;98:41-45.
141. King B et al. Endotracheal tube selection in children: a comparison of four methods. *Ann Emerg Med*. 1993;22:530-534.
142. Weiss M et al. Shortcomings of cuffed paediatric tracheal tubes. *Br J Anaesth*. 2004;92:78-88.
143. Marino E et al. A comparison of three methods for estimating appropriate tracheal tube depth in children. *Pediatric Anaesth*. 2005;15:846-851.
144. Stocks J. Prolonged intubation and subglottic stenosis. *BMJ*. 1966;2:1199-1200.
145. Schwartz R et al. Tracheal tube leak test—is there inter-observer agreement? *Can J Anaesth*. 1993;40:1049-1052.
146. Marley R. Postextubation laryngeal edema: a review with consideration for home discharge. *J Perianesth Nurs*. 1998;13:39-53.
147. Suominen P et al. Optimally fitted endotracheal tubes decrease the probability of postextubation adverse events in children undergoing general anesthesia. *Pediatr Anaesth*. 2006;16:641-647.
148. Werkhaven J. Microlaryngoscopy-airway management with anaesthetic techniques for CO_2 laser. *Paediatr Anaesth*. 2004;14:90-94.
149. Orliaguet G et al. Postal survey of cuffed or uncuffed tracheal tubes used for pediatric tracheal intubation. *Pediatr Anaesth*. 2001;11:277-281.
150. Hawkins D. Glottic and subglottic stenosis from endotracheal intubation. *Laryngoscope*. 1977;87:339-346.
151. Honig E. Persistent tracheal dilation: onset after brief mechanical ventilation with a "soft-cuff" endotracheal tube. *South Med J*. 1979;72:487-490.
152. Dullenkopf A et al. Fit and seal characteristics of a new paediatric tracheal tube with high volume-low pressure polyurethane cuff. *Acta Anaesthesiol Scand*. 2005;49:232-237.
153. Khine H et al. Comparison of cuffed and uncuffed endotracheal tubes in young children during general anesthesia. *Anesthesiology*. 1997;86:627-631.
154. Newth C et al. The use of cuffed versus uncuffed endotracheal tubes in pediatric intensive care. *Pediatrics*. 2004;144:333-337.
155. Browning D, Graves SA. Incidence of aspiration with endotracheal tubes in children. *Pediatrics*. 1983;102:582-584.
156. Tonnenson A et al. Endotracheal tube cuff residual volume and lateral wall pressure in a tracheal model. *Anesthesiology*. 1981;81:680-683.
157. Seegobin R, Hasselet GL. Endotracheal tube pressure and tracheal mucosal blood flow: endoscopic study of effects of four volume cuffs. *BMJ*. 1984;288:965-968.
158. Felton M et al. Endotracheal tube cuff pressure is unpredictable in children. *Anesth Analg*. 2003;97:1612-1616.
159. Dullenkopf A et al. Nitrous oxide diffusion into tracheal tube cuffs: comparison of five different tracheal tube cuffs. *Acta Anaesthesiol Scand*. 2004;48:1180-1184.
160. Algren J et al. The effect of nitrous oxide diffusion on laryngeal mask airway cuff inflation in children. *Pediatr Anaesth*. 1998;8:31-36.
161. Spielman F. Complete separation of the tube from the mask during removal of a disposable laryngeal mask airway. *Can J Anaesth*. 2002;49:990-992.
162. Devys J et al. Biting the laryngeal mask: an unusual cause of negative pressure pulmonary edema. *Can J Anaesth*. 2000;47:176-178.
163. Baird M et al. Removal of the laryngeal mask airway: factors affecting the incidence of postoperative adverse respiratory events in 300 patients. *Eur J Anaesthsiol*. 1999;16:251-256.
164. Sinha A, Sood J. Safe removal of LMA in children—at what BIS. *Pediatr Anaesth*. 2006;16:1144-1147.
165. Litman R. *Pediatric Anesthesia: The Requisites in Anesthesiology*. Philadelphia: Mosby; 2004.
166. Bain J. The Bain anesthesia circuit. *Int Anesthesiol Clin*. 1982;20:149-157.
167. Bain J, Spoerel WE. A streamlined anaesthetic system. *Can J Anaesth*. 1979;19:426.
168. Pethick S. Letter to the editor. *Can J Anaesth*. 1975;22:115.
169. Cotes CJ. Pediatric equipment. In: Cote CJ et al, eds. *Practice of Anesthesia for Infants and Children*. 3rd ed. Philadelphia: Saunders; 2001:715-738.
170. Conterato J et al. Assessment of spontaneous ventilation in anesthetized children with the use of a pediatric circle or Jackson-Rees system. *Anesth Analg*. 1989;69:490-584.
171. Maxwell L. Age-associated issues in preparative evaluation, testing, and planning: pediatrics. *Anesthesiol Clin North America*. 2004;22:27-43.
172. Hanallah R et al. Preoperative investigations. *Pediatr Anaesth*. 1995;5:325-329.
173. Hackmann T et al. Anemia in pediatric day-surgery patients: prevalence and detection. *Anesthesiology*. 1991;68:361-368.
174. Azarnoff P, Woody PD. Preparation of children for hospitalization in acute care hospitals in the United States. *Pediatrics*. 1981;68:361-368.
175. Warner M et al. Perioperative pulmonary aspiration in infants and children. *Anesthesiology*. 1999;90:66-71.
176. Roberts R, Shirley MA. Reducing the risk of acid aspiration during cesarean section. *Anesth Analg*. 1974;53:859-868.
177. Olsson G et al. Aspiration during anesthesia: a computer-aided study of 185,353 anaesthetics. *Acta Anaesthesiol Scand*. 1986;30:84-92.
178. Splinter W, Schreiner MA. Preoperative fasting in children. *Anesth Analg*. 1999;89:80-89.
179. Ljungqvist O, Soreide E. Preoperative fasting. *Br J Surg*. 2003;90:400-406.
180. Cook-Sather S et al. A liberalized fasting guideline for formula-fed infants does not increase average gastric fluid content volume before elective surgery. *Anesth Analg*. 2003;96:965-969.
181. Litman R et al. Gastric volume and pH in infants fed clear fluids and breast milk prior to surgery. *Anesth Analg*. 1994;79:482-485.
182. Fishkin S, Litman RS. Current issues in pediatric ambulatory anesthesia. *Anesthesiol Clin North America*. 2003;21:305-311.
183. Tait A et al. Perioperative considerations for the child with an upper respiratory tract infection. *J Perianesth Nurs*. 2000;15:392-396.
184. Tait A et al. Risk factors for perioperative adverse respiratory events in children with upper respiratory tract infections. *Anesthesiology*. 2001;95:283-285.
185. Murat I et al. Perioperative anesthetic morbidity in children: a database of 24,165 anaesthetics over a 30-month period. *Pediatr Anaesth*. 2004;14:158-166.
186. Olsson G. Bronchospasm during anaesthesia. *Acta Anaesthesiol Scand*. 1987;31:244-252.
187. Smythe J et al. Initial evaluation of heart murmurs: are laboratory tests necessary? *Pediatrics*. 1990;86:497-500.
188. Pelech A. Evaluation of the pediatric patient with a cardiac murmur. *Pediatr Clin North Am*. 1999;46:2.
189. Tobias J. Anesthesia for minimally invasive surgery in children. *Best Pract Res Clin Anaesthesiol*. 2002;16:115-120.
190. Dawson B et al. Use of anesthesia: implications of day-care surgery and anaesthesia. *BMJ*. 1980;281:212-214.

191. Brett C. Pediatrics. In: Stoelting R, et al, eds. *Basics of Anesthesia*. Philadelphia: Churchill Livingstone; 2007:504-517.
192. Eckenhoff J. Relationship of anesthesia to postoperative personality changes in children. *Am J Dis Child*. 1953;86:587-591.
193. Levine M et al. Oral midazolam premedication in children with congenital cyanotic heart disease undergoing cardiac surgery. *Can J Anaesth*. 1993;40:934-938.
194. Cote C et al. A single-blinded study of combined pulse oximetry and capnography in children. *Anesthesiology*. 1991;74:980-987.
195. Bagwell J et al. End-tidal P_{CO_2} sampled at the distal and proximal ends of the endotracheal tube in infants and children. *Anesth Analg*. 1987;66:959-964.
196. Bagwell J, Heavener JE. End-tidal carbon dioxide pressure in neonates and infants measured by aspiration and flow-through capnography. *J Clin Monit*. 1991;7:285.
197. Swan H et al. Additive contribution of nitrous oxide to sevoflurane minimum alveolar concentration for tracheal intubation in children. *Anesthesiology*. 1999;91:667-671.
198. Politis G et al. Tracheal intubation of healthy pediatric patients without muscle relaxant: a survey of technique utilization and perceptions of safety. *Anesth Analg*. 1999;88:737-741.
199. Bauchner H et al. Pediatric procedures: do parents want to watch? *Pediatrics*. 1989;84:907-909.
200. Ryder I, Spargo P. Parents in the anesthetic room: a questionnaire survey of parents' reactions. *Anaesthesia*. 1991;46:977-979.
201. Henderson M et al. Parental attitudes to presence at induction of pediatric anaesthesia. *Anesth Intensive Care*. 1993;46:324-327.
202. Kain Z et al. Parental presence during induction of anesthesia versus sedative premedication: which intervention is more effective? *Anesthesiology*. 1998;89:1147-1156.
203. Kain Z et al. Trends in the practice of parental presence during induction of anesthesia and the use of preoperative sedative premedication in the United States, 1995-2002: results of a follow-up national survey. *Anesth Analg*. 2004;98:1252-1259.
204. Hanallah R, Patel RI. Low dose intramuscular ketamine for anesthesia pre-induction in young children undergoing brief outpatient procedures. *Anesthesiology*. 1989;70:598.
205. Wyant G. Intramuscular ketalar in pediatric anaesthesia. *Can J Anaesth*. 1971;18:72-83.
206. Tiret L et al. Complications related to anaesthesia in infants and children. *Br J Anaesth*. 1988;61:263-269.
207. Isono S. Developmental changes of pharyngeal airway patency: implications for pediatric anesthesia. *Paediatric Anaesth*. 2006;16:109-122.
208. Butz R Jr. Length and cross-section growth patterns in the human trachea. *Pediatrics*. 1968;42:336-341.
209. Remmers J et al. Pathogenesis of upper airway occlusion during sleep. *J Appl Physiol*. 1978;44:931-938.
210. Brouillette R, Thach BT. A neuromuscular mechanism maintaining extrathroacic airway patency. *J Appl Physiol*. 1979;46:772-779.
211. Stalford K. The Starling resistor: a model for explaining and treating obstructive sleep apnea. *AANA J*. 2004;72:133-137.
212. Wheatley J et al. Influence of sleep on response to negative airway pressure of tensor palatini muscle and retropalatal airway. *J Appl Physiol*. 1993;75:2117-2124.
213. Parisi R et al. Correlation between genioglossal and diaphragmatic responses to hypercapnia during sleep. *Am Rev Respir Dis*. 1987;135:378-382.
214. Parisi R et al. Genioglossal and diaphragmatic EMG responses to hypoxia during sleep. *Am Rev Respir Dis*. 1988;138:610-616.
215. Van Lunteren E et al. Nasal and laryngeal reflex responses to negative upper airway pressure. *J Appl Physiol*. 1984;56:746-752.
216. Nishino T et al. Comparison of changes in the hypoglossal and phrenic nerve activity in response to increasing depth of anesthesia in cats. *Anesthesiology*. 1984;60:19-24.
217. Ochiai R et al. Differential sensitivity to halothane anesthesia of the genioglossus, intercostals, and diaphragm of kittens. *Anesth Analg*. 1992;74:338-344.
218. Eastwood P et al. Collapsibility of the upper airway during anesthesia with isoflurane. *Anesthesiology*. 2002;97:786-793.
219. Wilson S et al. Upper airway patency in the human infant: influence of airway pressure and posture. *J Appl Physiol*. 1980;48:500-504.
220. Hammer J et al. Effect of jaw-thrust and continuous positive airway pressure on tidal breathing in deeply sedated infants. *Pediatrics*. 2001;138:826-830.
221. Reber A et al. Effect of airway opening maneuvers on thoraco-abdominal asynchrony in anaesthetized children. *Eur Respir J*. 2001;17:1239-1243.
222. Isono S et al. Lateral position decreases collapsibility of the passive pharynx in patients with obstructive sleep apnea. *Anesthesiology*. 2002;97:780-785.
223. Olsson G et al. Laryngospasm during anaesthesia. A computer-aided incidence study in 136,929 patients. *Acta Anaesthesiol Scand*. 1984;28:567-575.
224. Lakshmipathy N, Bokesch PM. Environmental tobacco smoke: a risk factor for pediatric laryngospasm. *Anesth Analg*. 1996;82:724-727.
225. Fink B. The etiology and treatment of laryngospasm. *Anesthesiology*. 1951;17:569-577.
226. Johnstone R. Laryngospasm treatment—an explanation [letter]. *Anesthesiology*. 1991;91:581-582.
227. Larson C. Laryngospasm—the best treatment [letter]. *Anesthesiology*. 1998;89:1293-1294.
228. Rajan G. Supraglottic obstruction versus true laryngospasm: the best treatment [letter]. *Anesthesiology*. 1999;91:581.
229. Suzuki M, Sasaki CT. Laryngeal spasm: a neurophysiological redefinition. *Ann Otol Rhinol Laryngol*. 1977;86:150-157.
230. Gregory G, Rizal J. Classification and assessment of the difficult pediatric airway. *Anesthesiol Clin North America*. 1998;16:729-741.
231. Oyama T et al. Plasma levels of antidiuretic hormone in man during halothane anesthesia and surgery. *Can Anaesth Soc J*. 1971;18:614.
232. Bozkurt P et al. Effects of systemic and epidural morphine on antidiuretic hormone levels in children. *Pediatr Anaesth*. 2003;13:508-514.
233. Friis-Hansen B. Body water compartments in children: changes during growth and related changes in body composition. *Pediatrics*. 1961;28:169-181.
234. Holiday M, Segar WE. The maintenance need for water in parenteral fluid therapy. *Pediatrics*. 1957;19:823-832.
235. Furman E et al. Specific therapy in water, electrolyte and blood-volume replacement during pediatric surgery. *Anesthesiology*. 1975;42:187-193.
236. Sieber F et al. Glucose: a reevaluation of its intraoperative use. *Anesthesiology*. 1987;67:72-81.
237. Aun C, Panesar NS. Pediatric glucose homeostasis during anaesthesia. *Br J Anaesth*. 1990;64:413-418.
238. van der Walt J, Carter JA. The effect of different preoperative regimens on plasma glucose and gastric volume and pH in infancy. *Anaesth Intensive Care*. 1986;14:352-359.
239. Ayers J, Graves SA. Perioperative management of total parenteral nutrition, glucose containing solutions, and intraoperative glucose monitoring in paediatric patients: a survey of clinical practice. *Pediatr Anaesth*. 2001;11:41-44.
240. Lanier W et al. The effect of glucose infusion and head position on neurologic outcome after complete cerebral ischemia in primates: examination of a model. *Anesthesiology*. 1987;66:39-48.
241. Anand K, Carr DB. The neuroanatomy neurophysiology and neurochemistry of pain, stress analgesia in newborn and children. *Pediatr Clin North Am*. 1989;36:795-821.
242. McNeeley J et al. Epidural analgesia improves outcome following pediatric fundoplication: a retrospective analysis. *Reg Anesth*. 1997;22:16-23.
243. Bromage P, Benumof JL. Paraplegia following intracord injection during attempted epidural anesthesia under general anesthesia. *Reg Anesth Pain Med*. 1998;23:104-107.
244. Krane E et al. The safety of epidurals placed during general anesthesia. *Reg Anesth Pain Med*. 1998;23:433-438.
245. Booker P et al. Perioperative changes in alpha-1 acid glycoprotein concentrations in infants undergoing major surgery. *Br J Anaesth*. 1996;76:365-368.
246. Desparmet J et al. Efficacy of epidural test dose in children anesthetized with halothane. *Anesthesiology*. 1990;72:249-251.
247. Tanaka M, Nishikawa T. Simulation of an epidural test dose with intravenous epinephrine in sevoflurane-anesthetized children. *Anesth Analg*. 1998;86:952-957.
248. Fisher Q et al. Detection of intravascular injection of regional anaesthetics in children. *Can J Anaesth*. 1997;44:592-598.

CHAPTER 50

GERIATRICS AND ANESTHESIA PRACTICE

Carmencita Ford-Fleifel

PERSPECTIVES ON AGING

The geriatric segment of the population continues to grow significantly (Figure 50-1). In the year 2006, nearly 37.3 million people in the United States were more than 65 years of age and made up 12.4% of the general population. Persons reaching age 65 now have an average life expectancy of an additional 18.4 years—19.8 years for females and 16.8 years for males.[1] Providing anesthesia care to elderly individuals with diverse and variable age-induced physiologic changes constitutes a major part of modern adult anesthesia practice.

Although an absolute definition of who is elderly places an arbitrary marker on chronologic age, and because a concise definition has not been agreed on, individuals who are 65 years of age and older generally are considered to be part of the geriatric cohort. Aging is now viewed as a physiologic continuum rather than chronologic age.[2] It is a progressive process with a diminishing ability to adjust to stressful events. Over half the members of this population will have at least one surgical procedure and anesthesia during their lifetime.[3] Despite conflicting data, the geriatric patient who undergoes anesthesia and surgery may be at increased risk for perioperative morbidity and mortality as a result of continuous physiologic aging processes and concomitant diseases. Anesthesia and surgery-related morbidity and mortality are likely to increase if the geriatric patient requires emergency surgery. When the anesthesia provider plans the perioperative management for the geriatric patient, it is important to understand the influence that aging and disease processes have on patient outcome.

It should be noted that the extent to which systemic changes occur in the geriatric patient is not consistent across the population. For instance, individuals who maintain physical fitness may be less affected than patients who lead a sedentary lifestyle. The following sections discuss system changes that are predictable as functions of aging and of the decreased capacity for adaptation associated with it.

EXPECTED ANATOMIC AND PHYSIOLOGIC CHANGES

Over the past few decades, anesthesia providers have identified changes in the physiology and pharmacology of aging.[4] Aging is associated with structural changes of cells and organs. At the cellular level, a genetically controlled number of cell divisions limits the number of human fibroblasts. After the maximum number of cell divisions has been reached, cells fail to grow and then die, despite apparent uniformity in the environment. The accumulation of random errors in the replication of deoxyribonucleic acid (DNA) and ribonucleic acid (RNA) and in protein synthesis is superimposed on the limitation of cellular division. When a sufficient number of cells fail to function,

the organs eventually become unable to function effectively (Box 50-1).[5]

Human organ function shows a linear decline with age. The rate constant for this decline is slightly less than 1% per year of the functional capacity present at age 30 years. As a consequence, a 70-year-old geriatric patient may have a 40% decrease in the function of any specific organ compared with that present at the age of 30 years. Fortunately the healthy adult patient at age 30 years has 4 to 10 times the organ function required for maintenance of homeostasis.[6]

The degree of physiologic function that remains with increasing age varies. Changes in organ function manifest as decreased margins of reserve. Geriatric patients may be able to maintain homeostasis but become increasingly less able to restore it when they are subjected to trauma, disease, or drugs. For example, the response to a decrease in arterial oxygen tension or pH or to an increase in arterial carbon dioxide (CO_2) tension should be an increase in ventilation and heart rate. The response to hypoxemia and hypercarbia is blunted by aging and by residual anesthesia and narcotics. Postoperatively the geriatric patient may lack the reserve required to meet the added demands residual anesthetics place on ventilatory capability. As a result, the patient may be predisposed to hypoxemia and respiratory failure.

As a person ages, changes in body composition may have a significant effect on anesthetic patient-care management. Overall, a loss of skeletal muscle (lean body mass) and a 20% to 30% reduction in blood volume can be expected. The essentially contracted state of the vasculature may produce a higher than anticipated initial plasma concentration when anesthetic agents are administered. An increase in the amount of body fat also develops, with an increased availability of lipid storage sites and a greater reservoir for deposition of lipid-soluble anesthetic agents. As a consequence, it is likely that a greater than expected time period is required for lipid-soluble agents to be eliminated from storage sites, a prolonged effect may be seen, and hypotension can be anticipated.[7]

Thermoregulation and positioning are important considerations for the elderly patient. Thermoregulation in the elderly patient is impaired; therefore, body temperature conservation measures must be used even for short periods of time. Hypothermia is more pronounced and lasts longer because of a lower basal metabolic rate, hypothyroidism, a high ratio of surface area to body mass, and less effective peripheral vasoconstriction. Shivering increases oxygen consumption up to 400%, which leads to hypoxia, acidosis, and cardiopulmonary compromise.[8,9] Younger patients shiver at 36.1° C, but patients older than 80 years will not shiver until core body temperature decreases to 35.2° C.[10] Elderly patients in whom intraoperative normothermia

**Increasing numbers of persons
65 years and older from 1900 to 2030**

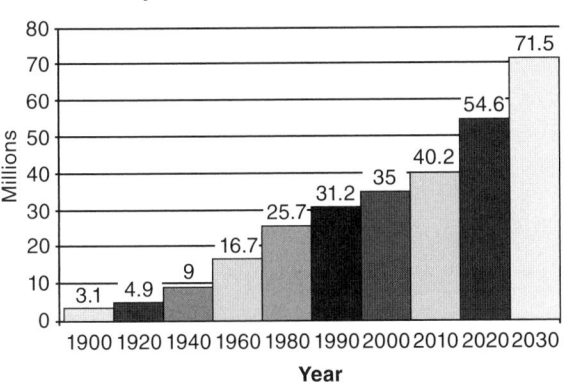

FIGURE **50-1** Increasing numbers of persons age 65 and older from 1900 to 2030. (*From Greenberg S. A Profile of Older Americans: 2006. Washington, DC: U.S. Department of Health and Human Services Administration on Aging; 2006.*)

BOX **50-1**

Common Age-Related Anatomic and Physiologic Changes

- Decreased organ function
- Increased body fat
- Decreased blood volume
- Loss of protective reflexes
- Decreased ability to retain body heat
- Decreased lean body mass
- Decreased skin elasticity
- Collagen loss
- Decreased intracellular water

BOX **50-2**

Common Age-Related Cardiovascular Anatomic and Physiologic Changes

- Impaired pump function
- Prolonged circulation time
- Myocardial fiber atrophy
- Hypertension
- Impaired cardiac adrenergic receptor quality
- Increased peripheral vascular resistance
- Decreased cardiac output
- Decreased organ perfusion
- Left ventricular hypertrophy
- Coronary artery disease

---

is difficult to control have a greater incidence of shivering on arrival to the postanesthesia care unit and are prone to the development of significant postoperative protein catabolism.[11]

Positioning and padding of the elderly patient requires extra care and attention because of fragile skin, decreased subcutaneous fat, and poor skin turgor.[8] Great care must be taken to prevent trauma to skin and bony prominences when the geriatric patient is positioned for surgery on the operating table. Collagen loss and decreased elasticity of tissue make the skin more sensitive to damage from tape, monitoring devices, and contact with hard table surfaces. There may be musculoskeletal limitations preventing specific positions on the operating room table.

Protein catabolism may be compounded by nutritional deficiencies that occur in the elderly; these deficiencies are associated with a reduction in intracellular water and in potassium. The loss in total body water that renders the patient vulnerable to hypotension during anesthesia also makes it difficult for him or her to compensate for changes in position and posture.[12]

Cardiovascular System

Cardiac function declines by 50% between the ages of 20 and 80 years.[2] Age-related changes within the peripheral vascular system and myocardium are important to asses prior to any

anesthesia (Box 50-2). Changes in the peripheral vasculature include an increase in wall thickness and diameter and a stiffening of the aorta and large arteries.[9] These changes ultimately lead to a decrease in vasodilation of the systemic vasculature. Myocardial changes include an increase in left ventricular wall thickness, decreased myocardial compliance, and thickening of the aortic valve cusps, commonly heard as a midsystolic ejection murmur.[9] Left ventricular hypertrophy results from the related chronic increase in afterload to left ventricular ejection imposed by elevations in peripheral vascular resistance.

Impaired myocardial pump function and reduced cardiac output in the elderly prolong circulation time and decrease the perfusion of such vital organs as the brain, heart, and liver. Prolonged circulation time may delay the onset of drug effects. This in turn may be reflected in delayed induction time and slow onset of drug action. Backlund and colleagues noted no significant difference in cardiac output in response to exercise in elderly patients who were free of coronary artery disease and other complicating illnesses when compared with a population of younger patients.[13] Elderly patients, however, appear to be more dependent on an increase in end-diastolic volume than an increase in heart rate to produce an increase in cardiac output.[14] These factors make the geriatric patient more prone to congestive heart failure when large volumes of intravenous fluid are administered in the presence of anesthetic-induced myocardial depression and hypotension.

Variable degrees of myocardial fiber atrophy occur as the fibers become replaced by connective tissue during the aging process. Loss of elasticity also is seen throughout the arterial vasculature, along with progressive loss of arterial distensibility. Because increases in peripheral vascular resistance are greater than the decreases seen in cardiac output, and because blood vessels are poorly compliant, general systemic hypertension is common.

Replacement of elastic tissue by less resilient fibrous connective tissue also occurs in the coronary arteries. Coronary artery disease progressively increases in severity over the entire adult age span, but clinical symptoms may not be seen until a critical threshold is reached. The fact that coronary artery disease may be occult in many elderly patients should guide anesthetic patient care management in this population.

Cardiovascular function is altered with aging, even in the absence of arteriosclerotic, calcific, or hypertensive disease. The aging myocardium becomes thicker in both systole and diastole; an increase in the size and number of individual muscle fibers and

---

BOX **50-3**

Common Age-Related Pulmonary Anatomic and Physiologic Changes

- Increased lung compliance
- Decreased forced expiratory volume
- Increased closing volume
- Decreased resting arterial oxygen tension
- Increased alveolar-arterial difference
- Ventilation-perfusion mismatch
- Decreased functional residual capacity
- Decreased total lung capacity

BOX **50-4**

Common Age-Related Central Nervous System Anatomic and Physiologic Changes

- Decreased activity
- Decreased oxygen consumption
- Reduced number of functioning receptors
- Reduced production of neurotransmitters
- Neuron loss
- Decreased cerebral blood flow

---

in adipose tissue occurs. Atrial contraction, which normally produces 20% of the left ventricular end-diastolic volume, becomes even more important to the filling of these stiffer ventricles. Loss of the "atrial kick" in a nodal rhythm under anesthesia can cause a drop in systolic pressure.

Although the resting heart rate and heart response exercise loads in the elderly are similar to those seen in younger patients, the maximum heart rate that can be generated by an elderly patient is considerably lower. An age-related decrease in target-organ responsiveness to the regulation of chronotropic and inotropic cardiac function results from impaired quality of adrenergic receptors in the heart. As a result, catecholamine effects that enhance calcium ion transport in the myocardium and improve calcium ion availability are less pronounced in the elderly.[14,15]

Respiratory System

The effect of aging on the lung parenchyma can be described as a generalized reduction of elastic tissue and an increase in the amount of collagen. As a result, there is a 15% reduction of the functional alveolar surface area available for gas exchange by 70 years of age.[9] In elderly patients, even in the absence of disease, emphysema-like decreases in lung compliance impair the matching of ventilation and perfusion, physiologic shunt is increased, and the efficiency of oxygen exchange is reduced at the alveolar level (Box 50-3).

Functional efficiency also is impaired at the skeletal muscle level. A progressive decrease in forced expiratory volume in 1 second and forced vital capacity is caused by loss of elastic tissue around the alveoli and lung ducts. This loss of elasticity allows the alveoli to remain more distended at rest and less distensible at inspiration. The overall closing volume (i.e., the volume at which the small airways collapse) increases.[16] In the anesthetized elderly patient, closing capacity is much greater than functional residual capacity, more dependent airways are collapsed, and more of the tidal volume is distributed to areas of the lung that are less perfused. These changes manifest as atelectasis in the dependent lung areas.[9]

Total lung capacity declines approximately 10% by 70 years of age, reflecting a loss of height due to deterioration of intervertebral disks. Increased stiffness of the thoracic cage and progressive dorsal kyphosis are accompanied by upward and anterior rotation of the ribs and sternum, which leads to an increase in the anterior-to-posterior diameter of the chest and in restricted chest expansion.[16]

Other major contributors to the decline in gas exchange efficiency include a reduction in the surface area of the alveoli, an increase in the alveolocapillary membrane thickness, and a reduction in pulmonary capillary blood volume. As a result, resting arterial oxygen tension (PaO_2) normally declines with age in accordance with the following equation:

Equation 50-1

$$PaO_2 = 100 - (0.4 \text{ age [years]}) \text{ mm Hg}$$

The alveolar-arterial difference for oxygen increases from approximately 8 mm Hg at 20 years of age to more than 20 mm Hg at 70 years of age, and the PaO_2 decreases 0.5 mm Hg per year after 20 years of age.[17,18] Because of the changes in pulmonary function that occur with age, elderly patients must be observed closely after surgery and anesthesia to ensure that they do not develop hypoxia and hypercarbia in the postoperative period. In addition, members of this population may require higher inspired intraoperative concentrations of oxygen because of their lower PaO_2 values and reduced efficiency of gas exchange. The respiratory changes result in a higher incidence of mechanical ventilation, acute lung injury, a longer intensive care unit stay and high morbidity.[2]

Waugaman and Rigor[12] point out that the airway of the geriatric patient may present several challenges to the anesthetist during patient-care management. A progressive decrease in the reactivity of protective airway reflexes, such as coughing and swallowing, can be expected with aging secondary to diminished laryngeal and pharyngeal responses.[9] The risk of pulmonary aspiration is therefore increased. Because the elderly often are edentulous, a sealed fit with the anesthetic face mask may be difficult. These factors may increase the likelihood of regurgitation of gastric contents, with aspiration of vomitus into the lungs. The changes that accompany cervical arthritis and osteoarthritis, limiting extension and flexion of the neck, often make endotracheal intubation difficult.

Central Nervous System

The extent to which central nervous system (CNS) function declines with age is debated in the literature. On average, 30% of total brain mass is lost by 80 years of age.[9] It has been thought that aging is associated with a progressive decline in CNS activity and a loss of neurons, particularly in the cerebral cortex. The decreased CNS activity is related to a decrease in neuronal density, a decrease in cerebral metabolic oxygen consumption, a decrease in blood flow, a reduction in the number of receptor sites for neurotransmitter action, and a decrease in the rate of synthesis of neurotransmitters. Gradually the conduction velocity in peripheral nerves slows, and a reduction in the number of fibers in spinal cord tracts may occur (Box 50-4).[12,19]

Structural changes within the CNS are not automatically associated with a decline in cognitive function; however, postoperative delirium and cognitive dysfunction are higher in the elderly population.[9] Postoperative delirium and postoperative cognitive dysfunction are distinctly separate conditions.[20] *Postoperative delirium* is a transient and fluctuating disturbance of consciousness that occurs shortly after surgery. *Postoperative cognitive dysfunction* is a more persistent change in cognitive performance diagnosed by neuropsychological tests. Transient postoperative neurologic impairment was found to be as frequent as 44% to 61% in elderly patients undergoing orthopedic surgery.[21]

Postoperative delirium (PD) in the elderly leads to increased morbidity, delayed functional recovery, prolonged hospital stay, nursing home placement, and mortality.[22] PD tends to occur between postoperative day 1 and day 3 and usually resolves anywhere from hours to days. PD symptoms may persist for weeks to months. Patients at risk for postoperative delirium are listed in Box 50-5.[22] Sedative hypnotics, narcotics, and anticholinergics have been identified as the classes of drugs associated with PD.

Protocols have been developed with effective interventions to decrease PD. A study identified that the average additional in-hospital cost per surgical patient with PD was $2947, which equates to more than $2 billion additional health care dollars per year in the United States.[22] Haloperidol has been successfully used in the treatment of immediate agitation. Benzodiazepines tend to worsen agitation unless the cause of delirium has been identified as alcohol withdrawal.

The existence of an age-related decline in cerebral function does not appear to be conclusive. Much of the cognitive loss associated with aging may in fact be related to (1) the degree to which the elderly exercise their mental functions and (2) nutritional changes that occur as people age, rather than to the aging process itself. Cognitive loss may be preventable with better nutrition and stimulation of mental function in the elderly as a group.

Although the age-induced changes in CNS function remain controversial, the nervous system is the target organ for virtually every anesthetic agent administered to the patient. It is generally agreed that the geriatric patient has a reduced requirement for anesthetic agents. The variability of effect of the anesthetic agents may not be distinguishable in any given patient but has been observed between elderly patients and younger ones.[5,7]

Anesthetic requirements for the inhalation anesthetic agents decrease linearly with age as the minimum alveolar concentration (MAC) required falls. This applies not only to the inhalation agents but also to local anesthetics, opioids, barbiturates, benzodiazepines, and other intravenous agents. A comparable level of sedation at diazepam plasma concentrations significantly lower than that required for younger adults has been demonstrated in elderly patients.[23] Equivalent electroencephalographic suppression occurs at a lower plasma concentration of both fentanyl and alfentanil.[24]

Renal System

Aging has a profound effect on the renal vasculature and therefore exerts great influence on renal function (Box 50-6). The glomerular filtration rate decreases approximately 6% to 8% per decade. Although the ability to concentrate urine and conserve water is progressively impaired, reduction in plasma flow is the primary source of loss of renal function with age. Renal blood flow decreases 1% to 2% each year after the age of 25 and is decreased 40% to 50% by the age of 65 years.[25] Declines in renal blood flow are due to decreases in cardiac output that accompany aging, as well as to reductions in the size of the renal vascular bed.

Renal function is sufficient for gross azotemia or uremia to be avoided, but the renal functional reserve needed to withstand water and electrolyte imbalance in elderly patients is minimal. The combination of decreased renal and reduced cardiac function makes geriatric patients prone to fluid overload. In addition, renal elimination of drugs may be impaired.

Hepatobiliary System

Hepatic blood flow decreases with age, paralleling reductions in cardiac output; nevertheless, hepatocellular function changes little. In normal individuals, microsomal activity and nonmicrosomal activity appear well preserved, although some evidence suggests that plasma clearance of drugs known to be extensively metabolized in the liver is reduced (Box 50-7).[26]

The effect of an age-associated reduction of hepatic blood flow and a potential reduction in microsomal enzyme function impairs the liver's ability to metabolize anesthetics and nondepolarizing neuromuscular blocking agents. Reduced liver function, combined with the reduced filtration and excretory capacity of the aging kidney, results in a gradual decline in the plasma concentration of drugs and may contribute to a prolonged duration of drug effect.

Common Age-Related Endocrine Anatomic and Physiologic Changes

- Decreased pancreatic function
- Increased incidence of diabetes
- Decreased tolerance to glucose load

TABLE **50-1**	Age-Related Changes and Pharmacokinetics
Change	**Effect**
Contracted vascular volume	High initial plasma concentration
Decreased protein binding	Increased availability of free drug
Increased total body lipid storage sites	Prolonged action of lipid-soluble drugs
Decreased renal and hepatic blood flow	Prolonged action of drugs dependent on kidney and liver elimination

Endocrine System

Pancreatic function declines during aging, and the incidence of diabetes mellitus increases as the ability to metabolize glucose load becomes impaired. Elderly patients have demonstrated an age-related increase in postprandial blood glucose levels. Mechanisms responsible for these alterations include a sluggish liberation of insulin in response to hyperglycemia and resistance to the effects of insulin at peripheral sites (Box 50-8).[27,28]

Because insulin responsiveness varies from patient to patient, the anesthetist may be required to include the administration of exogenous insulin as part of perioperative patient care management. In addition, because intolerance to a glucose load is common, limitation of the administration of intravenous solutions that contain glucose also may be required for many surgical patients. Frequent intraoperative evaluation of blood glucose levels may be beneficial in the estimation of a patient's status.

Metabolic Rate

Maintaining normothermia during a general anesthetic in the elderly patient is difficult because of a decrease in metabolic rate associated with aging. Hypothermia may lead to slower metabolism and excretion of drugs

PHARMACOKINETIC AND PHARMACODYNAMIC CONSIDERATIONS

The term *pharmacokinetics* of anesthetic agents used during patient care management refers to the physiologic processes of drug absorption, tissue distribution, metabolism, and elimination. Plasma protein binding, the percentage of lean and fat body mass, and circulating blood volume have an effect on pharmacokinetics. *Pharmacodynamics* refers to the relationship between drug quantity and drug effect. Physiologic changes occur during aging that affect the disposition and clearance of pharmacologic agents and the typical dose-response relationship produced. However, it is important to remember that the circumstances in which pharmacodynamics and pharmacokinetics interact reflect significant variability among patients.

Pharmacokinetics

The disposition and clearance of pharmacologic agents employed during anesthetic patient care management are characterized by age-related changes. However, the extent to which each process changes with age is debated in the literature.

Lee[29] points out that a reduction in plasma concentration in the elderly may produce clinically important changes in the amount of unbound drug in plasma after intravenous administration. The role that aging has in modifying the oral or parenteral uptake of drugs also is important. Changes in vascular volume, plasma protein binding, the percentage of body mass that is adipose or lean tissue, and the efficiency of metabolism and

elimination of drugs are likely to affect an individual patient's response to anesthetic agents (Table 50-1).

The relatively contracted blood volume of the elderly patient leads to higher than expected initial plasma drug levels after the administration of standard doses of drugs on the basis of calculated body weight. A reduced plasma protein-binding capacity results in an increase in the amount of the free form of drug able to penetrate the blood-brain barrier. Significant increase in total body adipose tissue into which lipid-soluble drugs must be dispersed prolongs elimination, because the volume of drug that must be cleared is increased. Drug disposition also is altered as a result of reduced renal and hepatic function, slowing the elimination of drugs cleared through these pathways.

Pharmacodynamics

Pharmacodynamic factors determine the relationship between the concentration of the drug at the site of action and the intensity of the effect produced. Although the exact mechanisms responsible have not been clearly described, a reduced need for anesthetic drugs, including reduced MAC requirements of the volatile anesthetic agents, is well established in the elderly. Possible responsible mechanisms elucidated are reductions in brain mass, absolute brain blood flow, and the number of neurons and axons in the CNS and peripheral nervous system. In addition, neurotransmitter activity and nervous system functional reserve also may be involved.

Clinically, the induction dose of barbiturates is reduced 30% to 40% in members of the geriatric population, compared with younger patients. The sensitivity may be explained on the basis of a higher plasma concentration after administration of barbiturates. Similarly, the dose of propofol required for induction is reduced. Significant hypotension may be seen if standard induction doses are administered.

The MAC of potent inhalation anesthetic agents decreases with age by approximately 4% for each decade of life after the age of 40. The age-related CNS changes discussed previously emphasize the pharmacodynamic correlation between cerebral metabolic function and anesthetic requirements for the potent inhalation anesthetic agents.[30] In addition, the contemporary inhalation anesthetic agents undergo little metabolism, have low solubility in blood, and produce less depression of myocardial contractility and left ventricular ejection fraction; these characteristics may make them well suited for use in elderly patients.

Because nondepolarizing muscle relaxants are usually highly polarized, relatively fat insoluble, and dependent on urinary excretion for elimination (with the exception of cisatracurium), a reduction in clearance and increased elimination half-life are seen in elderly patients. No significant age-related changes have been found for cisatracurium. Succinylcholine may produce a longer effect in elderly men, because they appear to have a median effective dose that is significantly less than that in younger patients, as well as reduced levels of plasma cholinesterase.[31]

PREOPERATIVE ASSESSMENT

Preparing a plan of anesthetic management for the geriatric patient requires that the anesthetist consider factors that may influence patient outcome. Those factors discussed previously include the anatomic and physiologic changes that occur with aging and the pharmacokinetic and pharmacodynamic processes that affect uptake, distribution, elimination, and the end-organ effect of pharmacologic agents used during the anesthetic procedure. In addition, the anesthetist must tailor the anesthetic plan according to individual patient needs and predispositions, especially taking into account the effect of concomitant diseases (Box 50-9).

Patient History and Physical Examination

Even for a minor procedure, information pertinent to the history and status of the patient should be obtained directly from the patient, the patient's family, and others involved in caregiving. It is not uncommon to find patients who are reluctant to ask the anesthetist questions because of cultural predispositions or who are unable because of anxiety to understand questions asked of them. In addition, elderly patients may be unable to clearly hear the questions posed to them.

Current Medications

It should be determined what prescription and over-the-counter medications the patient is currently receiving. It is likely that the geriatric patient is taking several different medications that have the potential to affect or interact with pharmacologic agents used during the anesthetic process. Medications frequently taken by elderly patients include diuretics, antihypertensives, β-adrenergic antagonists, cardiac antidysrhythmics, digitalis, tricyclic antidepressants, antibiotics, oral hypoglycemics, nonopioid and nonsteroidal analgesics, antiinflammatory medications, antibiotics, and alcohol.[13] Nonopioid and nonsteroidal analgesics and antiinflammatory medications may prolong bleeding time, produce renal and hepatic dysfunction, and precipitate allergic reactions. Diuretics may result in hypokalemia and hypovolemia. β-Adrenergic antagonists may decrease autonomic nervous system activity, decrease anesthetic requirements, and result in bronchospasm and bradycardia. Sympathomimetics with β-adrenergic agonist effects, as well as pancuronium, may increase the likelihood of cardiac dysrhythmias in the presence of cardiac glycosides. Patients being treated with antihypertensive agents may display attenuated sympathetic activity and a modified response to sympathomimetic drugs and sedation.[30] Cardiac antidysrhythmics may potentiate neuromuscular blocking agents. Digitalis may result in cardiac dysrhythmias and cardiac conduction disturbances. Tricyclic antidepressants may result in anticholinergic effects. Antibiotics may potentiate neuromuscular blocking agents. It is important to ask about medication use during the review of systems; patients may fail to respond positively to a general question about what medications they use but may respond affirmatively, for example, to a direct question asking if they use eye drops. As a guideline, all antihypertensive and cardiac medications should be continued until surgery, with the exception of diuretics.[9] Some of the literature, however, states that angiotensin-converting enzyme (ACE) inhibitors

---

> ### BOX **50-9**
> #### Common Coexisting Diseases in Elderly Patients
> - Systemic hypertension
> - Coronary artery disease
> - Congestive heart failure
> - Peripheral vascular disease
> - Chronic obstructive pulmonary disease
> - Anemia
> - Renal disease
> - Liver disease
> - Diabetes mellitus
> - Arthritis
> - Dementia

and angiotensin-receptor antagonists should be discontinued prior to surgery.[32] The benefits versus risks must be taken into consideration for those patients taking aspirin or warfarin. In the case of an emergency, fresh frozen plasma or vitamin K may be given to reverse the effects of warfarin.[9]

Laboratory Results

Requests for specific laboratory data depend on the patient's overall state of health, nutritional status, and current drug regimen. The extent and duration of surgery and anesthesia also should be considered. Patients who have chronic diseases, such as diabetes mellitus and hypertension, may require electrolyte and glucose screening.

Cardiac Evaluation

In patients with chronic obstructive pulmonary disease and coronary artery disease, chest radiography and electrocardiography may be appropriate. Although not the overriding factor, a cost-benefit balance must be reached between "routine" laboratory screening tests and tests performed for recognizable indications. It is important to note that researchers continue to debate which screening tests are integral components of the assessment of the elderly patient and how they affect outcome.[33]

ANESTHETIC MANAGEMENT
Perioperative Period
Premedication

Much controversy exists regarding the use of premedication in the geriatric population. After careful patient assessment has been performed, if a patient requires anxiety relief, administration of medication should be guided by the pharmacokinetic and pharmacodynamic concepts discussed previously in this chapter. Unwanted confusion, agitation, and prolonged duration of action may develop after administration of benzodiazepines because of their sedative-anxiolytic properties. The hepatic clearance of midazolam, for example, is decreased in the elderly, and the elimination half-life is 6 hours, compared with 2 hours in younger patients.[24] Reduced dose requirements are necessary for preventing these centrally active sedatives and analgesics from producing a prolonged effect.[4]

Many advocate the routine administration of prophylactic oral antacids to all patients in whom general anesthesia is anticipated, because elderly patients may be at increased risk for aspiration pneumonitis as a result of decreased reactivity of the protective airway reflexes, increased gastric residual volume, and dysfunction of the lower esophageal sphincter. Others note that healthy geriatric patients are not at an increased aspiration risk, and administration of multiple unnecessary drugs should be discouraged.[34]

Monitoring

All standard noninvasive monitors should be used in the elderly surgical patient. Standard noninvasive monitors include electrocardiogram (ECG), pulse oximetry, temperature and blood pressure measurement, and end-tidal CO_2 determination. Studies report that placement of an arterial line or central venous catheter may allow for earlier recognition and treatment of intraoperative problems and lower the incidence of morbidity and mortality, particularly for major surgical procedures. Other researchers question whether the use of invasive monitors has any effect on patient outcome overall, because definitive studies of patient outcome have not been conclusive.[35]

Anesthetic Technique

As with the selection and administration of preoperative medication, the choice of anesthetic technique should be based on the changes in organ system function in the patient, the pharmacokinetic and pharmacodynamic effects anticipated, the surgical requirements, and the needs and predisposition of the patient. As a rule, the geriatric patient is likely to be predisposed to hypotension due to reduced activity of the sympathetic nervous system and decreased intravascular volume. Decreased cardiac output and delayed drug clearance are likely to prolong the onset of drug effects and prolong the duration of action.

Regional, general, and MAC techniques are appropriate selections for the geriatric patient. The use of shorter-acting anesthetic and analgesic drugs may contribute to less postoperative cognitive impairment and confusion in elderly patients.[21] No conclusive study has demonstrated the superiority of any one specific anesthetic technique. In one study, however, elderly patients were found to recover faster and earlier with desflurane than sevoflurane after total knee or hip replacement procedures, although postoperative recovery of cognitive function was similar for both volatile anesthetics.[21] With regional and local techniques, maintenance of consciousness during the surgical procedure may be associated with less confusion during the postoperative period.

The past few years have seen significant increases in gastroenterology and gastrointestinal endoscopy procedures. More and more hospitals and outpatient surgical facilities are seeing patients for endoscopic therapy. The rate of hospitalization resulting from complications of cholelithiasis has doubled in the elderly over the past 30 years.[36] Patients' expectations include "painless" endoscopy, but anesthesia providers must keep in mind that oversedation in the elderly population can produce respiratory depression and delayed recovery, especially for those with cardiovascular and or pulmonary dysfunction. Safe guidelines for sedation for endoscopic procedures in the elderly population include a lower dose titrated slowly to effect.

Inhalation Agents

Minimum alveolar concentration (MAC) for inhaled anesthetics is decreased by approximately 6% per year after 40 years of age.[9] Inhalation agents cause a larger decrease in blood pressure in elderly patients as compared with younger patients, so the rate of induction should be slow.[9]

Intravenous Anesthetic Agents

Propofol and etomidate are commonly used general anesthetic induction agents. Decreased dose requirements or slow titration of propofol is recommended in the elderly population[9] because this agent may result in dramatic decreases in systemic blood pressure. With respect to cognitive function, propofol may offer a quicker recovery. Etomidate is used as an induction agent for patients with cardiovascular instability.

Narcotics

Elderly patients have a decreased volume of distribution and protein binding that decreases their requirement for narcotics.[10] Elimination half-life is prolonged, resulting in depressed ventilation and prolonged analgesia, and decreased hepatic clearance may prolong the effects of narcotics.[9] Meperidine protein binding decreases with increasing age, thereby generating more unbound drug.

Neuromuscular Blocking Agents

Current literature states the effects of depolarizing and nondepolarizing neuromuscular blocking agents are not altered in the elderly.[9] Some believe the elderly should only be given short- and intermediate-acting neuromuscular blocking agents for cases in which extubation is planned.[10]

Regional Anesthesia versus General Anesthesia

Most agree that the anesthetic plan for the elderly population should remain as simple as possible. In the 1980s, studies suggested that general anesthetics placed patients at a higher risk for postoperative cognitive dysfunction. More recent studies have concluded that choice of anesthesia does not influence the incidence of postoperative cognitive dysfunction.[22] The conclusion of another study found that the use of 8% sevoflurane on induction was associated with less frequent apnea and hypotension as compared with a propofol induction.[37]

Challenges in the Postanesthesia Care Unit

Postoperative complications in the elderly population are often related to cardiac and pulmonary dysfunction and decreased reserves. Monitoring with a pulse oximeter may permit detection of the need for supplemental oxygenation or ventilation during the postoperative period, because ventilation-perfusion mismatch is common in geriatric patients. The elderly patient may be especially prone to regurgitation and aspiration from a reduction in airway reflexes. Rapid response on the part of anesthesia and postanesthesia care unit staff to changes in patient status is especially important for the prevention of rapid deterioration.

In addition, renal and hepatic dysfunction may prolong the duration of action of pharmacologic agents administered to the patient. It is not uncommon to find ventilatory depression from the presence of residual anesthetic during the postoperative period. Postoperatively the patient may be less able to handle the fluid load administered during surgery and should be observed for signs of congestive failure.

The elderly patient also is prone to postoperative heat loss. To ensure rewarming and prevent problems associated with shivering, the patient should be placed in a warmed environment.

Finally, the geriatric patient may require special assistance in being oriented to time and place. Prolonged anesthetic effect may compound disorientation to an unfamiliar environment.

Development and implementation of a plan of anesthetic management for the geriatric patient must reflect an appreciation of the fact that the geriatric patient who undergoes surgery and anesthesia may be at increased risk for perioperative morbidity and mortality as a result of continuous physiologic aging processes and concomitant diseases. A thorough understanding of these changes, their effect on the anesthetic process, and variability among the cohort are essential components of continuous quality improvement directed toward decreasing morbidity and mortality in this ever-growing patient population.

SUMMARY

As noted in this chapter, there are numerous medical challenges unique to the geriatric patient. As the population ages, we will encounter an ever-increasing number of geriatric patients requiring surgical procedures. A large percentage of our daily practice will encompass the anesthesia management of this special population. Guiding the elderly patient through the perioperative period is a rewarding part of our care.

REFERENCES

1. Greenberg S. *A Profile of Older Americans: 2006.* Washington, DC: U.S. Department of Health and Human Services Administration on Aging; 2006:1-16.
2. Lewis M et al. Geriatric trauma: special considerations in the anesthetic management of the injured elderly patient. *Anesthesiol Clin.* 2007;25:75-90.
3. Beliveau MM, Multach M. Perioperative care for the elderly patient. *Med Clin North Am.* 2003;87:273-289.
4. Rooke G, Reves J. Anesthesiology and geriatric medicine: mutual needs and opportunities. *Anesthesiology.* 2002;96:2-4.
5. Calabrese V et al. Mitochondrial involvement in brain function and dysfunction: relevance to aging, neurogenic disorders and longevity. *Neurochem Res.* 2001;26:739-764.
6. Muravchick S. Preoperative assessment of the elderly patient. *Anesthesiol Clin North America.* 2000;18:71-89.
7. Kirkbride DA et al. Induction of anesthesia in the elderly ambulatory patient: a double-blinded comparison of propofol and sevoflurane. *Anesth Analg.* 2001;93:1185-1187.
8. Monarch S, Wren K. Geriatric anesthesia implications. *J Perianesth Nurs.* 2004;19:379-384.
9. Leung J. Elderly patients. In: Stoelting R Miller R, eds. *Basics of Anesthesia.* 5th ed. Philadelphia: Churchill Livingstone; 2007:518.
10. Sophie S. Anaesthesia for the elderly patient. *J Pak Med Assoc.* 2007;57: 196-201.
11. Nesher N et al. A new thermoregulation system for maintaining perioperative normothermia and attenuating myocardial injury in off-pump coronary artery bypass surgery. *Heart Surg Forum.* 2002;5:373-380.
12. Waugaman W, Rigor B. Geriatrics in anesthesia. In: Waugaman WR et al, eds. *Principles and Practice of Nurse Anesthesia.* 3rd ed. Norwalk, CT: Appleton & Lange; 1999:283.
13. Backlund M et al. Factors associated with post-operative myocardial ischaemia in elderly patients undergoing major non-cardiac surgery. *Eur J Anaesthesiol.* 1999;16:826-833.
14. Rooke GA. Autonomic and cardiovascular function in the geriatric patient. *Anesthesiol Clin North America.* 2000;18:31-51.
15. Priebe HJ. The aged cardiovascular risk patient. *Br J Anaesth.* 2001;86: 897-898.
16. Zaugg M, Lucchinetti E. Respiratory function in the elderly. *Anesthesiol Clin North America.* 2000;18:47-58.
17. Raine J, Bishop M. Differences in O_2 tension and physiologic dead space in normal man. *J Appl Physiol.* 1963;18:284-288.
18. Kitamura H et al. Postoperative hypoxemia: the contribution of age to the maldistribution of ventilation. *Anesthesiology.* 1972;36:244-252.
19. Rasmussen LS, Moller JT. Central nervous system dysfunction in the geriatric patient. *Anesthesiol Clin North America.* 2000;18:59-70.
20. Newman S et al. Postoperative cognitive dysfunction after noncardiac surgery. *Anesthesiology.* 2007;106:572-589.
21. Chen X et al. The recovery of cognitive function after general anesthesia in elderly patients: a comparison of desflurane and sevoflurane. *Anesth Analg.* 2001;93:1489-94.
22. Silverstein J et al. Central nervous system dysfunction after noncardiac surgery and anesthesia in the elderly. *Anesthesiology.* 2007;106:622-628.
23. Bjorkman S et al. Prediction of the disposition of midazolam in surgical patients by a physiologically based pharmacokinetic model. *J Pharm Sci.* 2001;90:1226-1241.
24. Shafer SL. The pharmacology of anesthetic drugs in elderly patients. *Anesthesiol Clin North America.* 2000;18:1-29.
25. Kumle B et al. The influence of different intravascular volume replacement regimens on renal function in the elderly. *Anesth Analg.* 1999;89:1124-1130.
26. Suttner SW et al. Low-flow desflurane and sevoflurane anesthesia minimally affect hepatic integrity and function in elderly patients. *Anesth Analg.* 2000;91:206-212.
27. Bailes BK. Hypothyroidism in the elderly. *AORN J.* 1999;69:1026-1030.
28. Bailes BK. Hyperthyroidism in the elderly. *AORN J.* 1999;69:254-258.
29. Lee M. Drugs in the elderly: do you know the risks? *Am J Nurs.* 1996;96:25-31.
30. Stoelting R, Hillier SC. *Pharmacology and Physiology in Anesthesia Practice.* 4th ed. Philadelphia: Lippincott Williams & Wilkins; 2006:42-86.
31. Jones AG, Hunter JM. Anaesthesia in the elderly, special considerations. *Drugs Aging.* 1996;9:319-331.
32. Bruessel T. Co-medications, pre-medication and common diseases in the elderly. *Best Pract Res Clin Anaesthesiol.* 2003;17:179-190.
33. Muravchick S. Preoperative assessment of the elderly patient. *Anesthesiol Clin North America.* 2000;18:71-89.
34. Nagelhout JJ. Aspiration prophylaxis: is it time for changes in our practice? *AANA J.* 2003;71:299-303.
35. O'Hara DA et al. The effect of anesthetic technique on postoperative outcomes in hip fracture repair. *Anesthesiology.* 2000;92:947-957.
36. Ladas S et al. Ethical issues in endoscopy: patient satisfaction, safety in elderly patients, palliation, and relations with industry. *Endoscopy.* 2007;39:556-565.
37. Shao G, Zhang G. Comparison of propofol and sevoflurane for laryngeal mask airway insertion in elderly patients. *South Med J.* 2007;100:360-365.

CHAPTER 51

POSTANESTHESIA RECOVERY

Jan Odom-Forren

The term *perianesthesia patient care* reflects a continuum of care, because the patient is moved from the preanesthesia holding or admitting area to the operating room (OR) and then to the postanesthesia care unit (PACU). *Postanesthesia recovery* refers to those activities undertaken to manage the patient after completion of a surgical or nonsurgical procedure in which anesthesia, analgesia, or sedation was administered. The primary purpose of postanesthesia recovery is critical assessment and stabilization of patients after these procedures, with an emphasis on prevention and detection of complications.[1] Care in the postanesthesia Phase I unit focuses on providing postanesthesia nursing care and transitioning the patient to the intensive care setting, the surgical floor setting, or Phase II outpatient care.[2] The focus of this chapter is on the postanesthesia care of patients with the goals of improving postanesthetic safety and quality of life, reducing postoperative adverse events, providing a uniform assessment of recovery, and streamlining postoperative care and discharge criteria.

POSTANESTHESIA CARE UNIT ADMISSION

Before the patient is transferred, PACU personnel should be notified not only to expect the transfer but also to have any necessary equipment (e.g., ventilator, nebulizer, invasive monitoring equipment, pharmacologic infusions) ready and waiting. Knowledge of the patient's acuity enables the PACU staff to best plan the patient's care and assign that care to an appropriately experienced practitioner.

Both the anesthesia provider and the PACU nurse should collaborate in the patient's admission to the PACU. The immediate priority is evaluation of respiratory and circulatory adequacy. During this initial assessment, any signs of inadequate oxygenation or ventilation are identified (Boxes 51-1 and 51-2). Although many of the signs of respiratory compromise could have multifactorial explanations, assessment of the adequacy of oxygenation and ventilation ensures that respiratory inadequacy is not contributory. Any evidence of respiratory compromise requires immediate correction.

Electrocardiographic (ECG) monitoring is initiated for determination of cardiac rate and rhythm. Any deviation from preoperative or intraoperative findings is noted and evaluated. Also, blood pressure is measured, and adequacy of organ perfusion is determined (Box 51-3). Any invasive monitoring, such as an arterial line, is initiated. Any evidence of cardiocirculatory compromise requires immediate correction.

The anesthesia provider should be active during the patient's transfer and stabilization in the PACU. Assistance in the initiation of oxygen therapy, maintenance or verification of airway adequacy, and assessment of circulatory status familiarizes PACU personnel with the patient and fosters a smooth transfer of care. After initially stabilizing the patient, the anesthesia provider can communicate relevant preoperative and intraoperative data to the PACU nurse.

ANESTHESIA REPORT

To ensure patient safety and continuity of care, the anesthesia provider must give a verbal report to the PACU nurse that specifies the details of the surgical and anesthetic course, the preoperative conditions that warrant or influence the surgical and anesthetic outcome, and the PACU treatment plan, including suggested interventions and end-points. Transfer of the patient from the OR to the PACU is a critical patient handoff and should include an opportunity for the PACU nurse to ask questions and the anesthesia provider to respond.[3] A coherent order for the presentation of this information is presented in Box 51-4.

The importance of the anesthesia report is reflected in the American Association of Nurse Anesthetists (AANA) guideline from the AANA *Scope and Standards for Nurse Anesthesia Practice*: "Standard VII: Transfer the responsibility for care of the patient to other qualified providers in a manner which assures continuity of care and patient safety."[4] The American Society of Anesthesiologists (ASA) point to the importance of a verbal report to the responsible PACU nurse but also go on to state, "The member of the Anesthesia Care Team shall remain in the PACU until the PACU nurse accepts responsibility for the nursing care of the patient."[5]

INITIAL POSTANESTHESIA CARE UNIT ASSESSMENT

Many postanesthesia assessment approaches (e.g., head-to-toe, major body systems assessments and scoring systems) are currently used in PACUs, and each approach has its benefits and limitations. The assessment approach should accomplish the following:

1. Determine the patient's physiologic status at the time of admission to the PACU
2. Allow the periodic reexamination of the patient so that physiologic trends become obvious
3. Establish the patient's baseline level so that the effect of previous medical conditions can be assessed and predicted as they affect current physiology
4. Assess the ongoing status of the surgical site and its effect on any preexisting conditions and recovery
5. Assess the patient's recovery from anesthesia and note residual effects

BOX 51-1

Signs and Symptoms of Inadequate Oxygenation

Central Nervous System
Restlessness, agitation, confusion, coma
Muscular twitches or seizures

Cardiovascular System
Hypertension, tachycardia (sympathetic nervous system mediated)
Hypotension, bradycardia (direct hypoxic effect)
Dysrhythmias

Skin
Cyanosis (absent in severe anemia and vasoconstriction)
Poor capillary refill

Pulmonary System
Increased to absent respiratory efforts
Decreased Pao_2*
Oximetry saturation <90%

Modified from Litwack K. Immediate postoperative care: a problem-oriented approach. In: Vender J, Spiess B, eds. Post-Anesthesia Care. Philadelphia: Saunders; 1992:2.
Pao_2, *Partial pressure of arterial oxygen.*
*Not standard practice to obtain during initial assessment.

BOX 51-3

Signs of Adequate Organ Perfusion

Central Nervous System
Appropriate mentation
Intact sensation, motor function, reflexes
Electroencephalographic and evoked potential results appropriate for residual anesthetic exposure*

Cardiovascular System
Electrocardiography shows normal sinus rhythm without signs of ischemia
Cardiac output appropriate for preload and metabolic acuity*

Skin
Warm and dry with good color and capillary refill

Renal System
Urine production >0.5 mL/kg/hr (of appropriate specific gravity and composition)*
No evidence of osmotic diuresis
No evidence of postobstructive diuresis

Pulmonary System
Normal arterial blood gas results*
Normal intrapulmonary shunt activity*

Modified from Litwack K. Immediate postoperative care: a problem-oriented approach. In: Vender J, Spiess B, eds. Post-Anesthesia Care. Philadelphia: Saunders; 1992:2.
*Not standard practice to obtain during initial assessment.

BOX 51-2

Signs and Symptoms of Inadequate Ventilation

Spontaneous Ventilation
Increased or decreased respiratory frequency
Nasal flaring
Suprasternal or intercostal retractions
Decreased to absent movement of air at mouth, nares, or endotracheal tube
Abnormal airway sounds
Decreased to absent breath sounds
Diminished chest movement
Diaphragmatic breathing
Abnormal $ETCO_2$ or $Paco_2$ values*
Signs of inadequate oxygenation (see Box 51-1)

Assisted or Controlled Ventilation
Increased frequency of respiratory efforts
Decreased chest expansion and contraction during ventilatory cycle
Abnormally high inflation pressures
Decreased to absent air movements in endotracheal tube
Decreased to absent breath sounds
Decreased air movement as assessed by monitors (apnea, capnography)
Abnormal $ETCO_2$ or $Paco_2$ values*
Signs of inadequate oxygenation (see Box 51-1)

Modified from Litwack K. Immediate postoperative care: a problem-oriented approach. In: Vender J, Spiess B, eds. Post-Anesthesia Care. Philadelphia: Saunders; 1992:2.
$ETCO_2$, *End-tidal carbon dioxide;* $Paco_2$, *partial pressure of arterial carbon dioxide.*
*Not standard practice to obtain during initial assessment.

BOX 51-4

Anesthesia Admission Report

General Information
Patient name
Patient age
Surgical procedure
Name of surgeon and anesthesia provider(s)
Type of procedure

Patient History
Acute (indication for surgery)
Chronic (medical history, medication use, allergies)

Intraoperative Management
Anesthetic agents, including dose and technique
Time of last opioid administration
Use of reversal agents
Intraoperative medications (antibiotics, antiemetics, vasopressors)
Estimated blood loss
Fluid and blood administration
Urine output

Intraoperative Course
Unexpected response to anesthetic administration
Unexpected surgical course
Laboratory results (arterial blood gas, glucose, hemoglobin)

Postanesthesia Care Unit Plan
Potential and expected problems
Suggested interventions
Limits of acceptability of laboratory tests
Discharge criteria
Responsible contact person

BOX 51-5

Postanesthesia Recovery Score

Activity

0 = Unable to lift head or move extremities voluntarily or on command.

1 = Moves two extremities voluntarily or on command and can lift head.

2 = Able to move four extremities voluntarily or on command. Can lift head and has controlled movement. Exceptions: patients with a prolonged block such as with bupivacaine (Marcaine), who may not move an affected extremity for as long as 18 hours; patients who were immobile preoperatively.

Respiration

0 = Apneic; condition necessitates ventilator or assisted respiration.

1 = Labored or limited respirations. Breathes by self but has shallow, slow respirations. May have an oral airway.

2 = Can take a deep breath and cough well; has normal respiratory rate and depth.

Circulation

0 = Has abnormally high or low blood pressure; blood pressure within 50 mm Hg of preanesthetic level

1 = Blood pressure within 20-50 mm Hg of preanesthetic level

2 = Stable blood pressure and pulse. Blood pressure 20 mm Hg of preanesthetic level (minimum 90 mm Hg systolic). Exception: patient may be released by anesthesia provider after drug therapy.

Neurologic Status

0 = Not responding or responding only to painful stimuli.

1 = Responds to verbal stimuli but drifts to sleep easily.

2 = Awake and alert; oriented to time, place, and person.

O_2 Saturation

0 = O_2 saturation <90%, even with O_2 supplement

1 = Needs O_2 inhalation to maintain O_2 saturation >90%

2 = Able to maintain O_2 saturation >92% on room air

Modified from Aldrete J, Kroulik D. A post anesthetic recovery score. Anesth Analg. 1970;49:924-933; Aldrete JA. Discharge criteria. Bailliere's Clin Anaesthesiol. 1994;8:763-773; and DeFazio Quinn D. Management and policies. In: Drain CB, Odom-Forren J, eds. Perianesthesia Nursing: A Critical Care Approach. 5th ed. St Louis: Saunders; 2009:32-42.

6. Prevent or immediately treat complications that occur

7. Provide a safe environment for the patient who is impaired either physically, mentally, or emotionally

8. Allow the compilation and trend analysis of patient-specific characteristics that relate to discharge or transfer criteria[6,7]

Anesthesia personnel must assist in management of the patient until PACU providers secure admission vital signs and attach appropriate monitors. To optimize safety, the anesthesia provider cannot shift responsibility to PACU personnel until the patient's airway status, ventilation, and hemodynamics are appropriate.

Aldrete Scoring System

The most commonly used assessment approach is a combination of the Aldrete scoring system[8] and the major body systems assessment. The Aldrete scoring system evaluates the patient's activity, respiration, circulation, consciousness, and oxygen saturation level (Box 51-5). Patients receive a numeric score of 0, 1, or 2 in each area, with 2 representing the highest level of function. The Aldrete postanesthetic scoring system is the most widely used scoring system in PACUs, although its predictive value in determining recovery from anesthesia has not been studied prospectively.

Major Body Systems

The major body systems assessment systematically evaluates the body systems that are most affected by anesthesia and the surgical procedure. After the patient is admitted to the PACU, an assessment of cardiorespiratory stability and a more in-depth cardiac assessment are performed. Respiratory assessment comprises rate, depth of ventilation, auscultation of breath sounds, and oxygen saturation level. Type of oxygen delivery system and presence of any artificial airway should be noted.[9] The heart is auscultated, and the quality of heart sounds, the presence of any adventitious sounds, and any irregularities in rate or rhythm are noted. Unexpected findings are compared with preoperative data. Arterial pulses are evaluated for strength and equality. An ECG strip is obtained on admission to the PACU and compared with the preoperative ECG. In addition, body temperature and skin color and condition are assessed and the findings documented.

After respiratory and cardiac assessments are completed, the neurologic system is evaluated, with a focus on the level of consciousness, orientation, sensory and motor status, and pupil size, equality, and reactivity.

The renal system assessment focuses on fluid intake and output (blood, crystalloids, and colloids), as well as on volume and electrolyte status. The anesthesia provider relates intraoperative fluid totals in the verbal report, and the PACU nurse notes and documents all intravenous (IV) lines, irrigation solutions, and infusions that enter the patient. All output devices, including drains, catheters, and tubes, are inspected, and the color and consistency of any drainage are noted.

The surgical site is examined. The amount and color of any drainage on the bandage are noted. The patient is also assessed for pain or discomfort, such as nausea, with appropriate interventions.

All data obtained in the admission assessment should be documented in a manner that facilitates data collection, trend analysis, and retrieval. Recommended criteria for the initial assessment of a patient in the PACU are included in Box 51-6.

ONGOING ASSESSMENT

Perioperative and postanesthetic management of the patient includes periodic assessment and monitoring of the following[5]:

- Respiratory function (e.g., obstruction, hypoxemia, hypercarbia)
- Cardiovascular function (e.g., hypotension, hypertension, dysrhythmias)
- Neuromuscular function (e.g., inadequate reversal of neuromuscular blockade)
- Mental status (e.g., delayed awakening, emergence delirium)
- Pain
- Temperature (e.g., hypothermia)

The goal for the relief of a tongue obstruction is a patent airway. Treatment consists of a series of interventions. The initial intervention may be as simple as stimulating the patient to take deep breaths, or it may require repositioning of the airway via a jaw thrust or a chin lift. Placement of an oral or a nasal airway may be required. The nasal airway is tolerated much better by patients emerging from general anesthesia, and unlike the oral airway, it is unlikely to cause gagging or vomiting. If the obstruction remains unrelieved, reintubation may be required, with or without adjunctive mechanical ventilation.

Laryngeal obstruction may occlude the airway as a result of partial or complete spasm of the intrinsic or extrinsic muscles of the larynx. Laryngospasm may be the result of a reflex closure of the glottis (intrinsic muscles) or the larynx (extrinsic muscles).[10] Glottic closure usually manifests as intermittent obstruction; laryngeal closure manifests as complete obstruction. Airway irritation that predisposes a patient to laryngospasm may be the result of laryngoscopy, secretions, vomitus, blood, artificial airway placement, coughing, bronchospasm, or frequent suctioning. Symptoms that suggest laryngospasm include agitation, decreased oxygen saturation, absent breath sounds, and acute respiratory distress. Incomplete obstruction may manifest as a crowing sound or stridor.

Treatment of laryngospasm must be immediate. Positive-pressure ventilation with 100% oxygen is the initial intervention. If this intervention is ineffective, a subparalytic dose of IV succinylcholine (0.1 mg/kg) may be given. If succinylcholine is administered, assisted ventilation for 5 to 10 minutes is required, even if the obstruction has been relieved. Reintubation should be performed only if severe airway edema is present or if the obstruction persists despite treatment interventions. During the crisis, the anesthesia provider should consider medication for sedation, such as midazolam, to alleviate high anxiety of an awake or partially awake patient.

Steroids and topical or IV lidocaine have been included in the prevention and management of airway irritability. Other preventive strategies include obtaining meticulous hemostasis during surgery, suctioning the oropharynx before extubation to clear any retained blood or secretions, and extubating the patient when he or she is in either a very deep plane of anesthesia or the awake state.[10] When obstruction occurs, rapid intervention is imperative because the arterial carbon dioxide pressure ($PaCO_2$) increases 6 mm Hg in the first minute of total obstruction and an additional 3 to 4 mm Hg each minute thereafter.[11]

Hypoxemia

Hypoxemia, defined as low arterial oxygen pressure (PaO_2) (usually <60 mm Hg), is characterized by nonspecific signs and symptoms ranging from agitation to somnolence, hypertension to hypotension, and tachycardia to bradycardia. Pulse oximetry may confirm low oxygen saturation (<90%); arterial blood gas analysis may confirm a PaO_2 of less than 60 mm Hg. Hypoxemia, if untreated, can result in organ ischemia.

Hypoxemia can be the result of a delivered low concentration of oxygen, hypoventilation, impaired alveolar-capillary diffusion, ventilation-perfusion mismatches, or increased intrapulmonary shunting.[12] The most common causes of hypoxemia in the PACU include atelectasis, pulmonary edema, pulmonary embolism, aspiration, bronchospasm, and hypoventilation. A brief explanation of these pathologic states follows.

Clinical issues with pulse oximetry have to be considered when used to determine oxygen saturation levels. The relationship

---

BOX **51-6**

Criteria for Initial Assessment: Phase I PACU

Initial assessment and documentation include:
1. Integration of data received at transfer of care
2. Vital signs
   a. Respiratory status—airway patent, breath sounds, type of artificial airway, mechanical ventilatory settings, oxygen saturation, end-tidal CO_2 (if ordered)
   b. Blood pressure—cuff or arterial line
   c. Pulse—apical, peripheral
   d. Cardiac monitor, rhythm documented
   e. Temperature/route
   f. Hemodynamic pressure readings: central venous, pulmonary artery, and wedge; intracranial pressure as indicated
3. Pain and comfort level, level of emotional comfort
4. Neurologic function to include level of consciousness. Pupillary response as indicated.
5. Sensory and motor function as appropriate
6. Position of patient
7. Condition and color of skin
8. Patient safety needs
9. Neurovascular: peripheral pulses and sensation of extremity(ies) as applicable
10. Condition of dressings and visible incisions
11. Type and patency of drainage tubes, catheters, and receptacles; effectively secured
12. Amount and type of drainage
13. Fluid therapy: location of lines, condition of IV site, and amount of solution infusing
14. Procedure-specific assessment (i.e., firmness of abdomen)
15. Postanesthesia scoring system if used

Modified from American Society of Perianesthesia Nurses. 2006-2008 Standards of Perianesthesia Nursing Practice. Cherry Hill, NJ: ASPAN; 2006.

- Nausea and vomiting
- Fluids
- Urine output and voiding

Respiratory Function

In postoperative patients, airway problems that interfere with oxygenation and ventilation are always related to an increase in the resistance to gas flow somewhere in the airways.[10]

Obstruction

In postanesthesia patients, the tongue causes most upper airway obstructions. Obstruction occurs when the tongue falls back into a position that occludes the pharynx and blocks the flow of air into and out of the lungs. Signs and symptoms of an upper airway obstruction include snoring and activation of accessory muscles of ventilation. Intercostal and suprasternal retractions may be noted. However, patients are usually somnolent and may be difficult to arouse. Risk factors for an upper airway obstruction include anatomy (obesity, large neck, or short neck), poor muscle tone (secondary to opioids, sedation, residual neuromuscular blockade, or neuromuscular disease), or swelling (secondary to surgical manipulation, edema, or anaphylaxis).

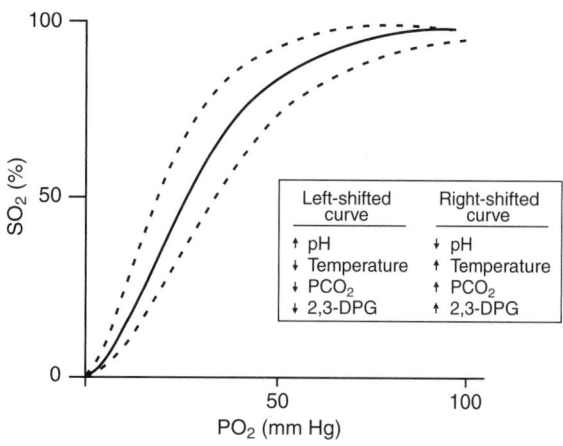

FIGURE **51-1** Normal oxyhemoglobin dissociation curve. *(From Drain CB, Odom-Forren J. Perianesthesia Nursing: A Critical Care Approach. 5th ed. St Louis: Saunders, 2009:365.)*

between SaO_2 and PaO_2 is symbolized by the oxyhemoglobin dissociation curve (Figure 51-1). Shifts in the curve are caused by abnormal values of pH, temperature, partial pressure of carbon dioxide, and 2,3-diphosphoglycerate. The patient's level of hemoglobin must also be considered, because if too low, even fully saturated hemoglobin is not adequate to meet tissue needs.[1]

Atelectasis

Atelectasis is the most common cause of postoperative arterial hypoxemia and can lead to an increase in right-to-left shunt. Atelectasis may be the result of bronchial obstruction caused by secretions or decreased lung volumes. Hypotension and low cardiac output conditions can also contribute to the development of decreased perfusion and atelectasis. Treatment includes the use of humidified oxygen, coughing, deep breathing, postural drainage, and increased mobility. Incentive spirometry and intermittent positive-pressure ventilation may also be used.[13]

Pulmonary Edema

Pulmonary edema, which is caused by fluid accumulation within the alveoli, may be the result of an increase in hydrostatic pressure, a decrease in interstitial pressure, or an increase in capillary permeability.

An increase in hydrostatic pressure is usually the result of fluid overload, left ventricular failure (especially in the presence of systolic hypertension), mitral valve dysfunction, or ischemic heart disease. Increased capillary permeability may be the result of sepsis, aspiration, transfusion reaction, trauma, anaphylaxis, shock, or disseminated intravascular coagulation and is frequently referred to as *adult respiratory distress syndrome*.[10]

A decrease in interstitial pressure is often seen after prolonged airway obstruction, such as laryngospasm. Acute pulmonary edema that occurs shortly after relief of severe upper airway obstruction is called *postobstruction* or *negative-pressure pulmonary edema* or *noncardiogenic pulmonary edema*. The airway obstruction causes extreme negative intrapleural pressure that increases the pulmonary transvascular hydrostatic pressure gradient. The rapid movement of fluid from pulmonary vasculature to interstitium exceeds the clearing capacity of the pulmonary lymphatic system, and the alveoli become flooded.[14] Other causes of noncardiogenic pulmonary edema are bolus dosing with naloxone, incomplete reversal of neuromuscular blockade, or a significant period of hypoxia.[15]

Pulmonary edema is characterized by hypoxemia, cough, frothy sputum, rales on auscultation, decreased lung compliance, and pulmonary infiltrates seen on chest radiography. Treatment of pulmonary edema is directed toward identification of the cause and reduction of hydrostatic pressure within the lungs. Oxygenation must be maintained (particularly in the presence of profound hypoxemia) via oxygen mask or continuous positive airway pressure (CPAP) with mask, or if necessary, intubation, mechanical ventilation, and the addition of positive end-expiratory pressure (PEEP) ventilation. Diuretics (most commonly furosemide) and fluid restriction are a part of treatment. Dialysis may be used if the fluid retention results from renal failure. Afterload reduction, which is achieved through the use of nitroglycerin or sodium nitroprusside, may be used to decrease myocardial work.[10] Patients with noncardiogenic pulmonary edema usually recover quickly after the acute phase and have no permanent sequelae.[15]

Pulmonary Embolism

Pulmonary embolism is a leading cause of morbidity and mortality, accounting for 50,000 to 90,000 deaths annually in the United States. Most cases of pulmonary embolism are not fatal; however, two thirds of all deaths caused by a pulmonary embolism occur within 30 minutes of an acute event.[16]

Patients can be considered to be at risk for pulmonary embolism if three conditions, known as *Virchow's triad*, exist: venous stasis, hypercoagulability, and abnormalities of the blood vessel wall. These conditions are accentuated in the presence of obesity, varicose veins, immobility, malignancy, congestive heart failure, and increased age and after pelvic or long-bone surgery or injury. However, 90% of all pulmonary emboli arise from deep veins in the legs.[16-17] Thrombosis in postoperative patients seems to be related to surgical tissue trauma and liberation of tissue factor that leads to thrombin formation. Leukocyte reactivity and surgery-induced hemostatic changes may also contribute[18] (Box 51-7).

A pulmonary embolism should be suspected in a patient who complains of or whose presenting signs include acute-onset tachypnea, dyspnea, and tachycardia, particularly when the patient is already receiving oxygen therapy. Signs and symptoms may also include chest pain, hypotension, hemoptysis, dysrhythmias, and congestive heart failure. Although the clinical symptomatology may be suggestive of a pulmonary embolism, confirmation requires pulmonary angiography. Pulmonary angiography is infrequently performed because of its high risk and associated mortality. A ventilation-perfusion scan may also prove useful.

Treatment of a pulmonary embolism is directed toward the correction of hypoxemia and support of hemodynamic stability. Preventive measures may include the use of antiembolic stockings or sequential compression devices. Subcutaneous heparin therapy may also be initiated. Once the occurrence of a pulmonary embolism has been confirmed, IV heparin therapy is started for the prevention of further clot formation. The goal of heparin therapy is an activated partial thromboplastin time that is 1.5 to 2 times the control value.

Aspiration

Aspiration is a potentially serious airway emergency that can compromise patient safety and stability on the induction of, or

BOX **51-7**

Surgery-Induced Hemostatic Changes

Increased Platelet Reactivity

↑ Aggregation
↑ Dense granule release

Increased Leukocyte Reactivity

↑ Free-radical release
↑ Surface adhesion molecules

Increased Coagulation Cascade Activation

↑ Fibrinogen
↑ Factor VIII
↑ Von Willebrand factor
↑ Thrombin formation

Decreased Endogenous Anticoagulants

↓ Antithrombin III
↓ Heparin cofactor II
↓ Tissue factor pathway inhibitor
↓ Protein C, protein S

Decreased Fibrinolysis

↑ Plasminogen activator inhibitor-1

From Patel K, Chaney MA. Hypercoagulable states: thrombosis and embolism. In: Atlee JL. Complications in Anesthesia. 2nd ed. Philadelphia: Saunders; 2007.

the emergence from, anesthesia. Aspiration may occur in the OR, in the PACU, or at any time during transfer. Patients may aspirate foreign matter (e.g., a tooth, food), blood, or gastric contents. Each type of material is associated with a characteristic clinical presentation.

Foreign matter aspiration may result in cough, airway obstruction, atelectasis, bronchospasm, and pneumonia. A profound reflex sympathetic nervous system (SNS) response might also cause hypertension, tachycardia, and dysrhythmias. In the absence of complete upper airway obstruction, complications are often localized and treated with supportive care once the foreign matter has been expelled or removed by bronchoscopy.[16]

Aspiration of blood may result from trauma or surgical manipulation and may also cause minor airway obstruction that is rapidly cleared by cough, resorption, and phagocytosis. Massive blood aspiration interferes with gas exchange through mechanical blockage of airways and leads to chronic fibrinous changes in air spaces or pulmonary hemochromatosis from iron accumulation in phagocytic cells. Aspiration of blood may result in infection, particularly if particles of soft tissue are aspirated along with the blood.[19] Treatment involves correction of hypoxemia, maintenance of airway patency, and initiation of antibiotic therapy, if indicated.

Aspiration of gastric contents is the most severe form of aspiration and may result in a chemical pneumonitis. Patients have diffuse bronchospasm (secondary to reflex airway closure), hypoxemia (compromised alveolar-capillary membrane), atelectasis (loss of surfactant), interstitial edema (loss of capillary integrity), hemorrhage, and adult respiratory distress syndrome. Gastric aspiration may also cause laryngospasm, infection, and pulmonary edema.

For this reason, the prevention of gastric aspiration, rather than its treatment, is the goal. Patients who are at risk for gastric

aspiration (e.g., obese or pregnant patients or those with a history of hiatal hernia, peptic ulcer, or trauma) may be given histamine-2 (H_2) blockers, gastrokinetic agents, nonparticulate antacids, or anticholinergics before anesthesia induction.[19] Rapid-sequence induction is likely used. Intraoperatively a nasogastric tube may be inserted and is usually then removed to decrease gastric volume and decompress the stomach. Postoperatively the patient should be left intubated until airway reflexes return.

Treatment of gastric aspiration is directed toward correction of hypoxemia and maintenance of hemodynamic stability. Antibiotics are indicated only if signs of infection (e.g., fever, leukocytosis, positive culture results) are present. No beneficial effect of corticosteroids has been determined. Corticosteroids may have an indication with inflammatory pneumonitis, but the immunosuppressant effect may exacerbate any secondary bacterial pneumonia.[20]

If aspiration causes hypoxemia, increased airway resistance, atelectasis, or pulmonary edema, institution of support with supplemental oxygen, PEEP, or CPAP and mechanical ventilation is often necessary. Pulmonary edema is usually secondary to increased capillary permeability, so diuretics should not be used to decrease intravascular volume. Bacterial infection does not always occur, so prophylactic antibiotics might merely promote colonization by resistant organisms. If evidence of secondary bacterial infections appears, specific antibiotic therapy is instituted, based on sputum samples obtained for Gram stain and culture or on prevailing colonization experience within the institution.[19]

Bronchospasm

Bronchospasm results from an increase in bronchial smooth muscle tone, with resultant closure of small airways. As a result of the strong increase in inspiratory force against these closed airways, airway edema develops, causing secretions to build up in the airway. Clinically, the patient demonstrates wheezing, dyspnea, use of accessory muscles, and tachypnea. Airway resistance is increased, and increased peak inspiratory pressures are noted if the patient is receiving mechanical ventilation.[10,21]

Bronchospasm may result from aspiration, pharyngeal or tracheal suctioning, endotracheal intubation, histamine release secondary to medications, or an allergic response, and it may be seen in greater frequency in patients with a history of asthma or chronic obstructive pulmonary disease.

Treatment of bronchospasm requires confirmation and removal of the precipitating cause. Pharmacotherapy is instituted, with the goals of decreasing airway irritability and promoting bronchodilation. Medications used in the management of bronchospasm include salmeterol (Serevent) and β_2-agonists such as albuterol (Proventil, Ventolin), salbutamol, and terbutaline and, if the condition is life threatening, IV epinephrine.[6] Cholinergics such as atropine sulfate and glycopyrrolate have been given via nebulization in order to decrease secretions. Both IV and inhaled lidocaine attenuate histamine-induced bronchospasm; however, inhaled lidocaine works at a lower serum level than IV lidocaine.[21] Steroids have been used if the underlying cause is an inflammatory disease such as asthma.

Hypoventilation

Hypoventilation is a common, easily recognizable complication in the PACU. It is manifested clinically by a decrease in respiratory rate that results in an increase in $PaCO_2$ secondary to a decrease in alveolar ventilation. This may occur because of a decrease in central respiratory drive, poor respiratory muscle function, or a combination of both.[11]

Depression of central respiratory drive can occur with both IV and inhalation anesthetics. Central respiratory depression is most profound on admission to the PACU, although the time and route of anesthetic administration may suggest otherwise. For example, an IV dose of fentanyl given just before the patient emerges from anesthesia may not peak until later in the PACU. An intramuscular dose of an opioid takes substantially longer to peak than does an IV dose.[16]

Patients may also demonstrate a secondary stage of respiratory depression once certain stimuli are removed. For example, a patient may be admitted awake and breathing to the PACU with an endotracheal tube in place. After extubation, because of the loss of stimulation from the endotracheal tube, the patient may become hypercarbic secondary to residual opioid effects and hypoventilation.[10] Verbal and tactile stimulation, deep breaths, and repositioning the patient may increase ventilatory function and decrease carbon dioxide. Capnography may be of use in patients at risk.[15]

Poor respiratory muscle function can result from many conditions. Some of the most common situations are inadequate reversal of neuromuscular blocking agents, surgery involving the upper abdomen, positioning, obesity, and diseases involving the neuromuscular system.

Inadequate reversal of neuromuscular blocking agents can result in hypoventilation secondary to respiratory muscle weakness. Factors that can adversely affect neuromuscular blockade and reversal include certain medications, hypokalemia, hypermagnesemia, hypothermia, and acidosis.[22]

Medications that have been associated with prolongation of blockade include the aminoglycoside antibiotics (gentamicin, clindamycin, and neomycin), as well as furosemide and propranolol. Hypermagnesemia and hypothermia may potentiate neuromuscular blockade. Hypokalemia and respiratory acidosis inhibit reversal.[23]

Upper abdominal surgery can also affect respiratory muscle function. Hypoventilation occurs because of a reduced vital capacity secondary to poor diaphragmatic function. A reduction in vital capacity of up to 60% has been noted on the first postoperative day.[11] Obesity, especially when combined with upper abdominal surgery, further contributes to hypoventilation because of the increased intraabdominal pressure in obese patients.

Diseases of the neuromuscular system can also affect ventilation. Patients with muscular dystrophy, myasthenia gravis, Eaton-Lambert syndrome, Guillain-Barré syndrome, or other muscle diseases can exhibit postoperative muscle weakness. Patients with severe scoliosis also exhibit poor respiratory muscle function. It is often in the best interests of patients with these disorders that they remain intubated in the PACU until complete return of function occurs, and any residual anesthetic effects are absent.

Cardiovascular Function
Hypotension

Classically, *hypotension* has been defined as a blood pressure of less than 20% of the baseline or preoperative blood pressure. However, the clinical signs of hypoperfusion, rather than numeric values, should be the indicators of compromise. Because the autonomic nervous system preferentially maintains blood flow to the brain, heart, and kidneys, signs of hypoperfusion to these organs (including disorientation, nausea, loss of consciousness, chest pain, oliguria, and anuria) reflect the failure of physiologic compensation. Hypoxia, which results from hypoperfusion, may cause lactic acidosis. Intervention must be implemented in a timely fashion so that cerebral ischemia, cerebrovascular accident (CVA), myocardial infarction or ischemia, renal ischemia, bowel infarction, and spinal cord damage do not develop.[24]

Hypotension in the PACU is most commonly caused by hypovolemia secondary to inadequate replacement of intraoperative fluid and blood loss. As a result, initial treatment should focus on restoring circulating volume. A 300- to 500-mL fluid bolus of physiologic saline or lactated Ringer's solution should be given. If no response is noted, myocardial dysfunction should be considered the cause of hypotension.

Primary cardiac dysfunction, as is the case with myocardial infarction, tamponade, or embolism, results in an acute fall in ventricular emptying and cardiac output. Secondary cardiac dysfunction occurs as a result of the negative chronotropic and negative inotropic effects of medications.

Low systemic vascular resistance (SVR) can also contribute to hypotension. Numerous anesthetic agents cause histamine release with subsequent vasodilation (e.g., barbiturates, morphine, atracurium), whereas others cause vasodilation by directly relaxing arterial smooth muscle (volatile inhalation anesthetics, local anesthetics used for producing spinal anesthesia). Sensitivity to vasodilators such as hydralazine, sodium nitroprusside, and nitroglycerin can also produce profound hypotension. Sepsis may be another cause of low SVR.

Dysrhythmias that interfere with cardiac conduction and subsequently compromise cardiac output can also produce hypotension. Tachydysrhythmias prevent optimal ventricular filling and emptying. Conduction blocks compromise myocardial effectiveness, resulting in a lowered cardiac output and hypotension.

Intervention should always include supplemental oxygen therapy while the cause of the hypotension is investigated. Volume status should be evaluated, and preoperative and intraoperative fluid administration should be considered. Hypotension caused by artifact of the measurement system should also be considered—for example, a blood pressure cuff that is too large or too small or an inappropriate transducer height. The presence of hypotension secondary to myocardial dysfunction suggests the need for coronary vasodilators, inotropic therapy, and afterload reduction (e.g., through nitroglycerin therapy, dobutamine therapy, or both). Secondary myocardial dysfunction may require that administration of the causative medications be discontinued. Vasodilation resulting in lower SVR and symptomatic hypoperfusion can be treated with vasoconstrictive agents, either by IV bolus (ephedrine) or by infusion (dopamine or epinephrine).

Hypertension

Hypertension, defined as a 20% to 30% increase relative to the baseline blood pressure, is a common finding in the PACU and can be caused by stimulation of the SNS and pain, respiratory compromise, visceral distention, and significant increases in plasma catecholamine levels that produce vasoconstriction.

Pain remains the leading cause of hypertension and tachycardia in the PACU and results in stimulation of the somatic afferent nerves, producing a pressor response known as the *somatosympathetic reflex*.[24] The use of analgesics attenuates the sympathetic response, thereby normalizing blood pressure.

Hypoxemia and hypercarbia cause direct stimulation of the vasomotor area of the medulla, resulting in increased vasomotor tone, increased arteriolar constriction, and increased blood pressure.[24] Correction of the respiratory compromise should result in normalization of blood pressure.

Distention of the bladder, bowel, or stomach causes stimulation of afferent fibers of the SNS, producing an increase in plasma catecholamine levels. Catheterization of the bladder and decompression of the bowel or stomach remove the offending stimulus.

Hypertension may also develop as a sequela of hypothermia. Increased catecholamine secretion is an important endocrine response to cold.[24] As cooling occurs, blood vessels become more sensitive to catecholamines, resulting in arteriolar and venous constriction. Rewarming reverses the process. As vasodilation occurs, reperfusion of the extremities and skin decreases systemic elevations in pressure.

Preexisting hypertension exists in many of the patients who develop hypertension in the PACU. The degree of elevation in pressure is greater if preoperative antihypertensive medications are withdrawn suddenly. Ideally, patients receive their antihypertensive medications on the day of surgery.

Hypertension may also be seen secondary to revascularization and baroreceptor stimulation after vascular or cardiac surgery, including carotid endarterectomy. Pharmacologic intervention is required for the protection of graft sites and the prevention of hemorrhage. Sodium nitroprusside and nitroglycerin are agents of choice for vasodilation.

Agents that may be used for the reduction of blood pressure include hydralazine and labetalol hydrochloride. Hydralazine relaxes vascular smooth muscle, preferentially favoring the arteriolar circulation. Labetalol is both an α- and a β-blocking agent, causing peripheral vasodilation and slowing of the heart rate. Many other agents are available and may include the patient's usual prescription antihypertensive for mild increases.

Dysrhythmias

Dysrhythmias seen in the PACU most commonly have an identifiable cause that is not an actual myocardial injury. The major postanesthetic and surgical factors that lead to a relatively high incidence of perioperative dysrhythmias include hypokalemia, hypoxia, hypercarbia, altered acid-base status, circulatory instability, and preexisting heart disease.

Arterial desaturation is a common postoperative complication that may result from obstruction or hypoventilation or less commonly from pulmonary embolism, pulmonary edema, or aspiration. A direct consequence of hypoxia is myocardial ischemia and depression of cardiac contractility. Signs of cardiac irritability may be manifested by atrial and ventricular dysrhythmias, conduction delays, and heart block.

Hypercarbia caused by reduced alveolar ventilation results in elevation of the arterial carbon dioxide tension, which in turn stimulates the SNS and sensitizes the myocardium to the arrhythmic effects of endogenous catecholamines. Among the earliest signs of hypercarbia are tachycardia and hypertension, which may progress to ventricular dysrhythmias.

Hypokalemia may occur secondary to hyperventilation, respiratory alkalosis, gastric suctioning, insulin administration, and diuretic use. The ECG may demonstrate widening of the QRS complex, U waves, and ST-segment abnormalities that may progress into premature ventricular complexes, ventricular tachycardia, and ventricular fibrillation.

Acid-base disturbances may occur as a result of alterations in ventilation, gastrointestinal losses, and lactic acid production during hypotension or shock. The cardiovascular effects include increased cardiac excitability and irritability.

Hypotension may result in impaired oxygen transport and compromised coronary circulation, leading to myocardial ischemia with associated conduction deficits. The use of vasoconstrictive medications designed to treat the hypotension may also contribute to the development of dysrhythmias. Patients with preexisting heart disease, particularly those who have a history of myocardial infarction, are at continued risk for myocardial ischemia throughout the perioperative period.

Hypothermia prolongs the refractory period, contributing to the development of sinus bradycardia and atrial fibrillation. Conduction deficits may progress to atrioventricular block and eventually to ventricular fibrillation.[25]

Vagal reflexes are usually transient and are produced by the Valsalva maneuver or direct eye, vagal nerve, or carotid sinus pressure. Severe sinus bradycardia with possible ventricular escape beats may occur. Vagotonic medications, such as neostigmine or pyridostigmine, can also produce these dysrhythmias.

The presence of residual anesthetics in both blood and tissue in patients admitted to the PACU may contribute to dysrhythmias. Ketamine may contribute to sympathetic stimulation, resulting in tachyarrhythmias and hypertension, as can vagolytic drugs such as atropine and glycopyrrolate.[26,27] Opioids such as morphine, fentanyl, and sufentanil may result in the indirect development of dysrhythmias. Respiratory depression, a potential side effect of opioids, may result in hypoxemia and hypercarbia, both of which are known to be dysrhythmogenic. Anticholinesterase agents may produce severe bradyarrhythmias or heart block.[26]

Surgical stress and pain can significantly increase plasma catecholamine levels. Although this sympathetic response may be mitigated by anesthetic administration, norepinephrine and epinephrine concentrations are consistently elevated in PACU patients who are in pain. Administration of analgesic medications may blunt this sympathetic response; however, cardiac irritability, tachycardia, and conduction dysrhythmias may occur.

Neuromuscular Function
Reversal of Neuromuscular Blockade

Incomplete reversal of neuromuscular relaxation can lead to postoperative airway obstruction and hypoventilation. Residual paralysis compromises cough, airway patency, ability to overcome airway resistance, and airway protection. Intraoperative use of shorter-acting relaxants might decrease the incidence of residual paralysis but does not eliminate the problem.[28] Marginal reversal can be more dangerous than near total paralysis, because an agitated patient exhibiting uncoordinated movements and airway obstruction is more easily identified. A somnolent patient exhibiting mild stridor and shallow ventilation from marginal neuromuscular function might be overlooked. Insidious hypoventilation leading to respiratory acidemia or regurgitation with aspiration can occur later into recovery. Patients with coexisting neuromuscular abnormalities such as myasthenia gravis, Eaton-Lambert syndrome, or muscular dystrophies exhibit exaggerated or prolonged responses to muscle relaxants. Even without muscle relaxant administration, such patients can exhibit postoperative respiratory insufficiency from inadequate neuromuscular reserves.

Simple bedside tests help assess mechanical ability to ventilate. Forced vital capacity of 10 to 12 mL/kg and inspiratory pressure more negative than −25 cm H_2O imply that strength of ventilatory muscles is adequate to sustain ventilation. Sustained head elevation in a supine position, hand grip, and ability to bite down, swallow, and stick out the tongue are easily assessed parameters. These measures, along with tactile train-of-four and double-burst stimulation assessment, accurately predict a patient's ability to maintain sustained ventilation.

Mental Status
Emergence Delirium

Postoperatively, emergence delirium is the alteration in neurologic functioning that causes the most concern to the practitioner. *Delirium* is defined as a condition that is characterized by extreme disturbances of arousal, attention, orientation, perception, intellectual function, and affect and is most commonly accompanied by fear and agitation.[29] There have been recent attempts to differentiate emergence delirium from agitation,[30-31] with *agitation* defined as mild restlessness and mental distress. Agitation can be due to pain, physiologic compromise, or anxiety. Delirium can be confused with agitation or the source of agitation, and can be very difficult to differentiate.[31] The incidence of postoperative delirium has been described to be 3% to 20%; with some procedures, the incidence may be as high as 75%. A recent study found an incidence of 4.7% in adult PACU patients.[32] The causes of postoperative delirium have been classified into four categories: withdrawal psychosis, toxic psychosis, circulatory and respiratory origin, and functional psychosis.[29]

Withdrawal psychosis is caused by withdrawal of various substances such as alcohol and illicit drugs. Alcohol withdrawal can be dangerous because it can cause delirium tremens. Clinical symptoms of delirium tremens may include hallucinations, extreme combativeness, and confusion.[29]

Amphetamine-induced delirium usually appears 1 hour after amphetamine use and disappears within 6 hours of use. Cocaine-induced delirium results from alteration of neurotransmitters. Management of withdrawal psychosis may include protection of patient safety and use of benzodiazepines or other sedatives.[29]

Toxic psychosis is caused by exposure to toxins, including toxic fumes that may occur in the OR, as from a malfunctioning laser. The Occupational Safety and Health Administration's regulations and its mandates on monitoring help to limit the occurrence of these events.[33]

Circulatory and respiratory causes of emergence delirium most commonly include hypoxemia and hypercarbia, which may be the result of central respiratory depression, airway obstruction, or perfusion deficits. The primary cause of postoperative emergence delirium is always considered to be hypoxemia until proved otherwise. As a result, sedation of the agitated patient should never be considered until hypoxemia has been ruled out as the cause of agitation.

Functional psychosis is defined as a brief reaction of paranoia and other changes not caused by an organic abnormality. This diagnosis is made by exclusion after known organic causes have been ruled out.[33]

Although this classification is useful, other more frequently occurring causes of emergence delirium may be seen in the PACU. Confusion and agitation are common during recovery from inhalation anesthetics. Sevoflurane in particular has been associated with emergence delirium in children.[30] Many drugs used during the perioperative period have been reported to contribute to postoperative delirium. Ketamine, a phencyclidine derivative, is associated with hallucinations, delirium, and unpleasant dreams, particularly in patients between 16 and 65 years of age. Local anesthetics can cross the blood-brain barrier and may cause postoperative delirium. Nitrous oxide may cause acute mental status changes with prolonged exposure. Other anesthetic adjuncts associated with delirium include butyrophenones (e.g., droperidol), naloxone, and muscle relaxants, which can cause dissociative reactions, heightened pain perception, and hypoxemia, respectively. Delirium has also been reported as a side effect of antibiotic therapy (e.g., cefazolin, penicillin, streptomycin, chloramphenicol), antituberculosis drugs (e.g., isoniazid, cycloserine), antiviral agents (e.g., acyclovir), anticonvulsant medications (e.g., carbamazepine, phenytoin), and antiparkinsonian agents (e.g., levodopa, bromocriptine). Adverse reactions to medications that result in delirium have been reported with digitalis, antidysrhythmics (e.g., amiodarone, flecainide, lidocaine, mexiletine), β-blockers, calcium channel blockers, contrast dye, corticosteroids, chemotherapeutic agents, immunosuppressants, H_1 and H_2 blockers, antipsychotic medications, and clonidine.[34]

Premedicants, including anticholinergics, benzodiazepines, and opioids, may induce untoward reactions. Anticholinergics, specifically atropine and scopolamine, have been noted to cause central anticholinergic syndrome. These drugs cross the blood-brain barrier, altering the neurotransmitter balance and causing agitation, combativeness, and lack of cooperation. Benzodiazepines may contribute to postoperative delirium, especially in the elderly.[35] Flumazenil (Romazicon) remains the only benzodiazepine antagonist available to reverse the effects of benzodiazepine-induced delirium. Opioids, particularly morphine, have been cited as a contributing factor to postoperative delirium secondary to respiratory depression and hypoxemia. In patients with renal failure, meperidine may cause excitation because of accumulation of normeperidine, a neuroexcitatory metabolic by-product.

Metabolic disturbances associated with postoperative delirium include acidosis and alkalosis, electrolyte imbalance (magnesium, calcium, sodium), and porphyria. Treatment is directed at correction of the cause.[34]

Other causes of postoperative delirium include pain, visceral distention (bowel and bladder), anxiety (including separation anxiety in children), hyperthermia, and hypothermia.[34] Again, treatment is directed at correction of the cause. In a study of adult postanesthesia patients, the most common causes of emergence delirium were presence of an endotracheal tube, pain, and anxiety.[32] In children, determination of cause and treatment of delirium is complex, with pain and anxiety more easily recognized and treated than other anesthetic-related causes. Voepel-Lewis and colleagues developed an algorithm for assessment, reassessment, and treatment decisions in children with emergence delirium.[36]

Once hypoxemia has been eliminated as a cause of postoperative delirium, and all known causes have been evaluated, sedation may prove useful in controlling the agitation and providing for patient safety. Most events are time limited to the PACU and are resolved before discharge. Figure 51-2 summarizes the factors that contribute to postoperative delirium and treatment options.

Delayed Awakening

Delayed awakening is a common, often easily explained postoperative finding and can be defined as a clinician's expectation in a specific circumstance that the patient "should be awake by now" but is not. Although delayed awakening may slow turnover of PACU beds and delay patient discharge from the PACU, the causes and consequences of delayed awakening are rarely serious. The most common causes of delayed awakening are:

1. Prolonged action of anesthetic drugs
2. Metabolic causes
3. Neurologic injury

Prolonged action of anesthetic drugs is the most common cause of delayed awakening. This may occur secondary to alterations in drug pharmacokinetics and pharmacodynamics. Pharmacokinetic alterations include changes in drug distribution secondary to

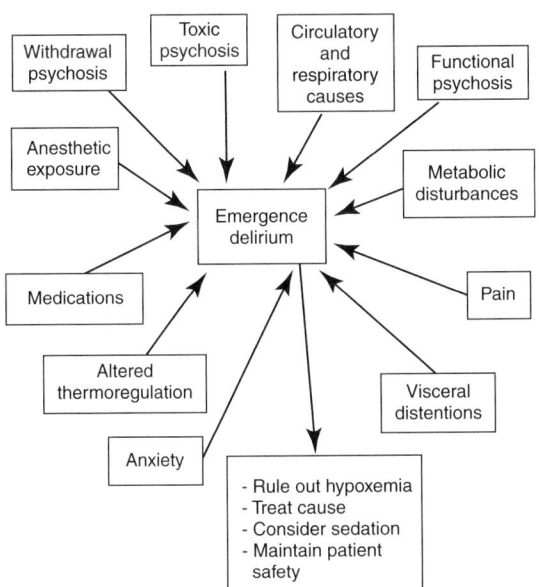

FIGURE **51-2** Emergence delirium in the postanesthesia care unit: contributing factors and treatment.

mobilization of drugs from body tissue stores, redistribution, or decreased protein binding; changes in metabolism; and excretion secondary to renal or hepatic dysfunction. Pharmacodynamic alterations include increased patient sensitivity to drug effects because of extremes of age, hypothermia, or concomitant alcohol and drug use. Other patients at risk for delayed awakening are those with preexisting cognitive or psychiatric disorders, patients who chronically take sedative medications, patients who were intoxicated with alcohol or illicit drugs at the time of anesthesia, and those who were physically exhausted prior to surgery.[37]

Prolonged effects of inhalation anesthetics may be seen secondary to alterations in ventilation. Hypoventilation limits exhalation and prolongs elimination of inhalation agents.[38] Retention of carbon dioxide contributes to narcosis, particularly in the presence of inhalation agents, and compounds the problem.

The potentiating effects of combining inhalation agents with IV anesthetics and opioids can also contribute to delayed awakening.[39] Premedications, particularly the long-acting benzodiazepines diazepam and lorazepam, may contribute to delayed awakening, especially in the elderly.[39] Prolonged effects of inhalation and IV agents may also occur secondary to accidental or intentional overdose and multiple drug interactions. Prolonged neuromuscular blockade may mean the patient is awake but unable to move.[40] Some herbal supplements have the potential to cause delayed awakening, especially kava kava, St. John's wort, and valerian.[37]

Metabolic causes of delayed awakening include hypoglycemia, hyperglycemia, and electrolyte disturbances. Diabetic patients have an increased risk of postoperative hypoglycemia. Taking the usual insulin dose (or half the dose) on the morning of surgery, the patient's nothing-by-mouth (NPO) status, and the stress of surgery all contribute to the development of hypoglycemia.[39] It is important to monitor serum glucose levels intraoperatively and postoperatively. Central nervous system changes may occur as blood glucose levels fall below 50 mg/dL.[41] It is good practice to obtain a baseline blood glucose level of all diabetic patients before they are admitted to surgery. Blood glucose levels of

greater than 600 mg/dL can produce hyperosmolar, nonketotic, hyperglycemic coma. Approximately half of these patients have type 2 diabetes, but the syndrome can occur with severe dehydration (especially in the elderly), uremia, pancreatitis, sepsis, pneumonia, CVA, and large surface burns.[39]

Electrolyte disturbances, specifically alterations in sodium, calcium, and magnesium, can prolong awakening. Dilutional hyponatremia, occurring secondary to water intoxication, may develop after transurethral prostate resection surgery, producing sedation, coma, or even hemiparesis. Hypocalcemia, seen after parathyroidectomy and occasionally thyroidectomy, may delay awakening. Hypermagnesemia, which may occur after prolonged administration of magnesium sulfate to women with eclampsia or preeclampsia, may result in sedation and muscle weakness after general or regional anesthesia for cesarean section.[41]

Neurologic injury is a rare cause of delayed awakening of the nonneurosurgical patient. Potential causes of neurologic injury include CVA, intracranial hemorrhage, increased intracranial pressure, uncontrolled extreme hypertension (especially in the anticoagulated patient), air or fat emboli, and uncontrolled hypotension (especially in patients with hypertension or occlusive carotid disease).[40,41]

Evaluation of the patient who fails to awaken begins with an assessment of the patient's preoperative status and a review of intraoperative events. Oxygenation and gas exchange must be assessed and verified with pulse oximetry, physical assessment, and arterial blood gas analysis. When prolonged drug effects are suspected as the cause of delayed awakening, care must be taken to ensure the adequacy of ventilation and oxygenation through appropriate patient monitoring.

Residual drug effects should be considered. If possible and not contraindicated, reversal of medications should be attempted. Flumazenil reverses benzodiazepines, and naloxone reverses the opioids.[37]

If other contributing factors are found, intervention should be initiated. Hypothermia necessitates rewarming, and electrolyte disturbances require correction. Hypoglycemia and hypocalcemia are treated with the IV administration of glucose and calcium, respectively. Hyperglycemia is treated with IV insulin to lower blood glucose levels and 0.5% normal saline to correct dehydration.

A neurologic cause of delayed awakening is usually either a diagnosis that is initially expected because of patient status or known intraoperative events or a diagnosis of exclusion (i.e., suspected after all other causes have been ruled out). At this point, a CT scan and neurologic consultation are warranted for a more in-depth evaluation.[37]

Pain

Relief of surgical pain with minimal side effects is a primary goal of PACU care and a very high priority for both anesthesia provider and patient. Patients should be assessed on admission to PACU and at frequent intervals using a verbal rating scale or visual analogue scale to assess for severity of pain (Figure 51-3).[9] When prioritizing pain assessment, the patient's self-report of pain is the most important measure of pain. Other measures to assess pain intensity include the patient's exposure to painful procedures; behavioral signs, such as crying or agitation; a proxy pain rating by someone who knows the patient well; and physiologic indicators, such as elevated vital signs.[42] Inadequate postoperative analgesia is a major source of preoperative fear and postoperative dissatisfaction in surgical patients. Apfelbaum and colleagues[43] found that approximately 80% of postoperative

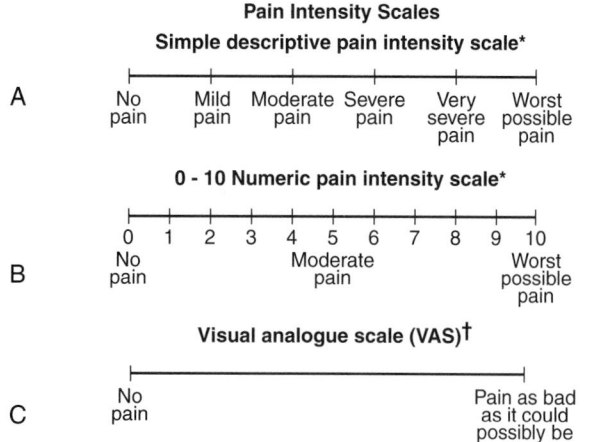

Pain Intensity Scales

Simple descriptive pain intensity scale*

A

| No pain | Mild pain | Moderate pain | Severe pain | Very severe pain | Worst possible pain |

0 - 10 Numeric pain intensity scale*

B

0 1 2 3 4 5 6 7 8 9 10
No pain   Moderate pain   Worst possible pain

Visual analogue scale (VAS)†

C

No pain   Pain as bad as it could possibly be

* If used as a graphic rating scale, a 10-cm baseline is recommended.
† A 10-cm baseline is recommended for VAS scales.

Which face shows how much hurt you have now?

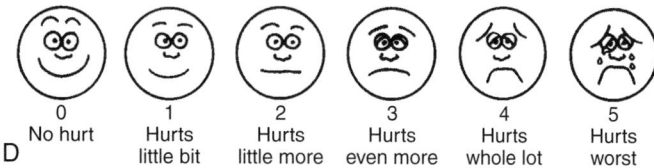

D

| 0 No hurt | 1 Hurts little bit | 2 Hurts little more | 3 Hurts even more | 4 Hurts whole lot | 5 Hurts worst |

FIGURE **51-3** Pain intensity scales. (**A-C** *From Acute Pain Management Guideline Panel.* Acute Pain Management in Adults: Operative Procedures: Quick Reference Guide for Clinicians *[AHCPR Publication No. 92-0019]. Rockville, MD: Agency for Health Care Policy and Research; 1992;* **D** *from Hockenberry MJ, Wilson D.* Wong's Nursing Care of Infants and Children. *8th ed. St Louis: Mosby; 2007:210.*)

patients experienced acute pain, with most of the patients experiencing pain they described as moderate, severe, or extreme. In addition to improving patient comfort, relief of pain reduces SNS response and helps avoid hypertension, tachycardia, and dysrhythmias.

Incisional pain may be effectively treated with careful titration of IV opioids with frequent cardiorespiratory assessments. Short-acting IV opioids are useful to expedite discharge and minimize nausea in ambulatory settings. Ketorolac is an effective analgesic with antiinflammatory characteristics that lower opioid requirements, although the possibility of hemorrhage resulting from its antiplatelet properties must be considered.[44]

Other analgesic modalities provide effective pain relief beyond the PACU. IV opioid loading in the PACU is important for smooth transition to patient-controlled analgesia. Injection of opioids into the epidural or subarachnoid space during anesthesia or in the PACU often yields prolonged postoperative analgesia.[44] Epidural opioid analgesia is effective after thoracic and upper abdominal procedures and helps wean patients with obesity or chronic obstructive pulmonary disease from mechanical ventilation. Epidural analgesia may also improve surgical outcomes after orthopedic and urologic procedures. With epidural or intrathecal opioid administration, immediate and delayed ventilatory depression can occur, along with other side effects such as nausea and pruritus.

Patient-controlled analgesia (PCA) allows patients to administer their own pain medication. The most commonly used methods of PCA are intravenous or epidural. Patient therapy should be initiated in the PACU after the patient's initial pain

level is under control. Oral opioids are used often with outpatients and have been studied in appropriate orthopedic patients with success. A new device called the *MOD* (Medication on Demand) allows patients to access oral analgesics at the bedside. Another addition to the pain management arsenal is PCA fentanyl delivered intradermally by iontophoresis with a device called the *IONSYS* (Ortho McNeil, Titusville, NJ). The patient can push a button on the device that is attached to the patient's chest or upper arm. Forty micrograms of fentanyl is delivered by indiscernible, mild, battery-generated electric currents over a 10-minute period. The active transport allows a much faster delivery than the fentanyl patches used for chronic pain. The IONSYS is self-contained and does not require a pump or tubing.[45]

Placement of long-acting regional analgesic blocks reduces pain, controls SNS activity, and often improves ventilation. For example, interscalene block yields almost complete pain relief from shoulder or upper extremity procedures, with only moderate inconvenience from motor impairment. Paralysis of the ipsilateral diaphragm can impair postoperative ventilation in patients with marginal respiratory reserve. Caudal analgesia is effective in children after inguinal or genital procedures, whereas infiltration of local anesthetic into joints, soft tissues, or incisions decreases the intensity of pain. Other uses of local anesthesia include continuous wound infusion, in which the catheter is inserted at the end of the case by the surgeon, and perineural infusions, in which the anesthesia provider inserts the catheter near the affected peripheral nerves or a nerve plexus.[45]

Opioid treatment for postoperative or chronic pain is frequently associated with adverse effects, the most common being dose-limiting and debilitating bowel dysfunction. Postoperative ileus, although attributable to surgical procedures, is often exacerbated by opioid use during and after surgery. Postoperative ileus is marked by increased inhibitory neural input, heightened inflammatory responses, decreased propulsive movements, and increased fluid absorption in the gastrointestinal tract. The current management of opioid-induced bowel dysfunction among patients receiving opioid analgesics consists primarily of nonspecific ameliorative measures. Clinical studies with the agent alvimopan suggest that it may normalize bowel function without blocking systemic opioid analgesia in abdominal laparotomy patients with opioid-related postoperative ileus.[46]

Nonpharmacologic interventions may include positioning for comfort, verbal reassurance, touch, applications of heat or cold, massage, transcutaneous electrical nerve stimulation, relaxation techniques, imagery, biofeedback controlled breathing, and use of the patient's support system (e.g., parent or significant other), particularly in children. Nonpharmacologic interventions should supplement and not replace pharmacologic therapy.[9]

Most of the current guidelines for pain management are very general and do not offer specific guidelines associated with different types of surgery.[47] The newest outlook for evidence-based guidelines in the field of pain management are procedure-specific guidelines offered via a web-based program called "PROSPECT" (Procedure Specific Postoperative Pain Management).[48,49] An international panel of surgeons and anesthesiologists reviews procedure-specific pain research and grades the evidence.[48] Then clinical practice guidelines and recommendations are developed after consensus by the working group (Figure 51-4). The PROSPECT website offers procedure-specific guidelines for managing pain associated with abdominal hysterectomy, herniorrhaphy, open colon resection, laparoscopic cholecystectomy,

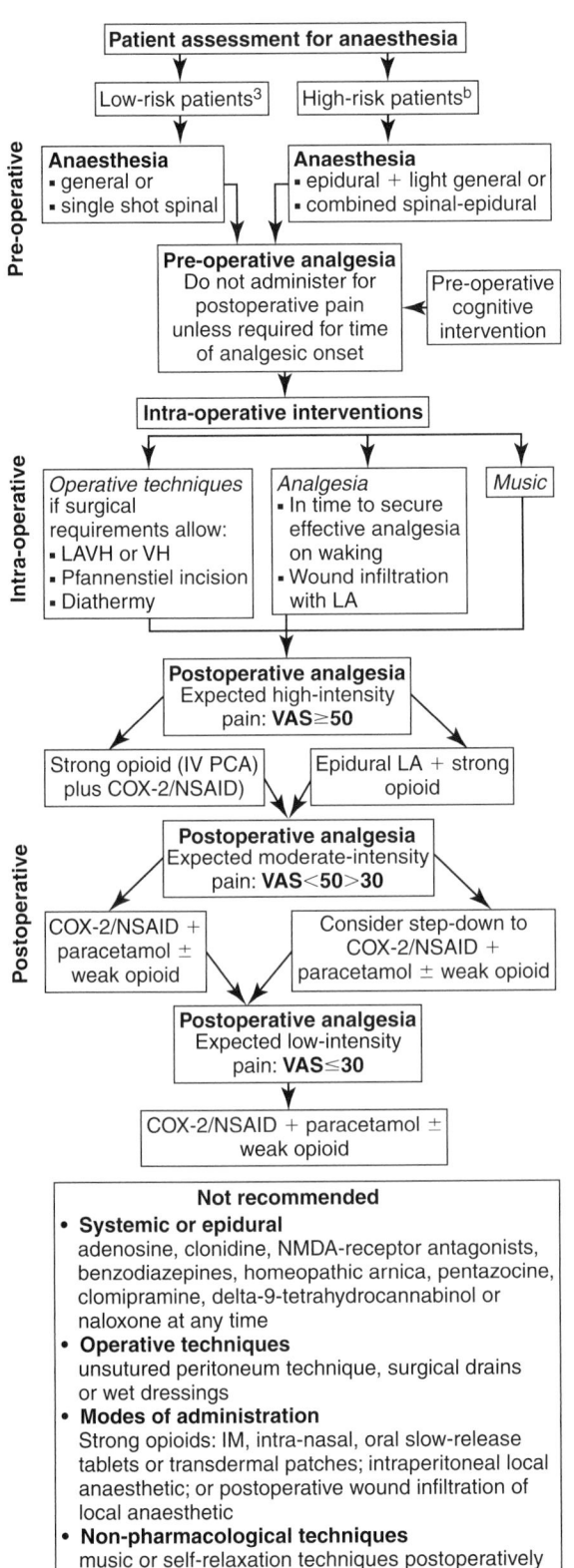

Patient assessment for anaesthesia

Low-risk patients[a] / High-risk patients[b]

Pre-operative

Anaesthesia
- general or
- single shot spinal

Anaesthesia
- epidural + light general or
- combined spinal-epidural

Pre-operative analgesia
Do not administer for postoperative pain unless required for time of analgesic onset

Pre-operative cognitive intervention

Intra-operative interventions

Intra-operative

Operative techniques
if surgical requirements allow:
- LAVH or VH
- Pfannenstiel incision
- Diathermy

Analgesia
- In time to secure effective analgesia on waking
- Wound infiltration with LA

Music

Postoperative analgesia
Expected high-intensity pain: **VAS≥50**

Strong opioid (IV PCA) plus COX-2/NSAID) / Epidural LA + strong opioid

Postoperative

Postoperative analgesia
Expected moderate-intensity pain: **VAS<50>30**

COX-2/NSAID + paracetamol ± weak opioid / Consider step-down to COX-2/NSAID + paracetamol ± weak opioid

Postoperative analgesia
Expected low-intensity pain: **VAS≤30**

COX-2/NSAID + paracetamol ± weak opioid

Not recommended
- **Systemic or epidural**
adenosine, clonidine, NMDA-receptor antagonists, benzodiazepines, homeopathic arnica, pentazocine, clomipramine, delta-9-tetrahydrocannabinol or naloxone at any time
- **Operative techniques**
unsutured peritoneum technique, surgical drains or wet dressings
- **Modes of administration**
Strong opioids: IM, intra-nasal, oral slow-release tablets or transdermal patches; intraperitoneal local anaesthetic; or postoperative wound infiltration of local anaesthetic
- **Non-pharmacological techniques**
music or self-relaxation techniques postoperatively

FIGURE **51-4** Algorithm for the management of postoperative pain—abdominal hysterectomy. (*From PROSPECT: Procedure-Specific Postoperative Pain Management website. http://www. postoppain.org.*)

thoracotomy, total hip arthroplasty, and total knee arthroplasty.[49]

Hypothermia

Hypothermia is a condition marked by an abnormally low internal body temperature (below 36° C), that occurs when systemic heat loss exceeds heat production.[50] Many patients are admitted into the PACU with hypothermia, which can prolong recovery, compromise physiologic stability, and contribute to postoperative morbidity. The patient's interaction with the environment determines the degree of heat loss. Heat loss may occur via radiation, convection, conduction, or evaporation.

Radiant heat loss involves the loss of heat from a warm or hot surface (the body) to a cooler one (the environment). It does not require that the two surfaces be in direct contact with each other. Radiant heat loss accounts for 40% to 60% of heat loss to the environment. It is especially profound in the elderly, debilitated, and neonatal populations.[51,52]

Convective heat loss depends on the existence of a temperature gradient between the body and the ambient air. This type of heat loss may occur in the OR, particularly in laminar flow rooms, and accounts for 25% to 50% of heat loss.[51,52]

Conductive heat loss involves loss of heat from a warm surface that comes into contact with a cooler one; it accounts for as much as 10% of heat loss in the OR, where patients lose heat to cooler OR tables, sheets, drapes, skin preparation fluids, and IV fluids or irrigants.[51,52]

Evaporative heat loss involves transfer of heat during the change from a liquid to a gas. Evaporative heat loss occurs via perspiration, respiration, or exposed viscera during surgery. Evaporation accounts for as much as 25% of heat loss in the OR.[51,52]

Patients at high risk for the development of hypothermia can be identified. Elderly patients are at risk because of their decreased subcutaneous fat and alterations in their hypothalamic function. Neonates are at risk because of their immature thermoregulatory center and their high surface-to-volume ratio. Intoxicated individuals are at risk because of vasodilation and depression of their heat regulatory center. Patients taking vasodilators, nonsteroidal antiinflammatory agents, and phenothiazines have alterations in thermoregulation that are caused by either vasodilation or suppression of the thermoregulatory center.[53] Other risk factors are female gender, decreased ambient room temperature, length and type of surgery, preexisting conditions such as peripheral vascular disease or burns, use of cold irrigants, and use of general or regional anesthesia.[50,51,53,54]

General anesthetics depress the thermoregulatory center, with a usual temperature drop of 1° to 3° C. General anesthesia reduces the vasoconstriction threshold; general anesthesia and regional anesthesia both cause peripheral vasodilation, which results in a core-to-peripheral redistribution of heat.[55] Opioids and muscle relaxants depress voluntary shivering as a mechanism for the generation of heat. Any patient in whom a body cavity is entered may lose heat via convection and evaporation. Irrigation solutions used in genitourinary procedures or with cardioplegia in cardiac surgery cause internal cooling.[56]

Physiologically, hypothermia results in decreased oxygen availability by shifting of the oxyhemoglobin dissociation curve to the left. Shivering may increase oxygen demand by 400% to 500%.[57] Metabolically dependent processes slow, thereby decreasing drug biotransformation. Renal transport processes are slowed, thereby decreasing glomerular filtration. Cardiac rate and rhythm disturbances, including bradydysrhythmias and premature ventricular contractions, may occur. Central nervous system depression may be profound.[57] Other adverse effects of perioperative hypothermia include patient discomfort, increased adrenergic stimulation, coagulopathy, impaired wound healing, surgical site infection, and increased hospital costs.[50,51,54,58,59]

Treatment of hypothermia should ideally be focused on prevention. Assessment of the patient's need for prewarming begins preoperatively, and active warming measures can be instituted for hypothermic patients.[9,50] As a result of positioning, operating time, and anesthetic exposure, therapeutic intervention most often begins in the PACU. Every patient in the PACU should be assessed for hypothermia and care provided as suggested in the multidisciplinary ASPAN Clinical Guideline for the Prevention of Perioperative Hypothermia (Figure 51-5).[50] Passive rewarming is designed to maximize basal heat production. Active rewarming consists of the use of external rewarming techniques and may include the use of heated blankets, heated water blankets, and radiant warmers. Forced-air rewarming systems are the most effective method for treating hypothermia.[5]

Postoperative shivering consists of muscular tremor and rigidity. It is often associated with body heat loss, although hypothermia alone does not fully explain the occurrence of shivering. Shivering is self-limiting, never becomes chronic, and is rarely associated with major morbidity. However, it affects the comfort of patients and may sometimes lead to more serious complications.[60] Treatment is rewarming. However, when clinically indicated, meperidine can be effective in the treatment of shivering during emergence and recovery.[61]

Nausea and Vomiting

In 1914, the first journal devoted solely to the topic of anesthesia featured an original article titled "Prophylaxis of Postanesthetic Vomiting."[62] More than 90 years later, postanesthetic vomiting is still one of the major problems faced in the PACU. Postoperative nausea and vomiting (PONV) affects 20% to 30% of all surgical patients, and the chance for PONV can be as high as 70% to 80% for high-risk patients.[63] Risk factors can be divided into three categories: patient-specific, anesthetic-related, and surgery-related (Box 51-8).[64]

The patient-specific risk factors listed in Box 51-8 are independent predictors for PONV. Females experience PONV two to three times more often than males, although these differences do not show up until after puberty. Being a nonsmoker and having a history of motion sickness or PONV are also independent predictors of PONV. Other associated factors are migraines, better health status as defined by the ASA risk classification, and anxiety. Children ages 11 to 14 experience an increased incidence of PONV. The highest rate occurs in young adults but decreases in older adults.[63-66]

FIGURE **51-5** Postoperative Patient Management: Phase I PACU. (*From the American Society of PeriAnesthesia Nurses. Clinical Guidelines for the Prevention of Unplanned Perioperative Hypothermia: ASPAN 2002 Standards of Perianesthesia Nursing Practice. Cherry Hill, NJ: American Society of PeriAnesthesia Nurses; 2002.*)

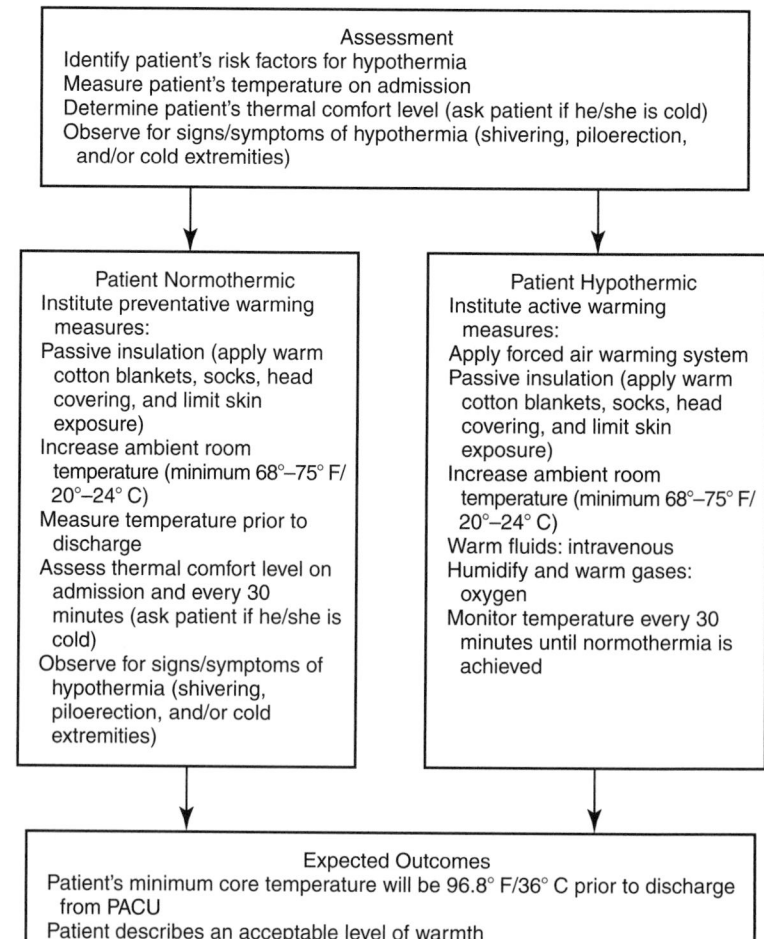

Postoperative Patient Management: Phase I PACU

Assessment
Identify patient's risk factors for hypothermia
Measure patient's temperature on admission
Determine patient's thermal comfort level (ask patient if he/she is cold)
Observe for signs/symptoms of hypothermia (shivering, piloerection, and/or cold extremities)

Patient Normothermic
Institute preventative warming measures:
Passive insulation (apply warm cotton blankets, socks, head covering, and limit skin exposure)
Increase ambient room temperature (minimum 68°–75° F/ 20°–24° C)
Measure temperature prior to discharge
Assess thermal comfort level on admission and every 30 minutes (ask patient if he/she is cold)
Observe for signs/symptoms of hypothermia (shivering, piloerection, and/or cold extremities)

Patient Hypothermic
Institute active warming measures:
Apply forced air warming system
Passive insulation (apply warm cotton blankets, socks, head covering, and limit skin exposure)
Increase ambient room temperature (minimum 68°–75° F/ 20°–24° C)
Warm fluids: intravenous
Humidify and warm gases: oxygen
Monitor temperature every 30 minutes until normothermia is achieved

Expected Outcomes
Patient's minimum core temperature will be 96.8° F/36° C prior to discharge from PACU
Patient describes an acceptable level of warmth
Signs/symptoms of hypothermia will be absent

The choice of anesthetic agent may influence the incidence of PONV. Early vomiting in the PACU is usually the result of anesthetic agents.[67] PONV occurs twice as often with inhalation anesthetics as with propofol anesthesia, and the risk of PONV decreases significantly after regional anesthesia. The use of nitrous oxide has been associated with PONV, but its relationship may not be as important as originally thought.[64] Desflurane, isoflurane, and sevoflurane have not shown significant differences in the incidence of nausea and vomiting after their use. Propofol, used as an induction agent and IV anesthetic, is associated with a lower incidence of postoperative nausea and vomiting, whereas etomidate and ketamine may increase this adverse effect.[68] Postoperative use of opioids is strongly correlated with PONV, although the effect of intraoperative opioids is not as well defined.[64]

The duration of surgery contributes to the incidence of PONV. Longer procedures are associated with a longer exposure to inhalation agents and possibly a larger dose of opioids during the surgery. The type of surgical procedure has also been cited as a contributing factor in PONV, although the evidence is conflicting about site and types of surgeries.[64,66] In children, strabismus and orchiopexy surgery are associated with a higher incidence of PONV. Patients undergoing tonsillectomy and adenoidectomy have a high incidence of nausea and vomiting as a result of swallowed blood.[69] In adults, an increased incidence of nausea and vomiting has been noted in patients undergoing diagnostic laparoscopy procedures, breast surgery, gynecologic surgery, intracranial/neurosurgery, and otologic and ophthalmic procedures.[15,64,66]

Simplified risk-assessment instruments are available that that identify patients' risk for PONV. One tool in widespread use is Apfel's risk assessment tool.[63] The patient is scored based on four risk factors: gender, smoking status, history of PONV or motion sickness, and postoperative use of opioids. A patient's risk increases with the number of risk factors present. An assessment of risk factors should be done preoperatively and the management of patients at risk guided by number of risk factors and chance of PONV. Figure 51-6 offers

---

BOX **51-8**

Primary Risk Factors Associated with PONV

Patient Specific
Female gender
Nonsmoker
History of PONV
History of motion sickness

Anesthetic Related
Use of volatile anesthetics
Use of nitrous oxide
Postoperative use of opioids

Surgery Related
Duration of surgery
Type of surgery

Data from Murphy MJ et al. Identification of risk factors for postoperative nausea and vomiting in the perianesthesia patient. J Perianesth Nurs. 2006;21:377-384; Gan TJ et al. Society for Ambulatory Anesthesia guidelines for the management of postoperative nausea and vomiting. Anesth Analg. 2007;105:1615-1628.

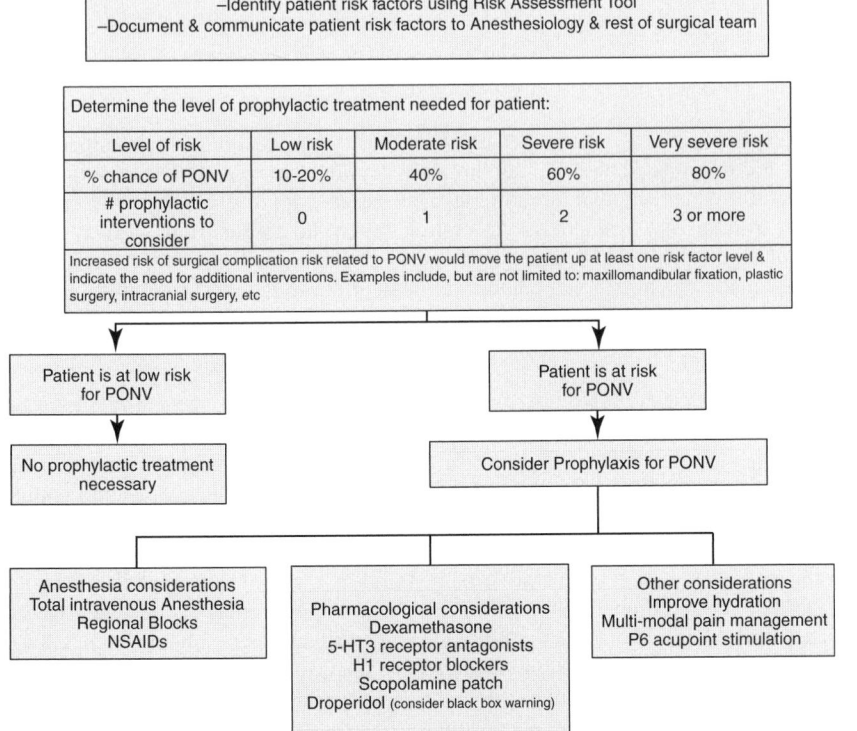

FIGURE **51-6** Preoperative patient management. *(From American Society of PeriAnesthesia Nurses. J Perianesth Nurs. 2006;21:243.)*

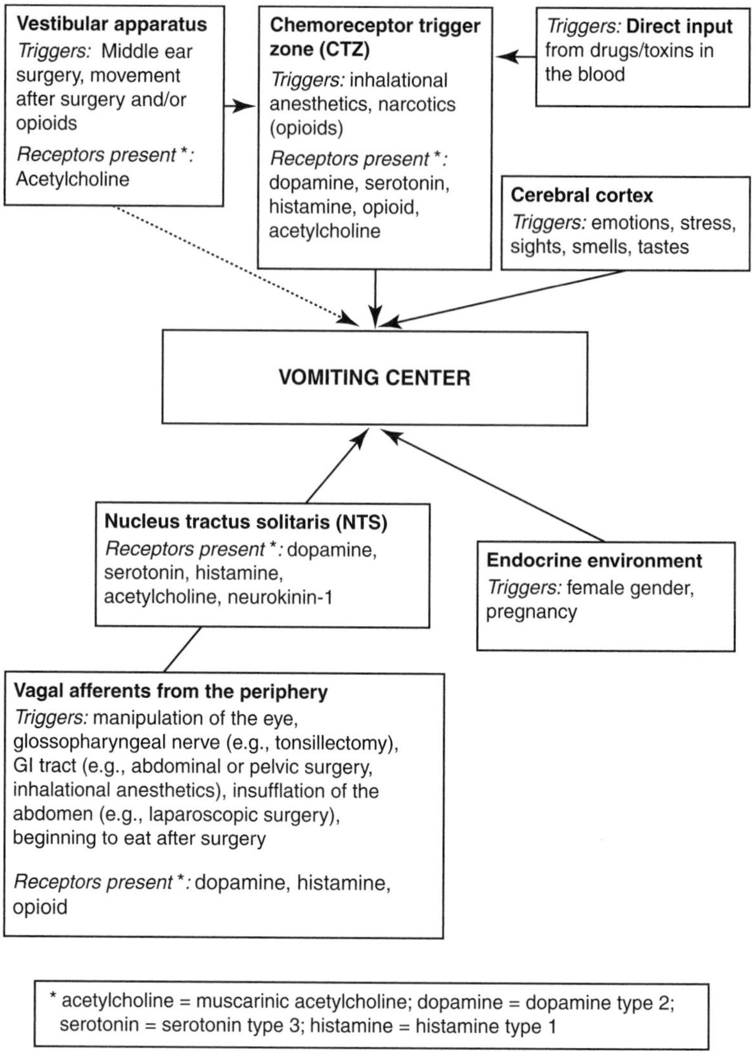

FIGURE **51-7** Mechanisms and neurotransmitter systems of PONV. (*From Drain CB, Odom-Forren J. Perianesthesia Nursing: A Critical Care Approach. St Louis: Saunders, 2009:414.*)

recommendations for preoperative antiemetic prophylaxis from ASPAN's Evidence-Based Clinical Practice Guideline for the Prevention and/or Management of PONV/PDNV.

Management of nausea and vomiting should originate from a prophylactic rather than a therapeutic approach, particularly in patients identified as at risk. Figure 51-7 provides a schematic view of some of the mechanisms that cause nausea and vomiting and neurotransmitter systems.

The patient who experiences PONV may begin with nausea, a subjective feeling of discomfort or need to vomit.[64] Nausea can be rated on a verbal descriptor scale or numeric rating scale to determine its severity. A rescue antiemetic that targets a different receptor site than the prophylactic agent given should be administered.[65,66,70] Other rescue interventions should be implemented, including verification of hydration and appropriate nonpharmacologic therapy such as aromatherapy.[65] Figure 51-8 presents strategies for postoperative management of PONV.

Drugs that block the serotonin receptors (5-HT3) are ondansetron, dolasetron, granisetron, and palonestron. Droperidol blocks the dopamine (D_2) receptor sites (although the FDA black box warning about QT prolongation and required ECG monitoring must be kept in mind). Other D_2-blocking agents are prochlorperazine or metoclopramide. For histamine receptors, promethazine or diphenhydramine can be used. Glycopyrrolate or scopolamine patches may be used for the muscarinic receptors. Dexamethasone is often given in conjunction with a 5-HT^3 blocking agent or droperidol. Substance P is another neurotransmitter that belongs to the neurokinin family of neurotransmitters. Substance P has affinity for neurokinin 1 (NK-1) receptors. The only medication available at the present time is aprepitant, which can be given orally as a prophylactic agent.[15,70]

Side effects (e.g., agitation, restlessness, drowsiness) may be associated with the use of some antiemetics. Prophylaxis using a combination of antiemetic drugs has been suggested as an effective strategy for minimizing postoperative nausea and vomiting.[66,70,71] Ephedrine has also been used for maintaining systemic blood pressure, thereby minimizing cerebral ischemia and preventing postoperative nausea and vomiting.[66] The FDA warning for droperidol is intended to increase awareness of the potential for cardiac dysrhythmias during drug administration and to encourage consideration of alternative medications for patients at high risk for cardiac dysrhythmias.[72] Droperidol currently carries a warning about cases of sudden death at high doses (greater than 25 mg) in patients at risk for cardiac dysrhythmias. Recent research has

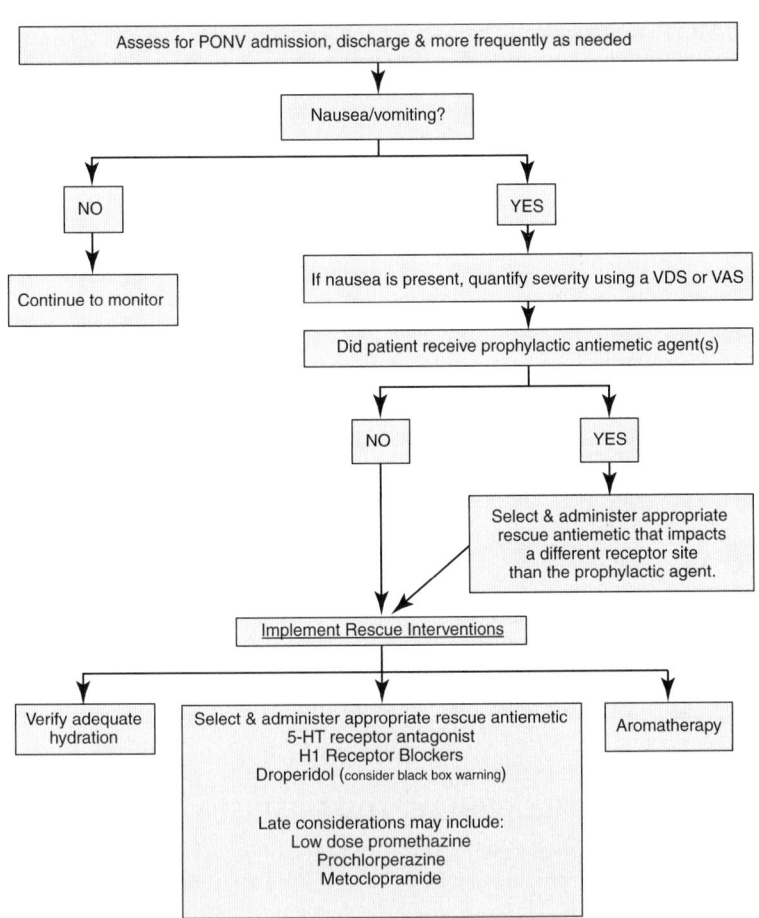

FIGURE **51-8** Postoperative patient management. (*From American Society of PeriAnesthesia Nurses.* J Perianesth Nurs. *2006;21:244*)

shown QT prolongation (delayed recharging of the heart between beats) within minutes after injection of a dose of droperidol at the upper end of the labeled dose range. Prolonged QT is dangerous because it can cause a fatal heart arrhythmia known as *torsades de pointes.* Historically the typical dose of droperidol given to adults with symptoms of postoperative nausea and vomiting has been 0.625 to 2.5 mg IV.[73]

Nonpharmacologic interventions may also be appropriate for the patient with PONV in addition to pharmacologic interventions.[15,65,66,74] Acupuncture, transcutaneous electrical nerve stimulation, acupoint stimulation, and acupressure have been shown to be effective in reducing the incidence of PONV and need for rescue medication. P6 stimulation has been shown to be effective, as well as Korean hand acupoints.[65,66,74] Aromatherapy (e.g., isopropyl alcohol or peppermint oil) has been used to treat PONV.[15,74,75] There are limited studies to date, but some show improvement in PONV. Aromatherapy was identified by the ASPAN guideline as an option with limited evidence but little risk to the patient.[65]

Postdischarge nausea and vomiting (PDNV), nausea and vomiting experienced after discharge from a health-care facility after outpatient surgery, continues to affect 20% to 30% of patients.[76] In a review of the literature, one author looked at evidence for treatment modalities with PDNV. Based on the evidence, certain prophylactic antiemetics and combination medications work significantly better than placebo, with some evidence available for ondansetron dissolving tablets and scopolamine patches. It is not likely that the type of anesthetic agent has an effect on PDNV. Inhalation agents seem to have more effect on PONV

than PDNV. It does seem that acupuncture and acustimulation may work. More research needs to be conducted to find appropriate treatment modalities, pharmacologic and nonpharmacologic, that prove effective in this patient population.[65,66,76] Figure 51-9 illustrates management of PDNV guidelines.

Fluids

According to the ASA practice guidelines,[5] routine perioperative assessment of patients' hydration status and fluid management reduces adverse outcomes and improves patient comfort and satisfaction. On the patient's admission to the PACU, intravascular volume is estimated, with consideration given to preoperative status, type and duration of surgery, estimated blood loss, fluid replacement, and hemostasis. Monitoring urine output as an index of intravascular volume can be misleading. Surgery and anesthesia impair renal tubular concentrating ability, and glycosuria causes osmotic diuresis, each falsely indicating that intravascular volume is adequate. Central venous, pulmonary arterial pressure, or transesophageal ultrasound monitoring can help to clarify volume status.

A reduction in circulating intravascular volume decreases ventricular filling and cardiac output. SNS-mediated tachycardia, increased SVR, and venoconstriction might compensate for a 15% to 20% loss of intravascular volume. Greater deficits can cause hypotension. Failure to replace preoperative fluid deficit and fluid or blood lost during surgery frequently causes hypovolemia. In the PACU, ongoing hemorrhage, sweating, and exudation of fluid into tissues (third-space losses) exacerbate hypovolemia. Blood loss is often occult, as with retroperitoneal bleeding, diffuse oozing related to coagulopathy, or hemorrhage into muscle after trauma or orthopedic procedures. Third-space losses can continue for up to 48 hours after surgery and can be massive during high-permeability pulmonary edema or accumulation of ascites. In a hypothermic, venoconstricted patient, a low intravascular volume might maintain cardiac output on PACU admission but cause hypotension when venous capacity increases during rewarming.[52]

Urinary Output and Voiding

Monitoring kidney function during recovery reduces morbidity in patients with marginal cardiovascular or renal status. The ability to void after spinal or epidural anesthesia should be assessed, because autonomic effects of regional anesthetics or opioids interfere with sphincter relaxation and promote urine retention.[77] Urinary retention is common after urologic, inguinal, and genital surgery and frequently delays discharge. It is reasonable to discharge inpatients to a surgical floor and selected ambulatory surgical patients from the facility before they void.[5] However, it is important to ensure that urine output is monitored after discharge from the PACU to avoid urinary retention. It is prudent to give ambulatory patients who are discharged without voiding a specific time interval in which to void (e.g., 10 to 12 hours after discharge). If retention persists, the patient should be instructed to contact a health-care facility. Patients with indwelling catheters should have urinary output recorded hourly.

Urine color is not useful for assessment of renal tubular function such as concentrating ability, but color can signal hematuria, hemoglobinuria, or pyuria. Urine osmolarity is a more reliable index of tubular function than specific gravity, which is affected by molecular weight.

Oliguria (<0.5 mL/kg/hr) occurs frequently during recovery and usually reflects an appropriate renal response to hypovolemia or systemic hypotension. However, a decreased urine output might indicate abnormal renal function. The acceptable degree and duration of oliguria vary with underlying renal status, the surgical procedure, and the anticipated postoperative course. If events related to the surgical procedure could jeopardize renal function (e.g., aortic cross-clamping, severe hypotension, massive transfusion), oliguria must be aggressively evaluated. In patients without catheters, bladder volume and interval since last voiding should be checked to help differentiate between oliguria and inability to void. Urinary catheters should be checked for kinking and obstruction by blood clots or debris. Patient position might also place the catheter tip above the urinary level in the bladder.[52]

Polyuria, a state of profuse urine output, usually reflects generous intraoperative fluid administration. Osmotic diuresis caused by hyperglycemia and glycosuria is another cause, particularly if glucose-containing crystalloid solutions have been infused. Polyuria might also reflect intraoperative diuretic administration. Sustained polyuria (4 to 5 mL/kg/hr) can indicate abnormal regulation of water clearance, especially if urinary losses compromise intravascular volume and systemic blood pressure. Polyuria related to diabetes insipidus occurs secondarily to intracranial surgery, pituitary ablation, head trauma, increased intracranial pressure, and inadvertent omission of preoperative vasopressin. The diagnosis is made by comparing urine and serum electrolytes and osmolarity. High-output renal failure should also be considered as a cause.[16]

DISCHARGE FROM THE POSTANESTHESIA CARE UNIT

The patient leaving the PACU may be discharged to home, an ambulatory surgical unit, a surgical inpatient unit, or an intensive care unit. The choice of a discharge facility should depend on the patient's need and physical status and the availability of appropriate resources.

When possible, before discharge, each patient should be sufficiently oriented to assess his or her physical condition and be able

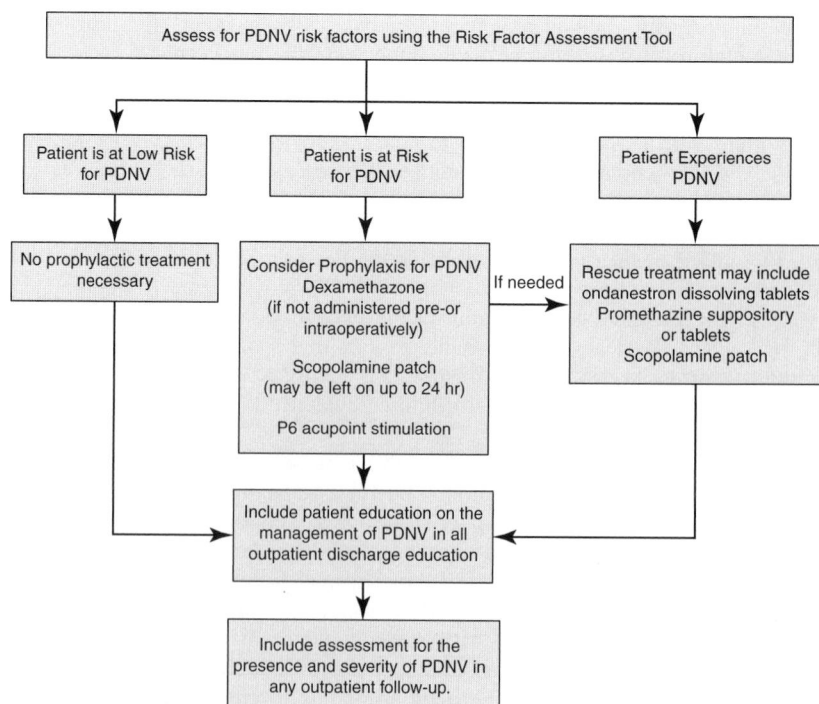

FIGURE **51-9** Management of PDNV. (*From American Society of PeriAnesthesia Nurses. J Perianesth Nurs. 2006;21:245.*)

to summon assistance. Airway reflexes and motor function must be adequate to prevent aspiration. Ventilation and oxygenation should be acceptable and demonstrate sufficient reserve to safely cover minor deterioration in unmonitored settings. To detect hypoxemia, oxygen saturation should be monitored for an appropriate period of time after discontinuation of supplemental oxygen. Before discharge, patients should be observed for a period of time after the last IV opioid or sedative is administered to assess peak effects, as well as side effects. Hemodynamic measurement and indexes of peripheral perfusion should be relatively constant. Achievement of normal body temperature should occur before discharge home or to a medical floor; ICU can continue an active warming process. Resolution of shivering is important. Acceptable analgesia must be achieved and vomiting

appropriately controlled. Likely surgical complications must be determined (e.g., bleeding, vascular compromise, pneumothorax, complications of coexisting diseases such as coronary artery disease, diabetes, hypertension, or asthma). The results of postoperative diagnostic tests should be reviewed. The routine requirement for urination before discharge should not be part of a discharge protocol and may be necessary only for selected day-surgery patients.[5] Likewise, the requirement of drinking clear fluids should not be a part of a discharge protocol and may be necessary only for selected patients (e.g., diabetic patients) and determined on a case-by-case basis.[5]

The Joint Commission requires the use of outcome indicators as the basis for quality monitoring.[3] Outcome indicators applied to discharge criteria should be written with a patient focus—for example, "Before discharge, the patient will maintain vital signs within the preoperative range." Examples of discharge criteria are found in Box 51-9. The patient's ability to meet these criteria constitutes clearance for discharge from the PACU but does not imply readiness for discharge to home. Two clinicians, Aldrete[78] and Chung,[79] have piloted scoring systems designed to evaluate the patients for outpatient discharge.

The Aldrete modified postanesthesia recovery (PAR) score is a modification of the original Aldrete score for PAR (Table 51-1). This modification of the scoring system changed assessment of "color" to assessment of "oxygen saturation." This scoring system is for use when patients are discharged from PACU Phase I. This further modification of the Aldrete scoring system for outpatients' street fitness is given in Table 51-2.

Chung and colleagues developed the Postanesthesia Discharge Scoring system as a simple, objective tool to assess the readiness of patients to be discharged to home (Box 51-10). A score of 9 is needed for the patient to be discharged. Although studied retrospectively, the scoring system has yet to be tried as a predictive index in a widespread clinical trial. Regardless of the method used to assess readiness for discharge, the

---

BOX **51-9**

Postanesthesia Care Unit Discharge Criteria

- Regular respiratory pattern
- Respiratory rate appropriate for age
- Absence of restlessness and confusion
- Vital signs within preoperative range
- Pulse oximetry indicates 95% saturation* or value equal to preoperative saturation
- Arterial blood gas values within normal limits†
- Ability to maintain patent airway
- Surgical stability of operative site or system

*Unit policies may dictate another number needed for oxygen saturation on discharge. There is no known accepted saturation level for discharge; most units require at least 92%.
†Not routinely obtained before discharge.

TABLE **51-1**   Aldrete Postanesthesia Scoring System

			Admit	15 min	30 min	45 min	60 min
Activity	Able to move voluntarily on command	Four Extremities	2	2	2	2	2
		Two Extremities	1	1	1	1	1
		No Extremities	0	0	0	0	0
Respiration	Able to breathe deeply, cough freely		2	2	2	2	2
	Dyspnea or limited breathing		1	1	1	1	1
	Apnea		0	0	0	0	0
Circulation	BP ± 20 mm Hg of preanesthesia level		2	2	2	2	2
	BP ± 20-50 mm Hg of preanesthesia level		1	1	1	1	1
	BP ± 50 mm Hg of preanesthesia level		0	0	0	0	0
Consciousness	Fully awake		2	2	2	2	2
	Arousable on calling		1	1	1	1	1
	Not responding		0	0	0	0	0
O₂ Saturation	Able to maintain O₂ saturation >90% on room air		2	2	2	2	2
	Needs O₂ inhalation to maintain O₂ saturation >90%		1	1	1	1	1
	O₂ saturation <90% even with O₂ supplementation		0	0	0	0	0

From Marshall S, Chung F. Assessment of 'home readiness' discharge criteria and post-discharge complications. Curr Opin Anesthesiol. 1997;10:445-480.
BP, *Blood pressure;* O₂, *oxygen.*

TABLE **51-2**	Modified Postanesthesia Recovery Score for Outpatients' Street Fitness	
Activity	Able to move four extremities voluntarily on command	2
	Able to move two extremities voluntarily on command	1
	Able to move no extremities voluntarily on command	0
Respiration	Able to breathe deeply and cough freely	2
	Dyspnea or limited breathing	1
	Apneic	0
Circulation	BP ± 20 mm Hg of preanesthetic level	2
	BP ± 21-49 mm Hg of preanesthetic level	1
	BP + 50 mm Hg of preanesthetic level	0
Consciousness	Fully awake	2
	Arousable on calling	1
	Not responding	0
O_2 saturation	Able to maintain O_2 saturation >92% on room air	2
	Needs O_2 inhalation to maintain O_2 saturation >90%	1
	O_2 saturation <90% even with O_2 supplement	0
Dressing	Dry	2
	Wet but stationary	1
	Wet but growing	0
Pain	Pain free	2
	Mild pain handled by oral medications	1
	Pain requiring parenteral medications	0
Ambulation	Able to stand up and walk straight*	2
	Vertigo when erect	1
	Dizziness when supine	0
Fasting and feeding	Able to drink fluids	2
	Nauseated	1
	Nausea and vomiting	0
Urine output	Has voided	2
	Unable to void but comfortable*	1
	Unable to void and uncomfortable	0

From Aldrete JA. *The postanesthesia recovery score*. Anesth News. 1995;7:89-91.
May be replaced by Romberg's test or picking up 12 clips in one hand.

assessment should be documented in an objective manner using criteria agreed on by the departments of anesthesia, nursing, and surgery.

Fixed PACU discharge criteria must be used with caution, because variability among patients is tremendous. Scoring systems that quantify physical status or establish thresholds for vital signs are useful for assessment but cannot replace individual evaluation.

BOX **51-10**

Postanesthesia Discharge Scoring System

Vital Signs
2 = Within 20% of preoperative value
1 = 20%-40% of preoperative value
0 = >40% of preoperative value

Activity and Mental Status
2 = Oriented 3 separate times and a steady gait
1 = Oriented 3 separate times or a steady gait
0 = Neither

Pain, Nausea, Vomiting
2 = Minimal
1 = Moderate, requiring treatment
0 = Severe, requiring treatment

Surgical Bleeding
2 = Minimal
1 = Moderate
0 = Severe

Intake and Output
2 = Postoperative fluids and void
1 = Postoperative fluids or void
0 = Neither

From Chung F et al. *A post-anesthetic discharge scoring system for home-readiness after ambulatory surgery.* J Clin Anesth. 1995;7:500-506.

Fast-tracking outpatients after general anesthesia has assumed increased importance in ambulatory anesthesia because of the cost-savings potential when patients are transferred directly from the OR to the less labor-intensive Phase II recovery area. Given the inherent risks of complications associated with bypassing the PACU, effective and reliable fast-track criteria that allow anesthesia providers to rapidly assess a patient's postoperative alertness, physiologic stability, and comfort level immediately before transferring the patient from the OR are clearly needed.[80] With the availability of shorter-acting anesthetics, some patients may be eligible for safe discharge directly from the OR to home. An outpatient should be discharged to a responsible adult, who will accompany the patient home and be able to report any postprocedure complications. In addition, outpatients should be provided with written instructions regarding postprocedure diet, medications, activities, and a phone number to be called in case of emergency.[1]

Ideally, each patient should be evaluated for discharge by a qualified anesthesia provider using a consistent set of criteria that take into consideration the severity of the underlying disease, the anesthetic and recovery course, and the level of care at the destination, especially for ambulatory patients.

SUMMARY

Postanesthesia care units are vital to the safe recovery of patients from surgery and anesthesia. Nurses provide the skillful bridge to ensuring a successful perioperative experience. They monitor patients for residual anesthetic effects and surgical complications and reinstitute care for preexisting medical problems. Integrating their care with that of the anesthesia and surgical teams is essential in the modern surgical center.

REFERENCES

1. Schick L. Assessment and monitoring of the perianesthesia patient. In: Drain CB, Odom-Forren J, eds. *Perianesthesia Nursing: A Critical Care Approach.* St Louis: Saunders; 2009.
2. American Society of PeriAnesthesia Nurses. *2006-2008 Standards of Perianesthesia Nursing Practice.* Cherry Hill, NJ: ASPAN; 2006.
3. The Joint Commission on Accreditation of Healthcare Organizations. *Comprehensive Accreditation Manual for Hospitals: The Official Handbook.* Oakbrook Terrace, IL: TJC; 2008.
4. American Association of Nurse Anesthetists. *Postanesthesia Care Standards for the Certified Registered Nurse Anesthetist.* 2001. Available at: http://www.aana.com/resources.aspx?ucNavMenu_TSMenuTargetID=51&ucNavMenu_TSMenuTargetType=4&ucNavMenu_TSMenuID=6&id=782. Accessed July 29, 2008.
5. American Society of Anesthesiologists. *Standards for Postanesthesia Care.* 2004. Available at: http://www.asahq.org/publicationsAndServices/standards/36.pdf. Accessed July 29, 2008.
6. Litwack K. Immediate postoperative care: a problem-oriented approach. In: Vender J, Spiess B, eds. *Post Anesthesia Care.* Philadelphia: Saunders; 1992.
7. Ferrara-Love R. Immediate postoperative assessment. In: Quinn DMD, Schick L, eds. *PeriAnesthesia Nursing Core Curriculum.* St Louis: Saunders; 2004:608-650.
8. Aldrete JA. Modifications to the postanesthesia score for use in ambulatory surgery. *J Perianesth Nurs.* 1998;13:148-155.
9. Odom-Forren J: Postoperative patient care and pain management. In: Rothrock J, ed. *Alexander's Care of the Patient in Surgery.* St Louis: Mosby; 2007:246-270.
10. Mecca R. Postoperative airway problems. *Curr Rev Nurse Anesth.* 2002;25:3-11.
11. Feeley TW, Macario A. The postanesthesia care unit. In: Miller R, ed. *Anesthesia.* 6th ed. New York: Churchill Livingstone; 2004:2703-2726.
12. Mecca R. Supplemental oxygen after anesthesia: risks, misconceptions, and recommendations. *Curr Rev Nurse Anesth.* 2001;24:87-93.
13. Strandberg A et al. Constitutional factors promoting development of atelectasis during anesthesia. *Acta Anaesthesiol Scand.* 1987;31:21-24.
14. Travis KW, Atlee JL. Postobstruction pulmonary edema. In: Atlee JL, ed. *Complications in Anesthesia.* 2nd ed. Philadelphia: Saunders; 2007.
15. O'Brien D. Postanesthesia complications. In: Drain CB, Odom-Forren J, eds. *Perianesthesia Nursing: A Critical Care Approach.* St Louis: Saunders; 2009.
16. Mecca R. Postanesthesia recovery. In: Barash P, et al, ed. *Clinical Anesthesia.* 5th ed, Philadelphia: Lippincott; 2006:1374-1404.
17. Ginsberg JS. Management of venous thromboembolism. *N Engl J Med.* 1996;335:1816-1828.
18. Patel K, Chaney MA. Hypercoagulable states: thrombosis and embolism. In: Atlee JL. *Complications in Anesthesia.* 2nd ed. Philadelphia: Saunders; 2007.
19. American Society of Anesthesiologists. Practice guidelines for preoperative fasting and the use of pharmacologic agents to reduce the risk of pulmonary aspiration: application to healthy patients undergoing elective procedures. *Anesthesiology.* 1999;90:896-905.
20. Tasch MD. Pulmonary aspiration. In: Atlee JL, ed. *Complications in Anesthesia.* 2nd ed. Philadelphia: Saunders; 2007:186-188.
21. Benca J. Bronchospasm. In: Atlee JL. *Complications in Anesthesia.* 2nd ed. Philadelphia: Saunders; 2007:189-192.
22. Bevan DR. Monitoring and reversal of neuromuscular block. *Am J Health Syst Pharm.* 1999;56(suppl 1):S10-S13.
23. Drain CB. Neuromuscular blocking agents. In: Drain CB, Odom-Forren J. *Perianesthesia Nursing: A Critical Care Approach.* St Louis: Saunders; 2009:318-337.
24. Ganong W. *Review of Medical Physiology.* 21st ed. Norwalk, CT: Appleton & Lange; 2003.
25. Sessler DI. Perioperative heat balance. *Anesthesiology.* 2000;92:578-596.
26. Dunn PF: *Clinical Anesthesia Procedures of the Massachusetts General Hospital.* 7th ed. Boston: Lippincott Williams & Wilkins; 2007.
27. White P. Ketamine update: its clinical uses in anesthesia. *Semin Anesth.* 1988;7:111-126.
28. Berg H et al. Residual neuromuscular block is a risk factor for postoperative pulmonary complications: a prospective, randomized, and blinded study of postoperative pulmonary complications after atracurium, vecuronium, and pancuronium. *Acta Anaesthesiol Scand.* 1997;41:1095.
29. O'Brien D. Acute postoperative delirium: definitions, incidence, recognition and interventions. *J Perianesth Nurs.* 2002;17:384-392.
30. Moos DD. Sevoflurane and emergence behavioral changes in pediatrics. *J Perianesth Nurs.* 2005;20:13-18.
31. Vlajkovic GP, Sindjelic RP. Emergence delirium in children: many questions, few answers. *Int J Anesth.* 2007;104:84-91.

32. Lepouse C et al. Emergence delirium in adults in the post-anaesthesia care unit. *Br J Anaesth.* 2006;96:747-753.
33. Sikich N, Lerman J. Emergence delirium: statistically significant or not? *J Clin Anesth.* 2001;13:157-158.
34. Haynes C. Emergence delirium: a literature review. *Br J Theatre Nurs.* 1999;9:502-503, 506-510.
35. Madi-Jebara S et al. The central anticholinergic syndrome: a rare cause of uncontrollable agitation after coronary artery bypass graft surgery. *J Cardiothorac Vasc Anesth.* 2002;16:665-666.
36. Voepel-Lewis T et al. Nurses' diagnosis and treatment decisions regarding care of the agitated child. *J Perianesth Nurs.* 2005;20:239-248.
37. McClain DA. Delayed emergence. In: Atlee J, ed. *Complications in Anesthesia.* 2nd ed. Philadelphia: Saunders; 2007:885-888.
38. Nagelhout JJ. Inhaled anesthetics in essentials of nurse anesthesia. In: McIntosh LW, ed. *Essentials of Nurse Anesthesia.* New York: McGraw-Hill; 1997:71-80.
39. Benumof J. *Anesthesia and Perioperative Complications.* 2nd ed. Chicago: Year Book; 1999.
40. Carlson K. Perianesthesia complications. In: Quinn DMD, Schick L, eds. *PeriAnesthesia Nursing Core Curriculum.* St Louis: Saunders; 2004:651-684.
41. Kortilla K. Postanesthesia cognitive and psychomotor impairment. *Int Anesthesiol Clin.* 1986;24:59-74.
42. Pasero C. The challenge of pain assessment in the PACU. *J Perianesth Nurs.* 2002;17:348-350.
43. Apfelbaum J et al. Postoperative pain experience: results from a national survey suggest postoperative pain continues to be undermanaged. *Anesth Analg.* 2003;97:534-540.
44. Pavlin DJ et al. Pain as a factor complicating recovery and discharge after ambulatory surgery. *Anesth Analg.* 2002;95:627-634.
45. Pasero C, McCaffery M. Orthopaedic postoperative pain management. *J Perianesth Nurs.* 2007;22:160-174.
46. Kurz A, Sessler DI. Opioid-induced bowel dysfunction: pathophysiology and potential new therapies. *Drugs.* 2003;63:649-671.
47. Kehlet H et al. PROSPECT: Evidence-based, procedure-specific postoperative pain management. *Best Pract Res Clin Anaesthiol.* 2007;21:149-159.
48. Pasero C. Procedure-specific pain management: PROSPECT. *J Perianesth Nurs.* 2007;22:335-340.
49. PROSPECT: *Procedure-Specific Postoperative Pain Management.* Available at: http://www.postoppain.org. Accessed July 29, 2008.
50. American Society of PeriAnesthesia Nurses. *Clinical Guideline for the Prevention of Unplanned Perioperative Hypothermia.* Available at: http://www.aspan.org/PDFfiles/HYPOTHERMIA_GUIDELINE10-02.pdf. Accessed July 29, 2008.
51. Hooper VD. Care of the patient with thermal imbalance. In: Drain CB, Odom-Forren J, eds. *Perianesthesia Nursing: A Critical Care Approach.* St Louis: Saunders; 2009:748-759.
52. Sessler DI. Perioperative heat balance. *Anesthesiology.* 2000;92:578-596.
53. Macario A, Dexter F. What are the most important risk factors for a patient's developing intraoperative hypothermia? *Anesth Analg.* 2002;94:215-220.
54. Wagner DV. Unplanned perioperative hypothermia. *AORN J.* 2006;83:470.
55. Hooper VD. Thermoregulation. In: Quinn DMD, Schick L. *PeriAnesthsia Nursing Core Curriculum: Preoperative, Phase I and Phase II PACU Nursing.* St Louis: Saunders; 2004:444-466.
56. De Witte J, Sessler DI. Perioperative shivering: physiology and pharmacology. *Anesthesiology.* 2002;96:467-484.
57. Buggy DJ, Crossley AW. Thermoregulation, mild perioperative hypothermia and postanesthetic shivering. *Br J Anaesth.* 2000;84:615-628.
58. Sessler DI, Akca O. Nonpharmacological prevention of surgical wound infections. *Healthcare Epidemiol.* 2002;35:1397-1404.
59. Mahoney C, Odom J. Maintaining intraoperative normothermia: a meta-analysis of outcomes with costs. *AANA J.* 1999;67:155-164.
60. Kranke P et al. Postoperative shivering in children: a review on pharmacologic prevention and treatment. *Paediatr Drugs.* 2003;5:373-383.
61. Alfonsi P. Postanesthetic shivering. Epidemiology, pathophysiology and approaches to prevention and management. *Minerva Anestesiol.* 2003;69:438-442.
62. Buckler H. Prophylaxis of postanesthetic vomiting. *Am J Surg Q.* 1914.
63. Apfel CC et al. A simplified risk score for predicting postoperative nausea and vomiting. *Anesthesiology.* 1999;91:693-700.
64. Murphy MJ et al. Identification of risk factors for postoperative nausea and vomiting in the perianesthesia patient. *J Perianesth Nurs.* 2006;21:377-384.
65. American Society of PeriAnesthesia Nurses. ASPAN's evidence-based clinical practice guideline for the prevention and/or management of PONV/PDNV. *J Perianesth Nurs.* 2006;21:230-242.

66. Gan TJ et al. Society for ambulatory anesthesia guidelines for the management of postoperative nausea and vomiting. *Anesth Analg.* 2007;105:1615-1628.

67. Verheecke G. Early postoperative vomiting and volatile anaesthetics or nitrous oxide. *Br J Anaesth.* 2003;90:109.

68. Kovac AL. Prevention and treatment of postoperative nausea and vomiting. *Drugs.* 2000;59:213-243.

69. Rose JB, Watcha MF. Postoperative nausea and vomiting in pediatric patients [review]. *Br J Anaesth.* 1999;83:104-117.

70. Golembiewski J, Tokumaru S. Pharmacological prophylaxis and management of adult postoperative/postdischarge nausea and vomiting. *J Perianesth Nurs.* 2006;21:385-397.

71. Tang J et al. Antiemetic prophylaxis for office-based surgery: are the 5-HT3 receptor antagonists beneficial? *Anesthesiology.* 2003;98:293-298.

72. Nuttall GA et al. Does low-dose droperidol administration increase the risk of drug-induced QT prolongation and torsades de pointes in the general surgical population? *Anesthesiology.* 2007;107(4):531-536.

73. Norred C. Antiemetic prophylaxis: pharmacology and therapeutics. *AANA J.* 2003;71:2.

74. Mamaril ME et al. Prevention and management of postoperative nausea and vomiting: a look at complementary techniques. *J Perianesth Nurs.* 2006;21:404-410.

75. Winston A et al. Comparison of inhaled isopropyl alcohol and intravenous ondansetron for treatment of postoperative nausea. *AANA J.* 2003;71:2.

76. Odom-Forren J et al. Evidence-based interventions for postdischarge nausea and vomiting: a review of the literature. *J Perianesth Nurs.* 2006;21:411-439.

77. Kamphuis ET et al. Recovery of storage and emptying functions of the urinary bladder after spinal anesthesia with lidocaine and with bupivacaine in men. *Anesthesiology.* 1998;88:310-316.

78. Aldrete JA. The post-anesthesia recovery score revisited. *J Clin Anesth.* 1995;7:89-91.

79. Chung F et al. A post-anesthetic discharge scoring system for home readiness after ambulatory surgery. *J Clin Anesth.* 1995;7:500-506.

80. White PF, Song D. New criteria for fast-tracking after outpatient anesthesia: a comparison with the modified Aldrete's scoring system. *Anesth Analg.* 1999;88:1069-1072.

CHAPTER 52

PAIN MANAGEMENT

Margaret Faut-Callahan, Walter R. Hand, Jr.

The nature and incidence of unrelieved pain are major concerns as we enter the 21st century. As providers of anesthesia care in the United States, certified registered nurse anesthetists (CRNAs) are integral to the study and management of acute, chronic, and cancer-related pain. CRNAs have often been removed from the decision-making processes related to pain management. Only recently have CRNAs been recognized as experts in the area of pain management, and their knowledge and skills are needed to address this major societal health-care problem. So important is the issue of unrelieved pain in the United States that the Agency for Healthcare Research and Quality (AHRQ), a federally funded agency, chose pain as one of its initial health-care issues to address. Unrelieved pain associated with operative and medical procedures and trauma,[1] oncology,[2] and pediatric patients[3] has been thoroughly studied. Recommendations from the various study groups are being integrated throughout the health-care system. CRNAs must be fully aware of the issues that were addressed in these important studies.

Fundamentally the members of the study panels found that undermedication of patients in moderate to severe pain has been well documented in the literature for decades.[4-11] Many centers have tried to address this serious health issue through major interventional programs. Despite the implementation of various interventions, the problem of inadequately managed pain remains. Loeser and Egan,[12] experts in pain management, suggested a model of care that described the complexity of the phenomenon. Donovan and colleagues[13] modified this model to include an additional element, system response (Figure 52-1). The system response, or those of us in a position to intervene in a pain management situation, has been underemphasized. CRNAs must assume responsibility for being key members of the pain management team.

The role of health-care providers in the management of acute and chronic pain has become the focus of many professional and regulatory groups. The Joint Commission has focused on the adequacy of pain management for a number of years. They developed pain management standards and implemented them on January 1, 2001. The standards were developed through an effort of The Joint Commission and the University of Wisconsin, Madison, through a grant from the Robert Wood Johnson Foundation. The significance of this move by a regulatory agency is great and has had far-reaching effects. The Joint Commission clearly outlined the responsibilities of hospitals, home-care agencies, nursing homes, behavioral health facilities, outpatient clinics, and health plans. The responsibilities are:

- Recognize the right of patients to appropriate assessment and management of pain.

- Assess the existence of pain and if present its nature and intensity in all patients.
- Record the results of the assessment in a way that facilitates regular reassessment and follow-up.
- Determine and ensure staff competency in pain assessment and management, and address pain assessment and management in the orientation of all new staff.
- Establish policies and procedures that support the appropriate prescription or ordering of effective pain medications.
- Educate patients and their families about effective pain management.
- Address patient needs for symptom management in the discharge-planning process.[14]

Assessment of these standards includes review of policy and procedures, protocols, documentation, educational materials, and interviews with patients, families, and clinicians. The Joint Commission has published three documents that explicitly define the agency's initiatives. *Pain: Current Understanding of Assessment, Management and Treatment* was published in December 2001.[15] *Improving the Quality of Pain Management through Measurement and Action* was published in March 2003.[16] In 2003, The Joint Commission published *Approaches to Pain Management: An Essential Guide for Clinical Leaders*.[17] This text provides advice regarding the development of a comprehensive pain-management strategy for health-care organizations.

The American Pain Society (APS), a respected professional organization dedicated to the effective management of pain, developed standards for the relief of both acute and cancer-related pain. Key elements of the standards are as follows:
1. Recognize and treat pain promptly.
   - Chart and display pain and relief (process).
   - Define pain and relief levels to trigger review (process).
   - Survey patient satisfaction (outcome).
2. Make information about analgesia readily available (process).
3. Promise patients attentive analgesic care (process).
4. Define explicit policies for use of advanced analgesic technologies (process).
5. Monitor adherence to standards (process).[18]

Further evidence of the importance now placed on effective management of pain is the introduction of a national strategy to alleviate pain in the United States. HR 1863, the National Pain Care Policy Act of 2003, was introduced. The purpose of the legislation is to provide resources for pain-care research, education, and the establishment of treatment plans within federally funded health-care programs. This follows the declaration by Congress that 2000 to 2010 is the "Decade of Pain Control."

The APS has developed guidelines for practitioners treating both acute and chronic pain. *The Guideline for the Management of*

Conceptual Framework

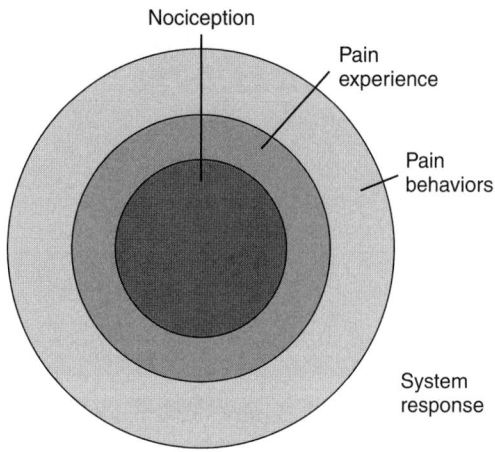

FIGURE **52-1**   Model for pain management. (*Modified from Loeser J, Egan D. Managing the Chronic Pain Patient. Theory and Practice at the University of Washington Multidisciplinary Pain Clinic. New York: Raven; 1989:6.*)

Cancer Pain in Adults and Children,[19] *Guideline for the Management of Fibromyalgia Syndrome Pain in Adults and Children,*[20] *Guideline for the Management of Pain in Osteoarthritis, Rheumatoid Arthritis and Juvenile Arthritis,*[21] and *Guideline for the Management of Acute and Chronic Pain in Sickle-Cell Disease*[22] are excellent resources for the CRNA. Two clinical reference guides assist the practitioner at the bedside with current practice information: *Principles of Analgesic Use in the Treatment of Acute and Pain and Cancer Pain*[23] and *Pain Control in the Primary Care Setting.*[24] Further, APS has developed many electronic resources that are of value to educators. The organization's commitment to practitioners is evident by the extensive resources that have been developed.

The complex issues related to effective pain management include an understanding of the physiologic, pathophysiologic, pharmacologic, and behavioral principles that occur. This chapter reviews the scientific foundation of the management of acute and cancer-related pain and the current methods of assessment, planning, implementation, and evaluation of a pain-management plan.

PAIN

Definition

The International Association for the Study of Pain and the APS developed a definition of pain. This was necessary because there was reluctance to look beyond the physiologic components of pain. *Pain* was defined as "an unpleasant sensory and emotional experience associated with actual or potential tissue damage or described in terms of such damage."[25] Although it is unquestionably a sensation in part or parts of the body, it is always unpleasant and therefore an emotional experience"[26] These definitions remind us that pain is both a physiologic and a behavioral phenomenon.[27]

It is necessary to clarify terms associated with the understanding of pain. *Nociception* is the process of transduction, transmission, perception, and modulation of pain.[28] Two general categories of pain exist: nociceptive and neuropathic. Nociceptive pain is associated with the stimulation of specific nociceptors and can be either somatic or visceral. *Somatic pain* refers to pain that has an identifiable locus and follows the distribution of a somatic nerve. In addition, somatic pain is well

localized, sharp in nature, and generally hurts at the point or area of stimulus. Conversely, visceral pain is diffuse, can be referred to another area, and is often described as dull and vague in nature. *Visceral pain* is often associated with the distention of an organ capsule or the obstruction of a hollow viscus. In contrast, *neuropathic pain* is caused by abnormal processing of painful stimuli. It is a dysfunction of the central nervous system (CNS) that allows for spontaneous excitation leading to severe pain. Neuropathic pain can be generated centrally or peripherally and is difficult to treat.[28] Patients describe their pain as burning, tingling, or shocklike.

Physiology

Pain is most commonly defined in terms of four processes: transduction, transmission, perception, and modulation. A noxious stimulus, be it chemical, mechanical, or thermal, is transformed into electrical energy during *transduction*. The electrical energy produces signals that are transmitted from the periphery to the CNS, and this process is called *transmission*. *Perception* occurs once the signal is recognized by the brain. *Modulation* occurs through descending mechanisms that modulate signal transmission in the spinal cord. Understanding of these distinct processes involved in the pain experience has allowed for the development of specific treatments to manage pain.

When peripheral tissues such as skin, bone, and viscera receive chemical, thermal, or mechanical stimuli or are traumatized by either surgery or injury, a series of biochemical events takes place. These events include the release of a number of endogenous chemicals (neurotransmitters) such as bradykinin, serotonin, and substance P. The most well-known neurotransmitter as it relates to pain is substance P. As this process continues, the arachidonic acid cascade is activated. Collectively these substances generate an action potential that stimulates peripheral nerve receptors, causing nociceptive stimulation. This nociceptive stimulation results in a transduction of nociceptive impulses. Because the suspected chemical reactions have such far-reaching influence throughout the body, it is necessary to trace the effects (Figure 52-2).

The stimuli are then transmitted to the dorsal horn of the spinal cord, where a sympathetic reflex response is created. Afferent nerve fibers are classified as type A, B, or C. Type A fibers are further defined as alpha, beta, gamma, or delta. Type A and B fibers are known to be myelinated, whereas type C fibers are nonmyelinated.[28] In the spinal cord are several receptor systems that function as modulators in the neurotransmission of nociceptive impulses.[27] Information is transmitted via ascending tracts to the supraspinal sites, where it is then processed. Such sites include the cerebral cortex, hypothalamus, and periaqueductal gray matter. The neurochemical mechanisms of pain and nociception are complex. In recent years, several categories of pain receptors have been identified.

Both *N*-methyl-D-aspartate (NMDA) and α-amino-acid-3-hydroxyl-5-methyl-4-isoxazole propionic acid (AMPA) receptors are located throughout the brain and spinal cord.[29] However, their interaction in the transmission of pain is predominantly at the level of the dorsal horn. Both receptor subtypes are ionotropic glutamate receptors located postsynaptically on the second-order neuron. When glutamate (excitatory neurotransmitter) is released from the depolarized primary afferent nerve terminals, it binds postsynaptically to these glutamate receptors to depolarize the second-order neuron and continue transmission of the nociceptive impulse to the CNS. NMDA and AMPA antagonists are newer additions to pain-management strategies.

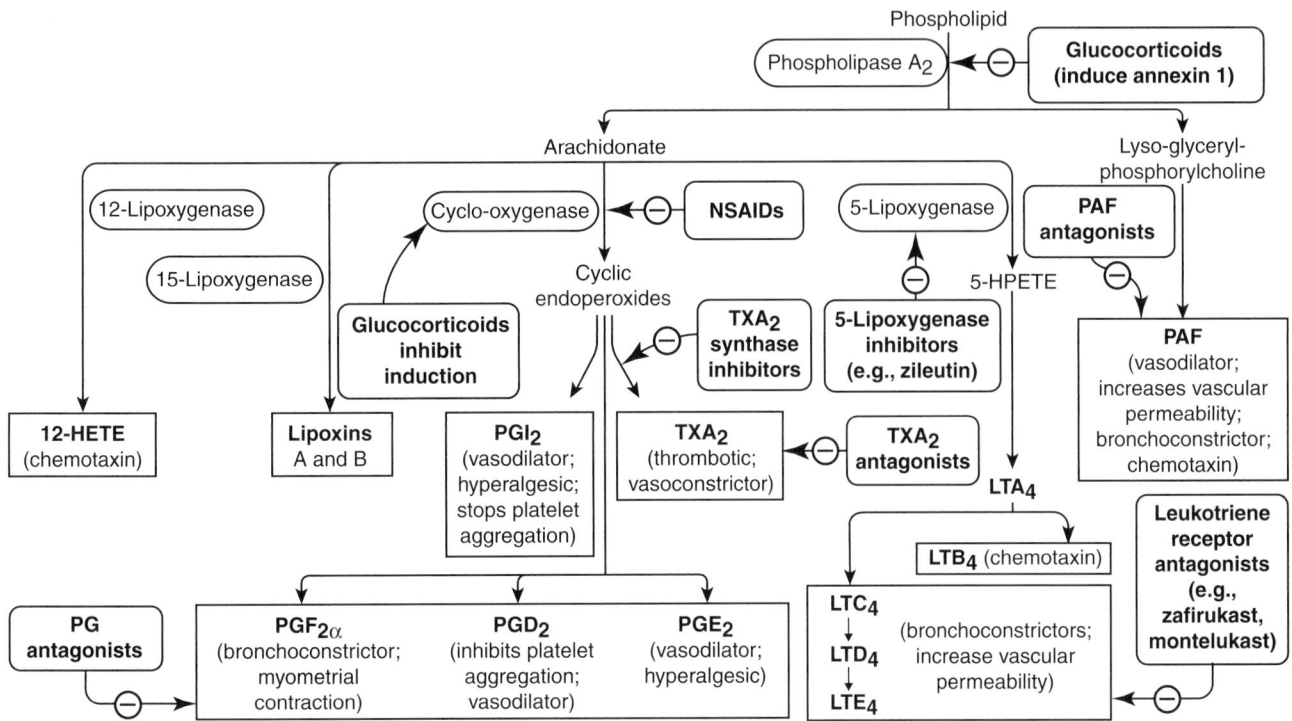

FIGURE **52-2** Summary diagram of the inflammatory mediators derived from phospholipids, with an outline of their actions and the sites of action of antiinflammatory drugs. (*From Rang HP, Dale MM et al. Pharmacology. 6th ed. London: Churchill Livingstone; 2007.*) *HETE,* Hydroxyeicosatetraenoic acid; *HPETE,* hydroperoxyeicosatetraenoic acid; *LT,* leukotriene; *PAF,* platelet-activating factor; *PGI₂,* prostacyclin; *TX,* thromboxane.

Pathophysiology

Pathophysiologic alterations related to pain may complicate existing disease and alter outcome.[1] Inadequately relieved or unrelieved pain is a source of fear, anxiety, helplessness, depression, and demoralization. Pain management unfortunately is still given a low priority and is associated with myths, misconceptions, and knowledge deficit among some health-care providers.[30] We have learned a great deal about the effects of pain on the human body. In addition, factors such as the extent of the trauma or surgical field, the number of pain receptors involved in the particular area, bleeding, infection, anxiety, and physiologic stress accelerate the endocrine stress response to trauma (Figure 52-3).

Cardiovascular System

The stress of pain resulting from surgery or trauma causes many cardiovascular responses. The most significant of these is the activation of the sympathetic nervous system. Release of substances such as catecholamines, cortisol, and angiotensin II occurs. Common cardiovascular symptoms associated with unrelieved pain are increased heart rate, increased cardiac output, increased myocardial oxygen consumption, and increased vascular resistance (peripheral, systemic, and coronary). Hypertension, hypercoagulation, and deep vein thrombosis can be seen. These factors may negatively affect postoperative outcome. Aggressive pain management may reduce the postoperative incidence of cardiac complications.[30]

Respiratory System

The presence of pain can have a tremendous effect on the respiratory system. This effect is most pronounced in those patients having surgery or trauma in the area of the upper abdomen and thorax. Pain causes a measurable decrease in tidal volume because of limited thoracic and abdominal movement. Specifically, decreases in vital capacity, inspiratory capacity, and functional residual capacity, as well as a decreased physical ability to clear the airway, are the result of unrelieved pain. Muscle spasm below and above the site of injury caused by the noxious stimuli promotes limited movement of the respiratory muscles. Patients also voluntarily decrease the movement of the thorax and abdomen in an attempt to limit pain. Furthermore, patients are reluctant to breathe deeply and to cough, enhancing their respiratory compromise. As a result, atelectasis and pneumonia are common postoperative complications.[31,32] These alterations may be aggravated in those with preexisting pulmonary dysfunction (e.g., asthma, chronic obstructive pulmonary disease). Successful strategies to manage pain must include precautions against further respiratory compromise.

Gastrointestinal and Genitourinary System

Increased sympathetic activity results in a delay in gastric emptying and decreased intestinal motility. Intestinal secretions and smooth-muscle sphincter tone increase. Paralytic ileus with nausea and vomiting is a common problem related to postoperative pain. In addition to the physiologic consequences of pain, some commonly used analgesics also alter gastrointestinal functioning. Systemic opioids may cause delayed gastric emptying and contribute to the development of paralytic ileus. In cases in which the speed of gastrointestinal recovery is of importance, local anesthetics have been shown to be beneficial.[32]

Pain can also result in hypomotility of the urethra and bladder, resulting in difficulty with urination. This increases the likelihood of having to catheterize the patient because of inability to void.[33]

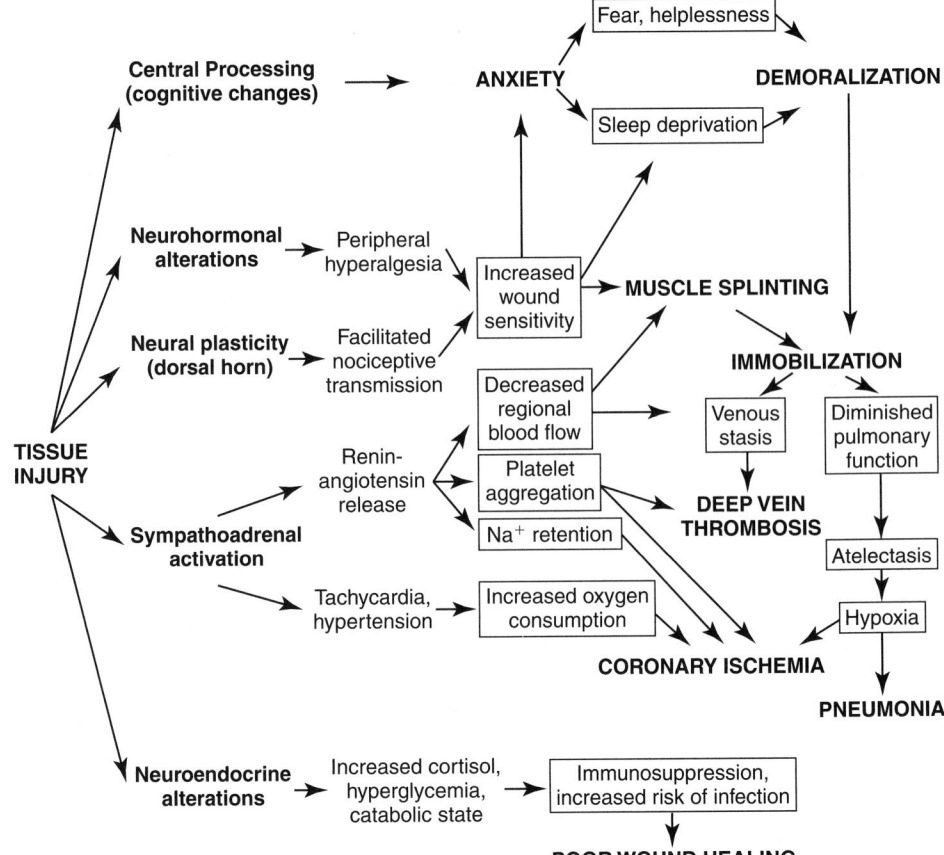

FIGURE **52-3** Outline of pathophysiologic responses associated with surgical trauma and their effect on key target organs.

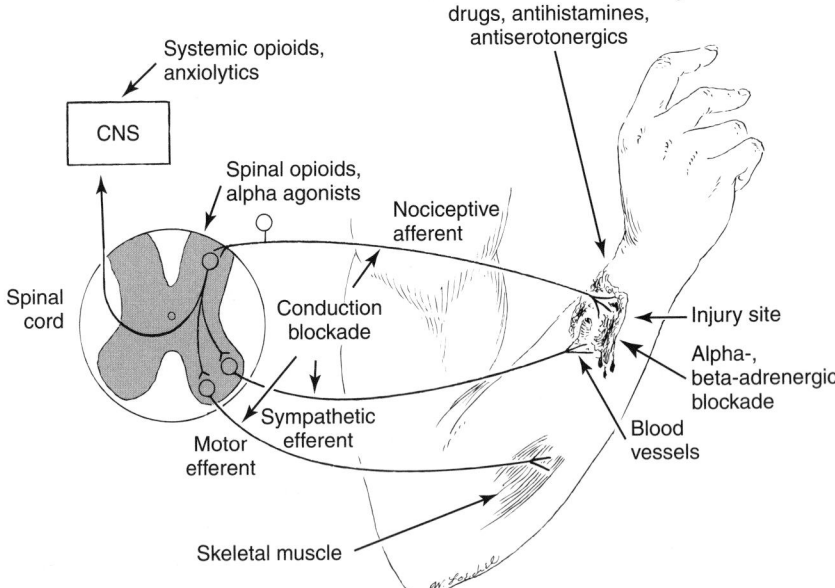

FIGURE **52-4** Sympathoadrenal response occurring because of the increased release of norepinephrine from the sympathetic nerve endings.

Endocrine System

The neurohormonal response to pain is complex and involves an array of both anabolic and catabolic hormones. The endocrine response to pain is characterized by an increase in the secretion of hormones such as adrenocorticotropic hormone, cortisol, antidiuretic hormone, growth hormone, and glucagon. Insulin and testosterone secretion is decreased.[30] In addition, hormones such as prolactin, vasopressin, and thyroxin are released as part of the endocrine response to pain.

Effective pain management decreases the neuroendocrine response to surgery or trauma. The timing of drug administration plays a major role in the blockade of the neuroendocrine response. In addition to the neuroendocrine response, a sympathoadrenal response and pathophysiologic change occur as a result of the increased release of norepinephrine from the sympathetic nerve endings (Figure 52-4).

Immune System

Pain, surgery, and trauma affect the competence of the immune system through neuroendocrine pathways. It is known that the degree of immunosuppression is closely linked to the magnitude of tissue damage.[34] Immunosuppression seen in the postoperative period may last as long as 1 to 2 weeks in healthy patients. Patients who are at higher risk for immunocompromise may experience more severe problems associated with immune dysfunction. Limiting pain and causes of surgical stress and infection is critical in these patients.

Psychological Effects

The psychological nature of pain must be recognized. The complex, subjective nature of pain is often difficult to comprehend.[35] The presence of pain can be a major source of fear and anxiety for the patient. An adversarial relationship may develop between the patient and doctors and nurses when pain is prolonged. This relationship may develop because the patient may perceive that the hospital staff is withholding pain relief, that the staff does not place a high priority on pain management, or that the staff believes that the patient's complaints of pain are exaggerated or contrived. Every effort must be made to reassure the patient that his or her pain relief is important to the staff. The patient should know that complaints of pain will be addressed in a timely and definitive manner.

ACUTE PAIN MANAGEMENT

General Aspects

Preoperative planning should include a discussion of the patient's expectations of postoperative pain and its management. Goals for pain management should be set by both the patient and care providers. The patient should be informed about the modalities available and should be given instructions on how to quantify pain intensity with instruments such as a verbal numeric scale, a visual analogue scale, or another instrument appropriate to the individual's cognitive skills. CRNAs should always be cognizant of the fact that pain in a multidimensional phenomenon. Although the presence or absence of pain is the initial step, there can be other factors contributing to the patient's perception of that pain. The patient should be encouraged to make use of simple nonpharmacologic techniques such as relaxation, simple imagery, and music.[1]

Regardless of the cause of the acute pain, a thorough patient interview, physical assessment, and review of the medical record (laboratory results, diagnostic studies, and so on) must be completed before the implementation of a plan to manage the patient's pain. The goal of the patient interview is to determine the existence of any history of pain, either malignant or nonmalignant (e.g., arthritis, chronic back pain). Patients should be asked if they have been taking any prescription or nonprescription medications to treat pain. A specific question regarding the use of any over-the-counter analgesics should be asked. In addition, CRNAs should know that there are a number of prescriptive adjunctive medications used to treat pain. It should not be assumed that a patient is being treated for a seizure disorder or depression because the patient is taking anticonvulsants or tricyclic antidepressants, both of which can effectively be used to treat different types of neuropathic pain. During the interview, every effort should be made to try to determine what type of pain the patient is experiencing. Opioids are not as effective at alleviating neuropathic pain as they are in treating either somatic or visceral pain. Furthermore, the patient's perception, psychological response, and behavioral and cognitive responses to the pain should be assessed. The perception should include location, description (qualitative), and intensity (via a verbally administered numeric rating scale), as well as factors that aggravate or relieve the pain.

Every assessment of a patient's pain should be accompanied by a physical assessment of the suspected locus of the pain. A visual inspection of the area may reveal signs and symptoms of infection, pressure, and so on. During the postoperative period, it should not be assumed that the pain is related to the surgical procedure. The cause of the pain could be a burn from the electrocautery pad, an infiltrated intravenous (IV) line, angina, and so on.

Finally, a review of the medical record should be completed. A nursing summary or assessment completed when the admitting nurse interviews the patient or family can provide a wealth of information. This summary can be particularly useful when patients are poor historians or simply cannot remember information secondary to the presence of pain or the effects of medications. Laboratory and radiologic data can provide invaluable information regarding the cause of the pain (e.g., infection, tumor).

If optimal analgesic care is to be provided to the patient in pain, assessment and reassessment play a vital role. Assessment should be done at regular intervals and should be simple. Key to the success of a treatment plan are adequate documentation and communication among all care providers. Evidence suggests that the addition of a simple flowchart documenting the patient's pain increases successful management.[1]

Pharmacologic Aspects

A clear understanding of the physiology of pain has led to the development of improved treatment modalities. Because pain is a complex phenomenon, the effective management of pain can be extremely difficult. Despite increasing knowledge in the area of pain physiology and pharmacology, many providers continue to treat the problem as if it is unidimensional. The use of multiple strategies to control pain is essential. Research in basic sciences and pharmacology continues to suggest that the use of analgesic drugs in combination remains the most logical and efficient way to manage or decrease postoperative pain.[36-39] The optimal strategy for pharmacologic management of pain should include a combination of analgesics and nonpharmacologic strategies as determined through individual patient assessment.

Preemptive Analgesia

Preemptive analgesia is a concept first postulated approximately 100 years ago. It is postulated that pain perception can be decreased through the use of analgesics capable of inhibiting CNS sensitization before the painful stimulus occurs.[40,41]

After injury or surgery, the tissue damage elicits peripheral sensitization and central sensitization. This causes a decrease in the pain threshold, hypersensitivity, and increased response to pain. Preemptive analgesia purports to prevent the sensitization of the CNS and may alter the overall pain response. The use of preemptive analgesia to limit central sensitization remains controversial, and some studies suggest that intraoperative administration of analgesics has little effect.

Although the use of preemptive analgesia has not been proved effective in decreasing central desensitization, research continues to evaluate the use of drugs that limit sensitization in the periphery. However, animal studies provide some evidence that this is an area for further study. Because many analgesics work in the periphery, it is postulated that they may be helpful in limiting peripheral sensitization. The use of nonsteroidal antiinflammatory drugs (NSAIDs), opioids, and local anesthetics is being studied. Reuben and Connelly found that preemptive use of cyclooxygenase (COX)-2 inhibitors decreased the use of morphine in a postoperative spinal fusion population.[42] Helmy and Bali found that the use of dextromethorphan (120 mg intramuscular [IM]) preincision decreased postoperative merperidine consumption.[43] The administration preoperatively of rofecoxib to arthroscopic knee surgery patients reduced postoperative pain.[44] Buvanendran and colleagues studied 70 randomized patients who underwent total knee replacement and found that preoperative administration of rofecoxib, followed by postoperative continuation, reduced opioid consumption and improved clinical outcomes.[45] Gramke and colleagues [46] studied the preoperative use of sublingual piroxicam in a double-blind study and recommended that use is more effective than when given in the postoperative period. They caution that both the control and study groups had low pain scores and futher study is needed. Yamashita and colleagues. demonstrated that the preoperative administration of intravenous fluribiprofind provided analgesia and opioid-sparing effects in the early postoperative period.[47]

Skinner and Shintani [39] found that the use of multiple non-narcotics in a stacked regimen significantly reduces postopertive pain. However, Kehle and Dahl reviewed 40 clinical studies and found little support for the use of preemptive analgesia.[36] More recently, Møiniche, and colleagues[48] conducted a meta-analysis of 93 randomized clinical trials of preincisional versus postincisional analgesia. Ultimately, 80 trials met the rigid inclusion criteria, representing 3761 patient encounters. The authors concluded that there is no benefit to preemptive analgesia but advocate that aggressive perioperative analgesic regimens be studied. Grape and Tramèr[37] and Pogatzki-Zahn and Zahn[38] suggest that extending a multimodal analgesic plan into the recovery period may result in better postoperative pain control. Adachi and colleagues recommend that anesthetists use multimodal analgesic techniques.[49] Critics of the preemptive analgesia technique suggest that the use of NSAIDs in a surgical population, with limited evidence that preemptive analgesia is effective, does not warrant potential complications. Postoperative bleeding is a concern in a surgical population.

DRUGS USED IN PAIN MANAGEMENT

Nonsteroidal Antiinflammatory Drugs and Acetaminophen

NSAIDs are best known for their use in the management of mild to moderate postoperative pain and pain related to inflammatory conditions. They represent a variety of chemical substances that inhibit the action of COX and thereby prevent conversion of arachidonic acid to prostaglandins; as a result, the nociceptive response to endogenous mediators of inflammation is attenuated. Prostaglandins are responsible for sensitizing and amplifying peripheral nociceptors to the inflammatory mediators (substance P, bradykinin, and serotonin) released when tissue is traumatized.

COX exists in two isoforms: COX-1 and COX-2. COX-1 is constitutive, widespread throughout the body, and necessary for homeostasis. It is located particularly in the kidneys, gastric mucosa, platelets, and endothelium. Conversely, COX-2 is normally present in the kidneys and central nervous system, and synthesis is induced in the presence of inflammation. Until recently, all of the NSAIDs were nonselective in their COX inhibition. As a result, in addition to the analgesia that results from the inhibition of the COX-2 isoform, inhibition of COX-1 leads to the detrimental side effects of gastric irritation, renal microvasculature constriction, and platelet inhibition. Presently there is one COX-2 selective NSAID, celecoxib. Others have been withdrawn from the market because of concerns over

cardiovascular side effects. Postsurgical pain can now be successfully treated with the judicious use of celecoxib because it does not inhibit COX-1 platelet aggregation, which has been a limiting factor in the use of traditional NSAIDs in postsurgical patients. Buvanendran and colleagues did not find any bleeding complications in a postsurgical population.[45] In addition to the antiinflammatory properties of these drugs, recent research suggests that NSAIDs also work at the spinal and supraspinal levels.[50-53]

When an NSAID is used as part of a postoperative pain regimen, nociception is diminished at the peripheral level. Evidence suggests that if an optimal dose of an NSAID is combined with an opioid, it produces an additive analgesic effect greater than that obtained by doubling the dose of either constituent.[54,55] The best time to initiate therapy is controversial. Research suggests that beginning NSAID therapy before activation of the inflammatory process and including NSAIDs as part of a preemptive analgesia regimen are effective.[36,53]

Some clinicians believe that the undesirable side effects of nonselective NSAIDs (gastrointestinal discomfort, the possibility of gastrointestinal bleeding, decreased platelet aggregation, potential renal insufficiency, and delayed wound healing) are sufficient grounds for avoiding their use in surgical patients, even for short periods. However, the short-term use of NSAIDs (<1 week) has not been shown to increase bleeding during surgery or to cause other major side effects.[56] NSAIDs are available primarily in oral form. Some are available as suppositories and can therefore be administered to patients denied oral intake. Ketorolac and indomethacin are available for parenteral administration. Ketorolac's analgesic potency is disproportionate to its antiinflammatory potency; however, its side-effect profile is similar to that of any other NSAID (Table 52-1).

Opioids

Opioids remain the drugs of choice for treatment of moderate to severe pain. Opioids are characterized on the basis of their specific affinity for the opioid receptors. Specific pharmacology is discussed in Chapter 12.

Adequate pain control may be hampered by fears of respiratory depression or hypotension. These misconceptions have little foundation, provided that the dose, route of administration, and choice of drug are appropriate for the situation and that the pain management is based on thorough assessment and reassessment of the patient. Table 52-2 lists the opioids and opioid antagonists that are used for pain control.

The continued development of opioids indicates the focus the health-care industry has placed on the optimal management of pain. Many effective opioids are available, including meperidine, a commonly used opioid. It should be noted that meperidine has a neurotoxic metabolite, normeperidine, which has a half-life of 15 to 24 hours. The neurotoxic side effects of normeperidine (shakiness, tremor, twitches, multifocal myoclonus, and grand mal seizures)[57-60] are not reversible with naloxone. Although a small dose of meperidine (12.5 to 25 mg) may be beneficial to treat postoperative rigors, its use in acute and cancer pain management is not recommended by the American Pain Society. Additionally, the risk of normeperidine toxicity is increased in those patients with preexisting renal or CNS disease, patients receiving greater than 600 mg/24 hours, or those using meperidine for more than 24 hours.[57]

A stigma is still associated with the prescription and administration of opioids because of the risk of psychological dependence. This phenomenon was referred to as "opiophobia" by Morgan,[61] who defined it as "undocumented fear that appropriate

Text continued on p. 1250

TABLE 52-1	Nonsteroidal Antiinflammatory Agents				
Agent	**Potency**	**Dose**	**Onset**	**Duration**	**Comments**
Acetaminophen (Tylenol, Panadol, Phenaphen, Tempra; in Anacin-3, Excedrin, Vicodin, Tylox, Percocet, Darvon-N)	1	PO or rectal 325-650 mg (6-12 mg/kg) q4h	PO 5-30 min	PO 3-7 hr	Most commonly available analgesic. Does not produce gastric irritation, does not interfere with platelet function.
Aspirin (in Bufferin, Buffaprin, Alka-Seltzer, Anacin, Percodan, Talwin)	1	PO 325-650 mg (6-12 mg/kg) q4-8h	PO 5-30 min	PO 3-7 hr	Irreversibly inhibits platelet aggregation for the life of the platelet (7-10 days) and prolongs bleeding time. Enhances urinary excretion of uric acid and is useful for treatment of gout. May prevent arterial and possibly deep venous thrombosis. Increased risk of development of Reye syndrome if used in children with influenza or chickenpox.
Celecoxib (Celebrex)	1-2	PO 100-200 mg bid	PO <45 min	PO 4-6 hr	NSAID that exerts its effect by selective inhibition of COX-2. GI effects and development of ulcers are reported to be less with this class of drugs. Avoid during pregnancy.
Choline salicylate (Arthropan)	1	PO 435-870 mg or 2.5-5 mL (8-16 mg/kg or 0.05-0.1 mg/kg) q4h	PO 5-30 min	PO 3-7 hr	Does not inhibit platelet aggregation. Useful in patients with GI intolerance to aspirin.
Diclofenac sodium (Voltaren)	15	PO 100-200 mg (2-4 mg/kg) daily in two to four divided doses	PO 15-30 min	PO 4-6 hr	Structurally related to mefenamic acid but more potent.
Diflunisal (Dolobid)	3.5-13	PO 1 g, then 500 mg q8-12h	PO <60 min	PO 3-7 hr	May be administered twice daily. In contrast to the prolonged effects of aspirin, platelet aggregation returns to normal within 24 hours.
Etodolac (Lodine)	3	PO 200-400 mg (4-8 mg/kg) q6-12h	PO 15-30 min	PO 4-6 hr	Better tolerated than indomethacin, naproxen, or ibuprofen; equipotent doses are associated with fewer gastric mucosal abnormalities.
Fenoprofen calcium (Nalfon)	3	PO 200 mg (4 mg/kg) q4-6h	PO 15-30 min	PO 4-6 hr	Better tolerated than aspirin; equipotent doses are associated with fewer gastric mucosal abnormalities.
Ibuprofen (Advil, Motrin)	M	PO 200-800 mg (8-16 mg/kg) q6h	PO 30 min	PO 6-8 hr	Better tolerated than aspirin or naproxen; equipotent doses are associated with fewer gastric mucosal abnormalities.
Indomethacin (Indocin)	20	PO 25-50 mg (0.5-1 mg/kg) q6-12h	PO 15-30 min	PO 4-6 hr	Potent NSAID. More effective than aspirin in relieving the pain of primary dysmenorrhea. Indomethacin has antiinflammatory effects comparable with those of colchicine in the treatment of gouty arthritis.
Ketoprofen (Orudis)	20	PO 25-50 mg (0.5-1 mg/kg) q6-8h	PO 15-30 min	PO 3-4 hr	Potent NSAID. Better GI tolerance than indomethacin or aspirin.

Data from Mosby's Drug Consult. St Louis: Mosby; 2007; Boyce EG, Breen GA. Celecoxib: a COX-2 inhibitor for osteoarthritis and rheumatoid arthritis. Formulary. 1999;34:405-417; Drugs for pain. Med Lett Treat Guidel. 2007;56:23-32.

Continued

TABLE 52-1   Nonsteroidal Antiinflammatory Agents—cont'd

Agent	Potency	Dose	Onset	Duration	Comments
Ketorolac tromethamine (Toradol)	60 (PO)	Loading: IM or IV 30-60 mg (0.5-1 mg/kg) Maintenance: IM or IV 15-30 mg (0.25-0.5 mg/kg) PO 10 mg q4-6h	IV <1 min IM <10 min PO <1 hr	IV 3-7 hr IM 3-7 hr PO 3-7 hr	The only NSAID approved for parenteral administration for analgesia. To minimize serious adverse effects, duration of use should not exceed 5 days for parenteral and 14 days for oral administration.
Meclofenamate sodium (Meclomen)	3	PO 200-300 mg (4-6 mg/kg) daily in three or four divided doses	PO 30-60 min	PO 3-7 hr	Structurally related to mefenamic acid but fewer incidences of hematologic abnormalities
Mefenamic acid (Ponstel)	3	PO 500 mg (10 mg/kg), then 250 mg (5 mg/kg) daily q6h	PO 30-60 min	PO 3-7 hr	May be associated with hematologic abnormalities (e.g., decreased hematocrit, leukopenia, agranulocytosis, and pancytopenia).
Naproxen (Naprosyn, Aleve)	3	PO 500 mg (10 mg/kg), then 250 mg (5 mg/kg) q6-12h	PO 30-60 min	PO 3-7 hr	Medium-potency NSAID. Better GI tolerance than aspirin. Available over the counter in the United States.
Oxyphenbutazone (various)	20	Initial: PO 300-600 mg (6-12 mg/kg) daily in three or four divided doses Maintenance: PO 100-400 mg (2-8 mg/kg) daily in three or four doses	PO 15-30 min	PO 4-6 hr	Potent NSAID, may cause serious adverse effects. Should not be used as a simple analgesic or antipyretic. May compete with thyroxine for protein-binding sites and may reduce the uptake of iodine by thyroid gland. May cause significant sodium retention.
Parecoxib (Dynastat)	10	IV or IM 20-40 mg	10-20 min	6-8h	COX-2 inhibitor for perioperative use. Allergic and anaphylactic responses have been reported.
Phenylbutazone (Butazolidin)	20	Initial: PO 300-600 mg (6-12 mg/kg) daily, in three or four divided doses Maintenance: PO 100-400 mg (2-8 mg/kg) daily in three or four doses	PO 15-30 min	PO 4-6 hr	Potent NSAID, may cause severe adverse effects; used only as a second-line agent. Has mild uricosuric activity and decreases tubular reabsorption of uric acid.
Piroxicam (Feldene)	3	PO 20-40 mg (0.4-0.8 mg/kg) daily, in one or two divided doses	PO 30-60 min	PO 48-72 hr	May be administered once daily. Structurally unrelated to other NSAIDs. Medium potency and long duration of action.
Salsalate (Disalcid, Argesic)	1	PO 2-4 g (40-80 mg/kg) daily in two or three divided doses	PO 5-30 min	PO 3-7 hr	Useful in patients with GI intolerance to aspirin. Does not inhibit platelet aggregation. Increased risk of developing Reye syndrome if used in children with influenza or chickenpox.
Sulindac (Clinoril)	20	PO 150-200 mg (3-4 mg/kg) bid	PO 15-30 min	PO 3-4 hr	Equipotent to indomethacin but associated with fewer gastric mucosal abnormalities.
Tolmetin sodium (Tolectin)	20	PO 400-600 mg (8-12 mg/kg) q8h	PO 15-30 min	PO 3-4 hr	Equipotent to indomethacin but associated with fewer gastric mucosal abnormalities

TABLE 52-2 Opioids and Opioid Antagonists					
Agent	**Potency***	**Dose**	**Onset**	**Duration**	**Comments**
Buprenorphine HCl (PA) (Buprenex)	30	IV, IM, SL 0.3-0.6 mg (6-12 mcg/kg) q4-6h; Epidural 50-60 mg (1 mg/kg)	IV <1 min; IM 1 hr	IV, IM, SL 6 hr	Binds avidly to opioid receptors. Respiratory depression may not respond to naloxone; doxapram may be more suitable.
Butorphanol tartrate (Ag-An) (Stadol)	3.5-7	IV 0.5-2 mg (0.010.04 mg/kg) q3-4h; IM 1-4 mg (0.02-0.08 mg/kg) q3-4h; Nasal 1 mg; Epidural 1-2 mg 20-40 mcg/kg)	IV 1-5 min; IM 10 min; Nasal <15 min	IV 2-4 hr; IM 3-4 hr; Nasal 4-5 hr; Epidural 3-4 hr	May be administered by epidural route for acute and chronic pain.
Codeine phosphate or sulfate (Ag) (Tylenol with codeine, Phenaphen with codeine)	1/30-1/8	PO, IM, IV 15-60 mg (0.5 mg/kg) q4h	PO 15-30 min	PO 3-6 hr	May be used with acetaminophen or aspirin for mild to moderate pain. Has analgesic and antitussive properties.
Fentanyl citrate (Ag) (Sublimaze)	75-125	Oral (transmucosal) 200-400 mcg (5-15 mcg/kg) q4-6h; IV, IM 25-100 mcg (0.7-2 mcg/kg); Epidural 50-100 mcg (1-2 mcg/kg); Spinal 5-20 mcg (0.1-0.4 mcg/kg); Transdermal 25-100 mcg/hr	Oral 5-15 min; IV <30 sec; IM <8 min; Epidural 4-10 min; Spinal 4-10 min; Transdermal 12-18 hr	Oral 1-2 hr; IV 30-60 min; IM 1-2 hr; Epidural 4-8 hr; Spinal 4-8 hr; Transdermal 3 days	Potent opioid. Related to meperidine. Transdermal and oral transmucosal forms useful in chronic pain.
Hydrocodone HCl (Ag) (Lortab, Lorcet, Co-Gesic, Vicodin)	1/30-1/8	PO 5-10 mg q4-6h	PO 15-30 min	PO 4-8 hr	Mild analgesic. Potency similar to codeine. Used in combination with aspirin or acetaminophen.
Hydromorphone HCl (Ag) (Dilaudid)	7	PO 2-4 mg q4-6h; IM, subQ 2-4 mg (0.04-0.08 mg/kg); Slow IV 0.5-2 mg (0.01-0.04 mg/kg); Epidural 1-2 mg (20-40 mcg/kg)	PO, IM, subQ 15-30 min; IV <30 sec; Epidural 5 min	PO, IM, subQ 4-6 hr; IV 2-4 hr; Epidural 10-16 hr	Potent, short-acting opioid. Used for breakthrough pain in conjunction with long-acting opioid (e.g., morphine). May be administered parenterally, rectally, or subcutaneously.
Levorphanol tartrate (Ag) (LevoDromoran)	5	PO, subQ 2-4 mg q4-6h; Slow IV 1 mg (0.02 mg/kg)	IV 10-15 min	subQ 6-8 hr; IV 6-8 hr	Highly concentrated. Useful for subcutaneous infusions requiring small volumes.

Data from Drugs for pain. Med Lett Treat Guidel. 2007;56:23-32; Mosby's Drug Consult. *St Louis: Mosby; 2007.*
Ag, Agonist; Ag-An, agonist-antagonist; An, antagonist; IM, intramuscular; IV, intravenous; NA, not applicable; PA, partial agonist; PO, by mouth; subQ, subcutaneous; SL, sublingual.
Compared with oral morphine sulfate.

Continued

TABLE **52-2**   Opioids and Opioid Antagonists—cont'd

Agent	Potency*	Dose	Onset	Duration	Comments
Meperidine HCl (Ag) (Demerol)	0.1	PO, IM. IV, subQ 50-150 mg (1-3 mg/kg) Slow IV 25-100 mg (0.5-2 mg/kg) Epidural 50-100 mg (1-2 mg/kg) Spinal 0.2-1 mg (4-20 mcg/kg)	PO 10-45 min IM 1-5 min IV <1 min Epidural 2-12 min Spinal 2-12 min	IV, IM, PO 2-4 hr Epidural 1-8 hr Spinal 1-8 hr	Only opioid with local anesthetic properties and direct myocardial depressant effects.
Methadone HCl (Ag) (Dolophine)	1-3	PO, IM, subQ 2.5-10 mg (0.05-0.1 mg/kg) q3-4h, then 5-20 mg/hr, q6-8h Epidural 1-5 mg (20-100 mcg/kg)	PO 30-60 min IV 1 min IM 1-5 min Epidural 5-10 min	IV, IM 4-6 hr PO 22-48 hr Epidural 6-10 hr	Long-acting opioid analgesic; accumulates with use, and administration frequency may be decreased.
Morphine sulfate (Ag) (Morphine, MS Contin, Duramorph, Astramorph)	1	PO 10-60 mg q4h PO (MS Contin) 15-100 mg q12h IM, subQ 2.5-20 mg q4h Rectal 10-20 mg q4h IV 2.5-15 mg Epidural 2-5 mg (40-100 mcg/kg) Spinal 0.2-1 mg (4-20 mcg/kg)	PO <60 min IM 1-5 min IV 1 min Epidural 15-60 min Spinal 15-60 min	IV, IM, subQ 2-7 hr Epidural 6-24 hr Spinal 6-24 hr	Principal alkaloid of opium. Prototype of the opiate agonists. Long-acting preparation used for chronic pain.
Nalbuphine HCl (Ag-An) (Nubain)	1	IV, IM, subQ 5-10 mg (0.1-0.3 mcg/kg) q3-6h	IV 2-3 min IM, subQ 15 min	IV, IM, subQ 3-6 hr	Effective in reversing ventilatory depression of agonist opioids (e.g., morphine) while maintaining reasonable analgesia.
Nalmefene (Revex)	NA	IV 0.25 mcg/kg, repeat as necessary in 2- to 5-min intervals up to a total dose of 1 mcg/kg	IV 1-3 min	IV 6-8 hr	Reverses the side effects (e.g., respiratory depression and pruritus) of opioid agonists and the psychotomimetic and dysphoric effects of agonists-antagonists (e.g., pentazocine).

Drug		Dose/Route	Onset	Duration	Comments
Naloxone HCl (Narcan)	NA	IV, IM, subQ 0.1-2 mg (10-100 mcg/kg)	IV 1-2 min IM, subQ 2-5 min	IV, IM, subQ 1-4 hr	Reverses the side effects (e.g., respiratory depression and pruritus) of opioid agonists and the psychotomimetic and dysphoric effects of agonists-antagonists (e.g., pentazocine).
Naltrexone HCl (Ant) (Trexan)	NA	PO 12.5-50 mg daily	PO 15-30 min	PO 24-72 hr	May reverse the hypotension and cardiovascular instability secondary to endogenous endorphins (potent vasodilators) released in patients with septic or cardiogenic shock.
Oxycodone HCl (Ag) (Roxicodone; in Percocet, Percodan, Roxicet, Tylox)	2	PO 5-10 mg q4-6h	PO 10-15 min	PO 3-6 hr	Potency similar to morphine. Used often in combination with aspirin and acetaminophen.
Oxymorphone HCl (Ag) (Numorphan)	10	IV 0.5 mg q4-6h IM, subQ 0.5-1.5 mg q4-6h Rectal 5 mg q4-6h	IV 5-10 min IM, subQ 10-15 min	IV, IM 3-6 hr	Derivative of hydromorphone with similar effects.
Pentazocine HCl (Ag-An) (Talwin)	1/3	PO 50-100 mg (1-2 mg/kg) q3-4h IM, subQ 30-60 mg (0.5-1 mg/kg) q3-4h IV 15-30 mg (0.3-0.5 mg/kg) q3-4h	PO 15-30 min IM, subQ 15-20 min IV 2-3 min	PO 3-6 hr IM 2 hr IV 1 hr	Oldest agonist-antagonist opioid. Like other agonist-antagonists, may be associated with psychotomimetic effects.
Propoxyphene HCl (Ag) (Darvon; in Genagesic, Wygesic)	1/50-1/25	PO 65 mg q4h	PO 15-60 min	PO 4-6 hr	Derivative of methadone. Weak analgesic. Used in combination with other analgesics (e.g., acetaminophen).
Sufentanil citrate (Ag) (Sufenta)	500-700	IV, IM 10-30 mcg (0.2-0.6 mcg/kg) Epidural 10-30 mcg (0.2-0.6 mcg/kg) Spinal 1-4 mcg (0.02-0.08 mcg/kg)	IV 1-3 min Epidural 4-10 min Spinal 4-10 min	IV 20-45 min IM 2-4 hr Epidural 2-4 hr Spinal 2-4 hr	Most potent opioid in clinical use, 700 times more potent than morphine. Administered via epidural or spinal route for chronic pain. Parenteral route used for general anesthesia.

use of opioids causes addiction." Although the risk of iatrogenically induced psychological dependence to opioids is thought to be relatively low, there are no recent definitive studies to substantiate this claim.[62]

Misconceptions exist among health professionals and patients about the principles of tolerance, pseudoaddiction, physiologic dependence, and psychological dependence. Unfortunately, these misconceptions can result in the inappropriate labeling of patients as addicts.

Tolerance refers to a change in the dose-response relationship induced by exposure to the drug and manifested as a need for a higher dose to maintain an effect. The development of tolerance to an opioid is a normal physiologic response.

Pseudoaddiction is often confused with psychological dependence because the behavior of the patients can be the same. That is, patients with both of these conditions exhibit what appears to be drug-seeking behavior. However, in the patient who is "pseudoaddicted," the origin of the behavior is inadequate analgesia. When these patients receive adequate analgesia, they no longer demonstrate drug-seeking behavior.

Physiologic dependence is a pharmacologic property of opioid drugs defined by the occurrence of an abstinence (withdrawal) syndrome after abrupt discontinuation of the drug or the administration of an opioid antagonist. Physiologic dependence should always be assumed to exist after repeated administration of an opioid for more than a few days.[63,64] To avoid this abstinence syndrome, opioids should always be tapered before being discontinued.

Psychologic dependence is characterized by the craving for an opioid drug to achieve a psychological effect, resulting in the continual use of the drug despite harm to self or others. Iatrogenically induced psychological dependence on opioids is rare when they are taken for medicinal reasons.[61]

Coanalgesics

The use of adjuvant therapy can be beneficial for patients experiencing neuropathic pain. Anesthesia providers must be aware of this type of therapy, because patients may be on complex pharmacologic regimens that must be evaluated for effectiveness and maintained if appropriate. In addition, the anesthetist may need to add these agents to the armamentarium. It may be useful to use adjuvant drugs such as tricyclic antidepressants, anticonvulsants, corticosteroids, muscle relaxants, and local anesthetics.

The tricyclic antidepressants block the reuptake of serotonin and norepinephrine at the neuronal membrane. Although small doses (compared with the doses used for their primary indication) are effective, they produce anticholinergic effects, such as dry mouth; CNS effects, such as sedation and fatigue; and cardiovascular effects, such as orthostatic hypotension, arrhythmias, and tachycardia. The onset of the analgesic effect may not occur until 4 to 10 days after initiation of the treatment (Table 52-3).

Anticonvulsant drugs are used to alter the ion channels along the nerve fiber, thereby blocking pain stimuli by blocking the action potential. Carbamazepine, phenytoin, gabapentin, and clonazepam have been used. Common side effects include sedation and dizziness (Table 52-4).

Corticosteroids are used in the management of complex pain syndromes and work to reduce inflammation and swelling. Commonly used in the care of cancer patients, steroids may be indicated in other surgical and disease situations. Edema associated with tumors and the reduction of inflammatory mediators (e.g., prostaglandins and leukotrienes) is often associated with the use of corticosteroids (see Table 52-4).

The use of muscle relaxants in pain management is common. Some practitioners suggest that easing the tension of muscle spasm reduces various types of discomfort such as back pain, acute trauma, and surgical incision pain. Some clinicians do not believe that these drugs relieve muscle spasm but provide analgesia through a mechanism not yet understood.[65]

NMDA receptor antagonists have been used for many years. Ketamine and dextromethorphan are common NMDA receptor antagonists. Ketamine has been used in the treatment of various neuropathic pain syndromes. Dextromethorphan has been used successfully in the treatment of diabetic neuralgia.[66]

Like clonidine, dexmedetomidine is an α_2-adenoreceptor agonist. However, dexmedetomidine (Precedex) is a second-generation formulation of the medication. α_2-Receptors are located on or near the terminals of unmyelinated peripheral nerves and postsynaptically within the dorsal horn. Dexmedetomidine inhibits nociceptive neuron firing and the release of substance P centrally. Clinically, dexmedetomidine administered during the perioperative period has demonstrated anesthetic as well as opioid-sparing effects.[67,68] Patients undergoing off-pump coronary artery bypass[67] and bariatric surgery[68] have benefited from the administration of dexmedetomidine intraoperatively.

γ-Aminobutyric acid (GABA) is an inhibitory transmitter. Several GABA receptor agonists have been identified. The most commonly used drug is Baclofen, which acts in the spinal cord to prevent the release of excitatory neurotransmitters. Baclofen has been used in the treatment of trigeminal neuralgia.[69]

MODE OF ADMINISTRATION

Previously, the most common approach to postoperative pain relief was IM injection of an opioid, administered as needed. However, this modality is painful and is associated with unpredictable absorption and peaks and valleys in blood levels, creating inconsistent pain relief.[53] Today we know that pain medication should be administered around the clock via an IV or oral route in doses based on the assessment, dose response, and reassessment of the patient.[70]

The most reliable indicator of the existence and intensity of pain is the patient's own self-report. Opioids are often administered at fixed doses at arbitrary time intervals rather than on a dose-response basis. Correlation appears to be lacking between the opioid dose and subjective pain relief.

Of the less invasive modalities, the IV route is preferred for the administration of postoperative opioid therapy, with the sublingual or rectal route used as a secondary option.[1] Treatment of postoperative pain via subcutaneous (subQ) or IM administration should not be considered as a primary choice. Newer modalities, such as buccal or intranasal administration and perhaps the transdermal patch, may be considered when the traditional approaches fall short. The rationale behind this order of priority is to promote the titration of the opioid until pain relief is achieved and to avoid the unpredictability of absorption through the tissue.[1]

Patients should be switched to oral pain medication in equipotent doses as soon as the general condition permits or the patient is permitted to take food by mouth. When the oral route is chosen, the appropriate dose must be calculated on the basis of bioavailability and equipotency.[1] The importance of this point cannot be overstated. Too often patients are switched to oral medications too early or with little concern about required doses.

Patient-controlled analgesia was developed in the early 1970s with the advent of microprocessor technology. The administration technique has changed the face of pain management. It uses

Text continued on p. 1255

TABLE **52-3**	Antidepressant Agents				
Agent	**Dose**	**Onset**	**Peak**	**Duration**	**Comments**
Amitriptyline HCl (Elavil)	*Pain:* Initial PO 10-25 mg (0.2-0.5 mg/kg) daily at bedtime Titrate up q3-4wk by 10-25 mg as necessary Maintenance: PO 10-150 mg (0.2-3 mg/kg) daily at bedtime	Analgesic: PO 5 days			Classic tricyclic antidepressant. Like other tricyclics, may produce anticholinergic, antihistaminic, and sedating effects. Potentiates analgesic effects of opioids. May enhance ulcer healing (antihistaminic effect).
	Depression: Initial PO 75-100 mg (1.5-2 mg/kg) daily in one to four doses Maintenance: PO 25-150 mg/kg (0.5-3 mg/kg) daily in one to four doses IM 20-30 mg qid, then replace with oral Do not use intravenously	Antidepressant: PO 1-2 wk	PO 2-4 wk	PO variable	
Amoxapine HCl (Asendin)	*Pain:* Initial PO 50-150 mg (1-3 mg/kg) daily at bedtime Titrate dose up q3-4wk by 25-50 mg as necessary Maintenance: PO 50-300 mg (1-6 mg/kg) daily at bedtime	Analgesic: PO <5 days			Tricyclic antidepressant. Moderately sedating and has little anticholinergic effect. Rapid onset of activity. May be associated with development of extrapyramidal symptoms. Toxic levels produce CNS manifestations rather than cardiovascular effects (as compared with other tricyclics).
	Depression: Initial PO 100-150 mg (2-3 mg/kg) daily in one to three doses Maintenance: PO 100-400 mg (2-8 mg/kg) daily in one to three doses Doses >300 mg should be administered in two or three doses	Antidepressant: PO 4-7 days	PO 2-4 wk	PO variable	
Citalopram (Celexa)	*Pain:* Initial PO 20 mg daily	Analgesic: PO 1 wk	PO 2-4 wk	PO variable	Selective serotonin reuptake inhibitor. Antidepressant activity is comparable with that of fluoxetine and superior to that of doxepin or trazadone with fewer adverse effects. Unlike the tricyclics, sedating, anticholinergic, and cardiovascular effects are minimal.

Data from Formulary. 31:1999;4:405-417; Med Lett Drugs Ther. 1998;40:113-114; Mosby's Drug Consult. St Louis: Mosby; 2007.
CNS, *Central nervous system;* IM, *intramuscular;* PO, *by mouth;* qid, *four times a day;* tid, *three times a day.*

Continued

TABLE 52-3 Antidepressant Agents—cont'd

Agent	Dose	Onset	Peak	Duration	Comments
	Depression: PO 20-60 mg daily; dose increases are recommended at a rate of 20 mg/wk	Antidepressant: PO 1-2 wk	PO 2-4 wk	PO variable	
Desipramine HCl (Pertofrane)	*Pain:* Initial PO 50-100 mg (1-2 mg/kg) daily at bedtime; Titrate dose up q3-4wk by 25-50 mg as necessary; Maintenance: PO 50-200 mg (1-4 mg/kg) daily at bedtime	Analgesic: PO 5 days			Tricyclic antidepressant. Compared with the parent drug (imipramine), has fewer side effects (e.g, orthostatic hypotension, urinary retention). Used in patients who cannot tolerate the parent drug (imipramine).
	Depression: Initial PO 75-100 mg daily in one to four doses; Maintenance: PO 50-300 mg in one to four doses; Doses >200 mg not recommended for outpatients; IM 100 mg daily in divided doses, then replace with oral	Antidepressant: PO 2-5 days	PO 2-3 wk	PO variable	
Fluoxetine (Prozac)	*Pain and depression:* Adults: 20 mg/day (two 10-mg capsules) in the morning; may increase after 4 wk in 10-20 mg/day increments; maximum: 80 mg/day; doses >20 mg should be divided into two daily doses. Note: Lower doses of 10 mg/day have been used for initial treatment.	PO 1-2 wk	PO 2-4 wk	PO variable	Selective serotonin reuptake inhibitor. Antidepressant activity is comparable with that of paroxetine and superior to that of doxepin or trazadone with fewer adverse effects. Unlike the tricyclics, sedating, anticholinergic, and cardiovascular effects are minimal.
Nortriptyline HCl (Pamelor)	*Pain:* Initial PO 10-50 mg (0.5-1 mg/kg) daily at bedtime; Titrate dose up q3-4wk by 10-25 mg as necessary; Maintenance: PO 10-150 mg (0.2-3 mg/kg) daily at bedtime	Analgesic: PO 5 days			Compared with parent drug (amitriptyline), nortriptyline has fewer side effects. Only tricyclic antidepressant with a therapeutic window for serum levels (50-150 ng/mL).
	Depression: Initial PO 50-100 mg (1.5-2 mg/kg) daily in one to four doses; Maintenance: PO 50-150 mg (1-3 mg/kg) daily in one to four doses; Monitor serum levels with doses >100 mg daily	Antidepressant: PO 1-2 wk	PO 2-4 wk	PO variable	

Drug	Dosage	Onset	Comments
Paroxetine HCl (Paxil)	*Pain:* Initial PO 10-20 mg daily, preferably in the morning. Titrate dose up every week by 10 mg as necessary. Maintenance: PO 10-50 mg daily in the morning	Analgesic: PO 5 days	Selective serotonin reuptake inhibitor. Antidepressant activity is comparable with that of fluoxetine and superior to doxepin or trazadone with fewer adverse effects. Unlike tricyclics, sedating, anticholinergic, and cardiovascular effects are minimal.
	Depression: Initial PO 20 mg daily, preferably one dose in morning. Titrate dose up by 10 mg/day by weekly intervals as necessary. Maintenance: PO 20-50 mg daily in one dose in morning	Antidepressant: PO 1-2 wk PO 3-4 wk PO variable	
Protriptyline HCl (Vivactil)	*Pain:* Initial PO 5 mg (0.1 mg/kg) tid. Maintenance: PO 5-10 mg (0.1-0.2 mg/kg) tid	Analgesic: PO 5 days	Tricyclic antidepressant. Protriptyline may have a more rapid onset of action than imipramine or amitriptyline. Like other secondary amines (e.g., amoxapine, nortriptyline, and desipramine), it is more effective in patients with low norepinephrine levels compared with serotonin-deficient patients.
	Depression: Initial PO 5 mg (0.1 mg/kg) tid. Maintenance: PO 5-20 mg (0.1-0.4 mg/kg) tid	Antidepressant: PO 7 days PO 2-4 wk PO variable	
Sertraline (Zoloft)	*Pain and depression:* Initial PO 50 mg/day (half of a 100-mg tablet) as a single dose; dose may be increased at intervals of at least 1 wk to a maximum recommended dose of 200 mg/day	PO 1 week PO 1-3 wk PO variable	Selective serotonin reuptake inhibitor. Antidepressant activity is comparable with that of fluoxetine and superior to that of doxepin or trazadone with fewer adverse effects. Unlike the tricyclics, sedating, anticholinergic, and cardiovascular effects are minimal.
Trimipramine maleate (Surmontil)	*Pain:* Initial PO 25-100 mg (0.5-2 mg/kg) daily at bedtime. Titrate dose up q3-4wk by 25-50 mg as necessary. Maintenance: PO 25-200 mg (0.5-4 mg/kg) daily at bedtime	Analgesic: PO 5 days	Tricyclic antidepressant. Structurally related to imipramine.
	Depression: Initial PO 75-100 mg daily in one to four doses. Maintenance: PO 50-300 mg daily in one to four doses. Doses of >200 mg daily are not recommended for outpatients. Do not administer intravenously	Antidepressant: PO 1-2 wk PO 2-4 wk PO variable	

TABLE 52-4   Adjuvants Used in Pain Management

Drug Class	Indications	Drug and Routes	Starting Dose (mg/day)	Administration Schedule	Comments
Anticonvulsants	Multipurpose for chronic pain	Tizanidine PO (Zanaflex)	6	bid	
		Carbamazepine PO (Tegretol)	200	q6-8h	
		Clonazepam PO (Klonopin)	0.5	q8h	
	First-line for paroxysmal or "shooting" pain; second-line for nonparoxysmal pain	Divalproex sodium PO (Depakote)	500-1000	Daily	
		Phenytoin PO (Dilantin)	300	Daily	
		Phenytoin IV (Dilantin)	15-18 in divided doses	One to three doses	IV dose used for escalating neuropathic pain
		Valproate sodium IV (Depacon)	10-15 mg/kg/day	One to three doses	IV dose used for escalating neuropathic pain followed by PO doses
	Multipurpose for all types of neuropathic pain	Gabapentin PO (Neurontin)	900-1800	Three doses	May increase dose daily
Corticosteroids	Multipurpose analgesics	Dexamethasone PO (Decadron)	Low dose: 1-2	Daily or bid	May also improve appetite, nausea, and malaise; used when pain persists after optimal opioid dose
			High dose: 100	qid	High doses used for acute episodic pain unresponsive to opioids; risk of serious toxicity increases with dose, duration of therapy, and NSAIDs
GABA-ergic	"Shooting" neuropathic pain	Baclofen PO (Lioresal)	15	q8h	
Local anesthetics	Neuropathic pain of any type	Lidocaine IV	Brief infusion: 2-5 mg/kg over 20-30 min		
		Lidocaine subQ, IV	Continuous infusion: 2.5 mg/kg/hr		

Modified from McCaffery M, Pasero C. Pain: Clinical Manual. St Louis: Mosby; 1999:342-344.
bid, Twice daily; GABA, γ-aminobutyric acid; IV, intravenous; NSAIDs, nonsteroidal antiinflammatory drugs; PO, by mouth; subQ, subcutaneous.

TABLE **52-5**	Guidelines for Patient-Controlled Intravenous Opioid Administration for Adults with Acute Pain			
Dose*	Usual Starting Dose After Loading	Usual Dose Range	Usual Starting Lockout (minutes)	Usual Lockout Range (minutes)
Morphine (1mg/mL)	1 mg	0.5-2.5 mg	8	5-10
Hydromorphone (0.2 mg/mL)	0.2 mg	0.05-0.4 mg	8	5-10
Fentanyl (50 mcg/mL)	10 mcg	10-50 mcg	6	5-8

From Principles of Analgesic Use in the Treatment of Acute Pain and Cancer Pain. 5th ed. American Pain Society; 2003.
*Standard concentration for most PCA machines is listed in parentheses.

electronic devices programmed to inject set doses and incorporates lockout intervals, with or without basal infusions, and other built-in limitations to prevent peaks and valleys in analgesic blood levels. This technique makes the patient less dependent on the caregivers (within certain limits) for administration of the medication. The drugs most frequently used in these devices are morphine sulfate, hydromorphone, and fentanyl (Table 52-5). Meperidine use with patient-controlled analgesia is not recommended for the reasons cited earlier.

A new noninvasive patient-controlled analgesia delivery system is currently being evaluated and is demonstrating promise. The transdermal system was tolerated well by patients in this double-blind study.[71,72]

Local Anesthetics
Over the past few decades, the use of local anesthetics administered as single injections or via continuous catheter techniques has gained popularity. Most peripheral nerve blocks consist of a bolus dose of local anesthetic injected to cause infiltration of an area or are applied at a peripheral nerve site. These techniques are primarily used for analgesia for minor surgical procedures, although they often provide pain relief in the immediate postoperative period as well.

The use of continuous local anesthetic techniques is becoming increasingly popular. These techniques may be applied where an anatomic structure allows the insertion of a temporary catheter adjacent to a nerve. The most commonly used technique is the brachial plexus block. Catheters can also be placed to provide nerve blocks in the intercostal, femoral, sciatic, and other major peripheral nerves.

Because nerve blocks only limit the path of nociceptive impulses, some clinicians favor adding an antiinflammatory agent to decrease inflammation at the peripheral (trauma) site. Several peripheral blocks are briefly discussed in this chapter.

Intercostal Blocks
Intercostal blocks have been used successfully as a means of pain relief for rib fractures. They are relatively easy to apply in the form of an injection but carry a potential risk of pneumothorax with repeated injections. Intercostal blocks may also be applied via a catheter after thoracic or upper-quadrant abdominal surgery or trauma. Intercostal local anesthetics can be administered as bolus injections as required.

Intrapleural Analgesia
Intrapleural analgesia is a modality that can be used for thoracic and upper abdominal surgery. A catheter can be placed in the intrapleural cavity for bolus injections or continuous infusion.

This modality has the advantage of avoiding blockade of the sympathetic nervous system. It may not be as useful in thoracotomies with pleural drainage because of the unpredictable distribution and uptake of the local anesthetic agent. Cases of toxicity have been reported to result from systemic uptake. Other potential sequelae of continuous pleural analgesia include pneumothorax and ventilatory problems while the chest tube is clamped during equilibration in the pleural cavity.

Continuous Epidural Analgesia
A combination of a low-dose opioid and a low-concentration local anesthetic via an epidural route is an efficient treatment modality for postoperative pain. Continuous epidural analgesia was used in the late 1940s but lost popularity.[73] It regained popularity in the 1980s.[74,75]

Neuraxial blockade has been found to be useful in the management of postoperative pain. Because it provides profound analgesia, some clinicians also use the epidural technique with light general anesthesia during the surgical procedure. At the end of the procedure, the epidural catheter is left in place for postoperative pain management. Drugs can then be administered as bolus injections or continuous infusion or via a patient-controlled device. The continuous epidural technique can be used for thoracic, abdominal, and lower-extremity surgery, including trauma.

This technique is a powerful tool in the management of pain. Unfortunately, its implementation ideally requires that a pain-management service be available for training the care providers and for coordination of pain management.

Analgesia is provided through the administration of a local anesthetic or an opioid alone or the combination of a diluted concentration of a local anesthetic and an opioid. The purpose of combining the two drugs is the use of the different sites of action and the provision of synergy.[76-78] If one of the agents is used alone, tachyphylaxis may develop. This is characterized by blockade of fewer dermatomes, despite the injection of an increased amount of local anesthetic in identical concentration, as well as regression of a stable analgesic dermatomal level during continuous epidural infusion. Scott and co-workers[78] have reported evidence of a synergistic effect of the opioid–local anesthetic combination. Some clinicians advocate concomitant use of NSAIDs with the epidural modality to decrease inflammation at the peripheral site.

The analgesic solution can be administered either as a bolus or as a continuous infusion via a programmable pump. The placement of the epidural catheter and the initiation of treatment may vary. Some clinicians prefer to insert the catheter and start the treatment as part of the preoperative preparation; others insert it in the postoperative phase.

TABLE 52-6	Epidural Analgesic Dosing Guidelines for Acute Pain in Adults*			
Drug*	Single Dose†(mg)	Infusion Rate‡ (mg/hour)	Onset (minutes)	Duration of Single Dose (hours)
Epidural				
Morphine	1.0-60	0.10-1.0	30	6-24
Fentanyl	0.025-0.100	0.025-0.100	5	4-8
Clonidine§	—	0.30	—	—
Hydromorphone	0.8-1.5	0.15-0.3	5-8	4-6

From Principles of Analgesic Use in the Treatment of Acute Pain and Cancer Pain. 5th ed., American Pain Society; 2003.
*Infusions injected into the epidural space must be preservative-free.
†A clinician experienced in using epidural drugs should adjust doses for age, injection site, patient's medical condition, and degree of tolerance to opioids.
‡If a local anesthetic is used in conjunction with an infusion, 0.06% bupivacaine is recommended.
§Recently approved by FDA for severe pain in cancer patients in combination with opioids. Available as a preservative-free preparation (100 mcg/mL) in 10-mL vials.

Individual preferences vary with regard to the level at which the epidural catheter should be placed. The following guideline is advocated by Lubenow[79]:

Procedure	Vertebral Range
Thoracic surgery	T2 through T8
Upper abdominal surgery	T4 through L1
Renal surgery	T6 through L1
Hip surgery	T12 through L3
Lower abdominal and gynecologic surgery	T10 through L3

The protocols used for monitoring patients with continuous epidural analgesia vary a great deal. Some institutions have the patients fully monitored in a critical care setting, whereas others have well-trained staff that care for these patients on regular floors. In many institutions with an acute pain management service, standard order sheets are used. The orders include drugs used, vital signs (including level of consciousness), and assessment of pain. Orders for treatment of respiratory depression, breakthrough pain, nausea, and itching should be available. It is important to instruct the nurses who provide bedside care to inspect the epidural catheter site when assessing for progressive loss of sensation or motor function and when evaluating for side effects of opioids.

Two commonly occurring side effects of epidural therapy are nausea, with or without vomiting, and pruritus.[80] Nausea is related to the opioid level at the chemoreceptor zone in the medulla. Opioid-induced nausea can be reduced with commonly used antiemetics, such as phenothiazines. Also, intermittent low-dose naloxone (0.4 to 1 mg) may be administered intermittently via an IV route. If the nausea persists, a continuous infusion of naloxone (1 mcg/kg/hr) may be used, with the dose increased until effective.

Although histamine plays a minimal role in pruritus caused by epidurally administered opioids, antihistamines such as diphenhydramine may be used to treat itching. For severe cases of itching, naloxone in doses similar to those used in the treatment of nausea may be administered.

Urinary retention is a well-recognized side effect of epidural pain management. The condition may be reversed with incremental doses of naloxone, although catheterization of the bladder often is the treatment of choice.

Local anesthetics in the epidural infusion, although diluted, may cause hypotension, as well as sensory and motor block.

The side effect of epidural opioids that causes the most concern is respiratory depression. This is caused by the rostral spread of the opioid and its subsequent effect on the respiratory control center in the brainstem. The poorer the opioid's lipid solubility, the greater the risk for delayed respiratory depression. When patients are treated with epidural opioids, equipment for airway management and assisted ventilation must be available. A patient who becomes apneic from epidural analgesia is treated with manual ventilation and incremental doses of naloxone. Alternatively, an infusion of naloxone (1 mcg/kg/hr) may be begun. The use of this modality may necessitate admission to a critical care or an intermediate care unit for observation.

Some controversy exists with regard to whether apnea or other monitors should be used as part of the protocol for the epidural treatment. This addition makes the modality extremely resource consuming. It is vital that nurses at the bedside be well trained in the observation of patients with epidural catheters. Lubenow states that the observation of vigilant nurses is paramount, and that it should be the complete responsibility of the pain-management service to manage the analgesia and sedation.[79,81] Dosing guidelines for epidural analgesics in adults are given in Table 52-6.

PAIN MANAGEMENT IN CHILDREN

The pediatric patient in pain poses numerous challenges. The anesthetist must keep in mind that both the patient and the family member responsible for the child should be included in the development of the pain management plan. Unfortunately, some health-care providers still believe that children do not have pain, and undermedication is more the rule than the exception. As with adult patients, several myths and misconceptions are related to the lack of adequate management of pediatric pain.[82-84]

One difficulty in providing adequate pain control in children is assessment and evaluation, owing to the child's cognitive development and individual emotions and reactions to pain. However, skilled pediatric nursing staff are still capable of providing adequate observation of the pediatric patient in discomfort or pain, as well as assessing the response to analgesics. Several scales are available for the quantification of pediatric pain and assessment of relief.

The modality and drugs of choice for the pediatric patient depend largely on (1) the knowledge and skills of the staff involved in the care and (2) the age of the child. The choices are the same as those available for the adult, with different

TABLE 52-7	Local Anesthetics for Pediatric Regional Anesthesia				
Drug	**Techniques**	**Concentration**	**Dose**	**Duration (min)**	
Bupivacaine (Marcaine)	Epidural or caudal	0.25%	2.5 mg/kg or 0.5-1 mL/kg	120-240	
	Spinal*	Hyperbaric: 0.5% in 8% dextrose	<5 kg: 0.5 mg/kg 5-15 kg: 0.4 mg/kg >15 kg: 0.3 mg/kg	30-60	
	Brachial plexus	0.25%	0.7 mL/kg up to 50 kg	150-360	
Mepivacaine (Carbocaine)	Brachial plexus	0.5%-2%	5 mg/kg (maximum 8 mg)	60-90	
	Caudal	0.5-1.5%	0.5 mg/kg	120-360	
Lidocaine (Xylocaine)	Epidural or caudal	1%-2%	5 (7) mg/kg†	30-60	
	Brachial plexus	0.5%-2%	5 (7) mg/kg†	45-160	
	Spinal	5% with 7.5% dextrose	2 mg/kg	Variable	
Tetracaine (Pontocaine)	Spinal*	0.5% in 10% dextrose	<5 kg: 0.4-0.8 mg/kg 5-15 kg: 0.4-0.8 mg/kg >15 kg: 0.3 mg/kg	60-90	

From Kremer M, Faut-Callahan M. Regional anesthesia and pain management. In: Zaglaniczny K, Aker J, eds. Clinical Guide to Pediatric Anesthesia. Philadelphia: Saunders; 1999:369.
*Indications: patient <60 wk postconceptional age, high risk for apnea and bradycardia.
†Without (with) epinephrine.

dosages used because of the different pharmacokinetics (Tables 52-7 and 52-8).

One goal of management of acute pain in children is minimizing the emotional trauma associated with treatment through a reliable method of administration. The pain experience of a pediatric patient largely influences the individual's future experiences with pain.

The fear of psychological dependence in children is often a deterrent to adequate pain management. However, no evidence exists that children with moderate to severe postoperative pain, treated adequately, are likely to become drug dependent or craving.

The modality chosen should be as atraumatic as possible. Many children would rather suffer in silence than receive an IM injection. Because most children have IV access postoperatively, it is logical to give opioids intravenously. The technique depends on the age of the child. Older children may be able to use patient-controlled analgesia with or without a basal infusion. The determining factor for the implementation should be the cognitive development rather than the age. For younger children, an alternative is continuous infusion, which provides a uniform level of analgesia. Some may be reluctant to use this technique out of fear of side effects from the opioids, but the literature provides very little evidence of complications associated with this particular technique.

Intermittent IV bolus injections are an alternative; however, they are associated with high peaks that are short lived, and they are just as labor intensive as IM injections. Respiratory depression may be more of a problem with this approach. If the patient still has the need for opioids when IV access is removed, oral medication should be strongly considered.

Postoperative pain relief should commence at the induction of the anesthesia whenever applicable. Use of local anesthetics at the surgical site before incision has proven effective. The combination of regional analgesia and general anesthesia has also been promoted for management of pediatric postoperative pain.

Although limited by the lack of qualified providers, the use of regional analgesia in children is growing in popularity. Regional analgesia with the administration of local anesthetics or opioids modulates the transmission of afferent nociceptive impulses. Minimal side effects have been reported, and pain management is highly effective.[85]

Local infiltration of the surgical site and a variety of peripheral nerve blocks can be used in the pediatric population. Wrist, ankle, femoral, and axillary blocks are common. Intercostal blocks have been used for thoracotomy and nephrectomy. Spinal, caudal, and epidural analgesia have also been used successfully. Local anesthetics can be used safely, provided close attention to dosage is maintained (see Table 52-7). It is unlikely that a child will tolerate the placement of a regional anesthetic. However, placement of a regional block may be done under sedation or once the child is anesthetized. This should be done very judiciously because when major conduction anesthesia is used (femoral, axillary, intercostal, or epidural), it can be very difficult to diagnose intraneural and intravascular injections in children who are heavily sedated or anesthetized.

CANCER-RELATED PAIN

Cancer and cancer-related pathology are responsible for 20% of deaths annually in the United States and 10% of deaths worldwide. Presently, more than 8 million Americans have cancer, and another 1.2 million are diagnosed yearly. At the time of their cancer diagnosis, 20% to 75% of adult patients are experiencing pain.[86] Pain often accompanies the diagnosis and treatment of cancer; 17% to 57% of cancer patients undergoing active therapy and 23% to 100% of those with advanced disease experience pain.[87] Studies have demonstrated that 70% to 90% of cancer-related pain can be effectively managed with pharmacotherapy alone. More sobering, however, is the fact that surveys suggest that 40% to 50% of patients experiencing cancer-related pain do not receive effective analgesia.[88] Numerous barriers prevent the achievement of this goal. All of the barriers can in some way be attributed to health professionals, the patients and family

TABLE 52-8	Pharmacologic Management of Cancer Pain—Relative Potency, Half-Life, and Duration of Action of Commonly Used Opioid Drugs				
Drug	Half-Life (hr)	Equianalgesic Intramuscular Dose (mg)	Intramuscular or Oral Potency	Starting Oral Dose Range (mg)	Comments
Morphine	2-3	10	3 (Repeated dose)	15-30	Standard of comparison for opioid analgesics; multiple routes of administration; controlled-release available; morphine-6-glucuronide accumulation in patients with renal failure; lower doses for the elderly
Hydromorphone	2-3	1.5	5	4-8	Useful alternative for morphine; no known active metabolite; multiple routes available
Methadone	15-190	10	2	5-10	May accumulate with repetitive administration
Levorphanol	12-15	2	2	2-4	May accumulate with repetitive administration
Meperidine	2-3	75	4	Not recommended	Central nervous system excitatory toxic metabolite, normeperidine; contraindicated for repetitive administration, for patients with renal failure, and for patients receiving monoamine oxidase inhibitors
Fentanyl	2	N/A	N/A	N/A	Short half-life; parenteral use by infusion; clinical experience suggests 2 mg morphine sulfate/hr = 100 mcg transdermal patch; patches available to deliver 25, 50, 75, 100 mcg/hr
Oxycodone	2-3	15	2	5-10	Available in liquid or tablet preparations; also in combination with a nonopioid
Codeine	2-3	130	1.5	30-60	Used orally for less severe pain; usually combined with a nonopioid

N/A, *Not applicable.*

members, or the health-care system. By obtaining the necessary knowledge and sharing this information with their colleagues, educating patients and families, and initiating or becoming involved in institutional pain management programs and palliative care, CRNAs can have a significant effect on all three of these areas.

Untreated pain in patients with cancer can be psychologically devastating. Not only can pain cause unnecessary suffering, but many patients view the presence of pain as a constant reminder of the disease. In addition, patients who receive adequate analgesia are more likely to comply with potentially curative treatments and participate in activities of daily living.[89] Clearly, inadequate pain management affects patients' quality of life.

In 1994, the AHRQ established clinical practice guidelines for the management of cancer pain.[89] These guidelines were reviewed and revised in 2004 by a Clinical Practice Guideline Committee of the American Pain Society. These practice guidelines provide a framework for CRNAs to accurately assess and effectively manage cancer-related pain. Despite the promulgation of these guidelines, CRNAs may lack the assessment skills and

pharmacologic knowledge base necessary to alleviate pain and suffering in patients with cancer. Although nurse anesthetists are proficient at the perioperative assessment of pain and opioid administration, they can no longer confine their practice to the perioperative period. As nurses in advanced practice, CRNAs should possess the knowledge to effectively assess and manage cancer-related pain during the preoperative and postoperative periods.

In a survey of 1777 cancer specialists, only 51% reported that patients in their treatment settings attained adequate relief.[89] Because the number of comprehensive cancer centers is small, CRNAs in smaller and rural hospitals must become involved in the pain management of these patients. This section provides the practicing CRNA with the rudimentary information necessary to effectively assess and pharmacologically manage patients with pain related to cancer. Other treatment modalities are mentioned for the sake of completeness, but the reader is cautioned that the information contained herein should be supplemented with additional reading and clinical exposure to affected patients.

In May 2004, the National Consensus Project[90] —overseen by the American Academy of Hospice and Palliative Care, Center to Advance Palliative Care, Hospice and Palliative Nurses Association, Last Acts Partnership, and National Hospice and Palliative Care Organization—reported on "clinical guidelines" for palliative care. Each year in the United States, an estimated 1.5 million people, including 250,000 children and adults with cancer, die without the benefit of palliative care services.[91-97] To alleviate needless physical and emotional suffering, these individuals require and should receive comprehensive and compassionate palliative care.[91,92]

Pain management and palliative care are beginning to receive more attention from regulatory agencies and quality watchdogs such as The Joint Commission, the National Quality Forum (NQF), and the University Health Consortium (UHC), but the need for expanded services remains.[93,94] CRNAs must take the lead in developing the knowledge and skills to be members of these teams. One such project includes adding a required interdisciplinary palliative care course to the nurse anesthesia curriculum.[98]

Assessment of Cancer Pain

One of the greatest barriers to effective pain management is poor pain assessment.[99] The ability to complete a thorough assessment of pain in patients with cancer is an essential step. Initial assessment of the cancer pain must be comprehensive and completed in a stepwise fashion, beginning with data collection and finishing with a patient-oriented problem list and a strategy for pain management. The evaluation should be guided by the ability to conduct thorough physical and neurologic examinations. In addition, the CRNA should have knowledge of common pain syndromes, oncologic emergencies, and modalities available to treat a pain crisis. Ultimately, the two main goals of the assessment are to gain an accurate characterization of the pain, including the pain syndrome and inferred pathophysiology, and to evaluate the effect of the pain and the role it plays in the overall suffering of the patient.[88]

Cancer-related pain can result from any of the following: (1) tumor invasion into bone, joint, muscle, or connective tissue; (2) diagnostic or therapeutic procedures (lumbar punctures, chemotherapy, radiation); and (3) unrelated pain (e.g., preexisting arthritis, infection). The overall incidence of pain in patients with cancer depends on the type and stage of the disease. When cancer is diagnosed at early and intermediate stages, 30% to 45% of patients experience pain, whereas nearly 23% to 100% of patients with advanced cancer have pain.[89]

The complete assessment of the patient with cancer-related pain has four facets[88]: (1) detailed pain history, (2) psychosocial assessment, (3) physical and neurologic examinations, and (4) diagnostic evaluation. Evaluation of the intensity, quality, distribution, and temporal relationships of the pain can be beneficial in identification of cancer pain syndromes. Evaluating the intensity of the pain is critical, because it indicates the urgency with which pain relief is needed. Patient self-report should be the primary source of information regarding pain intensity. The use of validated and reliable tools, such as the numeric rating scale (0 through 10), the categoric scale (none, mild, moderate, severe, worst possible), or the Brief Pain Inventory or the McGill Pain Questionnaire,[100] enables the clinician to assess pain intensity, as well as pain relief. Every effort should be made to assess the character of the pain; the location; onset and duration; aggravating and relieving factors; past treatments, including what was effective or ineffective; and how the pain has affected the patient's physical and social functioning. As mentioned earlier in the chapter, and more so with cancer-related pain, CRNAs should always be cognizant of the fact that pain is a multidimensional phenomenon. Although the presence or absence of pain is the intial step, other factors can contribute to the patient's perception of that pain. In addition, assessment of pain intensity helps in selecting the analgesic drug to be used, the route of administration, and the rate at which the medication is titrated. Determination of pain intensity also may be beneficial in identifying the cause of the underlying syndrome. For example, nerve injury after radiation is rarely severe; however, severe pain in a previously irradiated region is suggestive of recurrent neoplasm.[88]

Assessing the quality of the patient's pain is crucial because it can suggest the pathophysiology of the pain. Somatic pain is described as sharp, aching, throbbing, or pressure-like. Pain that is described as gnawing or cramping is most often visceral in nature, secondary to obstruction of a hollow viscus. Visceral pain can be sharp or throbbing when it is associated with organ capsules or mesentery. Pain experienced as burning, tingling, or shocklike—particularly when it is associated with subjective numbness, loss of sensation, and weakness—is likely to have a neuropathic origin.[88]

The distribution of the pain is particularly important when pain is experienced at a location with no evidence of pathology, when there is more than one site of pain, or when the patient complains of generalized pain. For example, patients can have referred pain in the iliac crest from a lesion at spinal cord level T12. Frequently, patients with advanced cancer experience pain at two or more sites. Complaints of diffuse, dull, aching pain can often indicate bone metastases.

The psychosocial assessment encompasses the meaning of pain to the patient and his or her family, as well as how the individual and caregivers are coping with cancer and the pain that may be associated with the diagnosis. In addition, the patient's level of understanding with regard to expectations of treatment and opioid therapy must be addressed. Last, the nurse anesthetist must try to assess what provisions the patient and family have for dealing with the economic effect the disease will inevitably have on their lives.

The physical and neurologic examination should be focused and evaluate common referral of pain to other areas of the body. The diagnostic evaluation attempts to evaluate the recurrence or progression of disease or tissue injury related to cancer treatment. Appropriate radiologic studies and blood tests are performed and their results correlated with the physical and neurologic examination. Every effort should be made to provide the patient with analgesia during the initial assessment and diagnostic evaluation. Patient comfort will improve compliance and will not result in an inadequate examination.[88]

The assessment of the patient's pain and the effectiveness of the treatment is an ongoing process. Results of evaluations should be continually documented so that all people involved in the patient's care have access to the information. This ensures that all caregivers are aware of the current status of the patient's pain and the efficacy of the present analgesic therapy. Patients are encouraged to report changes in pain patterns or new pain. These reports should trigger a diagnostic evaluation, because when patients have stable, controlled cancer pain, new complaints of pain are generally associated with progressive disease rather than opioid tolerance.[101,102]

The assessment of the patient is not complete without an attempt to quantify the effect of the entire cancer experience on the patient. This includes not only the physical pain the

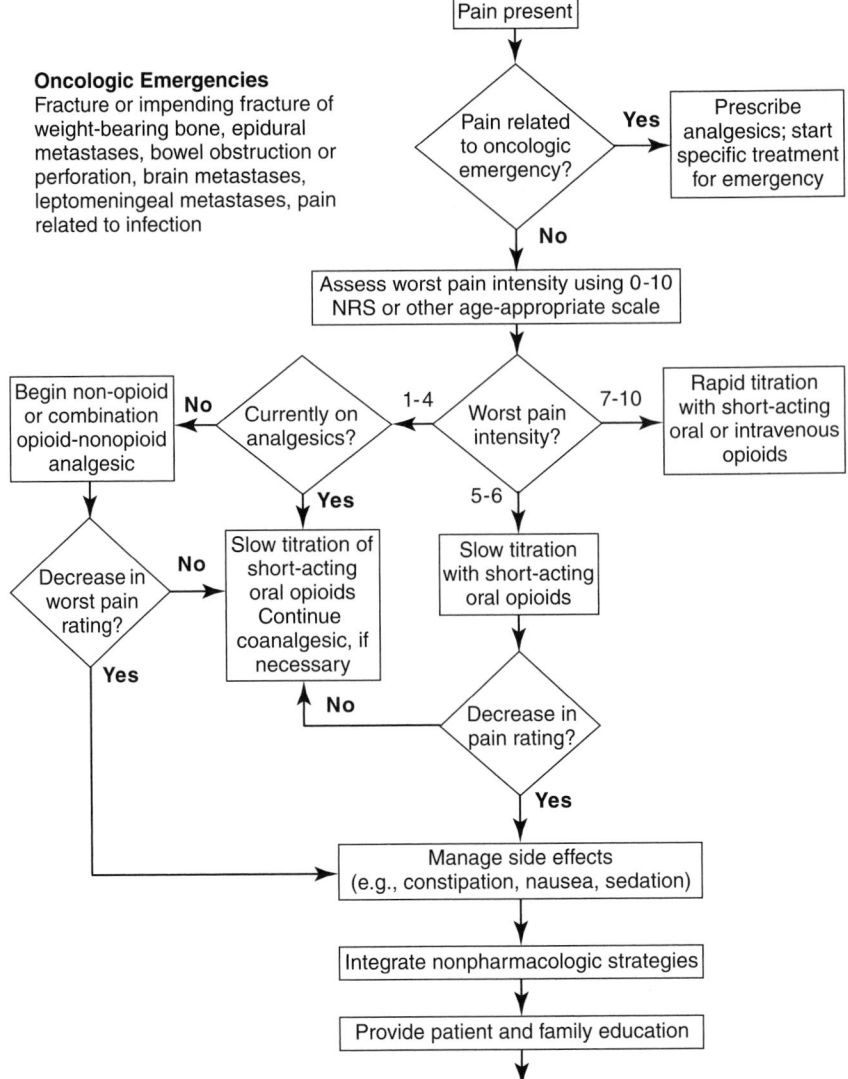

FIGURE **52-5** Initial treatment of cancer pain. *NRS,* Numeric rating scale. (From *Guidelines for the Management of Cancer Pain in Adults and children.* Copyright 2005. American Pain Society.)

patient may be experiencing, but also the amount of suffering the pain and disease process have inflicted on the patient and the family. The CRNA must understand that pain and suffering are not synonymous. It is possible for a patient to experience suffering without pain. For example, the loss of a loved one can cause suffering without the perception of nociception (i.e., pain). The converse is also true. Determining whether a patient is suffering in addition to being in pain is important, because the presence of suffering undermines the patient's quality of life. However, determining whether a patient is suffering in addition to being in physical pain can be difficult. Establishing a relationship with the patient and family whereby they are comfortable discussing their financial concerns, their interactions with one another, and their fears can aid in this assessment. In addition, evaluation of the patient's appetite, sleep patterns, interactions with family, socioeconomic status, and so on is an integral part of this assessment.

Although the management of the patient's pain and suffering may seem like a daunting task, it is important to note that the comprehensive care of patients with cancer requires a multidisciplinary approach. The addition of pharmacists, physicians,

clerics, psychologists, and social workers to the pain management team is invaluable.

Management of Cancer Pain

Comprehensive management of cancer pain incorporates primary therapy, pharmacologic therapy, and if necessary psychological interventions and invasive therapies.[88] The initial management of the pain should never be delayed while diagnostic tests are being performed. Effective pain management during the initial stages of the diagnostic workup does not interfere with or lead to erroneous data from the tests. Tremendous benefit can be derived from primary therapy, but most patients eventually require some form of analgesic therapy. Pharmacologic therapy is the mainstay of analgesic therapy.

As CRNAs move into the realm of chronic pain management and palliative care, in-depth knowledge of pharmacologic interventions is needed. A number of algorithms have been developed for CRNAs to optimally manage cancer-related pain (Figures 52-5 through 52-8). This algorithm-based approach is recommended because of the continually evolving nature of the disease process and the pain associated with it. These algorithms

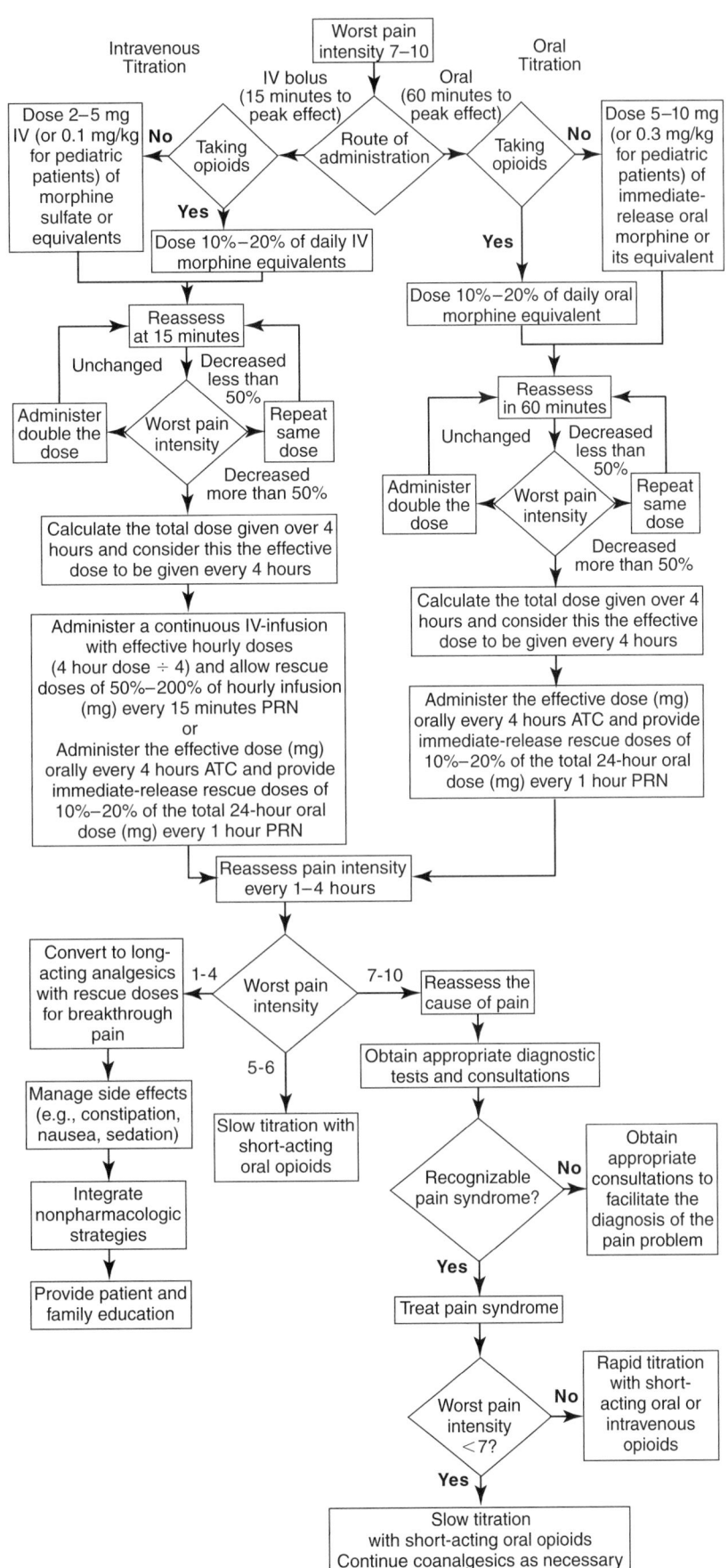

FIGURE **52-6** Rapid titration with short-acting oral or intravenous opioids. (*From Guidelines for the Management of Cancer Pain in Adults and children.* Copyright 2005. American Pain Society.)

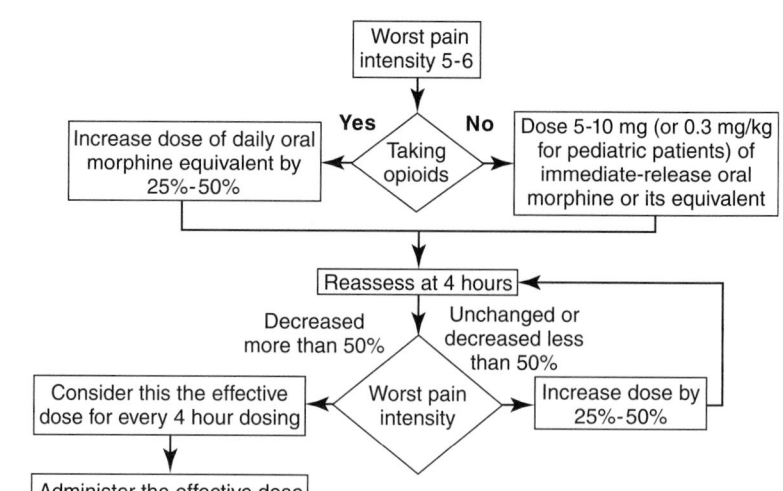

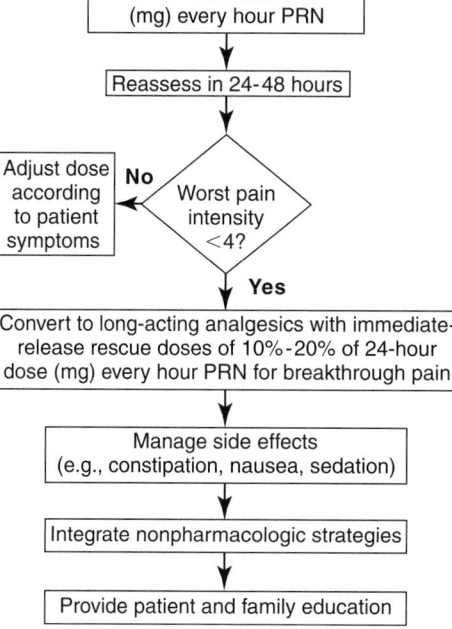

FIGURE **52-7** Slow titration with short-acting oral opioids. (From *Guidelines for the Management of Cancer Pain in Adults and children.* Copyright 2005. American Pain Society.)

provide a guideline and can be modified based on the intensity of the patient's pain, age, and the treatment setting.

Nonopioid Analgesics

Nonopioid analgesics are useful in the treatment of mild pain or in combination with opioids or adjuvant drugs for the treatment of moderate to severe pain. Unlike opioid analgesics, these drugs have a "ceiling effect," whereby no additional analgesic effects can be derived from escalation of the dose past the recommended maximum daily amount. They also do not produce tolerance or physical dependence. Nonopioid analgesics are divided into numerous subclasses.[56] Aspirin and other NSAIDs exert their analgesic effect by inhibiting the enzyme cyclooxygenase. Inhibition of this enzyme blocks the synthesis of prostaglandins, inflammatory mediators known to sensitize peripheral nociceptors. A central mechanism of action is also thought to

contribute to NSAID analgesia and probably predominates with acetaminophen-induced analgesia.

To maximize the benefits of these drugs, the CRNA must have a thorough understanding of their pharmacologic profiles, dosage guidelines, and potential adverse effects. Adverse effects secondary to nonselective NSAIDs include bleeding, renal failure, gastric ulceration, and hepatic dysfunction. Caution is required when administering these medications to patients at increased risk, including elderly patients; patients with blood-clotting disorders, ulcer diathesis, or impaired renal function; and patients concurrently taking corticosteroids. Proton-pump inhibitors have been shown to provide the greatest gastroprotection against nonselective NSAID-induced gastric mucosal damage. In addition, some of the potential adverse effects associated with nonselective NSAIDs can be avoided with the use of COX-2–selective drugs. Although no comparative studies

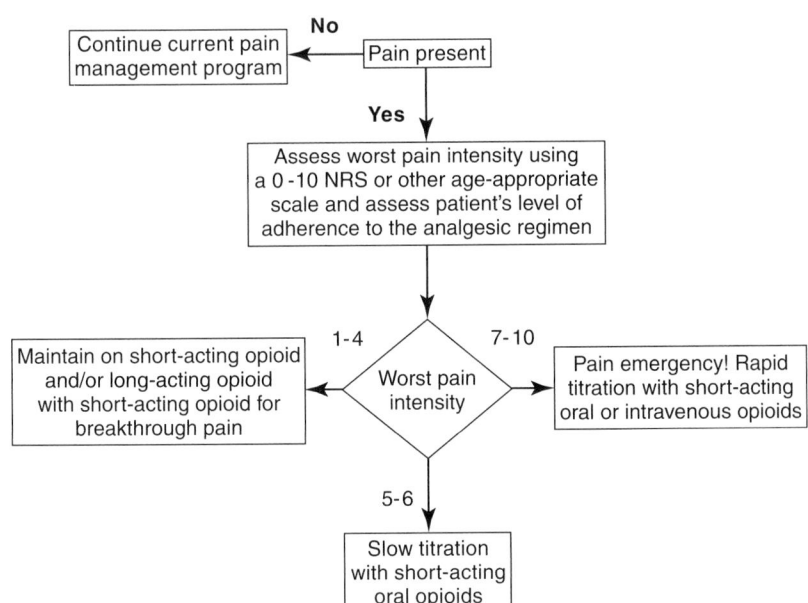

FIGURE **52-8** Ongoing treatment of pain in patients with cancer. *NSR*, Numeric rating scale. (From *Guidelines for the Management of Cancer Pain in Adults and children.* Copyright 2005. American Pain Society.)

demonstrate the analgesic efficacy of nonselective NSAIDs and COX-2 selective NSAIDs in cancer patients, an initial trial of a COX-2 selective drug may be indicated in patients at risk for development of adverse reactions.

The nonacetylated salicylates, choline magnesium trisalicylate and salsalate, have less effect on platelet function and do not affect bleeding times when administered at usual clinical doses. Acetaminophen doses in excess of 4000 mg/day can induce hepatic toxicity, particularly in patients with preexisting liver disease.

Opioid Analgesics

Expertise in opioid therapy is the single most important factor in the successful management of cancer-related pain.[103] This expertise should extend from the pharmacologic profiles of the opioids to the principles of tolerance, pseudoaddiction, physiologic dependence, and psychological dependence. Opioids exert their analgesic effects through supraspinal, spinal, and possibly peripheral mechanisms by binding to the mu, delta, and kappa receptors.[104] For cancer pain management, the pure opioid analgesic drugs are most commonly used. The use of mixed agonist-antagonist and partial agonist opioids is of limited value in this setting because of their ceiling effect for analgesia, ability to precipitate withdrawal symptoms in patients physiologically dependent on pure opioid drugs, and a higher incidence of psychomimetic side effects than pure opioids. Pure opioid analgesic drugs do not have a ceiling effect. Their ability to provide effective analgesia with escalating doses is limited only by the development of unmanageable or intolerable side effects.

Coanalgesics

The American Pain Society recommends the use of coanalgesic drugs when indicated with nonopioid and opioid medications. Coanalgesics are those drugs that have a primary indication other than the treatment of pain but have analgesic properties in certain painful conditions. Their use is indicated for specific painful conditions or when the adverse effects of opioid therapy become intolerable or unmanageable. The addition of a coanalgesic may have an opioid-sparing effect and may allow the

CRNA to decrease the total dose of opioid. There are a number of coanalgesic drugs, and they are classified based on their drug class or physiologic effect. The following are coanalgesic drugs available: anticonvulsants, antidepressants, oral local antiarrhythmics, corticosteroids, N-methyl-D-aspartate (NMDA) antagonists, sympatholytic agents, topical agents, local anesthetic topical drugs, and capsaicin. The interpatient response varies greatly with coanalgesic medications, so numerous trials of several drugs may be necessary before any analgesia is appreciated. A list of the drugs, indications, and dosage regimens can be found in Tables 52-1, 52-3, and 52-4).

Corticosteroids are the most common multipurpose coanalgesic used to treat cancer pain. In addition to their ability to provide analgesia, corticosteroids have a beneficial effect on appetite, nausea, and mood. This class of drugs is most beneficial for pain secondary to metastatic bone disease, increased intracranial pressure, acute spinal cord compression, superior vena cava syndrome, neuropathic pain resulting from infiltration or compression by tumor, symptomatic lymphedema, and hepatic capsular distention.

Much success has been enjoyed in the treatment of neuropathic pain. Although numerous drugs can provide analgesia for this type of pain, anticonvulsants and antidepressants are the mainstays of the therapy. To select the drug most likely to yield positive results, it is imperative for the CRNA to determine whether the neuropathic pain is continuous, lancinating, or sympathetically mediated.

The effective treatment of bone pain often requires a combination of opioid therapy and coanalgesic therapies. The addition of NSAIDs or corticosteroids to opioid therapy can have tremendous benefits for patients suffering from bone pain. Bone pain that is localized to one area may respond to primary radiation therapy. However, if bone pain is multifocal and poorly controlled with opioids, bisphosphonates, calcitonin, or the radiopharmaceutical strontium 89 may be indicated.

Drug Selection

For young, healthy patients and patients without major organ system dysfunction, any of the opioid-agonist drugs can be used.

Initial drug selection should be based on a thorough assessment of the pain, the severity, etiology, and the patient's experience with opioid medications. Opioids with a short half-life (e.g., morphine, hydromorphone, oxycodone) are used to initiate therapy because they are easier to titrate than opioids with a longer half-life (e.g., methadone, levorphanol), which take longer to achieve a steady-state plasma concentration.

Particular caution must be used when initiating opioid therapy in patients with impaired renal function. These patients can accumulate the active metabolites of morphine sulfate (morphine-6-glucuronide), meperidine (normeperidine), and propoxyphene (norpropoxyphene). As discussed, normeperidine has the most potentially detrimental side effects. This metabolite is twice as potent a convulsant as its parent compound. Accumulation of this metabolite can lead to CNS excitability manifested by irritability, myoclonus, and occasionally seizures. For these reasons the use of meperidine for the treatment of cancer pain is not recommended.

Knowing how the patient has responded to previous trials of opioids is imperative. A particular opioid should be continued as long as effective analgesia can be maintained and unmanageable side effects are avoided. However, rotating to a different opioid should be considered when escalating doses become ineffective or when adverse effects become intolerable or unmanageable. Consequently, CRNAs must be familiar with several different opioids and possess the knowledge to initiate therapy with another opioid, based on equianalgesic dosage data[24] and the incomplete cross-tolerance between opioids (see Table 52-8).

Other medications the patient is taking must be considered when one initiates opioid therapy. The metabolism and bioavailability of morphine can be altered by other medications. In addition, opioids are often indicted for causing excessive sedation, when in fact it may be other centrally acting drugs or their interaction with the opioids.

Route of Administration

When considering which route of administration to use, the clinician must determine the least invasive, most convenient, and most fiscally responsible method of providing effective analgesia. In the majority of cases, this is the oral route. However, in patients in whom this route is precluded, opioids can also be administered via the rectal, sublingual, transdermal, parenteral, and intraspinal routes.

The oral route is the most convenient and economic method of providing analgesia for cancer patients. In addition, most patients tolerate orally administered opioids throughout the course of the illness. Immediate-release preparations are available in both pill and syrup forms and have a peak onset of 45 to 60 minutes. Controlled-release opioids provide added convenience because of the 8-, 12-, or 24-hour doses and achieve their peak effectiveness within 3 to 5 hours, for those medications administered every 8 to 12 hours, and within 8 to 10 hours, for those medications administered every 24 hours.

Rectal preparations of morphine, hydromorphone, and oxymorphone are available in the United States. Dosage of rectally administered opioids is approximately the same as that for oral medications.[105]

The sublingual route of administration, although not frequently used, provides an alternative route for those patients who lose their ability to take oral preparations for a short period of time. Bioavailability is limited with hydrophilic opioids (morphine), but lipophilic preparations (fentanyl and methadone) are well absorbed.[106]

Fentanyl is the only currently available opioid capable of being delivered via the transdermal route. Because interindividual pharmacokinetic variability is large, the administration interval can range from 48 to 72 hours. Transdermal fentanyl can be used only to treat stable pain, which necessitates that a short-acting opioid be provided to treat breakthrough pain.

The parenteral route encompasses IM, subQ, and IV routes of administration. IM administration should be discouraged, because repetitive IM injections are painful, and absorption is unreliable. Both the subQ and IV routes can be used for bolus injections and continuous infusions. Bolus injections provide for rapid titration but can be associated with adverse effects at peak levels (excessive sedation) and trough levels (pain). Continuous infusions avoid bolus effects and can be administered via the subQ or IV route. Opioids that are soluble, nonirritating, and well absorbed can be given subcutaneously via a needle that can remain in place for up to 1 week. Infusion rates should not exceed 5 mL/hr, and dosage is the same as IV. subQ infusions are particularly beneficial in ambulatory patients and in patients in whom IV access is unavailable. Continuous infusions of morphine subQ can be problematic secondary to local histamine release. This reaction can be avoided by using fentanyl or hydromorphone subQ. IV infusions should be used when available and are recommended when large amounts of fluid are infused.

Intraspinal opioids can be administered in the intrathecal or epidural space. This route of administration is beneficial in a small number of cancer patients.

Dosage Schedule

Patients with continuous or frequently occurring pain should receive opioids "around the clock" (ATC). This type of administration provides the patient with opioids at regular, fixed intervals. When immediate-release opioids are used, they should be administered every 3 to 4 hours. Controlled-release oral preparations (morphine, oxycodone, hydromorphone) are the most convenient form, because they reach peak serum levels in 3 to 5 hours, and their analgesic half-life is 8 to 12 hours. Patients undergoing this regimen should also have access to an immediate-release form of the drug to treat breakthrough pain ("rescue dose"). Rescue doses are equivalent to 10% to 20% of the 24-hour baseline dose and offered every hour.[19] IV or subQ rescue doses can be given every 15 to 30 minutes at an equivalent dose of 50% to 200% of the hourly infusion rate. "As needed" (prn) administration may be useful in opioid-naive patients beginning therapy or in those patients in whom rapid titration is necessary. This form of administration is not recommended in the routine management of continuous pain, because the patient can suffer needlessly if a time lag occurs between when the request is made and when the opioid is actually administered.

A patient in severe pain and beginning opioid therapy should receive a dose equivalent to 5 to 10 mg of IV morphine every 4 hours, with rescue doses of 6 to 12 mg every hour (i.e., 15 to 30 mg PO every 4 hours with rescue doses of 18 to 36 mg every hour). If pain continues to be intolerable despite escalating doses, or if adverse effects become unmanageable, rotation to another opioid should be considered. Equianalgesic dose charts are used to guide the conversion to the new drug. The starting dose of the new drug should be decreased by 50% to account for the incomplete cross-tolerance between opioids. If the new opioid is methadone, the dose should be decreased by 75% to account for the prolonged half-life of the drug.

Dose Titration

The severity of the pain should dictate the rate of dose titration. For patients with severe pain, parenteral administration of an opioid with a short half-life is the preferred method of dose titration. Doses can be administered intravenously every 15 to 30 minutes until adequate analgesia is obtained. Once analgesia is achieved, the patient should receive a continuous infusion of the same opioid or an equivalent dose every 4 hours. During the titration process, doses can become quite high before adequate analgesia is obtained. CRNAs must understand that the total dose of opioid is immaterial as long as analgesia is obtained and adverse effects are not intolerable or unmanageable.

After effective analgesia is obtained, patients usually remain on a stable dose of opioid for pain control. Nurse anesthetists should not let their concern about tolerance deter the use of opioids early in the treatment of cancer pain. New complaints of pain and the need for continued dose escalation are seldom the result of analgesic tolerance. New pain or worsening pain should be aggressively pursued diagnostically, because once a stable dose of opioid has been achieved, worsening pain is often indicative of disease progression.[101,102]

Adverse Effects and Management

Successful cancer pain management mandates that the CRNA possess the skills necessary to assess and manage the adverse effects associated with opioid therapy. Clearly, the objective is for the analgesic effects of the opioid to outweigh the treatment-related adverse effects. The most common adverse effects of chronic opioid use are constipation, nausea, vomiting, sedation, and cognitive impairment. Also possible, but to varying degrees, are dysphoria, myoclonus, urinary retention, and respiratory depression.

The incidence of opioid-related constipation is extremely high, and tolerance to this side effect occurs very slowly, if at all. Patients who are dehydrated and immobile, with advanced age or abdominal disease, are particularly predisposed to this side effect. All patients receiving opioids should be on some type of bowel regimen. The aggressiveness of the regimen is dictated by the severity of the constipation, but patients should receive both a cathartic and a stool softener.

Nausea and vomiting are common adverse effects of opioid therapy, with an estimated incidence of between 10% and 40%. A treatment approach should be initiated based on the suspected cause. Opioid-induced nausea and vomiting can be mediated by the chemoreceptor trigger zone, vestibular sensitivity, and increased gastric tone.[107] Patients with nausea and vomiting secondary to enhanced vestibular sensitivity can be treated with scopolamine or meclizine. When nausea and vomiting are associated with increased gastric tone or delayed gastric emptying, prokinetic medications such as metoclopramide are indicated. Centrally induced nausea and vomiting can be treated with ondansetron, droperidol, haloperidol, benzodiazepines, metoclopramide, or chlorpromazine. Tolerance to opioid-induced nausea and vomiting generally develops very quickly.

Sedation generally occurs when opioid therapy is initiated, but patients become tolerant to this adverse effect rapidly. When sedation cannot be controlled by decreasing the dose of opioid and eliminating other centrally depressing drugs, psychostimulants such as caffeine, methylphenidate, dextroamphetamine, or modafinil may be added. If sedation persists, administration of opioid-sparing drugs (NSAIDs or adjuvant) or rotation to a different opioid should be considered.

Respiratory depression is rare in cancer patients undergoing opioid therapy. If clinically significant respiratory depression is related to the opioid, other signs of CNS depression will be present (sedation and mental clouding). When respiratory depression is accompanied by tachypnea and anxiety, other causes must be sought (pneumonia or pulmonary embolism).[107]

Anesthetic Implications

Providing an anesthetic to a patient receiving chronic opioid therapy for cancer-related pain presents numerous challenges for the nurse anesthetist. First, one may assume that patients on chronic opioid therapy are physiologically dependent on the medication. As a result, patients scheduled for surgery should continue their opioids up to and including the morning of surgery with a sip of water. Failure to do so could result in the manifestation of an abstinence syndrome. In addition, these patients normally develop some degree of tolerance to opioids. This understanding may lead to increasing the amount of opioids needed for opioid-based anesthetic procedures.

Comprehensive pain management for cancer patients can be both challenging and rewarding. With a select number of specialized cancer treatment hospitals available, CRNAs are in the ideal position to become actively involved with the management of pain in patients with cancer. Cancer pain management is much more than merely managing symptoms. All management must begin with a thorough assessment of the patient. This involves assessment of the pain itself, a complete physical and neurologic examination, and evaluation of the diagnostic findings. Equally important is the psychosocial effect of the pain on the patient and his or her family.

To effectively achieve the ultimate goal of pain relief, CRNAs must have an in-depth knowledge of the pharmacodynamics and pharmacokinetics of at least three different opioids, as well as adjuvant medications. In addition, the nurse anesthetist must know various routes of administration, equianalgesic dosages, and management of adverse effects of opioids.

SUMMARY

As advanced practice nurses, CRNAs not only should learn how to effectively manage pain but also should share this information with their anesthesia colleagues and primary care nurses. CRNAs are in a unique position to participate in the treatment of pain across the life span and across disease states. When patients receive effective analgesia, they are inclined to participate in treatment protocols and empowered to participate in decisions that influence the plan of care.

REFERENCES

1. Acute Pain Management Panel. *Acute Pain Management: Operative or Medical Procedures and Trauma. Clinical Practice Guidelines.* USDHS Publication No. 92-0032. Rockville, MD: Agency for Health Care Policy and Research, Public Health Service, U.S. Department of Health and Human Services; 1992.
2. Acute Pain Management Panel. *Acute Pain Management in Oncology.* USDHS Publication No. 94-0592. Rockville, MD: Agency for Health Care Policy and Research, Public Health Service, U.S. Department of Health and Human Services; 1994.
3. Acute Pain Management Panel. *Acute Pain Management in Infants, Children and Adolescents: Operative and Medical Procedures.* USDHS Publication No. 92-0020. Rockville, MD: Agency for Health Care Policy and Research, Public Health Service, U.S. Department of Health and Human Services; 1992.
4. Marks R, Sachar E. Undertreatment of medical patients with narcotic analgesics. *Ann Intern Med.* 1973;78:173-181.

5. Cohen F. Postsurgical pain relief: patients' status and nurses' medication choices. *Pain*. 1980;9:265-274.

6. Sriwantanakul I et al. Analysis of narcotic usage in the treatment of postoperative pain. JAMA. 1983;250:926-929.

7. Donovan M et al. Incidence and characteristics of pain in a sample of medical surgical in-patients. *Pain*. 1987;30:69-78.

8. Paice JA et al. Factors associated with adequate pain control in hospitalized post-surgical patients diagnosed with cancer. *Cancer Nursing*. 1991;14(6): 298-305.

9. Paice JA et al. Pain control in hospitalized postsurgical patients. *Med Surg Nurs*. 1995:4(5):367-372.

10. Ballentyne J. Standards of treatment: American Pain Society quality assurance standards for relief of acute pain and cancer. In: *Massachusetts General Hospital Handbook of Pain Management*. Philadelphia: Lippincott Williams & Wilkins; 2001:539-541.

11. Ward S, Gordon D. Patient satisfaction and pain severity as outcomes in pain management: a longitudinal view of one setting's experience. *J Pain Symptom Manage*. 1996;11:242-251.

12. Loeser J, Egan D. *Managing the Chronic Pain Patient: Theory and Practice at the University of Washington Multidisciplinary Pain Center*. New York: Raven; 1989.

13. Donovan M et al. Factors associated with inadequate management of pain. In: *Proceedings of the Eighth Annual Scientific Meeting of the American Pain Society*. Glenville, IL: American Pain Society; 1989.

14. Sawyer P et al. Pain and pain medication use in community-dwelling older adults. *Am J Geriatr Pharmacother*. 2006;4(4):316-324.

15. Joint Commission on Accreditation of Healthcare Organizations. *Pain: Current Understanding of Assessment, Management and Treatment*. Oak Brook, IL: JCAHO; 2001.

16. Joint Commission on Accreditation of Healthcare Organizations: *Improving the Quality of Pain Management through Measurement and Action*. Oak Brook, IL: JCAHO; 2003.

17. Joint Commission on Accreditation of Healthcare Organizations: *Approaches to Pain Management: an Essential Guide for Clinical Leaders*. Oak Brook, IL: JCAHO; 2003.

18. American Pain Society Quality of Care Committee. Quality improvement guidelines for the treatment of acute pain and cancer pain. JAMA. 1995;274:1874-1880.

19. American Pain Society. *Guideline for the Management of Cancer Pain in Adults and Children*. Glenview, IL: APS; 2005.

20. American Pain Society. *Guideline for the Management of Fibromyalgia Syndrome Pain*. Glenview, IL: APS; 2005.

21. American Pain Society. *Guideline for the Management of Pain in Osteoarthritis, Rheumatoid Arthritis and Juvenile Chronic Arthritis*. Glenview, IL: APS; 2002.

22. American Pain Society: *Guideline for the Management of Acute and Chronic Pain in Sickle-Cell Disease*. Glenview, IL: APS; 1999.

23. American Pain Society. *Principles of Analgesic Use in the Treatment of Acute and Cancer Pain*. 5th ed. Glenview, IL: APS; 2003.

24. American Pain Society. *Pain Control in the Primary Care Setting*. Glenview, IL: APS; 2006.

25. Merskey H. Classification of chronic pain: description of chronic pain syndromes and definitions of pain terms. *Pain*. 1979;Suppl3:S217.

26. Bonica J. Importance of effective pain control. *Acta Anaesthesiol Scand*. 1989;85:1-16.

27. Fields HL. *Pain: Mechanisms and Management*. 2nd ed. New York: McGraw-Hill; 2007.

28. Heavener J, Wells W. Pathways: anatomy and physiology. In: Raj P, ed. *Pain Medicine: A Comprehensive Review*. 2nd ed. St Louis: Mosby; 2003:.

29. Childers WE Jr, Baudy RB. N-methyl-D-aspartate antagonists and neuropathic pain: the search for relief. *J Med Chem*. 2007;50(11):2557-2562.

30. McCaffery M, Pasero C. *Pain. Clinical Manual*. St Louis: Mosby; 1999.

31. Terman G, Bonica J. Spinal mechanisms and their modulation. In: *Bonica's Management of Pain*. 3rd ed. Hagerstown, MD: Lippincott Williams & Wilkins; 2003.

32. Cousins M. Acute postoperative pain. In: Wall PD, Melzack R, eds. *Textbook of Pain*. 4th ed. New York: Churchill Livingstone; 2005.

33. Wu CL. Acute postoperative pain. In: Miller RD, ed. *Anesthesia*. 6th ed, Philadelphia: Churchill Livingstone; 2005:2729-2762.

34. Kremer MJ. Surgery, pain, and immune function. CRNA. 1999;10:94-100.

35. Chapman CR, Turner J. Psychological aspects of pain. In: *Bonica's Management of Pain*. 3rd ed, Hagerstown, MD: Lippincott Williams & Wilkins; 2003:180-190.

36. Kehlet H, Dahl JB. The value of "multimodal" or "balanced analgesia" in postoperative pain treatment. *Anesth Analg*. 1993;77(5):1048-1056.

37. Grape S, Tramèr MR. Do we need preemptive analgesia for the treatment of postoperative pain? *Clin Anesthesiol*. 2007;21(1):51-63.

38. Pogatzki-Zahn E, Zahn P. From preemptive to preventive analgesia. *Curr Opin Anesthesiol*. 2006;19(5):551-555.

39. Skinner H, Shintani E. Results of a multimodal analgesic trial involving patients with total hip or total knee arthroplasty. *Am J Orthop*. 2004;33(4):85-92.

40. Gottschalk A et al. Current treatment options for acute pain. *Exp Opin Pharmacother*. 2002;3:1599-1611.

41. Gottschalk A et al. Preemptive analgesia: what do we do now? *Anesthesiology*. 2003;98(1):280-281.

42. Reuben SS, Connelly NR. Postoperative analgesic effects of celecoxib or rofecoxib after spinal fusion surgery. *Anesth Analg*. 2000;91:1221-1225.

43. Helmy SA, Bali A. The effect of preemptive use of the NMDA receptor antagonist dextromethorphan on postoperative analgesic requirements. *Anesth Analg*. 2001;92:739-744.

44. Reuben SS et al. The preemptive analgesic effect of rofecoxib after ambulatory arthroscopic knee surgery. *Anesth Analg*. 2002;94:55-59.

45. Buvanendran A et al. Effects of perioperative administration of a selective cyclooxygenase 2 inhibitor on pain management and recovery of function after knee replacement: a randomized controlled trial. JAMA. 2003;290:2411-2418.

46. Gramke H et al. Sublingual piroxicam for postoperative analgesia: preoperative versus postoperative administration: a randomized, double-blind study. *Anesth Analg*. 2006;102(3):755-758.

47. Yamashita K et al. Preoperative administration of intravenous flurbiprofen axetil reduces postoperative pain for spinal fusion. *J Anesth*. 2006;20:92-95.

48. Møiniche S et al. A qualitative and quantitative systematic review of preemptive analgesia for postoperative pain relief: the role of timing of analgesia. *Anesthesiology*. 2002;96(3):725-741.

49. Adachi YU et al. Preemptive analgesia by preoperative administration of nonsteroidal anti-inflammatory drugs. *J Anesth*. 2007;20(2):92-95.

50. Ruoff G, Lema M. Strategies in pain management: new and potential indications for COX-2 specific inhibitors. *J Pain Symptom Manage*. 2003; 25(Suppl 2):S21-S31.

51. Yaksh T. Central sites and mechanisms of actions of NSAID drugs. In: *American Pain Society Twelfth Annual Scientific Meeting*. Palm Desert, CA: Convention Cassettes; 1993.

52. Rowlingson JC, Rawal N. Postoperative pain guidelines: targeted to the site of surgery. *Reg Anesth Pain Med*. 2003;28:265-267.

53. Yaksh TL, Abram SE. Preemptive analgesia: a popular misnomer, but a clinically relevant truth? *APS J*. 1993;2:116-121.

54. Dahl JB, Kehlet H. Non-steroidal anti-inflammatory drugs: rationale for use in severe postoperative pain. *Br J Anaesth*. 1991;66:703-712.

55. Dupuis R et al. Preoperative flurbiprofen in oral surgery: a method of choice in controlling postoperative pain. *Pharmacotherapy*. 1988;8:193-200.

56. Kaye AD et al. Pharmacology of cyclooxgenase-2 inhibitors and preemptive analgesia in acute pain management. *Curr Opin Anaesthesiol*. 2008;21(4): 439-445.

57. Miller RR, Jick J. Clinical effects of meperidine in hospitalized medical patients. *J Clin Pharmacol*. 1978;18:180-189.

58. Kaiko RF et al. Central nervous system excitatory effects of meperidine in cancer patients. *Ann Neurol*. 1983;13:180-185.

59. Marlowe KF, Chicella MF. Treatment of sickle cell pain. *Pharmacotherapy*. 2002;22:484-491.

60. American Pain Society. *Principles of Analgesic Use in the Treatment of Acute and Cancer Pain*. 5th ed. Glenview, IL: APS; 2003.

61. Morgan JP. American opiophobia: customary underutilization of opioid analgesics. *Adv Alcohol Subst Abuse*. 1985/1986;5:163-173.

62. Wasan AD et al. Iatrogenic addiction in patients treated for acute or subacute pain: a systematic review. *J Opioid Manag*. 2006;2(1):16-22.

63. Porter J, Jick H. Addiction rare in patients treated with narcotics. *N Engl J Med*. 1980;302:123.

64. McGuire DB et al: *Cancer Pain Management*. 2nd ed, Boston: Jones & Bartlett; 1995.

65. Portenoy R, McCaffery M. Adjuvant analgesics. In: McCaffery M, Pasero C, eds. *Pain: Clinical Manual*. 2nd ed. St Louis: Mosby; 1999:300-361.

66. Wall PD, Melzack R. *Textbook of Pain*. 5th ed. New York: Churchill Livingstone; 2005.

67. Horswell JL et al. *Use of dexmedetomidine as an adjunct to pain control following OPCAB: a randomized, double-blind study*. ASA Meeting Abstracts. Philadelphia: Lippincott Williams & Wilkins; 2002.

68. Walker G et al. *Dexmedetomidine in bariatric surgery patients*. ASA Meeting Abstracts. Philadelphia: Lippincott Williams & Wilkins; 2002.

69. Zakrzewska J. Trigeminal eye and ear pain. In: Melzcak R, Wall PD, eds. *Handbook of Pain Management*. New York: Churchill Livingstone; 2003: 598-620.

70. Austin KL et al. Multiple injections: a major source of variability in analgesic response to meperidine. *Pain*. 1980;8:47-62.

71. Viscusi ER et al. Evaluation of a non-invasive patient-controlled analgesia delivery system for the treatment of acute postoperative pain:

a double-blind, multicenter, placebo-controlled trial incorporating JCAHO pain management standards. *ASA Meeting Abstracts*. Philadelphia: Lippincott Williams & Wilkins; 2003.

72. Viscusi ER. Patient-controlled drug delivery for acute postoperative pain management: a review of current and emerging technologies. *Reg Anesth Pain Med*. 2008;33(2):146-158.

73. Cleland JG. Continuous peridural analgesia in surgery and early ambulation. *Northwest Med*. 1949;48:26.

74. El-Baz NM et al. Continuous epidural infusion of morphine for treatment of pain after thoracic surgery: a new technique. *Anesth Analg*. 1984;63:757-764.

75. Hjorts NC et al. Epidural morphine improves pain relief and maintains sensory analgesia during continuous epidural bupivacaine after abdominal surgery. *Anesth Analg*. 1986;65:1033-1036.

76. Bonnet F, Marret E. Postoperative pain management and outcome after surgery. *Best Pract Res Clin Anaesthesiol*. 2007;21(1):99-107.

77. White PF. Multimodal analgesia: its role in preventing postoperative pain. *Curr Opin Investig Drugs*. 2008;9(1):76-82.

78. Scott NB et al. Continuous thoracic extradural 0.05% bupivacaine with or without morphine: effect on quality of blockade, lung function and the surgical stress response. *Br J Anaesth*. 1989;62:253-257.

79. Lubenow T. Epidural analgesia: considerations and delivery methods. In: Sinatra RS et al, eds. *Acute Pain Mechanisms and Management*. St Louis: Mosby; 1992:233-242.

80. Waxler B et al. Primer of postoperative pruritus for anesthesiologists. *Anesthesiology*. 2005Jul;103(1):168-178.

81. Lubenow TR et al. Management of acute postoperative pain. In: Barash PG et al, eds. *Clinical Anesthesia*. 5th ed. Philadelphia: Lippincott Williams & Wilkins; 2006:1405-1440.

82. Schecter NL. The undertreatment of pain in children: an overview. *Pediatr Clin North Am*. 1989;36:781-794.

83. Kliegman R et al. *Nelson Textbook of Pediatrics*. 18th ed. Philadelphia: Saunders; 2007.

84. Schecter NL et al: *Pain in Infants, Children and Adolescents*. Philadelphia: Lippincott Williams & Wilkins; 2003.

85. Kremer M, Faut-Callahan M. Regional anesthesia and pain management. In: Zaglaniczny K, Aker J, eds. *Clinical Guide to Pediatric Anesthesia*. Philadelphia: Saunders; 1999:359-382.

86. Tycross RG. Cancer pain syndromes. In: Sykes N et al, eds. *Clinical Pain Management: Cancer Pain*. New York: Oxford University Press; 2003:4-19.

87. Gosney M. Elderly cancer. In: Sykes N et al, eds. *Clinical Pain Management: Cancer Pain*. New York: Oxford University Press; 2003:21-32.

88. Fisch M, Burton A. *Cancer Pain Management*. New York: McGraw-Hill; 2006.

89. Trescot AM et al. Opioids in the management of chronic non-cancer pain: an update of American Society of the Interventional Pain Physicians' (ASIPP) Guidelines. *Pain Physician*. 2008;11(2 Suppl):S5-S62.

90. American Academy of Hospice and Palliative Medicine, Center of Advanced Palliative Care, Hospice and Palliative Nurse Association, Last Acts Partnership, National Hospice and Palliative Care Organization. National Consensus Project for Quality Palliative Care: Clinical practice guidelines for quality palliative care, executive summary. *J Palliat Med*. 2004; 7(5):611-627.

91. Hospice Association of America. *Hospice Facts and Statistics*. National Association for Home Care and Hospice website. http://www.nahc.org/Consumer/hpcstats.html. Accessed December 17, 2004.

92. Ferrell B et al. The national agenda for quality palliative care: the National Consensus Project and the National Quality Forum. *J Pain Symptom Manage*. 2007;33(6):737-744.

93. Lorenz KA et al. Evidence for improving palliative care at the end of the life: a systematic review. *Ann Intern Med*. 2008;148(2):147-159.

94. Lorenz KA et al. Quality measures for symptoms and advance care planning in cancer: a systematic review.

95. Qaseem A et al. Evidence-based interventions to improve the palliative care of pain, dyspnea, and depression at the end of life: a clinical practice guideline from the American College of Physicians. *Ann Intern Med*. 2008;148(2):141-146.

96. Wolfe J et al. Easing of suffering in children with cancer at the end of life: is care changing? *J Clin Oncol*. 2008;26(10):1717-1723.

97. Liben S et al. Paediatric palliative care: challenges and emerging ideas. *Lancet*. 2008;371(9615):852-864.

98. Faut-Callahan M, Breakwell S. Interdisciplinary Palliative Care Education. Washington, DC: National Institutes of Health, National Cancer Institute; 2005.

99. Von Roenn JH et al. Physicians' attitudes and practice in cancer pain management: a survey from the Eastern Cooperative Oncology Group. *Ann Intern Med*. 1993;119:121-126.

100. McDonald DD, Weiskopf CS. Adult patients' postoperative pain descriptions and responses to the Short-Form McGill Pain Questionnaire. *Clin Nurs Res*. 2001;10(4):442-452.

101. Coyle N et al. Disease progression and tolerance in the cancer pain patient. Second International Congress on Cancer Pain. *J Pain Symptom Manage*. 1988;3:S25.

102. Davis MP et al. Practical guide to opioids and their complications in managing cancer pain. What oncologists need to know. *Oncology*. 2007;21(10):1229-1238;discussion 1238-1246, 1249.

103. Portenoy RK. Management of cancer pain: opioid and adjuvant pharmacotherapy. In: Portenoy RK, ed. *Real Patients, Real Problems: Optimal Assessment and Management of Cancer Pain*. Glenview, IL: American Pain Society; 1997.

104. Gutstein HB, Akil H. Opioid analgesics. In: Brunton LL et al, eds. *Goodman & Gillman The Pharmacological Basis of Therapeutics*. 11th ed, New York: McGraw-Hill; 2006:547-590.

105. Hanning CD. The rectal absorption of opioids. In: Benedette C et al, eds. *Opioid Analgesia. Advances in Pain Research and Therapy*. Vol 14. New York: Raven; 1990:259-269.

106. Weinberg DS et al. Sublingual absorption of selected opioid analgesics. *Clin Pharmacol Ther*. 1988;44:335-342.

107. Cherny NI, Foley KM. Nonopioid and opioid analgesic pharmacotherapy of cancer pain. *Hematol Oncol Clin North Am*. 1996;10:79-102.

CHAPTER 53

ANESTHESIA FOR THERAPEUTIC AND DIAGNOSTIC PROCEDURES

Allan J. Schwartz

Although most anesthetics were traditionally administered in the operating room, it is no longer unusual to provide services outside the operating suite in a variety of settings far from the traditional setting. There are estimates today that up to 40% of the procedures requested of the anesthesia service are taking place outside the conventional operating room.[1] Box 53-1 provides a current and comprehensive list of such procedures.[2] Patients treated in these new settings deserve the same safe, vigilant attention, anesthetic administration, and recovery as those patients treated in the operating suite. The key for the anesthesia provider is to make sure the therapeutic and diagnostic environment where anesthesia is to be performed is as familiar, as well equipped, and as safe as in the operating room.

Although certain therapeutic and diagnostic procedures are sometimes performed without anesthesia, the patient's condition or the requirements of the test or procedure may necessitate administration of an anesthetic. Anesthesia could range from local anesthetic infiltration and regional anesthesia techniques to monitored anesthesia care involving enteral minimal sedation, parenteral moderate sedation/analgesia, deep sedation/analgesia, or general anesthesia. Patients can range in age from pediatric to geriatric. In remote locations, patients who require anesthesia could be confused or disoriented, uncooperative, unwilling or unable to understand the requirements of the procedure, claustrophobic, anxious, or mentally disabled. As medical technology rapidly progresses, more patients will be seen outside the operating room for therapeutic and diagnostic procedures. Older and medically higher-risk patients are being treated more often in this environment.[3] The therapeutic or diagnostic procedure might require the patient to lie still for an extended length of time or cause moments of painful, visual, and audio stimulation alternating with long periods of no stimulation, which makes anesthesia delivery challenging for the anesthetist.

Given the rapid advances in medical knowledge and technology, coupled with a strong societal impetus to reduce health-care costs, more therapeutic and diagnostic procedures will be performed in remote locations.[1,2]

ADMINISTRATION OF ANESTHESIA IN REMOTE LOCATIONS

Special Considerations

The operating room provides an ideal environment for the administration of anesthesia and the performance of surgical procedures because of its familiarity and the rapid availability of needed anesthesia equipment, medications, supplies, and well-trained adjunct personnel. The anesthesia setting in a remote location must possess the same level of safety and high standards. Many considerations and plans must be made before a patient can safely receive anesthesia for a therapeutic or diagnostic procedure

in a remote location. Box 53-2 provides a comprehensive checklist of the requisites that will facilitate planning and gathering needed equipment, supplies, and medications.

A policy must be developed that outlines the organization of emergency services for either in-hospital or office-based facilities. Office-based facilities should have a plan for regular emergency training of personnel, interoffice communication during an emergency, communication with emergency medical personnel, and transportation to the nearest hospital emergency department.

An anesthesia machine and portable anesthesia cart with the listed equipment, supplies, and medications should be dedicated strictly for use in remote locations. This can save preparation time whenever a procedure is required in a remote location. It also increases patient safety and decreases the risk of a mishap resulting from lack of necessary equipment and materials.

As part of the planning process before patient treatment, it is important to familiarize oneself with the personnel and the work area in the remote environment. The workplace allotted for anesthesia care may be small, crowded, and different from the usual operating room setting. Pre-planning is important to make this *different* location *familiar* to the anesthetist and safe for the patient to receive the anesthetic and therapeutic or diagnostic procedure. Some have advocated the use of total intravenous anesthesia (TIVA) in small workplaces in which the use of excessive equipment and supplies and an anesthesia machine with a ventilator, along with the handling of fresh and waste anesthetic gases, would be too costly or prohibitive.[4,5] No remote location should ever limit the ability to manage these anesthetic procedures or prevent equipment, medications, supplies, positive-pressure ventilation, resuscitation, and suction from being readily available.

The Anesthesia Patient Safety Foundation is a good resource to seek information regarding new anesthesia-related developments, new anesthesia products, and discussion of safety issues.

The American Association of Nurse Anesthetists (AANA),[6] the American Society of Anesthesiologists (ASA),[7,8] The Joint Commission,[9-11] and other sources[12-14] have established written standards and professional commentary to provide for the basic rights and safety of patients, along with the safety of anesthesia providers and ancillary personnel. As technology advances, these standards are adapted.

Licensed registered nurses who are not qualified anesthesia providers have become involved in the monitoring of patients and the administration of medications for procedural sedations involving therapeutic and diagnostic procedures, as well as for certain surgical procedures.

BOX **53-1**

Comprehensive List of Procedures That May Require Anesthesia Outside the Operating Room

Cardiology and Vascular Procedures
Diagnostic angiography
Automatic implantable cardiac defibrillator (AICD) insertion
Cardiac catheterization
Percutaneous coronary intervention (PCI)
Cardioversion
Cryoablation
Electrophysiologic mapping
Exclusion of thoracic or abdominal aortic aneurysms
Femoral arterial sheath removal
Pacemaker insertion
Percutaneous ventricular assist device insertion
Radiofrequency catheter ablation (RFCA) for certain cardiac
  dysrhythmias
Transcatheter closure of atrial septal defects
Valvuloplasty
Venous filter insertion

Emergency Department Procedures
Diagnostic peritoneal lavage
Central venous catheter insertion
Emergency endotracheal intubation
Insertion of intracranial pressure monitor
Orthopedic manipulations
Pericardiocentesis
Thoracocentesis
Tube thoracotomy
Vascular "cut down"

Gastroenterology Procedures
Colonoscopy
Endoscopic retrograde cholangiopancreatography (ERCP)
Esophagogastroduodenoscopy (EGD)
Liver biopsy
Percutaneous endoscopically placed gastrostomy
Radiofrequency ablation of colorectal liver metastases
Upper endoscopy
Lower endoscopy

Gynecology Procedures
Assisted reproductive technologies (ART)
Gamete intrafallopian transfer (GIFT)
In vitro fertilization (IVF)
Ovular transvaginal withdrawal
Peritoneal oocyte and sperm transfer (POST)
Tubal embryo transfer (TET)
Zygote intrafallopian transfer (ZIFT)

Hematology and Oncology Procedures
Bone marrow aspiration and biopsy
Infusion therapy
Lumbar puncture
Pediatric spinal tap for patients with blood dyscrasias
Radiotherapy procedures
Removal of indwelling central venous catheters

Intensive Care Procedures
Bronchoscopy
Cardioversion

Central venous catheter insertion
Diagnostic peritoneal lavage
Endotracheal intubation
Percutaneous endoscopic gastrostomy
Percutaneous tracheostomy
Thoracocentesis
Thoracotomy and tube thoracotomy
Vascular "cut down"
Ventriculostomy

Office-Based Procedures
Neurophysiology Laboratory
Brainstem auditory–evoked responses

Office-Based Surgeries
Dental surgery
  Pedodontics
  Pediatric dentistry
  Oral and maxillofacial surgery
  Periodontics
  Endodontics
  Prosthodontics
  General dentistry
  Dental hygiene
Plastic surgery
  Removal of superficial skin lesions
  Rhizotomy
  Liposuction
Ophthalmology
  Electroretinography
  Examination under anesthesia
  Retinoscopy and tonometry
  Various ocular surgical procedures

Orthopedic Procedures
Cast changes
Hardware removal
Joint aspiration

Psychiatric Procedures
Electroconvulsive therapy (ECT)

Radiology and Diagnostic Procedures
Biliary drainage and dilation
Brachytherapy
Computed tomography (CT)
Embolization
Functional brain imaging
Interventional neuroradiology
Interventional radiology (vascular and nonvascular)
Intraoperative radiotherapy
Magnetic resonance imaging (MRI)
Positron emission tomography (PET)
Radiosurgery
Stereotactic radiosurgery
Radiotherapy and imaging procedures
Teletherapy
Transjugular intrahepatic portosystemic shunt placement
Ultrasound-guided diagnostic and therapeutic procedures

*Modified from Kotob F, Twersky RS. Anesthesia outside the operating room: general overview and monitoring standards. Int Anesthesiol Clin.
2003;41:1-15.*

Continued

BOX 53-1

Comprehensive List of Procedures That May Require Anesthesia Outside the Operating Room–cont'd

Urology Procedures
Cystoscopy procedures
Extracorporeal shock-wave lithotripsy
Percutaneous sclerotherapy and drainage of renal cysts
Prostate biopsies
Renal and drainage and dilation

Other Procedures
Anesthesia in military bases and war fields
Remote anesthetic monitoring using telecommunications technology
Veterinary anesthesia

BOX 53-2

Requisites for Administration of Anesthesia in Remote Locations

Utilities
Adequate workspace
Adequate overhead lighting
Adequate numbers and current-carrying capacity of electrical outlets
Electrical service with either isolated electric power or ground fault circuit interrupters
Uncluttered floor space
Two-way communication devices—telephone, intercom, Internet availability (instant messaging), personal digital assistant (PDA) device, two-way radios. Consider devices with power independent of the electrical service.
Backup power
Suitable area for post-procedure recovery (All building codes, fire codes, safety codes, and facility standards must be met.)

Equipment
Local infiltration, intravenous sedation, regional and general anesthesia
Patient chair, cart, or operating surface that can be quickly placed into Trendelenburg position
Regularly serviced and functioning equipment
Patient monitors
Pulse oximeter
Electrocardiograph
Blood pressure monitor with a selection of adequate-sized cuffs
Capnograph
Anesthesia awareness/level of consciousness/anesthesia-depth monitor
Body temperature monitor
Oxygen supplies
Minimum of two oxygen sources must be available with regulators attached (compressed oxygen should be the equivalent of an E cylinder)
Positive-pressure ventilation sources, including a self-inflating resuscitator bag capable of delivering at least 90% oxygen and a mouth-to-mask unit
Defibrillator—manual biphasic or automatic external defibrillator (AED) (charged, ready, and easily accessible)
Suction source or a suction machine (electric-powered suction, battery-powered suction, or foot pump suction devices are available), tubing, suction catheters, and Yankauer suctions

Lockable anesthesia cart to permit organization of supplies, including endotracheal equipment, laryngeal mask airways, dental laryngeal mask airways, tube of water-soluble lubricating jelly, Combitubes, an assortment of various sized disposable face masks, nasal cannulas, Connell airways, disposable face masks with oxygen tubing, oral and nasal airways, syringes (1 mL tuberculin syringe, 3 mL, 5 mL, 10 mL, 20 mL, 60 mL), needles, intravenous catheters, tourniquet, intravenous fluids and tubing, alcohol pads, adhesive tape, sterile intravenous site covers, disposable gloves, stethoscopes, precordial stethoscope with monaural earpiece and extension tubing, precordial stethoscope adhesive disks, and appropriate anesthetic medications
Battery-powered flashlight for the illumination of the patient, the anesthesia machines, and the monitors along with spare batteries
Syringe pump, wall plug/transformer and spare batteries
Warm blankets, electric blanket (check with hospital policy before using an electric blanket), or forced-air warming devices with the appropriate blanket; towels or hat to cover the patient's head to preserve body warmth
Blankets, towels, or foam for padding for protection of skin integrity, bony prominences, and body extremities
Emergency medications to include, at a minimum: adenosine, aminophylline, amiodarone, atropine, dextrose 50%, diphenhydramine, ephedrine, epinephrine, flumazenil, hydrocortisone, lidocaine, naloxone, nitroglycerin, phenylephrine, succinylcholine, verapamil, and a bronchial dilator inhaler such as albuterol or nebulized epinephrine (such as Primatene mist)
Preoperative anesthesia evaluation forms
Anesthesia consent form
Anesthesia charts, clipboard, black ink pens, indelible ink pens

Additional Requirements for General Anesthesia:
Oxygen fail-safe system
Oxygen analyzer
Waste gas exhaust scavenging system
End-tidal carbon dioxide ($ETCO_2$) analyzer, extra $ETCO_2$ filter and extension sample tubing
Vaporizers—calibration and exclusion system
Respiratory monitoring apparatus (for the anesthesia circuit reservoir bag)
Alarm system

BOX 53-2

Requisites for Administration of Anesthesia in Remote Locations—cont'd

Anesthetic medications (Note that some anesthetic medications must be kept refrigerated until ready for use. To have fresh and active medications, check with the drug manufacturer's package insert or the bottle label.)

In addition to the emergency medications listed above, consider the following:

Premedication drugs—midazolam, pentobarbital, ketamine, nitrous oxide, diazepam, chloral hydrate

Induction drugs—propofol, etomidate, methohexital, thiopental, ketamine

Maintenance drugs—bottles of sevoflurane, isoflurane, desflurane, propofol, ketamine, dexmedetomidine

Narcotics—midazolam, diazepam, fentanyl, alfentanil, sufentanil, remifentanil

Muscle relaxants—succinylcholine, rocuronium, cisatracurium, atracurium, vecuronium

Muscle relaxant reversal agents—edrophonium, neostigmine, atropine, glycopyrrolate

Cardiovascular drugs—labetalol, esmolol, verapamil, hydralazine

Narcotic reversal drugs—naloxone, flumazenil

Antiemetic drugs—ondansetron, dolasetron, granisetron, metoclopramide, droperidol*

Emergency cart and equipment

Basic airway equipment (adult and pediatric)

Nasal and oral airways

Face mask (appropriate for patient)

Laryngoscope handle assortment with spare batteries

Assortment of laryngoscope blades and spare light bulbs, endotracheal tubes (adult and pediatric), laryngeal mask airways (LMAs), and dental LMAs

Combitube

Self-inflating resuscitator bag (Ambu bag)

Difficult airway equipment

Laryngeal mask airway

Light wand

Emergency cricothyrotomy kit

Defibrillator—manual biphasic defibrillator or automatic external defibrillator (AED)

Supplemental oxygen and nitrous oxide tanks with attached and functional regulators; allow for safe transportation and storage of tanks

Emergency medications

Cardiopulmonary resuscitation (CPR) compression board

Suction equipment (suction catheter, Yankauer type)

Malignant hyperthermia emergency drugs, equipment, and the phone number for the Malignant Hyperthermia Association of the United States (MHAUS) for live help during the treatment of malignant hyperthermia on-site. (United States and Canada: 1-800-MH HYPER or 1-800-644-9737. Outside the United States and Canada: 001-1-315-464-7079.) More information is available at the Malignant Hyperthermia Association of the United States website at: http://www.mhaus.org.

Be aware of droperidol use in patients with prolonged QT syndrome.

The AANA and the ASA together have issued a joint statement in regard to criteria (Box 53-3) that must be met to protect the safety and well-being of the patient.[15]

Standards for the Delivery of Anesthesia in a Remote Location

A. Perform a complete preanesthesia assessment. The patient, parent(s), or legal guardian(s) must be thoroughly and unhurriedly interviewed before the performance of an anesthetic procedure. The preanesthesia assessment should be performed in consideration of the patient's right to privacy and confidentiality and which safeguards their dignity and respects aspects of their psychological, cultural, and spiritual values. During this assessment, information is obtained regarding the patient's medical history (prior allergy must be assessed), anesthesia history (noting any prior complications and responses to prior anesthetic experiences), surgical history, and medication history (including tobacco, alcohol, and any substance abuse). A complete physical assessment of the patient is made, along with inspection of the head, neck, mouth, and airway. The anesthetist's head and neck assessment can be especially beneficial to the patient's well-being, because common oral conditions and suspicious head/neck, skin, and oral pathologic lesions can be detected and referred for further evaluation by a dentist or a physician. Knowledge of the appearance of healthy and pathology-free tissues can alert the anesthetist when deviations from normal are observed, warranting further investigation. Early referral for diagnosis and treatment of disease contributes to patient cure and recovery to wellness, as well as reduced morbidity and mortality.[16] Lung and heart sounds are auscultated. Review is made of objective diagnostic data such as patient laboratory values, radiographs, and electrocardiogram (ECG). Important findings are noted in the patient's anesthesia record. A physical status classification is then assigned the patient.

Box 53-4 outlines specific patient conditions which alert the anesthetist to a need for special attention and care for anesthetics provided for therapeutic and diagnostic procedures.

B. Obtain informed consent for the planned anesthetic intervention from the patient or legal guardian. The anesthesia provider should discuss the course of the anesthetic care and enumerate the following in understandable terms appropriate for the patient or guardian:

- How the anesthetic procedure will be performed
- Possible risks of the anesthetic procedure
- Pertinent possible reactions or complications the patient might expect while receiving a typical anesthetic, along with informing the patient or guardian that the anesthetist has permission to make changes or adjustments as deemed necessary in his or her professional judgment
- Possible options to the type of anesthetic to be received by the patient
- The ability for the patient/parent(s)/guardian(s) to have any concerns addressed and questions answered

At times, anesthesia for therapeutic and diagnostic procedures will only require minimal, moderate, or deep sedation, which by definition may not include patient amnesia. Only general

---

BOX 53-3

Criteria for the Management and Monitoring of Patients Undergoing Sedation Delivered for Therapeutic or Diagnostic Procedures by Non-Qualified Anesthesia Providers

- Guidelines for patient monitoring, drug administration, and protocols are available for dealing with potential complications or emergency situations, developed in accordance with accepted standards of anesthesia practice.
- A qualified anesthesia provider or attending physician selects and orders the agents to achieve sedation and analgesia.
- Registered nurses who are not qualified anesthesia providers should not administer agents classified as anesthetics, including but not limited to ketamine, propofol, etomidate, sodium thiopental, methohexital, nitrous oxide, and muscle relaxants. (A computer-assisted personalized sedation device [CAPS] is being developed to enable a non-qualified anesthesia provider [physician-nurse team] to safely and effectively administer propofol for colonoscopy or esophagogastroduodenoscopy EGD procedures.)
- The registered nurse managing and monitoring the patient receiving and analgesia sedation shall have no other responsibilities during the procedure.
- Venous access shall be maintained for all patients having sedation and analgesia.
- Supplemental oxygen shall be available for any patient receiving sedation and analgesia and when appropriate in the postprocedure period.

- Documentation and monitoring of physiologic measurements including but not limited to blood pressure, respiratory rate, oxygen saturation, cardiac rate and rhythm, and level of consciousness should be recorded at least every 5 minutes.
- An emergency cart must be immediately accessible to every location where analgesia sedation is administered. This cart must include emergency resuscitative drugs, airway and ventilatory adjunct equipment, defibrillator, and a source for administration of 100% oxygen. A positive-pressure breathing device, oxygen, suction and appropriate airways must be placed in each room where analgesia sedation is administered.
- Back-up personnel who are experts in airway management, emergency intubations, and advanced cardiopulmonary resuscitation must be available.
- A qualified professional capable of managing complications is present in the facility and remains in the facility until the patient is stable.
- A qualified professional authorized under institutional guidelines to discharge the patient remains in the facility to discharge the patient in accordance with established criteria of the facility.

BOX 53-4

Specific Patient Conditions That Warrant Anesthesia-Care Vigilance

- Mental impairment with no possibility of cooperation
- Severe gastroesophageal reflux; delayed gastric emptying; aspiration risk
- Gastroparesis secondary to diabetes mellitus
- Orthopnea; obstructive sleep apnea
- Decreased level of consciousness; depression of airway protection reflexes
- Increased intracranial pressure
- Known difficult intubation; assessed oral, dental, craniofacial, cervical, or thoracic abnormalities that could preclude airway access and maintenance
- Respiratory tract infection; unexplained fever
- Morbid obesity
- Therapeutic or diagnostic procedures that impede access to the airway
- Therapeutic or diagnostic procedures that are complex, lengthy, painful, or invasive
- Positioning that is complex, atypical, painful; prone position
- Patient suffering acute trauma
- Patients at extremes of age
- Prematurity
- Physical status 3 or 4

anesthesia ensures amnesia as a standard of care. Therefore, discussion of what the patient can reasonably expect should take place at this time.[17,18] It is far easier to discuss these points with the patient before the anesthetic procedure than to explain these points after the fact. Box 53-5 displays a sample patient informed consent for anesthesia services, which can serve as a starting point for further discussion between the patient and the anesthetist.[19]

C. Formulate a patient-specific plan for anesthesia care. The art and science of anesthesia mandate that the safest and least invasive anesthetic technique be administered to the patient to simplify delivery of the anesthetic and to avoid complications for the patient while in the remote location.

D. Implement and adjust the anesthesia care plan based on the patient's physiologic response. Immediately before implementation of anesthesia, reassess the patient (vital signs, airway status, and response to preprocedure medications given), and document a reassessment note in the anesthesia record. The Joint Commission defines "immediately" as the moments just before the sedation is administered. Also, make sure all anesthesia equipment, supplies, and medications are checked and immediately available in case the patient needs a change in the anesthetic plan.

E. Properly prepare, dispense, and label all medications to be used for the patient. All medications drawn up prior to the case must be labeled with the drug name, strength (concentration), amount (if not apparent from the container), and expiration date (if not used within 24 hours). Medications drawn up and used immediately for the procedure do not require labeling.

F. Adhere to appropriate safety precautions, as established with the institution, to minimize the risks of fire, explosion, electrical shock, and equipment malfunction. This standard is

---

BOX **53-5**

Sample Consent for Anesthesia Services

Consent for Anesthesia Services

I, _____, acknowledge that my doctor has explained to me that I will have an operation, diagnostic, or treatment procedure. My doctor has explained the risks of the procedure, advised me of alternative treatments and told me about the expected outcome and what could happen if my condition remains untreated. I also understand that anesthesia services are needed so that my doctor can perform the operation or procedure.

It has been explained to me that all forms of anesthesia involve some risks, and no guarantees or promises can be made concerning the results of my procedure or treatment. Although rare, unexpected *severe complications* with anesthesia can occur and include the remote possibility of *infection, bleeding, drug reactions, blood clots, loss of sensation, loss of limb* function, paralysis, stroke, brain damage, heart attack, or death. I understand that these risks apply to all forms of anesthesia and that additional or specific risks have been identified below as they may apply to a specific type of anesthesia. I understand that the type(s) of anesthesia service checked below will be used for my procedure and that the anesthetic technique to be used is determined by many factors, including my physical condition, the type of procedure my doctor is to do, his or her preference, as well as my own desire. It has been explained to me that sometimes an anesthesia technique that involves the use of local anesthetics, with or without sedation, may not succeed completely, and therefore another technique may have to be used including general anesthesia.

Modified from American Association of Nurse Anesthetists. Consent for Anesthesia Services. *Available at the AANA website: http://www.aana.com/ Resources.aspx?ucNavMenu_TSMenuTargetID=51&ucNavMenu_TSMenuTargetType=4&ucNavMenu_TSMenuID=6&id=756. Accessed April 24, 2007.*

---

important for the patient, the anesthesia provider, and ancillary personnel for the prevention of accidents and injury. It is also important from a medicolegal standpoint. The anesthesia provider should also be an integral part of the team involved with protocols for preventing wrong site, wrong procedure and wrong person surgery, also known as the *Universal Protocol* established by The Joint Commission.[20-24] Safety must be a consideration for scheduling obligations of anesthesia personnel because anesthesia for therapeutic and diagnostic procedures is often more involved and complex when compared with anesthesia delivered in the operating room.

G. Monitor and document the patient's physiologic condition as appropriate for the type of anesthesia and specific patient needs.[25]

Monitor ventilation continuously. Ventilation may be monitored in the patient undergoing mild, moderate, or deep sedation with a precordial stethoscope or by direct auscultation of the patient's ventilatory effort. Verify intubation of the trachea by auscultation, chest excursion, and confirmation of carbon dioxide in the expired gas. Continuously monitor end-tidal carbon dioxide ($ETCO_2$) during controlled, assisted, or spontaneous ventilation, including any anesthesia or sedation technique requiring artificial airway support. Use spirometry and ventilatory pressure monitors as indicated.

Monitor oxygenation continuously by clinical observation, pulse oximetry, cerebral oximetry, and, if indicated, arterial blood gas analysis.

Monitor cardiovascular status continuously via electrocardiography and heart sounds. Record blood pressure and heart rate at least every 5 minutes.

Consider the use of a monitor of anesthesia awareness/level of consciousness/depth of sedation via electroencephalographic processing for procedures intended to produce loss of consciousness.[25,26]

Monitor body temperature continuously in all patients when clinically significant changes in body temperature are intended, anticipated, or suspected. Maintenance of normothermia must be an integral part of the anesthetic plan to preserve

BOX **53-6**

Reasons for Maintaining Normothermia for Therapeutic and Diagnostic Procedures

- To decrease sympathetic activity related to vasoconstriction while hypothermic
- To decrease cardiac morbidity and cardiac demand during recovery from hypothermia
- To minimize patient morbidity and discomfort related to being cold and shivering
- To maintain the normal pharmacokinetics of administered medications. Hypothermia decreases the normal metabolism of medications.
- To decrease anesthesia recovery time. Hypothermia impairs the rapid recovery from anesthesia.
- To maintain bodily metabolic functions. The enzymes involved in body metabolic chemical reactions function ideally at normothermia.
- To maintain normal blood coagulation and to decrease blood loss. The coagulation cascade is impaired or delayed during hypothermia.
- To decrease the incidence of wound infection
- To decrease the incidence of complications that may require hospitalization

essential body functions (Box 53-6) and to prevent complications leading to patient morbidity and mortality.[27,28] Temperature monitoring is a standard of care when delivering general anesthesia to the patient and optional while performing mild, moderate, or deep sedation.

Monitor neuromuscular function and status prior to the procedure and recovery when neuromuscular blocking agents are administered.

Monitor and assess patient positioning and protective measures at frequent intervals. Periodic assessment of eye protection, skin, bony prominences, and extremities is necessary.

Perform a complete anesthesia equipment safety check daily and document in the patient's medical record. An abbreviated check of all equipment is acceptable before each subsequent anesthetic is administered.

H. Precautions shall be taken to minimize the risk of infection to the patient, the operator, and ancillary personnel. Clean equipment and fresh medications and supplies (to include personal protective equipment and supplies) should be used to ensure safety.

I. There shall be complete, accurate, and time-oriented documentation of pertinent information on the patient's anesthesia record. Document baseline patient vital signs before the anesthetic procedure and the therapeutic or diagnostic procedure has begun. Documentation must be made of all vital signs: heart rate, blood pressure, pulse oximeter readings, patient temperature, and the presence of ETCO$_2$. Also, documentation must be made of all fluids administered and the names and quantities of all drugs and agents administered. A narrative must be written concerning the technique(s) of anesthesia used and any unusual events that occurred during the anesthetic period. An anesthesia form approved by the AANA is available at their website.

J. After the anesthetic treatment for therapeutic or diagnostic procedures, transfer the responsibility for care of the patient to other qualified personnel in a manner that ensures continuity of care and patient safety. Anesthesia care does not end with the completion of the therapeutic or diagnostic procedure. The patient may receive postanesthesia care at the site of the therapeutic or diagnostic procedure. Those sites that preclude postanesthesia recovery at that particular location must be safely transported to a separate area for postanesthesia care. From there patient care can be transferred to another qualified health-care provider along with a full verbal report. Document to whom the report was given. The transported patient must be accompanied by a person capable of initiating basic life support (CPR) and possessing access to portable anesthesia monitors, equipment, and supplies, especially if transport will require some time and/or distance. Recovery from anesthesia can be divided into three phases. Phase I recovery encompasses the recovery from sedation, during which assessment is made of adequate patient oxygenation and respirations, cardiovascular function, neuromuscular function, mental status, body temperature, pain, postoperative nausea and vomiting (PONV), fluid status, urine output, the ability to void, and any bleeding or drainage, which must be noted and continually assessed. Treatments may be administered as necessary for any adverse signs or symptoms elicited by the patient. Phase II recovery encompasses the adequate resumption of psychomotor functions, such as the ability to communicate, ambulate, and consume fluids. Finally, before discharge from this area, a responsible individual must be present to escort the patient home and be available to observe and assist the patient for the next 24 hours. In phase III recovery, the patient regains full preanesthetic psychological and physical recovery.[29] It is important to remember that phase III may occur several hours or days later, depending on the anesthetic technique and patient variables, but with newer anesthetics, recovery time has dramatically decreased. Postanesthesia recovery and discharge guidelines are discussed in Chapter 51.

K. Reimbursement. Third-party payers of anesthesia services may require documentation of the necessity for anesthetic services for therapeutic and diagnostic procedures. Box 53-7 lists some patient indications that can require the need for anesthesia in remote locations.

BOX 53-7

Patient Indications for the Necessity of Anesthesia in Remote Locations

Central Nervous System
Presenile dementia
Drug-induced mental disorders
Major depressive disorders or schizophrenia
Hysteria, unspecified (includes fear of pain)
Phobic disorders, unspecified (claustrophobia)
Transient cerebral ischemia
Cerebrovascular disease, other and ill-defined

Cardiovascular
Hypertensive heart disease, malignant, benign, unspecified
Ischemic heart disease, acute or subacute forms
Old myocardial infarction
Coronary atherosclerosis, bundle branch block, other and unspecified cardiac dysrhythmias
History of atrial or ventricular fibrillation or flutter

Pulmonary
Bronchitis, acute, chronic, or unspecified
Chronic airway obstruction
Radiation-induced pulmonary disease, acute or chronic

Other
Acquired hypothyroidism
Electrolyte imbalance
Morbid obesity
Adverse effects not classified elsewhere
Opioid, barbiturate, cocaine, cannabis, amphetamine, or unspecified drug dependence
Combative patient
Patient with low pain thresholds or experiencing severe pain
Chronic liver disease or cirrhosis
GI tract hemorrhage, unspecified

Modified from Arens JF, MacLachlan AA. Billing for Offsite Anesthesia Services. Available at the American Society of Anesthesiologists website: http://www.asahq.org/Newletters/2004/03_04/arensMaclach03_04.html. Accessed July 31, 2008.

L. Conclusion. The standards listed in this section describe the minimum requirements for treatment and monitoring of any patient who requires anesthesia care. The standards must be followed wherever and whenever anesthesia is given. Standards are considered essential in a malpractice case, and an anesthetic incident will be judged according to those standards.[30] The omission of any monitoring standard should be documented and the reason stated on the patient's anesthesia record. Any anesthetic procedure, including those performed in a remote location, should not begin until the anesthetist feels sufficiently comfortable, safe, and well prepared to deliver the anesthetic treatment required for the patient.

Guidelines for Sedation

Therapeutic and diagnostic and procedures can be performed with various types of sedation. Sedation is possible with enteral, parenteral (intravenous), and inhaled medications. It is important to remember that the depth of sedation in a patient is a continuum of progressive changes in cognition, respirations, and protective reflexes.[31-33] Sedation does not have strict boundaries. The patient

---

BOX 53-8

Considerations and Requirements of Ancillary Personnel for Areas of Anesthesia Delivery for Therapeutic or Diagnostic Procedures in Remote Locations

Training in basic life support
Awareness of and training in emergency protocols
Familiarity with anesthesia responsibilities; to serve as an assistant
Assist with patient positioning and comfort
Training in postprocedure observation and recovery

Modified from Robbertze R et al. Closed claims review of anesthesia for procedures outside the operating room. Curr Opin Anaesthesiol. 2006;19:436-442; Stensrud PE. Anesthesia at remote locations. In: Miller E, ed Anesthesia. 6th ed. Philadelphia: Churchill Livingstone; 2005:2637-2663.

may quickly progress from one level of sedation/anesthesia to another; therefore, it is essential that the competent anesthesia provider is able to rescue patients in each level, as well as have quick access to vital equipment, supplies, and trained and qualified ancillary personnel who are familiar with anesthesia delivery, emergencies, and monitoring.[3,32-34]

Box 53-8 lists ancillary personnel requirements the anesthetist should consider during the planning stages of anesthesia for therapeutic and diagnostic procedures.

The Joint Commission and the ASA publish definitions for the four levels of sedation and anesthesia in their *Comprehensive Accreditation Manual for Hospitals: The Official Handbook (CAMH)*.[32] Box 53-9 lists The Joint Commission's definitions of the four levels of sedation and anesthesia. Figure 53-1 illustrates the continuum of sedation described by The Joint Commission. From these definitions, standards are provided to practitioners for the administration of safe and high-quality care to patients.[33] The Joint Commission's standards do not cover minimal sedation (anxiolysis) but do cover patients undergoing moderate sedation/analgesia and deep sedation/analgesia.[32]

Accepted standards for moderate sedation/analgesia and deep sedation/analgesia state the following[11,25,32,33,35]:

1. The process from minimal sedation (anxiolysis) to general anesthesia is a continuum, and individuals vary in their responses to medications.
2. Qualified individuals with appropriate credentials (nurses, certified registered nurse anesthetists [CRNAs], anesthesiologists, dentists) who are trained in professional standards and techniques do the following:
   a. May administer pharmacologic agents to achieve a desired level of sedation
   b. Must monitor patients carefully to maintain the patient's vital functions at the desired level of sedation. Appropriate equipment must be available for monitoring heart rate via ECG, respiratory rate and adequacy of pulmonary ventilation, oxygenation via pulse oximetry, and blood pressure measurement at regular intervals (at least every 5 minutes)
   c. Must be competent to evaluate the patient before performing the moderate sedation/analgesia and deep sedation/analgesia
   d. Must be competent to support the patient's psychological functions and physical comfort
   e. Must be competent in the administration of sedatives, analgesics, hypnotics, and other medications to produce

---

BOX 53-9

The Continuum of Depth of Sedation: The Four Levels of Sedation and Anesthesia

Minimal Sedation (formerly known as anxiolysis)
A drug-induced state during which patients respond normally to verbal commands. Although cognitive function and coordination may be impaired, ventilatory and cardiovascular functions are unaffected.

Moderate Sedation/Analgesia (formerly known as conscious sedation)
A drug-induced depression of consciousness during which patients respond purposefully to verbal commands, either alone or accompanied by light tactile stimulation. No interventions are required to maintain a patent airway, and spontaneous ventilation is adequate. Cardiovascular function is usually maintained. (Note: Reflexive withdrawal from a painful stimulus is not considered a purposeful response.)

Deep Sedation/Analgesia
A drug-induced depression of consciousness during which patients cannot be easily aroused but respond purposefully after repeated or painful stimulation. The ability to independently maintain ventilatory function may be impaired. Patients may require assistance in maintaining a patent airway, and spontaneous ventilation may be inadequate. Cardiovascular function is usually maintained.

Anesthesia (General Anesthesia)
Consists of general anesthesia and spinal or major regional anesthesia. It does not include local anesthesia. General anesthesia is a drug-induced loss of consciousness during which patients are not arousable, even by painful stimulation. The ability to independently maintain ventilatory function is often impaired. Patients often require assistance in maintaining a patent airway, and positive-pressure ventilation may be required because of depressed spontaneous ventilation or drug-induced depression of neuromuscular function. Cardiovascular function may be impaired.

Modified from The Joint Commission. Comprehensive Accreditation Manual for Hospitals. The Official Handbook (CAMH). Chicago: The Joint Commission, refreshed core; 2007; and American Society of Anesthesiologists. Continuum of Depth of Sedation, Definitions of General Anesthesia, and Levels of Sedation/Analgesia. Available at the ASA website: http://www.asahq.org/publicationsAndServices/standards/20.pdf. Accessed July 21, 2008.

and maintain moderate sedation/analgesia and deep sedation/analgesia
   f. Must be competent to rescue the patient who unavoidably or unintentionally moves into a deeper than desired level of sedation and analgesia. In the case of the CRNA, competency is mandatory for all levels of the sedation continuum. This includes competency in management of a compromised airway, the provision of oxygen, and the initiation of emergency rescue procedures such as basic life support (BLS), advanced life support (ACLS), or pediatric advanced life support (PALS). In addition, for patients undergoing deep sedation/analgesia, one must also have competency to manage an unstable cardiovascular system.

The Joint Commission Continuum of Sedation and Anesthesia

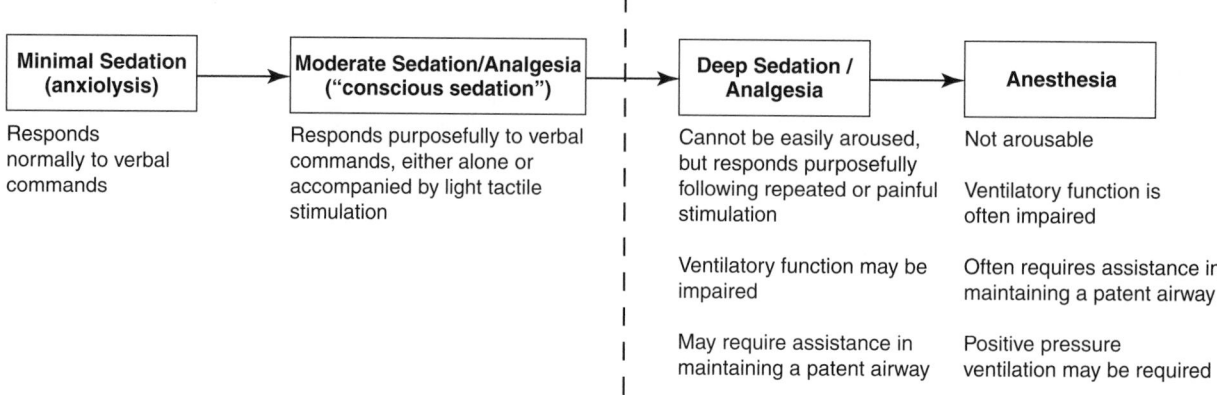

FIGURE **53-1** The Joint Commission's continuum of sedation and anesthesia. (*From Kaplan RF, Yang CI. Sedation and analgesia in pediatric patients for procedures outside the operating room. Anesthesiol Clin North America. 2002;20:181-194.*)

g. Must be competent to assess and treat problems the patient may attain related to the therapeutic or diagnostic procedure they are having performed

h. Must properly document the patient's response to care

i. Must supervise recovery of the patient after the sedation in a postsedation area or a postanesthesia recovery area

j. Must discharge the patient. This may be done in consultation with qualified personnel and/or the physician, surgeon, or dentist.

3. Adequate numbers of qualified and competent personnel must be present during the performance of moderate sedation/analgesia, deep sedation/analgesia, and general anesthesia to serve as a skilled second pair of hands if necessary. This should include not only qualified anesthesia providers as described above but nurses, assistants, technicians, and other office staff to meet the needs of the patient.[32]

The Pediatric Patient

The pediatric population can pose complex challenges for the delivery of anesthesia (Box 53-10). Pediatric patient behavior and degree of cooperation can range from very helpful to extremely anxious. Fortunately, several common anesthetic medications can help patients with slight to high levels of anxiety. Pediatric sedation and anesthesia increases the quality of care the patient receives by greatly reducing anxiety and by eliminating movement when necessary for therapeutic or diagnostic procedures.

First and foremost in the practice of nurse anesthesia are patient safety and guardianship of patient welfare. Important lessons can be learned from the literature regarding anesthesia in pediatric patients. Children ages 1 to 5 years seem to be at the greatest risk for adverse events, even with no underlying disease. Adverse events have occurred more commonly with the use of multiple drugs, especially sedative medications.[36-38] The problems encountered most frequently are respiratory events: respiratory depression, respiratory obstruction, and apnea.[36,37]

Adverse events can be reduced by proper adherence to patient selection and a comprehensive preoperative assessment, proper

---

BOX **53-10**

Goals of Pediatric Anesthesia

- Foremost, to provide safety and welfare to the patient
- To minimize physical discomfort/pain or to provide more profound analgesia when necessary to the patient
- To minimize negative psychological consequences of the therapeutic or diagnostic procedure for both the pediatric patient and the parent(s)/guardian(s). This can be accomplished by the provision of proper preprocedure discussions along with sedative medications, analgesics, and amnestic agents for the patient
- To ideally obtain patient cooperation and safely control uncooperative or endangering behavior
- To obtain immobility of the patient to achieve therapeutic or diagnostic procedure goals
- To provide the patient a safe discharge to the guardian and to home
- To minimize or eliminate patient complications from applied therapeutic or diagnostic procedures and administered anesthetic medications

Modified from Kaplan RF, Yang CI. Sedation and analgesia in pediatric patients from procedures outside the operating room. Anesthesiol Clin North Am. 2002;20:181-194.

dosage of medications to minimize unexpected responses, proper monitoring, skilled administration of anesthesia, and proper recovery time. The anesthesia provider must plan to minimize the possibility of adverse reactions.[25,36,39,40] General patient selection criteria to help minimize the possibility of adverse events are seen with patients 6 months of age and older and applied during the preoperative assessment. It is during this time that the temperament of the child can be

TABLE **53-1**	Common Pediatric Premedications and Doses			
Medication	**Dose**	**Route**	**Onset**	**Duration**
Analgesics (non-narcotic)				
Acetaminophen (APAP)	20-40 mg/kg	PO	<60 min	2-8 h
Ibuprofen	(Use lowest dose possible; maximum 30-40 mg/kg/day)	PO	<60 min	5 h
Benzodiazepines				
Midazolam	0.1-0.15 mg/kg up to 10 mg	IM	5-10 min	0.5-2 h
	0.2 mg/kg	IN	10 min	0.5-2 h
	0.025-1 mg/kg	IV	1-3 min	0.5-2 h
	0.25-1 mg/kg up to 20 mg	PO	15-30 min	0.5-2 h
	0.3-1 mg/kg	PR	10-20 min	0.5-2 h
Diazepam	0.1-0.5 mg/kg	IM, PO, PR	60 min	>24 h
Narcotics				
Fentanyl	1-3 mcg/kg	IM	5-15 min	30-60 min
	0.5-1 mcg/kg	IV	1-3 min	30-60 min
	5 mcg/kg	OT	5-30 min	30-60 min
Sufentanil	1.5-4.5 mcg/kg	IN	7-10 min	30-60 min
Morphine sulfate	0.1-0.2 mg/kg	IM	30-45 min	4-5 h
	0.05-0.1 mg/kg	IV	3-10 min	
Dissociative Anesthesia				
Ketamine	1-2 mg/kg	IM	30sec-2 min	12-25 min
	3 mg/kg	IN	20 min	
	0.2-1 mg/kg	IV	30sec-1 min	
	6-10 mg/kg	PO	10-20 min	
	10 mg/kg	PR	10 min	
Reversal Agents				
Flumazenil	Adult 0.2 mg	IV	>15 seconds; wait 45 sec; if necessary give 0.2 mg; repeat at 60-sec intervals; maximum dose 3 mg/kg	
	Child 10 mcg	IV	Up to 1 mg cumulative dose	
Naloxone	Adult 0.4-2 mg	IV, subQ, IM	Repeat in 2-3 min if needed	
	Child 0.5-2 mcg/kg	IV, subQ, IM	Repeat in 1 min if needed	

Data from Mosby Drug Consult 2007. St Louis: Mosby; 2008; Skidmore-Roth L. 2008 Mosby's Nursing Drug Reference. St Louis: Mosby; 2008; White PF. Perioperative Drug Manual. 2nd ed. Philadelphia: Saunders; 2005.
IM, *Intramuscular;* IN, *intranasal;* IV, *intravenous;* OT, *oral transmucosal;* PO, *by mouth;* PR, *by rectum;* subQ, *subcutaneous.*

assessed.[41] Consideration must be made for the type of procedure to be performed, past medical history, past sedation/anesthesia history, current medication therapy, allergies, and respiratory or airway difficulties.[42,43] Will there be a great degree of patient stimulation, a large amount of blood loss, an inability to maintain normothermia, an inability to have close contact in which to monitor the patient during the therapeutic or diagnostic procedure? It is found that adverse reactions are reduced with procedures that last less than 1 hour.[39] Clear communication with the technician and the medical practitioner is essential to clarify the requirements for the patient to be safe and properly anesthetized for the procedure.

The pediatric patient and the parent or legal guardian must be properly prepared for the planned therapeutic or diagnostic procedure. Clear explanation of the entire anesthetic process to the parent or guardian is based on the developed treatment plan and is offered in age-appropriate terms for the pediatric patient.[41] "Inform before you perform."

Fasting times are constantly being reevaluated in clinical anesthesia and must be stringently adhered to. Fasting guidelines are discussed in Chapters 20 and 49.

Premedication with oral, intranasal, or rectal sedatives may be necessary. Common pediatric premedications and doses are listed in Table 53-1. Other sedative premedications reported in the literature are pentobarbital[44,45] and chloral hydrate.[42,44]

It is essential to have qualified personnel to assist in the safe care of pediatric patients receiving anesthesia in remote locations for therapeutic or diagnostic procedures. An extra pair of trained hands enhances the ability for the patient to receive safer care throughout the entire procedure.

Knowledge of the most common causes of adverse pediatric anesthesia events can help the anesthetist plan for and avoid these events (Box 53-11).[46]

Most anesthesia adverse events are caused when multiple anesthetic agents are used.[46,47] Adverse events are not dependent on the class of the drug (opioids, benzodiazepines, barbiturates,

BOX **53-11**

Most Common Causes of Pediatric Anesthesia Adverse Events for Therapeutic or Diagnostic Procedures

- Drug overdose
- Nitrous oxide in combination with any other sedative medication
- Inability to rescue the patient from an adverse anesthetic event
- Unmet monitoring standards—especially respiration, oxygenation
- Respiratory depression/hypoventilation/apnea
- Airway obstruction
- Bradycardia secondary to hypoxia
- Laryngospasm/stridor
- Vomiting, aspiration, diarrhea
- Hypotension
- Inadequate sedation/paradoxical excitation (sustained irritability or combativeness)
- Prolonged sedation after the procedure

antihistamines, local anesthesia, intravenous anesthesia, inhaled anesthesia) or the route of administration (oral, rectal, nasal, intramuscular, intravenous, local infiltration, inhalation).[48]

The Geriatric Patient

As a result of a number of factors, including better nutrition, more physical activity, less tobacco and alcohol use, improved medical care and medical technologies, more Americans are living longer. The U.S. Social Security Administration states that 12% of the total population is age 65 or older and that 23% of the population will be 65 or older by 2080, with increased life expectancy.[49,50] The increasing elderly population is going to place many demands on the public health-care system. Medical technology is advancing, and therefore more procedures requiring anesthesia will be performed in elderly patients. It is estimated that 20% to 40% of anesthesia cases may be performed outside of the traditional operating room and that the elderly prefer ambulatory settings, with trends pointing toward more invasive therapeutic or diagnostic procedures.[51,52] Perioperative complications can increase with age. Special considerations related to the physiology of aging are necessary if anesthetic treatment is to be performed safely.[53]

The elderly have a greater prevalence of atherosclerosis, infections, autoimmune diseases, chronic disorders, and cancer. The immune system gradually and slowly diminishes in function with age. Therefore, the ability to heal and fight foreign bacteria, viruses, and malignant cells diminishes. There are no fewer T cells than at a younger age, but T-cell function is decreased. Many of the body's cells begin to diminish in function or to function abnormally. Cells also may have increasing difficulty in membrane transfer of nutrients and waste.[53]

The normal aging process results in an increase in the ratio of adipose tissue to aqueous body tissues.[31,41,53,54] This means more lipid-soluble anesthetic drug is stored. Basal metabolic rate decreases with age.[54] Liver and kidney functions decrease with age. This results in a decrease in the rate of metabolism and excretion of anesthetic drugs. Nervous system function generally produces decreases in the perception of sight, hearing, touch,

smell (taste), pain, and temperature sensations. Cerebral atrophy occurs with aging, resulting in an overall loss of neurons in the neocortex.[54] This suggests increased sensitivity to anesthetic medications. The elderly are at an increased risk for perioperative delirium and postoperative cognitive dysfunction.[52] Therefore, the dosage requirements for anesthetic drugs usually are decreased. Cardiovascular function is a function of the level of activity of the patient and generally decreases with age, with generally limited physiologic reserves. Patients may be restricted in their activity because of arthritis or other debilitation. Circulation time is decreased. Skeletal muscle size is decreased with decreases in physical activity, which decreases total oxygen consumption and blood-flow needs to the muscles, resulting in decreased cardiac output.[54] The ability of the cardiovascular system to respond to the effects of anesthetic drugs, fluid administration, and the stresses of therapeutic and diagnostic procedures can cause decreased cardiac function, resulting in hemodynamic instability and reduced circulation to vital organs.[31,41,52,54] Tissue oxygenation can decrease because of changes in ventilation ability and lung tissue. Lung compliance is decreased, resulting in ventilation-perfusion mismatch. Aging itself brings on the increasing inability to respond to hypoxia and hypercapnia, especially while experiencing the effects of anesthesia. Therefore, the anesthetist must always ensure and constantly monitor the supply of adequate amounts of oxygen to the elderly patient and be ready to offer needed respiratory support.[52] The ability to thermoregulate is also decreased with age.[31] Body metabolism, enzyme function, and the coagulation cascade best function at 37° C. Changes in mental status or even delirium can occur more frequently in geriatric patients. All of these factors must be taken into consideration when one provides anesthesia to all patients, but especially to geriatric patients.

Significant variability exists in each of these vital functions among patients. Geriatric patients who are more physically fit have a decreased mortality, reduced incidence of cardiovascular disease, lower blood pressure, reduced blood cholesterol, and most important, better bodily reserves when they become surgically challenged or sick.[53] A thorough and comprehensive preanesthetic assessment is necessary, from which a plan of treatment can be deduced.[52]

Complications related to anesthesia can be linked to poor preoperative planning and preparation of the patient. To prevent confusion, delirium, or cognitive impairment in the elderly, agents with short half-lives are ideal.[51,52] Carefully consider the use of drugs that are synergistic or antagonistic in their effects. Such drugs as propofol, midazolam, fentanyl, alfentanil, remifentanil, and local anesthetics are ideal because doses are calculated and titrated according to the patient's responses. The literature reports no difference of outcome in the elderly as a result of anesthetic choice when either a regional anesthetic or general anesthesia is used.[52]

There are several electroencephalographic (EEG) processing monitors available that help in assessment of patient responses to anesthetic medications (Table 53-2). These devices monitor anesthesia awareness/level of consciousness/depth of sedation and response to anesthetic medications, which allows for more precise titration of anesthetic medications according to the patient's needs.[51] Care must be taken to preserve body warmth and ensure the continual delivery of adequate warmth when necessary. Ensure the protection of the eyes, skin, and the extremities while moving the patient and during the procedure by skin padding of bony prominences.[41,51] Consideration must also be given to the preprocedure, and postoperative care of the elderly patient

TABLE **53-2**	Current Common Anesthesia Awareness/Level of Consciousness/Depth of Sedation Monitors	
Monitor	**Physiologic Basis**	**Technology**
Aspect BIS	EEG	Bispectral array of global activity
Hospira SEDLine	EEG	Algorithm interpretation of multichannel EEG activity
Narcotrend	EEG	Algorithm interpretation of dual-channel EEG activity
Entropy	EEG derived state entropy	Algorithm interpretation of EEG activity
Auditory evoked potential	EEG response to an auditory stimulus	Algorithm interpretation of EEG activity

Modified from Cravero JP, Blike GT. Pediatric sedation: update for clinicians. Anesth Today. 2006;17:12-18.

in regard to possible malnutrition, depression, immobility, cognitive dysfunction, pulmonary difficulty, dehydration, acute pain, and chronic pain.[52] Finally, consider verbal and written postoperative instructions to both the elderly patient and caregivers/significant others who will accompany the patient and be present to both monitor and care for the elderly patient after a therapeutic or diagnostic procedure.[51]

There are two new formulations of propofol that may better add to its use in anesthesia for therapeutic and diagnostic procedures. Fospropofol, a water-soluble prodrug that is enzymatically converted to propofol, is a formulation in Phase III clinical studies. Cyclodextran-encased propofol is being developed, which will more easily solubilize the propofol molecule and make it less painful on administration.[55-57]

ANESTHESIA FOR SPECIFIC PROCEDURES IN REMOTE LOCATIONS

Cardiology Procedures

Automatic Implantable Cardiac Defibrillator and Cardiac Pacemaker

Procedure Overviews. Patients who experience sudden cardiac death are usually approximately 60 years of age, and their most common underlying rhythm is pulseless ventricular tachycardia (VT) or ventricular fibrillation (VF).[58]

Defibrillation is the application of a flow of electric current through the appropriate chambers of the heart to completely depolarize the entire myocardium to restore a suitable heart rhythm to sustain life.[59-62] If enough stores of high-energy adenosine triphosphate molecules remain and are available within the myocardium, automaticity can resume. Fibrillating myocardium rapidly consumes high-energy phosphate molecules.[54,62] It has been proved that early defibrillation, along with cardiopulmonary resuscitation, can result in high long-term survival rates. The automatic implantable cardiac defibrillator (AICD) was conceived by Mirowski and co-workers to bypass the delay patients experienced before receiving defibrillation.[59] The AICD is composed of two basic parts: a pulse generator and a lead electrode for detection of dysrhythmias, delivery of a defibrillating shock, cardiac pacing, telemetry, and provision of diagnostic data. The pulse generator is a hermetically sealed titanium can that contains a computer microprocessor, resistors, transformers, capacitors, and a battery. The battery is designed to deliver 120 shocks and usually lasts for 3 to 6 years. The computer is programmed with algorithms to detect VT and VF. If VF occurs, an electric shock is administered within 10 to 15 seconds of detection (much of the time delay results from the charging of the capacitor). VT is treated with overdrive pacing called *antitachycardia pacing* (ATP). ATP is an extremely successful procedure. AICD implantation has been a crucial technique for prevention of sudden cardiac death.[63]

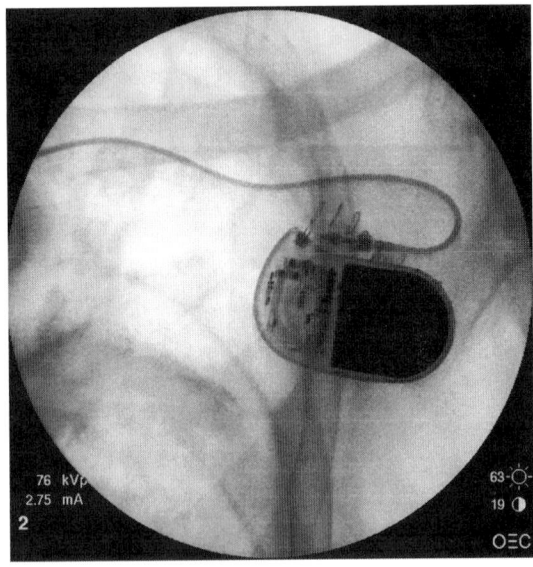

FIGURE **53-2** Radiograph of a pacemaker pulse generator, computer, and battery inserted into a patient.

A cardiac pacemaker is used to treat bradycardia, atrioventricular block, sinus nodal dysfunction, and other dysrhythmias. The pacemaker is used concurrently with other therapies for management of dysrhythmia and hemodynamics. The pacemaker consists of a pulse generator containing a computer and a battery that is designed to last 6 to 10 years. Attached to the pulse generator is a lead, which delivers the current used to depolarize the myocardium, and an anode, which completes the electrical circuit. Two different types of pacemaker leads are available. A unipolar pacemaker lead uses one lead as the cathode and the pulse generator as the anode. Unipolar leads are less likely to fail. A bipolar pacemaker lead uses two separate leads that are close together, the advantage of which is a sharper signal with less noise. The leads are inserted under fluoroscopic guidance via the cephalic vein or the subclavian vein into the cardiac chamber, usually the right ventricle in the case of an AICD and the right atrium and right ventricle for a cardiac pacemaker. The leads are then tunneled and connected to the pulse generator, which is then inserted into a subcutaneous pocket in the patient's pectoral region or into a subpectoral muscle pocket.[63] Figure 53-2 shows a postoperative radiograph of a pacemaker pulse generator, computer, and battery inserted into a patient. Figure 53-3 shows a postoperative radiograph of a unipolar pacemaker lead inserted into the right ventricle of a patient. Research and continual improvements allow more people to receive better and more reliable AICD and cardiac pacemaker therapy.

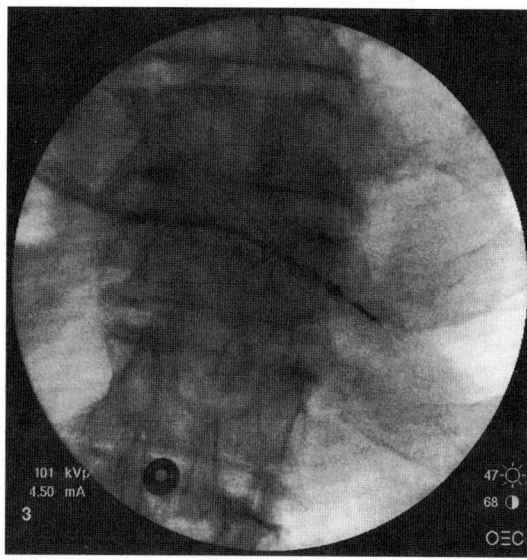

FIGURE **53-3** Radiograph of a unipolar pacemaker lead inserted into the right ventricle of a patient.

Anesthetic Considerations. The AICD or cardiac pacemaker procedure may be performed in the operating room, in a special cardiac procedure room, or in the cardiac catheterization suite by a cardiologist or other physician.[64] Routine monitors are attached to the patient, with special attention paid to a properly functioning five-lead ECG. The ECG monitor screen must be available to the anesthesia team, the operating physician, and the AICD or pacemaker manufacturer's technical service representative, who is always present during insertion. The procedures are usually adequately performed with local anesthetic and moderate sedation/analgesia or deep sedation/analgesia, although some clinicians prefer a general anesthetic.[63]

AICD insertion requires purposeful triggering of VF in an attempt to test thresholds and functioning of the AICD.[65] General anesthesia with inhaled agents such as halothane and isoflurane along with fentanyl can increase the amount of energy needed for defibrillation after the induction of ventricular fibrillation during insertion of the AICD.[66] Lidocaine with propofol anesthetic caused no significant increase in the threshold energy needed for defibrillation.[67] As in all anesthetic procedures, endotracheal intubation may be required to secure the airway should a cardiac emergency arise.

After insertion of the cardiac pacemaker and before wound closure, the device is threshold tested by the pacemaker manufacturer's technical service representative to ensure adequate contact between the leads and the myocardium.[63] After wound closure and dressing application, all computer-function programming of either the AICD or the cardiac pacemaker can then be performed with a pacemaker programmer that connects to a portable wand. The wand is placed within close proximity to the implanted pulse generator by the manufacturer's technical service representative; it allows a telemetric connection to properly program or interrogate the AICD or cardiac pacemaker.

Postanesthesia Care. When the procedure is completed, the patient is transported to the recovery room with oxygen and observed for any hemodynamic or cardiovascular ECG changes.

AICDs are generally well tolerated by patients. Some patients display anxiety or depression because of the possibility of sudden cardiac death, device failure, inappropriate shocks, and recalls of certain devices.[63] Shocks from the AICD are described as a

sudden, heavy blow to the chest. Medical technology is ever improving, and the demand for AICDs and cardiac pacemakers increases annually.

Cardioversion

Procedure Overview. Cardioversion is the discharge of electrical energy, synchronized to the R wave of the QRS complex of the electrocardiogram, to convert hemodynamically unstable supraventricular rhythms such as atrial flutter or atrial fibrillation or hemodynamically stable VT.[63,66] These rhythms can be life threatening if left untreated. Atrial flutter and atrial fibrillation are associated with the development of congestive heart failure and with the formation of thromboemboli, which can lead to stroke.[63] The patient may also have symptoms of chronic fatigue.[66] Cardioversion is usually a scheduled and planned procedure. At times, patient optimization is not possible because of the urgency for cardioversion as a result of hemodynamic instability. Much less electrical energy is required to synchronously cardiovert a patient when compared with asynchronous defibrillation.[61] Defibrillation is an unplanned and usually emergent application of unsynchronized electrical energy. Cardioversion is believed to be therapeutic because it closes an excitable gap in the myocardium, which causes currents to reenter and excite the electrical system of the heart.[63]

Anesthetic Considerations. Because cardioversion is usually a nonemergent and planned procedure, patient conditions usually can be optimized. Proper nothing-by-mouth (NPO) status must be observed unless the cardioversion is deemed urgent or emergent. Standard monitors are applied, with special attention paid to the ECG.[66] A monitor of anesthesia awareness/level of consciousness/depth of sedation via electroencephalographic processing can be used to assess consciousness during cardioversion.[68,69] Intravenous access is necessary. The energy required for cardioversion is measured in joules (watt-seconds). The cardiologist or physician uses a cardioverter-manual monophasic or biphasic defibrillator for the procedure. The optimal shock dose for cardioversion of atrial flutter and other supraventricular tachycardias is 50 to 100 J.[60,63] The operator applies cardioversion-defibrillator paddles with conduction gel or defibrillator patches to the patient's skin. One paddle or patch is placed parasternally over the second and third intercostal space. The other paddle or patch is placed over the area of the apex of the heart. The cardioverter-defibrillator is set to the synchronized (sync) mode. Visible synchronization marks are placed by the cardioverter atop the tallest R waves of the ECG. Energy shocks are delivered initially at 50 to 100 J and are titrated progressively, up to 360 J as necessary, after observation of the effectiveness of the synchronized shock.[61,63]

Midazolam may be administered as both a sedative and amnestic agent before cardioversion.[70] The patient is then assisted in breathing oxygen via face mask and Ambu bag with high-flow oxygen. Because of the intense and brief pain of cardioversion, an ultra-short-acting general anesthetic such as propofol, thiopental, or methohexital is administered. After the loss of eyelash reflex occurs, an "all-clear" signal is given by the operator. Positive-pressure respirations are temporarily suspended, with care taken not to touch any part of the patient or the patient's bed. Then the synchronized shock or shocks are administered.[66,69] Muscle relaxation is not necessary. As always, an assortment of oral airways, nasal airways, laryngeal mask airways (LMAs), endotracheal tubes, and laryngoscopes with blades and suction should be readily available in case complications occur. If cardioversion is required in a patient who has not fasted, general anesthesia with tracheal intubation is necessary to prevent aspiration of gastric contents.[69]

Postanesthesia Care. It is hoped that the patient's heart is now beating in a desirable cardiac rhythm and that the patient's blood pressure is stable. Spontaneous respirations return, along with swallowing and coughing reflexes. The patient is observed for any reactions to the anesthetic, and care is turned over to the nurse accompanying the patient.

Radiofrequency Catheter Ablation

Procedure Overview. Radiofrequency catheter ablation (RFCA) uses a catheter with an electrode at its tip, which is guided under fluoroscopy to an area of heart muscle that has demonstrated accessory electrical conductive pathways.[66] RFCA has all but replaced arrhythmia surgery and is now considered the foremost therapy for the treatment of many arrhythmias in pediatric and adult patients.[71,72] Supraventricular tachycardia is the most common tachyarrhythmia in children, and symptomatic supraventricular tachydysrhythmias are most often treated by RFCA.[73,74] Accessory electrical conductive pathways are distributed unevenly along the right and left atrioventricular valve annuli. Left-sided accessory pathways are most common, but both right- and left-sided accessory electrical pathways can be accessed and ablated.[71,73] Other treatments possible with RFCA are modification of the sinus node or AV node, ablation of atrial flutter and atrial tachycardia, and ablation of focal atrial fibrillation and VT foci.[63,66] Patients must undergo electrophysiologic studies to determine the origin and pathway of the arrhythmia, as well as the mechanism of action, before RFCA can be chosen as a therapy.

Cryoablation is now being used prior to RFCA, or in place of RFCA. Liquid nitrous oxide is circulated through the catheter tip to cause temperatures at the tip of $-22°$ C to $-75°$ C. At a higher temperature ($-22°$ C or lower), tissue can be temporarily "ice mapped," which is a trial to see if this nonpermanent freezing of the tissue will successfully eliminate the dysrhythmia. If the ice mapping is successful, then the probe is further cooled, causing permanent destruction of the arrhythmogenic tissue. Cryoablation causes less discomfort and is being found safer to use in dysrhythmias in the area of the atrioventricular (AV) node, where iatrogenic complete AV heart block can be caused. Iatrogenic AV block is relatively common, and may require placement of a transvenous pacemaker.[75]

RFCA is an extremely safe and successful procedure, with success rates of 95% overall. Many patients no longer need their antiarrhythmic medications soon after therapy.[66]

RFCA is now being used as treatment for liver metastases from colorectal cancer. RFCA is providing a new treatment options for those patients with high risks for surgery but who would be at a lesser risk for the less invasive RFCA.

Anesthetic Considerations. Electrophysiologic studies before RFCA are time-consuming procedures that may require moderate sedation in adults or general anesthesia in children. RFCA can be performed in the operating room, in a special cardiac procedure room, or in the cardiac catheterization suite by a cardiologist. The electrode catheter is guided via the femoral artery and vein to the area of the accessory electrical pathway or an area of arrhythmogenic focus.[75,76] The internal jugular vein also may be used. The electrode is then energized with radiofrequency energy, and cells within the path of the electrode are obliterated. The procedure can produce brief periods (<1 to 2 minutes) of mild to moderate retrosternal, angina-like pain.[75]

RFCA is a short procedure. Patients must remain perfectly still, except for respiratory movement, during the procedure.[74] Many adults can be anesthetized with moderate sedation/analgesia along with local anesthetic applied by the operator.[74] Children may be best treated with general endotracheal anesthesia using either an LMA or an endotracheal tube to secure the airway. If general endotracheal anesthesia is used, the patient may be held apneic for a short period of time while the catheter is accurately directed and the ablation procedure performed.[75] Full monitors and an intravenous catheter are necessary. Total intravenous anesthesia (TIVA) using propofol as the key medication has been used. Midazolam and thiopental, as well as a potent inhaled anesthetic gas such as isoflurane, have been used successfully for RFCA. TIVA with propofol and ondansetron has a much lower rate of nausea (PONV) than does use of isoflurane and an antiemetic. Careful attention must be paid to the ECG, because the patient must stop taking any antiarrhythmic drugs before the electrophysiologic study and RFCA are performed.[76-78]

There is currently concern of possible thermal injury to the esophagus during RFCA of the left atrium. Insertion and use of an esophageal temperature probe are essential, as is the position of the probe. The probe should be inserted so that it is alongside the esophageal tissues with no space in between.

Postanesthesia Care. Patients must be monitored during recovery from administered anesthetics after RFCA. Patients must also be observed for possible RFCA procedural complications such as bleeding, ECG changes, cerebrovascular accidents, cardiac tamponade, or damage to the aortic valve.[63]

Percutaneous Coronary Intervention

Procedure Overview. Percutaneous coronary intervention (PCI) encompasses a wide variety of procedures performed in the cardiac catheter laboratory (CCL). PCI is being performed on adults and is now more commonplace on younger and sicker patients. The CCL is generally located remotely from the operating rooms and the blood bank. It consists of a large procedural area with a small control room. PCI procedures use x-radiation/fluoroscopy doses "as low as reasonably achievable" (the ALARA principle), as well as the use of intravenous radiocontrast media. The heart is commonly accessed via the femoral artery (although the brachial or radial artery can be used). The right heart and pulmonary circulation are commonly accessed via the femoral vein.

Anesthetic Considerations. PCI necessitates access to major blood vessels and the heart itself. Box 53-12 lists possible PCI complications that affect the safety of the anesthetic and may require interventions from the anesthetist. Consideration for rapid access to competent anesthesia help has to be prepared well in advance of PCI anesthesia. Anesthesia techniques can range from intravenous moderate sedation/analgesia, deep sedation/analgesia, or general anesthesia, aided with local anesthetic infiltration (such as levobupivacaine) at the insertion site and alongside the major vein (usually the femoral vein) used for insertion of the PCI armamentaria.

Postanesthesia Care. Care of the patient undergoing PCI usually does not end with the end of the PCI procedure. Arrangements can be made for observation and ongoing care of the patient in a telemetry environment or in the intensive care unit, depending on the criticality of the patient. Immediate postanesthesia concerns are continuing dysrhythmias, hypothermia, current fluid status, changes in fluid status, PONV, hemodynamic status related to hemorrhage, and analgesia.

PCI Complications That May Affect the Delivered Anesthetic and Require Anesthetist Intervention

- Supraventricular dysrhythmias
- Ventricular dysrhythmias
- Severe and rapid hemorrhage
- Pain
- Anaphylaxis related to administration of intravenous contrast media
- Vasovagal response
- Cardiac arrest
- Thromboembolic events
- Hypotension/hypertension
- Respiratory instability

Adapted from Joe RR, Diaz LK. Anesthesia in the Cardiac Cath Lab: Catheter and EPS, Therapeutic Procedures for Pediatrics and Adults. Available at American Society of Anesthesiologists website: http://www.asahq.org/Newletters/2003/10_03/joe.html. Accessed July 29, 2008. PCI, Percutaneous coronary intervention.

Gastroenterology Procedures
Colonoscopy, EGD, and ERCP

Procedure Overview. Endoscopy came into popular use in the early 1960s with the invention of a snare for collecting intestinal polyps for biopsy. Endoscopy for gastrointestinal procedures is the use of a flexible fiberoptic endoscope that transmits brilliant, coherent, high-resolution, magnified, direct visual images to the operator. The operator can then examine, biopsy, dilate, or cauterize portions of the gastrointestinal tract. The endoscopist may pass accessory devices down the endoscope such as biopsy forceps, dilation devices, cytology brushes, measuring devices, needles for injection, Doppler probes, ultrasound probes, and probes to measure electrical activity and pH. Even foreign bodies may be removed with the aid of a snare passed through an endoscope. Endoscopes are available in different diameters for use in pediatric to adult patients.[79]

An upper endoscopy, such as an esophagogastroduodenoscopy (EGD), is an accurate way for the operator to evaluate the mucosa of the esophagus, stomach, and duodenum. A colonoscopy allows total diagnostic visualization of the mucosa of the tortuous colon from the anus to the cecum. Endoscopic retrograde cholangiopancreatography (ERCP) is used for the diagnosis of obstructive, neoplastic, or inflammatory pancreatobiliary structures. The use of ERCP is decreasing because of the availability of less-invasive and noninvasive techniques. Box 53-13 provides a brief list of indications for colonoscopy, EGD, and ERCP.[79]

Endoscopy for gastrointestinal procedures may be performed by a gastroenterologist, a general surgeon, a family practitioner, or a proctologist. The endoscope is passed into the gastrointestinal tract with the aid of lubricant. The endoscope has controls to change the direction of the flexible tip, allow flushing with water, apply suction, or insufflate air or carbon dioxide within the portion of the gastrointestinal tract being observed.

Anesthetic Considerations. Because of the expectations of patients, endoscopically caused discomfort, and the desirability for no patient movement, moderate sedation, deep sedation, and in some cases general endotracheal anesthesia are used. A proper preanesthetic assessment of the patient must be performed, focusing on the areas of age, ability to cooperate, level of anxiety,

Indications for Colonoscopy, Esophagogastroduodenoscopy, and Endoscopic Retrograde Cholangiopancreatography, with Anesthetic Implications

Colonoscopy
Gastrointestinal bleeding and occult bleeding
Evaluation of an abnormality on barium enema
Polypectomy
Unexplained iron deficiency anemia
Significant diarrhea
Chronic inflammatory bowel disease
Malignancy
Dilation of stenotic lesions
Foreign body removal

Esophagogastroduodenoscopy
Persistent and recurrent dyspepsia (heartburn)
Persistent nausea or vomiting (PONV)
Dysphagia (difficulty swallowing)
Chest pain with a negative cardiac evaluation
Iron deficiency anemia
Suspected small bowel malabsorption
Malignancy
Stomach or esophageal ulcer
Control of bleeding
Ligation or sclerosis of varices
Dilation of strictures
Percutaneous gastrostomy
Polypectomy
Removal of foreign body

Endoscopic Retrograde Cholangiopancreatography (ERCP)
Suspected biliary ductal disorder
Suspected pancreatic ductal disorder
Biliary drainage
Pancreatic drainage
Biopsy
Bile or pancreatic juice collection
Mapping of the pancreatic duct before intended surgery
Manometry of the sphincter of Oddi or other ductal mapping

Data from Waye JD, Williams CB. Colonoscopy and flexible sigmoidoscopy. In: Textbook of Gastroenterology. Philadelphia: Lippincott Williams & Wilkins; 2003:2851-2865; Sherman S, Lehman GA. Endoscopic retrograde cholangiopancreatography, endoscopic sphincterotomy and stone removal, and endoscopic biliary and pancreatic drainage. In: Yamada T, ed. Textbook of Gastroenterology. Yamada T, ed. Philadelphia: Lippincott Williams & Wilkins; 2003:2866-2892.

mental disability, allergies, fluid status, laboratory electrolyte values, cardiac history, hypertension, bleeding history, clotting status, respiratory status, obesity, drug and alcohol abuse, gastroesophageal reflux, and pregnancy.[31]

Endoscopy has been safely performed in pregnant patients.[79] Consideration should be given to any anesthetic drugs administered to the parturient, because transfer can occur through the placenta to the fetus. Rarely, elective procedures should be reconsidered and performed only after consultation with the patient's physician or obstetrician. Urgent endoscopic procedures must be performed. None of the common sedative drugs such as propofol or the opioid fentanyl have been demonstrated to cause terato-genic changes in the fetus. Studies of the obstetric effect of anesthetic drugs are limited because of the infrequent requirements for surgery during pregnancy and the ethical difficulties associated with performing controlled trials. Midazolam crosses the placenta, causing neonatal central nervous system depression; therefore, it is not recommended for obstetric use.[80] Regional anesthesia may expose the parturient to the fewest anesthetic drugs.[81]

Patients must adhere to proper NPO guidelines. Bacteremia is possible as a result of endoscopic procedures. Necessary medications may be given, such as cardiac medications, antihypertensives, and antibiotics.[79] Preemptive analgesia with gargled flavored viscous lidocaine helps patient acceptance of the procedure.[82] Moderate sedation/analgesia is usually accomplished with the short-acting sedatives midazolam or propofol and analgesics such as remifentanil, alfentanil, or fentanyl. Deep sedation can be achieved with titration of propofol until effective along with an analgesic medication.[31,44,80] Upper endoscopy may necessitate the use of any antisialagogue such as glycopyrrolate.[82]

Colonoscopy requires thorough cleansing of the lumen of the colon of fecal material. The colon may be partly prepared with a cleansing enema. Full preparation of the colon is accomplished commonly with orally administered balanced electrolyte solutions in a volume of up to 4 L. Other types of solutions are also available.[83] Patients often find this the most distressing portion of the procedure. After the preparation can come abdominal cramping, diarrhea, weakness, and nausea. Patients who arrive for the procedure require reassessment and the insertion of an intravenous catheter with intravenous fluid, usually lactated Ringer's solution or normal saline. Patients are usually left reclining for the procedure in the transport cart. Conventional monitors, including pulse oximeter, noninvasive blood pressure monitor, and electrocardiograph, are attached. The patient is supplied with oxygen through a disposable nasal cannula or disposable face mask. The procedure is usually performed with the patient positioned in a lateral decubitus position, with the body flexed, the head and back bent downward toward the knees, and the legs bent upward toward the abdomen. Patient anxiety, distention because of insufflation, and acute discomfort during the maneuvering of the endoscope usually necessitates the administration of deep sedation or a general anesthetic in some cases.[84] The depth of sedation required may be titrated with the use of an available monitor of anesthesia awareness/level of consciousness/depth of sedation via electroencephalographic processing.[85] Strong vagal nerve stimulation can occur as a result of distention of the colon. This may cause hypotension, bradydysrhythmia, and electrocardiographic changes.[79]

EGD requires a general patient assessment with special emphasis on any cardiac history, hypertension, bleeding disorders, nausea (PONV), dysphagia, and gastroesophageal reflux. The patient must be NPO according to guidelines. Most patients are able to have EGD performed with a spray or gargle of topical anesthetic such as Cetacaine, benzocaine, or 4% lidocaine liquid.[86] Rapid absorption of highly concentrated local anesthetics, applied topically over highly vascular and absorptive mucosal tissues, can lead to possible toxicity reactions whose symptoms could be masked while the patient is receiving sedative anesthesia.[87] Topical benzocaine can pose a small risk of methemoglobinemia if overused. Occasionally, patients require moderate sedation or deep sedation because topical anesthesia and even hypnosis have been found less effective.[88-90] An intravenous catheter is inserted, with fluids such as lactated Ringer's or

normal saline attached. The patient is connected to standard monitors. Oxygen can be supplied through a disposable nasal cannula or a disposable face mask. EGD is generally performed with the patient positioned supine. After the patient is adequately sedated, the operator inserts a hollow oral airway gently into the patient's mouth, and the endoscope is advanced through this airway, allowing direct visualization of the larynx, hypopharynx, esophagus and stomach, and through the pylorus into the duodenal bulb.[79]

ERCP requires thorough assessment of the patient, including a review of laboratory values of a complete blood count, serum liver chemistries and amylase or lipase levels to evaluate liver function, and clotting studies. Patients must also be evaluated for anticoagulant medications, bleeding history, and prosthetic heart valves.[79] Allergies must be evaluated, especially those to iodinated contrast media.[91] Patients who require ERCP are usually more ill than patients seen routinely for colonoscopy or EGD. The patient must be NPO according to guidelines. Intravenous access is obtained and fluid is administered. Standard monitors are applied, and oxygen is supplied to the patient via a disposable face mask. The procedure requires that the patient be in a prone or slightly left lateral decubitus position. Deep sedation is generally required, although painful or complex ERCP may require general anesthesia.[92,93]

Pediatric endoscopy has been performed with patients under deep intravenous sedation with agents such as propofol, midazolam, and alfentanil (when the patient will allow placement of the intravenous catheter) and under general endotracheal anesthesia.[94-97] Propofol has been found to provide anterograde amnesia during the procedure with no provided retrograde amnesia.[98] The use of a eutectic mixture of local anesthetics lidocaine and prilocaine (EMLA cream) facilitates the placement of the IV catheter. EMLA must be applied to undamaged skin, under an occlusive dressing for a period of 45 to 60 minutes, before the IV catheter is inserted.[99] When general anesthesia is administered, a sturdily secured endotracheal tube should be considered because of relative inaccessibility to the airway, as in the patient position required for pediatric colonoscopy or for EGD in which the oral cavity will be shared with the operator.

These procedures can cause bowel rupture or duct rupture. One must be ready with immediate airway and hemodynamic support as necessary, along with monitored emergency transport to the operating room for surgical intervention.

Postanesthesia Care. Postprocedure morbidity differs with each of the described procedures. All patients must be monitored in a postanesthesia care area until they have recovered from the sedation or general anesthetic.

Colonoscopy patients have intestinal distention, which is relieved with encouragement to pass flatus. Rectal bleeding, nausea (PONV), hypotension, and vomiting also may be seen. Administration of a bolus of intravenous fluids along with an intravenous antiemetic agent, such as ondansetron, dolasetron, or granisetron is indicated.

EGD morbidity relates to bleeding, nausea, vomiting (PONV), aspiration, dysphagia, and hypotension. Treatments such as those used for colonoscopy may be indicated.

ERCP morbidity relates to possible reactions to iodinated contrast media. Patient reactions can be mild (such as PONV, pruritus, diaphoresis, flushing, or mild urticaria), moderate (such as faintness, severe vomiting, profound urticaria, mild bronchospasm, mild hypotension, mild tachycardia, or bradycardia) or severe (hypotensive shock, angioedema, respiratory arrest, cardiac arrest, convulsions, or death).[91] Postprocedure bleeding, nausea, and vomiting (PONV) are possible and can be treated as described previously.

Gynecology Procedures

Assisted Reproductive Technologies

Procedure Overview. *Assisted reproductive technologies* (ARTs) refers to all techniques used to retrieve and fertilize the human oocyte. In vitro fertilization (IVF) is the most common technique used to artificially fertilize the human oocyte.[100,101] Research by reproductive endocrinologists has advanced technology since the first "test-tube baby" was born in 1978 and continues to result in new and more effective techniques.[31] In 2003, 122,872 cycles of ART resulted in the birth of 48,756 neonates, and the numbers of ART procedures continues to grow.[102] The procedure, which takes approximately 20 to 30 minutes to complete, is generally performed by a gynecologist who has had an advanced training fellowship in reproductive endocrinology and infertility.

The procedure is performed by initially stimulating maturation of the follicle with a gonadotropin-releasing hormone agonist, which induces pituitary-gland suppression and creates quiescent ovaries to prevent the production of a single dominant follicle. Follicle stimulating hormone (FSH) and human menopausal gonadotropin are then administered, which induces 10 to 15 ovarian follicles. The patient is then given human chorionic gonadotropin (HCG), which induces the follicle to mature and move into the follicular fluid. The oocyte is retrieved transvaginally, transabdominally, or via laparoscopy with an ultrasonically guided probe 34 to 36 hours after HCG administration. All visible follicles are collected, washed, incubated for 4 to 6 hours in a culture medium, and examined microscopically. Most follicles contain only one oocyte.[102] Fertilization occurs in the IVF laboratory. The oocyte is identified and has minimal exposure to ambient room temperature, room air, and especially any chemical odors. Sperm are washed and centrifuged. Fresh media is added next to the centrifuged sperm, and those sperm that swim to the media, which can number 50,000 sperm, are placed with the oocyte. Male factor infertility, which affects 37% of couples seeking ART procedures, requires direct intracytoplasmic injection of sperm; 16 to 20 hours later, the fertilized oocytes are examined for evidence of fertilization. Within 3 to 5 days after fertilization is verified, the embryo (which has developed into 8 to 10 cells) is transferred into either the fallopian tube or (more commonly) the uterus. Timing must be coordinated with proper maturation of the uterine endometrium.[100,102] ART is found to increase the risk of multiple gestations. Also, it has been reported that atypical implantations of the fertilized ovum or zygote, such as abdominal, cervical, ovarian, or tubal pregnancy, occur more frequently with ART.[103] Common ART techniques are listed in Table 53-3. IVF was first performed nearly 25 years ago and is accepted because of increased success rates, currently at 25%.[100,103] Infertility affects approximately 20% of couples.[103]

Patients are assessed for antibodies to human immunodeficiency virus types 1 and 2 (HIV-1, HIV-2) and human T-cell lymphotropic virus type 1 (HTLV-1), hepatitis B antigen, and antibodies to hepatitis B and C. Patients are also tested for chlamydia, syphilis, gonorrhea, and cytomegalovirus. Smokers require twice as many attempts at successful IVF than nonsmokers, so smoking is extremely discouraged.[100]

Anesthetic Considerations. IVF is generally performed on patients who are ASA class 1 or 2 in their third or fourth decade of life. Although IVF is a relatively simple procedure for the reproductive endocrinologist to perform, especially

TABLE **53-3**	Common Assisted Reproductive Technology Techniques
In vitro fertilization (IVF)	Oocytes are removed, fertilization occurs in the laboratory, and the embryo is placed transcervically into the uterus or into the distal portion of the fallopian tube(s).
Gamete intrafallopian transfer (GIFT)	Oocytes and sperm are transferred into one or both fallopian tubes for fertilization. Advantage: Oocyte retrieval and gamete transfer occur with a single procedure. Disadvantages: Requires at least one patent fallopian tube and laparoscopic surgery. Fertilization cannot be confirmed.
Zygote intrafallopian transfer (ZIFT)	Fertilized embryos are placed into the fallopian tube. Advantages: Fertilization is confirmed. Laparoscopic surgery can be avoided if fertilization has not occurred. The embryos can be transferred at an appropriate developmental stage. Disadvantage: Requires a two-stage procedure, with added risks and costs. Requires at least one patent fallopian tube.
Tubal embryo transfer (TET)	Cleaving embryos are placed into the fallopian tube.
Peritoneal oocyte and sperm transfer (POST)	Oocytes and sperm are placed into the pelvic cavity.

Modified from Speroff L et al. Clinical Gynecologic Endocrinology and Infertility. 6th ed. Baltimore: Lippincott Williams & Wilkins; 1999: 1133-1148; and Tsen LC. Anesthesia for assisted reproductive technologies. Int Anesthesiol Clin. 2007;45:99-113.

outside the operating room, IVF is an uncomfortable procedure and requires that patients do not move while the probe is guided for retrieval and later reimplantation. The vaginal wall must be pierced for the desired ovary to be accessed. Also, major blood vessels are present in the proximity of the ovaries, and their injury could lead to complications.[31]

Anesthesia requirements vary with the individual needs of the patient and the reproductive endocrinologist.[104] Multiple ART procedures may need to be performed until one of them is successful, so safe yet inexpensive anesthetic techniques are desirable.[31] Minimal sedation, moderate sedation/analgesia, regional intrathecal anesthesia, paracervical block, or general anesthesia can be administered to assist in making the procedure as comfortable and successful as possible.[31,101,105-108] Moderate sedation with analgesia is usually sufficient for most patients. None of the anesthetic procedures causes differences in reproductive outcome.[101,106,107] Anesthetic medications generally considered safe for use in anesthesia for ART are listed in Box 53-14. Anesthetists should consider using safe anesthetic techniques with quick onset and a short duration. It should be noted that propofol, lidocaine, thiopental, thiamylal, and alfentanil have been shown to accumulate in the follicular fluid. Although no deleterious effects of any anesthetics have been identified, this

BOX **53-14**

Anesthetic Medications Used for Assisted Reproductive Technologies

Intrathecal
Bupivacaine
Lidocaine
Fentanyl
Morphine

Paracervical Block
Bupivacaine
Lidocaine
Mepivacaine

Intravenous Sedation or Total Intravenous Anesthesia
Fentanyl
Alfentanil
Remifentanil
Meperidine
Ketamine
Midazolam
Propofol

Inhalation Agents
Nitrous oxide

BOX **53-15**

Common Anesthetic Agents That Could Cause Problems with Assisted Reproductive Technologies

Morphine
Sevoflurane
Desflurane
NSAIDs—ibuprofen, indomethacin, ketoprofen, ketorolac, meloxicam, naproxen, oxaprozin
Droperidol
Metoclopramide
Postanesthesia care:
As in all cases of anesthetic administration, the patient is assessed in a postanesthetic recovery area. Vital signs and pulse oximetry are assessed and must be stable. If intrathecal anesthesia was used, the patient must have a recovery of sensorium, be able to ambulate, and be able to void. All patients must be free of nausea.

NSAIDs, *Nonsteroidal antiinflammatory drugs.*

area continues to be studied.[101,102,107] No data from human trials have ever condemned the use of local anesthetic agents for oocyte retrival.[102] Morphine has been shown to adversely affect fertilization of sea urchin eggs in vitro by allowing more than one sperm to enter the oocyte in 30% of cases, so it is not used because of the existence of safe alternatives such as fentanyl, alfentanil, remifentanil and meperidine.[102] Midazolam, when titrated in small doses to provide mild to moderated sedation and anxiolysis has been shown to be safe, with no accumulation in follicular fluid or being a teratogen.[102] Ketamine (0.75 mg/kg) with midazolam (0.06 mg/kg) moderate sedation/analgesia has been safely used as an alternative to general anesthesia with isoflurane.[102] The literature has suggested the use of caution if the anesthetist desires to select a potent inhaled agent (especially sevoflurane and desflurane) because of possible negative effects to ART outcomes.[102] Nonsteroidal antiinflammatory agents such as ibuprofen, indomethacin, ketoprofen, ketorolac, meloxicam, naproxen, or oxaprozin are avoided owing to inhibition of prostaglandin synthesis and possible effects on embryo implantation.[44,80,102] Droperidol and metoclopramide have been shown to induce rapid hyperprolactinemia and should be avoided. Low plasma prolactin levels are associated with higher incidences of pregnancy.[102] Box 53-15 lists common anesthetic agents that could cause problems with ART. The necessity for any medication given to the patient should be carefully considered, and the anesthetic technique should be kept simple and basic.

Office-Based Surgery
General Dental Procedures

Procedure Overview. Anesthesia for dental procedures and dental surgery can present many challenges. The demand for dental care and visits from patients are increasing. Dentistry has changed from a role of therapeutic treatment of dental disease to a role of prevention. The old mainstay was that 50% of the population never visited a dentist. This group used dentistry only for treatment of extreme pain or in an emergency. Latest demographic statistics show that this has changed for the better. Overall, rates vary drastically across the U.S. population, with more than 60% of the population visiting a dentist at least once annually. More women see dentists annually than men, and as employment status, income, and educational levels increase, so do the number of annual visits to the dentist. Also, children ages 6 or younger and adults ages 65 or older are seeing dentists more frequently than in the past.[109-111]

Dental procedures may be performed in an operating room, a specially equipped hospital suite, an ambulatory surgical center, or a dental office operatory (dental surgical area). Anesthesia may be required for dental procedures in the following areas of dentistry[112]:

Pediatric dentistry—an age-defined specialty that provides primary and comprehensive preventive and therapeutic oral health care for infants and children through adolescence, including those with special health care needs.

Oral and maxillofacial surgery—the specialty that includes the diagnosis, surgical and adjunctive treatment of diseases, injuries, and defects involving both the functional and esthetic aspects of the hard and soft tissues of the oral and maxillofacial region.

Periodontics—the specialty that encompasses the prevention, diagnosis, and treatment of diseases of the supporting and surrounding tissues of the teeth, or their substitutes, and the maintenance of the health, function, and esthetics of these structures and tissues.

Endodontics—the specialty that is concerned with the etiology, diagnosis, prevention, and treatment of diseases and injuries of the pulp and associated periradicular (concerning the root of the tooth) conditions.

Prosthodontics—the dental specialty involved with the diagnosis, treatment planning, rehabilitation, and maintenance of oral functions, comfort, appearance, and patient health associated with clinical conditions of missing or deficient teeth and/or oral and maxillofacial tissues along with biocompatible substitutes.

General dentistry—encompasses the etiology, diagnosis, and treatment of conditions of oral, head, and neck tissues; the general dentist may perform procedures that encompass any or all of the dental specialty areas, depending on the training, abilities and experiences of the general dentist.

Dental hygiene—a licensed oral health professional trained to treat patients by the removal of dental plaque and calculus (tartar) above or below the gingiva.[113,114]

Anesthetic Considerations. Important considerations that must be part of the anesthesia treatment plan for the dental setting are outlined in Box 53-16. The patient may require minimal sedation, moderate sedation/analgesia, deep sedation/analgesia, or general anesthesia for dental surgery. The anesthesia required depends on the patient-related factors of fear, anxiety, age, medical condition, level of cooperation and behavior, gagging, ineffective local anesthesia in the past, mental impairment, and physical disability. A thorough, documented patient assessment along with appropriate laboratory studies and possible physician consultation regarding patient clearance for physically and/or psychologically stressful dental surgery are necessary.[115-117] In pediatric dentistry, a comprehensive and personalized discussion with the parent or guardian (with or without the patient present) of what the anesthetic procedure will entail, coupled with an opportunity for the parent or patient to engage in dialogue and ask questions, can alleviate the stress of the upcoming procedures for all parties.

The dental operatory must be of adequate size for both access and egress of both the patient and personnel. Proper considerations and advanced planning must be made to accommodate patients according to the Americans with Disabilities Act.[118-120] Also, the anesthetist must have full and rapid access to both the patient and all required equipment and supplies. Full monitors are necessary. Consider the use of the antisialogogue glycopyrrolate, because dental surgery can stimulate the flow of saliva. Excess salivation can lead to coughing, choking,

laryngospasm, or aspiration in the sedated patient. Delivery of anesthesia in the dental operatory should be as familiar as if it were in an operating room. Postoperative problems in dentistry generally are minimal but can involve pain, swelling, bleeding, PONV, the vasovagal response, airway problems, hypoxemia, or hypothermia, as a result of anesthetic procedures other than local anesthesia administered. Hypothermia can be addressed by the use of an electric blanket; forced-air warming may not be feasible for the dental operatory.

General dentists and board-certified dental specialists are also trained to administer intraoral local anesthesia, which is a cardiac depressant and may cause either central nervous system depression or excitation. Local anesthesia for dentistry is commonly administered with an aspirating syringe/needle system. Local anesthetic is available in 1.8-mL glass carpules, both with and without epinephrine, or levonordefrin (neo-Cobefrin) as a vasoconstrictor.

Dental specialists and specially trained general dentists can be licensed by state dental boards to administer the continuum of anesthesia, from minimal sedation to general anesthesia while performing the dental surgery. The dental literature reports good long-standing success rates and safety, but caution is necessary.[121-125]

Each dental specialty has particular anesthetic considerations, which are discussed in the following sections.

Pediatric Dentistry. Pediatric dental patients can require the continuum of anesthesia from enteral minimal sedation to parenteral moderate sedation/analgesia, deep sedation/analgesia, or general anesthesia if the patient is behaviorally uncooperative, immature, frightened, or mentally disabled or because of the necessity to perform all necessary dental surgery in one session. Pediatric dentists may have a patient immobilization device available, commonly called a *papoose board*, to safely restrain the patient until anxiolytic anesthesia can be administered. Anesthetic choices such as oral or intravenous ketamine; a mixture of oral chloral hydrate, meperidine, and hydroxyzine; intravenous diazepam; midazolam; and propofol have been used with success.[122,123,126-129] Premedication with orally administered midazolam dissolved in a small amount of the liquid forms of acetaminophen, ibuprofen, aspirin, or low-sugar clear juice is commonly used. For the liquid forms of acetaminophen, ibuprofen, or aspirin, the anesthesia provider should refer to the package insert for the proper dosing based on the patient's weight. Intranasal or rectal midazolam can be used alone or given before general endotracheal anesthesia and has proved as effective as nitrous oxide for sedation.[127-131] Oral transmucosal fentanyl citrate has been used as an effective preoperative sedative.[132] After an inhaled mask or intravenous induction, insertion of a dental LMA, or oronasal endotracheal intubation can be performed to allow the pediatric dentist full access to the mouth. The dental LMA, will allow the pediatric dentist the benefits of the LMA (less trauma and less stimulation when compared with endotracheal intubation) with the added benefit of being able to check occlusion (the bite) while the patient remains anesthetized. In one study, 68% of children found induction to be an upsetting factor in their care.[133] Pediatric dentists allow a secured dental LMA or oral endotracheal tube and are very cognizant of the importance of sharing the airway during surgery. Typical pediatric dental procedures include restorative dentistry, such as fillings of amalgam or composite, and placement of stainless steel crowns for posterior teeth, polycarbonate crowns, composite crowns, or stainless steel crowns with porcelain for anterior teeth, pulpotomies, tooth extractions, and

BOX **53-16**

Considerations Related to Anesthesia in the Dental Setting

- Anesthesia may be administered in an unfamiliar area. Carefully plan, equip, and set up the operatory so that it is as familiar and comfortable as in an operating room.
- The established airway will be shared with the dental surgeon.
- The potential exists for heavy bleeding because of the vast blood supply to the head and neck region.
- There could be the use of small instruments, burs (dental drill bits), files, implants, and filling materials in the mouth, with the potential of falling into the oropharynx or being aspirated.
- Patients may be receiving dental prosthetic devices such as crowns, bridges, or full or partial dentures, which can also affect the airway.
- There exists the possibility of intense pain, transmitted primarily by the maxillary and mandibular divisions of the trigeminal nerve.
- Patients usually display a high level of anxiety, and adequate time must be incorporated into the schedule to allow for safe anesthetic treatment.

space maintainers. Successful treatments can be provided along with stress reduction for the patient, parents or guardians, and for the health-care providers with appropriate airway maintenance and under deep sedation. A study has shown that stainless steel crowns are more successful when the procedure is performed with the patient under general anesthesia.[134]

Oral and Maxillofacial Surgery. Procedures performed within the specialty of oral and maxillofacial surgery (OMS) are among the most invasive in dentistry. Oral surgeons perform uncovering of teeth for orthodontic treatment; extraction of impacted, severely carious, and multiple teeth; insertion of dental implants, treatment of infections of the head and neck; surgical remodeling of maxillary and mandibular alveolar bone; facial cosmetics; and removal of soft-tissue or bony tumors, as well as many other procedures. These procedures can produce both severe pain and heavy bleeding. Many OMS procedures are performed within the office setting. Oral and maxillofacial surgeons receive 6 years of postdoctoral training and become licensed by the state dental board to perform the continuum from minimal sedation to anesthesia (general anesthesia) care. Patients can have challenging physical and mental conditions; therefore, a thorough preanesthetic assessment is necessary.[135] The patient's airway is shared with the oral surgeon; therefore, nasal intubation may be necessary. It may be possible to perform some oral surgical procedures while carefully working around an unsecured tube or with a standard or reinforced LMA.[135-137] Local anesthesia in combination with intravenous sedation (propofol, midazolam), inhalation sedation (nitrous oxide), inhaled potent endotracheal anesthetics, and total intravenous general anesthesia are techniques available for office-based OMS.[135,138-140] Remifentanil has become a useful adjunct with the techniques listed, to counteract the intense stimulation of OMS.[141,142] An anesthesia awareness/level of consciousness/depth of sedation monitor is also useful for careful anesthetic titration.[133,143]

Periodontics. Periodontal procedures can involve painful stimulation. Periodontists generally work in a particular quadrant of the patient's mouth and administer local anesthetic for the particular area of surgery. Periodontal treatment involves surgery of the teeth, gingiva, connective tissue, periodontal ligament, and alveolar bone, as well as insertion and maintenance of dental implants. Local anesthetics are administered with a normal epinephrine 1:100,000 concentration, unless contraindicated, along with greater than normal epinephrine concentrations (1:50,000) injected directly into the gingiva because of its local anesthetic ability and for hemostasis. Periodontal surgery can involve lengthy procedures with moderate amounts of hemorrhage, and can be well managed with minimal sedation (both enteral or with inhalation sedation) or moderate sedation/analgesia.[116] A full array of monitors is necessary. Midazolam with a propofol infusion helps achieve the goals of safety and comfort for periodontal surgical patients.[144]

Endodontics. Anesthesia for endodontic procedures is similar to that described for periodontal surgery. Local anesthesia provides adequate comfort, but in the presence of patient anxiety related to the length of endodontic procedures, minimal sedation (both enteral or with inhalation sedation) or moderate sedation/analgesia can make the procedure tolerable and less anxiety producing for the patient. A dental dam is usually applied around the tooth and held in place with a special clamp to prevent aspiration of dental burs and endodontic files.

General Dentistry and Prosthodontics. General dentistry can encompass all procedures from all of the dental specialties,

depending on the interest and training of the general dentist. Anesthesia can be delivered along the continuum of care to ensure safety for the patient and to fill the requirements of the particular dental procedure.[124,145,146]

Dental Hygiene. Dental hygienists are also involved with providing dental care to patients who may require anesthesia along the continuum from minimal sedation/analgesia to deep sedation/analgesia with combinations of inhalation nitrous oxide/oxygen, local anesthesia, and intravenous medications. Thorough treatment can generate tooth or gingival sensitivity and pain. Procedures range from routine hygiene to deep scaling and root planing of teeth with heavy dental accretions.

Postanesthesia Care. Patients recover in a quiet, monitored environment. Intravenous access allows the titration of additional analgesia or antiemetics as necessary. Fortunately, patient morbidity from general anesthesia for dental procedures is low.[147] Patients who receive inhaled sedation are less stressed postoperatively than those who receive general anesthesia, but TIVA procedures with proper airway maintenance and supplemental oxygen also prove great success.[148]

Invasive dental procedures can be another source of distress in children, which can lead to crying, nausea, vomiting (PONV), and bleeding postoperatively.[149] The addition of the potent opioid morphine, ketorolac, or both greatly aids patient comfort in the postsurgical anesthesia recovery area. The use of oral minimal to moderate sedation in pediatric patients ages 2 to 34 months has been found to have no effect on behavior when the individual requires treatment later.[150] Adolescents who have undergone sedation for childhood dental therapy are found to possess a high level of anxiety regarding dentistry, when compared with adolescents without that history.[151]

Psychiatric Procedures
Electroconvulsive Therapy
Electroconvulsive therapy (ECT) is the intentional inducement of a generalized seizure of the central nervous system for an adequate duration of time to treat patients with certain severe neuropsychiatric disorders.[152] In 2001, the American Psychiatric Association Committee on Electroconvulsive Therapy published a report approving ECT as a safe and effective treatment for severe and medication-resistant major depression, with response rates of 80% to 90% as a first-line treatment and 50% to 60% in patients unresponsive to adequate trials of antidepressant medications such as a combination of nortriptyline and lithium carbonate. This report was reaffirmed in both 2006 and 2007 in a comparison with new therapies for major depression.[153-156] Antidepressant medication administration, along with ECT, is well tolerated by patients, and both therapies can be beneficial to the patient. Most patients receive three treatments per week and can undergo a total of 6 to 12 treatments overall.[157] Clinical improvement is seen within the first three to five treatments, and positive response to treatment is seen in 50% to 90% of patients, even those who had been treatment resistant.[158] ECT treatments exceed the total numbers of coronary revascularizations, herniorrhaphy, and appendectomy procedures performed in the United States.[157] Death from ECT itself is possible but is rare. ECT is also used in certain patients who experience mania, catatonia, vegetative dysregulation, inanition, suicidal drive, and schizophrenia with affective disorders.[152,157]

ECT is one of the most controversial and invasive treatments in medicine. The first documented use of ECT was in 1938. Early ECT was performed without anesthesia, with the occurrence of many adverse effects such as bitten tongues, broken bones, and

TABLE 53-4	Anesthetic Medications Used for Electroconvulsive Therapy	
Drug	**Dose**	
Anticholinergics		
Atropine	0.4-1 mg IV or IM	
Glycopyrrolate	0.005 mg/kg IV or IM	
Anesthetics		
Alfentanil	0.2-0.3 mcg/kg IV	
Etomidate	0.1-0.3 mg/kg IV	
Ketamine	0.5-1 mg/kg IV	
Methohexital	0.5-1 mg/kg IV	
Propofol	0.75-1.5 mg/kg IV	
Thiopental	1.5-2.5 mg/kg IV	
Muscle Relaxants *Depolarizing*		
Succinylcholine	0.75-1.5 mg/kg IV	
Nondepolarizing		
Cisatracurium	0.15-0.25 mg/kg IV (onset 1-2 minutes)	
Atracurium	0.3-0.4 mg/kg IV (onset 6 minutes)	
Rocuronium	0.3-0.9 mg/kg IV (onset 1-2 minutes)	

Modified from Ding Z, White PF. Anesthesia for electroconvulsive therapy. Anesth Analg. 2002;94:1351-1364; White PF. Perioperative Drug Manual. 2nd ed. Philadelphia: Saunders; 2005; Wagner KJ et al. Guide to anaesthetic selection for electroconvulsive therapy. CNS Drugs. 2005;19:745-758.
IM, Intramuscular; IV, intravenous.

broken teeth. Treatment involves placement of electrodes with a conducting gel, either right-sided unilaterally or bitemporally bilaterally. An alternating current of electricity is passed through the electrodes.[152] Theories for the mechanism of ECT are related to profound changes in brain chemistry, such as enhancement of dopaminergic, serotonergic, and adrenergic neurotransmission. Another theory postulates the release of hypothalamic or pituitary hormones, which have antidepressant effects. Finally, ECT produces anticonvulsant effects that raise the seizure threshold and decrease seizure duration, exerting a positive effect on the brain.[152]

Anesthetic Considerations. Anesthesia for ECT involves the administration of an ultra-brief general anesthetic to provide lack of consciousness to the patient for the procedure (Table 53-4).

A thorough preanesthetic assessment must be performed, with consideration given to the possible great physiologic hemodynamic responses generated by the induced seizure activity. Box 53-17 lists possible physiologic effects as a result of ECT.

Few absolute and relative contraindications to ECT exist (Box 53-18).[152,157,159]

Patients may have results of laboratory studies, a pharmacologic regimen, and ECG readily available because of their psychiatric hospitalization. Informed consent is obtained whenever possible from the patient or legal guardian. An intravenous catheter is inserted in a peripheral vein. The patient is monitored with a pulse oximeter, ECG, noninvasive blood pressure monitor, temperature-monitoring device, and peripheral nerve stimulator. Use of $ETCO_2$ monitoring has been suggested because hypercarbia and hypoxia shorten seizure duration. Suction, oxygen, a positive-pressure Ambu bag and face mask, and rubber bite protectors

BOX 53-17

Possible Physiologic Effects of Electroconvulsive Therapy

Cardiovascular
Parasympathetic Response During Tonic Phase of Seizure:
Decreased heart rate
Hypotension
Bradydysrhythmias

Sympathetic Response During Clonic Phase of Seizure:
Tachycardia
Hypertension
Tachydysrhythmias

Cerebral
Increased cerebral blood flow (increases of 100% to 400% above baseline are possible)
Increased intracranial pressure

Other
Increased intraocular pressure
Increased intragastric pressure

Adapted from Lee M. Anesthesia for electroconvulsive therapy. In: Atlee JL, ed. Complications in Anesthesia. 2nd ed. Philadelphia: Saunders: 2007:903-905.

BOX 53-18

Absolute and Relative Contraindications to Electroconvulsive Therapy

Absolute Contraindications to ECT
Pheochromocytoma
Recent myocardial infarction (<4-6 weeks ago)
Recent cerebrovascular accident (≤3 months ago)
Recent intracranial surgery (≤3 months ago)
Intracranial mass lesion
Unstable cervical spine

Relative Contraindications to ECT
Angina
Congestive heart failure
Cardiac rhythm management device (pacemaker, automatic internal cardiac defibrillator [AICD])
Severe pulmonary disease
Major bone fracture
Glaucoma
Retinal detachment
Thrombophlebitis
Pregnancy

Modified from Lee M. Anesthesia for electroconvulsive therapy. In: Atlee JL, ed. Complications in Anesthesia. 2nd ed. Philadelphia: Saunders: 2007:903-905.

must be present, as well as necessary airway and cardiovascular resuscitation equipment, medications, and supplies. ECT is usually performed in a dedicated psychiatric suite or special treatment room.

The patient is preoxygenated before induction. Anticholinergics may be administered as an antisialagogue or to prevent asystole.[157] The induction agent is administered intravenously. Methohexital is the standard agent used for ECT. Methohexital produces rapid induction of general anesthesia, is associated with rapid recovery, and has convulsive properties because of its unique oxybarbiturate structure with a methyl radical.[160] Propofol, etomidate, thiopental, and ketamine have also been used, although an enhanced hemodynamic response and increased intracranial pressure are possible after using ketamine.[161-164] After loss of consciousness, positive-pressure ventilation is applied to the patient via the breathing bag and a face mask and is continued until after treatment is completed and spontaneous respirations resume. To assess the duration of the induced convulsion, the psychiatrist usually applies a tourniquet (or manual blood pressure cuff inflated to slightly greater than the systolic blood pressure) above a lower extremity so that the muscle relaxant cannot reach the skeletal muscle in the extremity. A rubber bite block is gently placed in the patient's mouth to prevent biting of the teeth, lips, and tongue, and an ultra-short-acting muscle relaxant is administered. Atracurium use has been described most often among the nondepolarizing relaxants, although the depolarizing relaxant succinylcholine is also used.[157,164] A nerve stimulator must be used, and appropriate neuromuscular blockade reversal agents should be administered if necessary. The electrodes are applied, the proper waveform and current level are selected, and the electroconvulsive seizure is induced. The seizure lasts from 30 to 90 seconds; the motor seizure is shorter than the seizure duration as seen on an electroencephalogram (EEG). Use of an anesthesia awareness/level of consciousness/depth of sedation monitor correlates with the EEG, and it can be a useful tool for the anesthetist and the psychiatrist.[165] The level of sedation displayed by this monitor correlates with the proper point to induce seizure, the duration of seizure, and the potential for awareness during the ECT procedure.[166-171] At the end of the seizure, spontaneous respirations resume, the patient is transferred to a recovery area, and vital signs are continually monitored until the patient is determined to be stable and able to be safely discharged.[152,172] Certain anesthetic medications and techniques such as hyperventilation can affect seizure duration (Box 53-19).

Adult patients about to undergo ECT should follow fasting guidelines of at least 6 hours for solids and 2 hours for liquids.[57,60,69] Necessary bronchodilators may be taken.[69] Oral medications, such as antihypertensives, cardiac medications, anticoagulants, and thyroid medications, may be taken with a sip of water up to 1 hour before the procedure.[57,69] Rapid-sequence induction of general anesthesia with applied cricoid pressure and endotracheal intubation can be performed. One must take into consideration the total number of ECT treatments to be received, weighed against the necessity for repeated intubations and the fact that most patients, even obese patients, have rarely been found to aspirate as a result of ECT.[173] The CRNA may perform a rapid-sequence induction and apply cricoid pressure until the protective reflexes return and the danger of aspiration is eliminated, rather than intubating the patient.

Postanesthesia Care. The intentional creation of central nervous system convulsions has profound effects on the patient's physiology. Patients usually experience temporary cognitive and memory impairment after ECT.

The first type of impairment that may be seen is postictal confusion, in which the patient is transiently restless, confused, and agitated immediately after the convulsive episode and for approximately 30 minutes. The agitation can be difficult to manage for the recovery nurse. Some patients require physical

---

BOX 53-19

Effects of Common Medications and Conditions on Seizure Duration

Medications That Can Prolong Seizure Duration
Alfentanil with methohexital or propofol
Aminophylline
Caffeine
Clozapine
Etomidate
Ketamine (a proconvulsant)
Methohexital (some proconvulsant properties) with remifentanil

Conditions That Can Prolong Seizure Duration
Hyperventilation/hypocapnia

Medications That Can Shorten Seizure Duration
Diltiazem
Diazepam
Fentanyl
Lidocaine
Lorazepam
Midazolam
Propofol
Sevoflurane
Thiopental

Medications with No Apparent Effect on Seizure Duration
Clonidine
Dexmedetomidine
Esmolol (may possibly shorten seizure duration)
Labetalol (may possibly shorten seizure duration)
Nicardipine
Nifedipine
Nitroglycerin
Nitroprusside
Trimethaphan

Modified from Ding Z, White PF. Anesthesia for electroconvulsive therapy. Anesth Analg. 2002;94:1351-1364; Stensrud PE. Anesthesia at remote locations. In: Miller, RD, ed. Miller's Anesthesia. 6th ed. Philadelphia: Churchill Livingstone; 2005:2655-2656; Wagner KJ et al. Guide to anaesthetic selection for electroconvulsive therapy. CNS Drugs. 2005;19:745-758.

restraint or sedation with a benzodiazepine such as lorazepam or diazepam or an antipsychotic medication such as haloperidol. Researchers have recently hypothesized that high plasma lactate levels cause this agitation.[156] The authors suggest that this is caused by inadequate neuromuscular blockade and that increasing the dose of muscle relaxant is necessary.[156,157]

A second type of cognitive impairment that may be seen later is anterograde memory dysfunction, in which the patient may rapidly forget new information. The patient may not remember things that he or she does or is told in the days after ECT. Anterograde amnesia usually subsides within days or a few weeks. However, it can be frightening to the patient. A third cognitive dysfunction is retrograde memory dysfunction, which is the forgetting of memories from several weeks to several months before the ECT treatment. No evidence suggests that ECT causes any brain damage, nor does it impair the long-term ability for the patient to learn and retain new information. The cognitive effects described vary depending on the frequency and the number of ECT treatments the patient has received. The quantities of energy used to elicit the convulsions and the placement of the electrodes are also factors. Even the type of anesthetic drugs used is believed to be involved.[152,172]

Cardiovascular stimulation also occurs with ECT. The sympathetic and parasympathetic nervous systems are stimulated sequentially. Therefore, the patient may experience an increase in heart rate and blood pressure, followed by a period of bradycardia or even asystole. This can lead to increases in myocardial oxygen demand, arrhythmias, and transient ischemic changes in susceptible individuals. Transient cardiac changes can be managed before ECT with anticholinergics, intravenous local anesthetics such as lidocaine, or intravenous narcotics such as remifentanil.[157,174] Changes after ECT can be managed with β-blockers such as esmolol or labetalol, calcium channel blockers such as verapamil or nifedipine, or other antihypertensives such as nitroprusside or nitroglycerin.[154,158,175]

Finally, patients may also experience headache, muscle aches, or nausea. Symptoms of headache or muscle ache respond well to acetaminophen, aspirin, or nonsteroidal antiinflammatory agents such as intravenous or intramuscular ketorolac or oral ibuprofen.[157,172] Nausea can be caused by the stress and anxiety before the ECT treatment, the anesthetic agents used, the seizure itself, or air in the stomach from assisted ventilation. Nausea can be treated with agents such as ondansetron, dolasetron, granisetron, or metoclopramide.[157,172]

New Therapies for Major Depressive Disorders

Two new therapies for severe major depressive disorders are now available, which require anesthetic treatment: repetitive transcranial magnetic stimulation (rTMS) and vagus nerve stimulation (VNS).[158] Neuroanatomic studies have suggested that patients with major depressive disorder (MDD) have dysfunction within the frontal cortical-subcortical-brainstem neural network, specifically the dorsolateral prefrontal cortices (DLPFC). ECT and antidepressant medications do not act in these discrete areas of the brain, but new therapies stimulating these focal areas of the brain are now approved and in use in the United States.

Repetitive Transcranial Magnetic Stimulation and Magnetic Seizure Therapy. Repetitive transcranial magnetic stimulation (rTMS) uses electric current passing through an electromagnetic coil that has been placed on the scalp. The coil delivers brief, rapidly changing magnetic field pulses to specific areas of the brain. These bursts of pulses are called a "train" of stimuli. Multiple trains of rTMS may be delivered in one session. The scalp and skull are transparent to magnetic fields, an advantage over ECT, in which the scalp and skull are resistors to the electrical stimulation.[158,176] To produce antidepressant effects, a convulsion must be initiated by trains of rTMS, because subconvulsive trains of rTMS are ineffective.[172]

Convulsive magnetic energy levels are determined by the use of motor threshold (MT). MT is the point at which a single pulse of magnetic energy begins to elicit an electromyographic response, that is, a twitch, usually of the abductor pollicis brevis muscle of the thumb or first dorsal interosseous muscle of the index finger.[158,176,177] Treatment with rTMS is safe and well tolerated, with reduced cognitive side effects when compared with ECT. Patients are found to recover much more rapidly from rTMS or MST therapy as compared with ECT.[178]

Magnetic seizure therapy (MST) uses a higher intensity, more frequent, and longer-duration magnetic seizure-inducing dose when compared with the magnetic dose required for rTMS. MST can stimulate tonic-clonic seizures in more localized and focal regions of the prefrontal cerebral cortex when compared with ECT, as well as generalized tonic-clonic seizures that resemble ECT.[158,178] MST does not produce the rigid bilateral masseter muscle contractions noted during ECT but can produce elevations in blood pressure and heart rate similar to ECT.[178]

After rTMS some patients experience mild headache, disorientation and inattention (although patients become reoriented much more quickly than with ECT), retrograde amnesia, some anterograde amnesia, transient auditory threshold increases due to the high-frequency clicking sound heard during coil discharge (which can be alleviated with the use of foam earplugs), and (rarely) generalized seizure.[158,176] A single TMS treatment may be all that is necessary for treating certain severe MDD nonpsychotic patients along with their medications, although rTMS may be necessary.[153]

The literature describes anesthesia requirements for rTMS or MST from none needed to ultra-brief general anesthesia as for ECT.[158,176,179] A patent and secure intravenous catheter is established, and full monitors are applied. Glycopyrrolate 0.004 mcg/kg is administered as an antisialagogue along with ketorolac, 0.4 mg/kg, 2 to 3 minutes prior to induction of ultra-brief general anesthesia. Etomidate 0.15 to 0.2 mg/kg can be used for induction, as well as methohexital, 1 to 2 mg/kg, or propofol, 1 to 2.5 mg/kg. Succinylcholine, 0.5 to 1 mg/kg, can be used as the muscle relaxant after isolation of a lower extremity for observation of seizure duration. Use the smallest amount of muscle relaxant necessary to enable recovery from paralysis prior to the return of consciousness. The anesthetist can then manually hyperventilate the patient's lungs with a face mask to an ETCO$_2$ value of 30 to 34 torr. At this point, the magnetic stimulus may be applied.[44,178]

Vagus Nerve Stimulation. VNS requires surgical implantation of a programmable battery-powered electrical stimulator that connects with the patient's left vagus nerve (cranial nerve X). The stimulator is usually implanted in the patient's chest with minimal sedation, moderate sedation/analgesia, deep sedation/analgesia, or under general anesthesia. Because of the delicacy of the surgery and its proximity to vital structures, no extraneous patient movement is permitted. Although originally approved for treatment-resistant epilepsy, the VNS is now approved for major depressive episodes that have not responded to four antidepressant medication trials.[153,158]

Radiologic and Diagnostic Procedures

Medical science has been able to use the sciences of physics, chemistry, and computers to produce remarkably accurate images of the internal structure and function of the body to aid medical diagnosis. Energy is transmitted to the patient and interacts with patient tissues. This energy is then detected, processed, and displayed on a computer console, which allows images to be selected for further investigation and diagnosis. Some medical images are created in real time and allow observation of flow or changes in tissue resulting from treatment.[180]

Procedure Overviews

Computed Tomography. Computed tomography (CT) uses x-rays generated from a rotating anode x-ray generator. The patient is placed supine on a flat, wooden, wheeled platform and moved inside the scanning gantry. X-rays are then projected through the patient at different angles, penetrating tissues differently according to the atomic numbers of the atoms within the tissue. Dense tissue such as bone attenuates (reduces the energy of) the x-ray beam more than less dense tissue such as muscle, yielding high-resolution images of the scanned tissue. The patient images are then detected, and the computer acquires the image data. Finally, an image analyzer projects the analyzed data in the form of a tomogram or body section slice onto an operator console and a physician-viewing console. CT is excellent for imaging bone. The diagnostic quality of a CT scan is enhanced with the injection of intravenous contrast media (ICM).[181] Contrast media containing iodine may be administered to the patient enterally or parenterally to further attenuate the x-ray beam to enhance the images for CT vascular or gastrointestinal studies.[180,181]

Magnetic Resonance Imaging. Magnetic resonance imaging (MRI) uses the dipole moment (the ability of the atomic nucleus to behave as a magnet) of the hydrogen atom. The patient is placed supine within the scanning gantry or bore of the magnet. The magnet used for MRI can be a permanent magnet or a powerful superconducting electromagnet cooled with liquid helium to 4° kelvin. Magnetic strength is measured in teslas (T); 1 T is equivalent to 10,000 gauss or oersted. MRI magnets can generate field strengths of 0.15 to 4 T, although MRI magnetic field strength generally ranges from 0.15 to 2 T. The quality of the MRI image is directly related to the strength of the magnetic field.[182] The spin of the electron in hydrogen will align the hydrogen atoms parallel to this powerful magnetic field. The patient's water-containing tissues are then excited with variable radiofrequency pulses. After the proton in hydrogen receives this radiofrequency energy, it emits radiofrequency energy with three-dimensional appearing spatial information. MRI technology now allows its use within the operating room with an open bore, portable, 0.12-T, low-intensity magnet to assist the neurosurgeon with diagnostic decisions.[183] Contrast media are also used in MRI studies to enhance the patient's tissues and allow the scan to provide further diagnostic information. MRI contrast is most commonly gadopentetate dimeglumine, which contains the element gadolinium bound as a chelated structure and administered primarily parenterally but rarely enterally.[182,184-186]

The U.S. Food and Drug Administration (FDA) classifies the MRI as a Class II device. Class II devices require special labeling, mandatory performance standards, and post-market surveillance by the FDA. The electromagnetic energy greatly drops off just outside the margins of the bore of the electromagnet. This is called the *fringe field*. There are no known reports of harmful physiologic effects from magnetic fields.[182,184]

Because of the potential of danger of the powerful electromagnetic attraction of ferromagnetic objects to both the patient and health-care personnel, the American College of Radiology divides the MRI suite into four zones:

- Zone 1 has public access and no supervision, such as the hallway outside the MRI suite.
- Zone 2 has public access and limited supervision, such as the entrance into the MRI suite.
- Zone 3 has limited access and explicit supervision, such as immediately outside the MRI scanner room where MRI controls may be located.
- Zone 4 is the MRI scanner room itself, and has strict and controlled access which is under constant supervision.[187]

Interventional Radiology (Vascular and Nonvascular) and Radiotherapy or Radiosurgery. Interventional radiology (IR) involves minimally invasive procedures and therapies performed by radiologists, especially in patients at high medical risk.[37,188,189] Major IR therapies include angiography, the embolization of blood vessels such as arteriovenous malformations or for epistaxis, the delivery of chemical or physical vascular occlusive devices,

---

BOX **53-20**

Indications for Endovascular Embolization

Arteriovenous malformation
Arteriovenous fistula
Intracranial aneurysm
Recurrent epistaxis
Hemoptysis
Traumatic solid organ hemorrhage
Preoperative major organ tumor embolization for blood loss reduction
Gastrointestinal hemorrhage
Uterine leiomyoma (fibroid)
Uterine hemorrhage
Pelvic fracture hemorrhage
Postoperative hemorrhage after prosthetic hip or knee replacement
Varicocele

From Higgins GA. Embolization procedures. In: Atlee JL, ed. Complications in Anesthesia. 2nd ed. Philadelphia: Saunders; 2007:912-914.

---

the removal of thrombi, ablation of aneurysms, and angioplasty of blood vessels with stent placement.[37,190,191] Box 53-20 lists indications for endovascular embolization procedures. See Chapter 26 for a discussion of interventional vascular surgery.

Radiation is a treatment itself for both benign tumors (low-grade astrocytoma, meningioma, pituitary adenoma, craniopharyngioma, schwannoma, pineocytoma, chemodectoma, low-grade papillary neoplasms) and aggressive tumors (germinoma, primitive neuroectodermal tumor, chordoma, intermediate-grade pineal tumor, immature teratoma, undifferentiated sarcoma, anaplastic oligoastrocytoma, and metastatic tumors). Radiation surgery is the delivery of a single massive dose of radiation to the target tissue. Radiation therapy is the delivery of smaller doses of radiation over several sessions.

Gamma radiation is used for radiotherapy and radiosurgery. The gamma radiation is introduced to the patient by the use of either a GammaKnife or a CyberKnife. Each uses beams of gamma rays obtained from the radioactive decay of cobalt 60 or from a linear accelerator. The CyberKnife is used by first obtaining stereotactic three-dimensional images, which then allow computer-controlled robot arm guidance of the CyberKnife. The CyberKnife therapy delivers a sequence of many hundreds of gamma beams to the cancerous tumor from many different directions. GammaKnife therapy delivers gamma radiation to the cancerous tumor simultaneously in a single dose.[192,193]

Interventional Neuroradiology. Interventional neuroradiology (INR) is the diagnosis and treatment of CNS diseases endovascularly to deliver therapeutic medications or devices.[188] INR was first used in the early 1980s, when digital subtraction angiography was developed.[194,195] Digital subtraction angiography first uses an original angiograph of the blood vessels to be studied. Then a contrast medium is injected into the same blood vessels, and opaque structures such as bone and tissues can be digitally subtracted or removed from the angiographic image, leaving a clear picture of the blood vessels.[180]

Improvements in vascular access techniques, new thin and flexible catheters and guide wires, and the development of innovative coils and therapeutic medications have made new treatments possible. Conditions that once required extensive surgery, with accompanying patient morbidity and mortality, can now be performed less invasively.[196] Some major procedures performed with INR are mechanical or chemical removal of emboli or thrombi that cause stroke, the physical occlusion of malformed vascular structures such as arteriovenous malformations with chemicals or flow-directed balloons, dilation of stenotic blood vessels, and embolization (blocking blood flow) of cerebral vascular aneurysms using catheter-deployed coils.[196-199]

Box 53-21 lists some current uses for each of the above radiologic and diagnostic procedures. As technology advances, more uses will be seen.

Anesthetic Considerations

Computed Tomography. CT scans require that the patient remain as motionless as possible for several minutes to an hour. Patient motion can produce artifacts in the diagnostic images to be read by the radiologist. Patients must lie on a flat, lightly padded wheeled platform, which is rolled into the short bore scanning gantry of the CT scanner. Although the majority of patients are able to cooperate and tolerate CT, others may not be able because of extremes in age, concurrent medical conditions, or mental disability. The CT scan is neither physically invasive nor painful. Patients enter the CT scanner without precautions for ferromagnetic objects as for an MRI scan. CT is more rapidly performed than an MRI scan, especially if a spiral CT scanner is used.

The patient may require anesthesia anywhere along the continuum from minimal sedation to general anesthesia. Use of ferromagnetic anesthesia equipment and supplies around the CT scanner is not a concern. A standard anesthesia machine, laryngoscope and blades, and intravenous infusion pumps can be used as if in the operating room. An LMA is an appropriate alternative choice as a minimally invasive and secure airway in the patient without contraindications to its use. An LMA is contraindicated in patients with gastroesophageal reflux disease or a full stomach. Attention must be paid to securing the airway, and the anesthesia breathing circuit, the leads for the ECG, the noninvasive blood pressure cuff, the intravenous line, and the pulse oximeter must extend into the scanning gantry. The anesthetist must allow for extra lengths of anesthesia circuitry and electrical monitoring leads because of patient movement that will occur during intermittent repositioning of the mechanized table that positions the patient within the scanning gantry.[194]

Sedation can be performed with a variety of agents, including midazolam, chloral hydrate, pentobarbital, diazepam, or propofol. General anesthesia can be performed with TIVA, such as with intravenous propofol, or with potent inhaled agents.

All personnel must be aware of the use of ionizing radiation during the CT scan and should take precautions to be shielded from any exposure to the radiation. Radiation exposure is cumulative over a lifetime, and every precaution must be made to protect oneself from any unnecessary doses of radiation, which can cause genetic mutation and may lead to cancer. Protection can be accomplished with the use of a lead glass barrier, a lead apron, a lead thyroid collar, and lead-glass safety glasses. Radiation dose badges are available that attach to clothing. The badge monitors the dose of radiation received and is evaluated monthly.[194] Federal technical information and guidelines for working in conjunction with radiation is available from the U.S. Environmental Protection Agency.[200]

ICM can cause an unexpected allergic reaction in some patients, varying from itching with hives to severe, life-threatening anaphylactoid and anaphylactic reactions that have led to

---

BOX **53-21**

Some Indications for Radiologic and Diagnostic Procedures

Computed Tomography
Assessment of the airway with neck or thoracic tumors
Assessment of bony trauma, especially the spine
Assessment of head trauma
Assessment of increased intracranial pressure
Assessment of neoplasms
Imaging of brain tumors
Imaging of intracerebral hemorrhage

Magnetic Resonance Imaging
Central nervous system imaging
Imaging of the blood-brain barrier
Kidney imaging
Liver imaging
Urinary bladder imaging

Interventional Radiology (Vascular and Nonvascular), Radiotherapy, and Radiosurgery
Angiography
Catheterization of ducts, and vascular lesions for drainage of cysts or hemangiomas (e.g., liver hydatid cyst, renal cyst, soft tissue hemangiomas)
Catheterization of tumors for delivery of chemotherapy directly to tumors (e.g., liver tumors)
Embolization or embolectomy or thrombofragmentation of vascular lesions and tumors (pulmonary thrombi or emboli)
Radiosurgery
Stereotactic radiosurgery
Radiotherapy
Transluminal dilation, angioplasty, and stent insertion for vascular stenosis, biliary stenosis, or tracheal malacia

Interventional Neuroradiology
Angioplasty and stent placement for an atherosclerotic lesion
Angioplasty or endovascular ablation of cerebral vasospasm from aneurysmal subarachnoid hematoma
Balloon angioplasty of cerebral vasospasm
Brain arteriovenous malformation embolization
Carotid artery stenting
Carotid cavernous fistula and vertebral fistula treatment
Carotid test occlusion
Dural arteriovenous malformation embolization
Embolization of highly vascularized intracranial tumors
Glomus tumor treatment
Intracranial aneurysm ablation
Juvenile nasopharyngeal angiofibroma treatment
Meningioma treatment
Sclerotherapy of venous angiomas
Spinal cord lesion embolization
Therapeutic carotid occlusion
Thrombolysis of acute thromboembolic stroke
Trigeminal nerve rhizotomy or glycerol injection
Vein of Galen malformation treatment
Vertebroplasty for back pain/vertebral body fractures

Considerations and Treatment Protocols for Preventing Intravenous Contrast Medium Extravasation

Considerations
- Use intravenous catheters (as opposed to metal needles or butterfly needles).
- Avoid use of the same vein if the first attempt at intravenous catheterization was missed.
- Ensure the intravenous catheter is patent and is free-flowing.

Treatments
- Attempt to aspirate as much ICM as possible.
- Elevate the affected limb.
- Apply ice packs for 20 to 60 minutes until swelling resolves.
- A heating pad may be necessary in place of ice for swelling.
- Observe the patient for possible tissue damage related to continual contact with ice or heat.
- Observe the patient for 2 to 4 hours before discharge; consider medical/surgical consultation if necessary.
- Follow up with patient assessing for residual pain, increased or decreased temperature, hardness, change in sensation, redness, or blistering.

Modified from Sum W, Ridley LJ. Recognition and management of contrast media extravasation. Australas Radiol. 2006;50:549-552.
ICM, *Intravenous contrast medium.*

patient death.[181,193,201-204] ICM can also cause renal toxicity, as well as well as local tissue sloughing and necrosis if the ICM extravasates from the vein into the surrounding tissue.[201,205] The anesthetist will be involved with patient care related to ICM extravasation and should be familiar with treatment protocols to minimize patient morbidity (Box 53-22).

ICM is typically a water-soluble, iodine-containing solution of two available types: media that can dissociate into ions in solution and media that will remain in a neutral state in solution. ICM is also formulated as high-osmolar contrast media (HOCM), which contain few dissolved particles and iodine atoms, and low-osmolar contrast media (LOCM), which contain greater numbers of dissolved particles with iodine. An HOCM solution causes fluid shift from the cell to the vein with the ICM, whereas an LOCM solution is closely iso-osmolar, inducing less fluid shift from the cell.[111] Nonionized LOCM is a more costly contrast medium for the patient. Some advocate that it should be the only contrast medium used for CT with dye studies.[201]

Reactions are possible with either type of ICM solution, although fewer reactions occur with LOCM.[201,206] Some reactions may present anywhere from a half hour to a week after the administration of the ICM. Reactions to ICM are theorized to be caused by the ICM molecule's serving as an antigen and affixing itself to either mast cells or basophils. This causes release of mediators such as histamine and tryptase, which can inhibit coagulation, dilate blood vessels, release complement, or even stimulate an IgE-modulated immune reaction.[181,202]

A new ICM using gold nanoparticles is available and undergoing tests prior to use in humans. It has many advantages over iodinated ICM, such as higher radiation absorption, yielding better images with lower x-ray dose; low allergenic response; and longer imaging times due to its nanoparticle size.[207]

A thorough preanesthetic assessment for a patient about to undergo CT should include questions pertaining to asthma,

allergies, and any previous reactions to any contrast media. Other patients at risk for reactions to ICM are patients with multiple medical problems, especially those with cardiac disease or with preexisting azotemia, patients of advanced age, and patients being treated with nephrotoxic agents such as the aminoglycoside antimicrobials gentamicin, tobramycin, streptomycin, amikacin, kanamycin, and neomycin or nonsteroidal antiinflammatory agents. ICM is contraindicated in pregnant patients.[160,201]

Clinicians may use preventive measures in patients who may be at risk for a reaction to ICM. The radiologist should use the smallest amount of contrast agent necessary. To safeguard against the possibility of renal failure, the patient should be adequately hydrated beginning 1 hour before the procedure and continuing for another 24 hours. Patients who are at risk for possible anaphylactoid reactions should be pretreated with corticosteroids such as methylprednisolone or prednisone administered by mouth or intravenously. In cases of moderate or severe previous ICM reactions, a histamine-1 (H_1) blocker such as diphenhydramine and an H_2-blocker such as cimetidine or ranitidine should be given together either intravenously or by mouth.[181,193,201]

ICM is probably the most frequently used agent that causes anaphylactoid reactions. *Anaphylaxis* is an immediate hypersensitivity reaction caused by immunoglobulin E (IgE)–mediated release of pharmacologically active substances that produce signs and symptoms of anaphylaxis. Anaphylactoid reactions produce very similar signs and symptoms but are not mediated by IgE or an antigen-antibody process. Anaphylactoid and anaphylactic reactions are rapidly life threatening and must be promptly recognized and treated (Boxes 53-23 and 53-24). As little as 1 mL of ICM can initiate these reactions. Control of the airway is imperative.

The goals of treatment for anaphylactoid or anaphylactic reaction are to provide an airway, increase heart rate and contractility, and support blood pressure.[159,201,208]

Magnetic Resonance Imaging. MRI can take up to an hour or longer. During this time, the patient must remain extremely still to reduce motion artifacts. These artifacts can cause unfaithful representations of the tissues being studied. The motions of breathing, the heart, blood flow, swallowing, and even cerebral spinal fluid flow produce artifacts in a highly sensitive MRI scan.

Patients must remain within the bore of the magnet for an MRI scan for longer periods of time than for a CT scan. During this time, the MRI suite's ambient temperature is cold.

The patient is exposed to varying magnetic fields of up to 4 T, along with additional exposure to variable radiofrequency radiation. Blood flow is decreased by strong magnetic fields, and blood pressure compensates by rising. Patients also have reported symptoms of vertigo, nausea, headache, and visual sensations.[180]

The MRI machine produces loud vibratory and knocking noises as coils are switched on and off during the course of the study. The size of the MRI magnet bore may preclude the morbidly obese or claustrophobic patient from MRI scanning, although a more open bore MRI is available. Most patients are content with an explanation of what to expect during the procedure and with reassurance. Some patients need minimal or moderate sedation. Patients with claustrophobia or those who cannot or will not remain motionless during the study, as well as critically ill patients, may require deep sedation or general endotracheal anesthesia.[37,180,193,209-211] MRI is not painful, so opioids are not usually required. Sedation has been performed with oral and intravenous midazolam, ketamine, pentobarbital, chloral hydrate, and propofol.[37,202,210,212,213] Minimal sedation

BOX 53-23

Signs and Symptoms of Anaphylaxis

Cardiovascular
- Dizziness
- Malaise/confusion
- Retrosternal pressure
- Diaphoresis
- Hypotension
- Tachycardia
- Dysrhythmias
- Reduced systemic vascular resistance
- Pulmonary hypertension

Cutaneous
- Pruritus
- Burning
- Tingling
- Urticaria (hives)
- Angioedema
- Erythema (redness, flushing)
- Periorbital and/or facial edema

Respiratory
- Nasal stuffiness
- Dyspnea; tachypnea; acute respiratory distress
- Chest tightness; intercostal and/or substernal retractions
- Coughing; sneezing; wheezing
- Hoarseness
- Perioral and/or intraoral edema
- Laryngeal edema; stridor
- Cyanosis
- Reduced pulmonary compliance
- Pulmonary edema

Other
- Aura; feeling of impending doom
- Nausea
- Abdominal pain
- Vomiting
- Diarrhea
- Acute intravascular coagulation

BOX 53-24

Treatments for Anaphylactoid or Anaphylactic Reactions

Remember that this is a crisis situation, and immediate response is imperative.

Mild Allergic Reactions
- Discontinue the causative agent immediately.
- Assess and aggressively manage the airway if necessary.
- Administer diphenhydramine 50-100 mg IV.
- Consider administration of inhaled nebulized epinephrine (Primatene Mist).
- Continuously monitor and document patient vital signs; consider the administration of IV fluids

Moderate to Severe Reactions
- Terminate administration of the causative agent immediately.
- Administer 100% O_2 with ventilatory support.
- Discontinue all anesthetic medications immediately.
- Administer a wide-open massive fluid bolus.
- Administer α-adrenergic agents as necessary to reverse severe hypotension:
  - Epinephrine in 5- to 10-mcg boluses or as an intravenous drip of 0.05-0.1 mcg/kg/min titrated to effect an acceptable blood pressure
  - Norepinephrine drip of 0.5-30 mcg/min IV for systolic BP <70 torr
  - Dopamine 5-15 mcg/kg/min IV for systolic BP 70-100 torr with signs and symptoms of shock
  - Dobutamine 2-20 mcg/kg/min IV for systolic BP 70-100 torr with no signs or symptoms of shock
- Administer bronchodilators as necessary
- Aminophylline 5-6 mg/kg
- Corticosteroids have been shown to have some positive effect in treatment of bronchospasm but have not been shown to be of help in an acute anaphylactoid or anaphylactic reaction.
- Continuously monitor and document patient vital signs

Modified from Bjoraker DG. Anaphylaxis and anaphylactoid reactions. In: Atlee JL, ed. Complications in Anesthesia. 2nd ed. Philadelphia: Saunders; 2007:97-100; Malamed SF. Allergy. In: Medical Emergencies in the Dental Office. 6th ed. St Louis: Mosby; 2007:397-428.

BP, *Blood pressure*; IV, *intravenous*; O_2, *oxygen*.

requires full monitoring. Deep sedation or general anesthesia requires intravenous access and full monitoring.[25] The LMA has served as an excellent, relatively noninvasive airway for MRI. Some anesthesia providers prefer general endotracheal intubation.[37] Children who cannot or will not cooperate experience better MRI scans with general endotracheal anesthesia in shorter periods of time, despite longer recovery times, when compared with sedation.[209-213]

Because of the intense magnetic field always present in the MRI suite, anesthesia providers must be aware of every item on their persons and every item that is to be used in conjunction with anesthesia administered to the patient. Ferromagnetic (iron-containing) substances are attracted at astonishing rates of speed into the bore of the magnet. Personal items such as pens, certain types of eyeglasses, jewelry, watches, pagers, personal computers, calculators, name badges, coins, audiotapes, videotapes, and credit cards are some of the items that should never enter the MRI suite, as well as any ferromagnetic anesthesia equipment,

medication vials, and supplies. If a patient were present within the bore of the MRI, injury or death could be possible from the missile created.[193,214] As newer and more powerful 3T MRI scanners become more prevalent, previously "safe" items could cause injury.[215] Metals known to be safe within the proximity of the MRI bore are stainless steel, nonferrous alloys, nickel, and titanium. Materials and equipment constructed of plastic are safe.[191]

Patients possessing certain medical therapeutic devices may be prohibited from an MRI scan. MRI lists devices or metal that patients may possess that could be affected by the MRI and cause patient morbidity or mortality (Box 53-25).[25,180,182,187,216] Further investigation by the anesthetist in concert with the radiologist or MRI technician regarding the metal content and MRI compatibility of these metal items is necessary.

BOX 53-25

Potentially Harmful Items When in Proximity to MRI

- Automatic implantable cardiac defibrillators (AICD)
- Cardiac pacemakers
- Certain mechanical heart valves
- Cochlear implants
- Deep brain neurostimulators
- Dorsal column stimulators
- Pacing wires
- Penile implants
- Permanent eyeliner or tattoos
- Prostheses (including dental prostheses)
- Implanted pumps (such as baclofen, narcotic, or insulin pumps)
- Internal plates, wires, or screws
- Metallic aneurysm clips (clips manufactured after 1995 and certified MRI compatible can be scanned)
- Certain metallic implants (history of recent orthopedic implants inserted within 3 months, dental implants)
- Metallic sutures
- Shrapnel and metal fragments (especially intraocular metal shrapnel)
- Tissue expanders with metallic ports

MRI; *Magnetic resonance imaging.*

BOX 53-26

List of Available MRI-Compatible Equipment and Supplies

MRI-compatible anesthesia machine
Pulse oximeter
Intravenous bag pole
Liquid crystal temperature monitoring strip
Thermocouple temperature probe with radiofrequency (RF) filter
Respiratory rate monitor
Noninvasive blood pressure monitor
Pulse oximeter
Electrocardiograph
Electrocardiograph patches
Electrocardiograph cable
Capnograph
Laryngoscope with lithium batteries and aluminum spacers
Laryngoscope blades
Nerve stimulator
Intravenous infusion pump
Oxygen tanks
Precordial stethoscope
Esophageal stethoscope
Patient carts
Tables and trays

MRI; *Magnetic resonance imaging.*

Cardiac pacemakers may be effected several ways by the electromagnetic field: reprogramming may occur, the pacemaker may be inhibited, it may revert to an asynchronous mode, it may have the reed switch close, it may become dislodged, or it may become heated by the magnetic field.[184]

Manufacturers have developed a host of MRI-compatible anesthesia equipment and supplies (Box 53-26). This host of equipment and supplies allows performance of the anesthetic procedure directly within the MRI suite. Be aware that some equipment designated by the manufacturer as MRI compatible may not be compatible as magnet strengths increase.[214]

Facilities that cannot afford MRI-compatible equipment and supplies can provide anesthetic services to their patients by inducing anesthesia outside the MRI suite. The patient is placed on an MRI-compatible cart or a detachable MRI scanning table that fits within the bore of the electromagnet, where anesthesia may be then induced. With the aid of extra-long circuits, extension intravenous tubing, and properly insulated monitor cables, the anesthesia can be maintained with full monitors and a standard anesthetic machine outside the MRI suite. The patient is then carefully moved on a flat, relatively hard, wheeled platform into the bore of the electromagnet. Attention should be paid to isolate any monitor leads or intravenous tubing from touching the skin of the patient. Any monitor leads and intravenous tubing should be kept in straight alignment, because the intense magnetic fields in the MRI suite can induce current flow in coiled leads or tubing, and severely burn the patient.[25] Flexible LMAs and endotracheal tubes that contain wire windings can also be sources of burns. The American College of Radiology recommends strong attention to and the elimination of induced current, which can be large tissue loops, such as the loop created by the hand touching the hip or thigh, or the loop created when the feet or calves of the legs touch.[187]

Consideration must be given to the MRI contrast media administered to patients. Fortunately, the dyes used for MRI contrast are nonionic gadolinium chelates and have extremely low allergy rates.[180,185,186] Nausea is a common side effect. Urticaria (hives) and anaphylactoid reactions occur in less than 1% of patients.[185] The risk of a reaction to MRI dye is increased in patients with a history of asthma or other allergies or drug sensitivities, especially to iodinated contrast dyes.[185,186] Proper equipment, medications, and supplies must be immediately available for management of a reaction if one occurs. Treatments for anaphylactoid and anaphylactic reactions are discussed in Box 53-24.

Although MRI does not use ionizing radiation, patients and personnel are exposed to constant levels of magnetic force while in the MRI suite. Acute exposure to magnetic fields under 2.5 T have not been shown to have adverse effects in humans. All care providers must make their own determinations regarding how much magnetic exposure they will accept during a patient's MRI scan. Doses both to the patient and to all personnel should be minimized.[180] Pregnant anesthesia personnel have no restrictions on presence in the MRI scanner room during all of the required anesthesia preparations necessary to treat the patient, but the American College of Radiology recommends that personnel not be present in the MRI scanner room during the scan. Pregnant patients should discuss risks and benefits with their physician.[187]

If the anesthesia provider is away from the patient during the procedure, it should be ensured that all airway circuitry, monitoring leads, and intravenous connections are secure and tight. A respiratory monitoring apparatus (RMA) built into the anesthesia circuit reservoir bag will soon be available to monitor respiration with both visual and audible signals pertaining to movement of the RMA relative to the patient's respiratory rate and tidal volume.[217,218]

When the environment could pose physical danger, anesthetists must be cognizant of their own safety and physical well-being while administering anesthesia for patients, especially during repeated exposures of radiation and/or chemicals. Therefore, a means for remote observation and monitoring either via a clear window, a camera, or telemetry must be available, although controversies regarding the traditional standards of physical presence during the conduct of anesthesia exist.[219-223] In conjunction with recognized standards of safety, the anesthetist must use monitors with both audible and visual alarms and have clear and continual view of the patient and the anesthesia monitors. Consideration must be made for safe and rapid access to the patient should the need exist.[25,224,225]

The functional MRI (fMRI) is a tool used to better differentiate residual pathologic tissue from normal healthy tissue to perform higher quality tumor resection. An fMRI scan requires the patient to remain motionless and cooperative to avoid artifact. It is known that anesthetic agents can alter cerebral blood flow and cerebral oxygen metabolism, which can affect the interpretation of the fMRI scan. Therefore fMRI use for uncooperative or pediatric patients may preclude its use in this cohort of patients. Anesthesia research will provide the anesthetist tools to enable this population to receive both an anesthetic and needed fMRI.[226]

Positron Emission Tomography (PET) Scan. PET scan is used for the imaging and detection of malignant disease, neurologic function, and cardiovascular disease. The isotope fluorodeoxyglucose (FDG) is injected and is then absorbed into metabolically active cells. The absorbed isotope emits minute amounts of positron antimatter, which are detected and produce high-resolution images of diseased tissue.[227] The patient must remain still for about an hour after the injection of FDG to minimize the amount of the amount of muscle uptake of this glucose-like molecule. The patient must have fasted to minimize blood glucose levels. Any sedation medications containing sugar should also be avoided.[227]

New Imaging Techniques. Table 53-5 lists new imaging techniques that may require anesthesia for patients requiring these services in the near future.

Interventional Radiology (Vascular and Nonvascular), Radiotherapy, Stereotactic Radiosurgery, Interventional Neuroradiology. As skills, techniques, and technology progress, more procedures will be performed with radiation or under radiologic guidance.[188,189,195] These procedures all require the absolute immobility of the patient, with periods of controlled apnea, which assist in the viewing or treatment of the targeted area of the patient, especially during whole-body therapeutic radiation treatment.[37,189,228] These procedures are also time consuming, taking up to several hours to complete. Procedures may be necessary in patients of various age groups from infants to geriatrics and in all states of health.[37,188] A thorough preanesthetic assessment is imperative.[188]

With the exceptions of angiography or radiotherapy, procedures for IR are painful, are physically invasive to the patient, and may need to be accomplished over several treatment sessions. Treatment may be required electively or urgently.[37] Patients may require anesthesia along the continuum from minimal or moderate sedation/analgesia, local or regional anesthesia, with the trend moving toward general anesthesia because of the superior image quality obtained in a motionless patient, especially if the patient is held apneic for a brief period of time by the anesthetist.[52,190] Full monitors and intravenous access are required.[38,228,229] Additional catheterization and monitoring of arterial pressure and central venous pressure may be

TABLE 53-5	Emerging Imaging Techniques that May Require Anesthesia Services
Technique	**Uses**
Ultrasound Biomicroscopy	Dermatologic imaging Intravascular imaging Possible dynamic imaging of blood vessel morphology Possible use in study of blood vessel plaque formation Possible use in real-time guidance of microsurgical instrumentation
Micro Single Photon Emission Tomography	Determine the area of myocardial infarction
Combined PET/CT and PET/MRI	Determine recovered function in myocardial tissue treated with local therapy
Near-Infrared Fluorescence Imaging	Observe and examine the morphology and function of blood vessels and myocardial perfusion
Quantum Dots (QD)	Use of semiconductor crystals to tissue graft acceptance or rejection by imaging capillaries and capillary blood flow. Further applications allow QD to enter cells of various tissues for study.

Modified from McVeigh ER. Emerging imaging techniques. Circ Res. 2006;98:879-886.

necessary.[37,188] Certain procedures require monitoring of the patient's neurophysiologic status for changes. The patient may also need to be assessed awake and then resedated at times during the procedure.[37,188,190,228] Anesthetics that can be used are midazolam, propofol, ketamine, isoflurane, and the other potent inhaled general anesthetics.[37,230] Dexmedetomidine, a selective α_2-adrenoreceptor agonist is also being explored for its reduction of intraprocedure and postprocedure anesthetic requirments.[190] To assess and monitor the patient's neurologic functioning, rapid recovery from anesthesia at the end of the case is ideal.[192]

It may be necessary to manipulate or manage normal systemic blood flow, normal cerebral blood flow, or other regional blood flow. The anesthetist may be called on to control deliberate hypertension or deliberate hypotension, manage anticoagulation, and manage unexpected procedural complications.[37,190,221,228]

Intraoperative radiation therapy (IORT) is the delivery of radiation to the patient via a linear accelerator, at times in conjunction with tumor surgery. If surgery is performed coincidental to the dose of radiation, normal tissues may be able to be moved away from the ionizing radiation beam. Normal tissues and organs can be shielded with lead beforehand. Some facilities use a dedicated IORT suite, whereas others use an operating room with transport of the patient to the radiation oncology suite. General anesthesia is performed if the surgical and radiation procedures are concurrent. All personnel must leave the room during IORT and stereotactically guided GammaKnife or CyberKnife surgery so that high-dose radiation can be delivered to the patient while personnel are protected from the scattered radiation. The radiation oncology suite is heavily shielded and has a lead or iron door that can take from 30 to 60 seconds to open. The patient is monitored via closed-circuit video and hands-off anesthesia delivery during treatment.[194]

Complications can occur rapidly and be life threatening. Foremost is the possible complication of hemorrhage. A sedated patient experiencing hemorrhage may show sudden signs of headache, nausea and vomiting, and vascular pain. A patient under general anesthesia may experience sudden bradycardia. The airway must be secured first if necessary, followed by support of the cardiovascular system, discontinuation of heparin, and administration of protamine (1 mg/100 units of total heparin dose administered).[193] Other possible complications are radiocontrast reactions, embolization of particles or tissue, perforation of an aneurysm, and obliteration of unintended physiologically necessary arteries.[37,228] Patient safety necessitates skilled and competent staff assistance in treatment of complications.[229] Complications may necessitate the safe transfer of the patient to the operating room.

Postanesthesia Care

Physiologic stability is the goal in any patient undergoing a radiologic or diagnostic procedure. The patient must be observed for possible reactions to dyes administered by the radiologist. The patient must be relieved of pain. Cardiovascular status must be stable. Hospital admission may be necessary for observation after any complication experienced by the patient or suspected to have occurred. One should always err on the side of patient safety and patient welfare.

REMOTE ANESTHETIC MONITORING USING TELECOMMUNICATIONS TECHNOLOGY

Communications technology in conjunction with reliable and accurate electronic monitoring (telemonitoring) have made it possible to perform anesthetic monitoring with the anesthetist in one location and the therapeutic or diagnostic procedure in another physically remote, geographically isolated, or environmentally extreme environment.

The anesthetist may be involved with communication and monitoring involving land-line telephone, cellular telephone, wireless walkie-talkies, amateur (ham) radio communications, satellite communications, real-time audio and video, computer/monitor interlinks, the Internet, and videoconferencing software.

The purposes of telemonitoring are the benefits to patients requiring therapeutic or diagnostic procedures with the added safety of available expert care to assist the anesthetist in performing anesthesia in a challenging environment. Anesthetists can collaborate and use their combined skills during the entire anesthetic procedure—from preoperative planning to postprocedure care and eventual discharge. Telemonitoring also provides a tool for mentoring and teaching.[231,232]

MORBIDITY AND MORTALITY RELATED TO THERAPEUTIC AND DIAGNOSTIC PROCEDURES

Patient morbidity can occur without careful attention to the standards of care previously discussed. Box 53-27 outlines likely sources of consideration and concern that the anesthetist can

> ### BOX **53-27**
>
> **Anesthetic Considerations and Concerns for Preventing Patient Morbidity and Mortality**
>
> - Small and unfamiliar surroundings for the anesthetist
> - Inadequate access to the patient
> - Lack of adequately trained ancillary personnel
> - Insufficient staffing
> - Insufficient lighting
> - Limited electrical supply
> - Hypothermia
> - Hypovolemia
> - Allergies and/or anaphylaxis
> - Aspiration
> - Airway management difficulties
> - Falls, slips, improper positioning
> - Pain
> - Postprocedure nausea and vomiting
> - Awareness
> - Lack of scavenging of waste anesthetic gases

address to ward off patient morbidity and mortality with proper planning and care. This table summarizes situations that can and have occurred to patients undergoing therapeutic and diagnostic procedures. Some of the considerations listed are based on closed claim reviews.[3] Pediatric considerations surrounding adverse events can be found in Box 53-10.

SUMMARY

New procedures and patient treatments are evolving and moving out of the traditional operating room. This demands evolution of anesthesia providers, equipment, and techniques for the provision of anesthesia services to patients in need of such service. Those providing anesthesia for therapeutic and diagnostic procedures should adhere to the same standards of care in a remote location as they would in the operating room. An anesthetic procedure should be performed only when the provider is absolutely comfortable that all required equipment, medications, and supplies are available, as would be true in a typical, fully equipped operating room. It is easier and safer to prepare beforehand than to gather the items needed for safe anesthesia delivery later or go without them. Cases of minor surgery (patient interventions) exist, but cases of minor anesthesia do not.

ACKNOWLEDGMENTS

For their devoted assistance in the preparation of this chapter, the author would like to acknowledge and thank Anita Schwartz; David Brodsky; Judy Feintuch, MA, MLS; The J. Otto Lottes Health Sciences Library at the University of Missouri, Columbia; Boone Hospital Center Medical Library, Columbia, Missouri; John (Jack) Gay, MD, MPH; Barbara Tellerman, MD; Carol Hoepner; ProDental, Columbia, Missouri; and Heartland Dental Care, Effingham, Illinois.

REFERENCES

1. Leak JA. *Hospital-Based Anesthesia Outside of the Operating Room.* Available at the American Society of Anesthesiologists website: http://www.asahq.org/Newletters/2003/10_03/leakIntro.html. Accessed July 29, 2008.

2. Kotob F, Twersky RF. Anesthesia outside the operating room: general overview and monitoring standards. *Int Anesthesiol Clin.* 2003;41:1-15.

3. Robbertze R et al. Closed claims review of anesthesia for procedures outside the operating room. *Curr Opin Anaesthesiol.* 2006;19:436-442.

4. Saissy JM. Simplified use of mixed propofol and alfentanil for anesthesia in remote locations. *Mil Med.* 2000;165:195-199.

5. Van de Velde M. Pediatric anesthesia and sedation in remote locations. *Acta Anaesthesiol Belg.* 2001;52:187-190.

6. American Association of Nurse Anesthetists. *Standards for Office-Based Anesthesia Practice.* Available at the AANA website: http://www.aana.com/crna/prof/obstandards.asp. Accessed March 19, 2007.

7. American Society of Anesthesiologists. *Guidelines for Office-Based Anesthesia.* Available at the ASA website: http://www.asahq.org/publicationsAndServices/standards/12.pdf. Accessed April 23, 2007.

8. American Society of Anesthesiologists Task Force on Postanesthetic Care. Practice guidelines for postanesthetic care. *Anesthesiology.* 2002;96:742-752.

9. The Joint Commission. *Pre-induction Assessment for Sedation and Anesthesia,* 2005. Available at: http://www.jointcommission.org/AccreditationPrograms/Hospitals/Standards/FAQs/Provision+of+Care/Assessment/Pre_Induction.htm. Accessed April 2, 2007.

10. The Joint Commission. *Labeling Medication for Anesthesia,* 2005. Available at: http://www.jointcommission.org/AccreditationPrograms/Hospitals/Standards/FAQs/Medication+Management/Preparing+and+Dispensing/Label_Med_Anesthesia.htm. Accessed April 2, 2007.

11. The Joint Commission. *Office-Based Surgery Standards Sampler,* 2006. Available at: http://www.jointcommission.org/AccreditationPrograms/Office-BasedSurgery/Standards/standards_sampler.htm. Accessed April 2, 2007.

12. American Society of Anesthesiologists. *JCAHO Compliance Toolkit: Sedation Model Policy.* Available at the ASA website: http://www.asahq.org/clinical/toolkit/sedmodelfinal.htm. Accessed March 24, 2005.

13. American Society of Anesthesiologists. *Standards for Basic Anesthetic Monitoring.* Available at the ASA website: http://www.asahq.org/publicationsAndServices/standards/02.pdf. Accessed June 20, 2007.

14. Gravenstein JS. Safety in anesthesia. *Anaesthetist.* 2002;51:754-759.

15. American Association of Nurse Anesthetists. *Considerations for Policy Guidelines for Registered Nurses Engaged in the Administration of Sedation and Analgesia.* Available at the AANA website: http://www.aana.com/resources.aspx?ucNavMenu_TSMenuTargetID=51&ucNavMenu_TSMenuTargetType=4&ucNavMenu_TSMenuID=6&id=706. Accessed July 31, 2008.

16. Palo Alto Medical Foundation. *Early Disease Detection.* Available at the Palo Alto Medical Foundation website: http://www.pamf.org/health/healthinfo/index.cfm?A=C&hwid=tc4037. Accessed May 21, 2007.

17. American Association of Nurse Anesthetists. *Conscious Sedation: What Patients Should Expect.* Available at the AANA website: http://www.aana.com/forpatients.aspx?ucNavMenu_TSMenuTargetID=68&ucNavMenu_TSMenuTargetType=4&ucNavMenu_TSMenuID=6&id=298. Accessed April 24, 2007.

18. American Association of Nurse Anesthetists. *Consent for Anesthesia Services.* Available at the AANA website: http://www.aana.com/Resources.aspx?ucNavMenu_TSMenuTargetID=51&ucNavMenu_TSMenuTargetType=4&ucNavMenu_TSMenuID=6&id=756#. Accessed April 24, 2007.

19. Dexter F et al. Staffing and case scheduling for anesthesia in geographically dispersed locations outside of operating rooms. *Curr Opin Anaesthesiol.* 2006;19:453-458.

20. The Joint Commission. *Implementation Expectations for the Universal Protocol for Preventing Wrong Site, Wrong Procedure and Wrong Person Surgery.* Available at The Joint Commission website: http://www.jointcommission.org/NR/rdonlyres/DEC4A816-ED52-4C04-AF8C-FEBA74A732EA/0/up_guidelines.pdf. Accessed June 20, 2007.

21. The Joint Commission. *Procedures Requiring Surgical Site Marking.* Available at The Joint Commission website:http://www.jointcommission.org/AccreditationPrograms/Hospitals/Standards/FAQs/Provision+of+Care/Operative_HRP_Sed_Anesth/Surgical_Site_Marking.htm. Accessed June20, 2007.

22. The Joint Commission. *Universal Protocol for Preventing Wrong Site, Wrong Procedure, Wrong Person Surgery.* Available at The Joint Commission website: http://www.jointcommission.org/NR/rdonlyres/E3C600EB-043B-4E86-B04E-CA4A89AD5433/0/universal_protocol.pdf. Accessed June 20, 2007.

23. The Joint Commission. *Frequently Asked Questions About the Universal Protocol for Preventing Wrong Site, Wrong Procedure, Wrong Person Surgery.* Available at The Joint Commission website:http://www.jointcommission.org/PatientSafety/UniversalProtocol/up_faqs.htm. Accessed June 20, 2007.

24. Association of Operating Room Nurses. *Guidelines for Implementing JCAHO Universal Protocol to Promote Correct Site Surgery.* Available at the AORN website: http://www.aorn.org/toolkit/pdf/Laminatecard.pdf. Accessed June 20, 2007.

25. Alspach D, Falleroni M. Monitoring patients during procedures conducted outside the operating room. *Int Anesthesiol Clin.* 2004;42:95-111.

26. McKibban T et al. *Considerations for Policy Development: Unintended Intraoperative Awareness.* Available at the American Association of Nurse Anesthetists website: http://www.aana.com/news.aspx?ucNavMenu_TSMenuTargetID=62&ucNavMenu_TSMenuTargetType=4&ucNavMenu_TSMenuID=6&id=712. Accessed June 21, 2007.

27. Fiedler MA. Thermoregulation: anesthetic and perioperative concerns. *AANA J.* 2001;69:485-491.

28. Insler SR, Sessler DI. Perioperative thermoregulation and temperature monitoring. *Anesthesiol Clin.* 2006;24:823-837.

29. Henrichs BM. Discharge criteria: cognitive functioning, monitoring, and legal and ethical considerations. *Anesth Today.* 2003;14:5-10.

30. Mannino MJ. Legal aspects of nurse anesthesia practice. *Nurs Clin North Am.* 1996;31:581-589.

31. Wiener-Kronish JP, Gropper MA. *Conscious Sedation.* Philadelphia: Hanley & Belfus; 2001:31-43, 45-57, 89-103, 105-115, 135-142.

32. The Joint Commission. *Comprehensive Accreditation Manual for Hospitals. The Official Handbook (CAMH)* PC-41-45. Chicago, IL: The Joint Commission, refreshed core, January 2007.

33. American Society of Anesthesiologists. *Continuum of Depth of Sedation, Definitions of General Anesthesia and Levels of Sedation/Analgesia.* Available at the ASA website: http://www.asahq.org/publicationsAndServices/standards/20.pdf. Accessed June 21, 2007.

34. The Joint Commission. *Permission to Administer Moderate Sedation.* Available at The Joint Commission website: http://www.jointcommission.org/AccreditationPrograms/Hospitals/Standards/FAQs/Provision+of+Care/Operative_HRP_Sed_Anesth/Moderate_Sedation.htm. Accessed June 21, 2007.

35. American Society of Anesthesiologists. *Position on Monitored Anesthesia Care.* Available at the ASA website: http://www.asahq.org/publicationsAndServices/standards/23.pdf. Accessed June 21, 2007.

36. Kaplan RF, Yang CI. Sedation and analgesia in pediatric patients for procedures outside the operating room. *Anesthesiol Clin North America.* 2002;20:181-194.

37. Osborn IP. Anesthesia for diagnostic and interventional radiology. *American Society of Anesthesiologists Annual Meeting Refresher Course Lectures.* 145:pp 1-4, October 2006.

38. Mace SE et al. Clinical policy: evidence-based approach to pharmacologic agents used in pediatric sedation and analgesia in the emergency department. *Ann Emerg Med.* 2004;44:342-377.

39. Kinder Ross A, Eck JB. Office-based anesthesia for children. *Anesthesiol Clin North America.* 2002;20:195-210.

40. Twite MD, Friesen RH. Pediatric sedation outside the operating room: the year in review. *Curr Opin Anaesthesiol.* 2005;18:442-446.

41. Kirby RR et al. *Clinical Anesthesia Practice.* 2nd ed. Philadelphia: Saunders; 2002:1-22.

42. Shankar V, Deshpande JK. Procedural sedation in the pediatric patient. *Anesthesiol Clin North America.* 2005;23:635-654.

43. Levati A et al. SIAARTI-SARNePI guidelines for sedation in pediatric neuroradiology. *Minerva Anestesiol.* 2004;70:675-715.

44. White PF. *Perioperative Drug Manual.* 2nd ed. Philadelphia: Saunders; 2005: 83, 92,371,374.

45. Mason KP et al. Infant sedation for MR imaging and CT: oral versus intravenous pentobarbital. *Radiology.* 2004;233:723-728.

46. Serafini C et al. Anesthesia for MRI in the pediatric patient. *Minerva Anestesiol.* 2005;71:361-366.

47. Sanborn PA et al. Adverse cardiovascular and respiratory events during sedation of pediatric patients for imaging examinations. *Radiology.* 2005;237:288.

48. Cote CJ et al. Adverse sedation events in pediatrics: analysis of medications used for sedation. *Pediatrics.* 2000;106:633-644.

49. Reznik GL et al. *Coping with the Demographic Challenge: Fewer Children and Living Longer.* Available at the United States Social Security Administration Office of Policy website:http://www.ssa.gov/policy/docs.ssb/v66n4/v66n4p37.html. Accessed June 13, 2007.

50. United States Social Security Administration. *Actuarial Publications: Period Life Expectancy.* Available at the USSSA website: http://www.ssa.gov/OACT/TR07?lr5A3.html. Accessed June 13, 2007.

51. Shaughnessy TE. Safe *Sedation of the Elderly Outside the Operating Room.* Available at the American Society of Anesthesiologists website: http://www.a-sahq.org/clinical/geriatrics/safe.htm. Accessed June 21, 2007.

52. Sieber FE, Pauldine R. Anesthesia for the elderly. In: Miller RD, ed. *Anesthesia.* 6th ed. Philadelphia: Churchill Livingstone; 2005:2435-2449.

53. Tonner PH et al. Pathophysiological changes in the elderly. *Best Pract Res Clin Anaesthesiol.* 2003;17:163-177.

54. Guyton AC, Hall JE. *Textbook of Medical Physiology.* 11th ed. Philadelphia: Saunders; 2006:232, 237,250-251,889-901.

55. MGI Pharma. *MGI Pharma Announces Positive Results from a Pivotal Phase 3 Study of Aquavan® Injection in Patient Undergoing Bronchoscopy.* Available at

the MGI Pharma website: http://investors.mgipharma.com/phoenix.zhtml?c=73842&p=irol-newsArticle&ID=1006013&highlight=. Accessed June 25, 2007.

56. Clinical Trials.gov. *A Safety Study of Aquavan® (fospropofol disodium) Injection for Sedation During Minor Surgical Procedures.* Available at the ClinicalTrials.gov website at: http://clinicaltrials.gov/ct/show/NCT00327392?order=1. Accessed June 25, 2007.

57. Welliver M. Update for nurse anesthetists: part 3—cyclodextrin introduction to anesthesia practice: form, function, and application. *AANA J.* 2007;75:(4):289-296.

58. Goldberger JJ. Prevention of sudden cardiac death. *Heart Dis.* 2000;2:305-313.

59. Heilman MS. collaboration with Michael Mirowski on the development of the AICD. *Pacing Clin Electrophysiol.* 1991;14(5Pt 2):910-915.

60. American Heart Association. Highlights of the 2005 American Heart Association guidelines for cardiopulmonary resuscitation and emergency cardiovascular care. *Currents.* 2005;16:1-27.

61. Field JM, ed. The ACLS core cases: VF treated with CPR and AED. In: *Advanced Cardiovascular Life Support Provider Manual.* Dallas: American Heart Association; 2006:34-35.

62. Cummins RO, ed. VF treated with CPR and automated external defibrillation. In: *Advanced Cardiovascular Life Support Provider Manual.* Dallas: American Heart Association; 2002:66.

63. Reynolds MR et al. Sudden cardiac death. In: Fuster V, et al, eds. *Hurst's The Heart.* 12th ed, New York: McGraw-Hill; 2008:1161-1186.

64. Wolpert C, Borggrefe M. The implantable cardioverter defibrillator. In: Fuster V et al, eds. *Hurst's the Heart.* 12th ed. New York: McGraw-Hill; 2008:1109-1120.

65. Olgin JE, Zipes DP. Specific arrhythmia: diagnosis and treatment. In: Libby B et al, eds. *Braunwald's Heart Disease: A Textbook of Cardiovascular Medicine.* 8th eds. Philadelphia: Saunders; 2008:863-932.

66. Weinbroum AA et al. Halothane, isoflurane, and fentanyl increase the minimally effective defibrillation threshold of an implantable cardioverter defibrillator: first report in humans. *Anesth. Analg.* 2002;1147-1153.

67. Franckowiak M, Nader ND. Cardioversion. In: Atlee JL, ed. *Complications in Anesthesia.* 2nd ed. Philadelphia: Saunders; 2007:906-908.

68. Baker GW et al. Electroencephalographic indices related to hypnosis and amnesia during propofol anaesthesia for cardioversion. *Anaesth Intensive Care.* 2000;28:386-391.

69. James S, Broome IJ. Anaesthesia for cardioversion. *Anaesthesia.* 2003;58:291-292.

70. Hubner PJ et al. Simplified cardioversion service with intravenous midazolam. *Heart.* 2004;90:1447-1449.

71. Blaufox AD, Saul JP. Radiofrequency ablation of right-sided accessory pathways in pediatric patients. *Prog Pediatr Cardiol.* 2001;13:25-40.

72. Manolis AS et al. Radiofrequency ablation in pediatric and adult patients: comparative results. *J Interv Card Electrophysiol.* 2001;5:443-453.

73. Etheridge SP. Radiofrequency catheter ablation of left-sided accessory pathways in pediatric patients. *Prog Pediatr Cardiol.* 2001;13:11-24.

74. Kugler JD et al. Pediatric radiofrequency catheter ablation registry success, fluoroscopy time, and complication rate for supraventricular tachycardia: comparison of early and recent eras. *J Cardiovasc Electrophysiol.* 2002;13:336-341.

75. Williams GD. Catheter ablation for arrhythmias. In: Atlee JL, ed. *Complications in Anesthesia.* 2nd ed. Philadelphia: Saunders; 2007:915-917.

76. Erb TO et al. Comparison of electrophysiologic effects of propofol and isoflurane-based anesthetics in children undergoing radiofrequency catheter ablation for supraventricular tachycardia. *Anesthesiology.* 2002;96:1386-1394.

77. Lai LP et al. Usefulness of intravenous propofol anesthesia for radiofrequency catheter ablation in patients with tachyarrhythmias: infeasibility for pediatric patients with ectopic atrial tachycardia. *Pacing Clin Electrophysiol.* 1999;22:1358-1364.

78. Erb TO et al. Postoperative nausea and vomiting in children and adolescents undergoing radiofrequency catheter ablation: a randomized comparison of propofol and isoflurane-based anesthetics. *Anesth Analg.* 2002;95:1577-1581.

79. Waye JD, Williams CB. Colonoscopy and flexible sigmoidoscopy. In: Yamada T, ed. *Textbook of Gastroenterology.* Philadelphia: Lippincott Williams & Wilkins; 2003:2851-2865.

80. Abernethy DR, ed. *Mosby's Drug Consult, 2007.* St Louis: Mosby; 2007:ii-1920, ii-2424-ii-2425.

81. Naughton NN, Cohen SE. Nonobstetric surgery during pregnancy. In: Chestnut DH, ed. *Obstetric Anesthesia.* 3rd ed. Philadelphia: Mosby; 2004:255-274.

82. Leak JA. *Endoscopy, Diagnostic Imaging and Therapeutic Radiation Suites.* Available at American Society of Anesthesiologists website: http://www.asahq.org/Newsletters/2003/10_03/leak.html. Accessed June 25, 2007.

83. Barkun A et al. Commonly used preparations for colonoscopy: efficacy, tolerability, and safety—a Canadian association of gastroenterology position paper. *Can J Gastroenterol.* 2006;20:699-710.

84. Theodorou T et al. Total intravenous versus inhalational anaesthesia for colonoscopy: a prospective study of clinical recovery and psychomotor function. *Anaesth Intensive Care.* 2001;29:124-136.

85. Leslie K et al. Closed loop control of sedation for colonoscopy using the Bispectral Index. *Anaesthesia.* 2002;57:693-697.

86. Soma Y et al. Evaluation of topical pharyngeal anesthesia for upper endoscopy including factors associated with patient tolerance. *Gastrointest Endosc.* 2001;53:14-18.

87. McLure HA, Rubin AP. Review of local anesthetic agents. *Minerva Anestesiol.* 2005;71:59-74.

88. Swaroop VS. Topical pharyngeal anesthesia for upper gastrointestinal endoscopy. *Am J Gastroenterol.* 2000;95:1360.

89. Davis DE et al. Topical pharyngeal anesthesia does not improve upper gastrointestinal endoscopy in conscious sedated patients. *Am J Gastroenterol.* 1999;94:1853-1856.

90. Conlong P, Rees W. The use of hypnosis in gastroscopy: a comparison with intravenous sedation. *Postgrad Med J.* 1999;75:223-225.

91. Draganov P, Cotton PB. Iodinated contrast sensitivity in ERCP. *Am J Gastroenterol.* 2000;95:1398-1401.

92. Raymondos K et al. Evaluation of endoscopic retrograde cholangiopancreatography under conscious sedation and general anesthesia. *Endoscopy.* 2002;34:721-726.

93. Cocking JB et al. Short-acting general anaesthesia facilitates therapeutic ERCP in frail elderly patients with benign extra-hepatic biliary disease. *Eur J Gastroenterol Hepatol.* 2000;12:451-454.

94. Kaddu R et al. Propofol compared with general anesthesia for pediatric GI endoscopy: is propofol better? *Gastrointest Endosc.* 2002;55:27-32.

95. Sabra S et al. Oxygen saturation during esophagogastroduodenoscopy in children: general anesthesia versus intravenous sedation. *J Pediatr Gastroenterol Nutr.* 1999;28:455.

96. Koh JL et al. Experience with an anesthesiologist interventional model for endoscopy in a pediatric hospital. *J Pediatr Gastroenterol Nutr.* 2001;33:314-318.

97. Hammer GB et al. Determination of the median effective concentration (EC50) of propofol during esophagogastroduodenoscopy in children. *Paediatr Anaesth.* 2001;11:549-553.

98. Rich JB et al. Anterograde and retrograde memory in children anesthetized with propofol. *J Clin Exp Neuropsychol.* 1999;21:535-546.

99. Bouchut JC. Deep sedation for upper gastrointestinal endoscopy in children. *J Pediatr Gastroenterol Nutr.* 2001;32:108.

100. Speroff L et al. *Clinical Gynecologic Endocrinology and Infertility.* 6th ed. Baltimore: Lippincott Williams & Wilkins; 1999:1133-1148.

101. Kim WO et al. Effects of general and locoregional anesthesia on reproductive outcome for in vitro fertilization: a meta-analysis. *J Korean Med Sci.* 2000;15:68-72.

102. Tsen LC. Anesthesia for assisted reproductive technologies. *Int Anesthesiol Clin.* 2007;45:99-113.

103. Cunningham FG et al. *Ectopic pregnancy. Williams Obstetrics.* 21st ed. New York: McGraw-Hill; 2001:16, 771, 883-911.

104. Hong JY, Luthardt FW. Comparison of conscious sedation for oocyte retrieval between low-anxiety and high-anxiety patients. *J Clin Anesth.* 2005;17:549-553.

105. Tsen LC et al. Intrathecal low-dose bupivacaine versus lidocaine for in vitro fertilization procedures. *Reg Anesth Pain Med.* 2001;26:52-56.

106. Pellicano M et al. Conscious sedation versus general anaesthesia for mini laparoscopic gamete intra-fallopian transfer: a prospective randomized study. *Hum Reprod.* 2001;16:2295-2297.

107. Martin R et al. Anesthesia for in vitro fertilization: the addition of fentanyl to 1.5% lidocaine. *Anesth Analg.* 1999;88:523-526.

108. Eige S et al. Anesthesia for office endoscopy. *Obstet Gynecol Clin North Am.* 1999;26:99-108.

109. Manski RJ et al. Dental services: an analysis of utilization over 20 years. *J Am Dent Assoc.* 2001;132:655-663.

110. Brown LJ, Lazar V. Dental care utilization: how saturated is the patient market? *J Am Dent Assoc.* 1999;130:573-580.

111. American Dental Association. *The Future of Dentistry.* Chapter 3: 30-76. Available at the ADA website: http://www.ada.org/prof/resources/topics/futuredent/index.asp#future. Accessed June 25,2007.

112. American Dental Association. *Definitions of Recognized Dental Specialties.* Available at the ADA website: http://www.ada.org/prof/ed/specialties/definitions.asp. Accessed June 26, 2007.

113. American Dental Hygienists' Association. *Important Facts About Dental Hygienists.* Available at the American Dental Hygienists' Association website: http://www.adha.org/careerinfo/dh_facts.htm. Accessed June 26, 2007.

114. American Dental Hygienists' Association. *Professional Roles of the Dental Hygienist.* Available at the American Dental Hygienists' website: http://www.adha.org/careerinfo/roles.htm. Accessed June 26, 2007.

115. Haug RH, Reifeis RL. Prospective evaluation of the value of preoperative laboratory testing for office anesthesia and sedation. *J Oral Maxillofac Surg.* 1999;57:16-20.

116. Committee on Research, Science and Therapy, the American Academy of Periodontology. Guidelines: in-office use of conscious sedation in periodontics. *J Periodontol.* 2001;72:968-975.

117. Ghezzi EM et al. General anesthesia protocol for the dental patient: emphasis for older adults. *Spec Care Dentist.* 2000;20:81-92.

118. United States Department of Justice. *Americans with Disabilities Act: Questions and Answers.* Available at the United States Department of Justice website: http://www.usdoj.gov/crt/ada/q%26aeng02.htm. Accessed May 14, 2007.

119. United States Department of Justice. *Americans with Disabilities Act Accessibility Guidelines (ADAAG); Checklist for Buildings and Facilities.* Available at the United States Department of Justice website: http://www.usdoj.gov/adaag/checklist/a16.html. Accessed May 14, 2007.

120. United States Department of Justice. *Americans with Disabilities Act; Survey from 24:Medical Care Facilities.* Available at the United States Department of Justice website:http://www.access-board.gov/adaag/checklist/Medical.html. Accessed May 14, 2007.

121. Malamed SF. *Handbook of Local Anesthesia.* 5th ed. St Louis: Mosby; 2004:55-81, 99-102, 109-117, 123-135.

122. Manley MCG et al. Dental treatment for people with challenging behaviour: general anaesthesia or sedation. *Br Dent J.* 2000;188:358-360.

123. Webb MD, Moore PA. Sedation for pediatric dental patients. *Dent Clin North Am.* 2002;46:803-814.

124. Cote CJ et al. Adverse sedation events in pediatrics: a critical incident analysis of contributing factors. *Pediatrics.* 2000;105:805-814.

125. Rodgers SF. Safety of intravenous sedation administered by the operating oral surgeon: the first 7 years of office practice. *J Oral Maxillofac Surg.* 2005;63:1478-1483.

126. Wilson S et al. A retrospective study of chloral hydrate, meperidine, hydroxyzine, and midazolam regimens used to sedate children for dental care. *Pediatr Dent.* 2000;22:107-112.

127. Bergman SA. Ketamine: review of its pharmacology and its use in pediatric anesthesia. *Anesth Prog.* 1999;46:10-20.

128. Coetzee JF, Coetzer M. Propofol in paediatric anaesthesia. *Curr Opin Anaesthesiol.* 2003;16:285-290.

129. Wilson KE et al. A randomised, controlled, crossover trial of oral midazolam and nitrous oxide for paediatric dental sedation. *Anaesthesia.* 2002;57:860-867.

130. al-Rakaf H et al. Intra-nasal midazolam in conscious sedation of young paediatric dental patients. *Int J Paediatr Dent.* 2001;11:33-40.

131. Jensen B, Matsson L. Oral versus rectal midazolam as a pre-anaesthetic sedative in children receiving dental treatment under general anaesthesia. *Acta Paediatr.* 2002;91:920-925.

132. Moore PA et al. Oral transmucosal fentanyl pretreatment for outpatient general anesthesia. *Anesth Prog.* 2000;47:29-34.

133. Vinckier F et al. Comprehensive dental care for children with rampant caries under general anaesthesia. *Int J Paediatr Dent.* 2001;11:25-32.

134. Al-Eheideb AA, Herman NG. Outcomes of dental procedures performed on children under general anesthesia. *J Clin Pediatr Dent.* 2003;27:181-183.

135. Ganzberg SI, Weaver JM. Anesthesia for office-based oral and maxillofacial surgery. *Dent Clin North Am.* 1999;43:547-562.

136. George JM, Sanders GM. The reinforced laryngeal mask in paediatric outpatient dental surgery. *Anaesthesia.* 1999;54:546-551.

137. Todd DW. A comparison of endotracheal intubation and use of the laryngeal mask airway for ambulatory oral surgery patients. *J Oral Maxillofac Surg.* 2002;60:2-4.

138. Cillo JE. Propofol anesthesia for outpatient oral and maxillofacial surgery. *Oral Surg Oral Med Oral Pathol Oral Radiol Endod.* 1999;87:530-538.

139. Fujii Y et al. Small dose of propofol for preventing nausea and vomiting after third molar extraction. *J Oral Maxillofac Surg.* 2002;60:1246-1249.

140. Leitch JA et al. Patient-maintained sedation for oral surgery using a target-controlled infusion of propofol—a pilot study. *Br Dent J.* 2003;194:43-45.

141. Ganzberg S et al. Remifentanil for use during conscious sedation in outpatient oral surgery. *J Oral Maxillofac Surg.* 2002;60:244-250.

142. Pendeville PE et al. Use of remifentanil in combination with desflurane or propofol for ambulatory oral surgery. *Acta Anaesthesiol Belg.* 2001;52:181-186.

143. Sandler NA, Sparks BS. The use of bispectral analysis in patients undergoing intravenous sedation for third molar extractions. *J Oral Maxillofac Surg.* 2000;58:364-368.

144. Craig DC et al. A sedation technique for implant and periodontal surgery. *J Clin Periodontol.* 2000;27:955-959.

145. Jackson DL, Johnson BS. Conscious sedation for dentistry: risk management and patient selection. *Dent Clin North Am.* 2002;46:767-780.

146. Jackson DL, Johnson BS. Inhalational and enteral conscious sedation for the adult dental patient. *Dent Clin North Am.* 2002;46:781-802.

147. Enever GR et al. A comparison of post-operative morbidity following outpatient dental care under general anaesthesia in paediatric patients with and without disabilities. *Int J Paediatr Dent.* 2000;10:120-125.

148. Arch LM et al. Children choosing between general anaesthesia or inhalation sedation for dental extractions: the effect on dental anxiety. *Int J Paediatr Dent.* 2001;11:41-48.

149. Bridgman CM et al. An investigation of the effects on children of tooth extraction under general anaesthesia in general dental practice. *Br Dent J.* 1999;186:245-247.

150. McComb M et al. The effects of oral conscious sedation on future behavior and anxiety in pediatric dental patients. *Pediatr Dent.* 2002;24:207-211.

151. Koroluk LD. Dental anxiety in adolescents with a history of childhood dental sedation. *ASDC J Dent Child.* 2000;67:200-205.

152. Sadock BJ, Sadock VA. *Comprehensive Textbook of Psychiatry.* 7th ed. Philadelphia: Lippincott Williams & Wilkins; 2000:2503-2515.

153. Nemeroff CB. The burden of severe depression: a review of diagnostic challenges and treatment alternatives. *J Psychiatric Res.* 2007;41:189-206.

154. Eranti S et al. A randomized, controlled trial with 6-month follow-up of repetitive transcranial magnetic stimulation and electroconvulsive therapy for severe depression. *Am J Psychiatry.* 2007;164:73-81.

155. McLoughlin DM et al. The clinical effectiveness and cost of repetitive transcranial magnetic stimulation versus electroconvulsive therapy in severe depression: a multicentre pragmatic randomized controlled trial and economic analysis. *Health Techno Assess.* 2007;11:1-54.

156. Auriacombe M et al. Post-ECT agitation and plasma lactate concentrations. *J ECT.* 2000;16:263-267.

157. Ding Z, White PF. Anesthesia for electroconvulsive therapy. *Anesth Analg.* 2002;94:1351-1364.

158. Holtzheimer PE, Nemeroff CB. Advances in the treatment of depression. *NeuroRx.* 2006;3:42-56.

159. Lee M. Anesthesia for electroconvulsive therapy. In: Atlee JL, ed. *Complications in Anesthesia.* 2nd ed. Philadelphia: Saunders; 2007:903-905.

160. Stoelting RK: *Pharmacology and Physiology in Anesthetic Practice.* 4th ed. Philadelphia: Lippincott Williams & Wilkins; 2006:127-139.

161. Zaidi NA, Khan FA. Comparison of thiopentone sodium and propofol for electroconvulsive therapy (ECT). *J Pak Med Assoc.* 2000;50:60-63.

162. Sa Rego MM et al. The cost-effectiveness of methohexital versus propofol for sedation during monitored anesthesia care. *Anesth Analg.* 1999;88:723-728.

163. Kadoi Y et al. The comparative effects of propofol versus thiopentone on left ventricular function during electroconvulsive therapy. *Anaesth Intensive Care.* 2003;31:172-175.

164. Wagner KJ et al. Guide to anaesthetic selection for electroconvulsive therapy. *CNS Drugs.* 2005;19:745-758.

165. White PF et al. Can the bispectral index be used to predict seizure time and awakening after electroconvulsive therapy? *Anesth Analg.* 2003;96:1636-1639.

166. Lemmens HJ et al. The timing of electroconvulsive therapy and bispectral index after anesthesia induction using different drugs does not affect seizure duration. *J Clin Anesth.* 2003;15:29-32.

167. Nashihara F, Saito S. Preictal bispectral index has a positive correlation with seizure duration during electroconvulsive therapy. *Anesth Analg.* 2002;94:1249-1252.

168. Nishihara F, Saito S. Adjustment of anaesthesia depth using bispectral index prolongs seizure duration in electroconvulsive therapy. *Anaesth Intensive Care.* 2004;32:661-665.

169. Ochiai R et al. Bispectral index as an indicator of seizure inducibility in electroconvulsive therapy under thiopental anesthesia. *Anesth Analg.* 2004;98:1030-1035.

170. White PF et al. Can the bispectral index be used to predict seizure time and awakening after electroconvulsive therapy? *Anesth. Analg.* 2003;96(6):1636-1639.

171. Gajwani P et al. Awareness under anesthesia during electroconvulsive therapy treatment. *J ECT.* 2006;22:158-159.

172. Folk JW et al. Anesthesia for electroconvulsive therapy: a review. *J ECT.* 2000;16:157-170.

173. Kadar AG et al. Anesthesia for electroconvulsive therapy in obese patients. *Anesth Analg.* 2002;94:360-361.

174. Recart A et al. The effect of remifentanil on seizure duration and acute hemodynamic responses to electroconvulsive therapy. *Anesth Analg.* 2003;96:1047-1050.

175. Wajima Z et al. Intravenous verapamil blunts hyperdynamic responses during electroconvulsive therapy without altering seizure activity. *Anesth Analg.* 2002;95:400-402.

176. Lisanby SH et al. Safety and feasibility of magnetic seizure therapy (MST) in major depression: randomized within-subject comparison with electroconvulsive therapy. *Neuropsychopharmacology.* 2003;28:1852-1865.

177. Clemente CD. *Anatomy: A regional Atlas of the Human Body.* Philadelphia: Lea and Febiger; 1975.

178. White PF et al. Anesthetic considerations for magnetic seizure therapy: a novel therapy for severe depression. *Anesth Analg.* 2006;103:76-80.

179. Kosel M et al. Magnetic seizure therapy improves mood in refractory major depression. *Neuropsychopharmacology.* 2003;28:2045-2048.

180. Hobbs G, Mahajan R. *Imaging in Anaesthesia and Critical Care.* London: Churchill Livingstone; 2000:1-10.

181. Howatson-Jones I. Adverse reactions to contrast media. *Prof Nurse.* 2000;15:771-774.

182. Gooden CK, Dilos B. Anesthesia for magnetic resonance imaging. *Int Anesthesiol Clin.* 2003;41:29-37.

183. Berkenstadt H et al. Anesthesia for magnetic resonance guided neurosurgery: initial experience with a new open magnetic resonance imaging system. *J Neurosurg Anesthesiol.* 2001;13:158-162.

184. Gooden CK. Anesthesia for magnetic resonance imaging. *Curr Opin Anaesthesiol.* 2004;17:339-342.

185. Runge VM. Safety of approved MR contrast media for intravenous injection. *J Magn Reson Imaging.* 2000;12:205-213.

186. Runge VM. Safety of magnetic resonance contrast media. *Top Magn Reson Imaging.* 2001;12:309-314.

187. Hushek SG et al. Safety protocols for interventional MRI. *Acad Radiol.* 2005;12:1143-1148.

188. Lai YC, Manninen PH. Anesthesia for cerebral aneurysms: a comparison between interventional neuroradiology and surgery. *Can J Anaesth.* 2001;48:391-395.

189. Watkinson AF et al. Commentary: the role of anaesthesia in interventional radiology. *Br J Radiol.* 2002;75:105-106.

190. See JJ, Manninen PH. Anesthesia for neuroradiology. *Curr Opin Anaesthesiol.* 2005;18:437-441.

191. Young WL. New age neurosurgery: avoiding complications in interventional neuroradiology. *American Society of Anesthesiologists annual meeting refresher course lectures,* 311:pp 1-6, October 2006.

192. Higgins GA. Embolization procedures. In: Atlee JL. ed. *Complications in Anesthesia.* 2nd ed, Philadelphia: Saunders; 2007:912-914.

193. Litt L, Young WL. Procedures performed outside the operating room. In: Stoelting RK, ed. *Basics of Anesthesia.* 5th ed. Philadelphia: Churchill Livingstone; 2007:550-560.

194. Huncke K. Radiation oncology. In: Atlee JL, ed. *Complications in Anesthesia.* 2nd ed. Philadelphia: Saunders; 2007:909-911.

195. Strother CM. Interventional neuroradiology. *AJNR Am J Neuroradiol.* 2000;21:19-24.

196. Nakstad PH. Interventional neuroradiology. *Acta Radiol.* 1999;40:344-359.

197. Wikholm G. Transarterial embolectomy in acute stroke. *AJNR Am J Neuroradiol.* 2003;24:892-894.

198. van der Schaaf IC et al. Endovascular treatment of aneurysms in the cavernous sinus: a systematic review on balloon occlusion of the parent vessel and embolization with coils. *Stroke.* 2002;33:313-318.

199. Lusseveld E et al. Endovascular coiling versus neurosurgical clipping in patients with a ruptured basilar tip aneurysm. *J Neurol Neurosurg Psychiatry.* 2002;73:591-593.

200. United States Environmental Protection Agency. *Technical Reports: Radiation Protection Program.* Available at the USEPA website: http://www.epa.gov/radiation/federal/techdocs.htm. Accessed May 22, 2007.

201. Maddox TG. Adverse reactions to contrast material: recognition, prevention, and treatment. *Am Fam Physician.* 2002;66:1229-1234.

202. Laroche D et al. Anaphylactoid and anaphylactic reactions to iodinated contrast material. *Allergy.* 1999;54(Suppl):13-16.

203. Hong SJ et al. Reactions to radiocontrast media. *Allergy Asthma Proc.* 2002;23:347-351.

204. Nakamura I et al. Cardiopulmonary arrest induced by anaphylactoid reaction with contrast media. *Resuscitation.* 2002;53:223-226.

205. Sum W, Ridley LJ. Recognition and management of contrast media extravasation. *Australas Radiol.* 2006;50:549-552.

206. Webb JA et al. Late adverse reactions to intravascular iodinated contrast media. *Eur Radiol.* 2003;13:181-184.

207. Hainfeld JF et al. Gold nanoparticles: a new x-ray contrast agent. *Br J Radiol.* 2007;80:248-253.

208. Hazinski MF et al. *2000 Handbook of Emergency Cardiovascular Care for Healthcare Providers.* Dallas: American Heart Association; 2000:21.

209. Sutherland P, Platt M. Sedation and general anaesthesia in children undergoing MRI and CT. *Br J Anaesth.* 2000;85:803-880.

210. Malviya S et al. Sedation and general anaesthesia in children undergoing MRI and CT: adverse events and outcomes. *Br J Anaesth.* 2000;84:743-748.

211. Davis C et al. Sedation versus general anesthesia for MRI scanning in children. *Arch Dis Child.* 2000;83:276.

212. Haeseler G et al. Anaesthesia with midazolam and S-(+)-ketamine in spontaneously breathing paediatric patients during magnetic resonance imaging. *Paediatr Anaesth.* 2000;10:513-519.

213. Auden SM. This little piggy went to MRI: the tale of the toe test. *Anesth Analg.* 2001;93:241.

214. Farling P et al. Magnetic resonance compatible equipment: read the small print. *Anaesthesia.* 2003;58:86-87.

215. Feldman JM, Kalli I. Equipment and environmental issues for nonoperating room anesthesia. *Curr Opin Anaesthesiol.* 2006;19:450-452.

216. Gautam HM, Heard CMB. Magnetic resonance imaging. In: Atlee JL, ed. *Complications in Anesthesia.* 2nd ed. Philadelphia: Saunders; 2007:918-920.

217. Schwartz AJ. Randall Pauley and the respiratory monitoring apparatus. *AANA Newsl.* 2003;57:30.

218. Patent Storm. *Respiratory Monitoring Apparatus.* Available at Patent Storm website: http://www.patentstorm.us/patents/5975078-fulltext.html. Accessed April 24, 2007.

219. Kempen PM. Stand nearby in the MRI. *APSF Newsl.* 2005;20:32,36.

220. Flowerdew RM. Radiation prevents presence in room. *APSF Newsletter.* 2006;21:19.

221. ICU patients need careful monitoring in the MRI. *APSF Newsl.* 2006;21:37.

222. DeLeo BC. MRI monitoring done within the room. *APSF Newsl.* 2005;20:57.

223. Martin TW. Radiation therapy removes anesthesia provider from the treatment room. *APSF Newsl.* 2005;20:57.

224. Missant C, Van de Velde M. Morbidity and mortality related to anaesthesia outside the operating room. *Curr Opin Anaesthesiol.* 2004;17:323-327.

225. Melloni C. Morbidity and mortality related to anesthesia outside the operating room. *Minerva Anestesiol.* 2005;71:325-334.

226. Taghon TA et al. Pediatric radiology sedation and anesthesia. *Int Anesthesiol Clin.* 2006;44:65-79.

227. McVeigh ER. Emerging imaging techniques. *Circ Res.* 2006;98:879-886.

228. Hashimoto T et al. Interventional neuroradiology—anesthetic considerations. *Anesthesiol Clin North America.* 2002;20:347-359.

229. Martin ML, Lennox PH. Sedation and analgesia in the interventional radiology department. *J Vasc Interv Radiol.* 2003;14:1119-1128.

230. Munte S et al. General anesthesia for interventional neuroradiology: propofol versus isoflurane. *J Clin Anesth.* 2001;13:186-192.

231. Cone SW et al. Case report of remote anesthetic monitoring using telemedicine. *Anesth Analg.* 2004;98:386-388.

232. Cone SW et al. Remote anesthetic monitoring using satellite telecommunications and the internet. *Anesth Analg.* 2006;102:1463-1467.

ANESTHESIA COMPLICATIONS

Henry C. Talley

The lack of consistent taxonomy and a universal classification for "acceptable risk" during the course of anesthesia complicate the development of a definition for an "anesthetic complication." Any type of anesthesia involves some degree of risk; however, major side effects and complications resulting from the administration of anesthesia are uncommon. Complications and risks depend on many factors: the patient's health, the type of anesthesia delivered, and the patient's response to the anesthetic. It is important to note that not all complications result in actual harm to the patient. A comprehensive review of all complications that may arise during the course of anesthesia is beyond the scope of this text. Therefore, this chapter is limited to a brief discussion of some of the more common complications associated with anesthesia.

The term *prevalence of complications* provides data on the estimated population of people who are managing anesthesia complications at any given time. Prevalence measures are proportions—as such they are dimensionless and must not be expressed as rates. The term *incidence of complications* refers to the annual diagnosis rate, or the number of new occurrences, of anesthesia complications diagnosed each year. Consequently, these two statistics types can differ. A short-lived complication like laryngospasm can have high annual incidence but low prevalence, whereas emergency tracheotomy may have a low annual incidence but high prevalence for "can't ventilate–can't intubate" situations. It is hoped that the anesthetist will become more aware of the potential for complications and remain vigilant throughout the course of anesthesia and surgery.

Many complications that occur during anesthesia cannot be prevented; anesthesia administration is never risk-free. However, rapid identification and aggressive treatment of anesthesia complications may prevent them from leading to irreversible damage and death. From 2001 to 2004, there was overall significant improvement in the death rates following complications of anesthesia care (from 140 per 1000 in 2001 to 122.6 per 1000 in 2004).[1] Although the safety and efficacy of anesthesia have markedly increased over the years, management of the course of anesthesia still relies on the motto: Anesthetic agents are best used where and when they are indicated.

Anesthesia is used for many invasive and noninvasive procedures and requires a complete range of drugs from which an anesthetic plan can be implemented to achieve the desired anesthetic effect. Serious complications of anesthesia are uncommon in people who are otherwise healthy. However, because anesthesia can affect the entire body, complications are likely. Fortunately, most complications of anesthesia are minor and can be managed without difficulty. Proper management of an anesthetic requires high-quality care and vigilance, and a basic working knowledge of numerous physiologic and pathologic states of balance and imbalance are necessary to appropriately treat the cause and consequence of anesthesia-related complications.

EYE INJURY

Eye injury during the perioperative period is a rare but important complication for anesthesia providers. Sixty percent of the total indemnity paid to a group of patients who brought lawsuits against ophthalmologists for complications related to eye injury was for claims involving anesthesia.[2-4] Complications of anesthesia had the highest ratio of indemnification per claim of any type. Blindness was a frequent occurrence, with most occurring during general anesthesia, occasionally under monitored anesthesia care. Complications during the administration of anesthesia for ophthalmic surgery are relatively uncommon, but the losses from these procedures involve significant loss of vision, serious physical disability, or (rarely) death.

Corneal Abrasion

Corneal injury is an infrequent occurrence during anesthesia. The cornea is a tough, transparent, dome-shaped surface covering the eye and serves as a barrier to infection and trauma in this highly-exposed organ. The cornea is a continuation of the sclera, the "white" connective tissue layer of the eye, and consists of five distinct layers: the epithelial layer, Bowman's membrane, stroma, Descemet's membrane, and an endothelium layer. The cornea contains no blood vessels, causing it to remain clear. It covers the iris, and its main function is to focus light into the eye (Figure 54-1). Corneal abrasions are superficial defects of the corneal epithelium. Application of a short-acting topical anesthetic prior to assessment will facilitate an examination. Visual acuity is usually normal unless the abrasion includes the visual axis or if there is considerable edema. There may be miosis caused by ciliary spasm and blepharospasm (marked by an uncontrollable, forcible closure of the eyelids) of the affected eye as a result of photophobia.[5] The cornea may also appear hazy if edema is present.

A corneal abrasion, although infrequent, is the foremost injury after general anesthesia[6,7] and may occur during other types of anesthesia (monitored anesthesia care and major conduction block)[8] when something strikes the eye. For example, while intubating, if the practitioner has an object hanging from the neck (e.g., identification badge, stethoscope), it could scratch the patient's eye, causing an abrasion to the cornea. Corneal injury may also occur if something gets into an uncovered or unprotected eye (i.e., prior to taping the eyes shut during general anesthesia). The substance may lodge under the lid and scratch the corneal surface, causing an abrasion or corneal defect once the offending substance is removed. Corneal abrasions cause tearing, sensations of a foreign body, photophobia, reduced visual acuity, and eye pain. Postoperative corneal injuries can lead to significant morbidity and lost productivity.[2]

Drying of an exposed cornea or patient movement during ophthalmic surgery (e.g., coughing, turning) can lead to abrasion of the cornea, with subsequent poor surgical outcomes. Keratoconjunctivitis sicca, also called *dry eye disease* (DED) and dysfunctional tear syndrome, is a multifactorial disorder of the tear film and ocular surface involving multiple interacting mechanisms.[9] Although recent research has made some progress

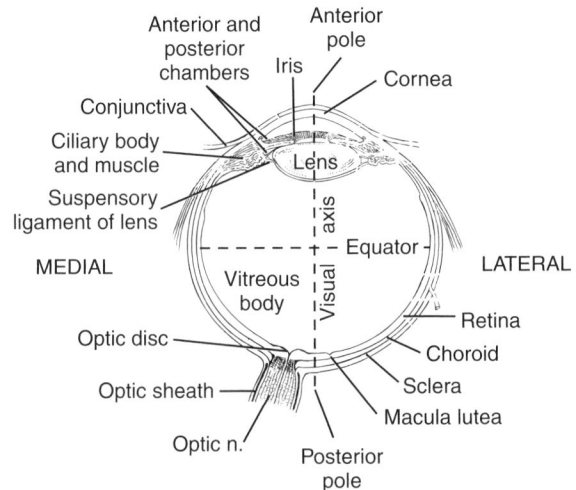

FIGURE **54-1** Cross-sectional view of the ocular globe.

in clarifying DED pathophysiology, presently there are no uniform diagnostic criteria; however, symptoms include eye discomfort, visual disturbance, and often ocular surface damage.

Likewise, pressure on the eye (e.g., prone position, leaning on the face) may result in occlusion of choroidal blood flow and reduction of blood flow to the cornea. Because the cornea contains no blood vessels, oxygen delivery is accomplished through diffusion. As a result, reduced blood flow to the cornea leads to a reduction in oxygen availability, with subsequent corneal edema. Together with the avascular nature of the cornea and a dry environment, pressure leads to desquamation of the epithelium of the eye and corneal abrasion.[2,8]

The diagnosis of corneal abrasion is confirmed by green fluorescence in damaged areas of the cornea seen under a Wood's lamp or cobalt blue light on slit-lamp examination after the application of fluorescein.[5] The treatment of corneal abrasion varies; however, occlusion of the affected eye is often recommended.[10-12] Occlusion of the affected eye is frequently augmented with topical application of antibiotic ointment or nonsteroidal medications. Patching the affected eye has often been embraced; however, in a recent study, patients with traumatic corneal abrasions healed significantly faster, had better compliance, had less pain, and had fewer reports of "blurred vision" when a patch was not worn.[10] Current treatment for corneal abrasions is largely based on theoretic benefit and general consensus.[5,11,12] Primary goals of therapy are pain control, prevention of infection, and rapid healing of the corneal epithelium. Most corneal abrasions heal within 1 to 3 days; however, defects involving greater than half of the corneal surface may require 4 to 5 days to fully heal.[5,13]

Prevention of corneal abrasion is a primary focus during the course of anesthesia. Although no method is guaranteed to be 100% effective, care and vigilance are required to reduce the associated morbidity (Table 54-1) of this disturbing complication.

TABLE **54-1**	Commonly Used Methods to Protect Eyes During General Anesthesia	
Method	**Strengths**	**Weaknesses**
Manual closure	Prevents trauma to globe and lids Prevents injury associated with introduction of agents onto the eye (ointments, tape)	Inappropriate when surgery involves head or neck Incompatible with prone or lateral position; may cause greater harm to the eye
Taping the eyelids	Prevents exposure keratopathy and injury associated with introduction of agents onto the eye	Incorrect placement leads to exposure keratopathy May cause corneal abrasion if tape is placed directly onto cornea Inappropriate when surgery involves head or neck Incompatible with prone or lateral position; may cause greater harm to the eye May cause injury when removing tape at end of procedure
Ophthalmic ointments, methylcellulose, and hydrogels	Equally effective as taping to prevent corneal abrasion Prevents drying of eyes for extended periods Permits continuous perioperative monitoring of eyes during certain procedures	Postoperative sensation of foreign body in some patients Causes blurred vision and confusion in some patients May cause allergic reactions following use of ointments containing methylparaben, chlorobutanol, and other preservatives May require reassessment during long procedures.
Eye shields and pads	Reduces risk of mechanical injury May be used in prone and lateral positions Equally effective as taping and ointments at preventing corneal abrasion	Must include taping eyelids or applying ointment

Blindness

Blindness as a complication of anesthesia during nonocular surgery is a rare but devastating risk and a medicolegal concern for the surgical team (anesthesia provider, surgeon, and nursing staff). The incidence of perioperative blindness ranges from 0.002% of all surgeries to as high as 0.2% of cardiac and spine surgeries.[14,15] Any portion of the visual pathways may be involved, but the most common site of permanent injury is the optic nerve, and the most often presumed mechanism is ischemia.[14,15] With more than 1.2 billion myelinated nerve fibers arising from the cell bodies of cells in the retina, ischemia can be an immense problem, resulting in axonal swelling of these fibers and blindness. In 1999, the American Society of Anesthesiologists (ASA) established the Postoperative Visual Loss Registry (as part of the Closed Claims study) in an attempt to identify risk factors that predispose patients to visual deficits within 7 days after nonophthalmic surgery. Notable risk factors include estimated blood loss of 2.3 L and hematocrit less than 25% (anemia), prolonged venous congestion of the head and neck (i.e., prone position), hypotension and the resulting decrease in oxygen delivery to the optic nerve, advanced age, atherosclerosis, diabetes mellitus, hypertension, morbid obesity, a history of smoking, surgical procedure, and anesthetic technique.[16]

Multiple factors have been proposed as risk factors for perioperative blindness, including spinal anesthesia, prone position (greater than 6 hours), excessive blood loss, hypotension, anemia, hypoxia, excessive fluid replacement, use of vasoconstricting agents, elevated venous pressure, head-down positioning, and a patient-specific vascular susceptibility that may be anatomic or physiologic.[14,15,17]

Treatment and prevention of perioperative blindness, especially as a complication of anesthesia, are difficult. Immediate consultation is imperative for the patient with perioperative blindness. If an obvious ocular cause is not apparent, urgent neuroimaging should be obtained to rule out intracranial pathology.[15] Currently, the pathogenesis of perioperative blindness remains uncertain, and preventive and therapeutic measures remain indefinable. Guidelines for prevention of postoperative vision loss are listed in Box 54-1.

A better understanding of the causes of these two complications of anesthesia, corneal abrasion and blindness, is needed so that anesthesia providers can help prevent their occurrence or reduce the incidence by altering the perioperative management (e.g., avoid prolonged hypotension, protect eyes from trauma and drying) of these complications. Further research is needed to improve our understanding of perioperative blindness and to help clarify the mechanisms of this devastating complication. Furthermore, aggressive treatment of recognized complications will help avoid extending the visual assault.

CARDIOPULMONARY COMPLICATIONS

Progress in perioperative care has become increasingly significant with improvements in pharmacology and monitoring modalities available to anesthesia providers. The Scope and Standards of Practice for anesthetists includes the management of the patient's airway and pulmonary status, as well as continuous monitoring of the cardiovascular status.[18] However, cardiopulmonary mishaps continue to be a significant hazard during anesthesia and complicate patient care.[19-22] Although surgical progress is an important concern during adverse cardiopulmonary incidents, anesthesia providers must carefully consider the risks associated with these occurrences in light of the treatment options available.

BOX 54-1

Anesthesia Guidelines for Prevention of Postoperative Vision Loss

Preoperative Considerations

Identification of Patient Risk Factors
Anemia
Vascular disease: hypertension
Glaucoma
Diabetes
Smoking obesity

Identification of Surgical Risk Factors
Prolonged surgical procedures (>6 hours)
Large blood loss (>40% of blood volume)
Procedures in the prone position
Patient education and informed consent if high-risk patient

Intraoperative Considerations

Blood Pressure Management
Maintain normal range of blood pressures
Avoid prolonged episodes of hypotension and/or hypertension

Fluid Management
Careful titration of crystalloid and blood therapy
Use central venous pressure or pulmonary artery catheters for hemodynamic monitoring in high-risk patients

Management of Anemia
Monitor hemoglobin and hematocrit during surgery
  Large amounts of blood loss
  Borderline preoperative levels
  Consider early transfusion in high-risk patients

Patient Positioning
Avoid pressure on eyes in all positions
Cognizant monitoring and documentation throughout surgical procedure
Maintain head in neutral position avoiding neck flexion, extension, lateral position, or rotation
If possible position the head above the heart to decrease facial edema

Surgical Procedures
Consider length of procedures (<6 hours)
Consider staging surgical procedures if possible for high risk
Consider combination of long surgery, prone position, and large blood loss and increased risk for development

Postoperative Considerations
Assess for occurrence when patient has awakened
Initiate immediate measures if present
  Ophthalmology consult
  Optimize hemoglobin and hematocrit levels
  Maintain hemodynamic stability
  Ensure adequate oxygenation

Modified from Practice Advisory for Perioperative Visual Loss Associated with Spine Surgery. A Report by the ASA Task Force on Perioperative Blindness Anesthesiology. 2006;104(6):1319-1328.

Hypertension/Hypotension

Hypertension and its management have been thoroughly addressed as a topic in Chapter 24; however, hypotension as a possible complication of anesthesia is an ongoing concern to the anesthesia provider. The definition of hypotension is somewhat inconsistent, with ranges of greater than 33%, 30%, 20% and 40 mm Hg reductions in preoperative systolic blood pressure. Anesthesia plan and surgical position may affect cardiac vasculature and influence blood pressure.

Hypotension as a complication of anesthesia may be a result of decreases in cardiac index and stroke volume, with little change in heart rate.[23] It can also be a consequence of obstruction of the inferior vena cava, anesthesia pharmacokinetics, or (often overlooked) pooling during prolonged surgery. Hypotension during the course of anesthesia and surgery is usually self-limiting, but if it is not adequately recognized and corrected when appropriate, it may lead to permanent damage to the vital organs (brain, liver, kidneys) and to the fetus in the pregnant patient.

Hypotension is often associated with hypovolemia and changes in other vital signs and may lead to hypoxia and hypercarbia due to the inability for adequate gas exchange. Hypotension is also a sequel to bradyarrhythmia, tachyarrhythmias, and cardiac arrest. Management of perioperative hypotension varies. Intravenous volume loading, physical interventions like leg wrapping to prevent blood pooling, prophylactic use of vasopressors, and perioperative use of vasopressors have all been used with varying success.[24-28]

It is difficult to infer meaning to the various causes of hypotension as a complication of anesthesia because of the different patient populations that exhibit this problem (i.e., obstetric, elderly, cardiac). For instance, vasovagal syncope is a common type of syncope seen in older patients and is characterized by an exaggerated sympathetic nervous response followed by excessive stimulation of the pneumogastric nerve, resulting in acute blood pressure drops. Most patients with vasovagal syncope have no organic cardiovascular system disease, but they are hypersensitive to autonomic nervous system stimulus.[29] The hallmark of treatment for the patient with hypotension is recognition and definitive support for circulatory and respiratory function to avoid end-organ hypoperfusion.

A better understanding of the causes of perioperative hypotension as a complication of anesthesia will contribute to a decrease in associated crisis interventions (i.e., acute and chronic renal dysfunction, fluid overload) and more effective treatment and better outcomes for surgical patients. Research suggests that prevention of perioperative hypotension substantially decreases the associated complications attributed to this phenomenon.[26,30-32] However, the physiologic consequences of hypotension exhibited by the younger patient are far different from those exhibited by the older patient with preexisting comorbidities.

Cardiac Arrest

In clinical settings, the prevalence of cardiac arrest is somewhere between 300,000 and 400,000 occurrences,[33] with an annual incidence rate of cardiac death reported at 5.6%.[34,35] Cardiac arrest as an anesthesia complication is a constant danger as a result of the compromised physiology and comorbid pathophysiologic processes in populations seen in the operating room for surgery. Table 54-2 summarizes the mechanisms, patient disease/conditions, and surgical factors attributing to cardiac arrest in surgical patients. For this chapter, *cardiac arrest* refers to the abrupt disruption of cardiac function or cessation of effective cardiac pumping as a consequence of ineffective ventricular

TABLE **54-2**	Mechanisms, Patient Disease/Conditions and Surgical Factors Attributing to Cardiac Arrest in Surgical Patients	
Mechanism	**Patient Disease/Condition**	**Surgical Factor**
Cardiovascular Hemorrhage/transfusion Fluid management Arrhythmia Hyperkalemia Embolic episode Pacemaker malfunction	Sepsis/multiorgan failure Trauma (MVA, GSW, stab wound, electrocution) Complications related to CHD	Massive hemorrhage or exsanguination Complications from cardiopulmonary bypass
Respiratory Laryngospasm Obstruction Complication during intubation Inadequate oxygenation Unintended extubation	Pulmonary embolus Perioperative infarction	Ruptured aneurysm (thoracic or abdominal) Complications related to radical procedures for cancer
Medication Inhalation agent Intravenous medication reaction/error		End-stage liver disease/liver transplant complications
Equipment Invasive catheter line Breathing circuit Peripheral IV catheter		

CHD, *Coronary heart disease;* GSW, *gun shot wound;* MVA, *motor vehicle accident.*

rhythm (mechanical or electrical). Recent changes in the American Heart Association guidelines for resuscitation exemplify the heightened readiness anesthesia providers must observe when providing care to patients (Figure 54-2).

Unexplained

Although knowledge of the pathophysiology of cardiac arrest has advanced, unexplained cardiac arrest still occurs in approximately 5% of fatalities of sudden death, indicating that sudden death in the absence of organic heart disease is more common than previously recognized.[36] The lack of standardized criteria to define and diagnose unexplained cardiac arrest does not permit meaningful comparison of data collected by different investigators. However, risk of unexplained cardiac arrest in this population must be addressed by anesthesia practitioners when it occurs. Genetics (e.g., hypertrophic cardiomyopathies are inherited conditions of gene encoding),[37-40] left ventricular function, long–QT-interval syndrome (response to exercise triggers, arrhythmias, and unexplained cardiac arrest),[41,42] and individual health practices are all potential contributors to unexplained cardiac arrest. Cardiac arrest with preserved left ventricular function may result from rare genetic conditions.[43] Risk stratification and extensive preoperative assessment, although impractical, may be valuable in clarifying the etiology of unexplained cardiac arrest.

Many unexplained cardiac arrests may be attributed to vagal predominance. The evidence for a vagal-linked circulatory mechanism for these arrests has been investigated, and the characteristics that are associated with an increased risk for cardiac arrest during certain anesthetic procedures have been identified.[44,45] Unexplained cardiac arrest following neuraxial block has been described as being relatively common.[46-48] Multiple factors may be responsible for cardiac arrest during neuraxial block, but vagal stimulation is the reason that most predominates. Patients prone to increased vagal stimulation (i.e., patients with "vagotonia"), when exposed to circumstances that trigger further increases in vagal activity, are at risk and should be thoroughly assessed for fluid volume balance prior to anesthesia (adequate preload is essential if sympathetic block is anticipated). Likewise, when significant blood loss or the use of vasodilators is anticipated, neuraxial block may not be the technique of choice.[44]

As previously stated, perioperative cardiac arrest data vary, depending on study methodologies. It is therefore difficult to discern whether reports of unexpected perioperative cardiac arrests during anesthesia accurately fault anesthesia as a direct cause or if anesthesia is only a contributing factor.[33,49,50] As a consequence of the concurrent monitoring and pharmacologic environment in the operating room, the manner in which unexpected cardiac arrest is managed during the perioperative period may differ significantly from management outside the operating room and post anesthesia care unit (PACU).

The three most recurrent reasons for cardiac arrest are overdose, hypovolemia and hypoxemia.[21,51-57] The most frequent

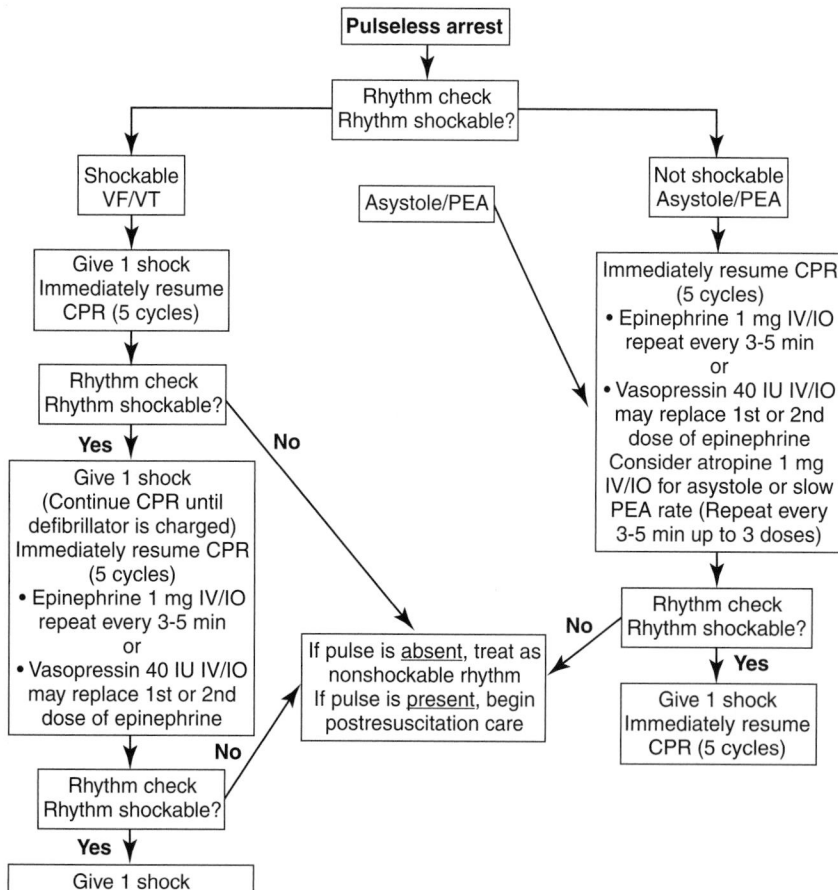

FIGURE **54-2** Algorithm for advanced cardiovascular life support (ACLS) after pulseless arrest. *CPR,* Cardiopulmonary resuscitation; *IO,* intraosseous; *IU,* International Units; *IV,* intravenous; *PEA,* pulseless electrical activity; *VF,* ventricular fibrillation; *VT,* ventricular tachycardia. (*Modified from American Heart Association. Part 7.2: Management of cardiac arrest. ACLS Pulseless Arrest Algorithm. Circulation. 2005;112(24 Suppl):IV58-66.*)

cause of anesthesia-related cardiac arrest is hypoxemia.[58,59] Hypoxemia during anesthesia is usually a result of unrecognized esophageal intubation or inadequate patient ventilation. Each of these causes has as its basis human error. Human error as a cause of anesthesia complications and cardiac arrest is not new.[58-63] Furthermore, most of the anesthesia-related causes of cardiac arrest are preventable, given adequate vigilance and resources. Anesthesia technique, surgical procedure, patient physiology, and pathophysiology all contribute to the possibility of cardiac arrest during anesthesia.

The prevalence of cardiovascular disease in patients undergoing anesthesia and surgery is increasing. This frequency among pediatric patients is greater, reported to be between 1.4 and 4.6 per 10,000.[22] Treatment of unexpected cardiac arrest must be immediate and aggressive to improve patient outcomes.[60,61] As such, overzealous treatment may be detrimental. Hyperventilation of the surgical patient in cardiac arrest increases intrathoracic pressures, leading to decreased coronary perfusion pressures, the inability to adequately diffuse oxygen to the coronary musculature because of the perfusion pressure gradient. The results are decreased perioperative survival rates.

Because the majority of persons who suffer cardiac arrest have coronary heart disease, there is a significant parallel between the epidemiology of cardiac arrest and that of coronary heart disease. Efforts must be made to improve preoperative assessment of the surgical patient as the first line of defense for prevention of this complication. Recognition of potential cardiac disorders during the perioperative period may be addressed during the initial assessment, at which time predisposing factors can be identified. Although cardiac arrest is a devastating event, it can be minimized through proper assessment, adequate resources, and practitioner vigilance.

Airway Management

Management of the airway is a primary focus of anesthesia practice. Several studies have reported that the inability to properly manage the airway contributes to both morbidity and mortality.[62-64] Inadequate control or loss of control of the airway occurs infrequently, and failure to secure an airway is rare. Failure to establish an adequate airway, if it occurs, can be devastating to the anesthesia provider, resulting in severe physical and emotional morbidity and possibly death.[65] An adequate airway, once obtained, must be managed appropriately if the course of anesthesia is to be successful. Although anesthesia management of the airway is understood to be essential to a successful anesthetic, several complications can occur during the management process.

Complications associated with airway management is a well-known cause of anesthesia-related morbidity and mortality.[66-69] Endotracheal intubation is the benchmark against which control of the airway is measured; however, although several recent advances in airway devices have resulted in fewer airway complications, more unusual complications resulting from the use of these devices should be anticipated. Airway management in anesthesia usually begins with face mask ventilation. Mask ventilation is a crucial constituent during induction of anesthesia and in the maintenance of anesthesia if this technique is chosen to deliver the anesthetic. Whereas maintenance of airway patency and oxygenation are the main objectives of face mask ventilation, there are associated complications, including temporomandibular joint (TMJ) subluxation.[70] Potential factors contributing to complications during face mask ventilation include large body mass index (>26 kg/m^2), age (very young and very old),

macroglossia, beard, lack of teeth, history of snoring, increased Mallampati grade, and lower thyromental distance, causing mucosal swelling, skin and eye injury, and in extreme cases, nerve injury and death.[70]

Complications involving supraglottic airway devices and infraglottic airway procedures may include ventilatory impedance, soft-tissue edema, sore throat, cuff pressure (as a result of overinflation) vascular stasis, aspiration and epiglottitis.[71-73] Aspiration is well known to be a potential life-threatening occurrence during airway control. Epiglottitis, although rare and often occurring in children, can also be a life-threatening condition. Acute epiglottitis results from inflammation, usually as a result of infection. The epiglottis and surrounding tissue, including the aryepiglottic folds, the arytenoids, and the supraglottic larynx, are affected.[74-76]

Additional airway-management complications are associated with the more commonly used devices and procedures (laryngoscopy, endotracheal and nasotracheal tube placement). Treatments of these complications are directly related to the precipitating factors causing the complication. In difficult-to-intubate and trauma patients, care must be taken to prevent lip and dental injury, injury to the uvula, arytenoid dislocation and subluxation, and larynx and vocal cord trauma. Although complications occurring during management of the airway are somewhat uncommon, the large investments made to improve control of the airway while decreasing the chances of complications have the accompanying ethical responsibility to continue investigating the causes of complications and reporting the incidences to improve care to the patient awaiting anesthesia.

Laryngospasm

The difficult airway algorithm of the ASA provides recommendations associated with preventing and treating the difficult airway. Laryngospasm, as a separate entity, is not directly addressed in this recommendation. *Laryngospasm* is usually defined as the closure of the glottis as a result of reflex constriction of the laryngeal muscles. It occurs more frequently in pediatric patients than in the general population.[77-79]

Laryngospasm, in its truest form, is accompanied by complete spasmodic closure of the larynx as a consequence of an outside stimulus. Stimuli range from secretions on the vocal cords to tracheal extubation after general anesthesia. Because complete closure of the larynx is not always seen in the clinical area, laryngospasm is usually described as either complete or partial. Complete laryngospasm is accompanied by silent, paradoxical movement of the chest, tracheal tug, and no ventilation. Partial laryngospasm manifests as a "crowing" noise, with a mismatch between respiratory effort and ventilatory effectiveness.[78] General anesthesia can precipitate a laryngospasm as a result of glottic reflex inhibition due to inadequate central nervous system depression and increased stimulation of the larynx from secretions or manipulation.[66,78]

Although the majority of laryngospasms are self-limiting, laryngospasm can sometimes persist and if not appropriately treated result in serious complications and death. Because hypoxia is one of the leading causes of death and neurologic complications related to anesthesia, management of laryngospasm continues to garner interest in anesthesia practice.[78,80] Stridorous respirations, tachypnea, tracheal tug, paradoxical chest movement, and oxygen desaturation are signs and symptoms of laryngospasm.[77,78,80,81] This is a complication of anesthesia that usually occurs during emergence[77,78,80,81]; however, it can also arise during induction and maintenance of anesthesia. Anesthetic technique and airway management may be contributing factors.

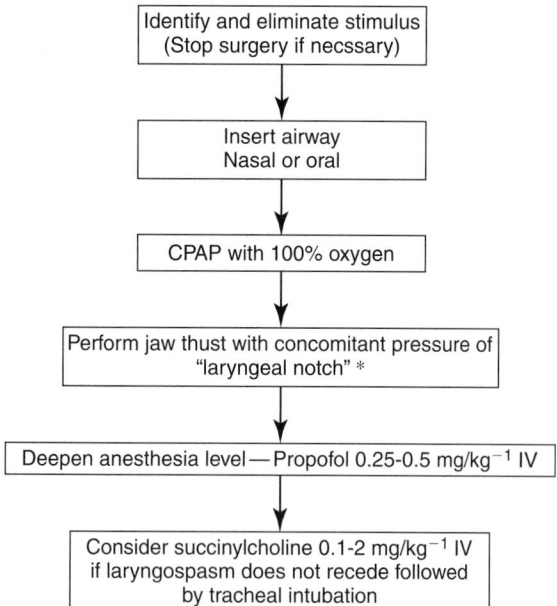

FIGURE **54-3** Algorithm for managing perioperative laryngospasm. CPAP, Continuous positive airway pressure. *The "laryngeal notch" is bounded by the ascending ramus of the mandible anteriorly, adjacent to the condyle; by the mastoid process of the temporal bone posteriorly; by the base of the skull cephalad and just behind the pinna of the ear. If the laryngospasm subsides with any of the above interventions, then no further steps in the intervention will be necessary. If at any time the airway is secured, consider continuing the procedure. If there is no improvement, cardiopulmonary resuscitation (CPR) and advanced cardiovascular life support (ACLS) may be indicated. (*Data from Young ER. Anesthesia and patient risk: the debate continues.* J Can Dent Assoc. 1991;57(9):711-712; *Woodall NM et al. Complications of awake fiberoptic intubation without sedation in 200 healthy anaesthetists attending a training course.* Br J Anaesth. 2008;100[6]:850-855; *and Siddiqi N et al. Interventions for preventing delirium in hospitalised patients.* Cochrane Database Syst Rev. 2007[2]:CD005563.)

During mask induction (especially in pediatric patients), laryngospasm can be easily differentiated from soft-tissue obstruction by using a nasal or oral airway (a nasal airway can also be placed along the side of the tongue into the oropharynx to bypass a mild obstruction). If a partial laryngospasm occurs during induction or emergence, the anesthesia practitioner should first identify and then remove the offending stimulus (remove airway and suction secretions). Continuous positive-airway pressure (>15 cm H_2O) will usually be adequate to resolve a partial laryngospasm, but excessive positive pressure (>40 cm H_2O) may in itself cause laryngospasm. Oxygen at 100% will ensure adequate oxygenation once the laryngospasm is overcome. If the obstruction is not remedied, complete laryngospasm should be suspected, and the practitioner should call for assistance while deepening the anesthetic.[80] Because of its rapid and predictable action, propofol has been shown to have little cardiovascular depression when used in doses of 0.5 mg/kg for treatment of laryngospasm.[80,82] If a subhypnotic dose of propofol is unsuccessful, then a small dose of succinylcholine (0.1 to 3 mg/kg) to treat the obstruction will permit abduction of the vocal cords. This should be followed by mask ventilation and/or tracheal intubation and nasogastric tube placement to decompress the stomach of air from mask ventilation.

There are several ways to reduce or prevent the incidence of laryngospasm, yet no definitive protocol for managing this complication exists. Early recognition and prevention of further complications, including bronchospasm, are essential. Prompt and aggressive intervention is essential when faced with a laryngospasm (Figure 54-3).

Bronchospasm

Anesthesia predisposes the patient to many conditions that have little relationship to bronchial smooth muscle constriction. Bronchospasm is caused by the spasmodic constriction of the bronchial smooth muscle. It usually manifests as prolonged expiration and/or high inflation pressures with intermittent positive-pressure ventilation (IPPV) and expiratory wheezing during anesthesia.[83] Bronchospasm leads to narrowing of airway passages and increases airway resistance. Bronchoconstriction is a result of stimulation of muscarinic receptors or vagus nerve activity,[84] causing exponential changes in bronchial airway lumen diameter because of the relationship between pressure and flow (Poiseuille's law: $R = 8\eta L/\pi r^4$, where r is the radius of the tube, L is its length, and η is the viscosity of the fluid; 8 and π are geometric constants).[85] Therefore, if bronchial airway constriction reduces the lumen by half, there is a 16-fold increase in airway resistance. The American Society of Anesthesiologists Closed Claims study suggests that severe bronchospasm can result in death or brain injury in patients undergoing anesthesia. Bronchospastic disease can lead to bronchospasm; however, many other conditions may mimic bronchospasm during anesthesia (Box 54-2).

Signs and symptoms of bronchospasm include wheezing, decreased breath sounds, increased airway pressures during positive-pressure ventilation, prolonged expiration, and subsequent decrease in oxygen saturation. Carbon dioxide concentration may be reduced due to ventilation-perfusion mismatch. Two percent of the 1991 ASA Closed Claims study cases involved bronchospasm, and 90% of these cases resulted in brain injury or death. A structured approach to discern the causes of bronchospasm and wheezing during anesthesia should be part of the practitioner's diagnosis and management protocol.

Bronchospasm is not confined to patients with a history of severe bronchial hyperreactivity, but patients with a history of hyperreactivity should receive bronchodilators and perhaps be considered for steroids before the induction of anesthesia. As a preoperative precaution, respiratory depressants (narcotics, benzodiazepines, hypnotics) should be avoided, except in patients who are closely monitored. Risk factors include tobacco smoke exposure, asthma, upper respiratory infection, and recent reactive pulmonary symptoms. In 1997, the National Heart, Lung, and Blood Institute's Expert Panel on Asthma suggested guidelines for the treatment of asthmatic patients (Box 54-3). Other preanesthesia interventions include lidocaine (intravenous,

---

BOX **54-3**

Guidelines for the Treatment of Asthmatic Patients

Reduce Impairment
- Prevent chronic symptoms (coughing or breathlessness)
- Infrequent use of inhaled, short-acting β_2-agonist
- Maintain pulmonary function (near normal)
- Maintain normal activity

Reduce Risk
- Prevent recurrent exacerbations
- Minimize need for visits to emergency department
- Prevent progressive loss of lung function
- Prevent reduced lung growth in children
- Provide optimal pharmacotherapy

Gain and Maintain Control of Symptoms
- Severity should dictate medication scheduling
- Level of asthma control should drive therapy

Monitor and Follow Up
- After initiating therapy, monitor every 2-6 weeks
- Regular follow-up contacts should occur every 1-6 months
- Written action plan
- Refer to asthma specialist for consultation or co-management

TABLE **54-3**	Categories of Pulmonary Edema
Type	**Causes and Associated Factors**
Hydrostatic pulmonary edema	Volume overload Left ventricular failure Valvular heart disease Lymphatic insufficiency
Alveolar capillary leak (permeability pulmonary edema)	Systemic inflammatory response syndrome (SIRS) Pulmonary contusion Thermal injury Fat embolism Closed-head injury Infectious agents Near-drowning Inhaled toxins Pancreatitis Drug ingestion Multiple transfusions
Mixed pulmonary edema	Combination of both hydrostatic pulmonary edema and alveolar capillary leak
Neurogenic pulmonary edema	Occurs acutely shortly after a central neurologic insult Presents without preexisting cardiovascular or pulmonary pathology May have a coexisting effect of neurologic insult on myocardial function

nebulized, or intratracheal) and nebulized β-agonists (e.g., albuterol, ipratropium, salbutamol, epinephrine). Even with treatment, bronchospasm may still occur. Slow, careful, meticulous attention to detail in patients with hyperreactive pulmonary disorders is imperative. Use of potent inhalational anesthetics to deepen an anesthetic in these patients may not always be successful and may exacerbate the condition. If a severe bronchospasm occurs, a decision should be made whether to cancel the surgical procedure and awaken the patient or to continue using alternative ventilatory techniques (jet ventilation or surgical airway). The most essential aspect of care for these complications is to prevent laryngospasm and bronchospasm during the course of anesthesia by providing a depth of anesthesia sufficient for airway manipulation, tracheal intubation, and subsequent extubation. If these complications do occur, a complete explanation should be given to the patient regarding the incident. Documentation of the incident in the anesthesia record should be comprehensive, and the patient should be given a MedicAlert bracelet to warn future providers of the occurrence, specifying the precipitating stimulus and subsequent useful actions to resolve the crisis.[83]

Bronchospasm may be a component of other problems (i.e., anaphylaxis) and often includes a variety of different conditions causing wheezing during anesthesia; however, the prototypical conditions that most concern the anesthesia practitioner are chronic bronchitis and asthma. Bronchitis and asthma commonalities include bronchial hyperreactivity to physical, pharmacologic, and chemical stimuli. Both conditions will cause audible wheezing with or without auscultation if gas flow occurs in the patient's airways. Otherwise, in the case of severe bronchospasm, the auscultations are not heard, and the diagnosis relies on proper assessment of increased inflation pressures.[83] Bronchospasm is an anesthetic emergency and requires early recognition and

treatment. Left untreated, bronchospasm will lead to hypoxemia, hypotension, neurologic damage, and death.

Although desaturation is not a definitive sign of bronchospasm, saturation changes are a useful guide in the course of treatment. Desaturation in the anesthetized patient is a call for alarm. Emergency management should include oxygen administration at 100%, request for immediate assistance, and differential diagnosis of the stimulus and pharmacologic intervention when appropriate. Prevention relies on identifying the possible causes of bronchospasm and removing or avoiding the offending stimulus whenever possible.

Pulmonary Edema

Pulmonary edema is a common descriptive term for fluid accumulation within the interstitial or alveolar spaces of the lungs. The causes are numerous, owing in part to disturbances in the normal Starling equation describing fluid exchange through capillary walls.

Equation 54-1

$$J = K_f(P_c - P_i) - (\pi_c - \pi_i)$$

where J is equal to the total transcapillary fluid exchange, K, the capillary hydraulic conductivity, and f, the capillary surface area times the differences between the hydrostatic and oncotic forces between the capillary lumen and interstitial space.[86,87]

The Starling equation (also known as the *Starling-Landis equation*) states that the overall flow of fluid, expressed in units of volume per time in a given mass of tissue is equal to the K_f times the differences between the hydrostatic and oncotic forces between the capillary lumen and interstitial space.[86,87] A high value correlates with fluid filtration from the vasculature into the tissues (transudation), and a low or negative value indicates fluid resorption.[86] Therefore, the Starling equation implies that the combination of increased hydrostatic pressure, increased permeability, and osmotic imbalance together can lead to the development of pulmonary edema.

Pulmonary edema is classified into different categories (Table 54-3). The classic techniques of diagnosis may not be reliable during intraoperative management, but they are important in the perioperative period. They include physical examination, chest radiography, laboratory findings, and CVP monitoring. The underlying pathology is usually low cardiac output or fluid accumulation in excess of the ability of the heart and kidneys to compensate.

Treatment of pulmonary edema ranges from supportive to endotracheal intubation with mechanical ventilation.[88] Because the most common cause revolves around low cardiac output and fluid accumulation, treatment should be aimed at these factors. Perioperatively, central line catheterization (CVP or pulmonary artery catheter) should be considered in poorly controlled patients and those presenting with renal disease or a history of low cardiac output. Fluid administration should be judiciously monitored in these patients as well.

Increased F_{IO_2} to treat hypoxemia, continuous positive airway pressure (CPAP), osmotic or loop diuretics, dobutamine and α-adrenergic blockers have been described as possible treatment options. Prevention includes performing a careful preoperative evaluation to assess and address the extent of the control factors for pulmonary edema.

Negative-pressure pulmonary edema (NPPE) is a rare but life-threatening complication that anesthesia practitioners must be acutely aware of during their clinical practice. NPPE usually results from attempts to ventilate against an acutely obstructed upper airway. It typically occurs immediately after the obstruction is relieved but may be delayed for several hours. NPPE often occurs during the perioperative period when increased negative intrathoracic pressure develops as a result of the obstructed airway (causing increased preload) and is followed by forced expiratory attempts (causing stress failure of capillary membranes). Causes of NPPE during the perioperative period are laryngospasm, endotracheal tube obstruction, spontaneously breathing patients attempting to ventilate against a completely collapsed breathing bag, and postextubation airway compromise.[89-91]

As stated, Starling forces govern the movement of capillary fluids and are usually in balance during normal ventilation as a net result of opposing hydrostatic and oncotic pressures between tissue and capillaries. Changes in these pressures, as would occur once the obstruction is relieved, permits unrestricted increase in venous hydrostatic pressure, transudation of fluid into the alveoli, and the subsequent development of pulmonary edema because of residual exudates remaining in the lungs.

The diagnosis of NPPE during the perioperative period is made on the basis of acute changes in vital signs. Cardinal signs include tachypnea, dyspnea, tachycardia, hypercapnia, hypoxemia, and the production of pink, frothy pulmonary secretions once the obstruction is relieved.[89-91] Treatment of NPPE varies. Because NPPE occurs secondary to acute airway obstruction and changes in oncotic and hydrostatic pressures, usual treatment results with diuretics and positive end-expiratory pressure (PEEP) is uncertain; however, the need to maintain a patent airway, provide airway support, and monitor oxygen saturation is unquestionable.

Pulmonary Embolism

The true incidence of thromboembolic complications is unknown; however, deep vein thrombosis and pulmonary embolism are major causes of morbidity and mortality during surgery, especially in long orthopedic procedures.[92-94] Orthopedic thromboembolic complications usually begin in the lower leg veins as deep vein thromboses (DVTs) and progress proximally to the deep thigh veins before eventually embolizing to the right heart and pulmonary circulation.[92] Orthopedic events differ from arterial thromboembolic and vasoocclusive events in that the former primarily affects the venous system and is associated with endothelial damage, venous stasis, and hypercoagulability (Virchow's triad).[92] It is estimated that DVTs and pulmonary embolisms (PEs) account for more than 250,000 hospitalizations per year in the United States, and PEs account for approximately 200,000 deaths annually and 10% of hospital deaths.[95,96]

Surgical procedures that are prolonged, as in the case of long orthopedic procedures, prevent venous return from the legs via (1) contraction of the calf muscles, which ordinarily propels blood upward from the extremities, and (2) action of the venous valves, which are responsible for preventing pooling in the lower extremities.[94] Long orthopedic cases, in particular, predispose the surgical patient to the development of thrombi by allowing stagnation of the blood, with related limited hypoxia stimulating endothelial cell release of an activator of factor X.[94,97] Furthermore, greater than 90% of thromboemboli begin in the popliteal or iliofemoral veins. Other risk factors include low cardiac output states (congestive heart failure and myocardial infarction), obesity, previous DVTs or PEs, surgery lasting longer that 70 minutes, hypothermia, hypotension, and indwelling central venous catheters.[92] Most thromboembolic complications occur within the first hour to 48 hours postoperatively. Because these embolic complications include high mortality and morbidity risks, prophylaxis is warranted in these patients when possible.

Symptoms of pulmonary emboli include chest pain, tachypnea, dyspnea, anxiety, tachycardia, cough, hemoptysis, and cardiac dysrhythmias.[93,95,96] Therefore, the management of pulmonary thromboembolic complications is primarily supportive, owing to the fact that the differential diagnosis cannot be readily confirmed with any certainty during anesthesia. The purpose of treatment is to preserve cardiopulmonary function.

Surgical patients do not need to concern themselves with aspirin, because other measures are more effective and readily available. In low-risk surgical procedures on patients younger than 40 years of age presenting with no clinical risk factors, the recommendation is that no specific prophylaxis other than early ambulation be used. Measures to support cardiopulmonary function include volume support of right ventricular preload, administration of inotropic drugs, reduction of afterload for the right ventricle, and increasing the fraction of inspired oxygen.[92] If cardiac arrest or persistent hypotension and hypoxemia occur, emergency operative embolectomy requiring cardiopulmonary bypass, bilateral thoracotomy and massage of the pulmonary vessels, interventional radiographic attempts to extract the thrombus, or catheter-directed fibrinolytic therapy may be necessary.[92] The choice of regional anesthesia over general anesthesia to reduce the risk of pulmonary thromboembolic complications is supported by a five-fold decreased incidence of DVT. The most convincing evidence against the use of regional anesthesia during orthopedic surgery concerns the use of heparin and the risk of spinal or epidural hematoma. Likewise, the use of unfractionated or low-molecular-weight heparin during regional anesthesia is questionable because of its long half-life.

There are several well-established protocols for managing adverse cardiopulmonary complications during anesthesia.* Once a complication is recognized, prompt treatment must follow. Most cardiopulmonary complications resulting from anesthesia are unpredictable. However, a thorough preoperative evaluation of the patient's cardiovascular and pulmonary systems is absolutely essential if preexisting or predisposing factors are known or suspected. Prevention of cardiopulmonary complications cannot be certain. However, proper preparation on the part of the anesthesia provider can thwart some of the crisis and help manage associated problems. Every anesthesia provider must have a preformed plan for dealing with complications involving the cardiopulmonary system. Vigilance and attention to detail are crucial in the management and prevention of cardiopulmonary-associated complications of anesthesia.

COGNITIVE IMPAIRMENT

Impairments in cognitive functioning from disturbances in the brain's physiology can easily occur in the surgical patient. Neurologic impairment can be devastating in the postanesthesia patient in terms of quality of life and activities of daily living. Cognitive functioning is a broad construct that includes a number of categories: attention span, concentration, judgment, memory, orientation, perception, psychomotor ability, reaction time, and social adaptability. The assessment of cognitive functioning does not embrace all of these dimensions, but typical screening instruments include many of them and give the clinician an important indication of whether cognitive impairment is present. The prevalence of adverse neurologic impairment in surgical patients often results from organic brain disorders; the most common incidences are confusion, delirium, awareness, and infrequently, coma.

Postoperative Cognitive Dysfunction

The neurobiology of cognition has become increasingly complex as measuring techniques become more sophisticated, and opportunities to explore connections between different areas of the brain are refined.[98] The measurement techniques have led to a better understanding of dysfunctions of cognition during the perioperative period. *Postoperative cognitive dysfunction* (POCD) is of particular interest to anesthesia providers. POCD is characterized by persistent deterioration of cognitive performance after anesthesia and surgery.[99] Conceptually, patients with preoperative cognitive impairment would seem to be most at risk for the development of further cognitive impairment after anesthesia and surgery because they are already compromised, and their potential vulnerability during the postoperative period increases.[98,100]

POCD is often associated with cardiac and orthopedic surgery but can also accompany other surgical procedures.[98,101,102] Cognitive dysfunction in both cardiac and noncardiac surgery has largely focused on older adults, who might have a greater vulnerability to neurologic deterioration as a consequence of the aging process.[99,101-103] Studies on normal aging have shown that abrupt declines in cognitive function in older adults are associated with early death; however, the relation between POCD and mortality has not been reported.[101-103] Although the cognitive effects of anesthesia and surgery in younger adults are poorly understood, the difficulty of determining whether

advancing age is the primary risk factor for this complication supports the need for further exploration.

Confusion

The term *confusion* is used to describe the general affect and behaviors of patients. It is not specific and appears to have a great deal in common with delirium. Both confusion and delirium share one main characteristic: information reception with varying degrees of perception. It is the degree of perception of self and the environment that differentiates the two conditions and makes treatment challenging for the anesthesia provider. Assessment of behavior and discrimination of terms are important for planning appropriate anesthesia care of all patients with any degree of cognitive disorder. Confusion after anesthesia relates to disorders of orientation and is usually a relatively short-lived transient dysfunction of cognition. Confusion after anesthesia is a normal occurrence, and it is suggested that patients refrain from engaging in activities requiring rapid responses for at least 48 hours postanesthesia.

Postoperative Delirium

It was not until the publication of the *Diagnostic and Statistical Manual of Mental Disorders*, 3rd edition (DSM-III), that the core figures of delirium, disturbances of consciousness, and impairment of cognition were brought together.[104,105] Delirium, or acute mental confusion, is transient, often abrupt and fluctuating, typically reversible, and related to increased risk of postoperative adverse reactions (i.e., pulmonary edema, myocardial infarction, respiratory failure, pneumonia, and death), increased length of hospital stay, increased health care costs, and poor functional and cognitive recovery.[106-108] Key symptoms include anxiety, incoherent or disorganized thinking and perceiving, reduced ability to sustain and shift attention to new external stimuli, and agitated behavior. There is sensory misperception, a disordered stream of thought, and difficulty in shifting, focusing, and sustaining attention to both external and internal stimuli. Irrelevant stimuli can easily distract the delirious individual. Also common are perceptual disturbances that result in misinterpretations, illusions, and hallucinations. In addition, disturbances of sleep/wakefulness and psychomotor activity are present. Precipitants are related to physical illness (e.g., cardiovascular disease), infection, hormone disorders, or nutritional deficiencies. Most frequent precipitants are metabolic disturbances, fluid and electrolyte imbalances, drug and alcohol toxicity, and unfamiliar and excessive sensory-environmental stimuli.[109,110] Delirium may be life threatening and is a medical emergency.[111] Delirium occurs in about 20% of elderly surgical patients[112] and is more common in patients undergoing orthopedic procedures (i.e., femoral fractures), with an incidence of 28% to 60% in this surgical population.[103,107] Thirty-two percent of patients who had coronary artery bypass surgery reported postoperative delirium.[113]

Early identification and prompt treatment of the causes of delirium prevent irreversible dementia and death, with interventions targeted to reversing physiologic disturbances and preventing sensory deprivation.[114-119] Limited evidence suggests efficacy for reality orientation, perioperative management of hypoxia and orthostatic hypotension, postoperative pain management, and curtailment of excessive or meaningless stimuli.[117-119]

Most mental status exams are measures of general cognitive impairment. Anesthesia providers are challenged to develop, systematically evaluate, and use nonrestrictive strategies for responding to the behaviors associated with cognitive impairment experienced by older adults in all settings.

*References 60, 61, 77, 80, 81, 93.

Awareness

Awareness, a feared complication of general anesthesia, has been recognized as a complication since 1846, when Dr. William Morton administered ether anesthesia to Gilbert Abbot to remove a tumor from his jaw.[120,121] However, in 1960, Ruth Hutchinson[122] published the pioneer study on the incidence of awareness. During routine postoperative visits, she asked patients about the last things they remembered before and the first things they remembered after their surgery. *Awareness*, the unambiguous recall of events during general anesthesia, reveals incidences of 0.18%[123] and 0.12%[124] in the United States and Europe, respectively. In anesthesia practice, awareness differs from dictionary definitions and its use in psychology-based literature.[125] Malpractice claims for awareness under anesthesia form a relatively small proportion of mismanagement claims, but acute perioperative distress during wakefulness can lead to long-standing, persistent mental symptoms postoperatively. The term *recall*, the ensuing retention of an event after it occurs, is a better description of the phenomenon; however, episodes of awareness are strong predictors of dissatisfaction with anesthesia care.[121,124,126]

There are approximately 40 million anesthetics administered to patients in North America each year. Although the risk of major complications continues to decrease, patients scheduled for anesthesia continues to express concerns surrounding the threat of having perioperative recall or awareness of the operative event.[127,128] For every 1000 adult patients who receive a general anesthetic, as many as 1 or 2 will express the occurrence of awareness or recall, and this figure is higher in children.[123,124,128,129] Inadequate depths of anesthesia may lead to the experience. Accounts rely on patient recollection, and most reports do not include recalling pain during the procedure. Instead, patients report "dreamlike" experiences and auditory remembrance in which they are not in distress. However, reports of intraoperative awareness should be addressed immediately and thoroughly evaluated to obtain information for quality assurance. Furthermore, management of awareness begins when patients are given an opportunity to discuss the causes of the event with the anesthesia provider to gain (1) a clearer understanding of the circumstances surrounding the experience and (2) follow-up consultation. Information gathered from closed claims reports of the ASA suggests that unintentional awareness accounts for roughly 2% of claims against anesthesia providers.[130] The awareness experience is certainly a distressing event and outside normal operative occurrences. These stressful events may lead to nightmares and sleep disturbances, intrusive memories and avoidance behavior, emotional numbing and forgetting, and other diagnostic criteria for posttraumatic stress disorder (PTSD).[121] A study by Sandin[124] identified 18 prospective patients with explicit recall; 9 of the 18 were interviewed 2 years after surgery regarding persistent problems and diagnostic criteria for PTSD.[131] Four of the 9 patients were still severely disabled due to psychological and/or psychiatric symptoms, 3 of these patients had transient mental symptoms that did not disrupt their daily life, and 2 had long-standing psychiatric outcomes.[121] In 2004, The Joint Commission released a Sentinel Event Alert addressing prevention and management of the effect anesthesia awareness has on patients.[132]

The causes of intraoperative awareness are diverse and include factors like chronic medication use, causing tolerance to anesthetic agents, and the hemodynamic instability witnessed in certain procedures associated with hypotension (cardiac surgery, acute trauma, emergency cesarean section). Patients who have liver enzyme induction and the associated effect of the cytochrome CYP 450 system (the cytochrome CYP 450 system is responsible for metabolizing many anesthetic agents) may also be vulnerable to recall under anesthesia.[120,133,134] Awake paralysis, one of the most feared causes (possibly because of the effect Hollywood and the media have on the public and this subject) is possibly the most preventable. Awake paralysis is related to lapses in practitioner vigilance and can lead to out-of-sequence neuromuscular blockade administration and medication error.[130]

Prevention of awareness is the best treatment for awareness. The American Association of Nurse Anesthetists (AANA) has an awareness policy that helps identify at-risk patients and offers measures to address and possibly avoid perioperative awareness[135]:

- During preanesthesia assessment, the risk of awareness should be assessed, and those risks discussed during informed consent.
- Proper function of all anesthesia equipment should be verified to ensure adequate delivery of anesthetic agents to the patient.
- If appropriate, the anesthesia care plan should include pharmacologic agents, anesthesia techniques, and patient monitoring techniques considered beneficial in reducing the incidence of unintended awareness.
- Brain function monitoring, if available, should be considered, particularly in situations in which the risk of intraoperative awareness is increased.
- Patients should be appropriately assessed to identify the possible occurrence of unintended awareness. Any such cases should be promptly managed to minimize the potential for psychological injury.

Although awareness and recall of some of the anesthesia experience are impossible to prevent in all patients, vigilance on the part of the anesthesia practitioner (close attention to monitoring modalities and anesthetic levels) should decrease the incidence substantially. Patients do not routinely convey their concerns about potential recall or awareness during the perioperative period to the anesthesia provider; therefore, providers should never tell patients that they "will be unaware" of any part of the anesthesia or surgical experience. Although some providers may be hesitant to discuss this issue with patients, fearing that patients would then enter the operative experience more apprehensively, evidence that actual awareness or recall is greater in patients who speak openly about awareness and recall is lacking. Awareness and recall are complex constructs. There are several components to recall, and research suggests that just because a patient cannot recount clear details of intraoperative events, this doesn't mean that he or she was deeply unconscious. Also, it is important to remember that under general anesthesia, practitioners should be "aware" of MAC-awake values, as well as the contributions of benzodiazepines and scopolamine in achieving amnesia in high-risk patients (obstetrics, trauma, hypovolemia, and the like). Reassuring patients that everything will be done to keep them safe, comfortable, and amnesic avoids undeliverable promises of the impossible.

Stroke ("Brain Attack")

Cerebral neurons are extremely sensitive to changes in their environment and decreases in oxygen, such as that which occurs during acute cerebral ischemic stroke, a result of a higher basal metabolic rate. This change in cellular environment can lead to transient or permanent injury by affecting the cells' pump function, energy requirements, membrane integrity, or overall cellular surroundings.[136] Stroke caused by acute ischemia during the perioperative period is a particularly cruel and devastating complication depleting many patient, family, and health-care facility resources. *Stroke* has been defined as an acute neurologic deficit that persists for longer than 24 hours. The incidence of acute perioperative ischemic stroke is low and uncommon, whereas the overall mortality is high, with roughly 80% occurring as a consequence of thromboembolic mechanisms. The major causes include combined cardiac procedures, vascular procedures, lacunar or cerebellar infarction, and hemorrhage. Risk factors include male gender, past history of transient ischemic attacks, and cigarette smoking. Perioperatively, the incidence depends mainly on the type and complexity of the surgical procedure.[137] Slightly fewer than half of all perioperative strokes are recognized within the first postsurgical day, and the remaining cases occur after an uneventful postsurgical recovery period, usually from the second postoperative day forward.[94,136-140]

The stress of surgery results in hypercoagulability and activation of the hemostatic system, with a resulting reduced fibrinolysis after surgery.[137] Perioperative withholding of antiplatelet and anticoagulant agents can exacerbate surgery-induced hypercoagulability and add to the risk of perioperative stroke.[137] The neurologic deficit may be mild and transient, often going unnoticed depending on the extent of the infarct. Hemodilution has been suggested as a neurologic protectant in animal studies, but this finding is inconclusive in clinical studies.[139,141-144] Moreover, Reich and colleagues found that specific intraoperative hemodynamic abnormalities were independently associated with stroke.[145] These finding are of particular importance to the anesthesia provider because of the control on intraoperative fluid-volume shifts and hemodynamic variables delegated to the anesthesia provider during surgery, aside from the patient's preoperative risk factors.

The American Heart Association guidelines suggest the use of systemic thrombolysis using alteplase (ft-PA) within 3 hours of the onset of stroke.[38] Although mortality is unchanged, the use of thrombolytic therapy has been shown to support carotid and vertebrobasilar recanalization in approximately 25% of cases when given within 3 hours of symptoms and shown to improve 3-month neurologic outcomes. Intraarterial thrombolysis has not been shown to be better than the intravenous route, and intravenous streptokinase is not indicated for acute ischemic stroke. Stroke in patients with sickle cell disease is often fatal, particularly in children between the ages of 4 and 15 years. There is a 300-fold increased risk of stroke in these patients, making it the most common cause of childhood stroke.[146] Research also suggests that nitric oxide as a treatment for sickle cell–disease stroke may be beneficial because of its ability to improve blood flow and oxygenation as a result of preventing erythrocyte, platelet, and leukocyte adhesion to the vascular endothelium.[147] Nitric oxide for the treatment of stroke is experimental and should be interpreted with caution.

Surgery and anesthesia have been shown to be independent risk factors for the development of acute ischemic stroke perioperatively.[140] Research has shown that a previous stroke is important for the adjusted risk of neurologic injury in men compared with women.[148] Acute ischemic stroke has a high mortality rate, and in certain instances of intractable intracranial hypertension, hemicraniectomy or decompressive surgery of the posterior fossa could be lifesaving.[149] The risk of acute ischemic stroke, or brain attack, continues to be a devastating complication during the perioperative period. Practitioner understanding of the pathologic mechanism of stroke after anesthesia and surgery is vital and requires additional investigation to prevent its occurrence.

OPERATING ROOM FIRE

Fortunately, fires in the operating room are a relatively rare event. Although ether and cyclopropane are no longer operating room hazards, fire in the operating room continues to be a potential perioperative complication. On June 24, 2003, The Joint Commission issued a Sentinel Event Alert related to operating room fires.[150] The alert was issued in response to an alarming number of surgical fires occurring in the United States each year. The classic fire triangle requires the presence of three elements: fuel, ignition source, and oxidizing agent (gas that supports combustion). In 74% of the approximately 100 surgical fires reported in the United States each year, an oxygen-enriched environment (oxidizing agent) was a contributing factor. In all cases that require anesthesia involvement (general, local-MAC, regional), the source of oxygen is historically under the direct control of the anesthesia provider. Of the approximately 100 surgical fires reported each year, approximately 20 cause major thermal injuries; however, one or two of these fires result in death. The most common ignition sources are electrosurgical equipment (68%) and lasers (13%). High-intensity light cords have also been reported to be a source of ignition. The most common locations of these fires are in the airway (34%), about the head or face (28%), and several other areas of the patient's body (38%).

Fuels commonly found in the OR consist of alcohol, solvents, sheets and drapes (cloth and disposable paper), and plastic or rubber materials (including endotracheal tubes). Oxygen is by far the most common oxidizing agent, although nitrous oxide can also support combustion. Materials that are only marginally combustible in air can produce a massive flame in the presence of high oxygen concentration. Lasers and electrocautery devices are the most common sources of ignition.

The entire surgical team (surgeons, anesthesia personnel, and surgical nurses) all have a part in reducing operating room fires. Surgeons generally control the ignition sources; anesthesia personnel generally control the oxidizing agents (air, oxygen, and nitrous oxide); and surgical nurses generally control the fuel source (flammable prep solutions and solvents, sheets, drapes). The simultaneous presence of these three factors (ignition source, oxidizers, and fuel) is needed to initiate a fire.

Fire Precautions and Prevention

The risk of ignition of combustible materials is progressively increased as oxidizing agents build in the operating room. Oxygen levels should be kept as low as can be safely done, and leaks to the ambient air should be kept to a minimum—with special attention to oxygen and nitrous oxide leaks from the anesthesia mask and nasal cannula. Providers should reduce the oxygen concentration when a heat-producing device, such as a cautery unit or fiberoptic light source, is used. Although fiberoptic light is often called "cool light," heat is generated. Excessive oxygen can accumulate under the patient drape or about the operative site, creating an enriched oxygen environment. If a spark is created in these areas, a flash-fire can rapidly spread out of control.

Procedures near the head and neck are more likely to be associated with fires, owing to the frequent presence of enriched oxygen and nitrous oxide. The total oxygen liter-per-minute flow should be kept as low as possible, consistent with the patient's status and response as monitored by standard physiologic monitors, with special attention to the SaO$_2$ values as compared with the patient's baseline values. Avoid petroleum-based ointments in the vicinity of surgery. This would include petroleum-based ophthalmic ointments when surgery is in the vicinity of the face.

When electrocautery is used and open oxygen is administered by nasal cannula, a surgical site above the xyphoid process should be surrounded by cloth towels wetted with sterile water. The wet surgical towels reduce the likelihood of a flash fire being precipitated by cautery. During a well-conducted local-MAC technique, the patient is not necessarily oblivious to his or her circumstances, so fire precautions should be explained to the patient and surgeon in advance of the contemplated procedure.

Obtain and document the patient's baseline oxygen saturation value with pulse oximetry prior to the administration of opioids and sedative drugs and strive to maintain the oxygen saturation value during sedation at a similar value. Administer higher levels of inspired oxygen during the preparation and local anesthetic infiltration if needed, then reduce the inspired oxygen to the lowest possible level consistent with the patient's condition during the use of electrosurgery, electrocautery, or laser units (drills, defibrillators, static electricity).

When surgical drapes are placed over the face (e.g., eye surgery) during local or local-MAC techniques, consider active evacuation of the ambient gases given off by nasal cannulas or face masks. This can be achieved by the placement of a funnel-like collection device that evacuates the gases by way of the hospital suction system. Consider giving an oxygen-air blend to the patient with an FIO_2 of 0.3 or less. This can be done by administering nasal O_2 via O_2 tubing connected with an approximately 5-mm endotracheal tube connector placed at the Y-connection outlet from the circle system anesthesia circuit. In this manner, a mixture of oxygen and medical-grade air can be blended from the anesthesia machine flowmeters while using the oxygen analyzer to regulate the O_2 level of (ideally) 0.3 or less.

The use of an incise drape (clear vinyl drape that is placed over the proposed surgical site so that the incision is made through the clear drape) has been recommended by some sources to keep the oxygen concentrated below the incision. This should not be considered a totally effective method of keeping the oxygen concentration low in the surgical field. Channeling of oxygen can occur through any small opening in the area between the incise drape and the skin. If the oxygen is concentrated below the drape, any breach of the incise drape with an instrument or the electrosurgical cautery tip would have the potential of causing a catastrophic flash-fire below the drapes and directly on the skin. The hot tip of an electrocautery unit laid on a drape can cause ignition of the drapes. The cautery hand unit is placed in its holster when not in use. Activate heat sources only when the tip is in view and deactivate before the tip leaves the surgical site.

During surgical procedures in the head, neck, and upper-chest areas, consider using blended supplemental oxygen/air by use of the anesthesia machine final gas outlet at the Y-piece of the anesthetic circuit. This allows for monitoring FIO_2 by way of the machine's oxygen cell monitor.[151] If possible, stop oxygen administration for a minimum of 1 minute prior to the use of electrosurgical units (cautery).

Arrange drapes to allow ready access to the patient's face to facilitate observation, permit maximal exchange of ambient room air, increase communications with the patient, and have ready access for possible airway manipulations. Oxygen and nitrous oxide are heavier than room air, causing these gases to gravitate down over the patient in a manner similar to that of water poured over a surface. Heavier-than-air gas tends to spread and become concentrated under the drapes. It also contributes to a phenomenon called *surface fiber flame propagation* (SFFP). When oxygen

coats the fine fibers of a surface such as draping fabrics or even the fine facial (vellus) hair and other body hair surfaces, an enriched oxygen environment can cause the flames to rapidly spread by means of these fibers igniting rapidly in the presence of oxygen enrichment. Facial hair or any other hair should be coated with a water-soluble gel if it is in the area of surgery when cautery use is anticipated.

Fire Management

If a fire starts, immediately cut or tear off any burning drapes or other materials from the patient. Water should be readily available to extinguish fire, especially in the mouth or other open body cavities. Because many drapes (especially disposable ones) are liquid resistant, water will tend to bead up rather than soak the material to reduce flame propagation. Water mist extinguishers are also an option for extinguishing a surgical fire. Water mist canisters may decrease the risk of electrocution, because the mist will not pool as readily as water spray. If tearing the material away is difficult or ineffective, use a CO_2 fire extinguisher. Fire blankets should be available to smother flames if they occur. However, if there is a concern that the fire started under a surgical drape due to an oxygen-enriched environment, a fire blanket may not be able to smother the fire, and the fire could actually continue to thermally injure the patient.

Sponges, gauze, pledgets, and strings should be wet and kept moistened when in use in the area of surgery to help prevent airway fires. The anesthesia provider must be ever vigilant to prevent OR fires by treating oxygen and nitrous oxide as potentially dangerous elements in the fire triangle of fuel, ignition source, and oxidizing agent. Patient safety will be enhanced by keeping the oxygen concentration as low as possible consistent with the patient's condition. Displaying prevention reminders, posters, recommendations, guidelines, and information on fire safety where they are readily available for OR staff to read and review emphasizes the importance of vigilance with this potential anesthesia complication.

SUMMARY

Anesthesia involves some degree of risk; however, complications and risks depend on many factors. When complications occur, oftentimes the anesthesia provider is thought to have been associated with a failure to maintain vigilance or with substandard care. Box 54-4 summarizes some of the more common claims associated with substandard care. Recognition and management of complications should be the primary goal of treatment. Successful recognition and management of anesthesia complications are critical elements in the control of anesthesia complications and will prove to be of benefit to thoughtful anesthesia practitioners. The systematic study of complications in anesthesia

---

BOX **54-4**

Claims Associated with Substandard Care

- Failure to monitor properly
- Negligent administration of oxygen
- Leaving patient unattended
- Deactivating monitoring alarms
- Failure to recognize complications
- Medication errors
- Improper charting

began in 1984 with the ASA review of closed medical malpractice claims.[152] If a complication occurs, it is indeed a rare event. As a result, severe morbidity and mortality related to anesthesia have decreased. Vigilance in patient monitoring and evaluation during anesthesia is by far the best way to ward off an anesthesia complication.[75,153] Preventing further harm to the patient is the priority. After an anesthesia complication, particularly when a patient has the potential to be harmed, there are a number of issues to be addressed: the continued care of the patient; thorough documentation of the anesthesia complication; investigation of the causes and other precipitating factors; completion of internal and external reports for quality improvement and root-cause analysis; and consultation with the patient and/or the next

of kin for psychological support, apologies, and expressions of regret. The scope and depth of the follow-up depend on what if any impairment may have ensued. This may constitute completion of an incident report; warning of an equipment failure; consultations with a mental health professional to manage psychological consequences (especially following an awareness or recall incident); or if a death occurred, a full medicolegal debriefing. The most important step in dealing with a complication of anesthesia is to first determine whether the patient has suffered any harm. This harm may be physical or mental, actual or potential[154]; it doesn't matter. The ultimate goal is to make sure that it never happens to anyone else.

REFERENCES

1. Agency for Healthcare Research and Quality. National Healthcare Disparities Report. In: U.S. Department of Health and Human Services AfHRaQ, ed. Rockville, MD: USDHHS; 2007.
2. White E, Crosse MM. The aetiology and prevention of peri-operative corneal abrasions. *Anaesthesia.* 1998;53(2):157-161.
3. Mozaffarieh M, Wedrich A. Malpractice in ophthalmology: guidelines for preventing pitfalls. *Med Law.* 2006;25(2):257-265.
4. Kraushar MF. Medical malpractice experiences of vitreoretinal specialists: risk prevention strategies. *Retina.* 2003;23(4):523-529.
5. Dargin JM, Lowenstein RA. The painful eye. *Emerg Med Clin North Am.* 2008;26(1):199-216, viii.
6. Gild WM et al. Eye injuries associated with anesthesia. A closed claims analysis. *Anesthesiology.* 1992;76(2):204-208.
7. Jordan LM et al. Data-driven practice improvement: the AANA Foundation closed malpractice claims study. *AANA J.* 2001;69(4):301-311.
8. Moos DD, Lind DM. Detection and treatment of perioperative corneal abrasions. *J Perianesth Nurs.* 2006;21(5):332-338; quiz 339-341.
9. Perry HD. Dry eye disease: pathophysiology, classification, and diagnosis. *Am J Manag Care.* 2008;14(3 Suppl):S79-S87.
10. Kaiser PK. Corneal Abrasion Patching Study Group. A comparison of pressure patching versus no patching for corneal abrasions due to trauma or foreign body removal. *Ophthalmology.* 1995;102(12):1936-1942.
11. Kaiser PK, Pineda R II. A study of topical nonsteroidal anti-inflammatory drops and no pressure patching in the treatment of corneal abrasions. Corneal Abrasion Patching Study Group. *Ophthalmology.* 1997;104(8):1353-1359.
12. Turner A, Rabiu M. Patching for corneal abrasion. *Cochrane Database Syst Rev.* 2006(2):CD004764.
13. Aslam SA et al. Emergency management of corneal injuries. *Injury.* 2007;38(5):594-597.
14. Ho VT et al. Ischemic optic neuropathy following spine surgery. *J Neurosurg Anesthesiol.* 2005;17(1):38-44.
15. Newman NJ. Perioperative visual loss after nonocular surgeries. *Am J Ophthalmol.* 2008;145(4):604-610.
16. Nuttall GA et al. Risk factors for ischemic optic neuropathy after cardiopulmonary bypass: a matched case/control study. *Anesth Analg.* 2001;93(6):1410-1416.
17. Sadda SR et al. Clinical spectrum of posterior ischemic optic neuropathy. *Am J Ophthalmol.* 2001;132(5):743-750.
18. American Association of Nurse Anesthetists. *Scope and Standards for Nurse Anesthesia Practice.* Park Ridge, IL: American Association of Nurse Anesthetists; 2007.
19. Bragg K et al. Cardiac arrest under anesthesia in a pediatric patient with Williams syndrome: a case report. *AANA J.* 2005;73(4):287-293.
20. Runciman WB et al. Crisis management during anaesthesia: cardiac arrest. *Qual Saf Health Care.* 2005;14(3):e14.
21. Biboulet P et al. Fatal and non fatal cardiac arrests related to anesthesia. *Can J Anaesth.* 2001;48(4):326-332.
22. Odegard KC et al. The frequency of anesthesia-related cardiac arrests in patients with congenital heart disease undergoing cardiac surgery. *Anesth Analg.* 2007;105(2):335-343.
23. Edgcombe H et al. Anaesthesia in the prone position. *Br J Anaesth.* 2008;100(2):165-183.
24. Alahuhta S et al. Ephedrine and phenylephrine for avoiding maternal hypotension due to spinal anaesthesia for caesarean section. Effects on uteroplacental and fetal haemodynamics. *Int J Obstet Anesth.* 1992;1(3):129-134.
25. Glosten B. Obstetric anesthesia risk: a review of recent literature. *Int J Obstet Anesth.* 1994;3(1):7-12.

26. Morgan P. The role of vasopressors in the management of hypotension induced by spinal and epidural anaesthesia. *Can J Anaesth.* 1994;41(5 Pt 1):404-413.
27. Mulroy M, Glosten B. The epinephrine test dose in obstetrics: note the limitations. *Anesth Analg.* 1998;86(5):923-925.
28. van Bogaert LJ. Lumbar lordosis and the spread of subarachnoid hyperbaric 0.5% bupivacaine at cesarean section. *Int J Gynaecol Obstet.* 2000;71(1):65-66.
29. Han Y et al. Serious response during tilt-table test in elderly and its prophylactic management. *J Zhejiang Univ Sci B.* 2005;6(4):304-306.
30. Cyna AM et al. Techniques for preventing hypotension during spinal anaesthesia for caesarean section. *Cochrane Database Syst Rev.* 2006(4):CD002251.
31. Hofmeyr G et al. Prophylactic intravenous preloading for regional analgesia in labour. *Cochrane Database Syst Rev.* 2004;(4):CD000175.
32. Morioka T et al. Cerebrospinal fluid leakage in intracranial hypotension syndrome: usefulness of indirect findings in radionuclide cisternography for detection and treatment monitoring. *Clin Nucl Med.* 2008;33(3):181-185.
33. Zipes DP, Wellens HJ. Sudden cardiac death. *Circulation.* 1998;98(21):2334-2351.
34. Chugh SS et al. Current burden of sudden cardiac death: multiple source surveillance versus retrospective death certificate-based review in a large U.S. community. *J Am Coll Cardiol.* 2004;44(6):1268-1275.
35. Rea TD et al. Incidence of EMS-treated out-of-hospital cardiac arrest in the United States. *Resuscitation.* 2004;63(1):17-24.
36. Survivors of out-of-hospital cardiac arrest with apparently normal heart. Need for definition and standardized clinical evaluation. Consensus Statement of the Joint Steering Committees of the Unexplained Cardiac Arrest Registry of Europe and of the Idiopathic Ventricular Fibrillation Registry of the United States. *Circulation.* 1997;95(1):265-272.
37. Maron BJ. Hypertrophic cardiomyopathy. *Lancet.* 1997;350(9071):127-133.
38. Spirito P et al. The management of hypertrophic cardiomyopathy. *N Engl J Med.* 1997;336(11):775-785.
39. Adabag AS et al. Occurrence and frequency of arrhythmias in hypertrophic cardiomyopathy in relation to delayed enhancement on cardiovascular magnetic resonance. *J Am Coll Cardiol.* 2008;51(14):1369-1374.
40. Maron BJ et al. Sudden cardiac arrest in hypertrophic cardiomyopathy in the absence of conventional criteria for high risk status. *Am J Cardiol.* 2008;101(4):544-547.
41. Roden DM. Clinical practice. Long-QT syndrome. *N Engl J Med.* 2008;358(2):169-176.
42. Patel C et al. A rare cause of 2:1 AV block: long QT syndrome. *J Cardiovasc Electrophysiol.* 2008;Feb 12 [Epub]. PMID: 18284491.
43. Krahn AD et al. Diagnosis of unexplained cardiac arrest: role of adrenaline and procainamide infusion. *Circulation.* 2005;112(15):2228-2234.
44. Pollard JB. Cardiac arrest during spinal anesthesia: common mechanisms and strategies for prevention. *Anesth Analg.* 2001;92(1):252-256.
45. Pollard JB. Common mechanisms and strategies for prevention and treatment of cardiac arrest during epidural anesthesia. *J Clin Anesth.* 2002;14(1):52-56.
46. Caplan RA et al. Unexpected cardiac arrest during spinal anesthesia: a closed claims analysis of predisposing factors. *Anesthesiology.* 1988;68(1):5-11.
47. Geffin B, Shapiro L. Sinus bradycardia and asystole during spinal and epidural anesthesia: a report of 13 cases. *J Clin Anesth.* 1998;10(4):278-285.
48. Joshi GP et al. Ruptured aortic aneurysm and cardiac arrest associated with spinal anesthesia. *Anesthesiology.* 1997;86(1):244-247.
49. Newland MC et al. Anesthetic-related cardiac arrest and its mortality: a report covering 72,959 anesthetics over 10 years from a US teaching hospital. *Anesthesiology.* 2002;97(1):108-115.

50. Sawasdiwipachai P et al. Cardiac arrest after neuromuscular blockade reversal in a heart transplant infant. *Anesthesiology.* 2007;107(4):663-665.

51. Young ER. Anesthesia and patient risk: the debate continues. *J Can Dent Assoc.* 1991;57(9):711-712.

52. Zanette G et al. Cardiac arrest during continuous psoas compartment block for hip surgery. *Anaesth Intensive Care.* 2007;35(1):143-144.

53. Sprung J et al. Predictors of survival following cardiac arrest in patients undergoing noncardiac surgery: a study of 518,294 patients at a tertiary referral center. *Anesthesiology.* 2003;99(2):259-269.

54. Posner KL et al. Unexpected cardiac arrest among children during surgery, a North American registry to elucidate the incidence and causes of anesthesia related cardiac arrest. *Qual Saf Health Care.* 2002;11(3):252-257.

55. Barreiro G et al. Unexpected cardiac arrest in spinal anaesthesia. *Acta Anaesthesiol Belg.* 2006;57(4):365-370.

56. Bhananker SM et al. Anesthesia-related cardiac arrest in children: update from the Pediatric Perioperative Cardiac Arrest Registry. *Anesth Analg.* 2007;105(2):344-350.

57. Keenan RL, Boyan CP. Cardiac arrest due to anesthesia. A study of incidence and causes. *Jama.* 1985;253(16):2373-2377.

58. Eti Z et al. An uncommon complication of thoracic epidural anesthesia: pleural puncture. *Anesth Analg.* 2005;100(5):1540-1541.

59. Jagadeesan J et al. Ventricular standstill: a complication of intrapleural anesthesia using bupivacaine in a patient with free transverse rectus abdominus myocutaneous flap breast reconstruction. *Ann Plast Surg.* 2007;59(4):445-446.

60. Bell DD et al. Management following resuscitation from cardiac arrest: recommendations from the 2003 Rocky Mountain Critical Care Conference. *Can J Anaesth.* 2005;52(3):309-322.

61. Kaluski E et al. Management of cardiac arrest in 2005: an update. *Isr Med Assoc J.* 2005;7(9):589-594.

62. Gentleman D, Jennett B. Hazards of inter-hospital transfer of comatose head-injured patients. *Lancet.* 1981;2(8251):853-854.

63. Hussain LM, Redmond AD. Are pre-hospital deaths from accidental injury preventable? *BMJ.* 1994;308(6936):1077-1080.

64. von Ungern-Sternberg BS et al. Laryngeal mask airway and children's risk of perioperative respiratory complications: randomized controlled studies are required to discriminate cause and effect. *Anesthesiology.* 2008;108(6):1155.

65. Vasdev GM et al. Management of the difficult and failed airway in obstetric anesthesia. *J Anesth.* 2008;22(1):38-48.

66. Flick RP et al. Risk factors for laryngospasm in children during general anesthesia. *Paediatr Anaesth.* 2008;18(4):289-296.

67. Hove LD et al. Analysis of deaths related to anesthesia in the period 1996-2004 from closed claims registered by the Danish Patient Insurance Association. *Anesthesiology.* 2007;106(4):675-680.

68. Mhyre JM et al. A series of anesthesia-related maternal deaths in Michigan, 1985-2003. *Anesthesiology.* 2007;106(6):1096-1104.

69. Woodall NM et al. Complications of awake fibreoptic intubation without sedation in 200 healthy anaesthetists attending a training course. *Br J Anaesth.* 2008;100(6):850-855.

70. Ovassapian A et al. The unexpected difficult airway and lingual tonsil hyperplasia: a case series and a review of the literature. *Anesthesiology.* 2002;97(1):124-132.

71. Abdi W et al. Evidence of pulmonary aspiration during difficult airway management of a morbidly obese patient with the LMA CTrach. *Br J Anaesth.* 2008;100(2):275-277.

72. Kubo K et al. An unusual case of airway obstruction at the tip of an endotracheal tube caused by insertion of a nasogastric tube. *J Anesth.* 2008;22(1):52-54.

73. Ozdemir Kol I et al. Open-label, prospective, randomized comparison of propofol and sevoflurane for laryngeal mask anesthesia for magnetic resonance imaging in pediatric patients. *Clin Ther.* 2008;30(1):175-181.

74. Iguchi H et al. Orotracheal intubation with an AirWay Scope in a patient with Treacher Collins syndrome. *J Anesth.* 2008;22(2):186-188.

75. Masursky D et al. Long-term forecasting of anesthesia workload in operating rooms from changes in a hospital's local population can be inaccurate. *Anesth Analg.* 2008;106(4):1223-1231.

76. Wheeler DS et al. An infant with fever and stridor. *Pediatr Emerg Care.* 2008;24(1):46-49.

77. Burgoyne LL, Anghelescu DL. Intervention steps for treating laryngospasm in pediatric patients. *Paediatr Anaesth.* 2008;18(4):297-302.

78. Hampson-Evans D et al. Pediatric laryngospasm. *Paediatr Anaesth.* 2008;18(4):303-307.

79. Obholzer RJ et al. An approach to the management of paroxysmal laryngospasm. *J Laryngol Otol.* 2008;122(1):57-60.

80. Alalami AA et al. Laryngospasm: review of different prevention and treatment modalities. *Paediatr Anaesth.* 2008;18(4):281-288.

81. Ahmad I, Sellers WF. Prevention and management of laryngospasm. *Anaesthesia.* 2004;59(9):920.

82. Batra YK et al. The efficacy of a subhypnotic dose of propofol in preventing laryngospasm following tonsillectomy and adenoidectomy in children. *Paediatr Anaesth.* 2005;15(12):1094-1097.

83. Westhorpe RN et al. Crisis management during anaesthesia: bronchospasm. *Qual Saf Health Care.* 2005;14(3):e7.

84. Linck SL. Use of heliox for intraoperative bronchospasm: a case report. *AANA J.* 2007;75(3):189-192.

85. Rooke T, Sparks H. An overview of the circulation and hemodynamics. In: Rhoades R, Tanner G, eds. *Medical Physiology.* Baltimore: Lippincott Williams & Wilkins; 2003.

86. Seifter J et al. *Concepts in Medical Physiology.* Baltimore: Lippincott Williams & Wilkins; 2005.

87. Thiagarajan RR, Laussen PC. Negative pressure pulmonary edema in children—pathogenesis and clinical management. *Paediatr Anaesth.* 2007;17(4):307-310.

88. Tan CK, Lai CC. Neurogenic pulmonary edema. *CMAJ.* 2007;177(3):249-250.

89. Louis PJ, Fernandes R. Negative pressure pulmonary edema. *Oral Surg Oral Med Oral Pathol Oral Radiol Endod.* 2002;93(1):4-6.

90. Noble KA. Physically powerful can be hazardous: negative pressure pulmonary edema. *J Perianesth Nurs.* 2007;22(2):132-135.

91. Tarrac SE. Negative pressure pulmonary edema—a postanesthesia emergency. *J Perianesth Nurs.* 2003;18(5):317-323.

92. Atlee J. Thromboembolic complications. In: Helfand R, ed. *Complications in Anesthesia.* Philadelphia: Saunders; 2007.

93. Haas S, Spyropoulos AC. Primary prevention of venous thromboembolism in long-term care: identifying and managing the risk. *Clin Appl Thromb Hemost.* 2008;14(2):149-158.

94. Merli GJ. Pathophysiology of venous thrombosis and the diagnosis of deep vein thrombosis-pulmonary embolism in the elderly. *Cardiol Clin.* 2008;26(2):203-219.

95. Anderson FA et al. A population-based perspective of the hospital incidence and case-fatality rates of deep vein thrombosis and pulmonary embolism. The Worcester DVT Study. *Arch Intern Med.* 1991;151(5):933-938.

96. Kim V, Spandorfer J. Epidemiology of venous thromboembolic disease. *Emerg Med Clin North Am.* 2001;19(4):839-859.

97. Ogawa S et al. Hypoxia modulates the barrier and coagulant function of cultured bovine endothelium. Increased monolayer permeability and induction of procoagulant properties. *J Clin Invest.* 1990;85(4):1090-1098.

98. Silverstein JH et al. Postoperative cognitive dysfunction in patients with preoperative cognitive impairment: which domains are most vulnerable? *Anesthesiology.* 2007;106(3):431-435.

99. Moller JT et al. Long-term postoperative cognitive dysfunction in the elderly. ISPOCD1 study. ISPOCD investigators. International Study of Post-Operative Cognitive Dysfunction. *Lancet.* 1998;351(9106):857-861.

100. Richards M, Deary IJ. A life course approach to cognitive reserve: a model for cognitive aging and development? *Ann Neurol.* 2005;58(4):617-622.

101. Newman MF et al. Longitudinal assessment of neurocognitive function after coronary-artery bypass surgery. *N Engl J Med.* 2001;344(6):395-402.

102. Selnes OA et al. Neurobehavioural sequelae of cardiopulmonary bypass. *Lancet.* 1999;353(9164):1601-1606.

103. Williams-Russo P et al. Post-operative delirium: predictors and prognosis in elderly orthopedic patients. *J Am Geriatr Soc.* 1992;40(8):759-767.

104. American Psychiatric Association. *Diagnostic and Statistical Manual of Mental Disorders (DSM-III).* Washington, DC: APA; 1980.

105. Siddiqi N et al. Interventions for preventing delirium in hospitalised patients. *Cochrane Database Syst Rev.* 2007;(2):CD005563.

106. Francis J, Kapoor WN. Prognosis after hospital discharge of older medical patients with delirium. *J Am Geriatr Soc.* 1992;40(6):601-606.

107. Marcantonio ER et al. A clinical prediction rule for delirium after elective noncardiac surgery. *JAMA.* 1994;271(2):134-139.

108. Tonner PH et al. Pathophysiological changes in the elderly. *Best Pract Res Clin Anaesthesiol.* 2003;17(2):163-177.

109. Eden BM et al. Delirium: comparison of four predictive models in hospitalized critically ill elderly patients. *Appl Nurs Res.* 1998;11(1):27-35.

110. Martin NJ et al. Development of delirium: a prospective cohort study in a community hospital. *Int Psychogeriatr.* 2000;12(1):117-127.

111. Neitzel J et al. Delirium in the orthopaedic patient. *Orthop Nurs.* 2007;26(6):354-363;quiz 364-355.

112. Beliveau MM, Multach M. Perioperative care for the elderly patient. *Med Clin North Am.* 2003;87(1):273-289.

113. Rolfson DB et al. Incidence and risk factors for delirium and other adverse outcomes in older adults after coronary artery bypass graft surgery. *Can J Cardiol.* 1999;15(7):771-776.

114. Brown S et al. Delirium dichotomy: a review of recent literature. *Contemp Nurse.* 2007;26(2):238-247.
115. Heidrich DE. Delirium: an under-recognized problem. *Clin J Oncol Nurs.* 2007;11(6):805-807.
116. Inott T. Is it delirium, dementia, or depression? *Nursing.* 2007;37(11):65.
117. Kirshner HS. Delirium: a focused review. *Curr Neurol Neurosci Rep.* 2007;7(6):479-482.
118. Ely EW et al. The impact of delirium in the intensive care unit on hospital length of stay. *Intensive Care Med.* 2001;27(12):1892-1900.
119. Schofield I. Delirium: challenges for clinical governance. *J Nurs Manag.* 2008;16(2):127-133.
120. Cork RC. Awareness under anesthesia. *J Perianesth Nurs.* 2006;21(4):288-290.
121. Lennmarken C, Sydsjo G. Psychological consequences of awareness and their treatment. *Best Pract Res Clin Anaesthesiol.* 2007;21(3):357-367.
122. Hutchinson R. Awareness during surgery. A study of its incidence. *Br J Anaesth.* 1960;33:463-469.
123. Sebel PS et al. The incidence of awareness during anesthesia: a multicenter United States study. *Anesth Analg.* 2004;99(3):833-839.
124. Sandin RH et al. Awareness during anaesthesia: a prospective case study. *Lancet.* 2000;355(9205):707-711.
125. Ghoneim MM. Incidence of and risk factors for awareness during anaesthesia. *Best Pract Res Clin Anaesthesiol.* 2007;21(3):327-343.
126. Myles PS. Prevention of awareness during anaesthesia. *Best Pract Res Clin Anaesthesiol.* 2007;21(3):345-355.
127. McCleane GJ, Cooper R. The nature of pre-operative anxiety. *Anaesthesia.* 1990;45(2):153-155.
128. Orser BA. Depth-of-anesthesia monitor and the frequency of intraoperative awareness. *N Engl J Med.* 2008;358(11):1189-1191.
129. Lopez U et al. Intra-operative awareness in children: the value of an interview adapted to their cognitive abilities. *Anaesthesia.* 2007;62(8):778-789.
130. Kent CD, Domino KB. Awareness: practice, standards, and the law. *Best Pract Res Clin Anaesthesiol.* 2007;21(3):369-383.
131. Lennmarken C et al. Victims of awareness. *Acta Anaesthesiol Scand.* 2002;46(3):229-231.
132. Preventing, and managing the impact of, anesthesia awareness. *Sentinel Event Alert.* 2004;(32):1-3.
133. Geisz-Everson M, Wren KR. Awareness under anesthesia. *J Perianesth Nurs.* 2007;22(2):85-90.
134. Heier T, Steen PA. Awareness in anaesthesia: incidence, consequences and prevention. *Acta Anaesthesiol Scand.* 1996;40(9):1073-1086.
135. American Association of Nurse Anesthetists. *Position Statement 2.12: Unintended Awareness Under General Anesthesia, 2002.* Available at AANA Web site: http://www.aana.com/resources.aspx?ucNavMenu_TSMenuTarget ID=51&ucNavMenu_TSMenuTargetType=4&ucNavMenu_TSMenuID=6 &id=1747. Accessed March 28, 2008.
136. del Zoppo GJ. Stroke and neurovascular protection. *N Engl J Med.* 2006;354(6):553-555.
137. Selim M. Perioperative stroke. *N Engl J Med.* 2007;356(7):706-713.
138. The National Institute of Neurological Disorders and Stroke rt-PA Stroke Study Group. Tissue plasminogen activator for acute ischemic stroke. *N Engl J Med.* 1995;333(24):1581-1587.
139. Ginsberg MD. Neuroprotection for ischemic stroke: Past, present and future. *Neuropharmacology.* 2008;55(3):363-389.
140. Wong GY et al. Risk of surgery and anesthesia for ischemic stroke. *Anesthesiology.* 2000;92(2):425-432.
141. Chang CK et al. Oxidative stress and ischemic injuries in heat stroke. *Prog Brain Res.* 2007;162:525-546.
142. Lee SH et al. Optimum degree of hemodilution for brain protection in a canine model of focal cerebral ischemia. *J Neurosurg.* 1994;80(3):469-475.
143. O'Dwyer C et al. Determinants of cerebral perfusion during cardiopulmonary bypass. *J Cardiothorac Vasc Anesth.* 1996;10(1):54-64;quiz 65.
144. Williams GD, Ramamoorthy C. Brain monitoring and protection during pediatric cardiac surgery. *Semin Cardiothorac Vasc Anesth.* 2007;11(1):23-33.
145 Reich DL et al. Intraoperative hemodynamic predictors of mortality, stroke, and myocardial infarction after coronary artery bypass surgery. *Anesth Analg.* 1999;89(4):814-822.
146. Ohene-Frempong K et al. Cerebrovascular accidents in sickle cell disease: rates and risk factors. *Blood.* 1998;91(1):288-294.
147. Montero-Huerta P et al. Inhaled nitric oxide for treatment of sickle cell stroke. *Anesthesiology.* 2006;105(3):619-621.
148. Hogue CW et al. The importance of prior stroke for the adjusted risk of neurologic injury after cardiac surgery for women and men. *Anesthesiology.* 2003;98(4):823-829.
149. Treggiari M, Deem S. Anesthesia and critical care medicine. In: Barash P et al, eds. *Clinical Anesthesia.* 5th ed. Philadelphia: Lippincott Williams & Wilkins; 2006.
150. Preventing surgical fires. *Sentinel Event Alert.* 2003;(29):1-2.
151. A clinician's guide to surgical fires. How they occur, how to prevent them, how to put them out. *Health Devices.* 2003;32(1):5-24.
152. Fitzgibbon DR et al. Chronic pain management: American Society of Anesthesiologists Closed Claims Project. *Anesthesiology.* 2004;100(1):98-105.
153. Leedal JM, Smith AF. Methodological approaches to anaesthetists' workload in the operating theatre. *Br J Anaesth.* 2005;94(6):702-709.
154. Bacon AK et al. Crisis management during anaesthesia: recovering from a crisis. *Qual Saf Health Care.* 2005;14(3):e25.

INDEX